Critical Care Toxicology

Critical Care Toxicology

Diagnosis and Management of the Critically Poisoned Patient

Jeffrey Brent, MD, PhD
Clinical Professor of Medicine and Pediatrics
Associate Clinical Professor of Surgery
University of Colorado Health Sciences Center
Toxicology Associates, Prof LLC
Denver, Colorado

Kevin L. Wallace, MD
Clinical Associate Professor of Emergency Medicine
University of Arizona College of Medicine
Tucson, Arizona
Faculty Member
Medical Toxicology Fellowship
Good Samaritan Regional Medical Center
Phoenix, Arizona

Keith K. Burkhart, MD
Professor of Clinical Emergency Medicine
Pennsylvania State University College of Medicine
Hershey, Pennsylvania
Regional Medical Toxicologist
Division of Regional Operations
Agency for Toxic Substances and Disease Registry
Philadelphia, Pennsylvania
State Medical Toxicologist
Division of Environmental Health Epidemiology
Harrisburg, Pennsylvania

Scott D. Phillips, MD
Associate Clinical Professor of Medicine and Surgery
University of Colorado Health Sciences Center
Faculty
Rocky Mountain Poison and Drug Center
Denver, Colorado

J. Ward Donovan, MD
Professor Emeritus of Emergency Medicine
Pennsylvania State University College of Medicine
Hershey, Pennsylvania
Medical Director and Chief, PinnacleHealth
Toxicology Center
Harrisburg Hospital
Harrisburg, Pennsylvania

Illustrations Editor: Robert B. Palmer, PhD

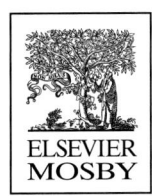

ELSEVIER
MOSBY

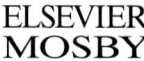

ELSEVIER
MOSBY

The Curtis Center
170 S Independence Mall W 300E
Philadelphia, Pennsylvania 19106

CRITICAL CARE TOXICOLOGY: Diagnosis and Management
of the Critically Poisoned Patient   0-8151-4387-7

NOTICE

Toxicology is an ever-changing field. Standard safety precautions must be followed but as new research
and clinical experience broaden our knowledge, changes in treatment and drug therapy may become
necessary or appropriate. Readers are advised to check the most current product information provided by
the manufacturer of each drug to be administered to verify the recommended dose, the method and
duration of administration, and contraindications. It is the responsibility of the treating physician, relying
on experience and knowledge of the patient, to determine dosages and the best treatment for each
individual patient. Neither the Publisher nor the authors assumes any liability for any injury and/or damage
to persons or property arising from this publication.

The Publisher

Library of Congress Cataloging-in-Publication Data

Critical care toxicology: diagnosis and management of the critically poisoned patient/
    Jeffrey Brent . . . [et al.].—1st ed.
        p.   ; cm.
    ISBN 0-8151-4387-7
    1. Toxicological emergencies.   I. Brent, Jeffrey.
    [DNLM: 1. Poisoning—diagnosis. 2. Antidotes. 3. Critical Care. 4. Poisoning—therapy.
    5. Poisons. 6. Toxins.   QV 600 C934 2005]
RA1224.5.C75 2005
615.9′08—dc22   2004040338

Publisher: Natasha Andjelkovic
Developmental Editor: Anne Snyder
Publishing Services Manager: Tina Rebane
Project Manager: Amy Norwitz
Design Manager: Gene Harris
Design Supervisor: Steven Stave

Printed in the United States of America

Last digit is print number: 9   8   7   6   5   4   3   2   1

We dedicate this book to our patients from whom we have learned both the science and art of medical toxicology. It has been our privilege to serve you.

The Editors

Contributors

Cynthia K. Aaron, MD
Associate Professor of Emergency Medicine and Pediatrics
Wayne State University School of Medicine
Director of Medical and Clinical Toxicology Education
Associate Fellowship Director, Michigan Poison Center at
  Children's Hospital
Detroit, Michigan

Timothy E. Albertson, MD, PhD, MPH
Professor of Medicine, Anesthesia and Pharmacology
Division of Pulmonary and Critical Care Medicine and
  Emergency Medicine
University of California, Davis, School of Medicine
Sacramento, California

Christopher S. Amato, MD
Attending Physician
Department of Emergency Medicine
Morristown Memorial Hospital
Morristown, New Jersey

Yona Amitai, MD, MPH
Associate Professor in Pediatrics
Hadassah Medical Center
Hebrew University
Director, Department of Mother, Child and Adolescent Health
Ministry of Health
Jerusalem, Israel

Bruce D. Anderson, PharmD
Associate Professor of Pharmacy Practice and Science
University of Maryland School of Pharmacy
Director, Maryland Poison Center
Baltimore, Maryland

Kia Balali-Mood, BSc, MSc, PhD
Lecturer, Biology Teaching Organization
University of Edinburgh
Edinburgh, Scotland
United Kingdom

Mahdi Balali-Mood, BSc, MD, PhD
Professor of Medicine and Clinical Toxicology
Mashhad University of Medical Sciences, School of Medicine,
Physician in Charge and Director, Medical Toxicology Center
Imam Reza Hospital
Mashhad, Khorassan
Iran

Ronald Balkissoon, MD, DIH
Associate Professor
University of Colorado School of Medicine and National
  Jewish Hospital and Research Center
Denver, Colorado

Donald G. Barceloux, MD, FACEP, FAACT
Clinical Professor of Medicine
University of California, Los Angeles
David Geffen School of Medicine
Los Angeles, California
Staff Physician
Department of Emergency Medicine
Pomona Valley Hospital Medical Center
Pomona, California

D. Nicholas Bateman, MD, FRCP, FRCP(E)
Reader in Clinical Pharmacology
Consultant Physician
Scottish Poisons Information Bureau
Royal Infirmary of Edinburgh
Edinburgh, Scotland
United Kingdom

Nicola Bates, BSc (Brunel), BSc (Open), MSc, MA
Specialist in Poisons Information
Medical Toxicology Unit
London, England
United Kingdom

Frédéric J. Baud, MD
Professor of Critical Care Medicine
University Paris 7
Faculty of Medicine
Lariboisière St. Louis Hospitals
Head, Medical and Toxicological Critical Care
  Department
Hôpital Lariboisière
Paris, France

Carl R. Baum, MD, FAAP, FACMT
Assistant Professor of Pediatrics
Yale University School of Medicine
Director, Center for Children's Environmental
  Toxicology
Attending Physician, Pediatric Emergency Medicine
Yale-New Haven Children's Hospital
New Haven, Connecticut

Neal Benowitz, MD
Professor of Medicine
Chief, Division of Clinical Pharmacology and
  Toxicology
University of California, San Francisco
Associate Medical Director
California Poison Control System
San Francisco Division
San Francisco, California

Blaine E. Benson, PharmD
Associate Professor
University of New Mexico College of Pharmacy
Director, New Mexico Poison and Drug Information Center
University of New Mexico
Albuquerque, New Mexico

Jeffrey N. Bernstein, MD, FACEP, FACMT
Medical Director, Florida Poison Information
   Center/Miami
Voluntary Associate Professor of Pediatrics and Medicine
University of Miami
Attending Physician, Emergency Care Center
Jackson Memorial Hospital
Miami, Florida

Michael Beuhler, MD
Clinical Instructor of Emergency Medicine
University of North Carolina at Chapel Hill
Medical Director, Carolinas Poison Center
Carolinas Medical Center
Charlotte, North Carolina

Stephen W. Borron, MD
Associate Clinical Professor of Emergency Medicine and
   Medicine (Occupational and Environmental Health)
George Washington University School of Medicine
Washington, DC
Associate Professor of Therapeutics
Hospital Practitioner
University of Paris XIII
Bobigny, France

Edward M. Bottei, MD
Assistant Clinical Professor of Pulmonary and Critical Care
   Medicine
University of Iowa
Iowa City, Iowa
Medical Director, Iowa Statewide Poison Control Center
Sioux City, Iowa
State Medical Toxicologist
Iowa Department of Public Health
Des Moines, Iowa

Sally M. Bradberry, BSc, MB, MRCP
Assistant Director, National Poisons Information Service
   (Birmingham Centre)
City Hospital
Birmingham, England
United Kingdom

George Braitberg, MBBS, FACEM, GRAD Dip Clinical Epidemiology and Biostatistics
Associate Professor of Medicine
University of Melbourne
Parkville, Victoria
Director of Emergency Medicine
Co-Director of Medical Toxicology
Austin Health
Heidelberg, Victoria
Australia

Jeffrey Brent, MD, PhD
Clinical Professor of Medicine and Pediatrics
Associate Clinical Professor of Surgery
University of Colorado Health Sciences Center
Toxicology Associates, Prof LLC
Denver, Colorado

Daniel E. Brooks, MD
Assistant Professor of Emergency Medicine and Medical
   Toxicology
Department of Emergency Medicine
University of Pittsburgh Medical Center
Co-Medical Director
Pittsburgh Poison Control Center
Pittsburgh, Pennsylvania

Sean M. Bryant, MD
Assistant Professor of Emergency Medicine
University of Cincinnati
Cincinnati, Ohio

Jefferey L. Burgess, MD, MPH, FACMT
Associate Professor, Environmental and Occupational
   Health
University of Arizona
Tucson, Arizona

Keith K. Burkhart, MD, FACMT, FAACT, FACEP
Professor of Clinical Emergency Medicine
Pennsylvania State University College of Medicine
Hershey, Pennsylvania
Regional Medical Toxicologist
Division of Regional Operations
Agency for Toxic Substances and Disease Registry
Philadelphia, Pennsylvania
State Medical Toxicologist
Division of Environmental Health Epidemiology
Harrisburg, Pennsylvania

Michael J. Burns, MD
Assistant Professor of Medicine
Harvard Medical School
Co-Director, Division of Medical Toxicology
Department of Emergency Medicine
Beth Israel Deaconess Medical Center
Boston, Massachusetts

Michael V. Callahan MD, DTM&H (UK), MSPH
Biological Threat Defense and Mass Casualty Care
CIMIT/Division of Infectious Diseases
Massachusetts General Hospital
Boston, Massachusetts
Medical Director, Rescue Medicine—Southeast Asia
Bangkok, Thailand

João Luiz Costa Cardosa, MD
Assistant Professor of Dermatology
School of Medicine, University of Taubaté
Taubaté, São Paulo
Brazil

Andrea Carlson, MD
Department of Emergency Medicine
Advocate Christ Medical Center
Oak Lawn, Illinois

Gregory L. Carter, MBBS, FRANZCP, Cert. Child Psychiatry
Senior Lecturer
Faculty of Health Sciences
University of Newcastle
Head, Suicide Prevention Research Unit
Centre for Mental Health Studies
Acting Director
Department of Consultation-Liaison Psychiatry
Newcastle Mater Hospital
Newcastle, New South Wales
Australia

Edward W. Cetaruk, MD
Clinical Assistant Professor of Medicine
Division of Toxicology and Pharmacology
University of Colorado Health Sciences Center
Toxicology Associates, Prof LLC
Denver, Colorado

Youngsoo Cho, MD
Brown University School of Medicine
Rhode Island Hospital
Department of Medicine
Providence, Rhode Island

Richard F. Clark, MD
Professor of Medicine
University of California, San Diego
School of Medicine
Director, Division of Medical Toxicology
University of California, San Diego, Medical Center
Medical Director, California Poison Control System,
    San Diego Division
San Diego, California

Jack Clifton II, MD
Assistant Professor of Pediatrics and Internal Medicine
Section of Clinical Toxicology
Rush University Medical Center
Attending Physician
Rush Children's Hospital
Attending Physician
Cook County Hospital
Chicago, Illinois

Daniel J. Cobaugh, PharmD
Director of Research
ASHP Research and Education Foundation
Bethesda, Maryland

Kirk L. Cumpston, DO
Assistant Professor of Emergency Medicine,
    School of Medicine
Assistant Professor, School of Pharmacy
University of New Mexico
Associate Medical Director
New Mexico Poison Center
Albuquerque, New Mexico

Steven C. Curry, MD
Associate Professor of Clinical Medicine
University of Arizona College of Medicine
Director, Department of Medical Toxicology
Banner Good Samaritan Medical Center
Phoenix, Arizona

Frank F. S. Daly, MBBS, FACEM
Clinical Senior Lecturer
University of Western Australia
Consultant Clinical Toxicologist
Staff Specialist, Emergency Medicine
Royal Perth Hospital
Perth, Western Australia
Australia

Irma de Vries, MD
Medical Director, Department of Intensive Care and Clinical
    Toxicology
Utrecht University Hospital
Associate Director, National Poisons Information
    Center
National Institute of Public Health and the Environment
Bilthoven, The Netherlands

Jou-Fang Deng, MD
Associate Professor of Medicine
National Yang-Ming University, School of Medicine
Director, Division of Clinical Toxicology
Department of Medicine
Taipei Veterans General Hospital
Taipei, Taiwan

Mark Donnelly, MD
University of Rochester
School of Medicine
Strong Memorial Hospital
Rochester, New York

J. Ward Donovan, MD, FACMT, FACEP
Professor Emeritus of Emergency Medicine
Pennsylvania State University College of Medicine
Hershey, Pennsylvania
Medical Director and Chief, PinnacleHealth Toxicology
    Center
Harrisburg Hospital
Harrisburg, Pennsylvania

Stephen C. Dreskin, MD, PhD
Associate Professor of Medicine
Division of Allergy and Clinical Immunology
University of Colorado School of Medicine
Director of Allergy and Rheumatology Practices
University of Colorado Health Sciences Center
University of Colorado Hospital
Denver, Colorado

Michael P. Dubé, MD
Associate Professor of Medicine
Indiana University School of Medicine
Medical Director
HIV Outpatient Care Clinic
Wishard Memorial Hospital
Indianapolis, Indiana

K. Sophia Dyer, MD
Assistant Professor of Emergency Medicine
Boston University School of Medicine
Attending Physician
Boston Medical Center
Medical Toxicologist
Boston Police, Fire, and EMS
Boston, Massachusetts

Andrew Erdman, MD
Medical Toxicologist
Postdoctoral Clinical Pharmacology Fellow
University of California, San Francisco
San Francisco, California

Timothy B. Erickson, MD, FACEP, FACMT, FAACT
Associate Professor of Emergency Medicine
Emergency Medicine Residency Program Director
Director, Division of Clinical Toxicology
University of Illinois at Chicago
Chicago, Illinois

Peter Eyer, MD
Senior Professor
Walther Straub Institute of Pharmacology and Toxicology
Ludwig Maximilians University
Munich, Germany

Frederick W. Fiesseler, DO, FACEP
Clinical Assistant Professor of Surgery
UMDNJ/New Jersey Medical School
Newark, New Jersey
Attending Physician
Department of Emergency Medicine
Morristown Memorial Hospital
Morristown, New Jersey

R. Brent Furbee, MD, FACMT
Associate Clinical Professor of Emergency Medicine
Indiana University School of Medicine
Medical Director, Indiana Poison Center
Indianapolis, Indiana

Hernan F. Gomez, MD, ACMT
Clinical Associate Professor
University of Michigan Health System
Ann Arbor, Michigan

Kimberlie A. Graeme, MD
Senior Associate Consultant
Vice Chair, Research
Department of Emergency Medicine
Mayo Clinic Hospital
Phoenix, Arizona

James Groff, DO
Clinical Assistant Professor of Medicine
Pennsylvania State University College of Medicine
Hershey, Pennsylvania
Hypertension and Kidney Specialists
Lancaster, Pennsylvania

In-Hei Hahn, MD
Assistant Clinical Professor of Medicine
Columbia University College of Physicians and Surgeons
Associate Attending in Emergency Medicine
Assistant Director of Research
St. Luke's-Roosevelt Hospital Center
New York, New York

Philippe Hantson, MD, PhD, FACMT
Associate Professor
Université Catholique de Louvain
Department of Intensive Care
Cliniques Universitaires St. Luc
Brussels, Belgium

Henrietta Harrison, BSc, MSc, Dip Toxicol
Environmental Hazards Project Officer
London, England
United Kingdom

Kennon Heard, MD
Assistant Professor of Surgery and Medicine
University of Colorado Health Sciences Center
Denver, Colorado

Mary Beth Hines, DO
Former Director of Medical Toxicology
Ingham Regional Medical Center
Lansing, Michigan
Former Assistant Director of Education
Michigan State University Emergency Medicine
    Residency Program
Lansing, Michigan

Robert J. Hoffman, MD
Albert Einstein College of Medicine
Bronx, New York
Research Director, Department of Emergency Medicine
Beth Israel Medical Center
New York, New York

Robert S. Hoffman, MD
Associate Professor of Emergency Medicine and Medicine
New York University School of Medicine
Director, New York City Poison Center
New York, New York

Michael G. Holland, MD, FACMT, FACOEM, FACEP
Occupational Physician
Glens Falls Hospital
Glens Falls, New York

Christopher P. Holstege, MD
Assistant Professor of Emergency Medicine
University of Virginia
Medical/Managing Director
Blue Ridge Poison Center
University of Virginia Health System
Charlottesville, Virginia

Dag Jacobsen, MD, PhD
Professor of Medicine and Clinical Toxicology
University of Oslo
Director, Department of Acute Medicine
Ullevaal University Hospital
Oslo, Norway

Heath A. Jolliff, DO
Clinical Assistant Professor of Emergency Medicine
Ohio University College of Osteopathic Medicine
Athens, Ohio
Director, Medical Toxicology
Doctors Hospital
Columbus, Ohio

Alison L. Jones, BSc (Hons), MD, FRCPE, FRCP, FiBiol
Senior Lecturer in Clinical Pharmacology
University of London
Director of Toxicology
Consultant Physician and Clinical Toxicologist
National Poisons Information Service (London Centre)
Guy's and St. Thomas' NHS Trust
London, England
United Kingdom

Louise W. Kao, MD
Clinical Assistant Professor of Emergency Medicine
Associate Fellowship Director
Medical Toxicology Fellowship Program
Indiana University School of Medicine
Assistant Medical Director
Indiana Poison Center
Methodist Hospital
Indianapolis, Indiana

Christine Karlson-Stiber, MD
Senior Consultant in Clinical Toxicology
Swedish Poisons Information Centre
Karolinska Hospital
Stockholm, Sweden

Kenneth D. Katz, MD
Director, Medical Toxicology Fellowship
University of Pittsburgh Medical Center
Pittsburgh, Pennsylvania

Fergus Kerr, MBBS, FACEM, MPH
Emergency Physician and Clinical Toxicologist
Austin Hospital
Melbourne, Victoria
Australia

Laura J. Klein, MD
Psychiatric Evaluations, Inc.
Denver, Colorado

Paul Kolecki, MD
Assistant Professor of Emergency Medicine
Thomas Jefferson University Hospital
Consultant for the Philadelphia Poison Control Center
Philadelphia, Pennsylvania

Michael J. Kosnett, MD, MPH
Associate Clinical Professor of Medicine
Division of Clinical Pharmacology and Toxicology
University of Colorado Health Sciences Center
Denver, Colorado

Edward P. Krenzelok, PharmD
Professor of Pharmacy and Pediatrics
University of Pittsburgh
Director, Pittsburgh Poison Center
Children's Hospital of Pittsburgh
Pittsburgh, Pennsylvania

Ken Kulig, MD
PorterCare Memorial Hospital
Denver, Colorado

Hugo Kupferschmidt, MD
Medical Director, Swiss Toxicological Information Centre
Zurich, Switzerland

Frédéric Lapostolle, MD
University Paris XIII
Bobigny, France

Charles Lee, MD
Teaching Fellow
Division of Pulmonary, Critical Care, and Sleep Medicine
Brown University School of Medicine
Rhode Island Hospital
Providence, Rhode Island

Melissa Dilanni Lee, MD
Pulmonary Critical Care Fellow
Brown University
Providence, Rhode Island

Jerrold B. Leikin, MD
Professor of Medicine
Feinberg School of Medicine
Northwestern University
Professor of Medicine, Pharmacology, and Health Systems
    Management
Rush Medical College
Chicago, Illinois
Director of Medical Toxicology
Evanston Northwestern Healthcare—OMEGA
Glenbrook Hospital
Glenview, Illinois

Christopher H. Linden, MD
Professor
Division of Medical Toxicology
Department of Emergency Medicine
University of Massachusetts Medical School
Worcester, Massachusetts

Ruth Lopert, BSc, BMed, MMed Sc
Research Academic
Discipline of Clinical Pharmacology
Faculty of Medicine and Health Sciences
University of Newcastle,
Callaghan, New South Wales
Medical Advisor
Pharmaceutical Benefits Branch
Department of Health and Ageing
Canberra, ACT
Australia

Frank LoVecchio, DO, MPH
Associate Professor
Arizona College of Osteopathic Medicine
Glendale, Arizona
Medical Director, Banner Good Samaritan Regional Poison
    Center
Research Director, Maricopa Medical Center
Department of Emergency Medicine
Phoenix, Arizona

Jennifer A. Lowry, MD, FAAP
Clinical Assistant Professor of Pediatrics
University of Kansas School of Medicine
Medical Director, Mid-America Poison Control Center
University of Kansas Medical Center
Kansas City, Kansas

Barbarajean Magnani, MD, PhD
Associate Professor of Pathology and Laboratory
    Medicine
Boston University School of Medicine
Chief, Department of Laboratory Medicine
Medical Director, Clinical Chemistry
Boston Medical Center
Boston, Massachusetts

Anthony S. Manoguerra, PharmD
Professor of Clinical Pharmacology
University of California, San Diego
School of Pharmacy and Pharmaceutical Sciences
La Jolla, California

Thomas G. Martin, MD, MPH, FACMT, FAACT, FACEP
Associate Professor of Medicine, Division of Emergency
    Medicine
University of Washington
Director, UW-Medical Toxicology Consult Service
Associate Medical Director
Washington Poison Center
Attending Physician in Emergency Medicine
University of Washington Medical Center
Seattle, Washington

George Mathew, MD
Assistant Clinical Professor of Medicine
Indiana University School of Medicine
Indianapolis, Indiana

Patrick E. McKinney, MD*
Formerly, University of New Mexico School of Medicine
University of New Mexico Medical Center
New Mexico Poison Control Center
Albuquerque, New Mexico

Steven A. McLaughlin, MD
Assistant Professor of Emergency Medicine
University of New Mexico
Albuquerque, New Mexico

Kenneth McMartin, PhD
Professor of Pharmacology
Louisiana State University Health Sciences Center
Shreveport, Louisiana

Bruno Mégarbane, MD
Assistant Professor
Université Paris VII
Physician
Hôpital Lariboisière
Réanimation Médicale et Toxicologique
Paris, France

Jan Meulenbelt, MD, PhD
University Senior Teacher in Intensive Care
    and Clinical Toxicology
Utrecht University
Internist, Intensivist, Toxicologist
Department of Intensive Care and Clinical Toxicology
University Medical Center Utrecht
Utrecht, The Netherlands

___

*Deceased

Jordan Miller, MD
Associate Professor of Anesthesiology
Director, Malignant Hyperthermia Program
David Geffen School of Medicine at UCLA
Los Angeles, California

Kirk C. Mills, MD, FACMT, FACEP
Clinical Assistant Professor of Emergency Medicine
Detroit Receiving Hospital
Medical Toxicologist
Detroit Medical Center
Detroit, Michigan

Anthony Morkunas, PharmD
Associate Professor
A.T. Still University of Health Science
Mesa, Arizona
Clinical Pharmacy Specialist
Carl T. Hayden VA Medical Center
Phoenix, Arizona

William D. Morris, MD
Attending Physician
Harrison Hospital
Bremerton, Washington

Gert J. Muller, MB ChB, MMed (Anesth), PhD
Senior Lecturer, Department of Pharmacology
Faculty of Health Sciences
University of Stellenbosch
Senior Specialist (Pharmacology)
Head, Tygerberg Poison Information Centre
Tygerberg Hospital
Tygerberg, South Africa

Stephen Munday, MD, MPH
Clinical Assistant Professor
University of California, San Diego
Staff Physician
San Diego Division, California Poison Control System
Assistant Medical Director, Occupational Health Services
Sharp Rees-Stealy Medical Group
San Diego, California

Lewis S. Nelson, MD
Assistant Professor of Emergency Medicine
Fellowship Director, Medical Toxicology
New York University School of Medicine
Attending Physician
New York University Medical Center
Bellevue Hospital
New York, New York

Kathleen Northrup, MD
Attending Physician
Milford Regional Hospital
Milford, Massachusetts

Ruben Olmedo, MD
Assistant Professor of Emergency Medicine
Mount Sinai School of Medicine
Director, Division of Toxicology
Mount Sinai Medical Center
New York, New York

Michael J. Pali, MD
Fellow in Toxicology
Division of Pulmonary and Critical Care Medicine
University of California, Davis, School of Medicine
Sacramento, California

Robert B. Palmer, PhD, DABAT
Assistant Clinical Professor, Department of Surgery
University of Colorado Health Sciences Center
Associate Professor (Adjunct), School of Pharmacy
University of Wyoming
Laramie, Wyoming
Rocky Mountain Poison and Drug Center
Toxicology Associates, Prof LLC
Denver, Colorado

Michael Parra, MD
Assistant Clinical Professor of Medicine
University of Colorado School of Medicine
Denver, Colorado

Manish M. Patel, MD
Assistant Professor of Emergency Medicine
Emory School of Medicine
Medical Toxicologist
Centers for Disease Control and Prevention
Atlanta, Georgia

Holly E. Perry, MD
Assistant Professor
University of Connecticut
Farmington, Connecticut
Attending Physician
Connecticut Children's Medical Center
Hartford, Connecticut

Hans Persson, MD
Senior Consultant in Clinical Toxicology
Swedish Poisons Information Centre
Stockholm, Sweden

Scott D. Phillips, MD, FACP, FACMT
Associate Clinical Professor of Medicine and Surgery
University of Colorado Health Sciences Center
Faculty
Rocky Mountain Poison and Drug Center
Denver, Colorado

Alex T. Proudfoot, BSc, MB, FRCP, FRCPE
Consulting Clinical Toxicologist
National Poisons Information Service (Birmingham Centre)
City Hospital
Birmingham, England
United Kingdom

Cyrus Rangan, MD
Clinical Instructor in Pediatrics
University of Southern California Keck School of Medicine
Director of Los Angeles Medical Toxicology Education
 Program
California Poison Control System
Director of Toxics Epidemiology Program
Los Angeles County Department of Health Services
Attending Staff
Children's Hospital Los Angeles
Los Angeles, California

Robert A. Raschke, MD
Associate Professor of Clinical Medicine
University of Arizona College of Medicine
Department of Critical Care Medicine
Banner Good Samaritan Regional Medical Center
Phoenix, Arizona

Joseph G. Rella, MD
Assistant Professor, Division of Emergency Medicine
Department of Surgery
University of Medicine and Dentistry of New Jersey
New Jersey Medical School
Attending Physician
The University Hospital
Newark, New Jersey

Thomas Riley, MD
Associate Professor of Medicine
Pennsylvania State University College of Medicine
Milton S. Hershey Medical Center
Hershey, Pennsylvania

George C. Rodgers, Jr., MD, PhD
Professor of Pediatrics and Pharmacology/Toxicology
University of Louisville School of Medicine
Louisville, Kentucky

Daisy Schwab Rodrigues, MPH
Director, Centro Informações Antivenedo da Bahia (Ciave)
State Secretary of Health
Salvador, Bahia
Brazil

S. Rutherfoord Rose, PharmD
Associate Professor of Emergency Medicine
Virginia Commonwealth University
Director, Virginia Poison Center
Virginia Commonwealth University Medical Center
Richmond, Virginia

Henry Rosenberg, MD, CPE
Professor of Anesthesiology
Mount Sinai School of Medicine
New York, New York
Director, Department of Medical Education and Clinical
 Research
Saint Barnabas Medical Center
Livingston, New Jersey

Mitchell P. Ross, MD
Partner, Pediatric Critical Care of Arizona
Pediatric Faculty, Residency Program
St. Joseph's Hospital and Medical Center
Phoenix, Arizona

Anne-Michelle Ruha, MD
Associate Fellowship Director, Department of Medical
 Toxicology
Maricopa Medical Center
Emergency Medicine Residency Program
Banner Good Samaritan Regional Medical Center
Phoenix, Arizona

Daniel E. Rusyniak, MD
Assistant Professor of Emergency Medicine
Indiana University School of Medicine
Indianapolis, Indiana

Amit Sadana, MD
Fellow in Gastroenterology
Pennsylvania State University College of Medicine
Milton S. Hershey Medical Center
Hershey, Pennsylvania

Anthony Santilli, MD
Department of Medicine
Rhode Island Hospital
Providence, Rhode Island

Daniel Savitt, MD
Emergency Department
The Miriam Hospital
Providence, Rhode Island

Anthony J. Scalzo, MD, FAAP, FACMT, FAACT
Professor of Pediatrics and Internal Medicine
Director, Division of Toxicology
Saint Louis University School of Medicine
Medical Director
Missouri Regional Poison Center
Cardinal Glennon Children's Hospital
Saint Louis, Missouri

Donna L. Seger, MD
Assistant Professor of Medicine and Emergency Medicine
Vanderbilt University Medical Center
Medical Director, Tennessee Poison Center
Nashville, Tennessee

Steven A. Seifert, MD, FACMT, FACEP
Professor of Surgery
Section of Emergency Medicine
University of Nebraska Medical Center
Medical Director
Nebraska Regional Poison Center
Omaha, Nebraska

Michael Shannon, MD, MPH
Associate Professor
Harvard University School of Medicine
Children's Hospital Boston
Boston, Massachusetts

Adhi N. Sharma, MD
Assistant Professor of Emergency Medicine
Mount Sinai School of Medicine
New York, New York
Director, Division of Toxicology
Department of Emergency Medicine
Elmhurst Hospital Center
Elmhurst, New York

Richard D. Shih, MD
Associate Professor of Surgery
Attending Toxicologist, NJ Poison Center
New Jersey Medical School
Newark, New Jersey
Emergency Medicine Residency
    Program Director
Morristown Memorial Hospital
Morristown, New Jersey

George W. Skarbek-Borowski, MD, MPH
Clinical Instructor of Emergency Medicine
Brown University
Providence, Rhode Island

Dorsett D. Smith, MD, FACP, FCCP, PACOEM
Clinical Professor of Medicine
Division of Respiratory Diseases and
    Critical Care
University of Washington Medical School
Seattle, Washington

Wayne R. Snodgrass, MD, PhD
Professor
University of Texas Medical Branch
Galveston, Texas
Head, Clinical Pharmacology–Toxicology Unit
Medical Director, Texas Poison Center–Houston/
    Galveston
Galveston, Texas

Curtis P. Snook, MD
Associate Professor of Clinical Emergency Medicine
University of Cincinnati Medical Center
Attending Emergency Physician
The University Hospital
Cincinnati, Ohio

Lisa K. Snyder, MD
Emergency Medicine Physician
Air National Guard–Flight Surgeon
Hancock Memorial Hospital
Greenfield, Indiana

Christine M. Stork, PharmD
Associate Professor of Emergency Medicine
Section of Clinical Pharmacology,
    Department of Medicine
SUNY Upstate Medical University
Clinical Director, Central New York Poison Center
University Hospital
Syracuse, New York

Jeffrey R. Suchard, MD
Associate Clinical Professor of Emergency Medicine
Director of Medical Toxicology
University of California, Irvine, Medical Center
Orange, California

Daniel Sudakin, MD, MPH
Assistant Professor of Environmental and Molecular
    Toxicology
Oregon State University
Corvallis, Oregon
Volunteer Clinical Faculty
Oregon Health and Science University
Department of Emergency Medicine
Portland, Oregon

Alan Talbot, MD
Director, Department of Critical Care Medicine
Changhua Christian Hospital
Changhua, Taiwan

R. Steven Tharratt, MD, MPVM
Professor of Medicine and Anesthesiology
Division of Pulmonary Medicine and Critical Care
University of California, Davis, School of Medicine
Medical Science Advisor
California Governor's Office of Emergency Services
Sacramento, California

Stephen R. Thom, MD, PhD
Professor of Emergency Medicine
University of Pennsylvania School of Medicine
Philadelphia, Pennsylvania

Anthony J. Tomassoni, MD
Associate Professor
University of Vermont College of Medicine
Burlington, Vermont
Medical Director, Northern New England Poison
    Center
Maine Medical Center, Department of
    Emergency Medicine
Portland, Maine

Marianne de Tourtchaninoff, MD
Université Catholique de Louvain
Department of Neurology
Cliniques Universitaires St. Luc
Brussels, Belgium

J. Allister Vale, MD, FRCP, FRCPE, FRCPG, FFOM, FAACT
Director, National Poisons Information Service (Birmingham Centre) and West Midlands Poisons Unit
City Hospital
Birmingham, England
United Kingdom
President, British Toxicology Society
Past President, European Association of Poison Centres and Clinical Toxicologists

Javier Waksman, MD
Assistant Clinical Professor of Medicine
Division of Clinical Pharmacology and Toxicology
University of Colorado Health Sciences Center
Faculty Member
Rocky Mountain Poison and Drug Center
Denver, Colorado

Kevin L. Wallace, MD, FACMT
Clinical Associate Professor of Emergency Medicine
University of Arizona College of Medicine
Tucson, Arizona
Faculty Member
Medical Toxicology Fellowship
Good Samaritan Regional Medical Center
Phoenix, Arizona

Richard Y. Wang, DO
Attending Physician
Grady Memorial Hospital
Emory University School of Medicine
Atlanta, Georgia

Gary S. Wasserman, DO, FAAP, FACMT, FAACT
Professor of Medicine
Department of Pediatrics
University of Missouri-Kansas City School of Medicine
Chief, Section of Medical Toxicology
Children's Mercy Hospitals and Clinics
Kansas City, Missouri

William A. Watson, PharmD
Adjunct Clinical Professor
School of Pharmacy
University of Missouri-Kansas City
Kansas City, Missouri
Associate Director, Toxicosurveillance
American Association of Poison Control Centers
Washington, DC

Barbara E. Watt, MSc, PhD
Senior Clinical Scientist
National Poisons Information Service (Birmingham Centre)
City Hospital
Birmingham, England
United Kingdom

Paul Wax, MD
Professor of Clinical Emergency Medicine
University of Arizona School of Medicine
Managing Director
Banner Poison Center
Banner Samaritan Regional Medical Center
Phoenix, Arizona

Lindell K. Weaver, MD
Professor of Medicine
University of Utah School of Medicine
Medical Director, Hyperbaric Medicine
Medical Co-Director, Shock-Trauma Respiratory ICU
LDS Hospital
Salt Lake City, Utah

Robert Wennig, PhD
Professor
University of Luxembourg
Laboratoire National de Santé–Toxicologie
Centre Universitaire de Luxembourg
Luxembourg, Luxembourg

Julian White, MD, FACTM
Professor of Paediatrics
University of Adelaide Medical School
Professor, School of Pharmacy
University of South Australia
Head of Toxinology
Women's and Children's Hospital
North Adelaide, South Australia
Australia

James F. Winchester, MD, FRCP (Glasgow), FACP
Adjunct Professor of Medicine
SUNY Health Science Center at Brooklyn
Clinical Professor of Medicine
Albert Einstein College of Medicine
Senior Lecturer, Mailman School of Public Health
Columbia University
Chief Medical Officer
RenalTech International
New York, New York

Alan D. Woolf, MD, MPH
Associate Professor of Pediatrics
Harvard Medical School
Director, Program in Pediatric Environmental Medicine
Division of General Pediatrics
Children's Hospital
Boston, Massachusetts

Anthony Wong, MD, PhD
Associate Professor of Pediatrics and Clinical Toxicology
Director, Poison Control Center
Instituto da Criança do Hospital das Clinicas
School of Medicine, University of São Paulo
São Paulo, Brazil

Chen-Chang Yang, MD, MPH, DrPH
Associate Professor of Medicine
National Yang-Ming University, School of Medicine
Adjunct Attending Physician
Division of Clinical Toxicology
Department of Medicine
Taipei Veterans General Hospital
Taipei, Taiwan

Thomas Zilker, MD, PhD, PRDF
Lecturer in Clinical Toxicology, Internal Medicine
Technical University
Director of the Toxicological Department
Klinikum Rechts der Isar
Munich, Germany

Foreword

In the last two decades in particular, a substantial number of textbooks on clinical toxicology have been published, though none has focused on the critical care management of the poisoned patient. Equally, many excellent books on critical care medicine have been published but, of necessity, the sections on clinical toxicology have been limited in length and scope. Thus, *Critical Care Toxicology* is a unique text and will be of immense value both to clinical toxicologists and to critical care physicians and intensivists who care for seriously poisoned patients.

Those involved in the critical care management of poisoned patients have undergone specialized training in critical care medicine and clinical toxicology and have acquired an understanding of the toxicokinetics of the drugs and chemicals involved in cases of poisoning. For reasons of continuing professional development, however, they will also require an in depth and up-to-date knowledge of the substantial literature on clinical toxicology. *Critical Care Toxicology* details the present state of knowledge in the field and will therefore be valuable as an aid to professional development, as well as providing timely advice to all who seek to offer optimal care to their patients.

Even though the prime focus of this new book is the management of severely poisoned patients admitted to a critical care unit, clinical toxicologists generally, including those who offer expert advice to other health care providers via a poison center, will find substantial academic and clinical benefit from reading *Critical Care Toxicology*.

Critical Care Toxicology not only covers the general management of the critically poisoned patient but also reviews the toxic syndromes with which poisoned patients may present. Some 70 chapters are devoted to specific drugs and other chemicals, and there is comprehensive coverage of biologic toxins including snake venom, arthropod venom, marine toxins, mushrooms, and plants. Chapters on those chemical and biologic agents that are likely to be involved in terrorist activity are also included. The concluding 25 chapters are on individual antidotes.

In their preface, the Editors describe their personal and professional passion for critical care toxicology. As readers face the clinical challenges of caring for critically poisoned patients, they will be very grateful for the passion and commitment that has led to the creation of a book of this depth and comprehensiveness. They will also be much in debt to the many critical care toxicologists worldwide who have contributed their expertise in the 160 chapters.

J. Allister Vale, MD, FRCP,
FRCPE, FRCPG, FFOM, FAACT

Preface

To us, this book is about passion. It is the result of the passion we share for the clinical challenges we face every day in caring for critically poisoned patients and in understanding their unique and enchanting pathophysiology and its therapeutic implications. This is a passion we hope to elicit in all who venture into the world of clinical toxicology as they read this book. To the medical toxicologist, the care of the seriously poisoned patients merges the diverse worlds of critical care, emergency medicine, pharmacology, altered drug pharmacokinetics (hence the term "toxicokinetics"), diagnostic challenges, multisystem involvement in often otherwise healthy patients, and the use of specific and often esoteric treatment strategies and antidotes.

Before embarking on the extraordinarily labor-intensive activity of generating a book of this depth and complexity, we queried the importance of producing another clinical toxicology textbook. We are aware of several excellent general clinical toxicology textbooks on the market and appreciate their attempts to achieve a far greater breadth than the present work. However, toxicology is such a broad field that general textbooks encompassing all of clinical toxicology necessarily must limit the extent of their coverage of the intensive care unit management of major poisonings. Thus, the intensivist, and critically poisoned patients, deserve a reference that specifically addresses their needs. This need is made all the more important by the life-threatening nature of many of these poisonings. Stark evidence of the complexity of just these issues is that to cover them adequately required 160 chapters and 1633 pages.

Our goal was to have the most knowledgeable and experienced medical toxicologists author relevant chapters. In order to achieve this goal we drafted our colleagues with unique experience and expertise worldwide. As witnessed by our contributor list, all continents, except Antarctica, are represented. We proudly boast that our collective chapter authors represent a significant proportion of the most expe-rienced critical care toxicologists in the world. Medical toxicologists interested in acute care tend to be domiciled at the bedside, in poison centers, or both. Because of the highly clinical nature of this book, we selected authors with a predominantly bedside care orientation.

With the ready access to facts and data via the internet, the very nature of hard copy books has changed dramatically. No longer is it necessary for books to be compendia of facts. However, electronic databases cannot convey the reasoned clinical approaches and the synthesis of pathophysiology with clinical effects and treatment that characterizes the pages that follow. Certainly, important physiologic and monitoring parameters as well as drug dosages are amply provided. The degree to which they are included represents our view of the best balance between those that are important to know and the desire to dedicate as much space as necessary to an elucidation of relevant concepts and a critical discussion of therapeutic controversies. We have embraced rather than glossed over controversies. The reader will find that this is not simply a "how to" handbook. Our aim is to provide the practitioner with the data needed to care for his or her individual patients. As an aid to those who choose to delve more deeply into the concepts, approaches, and controversies in this book, chapters are well referenced with primary source citations.

It is our hope and expectation that this book will evoke the same passion in the reader that the subject does for us.

Jeffrey Brent, MD, PhD
Kevin L. Wallace, MD
Keith K. Burkhart, MD
Scott D. Phillips, MD
J. Ward Donovan, MD
Robert B. Palmer, PhD

Acknowledgments

I cannot possibly overstate my gratitude to my wife, Laura Klein Brent, MD, and my son, Zachary R.B. Brent, for graciously tolerating the years of evenings and weekends I spent at my office editing this book. They were my inspiration.

Jeffrey Brent

I give my deep, heartfelt thanks to those whose love, support, and guidance have made my contributions to this work possible: my wife, Marialice; my children, Lindsey, Ian, Hannah, and Jenna; my parents, James and Rose; my brother, Bruce; and to all the students, teachers, and advisors I have been fortunate to encounter over the years.

Kevin L. Wallace

To Christina Pugliese Burkhart, MD, my wife, and my children, Kyle Peter Burkhart, Karly Elisa Burkhart, and Christopher Keith Burkhart, for their support and understanding of the commitment required to edit this book. But especially, I thank my family for tolerating the phone calls through so many nights of call and for their understanding when I was not with them, but at the bedside treating the patients described in this book. Their love is my strength and inspiration.

Keith K. Burkhart

I would like to acknowledge and to thank my teachers and colleagues, for it has been a privilege to have such inspirational mentors. Through their devotion and intellectual curiosity, I have learned the challenges and deeply gratifying rewards of medicine and toxicology. I am grateful to them for sharing the gift of medical knowledge and for creating a community of scholars of which I am proud to be a part.

Scott D. Phillips

To my physician father, who inspired me; my mother, who encouraged me; and my family, Joan, Ryan, and Erin, who tolerated me and my career.

J. Ward Donovan

To my parents, Robert L. Palmer, MD, and Linda J. Palmer, RN, for encouraging my curiosity. To my wife, Pamela Baxter Palmer, PhD, and our daughter, Abigail J. Palmer—the only 5-year-old ever to tell an entire pre-kindergarten class that "A methyl group has only one big 'C',"—for the numerous oddly timed meticulous discussions of scientific minutiae, and especially for the love, support, and big hugs.

Robert B. Palmer

Although there were many individuals who gave of their time, effort, and heart in the development and production of this book, we wish to express a special thanks to Su Dierbeck for the many hours of meticulous processing of edited chapters, chasing down and acquiring large numbers of references, and procuring necessary information from contributors and editors in her firm, yet always friendly and positive way.

All of the Editors

Contents

*Deceased

Color Figures

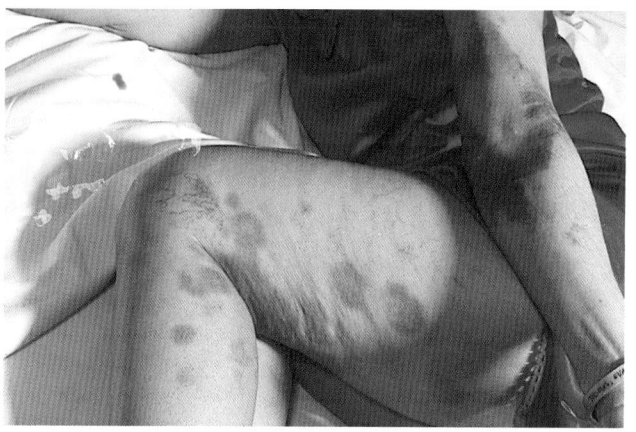

COLOR FIGURE 2-1

Diffuse ecchymoses after long-acting anticoagulant ingestion. *(Courtesy of J. Ward Donovan, MD.)*

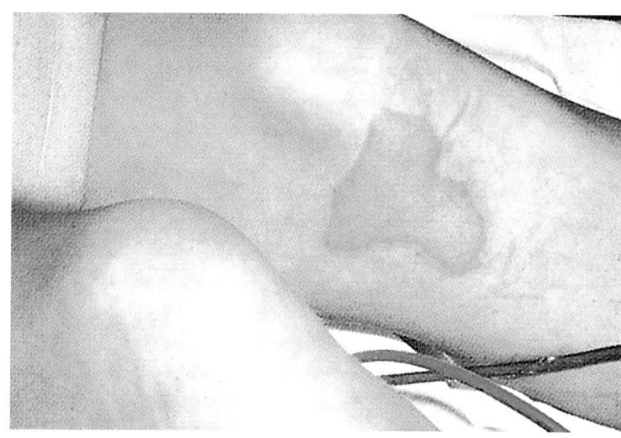

COLOR FIGURE 2-2

Skin lesion on medial knee after prolonged coma ("barbiturate burns"), early phase. *(Courtesy of J. Ward Donovan, MD.)*

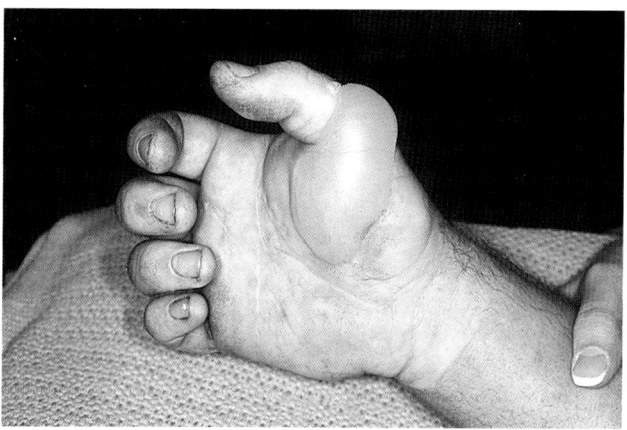

COLOR FIGURE 2-3

Hand blisters after prolonged coma ("barbiturate burns"), late phase. *(Courtesy of J. Ward Donovan, MD.)*

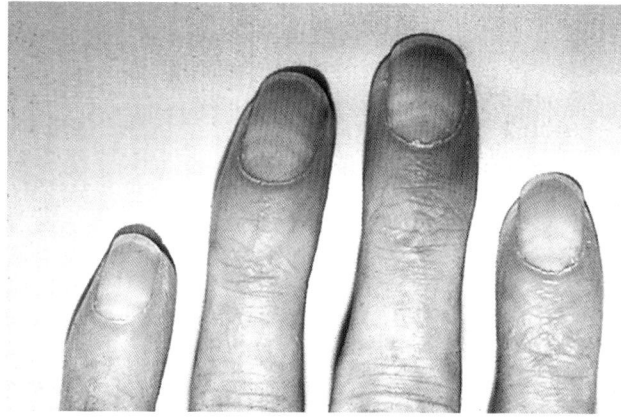

COLOR FIGURE 2-4

Mees' lines due to arsenic poisoning. *(Courtesy of J. Ward Donovan, MD.)*

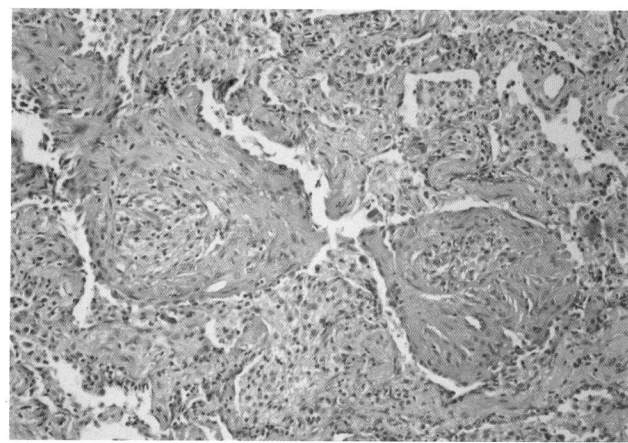

COLOR FIGURE 27-3

Cryptogenic organizing pneumonia. This high-power photomicrograph shows two nodules of young connective tissue (Masson bodies) in alveoli. Surrounding lung shows chronic inflammation. *(Courtesy of Richard Sobonya, MD, University of Arizona.)*

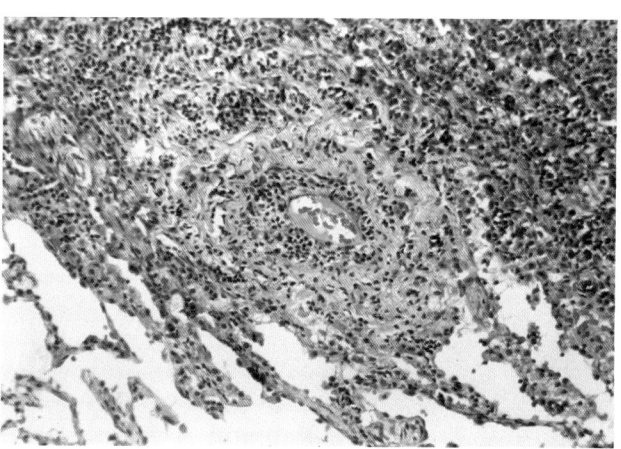

COLOR FIGURE 27-4

Wegener's granulomatosis. A small blood vessel shows infiltration by lymphocytes (vasculitis). Surrounding lung tissue shows chronic inflammation. *(Courtesy of Richard Sobonya, MD, University of Arizona.)*

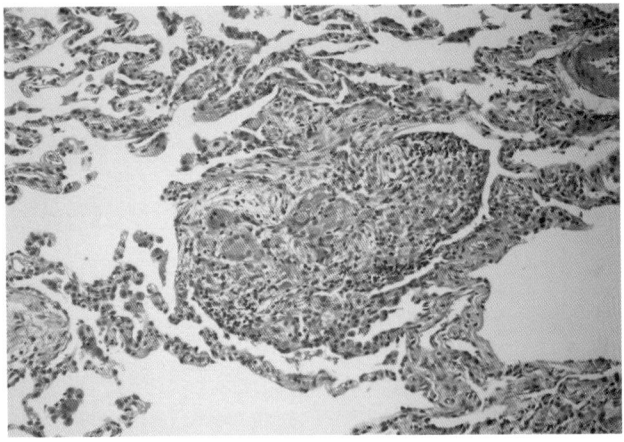

COLOR FIGURE 27-5

Hypersensitivity pneumonitis. A few poorly formed granulomas are present in the lung, associated with lymphocytic inflammation. *(Courtesy of Richard Sobonya, MD, University of Arizona.)*

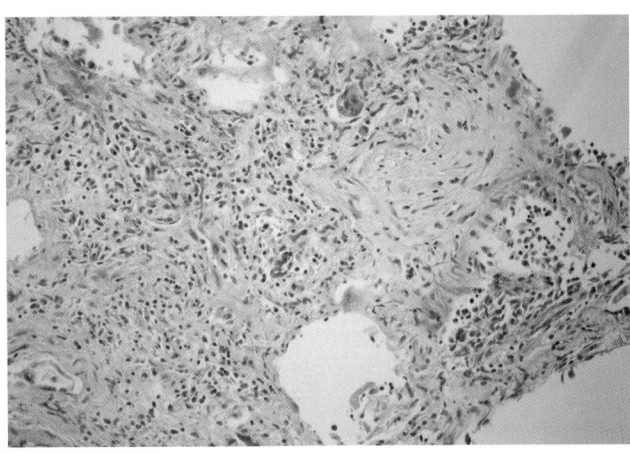

COLOR FIGURE 27-6

Interstitial fibrosis due to bleomycin. Nonspecific chronic inflammation and fibrosis with atypical reactive pneumocytes are present in the lung. *(Courtesy of Richard Sobonya, MD, University of Arizona.)*

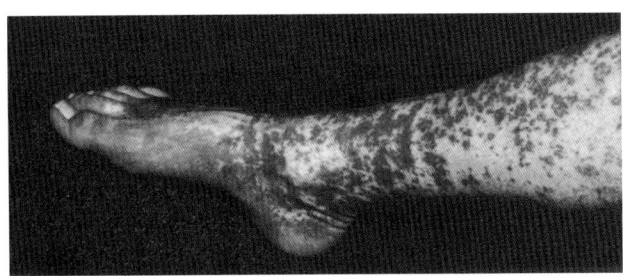

COLOR FIGURE 102-6

Serum sickness manifested as a diffuse maculopapular rash. *(Courtesy of Ken Kulig, M.D.)*

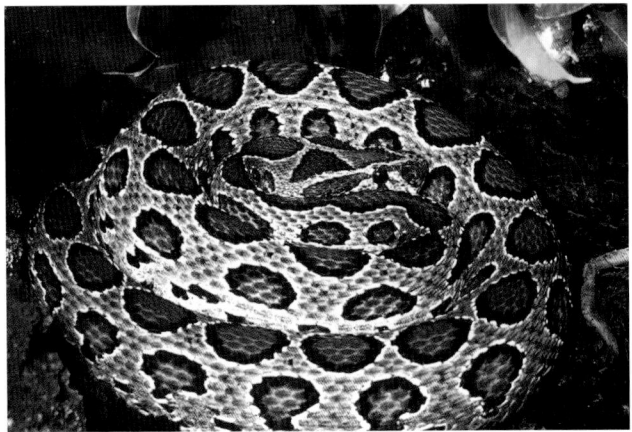

COLOR FIGURE 106-1

Daboia. This wide-ranging species possesses venom that induces largely neurotoxic symptoms, coagulopathies, and myonecrotic effects or combinations of these. *(Courtesy of Dr. Beat Akeret.)*

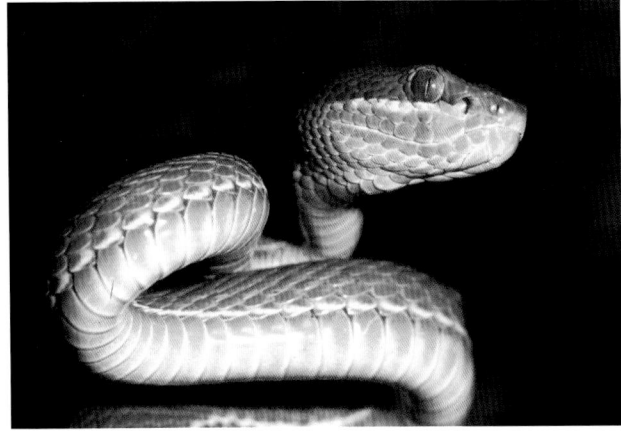

COLOR FIGURE 106-2

Trimeresurus. These Old World vipers are found throughout tropical Asia. Most species are arboreal, so bites of the hands are more common. The predominant symptoms are local tissue swelling, myonecrosis, and coagulopathy. *(Courtesy of Dr. Beat Akeret.)*

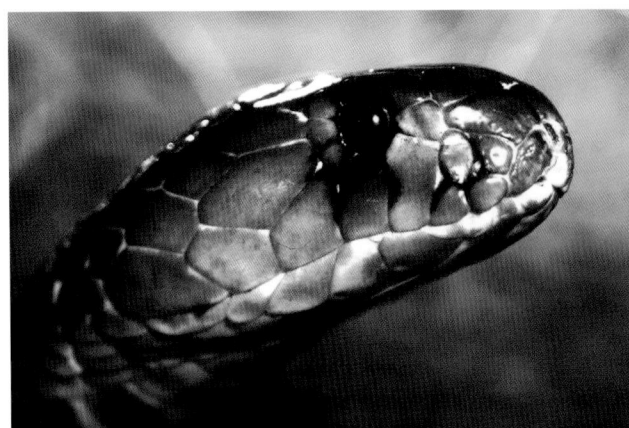

COLOR FIGURE 106-3

Naja. In contrast to many reports, members of the cobra family frequently cause significant local tissue destruction. Mixed neurotoxicity and myonecrosis is common. In contrast to kraits, few cobras possess pure neurotoxic activity. *(Courtesy of Dr. Beat Akeret.)*

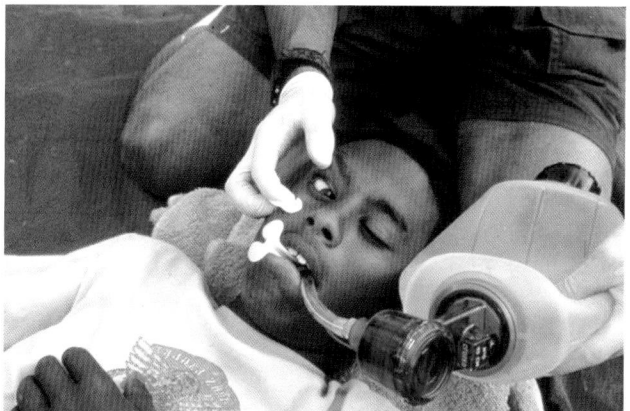

COLOR FIGURE 106-4

Severe envenoming. The patient was a 13-year-old boy with respiratory paralysis 9 hours after being bitten by an unknown krait (*Bungarus*). He received antivenom after symptoms appeared without effect, but he made a full recovery after 6 days of ventilation support. Note bulbar palsy.

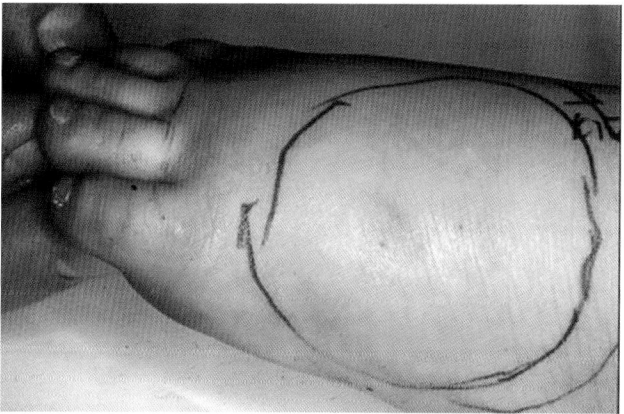

COLOR FIGURE 106-6

Minimal envenoming. The patient was a 9-year-old girl with s *Trimeresurus* bite to the foot. Note ecchymosis around fang marks and minimal swelling. The patient was observed overnight. No antivenom was given.

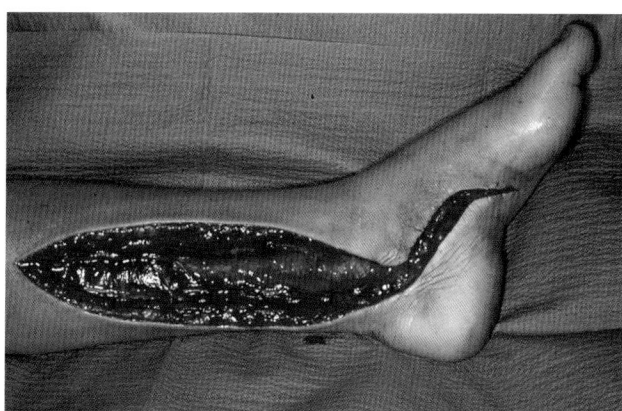

COLOR FIGURE 106-8

Fasciotomy for compartment syndrome may be suggested by excessive swelling of soft tissue; however, compartment pressures rarely are elevated significantly. Prophylactic fasciotomy is based on the belief that it protects against compartment syndrome. Such practices are unnecessary and can be catastrophic in venom-defibrinated patients.

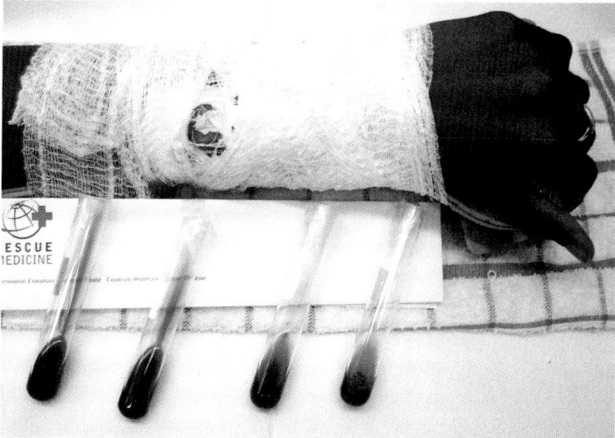

COLOR FIGURE 106-5

A 23-year-old woman with severe envenoming by *Daboia russelii*. The splint and gauze bandage help to stabilize the bitten extremity. Coagulopathy is checked using the whole-blood clotting test. The two tubes on the left, collected at 0 and 2 hours, lack clot formation. The two tubes on the right, collected at 5 and 10 hours after antivenom treatment, show return of clot formation. Note continued bleeding from the fang wounds to the forearm.

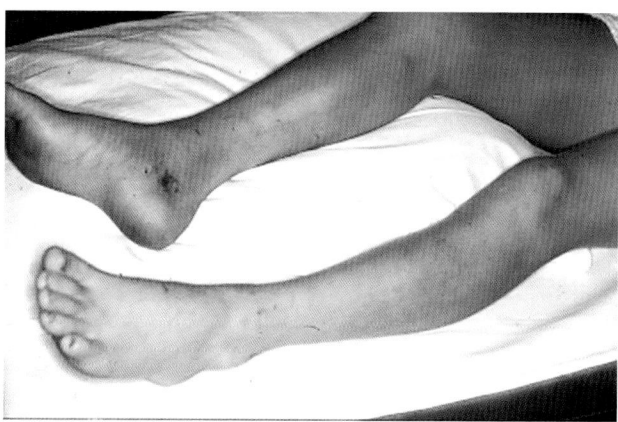

COLOR FIGURE 106-7

Moderate envenoming. The patient was a 15-year-old female tourist with bite to right ankle. Note ecchymosis and swelling involving the lower leg (species unknown).

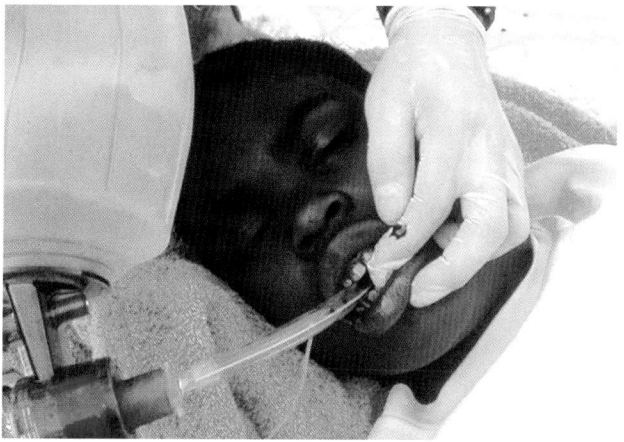

COLOR FIGURE 106-9

Caregivers should be vigilant for evidence of systemic anticoagulation, as occurred in this critically envenomed *Echis* bite. Note gingival bleeding after field intubation.

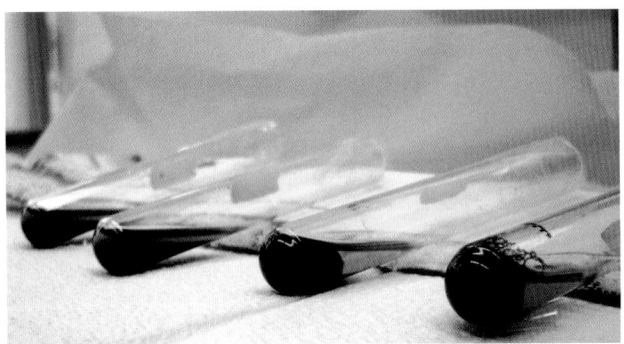

COLOR FIGURE 106-10

The whole-blood clotting test is a simple bedside test to measure anticoagulation. Clean glass tubes are filled with 5 mL of blood and left undisturbed for 20 minutes. Coagulopathy is present if blood flows down the tube (left two tubes). Antivenom usually produces a rapid but often transient return of clotting function (right two tubes).

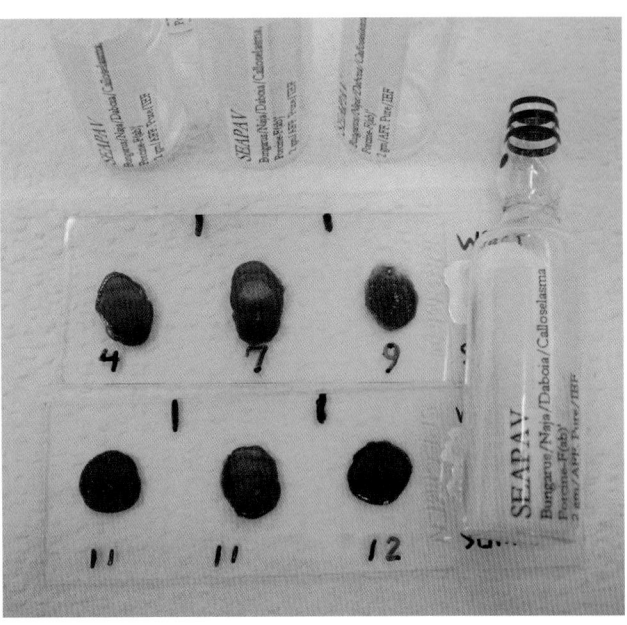

COLOR FIGURE 106-11

Rapid clot test. A simple test to guide antivenom use in austere settings. Blood (100 μL) is placed on a clean glass slide that is elevated 2 mm by resting the edge on top of another slide. Black numerals refer to the number of vials of antivenom administered. Defibrinated blood pools dependently or drips off the slide (four and seven vials). Note return of coagulopathy after 11 vials, requiring additional treatment (12 vials total).

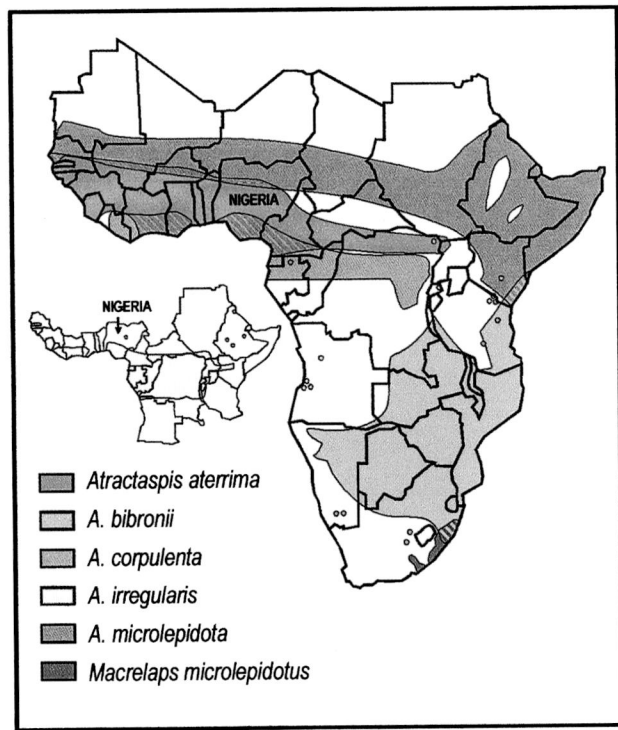

COLOR FIGURE 108-1

Distribution of Atractaspididae and the Natal black snake (*Macrelaps*). *(From Spawls S, Branch B: The Dangerous Snakes of Africa. London, 1995, Southern Book Publishers.)*

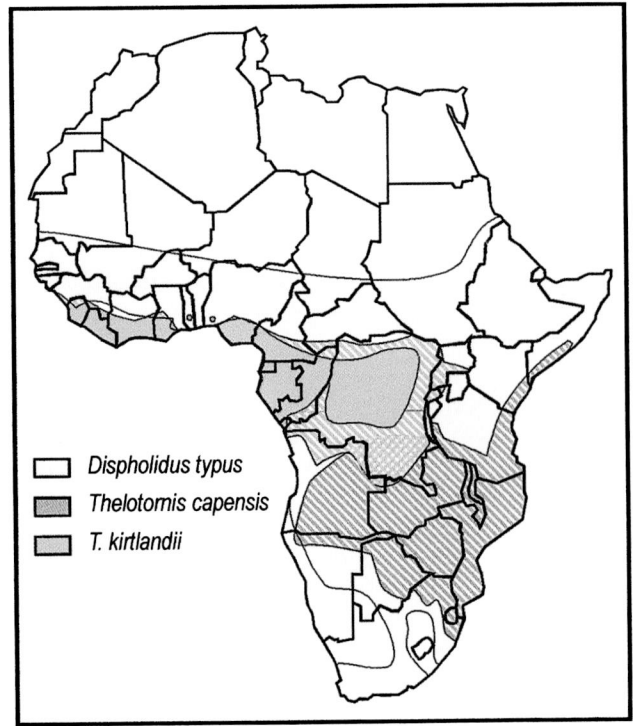

COLOR FIGURE 108-2

Distribution of selected Colubridae (*Dispholidus* and other hemotoxic species). *(From Spawls S, Branch B: The Dangerous Snakes of Africa. London, 1995, Southern Book Publishers.)*

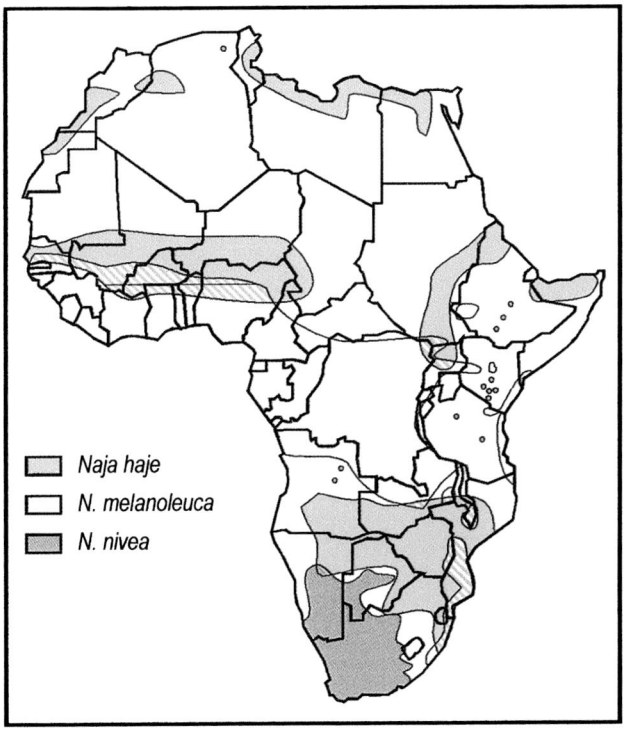

COLOR FIGURE 108-3

Distribution of the neurotoxic cobras (*Naja haje* and related species). *(From Spawls S, Branch B: The Dangerous Snakes of Africa. London, 1995, Southern Book Publishers.)*

Legend:
- Naja haje
- N. melanoleuca
- N. nivea

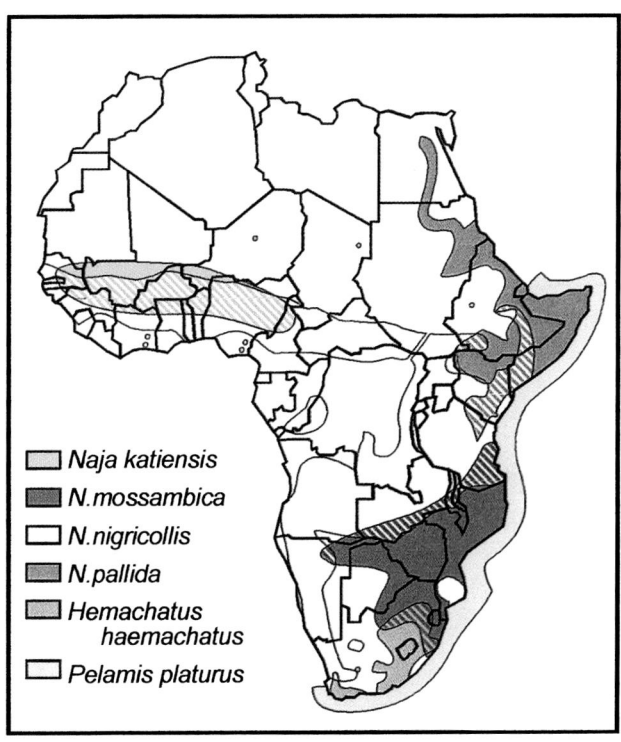

COLOR FIGURE 108-4

Distribution of the spitting cobras, rinkhals (*Hemachatus haemachatus*) and the sea snake (*Pelamis platurus*). *(From Spawls S, Branch B: The Dangerous Snakes of Africa. London, 1995, Southern Book Publishers.)*

Legend:
- Naja katiensis
- N. mossambica
- N. nigricollis
- N. pallida
- Hemachatus haemachatus
- Pelamis platurus

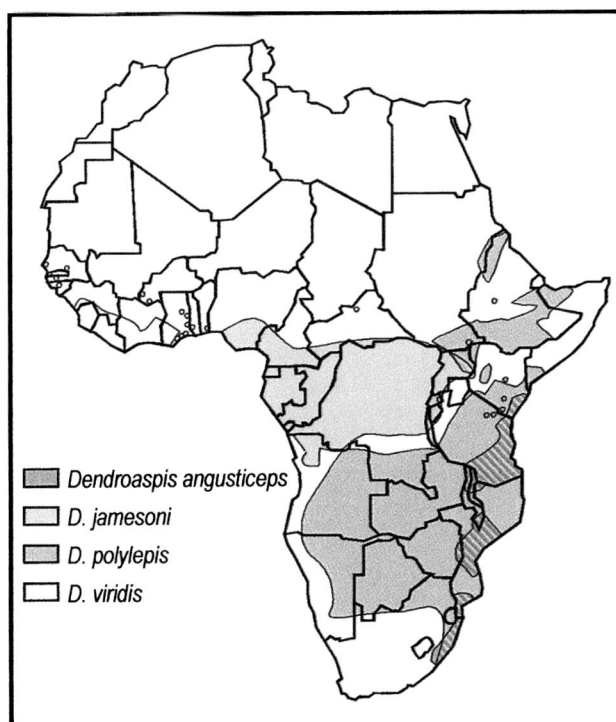

COLOR FIGURE 108-5

Distribution of mambas (*Dendroaspis* spp.). *(From Spawls S, Branch B: The Dangerous Snakes of Africa. London, 1995, Southern Book Publishers.)*

Legend:
- Dendroaspis angusticeps
- D. jamesoni
- D. polylepis
- D. viridis

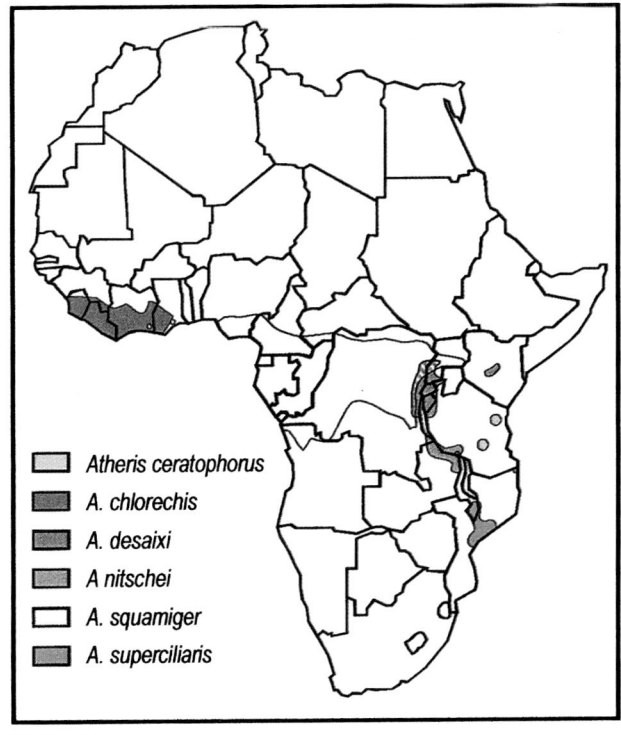

COLOR FIGURE 108-6

Distribution of the bush vipers (*Atheris* spp.). *(From Spawls S, Branch B: The Dangerous Snakes of Africa. London, 1995, Southern Book Publishers.)*

Legend:
- Atheris ceratophorus
- A. chlorechis
- A. desaixi
- A. nitschei
- A. squamiger
- A. superciliaris

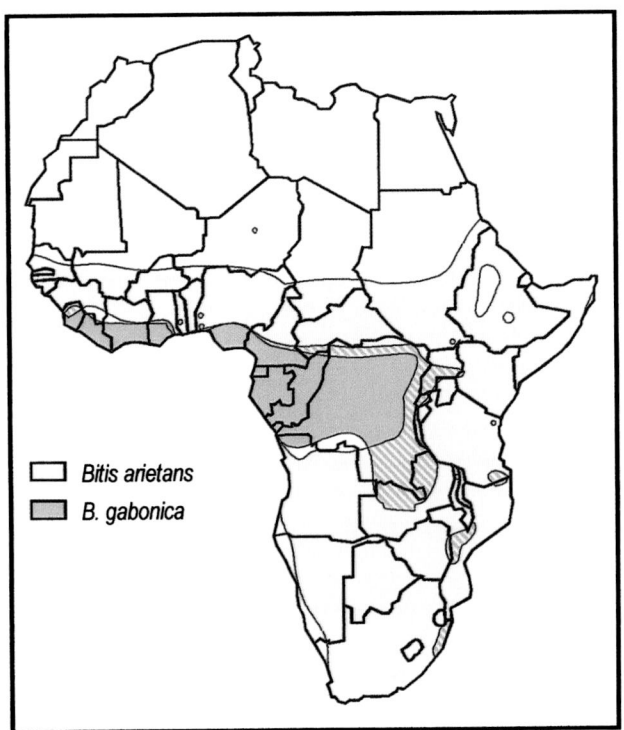

COLOR FIGURE 108-7

Distribution of the puff adder (*Bitis arietans*) and gaboon adder (*Bitis gabonica*). *(From Spawls S, Branch B: The Dangerous Snakes of Africa. London, 1995, Southern Book Publishers.)*

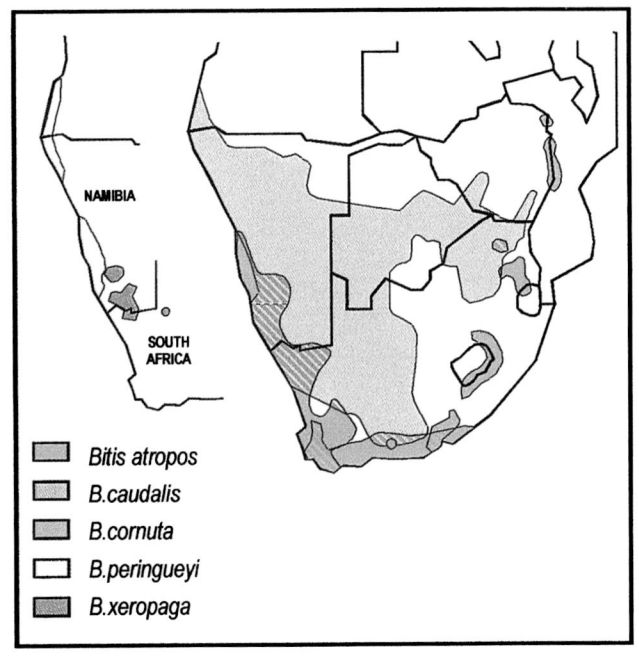

COLOR FIGURE 108-8

Distribution of the *Bitis atropos* and other dwarf adders of southern Africa. *(From Spawls S, Branch B: The Dangerous Snakes of Africa. London, 1995, Southern Book Publishers.)*

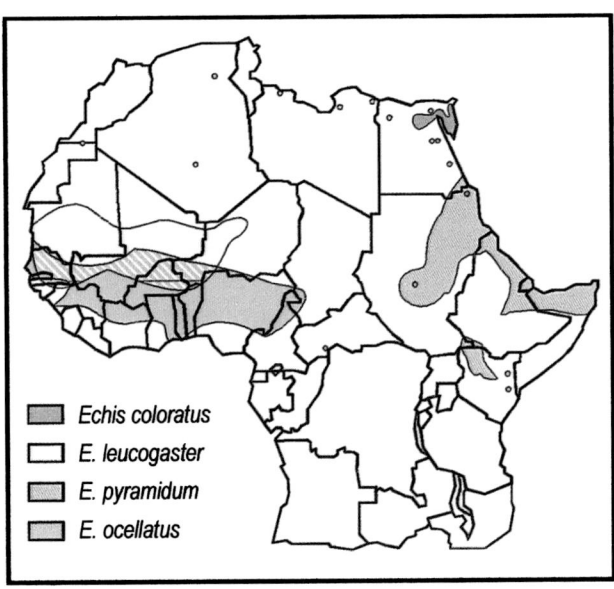

COLOR FIGURE 108-9

Distribution of carpet or saw-scaled vipers (*Echis* spp.). *(From Spawls S, Branch B: The Dangerous Snakes of Africa. London, 1995, Southern Book Publishers.)*

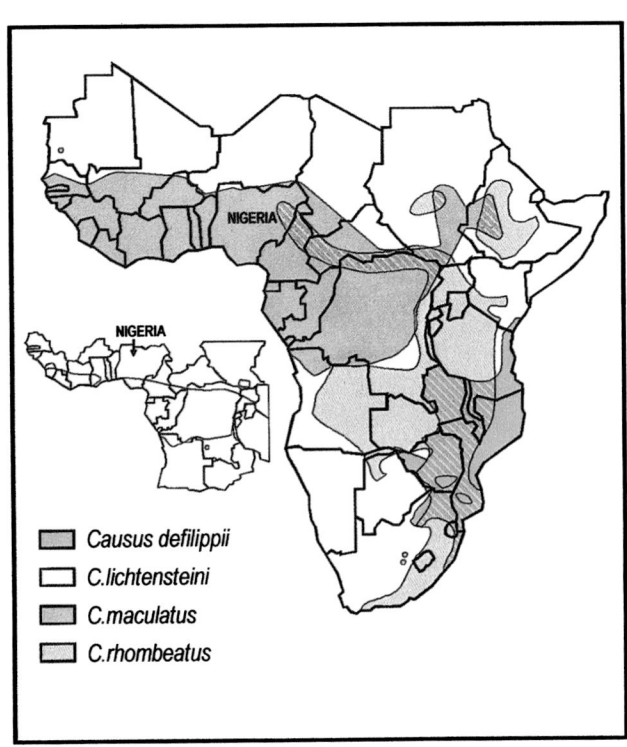

COLOR FIGURE 108-10

Distribution of the night adders (*Causus* spp.). *(From Spawls S, Branch B: The Dangerous Snakes of Africa. London, 1995, Southern Book Publishers.)*

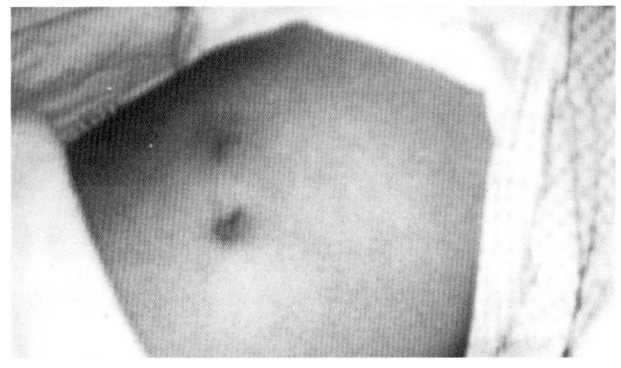

COLOR FIGURE 111-1

Target lesion after the bite of a *Latrodectus* spider.

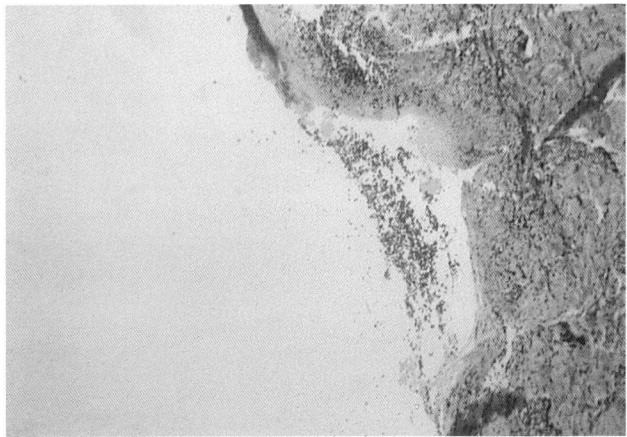

A

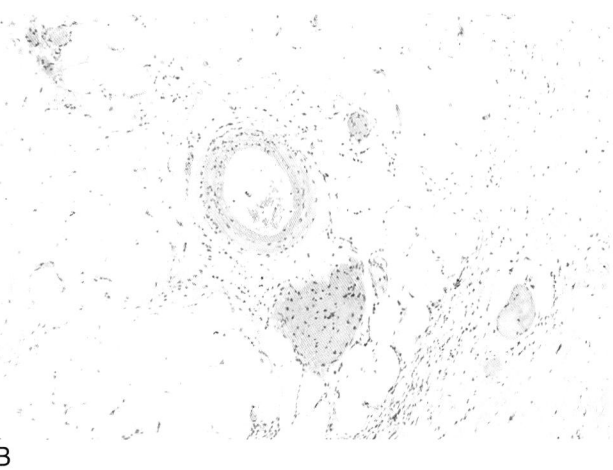

B

COLOR FIGURE 112-2

Dermatitis, panniculitis, and vasculitis. **A,** Skin biopsy specimen from an 18-month-old boy shows polymorphonuclear inflammatory response, 1-cm diameter necrotic crater, and probably fang mark. **B,** Skin biopsy specimen from autopsy of a 7-year-old girl who had hemolysis, disseminated intravascular coagulation, and dysrhythmias. There is superficial edema, fibrin thrombi, and moderate polymorphonuclear infiltration in the dermis, subcutaneous tissue, and large vessel wall.

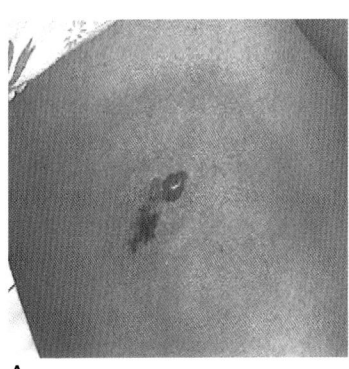

A

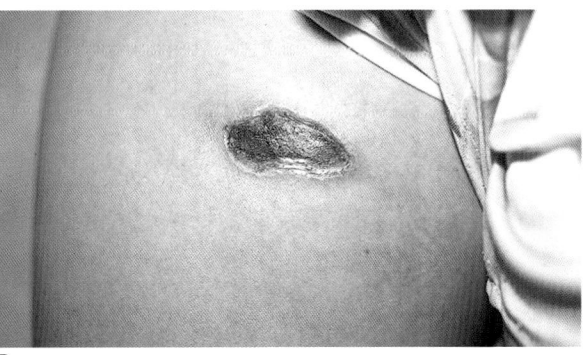

B

COLOR FIGURE 112-3

A, A 10-year-old girl as seen on day 2 postenvenomation. Note the blister indicating the puncture site, irregular necrosis (inferolaterally) representing venom spread by gravity, ecchymosis measuring 3.5 × 2 cm, and large area of inflammation. **B,** On day 7 postenvenomation, the entire original area of ecchymosis became necrotic and now is seen with eschar. Healing took 3 months with basic wound care.

COLOR FIGURE 112-4

"Halo" skin lesion on the forearm of a 9-year-old girl, day 3 postbite. She also had fever, abdominal pain, and hemolysis. Note the small blister, surrounded by an irregular area of ecchymosis, which is outlined with pallor (ischemia), then normal skin. Only the blister site became necrotic and healed in 6 weeks.

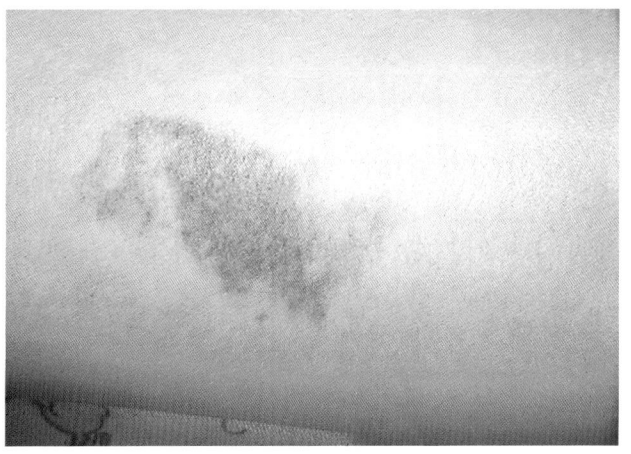

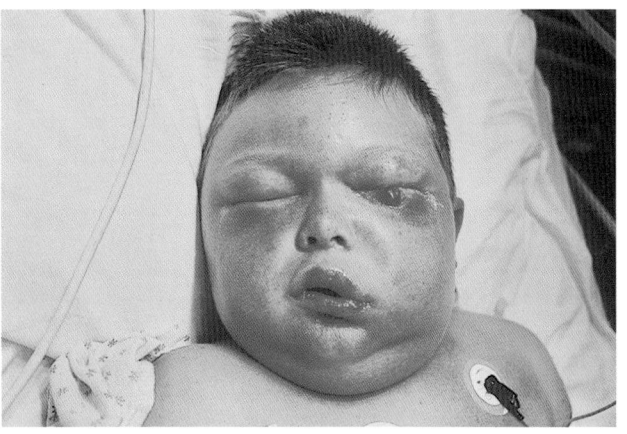

COLOR FIGURE 112-5

A 21-month-old boy bitten on the lower left eyelid. Note the extent of facial edema, which includes the neck and potentially the airway.

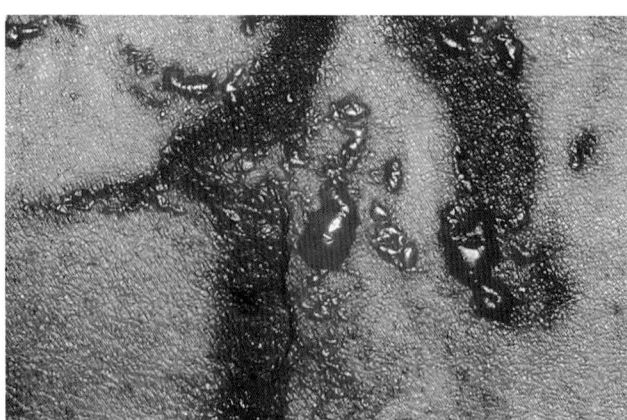

COLOR FIGURE 115-3

Incipient necrosis and blistering within 24 hours of box-jellyfish (*Chironex fleckeri*) envenomation. *(Courtesy of John Williamson, MD. From Auerbach PS: Envenomation by aquatic invertebrates. In Auerbach PS [ed]: Wilderness Medicine, 4th ed. Philadelphia, Mosby, 2001, p 1469.)*

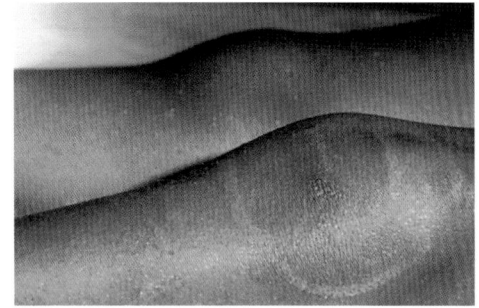

A

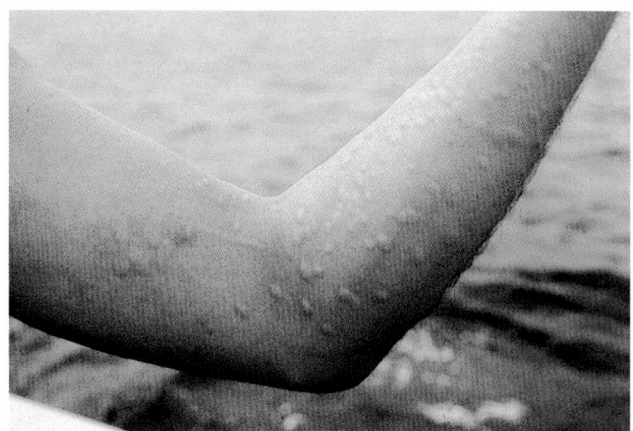

COLOR FIGURE 115-6

Hydroid sting on arm of a diver. *(Photo by Neville Coleman. From Auerbach PS: Envenomation by aquatic invertebrates. In Auerbach PS [ed]: Wilderness Medicine, 4th ed. Philadelphia, Mosby, 2001, p 1461.)*

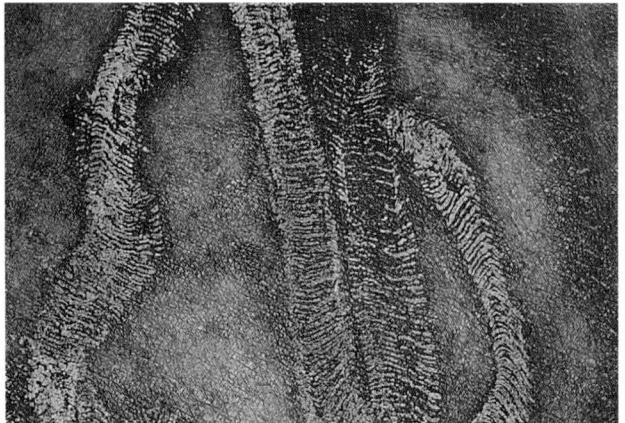

B

COLOR FIGURE 115-4

A, Frosted crosshatched pattern pathognomonic for a box-jellyfish envenomation. The victim of this sting died rapidly. **B,** The enhanced frosted appearance is a result of application of a spray of aluminum sulfate. *(Courtesy of John Williamson, MD. From Auerbach PS: Envenomation by aquatic invertebrates. In Auerbach PS [ed]: Wilderness Medicine, 4th ed. Philadelphia, Mosby, 2001, p 1469.)*

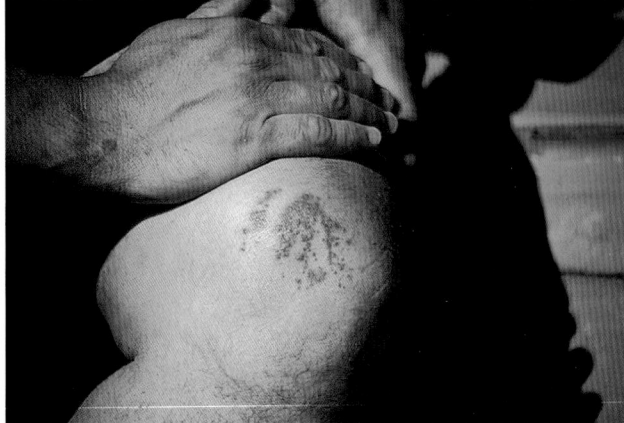

COLOR FIGURE 115-7

Fernlike hydroid print on the knee of a diver. *(Photo by Paul Auerbach, MD. From Auerbach PS: Envenomation by aquatic invertebrates. In Auerbach PS [ed]: Wilderness Medicine, 4th ed. Philadelphia, Mosby, 2001, p 1461.)*

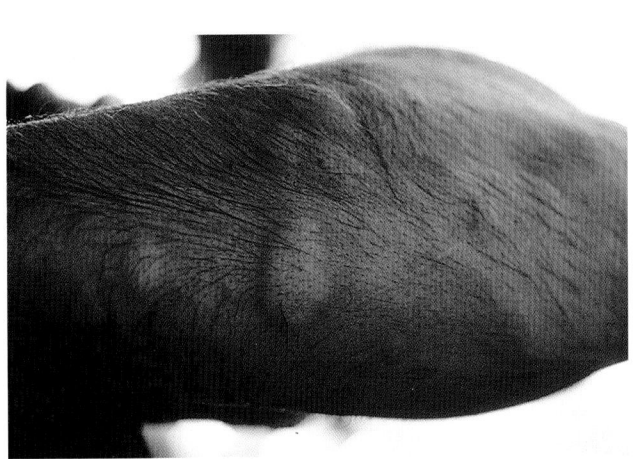

COLOR FIGURE 115-8

Fire coral sting. *(Photo by Kenneth Kizer, MD. From Auerbach PS: Envenomation by aquatic invertebrates. In Auerbach PS [ed]: Wilderness Medicine, 4th ed. Philadelphia, Mosby, 2001, p 1462.)*

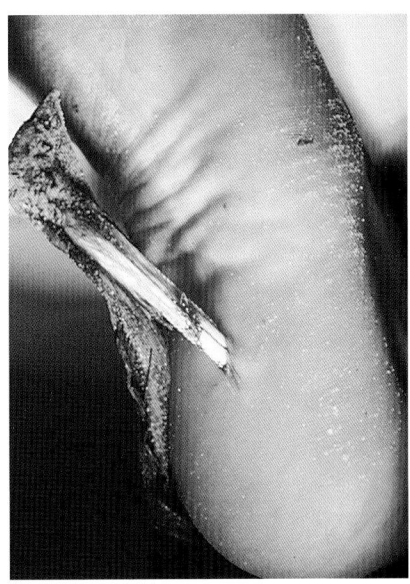

COLOR FIGURE 115-11

Stingray spine tip broken off into the heel of a victim. *(Photo by Robert D. Hayes. From Auerbach PS: Envenomation by aquatic invertebrates. In Auerbach PS [ed]: Wilderness Medicine, 4th ed. Philadelphia, Mosby, 2001, p 1490.)*

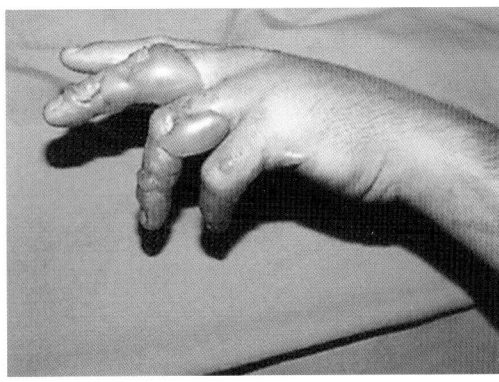

COLOR FIGURE 115-13

Vesiculation of the hand 48 hours after the sting of a lionfish. *(Photo by Howard McKinney. From Auerbach PS: Envenomation by aquatic invertebrates. In Auerbach PS [ed]: Wilderness Medicine, 4th ed. Philadelphia, Mosby, 2001, p 1495.)*

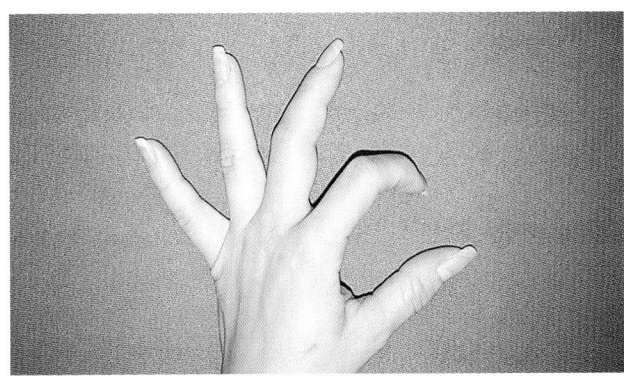

COLOR FIGURE 115-17

Finger swelling from sea urchin puncture. A single spine entered the palm over the third metacarpal bone. Swelling was severe in the second and third digits. *(Photo by Paul Auerbach, MD. Courtesy of John Williamson, MD. From Auerbach PS: Envenomation by aquatic invertebrates. In Auerbach PS [ed]: Wilderness Medicine, 4th ed. Philadelphia, Mosby, 2001, p 1478.)*

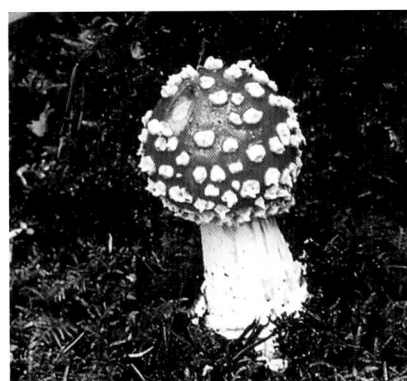

COLOR FIGURE 119-5

Amanita muscaria. *(From Schneider S, Donnelly M: Mushroom toxicity. In Auerbach PS [ed]: Wilderness Medicine, 4th ed. Philadelphia, Mosby, 2001, p 1148.)*

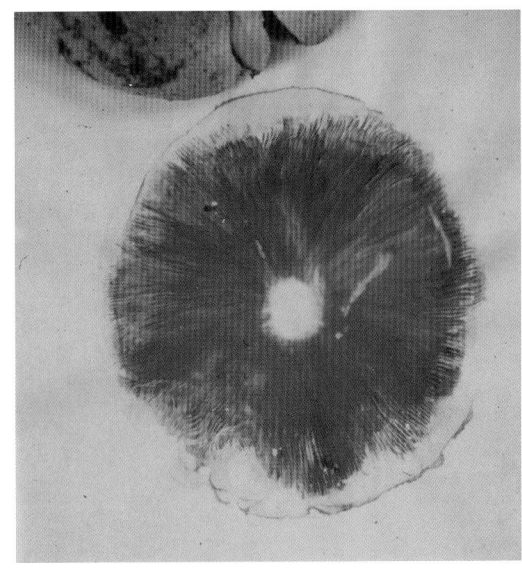

COLOR FIGURE 119-8

Chlorophyllum molybdites spore print.

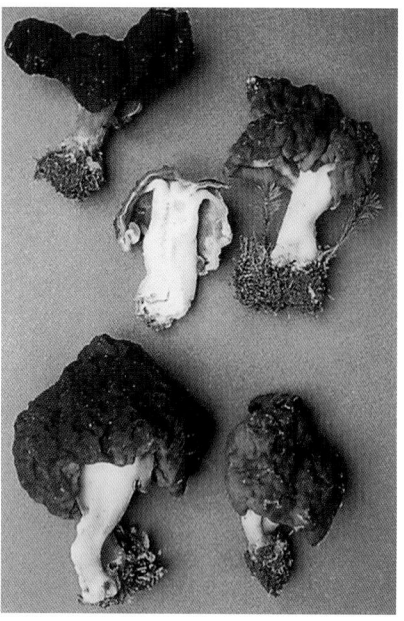

COLOR FIGURE 121-1

Gyromitra esculenta, which contains the hepatoxin gyromitrin. *(From Phillips R: Mushrooms of North America. Boston, Little Brown, 1991.)*

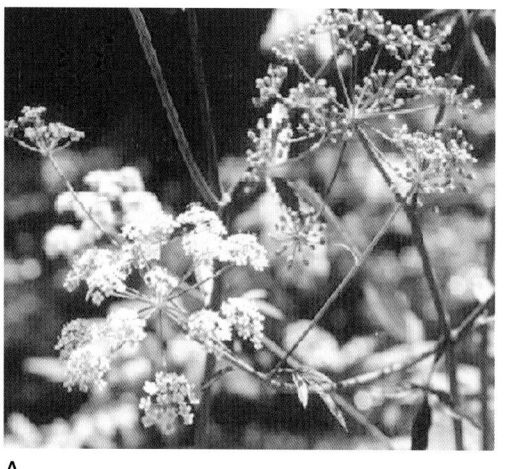

A

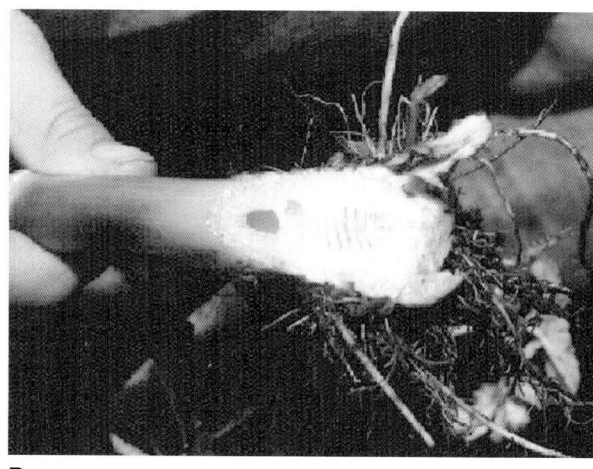

B

COLOR FIGURE 123-1

A, *Cicuta* spp. umbels typical of the Umbelliferea family. **B,** Chambered root characteristic of *Cicuta* spp. *(Photos courtesy of Steven Curry, MD. From Graeme KA, Braitberg G, Kunkel DB, Adler M: Toxic plant ingestions. In Auerbach PS [ed]: Wilderness Medicine. St. Louis, Mosby, 2001.)*

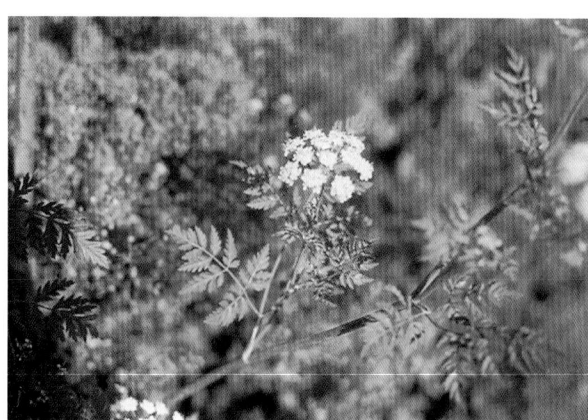

COLOR FIGURE 124-1

Poison hemlock (*Conium maculatum*). *(From Graeme KA, Braitberg G, Kunkel DB, et al: Toxic plant ingestions. In Auerbach PS [ed]: Wilderness Medicine, 4th ed. Philadelphia, Mosby, 2001, p 1114.)*

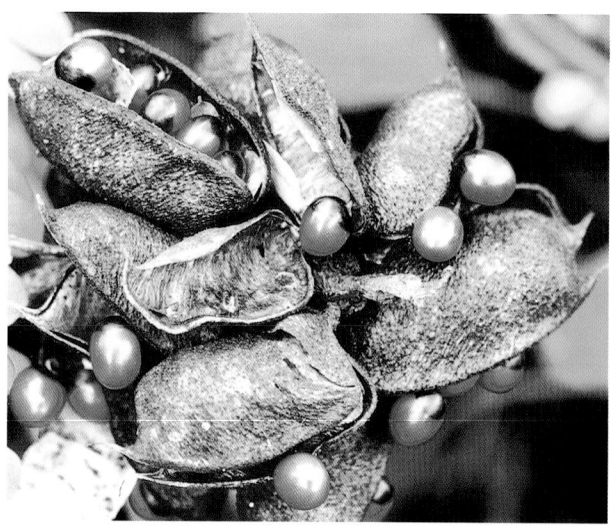

COLOR FIGURE 127-2

Abrus precatorius seeds. *(From New Leaf Graphics, Port St. Lucie, FL.)*

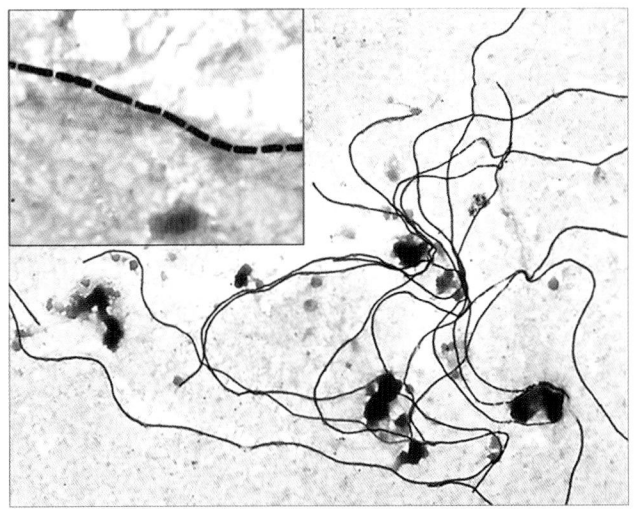

COLOR FIGURE 132-2

Gram-positive vegetative *Bacillus anthracis* growing in characteristic long chains in culture (original magnification 20%). *Inset*, Enlargement shows "jointed bamboo rod" of *B. anthracis* in culture (original magnification 100%). *(From Borio L, Frank D, Mani V, et al: Death due to bioterrorism-related inhalational anthrax: Report of 2 patients. JAMA 286:2554–2559, 2001.)*

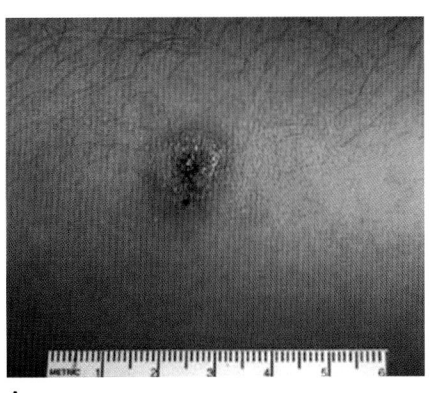
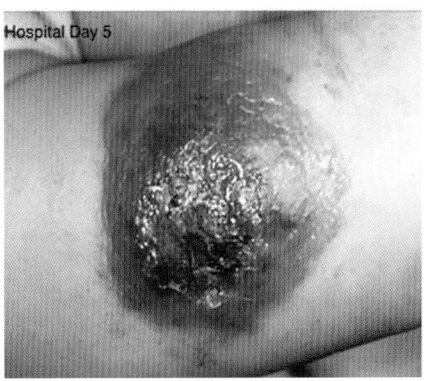
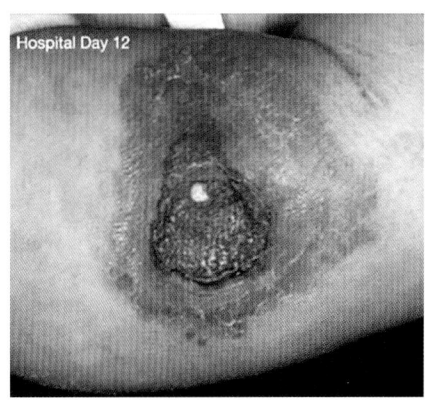

A   B   C

COLOR FIGURE 132-4

A, Cutaneous anthrax on forearm of a 34-year-old mail handler. **B,** Cutaneous anthrax on upper arm of a 7-month-old infant. **C,** Same patient as in **B** after antibiotic therapy. *(A from Gallagher TC, Strober BE: Cutaneous Bacillus anthracis infection. N Engl J Med 345:1646, 2001. B and C from Freedman A, Afonja O, Chang MW, et al: Cutaneous anthrax associated with microangiopathic hemolytic anemia and coagulopathy in a 7-month-old infant. JAMA 287:869–874, 2002.)*

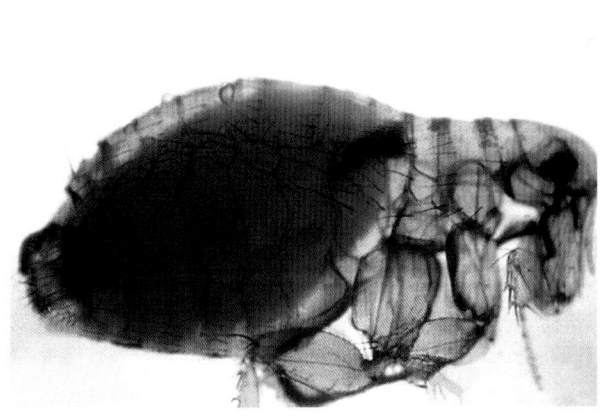

COLOR FIGURE 133-2

Xenopsylla cheopis, Oriental rat flea, with a proventricular plague mass. During feeding, the flea draws viable *Yersinia pestis* organisms into its esophagus, which multiply and block the proventriculus just in front of the stomach, later forcing the flea to regurgitate infected blood onto the host when it tries to swallow. *(From U.S. Centers for Disease Control, Public Health Image Library ID 2025.)*

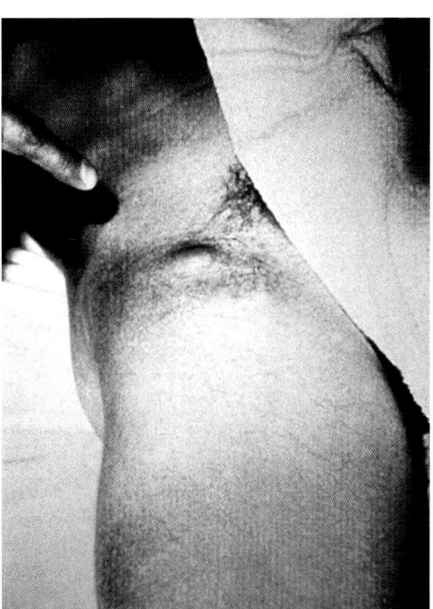

COLOR FIGURE 133-5

This plague patient shows symptoms that include a swollen inguinal lymph node, or bubo. *(From U.S. Centers for Disease Control, Public Health Image Library ID 2044.)*

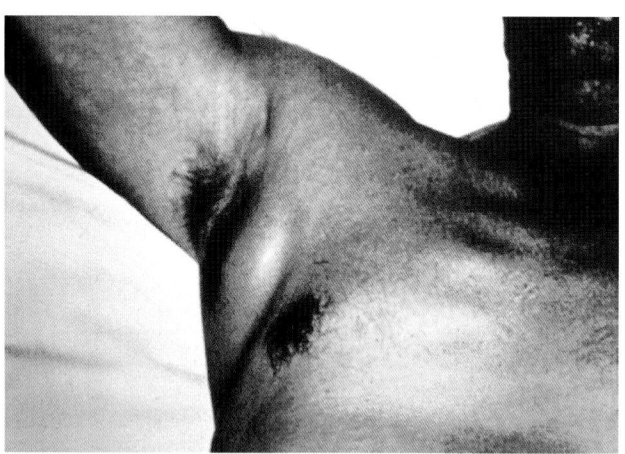

COLOR FIGURE 133-6

Plague patient displaying a swollen axillary lymph node. *(From U.S. Centers for Disease Control, Public Health Image Library ID 2045.)*

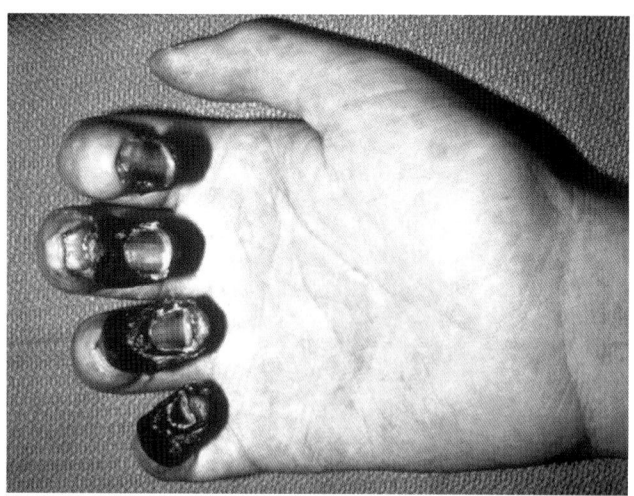

COLOR FIGURE 133-8

Right hand of a plague patient displaying acral gangrene. *(From U.S. Centers for Disease Control, Public Health Image Library ID 1957.)*

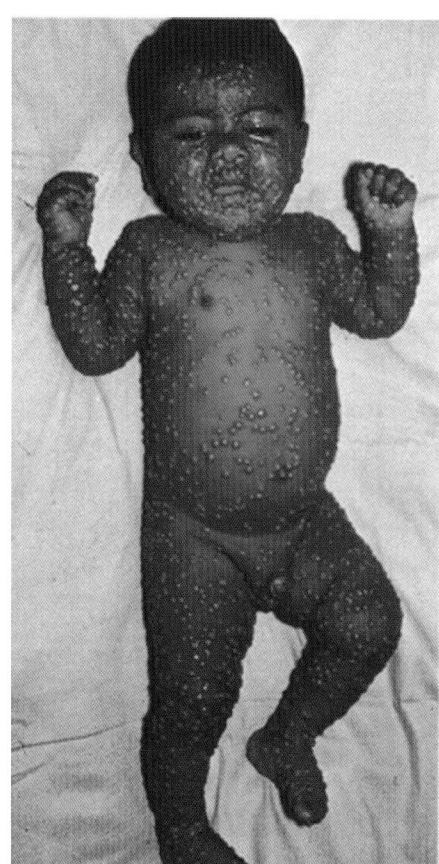

A

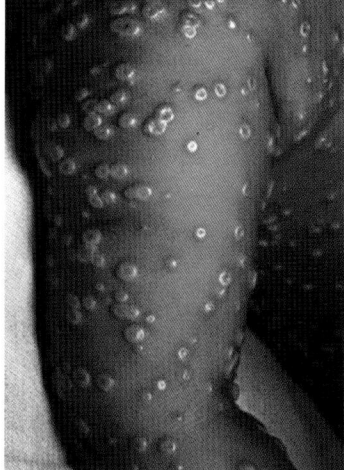

B

COLOR FIGURE 134A-2

A, A 9-month-old infant with discrete ordinary-type smallpox, day 9 of rash. **B,** Umbilicated lesions from the same patient, day 8 of rash. *(Fom Senkevich T, Wolffe EJ, Buller ML: Ectromelia virus RING finger protein is localized in virus factories and is required for virus replication in macrophages. J Virol 69:4103–4111, 1995.)*

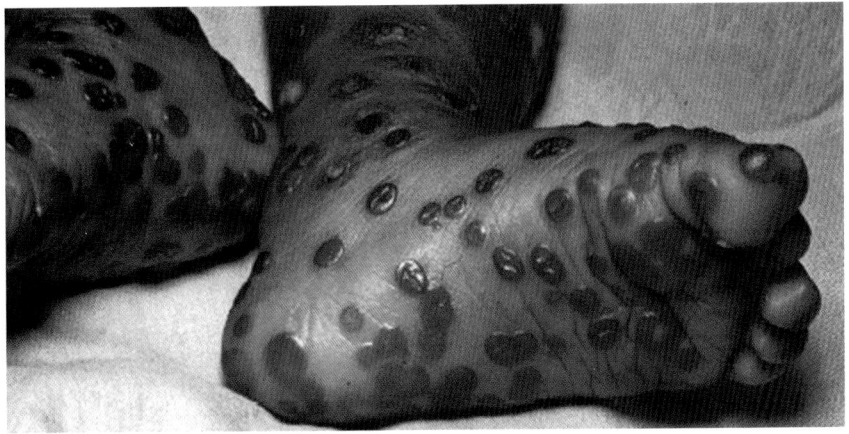

A

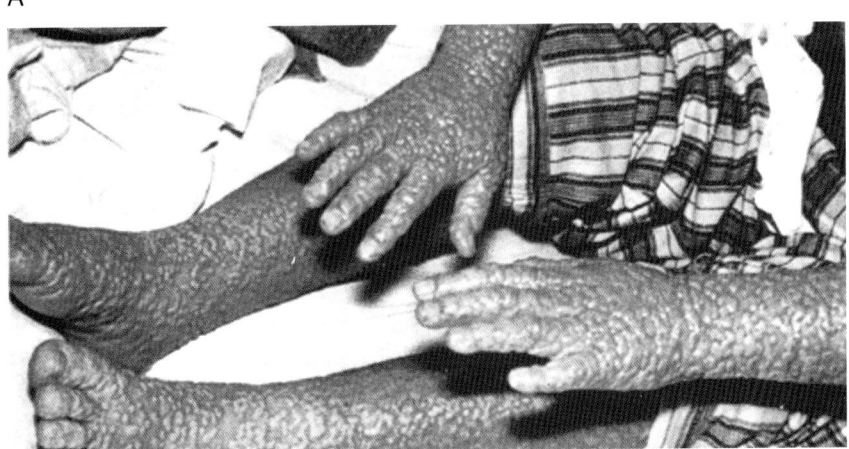

B

COLOR FIGURE 134A-3

A, Smallpox lesions on soles of feet. B, Confluent ordinary-type smallpox. *(Fom Senkevich T, Wolffe EJ, Buller ML: Ectromelia virus RING finger protein is localized in virus factories and is required for virus replication in macrophages. J Virol 69:4103–4111, 1995.)*

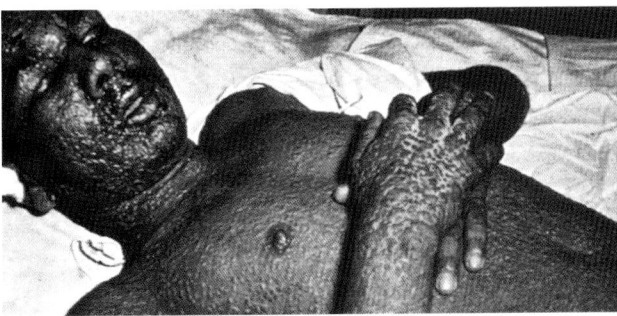

A

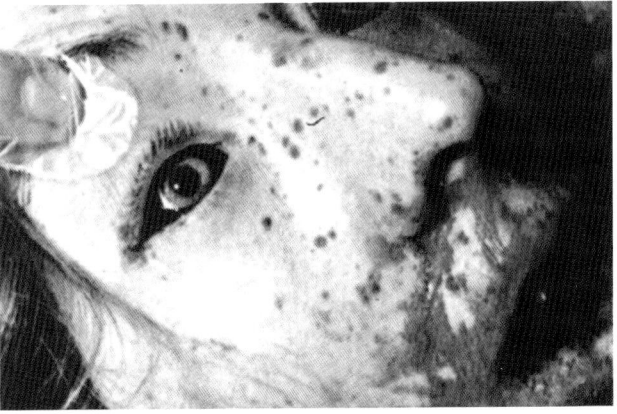

C

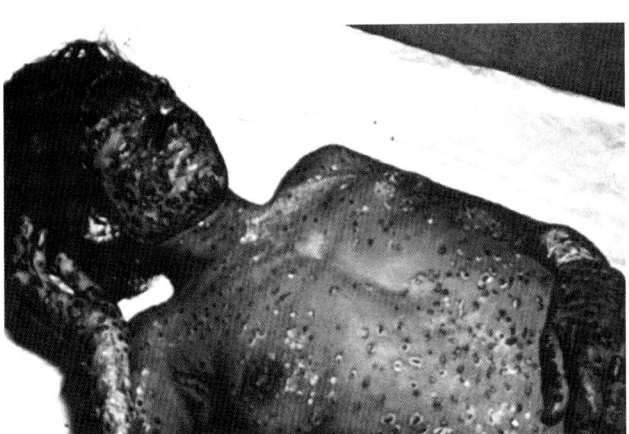

B

COLOR FIGURE 134A-4

A, Confluent flat-type smallpox; note lack of papular or vesicular lesions and severely toxic appearance. B, Late hemorrhagic-type smallpox; note well-evolved lesion with hemorrhages into lesions and severely toxic appearance. C, Early hemorrhagic-type smallpox; note conjunctival hemorrhages, poorly evolved lesions, and severely toxic appearance. *(Fom Senkevich T, Wolffe EJ, Buller ML: Ectromelia virus RING finger protein is localized in virus factories and is required for virus replication in macrophages. J Virol 69:4103–4111, 1995.)*

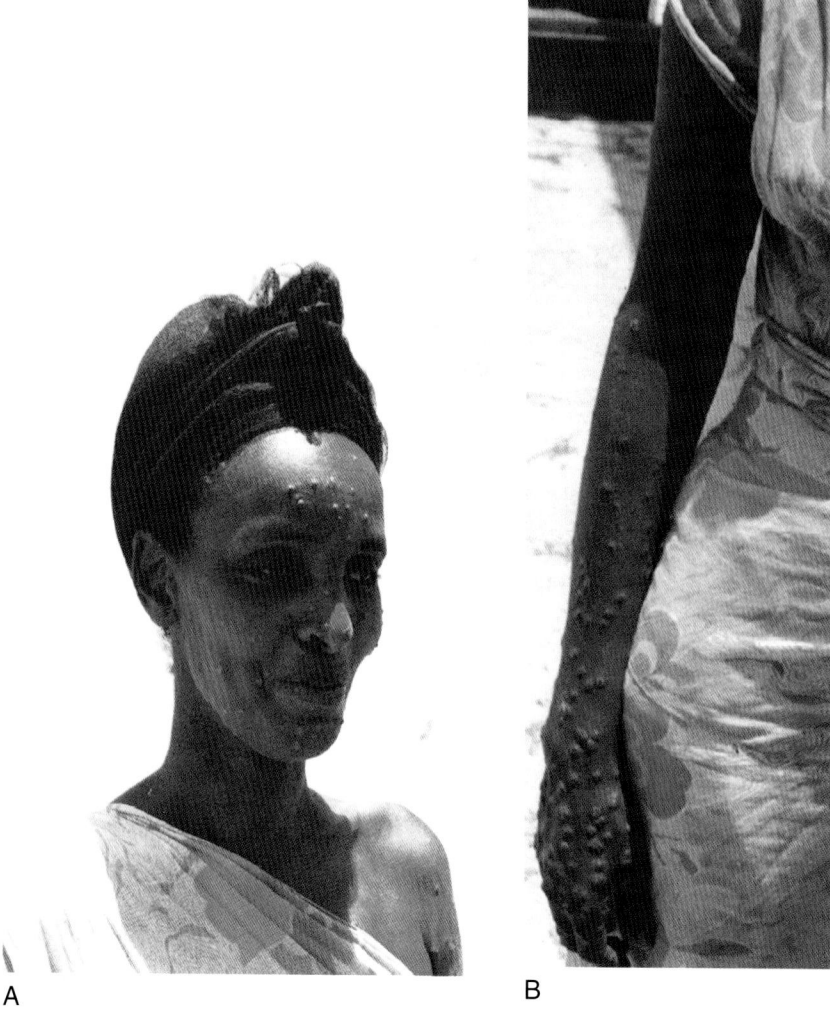

A   B

COLOR FIGURE 134A-5

Variola minor in an unvaccinated 30-year-old woman (12 days after rash eruption). The patient was not toxic throughout course of illness. Lesions are sparse on the face **(A)** and evolved more rapidly than lesions on the extremities **(B)**. *(Fom Senkevich T, Wolffe EJ, Buller ML: Ectromelia virus RING finger protein is localized in virus factories and is required for virus replication in macrophages. J Virol 69:4103–4111, 1995.)*

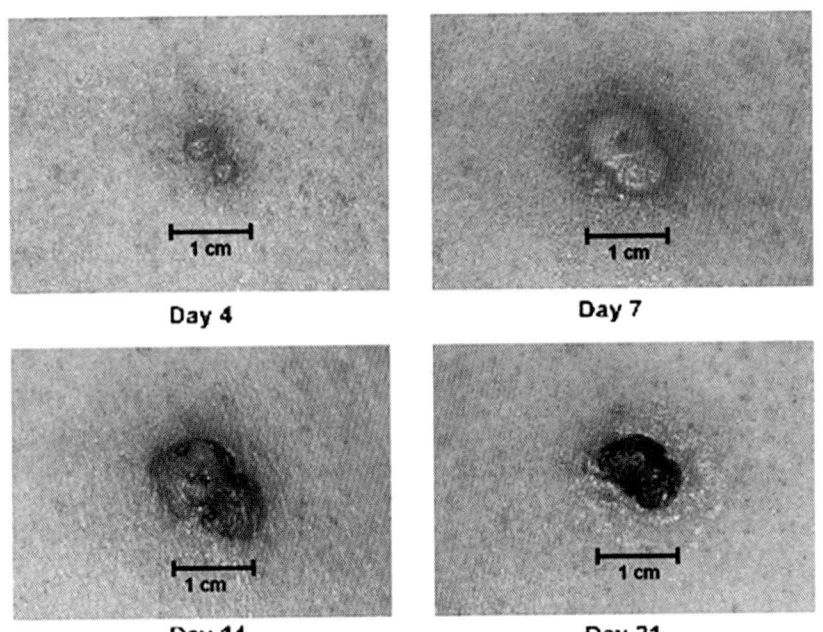

Day 4

Day 7

Day 14

Day 21

COLOR FIGURE 134A-6

Major (primary) reaction. Expected vaccine site reaction and progression after primary smallpox vaccination or revaccination after a prolonged period between vaccinations. Multiple pressure vaccination technique was used. *(From U.S. Centers for Disease Control and Prevention. Available at: http://www.bt.cdc.gov/agent/smallpox/vaccineimages.asp.)*

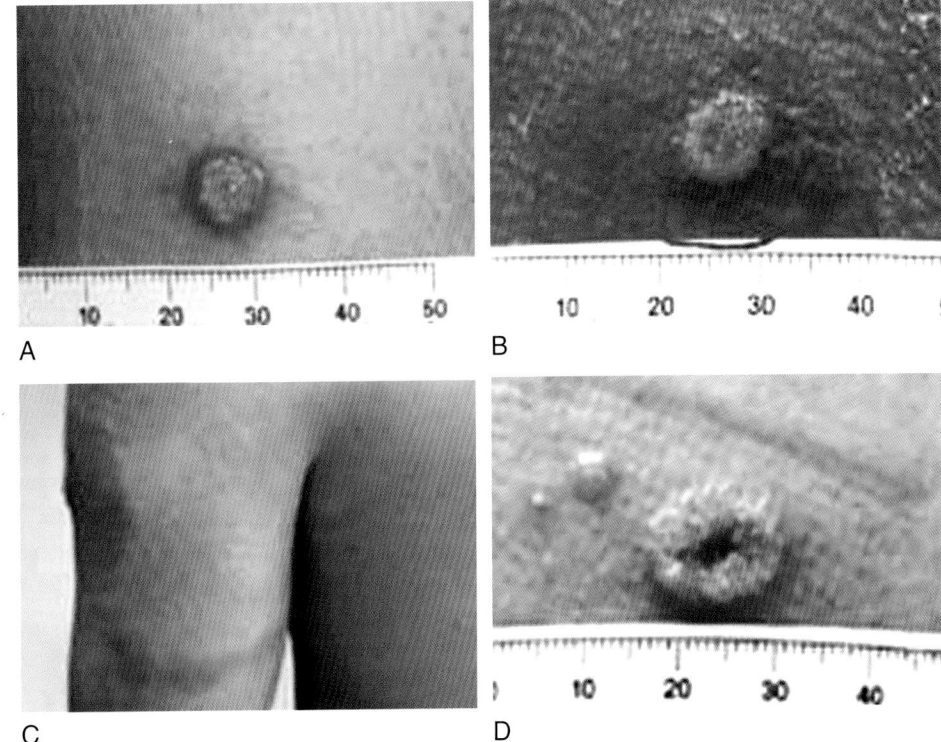

A

B

C

D

COLOR FIGURE 134A-7

A and **B**, Normal vaccination reactions. **C**, Normal reaction with lymphangitis. **D**, Normal reaction with satellite lesions. *(From U.S. Centers for Disease Control and Prevention. Available at: http://www.bt.cdc.gov/training/smallpoxvaccine/reactions/default.htm.)*

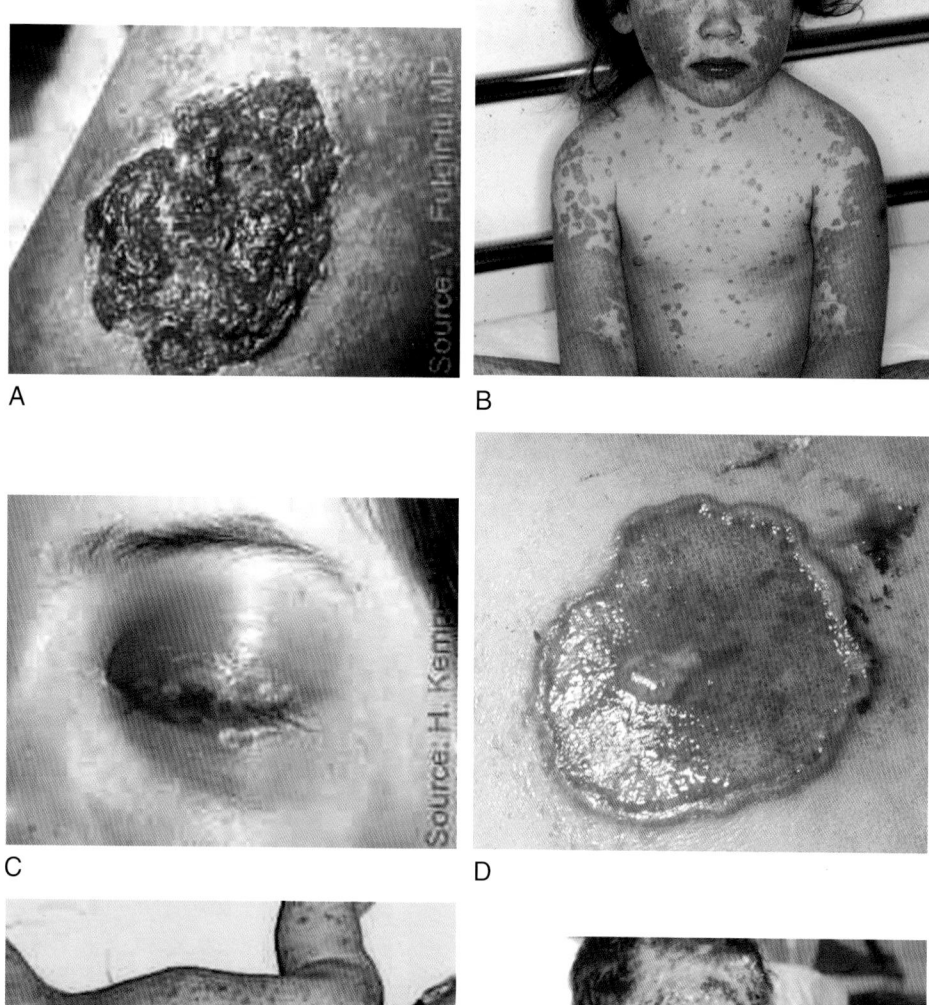

A

B

C

D

E

F

COLOR FIGURE 134A-8

Complications of vaccination. **A,** Secondary bacterial infection at vaccination site. **B,** Erythema multiforme. **C,** Autoinoculation. **D,** Progressive vaccinia (vaccinia gangrenosum). **E,** Generalized vaccinia. **F,** Eczema vaccinatum. (*A-E* from U.S. Centers for Disease Control and Prevention. Available at: http://www.bt. cdc.gov/agent/smallpox/vaccination/clinicians.asp; *F* from Anonymous: Human monkeypox in Kasai Oriental, Zaire [1996–1997]. Wkly Epidemiol Rec 72:101–104, 1997.)

PART 1

General Management of the Critically Poisoned Patient

CHAPTER **1**

The Critically Poisoned Patient

J. Ward Donovan ▪ Keith K. Burkhart ▪ Jeffrey Brent

The disciplines of critical care medicine and medical toxicology have been intertwined throughout medical history. Texts combining the principles of these closely related specialties may be traced to medieval times; Maimonides wrote his *Treatise on Poison and Their Antidotes* in 1198.[1] In his *Treatise*, Maimonides outlined the classification, diagnosis, and antidotal therapy of poisonings and described some resuscitation methods of the age. He also, in undoubtedly what was among the first attempts to evaluate therapies critically, refuted many of the then-popular treatments. The need to continually reevaluate—and commonly refute—generally accepted therapies continues to this day. This book continues this tradition in the spirit established by Maimonides, except, of course, with a more data-driven approach.

Descriptions of the use of specific antidotal therapy dates back to Homer's *Odyssey*, in which Ulysses was advised to use "moly," likely a natural cholinesterase inhibitor, to treat poisoning from anticholinergic plants such as *Datura stramonium*.[2] Other publications from ancient times addressing the use of poisoning therapies include Nicander's *Alexipharmaca*, or "that which keeps off poisons"; Dioscordes' *Materia Medica*; and Galen's *DeAntidotis* and *De Theriaca ad Pisonem*.[3,4]

The identification, diagnosis, and therapy of poisons began in Greek and Roman times, with classifications by Dioscordes of poisonings by source and speed of action.[3] The Greek Nicander and King Mithridates of Pontus described the use of "theriacs" and "alexipharmacas" as universal antidotes and red clay ingestion or induction of emesis with feathers or oil to prevent toxin absorption.[3] In addition to his general description of poisons, Maimonides suggested emesis by ingesting oil, water, and honey.[1] Antimony salt, also known as tartar emetic, was widely used to induce stomach emptying and functioned as a sedative and cathartic in the 19th century, but it was replaced in the early 20th century by saltwater emetics, mustard powder, mechanical throat stimulation, copper sulfate, and apomorphine.[5,6] Ipecac syrup was first employed to induce emesis in the 17th century and became the emetic of choice in the 20th century. Gastric lavage was first advocated by Munro

in 1769 and supported by the physicians Physik of Philadelphia, Jukes of Britain, Dupuytren of France, and Bryce of Edinburgh.[7] In the 16th century, Paracelcus emphasized the fundamental importance—and to this day, the often overlooked—dose relationship of chemicals and drugs and the need for scientific study of toxins. Charcoal to adsorb toxins was described in the 18th century and employed in self-experiments by Bertrand and Touery, who publicly ingested toxins followed by a dose of charcoal.[8] The "universal antidote" of magnesium oxide, tannic acid, and activated charcoal was touted as the definitive adsorbent of toxins throughout the 20th century, until it was recognized to be inferior to activated charcoal alone.[5] Activated charcoal ultimately replaced other means of gastric decontamination beginning in the 1970s.[8]

Textbooks establishing medical toxicology as a unique scientific specialty began to appear in the 19th century, with the publication of Orfila's *Traite des Poisons* in Paris in 1814, which emphasized experimental and forensic toxicology, followed by his student Christison's writing the first of several editions from Edinburgh of *Treatise on Poisons* in 1829.[9] Christison reportedly first highlighted the lifesaving properties of artificial respiration in opium poisoning, showing the close relationship between medical toxicology and critical care medicine.[7] Other texts of that era were Costill's *A Practical Treatise on Poisons* and Taylor's *On Poisons*, both published in 1848. Early texts of the 20th century on clinical toxicology include Leschke's *Clinical Toxicology*; Driesbach's *Handbook of Poisoning*; Gleason, Gosselin, and Hodge's *Clinical Toxicology of Commercial Products*; and Jay Arena's *Poisoning*. Historical toxicology reference texts are listed in Table 1-1.

More specific therapies and antidotes to treat poisonings also date back in history. Beginning with Maimonides, some examples include the use of natural anticholinesterase inhibitors to treat anticholinergic poisoning, *Strychnos nuxvomica* (strychnine) as an arousal and emetic agent, and in the 1800s the use of rabbit brain to protect against *Amanita phalloides* mushroom poisoning.[1,6] Physostigmine,

TABLE 1-1 Historical Toxicology Reference Texts

TEXT	AUTHOR	DATE	CITY
A Treatise on Poisons	M.C. Cooke	1770	London
Traite des Toxicologie	H.J.B. Orfila	1813	Paris
A Treatise on Poisons	Robert Christison	1829	Edinburgh
On Poisons	Alfred Taylor	1848	London
A Practical Treatise on Poisons	O.H. Costill	1848	Philadelphia
Micro-Chemistry of Poisons	Theodore Wormley	1869	New York
What to Do in Cases of Poisoning	William Murrell	1884	New York
A Manual of Medical Jurisprudence, General Toxicology	M.D. Ewell	1887	Boston
A Manual of Medical Jurisprudence and Toxicology	Henry Chapman	1896	Philadelphia
Handbuch der Toxicologie	A.K. Kunkel	1899	Jena
Manual of Toxicology	R.A. Witthaus	1911	New York
Handbook of Poisoning	R.H. Driesbach	1955	Los Altos, CA
Clinical Toxicology	C.H. Thienes	1955	Philadelphia, PA
Clinical Toxicology of Commercial Products	Gleason, Gosselin & Hodge	1957	Baltimore
Poisoning	J.M. Arena	1963	Springfield, IL

an anticholinesterase inhibitor from the Calabar bean, reportedly was advocated for atropine poisoning by Christison's successor to the Chair of Medical Jurisprudence in Edinburgh, Thomas Fraser.[7] Arousal of the patient affected by opiate or sedative toxicity was popularized in the 19th and 20th centuries, first by mechanical stimulation and later by the use of analeptics.[7] The latter included natural agents, such as caffeine, strychnine, cocaine, camphor, picrotoxin, and lobeline, and later synthetic agents, such as pentylenetetrazol, nikethamide, methylphenidate, and bemegride.[10] The use of analeptics eventually was recognized to cause serious complications, such as hyperthermia, seizures, delirium, and increased mortality.[10] One of the most important advances in medical toxicology occurred in Scandinavia in the 1940s, when intensive supportive care with mechanical ventilation and cardiovascular support instead of analeptics was shown to reduce mortality from barbiturate poisoning from 20% to 2%.[9,10] The overlap of critical care medicine and medical toxicology again was reinforced. This overlap further included the advocacy for poisoned patients of close observation and monitoring; airway protection; frequent pulmonary toilet; and careful attention to fluid and electrolyte balance, cardiovascular status, and position changes.

Later advances in toxicology in the 20th century included the discovery of the opiate antagonists/agonists nalorphine and levallorphan and the pure antagonist naloxone, the development of highly specific and sensitive assays for drugs and chemicals, greater understanding of pharmacokinetic principles, refinement of the principles of urinary pH manipulation to enhance drug excretion, and implementation of extracorporeal removal techniques. More recently, progress has been made in the application of immunotherapies as antidotes, the development of additional antidotes to reverse specific drug effects, the wide availability of toxicology information via computer software and the Internet, and the early use of toxicogenetics to determine individual variations in responses to toxins and treatments.

EPIDEMIOLOGY

Incidence

The incidence of poisonings is about 1470 per 100,000 population in the United States, with 2.4 million exposures per year. As the cause of 11% of all injury deaths, poisoning is the third leading cause of injury-related mortality in the United States.[11,12] The U.S. National Center for Health Statistics recorded 16,527 poisoning deaths in 1994.[13] Between 1993 and 1996, there were 1 million emergency department visits for poisonings in the United States each year[12,14]; this represents 590 emergency department visits and 1 death for poisonings per 100,000 population.[12] The death rate was 160 per 10,000 population in the 35- to 44-year age group. In the United Kingdom, there is a reported incidence of 310 poisonings per 100,000 population, or 170,000 annual hospital visits, much lower than the U.S. rate.[15] Overdoses account for one fourth of all suicide attempts in England.[16]

Poisonings typically represent 1% to 3% of all emergency department visits and account for 10% of all admissions for injuries.[17,18] The incidence of hospital admissions for poisonings in the United States is about 130 per 100,000 population, or about 220,000 poisoning admissions in the United States each year.[12] There are a reported 80,000 poisonings admissions each year in England, which result in about 400 deaths, or 0.5% of all such admissions.[16] According to another report, for all of the United Kingdom, the total admissions are about 170,000 annually.[15]

Emergency department reporting of poisoning cases is highly variable. In one study, an academic tertiary care emergency department called its regional poison control center (PCC) on 26% of its cases.[19] In many poisoning cases, the exposure was highly reported to the PCC (e.g., 95% for cyclic antidepressants), in contrast to cases of drug abuse (e.g., 5% for cocaine or heroin poisoning), which are not often reported to poison control centers. A review of an entire state's hospital admissions for poisoning indicated that the Oregon Poison Center was contacted for 54%, or 1352, of 2486 admissions in 1989.[20]

Drug overdoses typically account for approximately 2.5% to 5% of all intensive care unit (ICU) admissions in the United States,[21–23] with an average length of stay (LOS) of 2.5 to 3.5 days.[21,24,25] Poisonings have been reported to represent 11% to 14% of all ICU admissions in some countries.[24,26] Mortality rates in the ICU for poisoning admissions range from 3% to 6% according to most reports.[21,25]

Toxins

Reports from Edinburgh describe the evolving patterns of admissions from the 1960s into the 1980s. In 1966, 60% of the admissions to the Royal Infirmary of Edinburgh were for barbiturate poisoning.[27] Only in the teenage group did aspirin surpass barbiturates as a cause of toxicity. In this time period, poisoning accounted for 10% of hospital admissions. In 1968, 74% of the patients had an LOS of 2 days or less.[28] Proudfoot[9] reported on the subsequent 20-year trend (1967 through 1986) at the same center. During this period, barbiturate poisonings decreased from 30% of admissions in the 1970s to a rare occurrence. Methaqualone was initially responsible for 10% of admissions but by the mid-1970s was almost no longer seen. A predominance of benzodiazepine overdoses subsequently replaced barbiturates and methaqualone, their incidence increasing from 10% to approximately 40% of admissions in the 1970s. Throughout the 1970s, there was also a rapidly increasing admission percentage for paracetamol (acetaminophen), whereas there was a slightly decreasing trend for salicylates.

Benzodiazepines were reported as the predominant ICU admission for poisonings in Stockholm, Sweden, from 1972 through 1985, increasing from 17% to 28% of the total number.[29] In 51% of cases, a benzodiazepine was part of a polydrug overdose, and in 21% of cases, benzodiazepines were the single ingestant. Benzodiazepine-alone admissions were intubated in 37% of cases, whereas the intubation rate was 47% if benzodiazepines were consumed with alcohol or as part of a polydrug overdose. Of the 702 ICU admissions, the complication rate was 9.8%. There were five fatalities related to respiratory insufficiency or aspiration pneumonia or both.

During the 1980s and 1990s, cyclic antidepressant poisoning was a predominant ICU admission diagnosis. In the Netherlands from 1994 through 1998, cyclic antidepressants constituted 33.3% of the total intoxication admissions and 2.4% of total admissions. The average LOS was 3.1 days. Of these patients, 40% were intubated, and seven (2.7%) died.[22]

In New Zealand in 1992, there was a similar experience. Of all emergency department visits, 1.2% were poisoning related, yet these cases constituted 11% of ICU admissions. The incidence was 17 per 100,000 population. The most common agents ingested were cyclic antidepressants (19.6%), benzodiazepines (18%), acetaminophen (16.9%), and various antipsychotics. The average LOS was 2.4 days.[26] A 6-year review (1986 through 1991) of ICU admissions for poisoning was published in Australia. Poisonings accounted for 13.8% of all admissions. The most common agents were benzodiazepines, ethanol, tricyclic antidepressants, acetaminophen, phenothiazines, and antihistamines. The mean age was 32, the mortality rate was 2%, and 6 of the 14 fatalities were from nonmedicinal products.[24]

The introduction of flumazenil, a benzodiazepine antagonist at the γ-aminobutyric acid receptor site, reportedly had an impact on ICU care and LOS in Israel. Leykin and colleagues[30] described acute poisonings treated in the ICU from 1982 through 1984. The predominant intoxicants were benzodiazepines (51%), tricyclics (25%), barbiturates (21%), and narcotics (11%). Flumazenil was believed to have contributed to a decreased ventilator time and LOS (from 4.8 to 3.1 days). The introduction of the safer antidepressants, selective serotonin reuptake inhibitors, also markedly reduced the ICU admission rate, LOS, and cost of care.[31]

In many countries, nonmedicinals such as plants and pesticides remain a significant cause for ICU admissions and fatalities. Over a 15-year period in Hong Kong during the 1980s and 1990s, rates of medicinal poisoning admissions per 100,000 population ranged from 57.3 to 80.9.[32] In the more recent years of the report, admissions for nonmedicinal poisonings decreased from 53 to 22 per 100,000 population. Overall, poisoning fatality rates have ranged from 2 to 4 per 100,000 population, with an increasing rate into the 1990s.

The climate can have an impact on environmental exposures. In South Africa, 15.5% of toxicology consultations are for plant, spider, snake, scorpion, mushroom, and insect poisoning.[33] In addition, frequent consultations occur for household, agricultural, and industrial agents, including cholinesterase inhibitors and other pesticides, volatiles, corrosives, and soaps. The pattern of pharmaceutical exposures is similar to that in many other countries, however. Acetaminophen is the most common (14.6%), followed by benzodiazepines (13.1%), aspirin and nonsteroidal antiinflammatory drugs (9.4%), antidepressants (6.7%), and cardiovascular agents (5.5%).

In a report from Ecuador, only 26% of the reported poisoning cases were drug related.[34] The leading drugs were benzodiazepines (24%), acetaminophen (23%), aspirin (22%), and carbamazepine (11%). Except for carbamazepine, this experience is not too different from that in many other countries. The top four categories of nonmedicinal substances were organophosphate pesticides, which constituted 18% of all poisonings, followed by phosphorus (14%), rat poison (10%), and solvents (6%). Pesticides are often a leading category of poisoning in some developed and many underdeveloped countries. In one hospital in Turkey, pesticides followed analgesics as the second most common poisoning.[35]

A few reports have focused on pediatric poisoning admissions. In a study from Boston during 1981 and 1982, 90 acute poisonings (52 accidental and 38 suicidal) constituted 1.1% of the 8296 total admissions[36]; 64% were medical ICU admissions, 4.5% of total medical ICU admissions. The average LOS was 2.2 days. There was one fatality due to diphenoxylate. The most frequent agents responsible were alcohol (11), barbiturates (9), cyclic antidepressants (9), theophylline (8), aspirin (8), and benzodiazepines (8). A review of pediatric hospitalizations from the same children's hospital approximately a decade later (over a 4-year period from 1992 to 1995) documented a 0.9% admission rate for poisoning.[37] Two thirds of the 638 admissions for poisonings were medication related. Toddlers, age 1 to 5 years, accounted for 42% of admissions, and adolescents older than 12 years accounted for 45% of admissions. In the toddlers, lead, caustic agents, and benzodiazepines were the most common agents, whereas acetaminophen predominated in the adolescents. Antidepressants, antihistamines, and salicylates also accounted for a significant number of admissions. The LOS over this period decreased from 5.85 days to 3.45 days.

The state of Washington reviewed all hospital pediatric discharges over an 11-year period.[38] The incidence was 45 per 100,000 children per year. Intoxication accounted for 0.06% of the hospitalizations. Children age 12 to 18 accounted for 75% of the admissions, whereas toddlers (age $\leq$5 years) accounted for 20% of the admissions. The fatality rate was 0.2%. The average LOS was 1 day (range 1 to 3 days). ICU issues related to pediatric poisoning are discussed in detail in Chapter 10.

Fatalities

Carbon monoxide is the most common cause of poisoning fatality. In the 1950s and 1960s in Scotland, England, and Wales, barbiturates were second. In 1962, there were 4208 carbon monoxide deaths and 1987 barbiturate, sedative, and salicylate deaths combined.[27] In 1968, the fatality rate for all poisoning admissions at The Royal Infirmary of Edinburgh was 0.7%.[28]

The Massachusetts Poison Control System reviewed 1986 and 1987 fatality reports from three sources: death certificates, medical examiner reports, and poison center cases.[39] Of the 714 fatalities, 77% were prehospital deaths, whereas 163 (23%) were hospital deaths. Carbon monoxide was the leading cause of prehospital deaths. The other poisonings included opiates alone (21%), opiates combined with other agents (11%), and cocaine (11%). The leading causes of in-hospital deaths were polydrug (19%), cyclic antidepressant (12%), and opiate (9%) poisoning. The PCC was consulted on 86 (53%) of these cases. The poison center database and death certificate files identified 69 hospital deaths that were not in the medical examiner files.

The Rhode Island Poison Center reviewed and compared its fatality reports with reports of the medical examiner for a 4-year period (1986 to 1989).[40] Carbon monoxide was the most common cause of fatality, accounting for 98 of the 369 fatalities. After excluding cases of patients pronounced dead at the scene or dead on arrival, there were 112 cases in which the PCC could have been called; however, they were called on only 33 of these cases. In 10 of these cases, the poison center determined that they would have had additional recommendations that may have altered the outcome.

The San Francisco Bay Area Regional Poison Control Center compared its 10 fatality reports with the 358 poisoning and drug fatalities reviewed by the San Francisco City and County Medical Examiner's office for 2 years (1988 and 1990).[41] Of the medical examiner cases, 245 (68%) were prehospital deaths. Only 5 of the 113 emergency department cases were reported to the PCC. Of the cases, 89% involved illicit drugs, narcotics, or sedative-hypnotics. Specifically, heroin accounted for 31%; cocaine accounted for 17%; and amphetamines, codeine, barbiturates, and benzodiazepines accounted for 1% to 4% each. In this time period, among prescription medications, cyclic antidepressants accounted for 12% of the deaths. There were also discrepancies between the PCC and the medical examiner regarding whether the fatalities were drug related.

In Australia, deaths due to poisonings in 1989 and 1990[42] had an average victim age of 36 years. Opiates primarily accounted for 40% of the cases, cyclic antidepressants accounted for 14%, and benzodiazepines accounted for 6.5%. Only 25 of the 231 patients reached the hospital alive. In a later Australian report, the Hunter Area Toxicology Service reported a 0.6% mortality rate from 1987 to 1995.[43]

Aspiration syndrome after drug overdose is a common complication and reason for ICU admission. In a study from 1987 through 1995, 39% of all community-acquired aspiration syndromes admitted to the ICU were secondary to drug overdose.[44] The overall mortality rate was 22%, but it was unclear how many of these fatalities followed drug overdose. Medical complications of poisoning are discussed in detail in Chapter 8.

The aforementioned reports show that poisoning fatalities, mostly suicidal, continue to be a leading cause of death, especially in young adults. In North America, most of these fatalities occur out of the hospital and are reported by coroners. In-hospital fatalities continue to occur, however. Although some deaths are unavoidable (e.g., post–cardiac arrest or hypoxic brain injury occurring before hospital arrival), avoidable deaths still occur. A validated assessment or predictive tool for poisoned patients does not exist. It is difficult to envision the development of such a tool because of the variability of each potential intoxicant and the diverse pharmacokinetic profiles of drugs and other chemical substances. The time of ingestion and dose taken can be used to predict the course of intoxication. This evaluation must be done individually in each case, however. The medical toxicologist and PCC are resources to help predict severity for each individual case and to provide specific information that may attenuate the severity.

The mental health and social issues that lead to poisoning fatalities need further studies and resources to help reduce poisoning fatality rates. Stern and associates[45] followed 104 consecutive ICU admissions for poisonings. Of these, 88 were followed for 5 to 24 months. The follow-up mortality rate was 6% by another overdose; 42% were readmitted for another overdose or psychiatric illness.

Ojehagen and colleagues[46] analyzed the repeat overdose patients and the nonrepeaters in a total of 79 patients admitted to a Swedish ICU over an 18-month period. The predominant psychiatric diagnoses were adjustment disorder (31%), alcohol abuse (22%), major depression (19%), dysthymia (14%), and psychosis (9%). Of the patients, 66% were receiving psychiatric care. Repeaters were 58% of the sample and were less educated, had a higher rate of unemployment, and were more likely to be taking psychopharmacologic therapy. In many other series of patients from other countries or regions, the rates of repeaters have been much lower. The psychiatric care of critically poisoned patients is discussed in greater detail in Chapter 9.

MEDICAL TOXICOLOGY TRAINING

Training of health care professionals in toxicology has lagged behind that of other disciplines around the world.[47] Academic toxicology programs are lacking in most countries, although veterinary and pharmacy students receive some background in the field.[47,48] It became apparent in recent years in the United States that the fields of emergency medicine, critical care medicine, internal medicine, pediatrics, pharmacology, and occupational medicine could collaborate their basic and clinical science curricula to train physicians in the subspecialty of medical toxicology.[49] Success has been limited so far, owing to inadequate resources in faculty, curriculum guidelines, and clinical training centers. Despite this, in the United States there is a clearly evolving trend of medical toxicology inpatient services, either as primary admitting or as consulting services.

Medical Students

A 1990 survey of Canadian and U.S. medical schools[47] found that although 88% of U.S. schools reported teaching medical toxicology, only 5% had formal toxicology courses. In Canada and the United States, medical schools averaged only 5 hours of didactic toxicology teaching. An MD or PhD toxicologist was on staff at only 51% of the schools. This report represented an improvement, however, from an earlier survey of undergraduate U.S. education.[50] Of Britain's 24 medical schools, 22 reported formal toxicology teaching for a median of 5 hours (range 1 to 12 hours).[51] Many medical schools have moved away from traditional lecture-based curricula to problem-based, facilitator-guided learning formats. Toxicology is often covered in the neuroscience or pharmacology block in the second year.[52]

Residency Training

The experience in medical toxicology obtained in residency programs is highly variable. The formalization of training in medical toxicology varies greatly among countries. In the United States, medical toxicology is a core content area for emergency medicine residencies, so these postgraduate programs provide the most training in the field. Nonetheless, only 26% of the programs in a 1990 survey of U.S. emergency medicine residencies had a board-certified medical toxicology faculty member, and 19% offered no toxicology rotations at all.[53] Of the programs, 43% required toxicology training outside of the emergency department, but most of this was at poison information centers rather than bedside experiences. A 2000 survey of emergency medicine residencies documented an increase in toxicology faculty to 63% of the programs.[54] A toxicology rotation was required at 76% and was an elective at 19%. The experience was widely variable, however, with most still receiving the training primarily at a PCC rather than in patient care.[54] PCC training has been shown to modestly increase test scores in toxicology.[55] Poison information center experience, however, is limited in its ability to provide the skills necessary to treat critically poisoned patients.

In other U.S. residency training programs, clinical toxicology education is highly variable and often lacking. Only 4% of pediatric and psychiatry programs offer a clinical toxicology rotation, yet only 11% of the pediatric residency directors believed that their residents needed improvement in toxicologic management.[56,57] Only 41% of psychiatry programs have didactics in toxicology, and only two programs had a toxicology elective.[57]

Fellowship Training

In the United States, medical toxicology is a formally recognized subspecialty by the American Board of Medical Specialties, the regulatory authority for specialty and subspecialty certification. Postresidency fellowship training programs in medical toxicology emerged in the 1970s in the United States. In 1974, the American Board of Medical Toxicology (ABMT) was established by the American Academy of Clinical Toxicology (AACT)[49] to set standards in care and training. A primary function of the ABMT was offering a certifying examination in medical toxicology to physicians. In 1989, the ABMT published guidelines for fellowship training in medical toxicology[50] and continued to certify physicians until 1992, when the American Board of Medical Specialties officially recognized medical toxicology as a subspecialty. This new subspecialty board was developed and sponsored by the American Boards of Emergency Medicine, Preventive Medicine, and Pediatrics.[49]

Medical toxicology fellowship training requirements in the United States have been developed under the auspices of the American College of Graduate Medical Education. Primary certification is required in a medical specialty, and subspecialty medical toxicology training requires 2 years of full-time fellowship in a certified program. The certification examination was first offered in 1994, and accreditation of training programs began in 1999.[59] In 2004, there were 28 medical toxicology fellowships in the United States and Canada, listed on the American College of Medical Toxicology (ACMT) website (www.acmt.net). Clinical experience is still variable in many programs, however. Bedside experience in most programs includes consultations on adult and pediatric patients. A few programs have inpatient admitting referral services, but the number is growing. Experience in PCC telephone consultation is also now a program requirement. Pediatric emergency medicine offers a combined fellowship with medical toxicology.[60,61] In the United Kingdom, medical registrars receive training in medical toxicology at the regional poison treatment centers, in preparation to be consultants in the specialty.

Medical Toxicologists

There were 209 physician toxicologists certified by the ABMT between 1974 and 1992, having qualified by fellowship training, practice experience, or a combination of both, but by 1992 there were only 183 still practicing in this field.[62] Fewer than half spent more than 25% of their professional time in medical toxicology at that time, but 80% provided direct patient care, some outside the United States.[63] By 2002, there were 315 members of the ACMT, who were certified by the ABMT or the new subspecialty board. They represented 55 solo or group practices serving 125 hospitals in the United States.[64] The average number of in-hospital patients treated annually was 228 per group practice, and 36 of these groups were affiliated with a poison treatment center. Of the estimated 220,000 poisoning hospitalizations in the United States each year, only about 12,540 (0.6%) are seen by a medical toxicologist.[12,64] Most critically poisoned patients are cared for not by medical toxicologists but by intensivists, hospitalists, or primary care physicians.

Other Health Care Professionals

Additional training in medical toxicology is needed for other health care professionals worldwide. Critical care and emergency department nurses scored only about 50% on a questionnaire about antidote dosing and indications.[65]

Paramedic training programs in the United States devote only 2% of their time to toxicology, and only 11% have a designated experience at a poison center.[66] Poison centers and regional toxicology treatment centers are rich resources for continuing education for health care professionals. These centers have filled this role in industrialized nations and in developing countries, such as Zimbabwe.[67] The poison center may function as a multidisciplinary training site where medical, pharmacy, nursing, paramedic, and school of public health students work together with residents and toxicology fellows in the delivery of clinical advice.[68] Clinical pharmacology has been combined with clinical toxicology in some institutions.[69]

STANDARDS IN MEDICAL TOXICOLOGY

Practitioners

The provision of poisoning treatment throughout the world generally is the responsibility of emergency physicians, pediatricians, internists, occupational physicians, and intensivists. They are supported by a relatively small group of trained clinical toxicologists, consisting of medical toxicologists and pharmacologists, who usually are located at large academic centers or poison centers. In such centers, a medical toxicologist often functions as the primary attending physician for poisoned patients. In the absence of locally available specialists in the field, physicians are forced to rely on telephone consultation, computerized data information systems, or standard texts. The now-disbanded World Federation of Associations of Clinical Toxicology Centers and Poison Control Centers in the 1960s advocated that poison information centers be available and provide the physician with advice tailored to the individual case, but this is not always practical.[9] The American College of Emergency Physicians (ACEP) has stated that poison treatment and information should include consultation with a medical toxicologist or PCC and that there should be regional centers for poison treatment for serious poisonings.[70] Many professional societies, such as the AACT, the European Association of Poison Centres and Clinical Toxicology, the Society of Critical Care Medicine, the ACEP, and the American Heart Association, have published clinical guidelines for the treatment of poisonings, and these principles are outlined in chapters throughout this book.[11,71,72]

There are multiple demonstrated weaknesses in providing poisoning care with the frequently employed model of care by generalists, such as lack of available medical toxicology care or consultation. Treatment recommended by emergency departments in simulated cases of drug overdoses was found to be correct in only 68% of cases, including in only 50% of the cases presented to a teaching hospital and in only 22% of cases when the emergency physician was consulted.[73] A study of poisoning deaths in Massachusetts found that 29 of 60 deaths (48%) had errors in management as judged by an expert panel.[39] In two other studies, it was judged that 20% to 24% of in-hospital poisoning deaths could have been prevented if a medical toxicologist had been consulted.[40,42] In England and in the United States, one fourth of all poisoning deaths occur after hospitalization, suggesting that better prehospital or in-hospital care might prevent some of them.[16,39]

An evaluation of the Acute Physiology and Chronic Health Evaluation (APACHE) III showed APACHE III to underpredict drug overdose mortality.[74] In this observational cohort study, APACHE III was used to predict mortality for 1032 drug overdose admissions to 161 U.S. hospitals. The predicted mortality from APACHE III was 7 (0.7%), but the actual mortality was 25 (2.4%) ($P < .0001$). This study suggests that in-hospital poisoning deaths are a greater risk than the APACHE III score can predict or that there is need for improvement in toxicologic care.

A report from England showed significant variability in the management of poisoned patients. Thomas and coworkers[17] reported this finding by comparing six hospitals in northeastern England over 12 weeks. The catchment area included 1.52 million people. The admission rates for patients presenting to the accident and emergency wards varied from 50% to 87% (average 73%). The LOS varied from 0.8 to 2.1 days. Reasons for this variability were not presented. Only 12% of the patients had an LOS greater than 2 nights. Being elderly and ingesting benzodiazepines, acetaminophen, or antidepressants seemed to predict a longer LOS. Of the 690 admissions, there were 3 fatalities (0.4%).

TOXICOLOGY RESOURCES

References for toxicology information in the mid-1900s were card files of individuals, poison centers, and the U.S. National Clearinghouse for Poison Control Centers, followed by a computerized version of the Clearinghouse cards.[68,75] In the 1970s, microfiche technology allowed for the storage and retrieval of larger toxicology databases, which eventually were replaced by computerized information database systems, such as the POISINDEX, which has become one of the standard references for clinicians and poison centers in the United States.[68] In the United Kingdom, the TOXBASE Internet database system is available to emergency departments and individual physicians at www.spib.axl.co.uk.[9] Both database systems contain extensive information on the features and management of pharmaceuticals and toxins.

Clinical toxicology textbooks are another resource for clinicians, although their reliability has been variable. To our knowledge, none before this book has comprehensively focused specifically on critically poisoned patients. The *Physician's Desk Reference* is a frequent source of drug overdose information for 50% of U.S. physicians according to one survey, yet it was judged to include deficient treatment recommendations in 80% of the drugs reviewed, and in 35% of the drug outlines, contraindicated or potentially harmful advice was included.[76]

It is often thought that contacting a PCC provides the local physician with reliable assistance in treating poisoned patients, avoiding transfer to a specialty center; some medical organizations even recommend that this be a standard of care.[77,78] Contacting a PCC has been shown to be possible in cases of minor poisonings and drug or toxin identification, in which PCCs gave correct information 75% of the time in one study.[79] Physicians contact a PCC in only 19% to 29% of serious cases, however, and even then the recommendations are followed less than half of the time.[39,40,80,81] Although advice from PCCs regarding specific poisonings is generally excellent, the pharmacists or nurses giving most consultations from PCCs are not fully prepared to advise on issues related to the care of seriously ill patients. Contacts with PCCs are increased if a physician toxicologist is available, but experts are infrequently available or accessed for individual cases, and their advice still is followed only in about two thirds of these cases.[80,82] Consultations by telephone have been known to be fraught with hazard, which may account for some of this reluctance. Clinical data recorded at hospitals are often unavailable to PCCs or are significantly different from that provided, and the physician at the bedside is often in a better position to assess and act on the patient's status than a telephone consultant.[9,83] For this reason, the ACEP states, "Most medical conditions cannot be accurately diagnosed over the telephone."[78] The ACEP further recommends "emergency departments do not attempt medical assessment or management over the telephone."[78] The assessment of the circumstantial, laboratory, and clinical evidence requires a high level of clinical and toxicologic expertise on the part of the consultant at the PCC, who is often a nonphysician.[9] Limitations of this model of poison care delivery are best exemplified by a study in which treatment advice was sought from U.S. PCCs in a simulated case of serious antidepressant poisoning. The advice was deemed to be correct from only 42% of all the PCCs contacted and from only 60% of the regional centers certified by the AAPCC.[79]

The lack of adequate resources also hampers hospitals in providing care to poisoned patients. Pharmacy stocking of emergency antidotes has been found to be adequate in a wide range of hospitals surveyed (2% to 98%), depending on the antidote, but only about 1% of hospitals have adequate supplies of all antidotes in amounts necessary to treat even one patient.[84,85] Most health care facilities have on-site access to qualitative urine drug assays for only a few drugs of abuse and must rely on distant toxicology reference laboratories for more comprehensive drug screens and many necessary quantitative analyses.[64] Specialty poisoning treatment units are available in major cities in some countries, but this is not universally true.

Sites of Care

An ICU is usually recommended to be the most appropriate location for management of poisoned patients requiring hospital admission because of the availability of rapid diagnostic procedures, intense observation and monitoring, and complex treatment modalities.[86] Caution must be employed in triaging patients with altered mental status to other sites. One study found that 69% of patients with unrecognized medical emergencies inappropriately admitted to a psychiatric unit had a drug overdose or intoxication or severe drug/alcohol withdrawal.[87]

The Society of Critical Care Medicine recommends that overdose patients be admitted to an ICU if they have cardiovascular instability, altered level of consciousness with airway compromise, or seizures.[88] One study found that ICU admission was necessary if in the emergency department the patient required mechanical ventilation or had seizures, coma, a partial pressure of carbon dioxide greater than 45 mm Hg, arrhythmias, high atrioventricular block, a QRS greater than 0.11 second, or systolic blood pressure less than

80 mm Hg.[89] The Glasgow Coma Scale has been used to predict the need for ICU admission, with a score of less than 13; intubation; or the presence of infectious, cardiovascular, or electrocardiogram complications being sensitive and specific for needing ICU interventions in one study.[90] A smaller study suggested that nonintubated patients with a Glasgow Coma Scale score greater than 6 did not require ICU admission and could be handled on the general medical floors.[21] Intensive care for poisoned patients also may be delivered in an emergency department observation unit with respiratory care capabilities and can result in fewer complications and shorter LOS compared with admission to a general medical floor.[91–93]

In severe cases, local resources may be inadequate to meet the patient's needs. Transfer of seriously ill patients to specialty centers is supported in policy statements of the ACEP, ACMT, and Society of Critical Care Medicine.[94–96] Transfer is often necessary to provide access to experienced medical toxicologists, antidotes, and analytic laboratory services not available elsewhere. Specialty poison treatment centers are available in a few cities around the world (see later section on poison centers).

Recommended Equipment and Resources

Care of the seriously poisoned patient requires medical and nursing expertise, an emergency department and critical care unit, analytic toxicology laboratory support, an adequate supply of antidotes, and psychosocial services.[28,97] Available services should include hemodialysis, a clinical laboratory able to perform routine analyses, plus at least the emergency toxicology laboratory tests listed in the ACMT facility guidelines, a 24-hour pharmacy, radiology, respiratory care, and psychiatric and social services.[98]

The ACEP has published a clinical policy for the care of patients with toxic exposures, including recommended laboratory tests and common necessary emergency antidotes.[72] Although intended for facilities serving as regional poison treatment centers, the guidelines of the ACMT also outline the resources deemed necessary in any hospital caring for poisoned patients.[98] The minimal qualitative urine drug assays recommended are listed in Table 1-2, and the quantitative tests necessary for immediate care are listed in Table 1-3. In addition to these drug assays, the hospital laboratory must be able to perform rapidly arterial blood gases, a comprehensive

---

TABLE 1-2 Recommended Analytes to Be Available on Qualitative Urine Screening Assays*

Amphetamines
Barbiturates
Benzodiazepines
Cannabinoids
Cocaine
Cyclic antidepressants
Opiates
Phencyclidine

---

*This is a recommended list for hospitals in the United States and Canada. It should be modified based on the regional drug use patterns in other locations.

TABLE 1-3 Recommended Analytes to Be Available for Emergency Quantitative Drug Assays (Available within 2 Hours)*

Acetaminophen	Lithium
Carbamazepine	Methanol
Carboxyhemoglobin	Methemoglobin
Digoxin	Phenobarbital
Ethanol	Phenytoin
Ethylene glycol	Salicylate
Iron	Theophylline
Isopropanol	Valproic acid

*This is a recommended list for hospitals in the United States and Canada. It should be modified based on the regional epidemiology of poisoning.

metabolic panel, coagulation studies, serum osmolality, acetone, and lactate. Antidote needs may vary based on geography and setting; the minimal required antidotes are listed in Table 1-4.

POISON CENTERS

The proliferation of accidental and intentional poisonings in the 1940s led to the development of centers for poison information dissemination and treatment around the world. The infancy of such centers was in Copenhagen, the Netherlands, Edinburgh, and Chicago. These specialty centers serve as resources for poison information, public and heath professional education, poison prevention, research, and in some cases tertiary patient care. The increasing number of childhood accidental poisonings and deaths and physicians' general lack of knowledge and resources about drug and chemical ingredients initially highlighted the need for poison centers.

Poison Information Centers

The first poison information service is thought to have been established in the Netherlands in 1949, followed in

TABLE 1-4 Recommended Emergency Antidotes

Activated charcoal	N-Acetylcysteine
Amyl nitrate	Naloxone
Antivenin, Crotalidae*	Physostigmine
Calcium chloride	Polyethylene glycol electrolyte
Calcium gluconate gel	solution
Deferoxamine mesylate	Pralidoxime hydrochloride
Digoxin immune Fab	Protamine sulfate
Ethanol	Pyridoxine
Folic acid	Sodium bicarbonate
Fomepizole	Sodium nitrite 3%
Flumazenil	Sodium thiosulfate
Glucagon	Succimer
Leucovorin	Thiamine hydrochloride
Methylene blue 1%	Vitamin K_1

*For crotaline endemic areas.

Europe by similar centers in Paris in 1959, London and Edinburgh in 1962, and Zurich in 1966.[9,48] The first information center, or PCC, in the United States was established in Chicago in 1953 and had been preceded by an informal information service in the pharmacy of St. Luke's Hospital.[75] The first PCC was intended to provide information to physicians on ingredient and toxicity information, and the database was a set of small cards. Subsequently a manual was developed outlining the ingredients of common household products and distributed to emergency departments. Similar centers began to appear across the United States, and by 1957 there were 17 PCCs, which now also were taking calls from the public.[75] An initial barrier was the lack of reliable data sources and data collection, so the U.S. Surgeon General designated the National Clearinghouse for Poison Control Centers, which distributed index cards of poison information and collected poison data from centers.[75] There was an uncontrolled growth of PCCs in the United States during the 1960s and 1970s, resulting in 661 PCCs of variable quality.[75] The AAPCC was established in 1958 primarily by pediatricians to develop public and professional education programs, promote cooperation between centers, and set standards for operation. In 1978, the AAPCC published standards for PCCs, and as a result the number of PCCs declined to 91 in 1995 and to 73 in 1998.[99] These centers are staffed around the clock by nurses and pharmacists and usually are directed by pharmacists with some medical direction provided by part-time medical toxicologists.[99] Some centers do not have adequate medical toxicologist availability, and most cases do not involve physician consultation.[81,99] PCCs have been shown to reduce unnecessary hospital visits and health care expenses, however, and serve as a resource for education, research, poison prevention efforts, and data collection.[99,100] They also have been shown to be a reliable source of first aid and triage advice for the public and hospitals in cases of non–life-threatening toxic exposures.[73,79] Poison center services in the United States to physicians caring for poisoned patients have evolved over the years. Initially, PCCs were primarily consulted for ingredient information. The lack of availability of medical toxicologists at most hospitals has rendered PCCs as the default source of treatment recommendations. Most of this advice comes from nonphysicians working in PCCs, however. The need for medical toxicology resources for information on the treatment of critically poisoned patients is evident.

Likewise, in Europe the European Association of Poison Centres and Clinical Toxicology was formed in 1964 to share knowledge and to identify toxic hazards. There are now approximately 80 European PCCs.[48] Networks of multiple centers operate in France, Germany, Italy, and the United Kingdom.[48] In the United States, poison centers can be contacted by the public and health care professionals at 1-800-222-1222, and in the United Kingdom the National Poisons Information Service is available to health care professionals and emergency departments at 0870-600-6266. Health officers, medical toxicologists, and pharmacists staff the centers, and they are often affiliated with poison treatment centers, ICUs, or emergency departments.[48] It has been advocated that these centers be part of a larger toxicology center that includes an analytic laboratory, inpatient treatment center, outpatient services, adverse drug reaction and occupational exposure advice, research, an expanded medical staff, and training.[97,101]

In addition to the United States and Europe, there are poison information centers operating on every continent worldwide except Antarctica. Many of these centers are still in the early stages of development. The Japan Poison Information Center was established in 1986 to serve a population of 124 million and received only about 35,000 calls in 1994.[102] This represents a case volume of only 27 per 100,000 population, in contrast to the United States's call volume of 920 calls per 100,000 at that time.[102] Before its dissolution, the World Federation of Associations of Poison Centers and Clinical Toxicologists issued a directory (Yellowtox) of worldwide poison information centers and analytic toxicology services, which still can be found at www.intox.org/pagesource/yellowtox/yellowtoxhtm.

Poison Treatment Centers

Poison treatment centers are highly specialized inpatient units directed by medical toxicologists and are capable of caring for the most complex cases of poisonings. Strong centralized regional poison treatment centers have flourished in some countries and serve as specialty care centers and institutes for toxicologic research, treatment advances, and education. Their origin probably is based in Scotland, where a "delirium ward" was established at the Royal Infirmary of Edinburgh in 1879.[27] This unit gradually evolved into the Regional Poisoning Treatment Centre of Edinburgh, and by 1964 it cared for more than 90% of overdose patients in the Edinburgh area.[27] Another formal treatment center in Europe was founded in 1949 in Copenhagen, followed by other centers in Paris and in Romford, Essex, in the late 1950s.[9,27,28] The impetus for further development of centers in the United Kingdom in Birmingham, Dublin, Belfast, Cardiff, and London was the Atkins Report of 1962 and the Hill Report of 1968, in which the United Kingdom Ministry of Health recommended the establishment of regional poisoning treatment centers with consultants in toxicology and associated psychiatric and chemical toxicology laboratory services.[28] Other such centers developed in Europe and Russia in the 1960s and more recently in the United States and Australia.[43,64,98,103]

In 1993, the AACT published standards for toxicology treatment centers[104]; subsequently the ACMT refined and promoted those standards.[98] The Center for Poison Treatment Facility Assessment Guidelines can be found at www.acmt.net. The rationale for the existence of these treatment centers is cited as the need for a dedicated professional staff to develop expertise, to assess and manage more efficiently medical and psychiatric issues, to advance knowledge rapidly by concentrating patients at dedicated sites for education and research, to focus psychosocial support for the patients' special needs, and to make it efficient to provide analytic laboratory support on-site.[27,28,43,97] It was reported that in the first year of operation, the Copenhagen center reduced poisoning mortality by half by centralizing care.[27] The average LOS also has been reported to decrease, compared with general ICU or hospital ward admissions. In Australia, there was a reduction of 2 to 3 days in hospital stays for complicated poisoning cases at two toxicology cen-

ters, but there was only a statistically insignificant reduction in mortality.[43,105] Use of health care resources also has been shown to decrease at these centers without compromising patient care, and the coupling of a treatment center with an aviation medicine service allows for efficient access to therapies unavailable in rural regions.[106,107] Transfer of such seriously ill patients to specialty centers is supported in a policy statement of the ACEP, which states, "Patients should be transferred to a health care facility that meets their needs."[94] Transfer is often necessary to provide access to experienced medical toxicologists, antidotes, and analytic laboratory services not available elsewhere.

Regional poison treatment centers care for a highly variable number of patients annually. Admissions to the Edinburgh center peaked at about 2200 admissions per year, then declined to about 1500 annual admissions in 1986.[9] Two centers in Australia admitted 736 and 192 patients in years reported in the mid-1990s.[43,105] In the United States, centers in Pennsylvania, Colorado, and Utah each had about 500 annual admissions.[64] A center in St. Petersburg, Russia, serves about 7 million people and reported more than 5500 admissions per year.[103]

REFERENCES

1. Rosner F: Moses Maimonides' treatise on poisons. JAMA 205:98–100, 1968.
2. Plaitikis A, Duvoisin RC: Homer's moly identified as galanthus nivalis: Physiologic antidote to stramonium poisoning. Clin Neuropharmacol 6:1–5, 1983.
3. Timbrell JA: Introduction to Toxicology. London, Taylor & Francis, 1989.
4. Jarco S: Medical numismatic notes. Bull N Y Acad Med 48:1059–1064, 1972.
5. Picchioni AL, Chin L, Verhulst HL, Dieterle B: Activated charcoal vs universal antidote as an antidote for poisons. Toxicol Appl Pharmacol 8:447–454, 1966.
6. Leschke E: Clinical Toxicology: Modern Methods in the Diagnosis and Treatment of Poisoning. Baltimore, William Wood, 1934.
7. Proudfoot AT: The development of clinical toxicology in Edinburgh. In Passmore R (ed): Proceedings of the Royal College of Physicians of Edinburgh Tercentenary Congress. Edinburgh, Royal College of Physicians of Edinburgh, 1982.
8. Holt LE, Holz PH: The black bottle: A consideration of the role of charcoal in the treatment of poisoning in children. J Pediatr 63:306–314, 1963.
9. Proudfoot AT: Clinical toxicology—past, present, and future. Hum Toxicol 7:481–487, 1988.
10. Clemmesen C, Nillson E: Therapeutic trends in the treatment of barbiturate poisoning: The Scandinavian method. Clin Pharmacol Ther 2:220–229, 1961.
11. American Heart Association: ECC guidelines part 8: Advanced challenges in resuscitation. Circulation 102:I-223–228, 2000.
12. McKaig LF, Burt CW: Poisoning-related visits to emergency departments in the United States, 1993–1996. Clin Toxicol 37:817–826, 1999.
13. Hoppe-Roberts JM, Lloyd LM, Chyka PA: Poisoning mortality in the United States: Comparison of national mortality statistics and poison control center reports. Ann Emerg Med 35:440–448, 2000.
14. Fingerhut LA, Cox CS: Poisoning mortality, 1985–1995. Public Health Rep 113:218–233, 1998.
15. Kapur N, House A, Creed F, et al: Management of deliberate self poisoning in adults in four teaching hospitals: Descriptive study. BMJ 316:831–832, 1998.
16. Gunnell D, Ho D, Murray V: Medical management of deliberate drug overdose: A neglected area for suicide prevention? Emerg Med J 21:35–38, 2004.
17. Thomas SHL, Lewis S, Bevan L, et al: Factors affecting hospital admission and length of stay of poisoned patients in the North East of England. Hum Exp Toxicol 15:915–916, 1996.

18. Strotmeyer SJ, Weiss HB: Injuries in Pennsylvania: Hospital discharges, 1999. Pittsburgh, PA, Center for Injury Research and Control, Department of Neurologic Surgery, University of Pittsburgh, 2000.

19. Harchelroad F, Clark RF, Dean B, Krenzelok EP: Treated vs. reported toxic exposures: Discrepancies between a poison control center and a member hospital. Vet Hum Toxicol 32:156–159, 1990.

20. Giffin S, Steele P: Utilization of the uniform hospital discharge data set (UHDDS) to evaluate poisoning incidence. Vet Hum Toxicol 33:376, 1991.

21. Heyman EN, LoCastro DE, Gouse LH, et al: Intentional drug overdose: Predictors of clinical course in the intensive care unit. Heart Lung 25:246–252, 1996.

22. Bosch TM, van der Werf TS, Uges DRA, et al: Antidepressants self-poisoning and ICU admissions in a university hospital in the Netherlands. Pharm World Sci 22:92–95, 2000.

23. Zimmerman JE, Wagner DP, Draper EA, et al: Evaluation of acute physiology and chronic health evaluation: III. Predictions of hospital mortality in an independent database. Crit Care Med 26:1317–1326, 1998.

24. Henderson A, Wright M, Pond SM: Experience with 732 acute overdose patients admitted to an intensive care unit over six years. Med J Aust 158:28–30, 1993.

25. Strom J, Thisted B, Krantz T, Sorensen MB: Self-poisoning treated in an ICU: Drug pattern, acute mortality and short-term survival. Acta Anaesthesiol Scand 30:148–153, 1986.

26. Hall AK, Curry C: Changing epidemiology and management of deliberate self poisoning in Christchurch. N Z Med J 107:396–399, 1994.

27. Matthew H: Acute poisoning. Scott Med J 11:1–6, 1966.

28. Matthew H, Proudfoot AT, Brown SS, Aitken RCB: Acute poisoning: Organization and work-load of a treatment center. BMJ 3:489–493, 1969.

29. Hojer J, Baehrendtz S, Gustafsson L: Benzodiazepine poisoning: Experience of 702 admissions to an intensive care unit during a 14-year period. J Intern Med 226:117–122, 1989.

30. Leykin Y, Halpern P, Silbiger A, et al: Acute poisoning treated in the intensive care unit: A case series. Isr J Med Sci 25:98–102, 1989.

31. Ramchandani P, Murray B, Hawton K, House A: Deliberate self poisoning with antidepressant drugs: A comparison of the relative hospital costs of cases of overdose of tricyclics with those of selective-serotonin re-uptake inhibitors. J Affect Disord 60:97–100, 2000.

32. Chan TYK: Trends in hospitalizations and mortality due to medicinal or non-medicinal poisonings in Hong Kong. Vet Hum Toxicol 39:372–373, 1997.

33. Muller GJ, Hoffman BA, Lamprecht: Drug and poison information—the Tygerberg experience. S Afr Med J 83:395–39, 1993.

34. Brito MA, Reyes RM, Arguello JR, Spiller HA: Principal causes of poisoning in Quito, Ecuador: A retrospective epidemiology study. Vet Hum Toxicol 40:40–42, 1998.

35. Pinar A, Fowler J, Bond GR: Acute poisoning in Ismir, Turkey—a pilot epidemiologic study. Clin Toxicol 31:593–601, 1993.

36. Frazen LE, Lovejoy FH, Crone RK: Acute poisoning in a children's hospital: A 2-year experience. Pediatrics 77:144–151, 1986.

37. Woolf A, Wieler J, Greenes D: Costs of poison-related hospitalizations at an urban teaching hospital for children. Arch Pediatr Adolesc Med 151:719–723, 1997.

38. Gauvin F, Bailey B, Bratton SL: Hospitalizations for pediatric intoxication in Washington State, 1987–1997. Arch Pediatr Adolesc Med 155:1105–1110, 2001.

39. Soslow AR, Woolf AD: Reliability of data sources for poisoning deaths in Massachusetts. Am J Emerg Med 10:124–127, 1992.

40. Linakis JG, Frederick KA: Poisoning deaths not reported to the regional poison control center. Ann Emerg Med 22:42–48, 1993.

41. Blanc PD, Kearney TE, Olson KR: Underreporting of fatal cases to a regional poison control center. West J Med 162:505–509, 1995.

42. Coleridge J, Cameron PA, Drummer OH, McNeil JJ: Drug overdose deaths in Victoria, Australia. Med J Aust 157:459–462, 1992.

43. Whyte IM, Dawson AH, Buckley NA, et al: A model for the management of self poisoning. Med J Aust 167:142–146, 1997.

44. Leroy O, Vendenbussche C, Coffinier C, et al: Community-acquired aspiration pneumonia in intensive care units. Am J Respir Crit Care Med 156:1922–1929, 1997.

45. Stern TA, Mulley AG, Thibault GE: Life-threatening drug overdose. JAMA 251:1983–1985, 1984.

46. Ojehagen A, Regnell G, Traskman-Bendz L: Deliberate self-poisoning: Repeaters and nonrepeaters admitted to an intensive care unit. Acta Psychiatr Scand 84:266–271, 1991.

47. Hays EP, Schumacker C, Ferrario CG, et al: Toxicology training in US and Canadian medical schools. Am J Emerg Med 10:121–123, 1992.

48. Descotes J: The status and future of toxicology in Europe. Vet Hum Toxicol 36:142–143, 1994.

49. Goldfrank LR: Medical toxicology training and certification. Acad Emerg Med 1:124–126, 1994.

50. Sanders AB, Criss E, Witzke D: Core content survey of undergraduate education in emergency medicine. Ann Emerg Med 15:6–11, 1986.

51. Dayan AD: Who needs toxicology? Roy Soc Med 82:320–322, 1989.

52. Sivam SP, Iatridis PG, Vaughn S: Integration of pharmacology into a problem-based learning curriculum for medical students. Med Educ 29:289–296, 1995.

53. Caravati EM, Ling LJ: Toxicology education in emergency medicine residency programs. Am J Emerg Med 10:169–171, 1992.

54. Hantsche CE, Mullins ME, Pledger D, Bexdicek KM: Medical toxicology experience during emergency medicine residency. Acad Emerg Med 7:1170, 2000.

55. Cobaugh DJ, Goetz CM, Lopez GP, et al: Assessment of learning by emergency medicine residents and pharmacy students participating in a poison center clerkship. Vet Hum Toxicol 39:173–175, 1997.

56. Trainor JL, Krug SE: The training of pediatric residents in the care of acutely ill injured children. Arch Pediatr Adolesc Med 154:1154–1159, 2000.

57. Ingels M, Marks D, Clark RF: A survey of medical toxicology training in psychiatry residency programs. Acad Psychiatry 27:50–53, 2003.

58. ABMT: Guidelines for fellowship in medical toxicology. Vet Hum Toxicol 31:486–488, 1989.

59. Wax PM, Donovan JW: Fellowship training in medical toxicology: Characteristics, perceptions, and career impact. J Toxicol Clin Toxicol 38: 637–642, 2000.

60. Shannon M, Fleisher GR, Woolf A: The pediatric emergency medicine—clinical toxicology combined fellowship. Pediatr Emerg Care 7:30–31, 1991.

61. Tenenbein M: The combined pediatric emergency medicine—clinical toxicology fellowship. Pediatr Emerg Care 7:38–39, 1991.

62. Donovan JW: Survey of medical toxicologist practice characteristics, specialty certifications, and manpower needs. Vet Hum Toxicol 34:336, 1992.

63. Donovan JW, Martin TG: Regional poisons systems—roles and titles. J Toxicol Clin Toxicol 31:221–222, 1993.

64. McKay CA: The current practice of bedside medical toxicology in the United States. Int J Med Toxicol 5:2, 2002.

65. Swanson-Biearman B, Mrvos R, Dean BS, Kenzelok EP: Critical care nurses' limited knowledge about drugs in toxicology. Vet Hum Toxicol 32:378, 1990.

66. Davis CO, Cobaugh DJ, Leahey NF, Wax PM: Toxicology training of paramedic students in the United States. Am J Emerg Med 17:138–140, 1999.

67. Kasilo OJ, Nhachi CF: Recommendations for establishing a drug and toxicology information center in a developing country. Ann Pharmacol 25:1379–1383, 1991.

68. Lovejoy FH: Clinical toxicology: Built better than they knew: Reflections on yesterday, today, and tomorrow. Vet Hum Toxicol 43:113–116, 2001.

69. Wilson JT: Concepts to facilitate a combined program of clinical pharmacology and clinical toxicology. Clin Toxicol 16:371–376, 1980.

70. American College of Emergency Physicians: Poison information and treatment systems. Ann Emerg Med 37:370, 2001.

71. Albertson TE, Dawson A, deLatorre F, et al: Tox-ACLS: Toxicologic oriented advanced cardiac life support. Ann Emerg Med 37:S78-S90, 2001.

72. American College of Emergency Physicians: Clinical policy for the initial approach to patients presenting with acute toxic ingestion or dermal or inhalation exposure. Ann Emerg Med 33:735–761, 1999.

73. Wigder HN, Erickson T, Morse T, Saporta V: Emergency department poison advice telephone calls. Ann Emerg Med 25:349–352, 1995.

74. Zimmerman JE, Knause WA, Judson JA, et al: Patient selection for intensive care: A comparison of New Zealand and United States hospitals. Crit Care Med 16:318–326, 1988.

75. Burda AM, Burda NM: The nation's first poison control center: Taking a stand against accidental childhood poisoning in Chicago. Vet Hum Toxicol 39:115–119, 1997.

76. Mullen WH, Anderson IB, Kim SY, et al: Incorrect overdose management advice in the Physician's Desk Reference. Ann Emerg Med 29:255–261, 1997.

77. Dean BS, Krenzelok EP: The Pittsburgh poison center and its member hospital network. Vet Hum Toxicol 28:66–67, 1986.

78. American College of Emergency Physicians: Providing telephone advice from the emergency department. Policy Statement #400100, Dallas, TX, July 2000.

79. Geller RJ, Fisher JG, Leeper JD, et al: Poison centers in America: How well do they perform. Vet Hum Toxicol 32:240–245, 1990.

80. Schneider SM, Dean BS, Krenzelok EP: The effectiveness of medical toxicology consultations from a regional poison information (Abstract). Ann Emerg Med 21:663, 1992.

81. Caravati EM, McElwee NE: Use of clinical toxicology resources by emergency physicians and its impact on poison control centers. Ann Emerg Med 20:147–150, 1991.

82. Chyka PA, Butler AY: Utilization of expert consultants by poison centers in the United States. Vet Hum Toxicol 37:369–370, 1995.

83. Hoyt B, Rasmussen R, Giffin S, et al: Poison center data accuracy: A comparison of rural hospital chart data with the TESS database. Acad Emerg Med 6:851–855, 1999.

84. Dart RC, Stark Y, Fulton B, et al: Insufficient stocking of poisoning antidotes in hospital pharmacies. JAMA 276:1508–1510, 1996.

85. Teresi WM, King WD: Survey of the stocking of poison antidotes in Alabama hospitals. South Med J 92:1151–1156, 1999.

86. Kulling P, Persson H: Role of the intensive care unit in the management of the poisoned patient. Med Toxicol 1:375–386, 1986.

87. Reeves RR, Pendarvis EJ, Kimble R: Unrecognized medical emergencies admitted to psychiatric units. Am J Emerg Med 18:390–393, 2000.

88. Society of Critical Care Medicine: Guidelines for ICU admission, discharge, and triage. Crit Care Med 27:633–638, 1999.

89. Brett AS, Rothschild N, Gray R, Perry M: Predicting the clinical course in intentional drug overdose. Arch Intern Med 147:133–137, 1987.

90. Hamad AE, Al-Ghadban A, Carcounis CP, et al: Predicting the need for medical intensive care monitoring in drug-overdosed patients. J Intensive Care Med 15:321–328, 2000.

91. Piper KW, Griner PF: Suicide attempts with drug overdose. Arch Intern Med 134:703–706, 1974.

92. Dribben W, Welch J, Dunn D, et al: The utilization of emergency department observation units for the poisoned patient (Abstract). J Toxicol Clin Toxicol 37:586, 1999.

93. Gummin DD, Butler JR, Roberts RR, et al: Utilization of emergency department observation units for acute intoxications (Abstract). J Toxicol Clin Toxicol 37:586–587, 1999.

94. American College of Emergency Physicians: Principles of appropriate patient transfer. Ann Emerg Med 19:337–338, 1990.

95. Guidelines Committee of the American College of Critical Care Medicine: Guidelines for the transfer of critically ill patients. Crit Care Med 21:931–937, 1993.

96. Martin TG: ACMT position statement: Care of poisoned patients. American College of Medical Toxicology, 2002. Available at: http://www.acmt.net/resources/position_care of poisoned.htm.

97. Vale JA, Meredith TJ: Clinical toxicology in the 1990s: The development of clinical toxicology centers—a personal view. J Toxicol Clin Toxicol 31:223–227, 1993.

98. American College of Medical Toxicology: Center for poison treatment facility assessment guidelines. Fairfax, VA, May 21, 2003. Available at: http://www.acmt.net.

99. Youniss J, Litovitz T, Villanueva P: Characterization of US Poison Centers: A 1998 survey conducted by the American Association of Poison Control Centers. Vet Hum Toxicol 42:43–53, 2000.

100. Darwin J, Seger D: Reaffirmed cost-effectiveness of poison centers. Ann Emerg Med 41:159–160, 2003.

101. Bonfiglio JF, Clark CS, Sigell LT, et al: Poison centers: A resource for occupational health services. Vet Hum Toxicol 30:569–571, 1988.

102. Akahori F, Shintani S: The status and future of toxicology in Japan and the Pacific Rim. Vet Hum Toxicol 36:144–151, 1994.

103. Afansiev VV, Blair TN, Rondeau ES: The organization of a toxicological service in St. Petersburg. Vet Hum Toxicol 34:346, 1992.

104. American Academy of Clinical Toxicology: Facility assessment guidelines for regional toxicology treatment centers. Clin Toxicol 31:211–217, 1993.

105. Lee V, Kerr JF, Braitberg G, et al: Impact of a toxicology service on a metropolitan teaching hospital. Emerg Med 13:37–42, 2001.

106. Clark RF, Williams SR, Nordt SP, et al: Resource-use analysis of a medical toxicology consultation service. Ann Emerg Med 31:705–709, 1998.

107. Dubin M, Kunst D: Transporting the overdose patient. Hosp Aviat 9:11–14, 1989.

CHAPTER 2

Diagnosis of Poisonings

Alex T. Proudfoot ▪ J. Ward Donovan

DIAGNOSTIC PROCESS IN CLINICAL TOXICOLOGY

Establishing that a patient's symptoms and signs are the result of exposure to one or more chemical substances rather than to some other disease process is of prime importance. Ideally the physician would wish to know the following:

To what substance or substances was the person exposed?
By what route or routes was the person exposed?
To what dose or doses was the person exposed?
At what time and over what period did exposure occur?

Answers to these questions would allow anticipation of the hazards likely to be encountered; assessment of the risk (the likelihood of the hazards' occurring); prediction of the course of poisoning, particularly its duration and outcome; and initiation of therapeutic interventions. Clinical reality is far from ideal, however. Even with the simplest poisoning scenario—a single exposure by one route to one substance at a discrete point in time—the route is often the only factor that is known with any certainty. The name of the substance, the dose, and the time of exposure are frequently not available or at best are only rough approximations. How can clinicians be reassured that they are managing poisoning appropriately and not missing the presence of potentially lethal toxins that are eminently treatable? Expecting the laboratory to identify the toxins involved in every case is unrealistic. Although reliable analytic techniques are available for many chemicals, hospital laboratories are equipped to identify and quantify readily only a small fraction of the drugs commonly encountered in clinical practice.[1] Managing patients who are possibly poisoned is often an uncomfortable experience. Unless clinicians have compelling reasons to the contrary, they have little choice but to proceed on the basis that the evidence available, incomplete and unsatisfactory though it may be, is correct in essence. In doing so, clinicians obtain reassurance from the following:

Ensuring that the evidence is as accurate and complete as possible.
Finding clinical, laboratory, and other features that are compatible with poisoning with the substance thought to be involved.
Obtaining results of limited laboratory toxicologic screening.

The clinician must ensure, as far as possible, that other disease processes are reasonably excluded and must be prepared to reconsider the diagnosis in the light of clinical progress. The evidence that can lead to a diagnosis of acute poisoning is shown in Table 2-1. Although it is often stated that the history of exposure is unreliable, historical information from the patient and others, coupled with the physical examination and routine laboratory studies, can be quite accurate in determining the diagnosis.[2]

HISTORY

Most adults and children who are exposed to poisons are conscious or drowsy when they arrive at the emergency department, and most volunteer information about what has happened. Establishing a diagnosis of poisoning rather than some other disease process should not be difficult in these cases. Even when individuals have deliberately poisoned themselves, only a few do not disclose the reason for their presentation. The reliability of their statements is often suspect, however. Although approximately 60% of self-poisonings involve drugs prescribed for the individual or for a close relative, the patient may be uncertain or completely ignorant of the drug names. In addition, drug overdoses commonly are taken by individuals whose mental functions are clouded by prior consumption of ethanol, and the impulse of the moment ends in ingestion of the contents of the first bottle that comes to hand. These factors may explain why comparison of what patients say they have taken with drug analysis of blood or urine reveals major disparities in half the cases.[3–6] For the same reasons, patient estimates of the amounts ingested are usually even less accurate. Tablets and capsules tend to be taken by the handful or bottleful; few patients count them before swallowing them. Counts of pills missing or remaining in the bottle often are not reliable because of spillage or the frequent practice of exchanging tablets between containers. It is important to obtain what corroboration is possible from the circumstantial evidence, the clinical features manifested, and, if possible, the laboratory.

In cases of potential therapeutic drug errors or interactions, it is crucial to obtain a careful and detailed history of medication doses, prescription changes, and use of over-the-counter or herbal products. Likewise, detailed information about job practices and environmental factors is crucial in cases of possible environmental or occupational poisoning.

The age distribution of accidental exposure to potential poisons in children (predominantly 9 months to 4 years) means that a clear history of exposure may not be forthcoming, much less the nature and amount of the exposure. Circumstantial evidence or the accounts of witnesses of the event may be the only source of diagnostic information.

TABLE 2-1 Diagnostic Process

History
    Patient
    Witnesses
    Emergency services staff
Circumstantial evidence
    Suicide notes
    Containers and potential toxins at scene of discovery
    Circumstances surrounding discovery
Physical examination findings
Biochemical abnormalities
Electrocardiogram abnormalities
Radiology
Toxicologic screening

CIRCUMSTANTIAL EVIDENCE

Young children, unconscious individuals, individuals with learning difficulties, and individuals with memory impairment, to varying degrees, are unable to provide accurate information. Circumstantial evidence then becomes important.

In young adults with no preexisting health concerns or external evidence of trauma, self-poisoning is probably the most important cause of unexplained coma.[3,7] Although family members are likely to deny the possibility, they are often wrong. When unconscious adults are found with empty drug containers or tablets nearby, it is reasonable to assume that the drugs may be the cause of the coma. Occasionally, tablet particles staining the mouth or clothing or a suicide note is found to support the assumption. The note may state explicitly what has been taken in addition to indicating the writer's objective or the nature of his or her emotional distress. Other useful sources, if available, are the patient's medical or pharmacy records, which at least reveal the medications ordinarily used and a likely cause of the poisoning. These records are particularly important in cases of therapeutic drug errors or interactions.

Less commonly, an adult is found unconscious or dead in some remote location, either in the open or in an automobile. In the absence of evidence of violence or the more obvious clue of a hose leading from the vehicle exhaust to its interior, poisoning should be suspected.

In young children, circumstances are often important in suspecting exposure to a substance. Such events commonly occur when children escape the direct observation of caretakers. A common scenario is that of a parent finding that an unsupervised child has been quietly exploring his or her environment and now has some substance in his or her mouth or on the skin or is surrounded by it. The natural concern is that some of the substance has been swallowed.

SYMPTOMS AND SIGNS

There is no symptom that cannot be explained by some toxin, and symptoms are often so nonspecific that there is little value in determining their cause. Physical signs are of greater diagnostic value. Frequently the clinician must rely on the findings on physical examination to establish the diagnosis, even though the findings may conflict with the available exposure history.

GENERAL FEATURES

The general appearance of the patient, including skin color and lesions, skin and breath odors, vital signs, and urine color, may yield important diagnostic clues to focus the examination and laboratory investigations. Although many such findings have been described, only those likely to be found in seriously ill poisoned patients are described here.

Odors

The possibility of poisoning may be suggested by the smell of a patient's clothing and breath (Table 2-2). Alcohol is the most common odor detected in intoxicated patients. Smoke from domestic fires, phenol, some organic solvents, and clomethiazole (which has a sweet smell) are among other immediately recognizable odors. Heredity ensures that not everyone is capable of recognizing the bitter almond odor of cyanide poisoning, not to mention the infrequency of this type of poisoning. A garlic-like smell suggests exposure to arsenic, organophosphate insecticides, thallium, or phosphorus[8]; the smell of wintergreen suggests methyl salicylate poisoning; and the familiar fruity odor of acetone may be

---

TABLE 2-2 Odors of Drugs and Toxins

ODOR	TOXIN	ODOR	TOXIN
Acetone	Alcoholic ketoacidosis	Mothballs	Camphor
	Isopropyl alcohol		Naphthalene
Acrid (pearlike)	Paraldehyde		Paradichlorobenzene
	Chloral hydrate	Solvent/glue	Toluene
Bitter almonds	Cyanide		Xylene
Disinfectant	Phenol		Trichloroethane
Garlic	Arsenical insecticides		Tetrachloroethylene
	Organophosphate insecticides	Smoke	Carbon monoxide
			Cyanide
	Selenium		Clomethiazole
	Thallium	Wintergreen	Methyl salicylate
	Phosphorus	Rotten eggs	Hydrogen sulfide

---

from isopropyl alcohol ingestion or alcoholic ketoacidosis. A pearlike odor was described from paraldehyde and chloral hydrate, agents no longer commonly encountered. A rotten egg or sewage odor is consistent with hydrogen sulfide poisoning. Solvents and glues are often abused by teenagers, and their odor and stains may be encountered on the breath and skin. Factors such as a hospital's own odors (emesis, antiseptics, perspiration) and patient removal from the toxic environment limit the diagnostic value of odors.

Skin

Changes in the skin, such as color and staining, diaphoresis or dryness, bruising, the presence of needle tracks, lesions representing skin compression and breakdown, and hair loss, may yield diagnostic clues to poisoning.

COLOR

Patients poisoned with cyanides have a pink appearance because they are incapable of using the oxygen in their blood. Although carboxyhemoglobin is widely believed to impart a skin color similar to that of patients poisoned with carbon monoxide, it is rarely, if ever, encountered in vivo. More often, the patient is pale from hypotension or cyanotic from respiratory depression. Jaundice is a relatively late feature (usually ≥48 hours) of hepatotoxins, such as acetaminophen or cyclopeptide mushrooms, particularly those of the *Amanita* family, and is of limited diagnostic value initially. Exposure to dinitrophenol compounds may stain the skin yellow, whereas the skin, sweat, and urine of a patient may become pink or red after ingestion of a large dose of rifampicin—the so-called red man syndrome.[2] Flushed skin suggests anticholinergic poisoning, serotonin syndrome, alcohol-disulfiram reaction, monosodium glutamate exposure, scombroid fish poisoning (histamine release), or α-blocking agents such as phenothiazines or the atypical neuroleptics.[2] A patient who is disproportionately well despite intense cyanosis that has not been reversed by oxygen therapy almost certainly has methemoglobinemia. Common toxic causes include aniline, dapsone, chlorates, local anesthetics, nitrites (particularly the inorganic varieties), and some urea herbicides such as linuron and monolinuron that are metabolized to aniline derivatives. In such cases, the patient's blood may show a characteristic chocolate-brown color. Some of these agents also cause intravascular hemolysis, with the serum and urine becoming brownish owing to the presence of free hemoglobin. Methemoglobinemia is discussed in detail in Chapter 28.

DIAPHORESIS

Diaphoresis is found commonly in salicylate, sympathomimetic, phencyclidine, and organophosphate toxicity. It also is found in hypoglycemia, hyperthyroidism, serotonin syndrome, neuroleptic malignant syndrome, alcohol or sedative withdrawal, and shock. The presence of diaphoresis is particularly useful in excluding anticholinergic poisoning, which characteristically presents with dry skin and mucous membranes.

BRUISING

Skin bruising is common in patients who poison themselves. Commonly, bruising is due to falling while under the influ-

ence of ethanol or psychotropic drugs or violent exchanges with others. Diffuse ecchymosis also is commonly found, however, in anticoagulant poisoning, especially with second-generation rodenticides, such as difenacoum and brodifacoum (Fig. 2-1). More local ecchymosis along with edema is found in envenomations but may take 24 hours or longer to become apparent.

NEEDLE TRACKS

The presence of needle tracks should alert the physician to the possibility of intravenous abuse of opiates, amphetamines, and cocaine as an explanation for the patient's clinical state. The tracks may be immediately apparent or hidden in areas such as the groin or interdigital spaces.

BLISTERS

The skin lesions that are found in some poisoned patients who have been unconscious for about 6 hours or longer have fascinated clinicians over the years.[9–23] The lesions start as erythematous patches that may be discoid or highly irregular in shape. As the vessels in the lesion leak fluid into the intercellular space, they become raised with a dimpled surface caused by the hairs that are anchored deeper in the dermis and have a red halo of varying width. Frank blistering is the final stage of development. Although the location of many, but not all, of these lesions over bony prominences in the limbs testifies to the role of pressure in their etiology, there is evidence to suggest that a direct effect of the toxin on blood vessels[23] and sweat gland necrosis[10,11,21] also may be involved.

Skin lesions of this type began to be reported within a few years of the clinical use of barbiturate sedatives,[9] and by the 1960s they were considered virtually diagnostic of barbiturate overdose, being present in some 6% of these cases.[10] The lesions were referred to as "barbiturate burns" because of their resemblance to thermal burns (Figs. 2-2 and 2-3), but later experience revealed their association with virtually any poison that leads to coma, including carbamazepine,[19] amitriptyline,[17] carbon monoxide,[18,20] oxazepam,[17,22] and diazepam.[16] The lesions are of no value in differentiating among different toxins, but they occur sufficiently infrequently in patients unconscious from nontoxic causes that

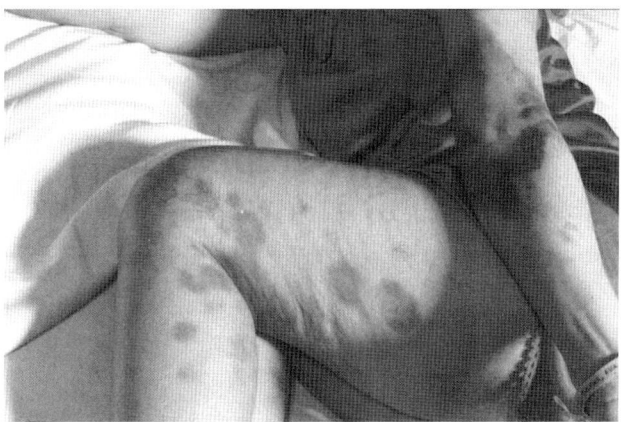

FIGURE 2-1

Diffuse ecchymoses after long-acting anticoagulant ingestion. *(Courtesy of J. Ward Donovan, MD.)* **See Color Fig. 2-1.**

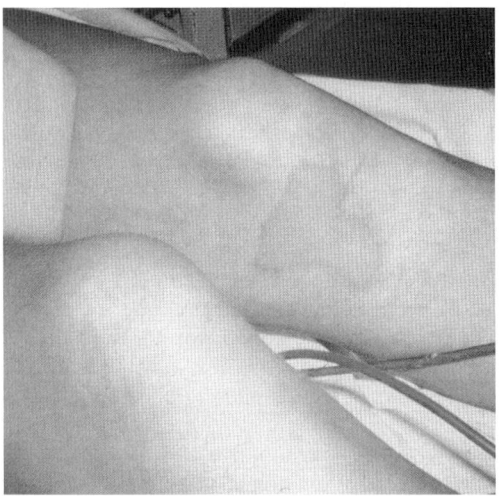

FIGURE 2-2

Skin lesion on medial knee after prolonged coma ("barbiturate burns"), early phase. *(Courtesy of J. Ward Donovan, MD.)* See Color Fig. 2-2.

they are of some diagnostic value.[12] Their presence also should alert the physician to possible later development of rhabdomyolysis, compartment syndromes, and axonopathies (especially involving the radial and common peroneal nerves) that also complicate prolonged immobilization, particularly against hard surfaces.

HAIR

Hair loss is well known from chemotherapeutic agents and less often is due to metal poisonings or colchicine. Alopecia is commonly seen about 1 week after exposure to thallium or arsenic, and its association with gastroenteritis and peripheral neuropathy is pathognomonic of these toxins. Another delayed skin finding in thallium and arsenic poisoning is the development of horizontal white lines in the nails (Mees' lines) in the weeks after exposure (Fig. 2-4).

Urine Color

A common urine discoloration in poisoned patients is the characteristic red or muddy brown color of myoglobinuria, secondary to rhabdomyolysis, which can be caused by any

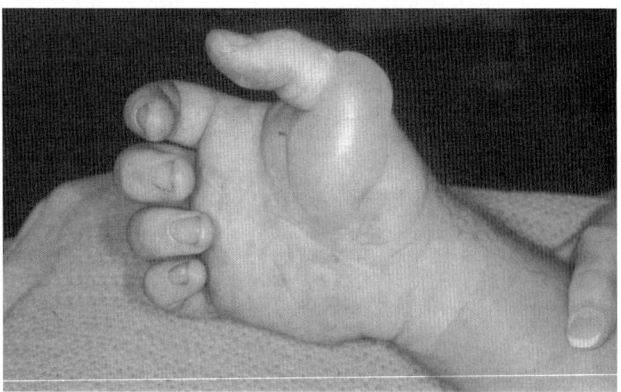

FIGURE 2-3

Hand blisters after prolonged coma ("barbiturate burns"), late phase. *(Courtesy of J. Ward Donovan, MD.)* See Color Fig. 2-3.

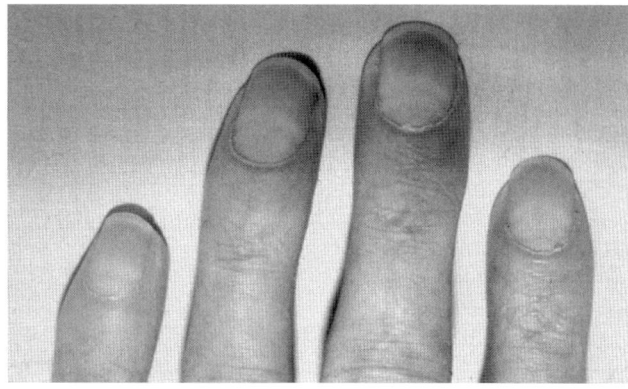

FIGURE 2-4

Mees' lines due to arsenic poisoning. *(Courtesy of J. Ward Donovan, MD.)* See Color Fig. 2-4.

drug or toxin that causes prolonged coma, intense myoclonus, or seizures. Brownish discoloration of the urine also can be due to metabolites of acetaminophen and not bilirubin. The red urine color of rifampicin overdose was noted earlier, associated with pink/red skin and sweat. The urine color also may become red (*vin rosé*) in patients who have been given deferoxamine for the treatment of iron poisoning. Urine color becomes green if patients receive methylthioninium chloride (methylene blue) for the treatment of methemoglobinemia. Crystalluria is a possible feature of ethylene glycol poisoning and primidone overdose. Other changes in urine color associated with drug and toxin exposures are listed in Table 2-3.[25–27]

VITAL SIGNS

Vital signs coupled with mental status can provide significant clues to the drug or toxin involved in acute poisoning and at least can narrow the differential diagnosis. Vital signs are influenced by many other nontoxic factors, however, such as body temperature, dehydration, endocrine status, oxygenation, infection, psychological state, and other preexisting disorders, so they also may be misleading. Although alterations in individual vital signs as outlined subsequently can be helpful, it is more useful to consider them together. Serial changes in vital signs also can provide additional information about the cause, especially if the time of exposure is known. Additionally, some abnormalities in vital signs can suggest the time and the type of exposure. Hypothermia and hypotension are consistent with late presentation of opiate and sedative-hypnotic overdose, and marked sinus tachycardia with hyperthermia may be seen in recent anticholinergic, amphetamine, or cocaine toxicity. If the vital signs are available, it is also useful to review the sequence of vital signs in the prehospital setting and before any therapy.

Heart Rate and Blood Pressure

Drugs and toxins affect the heart rate directly through changes in the sympathetic or parasympathetic nervous system; by central nervous system (CNS) depression or stimulation; or indirectly through changes in intravascular volume, vasodilation, oxygenation, or body temperature. Changes in

TABLE 2-3 Urine Colors

COLOR	DRUG/TOXIN	COLOR	DRUG/TOXIN
Brown	Metronidazole	Smoky	Phenols
	Levodopa	Pink	Cephalosporins
	Quinine		Phenothiazines
	Phenacetin		Ampicillin
	Myoglobin		Phenytoin
	Carbon tetrachloride	Green/blue	Copper sulfate
	Niridazole		Amitriptyline
	Aniline		Methylene blue
	Methyldopa		Methemoglobin inducers
	Nitrofurantoin		Boric acid
	Chloroquine	Green	Propofol
Black	Phenazopyridine		Indomethacin
	Cresols		Methocarbamol
	Methyldopa	Orange	Phenazopyridine
	Naphthalene		Mercury
	Phenols		Fluorescein
	Methocarbamol		Rifampin
Red	Phenolphthalein		Lead (chronic)
	Phenazopyridine	Luminescent	Phosphorus
	Deferoxamine	Fluorescent	Ethylene glycol
	Phenothiazines		(antifreeze)
	Rifampin		Triamterene
	Aniline	Crystalluria	Ethylene glycol
	Methyldopa		Sulfonamides
	Phenytoin		Primidone

cardiac conduction or membrane depressant effects also may induce sinus node, supraventricular, or ventricular arrhythmias that are likely to influence blood pressure, so it is most helpful to consider both of these vital signs together, as outlined in Tables 2-4 and 2-5.[2]

TABLE 2-4 Compounds Inducing Hypertension

Hypertension with Tachycardia

Adrenergic agonists
  Adrenaline (epinephrine)
  Amphetamines
  Bretylium (initial response)
  Cocaine
  Ephedrine
  Hypnosedative or alcohol
  Levodopa
  LSD
  MAO inhibitors (phenelzine and tranylcypromine)
  Marijuana
  Phencyclidine
  Pseudoephedrine

Anticholinergic agents
  Antihistamines
  Antipsychotic agents
  Tricyclic antidepressants
  Many others
Cholinergic agents
  Nicotine
  Organophosphate insecticides
  Other cholinesterase inhibitors

Hypertension with Normal or Slowed Pulse
Adrenaline (epinephrine)
Clonidine
Ergot derivatives
Noradrenaline (norepinephrine)
Other sympathomimetic amines
Phenylpropanolamine

LSD, lysergic acid diethylamide; MAO, monoamine oxidase.
Adapted from Olson KR, Pentel PR, Kelley MT: Physical assessment and differential diagnosis of the poisoned patient. Med Toxicol 2:56, 1987.

BRADYCARDIA AND HYPOTENSION

Depression of heart rate and blood pressure in present-day toxicology suggests exposure to sympatholytic agents, drugs with membrane-depressant actions, parasympathomimetic or central α_2-agonist agents, or CNS depressants. Drugs that most commonly cause these effects are calcium channel–blocking or β-blocking drugs, opiates, cardiac glycosides, sedative-hypnotics, and sodium channel–blocking drugs, as in massive cyclic antidepressant overdose. Severe hypoxemia induced by respiratory depression or cellular hypoxia, as in cyanide toxicity, also can cause bradycardia and hypotension. The inhibition of acetylcholinesterase by organophosphate and carbamate insecticides also would be expected to cause bradycardia owing to their muscarinic effects and hypotension from fluid loss. The heart rate conversely may be increased by nicotinic stimulation.

BRADYCARDIA AND HYPERTENSION

Drug-induced hypertension from intense vasoconstriction can produce reflex bradycardia seen most often in sympathomimetic toxicity, particularly with phenylpropanolamine. Central α_2-agonists, such as clonidine and the imidazolines, also may cause initial hypertension despite bradycardia, secondary to vasoconstriction from stimulation of peripheral α_1-receptors. Intracranial hemorrhage from cocaine or sympathomimetic-induced hypertensive crisis also could result in this combination of vital signs.

TACHYCARDIA AND HYPOTENSION

Hypovolemia caused by fluid loss or vasodilation from sepsis, peripheral α_1 blockade, or β_2 stimulation leads to tachycardia

TABLE 2-5 Compounds Inducing Hypotension

Hypotension with Bradycardia

α_2-Agonists
  Clonidine
  Tetrahydrozoline
β-Blockers
Bretylium (after initial
  hypertension)
Calcium channel blockers
Cyanide
Dextropropoxyphene
Fluoride
Hypnosedative agents (e.g.,
  barbiturates, benzodiazepines)
Hypothermia inducers
Narcotics
Nicotine
Organophosphate insecticides
Sympatholytic antihypertensives
  (e.g., reserpine, methyldopa)
Tricyclic antidepressants*
Vacor†

Hypotension with Tachycardia

Fluid Loss or Third Spacing
Amatoxin-containing mushrooms
Arsenic

Colchicine
Hyperthermia
Iron
Numerous plant toxins
2,4-Dichlorophenoxyacetic acid

*Peripheral Arteriolar Dilation
with Reflex Compensation*
Antipsychotic agents
β_2 stimulants (e.g., terbutaline,
  orciprenaline [metaproterenol])
Caffeine
Disulfiram-ethanol interaction
Hydralazine
Hyperthermia
Nitrites
Phenothiazines
Sodium nitroprusside
Theophylline
Tricyclic antidepressants‡

*Toxin-Induced Tissue
Hypoxia*
Carbon monoxide
Cyanide

*Late, severe/fatal cases.
†N-3 pyridylmethyl-N′ 4 nitrophenyl urea.
‡Also, direct cardiac depression.
Adapted from Olson KR, Pentel PR, Kelley MT: Physical assessment and differential
diagnosis of the poisoned patient. Med Toxicol 2:57, 1987.

with hypotension, presuming that the cardiovascular reflexes are intact. Toxins likely to cause massive fluid loss include iron salts, colchicine, paraquat, plants and mushrooms that target the gastrointestinal tract, insecticides, salicylates, and heavy metals. Peripheral α_1 blockade is seen with nitrites, phenothiazines, and the newer atypical neuroleptics. Toxins that cause myocardial depression, vasodilation, or tachyarrhythmias also can cause this combination of features and include cyclic antidepressants, antipsychotic agents, caffeine, theophylline, and pure β_2 stimulants such as terbutaline. The dihydropyridine calcium channel antagonists amlodipine and nifedipine cause vasodilation and a reflex tachycardia, in contrast to the other calcium channel blockers, which cause bradycardia. Alcohol withdrawal associated with intravascular volume depletion or acid-base disturbances (as in alcoholic ketoacidosis) or both results in tachycardia and hypotension. The anticholinesterase insecticides also can cause this combination when muscarinic effects produce volume losses, but nicotinic effects on the heart predominate. The tachycardia can be exacerbated by hypoxia from bronchorrhea, bronchoconstriction, and respiratory depression. Cellular toxins, such as cyanide, and tissue hypoxia from methemoglobinemia or carboxyhemoglobinemia are other potential causes. The serotonin and neuroleptic malignant syndromes typically cause tachycardia and can be associated with either hypotension or hypertension.

TACHYCARDIA AND HYPERTENSION

Drugs and toxins that stimulate the sympathetic nervous system and the indirect-acting sympathomimetic drugs cause vasoconstriction and cardiac stimulation. These include amphetamines, cocaine, and phenylephrine. The hallucinogens phencyclidine and lysergic acid diethylamide (LSD) also are adrenergic agents, which commonly elevate the blood pressure and heart rate. Monoamine oxidase inhibitors in overdose or when taken with sympathomimetics or tyramine-containing foods typically cause initial hypertension and tachycardia followed by hypotension and bradycardia resulting from eventual depletion of catecholamines. This sequence also can be seen in cyclic antidepressant toxicity. Anticholinergic agents such as antihistamines and plants such as Jimson weed (*Datura stramonium*) cause a marked tachycardia but only mild hypertension.

Respiratory Rate

The respiratory rate or depth can be affected by acid-base status, drugs or toxins affecting the CNS, or neuromuscular agents. Any compound that causes metabolic acidosis of whatever etiology causes hyperventilation. Likewise, cellular hypoxia from carbon monoxide or cyanide toxicity also induces compensatory hyperventilation. Hypoxia from aspiration pneumonitis or noncardiogenic pulmonary edema (both commonly encountered in drug overdose) or inhalation of pulmonary irritants such as chlorine results in tachypnea. Stimulants, including amphetamines, cocaine, sympathomimetics, and hallucinogens, increase the respiratory rate and depth directly, whereas salicylates and phenols cause tachypnea resulting from direct stimulation of the respiratory center and increased oxygen consumption from uncoupling of oxidative phosphorylation. Phenoxyacetate (chlorophenoxy) herbicides and pentachlorophenol also cause hyperventilation secondary to uncoupling of oxidative phosphorylation. The methylxanthines caffeine and theophylline also are direct respiratory center stimulants. CNS arousal during withdrawal from alcohol, opiates, or sedative-hypnotics also results in tachypnea and hyperpnea.

Respiratory depression due to drugs most commonly involves CNS depressants, such as opiates, barbiturates, other sedatives, and alcohol. Respiratory muscle weakness follows poisoning with neuromuscular blockers, as in strychnine, venoms, tetrodotoxin, and botulinum, and depolarization of nicotinic receptors by organophosphate and carbamate insecticides. Table 2-6 lists compounds that typically affect the rate or depth of respiration.

Body Temperature

Changes in body temperature alone are unlikely to aid the diagnosis of poisoning but can provide support for suspected toxins or syndromes. Measurement of temperature is often forgotten during initial resuscitation, but recognition of extreme changes in both directions is important in regard to suggesting possible toxic causes and appropriate treatment. Temperature changes also give clues to the time that has elapsed since exposure and the presence of comorbid conditions. Hypothermia in poisoning most often occurs due to prolonged coma, even in warm environments and particularly when sedatives, opiates, and ethanol are involved. Phenothiazines and other α-antagonists cause heat loss owing to vasodilation. Nontoxic conditions include environmental exposure, hypothyroidism, and hypoglycemia, although the last-mentioned may be drug-induced.

TABLE 2-6 Drugs and Toxins Affecting Respiratory Rate

Respiratory Depression	Hyperventilation (Tachypnea or Hyperpnea)
Central Nervous System Depressants	Amphetamines
Barbiturates	Caffeine
Benzodiazepines	Cocaine
Carbon monoxide	Drugs causing tissue hypoxia
Clonidine	(carbon monoxide, cyanide,
Cyanide	hydrogen sulfide, methemo-
Cyclic antidepressants	globin inducers)
Opiates	Drugs/toxins causing hepatic
Phenothiazines	encephalopathy
Sedative-hypnotics	Drugs/toxins causing
Zolpidem	metabolic acidosis
	Hallucinogens
Respiratory Muscle Weakness	Nicotine
Botulinum toxin	Phenols
Neuromuscular blockers	Phenoxyacetate
Nicotine	herbicides
Organophosphate insecticides	Salicylates
Paralytic shellfish poisoning	Sympathomimetics
Poison hemlock	Theophylline
Snake venom	
Strychnine	

Hyperthermia may result from increased heat production secondary to muscle rigidity; seizures; agitation; vasoconstriction caused by agents such as amphetamines, cocaine, and hallucinogens; and the serotonin and neuroleptic malignant syndromes. Anticholinergic compounds, such as cyclic antidepressants and first-generation antihistamines, have dual actions; they increase heat production by inducing agitation and by inhibiting sweating. An increased metabolic rate due to uncoupling of oxidative phosphorylation by salicylates and phenols also can cause temperature elevation. Direct effects of drugs and toxins can cause fever, as in metal fume fever. The most common cause of fever in poisoned patients is probably aspiration pneumonitis, from loss of airway protection or hydrocarbons. Table 2-7 shows examples of temperature changes secondary to toxic exposures.

TABLE 2-7 Compounds and Toxidromes Affecting Body Temperature

HYPOTHERMIA	HYPERTHERMIA
Barbiturates	Alcohol withdrawal
Benzodiazepines	Amphetamines
Carbon monoxide	Anticholinergic agents
Clonidine	Cocaine
Cyclic antidepressants	Hallucinogens
Ethanol	Malignant hyperthermia
Hypoglycemic agents	MAO inhibitors
Isopropyl alcohol	Metal fume fever
Opiates	Neuroleptic malignant syndrome
Phenothiazines	Phenols
Sedative-hypnotics	Salicylates
	Sedative-hypnotic withdrawal
	Thyroid hormone

MAO, monoamine oxidase.

TOXIDROMES

It is highly improbable that single abnormalities detected on examination of poisoned patients would definitively differentiate poisoning from other causes of illness or point the clinician in the direction of a specific toxin or group of toxins. Toxidromes—clusters of symptoms and signs in the same patient—are of considerable diagnostic value, however, especially when considered in the context of the poisonings that occur commonly in a given community. Individual toxidromes are discussed in detail in Part 2 of this textbook (Chapters 17 through 32). It is sufficient here to summarize the toxidromes due to opioids, anticholinergics, cholinergics, amphetamines, and salicylates that are most readily recognizable.

Opioid poisoning is characterized by impaired consciousness (often deep coma) in association with pupils that are constricted to pinpoint diameter and hypoventilation. When hypoventilation is manifested by a reduced respiratory rate, as it commonly is, the cause is in little doubt. General depression of all neurologic functions with coma, hypoventilation (usually without bradypnea), reduced muscle tone and tendon reflexes, and normal or absent plantar responses formerly would have suggested barbiturates as the responsible toxins, but in present-day society severe intoxication with tricyclic antidepressants (TCA), alone or in combination with other CNS depressants, is more likely. Other possible causes of depressed consciousness and respiration include overdose of muscle relaxants such as carisoprodol (see Chapter 53), anxiolytics and sedative-hypnotics (see Chapter 47), and occasionally anticonvulsants (see Chapters 49 through 51).

TCA poisoning (see Chapter 42) severe enough to resemble opiate toxicity is uncommon, and the toxidrome that characterizes less severe TCA poisoning is more readily identifiable. It presents a mix of features suggesting simultaneous depression and stimulation of the nervous system, including dilated pupils; increased muscle tone and tendon reflexes; myoclonic jerks; convulsions; extensor plantar responses; sinus tachycardia, often with cardiac conduction disturbances; and varying degrees of coma. These clinical effects are produced by a combination of anticholinergic actions, sodium channel blockade, and impaired reuptake of catecholamines into nerve endings. The occurrence of convulsions and the finding of PR, QT_c, and QRS prolongation on the electrocardiogram (ECG), particularly when combined with a prominent terminal R wave in lead aVR, is supportive evidence of TCA overdose. Although overdoses of agents with catecholamine-like actions (e.g., amphetamines, cocaine) also would be expected to dilate the pupils, exaggerate muscle tone and reflexes, and increase the heart rate similarly, the failure to lose consciousness would differentiate poisoning with these drugs from poisoning with TCAs.

The opposite of the anticholinergic consequences of TCA poisoning is the cholinergic syndrome (see Chapter 23), commonly encountered in developing countries after exposure to cholinesterase-inhibiting organophosphate and carbamate insecticides (see Chapter 91). In these cases, the accumulation of acetylcholine at autonomic nerve endings results in hypersalivation, tearing, bronchorrhea, wheezing, bladder emptying, and tenesmus. Paradoxically, however, the bradycardia one would expect from knowledge of the mechanism of action of these agents is seen in only approximately 15% to

20% of cases.[28,29] Failure to hydrolyze acetylcholine at the neuromuscular junction leads to muscle weakness, hyporeflexia, and fasciculation and, in the brain, to impaired consciousness and reduced respiratory drive.

A further readily identifiable toxidrome is that of salicylate intoxication (see Chapter 57); although one would expect this condition to be suggested by an increased anion gap acidosis and diagnosed by laboratory testing, the toxidrome offers confirmation. Nausea, vomiting, tinnitus, impaired hearing, profuse sweating, and peripheral vasodilation in a fully conscious individual are diagnostic. Cinchonism, usually due to overdose of quinine (see Chapter 63), is the only other possibility but is much rarer and is commonly associated with impaired vision (see later), which precludes any confusion with salicylate poisoning.

NEUROLOGIC SIGNS

Coma is one of the most serious consequences of acute poisoning, and other neurologic signs are important in elucidating its cause, especially when a history is not available. In general, if an unconscious patient is found to have focal signs, the clinician should be extremely reluctant to accept poisoning as the cause unless the history has revealed some preexisting neurologic disease; individuals who have had strokes or have multiple sclerosis do poison themselves occasionally. Transient lateralizing signs have been described after overdoses of barbiturates[30] and phenytoin[31,32] but only in single cases.

Abnormalities of the Pupils

One lateralizing sign that is an exception and may result from poisoning is inequality of the size of the pupils or their reaction to light. There are no data on how often unequal pupils occur in the normal population, and few observers have commented on them in poisoned patients except with glutethimide[33,34] and ethylene glycol.[35] Clinical experience suggests that inequalities are not unusual and are seldom evidence of brainstem compression; virtually all patients exhibiting the sign recovery uneventfully. The greater the doubt about a diagnosis of poisoning, however, the more important it is to keep the pupil changes under frequent review and to perform imaging studies if the disparity increases.

The diameter of the pupils is also valuable in determining the substance responsible for unexplained coma. In developed countries, miosis is usually due to overdose of opioid analgesics, whereas in developing countries, a cholinergic syndrome secondary to poisoning with organophosphate and carbamate insecticides is the common cause. The converse, dilation of the pupils, is most likely to be due to intoxication with toxins such as TCAs that have marked anticholinergic actions or theophylline and others with sympathomimetic actions, including dopamine used therapeutically.[36] Dilation of the pupils also may be the first sign of visual impairment complicating intoxication with quinine[37] and methanol.

Although changes in pupil diameter can be useful, the extent and speed with which the pupils react to light is of no clinical value. Pupils that are either constricted or dilated due to toxins are unlikely to show much, if any, response to light.[38]

Pyramidal Tract Features

Pyramidal tract features, such as hypertonia, hyperreflexia, and extensor plantar responses, are found commonly in TCA poisoning, provided that it is not unduly severe (see earlier). Other drugs, including the first-generation antihistamines and some Parkinson's disease agents (especially orphenadrine), have similar actions. Drugs causing the serotonin syndrome (see Chapter 24) can produce similar physical findings, in addition to sustained ankle clonus and lower extremity rigidity. Similarly the neuroleptic malignant syndrome (see Chapter 26) presents with extreme muscle rigidity, but hyperreflexia is atypical.

Brainstem Function

It has been known for more than a century that the posture or movements of the eyes may be abnormal under anesthesia.[39] These abnormal movements indicate impaired brainstem functioning; a study showed that they occurred in 23 of 26 patients anesthetized with thiopentone and halothane.[40] It is only since the 1970s, however, that it has been appreciated that similar changes occur when individuals are poisoned with a variety of drugs.

STRABISMUS AND OPHTHALMOPLEGIA

Failure to maintain parallel optical axes manifests as strabismus, usually with divergence in the horizontal plane, but also occasionally in the vertical plane. This phenomenon, as with all the ocular abnormalities found in acute poisoning, may be transient and change over minutes. It has been described in association with carbamazepine,[41,42] in association with phenytoin,[43,44] and in about 29% of cases of TCA overdosage.[45] Occasionally, carbamazepine[46,47] and phenytoin[48,49] cause total external ophthalmoplegia when consciousness is no more than minimally impaired.

ROVING EYE MOVEMENTS

Roving eye movements also may be seen in unconscious poisoned patients if both eyes are observed for a time. These movements are often dysconjugate and have been reported in poisoning with TCAs, barbiturates, benzodiazepines, ethanol, phencyclidine, and phenothiazines.

OCULOVESTIBULAR REFLEXES

Occasionally, it is only when the oculovestibular reflexes are examined that dysconjugate eye movements become apparent. Syringing ice-cold water into the external auditory meatus should make both eyes turn to the side being syringed. Failure of one eye to deviate is evidence of internuclear ophthalmoplegia and a lesion of the medial longitudinal fasciculus. It has been reported in 10% of poisoned patients,[50] specifically with poisoning with cyclic antidepressants,[51,52] phenothiazines,[53] benzodiazepines, barbiturates, and ethanol.[50]

As with the development of divergent optic axes with anesthesia, so doll's eye reflexes also may be lost. This loss occurred in almost 50% of children anesthetized with thiopentone.[54] Similarly, the doll's eye and oculovestibular reflexes may be lost in patients acutely poisoned with carbamazepine,[55] phenytoin,[48,56] and TCAs.[46,57–61] Their loss should not be interpreted, however, as evidence of brainstem death until it can be shown that the drugs have been completely eliminated from the body. Similarly, decerebrate and decorticate movements of the limbs of patients who are unconscious owing to poisons are not signs of irreversible structural brain damage. The patients can be expected to make a full, uneventful recovery.

CONVULSIONS

Seizures can be induced by multiple drugs and toxins and are a common manifestation of therapeutic and recreational drug abuse and overdose. Antidepressants of the cyclic and serotonin reuptake inhibitor classes are a particularly high risk, as are the analgesics meperidine, propoxyphene, mefenamic acid, and occasionally salicylates. First seizures in adolescents and young adults always should raise the suspicion of cocaine or amphetamine abuse or an overdose of anticholinergic agents or antihistamines. Phenothiazines, chronic lithium toxicity, or the serotonin syndrome should be considered in patients on psychoactive agents. Seizures also may be the first manifestation of withdrawal from alcohol, benzodiazepines, or other sedative-hypnotics. Prolonged seizures that are difficult to control should suggest isoniazid, strychnine, or theophylline toxicity. Table 2-8 lists agents that should be considered in the differential diagnosis of drug-induced or toxin-induced seizures.

VISUAL IMPAIRMENT

Visual impairment is a useful diagnostic feature and is most often associated with methanol and quinine toxicity. In quinine toxicity, blurring of vision may be the only initial complaint; later acuity becomes reduced, often to the point of

TABLE 2-9 Drugs and Toxins Causing Visual Disturbances

Anticholinergics	Ethambutol
Botulinum toxin	Hydroxychloroquine
Carbon monoxide	Methanol
Chloroquine	Quinine
Ciguatera	Squill
Digitalis	

blindness.[62,63] Methanol (see Chapter 86) also poses a serious risk to vision, but other features of its toxicity, particularly the associated profound metabolic acidosis, pulmonary edema, and renal failure, readily differentiate it from quinine. Visual loss from these toxins usually is recovered, but some permanent loss may result, especially loss of peripheral and night vision in the case of quinine. In more severe cases, patients may be left with no more than tunnel vision. Other agents that characteristically can cause visual loss include ethambutol, carbon monoxide, cyclosporine, and vincristine. Visual disturbances also are a nonspecific finding in many cases of sedative-hypnotic and ethanol toxicity. Drugs and toxins potentially causing visual disturbances are listed in Table 2-9.[26]

HEARING IMPAIRMENT

Mild impairment of hearing, usually accompanied by tinnitus, is characteristic of acute salicylate toxicity and the early stage of quinine toxicity (cinchonism). There also have been sporadic reports of toxicity with acute heroin, carbon monoxide, and nonsteroidal drugs as a cause of temporary deafness.[64,65] The other agents listed in Table 2-10 may cause hearing loss with long-term use.[2,26]

INVOLUNTARY MOVEMENTS

Acute dystonic movements, including acute torticollis, orolingual dyskinesias, and oculogyric crises, are virtually diagnostic of exposure to metoclopramide[66] and, less commonly, droperidol, haloperidol, prochlorperazine, and trifluoperazine (or other dopamine antagonists). Rarely, such exposure may have disastrous consequences.[67] Choreoathetosis may be the presenting feature of poisoning with organophosphorous insecticides,[68,69] pemoline,[70] metronidazole,[71] and benztropine.[72]

TABLE 2-8 Drugs and Toxins Inducing Seizures

Alcohol (withdrawal)	Lithium
Amphetamines	MAO inhibitors
Anticholinergic drugs/plants	Mefenamic acid
Antihistamines	Meperidine (pethidine)
Baclofen	Nicotine
Benzodiazepine withdrawal	Organophosphate insecticides
Bupropion	Phenothiazines
Camphor	Phenylpropanolamine
Carbamazepine	Propoxyphene
Chlorinated hydrocarbons	Propranolol
Chloroquine	Salicylates
Cocaine	Sedative-hypnotic withdrawal
Cyclic antidepressants	Selective serotonin reuptake
Ergotamine	inhibitors
Ethylene glycol	Strychnine
Isoniazid	Theophylline
Lidocaine	Water hemlock plant
Lindane	(cicutoxin)

MAO, monoamine oxidase.

TABLE 2-10 Drugs and Toxins Causing Hearing Loss

Aminoglycosides	Heroin
Carbon monoxide	Nonsteroidal analgesics
Cisplatin	Potassium bromate
Erythromycin	Quinidine
Ethacrynic acid	Quinine
Furosemide	Salicylates

BIOCHEMICAL ABNORMALITIES

Changes in Electrolyte Concentrations

A change in the concentration of an electrolyte in serum or plasma can occasionally be helpful in suggesting the involvement of particular toxins. By itself, no concentration is diagnostic, but in the absence of other evidence, it may help reduce the number of substances under suspicion. In theory, electrolyte concentrations may be modified by many mechanisms, including changing the total body load of the electrolyte or the volume in which it is dissolved, altering its elimination, redistributing it between the intracellular and extracellular fluid compartments, and chelating it so that the effective total body load is reduced. Although all of these mechanisms occur in clinical toxicology, some are encountered more frequently than others, and because toxins commonly affect multiple systems, more than one mechanism may be operating simultaneously. An increase in the total body load of an electrolyte is possible only if a quantity is ingested or acquired in some other way. Loss of significant amounts, whether through the kidneys or through the gut, is more likely to occur over days than over hours. Acute changes are usually the result of redistribution or, much less commonly, chelation. The time scale over which concentrations change is vital in determining the morbidity that results. The profoundly low serum sodium concentrations associated with compulsive water drinking would be lethal if they developed over hours rather than weeks or months. Consequently, the greater the degree of deviation of an electrolyte concentration from the reference range and the more rapidly it develops, the more ominous is its significance in acutely poisoned individuals.

Hypernatremia

Hypernatremia is uncommon in clinical toxicology and is most likely to be the result of excessive intake in the form of common salt as an emetic or ingestion of some bleaches.[73] It also may complicate therapeutic interventions, however, such as large doses of sodium bicarbonate for TCA overdose or correction of life-threatening acidosis from methanol or ethylene glycol toxicity. Even "maintenance" administration of normal saline can cause significant hypernatremia in individuals with toxin-induced (usually lithium) diabetes insipidus.

Hyponatremia

Hyponatremia is rare in acute poisonings and when it does occur is caused by dilution rather than reduction of total body load. The syndrome of inappropriate secretion of antidiuretic hormone with water retention, as occurs in some users of Ecstasy (3,4-methylenedioxymethamphetamine), is perhaps the best-known example. Rarely, severe and fatal hyponatremia is due to ingestion of vast amounts of water over a short time.

Hyperkalemia

Acute changes in serum potassium concentrations are potentially of much greater clinical significance than changes in sodium concentrations because relative concentration of potassium across the membranes of some cells, especially cardiac myocytes, determines their excitability. Potentially lethal arrhythmias may develop if potassium concentrations change significantly over a short time. Hyperkalemia is only occasionally the result of ingestion of potassium salts, alone or as formulated with diuretics. Much more commonly in toxicology, hyperkalemia is due to redistribution of potassium from cells to the extracellular and intravascular spaces. The shift may occur for many reasons. Massive cell damage, particularly rhabdomyolysis, is an important cause, whereas some toxins, such as digoxin and similar cardiac glycosides (see Chapter 33), inhibit the adenosine triphosphatase–dependent membrane sodium-potassium pump with subsequent leakage of potassium from cells. Hyperkalemia is a feature of massive acute digoxin intoxication, whereas hypokalemia is the usual finding in longer term therapeutic overdose. Potassium supplements given to correct hypokalemia (e.g., as in theophylline overdose) also can cause severe rebound hyperkalemia as the effects of the toxin on the cell membranes decline during recovery. Metabolic acidosis, a common accompaniment of serious poisoning, is unlikely to lead by itself to significant hyperkalemia but may be a significant background factor. Toxins causing renal failure, such as ethylene glycol, indirectly result in hyperkalemia.

Hypokalemia

As with hyperkalemia, hypokalemia complicating acute poisoning is usually due to redistribution of potassium, in this case from the extracellular to the intracellular compartment. Redistribution is mediated by stimulation of the membrane sodium-potassium pump or inhibition of phosphodiesterase within the cells. Drugs such as theophylline, amphetamines, and sympathomimetics that increase catecholamine activity are most likely to induce hypokalemia. Normokalemia in severe theophylline intoxication suggests that the movement of the potassium into some cells is being balanced by efflux from others and that there is underlying rhabdomyolysis. Hypokalemia also occurs with overdose of insulin and oral hypoglycemic agents, particularly chlorpropamide. Alkalosis, whether induced by hyperventilation or by administration of alkali (e.g., to induce an alkaline urine), causes hypokalemia by virtue of increased urine loss.

Hyperchloremia

An increase in serum chloride concentrations has been reported occasionally after ingestion of massive quantities of bleach; there is usually an associated alkalosis.[73] It also may be a clue to bromide poisoning but, in this case, depends on the use of ferricyanate in the analytic method. This method does not differentiate bromide from chloride, yielding an apparent hyperchloremia and a decrease in the anion gap (see later).[74]

Hypocalcemia

Hypocalcemia is uncommon in acutely poisoned patients but is potentially of great significance because it enhances the excitability of the myocardium, skeletal muscle cells, and neurons. The primary reason for reduced serum calcium concentrations is binding to toxins or their metabolites. Fluoride ions (usually from hydrofluoric acid) are a potent direct cause of hypocalcemia. In contrast, the metabolites of ethylene glycol and sodium fluoroacetate (oxalic acid and fluorocitrate) bind calcium and reduce serum concentrations. In the case of ethylene glycol, crystals of calcium oxalate may be deposited in tissues or excreted in the urine. Intravenous administration of phosphates also may lead to hypocalcemia, whereas concentrations may decrease later if calcium is sequestered in necrotic tissue, usually skeletal muscle.

Alterations in Blood Glucose Concentrations

Blood glucose concentrations are altered in a variety of poisonings. Overdose of insulin and oral hypoglycemic agents would be expected to induce hypoglycemia (see Chapter 70). Hypoglycemia is also an occasional finding, however, in poisoning with β-adrenoceptor blocking drugs, ethanol,[75] and salicylates, in addition to being a common feature of acute hepatic necrosis induced by massive amounts of acetaminophen and iron salts.

Hyperglycemia is induced by drugs such as theophylline that stimulate catecholamine release and glycogenolysis. It also has been reported in poisoning with such varied substances as acetaminophen, acetone, calcium channel–blocking drugs, isoniazid, and organophosphate insecticides and in 50% or more of cases of poisoning with the herbicide amitraz,[76] although the mechanism is not always clear.

ACID-BASE DISTURBANCES

Metabolic Acidosis

Before thinking a metabolic acidosis to be of potential diagnostic value in a poisoned patient, it is essential to consider possible confounding factors. Among these factors, the most important are hypoxia and peripheral circulatory failure, both of which may result in anaerobic glycolysis and lactic acidosis. It is also important to know the timing of the sample in which the acidosis was reported in relation to other events; the results of blood gas analysis of samples taken within minutes of convulsions may be seriously misleading. Less commonly, ketoacidosis due to starvation (if the patient has been unconscious for 1 or 2 days before presentation), alcoholic ketoacidosis, or ketoacidosis in a poisoned diabetic may be a possibility. Acute renal tubular damage complicating poisoning also may contribute to acidosis. Metabolic acidosis that may be of diagnostic value in clinical toxicology is one that persists after elimination of confounding factors.

Some degree of acidosis is common in symptomatic poisonings of many types, and minor deviations from normal are of no diagnostic value. Severe acidosis may suggest the involvement of certain toxins, however. It is only rarely due to massive ingestion of an acid. Even when found in patients with aspirin (acetylsalicylic acid) overdose, the acid radical contributes only a little to the acidosis. Accumulation of the acidic metabolites of toxins can cause profound acidosis; formic and oxalic acids from metabolism of methanol and ethylene glycol are the most obvious examples. Severe lactic acidosis can result from serious poisoning with cyanide, isoniazid, and strychnine. Toxin-induced acid-base disturbances are described in more detail in Chapter 29.

Other Acid-Base Disturbances

Acid-base disturbances other than metabolic acidosis, although common, are of less diagnostic importance. Salicylates and drugs such as theophylline and amphetamines directly stimulate the respiratory center and are the most common toxic causes of a primary respiratory alkalosis. Hyperventilation secondary to emotional distress is another possible explanation. Uncompensated metabolic alkalosis is rare and not likely to be encountered in acute poisoning except in misuse of antacids.

Anion Gap

Measurement of the anion gap is intended to identify the presence of unmeasured cations or anions in serum or plasma. It has two main uses: first, the differentiation of the cause of a metabolic acidosis, and second, monitoring the effects of its treatment. Many equations have been proposed for estimating the anion gap. One in which all the units of measurement for concentrations are in mmol/L is as follows:

$$\text{Anion gap} = \{Na^+\} - (\{Cl^-\} + \{HCO_3^-\})$$

The normal gap is generally accepted to be 10 to 14 mmol/L. Calculation of the anion gap is a problem when hospital laboratories measure only serum or plasma chloride concentration and do not include total carbon dioxide as a component of the standard electrolyte profile, but the value determined by blood gas analysis can be used in the above-noted equation. Alternative equations include potassium as a cation, but its variation is so insignificant that it is usually excluded.

In clinical toxicology, the most common reason for an elevated anion gap is the presence of an increased amount of unmeasured anion. It may derive from the toxin (e.g., salicylates) or its metabolites (as with methanol, ethylene glycol) or from accumulation of increased amounts of ketones (e.g., acetoacetic acid and hydroxybutyrate) and lactate secondary to anaerobic metabolism. Serum lactate and acetone should always be measured if the cause of a high anion gap is not clear. When lactic acidosis and ketoacidosis have been eliminated, a high anion gap acidosis is likely to be due to toxins such as cyanides, ethylene glycol, methanol, paraldehyde, salicylates, acetaminophen, or toluene. Drugs or toxins causing an elevated anion gap metabolic acidosis are listed in Table 2-11, with associated findings. Other than poisoning with lithium, it is rare for an unmeasured cation to decrease the anion gap. Acid-base disturbances are discussed in greater detail in Chapter 29.

Osmolar Gap

The osmolar gap detects the presence of osmotically active substances in serum or plasma. Because the standard deviation of the normal gap is of the order of ± 10 mmol/L, only major changes, such as those induced by large concentrations of small molecules, are likely to be detected with certainty. The best-known example is ethanol, but methanol, isopropanol, and ethylene glycol also increase the gap if present in sufficient amounts. The osmolar gap is no more than a screening test, but serum osmolality measurement is more readily available than definitive analyses for ethanol,

TABLE 2-11 Differential Diagnosis of Anion Gap Acidosis

SUBSTANCES/CONDITION	ACRONYM	SYMPTOMS/SIGNS	OSMOLAR GAP
Acetaminophen	A	Hepatic/renal failure	
Methanol	M	Visual defects, dilated pupils, blurred disks	+ +
Uremia	U	Myoclonus, seizures	
Diabetic/alcoholic ketoacidosis	D	Dehydration, acetonemia	+
Paraldehyde	P	Gastric/respiratory distress	
Phenformin/metformin		Renal insufficiency	
Iron	I	Gastritis, melanotic diarrhea	
Isoniazid		Seizures	
Isopropyl alcohol		Gastritis, hypotension	+ +
Ibuprofen/NSAIDs		Abdominal pain, nausea/vomiting, lethargy	
Lactic acidosis	L	Hypotension or seizures	+
Ethylene glycol	E	Renal failure; oxalate crystals	+ +
Salicylates	S	Gastritis, tinnitus, tachypnea	

NSAIDs, nonsteroidal antiinflammatory drugs.

methanol, and ethylene glycol and is more readily performed. Finding an abnormal gap is an indication to undertake more specific assays, particularly if poisoning with methanol or ethylene glycol is suspected. Other potential causes of an increased osmolar gap are acetonemia and the presence of mannitol or propylene glycol. Table 2-12 lists reported causes of an increased osmolar gap.[2]

Two values are required to estimate the osmolar gap: first, a measurement of actual osmolality (usually determined by depression of the freezing point of serum/plasma) and second, a calculated osmolality. Although the former measures extraneous and endogenous substances that normally contribute to osmolality, the latter is an estimate of the contributions of endogenous substances alone. The osmolar gap is the difference between the two values. Many formulas have been proposed for deriving the calculated osmolality. A typical example (in which the units of measurement are mmol/L) is as follows:

$$\text{Calculated osmolality} = 2\ \{Na^+\} + \{urea\} + \{glucose\} + ethanol$$

If the values are in mass units, the equation is

$$\text{Calculated osmolality} = 2\{Na\} + urea/2.8 + glucose/18 + ethanol/4.6$$

TABLE 2-12 Drugs and Toxins Causing Increased Osmolar Gap

Acetone
Ethanol
Ethyl ether
Ethylene glycol
Mannitol
Methanol
Propylene glycol
Trichloroethane

The amount of common osmotically active toxins can be estimated by multiplying the entire osmolar gap by the values listed in Table 2-13.[77]

LIVER FUNCTION TESTS

Acetaminophen is now the most common cause of fulminant hepatic failure in some developed countries, so unexplained jaundice in conjunction with serum alanine or aspartate aminotransferase activities exceeding 5000 U/L is a strong pointer to undisclosed overdose.

TRIALS OF ANTIDOTES

When overdose of an opioid or benzodiazepine is suspected, confirmation of the diagnosis may be obtained from improvement in the patient's clinical condition within 1 to 2 minutes of giving an intravenous bolus dose of naloxone[78] or flumazenil.[79,80] The use of these antidotes in this way is possible by virtue of the fact that both have a low incidence of adverse reactions and, if the diagnosis is correct, produce dramatic change for the better. The use of these antidotes for diagnostic purposes requires several caveats, however. The first and most important is that they compete with their agonist for receptor sites. In general, it is reasonable to assume that the more

TABLE 2-13 Osmolar Gap Calculations

EACH 1 mOsm CAUSED BY	=	SERUM LEVEL (mg/dL)
Acetone		5.5
Ethanol		4.6
Ethylene glycol		5.0
Isopropyl alcohol		5.9
Methanol		2.6

severe the poisoning, the greater the number of agonist molecules occupying receptors, and a correspondingly larger amount of antidote may have to be given to induce clinically detectable improvement. The second pertains only to naloxone, which has been claimed to reverse toxicity in patients poisoned with substances other than opioid analgesics. Any improvement is unlikely to be as dramatic as when opioid overdose is reversed, however. Another concern is that sudden reversal of sedation from opiates or benzodiazepines may precipitate agitation or seizures, either from acute withdrawal or by unmasking the toxic effects of coingestants. Reports suggest that these effects are uncommon, however, particularly if the use of these antidotes is judicious and limited to suspected isolated exposures to the target drug.[78,80]

Previously, it was suggested that administration of a single parenteral dose of deferoxamine could be used as a diagnostic test for acute iron overload.[81] In this context, the criterion of success was not clinical improvement but a change in the color of the urine over the ensuing period. The diagnosis depended on deferoxamine's binding circulating free iron (concentrations greater than the serum total iron binding capacity) to form ferrioxamine, which is excreted in the urine, turning it orange-red (*vin rosé*). False-negative results are so frequent that the diagnostic use of deferoxamine cannot be recommended. Freeman and Manoguerra[82] failed to find any change in urine color at any stage in the treatment of a sick child with a peak serum iron concentration of 19.89 mg/L (356 µmol/L), and Villalobos[83] found that of 12 patients with serum iron concentrations greater than 3.5 mg/L (>63 µmol/L), only 3 developed urine color change after being given desferrioxamine. Chyka and Butler[84] reported that only 8 of 26 children with serum iron concentrations greater than total iron-binding capacity and given desferrioxamine developed *vin rosé* urine and, conversely, that the urine color changed in some patients who should have had no free iron. The conclusion was that there was no correlation between the presence of *vin rosé* urine and iron levels greater than total iron-binding capacity, a view shared by Klein-Schwartz and colleagues.[85] Decreased urine output in the hours after administration of the antidote was a factor in delaying detection of the color change in some cases,[83] but failure of the *vin rosé* color to develop under circumstances when one would have expected it to do so was more important.

ELECTROCARDIOGRAM ABNORMALITIES

Although many toxins induce changes in the ECG, they are usually so nonspecific that they are of no diagnostic value. The most readily recognizable ECG abnormalities are those of TCA overdose, in which, after an initial sinus tachycardia, there is elevation of the terminal R wave in lead aVR, prolongation of the QT_c interval, and widening of the PR and QRS intervals to the extent that the P wave may seem to disappear into the preceding T wave. In the most severe cases, the QRS complex increasingly resembles a sine wave. Other common causes of QRS prolongation include diphenhydramine, quinidine, and quinine. Cardiac conduction abnormalities also may result from β-blockers, calcium channel blockers, increased cholinergic tone, or inhibition of the fast sodium channel. Alterations in T-wave morphology also may occur owing to toxins, particularly in chronic lithium toxicity, in which flattening and inversion are

---

TABLE 2-14 Electrocardiogram Changes Related to Drugs and Toxins

Bradycardia or Atrioventricular Block	Theophylline	Procainamide	Fosphenytoin
α-Agonists (reflex)	Thyroid hormone	Propoxyphene	Haloperidol
Barbiturates		Quinidine	Levofloxacin
β-Blockers	**Ventricular Tachycardia/ Fibrillation**	Quinine	Lithium
Calcium channel blockers	Amphetamines	Thioridazine	Maprotiline
Carbamate insecticides	Caffeine		Nicardipine
Cardiac glycosides	Cardiac glycosides	**QT_c Prolongation/Torsades de Pointes**	Olanzapine
Chloroquine	Chloral hydrate		Ondansetron
Cyclic antidepressants (severe)	Chlorinated hydrocarbon solvents	Amantadine	Organophosphate insecticides
	Chloroquine	Amiodarone	Pentamidine
Supraventricular Tachycardia	Cocaine	Arsenic	Pimozide
Alcohol withdrawal	Cyclic antidepressants	Astemizole	Procainamide
α-Antagonists (reflex)	Digitalis	β-Agonists	Prochlorperazine
Amphetamines	Diphenhydramine	Bupropion	Quetiapine
Anticholinergics	Quinidine	Carbamazepine	Quinidine
Antidepressants	Theophylline	Chloroquine	Risperidone
Antihistamines	Thioridazine	Chlorpromazine	Sertindole
Atypical neuroleptics		Cisapride	Sertraline
Caffeine	**QRS Prolongation**	Citalopram	Sotalol
Carbon monoxide	Amantadine	Clarithromycin	Tacrolimus
Cocaine	β-Blockers	Clozapine	Terfenadine
Neuroleptic malignant syndrome	Chloroquine	Cyclic antidepressants	Thallium
Phenothiazines	Cyclic antidepressants	Diphenhydramine	Thioridazine
Salicylates	Diphenhydramine	Droperidol	Trazodone
Sedative-hypnotic withdrawal	Disopyramide	Erythromycin	Venlafaxine
Serotonin syndrome	Flecainide	Escitalopram	Ziprasidone
Sympathomimetics	Maprotiline	Flecainide	
		Fluoxetine	

characteristic. Table 2-14 lists common ECG findings of drugs and toxins.[2,86–88] ECG findings are discussed in more detail in Chapter 21.

RADIOLOGY

Neither radiographs[89–91] nor ultrasound studies[92] are particularly helpful diagnostic investigations in clinical toxicology. They can be useful in confirming ingestion of metallic objects or packets of heroin or cocaine (body packing) and the subcutaneous injection of metallic mercury[93] or its embolization to the lungs.[94] Occasionally, when a hydrocarbon solvent has been ingested, it can be seen floating on top of the gastric contents when a radiograph of the patient in the erect posture is obtained.[95] Some drugs, such as formulations of iron salts and potassium supplements, are also radiopaque so that a radiograph of the abdomen taken 1 to 2 hours after may confirm ingestion (Fig. 2-5).[96] Most medicines are not radiopaque, however.

TOXICOLOGIC SCREENING

For most substances, precise knowledge of their nature or their concentrations in serum or plasma is of no relevance whatsoever to determining appropriate therapeutic intervention or influencing outcome. Toxicologic screening has long been a source of tension between clinicians and technicians providing hospital laboratory services. Laboratory staff argue, not unreasonably, that clinicians, especially the less experienced with their inherent wish to act "on the safe side," have unrealistic expectations of screening for poisons and tend to request it almost as a reflex action rather than with specific objectives in mind. Clinicians are mindful of the clinical, professional, and legal consequences of missing a toxicologic diagnosis for which there is a specific and, perhaps, lifesaving treatment. It is an inescapable fact, however, that even in the world's most developed countries, analytic toxicology laboratories are often not readily available. The overall result is a curious compromise in which laboratories provide limited screens from which clinicians seem

to draw unwarranted comfort—a phenomenon that testifies to their irrelevance.

In general, screening for toxins is justified only when the result is likely to influence treatment. In developed societies today, the prime example is acetaminophen. A low threshold for screening is undoubtedly justified by its common ingestion, the availability of an effective antidote, and the potentially serious consequences if administration of the antidote is not implemented expeditiously. It is generally advised to screen for acetaminophen in overdose patients because it is inexpensive and readily available. Screening for salicylates in the absence of a history of ingestion or an unexplained metabolic acidosis is no more justified than was screening for barbiturates decades ago. Emergency analysis of these drugs does not pose problems for laboratories, and they generally proceed directly to quantitative measurement. Lithium is another toxin whose serum concentration might alter management (i.e., dialysis), and its analysis, too, is generally available on an emergency basis. It is also relatively easy to obtain emergency quantitative assays of drugs whose concentrations require regular monitoring. The situation is more difficult, however, in respect to iron salts, methanol, and ethylene glycol, in which serum concentrations might determine treatment. These analyses are comparatively rarely requested, and laboratories have difficulties in ensuring that suitably experienced staff and validated methods are available at all times. Table 2-15 lists drugs for which quantitative analysis affects treatment and that should be readily available.[97]

A more difficult situation for screening is when a patient is ill and his or her condition is deteriorating without a clear cause having been established. It is then only a short time until the possibility of poisoning is raised. To be of value in this context, screening has to be focused and ought to be the outcome of thoughtful discussion between clinician and analyst. Appropriate body fluids have to be selected, and confounding factors, such as agents given therapeutically, need to be identified. Usually urine is the most appropriate fluid to screen for toxins. It is usually available in greater quantity than blood, and the concentrations of drugs in it are likely to be much higher than in blood. The closer the timing of the urine used to the onset of the illness, the better. Rapid screening tests are available for the drugs that are commonly abused, and they are easily detected or eliminated. It is customary to extract some of the urine into alkaline and acid media, analyzing each for acidic and basic drugs. Laboratory qualitative and quantitative drug testing is discussed in more detail in Chapter 4.

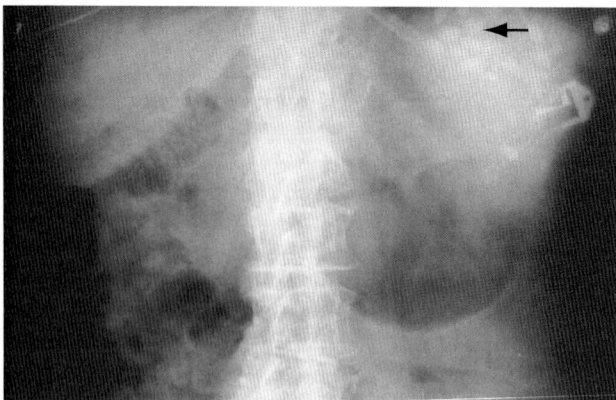

FIGURE 2-5

Radiopaque potassium chloride tablets in the stomach (*arrow*). *(Courtesy of J. Ward Donovan, MD.)*

TABLE 2-15 Recommended Emergency Quantitative Drug Assays

Acetaminophen (paracetamol)	Lithium
Acetone	Methanol
Carboxyhemoglobin	Methemoglobin
Digoxin	Phenobarbital
Ethylene glycol	Salicylate
Iron	Theophylline
Isopropanol	

REFERENCES

1. Badcock NR: Detection of poisoning by substances other than drugs: A neglected art. Ann Clin Biochem 37:146–157, 2000.
2. Olson KR, Pentel PR, Kelley MT: Physical assessment and differential diagnosis of the poisoned patient. Med Toxicol 2:52–81, 1987.
3. Helliwell M, Hampel G, Sinclair E, et al: Value of emergency toxicological investigations in differential diagnosis of poisoning. BMJ 2:819–821, 1979.
4. Mahoney JD, Gross PL, Stern TA, et al: Quantitative serum toxic screening in the management of suspected drug overdose. Ann Emerg Med 8:16–22, 1990.
5. Pohjola-Sintonen S, Kivisto KT, Vuori E, et al: Identification of drugs ingested in acute poisoning: Correlation of patient history with drug analysis. Therap Drug Monit 22:749–752, 2000.
6. Montague RE, Grace RF, Lewis JH, Shenfield GM: Urine drug screens in overdose patients do not contribute to immediate clinical management. Therap Drug Monit 23:47–50, 2001.
7. Safranek DJ, Eisenberg MS, Larsen MP: The epidemiology of cardiac arrest in young adults. Ann Emerg Med 21:1102–1106, 1992.
8. Goldfrank L, Weisman R, Flomenbaum N: Teaching the recognition of odors. Ann Emerg Med 11:684–686, 1982.
9. Holten C: Cutaneous phenomena in acute barbiturate poisoning. Acta Dermatovenereol 32:162–168, 1952.
10. Beveridge GW, Lawson AAH: Occurrence of bullous lesions in acute barbiturate intoxication. BMJ 1:835–837, 1965.
11. Leavell UW: Sweat gland necrosis in barbiturate poisoning. Arch Dermatol 100:218–221, 1969.
12. Groschel D, Gerstein AR, Rosenbaum JR: Skin lesions as a diagnostic aid in barbiturate poisoning. N Engl J Med 283:409–410, 1970.
13. Mandy S, Ackerman ABA: Characteristic traumatic skin lesions in drug-induced coma. JAMA 213:253–256, 1970.
14. Hoffbrand BI, Ridley CM: Bullous lesions in poisoning. BMJ 2:295, 1972.
15. Holden CEA: Cutaneous bullae in coma due to poisoning. Anaesthesia 32:554–555, 1977.
16. Varma AJ, Fisher BK, Sarin MK: Diazepam-induced coma with bullae and eccrine sweat gland necrosis. Arch Intern Med 137:1207–1210, 1977.
17. Herschthal D, Robinson MJ: Blisters of the skin in coma induced by amitriptyline and clorazepate dipotassium. Arch Dermatol 115:499, 1979.
18. Najy R, Greer KE, Harman LE Jr: Cutaneous manifestations of acute carbon monoxide poisoning. Cutis 24:381–383, 1979.
19. Godden DJ, McPhie JL: Bullous skin eruption associated with carbamazepine overdosage. Postgrad Med J 59:336–337, 1983.
20. Myers RAM, Snyder SK, Majerus TC: Cutaneous blisters and carbon monoxide poisoning. Ann Emerg Med 14:119–123, 1985.
21. Rocamora A, Matarredona J, Sendagorta E, Ledo A: Sweat gland necrosis in drug-induced coma. J Dermatol 13:49–53, 1986.
22. Moshkowitz M, Pines A, Finkelstein A, et al: Skin blisters as a manifestation of oxazepam toxicity. Clin Toxicol 28:383–386, 1990.
23. Taniguchi Y, Wada Y, Takahashi M, et al: Multiple bullae and paresis after drug-induced coma. Acta Derm Venereol 71:536–538, 1991.
24. Cotliar RW, Stringham R, Leavell UW: Dermographism, erythema and flare: Clinical signs of drug overdose in the comatose patient. South Med J 66:1277–1278, 1973.
25. Thoman M: Discolored urine. Vet Hum Toxicol 24:55, 1982.
26. Done AK: The toxic emergency: Signs, symptoms and sources. Emerg Med 42–77, 1982.
27. Erikson TB: Dealing with the unknown overdose. Emerg Med 8:74–89, 1996.
28. Zwiener RJ, Ginsburg CM: Organophosphate and carbamate poisoning in infants and children. Pediatrics 81:121–126, 1988.
29. Sofer S, Tal A, Shahak E: Carbamate and organophosphate poisoning in early childhood. Pediatr Emerg Care 5:222–225, 1989.
30. Carroll BJ: Barbiturate overdosage: Presentation with focal neurological signs. Med J Aust 1:1133–1135, 1969.
31. Sandyk R: Transient hemiparesis caused by phenytoin toxicity. S Afr Med J 64:493, 1983.
32. Sandyk R: Transient hemiparesis—a rare complication of phenytoin toxicity. Postgrad Med J 59:601–602, 1983.
33. Mayer JF, Schreiner GE, Westervelt FB: Acute glutethimide intoxication. Am J Med 33:70–81, 1962.
34. Brown DG, Hammill JF: Glutethimide poisoning: Unilateral pupillary abnormalities. N Engl J Med 285:806, 1971.
35. Linnanvuo-Laitinen M, Huttunen K: Ethylene glycol intoxication. J Toxicol Clin Toxicol 24:167–174, 1986.
36. Ong GL, Bruning HA: Dilated fixed pupils due to administration of high doses of dopamine hydrochloride. Crit Care Med 9:658–659, 1981.
37. Smilkstein MJ, Kulig KW, Rumack BH: Acute toxic blindness: Unrecognized quinine poisoning. Ann Emerg Med 16:98–101, 1987.
38. Mallampalli R, Pentel PR, Anderson DC: Nonreactive pupils due to monoamine oxidase inhibitor overdose. Crit Care Med 15:536–537, 1987.
39. Mercier C: Independent movements of the eye in coma. BMJ 1:292, 1877.
40. Mazzia VDB, Randt C: Amnesia and eye movements in first stage anesthesia. Arch Neurol 14:522–525, 1966.
41. Salgman M, Pippenger CE: Acute carbamazepine encephalopathy. JAMA 231:915, 1975.
42. May DC: Acute carbamazepine intoxication: Clinical spectrum and management. South Med J 77:24–26, 1984.
43. Manaplaz JS: Abducens nerve palsy in dilantin intoxication. J Pediatr 55:73–77, 1959.
44. Blair AAD, Hallpike JF, Lascelles PT, Wingate DL: Acute diphenylhydantoin and primidone poisoning treated by peritoneal dialysis. J Neurol Neurosurg Psychiatry 31:520–523, 1968.
45. Proudfoot AT: Diagnosis and Management of Acute Poisoning. Oxford, Blackwell Scientific, 1982.
46. Miadinich EK, Carlow TJ: Total gaze paresis in amitriptyline overdose. Neurology 27:695, 1977.
47. Ng K, Silbert PL, Edis RH: Complete external ophthalmoplegia and asterixis with carbamazepine toxicity. Aust N Z J Med 21:886–887, 1991.
48. Spector RH, Davidoff RA, Schwartzman RJ: Phenytoin-induced ophthalmoplegia. Neurology 26:1031–1034, 1976.
49. Teta D, Uldry P-A, Regli F: Ophtalmoplegie, syndrome cerebelleux et troubles de la vigilance reversibles apres intoxication a la phenytoine. Schweiz Med Wschr 120:1504–1507, 1990.
50. Barret LG, Vincent FM, Arsac PL, et al: Internuclear ophthalmoplegia in patients with toxic coma: Frequency, prognostic value, diagnostic significance. J Toxicol Clin Toxicol 20:373–379, 1983.
51. Hotson HR, Sachdev HS: Amitriptyline: Another cause of internuclear ophthalmoplegia with coma. Ann Neurol 12:62, 1982.
52. Pulst SM, Lombrosco CT: External ophthalmoplegia, alpha and spindle coma in imipramine overdose: Case report and review of the literature. Ann Neurol 14:587–590, 1983.
53. Cook FF, Davis G, Russo LS: Internuclear ophthalmoplegia caused by phenothiazine intoxication. Arch Neurol 38:465–466, 1981.
54. Grattan-Smith P, Butt W: Suppression of brainstem reflexes in barbiturate coma. Arch Dis Child 69:151–152, 1993.
55. Kalaawi MH, Auger LT, Carroll JE, Angelo-Khattar M: Encephalopathy and brain stem dysfunction in an infant with non-accidental carbamazepine intoxication. Clin Pediatr 30:385–386, 1991.
56. Orth DN, Almeido H, Walsh FB, Honda M: Ophthalmoplegia resulting from diphenylhydantoin and primidone intoxication. JAMA 201:225–227, 1967.
57. Smith MS: Amitriptyline ophthalmoplegia. Ann Intern Med 91:793, 1979.
58. Delaney P, Light R: Gaze paresis in amitriptyline overdose. Ann Neurol 9:513, 1981.
59. LeWitt PA: Transient ophthalmoparesis with doxepin overdosage. Ann Neurol 9:618, 1981.
60. White A: Overdose of tricyclic antidepressants associated with absent brain-stem reflexes. Can Med Assoc J 139:133–134, 1988.
61. Yang KL, Dantzker DR: Reversible brain death: A manifestation of amitriptyline overdose. Chest 99:1037–1038, 1991.
62. Mackie MA, Davidson J, Clark J: Quinine—acute self-poisoning and ocular toxicity. Scot Med J 42:8–9, 1997.
63. Nordt SP, Clark RF: Acute blindness after severe quinine poisoning. Am J Emerg Med 16:214–215, 1998.
64. Lee C, Robinson P, Chelladurai J: Reversible sensorineural hearing loss. Int J Pediatr Otorhinolaryngol 66:297–301, 2002.
65. Polpathapee S, Tuchinda P, Chiwapong S: Sensorineural hearing loss in a heroin addict. J Med Assoc Thailand 67:57–60, 1984.
66. Bateman DN, Rawlins MD, Simpson JM: Extrapyramidal reactions with metoclopramide. BMJ 291:930–932, 1985.
67. Pollera CF, Cognetti F, Nardi M, Mazza D: Sudden death after acute dystonic reaction to high-dose metoclopramide. Lancet 2:460–461, 1984.

68. Joubert J, Joubert PH, ven der Spuy M, van Graan E: Acute organophosphate poisoning presenting with choreo-athetosis. J Toxicol Clin Toxicol 22:187–191, 1984.

69. Moody SB, Terp DK: Dystonic reaction possibly induced by cholinesterase inhibitor insecticides. Drug Intell Clin Pharm 22:311–312, 1988.

70. Brisco JG, Curry SC, Gerkin RD, Ruiz RR: Pemoline-induced choreoathetosis and rhabdomyolysis. Med Toxicol 3:72–76, 1988.

71. Kirkham B, Gott J: Oculogyric crisis associated with metronidazole. BMJ 292:174, 1986.

72. Howrie DL, Rowley AH, Krenzelok EP: Benztropine-induced acute dystonic reaction. Ann Emerg Med 15:594–596, 1986.

73. Ward MJ, Routledge PA: Hypernatraemia and hyperchloraemic acidosis after bleach ingestion. HumToxicol 7:37–38, 1988.

74. Oh MS, Carrol HJ: The anion gap. N Engl J Med 297:814–817, 1977.

75. Ernst AA, Jones K, Bick TG, Sanchez J: Ethanol ingestion and related hypoglycemia in a pediatric emergency department population. Acad Emerg Med 3:46–49, 1996.

76. Yaramis A, Soker M, Bilici M: Amitraz poisoning in children. Hum Exp Toxicol 19:431–433, 2000.

77. Kulig K, Duffy JP, Linden CH, et al: Methanol, ethylene glycol, and isopropyl alcohol poisoning. Top Emerg Med 84:14–29, 1984.

78. Yealey DM, Paris PM, Kaplan RM, et al: The safety of prehospital naloxone administration by paramedics. Ann Emerg Med 19:902–905, 1990.

79. Winkler E, Almog S, Kriger D, et al: Use of flumazenil in the diagnosis and treatment of patients with coma of unknown etiology. Crit Care Med 21:538–542, 1993.

80. Weinbroum A, Rudick V, Sorkine P, et al: Use of flumazenil in the treatment of drug overdose: A double blind and open clinical study in 110 patients. Crit Care Med 24:199–206, 1996.

81. Henretig FM, Temple AR: Acute poisoning in children. Emerg Med Clin North Am 2:121–132, 1984.

82. Freeman DA, Manoguerra AS: Absence of urinary color change in a severely poisoned child treated with deferoxamine. Vet Hum Toxicol 23:351, 1981.

83. Villalobos D: Reliability of urine color change after deferoxamine challenge. Vet Hum Toxicol 34:330, 1992.

84. Chyka PA, Butler AY: Assessment of acute iron poisoning by laboratory and clinical observations. Am J Emerg Med 11:99–103, 1993.

85. Klein-Schwartz W, Oderda GM, Gorman RL, et al: Assessment of management guidelines: Acute iron ingestion. Clin Pediatr 29:316–321, 1990.

86. Rothenhausler HB, Hoberl C, Ehrentrout S, et al: Suicide attempt by pure citalopram overdose causing long-lasting severe sinus bradycardia, hypotension and syncopes. Pharmacopsychiatry 33:150–152, 2000.

87. Deponti F, Poluzzi E, Montanaro N: Organizing evidence on QT prolongation and occurrence of torsades de pointes with non-antiarrhythmic drugs: A call for consensus. Eur J Clin Pharmacol 57:185–209, 2001.

88. Goodnick PJ, Jerry J, Parra F: Psychotropic drugs and the ECG: Focus on the QTc interval. Exp Opin Pharmacother 3:479–498, 2002.

89. Jaeger RW, Decastro FJ, Barry RC, et al: Radiopacity of drugs and plants in vivo—limited usefulness. Vet Hum Toxicol 23(Suppl):2–4, 1981.

90. O'Brien RP, McGeehan PA, Helmeczi AW, Dula DJ: Detectability of drug tablets and capsules by plain radiography. Am J Emerg Med 4:302–312, 1986.

91. Savitt DL, Hawkins HH, Roberts JR: The radiopacity of ingested medications. Ann Emerg Med 16:331–339, 1987.

92. Amitai Y, Silver B, Leikin JB, Frischer H: Visualization of ingested medications in the stomach by ultrasound. Am J Emerg Med 10:18–23, 1992.

93. Zillmer EA, Lucci K-A, Barth JT, et al: Neurobehavioral sequelae of subcutaneous injection with metallic mercury. J Toxicol Clin Toxicol 24:91–110, 1986.

94. Rodrigues IMA, Hopkinson ND, Harris RI: Pulmonary embolism associated with self-administration of mercury. Hum Toxicol 5:287–289, 1986.

95. Mathieson FW, Williams G, MacSweeney JE: Survival after massive ingestion of carbon tetrachloride treated by intravenous infusion of acetylcysteine. Hum Toxicol 4:627–631, 1985.

96. Lacouture PG, Wason S, Temple AR, et al: Emergency assessment of severity in iron overdose by clinical and laboratory methods. J Pediatr 99:89–91, 1981.

97. American Academy of Clinical Toxicology: Facility assessment guidelines for regional toxicology treatment centers. J Toxicol Clin Toxicol 31:211–217, 1993.

CHAPTER 3

Therapeutic Approach to the Critically Poisoned Patient

Edward M. Bottei ■ Donna L. Seger

Certain therapeutic issues are unique to the poisoned patient in the intensive care unit (ICU). Although supportive care is the mainstay for all ICU patients, the usual therapeutic approach (i.e., airway management, ventilator management, choice of pressors, use of pulmonary artery catheters [PACs], sedation and paralysis) must be reassessed in the poisoned patient. Subsequent chapters describe therapeutic decisions unique to particular drugs and toxins.

GENERAL APPROACH TO PATIENT DATA FOR THE POISONED PATIENT

Organization of data may be problem based (e.g., phenytoin overdose or hydrocarbon aspiration) or system based (i.e., pulmonary, cardiovascular, renal, or hematologic). The system-based approach, typically used for critical care patients, better organizes large quantities of data (e.g., liver failure following acetaminophen ingestion causing coagulopathy, increased intracranial pressure, and hepatopulmonary syndrome). For the toxicology patient, however, substance-specific problems and therapies also should be noted. The system-based approach prevents important therapeutic and organizational issues from being overlooked (Table 3-1). The system-based approach clearly identifies the number of organ system failures, a criterion used to determine need for ICU admission and to predict ICU mortality.[1]

DURATION OF INTENSIVE CARE UNIT ADMISSION

The American Association of Poison Control Centers (AAPCC) Toxic Exposure Surveillance System (TESS) reported 61,510 exposure-related ICU admissions (2.8% of all toxicant exposures) in 1999.[2] Of these patients, 77% had clinical effects lasting less than 24 hours. Of poisoned patients arriving in the ICU, 75% were ready for transfer within 24 to 36 hours; however, 23% of patients had clinical effects lasting greater than 24 hours and presumably remained in the ICU for a longer period. Of all the patients admitted to ICUs, 15% had medical outcomes classified as "major effect." Major effect is defined by TESS as the patient's exhibiting signs or symptoms that were life-threatening or resulted in significant residual disability or disfigurement. Examples include repeated

seizures or status epilepticus, respiratory compromise requiring intubation, ventricular tachycardia, hypotension, cardiac or respiratory arrest, esophageal stricture, and disseminated intravascular coagulation. Major effect and duration of effect greater than 3 days occurred in 3.5% of the poisoned patients. West Virginia Poison Center data revealed that 4.6% of the 53,691 exposures reported over a 21-month period were admitted to ICUs. Forty-four patients (1.8% of ICU admissions) were older than 40 years old and had major clinical effects lasting longer than 3 days. Although many healthy, young, poisoned patients leave the ICU expeditiously, older critically poisoned patients may remain in the ICU for several days.

INITIAL ASSESSMENT

As with any unstable or critically ill patient, the ABCs (airway, breathing, circulation) of basic life support take priority. In the poisoned patient, therapeutic interventions and diagnostic evaluation often are initiated simultaneously (see Chapter 2). Findings on physical examination often guide the initial therapy. Airway patency and ventilatory drive frequently are compromised in patients with decreased mental status and may need immediate intervention. The decision to use the coma cocktail, which variably may include thiamine, glucose, naloxone, flumazenil, and possibly physostigmine, is made early in the diagnostic stage before ICU management. Although naloxone and flumazenil may obviate the need for intubation in some selected patients, flumazenil should not be administered to patients who may have long-term benzodiazepine use or to patients who have coingested a benzodiazepine and a drug that lowers the seizure threshold. Further discussions of benzodiazepine poisoning and flumazenil are found in Chapters 47 and 138. For further discussion about the controversial role of physostigmine, see Chapters 22 and 153. Diagnostic tests often need to be repeated to follow the ongoing effects of the toxin (acid-base status in ethylene glycol ingestion) or to determine effectiveness of treatment (electrocardiogram after each administration of $NaHCO_3$ or establishment of an induced respiratory alkalosis for wide QRS in tricyclic antidepressant [TCA] overdose). Toxicology laboratory screening often is performed, and proper interpretation of the results is essential to making appropriate therapeutic decisions. Chapter 2 on the diagnostic approach and Chapter 4 on

---

TABLE 3-1 System-Based Approach to the Poisoned Intensive Care Unit Patient

General
Vital signs: current HR, BP, RR, temperature
Avoid giving vital sign ranges (e.g., "systolic BP ranging from 50–180"),
    as this can be misleading and counterinformative
State vital signs that are "out of normal" (e.g., fever spikes, hypotension)
Intakes and outputs/weight

Cardiovascular
Cardiac enzymes and ECG
Pressors: dopamine, dobutamine, norepinephrine, glucagon
Pulmonary artery catheter data: CVP, PAP, PCWP, CO, SVR, SvO_2, stroke
    volume
Echocardiogram

Pulmonary
Ventilator settings
    Mode and rate, V_T (tidal volume), PEEP, FiO_2
    Pressure support, if added to SIMV or CPAP modes
Report the patient's actual RR, V_T, and V_E (minute volume)
Airway peak and plateau pressures, auto-PEEP
Arterial blood gases: pH, PCO_2, PO_2, SaO_2
Liberation parameters: NIF (MIP), rapid shallow breathing index
Chest x-ray findings

Gastrointestinal
Liver function tests, amylase and lipase
Bowel function/elimination

Renal
Electrolytes, BUN, creatinine, anion gap

Infectious Diseases
Maximum temperature (minimum temperature when low), antibiotics
    (day number), positive cultures, cultures outstanding
WBC and bands

Neurologic
Sedation and paralysis

Hematologic
Coagulation studies, platelet count, DIC information

Endocrine
Blood glucose, thyroid function

ICU Housekeeping
Stress ulcer and DVT prophylaxis
Nutritional support (tube feedings or TPN)
Central venous and arterial catheters
Daily chest x-ray when the patient is intubated or has a pulmonary artery
    catheter

Toxicology
Toxin or drug exposed to and route of exposure
Ongoing diagnostic testing (e.g., follow-up renal function, ECG)
Specific therapy or antidote

BP, blood pressure; BUN, blood urea nitrogen; CO, cardiac output; CPAP, continuous positive airway pressure; CVP, central venous pressure; DIC, disseminated intravascular coagulation; DVT, deep venous thrombosis; ECG, electrocardiogram; FiO_2, fraction of inspired oxygen; HR, heart rate; ICU, intensive care unit; MIP, maximum inspiratory pressure; NIF, negative inspiratory force; PAP, pulmonary artery pressure; PCO_2, partial pressure of carbon dioxide; PCWP, pulmonary capillary wedge pressure; PEEP, positive end-expiratory pressure; PO_2, partial pressure of oxygen; RR, respiratory rate; SaO_2, oxygen saturation in arterial blood; SIMV, synchronized intermittent mandatory ventilation; SvO_2, mixed venous oxygen saturation; SVR, systemic vascular resistance; TPN, total parenteral nutrition; WBC, white blood cell count.

---

toxicology laboratory testing thoroughly review the role of the toxicology laboratory and screens. Although gastrointestinal (GI) decontamination is initiated in the emergency department, the decision to continue GI decontamination in the ICU is usually toxin specific (see Chapters 5 and 6).

SUPPORTIVE CARE DECISIONS

Airway Maintenance

The loss of airway-protective reflexes or the presence of respiratory failure dictates the need to secure the airway. Securing the airway should be accomplished by tracheal intubation because noninvasive ventilation is contraindicated in patients with hemodynamic instability, patients with inability to protect the airway, and patients with a full stomach (including pregnancy and obesity).[3] Orotracheal intubation is preferred over nasotracheal intubation for many reasons. Nasotracheal intubation causes a statistically significant increase in sinusitis,[4–7] purulent and serous otitis,[8] ventilator-associated pneumonia,[9] and sepsis[10] compared with orotracheal intubation. Typically a 6.0- or 6.5-mm endotracheal tube is used for nasotracheal intubation. These narrow tubes have increased airflow resistance compared with the larger diameter tubes used for orotracheal intubation. Airflow resistance increases

after several days of intubation as secretions harden inside the tube and decrease the tube's diameter.[11] Increased airflow resistance can increase respiratory workload significantly. Should bronchoscopy be required (e.g., new infiltrates on chest x-ray or mucus plugging), the narrower, longer nasotracheal tube makes it more difficult, if not impossible, to pass a flexible bronchoscope.

Ingestion of caustic agents, with concomitant injury to the respiratory tract and oropharynx, requires special consideration in airway maintenance. Although airway obstruction is rare in patients who ingest caustic agents,[12] airway patency is more at risk with the ingestion of solid rather than liquid caustic agents.[13] Only 11 of 33 children (33%) with either acid or alkali ingestions required intubation.[14] Seven children required immediate intubation for respiratory distress or airway obstruction, and the other four had minimal or no respiratory symptoms but were intubated after endoscopic findings of supraglottic edema. Most intubations after caustic ingestion can be done under direct vision using standard direct laryngoscopic techniques. The equipment for alternative methods of securing the airway should be in place before any paralytic or induction agent is given, however, in case the normal visual landmarks are obscured and orotracheal intubation cannot be accomplished. In the 11 intubated pediatric patients described, no adverse consequences occurred as a result of the orotracheal intubations.[14]

Respiratory Function

Adequacy of respiratory function must be assessed immediately after the airway is secured. The causes of respiratory failure can be divided into four groups (Table 3-2), as follows:[15]

1. Hypoxemic (type I) respiratory failure arises from the flooding or collapse of alveoli, resulting in intrapulmonary shunting.
2. Hypercapnic (type II) respiratory failure is caused by inadequate alveolar ventilation from either decreased respiratory drive or an imbalance between respiratory load and respiratory muscle strength.
3. Postoperative (type III) respiratory failure is caused by pain leading to shallow breathing, atelectasis, hypoxemia, or narcotic administration (which decreases respiratory drive and worsens atelectasis).
4. Shock-related (type IV) respiratory failure is caused by a combination of inadequate oxygen delivery to respiratory muscles and increased total-body metabolic demands.

Type I respiratory failure in the overdose patient typically is caused by aspiration. Type II respiratory failure can be caused by ingestion of drugs that decrease respiratory drive (e.g., narcotic overdose) or cause respiratory muscle weakness (e.g., botulism). Type IV respiratory failure can be associated with any drug ingestion that causes myocardial depression or shock, such as calcium channel antagonists. Type III respiratory failure is not applicable to the overdose patient.

The therapeutic approach to each type of respiratory failure is determined by its pathophysiology. Type I respiratory failure is treated with a high fraction of inspired oxygen (FiO_2) and the judicious use of positive end-expiratory pressure (PEEP). Some focal lung lesions, such as lesions that may be seen in hydrocarbon aspiration, may not be PEEP responsive, however. In these situations, high levels of PEEP

(>10 cm H_2O) may worsen the patient's condition by decreasing venous return (preload) and causing hypotension. When type II (hypercapnic) respiratory failure is caused by decreased respiratory drive, minute volume (V_E) provided by the ventilator must be sufficient to maintain alveolar ventilation. Respiratory load and respiratory muscle strength are connected inseparably. Bronchoconstriction and increased secretions increase respiratory load. Impaired neuromuscular transmission or respiratory muscle problems (e.g., botulism, myopathy, or overuse fatigue) decrease respiratory muscle strength. If respiratory load increases or strength decreases to the point at which load is greater than strength, type II respiratory failure ensues. Treatment of increased respiratory load includes the use of bronchodilators and frequent suctioning. Muscle strength can be increased by treatment of underlying causes and ventilator support until respiratory muscle strength has returned. Therapy for type IV respiratory failure is to provide ventilatory assistance while treating the shock state.

The ventilator mode to be used is dictated by the type of respiratory failure. In general, patients with type I (hypoxemic) or type IV (shock) respiratory failure should be managed with an assist/control (A/C) or continuous mandatory ventilation (CMV) mode, which decreases the patient's work of breathing. Use of A/C or CMV decreases but does not eliminate respiratory muscle work and decreases the patient's oxygen requirements. This decrease in oxygen requirements is particularly important when oxygen transfer from the airways to the blood is impaired (aspiration) or there is inadequate oxygen delivery (shock). Type II (hypercapnic) respiratory failure typically is seen with drug-induced coma or paralysis and is managed with either a CMV or a synchronized intermittent mandatory ventilation (SIMV) mode.

Patient workload in a patient-triggered SIMV mode has been shown to range from 49% to 118% of the workload expected from a spontaneously breathing subject.[16,17] This

---

TABLE 3-2 Classification of Respiratory Failure

	TYPE I: ACUTE HYPOXEMIC RESPIRATORY FAILURE	TYPE II: HYPERCAPNIC	TYPE III: POSTOPERATIVE	TYPE IV: SHOCK
Pathophysiology	Alveolar flooding Alveolar collapse	Decreased respiratory drive Increased respiratory workload Decreased respiratory muscle strength	Atelectasis (pain) Decreased respiratory drive (narcotics)	Inadequate respiratory muscle perfusion with increased metabolic demands
Therapy	High FiO_2 PEEP Decrease lung water Treat pneumonia	Wake up/allow drugs to wear off Bronchodilators and suctioning Increase respiratory muscle endurance Correct metabolic problems	Pain control Chest physical therapy Elevate head of bed	Treat underlying cause of the shock state Ventilator support
Overdose scenarios	Hydrocarbon aspiration	Narcotic overdose Benzodiazepine overdose Bronchospasm Botulism	Not applicable	CCB overdose Sepsis

CCB, calcium channel blocker; FiO_2, fraction of inspired oxygen; PEEP, positive end-expiratory pressure.

is important because if the patient's type II (hypercapnic) respiratory failure is from muscular weakness, use of the SIMV mode can exacerbate the muscular weakness and prolong time on the ventilator.

If there is increased respiratory load from bronchoconstriction, care must be taken to avoid air trapping within the lung. Commonly called *auto-PEEP*, this dynamic hyperinflation of the lung occurs when a breath is delivered to the patient before the previous breath is completely exhaled. Adverse effects of auto-PEEP include hypotension and pulmonary barotrauma (pneumothorax). Auto-PEEP can be minimized by decreasing inspiratory time and maximizing expiratory time and use of small tidal volumes (V_T), slow respiratory rates, and increased flow rates.

When the patient has been intubated and initial ventilator settings chosen, further information may be obtained from arterial blood gas measurements, bedside observations, and patient-ventilator interactions. Arterial blood gases assess the patient's acid-base status, arterial oxygenation, and ventilation. Initiation of mechanical ventilation may cause rapid deterioration in some poisoned patients if appropriate V_E, $PaCO_2$, and pH are not maintained. Intoxicants such as salicylates, methanol, and ethylene glycol produce severe life-threatening acidosis for which the patient tries to compensate by creating a respiratory alkalosis. If the patient is well sedated or paralyzed, he or she may not be able to increase V_E to compensate for either respiratory or metabolic acidosis. When the amount of V_E set on the ventilator is less than the V_E the patient was maintaining before intubation, significant acid-base changes may occur and precipitate disastrous events. Loss of compensatory respiratory alkalosis in salicylate intoxication causes acidemia and further movement of salicylate into the central nervous system that may precipitate seizures and death. This is not a reason to forgo intubation; the physician must remember to adjust the ventilator settings to maintain appropriate ventilation. It is important to monitor arterial blood gases and make appropriate ventilator changes to keep pH, $PaCO_2$, and PaO_2 in the desired ranges.

Frequent physical examination is necessary to evaluate the patient's comfort and interactions with the ventilator. If the patient is not synchronizing well with the ventilator, the cause of the patient's discomfort should be determined. Ventilator settings must be adjusted to stabilize and comfort the patient rather than reflexively increase sedation or paralyze the patient. Much information can be obtained by observing the patient's pattern of breathing. Most ventilators display airway pressure versus time and flow versus time waveforms. Careful analysis of these waveforms yields important clues as to the cause of the patient's discomfort.[18] Waveform analysis is beyond the scope of this chapter and can be achieved best with the help of an experienced intensivist. Some maneuvers that can make the patient more comfortable on the ventilator include increasing V_E (by increasing V_T, respiratory rate, or both), decreasing triggering sensitivity or switching to flow triggering, and increasing flow rates.[17] Other maneuvers include treating pain, anxiety, and derangements of gas exchange or respiratory mechanics.[18] When these changes fail to match the ventilator to the patient, judicious use of sedation is required. Paralysis in poisoned patients usually is reserved for specific indications (see later).

Circulation and Hemodynamics

After establishing an airway and supporting respiratory function, the next priority is assessment of circulatory status. In the poisoned patient, cardiovascular abnormalities commonly seen are hypertension, hypotension, cardiac arrhythmias, or conduction disturbances.

HYPERTENSION

Elevated blood pressure in the poisoned patient may or may not be the result of exposure to any one of many substances (Table 3-3). Other causes of elevated blood pressure should be considered and include (1) withdrawal (i.e., benzodiazepine or ethanol withdrawal); (2) the discontinuation of a therapeutically prescribed medication, such as clonidine or minoxidil, causing rebound hypertension; and (3) inadequately treated or untreated essential hypertension.

Treatment of hypertension is determined by its underlying cause. When hypertension is caused by overdoses of drugs with direct adrenergic activity, such as amphetamines, ephedrine, or pseudoephedrine, direct vasodilators, such as phentolamine or nitroprusside,[19] may be required. When hypertension is caused by drugs with indirect adrenergic activity or by drug-of-abuse withdrawal, sedation with benzodiazepines[20,21] may be the treatment of choice. Pharmaceutical drug withdrawal can be treated by reinstitution of the causative agent or use of another agent that attenuates the signs and symptoms. The physiology and treatment of withdrawal states are described in detail in Chapter 30. Combining direct vasodilators, such as oral nifedipine or parenteral nitroprusside, and sedatives may be necessary in cases of severe hypertension resulting from any cause. For sympathomimetic-induced hypertension, such as seen with cocaine or amphetamines, administration of a β-adrenergic blocker alone may cause unopposed α-adrenergic stimulation and worsen hypertension.

HYPOTENSION AND SHOCK

Clinically, shock is defined as the constellation of hypotension, tachycardia, decreased mentation, and oliguria or anuria. A more physiologic definition of shock is inadequate oxygen delivery (QO_2) to the tissues.[22] Of patients who receive fluid resuscitation for shock, 85% have inadequate oxygen delivery to the tissues despite normalization of vital signs and urine output.[23] The goal of circulatory resuscitation is to return oxygen delivery to normal and not simply to "fix the vital signs."

The initial assessment of the poisoned patient in shock is to determine the physiologic cause of the inadequate QO_2. QO_2 is the product of arterial oxygen content (CaO_2) and cardiac output (Q_T):

$$QO_2 = CaO_2 \times Q_T$$

CaO_2 is determined primarily by hemoglobin concentration and saturation:

$$CaO_2 = (1.39 \text{ mL } O_2/\text{g hemoglobin} \times \text{g hemoglobin/dL} \times SaO_2) + (0.0031 \text{ mL/dL/mm Hg} \times PaO_2)$$

Cardiac output is the product of heart rate (HR) and stroke volume (SV):

$$Q_T = HR \text{ (beats/min)} \times SV \text{ (mL/beat)}$$

TABLE 3-3 Common Examples of Toxins Causing Hypertension

Direct Adrenergic Agonists
Albuterol
Epinephrine
Isoproterenol
Norepinephrine
Phenylephrine
Methoxamine
Midodrine
Ergotamines

Indirect Adrenergic Agonists
Monoamine oxidase inhibitors
Amphetamine and derivatives
LSD
Cocaine
PCP
Methylphenidate
Serotonin syndrome

Mixed Direct and Indirect Adrenergic Agonists
Ephedrine
Ergotamine derivatives
Pseudoephedrine
Phenylpropanolamine
Oxymetazoline
Tetrahydrazoline

Anticholinergic Agents
Tricyclic antidepressants
First-generation antihistamines
Atropine and derivatives

Other Agents
Nicotine
Scorpion venom

Drug-of-Abuse Withdrawal
Ethanol
Benzodiazepines

Pharmaceutical Drug Withdrawal
Clonidine
Minoxidil
Propranolol
Metoprolol
Methyldopa
Benzodiazepines

LSD, lysergic acid diethylamide; PCP, phenylcyclohexyl piperidine.

SV is determined by the left ventricular preload, contractility, and afterload. Physiologic causes of inadequate QO_2 in the poisoned patient may be the result of decreased hemoglobin concentration or saturation, decreased left ventricular preload (hypovolemia), decreased afterload (vasodilation), or impaired cardiac contractility.

Interruption of oxygen use at the molecular level is another cause of inadequate QO_2 in the poisoned patient. Specifically, abnormal hemoglobins (methemoglobin, sulfhemoglobin, or carboxyhemoglobin[24–26]) and toxins that disrupt the mitochondrial electron transport chain (cyanide, hydrogen sulfide, or sodium azide[27–29]) prevent the use of oxygen on the molecular level. Lactic acidosis is often a marker of these toxicities.

Ineffective oxygen use also may occur from the disruption of metabolic processes, such as the uncoupling of oxidative phosphorylation (salicylate and dinitrophenol ingestions).

Decreased hemoglobin concentration may be the result of GI bleeding (e.g., gastric erosions from iron or nonsteroidal antiinflammatory drug ingestion), intravascular hemolysis (arsine gas exposure), or various chronic medical conditions (renal failure or cancer). Hemoglobin concentration is measured easily, and when the evaluation of the cause of decreased hemoglobin is initiated, blood transfusion may be required. Causes and therapy of decreased hemoglobin saturation were addressed previously in the discussion of type I respiratory failure (see Table 3-2).

Hypovolemia in the poisoned patient may be caused by GI losses (organophosphates or cathartics), renal losses (lithium or diuretics), redistribution (caustic burns or snake bites), or increased insensible losses (fever from methamphetamine or its derivatives). Vasodilation from overdoses of angiotensin-converting enzyme inhibitors, nitrates, or hydralazine causes a relative hypovolemia. Signs of hypovolemia include dry mucous membranes, narrow pulse pressure, and low cardiac output. Certain vasodilated shock states, such as liver failure (acetaminophen overdose or *Amanita* mushroom poisoning) or thyroid storm (thyroxine overdose), present a clinical picture more consistent with sepsis: hypotension, warm extremities, a wide pulse pressure, and a high cardiac output.

CARDIAC DYSRHYTHMIAS AND CONDUCTION ABNORMALITIES

Cardiac depression, dysrhythmias, cardiac conduction abnormalities, or a combination of all three may cause shock from *impaired cardiac contractility*. Impaired cardiac contractility may be caused by β-blocker overdoses or cocaine-induced myocardial ischemia and is manifested by hypotension, narrow pulse pressure, low cardiac output, jugular venous distention, a gallop rhythm, and crackles in the lungs.

An electrocardiogram should be obtained to assess for dysrhythmias, cardiac conduction defects, heart rate, and wave intervals (PR, QRS, QT), which may give clues as to the poison, the severity of the poisoning, and the treatment. See Chapters 2 and 31 for a detailed review. The relationships between heart rate, QRS duration, and possible causes are listed in Table 3-4. Specific therapies are reviewed in Chapter 21 and in chapters dealing with individual toxins.

Torsades de pointes, a form of ventricular tachycardia associated with a long QT interval, also may impair cardiac output. Although other causes exist, torsades de pointes is most often drug related. Medications that can cause torsades de pointes, its pathophysiology, and treatment are reviewed in Chapter 21 (Table 3-5).

FLUID RESUSCITATION

Fluid resuscitation of the poisoned patient must be individualized. Many patients, especially patients found in coma many hours after their ingestion, may be volume depleted (e.g., GI losses, fever, insensible losses). Volume depletion usually is not the cause of shock, however, in poisoned patients who present with shock soon after their overdose. Shock may be caused by vasodilation, myocardial depression, chemically induced hemoglobinopathy, or a combination of these. The usual approach of administering fluids until clinical improvement (e.g., improved blood pressure,

TABLE 3-4 Toxin Association Between Heart Rate and QRS Duration

HEART RATE	NARROW QRS COMPLEX	WIDE QRS COMPLEX
Tachycardia	Cocaine Amphetamines α-Adrenergic agonists Theophylline Anticholinergic agents	Tricyclic antidepressants Antihistamines Thioridazine Propoxyphene Aberrant conduction Sodium channel blockers
Bradycardia	Cardiac glycosides β-Adrenergic blocking agents Calcium channel blockers Tetrodotoxin Ciguatoxin Class Ia antiarrhythmics α-Adrenergic lytic agents	Calcium channel blockers β-Adrenergic blockers Hyperkalemia

mentation) or development of a complication (pulmonary edema or worsening gas exchange) should be modified in the poisoned patient. Initial resuscitation measures should include the administration of intravenous crystalloid fluid, but when appropriate, vasopressor infusion should be started early in the course of the resuscitation. Vasopressors may be

TABLE 3-5 Toxic Causes of Torsades de Pointes

Antiarrhythmics
Amiodarone
Moricizine
Procainamide
Quinidine
Sotalol

Antipsychotics
Haloperidol
Chlorpromazine
Perphenazine
Thiothixene
Thioridazine
Trifluoperazine

Tricyclic Antidepressants
Amitriptyline
Amoxapine
Desipramine
Doxepin
Imipramine
Nortriptyline

Miscellaneous
Arsenic
Astemizole
Chloroquine
Cisapride
Diphenhydramine
Erythromycin
Indapamide
Syrup of ipecac
Organophosphates
Pentamidine
Prochlorperazine
Terfenadine
Thallium

more appropriate than continued fluid administration in patients poisoned with direct vasodilators or negative inotropes. Some patients require the placement of a central venous or PAC to determine cardiac filling status and to optimize fluid and vasopressor therapy.

The debate regarding the most effective resuscitation fluid to use for poisoned patients parallels the debate in critical care medicine in general.[30–33] Fluids that provide oncotic pressure (e.g., albumin, fresh frozen plasma, hetastarch) and stay in the intravascular space longer than crystalloids[34] theoretically are preferred for resuscitation. The infusion of packed red blood cells in patients with decreased hemoglobin concentrations increases plasma volume, CaO_2, and QO_2. Crystalloids are used more frequently in poisoned patients, however, because they are readily available, are much cheaper, do not carry the risk of disease transmission seen with blood products, and have not been shown to be less efficacious than oncotic agents.

VASOACTIVE AGENTS

The usual ICU approach to a patient with adequate fluid resuscitation and inadequate cardiac contractility is the administration of dobutamine or dopamine, the former being more desirable based on its β_1-adrenergic specificity. The vasodilator properties of dobutamine may worsen hypotension in a hypovolemic patient, however; this again stresses the need for optimal fluid resuscitation. If cardiac output is adequate, and the patient is still in shock, norepinephrine increases mean arterial pressure. The increased afterload produced by infusion of norepinephrine may decrease cardiac output, however. Theoretically, dopamine may not be the agent of choice for treating depressed cardiac contractility owing to its mixed α and β effects and indirect actions. Dopamine stimulates different adrenergic receptors at different infusion rates: dopaminergic at 1 to 3 μg/kg/min, β-adrenergic at 5 to 10 μg/kg/min, and α-adrenergic at 10 to 20 μg/kg/min. Further individual variability in response to dopamine infusions precludes the ability to predict which subset of adrenergic receptors would be stimulated at a given dose of dopamine in a specific individual. Because part of dopamine's pressor effect is through release of norepinephrine, dopamine has a decreased effect in norepinephrine-depleted states, such as cyclic antidepressant toxicity.[35] If stimulation of β-receptors is desired, dobutamine is theoretically advisable. Norepinephrine or phenylephrine may be used selectively to stimulate α-receptors. Despite these considerations, the agent of choice is the one that works best for the individual patient and may not be predicted based on the above-mentioned theoretical considerations. "Renal dose" dopamine is addressed in Chapter 18.

There are almost no data regarding the optimal adrenergic vasoactive agents in poisoned patients.[36] Case reports[37] and retrospective case series[38] imply that TCA-related hypotension may be more responsive to norepinephrine than dopamine. In a dog model, TCA-induced hypotension was equally responsive to dopamine and norepinephrine. Only high-dose dopamine infusions of 15 μg/kg/min or higher (α range) were as effective, however, as low doses of norepinephrine (0.25 μg/kg/min).[39] There is some evidence that norepinephrine may be the initial vasopressor of choice for TCA-induced hypotension. Because of its ready availability and familiarity of use, many toxicologists start with a trial of dopamine for TCA-induced hypotension. If there is not a rapid response, however, the patient should be treated with norepinephrine.

Because of lack of data, the choice of pressor must be made on clinical and theoretical grounds. Considerations for each toxin are reviewed in their respective chapters.

Nonadrenergic vasoactive drugs may be the most effective therapy for shock caused by β-adrenergic blockers and calcium channel blockers. Glucagon stimulates adenyl cyclase, which increases intracellular cyclic adenosine monophosphate (cAMP) through a nonadrenergic mechanism. This increased cAMP causes an increase in intracellular calcium, which leads to positive chronotropic and inotropic actions. Glucagon improves cardiac index, urine output, and symptoms in patients with chronic congestive heart failure.[40] Numerous case reports and laboratory investigations describe glucagon's effectiveness in reversing hypotension caused by overdoses of β-blockers and calcium channel blockers.[41–44] There are also reports of glucagon reversing TCA-induced hypotension.[45,46] In overdose patients, glucagon should be considered in hypotension unresponsive to the usual pressors. A glucagon dose of 10 mg administered intravenously over 10 minutes should be followed by a glucagon infusion (1 to 5 mg/hr). An infusion of 3 mg/hr is unlikely to cause emesis, a frequent side effect of glucagon administration. Amrinone, a phosphodiesterase type III inhibitor, prevents the breakdown of intracellular cAMP. Amrinone administration has been reported to reverse hypotension in overdoses of calcium channel antagonists,[47] chloroquine,[48] and propranolol.[49] It also has reversed hypotension in experimental calcium channel antagonist overdose in animals.[50,51] Because amrinone has direct peripheral vasodilatory properties, however, further worsening of hypotension may occur. Amrinone should be used cautiously with continuous bedside monitoring, if at all.

Insulin and glucose have been administered to treat calcium channel antagonist–induced hypotension that is refractory to adrenergic agonists and glucagon. In overdose, calcium channel antagonists decrease insulin release from pancreatic β cells, cause insulin resistance in the myocardium, and change myocyte metabolism from fatty acid to carbohydrate use.[52] In the laboratory, insulin infusions increase myocardial contractility, possibly through increases in intracellular calcium.[53] Compared with calcium chloride, epinephrine, and glucagon, insulin-glucose infusions decreased mortality in dogs poisoned with verapamil.[52–54] To prevent hypoglycemia, glucose infusions should accompany insulin infusions. Limited case reports support the efficacy of insulin for calcium channel antagonist poisoning. Insulin-glucose therapy improved hemodynamic parameters in five patients with calcium channel antagonist overdose who had been persistently hypotensive despite multiple therapies (calcium, atropine, glucagon, adrenergic agonists).[55] All five patients survived. The value of insulin-glucose therapy for calcium channel antagonist (or β-blocker) toxicity has not been prospectively validated. Based on current knowledge, insulin and glucose infusion should be used in shock caused by calcium channel antagonists and β-blockers that is unresponsive to fluid resuscitation, adrenergic agonists, and glucagon.

Overdose and Cardiac Arrest

Few data specifically address the issue of cardiac arrest as a direct consequence of poisonings. In 1999, the AAPCC reported only 873 deaths and 13,500 major effects out of 2,201,156 exposures.[2] This report did not specify how many of the 14,373 exposures classified with either "major effect" or "death" involved a prehospital or in-hospital cardiac arrest. Of the 78 death cases abstracted in the 1999 AAPCC annual report, cardiac arrest occurred in 15 patients in either the prehospital setting or soon after arrival at the emergency department. Only three of these patients were resuscitated initially. The only data regarding frequency and survivability of cardiac arrest after overdose are descriptive reports of prehospital cardiac arrest after overdose. Among 84 patients younger than 39 years old who experienced prehospital nontraumatic cardiac arrest,[56] 21 (25%) cases were due to overdose. Only 1 of the 21 patients survived to hospital discharge. Five of 353 (1.4%) nontraumatic, prehospital cardiac arrests were caused by overdose in patients younger than 17 years old. Only one patient survived to hospital discharge.[57] Of 252 (24%) cardiac arrests in the 18- to 35-year-old age group, 60 were caused by overdose, and 10 patients survived. Of 7749 (0.7%) nontraumatic cardiac arrests in patients older than 35 years, 52 were caused by overdose; 6 of the 52 patients survived. Most cardiac arrests due to drug poisoning occur in patients 18 to 35 years old, and mortality is high.

A significant proportion of cardiac arrests caused by poisoning are due to TCAs and have a poor prognosis. In a retrospective study, 7 of 22 overdose-related cardiac arrests were caused by TCAs.[58] None of these patients survived. The second most common cause of cardiac arrest was polydrug overdose (5 of 22). Another retrospective study revealed 12 of 83 nontraumatic cardiac arrests were caused by overdose.[59] Three of the 12 patients had ingested TCAs, and only 1 patient survived.

Autopsy findings revealed that 76% of older adults and 25% of young adults had atherosclerotic coronary artery disease as a cause of cardiac arrest. This finding should influence the medical management of drug-induced cardiac arrest. Advanced Cardiac Life Support (ACLS) algorithms[60] should be altered when cardiac arrest, ventricular tachycardia, or ventricular fibrillation is caused by drug overdose because the mechanisms for these arrests are significantly different from the cardiovascular events for which ACLS protocols were created. Specific therapies, such as sodium bicarbonate, glucagon, and insulin-glucose infusions, should be considered. A working group has been created specifically to address treatment of cardiac arrest and arrhythmias resulting from toxicologic causes.

Use of the Pulmonary Artery Catheter

When a patient remains in a persistent shock state despite optimal initial therapy, further information may be obtained from a PAC. Data obtained from a PAC includes central venous pressure, right ventricular pressure, pulmonary artery pressure, and left atrial pressure via the pulmonary capillary wedge pressure. Other data that can be obtained include oxygen saturation of mixed venous blood (SvO_2), thermodilution Q_T, systemic and pulmonary vascular resistance, QO_2, shunt fraction (Q_S/Q_T), and oxygen consumption (VO_2).

Some situations in which PACs are useful are listed in Table 3-6. Because most overdose patients leave the ICU in 1 to 2 days, they rarely require a PAC. The PAC may add useful data in some overdose situations, as follows: (1) assessment of left heart filling pressures when persistent pulmonary edema is present (hydrocarbon aspiration or adult respiratory distress syndrome) and (2) assessment of myocardial contractility (cardiac output and stroke volume) to determine the severity of myocardial depression and efficacy of therapy (i.e., calcium channel antagonist overdose). Also, older overdose patients with underlying medical conditions or patients developing sepsis during their ICU stay may benefit from PAC placement. With data gathered from placement of the PAC, it is possible to assess the effect of therapy on specific physiologic parameters. Volume replacement can be optimized with the aforementioned information. Although several case reports describe the use of a PAC in calcium channel antagonist overdose,[41,48,61–63] no studies address either the indications for placement or

whether information obtained from the pulmonary catheter changes outcome.

There are risks associated with the insertion of a PAC. Common complications are listed in Table 3-7.[64] Minor complications of PAC (incidence of 26% reported in one study) include multiple needle sticks attempting to locate the vessel, hematomas, and premature atrial contractions.[65] Major complications (4.4%) include ventricular tachycardia, wedge-shaped pulmonary infiltrates/pulmonary infarct, sepsis, and hemoptysis. Pulmonary artery rupture, the most feared complication, has been estimated to occur in about 0.2% of cases.[66]

A frequent "complication" of PAC use is misinterpretation of waveforms generated from the catheter. Of 282 attempts to obtain a pulmonary capillary wedge pressure waveform, 33% were complicated by technical problems.[67] Approximately 50% of physicians cannot interpret accurately the waveform tracings obtained from the PAC.[68,69] If the medical staff is unaware of the technical pitfalls associated with obtaining accurate PAC waveforms or incorrectly interprets the waveforms obtained, erroneous information may be used to determine treatment.

Sedation and Paralysis

When a patient is intubated and in the ICU, sedation and analgesia are important to minimize discomfort. Some patients have vivid recall of events that occurred in the ICU.[70] These events (discomfort, being in unfamiliar surroundings, invasive procedures performed by total strangers) can be terrifying because the patient's consciousness is clouded

---

TABLE 3-6 Clinical Uses of the Pulmonary Artery Catheter

Determine etiology of shock state and assess efficacy of therapy
Assess intravascular volume
  Renal failure, hypovolemia
Assess cardiac contractility
  Cardiac output, mixed venous saturation (i.e., efficacy of therapy in CCB overdose)
Diagnosis of constrictive pericarditis or pericardial effusion
  Waveform analysis
Measurement of pulmonary artery pressure
  Pulmonary hypertension
Determine PCWP in the setting of pulmonary edema
  High pressure (CHF) versus low pressure (ARDS) (i.e., hydrocarbon aspiration, toxic gas inhalation)

ARDS, adult respiratory distress syndrome; CCB, calcium channel blocker; CHF, congestive heart failure; PCWP, pulmonary capillary wedge pressure.

TABLE 3-7 Complications from Pulmonary Artery Catheterization

Placement Related
Arterial puncture or placement
Pneumothorax
Thoracic duct injury
Nerve injury
  Recurrent laryngeal nerve
  Brachial plexus
  Cranial nerves XI and XII
Arrhythmias
  Ventricular tachycardia
  Bundle branch block
  Asystole
Venous air embolism

Catheter Related
Pulmonary artery rupture
Cardiac perforation
Valvular hemorrhage or rupture
Infective endocarditis
Aseptic valvular vegetations
Catheter or insertion site infection
Knotting of catheter
Catheter or balloon embolization
Pulmonary infarction
Clot formation or embolization
Latex allergy
Heparin-induced thrombocytopenia

from illness and partial sedation. Worse yet is being paralyzed without adequate sedation or analgesia and being unable to communicate.[71] For overdose patients, the patient's underlying emotional instability may complicate management further (see Chapter 9).

Sedation typically is achieved via benzodiazepine administration (continuous infusion or intermittent around-the-clock dosing) or by continuous propofol infusion. Continuous infusion provides a constant serum drug concentration and decreases the chance of the patient awakening or becoming agitated.[72,73] Continuous sedative infusions, compared with intermittent dosing, prolong ventilator time and ICU time, however, as a result of overmedication.[74]

For patients requiring sedation, lorazepam and propofol are common choices. Continuous infusion midazolam, compared with continuous infusion propofol or lorazepam, lengthens time until the patient is awake and extubated after sedation has been stopped.[75–77] In critically ill patients, the midazolam half-life and volume of distribution are increased.[78] The half-life is prolonged further in renal failure.[79] Although midazolam is less expensive than propofol, costs of using these two agents are comparable because awakening times and stays in the ICU are less in propofol-treated patients.[75,80] Haloperidol also can be used as adjunctive therapy. Independent of which sedative agents are used, daily interruption of sedation to assess the patient's neurologic status shortens the duration of mechanical ventilation and ICU stay.[81]

In postoperative patients, the use of topical anesthetics to the pharyngeal, laryngeal, and tracheal mucosa statistically decreases the amount of sedation required.[82] As patients begin to regain consciousness and are uncomfortable from an endotracheal tube, the use of topical anesthetics may relieve discomfort without requiring consciousness-altering medications. This may be true of nonsurgical intubated patients as well. Topical anesthetics must be administered judiciously because overzealous administration may cause significant methemoglobinemia.

For poisoned patients, as for all ICU patients, analgesia is as important as sedation. Benzodiazepines and propofol have no analgesic properties. Narcotic analgesics, such as fentanyl and morphine, may decrease the pain and discomfort patients experience from intubation, having invasive devices in place, and inability to move. Combining narcotics with sedative-hypnotics decreases the amount of sedative-hypnotics required for comfort.[83] Simultaneous administration of opiates and propofol may cause hypotension, especially if large doses are used. Caution is warranted in patients who are poisoned by cardiovascular agents and prone to hypotension.

In the overdose patient, the issue of sedation is often less problematic because most patients have taken central nervous system depressants and usually require intubation for fewer than 24 hours. In these cases, if additional sedation is required, intermittent administration of benzodiazepines, combined with the use of topical anesthetics, may be the best choice. This combination avoids oversedation and allows for continuous assessment of the patient's mental status and clinical signs and symptoms indicating that the patient is ready to be liberated from the ventilator. Overdose patients with depressed mental status may not require

sedation. When the clinical effects of the overdose begin to resolve, either further sedation or ventilator liberation must be performed. Many patients, especially polydrug-overdose patients, have persistent delirium or a fluctuating level of alertness that may benefit from small amounts of sedation. In general, if the patient is sufficiently awake, can protect the airway, and is not a threat to himself or herself, rapid ventilator liberation and extubation is appropriate. For generally healthy overdose patients, extubation usually can be accomplished safely without a "wean."

Neuromuscular blocking agents (NMBAs) should be used in only two circumstances in the poisoned patient: (1) in patients who, despite adequate sedation, still have a high oxygen demand owing to the work of respiratory muscles and (2) in patients poisoned with chemicals such as strychnine. Normally, about 5% of oxygen consumed by the body (VO_2) is used by the respiratory muscles. In critically ill patients, this can be 25% or greater.[84] Although therapeutic paralysis decreases VO_2, it has been shown that administering an NMBA to patients who are adequately sedated does not decrease VO_2 further.[85] Critically ill patients who have received NMBAs may develop persistent muscular weakness after discontinuation of the NMBA,[86–88] even after short-term or intermittent NMBA administration.[89] The effect may last for weeks or months. The presence of renal dysfunction allows for the accumulation of active metabolites from some NMBAs (e.g., vecuronium). Addition of steroids (e.g., in patients with either upper airway obstruction or lower airway bronchospasm) increases the risk and severity of prolonged muscular weakness.[86] NMBAs should be administered only if the patient can benefit from decreasing VO_2 requirements. NMBAs should never be used to control an agitated patient without first evaluating the patient, attempting other therapeutic maneuvers (i.e., ventilator manipulation), and providing adequate sedation and pain relief. Paralysis should not be used as a punitive intervention or to absolve the physician from the need to sedate an active patient. A poisoned patient seldom requires the use of an NMBA, unless adult respiratory distress syndrome, sepsis, or an intoxicant such as strychnine is part of the clinical picture.

Ventilator Liberation

When the patient begins to show improvement, the issue of ventilator liberation arises. *Liberation* is a more desirable term, and a better mind set, than *weaning* for discontinuing ventilatory support. Weaning implies a gradual withdrawal of ventilator support, and most patients do not need to be "weaned" from the ventilator. Of 456 patients evaluated for participation in a trial designed to compare ventilator modes during liberation, 347 (76%) were liberated after an initial 2-hour, spontaneous-breathing T-piece trial.[90] These findings have been confirmed in other studies.[91] In most cases, "the most easily effected plan for discontinuation of mechanical ventilation is to wheel the machine out of the room."[92] This is particularly true of overdose or poisoned patients who, in general, tend to be younger and healthier than the general ICU population.

The conditions that led to the patient's being intubated and ventilated need to be resolved. In the case of overdoses, most respiratory failure is type II (hypercapnic) from decreased mental status and respiratory drive. When the patient regains his or her respiratory drive and the ability to protect the airway, ventilator liberation should proceed rapidly. If type I (hypoxemic) respiratory failure was involved, adequate oxygenation on 40% FiO_2 and PEEP of less than 5 cm H_2O should be present before liberation is attempted.[92] In type IV (shock) respiratory failure, the patient should be hemodynamically stable and metabolic abnormalities corrected. If type II (hypercapnic) respiratory failure from respiratory muscle weakness has complicated the clinical course, liberation may require the more thoughtful approach outlined subsequently.

Indices previously used to determine whether respiratory muscle strength was adequate for liberation have included a negative inspiratory force less than -20 cm H_2O, respiratory rate less than 35 breaths/min, V_T greater than 5 mL/kg, V_E less than 10 L, and forced vital capacity greater than 10 mL/kg.[93,94] All of these parameters are moderately sensitive but poorly specific.[95] Their utility in the overdose or poisoned patient population has not been evaluated.

The rapid-shallow breathing index (RSBI) was developed to assist in the bedside assessment of patients who are potentially ready for ventilator liberation.[96] The RSBI quantifies what we intuitively know about patients' breathing patterns: Patients who take deep breaths at a slow rate are ready for ventilator liberation, whereas patients panting rapidly are unlikely to be liberated. The RSBI is performed while the patient is spontaneously breathing for 1 minute without any ventilator assistance. The respiratory rate is divided by the spontaneous V_T in liters. Patients with an RSBI greater than 105 have a greater chance of failing ventilator liberation. The RSBI is highly sensitive (0.97) and moderately specific (0.64) in medical ICU patients.[96] Further studies have shown a sensitivity and specificity equal to the original study when the RSBI is performed after 30 minutes of spontaneous breathing.[97] The RSBI has been shown to be valid for surgical patients as well.[98] Analysis of patients failing liberation with RSBIs less than 100 found that most fail because of problems not related to the original pulmonary process, such as new-onset congestive heart failure, upper airway obstruction, and aspiration.[99] The utility of the RSBI in overdose or poisoned patients has not been studied.

Questions arise about which ventilator mode to use during ventilator liberation. As mentioned previously, use of the SIMV mode can increase the work of breathing. For the general ICU population, once-daily trials of spontaneous breathing lead to extubation three times faster than SIMV and two times faster than pressure support ventilation.[91] It is not known whether this applies to toxicology patients.

If there is concern that the patient may not be ready for ventilator liberation, a simple five-step procedure can be followed:[95]

1. Ensure that all underlying abnormalities that led to intubation have been corrected.
2. Assess the RSBI. If the RSBI is greater than 105, therapy to decrease respiratory workload and increase respiratory muscle strength should be employed.
3. For patients with an RSBI less than 105, perform a 2-hour spontaneous breathing trial (SBT). This is accomplished

by placing the patient on a T-piece or on continuous positive airway pressure with minimal or no pressure support.
4. Evaluate the patient during the SBT. Failure of an SBT can be manifested by diaphoresis, tachypnea, desaturation, tachycardia, hypotension, or arrhythmias.
5. If the patient tolerates a 2-hour SBT, he or she is ready to be liberated from the ventilator.

Ventilator liberation does not imply that extubation should be performed, just as inability to protect the airway does not imply respiratory failure. Other factors need to be considered, especially in cases of upper airway injury. Bedside assessment of airway adequacy may be determined by endotracheal tube "cuff-leak." The cuff-leak test can be performed in one of two ways. The first way is to disconnect the patient from the ventilator, deflate the endotracheal tube's cuff while it is still in place, occlude the end of the tube, and listen for air passing around the tube. The second way is to leave the endotracheal tube connected to the ventilator, deflate the cuff, and measure the difference between the V_T delivered by the ventilator and the V_T returned to the ventilator. Prospective evaluation of 72 patients with upper airway obstructions using the first method led to successful extubation in 89% of patients with a cuff-leak.[100] Using the second method, patients who did not develop stridor on extubation averaged 360 mL cuff-leak with average V_T of 650 mL. Patients who did develop stridor, given the same average V_T, had cuff-leaks of only 180 mL.[101] These data, along with direct visualization of the upper airway, can assist the clinician in deciding whether patients with upper airway obstruction (e.g., patients who have ingested caustics) are ready for extubation.

ANCILLARY ISSUES IN THE INTENSIVE CARE UNIT MANAGEMENT OF POISONED PATIENTS

Certain management issues need to be addressed in all patients who enter the ICU. Any patient who is critically ill, is intubated, or has a PAC in place needs to have a daily chest x-ray performed. New findings are discovered in 15% to 45% of daily chest x-rays[102–105]; 8% had findings of "major" clinical significance (e.g., pneumothorax, improperly positioned endotracheal tube), and 42% of these findings (3.3% of total) were not suspected previously from bedside assessment.[106]

Critically ill poisoned patients are at increased risk of GI bleeding. Of ICU patients, 75% have endoscopic evidence of gastric mucosal injury by 18 hours after admission. About 5% of patients develop overt bleeding.[107] GI bleeding prophylaxis should be started on admission to the ICU and can be achieved best through the use of histamine$_2$-receptor antagonists or proton-pump inhibitors.[108]

Poisoned ICU patients are at risk for venous thromboembolic disease if they have a prolonged course. Approximately 33% of all ICU patients develop ultrasonographically detectable deep venous thrombosis despite receiving prophylaxis. Meta-analyses have shown that the use of heparin or pneumatic compression stockings decreases the incidence of deep venous thromboses by at least 50%.[109] Deep venous thrombosis prophylaxis should be initiated with unfractionated heparin, low-molecular-weight heparin, or compression devices as soon as the patient is admitted to the ICU if a prolonged stay is anticipated.

The goal of nutritional support is to meet the patient's nutritional needs without overfeeding. This may be difficult because critically ill patients can be catabolic with a negative nitrogen balance. Exact caloric requirements can be determined through indirect calorimetry ("metabolic cart"). Overfeeding should be avoided because excess carbohydrates can lead to increased carbon dioxide production, which leads to higher minute ventilation needs. The increased ventilation needed to blow off the excess carbon dioxide may prevent liberation from the ventilator. Enteral feedings, which help maintain integrity of the gut's mucosal barrier, are preferred over the parenteral route. If a prolonged stay is anticipated, feedings optimally should be initiated within the first 24 hours after admission. If ventilator liberation is anticipated within the first day, however, as is typical of many poisoned patients, enteral feedings are not necessary.

DECONTAMINATION AND ENHANCED DRUG REMOVAL

GI decontamination with single-dose activated charcoal or gastric lavage is unlikely to be an issue when the patient has arrived in the ICU because this situation generally is addressed in the emergency department. Decontamination issues that might arise in the ICU are skin decontamination, multiple-dose activated charcoal, whole-bowel irrigation, and extracorporeal drug removal. Chapters 5, 6, and 7 provide in-depth discussion of these modalities.

ANTIDOTES

Overwhelmingly, most poisoned patients can be treated with standard supportive care, as detailed earlier. In certain instances, specific therapy or antidotes are required. The specific therapies are described in the chapters dealing with specific substances. The pharmacology of the antidotes is given in the chapters at the end of the book. Some antidotes that may be administered in the ICU are listed in Table 3-8.

SUBSPECIALTY CARE

In the United States, medical toxicology is now a recognized subspecialty by the American Board of Medical Specialties. There are currently 200 to 300 board-certified practicing medical toxicologists in the United States. These individuals have the greatest experience in the care of critically poisoned patients. When available, on-site consultation is recommended. In some areas of the United States, highly specialized regional poison treatment centers have been established to which critically poisoned patients may be transferred. When neither of these options is available, consultation with an AAPCC certified poison center is recommended.

TABLE 3-8 Common Toxins and Antidotes

TOXIN/POISON	ANTIDOTES
Acetaminophen	*N*-acetylcysteine
Anticholinergic agents (not TCAs)	Physostigmine
Benzodiazepines	Flumazenil (with caution)
Black widow	*Latrodectus* antivenin
Botulism	Botulin antitoxin
Calcium channel antagonists	Glucagon
	Insulin and glucose
Carbamate insecticides	Atropine
Carbon monoxide	Oxygen or HBO
Cyanide	Amyl and sodium nitrites
	Thiosulfate
	Hydroxycobalamin
Digoxin/digitoxin	Antidigoxin antibodies
Dystonic reactions	Diphenhydramine
	Benztropine
Ethylene glycol	Ethanol
	4-Methylpyrazole
	Thiamine and pyridoxine
Fluoride	Calcium salts
Heparin	Protamine
Heavy metals	Dimercaprol (BAL)
	Penicillamine
	Dimercaptosuccinic acid (DMSA)
	EDTA
	DMPS
Isoniazid/Hydra-Zide	Pyridoxine
Iron	Deferoxamine
Methanol	Ethanol
	4-Methylpyrazole
	Folate or folinic acid
Methemoglobinemia	Methylene blue
Methotrexate, trimethoprim, pyrimethamine	Folinic acid
Opiates	Naloxone/naltrexone
Oral hypoglycemics	Glucose infusion
	Octreotide
Organophosphate insecticides	Pralidoxime/obidoxime
	Atropine
Rattlesnake envenomation	*Crotalidae* antivenin
Sodium channel blockade (TCAs, type I antiarrhythmics)	Sodium bicarbonate
Warfarin	Vitamin K

DMPS, dimercaptopropane sulfonic acid; EDTA, ethylene diaminetetraacetic acid; HBO, hyperbaric oxygen; TCAs, tricyclic antidepressants.

REFERENCES

1. Zimmerman JE, Knaus WA, Wagner DP, et al: A comparison of risks and outcomes for patients with organ system failure: 1982–1990. Crit Care Med 24:1633–1641, 1996.
2. Litovitz TL, Klein-Schwartz W, White W, et al: 1999 annual report of the American Association of Poison Control Centers toxic exposure surveillance system. Am J Emerg Med 18:517–574, 2000.
3. O'Connor MF, Hall JB, Schmidt GA, Wood LDH: Acute hypoxemic respiratory failure. In Hall JB, Schmidt GA, Wood LDH (eds): Principles of Critical Care, 2nd ed. New York, McGraw-Hill, 1998.
4. Gabbott DA, Baskett PJF: Management of the airway and ventilation during resuscitation. Br J Anaesth 79:159–171, 1997.
5. Bach A, Boehrer H, Schmidt H, et al: Nosocomial sinusitis in ventilated patients, nasotracheal versus orotracheal intubation. Anaesthesia 47:335–339, 1992.

6. Michelson A, Schuster B, Kamp HD: Paranasal sinusitis associated with nasotracheal and orotracheal long-term intubation. Arch Otolaryngol Head Neck Surg 118:937–939, 1992.
7. Salord F, Gaussorgues P, Marti-Flich J, et al: Nosocomial maxillary sinusitis during mechanical ventilation: A prospective comparison of orotracheal versus the nasotracheal route for intubation. Intensive Care Med 16:390–393, 1990.
8. O'Connor MF, Keamy M, Hall JB: Airway management. In Hall JB, Schmidt GA, Wood LDH (eds): Principles of Critical Care, 2nd ed. New York, McGraw-Hill, 1998.
9. Holzapfel L, Chevret S, Madinier G, et al: Influence of long-term oro- or nasotracheal intubation on nosocomial maxillary sinusitis and pneumonia: Results of a prospective, randomized, clinical trial. Crit Care Med 21:1132–1138, 1993.
10. Aebert H, Hunefeld G, Regel G: Paranasal sinusitis and sepsis in ICU patients with nasotracheal intubation. Intensive Care Med 15:27–30, 1988.
11. Wright PE, Marini JJ, Bernard GR: In vitro versus in vivo comparison of endotracheal tube airflow resistance. Am Rev Respir Dis 140:10–16, 1989.
12. Friedman EM, Lovejoy FH: The emergency management of caustic ingestions. Emerg Med Clin North Am 2:77–86, 1984.
13. Howell JM: Alkaline ingestions. Ann Emerg Med 15:820–825, 1986.
14. Moulin D, Bertrand JM, Buts JP, et al: Upper airway lesions in children after accidental ingestion of caustic substances. J Pediatr 106:408–410, 1985.
15. Wood LDH, Schmidt GA, Hall JB: Principles of critical care of respiratory failure. In Murray JF, Nadel JA (eds): Textbook of Respiratory Medicine, 3rd ed. Philadelphia, WB Saunders, 2000.
16. Marini JJ, Rodriguez M, Lamb V: The inspiratory workload of patient-initiated mechanical ventilation. Am Rev Respir Dis 134:902–909, 1986.
17. Marini JJ, Capps JS, Culver BH: The inspiratory work of breathing during assisted mechanical ventilation. Chest 87:612–618, 1985.
18. Schmidt GA, Hall JB: Management of the ventilated patient. In Hall JB, Schmidt GA, Wood LDH (eds): Principles of Critical Care, 2nd ed. New York, McGraw-Hill, 1998.
19. Murphy C: Hypertensive emergencies. Emerg Med Clin North Am 13:973–1007, 1995.
20. Grossman E, Messerli FH: High blood pressure: A side effect of drugs, poisons, and food. Arch Intern Med 155:450–460, 1995.
21. Olmedo R, Hoffman RS: Withdrawal syndromes. Emerg Med Clin North Am 18:273–287, 2000.
22. Walley KR, Wood LDH: Shock. In Hall JB, Schmidt GA, Wood LDH (eds): Principles of Critical Care, 2nd ed. New York, McGraw-Hill, 1998.
23. Porter JM, Ivatury RR: In search of optimal end points of resuscitation in trauma patients: A review. J Trauma 44:908–914, 1998.
24. Griffin JP: Methaemoglobinaemia. Adverse Drug React Toxicol Rev 16:45–63, 1997.
25. Park CM, Nagel RL, et al: Sulfhemoglobin properties of partially sulfurated tetramers. J Biol Chem 261:8805–8810, 1986.
26. Hardy KR, Thom SR: Pathophysiology and treatment of carbon monoxide poisoning. J Toxicol Clin Toxicol 32:613–629, 1994.
27. Agency for Toxic Substances and Disease Registry: Cyanide toxicity. Am Fam Physician 48:107–114, 1993.
28. Smith RP, Gosselin RE: Hydrogen sulfide poisoning. J ICU Med 21:93–97, 1979.
29. Abrams J, El-Mallakh RS, Meyer R: Suicidal sodium azide ingestion. Ann Emerg Med 16:1378–1380, 1987.
30. Velanovich V: Crystalloid versus colloid fluid resuscitation: A meta-analysis of mortality. Surgery 105:65–71, 1989.
31. Schierhout G, Roberts I: Fluid resuscitation with colloid or crystalloid solutions in critically ill patients: A systematic review of randomized trials. BMJ 316:961–964, 1998.
32. Shoemaker WC, Monson DO: The effect of whole blood and plasma expanders on volume-flow relationships in critically ill patients. Surg Gynecol Obstet 137:453–457, 1973.
33. Cochrane Injuries Group Albumin Reviewers: Human albumin administration in critically ill patients: Systematic review of randomised controlled trials. BMJ 317:235–240, 1998.
34. Shoemaker WC: Comparison of the relative effectiveness of whole blood transfusions and various types of fluid therapy in resuscitation. Crit Care Med 4:71–78, 1976.
35. Murray P, Wylam ME: Dopamine, dobutamine, and dopexamine. In Leff AR (ed): Pulmonary and Critical Care Pharmacology and Therapeutics. New York, McGraw-Hill, 1996, p 242.
36. Hannemann L, Reinhart K, Grenzer O, et al: Comparison of dopamine to dobutamine and norepinephrine for oxygen delivery and uptake in septic shock. Crit Care Med 23:1962–1970, 1995.
37. Teba L, Schiebel F, Dedhia H, et al: Beneficial effect of norepinephrine in the treatment of circulatory shock caused by tricyclic antidepressant overdose. Am J Emerg Med 6:566–568, 1988.
38. Tran TP, Panacek EA, Rhee KJ, et al: Response to dopamine vs norepinephrine in tricyclic antidepressant-induced hypotension. Acad Emerg Med 4:864–868, 1997.
39. Vernon DD, Banner W, Garrett JS, et al: Efficacy of dopamine and norepinephrine for treatment of hemodynamic compromise in amitriptyline intoxication. Crit Care Med 19:544–549, 1991.
40. White CM: A review of potential cardiovascular uses of intravenous glucagon administration. J Clin Pharmacol 39:442–447, 1999.
41. Doyon S, Roberts JR: The use of glucagon in a case of calcium channel blocker overdose. Ann Emerg Med 22:1229–1233, 1993.
42. Walter FG, Frye G, Mullen JT, et al: Amelioration of nifedipine poisoning associated with glucagon therapy. Ann Emerg Med 22:1234–1237, 1993.
43. Stone CK, May WA, Carroll R: Treatment of verapamil overdose with glucagon in dogs. Ann Emerg Med 25:369–374, 1995.
44. Salzberg MR, Gallagher EJ: Propranolol overdose. Ann Emerg Med 9:26–27, 1980.
45. Sensky PR, Olczak SA: High-dose intravenous glucagon in severe tricyclic poisoning. Postgrad Med J 75:611–612, 1999.
46. Sener EK, Gabe S, Henry JA: Response to glucagon in imipramine overdose. J Toxicol Clin Toxicol 33:51–53, 1995.
47. Wolf LR, Spadafora MP: Use of amrinone and glucagon in a case of calcium channel blocker overdose. Ann Emerg Med 22:1225–1228, 1993.
48. Hantson P, Fonveau JL, DeConinck B, et al: Amrinone for refractory cardiogenic shock following chloroquine poisoning. Intensive Care Med 17:340–431, 1991.
49. Whitehurst VE, Vick JA, Alleva FR, et al: Reversal of propranolol blockade of adrenergic receptors and related toxicity with drugs that increase cyclic AMP. Proc Soc Exp Biol Med 221:382–385, 1999.
50. Koury SI, Stone CK, Thomas SH: Amrinone as an antidote in experimental verapamil overdose. Acad Emerg Med 3:762–767, 1996.
51. Tuncok Y, Apaydin S, Gidener S, et al: The effects of amrinone and glucagon on verapamil-induced myocardial depression in a rat isolated heart model. Gen Pharmacol 28:773–776, 1997.
52. Kilne JA, Leonova E, Raymond RM: Beneficial myocardial metabolic effects of insulin during verapamil toxicity in the anesthetized canine. Crit Care Med 23:1251–1263, 1995.
53. Kline JA, Tomaszewski CA, Schroeder JD, et al: Insulin is a superior antidote for cardiovascular toxicity induced by verapamil in the anesthetized canine. J Pharmacol Exp Ther 267:744–750, 1993.
54. Kline JA, Raymond RM, Leonova ED, et al: Insulin improves heart function and metabolism during non-ischemic cardiogenic shock in awake canines. Cardiovasc Res 34:289–298, 1997.
55. Yuan TH, Kerns WP, Tomaszewski CA, et al: Insulin-glucose as adjunctive therapy for severe calcium channel antagonist poisoning. J Toxicol Clin Toxicol 37:463–474, 1999.
56. Clinton JE, McGill J, Irwin G, et al: Cardiac arrest under age 40: Etiology and prognosis. Ann Emerg Med 13:1011–1015, 1984.
57. Safranek DJ, Eisenberg MS, Larsen MP: The epidemiology of cardiac arrest in young adults. Ann Emerg Med 21:1101–1106, 1992.
58. Ng AY, Clinton JE, Peterson G: Nontraumatic prehospital cardiac arrest ages 1 to 39 years. Am J Emerg Med 8:87–91, 1990.
59. Raymond JR, van den Berg EK, Knapp MJ: Nontraumatic prehospital sudden death in young adults. Arch Intern Med 148:303–308, 1988.
60. Richman PB, Nashed AH: The etiology of cardiac arrest in children and young adults: Special considerations for ED management. Am J Emerg Med 17:264–270, 1999.
61. Proano L, Chiang WK, Wang RY: Calcium channel blocker overdose. Am J Emerg Med 13:444–450, 1995.
62. Quezado Z, Lippmann M, Wertheimer J: Severe cardiac, respiratory and metabolic complications of massive verapamil overdose. Crit Care Med 19:436–438, 1991.
63. Brass BJ, Winchester-Penny S, Lipper BL: Massive verapamil overdose complicated by noncardiogenic pulmonary edema. Am J Emerg Med 14:459–461, 1996.

64. Coulter TD, Wiedemann HP: Complications of hemodynamic monitoring. Clin Chest Med 20:249–267, 1999.
65. Boyd KD, Thomas SJ, Gold J, et al: A prospective study of complications of pulmonary artery catheterizations in 500 consecutive patients. Chest 84:245–249, 1983.
66. Tarnow J: Swan-Ganz catheterization: Application, interpretation and complications. Thorac Cardiovasc Surg 30:130–136, 1982.
67. Morris AH, Chapman RH, Gardner RM: Frequency of wedge pressure errors in the ICU. Crit Care Med 13:705–708, 1985.
68. Gnaegi A, Feihl F, Perret C: Intensive care physicians' insufficient knowledge of right-heart catheterization at the bedside: Time to act? Crit Care Med 25:213–220, 1997.
69. Iberti TJ, Fischer EP, Leibowitz AB, et al: A multicenter study of physicians' knowledge of the pulmonary artery catheter. JAMA 264:2928–2932, 1990.
70. Schelling G, Stoll C, Haller M, et al: Health-related quality of life and posttraumatic stress disorder in survivors of the acute respiratory distress syndrome. Crit Care Med 26:651–659, 1998.
71. Jones JG: Perception and memory during general anesthesia. Br J Anaesth 73:31–37, 1994.
72. Shapiro BA, Warren J, Egol AB, et al: Practice parameters for intravenous analgesia and sedation for adult patients in the intensive care unit: An executive summary. Crit Care Med 23:1596–1600, 1995.
73. Young C, Knudsen N, Hilton A, et al: Sedation in the intensive care unit. Crit Care Med 28:854–866, 2000.
74. Kollef MH, Levy NT, Ahrens TS, et al: The use of continuous IV sedation is associated with prolongation of mechanical ventilation. Chest 114:541–548, 1998.
75. Barrientos-Vega R, Sanchez-Soria MM, Morales-Garcia C, et al: Prolonged sedation of critically ill patients with midazolam or propofol: Impact on weaning and costs. Crit Care Med 25:33–40, 1997.
76. Kress JP, O'Connor MF, Pohlman AS, et al: Sedation of critically ill patients during mechanical ventilation: A comparison of propofol and midazolam. Am J Respir Crit Care Med 153:1012–1018, 1996.
77. Pohlman AS, Simpson KP, Hall JB: Continuous intravenous infusions of lorazepam versus midazolam for sedation during mechanical ventilatory support: A prospective, randomized study. Crit Care Med 22:1241–1247, 1994.
78. Malacrida R, Fritz ME, Suter PM, et al: Pharmacokinetics of midazolam administration by continuous intravenous infusion to intensive care patients. Crit Care Med 20:1123–1126, 1992.
79. Fragen RJ: Pharmacokinetics and pharmacodynamics of midazolam given via continuous intravenous infusion in intensive care units. Clin Ther 19:405–419, 1997.
80. Carrasco G, Molina R, Costa J, et al: Propofol vs midazolam in short-, medium-, and long-term sedation of critically ill patients: A cost-benefit analysis. Chest 103:557–564, 1993.
81. Kress JP, Pohlman AS, O'Connor MF, et al: Daily interruption of sedative infusions in critically ill patients undergoing mechanical ventilation. N Engl J Med 342:1471–1477, 2000.
82. Mallick A, Smith SN, Bodenham AR: Local anaesthesia to the airway reduces sedation requirements in patients undergoing artificial ventilation. Br J Anaesth 77:731–734, 1966.
83. Wheeler AP: Sedation, analgesia, and paralysis in the intensive care unit. Chest 104:566–577, 1993.
84. Marik PE, Kaufman D: The effects of neuromuscular paralysis on systemic and splanchnic oxygen utilization in mechanically ventilated patients. Chest 109:1038–1042, 1996.
85. Pohlman A, O'Connor M, Olsen D, et al: Sedation with propofol lowers VO$_2$ in critically ill patients. Am J Respir Crit Care Med 151:A325, 1995.
86. Hansen-Flaschen J, Cowen J, Raps EC: Neuromuscular blockade in the intensive care unit: More than we bargained for. Am Rev Respir Dis 147:234–236, 1993.
87. Segredo V, Caldwell JE, Matthay MA, et al: Persistent paralysis in critically ill patients after long-term administration of vecuronium. N Engl J Med 327:524–528, 1992.
88. Shapiro BA, Warren J, Egol AB, et al: Practice parameters for sustained neuromuscular blockade in the adult critically ill patient: An executive summary. Crit Care Med 23:1601–1605, 1995.
89. Watling SM, Dasta JF: Prolonged paralysis in intensive care unit patients after the use of neuromuscular blocking agents: A review of the literature. Crit Care Med 22:884–893, 1994.
90. Brochard L, Rauss A, Benito S, et al: Comparison of three methods of gradual withdrawal from ventilatory support during weaning from mechanical ventilation. Am J Respir Crit Care Med 150:896–903, 1994.
91. Esteban A, Frutos F, Tobin MJ, et al: A comparison of four methods of weaning patients from mechanical ventilation. N Engl J Med 332:345–350, 1995.
92. Hall JB, Wood LDH: Liberation of the patient from mechanical ventilation. JAMA 257:1621–1628, 1987.
93. Millbern SM, Downs JB, Jumper LC, et al: Evaluation of criteria for discontinuing mechanical ventilatory support. Arch Surg 113:1441–1443, 1978.
94. Sahn SA, Lakshminarayan S: Bedside criteria for discontinuation of mechanical ventilation. Chest 63:1002–1005, 1973.
95. Manthous CA, Schmidt GA, Hall JB: Liberation from mechanical ventilation, a decade of progress. Chest 114:886–901, 1998.
96. Yang KL, Tobin MJ: A prospective study of indexes predicting the outcome of trials of weaning from mechanical ventilation. N Engl J Med 324:1445–1450, 1991.
97. Chatila W, Jacob B, Guaglionone D, et al: The unassisted respiratory rate-tidal volume ratio accurately predicts weaning outcome. Am J Med 101:61–67, 1996.
98. Jacob B, Chatila W, Manthous CA: The unassisted respiratory rate/tidal volume ratio accurately predicts weaning outcome in postoperative patients. Crit Care Med 25:253–257, 1997.
99. Esteban A, Alia I: Clinical management of weaning from mechanical ventilation. Intensive Care Med 24:999–1008, 1998.
100. Fisher MM, Raper RF: The "cuff-leak" test for extubation. Anaesthesia 47:10–12, 1992.
101. Miller RL, Cole RP: Association between reduced cuff leak volume and postextubation stridor. Chest 110:1035–1040, 1996.
102. Brainsky A, Fletcher RH, Glick HA, et al: Routine portable chest radiographs in the medical intensive care unit: Effects and costs. Crit Care Med 25:801–805, 1997.
103. Strain DS, Kinasewitz GT, Vereen LE, et al: Value of routine daily chest x-rays in the medical intensive care unit. Crit Care Med 13:534–536, 1985.
104. Greenbaum DM, Marschall KE: The value of routine daily chest x-rays in intubated patients in the medical intensive care unit. Crit Care Med 10:29–30, 1982.
105. Bekemeyer WB, Crapo RO, Calhoon S, et al: Efficacy of chest radiography in a respiratory intensive care unit: A prospective study. Chest 88:691–696, 1985.
106. Hall JB, White SR, Karrison T: Efficacy of daily routine chest radiographs in intubated, mechanically ventilated patients. Crit Care Med 19:689–693, 1991.
107. Liolios A, Oropello JM, Benjamin E: Gastrointestinal complications in the intensive care unit. Clin Chest Med 20:329–345, 1999.
108. Cook D, Guyatt G, Marshall J, et al: A comparison of sucralfate and ranitidine for the prevention of upper gastrointestinal bleeding in patients requiring mechanical ventilation. N Engl J Med 338:791–797, 1998.
109. Legere BM, Dweik RA, Arroliga AC: Venous thromboembolism in the intensive care unit. Clin Chest Med 20:367–384, 1999.

CHAPTER 4

The Role of the Toxicology Laboratory in the Management of the Acutely Poisoned Patient

Robert Wennig

Many new developments in analytic technologies have occurred over the years, such as the ability to detect and to quantify trace amounts of toxicants in body tissues, the determination of metabolic pathways, and the understanding of pharmacokinetic and toxicokinetic parameters. These advances have contributed to the growing number of toxicology laboratories. The most important tasks of modern analytic toxicology laboratories can be summarized as follows:

Identification and quantification of toxicants potentially responsible for the intoxication of an emergency department patient
Confirmation or exclusion of poisoning diagnoses in emergency cases
Grading and prognosis of an intoxication
Monitoring of elimination therapies
Testing for drugs-of-abuse
Exclusion of the presence of central depressants before organ explantation or discontinuation of life support
Checking the compliance of patients with prescribed drug therapy
Therapeutic drug monitoring (TDM)

Is there a need for toxicology screening? Many investigators[1-8] have tried to answer this question. A common conclusion is that toxicology screening results are not obtained rapidly enough to be useful. The term *toxicology screening* is misleading. It often has a different meaning to different people. A consultation between clinicians and analytic toxicologists is always recommended. In many cases the toxicology screening seems of limited utility, but in others it may be extremely useful if the health care professionals do not know the poison ingested (e.g., in intoxication of young children or comatose patients). In these situations, the detection and the exclusion of drugs or drugs of abuse are important and guide the physician in the treatment of patients. Not all poisons are easily detected, however. A toxicology screening includes or excludes only toxicants that can be detected by the analytic techniques that are used. The claim of Stewart[9] that clinicians can deal with poisoned patients without analytic toxicologic investigations is true only in certain circumstances. Schäfer and Maurer[10] do see a need for toxicology screening because of the current underdiagnosis of poisoning. In a case of intoxication by several toxicants, the treatment of the patients may be handled differently and more efficiently when all the poisons to which the patient has been exposed are known.

The analytic approach to a poisoning case may be divided into preanalytic, analytic, and postanalytic phases. These different phases and the pros and cons of the techniques used are discussed in this chapter.

ANALYTIC TOXICOLOGY

Preanalytic Phase

The preanalytic phase deals with the acquisition or sampling of the biologic specimens, the storage of the specimens before analysis, the transportation of the specimens to the analytic laboratory, and the request by the physician. Clinical personnel play an important role in the preanalytic phase and consequently in the outcome of the entire analytic process. Besides the specimens, it is recommended that the toxicology laboratory be provided with a summary of the most relevant clinical information available. This procedure makes the analytic toxicologic investigation more efficient.

Sampling is a crucial step for analytic toxicology, and the choice of biologic specimens is essential. Depending on the toxicologic investigations needed, the following choices exist:

Whole blood—most commonly for determination of carboxyhemoglobin, methemoglobin, and cholinesterase inhibition.
Serum/plasma—detection and quantification of most toxicants.
Urine—screening and identification of most toxicants.
Gastric content—identification of toxicants after oral ingestion in some special cases.
Alternative matrices—hair, saliva, and sweat are rarely useful for acute poisoning[11-13]; they might be useful for the determination of the patient's drug history.
Paraphernalia—poisons, containers, spoons, and syringes found at the scene of poisoning. Experts may identify mushrooms and plants easily. All these items may give important clues to the physician.

The minimal sampling for a toxicology screen at most laboratories is the following: serum, 5 mL; plasma, 5 mL; whole blood, 10 mL, if necessary; urine, 20 mL; and gastric content, 10 mL. According to the position statement of the American Academy of Clinical Toxicology and the

European Association of Poison Centers and Clinical Toxicologists (EAPCCT), gastric specimens are no longer frequently collected.[14] Gastric content may be useful, however, for identification of pesticides (because plasma concentrations may be too low) and mineral elements, such as arsenic and thallium. All specimens must be obtained in clean containers. Specimens should be shipped immediately to the toxicology laboratory with a precise description of the analyses needed and a short outline of the major clinical symptoms of the patient. If the samples need to be stored before analysis, this should be done at 0° to 4°C.

Because the exact nature of the toxicants is often unknown to the physician or health care personnel, the toxicology laboratory usually needs more specimen than the clinical chemistry laboratory. Splitting of specimens and sending them to different laboratories is not recommended. This practice reduces the volume of specimens available and diminishes the opportunity of any one laboratory to develop a coherent and complete elucidation of the intoxication case. Figure 4-1 shows a toxicology screening request form that facilitates the laboratory's role.

Analytic Phase

For routine toxicology screening and if information concerning the patient is not available, the following investigations are recommended:

Drugs frequently encountered in the geographic area where the intoxication took place; should be detected in serum and urine by immunoassays (IAs)

Alcohol and solvents in serum and urine by head-space gas chromatography coupled with mass spectrometry (HS-GC/MS)

Serum acetaminophen (paracetamol)

Paraquat by spot tests in urine (if this toxicant is prevalent in the geographic area)

Acidic, basic, and neutral toxicant extracts in serum, urine, and gastric content (if necessary) for "general unknown screening" by GC/MS

Quantification of the implicated toxicants by high-performance liquid chromatography (HPLC), GC/MS–selected ion monitoring (SIM) mode, or by any other suitable techniques, if possible and if needed

A comparison of the performances of analytic techniques is summarized in Table 4-1.

Precise quantitative results may not be required for clinical purposes in acute intoxication cases, but the indication of qualitative results may suggest to the physician that the patient is intoxicated when therapeutic or even subtherapeutic quantities of a substance have been "detected." Semiquantitative results may be considered a good compromise between rapidity, accuracy, and precision.

Tests for the most relevant drugs or poisons that may be requested in emergency situations and for which there are implications for treatment are listed in Table 4-2. All analytic toxicology laboratories should be able to detect and quantify at least these substances. In general, the analytic methodology can be divided into two different categories of methods: (1) nonseparation methods (spot tests, IAs), in which the different drugs or groups of drugs (benzodi-

azepines, opiates) are analyzed without a separation step of the compounds; and (2) separation methods (thin-layer chromatography [TLC], GC, HPLC, capillary electrophoresis [CE]), in which the different compounds are separated before identification by more or less specific color reactions (for TLC) or by MS, ultraviolet (UV), or any other suitable detectors in the instrumental methods. Other analytic techniques may be useful in some circumstances, as follows:

Dräger detection systems for gases in the expired air or in the air of a room

Spectrophotometry for carboxyhemoglobin, methemoglobinemia, and salicylates

Emission photometry and atomic absorption spectrometry for lithium and other metals

X-ray fluorescence for metals and some toxic anions if at relatively high amounts in gastric content

Specific electrode potentiometry for lithium and anions such as cyanide or fluoride

Several standard books[11,15–18] and more recent reviews[4,19] concerning analytic toxicology are available. A selection of analytic methods is available for detection and quantification of particular drugs or poisons frequently encountered (barbiturates, benzodiazepines,[20–22] heroin, cocaine, amphetamines, cannabinoids and designer drugs,[23–25] hallucinogens,[26,27] alcohol,[28] γ-hydroxybutyrate,[29,30] β-agonists,[31] plant poisons,[32] ethylene glycol,[33] pesticides,[11,17,34–36] quaternary ammonium compounds such as surfactants[37] or succinylcholine[38]).

Most toxicologic analyses start with specimen pretreatment, such as centrifugation, protein precipitation, acidic or enzymatic hydrolysis of conjugates,[39] and enzymatic digestion. Several extraction techniques are used currently, including liquid-liquid extractions,[40] back-extractions at different pHs,[41] Kieselgur clean-up or solid-phase extraction with C18 columns,[42,43] ion-exchange columns and preconcentration steps on special disks,[44] and solid-phase microextraction.[45,46]

NONSEPARATION METHODS

Immunoassays. In most laboratories, a "general unknown" screen starts with a batch of IAs. No special pretreatment of the specimens is necessary, and results are rapidly obtainable.

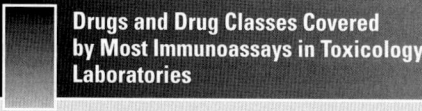
Drugs and Drug Classes Covered by Most Immunoassays in Toxicology Laboratories

Acetaminophen
Amphetamines
Barbiturates
Benzodiazepines
Cannabinoids
Cocaine
Methadone
Opiates
Phencyclidine (PCP)
d-Propoxyphene
Tricyclic antidepressants

TOXICOLOGY SCREENING REQUEST

Last Name and First Name of Patient (or self-adhesive label)	Physician Requesting	Analyze Number or Bar Code
	Telephone Extension	**Specimen Obtained** Serum/Blood Urine
Age / **Sex**		
State of Consciousness: AWAKE LETHARGIC BELLIGERENT DELIRIOUS		**Comatose Stage:** 1 2 3 4

Suspected Drug or Poison	What Drugs?	Current Drug Therapy	Chronic Drug User YES NO	Anamnesis

---

All SCREENING results are to be considered PRESUMPTIVE until confirmed by further testing at a slower turnaround time.

Check Tests Requested	For Laboratory Use Only Do not write below this line	Results	WARD CALLED date: hour:
SERUM* and URINE ☐ (Send 2 red top tubes of blood) and 20 mL random urine sample) **Qualitative Screening** ☐ If quantitation **ONLY** of a specific drug in this group is desired, please list under **OTHER** below SCREENING includes: cf local practice **Confirmed positives in serum/whole blood will be quantitated and a supplementary report issued** **ONLY** if urine is also received. URINE RECEIVED? YES ☐ NO ☐			
URINE (Send 2 mL random urine sample) **DOA Screening** ☐			
OTHER Type of Specimen Test Requested			

FIGURE 4-1

Sample toxicology screening request.
*For cyanides, carboxyhemoglobin, and methemoglobin, whole blood is needed.

TABLE 4-1 Comparison of Analytic Techniques for Screening Chromatographic and Immunologic Methods

	TLC	GC/MS	IAs (6–8 TESTS)	LC-DAD	LC-MS/MS
Test/8 hr/technician	60	15	30–300	15	15
Turnaround time for 1 test	0.5 hr	1 hr	2–20 min	1 hr	1 hr
Material costs/test	$3	$3	$6–20	$3–4	$5–10
Equipment costs	$1000	$100,000	$100,000	$80,000	$150,000
Equipment maintenance/yr	—	$10,000	$5000	$5000	$15,000
Objectivity	Depends on amount of drug present	Very good	Good	Good	Very good
Sensitivity	100–500 μg/L	2–10 μg/L	5–100 μg/L	10–20 μg/L	0.5–5 μg/L
Specificity	Poor	Very good	Cross reactions with other metabolites/ substances	Good	Very good

GC/MS, gas chromatography with mass spectrometry; IAs, immunoassays; LC-DAD, liquid chromatography with diode array detector; LC-MS, liquid chromatography with mass spectrometry; MS, mass spectrometry; TLC, thin-layer chromatography.

Many IA systems are available now and include kits for instrumental analyses and on-site testing kits (Table 4-3). These kits do not have comparable performances. Because automation and batch processing is possible, noncomprehensive screening tests can be done quickly. Technologists doing routine clinical chemistry testing can be easily trained to use these kits. Detection thresholds are relatively low and can be tailored to meet the requirements to enhance detection rates. IAs are relatively inexpensive (except if large panels are performed), and most IAs do not require a specialized laboratory. Several disadvantages are specific to IAs, however, as follows:

Adulteration of urine specimens is done easily by the addition of common household chemicals,[47] leading to false-negative results.

Most IA tests are useful for detecting classes of drugs. The specificity for individual drugs within a given class may be weak, however. The opiate tests do not identify the exact nature of the different opiates. The distinction between an overdose and a therapeutic codeine concentration is not possible in urine testing. In addition, these tests are not specific for heroin metabolites, and not all opioids cross-react in opiate IAs, such that buprenorphine, tilidine, d-propoxyphene, bezitramide, piritramide, dextromoramide, meperidine (pethidine), fentanyl, and pentazocine are not detected.

Amphetamine tests may give positive results owing to interference with ephedrine, norpseudoephedrine, or norephedrine. Many designer drugs, such as methylenedioxymethamphetamine, are not detected by IAs. Some metabolites from common legal drugs may give positive IA results.

Benzodiazepine tests generate many interpretation problems. An IA result in serum of 0.20 mg/L would be considered subtherapeutic if it is diazepam, but if it is flunitrazepam or lormetazepam, this may be a toxic concentration.

A low therapeutic result in serum on a theophylline test may correspond to a large overdose of caffeine.

A low therapeutic result in the serum for a barbiturate test may be a fatal concentration of cyclobarbital.

It is impossible to apply a detection threshold (cutoff) in the case of the unknown exact nature of analyte in serum or urine. Benzodiazepines, opiates, and amphetamines have different within-class cross-reactivities. This is a real dilemma because the exact chemical entity cannot be identified by IAs. IA test results should be "confirmed" by a second non-IA technique to identify the analytes responsible for the positive test result. It also must be

TABLE 4-2 Selection of Prominent Drugs and Classes of Drugs for Which Tests Should Be Available in All Toxicologic Laboratories in Emergency Cases

Acetaminophen
Amphetamines
Antidepressant drugs
Barbiturates
Benzodiazepines
Carbamazepine
Carboxyhemoglobin
Cocaine
Cyanide and thiocyanate
Digoxin
Ethanol
Ethanediol (ethylene glycol)
Isopropanol
Iron
Lithium
Methanol
Methemoglobin
Opioids
Paraquat
Phencyclidine
Phenytoin
Salicylates
Theophylline
Valproic acid

TABLE 4-3 Different Immunoassay Systems

Abusign Princeton Biomedical
Accupinch
Accusign
Autolyte Drug Screens STC-Diagnostics
Card Test
Cedia Microgenics
Clinical Assays (Incstar)
Dart
dBest
EMIT Syva/Dade-Behring
EZ-Screen
FPIA Abbott
Frontline/Boehringer-Roche Diagnostics
Insta Test
KIMS-On Line Roche
Milena DPC
Ontrak Roche/Testcup
Quickscreen Instant Diagnostics
Rapid Drug Screen
Rapitest-Morwell
RIA Abuscreen Roche
Roche Test-cup
Syva-Rapid Test
Toxiquick
Triage Biosite
Verdict
Visualine II Monotests

emphasized that the original cutoff concept was intended only for urine testing of the so-called NIDA-5 substances (amphetamines, cannabinoids, cocaine, opiates, and phencyclidine [PCP]), for drugs-of-abuse testing to avoid false-positive results. The cutoff concept was *not* intended for drugs such as benzodiazepines or tricyclic antidepressants encountered in cases of acute intoxication. The word *confirmation* was not well chosen; *identification* would be better.

Because antibodies are generated from laboratory animals, there can be lot-to-lot or batch-to-batch variation in the antibody reagents.

Only one single drug with its metabolites can be tested at one time. This leads to high costs compared with chromatographic methods if a large panel is performed.

No real quantitative results can be expected without a prior analytic separation step because cross-reacting drug metabolites always occur.

Negative results often are not confirmed. There may be some false-negative results due to low cross-reactivities.

Nonsteroidal antiinflammatory drugs and ritodrine have been known to interfere with cannabinoid tests. Nonsteroidal antiinflammatory drugs also use methylation reagents in GC/MS and avoid confirmation of cannabinoids. The antiemetic nabilone does not cross-react in the IA test, but dronabinol (Δ^9-tetrahydrocannabinol [THC]) does.

To improve limit of detection (LOD) or limit of quantification (LOQ), radioimmunoassay may be an alternative to the "cold" IAs. Radioimmunoassay requires compliance with special licensing procedures, however (e.g., use of gamma counters to measure radioactivity and disposal of the radioactive waste).

SEPARATION METHODS

Thin-Layer Chromatography. TLC[17] is an easy, noninstrumental technique, but interpretation of the test results is subjective; training and a long professional experience of the technologist are crucial. The technique is inexpensive, and results are obtained quickly. TLC is an older technique being replaced today by HPLC and GC. It is simple to perform, but identification and resolving power are too weak for most toxicants. LOD and LOQ tests are difficult to establish and usually not adequate.

Gas Chromatography and High-Pressure Liquid Chromatography. For GC and HPLC,[48] equipment costs are high, depending on the type of detector and automation selected. These are the techniques of choice, however, for quantification. HPLC combines separation of the compounds by selective separation of substances between a stationary and a liquid phase and, at the end of the column, an identification and quantification. Compared with GC, HPLC has the advantages that relatively large amounts of extracts can be deposited on the column and no derivatization step is needed. Even small amounts of toxicants can be detected and quantified. The major drawback of HPLC is the relatively weak identification power by UV detection. Many compounds (especially drugs belonging to the same class, benzodiazepines and amphetamines) have similar UV spectra.

Mass Spectrometry. For GC/MS, liquid chromatography (LC) coupled with MS (LC/MS), and LC coupled with tandem MS (MS/MS),[48–54] equipment costs may be the highest, depending on the degree of sophistication required. Because of the complexity of the instruments, highly trained technologists are necessary to run them. The results of these techniques are the most reliable, however. MS has an unmatched identification power for many organic substances, including most drugs and substances of abuse. MS coupled with separative techniques such as GC or LC is the most important identification and quantification technique, giving reliable results in a reasonable amount of time. LC/MS and LC/MS/MS are relatively new techniques that combine the advantages of HPLC (injection of relatively large quantities of extracts and no derivatization needed) and the advantages of MS (unambiguous identification). These techniques have been applied in many toxicology laboratories.

Capillary Electrophoresis. CE[48,55,56] has been introduced more recently to the toxicology laboratory. This technique has the advantage of being fast, and only minute amounts of extracts are needed for analysis. Because detection also is made mostly by UV-photometry, it has the same disadvantages as HPLC. Many parameters have to be controlled when performing CE, and reproducibility still is a major problem. Toxicology screening by CE has become more widely used but has not yet been generally accepted, such that GC and LC (both coupled with MS) remain the most important separation and identification techniques in analytic toxicology.

Gas Chromatography–Mass Spectrometry. GC/MS is the most popular analytic technique routinely used for the detection of many toxicants owing to its good separation capacity and identification power. This technique is also of great value for the quantification of toxicants by using full-scan or by using the SIM mode for drugs at a low concentration range. For GC/MS, as for most separation methods, it is necessary to extract the drugs or toxicants from the biologic matrices. In many cases, a chemical derivatization to obtain sufficiently volatile analytes also is necessary.

The common derivatization reactions have been reviewed.[57] The most popular are acetylation by acetic anhydride/pyridine; methylation by diazomethane; trimethylsilylation by *N*-methyl-*N*-trimethylsilyl-trifluoroacetamide *N,O-bis*-trimethylsilyl-trifluoroacetamide or trimethylchlorosilane; and multifluorination by pentafluoropropionic anhydride/pentafluoropropanol and heptafluorobutyric anhydride. For derivatization of chiral compounds, the reagent S-trifluoroacetylprolyl chloride[58] may be used to separate R and S enantiomers without changing the GC column. After derivatization and evaporation of the derivatization reagent, the residue is taken up in a solvent and injected into the GC/MS instrument.

GC/MS screening allows a large panel of toxicants to be detected. Caution is necessary, however, because not all drugs or poisons are detected in a single run. Different derivatization methods may be necessary. The most important drug families detected by comprehensive GC/MS screening after derivatization with acetic anhydride/pyridine are listed in Table 4-4.

Some substances or drug families are detected by GC/MS only after special treatment. To be detected, the nature of the suspected compounds has to be known to the toxicology laboratory (Table 4-5). Finally, comprehensive GC/MS screening does not detect all substances. Substances not detected as such by GC/MS are listed in Table 4-6.

A major drawback to the new sophisticated technologies such as GC/MS is that they are labor intensive, and highly trained staff is needed for their operation. This makes it

TABLE 4-4 Most Important Drug Families Detected by Gas Chromatography with Mass Spectrometry after Derivatization with Acetic Anhydride/Pyridine

Alkaloids (most)
Analgesics
Antihistaminics
Antiarrhythmics
Anticonvulsants
Antidepressants
Antiparkinsonians
Benzodiazepines
β-Blockers
Butyrophenones
Calcium antagonists
Designer drugs
Local anesthetics
Opioids
Phenothiazines
Stimulants (xanthines, cocaine)
Tranquilizers

TABLE 4-5 Substances Detected by Gas Chromatography with Mass Spectrometry only after Special Treatment and if the Nature of the Compounds Is Known

Angiotensin-converting enzyme inhibitors
Anticoagulants
Chloral hydrate
Chloralose
Diuretics
LSD
Pesticides
Solvents (including ethylene glycol)
Sulfonamides
THC-COOH
Valproate

LSD, lysergic acid diethylamide; TCH-COOH, cannabis THC metabolite.

TABLE 4-6 Substances Not Detected as Such by Gas Chromatography with Mass Spectrometry

α-Amanitin
Antibiotics
Polypeptides (insulin)
Cytostatic drugs
Anthraquinone laxatives
Gases (CO, HCN)
Digoxin
Mineral substances (lithium, arsenic, titanium)
Oral antidiabetics

CO, carbon monoxide; HCN, hydrogen cyanide.

difficult to maintain a full toxicology service with professional competence operational 24 hours a day. Although these techniques are rather specific, confirmation still may be desirable on some occasions by means of a second independent method (especially HPLC or LC/MS). Even a combination of powerful techniques does not guarantee a failure-free screening, and missing toxicants is always possible. Toxicants may be missed owing to thermal instability of analytes, low concentrations, unsuitable libraries used for spectral identification, and low cross-reactivities in IAs not included in the confirmation identification procedures. Measurements always are a compromise between rapidity and precision. To obtain expeditious results, precision may have to be sacrificed.

Postanalytic Phase

INTERPRETATION OF ANALYTIC FINDINGS

Today, spectral databases ("libraries") have become standard equipment in toxicology laboratories. Interpretation of the qualitative analytic findings is facilitated greatly but is still not easy. Not all toxicants are included in these databases.

IAs are useful for drugs-of-abuse testing because they avoid useless identification or confirmation of other drugs.

There may be problems, however, in the diagnosis of acute intoxication cases. In general, at most semiquantitative results can be expected. These results may be acceptable in the acute situation. The following statements summarize some of the major disadvantages: Not all opioids cross-react, such that some of these compounds may be missed. Certain barbiturates and benzodiazepines react poorly with the antibodies and may suggest a therapeutic concentration when toxic amounts are present. High concentrations of carbamazepine, phenothiazines, or prothipendyl may be identified mistakenly as low therapeutic concentrations of tricyclic antidepressants.

INTERPRETATION OF TOXICOLOGIC TEST RESULTS

A second step in interpretation is one of the most difficult tasks in analytic toxicology: the interpretation of quantitative test results, which usually can be done only on plasma or serum or occasionally whole blood. Therapeutic and toxic plasma concentrations found in the literature should be used with caution because they often were generated under noncomparable conditions. Several useful publications are available[59-62] in the literature and on the Internet (e.g., D.R.A. Uges on the TIAFT-net: http://www.tiaft.org). Examples illustrating the wide range of concentrations encountered in toxicology are provided in Table 4-7.

It is not always possible to relate symptoms and blood concentrations of drugs or poisons. In many cases, it is better to monitor biochemical parameters instead of drug concentrations in the management of poisoned patients. The best tests to follow in organophosphate poisoning are cholinesterase levels. Common specific problems that may occur in the interpretation of certain drug assays include the following:

In cases of positive urinary amphetamine detection, drugs that have methamphetamine or amphetamine as major metabolites also must be considered. Methamphetamine can be formed by biotransformation from benzphetamine, furfenorex, dimethylamphetamine, selegiline,[58] and famprofazone. Amphetamine may be a metabolite of fenetylline, ethylamphetamine, clobenzorex, mefenorex, fenproporex, prenylamine, amphetaminil, or fencamine. The suspected designer drug methoxyethylamphetamine also may simply be a metabolite of the antispasmodic mebeverine.[63,64]

Benzodiazepines create a confusing situation because several drugs in this class have common metabolites. Some benzodiazepine metabolites also may be used as therapeutic drugs. Nordazepam is available as the drug nordiazepam but also is a metabolite from chlordiazepoxide, demoxepam, diazepam, halazepam, ketazolam, medazepam, oxazolam, pinazepam, and prazepam and is an artifact from potassium clorazepate. It sometimes may be difficult to identify the drug that was administered.

Automobile drivers use not only alcohol but also drugs that may lead to accidents, hospital admissions, and forensic cases.[19,65-69] Although cannabis generally may not play an important role in acute intoxications, a positive THC-COOH test result may occur in urine from a legally cultivated hemp product's consumption.[70]

Distinguishing between active and inactive metabolites, such as opiate glucuronides, sometimes may be important in the interpretation of the analytic results.[71] Cytochrome P-450 isoenzyme polymorphism leads to alterations in drug metabolism.[72,73] This polymorphism is due to genetic differences among individuals or among different ethnic populations (Table 4-8).

DOCUMENTATION AND COMMUNICATION OF TOXICOLOGY LABORATORY RESULTS

As soon as results become available to the laboratory, they should be communicated (by phone, fax, or e-mail) to the physician. It also should be discussed whether other quantitative or qualitative assays are necessary. A written report

TABLE 4-7 Therapeutic and Toxic Ranges of Some Drugs

	THERAPEUTIC RANGE	TOXIC RANGE*
Amitriptyline	50–200 ng/mL 180–720 nmol/L	>1000 ng/mL >3610 nmol/L
Butalbital	1–10 mg/L 4.46–44.6 μmol/L	7–15 mg/L 31.2–62.4 μmol/L
Diazepam	100–800 ng/mL 0.35–2.8 μmol/L	>10,000 ng/mL >35.1 μmol/L
Digitoxin	<20 μg/L <26.2 nmol/L	>30 μg/L >39.2 nmol/L
Digoxin	<2 μg/L <2.56 nmol/L	>4 μg/L >5.12 nmol/L
Ethanol	<0.1 g/L <2170 μmol/L	>0.3 g/L >6510 μmol/L
Lead	<30 μg/dL <1.45 μmol/L	>50 μg/dL >2.42 μmol/L
Meprobamate	<10 mg/L <45.8 μmol/L	>50 mg/L >229 μmol/L
Morphine (from heroin)	<0.05 mg/L <0.76 μmol/L	>0.15–2.0 mg/L >0.52–7.0 μmol/L
Paracetamol (acetaminophen)	<20 μg/mL <132 μmol/L	>100 μg/mL >662 μmol/L
Phenobarbital	<30 μg/mL <130 μmol/L	60–80 μg/mL 260–345 μmol/L
Salicylates	<25 mg/dL <1.8 mmol/L	>100 mg/dL >7.24 mmol/L
Triazolam	10–100 ng/mL 0.029–0.29 μmol/L	10–600 ng/mL 0.029–1.75 μmol/L

*Toxic concentrations should be considered only in the context of the complete clinical presentation of the patient. See individual chapters for more information.

TABLE 4-8 Proportions of Cytochrome P-450 Isoenzyme Deficiencies in Different Populations

POPULATION GROUP	CYP2D6 (%)	CYP2C19 (%)
Whites	7	3
Asians	1	22
Blacks	2 (1–15)	3
Arabs	1	1
Vanuatu (Aborigines)	—	70

should always be sent to the physician. This report should contain the following:

1. Date and time of the sampling of the specimens
2. Date and time of the arrival of the specimens at the toxicology laboratory
3. Analysis requested by the physician
4. Results of all tests performed, with a short interpretation of positive results

After the analysis, the specimens should be kept at $-18\,^{\circ}C$ for 2 weeks, in case other investigations or a confirmation of the results is needed. It is important to maintain well-organized documentation of every individual case.

QUALITY ASSURANCE FOR TOXICOLOGY LABORATORIES

It generally has become accepted that in analytic toxicology laboratories quality assurance is as important as in any other clinical laboratory. This concept is much more difficult to organize, however. Clinical and toxicology laboratories are fundamentally different. The toxicology laboratory must first identify the unknown intoxicants before quantifying them. The respect of the chain of custody, clear quality policy concepts, standard operating procedures, external quality assurance by proficiency testing, equipment maintenance, documentation, and performance monitoring of analytic methods after adequate validation procedures are compulsory. An adequate quality assurance program helps address the following questions:

What are the reasons for false-negative results?
In greater than 90% of the cases, the concentrations of the analytes are below the cutoff values. This fact is not as clinically relevant for acute intoxication. In some cases, the wrong specimen is analyzed. Sometimes a positive analytic result is missed. There may be reporting errors. Another explanation is that there may be an assay incompatibility (e.g., designer amphetamines or benzodiazepines that lack specificity or have low cross-reactivity).

What are the reasons for false-positive results?
Reasons may include all the following: carryover contamination from highly concentrated specimens processed before the actual analysis, failure to dilute, methamphetamine generated from ephedrine during GC/MS analysis, or incorrect reporting of results.

What should be done for analytic method validation?
The following parameters are important to have reliable analytic methods: accuracy, LODs and LOQs of the most relevant toxicants, linearity, interferences, imprecision (within-day, day-to-day), specificity, carryover, recovery, ruggedness. Sometimes metabolite standards are not readily available. In these cases, it may be necessary to obtain them from the manufacturer or by preparation in the laboratory (e.g., in vitro production of phase I metabolites using rat microsomes containing cytochrome P-450 enzymes or phase II metabolites using UDP-glucuronosyl transferases[74] or by synthesis[63]).

CONCLUSIONS

This chapter has explained the role of analytic toxicology in the management of acutely poisoned patients. In general, correct documentation of a poisoned patient is not complete without analytic toxicology. Analytic toxicology is for the toxicologist the equivalent to radiologic imaging for the surgeon. Analytic toxicology also may be necessary for forensic reasons because any intoxication may have a criminal origin.

Sufficient routine work is needed for training purposes of the laboratory personnel. Without this routine experience, the toxicology laboratory would be unable to perform correct and complex analyses in situations in which results are crucial. In cases of mixed drug poisonings, the simultaneous presence and interaction of different drugs may mask some toxic signs and symptoms. Even though a patient initially responds to a specific antidote (e.g., naloxone in heroin overdose), further testing may be warranted because of multiple intoxicants.

Analytic toxicology is needed not only for the diagnosis of poisoning but also in the follow-up of patients in cases of intensive care medicine and for pharmacokinetic or toxicokinetic studies. Although analytic toxicology has an important role in the treatment of intoxicated patients, the old adage "treat the patient, not the poison" is still the guiding principle of clinical toxicology. Interpretation of toxicology laboratory results with the available clinical data is crucial to the optimal care of poisoned patients in the intensive care unit.

REFERENCES

1. Ellenhorn MJ, Barceloux DG: Ellenhorn's Medical Toxicology. New York, Elsevier, 1997.
2. Jaeger A, Mangin P: Intérêt et limites de la recherche des toxiques en urgence-L'analyse toxicologique doit être ciblée par le clinicien. Rev Prat 125:287–292, 1992.
3. Hassoun A: The role of the laboratory of toxicology in the diagnosis and therapy of the poisoned patient. Acta Clin Belg 13(Suppl):48–50, 1990.
4. Wennig R: Laboratory diagnosis of poisonings. In Descotes J (ed): Human Toxicology. Amsterdam, Elsevier, 1996, pp 25–236.
5. Maurer HH: What are the appropriate analytical methods in clinical and forensic toxicology? IATDMCT News 1–2, 2000.
6. Durback LF, Scharman EJ, Brown BS: Emergency physicians' perceptions of drug screens at their own hospitals. Vet Hum Toxicol 40:234–237, 1998.
7. Montague RE, Grace RF, Lewis JH, Shenfield GM: Urine drug screens in overdose patients do not contribute to immediate clinical management. Ther Drug Monit 23:47–50, 2001.
8. Pohjola-Sintonen S, Kivistö KT, Vuori E, et al: Identification of drugs ingested in acute poisoning: Correlation of patient history with drug analyses. Ther Drug Monit 22:749–752, 2000.
9. Stewart M: Discussion contribution in Workshop of IVth International Congress of IATDMCT, Vienna, 1995.
10. Schäfer SG, Maurer HH: Erkennen und Behandeln von Vergiftungen. Mannheim, BI, Wissenschaftsverlag, 1993.
11. Kintz P (ed): Toxicologie et Pharmacologie Médicolégales. Amsterdam, Elsevier, 1998.
12. Sachs H, Kintz P: Testing for drugs in hair: Critical review of chromatographic procedures since 1992. J Chromatogr B Biomed Sci Appl 713:147–161, 1998.
13. Moeller MR: Hair analysis as evidence in forensic cases. Ther Drug Monit 18:444–449, 1996.
14. Position statement of AACT and EAPCCT. Clin Toxicol 35:711–719, 1997.
15. Baselt RC: Disposition of toxic drugs and chemicals in man. In Chemical Toxicology, 6th ed. Foster City, CA, Biomedical Publications, 2000.
16. Wong SHY, Sunshine I: Handbook of Analytical Therapeutic Drug Monitoring and Toxicology. Boca Raton, FL, CRC Press, 1997.

17. Brandenberger H, Maes RAA (eds): Analytical Toxicology for Clinical, Forensic and Pharmaceutical Chemists. Berlin, W de Gruyter, 1997.

18. Flanagan RJ, Braithwaite RA, Brown SS, et al: Basic Analytical Toxicology. Geneva, WHO, 1995.

19. Bogusz MJ (ed): Handbook of Analytical Separations Series, Vol 2. Forensic Science. Amsterdam, Elsevier Science, 2000.

20. Recommended Methods for the Detection and Assay of Barbiturates and Benzodiazepines in Biological Specimens.Vienna, UNDCP, 1997.

21. Drummer OH: Methods for the measurement of benzodiazepines in biological samples. J Chromatogr B Biomed Sci Appl 713:201–225, 1998.

22. Bogusz MJ, Maier RD, Krüger KD, Früchtnicht W: Determination of flunitrazepam and its metabolites in blood by high-performance liquid chromatography-atmospheric pressure chemical ionization mass spectrometry. J Chromatogr B Biomed Sci Appl 713:361–369, 1998.

23. Recommended Methods for the Detection and Assay of Heroin, Cannabinoids, Cocaine, Amphetamine and Ring-substituted Amphetamine Derivatives. Vienna, UNDCP, 1995,

24. Badia R, De la Torre R, Corcione S, Segura J: Analytical approaches of European Union laboratories to drugs of abuse analysis. Clin Chem 44:790–799, 1998.

25. Poortman AJ, Lock E: Analytical profile of 4-methylthioamphetamine (4-MTA), a new street drug. Forensic Sci Int 100:221–233, 1999.

26. Recommended Methods for the Detection and Assay of LSD, PCP, Psilocybin and Methaqualone in Biological Specimen. Vienna, UNDCP, 1998.

27. Schneider S, Kuffer P, Wennig R: Determination of lysergide (LSD) and phencyclidine in biosamples. J Chromatogr B Biomed Sci Appl 713:189–200, 1998.

28. Tagliaro F, Lubli G, Ghielmi S, et al: Chromatographic methods for blood alcohol determination. J Chromatogr 580:161–190, 1992.

29. Couper FJ, Logan BK: Determination of γ-hydroxybutyrate (GHB) in biological specimens by gas chromatography-mass spectrometry. J Anal Toxicol 24:1–7, 2000.

30. Elliott S: The presence of gamma-hydroxybutyric acid (GHB) in postmortem biological fluids. J Anal Toxicol 25:152, 2001.

31. Black SB, Hansson RC: Determination of salbutamol and detection of other β-agonists in human postmortem whole blood and urine by GC-MS-SIM. J Anal Toxicol 23:113–118, 1999.

32. Gaillard Y: Poisoning by plant material: Review of human cases and analytical determination of main toxins by HPLC-tandem mass spectrometry. J Chromatogr 733:181–229, 1999.

33. Porter WH, Rutter PW, Yao HH: Simultaneous determination of ethylene glycol and glycolic acid in serum by GC/MS. J Anal Toxicol 23:591–597, 1999.

34. Lin J, Suzuki O: Conditions of SPE for the mixture of organophosphates and synthetic pyrethroids in human body fluids. Forensic Sci Int 99:159–161, 1999.

35. Moriya F, Hashimoto Y, Kuo TL: Pitfalls when determining tissues distributions of organophosphorus chemicals: NaF accelerated chemical degradation. J Anal Toxicol 23:210–215, 1999.

36. Hamen J, Wennig R: Diagnosis of an acute parathion-intoxication and forensic consequences. Acta Clin Belg 1(Suppl):54–58, 1999.

37. Masami S, Reiko E, Akiko K, et al: Separation and determination of quaternary ammonium compounds by high-performance liquid chromatography with a hydrophilic polymer column and conductometry detection. J Chromatogr A 830:321–328, 1999.

38. Lagerwerf AJ, Valinthout LEH, Vree TB: Rapid determination of succinylcholine in human plasma by HPLC with fluorescence detection. J Chromatogr B Biomed Sci Appl 570:390–395, 1991.

39. Toennes SW, Maurer HH: Efficient cleavage of conjugates of drugs or poisons by immobilized β-glucuronidase and arylsulfatase in columns. Clin Chem 45:2173–2182, 1999.

40. Brau M, Vanbinst R, Hassoun A, Wallemacq PE: Simultaneous detection and quantification of acidic and basic drugs in serum toxicological screening: Use of ion-pairing technique in liquid-liquid extraction. Acta Clin Belg 1(Suppl):74–78, 1999.

41. Ma M, Cantwell FF: Solvent microextraction with simultaneous backextraction for sample cleanup and preconcentration: Quantitative extraction. Anal Chem 70:3912–3919, 1998.

42. Franke JP, de Zeeuw RA: Solid-phase extraction procedures in systematic toxicological analysis. J Chromatogr B Biomed Sci Appl 713:51–59, 1998.

43. Soriano T, Jurado C, Menéndez M, Repetto M: Improved solid-phase extraction method for systematic toxicological analysis in biological fluids. J Anal Toxicol 25:137–144, 2001.

44. Koole A, Jetten AC, Lino Y, et al: Rapid extraction of clenbuterol from human and calf urine using Empore C8 extraction disks. J Anal Toxicol 23:632–635, 1999.

45. Junting L: Solid phase microextraction (SPME) of drugs and poisons from biological samples. Forensic Sci Int 97:93–100, 1998.

46. Bermejo AM, Seara R, dos Santos Lucas AC, et al: Use of solid-phase microextraction (SPME) for the determination of methadone and its main metabolite EDDP in plasma by gas chromatography-mass spectrometry. J Anal Toxicol 24:66–69, 2000.

47. Coleman DE, Baselt RC: Efficacy of two commercial products for altering urine drug test results. Clin Toxicol 35:637–642, 1997.

48. Maurer HH (ed): Chromatography and capillary electrophoresis in forensic and clinical toxicology. J Chromatogr B Biomed Sci Appl 713:1–279, 1998.

49. Polettini A, Groppi A, Vignali C, Montagna M: Fully-automated systematic toxicological analysis of drugs, poisons, and metabolites in whole blood, urine, and plasma by gas chromatography-full scan mass spectrometry. J Chromatogr B Biomed Sci Appl 713:265–279, 1998.

50. Maurer HH: Liquid chromatography-mass spectrometry in forensic and clinical toxicology. J Chromatogr B Biomed Sci Appl 713:3–25, 1998.

51. Fitzgerald RL, Rivera JD, Herold DA: Broad spectrum drug identification directly from urine, using liquid chromatography-tandem mass spectrometry. Clin Chem 45:1224–1234, 1999.

52. Stimpfl Th, Vycudilik W: Identification of the general unknown: Application of mass selective detectors in forensic toxicology. J Anal Toxicol 24:32–35, 2000.

53. Marquet P, Lachâtre G: Liquid chromatography-mass spectrometry: potential in forensic and clinical toxicology. J Chromatogr B Biomed Sci Appl 733:93–118, 1999.

54. Rittner M, Pragst F, Bork WR, Neumann J: Screening method for seventy psychoactive drugs or drug metabolites in serum based on high-performance liquid chromatography-electrospray ionization mass spectrometry. J Anal Toxicol 25:115–124, 2001.

55. Tagliaro F, Turrina S, Pisi P, et al: Determination of illicit and/or abused drugs and compounds of forensic interest in biosamples by capillary electrophoretic/electrokinetic methods. J Chromatogr B Biomed Sci Appl 713:27–49, 1998.

56. Hudson JC, Golin M, Malcolm M, Whiting CF: Capillary zone electrophoresis in a comprehensive screen for drugs of forensic interest in whole blood: An update. Can Soc Forens Sci J 31:1–29, 1998.

57. Segura J, Ventura R, Jurado C: Derivatization procedures for gas chromatographic-mass spectrometric determination of xenobiotics in biological samples, with special attention to drugs of abuse and doping agents. J Chromatogr B Biomed Sci Appl 713:61–90, 1998.

58. Maurer HH, Kraemer T: Toxicological detection of selegiline and its metabolites in urine using fluorescence polarization immunoassay (FPIA) and gas chromatography-mass spectrometry (GC-MS) and differentiation by enantioselective GC-MS of the intake of selegiline from abuse of methamphetamine or amphetamine. Arch Toxicol 66:675–678, 1992.

59. Uges DRA: Therapeutic and toxic drug concentrations. Bull TIAFT 26(Suppl 1):1–34, 1996; and update on Internet website TIAFT.

60. Schulz M, Schmoldt A: Therapeutic and toxic blood concentrations of more than 800 drugs and other xenobiotics. Pharmazie 58:447–474, 2003.

61. Flanagan RJ: Guidelines for the interpretation of analytical toxicology results and unit of measurement conversion factors. Ann Clin Biochem 35:261–267, 1998.

62. Regenthal R, Krüger M, Köppel C, Preiss R: A review of therapeutic, toxic and lethal drug concentrations in plasma, serum and whole blood. Anästhesiol Intensivmed 40:129–144, 1999.

63. Marson C, Schneider S, Meys F, Wennig R: Structural elucidation of an uncommon phenylethylamine analogue in urine responsible for discordant amphetamine immunoassay results. J Anal Toxicol 24:17–21, 2000.

64. Kraemer T, Bock K, Wennig R, Maurer HH: The antispasmodic mebeverine leads to positive amphetamine results with the fluorescence polarization immuno assay (FPIA)—studies on the metabolism and the toxicological detection in urine by GC-MS and FPIA. Proceedings GTFCh-Mosbach Symposium 1999, pp 34–43.

65. Logan BK, Schwilke EW: Drug and alcohol use in fatally injured drivers in Washington State. J Forensic Sci 41:505–510, 1996.

66. Charlier C, Verstraete A, Maes V, et al: Narcotic drugs and traffic safety in Belgium. Toxicorama 10:27–31, 1998.
67. Marquet P, Delpla PA, Kerguelen S, et al: Prevalence of drugs of abuse in urine of drivers involved in road accidents in France: A collaborative study. J Forensic Sci 43:806–811, 1998.
68. Barbone F, McMahon AD, Davey PG, et al: Association of road-traffic accidents with benzodiazepine use. Lancet 352:1331–1336, 1998.
69. Logan BK: Methamphetamine and driving impairment. J Forensic Sci 41:457–464, 1996.
70. Kevin LW, Donald BK: Legal hemp products and urine cannabinoid testing. Clin Toxicol 37:897–898, 1999.
71. Aderjan RE, Skopp G: Formation and clearance of active and inactive metabolites of opiates in humans. Ther Drug Monit 20:561–569, 1998.
72. Alfaro C, Lam Y, et al: CYP2D6 status of extensive metabolizers after multiple-dose fluoxetine, fluvoxamine, paroxetine or sertraline. J Clin Psychopharmacol 19:155–163, 1999.
73. Bon MAM, Vermes I, van den Bergh FAJ, et al: Pharmacogenetics: A tool for TDM, a correlation study on CYP2D6 and nortriptyline. Clin Chem 44:198, 1998.
74. Bickeboeller-Friedrich J, Maurer HH: Developing of a GC-MS procedure for the detection of new psychotropic drugs in urine based on rat liver microsome studies. Proceedings GTFCh-Mosbach Symposium, 1999, pp 50–59.

CHAPTER 5

Gastrointestinal Decontamination

Edward P. Krenzelok   ▪   J. Allister Vale

A historical cornerstone in the management of poisoned patients has been the use of gastrointestinal (GI) decontamination to prevent the absorption of the poisons. Most commonly, patients in the emergency department were subjected to emesis, gastric lavage, or the administration of activated charcoal and a cathartic. Occasionally, additional doses of activated charcoal were administered after the patient had been transferred to the critical care unit. In severely poisoned patients who had ingested a poison associated with high morbidity and mortality, whole-bowel irrigation (WBI) also may have been employed, particularly if the poison involved (e.g., iron) was not adsorbed by activated charcoal. Are such therapeutic approaches valid and effective?

Pediatric exposures constitute approximately 50% of reported exposures.[1] Most cases do not necessitate the use of GI decontamination or hospital referral because they are poisoning scares rather than true poisonings. The pediatric critical care specialist is presented only rarely with the issue of whether to perform a decontamination procedure (see Chapter 10). In adult patients, there is often a substantial delay between the ingestion of a poison and presentation to the emergency department. Clinically significant gastric emptying of the poison into the small bowel is likely to have occurred during that interval, which renders evacuation of the stomach inappropriate and impractical. Time is the most important determinant—the longer the delay, the less likely that a poison will reside in the stomach and be accessible for removal by GI decontamination.[2-6] Because poison center data suggest that the overall mortality associated with poisoning is low (<0.5% in the general population and 0.002% in children ≤12 years old),[1] whether or not GI decontamination is employed, the routine use of GI decontamination in all poisonings, regardless of circumstances, is unjustifiable.

To assist physicians with the management of poisoned patients, the American Academy of Clinical Toxicology and the European Association of Poisons Centres and Clinical Toxicologists have published five position statements on the use of GI decontamination.[2-6] We were cochairs of the Position Statement Committee and authors of two of the position statements. With the permission of the publisher of *Journal of Toxicology–Clinical Toxicology*, we relied on these position statements heavily in developing the recommendations in this chapter, but readers are encouraged to refer to the position statements for a more comprehensive review of the literature.

IPECAC SYRUP–INDUCED EMESIS

Ipecac syrup (syrup of ipecacuanha) has long been promoted as a panacea for the management of acute poisoning. In the past, owing to the rapid onset of vomiting after administration of ipecac syrup, poison centers have recommended that it be made available in the home as a first-aid measure. In addition, the literature has extolled the virtues of ipecac syrup, although few studies have investigated adequately its impact on patient outcome.

Rationale

Ipecac syrup is available as a nonprescription drug at pharmacies in many countries and may be administered at home or at a health care facility shortly after an ingestion. Ipecac syrup contains two primary alkaloids, emetine and cephaeline, which induce vomiting through peripheral and central mechanisms, theoretically removing ingested poisons from the stomach. Emesis is noninvasive, uses a physiologic mechanism, and consumes little staff time.

Animal Studies

The value of ipecac in reducing marker (sodium salicylate, barium sulfate, acetaminophen) absorption was investigated in four studies.[7-10] In these studies, the mean recovery of ingested material was highly variable (17.5% to 62%), although generally the amount of ingested material removed by ipecac syrup–induced emesis depended on the time elapsed between dosing and the onset of emesis.

Volunteer Studies

Ten volunteer studies investigated the value of ipecac syrup in preventing the absorption of marker substances.[11-20] In these studies, the recovery of material was highly variable, although generally the amount of ingested material removed by ipecac syrup–induced emesis depended on the elapsed time between dosing and the onset of emesis. If ipecac syrup was administered 5 minutes after dosing, the mean recoveries in two studies using a ^{99m}Tc marker were 54.1%[20] and 83%.[17] In two other studies, the mean plasma concentrations for various drugs were reduced to 21% to 48% of control.[11,13] When ipecac syrup was administered at 10 minutes after dosing, the mean recoveries in two studies were 28.4% (cyanocobalamin marker)[14] and either 46.9% or 47.2% (cobalt marker).[19]

Ipecac syrup administered at 30 minutes after dosing resulted in a mean recovery of 59% of the ^{99m}Tc-labeled human albumin-sucralfate marker.[17] In another study,[11] in which ipecac was given at 30 minutes, the mean plasma concentrations of three drugs (acetaminophen, tetracycline, aminophylline) were 70% to 107% of control. When ipecac syrup was administered at 60 minutes, the mean areas under the curve (AUCs) were 79%[18] and 62%.[15] When mean total urine salicylate excretion was measured over 48 hours in volunteers administered ipecac syrup 60 minutes after aspirin dosing, 70.3%[12] (control 96.3%) and 55.6%[16] (control 60.3%) of the administered aspirin dose were recovered. In another study,[17] the mean recovery of marker at 60 minutes was 44%. Other studies suggested that tablet debris may be found in the stomach after administration of ipecac syrup and that ipecac syrup may propel material into the small intestine, increasing the probability of enhanced drug absorption.[21]

Clinical Studies

In a study in children with *nontoxic* acetaminophen (paracetamol) concentrations, the mean plasma acetaminophen concentrations decreased from 33.1 mg/L (2.40 mmol/L) to 15.7 mg/L (1.14 mmol/L), a 52.6% reduction, when emesis was induced 59 minutes after ingestion.[22] Two clinical studies[23,24] showed no benefit on patient outcome from the administration of ipecac syrup before activated charcoal compared with activated charcoal alone, regardless of the time of ipecac syrup administration. Most studies excluded the use of ipecac syrup in life-threatening intoxications, so it is difficult to determine the benefit of ipecac syrup in more severely poisoned patients.

Conclusions and Recommendations

Ipecac syrup should not be administered routinely in the management of poisoned patients. There is no evidence from clinical studies that ipecac syrup improves the outcome of poisoned patients, and its routine administration in critical care or emergency departments should be abandoned. In addition, ipecac syrup may delay the administration or reduce the effectiveness of activated charcoal, oral antidotes, or WBI. Ipecac syrup administration may increase the risk of complications in a patient who has a decreased level of consciousness, has an impending loss of consciousness, has ingested a corrosive substance or hydrocarbon with high aspiration potential, is elderly or debilitated, or has a medical condition that may be compromised further by the induction of emesis. The most common adverse effect of using ipecac syrup are diarrhea,[25–27] lethargy and drowsiness,[25–27] and prolonged (>1 hour) vomiting.[25,26] The last-mentioned effect renders the patient at risk for aspiration and, in small children, volume and electrolyte imbalance.

GASTRIC LAVAGE

Rationale

Gastric lavage involves the passage of an orogastric tube and the sequential administration and aspiration of small volumes of liquid with the intent of removing toxic substances present in the stomach. It has been used for nearly 200 years as a means of eliminating poisons from the stomach, yet few studies have investigated its impact on patient outcome. Proudfoot[28] articulated eloquently the need for review: "To advocate abandoning it [gastric lavage] is to attack one of the very pillars of management of poisoning by ingestion and cannot be supported lightly. However, endorsement by common usage should not blind physicians to its limitations or prohibit it from critical appraisal."

Technique

Gastric lavage should be undertaken by personnel who are experienced with the procedure. If the patient is conscious and alert, the procedure should be explained to the patient and verbal consent obtained. Because of the possibility of emesis, it is important that an appropriate suction device be available. If the patient cannot protect the airway adequately, endotracheal intubation should precede lavage.

Lavage should be undertaken with a large-bore tube (30G or 36F to 40F for adults, 24F to 28F for pediatric patients). The tube should be lubricated with a hydroxyethyl cellulose jelly and should be sufficiently pliable not to cause tissue injury, yet firm enough to pass into the stomach. There is no role for nasogastric lavage.

When tube placement is verified by either the auscultation of insufflated air or testing the pH of the aspirate, lavage should be undertaken with 200- to 300-mL aliquots of warm normal saline or water. For pediatric patients, 10-mL/kg aliquots of normal saline should be used. Young children may develop hyponatremia if lavaged with water. The end point of lavage is the clearance of visual gastric contents from the return fluid.

Animal Studies

Three studies[7–9] were performed in animals, but none showed substantial drug recovery, particularly if lavage was delayed for 60 minutes. If gastric lavage was undertaken within 15 to 20 minutes of dosing, the mean recovery of marker was 38% for sodium salicylate marker[7] and 29% for barium sulfate marker.[9] When lavage was performed at 30 minutes, the mean recovery of barium sulfate was 26%.[8] Gastric lavage undertaken at 60 minutes resulted in mean recoveries of 13%[7] and 8.6%.[8]

Volunteer Studies

Five volunteer studies provide insufficient support for the clinical use of gastric lavage: Three[14,20,29] were performed less than 20 minutes after dosing; two[15,16] were undertaken at 60 minutes. The recovery of marker was highly variable when lavage was undertaken less than 20 minutes after dosing. When gastric lavage was performed at 5 minutes, the mean recovery of a thiamine marker was 90%[29]; when it was performed at 10 minutes, the mean recovery of a cyanocobalamin marker was 45%[14]; and when it was undertaken at a mean time of 19 minutes, the mean recovery of a ^{99m}Tc-labeled marker was 30.3%.[20] In the studies performed at 60 minutes after dosing, the mean reduction in the AUC was 32% in one study,[15] and in the second study,[16] the mean reduction in salicylate excretion was 8%. Other studies suggested that tablet debris may be found in the stomach after lavage and that lavage may propel material into the small intestine, increasing the possibility of enhanced drug absorption.[21]

Clinical Studies

Clinical studies[30–33] have not confirmed the benefit of gastric lavage alone even when it was performed less than 60 minutes after poison ingestion, and there is the possibility that drug absorption may be enhanced by its use. In one study,[23] benefit from lavage was shown in a small subset (n = 16) of obtunded patients in whom lavage was undertaken and activated charcoal administered less than 60 minutes after ingestion; there were only three patients in the comparison group who received charcoal alone. Small group sizes and selection bias limit the conclusions that can be drawn from this study. In a similar although larger study,[24] benefit from gastric lavage was not confirmed regardless of the time postingestion. Although anecdotal reports indicate that occasionally impressive returns are achieved, there is no strong clinical evidence to support the view that, overall, gastric lavage benefits the poisoned patient. In one study,[33] gastric lavage was associated with an increased occurrence of aspiration and admission to an intensive care unit.

Conclusions and Recommendations

Gastric lavage should not be employed routinely in the management of poisoned patients. Based on experimental and clinical studies, it is unlikely that gastric lavage would be of value longer than 1 hour postingestion. Unless a patient is intubated, gastric lavage is contraindicated if airway protective reflexes are lost. It also is contraindicated if a hydrocarbon with high aspiration potential or corrosive substance has been ingested. Potential complications include aspiration pneumonia; laryngospasm; hypoxia and hypercapnia; mechanical injury to the throat, esophagus (potentially causing mediastinitis), and stomach; and fluid and electrolyte imbalance.

A long interval between the ingestion of a poison and admission to a critical care unit contraindicates the routine or even occasional use of gastric lavage. In general, gastric lavage has no role in the management of a poisoned patient who is being treated in a critical care unit. In the increasingly rare instance in which gastric lavage has been performed, the patient should be evaluated for the abovementioned complications.

SINGLE-DOSE ACTIVATED CHARCOAL

Rationale

Single-dose activated charcoal therapy involves the oral administration or instillation by nasogastric tube of an aqueous preparation of activated charcoal after the ingestion of a poison. Activated charcoal adsorbs a wide variety of poisons in the GI tract, decreasing absorption and reducing or preventing systemic toxicity.

The literature of the 1980s and early 1990s promoted the general and sole use of single-dose activated charcoal to reduce the absorption of poisons. In vitro and in vivo studies have shown that activated charcoal adsorbs a variety of compounds and reduces drug absorption. However, single-dose activated charcoal has not been shown to improve the outcome in a poisoned patient.

In Vitro and Animal Studies

Scores of compounds, including many drugs, have been shown to be adsorbed by activated charcoal to varying degrees.[34] The administration of activated charcoal in animal studies produced variable reduction in marker absorption.[34] Commonly encountered poisons that are not well adsorbed by activated charcoal are listed in Table 5-1.

Volunteer Studies

The results of 115 comparisons with 43 drugs indicate considerable variation in the absolute amount of charcoal used (0.5 to 100 g) and the time of administration ($\leq$240 minutes after ingestion). In these studies, when activated charcoal was administered 30 minutes or less after drug administration (Table 5-2), the mean bioavailability was reduced by 69.1%. When activated charcoal was administered 60 minutes after drug administration, the mean reduction in bioavailability was 34.4%. In 40 studies involving 26 drugs, using at least 50 g of activated charcoal, the mean reduction in drug absorption was 88.6% when charcoal was administered 30 minutes after dosing; the mean reduction at 60 minutes was 37.3% (Table 5-3). There are few reliable data that examine the efficacy of single-dose activated charcoal after 60 minutes, but it can be surmised that it would be even less effective owing to the absence of the poison in the stomach.

Clinical Studies

There are no satisfactorily designed clinical studies assessing benefit from single-dose activated charcoal. One study[33] of symptomatic patients who received activated charcoal and some form of gastric evacuation (gastric lavage, ipecac syrup, gastric aspiration) showed that patients receiving gastric aspiration and activated charcoal were less likely to be admitted to an intensive care unit than patients who received activated charcoal and either lavage or ipecac syrup.

TABLE 5-1 Drugs and Chemicals Bound Poorly to Activated Charcoal
Ethanol
Iron
Isopropanol
Lithium
Methanol
Heavy metals

TABLE 5-2 Summary of Reduction of Drug Absorption by Single-Dose Activated Charcoal (0.5–100 g) in Human Volunteer Studies (n = 115)*

% REDUCTION OF DRUG ABSORPTION	TIME (min) OF ADMINISTRATION OF CHARCOAL AFTER DRUG DOSING					
	0–5 (n = 81)[†]	*30 (n = 9)*	*0–30 (n = 92)*	*60 (n = 17)*	*0–60 (n = 110)*	*>60 (n = 5)*
Mean	70.86	51.74	69.12	34.36	64.03	33.2
SD	29.37	17.97	28.85	18.38	30.26	21.75
Median	85	49.4	77.15	29.7	64.65	37.5
Maximum	100	75	100	77.9	100	57
Minimum	10	28.8	10	5.7	5.7	8.4

*Comparisons involving 43 drugs at varying time intervals (0–240 minutes) after drug dosing.
[†]Number of studies.

TABLE 5-3 Summary of the Reduction of Drug Absorption by Single-Dose Activated Charcoal (at least 50 g) in Human Volunteer Studies (n = 40)*

% REDUCTION OF DRUG ABSORPTION	TIME (min) OF ADMINISTRATION OF CHARCOAL AFTER DRUG DOSING				
	0–5 (n = 25)[†]	*30 (n = 4)*	*0–30 (n = 29)*	*60 (n = 11)*	*0–60 (n = 40)*
Mean	94.08	54.22	88.59	37.34	74.49
SD	9.1	17.32	17.29	18.21	28.93
Median	98.2	51	97	29.9	87.05
Maximum	100	75	100	77.9	100
Minimum	63.5	39.9	39.9	12.9	12.9

*Comparisons involving 26 drugs at varying time intervals (0–60 minutes) after drug dosing.
[†]Number of studies.

Adverse Effects

Few serious adverse effects or complications from the use of single-dose activated charcoal have been reported in poisoned patients. After the administration of aqueous activated charcoal, emesis occurs infrequently. The incidence of emesis seems to be greater, however, when activated charcoal is administered with sorbitol.[35,36] With inadequate airway management, pulmonary aspiration has occurred after the administration of activated charcoal.[24] Aspiration of charcoal-containing povidone has occasionally led to major respiratory problems.[37] Corneal abrasions may occur on direct ocular contact.[38]

Conclusions and Recommendations

Single-dose activated charcoal should not be administered routinely in the management of poisoned patients, but it should be considered on an individual basis. The administration of activated charcoal should be considered if a patient has ingested a potentially toxic amount of a poison (that is known to be adsorbed to charcoal) 1 hour previously; there are insufficient data to support or exclude its use after 1 hour of ingestion. There is no evidence that the administration of activated charcoal improves clinical outcome. Unless a patient has an intact or protected airway, the administration of charcoal is contraindicated.

Single-dose activated charcoal use has not been validated as a means of improving patient outcome. Because activated charcoal generally is administered in emergency departments, it is unlikely that critical care specialists would need to consider the dose of charcoal to reduce poison absorption. The administration of multiple-dose activated charcoal to increase the elimination of a select number of poisons may be appropriate, however.[39] Multiple-dose activated charcoal therapy is reviewed in Chapter 6.

CATHARTICS

Cathartics are the least validated of the GI decontamination techniques. They have been used for decades in conjunction with activated charcoal in an attempt to enhance the elimination of the poison-activated charcoal complex and reduce the potential for desorption of a poison from activated charcoal. The two general types of osmotic cathartics used in poisoned patients are saccharide (sorbitol) and "saline" (magnesium citrate, magnesium sulfate, sodium sulfate) agents. Cathartics alone have been administered with the intent of decreasing the absorption of substances by accelerating their expulsion from the GI tract. Sorbitol improves the palatability of activated charcoal by imparting a sweet taste and by masking the grittiness of the charcoal.

In Vitro Studies

Seven studies investigated the effect of cathartics on the adsorption of drugs by activated charcoal. One study[40] evaluated the effect of magnesium citrate on the binding of salicylates to charcoal and found apparent pH-dependent changes in adsorption. At low pH, magnesium citrate interfered with salicylate adsorption, and at high pH, it enhanced salicylate adsorption. The statistical significance of this increase was not calculated. Four other studies[41–44] evaluated the impact of magnesium citrate at controlled pH on the adsorptive capacity of activated charcoal. At a pH of 1.2, magnesium citrate reduced the adsorptive capacity of charcoal by 15% ($P < .05$).[41] In a study conducted with a pH of 4.0, magnesium citrate significantly ($P < .01$) enhanced the adsorption of salicylate to charcoal, regardless of the initial salicylate concentration and the charcoal-to-salicylate ratio.[42] In another study in which the pH was unknown but controlled, the presence of magnesium citrate apparently increased the adsorption of carbon 14–labeled paraquat at charcoal-to-paraquat ratios of 10:1 and 20:1.[43] A study using simulated gastric fluid with an unstated pH showed an apparent decrease in the adsorption of aspirin to charcoal when magnesium citrate was added and an apparent increase in adsorption to charcoal when simulated intestinal fluid was used.[44]

Animal Studies

The combination of magnesium citrate and activated charcoal given to mice 30 minutes after paraquat administration increased survival from 31% (controls) to 94% ($P < .01$).[43] When sorbitol and mannitol were coadministered with activated charcoal to dogs, Van de Graaff and colleagues[45] showed that the AUC for acetaminophen (paracetamol) was 75% greater with cathartics plus charcoal compared with charcoal alone ($P = .07$), and the peak plasma acetaminophen concentration was 80.4% greater ($P = .012$) after cathartics and charcoal compared with charcoal alone.

In studies conducted in rats, the addition of activated charcoal to sorbitol reduced significantly the peak drug concentrations to 23.8% of control ($P < .001$) for chlorpheniramine, to 20.6% of control ($P < .001$) for chloroquine, to 25.6% of control ($P < .001$) for pentobarbital, and to 55.2% of control ($P < .001$) for aspirin.[46] Sodium sulfate and activated charcoal administered to rats reduced significantly ($P < .001$) peak plasma concentrations of salicylate, pentobarbital, chlorpheniramine, and chloroquine compared with control. The combination was significantly ($P < .001$) more effective than charcoal alone in reducing peak drug concentrations of salicylate, pentobarbital, and chloroquine.[47] Sodium sulfate, but not sorbitol, together with superactivated charcoal increased survival (2 of 11) and increased significantly ($P < .01$) survival times of rats that were given lethal doses of T-2 mycotoxin.[48]

Volunteer Studies

CATHARTICS ALONE

Magnesium sulfate did not alter significantly ($P > .10$) the serum concentrations of lithium and salicylate when administered 30 minutes after dosing.[49] Galinsky and Levy[50] showed that sodium sulfate did not significantly change the urinary recovery of acetaminophen and its metabolites (87% ± 8.3% [mean ± SD]) compared with control (89.6% ± 10.7%). After the administration of sorbitol, urine salicylate recovery (95.9% ± 14.4%) was not significantly reduced compared with control (100%).[51] Al-Shareef and coworkers[52] showed that the mean peak plasma theophylline concentration (7.8 mg/L [42.9 μmol/L]) was significantly ($P < .001$) greater in volunteers given sorbitol than in the control group (5.5 mg/L [30.5 μmol/L]). The mean time to peak concentration was significantly ($P < .01$) shorter (11.38 hours) in the sorbitol group than in the control group (16 hours). There was no difference in the mean $AUC_{0–24}$ hours between the sorbitol (116.6 mg/L/hr [647.1 μmol/L/hr]) and control (97.6 mg/L/hr [541.7 μmol/L/hr]) groups. In another study, Minton and Henry[53] found that sorbitol did not alter significantly the AUC of theophylline whether administered at 1 hour (142.2 mg/L/hr [789.2 μmol/L/hr]) or at 6 hours (124 mg/L/hr [688.2 μmol/L/hr]) after dosing compared with control (152.8 mg/L/hr [848 μmol/L/hr]).

SORBITOL PLUS ACTIVATED CHARCOAL

Sorbitol and activated charcoal significantly reduced ($P < .01$) the AUC of theophylline (85.5 ± 10 mgh/L) compared with charcoal (113 ± 5.7 mgh/L) and with no treatment (304.6 ± 18.8 mgh/L) groups.[54] Keller and associates[55] found that sorbitol and activated charcoal significantly reduced ($P < .05$) salicylate elimination (0.912 ± 0.18 g) in the urine compared with charcoal alone (1.26 ± 0.15 g). Al Shareef and coworkers[52] showed that sorbitol and activated charcoal did not significantly reduce ($P > .05$) the AUC of theophylline (7.48 mg/L/hr [41.5 μmol/L/hr]) compared with charcoal alone (10.46 mg/L/hr [58.1 μmol/L/hr]). Urinary salicylate excretion was not significantly reduced ($P > .05$) by the administration of sorbitol (43 g and 77 g) and activated charcoal (mean 63.8% and 61.5%) compared with activated charcoal alone (mean 62.3%).[56]

Clinical Studies

No clinical studies have been published to investigate the ability of cathartics, with or without activated charcoal, to reduce the bioavailability of drugs or to improve the outcome of poisoned patients.

Conclusions and Recommendations

The administration of a cathartic alone has no role in the GI decontamination of a poisoned patient. Experimental data regarding the use of cathartics in combination with activated charcoal are conflicting. No clinical studies have been published to investigate the ability of a cathartic, with or without activated charcoal, to reduce the bioavailability of drugs or to improve the outcome of poisoned patients. Based on available data, the routine use of a cathartic in combination with activated charcoal is not endorsed. If a cathartic is used, it should be limited to a single dose to minimize adverse effects. Potential complications of administering cathartics include nausea, abdominal cramps, vomiting, transient hypotension, dehydration, hypernatremia in patients receiving a sodium-containing cathartic, and hypermagnesemia in patients receiving a magnesium-containing cathartic.

WHOLE-BOWEL IRRIGATION

Rationale

WBI involves the use of large volumes of polyethylene glycol isosmotic solution, administered with the theoretical intention of flushing the bowel, enhancing elimination of poison from the gut. WBI is accomplished through the enteral administration of large amounts (infants and children 9 months old to 6 years old, 500 mL/hr; children 6 to 12 years old, 1000 mL/hr; children >12 years old and adults, 1500 to 2000 mL/hr) of an osmotically balanced polyethylene glycol electrolyte solution, which induces a liquid stool. WBI has the theoretical potential to reduce drug absorption by decontaminating the entire GI tract by physically expelling intraluminal contents.[57] The concentration of polyethylene glycol and electrolytes in polyethylene glycol electrolyte solution causes no net absorption or secretion of ions, so no significant changes in water or electrolyte balance occur.[58]

In Vitro Studies

In vitro studies show that activated charcoal does not produce a significant alteration in the osmolality of WBI solution.[59] Polyethylene glycol electrolyte solution may reduce the binding capacity of charcoal if both are administered concurrently.[59–61] In two other studies,[62,63] the binding of drug (mexiletine, imipramine) to charcoal was greater, however, in WBI solution than in a slurry of charcoal.

Animal Studies

Two studies were performed in dogs.[64,65] One study[64] showed a benefit from WBI. The mean total body clearance of paraquat was increased ($P < .05$) from 5.67 L/hr to 13.2 L/hr by WBI, and this procedure removed 68.9% of the ingested dose.[64] In an awake canine model, WBI used as an adjunct to multiple-dose activated charcoal did not reduce the terminal half-life of theophylline. This study did not have a no-treatment control group because of the large dose of sustained-release theophylline given to awake dogs.[65]

Volunteer Studies

Six volunteer studies investigated the value of WBI in reducing the absorption of ingested drugs.[66–71] Three studies involving dosing with ampicillin,[66] delayed-release aspirin,[67] and sustained-release lithium[68] showed significant reductions in bioavailability of 67%, 73%, and 67% (all $P < .05$). In a study designed to evaluate whether WBI enhanced the excretion of drugs during the postabsorptive phase, WBI did not reduce the bioavailability of aspirin.[69] Two studies[70,71] involving aspirin are difficult to interpret because one[70] lacked a control (no treatment) arm and because both the duration and the total volume of WBI were less than in other studies. A study of WBI using coffee beans as a marker failed to show enhanced expulsion from the GI tract.[72]

Clinical Studies

No controlled clinical studies have been performed. Eleven anecdotal reports of the use of WBI in 17 patients have been published.[73–83] Nine patients ingested iron,[73–77] and seven ingested other agents (sustained-release verapamil,[78] delayed-release fenfluramine,[79] latex packets of cocaine,[80] zinc sulfate,[81] lead oxide,[82] and arsenic[83]). No conclusions regarding the efficacy of WBI can be gleaned from these observations.

Adverse Effects

Nausea, vomiting, abdominal cramps, and bloating have been described when WBI was used in preparation for colonoscopy and barium enema.[84] There are insufficient clinical data to accurately describe the types and incidences of complications associated with the use of WBI for the treatment of potentially toxic ingestions. Nausea and vomiting may complicate the use of WBI.[67] Vomiting is more likely to occur if the patient has been treated recently with ipecac syrup[85] or if the patient has ingested an agent that produces vomiting. Patients with altered mental status or compromised and unprotected airways are at risk for pulmonary aspiration during WBI.

Conclusions and Recommendations

WBI should not be used routinely in the management of poisoned patients. No controlled clinical trials have been performed, and there is no conclusive evidence that WBI improves the outcome of poisoned patients. There are insufficient data to support or exclude the use of WBI for potentially toxic ingestions of iron, lead, zinc, or packets of illicit drugs; WBI remains a theoretical option for these ingestions. WBI is contraindicated in patients with bowel obstruction, perforation, and ileus and in patients with hemodynamic instability or compromised unprotected airways. WBI should be used cautiously in debilitated patients or in patients with medical conditions that may be compromised further by its use. A single dose of activated charcoal administered before WBI does not seem to decrease the binding capacity of charcoal or to alter the osmotic properties of WBI solution. Administration of charcoal during WBI seems to decrease the binding capacity of charcoal.[60,61,67]

REFERENCES

1. Litovitz TL, Klein-Schwartz W, White S, et al: 1999 Annual report of the American Association of Poison Control Centers Toxic Exposure Surveillance system. Am J Emerg Med 18:517–574, 2000.
2. American Academy of Clinical Toxicology, European Association of Poisons Centres and Clinical Toxicologists: Position statement: Ipecac syrup. J Toxicol Clin Toxicol 35:699–709, 1997.
3. American Academy of Clinical Toxicology, European Association of Poisons Centres and Clinical Toxicologists: Position statement: Gastric lavage. J Toxicol Clin Toxicol 35:711–719, 1997.

4. American Academy of Clinical Toxicology, European Association of Poisons Centres and Clinical Toxicologists: Position statement: Single-dose activated charcoal. J Toxicol Clin Toxicol 35:721–741, 1997.
5. American Academy of Clinical Toxicology, European Association of Poisons Centres and Clinical Toxicologists: Position statement: Cathartics. J Toxicol Clin Toxicol 35:743–752, 1997.
6. American Academy of Clinical Toxicology, European Association of Poisons Centres and Clinical Toxicologists: Position statement: Whole bowel irrigation. J Toxicol Clin Toxicol 35:753–762, 1997.
7. Arnold FJ Jr, Hodges JB Jr, Barta RA Jr, et al: Evaluation of the efficacy of lavage and induced emesis in treatment of salicylate poisoning. Pediatrics 23:286–301, 1959.
8. Abdallah AH, Tye A: A comparison of the efficacy of emetic drugs and stomach lavage. Am J Dis Child 113:571–575, 1967.
9. Corby DG, Lisciandro RC, Lehman RH, Decker WJ: The efficacy of methods used to evacuate the stomach after acute ingestions. Pediatrics 40:871–874, 1967.
10. Teshima D, Suzuki A, Otsubo K, et al: Efficacy of emetic and United States Pharmacopoeia ipecac syrup in prevention of drug absorption. Chem Pharm Bull 38:2242–2245, 1990.
11. Neuvonen PJ, Vartiainen M, Tokola O: Comparison of activated charcoal and ipecac syrup in prevention of drug absorption. Eur J Clin Pharmacol 24:557–562, 1983.
12. Curtis RA, Barone J, Giacona N: Efficacy of ipecac and activated charcoal/cathartic: Prevention of salicylate absorption in a simulated overdose. Arch Intern Med 144:48–52, 1984.
13. Neuvonen PJ, Olkkola KT: Activated charcoal and syrup of ipecac in prevention of cimetidine and pindolol absorption in man after administration of metoclopramide as an antiemetic agent. J Toxicol Clin Toxicol 22:103–114, 1984.
14. Tandberg D, Diven BG, McLeod JW: Ipecac-induced emesis versus gastric lavage. Am J Emerg Med 4:205–209, 1986.
15. Tenenbein M, Cohen S, Sitar DS: Efficacy of ipecac-induced emesis, orogastric lavage, and activated charcoal in acute drug overdose. Ann Emerg Med 16:838–841, 1987.
16. Danel V, Henry JA, Glucksman E: Activated charcoal, emesis, and gastric lavage in aspirin overdose. BMJ 296:1507, 1988.
17. Vasquez TE, Evans DG, Ashburn WL: Efficacy of syrup of ipecac–induced emesis for emptying gastric contents. Clin Nucl Med 13:638–639, 1988.
18. McNamara RM, Aaron CK, Gemborys M, Davidheiser S: Efficacy of charcoal cathartic versus ipecac in reducing serum acetaminophen in a simulated overdose. Ann Emerg Med 18:934–938, 1989.
19. Tandberg D, Murphy LC: The knee-chest position does not improve the efficacy of ipecac-induced emesis. Am J Emerg Med 4:267–270, 1989.
20. Young WF, Bivins HG: Evaluation of gastric emptying using radionuclides: Gastric lavage versus ipecac-induced emesis. Ann Emerg Med 22:1423–1427, 1993.
21. Saetta JP, March S, Gaunt ME, Quinton DN: Gastric emptying procedures in the self-poisoned patient: Are we forcing gastric content beyond the pylorus? J R Soc Med 84:274–276, 1991.
22. Bond GR, Requa RK, Krenzelok EP, et al: Influence of time until emesis on the efficacy of decontamination using acetaminophen as a marker in a pediatric population. Ann Emerg Med 22:1403–1407, 1993.
23. Kulig K, Bar-Or D, Cantrill SV, et al: Management of acutely poisoned patients without gastric emptying. Ann Emerg Med 14:562–567, 1985.
24. Pond SM, Lewis-Driver DJ, Williams GM, et al: Gastric emptying in acute overdose: A prospective randomised controlled trial. Med J Aust 163:345–349, 1995.
25. Chafee-Bahamon C, Lacouture PG, Lovejoy FH Jr: Risk assessment of ipecac in the home. Pediatrics 75:1105–1109, 1985.
26. Czajka PA, Russel SL: Nonemetic effects of ipecac syrup. Pediatrics 75:1101–1104, 1985.
27. Litovitz TL, Klein-Schwartz W, Oderda GM, et al: Ipecac administration in children younger than 1 year of age. Pediatrics 76:761–764, 1985.
28. Proudfoot AT: Abandon gastric lavage in the accident and emergency department? Arch Emerg Med 2:65–71, 1984.
29. Auerbach PS, Osterloh J, Braun O, et al: Efficacy of gastric emptying gastric lavage versus emesis induced with ipecac. Ann Emerg Med 15:692–698, 1986.
30. Allan BC: The role of gastric lavage in the treatment of patients suffering from barbiturate overdose. Med J Aust 2:513–514, 1961.
31. Comstock EG, Faulkner TP, Boisaubin EV, et al: Studies on the efficacy of gastric lavage as practiced in a large metropolitan hospital. J Toxicol Clin Toxicol 18:581–597, 1981.
32. Matthew H, Mackintosh TF, Tompsett SL, Cameron JC: Gastric aspiration and lavage in acute poisoning. BMJ 1:1333–1337, 1966.
33. Merigian KS, Woodard M, Hedges JR, et al: Prospective evaluation of gastric emptying in the self-poisoned patient. Am J Emerg Med 8:479–483, 1990.
34. Cooney DO: Activated Charcoal in Medical Applications. New York, Marcel Dekker, 1995.
35. Kornberg AE, Dolgin J: Pediatric ingestions: Charcoal alone versus ipecac and charcoal. Ann Emerg Med 20:648–651, 1991.
36. Harchelroad F, Cottington E, Krenzelok EP: Gastrointestinal transit times of a charcoal/sorbitol slurry in overdose patients. J Toxicol Clin Toxicol 27:91–99, 1989.
37. Menzies DG, Busuttil A, Prescott LF: Fatal pulmonary aspiration of oral activated charcoal. BMJ 297:459–460, 1988.
38. McKinney P, Phillips S, Gomez HF, Brent J: Corneal abrasions secondary to activated charcoal therapy. Vet Hum Toxicol 34:336, 1992.
39. American Academy of Clinical Toxicology, European Association of Poisons Centres and Clinical Toxicologists, Vale JA, Krenzelok EP, Barceloux DG: Position statement and practice guidelines on the use of multi-dose activated charcoal in the treatment of acute poisoning. J Toxicol Clin Toxicol 37:731–751, 1999.
40. Cooney DO, Wijaya J: Effect of magnesium citrate on the adsorptive capacity of activated charcoal for sodium salicylate. Vet Hum Toxicol 28:521–523, 1986.
41. Czajka PA, Konrad JD: Saline cathartics and the adsorptive capacity of activated charcoal for aspirin. Ann Emerg Med 15:548–551, 1986.
42. Ryan CF, Spigiel RW, Zeldes G: Enhanced adsorptive capacity of activated charcoal in the presence of magnesium citrate, N.F. J Toxicol Clin Toxicol 17:457–461, 1980.
43. Gaudreault P, Friedman PA, Lovejoy FH Jr: Efficacy of activated charcoal and magnesium citrate in the treatment of oral paraquat intoxication. Ann Emerg Med 14:123–125, 1985.
44. LaPierre G, Algozzine G, Doering PL: Effect of magnesium citrate on the in vitro adsorption of aspirin by activated charcoal. J Toxicol Clin Toxicol 18:793–796, 1981.
45. Van de Graaff WB, Thompson WL, Sunshine I, et al: Adsorbent and cathartic inhibition of enteral drug absorption. J Pharmacol Exp Ther 221:656–663, 1982.
46. Picchioni AL, Chin L, Gillespie T: Evaluation of activated charcoal–sorbitol suspension as an antidote. J Toxicol Clin Toxicol 19:433–444, 1982.
47. Chin L, Picchioni AL, Gillespie T: Saline cathartics and saline cathartics plus activated charcoal as antidotal treatments. J Toxicol Clin Toxicol 18:865–871, 1981.
48. Galey FD, Lambert RJ, Busse M, Buck WB: Therapeutic efficacy of superactive charcoal in rats exposed to oral lethal doses of T-2 toxin. Toxicon 25:493–499, 1987.
49. Sørensen PN, Lindkaer-Jensen S: The effect of magnesium sulfate on the absorption of acetylsalicylic acid and lithium carbonate from the human intestine. Arch Toxicol 34:121–127, 1975.
50. Galinsky RE, Levy G: Evaluation of activated charcoal–sodium sulfate combination for inhibition of acetaminophen absorption and repletion of inorganic sulfate. J Toxicol Clin Toxicol 22:21–30, 1984.
51. Mayersohn M, Perrier D, Picchioni AL: Evaluation of a charcoal-sorbitol mixture as an antidote for oral aspirin overdose. J Toxicol Clin Toxicol 11:561–567, 1977.
52. Al-Shareef AH, Buss DC, Allen EM, Routledge PA: The effects of charcoal and sorbitol (alone and in combination) on plasma theophylline concentrations after a sustained-release formulation. Hum Exp Toxicol 9:179–182, 1990.
53. Minton NA, Henry JA: Prevention of drug absorption in simulated theophylline overdose. J Toxicol Clin Toxicol 33:43–49, 1995.
54. Goldberg MJ, Spector R, Park GD, et al: The effect of sorbitol and activated charcoal on serum theophylline concentrations after slow-release theophylline. Clin Pharmacol Ther 41:108–111, 1987.
55. Keller RE, Schwab RA, Krenzelok EP: Contribution of sorbitol combined with activated charcoal in prevention of salicylate absorption. Ann Emerg Med 19:654–656, 1990.
56. Scholtz EC, Jaffe JM, Colaizzi JL: Evaluation of five activated charcoal formulations for the inhibition of aspirin absorption and palatability in man. Am J Hosp Pharm 35:1355–1359, 1978.
57. Tenenbein M: Whole bowel irrigation as a gastrointestinal decontamination procedure after acute poisoning. Med Toxicol 3:77–84, 1988.

58. Davis GR, Santa Ana CA, Morawski SG, Fordtran JS: Development of a lavage solution associated with minimal water and electrolyte absorption or secretion. Gastroenterology 78:991–995, 1980.

59. Kirshenbaum LA, Sitar DS, Tenenbein M: Interaction between whole-bowel irrigation solution and activated charcoal: Implications for the treatment of toxic ingestions. Ann Emerg Med 19:1129–1132, 1990.

60. Hoffman RS, Chiang WK, Howland MA, et al: Theophylline desorption from activated charcoal caused by whole bowel irrigation solution. J Toxicol Clin Toxicol 29:191–201, 1991.

61. Makosiej FJ, Hoffman RS, Howland MA, Goldfrank LR: An in vitro evaluation of cocaine hydrochloride adsorption by activated charcoal and desorption upon addition of polyethylene glycol electrolyte lavage solution. J Toxicol Clin Toxicol 31:381–395, 1993.

62. Arimori K, Deshimaru M, Furukawa E, Nakano M: Adsorption of mexiletine onto activated charcoal in macrogol-electrolyte solution. Chem Pharm Bull 41:766–768, 1993.

63. Arimori K, Furukawa E, Nakano M: Adsorption of imipramine onto activated charcoal and a cation exchange resin in macrogol-electrolyte solution. Chem Pharm Bull 40:3105–3107, 1992.

64. Mizutani T, Okubo N, Tanaka M, Naito H: Efficacy of whole bowel irrigation using solutions with or without adsorbent in the removal of paraquat in dogs. Hum Exp Toxicol 11:495–504, 1992.

65. Burkhart KK, Wuerz RC, Donovan JW: Whole-bowel irrigation as adjunctive treatment for sustained-release theophylline overdose. Ann Emerg Med 21:1316–1320, 1992.

66. Tenenbein M, Cohen S, Sitar DS: Whole bowel irrigation as a decontamination procedure after acute drug overdose. Arch Intern Med 147:905–907, 1987.

67. Kirshenbaum LA, Mathews SC, Sitar DS, Tenenbein M: Whole-bowel irrigation versus activated charcoal in sorbitol for the ingestion of modified-release pharmaceuticals. Clin Pharmacol Ther 46:264–271, 1989.

68. Smith SW, Ling LJ, Halstenson CE: Whole-bowel irrigation as a treatment for acute lithium overdose. Ann Emerg Med 20:536–539, 1991.

69. Mayer AL, Sitar DS, Tenenbein M: Multiple-dose charcoal and whole-bowel irrigation do not increase clearance of absorbed salicylate. Arch Intern Med 152:393–396, 1992.

70. Olsen KM, Ma FH, Ackerman BH, Stull RE: Low-volume whole bowel irrigation and salicylate absorption: A comparison with ipecac-charcoal. Pharmacotherapy 13:229–232, 1993.

71. Rosenberg PJ, Livingstone DJ, McLellan BA: Effect of whole-bowel irrigation on the antidotal efficacy of oral activated charcoal. Ann Emerg Med 17:681–683, 1988.

72. Scharman EJ, Lembersky R, Krenzelok EP: Efficiency of whole bowel irrigation with and without metoclopramide pretreatment. Am J Emerg Med 12:302–305, 1994.

73. Tenenbein M: Whole bowel irrigation in iron poisoning. J Pediatr 111:143–145, 1987.

74. Mann KV, Picciotti MA, Spevack TA, Durbin DR: Management of acute iron overdose. Clin Pharm 8:428–440, 1989.

75. Everson GW, Bertaccini EJ, O'Leary J: Use of whole bowel irrigation in an infant following iron overdose. Am J Emerg Med 9:366–369, 1991.

76. Kaczorowski JM, Wax PM: Five days of whole-bowel irrigation in a case of pediatric iron ingestion. Ann Emerg Med 27:258–263, 1996.

77. Turk J, Aks S, Ampuero F, Hryhorczuk DO: Successful therapy of iron intoxication in pregnancy with intravenous deferoxamine and whole bowel irrigation. Vet Hum Toxicol 35:441–444, 1993.

78. Buckley N, Dawson AH, Howarth D, Whyte IM: Slow-release verapamil poisoning—use of polyethylene glycol whole-bowel lavage and high-dose calcium. Med J Aust 158:202–204, 1993.

79. Melandri R, Re G, Morigi A, et al: Whole bowel irrigation after delayed release fenfluramine overdose. J Toxicol Clin Toxicol 33:161–163, 1995.

80. Hoffman RS, Smilkstein MJ, Goldfrank LR: Whole bowel irrigation and the cocaine body-packer: A new approach to a common problem. Am J Emerg Med 8:523–527, 1990.

81. Burkhart KK, Kulig KW, Rumack B: Whole-bowel irrigation as treatment for zinc sulfate overdose. Ann Emerg Med 19:1167–1170, 1990.

82. Roberge RJ, Martin TG: Whole bowel irrigation in an acute oral lead intoxication. Am J Emerg Med 10:577–583, 1992.

83. Lee DC, Roberts JR, Kelly JJ, Fishman SM: Whole-bowel irrigation as an adjunct in the treatment of radiopaque arsenic. Am J Emerg Med 13:244–245, 1995.

84. Ernstoff JJ, Howard DA, Marshall JB, et al: A randomized blinded clinical trial of a rapid colonic lavage solution (Golytely) compared with standard preparation for colonoscopy and barium enema. Gastroenterology 84:1512–1516, 1983.

85. Tenenbein M: Whole bowel irrigation for toxic ingestions. J Toxicol Clin Toxicol 23:177–184, 1985.

CHAPTER **6**

Multiple-Dose Activated Charcoal

Edward P. Krenzelok ▪ J. Allister Vale ▪ Donald G. Barceloux

The challenge for critical care physicians caring for poisoned patients is to identify at an early stage patients who are most at risk of developing serious complications and who potentially might benefit from elimination techniques, such as multiple-dose activated charcoal (MDAC), urine alkalization, hemodialysis, or hemoperfusion. Most poisoned patients are not poisoned severely, and few require the use of elimination techniques. MDAC therapy was used in only 7370 of 2,380,028 (0.0.31%) patients reported to the American Association of Poison Control Centers in 2002.[1] Even among seriously poisoned patients admitted to intensive care units, however, few are candidates for interventions, such as MDAC, aimed at achieving enhanced substance elimination.

RATIONALE

Single-dose activated charcoal therapy involves the oral administration or instillation by nasogastric tube of an aqueous preparation of activated charcoal after the ingestion of a poison with the intent of decreasing poison absorption and reducing or preventing systemic toxicity (see Chapter 5). In contrast, MDAC involves the administration of repeated doses of activated charcoal with the intent of enhancing drug elimination.[2] A variety of factors dictate whether the elimination of a substance can be enhanced with MDAC. Drugs with a low volume of distribution (preferably <1 L/kg) and a prolonged elimination half-life after overdose are particularly likely to have their elimination enhanced to a clinically significant degree by the use of MDAC. Other desirable characteristics include a pK_a that favors the undissociated form of the drug and low protein binding.

MECHANISMS OF ACTION

Two mechanisms of action may account for the effectiveness of MDAC. First, after absorption, some drugs are known to diffuse from the circulation into the gut lumen (Fig. 6-1). The rate of this passive diffusion process depends on the concentration of drug in the general circulation. Under conditions in which there is a high concentration of the drug in the blood, it diffuses along the concentration gradient into the gut. Drug continues to diffuse into the gut as long as the concentration gradient exists. MDAC adsorbs drug present in the gut lumen and prevents it from being reabsorbed, interrupting the enteroenteric circulation and

ensuring the persistence of the concentration gradient. This process is often called *gastrointestinal dialysis*.[3] The second proposed mechanism of action is the interruption of the less frequent dynamic of the enterohepatic circulation of drugs.

INDICATIONS

Based on experimental and clinical studies, MDAC should be considered if a patient has ingested a life-threatening amount of carbamazepine, dapsone, phenobarbital, quinine, or theophylline.[2] MDAC use has been suggested but not validated for the treatment of poisoning due to phenytoin, salicylates, meprobamate, phenylbutazone, digoxin, digitoxin, and sotalol.[2] Although there is no evidence that supports the use of MDAC when sustained-release pharmaceuticals have been ingested, MDAC is often used in this type of poisoning.

Carbamazepine

There is evidence from a volunteer study[4] and two clinical studies[5,6] that MDAC enhances the total body clearance of carbamazepine. A randomized crossover study involving five volunteers who were administered carbamazepine, 400 mg orally, showed a significant reduction ($P < .05$) in the carbamazepine elimination half-life from 32 ± 3.4 hours (standard error of the mean [SEM]) to 17.6 ± 2.4 hours (SEM) and a significant increase ($P < .05$) in the total body clearance from 22 ± 1.9 mL/min (SEM) to 40 ± 2.7 mL/min (SEM).[4]

Clinical research also supports the results of this volunteer study. Fifteen patients poisoned by carbamazepine and treated with MDAC (mean total dose 203 ± 58 g) had a mean carbamazepine elimination half-life of 8.6 ± 2.4 hours (standard deviation [SD]) and a total body clearance of 113 ± 44 mL/min (SD).[5] Eight patients who were administered a mean dose of 386 ± 72 g of charcoal had a mean half-life of 9.5 ± 1.9 hours and a mean total body clearance of 105.13 ± 20.4 mL/min.[6]

Although MDAC reduces the elimination half-life and increases the total body clearance of carbamazepine, a reduction in morbidity and mortality has not been shown. This fact should not discourage the use of MDAC in patients poisoned severely by carbamazepine, however, particularly because the clearances are comparable to those achieved with charcoal hemoperfusion (Table 6-1).

61

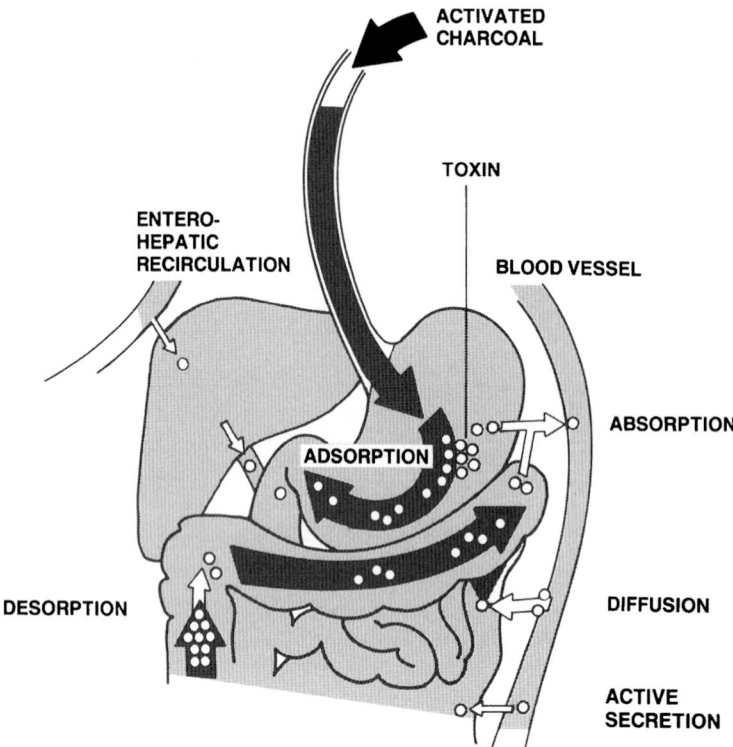

FIGURE 6-1

Mechanism of action of activated charcoal to reduce drug absorption and enhance elimination. Charcoal adsorbs drug from enteroenteric or enterohepatic secretion to prevent absorption and desorption as drug moves through the gastrointestinal tract.

Dapsone

Dapsone poisoning is an uncommon event, but it is associated with significant morbidity. In a volunteer study that involved five subjects who were administered dapsone over 4 days and MDAC (total dose 118 g), the mean elimination dapsone half-life was reduced from 20.5 ± 2 hours (SEM) to 10.8 ± 0.4 hours (SEM) ($P < .01$); the half-life of the primary metabolite (monoacetyldapsone) also was reduced significantly ($P < .001$).[10] In a clinical study by the same group, two patients with dapsone poisoning received MDAC (total dose 80 g and 160 g, respectively), and the dapsone elimination half-life was reduced from 88 to 13.5 hours.[10] In three other patients, the mean dapsone half-life was reduced from 77 ± 23 hours (SEM) to 12.7 ± 0.7 hours (SEM) by the use of MDAC (total dose 80 to 160 g).[11] Although MDAC produced an impressive increase in dapsone elimination, it is unknown whether intervention with MDAC would reduce or prevent the development of methemoglobinemia and hemolytic anemia.

TABLE 6-1 Comparison of Elimination Techniques in Carbamazepine Poisoning		
TREATMENT	**HALF-LIFE (hr)***	**CLEARANCE (mL/min)**
Hemoperfusion	8.6–10.7[7]	80–129[7–9]
MDAC	8.6 ± 2.4[5]	113 ± 44[5]
MDAC	9.5 ± 1.9[6]	105 ± 20[6]

*The normal plasma half-life of carbamazepine after initial dosing is 8 to 72 hours and 12 to 17 hours with multiple dosing.
MDAC, multiple-dose activated charcoal.

Phenobarbital

Phenobarbital has been studied extensively as a candidate for MDAC therapy because it has ideal pharmacokinetic characteristics. Evidence from volunteer[4,12,13] and clinical studies[14–17] supports the efficacy of MDAC in phenobarbital poisoning. Neuvonen and Elonen[4] gave five volunteers MDAC (total dose 101 g) after the oral administration of phenobarbital and found that its mean elimination half-life was reduced from 110 ± 23 hours (SEM) to 19.8 ± 1 hours (SEM) ($P < .05$). The total phenobarbital clearance was increased from 4.6 ± 0.9 mL/min (SEM) to 23 ± 3 mL/min (SEM) ($P < .05$).

In another study, six volunteers were given MDAC (total dose 180 g each) after the intravenous administration of 200 mg of phenobarbital.[12] The mean phenobarbital half-life was reduced from 110 ± 8 hours (SEM) to 45 ± 6 hours (SEM) ($P < .01$), mean total body clearance was increased from 4.4 ± 0.2 mL/kg/hr to 12 ± 1.6 mL/kg/hr ($P < .01$), and nonrenal clearance was increased from 52% to 80% of the total body clearance.

Using a nonrandomized crossover design, Frenia and colleagues[13] compared MDAC (initial dose 50 g, then 25 g every 4 hours) with urine alkalization in the enhancement of phenobarbital elimination in 12 volunteers who were administered phenobarbital intravenously. MDAC reduced the phenobarbital elimination half-life from 148.1 ± 332.1 hours to 18.87 ± 14.71 hours ($P < .005$) and increased the phenobarbital clearance from 2.79 ± 9.69 mL/kg/hr to 19.95 ± 11.55 mL/kg/hr compared with control ($P < .0005$); MDAC was superior to urine alkalization ($P < .0005$) in increasing elimination.

In a randomized study of 10 comatose patients who received either a single dose (50 g) of activated charcoal or MDAC (50 g immediately, then 17 g every 4 hours until extubation), the mean phenobarbital elimination half-life in the MDAC-treated patients was 36 ± 13 hours (SD) compared with 93 ± 52 hours (SD) in the patients who received a single dose of activated charcoal; however, there was no statistical evaluation for this result.[14] In another case series,[15] six patients with moderate-to-severe phenobarbital poisoning were treated with MDAC (the activated charcoal in three of the six patients contained sodium bicarbonate). During the MDAC treatment phase, the mean phenobarbital half-life was 11.7 ± 3.5 hours (SD). This finding is especially notable because the half-life of phenobarbital is extremely long—approximately 110 hours.[4] Additionally, the mean total body clearance was 84 ± 34 mL/min (SD), which is comparable to hemoperfusion, although high-efficiency dialysis was superior (Table 6-2).

Mohammed Ebid and Abdel-Rahman[17] described the impact of MDAC (total dose 275 g) and urine alkalization on phenobarbital elimination in 10 male patients poisoned with phenobarbital (mean plasma phenobarbital concentrations in the two groups were 103.2 ± 12.2 mg/L and 100.6 ± 12.6 mg/L). MDAC reduced the elimination half-life more than urine alkalization (38.6 ± 6.6 hours versus 81.1 ± 14.6 hours) and increased the clearance (10.8 ± 1.8 mL/kg/hr versus 5.1 ± 0.9 mL/kg/hr [equivalent to mean clearances of approximately 12.85 mL/min and 6.34 mL/min]). The mean durations of assisted ventilation (40.2 ± 12.5 hours [SD] versus 79.4 ± 2.9 hours [SD]), intubation (29.4 ± 10.3 hours [SD] versus 54.2 ± 12.8 hours [SD]), and coma (24.4 ± 9.6 hours [SD] versus 50.6 ± 12.5 hours [SD]) were significantly shorter in the group treated with MDAC than in the group treated with urine alkalization. Although this study did not include a control group or a statistical evaluation, MDAC seemed to be superior to urine alkalization.

The use of MDAC (0.7 g/kg) in a severely brain-damaged neonate decreased the serum phenobarbital half-life from a calculated 250 hours to 22 hours.[16] In the critical care setting, supportive care may be sufficient to manage most mild-to-moderate phenobarbital poisonings. In severe phenobarbital poisoning, MDAC is the preferred therapy because it enhances drug clearance without the need for urine alkalization. MDAC also avoids the invasiveness of hemodialysis and hemoperfusion, although high-efficiency hemodialysis gives superior phenobarbital clearances.

Quinine

Data on the effect of MDAC on quinine elimination are limited. One study evaluated the role of MDAC (total dose 200 g) in seven volunteers who were administered quinine bisulfate orally.[22] MDAC decreased the quinine elimination half-life from 8.23 ± 0.57 hours (SD) to 4.55 ± 0.15 hours (SD) (*P* < .001). The quinine clearance was increased from 11.8 ± 1.23 L/hr (SD) to 18.4 ± 2.8 L/hr (SD) (*P* < .001). Compared with a half-life of approximately 26 hours in patients receiving only supportive care,[23] five quinine-poisoned patients who received MDAC had a mean elimination half-life of 8.1 ± 1.1 hours (SD).

Despite the fact that quinine has a relatively large volume of distribution (1.5 to 1.8 L/kg) and is protein bound (70% to 90%), a less than desirable pharmacokinetic profile, MDAC seems to be an effective treatment intervention in quinine poisoning. It has not been determined, however, if morbidity and mortality associated with quinine poisoning are influenced favorably.

Theophylline

Severe theophylline poisoning is associated with significant morbidity and mortality, and MDAC should be considered if vomiting does not preclude its use. Volunteer studies[24–28] confirmed that MDAC decreases the theophylline elimination half-life and increases clearance significantly.

Clinical studies also have shown the effectiveness of MDAC in reducing the theophylline half-life and increasing total body clearance. In one series, the mean serum theophylline half-life was reduced from 23.30 ± 7.95 hours (SD) to 8.0 ± 3.95 hours (SD).[29] No statistical analysis of significance was provided, however. Other studies have reported theophylline half-lives of 4.9 ± 0.8 hours,[30] 2.2 hours,[31] 2.6 hours and 3.2 hours,[32] and 5.6 ± 2.5 hours (SD).[33] Similarly impressive reductions in half-life have been observed in infants.[34,35]

DOSAGE AND ADMINISTRATION

An aqueous slurry of activated charcoal (adults, 50 to 100 g; children, 10 to 25 g) should be administered to the patient as soon as possible.[2] This initial dose should be followed by oral doses at intervals of 1, 2, or 4 hours, depending on the ability of the patient to tolerate the activated charcoal.[2] The dose in adults could be 12.5 g every hour, 25 g every 2 hours, or 50 g every 4 hours. If the patient is not alert and awake, the airway should be protected before the administration of the MDAC via an orogastric tube. If a patient is unable to tolerate the MDAC because of vomiting, an antiemetic should be administered and the dose withheld until the vomiting has ceased. Smaller doses administered every hour instead of a large-volume bolus at 4-hour intervals may reduce the emetic response. Cathartics should *never* be administered during MDAC therapy. The use of cathartics is contraindicated because of the lack of any benefit and the risk of inducing profound fluid and electrolyte imbalance.[2]

COMPLICATIONS

MDAC results rarely in the development of clinically relevant adverse effects. Black stools are to be expected. Activated charcoal is inert pharmacologically, and systemic effects from

---

TABLE 6-2 Comparison of Elimination Techniques in Phenobarbital Poisoning

TREATMENT	CLEARANCE (mL/min)
Endogenous clearance	4[18]
Urine alkalization	7[19]
Hemodialysis	174[20]
Hemoperfusion	79[19,21]
MDAC	84[15]

MDAC, multiple-dose activated charcoal.

its use do no occur. Constipation may occur occasionally, and severe diarrhea may occur when sorbitol-containing activated charcoal products are used. Bowel obstruction has been reported most frequently.[36–39] Respiratory complications have occurred when activated charcoal was aspirated[2] or administered directly into the lungs.[40] Because aqueous activated charcoal does not contain a cathartic, fluid and electrolyte derangement is not expected. The coadministration of cathartics with MDAC therapy may have devastating consequences, however, especially in pediatric patients. Cathartics should not be used in children or adults.

CONCLUSIONS AND RECOMMENDATIONS

MDAC is a viable treatment intervention that has limited application in severely poisoned patients. The best evidence suggests that the elimination of carbamazepine, dapsone, phenobarbital, quinine, and theophylline may be enhanced with MDAC therapy. Although there is insufficient evidence to show that MDAC reduces morbidity and mortality, the elimination half-lives of these drugs are reduced significantly when MDAC therapy is implemented. The total body clearance is enhanced. It is possible that morbidity, mortality, and length of hospital stay may be reduced when MDAC is used appropriately.

REFERENCES

1. Watson WA, Litovitz TL, Rodgers GC, et al: 2002 Annual report of the American Association of Poison Control Centers Toxic Exposure Surveillance System. Am J Emerg Med 21:353–421, 2003.
2. American Academy of Clinical Toxicology, European Association of Poisons Centres and Clinical Toxicologists, Vale JA, Krenzelok EP, Barceloux DG: Position statement and practice guidelines on the use of multi-dose activated charcoal in the treatment of acute poisoning. J Toxicol Clin Toxicol 37:731–751, 1999.
3. Levy G: Gastrointestinal clearance of drugs with activated charcoal. N Engl J Med 307:676–678, 1982.
4. Neuvonen PJ, Elonen E: Effect of activated charcoal on absorption and elimination of phenobarbitone, carbamazepine and phenylbutazone in man. Eur J Clin Pharmacol 17:51–57, 1980.
5. Boldy DAR, Heath A, Ruddock S, et al: Activated charcoal for carbamazepine poisoning. Lancet 1:1027, 1987.
6. Montoya-Cabrera MA, Sauceda-Garcia JM, Escalante-Galindo P, et al: Carbamazepine poisoning in adolescent suicide attempters: Effectiveness of multiple-dose activated charcoal in enhancing carbamazepine elimination. Arch Med Res 27:485–489, 1996.
7. De Groot G, van Heijst ANP, Maes RAA: Charcoal hemoperfusion in the treatment of two cases of acute carbamazepine poisoning. J Toxicol Clin Toxicol 22:349–362, 1984.
8. Nilsson C, Sterner G, Idvall J: Charcoal hemoperfusion for treatment of serious carbamazepine poisoning. Acta Med Scand 216:137–140, 1984.
9. Leslie PJ, Heyworth R, Prescott LF: Cardiac complications of carbamazepine intoxication: Treatment by haemoperfusion. BMJ 286:1018, 1983.
10. Neuvonen PJ, Elonen E, Mattila MJ: Oral activated charcoal and dapsone elimination. Clin Pharmacol Ther 27:823–827, 1980.
11. Neuvonen PJ, Elonen E, Haapanen EJ: Acute dapsone intoxication: Clinical findings and effect of oral charcoal and haemodialysis on dapsone elimination. Acta Med Scand 214:215–220, 1983.
12. Berg MJ, Berlinger WG, Goldberg MJ, et al: Acceleration of the body clearance of phenobarbital by oral activated charcoal. N Engl J Med 307:642–644, 1982.
13. Frenia ML, Schauben JL, Wears RL, et al: Multiple-dose activated charcoal compared to urinary alkalinization for the enhancement of phenobarbital elimination. J Toxicol Clin Toxicol 34:169–175, 1996.
14. Pond SM, Olson KR, Osterloh JD, Tong TG: Randomized study of the treatment of phenobarbital overdose with repeated doses of activated charcoal. JAMA 251:3104–3108, 1984.
15. Boldy DAR, Vale JA, Prescott LF: Treatment of phenobarbitone poisoning with repeated oral administration of activated charcoal. QJM Mon J Assoc Physicians 61:997–1002, 1986.
16. Veerman M, Espejo MG, Christopher MA, Knight M: Use of activated charcoal to reduce elevated serum phenobarbital concentration in a neonate. J Toxicol Clin Toxicol 29:53–58, 1991.
17. Mohammed Ebid A-HI, Abdel-Rahman HM: Pharmacokinetics of phenobarbital during certain enhanced elimination modalities to evaluate their clinical efficacy in management of drug overdose. Ther Drug Monit 23:209–216, 2001.
18. Hardman JG, Limbird LE, Molinoff PB, et al (eds): Goodman and Gilman's The Pharmacological Basis of Therapeutics, 9th ed. New York, McGraw-Hill, 1996.
19. Jacobsen D, Wiik-Larsen E, Dahl T, et al: Pharmacokinetic evaluation of haemoperfusion in phenobarbital poisoning. Eur J Clin Pharmacol 26:109–112, 1984.
20. Palmer BF: Effectiveness of hemodialysis in the extracorporeal therapy of phenobarbital overdose. Am J Kidney Dis 36:640–643, 2000.
21. Raper S, Crome P, Vale A, et al: Experience with activated carbon-bead haemoperfusion columns in the treatment of severe drug intoxication: A preliminary report. Arch Toxicol 49:303–310, 1982.
22. Lockey D, Bateman DN: Effect of oral activated charcoal on quinine elimination. Br J Clin Pharmacol 27:92–94, 1989.
23. Bateman DN, Blain PG, Woodhouse KW, et al: Pharmacokinetics and clinical toxicity of quinine overdosage: Lack of efficacy of techniques intended to enhance elimination. QJM Mon J Assoc Physicians 54:125–131, 1985.
24. Lim DT, Singh P, Nourtsis S, Dela Cruz R: Absorption inhibition and enhancement of elimination of sustained-release theophylline tablets by oral activated charcoal. Ann Emerg Med 15:1303–1307, 1986.
25. Minton NA, Henry JA: Prevention of drug absorption in simulated theophylline overdose. J Toxicol Clin Toxicol 33:43–49, 1995.
26. Goldberg MJ, Spector R, Park GD, et al: The effect of sorbitol and activated charcoal on serum theophylline concentrations after slow-release theophylline. Clin Pharmacol Ther 41:108–111, 1987.
27. Berlinger WG, Spector R, Goldberg MJ, et al: Enhancement of theophylline clearance by oral activated charcoal. Clin Pharmacol Ther 33:351–354, 1983.
28. Mahutte CK, True RJ, Michiels TM, et al: Increased serum theophylline clearance with orally administered activated charcoal. Am Rev Respir Dis 128:820–822, 1983.
29. True RJ, Berman JM, Mahutte CK: Treatment of theophylline toxicity with oral activated charcoal. Crit Care Med 12:113–114, 1984.
30. Radomski L, Park GD, Goldberg MJ, et al: Model for theophylline overdose treatment with oral activated charcoal. Clin Pharmacol Ther 35:402–408, 1984.
31. Davis R, Ellsworth A, Justus RE, Bauer LA: Reversal of theophylline toxicity using oral activated charcoal. J Fam Pract 20:73–74, 1985.
32. Ohning BL, Reed MD, Blumer JL: Continuous nasogastric administration of activated charcoal for the treatment of theophylline intoxication. Pediatr Pharmacol (New York) 5:241–245, 1986.
33. Sessler CN, Glauser FL, Cooper KR: Treatment of theophylline toxicity with oral activated charcoal. Chest 87:325–329, 1985.
34. Amitai Y, Yeung AC, Moye J, Lovejoy FH Jr: Repetitive oral activated charcoal and control of emesis in severe theophylline toxicity. Ann Intern Med 105:386–387, 1986.
35. Shannon M, Amitai Y, Lovejoy FH Jr: Multiple dose activated charcoal for theophylline poisoning in young infants. Pediatrics 80:368–370, 1987.
36. Ray MJ, Padin DR, Condie JD, Halls JM: Small-bowel obstruction secondary to amitriptyline overdose therapy. Dig Dis Sci 33:106–107, 1988.
37. Atkinson SW, Young Y, Trotter GA: Treatment with activated charcoal complicated by gastrointestinal obstruction requiring surgery. BMJ 305:563, 1992.
38. Goulbourne KB, Cisek JE: Small-bowel obstruction secondary to activated charcoal and adhesions. Ann Emerg Med 24:108–110, 1994.
39. Gomez HF, Brent JA, Munoz DC, et al: Charcoal stercolith with intestinal perforation in a patient treated for amitriptyline ingestion. J Emerg Med 12:57–59, 1994.
40. Harris CR, Filandrinos D: Accidental administration of activated charcoal into the lung: Aspiration by proxy. Ann Emerg Med 22:1470–1473, 1993.

CHAPTER 7

Extracorporeal Removal of Toxic Substances

James F. Winchester

Mortality from poisoning is low if poisoning is appropriately managed, even at home.[1] Hospitalized patients, if managed with standard intensive care, also have a low mortality.[2] In certain groups of patients, severe poisoning contributes to a high mortality, however. This chapter discusses the role of alterations of urine pH, advances in dialysis techniques,[3] and specific criteria that should enable the clinician rationally to judge when these techniques should be used in the poisoned patient.

In the 1999 American Association of Poison Control Centers report, Litovitz and colleagues[1] reported that of 2,201,156 reported human exposure cases, decontamination by oral sorbents was used in 1,412,305 (64%) patients. Antidotes were used in 26,740 (1.2%) patients. To effect drug excretion, manipulation of urine pH was done in 7534 (0.34%) patients, and hemodialysis and hemoperfusion were performed in 1082 (0.05%) patients.

MANIPULATION OF URINE pH

Most drugs are weak acids or bases and in solutions exist as nonionized or ionized moieties. The nonionized species are lipid soluble and diffuse across the cell membrane by the process known as *nonionic diffusion*. The ionized form, in contrast, is unable to penetrate lipid membranes. This physical attribute is used to trap drugs within the renal tubule—so-called ion trapping. Glomerular filtration, tubule secretion, and passive tubule reabsorption are the main processes that determine drug excretion. The latter involves a bidirectional movement of drugs across the renal tubule epithelium, limited to lipid-soluble drugs and the nonionized fraction of the drugs that are weak electrolytes. Increasing the pH of tubule fluid increases the degree of ionization of weak acids (Fig. 7-1) and reduces passive free drug absorption by the tubule (Equation 1):

$$\text{HA (weak acid)} \rightarrow \text{A}^- \text{ (poorly absorbed)} + \text{H}^+ \qquad (1)$$

The reverse applies to weak bases (Equation 2):

$$\text{A}^- \text{ (weak base)} \rightarrow \text{AH (well absorbed)} \qquad (2)$$

Figure 7-2 is a schematic based on these chemical equations. The dissociation of a weak acid or base is determined by its dissociation constant (pK_a) (Table 7-1 and Fig. 7-3) and the pH gradient across the tubule membrane.

At a pK_a equal to the pH, the concentrations of nonionized drug and ionized drug are equal (see Fig. 7-1).

Elimination of weak acids with pK_a ranging from 3.0 to 7.5 by the kidney typically is increased, whereas elimination of weak bases is increased in acid urine if the pK_a is 7.5 to 10.5 (Fig. 7-4). This pH-induced increase in renal clearance results in a clinically significant increase in urinary excretion, however, only if the substance is removed substantially by the kidney at normal pH. For substances whose clearance is governed primarily by hepatic metabolism, it is unlikely that any increases in renal excretion, provoked by manipulation of urine pH, would have a marked effect on the amount eliminated from the body. Phencyclidine hydrochloride (PCP) is eliminated primarily by hepatic clearance with low renal elimination. Although acidifying the urine may increase renal elimination of PCP 10-fold, this has little effect on the total body clearance.

Urine alkalization typically is used in attempts to increase the renal clearance of phenobarbital, salicylate, and 2,4-dichloroacetic acid poisoning. Urine acidification may enhance the elimination of quinine, amphetamine, fenfluramine, and PCP. In the case of quinine, acidification may worsen cardiac conduction disturbances and cause dysrhythmias. In the case of amphetamines and PCP, rhabdomyolysis and myoglobinuria may develop. The risk of decreasing the solubility of myoglobin in the urine and precipitating acute renal failure and the small increases in total body clearance mitigates against the use of urine acidification.

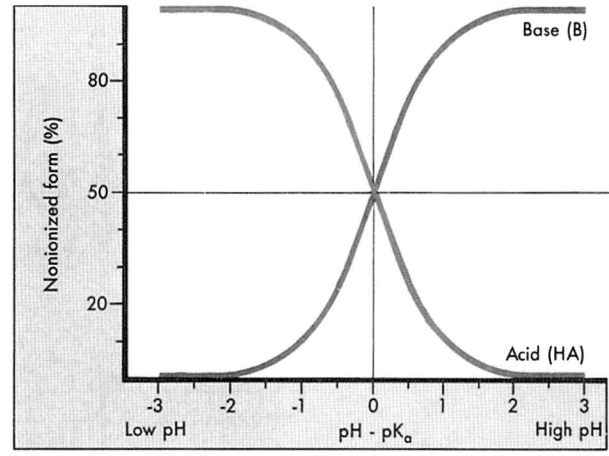

FIGURE 7-1

Degree of acidic or basic drug in nonionized (uncharged) form (B, base; HA, acid) at different pH values, with pH expressed relative to the drug pKa. *(From Brody TM, Larner J, Minneman KP: Human Pharmacology: Molecular to Clinical, 3rd ed. St. Louis, Mosby, 1998.)*

The use of "forced diuresis" may be complicated by the development of hyponatremia, fluid overload, pulmonary edema, cerebral edema, hypokalemia, and either alkalinemia or acidemia, depending on the agent used to promote the diuresis. Rhabdomyolysis with myoglobinuria may cause renal tubular injury in the setting of acidified urine. Severe alkalinemia may precipitate dysrhythmias.

Guidelines to the techniques of manipulation of urine pH have been published.[4] The concept of forced diuresis is based on the mistaken notion that urine volume has a substantial effect on the renal elimination of weak acids or bases. Rather, the major determinant of urinary clearance of these substances is urine pH. Urinary alkalization with intravenous potassium and bicarbonate, in the absence of forced diuresis, significantly enhances salicylate removal.[5] The intravenous fluid used to create an alkaline urine is created by mixing 150 mEq of sodium bicarbonate in 1 liter of 5% dextrose in water. The amount of sodium should not exceed 0.9%. Usually 10 to 20 mEq of potassium chloride also is added per liter. Each liter is given over 1 to 2 hours for the first few hours. Manipulation of urinary pH requires vigilance.[6] Urine pH should be measured at least hourly. Electrolytes should be assessed every 1 to 2 hours. The rate of fluid and bicarbonate administration can be slowed down when the target pH 7.5 or greater is achieved.

EXTRACORPOREAL TECHNIQUES FOR REMOVING POISONS

Techniques for removing substances from blood include dialysis (in its various forms), hemoperfusion, exchange blood transfusion, and plasmapheresis. Today extracorporeal removal is performed mostly for poisoning by methanol, ethylene glycol, lithium, theophylline, salicylates, and phenobarbital.

Principles of Dialysis

Factors governing drug removal are solute (or drug) size, the lipid-water partition coefficient (or lipid solubility), the degree to which the solute is protein bound, its volume of

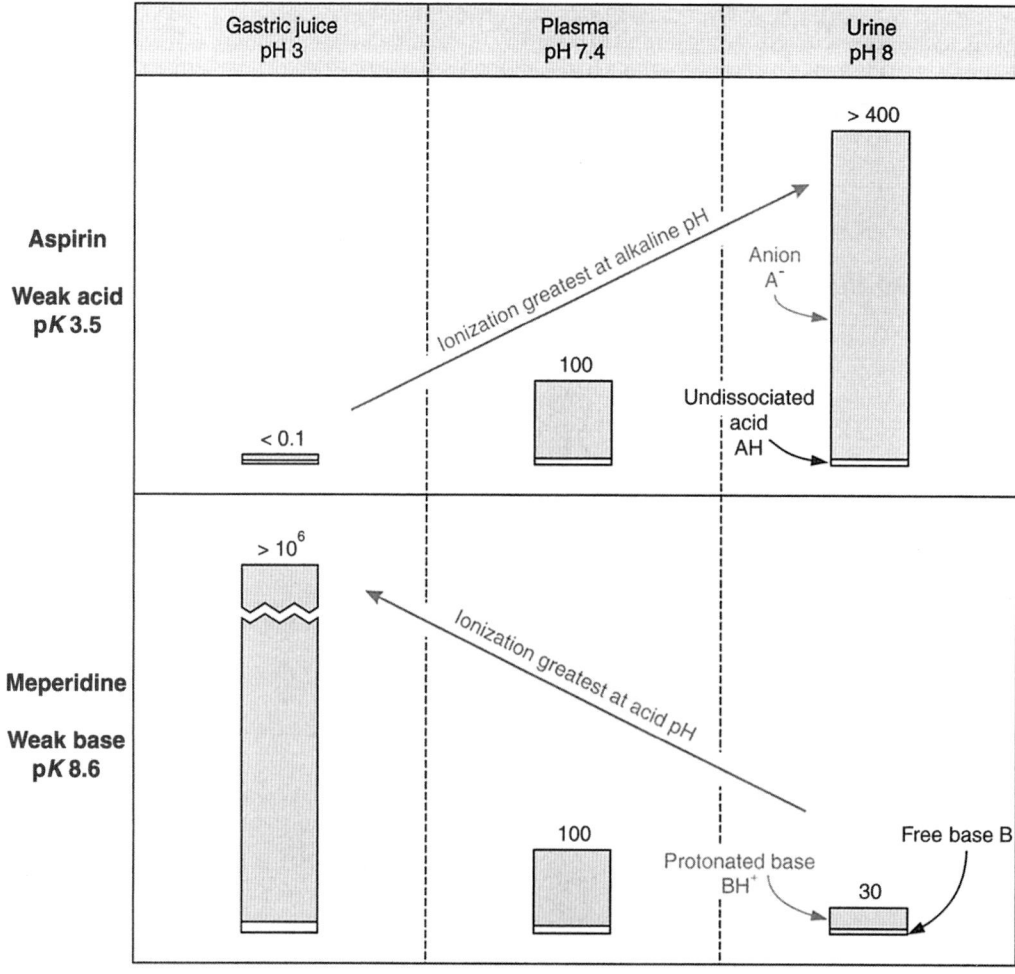

FIGURE 7-2

Theoretical partition of a weak acid (aspirin) and a weak base (meperidine) between aqueous compartments (urine, plasma, and gastric juice) according to the pH difference between them. Numbers represent relative concentrations (total plasma concentration = 100). It is assumed that the uncharged species in each case can permeate the cellular barrier separating the compartment and reach the same concentration in all three. Variations in the fractional ionization as a function of pH give rise to the large total concentration differences with respect to plasma. *(From Rang HP, Dale MM, Ritter JM, Gardner P et al: Pharmacology, 4th ed. New York, Churchill Livingstone, 2001.)*

TABLE 7-1 Dissociation Constants (pKa) of Drugs That Have Increased Urinary Excretion with pH Manipulation

ACIDS		BASES	
Drug	*PKa*	*Drug*	*pKa*
Acetylsalicylic acid	3.49	Amphetamine	9.9
Barbital	7.91	Fenfluramine	9.9
2,4-Dichlorophenoxyacetic acid	2.6	Phencyclidine	8.5
Pentobarbital	8.2	Quinidine	8.4
Phenobarbital	7.2	Quinine	8.4
Salicylic acid	3.0		

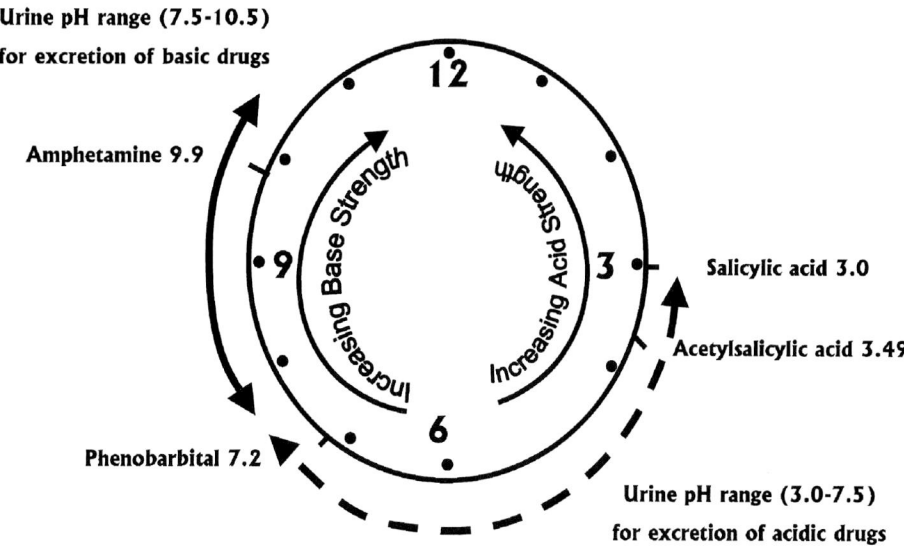

FIGURE 7-3

Values for pKa for some acidic and basic drugs. *(From Rang HP, Dale MM, Ritter JM, Gardner P et al: Pharmacology, 4th ed. New York, Churchill Livingstone, 2001.)*

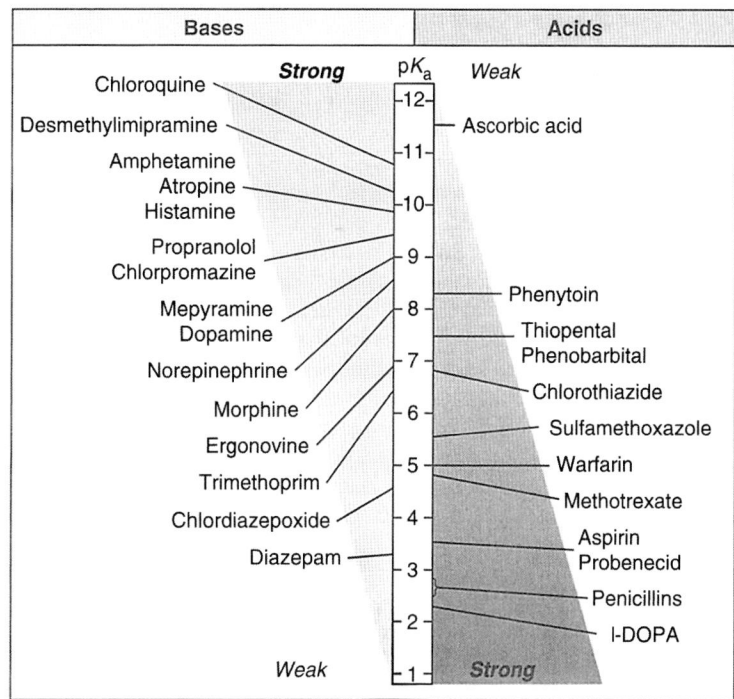

FIGURE 7-4

Urine pH ranges for enhanced excretion of weak acids and weak bases: pK$_a$ values for representative drugs are given. See Table 7-1.

distribution, and the maintenance of a concentration gradient.[7] Small uncharged molecular weight substances readily cross membranes and are usually dialyzable. Water-soluble substances with small volumes of distribution are contained in the blood compartment and are accessible for extracorporeal removal. Highly protein-bound substances may be removed more quickly by hemoperfusion.

Peritoneal dialysis uses the natural lining of the abdominal cavity; hemodialysis uses artificial semipermeable membranes to achieve solute (substance) removal. All forms of dialysis depend on the existence of a concentration gradient between plasma and dialysis fluid, which allows diffusion of substance into the dialysis fluid. Employing ultrafiltration of water through the membrane (with osmotic agents in peritoneal dialysis and hydraulic pressure in hemodialysis), substance removal accompanies the ultrafiltrate in the process of "solvent drag." Drug or chemical removal also may be increased by continuous arteriovenous hemofiltration (CAVH), continuous arteriovenous hemodialysis (CAVHD), continuous venovenous hemofiltration (CVVH), and continuous venovenous hemodialysis (CVVHD) modifications of the hemodialysis process, as follows: continuous (C), arterial (A) or venous (V) blood, hemofiltered/ultrafiltered (H) or ultrafiltered/dialyzed (D), at high rates through membranes that have a pore structure larger than conventional dialysis membranes,[8] rapidly or slowly over a continuous 24-hour period.[9] Peritoneal dialysis is much less efficient than hemodialysis.

Substance removal depends not only on the characteristics of the substance but also on physical factors of the specific dialyzer used. The physical factors governing substance removal by the dialyzer itself depend on blood flow rate through the dialyzer, dialysate flow rate, dialyzer surface area, and the characteristics of the specific membrane chosen. Substance removal is limited by the membrane area times the permeability. The clearance of solute from the blood is determined by Equation 3:

$$\text{Clearance} = Q_b \cdot (A - V)/A \qquad (3)$$

A is the arterial (inlet) concentration and *V* is the venous (outlet) concentration of drug going through the dialyzer. Q_b is the blood flow rate (mL/min) through the dialyzer. The ratio A − V/A also equates to the drug extraction ratio. In modern medicine, hemodialysis is performed with large-pore membrane dialyzers (as are CAVH, CAVHD, CVVH, and CVVHD, which rely on ultrafiltration for solute and fluid removal), which are highly efficient at removing drugs.[10] Highly porous membranes (e.g., polysulfone) may obviate the need for hemoperfusion because the pore structure more easily allows passage of the drug compared with conventional membranes (e.g., cuprophane).

Redistribution or rebound is a common phenomenon that may complicate extracorporeal removal. Using appropriate pharmacokinetic models, it has been shown that hemoperfusion increases drug elimination rates (k_{el}) in animals intoxicated with acetaminophen, amobarbital, ethchlorvynol, doxorubicin, digoxin, and digitoxin. In all these experiments and in clinical experience, it has been observed that "rebound" of drug concentration occurs after hemoperfusion as drug redistributes from the tissues back into the plasma after its removal from the plasma compartment. This phenomenon is consistent with pharmacokinetic handling of drugs after their removal from the central compartment, but

clinically the patient may return to coma, as occurs after hemoperfusion for glutethimide poisoning.

Peritoneal Dialysis

Because of its relative inefficiency, peritoneal dialysis should be used for treating dialyzable poisons only if the other methods are unavailable. One exception is the small infant in whom blood volume may be too small to allow hemodialysis or hemoperfusion. In most cases, however, using modern techniques, all but the smallest of infants can be hemodialyzed. In the poisoned hypothermic patient, peritoneal dialysis with preheated solutions increases core temperature.

Hemodialysis

Hemodialysis (Fig. 7-5) generally requires anticoagulation by heparin (most commonly), citrate, or prostacyclin. In certain situations, nonanticoagulated blood can be used, but this requires special skills on the part of the dialysis nurse and requires fairly high blood flow rates (>200 to 300 mL/min). Arterial or venous blood is pumped through the devices with a roller pump, or, in the case of CAVH, an arteriovenous shunt supplies blood at intraarterial blood pressure and flow rate.

Medications that are removed by hemodialysis (or hemoperfusion), such as most pressor agents, should be infused at sites distal to dialyzers (or hemoperfusion devices) to ensure bioavailability. Dialysate regeneration sorbent systems theoretically may become saturated with drugs, and for certain drugs removal rates then decrease over time. There may be a lower clearance rate for continuous dialysis methods than for standard episodic hemodialysis. Because continuous techniques may be used over prolonged periods, however, greater drug removal may be achieved *over time* compared with standard hemodialysis. This may not be a desirable clinical goal, however, if rapid reversal of a poison is necessary (e.g., reversal of coma or hypotension as a result of severe barbiturate or salicylate poisoning).

Sorbent Hemoperfusion

Hemoperfusion (see Fig. 7-5) is the method by which anticoagulated blood is passed through a column containing sorbent

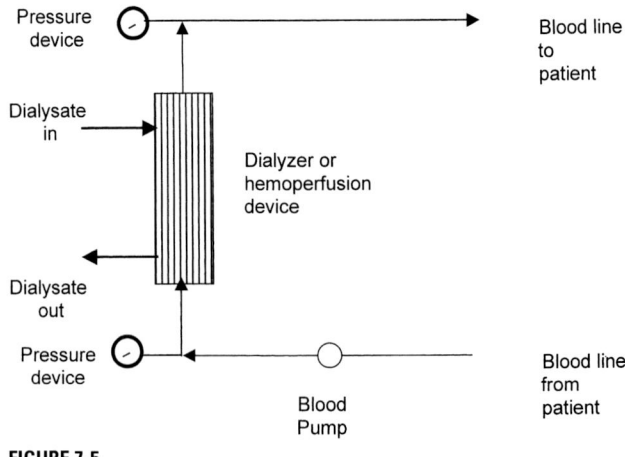

FIGURE 7-5

Typical dialysis or hemoperfusion circuit.

TABLE 7-2 Available Hemoperfusion Devices				
MANUFACTURER	**DEVICE**	**SORBENT TYPE**	**AMOUNT OF SORBENT**	**POLYMER COATING**
Clark (Folsom, LA)	Biocompatible system	Charcoal	50, 100, 250 mL	Heparinized polymer
Gambro (Stockholm, Sweden)	Adsorba	Norit	100 or 300 g	Cellulose acetate
Nextron Medical (Fairfied, NJ)	Hemosorba CH-350	Petroleum-based spherical charcoal	170 g	Polyhema

particles.[11–13] Activated charcoal particles and resin beads (with or without ligands) contained in the hemoperfusion devices have been used. In addition, antibiotic-coated fibers or antibody-coated or antigen-coated particle hemoperfusion devices have been constructed for the removal of specific toxins.[14–16] Platelet depletion is the main side effect of uncoated charcoal (carbon) hemoperfusion; substantial improvement is achieved by coating the particle surface with a thin hemocompatible membrane. Carbon is efficient at removing lipid-soluble and water-soluble drugs, whereas certain resins are most effective for removing lipid-soluble drugs. Clinically available hemoperfusion devices and their contained sorbents are listed in Table 7-2.

Hemoperfusion uses the physical process of drug adsorption for efficiency, and in many instances drug removal is superior to hemodialysis, peritoneal dialysis, or manipulation of urinary pH. Water-soluble and lipid-soluble substances with molecular weights ranging from 113 to 40,000 d may be adsorbed. Substances at higher molecular weights are adsorbed less efficiently if coated with a biocompatible polymer coating,[17] unless special techniques for coating are employed.[18]

Amanita phalloides and acetaminophen poisoning may result in fulminant hepatic failure.[19–21] Hemoperfusion has been used in the management of these patients (see Chapters 55 and 120 for a further discussion). Table 7-5 lists representative drugs that have been reported to be removed by dialysis or hemoperfusion; in many cases, enhanced drug elimination or decreased coma time in response to treatment has been observed.[22–25]

Using Hemodialysis or Hemoperfusion in Poisoning

The clinical criteria for considering hemodialysis are summarized in Table 7-3. Plasma concentrations above which hemodialysis or hemoperfusion should be considered are given in Table 7-4. Table 7-5 provides a more extensive list of substances that are at least theoretically dialyzable or adsorbable. Table 7-6 is a guide to choosing either hemoperfusion or hemodialysis. The indications for extracorporeal removal of specific substances are discussed further in other relevant chapters.

Plasma Exchange and Exchange Blood Transfusion

Plasma exchange (plasmapheresis)[26] is most applicable to strongly protein-bound drugs not well removed with hemodialysis (e.g., chromic acid and chromate poisoning).

Exchange blood transfusion has been used when hemolysis and methemoglobinemia have complicated the poisoning (e.g., sodium chlorate poisoning), whereas plasma exchange with subsequent plasma perfusion over sorbents has been used in a variety of poisons.

IMMUNOPHARMACOLOGY IN POISONING

Pharmaceutical poisoning treated by immunopharmacology presently is limited to digoxin poisoning, although immunotherapies for other poisonings are under development. In digoxin poisoning, the elimination half-time of digoxin in anephric patients can be reduced substantially with the addition of hemoperfusion. Potentially fatal cases of digoxin poisoning have been treated successfully by Fab antibody fragments, but failures also have been reported. The cost of treatment averages $1680 (range $175 to $7000).[27] Immobilized antibody on hemoperfusion devices may offer an alternative.[28] In dialysis patients (in whom vascular access facilitates interventional therapy), a judgment to use either hemoperfusion or Fab antibody fragments is required. Recrudescence of digoxin poisoning has been reported 24 to 48 hours after receiving Fab antibodies in renal failure patients[29] (see Chapter 33 for a more detailed discussion).

An experimental hemoperfusion system used immobilized avidin for selective removal of biotinylated therapeutic antibodies from rats.[30] Two antibodies, ovine antidigoxin Fab fragment and murine 8A1 against *Escherichia coli* J5 lipopolysaccharide endotoxin, were biotinylated using biotin-long-chain-*N*-hydroxysuccinimide ester. The half-lives and areas under the time versus concentration curves of

TABLE 7-3 Clinical Considerations for Hemodialysis or Hemoperfusion in Poisoning
Progressive deterioration despite intensive supportive therapy
Severe intoxication with depression of midbrain function leading to hypoventilation, hypothermia, and hypotension
Development of complications of coma, such as pneumonia or septicemia, and underlying conditions predisposing to such complications (e.g., obstructive airway disease)
Impairment of normal drug excretory function in the presence of hepatic, cardiac, or renal insufficiency
Intoxication with agents with metabolic and/or delayed effects (e.g., methanol, ethylene glycol, and paraquat)
Intoxication with an extractable drug or poison, which can be removed at a rate exceeding endogenous elimination by liver or kidney

TABLE 7-4 Plasma Concentration* of Common Poisons in Excess of Which Hemodialysis or Hemoperfusion Should Be Considered

DRUG	CONCENTRATION (μg/mL)	CONCENTRATION (mmol/L)	METHOD OF CHOICE
Phenobarbital	100	430	HP > HD
Other barbiturates	50	200	HP
Glutethimide	40	160	HP
Methaqualone	40	160	HP
Salicylates	800	5000	HD
Theophylline	400	2200	HP > HD
Paraquat	0.1	0.5	HP > HD
Ethylene glycol	50		HD
Methanol	50		HD
Lithium, long-term		2.0	HD
Lithium, short-term		4.0	HD

*Suggested concentrations only; clinical condition may warrant intervention at lower concentrations (e.g., in mixed intoxications).
HD, hemodialysis; HP, hemoperfusion.

TABLE 7-5 Drugs and Chemicals Removed with Dialysis and Hemoperfusion*

Barbiturates
Amobarbital
Butabarbital
Hexabarbital
Pentobarbital
Phenobarbital[†]
Quinalbital
Secobarbital
Thiopental
Vinalbital

Analgesics
Acetaminophen
Acetylsalicylic acid
Colchicine
d-Propoxyphyene
Methylsalicylate
Phenylbutazone
Salicylic acid

Nonbarbiturate Hypnotics and Tranquilizers
Carbromal
Chloral hydrate

Chlorpromazine
(Diazepam)
Diphenhydramine
Ethchlorvynol
Meprobamate
Methaqualone
Valproate

Inorganics and Alcohols
Ethanol
Ethylene glycol
Isopropanol
Methanol
Polychlorinated
  biphenyls
Paraquat
Parathion

Antimicrobials and Anticancer Agents
Ampicillin
Carbenicillin
Tetracycline

Isoniazid
Chloramphenicol
Chloroquine
Clindamycin
Dapsone
(Doxorubicin)
Carmustine

Cardiovascular
β-Blockers
Captopril
(Digoxin)
Diltiazem
(Disopyramide)
Flecainide
Metoprolol
N-Acetyl-procainamide
Procainamide
Quinidine

Antidepressants
(Amitriptyline)
(Imipramine)
(Tricyclics)[†]

Metals and Others
(Aluminum)
Cimetidine
Diquat
(Lead)
Lithium
Methylmercury
  complex
Paraquat
Sodium chlorate
Theophylline
(Phencyclidine)
Phenols
(Podophyllin)
Herbicides
Solvents, gases
Insecticides
Carbon tetrachloride
Amanitin
Ethylene oxide

Note. Agents in parentheses are not well removed or required a chelating agent.
*For more detail, see Winchester and Kitiyakara.[31]
[†]More recent clinical success with highly efficient dialysis or hemoperfusion.

TABLE 7-6 Choice of Hemodialysis or Hemoperfusion for Certain Drugs

HEMODIALYSIS	HEMOPERFUSION
Lithium	Lipid-soluble drugs
Bromide	Barbiturates
Ethanol	Nonbarbiturate hypnotics,
Methanol	sedatives, and tranquilizers
Ethylene glycol	Digitalis glycosides
Salicylates	

the biotinylated antibodies were reduced significantly after hemoperfusion over immobilized avidin. Future pharmaceuticals could be engineered such that they may be bioretrievable with such a hemoperfusion system.

CONCLUSION

Currently, extracorporeal removal rarely is required in the management of critically poisoned patients. Extracorporeal removal is a procedure with some risks associated with its use. When possible, it is recommended to consult with a nephrologist, medical toxicologist, or a regional certified poison center when considering any of these procedures in a critically poisoned patient.

REFERENCES

1. Litovitz TL, Klein-Schwartz W, White S, et al: 1999 Annual Report of the American Association of Poison Control Centers Toxic Exposure Surveillance System. Am J Emerg Med 18:517–574, 2000.
2. Clemmesen C, Nilsson E: Therapeutic trends in the treatment of barbiturate poisoning: The Scandinavian method. Clin Pharmacol Ther 2:220, 1961.
3. Jacobs C, Kjellstrand CM, Koch KM, Winchester JF (eds): Replacement of Renal Function by Dialysis, 4th ed. Dordrecht, Kluwer, 1996.
4. Winchester JF. Active methods for detoxification. In Haddad LM, Shannon MW, Winchester JF (eds): Clinical Management of Poisoning and Drug Overdose, 3rd ed. Philadelphia, WB Saunders, 1997, p 175.
5. Prescott LF, Balali-Mood M, Critchley JA, et al: Diuresis or urinary alkalinization in salicylate poisoning? BMJ 285:1383–1386, 1982.
6. Gabow PA, Peterson LN: Disorders of potassium metabolism. In Schrier RW (ed): Renal and Electrolyte Disorders, 2nd ed. Boston, Little, Brown, 1980, p 183.
7. Maher JF: Principles of dialysis and dialysis of drugs. Am J Med 62:475, 1977.
8. Henderson LW, Silverstein MAE, Ford CA, Lysaght MJ: Clinical response to maintenance hemodiafiltration. Kidney Int 7:S52, 1975.
9. Kaplan AA: Continuous arteriovenous hemofiltration and related therapies. In Jacobs C, Kjellstrand CM, Koch KM, Winchester JF (eds): Replacement of Renal Function by Dialysis, 4th ed. Dordrecht, Kluwer, 1996, p 390.
10. Palmer BF: Effectiveness of hemodialysis in the extracorporeal therapy of phenobarbital overdose. Am J Kidney Dis 36:640–643, 2000.
11. Hampel G, Crome P, Widdop B, Goulding R: Experience with fixed-bed charcoal haemoperfusion in the treatment of severe drug intoxication. Arch Toxicol 45:133, 1980.
12. Gelfand MC, Winchester JF, Knepshield JH, et al: Charcoal hemoperfusion in severe drug overdosage. Trans ASAIO 23:599, 1977.
13. Verpooten GA, De Broe ME: Combined hemoperfusion/hemodialysis in severe poisoning: Kinetics of drug extraction. Resuscitation 11:275, 1984.
14. Terman DS, Buffaloe G, Mattioli C, et al: Extracorporeal immunoabsorption: Initial experience in human systemic lupus erythematosus. Lancet 2:824, 1979.
15. Hakim RM, Milford E, Himmelfarb J, et al: Extracorporeal removal of anti-HLA antibodies in transplant candidates. Am J Kidney Dis 16:423–431, 1990.
16. Anspach FB, Petschl D: Membrane adsorbers for selective endotoxin removal from protein solutions. Process Biochem 35:1005–1012, 2000.
17. Denti E, Luboz MP, Tessore V: Adsorption characteristics of cellulose acetate coated charcoals. J Biomed Mater Res 9:143, 1975.
18. Ronco C, Brendolan A, Winchester JF, et al: First clinical experience with an adjunctive hemoperfusion device designed specifically to remove beta(2)-microglobulin in hemodialysis. Blood Purif 19:260–263, 2001.
19. Mullins ME, Horowitz BZ: The futility of hemoperfusion and hemodialysis in Amanita phalloides poisoning. Vet Hum Toxicol 42:90–91, 2000.
20. Kaplan AA, Epstein M: Extracorporeal blood purification in the management of patients with hepatic failure. Semin Nephrol 17:576–582, 1997.
21. Aji DY, Caliskan S, Nayir A, et al: Haemoperfusion in Amanita phalloides poisoning. J Trop Pediatr 41:371–374, 1995.
22. Maher JF, Schreiner GE: The dialysis of poison and drugs. Trans ASAIO 13:369, 1967.
23. Hadden J, Johnson K, Smith S, et al: Acute barbiturate intoxication: Concepts in management. JAMA 209:893, 1969.
24. Winchester JF, Gelfand MC, Tilstone WJ: Hemoperfusion in drug intoxication: Clinical and laboratory aspects. Drug Metab Rev 8:69, 1978.
25. Winchester JF, Rahman A, Tilstone WJ, et al: Will hemoperfusion be useful for cancer chemotherapeutic drug removal? Clin Toxicol 17:557–569, 1980.
26. Gurland HJ, Samtleben W, Lysaght MJ, Winchester JF: Extracorporeal blood purification techniques: Plasmapheresis and hemoperfusion. In Jacobs C, Kjellstrand CM, Koch KM, Winchester JF (eds): Replacement of Renal Function by Dialysis, 4th ed. Dordrecht, Kluwer, 1996, p 472.
27. Martiny SS, Phelps SJ, Massey KL: Treatment of severe digitalis intoxication with digoxin-specific antibody fragments: A clinical review. Crit Care Med 16:629, 1988.
28. Savin H, Marcus L, Margel S, et al: Treatment of adverse digitalis effects by hemoperfusion through columns containing antidigoxin antibodies bound to agarose polyacrolein microsphere beads. Am Heart J 113:1078, 1987.
29. Ujhelyi MR, Robert S, Cummings DM, et al: Disposition of digoxin immune Fab in patients with kidney failure. Clin Pharmacol Ther 54:388–394, 1993.
30. Burkhart KK, Beard D, Billingsley ML: Enhanced elimination of biotinylated antibodies by avidin-based hemoperfusion in rats. J Pharmacol Exp Ther 270:356–361, 1994.
31. Winchester JF, Kitiyakara C: Use of dialysis and hemoperfusion in treatment of poisoning. In Daugirdas JT, Blake PG, Ing TG (eds): Handbook of Dialysis, 3rd ed. Boston, Little, Brown, 2001, pp 263–277.

CHAPTER 8

Common Complications in the Critically Poisoned Patient

Donna L. Seger

Demographically, poisoned patients admitted to the intensive care unit (ICU) differ from other ICU patients. In general, poisoned patients are younger, have fewer comorbidities, and are free of traumatic or infectious complications. Poisoned patients are at risk, however, for a variety of secondary adverse effects related to their poisonings. This chapter provides a brief overview of the complications commonly encountered in poisoned patients. For an encyclopedic discussion of the various complications that may be encountered, the reader is referred to standard textbooks of intensive care medicine. A brief discussion of some of the more common complications in poisoned patients and treatment considerations follows.

ASPIRATION PNEUMONITIS

Aspiration pneumonitis occurs in approximately 10% of patients who are admitted to hospitals after an overdose.[1,2] The term *aspiration pneumonitis* is frequently confused with the term *aspiration pneumonia*, although clinically and pathophysiologically these are different syndromes with their own therapeutic implications. *Aspiration pneumonitis* refers to the acute pulmonary response that occurs after the pulmonary deposition of gastric contents. Originally called *Mendelson's syndrome* (based on the pioneering studies of Mendelson), aspiration pneumonitis is now known to be a consequence of a decreased level of consciousness.[3,4] Protection of the airway in patients who may have an inadequate gag reflex as a consequence of poisoning is paramount. This protection should be obtained by standard endotracheal intubation with a high-volume, low-pressure tube rather than by laryngeal mask airway because it is not known if the latter technique provides an equivalent measure of protection in these patients. Poisoned patients are at a higher risk than other critically ill intubated patients for the development of aspiration syndromes,[5] and aggressive airway management should be a primary objective in these patients. During mechanical ventilation, simply elevating the head of the bed provides some protection against aspiration of gastric contents.[6]

Gastric contents are generally sterile, and their aspiration is not typically associated with microbial infection. Gastric acid causes inflammation, however, which activates neutrophils and complement.[7] Acid aspiration can lead to widespread pulmonary injury characterized by pulmonary alveolar hemorrhage, exudation and edema, atelectasis, loss of airway epithelium (including that of the trachea) with consequent loss of normal ciliary defenses, neutrophil infiltration into the alveolar airspace, and necrosis of type I and type II alveolar cells.[8,9] The edema causes intrapulmonary shunting, hypoxemia, and decreased pulmonary compliance.

Acid aspiration and hypoxemia may cause pulmonary vasoconstriction and an abrupt increase in pulmonary vascular resistance. The pathophysiology of this response is complex and has been reviewed in detail by Boysen and Modell.[10] This rise in pulmonary vascular resistance may cause acute right-sided heart failure.

Aspirated food particles may serve as a nidus of infection and as foreign bodies capable of inducing an inflammatory response and granuloma formation. Larger particulates may cause airway obstruction. Significant food particulates should be removed bronchoscopically.

The classic studies done in the 1940s by Mendelson[11] on obstetric patients suggested that aspiration pneumonitis is due to the acidity of gastric contents. Acid-induced injury occurs immediately on contact, so there is no benefit from attempts to neutralize the pH. Subsequent studies reported that the two major factors determining the degree of aspiration pneumonitis are the gastric pH and the volume of aspirated material.[7] The consensus is that a volume of aspiration of at least 20 mL (or 0.4 to 0.8 mL/kg) and a pH less than 2.5 are required for aspiration pneumonitis to occur, although the absolutism implicit in these criteria has been questioned.[12]

Activated charcoal is frequently administered to poisoned patients. Because activated charcoal is an inert substance, it has been believed that lung injury occurring after aspiration in overdose patients was caused by gastric contents. Experimental data reveal that this is not the case, that charcoal itself may play a role. Earlier animal experiments showed that aspiration of gastric contents causes neutrophils to release neutrophil-elastase, which increases pulmonary vascular permeability.[13] More recent animal experiments show, however, that activated charcoal does not cause neutrophil-mediated lung injury.[14] In vitro evidence reveals that the process of phagocytosis of inorganic particles activates alveolar macrophages; this may be the case when activated charcoal is instilled in the lung. Alveolar macrophages are a potent source of oxygen radicals, proteases, and inflammatory leukokines.[15] After instillation of activated charcoal, lung histology reveals charcoal obstruction of small distal airways interspersed with unobstructed airways. Overdistention of alveolar segments in areas not occluded by charcoal leads to volutrauma in those areas, which increases microvascular permeability.[14] Charcoal aspiration should not be considered innocuous.

Although it is generally assumed that aspiration pneumonitis frequently leads to aspiration pneumonia and should be treated with antibiotics, this progression has not been studied in any detail. Diagnosis of true aspiration pneumonia is difficult because the inflammation associated with a nonbacterial pneumonitis syndrome can cause alveolar pulmonary infiltrates, elevated white blood cell counts, hypoxemia, respiratory alkalosis, and fever.[16] Severe aspiration pneumonitis may lead to adult respiratory distress syndrome (ARDS).[17] Antibiotics should be reserved for patients with clinical and radiographic signs of aspiration pneumonitis if it fails to resolve in 48 hours.[7]

Until more recently, anaerobic organisms were assumed to be responsible for aspiration pneumonia. More recent studies, reviewed by Marik,[7] have shown that aerobes are of greater importance. Recommendations for antibiotic therapy are presented in Table 8-1. Two multicenter randomized clinical trials have failed to show a beneficial effect of corticosteroids in the treatment of aspiration syndromes,[18,19] and they are not recommended. This lack of benefit of corticosteroids is supported by animal studies suggesting that this treatment may predispose to gram-negative pneumonia.[20] The treatment of aspiration pneumonitis should consist of endotracheal suctioning, mechanical ventilatory support, and bronchoscopy, if necessary. Bronchoscopy may be beneficial if there is evidence of significant atelectasis.[21] Endotracheal suctioning is most beneficial if done early, before the aspirated material disperses to distal airways and the alveoli.

Positive end-expiratory pressure (PEEP) or continuous positive airway pressure may improve oxygenation by reducing pulmonary edema and decreasing the intrapulmonary shunting. Although PEEP (or continuous positive airway pressure) may decrease systemic venous return and cardiac out-put, these measures also may increase lung volumes and oxygenation, decreasing pulmonary vascular resistance and enhancing pump performance. The response to these induced increases in airway pressures should be evaluated carefully in each patient, and adjustment should be made based on changes in oxygenation, cardiac parameters, and urine production. The use of PEEP and continuous positive airway pressure should be restricted to the minimum necessary to achieve adequate oxygenation. Patients with aspiration syndromes seem to be at enhanced risk of pulmonary barotrauma, possibly as a result of acid-induced tissue injury or overdistention of some alveoli secondary to foreign body.[20]

ADULT RESPIRATORY DISTRESS SYNDROME

Definition

ARDS is a clinical syndrome of acute lung injury. Historically, ARDS was defined as respiratory distress with cyanosis refractory to oxygen therapy, decreased lung compliance, and diffuse radiographic pulmonary infiltrates.[22,23] ARDS currently is defined by the following criteria:[24]

Acute onset
Arterial oxygen tension-to-fraction of inspired oxygen (FiO_2) ratio less than 200 mm Hg (regardless of PEEP)
Bilateral infiltrates on frontal chest radiograph
Pulmonary capillary wedge pressure less than 18 mm Hg when measured or no clinical evidence of left atrial hypertension[24]

Simply defined, ARDS is a syndrome of increased vascular permeability and progressive fibrosis in the lung.

Syndrome

Progressive respiratory distress is associated with distinct clinical, radiographic, and histologic manifestations. Acutely, arterial hypoxemia refractory to supplemental oxygen causes rapid onset of respiratory failure in a patient with risk factors for ARDS (Table 8-2). Pulmonary edema, the hallmark of the initial injury, is caused by endothelial injury and increased vascular permeability.[25] Surfactant activity and production are reduced. Chest radiograph reveals bilateral infiltrates with a ground-glass appearance (Figs. 8-1 and 8-2).[26]

If resolution does not occur, progressive fibrosing alveolitis causes ventilation/perfusion mismatching (shunting) and hypoxemia (Fig. 8-3). Hypercapnia replaces normocapnia (or hypocapnia) as dead space increases from bulla

TABLE 8-1 Recommended Treatment Regimens for Aspiration Pneumonia*

PATIENT	RECOMMENDED TREATMENT
Healthy community-dwelling	Levofloxacin or ceftriaxone
Resident of long-term care facility	Levofloxacin, piperacillin/tazobactam, or ceftazidime
Alcoholic, severe periodontal disease, putrid sputum	Piperacillin/tazobactam, imipenem or both *or* Levofloxacin, ciprofloxacin, or ceftriaxone[†]

*The following are recommended adult doses, which should be adjusted for patients with renal insufficiency:
Levofloxacin, 500 mg/day
Ceftriaxone, 1–2 g/day
Ciprofloxacin, 400 mg q12h
Piperacillin/tazobactam, 3.375 g q12h
Ceftazidime, 2 g q8h
Imipenem, 0.5–1 g q6–8h
Clindamycin, 600 mg q8h
Metronidazole, 500 mg q8h
[†]Clindamycin or metronidazole should be added.
Modified from Marik PE: Aspiration pneumonitis and aspiration pneumonia. N Engl J Med 344:665–671, 2001.

TABLE 8-2 Risk Factors for Adult Respiratory Distress Syndrome

DIRECT LUNG INJURIES	INDIRECT INJURIES
Gastric aspiration	Sepsis
Pneumonia	Trauma with shock
Near-drowning	Multiple transfusions
Pulmonary contusion	Drug overdose
Fat emboli	

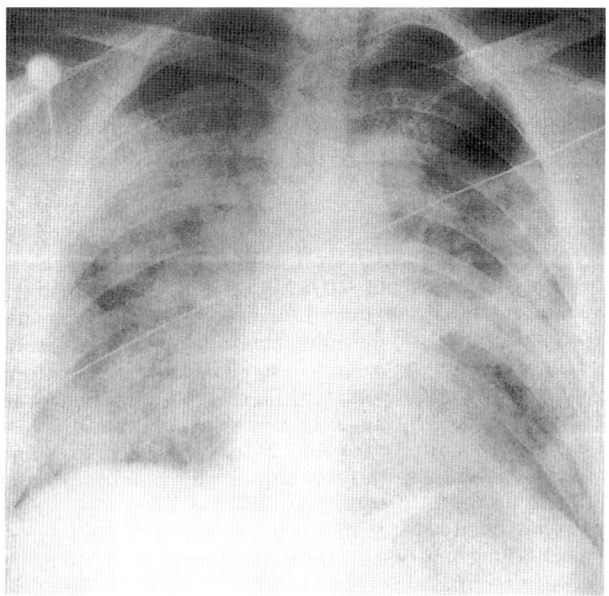

FIGURE 8-1

Early exudative phase of adult respiratory distress syndrome. This chest radiograph, obtained immediately before intubation, shows widespread, patchy, bilateral infiltrates. *(From Hansen-Flaschen JH: Adult respiratory distress syndrome: Clinical features. In Carlson RW, Geheb MA [eds]: Principles and Practice of Medical Intensive Care. Philadelphia, WB Saunders, 1993, p 822.)*

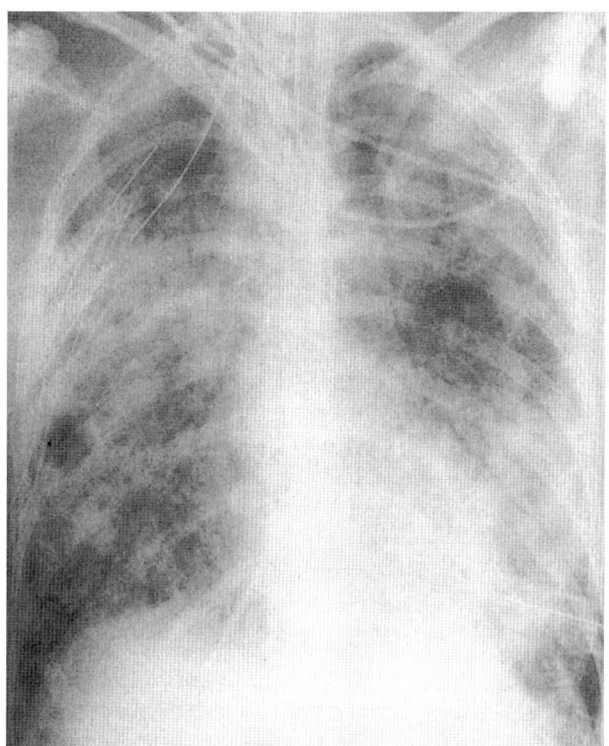

FIGURE 8-2

Proliferative and fibrotic phase of adult respiratory distress syndrome. Coarse, reticular infiltrates are seen in some areas; ground-glass opacities predominate in other areas. The right lower lobe contains a salt-and-pepper infiltrate. A small subpleural air cyst is present in the right midlung field. *(From Hansen-Flaschen JH: Adult respiratory distress syndrome: Clinical features. In Carlson RW, Geheb MA [eds]: Principles and Practice of Medical Intensive Care. Philadelphia, WB Saunders, 1993, p 823.)*

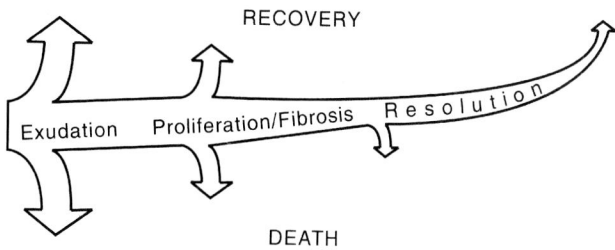

FIGURE 8-3

Adult respiratory distress syndrome tends to evolve along a similar pathway regardless of cause, although many patients leave this path along the way to recover or to die. *(From Hansen-Flaschen JH: Adult respiratory distress syndrome: Clinical features. In Carlson RW, Geheb MA [eds]: Principles and Practice of Medical Intensive Care. Philadelphia, WB Saunders, 1993, p 820.)*

formation, fibrosis, and vascular obliteration.[27] As the pulmonary capillary bed is obliterated, pulmonary hypertension may become severe. Chest radiograph then reveals linear opacities (fibrosis) and occasionally pneumothorax.[28]

Histologically, one initially sees alveolar edema, hemorrhage, hyaline membranes, neutrophilic alveolitis, and diffuse alveolar damage (Fig. 8-4). About 1 week later, a proliferative phase follows, characterized by inflammation, fibrosis, regional loss of lobular and alveolar architecture, cyst formation, and local emphysema (Figs. 8-5 through 8-7).[29]

Treatment

There are no specific treatments to decrease the vascular permeability and slow the progressive inflammatory process. Mechanical ventilation, changing patient position, and meticulous attention to fluid balance are aspects of supportive care that may improve outcome.

By reversing life-threatening hypoxemia and decreasing the work of breathing, mechanical ventilation allows the

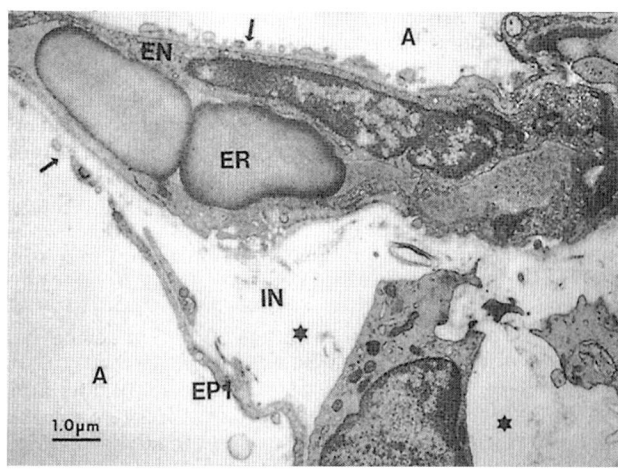

FIGURE 8-4

Exudative phase of adult respiratory distress syndrome. Electron micrograph shows fragmentation *(arrow)* of epithelial cells (EPI) and accumulation of edema fluid *(asterisk)* within the interstitial spaces (IN) of an alveolar wall. A, alveolar space; EN, endothelial cell; ER, erythrocytes within a capillary lumen. *(From Hansen-Flaschen JH: Adult respiratory distress syndrome: Clinical features. In Carlson RW, Geheb MA [eds]: Principles and Practice of Medical Intensive Care. Philadelphia, WB Saunders, 1993, p 821.)*

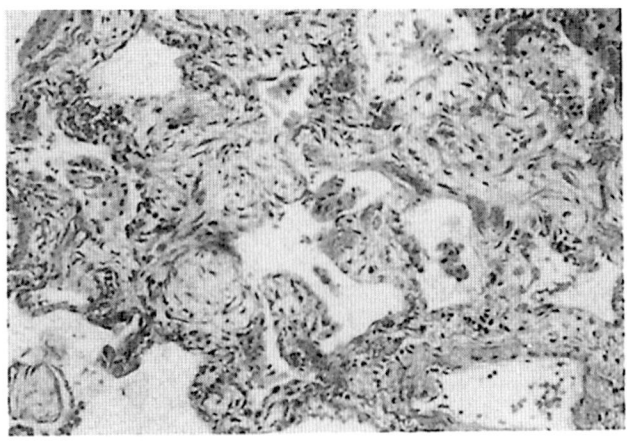 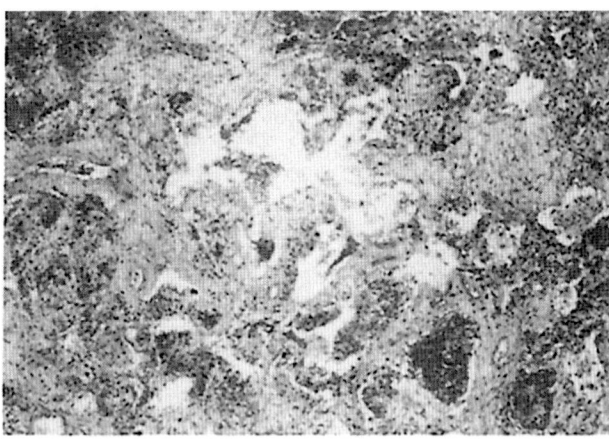

A   B

FIGURE 8-5

Proliferative and fibrotic stage of adult respiratory distress syndrome. Samples of an open-lung biopsy obtained 3 weeks after onset of respiratory failure. **A,** The alveolar architecture is distorted by proliferative changes and fibrosis. Note the whorls of granulation tissue filling some of the airspaces. **B,** Dense bands of fibrous tissue have replaced normal alveolar walls. Some distal airspaces are collapsed; a dilated alveolar duct also is seen. *(From Hansen-Flaschen JH: Adult respiratory distress syndrome: Clinical features. In Carlson RW, Geheb MA [eds]: Principles and Practice of Medical Intensive Care. Philadelphia, WB Saunders, 1993, p 823.)*

lungs time to heal. Mechanical ventilation also can cause alveolar rupture and hemorrhage, however, when high airway pressures are employed. PEEP, permissive hypercapnia, and inverse-ratio ventilation may improve outcome. Prevention (or reversal) of compression atelectasis is an important mechanism by which PEEP improves oxygenation. Low tidal volume ($\leq$6 mL/kg to reduce the plateau airway pressure to <30 cm H_2O) and higher PEEP (that required to maintain acceptable oxygenation with an FiO_2 <0.6) may improve survival and decrease the incidence of barotrauma.[30] Permissive hypercapnia from low tidal volumes and low end-expiratory pressures decreases mortality.[31] Inverse-ratio ventilation (inspiratory times equal to or greater than expiratory times), frequently accompanied by pressure control, theoretically increases recruitment of atelectatic

alveoli. These measures require sedation and neuromuscular blockade.[25] Oxygen concentrations greater than 60% cause the release of leukotrienes, lipid peroxidation, and neutrophil aggregation.[32,33] FiO_2 should be restricted to maintain acceptable oxygen saturation.[34]

Because lung infiltrates are *not* evenly distributed, changing patient position may improve gas exchange.[35] Prone positioning may be cumbersome, but there are few associated complications. Position change improves oxygenation rapidly in most patients; the improvement persists when the patient is placed supine again; turning the patient early in the course results in maximal improvement; and oxygenation may improve on subsequent prone positioning

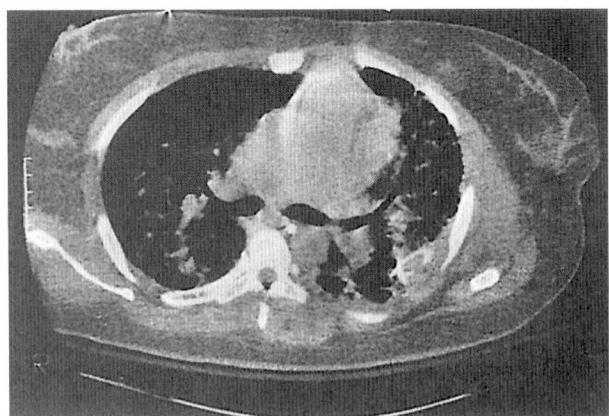 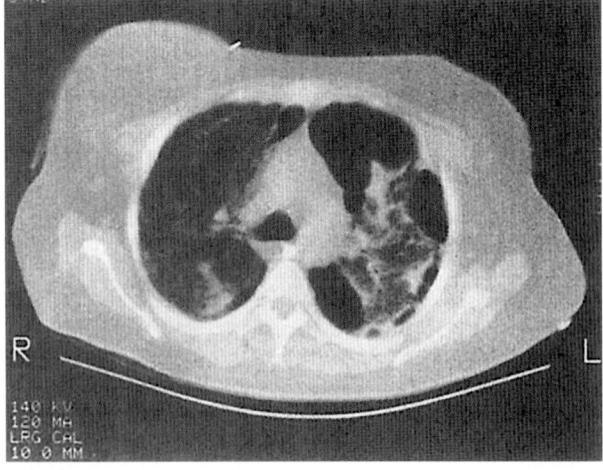

FIGURE 8-6

Proliferative and fibrotic phase of adult respiratory distress syndrome. High-resolution computed tomography scan obtained 3 weeks after onset of adult respiratory distress syndrome shows cystic airspaces and coarse, reticular infiltrates indicating fibrosis. *(From Hansen-Flaschen JH: Adult respiratory distress syndrome: Clinical features. In Carlson RW, Geheb MA [eds]: Principles and Practice of Medical Intensive Care. Philadelphia, WB Saunders, 1993, p 824.)*

FIGURE 8-7

Advanced proliferative and fibrotic phase of adult respiratory distress syndrome. Computed tomography scan shows multiple bilateral loculated pneumothoraces. Portions of the lung tissue appear fibrotic and cystic. *(From Hansen-Flaschen JH: Adult respiratory distress syndrome: Clinical features. In Carlson RW, Geheb MA [eds]: Principles and Practice of Medical Intensive Care. Philadelphia, WB Saunders, 1993, p 823.)*

even if there was not significant improvement on the first prone positioning. Prone positioning may be beneficial owing to the following: reduced pleural pressure gradient, more uniform alveolar ventilation, recruitment of dorsal regions of atelectasis, improved postural drainage, and redistribution of perfusion. Periodic changes in patient position should be considered.[36–38]

Fluids and diuretics should be used judiciously to attempt to achieve the lowest pulmonary artery occlusion pressure compatible with adequate blood pressure and cardiac output.[26] Persistent positive fluid balance has been associated with a poor outcome in ARDS.[39–40]

Trials with *N*-acetylcysteine, prostaglandin E₁, ketoconazole, nitric oxide, surfactant replacement, total/partial ventilation, antioxidant therapy, and nonsteroidal antiinflammatory drugs (NSAIDs) have not shown improved outcome.[34,41] There is some evidence that glucocorticoids may prevent fibrosis during the proliferative phase of ARDS.[37,42–45]

Mortality

Mortality ranges from 40% to 60%, and most deaths are a result of sepsis and multiorgan failure.[37] There are few quantitative data regarding risk factors that may lead to ARDS in poisoned patients. Hypotension and fluid overload may play a role. Many poisoned patients who are hypotensive in the emergency department receive massive fluid resuscitation, sometimes inappropriately. Fluid resuscitation should be judicious.

ACUTE RENAL FAILURE

Acute renal failure (ARF) is defined as a decline in the kidney's ability to clear nitrogenous waste that occurs over hours to days.[46] Although ARF is a common problem in critically ill patients, there are no defined criteria for this diagnosis. Examples of agents associated with ARF are acetaminophen, NSAIDs, ethylene glycol, radiocontrast agents, aminoglycosides, and amphotericin B. Clinically, plasma urea and creatinine concentrations increase, frequently with concomitant oliguria. ARF is termed *prerenal* if it is induced by hypoperfusion; *postrenal* if it is secondary to obstruction to urine flow; and *renal* if it is secondary to parenchymal insults, such as ischemia.[47,48] This discussion is limited to the issues related to ARF in poisoned patients.

Etiology

In poisoned patients, ARF is most frequently due to a decrease in extracellular fluid volume and renal hypoperfusion caused by drug-induced or chemical-induced vasodilation, drug-induced myocardial depression, or hypotension. Another cause of ARF in poisoned patients is rhabdomyolysis. Pressure necrosis of muscle due to prolonged coma (which also may cause a compartment syndrome) is the most common cause of rhabdomyolysis. Direct drug effect and intraarterial injection with subsequent ischemic necrosis also may cause rhabdomyolysis.[49]

Hypovolemia causes carotid baroreceptors to trigger a neuroendocrine cascade. Antidiuretic hormone is released as the sympathetic and renin-angiotensin systems are activated. Noradrenaline, angiotensin II, and antidiuretic hormone cause vasoconstriction and salt and water retention. Although there are several compensatory mechanisms that tend to maintain glomerular filtration rate (GFR), the kidneys are among the first organs to experience decreased perfusion during times of hypotension.[50,51]

Renal dysfunction may be readily reversible if perfusion is restored. A mean arterial pressure of less than 60 to 70 mm Hg for more than 30 minutes puts the patient at risk of renal injury.[48] If renal ischemia persists, renal failure occurs with histologic evidence of ischemic parenchymal injury. Ischemic tubular epithelial cells detach from the basement membrane and slough into the tubule lumen, forming urinary casts that obstruct the tubules. Acute tubular necrosis (ATN) can be seen after any episode of severe circulatory compromise. ATN is the clinical entity defined as renal failure after hypoperfusion or nephrotoxin exposure, tubular dysfunction evident on urinalysis, and expected recovery of renal function.[46]

Clinical Manifestations

Clinically, ARF may be oliguric or nonoliguric. Reduced tubular urine flow and increased tubular reabsorption of urea nitrogen result in a ratio of blood urea nitrogen to creatinine greater than 10:1. Because daily creatinine production is constant, an increasing creatinine implies that creatinine production has exceeded the GFR. A stable elevation of creatinine implies that the GFR has decreased, and a new steady state has been achieved. Renal dysfunction cannot be assessed until creatinine stabilizes. Kidney size is normal.[48]

The urine of a patient with "typical" ATN reveals a urinary sodium concentration less than 40 mEq/L, osmolality less than 400 mOsm/L, and fractional excretion of sodium greater than 1. The urine of these patients tends to contain tubular cells and casts. In prerenal failure, the urine reflects the response of the tubules to impaired perfusion. Urinalysis usually reveals only hyaline casts. The tubule reabsorbs sodium and water, leading to low urinary sodium and high urinary urea and creatinine concentrations. Urinary sodium is less than 20 mEq/L, osmolality is greater than 500 mOsm/L, and specific gravity is greater than 1.015. Fractional excretion of sodium is less than 1%. Urinary indices are of little clinical value because many intermediate values are common, and values do not predict renal prognosis. Treatment should not be dictated by urinary biochemical indices.[46,48]

Most patients regain renal function within a few days of the initial insult. Obstruction of the urinary tract must be considered in all patients with acute deterioration of renal function.[46] Common potential toxicologic causes of acute obstructive nephropathy are sulfonamides and methotrexate.

Prevention of Acute Renal Failure in Poisoned Patients

Attempts to prevent ARF are crucial because there is no specific therapy when ARF has occurred. Intravascular volume must be adequate for renal perfusion. Caution must be exercised in keeping ventilated patients "dry" to maintain oxygenation because this practice may predispose to prerenal azotemia. Central venous pressure measurement may aid in the assessment of volume status. Pulmonary capillary wedge pressure measurement may be valuable in selected cases, such as in older patients or patients with coexisting medical conditions. Fluid intake and output must be evaluated meticulously and constantly. Daily weights and frequent clinical assessment of volume status are indicated.[46,48]

> **Clinical Signs of Decreased Volume Status**
>
> Decreased blood pressure
> Increased heart rate
> Decreased peripheral perfusion
> Skin changes—cool mottled extremities, dry mucous membranes, skin tenting (age-induced reduction in skin elasticity is not as prominent on the forehead and sternum)
> Orthostatic changes—increased (15 beats/min) pulse or decreased (10 mm Hg) diastolic blood pressure indicates 5% loss of extracellular fluid volume

LOW-DOSE DOPAMINE

The efficacy of administering low-dose dopamine (0.5 to 3 mg/kg/min) to prevent ARF is controversial. When low-dose dopamine is administered, renal dopaminergic receptors are stimulated, causing renal vasodilation, natriuresis, and diuresis. When dopamine is administered to normal human subjects, there is a dose-dependent increase in renal blood flow,[52,53] sodium excretion, and GFR. This selective intrarenal vasodilation is maximal at a dose of 3 mg/kg/min and decreases at higher doses. Low-dose dopamine also limits adenosine triphosphate (ATP) use and oxygen requirements in nephron segments at risk for ischemia.[54] These actions of dopamine may prevent tubular ischemia. When ATN has developed, dopamine-induced natriuresis and diuresis (which washes out obstructing tubular casts) may hasten recovery of renal function. Anecdotes in clinical practice suggest increased urinary output in oliguric/anuric patients after administration of low-dose dopamine.

Studies evaluating the efficacy of low-dose dopamine have been done only in critically ill patients who had established ARF or were at high risk for developing ARF.[55–58] Although these studies have not shown any benefit, the patient population being evaluated is different from a population of poisoned patients. The use of low-dose dopamine in the oliguric or anuric, previously hypotensive poisoned patient has yet to be studied, and this research needs to be undertaken.

It is possible that dopamine may prevent ARF if administered prophylactically (i.e., after periods of hypotension before the development of anuria). Until data from overdose patients are obtained, based on the aforementioned data, I believe that it is reasonable to administer low-dose dopamine to previously healthy poisoned patients with adequate vascular volume who remain oliguric or anuric despite maximal diuretic therapy.

It is common to administer loop diuretics, such as furosemide, in conjunction with low-dose dopamine with a view to achieving a synergistic effect. Large doses of furosemide may increase urinary volume. Whether this increases clearance of metabolic wastes or affects outcome has not been determined.

In hypotensive poisoned patients, it is theoretically reasonable to add low-dose dopamine to pressor doses of norepinephrine to counter the effects of the latter drug on renal perfusion. In six healthy subjects, infusion of norepinephrine decreased renal blood flow from 1241 ± 208 mL/min/1.73 m^2 to 922 ± 143 mL/min/1.73 m^2. The addition of dopamine returned renal blood flow to baseline values. Urine output and GFR did not always increase when renal blood flow (measured by paraaminohippurate clearance) increased.[54] Urine output or measurements of GFR may not reflect renal function accurately.

Theoretical concerns of potentially detrimental effects of dopamine include a decrease in prolactin, thyroid-stimulating hormone, growth hormone, and T-cell proliferation; adverse effects on splanchnic blood flow, cardiopulmonary hemodynamics, and cardiac conduction pathways; acidosis; and hypophosphatemia.[51,55–61] Studies indicating these abnormalities, however, were done in critically ill patients who had multiple causes for endocrine and cardiopulmonary dysfunction.

Complications and Treatment of Acute Renal Failure

The treatment is the same whether the diagnosis is ARF or ATN. Management issues include assessment of volume status and treatment of life-threatening complications. Life-threatening complications of ARF include hyperkalemia and pulmonary edema (Table 8-3).[62,63] Clinical examination of a patient with hyperkalemia is frequently unremarkable. The diagnosis may be made by electrocardiogram and by serum potassium analysis. Chronologic electrocardiogram changes of hyperkalemia include tenting of the T wave, small P wave,

---

TABLE 8-3 Complications of Acute Renal Failure

Metabolic
  Hyperkalemia, acidosis, hypocalcemia, hyperphosphatemia, hyperuricemia, hypermagnesemia, insulin resistance, malnutrition
Cardiovascular
  Pulmonary edema, arrhythmias, hypertension, pericarditis
Neurologic
  Asterixis, myoclonus, confusion, somnolence, coma, seizures, nonspecific electroencephalographic changes
Gastrointestinal
  Nausea, vomiting, gastritis/duodenitis, anorexia, ileus
Hematologic
  Platelet dysfunction, factor VII dysfunction, anemia
Infectious
  Pneumonia, septicemia, urinary tract infection, indwelling catheter–related infection.

From Gehr TWB, Schoolwerth AC: Adult acute and chronic renal failure. Shoemaker WC, Ayres SM, Grenvik A, Molbrook PR (eds): Textbook of Critical Care, 4th ed. Philadelphia, WB Saunders, 2000.

TABLE 8-4 Modern Indications for Initiating Renal Replacement Therapy in Critically Ill Adult Patients*

1. Oliguria (urine output <200 mL/12 hr)
2. Anuria or extreme oliguria (urine output <50 mL/12 hr)
3. Hyperkalemia ([K+] >6.5 mmol/L and rising)
4. Severe acidemia (pH <7.1)
5. Azotemia ([urea] >30 mmol/L or [creatinine] >300 μcmol/L)
6. Pulmonary edema
7. Uremic encephalopathy
8. Uremic pericarditis
9. Uremic neuropathy or myopathy
10. Severe dysnatremia ([Na+] >160 or <115 mmol/L)
11. Hyperthermia
12. Drug overdose with filterable toxin (e.g., lithium, vancomycin, procainamide)
13. Anasarca
14. Diuretic-resistant cardiac failure
15. Imminent or ongoing massive blood product administration

*Note: The presence of one of these criteria is sufficient to initiate renal replacement therapy (RRT). The simultaneous presence of two of these criteria makes the prompt initiation of RRT highly desirable. The presence of three criteria makes the prompt initiation of RRT mandatory. In all of these cases, continuous RRT is the preferred approach.
From Silvester W, Chertow G, Ronco C, Bellono R: Renal replacement therapy in the intensive care unit. In Shoemaker WC, Ayres SM, Grenvik A, Holbrook PR (eds): Textbook of Critical Care, 4th ed. Philadelphia, WB Saunders, 2000.

increased PR interval, and widened QRS complex. The P wave subsequently disappears, and the QRS widens to become a sine wave.[46] Electrocardiogram changes that occur subsequent to tenting of the T wave require treatment. Initial management is administration of intravenous calcium gluconate (10 mL of 10%) to stabilize cardiac membranes, followed immediately by 10 U of regular insulin plus 50 mL of 50% glucose to drive potassium into the cells and intravenous sodium bicarbonate (50 mL). Calcium administration may worsen the inherent toxicity of cardiac glycosides or ethylene glycol, however. Administration of calcium should be judicious in these patients. Cation exchange resins (require hours until effect) and hemodialysis may be required, depending on the response to the initial measures to treat the hyperkalemia.[46]

In the setting of ARF, the cause of pulmonary edema is frequently iatrogenic salt and water overload. Clinical manifestations are those of hypoxia (e.g., restlessness, confusion, cyanosis, tachypnea, tachycardia, rales, wheezes, and a gallop heart rhythm). Chest radiograph reveals increased pulmonary markings. Morphine helps to relieve symptoms, but hemodialysis or hemofiltration may be required. Venesection of 100 to 200 mL of blood may be lifesaving while preparations are made for hemodialysis.[64,65] A controlled prospective clinical trial has shown that for patients requiring hemodialysis, daily treatments, instead of conventional alternate-day hemodialysis, is associated with reduced mortality without causing any adverse hemodynamic effects.[66] Indications for hemodialysis in patients with ARF are presented in Table 8-4. When hemodialysis for ARF is instituted, catheters may be placed in the femoral, subclavian, or internal jugular veins. Advantages and disadvantages of using these locations are listed in Table 8-5. When instituted, however, hemodialysis may slow the patient's recovery from ATN[67] because of the reaction to the material constituting the dialysis membrane.

Biochemical complications of ARF include acidosis, hypocalcemia, and hyperphosphatemia. Products of protein

TABLE 8-5 Advantages and Disadvantages of Percutaneous Venous Catheters

CHARACTERISTIC	FEMORAL VEIN	SUBCLAVIAN VEIN	INTERNAL JUGULAR VEIN
Duration catheter may be left in place	Must be removed within 24–72 hr	Can be left in place for several weeks	Can be left in place for several weeks
Patient's position when catheter inserted	Must lie flat while in place	Can be ambulatory	Can be ambulatory; limited neck mobility
Ease of insertion	Inserted easily	Requires a skilled operator	Requires intermediate skills
Position during insertion	Can be inserted in the semirecumbent position	Insertion should not be attempted if patient cannot lie flat	Insertion more difficult, but not impossible, if patient cannot lie flat
Complications	Usually minor: hematomas (groin, retroperitoneal)	Can be major and life-threatening: pneumothorax, hemothorax, brachial plexus injury, mediastinal hemorrhage, pericardial tamponade	Usually minor: low risk of pneumothorax
Risk of thrombosis and stricture of vein	No venographic data	High rate in the subclavian vein and superior vena cava	Low rate in the large veins
Rate of catheter-associated bacteremia	Low rate (provided that a new catheter is used for each treatment)	Relatively high rate	No reliable data
Use in bacteremic patients	May be used in bacteremic patients (new catheter for each treatment)	Should not be inserted in bacteremic patients because of risk of catheter seeding	Same as for subclavian catheters

From Shihab F, Kobrin SM: Intermittent renal replacement therapy in treating the critically ill patient with acute renal failure. In Carlson RW, Geheb MA (eds): Principles and Practice of Medical Intensive Care. Philadelphia, WB Saunders, 1993.

catabolism, such as sulfuric and phosphoric acids, usually are buffered with bicarbonate and excreted by the kidney. In ARF, acidosis is usually mild and does not require correction with sodium bicarbonate. Administration of sodium bicarbonate should be determined by severity of acidosis. Hypocalcemia occurs secondary to calcium malabsorption and disordered vitamin D metabolism. Although hypocalcemic patients are usually asymptomatic, seizures and tetany may be precipitated by rapid correction of acidosis, causing decreased ionized calcium.[63] The dose of many medications must be adjusted in patients with renal failure. Guidelines for these adjustments are given in Appendix C.

RHABDOMYOLYSIS

The first known reference to rhabdomyolysis is said to be in the Bible in the Book of Numbers,[68] in which an illness is described that occurred in Israelites after eating hemlock-fed quail. Rhabdomyolysis is a clinical and biochemical syndrome that occurs when skeletal muscle cell disruption causes release of muscle cell contents (creatine kinase, lactate dehydrogenase, aldolase, myoglobin, purines, potassium, and phosphates) into the interstitial space and plasma. Although direct mechanical trauma, compression, excessive muscle activity, and ischemia are frequent causes, nontraumatic rhabdomyolysis (which may be caused by certain drugs and chemicals) results from toxic insult to the cell membrane, affecting its ability to maintain ion gradients. Although rhabdomyolysis does not indicate irreversible necrosis of muscle, life-threatening illness and multiorgan failure may result.[64,65]

At the molecular level, rhabdomyolysis occurs when ATP production or consumption is impaired, or energy requirements exceed available ATP production in skeletal muscle. Resting and working muscle require ATP as a source of energy. As ATP concentrations decrease, the sodium-potassium transport pump malfunctions.[64,65] Sodium, chloride, and water move into the cell. Calcium ions, essential for the integrity of the muscle cell,[69] also move into the cell, causing cell lysis.[46]

Rhabdomyolysis may cause myoglobinuria. Myoglobin, a protein unique to myocytes, transports oxygen by a heme group. It has a much greater affinity for oxygen than does hemoglobin and does not release oxygen until ambient oxygen tension is low, such as occurs in working skeletal muscle. When myoglobin is released from myocytes, myoglobin becomes protein bound (50% at serum concentrations <23 mg/dL) and is rapidly metabolized to bilirubin.[70] Free myoglobin is rapidly filtered by renal glomeruli, with an elimination half-life of 1 to 3 hours and disappearance from the circulation within 6 hours of release.[71,73]

Drugs and Toxins

Examples of drugs or other agents and the mechanisms by which they may cause rhabdomyolysis are listed in Table 8-6.[49] Drug-induced agitation, seizures, withdrawal, and hyperthermia also may lead to rhabdomyolysis. Even in the absence of coma or seizures, ethanol ingestion (especially binge drinking) can cause muscle damage and rhabdomyolysis.[74] The mechanism is unknown, but theories include altered muscle ion homeostasis because of changes in sodium-potassium

TABLE 8-6 Examples of Drug-Induced or Chemical-Induced Rhabdomyolysis

PROLONGED UNCONSCIOUSNESS AND IMMOBILITY	INTRAARTERIAL INJECTION	DIRECT TOXIC EFFECT
Benzodiazepines	Heroin	Paint/glue sniffing
Major tranquilizers	Temazepam	Clofibrate
Methadone		Aminocaproic acid
Antidepressants		Cocaine
Carbon monoxide		Carbon monoxide
Barbiturates		Snake venom
		Bee venom
		Methadone
		Ethanol

Note: These are a few examples of the prodigious number of drugs or other chemicals capable of inducing rhabdomyolysis.

transport pump activity allowing increased sodium entry into the cell.[75,76] Nutritional deficiencies, hypophosphatemia, and hypokalemia may be coexistent risk factors for the development of rhabdomyolysis.[65,77] Cholesterol-lowering drugs of the statin class also have been associated with drug-induced rhabdomyolysis in the absence of other major clinical manifestations of toxicity.[78]

Clinical and Laboratory Manifestations

Clinical symptoms range from absence of symptoms to muscle weakness, tenderness, and swelling. Most patients complain of muscle soreness of the back and lower extremities. A gradual state of subjective and objective stiffness may ensue.[46]

The biochemical hallmarks of rhabdomyolysis are elevated serum creatine kinase (the most sensitive marker of muscle injury) and myoglobinuria. Creatinine phosphokinase is a sarcoplasmic enzyme present in striated and cardiac muscle and, to a lesser extent, in the tissues of the central nervous system.[79] Creatinine phosphokinase activity begins to increase 2 to 12 hours after injury and may continue to rise for more than 24 hours. Its serum half-life is 1.5 days. Creatinine phosphokinase isoenzyme analysis may be of value if there is a question of myocardial involvement.[46,63]

Serum myoglobin increases within a few hours of muscle injury, before the increase in serum creatine kinase. Because the metabolism of protein-bound myoglobin to bilirubin and the renal excretion of free myoglobin occur so rapidly, serum myoglobin concentrations are typically normal 1 to 6 hours after cessation of muscle injury in the presence of normal renal function.[77] Consequently, absence of myoglobinuria does not preclude the diagnosis of rhabdomyolysis. Variables that determine the presence of myoglobin in the urine are GFR, the concentration of plasma myoglobin, the degree of plasma protein binding, and the rate of urine production and flow.[79,80]

Dark brown urine, positive for blood on a reagent strip but without red blood cells on microscopic examination, indicates the presence of myoglobin.[46] Although the renal myoglobin threshold is 1 mg/dL, the urine does not become discolored until its urinary myoglobin concentration is 100 mg/dL. Urine dip-sticks containing orthotoluidine react with the globin fraction of hemoglobin and myoglobin. If red blood cells are present, the orthotoluidine reaction does not differentiate hemoglobin from myoglobin. Radioimmunoassay, immuno-electrophoresis, and hemagglutination are more specific than urine dip-stick but also significantly more expensive.[46]

Muscle cell disruption allows the release of potassium, phosphate, and urate. Acidosis and renal failure also cause potassium elevation. Hypocalcemia, the result of deposition of calcium in the damaged muscle, may be present with or without ARF. It is usually clinically insignificant, unless it occurs in the setting of severe hyperkalemia or ventricular dysfunction.[46] In approximately 30% of patients with ARF and rhabdomyolysis, hypercalcemia occurs in the subsequent diuretic phase of ARF. Parathormone concentrations are normal or low, but 1,25-dihydroxycholecalciferol concentrations are much greater in the hypercalcemic patients than in patients who do not develop hypercalcemia.[81]

Aldolase, lactate dehydrogenase, and aspartate transaminase (AST) activities are frequently elevated. Only aldolase is specific for muscle. Creatinine may be elevated not only from renal failure but also secondary to the release of creatine from muscle and its spontaneous hydration to creatinine.[46]

Complications

The primary complication, ARF, occurs in about 30% of patients with rhabdomyolysis. Risk factors for ARF in the presence of rhabdomyolysis include hyperkalemia, hyperphosphatemia, dehydration, sepsis, intravascular volume depletion, high serum myoglobin concentrations, and low myoglobin clearance. Compartment syndrome occurs infrequently.[75,82–86]

RHABDOMYOLYSIS-INDUCED ACUTE RENAL FAILURE

The contribution of heme pigments to ARF is not well understood. At urine pH less than 5.6, myoglobin dissociates into ferrihemate and globin. Ferrihemate depresses renal tubular transport mechanisms and causes a subsequent deterioration in renal function.[72,73] Myoglobin (molecular weight 17,500) may interfere with the endogenous vasodilator nitric oxide, causing a decrease in GFR. Myoglobin and other muscle constituents, such as urate, which is metabolized to uric acid, may plug the tubules. Other theories include the presence of oxygen free radicals. Animal experiments show that myoglobin causes renal damage when dehydration is present. Contributing factors seem to be concentrated urine with low urine flow and urine pH less than 5.6. Published clinical reviews conclude that patients with hyperkalemia, hyperphosphatemia, high serum myoglobin concentrations, and low myoglobin clearance seem to be at risk for development of ARF.[75,83–86]

Treatment

Hypovolemia occurs as a result of the movement of fluid into the traumatized muscle. Volume requirements can be large. Treatment begins with volume replacement. In severe cases, hemodialysis or continuous hemofiltration is necessary. Potentially nephrotoxic agents, such as aminoglycosides or NSAIDs, should be avoided.

The efficacy of administering bicarbonate or mannitol to achieve alkaline or osmotic diuresis to prevent rhabdomyolysis-induced ARF is unknown. Clinical reports[79] suggest that alkaline diuresis may be effective in preventing ARF, but there are no prospective randomized studies. There is even less convincing evidence for mannitol administration. Although many mechanisms have been postulated regarding the renoprotective effects of mannitol, prevention of heme protein trapping by diuretic action explains most of the data.[82] Extreme caution must be exercised to prevent hypovolemia from the osmotic diuresis. Determination of the prophylactic efficacy of bicarbonate and mannitol (if any) represents a further research need in poisoned patients.

In animals with rhabdomyolysis that had a low urinary pH, dehydration predisposed to renal injury, which was prevented by urinary dilution.[86–88] One of the goals of treatment is adequate urine output. One practice recommendation is to maintain urine flow rates of 2 mL/kg body weight/hr.[89] Volume administration (as determined clinically or with central venous pressure) must be adequate to maintain high urinary flow rates. If volume administration does not cause diuresis, furosemide (40 mg) may be administered; the dose may be doubled every 20 minutes to a maximum of 360 mg. Administration of bicarbonate may be considered, but systemic alkalosis should be avoided because it may worsen hypocalcemia.

Hyperkalemia may occur within a few hours of onset of rhabdomyolysis and may require treatment as described earlier.[89] Hyperphosphatemia may require the administration of phosphate binders. Treatment is dictated by the degree of serum phosphate elevation.

Hypocalcemia may occur early in the clinical course of rhabdomyolysis.[86] Calcium should not be administered unless hyperkalemia or ventricular dysfunction occurs. Calcium infusion may increase the deposition of calcium in injured muscle. The late hypercalcemia seen during the diuretic phase of ARF is usually self-limiting and requires only conservative treatment with fluid replacement.[90]

Disseminated intravascular coagulation occurs infrequently as a result of activation of the clotting cascade by muscle components.[91] Drug-induced hyperthermia may contribute to the development of disseminated intravascular coagulation.

COMPARTMENT SYNDROME

Muscle necrosis and resultant accumulation of fluid within a rigid fibro-osseous compartment causes increased tissue pressure, venous stasis, decreased capillary flow, and tissue hypoperfusion. Compartment syndrome is well recognized after trauma or coma with prolonged extremity immobilization, but diagnosis is more difficult in the atraumatic causes of compartment syndrome (such as may occur in the overdose patient), in which clinical parameters may not be evident. Intravenous injection may cause direct local vasotoxicity and vascular damage. Hypotensive patients, unconscious patients, and patients with altered mental status or psychosis are unable to express the pain that they feel in an extremity. All patients with snake bite–associated swelling should be evaluated for compartment syndrome.[92]

Clinical Manifestations and Treatment

Diagnosis of compartment syndrome is based on clinical suspicion. Clinical findings are edema, pain in the compartmental muscle when passively stretched, hypesthesia of areas of skin supplied by nerves running through the compartment, tenderness, and weakness. Sensory deficit usually precedes motor deficit. Decreased sensation is distal to the affected compartment.[93,94] A palpable arterial pulse does not exclude compartment syndrome because muscle and nerve necrosis may occur while distal pulses are maintained. If clinical diagnosis is uncertain, compartment pressures should be measured. When intracompartmental pressure is greater than 40 mm Hg or clinical signs are present, or both, surgical fasciotomy is the definitive treatment.[94,95] Normal muscle interstitial pressure is about 5 mm Hg. Although fasciotomy releases the pressure within the enclosed sheaths and restores perfusion, the procedure is not without risk because a closed necrotic muscle injury is converted into an open wound with potential dissemination of infection.[93] Indications for pressure monitoring are controversial, and practice (and availability of monitoring equipment) varies.[96] Administration of mannitol, to extract water from the compartment by extracellular fluid hyperosmolarity, has not been shown to change outcome.[97]

The most important factor in determining outcome is length of time to diagnosis. Complications include permanent atrophy, loss of sensation, infection, contracture, and amputation, all which may be disabling. Young men have the highest incidence of acute compartment syndrome, perhaps owing to relatively large muscle volumes. Compartment size does not change after growth is complete, leaving less space for swelling of muscle after injuries. Older people, in contrast, have small hypotrophic muscles and relatively higher blood pressure.[98]

In North America, extremity bites by snakes that may cause swelling (e.g., crotaline) must be evaluated frequently for symptoms and signs of a compartment syndrome (see Chapter 102). Progression of local edema as determined by circumferential measurements, temperature, and perfusion of the extremity should be documented. The area of the bite may be swollen and tender when palpated, making clinical evaluation of a compartment syndrome difficult. Fasciotomy is seldom necessary after snakebites, and it should be performed only when clinical symptoms and signs of a compartment syndrome and elevated compartmental pressures are present.[99]

The extremity of any patient receiving prophylactic low-molecular-weight heparin should be monitored for signs of compartment syndrome. Hemorrhagic risks also should be considered. The doses of low-molecular-weight heparin used in the United States are greater than doses previously used in Europe.[100] Frequent examination is paramount.

HEPATOTOXICITY

One of the causes of acute hepatic injury is toxin exposure. Xenobiotic-induced (drug and environmental chemical) hepatotoxicity is the second most common cause of hepatic injury, the most frequent cause being viral hepatitis. The liver may be one of multiple organs damaged by a toxin, or hepatic injury may be the primary manifestation of poisoning, such as with acetaminophen toxicity.

Liver

Ingested toxins are absorbed through the gastrointestinal tract and transported via the portal system to the liver. Histologically the liver is divided into multiple lobules. The center of each lobule is a hepatic vein from which cords of hepatocytes radiate concentrically. The outer boundary of the lobule is the portal triad (i.e., the hepatic artery, portal vein, and bile duct). The hepatocyte walls are penetrated by vascular sinusoids, which are lined by reticuloendothelial cells possessing immune function. The portal vein and the hepatic artery bring blood to the liver.

Functionally the liver is divided into acini. Each acinus consists of three concentric zones of hepatocytes radiating from a portal triad and terminating at an adjacent terminal hepatic venule. The zones are determined by distance from the triad. Zone 1 hepatocytes are closest to the portal triad, receive the most oxygen and nutrient–enriched blood, and are most resistant to injuries. As the distance from the triad increases, hepatocytes become more susceptible to ischemic or nutritional damage. Zone 3 hepatocytes, farthest from the triad, are the site of cytochrome P-450 enzyme activity, making them the most susceptible to xenobiotic-induced liver injury.[101,102]

Xenobiotics are highly lipophilic and are poorly excreted by the kidney. Biotransformation is the process by which polar groups are introduced during drug metabolism so that the drugs become water-soluble, allowing biliary or renal elimination. Detoxification consists of phase I reactions, in which polar groups are placed in the molecule, usually mediated by a cytochrome P-450 system, and phase II reactions, in which the molecule is conjugated to a water-soluble ligand.[101,103] Xenobiotics usually cause so-called intrinsic injury (dose-dependent zonal hepatocellular necrosis) or idiosyncratic injury (non–dose dependent, unpredictable regional cellular damage and necrosis or a mixed pattern). The latter may be immune mediated, but this is not universally so. Histologic examination of a liver biopsy may yield clues to the diagnosis.[103,104] Table 8-7 schematically portrays patterns of xenobiotic-induced liver injury.[105]

Biochemical Changes in Liver Injury

Elevations of serum concentrations of AST and alanine aminotransferase (ALT) activities indicate hepatocellular injury. ALT is specific for liver; AST is found in other tissue (e.g., muscle). The greatest increase of these enzyme activities occurs in xenobiotic-induced necrosis or acute viral hepatitis, with lesser elevations in alcoholic liver disease or cholestasis. Transaminase elevations into the thousands should always prompt the consideration of toxin-induced hepatic injury. Other possibilities are viral hepatitides, sepsis, hypoxia, and shock. Most commonly, the toxins to consider are acetaminophen or hepatotoxic mushrooms. Most drug-induced elevations return to normal when the drug is discontinued. The degree of increase does not correlate with the extent of liver injury and is not prognostic of outcome. Serum alkaline phosphatase (ALP) concentrations are affected by age and other physiologic variables. This enzyme

TABLE 8-7 Xenobiotic-Induced Liver Injury

	HEPATOTOXIN-INDUCED HEPATOCELLULAR NECROSIS	TOXIC HEPATITIS (INCLUDES IDIOSYNCRATIC AND AUTOIMMUNE)	STEATOSIS	CHOLESTASIS	HEPATIC VASCULAR INJURY	HEPATIC GRANULOMAS	HEPATIC TUMORS (MALIGNANT)
Signs and Symptoms	Nausea and vomiting Symptoms resolve 48–72 hr or progression to FHF (3–5 days)	Fever, nausea, rash, myalgia (similar to viral hepatitis)	Consistent with Reye's syndrome Gastrointestinal upset, mental status change	Malaise Flulike	Hepatomegaly, abdominal pain Jaundice	Malaise, jaundice, hepatomegaly	
Biochemical	↑ Hepatic aminotransferase enzymes ↑ Bilirubin ↑ PT→ (degree of coagulopathy and rapidity of development indicative of degree of hepatic injury) FHF ARF	Mild ↑ hepatic aminotransferase to FHF	↑ TG ↑ Aminotransferase (minimal)	↑ ALP ↑ Bilirubin (mild); ↑ transaminase (similar to profile seen with extrahepatic obstruction)	↑ Aminotransferase ↑ ALP	↑ ALP	
Agents Implicated*	Acetaminophen Methyldopa Hydralazine Amitriptyline Allopurinol Acetylsalicylic acid Baclofen Dantrolene Cocaine Ecstasy	Isoniazid Phenytoin Amiodarone Acetylsalicylic acid Cimetidine Diclofenac Methotrexate PTU Valproate Vitamin A	Valproic acid Tetracycline Amiodarone Methotrexate NSAID	Phenothiazine Especially Chlorpromazine TMP-SMX, rifampin Erythromycin (estolate) Captopril Amitriptyline	Azathioprine Pyrrolizidine alkaloids Actinomycin Oral contraceptive Vitamin A Methotrexate	Methyldopa Diltiazem Hydralazine Procainamide Quinidine Tolamide Chlorpropamide Tolbutamide Dapsone Isoniazid Carbamazepine Acetylsalicylic acid Chlorpromazine	Anabolic and androgenic steroids Oral contraceptives

*This list is not comprehensive. Although the listed agents have been implicated as causing hepatic injury, the strength of the data supporting these associations is variable.

ALP, alkaline phosphatase; ARF, acute renal failure; FHF, fulminant hepatic failure; NSAID, nonsteroidal antiinflammatory drug; PT, prothrombin time; PTU, propylthiouracil; TG, triglyceride; TMP-SMX, trimethoprim-sulfamethoxazole.

increases in most liver injuries, but it cannot be used to differentiate the cause of the elevation.[86,105] In adults, if ALP is the predominant enzyme elevated, cholestatic injury is the most likely cause.

Serum γ-glutamyltransferase correlates well with ALP. Increased ALP occurs in bone and liver disease, but γ-glutamyltransferase is increased only in liver disease. Significant isolated elevation of bilirubin may indicate hepatic injury but has no prognostic significance in acute injury. Serum albumin, a marker of hepatic synthetic function, has a half-life of 20 days and is not a reflection of acute injury.

Prothrombin time is an indirect measure of hepatic synthesis of clotting factors and has prognostic value in acute and chronic liver disease. In the setting of hepatocellular necrosis, markedly elevated prothrombin time is associated with an increased risk of liver failure. Vitamin K deficiency, use of warfarins, and acquired clotting factor deficiencies should be considered in the differential diagnosis of an elevated prothrombin time.

Hepatocellular damage is reflected by an increase in transaminases, cholestasis is reflected by an increase in ALP, and steatosis affects both equally. More severe liver injury is reflected by hyperbilirubinemia and an increase in prothrombin time. Hepatotoxicity is discussed in more detail in Chapter 17.

Examples of Specific Toxins

HERBS

Herbal remedies have become increasingly popular owing to a "back to nature" movement and the belief that what is natural cannot hurt you. Many commercially available herbs (and herbs grown in local gardens) can cause hepatotoxicity.[106,107]

Pyrrolizidine alkaloids are found in the plant species *Heliotropium, Senecio, Crotalaria,* and *Symphytum*. These toxic alkaloids may be ingested in teas, decoctions, or dietary supplements or administered as an enema. Veno-occlusive disease is the liver injury caused by pyrrolizidine alkaloids.[105] The hepatotoxicity is reproducible in laboratory animals and is dose related.[108]

Larrea tridentata is touted to contain antiviral properties and is frequently ingested by patients with human immunodeficiency virus in an attempt to induce remission.[109] Hepatocellular hepatitis has been reported after ingestion of this herb. The mechanism is unknown.[108,109]

Chinese herbal medicines are widely used in Asia and throughout the world. Acute hepatitis has been reported in people ingesting these herbs, but actual compositions of the ingested herbs were not tested.[110–112] A contaminant of Jin Bu Huan specifically has been implicated in causing a hepatotoxic syndrome.[113]

ANTICONVULSANTS

Owing to the frequency with which anticonvulsants are being prescribed, special mention should be made. Lamotrigine has been associated with hepatic failure. Risk factors may include multiple anticonvulsant therapies, rapid titration schedule, and additional medical problems. Fatal hepatotoxicity has been associated with felbamate and valproate therapy.[115–117]

ACETAMINOPHEN

Acetaminophen is the prototypic example of a dose-dependent hepatotoxin. Its toxicity is discussed in detail in Chapter 55.

REFERENCES

1. Daniels SK, Brailey K, Priestly DH, et al: Aspiration in patients with acute stroke. Arch Phys Med Rehabil 79:14–19, 1998.
2. Roy TM, Ossorio MA, Cipolla LM, et al: Pulmonary complications after tricyclic antidepressant overdose. Chest 96:852–856, 1989.
3. Adnet F, Baud F: Relation between Glasgow Coma Scale and aspiration pneumonia. Lancet 348:123–124, 1996.
4. Owens GR: Aspiration. In Carlson RW, Geheb MA (eds): Principles and Practice of Medical Intensive Care. Philadelphia, WB Saunders, 1993, p 872.
5. Whitman P, Zimmerman H, Burkhart K, et al: Pulmonary aspiration in the intubated overdose patient. Vet Hum Toxicol 36:364, 1994.
6. Torres A, Serra-Batlles J, Ros E, et al: Pulmonary aspiration of gastric contents in patients receiving mechanical ventilation: The effect of body position. Ann Intern Med 116:540–543, 1992.
7. Marik PE: Aspiration pneumonitis and aspiration pneumonia. N Engl J Med 344:665–671, 2001.
8. Greenfield LI, Singleton RP, McCaffree DR, et al: Pulmonary effects of experimental graded aspiration of hydrochloric acid. Ann Surg 170:74–86, 1969.
9. Wynne JW, Modell JH: Respiratory aspiration of stomach contents. Ann Intern Med 87:466–474, 1977.
10. Boysen PG, Modell J: Pulmonary aspiration. In Grenvik A, Ayres SM, Holbrook PR, Shoemaker WC (eds): Textbook of Critical Care. Philadelphia, WB Saunders, 2000, pp 1432–1439.
11. Mendelson C: Aspiration of stomach contents into the lungs during obstetric anesthesia. Am J Obstet Gynecol 52:191, 1946.
12. James CF, Modell JH, Gibbs CP, et al: Pulmonary aspiration: Effects of volume and pH in the rat. Anesth Analg 63:665–668, 1984.
13. Folkesson HG, Matthay MA, Herberbert CA, et al: Acid aspiration-inducing lung injury in rabbits is mediated by interleukin-8-dependent mechanism. J Clin Invest 96:107–116, 1995.
14. Arnold T, Willis B, Xiaao F, et al: Aspiration of activated charcoal elicits an increase in lung microvascular permeability. Clin Toxicol 37:9–16, 1999.
15. Cohen AB, Gold WM: Defense mechanisms of the lungs. Annu Rev Physiol 37:325–350, 1975.
16. Bynum LJ, Pierce AK: Pulmonary aspiration of gastric contents. Am Rev Respir Dis 114:1129–1136, 1976.
17. Bartlett J: Anaerobic bacterial infections of the lung. Chest 91:901, 1987.
18. Huxtable RJ: New aspects of the toxicology and pharmacology of pyrrolizidine alkaloids. Mol Pharmacol 10:159–167, 1979.
19. Kassler WJ, Blanc P, Greenblatt R: The use of medicinal herbs by human immunodeficiency virus-infected patients. Arch Intern Med 151:2281–2288, 1991.
20. Braun SR, Weiss FR, Keller AL, et al: Evaluation of the renal toxicity of heme pigments and their derivatives: A role in the genesis of acute tubular necrosis. J Exp Med 131:443–460, 1970.
21. Devins SS, Miller A, Herndon BL, et al: Effects of dopamine on T-lymphocyte proliferative responses and serum prolactin concentrations in critically ill patients. Crit Care Med 20:1644–1649, 1992.
22. Petty TL, Ashbauch DG: The adult respiratory distress syndrome: Clinical features, factors influencing prognosis and principles of management. Chest 60:233–239, 1971.
23. O'Connor MF, Hall JB, Wood LDH: Acute hypoxemia respiratory failure. In Hall JB, Schmidt GA, Wood LDH (eds): Principles of Critical Care, 2nd ed. New York, McGraw-Hill, 1998, 531–563.
24. Bernard GR, Artigas A, Brigham KL, et al: Report of the American-European Consensus Conference on Acute Respiratory Distress Syndrome: Definitions, mechanisms, relevant outcomes, and clinical trial coordination. J Crit Care 9:72–81, 1994.
25. Luce JM: Acute lung injury and the acute respiratory distress syndrome. Crit Care Med 26:369–374, 1988.
26. Keogh BF, Ranieri VM: Ventilatory support in the acute respiratory distress syndrome. Br Med Bull 1:140–164, 1999.
27. Hasle HC: Pathophysiology and pathogenesis in ARDS. In Warrell D, Cox T, Firth J (eds): Oxford Textbook of Medicine, 4th ed. Oxford, Oxford University Press, 2003, pp 1238–1249.

28. Ware LB, Matthay MA: Medical progress: The acute respiratory distress syndrome. N Engl J Med 342:1334–1349, 2000.

29. American Thoracic Society, European Society of Intensive Care Medicine, and Societe de Reanimation de Langue Francaise: International consensus conferences in intensive care medicine: Ventilatory-associated lung injury in ARDS. Approved by the ATS Board of Directors, July 1999. Intensive Care Med 25:1444–1452, 1999.

30. Amato MB, Barbas CS, Medeiros DM, et al: Effect of a protective-ventilation strategy on mortality in the acute respiratory distress syndrome. N Engl J Med 338:347–354, 1998.

31. Acute Respiratory Distress Syndrome Network: Ventilation with lower tidal volumes as compared with traditional tidal volumes for acute lung injury and the acute respiratory distress syndrome. N Engl J Med 342:1301–1308, 2000.

32. Griffith DE, Garcia JEN, James HL, et al: Hyperoxic exposure in humans: Effects of 50 percent oxygen on alveolar macrophage leukotriene B4 synthesis. Chest 101:392–397, 1992.

33. Risber B, Smith L, Örtenwall P: Oxygen radicals and lung injury. Acta Anaesth Scand 95(Suppl):106–118, 1991.

34. Lunn JL, Murray MJ: Acute respiratory distress syndrome. Yale J Biol Med 71:457–467, 1998.

35. Ward N: Effects of prone position ventilation in ARDS: An evidence-based review of the literature. Crit Care Clin 18:35–44, 2002.

36. Albet RK: Prone position in ARDS: What do we know, and what do we need to know? Crit Care Med 27:2574–2575, 1999.

37. Suchyta MR, Grissom CK, Morris AH: Epidemiology in ARDS. Intensive Care Med 25:538–539, 1999.

38. Gattioni L, Toognoni G: Effect of prone positioning on the survival of patients with acute respiratory failure. N Engl J Med 345:568–573, 2001.

39. Mitchell JP, Schuller D, Caladrino FS, et al: Improved outcome based on fluid management in critically ill patients requiring pulmonary artery catheters. Am Rev Respir Dis 145:990–994, 1992.

40. Schuster DP: Fluid management in ARDS: "Keep them dry" or does it matter? Intensive Care Med 21:101–103, 1995.

41. Wyncoll DLA, Evans TW: Acute respiratory distress syndrome. Lancet 354:497–501, 1999.

42. Meduri GU, Chinn AJ, Leeper KV, et al: Corticosteroid rescue treatment of progressive fibroproliferation in late ARDS: Patterns of response and predictors of outcome. Chest 105:1516–1527, 1994.

43. Masclans JR, Barbera JA, MacNee W, et al: Salbutamol reduces pulmonary neutrophil sequestration of platelet-activating factor in humans. Am J Respir Crit Care Med 154:529–532, 1996.

44. Newman V, Gonzalez RF, Matthay MA, Dobbs LG: A novel alveolar type I cell-specific biochemical marker of human acute lung injury. Am J Respir Crit Care Med 161:990–995, 2000.

45. Meduri GU, Headley AS, Golden E, et al: Effect of prolonged methylprednisolone therapy in unresolving acute respiratory distress syndrome: A randomized controlled trial. JAMA 280:159–165, 1998.

46. Hamemes M, Gillum DM, Brennan S: Acute renal failure. In Hall JB, Schmidt GA, Wood LDH (eds): Principles of Critical Care, 2nd ed. New York, McGraw-Hill, 1998, pp 1117–1132.

47. McDonald RH, Goldberg LI, McNay JL, Tuttle EP: Effects of dopamine in man: Augmentation of sodium excretion, glomerular filtration rate and renal plasma flow. Clin Invest 43:1116–1124, 1964.

48. Marini JJ, Wheeler AP: Acute renal failure and dialysis. In Marini JJ, Wheeler AP (eds): Critical Care Medicine: The Essentials, 2nd ed. Baltimore, Williams & Wilkins, 1997, pp 465–475.

49. Deighhan CJ, Wong KM, McLaughlin KJ, Harden P: Rhabdomyolysis and acute renal failure resulting from alcohol and drug abuse. QJM 93:29–33, 2000.

50. Power DA, Duggan J, Brady HR: Renal-dose (low-dose) dopamine for the treatment of sepsis-related and other forms of acute renal failure: Ineffective and probably dangerous. Clin Exp Pharmacol Physiol 26(Suppl):S23–S28, 1999.

51. Burton CJ, Tomson CRV: Can the use of low-dose dopamine for treatment of acute renal failure be justified? Postgrad Med J 75:269–274, 1999.

52. Goldberg LI: Cardiovascular and renal actions of dopamine: Potential clinical applications. Pharmacol Rev 24:1–29, 1972.

53. Ser I, Kone B, Gullans S, et al: Locally formed dopamine inhibits Na-K-ATPase activity in rat renal cortical tubule cells. Am J Physiol 255:F666–673, 1988.

54. Richer M, Robert S, Lebel M: Renal hemodynamics during norepinephrine and low-dose dopamine infusions in man. Crit Care Med 24:1150–1156, 1996.

55. Baldwin L, Henderson A, Hickman P: Effect of postoperative dopamine on renal function after elective major vascular surgery. Am J Nephrol 120:744–747, 1994.

56. Van den Bergh G, de Zegher F, Lauwers P: Dopamine and the sick euthyroid syndrome in critical illness. Clin Endocrinol 41:731–737, 1994.

57. Myles PS, Buckland MR, Schenk NJ, et al: Effect of "renal dose" dopamine on renal function following cardiac surgery. Anaesth Intensive Care 21:56–61, 1993.

58. Devins SS, Miller A, Herndon BL, et al: Effects of dopamine on T-lymphocyte proliferative responses and serum prolactin concentrations in critically ill patients. Crit Care Med 20:1644–1649, 1992.

59. Segal JM, Phang PT, Walley KR: Low-dose dopamine hastens onset of gut ischemia in a porcine model of hemorrhagic shock. J Appl Physiol 73:1159–1164, 1992.

60. Stephan H, Sonntag H, Henning H, Youshimine K: Cardiovascular and renal hemodynamic effects of dopexamine: Comparison with dopamine. Br J Anaesth 65:380–387, 1990.

61. Davis RF, Lappas DG, Kirklin JK, et al: Acute oliguria after cardiopulmonary bypass: Renal functional improvement with low-dose dopamine infusion. Crit Care Med 10:882–886, 1982.

62. Leier CV, Heban PT, Huss P, et al: Comparative systemic and regional hemodynamic effects of dopamine and dobutamine in patients with cardiomyopathic heart failure. Circulation 58:466–475, 1978.

63. Woodrow G, Brownjohn AM, Turney JH: The clinical and biochemical features of acute renal failure due to rhabdomyolysis. Renal Fail 17:467–474, 1995.

64. Brady HR, Brenner BM, Lieberthal W: Acute renal failure. In Brenner BM (ed): The Kidney, 5th ed. Philadelphia, WB Saunders, 1996.

65. Firth JD, Winerls CG: Acute renal failure. In Weatherall DJ, Ledingham JGG, Warrell DA (eds): Oxford Textbook of Medicine, 3rd ed. Oxford, Oxford University Press, 1996.

66. Schiffl H, Lang SM, Fischer R: Daily hemodialysis and the outcome of acute renal failure. N Engl J Med 346:305–310, 2002.

67. Conger J: Dialysis and related therapies. Semin Nephrol 18:533–540, 1998.

68. Billis AG: Acute renal failure after a meal of quail. Lancet 2:702, 1971.

69. Homsi E, Leme Barreiro FF, Orlando MC, Higa EM: Prophylaxis of acute renal failure in patients with rhabdomyolysis. Renal Fail 19:283–288, 1997.

70. Knochel JP: Rhabdomyolysis and myoglobinuria. Semin Nephrol 1:75–86, 1981.

71. Braun SR, Weiss FR, Keller AL, et al: Evaluation of the renal toxicity of heme pigments and their derivatives: A role in the genesis of acute tubular necrosis. J Exp Med 131:443–460, 1970.

72. Anderson WAD, Morrison DB, Williams EF Jr: Pathologic changes following injection of ferrihemate (hematin) in dogs. Arch Pathol 33:589–602, 1942.

73. Corcoran AC, Page IH: Renal damage from ferroheme pigments in myoglobin, hemoglobin, hematin. Tex Reprod Biol Med 3:528–544, 1945.

74. Muthukumar T, Jha V, Sud A, et al: Acute renal failure due to nontraumatic rhabdomyolysis following binge drinking. Renal Fail 21:545–549, 1999.

75. Ward MM: Factors predictive of acute renal failure in rhabdomyolysis. Arch Intern Med 148:1553–1557, 1988.

76. Perkoff GT, Dioso MM, Bleish V, Klinkerfuss G: A spectrum of myopathy associated with alcoholism: I. Clinical and laboratory features. Ann Intern Med 67:481–492, 1967.

77. Hojs R, Ekart R, Sinkovic A, Hojs-Fabja T: Rhabdomyolysis and acute renal failure in intensive care unit. Renal Fail 21:675–684, 1999.

78. Wombolt D, Jackson A, Punn R, et al: Case report: Rhabdomyolysis induced by mibetradil in a patient treated with cyclosporine and simvastatin. J Clin Pharmacol 39:310–312, 1999.

79. Haapanen E, Partanen J, Pellinen TJ: Acute renal failure following nontraumatic rhabdomyolysis. Can J Urol Nephrol 22:305–308, 1988.

80. Köppel C: Clinical features, pathogenesis and management of drug-induced rhabdomyolysis. Med Toxicol Adverse Drug Exp 4:108–126, 1989.

81. Stadhouders AM: Cellular calcium homeostasis, mitochondria and muscle cell disease. In Busch HFM, Jennekens FGI, Scholte HR (eds): Mitochondria and Muscular Diseases. Mefar b.v., 1981, pp 77–88.

82. Poel PJE, Gabreëls FJM: Rhabdomyolysis: A review of the literature. Clin Neurol Neurosurg 95:175–192, 1993.

83. Horowitz BZ, Panacek EA, Jouriles NJ: Severe rhabdomyolysis with renal failure after intranasal cocaine use. J Emerg Med 15:833–837, 1997.

84. Visweswaran P, Guntupalli J: Rhabdomyolysis. Environ Emerg 15:415–428, 1999.

85. Knochel JP: Mechanism of rhabdomyolysis. Curr Opin Rheumatol 5:725–737, 1993.

86. Sandhu JS, Sood A, Midha V, et al: Non-traumatic rhabdomyolysis with acute renal failure. Renal Fail 22:81–86, 2000.

87. Ferguson E, Blachley Y, Carter N, Knochel JD: Derangements of muscle composition, ion transport and oxygen consumption in clinically alcoholic dogs. Am J Physiol 246:700–709, 1984.

88. Gabow PA, Kaehny WD, Kelleher SP: The spectrum of rhabdomyolysis. Medicine 61:141–152, 1982.

89. Curry SC, Chang D, Connor D: Drug- and toxin-induced rhabdomyolysis. Ann Emerg Med 18:1068–1084, 1989.

90. Greenberg MI: The clinical settings and physical findings of rhabdomyolysis. EMN December 1997, pp 19–20.

91. Akmal M, Bishop J, Telfer N, et al: Hypocalcemia and hypercalcemia in patients with rhabdomyolysis with and without acute renal failure. J Clin Endocrinol Metabol 63:137–142, 1986.

92. Johnson GE, Downs AR: Extremity and pelvic trauma. In Hall JB, Schmidt GA, Wood LDH (eds): Principles of Critical Care, 2nd ed. New York, McGraw-Hill, 1998.

93. Franc-Law JM, Rossignol M, Vernec A, et al: Poisoning-induced acute atraumatic compartment syndrome. Am J Emerg Med 18:616–621, 2000.

94. Johnson IAT, Andrzejowski JC, Currie JSA: Lower limb compartment syndrome resulting from malignant hyperthermia. Anaesth Intensive Care 27:292–294, 1999.

95. Cara JA, Narvaez A, Bertrand mL, Guerado E: Acute atraumatic compartment syndrome in the leg. Int Orthop 23:61–62, 1999.

96. Williams PR, Russell ID, Mintowt-Czyz WJ: Compartment pressure monitoring current—UK orthopedic practice. Injury 29:229–232, 1998.

97. Daniels M, Reichman J, Brezis M: Mannitol treatment for acute compartment syndrome. Nephron 78:492–493, 1998.

98. McQueen MM, Gaston P, Court-Brown CM: Acute compartment syndrome. J Bone Joint Surg Br 82:200–203, 2000.

99. Bond GR: Snake, spider, and scorpion envenomation in North America. Pediatr Rev 20:147–151, 1999.

100. McLaughlin JA, Paulson MM, Rosenthal RE. Delayed onset of anterior tibial compartment syndrome in a patient receiving low-molecular weight heparin: A case report. J Bone Surg Am 80:1789–1790, 1998.

101. Sturgill MG, Lambert GH: Xenobiotic-induced hepatotoxicity: Mechanisms of liver injury and methods of monitoring hepatic function. Clin Chem 43:1512–1526, 1997.

102. Shah RR: Drug-induced hepatotoxicity: Phamacokinetic perspectives and strategies for risk reduction. Adverse Drug React Toxicol Rev 18:181–233, 1999.

103. Lee WM: Drug-induced hepatotoxicity. N Engl J Med 333:1118–1129, 1995.

104. Losser MR, Payen D: Mechanisms of liver damage. Semin Liver Dis 16:357–367, 1996.

105. Neuberger J: Drugs and liver damage. In Warrell D, Cox T, Firth J, (eds): Oxford Textbook of Medicine, 4th ed. Oxford, Oxford University Press, 2003, pp 764–770.

106. Larrey D: Hepatotoxicity of herbal remedies. J Hepatol 26(Suppl 1): 47–51, 1997.

107. Brent J: Three new herbal hepatotoxic syndromes. Clin Toxicol 37:715–719, 1999.

108. Katz M, Saibil F: Herbal hepatitis: Subacute hepatic necrosis secondary to chaparral leaf. J Clin Gastroenterol 12:203–206, 1990.

109. Chaparral-induced toxic hepatitis—California and Texas. MMWR Morb Mortal Wkly Rep 41:812–814, 1992.

110. Sheehan MP, Atherton DJ: One year follow-up of children with atopic eczema treated with traditional Chinese medicinal plants. Br J Dermatol 127(Suppl 40):13, 1992.

111. Graham-Brown R: Toxicity of Chinese herbal remedies. Lancet 340:673–674, 1992.

112. Perharic-Walton L, Murray V: Toxicity of Chinese herbal remedies. Lancet 340:674, 1992.

113. Woolf GM, Petrovic LM, Rojter SE, et al: Acute hepatitis associated with the Chinese herbal product Jin Bu Huan. Ann Intern Med 121:729–735, 1994.

114. Fayad M, Choueiri R, Mikati M: Potential hepatotoxicity of lamotrigine. Pediatr Neurol 22:49–52, 2000.

115. Bourgeois B: New antiepileptic drugs. Arch Neurol 55:1181–1183, 1998.

116. Pellock JM: Felbamate in epilepsy therapy: Evaluating the risks. Drug Safety 21:225–239, 1999.

117. Zimmerman HJ, Ishak KG: Valproate-induced hepatic injury: Analysis of 23 fatal cases. Hepatology 2:591–597, 1982.

CHAPTER 9

Psychiatric Issues in the Critically Poisoned Patient

Gregory L. Carter ■ Ruth Lopert

The care of the seriously poisoned patient is usually multidisciplinary, involving various medical specialists, including emergency physicians, anesthesiologists, intensivists, and toxicologists. The role of the psychiatrist sometimes is overlooked, especially in texts that focus on the ABCs (airway, breathing, circulation) of toxicologic management. Reviews of the topic often make little or no mention of the psychiatric management of these patients.[1] Yet patients who deliberately overdose have a high prevalence of preexisting psychiatric disorder,[2] and it is common for patients admitted to intensive care units (ICUs) to develop a psychiatric disturbance (delirium) during their admission, regardless of their premorbid psychiatric state.[3] This chapter describes the important role of the psychiatric service in the management of seriously poisoned patients.

BURDEN OF ILLNESS

Serious poisoning has a spectrum of etiologies. Various informal classifications exist (Table 9-1). Despite a lack of consensus in classification, it is well recognized that deliberate self-poisoning (DSP), recreational drug use, iatrogenic poisoning, and accidental poisoning in children account for most cases requiring hospitalization and treatment. One of the most widely accepted definitions of DSP is as follows:

> The deliberate ingestion of more than the prescribed amount of medicinal substances, or ingestion of substances never intended for human consumption, irrespective of whether harm was intended. This definition takes an epidemiological stance, defining attempted suicide on the basis of behaviour alone, rather than by an inference about intention.[3a]

There is still incomplete agreement, however, concerning the definitions used. Some large-scale studies[4] have preferred the term *parasuicide*.[5] Attempts have been made to operationalize the definitions for all types of self-harming behavior[6] and for suicide.[7]

The personal motivations of the DSP patient are more difficult to classify. Studies of personal motivation tend to suggest that communicating hostility, influencing others, relieving an unpleasant state of mind, and suicidality are the most common. Patients with significant suicidal intent often disclose this early in assessment interviews.[8]

In the United States, the National Co-morbidity Study reported a lifetime suicide attempt rate of 4.6%,[9] and a

Canadian study of school-age adolescents reported an attempt rate of 3.5%.[10] It is unknown what proportion of these attempts result in a presentation to the hospital. A study conducted in the mid-1980s reported that 5% of all ICU admissions in a U.S. center resulted from a drug overdose,[11] but this is likely to vary as a consequence of service mix and admission practices. Deliberate self-harm (DSH) is a common reason for general hospital admission and treatment, and DSP or overdose is overwhelmingly the most common form of DSH.[12] In a year-long survey of 15 European centers of all adult parasuicides treated in the hospital, mean admission rates of 167/100,000/yr for men and 222/100,000/yr for women were reported, although there was wide variation among centers.[13] An epidemiologic center in Oxford, United Kingdom, estimated the national DSH admission rate at approximately 400/100,000/yr.[14,15] DSH is one of the five leading causes of hospital admission for men and women in the United Kingdom, with DSP resulting in 150,000 hospital referrals a year.[14,16] In the United States, DSP has been reported to account for 1% of all emergency department (ED) presentations, with a subsequent admission rate twice that for all other ED patients.[17] In Australia, one regional catchment center estimated a rate of approximately 200/100,000/yr[18] for hospital-treated DSP. DSP accounts for more than 5% of Australian general hospital admissions and almost 20% of all ICU admissions.[19]

Not all cases of poisoning result in serious toxicity. Some units admit all presentations of DSP as a matter of policy, but this is by no means universal. In a New Zealand survey, 69% of all patients presenting with DSP were admitted to the hospital, with 10% admitted to the ICU.[20] There may be threefold to fourfold differences in the rate of direct discharge (nonadmission), however, from EDs in different settings, with 50% of patients with such presentations not admitted in the United Kingdom.[14] ED staff are more likely to discharge patients without admission or psychiatric assessment when the presentation occurs before or after daytime business hours or on weekends,[12] and more than 50% of cases may present during these times.[12,21] Definitions of toxicologically or medically serious cases also vary, although there is at best only a modest association between toxicologic severity and suicidal intent.[22] In New Zealand, a study of adolescents and young adults defined a "medically serious attempt" (at suicide) as one requiring hospitalization for at least 24 hours and at least one of the following: treatment in ICU, hyperbaric unit, or burns unit; surgery under general anesthetic; or medical treatment

TABLE 9-1 Classification of Poisoning Types from Two Australian Centers

CLASSIFICATION OF OVERDOSE*	CLASSIFICATION OF POISONINGS AND ENVENOMATIONS†
Accidental	Deliberate self-harm
Suicidal behavior	Recreational
Recreational/experimentation	Accidental
Compulsive	Iatrogenic
Indeterminate	Envenomations
	Other

*From Reilly et al (1987).[201]
†From Whyte et al (1997).[21]

beyond gastric lavage, activated charcoal, or routine neurologic observations.[23] Older studies defined *medically serious* differently, reflecting the poisonings common at the time and a simpler approach to classification (e.g., a coma level of 3 or 4, serum salicylate >50 mg/100 mL, or carboxyhemoglobin >30%),[22] or simply considered admission to the ICU or critical care unit (CCU) as appropriate to define a *serious poisoning*.[24]

Recreational poisonings in adults are second in frequency to DSP, with alcohol and opioids being the most common agents used. Benzodiazepines, anticholinergics, cocaine, amphetamines, phencyclidine hydrochloride, and hallucinogens (LSD) also are used recreationally and occasionally result in serious toxicity. Other therapeutic compounds, such as neuroleptics, antidepressants, dopamine agonists, and dopamine antagonists, also are used, albeit infrequently, as recreational compounds or drugs of abuse and occasionally may result in serious toxicity. In some instances, there may be serious long-term toxic effects from drugs used recreationally (e.g., former users of 3,4-methylenedioxymethamphetamine may have memory impairment, which is related to the degree of exposure[25]), although these cases rarely require toxicologic assessment.

Iatrogenic poisonings may be a less commonly recognized occurrence, but their potential seriousness should not be underestimated. Psychopharmacologic agents frequently are implicated in iatrogenic poisoning and may give rise to potentially fatal toxidromes, such as lithium toxicity,[26] neuroleptic malignant syndrome,[27] serotonin syndrome,[28,29] and anticholinergic toxicity,[30] and other serious systemic effects (e.g., cardiac arrhythmias, seizures, catatonia, pseudotumor cerebri, ataxia, nephrotic syndrome, priapism, or agranulocytosis).[31] Psychopharmacologic drugs of almost any class can produce serious toxicity in therapeutic use[32] and occasionally may give rise to a serious withdrawal syndrome,[33] which may complicate further an admission for self-poisoning.

There is a degree of interplay between psychiatric illness and toxicity. Commonly a patient with a psychiatric illness is started on a new drug or an increased dose of an existing drug and subsequently develops toxicity. The result is a mixture of psychiatric symptoms and toxicity effects that add a layer of complexity to the patient's management. This mixture can occur in a depressed patient whose therapy is changed from a tricyclic antidepressant to a specific serotonin reuptake inhibitor, with an inadequate washout period, leading to a serotonin syndrome and a mixed affective state (mania and depression). Another example is a schizophrenic patient treated with a neuroleptic who develops a neuroleptic malignant syndrome and who presents with symptoms of neuroleptic malignant syndrome and psychosis but still needs bromocriptine, which may worsen the psychosis.

Childhood poisoning is usually accidental and tends to be associated with less morbidity and mortality than poisoning in adults, which is usually deliberate (suicide or parasuicide).[34] Nevertheless, a study of child psychiatric patients (<13 years old) found a substantial rate of self-reported suicide attempts,[35] so an appropriate level of clinical suspicion is warranted. Children only rarely require admission to an ICU as a result of toxicity,[36] although an increase in the ingestion of drugs such as clonidine may increase the need for ICU admission.[37]

Although childhood poisoning is usually accidental, it remains alarmingly common. In the United States, poisonings result in a hospitalization rate of 65/100,000/yr in children younger than 10 years old,[38] and in the southeastern United States, unintentional poisoning is one of the six most common causes of injury resulting in hospital treatment in children younger than 15 years old.[39] In the United Kingdom, poisoning in children younger than 6 years old occurs at a rate of 333/100,000/yr,[40] whereas in Australia rates of 210/100,000/yr are reported in children younger than 5 years old.[41] Rarer types of poisoning include poisoning resulting from factitious disorders, especially Munchausen syndrome or Munchausen syndrome by proxy. Although rare phenomena, these disorders can result in serious toxicity, especially if the agents used are insulin,[42] anticonvulsants, opiates,[43] or laxatives.[44] The epidemiology of these rarer conditions is harder to establish. A 2-year prospective study in the United Kingdom and Ireland established 128 cases of Munchausen syndrome by proxy, nonaccidental poisoning, and nonaccidental suffocation in children younger than 16 years old, with an estimated rate of 0.5/100,000/yr and a rate greater than 2.8/100,000/yr in children younger than 12 months old.[43] Even the clinical classification of "accidental" childhood poisoning needs to be approached with some caution. A study of 50 childhood poisonings from a U.S. poison control center reported substantial recording of "accidental" cases as "suicidal," "intoxication," and one attempted homicide with only a few remaining as "accidental."[45]

Poisonings—especially poisonings that are deliberate, recreational, or accidental—are a common cause of presentation and admission to the hospital and represent a large burden on the health care sector. Nevertheless, a 1993 review of four measures of poisoning incidence suggested that as there is no gold standard for determining incidence, common surveillance measures of poisoning and drug overdose systematically might undercount morbidity.[46] There also have been calls for improved morbidity-based injury surveillance systems for children rather than the continued reliance on mortality-based data.[39]

Most poisoning deaths occur out of the hospital.[47] Two Australian studies reported an in-hospital death rate of 0.6% for all DSP admissions,[19,21] which reflects the death rate resulting from the initial out-of-hospital poisoning, rather than from suicidal actions taken after admission. Suicide among inpatients of general hospital medical or surgical units is an extremely rare event.[48,49]

ROLE OF CONSULTATION-LIAISON PSYCHIATRY

Consultation-liaison psychiatry is the subspecialty that manages the psychiatric needs of patients in the general hospital setting.[50,51] This subspecialty aims to maintain a bridge between psychiatry and medicine to provide biopsychosocial care to patients in nonpsychiatric settings.[50] Among patients in whom deliberate self-poisoning is certain or suspected, psychiatric management is desirable, but even patients who have been poisoned in recreational circumstances may benefit from some degree of involvement in their care from the psychiatry service; this is especially true of excessive users of alcohol, opioids, cocaine, amphetamines, and other drugs of addiction. Toxicologists and other clinicians managing poisoned patients may choose to involve available consultation-liaison psychiatry services in patient care, or they may manage these patients entirely without psychiatric input. There are now many examples of the multidisciplinary approach documented in the literature.

The Oxford, United Kingdom, regional poisoning service has reported a sizeable reduction in hospital stay in part as a result of the availability of a psychiatric service for assessment and ongoing treatment arrangements.[52] In Australia, an integrated centralized multidisciplinary model for the management of poisoned patients has shown a substantial reduction in length of stay and hospital costs.[21] More than 50% of poisoning presentations occur after regular daytime business hours, and the organization of services should reflect this.[21] A staff consisting of a senior psychiatrist, a psychiatric registrar (resident), two or three nurses, and a social worker has been suggested as sufficient to service 750 to 1000 DSH patients per year.[52]

Consultation-liaison psychiatry has two basic modes of operation. *Consultation psychiatry* generally refers to direct involvement in the clinical care and assessment of individual cases. *Liaison psychiatry* takes a more indirect approach, in which a psychiatrist interacts with and advises the treating team or service, sometimes without direct clinical contact with the patient.[53–55] In most clinical situations, a blend of these two modes is employed. Some authorities suggest that the term *consultation psychiatry* is sufficient to encompass the entire spectrum of activity and that *liaison* is now essentially redundant.[54]

Psychiatric care also is important in other circumstances involving poisoned patients. Chronic psychiatric sequelae sometimes can follow serious poisonings (e.g., with agents such as carbon monoxide[56] and organophosphates[57]). Patients with chronic illness states arguably attributable to various toxicities,[58] such as "multiple chemical sensitivity,"[59] also may benefit from psychiatric input. Occasionally a psychotic patient, believing himself or herself to be seriously poisoned, may enter the treatment system as a toxicology patient and present a clinical challenge.[60] Some poisonings (e.g., carbon monoxide, lead, and mercury) may present with essentially psychiatric symptoms,[61] and recognition of the toxicity may be delayed. A discussion of these specific examples is beyond the scope of this chapter.

STANDARDS OF CARE

In the United Kingdom, the Royal College of Psychiatrists has developed consensus guidelines for facilities, supervision, training, and practice of assessment and aftercare for DSH patients.[62] These guidelines require all DSH patients to have a psychiatric assessment at the time of presentation. Similar guidelines and mandatory service practices have been developed in other countries.[63] The extent to which these standards are achievable in clinical practice is difficult to establish. Reviews from the United Kingdom suggested that only half of the DSH patients who presented to the hospital received a specialist psychosocial assessment before discharge.[14,64] By contrast, a major regional service in Australia reported that 97.2% of DSP patients were assessed psychiatrically.[21] A study of attempted suicide patients in the United States, which used a computerized medical record system for case finding, reported that 78% of all attempters received a psychiatric assessment before discharge.[65] Most of these attempters were cases of "overdose," and 75% of all the overdose patients received a psychiatric assessment before discharge.

The usefulness of psychiatric assessment has been questioned largely because there has been no demonstrated effect on subsequent completed suicide or repetition of DSP/DSH.[66,67] There also has been justifiable criticism of the disorganized and inequitable nature of psychiatric services provided for these patients in the United Kingdom.[64] Psychiatric disorders,[14] substance-related problems,[68] and personality disorders in adults[19,69,70] and adolescents[71] are common in populations of DSP patients, although the patterns of illness may be different at different centers.[72] These patients also may experience relationship problems or psychosocial disadvantage.[73,74] Repeaters may have a higher general burden of psychopathology,[75] with greater risk of psychosis or personality disorder[76] or of a personality disorder and relationship problems.[77] A similar pattern of psychiatric and social problems is reported for adolescent repeaters.[78] Repetition also may constitute a behavioral response to stressful situations.[19] Psychiatric assessment of these patients seems warranted on the grounds of psychological morbidity and current personal crisis even when no benefit for subsequent suicidal behavior has been shown.

Delirium[79] is the most frequent psychiatric condition complicating a serious poisoning. Delirium is often due to drug effects, but aspiration, acidosis, cardiac arrhythmia, seizures, and drug or alcohol withdrawal may play a role. The management of a delirious patient after serious overdose is one of the most common tasks undertaken by the consultation psychiatry service. Guidelines have been developed for the treatment of patients with delirium of all causes[80] and suicidal patients with delirium,[81] and specific reviews are available for the treatment of drug-induced delirium.[82]

OUTCOMES OF DELIBERATE SELF-POISONING

Of the range of potential outcomes of DSP, there are three that are most important: subsequent completed suicide, repetition of DSP, and psychiatric hospitalization.

A review of 24 outcome studies concluded that an episode of DSH has a 1-year outcome of completed suicide of 6% (median 1%), approximately 100 times the general population risk.[14] The suicide risk is highest in the 12 months after an episode of DSH but remains substantially elevated over the general population risk for more than 10 years.[14] About a quarter of all suicides are treated at a hospital for an episode of DSH in the year before they die.[83,84]

Repetition of DSH, predominantly hospital-treated DSP, has been reported to have annual rates of 6% to 30% (median 16%).[14] It is not yet clear the extent to which particular models of service provision affect repetition rates. There may be benefit in admitting all patients rather than making discharge decisions based purely on toxicologic severity or on the apparent absence of psychological risk factors for repetition.[14] Three reviews of randomized controlled trials evaluating specific interventions aimed at reducing repetition are of interest.[14,85,86] Although substantial psychosocial benefits have been shown, few studies have shown a reduction in subsequent suicidal behavior. These results are due, at least in part, to methodologic problems, such as small sample sizes, the exclusion of high-risk subjects, short follow-up, and confusing outcome measures.[87] Among several trials included in a systematic review,[85] the largest effect size was shown in two trials in patients with personality disorders. The first trial treated male and female patients with personality disorder with a depot neuroleptic (flupenthixol).[88] The second trial treated women with borderline personality disorder[89] using dialectical behavior therapy, a specialized form of cognitive behavioral therapy. Other treatments, such as cognitive therapy emphasizing improved problem-solving strategies and a contact card offering contact with a psychiatric registrar (resident), also were thought to be promising by the authors of the review.[85] In a randomized controlled trial, a subgroup of subjects with predominantly cluster B personality disorders treated with paroxetine showed a reduction in repetition independent of depression status.[90]

Psychiatric hospitalization may be necessary after an episode of DSP, and this may be voluntary or involuntary. When toxicology patients are transferred to an appropriate center, their medical needs must be considered. Patients with acute medical problems that may delay a transfer to a psychiatric facility require appropriate standards of psychiatric care to be instituted in the interim within the ICU, CCU, or general ward. The availability of appropriate resources to meet a reasonable standard of psychiatric care varies. Hospitalization most commonly is instigated to protect the patient from an ongoing risk of self-harm, to reduce the risk of harm to others, to treat a psychiatric disorder or personality disorder, or for a combination of these reasons. The rates of psychiatric admission directly after an episode of DSH are less certain, although a range of 5% to 10% has been reported in the United Kingdom,[14] whereas another study reported a rate of 28% in a U.S. unit,[17] and a Swedish study found a rate of 57%.[91]

It is to be hoped that because suicide attempters frequently have a psychiatric disorder, have psychiatric symptoms, or at least are making a "cry for help," appropriate aftercare can be provided. Studies of depressed[92] and alcohol-dependent patients[93] who have made a suicide attempt suggest, however, that treatment before and after the suicide attempt is frequently inadequate. Attendance or compliance with psychiatric follow-up when offered after a poisoning episode has been reported as 16%.[94]

LEGAL ISSUES

"Clinicians should anticipate that there may be a conflict between the clinical and legal standards of care, in which the clinical standard might lean more toward the forensically riskier course of outpatient care and less toward the use of hospitalization."[95] The problem of adequately caring for patients with a variable degree of suicidal intent; patients who present with a deliberate, toxicologically serious poisoning requiring specific intervention; and patients who refuse to accept treatment is a recurrent clinical and legal dilemma facing clinicians. Staff can be immobilized by the threat of litigation—of being found negligent for failing to treat a patient in need of but refusing treatment—or of assault—for treating a patient without his or her consent. The available advice on how to proceed can be conflicting. Legislation and common law may vary in different jurisdictions, and a clinician's capacity to navigate the legal complexities may be inadequate. Treatment models that use psychiatric and other staff or relatives to improve compliance with procedures may be useful,[21] but a few patients may not be persuaded to accept toxicologic treatment. It is important to understand certain legal principles when determining an approach to the treatment of a poisoned patient. A detailed examination of the clinical and legal standards for the care of suicidal patients in the United States is available.[95]

In a review of standards of care for patients at risk of suicide in the United States, the authors noted that reasonable care must be shown by certain affirmative precautions, with standards equivalent to those prevailing in the community, and that the duty of care is proportionate to the patient's needs.[96] The most common legal action brought is for the failure to protect patients from harming themselves, and courts impose much stricter standards on inpatient than on outpatient care.[96] Psychiatrists who follow the procedures of the civil commitment laws are likely to have a broad protection from liability,[97] although psychiatrists who work in the public sector may be more likely to face lawsuits in regard to involuntary commitment.[98]

Consent to treatment requires that the patient understand the risks and benefits of the proposed treatment and those of alternative treatments or of no treatment.[99] Patients should give informed consent for *any* specific treatment; when a patient is incompetent, an appointed guardian may give consent. When a patient is legally competent but lacks the capacity to consent (e.g., comatose or delirious patients) or refuses to give consent, the legal position is less clear.[99] When a medical emergency exists in a delirious patient, the patient can be treated under the common law of implied consent.[100] In addition, there is the common-law principle of a duty of care to consider. Not all countries or provinces have an English common-law tradition, however. A duty of care exists when a physician undertakes the care of a patient; the physician must exercise a standard of care that would minimize the risk of injury to the patient. The standard of care to be expected is that of a "reasonable person" possessing the special skills and knowledge of the professional involved.[101] In emergency situations in which life-saving measures must be employed, physicians may institute treatment immediately without fear of incurring legal liability.[99] A review of the law in relation to suicide suggested that "it appears that there is a judicial assumption that there is a duty to take reasonable steps to prevent the suicide of a competent, informal (voluntary) patient in both psychiatric and ordinary health care settings."[102]

> The common law recognizes that a reasonable person would want to receive treatment in a true medical emergency, even if his impaired awareness at the time of the emergency precluded giving informed consent (. . .) practically this doctrine holds that the physician cannot be found legally liable for performing a procedure to which the patient has not consented, provided the situation is truly an emergency and the treatment itself is medically appropriate.[100]

An article from the United Kingdom outlining the legal issues affecting the care of DSH patients emphasized the concept of competence as the principal determining factor in decisions concerning treatment; however, such a narrow "rights"-based view of competency in suicidal patients has been challenged in a review of case law in relation to suicide.[102] It also has been suggested that because competence is a legal and not a clinical construct, clinicians are unable to apply such principles correctly.[103] Others have suggested that particular clinicians (e.g., psychiatrists) might be able to render an opinion as to a patient's competency[99] and that psychiatrists are able to detect subtle forms of incompetence more readily than other physicians.[104,105] Although competency assessments usually involve cognitive criteria and processes, affective disorders,[99,106] paranoid states, and even anorexia nervosa also may affect a patient's competence.[105]

> As the uncertainties of competency assessment are acknowledged, it is no longer possible to easily say that its determination should be left to the patient's therapist, the hospital's treatment staff, or the courts. Due process may sometimes require an independent, clinically trained person or persons.[105a]

Competency and *committability* are two different concepts legally and clinically.[99] Regardless of whether a patient is *committable* under the relevant civil legislation, a patient still must be presumed initially *competent* to refuse potentially lifesaving, anxiety-provoking, or merely inconvenient medical treatment. Specific procedures have been developed to assess psychiatric patients' competency to agree to treatment plans,[107] although these have not been adopted or accepted universally by the courts in the United States.[108] One of the key components of these procedures involves establishing that the patient understands the risks and benefits of withholding important information needed for assessment or appropriate treatment. Specifically in the case of a patient at risk for suicide, the withholding of dangerous thoughts or plans about self-injury or suicide needs to be understood by the patient as reducing the capacity of the treatment service to adequately protect him or her. Should the patient subsequently harm himself or herself after demonstrating this area of competence, the clinician may be able to show to a court that the patient's act was by deliberate rational choice or at least to have a defense against a charge of negligence.[107] If a patient was unable to show that he or she could understand the importance of withholding such clinical information, however, he or she would require more conservative management.[108] If patients are thought to be incompetent (either generally or in regard to consent to treatment), they may require presentation to a

judicial officer or some form of judicial process to be declared incompetent and so have the necessary treatment given. This situation is untenable when urgent treatment is required for the prevention of serious disability or death.

The position concerning *involuntary detention* or *psychiatric or civil commitment* is more clear-cut. Specific legislation usually defines the circumstances in which a person may be detained involuntarily. Details vary among jurisdictions, but typically the patient must be "mentally ill" and dangerous to either self or others. This judgment involves a prediction concerning the likelihood of such dangerousness or harm and an accepted threshold for such a prediction.[109] The clinical task often involves an evaluation of the balance between civil liberty and benevolence.[110]

In 1983, "a model state law on civil commitment of the mentally ill"[111] was proposed in the United States, suggesting four criteria necessary for involuntary commitment. A later summary of commitment legislation suggested six common criteria (Table 9-2).[112] An important focus of these developments was the need to place the patient's interests first, especially the need to treat psychiatric conditions likely to respond to treatment and not to consider dangerousness as the only criterion for commitment.[111] Similar principles have been incorporated into mental health legislation in other countries.[113–115] In a review of all statutory requirements[116] for involuntary hospitalization in the United States, it was found that each jurisdiction requires a person to have a mental illness and be dangerous to himself or herself, and 85% of jurisdictions require the dangerousness to be a result of the mental illness. Only two jurisdictions require, however, that an attempt be made to involuntarily commit a person in imminent danger to himself or herself. These findings were similar to an older review.[117] It has been suggested that clinicians rely particularly on the "dangerousness" criterion in seeking a commitment while being sensitive to the patient's need for treatment.[118] Even after involuntary referral to a psychiatric hospital, the patient may not be admitted or may be admitted only briefly. The process of admission to the hospital in two U.S. psychiatric hospitals has been reported to be influenced by factors from four categories: (1) characteristics of patients, (2) characteristics of admitting personnel, (3) system factors, and (4) the patient assessment.[119] Evaluations of the decision making by the judge in civil commitment decisions have shown that statutory and nonstatutory variables affect the process, with the

TABLE 9-2 Eligibility for Involuntary Hospitalization from Two Studies

STROMBERG AND STONE (1983)[111]	BEDNAR ET AL (1991)[112]
A severe mental disorder is present	Mental illness
Lacks the capacity to make a reasoned treatment decision	Danger to self or others or grave disability
Has a treatable condition	Refusal to consent
Likely to harm self or others	Treatable condition
	Lack of capacity to decide on treatment
	Use of the least restrictive treatment

patient's family favoring commitment being an important issue.[120] The decision to discharge a patient who has been committed involuntarily is difficult, and special procedures have been suggested to ensure that release decisions are competent and defensible (Table 9-3).[121]

Clinical decisions concerning the management of poisoned patients may be influenced by the fear of other forms of litigation. In addition to the issues already discussed, the psychiatrist (and other physicians) must deal with the legal implications of acts of violence, injuries resulting from negligent treatment, faulty treatment processes, and liability arising from inadequate supervisory relationships.[122] Occasionally there may be a duty to warn others of the risk of harm from a dangerous patient. A U.S. study found that this duty rarely is discharged by clinicians and that only 52% of dangerous patients were civilly committed.[123] Conversely, some authors have suggested that a fear of litigation may lead to some patients' being unnecessarily hospitalized because of a perceived risk of violence.[124]

ETHICAL ISSUES

Legal issues cannot be considered in isolation from ethical issues. Legislation concerning involuntary detention commonly incorporates the legal notion of a "least restrictive setting." It has been argued that this principle does not require positive results for the patient—that it tolerates neglect and is at odds with the medical goals of reducing suffering or improving function.[125] The decision to hospitalize involuntarily also should include the ethical consideration of being in the patient's "best interests."[109] It has been suggested that the ethical values of the law and medicine may be inherently in conflict in this clinical setting, especially when the possibility of involuntary psychiatric treatment is concerned.[125] It also has been suggested that in the treatment of psychiatrically ill patients, initial coercion can lead to greater freedom[125]; in other words, a greater benefit may accrue to the patient because of the insistence on legally applying appropriate psychiatric treatment.

BEHAVIORAL CONTROL

Seriously poisoned patients may exhibit a range of behavioral disturbance resulting from delirium, agitation, anxiety, suicidal ideation, relationship problems with staff or family, personality traits, persecutory delusions, hallucinatory phenomena, misunderstandings, pain, or a combination of these and other factors. For patient comfort, treatment requirements, and staff safety, there may be occasions when it is necessary to reduce the degree of behavioral disturbance. Understanding of the principles of "abnormal illness behavior"[60,126] and "abnormal treatment behavior"[127] may be useful. An important point to consider is that these patient behaviors usually involve some degree of interaction with the behavior of the service providers; they do not exist in a psychosocial vacuum. This understanding may suggest strategies for change within the treatment system and opportunities for direct, nonpharmacologic management of the patient; this has been expressed best in relation to borderline personality disorder. "In the medical setting, psychoanalytic interpretations of the unconscious are destined to fail; non-interpretive behavioral approaches are the ones that work."[127a]

Cognitive and behavioral interventions are common modes of effective nonpharmacologic intervention currently used. The more sophisticated forms of these psychological interventions are not generally applicable while the patient is in the ICU and are deployed more usefully during the recovery phase. Practical, nonpharmacologic interventions are usually of greater use during the period of treatment for severe toxicity.

NONPHARMACOLOGIC MANAGEMENT OF PSYCHOLOGICAL DISTURBANCE IN THE INTENSIVE CARE UNIT

The nonmedical aspects of management of the self-poisoned patient in the intensive care setting—the aspects of care that relate to the patient's emotional and psychological state, as opposed to the requirement to address the ABCs of emergency management and detoxification—are important. Psychological disturbance associated with ICU admission is well described even in patients without prior psychiatric morbidity. Disorientation, restlessness, agitation, confusion, and frank delirium are seen frequently in the ICU patient regardless of the reason for admission. Many aspects of the intensive care environment are in themselves sufficient to produce psychological disturbance. The ICU is an intrinsically frightening environment—it is difficult to imagine a more disturbing experience than the gradual or sudden regaining of consciousness coupled with the realization of the presence of an endotracheal tube and mechanical ventilation. ICUs often do not respect the distinction between

---

TABLE 9-3 Special Procedures for the Discharge of Involuntarily Committed Patients

Demonstrating Diligence in Release Decisions
Special policy development
  Adequate legal consultation in release policy drafting process
  Explicit documentation of violence assessment
  Systematically develop and document information pertinent
    to the assessment of the patient's potential for violence
  Hierarchical review (or "second opinion")
  Release procedures written so that the proposal to release is
    reviewable by senior staff or review committee

Meeting the Professional Standard of Care Criterion
Consultant health professional review of institution's policies regarding
    release (at the time of policy development)
  Enables feedback to ensure that policies meet professional standard of care
  Provides evidence of diligence in policy development process

Projecting a Positive Image of the Released Patient
Videotaped exit interviews conducted by skilled clinical staff at or near
    release date

Adapted from Poythress NG Jr: Avoiding negligent release: Contemporary clinical and risk management strategies. Am J Psychiatry 147:994–997, 1990.

day and night; they may be uncomfortable, confusing, and disorienting places, which can contribute easily to a patient's sense of depersonalization.

In considering the causes of psychological disturbance in the poisoned patient, the full panoply of organic comorbidities and the effects of their treatment must be considered in addition to the primary reason for admission. Recognition of and attendance to reversible causes of anxiety also should not be overlooked; in addition to the pathophysiologic effects of poisoning, these patients equally can be in pain, cold, or septic; have blocked catheters; or be in alcohol or other drug withdrawal.

ICU staff may be able to manage psychological disturbance[128] without particular need for formal psychiatric input. There are many simple, nonpharmacologic strategies that may be employed in the critical care setting to minimize psychological stress to the patient. Fundamental to these environmental strategies are the goals of orientation and reassurance. Key supportive measures include minimizing noise and sleep disturbance, clustering interventions, arranging appropriate ambient lighting or proximity to natural light, and displaying personal objects and photographs of familiar faces. In addition, ensuring consistency of staff members; facilitating communication with symbols, charts, whiteboards, and pointing devices for a delirious or intubated patient; simple and repeated explanations and reassurance by staff; and flexible visiting schedules to facilitate family and social supports all are valuable techniques that may be employed to help minimize anxiety.[129] Where possible, patients' relatives or significant others should be encouraged to participate in communicating with and reassuring the patient.

It is essential that ICUs have appropriate designated spaces for promoting effective communications with families—comfortable, nonthreatening places offering quiet and privacy, physically removed but not too distant from the unit. Attitudes of relatives are difficult to optimize in ICUs that lack appropriate places where relatives are able to speak with patients or staff. Relatives are frequently upset and when upset are more likely to misinterpret communications with staff.[130]

Historically the use of physical restraint for management of behaviorally disturbed patients with delirium (of any type) was far more common than it is today. Most mental health legislation and case law emphasize the principle of the "least restrictive alternative" form of care. The American Psychiatric Association Task Force's report on seclusion and restraint has suggested possible indications for use, as follows: the prevention of imminent harm to self or others when other methods are ineffective; the prevention of substantial damage to the physical environment; the prevention of serious disruption to the treatment program; as a contingency in the behavior therapy of dangerous behaviors; to decrease stimulation; and at the patient's request.[131] Although these indications are not universally agreed on, several of these indications might be relevant to seriously poisoned patients. Restraints are not without their proponents and probable usefulness, although a balance between the possible benefits and risks should be made in light of available evidence.[132] Perhaps the best indications for effectiveness are for the prevention of injury and reduction of agitation in inpatient psychi-

atric settings.[132] The usefulness of restraint in medical settings may be less than in psychiatric settings, and the indications for use may be less clear. A review of physical restraint in medical settings suggested that there is a strong likelihood of death's being underreported, with death or injury commonly due to strangulation, circulatory damage, and neuronal damage.[133]

In addition to physical injuries, adverse psychological effects on patients[133] and staff have been recognized.[132] Staff training in the prediction and prevention of violence may be valuable[134] in reducing the rates of usage and untoward effects of restraint.[132] Physicians and patients in a psychiatric setting reportedly favored psychotropic medication over physical restraint.[135] There is a reported continuing decline in the use of physical restraint in CCUs in response to ethical and clinical concerns,[136,137] although the rates of usage in psychiatric hospitals may be unchanged.[138] The opportunity for psychiatric staff to positively influence disturbed behavior has been expanded beyond restraint to include the manipulation of the patient's environment and psychological and pharmacologic strategies.

Patients may experience significant anxiety after self-poisoning, and this may arise from a delirium; as a direct effect of the toxic ingestion; as a result of the stressful experiences of resuscitation and hospitalization; because of a preexisting anxiety, depressive, or psychotic disorder; or some combination of these factors. Many of the management principles are similar to those for delirium,[80] and recommendations for recognition, assessment, and treatment of anxiety in CCUs are available.[129]

It is thought that most patients have little or no memory of their stay in the ICU[3]; among patients who do have recall, some may develop a posttraumatic stress disorder that will require long-term follow-up. Some types of poisoning (e.g., organophosphate poisoning, colchicine overdose, lithium toxicity) may lead to a prolonged stay in the ICU and require a range of invasive procedures. This prolonged exposure to traumatic events may increase the risk of long-term psychological sequelae.

PHARMACOLOGIC MANAGEMENT OF DELIRIUM, ANXIETY, AGGRESSION, AND AGITATION

There is far from a consensus on the appropriate drug, dose, or route of administration to be used for the management of disturbed behavior, whether associated with delirium or other psychiatric disturbance. There are few randomized controlled trials with clearly defined DSP patient samples. There should be clearly defined indications for the use of pharmacologic interventions because not all delirious patients require them.[82] Suggested indications include aggression, risk of harm to self or others,[139] hallucinations, distress, and perhaps insomnia.[82]

The most commonly used medications, by class, include neuroleptics, benzodiazepines, narcotics, anticonvulsants, and general anesthetics.[140–142] Haloperidol and the benzodiazepines, alone or in combination, have been suggested as the drugs of choice for the treatment of acute agitation and delirium in critically ill patients.[141] Within each drug class, there are often several candidate drugs to consider. Benzo-diazepines are sedating, are available in parenteral forms, have a high level of safety, and are pharmacologically reversible. Diazepam, lorazepam, and midazolam have been chosen most commonly. Neuroleptic drugs used most commonly are haloperidol, chlorpromazine, and droperidol, all of which have parenteral forms and high relative safety. Haloperidol probably has been the most popular, although it is relatively nonsedating and has substantial risk of extrapyramidal side effects. Droperidol has similar properties to haloperidol and traditionally has been used in many ICU settings. Chlorpromazine may have advantages over haloperidol in some settings; it is more sedating, has lower risk of extrapyramidal effects, is probably useful in treating withdrawal states, and is an effective treatment for the acute phase of serotonin syndrome.[143] More recently, risperidone has been used as an alternative to the older neuroleptics because of lower rates of extrapyramidal effects.

A consensus process involving more than 40 experts from the membership of the American College of Critical Care Medicine and the Society of Critical Care Medicine recommended midazolam or propofol for the short-term (<24 hours) treatment of anxiety, lorazepam for the prolonged treatment of anxiety, and haloperidol for the treatment of delirium in critically ill adults.[144] A review of ICU management has suggested pharmacologic strategies of using haloperidol, midazolam, or both, or midazolam (or lorazepam), fentanyl, or both.[145]

ATTITUDES AND SKILLS OF STAFF

The attitudes of ICU staff toward their patients are important to the success of the therapeutic relationship. Patients who have attempted suicide present a set of conflicts and contradictions. The ICU is the repository of finely honed lifesaving skills and high-technology equipment; yet these often limited resources are expended at times, in apparent paradox, in the care of patients who have expressed a wish to die. There may be a tendency for staff to consider aggressive lifesaving treatment in these patients as antithetical to the purpose of the ICU.[146] This attitudinal set represents not only a lack of compassion but also a failure to understand the patient's motives. Even repeat attempters are not necessarily intent on ending their lives. Rather, they may be seeking relief or escape from intolerable feelings of hopelessness and despair, often complicated by problems of (negative) cognitive distortion and impaired problem-solving abilities,[147] which may have their origins in childhood neglect[148]; physical or sexual abuse[149–151]; parental loss[152]; family violence[152]; or family history of depression, substance abuse, and parent-child discord[153]—all thought to be risk factors for suicidal behavior in later life.

Although health care professionals may be less likely than laypersons to be judgmental in their attitudes toward attempted suicide, it also has been reported that nursing staff may view attempted suicide as attention-seeking behavior.[154] In a study of almost 300 critical care nurses and more than 80 physicians working in Australian EDs and ICUs, it was found that both groups were frequently negative in their attitudes toward patients who had attempted suicide, with more than half considering parasuicide patients as manipu-

lative.[146] Almost two thirds indicated that they did not enjoy caring for these patients. The results seemed to be independent of the gender or professional status (i.e., nurse or physician) of the respondent and of the number of years of experience in the critical care environment. A sense of frustration was a theme frequently conveyed through individual comments. This study suggests that it is common for physicians and nurses to have attitudes that would work against the establishment of a sound therapeutic relationship with these patients. Similar negative attitudes to DSP patients have been found in studies of junior physicians and nursing staff in the United Kingdom.[155] A Scandinavian study of 40 consecutive suicide attempters admitted to the ICU found that the ICU personnel did not observe the patient's underlying feelings but responded to observable behavior, with reactions ranging from empathy to distancing and even to aggression.[130] Other factors that have been reported as contributing to negative attitudes in ICU staff are perceptions of poor institutional support, a lack of positive reinforcement from the patients themselves, and inadequate educational preparation to provide optimal care for these patients,[156] the lack of which conceivably could reinforce misconceptions and stereotypes that prevail in the professional and the lay communities.

Appropriate nursing goals in the care of suicidal patients in CCUs have been identified and disseminated: developing an understanding of the patient's response after a suicide attempt, accepting the patient in the unit, developing trust, conveying a sense of hope, providing psychosocial support, preparing the patient for discharge or transfer from the CCU, and managing problematic patient behavior.[157] Goals require appropriate education, training, support, and reinforcement if they are to be more than mere ideals. Consultation-liaison psychiatry nursing staff may be invaluable in helping ICU nursing staff to develop these skills.

ATTITUDES OF FAMILY

Patients in the critical care setting may be isolated abruptly and effectively from their usual social support systems and may have a reduced or diminished capacity to comprehend their circumstances or process new information.[129,158] They may be more likely to rely on support from friends and family rather than staff members. Where possible, staff should allow some flexibility in visiting schedules and should keep family and friends apprised of the patient's support needs.[129,159]

For patients who have attempted suicide, relationships with family or significant others may be strained by the events preceding the suicide attempt or may be frankly dysfunctional. Significant others may express ambivalence or hostility and aggression toward the patient and be unable or unwilling to provide even limited support.[160] Family members may withdraw support from the patient or even file "do not resuscitate" orders—sometimes a form of "passive euthanasia."[161] This may reflect ambivalence in the preexisting relationship or the inability to deal with a deteriorating depression and suicidality that preceded the self-poisoning episode. Even when this is not the case, the patient who *perceives* his or her social or familial support as inadequate or falling short of what the patient feels he or she needs may reject or frustrate further efforts to support him or her and engender feelings of rejection or indifference or the discontinuation of contacts, exacerbating the patient's sense of isolation.[129,162]

RATING SCALES

Suicidal Risk

Traditionally, clinical assessment has been used for assessment of immediate and long-term suicidal risk. This assessment is guided by many factors; a summary of the single variables that best predict suicide can be found in Table 9-4. Perhaps the most important aspect of the clinical assessment in determining short-term suicidal risk is the three-stage empathic enquiry:

1. What is the strength of your suicidal thinking at the moment?
2. What plans have you made to put these thoughts into action?
3. What would have to happen or go wrong from here that would make you likely to activate these plans?

More detailed material on the clinical assessment of the suicidal patient is available from several sources.[81,163–168]

The use of rating scales for the clinical assessment of various aspects of the suicidal actions of self-poisoning patients probably is not widely practiced, but many instruments are available for different purposes and clinical populations (Table 9-5). Some authors[169,170] recommend the use of particular scales, including the Scale for Suicide Ideation (for ideators), the Hopelessness Scale, the Suicide Intent Scale (for attempters), the Los Angeles Suicide Prevention Center Scale, the Scale for Assessing Suicidal Risk, and the Risk-Rescue Rating. Reviews of the psycho-

metric properties and usefulness of instruments concerned with suicide evaluation are available for all ages[171,172] and specifically for adolescents and young adults.[173]

The prediction of future suicide is difficult whether clinical assessments or rating scales are used. Both methods tend to produce a high rate of false-positive predictions and fail to predict some subsequent suicides.

Delirium

The presence of cognitive impairment, usually the result of a delirium, is common in seriously poisoned patients, and the severity of the impairment may have treatment and prognostic significance. There is a large range of instruments that measure cognitive impairment, screen for delirium, diagnose delirium, or rate the severity of delirium symptoms. Reviews may be useful in selecting the appropriate instrument for a given clinical setting.[174,175] Perhaps the most widely used are the mini-mental status examination[176] and the standardized mini-mental status examination,[177] which are screening instruments for cognitive impairment. The abbreviated mental status examination has been evaluated specifically in overdose patients and found to be clinically useful, with strong correlation to Glasgow Coma Scale. It also seems to have acceptable psychometric properties and to be a sensitive prognosticator of adverse outcome.[178] The American Psychiatric Association guidelines for the treatment of patients with delirium suggest that clinical assessment is usually sufficient for the diagnosis of delirium but also make suggestions for the use of delirium instruments and routine diagnostic investigations.[80]

Other Conditions

Apart from suicidal risk and delirium, there may be circumstances in which screening instruments for various conditions are used less frequently. Examples of these might include various bedside tests of other cognitive functions.[159] Similarly, depression and anxiety are relatively common, and suitable instruments include the Hospital Anxiety and Depression Scale,[179] which has been used in a variety of hospital-treated patients.[180]

CHILDREN AND ADOLESCENTS

Poisonings in young children, whether toxicologically significant or not, usually are considered to be "accidental," in the sense of there being no deliberate intent on the part of the child to harm himself or herself. Most primary prevention programs aim to reduce the morbidity and mortality of these poisonings through educational programs and packaging modifications (sublethal doses and the use of child-resistant closures). It has been suggested, however, that the factor most closely associated with childhood poisoning is the general level of psychological adjustment in the child and the family.[181] Perhaps 25% of all child patients repeat the poisoning, and although few studies have focused on these repeater populations, it would seem that child behavioral disturbance and family dysfunction are highly relevant.[181] In a series of clonidine poisonings reported in

---

TABLE 9-4 Single Predictors of Suicide

1. Depressive illness, mental disorder
2. Alcoholism, drug abuse
3. Suicide ideation, talk, preparation; religious ideas
4. Prior suicide attempts
5. Lethal methods
6. Isolation, living alone, loss of support
7. Hopelessness, cognitive rigidity
8. Older, white, man
9. Contact with suicide, family suicide
10. Work, financial problems, occupation
11. Marital problems, family pathology
12. Stress, life events
13. Anger, aggression, irritability, abnormalities of central nervous system 5-hydroxytryptamine (serotonin) metabolism
14. Physical illness
15. Repetition and comorbidity of factors 1–14

Adapted from Maris RW: Overview of suicide assessment and prediction. In Maris RW, Berman AL, Maltsberger JT, et al (eds): Assessment and Prediction of Suicide. New York, Guilford Press, 1992, pp 3–24.

TABLE 9-5 Suicide Prediction Scales

SCALE	AUTHOR	YEAR	TYPE
Subject as Informant			
Hopelessness Scale	Beck et al	1974	20 true-false questions
Index of Potential Suicide	Zung	1974	69 items, Likert scale
Rorschach Suicide Constellation	Exner and Wylie	1977	12 ratios from Rorschach
Suicide Probability Scale	Cull and Gill	1982	36 items, Likert scale
Reasons for Living Inventory	Linehan et al	1983	48 true-false questions
Suicide Risk Measure	Plutchick et al	1989	14 yes-no questions
Second Party as Informant			
Instrument for the Evaluation of Suicide Potential*	Cohen et al	1966	14 yes-no items
Suicide Potential Scale	Dean	1967	26-item checklist
Scale for Assessing Suicide Risk	Tuckman and Youngman	1968	14-item checklist
Los Angeles Suicide Prevention Center Scale	Beck et al	1974	65 items, 0–9 severity score
Neuropsychiatric Hospital Suicide Prevention Schedule*	Farberow and MacKinnon	1974	11 items
Suicide Intent Scale*	Beck et al	1974	20 items, 0–2 severity score
Suicidal Death Prediction Scale (Long and Short)	Lettieri	1974	Variable items, 0–2 severity score
Scale for Predicting Subsequent Suicidal Behavior*	Buglas and Horton	1974	6 present-absent items
Intent Scale*	Pierce	1977	12 items, Likert scale
Short Risk Scale*	Pallis et al	1982	6 items
SAD PERSONS	Patterson et al	1983	10-item checklist
Clinical Instrument to Estimate Suicide Risk	Motto et al	1985	15-item checklist

*Developed in or applied to hospital-treated deliberate self-harm populations.
Adapted from Rothberg JM, Geer-Williams C: A comparison and review of suicide prediction scales. In Maris RW, Berman AL, Maltsberger JT, et al (eds): Assessment and Prediction of Suicide. New York, Guilford Press, 1992, pp 202–217.

Australia, it was noted that the child's own medication, for the treatment of a behavioral disorder, was the source of ingested medication.[37]

These findings suggest that psychiatric assessment in cases of accidental childhood poisoning cases may be worthwhile to identify possible remedial factors. We are not aware, however, of any consultation psychiatry studies or programs in the clinical area specifically directed at this population.

Within the hospital setting, health professionals caring for children experience clinical and ethical problems similar to those of professionals involved in the care of poisoned adults, with some additional complexity. Delirium in children is often drug induced and is usually the result of accidental poisoning but occasionally may be deliberate or iatrogenic. A delirious child may interfere with intravenous lines and endotracheal tubes or present hostile behavior, and the psychiatric assessment and management of children at an early stage in delirium is recommended.[182] In the ICU in particular, the presence of a parent may be one of the most useful interventions for reassurance and behavioral control.[183]

Particular clinical scenarios require mention. Munchausen syndrome by proxy is a form of factitious disorder in which an adult, usually a parent, presents a child for hospital treatment. The child may be gravely ill, particularly if a poisoning has engendered the clinical presentation. A poisoning in this context is particularly stressful and warrants psychiatric involvement as part of a multidisciplinary approach.[184] Child and parental deaths have been known to occur in this disorder.

Adolescent suicide, DSH, and DSP have been reported to be increasing in recent years. Substantial numbers of middle school–age children involved in recreational drug use resulting in treatment also have been reported.[185] The assessment of the adolescent DSH patient may present particular difficulties, and the provision of and compliance with appropriate aftercare may be an even more difficult task, one that falls in large part to psychiatry services. Important elements of treatment may include addressing potential sources of noncompliance, determining proper intensity of treatment, providing family psychoeducation, treating concurrent psychopathology, and remediating social skills and problem-solving deficits.[186] The assessment of suicidal adolescents should begin in the ED and continue into a general hospital stay using predictors derived from adolescent suicides[187] or attempters.[188] Overviews of the general assessment and treatment of the suicidal adolescent[164] are applied usefully to the specific circumstance of the self-poisoned adolescent. Staff from the psychiatric service may be able to provide consultation services for the patient and liaison services for the staff.[189] Psychiatric disorders are as common in child and adolescent suicide attempters as they are in adult patients, although the pattern of disorder is different.[190–193] In addition to psychiatric disorders, self-poisoning patients frequently have difficulties in relationships with parents, boyfriends or girlfriends, school, work, or physical health.[194] Attendance for psychiatric follow-up may be low[195] even among children of school age.[196] Attempts to use a home-based treatment program were evaluated in a randomized controlled trial but failed to produce differences in the main outcome variables.[197] Good outcomes in the longer term may be related in part to improvements in home circumstances and in relationships with supportive and well-functioning adults.[192]

FUTURE RESEARCH AREAS

The opportunities for future research at the toxicology/psychiatry interface are as limitless as the possibilities for scientific evaluation of antidotes for specific poisonings.

Some issues are more important because of their relevance to the seriously poisoned patient.

1. What is the optimal pharmacologic management of delirium?

There is a need for randomized controlled trials, with clearly defined populations, that evaluate drug and dosage regimens and use standardized instruments relevant to the aspects of delirium or attendant behavioral disturbance to measure outcomes.

2. What are the optimal pharmacologic treatments of the toxidromes—neuroleptic malignant syndrome, serotonin syndrome, and anticholinergic delirium?

There is a need for randomized controlled (multicenter) trials. It may be necessary to develop suitable instruments to evaluate treatment response in these specific conditions.

3. What is the cost-effectiveness of service delivery systems for seriously poisoned patients?

There is a need to develop an appropriate methodology for evaluating the cost-effectiveness of multidisciplinary or psychiatric services to these patient groups; this would enable the evaluation of competing models of service delivery.

4. Can repetition of deliberate self-poisoning be reduced?

The repetition of DSP is an important phenomenon for which the epidemiology is reasonably well described, at least in some countries and regions. The field requires the evaluation of new or promising interventions, using randomized controlled trials, with sufficient sample sizes and with the inclusion of high-risk subjects.[85,198]

5. Which patients are referred for psychiatric hospitalization; what are their diagnoses; which patients benefit from psychiatric hospitalization?

These are important questions and have not been addressed adequately. There are considerable limitations because of ethical constraints and practical difficulties in recruiting subjects. A practical approach would be to conduct prospective, long-term, naturalistic cohort studies of clinical populations referred for psychiatric hospitalization. Outcome measures should include completed suicide, repeat DSP, service utilization, disability, quality of life, and social function.

FUTURE DEVELOPMENTS

There have been calls by the U.S. Surgeon-General for a systematic public health approach at a national level to reduce the frequency of suicide and suicidal behavior.[199] It also has been suggested that a comprehensive strategy aimed at preventing suicidal behavior should include a national collection of information on DSH and interventions, improved services in dealing with persons with suicidal behavior or at high risk for such behavior, the provision of information to and training of professionals and the public, and the provision of special services to high-risk groups.[200] There is ample opportunity for future collaboration between toxicologists and psychiatrists on many aspects of the management of poisoned patients. Restriction of these interests only to suicidal or DSP patients is unnecessary.

REFERENCES

1. Kulling P, Persson H: Role of the intensive care unit in the management of the poisoned patient. Med Toxicol 1:375–386, 1986.
2. Beaumont G, Hetzel W: Patients at risk of suicide and overdose. Psychopharmacology 106(Suppl):S123-S126, 1992.
3. Lloyd GG: Psychological problems and the intensive care unit. BMJ 307:458–459, 1993.
3a. Bancroft J, Skrimshire A, Reynolds F, et al: Self poisoning and self injury in the Oxford area: Epidemiological aspects 1969–1973. Br J Prev Soc Med 29:170–177, 1975.
4. Bille-Brahe U, Schmidtke A, Kerkhof AJ, et al: Background and introduction to the WHO/EURO Multicentre Study on Parasuicide. Crisis 16:72–78, 1984.
5. Kreitman N, Philip AE, Greer S, et al: Parasuicide. Br J Psychiatry 115:746–747, 1969.
6. O'Carroll PW, Berman AL, Maris RW, et al: Beyond the Tower of Babel: A nomenclature for suicidology. Suicide Life Threat Behav 26:23–39, 1996.
7. Rosenberg ML, Davidson LE, Smith JC, et al: Operational criteria for the determination of suicide. J Forensic Sci 33:1445–1456, 1988.
8. Bancroft J, Hawton K, Simkin S, et al: The reasons people give for taking overdoses: A further inquiry. Br J Med Psychol 52:353–365, 1979.
9. Kessler RC, Borges G, Walters EE: Prevalence of and risk factors for lifetime suicide attempts in the national comorbidity survey. Arch Gen Psychiatry 56:617–626, 1999.
10. Pronovost J, Cote L, Ross C: Epidemiological study of suicidal behaviour among secondary-school students. Canada Mental Health 38:9–14, 1990.
11. Stern TA, Mulley AG, Thibault GE: Life-threatening drug overdose: Precipitants and prognosis. JAMA 251:1983–1985, 1984.
12. Dennis M, Beach M, Evans PA, et al: An examination of the accident and emergency management of deliberate self harm. J Accid Emerg Med 14:311–315, 1997.
13. Platt S, Bille-Brahe U, Kerkhof A, et al: Parasuicide in Europe: The WHO/EURO multicentre study on parasuicide: I. Introduction and preliminary analysis for 1989. Acta Psychiatr Scand 85:97–104, 1992.
14. House A, Owens D, Patchett L: Deliberate self-harm. Effective Health Care 4:1–12, 1998.
15. House A, Owens D, Storer D: Psycho-social intervention following attempted suicide: Is there a case for better services? Int Rev Psychiatry 4:15–22, 1992.
16. Hawton K, Fagg J: Trends in deliberate self poisoning and self injury in Oxford, 1976–90. BMJ 304:1409–1411, 1992.
17. Stern TA, Gross PL, Pollack MH, et al: Drug overdoses seen in the emergency department: Assessment, disposition, and follow-up. Ann Clin Psychiatry 3:223–231, 1991.
18. Carter GL, Whyte IM, Ball K, et al: Repetition of deliberate self-poisoning in an Australian hospital-treated population. Med J Aust 170:307–311, 1999.
19. McGrath J: A survey of deliberate self-poisoning. Med J Aust 150:317–322, 1989.
20. Weir P, Ardagh M: The epidemiology of deliberate self poisoning presenting to Christchurch Hospital Emergency Department. N Z Med J 111:127–129, 1998.
21. Whyte IM, Dawson AH, Buckley NA, et al: A model for the management of self-poisoning. Med J Aust 167:142–146, 1997.
22. Rosen DH: The serious suicide attempt: Five-year follow-up study of 886 patients. JAMA 235:2105–2109, 1976.
23. Beautrais AL, Joyce PR, Mulder RT: Risk factors for serious suicide attempts among youths aged 13 through 24 years. J Am Acad Child Adolesc Psychiatry 35:1174–1182, 1996.
24. Frati ME, Marruescos L, Porta M, et al: Acute severe poisoning in Spain: Clinical outcome related to the implicated drugs. Hum Toxicol 2:625–632, 1983.
25. Bolla KI, McCann UD, Ricaurte GA: Memory impairment in abstinent MDMA ("Ecstasy") users. Neurology 51:1532–1537, 1998.
26. Minden SL, Bassuk EL, Nadler SP: Lithium intoxication: A coordinated treatment approach. J Gen Intern Med 8:33–40, 1993.
27. Pearlman CA: Neuroleptic malignant syndrome: A review of the literature. J Clin Psychopharmacol 6:257–273, 1986.
28. Sternbach H: The serotonin syndrome. Am J Psychiatry 148:705–713, 1991.

29. Gillman PK: Serotonin syndrome—history and risk. Fundam Clin Pharmacol 12:482–491, 1998.

30. Lipowski ZJ: Intoxication with medical drugs. In Delirium: Acute Confusional States. New York, Oxford University Press, 1990, pp 229–276.

31. Tueth MJ: Emergencies caused by side effects of psychiatric medications. Am J Emerg Med 12:212–216, 1994.

32. Meredith TJ, Vale JA: Poisoning due to psychotropic agents. Adverse Drug React Acute Poison Rev 4:83–126, 1985.

33. Dilsaver SC, Alessi NE: Antipsychotic withdrawal symptoms: Phenomenology and pathophysiology. Acta Psychiatr Scand 77:241–246, 1988.

34. Meredith TJ: Epidemiology of poisoning. Pharmacol Ther 59:251–256, 1993.

35. Milling L, Campbell NB, Davenport CW, et al: Suicidal behavior among psychiatric inpatient children: An estimate of prevalence. Child Psychiatry Hum Dev 22:71–77, 1991.

36. Wiseman HM, Guest K, Murray VS, et al: Accidental poisoning in childhood: A multicentre survey: 1. General epidemiology. Hum Toxicol 6:293–301, 1987.

37. Erickson SJ, Duncan A: Clonidine poisoning—an emerging problem: Epidemiology, clinical features, management and preventative strategies. J Paediatr Child Health 34:280–282, 1998.

38. Rodriguez JG, Sattin RW: Epidemiology of childhood poisonings leading to hospitalization in the United States, 1979–1983. Am J Prev Med 3:164–170, 1987.

39. King WD: Pediatric injury surveillance: use of a hospital discharge data base. South Med J 84:342–348, 1991.

40. Ferguson JA, Sellar C, Goldacre MJ: Some epidemiological observations on medicinal and non-medicinal poisoning in preschool children. J Epidemiol Community Health 46:207–210, 1992.

41. Hoy JL, Day LM, Tibballs J, et al: Unintentional poisoning hospitalisations among young children in Victoria. Inj Prev 5:31–35, 1999.

42. Kaminer Y, Robbins DR: Insulin misuse: A review of an overlooked psychiatric problem. Psychosomatics 30:19–24, 1989.

43. McClure RJ, Davis PM, Meadow SR, et al: Epidemiology of Munchausen syndrome by proxy, non-accidental poisoning, and non-accidental suffocation. Arch Dis Child 75:57–61, 1996.

44. Krahn LE, Lee J, Richardson JW, et al: Hypokalemia leading to torsades de pointes: Munchausen's disorder or bulimia nervosa? Gen Hosp Psychiatry 19:370–377, 1997.

45. McIntire MS, Angle CR: Psychological "biopsy" in self-poisoning of children and adolescents. Am J Dis Child 126:42–46, 1973.

46. Blanc PD, Jones MR, Olson KR: Surveillance of poisoning and drug overdose through hospital discharge coding, poison control center reporting, and the Drug Abuse Warning Network. Am J Emerg Med 11:14–19, 1993.

47. Buckley NA, Whyte IM, Dawson AH, et al: Self-poisoning in Newcastle, 1987–1992. Med J Aust 162:190–193, 1995.

48. Litman RE, Farberow NL: Suicide prevention in hospitals. In Schneidman ES (ed): Psychology of Suicide. New York, Science House, 1970, pp 461–473.

49. Reich P, Kelly MJ: Suicide attempts by hospitalized medical and surgical patients. N Engl J Med 294:298–301, 1976.

50. Lipowski Z: Consultation-liaison psychiatry 1990. Psychother Psychosom 55:62–68, 1991.

51. Lipowski ZJ: Consultation-liaison psychiatry at century's end. Psychosomatics 33:128–133, 1992.

52. Hawton K, Gath D, Smith E: Management of attempted suicide in Oxford. BMJ 2:1040–1042, 1979.

53. Lipowski Z: Consultation-liaison psychiatry: The first half century. Gen Hosp Psychiatry 8:305–315, 1988.

54. Hackett TP, Cassem NH, Stern TA, et al: Beginnings: Consultation psychiatry in a general hospital. In Cassem NH (ed): Massachusetts General Hospital Handbook of General Hospital Psychiatry, 3rd ed. St Louis, Mosby-Year Book, 1991, pp 1–8.

55. Pilowsky I: General principles in the practical management of AIB. In Abnormal Illness Behaviour. New York, John Wiley & Sons, 1997, pp 94–104.

56. Deckel AW: Carbon monoxide poisoning and frontal lobe pathology: Two case reports and a discussion of the literature. Brain Inj 8:345–356, 1994.

57. Rosenstock L, Daniell W, Barnhart S, et al: Chronic neuropsychological sequelae of occupational exposure to organophosphate insecticides. Am J Ind Med 18:321–325, 1990.

58. Kurt T: Multiple chemical sensitivities—a syndrome of pseudotoxicity manifest as exposure perceived symptoms. Clin Toxicol 33:101–105, 1995.

59. Simon G, Daniell W, Stockbridge H, et al: Immunologic, psychological, and neuropsychological factors in multiple chemical sensitivity. Ann Intern Med 19:97–103, 1993.

60. Pilowsky I: Abnormal illness behaviour: Definition. In Abnormal Illness Behaviour. West Sussex, UK, John Wiley & Sons, 1997, pp 25–64.

61. Hartman DE: Missed diagnoses and misdiagnoses of environmental toxicant exposure: The psychiatry of toxic exposure and multiple chemical sensitivity. Psychiatr Clin North Am 21:659–670, 1998.

62. Royal College of Psychiatrists: The General Hospital Management of Adult Deliberate Self-Harm: A Consensus Statement on Standards for Service Provision. London, Royal College of Psychiatrists, 1994.

63. Guidelines for the Management of Deliberate Self Harm in Young People. Australasian College for Emergency Medicine (ACEM) and The Royal Australian and New Zealand College of Psychiatrists (RANZCP). Melbourne, Australia, June, 2000.

64. Kapur N, House A, Creed F, et al: General hospital services for deliberate self-poisoning: An expensive road to nowhere? Postgrad Med 75:599–602, 1999.

65. McFarland BH, Beavers DJ: Psychiatric consultation following attempted suicide. J Am Osteopath Assoc 86:743–750, 1986.

66. Kessel N: Patients who take overdoses. BMJ Clin Res 290:1297–1298, 1985.

67. Proudfoot AT: Clinical toxicology—past, present and future. Hum Toxicol 7:481–487, 1988.

68. Hawton K, Simkin S, Fagg JN: Deliberate self-harm in alcohol and drug misusers: Patient characteristics and patterns of clinical care. Drug Alcohol Rev 16:123–129, 1997.

69. Casey PR: Personality disorder and suicide intent. Acta Psychiatr Scand 79:290–295, 1989.

70. Gupta B, Trzepacz P: Serious overdosers admitted to a general hospital: Comparison with nonoverdose self-injuries and medically ill patients with suicidal ideation. Gen Hosp Psychiatry 19:209–215, 1997.

71. Crumley FE: The adolescent suicide attempt: A cardinal symptom of a serious psychiatric disorder. Am J Psychother 36:158–165, 1982.

72. Grootenhuis M, Hawton K, van Rooijen L, et al: Attempted suicide in Oxford and Utrecht. Br J Psychiatry 165:73–78, 1994.

73. Morgan HG, Pocock H, Pottle S: Deliberate self harm: Clinical and socio-economic characteristics of 368 patients. Br J Psychiatry 127:564–574, 1975.

74. Beautrais AL, Joyce PR, Mulder RT: Precipitating factors and life events in serious suicide attempts among youths aged 13 through 24 years. J Am Acad Child Adolesc Psychiatry 36:1543–1551, 1997.

75. Rudd MD, Joiner T, Rajab MH: Relationships among suicide ideators, attempters, and multiple attempters in a young-adult sample. J Abnorm Psychol 105:541–550, 1996.

76. Peterson LG, Bongar B: Repetitive suicidal crises: Characteristics of repeating versus nonrepeating suicidal visitors to a psychiatric emergency service. Psychopathology 23:136–145, 1990.

77. Lipowska-Teutsch A, Reder V, Pach J: Motives and circumstances of repeated suicidal attempts by taking drugs. Przegl-Lek 47:505–508, 1990.

78. Kotila L, Lonnqvist J: Adolescents who make suicide attempts repeatedly. Acta Psychiatr Scand 76:386–393, 1987.

79. Diagnostic and Statistical Manual of Mental Disorders (DSM-IV), 4th ed. Washington, DC, American Psychiatric Association, 1994.

80. Practice guideline for the treatment of patients with delirium. Am J Psychiatry 156(5 Suppl S):1–20, 1999.

81. Bongar BM: Suicide: Guidelines for Assessment, Management, and Treatment. New York, Oxford University Press, 1992.

82. Carter GL, Dawson AH, Lopert R: Drug-induced delirium: Incidence, management and prevention. Drug Saf 15:291–301, 1996.

83. Foster T, Gillespie K, McClelland R: Mental disorders and suicide in Northern Ireland. Br J Psychiatry 170:447–452, 1997.

84. Owens D, House A: General hospital services for deliberate self-harm: Haphazard clinical provision, little research, no central strategy. J R Coll Physicians Lond 28:370–371, 1994.

85. Hawton K, Arensman E, Townsend E, et al: Deliberate self harm: Systematic review of efficacy of psychosocial and pharmacological

treatments in preventing repetition. BMJ Clin Res 317:441–447, 1998.

86. Van der Sande R, Buskens E, Allart E, et al: Psychosocial intervention following suicide attempt: A systematic review of treatment interventions. Acta Psychiatr Scand 96:43–50, 1997.

87. Cantor CH: Clinical management of parasuicides: Critical issues in the 1990s. Aust N Z J Psychiatry 28:212–221, 1994.

88. Montgomery SA, Montgomery DB, Jayanthi-Rani S: Maintenance therapy in repeat suicidal behaviour: A placebo controlled trial. Proceedings of the 10th International Congress for Suicide Prevention and Crisis Intervention. Ottowa, 227–229, 1979.

89. Linehan MM, Armstrong HE, Suarez A, et al: Cognitive-behavioral treatment of chronically parasuicidal borderline patients. Arch Gen Psychiatry 48:1060–1064, 1991.

90. Verkes RJ, Van der Mast RC, Hengeveld MW, et al: Reduction by paroxetine of suicidal behavior in patients with repeated suicide attempts but not major depression. Am J Psychiatry 155:543–547, 1998.

91. Runeson B, Wasserman D: Management of suicide attempters: What are the routines and the costs? Acta Psychiatr Scand 90:222–228, 1994.

92. Suominen KH, Isometsa ET, Henriksson MM, et al: Inadequate treatment for major depression both before and after attempted suicide. Am J Psychiatry 155:1778–1780, 1998.

93. Suominen KH, Isometsa ET, Henriksson MM, et al: Treatment received by alcohol-dependent suicide attempters. Acta Psychiatr Scand 99:214–219, 1999.

94. Vidalis AA, Jungalwalla HN, Baker GHB: Self poisoning: could psychiatric management be improved? Int J Soc Psychiatry 33:312–315, 1987.

95. Bongar B: The Suicidal Patient: Clinical and Legal Standards of Care. Washington, DC, American Psychological Association, 1991.

96. Bongar B, Maris RW, Berman AL, et al: Inpatient standards of care and the suicidal patient: Part I. General clinical formulations and legal considerations. Suicide Life Threat Behav 23:245–256, 1993.

97. Knapp S, Van de Creek L: A review of tort liability in involuntary civil commitment. Hosp Community Psychiatry 38:648–651, 1987.

98. Miller RD: Grievances and law suits against public mental health professionals: Cost of doing business? Bull Am Acad Psychiatry Law 20:395–408, 1992.

99. Deaton RJ, Colenda CG, Bursztajn H: Medical-legal issues. In Stoudemire A, Fogel B (eds): Psychiatric Care of the Medical Patient. New York, Oxford University Press, 1993, pp 929–938.

100. Fogel BS, Mills MJ, Landen JE: Legal aspects of the treatment of delirium. Hosp Community Psychiatry 37:154–158, 1986.

101. Plueckhahn VD, Breen KD, Cordner SM: The professional liability of doctors. In Plueckhahn VD, Breen KD, Cordner SM (eds): Law and Ethics in Medicine. Geelong, Australia, Henry Thacker Print Group, 1994, pp 81–87.

102. Wheat K: The law's treatment of the suicidal. Med Law Rev 8:182–209, 2000.

103. Appelbaum PS: The right to refuse treatment with antipsychotic medications: Retrospect and prospect. Am J Psychiatry 145:413–419, 1988.

104. Mahler JC, Perry S, Miller F: Psychiatric evaluation of competency in physically ill patients who refuse treatment. Hosp Community Psychiatry 41:1140–1141, 1990.

105. Gutheil TG, Bursztajn H: Clinicians' guidelines for assessing and presenting subtle forms of patient incompetence in legal settings. Am J Psychiatry 143:1020–1023, 1986.

105a. Brody EB: Patients' rights: A cultural challenge to Western psychiatry. Am J Psychiatry 142:58–62, 1985.

106. Bursztajn HJ, Harding HPJ, Gutheil TG, et al: Beyond cognition: The role of disordered affective states in impairing competence to consent to treatment. Bull Am Acad Psychiatry Law 19:383–388, 1991.

107. Gutheil TG, Bursztajn H, Brodsky A: The multidimensional assessment of dangerousness: Competence assessment in patient care and liability prevention. Bull Am Acad Psychiatry Law 14:123–129, 1986.

108. Galen KD: Assessing psychiatric patients' competency to agree to treatment plans. Hosp Community Psychiatry 44:361–364, 1993.

109. Kerridge I, Lowe M, McPhee J: Psychiatry. In Kerridge I, Lowe M, McPhee J (eds): Ethics and Law for the Health Professions. Katoomba, Australia, Social Science Press, 1998, pp 218–237.

110. Hiday VA: Civil commitment: A review of empirical research. Behav Sci Law 6:15–43, 1988.

111. Stromberg CD, Stone AA: A model state law on civil commitment of the mentally ill. Harv J Legislation 20:275–396, 1983.

112. Bednar RL, Bednar SC, Waite DR: Psychotherapy with High-Risk Clients: Legal and Professional Standards. Pacific Grove, CA, Brooks/Cole Publishing, 1991.

113. Overview of Mental Health Legislation in Canada. Ottowa, Mental Health Division, Health Canada, 1994.

114. Freckelton I: Decision-making about involuntary psychiatric treatment: An analysis of the principles behind Victorian practice. Psychiatry Psychol Law 5:249–264, 1998.

115. Errington MR: The operation of the Mental Health Act, 1983 (NSW). Aust N Z J Psychiatr 20:278–292, 1986.

116. Werth JL Jr: U.S. involuntary mental health commitment statues: Requirements for persons perceived to be a potential harm to self. Suicide Life Threat Behav 31:348–357, 2001.

117. Gove WR: Involuntary psychiatric hospitalization: A review of the statutes regulating the social control of the mentally ill. Deviant Behav 6:287–318, 1985.

118. Bursztajn H, Gutheil TG, Hamm RM, et al: Parens patriae considerations in the commitment process. Psychiatr Q 59:165–181, 1988.

119. Solomon P: The admissions process in two state psychiatric hospitals. Hosp Community Psychiatry 32:405–408, 1981.

120. Bursztajn HJ, Hamm RM, Gutheil TG: Beyond the black letter of the law: An empirical study of an individual judge's decision process for civil commitment hearings. J Am Acad Psychiatry Law 25:79–94, 1997.

121. Poythress NG Jr: Avoiding negligent release: Contemporary clinical and risk management strategies. Am J Psychiatry 147:994–997, 1990.

122. Menninger WW: The impact of litigation and court decisions on clinical practice. Bull Menninger Clin 53:203–214, 1989.

123. McNiel DE, Binder RL, Fulton FM: Management of threats of violence under California's duty-to-protect statute. Am J Psychiatry 155:1097–1101, 1998.

124. Appelbaum PS: The new preventive detention: Psychiatry's problematic responsibility for the control of violence. Am J Psychiatry 145:779–785, 1988.

125. Peele R, Chodoff P: The ethics of involuntary treatment and deinstitutionalization. In Bloch S, Chodoff P, Green SA (eds): Psychiatric Ethics, 3rd ed. Oxford, Oxford University Press, 1999, pp 423–440.

126. Pilowsky I: Abnormal illness behaviour: "A dangerous idea." In Abnormal Illness Behaviour. New York, John Wiley & Sons, 1997, pp 238–243.

127. Singh B, Nunn K, Martin J, et al: Abnormal treatment behaviour. Br J Med Psychol 54:67–73, 1981.

127a. Groves JE: Patients with borderline personality disorder. In Cassem NH (ed): Massachusetts General Hospital Handbook of General Hospital Psychiatry, 3rd ed. St Louis, Mosby-Year Book, 1991, pp 191–215.

128. Adam S, Forrest S: ABC of intensive care. BMJ 319:175–178, 1999.

129. Bone RC, Hayden WR, Levine RL, et al: Recognition, assessment, and treatment of anxiety in the critical care patient. Dis Mon 41:293–359, 1995.

130. Wolk-Wasserman D: The intensive care unit and the suicide attempt patient. Acta Psychiatr Scand 71:581–595, 1985.

131. American Psychiatric Association Task Force Report 22: Seclusion and Restraint: The Psychiatric Uses. Washington, DC, American Psychiatric Association, 1985.

132. Fisher WA: Restraint and seclusion: A review of the literature. Am J Psychiatry 151:1584–1591, 1994.

133. Marks W: Physical restraints in the practice of medicine: Current concepts. Arch Intern Med 152:2203–2206, 1992.

134. Blumenreich P, Lippmann S, Bacani-Oropilla T: Violent patients: Are you prepared to deal with them? Postgrad Med 90:201–206, 1991.

135. Sheline Y, Nelson T: Patient choice: Deciding between psychotropic medication and physical restraints in an emergency. Bull Am Acad Psychiatry Law 21:321–329, 1993.

136. Kapp MB: Physical restraint use in critical care: Legal issues. AACN Clin Iss 7:579–584, 1996.

137. Reigle J: The ethics of physical restraints in critical care. AACN Clin Iss 7:585–591, 1996.

138. Crenshaw WB, Cain KA, Francis PS: An updated national survey on seclusion and restraint. Psychiatr Serv 48:395–397, 1997.

139. Inouye SK: Delirium in hospitalized elderly patients: Recognition, evaluation, and management. Conn Med 57:309–315, 1993.

140. Crippen DW: The role of sedation in the ICU patient with pain and agitation. Crit Care Clin 6:369–392, 1990.

141. Fish DN: Treatment of delirium in the critically ill patient. Clin Pharm 10:456–466, 1991.

142. Levine RL: Pharmacology of intravenous sedatives and opioids in critically ill patients. Crit Care Clin 10:709–731, 1994.

143. Gillman PK: The serotonin syndrome and its treatment. J Psychopharmacol 13:100–109, 1999.

144. Shapiro BA, Warren J, Egol AB, et al: Practice parameters for intravenous analgesia and sedation for adult patients in the intensive care unit: An executive summary. Society of Critical Care Medicine. Crit Care Med 23:1596–1600, 1995.

145. Crippen DW: Pharmacologic treatment of brain failure and delirium. Crit Care Clin 10:733–766, 1994.

146. Bailey S: Critical care nurses' and doctors' attitudes to parasuicide patients. Aust J Adv Nurs 11:11–17, 1994.

147. Weishaar ME, Beck AT: Clinical and cognitive predictors of suicide. In Maris RW, Berman AL, Maltsberger JT, et al (eds): Assessment and Prediction of Suicide. New York, Guilford, 1992, pp 467–483.

148. Brown J, Cohen P, Johnson JG, et al: Childhood abuse and neglect: specificity of effects on adolescent and young adult depression and suicidality. J Am Acad Child Adolesc Psychiatry 38:1490–1496, 1999.

149. Santa Mina EE: Childhood sexual and physical abuse and adult self-harm and suicidal behaviour: A literature review. Can J Psychiatry 43:793–800, 1998.

150. van Egmond M, Garnefski N, Jonker D, et al: The relationship between sexual abuse and female suicidal behavior. Crisis 14: 129–139, 1993.

151. Lipschitz DS, Winegar RK, Nicolau AL, et al: Perceived abuse and neglect as risk factors for suicidal behavior in adolescent inpatients. J Nerv Ment Dis 187:32–39, 1999.

152. Botsis AJ, Plutchik R, Kotler M, et al: Parental loss and family violence as correlates of suicide and violence risk. Suicide Life Threat Behav 25:253–260, 1995.

153. Brent DA, Perper JA, Moritz G, et al: Familial risk factors for adolescent suicide: A case-control study. Acta Psychiatr Scand 89:52–58, 1994.

154. Platt S, Salter D: A comparative investigation of health workers' attitudes towards parasuicide. Soc Psychiatry 22:202–208, 1987.

155. Patel AR: Attitudes towards self-poisoning. BMJ 2:426–429, 1975.

156. Bailey SR: An exploration of critical care nurses' and doctors' attitudes towards psychiatric patients. Aust J Adv Nurs 15:8–14, 1998.

157. Perrin KO, Williams-Burgess C: The suicidal patient in the CCU: Nursing approaches. Crit Care Nurse 10:59–64, 1990.

158. Constantino RE, Boneysteele G, Gesmond SA, et al: Restraining an aggressive suicidal, paraplegic patient: a look at the ethical and legal issues. Dimensions Crit Care Nurs 16:144–151, 1997.

159. Trzepacz PT: The Psychiatric Mental Status Examination. New York, Oxford University Press, 1993.

160. Wolk-Wasserman D: Suicidal communication of persons attempting suicide and responses of significant others. Acta Psychiatr Scand 73:481–499, 1986.

161. Wasserman D: Passive euthanasia in response to attempted suicide: One form of aggressiveness by relatives. Acta Psychiatr Scand 79:460–467, 1989.

162. Kunisaki TA, Augenstein WL: Drug- and toxin-induced seizures. Emerg Med Clin N Am 12:1027–1056, 1994.

163. Peterson LG, Bongar B: Training physicians in the clinical evaluation of the suicidal patient. In Hale MS (ed): Methods in Teaching Consultation-Liaison Psychiatry. Basel, Switzerland, Karger, 1990, pp 89–108.

164. Berman AL, Jobes DA: Treatment of the suicidal adolescent. Death Stud 18:375–389, 1994.

165. Donnan AE, Hetzel BS, Oliver RG: Early psycho-social assessment of overdose patients in a casualty department. Aust N Z J Psychiatry 11:133–135, 1977.

166. Hall RC, Platt DE: Suicide risk assessment: A review of risk factors for suicide in 100 patients who made severe suicide attempts: Evaluation of suicide risk in a time of managed care. Psychosomatics 40:18–27, 1999.

167. Hawton K: Assessment of suicide risk. Br J Psychiatry 150:145–153, 1987.

168. Motto JA: An integrated approach to estimating suicide risk. In Maris RW, Berman AL, Maltsberger JT, et al (eds): Assessment and Prediction of Suicide. New York, Guilford Press, 1992, pp 625–639.

169. Bassuk EL: Emergency care of suicidal patients. In Bassuk EL, Schoonover S, Gill S (eds): Lifelines: Clinical Perspectives on Suicide. New York, Plenum, 1982, pp 97–125.

170. Sletten IW, Barton JL: Suicidal patients in the emergency room: A guide for evaluation and disposition. Hosp Community Psychiatry 30:407–411, 1979.

171. Range LM, Knott EC: Twenty suicide assessment instruments—evaluation and recommendations. Death Stud 21:25–58, 1997.

172. Rothberg JM, Geer-Williams C: A comparison and review of suicide prediction scales. In Maris RW, Berman AL, Maltsberger JT, et al (eds): Assessment and Prediction of Suicide. New York, Guilford Press, 1992, pp 202–217.

173. Garrison CZ, Lewinsohn PM, .Martseller F, et al: The assessment of suicidal behavior in adolescents. Suicide Life Threat Behav 21:217–230, 1991.

174. Trzepacz PT: A review of delirium assessment instruments. Gen Hosp Psychiatry 16:397–405, 1994.

175. Smith MJ, Breitbart WS, Platt MM: A critique of instruments and methods to detect, diagnose, and rate delirium. J Pain Sympt Manage 10:35–77, 1995.

176. Folstein MF, Folstein SE, McHugh PR: "Mini-mental state": A practical method for grading the cognitive state of patients for the clinician. J Psychiatr Res 12:189–198, 1975.

177. Molloy DW, Alemayehu E, Roberts R: Reliability of a standardized mini-mental state examination compared with the traditional mini-mental state examination. Am J Psychiatry 148:102–105, 1991.

178. Merigian KS, Hedges JR, Roberts JR, et al: Use of abbreviated mental status examination in the initial assessment of overdose patients. Arch Emerg Med 5:139–145, 1988.

179. Zigmond AS, Snaith RP: The hospital anxiety and depression scale. Acta Psychiatr Scand 67:361–370, 1983.

180. Herrmann C: International experiences with the hospital anxiety and depression scale: A review of validation data and clinical results. J Psychosom Res 42:17–41, 1997.

181. Flagler SL, Wright L: Recurrent poisoning in children: A review. J Pediatr Psychol 12:631–641, 1987.

182. Stoddard FJ, Wilens TE: Delirium. In Jellinek MS, Herzog DB (eds): Psychiatric Aspects of General Hospital Pediatrics. Chicago, Year Book Medical Publishers, 1990, pp 254–259.

183. Herzog DB, Jellinek MS, Todres ID: The intensive care units. In Jellinek MS, Herzog DB (eds): Psychiatric Aspects of General Hospital Pediatrics. Chicago, Year Book Medical Publishers, 1990, pp 41–50.

184. Sugar J: Munchausen syndrome by proxy. In Jellinek MS, Herzog DB (eds): Psychiatric Aspects of General Hospital Pediatrics. Chicago, Year Book Medical Publishers, 1990, pp 198–201.

185. Perry PA, Dean BS, Krenzelok EP: A regional poison center's experience with poisoning exposures occurring in schools. Vet Hum Toxicol 34:148–151, 1992.

186. Brent DA: The aftercare of adolescents with deliberate self-harm. J Child Psychol Psychiatry 38:277–286, 1997.

187. Gould M, Fisher P, Parides M, et al: Psychosocial risk factors of child and adolescent completed suicide. Arch Gen Psychiatry 53:1155–1162, 1996.

188. Gould MS, King R, Greenwald S, et al: Psychopathology associated with suicidal ideation and attempts among children and adolescents. J Am Acad Child Adolesc Psychiatry 37:915–923, 1998.

189. Adler R, Jellinek MS: Suicide. In Jellinek MS, Herzog DB (eds): Psychiatric Aspects of General Hospital Pediatrics. Chicago, Year Book Medical Publishers, 1990, pp 324–330.

190. Trautman PD, Rotheram-Borus MJ, Dopkins S, et al: Psychiatric diagnoses in minority female adolescent suicide attempters. J Am Acad Child Adolesc Psychiatry 30:617–622, 1991.

191. Andrews JA, Lewinsohn PM: Suicidal attempts among older adolescents: Prevalence and co-occurrence with psychiatric disorders. J Am Acad Child Adolesc Psychiatry 31:655–662, 1992.

192. Angle CR, O'Brien TP, McIntire MS: Adolescent self-poisoning: A nine-year followup. J Dev Behav Pediatr 4:83–87, 1983.

193. Beautrais AL, Joyce PR, Mulder RT: Psychiatric illness in a New Zealand sample of young people making serious suicide attempts. Aust N Z Med J 111:44–48, 1998.

194. Hawton K, O'Grady J, Osborn M, et al: Adolescents who take overdoses: Their characteristics, problems and contacts with helping agencies. Br J Psychiatry 140:118–123, 1982.

195. Clarke CF: Deliberate self poisoning in adolescents. Arch Dis Child 63:1479–1483, 1988.

196. Taylor EA, Stansfeld SA: Children who poison themselves: II. Prediction of attendance for treatment. Br J Psychiatry 145:132–135, 1984.
197. Harrington R, Kerfoot M, Dyer E, et al: Randomized trial of a home-based family intervention for children who have deliberately poisoned themselves. J Am Acad Child Adolesc Psychiatry 37:512–518, 1998.
198. Linehan MM: Suicide update address: Is anything effective for reducing suicidal behavior? Washington, DC, American Association of Suicidology, 1998, pp 17–18.
199. Satcher D: Bringing the public health approach to the problem of suicide. Suicide Life Threat Behav 28:325–327, 1998.
200. Diekstra RFW: Suicide and the attempted suicide: an international perspective. Acta Psychiatr Scand 80(Suppl 354):1–24, 1989.
201. Reilly DK, Ray JE, Day RO, et al: Classification of overdose/self-poisoning presentations to an accident and emergency department. Int J Addict 22:941–955, 1987.
202. Maris RW: Overview of suicide assessment and prediction. In Maris RW, Berman AL, Maltsberger JT, et al (eds): Assessment and Prediction of Suicide. New York, Guilford Press, 1992, pp 3–24.

CHAPTER **10**

Intensive Care of Pediatric Poisoning Patients

George C. Rodgers, Jr. ▪ Mitchell P. Ross

Of the estimated 200 admissions to critical care units per 100,000 children, 3% are thought to be related to poisoning.[1] An older study, based on data from 1979 through 1983, calculated a hospitalization rate of 65.1/100,000 for poisoning in children aged 0 to 9 years.[2] Some children already admitted to critical care units for other reasons become toxicologic cases as a result of therapeutic misadventures or adverse drug reactions (ADRs) occurring in the unit. Other children are admitted to critical care units with uncertain diagnoses that subsequently may be proved to be toxicologic. This chapter defines a critical care unit in the broadest sense, that is, any unit providing intensive care for newborns or children. This may be a true pediatric intensive care unit (PICU); a neonatal intensive care unit (NICU); a surgical intensive care unit; or, in a less specialized facility, a general intensive care unit (ICU), which may care for children and adults. Children admitted to any of these units require special care from a physician familiar with the care of critically ill children and their special needs. These children often also require the services of a medical toxicologist with the special skills required to care optimally for children exposed to toxins. Finally, particularly in the absence of a medical toxicologist, consultation with a regional poison control center is crucial.

EPIDEMIOLOGY OF PEDIATRIC POISONING

Most pediatric poisonings are not serious enough to require either hospital admission or intensive care. According to the American Association of Poison Control Centers Toxic Exposure Surveillance System (TESS) database for 1999, poisoning in persons younger than age 20 accounts for 67% of the 2.24 million cases reported by United States poison control centers.[3] Of these almost 1.5 million pediatric cases, 14.6% were treated in or admitted to a hospital. This compares with a 35.3% rate for persons older than age 20. Table 10-1 lists the number of pediatric poisonings, critical care admissions, deaths, and patients with major effects reported to the 1999 TESS database by age. Of the 61,723 people in the whole database reported to have been admitted to critical care units, 26% were younger than age 20. These figures equate to a 1.1% admission rate to critical care for children younger than age 20 exposed to toxins as opposed to a 6.2% critical care admission rate for adult poisoning patients. In an older study, 64% of hospitalized pediatric poisoning patients were admitted to a critical care unit.[4] The need for hospitalization and critical care is age dependent. ICU admission rates in the pediatric age range,

based on the 1999 TESS database, were 0.4% for children younger than 6 years old, 0.7% for children 6 to 12 years old, and 6.4% for children 13 to 19 years old.[5] Using recent U.S. census estimates, the above-mentioned overall PICU admission rate, and the 1999 TESS data, the percentage of ICU patients who are admitted because of a toxicologic problem may be 10%.[1,5]

Table 10-2 shows the reason for the exposures in the pediatric patients requiring ICU admission. Although most are unintentional, including medication errors, there are a significant number of intentional exposures and adverse reactions to medications. Table 10-3 shows the specific toxic agents involved. In addition to the 85 pediatric deaths reported by TESS in 1999, 2694 children were reported to have had major effects from their exposure. Major effects in the TESS database are defined as life-threatening effects, significant residual disability, and disfigurement. Most of these patients (58%) were cared for in a critical care unit. Of the 85 reported deaths, 59 occurred in critical care units.

Most intentional poisonings in children are suicide attempts or gestures. Although most of these cases occur in the teenage years, we have seen cases in 6-year-old children. An undetermined number of cases of intentional poisoning represent criminal poisoning or Munchausen syndrome by proxy (MSBP). MSBP involves the intentional injury of a child by an adult perpetrator, usually the mother, for the purpose of attracting attention to the perpetrator.[6,7] MSBP has been classified as a psychiatric disorder.[8] Although many such cases have been reported, the actual incidence in the United States is unknown, and the diagnosis often may be missed.[9] Likewise, there seem to be no reliable data on the incidence of criminal poisoning of children. The number of such cases is probably small. In one British study looking at the epidemiology of MSBP, intentional poisoning and intentional suffocation data from all consultant pediatricians in the United Kingdom and the Republic of Ireland were analyzed for a 2-year period.[10] A total of 128 cases were identified. Sixteen cases of intentional poisoning without the presence of MSBP and 28 cases in which both were present were identified. In the study as a whole, the perpetrator was the mother in 85% of cases, similar to what has been observed in other studies.[11] The median age of the children involved was 20 months; eight of the children had severe illness, and eight died. Among the poisoning cases, the most frequent agents were anticonvulsants and opiates. The annual incidences in the United Kingdom and Ireland were 0.06/100,000 for intentional poisoning alone and 0.1/100,000 for MSBP and poisoning.[10] It is likely that

103

TABLE 10-1 1999 TESS Data Reports of Pediatric Poisoning, Critical Care Admissions, Deaths, and Major Effects by Age

AGE RANGE	EXPOSURE CASES REPORTED	CRITICAL CARE UNIT ADMISSIONS	DEATHS	MAJOR EFFECTS
<6	1,154,799	4718	24	728
6–12	154,606	1091	8	261
13–19	157,993	10,341	53	1705
Total	1,467,398	16,150	85	2694

From Litovitz TL, Klein-Schwartz W, White S, et al: 1999 Annual report of the American Association of Poison Control Centers Toxic Exposure Surveillance System. Am J Emerg Med 18:517–574, 2000.

these are underestimates, considering the way in which data were collected. No data exist on the number of children with MSBP or intentional poisoning who require critical care, although it is highly likely that many of the latter group require ICU admission because the intent is often the death of the child.[12] Some children's hospitals now have specially modified rooms where parental interaction with a child can be observed with hidden cameras if MSBP is suspected. This observation must be done in conjunction with local police and judicial involvement.

The third most common reason for poison control center calls is ADRs to medication. There are no reliable data related to the overall incidence of ADRs in children. In adults, ADRs are thought to represent the most common cause of iatrogenic disease.[13] It is estimated that ADRs result in 300,000 hospital admissions per year and that the chances of having a serious ADR in hospitalized patients is about 0.4% per course of drug therapy.[13] These data relate primarily to adults. It is likely that comparable data for children would show less of a problem because fewer children take medications, and the drugs commonly used in children tend to have more favorable safety profiles. How many of these cases require critical care is unknown.

There are few good data on medication errors in children as a cause of hospitalization, need for critical care admission, or death.[14] The U.S. Institute of Medicine has called attention to the prevalence and importance of medication errors.[14,15] There is good reason to believe that the incidence of medication errors is greater in hospitalized children than in hospitalized adults, perhaps three times as great.[16] In this study,

conducted in two hospitals with pediatric units, including NICUs and PICUs, more than 10,000 medication orders were reviewed. Serious medication errors were identified in 1.1% of orders. In a previous study done in the same geographic area, using an identical study design, serious medication errors were found in 0.40% of adult medication orders.[17] In another study looking at medication errors in two children's hospitals, a total of 479 errors were identified out of 101,022 medication orders written.[18] The frequencies at the two hospitals were 4.9/1000 orders and 4.5/1000 orders. Of these errors, 27 were believed to be potentially lethal. In a separate study of 2147 admissions to a PICU and NICU, 315 medication errors resulting in injury were identified.[19] In this study, the risk of a drug-related injury to a patient in one of the units was 3.1%. The primary reason for an increased risk of medication errors in children is thought to relate to the need to calculate individualized doses based on age and weight.[20-23]

The neonatal abstinence syndrome has become a frequently encountered problem in NICUs.[24] Although the incidence of neonatal abstinence syndrome has not been reported, one large study using urine drug screens found a 44% incidence of illicit drug use in pregnant women near the time of delivery[25]; this contrasted with an 11% rate by self-reporting. The neonatal abstinence syndrome also can occur when the mother has been medicated intentionally with certain drugs during pregnancy. Table 10-4 lists agents commonly causing neonatal abstinence syndrome. Although withdrawal symptoms usually present within 24 to 48 hours of birth, they may be delayed for many days if the drug involved has a long half-

TABLE 10-2 Reason for Toxic Exposure by Age

AGE RANGE	REASONS			
	Unintentional	*Intentional*	*Adverse Reaction*	*Other/Unknown*
<6	1,148,693	688	3888	1530
6–12	142,085	7661	2626	2234
12–19	86,757	64,574	3663	2999
Total	1,377,535	72,923	10,177	6763

From Litovitz TL, Klein-Schwartz W, White S, et al: 1999 Annual report of the American Association of Poison Control Centers Toxic Exposure Surveillance System. Am J Emerg Med 18:517–574, 2000.

TABLE 10-3 Toxins Associated with Pediatric Admission to a Critical Care Unit

TOXIN	REPORTED CASES (% OF REPORTS) BY AGE		
	<6 Years	6–12 Years	13–19 Years
Drug Classes			
Analgesics	307 (5.7)	140 (11)	4448 (31.8)
Anticonvulsants	318 (5.9)	116 (9.1)	742 (5.3)
Antidepressants	373 (6.8)	172 (13.5)	2145 (15.3)
Antihistamines	166 (3.1)	50 (3.9)	675 (4.8)
Antimicrobials	62 (1.1)	19 (1.5)	206 (1.5)
Cardiovascular agents	1273 (23.5)	163 (13.2)	453 (3.2)
Cough/cold	140 (2.6)	25 (2)	589 (4.2)
Hormones/hypoglycemics	317 (5.9)	14 (1.1)	136 (0.97)
Muscle relaxants	46 (0.85)	22 (1.7)	273 (2)
Sedative-hypnotics	331 (6.1)	118 (9.3)	1111 (7.9)
Abuse drugs/stimulants	204 (3.8)	79 (6.2)	976 (7)
Others			
Ethyl alcohol	12 (0.22)	15 (1.2)	381 (2.7)
Glycols/other alcohols	70 (1.2)	11 (0.86)	52 (0.37)
Snakes/spiders	49/12 (1.1)	72/10 (6.5)	84/8 (0.66)
Miscellaneous chemicals	83 (1.5)	14 (1.1)	63 (0.45)
Cleaning agents	168 (3.1)	16 (1.3)	117 (0.84)
Carbon monoxide	16 (0.3)	11 (0.86)	11 (0.08)
Hydrocarbons	259 (4.8)	18 (1.4)	43 (0.31)
Insecticides	90 (1.7)	20 (1.6)	22 (0.16)
Plants/mushrooms	8/15 (0.43)	18/3 (1.6)	160/62 (1.5)
Total Reported Toxins*	5407	1273	13,993

*Number of toxins exceeds number of patients because some patients were exposed to more than one toxin.
From Litovitz TL, Klein-Schwartz W, White S, et al: 1999 Annual report of the American Association of Poison Control Centers Toxic Exposure Surveillance System. Am J Emerg Med 18:517–574, 2000.

life. The neonatal abstinence syndrome may be seen in either the NICU or with a later readmission in the PICU. Symptoms, which may relate to elevated catecholamine and β-endorphin levels seen in these infants, may be misdiagnosed if drug use by the mother is not suspected.

INDICATIONS FOR INTENSIVE CARE UNIT ADMISSION

Considering the cost and resource intensity of an ICU admission, it is prudent for physicians to exercise good judgment in deciding which poisoned patients appropriately

TABLE 10-4 Drugs Associated with Neonatal Abstinence Syndrome

Amphetamines	Marijuana
Barbiturates	Methadone
Benzodiazepines	Nicotine
Caffeine	Opioids
Chlordiazepoxide	Pentazocine
Cocaine	Phencyclidine
Diphenhydramine	Propoxyphene
Ethanol	

need an intensive care setting. Likewise, because of the potentially acute and often devastating effects of some toxins, it generally is wise to be conservative in selecting an appropriate hospital setting for poisoned children. In discussing intensive care settings, it is understood that some institutions combine true ICUs with step-down or transitional care units. Reference to *intensive care* in this chapter should be understood to refer to whichever type of unit is most appropriate for the patient's condition and consistent with institutional guidelines.

The most common reason to admit a pediatric poisoning patient to an ICU is organ system dysfunction or the perception that significant organ dysfunction is acutely eminent. The organ systems of primary concern are those that can lead to rapid death, specifically the respiratory, cardiovascular, and neurologic systems. Occasionally, patients are admitted to the ICU primarily for psychiatric observation after an intentional overdose if other appropriate facilities offering close patient observation are not immediately available.

Many drugs are known to adversely affect the cardiovascular system in an overdose, including most commonly cyclic antidepressants, dysrhythmic agents, antihypertensives, and sympathomimetics. Patients who are experiencing blood pressure abnormalities (increased or decreased) or instability should be admitted to an ICU for observation and possible intervention. Likewise, patients with significant or new-onset cardiac dysrhythmias (other than simple sinus tachycardia)

Indications for Pediatric ICU Admission Relevant to Toxic Exposures

1. Acute respiratory or ventilatory failure as manifested by one or more of the following:
   a. Need for mechanical ventilation or emergency tracheostomy
   b. Marked respiratory distress as indicated by
      (1) RR ≤ 20 or ≥ 60 for infants ≤ 1 year old
      (2) RR ≤ 12 or ≥ 60 for patients >1 year old
      (3) SpO_2 $\leq 92\%$ or 100% oxygen by a nonrebreather mask or tracheostomy collar
      (4) PaO_2 <80 mm Hg on 100% oxygen by nonrebreather mask
   c. Rapidly progressive deterioration in respiratory status
   d. Respiratory acidosis with $PaCO_2$ >60 mm Hg and pH <7.25
   e. Airway obstruction treated with heliox
   f. Need for continuous terbutaline or isoproterenol infusion
   g. Apnea
   h. Anaphylaxis
2. Hemodynamic instability or circulatory failure as manifested by one or more of the following:
   a. Shock as indicated by
      (1) Capillary refill >4 seconds
      (2) Nonpalpable distal or proximal pulses
      (3) Systolic blood pressure $<$ lower limit for age and/or MAP <50 mm Hg (neonates <40 mm Hg)
      (4) Acute metabolic acidosis with pH <7.25, base deficit >-10 or serum bicarbonate ≤ 10 mEq/L
      (5) Need to monitor central pressure (venous, pulmonary artery, or wedge), cardiac output, or mixed venous saturation
   b. Unstable or newly abnormal cardiac rhythm
   c. Need for continuous infusion of cardiac drugs
   d. ECG showing changes consistent with ischemia
   e. Acute congestive heart failure
   f. Unstable vascular volume as indicated by
      (1) Need for 40 mL/kg fluid bolus in 4 hours
      (2) Need for >1 RBC transfusion in <24 hours in a nononcology patient

      (3) Hemoglobin <8 g/dL in a bleeding or hemolyzing patient
      (4) Platelet count $<20,000$ with active bleeding
      (5) INR >2 with active bleeding
   g. Need for cardioversion
   h. Malignant hypertension
3. Neurologic instability as manifested by one or more of the following:
   a. Acute neurologic deterioration as indicated by
      (1) Glasgow Coma Scale score ≤ 10
      (2) Severe irritability
      (3) Hallucinations
      (4) Lethargy
      (5) Posturing
   b. Need for ICP monitoring
   c. Intracranial hemorrhage
   d. Evidence of increased ICP
4. Metabolic derangements placing patients at risk of serious complications as evidenced by one or more of the following:
   a. Serum sodium <125 mmol/L or >160 mmol/L
   b. Serum potassium <3 mmol/L or >6.5 mmol/L (nonhemolyzed)
   c. Blood glucose <30 mg/dL or >400 mg/dL (1.7 mmol/L or 22.2 mmol/L)
   d. Ionized calcium <0.8 mEq/L
   e. Base deficit >-10
5. Other patients displaying evidence of acute or developing failure of an essential organ system
6. Patients with a toxic exposure in which none of the above are present but in which
   a. One of the above admission criteria can be expected to develop within a few hours based on the nature of the exposure
   b. The patient is suicidal, and no other safe area of medical and psychiatric observation exists

ECG, electrocardiogram; ICP, intracranial pressure; INR, international normalized ratio; MAP, mean arterial blood pressure; PaO_2, arterial oxygen partial pressure; $PaCO_2$, arterial carbon dioxide partial pressure; RBC, red blood cell; RR, respiratory rate; SpO_2, arterial oxygen saturation.

also merit admission for observation. Patients with evidence of inadequate cardiac output (shock) also require ICU admission and prompt therapy.

Central nervous system (CNS) changes are another common manifestation of many poisonings. Some degree of CNS depression probably is the most common reason for ICU admission of poisoned patients. Drugs commonly presenting in this way and leading to ICU admission include cyclic antidepressants, ethyl alcohol, sedative-hypnotics, and anticonvulsants. These changes can be in the form of CNS depression or agitation, including seizures. The obvious concern with CNS depression is that it may progress to respiratory or cardiovascular instability or may be associated with seizures.

Respiratory depression or respiratory distress alone is a less frequent cause of ICU admission. The latter may be associated with aspiration if the patient has vomited as a result of either the poison or the therapy provided (e.g., ipecac syrup, activated charcoal, or gastric tube placement). Also included in the latter category are smoke inhalation

cases. Respiratory depression usually is associated with concomitant CNS depression.

Hepatic, renal, gastrointestinal, and dermatologic dysfunction also may result from poisoning but rarely leads to acute ICU admission because acute threats to life are unlikely. Hepatic and renal failure may occur from poisoning, and both eventually may present life-threatening situations, but these develop gradually over days and generally do not require initial management in an ICU. Acute gastrointestinal toxicity may be severe but usually can be managed adequately by fluid replacement therapy outside of an ICU. Rarely, fluid and electrolyte abnormalities may mandate ICU admission for observation or corrective action. Chemically induced skin burns may be sufficiently severe to require admission to a burn unit or ICU, but these cases in children are rare.

Perhaps the most difficult decision in deciding where to place a child requiring hospitalization is assessing the potential risk that a presently stable patient will deteriorate rapidly to the point of requiring intensive care. Patients who are perceived to be at significant risk for rapid deterioration should be placed in an ICU for observation so that lifesaving measures, such as intubation, pacing, or cardiovascular support, can be provided rapidly if the need arises. The adequate assessment of this risk depends on a good history of the exposure, good knowledge of the toxins involved, and good clinical judgment based in part on experience. The resources of a regional poison control center or a medical toxicologist should be employed. When uncertainty exists, it generally is better to err on the side of ICU admission. If the patient remains stable for a few hours, he or she can be transferred out of the ICU. In my experience, most pediatric poisoning patients admitted to the ICU have stays of 24 hours or less, distinctively different from the general pediatric ICU population.

GENERAL INTENSIVE CARE UNIT TREATMENT

The mainstay of the ICU management of a poisoned pediatric patient is supportive care. There are several unique aspects to the treatment of these patients, however. Although not all of these have been studied formally, the following is a compilation of the generally accepted toxicologic treatments of poisoned children. Appropriate, new, and experimental therapies are described.

Decontamination (gastrointestinal or otherwise) of the exposed patient, when appropriate, generally should have been accomplished or begun in the emergency department before arrival in the ICU. For a few toxins, there is demonstrable therapeutic value in the use of multiple doses of activated charcoal (see Chapter 6). These may be given in the ICU. Repeat doses of activated charcoal usually are given via a nasogastric tube because these patients are usually too sick to take activated charcoal by mouth. Chapter 5 provides a thorough review of appropriate gastrointestinal decontamination techniques.

The general ICU care of most poisoned patients is not any different from the care received by other ICU patients with a comparable level of severity and similar symptoms.[26,27] All PICU patients should have continuous monitoring of heart rate and respiratory rate and pulse oximetry. The frequency of nursing assessment and vital signs depends on the stability of the patient, the problems present or anticipated, and unit protocols. The frequency may vary from every few minutes to every 4 hours and should be appropriate for the patient and the circumstances.

Any patient admitted to an ICU should have stable intravenous access. Whether a peripheral intravenous catheter or a central line is required depends on the stability of the patient and the problems anticipated for the patient. If major organ system instability is present or likely, central access or multiple peripheral intravenous lines generally should be placed. A single peripheral intravenous line is not adequate for a severely ill patient and is not adequate to initiate lifesaving therapies. Central lines can be placed in subclavian, internal jugular, or femoral vessels. In newborns, the umbilical vein my be available and can be used. If lines are properly placed in either the superior or the inferior vena cava, they should be transduced to provide central venous pressure measurement. Because improperly placed lines can give incorrect and misleading information, place-

ment should be verified by radiograph before the lines are transduced. In unstable patients, particularly patients with cardiac or respiratory symptoms, the placement of a Swan-Ganz catheter should be considered. Arterial catheters for arterial blood sampling and continuous blood pressure monitoring should be inserted in any patient with significant respiratory or cardiovascular symptoms secondary to a toxic exposure and in patients intubated because of CNS depression.

Patients who are comatose or have a rapidly declining level of consciousness generally should be intubated prophylactically. If the diagnosis of a toxic exposure is uncertain, a cranial computed tomography scan should be considered in patients with neurologic symptoms. Patients in whom cerebral edema is suspected also should receive a cranial computed tomography scan.

The use of laboratory monitoring, including arterial blood gas measurements, should be dictated by the status of the patient, the initial values obtained, and the anticipated problems. Sequential measurement of drug or toxin levels may be valuable in selected cases as either a marker of therapeutic efficacy or a predictor of likely toxic effects.

Cardiovascular Toxicity

Cardiovascular compromise resulting from intoxication is a serious complication of poisoning that requires prompt critical care management and monitoring. A thorough understanding of the derangements produced by individual toxins and a sophisticated understanding of cardiovascular assessment and supportive care and monitoring techniques are essential for successful treatment of these critically ill patients. Cardiovascular function is the end result of a complex interaction between the heart and the peripheral vascular system. When functioning properly, this interaction provides for adequate cardiac output and appropriate distribution of cardiac output to specific organs and tissues to ensure optimal function. Cardiac function is regulated by specific neural and hormonal feedback mechanisms that monitor and modulate cardiac rate and contractility, peripheral vascular resistance and venous capacitance, and specific organ and tissue blood flows. A toxin may harm the heart or vascular smooth muscle directly; have neurogenic effects on the sympathetic or parasympathetic regulation of heart rate, contractility, or vascular resistance; or cause changes in intravascular volume, metabolic disturbances such as hypoglycemia, or electrolyte disturbances.

Evaluation of an intoxicated child at risk for cardiovascular compromise requires a thorough physical examination. Assessment of vital signs and autonomic findings, such as pupillary dilation or constriction, skin flushing or pallor, lacrimation, and salivation, provides useful information regarding cardiovascular status and may aid in identifying the type of intoxication. Evaluation of intravascular volume (performed by assessment of jugular venous distention, skin turgor, and moistness of mucous membranes) and liver size directs initial resuscitative management.

The adequacy of cardiac output is assessed indirectly by the assessment of organ and tissue function. The patient's mental status, depth and frequency of respirations (increased in metabolic acidosis), volume of urine output, and estimation of peripheral perfusion (via palpation of central and peripheral pulses, capillary refill time, and peripheral warmth and skin color) reflect cardiac output. After initial assessment, reexamination at frequent intervals identifies changes in the examination associated with alterations in cardiovascular stability, directing further resuscitative care.

In addition to assessment of physical findings, laboratory abnormalities should be addressed. Evaluation of acid-base status with arterial blood gases; measurement of electrolytes, including calcium, magnesium, and glucose; and baseline assessment of hepatic and renal function provide a basis for correction of metabolic derangements. In addition, if the intoxicant is known, plasma or serum concentrations of the intoxicating agent in selected cases may provide information regarding the severity of intoxication and aid in treatment decisions. Electrocardiograms and radiographs also may be indicated in cases of suspected intoxication with cardiovascular instability.

Patients requiring ICU admission for significant hemodynamic compromise and patients with a known ingestion with the potential for cardiovascular effects need cardiovascular monitoring. Critical care monitoring frequently includes placement of an arterial catheter for continuous direct measurement of blood pressure. The arterial catheter also allows painless arterial blood sampling for blood gases, enabling frequent monitoring of acid-base status and cardiorespiratory function. Placement of a central venous catheter may provide additional information about central venous filling pressures, which may be useful in decisions regarding fluid resuscitation and the use of inotropic agents. Central venous access also provides for the reliable administration of cardioactive agents, such as inotropes, vasoconstrictors, and vasodilators, as needed.

In patients with severe cardiovascular compromise or with combined cardiac and respiratory compromise requiring assisted ventilation and in patients in whom hemodynamic function fails to improve despite aggressive resuscitation with fluid administration and inotropic drugs, the addition of a pulmonary artery catheter may be indicated. Use of pulmonary artery catheters allows determination of cardiac output by thermodilution techniques, estimation of left ventricular end-diastolic pressure via measurement of the pulmonary artery occlusion pressure, and calculation of systemic and pulmonary vascular resistance indices. The measurement of paired samples of arterial and mixed venous blood from the pulmonary artery allows calculation of systemic oxygen availability and oxygen consumption, providing more detailed information regarding cardiac function and oxygen delivery. These data can be used to create a more targeted treatment plan for a hemodynamically unstable patient in whom the ingested substance is unknown and the hemodynamic derangements are more difficult to predict and in patients with multiple ingestants, in which more complex cardiopulmonary interactions may occur.

INITIAL MANAGEMENT

Initial management of cardiovascular dysfunction is focused on correction of vital sign abnormalities, restoration of cardiac output and organ system perfusion, and correction of metabolic and electrolyte disturbances. Early in the course of cardiovascular instability, the body's compensatory mechanisms may keep vital signs relatively normal. These compensatory mechanisms causing diminution in cardiac output include an increase in sympathetic tone, resulting in an increase in heart rate and peripheral vascular resistance, minimizing changes in blood pressure. Hypotension results only when compensatory mechanisms are exhausted or when the intoxicating substance directly interferes with these mechanisms. One example is tricyclic antidepressant intoxication, in which α-adrenergic receptor blockade interferes with peripheral vasoconstriction and with the direct cardiovascular effects of the drug diminish cardiac output. Drugs commonly associated with inadequate cardiac output and hypotension are listed in Table 10-5.

Initial correction of inadequate cardiac output often occurs before identification of an intoxicating substance. Identification of an intoxicating substance may simplify management if the intoxicant's common effects are known, allowing specific intervention for these effects. In the absence of this knowledge, initial resuscitation involves administration of intravenous fluids to ensure adequate intravascular volume. Initial rapid administration of isotonic fluids, usually crystalloid, such as normal saline or Ringer's lactate, in increments of 20 mL/kg body weight given over 10 to 15 minutes is used to reestablish sufficient intravascular volume. After initial fluid administration, reassessment of vital signs and physical examination are performed, and additional fluids are administered if reestablishment of intravascular volume is incomplete. Repletion of intravascular volume may result in restoration of vital signs and tissue perfusion to normal, with improvement in mentation, urine output, and peripheral pulses and perfusion. In patients in whom intrinsic cardiac function is impaired, expansion of intravascular volume may result in fluid overload, with an increase in liver size, evidence of pulmonary edema, jugular venous distention, or an increase in heart size on chest radiograph, without improvement in vital signs and tissue perfusion. In these patients, the addition of an inotropic agent may be necessary to improve cardiac function and tissue oxygen delivery. The choice of inotrope for a given circumstance depends on the cardiovascular derangements present. Inotropic drug effects depend on the drug's site of action (e.g., α-adrenergic versus β-adrenergic effects), and choosing a specific agent depends on matching the expected effects of a drug to the hemodynamic derangement requiring correction. The effects of various inotropic drugs on different aspects of cardiovascular function are outlined in Table 10-6.

HYPERTENSION

Hypertension is significantly less common than hypotension in a poisoned patient but may present as a medical emergency. Drugs responsible for arterial hypertension predominantly act via peripheral α-adrenergic receptors by direct stimulation of the receptor (e.g., phenylephrine), or indirectly by stimulation of release or inhibition of reuptake of endogenous norepinephrine or epinephrine (e.g., cocaine, cyclic antidepressants). Other agents may act via alternative pathways, such as the renin-angiotensin system. Drugs and toxins associated with significant hypertension are listed in Table 10-7.

Most patients with drug-induced or toxin-induced hypertension require minimal therapy. The need for treatment may be determined by the magnitude of the blood pressure, the

TABLE 10-5 Agents Commonly Causing Hypotension or Decreased Intravascular Volume

DRUGS CAUSING HYPOTENSION	DRUGS CAUSING DECREASED INTRAVASCULAR VOLUME
Myocardial Depressants	**Gastrointestinal Losses**
Antidysrhythmics	Abrin
β-Blockers	Arsenic
Calcium channel blockers	Bacterial toxins
Carbamazepine	Cathartics
Carbon monoxide (ischemic)	Caustics (acids, alkali)
Cardiac glycosides (digoxin, oleander, foxglove, yew)	Cholinergics
Chloroquine	Colchicine
Cyanide (ischemic)	Iron
Iron	Mercury
Quinine	Mushroom toxins (various)
Scorpion and snake envenomation (selected species)	Ricin
Sedative-hypnotics	**Renal Losses**
Tricyclic antidepressants	Cholinergics
Arrhythmics: see Table 10-8	Diuretics
Vasodilators	Ethanol
α₁-Blockers	Lithium
α₂-Agonists	Mercury
Angiotensin-converting enzyme inhibitors	Methyl xanthines
Calcium channel blockers	Salicylates
Diazoxide	**Insensible Losses**
Hydralazine	Cocaine
Nitrates	Cholinergics
Nitroprusside	Salicylates
Opioids	Dinitrophenol
Phenothiazines	Sympathomimetics
Sedative-hypnotics	Methyl xanthines

expected duration of action of the drug or toxin involved, and the associated symptoms. In poisoning in which the hypertension is mediated by release of endogenous catecholamines (e.g., cocaine), sedation with benzodiazepines is usually sufficient to control agitation and hypertension until drug effects resolve. For drugs with severe hypertensive effects (e.g., massive epinephrine overdose), the use of a direct-acting vasodilator (e.g., nitroprusside) or a specific receptor-blocking agent (e.g., phentolamine for α-receptor agonist overdose) is

TABLE 10-6 Effects of Various Inotropic Drugs on Cardiovascular Parameters

	HR	BP	SVR	CO
Dopamine				
<5 µg/kg/min	+/−	+/−	+/−	+/−
5–10 µg/kg/min	+ +	+	+/−	+ +
>10 µg/kg/min	+ + +	+ +	+ +	+ +
Dobutamine	+ + +	+/−	+/−	+ + +
Epinephrine	+ +	+ + +	+ +	+ + + +
Norepinephrine	+	+ + + +	+ + + +	+ +
Phenylephrine	+/−	+ + + +	+ + + +	+/−
Amrinone	+/−	+/−	− − −	+ + +
Milrinone	+/−	+/−	− − −	+ + +
Digoxin	− −	+	+/−	+ +
Glucagon	+	+ +	+/−	+ +

BP, blood pressure (arterial); CO, cardiac output; HR, heart rate; SVR, systemic vascular resistance.

TABLE 10-7 Agents Producing Hypertension

Direct α-Adrenergic Agonists	
Clonidine (massive)	Monoamine oxidase inhibitors
Dopamine	Phencyclidine
Epinephrine	Serotonin reuptake inhibitors
Naphazoline	Tricyclic antidepressants
Norepinephrine	Tyramine
Oxymetazoline	Yohimbine
Phenylephrine	Ethanol withdrawal
Phenylpropanolamine	Gamma hydroxybutyrate withdrawal
Pseudoephedrine	
Tetrahydrozoline	**Nonadrenergic Effects**
Scorpion envenomation	Cadmium
	Corticosteroids
Indirect α-Adrenergic Effects	Lead
Amphetamines	Mercury
Cocaine	Nicotine
Carbamazepine	Thallium
Diphenhydramine	Vincristine
Dopamine	Vasopressin
Ketamine	Zinc

indicated. Agents with a short duration of action are preferred so that as the hypertensive effects of the overdose resolve, treatment can be tapered rapidly as blood pressure normalizes. Many studies have suggested that in sympathomimetic overdoses, the use of β-adrenergic blocking agents is contraindicated because blocking of β-receptors may allow unopposed action at α-adrenergic receptors, resulting in increased hypertension and the potential for coronary artery vasospasm, especially in cases of cocaine overdose.[28,29]

DYSRHYTHMIAS

A common complication of poisoning with cardiovascular agents is the development of dysrhythmias. Dysrhythmogenic drugs may produce their actions by directly affecting the electrical conduction system of the heart, by changing the electrical potential of individual myocardial cells, by indirectly influencing the cardiac conduction system via the autonomic nervous system or CNS, or by inducing electrolyte and metabolic disturbances that affect electrical activity within the heart. Table 10-8 lists drugs commonly associated with dysrhythmias in pediatric patients.

Bradydysrhythmias occur as a result of agents that decrease sympathetic outflow from the CNS, such as opioids, benzodiazepines, and barbiturates, and as a result of drugs that decrease the chronotropic activity of the conduction system, including agents such as calcium channel blockers and class I antidysrhythmic drugs. Severe overdose of any of these agents may result in asystole and cardiac arrest.

Treatment of bradydysrhythmia resulting from an unknown ingestant is supportive. Administration of atropine or inotropic agents with positive chronotropic effects (e.g., dopamine, epinephrine) may be corrective. If the causative agent of the ingestion is known, therapies directed at antagonism of the toxic effects (e.g., calcium chloride administration for calcium channel blocker overdose) may be beneficial. In severe cases of bradydysrhythmia or heart block unresponsive to pharmacologic therapy, direct transthoracic pacing or transvenous pacing may be necessary (see subsequent section).

Tachydysrhythmias are commonly seen after poisoning. Sinus tachycardia may occur as a result of increased sympathetic tone after ingestion of CNS stimulants, as a result of ingestion of agents that block catecholamine reuptake at sympathetic nerve terminals (e.g., methamphetamine, cocaine), or as a result of ingestion of drugs with anticholinergic properties. Halogenated hydrocarbons, such as chloral hydrate, may sensitize the myocardium to the effects of endogenous catecholamines, increasing the risk of tachydysrhythmias, including supraventricular and ventricular tachycardia.[30,31] Overdose with antidysrhythmic agents, particularly class Ia agents, may result in supraventricular or ventricular tachycardia. Tricyclic antidepressants, carbamazepine, and diphenhydramine, all of which share structural similarities and have cell membrane effects similar to quinidine and other class Ia antidysrhythmics, have similar propensities to develop widecomplex ventricular dysrhythmias.

Torsades de pointes is a unique form of ventricular tachycardia that is seen with selected overdoses. Torsades de pointes may occur after ingestion of any drug associated with ventricular tachycardia, such as the class Ia and class Ic antidysrhythmics. It also has been identified after overdose or accumulation due to competitive inhibition or elimination of the antihistamines terfenadine and astemizole and with pentamidine for treatment of *Pneumocystis carinii* pneumonia.[32–35]

Treatment of tachydysrhythmias associated with poisoning is generally the same as in other circumstances, with some unique exceptions. The treatment of dysrhythmias associated with a specific antidysrhythmic or class of antidysrhythmic agents should avoid using another drug in the same class. The use of procainamide or other class Ia agents to treat dysrhythmias associated with quinidine overdose is contraindicated. Treatment of supraventricular tachycardia of hemodynamic significance may be benefited by the use of adenosine, although the short half-life of adenosine and the persistent presence of a dysrhythmogenic toxin make the utility of short-acting agents uncertain. The use of drugs of general utility, such as lidocaine and amiodarone, may be preferred in this setting, unless it is contraindicated on electrophysiologic grounds in specific intoxications.

A unique situation seen with dysrhythmias associated with overdose of tricyclic antidepressants and other agents with sodium channel activity, such as class Ia antidysrhythmic agents, is the use of sodium bicarbonate in the treatment of these dysrhythmias. Numerous studies have investigated the antidysrhythmic effects of sodium bicarbonate in these life-threatening overdoses. Sodium bicarbonate has been shown consistently to reverse wide-complex tachydysrhythmias associated with tricyclic antidepressant poisoning.[36–38] The mechanism of this effect is incompletely resolved, but the most consistent data suggest that acute increases in extracellular sodium concentration after sodium bicarbonate administration may overcome the sodium channel blockade that occurs in

TABLE 10-8 Agents Producing Dysrhythmias

Bradydysrhythmias

α₂-Adrenergic agonists
Aconitine
Antidysrhythmics
β-Adrenergic blockers
Calcium channel blockers
Carbamates
Cocaine (late)
Cholinomimetics
Digoxin
Jin bu huan
Opioids
Organophosphates
Plants containing cardiac
   glycosides (foxglove, lily of
   the valley, oleander, yew)
Sedative-hypnotics
Tricyclic antidepressants (late or
   massive ingestion)

Tachydysrhythmias

α-Adrenergic agonists
Aluminum phosphide
Amantadine
Antidysrhythmics
Anticholinergics
Antihistamines
Astemizole
β-Adrenergic agonists
Carbamazepine
Cisapride
Chloral hydrate
Chloroquine
Cholinomimetics
Digitalis glycosides
Hydrocarbons/solvents—
   "huffing"
Inhalational anesthetics
Ecstasy (3,4-methylene-
   dioxymethamphetamine)
Orphenadrine
Pentamidine
Plants containing cardiac
   glycosides (foxglove, lily of
   the valley, oleander, yew)
Phenothiazines
Phosphodiesterase inhibitors
   (methyl xanthines, amrinone,
   milrinone)
Propoxyphene
Scorpion envenomation
Selenium—"gun blue"
Snake envenomation
Sympathomimetics
   (amphetamines, cocaine,
   phencyclidine)
Terfenadine
Theophylline
Tricyclic antidepressants

this ingestion.[36,39–41] Similar but less consistent reversal of dysrhythmias has occurred with sodium bicarbonate in the treatment of dysrhythmias associated with quinidine and other class Ia antidysrhythmics and in dysrhythmias associated with carbamazepine and diphenhydramine.[41–44]

Treatment of a pediatric patient with torsades de pointes associated with overdose is similar to that seen with torsades de pointes in any other circumstance. Correction of electrolyte and other metabolic disturbances is crucial, followed by administration of magnesium sulfate, which seems to be the only consistently effective therapy for this difficult-to-control dysrhythmia.[45–47] Electrical cardioversion frequently is unsuccessful in converting torsades de pointes. See Chapter 21 for a more detailed review of cardiotoxicity and its management.

In pediatric patients with massive overdose with a cardiotoxic agent, dysrhythmias may be completely unresponsive to pharmacologic therapy, and electrical cardioversion may be unsuccessful or only temporarily successful in converting the patient back to a sinus rhythm. For these patients, temporary ventricular pacing may be the only solution to the dysrhythmia. Available methods of pacing include transcutaneous pacing, transvenous pacing, and transesophageal pacing. Transcutaneous pacing, although uncomfortable in a conscious patient, is the most readily available modality for cardiac pacing. This approach may be lifesaving while alternative therapies are initiated, such as transvenous pacing, initiation of effective pharmacologic measures, or cannulation for extracorporeal membrane oxygenation (ECMO) support.

Transvenous pacing, by way of a catheter placed into the heart via central venous access, is an alternative to transcutaneous pacing for patients large enough to accommodate a pacing catheter. This modality is more technically difficult, requiring availability of fluoroscopic guidance for effective catheter placement, and requires more time in its placement. Adverse effects are minimal when the catheter is placed appropriately, and the transvenous approach is tolerated better by the patient and may be used for a longer time than transcutaneous pacing.

Transesophageal pacing is useful for overdrive pacing of patients with atrial tachydysrhythmias only. Ventricular pacing is not possible via the transesophageal route, and patients with bradydysrhythmias associated with atrioventricular blocks are not benefited by this approach.

MECHANICAL CIRCULATORY SUPPORT

Children with massive overdoses of drugs with cardiac depressant, proarrhythmic, or vasodilator effects may be unresponsive to fluid resuscitation, inotropic therapy, vasoconstrictor therapy, and temporary pacemaker therapy. For these patients, mechanical support of the circulation may be the only alternative to mortality. In these patients, preexisting cardiac function and respiratory function are normal, the heart is free of preexisting arteriosclerotic disease, and the cause of the child's myocardial dysfunction is potentially self-limited, resolving with clearance of the intoxicant. For these patients, a range of mechanical supportive devices may be available in selected circumstances.

EXTRACORPOREAL MEMBRANE OXYGENATION

The most commonly available, most invasive, and probably most effective mechanical supportive device is ECMO. In ECMO, the patient's blood is removed from the body; pumped through a membrane oxygenator, which adds oxygen and removes carbon dioxide from the blood; and returned to the body. ECMO is a treatment with substantial risk because it requires systemic anticoagulation and is technically sophisticated, requiring the expertise of a center familiar with and prepared to perform ECMO regularly. Complications of ECMO, even in centers that perform ECMO regularly, include life-threatening hemorrhage, embolic complications including cerebrovascular accidents, development of multisystem organ failure, and risk of systemic infection. ECMO should be used only in situations in which the risk of mortality is great and only in centers with established experience.

Two forms of ECMO are available. Venoarterial ECMO, in which cannulae are placed in a central vein (usually jugular vein) and central artery (usually carotid artery), provides complete cardiorespiratory replacement for the duration of time necessary for clearance of an intoxicant and recovery of cardiac and respiratory function. Venovenous ECMO, in which either two venous cannulae (usually femoral vein and jugular vein) or one double-lumen venous cannula is placed, primarily provides replacement of respiratory function and requires adequate native cardiac output for adequate tissue perfusion. Venoarterial ECMO is most useful if the primary problem is myocardial dysfunction and poor cardiac output or combined cardiorespiratory failure, and venovenous ECMO may be considered if the primary problem is pulmonary, as in hydrocarbon aspiration or smoke inhalation associated with carbon monoxide poisoning. The advantage of venovenous ECMO in this circumstance is the avoidance of return flow into the arterial circulation, hence decreasing the risk of thromboembolic complications, such as cerebrovascular accidents and peripheral arterial embolism. ECMO has been used in selected circumstances with ready availability of this specialized technology in a timely fashion during the acute deterioration of a patient after a lethal ingestion. The successful use of ECMO has been reported in patients with overdoses with desipramine, quinidine, propranolol, and acebutolol and in patients with severe respiratory failure due to hydrocarbon aspiration, paraquat ingestion, and smoke inhalation injuries.[48–54]

CIRCULATORY ASSIST DEVICES

Two alternative, less invasive therapies are used in the management of patients with severe hemodynamic compromise unresponsive to less invasive medical management. The intraaortic balloon pump (IABP) and ventricular assist device (VAD) are widely used as cardiovascular assistive devices in adults with intractable cardiac failure, in most cases after cardiac surgery, after myocardial infarction, or as a bridge to transplant in patients with congestive cardiomyopathy. Technologic advances with both modalities have increased the application of these modes of mechanical cardiac assistance to small children and infants, particularly after surgery for congenital heart disease.

VADs provide augmentation of cardiac output by direct pump assistance to ventricular function. Early use of VADs in children was limited by the large size of the device and the risk of thromboembolic complications. In more recent years, heparin coating of the device to minimize thrombogenesis and production of devices in smaller sizes for small children and infants have resulted in greater success and fewer complications with VAD support, leading to its increased use. Although use of the VAD is widespread in patients with ventricular dysfunction from other causes, its use after poisoning has not been reported.

The IABP uses the timed inflation of a balloon placed in the aorta to provide diastolic augmentation of cardiac output, improving coronary artery perfusion and forward systemic cardiac output. The use of the IABP has been limited in children, particularly by the difficulty of appropriate timing of balloon inflation to achieve proper augmentation of cardiac output. Technical advances, including the use of M-mode echocardiography for timing of balloon inflation, may make IABP use more feasible in infants and children.[55,56] The use of the IABP has been associated with many complications, including aortic dissection, arterial injury at the site of insertion, infection, and thromboembolism.[57–60] IABP use has been reported after overdoses of dextropropoxyphene, disopyramide, and combined overdose of verapamil and atenolol in adults.[27] Its use in pediatric poisoning cases has not been reported.

Despite the logical utility of the use of mechanical cardiac support such as ECMO, VAD, or IABP in severely cardiotoxic patients, the application of these technologies in toxicology has been limited. The presentation of a patient with profound cardiotoxicity unresponsive to good supportive care to a center in which advanced mechanical support of the circulation is readily available is rare. Further research may refine these techniques, making the use of these invasive modalities possible for pediatric patients.

Respiratory Toxicity

Respiratory distress and the potential for respiratory failure are common reasons for ICU admission of children after intoxication. Respiratory insufficiency may develop as a result of ingestion of CNS depressant drugs, resulting in impairment of respiratory drive. Drugs and toxins that impair respiratory drive (e.g., opioids, barbiturates, benzodiazepines) may diminish respiratory rate, depth of respiration, or both, with resulting hypoventilation, causing hypercarbia or hypoxia or both. Alternatively, other drugs may stimulate respiration by increasing central respiratory drive (e.g., salicylates, theophylline), inducing a respiratory alkalosis. Patients ingesting such drugs are at risk for eventual respiratory embarrassment if excessive respiratory drive results in respiratory muscle exhaustion.

CNS depressants also may impair the function of pharyngeal and hypopharyngeal musculature, resulting in obstruction of the upper airway by the tongue or other pharyngeal structures. Upper airway obstruction also may occur after exposure to agents (e.g., organophosphates, carbamates, scorpion envenomation) that increase pharyngeal and tracheobronchial secretions, obstructing either the hypopharynx or glottic apparatus or the tracheobronchial tree with secretions. Caustic agents and thermal injuries to the airway may cause airway obstruction due to the development of airway edema. The pediatric airway, with the characteristic narrowing that occurs in the subglottic region, is at great risk for obstruction from airway edema or increased airway secretions.

Respiratory failure also may occur owing to a wide variety of problems involving the lower respiratory tract. Airway obstruction may occur secondary to increased tracheobronchial secretions or the development of bronchospasm due to the effects of airway irritants on bronchial smooth muscle. Aspiration of asphyxiant gases (e.g., volatile hydrocarbons, carbon dioxide) may interfere with oxygenation, with resulting CNS and organ system hypoxia.

Aspiration, inhalation, parenteral injection, or ingestion of a broad range of intoxicants may be responsible for parenchymal lung injury. A variety of trigger events, including hydrocarbon aspiration, inhalation of smoke or toxic gases, drowning, and a broad range of nonpulmonary triggers such as narcotic overdose, have been associated with the development of noncardiogenic pulmonary edema. Alteration in pulmonary alveolar and capillary permeability allows leakage of proteinaceous fluid from alveolar capillaries into the alveolar airspaces. The resulting alterations in alveolar diffusing capacity for oxygen and carbon dioxide, loss of surfactant, and development of pulmonary parenchymal inflammation are the hallmarks of acute lung injury and adult respiratory distress syndrome (ARDS). ARDS is defined as a syndrome of acute lung injury in which there is the presence of bilateral diffuse pulmonary infiltrates; no evidence of primary cardiac dysfunction as the cause of the pulmonary edema; and severe hypoxemia, defined by a ratio of arterial oxygen partial pressure (PaO_2) to fractional concentration of oxygen in inspired gas (FiO_2) of less than 200.[61] Progressive loss of respiratory system compliance results in progressive respiratory failure. Despite aggressive supportive care and significant advances in ventilatory management of patients with ARDS, mortality remains high, approaching 50%.[61] Table 10-9 lists drugs and toxins that have been associated with the development of ARDS.

Treatment of respiratory crises requires vigilant critical care monitoring. In addition to assessment of the patient's respiratory rate and work of breathing, continuous pulse oximetry is required for ongoing assessment of oxygenation of the blood. Supplemental oxygen is administered to ensure adequate tissue oxygenation if oxygen saturations decline to less than normal, usually considered to be 93% oxygen saturation. Intermittent monitoring of blood gases is

TABLE 10-9 Agents Triggering Adult Respiratory Distress Syndrome

Activated charcoal	Mercury inhalation
Aluminum phosphide	Nitrogen dioxide
Amphetamines	Nonsteroidal antiinflammatory
Amphotericin	drugs
Antidysrhythmics	Opioids
Cadmium inhalation	Organophosphates
Calcium channel blockers	Paraquat
Carbon monoxide	Quinine
Cocaine	Salicylates
Deferoxamine	Scorpion envenomation
Diphenhydramine	Sodium oleate
Ethchlorvynol	Smoke inhalation
Ethylene glycol	Snake envenomation
Haloperidol	Tricyclic antidepressants
Hydrocarbon aspiration	Zinc inhalation
Lithium	

essential to evaluate ventilation and oxygenation fully. In children with mild respiratory illness, capillary blood gases in conjunction with pulse oximetry may be sufficient to monitor respiratory function. For patients with more severe respiratory dysfunction, requiring more frequent blood gas analysis, placement of an arterial catheter for repeated blood gas monitoring allows direct measurement of PaO_2 and arterial carbon dioxide partial pressure ($PaCO_2$), providing the most accurate assessment of the patient's respiratory status.

As a child reaches a state of respiratory exhaustion, work of breathing and respiratory rate may seem to improve, while the child's ventilation and $PaCO_2$ are deteriorating. It is desirable to perform intubation electively at this point to avoid an emergent situation requiring immediate intubation. According to TESS data, approximately 5% of poisoned children admitted to critical care settings require assisted ventilation.[5]

Appropriate guidelines for intubation should take into account the patient's physiologic condition, findings on blood gas analysis, and the patient's current phase of illness. Similar blood gas findings may have much different meanings in a patient deteriorating in the first hours after a massive opioid ingestion and a patient recovering from a moderate overdose. Clinical judgment plays an essential role in these decisions.

Indications for Endotracheal Intubation

1. Upper airway obstruction
2. Altered mental status (Glasgow Coma Scale score ≤ 7)
   a. Absence of gag and cough reflexes
   b. Maintenance of normocarbia/mild hypocarbia (ICP prophylaxis after head injury)
3. Actual or impending respiratory failure
   a. Hypoxia (PaO_2 <60 mm Hg or oxygen saturation <90% on FiO_2 >0.6)
   b. Respiratory acidosis ($PaCO_2$ >50 mm Hg with pH <7.30)
4. Cardiovascular instability with hypotension, inadequate cardiac output, metabolic acidosis
5. Excessive airway secretions inadequately cleared with cough/pharyngeal suctioning
6. Treatment of pulmonary hypertension

FiO_2, fractional concentration of oxygen in inspired gas; ICP, intracranial pressure; PaO_2, arterial oxygen partial pressure; $PaCO_2$, arterial carbon dioxide partial pressure.

Patients undergoing endotracheal intubation associated with intoxication are often in a state of disorientation that makes their ability to cooperate with endotracheal intubation unlikely. Provision of sedation and analgesia and the use of a neuromuscular blocking agent to allow complete muscle relaxation before intubation are desirable in most patients to minimize the risk of traumatic intubation. The use of neuromuscular blocking agents, which by necessity result in apnea and complete loss of airway protective reflexes, requires that the airway manager have excellent airway skills to ensure that prompt intubation occurs without complications. Table 10-10 lists pharmacologic agents commonly used to aid in intubation.

TABLE 10-10 Pharmacologic Agents for Endotracheal Intubation

DRUG	DOSE	DURATION OF EFFECT
Sedation/Anesthesia		
Midazolam	0.1–0.2 mg/kg	45–90 min
Diazepam	0.1–0.2 mg/kg	2–3 hr
Ketamine	0.5–2 mg/kg	15–30 min
Thiopental	5 mg/kg	5–10 min
Fentanyl	2–5 μg/kg	30–60 min
Neuromuscular Blockers		
Vecuronium	0.1–0.2 mg/kg	30–60 min
Cisatracurium	0.15 mg/kg	30–60 min
Pancuronium	0.1–0.2 mg/kg	60–90 min
Rocuronium	0.5–1 mg/kg	15–30 min
Succinylcholine	1–2 mg/kg	5–10 min
Anticholinergic		
Atropine	0.02 mg/kg*	2–3 hr

*Minimum dose for small infants is 0.1 mg.

Intubation in pediatric patients requires a broad range of equipment sizes to allow for intubation of patients ranging in weight from less than 3 kg to greater than 100 kg. Knowledge of appropriate sizing of endotracheal tubes, nasogastric tubes, laryngoscope blades, and other equipment is crucial to successful intubation. An age-based size guide for intubation equipment is provided in Table 10-11.

MECHANICAL VENTILATION

After endotracheal intubation, appropriate ventilatory assistance is required. The choice of ventilator, mode of ventilation, and assisted breathing rate depends on the age and size of the patient and the clinical circumstances. Patients in whom the lungs are functionally normal and who are intubated for airway protection or the provision of hyperventilation are managed much differently than patients with hydrocarbon aspiration and evolving ARDS. Although detailed discussion of ventilator management is beyond the scope of this chapter, some general issues are discussed here.

The goal of mechanical ventilation is to provide sufficient exchange of oxygen and carbon dioxide to provide for the metabolic needs of a patient with a minimum of adverse effects. In patients intubated primarily for airway protection and in whom the lungs are essentially normal, minimal ventilatory assistance is required. Little resistance to air entry exists, and compliance is normal, allowing air to enter and escape from the lungs with minimal ventilator pressure. No barrier to gas exchange exists, and oxygen crosses the alveolar epithelial and pulmonary capillary membranes easily.

For patients with significant lung disease, hyaline membranes are present within the airspaces of the lung, providing a barrier to gas exchange. If interstitial edema and inflammation reduce pulmonary compliance and increase airway resistance, air exchange occurs with more difficulty. The increase in resistance to airflow and decreased compliance require greater pressure to force gases into the airway, and an increase in FiO_2 is required to provide the gradient of

TABLE 10-11 Equipment for Endotracheal Intubation			
AGE	**UNCUFFED ETT SIZE***	**ETT INSERTION DEPTH (cm)†**	**NG TUBE SIZE (F)**
Newborn (>2 kg)	3.5	9–10	10
1–6 mo	3.5	10–11	10
1 yr	4.0	12–13	12
2–3 yr	4.5	13–14	12–14
4–5 yr	5.0	14–16	14
6–7 yr	5.5	16–18	14–16
8–9 yr	6.0	17–19	16
10–11 yr	6.5	18–20	16–18
12–13 yr	7.0	19–21	18
14–15 yr	7.5	20–22	18–20

*External diameter of a cuffed ETT is equivalent to an uncuffed ETT a half-size larger (e.g., 5.0 cuffed = 5.5 uncuffed).
†ETT insertion depths are for oral insertion in a child of normal size for age.
ETT, endotracheal tube; NG, nasogastric.

oxygen concentration necessary to overcome the barrier to gas exchange provided by the proteinaceous debris in the alveolus. This increase in ventilator pressure (barotrauma) and oxygen concentration (oxygen toxicity) results in further injury to the lung. In these patients, the goal is to provide sufficient respiratory support to maintain vital functions, while minimizing further injury to the lungs.

Conventional ventilatory support provides respirations that mimic normal tidal breathing, providing a physiologically appropriate number of breaths of appropriate size and duration for age. Modern ventilators are designed to synchronize respirations with the patient's own breathing efforts (synchronized intermittent mandatory ventilation) in an effort to minimize the discomfort that the patient experiences with assisted ventilation. The various modes of conventional ventilation can be distinguished according to the method by which individual breaths are limited. In pressure-cycled ventilation, the peak inspiratory pressure is preset, providing for inspiratory airflow up to a predetermined maximum, with the size of individual breaths determined by peak inspiratory pressure, the rate of airflow, inspiratory time, and airway resistance and chest compliance. The size of individual breaths varies with changes in resistance and compliance. In volume-cycled modes of ventilation, air fills the lungs to a preset tidal volume at a flow rate determined by the tidal volume and a preset total inspiratory time. The pressure required to provide any given breath depends on and varies with changes in airway resistance and chest compliance. In both forms of ventilation, the desired goal is the achievement of stable minute ventilation (the product of tidal volume and respiratory rate). As the severity of lung disease increases and as pulmonary compliance worsens, the peak inspiratory pressure required to provide a given tidal volume increases. Excessive ventilator pressures have been associated with the development of ventilator-associated lung injury, or barotrauma. Maintaining peak inspiratory pressure at the minimum value necessary to provide adequate ventilation and oxygenation is essential to successful ventilator management. As a rule of thumb, peak inspiratory pressure greater than 40 cm H_2O pressure is associated with an increased risk of air leak (pneumothorax, pneumomediastinum) and should be avoided whenever possible.

In patients with significant parenchymal lung disease, alveolar collapse and ventilation/perfusion mismatching result in failure of oxygenation of the blood, with resulting desaturation of arterial blood and tissue hypoxia. FiO_2 should be adjusted to maintain adequate PaO_2 and hemoglobin oxygen saturation. The use of high levels of supplemental oxygen (FiO_2 >0.5) is associated with the development of pulmonary oxygen toxicity. Maintenance of adequate lung volume, which minimizes ventilation/perfusion mismatching within the lung, minimizes the need for supplemental oxygen. Lung volume is maintained best by the addition of positive end-expiratory pressure in the ventilator circuit. The appropriate level of positive end-expiratory pressure is determined by the severity of lung disease and the degree to which ventilation/perfusion inequality exists within the lung. The optimal level of positive end-expiratory pressure must be individualized to the specific situation and is the level of positive end-expiratory pressure that maintains alveolar patency without overdistention and that allows maintenance of FiO_2 at nontoxic levels (FiO_2 <0.6).[61,62]

Severe acute lung injury or ARDS causes a diminution in pulmonary compliance, requiring substantially elevated ventilator pressures to maintain adequate oxygenation and ventilation. A major contributor to morbidity and mortality in ARDS is the development of pulmonary air leak, with resulting pneumothorax or pneumomediastinum or both. Many studies have suggested that high ventilator pressures and high oxygen concentrations are significant contributors to lung injury in ARDS, and by the stimulatory release of inflammatory cytokines, they also may contribute to multiorgan system failure and nonpulmonary mortality in ARDS. Strategies to minimize barotrauma and oxygen toxicity may have a salutary effect on morbidity and mortality from ARDS. Lung protective strategies that emphasize low-pressure, low-volume ventilation with tolerance of respiratory acidosis (pH 7.20, $PaCO_2$ 120 mm Hg) and hypoxia (oxygen saturations >85%) have been suggested in an effort to minimize iatrogenic lung injury. This strategy is termed *permissive hypercapnia*. Uncontrolled studies have touted reductions in mortality in patients managed with permissive hypercapnia, and these lung protective strategies are used widely. Well-controlled clinical trials so far have failed to show consistently a change in long-term morbidity and mortality with this ventilatory strategy.[63–65]

For some patients with severe lung injury, despite lung protective strategies, conventional ventilation may be insufficient to provide adequate oxygenation and ventilation or may result in an unacceptable incidence of pulmonary air leak. For these patients, alternative strategies of cardiorespiratory support must be considered. These strategies include high-frequency ventilation and ECMO. Published information regarding the use of alternatives to conventional ventilation in poisoned children is limited. The common pathophysiology of ARDS allows extrapolation of data from nontoxicologic causes of ARDS to the poisoned patient, however.

HIGH-FREQUENCY VENTILATION

High-frequency ventilation is an alternative to conventional ventilation in which small volumes of air are injected into the airway at high frequencies. Two primary modes of high-frequency ventilation are currently in use. In high-frequency jet ventilation, jets of air are delivered into the airway via a high-velocity injector port at rates of 100 to 600 breaths/min. Inhalation in this mode of ventilation is active, whereas exhaled gases are expelled passively. Total lung inflation is controlled primarily by adjustment of tidal volume and inspiratory time. The precise mechanism of gas exchange in high-frequency jet ventilation is poorly understood. High-frequency oscillatory ventilation is an alternative to high-frequency jet ventilation; a piston or diaphragm actively oscillates air into and out of the lung at high frequencies, generally at oscillatory frequencies ranging from 6 to 12 Hz. It is hypothesized that at high frequencies resonance occurs within the lung, facilitating gas exchange. The mechanism of gas exchange in high-frequency oscillatory ventilation is similarly poorly understood. The purported advantage of high-frequency ventilation lies in the small tidal volumes (generally 1 to 3 mL/kg) used, which result in lower peak airway pressure and less ventilator-associated airway injury. In patients with significant alterations in compliance and in patients with significant air leak, high-frequency ventilation provides a theoretically less traumatic alternative to conventional ventilation. In patients with severe ARDS, early initiation of high-frequency ventilation has been shown to result in lower mortality than conventional ventilation.[66–68] Published reports have documented its successful use in patients with hydrocarbon aspiration and mercury inhalation.[69,70]

EXTRACORPOREAL MEMBRANE OXYGENATION

For patients with intractable respiratory failure in whom conventional ventilation and high-frequency ventilation fail to provide sufficient respiratory support, ECMO may be lifesaving. Reports of its successful use after respiratory failure, smoke inhalation and carbon monoxide poisoning, and hydrocarbon aspiration have been published.[52,54] Overall survival in pediatric patients with ARDS treated with ECMO has been reported to be 30% to 50%.[61] ECMO was discussed in detail earlier.

EXPERIMENTAL THERAPIES

Many experimental therapies have been considered in the treatment of ARDS in children. Given that a large part of the pathophysiology of ARDS results from loss of endogenous surfactant, replacement of surfactant has been considered

and tried in many children and adults with ARDS. A trial of calf lung surfactant administration in pediatric patients with ARDS has shown improvement in survival and decreased duration of mechanical ventilation and ICU stay.[71]

A second experimental therapy that has been used in the research setting is perfluorocarbon for partial liquid ventilation in patients with ARDS. Perfluorocarbons are liquids with unique surfactant qualities into which oxygen and carbon dioxide are highly soluble. Experimental studies have investigated the use of perfluorocarbon-assisted partial liquid ventilation in animal models of ARDS. These studies have shown improvement in pulmonary mechanics and improved gas exchange in animals treated with partial liquid ventilation.[72,73] Anecdotal pediatric studies have shown similar improvements in these variables, but controlled trials have not yet shown a survival advantage with partial liquid ventilation.

Neurologic Toxicity

Derangement of neurologic function associated with intoxication is a common reason for PICU admission. Common neurologic changes resulting from intoxication include altered mental status, with a depressed level of consciousness, agitation and delirium, or seizures. A detailed discussion of these topics is beyond the scope of this chapter, but some basic issues of critical care assessment and initial management strategies are discussed.

A diminished level of consciousness may result from intoxication, metabolic derangements, structural neurologic insults such as trauma, intracranial hemorrhage, focal ischemic injury or stroke, infection, or psychiatric disorders. Sometimes more than one of these categories simultaneously may be responsible for mental status change, as in a patient with ethanol toxicity accompanied by hypoglycemia. A detailed history of the evolution of the child's mental status change often suggests a cause, leading to diagnostic studies that confirm the diagnosis. Historical features suggesting intoxication as the cause of mental status alteration in a child may include an abrupt change in mentation in a previously normal child, a period of unsupervised time in which the child had access to an intoxicating substance, and the absence of antecedent trauma or prodromal symptoms suggesting infection. Altered mental status resulting from toxic and metabolic causes differs from mental status alteration from other causes in that brain structure is not altered, and neurologic pathways are intact. Clouding of consciousness usually is not associated with focal neurologic findings and is reflected in global encephalopathic change. Physical findings on neurologic examination after ingestion of a CNS depressant (e.g., benzodiazepine, opioid, or barbiturate) usually include diminution in the magnitude of response rather than loss of response, unless the overdose is large enough to induce coma. Pupillary response generally is preserved, although commonly it is sluggish and diminished in intensity. Toxic or metabolic encephalopathy also may result in diminution of control of brainstem functions, such as respiratory drive, resulting in hypoventilation or apnea, or control of peripheral vascular tone, resulting in vasodilation and hypotension. Loss of motor tone in skeletal musculature may result in bulbar and hypopharyngeal muscle dysfunction, causing upper airway obstruction and loss of airway protective reflexes, or may result in a decrease in respiratory muscle function, with resulting hypoventilation.

ASSESSMENT

Assessment of a child who presents with an unexplained alteration in level of consciousness begins with an assessment of airway patency and protective reflexes, adequacy of respiratory effort and function, and adequacy of the circulation and systemic oxygenation. When these vital functions are ensured, further assessment generally includes, in addition to a thorough history and physical examination, laboratory studies including electrolytes, glucose, renal and hepatic function studies, serum ammonia, complete blood count, and arterial blood gases to assess the adequacy of ventilation and oxygenation. If there is fever or any history suggesting infection, lumbar puncture to rule out meningitis is recommended. Computed tomography of the brain to rule out structural lesions and cerebral edema frequently is done. An electroencephalogram may be required to rule out subclinical status epilepticus. Toxicologic studies, focused by thorough history, also should be sent to aid in the diagnosis.

MANAGEMENT

Initial management of a child presenting with stupor or coma includes any measures necessary to secure an adequate airway, breathing, and circulation. Empirical administration of naloxone and glucose is recommended to ensure that easily reversible causes of altered mental status are ruled out. Thiamine, although widely recommended in adults because of the high incidence of thiamine deficiency in alcoholic and nutritionally depleted patients, is not recommended routinely for children because thiamine deficiency is rare in this population. Additional care of these patients is supportive, with close neurologic monitoring intended to prevent secondary injury while the intoxicant is metabolized and cleared.

An alternative presentation of an intoxicated child is agitation and delirium. This presentation may be accompanied by depression of consciousness, as may be seen in children with tricyclic antidepressant ingestion, who may manifest anticholinergic delirium or psychosis accompanied by mental status depression. Alternatively, children may present without sedation, as is seen in anticholinergic hallucinosis after Jimson weed ingestion. A patient presenting with toxin-induced agitation and delirium may be difficult to distinguish from a patient presenting with acute psychiatric illness. The relative infrequency of delusional psychiatric disorders in children makes this distinction easier in children than in adults. Toxins commonly presenting with agitation or delirium are listed in Table 10-12.

A history of acute onset of disorientation, delusion, and agitation in a child or adolescent, especially if alteration in level of consciousness is present, strongly suggests a toxic or metabolic cause because psychiatric illness rarely presents with alteration in level of consciousness. Presence of a prodromal aura or visual disturbance, complaint of current headache, or past history of headache may suggest acute confusional migraine as an alternative diagnosis. Visual or tactile hallucinations further support a toxic/metabolic etiology because psychiatric illness more typically presents with auditory hallucinations.

Assessment of airway patency and respiratory function is necessary to ensure adequate ventilation. Some intoxications that present with agitation and delirium, such as scorpion

TABLE 10-12 Toxins Causing Agitation or Delirium in Children	
Amphetamines	Ketamine
Anticholinergics	Lithium
Antiepileptics	Lysergic acid diethylamide (LSD)
Benzodiazepines (emergence)	Ecstasy (3,4-methylenedioxy-
Chloroquine	methamphetamine)
Cocaine	Opioids
Corticosteroids	Phencyclidine
Fluoroquinolones	Phenothiazines
Gamma hydroxybutyrate	Sympathomimetics
(emergence)	Volatile hydrocarbon/solvent "huffing"

envenomation with *Centruroides exilicauda* or organophosphate exposure, also may cause an increase in airway secretions, resulting in tracheal obstruction and prompting endotracheal intubation.

On physical examination, patients with toxic or metabolic disturbances rarely have focal neurologic findings, as discussed previously. The presence of focal neurologic findings or evidence of trauma should prompt aggressive investigation for a structural/neurologic cause. Laboratory studies, similar to those outlined earlier for patients with depressed mentation, should be sent to rule out metabolic etiologies and to allow for correction of any secondary metabolic disturbances. Increased motor activity and increased risk of musculoskeletal trauma in delirious or agitated patients place these individuals at increased risk for muscle injury. Measurement of creatine phosphokinase to assess for rhabdomyolysis is important because of the risk of myoglobinuria and renal impairment in these patients.

Treatment of a child who presents with agitation is primarily supportive and protective. Provision of sedation with benzodiazepines, accompanied by a supportive, low-stimulation environment, is usually sufficient to allow metabolism and clearance of the intoxicating substance and recovery. Protection of the patient from self-harm is important, and restraints may be necessary to minimize the risk of falls and inadvertent discontinuation of intravenous and bladder catheters.

SEIZURES

The development of seizures with toxic encephalopathy is relatively common. A broad range of toxins may induce seizures, and toxin-related seizures may be difficult to control. A detailed discussion of the neuropharmacology of seizures in poisoned patients is beyond the scope of this chapter (see Chapter 20). Seizure control is a primary issue in the management of a poisoned child in the ICU, however, and is addressed here.

Seizures in the intoxicated patient may result from a direct reduction in seizure threshold by the intoxicating substance (e.g., theophylline). Seizures associated with toxic ingestions may be difficult to control and may be recurrent or result in status epilepticus. Status epilepticus, defined as a seizure lasting greater than 30 minutes, is associated with a severalfold increase in cerebral metabolic demand and may be associated with insufficient respiratory effort, resulting in decreased oxygenation and ventilation. This combination of increased oxygen requirement by the brain and diminished oxygen delivery is a risk factor for secondary injury resulting from cerebral ischemia. Aggressive management of seizures associated with poisoning is crucial to unimpaired recovery.

Management of seizures associated with intoxication requires prompt attention to the adequacy of airway patency, respiratory effort, and oxygenation. Prompt administration of oxygen at the onset of a seizure, maintenance of the patency of the airway, placing the child on his or her side to avoid upper airway obstruction, and, if the seizure is prolonged, endotracheal intubation to ensure airway patency are recommended. Assessment of electrolytes and glucose and correction of hypoglycemia and electrolyte disturbances should be performed promptly. Monitoring of oxygen saturation continuously during the seizure episode and monitoring of arterial blood gases to assess oxygenation and ventilation if the seizure is prolonged, with aggressive intervention in patients with marginal respiratory status, ensure adequacy of oxygen delivery.

Anticonvulsant management of toxin-induced seizures usually can be achieved with benzodiazepines. My preferred agent, based on its rapid penetration of the CNS and its relatively long half-life, is lorazepam. Administration of repeated incremental doses of lorazepam controls seizures associated with poisoning in most cases. If lorazepam is insufficient, addition of a second anticonvulsant is required. Phenytoin, which is usually the second-line drug of choice for status epilepticus, may be contraindicated in tricyclic antidepressant–induced seizures because of the potential for prodysrhythmic effects. Phenobarbital and intravenous valproic acid may be considered useful additional agents for control of seizures if benzodiazepines fail to control seizures adequately and for seizure prophylaxis if the seizure is prolonged or recurrent. Patients who fail to respond to multiple anticonvulsants may require initiation of general anesthesia, either with inhalational agents or with intravenous pentobarbital, to control seizures and reduce cerebral metabolic demands.

An additional consideration in a patient with uncontrollable seizures may be ingestion of hydrazines, such as the drug isoniazid. Seizures in these children are the result of depletion of pyridoxine (see Fig. 61-3) and are generally unresponsive to conventional anticonvulsants. The availability of mushrooms, use of isoniazid, or the presence of individuals with tuberculosis in the child's home may be implicated. These patients generally respond promptly to intravenous replacement of pyridoxine with cessation of seizures. Large doses of pyridoxine (70 mg/kg to a maximum empirical dose of 5 g) frequently are required to stop seizures, followed by repeat dosing if seizures recur. The clinical pharmacology of pyridoxine is discussed in detail in Chapter 147. After control of the seizure event in this circumstance, neuroimaging of the head should be considered to rule out the development of cerebral edema and intracranial hemorrhage or focal neurologic abnormalities not previously evident.

Renal Toxicity and Extracorporeal Removal of Toxins

Renal insufficiency or renal failure is an unusual complication of poisoning in children because children uncommonly encounter many of the drugs and chemicals known to cause renal damage. Table 10-13 lists toxins associated with renal compromise in pediatric patients. Renal compromise also may occur secondary to other organ system failure, particularly in patients experiencing shock. Electrolyte and pH

TABLE 10-13 Drugs and Toxins Associated with Acute Renal Insufficiency in Children	
Drugs	**Other Toxins**
Acyclovir	Aristolochic acid
Aminoglycosides	Diethylene glycol
Cyclosporine	Ethylene glycol
Cytolytic agents	Hemoglobin/myoglobin
Nonsteroidal antiinflammatory drugs	Mercuric salts

imbalance secondary to renal failure and fluid loss occurs more easily in infants and small children than in adults because of the limited capacity of the body to buffer acute changes. Interventional dialysis for correction of metabolic abnormalities may be necessary in children under circumstances that adults might tolerate without dialysis.

The use of extracorporeal methods for toxin removal is unusual in the PICU. The 1999 TESS database shows that of the 16,150 pediatric critical care patients, 74 received hemodialysis, 2 were hemoperfused, and 4 were treated with other methods of extracorporeal toxin removal.[5] TESS data indicate that hemodialysis and hemoperfusion are about five times more likely to be used in an adult poisoning patient admitted to critical care than in a pediatric poisoning patient admitted to critical care. This finding probably relates, at least in part, to the epidemiology of pediatric and adult poisoning. Many of the agents for which

Indications for Use of Extracorporeal Method in a Poisoned Pediatric Patient

Renal failure
Severe electrolyte imbalance
Fluid overload in the face of renal insufficiency
Removal of a dialyzable toxin present in sufficient quantity potentially to cause serious organ system damage or instability

extracorporeal removal may be appropriate are ingested in large quantities less commonly in children. Table 10-14 presents toxins that reportedly have been treated with an extracorporeal method in children and the method used.

All of the various methods of extracorporeal removal, including hemodialysis, hemoperfusion, peritoneal dialysis, plasmapheresis, exchange transfusion, and the various methods of continuous dialysis or filtration, can be and have been used in children.[74–77] It is presumed that the relative efficacies of these methods in pediatric patients are similar to those reported in adults, although there are few data comparing them in pediatric patients. Many technical problems, including line size and circuit volume, make the use of techniques requiring vascular access more difficult in newborns and infants.[74] For these reasons, peritoneal dialysis has frequently been used in these patients, although its effectiveness at removing toxins is undoubtedly less than that of hemodialysis or hemoperfusion. In general, when vascular venous access is needed, the preferred site is the superior vena cava accessed via either a subclavian or an internal jugular line. Alternatively, femoral lines can be used. In newborns, the

TABLE 10-14 Toxins Reported to Have Been Removed by an Extracorporeal Method in Children

DRUG	METHOD	REFERENCES
Acetaminophen	HP	90
Amanita toxins	HP	91,92
Barbiturates	HP/HD	93
Boric acid	HD	94
Bromate	HD, PD, HP	95
Caffeine	PD	96
Carbamazepine	HP, PP, HD	97–99
Chloramphenicol	HP	100
Cupric sulfate	HP/HF	101
2,4-Dichlorophenoxyacetic acid	PP	102
Diethylene glycol	HD	103
Digitalis/digoxin	PD	104
Diltiazem	HP	105
Diphenylhydantoin	HD	106
Ethylene glycol	HD	107,108
Flecainide	HP	109
Fluoride	HD	110
Formic acid	HP	111
Isoniazid	HD	112
Lithium	HD, PD	77,113
Methanol	HD	114
Methotrexate	HF, HD/HP	115,116
Oleander	HP	117
Organophosphates	HD	118
Paraquat	HP/HD	119
Pentamidine	HP	120
Phenobarbital	ET, HD	121,122
Salicylic acid	HD, HP, PD	77,123,124
Sodium chloride	PD	125
Thallium	HD	126
Theophylline	HP, HD, PP	127–129
Trichloroethylene	PP, HP	130
Valproic acid	HP/HD	131
Vancomycin	HF, HD	132,133
Vincristine	PP	134

ET, exchange transfusion; HD, hemodialysis; HF, hemofiltration; HP, hemoperfusion; PD, peritoneal dialysis; PP, plasmapheresis.

umbilical vein still may be accessible. Various pediatric dialyzers designed for smaller (<20 kg) patients are available. These machines are designed for lower pump speeds and lower priming volumes. Likewise, hemofiltration cartridges come in sizes appropriate for infants and children.

The various methods of hemodialysis, hemoperfusion, and ultrafiltration pose several unique problems in infants and small children.[74] Because of their relatively low vascular volume relative to the volume of the dialyzer circuit, these patients are more susceptible to hypotension and hypothermia. Temperature and blood pressure need to be monitored closely. Children also are more likely to develop the dysequilibrium syndrome for unknown reasons.[74] To minimize the risk of the dysequilibrium syndrome, it is recommended that the serum sodium level in the dialysis solution be kept slightly higher than the plasma sodium level. Mannitol, used prophylactically, also may be used. Patients should be monitored closely for symptoms suggesting this syndrome during and for some time after dialysis. See Chapter 7 for additional information on hemodialysis and hemoperfusion.

Peritoneal dialysis, although less effective than either hemodialysis or hemoperfusion, offers some technical advantages in newborns or infants. It is relatively easy and fast to initiate, and the relatively large peritoneal membrane surface area compared with that in adults results in a more rapid equilibrium with the infused solute, leading to greater efficiency.[74] Peritoneal dialysis catheters for acute dialysis can be inserted easily at the bedside under local anesthesia. Catheters usually are inserted into a prefilled peritoneal cavity using the Seldinger technique. Alternatively, a Tenckhoff catheter can be placed. Exchange volumes of 40 to 50 mL/kg with a cycle time of 30 to 60 minutes generally are appropriate. Automated cyclers designed for pediatric patients are available.

Pharmacologic Considerations in Children

In toxicology, as in pharmacology, infants and children are not small adults. Many developmental, biochemical, and physiologic differences contribute to differences in the way that children may respond to toxic exposures.[78]

The biochemical and anatomic development of organ systems contributes to a significant age dependence in the metabolism of some drugs and chemicals. The activities of several liver enzyme systems involved in drug oxidation and conjugation are restricted severely at birth.[79] The activities of these enzyme systems mature during the first year of life at varying rates. Likewise, renal function is immature at birth but matures during the first year of life. Body composition differs significantly in newborns and young infants from that in adults.[79] Organs such as the liver and brain are significantly larger relative to body mass than in older children or adults. Infants have a much lower percentage of body fat and a much higher percentage of body water. Particularly in neonates, serum protein binding of most drugs is diminished.[79] All of these factors affect the rates at which many drugs or toxins are absorbed, distributed, and cleared from the body. In general, rates of metabolism and clearance increase during the first decade of life.[80] They then either plateau into adulthood or begin a slow decline toward adult values. Although these generalities apply to most drugs and toxins, there are significant variations from these generalities for some drugs and toxins. Commensurate with these changes, normal drug dosing and expected response to toxic doses of drugs change with age. Table 10-15 presents medications and doses commonly used in the PICU to treat poisoned patients.

One excellent example of age-dependent toxicity is offered by chloramphenicol, which has accentuated toxicity in the newborn period due to the limited drug-metabolizing ability of a newborn. Another medication with diminished toxicity in young children is acetaminophen because of the relative activation of their sulfate and glutathione conjugating enzyme systems, leading to ready detoxification of the drug.[81-83] Excellent reviews of this subject have been published.[84,85]

In the area of environmental toxins, numerous additional differences between younger children and adults affect the relative toxicities of chemicals in these two age groups. Within a given environment, many factors may contribute to increased exposure in children. The consumption of food

TABLE 10-15 Drugs Useful in Poisoned Patients

DRUG	PEDIATRIC DOSE	ROUTE
Anticonvulsants		
Diazepam	0.1–0.5 mg/kg/dose; may repeat every 10–15 min	IV/IO
	0.5–0.7 mg/kg/dose	PR
Lorazepam	0.05–0.15 mg/kg/dose; may repeat every 10–15 min	IV/IO
Paraldehyde	0.3 mL/kg every 2–4 hr in equal amounts of oil	PR
Phenobarbital	Load with 20 mg/kg; maintenance 4–8 mg/kg/day	IV/IO
Phenytoin	Load with 20 mg/kg; maintenance 5–10 mg/kg/day	IV/IO
Cardiac Drugs		
Adenosine	50–100 μg/kg/dose rapid push (maximum dose 12 mg) or 5–20 μg/kg/min CI	IV/IO
Amiodarone	5 mg/kg over 20–60 min (may repeat if needed), then 5–10 mg/kg/day CI	IV
Amrinone	Load with 2–4 mg/kg over 20–60 min, then 5–20 μg/kg/min CI	IV
Atropine	0.02 mg/kg/dose (minimum 0.1 mg; maximum 2 mg)	IV/IO
	0.04 mg/kg	ETT
Calcium chloride	20–25 mg/kg/dose over 20–30 min via central venous catheter (maximum 1 g)	IV/IO
Calcium gluconate	100 mg/kg/dose (maximum 3 g)	IV/IO
Diazoxide	1–6 mg/kg (maximum 150 mg); repeat every 5–15 min × 3 as needed	IV
Dobutamine	5–20 μg/kg/min CI	IV
Dopamine	3–20 μg/kg/min CI	IV
Epinephrine (1:10,000)	0.01–0.1 mg/kg/dose	IV/IO
Epinephrine (1:1000)	0.1–6 μg/kg/min CI	IV/IO
	0.1 mg/kg/dose	ETT
Esmolol	Load with 100–500 μg/kg over 1 min, then 100–300 μg/kg/min CI	IV
Hydralazine	0.1–0.3 mg/kg (maximum 20 mg); repeat every 0.5–4 hr (maximum 3.5 mg/kg/day)	IV
Isoproterenol	0.1–2 μg/kg/min CI	IV
Labetalol	0.1–0.5 mg/kg over 2 min; repeat every 10 min or 1–3 mg/kg/hr CI	IV
Lidocaine	1 mg/kg/dose or 10–50 μg/kg/min CI	IV/IO/ETT
Nitroglycerin	0.2–3 μg/kg/min CI	IV
Nitroprusside	0.5–10 μg/kg/min CI	IV
Norepinephrine	0.1–2 μg/kg/min CI	IV
Procainamide	Load with 15 mg/kg (maximum 300 mg) over 1 hr, then 1–4 mg/kg/hr CI (maximum daily dose 2 g)	IV
Diuretics		
Bumetanide	0.035–0.05 mg/kg/dose (maximum 2 mg) or 8–10 μg/kg/hr (maximum 10 mg/24 hr)	IV
Ethacrynic acid	1 mg/kg/dose	IV
Furosemide	0.5–2 mg/kg/dose (maximum 20 mg) or 0.05–0.1 mg/kg/hr	IV
Mannitol	0.25–1 g/kg/dose	IV
Metolazone	0.2–0.4 mg/kg every 12–24 hr	PO
Respiratory Drugs		
Albuterol (nebulization)	0.1–0.15 mg/kg/dose (maximum 10 mg) or 0.2–0.5 mg/kg/hr continuous nebulization	Inhalation
Aminophylline	Load with 6 mg/kg over 20 min, then 0.7 mg/kg/hr (6 mo–1 yr) or 1 mg/kg/hr (1–9 yr) or 0.8 mg/kg/hr (>9 yr)	IV
Atracurium	0.5–1 mg/kg/dose, then 1 mg/kg/hr CI	IV
Doxacurium	0.05–0.1 mg/kg/dose, then 0.1 mg/kg/hr CI	IV
Ipratropium	250 μg/dose every 1–6 hr	Inhalation
Succinylcholine	1–2 mg/kg/dose with pretreatment with atropine	IV/IO
Terbutaline	Load with 10 μg/kg over 3–10 min, then 0.5–10 μg/kg/min CI	IV
Vecuronium	0.1 mg/kg/dose, then 0.1 mg/kg/hr CI	IV
Sedation/Analgesics		
Chloral hydrate	25–100 mg/kg/dose	PR/PO
Fentanyl	1–5 μg/kg/dose, then 1–10 μg/kg/hr CI	IV
Midazolam	0.05–0.2 mg/kg/dose, then 0.05–0.2 mg/kg/hr CI	IV
Morphine	0.05–0.15 mg/kg/dose, then 0.1–0.15 mg/kg/hr CI	IV

CI, continuous infusion; ETT, via endotracheal tube; IO, intraosseous; IV, intravenous; PO, oral; PR, per rectum.

and water is greater on a per-kilogram basis in children than in adults.[86] Respiratory exposure (liters of air breathed per kilogram per day) and soil consumption also are greater in children than in adults.[86] Being shorter, children tend to inhale higher concentrations of vapors, fumes, and dusts because most of these are heavier than air and occur at higher concentrations closer to the ground. Children also have a larger relative surface area of skin, leading to an increased risk of dermal absorption.[87] All of these factors may lead to the delivery of a higher relative dose of an environmental toxin to a child than to an adult in a given environment.

There are few objective data in humans about the age dependence of receptor numbers, binding, and response. Limited human data and animal data indicate that the development of receptors and receptor response is likely an age-dependent process. It also is clear that the patterns of response to at least some toxins may be either qualitatively or quantitatively different in children from those in adults.[85] There is currently insufficient knowledge in this area, however, to be able to make useful predictive statements.

Numerous other age-dependent changes occurring during childhood are implicated in altered response to toxins. It is well known that young children are more susceptible to toxins producing metabolic acidosis, such as salicylate, because of the limited ability of their tissues to buffer an acid load.[88] Children also are more susceptible than adults to carbon monoxide[89]; this may be due to the altered oxygen dissociation curve in children, which leads to increased binding of carbon monoxide to hemoglobin.

REFERENCES

1. Zimmerman JJ: The pediatric critical care patient. In Fuhrman BP, Zimmerman JJ (eds): Pediatric Critical Care, 2nd ed. St. Louis, Mosby, 1998.
2. Rodriguez JC, Sattin RW: Epidemiology of childhood poisonings leading to hospitalization in the United States, 1979–1983. Am J Prev Med 3:164–170, 1987.
3. Litovitz TL, Klein-Schwartz W, White S, et al: 1999 Annual report of the American Association of Poison Control Centers Toxic Exposure Surveillance System. Am J Emerg Med 18:517–574, 2000.
4. Fazen LE III, Lovejoy FH, Crone RK: Acute poisoning in a children's hospital: A 2-year experience. Pediatrics 77:144–151, 1986.
5. Litovitz TL: Data from the American Association of Poison Control Centers 1999 TESS database. American Association of Poison Control Centers (personal communication).
6. Souid AK, Keith DV, Cunningham AS: Munchausen syndrome by proxy. Clin Pediatr 37:497–503, 1998.
7. Meadow R: Munchausen syndrome by proxy: The hinterland of child abuse. Lancet 2:343–345, 1977.
8. Rand DC, Feldman MD: Misdiagnosis of Munchausen syndrome by proxy: A literature review and four new cases. Harvard Rev Psychiatry 7:94–101, 1999.
9. Dine MS, McGovern ME: Intentional poisoning of children—an overlooked category of child abuse: Report of seven cases and review of the literature. Pediatrics 70:32–35, 1982.
10. McClure RJ, Davis PM, Meadow SR, et al: Epidemiology of Munchausen syndrome by proxy, non-accidental poisoning and non-accidental suffocation. Arch Dis Child 75:57–61, 1996.
11. Bools C, Neale B, Meadow R: Munchausen syndrome by proxy: A study of psychopathology. Child Abuse Negl 18:773–788, 1994.
12. Rosenberg D: Web of deceit: A literature review of Munchausen syndrome by proxy. Child Abuse Negl 11:457–563, 1987.
13. Jick H: Adverse drug reactions: The magnitude of the problem. J Allergy Clin Immunol 74:555–557, 1984.
14. Zimmerman E: Summary statement by the American Academy of Pediatrics. Presented at the Agency for Health Care Research and Quality and Center for Child Health Research Expert Meeting on Information Technology in Children's Health Care, Bethesda, MD, September 21–22, 2000.
15. Kohn LT, Conigan JM, Donaldson MS (eds): To Err Is Human: Building a Safer Health System. Washington, DC, National Academy Press, 2000.
16. Krushal R, Bates DW: How can information technology improve patient safety and reduce medication errors in children's health care? Presented at the Agency for Health Care Research and Quality and Center for Child Health Research Expert Meeting on Information Technology in Children's Health Care, Bethesda, MD, September 21–22, 2000.
17. Bates DW, Cullen D, Laird M, et al: Incidence of adverse drug events and potential adverse drug events: Implications for prevention. JAMA 271:29–34, 1995.
18. Foli HL, Pode RL, Benetz WE, et al: Medication error prevention by clinical pharmacists in two children's hospitals. Pediatrics 79:718–722, 1987.
19. Raju TMK, Kecskes S, Thornton JP, et al: Medication errors in neonatal and pediatric intensive care units. Lancet 2:374–376, 1989.
20. Koren G, Haslam RH: Pediatric medication errors: Predicting and preventing tenfold disasters. J Clin Pharmacol 34:1043–1045, 1994.
21. Perlstein PH, Callison C, White M, et al: Errors in drug computations during newborn intensive care. Am J Dis Child 133:375–379, 1979.
22. Lesar TS: Errors in the use of medication dosage equations. Arch Pediatr Adolesc Med 152:340–344, 1998.
23. Jonville A-PE, Autret E, Bavoux F, et al: Characteristics of medication errors in pediatrics. Ann Pharmacother 25:1113–1118, 1991.
24. Wagner CL, Katikaneni LD, Cox TH, et al: The impact of prenatal drug exposure on the neonate. Obstet Gynecol Clin North Am 25:169–194, 1998.
25. Ostrea EM, Brady M, Gause S, et al: Drug screening of newborns by meconium analysis: A large-scale, prospective, epidemiologic study. Pediatrics 89:107–113, 1992.
26. Banner W Jr: Concepts in toxicology review. Med Toxicol 1:225–235, 1986.
27. Banner W Jr, Timmons OD, Vernon DD: Advances in the critical care of poisoned paediatric patients. Drug Saf 10:83–92, 1994.
28. Lange RA, Cigarroa RG, Flores ED, et al: Potentiation of cocaine induced coronary vasoconstriction by beta-adrenergic blockade. Ann Intern Med 112:897–903, 1990.
29. Lange RA, Cigarroa RG, Yancy CW, et al: Cocaine induced coronary artery vasoconstriction. N Engl J Med 321:1557–1562, 1989.
30. Rokicki W: Cardiac arrhythmia in a child after the usual dose of chloral hydrate. Pediatr Cardiol 17:419–420, 1996.
31. Zahedi A, Grant MH, Wong DT: Successful treatment of chloral hydrate cardiac toxicity with propranolol. Am J Emerg Med 17:490–491,1999.
32. June RA, Nasr I: Torsades de pointes with terfenadine ingestion. Am J Emerg Med 15:542–543, 1997.
33. Pohjola-Sintonen S, Viitasalo M, Toivonen L, et al: Itraconazole prevents terfenadine metabolism and increases risk of torsades de pointes ventricular tachycardia. Eur J Clin Pharmacol 45:191–193, 1993.
34. Rao KA, Adlakha A, Verma-Ansil B, et al: Torsades de pointes ventricular tachycardia associated with overdose of astemizole. Mayo Clin Proc 69:589–593, 1994.
35. Otsuka M, Kanamori H, Sasaki S, et al: Torsades de pointes complicating pentamidine therapy of Pneumocystis carinii pneumonia in acute myelogenous leukemia. Intern Med 36:705–708, 1997.
36. McCabe JL, Cobaugh DJ, Menegazzi JJ, Fata J: Experimental tricyclic antidepressant toxicity: A randomized, controlled comparison of hypertonic saline solution, sodium bicarbonate, and hyperventilation. Ann Emerg Med 32(3 Pt 1):329–333, 1998.
37. Liebelt EL: Targeted management strategies for cardiovascular toxicity from tricyclic antidepressant overdose: the pivotal role for alkalinization and sodium loading. Pediatr Emerg Care 14:293–298, 1998.
38. Hoffman JR, Votey SR, Bayer M, et al: Effect of hypertonic sodium bicarbonate in the treatment of moderate-to-severe cyclic antidepressant overdose. Am J Emerg Med 11:336–341, 1993.
39. Pentel P, Benowitz N: Efficacy and mechanism of action of sodium bicarbonate in the treatment of desipramine toxicity in rats. J Pharmacol Exp Ther 230:12–19, 1984.
40. Sasyniuk BI, Jhamandas V, Valois M: Experimental amitriptyline intoxication: Treatment of cardiac toxicity with sodium bicarbonate. Ann Emerg Med 15:1052–1059, 1986.
41. Bou-Abboud E, Nattel S: Relative role of alkalosis and sodium ions in reversal of class I antiarrhythmic drug induced sodium channel blockade by sodium bicarbonate. Circulation 94:1954–1961, 1996.
42. Kim SY, Benowitz N: Poisoning due to class IA antiarrhythmic drugs: Quinidine, procainamide and disopyramide. Drug Saf 5:393–420, 1990.
43. Clark RF, Vance MV: Massive diphenhydramine poisoning resulting in a wide-complex tachycardia: Successful treatment with sodium bicarbonate. Ann Emerg Med 21:318–321, 1992.
44. Farrell M, Heinrichs M, Tilelli JA: Response of life threatening dimenhydrinate intoxication to sodium bicarbonate administration. J Toxicol Clin Toxicol 29:527–535, 1991.

45. Banai S, Tzivoni D: Drug therapy for torsade de pointes. J Cardiovasc Electrophysiol 4:206–210, 1993.
46. Faber TS, Zehender M, Just H: Drug-induced torsade de pointes: Incidence, management, and prevention. Drug Saf 11:463–476, 1994.
47. Bell D, Thoele DG, Mander G, et al: Effective use of magnesium for acquired torsade de pointes in a 4-month-old infant. Pediatr Cardiol 16:79–81, 1995.
48. Goodwin D, Lally K, Null D: Extracorporeal membrane oxygenation support for cardiac dysfunction from tricyclic antidepressant overdose. Crit Care Med 21:625–627, 1993.
49. Tecklenburg FW, Thomas NJ, Webb SA, et al: Pediatric ECMO for severe quinidine cardiotoxicity. Pediatr Emerg Care 13:111–113, 1997.
50. McVey FK, Corke CF: Extracorporeal circulation in the management of massive propranolol overdose. Anaesthesia 46:744–746, 1991.
51. Rooney M, Massey KL, Jamail F, et al: Acebutolol overdose treated with hemodialysis and extracorporeal membrane oxygenation. J Clin Pharmacol 36:760–763, 1996.
52. Scalzo AJ, Weber TR, Jaeger RW, et al: Extracorporeal membrane oxygenation for hydrocarbon aspiration. Am J Dis Child 144:867–871, 1990.
53. Klaff LJ, Levin PJ, Potgieter PD, et al: Treatment of paraquat poisoning with the membrane oxygenator. S Afr Med J 51:203–205, 1977.
54. McCunn M, Reynolds HN, Cottingham CA, et al: Extracorporeal support in an adult with severe carbon monoxide poisoning and shock following smoke inhalation: A case report. Perfusion 15:169–173, 2000.
55. Pantalos GM, Minich LL, Tani LY, et al: Estimation of timing errors for the intraaortic balloon pump use in pediatric patients. ASAIO 45:166–171, 1999.
56. Minich LL, Tani LY, McGough EC, et al: A novel approach to pediatric intraaortic balloon pump timing using M-mode echocardiography. Am J Cardiol 80:367–369, 1997.
57. Sakurai H, Maeda M, Sai N, et al: Aortic dissection in an infant caused by intraaortic balloon pumping. Pediatr Cardiol 20:373–374, 1999.
58. Gol MK, Bayazit M, Emir M, et al: Vascular complications related to percutaneous insertion of intraaortic balloon pumps. Am Surg 58:232–238, 1992.
59. Lazar JM, Ziady GM, Dummer SJ, et al: Outcome and complications of prolonged intraaortic balloon counterpulsation in cardiac patients. Am J Cardiol 69:955–958, 1992.
60. Funk M, Gleason J, Foell D: Lower limb ischemia related to use of the intraaortic balloon pump. Heart Lung 18:542–552, 1989.
61. Royall JA: Pulmonary edema and ARDS. In Fuhrmann BP, Zimmerman JJ (eds): Pediatric Critical Care, 2nd ed. St. Louis, Mosby, 1998.
62. Shapiro BA, Peruzzi WT: Changing practices in ventilator management: A review of the literature and suggested clinical correlations. Surgery 117:121–133, 1995.
63. Hickling KG, Walsh J, Henderson S, et al: Low mortality rate in adult respiratory distress syndrome using low-volume, pressure-limited ventilation with permissive hypercapnia: A prospective study. Crit Care Med 22:1568–1578, 1994.
64. Brochard L, Roudot-Thoraval F, Roupie E, et al: Tidal volume reduction for prevention of ventilator-induced lung injury in acute respiratory distress syndrome. The Multicenter Trial Group on Tidal Volume Reduction in ARDS. Am J Respir Crit Care Med 158:1831–1838, 1998.
65. Cooper AB, Ferguson ND, Hanly PJ, et al: Long-term follow-up of survivors of acute lung injury: Lack of effect of a ventilation strategy to prevent barotraumas. Crit Care Med 27:2616–2621, 1999.
66. Fedora M, Klimovic M, Seda M, et al: Effect of early intervention of high-frequency oscillatory ventilation on the outcome in pediatric acute respiratory distress syndrome. Bratisl Lek Listy 101:8–13, 2000.
67. Fort P, Farmer C, Westerman J, et al: High-frequency oscillatory ventilation for adult respiratory distress syndrome—a pilot study. Crit Care Med 25:906–908, 1997.
68. Arnold JH, Hanson JH, Toro-Figuero LO, et al: Prospective, randomized comparison of high-frequency oscillatory ventilation and conventional mechanical ventilation in pediatric respiratory failure. Crit Care Med 22:1530–1539, 1994.
69. Bysani GK, Rucoba RJ, Noah ZL: Treatment of hydrocarbon pneumonitis: High frequency jet ventilation as an alternative to extracorporeal membrane oxygenation. Chest 106:300–303, 1994.
70. Moromisato DY, Anas NG, Goodman G: Mercury inhalation poisoning and acute lung injury in a child: Use of high-frequency oscillatory ventilation. Chest 105:613–615, 1994.

71. Willson DF, Zaritsky A, Bauman LA, et al: Instillation of calf lung surfactant extract (calfactant) is beneficial in pediatric acute hypoxemic respiratory failure. Members of the Mid-Atlantic Pediatric Critical Care Network. Crit Care Med 27:188–195, 1999.
72. Leach CL, Fuhrman BP, Morin FC, et al: Perfluorocarbon-associated gas exchange (partial liquid ventilation) in respiratory distress syndrome: A prospective, randomized, controlled study. Crit Care Med 21:1270–1278, 1993.
73. Sukumar M, Bommaraju M, Fisher JE, et al: High-frequency partial liquid ventilation in respiratory distress syndrome: Hemodynamics and gas exchange. J Appl Physiol 84:327–334, 1998.
74. Fine RN, Tejani A: Dialysis in infants and children. In Dangerdas JT, Ing TS (eds): Handbook of Dialysis, 2nd ed. Boston, Little, Brown, 1996.
75. Parekh RS, Bunchman TE: Dialysis support in the pediatric intensive care unit. Adv Ren Replace Ther 3:326–336, 1996.
76. Peterson RG, Peterson LN: Cleansing the blood: Hemodialysis, peritoneal dialysis, exchange transfusion, charcoal hemoperfusion, forced diuresis. Pediatr Clin North Am 33:675–689, 1986.
77. Pond SM: Extracorporeal techniques in the treatment of poisoned patients. Med J Aust 154:617–622, 1991.
78. Rane A: Drug disposition and action in infants and children. In Yaffe SJ, Aronda JV (eds): Therapeutic Principles in Practice. Philadelphia, WB Saunders, 1992.
79. Blumer J, Reed MD: Principles of neonatal pharmacology. In Yaffe SJ, Aronda JV (eds): Therapeutic Principles in Practice. Philadelphia, WB Saunders, 1992.
80. Marselli PL: Drug Distribution During Development. New York, Spectrum, 1979.
81. Burns LE, Hodgman JE, Cass A: Fatal circulatory collapse in infants receiving chloramphenicol. N Engl J Med 621:1318–1321, 1959.
82. Sutherland JM: Fatal cardiovascular collapse in infants receiving large amounts of chloramphenicol. AMA J Dis Child 97:761–767, 1959.
83. Penna A, Buchanan N: Paracetamol poisoning in children and hepatotoxicity. Br J Clin Pharmacol 32:143–149, 1991.
84. Graeter LJ, Mortensen ME: Kids are different: Developmental variability in toxicology. Toxicology 111:15–20, 1996.
85. Bates N, Edwards N, Roper J, et al (eds): Paediatric Toxicology. New York, Stockton Press, 1997.
86. United States Environmental Protection Agency: Guidelines for Exposure Assessment. Washington, D.C., U.S. Government Printing Office, 1997.
87. Faustman EM, Silbernagel SM, Fenske RA, et al: Mechanisms underlying children's susceptibilities to environmental toxicants. Environ Health Perspect 108(Suppl 1):13–21, 2000.
88. Gaudreault P, Temple AR, Lovejoy FH Jr: The relative severity of acute versus chronic salicylate poisoning in children. Pediatrics 70:566–569, 1982.
89. White SR: Pediatric carbon monoxide poisoning. In Penney D (ed): Carbon Monoxide Toxicity. Boca Raton, FL, CRC Press, 2000.
90. Higgins RM, Goldsmith DJ, MacDiarmid-Gordon A, et al: Treating paracetamol overdose by charcoal haemoperfusion and long-hours high-flux dialysis. QJM 89:297–306, 1996.
91. Aji DY, Caliskan S, Nayir A, et al: Haemoperfusion in *Amanita phalloides* poisoning. J Trop Pediatr 41:371–374, 1995.
92. Sabeel AI, Kurkus J, Lindholm T: Intensive hemodialysis and hemoperfusion treatment of *Amanita* mushroom poisoning. Mycopathologia 131:107–114, 1995.
93. De Broe ME, Verpooten GA, Christiaens MA, et al: Clinical experience with prolonged combined hemoperfusion-hemodialysis treatment of severe poisoning. Artif Organs 81:59–66, 1981.
94. Litovitz TL, Klein-Schwartz W, Oderda GM, et al: Clinical manifestations of toxicity in a series of 784 boric acid ingestions. Am J Emerg Med 6:209–213, 1998.
95. De Vriese A, Vanholder R, Lameire N: Severe acute renal failure due to bromate intoxication: Report of a case and discussion of management guidelines based on a review of the literature. Nephrol Dial Transplant 12:204–209, 1997.
96. Walsh I, Wasserman GS, Mestad P, et al: Near-fatal caffeine intoxication treated with peritoneal dialysis. Pediatr Emerg Care 3:244–249, 1987.
97. Deshpande G, Meert KL, Valentini RP: Repeat charcoal hemoperfusion treatments in life threatening carbamazepine overdose. Pediatr Nephrol 13:775–777, 1999.
98. Tibbals J: Acute toxic reaction to carbamazepine: Clinical effects and serum concentrations. J Pediatr 121:295–299, 1992.

99. Schuerer DJ, Brophy PD, Maxvold NJ, et al: High-efficiency dialysis for carbamazepine overdose. J Toxicol Clin Toxicol 38:321–323, 2000.

100. Audet PR, Cupit GC, Norman M, et al: Resin hemoperfusion for chloramphenicol intoxication. Int J Pediatr Nephrol 7:51–54, 1986.

101. Takeda T, Yukioka T, Shimazaki S: Cupric sulfate intoxication with rhabdomyolysis, treated with chelating agents and blood purification. Intern Med 39:253–255, 2000.

102. Lankosz-Lauterbach J, Kaczor Z, Kacinski M, et al: Severe polyneuropathy in a 3-year-old child after dichlorophenoxyacetic herbicide—chwastox intoxication, treated successfully with plasmapheresis (PF). Przegl Lek 54:750–752, 1997.

103. Brophy PD, Tenenbein M, Gardner J, et al: Childhood diethylene glycol poisoning treated with alcohol dehydrogenase inhibitor fomepizole and hemodialysis. Am J Kidney Dis 35:958–962, 2000.

104. Berkovitch M, Akilesh MR, Gerace R, et al: Acute digoxin overdose in a newborn with renal failure: Use of digoxin immune fab and peritoneal dialysis. Ther Drug Monit 16:531–533, 1994.

105. Williamson KM, Dunham GD: Plasma concentrations of diltiazem and desacetyldiltiazem in an overdose situation. Ann Pharmacother 30:608–611, 1996.

106. Phelps SJ, Baldree LA, Boucher BA, et al: Neuropsychiatric toxicity of phenytoin: Importance of monitoring phenytoin levels. Clin Pediatr (Phila) 32:107–110, 1993.

107. Baum CR, Langman CB, Oker EE, et al: Fomepizole treatment of ethylene glycol poisoning in an infant. Pediatrics 106:1489–1491, 2000.

108. Saladino R, Shannon M: Accidental and intentional poisonings with ethylene glycol in infancy: Diagnostic clues and management. Pediatr Emerg Care 7:92–96, 1991.

109. Gotz D, Pohle S, Barckow D: Primary and secondary detoxification in severe flecainide intoxication. Intensive Care Med 17:181–184, 1991.

110. Berman L, Taves D, Mitra S, et al: Inorganic fluoride poisoning: treatment by hemodialysis (Letter). N Engl J Med 289:922, 1973.

111. Chan TC, Williams SR, Clark RF: Formic acid skin burns resulting in systemic toxicity. Ann Emerg Med 26:383–386, 1995.

112. Temmerman W, Dhondt A, Vandewoude K: Acute isoniazid intoxication seizures, acidosis and coma. Acta Clin Belg 54:211–216, 1999.

113. Jaeger A, Sauder P, Kopferschmitt J, et al: When should dialysis be performed in lithium poisoning? A kinetic study in 14 cases of lithium poisoning. J Toxicol Clin Toxicol 31:429–447, 1993.

114. Prabhakaran V, Ettler H, Mills A: Methanol poisoning: Two cases with similar plasma methanol concentrations but different outcomes. Can Med Assoc J 148:981–984, 1993.

115. Jambou P, Levraut J, Favier C, et al: Removal of methotrexate by continuous venovenous hemodiafiltration. In Sieberth HG, Stummvoll HK, Kierdorf H (eds): Continuous Extracorporeal Treatment in Multiple Organ Dysfunction Syndrome. Contribution to Nephrology Series, Vol 116. Basel, Karger, 1995, pp 48–52.

116. Grimes DJ, Bowles MR, Buttsworth JA, et al: Survival after unexpected high serum methotrexate concentrations in a patient with osteogenic sarcoma. Drug Saf 5:447–454, 1990.

117. Durakovic Z, Durakovic A, Durakovic S: Oleander poisoning treated by resin haemoperfusion. J Indian Med Assoc 94:149–150, 1996.

118. Novikova OV, Druzhinin NV, Kustovskii AV, et al: Use of hemodialysis in intensive care of organophosphorus insecticide poisoning. Anesteziol Reanimatol 1:74–76, 1997.

119. Tsatsakis AM, Perakis K, Koumantakis E: Experience with acute paraquat poisoning in Crete. Vet Hum Toxicol 38:113–117, 1996.

120. Watts RG, Conte JE Jr, Zurlinden E, et al: Effect of charcoal hemoperfusion on clearance of pentamidine isethionate after accidental overdose. J Toxicol Clin Toxicol 35:89–92, 1997.

121. Sancak R, Kucukodduk S, Tasdemir HA, et al: Exchange transfusion treatment in a newborn with phenobarbital intoxication. Pediatr Emerg Care 15:268–270, 1999.

122. Soylemezoglu O, Bakkaloglu A, Yigit S, et al: Haemodialysis treatment in phenobarbital intoxication in infancy. Int Urol Nephrol 25:111–113, 1993.

123. Halle MA, Collipp PJ: Treatment of methyl salicylate poisoning by peritoneal dialysis. N Y State J Med 69:1788–1789, 1969.

124. Snodgrass W, Rumack BH, Peterson RG, et al: Salicylate toxicity following therapeutic doses in young children. Clin Toxicol 18:247–259, 1981.

125. el-Dahr S, Gomez RA, Campbell FG, et al: Rapid correction of acute salt poisoning by peritoneal dialysis. Pediatr Nephrol 1:602–604, 1987.

126. Niehues R, Horstkotte D, Klein RM, et al: Repeated ingestion with suicidal intent of potentially lethal amounts of thallium. Dtsch Med Wochenschr 120:403–408, 1995.

127. Tenenbein M: Inefficacy of gastric emptying procedures. J Emerg Med 3:133–136, 1985.

128. Shannon MW: Comparative efficacy of hemodialysis and hemoperfusion in severe theophylline intoxication. Acad Emerg Med 4:674–678, 1997.

129. Laussen P, Shann F, Butt W, et al: Use of plasmapheresis in acute theophylline toxicity. Crit Care Med 19:288–290, 1991.

130. Sasdelli M, Vagnoli E, Duranti E: Treatment of acute "trilline" poisoning by plasmapheresis and hemoperfusion (Letter). Int J Artif Organs 9:195–196, 1986.

131. Roodhooft AM, Van Dam K, Haentjens D, et al: Acute sodium valproate intoxication: Occurrence of renal failure and treatment with haemoperfusion-haemodialysis. Eur J Pediatr 149:363–364, 1990.

132. Goebel J, Ananth M, Lewy JE: Hemodiafiltration for vancomycin overdose in a neonate with end-stage renal failure. Pediatr Nephrol 13:423–425, 1999.

133. Bunchman TE, Valenti RP, Gardner J: Treatment of vancomycin overdose using high-efficiency dialysis membranes. Pediatr Nephrol 13:773–774, 1999.

134. Pierga J-Y, Beuzeboc P, Dorval T: Favourable outcome after plasmapheresis for vincristine overdose (Letter). Lancet 340:184, 1992.

CHAPTER 11

Poisoning in Pregnancy

Kirk L. Cumpston ◼ Timothy B. Erickson ◼ Jerrold B. Leikin

The management of poisoning in pregnancy is often controversial and complicated by the fact that there are concerns for not only maternal but also fetal toxicity. Many of these controversies derive from the relative lack of data on poisoned pregnant patients. Questions often arise regarding not only treatment of maternal and fetal poisoning but also fetal complications and alterations of poison management specific to antidote administration. As a generally accepted rule, the best approach to all poisoned pregnant patients is to treat the mother in the same way as if she were not pregnant. It is assumed that maternal benefits would enhance the likelihood of fetal well-being.

This chapter discusses poisoning in pregnancy in critically ill patients. Epidemiology, physiologic changes in pregnancy, gastrointestinal (GI) decontamination, general management, administration of antidotes, and abortifacients are discussed. Specific poisonings in pregnancy that are well described in the literature, some unique case reports, and the toxic effects of several obstetric medications are reviewed.

EPIDEMIOLOGY

Poisoning in pregnancy can occur in four ways. First, the mother is exposed accidentally to a toxin. Second, the mother is suicidal and wants to end her own life along with the fetus. Third, an abortifacient is used to terminate the pregnancy. Fourth, the mother is involved in recreational drug use.

The leading causes of injury among pregnant women are motor vehicle–related (33.6%), falls (26.4%), and poisoning (16%).[1] One study compared injuries indicated by ICD-9-CM (*International Classification of Diseases–Ninth Revision–Clinical Modification*) codes between pregnant women and nonpregnant women (ages 15 to 44) from 1979 through 1990 and found poisoning to be the leading cause of hospitalization of pregnant women.[2] During pregnancy, suicide attempts with overdose are more common than gunshot wounds, self-mutilation, and jumping.[3] Of women making suicide attempts, 7% are likely to be pregnant.[4] Mortality is only 1% to 5%, but there may be significant morbidity.[3] The frequency of successful suicide in pregnancy has decreased in the United States since abortion was legalized. The successful suicide rate may have decreased, but the link between an unwanted pregnancy and overdose without suicidal success has been confirmed. Houston and Jacobson[5] reported that termination of pregnancy and overdose occur within 2 years of each other 73% of the time, with the act of overdose occurring first. This study was criticized for not including women older than age 34, not screening for prior psychiatric illness in the women who terminated pregnancy, and not showing a cause-and-effect relationship between termination of pregnancy and overdose.[6] Nevertheless, the cost of an unsuccessful maternal overdose may lead to the fetus's ultimately paying the price.

Most pregnant women who self-poison do so in the first trimester. According to a population-based prospective study by Czeizel and coworkers,[7] 61% of suicide attempts occurred before completion of the first trimester. Many of these attempts (38%) were early in the first month, and most of these were in the third and fourth weeks. The main reported reasons for the suicide attempts were either unwanted pregnancies and related tension or crisis. Of the case study group, 22% had early fetal loss compared with pregnant women without overdose, matched by maternal and gestational age. Mortality was 0.36% in the study group compared with 0.0% in controls.[7]

Knowledge of the outcome of these pregnancies after overdose is important because many of these women intend to harm the fetus. Flint and colleagues[8] observed the results of pregnancy in 61 women who overdosed during pregnancy. In this group, there was double the rate of miscarriages but no increased risk in congenital abnormalities or premature deliveries. Most of these women ingested acetaminophen (paracetamol), salicylates, psychotropics, or phenobarbital.

TERATOLOGY

The U.S. Food and Drug Administration (FDA) has a coding system for risk factors of possible teratogenicity to the fetus (see Appendix A). The key differentiation among the categories rests on the reliability of documentation and the risk-to-benefit ratio. Pregnancy risk category X (Table 11-1) is particularly notable in that if any data exist that may implicate a drug as a teratogen and the risk-to-benefit ratio is clearly negative, the drug is considered to be contraindicated in pregnancy. The FDA categorization must be interpreted with caution, particularly in the case of category C. This category can mean either that the drug has been found to have abnormal effects on the fetus in animals but has not been studied in humans, or that studies in humans and animals are not available. This category means that there is

TABLE 11-1 Drugs Rated as Pregnancy Risk Factor X

Amyl nitrite	Methyltestosterone
Castor oil	Methysergide
Clomiphene	Mifepristone
Danazol	Misoprostol
Diethylstilbestrol	Oxymetholone
Ergotamine	Oxytocin
Estazolam	Podophyllum resin
Estrogens	Pravastatin
Conjugated	Prazepam
Esterified	Quazepam
Ethinyl estradiol	Quinine
Etretinate	Ribavirin
Finasteride	Simvastatin
Flurazepam	Stanozolol
Fluvastatin	Temazepam
Isoretinoin	Testosterone
Levonorgestrel	Thalidomide
Lorazepam	Thiethylperazine
Lovastatin	Triazolam
Megestrol acetate	

Adapted from Leikin JB, Paloucek FP (eds): Leikin and Paloucek's Poisoning and Toxicology Handbook, 2nd ed. Hudson, OH, Lexi-comp, 1998.

a paucity of data. FDA pregnancy risk categories should not be considered to represent the most up-to-date interpretation of scientific literature. These categories are assigned at the time a drug is approved by the FDA and rarely are updated afterward; this is particularly true for data supporting a drug's safety in pregnancy. Information about potential adverse effects of a drug on the fetus has a greater likelihood of causing a change in FDA risk categories, however.

The fear of teratogenicity related to an acute drug overdose seems to be unwarranted according to two studies by Czeizel and colleagues.[9,10] The first study evaluated 1399 cases over a 30-year period and found no increase in congenital abnormalities in women with a "semilethal" (defined as patients who ingested an overdose amount sufficient to cause unconsciousness for 1 day).[9] A later study found no difference in teratogenicity in infants exposed to a drug overdose by the mother at 3 to 8 weeks of gestation.[10] Although the data are limited, it seems that the fetus in the "vulnerable phase" of 18 to 60 days of gestation either dies from the poisoning or survives without an increased risk for congenital abnormalities. These studies are based on a limited number of exposures; the potential for teratogenicity still must be considered for specific substances.

When abusing recreational drugs, such as cocaine or alcohol, the pregnant woman may not be trying intentionally to harm herself or the fetus, but she still is putting her fetus at risk of intrauterine growth retardation, premature delivery, premature fetal demise, placental abruption, and fetal alcohol syndrome.[11] It also has been shown that women with a positive screen for substances of abuse are at increased risk for being physically abused.[12,13]

PHYSIOLOGY OF PREGNANCY

Maternal Physiologic Changes

The physiologic changes in pregnancy can result in maternal exposures to toxins that are different from those of nonpregnant women at the same dose (Table 11-2). GI absorption is changed significantly by pregnancy. The hormonal effects of pregnancy cause delayed gastric emptying, decreased GI motility, and prolonged transit time. These changes lead to delayed but more complete absorption. These physiologic changes theoretically may make attempts at gastric decontamination more efficacious in overdose during pregnancy. As noted in Chapter 5, however, most studies in nonpregnant patients have not shown that attempts at GI decontamination in poisoned patients significantly affect their clinical course or outcome.

Because minute ventilation and tidal volume increase and residual capacity decreases, respiratory absorption of a poison can be increased in pregnancy. Inhalational exposures, such as those to carbon monoxide (CO), may be more serious in pregnant women because pregnant women also have less respiratory reserve to compensate for any respiratory insult.

The potential for dermal exposure is enhanced during pregnancy for two reasons. First, there is the increase in body surface area. Second, increased peripheral blood flow to the skin enhances the possibility of drug absorption.

Toxicopharmacokinetics also changes during pregnancy. The volume of distribution of most substances increases because of the expanded plasma volume and body fat stores. The albumin level decreases and the cardiac output increases during pregnancy, allowing for more free drug to distribute to target organs, including the placenta.

Changes in serum pH at different times during pregnancy cause the ionization of some drugs, leading to changes in tissue penetration and elimination. Early in pregnancy, the fetal pH is elevated compared with the maternal pH. Weak acids, such as salicylates, phenobarbital, valproic acid (VPA), trimethadione, phenytoin, thalidomide, warfarin, and isotretinoin, pass through the placenta in an electrically neutral state, but in the relatively alkaline fetal fluids, they may become ion trapped.[14] Late in gestation, the fetus's blood becomes more acidic than the mother's, and weak bases likewise diffuse into and become trapped within the fetus.

Late in gestation, maternal free fatty acids increase, displacing protein-bound drugs, such as diazepam and VPA, from serum proteins.[14] This displacement results in potentially greater toxicity by reducing the natural "chelator" effect of these proteins. In contrast, the hyperdynamic state of the pregnant patient causes glomerular filtration rate increases, and more renally cleared substances potentially can be excreted in the urine.

Placental Factors

The placenta acts similar to an internal dialysis unit, which can increase or decrease the likelihood of fetal toxicity. It allows most drugs to pass by simple diffusion along the natural maternal-to-fetal concentration gradient. Substances weighing less than 1000 d tend to have the

TABLE 11-2 Physiologic Changes of Pregnancy

General Physiologic Changes
↑ Body mass 25% by term
↑ Body water 7–8 L
↑ Body fat 20%
↑ Temperature 0.5°C

Specific Systems
Cardiovascular
↑ Cardiac output begins by 6 wk
↑ Cardiac output 35% by 10 wk
↑ Cardiac output 48% by 25 wk
↑ Heart rate 20%
↑ Stroke volume 10–32%
↓ Peripheral vascular resistance
↑ Peripheral flow
↓ Oxygen extraction
↑ Oxygen consumption
↓ Blood pressure by second trimester
     (10–15 mm Hg diastolic, 5–10 mm Hg
     systolic)

Respiratory
↑ Arterial PO₂ 10 mm Hg
↓ Arterial PCO₂ 10 mm Hg
↑ Minute volume 40–50%
↑ Respiratory rate 0–15%
↑ Tidal volume 40%
Vital capacity baseline
↓ Functional residual
     capacity 20%
↓ Expiratory reserve volume 20%
↓ Residual volume 20%
↓ Airway resistance 36%

Gastrointestinal
↑ Nausea and vomiting
↓ Lower esophageal sphincter tone
↑ Gastroesophageal reflux disease
↓ Mucus secretion
↓ Gastric acidity and small-bowel motility
↑ Stomach emptying time 0–160%
↑ or ↓ Hepatic metabolism

↑ Alkaline phosphatase secondary to
     placental production
Gallbladder emptying delayed

Urogenital
↑ Weight of uterus 400% by 10 wk
↑ Weight of uterus 2000% by term

Renal
↓ Urine concentration
Ureteral dilation secondary to hormonal
     relaxation or mechanical compression
↑ Aldosterone
↑ Antidiuretic hormone
↑ Plasma volume 45–50% with 70% in volume of
     extracellular fluid
↑ Glomerular filtration rate
↓ Serum creatinine, blood urea nitrogen

Hematopoietic
↑ Blood volume 35–40%
↑ Plasma volume 50%
↑ Red blood cells 20%, volume 300–400 mL
↓ Hematocrit 15%
↑ Reticulocyte count (small increase)
↓ Serum iron
↑ White blood cells 66%
↓ Total serum proteins 18% in third trimester
↓ Serum albumin 15–30%
↑ α-Globulin 0–20%
↑ Fibrinogen 40–200%
↑ Phospholipids, cholesterol, and free fatty acids
↓ Leukocyte function in second trimester
↑ Coagulation factors
↓ Platelets (small decrease)

Endocrine
Hyperinsulinemia
Fasting hypoglycemia
Thyroid function baseline

Neurologic
↓ Plasma cholinesterase 20%

capacity for passive diffusion across the placental membrane.[15] Drugs with small molecular weight, lipid solubility, neutral charge, and low protein binding are more apt to pass through the placenta. A common exception to this rule is iron, which enters the placenta by receptor-mediated endocytosis.[16–18]

Another important exception to the aforementioned generalizations is VPA. This drug is ionized predominantly at the mother's physiologic pH, but the small amount that is nonpolar is able to diffuse across the placental membrane.[19] The ionized and the nonionized VPA tend to approach equilibrium in the maternal serum. The ionized fraction, which is made greater by placental removal of un-ionized VPA, drives the equilibrium toward the un-ionized form in maternal serum. The latter can diffuse across the placenta. This maternal equilibrium process and the placental passive diffusion of the nonionized VPA continue cycling, leading to enhanced

fetal levels of valproate. Similar mechanisms may occur in other acidic drugs.

Fetal Factors

The fetus has physiologic characteristics that can protect it from or make it more susceptible to the toxic effects of maternal poisoning. The fetal oxygen-hemoglobin dissociation curve lies to the left of the mother's.[20] This position allows the fetus to bind oxygen at a lower PO₂. The fetus typically survives at a PCO₂ 10 to 15 mm Hg greater than the adult PCO₂. The hyperbolic shape of the fetal oxyhemoglobin curve also can be a disadvantage because fetal tissues are less able to extract oxygen from the hemoglobin. Also, because the curve is steep, a shift to the right because of acidemia results in decreased binding of fetal hemoglobin to oxygen at lower PO₂.

The fetus also has a physiologic reflex response to hypoxia. This response consists of apnea, bradycardia, systolic hypertension, peripheral vasoconstriction, and lactate production. The vagally mediated response to hypoxia causes a direct negative inotropic response, which can be reversed with atropine. The peripheral vasoconstriction allows shunting of the blood to critical organs, such as the heart, brain, adrenals, and placenta, theoretically increasing toxin delivery to these tissues.

TREATMENT OF POISONINGS IN PREGNANCY

The same aggressive supportive care that one would render to a nonpregnant poisoned patient should be administered to a pregnant patient. In general, if a toxin is causing seizures or hemodynamic instability in the mother, it also is having negative effects on the fetus. The optimal approach is to treat the mother; this is especially true in the critically poisoned patient. A remarkable report described a 27-year-old woman, 15 weeks pregnant, iatrogenically poisoned with intravenous lidocaine by the administration of a 1000-mg bolus (instead of 100 mg) for the treatment of bigeminy. This patient developed multiple arrhythmias, including electromechanical dissociation, asystole, and ventricular tachycardia, and status epilepticus over 23 minutes. Fetal heart tones were not heard for 14 minutes during resuscitation. The mother and fetus eventually did well. The infant was born at 40 weeks' gestation without complication and showed no developmental delays at age 9 months.[20]

Aggressive supportive care involves attention to airway, breathing, circulation, and neurologic disability. Maintenance of a patent airway, 100% oxygen administration, and, if the patient is hypotensive, left lateral decubitus positioning along with two large-bore intravenous lines and aggressive fluid management to restore hemodynamic status are crucial first steps. Moving the patient to the left lateral decubitus position prevents the enlarged uterine fundus from compressing the inferior vena cava, which can decrease the central venous pressure 30% to 70%. Cardiac drugs and 300 J during unsynchronized cardioversion have not been found to be harmful to the fetus. Open-chest cardiac massage has been suggested to reduce the required dose of epinephrine, which can cause vasoconstriction of the uteroplacental arteries.[20,21] In contrast to most other instances of open-chest cardiac resuscitation, however, it is crucial not to cross-clamp the aorta because doing so would interrupt immediately uteroplacental blood flow.

If there is a change in mental status, dextrose, naloxone, and thiamine may diagnose and treat the related causes of central nervous system depression. The benefit of reversing a mother's respiratory depression and hypoxia from an opiate overdose far outweighs the risk of opiate withdrawal in the fetus. Fetal heart monitoring, which could be instituted during maternal stabilization, is an important factor if the fetus is of a gestational age at which it is potentially viable if delivered.[22] Emergent cesarean section may be necessary if there is fetal distress in the later stages of pregnancy.

Decontamination

There is no approach to GI decontamination that could be applied empirically to all patients who overdose. Each patient must be assessed individually as to whether a particular method is indicated or contraindicated (see Chapter 5). This approach applies to pregnant patients as well, with some additional considerations.

Syrup of ipecac is relatively contraindicated in pregnant patients because of increased abdominal and thoracic pressure with repeated emesis.[23–25] There also may be teratogenic effects with syrup of ipecac.[26] The usual generalized absolute contraindications remain, such as mental status change, seizure, caustic ingestion, vomiting on presentation, cardiovascular instability, and aspiration risk. Currently, syrup of ipecac is rarely used in the treatment of poisonings in any population.

There are case reports of gastric lavage in the pregnant patient. The indications and contraindications are the same as those for nonpregnant patients (see Chapter 5). Its use is advocated occasionally in patients who present within 1 hour of ingestion on theoretical grounds. Because GI motility is slowed during pregnancy, gastric lavage after 1 hour may be useful if the patient has a potentially life-threatening ingestion. There are no data, however, to support a lavage-related change in outcome in these patients.

Activated charcoal (AC) can be an effective decontamination procedure, as it is in nonpregnant patients. There have been no reports of fetal toxicity from AC. Similar to gastric lavage in pregnant patients, slowed gut motility may allow AC to be effective even if given more than 1 to 2 hours after ingestion. Aspiration and bowel obstruction are the primary risks to the mother.

Cathartics, such as magnesium citrate and sorbitol, have a limited role in GI decontamination and should be administered with caution due to the potential for harmful outcome. In most cases, one dose is safe, but with repetitive use, multiple doses can cause electrolyte abnormalities and possibly induce premature labor.[23,27] Cathartics do not add to the efficacy of AC. Many medical toxicologists prefer to administer AC as an aqueous suspension with no cathartics. This approach is not known to increase the likelihood of any charcoal-related adverse effects.

Whole-bowel irrigation (WBI) has been reported in pregnant patients.[28,29] An iron overdose is one example in which this therapy may be used. In a report of an 18-year-old woman, 38 weeks pregnant, who ingested 55 tablets of prenatal iron, gastric lavage was attempted successfully, and the abdominal radiograph revealed tablets in the stomach. WBI with polyethylene glycol was started at 2 L/hr and continued until the rectal effluent was clear. Deferoxamine therapy was also initiated. Fetal heart tones were in the range of 130 to 140 beats/min. The patient did well and had a normal delivery of a healthy infant in 5 weeks.[28] The indications and contraindications for WBI are the same for pregnant and nonpregnant patients (see Chapter 5).

Antidotes

There is sparse literature on the beneficial or harmful effects of antidotal therapy in pregnancy (Table 11-3). Only case reports or case series give some insight on maternal-fetal effects or efficacy. These reports reveal little about the effect on the fetus but provide some observations about the effect on the mother. It is unlikely that a single exposure to antidotal therapy would cause harm. There are well-documented cases of maternal and fetal mortality caused by withholding an antidote because of fear of inducing fetal teratogenicity.[30,31]

TABLE 11-3 Antidotes Used in Pregnancy

ANTIDOTE	PREGNANCY RISK CATEGORY*	COMMENTS
Acetylcysteine[50,157]	B	Acetylcysteine can cross the human placenta
Ethyl alcohol[157]	X	In chronic use, >2 g/kg/day in the first trimester 2- to 3-fold higher risk for congenital malformations (about 10%)
	C	In acute therapy of toxic alcohol ingestion: use only if potential benefit outweighs the risks; ethanol crosses the placenta readily and enters fetal circulation
Amyl nitrite[157]	X	
Antitoxin botulinum A, B, E[157]	C	Use only if potential benefit outweighs the risks. It is unknown if the antitoxin antibodies cross the placenta
Antivenin (*Crotalidae*) polyvalent[157]	C	Pregnancy is not a contraindication for antivenin therapy
Antivenin (*Micurus fulvius*) North American coral snake[157]	C	Use only if potential benefit outweighs the risks. It is unknown if the antitoxin antibodies cross the placenta
Antivenin (*Crotalidae*) polyvalent (ovine) Fab[157]	C	Pregnancy is not a contraindication for antivenin therapy
Atropine[157]	C	Crosses the placenta; trace amounts appear in breast milk
Bromocriptine[157]	C	Use only if potential benefit outweighs the risks
Calcium chloride[157]	C	Crosses the placenta; appears in breast milk
Calcium gluconate[157]	C	Crosses the placenta; appears in breast milk
Charcoal[157]	C	
Deferoxamine[157]	C	Do not withhold chelation therapy for iron overdose solely due to pregnancy; has caused fetal abnormalities in animals
Digoxin immune Fab[157]	C	No animal studies conducted
Dimercaprol[157]	C	
Calcium EDTA[157]	C	
Flumazenil[157]	C	
Folic acid[157]	A (C if dose exceeds RDA)	400 μg/day needed to prevent neural tube defects
Glucagon[157]	B	
Hydroxycobalamin[157]	C	
Ipecac[157]	C	
Leucovorin[157]	C	
Levocarnitine[157]	B	
Methylene blue[157]	C (D if injected intraamniotically)	
Naloxone[157]	B	
Octreotide[157]	B	
Hyperbaric oxygen[157]		Indicated for the treatment of pregnant patients when symptomatic or with a carboxyhemoglobin level >20%
Penicillamine[157]	D	Correlated with cutis laxa in neonates
Physostigmine[157]	C	
Phytonadione[157]	C (X if used in third trimester)	
Polyethylene glycol (high molecular weight)[157]	C	
Pralidoxime[157]	C	
Pyridoxine[157]	A (C if dose exceeds RDA)	
Sodium bicarbonate[157]	C	
Sodium nitrite[157]	?	
Sodium thiosulfate[157]	C	
Succimer[157]	C	

EDTA, ethylenediaminetetraacetic acid; RDA, recommended daily allowance.
*Pregnancy risk categories are explained in Appendix A.

Enhanced Elimination

Although the supporting literature is limited, enhanced elimination with multiple-dose activated charcoal (MDAC) should be as effective and safe as single-dose AC in pregnant patients. As with single-dose AC, there is always the potential for aspiration. The few indications for possible MDAC therapy are the same as those in nonpregnant patients (e.g., ingestion of a potentially highly toxic amount of theophylline, phenobarbital, carbamazepine, dapsone, or quinine). MDAC for these drugs is supported in the literature because of effective "gut dialysis" or enterohepatic circulation in nonpregnant patients.[32] MDAC therapy is reviewed in detail in Chapter 6.

There are few reports of hemodialysis in pregnancy.[33,34] Premature labor and fetal growth retardation in pregnant patients on long-term dialysis have been documented. These cases have been attributed to the patients' underlying chronic diseases, however.[35,36] In a study of 16 infants born to mothers on long-term hemodialysis with some residual renal function, it was found that none of the offspring had abnormalities, and all were delivered spontaneously at term.[37] The authors concluded that careful blood pressure control, maintenance of good nutrition, and limitation of predialysis blood urea nitrogen levels allow for successful deliveries. If dialysis is indicated in a nonpregnant patient, it is indicated in a pregnant patient as well.

SPECIFIC AGENTS

Abortifacients

An abortifacient is any agent that a pregnant woman may use in an attempt to terminate her pregnancy. Many different substances have been used historically, including lead and qui-

nine.[38,39] Currently, in addition to over-the-counter medicines such as acetaminophen, aspirin, and iron with perceived abortifacient effects, herbal preparations are being used. Different cultures have their own contributions to the list of herbal abortifacients. Some representatives are cottonroot bark from Mexico; pulsatilla from India; and rue, apiol, cohosh, sage, and pennyroyal oil from the United States (Table 11-4).[40,41] In the United States, these herbal preparations are protected from scrutiny by the Dietary Supplement Health and Education Act of 1994, which designates herbal products as food. This allows them to be regulated in a less stringent fashion by the FDA than most other pharmaceuticals.

In a prospective observational study of 43 women who ingested known or perceived abortifacients, ingestions were most common in the first trimester (79%). Acetaminophen was the most common drug ingested (30.2%), and

TABLE 11-4 Abortifacients

AGENT	CLASS/ACTIVE COMPOUND	TOXIDROME	TOXICITY	COMMENTS
Angelica root—*Angelica archangelica*	Essential oil	Hypotension/shock	>1 mL ingested	Activated charcoal*; supportive therapy
Black cohosh—*Cimicifuga racemosa*	Alkaloids including methylcytosine and acetin	Bradycardia, dizziness, nausea, vomiting, tremors, headache	Not documented	Activated charcoal*; supportive therapy
Blue cohosh—*Caulophyllum thalictroides*	Alkaloid methyl cystine	Similar to nicotine: nausea, vomiting, muscle paralysis, seizures, tachycardia, hypotension	Not documented. Roasting eliminates toxicity	Activated charcoal*; supportive therapy
Buckthorn bark—*Rhamnus cathartica, R. frangula, R. alnifolia*	Frangulin (anthroquinone)	Nausea, vomiting, abdominal cramping, diarrhea, potential renal toxin in large doses	1-g berries, mild toxicity in children; 20 berries or chewing of bark is necessary for severe symptoms	Activated charcoal*; supportive therapy
Diethylcarbamazine	Antihelminthic-antifilarial agent that kills the parasite in the adult stage	Anorexia, dizziness, abdominal cramping, nausea, vomiting	>1 g	Gastric lavage if >10 mg/kg <1 hr in a life-threatening ingestion, activated charcoal; betamethasone can be used for hypersensitivity reactions; supportive care, multiple-dose charcoal may be useful for enhanced elimination
Ergotamine	Alkaloid; α-blocker; directly stimulates vasculature to vasoconstrict; serotonin antagonist	Tachycardia, hypertension, vasospasm, headache, seizure, hypotension, bradycardia, shock, peripheral vascular effects, nausea, vomiting, diarrhea	>1 mg/kg dose toxic; serum levels >1.8 ng/mL are toxic	Activated charcoal*; warm extremities; vasodilators; intraarterial phentolamine for vasospasm, aspirin for antiplatelet effect; prostaglandins; heparin for hypercoagulable state; hyperbaric oxygen for limb ischemia; cyproheptadine to reverse vasoconstriction; supportive care
Mifepristone; approved in France as an abortifacient (1988)	Antiprogestin agent acts on deciduous progesterone receptors, causing release of prostaglandin in the endometrium, resulting in uterine bleeding, contraction, and cervical dilation	Syncope, headache, nausea, vomiting, uterine pain, bleeding, rupture	A 600-mg dose can cause abortion of fetus within 56 days of amenorrhea	Activated charcoal; transfusion and curettage may be required for uterine bleeding; supportive care

	CLASS/ACTIVE			
AGENT	**COMPOUND**	**TOXIDROME**	**TOXICITY**	**COMMENTS**
Mistletoe—*Phoradendron falvescens, P. macrophyllum rubrum, P. serotinum, P. tomentosum, Viscum album*	Unknown	Nausea, vomiting, diarrhea, abdominal pain, bradycardia, ataxia, hypotension, seizures, cardiovascular collapse	>2–3 berries, teas, and extracts are toxic	Gastric lavage may be of value in recent ingestions of >3 berries or 2 leaves; activated charcoal; supportive care
Poison hemlock—*Conium maculatum*	Similar to nicotine; stimulation of autonomic ganglion, then depression	Nausea, vomiting, ataxia, burning sensation in throat, tachycardia followed by bradycardia, seizures, paralysis of skeletal muscles and diaphragm, rhabdomyolysis, renal failure	Ingestion of any part of the plant	Activated charcoal*; supportive care
Sodium chloride 20% by transabdominal intraamniotic injection	Causes fluid shift from intracellular to extracellular space, causing destruction of cells	Disseminated intravascular coagulation, renal necrosis, uterine and cervical lesions, pulmonary embolism, pneumonia, hemorrhage	Labor starts in 12–24 hr after injection	Supportive care
Misoprostol	Prostaglandin E_1 analogue	Hypertension, tachycardia, abdominal cramps, rhabdomyolysis, fever, tremor	3 mg—moderate; 6 mg—death	Activated charcoal*; supportive therapy
Pennyroyal—*Mentha pulegium/Hedeoma pulegioides*	Essential oil, pugelone; 22–98% active compound	Confusion, delirium, seizures, hepatic necrosis, renal failure, disseminated intravascular coagulation	5 mL toxic; 10–15 mL lethal; 50–100 g leaves = 1 mg oil	Activated charcoal*; supportive therapy; *N*-acetylcysteine may decrease hepatic damage
Windflower—*Anemone pulsatilla*	Ranunculin, metabolized protoanemonin	Mucosal irritation/ulceration, dizziness, paralysis, abdominal pain, diarrhea, vomiting, hypersalivation, renal injury	20 mg/kg can cause CNS and cardiac effects	Activated charcoal*; supportive therapy
Quinine	Alkaloid from cinchona bark	Cardiovascular toxicity the same as quinidine, within 8–24 hr; tinnitus, deafness, visual field constriction, blindness, vomiting, abdominal pain	>2 g	Multidose activated charcoal*; sodium bicarbonate for QRS widening; lidocaine for arrhythmias; avoid class IA–IC antidysrhythmics
Rue—*Ruta graveolens*	Pilocarpine, 1.4% quinoline alkaloids, furocoumarins, psoralens	Miosis, cholinergic crisis, headache, nausea, rash, hypotension	Not documented	Activated charcoal*; supportive therapy
Savin/juniper—*Juniperus sabina*	Oil of sabinol and other volatile oils	Agitation; one large dose can cause catharsis, but repeated small doses can cause personality changes and renal damage	Not documented	Activated charcoal*; supportive therapy
Mandrake—*Podophyllum peltatum*	Green fruit, foliage, roots contain podophyllum. Ripe fruit is nontoxic	Diarrhea, headache, respiratory stimulation, lethargy, coma in 12–24 hr	Not documented	Activated charcoal*; supportive therapy
Tansy—*Tanacetum/Chrysanthemum vulgare*	Thujone, tanacetin, boneol, camphor	Catharsis, personality changes, renal damage	Not documented	*Activated charcoal; supportive therapy

TABLE 11-4 Abortifacients—cont'd

*Gastric lavage may be helpful if the patient presents with a life-threatening overdose within 1 hour of ingestion.
CNS, central nervous system.

polysubstances were common (35%).[42] Five patients picked specific substances because they knew they were abortifacients. Minor toxicity generally was observed (81%) except in a tricyclic antidepressant overdose and a bupropion overdose. Fetal demise was not reported in a limited 3-day follow-up.

It has been questioned why women are using medical abortifacients when abortion is legal and accessible in many countries. The answer is thought to be the general movement away from traditional health care and toward herbal remedies.[40] Because of barriers to health care and increasing cost, a progressively greater proportion of the population is willing to try "self-help" remedies first. The dangers to women are the toxic effects of the agent on themselves, teratogenic effects if the fetus is carried to term, and complications from delaying a physician-assisted abortion when the abortifacient fails.

All women who present with an overdose should have a pregnancy test. If the pregnancy test is positive, the possibility of abortifacient usage should be addressed. Women who present with vaginal bleeding and pregnancy also should be questioned as to whether the vaginal bleeding was self-induced by an abortifacient.

Acetaminophen

Pregnant patients have wide accessibility to acetaminophen because it is considered "safe" in pregnancy when taken in therapeutic doses. Acetaminophen is contained in many other over-the-counter preparations. As a result, the chance of acetaminophen toxicity is increased in a poly-drug overdose.

Human and animal studies have shown that acetaminophen crosses the placenta.[43-45] The fetus is protected from acetaminophen toxicity in the first trimester by the immature cytochrome P-450 system, which is unable to form the toxic metabolite N-acetyl-p-benzoquinoneimine. The fetus begins to have cytochrome P-450 activity at approximately 14 weeks of gestation.[46] The ability of 19-week and 22-week fetal liver tissue to form oxides verifies cytochrome P-450 activity at this age of development.[47]

As with nonpregnant patients, N-acetylcysteine (NAC) is the treatment for maternal acetaminophen overdose. Pregnancy outcome is affected by time from ingestion until NAC administration. Spontaneous abortion was increased in pregnancies in which NAC was delayed in treating acetaminophen overdose.[46] One study in sheep showed that little NAC was able to penetrate the placenta.[48] However, NAC later was shown to cross the placenta in rats.[49] This discrepancy may be explained by the fact that sheep have a five-layer placenta and rats have a three-layered placenta similar to humans.[50]

Fetal cord blood concentrations of NAC were measured in four newborns with mothers who overdosed on acetaminophen alone. The average NAC concentration was 9.4 μg/mL, within the therapeutic range in healthy volunteers.[50,51] The use of intravenous NAC may be advantageous because oral NAC may induce emesis, and there is a greater maternal first-pass effect, which reduces the amount received by the fetus.[25,48] There is no clinical evidence, however, that the route of NAC administration alters efficacy.

The outcomes of the mother and fetus are generally good after an acetaminophen overdose. Multiple case studies show that the outcomes of the fetus and mother are better in the first and second trimesters than in the third trimester.[44,52-59] Even a massive 64-g ingestion at 15 weeks of gestation resulted in a good outcome,[52] whereas in the third trimester fetal infratentorial hemorrhage, fetal demise, and maternal and fetal death have been documented.[54-56] Two large studies of women exposed to acetaminophen during all trimesters found no correlation between toxicity and malformations or miscarriages.[60-62] There seems to be no indication for a mother to terminate pregnancy if she overdosed on acetaminophen.

Although most acetaminophen ingestions result in recovery in the mother with a resultant normal delivery, heroic measures have been suggested in extreme cases of toxicity. Some authors advocate emergent delivery of the fetus in the third trimester if the mother has documented toxic levels of acetaminophen, but there is little to support this approach in the absence of hepatic failure.[63] Early vaginal or cesarean delivery may avoid potential complications if the mother becomes encephalopathic and coagulopathic. If there is fetal demise, emergent delivery also may be indicated if the fetus is retained and the mother has evidence of disseminated intravascular coagulation.[54] Exchange transfusion does not seem to be efficacious in the acetaminophen-poisoned neonate.[44]

Treatment of pregnant patients for acetaminophen toxicity should be the same as that for nonpregnant patients, with some differences as noted previously. See Chapter 55 for an in-depth discussion of acetaminophen toxicity.

Salicylates

Similar to acetaminophen, salicylates can be found in combination with other drugs in many preparations.[64-66] There is potential harm from salicylates taken therapeutically during pregnancy. Because of effects on neonatal coagulation and premature closure of the ductus arteriosus, salicylates are contraindicated in the third trimester of pregnancy.[67] Salicylates freely cross the placental membrane.[68-71]

There are some variations from adult pharmacokinetics in the way the fetus reacts to the burden of a maternal salicylate overdose. Aspirin is hydrolyzed rapidly to salicylate. A small amount is excreted in the urine unchanged, whereas the remainder is metabolized to salicyluric acid, salicyl phenolic glucuronide, salicyl acyl glucuronide, and gentisic acid (Fig. 11-1). The largest fraction is converted to salicyluric acid, and the other pathways follow Michaelis-Menten kinetics. At low doses, salicylates are metabolized rapidly by first-order kinetics, whereas in higher doses, metabolism slows after a switch to zero-order kinetics. The mother and the fetus metabolize salicylate at a decreased rate after overdose.

The metabolism of salicylate was studied in the newborn of a mother who ingested 6.5 g of aspirin daily for the entire pregnancy.[68] The neonate metabolized a relatively larger fraction to salicyluric and gentisic acids, with little glucuronidation. As a result, salicylate elimination by the infant was much slower than that in the adult. Although it was noted that the elimination was delayed in large overdoses, when the amount of ingestion is decreased to 7 mg/kg, the elimination increased to adult rates.

The fetus is especially vulnerable to salicylate toxicity in the third trimester of development. In an overdose, the measured serum fetal salicylate level is greater than the maternal concentration.[72] A greater proportion of salicylate enters the fetal brain than the maternal central nervous system. The fetus also has decreased capacity to buffer salicylate-induced metabolic acidosis. Lastly, metabolism and excretion of salicylate are decreased in the fetus, as discussed earlier.[63,73] Treatment of the mother should be initiated at lower serum salicylate concentrations than one would initiate for a nonpregnant patient. Urinary alkalinization therapy might be warranted when serum salicylate

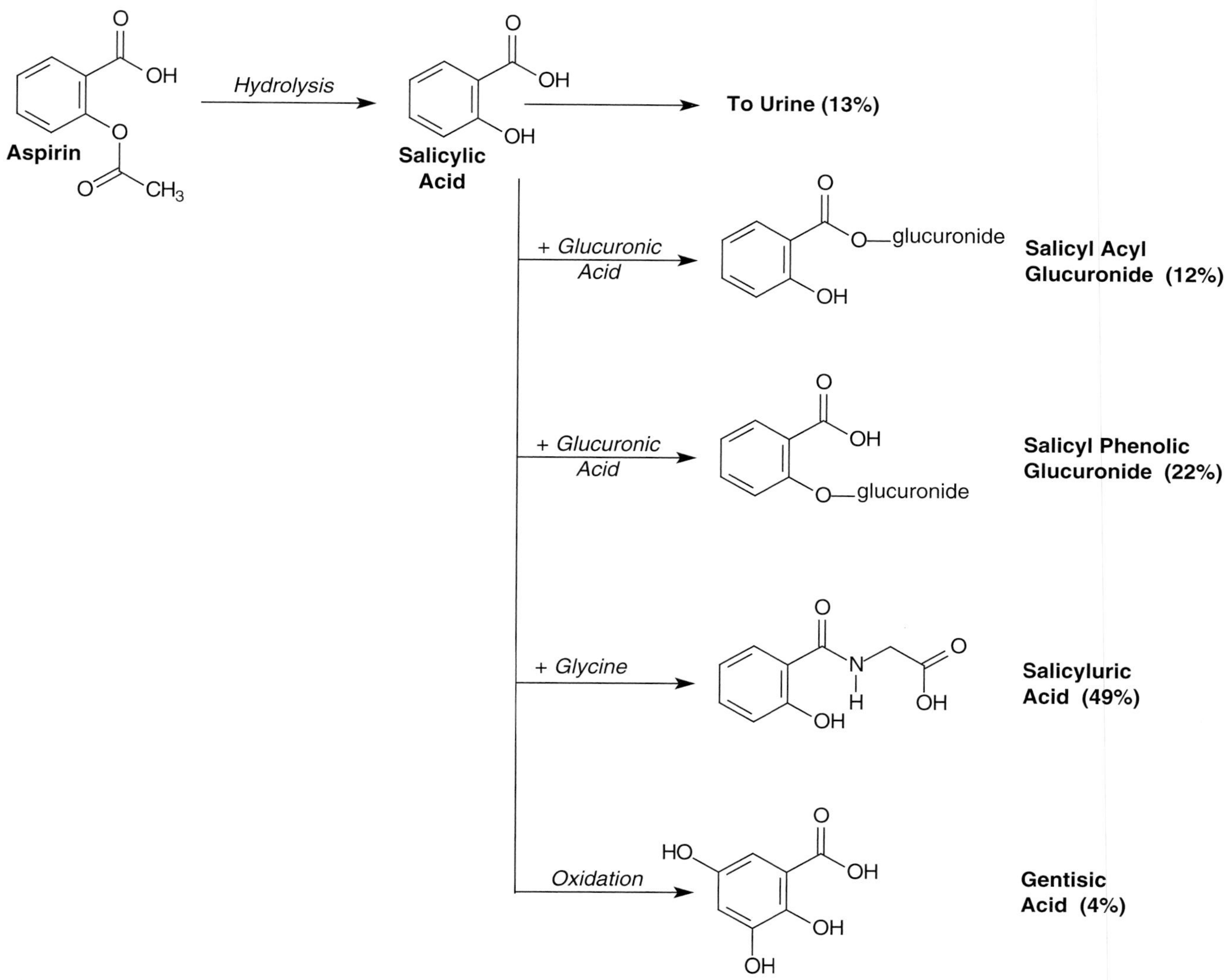

FIGURE 11-1

Disposition of the primary metabolite of aspirin, salicylic acid, at a single dose of 4 g (54 mg/kg body weight) in a healthy adult. The percentage values refer to the dose. Oxidation produces a mixture of *ortho-* and *para-* (relative to original OH group) isomers.

levels increase to greater than approximately 25 mg/dL (1.8 mmol/L).

Salicylate ingestion just before delivery can lead to maternal and fetal platelet dysfunction. After delivery, these neonates can have petechiae, purpura, cephalohematoma, GI bleeding, and intracranial bleeding.[74,75] Other effects on the fetus from maternal salicylate use are hyperbilirubinemia resulting from displacement from albumin, lower birth weight, and increased mortality.[76] Increased risk of congenital abnormalities and hypoglycemia are uncommon. It is believed that the antiprostaglandin effects of salicylates can cause complications in the mother as well.[77] The maternal effects of chronic salicylate ingestion include longer gestational periods, prolonged labor, increased risk of hemorrhage, and higher rates of cesarean.[72]

Treatment of pregnant patients with salicylate toxicity should be the same as that for nonpregnant patients, with the caveat discussed previously. In acute toxicity, GI decontamination should begin with AC, which is effective in binding salicylate. The total amount remains debatable, but at least a 1 g/kg dose generally is recommended. Multiple determinations of serum concentrations of salicylate are needed to monitor for continued absorption. Chapter 57 provides an in-depth discussion of the treatment of salicylate toxicity.

Because of the high toxicity of salicylate to the fetus, fetal monitoring may be needed to assist in the determination of the need for emergent delivery in a fetus of potentially viable gestational age. Emergent delivery is considered optimal treatment by some.[63] If the time of maternal overdose approximates the expected delivery date, the neonatologist should be alerted about the increased risk of platelet dysfunction.

Iron

Although accidental iron overdose has decreased substantially in the pediatric population because of changes in iron supplementation packaging, intentional overdose in the adult remains a serious ingestion. Iron is readily available to the pregnant woman because it is prescribed routinely during the prenatal period. As a result, it is a concern for potential overdose in pregnancy.

Iron toxicity assaults the human body through multiple mechanisms: peroxidation of biologic membranes, inhibition of oxidative phosphorylation, and formation of free hydrogen ions as a by-product of the change from the ferrous to the ferric state, causing metabolic acidosis.[78,79] Iron seems to have little direct toxicity to the fetus. It does not diffuse passively across biologic membranes but acts through a receptor-mediated endocytosis. A study of iron toxicity in pregnant sheep showed that elevated maternal serum iron concentrations are not reciprocated in the fetal circulation.[80] Human case reports also support this finding.[30,81] Iron does not affect the fetus directly but does so indirectly through poisoning of the mother. The placenta provides an effective barrier to iron, leaving the fetus reliant on the well-being of the mother for its survival.[82]

Two other components of general iron toxicity are present in pregnant patients. The peak serum iron concentration occurs in the range of 2 to 4 hours, and using the total iron-binding capacity to predict the severity of poisoning is inaccurate.[83] Treatment must focus on the sum of many different data points to determine what is most appropriate. Greater than 60 mg/kg ingestion, hypotension, mental status depression, metabolic acidosis, GI bleeding, shock, and serum iron level greater than 500 μg/dL (89 mM/L) all are signs of a severe iron poisoning and may be indications for deferoxamine administration.

GI decontamination after iron poisoning is controversial. Some authors support gastric lavage if a pregnant patient presents less than 1 hour after ingesting a potentially toxic dose. There are few data supporting the efficacy of this intervention, however, even when done early. Alternatively, WBI can be administered safely in the pregnant patient if iron-induced radiopacities are visualized on abdominal radiographs after recent ingestion. AC may be used if a coingestant is suspected, but it does not adsorb iron itself. Ultrasound may be the modality of choice for detecting pills in the stomach of a pregnant patient because it causes no ionizing radiation.[84] Pregnancy should not be a contraindication, however, to a flat plate of the abdomen in the case of an iron overdose. A kidney, ureter, and bladder film potentially could avoid toxicity from the mother and fetus by alerting the clinician to the diagnosis of iron toxicity, while guiding decontamination therapy with WBI. Adverse side effects from the amount of radiation are trivial compared with the potential threat of fetal toxicity after a substantial iron ingestion.

Deferoxamine is the antidote for iron poisoning. It chelates free iron and is excreted by the kidneys. The indications were listed previously, but some clinicians take a more conservative approach and treat a pregnant patient with a serum iron concentration greater than 350 μg/dL (62.5 mM/L).[82] The usual intravenous dose of 15 mg/kg/hr with the upper limit of 6 g in 24 hours is often quoted and still cited in the package insert.[85] The reason for this limit is to avoid hypotension and adult respiratory distress syndrome. A firm standard for the limits of deferoxamine therapy has yet to be shown in clinical trials.

Previously, deferoxamine was considered dangerous to give to the pregnant patient because of fears of teratogenicity. There have been reports of skeletal abnormalities in animals exposed to high doses of deferoxamine.[81,85] In contrast, reviews of multiple case studies have shown no

direct link between deferoxamine treatment in humans with iron toxicity and teratogenicity.[86–89] More reassurance of the safety of deferoxamine in pregnancy is provided by the fact that deferoxamine does not cross the placenta in the ovine model.[80] The clinical pharmacology of deferoxamine is discussed in detail in Chapters 65 and 143.

It follows that if iron itself has difficulty passing the placenta and if deferoxamine does not penetrate the placenta well, neither iron nor deferoxamine directly contributes to fetal injury. In this overdose, the mother has more potential morbidity than the fetus. The primary concern is the mother's clinical state. This constitutes a classic example of the dictum that the future of the mother and the fetus relies on optimal treatment of the mother. Iron toxicity is discussed in detail in Chapter 65.

Carbon Monoxide

CO is an endogenous by-product of heme degradation in humans (75% hemoglobin + 25% other blood pigments).[90] It is the number one cause of poisoning morbidity and mortality in the United States.[91] The clinical signs and symptoms of CO poisoning mimic the presentations of many illnesses, such as viral syndrome or gastroenteritis. The best way to diagnose CO poisoning is to consider it often in differential diagnoses. It cannot be overstated that one needs a high degree of suspicion to discover CO poisoning.

During a normal pregnancy, endogenous production of CO increases carboxyhemoglobin (COHb) 20% to 40% above normal levels.[90,92] Of this increase in maternal COHb, 30% to 40% is from an increase in maternal erythrocyte load. The fetus contributes 15% of the COHb increase. The instigator of this increase is progesterone, which induces the catabolism of hemoglobin by hepatic microsomal enzymes. The minute ventilation also increases during pregnancy. The baseline increased burden of CO and the increased minute ventilation make the pregnant woman more susceptible to CO poisoning.

The pathogenesis of CO toxicity is twofold: CO generates oxidative stress, and it binds to heme-containing proteins, such as hemoglobin, myoglobin, and cytochrome aa_3.[90] CO has an affinity for hemoglobin 250, 25, and 1 time greater than oxygen for hemoglobin, myoglobin, and cytochrome aa_3, respectively. This binding leads to systemic hypoxia and a shift of the oxygen-hemoglobin saturation curve to the left, with a transformation of the curve to a hyperbolic shape.[92] There may be direct toxicity to cardiac tissue as a result of the replacement of oxygen with CO in cardiac myocytes. Uncoupling of oxidative phosphorylation causes an increase in free hydrogen ions, leading to metabolic acidosis. Fetal hemoglobin complicates the situation because its oxygen binding curve is already hyperbola shaped and steep at low pressures of oxygen. Decreased ability of tissues to extract oxygen from the fetal hemoglobin and increased susceptibility to a precipitous drop in oxygen saturation result.

In acute maternal CO exposure, the CO slowly crosses the placenta by passive diffusion.[93] The fetal COHb concentration equals the maternal level in approximately 2 hours and eventually doubles the maternal percentage. In chronic maternal exposure, the COHb concentration increases rapidly in the first 2 to 3 hours and slows to a plateau in 7 to 8 hours. In humans, the fetal COHb concentration reaches maternal levels in 14 to 24 hours and a state of equilibrium in 36 to 48 hours, with percent fetal COHb 15% to 20% greater than the maternal percentage.[90,92,94] In acute exposure, death by anoxia occurs well before COHb concentrations increase.[95] In chronic CO exposure, the CO level in the fetus progressively increases, and the critical level seems to be 60%.[94] The CO elimination half-life is 2 hours in the mother and 7 hours in the fetus.

The sum of the effects from fetal hemoglobin, prolonged elimination, delayed peak in fetal COHb concentration, and elevated concentration of COHb in the fetus puts the fetus at greater risk for morbidity and mortality than the mother. There are multiple case reports of the mother's exhibiting minimal to no toxicity, with simultaneous significant adverse effects or death in the fetus.[94–97] Similar to the situation in nonpregnant patients, the CO level, expressed as percent COHb, does not correlate well with severity of toxicity. Fetal COHb levels are not realistically obtainable, making a history of exposure along with clinical signs and symptoms in the mother the only guide for therapy. Multiple sources point out that maternal symptoms of altered mental status, neurologic deficits, seizures, and coma are better predictors of fetal toxicity than are COHb concentrations.[93,94,98]

Teratogenicity varies with the timing of the exposure. Case reports suggest the possibility that exposure in the embryonic stage leads to neurologic, skeletal, and cleft palate deformities. During the fetal phase, anoxic encephalopathy and growth restriction may result. In the third trimester, premature delivery is reported and possibly decreased immunity, right-sided cardiomegaly, and delay in myelin formation.[90,99]

Primary treatment of CO toxicity involves removal of the mother from the source of exposure. The crucial therapeutic intervention is administration of 100% oxygen by facemask, possibly followed by hyperbaric oxygen (HBO) therapy.[100] HBO therapy has been advocated as the treatment of choice for pregnant patients exposed to CO.[90] HBO therapy can reduce the elimination half-life of CO from 4 to 6 hours to 20 minutes. Normobaric oxygen and HBO delivery increases dissolved oxygen, accelerates dissociation of CO from hemoglobin, and shifts the oxygen-hemoglobin curve back to the right. The efficacy of HBO therapy in the CO-poisoned pregnant patient has not been evaluated, however. Suggested indications for HBO therapy in the pregnant patient are a maternal COHb level greater than 20%, maternal neurologic signs or symptoms, and evidence of fetal compromise. If maternal or fetal signs of CO toxicity persist 12 hours after initial HBO therapy, a repeat session may be warranted.[90,101] It has been recommended that 100% oxygen continue five times longer in pregnant patients than standard treatment duration in nonpregnant patients to allow greater removal of CO from the fetal hemoglobin.[93,94,98] Some studies do not support HBO therapy as the ultimate therapy in any patient exposed to CO. In addition, there are specific areas of concern for the fetus treated with HBO. High PO_2 is known to be teratogenic and to cause retinopathy, cardiovascular defects, and premature closure of the ductus arteriosus.[101] An animal study showed similar adverse effects.[102] Several human case reports and studies strongly advocate HBO therapy in pregnant patients.[93,94,98,102–104] The safety of HBO therapy in pregnant patients was studied prospectively in 44 women, all of whom tolerated the procedure well, and no morbidity was seen in the mother or the fetus.[105]

In addition to the described standard therapy of CO poisoning, fetal heart monitoring is indicated in the late second and third trimesters. Poor variability and late decelerations are indications of fetal distress. One review article cautioned that immediate delivery of the fetus before HBO therapy carries a high risk of perinatal death. The authors concluded that HBO therapy should be considered before performing an emergency cesarean section.[90] This recommendation is based solely on theoretical considerations, however, and there are no data to support this from clinical trials.

Cocaine

Cocaine is a common drug of abuse in women of childbearing age.[106] One study found that 17% of urban women enrolled in prenatal care admitted to using cocaine once during their pregnancy.[107] Smoking crack cocaine is the most common route of exposure, and most pregnant women who use this substance do not receive any prenatal care.[108,109] Some women do not realize they are pregnant, whereas others surmise the pregnancy is lost and decide to continue using cocaine.[110] Still others falsely think that cocaine speeds labor. Cocaine can increase the length of labor, however, and exacerbates pain sensation.[111]

The manifestations of cocaine toxicity are the same as those in any nonpregnant patient. Hyperthermia, hypertension, tachycardia, agitation, seizures, stroke, myocardial infarction, intracerebral hemorrhage, and aortic dissection are possible results of cocaine use. The unique complications associated with cocaine use in pregnancy are abruptio placentae, decreased fetal growth, preterm labor, urinary congenital abnormalities, neurobehavioral abnormalities, and fetal demise.[112–114]

The pregnant patient theoretically is at enhanced susceptibility to cocaine poisoning due to reduced cholinesterase levels,[115] causing her to have decreased ability to metabolize cocaine. The fetus also has reduced levels of cholinesterase, but the placenta has sufficient activity to allow metabolism of some of the cocaine before it crosses the placenta and affects the fetus.[116] Cocaine administered to the pregnant ewe caused increased vascular resistance, decreased uterine flow, increased fetal heart rate and blood pressure, and lower fetal oxygen content.[117] Progesterone may increase cocaine's cardiovascular toxicity in the pregnant patient.[118]

Benzodiazepines are the medication of choice to treat the agitated, seizing, or tachycardic patient who is manifesting signs of cocaine toxicity. Diazepam and lorazepam are designated as class D in pregnancy (see Appendix A). Despite this warning, in the case of a pregnant woman with cocaine toxicity who presents with seizures, agitation, and hyperthermia, benzodiazepines are effective at diffusing cocaine toxicity and may decrease morbidity and mortality.[119] One source stated that no fetal malformations have been attributed to the administration of benzodiazepines during pregnancy.[66] There may be respiratory depression on delivery of a fetus from a mother treated with benzodiazepines, but the benefits outweigh the risks. If efforts to halt seizures are refractory to benzodiazepines, phenobarbital is recommended over phenytoin owing to the latter's known teratogenic effects on the fetus. Antihypertensives, such as nitroglycerin, may be used for hypertension, and rapid external cooling for hyperthermia is essential. If chest pain is present, investigation and treatment of possible myocardial ischemia are warranted. Cocaine toxicity is discussed in greater detail in Chapter 75.

Other Intoxications

There have been many reports of other poisonings and toxic syndromes in pregnancy. Some of these cases are summarized in Table 11-5.

Teratogens

For concerns about exposure to teratogens in pregnancy, it is useful to consult a medical toxicologist or a teratogen information service, if available.

TOXICITY OF PREGNANCY-RELATED MEDICATIONS

Magnesium Sulfate

Magnesium is an important cation used for many functions in the human body. It is involved in many physiologic reactions and regulation of ion channels. Most is stored in bone, leaving only 1% free in the serum. Magnesium sulfate is a commonly used anticonvulsant in pregnant patients with eclampsia or severe preeclampsia. In most cases, magnesium sulfate has been shown to be safe and effective.[132–134]

The true mechanism of magnesium's action is not documented clearly. It affects many different systems, which may contribute to the antiepileptic properties of this medication. Magnesium is a calcium antagonist and causes systemic and cerebral vasodilation. It increases cyclic guanosine monophosphate levels, which may act as a vasodilator by increasing nitric oxide levels and decreasing endothelin-1. Magnesium can slow conduction through the myocardium and decrease inotropy in high doses. It also can protect neuronal tissues from injury by blocking calcium channels directly in N-methyl-D-aspartate receptors. Finally, magnesium can decrease acetylcholine release from the motor end plate by causing hypocalcemia. The major importance of this effect is loss of diaphragm function.[132,134,135]

The toxicity of magnesium probably depends more on its rate of administration than the duration or the total dose, except in extreme circumstances. When magnesium administration exceeds its rate of renal clearance, its serum concentrations increase and may result in toxicity. There are many different regimens used in pregnancy, including regimens involving the intravenous and intramuscular routes with different target serum magnesium concentrations. At levels of 3.8 to 5 mmol/L, the patient may have flushing, headaches, blurred vision, nausea, nystagmus, lethargy, hypothermia, urinary retention, loss of the patellar reflex, or ileus. Respiratory muscle paralysis may occur at concentrations of 5 to 6.5 mmol/L. Cardiac conduction disturbances occur at magnesium serum concentrations of

7.5 mmol/L, and cardiac arrest may ensue at levels of approximately 12.5 mmol/L.[135]

Magnesium toxicity affects the mother and the fetus. For the mother, this toxicity typically occurs by an error in the rate of administration.[136] In a case report of a 23-year-old woman at 32 weeks' gestation, the patient had a cardiopulmonary arrest after 25 g had been administered instead of 1 g/min for a total dose of 4 g.[137] The mother also is in danger when magnesium therapy is combined with polarizing and nondepolarizing agents because of prolonged respiratory paralysis.[135] Hypotension can be a complication when magnesium is used with epidural blocks. Because of their calcium channel–blocking properties, magnesium combined with nifedipine can lead to profound hypotension.[135]

The effect of magnesium on the fetus is variable. The classic result in the neonate is hypotonicity, which may affect diaphragmatic function. Magnesium toxicity in the mother also increases the rate of perinatal mortality, even when there is little effect on the mother.[138] Magnesium therapy may be detrimental to the fetus in the scenario of maternal hemorrhage. A study of pregnant ewes at 123 days' gestation found increased mortality in the fetuses whose mothers were treated with magnesium therapy during maternal hemorrhage compared with saline therapy. The magnesium may have inhibited the natural response to hypoxemia in the fetus.[139] Another study in pregnant sheep found that magnesium did not impair cardiac output, however, or increase fetal death during maternal hemorrhage.[140]

The treatment of magnesium toxicity involves attention to airway, breathing, and cardiovascular status. Intubation and vasopressors with aggressive supportive care are the mainstays of treatment. Intravenous calcium may serve as an antidote to the effects of magnesium toxicity. Maintaining a urine output of at least 100 mL/4 hr also can ensure elimination of the magnesium.[135] Maternal hemodialysis may be indicated in cases of severe hypermagnesemia.

Methotrexate

Methotrexate (MTX) is used to abort ectopic pregnancies and to treat gestational trophoblastic disease. MTX destroys actively dividing cells because it acts as an analogue of folate (Fig. 11-2). MTX replaces folate at its binding site on dihydrofolate reductase and thymidylate synthetase (Fig. 11-3). The end result is inhibition of DNA synthesis, leading to cell death. MTX exhibits profound dose-dependent toxicity. It may cause nausea, vomiting, mucositis, pleuritis, pericarditis,[141,142] liver injury, renal failure, anemia, and leukopenia[143] at therapeutic doses.

MTX overdose has followed intravenous, oral, and intrathecal routes. Multiple doses of AC may be effective in lowering the serum MTX concentrations.[144] Urinary alkalinization may ion-trap MTX in the renal tubules and enhance its elimination. Leucovorin is the antidote of choice for MTX overdose. Its dosage depends on the serum MTX concentration. The standard dose is 10 mg/m² intravenously or orally every 6 hours. This antidote should not be delayed while waiting for an MTX level. Intrathecal MTX overdoses may be treated by cerebrospinal fluid drainage, exchange, or transfusion.[145] In a severe overdose,

TABLE 11-5 Poisonings in Pregnant Patients

TOXIN	CLINICAL COURSE/TREATMENT	OUTCOME	RECOMMENDATIONS
Methanol[120] Editorial: 1. Freely crosses the placenta 2. Alcohol dehydrogenase activity 10% in wk 10–16	See Chapter 86	?	1. Caution alcohol known teratogen 2. Blockade of alchohol dehydrogenase with ethanol and hemodialysis 3. Published before fomepizole 4. Emergent delivery if fetal distress
Ergotamine[121] Case report: 17-yr-old $G_1 P_0$, 35 wk gestation, ingested 20 mg of ergotamine 3 hr PTA and presented confused with normal vital signs	1. Gastric lavage 2. FHT 170 beats/min; NST 2 hr after arrival was reactive but unsatisfactory 3. Uterine contractions once/min	1. 8 hr later, fetal death and mother had myocardial ischemia 2. Fetal death presumed from uterine contractions and arterial spasm	1. Fetal death presumed from uterine contractions and arterial spasm 2. Early delivery because of deleterious fetal effects without morbidity to mother
Neuroleptic Malignant Syndrome[122] Case report: Mulitpara 25{6/7} weeks was in ICU for respiratory failure and pneumonia. She was treated with increasing doses of haloperidol for agitation	1. Haloperidol discontinued 2. Bromocriptine 2.5 mg tid 3. Dantrolene 40 mg pid 4. The above medications were discontinued in 12 days 5. Biweekly NST and weekly amniotic fluid tests	1. 4 wk after admission the patient was discharged 2. Healthy female infant born at 38{4/7} wk	1. Correct fluid, electrolytes, and fever 2. Bromocriptine is safe to use in pregnancy 3. Limited experience with dantrolene in the literature, but no neonatal effects noted in this case
Carbamazepine[123] Case report: Term breast-fed boy born to a mother on carbamazepine for epilepsy with asphyxia at birth and hepatic dysfunction in the first week of life. After recovery, at the 5th week of life, cholestatic hepatitis	1. Ruled out nontoxic etiologies 2. Liver biopsy showed bile duct lymphocytic infiltrates, hepatocellular cholestasis, and microvesicular fatty changes 3. Maternal carbamazepine level 12.4 mg/L 4. Fetal carbamazepine level 0.5 mg/L	No specific details of outcome	Consider drug-induced cholestatic hepatitis in a mother on carbamazepine during pregnancy and nursing
Snake Envenomation[124] Prospective observational study in Sri Lanka 1. 39 pregnant women 2. 62% snakes identified	26% received antivenom	1. 55.5% had adverse reactions (1 patient required epinephrine) 2. No maternal deaths 3. 29% abortions and 1 malformation (all abortions occurred <18 wk gestation)	1. Snake bite in first trimester with systemic envenomation results in a poor outcome (second trimester is better, and third trimester is the best outcome) 2. Did not find snake antivenom to be a risk factor for fetal death
Amanita phalloides[125] Case report: 22-yr-old, 11 wk gestation, ate mushrooms and 10 hr later gastrointestinal symptoms 36 hr AST/ALT = 663/607 U/L Peak AST/ALT = 4127/2903 U/L Factors V, II, VII, X decreased by 20%, 24%, 23%, 13%, respectively	1. Silybinin 20 mg/kg q 6 hr 2. Activated charcoal 3. NAC IV per protocol 4. Abdominal ultrasound 5. Fetal movements and cardiac activity monitored	1. Day 9 discharged 2. 38 wk delivered healthy infant 3. 2-year follow-up both patients doing well	1. During first trimester, invasive prenatal tests must be avoided 2. The therapy mentioned may be of benefit 3. Abortion is not recommended 4. Pregnancy is not a contraindication for transplant
Phenytoin[126] Case report: 18-yr-old, 8th mo of pregnancy, took 22 g of phenytoin and 2.4 g of phenobarbital. Presented alert with stable vital signs	1. Intubation 2. Gastric lavage 3. Hemodialysis 138 hr postingestion	Mother and infant did well	1. Hemodialysis did not seem to change clinical scenario 2. Questionable how much phenytoin or phenobarbital crosses the placenta
Vaginally Administered Cocaine[127] Case report: 21-yr-old $G_2 P_{1001}$, 16 wk gestation, presented	1. 0 pulse, 0 BP: intubation, CPR, dopamine	1. Mother died 8 mo after admission	1. Treatment of acidosis and seizures is a priority

Continued

TABLE 11-5 Poisonings in Pregnant Patients—cont'd

TOXIN	CLINICAL COURSE/TREATMENT	OUTCOME	RECOMMENDATIONS
unresponsive after boyfriend inserted 1.5 g of cocaine into vagina	2. Seizure: phenobarbital 3. Cocaine and benzylecgonine positive in urine and vaginal wash 4. Head CT: edema 5. Neonate delivered at 33 wk by cesarean section: betamethasone given, Apgar 1 and 4 at 1 and 5 min, respectively, hydrocephaly and no brainstem on brain CT	2. Fetus died on 10th day of life	2. Fatal dose in 70-kg person is 1.4 g intranasally, 750–800 mg SC, IV, or inhaled
Misoprostol[128] Case report: 19-yr-old $G_3 P_{1011}$, 31 wk gestation, ingested 30 tablets of misoprostol, 200 μg, and 4 tablets of trifluoperazine, 2 mg, 2 hr PTA	1. Gastric lavage and activated charcoal 2. 1 hr PTA no fetal movement by ultrasound 3. Uterine tetany, acidosis, hyperthermia, tachycardia, hypertension, hypoxemia treated with supportive care 4. Dead fetus delivered 2 hr postpresentation 5. CPK peaked at 5849 U/L 25 hr postingestion	1. Fetal death, autopsy remarkable for diffuse head and upper-body bruising 2. Maternal survival	1. Rapid onset of symptoms and resolution <12 hr consistent with misoprostol pharmacokinetics 2. 400 μg of misoprostol q 4 hr is the most administered to induce labor; ingestion of 6000 μg most likely led to fetal death. Uterine contractions and placental dysfunction probably led to death, but direct toxicity cannot be ruled out
Misoprostol[129] Case report: 25-yr-old $G_3 P_{0020}$, 36 wk gestation, intravaginally administered 6000 μg of misoprostol and ingested 600 μg, 3 hr PTA	1. Rapid chills, cramping, emesis, confusion, uterine contractions 2. 3.5 hr postingestion temperature 106°F, systolic BP 80 mm Hg 3. Ultrasound 3.5 hr postingestion, no fetal movement 4. Nonviable fetus delivered by cesarean section 5. Treatment of mother was supportive, including intubation with a paralytic to control agitation and hyperthermia	1. Fetal death, with normal anatomy and partial placental abruption 2. Maternal recovery in 16 hr	1. Activated charcoal if oral ingestion 2. Vaginal lavage with saline 3. Supportive care with benzodiazepines, fluids, cooling, paralysis
Diphenhydramine[130] Case report: 19-yr-old gravida 1, 26 wk gestation, ingested 35 25-mg diphenhydramine tablets, and acetaminophen	1. Hypertension, tachycardia treated supportively 2. 6-mg bolus followed by 3 mg/hr IV magnesium sulfate halted the uterine contractions	1. No comment on future delivery of the fetus, but no morbidity or mortality during monitoring in this case 2. Maternal recovery	1. Supportive care 2. IV tocolysis
Brodifacoum[131] Case report: 19-yr-old, 22 wk gestation, ingested a box of brodifacoum 8 days prior	1. Brodifacoum level of 220 ng/mL 2. PT >60 sec, INR >20 3. Transfusion of 2 U PRBCs, total of 70 mg phytonadione IV and 625 mg orally 4. FHT 150 beats/min	1. Discharged on hospital day 12 (21 days postingestion) 2. Fetus delivered term, no fetal hemorrhage, no abruption, no problems at 1-yr follow-up	1. No fetal hemorrhagic or teratogenic effects noted 2. Treatment supportive

AST/ALT, aspartate aminotransferase/alanine aminotransferase; BP, blood pressure; CPK, creatine phosphokinase; CPR, cardiopulmonary resuscitation; CT, computed tomography; FHT, fetal heart tones; ICU, intensive care unit; INR, international normalized ratio; IV, intravenous; NAC, N-acetylcysteine; NST, nonstress test; PRBCs, packed red blood cells; PT, prothrombin time; PTA, prior to arrival; SC, subcutaneous(ly).

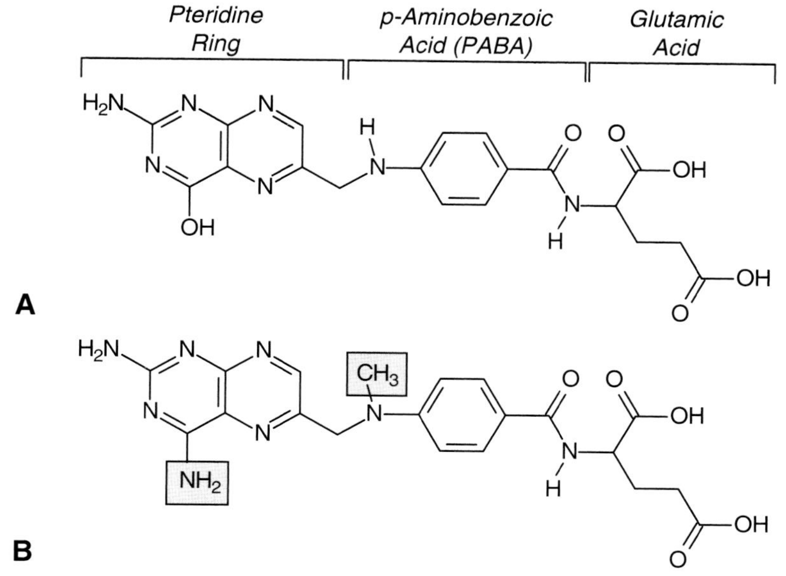

Pteridine Ring | p-Aminobenzoic Acid (PABA) | Glutamic Acid

A

FIGURE 11-2

Chemical structures of folic acid (**A**) and methotrexate (**B**). The positions at which methotrexate differs from folic acid are shaded.

B

granulocyte-macrophage colony-stimulating factor has been used to treat pancytopenia with apparent success.[146] MTX toxicity is described in detail in Chapter 60.

Vagotonics/Tocolytics

Vagotonics are medications used to increase contractions of the uterus. Methylergonovine in overdose can cause hypertension, chest pain, myocardial infarction, headache, vertigo, nausea, vomiting, and blurred vision. Fetal bradycardia may occur and may be treated with terbutaline.[146a] Standard treatment for possible myocardial infarction and stroke is the same as that for a nontoxic cause.

Oxytocin can cause fetal toxicity manifested by bradycardia, brain damage, neonatal jaundice, retinal hemorrhage, hypoxia, and death. In the mother, cardiac arrhythmias, hypertension, seizures, and the syndrome of inappropriate secretion of antidiuretic hormone (SIADH) have been

reported.[146a] Treatments for oxytocin toxicity include ritodrine to reverse oxytocin-induced labor and benzodiazepines for seizures. Because of the possibility of SIADH, serum sodium should be monitored.

Prostaglandins can cause tachycardia, hypertension, hyperthermia, chills, cramping, and possibly hypotension. In a case report, a 31-year-old woman of 35 weeks' gestation was administered 40 mg, instead of 1 to 5 mg, of prostaglandin $F_{2\alpha}$ inadvertently by intramyometrial injection to improve the contractility of the lower segment of the uterus after oxytocin failed to stop uterine bleeding. Three to four minutes after injection, she had no palpable blood pressure but was resuscitated successfully with intravenous fluids, red blood cells, and dopamine.[147]

Tocolytics are medications that are used to relax the uterus. These agents include magnesium, terbutaline, nifedipine, ritodrine, and indomethacin. Excluding magnesium, terbutaline is one of the more toxic agents in overdose. When comparing ritodrine, hexaprenaline, betamethasone, and terbutaline in mongrel dogs, terbutaline was found to be the most toxic.[148] Terbutaline overdose can lead to tremor, dizziness, palpitations, myocardial ischemia, and blood pressure changes.[149] Propranolol has been advocated as an antidote in a single case report but has not been studied formally.[150] Terbutaline can cross the placenta and cause injury to the fetus. Three out of the four newborns in a quadruplet pregnancy developed bradycardia, metabolic acidosis, poor tissue perfusion, and decreased urine output after 50 days of terbutaline therapy (total of 200 mg) to prevent labor.[151] It was suggested that the β_2-receptors were down-regulated by the prolonged therapy. All three neonates responded well to dobutamine administration.

Calcium channel antagonists are used widely for control of hypertension and tocolysis. The long-acting preparations seem to be safe and effective when used in these settings. When nifedipine has been administered with magnesium, however, severe hypotension has been described.[152] This association between magnesium and short-acting calcium channel blockers also has been studied in rhesus monkeys

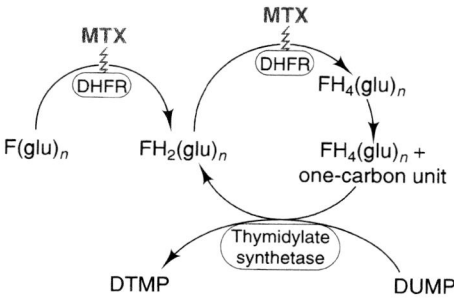

FIGURE 11-3

Simplified diagram of the action of methotrexate (MTX) on thymidylate synthesis. Tetrahydrofolate polyglutamate [$FH_4(glu)_n$] functions as a carrier of a one-carbon unit, providing the methyl group necessary for the conversion of 2′-deoxyuridylate (DUMP) to 2′-deoxythymidylate (DTMP) by thymidylate synthetase. This one-carbon transfer results in the oxidation of $FH_4(glu)_n$ to the dihydrofolate form $FH_2(glu)_n$. DHFR, dihydrofolate reductase. *(From Rang HP, Dale MM, Ritter JM, Gardner P: Pharmacology, 4th ed. New York, Churchill Livingstone, 2001, p 676.)*

and Sprague-Dawley rats. The results support the findings in the human case reports.[153,154] Treatment of calcium channel antagonist toxicity is described in detail in Chapter 35.

Ritodrine shares a similar toxicity with terbutaline because of its β_2-agonist properties, and ritodrine toxicity is treated in a similar fashion. Indomethacin may cause gastric irritation, ulcers, heartburn, and GI bleeding in the mother. In the fetus, it may cause premature closure of the ductus arteriosus, neonatal anuria, and bowel perforation.[155] There is a case report of maternal toxic epidermal necrosis after treatment with ritodrine, indomethacin, and betamethasone.[156] Treatment of the mother after indomethacin toxicity is supportive, whereas the treatment of the fetus is primarily preventive.

REFERENCES

1. Weiss HB: Pregnancy-associated injury hospitalizations in Pennsylvania, 1995. Ann Emerg Med 34:626–636, 1999.
2. Greenblatt JF, Dannenberg AL, Johnson CJ: Incidence of hospitalized injuries among pregnant women in Maryland, 1979–1990. Am J Prev Med 13:374–391, 1997.
3. Rayburn W, Aronow R, DeLancey B, et al: Drug overdose during pregnancy: An overview from a metropolitan poison control center. Obstet Gynecol 64:611–614, 1984.
4. Whitlock FA, Edwards JE: Pregnancy and attempted suicide. Compr Psychiatry 9:1–12, 1968.
5. Houston H, Jacobson L: Overdose and termination of pregnancy: An important association? Br J Gen Pract 46:737–738, 1996.
6. Gbolade BA: Overdose and termination of pregnancy. Br J Gen Pract 47:184, 1997.
7. Czeizel AE, Timar L, Susanszky E: Timing of suicide attempts by self-poisoning during pregnancy and pregnancy outcomes. Int J Gynecol Obstet 65:39–45, 1999.
8. Flint C, Larsen H, Gunnar LN, et al: Pregnancy outcome after suicide attempt by drug use: A Danish population-based study. Acta Obstet Gynecol Scand 81:516–522, 2002.
9. Czeizel A, Szentesi I, Molnar G: Lack of effect of self-poisoning on subsequent reproductive outcome. Mutat Res 127:175–182, 1984.
10. Czeizel AE, Tomcsik M, Timar L: Teratologic evaluation of 178 infants born to mothers who attempted suicide by drugs during pregnancy. Obstet Gynecol 90:195–201, 1997.
11. Thorp JM: Management of drug dependency, overdose, and withdrawal in the obstetric patient. Obstet Gynecol Clin North Am 22:131–142, 1995.
12. Dannenberg AL, Carter DM, Lawson HW, et al: Homicide and other injuries as causes of maternal death in New York City, 1987 through 1991. Am J Obstet Gynecol 172:1557–1564, 1995.
13. Reference omitted.
14. Fine JS: Reproductive and perinatal principles. In Goldfrank LR, Flomenbaum NE, Lewin NA, et al (eds): Goldfrank's Toxicologic Emergencies, 7th ed. New York, McGraw-Hill, 2002, pp 1606–1628.
15. Van Hoesen KB, Camporesi EM, Moon RE, et al: Should hyperbaric oxygen be used to treat the pregnant patient for acute carbon monoxide poisoning? A case report and literature review. JAMA 261:1039–1043, 1989.
16. Huebers HA, Clement AF: Transferrin: Physiologic behavior and clinical implications. J Am Soc Hematol 64:763–767, 1984.
17. Aisen P, Brown EB: The iron-binding function of transferrin in iron metabolism. Semin Hematol 14:31–52, 1977.
18. Curry SC, Bond GR, Raschke R, et al: An ovine model of maternal iron poisoning in pregnancy. Ann Emerg Med 19:632–638, 1990.
19. Nau H, Helge H, Luck W: Valproic acid in the perinatal period: Decreased maternal serum protein binding results in fetal accumulation and neonatal displacement of the drug and some metabolites. J Pediatr 104:627–634, 1984.
20. Selden BS, Burke TJ: Complete maternal and fetal recovery after prolonged cardiac arrest. Ann Emerg Med 17:346–349, 1988.
21. Krauer B, Krauer F, Hytten FE: Drug disposition and pharmacokinetics in the maternal-placental-fetal unit. Pharmacol Ther 10:301–328, 1980.
22. Gimovsky ML, Knee D: Fetal heart rate monitoring casebook. J Perinatol 15:246–248, 1995.
23. Jones JS, Dickson K, Carlson S: Unrecognized pregnancy in the overdosed or poisoned patient. Am J Emerg Med 15:538–541, 1997.
24. Graves HB, Smith EE, Braen CR, et al: Clinical policy for the initial approach to patients presenting with acute toxic ingestion or dermal or inhalation exposure. Ann Emerg Med 25:570–585, 1995.
25. Ford MD, Olshaker JS: Concepts and controversies in toxicology. Emerg Med Clin North Am 12:285–299, 1994.
26. Koren G: Maternal-Fetal Toxicology: A Clinician's Guide, 2nd ed. New York, Marcel Dekker, 1994.
27. D'Ascoli P, Gall SA: Common poisons. In Gleicher N (ed): Principles of Medical Therapy in Pregnancy. New York, Plenum Press, 1985.
28. Turk J, Aks SE, Ampuero F, et al: Successful therapy of iron intoxication in pregnancy with intravenous deferoxamine and whole bowel irrigation. Vet Hum Toxicol 35:441–444, 1993.
29. Van Ameyde KJ, Tennebein M: Whole bowel irrigation during pregnancy. Am J Obstet Gynecol 160:646–647, 1989.
30. Strom RL, Schiller P, Seeds AT, et al: Fatal iron poisoning in a pregnant female. Minn Med 59:483–489, 1976.
31. Manoguerra AS: Iron poisoning: Report of a fatal case in an adult. Am J Hosp Pharm 59:1088–1090, 1976.
32. Position statement and practice guidelines on the use of multi-dose activated charcoal in the treatment of acute poisoning. American Academy of Clinical Toxicology; European Association of Poisons Centres and Clinical Toxicologists. J Toxicol Clin Toxicol 37:731–751, 1999.
33. Vaziri DN, Kumar KP, Mirahmadi K, et al: Hemodialysis in treatment of acute chloral hydrate poisoning. South Med J 70:377–378, 1977.
34. Kurtz GG, Michael UF, Morosi HJ, et al: Hemodialysis during pregnancy. Arch Intern Med 118:30–32, 1966.
35. Trebbin WM: Hemodialysis in pregnancy. JAMA 241:1811–1812, 1979.
36. Hou S: Pregnancy in women requiring dialysis for renal failure. Am J Kidney Dis 9:368–373, 1987.
37. Report from the Registration Committee of the European Dialysis and Transplant Association: Successful pregnancies in women treated by dialysis and kidney transplantation. Br J Obstet Gynecol 87:839–845, 1980.
38. Hall A: The increasing use of lead as an abortifacient. BMJ 18:584–587, 1905.
39. Dannenberg AL, Dorfman SF, Johnson J: Use of quinine for self-induced abortion. South Med J 76:846–849, 1983.
40. Gold J: Herbal abortifacients. JAMA 243:1365–1366, 1980.
41. Netland KE, Martinez J: Abortifacients: Toxidromes, ancient to modern—a case series and review of the literature. Acad Emerg Med 7:824–829, 2000.
42. Perrone J, Hoffman RS: Toxic ingestions in pregnancy: Abortifacient use in a case series of pregnant overdose patients. Acad Emerg Med 4:206–209, 1997.
43. Ley G, Garretson LK, Soda DM: Evidence of placental transfer of acetaminophen. Pediatrics 55:895, 1975.
44. Roberts I, Robinson MZ, Mughal JG, et al: Paracetamol metabolites in the neonate following maternal overdose. Br J Pharmacol 18:201–206, 1984.
45. Wang, LH, Rudolph AM, Benet LZ: Pharmacokinetic studies of the disposition of acetaminophen in the sheep maternal placental unit. J Pharmacol Exp Ther 238:198–205, 1986.
46. Riggs BS, Bronsteine AC, Kulig KW, et al: Acute acetaminophen overdose during pregnancy. Obstet Gynecol 74:247–253, 1989.
47. Rollins DE, Glauman H, Moldeus P, Rane A: Acetaminophen: Potentially toxic metabolite formed by human fetal and adult liver microsomes and isolated fetal liver cells. Science 205:1414–1416, 1979.
48. Seldon BS, Curry SC, Clark RF, et al: Transplacental transport of N-acetylcysteine in an ovine model. Ann Emerg Med 20:1069–1072, 1991.
49. Ansai N, Kimura T, Chida S, et al: Studies on the metabolic fate of N-acetylcysteine in rats and dogs. Pharmacometrics 26:249–260,1983.
50. Horowitz RS, Dart RC, Jarvie DR, et al: Placental transfer of N-acetylcysteine following human maternal acetaminophen toxicity. J Toxicol Clin Toxicol 35:447–451, 1997.
51. Zed PJ, Krenzelok EP: Treatment of acetaminophen overdose. Am J Health Syst Pharm 56:1081–1089, 1999.
52. Ludmir J, Main DM, Landon MB, et al: Maternal acetaminophen overdose at 15 weeks of gestation. Obstet Gynecol 67:750–751, 1986.

53. Robertson RG, VanCleave BL, Collins JJ: Acetaminophen overdose in the second trimester of pregnancy. J Fam Pract 23:267–268, 1986.
54. Haibach H, Akhter JE, Muscato MS, et al: Acetaminophen overdose with fetal demise. Am J Clin Pathol 82:240–242, 1984.
55. Wang PH, Yang MJ, Lee WL, et al: Acetaminophen poisoning in late pregnancy. J Reprod Med 42:367–371, 1997.
56. Kurzel RB: Can acetaminophen excess result in maternal and fetal toxicity? South Med J 83:953–955, 1990.
57. Byer AJ, Traylor TR, Semmer JR: Acetaminophen overdose in the third trimester of pregnancy. JAMA 247:3114–3115, 1982.
58. Stokes IM: Paracetamol overdose in second trimester of pregnancy: Case report. Br J Obstet Gynaecol 91:286–288, 1984.
59. Rosevear SK, Hope PL: Favourable neonatal outcome following maternal paracetamol overdose and severe fetal distress: Case report. Br J Obstet Gynaecol 96:491–493, 1989.
60. McElhatton PR, Sullivan FM, Volans GN, et al: Paracetamol poisoning in pregnancy: An analysis of the outcomes of cases referred to the Teratology Information Service of the National Poisons Information Service. Hum Exp Toxicol 9:147–153, 1990.
61. McElhatton PR, Sullivan FM, Volans GN: Paracetamol overdose in pregnancy analysis of the outcomes of 300 cases referred to the Teratology Information Service. Reprod Toxicol 11:85–94, 1997.
62. Kozer E, Koren G: Management of paracetamol overdose: Current controversies. Drug Saf 24:503–512, 2001.
63. Tenebein M: Poisoning in pregnancy. In Koren G (ed): Maternal-Fetal Toxicology: A Clinician's Guide, 2nd ed. New York, Marcel Dekker, 1994, pp 223–252.
64. Litovitz T, Klein-Schwartz W, Rodgers GC Jr, et al: 2001 Annual report of the American Association of Poison Control Centers Toxic Exposure Surveillance System. Am J Emerg Med 20:391–452, 2002.
65. Bonassi S, Magnani M, Calvi A, et al: Factors related to drug consumption during pregnancy. Acta Obstet Gynecol Scand 73:535–540, 1994.
66. Corby DG: Aspirin in pregnancy: Maternal and fetal effects. Pediatrics 62(Suppl):930–937, 1978.
67. Koren G: Maternal-Fetal Toxicology: A Clinician's Guide, 2nd ed. New York, Marcel Dekker, 1994.
68. Gatterson LK, Procknal JA, Levy G: Fetal acquisition and neonatal elimination of a large amount of salicylate. Clin Pharmacol Ther 17:98–103, 1974.
69. Earle R: Congenital salicylate intoxication: Report of a case. N Engl J Med 265:1003–1004, 1961.
70. Lynd PA, Andreasen AC, Wyatt RJ: Intrauterine salicylate intoxication in a newborn. Clin Pediatr 15:912–913, 1976.
71. Rejent TA, Sung-ook Baik BA: Fatal in utero salicylism. J Forensic Sci 30:942–944, 1985.
72. Levy G, Procknal JA, Garrettson LK: Distribution of salicylate between neonatal and maternal serum diffusion equilibrium. Clin Pharmacol Ther 18:210–214, 1975.
73. Levy G, Garrettson LK: Kinetics of salicylate elimination by newborn infants of mothers who ingested aspirin before delivery. Pediatrics 53:201–210, 1974.
74. Haslam RH, Ekert H, Gillam GL: Hemorrhage in a neonate possibly due to maternal ingestion of salicylate. J Pediatr 84:556, 1974.
75. Karlowicz MG, White LE: Severe intracranial hemorrhage in a term neonate associated with maternal acetylsalicylic acid ingestion. Clin Pediatr 32:740–743, 1993.
76. Turner G, Collins E: Fetal effects of regular salicylate ingestion in pregnancy. Lancet 3:338–339, 1975.
77. Collins E: Maternal and fetal effects of acetaminophen and salicylates in pregnancy. Obstet Gynecol 58:57S–62S, 1981.
78. Reissman KR, Coleman TJ: Acute intestinal iron intoxication: II. Metabolic, respiratory and circulatory effects of absorbed iron salts. Blood 10:46–51, 1955.
79. Robotham JL, Troxler RF, Lietman PS: Iron poisoning: Another energy crisis. Lancet 2:664–665, 1974.
80. Curry SC, Bond GR, Raschke R, et al: An ovine model of maternal iron poisoning on pregnancy. Ann Emerg Med 19:632–638, 1990.
81. Rayburn WF, Donn SM, Wulf ME: Iron overdose during pregnancy: Successful therapy with deferoxamine. Am J Obstet Gynecol 147:717–718, 1983.
82. Lacoste H, Goyert GL, Goldman LS, et al: Acute iron intoxication in pregnancy: Case report and review of the literature. Obstet Gynecol 80:500–501, 1992.
83. Olenmark M, Biber B, Dottori O, et al: Fatal iron intoxication in late pregnancy. Clin Toxicol 25:347–359, 1987.
84. Andersen AC, Share JC, Woolf AD: The use of ultrasound in the diagnosis of toxic ingestions. Vet Hum Toxicol 32:355, 1990.
85. Blanc P, Hryhorczuk DO, Danel I: Deferoxamine treatment of acute iron intoxication in pregnancy. Obstet Gynecol 64:12S–14S, 1984.
86. McElhatton PR, Roberts JC, Sullivan FM: The consequences of iron overdose and its treatment with desferrioxamine in pregnancy. Hum Exp Toxicol 10:251–259, 1991.
87. Tran T, Wax JR, Philput C, et al: Intentional iron overdose in pregnancy: Management and outcome. J Emerg Med 18:225–228, 2000.
88. Tran T, Wax JR, Steinfeld JD, et al: Acute intentional iron overdose in pregnancy. Obstet Gynecol 92(Part 2):678–679, 1998.
89. Singer ST, Vichinsky EP: Deferoxamine treatment during pregnancy: Is it harmful? Am J Hematol 60:24–26, 1999.
90. Aubard Y, Magne I: Carbon monoxide poisoning in pregnancy. Br J Obstet Gynecol 107:833–838, 2000.
91. Cobb N, Etzel RA: Unintentional carbon monoxide-related deaths in the United States, 1979 through 1988. JAMA 266:659–663, 1991.
92. Longo LD: The biological effects of carbon monoxide on the pregnant woman, fetus, and newborn infant. Am J Obstet Gynecol 129:69–103, 1977.
93. Koren GK, Sharav T, Garrettson LK, et al: A mulitcenter prospective study of fetal outcome following accidental carbon monoxide poisoning in pregnancy. Reprod Toxicol 5:397–403, 1991.
94. Farrow JR, Davis GJ, Roy TM, et al: Fetal death due to nonlethal carbon monoxide poisoning. J Forensic Sci 35:1448–1452, 1990.
95. Cramer CR: Fetal death due to accidental maternal carbon monoxide poisoning. J Toxicol Clin Toxicol 19:297–301, 1982.
96. Muller GH, Graham S: Intrauterine death of the fetus due to accidental carbon monoxide poisoning. N Engl J Med 252:1075–1078, 1955.
97. Kopelman AE, Plaut TA: Fetal compromise caused by maternal carbon monoxide poisoning. J Perinatol 18:74–77, 1998.
98. Caravati EM, Adams CJ, Joyce SM, et al: Fetal toxicity associated with maternal carbon monoxide poisoning. Ann Emerg Med 17:714–717, 1988.
99. Hennequin Y, Blum D, Vamos E, et al: In-utero carbon monoxide poisoning and multiple fetal abnormalities. Lancet 341:240, 1993.
100. Weaver LK, Hopkins RO, Chan KJ, et al: Hyperbaric oxygen for acute carbon monoxide poisoning. N Engl J Med 347:1057–1067, 2002.
101. Silverman RK, Montano J: Hyperbaric oxygen treatment during pregnancy in acute carbon monoxide poisoning. J Reprod Med 42:309–311, 1997.
102. Van Hoesen KB, Camporesi EM, Moon RE, et al: Should hyperbaric oxygen be used to treat the pregnant patient for acute carbon monoxide poisoning? A case report and review of the literature. JAMA 261:1039–1043, 1989.
103. Brown DB, Mueller GL, Golich FC: Hyperbaric oxygen treatment for carbon monoxide poisoning in pregnancy: A case report. Aviat Space Environ Med 63:1011–1014, 1992.
104. Hollander DI, Nagey DA, Welch R, et al: Hyperbaric oxygen therapy for the treatment of acute carbon monoxide poisoning in pregnancy: A case report. J Reprod Med 32:615–617, 1987.
105. Elkharrat D, Raphael JC, Jars-Guincestre MC, et al: Acute carbon monoxide intoxication and hyperbaric oxygen in pregnancy. Intensive Care Med 17:289–292, 1991.
106. Hollander JE: The management of cocaine-associated myocardial ischemia. N Engl J Med 333:1267–1272, 1995.
107. Frank DA, Amaro H, Bauchner H, et al: Cocaine use during pregnancy: Prevalence and correlates. Pediatrics 82:888–895, 1988.
108. Bandstra ES, Burkett G: Maternal-fetal and neonatal effects of in utero cocaine exposure. Semin Perinatol 15:288–301, 1991.
109. Cherukui R, Minkoff H, Feldman J, et al: A cohort study of alkaloidal cocaine "crack" in pregnancy. Obstet Gynecol 72:147–151, 1988.
110. Little DR: Cocaine addiction and pregnancy: Education in primary prevention. Res Staff Physician 39:79–81, 1993.
111. Dombrowski MP, Wolfe HM, Welch RA, et al: Cocaine abuse is associated with abruptio placentae and decreased birth weight, but not shorter labor. Obstet Gynecol 77:139–141, 1991.
112. Meeker JE, Reynolds PC: Fetal and newborn death associated with maternal cocaine use. J Anal Toxicol 14:379–382, 1990.
113. Slutsker L: Risks associated with cocaine use during pregnancy. Obstet Gynecol 79:778–789, 1992.
114. MacGregor SN, Keith LG, Chasnoff IJ, et al: Cocaine use during pregnancy: Adverse prenatal outcome. Am J Obstet Gynecol 79:778–789, 1992.

115. Hoyme HE, Jones KL, Dixon SD, et al: Prenatal cocaine exposure and fetal vascular disruption. Pediatrics 85:743–747, 1990.

116. Roe DA, Little BB, Bawdon RE, et al: Metabolism of cocaine by human placentas: Implications for fetal exposure. Am J Obstet Gynecol 163:715–718, 1990.

117. Moore TR, Sorg J, Miller L, et al: Hemodynamic effects of intravenous cocaine on the pregnant ewe and fetus. Am J Obstet Gynecol 155:883–888, 1986.

118. Woods JR, Plessinger MA, Clark KE: Effect of cocaine on uterine blood flow and fetal oxygenation. JAMA 257:957–961, 1987.

119. Brent RL: Relationship between uterine vascular clamping, vascular disruption syndrome, and cocaine teratogenicity. Teratology 41:757–760, 1990.

120. Tenenbein M: Methanol poisoning during pregnancy: Prediction of risk and suggestions for management. Clin Toxicol 35:193–194, 1997.

121. Au KL, Woo JSK, Wong VCW: Intrauterine death from ergotamine overdosage. Eur J Obstet Gynecol Reprod 19:313–315, 1985.

122. Russell CS, Lang C, McCambridge M, et al: Neuroleptic malignant syndrome in pregnancy. Obstet Gynecol 98:906–908, 2001.

123. Frey B, Braegger CP, Ghelfi D: Neonatal cholestatic hepatitis from carbamazepine exposure during pregnancy and breast feeding. Ann Pharmacother 36:644–647, 2002.

124. Seneviratne SL, deSilva CE, Fonseka MMD, et al: Envenoming due to snake bite during pregnancy. Trans R Soc Trop Med Hyg 96:272–274, 2002.

125. Boyer JC, Hernandez F, Estorc J, et al: Management of maternal *Amanita phalloides* poisoning during first trimester of pregnancy: A case report and review of the literature. Clin Chem 47:971–974, 2001.

126. Theil GB, Richter R, Powell MR, et al: Acute dilantin poisoning. Neurology 10:138–142, 1960.

127. Greenland VC, Delke I, Minkoff HL: Vaginally administered cocaine overdose in a pregnant woman. Obstet Gynecol 74:476–477, 1989.

128. Bond GR, Van Zee A: Overdosage of misoprostol in pregnancy. Am J Obstet Gynecol 171:561–562, 1994.

129. Austin J, Ford MD, Rouse A: Acute intravaginal misoprostol toxicity with fetal demise. J Emerg Med 15:61–64, 1997.

130. Brost BC, Scardo JA, Newman RB: Diphenhydramine overdose during pregnancy: Lessons from the past. Am J Obstet Gynecol 175:1376–1377, 1996.

131. Zurawski JM, Kelly EA: Pregnancy outcome after maternal poisoning with brodifacoum, a long-acting warfarin-like rodenticide. Obstet Gynecol 90:672–674, 1997.

132. Anthony J, Johanson RB, Duley L: Role of magnesium sulfate in seizure prevention in patients with eclampsia and pre-eclampsia. Drug Saf 3:188–199, 1996.

133. Witlin AG, Sibai BM: Magnesium sulphate therapy in preeclampsia and eclampsia. Obstet Gynecol 92:883–889, 1998.

134. Raman NV, Rao CA: Magnesium sulfate as an anticonvulsant in eclampsia. Int J Gynecol Obstet 49:289–298, 1995.

135. Lu JF, Nightingale CH: Magnesium sulfate in eclampsia and pre-eclampsia. Clin Pharmacokinet 38:305–314, 2000.

136. Wax JR, Segna RA, Vandersloot JA: Magnesium toxicity and resuscitation—an unusual case of postcesarean evisceration. Int J Gynecol Obstet 48:213–214, 1995.

137. Swartjes JM, Schutte MF, Bleker OP: Management of eclampsia: Cardiopulmonary arrest resulting from magnesium sulfate overdose. Eur J Gynecol Obstet Reprod Biol 47:73–75, 1992.

138. Herschel M, Mittendorf R: Tocolytic magnesium sulfate toxicity and unexpected neonatal death. J Perinatol 21:261–262, 2001.

139. Reynolds JD, Chestnut DH, Dexter F, et al: Magnesium sulfate adversely affects fetal lamb survival and blocks fetal cerebral flow response during maternal hemorrhage. Anesth Analg 83:493–499, 1996.

140. Moon PF, Ramsay MM, Nathanielsz PW: Intravenous infusion of magnesium sulfate and regional redistribution of fetal blood flow during maternal hemorrhage in late-gestation ewes. Am J Obstet Gynecol 181:1486–1494, 1999.

141. Klein Z, Altaras M, Beyth Y, et al: Polyserositis as an unusual sign of methotrexate toxicity. Gynecol Oncol 61:446–447, 1996.

142. Sharma S, Jagdev S, Coleman RE, et al: Serosal complications of single-agent dose methotrexate used in gestational trophoblastic diseases: First reported case of methotrexate-induced peritonitis. Br J Cancer 81:1037–1041, 1999.

143. Isaacs JD, McGhee RP, Cowan BD: Life-threatening neutropenia following methotrexate treatment of ectopic pregnancy: A report of two cases. Obstet Gynecol 88:694–696, 1996.

144. Gadgil SD, Damle SR, Advani SH: Effect of activated charcoal on the pharmacokinetics of high dose methotrexate. Cancer Treat Rep 66:1169, 1982.

145. Erickson TB, Wahl M: Anticancer and other cytotoxic drugs. In Ford MD, Delaney KA, Ling LJ, Erickson TB (eds): Clinical Toxicology. Philadelphia, WB Saunders, 2001.

146. Steger GG, Mader RM, Gnant MFX, et al: GM-CSF in the treatment of a patient with severe methotrexate intoxication. J Intern Med 233:499–502, 1993.

146a. Leikin JB, Paloucek FP (eds): Leikin and Paloucek's Poisoning and Toxicology Handbook, 3rd ed. Hudson, OH, Lexi-comp, 2002.

147. Douglas MJ, Farquharson DF, Ross PLE, et al: Cardiovascular collapse following an overdose of prostaglandin F2 alpha: A case report. Can J Anesth 36:466–469, 1989.

148. Hankins GDV, Hauth JC: A comparison of the relative toxicities of beta-sympathomimetic tocolytic agents. Am J Perinatol 2:338–346, 1985.

149. Brandstetter RD, Gotz V: Inadvertent overdose of parenteral terbutaline. Lancet 1(8166):485, 1980.

150. Walden RJ: Management of terbutaline overdose. Lancet 1(8170):709, 1980.

151. Thorkelsson T, Loughead JL: Long-term subcutaneous terbutaline tocolysis: Report of possible neonatal toxicity. J Perinatol 11:235–238, 1991.

152. Davis WB, Wells SR, Kuller JA, et al: Analysis of the risks associated with calcium channel blockade: Implications for the obstetrician-gynecologist. Obstet Gynecol Surv 52:198–201, 1997.

153. Thorp JM, Spielman FJ, Valea FA, et al: Nifedipine enhances the cardiac toxicity of magnesium sulfate in the isolated perfused Sprague-Dawley rat heart. Am J Obstet Gynecol 163:655–656, 1990.

154. Ducsay CA, Thompson JS, Wu AT, et al: Effects of calcium entry blocker (nicardipine) tocolysis in rhesus macaques: Fetal plasma concentrations and cardiorespiratory changes. Am J Obstet Gynecol 157:1482–1486, 1987.

155. Demandt E, Legius H, Devliegger F, et al: Prenatal indomethacin toxicity in one member of monozygous twins: A case report. Eur J Obstet Gynecol Reprod Biol 35:267–269, 1990.

156. Claessens N, Delbeke L, Lambert J, et al: Toxic epidermal necrolysis associated with treatment for preterm labor. Dermatology 196:461–462, 1998.

157. Leikin JB, Paloucek FP (eds): Leikin and Paloucek's Poisoning and Toxicology Handbook, 2nd ed. Hudson, OH, Lexi-comp, 1998.

CHAPTER 12

Geriatric Poisoning

Kevin L. Wallace ▪ Anthony Morkunas

In 1999, it was estimated that approximately 12% of the U.S. population was older than age 65 years.[1,2] This age group is considered the fastest growing population in the United States and is expected to increase to 22% by 2050.[3] Drug consumption data in the United States suggest that elderly individuals are responsible for 30% of all prescription drug use and 40% of over-the-counter drug purchases.[1] The number of drugs prescribed per patient is related to the number of the patient's chronic medical conditions, which directly relates to age of the patient.[2] It is estimated that elderly individuals who are able to live independently use only three drugs per day, whereas elderly patients living in nursing homes receive about eight drugs per day.[1,2] With each new drug an elderly patient uses, the opportunity for untoward events increases.[4]

Data collected for the year 2000 by the American Association of Poison Control Centers (AAPCC) Toxic Exposure Surveillance System (TESS) for human exposures to pharmaceutical and nonpharmaceutical agents showed that although exposures occurring in individuals 60 years old or older represented only 4% of the approximately 2 million exposures reported for the year, the poisoning fatality rate within this age group, 0.16%, was 4 times higher than that occurring in younger individuals.[5] These findings are similar to those reported previously in regard to the epidemiology of poisoning in the elderly.[6] Of the 142 fatalities reported for the older age group, 40% were deemed to have resulted from suicidal exposure, whereas two thirds were attributed to poisoning by one or more pharmaceutical agents.[5] Of 95 deaths that occurred in this age group linked to pharmaceutical agents, more than one quarter were judged to have occurred as a result of therapeutic error or as an adverse reaction to therapy. The number of such therapeutic mishaps in this group represents more than half of this type of fatal poisoning occurrence recorded in the AAPCC TESS 2000 database. It is likely that the TESS data profoundly underestimate the morbidity and mortality of adverse drug effects in this age group.

It is conventional medical wisdom that the frequency of adverse drug-related events (ADEs) in the elderly, including medication errors and adverse drug reactions, is a function of the number of medications used per patient.[4,7] In a study of patients presenting to an urban emergency department, a notably positive exposure-effect relationship was observed between number of medications taken and frequency of ADEs.[8] Approximately 10% of emergency department visits in that study group were attributed to ADEs, most frequently associated with use of nonsteroidal antiinflammatory drugs

(NSAIDs), antibiotics, anticoagulants, diuretics, hypoglycemics, β-blockers, calcium channel blockers, or chemotherapeutic agents. A relationship also has been observed between the number of drugs prescribed and the number of diseases per patient and rate of hospitalization.[2,4]

General Themes in Geriatric Pharmacology and Toxicology

The elderly have

1. Age-related changes in physiologic/pharmacologic parameters
2. A high prevalence of chronic medical disorders
3. Frequent polypharmacy, associated with medication errors, adverse effects, and drug interactions

Drug-related problems in hospitalized patients, many of whom are elderly, are associated with increases in patient morbidity, length of hospital stay, and economic costs. The costs of medication errors alone have been estimated (1993 values) at greater than $4500 per adverse event and $2.8 million per year for a 700-bed teaching hospital, with an average associated increase in length of hospital stay of approximately 4.5 days.[9]

PHARMACOLOGY AND PATHOPHYSIOLOGY

The impact of advanced age on risk of toxic pharmaceutical or nonpharmaceutical exposure may be characterized in terms of several categories of determinants: (1) physiologic factor, such as age-related alteration in drug absorption or effect on myocardial function; (2) interactions among pharmaceutical and nonpharmaceutical agents resulting from the use of multiple medications for multiple medical problems; and (3) extrinsic, social, and behavioral factors, such as physician prescribing practice and patient compliance. The pharmacologic or toxicologic effects of exposure to a drug or other substance commonly are distinguished on the basis of whether they concern (1) the pharmacokinetic or toxicokinetic response to exposure (i.e., the disposition of that substance as a function of its absorption, distribution, metabolism, and elimination) or (2) the pharmacodynamic or toxicodynamic response (i.e., organ/system effects that result from the actions of a drug or other exogenous substance at tissue/organ effectors [e.g., cell membrane receptors, enzymes, or other components with cell signaling functions]).

The combination of age-related pharmacokinetic and pharmacodynamic changes and inappropriate exposure to drugs or other substances results in an increase in the incidence of untoward exposure events in older individuals. This increase is particularly true of pharmaceutical agents with narrow therapeutic indices (i.e., low therapeutic-to-toxic ratios), such as aminoglycosides, digoxin, lithium, metformin, phenytoin, salicylates, and theophylline. For many of these agents, their already low therapeutic index is reduced further by physiologic changes in the geriatric population. Older patients are at heightened risk of developing lithium toxicity with therapeutic use because their natural decline in renal function reduces their ability to excrete the drug. Iatrogenic events have a prominent causal role in mortality and morbidity from pharmaceutical exposure in all populations, but particularly in the elderly. Some types and examples of iatrogenic poisoning occurrences are listed in Table 12-1. For the reasons already described, the elderly population is at increased risk for all of these errors.

Pharmacokinetic Considerations

Much of the published data regarding pharmacokinetic characteristics of various drugs are based on volunteer studies in young, healthy individuals. Age-related physiologic changes may alter drug disposition significantly in elderly patients (Table 12-2) and should be considered in the prevention and treatment of toxicologic illness in elderly patients.

Several well-known, age-related changes within the gastrointestinal tract have been described. Increases in gastric pH and gastric emptying time have been observed along with decreases in gastrointestinal blood flow and mucosal absorptive surface area.[1,2,6] Despite these alterations, the extent of drug absorption typically does not change; however, there may be a significant decrease in the rate of absorption of some drugs. The net effect of these changes is hard to predict and does not allow for broad generalization, but with slowed absorption there may be a slower onset of action for some

drugs. This effect is particularly important for agents such as analgesics or sedatives, in which a rapid onset of drug effect is desirable. In addition, drugs that require an acidic environment for dissolution and absorption, such as ketoconazole or itraconazole, may be less bioavailable in the elderly.

Age-related changes in chemical, drug, or toxin distribution result from several factors. Reduction in body water and muscle mass along with an increase in body fat results in reduced volume of distribution (Vd) for substances that primarily distribute in water or lean body mass, such as digoxin and ethanol, whereas Vd is expanded for substances that distribute primarily in fat, such as diazepam. The time interval from first administration to attainment of steady state and the elimination half-life of a substance may be increased or reduced in elderly individuals depending on whether the substance is lipid soluble or water soluble. In elderly individuals started on regular doses of a fat-soluble drug such as diazepam, the onset of toxic effects may be delayed and their duration prolonged.

Serum albumin levels decline as a result of aging, disease, debilitation, and poor nutrition.[1] This change results in an increase in active, unbound fractions of drugs with characteristically high binding affinity to plasma proteins (e.g., salicylate, diazepam, warfarin, phenytoin, quinidine, theophylline) and an increase in the Vd. Under conditions of increased physiologic stress (e.g., acute myocardial infarction), the production and plasma content of α-acid glycoprotein (αAG), an acute-phase reactant, may be increased. The effect of an increase in αAG level in plasma is opposite to that of hypoalbuminemia (i.e., reduction in free drug fraction and amount of drug [e.g., lidocaine] available for target organ effect). These effects do not offset each other, however, because the drugs that bind to albumin frequently are different from the drugs that bind to αAG. Other disease states that are relatively common in elderly patients (e.g., sepsis) are associated with increased capillary permeability. This physiologic action may result in a dramatic increase in Vd of substances (e.g., gentamicin) that distribute into extracellular body water, requiring increased doses to maintain therapeutic blood levels.

The metabolism of a pharmaceutical or nonpharmaceutical compound may inactivate it (e.g., lidocaine), activate it (e.g., enalapril and several other angiotensin-converting enzyme inhibitor prodrugs), or prolong its activity (e.g., diazepam's conversion to its longer acting metabolite nordiazepam). The body's clearance of some drugs (e.g., lidocaine, propranolol) greatly depends on hepatic metabolism and on hepatic blood flow or enzyme activity. Aging-related declines in liver mass and cardiac output are associated with reduction in hepatic blood flow by 50% in individuals older than age 65, resulting in slowed metabolism of perfusion-dependent drugs (e.g., lidocaine).[10] Diseases such as congestive heart failure may compromise hepatic blood flow and clearance of perfusion-dependent drugs further.

Although experimental evidence suggests that their role, independent of other risk factors, in reduced drug clearance in elderly patients is relatively minor,[11] oxidative (phase I) enzymes that make lipid-soluble drugs more water soluble for excretion by the kidney may have reduced activity in the elderly. This reduced activity may result in reduced metabolism of active parent compounds (e.g., diazepam) and, in some instances, their active metabolites (e.g., nordiazepam).

TABLE 12-1 Types of Drug-Related Iatrogenic Disease

Predictable effects of a medication based on the known pharmacologic action (e.g., parkinsonism with metoclopramide)

Hypersensitivity reactions (e.g., penicillin-induced anaphylaxis)

Idiosyncratic (non–dose-related) reactions (e.g., NSAID-induced aseptic meningitis)

Overlapping pharmacology (e.g., anticholinergic toxicity from concomitant use of antihistamines and antidepressants)

Adverse effects related to metabolites (e.g., myoclonus and seizures secondary to accumulation of the meperidine metabolite normeperidine)

Drug interactions (e.g., inhibition of theophylline metabolism by cimetidine)

Inappropriate dosing (e.g., failure to adjust aminoglycoside maintenance dose for age-related decline in renal function)

Medication error (e.g., dispensing error based on similarity of drug names, such as Celexa [citalopram] and Celebrex [celecoxib])

NSAID, nonsteroidal anti-inflammatory drug.

TABLE 12-2 Pharmacokinetic Considerations in the Elderly

PARAMETER	AGE-RELATED CHANGE	IMPACT
Absorption		
Gastric pH	Increased	Reduced absorption (e.g., itraconazole)
Gastric emptying	Reduced	Reduced rate of absorption
Distribution		
Body fat	Increased	Increased Vd for lipophilic agents (e.g., diazepam)
Body water	Reduced	Reduced Vd for hydrophilic agents (e.g., lithium)
Plasma protein		
Albumin	Reduced	Increased free fraction (e.g., phenytoin)
α-Glycoprotein	Increased (illness)	Reduced free fraction (e.g., lidocaine)
Metabolism		
Hepatic mass/blood flow	Reduced	Reduced clearance (e.g., lidocaine)
Phase I enzyme activity	Reduced	Reduced clearance (e.g., diazepam, meperidine)
Elimination		
Liver metabolism	Reduced	Reduced elimination rate
Renal excretion		
GFR	Reduced	Reduced elimination rate

GFR, glomerular filtration rate; Vd, volume of distribution.

Age-related reduction in phase I enzyme activity may be compounded further by non–age-related genetic variation and exogenous influences, such as drugs (e.g., erythromycin) and dietary sources (e.g., grapefruit juice), that inhibit enzyme activity. Phase II reactions, involving attachment of large polar groups (e.g., glucuronide moiety) to drugs (e.g., lorazepam), inactivating them and further facilitating their excretion, seem to be affected minimally by aging. Drugs that normally are highly protein bound (e.g., phenytoin) may be subject to increased metabolism in the elderly as a result of the age-related decline in production of albumin and resultant increase in free drug available to the liver to be metabolized.

Perhaps the most important age-related physiologic determinant of ADEs is decline in renal clearance. Progressive diminution in renal perfusion, glomerular filtration, and tubular function commonly results in reduced clearance rates and potentially toxic accumulation of drugs or other exogenous substances. Most notable are agents that are highly dependent on renal elimination (e.g., lithium, digoxin, metformin, baclofen, normeperidine, aminoglycosides, penicillin). Serum creatinine levels may remain normal as creatinine production declines because of age-related reduction in muscle mass in parallel with decline in renal function. Estimates of renal function in elderly individuals that are based on serum creatinine level, including estimates that take age, weight, and gender into account (e.g., creatinine clearance = [(140 − age) × weight (kg)/(72 × serum creatinine)] × 0.85 [females])[2], should be viewed with caution and not overly relied on to assess renal-dependent drug clearance.

Pharmacodynamic Factors

Many pharmacodynamic factors are thought to influence the elderly individual's response to exposure to pharmaceutical and nonpharmaceutical agents. These factors include age-related changes in receptor tissue density; reduced capacity for compensatory response to physiologic change or stress; blunted homeostatic control (e.g., thermoregulatory and baroreceptor) mechanisms; and altered sensitivity to the effects of various agents, independent of their pharmacokinetic characteristics.[1] Data from experimental and clinical studies show significant age-dependent reduction in β-adrenergic receptor responsiveness to agonists and antagonists.[1,4] In general, however, elderly patients seem to be more sensitive than younger individuals to developing the adverse effects of various medications, including cognitive dysfunction (e.g., sedative agents), respiratory depression (e.g., opioid analgesics), dysrhythmia or conduction disturbance

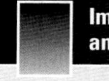

Important Geriatric Pharmacokinetic and Pharmacodynamic Characteristics

The elderly have

1. Altered drug/toxin distribution (increase or decrease in volume of distribution) of drugs depending on fat and water solubility and protein binding affinity
2. Reduced hepatic clearance of perfusion-dependent and phase I enzyme metabolized substances
3. Reduced elimination of drugs predominantly cleared by the kidney
4. Increased sensitivity to target organ/tissue effects
5. Reduced ability to compensate for the pathophysiologic effects of toxic exposure (age-related blunting of homeostatic control mechanisms or pathology associated with concurrent disease or both)

(e.g., digoxin, calcium channel blockers), postural hypotension (e.g., tricyclic antidepressants), gastrointestinal bleeding (e.g., NSAIDs), constipation (e.g., opioid analgesics), urinary retention (e.g., antihistamines), hyponatremia or hypokalemia (e.g., thiazide diuretics), hyperkalemia (e.g., trimethoprim), hypoglycemia (e.g., ethanol), renal failure (e.g., NSAIDs), and coagulopathy (e.g., warfarin).

Preexisting or comorbid medical conditions frequently amplify the elderly patient's sensitivity to the effects of various pharmaceutical and nonpharmaceutical agents. This familiar observation is well supported by marked age-related increases in prevalence of medical disorders such as various types of senile dementia, Parkinson's disease, hypertension, coronary artery disease, sick sinus syndrome, atrophic gastritis, prostatic hypertrophy, diabetes mellitus, hypothyroidism, malnutrition, sepsis, various malignant neoplastic diseases, and glaucoma.

Drug-Drug, Drug-Food, and Drug-Lifestyle Interactions

Toxic pharmacokinetic and pharmacodynamic interactions among various pharmaceutical and nonpharmaceutical (e.g., dietary) agents may be more likely to occur in elderly individuals, given their tendency to use multiple medications and their increased sensitivity to the effects of many agents. In a study of elderly emergency department patients, nearly one third were found to be at risk of adverse drug interaction based on a review of their drug regimens as recorded in the medical record.[8] A vigilant posture should be assumed in regard to rapid-onset, life-threatening drug-drug interactions (e.g., hyperkalemic cardiac arrest after administration of dantrolene to individuals taking verapamil[12,13]) that may occur in hospitalized elderly patients with multisystemic illness for which multiple medications may seem indicated.

Undesirable reduction in bioavailability of some drugs may occur in response to altered gastrointestinal pH or cation content or induction of phase I enzyme activity responsible for drug metabolism. The absorption of imidazole antifungal drugs (e.g., ketoconazole) is reduced when coadministered with drugs that raise gastrointestinal pH, such as antacids or proton-pump inhibitors, whereas the presence of increased gastrointestinal concentrations of cations (e.g., Fe^{++}, Ca^{++}, Mg^{++}) associated with consumption of iron supplements, milk, or antacids interferes with the absorption of some antibiotics (e.g., fluoroquinolones, tetracyclines). Another familiar example of a pharmacokinetic drug interaction is that involving cigarette smoking and theophylline; induction of a phase I isoenzyme involved in theophylline metabolism, cytochrome P-450 (CYP450) 1A2, by polycyclic aromatic hydrocarbons in tobacco smoke is believed to be responsible for the increased clearance of theophylline observed in individuals who smoke while taking theophylline.

Increased levels and prolonged effects of drugs metabolized by hepatic phase I enzymes (e.g., warfarin by CYP450 2C9 and diltiazem by CYP450 3A4) may occur in response to administration of drugs (e.g., amiodarone) or consumption of foods (e.g., grapefruit juice) that inhibit the activity of these enzymes. Other mechanisms responsible for toxic drug interactions include displacement of protein-bound drug (e.g., salicylate) by other drugs with high protein-binding affinity (e.g., warfarin); impaired renal elimination (e.g., NSAID-induced, angiotensin-converting enzyme inhibitor–induced, or thiazide-induced reduction in lithium clearance); and additive pharmacodynamic effects, such as those produced by central nervous system depressant medications (e.g., sedatives and opioid analgesics). The reader is referred to frequently updated reference sources for computerized searches,[14] tabulations,[15] and referenced discussions[16] of drug-drug interactions.

Social and Behavioral Factors

The increased prevalence of medical disorders in older individuals predisposes them to social, behavioral, and pharmacokinetic and pharmacodynamic risks of adverse exposure to pharmaceutical and nonpharmaceutical compounds. As previously noted, ADEs in this age group are related to individuals' tendency to use multiple medications. The causal basis for polypharmacy in the geriatric population seems to be multifactorial, involving not only an increased number of diagnoses but also deficiencies in health care professionals' education, attitudes (e.g., neglect), and prescribing practices (e.g., off-site management of nursing home patients, "standing" and "continuation" medication orders, tendency to add "blindly" to list of medications prescribed by other providers).

Iatrogenic medication errors (improper prescription, distribution, or administration) are an important cause of ADEs in all populations, but especially the elderly. The rates of medication errors and prescribing errors observed in hospitalized patients have been reported to vary between 1.7% and 59% and between 0.3% and 2.6%[9] The potential for therapeutic misadventure is compounded further by patient noncompliance, which may be intentional (e.g., on the basis of affective disturbance) or unintentional (e.g., on the basis of cognitive or perceptual dysfunction), resulting in subtherapeutic and supratherapeutic dosing.

In a 1994 study, it was determined that 25% of elderly individuals were prescribed at least one drug that was contraindicated in the elderly.[17] A more recent study showed that prescribers in a hospital ambulatory care center prescribed at least one potentially inappropriate medication during approximately 4% of encounters with elderly patients.[18] The most frequently prescribed drugs were diazepam, chlordiazepoxide, propoxyphene, dipyridamole, and amitriptyline. These medications accounted for 85% of outpatient visits that generated a pharmaceutical prescription.

In a review of 1996 data, researchers found that 16.6 million office or outpatient clinic visits by elderly patients resulted in a prescription for a psychotropic medication and that 4.5 million of these encounters resulted in prescription of a drug that was potentially dangerous.[19] Most of these prescriptions were written for amitriptyline and long-acting benzodiazepines.

CLINICAL PRESENTATION

Health care providers must be alert to the possibility that poisoning in the elderly individual may present in a manner that is chronic or subacute, subtle (e.g., mild sleep

1. Poisoning in a geriatric patient is often chronic, subacute, or subtle.
2. Neurobehavioral dysfunction is common.
3. Also relatively commonly occurring or life-threatening are cardiac dysrhythmia/conduction disturbance, postural hypotension, respiratory failure, pulmonary edema, gastrointestinal dysmotility, urinary retention, hypoglycemia, or bleeding diathesis.

TABLE 12-3 Examples of Drug Classes/Drugs that May Induce Neurobehavioral Dysfunction* in the Elderly

CLASS	SPECIFIC DRUGS
Antiarrhythmics	Digoxin, lidocaine, procainamide
Anticonvulsants	Phenytoin, carbamazepine, valproic acid
Antidepressants	Amitriptyline, fluoxetine
Antiemetics	Promethazine, metoclopramide
Antihypertensives	Clonidine, propranolol, verapamil
Antimicrobials	Penicillin, ciprofloxacin, isoniazid
Antiparkinsonians	Levodopa, amantadine
Antipsychotics	Thioridazine
Bronchodilators	Theophylline
Antineoplastics	Methotrexate, vincristine, procarbazine, cytarabine
Histamine receptor (H_1-, H_2-) antagonists	Diphenhydramine, cimetidine
Immunosuppressants	Corticosteroids, cyclosporine
Mood stabilizers	Lithium
Muscle relaxants	Carisoprodol, cyclobenzaprine, orphenadrine
Nonsteroidal anti-inflammatory drugs	Salicylate, mefenamic acid
Opioid analgesics	Meperidine/normeperidine
Sedative-hypnotics	Diazepam, phenobarbital, meprobamate

*Refer to specific chapters on relevant drug class (e.g., antihistamine) or toxic syndrome (e.g., anticholinergic poisoning) for detailed descriptions of the neurobehavioral and other systemic effects of the pharmaceutical agents of interest.

disturbance or intermittent decline in sensorium), indirect (e.g., fall or motor vehicle accident), or atypical compared with that seen in younger healthy individuals (e.g., focal neurologic abnormality). Obtaining an accurate history, with particular attention to prescribed, recently administered, or available medications or other health supplements, is paramount in making an accurate diagnosis and embarking on effective treatment for elderly individuals. The clinician's index of suspicion for a toxicologic basis for the presenting sign and symptom complex should be raised by the documented or suggested use of medications with low therapeutic indices (e.g., digoxin), preexisting disorders (e.g., dementia, depression, alcoholism, renal insufficiency), or history suggesting toxic exposure to non-pharmaceutical agents (e.g., ethanol, pesticides, carbon monoxide).

Elderly individuals are particularly vulnerable to the neurobehavioral effects of a broad array of pharmaceutical agents (Table 12-3; refer to specific chapters on relevant drug class [e.g., antihistamine] or toxic syndrome [e.g., anticholinergic poisoning] for detailed descriptions of the neurobehavioral and other systemic effects of the pharmaceutical agents of interest).[20,21] Cognitive disturbance is a common presentation for poisoning in older patients. Estimates of the occurrence of delirium in hospitalized elderly patients vary from approximately 15% to 55%, with a 15% prevalence noted at the time of hospital admission and significant incidence of mortality (10% to 75%) and morbidity (e.g., 55% permanent residual cognitive impairment) associated with its development.[21] Medication use has been established as the most common reversible cause of delirium, accounting for an estimated 22% to 39% of all cases.[21]

Evaluating health care providers should examine elderly patients with altered mental status for relatively common toxic syndromes. Anticholinergic poisoning (see Chapter 22) is associated with the use of many prescription and nonprescription medications, including tricyclic antidepressants, first-generation antihistamines, some antiarrhythmics, antiparkinsonian agents, antipsychotics, and muscle relaxants. Alcohol (see Chapters 47 and 30) or sedative-hypnotic drug (see Chapters 47 and 30) intoxication or withdrawal also produces mental status changes. A high index of suspicion for chronic salicylism should be maintained in elderly individuals who present with altered sensorium and a characteristic mixed acid-base disturbance (see Chapter 57). Delay in diagnosis of geriatric salicylate poisoning is common, in part because of its similarity to other disease processes.[22] Preexisting chronic or acute

drug (e.g., NSAID)-induced renal insufficiency may be an important contributing factor to the development of neurotoxicity, including seizures, from renally eliminated drugs, such as lithium and certain antibiotics, particularly among the fluoroquinolone (e.g., ciprofloxacin) and β-lactam antibacterials (e.g., penicillin, imipenem, cefazolin).[23]

Clinicians also should recognize that elderly individuals with underlying disorders such as atherosclerotic cerebrovascular disease may be more sensitive to insults such as sulfonylurea-induced or alcohol-induced hypoglycemia.[24-26] Acute-onset focal neurologic deficits may be more likely in elderly patients than in younger healthy individuals to represent the potentially reversible effects of a toxic insult, as opposed to progression of the primary disease process.

Although they are nonspecific, vital sign abnormalities that are more likely to occur in elderly individuals in response to a toxic insult include hyperthermia and hypothermia, orthostatic hypotension, and bradycardia. The reported prevalence of orthostatic hypotension in the geriatric population varies from 10% to 31%[27] and frequently is associated with the use of medications such as diuretics, calcium channel blockers, β-blockers, angiotensin-converting enzyme inhibitors, nitrates, antidepressants, and antipsychotics.

Presyncopal dizziness or frank syncope may reflect cardiac rhythm or conduction disturbance as an acute or chronic toxic effect of administration of drugs that directly (e.g., β-blockers, calcium channel blockers) or indirectly (e.g., digoxin) prolong atrioventricular nodal conduction, increase automaticity (e.g., digoxin), or cause repolarization abnormalities such as QT interval prolongation (e.g., type IA antidysrhythmics, tricyclic antidepressants, piperidine antipsychotics such as thioridazine and mesoridazine, and the newer atypical neuroleptics) (see Chapters 33–36, 42, and 45). Extracardiac manifestations of digoxin toxicity, such as anorexia, nausea, visual disturbance, and confusion, may support the diagnosis further but are so prevalent and nonspecific that their presence may not enhance clinical recognition.[28]

Pulmonary edema is more likely to occur in elderly individuals as a consequence of drug-induced negative inotropy combined with limited cardiac functional reserve capacity. Noncardiogenic pulmonary edema may be a manifestation of poisoning (e.g., chronic salicylism) and may not be associated with the presence of jugulovenous distention or S_3 gallop, typical features of cardiac failure. Gastrointestinal dysmotility disorders (e.g., constipation, adynamic ileus) and genitourinary dysfunction (e.g., urinary distention) are relatively common clinical presentations in the elderly for toxicity from drugs with narcotic (e.g., opioid analgesics) or anticholinergic (e.g., antihistamines) actions. The presence of a bleeding diathesis should suggest the possibility of warfarin-induced coagulopathy in individuals who have indications for or are known to be on anticoagulant treatment.

DIAGNOSIS

Although there is no substitute for a thorough and accurate history in making a timely diagnosis of poisoning in an elderly individual, the clinical laboratory can be of invaluable assistance to the clinician dealing with initially scant or unobtainable historical information. The limitations and caveats that apply to toxicologic analyses in general (see Chapter 4) apply to their role in the diagnosis and management of geriatric poisoning. Correlations between drug levels and the occurrence of toxicity may be even more limited in elderly patients, given their propensity to present well into the postdistribution phase after chronic, cumulative exposure to potentially toxic agents (e.g., salicylate, theophylline, digoxin, lithium) and their aging-altered drug distribution (e.g., increased free phenytoin fraction).

Routine clinical laboratory monitoring of serum electrolytes, glucose, and indices of renal function may be essential to the diagnosis and further prevention of untoward medication effects (e.g., digoxin-induced arrhythmia) in high-risk elderly patients, such as patients on diuretic or oral hypoglycemic therapy. Clinically significant abnormalities of serum sodium and potassium are particularly common among elderly individuals taking thiazide diuretics (hyponatremia, hypokalemia), whereas angiotensin-converting enzyme inhibitors, potassium-sparing diuretics, and trimethoprim may cause hyperkalemia.[29,30] As previously discussed, methods used to estimate drug clearance by the kidney that are based on serum creatinine should take into account age-related changes in muscle mass and creatinine excretion and otherwise be employed with caution.

In contrast to serum chemistry indices of renal function, quantitative serum values of hepatic enzymes (e.g., transaminases) and liver function tests (e.g., prothrombin time) are of little predictive value with regard to drug clearance. These analyses are used mainly to detect and monitor toxic hepatocellular injury (e.g., acetaminophen-induced hepatic necrosis) and effects on hepatic synthetic function (e.g., inhibition of vitamin K–dependent clotting factors by warfarin and salicylate). Quantitative serum drug assays generally are recommended if there is any clinical suspicion in elderly patients of salicylate or acetaminophen poisoning or for therapeutic monitoring of drug therapy involving agents with narrow therapeutic indices (e.g., digoxin, theophylline, lithium, aminoglycosides). Apart from routinely obtaining admission electrocardiograms and chest radiographs on all elderly patients requiring hospitalization for management of poisoning, indications for other diagnostic tests, such as abdominal radiographs and blood lead level, depend on the specific exposure (see pertinent chapter for substance-specific indications).

TREATMENT AND PREVENTION

Treatment of acute and chronic poisoning in elderly patients should be approached in much the same manner as for other age groups, with many added caveats that pertain to age-related pharmacokinetic and pharmacodynamic differences. Special attention should be directed at the potentially greater need for aggressive ventilatory support and for caution in fluid volume resuscitation in elderly individuals, given their greater sensitivity to the central depressant effects of some agents, greater likelihood of cardiac inotropic or chronotropic compromise, and tendency to develop life-threatening complications of such therapy (e.g., acute pulmonary edema). Clinicians also should recognize in older patients with chronic medical conditions the importance of considering blunted homeostatic (e.g., thermoregulatory) mechanisms, endocrine dysfunction (thyroid, adrenal), and nutritional deficiencies (e.g., limited vitamin and glucose stores) and address these with appropriate supportive measures (e.g., body warming or cooling, empirical thiamine administration). Although it may seem obvious, a frequently overlooked step in the initial management that may be of significant short-term or long-term benefit is temporary discontinuation of previously prescribed medications, particularly medications with narrow therapeutic indices or medications considered likely offenders (e.g., lithium, warfarin, digoxin, NSAIDs, anticholinergics, and serotoninergic drugs).

Administration of activated charcoal should be considered in instances in which recent acute ingestion of a toxic amount of a substance has occurred and no contraindications are present (see Chapter 6). The risks of orogastric lavage, repeated enteral doses of activated charcoal, or whole-bowel irrigation in elderly individuals, given their greater likelihood of gastrointestinal dysmotility disorder, should be weighed carefully against the unproven benefits of these interventions.

Hemodialysis as a method of enhanced elimination of drugs and toxins (see Chapter 7) plays an important role in the management of geriatric poisoning, particularly in instances in which the offending agent is of low molecular weight, low Vd, and low protein-binding affinity and undergoes predominantly renal elimination (e.g., lithium, salicylate, phenobarbital). The greater likelihood of impaired renal drug clearance and susceptibility to

> ### Key Points in the Management of Geriatric Poisoning
>
> 1. Medication history should be reviewed carefully for evidence of medication error, adverse effect, or drug interaction, and potentially offending medications should be discontinued.
> 2. Extra caution should be exercised during administration of supportive and antidotal therapy, urinary pH manipulation, and gastrointestinal decontamination.
> 3. Hemodialysis as a means of enhancing elimination may be warranted further in poisoned elderly individuals, given their age-related reduction in renal clearance or increased risks of other therapy.

complications from aggressive sodium and fluid loading in this age group provides a compelling argument in support of hemodialysis when it is indicated for toxicologic reasons.

In older individuals caution also should be exercised in the administration of antidotal agents such as physostigmine for anticholinergic poisoning in individuals at risk for cardiac conduction disturbance, antidigoxin antibodies for digitalis poisoning in patients with preexisting rapid atrial fibrillation, β-adrenergic antagonists for theophylline-induced tachydysrhythmias in individuals who may have underlying coronary artery or obstructive airway disease, and flumazenil for suspected benzodiazepine-induced central nervous system depression in individuals at risk for acute withdrawal from the latter agents. Antidotal agents that are cleared primarily by the kidney (e.g., the heavy metal chelator calcium sodium ethylenediamine tetraacetic acid) may be ineffective or contraindicated in individuals with renal insufficiency. Similarly the dosing of medications used to treat complicating or concurrent illness that are eliminated primarily via the renal route (e.g., aminoglycoside antibiotics, meperidine/normeperidine) should be adjusted for renal insufficiency. A guide to dosage adjustment of common medications in patients with renal insufficiency is given in Appendix C. Although the administration of an antidote in many of these circumstances still may be warranted, consultation with a medical toxicologist is recommended.

Prevention of toxic exposure in hospitalized elderly patients may be enhanced further through improved health care provider education, limited use or avoidance of certain pharmaceutical agents, computerized physician entry of medication orders, and pharmacy surveillance (computerized or on-site, pharmacist-staffed).[9,18,31]

REFERENCES

1. Woodard KW, Franklin RM: Treating elderly patients. US Pharmacist Aug: HS–7, 1999.
2. Chutka DS, Evans JM, Fleming KC, et al: Drug prescribing for elderly patients. Mayo Clin Proc 70:685–693, 1995.
3. Cody RJ: Physiological changes due to age: Implication for drug therapy of congestive heart failure. Drugs Aging 3:320–334, 1993.
4. Roberts J, Tumer N: Pharmacodynamic basis for altered drug action in the elderly. Clin Geriat Med 4:127–149, 1988.
5. Litovitz TL, Klein-Schwartz W, White S, et al: 2000 Annual report of the American Association of Poison Control Centers Toxic Exposure Surveillance System. Am J Emerg Med 19:337–395, 2001.
6. Klein-Schwartz W, Oderda GM: Poisoning in the elderly: Epidemiological, clinical and management considerations. Drugs Aging 1:67–89, 1991.
7. Pucino F, Beck CL, Seifert RL, et al: Review of pharmacogeriatrics. Pharmacotherapy 5:314, 1985.
8. Hohl CM, Dankoff J, Colacone A, Afilalo M: Polypharmacy, adverse drug-related events, and potential adverse drug interactions in elderly patients presenting to an emergency department. Ann Emerg Med 38:666–671, 2001.
9. van den Bemt PM, Egberts AC, Lenderink AW, et al: Risk factors for the development of adverse drug events in hospitalized patients. Pharm World Sci 22:62–66, 2000.
10. Iber FL, Murphy PA, Connor ES: Age-related changes in the gastrointestinal system: Effects on drug therapy. Drugs Aging 5:34–48, 1994.
11. Schmucker DL: Liver function and phase I drug metabolism in the elderly: A paradox. Drugs Aging 18:837–851, 2001.
12. Rubin AS, Zablocki AD: Hyperkalemia, verapamil, and dantrolene. Anesthesiology 66:246–249, 1987.
13. Saltzman LS, Kates RA, Corke BC, et al. Hyperkalemia and cardiovascular collapse after verapamil and dantrolene administration in swine. Anesth Analg 63:473–478, 1984.
14. Drug-Reax Interactive Drug Interactions. Micromedex Thomson Healthcare, vol III. Expiration March 2002.
15. Flockhart D: Cytochrome P450 drug interaction table. 2001. Available at: http://medicine.iupui.edu/flockhart/index.html. Accessed December 2001.
16. Hansten PD, Horn JR: Hansten and Horn's Drug Interactions Analysis and Management, St. Louis, Facts and Comparisons, 2001.
17. Wilcox SM, Hummelstein DU, Woolhandler S: Inappropriate drug prescribing for community dwelling elderly. JAMA 272:292–296, 1994.
18. Aparasu RR, Sitzman S: Inappropriate prescribing for elderly outpatients. Am J Health Syst Pharm 56:433–439, 1999.
19. Mort JR, Aparasu RR: Prescribing potentially inappropriate psychotropic medications to the ambulatory elderly. Arch Intern Med 160:2825–2831, 2000.
20. Anonymous: Drugs that may cause cognitive disorders in the elderly. Med Lett 42:111–112, 2000.
21. Lisi DM: Definition of drug-induced cognitive impairment in the elderly. Medscape Pharmacother Available at: www.medscape.com. Accessed June 2000. 2:1–22, 2000.
22. Durnas C, Cusack BJ: Salicylate intoxication in the elderly: Recognition and recommendations on how to prevent it. Drugs Aging 2:20–34, 1992.
23. Wallace KL: Antibiotic-induced convulsions. Crit Care Clin N Am 13:741–761, 1997.
24. Yoo J, Peter S, Kleinfeld M: Transient hypoglycemic hemiparesis in an elderly patient. J Am Geriatr Soc 34:479–481, 1986.
25. Khanna P: Hypoglycaemia as a cause of hemiplegia. Practitioner 232:298–301, 1988.
26. Wattoo MA, Lie HH: Alternating transient dense hemiplegia due to episodes of hypoglycemia. West J Med 170:170–171, 1999.
27. Mets TF: Drug-induced orthostatic hypotension in older patients. Drugs Aging 6:219–228, 1995.
28. Passmore AP, Johnston GD: Digoxin toxicity in the aged: Characterizing and avoiding the problem. Drugs Aging 1:364–379, 1991.
29. Baglin A, Boulard KC, Hanslik T, Prinseau J: Metabolic adverse reactions to diuretics: Clinical relevance to elderly patients. Drug Saf 12:161–167, 1995.
30. Marinella MA: Trimethoprim-induced hyperkalemia: An analysis of reported cases. Gerontology 45:209–212, 1999.
31. Beers MH, Ouslander JG: Risk factors in geriatric drug prescribing: A practical guide to avoiding problems. Drugs 37:105–112, 1989.

CHAPTER **13**

Critically Injured Workers

Michael G. Holland

Workplace exposures to toxins can cause severe illness and death similar to intentional poisonings and over-doses. In some cases, without a careful occupational history, the relationship between the job and the illness may be missed. Prolonged exposure to an insoluble gas, such as nitrogen dioxide after arc welding in a confined space, can cause a delayed pulmonary injury and adult respiratory distress syndrome (ARDS) that occurs 1 day later, when the link may go unnoticed. Careful questioning about the particular sequence of events is important when an illness occurs after performance of a common task. An example is exposure to phosgene gas after torch-cutting or welding metal that had been degreased recently with a chlorinated hydrocarbon solvent. Alternatively, a worker may experience a delayed illness such as metal fume fever (MFF) if he or she is performing another task near someone welding on galvanized metal. It is important to ask not only about the job of the ill worker but also about the nature of the workplace and the other processes being performed there.

The U.S. Department of Labor, Bureau of Labor Statistics, estimated that there were 5915 occupational fatalities in 2000, most caused by physical hazards, accidents, and falls. Of these fatalities, 8.1% were due to exposure to harmful substances or environments, and 3% were due to fires and explosions.[1] Of the 1.7 million nonfatal occupational illnesses and injuries involving lost work days, 4.5% were due to exposures to harmful substances.[2] The actual incidence may be higher because the connection between work and the illness may be missed.

Every poisoned worker should be considered to be an index case. It is crucial to ascertain whether other workers from the patient's environment have been injured or are at risk. Many countries have reporting requirements that mandate the clinician who becomes aware of workplace injuries to notify relevant governmental agencies.

Commensurate with the orientation of this book, this chapter highlights the most important occupational exposures that result in critical illness or death. A comprehensive review of all exposures is beyond the scope of this book. This chapter stresses the workplace-related issues regarding these exposures. More comprehensive discussions of the particular toxins involved may be found in their respective chapters. Minor illnesses, such as occupational dermatoses, and chronic diseases, such as asbestosis, beryllium disease, and coal workers' pneumoconiosis, are not addressed here.

OCCUPATIONAL PULMONARY TOXICOLOGY

Occupational Asthma

Occupational asthma is diagnosed when there is a work-related variable airway obstruction or airway hyperresponsiveness resulting from exposures encountered in the workplace. The asthma may be *caused by* the workplace exposure, or preexisting asthma may be *aggravated by* workplace exposures. Using this extremely broad definition, it has been estimated that 3% to 33% of all asthma cases may be considered work related,[3,4] but most authorities place the incidence at approximately 5%.[5] Occupational disease surveillance data indicate that occupational asthma is the most common occupational respiratory disease in industrialized nations.[3]

The two major types of occupational asthma are irritant-induced asthma (IIA) and sensitizer-induced asthma (SIA). Exposure to a significant dose of an irritating gas, dust, mist, or fume can cause IIA without an intervening latent period. This exposure may be a single isolated intense exposure or a lower-level exposure over months to years. The resulting asthmatic condition may be termed *reactive airways dysfunction syndrome* (RADS) or IIA. This condition may be short-lived or cause lifelong IIA/RADS and disability.[6] In these cases, there is generalized airway hyperresponsiveness but no specific responsiveness to any particular agent or antigen.

SIA is the classic form of occupational asthma and requires a variable amount of time between the first exposure and onset of illness, whereby the worker becomes sensitized to the offending agent. When the person is sensitized, minute quantities of the agent may cause significant signs and symptoms. Most SIA is caused by exposure to high-molecular-weight organic compounds that are considered "complete allergens." These include animal dander and plant proteins. The asthma is a type I, IgE-mediated immediate hypersensitivity reaction. Low-molecular-weight (LMW) compounds can cause SIA by acting as incomplete allergens or haptens (antibiotics, metals) or by other mechanisms that are poorly understood (e.g., toluene diisocyanates [TDI], trimellitic anhydride [TMA]). An important factor may be related to the chemical structure of the LMW agent: the requirement for the presence of at least two reactive groups with the ability to form bonds with native human macromolecules, such as albumin.[3] More than 200 LMW compounds have been implicated in the cause of occupational asthma, the most well known being plicatic acid in western red cedar, TDI, and colophony (resin).[3,7]

The physician evaluating a patient who presents with bronchoconstriction always must consider the possibility of work-related asthma, especially in a patient with no prior history of asthma, with asthma of recent onset, or with acute exacerbations of stable asthma. Careful questioning regarding the time of onset of symptoms as they relate to exposures at work can be helpful. SIA can have a biphasic or dual response, in which exposure to the allergen may induce an immediate bronchoconstriction, known as the *early response*, and a delayed or late response approximately 4 to 8 hours later. The early response often is self-limited, only to be followed later by the inflammation, airway hyperresponsiveness, and airway obstruction seen in the late response. Some workers may exhibit only the late response, becoming ill hours after leaving the workplace, when the causal relationship may not be apparent. The presence of the dual response may hinge on factors such as the type of compound, dose, length of exposure time, and concomitant use of medication. LMW agents seem more likely to induce an isolated late response, whereas high-molecular-weight "complete" allergens more commonly cause a dual response.[3,7]

Treatment of occupational asthma acutely is no different than conventional asthma treatment and consists of inhaled β-agonists, supplemental oxygen, and systemic corticosteroids as the condition dictates. Severe exacerbations associated with hypoxia or carbon dioxide retention or both require treatment in the intensive care unit. Long-term management hinges on identifying the sensitizer when possible and removing the patient from further exposure. IIA/RADS may have significant long-term sequelae that do not improve with removal from the workplace. Tables 13-1 and 13-2 list exposures and occupations known to be associated with occupational asthma.

Toxic Inhalant Injury

Many occupations have potential exposure to gases, and often these have significant potential for lung injury or systemic toxicity. Because oral ingestion of toxins in the workplace is uncommon, the primary routes of entry are pulmonary and dermal. Gases of toxicologic importance can be divided into three major categories: (1) simple asphyxiants, (2) toxic or chemical asphyxiants, and (3) irritant gases. Simple asphyxiants have no inherent toxicity other than displacing oxygen in inspired air, inducing anoxia. This toxicity is especially important in confined spaces, where the lack of air movement and ventilation may allow these gases to replace oxygen in the ambient air. Gases such as carbon dioxide are heavier than air and tend to accumulate in low areas. A victim who collapses to the floor is subjected to higher concentrations. On the other hand, a case report

TABLE 13-1 High-Molecular-Weight Sensitizing Agents and Jobs Associated with Occupational Asthma

HMW SENSITIZING AGENTS	ASSOCIATED OCCUPATIONS/INDUSTRIES
Animal dander	Animal handlers, veterinary workers, farmers
Pigeons (e.g., excreta, feathers)	Pigeon breeders
Chickens, turkeys	Poultry processing workers
Mice	Laboratory technicians
Guinea pigs	Laboratory technicians
Insects (bees, beetles, weevils, mites, silkworms, flies, others)	Many outdoor workers, silkworm farmers, insect research workers, granary workers, others
Grains (wheat, rye, buckwheat)	Farmers, grain mill workers, silo workers
Raw tobacco	Tobacco industry workers
Flours (wheat, rye)	Bakers, food processing workers
Enzymes	
Bacillus subtilis	Detergent manufacturers
Papain	Meat processing workers
Trypsin, pepsin	Pharmaceuticals workers
Wool	Wool workers, sorters
Marine organisms (prawns, crabs, oysters)	Prawn workers, oyster processing workers, crab processing workers
Foods (spices, grains, flours)	Chefs, food industry workers, food preparers
Natural rubber latex	Health care workers, rubber industry workers
Gums (acacia, arabic, tragacanth, karaya)	Pharmaceuticals workers, printers
Coffee beans, tea leaves	Coffee production workers, tea workers
Castor beans	Castor oil production workers
Seeds (flaxseed, cottonseed, linseed, psyllium seed)	Bakers, oil extraction workers, seed workers
Woods (oak, mahogany, California redwood, others)	Sawmill workers, carpenters, woodworkers
Hops	Brewery workers, farmers
Fungi, molds	Farmers, bakers, various industrial workers

HMW, high molecular weight.
Data from references 3, 8, 9, and 10.

TABLE 13-2 Selected Low-Molecular-Weight Sensitizing Agents and Jobs Associated with Occupational Asthma

LMW SENSITIZING AGENTS	ASSOCIATED OCCUPATIONS/INDUSTRIES
Antibiotics (penicillins, cephalosporins, tetracyclines)	Pharmaceuticals workers
Drugs (α-methyldopa, cimetidine, hydralazine, opiates, penicillamine, others)	Pharmaceuticals workers
Inorganic chemicals	
Ammonium persulfate	Beauticians, chemical production workers
Fluoride	Aluminum pot-room workers
Metals	
Aluminum	Aluminum smelting workers
Chromium salts	Leather tanning workers, metal plating workers, hard metal workers
Cobalt	Tungsten carbide hard metal workers
Nickel	Metal plating workers
Palladium	Metal plating workers, jewelers
Platinum	Platinum refining workers, electroplating workers, fluorescent screen manufacturers, jewelers
Vanadium	Ferrovanadium workers (hard metal workers)
Zinc	Metal plating workers
Organic chemicals	
Abietic acid (colophony-pine resin)	Soldering workers, electronics manufacturers
Acrylates	Glue workers
Aldehydes (formaldehyde, glutaraldehyde)	Hospital workers, laboratory technicians
Amines (ethanolamine)	Soldering workers, paint application workers, machining metal workers
Anhydrides (trimellitic anhydride, phthalic anhydride)	Plastics workers, epoxy resins workers
Dyes	Dye industry workers, fabrics workers
Insecticides (pyrethrins, organophosphates)	Farmers, insecticide applicators
Isocyanates	
Toluene diisocyanate	Polyurethane foam manufacturers
Diphenylmethane	Foundry workers, paint application workers
Plicatic acid (western red cedar)	Lumber workers, loggers, carpenters, cabinet-makers
Paraphenylenediamine	Fur dyers, chemical workers
Phenol	Chemical workers, laboratory workers
Piperazine	Chemical processing workers
Styrene	Chemical production workers, polymer industry workers

LMW, low molecular weight.
Data from references 3, 8, 9, and 10.

described a patient whose fall from a ladder after hydrogen sulfide exposure removed the patient from exposure and was lifesaving.[11] In the chemical production worker, confined spaces such as reactor vessels may contain no oxygen; entry for vessel cleaning requires self-contained breathing apparatus or other supplied air respirators.

SIMPLE ASPHYXIANTS

The simple asphyxiants commonly encountered by chemical workers include nitrogen, ethylene, propylene, carbon dioxide, butadiene, isobutylene, and hydrogen. When encountered in confined spaces, simple asphyxiants can cause anoxic central nervous system (CNS) injury due to oxygen deprivation. The degree of injury depends on the extent and duration of anoxia. Additionally, some simple asphyxiants, such as ethylene, propylene, butadiene, isobutylene, methane, and ethane, pose a significant explosive hazard. These confined-space exposures usually occur in the situation of inadequate safety training or lack of proper supervi-

sion. Treatment of simple asphyxiant exposure involves removing the victim from the source, ensuring adequate ventilation, and providing supplemental oxygen.

CHEMICAL ASPHYXIANTS

The gases considered chemical asphyxiants act either by decreasing the oxygen-carrying capacity of the blood (carbon monoxide) or by interfering with cellular utilization of oxygen (cyanide, hydrogen sulfide). These toxins are covered in detail in other chapters.

IRRITANT GASES

Irritant gases cause injury patterns directly related to their water solubility (Table 13-3). Highly soluble gases, such as hydrochloric acid, ammonia, sulfur dioxide, formaldehyde, and acid vapors, cause immediate irritation of the mucous membranes of the upper respiratory tract because they dissolve easily in the moisture of these tissues. These soluble gases first are deposited in the upper airways, making

TABLE 13-3 Relative Solubility of Common Irritant Vapors and Gases

GAS	CONVERSION FACTOR	MW (d)	RELATIVE VAPOR DENSITY (AIR = 1)	SOLUBILITY IN WATER	RELATIVE SOLUBILITY
Hydrofluoric acid (HF)	1 ppm = 0.82 mg/m³	20.006	1.86	Freely soluble in water	Very high
Hydrochloric acid (HCl)	1 ppm = 1.49 mg/m³	36.46	1.27	82.3 g/100 mL water	Very high
Chloramine (NH_2Cl): formed from bleach + NH_3		51.48	NA (liquid)	Freely soluble in water	Very high
Formaldehyde (CH_2O)	1 ppm = 1.23 mg/m³	30.03	1.04	55 g/100 mL water	High
Ammonia (NH_3)	1 ppm = 0.70 mg/m³	17.03	0.59	47 g/100 mL water	High
Fluorine (F_2)	1 ppm = 1.55 mg/m³	38	1.31	Reactive	Medium high
Acrolein (C=C–C=O)	1 ppm = 2.29 mg/m³	56.1	1.9	21 g/100 mL water	Medium high
Sulfur dioxide (SO_2)	1 ppm = 2.62 mg/m³	64.065	2.263	17.7 g/100 mL water	Medium high
Methyl isocyanate (MIC) (CH_3NCO)	1 ppm = 2.34 mg/m³	57.06	1.42	10 g/100 mL water	Medium high
Chlorine (Cl_2)	1 ppm = 2.90 mg/m³	70.9	2.47	1.46 g/100 mL water	Medium
Phosgene (carbonyl chloride [$COCl_2$])	1 ppm = 4.05 mg/m³	98.9	3.48	0.9 g/100 mL water	Low
Chlorine dioxide (ClO_2)	1 ppm = 2.76 mg/m³	67.46	2.33	0.3 g/100 mL water	Low
Nitrogen dioxide (NO_2)	1 ppm = 1.88 mg/m³	46	2.62	0.3 g/100 mL water	Low
Ozone (O_3)	1 ppm = 1.96 mg/m³	48	1.66	0.001 g/100 mL water	Very low

MW, molecular weight; NA, not applicable.
Data from references 12, 13, 14, and 15.

less concentration available to the lower respiratory tract. Also, the symptoms of burning in the eyes, nose, throat, and trachea tend to limit the exposure because the victim will rapidly exit an area causing these symptoms. The lack of these upper respiratory signs or symptoms rules out any significant exposure of a soluble gas and obviates the need for prolonged observation. Significant symptoms of upper respiratory tract burning and irritation associated with signs of mucosal and conjunctival inflammation, laryngeal symptoms, and cough indicate a possibility of lower respiratory tract injury and the need for admission and observation. Delayed pulmonary injury has been observed, with the onset of noncardiogenic pulmonary edema (ARDS) hours later. Long-term sequelae may include RADS/IIA, restrictive or obstructive defects, bronchiectasis, and bronchial stenosis.[6,16]

Phosgene, oxides of nitrogen, and ozone are poorly water-soluble gases. These insoluble gases cause little or no upper respiratory tract symptoms. Because there is no initial irritation, employees often are unaware of ongoing exposure. The exposures can be of longer duration, and the concentration reaching the lower airways is higher owing to lack of deposition in the upper airway mucosa. In these cases, delayed alveolar injury is possible, and onset of lower respiratory tract injury and pulmonary edema occurs hours after a significant exposure. Phosgene is encountered in chemical synthesis as an intermediate for isocyanate and pesticides or as a by-product when chlorinated hydrocarbons are burned or heated. Phosgene was a World War I warfare agent responsible for numerous deaths. Heavier than air, it accumulates in lower areas, making it an ideal agent for the trench warfare that was common during World War I. The only clue to phosgene exposure may be the reported odor of freshly mown hay. Nitrogen oxides are found in recently stored silage (silo filler's disease), from combustion products, and from oxidation of ambient nitrogen during high-temperature arc welding.

Because of the lack of upper respiratory tract irritation, patients often go home and develop these symptoms remote from the worksite. The clinical picture may present as ARDS, and sepsis or some other nonoccupational etiology may be suspected if an adequate occupational history is not obtained. Treatment consists of supplemental oxygen and ventilatory support as dictated by the clinical picture. Depending on the severity of injury, mortality rates from severe ARDS may be significant, and patients who recover may be left with permanent pulmonary impairment. Corticosteroids are probably useful to prevent the late sequelae of bronchiolitis obliterans fibrosa that is seen after nitrogen dioxide exposures. Their value in other toxic inhalational injuries is suggested by animal studies but is not proven in humans.[6]

Medium-solubility gases, such as chlorine, have dissolution rates in the upper airway moisture that are midway between highly soluble and poorly soluble irritant gases. Significant chlorine gas exposures can cause upper airway symptoms of burning and irritation, but these may be milder than the highly soluble gases and may progress to lower airway injury and delayed pulmonary edema. Clinical suspicion and careful evaluation are necessary when making disposition decisions after exposures to medium-solubility gases.

INHALATIONAL FEVERS

Inhaling a wide variety of organic and inorganic materials can cause a self-limited, flulike illness consisting of fever, chills, generalized body aches, and malaise. Patients frequently complain of headache, sore throat, chest pain, and cough and may have some dyspnea. There often is an elevated white blood cell count but generally no hypoxemia, radiographic abnormalities, or pulmonary infiltrates. The syndrome usually arises within a few hours after exposure and resolves within 1 day, with no residual effects. The mechanism seems to be an immunologic reaction in the alveolus, causing release of cytokines and immune mediators. Repeated exposures cause a "desensitization" or tachyphylaxis, whereby symptoms are worse at the beginning of the work week ("Monday morning fever"), and repeated exposures may elicit no symptoms at all.

Diagnosis is made based on the above-mentioned criteria, after ruling out influenza or other infectious causes. Treatment for inhalational fevers is supportive because this clinical entity is entirely self-limited. Proper education of the worker regarding the exposures that lead to this syndrome can prevent further episodes.

Many of the occupational settings where inhalational fevers occur also harbor risks of other acute lung injuries. Welding of stainless steel produces zinc oxide fumes responsible for MFF, welding metal with cadmium can produce acute lung injury, and high-temperature arc welding in a confined space can cause significant nitrogen dioxide (NO_2) exposure leading to ARDS. Farmers who unload silos may be exposed to silage that is contaminated with thermophilic bacteria and molds that can cause inhalational fever ("silo unloader's disease"), but exposure to freshly stored silage can cause silo filler's disease owing to liberation of NO_2 (acute lung injury). Farmers with moldy hay exposure may induce hypersensitivity pneumonitis as a result of exposure to the thermophilic bacteria that grow in wet hay.

In contradistinction to inhalational fevers, the acute lung injury due to hypersensitivity pneumonitis often is accompanied by cough, dyspnea, hypoxemia, and pulmonary infiltrates on chest radiographs. Although fever is required for the diagnosis of inhalational fevers, fever may also be present in hypersensitivity pneumonitis or in acute lung injury. The key distinguishing feature is that inhalational fevers have no chest x-ray abnormalities and usually no hypoxia, whereas chest x-ray abnormalities and hypoxia are prominent features of ARDS and of hypersensitivity pneumonitis. Repeated exposures to the causative agents of inhalational fevers cause a tolerance or significantly diminished response. Repeated insults of hypersensitivity pneumonitis and ARDS often cause pulmonary function abnormalities, however, and can lead to fibrosis and restrictive lung disease. Attack rates after typical exposures for inhalational fevers are often greater than 80%, whereas hypersensitivity pneumonitis occurs only in a small percentage of individuals exposed. Sensitization is required for the development of hypersensitivity pneumonitis, but this is not true for inhalational fevers. Repeated bouts of inhalational fevers due to certain materials (humidifier fever) may predispose individuals to the development of hypersensitivity pneumonitis.

Metal Fume Fever. Heating metals above their melting point, such as while welding, causes formation of solid aerosols (fumes), often with accompanying oxidation. The resultant particle size of 0.1 to 1.0 μm easily reaches the alveoli, where an acute inflammatory cell response causes release of cytokines, producing the constellation of symptoms. The classic syndrome involves a metallic taste in the mouth, fever, rigors, headache, chest pain, and dyspnea

with an abrupt onset 4 to 12 hours after exposure. Clinical tolerance to these effects occurs after regular exposure.[17] Zinc oxide fumes are the classic cause of MFF, and in the 18th century this was predominantly seen in brass foundries—hence the common name of *brasser's flu* or *brass founder's ague*. More recently, MFF has been seen after welding galvanized steel, from the heating of zinc in the galvanized coatings.[18,19] Limited epidemiologic evidence suggests that other metal fumes, such as the fumes produced when magnesium and copper are heated, can produce MFF.[20,21]

Polymer Fume Fever. Heating of polytetrafluoroethylene (PTFE, Teflon) causes formation of pyrolysis degradation products, the inhalation of which can lead to polymer fume fever. This fever occurs commonly when PTFE-coated metals are welded or flame cut. It also may occur after smoking cigarettes that are contaminated with PTFE resins from the hands of workers. This usually self-limited, flulike illness presents similarly to MFF, and diagnosis is based on the history of appropriate exposure. With prolonged exposures or when higher temperatures are involved, pulmonary involvement with accompanying chest x-ray findings of consolidation is possible.[22] There has even been a case of PFF from burning of the PTFE coating of a nonstick frying pan.[23]

Humidifier Fever. Humidifier fever is an inhalational fever caused by exposure to air contaminated by humidifier water that has excessive growth of microorganisms, most notably *Pseudomonas* and other gram-negative bacteria. It is a self-limited syndrome with features strikingly similar to MFF, and diagnosis usually is made after numerous workers from the same building present with the appropriate signs and symptoms. It occurs more often during winter months, when these humidification systems are commonly in use, and nonsmokers are more susceptible than smokers. Humidifier fever is not to be confused with humidifier lung, which is a type of hypersensitivity pneumonitis that occurs after long-term exposure to humidifier contaminants. There may be considerable overlap of these entities.[9]

Pontiac Fever. Pontiac fever can be thought of as a type of humidifier fever that is caused by exposure to water contaminated by *Legionella pneumophila*. In contrast to legionnaires' disease caused by the same organism, Pontiac fever is a self-limited, flulike illness that has occurred after common source exposure to buildings with contaminated air-conditioning systems (County Health Department Building in Pontiac, Michigan, in 1968, hence the name). It also has been seen after *Legionella* contamination of indoor fountains, whirlpools, and spas.[24,25]

Organic Dust Toxic Syndrome. Organic dust toxic syndrome (previously called *pulmonary mycotoxicosis*) is a catch-all term applied to a variety of inhalational fevers that occur after exposure to many different organic dust mixtures.[26,27] Many of these dusts are associated with agricultural industries and include bacteria, fungi, grains, silage, hay, animal danders, pollen, and other complex mixtures. Symptoms include fever, malaise, chest tightness, cough, and generalized aches. Hypoxia and chest x-ray abnormalities are typically absent, and the syndrome usually resolves without sequelae.[28] There is a strong overlap, however, with the causative agents of hypersensitivity pneumonitis, and in these exposure settings, hypersensitivity pneumonitis must be ruled out (see next).

Hypersensitivity Pneumonitis (Extrinsic Allergic Alveolitis). Hypersensitivity pneumonitis is an interstitial lung disease probably caused by a combination of type III (humoral or IgG-mediated) and type IV (cell-mediated) delayed hypersensitivity reactions that occur after exposure to a wide variety of antigens and some chemicals. Hypersensitivity pneumonitis most commonly has been associated with occupations with exposures to moldy organic materials, such as moldy hay in farmer's lung and moldy grain in grain handler's lung. It also can be seen in animal handlers secondary to exposure to animal proteins and excreta (pigeon breeder's lung). Exposures to various chemicals that also cause occupational asthma (e.g., TDI, TMA) also have been implicated in hypersensitivity pneumonitis.[29]

The pathophysiology of hypersensitivity pneumonitis involves immune complex deposition in the lung of sensitized individuals, with the resultant release of immune mediators and cytokines and inflammatory cell infiltration. Acutely, neutrophils are involved, but later lymphocytes predominate. The typical presentation occurs 4 to 6 hours after an intense inhalational exposure to the responsible antigen, and patients commonly have fever, chills, malaise, cough, and dyspnea. Chest x-rays are abnormal in greater than 80% of cases and often have a reticulonodular pattern or reveal patchy infiltrates. There is usually hypoxia, and patients have crepitant rales on auscultation of the chest. Pulmonary function testing can be normal or may show a restrictive defect and a decreased diffusion capacity. The acute episode usually resolves within 1 to 3 days, and corticosteroid treatment may be of some benefit. Repeated exposures often cause a worsening of the presentation; tolerance, such as that seen in inhalational fevers, does not occur. Repeated low-level exposures cause a progressive, often irreversible, pulmonary fibrosis. These patients may present from a typical occupational setting with the insidious onset of a constellation of signs and symptoms, including dyspnea, cough, weight loss, and fatigue. Chest x-rays may reveal increased interstitial markings and fibrosis, and pulmonary function testing usually shows restrictive disease and decreased diffusion capacity.

Treatment consists of administering oxygen and admission to the hospital when necessary. Corticosteroids are the only medications of any utility in the treatment of hypersensitivity pneumonitis. They have benefit in acute attacks; prednisolone, 1 mg/kg/day, is given. The mainstay of treatment is withdrawal from exposures, however, and prevention of any further contact with the inciting antigen or chemical.[29,30]

Miscellaneous Causes of Noncardiogenic Pulmonary Edema. Exposures to metal fumes, such as cadmium, manganese, and mercury, can induce an MFF-like illness, which then progresses hours later to acute chemical pneumonitis and pulmonary edema. This illness also can occur after exposure to gaseous metal compounds, such as nickel carbonyl, vanadium pentoxide, and zinc chloride.[20]

Toxins other than the above-described irritant gases can cause noncardiogenic pulmonary edema/ARDS by altering pulmonary capillary membrane permeability. Fluid can leak into the alveolar air spaces with subsequent pulmonary edema. Examples are the pesticides dinitrophenol and pentachlorophenol. These toxins act similarly to salicylates in that they uncouple oxidative phosphorylation, leading to a hypermetabolic state with fever, tachypnea, sweating, and pulmonary edema.[31] The acetylcholinesterase-inhibiting pesticides (organophosphates, carbamates) and nerve agents cause acetylcholine excess and can lead to cholinergic excess and muscarinic effects with copious pulmonary secretions and pulmonary edema. Neuromuscular blockade from the nicotinic effects of these insecticides can contribute to the respiratory failure and deaths associated with large exposures. Massive poisoning by a type II pyrethroid insecticide can cause pulmonary edema that has been mistaken for a reaction to an organophosphate. Subsequent atropine treatment was ineffective, and some deaths have occurred owing to atropine toxicity.[32] Aspiration of hydrocarbon solvents also can lead to pneumonitis and ARDS (see Chapter 84).

OCCUPATIONAL CARDIAC TOXICOLOGY

A variety of toxins encountered in the workplace can have deleterious effects on the heart (Table 13-4).

Myocardial Infarction

Carbon disulfide is the classic industrial toxin associated with accelerated atherosclerotic disease in workers. This property has been known for more than 100 years and was well described in the occupational literature.[33] The mechanism by which carbon disulfide causes accelerated atherosclerosis is poorly understood but may be mediated by its propensity to inhibit various enzyme systems. Workers exposed to carbon disulfide may have five times the incidence of coronary disease compared with nonexposed workers. Carbon disulfide also can cause peripheral neuropathies and neurobehavioral abnormalities.[34]

Carbon monoxide is the leading cause of toxic deaths in workers. Chronic exposure is believed to accelerate atherogenesis, and acute exposures to high levels can induce myocardial infarction, vasospasm, and sudden death. Mechanisms and treatment of carbon monoxide poisoning are described in Chapter 94.

Organic nitrates, such as nitroglycerin and ethylene glycol dinitrate, are used in the manufacture of explosives. Because they are well absorbed by inhalation and through the skin, workers can have significant systemic effects from simply handling or packing explosives. After a few years of exposure, the coronary vasodilatory effects of the nitrates are opposed by vasoconstriction. When organic nitrate exposure is withdrawn abruptly, the vasoconstriction is unopposed, and coronary vasospasm ensues with subsequent angina, myocardial infarction, or sudden death ("Monday morning angina"). Treatment is directed at reversing coronary vasospasm with calcium channel blockers and nitrates and prevention of further exposures.

TABLE 13-4 Serious Illnesses, Selected Causative Agents, and Associated Occupations/Workers*

ILLNESS	CAUSATIVE AGENT	ASSOCIATED OCCUPATIONS/WORKERS
ARDS (also possible late sequelae of RADS, BOF)	Irritant gases	
	Soluble gases	
	HCl, HF, H_2SO_4, HNO_3, NH_3, and other alkali and acid mists	Acid and alkali production workers; manure pit workers (NH_3)
	SO_2	Sulfuric acid production workers; air pollutant workers
	Tear gas	Law enforcement workers
	Isocyanates	Polyurethane industry workers, firefighters
	Insoluble gases	
	Phosgene	Polymer industry workers, welders, burning chlorinated metal degreasers
	NO_2	Silo fillers, high-temperature arc welders
	Medium-solubility gases	
	Chlorine	Water purification workers, paper pulp workers, swimming pool workers
	Acrolein	Polymer industry workers, firefighters (component of smoke)
	Smoke inhalation	Firefighters
	Pesticides	
	Organophosphates, carbamates, type II pyrethroids, dinitrophenol, pentachlorophenol (wood preservative), paraquat	Farmers, exterminators, crop dusters, pest control workers, lumber industry workers
	Metals and metal compounds	
	Cadmium, mercury, manganese, $Ni(CO)_4$	Smelters
Acute toxic encephalopathy		
	Lead	Lead-acid battery workers, HAZMAT site clean-up workers, lead reclamation workers, automobile radiator repair workers
	Mercury	Chlor-alkali workers (electrolytic production of chlorine and caustic soda), mercury-containing instrument manufacturers, fungicide users, topical antiseptics workers*
	Toluene, xylene, other hydrocarbon solvents	Painters, chemical production workers, solvent users (confined space)
	Simple asphyxiant gases (CO_2, CH_4, propane)	Gas production workers, various workers with confined space issues
	Cyanide	Metal plating workers, jewelers, firefighters (smoke inhalation)
	Hydrogen sulfide	Farmers (manure pits), sewer workers, petroleum refinery workers
	Carbon disulfide	Viscose rayon workers*, rubber manufacturers*
	Carbon monoxide	Garage workers, firefighters, paint strippers (methylene chloride) (any exposure to incomplete burning, improper ventilation, or exhaust)
Acute hemolysis		
	Chlorates	Match and explosive production workers, dye manufacturers, paper pulp bleach manufacturers (ClO_2)
	Arsine (AsH_3), stibine (SbH_3)	Workers with dopant gas for n-type semiconductors in the microelectronics industry
	Organic nitro and amino compounds	Synthetic dyes workers, leather and shoe industry workers, fabric dyers*
Cyanosis		
	Methemoglobin-forming agents: organic amino and nitro compounds*	Synthetic dyes workers, leather and shoe industry workers, fabric dyers*
	CNS depressants causing hypoventilation and hypoxia	Various workers (see acute toxic encephalopathy above)
Hyperthermia/fever		
	Pentachlorophenol—wood preservative	Lumber production workers
	Nitrophenol pesticides, chlorophenoxyacetic acid herbicides	Exterminators, pest control workers, agricultural workers, farmers, forestry workers, landscapers
	Inhalational fever syndromes	See fume fever syndromes below
Seizures		
	Metals	
	Arsenic	Copper smelters, leather tanning workers, pesticides workers
	Copper	Copper smelters, miners
	Lead	Lead-acid battery workers, Hazmat site clean-up workers, automobile radiator repair workers, lead reclamation workers

Continued

TABLE 13-4 Serious Illnesses, Selected Causative Agents, and Associated Occupations/Workers*—cont'd

ILLNESS	CAUSATIVE AGENT	ASSOCIATED OCCUPATIONS/WORKERS
	Manganese	Manganese miners, welders, chemical industry workers, metal refining workers
	Nickel	Workers in metal plating, coins, batteries, electronics, metal alloying industries
	Pesticides	
	Organochlorines* (lindane, cyclodienes, DDT), organophosphates, paraquat*, diquat (herbicides), pentachlorophenol, dinitrophenol, chlorophenoxyacetic acid herbicides	Farmers, agricultural workers, forestry workers, landscapers, pest control workers
	Rodenticides* (thallium, SMFA, strychnine, zinc phosphide, arsenic, methyl bromide)	Rodenticide users: granary workers, longshoremen, exterminators
	Phosphine, methyl bromide (fumigants)	Grain workers, pest control workers
	Any general CNS depressant producing hypoxia: toxic inhalants (CN, H_2S, carbon monoxide), simple asphyxiants (hydrocarbons, CO_2, He, N_2), chlorinated hydrocarbons	See acute toxic encephalopathy above
Rhabdomyolysis		
	Any agent causing seizures (see above)	See above
	Any agent causing hyperthermia associated with hypermetabolic state (pentachlorophenol, dinitrophenol, chlorophenoxy herbicides)	Farmers, lumber industry workers, pest control workers, exterminators
	Carbon monoxide (direct cellular toxicity)	Workers who have any exposure to incomplete burning, improper ventilation, or exhaust: garage workers, firefighters; paint strippers (methylene chloride)
	Any CNS depressants causing coma and inducing rhabdomyolysis from pressure	See acute toxic encephalopathy above
Fume fever syndromes		
	Metal fume fever	Welders (galvanized metal), foundry workers, smelting workers, metal refining workers
	Polymer fume fever	Welders (cutting through polytetrafluoroethylene coatings or polymer pipes), polymer workers
Organic dust toxic syndrome (ODTS) and other inhalational fevers		
	ODTS: Bioaerosols of fungi, bacteria, exotoxins	
	Moldy hay, moldy silage, compost	Farmers ("silo unloader's disease")
	Sewage sludge	Sewer workers, plumbers
	Grain dust	Grain mill workers (grain fever)
	Cotton dust	Cotton mill workers (mill fever)
	Animal confinement buildings	Veterinary workers, laboratory workers
	Other inhalational fevers	
	Contaminated humidifiers	Workers in any building with contaminated humidifiers (humidifier fever)
	Contaminated water cooling systems, spas, fountains	Workers in any building with contaminated cooling system or fountain (Pontiac fever)
	Contaminated wood dusts/chips/ bark (moldy wood chip exposure)	Sawmill workers, pulp and paper mill workers, landscapers ("wood-trimmer's disease")
Hypersensitivity pneumonitis		
	Organic antigen exposures	
	Moldy hay	Farmers (farmer's lung)
	Moldy compost	Mushroom workers (mushroom worker's lung)
	Contaminated humidifiers, dehumidifiers, HVAC	Office workers in any contaminated building (humidifier lung)

TABLE 13-4 Serious Illnesses, Selected Causative Agents, and Associated Occupations/Workers*—cont'd			
ILLNESS	**CAUSATIVE AGENT**	**ASSOCIATED OCCUPATIONS/WORKERS**
	Bagasse (moldy pressed sugarcane)	Sugarcane workers (bagassosis)
	Animal products (excreta, serum, feathers, dander)	Animal handlers (pigeon breeder's disease, duck fever)
	Chemicals	
	Trimellitic anhydride, phthalic anhydride	Painters, epoxy resin users
	Diisocyanates	Polyurethane foam industry workers
	Plicatic acid (red cedar)	Red cedar workers, lumber industry workers, carpenters
	Pyrethrum insecticides	Exterminators, pest control workers, insecticide manufacturers
	Sodium diazobenzene-sulfonate (Pauli's reagent)	Chromatographers
	Many others	Workers in varied industries
Myocardial infarction/ischemia		
	Carbon monoxide	Workers with exposure to exhaust or poorly ventilated combustion: miners, forklift operators, mechanics, firefighters
	Carbon disulfide	Viscose rayon workers*, rubber industry workers
Cardiac arrhythmias	Organic nitrates	Explosive industry (TNT) workers
Tachydysrhythmias		
	Chlorinated hydrocarbon	Mechanics, degreasers, dry cleaners
	Hydrocarbon solvents	Printers, painters, mechanics, degreasers, dry cleaners
	Carbon monoxide	Paint strippers (CH_3Cl), workers with exposure to exhaust or poorly ventilated combustion: miners, forklift operators, mechanics, firefighters
Bradydysrhythmias		
	Organophosphates, carbamates	Farmers, pest control applicators
Acute renal failure		
	Arsine, stibine (due to hemolysis)	Semiconductor industry workers
	Halogenated hydrocarbon solvents (many)	Dry cleaners, degreasers, plastics industry workers
	Toluene (ATN)	Painters
	Any agent associated with rhabdomyolysis	See rhabdomyolysis above
	Cadmium	Welders
Acute hepatic failure		
	CCl_4, CBr_4, $CHCl_3$, other halogenated hydrocarbons	Mechanics, degreasers, dry cleaners, plastics industry workers
	Solvents: 2-nitropropane, DMF	Painters
	Dimethylacetamide	Textile workers

*Many of the chemicals/toxins no longer may be used or manufactured in the United States, but still are in common use in other parts of the world. U.S. industries with modern industrial hygiene practices have limited or eliminated many exposures to industrial toxins, but workers in developing nations may remain at substantial risk.

ARDS, adult respiratory distress syndrome; ATN, acute tubular necrosis; BOF, bronchiolitis obliterans fibrosa; CN, cyanide; CNS, central nervous system; DDT, dichlorodiphenyltrichloroethane; HVAC, heating, ventilating, and air conditioning; RADS, reactive airways dysfunction syndrome; SMFA, sodium monofluoro acetate.

Data from references 9, 10, 12, 30, and 35.

Cardiac Dysrhythmia

Cardiac tachydysrhythmias can be caused by a variety of solvents, most notably chlorinated hydrocarbon solvents, such as trichloroethylene (TCE), but they also can occur with aromatics (xylene, toluene), aliphatic hydrocarbons (naphthas, gasoline), and chlorofluorocarbon refrigerants. These compounds sensitize the myocardium to the arrhythmogenic properties of catecholamines and in significant exposures can predispose the worker to tachydysrhythmias, syncope, and sudden death. Additionally, any toxin causing cellular hypoxia causes a subsequent tachycardia. This can include all the asphyxiants (carbon monoxide, hydrogen sulfide, cyanide, simple asphyxiants, irritant gases) and any

CNS depressant that causes hypoventilation and resultant hypoxia.

Cholinesterase-inhibiting pesticides, such as organophosphates, carbamates, and nerve agents, can cause effects secondary to an excess of acetylcholine and subsequent dysrhythmias. Depending on whether muscarinic or nicotinic effects predominate, tachycardia or bradycardia can be seen. There usually are other concomitant systemic signs of acetylcholine excess, such as *SLUDGE* (*s*alivation, *l*acrimation, *u*rination, *d*efecation, *g*astrointestinal cramping, and *e*mesis). There have been reports of QT prolongation and polymorphous ventricular tachycardia (torsades de pointes) associated with these insecticides. These agents are described in detail in Chapters 91 and 131. The heavy metals arsenic and thallium have been reported to cause QT prolongation and torsades de pointes as well (see Chapters 76 and 82).

OCCUPATIONAL HEPATIC TOXICOLOGY

Many toxins encountered in the workplace have effects on the liver (see Table 13-4) because these xenobiotics are metabolized by the same hepatic enzyme systems that metabolize pharmaceuticals. In many cases, such as with methanol, ethylene glycol, benzene, and *n*-hexane, the parent molecules are not toxic but are metabolized into toxic compounds or highly reactive intermediates. These metabolites exert the toxic effects in humans. In many cases, chronic ethanol intake is associated with an increased susceptibility to the hepatotoxic effects of these compounds, owing to P-450 enzyme induction. Many of the reported acute hepatotoxicities occur only after massive exposures. A wide variety of liver injury can be seen, however, after industrial exposures, including steatosis, cholestasis, hepatocellular necrosis, and vascular lesions.[36,37]

Halogenated Hydrocarbons

Halogenated hydrocarbons, primarily chlorinated hydrocarbons, are used mainly as solvents and degreasers. Many were used in the dry cleaning industry. The classic hepatotoxic chlorinated hydrocarbon is carbon tetrachloride. This compound is of historical interest because it was used widely as a solvent, degreaser, and fire extinguisher in the early 20th century. After large exposures, such as inhalation in a confined space or intentional suicidal ingestions, carbon tetrachloride caused a central lobular necrosis pattern similar to that seen with acetaminophen overdose. *N*-Acetylcysteine, the antidote for acetaminophen toxicity, has been used with success in carbon tetrachloride toxicity. Carbon tetrachloride is not used as widely today, having been replaced by other, less toxic products.[38] The main use of carbon tetrachloride is as a precursor for chlorofluorocarbons. Chloroform and carbon tetrabromide poisonings produce a similar pattern of hepatotoxicity. Other halogenated compounds, such as polychlorinated biphenyls and polybrominated biphenyls, have been associated with elevated liver enzymes and chloracne.[39]

The primary degreaser and dry cleaning agent in the United States today is tetrachloroethylene (perchloroethylene). In large exposures, it may be associated with acute hepatic injury.[40] Related compounds, TCE, trichloroethane, and tetrachloroethane, also are hepatotoxic in large doses.[41] All of these volatile compounds can cause CNS depression via a general anesthetic–type mechanism and can cause cardiac dysrhythmias (see earlier). Their thermal breakdown products include phosgene and hydrochloride (see earlier section on irritant gases).

Solvents

The solvent 2-nitropropane has been associated with acute hepatic failure after confined space exposures in painters.[42] *N,N*-Dimethylformamide can cause hepatic injury and a disulfiram-like reaction with ethanol ingestion.[12] Dimethylacetamide is a hepatotoxin used in acrylic fiber production.[43,44] Other petrochemicals have been implicated in liver injury.[45]

Miscellaneous Compounds

Trinitrotoluene (TNT), an explosive, and elemental white phosphorus have also been reported to cause acute hepatic injury. Compounds associated with chronic liver disease and hepatic angiosarcomas (vinyl chloride monomer, arsenic) occur in the workplace but are not of concern to the intensivist. Copper causes chronic hepatic injury, but only in individuals who are genetically predisposed.[21]

OCCUPATIONAL RENAL TOXICOLOGY

Acute Renal Failure

Many of the industrial hepatotoxic compounds also are injurious to the kidney, the most notable being carbon tetrachloride. Renal failure is usually a consequence of acute tubular necrosis due to volume depletion from the hepatotoxic effects. Because P-450 enzymatic metabolism of xenobiotics also occurs in the kidneys, there can be direct nephrotoxicity as well.[46] Toluene is metabolized to hippuric acid and can induce an elevated anion gap metabolic acidosis after significant intoxication, but this is seen primarily with intentional abuse and not workplace exposures. Renal failure has occurred secondary to acute tubular necrosis after toluene poisoning.[47] Other halogenated compounds associated with acute renal failure are chloroform, ethylene dichloride (solvent, fumigant), TCE, tetrachloroethane, vinylidene chloride (plastic intermediate), diesel fuel, and ethylene chlorohydrin (chemical intermediate).[48] Any compound that induces rhabdomyolysis can cause myoglobinuric renal failure (see Table 13-4). Treatment involves ensuring adequate urine volume and alkalinization of the urine to prevent pigment deposition in the renal tubular cells. Analogously, arsine and stibine gases cause acute renal failure because of hemoglobinuria induced by massive hemolysis. Exchange transfusions often are needed in addition to dialysis. Cadmium is associated with acute renal failure. Exposures in the industrial setting occur via torch-cutting or welding metals with cadmium coatings. Although chromium has been associated with acute tubular necrosis after massive oral exposures, these are not encountered in the workplace setting.[49] Arsenic, cadmium, and lead are known to induce chronic renal disease, and the effects of concomitant exposure to combinations needs further study.[50] By measuring LMW proteins (β-microglobulin, free retinol binding protein) in the urine of exposed workers, biomonitoring for early nephrotoxic effects is possible, but usually only as an epidemiologic tool.[51]

OCCUPATIONAL NEUROTOXICOLOGY

Central Nervous System

CNS depression caused by volatile solvents occurs commonly in the workplace and usually is due to inadequate ventilation or confined space issues. The CNS depression is due to the general anesthetic properties of these compounds. Any hydrocarbon or halogenated hydrocarbon can produce these effects, even chlorofluorocarbon refrigerants and Freon. Many workers have this type of exposure, including painters; mechanics; heating, ventilation, and air conditioning personnel; and workers in a varied assortment of occupations in which these solvents are used (Table 13-5). A purported chronic toxic encephalopathy due to long-term exposure to solvents, known as painter's syndrome, has been shown to be related to other factors, such as depres-

sion, low educational level, or chronic alcohol abuse, and not due to workplace exposures.[52] Many of these compounds, especially toluene and xylene, are inhaled intentionally for recreational use for their CNS depressant effects. Deaths have occurred in some cases owing to cardiac rhythm disturbances. Ethanol ingestion after TCE and trichloroethane exposure (and possibly other hydrocarbon

TABLE 13-5 Selected Occupations and Representative Possible Toxic Exposures*

OCCUPATIONS	POSSIBLE TOXIC EXPOSURES
Agriculturalist, farmer	Pesticides, H_2S, CH_4, NH_3, CO_2, NO_2; moldy hay (hypersensitivity pneumonitis), ODTS agents
Artist	Cadmium, toluene, other HC solvents, lead glazes as in ceramics
Battery manufacturer/reclamation	Lead, cadmium, mercury
Beautician/cosmetologist	Persulfates, phenylenediamine, thioglycolates
Carpenter/lumberjack	Plicatic acid (western red cedar), multiple wood dusts, wood preservatives (PCP, chromium-copper arsenate)
Chromatographer	Sodium diazobenzene-sulfonate (Pauli's reagent)
Construction worker	Asphalt, PAH, solvents, paints, glues, wood dusts, lead
Dentist/hygienist	Amalgams (silver, mercury), nitrous oxide
Electrician	PCBs, lead (cable splicing)
Electroplater	Chromium, copper, lead, Ni, cadmium, solvents
Firefighter	CO, CN, acrolein, phosgene, HCl, HF, NH_3, NO_2, SO_2, isocyanates, hydrocarbons, PAH, smoke
Forester/landscaper	Wood dusts, wood preservatives (PCP, copper arsenate), pesticides, herbicides
Foundry worker/smelter/metal refining	Zinc, copper, lead, mercury (gold and silver refining), cadmium (zinc smelting), acrolein, arsenic, selenium (copper refining by-product)
Health care worker	Ethylene oxide, mercury, natural rubber latex, formaldehyde, glutaraldehyde, radioisotopes, x-rays, chemotherapeutics, blood-borne pathogens, anesthetic gases
Heating, ventilation, and air conditioning personnel	Lead (solder), contaminated water coolant systems (Pontiac fever), contaminated humidifiers (humidifier fever), natural gas, PAH
Highway worker	PAH (coal tar fumes), HC solvents, CO (exhaust)
Jeweler	CN, zinc, lead, solvents
Law enforcement personnel	Lead (firing ranges), CO (traffic exhaust), tear gas
Machinist	Cutting oils, solvents
Mason	CaOH (lime)
Mechanic/gas station attendant	CO, trichloroethylene, gasoline (HCs, benzene, MTBE, ethanol), lead
Mortician	Embalming fluids: formaldehyde, methanol, glutaraldehyde, isopropanol
Painter	TDI, solvents: toluene, xylene, turpentine, VOCs, CH_3Cl, lead
Paper pulp industry worker	Chlorine dioxide, chlorine, H_2S, SO_2, methyl mercaptan
Pest control/exterminator	Pesticides: organophosphates, carbamates, pyrethroids; HC solvents, herbicides, wood preservatives (PCP, chromium-copper arsenate)
Petroleum refinery worker	Gasoline, benzene, MTBE, PAH, ethanol
Plumber	Sewage, lead (solder)
Printer	Solvents: naphthas, toluene, xylene
Semiconductor industry worker	Dopant gases: arsine (AsH_3), stibine (SbH_3); gallium arsenide, diborane, phosphine, solvents, HF
Shipbuilder	Styrene
Shoemaker/repairer	Hexacarbons: n-hexane, methyl n-butyl ketone; solvents: benzene, toluene, cyclohexane
Textile worker	DMF, PTFE, dimethylacetamide, dyes; CS_2 (viscose rayon)
Trucker	CO, diesel exhaust, lead
Veterinarians/animal handlers	Pesticides, animal dander
Welders	NO_2, phosgene, zinc oxide fumes (metal fume fever), polymer (polymer fume fever), lead, mercury, cadmium, chromium

*Many of the chemicals/toxins no longer may be used or manufactured in the United States but are still in common use in other parts of the world. U.S. industries with modern industrial hygiene practices have limited or eliminated many exposures to industrial toxins, but workers in developing nations may remain at substantial risk.
CN, cyanide; CO, carbon monoxide; DMF, N,N-dimethylformamide; HC, hydrocarbon; HF, hydrofluoric acid; MTBE, methyl-*tert*-butyl ether; ODTS, organic dust toxic syndrome; PAH, polycyclic aromatic hydrocarbons; PCB, polychlorinated biphenyls; PCP, pentachlorophenol; PTFE, polytetrafluoroethylene; TDI, toluene 2,4-diisocyanate; VOCs, volatile organic compounds.

solvents) induces a disulfiram-like reaction known as degreaser's flush, which may induce hypotension and subsequent syncope. Any asphyxiant gas can cause CNS depression secondary to oxygen deprivation, including the simple asphyxiants, such as carbon dioxide, methane, and nitrogen, and the toxic asphyxiants, such as carbon disulfide, cyanide, and hydrogen sulfide (see earlier section on pulmonary toxicology).

Some occupational toxicants have been shown to cause CNS stimulation and occasionally seizures; these include the organochlorine insecticides DDT, cyclodienes, chlordecone, lindane, and related compounds.[53,54] Although most no longer are registered with the U.S. Environmental Protection Agency and have been banned in Canada and Europe, developing nations still use these products extensively for pest control. Additionally, any agent that causes hypoxia or CNS depression to the point of hypoventilation can cause seizures by that mechanism (see Table 13-4).

Severe, acute poisoning by a few neurotoxins can induce a parkinsonian-like neurologic disorder. The most common such neurotoxin is carbon monoxide, which causes ischemic injury to the basal ganglia. Similarly manganese,[55] carbon disulfide, and methanol have been reported to cause this syndrome. Lead poisoning can cause an acute encephalopathy with coma or seizures or both, primarily seen in the pediatric population. The same blood levels associated with lead encephalopathy in children are well tolerated in adult workers after short-term exposures. Mercury is well known to exert most of its toxicity on the CNS.[27] The most toxic form, methylmercury, was the cause of severe permanent CNS impairment in children in Japan, termed *Minamata disease.* Mothers ate fish contaminated with methylmercury from industrial wastes dumped in Minamata Bay.[56] The potency of other organic mercurials cannot be discounted. A chemistry professor in New England suffered a fatal neurodegenerative disease after gloved-hand exposure to only a few drops of a related compound, dimethylmercury, used as a nuclear magnetic resonance reagent.[57] Ethylene oxide is used as a gas sterilant for surgical equipment. It can cause CNS depression and peripheral neuropathy.

Peripheral Neuropathy

A wide assortment of toxins have been associated with peripheral neuropathy, including the hexacarbons (hexane, methyl n-butyl ketone), carbon disulfide, acrylamide monomer, lead, arsenic, thallium, mercury, and ethylene oxide. Certain organophosphates that inhibit the enzyme neuropathy target esterase induce a delayed myeloneuropathy called *organophosphate-induced delayed neuropathy.* This was seen during Prohibition when alcoholics drank Jamaican ginger extracts contaminated with triorthocresyl phosphate. More recently, there have been reports of occupationally induced organophosphate-induced delayed neuropathy in the Chinese medical literature, mainly due to exposures to methamidophos.[58] Many older pesticides can cause chronic effects on the peripheral nervous system, owing to their heavy metal components, such as arsenic, lead, mercury, and thallium.[59]

OCCUPATIONAL HEMATOPOIETIC TOXICOLOGY

Methemoglobinemia and Hemolysis

Many aromatic amino and nitro compounds are strong oxidizing agents. They are used as chemical intermediates, in the production of aniline dyes, and as accelerators and antioxidants in rubber production. These compounds can oxidize the ferrous iron in hemoglobin, causing methemoglobinemia (see Chapter 28). Nitrates from fertilizers, TNT, and naphthalene are other compounds that have been shown to cause methemoglobinemia. Chlorates, used in match and explosive manufacturing, can cause oxidation of the hemoglobin and denaturing of the protein molecule. The end result is methemoglobinemia unresponsive to methylene blue, the antidote, and hemolysis frequently is seen. Arsine and stibine are semiconductor dopant gases that add a controlled amount of impurities to the silicon wafer to alter its electrical conductivity. Even brief exposures to these toxins can cause severe hemolysis, with subsequent acute renal failure and death in some cases.[20]

Aplastic Anemia

Benzene is a well-known bone marrow toxin, exerting these effects through its electrophilic reactive metabolite benzene epoxide. Exposures can cause depression of all blood cell lines, and it has been shown to be a cause of aplastic anemia and acute myeloblastic leukemia. Other marrow toxins shown to cause aplastic anemia are ionizing radiation and chemotherapeutic agents (alkylating agents and antimetabolites).

REFERENCES

1. U.S. Department of Labor: 2000 Census of fatal occupational injuries. Available at: http://www.bls.gov/iif/oshwc/cfoi/cftb132.txt. Accessed May 2002.
2. U.S. Department of Labor, Bureau of Labor Statistics: 1999 Lost-worktime injuries and illnesses. Available at: http://www.bls.gov/iif/oshwc/cfoi/cftb132.txt. Accessed May 2002.
3. Banks DE, Wang ML (eds): Occupational asthma. Occup Med State Art Rev 15:335–484, 2000.
4. Tarlo SB, Leung K, Broder I, et al: Asthmatic subjects symptomatically worse at work: Prevalence and characterization among a general asthma clinic population. Chest 118:1309–1314, 2000.
5. Malo JL: How much asthma can be attributed to occupational factors (revisited)? Chest 118:1232–1234, 2000.
6. Smith DC: Acute inhalation injury. Clin Pulm Med 6:224–235, 1999.
7. Chan-Yeung M, Malo J-L: Current concepts: Occupational Asthma. N Engl J Med 333:107–112, 1995.
8. Rabatin JT, Cowl CT: A guide to the diagnosis and treatment of occupational asthma. Mayo Clin Proc 76:633–640, 2001.
9. Rom WN (ed): Environmental and Occupational Medicine, 3rd ed. Philadelphia, Lippincott-Raven, 1998.
10. Zenz C (ed): Occupational Medicine, 3rd ed. St Louis, Mosby, 1994.
11. Gabbay DS, De Roos F, Perrone J: Twenty-foot fall averts fatality from massive hydrogen sulfide exposure. J Emerg Med 20:141–144, 2001.
12. National Library of Medicine: Hazardous substances database (HSDB). Available at: http://toxnet.nlm.nih.gov/. Accessed May 2002.
13. NIOSH pocket guide to chemical hazards. Available at: http://www.cdc.gov/niosh/npg/npgd0000.html-H. Accessed May 2002.
14. NIOSH international chemical safety cards. Available at: http://www.cdc.gov/niosh/ipcsneng/neng0000.html. Accessed May 2002.
15. New Jersey Department of Health and Senior Services: Right to know hazardous substance fact sheets. Available at: http://www.state.nj.us/health/eoh/rtkweb/ Accessed May 2002.

16. Taylor AJN: Occupational lung disease: 5. Respiratory irritants encountered at work. Thorax 51:541–545, 1996.
17. Fine JM, Gordon T, Chen LC, et al: Characterization of clinical tolerance to inhaled zinc oxide in naïve subjects and sheet metal workers. J Occup Environ Med 42:1085–1091, 2000.
18. Gordon T, Fine JM: Metal fume fever. Occup Med 8:504–517, 1993.
19. Barceloux DG: Zinc. Clin Toxicol 37:279–292, 1999.
20. Nemery B: Metal toxicity and the respiratory tract. Eur Respir J 3:202–219, 1990.
21. Barceloux DG: Copper. Clin Toxicol 37:217–230, 1999.
22. Shusterman DJ: Polymer fume fever and other fluorocarbon pyrolysis-related syndromes. Occup Med 8:519–531, 1993.
23. Blandford TB, Seamon PJ, Hughes R, et al: A case of polytetrafluoroethylene poisoning in cockatiels accompanied by polymer fume fever in the owner. Vet Rec 96:175–178, 1975.
24. Fang GD, Yu VL, Vickers, RM: Disease due to Legionellaceae (other than *Legionella pneumophila*): Historical, microbiological, clinical, and epidemiological review. Medicine 68:116–132, 1989.
25. Fields BS, Haupt T, Davis JP, et al: Pontiac fever due to *Legionella micdadei* from a whirlpool spa: Possible role of bacterial endotoxin. J Infect Dis 184:1289–1292, 2001.
26. Singh N, Davis GS: Review: Occupational and environmental lung disease. Curr Opin Pulm Med 8:117–125, 2002.
27. Hu H: Exposure to metals. Prim Care 27:983–996, 2000.
28. Von Essen S, Fryzek J, Nowakowski B, Wampler M: Respiratory symptoms and farming practices in farmers associated with an acute febrile illness after organic dust exposure. Chest 116:1452–1458, 1999.
29. Beckett WS: Current concepts: Occupational respiratory diseases. N Engl J Med 342:406–413, 2000.
30. Cormier Y, Desmeules M: Treatment of hypersensitivity pneumonitis (HP): Comparison between contact avoidance and corticosteroids. Can Respir J 1:223–228, 1994.
31. Jorens PG, Schepens PJC: Human pentachlorophenol poisoning. Hum Exp Toxicol 12:479–495, 1993.
32. He F, Wang S, Liu L, et al: Clinical manifestations and diagnosis of acute pyrethroid poisoning. Arch Toxicol 63:54–58, 1989.
33. Hamilton A: Exploring the Dangerous Trades. Beverly, MA, OEM Press, 1995.
34. Beauchamp RO, Bus JS, Popp JA: A critical review of the literature on carbon disulfide toxicity. Crit Rev Toxicol 11:169–278, 1983.
35. LaDou J (ed): Occupational and Environmental Medicine, 2nd ed. Stamford, CT, Appleton & Lange, 1997.
36. Zimmerman HJ, Lewis JH: Chemical- and toxin-induced hepatotoxicity. Gastroenterol Clin North Am 24:1027–1045, 1995.
37. Batt AM, Ferrari L: Manifestations of chemically induced liver damage. Clin Chem 41:1882–1887, 1995.
38. ATSDR Case Studies in Environmental Medicine: Carbon tetrachloride toxicity. Am Fam Physician 46:1199–1207, 1992.
39. Lemesh RA: Polychlorinated biphenyls: An overview of metabolic toxicologic and health consequences. Vet Hum Toxicol 34:256–260, 1992.
40. Lash LH, Parker JC: Hepatic and renal toxicities associated with perchloroethylene. Pharmacol Rev 53:177–208, 2001.
41. Zimmerman HJ: Hepatotoxicity. Dis Mon 39:675–787, 1993.
42. Harrison R, Letz G, Pasternak G, Blanc P: Fulminant hepatic failure after occupational exposure to 2-nitropropane. Ann Intern Med 107:466–468, 1987.
43. Baum SL, Surunda AJ: Toxic hepatitis from dimethylacetamide. Int J Occup Environ Health 3:1–4, 1997.
44. Spies GJ, Rhyne RH Jr, Evans RA, et al: Monitoring acrylic fiber workers for liver toxicity and exposure to dimethylacetamide: 2. Serum clinical chemistry results of dimethylacetamide-exposed workers. J Occup Environ Med 37:1102–1107, 1995.
45. Cotrim HP, Andrade ZA, Parana R, et al: Nonalcoholic steatohepatitis: A toxic liver disease in industrial workers. Liver 19:299–304, 1999.
46. Lock EA: Mechanism of nephrotoxic action due to organohalogenated compounds. Toxicol Lett 46:93–106, 1989.
47. Reisen E, Teicher A, Jaffe R, et al: Myoglobinuria and renal failure in toluene poisoning. Br J Ind Med 32:163–164, 1975.
48. Nelson NA, Robins TG, Port FK: Solvent nephrotoxicity in humans and experimental animals. Am J Nephrol 10:10–20, 1990.
49. Wedeen RP, Lifen Q: Chromium-induced kidney disease. Environ Health Persp 92:71–74, 1991.
50. Madden EF, Fowler BA: Mechanisms of nephrotoxicity from metal combinations: A review. Drug Chem Toxicol 23:1–12, 2000.
51. Lauwerys R, Bernard A, Cardenas A: Monitoring of early nephrotoxic effects of industrial chemicals. Toxicol Lett 64/65:33–42, 1992.
52. Albers JW, Berent S: Controversies in neurotoxicology. Neurol Clin 18:741–763, 2000.
53. Grutsch JF, Khasuwinah A: Signs and mechanisms of chlordane intoxication. Biomed Environ Sci 4:317–326, 1991.
54. Hayes WJ: Chlorinated hydrocarbon insecticides. In Hayes WJ, Lawes ER (eds): Pesticides Studied in Man. San Diego, Academic Press, 1991.
55. Barceloux DG: Manganese. Clin Toxicol 37:293–307, 1999.
56. Walker B: Neurotoxicity in human beings. J Lab Clin Med 136:168–180, 2000.
57. Nierenberg DW, Nordgren RE, Chang MB, et al: Delayed cerebellar disease and death after accidental exposure to dimethylmercury. N Engl J Med 338:1672–1676, 1998.
58. He F: Neurotoxic effects of insecticides—current and future research: A review. Neurotoxicology 21:421–433, 2000.
59. Keifer MC, Mahurin RK: Chronic neurologic effects of pesticide overexposure. Occup Med 12(2):291–304, 1997.

CHAPTER 14

Complications of Chronic Alcoholism That Affect Critical Illness

Alison L. Jones

The worldwide consumption of alcohol is increasing. For uniformity, the consumption of alcohol often is expressed in terms of *units* of ethanol ingested. Table 14-1 shows how units of alcohol routinely are calculated. Not everyone who abuses alcohol develops liver damage, however.[1,2] It is estimated that at least 80% of heavy drinkers show some features of fatty liver, 10% to 35% develop alcoholic hepatitis, and 10% develop cirrhosis.[1] A retrospective study in men showed that 50% of men with an average intake of alcohol of greater than 160 g (15 to 16 units) per day for 20 years developed cirrhosis.[2] Later studies showed risk levels with alcohol consumption of 40 g (7 units) per day for men.[3] The duration of alcohol abuse seems important because neither cirrhosis nor alcoholic hepatitis was seen in patients who consumed 160 g (28 units) of ethanol per day for less than 5 years, whereas 50% of patients consuming these levels for an average of 21 years developed cirrhosis.[2]

In many parts of the world, alcoholism is increasing among women as the social stigma surrounding drinking declines and the access to alcohol becomes easier. Women are less likely to be suspected of alcohol abuse, present at more advanced stage of disease, and are more likely to relapse after treatment. The increased vulnerability of women to alcohol-induced liver injury has been attributed to significantly higher alcohol concentrations and area under the concentration-time curve compared with men.[4,5] In addition, women often weigh less than men and have a lower volume of distribution for alcohol.[4] Following a brief description of the pathophysiology and clinical features of liver injury due to alcohol, this chapter reviews the major syndromes in ethanol abusers that may precipitate or complicate an intensive care unit admission.

PATHOPHYSIOLOGY AND CLINICAL FEATURES OF LIVER INJURY

Alcoholic liver injury seems to progress from fatty change through alcoholic hepatitis to cirrhosis.[6] Most individuals who abuse alcohol develop fatty change in the liver at some stage. The full progression from fatty liver to cirrhosis occurs in about 20% of individuals.[7] Alcoholic hepatitis develops in only a proportion of drinkers, even after several decades of alcohol abuse, and is assumed to be precirrhotic, although it is not essential for progression.[8]

A fatty liver is characterized histologically by microvesicles and macrovesicles of fat within the hepatocyte.[6] Although fat accumulation in liver occurs, it is not necessarily harmful. Most individuals with fatty liver are asymptomatic, although some have right upper quadrant pain or nausea, epigastric discomfort, or bowel disturbances.[6] Hepatomegaly is the most common physical finding. The most common biochemical abnormality is elevation of γ-glutamyl transferase and aspartate aminotransferase. Serum bilirubin may be mildly elevated in 20% to 30% of cases. Alkaline phosphatase is elevated in about half of cases. Macrocytosis commonly is observed. Most laboratory abnormalities show marked improvement, if not complete reversal, with abstinence in a few weeks. Liver biopsy shows accumulation of triglycerides that may be mild, moderate, or severe in extent but is not required for management purposes.

Alcoholic hepatitis is characterized by the presence of neutrophils in the lobules of the liver together with necrosis of hepatocytes.[6] The clinical presentation may vary from incidental hepatomegaly to jaundice, ascites, bleeding, and coma. Most patients with mild-to-moderate hepatitis on liver biopsy have anorexia, fatigue, lethargy, or epigastric pain.[6] Patients with severe hepatitis tend to present with jaundice, ascites, hemorrhage, or encephalopathy. On examination, patients may have ascites (60%) and splenomegaly (15%). Fever is a feature in 50% of patients. Cutaneous bruising may be marked. Serum γ-glutamyl transferase and asparate aminotransferase invariably are increased and higher than in other forms of alcoholic liver disease; 66% of patients have increased serum bilirubin and alkaline phosphatase. More than half of patients are anemic, and macrocytosis is prominent. Patients with hepatitis often show a marked deterioration in condition when admitted to the hospital.

Cirrhosis is defined as widespread fibrosis and nodule formation within the liver.[6] It follows hepatocellular necrosis due to a variety of insults and reflects the fact that the liver's response to necrosis is limited.[6] The fibrosis disrupts hepatic architecture, impeding exchange of oxygen and nutrients through the basement membranes between liver cells and the blood and causing portal hypertension.[9] Cirrhosis usually is believed to be irreversible, but fibrosis has been shown to regress in hemochromatosis and Wilson's disease.

The clinical spectrum in cirrhosis varies widely from asymptomatic hepatomegaly to profound hepatocellular

TABLE 14-1 Calculation of Units for Alcohol*

TYPE OF DRINK	% ALCOHOL BY VOLUME	VOLUME	ALCOHOL CONTENT (UNITS)
Beer/lager/cider			
Alcohol-free	<0.05	440 mL	0
Low-alcohol	0.5–1.0	440 mL	0.4
		1 pint	0.6
Standard strength	3.0–4.0	1 pint	1.7–2.3
Premium strength	5.0–6.0	1 pint	2.8–3.4
"Alcopops"	5.0–6.0	330 mL	1.7–2.0
Wine	8.0–13.0	750 mL	6.0–10.0
Fortified wines			
(e.g., sherry, vermouth)	14.0–20.0	750 mL	10.5–15.0
Spirits (e.g., gin, vodka, rum)	37.5–40.0	700 mL	26.3–28.0

*1 Unit = Volume % ethanol × 0.78.

failure and portal hypertension with ascites or variceal hemorrhage.[6] Patients with alcoholic cirrhosis who are actively abusing alcohol are more likely to present with features of decompensation, owing to superimposed hepatitis. The most common physical sign is irregular hepatomegaly. Features of portal hypertension, such as collateral veins, are present in at least 60% of patients. Features of encephalopathy may be present in one third of patients. Patients who are abstinent may show few laboratory abnormalities. Plasma albumin concentrations are low in approximately half of patients, and macrocytosis is common.

COAGULOPATHY

A reduced platelet count in alcohol abusers usually results from the hypersplenism of alcoholic cirrhosis. Very low platelet counts often accompany portal hypertension despite relatively normal liver function tests.[10] There also are direct toxic effects of alcohol on platelet production and function.[10] The risk of bleeding is higher, at a given platelet count, in patients with infection or coexistent abnormalities of coagulation.

The liver plays a major part in the control of hemostasis. It produces vitamin K–dependent clotting proteins; factors II, VII, IX, and X; and proteins C and S. The liver also has a role in fibrinolysis by protein generation and clearing from the blood active enzymes. An increased prothrombin time is seen in alcoholic cirrhosis, although not typically in hepatitis or fatty liver, owing to decreased synthesis of clotting factors and increased fibrinolytic activity.[11]

Bleeding can complicate invasive procedures, such as liver biopsy or invasive hemodynamic monitoring, in patients with alcoholic cirrhosis. The best policy is to undertake invasive tests only if they are absolutely necessary in management of the patient. In the presence of coagulopathy or thrombocytopenia, the insertion of invasive catheters or intracranial pressure monitors should follow prophylactic administration of fresh frozen plasma, together with platelets if the platelet count is less than 50,000/mm³.[11] In acute liver failure due to acetaminophen (paracetamol) poisoning, fresh frozen plasma should not be given, however, unless there is active bleeding.[12] This therapy impedes use of the prothrombin time or international normalized ratio (INR), which is one of the best guides for transplant decisions.[12] The risk of bleeding in any patient with a coagulopathy can be diminished by use of sites for insertion of catheters where pressure can be applied (e.g., external jugular insertion of central venous line, rather than a supraclavicular or subclavian approach). Transthoracic liver biopsies should not be done when the INR is greater than 1.2. Safer alternatives include direct-vision laparoscopic liver biopsy with subsequent coagulation, and transjugular liver biopsy, which can be carried out even with an INR greater than 3.[13] Particular care must be taken with arterial blood gas sampling, and often insertion of an arterial catheter saves several attempts and reduces the risk of bleeding. Intramuscular injections should be avoided. Recombinant factor VII is a therapeutic advance that can fully correct coagulation and platelet function defects in cirrhosis and allow invasive procedures to be performed safely.[14]

Stable patients who are not bleeding and are not undergoing invasive procedures generally do not require therapy for coagulopathy. Patients who are actively bleeding need blood component therapy, coagulation factor therapy, treatment aimed at elevating the platelet count to greater than 50,000/mm³, and measures to control the bleeding (see later). Fresh frozen plasma is effective for correcting most of the clotting factors associated with alcoholic liver disease because it contains coagulation factors, coagulation inhibitors, and fibrinolytic inhibitors; it should be given until the measured INR or prothrombin time ratio is less than 1.2.[15] It does not contain activated clotting factors and does not precipitate or worsen the disseminated intravascular coagulation that can be seen in these patients.[16]

HEMODYNAMIC EFFECTS OF CHRONIC ALCOHOLISM

Hepatic cirrhosis causes portal hypertension, which is thought to result from an increased resistance to portal venous blood flow through the liver (backward resistance hypothesis) or from increased portal venous blood flow through the liver (forward flow mechanism). When the portal circulation is obstructed by cirrhosis, a collateral circulation that returns portal blood into the systemic veins develops. Blood from the gastroesophageal collaterals and the retroperitoneal and venous systems of the abdomen reaches the superior vena cava via the azygos or hemiazygos vein. The presence of these collaterals implies the existence of portal hypertension. The connection between portal and systemic circulations at the gastroesophageal junction is complex. Turbulent flow in perforating veins between the varices and the periesophageal veins at the lower end of the stomach may explain why esophageal variceal rupture is frequent in this region.[17]

In portal hypertension, gastric vascularity is abnormal. Submucosal arteriovenous communications develop between the muscularis mucosae and dilated precapillaries and veins.[18] This congestive gastropathy places the alcoholic at a significant risk of bleeding, especially damage from aspirin or nonsteroidal antiinflammatory drugs. Bleeding can occur from gastric red spots.[18] These gastric changes may be increased after successful esophageal sclerotherapy.[18] Decreasing the portal pressure is the main intervention that stops bleeding.

Generalized systemic vasodilation is the characteristic hemodynamic change seen in alcoholic cirrhosis. Several vasoactive substances, including glucagon, bile acids, prostaglandins, 5-hydroxytryptamine, endothelins, and nitric oxide, are active. What is not clear, however, is how vasodilation leads to the state of permanent high cardiac output and increased regional blood flow. Typical hemodynamic values in cirrhosis indicate peripheral vasodilation and increased cardiac index.[19] The greater the degree of hepatic decompensation, the more pronounced the hyperdynamic changes. The increased cardiac output is often associated with normal filling pressures, but cirrhotic patients have decreased myocardial contractility, which becomes apparent when afterload is increased and the myocardium is stressed. This situation suggests that the heart in cirrhosis shows evidence of "cirrhotic cardiomyopathy," some of which may be due to the acute effects of alcohol.[20] Patients with alcoholic cardiomyopathy may show low-output cardiac failure. If surgery is contemplated in a patient with chronic liver disease, it is wise to assess cardiac function by echocardiography first. Some degree of mitral regurgitation may be evident in individuals with a hyperdynamic circulation. Multiple gated acquisition (MUGA) radionuclide scans at rest and during exercise may be helpful to detect wall-motion abnormalities and to assess ejection fraction. In patients with liver disease, direct measurement of arterial pressure and central venous pressure is essential for all but the most minor of procedures. A pulmonary artery catheter is indicated if there is significant evidence of abnormal cardiac function. In individuals with serum bilirubin greater than 2.7 mg/dL, measurement of oxygen saturation by pulse oximetry may be inaccurate.

The inotropic and chronotropic responses of the heart to β-adrenergic agonists are impaired in patients with cirrhosis. In one study, cirrhotics showed a nonsignificant increase in stroke volume with infusion of dobutamine.[21] The dose of isoproterenol required to increase the heart rate by 25 beats/min was three times higher in cirrhotics than in

controls.[22] β-Adrenergic receptor density is reduced in cirrhotics, and they may not manifest an appropriate tachycardia when hemorrhaging.[23]

Insertion of a transjugular intrahepatic portosystemic stent shunt (TIPSS) (see later) may impair cardiac function and hemodynamics in patients with cirrhosis.[24] These patients have increased pulmonary capillary wedge pressure, diastolic dysfunction of the hyperdynamic left ventricle, and decreased systemic vascular resistance. The shunt reduces systemic vascular resistance further by diversion through the splanchnic circulation. TIPSS insertion may unmask a coexisting preclinical cardiomyopathy in patients with alcoholic cirrhosis.[24]

GASTROINTESTINAL BLEEDING

Hematemesis from esophageal varices is the most common presentation of portal hypertension due to cirrhosis, although melena, without hematemesis, may occur from bleeding varices and portal hypertensive gastropathy (see earlier). The larger and redder an esophageal varix, the more likely it is to bleed.[25] Esophageal bleeding generally is localized to within 5 cm above the cardia.[25] This is the area in which sclerotherapy and band ligation, the treatment of choice for acutely bleeding varices, is directed.[25] Variceal bleeding is a medical emergency, and its management should be undertaken by an experienced team. Initial therapy is aimed at correcting hypovolemic shock and achieving hemostasis at the bleeding site, preventing complications associated with bleeding (airway aspiration, encephalopathy, infections by enteric organisms, hypoxemia, renal dysfunction). Excessive transfusion may occur with a consequent risk of continued bleeding or rebleeding.[26]

Full discussion of the pharmacologic and endoscopic treatment modalities for acute variceal hemorrhage is beyond the scope of this chapter, and the reader is referred to an excellent review.[27] Vasopressin has been used in the treatment of acute variceal hemorrhage, but it is a powerful vasoconstrictor of coronary arteries, and its use in acute bleeding is controversial.[28,29] Somatostatin reduces portal pressure without the adverse effects on coronary arteries.[28,29] It causes splanchnic vasoconstriction and decreases portal and collateral blood flow and portal pressure but is of unproven efficacy.[30] Octreotide also reduces portal pressure and collateral blood flow and is effective in reducing blood loss and transfusion requirements as initial intervention and as adjunctive therapy to endoscopic measures.[31] It can be started quickly, has a relatively rapid onset of action, and is free of significant adverse effects.[31] Balloon tamponade is aimed at achieving temporary hemostasis by direct compression of bleeding varices. It is effective in controlling bleeding temporarily, but fatal complications occur in 6% to 20% of treated patients, including aspiration pneumonia and airway obstruction.[32]

Mortality from esophageal bleeding is approximately 50% within 6 weeks of the bleed.[33] The risk of rebleeding during admission depends on the severity of the underlying liver disease and degree of portal hypertension. TIPSS placement (see later) leads to lower recurrent variceal bleeding rates and is more cost-effective in the short-term for prevention of recurrent esophageal variceal bleeding.[34]

ASCITES

Ascites is detectable free fluid in the peritoneal space. Portal hypertension due to cirrhosis is an important cause. Patients retain salt and water because homeostatic mechanisms become unbalanced, and the dysfunctional liver does not catabolize aldosterone efficiently.[35] In the later stages of cirrhosis, there may be absolute and relative reductions in renal blood flow and glomerular filtration rate as a result of vasoconstriction of the renal arteries. The kidney is less able to excrete free water because of reduced delivery of filtrate to the ascending loop of Henle and hypersecretion of antidiuretic hormone. Finally, an imbalance between the activity of endogenous vasoconstrictor systems, such as renin-angiotensin-aldosterone and sympathetic nervous systems, and the renal production of vasodilator substances, such as prostaglandins and renal kallikrein, may account more for the renal vasoconstriction.

The fact that patients with cirrhosis have hyperaldosteronism requires that particular caution be exercised in the amount of sodium given in food and intravenous fluids.[36] It is common to give too much saline in resuscitation, with the consequent development of ascites.

The treatment of ascites has been based on the combination of a low-sodium diet and the administration of diuretics, such as spironolactone (typically 100 mg/day). Paracentesis, with intravascular albumin repletion (40 mL of salt-poor albumin per liter of ascites removed), also has been effective management for ascites. Resistant ascites (and acute esophageal variceal bleeding) has been treated by radiographically guided insertion of a TIPSS.[37] The flow across the shunt can be monitored by Doppler ultrasound and revised if occlusion occurs. TIPSS seems to be superior to large-volume paracentesis, improves renal function, and can improve the chance of survival without liver transplantation in patients with refractory or recurrent ascites.[37]

HEPATORENAL SYNDROME

Hepatorenal syndrome is common in advanced cirrhosis and is characterized by renal failure due to marked renal hypoperfusion as the result of renal vasoconstriction and underfilling of the arterial circulation as a result of arterial vasodilation in the splanchnic circulation.[38] The diagnosis is by exclusion of nonfunctional causes of renal failure in a patient with advanced hepatic disease. The hepatorenal syndrome is characterized by a progressive increase in the plasma creatinine, oliguria, and low urinary sodium (usually <20 mmol/L) in the presence of normal-sized kidneys. The exact pathogenesis is not known but is probably due to intravascular volume depletion secondary to splanchnic arterial vasodilation.[39] Along with renal vasoconstriction, all other extrasplanchnic beds are vasoconstricted.

Prognosis in this condition is poor. A patient with hepatorenal syndrome should receive adequate rehydration. The role of dopamine is controversial.[39] TIPSS and hepatic transplantation have helped some patients.[40] The development of hepatorenal syndrome after spontaneous bacterial peritonitis (SBP) can be prevented effectively by the administration of albumin to patients who are hypoalbuminemic together with antibiotics (see the section on SBP for precise guidelines).[41,42] Splanchnic vasoconstrictors and V1 antagonists may improve renal function, according to preliminary studies.[43]

Acute tubular necrosis is often due to a combination of nephrotoxic drugs, such as aminoglycosides, and intravascular depletion.[42] Acute tubular necrosis is a more common cause of renal failure than hepatorenal syndrome in cirrhotic patients and should be excluded first.[42]

PULMONARY ABNORMALITIES ASSOCIATED WITH CHRONIC ALCOHOLISM

Patients with cirrhosis show a wide range of arterial oxygen tensions. The PO_2 may be normal, yet as a result of hypocapnia there is an increase in the alveolar/arterial PO_2 difference. Alternatively, some patients have mild-to-moderate hypoxemia—the hepatopulmonary syndrome. Patients with cirrhosis have pulmonary shunting, and this significantly increases cardiac work, but the exact form of shunting has been controversial. Many studies have failed to provide anatomic pathways for intrapulmonary shunts but implicate derangements of the pulmonary microcirculation sufficient to allow mixed venous blood to pass directly into the pulmonary veins. In addition, physiologic mechanisms almost certainly contribute to the hypoxemia of cirrhosis because a right shift in the oxygen dissociation curve occurs in many patients owing to an increase in 2,3-diphosphoglycerate.[44] This mechanism is insufficient, however, to explain the degree of hypoxemia. The multiple gas elimination technique has shown that ventilation/perfusion mismatching also may be responsible in some patients. Patients with lower pulmonary vascular resistance seem to have a greater mismatch.[45] Before anesthesia and surgery are contemplated, a complete assessment of the respiratory system of any patient with cirrhosis must be made. Many alcoholic cirrhotics are heavy cigarette smokers and develop bronchitis and emphysema, and as a result tidal volume, vital capacity, and functional residual capacity are reduced, and compensatory tachypnea may result in a respiratory alkalosis.

More severely hypoxic cirrhotic patients may show clinical evidence of dyspnea and cyanosis that improve with recumbency (platypnea). Standing increases the blood flow to dilated pulmonary vessels at the lung bases; these are poorly ventilated, so there is a further fall in PO_2. The combination of arterial hypoxemia and low pulmonary vascular resistance is unexplained but may be due to defective pulmonary vasoconstrictor response to hypoxia in some cirrhotics.[44]

Aspiration of blood or gastric secretions is particularly frequent in patients with impaired consciousness due to alcohol or hepatic encephalopathy. Prevention is based on well-trained nurses who position patients safely, intubation in comatose patients, and aspiration of gastric contents by nasogastric tubes. Times of particularly high risk are during hematemesis, emergency endoscopy, and placement of balloon tamponade tubes. Aspiration pneumonia should be treated with standard antibiotics when bacterial infection is suspected. Monitoring with pulse oximetry is recommended.

In addition to the usual causes in the critically ill alcoholic, adult respiratory distress syndrome has been associated with sodium morrhuate sclerotherapy.[46] This sclerosant contains several fatty acids that are toxic to the lung and may affect pulmonary hemodynamics with pulmonary hypertension associated with increased lymph flow of relatively protein-poor lymph.[46]

The incidence of pleural effusions is 5% to 6% in cirrhotics with ascites[47]; 67% are right-sided, and 17% are left-sided. Small holes have been detected in the diaphragm by several methods.[47,48] Pleural effusions usually respond to diuretics and salt and water restriction,[47] but when effusions are large, thoracentesis should be performed. Rarely, pleurodesis or TIPSS placement is necessary.[47] In any patient who abuses alcohol, but particularly in chronic alcoholics, pulmonary tuberculosis infection is common and must be excluded by chest x-ray and tuberculin testing.

SPONTANEOUS BACTERIAL PERITONITIS

SBP is a frequent complication in cirrhotic patients with ascites (incidence 7% to 23% of hospitalized cirrhotic patients) and has a mortality of 30% to 50%.[49] All hospitalized patients with ascites should have a diagnostic paracentesis performed even if they are in the hospital for an unrelated reason.

The diagnosis of SBP is made presumptively on the basis of abdominal pain or worsening ascites or a polymorphonuclear cell count in ascitic fluid greater than 250 cells/mm^3. The organism responsible is isolated in 60% to 70% of cases. This requires that samples be taken into blood culture bottles rather than sterile plastic universal tubes.[50] The treatment of choice is a third-generation cephalosporin. The remaining 30% are considered culture-negative but are treated with antibiotics anyway because of the risk of peritonitis and death if left untreated.[50] The SBP resolution rate ranges from 70% to 90%, and hospital survival is 50% to 70%. Despite the resolution of infection, SBP may trigger severe complications, such as renal failure, gastrointestinal bleeding, and hepatic insufficiency.[51] The development of hepatorenal syndrome after SBP in patients with cirrhosis can be prevented effectively by administration of albumin at a dose of 1.5 g/kg at the time of diagnosis, followed by 1 g/kg on day 3, together with antibiotics.[41] Prophylaxis against SBP can be undertaken with norfloxacin, but the incidence of quinolone-resistant organisms is increasing and may be a problem in the future.[50]

ENCEPHALOPATHY

Chronic hepatic encephalopathy is a neuropsychiatric disorder usually related to portosystemic shunts, dietary indiscretions, or accumulation of toxic substances not cleared by the failing liver. There also are changes to permeability in the blood-brain barrier and to neurotransmitter concentrations and cerebral metabolism. In patients who develop encephalopathy, it is important to exclude bacterial infections or gastrointestinal bleeding as a precipitant.[52] Most bacterial infections in cirrhotic patients are hospital acquired; urinary tract infections, SBP, respiratory tract infections, and bacteremia are the most frequent infections.[53] Encephalopathy is treated

with dietary protein restriction to less than 50 g/day and lactulose sufficient to achieve two or three soft bowel movements per day.[53] In the case of deep encephalopathy, oral intake is withheld for 24 to 48 hours, and intravenous glucose is given until improvement occurs. Enteral nutrition can be started if the patient appears unable to eat after this period; this is started at 0.5 g/kg/day and increased up to 1.5 g/kg/day gradually. The role of neomycin is controversial and requires careful monitoring.[54,55] Start neomycin at 250 mg orally two to four times per day up to 4 g/day. When anesthetizing these patients, it is appropriate to use a minimum of drugs.

ABNORMAL GLUCOSE METABOLISM

Most patients with cirrhosis show impaired glucose tolerance,[56] and there is a higher prevalence of overt diabetes than in the general population. Most cirrhotics are resistant to the effects of insulin, particularly on skeletal muscle. These patients also tend to have hyperinsulinemia[57] because of increased insulin secretion and reduced insulin clearance because of hepatocellular dysfunction or portosystemic shunting. Glucose intolerance is common in fatty liver associated with alcohol use.

Patients with postprandial hyperglycemia and minor increases of fasting blood glucose should be treated with a low-sugar diet. If persistent postprandial glucose elevations are 5.5 mmol/L (100 mg/dL) or greater, the patient should receive an oral hypoglycemic. Biguanides (e.g., metformin) should be avoided in patients with liver disease because they are at risk for serious drug-induced lactic acidosis. Sulfonylureas (e.g., tolbutamide and glipizide) can be used cautiously in alcoholic patients, but glibenclamide is best avoided because it can cause prolonged hypoglycemia. Patients who require insulin are managed best by injections of short-acting insulin 30 to 45 minutes before each meal. Patients with liver disease are more prone to fasting and nocturnal hypoglycemia, and longer-acting insulins should be avoided.

ALCOHOLIC KETOACIDOSIS

In alcoholic patients, metabolic acidosis can be due to lactic acidosis associated with sepsis or thiamine deficiency, alcoholic ketoacidosis (AKA), diabetic ketoacidosis, or methanol or ethylene glycol poisoning.[58] AKA occurs in alcoholics who have had a heavy drinking bout with subsequent vomiting, dehydration, starvation, and β-hydroxybutyrate–dominated ketoacidosis.[59] Awareness of the syndrome, a proper history, physical examination, and routine laboratory tests usually give the diagnosis.[59]

AKA and toxic alcohol ingestion can be difficult to distinguish on initial presentation. A high osmolar gap (e.g., >25 mmol/L) associated with increased anion gap acidosis is a strong indicator of methanol or ethylene glycol intoxication but is not specific, and history or analytic confirmation is crucial in determining cause.[59,60] Ethylene glycol and methanol poisoning are discussed in detail in Chapters 83 and 86, respectively.

In addition to a history of diabetes or alcoholism, patients with diabetic ketoacidosis are characterized by higher plasma glucose concentration (32 mmol/L [576 mg/dL] versus

6.6 mmol/L [119 mg/dL]) and lower β-hydroxybutyrate-to-acetoacetate and lactate-to-pyruvate ratios compared with patients with AKA.[61] If the serum glucose level (in mmol/L) is less than the anion gap, the diagnosis of AKA should be considered.[62] The initial hormone profile is characterized by decreased insulin levels in both conditions.

AKA is a cause of unexpected death in a chronic alcoholic with little or no alcohol in the blood, increased acetone concentration in the blood, and no specific features on autopsy or toxicology.[63] The diagnosis often is missed unless it is sought out specifically by analysis.

The treatment of AKA is replacement of fluid, glucose, electrolytes (especially potassium), and thiamine. Insulin or alkali should be avoided.[59] Some patients have serious co-existing acute illnesses, and treatment of these is essential.

ALTERED DRUG METABOLISM

Many factors determine the elimination of a drug, including its rate of absorption, distribution, plasma protein binding, and metabolism and elimination particularly by the liver and kidneys. The extraction ratio of a drug across an eliminating organ can be calculated by the clearance. Drugs are classified as highly cleared by the liver (>70% cleared at each passage through the liver), poorly cleared (<30%), or intermediate.[64] Hepatic clearance has an important effect on the extent to which drugs become available in the systemic circulation, particularly when given orally. Highly cleared drugs have high "first-pass" removal and low systemic availability.

Hepatic clearance of a drug is known to be a function of two factors[64]: (1) liver blood flow and (2) ability of the liver to remove the drug from the sinusoids. In the normal liver, the relative importance of each of these factors for a particular drug depends on its hepatic extraction ratio. For drugs with high extraction ratios, hepatic blood flow is the major factor determining its elimination.[64,65] In contrast, the elimination of drugs with low extraction ratios is determined by enzyme activity. This concept may be less important, however, in the presence of chronic liver disease than was previously

believed. Passayre and colleagues[66] showed that in cirrhosis, propranolol (a highly extracted drug in normal controls) no longer was highly extracted, and its hepatic clearance depended not only on liver blood flow but also, and predominantly, on the ability of the liver to remove drug from the blood. The main factor responsible for the reduced clearance of drugs metabolized by the liver in patients with cirrhosis seems to be impaired ability of the liver to remove the drug from the blood. Possible mechanisms are intrahepatic shunts, portasystemic shunts, reduced amounts of drug-metabolizing molecules, and reduced hepatic uptake of drugs. The metabolic capacity of the liver is not a homogeneous entity but depends on the metabolic pathways involved. Oxidation (phase I) takes place in the centrilobular location[67] and is more prone to hypoxia and more affected in liver disease than conjugation (phase II), which is periportal in location and well preserved in liver disease.[67]

Other mechanisms that could be responsible for altered drug kinetics in chronic liver disease include altered protein binding and acid-base or electrolyte changes. Many drugs commonly used in critical care units have reduced clearance or increased half-life in cirrhosis (Table 14-2). A significant increase in half-life calls for prolongation of the dosing interval, whereas a decrease in clearance calls for a reduction of dose (see Table 14-2). Whether a dose reduction is necessary also depends on the toxicity of a drug. For adequate antibiotic coverage in a patient with SBP, the dose of cephalosporin does not require reduction. For aminoglycosides, the dose and dosing interval must be reduced. In contrast, other drugs have high clearance in cirrhosis (Table 14-3).

Morphine and fentanyl have the most predictable narcotic effects and can be used safely in mild-to-moderate liver disease.[68] Pethidine (meperidine) should be used with care and reduced dosage.[69] Even moderate cirrhosis significantly reduces the clearance of alfentanil, which also must be used with care.[70]

The reduction of plasma pseudocholinesterase, which occurs with chronic liver disease, prolongs the duration of action of suxamethonium, but this seldom is clinically significant. Atracurium is the muscle relaxant of choice in liver disease, however, because its metabolism is independent of hepatic metabolism, occurring by Hoffman elimination and

TABLE 14-2 Drugs Whose Clearance Is Reduced in Cirrhosis

DRUG NAME	HALF-LIFE (CONTROL) (hr)	CLEARANCE (CONTROL) (mL/min)	RECOMMENDATION
Ampicillin	1.9 (1.3)	280 (324)	Normal dose
Chlordiazepoxide	63 (24)	9 (18)	Reduce dose by 50% and prolong interval to every other day or every third day
Cimetidine/ranitidine	3 (2.3)	460 (510)	Normal dose but inhibits CYP and interferes with metabolism of theophylline, propranolol, and anticoagulants
Diazepam	106 (47)	14 (27)	Prolong the dose interval
Furosemide	2 (1.2)	120 (140)	Efficacy may be decreased because of low albumin; dose should be increased
Lorazepam	32 (22)	57 (53)	Normal dose
N-Acetylcysteine	4.9 (2.7)	4.5 (6.5)	Normal dose

CYP, cytochrome P-450 enzymes.

TABLE 14-3 Drugs Whose Clearance Is Increased in Cirrhosis

DRUG NAME	HALF-LIFE (CONTROL) (hr)	CLEARANCE (mL/min)	RECOMMENDATION
Lidocaine	6 (1.8)	360 (640)	Dose reduction
Metoprolol	7 (4)	600 (800)	Normal dose
Morphine	2 (3)	1150 (1230)	Can be used safely in mild-to-moderate liver disease
Propranolol	11 (4)	600 (900)	Dose reduction
Verapamil	14 (3)	500 (1600)	Dose reduction

ester hydrolysis.[71] Vecuronium is well tolerated by cirrhotics in small doses, but with doses of 0.2 mg/kg, recovery is prolonged.[71] An increased volume of distribution means that a higher dose of most muscle relaxants may be needed.

Isoflurane is the inhalational anesthetic of choice because it undergoes minimal biotransformation, is least hepatotoxic, and maintains hepatic oxygen supply and uptake better than halothane or enflurane, although there have been reports of postoperative elevation in liver function tests even with this agent.[72] Halothane is best avoided because of its known hepatotoxicity, which, although rare, is unpredictable.[73]

There are many drugs with low hepatic clearance. Prednisolone, oxazepam, and warfarin have had no discernible differences detected in pharmacokinetics in the presence of liver disease.

Adverse drug reactions frequently occur in patients with liver disease, and it is important to consider carefully the use of all medications in these patients. Prostaglandin inhibitors, such as nonsteroidal antiinflammatory drugs, reduce renal perfusion, particularly in patients who are intravascularly depleted, and may precipitate renal failure.[74] Prostaglandin inhibitors should be used with great caution, if ever, in patients with cirrhosis and ascites. Aminoglycoside antibiotics are particularly nephrotoxic in patients with liver disease.[42] They should be used only when absolutely necessary, and their use must be stopped if nephrotoxicity due to acute tubular necrosis develops. An increase in serum creatinine concentration should prompt consider-

ation of discontinuing the aminoglycoside. The inadvertent use of sedatives, analgesics, or diuretics can precipitate encephalopathy, hepatorenal syndrome, and gastrointestinal hemorrhage in patients with liver disease.

ALCOHOL WITHDRAWAL

Alcohol abuse and dependence are common problems. It is estimated that more than 10 million Americans have problems with alcohol dependence that adversely affect their lives. Obtaining an alcohol consumption history is crucial in identifying individuals at risk from withdrawal. Anyone who drinks more than 2 to 3 units/day (see Table 14-1 for calculation of units) is at risk. The alcohol content of beers and lagers varies considerably, so 1 pint of beer may contain 2 to 5 units of alcohol, depending on its strength. In the United States, a standard drink of spirits contains 12 g of ethanol; in the United Kingdom and Europe, a standard drink contains 10 g of ethanol. One unit of alcohol is calculated from the formula

$$\% ABV \times 0.78 = \text{g alcohol/100 mL}$$

where %ABV is the alcohol content by volume percent. Heavier drinkers are at greater risk. Approximately 40% of individuals who drink excessive amounts of alcohol, if hospitalized, have the potential to experience symptoms of alcohol withdrawal.[75] The differential diagnosis of acute alcohol withdrawal from other conditions is given in Table 14-4.[75]

TABLE 14-4 Differentiation of Acute Alcohol Withdrawal from Other Events Altering Consciousness Levels

PARAMETER	ALCOHOL WITHDRAWAL	WERNICKE'S SYNDROME	SUBDURAL HEMATOMA	HYPOGLYCEMIA	HEPATIC ENCEPHALOPATHY
Consciousness level	Awake but agitated	Variable	Fluctuates	Variable	Reduced
Hallucinations	Yes	Yes	No	No	No
Anxiety	Yes	No	No	Yes	No
Speech	Rapid, incoherent	Slurred (cerebellar)	Normal	Slurred	Slurred
HR/BP	Raised	Tachycardia, BP normal	Slow pulse, hypertension	Tachycardia, hypotension	Normal
Sweating	Yes	No	No	Yes	No

BP, blood pressure; HR, heart rate.
Data from Mayo-Smith MF: Pharmacological management of alcohol withdrawal: A meta-analysis and evidence-based practice guideline. American Society of Addiction Medicine Working Group on Pharmacological Management of Alcohol Withdrawal. JAMA 278:144–151, 1997.

Most patients who drink heavily manifest a minor withdrawal symptom complex of hyperactivity, tremor, sweating, nausea, tachycardia, and hypertension. These symptoms usually peak between 10 and 30 hours and subside by 40 hours. Mild symptoms often do not require specific therapy but may be improved with benzodiazepines. The early administration of benzodiazepines may prevent progression of the alcohol withdrawal syndrome.

Seizures may occur in the first 12 to 48 hours and typically occur in bursts of two and can be treated successfully with diazepam (10 to 20 mg intravenously) or lorazepam (2 to 4 mg intravenously). Less frequently, frightening auditory and visual hallucinations arise and may last 5 to 6 days. Delirium tremens occurs in less than 5% of individuals withdrawing from alcohol and starts 60 to 80 hours after the last alcoholic beverage.[75] Delirium tremens is characterized by coarse tremors, agitation, fever, tachycardia, profound confusion, delusions, and hallucinations. Hyperpyrexia, ketoacidosis, and profound circulatory collapse may develop, and if untreated, the syndrome carries a mortality of 15%, versus 1% in patients who are treated.[75]

Benzodiazepines (chlordiazepoxide, diazepam, or lorazepam) are good pharmacologic treatments for alcohol withdrawal, including delirium tremens. The duration of action, rapidity of onset, metabolism, and cost of the specific agent determine the choice of agent. Dosage should be individualized, based on withdrawal severity, comorbid illness, and history of seizures.[76] As a guide, the daily doses employed in the early phase of management are chlordiazepoxide, 100 mg; diazepam, 40 mg; or lorazepam, 8 mg. After the third day, a daily dose reduction of at least 25% is recommended. Little or no modification of dose is needed in minimal liver disease, but if there is significant liver disease, the initial dose of longer acting benzodiazepines should be reduced by 25%. Benzodiazepines may be dosed on a fixed schedule for a predetermined number of doses, may be dosed on a tapering schedule over several days, or may be administered by front-loading.[76] Propofol has been used in the treatment of alcohol withdrawal but has not been studied systematically. β-Blockers, clonidine, carbamazepine, and neuroleptics may be used as adjunctive therapy to relieve some of the more distressing autonomic symptoms and delirium that accompany alcohol withdrawal.[76] There is ample evidence that pharmacologic management of alcohol withdrawal is effective.[75] Pharmacologic management of alcoholism, however, is only one component of the management of alcohol withdrawal. Provision of a calm, quiet environment; reassurance; and attention to fluid and electrolyte disorders and comorbidities are equally important.

Patients receiving treatment for alcohol withdrawal also should receive group B vitamins (intravenously or orally). The administration of vitamin B_1 (thiamine) prevents Wernicke's encephalopathy (characterized by confusion, ataxia, nystagmus, and short-term memory defects). Thiamine is discussed in greater detail in Chapter 158. Alcohol withdrawal is discussed further in Chapter 30.

REFERENCES

1. Grant BF, Dufour MC, Harford TC: Epidemiology of alcoholic liver disease. Semin Liver Dis 8:12–25, 1988.
2. Lelbach WK: Cirrhosis in the alcoholic and the relation to the volume of alcohol use. Ann N Y Acad Sci 252:85–105, 1975.
3. Batey RG, Burns T, Benson RJ, Blyth K: Alcohol consumption and the risk of cirrhosis. Med J Aust 156:413–416, 1992.
4. Morgan MY, Sherlock S: Sex related differences among 100 patients with alcoholic liver disease. BMJ 1:935–941, 1977.
5. Saunders JB, Davis M, Williams R: Do women develop alcoholic liver disease more readily than men? BMJ 282:1140–1143, 1981.
6. Lieber CS: Liver disease and alcohol: Fatty liver, alcoholic hepatitis, cirrhosis and their interrelationships. Ann N Y Acad Sci 252:63–84, 1975.
7. Leevy CM: Cirrhosis in alcoholics. Med Clin North Am 52:1445–1451, 1968.
8. Pares A, Caballeria J, Brugera M, et al: Histological course of alcoholic hepatitis: Influence of abstinence, sex and extent of hepatic damage. J Hepatol 2:33–42, 1986.
9. Shibayama Y, Nakata K: The role of sinusoidal stenoses in portal hypertension of liver cirrhosis. J Hepatol 8:60, 1989.
10. Mikhailidis DP, Jenkins WJ, Barradas MA, et al: Platelet function defects in chronic alcoholism. BMJ 293:715–718, 1986.
11. Denninger M-H: The liver and coagulation. In Bircher J, Benhamou J-P, McIntyre N, et al (eds): The Oxford Textbook of Clinical Hepatology. Oxford, Oxford Medical Publications, 1999, p 367.
12. Jones AL, Dargan PI: Churchill's Textbook of Toxicology. Edinburgh, Churchill Livingstone, 2001.
13. McCormack G, Nolan N, McCormick PA: Transjugular liver biopsy: A review. Ir Med J 94:11–12, 2001.
14. Papatheodoridis GV, Chung S, Keshav S, et al: Correction of both prothrombin time and primary hemostasis by recombinant factor VII during therapeutic alcohol injection of hepatocellular cancer in liver cirrhosis. J Hepatol 31:747–750, 1999.
15. Spector I, Corn M, Ticktin HE: Effect of plasma transfusions on the prothrombin time and clotting factors in liver disease. N Engl J Med 275:1032–1037, 1966.
16. Cederbaum AI, Blatt PM, Roberts HR: Intravascular coagulation with use of human prothrombin complex concentrates. Ann Intern Med 84:683–687, 1976.
17. McCormack TT, Rose JD, Smith PM, Johnson AG: Perforating veins and blood flow in oesophageal varices. Lancet 2:1442–1444, 1983.
18. Quintero E, Pique JM, Bombi JA, et al: Gastric mucosal vascular ectasias causing bleeding in cirrhosis. Gastroenterology 93:1054–1061, 1987.
19. Jones AL, Bangash IH, Bouchier IAD, Hayes PC: Portal and systemic haemodynamic action of N-acetylcysteine in patients with stable cirrhosis. Gut 35:1290–1293, 1994.
20. Spodick DH, Pigott VM, Chirife R: Preclinical cardiac malfunction in chronic alcoholism: Comparison with matched normal controls and with alcoholic cardiomyopathy. N Engl J Med 287:677–680, 1972.
21. Mikulic E, Munoz C, Putoni LE, Lebrec D: Hemodynamic effects of dobutamine in patients with alcoholic cirrhosis. Clin Pharmacol Ther 34:56–59, 1983.
22. Ramond MJ, Comoy E, Lebrec D: Alterations in isoprenaline sensitivity in patients with cirrhosis with evidence of abnormality of the sympathetic nervous system. Br J Clin Pharmacol 21:191–196, 1986.
23. Gerbes AL, Remien J, Jungst D, et al: Evidence for down-regulation of beta-2-adrenoceptors in cirrhotic patients with severe ascites. Lancet 1:1409–1411, 1986.
24. Huonker M, Schumacher YO, Ochs A, et al: Cardiac function and haemodynamics in alcoholic cirrhosis and effects of the TIPSS. Gut 44:743–748, 1999.
25. Johnston GW: Bleeding oesophageal varices: The management of shunt rejects. Ann R Coll Surg Engl 63:3–8, 1981.
26. McCormick PA, Jenkins SA, Mcintyre N, Burroughs AK: Why portal hypertensive varices bleed and bleed: A hypothesis. Gut 36:100–103, 1999.
27. Jalan R, Hayes PC: UK guidelines on the management of variceal haemorrhage in cirrhotic patients. British Society of Gastroenterology. Gut 46:III1–III15, 2000.
28. Kravetz D, Bosch J, Teres J, et al: Comparison of intravenous somatostatin and vasopressin infusions in treatment of acute variceal haemorrhage. Hepatology 4:442–446, 1984.
29. Bosch J, Kravetz D, Rodes J: Effects of somatostatin on hepatic and systemic haemodynamics in patients with cirrhosis of the liver: Comparison with vasopressin. Gastroenterology 80:518–525, 1981.
30. Burroughs AK, McCormick AA, Hughes MD, et al: Randomized, double-blind placebo-controlled trial of somatostatin for variceal bleeding: Emergency control and prevention of early variceal bleeding. Gastroenterology 11:1388–1395, 1990.

31. Erstad BL: Octreotide for acute variceal bleeding. Ann Pharmacother 35:618–626, 2001.

32. Chojkier M, Conn HO: Esophageal tamponade in the treatment of bleeding varices: A decade progress report. Dig Dis Sci 25:267–272, 1980.

33. Burroughs A, d'Heygere F, McIntyre N: Pitfalls in studies of prophylactic therapy for variceal bleeding in cirrhotics. Hepatology 6:1407–1413, 1986.

34. Russo MW, Zacks SL, Sandler RS, Brown RS: Cost-effectiveness analysis of transjugular intrahepatic portosystemic shunt (TIPS) versus endoscopic therapy for the prevention of recurrent esophageal variceal bleeding. Hepatology 31:358–363, 2000.

35. Arroyo V, Gines P: Mechanism of sodium retention and ascites formation in cirrhosis. J Hepatol 17(Suppl 2):S24-S28, 1993.

36. Bataller R, Gines P, Arroyo V: Practical recommendations for the treatment of ascites and its complications. Drugs 54:571–580, 1997.

37. Hidajat N, Vogl T, Stobbe H, et al: Transjugular intrahepatic portosystemic shunt: Experiences at a liver transplantation center. Acta Radiol 41:474–478, 2000.

38. Bataller R, Gines P, Arroyo V, Rodes J: Hepatorenal syndrome. Clin Liver Dis 4:487–507, 2000.

39. Gines P: Diagnosis and treatment of hepatorenal syndrome. Baillieres Best Pract Res Clin Gastroenterol 14:945–957, 2000.

40. Suzuki H, Stanley AJ: Current management and novel therapeutic strategies for recurrent acsites and hepatorenal syndrome. QJM 94:293–300, 2001.

41. Sort P, Navas M, Arroyo V, et al: Effect of intravenous albumin on renal impairment and mortality in patients with cirrhosis and spontaneous bacterial peritonitis. N Engl J Med 341:403–409, 1999.

42. Hampel H, Bynum GD, Zamora E, El-Serag HB: Risk factors for the development of renal dysfunction in hospitalised patient with cirrhosis. Am J Gastroenterol 96:2206–2210, 2001.

43. Planas R, Bataller R, Rodes J: Hepatorenal syndrome. Curr Treat Options Gastroenterol 3:445–450, 2000.

44. Rodriguez-Roisin R, Agusti AGN, Roca J: The hepatopulmonary syndrome: New name, old complexities. Thorax 47:897–902, 1992.

45. Evans JW, Wagner PD: Limits on V/Q distribution from analysis of experimental inert gas elimination. J Appl Physiol 42:889–898, 1977.

46. Monroe P, Morrow CF Jr, Millen JE, et al: Acute respiratory failure after sodium morrhuate esophageal sclerotherapy. Gastroenterology 85:693–699, 1983.

47. Conklin LD, Estrera AL, Weiner MA, et al: Transjugular intrahepatic portosystemic shunt for recurrent hydrothorax. Ann Thorac Surg 69:609–611, 2000.

48. Boz A, Cilli A, Yildiz A, et al: The diagnosis of peritoneo-pleural communication with Tc-99m MAA scintigraphy in the absence of ascites. Clin Nucl Med 25:935–936, 2000.

49. Thuluvath PJ, Morss S, Thompson R: Spontaneous bacterial peritonitis—in-hospital mortality, prediction of survival and health care costs from 1988–1998. Am J Gastroenterol 96:1232–1236, 2001.

50. Navasa M, Rimola A, Rodes J: Bacterial infections in liver disease. Semin Liver Dis 17:323–333, 1997.

51. Fernandez J, Bauer TM, Navasa M, Rodes J: Diagnosis, treatment and prevention of spontaneous bacterial peritonitis. Baillieres Best Pract Res Clin Gastroenterol 14:975–990, 2000.

52. Strauss E, de Costa MF: The importance of bacterial infections as precipitating factors of chronic hepatic encephalopathy in cirrhosis. Hepatogastroenterology 45:900–904, 1998.

53. Navasa M: Bacterial infection in patients with cirrhosis: Reasons, comments and suggestions. Dig Liver Dis 33:9–12, 2001.

54. Curiosos WH, Monkemuller KE: Neomycin should not be used to treat hepatic encephalopathy. BMJ 323:223, 2001.

55. Blei AT, Cordoba J: Hepatic encephalopathy. Am J Gastroenterol 96:1968–1976, 2001.

56. Conn HO, Schreiber W, Elkington SG: Cirrhosis and diabetes: II. Association of impaired glucose tolerance with portal-systemic shunting in Laennec's cirrhosis. Dig Dis 16:227–239, 1971.

57. Kaser S, Foger B, Waldenberger P, et al: Transjugular intrahepatic portosystemic shunt (TIPS) augments hyperinsulinaemia in patients with cirrhosis. J Hepatol 33:902–906, 2000.

58. Godet C, Hira M, Adoun M, et al: Rapid diagnosis of alcoholic ketoacidosis by proton NMR. Intens Care Med 27:785–786, 2001.

59. Hojer J: Severe metabolic acidosis in the alcoholic: Differential diagnosis and management. Hum Exp Toxicol 15:482–488, 1996.

60. Almaghamsi AM, Yeung CK: Osmolal gap in alcoholic ketoacidosis. Clin Nephrol 48:52–53, 1997.

61. Umpierrez GE, DiGirolamo M, Tuvlin JA, et al: Differences in metabolic and hormonal milieu in diabetic and alcohol-induced ketoacidosis. J Crit Care 15:52–59, 2000.

62. Marinella MA: Alcoholic ketoacidosis presenting with extreme hypoglycemia. Am J Emerg Med 15:280–281, 1997.

63. Iten PX, Meier M: Beta-hydroxybutyric acid—an indicator for an alcoholic ketoacidosis as cause of death in deceased alcohol abusers. J Forensic Sci 45:624–632, 2000.

64. Wilkinson GR, Shand DG: A physiological approach to hepatic drug clearance. Clin Pharmacol Ther 18:337–389, 1976.

65. Branch RA, James JA, Read AE: Proceedings: The influence of chronic liver disease on the elimination of d-propranolol, antipyrine, and indocyanine green. Gut 15:837–838, 1974.

66. Passayre D, Lebrec D, Descatoire V, et al: Mechanism for reduced drug clearance in patients with cirrhosis. Gastroenterology 74:566–571, 1978.

67. Callaghan R, Desmond PV, Paull P, Mashford ML: Hepatic enzyme activity is the major factor determining elimination rate of high clearance drugs in cirrhosis. Hepatology 18:54–60, 1993.

68. Shelley MP, Elston AC, Park GR: Sedative and analgesic drugs. In Park GR, Kang Y (eds): Anaesthesia and Intensive Care for Patients with Liver Disease. Oxford, Butterworth-Heinemann, 1995, pp 57–77.

69. Klotz U, McHorse TS, Wilkinson GR, Schenker S: The effect of cirrhosis on the disposition and elimination of meperidine in man. Clin Pharmacol Ther 16:667–675, 1974.

70. Ferrier C, Marty J, Bouffard Y, et al: Alfentanil pharmacokinetics in patients with cirrhosis. Anesthesiology 62:480–484, 1985.

71. Miller RD: Pharmacokinetics of atracurium and other non-depolarizing neuromuscular blocking agents in normal patients and those with renal or hepatic dysfunction. Br J Anaesth 58:11S-13S, 1986.

72. Gunza JT, Pashayan AG: Postoperative elevation of serum transaminases following isoflurane anesthesia. J Clin Anesth 4:336–341, 1992.

73. Lo SK, Wendon J, Mieli-Vergani G, Williams R: Halothane-induced acute liver failure: Continuing occurrence and use of liver transplantation. Eur J Gastorenterol Hepatol 10:635–639, 1998.

74. Boyer TD, Zia P, Reynolds TB: Effect of indomethacin and prostaglandin A1 on renal function and plasma renin activity in alcoholic lever disease. Gastroenterology 77:215–222, 1979.

75. Morgan M: Acute alcohol withdrawal. In Bircher J, Benhamou J-P, McIntyre N, et al (eds): Oxford Textbook of Hepatology. Oxford, Oxford University Press, 1999, p 1203.

76. Mayo-Smith MF: Pharmacological management of alcohol withdrawal: A meta-analysis and evidence-based practice guideline. American Society of Addiction Medicine Working Group on Pharmacological Management of Alcohol Withdrawal. JAMA 278:144–151, 1997.

CHAPTER **15**

Poisoning Fatalities

Philippe Hantson ▪ Marianne de Tourtchaninoff

EPIDEMIOLOGY OF TOXIC DEATHS

Acute poisoning is a common cause of emergency admission in developed countries. In 1995, poisoning was the third leading cause of injury mortality in the United States.[1] About three fourths of poisoning deaths are caused by drugs. The understanding of the epidemiology of poisoning deaths remains difficult, however. Many comorbid factors contribute to the outcome, including the patient's age, underlying medical condition, and the delay between exposure and treatment. There are limited statistical reports specifically addressing intensive care unit (ICU) mortality rates. The literature on poisoning deaths does not reflect the true prevalence. A major discrepancy exists between hospital and nonhospital deaths.[2]

The main sources of information in the United States are the data collected by the Toxic Exposure Surveillance System (TESS) of the American Association of Poison Control Centers and by the National Center for Health Statistics (NCHS).[1–3] There are marked differences between these two data sets.[2] In 1994, 16,527 poisoning deaths were recorded by the NCHS, and only 766 deaths were recorded by the TESS. In these data sets, the relative distribution of death circumstances differed for unintentional drug poisonings, unintentional nondrug poisonings, and intentional poisonings. There also was no statistical agreement in ranking of the 12 most frequent toxins associated with poisoning deaths. Most cases reported to poison control centers are not managed in a health care facility.[3] In 1998, of 2,241,082 human poison exposure cases, 61,386 (2.7%) were admitted to critical care units. On the same number of exposures, only 775 fatalities (0.0003%) were reported. Fatalities are underreported to poison control centers, and the NCHS data set gives a larger profile of poisoning deaths by reporting more out-of-hospital deaths. In recent years, a dramatic increase in death rates associated with opiates and cocaine among men 35 to 54 years old has been noted.[1,4]

Deaths due to specific substances (e.g., acetaminophen, dextropropoxyphene) are overrepresented in some countries for several reasons, such as availability, prescription versus nonprescription status, and pharmaceutical advertising and promotion.[5,6] New pharmaceuticals are being released onto the market continually. Antidepressant drugs now are represented mainly by selective serotonin reuptake inhibitors. Fatalities related to serotonin syndrome may be reported with an increasing frequency.[7] The mortality rate in ICUs approximates 1% to 2% for the most common pharmaceuticals (psychotropic, cardiotropic, and analgesic drugs) and

drugs of abuse.[8] This low rate is due mainly to supportive therapy rather than use of elimination techniques or specific antidotes. It is likely, however, that the mortality rate will remain significantly high with some household products (toxic alcohols) and industrial products or pesticides (mostly paraquat). In the United States and Northern Europe, carbon monoxide (CO) remains the leading cause of nondrug poisoning (accidental or intentional).[1]

MECHANISMS OF DEATH

Death may be the consequence of the direct or indirect action of a toxic substance on an isolated organ (target organ) or on the whole organism. The lung is the target organ in paraquat poisoning; progressive respiratory failure develops within a few days or weeks after exposure, with evident pathologic lesions. Mortality also exists, however, with toxins that do not have lesional effects. Outside the hospital, death due to acute poisoning is mainly the result of central nervous system (CNS) depression with subsequent cardiorespiratory failure. CNS depression is the mechanism of toxicity for opiates and most psychotropic drugs. Under these circumstances, death usually is related to the lack of early supportive treatment. Early cardiocirculatory failure, before hospital admission or a few hours after, is another common cause of toxic death. It is observed not only with cardiotropic drugs, such as calcium channel blockers and digoxin, but also with other substances, including cocaine, colchicine, and chloroquine. Delayed complications, such as infection, renal failure, hepatic failure, and respiratory failure, may account for late mortality in the ICU.

Brain death is encountered less commonly after acute poisoning. The early recognition of brain death by critical care physicians leads to major decisions, such as care withdrawal and organ donation. A first question to be answered is the possible mechanism of brain death in this setting. Brain death cannot be the sole consequence of anoxia due to unsuccessful resuscitation because pure anoxia seldom gives rise to brain death except when associated with brain edema leading to acute intracranial hypertension. In our experience, brain edema consistently preceded brain death in poisoned patients in whom a cerebral computed tomography scan was performed. Brain edema classically is said to be from a vasogenic or cytotoxic origin. The first mechanism is illustrated by hepatic encephalopathy in the case of acetaminophen poisoning

173

(Fig. 15-1).[9] Cytotoxic brain edema may be caused by numerous metabolic disorders. It has been documented after intoxications by some anoxic agents (CO) or following profound hypoglycemia in the case of insulin overdose.[10] Extremely severe metabolic acidosis is likely responsible for irreversible brain damage (with associated brain edema) in the case of methanol or ethylene glycol poisoning.[11,12] Ionic disorders and hyperthermia have been reported to contribute to cerebral edema associated with the use of 3,4-methylenedioxymethamphetamine (Ecstasy) or other substances leading to the serotonin syndrome.[13] The clinical picture usually is complicated by other disorders, such as autonomic instability or disseminated intravascular coagulation. Finally, epileptogenic substances may provoke irreversible brain injury after status epilepticus.

Intracranial hypertension also may be the result of focal anatomic lesions. Extensive neuronal destruction with hemorrhages was found at postmortem examination in an autopsy study of 28 patients who died from methanol poisoning.[14] In a personal observation of fatal methanol poisoning, extensive hemorrhagic necrosis originating from the basal ganglia was observed (Fig. 15-2). In methanol-poisoned patients investigated by magnetic resonance imaging, the putamen preferentially is involved.[11] The lesions can be edematous and fully reversible at the early stage or, in some instances, can become hemorrhagic and necrotic. These lesions are probably due to the combination effects of tissue acidosis and hypoxia-ischemia status. Cerebrovascular accidents, including subarachnoid hemorrhage, intracerebral hemorrhage, and cerebral infarction, have been reported with increasing

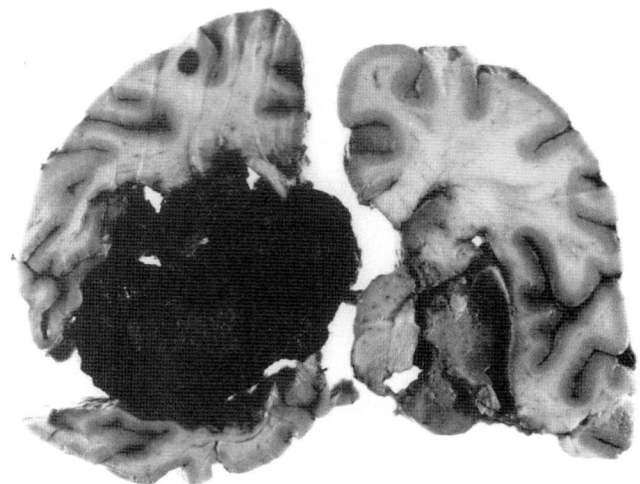

FIGURE 15-2

Extensive hemorrhagic necrosis originated from the basal ganglia in a 32-year-old man who died as a result of acute methanol poisoning.

frequency in association with cocaine use. Although most patients have evidence of underlying cerebrovascular disease, reports have failed to show underlying disease in some patients.[15–18] These observations illustrate the need to obtain brain imaging when irreversible brain damage is suspected after acute poisoning because functional disturbances are considerably more frequent than anatomic lesions.

DIAGNOSIS OF BRAIN DEATH IN POISONED PATIENTS

The accuracy of the brain death diagnosis is crucial in cases of poisoning.[19–22] With concurrent misleading conditions (hypothermia, drugs, metabolic disturbances), the brain death diagnosis should be improved by using a reliable, accurate, and safe confirmatory test. Even if brain death is basically a clinical diagnosis, confirmatory tests are required. In the case of brain death, the confirmatory tests show the absence of cerebral blood flow (four-vessel arteriography, radioisotopic technique, and transcranial Doppler) or the absence of electrocerebral activity (electroencephalogram [EEG], multimodality evoked potentials [MEPs]).

Cerebral four-vessel angiography remains for most authors the confirmatory test of choice to determine brain death. Cerebral angiography has a high accuracy because cerebral blood flow cannot be abolished completely by any toxic substance and gives clear-cut results in misleading conditions. Angiography cannot be performed at the bedside, however, and cannot be repeated easily. It can cause deleterious effects, which may be found ethically unacceptable if one considers that the prognosis of a patient presenting with barbiturate overdose with transient isoelectric EEG can be excellent.

Brain scintigraphy with ^{99m}Tc-HMPAO technique has been used in brain death diagnosis. Clinical conditions such as hypothermia or metabolic coma exhibit no or little effect on brain ^{99m}Tc-HMPAO uptake. Few data are available

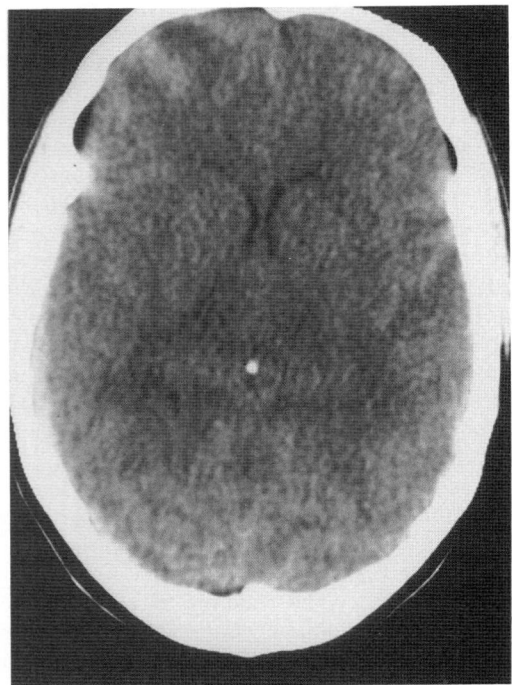

FIGURE 15-1

Major brain swelling in a 30-year-old woman who presented with fulminant hepatic failure after acetaminophen overdose.

concerning the use of cerebral angioscintigraphy for the diagnosis of brain death in poisoning.[23–25] Facco and colleagues[26] investigated 50 deeply comatose and brain-dead patients by single-photon emission computed tomography (SPECT). In 21 patients in whom brain death could not be diagnosed properly by EEG and clinical examination owing to the presence of associated factors (e.g., sedation, drug intoxication), SPECT showed brain perfusion arrest in 15 patients on the first test and in 6 patients on retesting.

Positron emission tomography has not been used to a significant extent in brain death diagnosis owing to practical difficulties. Only two reports have been found in the literature from 1988 to the present.[27,28] The reports showed the absence of significant intracerebral fludeoxyglucose uptake or retention in three cases and one obvious case of clinical brain death. In the second report, a slow rise of tracer was noted over time within the sagittal sinus, providing a false-negative scintigraphic evaluation for brain death diagnosis.

Transcranial Doppler is also a helpful method of estimating cerebral blood flow. This modality is more dependent on examiner skill and the patient's anatomic features, however. The results are not influenced by the action of sedative drugs.

EEG is by far the most often used confirmatory test for brain death diagnosis. Nevertheless, EEG is sensitive to hypothermia, drugs, and metabolic disorders and is of little help in the case of poisoning or other misleading conditions. The possible occurrence of reversible isoelectric EEG has been documented in hypothermia and with several drugs, including barbiturates, methaqualone, diazepam, meprobamate, and trichloroethylene.[29–37]

Evoked potentials may offer significant advantages over EEG. Evoked potentials are a minimally invasive technique largely used for many years in the operating room and in the ICU. Numerous conditions that may influence electrophysiologic testing have been studied extensively.[38] In all cases of suspected brain death, the general policy of our institution is to use the combination of EEG and MEPs (flash visual evoked potentials [VEPs], somatosensory evoked potentials [SEPs], and brainstem auditory evoked potentials [BAEPs]) to confirm brain death.[38–42] MEPs are recorded easily and rapidly at the patient's bedside and evaluate the brainstem and the cerebral cortex. The three-modality evoked potential pattern of brain death is highly specific and associates the disappearance of all cortical and brainstem activities to the persistence of retinal, peripheral, and spinal activities (Fig. 15-3). It is unequivocal in most situations mimicking brain death. Only the association of a bilateral optic nerve section, a spinal cord interruption at the cervical level, and a bilateral auditory nerve section could mimic the MEP pattern of brain death. MEPs can differentiate brain death from misleading factors, such as hypothermia, drugs, and metabolic disturbances, by the persistence of brainstem activities (waves from II to V in BAEPs and lemniscal P14 in median nerve SEPs).

Brain death diagnosis can be considered more difficult in infants than in children and adults, taking into account the immaturity of brainstem reactivity and EEG. The high proportion of anoxic encephalopathies in infants and the persistence of open fontanelles, which prevents transtentorial herniation, decrease the likelihood of a brain death occurrence in such comatose patients. BAEPs and VEPs are present in all premature infants older than 30 weeks. BAEPs are sensitive to pathologic conditions frequently encountered in infancy, such as anoxia (cochlea sensitivity) and hyperbilirubinemia (cochlea and brainstem sensitivity), that can give rise to null BAEPs. VEP alterations in anoxic infants are poorly documented. Cortical SEP components are inconstant, and their absence in normal term newborns is not pathological. After 6 months of age, the absence of cortical SEP components indicates a poor prognosis (death or severe neurologic sequelae). Consequently, MEPs should not be taken as a reliable brain death confirmatory test in these misleading conditions (anoxia, hyperbilirubinemia, and probably poisoning) in infants younger than 6 months old.[41]

The interpretation of MEPs in poisoning cases should take into account some specifics. Concerning VEPs, it is important to keep in mind that the same factors that provoke electrocerebral silence (CNS depressant intoxications, hypothermia) can abolish the VEPs. A completely abolished VEP has the same meaning as electrocerebral silence. The lower sensitivity to environmental artifacts due to the averaging process is a significant advantage over EEG and makes the interpretation easier.[41] Owing to the high toxicity to retina and optic nerve of formic acid, the main toxic metabolite after biotransformation of methanol, VEP interpretation in the case of methanol poisoning may not be reliable.[43] Early retinal dysfunction can be documented; it may or may not be followed by the development of optic neuropathy. In the case of disappearance of VEP activities in methanol poisoning, the preservation of BAEP and SEP components precludes the brain death diagnosis.

Hypothermia often is experienced in comatose patients secondary to poisoning or other causes. It has been shown that BAEPs also are less influenced by hypothermia and may help to rule out brain death diagnosis as long as the body temperature exceeds 20 °C to 22 °C.[44] From our experience in recording SEPs during profound hypothermia for surgical aorta repair, the lemniscal P14 of median nerve SEPs also is resistant to hypothermia and disappears only at temperatures less than 18 °C, whereas cortical SEP activities can be recorded at temperatures around 22 °C.[45] In most clinical situations, the hypothermia level is less marked and does not interfere with MEP interpretation.

There is a consensus among authors that SEPs and BAEPs can be considered relatively insensitive to CNS depressant drugs, and these evoked potentials are a good tool for examining brainstem function when these drugs are present.[46–48] Increased SEP latencies with increased central conduction time (as measured between cervical N13 and parietal N20) have been observed in amitriptyline, meprobamate, and nitrazepam overdose.[49] In the presence of CNS depressant drugs, BAEPs either are unchanged at therapeutic levels or are delayed at therapeutic or toxic levels. Amplitude or morphologic changes can occur with enflurane, cholinergic and serotoninergic agents, phentolamine, and propranolol.[50] Mauguière and colleagues[51] showed deep reversible BAEP alterations consecutive to the association of barbiturates and lidocaine in one case. In our experience, barbiturate intoxication sufficient to provoke a clinical and EEG pattern of brain death is associated with well-preserved BAEPs and persistent lemniscal P14 in median nerve SEPs (Fig. 15-4). The MEP

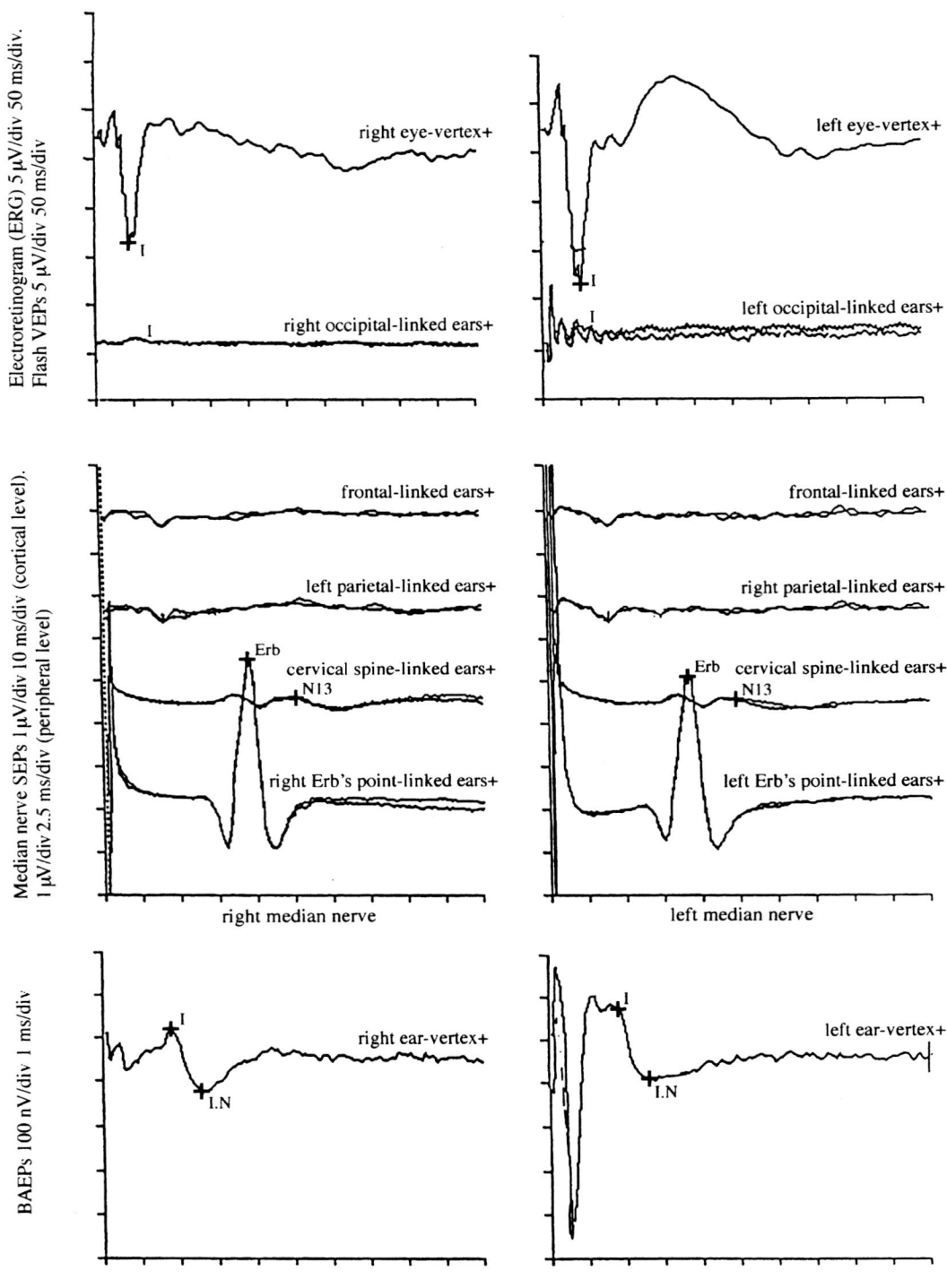

FIGURE 15-3

Multimodality evoked potential pattern in a brain death patient. Multimodality evoked potentials were recorded from a 33-year-old man. At the time of recording, clinical examination was consistent with brain death diagnosis. Flash visual evoked potentials (VEPs) show only a retinal component (wave I) on the cortical channel and the periocular recording. Median nerve somatosensory responses are represented only by peripheral (Erb) and spinal (N13) components, whereas brainstem and cortical components are bilaterally absent. Brainstem auditory evoked potentials (BAEPs) are limited to a cochlear nerve component (wave I). *(From de Tourtchaninoff M, Hantson P, Mahieu P, et al: Brain death diagnosis in misleading conditions. QJM 92:407–414, 1999.)*

pattern in brain death is clearly distinct from that observed in CNS depressant intoxication and allows clinicians to differentiate both states clearly. For most authors, evoked potentials might be included in brain death criteria even in clinically difficult conditions.[46,50,52] Drug intoxication cannot account for a complete MEP pattern of brain death if brain death is not really present. Subcortical (and even cortical) activities persist in high doses of CNS depressant drugs

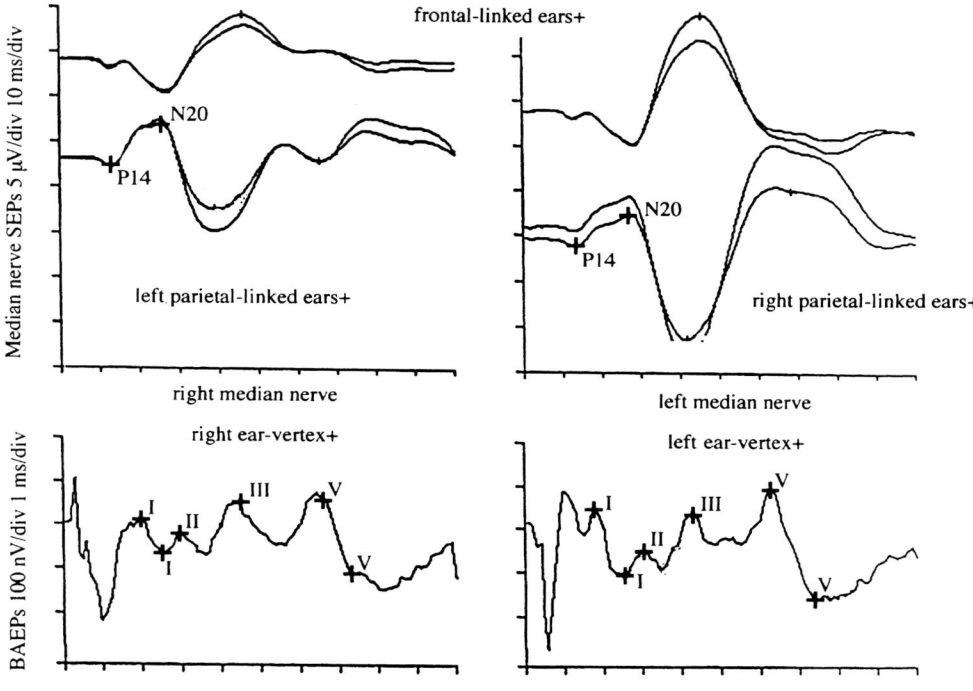

FIGURE 15-4

Electrophysiologic study in a 5-year-old epileptic girl under barbiturate. At the time of recording, blood level of thiopental was 53 μg/mL, and all cephalic reflexes were absent. The electroencephalogram was isoelectric during long periods. Median nerve somatosensory evoked potentials (SEPs) show delayed but recognizable lemniscal (P14) and cortical (N20) activities. Brainstem auditory evoked potentials (BAEPs) are well preserved but slightly delayed. *(From de Tourtchaninoff M, Hantson P, Mahieu P, et al: Brain death diagnosis in misleading conditions. QJM 92:407–414, 1999.)*

sufficient to give rise to a clinical and EEG pattern of brain death. The MEP pattern of brain death is encountered in other drug intoxications only when irreversible damage occurs at the brainstem and the cerebral cortex.[53]

ORGAN DONATION FROM POISONED DONORS

Organ donation after acute poisoning with evidence of brain death is a poorly documented topic.[54] The current shortage of grafts for organ transplantation should lead to consideration, in selected cases, of poisoned subjects as organ donors. Analysis of the more recent literature shows successful transplantation with grafts from donors poisoned by tricyclic antidepressants, benzodiazepines, barbiturates, insulin, CO, methanol, and other substances.[55–65] Experience indicates that in selected cases, the organs from such donors function as well in recipients as organs from more conventional sources. Some centers have a favorable experience in this setting.[57,66]

A first step is to exclude the risk of toxin transmission to the recipient by careful analysis of the toxicologic data (undetectable or nontoxic blood toxin levels). A second step is to check that the systemic consequences of acute poisoning are fully controlled. The routine biologic data are extremely helpful in excluding organ dysfunction (nonelevation of cardiac, hepatic, and pancreatic enzymes and normal serum creatinine). Morphologic analysis also is essential but is often possible only at organ harvest when biopsy also can exclude gross organ injury.

Heart Donation

Heart donation from poisoned donors is poorly studied.[66] Similar to the brain, the heart is extremely sensitive to hypoxic or ischemic injury. Some toxins may preclude donation, such as tricyclic antidepressants, dextropropoxyphene, cocaine, and ethylene glycol. Tricyclic antidepressants may accumulate in heart tissue.[67] Ultrastructural changes have been noted in the myocardia of patients who died from acute ethylene glycol and cocaine ovedose.[68,69] Cocaine interferes with cardiac biochemical functions, leading to oxidative stress, and with cellular calcium flux regulation.[70,71] Clear evidence of recovery from these toxicities must be shown. Heart donation after CO intoxication is still a matter of debate because fatal outcomes have been published.[59,72] Reversible cardiac dysfunction may be observed after CO exposure, prompting the hypothesis of myocardial stunning.[73] Ultrastructural myocardial changes, after acute CO exposure, also have been debated. Different factors may be involved in CO cardiotoxicity, such as individual susceptibility, duration of exposure, and type of exposure (e.g., smoke inhalation). In our opinion, CO poisoning remains a relative contraindication to heart donation. The influence of specific therapy (hyperbaric oxygen) has to be clarified. Heart donation after methanol poisoning also is controversial. Clinical experience is extremely limited.[65] Severe metabolic acidosis may contribute to myocardial dysfunction, but this has been poorly investigated in acute methanol poisoning. Methanol poisoning is a relative contraindication to heart donation, and more data should be collected on methanol-related cardiotoxicity (histopathology and tissue formic acid concentrations).

Echocardiography at the early stage would be helpful in showing the effect of severe metabolic acidosis on heart contractility.

Insulin and cyanide are good examples of functional toxins. Cyanide induces cellular hypoxia by inhibiting cytochrome oxidase. After cyanide exposure, successful cardiopulmonary resuscitation can be achieved by supportive therapy and antidote administration. Heart donation is possible after cyanide poisoning.[74] The main problem is to prevent cyanide intoxication of the recipient. It seems safe to wait until the donor's whole-blood cyanide concentration is less than 0.2 mg/L (7 μmol/L) and lactic metabolic acidosis has been corrected.

Fatal acetaminophen poisoning is particularly frequent in some countries. Heart donation seldom has been considered, however. According to the data in the literature, it is unlikely that acetaminophen is directly cardiotoxic.[60]

What criteria could be applied to minimize risk in heart donation after fatal poisoning? A normal electrocardiogram, intact left ventricular function (estimated by echocardiography), good hemodynamics with minimal inotropic support, and normal or near-normal cardiac enzymes would seem essential.[75] With CO poisoning, additional requirements might include relatively short ischemia time, favorable donor-to-recipient weight ratio, and avoidance of recipients with high pulmonary vascular resistance. It also is wise to avoid donors with prolonged CO exposure or sustained cardiocirculatory arrest.

Lung Donation

Lung transplantation from a poisoned donor has been described rarely.[63] A few toxins directly affect the lung (e.g., paraquat or bleomycin). Cardiogenic or noncardiogenic pulmonary edema may complicate some toxic deaths, however. CO poisoning illustrates the different mechanisms of lung injury. Caution should be exercised when lung donation is considered after smoke inhalation following fire hazard (associated chemical injury). In other cases, standard lung donation criteria can be applied.

Liver Donation

The liver is a target organ for some toxins (e.g., acetaminophen and some mushrooms) to the extent that liver transplantation is a successful therapy in the most severe cases.

Liver donation is possible in selected cases, and successful liver allografts have been reported after poisoning with benzodiazepines, methaqualone, barbiturates, cyclic antidepressants, insulin, CO, cyanide, methanol, cocaine, and lead.[55,57] Detectable alcohol concentrations are common in the blood of potential organ donors after motor vehicle accidents, intracranial hemorrhage, head injury, aspiration, and drug overdose; they are not a contraindication per se to liver harvesting. Many toxins might be expected to accumulate in the liver (e.g., tricyclic antidepressants); in practice, this has rarely proved the case. Risk can be minimized by a careful toxicokinetic analysis. The decision to harvest the liver should be guided mainly by donor history (chronic ethanol or drug abuse), liver function tests, serology, and liver morphology and biopsy at harvest.

Kidney Donation

The kidneys are relatively resistant to many hypoxic, ischemic, or toxic insults. Acute tubular necrosis, usually secondary to nontraumatic rhabdomyolysis, may occur in this setting but is generally reversible. The kidney is a target organ of acute ethylene glycol poisoning. Nevertheless, kidney transplantation has been performed with success after exposure to this substance, but this cannot be recommended routinely. There is experimental evidence that oxalate crystal deposition may lead to an inflammatory response with permanent epithelial cell injury, and some patients who survived acute ethylene glycol poisoning have developed chronic renal failure.[76,77] Clear evidence of recovery from the injury must be shown. In other instances, there is extensive experience with kidney grafts from poisoned donors, and the results are similar to those in the nonpoisoned donor population. The kidneys can be transplanted safely after fatal acetaminophen poisoning, even in the presence of acute tubular necrosis, a possible but rare complication of acetaminophen poisoning that probably could not be prevented by N-acetylcysteine administration.[78] Kidney donation may be considered safely after acute poisoning by most toxins that are not directly nephrotoxic. Renal function laboratory tests and pretransplant biopsy are mandatory.

Pancreas Donation

Pancreas transplantation from poisoned donors has been described rarely. Alcohol abuse is associated with acute and chronic pancreatitis. Several studies of the acute effects of ethanol administration have shown that the liver is affected significantly more often than the pancreas; no correlation is found between blood ethanol and serum amylase or lipase levels. Similar to ethanol, methanol is a possible cause of pancreatitis.[79] Pancreas injury may be exacerbated further by the ethanol therapy used as an antidote to methanol intoxication. The decision to harvest the pancreas should be based on laboratory indicators and organ morphology at surgery.

CONCLUSION

In-hospital death, particularly brain death, is a rare complication of acute poisoning compared with out-of-hospital deaths from a toxic origin. The diagnosis of brain death relies not only on the clinical examination but also on confirmatory tests, especially in poisoning cases. Among them, transcranial Doppler, brain scintigraphy, cerebral angiography, and overall MEPs are less susceptible to the influence of drugs or metabolic disorders than is EEG. Analysis of the more recent literature shows successful organ transplantations with grafts obtained from donors poisoned by various substances. Experience indicates that in selected cases, the organs from poisoned donors function in recipients as well as organs from more conventional sources. Physicians should be guided by the accurate knowledge of the target organs of poisoning; the analysis of the toxicokinetic data; and the results of laboratory investigations, functional tests, and morphologic studies before harvesting the organs.

REFERENCES

1. Fingerhut LA, Cox CS: Poisoning mortality 1985–1995. Public Health Rep 113:219–233, 1998.
2. Hoppe-Roberts JM, Lloyd LM, Chyka PA: Poisoning mortality in the United States: Comparison of national mortality statistics and Poison Control Centers reports. Ann Emerg Med 35:440–449, 1999.
3. Litovitz TL, Klein-Schwartz W, Caravati EM, et al: 1998 annual report of the Association of Poison Control Centers Toxic Exposure Surveillance System. Am J Emerg Med 17:435–487, 1999.
4. Gore SM: Fatal uncertainty: Death-rate from use of ecstasy or heroin. Lancet 354:1265–1266, 1999.
5. Jonasson U, Jonasson B, Saldeen T: Correlation between prescription of various dextropropoxyphene preparations and their involvement in fatal poisonings. Forensic Sci Int 103:125–132, 1999.
6. Makin AJ, Wendon J, Williams R: A 7-year experience of acetaminophen-induced hepatotoxicity (1987–1993). Gastroenterology 109:1907–1916, 1995.
7. Mueller PD, Korey WS: Death by "ecstasy": The serotonin syndrome? Ann Emerg Med 32:377–380, 1998.
8. Danel V, Bismuth Ch: Management of acute poisonings. In Descotes J (ed): Human Toxicology. Amsterdam, Elsevier, 1996, pp 5–24.
9. Flanagan RJ, Mant TGK: Coma and metabolic acidosis early in severe acute paracetamol poisoning. Hum Toxicol 5:179–182, 1986.
10. Dean BS, Verdile VP, Krenzelok EP: Coma reversal with cerebral dysfunction recovery after repetitive hyperbaric oxygen therapy for severe carbon monoxide poisoning. Am J Emerg Med 11:616–618, 1993.
11. Hantson P, Duprez T, Mahieu P: Neurotoxicity to the basal ganglia shown by brain magnetic resonance imaging (MRI) following poisoning by methanol and other substances. J Toxicol Clin Toxicol 35:151–161, 1997.
12. Morgan BW, Ford MD, Follmer R: Ethylene glycol ingestion resulting in brainstem and midbrain dysfunction. J Toxicol Clin Toxicol 38:445–451, 2000.
13. O'Connor A, Cluroe A, Couch R, et al: Death from hyponatremia-induced cerebral oedema associated with MDMA ("Ecstasy") use. N Z Med J 112:255–256, 1999.
14. Mittal BV, Desai AP, Khade KR: Methyl alcohol poisoning: An autopsy study of 28 cases. J Postgrad Med 37:9–13, 1991.
15. Lichtenfeld PJ, Rubin BD, Feldman RS: Subarachnoid hemorrhage precipitated by cocaine snorting. Arch Neurol 41:223–224, 1984.
16. Levine SR, Washington JM, Jefferson MF, et al: "Crack" cocaine-associated stroke. Neurology 37:1849–1853, 1987.
17. Iriye BK, Asrat T, Adashek JA, et al: Intraventricular haemorrhage and maternal brain death associated with antepartum cocaine abuse. Br J Obstet Gynaecol 102:68–69, 1995.
18. Wojak JC, Flamm ES: Intracranial hemorrhage and cocaine use. Stroke 18:712–715, 1987.
19. Guérit JM, de Tourtchaninoff M, Hantson P, et al: Multimodality evoked potentials in the differential diagnosis of brain death. In Machado C (ed): Recent Developments in Neurology: Brain Death. Amsterdam, Elsevier, 1995, pp 119–126.
20. Hantson P, de Tourtchaninoff M, Mahieu P, et al: Prélèvements d'organes consécutifs aux décès par intoxication: Expérience et problèmes diagnostiques. Réanim Urgences 9:197–209, 2000.
21. de Tourtchaninoff M, Hantson P, Mahieu P, et al: Brain death diagnosis in misleading conditions. QJM 92:407–414, 1999.
22. Hantson P, de Tourtchaninoff M, Guérit JM, et al: Multimodality evoked potentials as a valuable technique for brain death diagnosis in poisoned patients. Transplant Proc 29:3345–3346, 1997.
23. Schlake HP, Bottger IG, Grotemeyer KH, et al: Determination of cerebral perfusion by means of planar brain scintigraphy and ⁹⁹ᵐTc-HMPAO in brain death, persistent vegetative state and severe coma. Intensive Care Med 18:76–81, 1992.
24. Costa DC, Hubank M, Sinha A, et al: Influence of time, temperature, sodium-potassium pump inhibition and glutathione on the ⁹⁹ᵐTc-HMPAO uptake by cultured astrocytes. Eur J Nucl Med 15:584, 1989.
25. Nordlander S, Wiklund PE, Åsard PE: Cerebral angioscintigraphy in brain death and in coma due to drug intoxication. J Nucl Med 14:856–857, 1973.
26. Facco E, Zuchetta P, Munari M, et al: ⁹⁹ᵐTc-HMPAO SPECT in the diagnosis of brain death. Intensive Care Med 24:911–917, 1998.
27. Momose T, Nishikawa J, Watanabe T, et al: Clinical application of 18F-FDG-PET in patients with brain death. Kaku-Igaku 29:1139–1142, 1992.
28. Meyer MA: Evaluating brain death with positron emission tomography: Case report on dynamic imaging of 18F-fluorodeoxyglucose activity after intravenous bolus injection. J Neuroimaging 6:117–119, 1996.
29. Bird TD, Plum F: Recovery from barbiturate overdose coma with a prolonged isoelectric electroencephalogram. Neurology 18:456–460, 1968.
30. Haider I, Oswald I: Electroencephalographic investigation in acute drug poisoning. Electroencephalogr Clin Neurophysiol 29:105, 1970.
31. Jørgensen EO: The EEG during severe barbiturate intoxication. Acta Neurol Scand 46(Suppl 43):281, 1970.
32. Kirshbaum RJ, Carollo VJ: Reversible iso-electric EEG in barbiturate coma. JAMA 212:1215, 1970.
33. Mellerio F, Gaultier M, Fournier E, et al: Contribution of electroencephalography to resuscitation in toxicology. Clin Toxicol 6:271–285, 1973.
34. Mellerio F: EEG changes during intoxication with trichlorethylene. Electroencephalogr Clin Neurophysiol 29:101, 1970.
35. Mantz JM, Tempe JD, Jaeger A, et al: Silence électrique cérébral de vingt-quatre heures au cours d'une intoxication massive par 10 g de pentobarbital. Presse Med 79:1243–1246, 1971.
36. Powner DJ: Drug-associated isoelectric EEGs: A hazard in brain-death certification. JAMA 236:1123, 1976.
37. Haider I, Matthew H, Oswald I: Electroencephalographic changes in acute drug poisoning. Electroencephalogr Clin Neurophysiol 30:23–31, 1971.
38. García-Larrea L, Fischer C, Artru F: Effet des anesthésiques sur les potentiels évoqués sensoriels. Neurophysiol Clin 23:141–162, 1993.
39. Guérit JM (ed): Les Potentiels Évoqués. Paris, Masson, 1991.
40. Guérit JM, Mahieu P: Multimodality evoked potentials in the diagnosis of brain death. In Barko D, Gerstenbrand F, Turkani P (eds): Neurology in Europe—I. London, John Libbey, 1990, pp 373–378.
41. Guérit JM: Evoked potentials: A safe brain-death confirmatory tool? Eur J Med 1:233–243, 1992.
42. Guérit JM, de Tourtchaninoff M, Soveges L, et al: The prognostic value of three-modality evoked potentials in anoxic and traumatic comas. Neurophysiol Clin 23:209–226, 1993.
43. Hantson P, de Tourtchaninoff M, Simoëns G, et al: Evoked potentials investigation of visual dysfunction after methanol poisoning. Crit Care Med 27:2707–2715, 1999.
44. Guérit JM, Meulders M: Clinical applications of the quantification of the relationship between body temperature and brain-stem auditory evoked potentials. Electroencephalogr Clin Neurophysiol 52:S39-S40, 1981.
45. Guérit JM, Sovèges L, Baele P, et al: Evoked potentials in profound hypothermia for ascending aorta repair. Electroencephalogr Clin Neurophysiol 77:163–173, 1990.
46. Jones SJ: SEPs: Clinical observation and applications. In Halliday AM (ed): Evoked Potentials in Clinical Testing, 2nd ed. Edinburgh, Churchill Livingstone, 1993, pp 462–465.
47. Picton TW: Auditory evoked potentials. In Daly DD, Pedley TA (eds): Current Practice of Clinical Electroencephalography, 2nd ed. New York, Raven Press, 1990, pp 642–643.
48. Chiappa KH: BAEP: Methodology. In Chiappa KH (ed): Evoked Potentials in Clinical Medicine, 2nd ed. New York, Raven Press, 1990, pp 218–220.
49. Chiappa KH: Short-latency SEP: Methodology. In Chiappa KH (ed): Evoked Potentials in Clinical Medicine, 2nd ed. New York, Raven Press, 1990, pp 368–369.
50. Chiappa KH: BAEP: interpretation. In Chiappa KH (ed): Evoked Potentials in Clinical Medicine, 2nd ed. New York, Raven Press, 1990, pp 271–272.
51. Mauguière F, Garcia-Larrea L, Bertrand O: Utility and uncertainties of evoked potentials monitoring in the intensive care unit. In Grundi BL, Villani RM (eds): Evoked Potentials—Intraoperative and ICU Monitoring. Wien, Springer-Verlag, 1988, pp 153–167.
52. Chatrian GE: Coma, other states of altered responsiveness and brain death. In Daly DD, Pedley TA (eds): Current Practice of Clinical Electroencephalography, 2nd ed. New York, Raven Press, 1990, pp 425–487.
53. Hantson P, Mahieu P, de Tourtchaninoff M, et al: The problem of "brain death" and organ donation in poisoned patients. In Machado C (ed): Recent Developments in Neurology: Brain Death. Amsterdam, Elsevier, 1995, pp 127–134.
54. Jones AL, Simpson KJ: Drug abusers and poisoned patients: A potential source of organs for transplantation. QJM 91:589–592, 1998.

55. Leikin JB, Heyn-Lamb R, Erickson T, et al: The toxic patient as a potential organ donor. Am J Emerg Med 12:151–154, 1994.
56. Hantson P, Vekemans MC, Squifflet JP, et al: Successful pancreas-renal transplantation after cyanide poisoning. Clin Transplant 5:419–421, 1991.
57. Hantson P, Vekemans MC, Squifflet JP, et al: Outcome following organ removal from poisoned donors: Experience with 12 cases and a review of the literature. Transpl Int 8:185–189, 1995.
58. Hantson P, Kremer Y, Lerut J, et al: Successful liver transplantation with a graft coming from a methanol-poisoned donor. Transpl Int 9:437, 1996.
59. Hantson P, Vekemans MC, Squifflet JP, et al: Organ transplantation from victims of carbon monoxide poisoning. Ann Emerg Med 27:673–674, 1996.
60. Hantson P, Vekemans MC, Laterre PF, et al: Heart donation after fatal acetaminophen poisoning. J Toxicol Clin Toxicol 35:325–326, 1997.
61. Hantson P: The poisoned donors. Curr Opin Organ Transpl 4:125–129, 1999.
62. Hantson P, Mahieu P: Organ donation after fatal poisoning. QJM 92:415–418, 1999.
63. Evrard P, Hantson P, Ferrant E, et al: Successful double lung transplantation with a graft obtained from a methanol poisoned donor. Chest 115:1458–1459, 1999.
64. Hantson P, Vanormelingen P, Squifflet JP, et al: Methanol poisoning and organ transplantation. Transplantation 68:165–166, 1999.
65. Hantson P, Vanormelingen P, Lecomte C, et al: Fatal methanol poisoning and organ donation: Experience with seven cases in a single center. Transplant Proc 32:491–492, 2000.
66. Tenderich C, Koerner MK, Posival H, et al: Hemodynamic follow-up of cardiac allografts from poisoned donors. Transplantation 66:1163–1167, 1998.
67. Hanzlick R: Postmortem tricyclic antidepressant concentrations: Lethal vs nonlethal levels. Am J Forensic Med Pathol 10:326–329, 1989.
68. Karlson-Stiber C, Persson H: Ethylene glycol poisoning: Experience from an epidemic in Sweden. J Toxicol Clin Toxicol 30:565–574, 1992.
69. Tazelaar HD, Karch SB, Stephens BG, et al: Cocaine and the heart. Hum Pathol 18:195–199, 1987.
70. Devi BG, Chan AW: Effect of cocaine on cardiac biochemical functions. J Cardiovasc Pharmacol 33:1–6, 1999.
71. Bai H, Otsu K, Islam MN, et al: Direct cardiotoxic effects of cocaine and cocaethylene on isolated cardiomyocytes. Int J Cardiol 53:15–23, 1996.
72. Koerner MM, Tenderich G, Minami K, et al: Extended donor criteria: Use of cardiac allografts after carbon monoxide poisoning. Transplantation 63:1358–1360, 1997.
73. Tritapepe L, Macchiarelli G, Rocco M, et al: Functional and ultrastructural evidence of myocardial stunning after acute carbon monoxide poisoning. Crit Care Med 26:797–801, 1998.
74. Barkoukis TJ, Sarbak CA, Lewis D, et al: Multiorgan procurement from a victim of cyanide poisoning: A case report and review of the literature. Transplantation 55:1434–1436, 1993.
75. Smith JA, Bergin PJ, Williams TJ, et al: Successful heart transplantation with cardiac allografts exposed to carbon monoxide poisoning. J Heart Lung Transplant 11:698–700, 1992.
76. Tobbli JE, Ferder L, Angerosa M, et al: Effects of amlodipine on tubulointerstitial lesions in normotensive oxaluric rats. Hypertension 34:854–858, 1999.
77. Hylander B, Kjellstrand CM: Prognostic factors and treatment of severe ethylene glycol intoxication. Intensive Care Med 22:546–552, 1996.
78. Andrews PA, Koffman CG: Kidney donation after paracetamol overdose. BMJ 306:1129, 1993.
79. Hantson P, Mahieu P: Pancreatic injury following acute methanol poisoning. J Toxicol Clin Toxicol 38:297–303, 2000.

CHAPTER 16

The Treatment of Critically Ill Patients with Hyperbaric Oxygen Therapy

Lindell K. Weaver

Hyperbaric oxygen (HBO$_2$) therapy is defined by the Undersea and Hyperbaric Medical Society (UHMS) as the inhalation of 100% oxygen at pressures greater than 1.4 atmospheres absolute (atm abs).[1] There are 13 disease categories in which the scientific committee of the UHMS supports the use of HBO$_2$ therapy (Table 16-1). The inhalation of pure oxygen at increased ambient pressure is used in these disorders for specific physiologic purposes. Many of the patients who have the disorders listed in Table 16-1 could be critically ill, and the purpose of this chapter is to discuss pertinent issues regarding the treatment of critically ill patients with HBO$_2$.

If an HBO$_2$ unit anticipates referrals of critically ill patients, the unit needs to be equipped and configured as a critical care environment. The personnel assigned to the HBO$_2$ unit need to be skilled and trained in critical care. It is beyond the scope of this chapter to discuss critical care medicine in detail, but several important points related to the treatment of critically ill patients with HBO$_2$ therapy are covered.

TYPES OF CHAMBERS

There are two types of chambers in which patients are treated with HBO$_2$: the multiplace chamber (Fig. 16-1) and the monoplace chamber (Fig. 16-2). The multiplace chamber can be occupied by more than one individual. Multiplace chambers are filled with air. The patient breathes 100% oxygen delivered by a hood, mask, or endotracheal tube. Multiplace chambers require at least one inside attendant and at least one individual outside the chamber to operate the chamber. Multiplace chambers permit hands-on care of the patient. Information regarding the treatment of critically ill patients in the multiplace chamber can be found elsewhere.[2–5] A higher treatment volume is usually necessary to make a multiplace chamber economically viable.

The monoplace chamber generally is filled with oxygen, although the chamber may be filled with filtered, oil-free air while the patient breathes 100% oxygen similar to patients treated in the multiplace chamber. Monoplace chambers typically are made of acrylic cylinders and are mobile, although their weight can exceed 800 lb. A relatively long room is needed for the monoplace chamber because the patient is moved in and out of the chamber by use of a stretcher that attaches at the end of the chamber while the entry hatch is open. Information is available regarding critical care issues in the monoplace chamber as well.[6–8]

Patients compressed in hyperbaric chambers may be exposed to high partial pressures of oxygen, so fire safety is crucial.[9] Fires and explosions have occurred in multiplace and monoplace chambers, but hyperbaric medicine as practiced in the United States has been exceptionally safe. It is important that the patient be grounded and dressed in antistatic cotton and that no flammable materials enter the chamber. All physiologic monitoring must be satisfactorily grounded and all electrically operated apparatus must be intrinsically electrically safe.[7,9–12] Considerable detail about hyperbaric facility safety, including fire safety, is provided in another text.[12]

HISTORY OF HYPERBARIC OXYGEN THERAPY

Hyperbaric air therapy dates back to the time of Crenshaw in the 1660s in England. Hyperbaric air domiciliaries were available in several cities in Europe during the mid-1800s, and pressures of 4 atm abs were used in Junod's copper sphere. HBO$_2$ therapy first came into clinical use in the late 1950s and early 1960s by Boerema and colleagues[13] in the Netherlands, who treated life-threatening anaerobic infections and pioneered the use of HBO$_2$ to support life during asystolic cardiac arrest for surgery. HBO$_2$ therapy used for cardiac surgery was discarded when membrane oxygenators were developed in the 1970s. There was considerable enthusiasm for HBO$_2$ therapy in the mid to late 1960s, and the National Academy of Sciences published a report called *Fundamentals of Hyperbaric Oxygen*, which has been reprinted by the UHMS.[14] For various reasons, including some mishaps, enthusiasm for HBO$_2$ waned during the 1970s, but based on increasing evidence of its efficacy, HBO$_2$ therapy began to regain acceptance in the mid to late 1980s. Presently, there are more than 300 clinical hyperbaric medicine facilities in the United States, and the list continues to expand. Many HBO$_2$ centers in the United States are affiliated with problem wound centers because HBO$_2$ therapy is used for selected problem wounds.

PHYSIOLOGY AND MECHANISMS

HBO$_2$ therapy causes several physiologic effects (Table 16-2). According to Boyle's law (pressure × volume = constant), compression of a gas-filled space results in reduction of the

TABLE 16-1 Undersea and Hyperbaric Medical Society–Approved Indications for Hyperbaric Oxygen Therapy

Air or gas embolism
Carbon monoxide poisoning/carbon monoxide poisoning complicated by cyanide poisoning
Clostridial myositis and myonecrosis (gas gangrene)
Crush injury, compartment syndrome, and other acute traumatic ischemias
Decompression sickness
Enhancement of healing in selected problem wounds
Exceptional blood loss (anemia)
Intracranial abscess
Necrotizing soft tissue infections
Osteomyelitis (refractory)
Delayed radiation injury (soft tissue and bony necrosis)
Skin grafts and flaps (compromised)
Thermal burns

Data from Feldmeier JJ: Hyperbaric Oxygen 2003: Indications and Results. The Hyperbaric Oxygen Therapy Committee Report. Kensington, MD, Undersea and Hyperbaric Medical Society, 2003.

volume of the gas-filled space. HBO_2 causes high partial pressures of arterial oxygen and tissue oxygen tensions. High arterial oxygen tensions and tissue oxygen tensions may improve oxygen delivery to vital organs or tissues that are compromised by ischemia. Polymorphonuclear leukocytes require oxygen for optimal phagocytosis and oxidative burst mechanisms of microbial killing.[15] With HBO_2 therapy, white blood cell function can be enhanced, particularly if the infectious process is occurring in an anaerobic environment. HBO_2 therapy favorably modulates ischemia-reperfusion injury,[16] with evidence that CD11/18 polymorphonuclear leukocyte adherence is modulated,[17,18] and down-regulates endothelial expression of intracellular adhesion molecule-1.[19] Wound healing is influenced favorably by HBO_2 therapy, which can increase the number of growth factor receptor sites on human fibroblasts.[20,21] HBO_2 therapy can also sensitize tumors to radiation[22] and has been shown to be helpful as a radiosensitizing adjunct in the management of glioblastoma multiforme.[23]

INDICATIONS FOR HYPERBARIC OXYGEN THERAPY

There are several accepted indications for HBO_2 therapy per recommendations from the Hyperbaric Oxygen Therapy Committee of the UHMS (see Table 16-1).[1] Most of the disorders are associated with limitations in oxygen flow and delivery. All of the indications on the UHMS-approved list have been accepted based on strong physiologic and mechanistic reasons and convincing animal and human data. Only a few of the disorders have been subjected to the rigors of randomized clinical trials, however.[1,24] Some of the disorders could not be subjected to randomized clinical trials because they are uncommon (e.g., necrotizing fasciitis, clostridial myonecrosis, actinomycosis). Nevertheless, there is considerable information on efficacy for all of the disorders listed in Table 16-1, and the reader is encouraged to review the Hyperbaric Oxygen Therapy Committee Report.[1]

ASSESSMENT OF THE CRITICALLY ILL PATIENT REGARDING HYPERBARIC OXYGEN THERAPY

Just as with any treatment modality, the clinician continually must assess risk versus benefit with the application of treatment to the patient. This risk assessment is particularly true with HBO_2 therapy in a critically ill patient. Some HBO_2 departments are located considerable distances from the critical care unit, necessitating transport of the patient over relatively long distances within the hospital or occasionally even outside the confines of the hospital. One must consider possible risks to the patient related to transport.[25] Because the patient needs to be transported from the critical care environment to the chamber, a capable and experienced transport team needs to move the patient along with all necessary equipment. It is important that the level of care of the patient during transport (and during HBO_2)

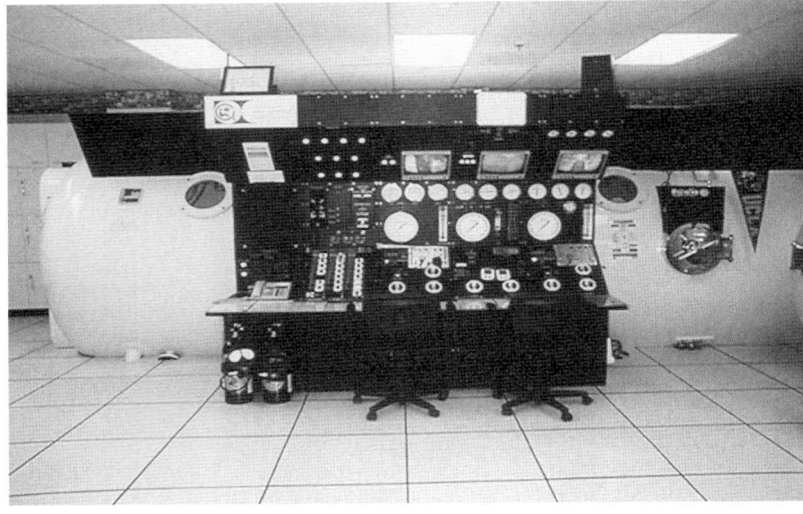

FIGURE 16-1

Multiplace hyperbaric chamber. *(Courtesy of OxyHeal Health Group, La Jolla, CA.)*

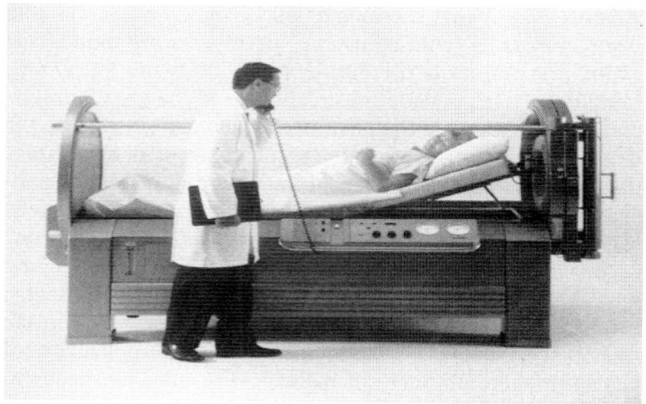

FIGURE 16-2

Sechrist 3200 monoplace hyperbaric chamber. *(Courtesy of Sechrist Industries, Inc, Anaheim, CA.)*

not be reduced compared with the level of care rendered in the intensive care unit (ICU). Specific issues that need to be addressed for HBO_2 therapy and transports are mechanical ventilation; maintenance of positive end-expiratory pressure (PEEP); adequate sedation and analgesia; and monitoring of physiologic variables, such as electrocardiogram, blood pressure, pulse oximetry, and occasionally end-tidal carbon dioxide.

If the risk of transport is believed to exceed the presumed benefit of therapy, the patient should not be moved from the ICU. It is important to ascertain the benefit of therapy so that the presumed benefit can be brought into the analysis. The benefit side of the equation is linked to the efficacy issue, which is addressed by the Hyperbaric Oxygen Therapy Committee Report.[1]

TABLE 16-2 Physiologic Properties of Hyperbaric Oxygen Therapy

Reduction in volume of gas-filled spaces
Hyperoxygenation of blood and tissue
    Sufficient oxygen dissolved in plasma to support life
    Increased oxygen diffusion distances
Reduction in edema
Enhanced host defense
    Enhanced neutrophil oxidative burst
    Bacteriostatic or bactericidal to several microorganisms
    Inactivates clostridial toxins
    Increased osteoclast activity
Neovascularization into previously irradiated, hypoxic tissue
Enhanced healing of hypoxic wounds
    Increased fibroblast production of collagen
    Increased strength of immature non–cross-linked collagen
    Increased growth factor receptor sites on fibroblasts
Modulation of ischemia-reperfusion injury
    Reduction of CD11/18-mediated neutrophil-endothelial adherence
    Down-regulation of endothelial ICAM-1 receptor sites
    Decreased arterial vasospasm after reperfusion
Tumor radiosensitization

ICAM-1, intercellular adhesion molecule-1.

HYPERBARIC DEPARTMENT

The staff members of the HBO_2 department need to be trained in critical care and be familiar with advanced cardiac life support if they are going to be treating critically ill patients. Ideally, the HBO_2 department should be near the critical care area or even within the confines of the critical care environment, if possible. As most HBO_2 facilities are economically viable because they treat problem wounds, which are predominantly treated as outpatients, the location and configuration of many HBO_2 departments are poorly suited for critically ill patients. If the unit anticipates treating critically ill patients, however, adequate space, personnel, and equipment must be available.

Suitable monitoring needs to be located in the unit. If the monitors in the HBO_2 unit are different from those in the critical care environment, suitable cables and connectors need to be available. Life-support resuscitation equipment needs to be immediately available, and the staff must be familiar with the equipment and their skills kept up to date.

Necessary equipment includes cardiac rhythm monitors, defibrillators, oxygen resuscitation masks, and various drugs, which might be used for airway protection and sedation. Other drugs include vasoactive agents (most of these drugs would be on a "crash cart"). The staff must be familiar with specific details of administering life-support drugs (e.g., lidocaine, dopamine).

The subject of defibrillation of a compressed patient seems to come up frequently, although in my experience, I have had to defibrillate or cardiovert only two patients decompressed from the chamber in more than 10 years. In the monoplace chamber, the patient can be withdrawn from the chamber quickly and can be defibrillated. The oxygen that filled the monoplace chamber pours out into the room, but by the time defibrillation pads are located on the patient and the defibrillator is charged, the risk of causing a fire if a spark were to occur is small. The patient's skin and clothing are saturated with oxygen, however, so positive contact with the paddles to the skin needs to be ensured. I have no personal experience with defibrillation in the multiplace chamber, although this technique has been described.[4,26,27]

Because the goal of HBO_2 therapy is to improve the patient's blood oxygen tension, lung efficiency needs to be optimal. Often, an increase in PEEP can reduce the right-to-left shunt fraction and venous admixture. We occasionally raise PEEP during HBO_2 therapy to try to increase oxygenation efficiency. However, a higher PEEP can cause hemodynamic instability, so airway pressure and blood pressure need to be monitored. Information is available regarding arterial oxygen tension measurements of critically ill patients with dysfunctional lungs.[28] From this work, potentially higher chamber pressures are necessary for the patient's arterial oxygen tension to approximate a similar oxygen tension as if he or she had relatively normal lungs.[28]

PEEP used in patients treated with HBO_2 needs to be monitored carefully and titrated occasionally. During HBO_2 therapy, gas density is greater than at atmospheric pressure. Most PEEP values exhibit a higher PEEP level than the stated value.[29] Experience with PEEP values is helpful for the therapist and clinicians to predict the PEEP the patient would be expected to have during HBO_2 therapy. PEEP can be titrated easily during multiplace chamber therapy and can be titrated during monoplace chamber therapy. During monoplace chamber therapy, an Emerson water column (J.H. Emerson Company, Cambridge, MA) can be used to apply PEEP. The water column (PEEP level) can be adjusted from outside the chamber by adding or removing water via an intravenous "pass-through."

It is common practice for a patient to be provided assisted breaths with a soft anesthesia bag during transport. During manually assisted ventilation, PEEP may decrease, and atelectasis could make the patient's lungs less efficient. It is generally important to maintain PEEP during transport and during HBO_2 to improve gas exchange efficiency. For this reason, it may be necessary to use portable transport ventilators or, if the patient's minute ventilation is not excessive (i.e., >15 L/min), to use a bag-valve system with PEEP applied. The measurement of airway pressures and tidal volumes should be monitored carefully during transport[30,31] and during HBO_2 therapy.[32]

PREPARING THE PATIENT FOR HYPERBARIC THERAPY

Critically ill patients often require sedation and occasionally require pharmacologic paralysis for HBO_2 therapy due to difficulties with matching the patient's ventilatory needs to the particular mechanical ventilator. Sedation and paralysis are required more often in treating mechanically ventilated patients in the monoplace chamber than in the multiplace chamber. Because hands-on capability is possible in the multiplace chamber, it may not always be necessary to paralyze the mechanically ventilated patient. There also are more ventilator choices for the multiplace chamber than the monoplace chamber. Several ventilators have been tested in the multiplace chamber,[33] including the Monoghan 225 ventilator[34] (Monoghan Medical Corp., Plattsburg, NY; production stopped in 1997 without continued parts or technical support) and the Penlon ventilator[4,35] (Penlon, Ltd., Oxford, England). Because all of these ventilators were designed for atmospheric pressure use, not HBO_2 therapy, their performance is reduced during HBO_2 use compared with their performance when used at atmospheric pressure. One must be mindful of pulmonary air trapping during HBO_2 therapy, and monitoring of the patient's airway pressures and hemodynamics during mechanical ventilation is important.

The choices for mechanical ventilation for monoplace chamber therapy include time-cycled pneumatic ventilators, such as the Sechrist 500A[36] (Sechrist Industries, Anaheim, CA) and the Omni-Vent[37,38] (Omni-Tech Medical, Inc., Topeka, KS). In a series of investigations, it was discovered that the Omni-Vent ventilator offers superior performance compared with the Sechrist 500A[36–38] during monoplace hyperbaric ventilation, but the Omni-Vent[37,38] ventilator requires considerable experience to titrate minute ventilation appropriately. Evidence of air trapping, associated hypotension, and possible barotrauma must be monitored carefully. The Sechrist 500A[36,38] and the Omni-Vent[37,38] can cause inverse-ratio ventilation if the ventilator operator is not observant and careful. An airway pressure monitor can be helpful during use of mechanical ventilation for monoplace therapy[32] (Tau Monitor; Core-M, Inc, Precision Instrument,

Allston, MA). This monitor displays airway pressures and ventilatory rates (with adjustable alarms) during monoplace ventilation. Controls for the Sechrist 500A and the Omni-Vent are located outside the chamber, and the ventilator circuit is located inside the chamber. If one chooses to use the Omni-Vent ventilator outside the chamber, it is *mandatory* that a one-way valve be located in the circuit inside the confines of the chamber.[38] The purpose of the one-way valve is to prevent potentially life-threatening pulmonary "squeeze" to the patient if there is a disconnection or pressure-reducing malfunction of the ventilator outside the chamber.[38] Presently, mechanical ventilation of critically ill patients treated in the monoplace chamber is a limitation for the application of HBO_2 in some critically ill patients. The clinician needs to have considerable experience regarding mechanical ventilation in these patients. Nevertheless, we have treated patients requiring 23 cm H_2O of PEEP and minute ventilations of 20 L/min (patients with acute respiratory distress syndrome and septic shock secondary to necrotizing fasciitis) who had satisfactory gas exchange shown by arterial blood gas measurements during HBO_2 therapy.

MONITORING

It is straightforward to monitor the electrocardiogram. Noninvasive blood pressure monitoring can be performed using the Oscillomate 1630[39] (CAS Medical Systems, Inc, Branford, CT). If the patient is critically ill, however, he or she often has an indwelling arterial catheter. For monoplace chamber therapy, an indwelling arterial catheter permitting continuous measurement of arterial pressure is important due to the level of sedation that often is needed and the limitations of mechanical ventilators (i.e., risk of air trapping resulting in hypotension).

Blood pressure is monitored in the multiplace and the monoplace chambers similarly to the way it is monitored in the ICU. Suitable connectors, all of which must be grounded, are used. The hospital's bioinstrumentation department can be a valuable resource regarding monitoring in the chamber. It is also possible to perform pulmonary arterial pressure, cardiac output, and arterial/venous oxygen content measurements.[40,41] Generally, it is clinically unnecessary to monitor Swan-Ganz catheter data during HBO_2 therapy. The technique of Swan-Ganz catheter monitoring has been described previously, and these techniques are beyond the scope of this chapter.[40,41] Monitoring of intracranial pressure[8,42] and intravascular pressure is possible through techniques identical to monitoring arterial blood pressure invasively. In the monoplace chamber, there is some limitation with the passing of electrical signals from inside the chamber to outside the chamber, and the bioengineering department needs to be engaged in the issues related to monitoring to provide suitable monitoring for monoplace chamber use.

Physiologic monitoring in the multiplace chamber is accomplished by sending the electrical signals outside the chamber, with monitors located outside the chamber. The monitors can be positioned so that personnel outside and inside the chamber may view the displays and the data.[4] A review article has summarized physiologic monitoring during HBO_2 therapy, including a comprehensive list of references.[43]

INTRAVENOUS THERAPY

Several intravenous infusion pumps are suitable for use with the monoplace chamber[44,45] and multiplace chamber.[4,5] Three intravenous infusion pumps are presently available for monoplace therapy: the reconditioned IVAC 530[44] (IVAC Corp., San Diego, CA), the Abbott Hyperbaric Pump[6] (Abbott Laboratories, Chicago, IL), and the Baxter Flo-Guard Pump[45] (Baxter Healthcare Corporation, Deerfield, IL). Data are limited regarding performance of these pumps. The Baxter pump is suitable for high-volume infusions, but the pressure alarm sensor needs to be adjusted by the hospital's bioinstrumentation department, or the pump will not operate at chamber pressures greater than 2 atm abs.[45] Many monoplace hyperbaric chamber units use the IVAC 530. This pump is a peristaltic pump and not a volumetric pump. The maximum infusion rate of the IVAC 530 is 297 mL/hr, whereas the Baxter pump maximum rate is 1999 mL/hr. The Abbott pump can infuse 800 mL/hr during HBO_2 therapy. The Baxter pump is suitable for infusion of blood products, whereas the Abbott pump is not, according to the manufacturer. The IVAC pump is poorly suited for infusion of blood products. The Baxter pump (after pressure sensor adjustment is made) seems to offer better performance than the IVAC and the Abbott pumps for monoplace applications. Intravenous infusions at 1 mL/hr or less exhibit lower-than-expected volumes during chamber compression and higher-than-expected volumes during chamber decompression.[45] This finding is clinically important for patients treated with pressors or insulin.[45]

The HBO_2 unit may need to have four to eight intravenous pumps, which could be dedicated for a single critically ill patient's treatment. If the patient requires multiple individual intravenous infusions, each infusion needs a dedicated high-pressure, hyperbaric-compatible pump. Also, the Baxter pump and the Abbott pump use special tubing, so the specific tubing may not be compatible with the current standard used in any particular hospital. Tubing requirements and sufficient numbers of pumps need to be considered if the HBO_2 unit anticipates treating critically ill patients who require multiple continuous intravenous infusions. Intravenous pass-throughs permit the intravenous line to penetrate the chamber. These pass-throughs incorporate one-way, back-check valves to prevent inadvertent blood loss if an intravenous line becomes disconnected or leaks outside the chamber.

PATIENT MANAGEMENT DURING HYPERBARIC OXYGEN THERAPY

Patient management during HBO_2 is similar to management of the patient in the critical care unit, with a few exceptions. Because patients who are intubated cannot equalize middle ear pressure, some hyperbaric medical practitioners recommend prophylactic myringotomies, whereas some do not (informal nonpublished telephone survey of approximately 20 HBO_2 centers in the United States and Canada). Our practice has been not to perform myringotomies of hyperbaric patients who are intubated, although we sedate and occasionally paralyze the patient before compression to facilitate passive eustachian tube opening during compression. There are no outcome data regarding the issue of whether myringotomies are mandatory in intubated patients receiving HBO_2 therapy. If hyperbaric unit personnel plan to perform myringotomies or to have an ear, nose, and throat (ENT) surgeons perform myringotomies, they need to have suitable equipment available (i.e., otoscopes or an ENT microscope) and training to perform the myringotomy or the immediate availability of ENT specialists who can do the myringotomies for their HBO_2-treated patients. For selected patients, prophylactic tympanostomy ventilation tubes are helpful if they can be placed before compression of an intubated or comatose patient.

If there is any doubt regarding the patient's ability to maintain the airway, the patient should be intubated for monoplace chamber therapy. Because intubation can be performed during multiplace chamber therapy, this requirement may be unnecessary for patients treated in the multiplace chamber. It takes at least 60 seconds to remove the patient from the monoplace chamber, so if there are concerns regarding aspiration or airway protection or about adequacy of ventilation or oxygenation, the patient should be intubated before HBO_2 treatment.

The endotracheal tube cuff needs to be filled with sterile saline before compression of the patient. If the cuff is not filled with sterile saline, the air-filled cuff becomes compressed as the chamber pressure increases, and the patient will develop a cuff leak. It is imperative to remove the sterile saline after each HBO_2 treatment to minimize excessive pressure transmitted from the endotracheal tube cuff to the patient's trachea.

Careful titration of mechanical ventilation is important. In selected patients, it may be important to assess arterial blood gases for adequacy of ventilation (carbon dioxide removal) and oxygenation (arterial oxygen tension). Techniques for withdrawing arterial blood from the monoplace chamber and analysis of the arterial carbon dioxide and oxygen tensions have been described previously.[28,46,47] If proper preanalytic technique is used and if the sample is maintained under firm pressure in a sealed blood gas syringe, representative data can be measured accurately by at least one instrument (ABL 330; Radiometer, Copenhagen, Denmark).[28,46,47]

Hypercapnia can increase the risk of central nervous system oxygen toxicity (seizures),[48] so careful titration and maintenance of a relatively normal arterial carbon dioxide tension ($PaCO_2$) during HBO_2 exposure is important. Because the ventilators used in monoplace chamber therapy are control mode only, the patient often needs to be sedated or pharmacologically paralyzed during HBO_2 therapy. Paralysis may be unnecessary in the multiplace chamber because there are more ventilator choices (as described previously) to ventilate the patient adequately.

HBO_2 can cause seizures,[48] although the mechanisms have not been elucidated. Fatality from arterial gas embolism in a patient with an HBO_2-induced seizure has been described.[49] Prophylactic anticonvulsants may be helpful for high-risk patients treated with HBO_2 therapy. Careful attention in following standard HBO_2-dosing schedules and control of the patient's $PaCO_2$ to prevent hypercapnia are general principles to reduce the likelihood of HBO_2-induced seizures. The incidence of HBO_2-induced seizures is 1/5000,[1] although in patients with carbon monoxide poisoning, the incidence of HBO_2-induced seizures increases to approximately 1%.[50] If a hyperoxic seizure occurs, the oxygen partial pressure should be reduced, and anticonvulsants may be given. Careful reduction in chamber pressures may be done only after the resolution of the tonic-clonic phase, unless the patient is intubated and has a patent airway. Barotrauma to the lung manifested as a pneumothorax during HBO_2 therapy is a rare possibility,[51,52] so the staff needs to be trained in the emergency placement of chest tubes and have the equipment for tube thoracostomy placement available.

Patients requiring vasoactive drugs (e.g., norepinephrine, dopamine, epinephrine) for maintenance of adequate blood pressure often experience a drop in blood pressure during compression in the monoplace chamber. Transiently increasing the vasopressor dose or even increasing the dose just before compression can treat these hypotensive episodes. We have observed that intravenous pumps decrease the amount of fluid infused into the patient during chamber compression, which is the most likely explanation for the observation of falling blood pressure during chamber compression.[45]

CONCLUSION

This chapter has reviewed some critical care issues regarding HBO_2 of critically ill patients. This brief chapter is not intended to replace specific training in critical care. If clinicians who treat HBO_2 patients anticipate receiving critically ill patients, sufficient training and experience in critical care are mandatory. HBO_2 exposes the patient to risks that the patient otherwise would not be exposed to regarding transport, possibility of seizures, and barotraumas, and a careful analysis of risk versus benefit must be ever present in the clinician's mind regarding applications of HBO_2 therapy to a given critically ill patient. Data for efficacy of HBO_2 therapy are important to facilitate this assessment. The UHMS scientific committee[1] has summarized pertinent data regarding the efficacy question of several disorders that are presently approved by the UHMS for HBO_2 therapy.

Acknowledgments
I greatly appreciate the assistance of Laura Ogaard and Kayla Deru in helping with preparation of this chapter.

REFERENCES

1. Feldman JJ: Hyperbaric Oxygen 2003: Indications and Results: The Hyperbaric Oxygen Therapy Committee Report. Kensington, MD, Undersea and Hyperbaric Medical Society, 2003.
2. Kindwall EP, Whelan HT: Hyperbaric Medicine Practice, 2nd ed. Flagstaff, AZ, 1999, Best Publishing Company.
3. Wattel F, Mathieu D, Neviere R: Management of HBO patients. In Oriani G, Marroni A, Wattel F (eds): Handbook on Hyperbaric Medicine. Milano, Italy, Springer-Verlag, 1996, pp 648–659.
4. Holcomb JR, Matos-Navarro AY, Goldmann RW: Critical care in the hyperbaric chamber. In Davis JC, Hunt TK (eds): Problem Wounds: The Role of Oxygen. New York, Elsevier Science, 1988, pp 187–209.
5. Moon RE, Hart BB: Operation use and patient monitoring in a multiplace hyperbaric chamber. Respir Care Clin N Am 5:21–49, 1999.
6. Weaver LK: Management of critically ill patients in the monoplace hyperbaric chamber. In Kindwall EP, Whelan HT (eds): Hyperbaric Medicine Practice. Flagstaff, AZ, Best Publishing Company, 1999, pp 245–322.
7. Weaver LK: Operational use and patient care in the monoplace hyperbaric chamber. Respir Care Clin N Am 5:51–92, 1999.
8. Rockswold GL, Ford E, Anderson JR, et al: Patient monitoring in the monoplace hyperbaric chamber. Hyperbaric Oxygen Review 6:161–168, 1985.
9. Sheffield PJ, Desautels DA: Hyperbaric and hypobaric chamber fires: A 73-year analysis. Undersea Hyperb Med 24:153–164, 1997.
10. Desautels DA: Guidelines for Clinical Multiplace Hyperbaric Facilities. Kensington, MD, 1994, Undersea and Hyperbaric Medical Society.
11. NFPA 99: Standard for Health Care Facilities, 1996 ed. Quincy, MA, 1996, National Fire Protection Agency.
12. Workman WT: Hyperbaric Facility Safety: A Practical Guide. Flagstaff, AZ, 2000, Best Publishing Company.
13. Boerema I, Meijne NG, Brummelkamp WH, et al: Life without blood. J Cardiovasc Surg 182:133–146, 1960.
14. Committee on Hyperbaric Oxygenation: Fundamentals of Hyperbaric Medicine. Kensington, MD, 1992, Undersea and Hyperbaric Medical Society.
15. Knighton DR, Halliday B, Hunt TL: Oxygen as an antibiotic. The effect of inspired oxygen on infection. Arch Surg 119:199–204, 1984.
16. Zamboni WA, Rogh AC, Russell RC, et al: Morphologic analysis of microcirculation during reperfusion of ischemic skeletal muscle and the effect of hyperbaric oxygen. Plast Reconstr Surg 91:1110–1123, 1993.
17. Thom SR, Mendiguren I, Hardy K, et al: Inhibition of human neutrophil $beta_2$-integrin-dependent adherence by hyperbaric O_2. Am J Physiol 273(3 Pt 1):C770-C777, 1997.
18. Chen Q, Banick PD, Thom SR: Functional inhibition of rat polymorphonuclear leukocyte β_2 integrins by hyperbaric oxygen is associated with impaired cGMP synthesis. J Pharmacol Exp Ther 276:929–933, 1996.
19. Buras JA, Stahl GL, Svoboda KK, et al: Hyperbaric oxygen down regulates ICAM-1 expression induced by hypoxia and hypoglycemia: The role of NOS. Am J Physiol Cell Physiol 278:C292-C302, 2000.
20. Reenstra WR, Dittmer C, Buras JA: Human dermal fibroblasts vary the expression of growth factor receptors in response to in vitro oxygen levels (Abstract). Undersea Hyperb Med 26(Suppl):71, 1999.
21. Bonomo SR, Davidson JD, Yu Y, et al: Hyperbaric oxygen as a signal transducer: Up regulation of platelet derived growth factor-beta receptor in the presence of HBO_2 and PDGF. Undersea Hyperb Med 25:211–216, 1998.
22. Overgarrd J, Horsman M: Modification of hypoxia-induced radioresistance in tumors by the use of oxygen and sensitizers. Semin Radiat Oncol 6:10–21, 1996.
23. Kohshi K, Kinoshita Y, Imada H: Effects of radiotherapy after hyperbaric oxygenation on malignant gliomas. Br J Cancer 80:236–241, 1999.
24. Bennett M: Randomized controlled trials. In Feldmeier JJ: Hyperbaric Oxygen 2003: Indications and Results. The Hyperbaric Oxygen Therapy Committee Report. Kensington, MD, Undersea and Hyperbaric Medical Society, 2003, pp 121–139.
25. Braman SS, Dunn SM, Amico CA, et al: Complications of intrahospital transport in critically ill patients. Ann Intern Med 107:469–473, 1987.
26. Martindale LG, Milligan M, Fries P: Test of an r-2 defibrillator adapter in a hyperbaric chamber. J Hyperb Med 2:15–25, 1987.
27. Swanson HT, Sheps S, Vanmeter KW: Use of defibrillators in the hyperbaric chamber (Abstract). Undersea Hyperb Med 26(Suppl):54, 1999.
28. Weaver LK, Howe S: Arterial oxygen tension of patients with abnormal lungs treated with hyperbaric oxygen is greater than predicted. Chest 106:1134–1139, 1994.
29. Youn BA, Houseknecht R, Deantonio A: Review of positive end-expiratory pressure and its application in the hyperbaric environment. J Hyperb Med 6:87–99, 1991.
30. Link J, Krause H, Wagner W, et al: Intrahospital transport of critically ill patients. Crit Care Med 18:1427–1429, 1990.
31. Stearley HE: Patients' outcomes: Intrahospital transportation and monitoring of critically ill patients by a specially trained ICU nursing staff. Am J Crit Care 7:282–287, 1998.
32. Hein S, Weaver LK, Howe S: Mechanical ventilator monitoring inside the monoplace hyperbaric chamber (Abstract). Undersea Hyperb Med 21(Suppl):34, 1994.
33. Stahl W, Calzia E, Radermacher P: Function of different ICU ventilators under hyperbaric conditions (Abstract). Undersea Hyperb Med 25(Suppl):15, 1998.
34. Moon RE, Bergquist LV, Conklin B, Miller JN: Monoghan 225 ventilator use under hyperbaric conditions. Chest 89:846–851, 1986.
35. Youn B, Houseknecht R: The Penlon Oxford ventilator: A second look. J Hyperb Med 6:255–261, 1991.
36. Weaver LK, Greenway L, Elliott CG: Performance of the Sechrist 500a hyperbaric ventilator in a monoplace hyperbaric chamber. J Hyperb Med 3:215–225, 1988.

37. Churchill S, Weaver LK, Haberstock D: Omni-vent: Another option for mechanical ventilation in the monoplace hyperbaric chamber (Abstract). Undersea Hyperb Med 25(Suppl):24, 1998.

38. Churchill S, Weaver LK, Haberstock D: Performance of the Omni-vent mechanical ventilator for use with the monoplace hyperbaric chamber (Abstract). Undersea Hyperb Med 26(Suppl):70–71, 1999.

39. Meyer GW, Hart GG, Strauss MB: Noninvasive blood pressure monitoring in the hyperbaric monoplace chamber: A new technique. J Hyperb Med 4:211–216, 1990.

40. Weaver LK: Technique of Swan-Ganz catheter monitoring in patients treated in the monoplace hyperbaric chamber. J Hyperb Med 7:1–18, 1992.

41. Moon RE, Baek PS, Lanzinger MJ, et al: Pulmonary hemodynamics and gas exchange at 40 m (Abstract). Undersea Hyperb Med 25(Suppl):26, 1998.

42. Sukoff MH, Ragatz RE: Hyperbaric oxygenation for the treatment of acute cerebral edema. Neurosurgery 10:29–38, 1982.

43. Roatsky GG, Shifrin EG, Mayevsky A: Physiologic and biochemical monitoring during hyperbaric oxygenation: A review. Undersea Hyperb Med 26:111–122, 1999.

44. Ziegler BA, Weaver LK: Intravenous infusion pumps: Evaluation for use with the monoplace hyperbaric chamber. Undersea Biomed Res 18(Suppl):91, 1991.

45. Ray D, Weaver LK, Churchill S, Haberstock D: Performance of the Baxter Flo-Gard 6201 infusion pump for use with the monoplace hyperbaric chamber. Undersea Hyperb Med 27:101–111, 2000.

46. Weaver LK, Howe S: Normobaric measurement of arterial oxygen tension in subjects exposed to hyperbaric oxygen. Chest 102:1175–1181, 1992.

47. Weaver LK, Howe S, Berlin SL: Normobaric measurement of O_2 tension of blood and saline tonometered under hyperbaric O_2 conditions. J Hyperb Med 5:29–38, 1990.

48. Clark JM: Oxygen toxicity. In Bennett P, Elliott D (eds): The Physiology and Medicine of Diving. London, 1993, WB Saunders, pp 121–169.

49. Bond GF: Arterial gas embolism. In Davis JC, Hunt TK (eds): Hyperbaric Oxygen Therapy. Kensington, MD, Undersea Medical Society, 1977, pp 141–152.

50. Hampson NB, Simonson SG, Kramer CC, et al: Central nervous system oxygen toxicity during hyperbaric treatment of patients with carbon monoxide poisoning. Undersea Hyperb Med 23:215–219, 1996.

51. Wolf HK, Moon RE, Mitchell PR, et al: Barotrauma and air embolism in hyperbaric oxygen therapy. Am J Forensic Med Pathol 111:49–53, 1990.

52. Murphy DG, Sloan EP, Hart RG, et al: Tension pneumothorax associated with hyperbaric oxygen therapy. Am J Emerg Med 9:176–179, 1991.

PART 2

Toxic Syndromes

CHAPTER 17

Drug-Induced Hepatic Failure

Thomas Riley ■ Amit Sadana

The sudden failure of a previously healthy and functioning liver is a dramatic and devastating event. Acute liver failure is the common final pathway of a multitude of conditions and insults, all of which result in massive hepatic necrosis or loss of normal hepatic function. The ensuing multiorgan system failure frequently has a fatal outcome, with mortality rates in most series ranging from approximately 55% to 95%.[1] Fulminant hepatic failure (FHF) knows no age boundaries, with many cases occurring in those younger than 30 years. Short of excellent intensive care unit (ICU) support and liver transplantation in selected cases, few viable treatment options are available. Over the past few decades, however, survival has been improved by anticipation, recognition, and early treatment of associated complications, as well as the application of prognostic criteria for early identification of patients requiring liver transplantation (along with improvement in the techniques and science of transplantation itself). Fortunately, FHF remains rare, with about 2000 cases being diagnosed annually in the United States. Acute viral hepatitis claims roughly 2000 lives on a yearly basis.[2] From 1980 to 1988, almost 7500 deaths from FHF occurred in the United States.[2] In 2002, an estimated 300 liver transplants were performed for FHF in the United States.

The aim of this chapter is to help clinicians recognize the presentation and clinical features of drug- or chemical-induced FHF, anticipate and appropriately manage the complications of FHF, and recognize the indications for timely referral for orthotopic liver transplantation (OLT). The pathophysiology, differential diagnosis, appropriate laboratory testing in the evaluation and treatment of FHF, and specific therapies available for certain etiologies of FHF will also be discussed. Current and future trends in liver transplantation will be described.

DEFINITIONS

The term "fulminant hepatic failure" was used in 1970 by Trey and Davidson[3] to describe patients without preexisting liver disease in whom hepatic encephalopathy developed

within 8 weeks of the first symptoms of liver injury. Since then, numerous changes in this definition and alternative nomenclatures have been proposed. In 1986, Bernuau and colleagues[4] suggested that FHF be applied to patients in whom encephalopathy would develop within 2 weeks of the onset of jaundice and that subfulminant hepatic failure be applied to those in whom this interval was 2 to 12 weeks. Gimson and coworkers[5] defined patients in whom encephalopathy developed between 8 and 26 weeks after the onset of jaundice as having late-onset hepatic failure. In 1993, O'Grady and associates[6] proposed the terms hyperacute, acute, and subacute liver failure based on whether the interval between the appearance of encephalopathy and jaundice was 0 to 7 days, 8 to 28 days, or 29 days to 12 weeks, respectively. Both Bernuau and O'Grady included cases of preexisting asymptomatic chronic liver conditions, thus eliminating Trey's original criterion of no previous liver disease.

These classification systems reflect important differences in the clinical course and prognosis observed between patient subgroups, thus facilitating earlier diagnosis and timely referral for OLT. For example, both the hyperacute and acute liver failure groups have a high incidence of cerebral edema. However, whereas patients in the hyperacute group are more likely to survive with medical management, patients in the acute liver failure group tend to die without liver transplantation.[6] The subacute failure group has a lower incidence of cerebral edema and a higher incidence of portal hypertension manifestations, including ascites and renal failure.[5,6] Mortality in this group remains high. O'Grady and colleagues found that the hyperacute failure group had a 36% survival rate, as opposed to 7% and 14% in the acute and subacute failure cohorts, respectively.[6] Of note, higher survival rates are now observed in similar patient populations with the widespread use of liver transplantation. Bernuau and coworkers also noted that those with the most rapid onset of encephalopathy had the best chance of survival.[4] Similar observations have been made in Japan.[7] However, it is important to note that although the interval between the onset of encephalopathy and jaundice was of prognostic significance in O'Grady's cohort,[1] it was not an independent prognostic factor in Brenuau's cohort,[8] thus raising doubts about its universal applicability. Application of the O'Grady classification to 423 prospectively studied patients from a tertiary care referral center in northern India failed to yield any prognostic differences between the groups.[9]

Although these classifications may be useful in highlighting differences in clinical course and prognosis among patient subgroups, the contribution of other independent prognostic indicators (etiology of FHF, patient age, prothrombin time, factor V level, renal function, mental status) should not be overlooked. In this text the original definition of FHF by Trey and coauthors will be used, with the recognition that no universally accepted nomenclature has been adopted and that there is heterogeneity and overlap in patient presentation and prognosis, regardless of the classification system used. Table 17-1 provides a summary of the various definitions of liver failure.

PATHOGENESIS

Measuring about 1500 mL in volume, the liver is the second largest organ in the body and plays a critical role in its homeostasis. At no time is this role more apparent than during an episode of acute injury. Derangements in synthetic function (hypoalbuminemia, decreased levels of clotting factors), gluconeogenesis (hypoglycemia), drug and toxin metabolism (sensitivity to narcotics and benzodiazepines, hyperammonemia), excretory function (hyperbilirubinemia), temperature regulation (hypothermia), and central nervous system function (encephalopathy) are the result of liver failure. Some of these parameters are used as prognostic factors and markers of severity of injury.

The exact mechanisms of injury and impairment in hepatocellular function that lead to FHF are poorly understood. Loss of integrity of the hepatocyte plasma membrane secondary to chemical, immunologic, or a wide variety of other insults is thought to represent the final common pathway that leads to cell necrosis and FHF.[10,11] Damage to the cell membrane permits leakage of enzymes, coenzymes, and electrolytes from the cytosol, followed by an influx of calcium ions, which eventually results in cell death. The importance of calcium is underscored by the finding that normally vulnerable hepatocytes in vitro do not succumb to the cytotoxic effects of membrane-active toxins when calcium ions are not included in the culture medium.[12]

New information is emerging on the role of growth factors and the inflammatory cascade in FHF. Transforming growth factor-β_1 (TGF-β_1) has been identified as exerting an inhibitory effect on hepatic regeneration, with its effects being counteracted by hepatocyte growth factor (HGF). In a recent study, FHF patients with non-A, non-B hepatitis demonstrated increased total TGF-β_1 with a less elevated HGF level, thus suggesting an imbalance in growth factor interplay as a cause of impaired hepatic regeneration.[13] This mechanism has also been suggested by research performed in posttransplant patients.[14] Studies suggest that activation of the cytokine network may represent the common final pathway for the development of FHF.[15] Although multiple inflammatory cascades come into play, interleukin-1, interleukin-6, and tumor necrosis factor-α have been identified as the more important mediators, along with endotoxin and nitric oxide. In response to the initial hepatic insult, interplay among these mediators sets into motion a vicious self-perpetuating cycle resulting in continued hepatic injury and multiorgan failure. Furthermore, higher levels of circulating interleukin-8 and interferon-γ have been demonstrated in patients with FHF than in healthy volunteers and those with chronic liver disease, thus suggesting a pathogenic role in acute hepatic injury. Although no relationship was found between the levels of these two markers and the clinical course, elevated levels of interleukin-10 were found to be predictive of improved outcome.[16]

ETIOLOGY AND DIFFERENTIAL DIAGNOSIS

The etiology of FHF can be determined in up to 60% to 80% of cases (Tables 17-2 and 17-3).[17] It warrants a diagnostic evaluation because the etiology can have prognostic implications (e.g., the prognosis is worse with Wilson's disease and idiosyncratic drug reactions, better with viral- and acetaminophen-induced FHF), influence treatment options (e.g., N-acetylcysteine [NAC] for FHF induced by acetaminophen [acetyl-para-aminophenol (APAP) or paracetamol]), and indicate the need for genetic testing of family members (e.g., Wilson's disease).[18] Etiologies of FHF can be divided into toxic and nontoxic. Toxic causes include pharmaceuticals, drugs of abuse, chemicals, and biologic agents. Nontoxic causes include, but are not limited to, infections, ischemia, metabolic derangements, malignancy, autoimmune problems, and primary graft failure after liver transplantation. Because FHF represents the common final pathway of injury, it is difficult to differentiate between the aforementioned causes based solely on clinical presentation and disease progression. A detailed patient history is invaluable, and a multitude of helpful diagnostic testing tools are available to help uncover the etiology of FHF in the majority of cases.

Frequency of Causes

Although the frequency varies geographically, the most common causes of FHF remain viral and drug-induced hepatitis. In London, paracetamol poisoning was responsible

---

TABLE 17-1 Definitions of Liver Failure

Trey (1970):	*Fulminant hepatic failure:* encephalopathy within 8 weeks of onset of symptoms with no preexisting liver disease
Bernuau (1986):	*Fulminant hepatic failure:* encephalopathy within 2 weeks of onset of jaundice
	Subfulminant hepatic failure: encephalopathy within 2–12 weeks of onset of jaundice
Gimson (1986):	*Late-onset hepatic failure:* encephalopathy within 8–26 weeks of onset of symptoms
O'Grady (1993):	*Hyperacute liver failure:* encephalopathy within 7 days of onset of jaundice
	Acute liver failure: encephalopathy within 8–28 days of onset of jaundice
	Subacute liver failure: encephalopathy within 5–12 weeks of onset of jaundice

TABLE 17-2 Etiology of Fulminant Hepatic Failure

INFECTIONS	TOXINS/CHEMICALS	VASCULAR	METABOLIC/OTHERS

Viral hepatitis
  HAV
  HBV
  HCV (rare, coinfection)
  HDV (coinfection)
  HEV (rare in USA)
  Herpesviruses (HSV/CMV/VZV/
    EBV in immunosuppressed)
  Yellow fever
Coxiella burnetii
Plasmodium falciparum
Amebic abscesses
Tuberculosis (disseminated)
Bacillus cereus
	Cyclopeptide mushrooms
	  A. phalloides
	  A. verna
	  A. virosa
	  A. tenuifolia
	  A. brunnescens
	  A. bisporigera
	  G. autumnalis
	  G. venenata
	  G. marginata
	  L. vosserandii
	  L. helveola
	Herbals
	  Kava
	  Chaparral
	  Gentian
	  Scutellaria
	  Germander
	  Alchemilla
	  Senna
	  Shark cartilage
	Sea anemone sting
	Carbon tetrachloride
	Aflatoxin
	Halogenated hydrocarbons
	Toluene
	Trichloroethylene
	Tetrachloroethane
	Chloroform
	Phosphorus
	Ethanol
	Drugs (see Table 17-3)
		Budd-Chiari syndrome
		VOD
		Heatstroke
		CHF
		Ischemia
		  MI, PE, tamponade, sepsis, intra-
		    operative hypotension, etc.
		Malignant infiltration
			Wilson's disease
			Fatty liver of pregnancy
			Reye's syndrome
			Galactosemia
			Hereditary fructose intolerance
			Hereditary tyrosinemia
			Jejunoileal bypass
			Autoimmune hepatitis
			Primary graft failure

A, *Amanita*; CHF, congestive heart failure; CMV, cytomegalovirus; EBV, Epstein-Barr virus; G, *Galerina*; HAV, hepatitis A virus;
HBV, hepatitis B virus; HCV, hepatitis C virus; HDV, hepatitis delta virus; HEV, hepatitis E virus; HSV, herpes simplex virus; L, *Lepiota*;
MI, myocardial infarction; PE, pulmonary embolism; VOD, vascular occlusive disease; VZV, varicella-zoster virus.

for 57% of FHF cases seen at King's College Hospital between 1973 and 1991, whereas in France, acetaminophen was identified as the etiology in only 2% of FHF cases between 1972 and 1990.[19] In the United States, a multicenter study of 295 patients in whom FHF was diagnosed between 1994 and 1996 found that the most common etiologies were APAP (20%), viral hepatitis (10% hepatitis B, 7% hepatitis A), cryptogenic (15%), and drug reactions (12%) (Fig. 17-1).[20]

Toxic Causes

PHARMACEUTICALS

Hepatotoxicity can result from therapeutic or toxic doses of many medications by a multitude of mechanisms. It can be manifested as asymptomatic elevations of liver enzymes, but some cases can progress to FHF. Hepatocyte injury can occur directly from disruption of intracellular function or membrane integrity or indirectly from immune-mediated membrane disruption. Drugs can also cause cholestasis, steatosis, idiosyncratic reactions, fibrosis, veno-occlusive disease, vasculitis, and granulomatous reactions. Categorization of these toxic reactions suggests the type and duration of exposure.

Acute APAP overdose (usually a suicide attempt) remains one of the most common causes of FHF in the United States and Great Britain (see Chapter 55). The maximum

TABLE 17-3 Examples of Drugs Commonly Implicated in Fulminant Hepatic Failure

Acetaminophen	Nonsteroidal antiinflammatory
Amiodarone	drugs
Carbon tetrachloride	Phenytoin
Gold	Rifampin
Halothane	Sulfonamides
Isoniazid	Tetracycline
Ketoconazole	Tricyclic antidepressants
Methyldopa	Valproic acid
Monoamine oxidase inhibitors	

Etiology of FHF (n = 295)

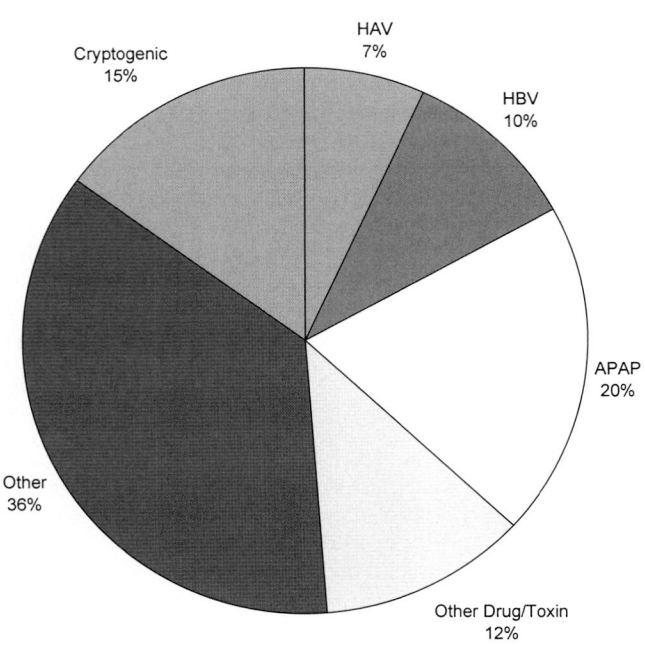

FIGURE 17-1

Etiology of fulminant hepatic failure (FHF). APAP, acetyl-*para*-aminophenol; HAV, hepatitis A virus; HBV, hepatitis B virus.

daily recommended dose of APAP is 80 mg/kg for children and 4 g for adults. The minimum dose for toxicity from a single ingestion is 150 mg/kg for children and 7.5 to 10 g for adults.[21] Doses greater than 350 mg/kg almost always result in severe hepatotoxicity.[22] However, APAP toxicity is increasingly being recognized as a cause of FHF even when used in supratherapeutic doses, and such "therapeutic misadventures" may represent the most common cause of FHF in the United States.[23] These cases usually occur when APAP is misused in the setting of chronic pain and alcohol use or less commonly with medications that induce the cytochrome P-450 system (e.g., isoniazid [INH], rifampin, phenytoin) or in the setting of starvation (depleted glutathione [GSH] stores).[24] High aminotransferase levels are typical of such cases, with values usually peaking above 4000 U/L and sometimes above 10,000 U/L. The case-fatality rate of alcohol-related acetaminophen toxicity is about 20%.[25]

The metabolic activation of certain drugs by the liver into hepatotoxic intermediates is an important phenomenon in drug-induced FHF. The resultant toxic metabolites co-valently bind to important macromolecular constituents of the cell and prevent normal functioning or cause necrosis of the cell. Acetaminophen metabolism (see Fig. 55-1) serves as a pertinent example. Most of the ingested APAP is conjugated with glucuronide or sulfate and excreted as a harmless metabolite.[26,27] In therapeutic doses, approximately 5% of APAP is oxidized by the P-450 system to *N*-acetyl-*p*-benzoquinoneimine (NAPQI), a toxic intermediate that is readily detoxified by reaction with GSH.[26,27] An APAP overdose overwhelms the sulfation and glucuronidation pathways and drives the formation of NAPQI, detoxification of which depletes GSH stores.[26,27] Once the binding capacity of GSH is exceeded, NAPQI covalently binds to key hepatocyte membrane and cellular proteins and causes necrosis.[26,27]

Concurrent use of certain medications can further amplify the production of hepatotoxic intermediates by induction of the cytochrome family responsible for metabolism of the parent drug. For example, alcohol,[28] INH,[29] and possibly phenytoin[30] cause induction of the P-450 system, which enhances the conversion of APAP to NAPQI. In addition, alcohol inhibits the synthesis of GSH, thereby decreasing clearance of NAPQI.[31] Chronic alcohol abusers are also more likely to be malnourished and have an antecedent fasting period, which also depletes GSH stores. Thus, supratherapeutic doses of APAP in conjunction with regular alcohol use can result in elevated NAPQI levels and subsequent hepatic injury—the so-called therapeutic misadventure.[32] It is important to note that starvation, a GSH-depleted state, is an independent risk factor for a therapeutic misadventure with APAP, regardless of concurrent alcohol use. Another example of synergistic toxicity is noted in patients treated with INH and rifampin, where rifampin-induced cytochrome induction can potentiate INH hepatotoxicity.[33]

Whereas APAP-induced injury is predictable and dose dependent, other drugs (e.g., valproic acid, troglitazone, amiodarone) can cause rare idiosyncratic and unpredictable hepatotoxic effects. Hypersensitivity reactions can occur with the use of phenytoin, *para*-aminosalicylate, chlorpromazine, and sulfonamides, with catastrophic results. Idiosyncratic reactions do not exhibit dose-related toxicity, and some can result in FHF with a single dose. They occur in a small fraction of susceptible individuals and are unpredictable. Patients with chronic liver disease may be at increased risk for such reactions. The formation of immunologically stimulating drug-protein complexes (neoantigens) with a resultant "innocent bystander" effect is thought to be one of the pathogenic mechanisms of injury.[34]

The halogenated anesthetics halothane, enflurane, methoxyflurane, and isoflurane have uncommonly been associated with the development of toxic hepatitis, but hepatic failure is rare. They usually develop after multiple exposures to these agents and are thought to be of combined toxic and allergic origin. Nonsteroidal antiinflammatory drugs, especially sulindac and diclofenac, have also been known to cause liver disease, with an incidence of 1.1 to 3.7 cases per 100,000 prescriptions.[35] The macrolide antibiotics erythromycin and clarithromycin are rare causes of hepatic failure that exhibit primarily cholestasis on biopsy and, uncommonly, hepatic necrosis.[36]

Tetracycline demonstrates yet another mechanism of hepatotoxicity. It is known to bind hepatocyte tRNA and impair apoprotein synthesis, thereby causing triglyceride buildup in the liver. It may also cause concurrent derangements in fatty acid uptake, formation, and oxidation by hepatocytes, which culminate in the loss of hepatic function secondary to acute microvesicular fatty infiltration.[37] Aspirin, valproic acid, amiodarone, and zidovudine are also known to cause microvesicular steatosis.[23]

HERBAL MEDICATIONS

Widespread use of herbal remedies in Europe and their ever-growing popularity in the United States have bought to light many case reports of associated hepatotoxicity. Herbals and alternative medications implicated include chaparral, gentian, germander, and senna, but they rarely result in liver failure.[38] Most recently, two case reports suggesting a causal relationship between kava (a herbal supplement used for the treatment of anxiety) and FHF requiring transplantation were published.[39] Twenty-four other reports of kava-related hepatotoxicity have led to a ban on kava in Switzerland and Germany. The U.S. Food and Drug Administration (FDA) currently has the supplement on so-called MedWatch alert status. Although virtually any drug can cause acute liver injury, more common examples are listed in Table 17-3.

DRUGS OF ABUSE

Severe liver injury and even hepatic failure can result from recreational drug use, including abuse of cocaine, 3,4-methylenedioxymethamphetamine (MDMA, or Ecstasy), and phencyclidine, or from recreational inhalation of solvents containing toluene or trichloroethylene.[40] Hepatic failure in these cases may be the result of liver ischemia, hypoxemia, severe hyperpyrexia, rhabdomyolysis, and/or direct hepatotoxic effect.

In addition to these effects, cocaine's hepatotoxicity is thought to be due primarily to ischemia from systemic arterial vasospasm and congestive heart failure, complicated by the occurrence of disseminated intravascular coagulation (DIC) and renal failure. The histologic pattern is both centrilobular necrosis and microvesicular steatosis. MDMA causes a syndrome similar to that of cocaine: hyperthermia, DIC, and rhabdomyolysis, complicated further by dehydration and acute renal failure. Toxic hepatitis may be immediate or delayed, and the histopathology is characterized by central and midzonal necrosis or by steatosis and eosinophilic infiltration.[40] The latter suggests an immune mechanism of MDMA hepatotoxicity, and liver transplantation has been required in some cases.[41]

CHEMICALS

Industrial exposure to cleaning solvents containing fluorinated or halogenated hydrocarbons is a well-documented cause of hepatic necrosis, fatty infiltration, and ultimately, FHF. Carbon tetrachloride's hepatotoxic effects, noted in the 1920s to 1940s, led to its abandonment as an anesthetic and anthelmintic by the FDA, but it is still used in the production of solvents, refrigerants, and aerosol propellants. The fluorinated hydrocarbon chloroform, a potent central nervous system depressant once used as an anesthetic, has also been banned by the FDA because of its hepatotoxicity, but it is still found in industrial use.

BIOLOGIC AGENTS

Hepatotoxicity secondary to accidental ingestion of poisonous mushrooms has been on the rise because of popular interest in gathering and eating uncultivated mushrooms.[42] An increase in the incidence of mushroom poisoning is usually seen after periods of heavy rainfall or during the fall, when the conditions for growth are optimal. Ingestion of cyclopeptide-containing mushrooms accounts for up to 90% of mushroom-related deaths worldwide.[42-46] The genus *Amanita* is the source of most of these poisonings, especially *A. phalloides* (death cap), *A. verna* (death angel), and *A. virosa* (destroying angel). *Galerina* and *Lepiota* species can also be hepatotoxic (see Table 17-2). *Amanita* species are found primarily in the temperate coastal regions of the west coast of the United States, but they have also adapted to the mid-Atlantic coast and the northeast. *A. phalloides* is the predominant hepatotoxic European mushroom. The mushroom itself has no distinct taste, smell, or appearance. Ingestion is usually followed 6 to 12 hours later by fever, nausea, vomiting, and severe diarrhea. Renal and hepatic impairment may become evident by 24 to 48 hours while the patient appears to be recovering clinically. However, renal failure and hepatic failure progress and tend to become severe by day 3 to 5, with the development of jaundice, encephalopathy, and possibly death. Liver transplantation has been carried out successfully for cases of severe *Amanita* poisoning.[45] Some *Amanita* mushrooms such as *A. muscaria* and *A. pantherina* do not contain hepatotoxins.

The cyclopeptide mushrooms contain two cyclic oligopeptide hepatotoxins: phallotoxins and amatoxins. Both are heat stable and resistant to drying.[44,46] Phallotoxins are not absorbed from the gastrointestinal (GI) tract and therefore are not thought to play a role in the symptoms associated with human poisoning.[47] α-Amanitin is a dialyzable octapeptide that inhibits RNA polymerase II, thus interfering with mRNA synthesis.[48] The cell is robbed of its ability to produce vital structural proteins and undergoes necrosis. Tissues with a high rate of protein synthesis (liver, kidneys, brain) suffer the most damage.[48] α-Amanitin is easily absorbed from the intestinal epithelium and enters the hepatocyte via bile transport carriers.[49] It demonstrates low plasma protein binding and is cleared from plasma in 36 hours.[48,49] Sixty percent is excreted into bile and undergoes enterohepatic circulation, whereas the rest is cleared renally.[48,49]

Case reports of FHF caused by other noninfectious biologic agents include one published in 1994 describing FHF secondary to a sea anemone sting.[50]

Nontoxic Causes

INFECTIONS

Viral hepatitis remains one of the most common causes of FHF worldwide.[19] It is unclear why fulminant failure develops in a select proportion of the infected population, but historical review of previous epidemics reveals that this number remains surprisingly constant at approximately 0.4%.[51] The hepatocellular necrosis seen in cases of FHF caused by hepatitis A and B is thought to be due in part to a direct cytopathic effect of the virus. This mechanism is supported by the relative lack of inflammation seen in the livers of patients with viral FHF. However, the normal humoral and cell-mediated response to a massively infected liver also plays a role. One study found that the amount of hepatitis A virus (HAV) isolated from the livers of patients with HAV-associated FHF was higher than titers from patients with nonfulminant HAV hepatitis.[52] In addition, CD8+ T lymphocytes isolated from the livers of two patients with acute HAV infection demonstrated the ability to kill

HAV-infected fibroblasts in culture, thus implying that the liver damage seen in virally induced FHF is in part cell mediated.[53]

FHF secondary to HAV infection is a rare event: 0.35% of HAV infections will progress to FHF.[54] Patients have a comparatively low mortality rate (<40%) and usually recover without liver transplantation. Acute hepatitis B infection progresses to FHF in approximately 1% of infected patients, thus making hepatitis B virus (HBV) the most common viral cause of FHF.[54] Its role may be underestimated when the impact of infection with a pre-core mutant (HBV viral infection that does not produce the surface [HBsAg] or e antigen) is taken into account, as demonstrated by a study in which it was found that 35% of patients who underwent transplantation for non-A, non-B hepatitis had evidence of HBV infection by polymerase chain reaction.[55] From one half to one third of patients with FHF secondary to HBV will clear HBsAg within a few days[56]; such rapid clearance is thought to be the result of a substantial immunologic response to HBV-laden hepatocytes. Interestingly, those who clear HBsAg rapidly have a more favorable prognosis (47% survival rate) than those with continued HBsAg positivity (17% survival rate).[8] Despite being an increasingly common cause of chronic liver disease, isolated infection with hepatitis C virus has yet to be definitively implicated in FHF.[2] Though rarely encountered in the United States, infection with hepatitis E virus in pregnant women carries a 40% mortality rate.[57] Infection with hepatitis delta virus has been implicated in about 30% of HBV-related FHF cases. In fact, the risk of FHF increases dramatically with any hepatitis virus coinfection.[58,59]

Infection with the viruses herpes simplex, Epstein-Barr, varicella-zoster, or cytomegalovirus occasionally causes FHF, though usually in an immunocompromised setting. Pediatric FHF in association with parvovirus B19 infection has been noted.

Case reports detailing other (rare) infectious causes of FHF have implicated *Coxiella burnetii*, *Plasmodium falciparum*, amebic abscesses, disseminated tuberculosis, and *Bacillus cereus* emetic toxin as causative agents.

VASCULAR EVENTS

The liver has a unique blood supply, with the portal vein supplying 70% of total blood flow and the hepatic artery making up the remaining 30%. Disruption of either the inflow or outflow of blood can lead to ischemia, hypoxia, and ultimately FHF. Examples include prolonged hypotension (intraoperative circulatory collapse, acute myocardial infarction, acute pulmonary embolism), gram-negative sepsis and shock, congestive heart failure, veno-occlusive disease (chemotherapy- or bone marrow transplant–related), Budd-Chiari syndrome, and hepatic artery thrombosis after OLT. Prolonged hypotension after an overdose of opiates or cardioactive drugs (e.g., β-receptor or calcium channel antagonists) or cardiac arrest from any agent may also produce hepatic failure. It is important to note that almost all cases of hepatic ischemia secondary to systemic hypotension are associated with very high aminotransferase levels and accompanying renal dysfunction. In contrast, patients with Budd-Chiari syndrome have aminotransferase levels between 100 and 600 U/L, although higher values are possible. Serum alkaline phosphatase is around 300 to 400 U/L, whereas bilirubin is usually less than

7 mg/dL (120 μmol/L) at onset. The disease commonly afflects women and causes severe right upper quadrant pain and hepatomegaly.

Exertional heatstroke is also an important cause of ischemic FHF and is usually seen in young unconditioned patients pursuing a new exercise program in high ambient temperature and humidity. Classic (nonexertional) heatstroke occurs in patients with multiple chronic medical problems or those taking anticholinergic medications, which leaves them susceptible to disruption of temperature regulatory mechanisms or incapable of escaping the heat. Heatstroke is usually manifested by hyperthermia (core body temperature >40.5°C [104.9°F]), mental status changes (including seizures), peripheral vasodilation, and a host of metabolic derangements. Leukocytosis may also be a prominent initial feature. Acute mortality was 21% in one series.[60] Adverse drug effects (e.g., neuroleptic malignant syndrome, veno-occlusive disease) can play a role in ischemic FHF. Disruption of sinusoidal blood flow by metastatic cancer has also been described as a cause of FHF. Gastric, breast, and oat cell carcinomas have been implicated, as have leukemia, carcinoid syndrome, and amyloidosis.

METABOLIC AND OTHER CAUSES

FHF can occur even without large-scale hepatic necrosis, as demonstrated by patients who suffer from liver failure secondary to acute fatty liver of pregnancy (AFLP), Reye's syndrome, or a fulminant manifestation of Wilson's disease. FHF as an initial feature of Wilson's disease is rare but carries a very high mortality rate without liver transplantation. A relatively low serum alkaline phosphatase level and a disproportionately elevated bilirubin level (up to 30 mg/dL [513 μmol/L]) characterize such a manifestation. The serum copper level is usually elevated.

Whereas loss of hepatocyte function in Wilson's disease is secondary to hepatic copper overload, AFLP results in FHF from an inherited defect in mitochondrial beta oxidation of long-chain fatty acids.[61] AFLP usually occurs in the third trimester and may be associated with preeclampsia. Serum aminotransferase levels usually stay below 1000 U/L unless the HELLP syndrome (hemolytic anemia, elevated liver function tests [LFTs], and low platelet count) is present. Infant mortality is high in either case.

Reye's syndrome has a similar pathogenesis and can be seen in pediatric cases with an antecedent viral illness treated with aspirin. Other rare metabolic anomalies that can cause FHF are listed in Table 17-2. Rarely, autoimmune hepatitis and primary graft failure after liver transplantation will be manifested as FHF.

DIAGNOSIS AND COMPLICATIONS

FHF is the common final pathway of a variety of insults, and thus the features remain remarkably similar regardless of the etiology. Nonspecific flulike symptoms, including fatigue, nausea, loss of appetite, and malaise, are the initial symptoms in previously healthy patients. These symptoms are followed by jaundice and then alteration of mental status with rapid progression to coma. Other helpful signs on physical examination include decreased or absent dullness to percussion in the right upper quadrant, indicative of reduced hepatic mass secondary to necrosis. Fetor hepaticus is usually present, but recognition of this condition is somewhat subjective. Ascites is more common with subfulminant hepatic failure. Stigmata of chronic liver disease do not support a diagnosis of FHF as per the classic definition. Low blood pressure (decreased systemic vascular resistance) and hypothermia may also be evident. Laboratory derangements include high serum aminotransferase levels, low blood glucose levels, and a prolonged prothrombin time. Respiratory alkalosis may be evident on arterial blood gas measurement. Complications seen in the course of the illness include cerebral edema; renal failure; cardiovascular, pulmonary, and metabolic derangements; and problems with infection, GI bleeding, and malnutrition. Multiorgan failure is commonly encountered. There is an inverse relationship between the presence and number of complications and patient survival, as shown in Figure 17-2. The diagnosis is often delayed without an appropriate index of suspicion, and such delay can have catastrophic implications inasmuch as early diagnosis and appropriate management are important to preserve the ability of these patients to receive a transplant should it become necessary. Overall, the presence of coagulopathy in a jaundiced patient with an altered mental status remains the hallmark of FHF.

Coagulopathy

Coagulopathy is universally present and can be the first sign of impending liver failure. It is due mainly to decreased hepatic synthesis of clotting factors.[62] Therefore, serial measurements of prothrombin time and factor V levels have prognostic significance and provide the best measure of whether hepatic function is improving or deteriorating. DIC and local fibrinolysis do occur in FHF, and though not usually severe, they can be exacerbated by infection or by the infusion of activated clotting factors.[63] Administration of fresh frozen plasma *in the absence of bleeding* is not recommended because it has not been shown to be of value[62] and will alter the prothrombin time, thus hindering patient assessment. Platelet function is altered (prolonged capillary

bleeding time), and thrombocytopenia secondary to bone marrow suppression, hypersplenism, and intravascular consumption is present in up to two thirds of patients.[64]

Encephalopathy

Unlike that seen with chronic hepatic disease, the encephalopathy associated with FHF can be manifested as agitated delirium, paranoid behavior, or even a psychotic state. Seizures may occur. The initial stages of encephalopathy are secondary to bilateral forebrain dysfunction, with the latter being secondary to brainstem impairment. Table 17-4 delineates the grading system used for acute hepatic encephalopathy; the presence of stupor or coma portends a poorer prognosis. Although the exact pathogenesis remains elusive, the encephalopathy is reversible and thought to be metabolic. Structural changes such as those seen with Alzheimer's disease are not part of the syndrome. It is postulated that elevated levels of neuroactive humoral substances secondary to decreased hepatic clearance cause the observed mental status changes. It is important to note that the blood-brain barrier is disrupted in FHF, and this increased permeability makes it unnecessary for a substance to be present in greater than normal concentration in plasma to affect cerebral function. In addition, with the blood-brain barrier demonstrating marked regional differences in permeability, the concentration of potentially encephalopathic agents at critical subcellular sites may be more important than their concentration in cerebrospinal fluid or plasma.[65] Studies have implicated increased GABAergic (transmitting or secreting γ-aminobutyric acid) tone, mediated by an endogenous benzodiazepine-like ligand, as a cause of the hepatic encephalopathy seen in FHF.[66] Treatment with flumazenil (a benzodiazepine receptor antagonist) has been shown to temporarily improve the coma grade of patients suffering from this syndrome.[67]

Cerebral Edema

Cerebral edema with resultant increased intracranial pressure (ICP) is a common complication of FHF, with up to 81% of patients demonstrating signs of increased ICP during the

FIGURE 17-2

Relationship between survival and complications of acute liver failure. *(From Walsh TS, Hopton P, Philips BJ, et al: The effect of N-acetylcysteine on oxygen transport and uptake in patients with fulminant hepatic failure. Hepatology 27:1332–1340, 1998.)*

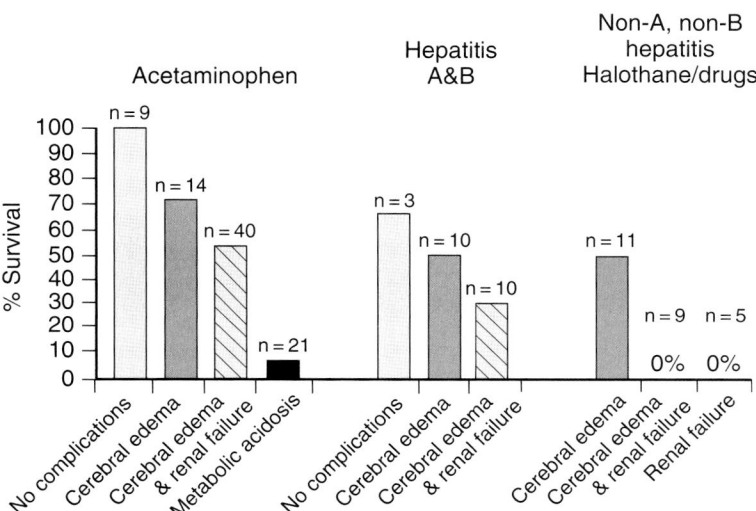

TABLE 17-4 Progressive Stages of Hepatic Encephalopathy

STAGE	LEVEL OF CONSCIOUSNESS	NEUROMUSCULAR CHANGES	BEHAVIORAL/INTELLECTUAL CHANGES
I	Reversal of sleep pattern Mild confusion	Mild asterixis Impaired handwriting	Euphoria/depression Short-term memory lapses
II	Slow responses Increasing drowsiness	Asterixis/ataxia Slurred speech	Inappropriate behavior Loss of time/amnesia
III	Disorientation Somnolence	Rigidity/spasticity Loss of continence	Stuporous/incoherent Marked confusion/paranoia

IV A/B	Comatose
	  A: responds to pain
	  B: no response to pain
		Decorticate/decerebrate
		Hyperreflexic
			Comatose

course of the illness.[68] Although it is a distinct entity, its signs and symptoms may be missed because of the presence of concurrent encephalopathy—often with deadly consequences. Herniation of the cerebellar tonsils or the uncinate process of the temporal lobe is a significant cause of death, and evidence of herniation is present in up to 25% to 30% of patients with cerebral edema.[69]

The causative metabolic and pathophysiologic derangements that lead to cerebral edema have yet to be fully elucidated. Research indicates a complex interplay among vasogenic (alterations in blood flow), cytotoxic (loss of osmoregulation), and hydrocephalic (extracellular expansion) factors. Even though earlier histologic studies of the brain revealed no abnormalities,[70] more recent data have found alterations in cell membrane integrity and blood-brain barrier permeability,[71,72] changes probably responsible for the increased water content and weight of the brain. Although patients with cirrhosis rarely have cerebral edema, a marked decrease in intracranial blood flow has been noted in those with acute or chronic encephalopathy.[73] This decreased blood flow, along with the systemic hypotension commonly found in FHF (see the next section) and the increased ICP secondary to cerebral edema, predisposes the brain to ischemic injury. Cerebral perfusion pressure (CPP = mean arterial pressure [MAP] − ICP) below 40 to 50 mm Hg is associated with ischemic brain injury and can have permanent consequences, even if the liver recovers fully. A persistent and refractory perfusion pressure of less than 40 mm Hg precludes transplantation.[74] Signs of increased ICP are noted in Table 17-5. Because they are manifested only late in the course of events (i.e., only if ICP is greater than 30 mm Hg), these signs cannot be used to gauge the need for therapeutic intervention.

Although computed tomography (CT) scans are often used to exclude intracerebral hemorrhage as a cause of a sudden change in mentation, their static nature in this rapidly evolving syndrome makes them unsuitable as a management guide. ICP monitoring provides reliable data on which treatment decisions can be made, and placement of a subdural or epidural transducer is indicated in patients being considered for transplantation. Patients should be transferred to a transplant center early in the course of the disease; transportation after the onset of cerebral edema and coma is fraught with danger because even positional changes can raise ICP with disastrous consequences. Factors that tend to increase ICP are noted in Table 17-6. Even without herniation, cerebral edema remains the most common cause of death in FHF.

Cardiovascular Derangements

Systemic hypotension occurs in most patients with FHF and is mediated in part by decreased systemic vascular resistance (resembling septic shock), bacteremia, hemorrhage, hypovolemia, and increased interstitial edema (increased capillary permeability) and ICP. An etiology is not found in up to 60% of cases.[75] Nearly all patients with stage IV encephalopathy suffer from arrhythmias. Although sinus tachycardia is most common, the spectrum includes heart block and cardiac arrest. ST segment and T wave changes may occur. Exacerbating factors include hypoxemia, acidosis, hyperkalemia, and cerebral edema.[76]

TABLE 17-5 Signs of Increased Intracranial Pressure in Fulminant Hepatic Failure

Brainstem respiratory pattern, apnea
Decerebrate posturing/rigidity
Focal seizures
Increased muscle tone
Loss of oculovestibular reflex
Myoclonus
Unequal, fixed, or abnormally reacting pupils

TABLE 17-6 Factors That Increase Intracranial Pressure

Arterial hypotension	Psychomotor agitation
Coughing	Respiratory suction
Fever	Seizures
Head and body movement	Severe hypoxemia
Hypercapnia	Shivering
Isometric muscle contraction	Sneezing
Neck vein compression	Trendelenburg position
Noxious stimuli	Valsalva maneuver
Positive end-expiratory pressure	Vasodilatory agents
	Vomiting

Renal Failure

Renal impairment is present in up to 75% of patients with FHF[77] and includes prerenal azotemia, hepatorenal syndrome, and acute tubular necrosis. Hepatorenal syndrome is a diagnosis of exclusion and is characterized by a serum creatinine concentration greater than 1.5 mg/dL (133 μmol/L), a urinary sodium concentration less than 10 mEq/L (without taking diuretics) and lack of improvement with volume expansion, and a bland urinary sediment.[78] Systemic hypotension and splanchnic vasodilation (probably nitric oxide driven) activate the renin-angiotensin axis, with resultant renal vasoconstriction. Renal vasoconstriction leads to a drop in renal perfusion pressure, which is reflected by a decreased glomerular filtration rate and increased sodium retention (causing ascites and edema). The presence of oliguric renal failure portends a poorer prognosis.[79] Renal impairment may also occur secondary to the toxic effects of substances that caused the FHF, such as APAP, hepatotoxic mushrooms, hydrocarbons, and MDMA.

Pulmonary and Ventilatory Derangements

Up to 30% of patients will have evidence of pulmonary edema during the course of their illness, especially those with cerebral edema.[80,81] Accurate determination of volume status by pulmonary artery pressure monitoring has been shown to improve survival.[82] Intrapulmonary arteriovenous shunting, peripheral capillary blockage with cellular debris from necrotic hepatocytes, or low-grade DIC, interstitial edema, and increased vasomotor tone ultimately lead to lactic acidosis secondary to anaerobic metabolism, which can exacerbate cerebral ischemia.[83,84] The use of NAC and prostacyclin to improve tissue oxygenation remains experimental and controversial.[84–86]

Infection

Metabolic inhibition of polymorphonuclear leukocytes, decreased opsonization, and impaired cell-mediated and humoral immunity greatly predispose patients with FHF to bacteremia and fungemia.[54,87] Patients have an increased risk of infection secondary to multiple indwelling catheters, antacid therapy, artificial ventilation, coma, and treatment with broad-spectrum antibiotics. Skin flora organisms (*Staphylococcus* and *Streptococcus* spp.) are most commonly isolated in patients with FHF.[88] In a prospective study of 50 patients with acute liver failure, infection was suspected in 45 patients and proved by positive cultures in 40.[89] However, prophylactic antibiotic treatment has not been shown to improve survival.[90]

Gastrointestinal Bleeding

The severe coagulopathy seen with FHF predisposes patients to hemorrhage from the GI tract, with the upper GI tract being the most frequent site of bleeding.[91] Diffusely hemorrhagic gastritis, esophagitis, and nasogastric tube trauma are common etiologies. Exacerbating factors include tissue hypoxia from hypotension, microcirculatory disruption, and hypoxemia, along with DIC, bacteremia, and ventilator-associated platelet dysfunction. Large episodes of bleeding lead to further hypotension and tissue (including cerebral) hypoxia and

can cause worsening renal failure as a result of prerenal azotemia, as well as exacerbating hepatic encephalopathy. Despite the numerous risk factors for hemorrhage, infusion of fresh frozen plasma or platelets for correction of coagulopathy or thrombocytopenia is not indicated in the absence of bleeding.

Metabolic Derangements

Electrolyte and acid-base disturbances are common in FHF and can exacerbate encephalopathy and cause arrhythmias. Despite renal retention of sodium, hyponatremia occurs frequently and is due to impaired renal free water excretion. Hypokalemia is present and can be profound; etiologies are multiple and include renal losses (secondary to hyperaldosteronism and sodium retention, as well as secondary to hydrogen ion resorption to compensate for respiratory alkalosis), GI losses (decreased intake, vomiting), and iatrogenic causes (e.g., diuretics, nasogastric tube suctioning, lactulose use). Hypophosphatemia, hypomagnesemia, and hypocalcemia can also occur. Complex acid-base disturbances with multiple processes at play are seen—respiratory alkalosis as a result of spontaneous hyperventilation is commonly present early in the course of the disease. However, with disease progression and depression of the central respiratory drive secondary to edema or circulating toxins, respiratory acidosis can develop. Hypokalemia is associated with metabolic alkalosis, whereas tissue hypoxia and massive hepatic necrosis give rise to metabolic acidosis with elevated levels of lactic acid, free fatty acid, and other organic acids. The presence of lactic acidosis is a poor prognostic indicator. Impaired glucose release, loss of glycogen reserves, and decreased gluconeogenesis are in combination responsible for severe hypoglycemia (blood glucose <40 mg/dL [2.2 mmol/L]) in up to 40% of patients. Decreased hepatic metabolism of insulin resulting in inappropriately elevated plasma insulin levels also plays a pathogenic role. If unrecognized and untreated, the fall in blood glucose can be rapid and may lead to irreversible brain injury.

DIAGNOSTIC STUDIES

Laboratory and radiographic testing should be performed to confirm the diagnosis, elucidate the etiology of FHF, evaluate for the presence of complications, and obtain data necessary for management, prognostication, and preparation of the patient for possible liver transplantation. See Table 17-7 for a list of recommended initial diagnostic tests for FHF. Serum glucose should be monitored frequently (every 2 hours), and other parameters such as electrolytes, hematocrit, and arterial blood gas should be monitored at least three times daily. Coagulation parameters and LFTs are usually checked twice a day. Further testing, such as tomographic studies of the head to rule out intracerebral hemorrhage as a cause of acute worsening of mental status, is performed as clinically indicated.

TREATMENT

Because of the unpredictable nature of the disease, the risk of acute decompensation, and the severity of the illness/complications, patients with FHF should be managed in an

TABLE 17-7 Initial Diagnostic Testing in Fulminant Hepatic Failure

PARAMETER	RATIONALE
Electrolytes and minerals	Imbalances are common; can cause arrhythmias, worsen encephalopathy. Hypophosphatemia is common in acetaminophen overdose
BUN/creatinine	Renal failure is typical, affects management and prognosis. Etiology (e.g., toxic effect of ingested substances) may alter therapy (e.g., hemodialysis)
Glucose	Hypoglycemia is common, can have permanent neurologic sequelae
CBC with platelets	Assess for sepsis (leukocytosis), GI bleeding (anemia), and risk of hemorrhage (thrombocytopenia)
Liver profile	Assess degree of damage, follow course of illness
Coagulation profile	Prognostic indicators (PT, factor V level), assess risk of hemorrhage
Arterial blood gases	Prognostic significance (lactic acidosis), derangements common
Blood group	Preparation for transplantation; type and crossmatch in anticipation of bleeding
Toxicology, virology, autoimmune panel, ceruloplasmin, medication history	Etiology affects management (e.g., NAC for acetaminophen, charcoal for *Amanita*) and prognosis. Refer to Table 17-2 for various etiologies of FHF
Blood and urine cultures	Surveillance for sepsis; aggressive treatment warranted if positive
ECG	May affect management, preparation for transplantation
Chest radiograph	Sepsis surveillance; evaluate for ARDS, pulmonary edema
Abdominal ultrasound	Evaluate for vascular thrombosis, preparation for transplantation
Pulmonary wedge pressure	Assess volume status if hypotension present
Intracranial pressure	Assess ICP if stage III-IV encephalopathy present. Cerebral edema is the most common cause of death

ARDS, adult respiratory distress syndrome; BUN, blood urea nitrogen; CBC, complete blood count; ECG, electrocardiogram; FHF, fulminant hepatic failure; GI, gastrointestinal; ICP, intracranial pressure; NAC, *N*-acetyl-L-cysteine; PT, prothrombin time.

ICU setting, preferably at a liver transplant center. Hospitals without liver transplant programs should transfer patients with FHF to such transplant centers as soon as possible because increased ICP and severe coagulopathy make transfer later in the course of the disease much more hazardous. Uncompromised ICU support is necessary to give these patients the best chance for survival. Specific treatment strategies for commonly encountered complications are discussed in the following sections.

Coagulopathy

Decreased synthesis of coagulation factors is a direct reflection of hepatic dysfunction and can be used as a prognostic indicator. Therefore, prophylactic correction of coagulopathy in a nonbleeding patient is not recommended because it does not influence mortality, can interfere with assessment of disease severity, and may predispose the patient to volume overload and worsening cerebral edema.[19,92] Blood products (fresh frozen plasma or, rarely, recombinant human factor VIIa) may be used to correct coagulopathy in cases of known hemorrhage/GI bleeding and for invasive procedures.[93]

Encephalopathy

Encephalopathy is part of the definition of FHF and as such plays a major role in the patient's clinical findings and course. Patients with grade 4 encephalopathy should be intubated for airway protection. Standard treatment with lactulose enemas or lactulose via a nasogastric tube, 30 mL three to four times a day, is instituted in an attempt to decrease the amount of nitrogenous waste (in the form of ammonia) absorbed from the gut lumen. Oral neomycin has traditionally been added if the encephalopathy is difficult to control,

but it has possible nephrotoxic and ototoxic side effects. Modern drugs of choice instead are metronidazole, 250 to 500 mg two to three times a day, aminopenicillins, 2 to 4 g/day, or vancomycin, 1 to 2 g/day.

Cerebral Edema

Cerebral edema (leading to elevated ICP, ischemic/hypoxic brain injury, and brainstem herniation) is the most common cause of death in FHF and is present in up to 80% of patients with grade 4 encephalopathy.[94] Given the deadly consequences of unrecognized cerebral edema and the difficulty in diagnosing it clinically, an epidural ICP monitor should be placed in all patients with grade 4 encephalopathy. This procedure has a 4% morbidity (infection, bleeding) rate and a 1% mortality rate and is thus safer than placement of a subdural, parenchymal, or intraventricular catheter.[95] Coagulopathy should be addressed before placement of an ICP monitor, and head CT should be considered to rule out other causes of acute mental status changes such as intracranial hemorrhage. The aim is to keep ICP lower than 20 mm Hg and CPP (MAP − ICP = CPP) higher than 50 mm Hg.[2]

Elevated ICP can be treated with mannitol boluses (0.5 to 1 g/kg to achieve a plasma osmolality between 310 and 325 mOsm/kg).[96] Clinicians should be vigilant for signs of volume overload with mannitol use; concurrent ultrafiltration or other dialysis methods may be needed to avoid hypervolemia. In addition, patients should be stimulated as little as possible because agitation can increase ICP. Sedatives should be used in the lowest dose possible so that the degree of encephalopathy can continue to be monitored. Short-acting drugs such as propofol should be used.[97] Elevating the head of the bed can decrease ICP, but it also causes CPP to fall and leads to paradoxical increases in ICP when elevation is above 30 degrees.[92] In the absence of ICP monitoring, the head of the bed should be elevated 10 to 20 degrees. The use of positive end-expiratory pressure during ventilation can also worsen cerebral edema.[98] Dexamethasone has been proved to be ineffective as treatment of cerebral edema and should therefore not be used.[99] Hyperventilation to lower PCO_2 has not been shown to be beneficial.[92]

Renal Failure

Most patients with FHF have evidence of acute renal failure, the presence of which carries a grave prognosis. Treatment is centered on prevention: the use of nephrotoxic drugs (e.g., aminoglycosides) is avoided, intravascular volume is optimized with judicious use of colloid supplementation in the form of packed red cells or salt-poor albumin, and MAP is maintained as close to normal as possible. A high index of suspicion should be entertained for renal failure secondary to the direct toxic effects of substances such as APAP or hepatotoxic mushrooms. Although urinary sodium values can be used to guide therapy, the blood urea nitrogen concentration may underestimate the renal dysfunction because of decreased hepatic urea production.

Infection

A decline in renal function or worsening/recalcitrant encephalopathy may be the first clues to an untreated infection in patients with FHF. Thus, a high index of suspicion must be maintained, with a low threshold for diagnostic testing (including blood, urine, and sputum cultures, chest x-ray, paracentesis) and empirical broad-spectrum antibiotic/antifungal coverage. The most common sites of infection include the respiratory system, the urinary tract, and blood.[100] Although prophylactic antibiotic use has not been shown to be helpful, a surveillance culture regimen with aggressive directed therapy if an infection is suspected is recommended.

Gastrointestinal Bleeding

All FHF patients deserve stress ulcer prophylaxis with oral/IV proton-pump inhibitors. Sucralfate may also be used. Coagulopathy and thrombocytopenia should be corrected in patients with bleeding from the GI tract, but not prophylactically. Large GI bleeds are investigated and treated endoscopically. If variceal bleeding is suspected, treatment with an octreotide IV drip should be initiated without delay for endoscopic confirmation.

Metabolic Derangements

The various metabolic derangements seen in FHF have been detailed earlier. As part of supportive ICU care, electrolytes should be checked and corrected at least twice a day. Hypoglycemia is common in FHF and needs closer attention. Hypertonic glucose solutions should be administered as an IV drip to keep blood glucose levels above 65 mg/dL. Restriction of free water may be needed to treat hyponatremia, but hypertonic saline is rarely required. Acetaminophen-induced FHF without renal impairment is commonly associated with hypophosphatemia, which may require therapy.

Nutrition

A diet low in protein is advocated for patients with FHF who are able to tolerate oral intake (grade 1 to 2 encephalopathy). Enteral low-protein tube feeding should be considered early in the course of the disease for the rest of the patients to prevent unnecessary catabolism and to optimize management before possible liver transplantation. Tube feeding should be administered into the distal duodenum/jejunum if possible to decrease the risk of aspiration.

Specific Antidotes

Two of the most common conditions for which specific treatment of FHF is available are APAP overdose and *Amanita* mushroom poisoning. Other rare treatable etiologies include AFLP (treated by delivery), shock liver (treated by optimizing hemodynamic status), acute Budd-Chiari syndrome (treatment considerations include transjugular intrahepatic portosystemic stent shunt versus surgical decompression versus thrombolysis), herpesvirus infection (treated with acyclovir), and autoimmune hepatitis (treated with steroids).

Chapter 55 provides detailed discussion on the treatment of APAP overdose, but in general, if severe acetaminophen toxicity is suspected, intravenous NAC should be administered without delay. Activated charcoal (1 g/kg) is also recommended if the patient is seen within 1 or 2 hours of ingestion. Plasma APAP concentrations should be determined in all suspected cases and values plotted against the established nomogram to determine whether NAC administration is indicated. However, those with liver injury and suspected acetaminophen toxicity, even in the absence of detectable APAP, should receive NAC treatment.

Mushroom poisoning can be established by isolating α-amanitin in serum or urine by radioimmunoassay. Its enterohepatic circulation can be interrupted by using repeated doses of activated charcoal, and possibly forced diuresis can increase the rate of renal clearance of the toxin (see Chapter 120). Silibinin and IV penicillin G have been used as specific therapies for *Amanita* poisoning. Silibinin is thought to impede the uptake of α-amanitin by hepatocytes and may be efficacious up to 48 hours after the ingestion of toxin.[49]

PROGNOSIS

Patients with FHF can be broadly divided into two categories—those who have enough hepatic reserve left to survive and recover with optimal medical care and those who have sustained an irreversible hepatic insult and will die despite supportive care. OLT is the best available option for the second cohort; it is not appropriate therapy for the first group. The difficulty lies in accurately categorizing patients into one of these two groups and doing so in a timely manner, before the complications associated with FHF preclude OLT as a therapeutic option. Overall, current estimates reveal that only about 10% of patients with FHF receive a transplant.[94] Posttransplant survival rates have been estimated at 55% to 75%,[101] although rates may improve to over 90% with stringent selection criteria.[96] As noted earlier, FHF without OLT is associated with very high mortality rates, and survival remains dismal for those who are listed for transplantation but do not receive an organ in time. In general, transplantation is recommended if the patient's survival rate is estimated to be below 20%.

A number of prognostic indicators have been identified to help clinicians predict the severity of FHF and identify patients who would benefit from transplantation. It is well known that the etiology and the presence/number of associated complications can influence the survival rate (see Figs. 17-2 and 17-3). Time from the onset of jaundice/symptoms to the development of hepatic encephalopathy can also predict a survival difference in certain cohorts, as mentioned in the discussion in the "Definitions" section of this chapter. The severity of encephalopathy at admission is inversely related to survival in patients with acetaminophen toxicity and acute liver failure.[20] Although age younger than 10 or older than 40 years has been shown to be a poor prognostic indicator in older studies, it did not play a role in survival rates from a more recent U.S. series.[20] Liver histology is not routinely used because it has not been proved to accurately predict outcome.[102]

The aforementioned variables (age, etiology, degree of encephalopathy, time to onset of symptoms, etc.), though identifying survival trends, do not allow for an accurate prediction of the need for transplantation. To better identify high-risk patients who would require liver transplantation for survival, a statistical model was developed by investigators at King's College in London. From a cohort of 588 patients managed medically between 1973 and 1985, a multivariate analysis was performed on a number of biochemical and clinical variables and their relationship to mortality, and recommendations for transplantation were based on the results. The negative prognostic indicators (also known as King's College criteria) for which transplantation is recommended are noted in Table 17-8.[1]

TABLE 17-8 King's College Criteria (Indications for Transplantation)

ACETAMINOPHEN TOXICITY	NON-ACETAMINOPHEN TOXICITY
pH <7.3 (irrespective of other factors)	PT >35 sec (U.S. units) or INR >7.7 (irrespective of degree of encephalopathy)
OR ALL 3 of the following:	*OR ANY 3 of the following*:
Grade III-IV encephalopathy	Age <10 or >40 yr
PT >100 seconds	Unfavorable etiology (non-A non-B hepatitis, idiosyncratic drug reaction, halothane hepatitis, Wilson's disease)
Serum creatinine >3.4 mg/dL (300 μmol/L)	Serum bilirubin >17 mg/dL (300 μmol/L)
	Time from jaundice to encephalopathy >7 days
	INR >4

INR, international normalized ratio; PT, prothrombin time.

The King's College Criteria have been validated at other centers and in a prospective manner. Patients with FHF but without APAP toxicity demonstrated a mortality rate of 80% with the presence of any one of the negative prognostic indicators; mortality rose to 95% with the association of three negative prognostic factors. Severe acidosis (pH <7.3) in patients with APAP toxicity was associated with a mortality rate of 95%. Excluding acidosis, the presence of any other adverse characteristic in this population resulted in a mortality rate of at least 55%. These mortality rates are much higher than those associated with liver transplantation; thus, patients with even one negative prognostic indicator should be considered for listing.[1]

Other predictive models have been developed to assess the degree of liver injury and identify patients who need liver transplantation for survival. A severity scoring system with a predictive value that is comparable to the King's College criteria has been proposed; however, it is cumbersome, involves complex arithmetic, and has not been validated prospectively.[103] Acute Physiology and Chronic Health Evaluation (APACHE) II scores were similar to the King's College criteria in identifying those needing transplantation, but patients were recognized earlier in a few cases.[104] Serum Gc-globulin and plasma factor V levels have been used independently to predict outcome; however, they are specialized laboratory tests that may not always be available and have not been shown to be any better than the King's College criteria.[105] Factor V levels vary by age; transplantation is recommended for a factor V level less than 20% in FHF patients younger than 30 years or for a factor V level less than 30% for those older than 30 years.[106] However, patients have recovered without transplantation with factor V levels less than 10%, in our experience. Although early recognition of patients most likely to benefit from transplantation is important, it is equally important to recognize those in whom liver transplantation is contraindicated (Table 17-9).

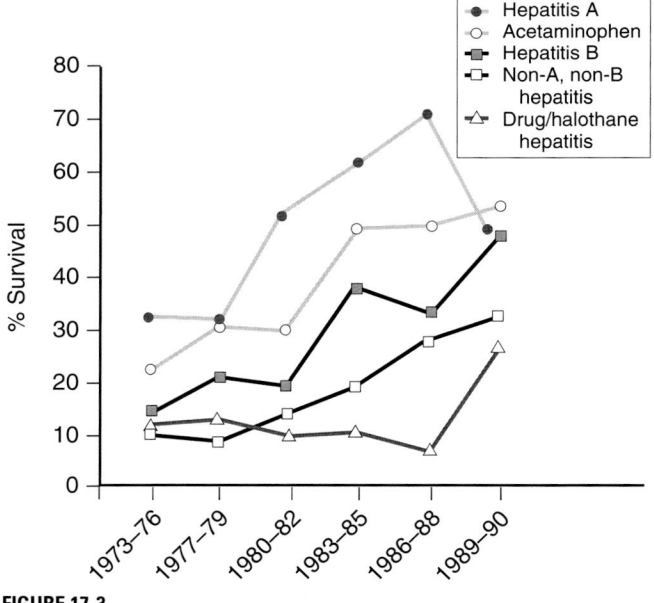

FIGURE 17-3

Survival based on the etiology of acute liver failure. *(From Hughes RD, Wendon J, Gimson AES: Acute liver failure. Gut Sep[Suppl]:S86–S91, 1991.)*

TABLE 17-9 Absolute Contraindications to Liver Transplantation
Severe cardiac or pulmonary disease
Severe pulmonary hypertension (PA systolic pressure ≥60 mm Hg)
Adult respiratory distress syndrome (FiO$_2$ >0.6)
Uncontrolled intracranial hypertension/irreversible brain damage
HIV infection/AIDS
Systemic sepsis
Extrahepatic malignancy
Portal and mesenteric vein thrombosis
Active alcohol or drug use
Severe psychological disorders
Inability to understand/commit to the procedure and the lifetime of responsibility it entails

AIDS, acquired immunodeficiency syndrome; HIV, human immunodeficiency virus; PA, pulmonary artery.

FUTURE TRENDS

The scarcity of donor livers has led to investigation of alternatives to transplantation not only for patients who need temporary support while their native liver recovers from the acute insult but also for those who need a "bridge" to transplantation. A number of novel and promising approaches have been tried, including auxiliary liver transplantation, liver dialysis systems, artificial hepatic assist devices, and xenotransplantation. All are in the research phase and need further study with controlled clinical trials to delineate their safety and efficacy. Liver dialysis systems have not met with great success. Hemodialysis, charcoal hemoperfusion, and blood and plasma exchange have been tried without any demonstrated alteration in outcome.[92]

Auxiliary liver transplantation involves placement of a partial liver graft in either a heterotopic location or a space provided by partial hepatectomy. Although the graft is not large enough to sustain the patient independently, it provides enough support to allow the native liver to recover. No indications for auxiliary transplantation have been established, and it still requires a donor source in the presence of the current organ shortage. However, a number of patients have recovered when auxiliary grafting is used as a bridge, thus obviating the need for whole-organ transplantation and lifelong immunosuppression.[107]

Xenotransplantation plus the use of animal livers for extracorporeal perfusion was reported in the 1960s and 1970s and was universally unsuccessful. Given the acute human donor liver shortage, however, research still continues to find ways to overcome the immunologic intolerance between the patient and the animal organ such that the xenotransplant can bridge the patient either to recovery or to transplantation with a human liver. However, interspecies transmission of infective agents remains a concern.

Early experiments of extracorporeal perfusion with animal organs led to the idea of hybrid artificial devices that would combine the efficacy and compatibility of a human liver with the ease of hemodialysis. These hybrids, known as extracorporeal liver assist devices (ELADs) and bioartificial livers, incorporate living human hepatocytes embedded around a nest of hollow fiber capillaries housed in a cartridge through which the patient's blood is transfused.[108] The device functions as an extracorporeal artificial liver, with the living hepatocytes performing all the functions of the native liver across the semipermeable capillary membrane. Recent research has focused on trying to reproduce the hepatic architecture in the ELAD cartridge, identifying the optimal hepatocyte mass needed to provide the best results, and determining the ideal perfusion time necessary for a favorable outcome.

REFERENCES

1. O'Grady JG, Alexander GJM, Hayllar KM, et al: Early indicators of prognosis in fulminant hepatic failure. Gastroenterology 97:439–445, 1989.
2. Hoofnagle JH, Carithers RL, Shapiro C, et al: Fulminant hepatic failure: Summary of a workshop. Hepatology 21:240, 1995.
3. Trey C, Davidson CS: The management of fulminant hepatic failure. Prog Liver Dis 3:282–298, 1970.
4. Bernuau J, Rueff B, Benhamou JP: Fulminant and subfulminant liver failure: Definitions and causes. Semin Liver Dis 6:97–106, 1986.
5. Gimson AES, O'Grady JC, Ede RJ, et al: Late onset hepatic failure: Clinical, serological and histological features. Hepatology 6:288–294, 1986.
6. O'Grady JG, Schalm SW, Williams R, et al: Acute liver failure: Redefining the syndromes. Lancet 342:273–275, 1993.
7. Takahashi Y, Shimizu M: Aetiology and prognosis of fulminant viral hepatitis in Japan: A multicenter study. J Gastroenterol Hepatol 6:159–164, 1991.
8. Bernuau J, Goudeau A, Poynard T, et al: Multivariate analysis of prognostic factors in fulminant hepatitis B. Hepatology 6:648–651, 1986.
9. Acharya SK, Dasarathy S, Tandon BN: Should we redefine acute liver failure? [letter]. Lancet 342:1421–1422, 1993.
10. Keppler D, Popper H, Bianchi L, et al (eds): Mechanisms of Hepatocellular Injury and Death. Lancaster, UK, MTP Press, 1984.
11. Schanne FAX, Kane AB, Young EE, et al: Calcium dependence of toxic cell death: A final common pathway. Science 206:700, 1979.
12. Popper H, Keppler D: Networks of interacting mechanisms of hepatocellular degeneration and death. Prog Liver Dis 8:209, 1986.
13. Miwa Y, Harrison PM, Farzaneh F, et al: Plasma levels and hepatic mRNA expression of transforming growth factor-beta$_1$ in patients with fulminant hepatic failure. J Hepatol 27:780–788, 1997.
14. Eguchi S, Okudaira S, Azuma T, et al: Changes in liver regenerative factors in a case of living-related liver transplantation. Clin Transplant 13:536–544, 1999.
15. Andus T, Bauer J, Gerok W: Effects of cytokines on the liver. Hepatology 13:364–375, 1991.
16. Yumoto E, Higashi T, Nouso K, et al: Serum gamma-interferon–inducing factor (IL-18) and IL-10 levels in patients with acute hepatitis and fulminant hepatic failure. J Gastroenterol Hepatol 17:285–294, 2002.
17. Lidofsky SD: Liver transplantation for fulminant hepatic failure. Gastroenterol Clin North Am 22:257, 1993.
18. White HM: Evaluation and management of liver failure. In Rippe JM (ed): Intensive Care Medicine, 3rd ed. Boston, Little, Brown, 1996.
19. O'Grady JG, Portmann B, Williams R: Fulminant hepatic failure. In Schiff L, Schiff R (eds): Diseases of the Liver. Philadelphia, JB Lippincott, 1993.
20. Schiodt FV, Atillasoy E, Shakil AO, et al: Etiology and outcome for 295 patients with acute liver failure in the United States. Liver Transpl Surg 5:29, 1999.
21. Lewis RK, Paloucek FP: Assessment and treatment of acetaminophen overdose. Clin Pharm 10:765, 1991.
22. Prescott LF: Paracetamol overdosage: Pharmacological considerations and clinical management. Drugs 25:290, 1983.
23. Lee WM: Drug-induced hepatotoxicity. N Engl J Med 333:1118, 1995.
24. Whitcomb DC, Block GD: Association of acetaminophen toxicity with fasting and ethanol use. JAMA 272:1845–1850, 1994.
25. Kumar K, Rex DK: Failure of physicians to recognize acetaminophen hepatotoxicity in chronic alcoholics. Arch Intern Med 151:1189–1191, 1991.
26. Mitchell JR, Jollow JD, Potter WZ, et al: Acetaminophen-induced hepatic necrosis: I. Role of drug metabolism. J Pharmacol Exp Ther 187:185, 1973.

27. Mitchell JR, Jollow JD, Potter WZ, et al: Acetaminophen-induced hepatic necrosis: IV. Protective role of glutathione. J Pharmacol Exp Ther 187:211, 1973.

28. Slattery JT, Nelson, SD, Thummel KE: The complex interaction between ethanol and acetaminophen. Clin Pharmacol Ther 60:241, 1996.

29. Murphy R, Swartz R, Watkins PB: Severe acetaminophen toxicity in a patient receiving isoniazid. Ann Intern Med 113:399, 1980.

30. Bray GP, Harrison PM, O'Grady JG, et al: Long term anticonvulsant therapy worsens outcome in paracetamol induced hepatic failure. Hum Exp Toxicol 11:265, 1992.

31. Lauterburg BH, Velez ME: Glutathione deficiency in alcoholics: Risk factor for paracetamol. Hepatology 29:1153, 1988.

32. Zimmerman HJ, Maddrey WC: Acetaminophen (paracetamol) hepatotoxicity with regular intake of alcohol: Analysis of instances of therapeutic misadventure. Hepatology 22:767, 1995.

33. Pessayre D, Bentata M, Degott C, et al: Isoniazid-rifampin fulminant hepatitis. A possible consequence of the enhancement of isoniazid hepatotoxicity by enzyme induction. Gastroenterology 72:284, 1977.

34. Riley TR 3rd, Smith JP: Ibuprofen-induced hepatotoxicity in patients with chronic hepatitis C: A case series. Am J Gastroenterol 93:1563–1565, 1998.

35. Garcia-Rodriguez LA, Williams R, Derby LE, et al: Acute liver injury associated with NSAIDs and the role of risk factors, Arch Intern Med 154: 311–316, 1994.

36. Shaheen N, Grimm IS: Fulminant hepatic failure associated with clarithromycin. Am J Gastroenterol 91:394–395, 1996.

37. Zimmerman HJ: Hepatotoxicity. The Adverse Effects of Drugs and Other Chemicals on the Liver. New York, Appleton-Century-Crofts, 1978.

38. Pratt DS, Kaplan MM: Evaluation of abnormal liver enzyme results in asymptomatic patients. N Engl J Med 342:1266–1271, 2000.

39. BMJ 322(7279):139, 2001, Dtsch Med Wochenschr 126(36):970–972, 2001. In Internal Medicine News, Jan 2002.

40. Scully RE, Mark EJ, McNeely WF, et al: Case records of the Massachusetts General Hospital. N Engl J Med 344:591–599, 2001.

41. Brauer RB, Heidecke CD, Nathrath W, et al: Liver transplantation for the treatment of fulminant hepatic failure induced by the ingestion of ecstasy. Transpl Int 10:229–233, 1997.

42. Bryson PD: Mushrooms. In Bryson PD (ed): Comprehensive Review in Toxicology for Emergency Clinicians, 3rd ed. Washington, DC, Taylor & Francis, 1996, pp 685–693.

43. Klein AS, Hart J, Brems JJ, et al: Amanita poisoning: Treatment and the role of liver transplantation. Am J Med 86:187–193, 1989.

44. Lampe KF, McCann MA: AMA Handbook of Poisonous and Injurious Plants. Chicago, American Medical Association, 1985.

45. Pinson CW, Daya MR, Benner KG, et al: Liver transplantation for severe *Amanita phalloides* mushroom poisoning. Am J Surg 159:493–499, 1990.

46. Kopple C: Clinical symptomatology and management of mushroom poisoning. Toxicon 31:1513–1540, 1993.

47. O'Brien B, Khuu L: A fatal Sunday brunch: *Amanita* mushroom poisoning in a Gulf Coast family. Am J Gastroenterol 91:581–583, 1996.

48. Faulstich H: New aspects of *Amanita* poisoning. Klin Wochenschr 57:1143–1152, 1979.

49. Wieland T, Faulstich H: Fifty years of *Amanita* review. Experientia 47:1186–1193, 1991.

50. Garcia PJ, Schein RMH, Burnett JW: Fulminant hepatic failure from a sea anemone sting. Ann Intern Med 120:665–666, 1994.

51. Lucke B: The fulminant form of epidemic hepatitis. Am J Pathol 22:867, 1946.

52. Mathieson LR, Linglof T, Moller AM, et al: Fulminant hepatitis A. J Infect Dis 11:303, 1979.

53. Vallbracht A, Maier K, Stierhof Y, et al: Liver-derived cytotoxic T cells in hepatitis A virus infection. J Infect Dis 160:209, 1989.

54. Fagan EA, Williams R: Fulminant viral hepatitis. Br Med Bull 46:462–480, 1990.

55. Wright TL, Mamish D, Combs C, et al: Hepatitis B and apparent non-A, non-B hepatitis. Lancet 339:952, 1992.

56. Saracco G, Macagno S, Rosina F, et al: Serologic markers with fulminant hepatitis in persons positive for hepatitis B surface antigen: A worldwide epidemiologic and clinical survey. Ann Intern Med 108:380–383, 1988.

57. Christie AB, Allam AA, Aref MK, et al: Pregnancy hepatitis in Libya. Lancet 2:827–829, 1976.

58. Chu CM, Yeh CT, Liaw YF: Fulminant hepatic failure in acute hepatitis C: Increased risk in chronic carriers of hepatitis B virus. Gut 45:613, 1999.

59. Smedile A, Verme G, Cargnel A, et al: Influence of delta infection on severity of hepatitis B. Lancet 2:945–947, 1982.

60. Dematte JE, O'Mara K, Buescher J, et al: Near-fatal heat stroke during the 1995 heat wave in Chicago. Ann Intern Med 129:173, 1995.

61. Sims HF, Brackett JC, Powell CK: The molecular basis of pediatric long chain 3-hydroxyacyl-CoA dehydrogenase deficiency associated with maternal acute fatty liver of pregnancy. Proc Natl Acad Sci U S A 92:841–845, 1995.

62. Pereira LMMB, Langley PG, Hayllar KM, et al: Coagulation factor V and VIII/V ratio as predictors of outcome in paracetamol induced fulminant hepatic failure: Relation to other prognostic indicators. Gut 33:98–102, 1992.

63. Hillenbrand P, Prabhoo SP, Jedrychowski A, et al: Significance of intravascular coagulation and fibrinolysis in acute hepatic failure. Gut 15:83, 1974.

64. O'Grady JG, Langley PG, Isola LM: Coagulopathy of fulminant hepatic failure. Semin Liver Dis 6:159–163, 1986.

65. Jones EA, Schafer DF, Ferenci P, et al: The neurobiology of hepatic encephalopathy. Hepatology 4:1235, 1984.

66. Mullen KD, Martin JV, Mendelson WB, et al: Could an endogenous benzodiazepine ligand contribute to hepatic encephalopathy? Lancet 1:457–459, 1988.

67. Grimm G, Ferenci P, Katzenschlager R, et al: Improvement of hepatic encephalopathy treated with flumazenil. Lancet 2:1392–1394, 1998.

68. Gimson AES, Braude S, Mellon PJ, et al: Earlier charcoal hemoperfusion in fulminant hepatic failure. Lancet 2:681, 1982.

69. Ware AJ, D'Agostino A, Combes B: Cerebral edema: A major complication of massive hepatic necrosis. Gastroenterology 61:877, 1971.

70. Berk PD, Popper H: Fulminant hepatic failure. Annotated abstracts of a workshop held at the National Institutes of Health, 1977. Am J Gastroenterol 69:349, 1978.

71. Traber PG, Dal Canto M, Ganger DR, et al: Electron microscopic evaluation of brain edema in rabbits with galactosamine induced fulminant hepatic failure: Ultrastructure and integrity of the blood-brain barrier. Hepatology 7:1272–1277, 1987.

72. Kato M, Hughes RD, Keays RT, et al: Electron microscopic study of brain capillaries in cerebral edema from fulminant hepatic failure. Hepatology 15:1060–1066, 1992.

73. Almdal T, Schroeder T, Ranek L: Cerebral blood flow and liver function in patients with encephalopathy due to acute and chronic liver diseases. Scand J Gastroenterol 24:229–303, 1989.

74. Lidofsky SD, Bass NM, Prager MC, et al: Intracranial pressure monitoring and liver transplantation for fulminant hepatic failure. Hepatology 16:1–7, 1992.

75. Trewby PN, Williams R: Pathophysiology of hypotension in patients with fulminant hepatic failure. Gut 18:1021, 1977.

76. Weston MJ, Talbot IC, Howorth PJN, et al: Frequency of arrhythmias and other cardiac abnormalities in fulminant hepatic failure. Br Heart J 38:1179, 1976.

77. O'Grady JG, Williams R: Management of acute liver failure. Schweiz Med Wochenschr 116:541, 1986.

78. Arroyo V, Gines P, Gerbes AL, et al: Definition and diagnostic criteria of refractory ascites and hepatorenal syndrome in cirrhosis. International Ascites Club. Hepatology 23:164–176, 1996.

79. Moore K, Taylor G, Ward P, et al: Etiology and management of renal failure in acute liver failure. In Williams R, Hughes RD (eds): Acute Liver Failure: Improved Understanding and Better Therapy. London, Miter Press, 1991, pp 47–53.

80. Warren R, Trewby PN, Laws JW, et al: Pulmonary complications in fulminant hepatic failure: Analysis of serial radiographs from 100 consecutive patients. Clin Radiol 29:346, 1978.

81. Trewby PN, Warren R, Contini S, et al: Incidence and pathophysiology of pulmonary edema in fulminant hepatic failure. Gastroenterology 74:859, 1978.

82. Wendon J, Alexander GJM, Williams R: Cardiovascular monitoring and local blood flow. In Williams R, Hughes RD (eds): Acute Liver Failure: Improved Understanding and Better Therapy. London, Miter Press, 1991, pp 39–41.

83. Bihari D, Gimson AW, Lindridge J, et al: Lactic acidosis in fulminant hepatic failure. Some aspects of pathogenesis and prognosis. J Hepatol 1:405, 1985.

84. Bihari D, Gimson AES, Waterson M, et al: Tissue hypoxia during fulminant hepatic failure. Crit Care Med 13:1043–1049, 1985.
85. Harrison PM, Wendon JA, Gimson AES, et al: Improvement by acetylcysteine of hemodynamic and oxygen transport in fulminant hepatic failure. N Eng J Med 324:1852–1857, 1991.
86. Walsh TS, Hopton P, Philips BJ, et al: The effect of *N*-acetylcysteine on oxygen transport and uptake in patients with fulminant hepatic failure. Hepatology 27:1332–1340, 1998.
87. Bailey RJ, Woolf IL, Cullens H, et al: Metabolic inhibition of polymorphonuclear leukocytes in fulminant hepatic failure. Lancet 1:1162–1163, 1976.
88. Wyke RJ, Canalese JC, Gimson AES, et al: Bacteremia in patients with fulminant hepatic failure. Liver 2:45–52, 1982.
89. Rolando N, Harvey F, Brahm J, et al: Prospective study of bacterial infection in acute liver failure: An analysis of fifty patients. Hepatology 11:49–53, 1990.
90. Rolando N, Gimson A, Wade J, et al: Prospective controlled trial of selective parenteral and enteral antimicrobial regimen in fulminant hepatic failure. Hepatology 17:196–201, 1993.
91. Gazzard BG, Portmann B, Murray-Lyon IM, et al: Causes of death in fulminant hepatic failure and relationship to quantitative histological assessments of parenchymal damage. Q J Med 44:615, 1975.
92. Caraceni P, van Thiel DH: Acute liver failure. Lancet 345:163, 1995.
93. Shami VM, Macik BG, Hespenheide EE, et al: Recombinant activated factor VII is superior to plasma alone in correcting the coagulopathy of fulminant hepatic failure [abstract]. Hepatology 34:327A, 2001.
94. Lee WM: Medical progress: Acute liver failure. N Engl J Med 329:1862–1872, 1993.
95. Blei AT, Olafsson S, Webster S, et al: Complications of intracranial pressure monitoring in fulminant hepatic failure. Lancet 341:157, 1993.
96. Ascher NL, Lake JR, Emond JC, et al: Liver transplantation for fulminant hepatic failure. Arch Surg 128:677, 1993.
97. Clinical practice guidelines for the sustained use of sedatives and analgesics in the critically ill adult. Am J Health Syst Pharm 59:150–178, 2002.
98. Munzo SJ: Difficult management problems in fulminant hepatic failure. Semin Liver Dis 13:395, 1993.
99. Canales J, Gimson AE, Davis C, et al: Controlled trial of dexamethasone and mannitol for cerebral oedema of fulminant hepatic failure. Gut 23:625, 1982.
100. Mas A, Rodes J: Fulminant hepatic failure. Lancet 349:1081, 1997.
101. Riegler JL, Lake JR: Fulminant hepatic failure review. Med North Am 77:1057–1083, 1993.
102. Hanau C, Munoz SJ, Rubin R, et al: Histopathological heterogeneity in fulminant hepatic failure. Hepatology 21:345, 1995.
103. Takahashi Y, Kumada H, Shimizu M, et al: A multicenter study on the prognosis of fulminant viral hepatitis: Early prediction for liver transplantation. Hepatology 19:1065, 1994.
104. Mitchell I, Bihari D, Chang R, et al: Earlier identification of patients at risk from acetaminophen-induced acute liver failure. Crit Care Med 26:279–284, 1998.
105. Pauwels A, Mostefa-Kara N, Floret C, et al: Emergency liver transplantation for acute liver failure. Evaluation of London and Clichy criteria. J Hepatol 17:124, 1993.
106. Schiodt FV, Bondesen S, Petersen I, et al: Admission levels of serum Gc-globulin: Predictive value in fulminant hepatic failure. Hepatology 23:713–718, 1996.
107. Chenard-Neu MP, Boudjema K, Bernuau J, et al: Auxiliary liver transplantation: Regeneration of the native liver and outcome in 30 patients with fulminant hepatic failure. Hepatology 23:1119–1127, 1996.
108. Nagamori S, Hasumura S, Matsuura T, et al: Developments in bioartificial liver research: Concepts, performance, and applications. J Gastroenterol 35:493–503, 2000.
109. Hughes RD, Wendon J, Gimson AES: Acute liver failure. Gut Sep: (Suppl):S86–S91, 1991.

CHAPTER 18

Toxin-Induced Renal Failure Syndromes

James Groff

The kidney plays a pivotal role in regulating many homeostatic functions. Alterations in body composition and volume are registered by a variety of chemoreceptors and stretch- and pressure-sensitive organelles throughout the body. The kidney is one of the most important final effector organs for these regulatory systems. Changes in ion content of the body are generally corrected by appropriate alterations in urinary excretion of these ions. Excess ion concentration promotes increased excretion, whereas deficiency provokes renal retention. Changes in body fluid volume also elicit a renal regulatory response, such as volume depletion resulting in sodium and water retention and volume expansion resulting in sodium and water excretion. The kidney is responsible for regulation of nitrogenous waste products from protein metabolism, including urea, creatinine, and uric acid. Regulation of blood pressure is yet another important function of the kidney.

Renal function and dysfunction certainly contribute to the morbidity and mortality of critically ill patients. Patients may have preexisting renal dysfunction, or renal dysfunction may develop after a variety of toxic or other insults. It is important to determine the etiology and time course of the renal dysfunction so that appropriate interventions can be made for these alterations in homeostasis. Many drugs and medications act as nephrotoxins, and the urinary tract is particularly susceptible to toxic injury. Physicians caring for a toxic or drug overdose patient need to have a fundamental understanding of renal pathophysiology, anatomy of the urinary tract system, and various forms of renal failure syndromes.

CLINICAL IMPORTANCE OF RENAL FAILURE SYNDROMES

Acute renal failure (ARF) is a common occurrence in the current practice of medicine. Prospective studies demonstrate that ARF will develop in approximately 3% to 5% of patients admitted to general medical and surgical wards.[1] In certain patient populations, such as those in medical/surgical intensive care units (ICUs), ARF develops in more than 20% of patients.[1] Modern renal replacement therapies (i.e., dialysis) have proved effective in correcting the life-threatening metabolic and volume-associated complications of ARF. However, the mortality rate for these patients is still as high as 40% to 80%, as reported in many recent studies. A study comparing the prognosis of ARF in ICU patients in two time periods (1977–1979 and 1991–1992) revealed a significantly improved rate of hospital survival (52%, versus 32% in the

earlier group) and 1-year survival (30%, versus 21% in the earlier group) in the later study group.[2] The mean Acute Physiology and Chronic Health Evaluation (APACHE) II score was the same in both study periods, but patients in the later group were older and had more chronic health problems. In the later study period, more patients had two or more factors contributing to the development of ARF, and preexisting cardiac prerenal azotemia and intravenous contrast studies were more frequent causes of ARF than in the earlier study group.[2]

There are several possible reasons for this apparent improvement in survival despite an older patient population with more preexisting chronic health problems. New sophisticated ICU support mechanisms such as better antimicrobial agents, improved mechanical ventilation, and parenteral nutrition are now available. There has also been a significant improvement in dialysis technology, including prevention of the common complication of hypotension. An ischemic kidney has deranged autoregulation of blood flow, and the hypotension associated with dialysis may induce additional ischemic injury. Hemodynamics can be improved with volumetric control of ultrafiltration and dialysate sodium profiles (a sodium content of 145 to 150 mmol/L early in the dialysis treatment promotes osmotic fluid shift into the intravascular space, after which it is tapered to 140 mmol/L). Lowering the dialysate temperature to 35°C to 36°C instead of the normal body temperature of 37°C may improve blood pressure and ultimately reduce the incidence of episodes of dialysis-associated hypotension.[3] Improved dialysis membranes may also contribute to improved survival. Dialysis membranes activate both complement and neutrophils. Bioincompatible membranes activate the immune system to a greater degree. Newer, biocompatible dialysis membranes are being used more frequently, and Hakim and colleagues have shown that patients dialyzed with the newer biocompatible membranes were more likely to have renal recovery.[4]

ANATOMY AND PHYSIOLOGY

The following is a simplified but practical review of the relevant renal anatomy and physiology. The normal kidney receives approximately one fifth of the cardiac output, or 1000 to 1200 mL/min in normal-sized adults. Nearly all of the kidney's blood supply passes through glomerular capillaries in the renal cortex. The ability of the kidneys to achieve their complex homeostatic function is made possible by the intricate microvascular system that regulates vascular resistance to maintain a physiologic intrarenal hemodynamic milieu. The functional unit of the kidney is the nephron, and it is designed to have both excretory and regulatory functions. The glomerulus is the basic filtering unit and is composed of an elegant capillary network that is primarily located in the cortex. This network has its origin at the level of the renal arteries. The renal arteries arise from the lateral region of the abdominal aorta at the level of the first and second lumbar vertebrae. Each artery divides into an anterior and posterior branch before traversing the renal hilus. Glomerular capillaries are derived from the afferent arteriole. The afferent arteriole divides into several primary capillary branches, each of which gives rise to an anastomosing capillary network. The nonanastomotic preglomerular arteriolar network delivers high blood flow to the glomeruli with nominal dissipation of the driving force. Interlobular arterial hydrostatic pressure may remain as high as 90% of aortic pressure, whereas glomerular capillary pressure is only about 55% of aortic pressure. Afferent arterioles provide the major preglomerular resistance. The afferent arteriole contains typical smooth muscle cells (responsive to neurohumoral stimuli) over most of its length. The terminal ends of the glomerular capillaries coalesce within the glomerulus to form the efferent arteriole and provide significant postglomerular resistance, which serves the dual role of maintaining high glomerular capillary pressure and low peritubular capillary pressure. The afferent and efferent arterioles each contribute to the regulation of glomerular blood flow and glomerular pressure in a unique manner. Changes in afferent arteriolar resistance produce directionally similar but quantitatively different changes in blood flow, glomerular filtration rate (GFR), and glomerular pressure. Alterations in efferent arteriolar resistance cause glomerular pressure and blood flow to change in the opposite direction.[5]

The glomerulus is enclosed by Bowman's capsule, the initial segment of the renal tubular system. Blood flowing from the afferent arteriole is "filtered" by the glomerular membrane. Normal adult kidneys produce approximately 150 L of filtrate per day, more than 99% of which is reabsorbed in the renal tubules to ultimately produce 1 to 2 L of urine per day. The glomerular filtrate (water and solutes) or ultrafiltrate of blood flows from Bowman's capsule into the proximal tubule. The ultrafiltrate passes into the descending loop of Henle and then into the distal tubule; the distal tubule joins with other tubules to form the cortical collecting ducts. The cortical collecting ducts ultimately drain into the renal pelvis, which in turn is drained by the ureters.

GFR is a measure of the function of the glomerulus and is defined as milliliters of ultrafiltrate produced per minute. The GFR is vital to the maintenance of acid-base, extracellular fluid, electrolyte, and metabolic homeostasis. The GFR directly parallels the hydrostatic pressure within the glomerulus (glomerular hydrostatic pressure), which itself is regulated by afferent and efferent arteriolar resistance across the glomerulus. In addition, the GFR parallels the ultrafiltration coefficient (Kf), which is a measure of the total surface area and permeability of the glomerulus.[6] Kf is regulated by circulation and intrarenal hormones. Alterations in GFR reflect the degree of renal dysfunction or injury caused by the underlying process. Clinical measurement of GFR becomes important in assessing renal injury, monitoring the response to therapy, and adjusting medications that are excreted by the kidneys.

The GFR, as measured by inulin clearance, is relatively constant in the same individual but varies among different people. Corrected for differences in body surface area, the mean GFR in young adults is approximately 130 mL/min in men and 120 mL/min in women. By approximately 1 year of age, the GFR (adjusted for body surface area) approximates that of an adult. Several studies have demonstrated a gradual decline in GFR of about 10 mL/min per decade beginning in the third to fourth decade.[7] The etiology of this decline appears to be glomerular obsolescence.

Renal autoregulation is an important concept to understand because many drugs, toxins, and physiologic states alter this homeostatic function. The kidneys are capable of maintaining GFR and renal blood flow (RBF) within narrow limits during a variety of conditions. Physiologic variations in GFR include diurnal variation, with the highest values occurring in the afternoon and the lowest values during the night. This variation may be explained by protein intake, which is generally highest during the day because of meals, and by protein loads, including infusions of amino acids, which are known to be associated with increases in GFR. Marked increases in GFR are seen in pregnancy (as much as 50%) and during the early stages of insulin-dependent diabetes mellitus. During periods of extracellular fluid volume expansion, the GFR temporarily increases. Exercise and volume depletion are noted to temporarily decrease GFR.

Autoregulation of GFR is characterized by changes in local feedback signals that modulate glomerular arteriolar tone. These alterations serve to maintain glomerular hydrostatic pressure and thus the hemodynamic factors governing the filtration process. Autoregulation can be viewed as a continuously operating negative feedback system that maintains an optimum filtered load in the presence of varying external influences. Autoregulatory responses are mediated primarily by alterations in smooth muscle tone of the afferent arteriole. GFR and RBF are highly autoregulated in response to changes in perfusion pressure. In addition, the intrarenal pressure in the glomerular and peritubular capillaries and in the proximal tubules exhibits autoregulatory responses. Direct observation of afferent arterioles during changes in perfusion pressure has confirmed that the major site of autoregulation is preglomerular.[5]

Currently, two hypotheses for autoregulation are advocated: the macula densa feedback hypothesis and the myogenic hypothesis.[5] The macula densa hypothesis evokes the tubuloglomerular feedback mechanism, which predicts that disturbances that increase distal tubular fluid flow past the macula densa will elicit vasoconstriction whereas decreased flow will cause vasodilation. For example, when RBF decreases, the concomitant fall in GFR results in delivery of less chloride ion to the macula densa, which then signals the afferent arteriole to dilate and thus restore GFR. Chloride ion may also influence efferent arteriolar tone. When GFR is reduced, decreased delivery of chloride ion to the juxtaglomerular apparatus triggers the release of renin, which ultimately results in the formation of angiotensin II. Angiotensin II produces efferent arteriolar constriction and increases glomerular filtration. When afferent and efferent arteriolar constriction occurs simultaneously, GFR will increase. The myogenic hypothesis is based on the premise that preglomerular arterioles can sense changes in vessel wall tension and respond to such changes with appropriate alterations in vascular tone. An increase in wall tension as might occur with elevations in arterial pressure is thought to stimulate a sensor element and start a series of events that result in vascular smooth muscle contraction. The opposite effect appears to occur with decreases in arterial pressure. Autoregulation of GFR and RBF occurs over a wide range of arterial pressures, but autoregulation of urine flow does not occur. There is a nearly linear relationship between mean arterial pressure above 50 mm Hg and urine output.[8]

PATHOPHYSIOLOGY

Renal Stress Response

Under conditions of stress, the kidney responds in a predictable manner to help maintain blood pressure and restore intravascular volume. RBF is markedly influenced by extrinsic stimuli such as stress, trauma, hemorrhage, pain, and exercise. Some of these conditions elicit increases in sympathetic nervous system activity that result in release of the α-adrenergic agonist norepinephrine, which directly increases renal vascular resistance. Norepinephrine also activates the renin-angiotensin-aldosterone system (RAAS) and thereby leads to release of antidiuretic hormone from the posterior pituitary gland. The RAAS plays an important role in regulating RBF and GFR. Renin release by the renal afferent arteriole may be triggered by hypotension/shock, increased tubular fluid chloride ion concentration, or sympathetic stimulation. Renin enhances angiotensin II production, which induces renal efferent arteriolar vasoconstriction. Angiotensin II plays a role in aldosterone release by the adrenal medulla. Activation of these systems, such as in some poisonings or shock, results in a shift of blood flow from the renal cortex to the medulla, avid sodium and water reabsorption, and decreased urine output. A further reduction in RBF and GFR may occur under conditions of greater stress as a result of afferent arteriolar constriction. Ischemic injury to the kidney and ARF may follow if the stress response is not reversed. Other renal insults contribute to ARF in patients with co-existing renal vasoconstriction from the stress response.[8]

Acute Renal Failure

ARF is characterized by a reduction in renal function over a period of hours to days, retention of nitrogenous waste products, and possibly fluid, electrolyte, and acid-base abnormalities. Even though a single unifying definition of ARF has not been established, it is commonly defined as an increase in serum creatinine greater than 0.5 mg/dL (44 μmol/L) over baseline or a reduction in calculated creatinine clearance of 50% or more.[9] By definition, this is a common occurrence in the hospital setting, especially in ICUs. ARF can further be divided into three groups: nonoliguric (>400 mL/day), oliguric (<400 mL/day), and anuric (<100 mL/day). These groups may give some clues regarding the etiology of ARF and will be discussed later in the chapter.

ARF is traditionally classified into three subgroups based on its pathophysiology. When ARF is due to a reduction in perfusion from any cause, it is termed *prerenal azotemia* or *prerenal failure*. ARF that is due to a primary intrarenal cause is termed *intrinsic renal failure*. When ARF is caused by an obstruction process, it is called *postrenal failure*. Although the former two types of ARF may commonly accompany toxic chemical exposure, the latter variety is uncommon. A prospective study by Hou and colleagues found prerenal azotemia to be the single most common cause (>40%) of ARF in a general medical-surgical hospital.[1] Prerenal failure accounts for nearly 70% of cases of ARF that occur outside the hospital.[10] Others have reported prerenal azotemia to account for 40% to 80% of all causes of ARF. However, ARF encountered in the ICU is most commonly due to intrinsic renal failure secondary to prolonged prerenal states, sepsis, profound hypotension, toxic insults, and multiple organ failure.

Prerenal azotemia is caused by hypoperfusion, and it is rapidly reversible if the underlying etiology is corrected. The kidney does not sustain any structural defect unless the insult is prolonged, at which point ischemic changes can occur. Any cause of real or perceived hypovolemia can result in prerenal azotemia (Table 18-1). Etiologies of real hypovolemia include blood loss/hemorrhage, vomiting, diarrhea, overdiuresis and osmotic diuresis (e.g., hyperglycemia), third spacing as seen with severe pancreatitis, diuretic overdose, and increased skin loss such as with thermal (not chemical) burns. Perceived hypovolemia or decreased effective circulatory volume results when changes in systemic hemodynamics result in decreased renal perfusion. Any condition that causes decreased cardiac output, including congestive heart failure, would fall into this category. Overdoses of cardiotoxic drugs such as tricyclic antidepressants, calcium channel antagonists, or β-blockers may cause ARF on this basis. Sepsis is associated with systemic vasodilatation and increased cardiac output; however, renal perfusion is reduced as a result of the renal vasoconstriction induced by the stress response. Many pharmacologic agents such as

---

TABLE 18-1 Major Causes of Prerenal Acute Renal Failure

Decreased Cardiac Output	Nonsteroidal antiinflammatory
Congestive cardiomyopathy	agents
Valvular heart disease	Angiotensin-converting enzyme
Pulmonary hypertension	inhibitors/angiotensin II
Cardiac tamponade	inhibitors
	Cyclosporine/tacrolimus
Decreased Cardiac Output with Normal or High Cardiac Output	Radiocontrast agents
Cirrhosis	**Intravascular Volume Depletion**
Sepsis syndrome	Burns
	Diarrhea
Drugs	Diuresis
Amphotericin B	Fever
Antihypertensive agents	Hemorrhage
Diuretics	Third spacing
Iron	Vomiting
Cathartics	

nonsteroidal antiinflammatory drugs (NSAIDs), angiotensin-converting enzyme (ACE) inhibitors, and angiotensin II receptor antagonists may affect renal hemodynamics directly, thereby causing apparent hypovolemia and prerenal azotemia.

Some basic aspects of the pathophysiology of prerenal ARF pertain to clinical practice. Conditions of low effective circulatory volume will result in the activation of central baroreceptors. Such activation leads to increases in angiotensin II, norepinephrine, and antidiuretic hormone, which cause vasoconstriction and salt and water retention in an attempt to preserve perfusion. Renal perfusion can be maintained with moderate degrees of hypovolemia because of the action of angiotensin II via increased efferent arteriolar resistance and stimulation of intrarenal vasodilatory prostaglandins. Severe hypoperfusion eventually overwhelms these compensatory mechanisms and ultimately causes renal ischemia and tubular injury.

The role of certain drugs in predisposing patients to prerenal azotemia and ARF is important. The most clinically important classes are NSAIDs, diuretics, ACE inhibitors, and angiotensin II receptor antagonists. NSAIDs affect afferent arterioles by inhibiting prostaglandin E_2 (a vasodilator), whereas ACE inhibitors and angiotensin II receptor antagonists (diminished vasoconstrictive effect of angiotensin II) affect efferent arterioles. By interfering with the autoregulatory mechanisms discussed earlier, these agents can induce prerenal azotemia and a reduction in GFR in patients with mild real or perceived hypovolemia. These classes of drugs must be used with great care in patients predisposed to or having low-flow states or hypotension. In this setting, the physician must monitor renal function closely and observe for signs of impaired renal function, at which point the use of these agents should be discontinued. Other drugs causing prerenal ARF are cyclosporine and tacrolimus, which are thought to inhibit prostaglandin-mediated vasodilation and cause afferent arteriolar vasoconstriction. Common drugs known to cause prerenal ARF are listed in Table 18-1.

Intrinsic renal failure reflects actual damage to the renal parenchyma (Table 18-2). This parenchymal damage may result from prolonged prerenal ARF, causing ischemia and, ultimately, necrosis of tubular epithelial cells resulting in acute tubular necrosis (ATN). Another etiology of ATN is insult by an extrinsic toxin (e.g., ethylene glycol). Finally, many renal or systemic diseases, such as interstitial nephritis or glomerulonephritis, can cause intrinsic renal failure. In hospitalized patients, ATN is the most common form of intrinsic ARF. Ischemic ATN is more prevalent than toxin-induced ATN.[11]

ATN is a natural consequence of prolonged renal ischemia and represents the far end of a continuum.[1,12] Ultimately, the ischemic tubular cells necrose and slough into the tubular lumen, which can result in tubular obstruction. These sloughed cells are the core of the coarsely granular or "muddy brown" casts seen in the urine in ATN. Profound intrarenal vasoconstriction is another contributor to the pathophysiology of ATN because it results in reduced total RBF. As a result of these hemodynamic disturbances, renal oxygen delivery is further compromised, contributing to the ischemic insult. Any condition that causes prolonged prerenal ARF may cause ATN if renal hypoperfusion is severe and prolonged. Therefore, cardiogenic shock, hemorrhage with hypovolemia, or septic shock may result in

TABLE 18-2 Major Causes of Intrarenal Acute Renal Failure	
Glomerulonephritis	Cephalosporins
Captopril	Cimetidine
Gold salts	Ciprofloxacin
Heroin	Clofibrate
Mercury compounds	Diuretics
Pentazocine	Infectious agents
	Infiltrative diseases
Ischemic Acute Tubular Necrosis	Isoniazid
	Methicillin
Cardiogenic, hypovolemic, or septic shock	Methyldopa
Hypotension	Nafcillin
Major surgery	NSAIDs
Prolonged prerenal physiology states	Phenobarbital
	Phenytoin
	Propranolol
Nephrotoxic Acute Tubular Necrosis	Rifampin
	Sulfamethoxazole
Acetaminophen	Sulfonamides
Aminoglycosides	Tetracyclines
Boric acid	
Chemotherapeutic agents	**Analgesic Nephropathy**
Colchicine	Acetaminophen
Ethylene glycol	Aspirin
Hemoglobinuria (hemolysis)	Cyclosporine
Lead	NSAIDs
Myoglobinuria (rhabdomyolysis)	Phenacetin
Pennyroyal oil	
Radiocontrast agents	**Other/Vascular**
Salicylates	Cholesterol embolization
	Crystal nephropathy
Acute Interstitial Nephritis	Granulomatous diseases
Allopurinol	Multiple myeloma
Amoxicillin	Thrombotic microangiopathy
Autoimmune diseases	Vascular compromise/ ischemia/infarction
Carbamazepine	
Carbenicillin	

parenchymal damage to the kidney if not corrected. Prolonged and severe ischemia may culminate in irreversible renal failure as a result of cortical necrosis.

After ischemia, nephrotoxins account for the largest number of cases of ARF. Aminoglycoside antibiotics, ethylene glycol, NSAIDs, and radiocontrast agents are the most common toxins encountered, but heme pigments, chemotherapeutic agents such as cisplatin, myeloma light chain proteins, and other drugs may be responsible. ARF caused by drugs can be due to direct tubular damage to tubular cells or various other mechanisms. Amphotericin B and cyclosporine cause both reduced RBF and direct tubular injury, the latter from either changes in cell permeability or necrosis of the epithelium of the proximal convoluted tubules.[13] Acetaminophen (paracetamol) has been reported to cause ATN even in the absence of hepatotoxicity, as well as acute interstitial nephritis (AIN).[13] Ethylene glycol poisoning is among the most common forms of toxin-induced ATN.

ARF secondary to AIN is most often due to an allergic reaction to a medication. Other less common etiologies are autoimmune diseases (e.g., lupus), infectious agents (e.g., hantavirus infection and legionnaires' disease), and infiltrative diseases (e.g., sarcoidosis).[9] It is characterized by an abrupt

TABLE 18-3 Pharmacologic Agents Used by Physicians or Patients That Cause Acute Renal Failure

DRUG	RENAL LESION
Acetaminophen	ATN
Aspirin	
Boric acid	
Bismuth salts	
Colchicine	
Lead	
Triamterene	
Uranium	
Heroin	GN
Acetaminophen	AIN/analgesic nephropathy
NSAIDs	
Alcohol	Myoglobinuric ATN
Amphetamines	
Barbiturates	
Cocaine	
Diazepam	
Doxepin	
Glutethimide	
Heroin	
Methadone	
Phencyclidine	
Phenylpropanolamine	
Strychnine	
Methamphetamine	Necrotizing vasculitis
Magnesium antacids	Nephrolithiasis
Calcium antacids	
Vitamin C	Oxalosis
Mannitol	Osmotic nephrosis

AIN, acute interstitial nephritis; ATN, acute tubular necrosis; GN, glomerulonephritis; NSAIDs, nonsteroidal antiinflammatory drugs.
Adapted from Abuelo JG: Renal failure caused by chemicals, foods, plants, animal venoms, and misuse of drugs. Arch Intern Med 150:505–510, 1990.

deterioration in renal function and histopathologically by inflammation and edema of the renal interstitium. Drug-induced AIN is classically associated with methicillin, although other antibiotics (e.g., cephalosporins, rifampin, sulfamethoxazole) and medications (e.g., NSAIDs and diuretics) have also been implicated (Tables 18-3 and 18-4).[13,14] The clinical picture of drug-induced AIN is classically described by the hypersensitivity triad of eosinophilia, fever, and rash. Despite the appearance of the full classic

TABLE 18-4 Inhaled or Cutaneously Absorbed Nephrotoxins

Acetone	Lysol
Boric acid	Methyl chloride
Cadmium	Mineral spirits
Carbon monoxide	Polyethylene glycol
Chromium	Povidone-iodine
Diethylene glycol	Toluene
Gasoline	Trichloroethylene
Hydrocarbons	

triad in some patients, the majority manifest only one or two features of the triad at the time of ARF. Renal failure secondary to AIN is often reversible after withdrawal of the offending medication. Renal recovery can occur over a period of days to weeks after discontinuation of the offending drug. One retrospective study suggested that a short course of steroids (i.e., prednisone 60 mg/day) with rapid tapering may shorten the course of ARF.[15]

Chronic use of analgesics can cause interstitial nephritis and papillary necrosis, referred to as analgesic nephropathy. This syndrome is primarily seen in middle-aged and older women who have used high doses of multiple analgesics for many years, and it is thought to be the result of toxic metabolites and medullary ischemia.[14] Acetaminophen (paracetamol) is a commonly implicated analgesic and is known to be oxidized to a toxic intermediate that binds to cellular macromolecules and causes cell necrosis. Whether acetaminophen, when used therapeutically, is nephrotoxic is a matter of debate. It has been hypothesized that concomitant use with NSAIDs or other drugs that inhibit prostaglandin synthesis results in decreased RBF and thus medullary ischemia because of the synergistic toxicity of these two common over-the-counter analgesics.[13] Slowly progressive renal insufficiency associated with defects in urine acidification, concentration, and sodium conservation could then develop.[13] A history of chronic pain, pyuria, hematuria, flank pain, and passage of necrotic papillary tissue characterizes the syndrome clinically. In addition to acetaminophen and NSAIDs, phenacetin and cyclosporine have been associated with this phenomenon.

Intrinsic ARF as a result of a glomerular disease is rarely seen in acutely hospitalized patients. (Glomerulonephritis usually causes admission to the hospital and generally does not occur or develop in the hospital setting.)

Glomerulonephritis can occur in an acute or subacute form. Serologic assays and immunopathologic examination of the kidney can identify specific causes of glomerulonephritis. Membranous glomerulonephritis has been associated with the use of gold salts and penicillamine for the treatment of rheumatoid arthritis.[13,16] In addition to causing nephrotoxicity on the basis of vascular changes, captopril in higher doses has infrequently been associated with membranous glomerulonephritis.[13] Minimal change glomerulonephritis has occurred after the chronic use of lithium and NSAIDs and in this case thought to be immunologically mediated.[13] It is crucial to diagnose glomerulonephritis quickly because the ARF may be reversible if treatment with immunosuppressive agents, plasma exchange, or both is initiated.

Chemical Toxins, Foods, and Plants

Inhalation, dermal exposure, envenomation from bites, or ingestion of numerous toxins can result in renal failure. The cause may be acute or chronic occupational exposure, suicidal ingestion, product misidentification, aberrant use of foods, inhalational solvent abuse, or accidental ingestion of toxic plants or mushrooms. The mechanism may be direct nephrotoxicity, hypotension, hemolysis, rhabdomyolysis, or a combination of these factors. Examples of occupational toxins that may result in exposure through inhalation include arsine gas, carbon tetrachloride, silica dust, and toluene.[17]

Ingestion of ethylene glycol for either suicidal intent or use as an alcohol substitute results in renal failure and should be strongly considered in any case of ARF, especially if associated with severe acidosis. Accidental or intentional ingestion of aniline dyes, heavy metals, organic solvents, pesticides, or insecticides is a less common cause.[18]

Ingestion of certain foods in very high quantity or some select plants and mushrooms can also be nephrotoxic. Examples include Vichy water, Worcestershire sauce, milk, licorice, rhubarb, or even small amounts of fava beans or djenkol beans in susceptible individuals.[17] Toxic plants that have been mistaken for edible varieties and ingested include water hemlock, *Cortinarius* and cyclopeptide mushrooms, rosary peas, and castor beans.

Worldwide, snakebites are the most common type of envenomation resulting in renal failure. The renal failure is due to a combination of hypotension, hemolysis, and direct tubular damage. Less often, arthropod stings are responsible. Potential chemical and biologic causes of renal failure are outlined in Table 18-5.

DIAGNOSIS

Careful evaluation of the patient's history and physical examination will generally uncover the etiology of the ARF. For example, recent exposure to intravenous iodinated contrast

TABLE 18-5 Chemicals/Toxins/Foods/Plants Causing Renal Failure

Chemicals

Acetone, aniline, arsenic, arsine gas, boric acid, cadmium, carbon monoxide, carbon tetrachloride, chlordane, chromium, copper sulfate, dichlorophenoxyacetic acid, diethylene glycol, diquat, ethylene dichloride, ethylene glycol, fluoride, germanium compounds, isopropyl alcohol, lead, lindane, Lysol, methylene chloride, mineral spirits, naphthalene, organic solvents, oxalic acid, paraquat, phenol, polyethylene glycol, potassium bromate, tetrachloroethylene, toluene, trichloroethylene

Foods

Djenkol beans, fava beans, grass carp bile, licorice, rhubarb, Vichy water (fluoride), Worcestershire sauce

Plants/Mushrooms

Amanita phalloides mushrooms, autumn crocus, castor bean, *Cortinarius* mushrooms, daphne, impila, rosary pea, water hemlock

Venom

Arthropods

African bee, brown recluse spider, Indian hornet, Oriental hornet, scorpion, South American house spider, yellow jacket

Snakes

Agkistrodons, Australian brown snake, black mamba, boomslang, copperhead, dugite, gwardar, jararaca, mamushi, puff adder, rattlesnakes, rough-scaled snake, Russell's viper, saw-scaled sand viper, sea snake, small African snake, small-eyed black snake, tiger snake, water moccasin

Adapted from: Abuelo GJ: Renal failure caused by chemicals, foods, plants, animal venoms, and misuse of drugs. Arch Intern Med 150:505–510, 1990.

agents or other known nephrotoxins and physical findings of intravascular volume depletion provide valuable diagnostic information. In the history, particular attention should be focused on the patient's volume status (e.g., thirst, orthostatic symptoms, sensible and insensible volume losses such as with diarrhea or fever) and current medications that may alter renal hemodynamics (e.g., NSAIDs, cyclosporine, ACE inhibitors, and angiotensin II antagonists) and thus predispose the patient to an ischemic insult. It is important to review all recent and current medications as possible nephrotoxic insults. Any radiologic procedure involving intravenous contrast agents should be suspect in the etiology of ARF if the time course of ARF is 24 to 48 hours after the exposure is documented. A thorough physical examination involving almost all the organ systems is extremely important. The patient's volume status can be assessed by evaluating for jugular venous distention, pulmonary rales, third heart sound, ascites, edema, and anasarca. Ischemic changes in an arm or leg might suggest rhabdomyolysis or thromboembolic disease. Palpable purpura, pulmonary hemorrhage, sinusitis, and synovitis should make the clinician consider systemic vasculitis. Rectal and vaginal masses and prostatic hypertrophy should raise the possibility of an obstructive process's being responsible for the ARF, especially in an anuric patient.

Careful examination of the urinary sediment and the use of urinary indices can help distinguish prerenal failure from intrinsic ARF. These studies are readily available and inexpensive. Common urine findings are shown in Table 18-6. Heme-positive urine, in the absence of erythrocytes, suggests the presence of myoglobin or hemoglobin and supports a clinical diagnosis of rhabdomyolysis or transfusion reaction. Cellular elements are important diagnostically because sterile pyuria or eosinophiluria may suggest AIN or atheroembolic ARF. Microscopic hematuria is nonspecific and has many possible etiologies, including but not limited to trauma (e.g., bladder catheterization), infection, calculi, anticoagulation, malignancy, and glomerulonephritis. Casts and their characteristics are useful diagnostically. Pigmented granular casts (e.g. "muddy brown") are typically seen in ischemic or toxic ATN. White cell casts are found in AIN and pyelonephritis, and red blood cell casts are found in glomerulonephritis.[19]

TABLE 18-6 Common Urinary Diagnostic Indices in Prerenal versus Intrinsic Renal Failure

PARAMETER	RENAL FAILURE	
	Prerenal	*Intrinsic*
Urinalysis	Hyaline casts	Abnormal, cellular or granular casts
Specific gravity	>1.020	Around 1.010
Urine osmolality	>500	<350
Urine sodium	<20	>20
FE sodium, %	<1	>1
BUN:creatinine ratio	>20:1	<20:1

BUN, blood urea nitrogen; FE, fractional excretion.

Urinary indices that measure urine osmolality, urinary sodium concentration, and fractional excretion of sodium help differentiate between prerenal azotemia and intrinsic renal failure. The use of urinary indices is based on the assumption that the capability of the renal tubules to reabsorb sodium and water and the concentrating ability of the tubules remain intact in prerenal ARF and preglomerular vascular lesions; however, these functions are impaired in ATN, glomerulonephritis, and tubulointerstitial diseases. In general, patients with ARF from prerenal causes have a urine osmolality greater than 500 mOsm/kg, a urinary sodium concentration below 20 mmol/L, and fractional excretion of sodium below 1.0%. The opposite is seen in patients with ATN and intrinsic ARF. They are not able to concentrate their urine. Urine osmolality is less than 350 mOsm/kg, the urinary sodium concentration is greater than 20 mmol/L, and fractional excretion of sodium is greater than 1.0%. These simple markers are not absolute but are supportive of these diagnoses. For example, urinary sodium and fractional excretion of sodium can be low early in the course of ATN and in contrast-induced ARF. To have diagnostic value, blood and urine specimens should be obtained simultaneously and before intravenous fluid replacement or the use of any diuretics.

Certain blood tests can be helpful in the differential diagnosis of ARF. A blood urea nitrogen–to–creatinine ratio greater than 20:1 is supportive of tubular reabsorption of urea nitrogen as a prerenal cause of ARF. Hypernatremia and metabolic alkalosis in a patient with ARF would be more consistent with a prerenal cause than with intrinsic renal lesions. With parenchymal damage, the kidney cannot excrete a free water load or acidify the urine, and hyponatremia and metabolic acidosis result. Hypercalcemia and hyperuricemia can point to a malignant condition associated with cell turnover or to a prerenal state because uric acid reabsorption in the proximal tubule is increased in prerenal states. Hypercalcemia can cause nephrogenic diabetes insipidus, leading to prerenal azotemia. Rapidly rising serum creatinine with a concurrent increase in creatinine kinase is suggestive of rhabdomyolysis. Eosinophilia in the presence of ARF should make the clinician consider allergic interstitial nephritis. These few simple and readily available blood tests are helpful in differentiating between the two most common etiologies of hospital-acquired ARF, prerenal and intrinsic renal causes.

One of the first causes of ARF to be excluded is that of postrenal. An abrupt onset of oliguria or anuria should make the clinician think of postrenal etiologies first. Bladder catheterization is a simple procedure that can quickly rule out urethral obstruction. Renal ultrasound is a relatively inexpensive and noninvasive method of diagnosing obstruction in the acute setting.

In the appropriate clinical setting with supportive information from urinalysis, urinary indices, and blood tests as just described, renal biopsy is generally unnecessary. In almost all cases of ARF secondary to prerenal azotemia and ATN, a histologic diagnosis would not be of additional value in the management of these patients. Renal biopsy should be considered in patients with unexplained ARF, ARF thought to be due to glomerulonephritis, hemolytic-uremic syndrome, and interstitial nephritis not responding to withdrawal of the offending agent, as well as in patients with renal transplants.

TREATMENT STRATEGIES IN ACUTE RENAL FAILURE

The first and most important aspect in managing patients with ARF is reversal of the underlying cause of the ARF. Other important considerations are correcting the metabolic, fluid, and electrolyte abnormalities. After the initial evaluation, it should be determined whether the patient needs renal replacement therapy.

For patients with prerenal azotemia, restoration of renal perfusion by definition will reverse the ARF. Patients with true intravascular volume depletion require intravenous volume resuscitation. Crystalloid solutions can be used in most situations; however, colloid products (e.g., albumin products and fresh frozen plasma) may be beneficial in certain settings such as patients with severe liver disease, active hemorrhage, or bleeding diatheses. Tenuous patients with prerenal azotemia caused by renal vasoactive medications will often require changes in the dose or possibly discontinuation of the drug. For example, patients taking NSAIDs and ACE inhibitors may demonstrate improved renal function by discontinuing the NSAID, thereby increasing afferent arteriolar flow. An acute overdose of agents causing prerenal ARF warrants a saline challenge of 1 to 2 L in adults. Patients with bilateral renal artery stenosis or renal artery stenosis in a solitary kidney frequently behave in a prerenal manner because of reduced preglomerular blood flow, and such patients ultimately require correction of the fixed lesion to restore or prevent further decline in renal function. In the critical care arena, invasive hemodynamic monitoring may be useful to guide the volume replacement therapy. It is important to note that diuretics may be detrimental in the setting of prerenal ARF. The clinician should use return to baseline renal function and improvement in metabolic and electrolyte status as end points for therapy.

The mainstay of therapy for intrarenal ARF, including ATN, is supportive and involves measures to control the complications of ARF (Table 18-7) until adequate renal function returns. The initial complications of ARF reflect the role of the kidneys as the primary regulator of volume and electrolyte status. In patients with severe ARF, the uremic syndrome develops because of the important role of the kidney in excreting nitrogenous waste products. This syndrome can have serious effects and must be managed carefully; renal replacement therapy is often required.

Considerable controversy has arisen regarding the benefits of conversion of oliguric to nonoliguric ARF. The potential benefits of conversion to a nonoliguric state include a

---

TABLE 18-7 Complications of Acute Renal Failure

Hyperkalemia
Hypermagnesemia
Hypernatremia
Hyperphosphatemia
Hypocalcemia
Hyponatremia
Metabolic acidosis
Symptomatic uremia: anemia, asterixis, bleeding diathesis, malnutrition, mental status changes, nausea/vomiting, pericarditis
Volume overload/pulmonary edema

decreased requirement for dialysis for volume overload and a decreased need for fluid and nutritional restriction. Some investigators believe that such conversion improves survival, although this hypothesis has not been proved. This line of reasoning is the basis of the rationale for using diuretics and dopamine in ARF.

Patients who are oliguric because of intrinsic ARF or ATN can possibly be converted to nonoliguric ARF with the administration of a loop diuretic. Klahr and Miller suggest an initial intravenous infusion of 100 to 200 mg of furosemide, whereas others have recommended a continuous infusion of 10 to 40 mg/hr. If urinary output does not increase within 1 to 2 hours, the dose may be doubled and a thiazide diuretic such as hydrochlorothiazide or metolazone added.[20] Caution must be used with high doses of loop diuretics because hearing impairment has been reported. If no response is noted after these interventions, the therapy should be discontinued. Mannitol, an osmotic diuretic administered intravenously at a dose of 12.5 to 25 g, can increase intratubular flow but must be used with extreme caution in oliguric patients because if it does not induce a diuretic response, volume overload, including pulmonary edema, may ensue. Mannitol is often recommended in addition to sodium bicarbonate and vigorous volume replacement therapy for the prevention and treatment of ARF from rhabdomyolysis.[21] Dopamine is another controversial agent. Dopamine dilates renal arterioles and increases RBF. It has been used for both the prevention and treatment of ARF in critically ill patients. Advocates of its use recommend a trial of low- or renal-dose dopamine (0.5 to 2.5 μg/kg/min) in patients with oliguric ARF.[22] If urinary output does not increase in the first 6 hours, administration of dopamine should be discontinued. Controlled studies supporting its use are lacking, and therefore it is no longer routinely recommended because of potential side effects, including tachyarrhythmias, gut or digital ischemia, extravasation injury, and pulmonary shunting. A randomized, multicenter trial comparing low-dose dopamine and placebo in critically ill patients showed no benefit of dopamine in protecting from renal dysfunction.[23]

Hypervolemia is a frequent complication of ARF, especially in patients who are oliguric. In such patients, fluid intake must be minimized and medications should be given with the least amount of fluid. As volume overload ensues, jugular venous distention, pulmonary rales, a third heart sound, and peripheral edema may develop. The use of loop diuretics such as furosemide can be justified to increase urine output for fluid management, but little data support the use of these agents to improve outcome. Thiazide diuretics given 30 to 60 minutes before a loop diuretic may improve urine output. Dopamine as described earlier has been a controversial agent. If ARF persists with oliguria in the presence of volume overload, renal replacement therapy is necessary to control volume and blood pressure.

A second major complication of ARF is hyperkalemia. The appearance in urine of more than 90% of all dietary potassium, ordinarily about 50 to 100 mEq/day, is the result of potassium secretion in the distal tubule and cortical collecting tubule. In the presence of ARF, potassium is retained and hyperkalemia ultimately results. Hyperkalemia can result in paresthesias, weakness, hyporeflexia, paralysis, heart block, ventricular tachycardia, and

fatal arrhythmias. Mild hyperkalemia without symptoms is often treated with loop diuretics, potassium restriction (1 mEq/kg/day), and potassium-binding resins (sodium polystyrene sulfate; 1 g binds approximately 1 mEq). Severe hyperkalemia (potassium greater than 6.5 mEq/L) requires prompt attention and treatment. Electrocardiographic changes associated with hyperkalemia include peaked T waves and widening of the QRS complex; emergency treatment with calcium gluconate, intravenous insulin and dextrose, β_2-agonists (e.g., inhaled albuterol), and sodium bicarbonate is required. These measures will stabilize the cardiac membrane and move the potassium to the intracellular compartment, which will allow time for definitive treatment. There are essentially two methods to remove potassium in ARF, binding resins and dialysis, both of which require time to be effective.

In patients with ARF, dialysis is used as an extension of the support mechanism. Dialysis is performed to control and correct excess extracellular volume, electrolyte abnormalities, uremic syndrome, and metabolic acidosis. Currently, no evidence has shown that dialysis shortens the time course of ARF. Some investigators believe that dialysis may prolong the period of recovery in certain patients.[24] The most common complication during acute hemodialysis is hypotension, which may perpetuate the renal injury and prolong the recovery phase. The selection of dialysis membranes may also be an important factor in determining the outcome of patients with ARF. Hakim and colleagues demonstrated that the widely used cellulose membranes prolong the time to renal recovery and that using biocompatible dialysis membranes improves the outcome after dialysis is initiated.[4]

Currently, three basic methods are used for acute renal replacement therapy: intermittent hemodialysis (e.g., daily or three times per week for 3 to 4 hours per treatment), continuous renal replacement therapy, and peritoneal dialysis. Intermittent hemodialysis causes rapid fluid shifts (e.g., 1 to 2 L can be removed per hour if blood pressure allows) and solute shifts (e.g., hypokalemia). Most patients tolerate these shifts well; however, critically ill patients are often hemodynamically unstable and are at high risk for hypotension or cardiac dysrhythmias. Continuous renal replacement therapy consists of continuous venovenous hemofiltration/hemodiafiltration (CVVH/CVVHDF). These procedures are generally performed by the critical care nursing staff at the patient's bedside over a period of 24 hours on a daily basis. Continuous renal replacement therapies are ideally suited for hemodynamically unstable patients with volume overload and azotemia. The last type of dialysis is acute peritoneal dialysis. This procedure involves the introduction of 1 to 3 L of a dextrose-containing salt solution (dialysis solution) into the peritoneal cavity. By diffusion and ultrafiltration, toxic substances are moved from the blood and surrounding tissue into the dialysate, which is then drained, and the procedure is repeated. Complications of acute peritoneal dialysis include those of the procedure itself (e.g., hyperglycemia from the dextrose load, peritonitis) and placement of the intraperitoneal catheter. Hemodynamically, peritoneal dialysis is well tolerated. Relative contraindications include recent abdominal surgery or abdominal trauma, bleeding diathesis, and ileus. For these reasons, this modality is not frequently used in the critical care setting. In critically ill toxicology patients, intermittent hemodialysis is most commonly used and most cited in the literature. Removal of various drugs and medications by this method is referenced in many sources. It is also the modality that can rapidly remove many toxic substances. Toxins most commonly requiring intermittent hemodialysis include methanol, ethylene glycol, lithium, theophylline, barbiturates, and salicylates. Extracorporeal removal of drugs and other chemicals is discussed in Chapter 7.

REFERENCES

1. Hou SH, Bushinsky DA, Wish JB, et al: Hospital acquired renal insufficiency: A prospective study. Am J Med 74:243–248, 1983.
2. McCarty JT: Prognosis of patients with acute renal failure in the intensive care unit: A tale of two eras. Mayo Clin Proc 71:117–126, 1996.
3. Daugirdal JT, Ing TS: Handbook of Dialysis, 2nd ed. Boston, Little, Brown, 1994, pp 155–156.
4. Hakim RM, Wingard RL, Parker RA: Effect of the dialysis membrane in the treatment of patients with acute renal failure. N Engl J Med 331:1338–1392, 1994.
5. Massery SG, Glassock RJ: Textbook of Nephrology, 3rd ed. Baltimore, Williams & Wilkins, 1995.
6. Guyton AC: Textbook of Medical Physiology, 5th ed. Philadelphia, WB Saunders, 1986, p 399.
7. Massery SG, Glassock RJ: Textbook of Nephrology, 2nd ed. Baltimore, Williams & Wilkins, 1995, p 1141.
8. Guyton AC: Textbook of Medical Physiology, 5th ed. Philadelphia, WB Saunders, 1986, p 411.
9. Thadhani R, Pascual M, Bonventre JV: Acute renal failure. N Engl J Med 334:1448, 1996.
10. Kauffman J, Dhakul M, Patel B, Hamburger R: Community acquired acute renal failure. Am J Kidney Dis 17:191–198, 1991.
11. Thadhani R, Pascual M, Bonventre JF: Acute renal failure. N Engl J Med 334:1449, 1996.
12. Myers BD, Morean SM: Hemodynamically mediated acute renal failure. N Engl J Med 314:97–105, 1986.
13. Hoitsma AJ, Wetzels JFM, Koene RAP: Drug-induced nephrotoxicity. Drug Saf 6:131–147, 1991.
14. Paller MS: Drug-induced nephropathies. Med Clin North Am 74:909–917, 1990.
15. Galpin JE, Shinaberger JH, Stanley TM, et al: Acute interstitial nephritis due to methicillin. Am J Med 65:753–765, 1978.
16. Koren G: The nephrotoxic potential of drugs and chemicals; pharmacological basis and clinical relevance. Med Toxicol 4:59–72, 1989.
17. Abuelo JG: Renal failure caused by chemicals, foods, plants, animal venoms, and misuse of drugs. An overview. Arch Intern Med 150:505–510, 1990.
18. Daniell WE, Couser WG, Rosenstock L: Occupational solvent exposure and glomerulonephritis. A case report and review of the literature. JAMA 259:2280–2283, 1988.
19. Anderson RJ, Schrier RW: Acute renal failure. In Schrier RW, Gottschalk CW (eds): Diseases of the Kidney, 6th ed. Boston, Little, Brown, 1997.
20. Klahr S, Miller SB: Acute oliguria. N Engl J Med 338:671–675, 1998.
21. Better OS, Stein JH: Early management of shock and prophylaxis of acute renal failure in traumatic rhabdomyolysis. N Engl J Med 322:825–829, 1991.
22. Flancbaum L, Choban PS, Dasta JF: Quantitative effects of low-dose dopamine on urine output in oliguric surgical intensive care unit patients, Crit Care Med 22:61–66, 1994.
23. Bellomo R, Chapman M, Finfer S, et al: Low-dose dopamine in patients with early renal dysfunction: A placebo-controlled randomized trial, Lancet 356:2139–2143, 2000.
24. Cogner JD: Hemodialysis in acute renal failure. Semin Dial 3:146–147, 1990.

CHAPTER 19

Alterations in Consciousness

Jerrold B. Leikin ■ Andrea Carlson

The central nervous system (CNS), with its large lipid content and extensive blood supply, is often the target organ of drugs or toxins (toxicants). Signs resulting from chemical effects on the CNS frequently include mental status changes often progressing to coma. Coma may be due to direct toxic effects, metabolic abnormalities, or anoxia. A review of the final diagnosis of 500 patients hospitalized with "coma of unknown etiology" found that 149 (30%) were due to the adverse effects of drugs.[1]

PATHOPHYSIOLOGY

Alterations in consciousness can be classified into several categories. *Lethargy* denotes an inability to maintain the wakeful state without external stimulation, whereas *stupor* is defined as arousability only in response to a noxious stimulus. Arousal usually does not outlast the stimulus application. *Delirium*, or acute cortical-subcortical neuronal encephalopathy, is a fluctuating condition characterized by confusion, irritability, and disorientation that develop over a short period. The mental status end point of impaired consciousness is *coma* (unresponsiveness that is not arousable by any stimulus). Seizures may occur at any point. Substance intoxication and withdrawal are common causes of delirium and can cause seizures or coma. Mental status changes due to drugs or toxins usually are characterized by three tenets: (1) a strong dose-response relationship; (2) occurrence either at the time of exposure or after a short latent period; and (3) neurologic improvement after cessation of exposure, unless secondary processes, such as the effect of prolonged hypoxia or seizures, supervenes.[2]

Disturbances in consciousness leading to coma directly due to drugs or toxins usually are due to the suppression of activity in the neurons located in the reticular activating system of the upper brainstem and throughout the cerebral cortex. The reticular activating system is interspersed through paramedian regions of the rostral pontine and midbrain tegmentum, in the thalamus and the midbrain.[3] Although damage to the dominant (language-producing) cerebral hemisphere can produce temporary coma, prolonged coma due to a toxic insult implies bilateral (global) hemispheric or midbrain (through the reticular activating system) involvement. Alteration in consciousness may result from direct effect of the toxicant on the neuronal membranes of the reticular activating system or cerebral cortex (e.g., ethanol and general anesthetics).

Drugs or toxins (e.g., organophosphate agents, nicotine, or barbiturates) also may interact with neuroreceptors and neurotransmitters.[3] Examples include the enhancement of γ-aminobutyric acid (GABA)–inhibitory influences on presynaptic and postsynaptic receptors, resulting in the opening of neuronal chloride channels. The resulting influx of chloride ions increases the negative resting potential, causing hyperpolarization, which stabilizes the nerve membrane, reducing neuronal firing rate.[4-6] Other drugs (e.g., benzodiazepines) increase the intracellular flux of chloride ions by enhancing GABA binding to other (GABA$_A$ receptors) neuroreceptor sites and by unmasking high-affinity GABA receptors.[6] Table 19-1 and Figure 19-1 present neurotoxic agents and their targets for disruption of neurosynaptic transmission. Metabolic neuronal disturbances (due to factors such as concomitant hypoxia, hyperkalemia, hypokalemia, acidosis, or vitamin deficiencies) are an additional mechanism for impaired consciousness. Hypoglycemia (serum glucose <40 mg/dL [2.2 mmol/L]) can result in cerebral cortex or brainstem dysfunction or both, occasionally also causing focal neurologic deficits.

An additional mechanism for coma production involves cerebral nitric oxide production through the enzyme nitric oxide synthase, which is involved in *N*-methyl-D-aspartate receptor activation. Neurodegeneration attributable to nitric oxide production is due to a peroxynitrite-induced oxidant stress, leading to endothelial damage in cerebral blood vessels, reversal of platelet aggregation, and cerebellar synaptic depression. This mechanism probably is involved in the mediation of carbon monoxide, glutamate, sodium nitrite, and paraquat toxicity. Other toxins involved in *N*-methyl-D-aspartate receptor activity include domoic acid and acute ethanol withdrawal.

Delirium can be caused by virtually any drug, but it is especially noted with anticholinergic drugs (Table 19-2). It can be considered as a disorder of neurotransmission in the cortical and subcortical regions of the brain involving acetylcholine, dopamine, GABA, and serotonin.[7-9]

CLINICAL CHARACTERISTICS

Delirium may be hypoactive, with inattention and decreased activity, or hyperactive, characterized by agitation and combativeness. It is a disorder of attention and arousal and can be detected easily using the confusion assessment method. The *Diagnostic and Statistical Manual of Mental Disorders, Fourth Edition*,[10] criteria specify three aspects of the clinical characteristics of delirium: (1) onset within hours or days, with fluctuation during the course of the day and usually worse at night; (2) cognition change (disorientation, memory deficit,

TABLE 19-1 Cellular Targets and Potentially Neurotoxic Agents

Acetylcholine	Organophosphate insecticides, triethylcholine, botulinum toxin, physostigmine
Adrenergic receptors	Clonidine and imidazolines, sympathomimetics, sympatholytics, ergot alkaloids, antipsychotic agents (chlorpromazine, haloperidol), yohimbine
Calcium ion channel	Calcium channel blockers (dihydropyridines, phenylalkylamines, benzodiazepines) calciseptine (black mamba snake) conotoxins (Cone snails), agatoxin (North American funnel web spider), octanol, flunarizine
Cannabinoid receptor	Cannabinoid (marijuana, hashish)
Dopamine receptors	Apomorphine, bromocriptine, antipsychotic drugs
GABA receptors	Benzodiazepine, cyclopyrrolones (zopiclone), imidazopyridines (zolpidem), barbiturates, ethanol, penicillin, muscimol (*Amanita muscaria*), bicuculline, neuroactive steroids (alphaxalone), flumazenil, baclofen
Glycine receptors	Strychnine, brucine, tetanus toxin, gelsemine
Histamine receptors	Antihistamines, TCAs
Membrane lipid	General anesthetic drugs (e.g., halothane)
MAO	MAO inhibitors (iproniazid, phenelzine, isocarboxazid)
Muscarinic receptors	Curare, *A. muscaria*, *Atropa belladonna*
Nicotinic receptors	Nicotine, neuromuscular blocking drugs, α-bungarotoxin
NMDA receptors	Arylcyclohexylamine (phencyclidine, ketamine), ethanol, domoic acid
Norepinephrine reuptake	TCAs, reserpine, amphetamine, cocaine
Opioid receptors	Opioid agonists (heroin, morphine, opium, meperidine, methadone) and antagonists (naloxone, naltrexone)
Potassium channels	Barium, 4-aminopyridine, tetraethylammonium ion, cesium, polypeptide toxins from scorpion (charybdotoxin), bee (apamin), snake (dendrotoxin), thallous salts, gossypol, quinidine, phencyclidine, Gaboon viper venom (*Bitis gabonica*)
Purine receptors	Adenosine, caffeine, theophylline
Purine/adenosine receptors	Caffeine, theophylline
Serotonin receptor	Atypical neuroleptics, buspirone, ondansetron, granisetron, LSD, mescaline, psilocybin, cyproheptadine, methysergide, khat
Serotonin reuptake	TCAs, selective serotonin reuptake inhibitors, nefazodone, venlafaxine
Sodium channels	Local anesthetics, (lidocaine, procaine), TCAs, tetrodotoxin (puffer fish), saxitoxin (paralytic shellfish), frog-skin poison (batrachotoxin), aconitine (monkshood), veratridine (Lillacae SP), scorpion anemone toxins, gray anotoxin (rhododendron), ciguatoxins

GABA, γ-aminobutyric acid; LSD, lysergic acid diethylamide; MAO, monoamine oxidase; NDMA, *N*-methyl-D-aspartate; TCAs, tricyclic antidepressants.
From Ford M, Delaney KA, Ling LJ, et al: Clinical Toxicology. Philadelphia, 2001, WB Saunders, p 135.

or language disturbance); and (3) disturbance of consciousness with a reduction of ability to focus, sustain, or shift attention. After recovery, the patient usually is amnestic about the delirium episode.

The general clinical characteristics of coma due to an acute toxic cause are an absence of meningeal irritation and a lack of focal neurologic signs (unless hypoglycemia is involved). Usually no discrete morphologic causative lesion can be detected on neuroimaging. In the absence of seizures, the patient often progresses to coma through varying stages of lethargy, confusion, and stupor, with these stages often noted on reemergence from the comatose state. Deep tendon reflexes and oculocephalic and oculovestibular reactions are also usually preserved except in intoxications involving sedative-hypnotics and anticonvulsant agents. Agents causing prolonged coma (possibly lasting for >100 hours) with intermittent periods of arousal are usually drugs that undergo enterohepatic or enteral-enteral recirculation of their active metabolites, resulting in cyclic coma (Table 19-3).

Ancillary clinical signs are essential in determination of the toxic etiology. An adequate ocular examination is crucial.[11] The salient feature of the ocular examination can be divided into three categories: pupillary size, pupillary reactivity, and assessment of the presence of nystagmus.

The pupillary size represents a constant balance between the autonomically innervated sphincter pupillae and the radi-ally arranged dilator muscle of the iris. In toxic cases, the pupillary size is symmetric, although 20% of normal individuals exhibit up to 0.5 mm of asymmetry.[3] Tables 19-4 and 19-5 list agents that may cause miosis (pupils <2 mm) and mydriasis (pupils >4 mm).[12] Pupil size can be variable in drug toxicity, however, due to multiple conflicting neurotransmitter responses in critical illness and is not a consistently reliable diagnostic finding.[13]

The pupillary light reflex usually is spared in coma of toxic origin; however, there are some exceptions. High-dose barbiturate poisoning and opiates can result in fixed miosis, whereas anticholinergic agents can cause fixed mydriasis that may not be reversible with physostigmine. Other causes of midrange-to-large, fixed pupils include methanol toxicity, hypothermia, and hypoxia.[3]

Drug-induced nystagmus (involuntary rhythmic eye movement) commonly results in "jerk nystagmus." In jerk nystagmus, the eye movements alternate between the slow component of initial (or induced) movement and the fast corrective component (jerk) in the opposite direction. Common causes for horizontal nystagmus include alcohol, anticonvulsants, sedative-hypnotics, solvents, and quinine. Lithium may cause downbeat nystagmus.[14] Phencyclidine, dextromethorphan, phenytoin, and sedative-hypnotics may cause a combination of vertical, horizontal, and rotary nystagmus. Sedative-hypnotics may cause disconjugate gaze. Opsoclonus (rapid, conjugate eye oscillations worsened

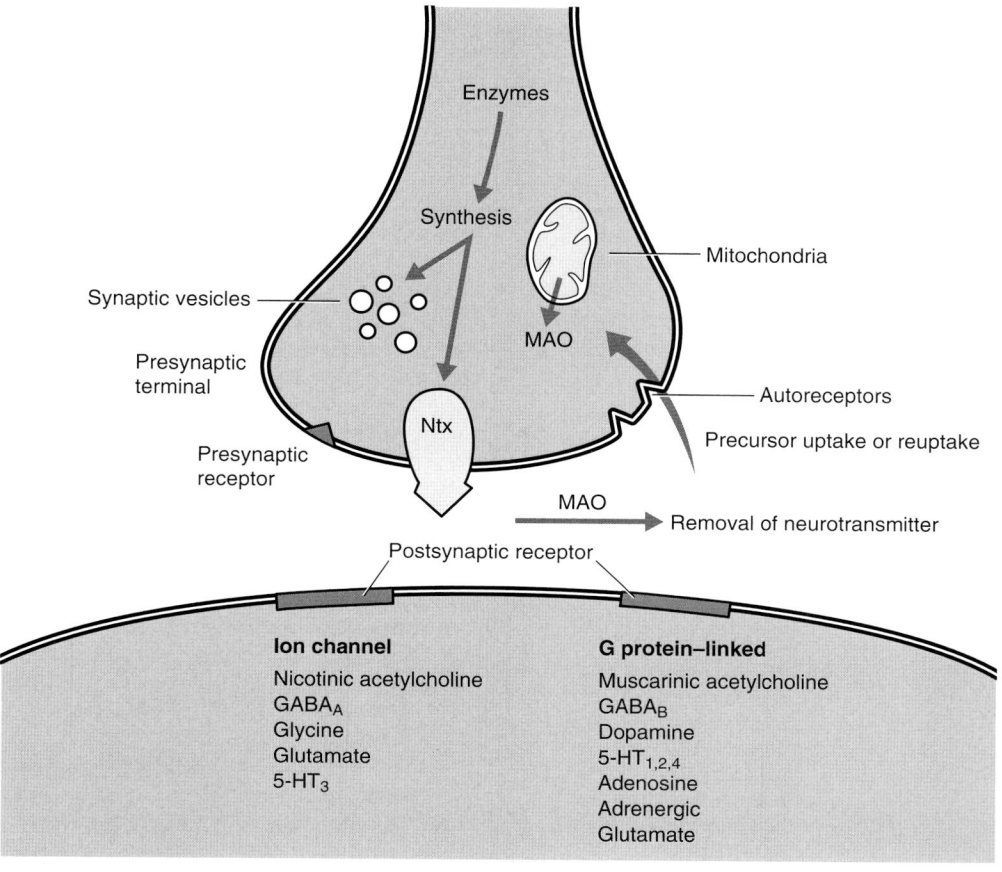

FIGURE 19-1

Schematic representation of a synapse showing the principal structures and sites of drug action. This synapse is a hybrid for the purpose of visualization; as outlined in the text, a neuron is typically highly specialized for a specific neurotransmitter system. GABA, γ-aminobutyric acid; 5-HT, 5-hydroxytryptamine; MAO, monoamine oxidase; Ntx, neurotransmitter. *(From Burkhart KK, Akhtar J: Clinical neurotoxicology. In Haddad LM, Shannon MW, Winchester JF [eds]: Clinical Management of Poisoning and Drug Overdose. Philadelphia, 1998, WB Saunders, p 135.)*

TABLE 19-2 Toxic Causes of Delirium

Medicinal Agents			
Acyclovir	Chlorpheniramine	Doxepin	Interferon alfa-2b
Aldesleukin	Chlorpromazine	Drug withdrawal	Interferon alfa-n3
Alfentanil	Choline magnesium trisalicylate	Ergotamine	Interferon beta-1b
Alprazolam	Cimetidine	Estazolam	Interferon gamma-1b
Aminophylline	Ciprofloxacin	Ethchlorvynol	Ipratropium
Amiodarone	Clomipramine	Ethyl alcohol	Isocarboxazid
Amitriptyline	Clonidine	Famotidine	Ketamine
Amoxapine	Clozapine	Fentanyl	Levodopa
Amphotericin B	Cocaine	Flumazenil	Levomethadyl acetate
Atropine	Codeine	Fluorouracil	hydrochloride
Belladonna	Colchicine	Fluoxetine	Levorphanol
Benztropine	Cortisone acetate	Fluphenazine	Lidocaine
Buprenorphine	Cyclobenzaprine	Glutethimide	Lithium
Bupropion	Cycloserine	Heroin	Loperamide
Butorphanol	Cyclosporine	Hydrocodone	Maprotiline
Butriptyline	Desipramine	Hydrocortisone	Mefloquine
Caffeine	Dextroamphetamine	Hydromorphone	Meperidine
Camphor	Dibenzepin	Hydroquinone	Mephentermine
Cantharidin	Dicyclomine	Hydroxyzine	Mesoridazine
Carbamazepine	Digitoxin	Hyoscyamine	Methadone
Chloral hydrate	Digoxin	Imipramine	Methamphetamine
	Diphenhydramine	Interferon alfa-2a	Methohexital

Continued

TABLE 19-2 Toxic Causes of Delirium—cont'd

Methotrexate	Promazine	Vigabatrin	Cathinone
Methyl salicylate	Promethazine	Vinorelbine	Chicken soup
Methyldopa	Propoxyphene	Vitamin A	Christmas cherry
Metoclopramide	Protriptyline	Zolpidem	*Claviceps purpurea*
Mianserin	Quinidine	**Nonmedicinal Agents**	Daphne
Midazolam	Ranitidine hydrochloride	2-Propanol	Deadly nightshade
Morphine sulfate	Rifampin	Arsenic	Foxglove
Nalbuphine	Salicylate	Benzene	Jimsonweed
Niacin	Salsalate	Bromates	Lantana
Nitroprusside	Scopolamine	Carbon dioxide	Marijuana (cannabis)
Nizatidine	Secobarbital	Carbon tetrachloride	Morning glory
Nortriptyline	Serotonin syndrome	Dichlorodiphenyl	Mushrooms, toxic
Opium alkaloids (hydrochlorides)	Sertraline	trichloroethane (DDT)	(group II)
Opium tincture	Sodium fluoride	Diethyltoluamide DEET)	monomethylhydrazines
Oxycodone	Sparfloxacin	Ethylene dichloride	Mushrooms, toxic
Oxymorphone	Stanozolol	Gasoline	(group III)
Para-aminosalicylate	Sufentanil	Lead	cholinergic
Paraldehyde	Tacrolimus	Lysergic acid diethylamide	Mushrooms, toxic (group V)
Paregoric	Theophylline	(LSD)	anticholinergic
Paroxetine	Thioridazine	Mercury	Mushrooms, toxic (group VI)
Pentazocine	Thiothixene	Nerve gases	psychedelic
Pentobarbital	Tocainide	Nickel carbonyl	Oleander
Perphenazine	Tramadol	Nitrous oxide	Pennyroyal oil
Phencyclidine	Tranylcypromine	Tetrachloroethane	Potato (leaves, stems,
Phenelzine	Trazodone	Thallium sulfate	tubercles)
Phenobarbital	Triamcinolone	Toluene	Sand brier
Phenylephrine	Trifluoperazine	Triethyltin	Scorpion fish
Phenytoin	Triflupromazine	**Biologic Agents**	Stonefish
Prazepam	Trimethaphan camsylate	Angel's trumpet	Turkey fish
Prednisolone	Trimipramine	Black nightshade	Woody
Procarbazine	Valacyclovir	Boxthorn	nightshade
Prochlorperazine	Venlafaxine		Wormwood

by voluntary movement) may be caused by intoxication with antidepressants, anticonvulsants, organophosphates, thallium, lithium, and haloperidol. Periodic gaze disturbances ("Ping-Pong" gaze) has been described with monoamine oxidase inhibitor intoxication.[15]

The nature of the respiratory response is a valuable clinical clue to ascertain a toxicologic cause in the patient with altered mental status. Slow, regular breathing (usually at a rate <12 breaths/min) indicates an opiate or sedative-hypnotic toxicity. These drugs inhibit the pontine and medullary respiratory centers, resulting in diminished responsiveness of these centers to increases in carbon dioxide tension.[16,17] Alternatively, sympathomimetic agents directly stimulate these respiratory centers, resulting in tachypnea with increased tidal volume.[3] Kussmaul respirations (rapid, regular respirations with large tidal volumes) are usually related to metabolic acidosis. Another typical respiratory pattern due to acute intoxication is

Cheyne-Stokes respiration. This pattern is characterized by periods of hyperpnea that regularly alternate with a shorter period of apnea. This abnormal pattern is due to neuronal metabolic disturbances, which isolate the respiratory center in the brainstem from the cerebral cortex. Pulmonary complications, such as noncardiogenic pulmonary edema (e.g., caused by salicylates, opioids, cyclic antidepressants, sedative-hypnotics) and aspiration pneumonitis, are indirect consequences of toxin-induced coma. Aspiration pneumonitis occurs in approximately 10% of patients hospitalized after a drug overdose and more frequently when mental status is depressed.[18]

Other clinical parameters to be evaluated in the patient with impaired consciousness due to toxins include cranial nerve dysfunction (Table 19-6). Examples include trichloroethylene causing trigeminal nerve sensory neuropathy and organophosphate exposure involving multiple cranial nerves. These cranial neuropathies are usually bilateral. Nonspecific neurologic signs, such as asterixis, fasciculation, and myoclonus, are associated with toxic delirium and are not caused by psychiatric conditions mimicking delirium (see Table 19-2).[19–21] Motor response to noxious stimuli is symmetric and nonfocal. Anticholinergic medications are associated specifically with an increase in delirium incidence and severity in elderly patients.[22] This increase is thought to be due to the frequency of anticholinergic drug prescribing in the elderly, age-related decrease in cholinergic neurotransmission,

TABLE 19-3 Drugs that Can Cause Cyclic Coma

Barbiturates	Glutethimide
Carbamazepine	Meprobamate
Ethchlorvynol	

TABLE 19-4 Drugs and Toxins Causing Miosis

Medicinal Agents

Aceclidine
Alfentanil
Ambenonium
Bethanechol
Bunazosin
Bupivacaine
Buprenorphine
Buspirone
Caffeine
Chloral hydrate
Chlorpromazine
Clonidine
Codeine
Dextromethorphan
Dezocine
Dihydroergotamine
Distigmine
Edrophonium
Fentanyl
Fluroxamine
Guanabenz
Guanidine
Heroin
Hydromorphone
Hydrocodone
Levomethadyl acetate hydrochloride
Levorphanol
Lidocaine

Loperamide
Melperone
Meperidine
Meprobamate
Meptazinol
Methadone
Methyprylon
Morphine sulfate
Nalbuphine
Neostigmine
Nicotine
Nilutamide
Opium alkaloids (hydro-
   chlorides)
Opium tincture
Oxycodone
Oxymorphone
Paregoric
Pentazocine
Phencyclidine
Phenobarbital
Phenylephrine
Phenoxybenzamine
Physostigmine
Pilocarpine
Piritramide
Procaine
Propoxyphene
Pyridostigmine

Rauwolfia serpentina
Reserpine
Risperidone
Tetracaine
Tilidine
Tramadol
Valproic acid and derivatives
Xylazine
Zolpidem

Nonmedicinal Agents

2,4-Dichlorophenoxyacetic acid
2-Methyl-4-chlorophenoxyacetic acid
Aldicarb
Amitraz
Bromoform
Bromophos
Carbamates
Carbaryl
Chenopodium oils
Chlorfenvinphos
Chlorpyrifos
Coumaphos
Diazinon
Dichlorvos
Dicrotophos
Dioxathion
Disulfoton
Endosulfan

Ethion
Fensulfothion
Fenthion
Isofenphos
Malathion
Methidathion
Methiocarb
Methomyl
Mevinphos
Nerve gases
Organophosphates
Parthion
Profenofos
Propoxur
Terbufos
Tetraethyl
   pyrophosphate

Biologic Agents

Betel nut
Castor bean
Eucalyptus oil
Fire-bellied toad
Mushrooms, toxic
   (group III) cholinergic
Nutmeg
Poison hemlock
Poison lily
Tetrodotoxin food poisoning

TABLE 19-5 Toxicants Typically Causing Mydriasis

Medicinal Agents

Acetaminophen
Acetophenazine
Amisulpride
Amitriptyline
Anisotropine
Apraclonidine
Atropine
Azatadine
Belladonna
Benztropine
Biperiden
Botulinum toxin type A
Bretylium
Bromides
Brompheniramine
Buclizine
Budipine
Buflomedil
Bupropion
Butriptyline
Butylscopalamine
Camphor
Carbamazepine
Carbinoxamine
Chlormezanone
Chlorprocaine
Chlorpheniramine
Chlorphenoxamine

Chlorpromazine
Chlorprothixene
Cimetidine
Clidinium
Clozapine
Cocaine
Cyclizine
Cyclobenzaprine
Cyproheptadine
Desipramine
Diazepam
Dibenzepin
Dicyclomine
Diethylpropion
Dimenhydrinate
Diphenhydramine
Disopyramide
Disulfiram
Dopamine
Doxapram
Doxepin
Doxylamine
Ephedrine
Estazolam
Ethchlorvynol
Ethyl alcohol and ethyl alcohol
   withdrawal
Fenfluramine
Fluoxetine

Flurazepam
Fosphenytoin
Glutethimide
Glycopyrrolate
Homatropine
Hyoscyamine
Imipramine
Ipratropium
Isocarboxazid
Isopropamide
Ivermectin
Lidocaine
Mecamylamine
Meclizine
Melperone
Meperidine
Meprobamate
Methamphetamine
Methantheline
Methscopolamine
Midazolam
Naphazoline
Nicotine
Nortriptyline
Opiate withdrawal
Otilonium
Oxybutynin
Papaverine
Paroxetine

Pemoline
Pentoxifylline
Phencyclidine
Phenelzine
Pheniramine
Phentermine
Phenylephrine
Phenylpropanolamine
Phenytoin
Pizotyline
Pralidoxime
Procaine
Procyclidine
Promethazine
Proparacaine
Propranolol
Protriptyline
Pseudoephedrine
Quinidine
Quinine
Reserpine
Scopolamine
Sertraline
Sodium fluoride
Tetrahydrozoline
Thioridazine
Thyroid
Tolazoline
Tridihexethyl chloride

Continued

TABLE 19-5 Toxicants Typically Causing Mydriasis—cont'd

Trimeprazine	Coumaphos	Phosdin	Khat
Trimethaphan camsylate	Cyanide	Profenofos	Lantana
Trimipramine	Diazinon	Propoxur	Lupine
Tripelennamine	Dichlorvos	Sodium azide	Marijuana (cannabis)
Trospium	Dicrotophos	Sodium monofluoroacetate	Mate
Yohimbine	Dioxathion	Terbufos	Mescaline
Zotepine	Disulfoton	Tetraethyl pyrophosphate	Morning glory
	Ethion	Thallium	Mushrooms, toxic
Nonmedicinal Agents	Ethylene glycol	Toluene	(group V)
1,2-Dibromoethane	Fanthion	Trichloroethylene	Mushrooms, toxic
2-Butoxyethanol	Fensulfothion	Turpentine oil	(group VI) psychedelic
3,4-Methylenedioxymeth-	Heptachlor		Neurotoxic shellfish poisoning
amphetamine	Hydrazine	**Biologic Agents**	Nutmeg
Aldcarb	Lysergic acid diethylamide (LSD)	Boxthorn	Peyote
Barium	Malathion	Burdock root	Sassafras oil
Benzene	Methaldehyde	Cathinone	Scotch broom
Bromophos	Methidathion	*Clostridium botulinum* food poisoning	Tetrodotoxin food poisoning
Carbaryl	Methiocarb	Corn lily (*Veratrum*)	Tyramine hydrochloride
Carbon monoxide	Methomyl	English ivy	food poisoning
Chenopodium oils	Methyl bromide	Ephedra	Valerian
Chlorfenvinphos	Methyl ethyl ketone	Golden chain tree	Water hemlock
Chloroform	Mevinphos	Goldenseal	Wild cucumber
Chloromethane	Parathion	Horse chestnuts	Woody nightshade
Chlorpyrifos	Pentachlorophenol	Jimsonweed	Yew

LABORATORY STUDIES

Diagnostic modalities used to determine the cause of altered mental status usually are focused on serum analysis rather than on acute neuroimaging studies. Any toxic cause of high anion gap metabolic acidosis requires investigation (see Chapters 2 and 29). The presence of a decreased anion gap suggests lithium or bromide exposure. The presence of an osmolar gap indicates ethanol, isopropanol, methanol, or ethylene glycol poisoning; diabetic ketoacidosis; sepsis; or alcoholic ketoacidosis. The osmolar gap is discussed in detail in Chapter 2. Pure respiratory acidosis is consistent with hypoventilation, a clue to possible intoxication with sedative-hypnotics or opioids. Although urinary immunoassay results may provide a clue to the cause of altered consciousness, they often yield misleading false-positive and false-negative results. Serum levels of specific drugs can be diagnostic and are more useful if available (Table 19-7). Tricyclic antidepressant intoxication can lead to electrocardiographic abnormalities with seizures (described in Chapter 42). Patients with QRS interval prolongation greater than 0.1 second with QRS axis shifted to the right (as is the axis in the terminal 40 msec of the QRS interval) may be at risk for neurologic complications[25]; this is seen most easily as a terminal R wave in lead AVR. For this reason, a screening electrocardiogram often is used in the initial assessment of patients with coma or seizures. Hair testing for the presence of drugs provides only qualitative interpretation and offers no utility in the acute investigative causes of coma.[26]

The electroencephalogram is useful in assessing cerebral cortical dysfunction and identifying seizure activity. Normal alpha with theta-delta (grade I) activity is compatible with a good prognosis, as is paradoxical monomorphic delta activity, whereas low-voltage delta activity (with alpha coma), alternating patterns, or isoelectric tracing (grades IV or V) is indicative of a poor prognosis.[27,28] Brainstem auditory evoked potentials correspond with brainstem dysfunction during coma and may be modified by anesthetics and barbituates.[33]

pharmacodynamic changes in cholinergic receptor sensitivity, and deficient drug metabolism and elimination.[23,24]

TABLE 19-6 Agents Causing Cranial Nerve Palsies

Aldicarb	Lead
Arizona bark scorpion	Malathion
Botulinum toxin type A	Mercury
Bromophos	Methdathion
Carbaryl	Methiocarb
Carbon disulfide	Methomyl
Chlorfenvinphos	Methotrexate
Diazinon	Mevinphos
Dementon-S-methyl	Parathion
1,1,-Dichloroethane	Phosdin
Dichlorvos	Pravastatin
Dicrotophos	Profenofos
Didanosine	Propoxur
Dioxathion	Rabies virus
Disulfoton	Terbufos
Ethion	Tetraethyl pyrophosphate
Ethylene glycol	Toluene
Fensulfothion	*Trichinella spiralis* food
Fenthion	poisoning
Ketoprofen	Trichloroethylene
King cobra venom	Vincristine

TABLE 19-7 Serum Levels of Specific Drugs or Toxins that Can Result in Coma

DRUG	CONVENTIONAL UNITS	SI UNITS	DRUG	CONVENTIONAL UNITS	SI UNITS
Acebutolol	20 mg/L	77.12 μmol/L	Glucose	800 mg/dL	44 mmol/L
Acetaminophen	300 mg/mL	1984 μmol/L	Glutethimide	10 mg/L	46 μmol/L
Acetone	500 mg/L	8.6 mmol/L	Iron	500 μg/dL	89.6 μmol/L
Amitriptyline	2 mg/L	7320 nmol/L	Isoniazid	20 mg/L	145.82 μmol/L
Amobarbital	43 mg/L	190 μmol/L	Lead	100 μg/mL	4.8 μmol/L
Baclofen	1 mg/L		Lidocaine	5 μg/mL	21.3 μmol/L
Barbital	160 mg/L		Lithium	3 mEq/L	3 μmol/L
Butabarbital	39 mg/L		Lorazepam	0.3 mg/L	
Caffeine	100 mg/L	516 μmol/L	Loxapine	0.7 mg/L	
Calcium	15 mg/dL	3.75 mmol/L	Meprobamate	60 mg/L	274.9 μmol/L
Carbamazepine	18 mg/L	13.77 μmol/L	Mephobarbital	40 mg/L	
Carboxyhemoglobin	30%		Methanol	100 mg/dL	31.2 μmol/L
Carisoprodol	30 mg/L	115.2 μmol/L	Methaqualone	8 mg/L	32 μmol/L
Cetirizine	2 mg/L		Methemoglobin	20%	
Chloral hydrate (trichloroethanol)	20 mg/L	134 μmol/L	Methyprylon	50 mg/L	272.9 μmol/L
			Nomifensine	10 mg/L	
Chlordiazepoxide	20 mg/L	67.2 μmol/L	Olanzapine	100 μg/L	
Chlormethiazole	7 mg/L		Orphenadrine	3 mg/L	
Chlormezanone	60 mg/L		Phenobarbital	65 mg/L	27,950 μmol/L
Chloroquine	1 mg/L	3.12 μmol/L	Phenytoin	40 mg/L	160 μmol/L
Chlorpromazine	0.5 mg/L	1.57 μmol/L	Propoxyphene	1 mg/L	2.946 μmol/L
Chlorprothixene	0.8 mg/L		Quetiapine	13 mg/L	
Cimetidine	10 mg/L		Quinine	12 μg/mL	
Clonazepam	0.07 mg/L		Salicylates	100 mg/dL	7.24 μmol/L
Clonidine	2 μg/L		Secobarbital	7 mg/L	
Clozapine	2 mg/L		Sodium	160 mEq/dL	
Codeine	5 mg/L		Theophylline	40 mg/L	222 μmol/L
Diazepam	20 mg/L	70.24 μmol/L	Tetrahydrocannabinol	180 μg/L	
Diethyltoluamide (DEET)	50 mg/L		Toluene	10 mg/L	
Digoxin	4 ng/L	5.124 μmol/L	Tramadol	2000 μg/L	
Dothiepin	1 mg/L		Tranylcypromine	1 mg/L	
Doxepin	0.4 mg/L	1431.6 μmol/L	Triazolam	31 μg/L	
Ethanol	300 mg/dL	65.13 mmol/L	Valproic acid	500 mg/L	3500 μmol/L
Ethchlorvynol	50 mg/dL	345.8 μmol/L	Venlafaxine	6 mg/L	
γ-Hydroxybutyrate	100 mg/L		Zopiclone	300 μg/L	

TREATMENT OF PATIENTS WITH ALTERED MENTATION

Respiratory compromise is the primary life threat in most toxic exposures causing alterations of consciousness. Initial stabilization (including endotracheal intubation, if warranted) must not be delayed by attempts at antidote administration or diagnostic testing.[34] A complete set of vital signs including temperature is mandatory. Supplemental oxygen should be administered if there is a suspicion of hypoxia or if carbon monoxide poisoning is suspected. Rapid determination of blood glucose should be performed.[35] If the patient is determined to be hypoglycemic, or if rapid measurement is unavailable, dextrose should be administered.[36]

Gastrointestinal decontamination with activated charcoal is of possible benefit in some toxic ingestions, especially if given early after ingestion. Multiple dosing of activated charcoal can enhance the elimination of a few drugs listed in Table 19-3. Whole-bowel irrigation with polyethylene glycol may be warranted in ingestions of drug packets or medications not found to bind to activated charcoal, such as lithium or iron tablets.[37] All of these techniques have possible morbidity, however, and none have been shown to alter outcome in poisoned patients. A full description of gastrointestinal decontamination modalities is given in Chapter 5.

After initial stabilization measures and decontamination, most overdoses may be managed expectantly. If the agent is known, specific antidotal therapy may be indicated (Table 19-8). Use of a series of agents—a "coma cocktail"— is often employed as a diagnostic and therapeutic strategy in a patient with altered mental status of unknown etiology. Dextrose with thiamine, supplemental oxygen, and naloxone are used widely in this setting. Two other antidotal agents, flumazenil and physostigmine, at one time also were considered components of the coma cocktail. Because of concern over the safety of these agents, however, many authors have discouraged their indiscriminate use in comatose patients with an unknown ingestion.[38–41] Familiarity with these agents, including risks and benefits of their use, is essential. The use of these agents in the initial evaluation and management of poisoned patients is discussed in Chapter 3.

TABLE 19-8 Agents Used to Reverse Coma or Encephalopathy of Toxic Etiology

AGENT	TOXIN
Naloxone	Opioids
	Clonidine
	Tetrahydrozoline
	Valproic acid
	Camylofin hydrochloride
Flumazenil	Captopril
	Benzodiazepines
	Zolpidem
	Baclofen
	Carbamazepine
	Chloral hydrate
Oxygen (100% or hyperbaric)	Zopiclone
	Carbon monoxide
Physostigmine	Hydrogen sulfide
	γ-Hydroxybutyrate
	Baclofen
Pyridoxine	Anticholinergic agents
	Isoniazid
Methylene blue	Hydrazine
Dextrose	Ifosfamide
Cyanide antidote kits or hydroxocobalamin	Hypoglycemic agents
Sodium thiosulfate	Cyanide
	Nitroprusside

Opioid Antagonists

Opioids produce alterations in consciousness via interaction with multiple opioid receptors (μ_1, μ_2, κ, and δ) located in the CNS. Stimulation of these receptors results in analgesia, euphoria, CNS and respiratory depression, and miosis. Although naloxone and nalmefene are structural analogues of morphine, they possess no agonist activity of their own. When administered, these agents antagonize the effect of opioids by competing for opioid receptor sites. Naloxone is the opioid antagonist most frequently used in the prehospital, emergency department, or postanesthesia setting. Its administration is indicated in patients with coma of suspected toxic etiology, particularly when signs of opioid intoxication (e.g., miosis, hypoventilation) are present. The use of opioid antagonists is discussed in detail in Chapter 56. Their clinical pharmacology is described in Chapter 137.

Several clinicians have reported a clinical response to naloxone in patients with various nonopioid drug intoxications. Improvement in mental status after naloxone has been reported in the setting of ethanol, clonidine and related imidazolines, valproate, and ibuprofen overdose.[42–46] The mechanism of this effect is unclear, but it is theorized that these agents have some degree of activity at the μ receptor. In clinical practice, however, response to naloxone with these overdoses has proved inconsistent, suggesting that in some cases the true mechanism may be one of coincidence, concomitant therapy, or nonspecific arousal.

Dosing practices for naloxone vary widely. An initial dose of 0.4 to 2.0 mg (0.01 mg/kg in pediatric patients) intravenously generally is recommended, although higher doses (10 mg) are needed in some cases.[17,47] The therapeutic index of naloxone is remarkable; 4 mg/kg has been administered to volunteers without adverse effect.[48] Use of this agent is not totally without risk, however. Precipitation of withdrawal can be a significant obstacle to patient management. If opioid dependency is suspected, a lower starting dose (0.1 to 0.2 mg) should be used to minimize the risk of this complication.[17] Seizures also have been reported rarely.[17] Although intravenous infusion is the most common route of administration, naloxone is also effective when given subcutaneously, intramuscularly, or endotracheally. Onset of action occurs in 1 to 2 minutes.

The elimination half-life of naloxone is 60 to 90 minutes, resulting in a duration of effect that may not extend beyond the duration of opioid toxicity. Naloxone-responsive patients must be monitored carefully because rebolus of naloxone may be required. In cases of intoxication with long-acting opioids (methadone, levomethadyl acetate), an option is to use a continuous naloxone infusion. One protocol recommends that two thirds of the response dose should be infused hourly.[17] A naloxone infusion always should be titrated to the desired clinical effect, however.

Nalmefene is a derivative of the opioid antagonist naltrexone, which differs in activity from naxolone only in its longer duration of action. The half-life of nalmefene after intravenous administration is 11 hours.[49] The typically recommended dose is 0.5 to 1.0 mg/70 kg body weight intravenously. In opioid-naive patients, 0.5 mg/70 kg body weight can be given intravenously as an initial dose, followed 2 to 5 minutes later by a second dose of 1 mg/70 kg body weight, if needed. Doses over 1.5 mg/70 kg body weight are unlikely to be of further benefit. Clinical response is expected within 5 minutes. Although nalmefene administration may be advantageous in the setting of toxicity from a long-acting opioid, special consideration must be given to the disadvantages of routine use of this agent. Opioid withdrawal produced by nalmefene is protracted compared with naloxone.[50,51] Additionally, emergency department discharge of substance abusers who are treated with nalmefene for opioid abuse is theoretically dangerous because the antagonist's persistent effects may compel the individual to use higher doses of illicit opioid to overcome the effect. If possible, diagnostic trials should be done with naloxone. If naloxone is unavailable, low-dose nalmefene (e.g., 1 mg) may be considered. Finally, substance abusers who receive nalmefene in the emergency department should be admitted for observation.[50]

Flumazenil

The benzodiazepine receptor antagonist flumazenil may be useful for reversal of benzodiazepine-induced sedation after general anesthesia, conscious sedation, or overdose.[41] Flumazenil is a nonspecific competitive antagonist at the benzodiazepine receptor. The effectiveness of flumazenil is well documented.[52–56] Its use can confirm quickly a clinical diagnosis of benzodiazepine receptor agonist–induced decreased level of consciousness, obviating the need for time-consuming, expensive investigations and interventions in patients with altered mental status.[46] In patients with pure benzodiazepine overdose, return to consciousness after flumazenil administration occurs within minutes. Its administration also results in faster return to baseline alertness in patients undergoing conscious sedation with benzodiazepines.[45] The intrinsic safety of flumazenil is remarkable; 100 mg intravenously has been given without significant adverse effects. Seizures and cardiac dysrhythmias have occurred after flumazenil administration, however.[52,53,57–61] In most cases, these effects are well tolerated and do not alter clinical outcome, but fatalities do occur.[58] Coingestion of drugs with proconvulsant properties (Table 19-9) is associated with an increased risk of seizure after flumazenil administration.[47] This risk presumably is due to loss of the benzodiazepine's protective anticonvulsant effect when the antagonist is administered. Combined overdose with tricyclic antidepressants accounts for 50% of these cases.[51] Other coingestants possessing proarrhythmic properties, such as carbamazepine and chloral hydrate, may increase the likelihood of cardiac effects by a similar mechanism.[53] Other risk factors contraindicating the use of flumazenil are summarized in Table 19-9. Using these criteria, stratification of patients into high-risk and low-risk categories can be done easily, but few patients are eligible for flumazenil if the criteria are strictly applied.[62] Nevertheless, flumazenil has been shown to safely reduce the need for ventilatory support and extensive diagnostic studies in selected patients, even when coingestants were involved.[61]

One common and important relative contraindication to flumazenil is regular abuse of benzodiazepines. Administering flumazenil to benzodiazepine-dependent patients may provoke severe benzodiazepine withdrawal, a condition that is characterized by agitation and potential seizures.[63]

Although flumazenil has been shown to be effective in reversing benzodiazepine-induced sedation, it does not reverse respiratory depression consistently.[64] Because the duration of action of flumazenil is short (0.7 to 1.3 hours), resedation occurs in 65% of patients and requires either redosing or continuous infusion.[52,65,66] In patients undergoing conscious sedation, use of lower doses of benzodiazepines may reduce this risk.[56] Any patient who has reversal of CNS depression with flumazenil must be monitored closely for a minimum of 1 hour for the possibility of resedation.

The usual recommended initial adult dose of flumazenil is 0.2 mg intravenously over 30 seconds. A second dose of 0.3 mg may be given, followed by 0.5-mg doses at 1-minute intervals, to a total dose of 3 mg. Most patients respond to less than 3 mg. In children, weight-based dosage of 0.01 mg/kg is recommended. Use of a continuous intravenous flumazenil infusion (0.25 to 1.0 mg/hr) after a loading dose may maintain better overall consciousness but does not decrease the rate of complications arising from severe benzodiazepine toxicity.[66]

Because of the aforementioned potential adverse effects, flumazenil should not be used indiscriminately in all patients with altered mental status. Flumazenil should not be used in place of standard support measures, including airway control, gastrointestinal decontamination, and hemodynamic stabilization. The clinical pharmacology of flumazenil is described in Chapter 138.

Physostigmine

Physostigmine is a short-acting acetylcholinesterase inhibitor used to reverse toxicity from anticholinergic agents. By competing with acetylcholine for metabolism via this enzyme, physostigmine effectively increases the concentration of acetylcholine in the synapse. The higher concentration of acetylcholine overcomes competitive postsynaptic muscarinic receptor blockade produced by anticholinergic agents. Use of physostigmine should be considered in the presence of signs and symptoms of anticholinergic toxicity, including tachycardia, fever, mydriasis, anhidrosis, gastrointestinal hypomotility, urinary retention, and altered mental status (Table 19-10). Other acetylcholinesterase inhibitors—pyridostigmine, neostigmine, and edrophonium—are ineffective due to an inability to penetrate the blood-brain barrier.[67] The anticholinergic syndrome is discussed in detail in Chapter 22.

Use of physostigmine in the appropriate setting of severe anticholinergic toxicity may have advantages over supportive care alone.[68] Clearing of signs of toxicity after administration of this antidote confirms the diagnosis and may obviate

---

TABLE 19-9 Use of Flumazenil

Indications
Isolated benzodiazepine overdose, nonhabituated user (e.g., accidental pediatric exposure)
Reversal of conscious sedation

Contraindications
Absolute
Known or suspected coingestant that lowers seizure threshold
Tricyclic antidepressants, cocaine, lithium, methylxanthines, isoniazid, propoxyphene, MAO inhibitors, buproprion, diphenhydramine, carbamazepine, cyclosporine, chloral hydrate
Patient taking benzodiazepine for control of potentially life-threatening condition
Concurrent sedative-hypnotic withdrawal
Seizure activity or myoclonus
Hypersensitivity to flumazenil or benzodiazepines
Patient with neuromuscular blockade

Relative
Chronic benzodiazepine user, not taking for control of life-threatening condition
Head injury
Panic attacks
Alcoholic patients

MAO, monoamine oxidase.
Data from Spivey WH: Flumazenil and seizures: Analysis of 43 cases. Clin Ther 14:292–305, 1992.

TABLE 19-10 Agents with Anticholinergic Effects

Antihistamines: diphenhydramine, doxylamine, cyproheptadine, hydroxyzine, brompheniramine
Antispasmodics: oxybutynin, hyoscyamine, atropine
Ipratropium bromide
Scopolamine
Diphenidol
Phenothiazines
Ophthalmic cycloplegics
Antiparkinsonian agents
Tricyclic antidepressants
Pirenzepine
Carbamazepine
Pizotifen hydrogen maleate
Botanicals: jimsonweed, deadly nightshade, angel's trumpet, black henbane, Paraguay tea, *Amanita muscaria* (mushroom)

the need for an intensive workup for altered mental status. Respiratory depression from severe intoxication may be reversed, avoiding the need for advanced airway management. Finally, a study suggested that physostigmine may control anticholinergic-induced agitation and delirium more adequately than benzodiazepines, which currently are the preferred agents to manage agitation in this setting.[69] Multiple doses of physostigmine were required in 58% of the patients, with side effects occurring in 11%.[69] Nevertheless, clinicians considering the use of physostigmine must have a thorough understanding of its pharmacologic effects and risks of its use. Administration of physostigmine in the absence of actual anticholinergic toxicity may produce cholinergic effects. Seizures after physostigmine administration have been reported, especially when concomitant intoxication with substances known to lower the seizure threshold has occurred.[70] Several drugs associated with seizures in overdose, such as tricyclic antidepressants, carbamazepine, and phenothiazines, also have anticholinergic effects that may render a misleading picture of pure anticholinergic overdose. Physostigmine has a parasympathomimetic effect, increasing vagal tone, which can lead to bradydysrhythmia. Asystole has been reported after use of physostigmine in a patient with poisoning from a tricyclic antidepressant.[71] Nevertheless, physostigmine has been shown to be safe and effective in large series and case reports when used appropriately.[69,72]

The use of physostigmine also has been reported to result in arousal of a series of patients with coma due to gamma hydroxybutyrate (GHB) intoxication.[73] The proposed, although unvalidated, mechanism is nonspecific CNS arousal. Two of the three patients in this series manifested cholinergic symptoms. Physostigmine should not be used routinely in cases of suspected intoxication by GHB or its congeners because of the risks of unrealized coingestants or precipitation of cholinergic symptoms (including emesis with risk for aspiration).[73] GHB intoxication generally resolves without sequelae after a few hours of supportive care and airway protection.[74,75] Intoxication with GHB or its congeners is discussed in detail in Chapter 71.

The usually recommended dose of physostigmine is 1 to 2 mg in adults or 0.02 mg/kg in children. Rapid intravenous bolus administration can be dangerous; slow infusion over approximately 2 to 4 minutes generally is recommended. Onset of the effect may be delayed for 10 to 15 minutes. Signs and symptoms of toxicity may recur because the duration of action of physostigmine is only 20 to 60 minutes. Repeat doses should be given with caution and are not usually necessary.[70] Some patients with otherwise hard-to-control anticholinergic delirium may benefit from repeat administration, however. The clinical pharmacology of physostigmine is discussed in detail in Chapter 153.

MANAGEMENT OF THE AGITATED PATIENT

Management of patients with violent behavior or agitation due to intoxication is often challenging to the clinician. Verbal attempts to de-escalate violent behavior in the intoxicated patient should remain the first approach, as should evaluation and treatment of any medical condition (e.g., hypoxia, pain) that may be contributing to the agitation. If these measures fail, use of restraint may be considered.

Physical restraint of violent patients with intoxications causing hyperadrenergic states or seizures (e.g., cocaine, amphetamines, phencyclidine, withdrawal from ethanol or benzodiazepines) may be dangerous, particularly if inadequate sedation is given. Pharmacologic management (i.e., "chemical restraint") also may be employed, but the clinician must remain mindful of potential side effects or drug interactions. Antipsychotics and benzodiazepines are the two most commonly used agents in this setting.

The butyrophenones (e.g., haloperidol) have emerged as the preferred antipsychotic agents because they manifest fewer anticholinergic and quinidine-like effects compared with the phenothiazines (e.g., chlorpromazine). Haloperidol has been shown repeatedly to be a safe and effective drug for acute control of agitation.[76] The commonly recommended dose is 5 to 10 mg deep intramuscularly (into the gluteal region) or intravenously every 10 to 30 minutes, titrated to the desired effect. Extrapyramidal side effects, such dystonia or akathisia, may occur in up to 16% of patients and should be treated with either benztropine, 1 to 4 mg intravenously or intramuscularly, or diphenhydramine, 50 mg (1 mg/kg in pediatric patients) intravenously or intramuscularly. Although the use of haloperidol has been shown to lower seizure threshold in animals, there are no reports of seizures clearly induced by haloperidol in humans. Droperidol differs from haloperidol in its faster onset of effect, shorter half-life, more pronounced sedation, and lower incidence of extrapyramidal side effects. Transient orthostatic hypotension has been reported after its use. The commonly recommended dose of droperidol is 2.5 to 10 mg intramuscularly.

Ziprasidone is an atypical antipsychotic agent that is a derivative of benzisothiazoyl piperazine. It is a serotonin (5-HT-2A) and dopamine (D$_2$) antagonist with fewer extrapyramidal effects than haloperidol. Prolongation of the QT/QT$_c$ interval on ECG may occur in a dose-related manner, but clinically relevant prolongation is rare (0.06%). Dose is 10 mg every 2 hours intramuscularly (or 20 mg every 4 hours) to a maximum daily dose of 40 mg.[77,78]

Benzodiazepines are the agents of choice in patients with ethanol or benzodiazepine withdrawal or in patients with hyperadrenergic states from sympathomimetic agents. Although many benzodiazepines have been shown to be effective, lorazepam has been studied most extensively. The usual recommended dose of lorazepam is 2 to 4 mg intravenously. Some studies suggest that combination therapy with a benzodiazepine plus a butyrophenone may control violent behavior more effectively.[76]

Patients with drug-induced or toxin-induced alterations in consciousness require close monitoring. Progressively worsening intoxication may lead to profound CNS depression and airway compromise. The propensity for these conditions to occur may be increased by the use of pharmacologic agents to achieve behavior control and sedation. Seclusion should never be employed unless some method of continuous observation (e.g., video monitoring) can be arranged.

PROGNOSIS

Generally, recovery from coma due to a toxic cause is much better than that from an anoxic cause. Mortality of coma due to a sedative drug intoxication is less than 1%.[79] Table 19-11

TABLE 19-11   Poor Neurologic Prognostic Signs for Recovery from Toxic Coma

Loss of pupillary reflexes (up to 1 week)
Absence of corneal reflexes after day 1
Lack of oculovestibular response
Absence of eye-opening response at day 3
Absence of bilateral cortical component of somatosensory evoked potential responses
Abnormal skeletal muscle tone
Absence of spontaneous eye movement
Low-voltage delta activity (with alpha coma) or isoelectric tracing on electroencephalogram

Data from Adams RD, Victor M, Ropper AH: Principals of Neurology, 6th ed. New York, 1997, McGraw-Hill, pp 344–366.

presents prognostic signs of worsening of coma and poor outcome.[2,80] Although these prognostic indicators generally have been studied in patients with hepatic encephalopathy, they seem to be a reasonable guideline for patients with a toxic cause of coma. Patients taking agents described in Table 19-3 resulting in cyclic coma can exhibit a full recovery despite these prognostic signs.[79,81] Full recovery from prolonged coma and loss of brainstem reflexes has been described after amitriptyline and doxepin overdose.[82,83] Short-term memory deficits and amnesia after coma usually are due to injury of the pyramidal neurons of the hippocampus (CA 1 subfield) and are possible sequelae of an anoxic injury or carbon monoxide toxicity.[84]

REFERENCES

1. Plum F, Posner JB: Diagnosis of Stupor and Coma, 3rd ed. Philadelphia, FA Davis,1980.
2. Spencer PS: Biological principles of chemical neurotoxicity. In Spencer PS, Schaumburg HH (eds): Experimental and Clinical Neurotoxicology, 2nd ed. New York, Oxford University Press, 2000, pp 3–54.
3. Adams RD, Victor M, Ropper AH: Principals of Neurology, 6th ed. New York, McGraw-Hill, 1997, pp 344–366.
4. DeFeudis FV: Overview-GABA A receptors. Ann N Y Acad Sci 585:231–240, 1990.
5. Snyder SH: Drug and neurotransmitter receptors: New perspectives with clinical relevance. JAMA 261:3126–3129, 1989.
6. Twyman RE, Rogers CJ, MacDonald RL: Differential regulation of gamma-aminobuteric acid receptor channels by diazepam and phenobarbital. Ann Neurol 25:213–220, 1989.
7. Crippen DW: Pharmacologic treatment of brain failure and delirium. Crit Care Clin 10:733–767, 1994.
8. Ely WE, Siegel MD, Ihouye SK: Delirium in the intensive care unit. Semin Resp Crit Care Med 22:115–126, 2001.
9. Murphy BA: Delirium. Emerg Med Clin North Am 18:243–252, 2000.
10. American Psychiatric Association: Diagnostic and Statistical Manual of Mental Disorders, 4th ed. Washington, DC, American Psychiatric Association, 1994, pp 122–138.
11. Oshika T: Ocular adverse effects of neuropsychiatric agents: Incidence and management. Drug Saf 12:256–263, 1995.
12. Leikin JB, Paloucek FP (eds): Symptoms Index in Poisoning and Toxicology Compendium. Hudson, OH, Lexicomp Publisher, 1998.
13. Starkey IR, Lawson AAH: Psychiatric aspects of acute poisoning with tricyclic and related antidepressants: A ten year review. Scott Med J 25:303–308, 1980.
14. Corbett JJ, Jacobson DM, Thompson HS, et al: Downbeat nystagmus and other ocular motor defects caused by lithium toxicity. Neurology 39:481–487, 1989.
15. Erich JL, Shih RD, O'Connor RE: Ping Pong gaze in severe monoamine oxidase inhibitor toxicity. J Emerg Med 13:653–655, 1995.
16. Hoffman JR, Schriger DL, Luo JS: The empiric use of naloxone in patients with altered mental status: A reappraisal. Ann Emerg Med 20:246–252, 1991.
17. Albertson TE, Dawson A, de Latorre F, et al: TOX-ACLS: Toxicologic-oriented advanced cardiac life support. Ann Emerg Med 37:578–590, 2001.
18. Marik PE: Aspiration pneumonitis and aspiration pneumonia. N Engl J Med 344:665–671, 2001.
19. Szlatenyi CS, Wang RY: Encephalopathy and cranial nerve palsies, caused by intentional trichloro-ethylene inhalation. Am J Emerg Med 14:464–466, 1996.
20. Delaney KA: Evaluation and management of the agitated patient in the intensive care unit. In Hoffman RS, Goldfrank LR (eds): Contemporary Management in Critical Care. New York, Churchill Livingstone, 1991, pp 147–177.
21. Lipowski ZJ: Delirium (acute confusional) states. JAMA 258:1789–1793, 1987.
22. Daniel DG, Rabin PL: Disguises of delirium. South Med J 78:666–670, 1985.
23. Han L, McCusker J, Cole M, et al: Use of medications with anticholinergic effect predicts clinical severity of delirium symptoms in older medical inpatients. Arch Intern Med 161:1099–1105, 2001.
24. Mintzer J, Burns A: Anticholinergic side effects of drugs in elderly people. J R Soc Med 93:457–462, 2000.
25. Boehnert MT, Lovejoy FH: Value of the QRS duration versus the serum drug level in predicting seizures and ventricular arrhythmias after an acute overdose of tricyclic antidepressants. N Engl J Med 313:474–480, 1985.
26. Paterson S, McLachlan-Throup N, Codero RN, et al: Qualitative screening for drugs of abuse in hair using GC-MS. J Anal Tox 25:203–208, 2001.
27. Syneck VM: Prognostically important EEG coma patterns in diffuse anoxic and traumatic encephalopathies in adults. J Clin Neurophysiol 5:161–165, 1988.
28. Maisese K, Caronna JJ: Coma in critical care medicine. In Parrillo JE, Bone RC (eds): Principles of Diagnosis and Management. St Louis, Mosby, 1995, pp 1157–1176.
29. Mellerio F: EEG in the prognosis of toxic coma: reflections apropos of unusual data. Rev Electroencephalogr Neurophysiol Clin 12:325–331, 1982.
30. Pulst SM, Lombroso CT: External ophthalmoplegia, alpha and spindle coma in imipramine overdose: Case report and review of the literature. Ann Neurol 14:587–590, 1983.
31. Pozzessere G, Valle E, Mollica MA, et al: Brainstem auditory evoked potentials in toxic, metabolic and anoxic coma. Riv Neurol 58:183–188, 1988.
32. Rumpl E, Prugger M, Battista HJ, et al: Short latency somatosensory evoked potentials and brain-stem auditory evoked potentials in coma due to CNS depressant drug poisoning: Preliminary observations. Electroencephalogr Clin Neurophysiol 70:482–489, 1988.
33. Garcia-Larrea L, Artu F, Bertrand D, et al: Transient drug-induced abolition of BAEPs in coma. Neurology 38:1487–1490, 1988.
34. American Heart Association: Adult advanced cardiac life support. JAMA 268:2199–2243, 1992.
35. Holstein A, Kuhne D, Elsing HG, et al: Practicality and accuracy of prehospital rapid venous blood glucose determination. J Emerg Med 18:690–694, 2000.
36. Kennedy J, Telford J: Altered mental status in salicylate poisoning: Reversal with I.V. glucose. J Toxicol Clin Toxicol 36:445, 1998.
37. Farmer JW, Chan SB, Beranek G, et al: Whole bowel irrigation for contraband bodypackers: A case series. Ann Emerg Med 36:585, 2000.
38. Burda A, Leikin JB, Fischbein C, et al: Emergency department use of flumazenil prior to poison center consultation. Vet Hum Toxicol 39:245–247, 1997.
39. Hoffman RS, Goldfrank LR: The poisoned patient with altered consciousness: Controversies in the use of a "coma cocktail." JAMA 274:562–569, 1995.
40. Doyon S, Roberts JR: Reappraisal of the "coma cocktail": Dextrose, flumazenil, naloxone, and thiamine. Emerg Med Clin North Am 12:301–316, 1994.
41. Mathieu-Noif M, Babe MA, Coquelle-Couplet V, et al: Flumazenil use in an emergency department: A survey. J Toxicol Clin Toxicol 39:15–20, 2001.
42. Dole VP, Fishman J, Goldfrank LR, et al: Arousal of ethanol-intoxicated comatose patients with naloxone, alcohol. Clin Exp Res 6:275–279, 1982.

43. Wedin GP, Edwards LJ: Clonidine poisoning treated with naloxone. Am J Emerg Med 7:343–344, 1989.

44. Holmes JF, Berman DA: Use of naloxone to reverse symptomatic tetrahydrozoline overdose in a child. Pediatr Emerg Care 15:193–194, 1999.

45. Alberto G, Erickson T, Popiel R, et al: Central nervous system manifestations of a valproic acid overdose responsive to naloxone. Ann Emerg Med 18:889–891, 1989.

46. Easley RB, Altemeier WA: Central nervous system manifestations of an ibuprofen overdose reversed by naloxone. Pediatr Emerg Care 16:39–41, 2000.

47. Handal KA, Schauben JL, Salmone FR: Naloxone. Ann Emerg Med 12:438–445, 1983.

48. Cohen MR, Cohen RM, Pickar D, et al: Behavioural effects after high-dose naloxone administration to normal volunteers. Lancet 2(8255): 1110, 1981.

49. Nalmefene: A long-acting injectable opioid antagonist. Med Lett 37:97–98, 1995.

50. Wang DS, Sternbach G, Varon J: Nalmefene: A long-acting opioid antagonist: Clinical applications in emergency medicine. J Emerg Med 16:471–475, 1998.

51. Gaeta TJ, Capodano RJ, Spevack TA: Potential danger of nalmefene use in the emergency department. Ann Emerg Med 29:193–194, 1997.

52. Sugarman JM, Paul RI: Flumazenil: A review. Pediatr Emerg Care 10:37–44, 1994.

53. Weinbroum AA, Flaishon R, Sorkine P, et al: A risk-benefit assessment of flumazenil in the management of benzodiazepine overdose. Drug Saf 17:181–196, 1997.

54. Spivey WH, Roberts JR, Derlet RW: A clinical trial of escalating doses of flumazenil for reversal of suspected benzodiazepine overdose in the emergency department. Ann Emerg Med 22:1813–1821, 1993.

55. Chern TL, Hu SC, Lee CH, Deng JF: The role of flumazenil in the management of patients with acute alteration of mental status in the emergency department. Hum Exp Toxicol 13:45–50, 1994.

56. Chudnofsky CR: Safety and efficacy of flumazenil in reversing conscious sedation in the emergency department: Emergency medicine conscious sedation study group. Acad Emerg Med 4:944–950, 1997.

57. Hojer J, Baehrendtz S, Matell G, Gustafsson LL: Diagnostic utility of flumazenil in coma with suspected poisoning: A double blind, randomized controlled study. BMJ 128:301:1308–1311, 1990.

58. Spivey WH: Flumazenil and seizures: Analysis of 43 cases. Clin Ther 14:292–305, 1992.

59. Haverkos GP, DiSalvo RP, Imhoff TE: Fatal seizures after flumazenil administration in a patient with mixed overdose. Ann Pharmacother 28:1347–1349, 1994.

60. Davis CO, Wax PM: Flumazenil associated seizure in an 11-month-old child. J Emerg Med 14:331–333, 1996.

61. McDuffee AT, Tobias JD: Seizure after flumazenil administration in a pediatric patient. Pediatr Emerg Care 11:186–187, 1995.

62. Gueye PN, Hoffman JR, Taboulet P, et al: Empiric use of flumazenil in comatose patients: Limited applicability of criteria to define low risk. Ann Emerg Med 27:730–735, 1996.

63. Mintzer MZ, Stoller KB, Griffins RR: A controlled study of flumazenil-precipitated withdrawal in chronic low-dose benzodiazepine users. Psychopharmacology 147:200–209, 1999.

64. Weinbroum A, Rudick V, Sorkine P, et al: Use of flumazenil in the treatment of drug overdose: A double-blind and open clinical study in 110 patients. Crit Care Med 24:199–206, 1996.

65. Shalansky SJ, Naumann TL, Englander FA: Effect of flumazenil on benzodiazepine-induced respiratory depression. Clin Pharmacol 12:483–487, 1993.

66. Chern CH, Chern TL, Wang LM, et al: Continuous flumazenil infusion in preventing complications arising from severe benzodiazepine intoxication. Am J Emerg Med 16:238–241, 1998.

67. Taylor P: Anticholinesterase agents. In Hardman JG, Limbird LE (eds): Goodman and Gilman's The Pharmacological Basis of Therapeutics, 10th ed. New York, McGraw-Hill, 2001, pp 175–192.

68. Beaver KM, Gavin TJ: Treatment of acute anticholinergic poisoning with physostigmine. Am J Emerg Med 16:505–507, 1998.

69. Burns MJ, Linden CH, Graudins A, et al: A comparison of physostigmine and benzodiazepines for the treatment of anticholinergic poisoning, Ann Emerg Med 35:374–381, 2000.

70. Shannon M: Toxicology reviews: Physostigmine. Pediatr Emerg Care 14:224–226, 1998.

71. Pentel P, Peterson CD: Asystole complicating physostigmine treatment of tricyclic antidepressant overdose. Ann Emerg Med 9:588–590, 1980.

72. Smilkstein MJ. Editorial (Letter). J Emerg Med 9:275–277, 1991.

73. Caldicott DG: Gamma-hydroxybutyrate overdose and physostigmine: Teaching new tricks to an old drug? Ann Emerg Med 37:99–102, 2001.

74. Boyer EW, Quang L, Woolf A, Shannon MW: Use of physostigmine in the management of gamma-hydroxy-butyrate overdose. Ann Emerg Med 38:346–347, 2001.

75. Chin RL, Sporer KA, Cullison B, et al: Clinical course of gamma-hydroxybutyrate overdose. Ann Emerg Med 31:716–722, 1998.

76. Hill S, Petit J: The violent patient. Emerg Med Clin North Am 18: 301–315, 2000.

77. Green B: Focus on ziprasidone. Curr Med Res Opin 17:146–150, 2001.

78. Camahan RM, Lund BC, Perry PJ: Ziprasidone: A new atypical antipsychotic drug. Pharmacotherapy 21:717–730, 2001.

79. Arieff AI, Friedman EA: Coma following nonnarcotic drug overdosage: Management of adult patients. Am J Med Sci 266:405–426, 1973.

80. Levy DE, Bates D, Caronna JJ: Prognosis in nontraumatic coma. Ann Intern Med 94:293–301, 1981.

81. Setter JG, Maher JF, Schreiner GE: Barbituate intoxication: Evaluation of therapy including dialysis in a large series selectively referred because of severity. Arch Intern Med 117:224–236, 1966.

82. White A: Overdose of tricyclic antidepressants associated with absent brainstem reflexes. Can Med Assoc J 139:133–134, 1988.

83. Roberge RJ, Krenzelok EP: Prolonged coma and loss of brainstem reflexes following amitriptyline overdose. Vet Hum Toxicol 43:42–43, 2001.

84. Nabeshima T, Katoh A, Ishimaru H, et al: Carbon monoxide induced delayed amnesia, delayed neuronal death and charge in acetylcholine concentration in mice. J Pharmacol Exp Ther 256:378–386, 1991.

CHAPTER 20

Toxin-Induced Seizures

Kevin L. Wallace

Seizures are a common feature of high-dose and, in some instances, minor or therapeutic exposure to a variety of drugs, chemicals, and toxins. Early and mid 20th century clinicians who used agents such as camphor, strychnine, and picrotoxin for their psychostimulant and analeptic effects (e.g., in the treatment of barbiturate poisoning) promoted the induction of life-threatening proconvulsant effects.[1] A statement from the 1937 edition of *The United States Dispensatory* suggests that at that time, convulsions were a targeted end point for analeptic therapy: "[I]n many cases it is essential to push the strychnine until marked exaggeration of the reflexes or even twitching of the muscle affords a warning that the patient is approaching the toxic stage."[2]

During the latter half of the 20th century, medical consensus regarding the clinical use of proconvulsant analeptics underwent a dramatic reversal, as noted in a 1959 review article that was highly critical of their use in the treatment of barbiturate poisoning: "[B]arbiturates detoxify convulsive poisons to a greater extent than convulsive poisons detoxify barbiturates."[3] Naturally occurring analeptics, such as picrotoxin, and synthetic ones, such as pentylenetetrazol, continue to be valuable to medical science because they still are used experimentally for their proconvulsant potency and specificity of central nervous system (CNS) effects, reflecting actions at γ-aminobutyric acid$_A$ (GABA$_A$) chloride channels, the brain's principal inhibitory ionophores.[4,5] The clinical use of analeptics largely has been abandoned.

In a prospective study of critically ill medical patients, seizures were found to be second only to metabolic encephalopathy as the most common neurologic complication encountered.[6] In addition to exhibiting a direct, dose-dependent relationship to exposure to various substances, seizures are characteristic of withdrawal from numerous drugs and chemicals with CNS depressant effects. Seizures may occur as a paradoxical effect of anticonvulsant medications, particularly after overdose or in seizure-prone individuals on accepted therapeutic regimens of these medications.[7,8]

Classes of agents frequently implicated in drug-induced, chemical-induced, and toxin-induced seizures (hereafter collectively referred to in this chapter as *toxicant-induced seizures* or *toxicant-induced convulsions*) include antidysrhythmics, anticonvulsants, antidepressants, antihistamines, antipsychotics, antimicrobials, antiasthmatics, antineoplastics, CNS stimulants, local anesthetics, opioid analgesics, sedative-hypnotics/alcohol (withdrawal), heavy metals (e.g., lead, alkylmercury), pesticides (e.g., insecticides, rodenticides), and certain alcohols (e.g., methanol).[9] Table 20-1 provides a more complete listing, by functional class, of

agents with proconvulsant potential. Olson and colleagues[10] observed that in 191 cases of seizures associated with poisoning and drug overdose reported to a West Coast U.S. regional poison control center, the most commonly implicated agents or class of agent were cyclic antidepressants (29%), cocaine (22%), diphenhydramine (7%), theophylline (5%), isoniazid (5%), and methamphetamine/amphetamine (3%).

Toxicant-induced convulsions, given the typically diffuse CNS distribution of proconvulsant substances and their highly specific neurochemical mechanisms, usually are generalized. They may be prolonged, recurrent, or both; they meet clinical and mechanistic definitions for status epilepticus (SE)[11]; and they may be remarkably refractory to widely recommended antiepileptic drug regimens. Definitions of SE, a condition of prolonged or recurrent seizure activity without interictal awakening, have incorporated critical time intervals for continuous seizure activity that range from 5[6,11] to 30 minutes.[12] Although there is little evidence to support these temporal cutoffs as thresholds beyond which seizure-induced CNS injury occurs, these definitions emphasize the apparent direct relationship between duration of seizure activity and clinicopathologic outcome and the paramount importance of anticonvulsant therapy in the management of sustained seizure activity.

Conservative estimates of the incidence of SE in the United States range from 60,000 to 160,000 patients per year.[12,13] The mortality associated with SE since the 1980s has been observed to be higher in adults (15% to 22%) than in children (3% to 15%) and greater than 10% if caused by drug toxicity.[14] Extremes of age and seizure duration of greater than 1 hour have been predictive of poor outcome.[11] In published case series of SE patients, the reported proportions of cases judged to be of toxic etiology (ethanol or drug related) range from 2.4% in patients younger than 16 years old[12] to 24% in older alcoholic individuals.[11]

Subtle[15] and *nonconvulsive* are descriptive terms that have been used to denote less than obvious or subclinical SE (i.e., ongoing electrical seizure activity shown by electroencephalography [EEG] with or without subtle convulsive movements, such as rhythmic muscle twitches or tonic eye deviation). Nonconvulsive SE, which may occur after pharmacologic neuromuscular blockade, has been an underrecognized cause of altered consciousness or behavior,[16] with coma at the time of diagnosis of SE predictive of fatal outcome.[17] In a study of 236 patients (age range 1 month to 87 years) with coma and no overt clinical seizure activity, 8% had at least 30 minutes of continuous electrographic seizure activity.[18]

The mortality rate associated with subtle SE in a multicenter trial comparing four drug treatments for generalized

TABLE 20-1 Proconvulsant Agents—Classification by Source and Use

CLASS	EXAMPLE(S)	CLASS	EXAMPLE(S)
Pharmaceuticals		**Nonpharmaceuticals**	
Analgesics	Meperidine/normeperidine, propoxyphene, pentazocine, salicylate, tramadol	Alcohols	Methanol, ethanol (withdrawal)
Anesthetics	Local anesthetics (lidocaine, benzocaine)	Antiseptics/preservatives	Ethylene oxide, phenol
Anticonvulsants	Carbamazepine	Biologic toxins	
Antidepressants	Tricyclics (amitriptyline/nortriptyline), amoxapine, bupropion, SSRIs (citalopram), venlafaxine	Marine animals	Domoic acid (shellfish [blue mussels])
		Mushrooms	Monomethylhydrazine (*Gyromitra* spp.)
Antihistamines	Diphenhydramine, doxylamine, tripelennamine	Plants	Conine (poison hemlock), virol A (water hemlock), camphor
Antimicrobials	Antibacterials (selected penicillins, cephalosporins, carbapenems, and fluoroquinolones), antimalarials (chloroquine), tuberculostatics (isoniazid)	Gases (naturally and/or anthropogenically occurring)	Carbon monoxide, hydrogen sulfide, hydrogen, cyanide
		Metals/organometallics	Alkyl mercurials (dimethylmercury), arsenic, lead, thallium, tetraethyl lead, organotins (trimethyltin)
Antineoplastics	Alkylating agents (chlorambucil, busulfan)	Metal hydrides	Pentaborane, phosphine
Antipsychotics	Clozapine, loxapine	Pesticides	
Asthma medications	Theophylline	Fungicides/herbicides	Dinitrophenol, diquat, glufosinate
Cardiovascular drugs	Propranolol, quinidine	Insecticides	Organochlorines (lindane, DDT), organophosphates (parathion), pyrethroids (type II), sulfuryl fluoride, alkyl halides (methyl bromide)
Cholinergics	Pilocarpine, bethanechol		
Muscle relaxants	Baclofen, orphenadrine		
NSAIDs	Mefenamic acid, phenylbutazone		
Psychostimulants/anorectics	Amphetamine, caffeine, cocaine, methamphetamine, MDMA	Molluscacides	Metaldehyde
		Rodenticides	Strychnine, zinc or aluminum phosphide
Vitamins/supplements	Vitamin A, iron salts (ferrous sulfate)		

MDMA, methylenedioxymethamphetamine; NSAIDs, nonsteroidal antiinflammatory drugs; SSRIs, selective serotonin reuptake inhibitors.

convulsive SE was 65%, versus 27% in patients with overt SE. Longer hospital stays also were associated with subtle SE.[15] There may be a rational basis for the concern that neuronal injury resulting from unrecognized subclinical SE is of equal or even greater severity than that occurring as a result of overt clinical SE. Understanding of the pathophysiology and prognosis of nonconvulsive SE is limited, however, by the current lack of controlled comparative data, difficulties with case definition, confounding factors (e.g., underlying neurologic disorder), and the highly anecdotal nature of available clinical data.[14,19]

The main objectives of this chapter are to provide a rational mechanistic approach to the evaluation and treatment of toxicant-induced convulsions. Emphasis is on the importance of considering nontoxic and primarily toxic causes of seizures and of employing an aggressive and more selective approach to anticonvulsant treatment than might be indicated in seizures of nontoxic origin.

PATHOPHYSIOLOGY

According to Schaumberg,[20] "The nature of the discharging lesion in toxin-induced seizures presumably is different in some respects from the lesion in most epileptic patients; the toxin-induced seizure usually originates in previously normal neurons, while the patient with epilepsy frequently has a focus in an abnormal cortical area." Other authorities on epilepsy note that the pathophysiology of posttraumatic or idiopathic seizures is characterized by the spread of electrical activity from a relatively isolated focus to neighboring cortical

regions when the intensity of seizure discharge overcomes the inhibitory influence of surrounding neurons.[21] In contrast, toxicant-induced seizures involve simultaneous increases in electrical discharge from susceptible neuronal populations in response to toxicant-induced neurochemical or other functional (e.g., metabolic) derangements or both.

Proconvulsant substances exert their neurotoxic effects through a variety of postulated mechanisms, for which there is a growing abundance of supporting experimental data.[22] A common theme that applies to most of these proconvulsant mechanisms is that in some manner they give rise to an imbalance in the normal neurochemical homeostasis of the CNS (i.e., they cause a disturbance in the balance between excitatory and inhibitory neurotransmission). This imbalance can result from increased excitatory tone, decreased inhibitory tone, or both, leading to a diffuse increase in neuronal excitability in typically dose-dependent fashion beyond the physiologic threshold for seizure activity. The remainder of this section focuses on the role that several major CNS neurotransmitter systems play in the genesis of toxicant-induced convulsions.

GABA Antagonism

GABA is the principal inhibitory central neurotransmitter, present in an estimated 30% of all central synapses. Substances that antagonize GABA activity produce CNS excitation and convulsions. Paradoxically, GABA is synthesized in the brain through the actions of glutamic acid decarboxylase on glutamate (Fig. 20-1), the brain's main excitatory neurotransmitter.

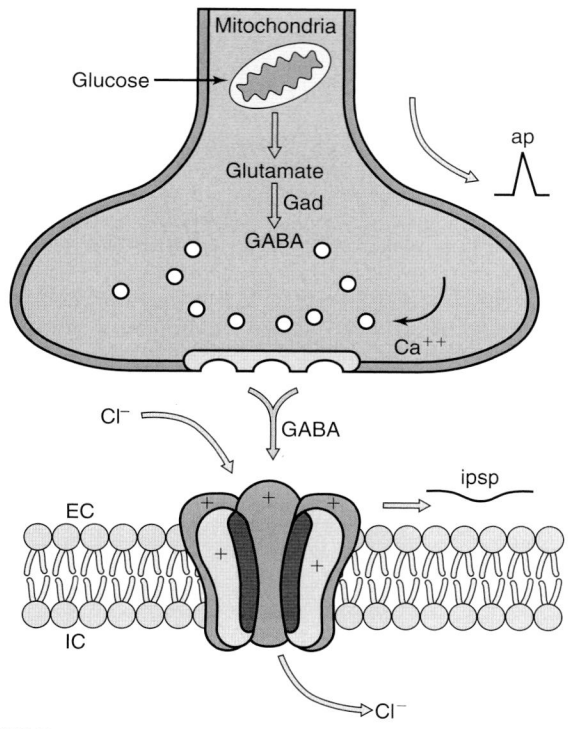

FIGURE 20-1

Presynaptic and postsynaptic elements. ap, action potential; Gad, glutamic acid decarboxylase; EC, extracellular; IC, intracellular; ipsp, inhibitory postsynaptic potential. *(From Brody TM, Larner J, Minneman KP [eds]: Human Pharmacology: Molecular to Clinical, 3rd ed. St Louis, Mosby, 1998, p 367.)*

GABA is stored in vesicles in presynaptic nerve terminals and is released into synapses in the brain and spinal cord via calcium (Ca^{2+})-dependent exocytosis. There are two main subtypes of transmembrane polypeptide receptors that bind GABA, designated *$GABA_A$* and *$GABA_B$*.

Antagonism of $GABA_A$ receptors has been implicated most frequently in the proconvulsant actions of drugs, chemicals, and toxins. The $GABA_A$ receptor complex (Fig. 20-2) is a ligand-gated chloride (Cl^-) channel that is integral to the postsynaptic neuronal membrane. When GABA binds to its receptor site on the complex, it triggers postsynaptic Cl^- influx, which results in membrane hyperpolarization and a decrease in postsynaptic neuronal excitability and impulse propagation (see Fig. 20-1).[23]

In addition, the $GABA_A$ Cl^- channel has multiple binding sites for exogenous and endogenous modulatory agents, including excitatory/proconvulsant drugs (e.g., penicillin, amoxapine, maprotiline[24-26]) and depressant/anticonvulsant drugs (e.g., benzodiazepines, barbiturates), which produce their actions through allosteric conformational enhancement or impairment of Cl^- influx in response to GABA binding.[27] Most of these drugs require that GABA itself bind to its receptor site on the $GABA_A$ complex for inhibitory or excitatory effects to occur and are termed *indirect* agonists and antagonists. Substances that exert their effects on the $GABA_A$ chloride ionophore by directly binding to the GABA receptor locus are termed *direct* agonists (e.g., muscimol) and antagonists (e.g., bicuculline).

Reduction in GABAergic neuroinhibitory tone also results from inhibition of GABA synthesis, such as that produced by isoniazid and other hydrazine compounds. Isoniazid lowers CNS GABA concentrations by several mechanisms, the main one being competitive inhibition of pyridoxine kinase, which results in depressed synthesis of pyridoxal phosphate, a cofactor needed for glutamic acid decarboxylase activity and GABA synthesis (see Fig. 20-1). Other mechanisms include direct inhibition of glutamic acid decarboxylase and increased urinary excretion of pyridoxine.[28,29]

Human and experimental data support direct and indirect antagonistic actions at the $GABA_A$ complex as the basis for the epileptogenic effects of members of several classes of antibiotics (penicillins, cephalosporins, carbapenems, and fluoroquinolones),[30] organochlorine compounds such as lindane and cyclodiene insecticides (e.g., dieldrin),[31] various antidepressants,[24-26] and virol A, a long-chain alcohol found in *Cicuta virosa*, a species of water hemlock.[32] Penicillin has been distinguished from other GABA antagonists on the basis of its multiple mechanisms of effect at $GABA_A$ chloride channels, including direct actions within the chloride channel itself (i.e., independent of its direct and indirect GABA agonist actions).[30] In addition, cefazolin, a first-generation cephalosporin antibiotic, and pentylenetetrazol, an analeptic compound that binds to the picrotoxin-binding site on the $GABA_A$ complex and is used widely in experimental epilepsy research, contain tetrazole moieties and are potent proconvulsants, consistent with a common structure-activity relationship.

Increases in the ratio of central neuroexcitatory to neuroinhibitory tone, resulting in convulsive activity, also can occur as a result of abrupt GABA agonist withdrawal after a chronic exposure period of sufficient duration to produce pharmacodynamic tolerance by down-regulating $GABA_A$ functional expression (see Chapter 47). Agents that possess $GABA_A$ agonist properties include ethanol, various benzodiazepines and barbiturate sedative-hypnotics, carisoprodol, meprobamate, zolpidem, and propofol.

Glycine Antagonism

Another type of neuroinhibitory ligand-gated ionophore, the glycine-gated chloride channel, has a well-established role in modulating efferent motor neuron activity at the level of the lower brainstem and spinal cord. Glycine functions as a postsynaptic inhibitory neurotransmitter in a manner that is analogous to GABA at $GABA_A$ chloride channels and prevents excessive lower motor neuronal electrical impulse propagation and reflex arc activation in response to afferent excitatory input. Strychnine antagonizes glycine's actions at these postsynaptic inhibitory chloride channels in the spinal cord and brainstem, resulting in polysynaptic motor neuronal disinhibition, and subsequent increase in motor tone and convulsive activity ("spinal convulsions") (see Chapter 93).[33]

Glutamate Agonism

As previously noted, glutamate is the main CNS excitatory neurotransmitter. It is synthesized in presynaptic nerve terminals from α-ketoglutarate or glutamine and released from storage vesicles as a result of the influx of calcium through voltage-gated presynaptic calcium channels in response to propagated electrical impulses. Its postsynaptic actions are mediated through receptor sites on ligand-gated

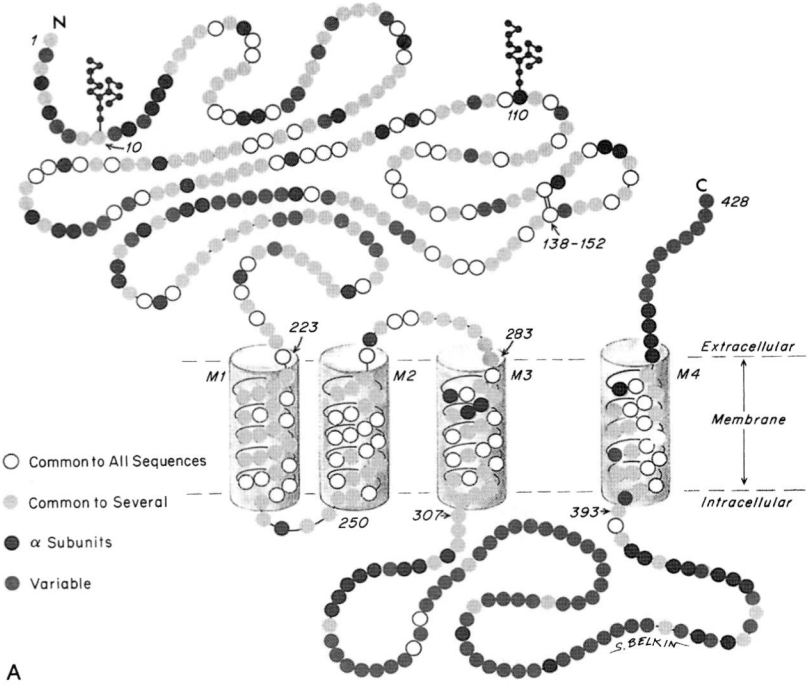

A

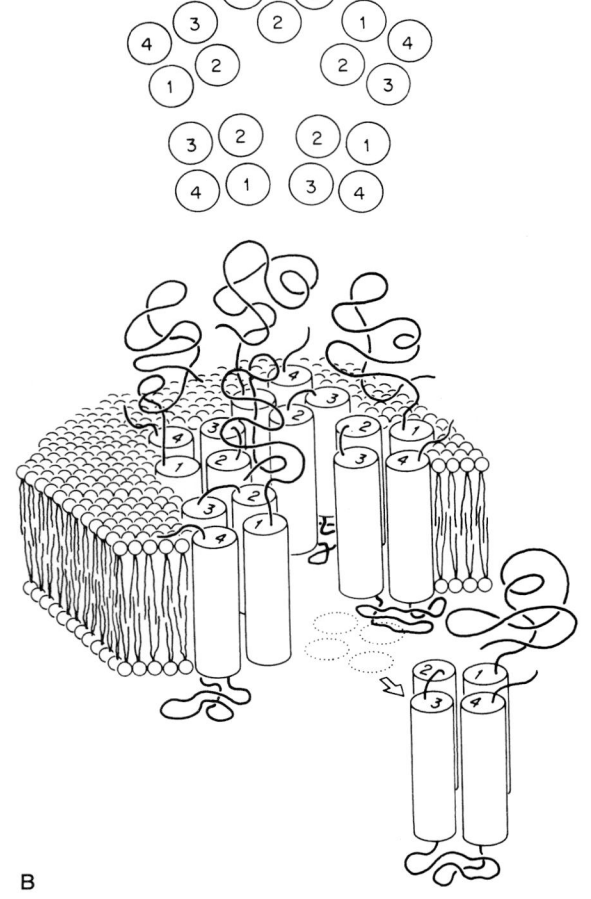

B

FIGURE 20-2

A, Generic GABA$_A$ receptor protein subunit sequence and putative topologic structure. The numbering follows that of the rat α_1 sequence used by Khrestchatisky and colleagues (Khrestchatisky M, MacLennan AJ, Chiang MY, et al: A novel alpha-subunit in rat brain GABA$_A$ receptors. Neuron 3:745–753, 1989). Note the NH$_2$ terminal (labeled N, residue 1) presumed extracellular domain, with probable sites for asparagine glycosylation (polymeric black circles at positions 10 and 110), and the cystine bridge (solid line connecting 138 and 152). Four putative membrane-spanning α-helical cylinders M1, M2, M3, and M4 are shown. The COOH-terminus (labeled C, residue 428) is extracellular. A large intracellular cytoplasmic loop between M3 and M4 is present. The shading indicates the degree of variability within the family of rat polypeptides published to date: α_1, α_2, α_4, β_1, β_2, β_3, γ_2, and δ. Amino acids that are identical in all the clones are shown in white, amino acids identical in two or more types are light gray, amino acids identical in all α but not in β, γ, and δ are black, and amino acids that vary between types are dark gray. **B**, Model of the GABA$_A$ receptor–chloride channel protein complex. The ligand-gated ion channel is proposed to be a heterooligomer composed of five subunits of the type shown in **A**. Each subunit has four membrane-spanning domains (cylinders numbered 1 through 4), one or more of which contribute to the wall of the ion channel. The structure is patterned after the well-characterized nicotinic acetylcholine receptor, another membrane of the same gene superfamily. The naturally occurring oligomers are composed of some of the α, β, γ, and δ polypeptides, but the exact subunit composition, stoichiometry, and number of subunits are not known at this time. (**A** from Smith CM, Reynard AM: Textbook of Pharmacology. Philadelphia, WB Saunders, 1992, p 278. **B** from Olsen RW, Tobin AJ: Molecular biology of GABA$_A$ receptors. FASEB J 4:1469–1480, 1990.)

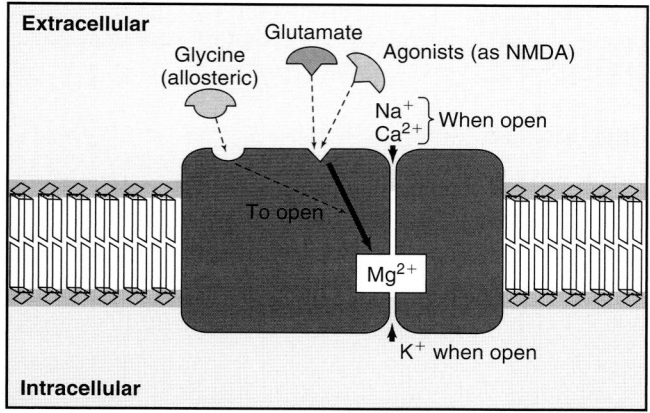

FIGURE 20-3

Suggested components of glutamate receptors in the central nervous system. Channel shown in resting stage. Depolarization by agonist binding or voltage gating releases blockade by magnesium ions and lets potassium ions pass outward and Na$^+$ and Ca^{2+} pass into the nerve cell. Glycine acts to augment agonist effect. *(From Brody TM, Larner J, Minneman KP [eds]: Human Pharmacology: Molecular to Clinical, 3rd edition. St Louis, Mosby, 1998, p 18.)*

Ca^{2+} channels that also have binding sites for other ligands, including glycine and *N*-methyl-D-aspartate (NMDA). When open, these NMDA-glutamate Ca^{2+} channels also permit sodium (Na$^+$) influx and, in some cases, potassium (K$^+$) efflux (Fig. 20-3). The pathophysiologic consequences of these transmembrane ion fluxes are postsynaptic neuronal membrane depolarization and enhanced electrical excitability and neuronal cytotoxicity as a result of increases in intracellular Ca^{2+} concentration. The clinical effects are agitation/seizures and persistent neurologic functional impairment.[34,35]

Proconvulsant substances that have direct agonist and neuroexcitatory actions at NMDA-glutamate receptors include the marine toxins, domoic acid and kainic acid,[36,37] and glufosinate, a broad-spectrum herbicide.[38] Chronic administration of NMDA-glutamate receptor antagonists (e.g., ethanol, meprobamate), which exert more potent anticonvulsant effects than GABA$_A$ agonists in some experimental models, results in up-regulation of glutamatergic neurotransmission and pharmacodynamic tolerance to the sedative effects.[39,40] Abrupt discontinuation of these agents is thought to result in increased NMDA-glutamate receptor complex–mediated ion flux, enhanced neuronal excitability, and increased risk of convulsions[35,41]; this, combined with evidence supporting

ethanol's actions at GABA$_A$ chloride channels, strongly suggests a dual and concordant effect of ethanol on the balance between excitatory and inhibitory neurotransmission.

Acetylcholine (Muscarinic) Agonism

Although their clinical importance is uncertain, other excitatory neurotransmitter systems are postulated to play a role in the proconvulsant actions of a variety of toxicants. The proconvulsant effects of the muscarinic agonist pilocarpine, used in experimental models of human epilepsy,[42,43] and the observation that stimulation of brain muscarinic receptors causes persistent tonic-clonic convulsions[44] suggest enhancement of muscarinic neurotransmission as a mechanism of induction of seizure activity by agents that inhibit neural acetylcholinesterase (e.g., organophosphate insecticides). It also has been suggested, however, that secondary GABAergic and glutamatergic mechanisms may be involved more directly in seizure production by these agents.[45]

Adenosine Antagonism

A third major mechanism of proconvulsant action involves interference with the normal modulation of presynaptic excitatory neurotransmitter (e.g., glutamate) release. Substantial evidence implicates adenosine as an endogenous anticonvulsant substance that is "released during seizure activity, exerts stabilizing effects on the epileptogenic focus and surrounding neural tissues and the accumulation of which terminates seizure activity while increasing the threshold for further seizure induction."[46] Prolonged clinical and electrographic seizure activity occurs when the anticonvulsant actions of adenosine are antagonized.[47]

Adenosine is released from the presynaptic nerve terminal in the brain along with other neurotransmitters, such as glutamate, then binds to G protein–coupled receptors on the same presynaptic terminal. The effect of stimulation of these so-named A$_1$ subtype adenosine receptors is a decrease in voltage-gated Ca^{2+} influx and inhibition of further presynaptic excitatory neurotransmitter release. When involved in negative feedback modulation of this sort, receptors commonly are referred to as *autoreceptors* (Fig. 20-4).

Adenosine-mediated spontaneous arrest of seizure activity is characterized by its alternating synaptic accumulation and clearance and is reflected in the ictal-interictal cycling that occurs during SE.[47] In addition, stimulation of a second adenosine receptor subtype, A$_2$, located on cerebral blood vessels, results in vasodilation and a compensatory increase

FIGURE 20-4

Presynaptic inhibition of excitatory neurotransmitter releases by adenosine. Agonism of the presynaptic inhibitory (also known as *autocoid*) A$_1$ receptor by adenosine attenuates voltage-gated Ca^{2+} release, reducing the release of excitatory neurotransmitters (e.g., glutamate).

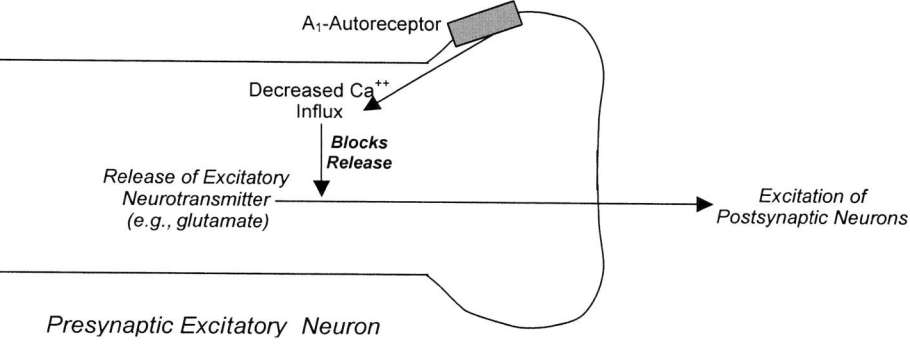

in cerebral blood flow during times of increased oxygen and nutrient requirements (e.g., during seizure).

Adenosine's anticonvulsant activity has been shown convincingly in experimental studies of its effects on seizures induced by adenosine antagonists, such as theophylline.[48] Many other drugs have been found to alter the excitatory/ inhibitory neurotransmitter balance through their effects on synaptic adenosine levels or more direct actions at adenosine receptors. There is evidence that benzodiazepines enhance neuroinhibitory tone, in part, through inhibition of presynaptic adenosine reuptake,[46] whereas carbamazepine

exhibits dose-dependent agonistic and antagonistic actions on adenosinergic modulation of excitatory neurotransmitter release.[46,49–51]

Other Mechanisms

Other neurotransmitter system components and mechanisms are postulated to play a contributory role in the proconvulsant effects of various pharmacologic agents, but supporting data are limited (Table 20-2). These mechanisms include the following:

TABLE 20-2 Mechanism of Action of Proconvulsant Drugs and Toxins

PRESUMPTIVE MECHANISM	EXAMPLES OF TOXIC AGENTS*
Neurochemical Effect	
GABAergic	
GABA$_A$ antagonism	
Direct	**Bicuculline, penicillin**
Indirect	**Lindane** (and other organochlorines), amoxapine, maprotiline, tricyclic antidepressants, **penicillin**, type II pyrethroids, cephalosporins, fluoroquinolones, virol A (*Cicuta virosa*, water hemlock), avermectin analogues (ivermectin)
Depressed GABA production	**Isoniazid**, monomethylhydrazine, cyanide
GABA$_B$ agonism (?)	Baclofen
Agonist tolerance/withdrawal	
GABA$_A$	**Ethanol, benzodiazepines, barbiturates**, carisoprodol, meprobamate, zolpidem
GABA$_B$ (?)	Baclofen
Glycinergic	
Antagonism (spinal cord)	**Strychnine**, picrotoxin
Agonism tolerance/withdrawal (brain NMDA-glutamate)	**Ethanol**
Glutamatergic agonism	**Domoic acid, kainic acid**, glufosinate
Adenosinergic antagonism	**Theophylline, caffeine**
Cholinergic agonism	
Acetylcholine release	Aminopyridines
Direct nicotinic receptor agonism	Nicotine (and other nicotinic alkaloids)
Direct muscarinic agonism	Pilocarpine, bethanechol alkaloids
Acetylcholinesterase inhibition	Organophosphates (sarin, diazinon)
Adrenergic agonism	Amphetamine, cocaine
Histaminergic antagonism	Diphenhydramine, tripelennamine
Sodium channel blockade (membrane-stabilizing effect)	Local anesthetics, cocaine, propranolol, carbamazepine, phenytoin, diphenhydramine
Metabolic or Cytotoxic Effect	
Hypoglycemia	Insulin, sulfonylureas, disopyramide, pentamidine, akee fruit
Hyponatremia (SIADH)	Carbamazepine, vinca alkaloids, chlorpropamide, phenothiazines
Direct mitochondrial dysfunction	
Uncoupling of oxidative phosphorylation	Salicylate, dinitrophenol
Cytochrome oxidase inhibition	Cyanide/cyanogens, carbon monoxide, hydrogen sulfide, iron, methanol/formate, azide (?), phosphine (?)
Krebs cycle inhibition	Arsenic, sodium monofluoroacetate
Cellular injury	
Nonspecific irritant/denaturant	Phenol
Alkylating injury	Busulfan, chlorambucil, ethylene oxide, methyl bromide, methyl chloride
Unknown	
	Bupropion, camphor, cicutoxin, chloroquine, gamma hydroxybutyrate, pyrimethamine, quinine/quinidine, mexiletine, tocainide, lithium, mefenamic acid, phenylbutazone, normeperidine, pentazocine, propoxyphene, tramadol, nonionic radiocontrast agents (intravenous/intrathecal metrizamide, iopamidol, iophendylate), propylene glycol, ethylene glycol (?), metaldehyde, organotins, pentaborane

*__Bold type__ = best supported by available evidence—see text for referenced discussion.
GABA, γ-aminobutyric acid; NMDA, *N*-methyl-D-aspartate; SIADH, syndrome of inappropriate diuretic hormone secretion.

Presynaptic and postsynaptic $GABA_B$ receptors as loci of action responsible for seizures observed in the setting of baclofen overdose[52] and withdrawal[53,54]

Presynaptic nerve terminal potassium channel blockade (e.g., by 4-aminopyridine),[55,56] resulting in membrane depolarization, opening of voltage-gated calcium channels, increased calcium influx, and increased release of excitatory neurotransmitters (e.g., acetylcholine)

Central histaminergic (H_1) receptor antagonism by antihistaminergic drugs (see Chapter 39) (although supporting experimental evidence for this as a proconvulsant mechanism of action of antihistamines is mixed[57])

Neuronal sodium channel blockade–mediated inhibition of presynaptic GABA release (e.g., by local anesthetics, such as lidocaine and procaine[58]) or disinhibition of excitatory neurons,[8] or both, as a basis for the paradoxical proconvulsant effects of anticonvulsants that possess sodium channel–blocking properties (e.g., phenytoin, carbamazepine)[7,8,59–61]

The mechanisms of seizure production of other proconvulsive agents less directly involve alterations in neurotransmitter balance and have more to do with effects on neuronal metabolism and maintenance of functional and structural integrity. These agents include the following:

Mitochondrial poisons that impair cellular adenosine triphosphate synthesis by uncoupling oxidative phosphorylation (e.g., salicylate, dinitrophenol) or inhibiting cellular respiration (e.g., cyanide, carbon monoxide)[62–64]

Agents that cause direct cytotoxic injury (e.g., alkylating agents, such as ethylene oxide and methyl bromide)[65]

Agents that cause fluid/electrolyte and other metabolic disorders, including hyponatremia, as a consequence of syndrome of inappropriate antidiuretic hormone (e.g., carbamazepine), hypoglycemia (e.g., sulfonylurea compounds), hypoglycorrhachia and neuroglycopenia (e.g., salicylate), and hypercalcemia (e.g., mithramycin)

The neurotoxic mechanisms of action for a large array of proconvulsant substances, including camphor, metaldehyde, cicutoxin, organotins, pentaborane, and tramadol, are unknown. The reader is referred to Table 20-2 for a mechanistically based listing of various drugs, chemicals, and natural toxins that can induce seizures.

Pathophysiology of Neurologic Sequelae and Systemic Complications

The development of neurologic sequelae of toxicant-induced convulsions, particularly when seizure activity is prolonged, likely involves excessive NMDA-glutamate–mediated influx and intracellular accumulation of calcium, which triggers events (e.g., apoptosis) that result in cell death. The relative importance of this mechanism, compared with the hypoxic-ischemic injury that might occur as a result of simple asphyxiation, is supported by the experimental occurrence of neuronal injury well before cerebral demand for oxygen exceeds supply.[14,66] Irreversible neuronal injury has been shown to occur within 1 hour of the onset of seizure activity,[12,14] whereas cerebral blood flow and oxygenation increase dramatically during the initial phase of SE and do not decline significantly until after several hours of seizure activity.[14]

Neuronal tissue necrosis, atrophy, and sclerosis can result from relatively prolonged seizure activity and tend to occur in areas of the hippocampus where NMDA-glutamate receptors are relatively concentrated. This tissue injury ultimately may result in the formation of an epileptic focus.[14] Cerebral edema, herniation, cerebral hypoperfusion, and brain death represent a common lethal sequence of events after severe, prolonged generalized SE.

Numerous other systemic complications may occur as a result of toxicant-induced convulsions, particularly when convulsions are prolonged.[14,67,68] Respiratory failure may occur as a result of central apnea, upper airway obstruction, aspiration, or noncardiogenic pulmonary edema secondary to persistent elevation of pulmonary vascular pressure. The consequences of marked, diffuse increase in skeletal muscle contractions include hyperthermia (also may be centrally mediated); rhabdomyolysis, with attendant hyperkalemia and myoglobinuric renal injury; and metabolic acidosis from increased consumption of oxygen and energy reserves.[69] The hyperadrenergic tone of the convulsing individual is manifested clinically by hypertension, cardiac tachydysrhythmias, and initial hyperglycemia. Experimental and clinical evidence support the notion that the hyperthermia, hypoxia, hypotension, and cerebral hypoperfusion that occur during relatively prolonged convulsive activity exacerbate neuronal injury and promote continuation of seizure activity.[66,67]

CLINICAL FEATURES

Toxicant-induced convulsions may occur with or without clinical "warning" symptoms (e.g., aura) or signs (e.g., altered mental status). Although seizures that occur after overdose of tricyclic antidepressant drugs commonly occur after decline in sensorium, seizures occurring as a result of acute supratherapeutic and, in some cases, chronic therapeutic exposure to some agents (e.g., bupropion) may occur without an obvious clinical prodrome. Other agents for which the clinical onset of proconvulsant effect is characteristically rapid, abrupt, or without obvious warning include isoniazid,[30] amoxapine, camphor, cicutoxin, cyanide, hydrogen sulfide, lidocaine, organochlorine insecticides such as lindane and toxaphene, and strychnine.

Most toxicant-induced seizures occur as generalized, tonic-clonic (grand mal) episodes,[20] with the relatively rare exception of focal seizure activity in individuals with preexisting epileptogenic foci.[21] Myoclonus (brief muscular contractions typically lasting <0.1 second)[21] may be the most frequently documented convulsant effect of some agents, such as penicillin,[70] normeperidine,[71,72] and selective serotonin reuptake inhibitors.[73] The convulsive episodes that occur as a result of strychnine's actions at inhibitory glycine-gated chloride channels in the spinal cord and lower brainstem are characterized by opisthotonos and tonic symmetric back and limb extensor spasm (spinal convulsions) without ictal or interictal change in sensorium. It is incumbent on the clinician to carefully distinguish between true seizure activity and abnormal motor activity resulting from voluntary and involuntary movement disorders, such as pseudoseizures, tremor, dystonia, akathisia, chorea, and athetosis (Table 20-3).[74]

TABLE 20-3 Differential Diagnosis of Toxicant-Induced Seizures

Toxic Neuromuscular Disorders That May Be Mistaken for Seizures
Serotonin syndrome*
Acute dystonia (butyrophenones)
Chorea (cocaine)
Akathisia (phenothiazines)
Strychnine†
Tetanus†
Neurotoxic scorpion envenomation (*Centruroides sculpturatus*)

Nontoxic Causes of Seizure Disorders
Stroke (hemorrhagic, nonhemorrhagic)
Subarachnoid hemorrhage
Traumatic brain injury (contusion, hemorrhage)
Intracranial neoplasm
Intracranial infection (abscess, meningitis, encephalitis)
Metabolic/electrolyte disorder (hypoxemia, hypoglycemia, uremia, hyponatremia, hypernatremia, hypocalcemia, hypomagnesemia)
Idiopathic (epilepsy)

---

*Although the neurologic presentation of serotonin syndrome commonly is limited to muscular rigidity and myoclonus, it also may include more clinically overt seizure activity.
†Strychnine-induced and tetanus-induced convulsions are mediated primarily by effects at the level of the spinal cord (hence the use of the term *spinal convulsions* to describe the seizure-like posturing and movements observed in the former) and are not considered true seizures.

As electrical seizure activity continues, the clinical features of such an episode may be more subtle or even absent.[75] The occurrence of nonconvulsive SE should be considered in an individual whose sensorium remains depressed after an overt convulsive episode. It has been estimated that at least 20% of SE episodes are nonconvulsive,[6] with an estimated prevalence of nonconvulsive SE by electrographic case definition of 26% among comatose patients and those with subtle convulsive movements, such as "muscle twitches or tonic eye deviation."[15] Nonconvulsive SE is even more likely to occur in the emergency department or intensive care unit than in other clinical settings, where pharmacologic masking of seizure activity frequently occurs owing to the use of neuromuscular blocking agents.

Seizure activity that is prolonged, recurrent, or refractory to initial treatment suggests poisoning by a member of a relatively select group of toxicants, notably theophylline, isoniazid, and certain antidepressant drugs (e.g., amoxapine). This observation was reflected in the findings of Olson and colleagues,[10] who reported in their series of nearly 200 toxicant-induced convulsive episodes the proportional occurrence of multiple or prolonged seizures (or both) after acute overdose of antidepressants (29%), theophylline (40%), and isoniazid (50%).

Olson and colleagues[10] also observed in their series of toxicant-induced convulsion cases that the most frequent complications were respiratory failure (34%), cardiac arrhythmias (22%), hypotension (16%), hyperthermia (7%), rhabdomyolysis (6%), and death (9%). Systemic complications typically are more severe and occur more commonly with prolonged seizure activity. Hyperthermia has been documented to occur in SE at case frequencies ranging from 28% to 79%.[66] Prolonged strychnine-induced convulsions in one reported case resulted in

hyperthermia (peak body temperature 43°C at 3 hours postexposure), metabolic acidosis (initial arterial pH 6.55), acute rhabdomyolysis (peak serum creatine phosphokinase 359,000 mU/mL [5983 μmol/L] approximately 2 days later), and myoglobinuria with transient acute renal insufficiency (peak serum creatinine 3.7 mg/dL [327 μmol/L]).[76] The same patient's clinical course subsequently was remarkable for diffuse weakness, severe myalgias, and transient upper and lower limb motor deficits consistent with acute, reversible compressive neuropathy. Postictal focal neurologic deficits of central origin may be transient (e.g., Todd's paralysis) or permanent in instances of irreversible cerebral insult.

DIAGNOSIS

Patient History

Obtaining a detailed history is crucial to effective decision making in the treatment of patients who have had toxic exposure to proconvulsant agents. A search for information regarding witnessed or possible unwitnessed exposure should include currently prescribed or available medications, nature of the occupational setting and presence of proconvulsant agents, and material evidence or history corroborating alcohol or illicit substance abuse. The presence of preexisting conditions, such as renal insufficiency, musculoskeletal disorders, epilepsy, and psychiatric illness, may lead to the early identification of a toxic convulsive etiology and prompt appropriate management decisions, including discontinuation of an offending pharmaceutical agent. Risk factors for toxicant-induced convulsions that may be discernible from a careful review of the patient's medical history include the following:

Drug or alcohol (or both) withdrawal (e.g., benzodiazepine or barbiturate sedative-hypnotics) and drug overdose, with the paradoxical inclusion of some anticonvulsants (e.g., phenytoin, carbamazepine)
Advanced age or demonstrated reduction in renal clearance (e.g., penicillins, cephalosporins,[30] normeperidine[72,77])
Impaired drug metabolism (e.g., isoniazid and slow acetylator status)
Drug-drug interaction (e.g., fluoroquinolone antibiotics, cyclosporine, and theophylline[78,79])
Preexisting or underlying seizure disorder
Intrathecal, intraventricular, or intravenous route of administration (e.g., penicillin and other antibiotics, bethanechol)[20,30,80]

Bedside Evaluation

The bedside evaluation of a patient at risk for onset or recurrence of toxicant-induced convulsions and associated complications should focus on the presence of other signs that may provide clues to the nature of the toxic exposure, such as tricyclic antidepressant–induced electrocardiographic abnormalities or organophosphate-induced cholinergic manifestations. The clinical approach should emphasize continued close monitoring for evidence of seizure activity (e.g., signs of adrenergic excess, including pupillary dilation, hypertension, and tachycardia) and should anticipate the development of complications of prolonged seizure activity, such as hypoxemia, respiratory failure, hyperthermia, hypoglycemia, and rhabdomyolysis.

Laboratory Evaluation

Appropriate laboratory evaluation includes routine monitoring of arterial blood gases, bearing in mind that arterial pH may be lower than 7.0 if measured during or immediately after a seizure episode. Other indicated studies include serum chemistries, with particular attention to bicarbonate, anion gap, glucose, sodium, calcium, and magnesium, and toxicologic analysis of urine or blood or both, particularly in instances in which the results support clinical decision making and treatment (e.g., in theophylline or tricyclic antidepressant poisoning) or are of forensic importance. The rapid urine drug immunoassays that commonly are employed in clinical treatment settings are severely limited in some cases by their low sensitivity or specificity or both. Rapid tricyclic antidepressant "screens" that have been commercially available have been notably false positive for a variety of other drugs, such as phenothiazines, diphenhydramine, carbamazepine, orphenadrine, and cyclobenzaprine, and have failed to detect the presence of other cyclic antidepressant drugs, such as amoxapine.[81]

Transient pleocytosis is a common, nonspecific finding in cerebrospinal fluid obtained during the early postictal interval, with total cerebrospinal fluid white blood counts ranging from $1/\mu L$ to $50/\mu L$ in about 15% of patients after seizure episodes.[21,82] It has been suggested that serum prolactin and adrenocorticotropic hormone levels, which have been observed to increase and stay elevated for 10 to 20 minutes after generalized seizures,[21] may help to differentiate seizure from pseudoseizure. These elevations also are recognized to be unreliable markers of seizure activity, however, because their specificity frequently is low in critically ill patients with multiple confounding disorders, and their sensitivity declines with increasing seizure frequency.[6]

Electroencephalogram

The most valuable test employed during the diagnostic evaluation and management of patients with documented or suspected toxicant-induced convulsions is EEG. A role for continuous, rather than intermittent, EEG monitoring is supported by continued uncertainty as to the "extent to which occasional seizures produce incremental neuronal damage in refractory SE."[6] This role is underscored further by observations that CNS injury can occur as a consequence of subclinical seizure activity within minutes of its onset and is supported by the argument that continuous EEG enhances the sensitivity and specificity of clinical seizure monitoring. Continuous EEG monitoring is especially applicable in instances in which the use of sedative-hypnotic agents or neuromuscular blockade blunts or abolishes the clinical seizure activity. Alternatively, the nonconvulsant (e.g., choreiform) effects of certain agents (e.g., cocaine) or manifestations of hypoxic-ischemic brain injury (e.g., decerebrate posturing) may be misinterpreted as seizures.[6]

Further appreciation of the role of EEG in critically ill patients is based on the observation that as documented electrical seizure activity becomes recurrent or prolonged, the clinical manifestations become more subtle (e.g., facial twitching, clonic ocular movements) or may be clinically indistinguishable from coma of nonictal origin.[66] In a study of patient transfers to a neurological intensive care unit with a transfer diagnosis of SE, only 14 of 26 (54%) patients satisfied the electrical definition for SE; of the remaining 12 patients, half were determined to be in drug-induced coma or were encephalopathic, and the other half were determined to have pseudoseizures.[83]

EEG monitoring should be instituted for any patient who is managed with relatively long-acting neuromuscular blockade, who does not regain consciousness after initial anticonvulsant treatment, or who requires prolonged treatment for refractory status.[66] SE may be defined and recognized readily on EEG as "continuous spike, sharp wave, or sharp and slow wave discharges with a generalized distribution persisting for all or most of a tracing lasting 20 minutes or longer."[17] Many electrographic patterns of seizure activity can occur, however, depending on the specific cause, neuroanatomy, and physiology involved, warranting formal interpretation by a qualified expert in most, if not all, instances.[21] Magnetic resonance imaging signal abnormalities in the hippocampus have been associated with SE[21]; however, the diagnostic utility of this and other imaging modalities in the evaluation and management of toxicant-induced convulsions has not been established.

Differential Diagnosis

The differential diagnosis of seizure-like activity that fails to fulfill the clinical and electrical definition of true seizure episode includes decorticate/decerebrate posturing, choreiform or athetoid movements, acute dystonic posturing, increased motor tone associated with hyperserotonergic states, pseudoseizure, posthypoxic myoclonus,[6,83] syncope, migraine, drop attacks, panic attacks, cataplexy, and hysterical pseudoseizures.[21] Nontoxic etiologies of convulsive episodes that meet accepted case definition for true seizure activity commonly are divided into two clinical subgroups on the basis of whether the seizure activity or associated neurologic deficits they cause are predominantly focal or nonfocal.

Key Points in the Evaluation of Toxin-Induced Seizures

1. The fundamental pathophysiology of toxicant-induced convulsions involves relatively diffuse changes in central nervous system neurotransmitter balance, favoring neuroexcitatory over neuroinhibitory tone.
2. Risk factors for toxicant-induced convulsions include patient age, drug overdose or withdrawal, parenteral route of exposure (e.g., antibiotics), underlying seizure disorder, and impaired drug clearance (e.g., normeperidine).
3. As seizure activity becomes more prolonged, the risks of neuronal injury and systemic complications increase, clinical manifestations become less pronounced, and responsiveness to anticonvulsant treatment tends to decline.
4. Common systemic complications of toxicant-induced seizures include respiratory failure, aspiration pneumonitis, hyperthermia, rhabdomyolysis, and metabolic acidosis.
5. Subclinical status epilepticus occurs in a high percentage (26%) of critically ill patients with altered sensorium. Continuous electroencephalogram monitoring is essential in the management of patients at high risk for this occurrence (e.g., patients receiving neuromuscular blockers).

TREATMENT

As generally applies to the management of ongoing or recurrent seizures of nontoxic origin, termination and suppression of further seizure activity are paramount in management of a patient with toxicant-induced convulsions. Stopping seizure activity may play an integral role in stabilizing the airway, ventilation, and circulatory status of the affected individual. In addition, *delay in termination of SE is associated with a marked decline in responsiveness to subsequent anticonvulsant treatment.* Lowenstein and Alldredge[66] observed an 80% response rate to first-line anticonvulsant treatment if it was initiated within 30 minutes of seizure onset and a decrease in response rate to less than 40% if treatment was begun 2 or more hours after onset of seizures.

The principal desired characteristics of an anticonvulsant regimen designed for use in a critical care setting are initial rapid onset of effect, subsequent prolonged duration of effect, marked enhancement in efficacy for instances when seizures prove refractory to initial treatment, and acceptably low acute and chronic adverse effect rates. Although some anticonvulsant drugs (e.g., phenytoin, fosphenytoin) are recommended widely for use in the general management of SE,[6,12,21,66] other choices may be more rational in the management of toxicant-induced convulsions, as discussed subsequently.

Initial Anticonvulsant Therapy

The ultimate goal of acute anticonvulsant drug treatment in the critical care setting is suppression of clinical and electrographic seizure activity or induction of a burst-suppression pattern on EEG, whichever occurs first.[66] Long-term anticonvulsant maintenance therapy usually is not indicated in patients in whom the sole cause of seizure activity is a transient metabolic or toxic disturbance (i.e., in the absence of a preexisting CNS structural disorder or seizure focus and without the development of a new and more permanent focus for recurrence).[12]

Although phenytoin and its phosphoester congener fosphenytoin may be appropriate choices for treatment of patients with idiopathic seizure disorders or patients with defined structural or electrical foci of seizure activity, they are not rational choices of therapy for toxicant-induced convulsions, which result from a diffuse lowering of neuronal seizure threshold, rather than a spread of electrical activity from a focal origin. Phenytoin frequently is recommended as a second-line and maintenance anticonvulsant in the treatment of SE of nontoxicant origin.[12,15,21,66] Phenytoin-induced blockade of voltage-dependent sodium channels inhibits the propagation of seizure activity from active electrical foci but has limited ability to elevate the threshold for seizures induced by GABA-antagonistic or glycine-antagonistic convulsant drugs (e.g., strychnine, picrotoxin, pentylenetetrazol).[84,85] Although it may be effective at preventing the spread of abnormal electrical activity from a CNS focus, phenytoin would not be expected to suppress the characteristically diffuse lowering of seizure threshold or oppose the increase in neuronal excitability induced by proconvulsant drugs, chemicals, and toxins.

A considerable body of experimental evidence exists indicating phenytoin's lack of anticonvulsant efficacy in the suppression of seizures induced by a variety of proconvulsant substances, including penicillin,[86–88] pilocarpine,[89,90] cocaine,[91] pyrethroids (deltamethrin, permethrin),[92] local anesthetics (e.g., procaine, lidocaine),[93,94] theophylline,[95–97] pentylenetetrazol,[98] picrotoxin,[98] strychnine,[98] NMDA,[22] and organophosphate insecticides.[45] There is evidence in animals that administration of phenytoin may enhance the proconvulsant potency of theophylline.[96] Phenytoin use in experimental animals has been reported to increase mortality rate in cyclic antidepressant toxicity.[99] One exception to phenytoin's apparent lack of anticonvulsant efficacy in toxicant-induced convulsions seems to be aminopyridine-induced seizures, wherein anecdotal clinical and experimental animal evidence suggests phenytoin is efficacious.[55,56] There also are ample clinical data to support the lack of efficacy of phenytoin in the treatment of alcohol withdrawal seizures.[100–102]

The clinical evidence available to support recommendations regarding the use of phenytoin in the management of toxicant-induced convulsions is far more limited. The Veterans Administration (VA) Status Epilepticus Cooperative Study Group compared the initial anticonvulsant efficacy of intravenous lorazepam, phenobarbital, phenytoin, and diazepam followed by phenytoin after treatments were assigned randomly to patients with generalized convulsive SE.[15] In this study, the definition of treatment success was cessation of clinical and electrical evidence of seizure activity within 20 minutes of the start of infusion, with no further seizure occurrence during the first hour after initiation of treatment. The 43.6% success rate for patients treated first with phenytoin was the lowest of any of the treatment groups and was significantly lower than that for lorazepam, 64.9% (p < 0.001). The significant difference between the lorazepam and phenytoin groups in the length of time required to complete drug infusion (mean infusion times—lorazepam, 4.7 minutes; phenytoin 33 minutes) might explain the observed overall difference in efficacy. Phenobarbital, which was infused over a mean interval of 16.6 minutes, was as effective as lorazepam, however, in patients with overt generalized convulsive SE, suggesting an alternative explanation (i.e., other than difference in infusion time) for the observed differences in treatment success.

Although the VA Cooperative Study included a group of patients whose episodes of SE were deemed to have resulted from the "toxic effects of therapeutic or recreational drug" exposure, the relevance of the study's conclusions to the current discussion is limited by the absence of comparisons made among the various treatments in this toxicologic substratum of patients. Given the small size of this group (n = 31), it is unlikely that meaningful comparisons could be made among its treatment subgroups.

In general, medications that cause neuronal hyperpolarization via increases in chloride influx (or potassium efflux) and that increase neuroinhibitory tone or reduce neuroexcitatory tone (or both) by suppressing NMDA-glutamate sodium and calcium influx are, in theory, rational choices of therapy for toxicant-induced convulsions. Consistent with this rationale and supported by previously cited clinical trial data,[15] widely accepted anticonvulsant regimens for the general treatment of SE begin with parenteral benzodiazepines (diazepam or lorazepam or both).[6,12,66] Phenobarbital, frequently a third-line agent in the broader treatment of SE, is a more appropriate second-line choice than phenytoin for toxicant-induced recurrent seizures or SE. This assertion is based on previously stated arguments against the use of phenytoin in toxicant-induced convulsions and on the rationale that barbiturates are more likely than phenytoin to act in an additive or synergistic manner with other GABA agonists, such as diazepam and lorazepam, to suppress toxicant-induced diffuse increases in neuronal electrical excitability.

Benzodiazepine compounds, such as diazepam and lorazepam, bind to the benzodiazepine receptor on the $GABA_A$ chloride ionophore to increase the binding affinity of GABA to its receptor and to increase the frequency of Cl^- channel opening in response to GABA binding. In addition, there is evidence that diazepam inhibits adenosine reuptake,[103,104] enhancing adenosinergic inhibition of excitatory neurotransmitter (e.g., glutamate) release. Lorazepam and diazepam exhibit a similar clinical response time (i.e., time to cessation of seizure activity); however, lorazepam has been shown to have a longer duration of anticonvulsant effect (12 to 24 hours versus 15 to 30 minutes) and is the preferred initial drug choice in SE management according to some authorities.[12] The successful use of lorazepam in the treatment of seizures, myoclonus, and other neurologic manifestations of serotonin syndrome is discussed in Chapter 24 and elsewhere.[105] Based on other, more toxicant-specific information sources, diazepam is the initial treatment of choice for convulsions caused by nerve agents (e.g., soman),[45,106] hydroxychloroquine,[107] or chloroquine overdose.[108] This recommendation simply may reflect the lack of experience to date with lorazepam treatment of these particular toxins.

Intravenous administration of antiepileptic drugs is the preferred route of treatment of SE. Recommended dosing for intravenous diazepam is 0.15 to 0.25 mg/kg in adults and 0.1 to 1 mg/kg in children at a rate no faster than 5 mg/min[13]; for intravenous lorazepam, recommended dosing is 0.05 to 0.2 mg/kg at a rate of 2 mg/min to a total initial dose of 8 mg. If intravenous access cannot be obtained, diazepam may be administered per rectum in the available gel form at a dose of 0.5 mg/kg to 20 mg,[6,66,67] although other, more efficacious alternatives to intravenous diazepam or lorazepam (e.g., intramuscular midazolam; see next section) may be available, depending on the treatment setting (i.e., prehospital, emergency department, or intensive care unit) and associated drug availability. Adverse acute effects of intravenous benzodiazepines include hypoventilation, depressed sensorium, and hypotension. With prolonged continuous infusion of propylene glycol–containing formulations of some drugs, such as diazepam (45% propylene glycol by volume) or lorazepam (80% propylene glycol by volume), coma, hyperosmolality, anion gap metabolic acidosis, and hyperlactatemia may occur.[109–111]

Barbiturates also bind to the $GABA_A$ complex, enhancing the binding of GABA and increasing the duration of Cl^- channel opening and Cl^- influx.[27] At high concentrations, some barbiturates directly open the Cl^- channel and exert a direct agonist action on chloride influx and neuronal hyperpolarization. Experimental evidence supports the superiority of phenobarbital over phenytoin in preventing theophylline-induced seizures and death.[96,97] Recommended dosing for phenobarbital as a second-line anticonvulsant after diazepam or lorazepam is 20 mg/kg intravenously infused at a rate of

50 to 75 mg/min. The time required for safe administration of an intravenous loading dose of phenobarbital, roughly 20 to 30 minutes in a 70-kg individual, is potentially a disadvantage compared with other agents (e.g., benzodiazepines or other barbiturates, such as thiopental or pentobarbital) in the initial treatment of sustained convulsive activity. As Treiman and colleagues[15] observed, however, there was no significant difference in the initial anticonvulsant success rate between phenobarbital-treated and lorazepam-treated patients with SE in their study. There also may be prophylactic anticonvulsant and other favorable (e.g., sedative) effects from administering phenobarbital to highly seizure-prone individuals, such as individuals who present with moderately severe theophylline toxicity (e.g., with agitation, tremor, tachycardia).[112] Potential acute adverse effects of therapy with parenteral phenobarbital and other barbiturates, especially the higher potency agents, such as thiopental and pentobarbital, include CNS and respiratory depression and hypotension.

From a pathophysiologic and therapeutic standpoint, isoniazid-induced convulsions represent a unique subset of toxicant-induced seizures. The underlying proconvulsant mechanism of isoniazid involves inhibition of GABA synthesis and decline in presynaptic and synaptic GABA. Anticonvulsant drugs that work via indirect GABA agonism and require the presence of GABA to exert an effect on $GABA_A$ chloride channel conductance are relatively ineffective in situations of synaptic GABA deficiency. Administration of pyridoxine, an essential cofactor in GABA synthesis, effectively restores GABA synthesis to adequate levels and promotes a return toward normal GABAergic neuroinhibitory tone.[30] Pyridoxine hydrochloride should be administered intravenously for acute isoniazid-induced neurotoxicity and given in gram-for-gram amounts if the toxicant dose is known or in 5-g incremental bolus doses if isoniazid dose is unknown. The experimental demonstration of synergism between diazepam and pyridoxine in treatment of acute isoniazid toxicity in dogs and rats[113,114] provides support for the administration of indirect GABA agonists such as diazepam along with pyridoxine to patients with isoniazid-induced convulsions. This combination may be particularly beneficial if the amount of pyridoxine available for use in the emergent treatment setting is limited (see Chapter 61).

Pharmacologic antagonists, such as naloxone and flumazenil, employed in the emergent reversal of toxic effects of CNS depressant agents, such as opiate μ receptor and benzodiazepine receptor agonists, may oppose, but more often enhance, the proconvulsant risks associated with administration and withdrawal of these drugs.[115] Although naloxone, based on experimental evidence, may antagonize the convulsant effects of propoxyphene,[116,117] it also has been observed to potentiate the proconvulsant effects of meperidine's major oxidative metabolite, normeperidine,[118] and of pentazocine[119] and should be used with caution in these settings. It has been well substantiated by clinical experience that the use of flumazenil (see Chapter 138) should be avoided in patients at risk for acute benzodiazepine antagonist–induced withdrawal or in whom the presence of benzodiazepine agonist effects may protect against the proconvulsant effects of other drugs (e.g., cyclic antidepressants).[120] Although some clinical studies suggest that flumazenil can be administered safely empirically in unclear cases of multiple-drug poisoning,[121,122] the conclusions reached by other investigators about the relative safety of this approach are limited by the confounding and neuroprotective presence of other anticonvulsant agents (e.g., phenobarbital).[123]

Treatment of Prolonged, Recurrent, or Refractory Toxicant-induced Convulsions and in Situations in Which Venous Access Is Unsuccessful

In addition to prompting questions as to the underlying etiology and appropriate selection of first-line treatment, prolonged or recurrent seizure activity may warrant increases in the potency, duration, and attendant risks of anticonvulsant therapy. This approach may require further provision of aggressive supportive measures before and during treatment (e.g., neuromuscular blockade, intubation, mechanical ventilation, external cooling, intravenous vasopressor therapy). Supportive care should include, when indicated, supplemental thiamine, if there is any reasonable risk of deficiency; intravenous dextrose, if objective evidence (e.g., rapid blood assay) or suspicion of hypoglycemia supports the need; intravenous bicarbonate for correction of severe metabolic acidosis; and maintenance of brisk urinary output, with urine pH greater than 6.5, in an effort to prevent myoglobinuric renal tubular injury. There are few data to support outcome benefit from selective employment of extracorporeal methods of enhanced elimination (e.g., hemodialysis or ventriculolumbar perfusion) in patients with prolonged, refractory toxicant-induced seizures. There may be at least some rationale, however, for the use of extracorporeal methods in individuals in whom impaired renal clearance may be an important pathophysiologic determinant (e.g., normeperidine toxicity)[124] or in whom intrathecal administration of a drug has resulted in life-threatening neurotoxicity.[30]

It is recommended in the general management of refractory SE that additional intravenous phenobarbital, 5 to 10 mg/kg, be administered if seizures continue after an initial 20-mg/kg load.[13] An alternative, more potent choice of barbiturate anticonvulsant that frequently is included in published regimens for refractory SE is pentobarbital, at a recommended intravenous loading dose of 10 to 15 mg/kg administered over 1 hour, followed by maintenance infusion at 0.5 to 1 mg/kg/hr.[66] The critical care provider should be prepared to institute pressor therapy, given the higher risk of hemodynamic compromise with high-potency barbiturate anticonvulsants (see Chapter 48).

Another recommended approach to refractory SE is the addition of midazolam, a potent, short-acting benzodiazepine, as an initial 0.2-mg/kg slow intravenous bolus followed by infusion at 0.75 to 10 μg/kg/min.[66] One of the advantages of this approach is that injectable formulations of midazolam do not contain propylene glycol and are not associated with propylene glycol toxicity during relatively prolonged infusion therapy. In patients with SE in whom venous access is unsuccessful, it is recommended that intramuscular midazolam be given as an effective alternative to intravenous administration of a benzodiazepine anticonvulsant. On the basis of published case experience and at least one prospective randomized study, termination of seizure activity was rapid (within 1 to 10 minutes) after intramuscular midazolam, 0.2 mg/kg (maximum 7 mg), and compared favorably with treatment with intravenous diazepam, 0.3 mg/kg (maximum 10 mg).[125]

Propofol is thought to act as a GABA agonist, with potent enhancement of chloride channel conductance in a manner that may be additive or synergistic with that of benzodiazepines or barbiturates.[126] A suggested propofol regimen for refractory SE that seems to be relatively widely endorsed by epileptologists consists of a 1- to 2-mg/kg loading dose, followed by infusion of 2 to 10 mg/kg/hr.[66] The advantages of propofol and midazolam over other anticonvulsants include their rapid onset and short duration of action, allowing for prompt, continuous suppression of seizure activity during infusion and rapid assessment of neurologic status after discontinuation of treatment. Potential disadvantages of treatment with propofol include the associated high cost and elevated risks for hypertriglyceridemia and neuroexcitatory events, such as dyskinesias and convulsive movements, the latter being reported more frequently at doses less than 3 mg/kg.[126] Supporting clinical data include a published report that showed that intravenous propofol bolus and maintenance infusion halted seizure activity in a 30-year-old woman who, after amoxapine overdose, had developed SE refractory to conventional therapy.[127]

Adverse effects such as hypotension and bradycardia may be associated less frequently with propofol than with barbiturate anesthetic agents. This suggestion is challenged, however, by the findings of one clinical investigation comparing propofol with high-dose pentobarbital in the treatment of refractory SE.[128] Efficacy with regard to seizure control was not significantly different when the propofol and pentobarbital groups were compared, although the mean time to propofol-induced EEG burst suppression, approximately 2.5 minutes, was significantly shorter than that for pentobarbital, approximately 2 hours. There was no significant increase in the incidence of adverse clinical effects, including hypotension, pneumonia, or prolonged intubation, in patients who received propofol compared with patients who received high-dose barbiturate treatment. The small number of patients (eight patients in each group) enrolled in this study and the severe systemic illness and multiorgan failure observed in both treatment groups limit interpretation of the outcome and dose-response data obtained in this study.[126]

Newer, investigational approaches that some day may become more routinely applicable to the anticonvulsant and neuroprotective treatment of patients with toxicant-induced convulsions include NMDA-glutamate Ca^{2+} antagonists, such as magnesium (Mg^{2+}), phencyclidine (PCP), MK-801, dextrorphan (dextromethorphan metabolite),[45] and adenosine agonists such as cyclohexyladenosine.[14]

Key Points in the Management of Toxin-Induced Seizures

1. Suppression of clinical and electrical seizure activity is the main goal of therapy.
2. Phenytoin has no rational role in the treatment of toxicant-induced seizures (possible exceptions are aminopyridine antimyasthenic drugs).
3. Benzodiazepine and barbiturate anticonvulsant drugs are the mainstays of pharmacologic treatment in patients with toxicant-induced convulsive disorders.

continued

SPECIAL POPULATIONS

Age-related differences in general SE-related incidence, features, treatment, and outcome have been discussed thoroughly in the medical literature.[67,129–131] There is little published information, however, regarding such differences among various age groups of patients with toxicant-induced convulsive disorders. Nevertheless, it is appropriate to approach the evaluation and management of pediatric and geriatric patients with relatively high suspicion that age-related differences in risk factors (e.g., impaired drug clearance) and dose-response thresholds may predispose individuals in these age groups to the development of toxicant-induced seizures and related complications. Examples of clinical settings in which seizure occurrence has been observed to be age dependent include narcotic withdrawal,[132] parenteral propylene glycol administration,[133] and parenteral antibiotic treatment.[30]

Recommendations for the treatment of toxicant-induced SE in pediatric patients, based on recommendations for general management of pediatric SE, are essentially the same as for adults.[67,130] Alternatives to intravenous anticonvulsant administration that are particularly appropriate considerations in younger pediatric patients include the intrarectal, intraosseous, and intramuscular (midazolam) routes.

REFERENCES

1. Wax PM: Analeptic use in clinical toxicology: A historical appraisal. J Toxicol Clin Toxicol 35:203–209, 1997.
2. Wood H, LaWall CH: The United States Dispensatory, 22nd ed. Philadelphia, JB Lippincott, 1937, pp 1038–1040.
3. Richards RK: Analeptics: Pharmacologic background and clinical use in barbiturate poisoning. Neurology 9:228–233, 1959.
4. Shih CL, Chen HH, Chie TH: Acute exposure to trichloroethylene differentially alters the susceptibility to chemoconvulsants in mice. Toxicology 162:35–42, 2001.
5. Kaminski RM, Mazurek M, Turski WA, et al: Amlodipine enhances the activity of antiepileptic drugs against pentylenetetrazole-induced seizures. Pharmacol Biochem Behav 68:661–668, 2001.
6. Bleck TP: Seizures. Balliere Clin Neurol 5:565–576, 1996.
7. Chua HC, Venketasubramanian N, Tan CB, Tjia H: Paradoxical seizures in phenytoin toxicity. Singapore Med J 40:276–277, 1999.
8. Perucca E, Gram L, Avanzin G, Dulac O: Antiepileptic drugs as a cause of worsening seizures. Epilepsia 39:5–17, 1998.
9. Zaccara G, Muscas GC, Messori A: Clinical features, pathogenesis and management of drug-induced seizures. Drug Safe 5:109–151, 1990.
10. Olson KR, Kearney TE, Dyer JE, et al: Seizures associated with poisoning and drug overdose. Am J Emerg Med 12:565–568, 1994.
11. Lowenstein DH: Status epilepticus: An overview of the clinical problem. Epilepsia 40(Suppl 1):S3–S8, 1999.
12. Working Group on Status Epilepticus: Treatment of convulsive status epilepticus: Recommendations of the Epilepsy Foundation of America's Working Group on Status Epilepticus. JAMA 270:854–859, 1993.
13. Cascino GD: Generalized convulsive status epilepticus. Mayo Clin Proc 71:787–792, 1996.
14. Fountain NB: Status epilepticus: Risk factors and complications. Epilepsia 41(Suppl 2):S23–S30, 2000.
15. Treiman DM, Meyers PD, Walton NY, et al: A comparison of four treatments for generalized convulsive status epilepticus. N Engl J Med 339:792–798, 1998.
16. Jagoda A, Riggio S: Nonconvulsive status epilepticus in adults. Am J Emerg Med 6:250–254, 1988.
17. Drislane FW, Schomer DL: Clinical implications of generalized electrographic status epilepticus. Epilepsy Res 19:111–121, 1994.
18. Towne AR, Waterhous EJ, Boggs JG, et al: Prevalence of nonconvulsive status epilepticus in comatose patients. Neurology 54:340–345, 2000.
19. Kaplan PW: Prognosis in nonconvulsive status epilepticus. Epileptic Disorders 2:185–193, 2000.
20. Schaumberg HH: Human neurotoxic disease. In Spencer PS, Schaumberg HH (eds): Experimental and Clinical Neurotoxicology, 2nd ed. New York, Oxford University Press, 2000, pp 55–82.
21. Victor M, Ropper AH: Epilepsy and other seizure disorders. In Adams and Victor's Principles of Neurology, 7th ed. New York, McGraw-Hill, 2001, pp 331–365.
22. Fisher RS: Animal models of the epilepsies. Brain Res Rev 14:245–278, 1989.
23. Olsen RW, DeLorey TM: GABA and glycine. In Siegel GJ, Agranoff BW, Albers RW, et al (eds): Basic Neurochemistry: Molecular, Cellular and Medical Aspects, 6th ed. Philadelphia, Lippincott Williams & Wilkins, 1999, pp 335–346.
24. Squires RF, Saederup E: Antidepressants and metabolites that block GABA_A receptors couple to 35S-t-butylbicyclophorothionate binding sites in rat brain. Brain Res 441:15–22, 1988.
25. Malatynska E, Knapp RJ, Ikeda M, Yamamura HI: Antidepressants and seizure-interactions at the GABA-receptor chloride-ionophore complex. Life Sci 43:303–307, 1988.
26. Pisani F, Spina E, Oteri G: Antidepressant drugs and seizure susceptibility: From in vitro data to clinical practice. Epilepsia 40(Suppl 10):S48–56, 1999.
27. Davies JA: Mechanisms of action of antiepileptic drugs. Seizure 4:267–272, 1995.
28. Miller J, Robinson A, Percy AK: Acute isoniazid poisoning in childhood. Am J Dis Child 134:290–292, 1980.
29. Oja SS, Kontro P: Neurochemical aspects of amino acid transmitters and modulators. Med Biol 65:143–152, 1987.
30. Wallace KL: Antibiotic-induced convulsions. Crit Care Clin North Am 13:741–762, 1997.
31. Narahashi T: Neuronal ion channels as the target sites of insecticides. Pharmacol Toxicol 79:1–14, 1996.
32. Uwai K, Ohashi K, Takay Y, et al: Virol A, a toxic *trans*-polyacetylenic alcohol of *Cicuta virosa*, selectively inhibits the GABA-induced Cl⁻ current in acutely dissociated rat hippocampal CA1 neurons. Brain Res 889:174–180, 2001.
33. Smith BA: Strychnine poisoning. J Emerg Med 8:321–325, 1990.
34. Dingledine R, McBain CJ: Glutamate and aspartate. In Siegel GJ, Agranoff BW, Albers RW, et al (eds): Basic Neurochemistry: Molecular, Cellular and Medical Aspects, 6th ed. Philadelphia, Lippincott Williams & Wilkins, 1999, pp 315–333.
35. Hoffman PL, Grant KA, Snell LD, et al: NMDA receptors: Role in ethanol withdrawal seizures. Ann N Y Acad Sci 654:52–60, 1992.
36. Cendes F, Andermann F, Carpenter S, Cashman NR: Temporal lobe epilepsy caused by domoic acid intoxication: Evidence for glutamate receptor-mediated exitotoxicity in humans. Ann Neurol 37:123–126, 1995.
37. Perl TM, Bedard L, Kosatsky T, et al: An outbreak of toxic encephalopathy caused by eating mussels contaminated with domoic acid. N Engl J Med 322:1775–1780, 1990.
38. Matsumura N, Takeuchi C, Hishikawa K, et al: Glufosinate ammonium induces convulsion through *N*-methyl-D-aspartate receptors in mice. Neurosci Lett 304:123–125, 2001.
39. Wirkner K, Poelchen LK, Muhlberg K, et al: Ethanol-induced inhibition of NMDA receptor channels. Neurochem Int 35:153–162, 1999.
40. Rho JM, Donevan SD, Rogawski MA: Barbiturate-like actions of the propanediol dicarbamate felbamate and meprobamate. J Pharmacol Exp Ther 280:1383–1391, 1997.
41. Tsai G, Coyle JT: The role of glutamatergic neurotransmission in the pathophysiology of alcoholism. Annu Rev Med 49:173–184, 1998.
42. Cavalheiro EA: The pilocarpine model of epilepsy. Ital J Neurol Sci 16:33–37, 1995.

43. Turski L, Ikonomidou C, Turski WA, et al: Cholinergic mechanisms and epileptogenesis: The seizures induced by pilocarpine: A novel experimental model of intractable epilepsy. Synapse 3:154–171, 1989.

44. Savolainen KM, Hirvonen MR: Second messengers in cholinergic-induced convulsions and neuronal injury. Toxicol Lett 64–65:437–445, 1992.

45. Lallement G, Dorandeu F, Filliat P, et al: Medical management of organophosphate-induced seizures. J Physiol 92:369–373, 1998.

46. Gupta YK, Malhotra J: Adenosinergic system as an endogenous anticonvulsant mechanism. Indian J Physiol Pharmacol 41:329–343, 1997.

47. Eldridge FL, Paydarfar D, Scott SC, Dowell RT: Role of endogenous adenosine in recurrent generalized seizures. Exp Neurol 103:179–185, 1989.

48. Shannon M, Maher T: Anticonvulsant effects of intracerebroventricular adenocard in theophylline-induced seizures. Ann Emerg Med 26:65–67, 1995.

49. Clark M, Post RM: Carbamazepine, but not caffeine, is highly selective for adenosine A1 binding sites. Eur J Pharmacol 164:399–401, 1989.

50. Skerlitt JH, Davies LP, Johnston GAR: A purinergic component in the anticonvulsant action of carbamazepine. Eur J Pharmacol 82:195–197, 1982.

51. Van Calker D, Steber R, Klotz K-N, Greil W: Carbamazepine distinguishes between adenosine receptors that mediate different second messenger responses. Eur J Pharmacol 82:195–197, 1991.

52. Lee TH, Chen SS, Su SL, Yang SS: Baclofen intoxication: Report of four cases and review of the literature. Clin Neuropharmacol 15:56–62, 1992.

53. Peng CT, Ger J, Yang CC, et al: Prolonged severe withdrawal symptoms after acute-on-chronic baclofen overdose. J Toxicol Clin Toxicol 36:359–363, 1998.

54. Kofler M, Leis AA: Prolonged seizure acitivity after baclofen withdrawal. Neurology 42:697–698, 1992.

55. Stork CM, Hoffman RS: Characterization of 4-aminopyridine in overdose. J Toxicol Clin Toxicol 32:583–587, 1994.

56. Yamaguchi S, Rogawski MA: Effects of anticonvulsant drugs on 4-aminopyridine seizures in mice. Epilepsy Res 11:9–16, 1992.

57. Hough LB: Histamine. In Siegel GJ, Agranoff BW, Albers RW, et al (eds): Basic Neurochemistry: Molecular, Cellular and Medical Aspects, 6th ed. Philadelphia, Lippincott Williams & Wilkins, 1999, pp 293–313.

58. Ikeda M, Dohi T, Tsujimoto A: Inhibition of gamma-aminobutyric acid release from synaptosomes by local anesthetics. Anesthesiology 58:495–499, 1983.

59. Stilman N, Masdeu JC: Incidence of seizures with phenytoin toxicity. Neurology 35:1769–1772, 1985.

60. Neufeld MY: Exacerbation of focal seizures due to carbamazepine treatment in an adult patient. Clin Neuropharmacol 16:359–361, 1993.

61. Snead OC, Hosy LC: Exacerbation of seizures in children by carbamazepine. N Engl J Med 313:916–921, 1985.

62. Yamamoto H: A hypothesis for cyanide-induced tonic seizures with supporting evidence. Toxicology 95:19–26, 1995.

63. Turchen SG, Manoguerra AS, Whitney C: Severe cyanide poisoning from the ingestion of an acetonitrile-containing cosmetic. Am J Emerg Med 9:264–267, 1991.

64. Herman LY: Carbon monoxide poisoning presenting as an isolated seizure. J Emerg Med 16:429–432, 1998.

65. Horowitz BZ, Albertson TE, O'Malley M, Swenson EJ: An unusual exposure to methyl bromide leading to fatality. J Toxicol Clin Toxicol 36:353–357, 1998.

66. Lowenstein DH, Alldredge BK: Status epilepticus. N Engl J Med 338:970–976, 1998.

67. Hanhan UA, Fiallos MR, Orlowski JP: Status epilepticus. Pediatr Clin North Am 48:683–694, 2001.

68. Walton NY: Systemic effects of generalized convulsive status epilepticus. Epilepsia 34(Suppl 1):S54–58, 1993.

69. Chin L, Sievers ML, Herrier RN, Picchioni AL: Convulsions as the etiology of lactic acidosis in acute isoniazid toxicity in dogs. Toxicol Appl Pharmacol 49:377–384, 1979.

70. Fossieck B, Parker RH: Neurotoxicity during intravenous infusion of penicillin: A review. J Clin Pharmacol 14:504–512, 1974.

71. Geller RJ: Meperidine in patient-controlled analgesia: A near-fatal mishap. Anesth Analg 76:655–657, 1993.

72. Kaiko RF, Foley KM, Grabinski PY, et al: Central nervous system excitatory effects of meperidine in cancer patients. Ann Neurol 13:180–185, 1983.

73. Mills KC: Serotonin syndrome: A clinical update. Crit Care Clin 13:763–783, 1997.

74. Gumnit RJ, Risinger M, Leppik IE, et al: The epilepsies and convulsive disorders. In Joynt RJ, Griggs RC (eds): Clinical Neurology, Vol 3. Philadelpia, Lippincott Williams & Wilkins, 1998, pp 1–95.

75. Lowenstein DH, Aminoff MJ: Clinical and EEG features of status epilepticus in comatose patients. Neurology 42:100–104, 1992.

76. Boyd RE, Brennan PT, Deng J-F, et al: Strychnine poisoning: Recovery from profound lactic acidosis, hyperthermia and rhabdomyolysis. Am J Med 74:507–512, 1983.

77. Szeto HH, Inturrisi CE, Houde R, Saal S: Accumulation of normeperidine, an active metabolite of meperidine, in patients with renal failure or cancer. Ann Intern Med 86:738–741, 1977.

78. Semel JD, Allen N: Seizures in patients simultaneously receiving theophylline and imipenem or ciprofloxacin or metronidazole. South Med J 84:465–468, 1991.

79. Hoffman A, Pinto E, Afargan M, Schattner A: Cyclosporine enhances theophylline neurotoxicity in rats. J Pharm Sci 83:559–561, 1994.

80. Read SL, Frazee J, Shapira J, et al: Intracerebroventricular bethanechol for Alzheimer's disease: Variable dose-related responses. Arch Neurol 47:1025–1030, 1990.

81. Miles MV, Greenwood RS, Hussey B: Diagnostic pitfalls associated with amoxapine overdose: A case report. Am J Emerg Med 8:335–337, 1990.

82. Simon RP: Physiologic consequences of status epilepticus. Epilepsia 26(Suppl 1):S58–66, 1985.

83. Walker MC, Howard RS, Smith SJ, et al: Diagnosis and treatment of status epilepticus on a neurological intensive care unit. QJM 89:913–920, 1996.

84. Tunnicliff G: Basis of the antiseizure action of phenytoin. Gen Pharmacol 27:1091–1097, 1996.

85. Rall TW, Schleifer LS: Drugs effective in the therapy of the epilepsies. In Gilman AG, Goodman LS, Gilman A (eds): Goodman and Gilman's the Pharmacological Basis of Therapeutics, 6th ed. New York, MacMillan, 1980, pp 448–474.

86. Williams JD (ed): Chemotherapy. New York, Plenum Press, 1976, pp 339–344.

87. Gerald MC, Massey JH, Spadaro DC: Comparative convulsant activity of various penicillins after intracerebral injection in mice. J Pharm Pharmacol 25:104–108, 1973.

88. Weihrauch TR, Rieger H, Kohler H, et al: Influence of diazepam and phenytoin on penicillin-induced cerebral convulsions. Arzneimittelforschung 26:379–382, 1976.

89. Sofia RD, Gordon R, Gels M, Diamantis W: Effects of felbamate and other anticonvulsant drugs in two models of status epilepticus in the rat. Res Commun Chem Pathol Pharmacol 79:335–341, 1993.

90. Turski WA, Cavalheiro EA, Coimbra C, et al: Only certain antiepileptic drugs prevent seizures induced by pilocarpine. Brain Res 434:281–305, 1987.

91. Derlet RW, Albertson TE: Anticonvulsant modification of cocaine-induced toxicity in the rat. Neuropharmacology 29:255–259, 1990.

92. Devaud LL, Szot P, Murray TF: PK 11195 antagonism of pyrethroid-induced proconvulsant activity. Eur J Pharmacol 121:269–273, 1986.

93. Sawaki K, Ohno K, Miyamoto K, et al: Effects of anticonvulsants on local anesthetic-induced neurotoxicity in rats. Pharmacol Toxicol 86:59–62, 2000.

94. Stone WE, Javid MJ: Anticonvulsive and convulsive effects of lidocaine: Comparison with those of phenytoin, and implications for mechanism of action concepts. Neurol Res 10:161–168, 1988.

95. Hoffman A, Pinto E, Gilhar D: Effect of pretreatment with anticonvulsants on theophylline-induced seizures in the rat. J Crit Care 8:198–202, 1993.

96. Blake KV, Massey KL, Hendeles L, et al: Relative efficacy of phenytoin and phenobarbital for the prevention of theophylline-induced seizures in mice. Ann Emerg Med 17:1024–1028, 1988.

97. Goldberg MJ, Spector R, Miller G: Phenobarbital improves survival in theophylline-intoxicated rabbits. J Toxicol Clin Toxicol 24:203–211, 1986.

98. Porter RJ, Cereghino JJ, Gladding GD, et al: Antiepileptic drug development program. Cleve Clin Q 51:293–305, 1984.

99. Callaham M, Schumaker H, Pentel P: Phenytoin prophylaxis of cardiotoxicity in experimental amitriptyline poisoning. J Pharmacol Exp Ther 245:216–220, 1988.

100. Alldredge BK, Lowenstein DH, Simon TP: Placebo-controlled trial of intravenous diphenylhydantoin for short-term treatment of alcohol withdrawal seizures. Am J Med 87:645–648, 1989.

101. Chance JF: Emergency department treatment of alcohol withdrawal seizures with phenytoin. Ann Emerg Med 20:520–522, 1991.

102. Rathlev NK, D'Onofrio G, Fish SS, et al: The lack of efficacy of phenytoin in the prevention of recurrent alcohol-related seizures. Ann Emerg Med 23:513–518, 1994.

103. Moritoki H, Fukuda H, Kotani M, et al: Possible mechanism of action of diazepam as an adenosine potentiator. Eur J Pharmacol 113:89–98, 1985.

104. Mehta AK, Kulkarni SK: Mechanism of potentiation by diazepam of adenosine response. Life Sci 24:81–86, 1984.

105. Brown TM, Skop BP, Mareth TR: Pathophysiology and management of the serotonin syndrome. Ann Pharmacother 30:527–533, 1996.

106. Sidell FR: Nerve agents In Sidell FR, Takafuji ET, Franz DR (eds): Medical Aspects of Chemical and Biological Warfare. Bethesda, MD, Uniformed Services University of the Health Sciences, 1997, pp 129–179.

107. Marquardt K, Albertson TE: Treatment of hydroxychloroquine overdose. Am J Emerg Med 19:420–424, 2001.

108. Riou B, Barriot P, Rimailho A, Baud FJ: Treatment of severe chloroquine poisoning. N Engl J Med 318:1–6, 1988.

109. Reynolds HN, Teiken P, Regan ME, et al: Hyperlactatemia, increased osmolar gap, and renal dysfunciton during continuous lorazepam infusion. Crit Care Med 28:1631–1634, 2000.

110. Cawley MJ: Short-term lorazepam infusion and concern for propylene glycol toxicity: Case report and review. Pharmacotherapy 21:1140–1144, 2001.

111. Arbour RB: Propylene glycol toxicity related to high-dose lorazepam infusion: Case report and discussion. Am J Crit Care 8:499–506, 1999.

112. Chyka PA, Hornfeldt CS, Howland MA, et al: Prophylaxis of seizures after theophylline overdose. Pharmacotherapy 17:1044–1045, 1997.

113. Chin L, Sievers ML, Laird HE, et al: Evaluation of diazepam and pyridoxine as antidotes to isoniazid intoxication in rats and dogs. Toxicol Appl Pharmacol 45:713–722, 1978.

114. Chin L, Sievers ML, Herrier R, Picchioni AL: Potentiation of pyridoxine by depressants and anticonvulsants in the treatment of acute isoniazid intoxication in dogs. Toxicol Appl Pharmacol 58:504–509, 1981.

115. Haverkos GP, DiSalvo RP, Imhoff TE: Fatal seizures after flumazenil administration in patient with mixed overdose. Ann Pharmacother 28:1347–1349, 1994.

116. Fiut RE, Picchioni AL, Chin L: Antagonism of convulsive and lethal effects induced by propoxyphene. J Pharm Sci 55:1085–1087, 1966.

117. Gilbert PE, Martin WR: Antagonism of the convulsant effects of heroin, d-propoxyphene, mepridine, normeperidine and thebaine by naloxone in mice. J Pharmacol Exp Ther 192:538–541, 1975.

118. Tortella FC, Cowan A, Adler MW: Studies on the excitatory and inhibitory influence of intracerebroventricularly injected opioids on seizure thresholds in rats. Neuropharmacology 23:749–754, 1984.

119. Dirksen R, Coenen AM, van Luijtelaar EL: Naloxone enhances epileptogenic and behavioral effects of pentazocine in rats. Pharmacol Biochem Behav 39:415–420, 1991.

120. Spivey WH, Roberts JR, Derlet RW: A clinical trial of escalating doses of flumazenil for reversal of suspected benzodiazepine overdose in the emergency department. Ann Emerg Med 22:1813–1821, 1993.

121. Winkler E, Almog S, Kriger D, et al: Use of flumazenil in the diagnosis and treatment of patients with coma of unknown etiology. Crit Care Med 21:538–542, 1993.

122. Hojer J, Baihrendtz S, Matell G, Gustafsson LL: Diagnostic utility of flumazenil in coma with suspected poisoning: A double blind, randomized controlled study. BMJ 301:1308–1311, 1990.

123. Weinbroum A, Rudick V, Sorkine P, et al: Use of flumazenil in the treatment of drug overdose: A double blind and open clinical study in 110 patients. Crit Care Med 24:199–206, 1996.

124. Hassan H, Gastan B, Gellens M: Successful treatment of meperidine neurotoxicity by hemodialysis. Am J Kidney Dis 35:146–149, 2000.

125. Towne AR, DeLorenzo RJ: Use of intramuscular midazolam for status epilepticus. J Emerg Med 17:323–328, 1999.

126. Brown LA, Levin GM: Role of propofol in refractory status epilepticus. Ann Pharmacother 32:1053–1059, 1998.

127. Merigian KS, Browning RG, Leeper KV: Successful treatment of amoxapine-induced refractory status epilepticus with propofol (diprivan). Acad Emerg Med 2:28–33, 1995.

128. Stecker MM, Kramer TH, Raps EC, et al: Treatment of refractory status epilepticus with propofol: Clinical and pharmacokinetic findings. Epilepsia 39:18–26, 1998.

129. Waterhouse IJ, DeLorenzo RJ: Status epilepticus in older patients: Epidemiology and treatment options. Drugs Aging 18:133–142, 2001.

130. Segeleon JE, Haun SE: Status epilepticus in children. Pediatr Ann 25:380–386, 1996.

131. DeLorenzo RJ, Towne AR, Pellock JM, Ko D: Status epilepticus in children, adults and the elderly. Epilepsia 33(Suppl 4):S15–S25, 1992.

132. Herzlinger RA, Kandall SR, Vaughan HG: Neonatal seizures associated with narcotic withdrawal. J Pediatr 91:638–641, 1977.

133. Macdonald MG, Getson PR, Glasgow AM, et al: Propylene glycol: Increased incidence of seizures in low birth weight infants. Pediatrics 79:622–625, 1987.

CHAPTER 21

Cardiac Conduction and Rate Disturbances

Manish M. Patel ▪ Neal Benowitz

Management of a critically ill patient with cardiovascular disturbances requires the clinician to consider that a cardiac toxin may be involved. This chapter emphasizes recognition of cardiac arrhythmias, conduction abnormalities, and specific electrocardiogram (ECG) findings that might suggest the involvement of a cardiovascular toxin. First, relevant cardiac physiology and the toxic mechanisms pertinent to poisonings and overdose are reviewed. Next, we describe a clinical approach to the recognition and management of patients with rate and rhythm disturbances from cardiovascular toxins. Lastly, we discuss some specific cardiovascular toxins that show how autonomic disturbances, membrane-depressant effects, triggered rhythms, and systemic influences produce the protean manifestations of a patient with cardiac poisoning.

CARDIAC PHYSIOLOGY

Understanding some basic principles of toxicity facilitates the management of critically poisoned patients with cardiovascular disturbances.

Myocardial Cell Physiology

Differing pharmacology of the three important transmembrane ion channels responsible for the cardiac cell action potential (AP) makes the myocardial cell unique with respect to therapeutic and toxic actions of drugs and toxins. The three channels are (1) fast sodium channels, (2) slow calcium channels, and (3) outward potassium channels.

The AP of the cardiac cell has five phases (Fig. 21-1).[1] When a cardiac cell AP reaches its threshold potential, opening of fast sodium channels results in a spikelike upward deflection due to the rapid influx of positive ions (phase 0). When the fast sodium channels begin to close (phase 1), opening of the slow calcium channels produces an influx of positive ions and a steady maintenance of the membrane potential (phase 2). The resultant plateau phase continues until the all the sodium and calcium channels are closed, and the outward potassium channels open to allow positive ions to leave the cell. The membrane potential subsequently returns to its baseline resting level (phase 3). The resting membrane potential is maintained (phase 4) until another impulse arrives to depolarize the cell or the cell spontaneously depolarizes. During phase 4, some cardiac fibers allow sodium ions to enter into the cell, raising the resting membrane potential, also known as spontaneous

diastolic depolarization. When the membrane potential reaches threshold, the fast sodium channels open, and another AP is generated.

Role of Calcium Ions in Myocardial Cells

Consideration of some regional electrophysiologic differences in the heart adds to the understanding of cardiotoxic actions of the various drugs. First, conduction in the His-Purkinje system and the atrial and ventricular myocardium depends on *sodium* entry via the fast sodium channels during phase 0. In contrast, conduction through the sinoatrial (SA) and atrioventricular (AV) nodes depends on *calcium* entry via the slow calcium channels during phase 0 (Fig. 21-2).[2] Additionally, myocardial contraction is initiated by calcium influx during the plateau phase 2; this calcium entry allows "excitation-contraction coupling," the mechanism by which the AP causes myocardial contraction.

Regulation of Cardiac Function

In addition to the regulation via the Frank-Starling mechanism, cardiac output also is controlled by the autonomic nervous system (ANS). In the ANS, impulses are transmitted from the brain via the preganglionic fibers that synapse with the postganglionic fibers and subsequently innervate an end organ. Transmission of the impulse occurs primarily through the release of the neurotransmitters acetylcholine and norepinephrine (Fig. 21-3).

SYMPATHETIC NERVOUS SYSTEM

Sympathetic fibers innervate most parts of the heart and increase heart rate, the rate of AV nodal conduction, and myocardial contractility. Postganglionic fibers release norepinephrine, which interacts with the β_1-adrenergic cardiac receptors to increase cells' permeability to sodium and calcium, increasing excitability, conduction, and contractility.[1,3]

PARASYMPATHETIC NERVOUS SYSTEM

In the heart, the vagus nerve provides the postganglionic parasympathetic fibers that cause the local release of acetylcholine. The parasympathetic nerves mainly innervate the sinus and the AV node. Vagal stimulation of the muscarinic receptors primarily decreases excitability of the atria and slows the conduction of impulse into the ventricles to a point where atrial arrest or complete blockade of transmission at the AV node is possible. Direct effects on myocardial contractility are modest.[3]

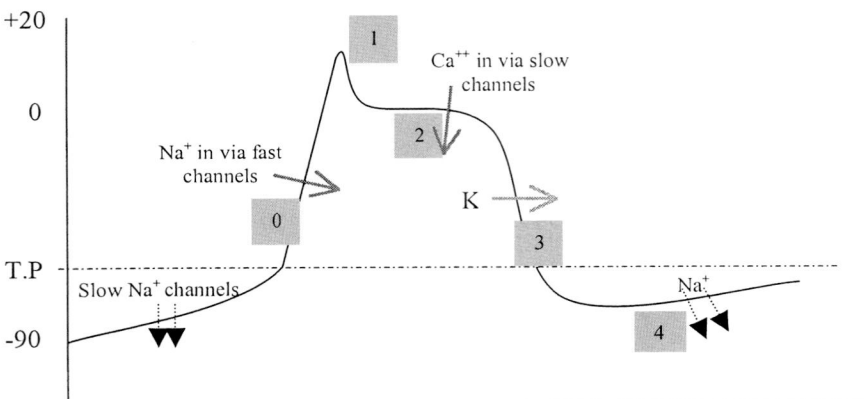

FIGURE 21-1

The five phases of transmembrane ion flow during action potential of an automatic myocardial cell with spontaneous diastolic depolarization. TP, threshold potential.

PATHOPHYSIOLOGY

As discussed later, various effects of drugs can result in cardiotoxicity. Considering arrhythmogenesis, three general mechanisms contribute to production and maintenance of arrhythmias: (1) abnormal impulse initiation, (2) triggered rhythms, and (3) abnormal impulse conduction.[4]

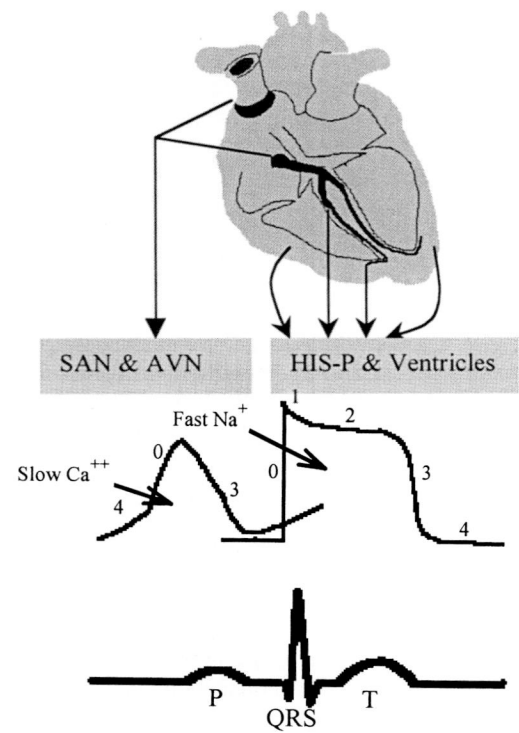

FIGURE 21-2

Schematic demonstration of the typical action potentials generated in the sinoatrial node (SAN) and atrioventricular node (AVN) versus the His-Purkinje and atrioventricular cells as a result of the variation in ion channels. The electrocardiogram (ECG) shows that atrial depolarization results in the P wave. The impulse spreads to the AV node, then to the ventricles via the bundle of His and the Purkinje fibers (HIS-P). The specialized AVN fibers delay the transmission to the ventricles, allowing atrial contraction to occur. This is indicated by the P-R interval on the ECG. The QRS complex represents ventricular muscle depolarization (phase 0, 1, 2), and the T wave indicates ventricular repolarization (phase 3). The QT interval represents phases 2 and 3 of the action potential.

Abnormal Impulse Initiation

The sinus node is the normal pacemaker because it has the fastest intrinsic firing rate. The intrinsic firing rate depends on four factors: (1) the resting potential, (2) the refractory period, (3) the threshold potential, and (4) the slope of diastolic depolarization (Fig. 21-4). An alteration in any of these four factors can cause normal atrial and ventricular working myocardial cells, which do not manifest automaticity, to generate automatic impulses. A new site of pacing results when the rate generated by this abnormal focus exceeds the sinus pacemaker rate.[4]

Triggered Rhythms

Triggered rhythms are abnormal initiations of impulses that occur as a result of afterdepolarizations (ADs) or oscillations in the AP during phases 2 through 4. Two types of ADs are categorized based on their temporal relationship with the repolarization phase of the AP: (1) early ADs and (2) delayed ADs (Fig. 21-5).[4,5]

Early ADs are the most common predecessors to triggered rhythms that result from poisoning. These result from outward potassium channel blockade (Fig. 21-5A). This blockade causes a surplus of positive ions intracellularly, resulting in delayed return of the AP to its baseline and upward oscillations in the AP above threshold. New APs resulting from early ADs are known as triggered activity, and torsades de pointes (TdP) may be precipitated by these triggered responses.[6] Delayed ADs occur when repolarization of the AP is complete or nearly complete (Fig. 21-5B). Delayed ADs are observed in conditions of intracellular calcium overload. In poisonings, this overload is associated most commonly with digitalis toxicity or excess catecholamine states. Delayed ADs also result in triggered activity and have been implicated in certain arrhythmias, especially digitalis-associated bigeminal and idioventricular rhythms.[7] In distinction to early ADs, the amplitude of triggered activity associated with delayed ADs increases with heart rate (see Fig. 21-5B).[7] It has been suggested that pacing-induced increase in heart rate may worsen digitalis toxicity in poisoned patients.[8,9] Basic science studies on delayed ADs supports this hypothesis.[7]

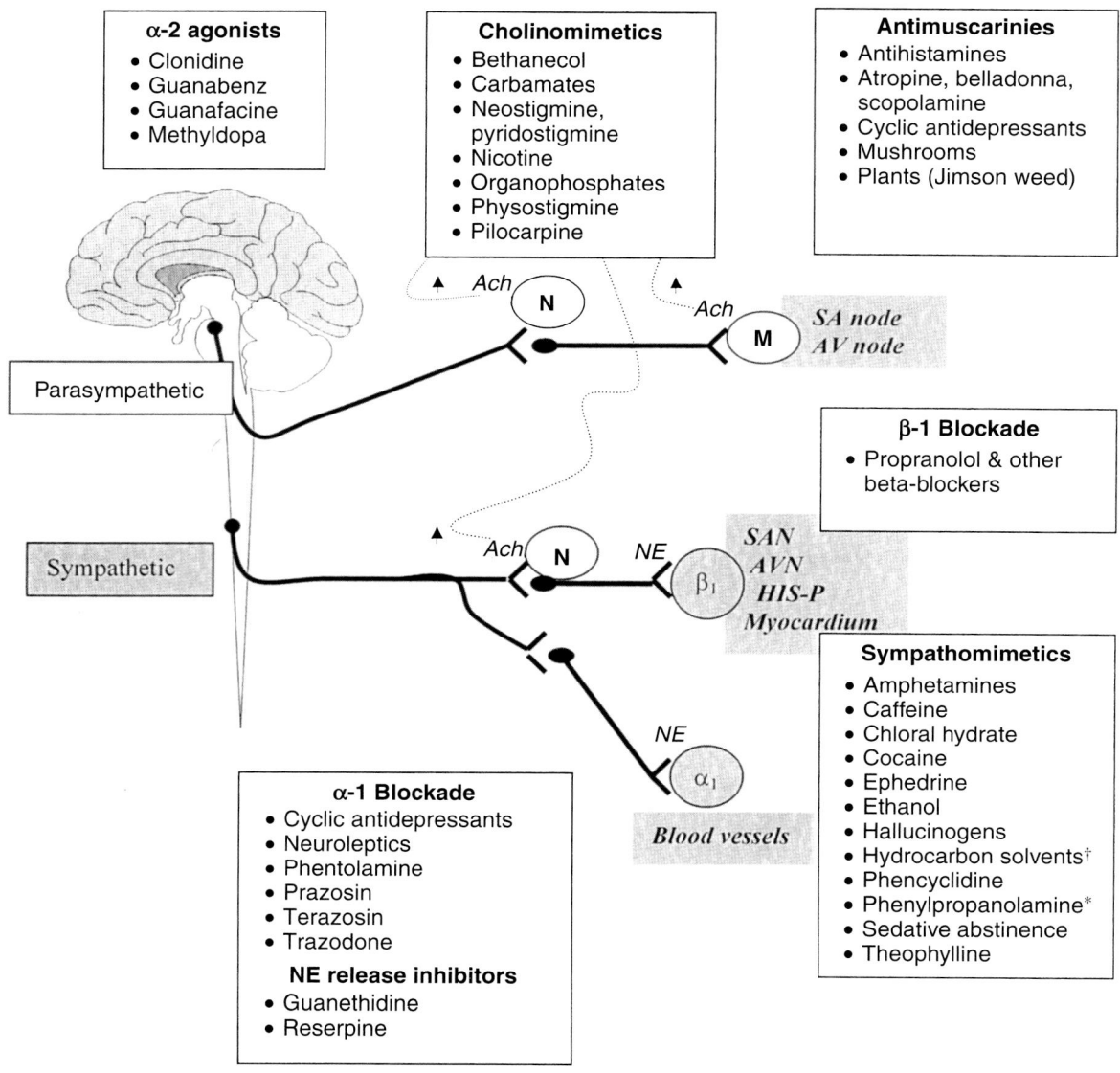

α-2 agonists
- Clonidine
- Guanabenz
- Guanafacine
- Methyldopa

Cholinomimetics
- Bethanecol
- Carbamates
- Neostigmine, pyridostigmine
- Nicotine
- Organophosphates
- Physostigmine
- Pilocarpine

Antimuscarinies
- Antihistamines
- Atropine, belladonna, scopolamine
- Cyclic antidepressants
- Mushrooms
- Plants (Jimson weed)

Parasympathetic

Ach N *Ach* M *SA node AV node*

β-1 Blockade
- Propranolol & other beta-blockers

Sympathetic

Ach N *NE* β₁ *SAN AVN HIS-P Myocardium*

α-1 Blockade
- Cyclic antidepressants
- Neuroleptics
- Phentolamine
- Prazosin
- Terazosin
- Trazodone

NE release inhibitors
- Guanethidine
- Reserpine

NE α₁

Blood vessels

Sympathomimetics
- Amphetamines
- Caffeine
- Chloral hydrate
- Cocaine
- Ephedrine
- Ethanol
- Hallucinogens
- Hydrocarbon solvents†
- Phencyclidine
- Phenylpropanolamine*
- Sedative abstinence
- Theophylline

FIGURE 21-3

The elements of the autonomic nervous system and its sites of cardiovascular action. The boxes list drugs or toxins that may influence the cardiovascular system through the autonomic nervous system at various sites.
*May cause reflex bradycardia.
†Sensitizes myocardium to catecholamines.
N, nicotinic receptors; M, muscarinic receptors; SAN, sinoatrial node; AVN, atrioventricular node; HIS-P, His-Purkinje system; Ach, acetylcholine; NE, norepinephrine.

Abnormal Impulse Conduction

Under normal conditions, an impulse initiated in the sinus node travels down the conducting tissues into the ventricles.[4] If an impulse arrives at an area of refractoriness or conduction block (ischemia, scar, or toxin-induced), it may travel down an alternative conduction pathway. If the impulse returns to the area that initially was refractory but is now excitable, a reentry "circuit" results (Fig. 21-6). Many cardiotoxins, particularly inhibitors of fast sodium channels, cause nonuniform slowing of conduction and shortening of the refractory period—forming a milieu for unidirectional block and reentry.[10] These reentry circuits are the source of many clinically significant tachyarrhythmias in nonpoisoned patients.

TOXIC MECHANISMS OF ARRHYTHMOGENESIS

A combination of membrane-depressant effects, autonomic disturbances, and systemic metabolic imbalances may occur during poisoning from cardiotoxins. Knowledge of various effects of drugs that contribute to arrhythmogenesis facilitates recognition and treatment of the manifestations of cardiotoxicity.

Membrane Depression

A toxin-induced block in conduction results in an inability of the propagating impulse to excite the tissue ahead of it. The manifestations of a conduction block vary depending on the toxin and its site of action.

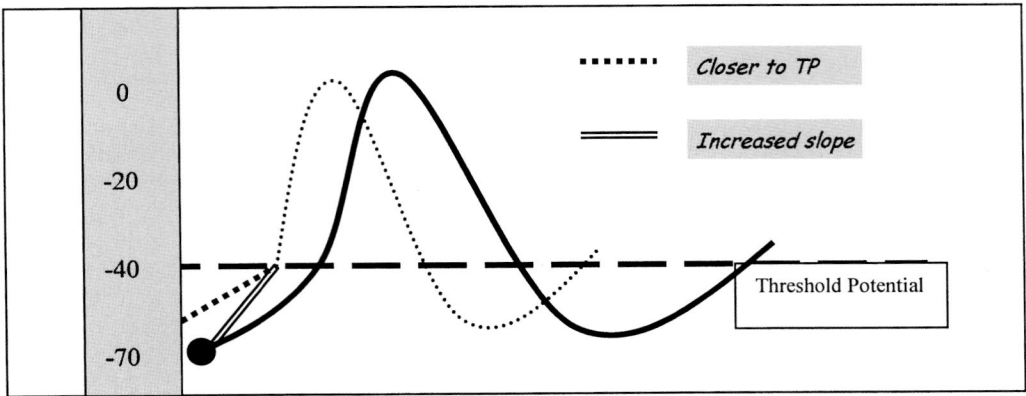

FIGURE 21-4

An example of enhanced automaticity *(dotted line)* by bringing resting potential closer to the threshold potential (TP) or increasing the slope of diastolic depolarization (DD). Conditions that make the resting potential more negative (away from the TP) or decrease the slope of DD depress automaticity and slow the pacemaker rate.

SODIUM CHANNEL BLOCKADE

Inhibition of the fast sodium channels (Fig. 21-7 and Table 21-1) decreases the maximum rate of rise and amplitude of the AP in Purkinje fibers and in atrial and ventricular myocardial cells. As a result, more stimulus current is needed to propagate an impulse throughout the His-Purkinje system and myocardium. Clinically the ECG may reveal QRS prolongation and, rarely, AV block. Nonuniform drug-induced depression of conduction may result in unidirectional block and reentry in the conduction system, resulting in tachyarrhythmias.[4,10]

SLOW CALCIUM CHANNEL BLOCKADE

In the pacemaker cells of the SA node and AV node, where the primary ion channel controlling depolarization is the slow calcium channel, inhibition of this channel results in a slowing or inability of the tissue to conduct a cardiac impulse (see Fig. 21-2).[2] Calcium channel inhibition results in depression of the SA node discharge rate (negative chronotropy) and slowing of conduction through the AV node (negative dromotropy). The ECG manifestations may include sinus bradycardia (delay at the SA node) or a prolonged P-R interval (delay at the AV node) or both.[11] Excessive delay prolongs AV conduction to the point of second-degree or complete heart block. Assuming that there is only isolated slow calcium channel inhibition of the pacemaker cells in an otherwise healthy heart, complete block in the pacemaker tissues is associated with an escape rhythm arising from the distal conduction tissues (His bundle, Purkinje fibers) or ventricular fibers. Conduction within the His-Purkinje cells, atrial myocytes, and ventricular myocytes depends on the fast sodium channels for phase 0 depolarization. Type I antiarrhythmics (e.g., lidocaine) are potentially harmful in a patient who has AV block with a ventricular rhythm because these drugs may abolish the only existing rhythm and cause asystole.[12] The slow calcium channels also are responsible for excitation-contraction coupling in the ventricular fibers. Impeding calcium entry into these cells results in a progressive depression of myocardial contractility (decreased inotropy). Similarly, vascular smooth muscle cells rely on calcium entry into the cells for contraction, and calcium blockade results in vasodilation. Decreased myocardial contractility and vasodilation result in hypotension.

OUTWARD POTASSIUM CHANNEL BLOCKADE

The significance of potassium channel blockade has been discussed in the previous section on triggered rhythms (see Fig. 21-5). Although our discussion focuses on drugs and toxins, various other conditions have been associated with triggered rhythms, including myocardial stretch, hypoxia, acidosis, hypothermia, hypokalemia, hypomagnesemia, and hypocalcemia (Table 21-2).[6]

SODIUM-POTASSIUM ATPase BLOCKADE

The energy-driven sodium-potassium ATPase pump maintains a high sodium and potassium concentration gradient across cell membranes by pumping sodium out of and potassium into the cell.[13,14] Inhibition of this pump by cardiac glycosides raises intracellular sodium concentrations, which increases intracellular calcium concentrations via the

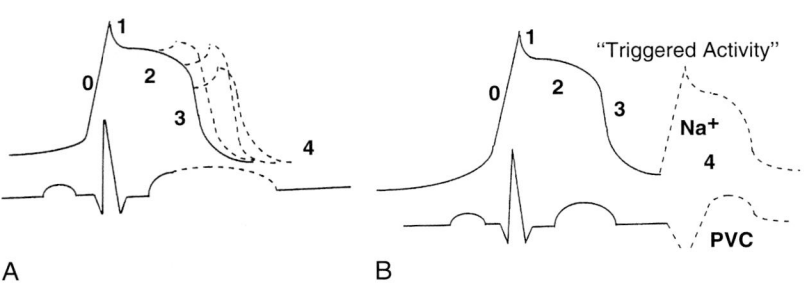

A   B

FIGURE 21-5

A, Cardiac action potential showing potassium flow blockade during phase 3 leading to membrane oscillations or *early afterdepolarizations.* Triggered activity occurs when oscillations reach threshold voltage. **B,** *Delayed afterdepolarizations* also result in triggered activity and dysrhythmias (i.e., premature ventricular contraction [PVC] and ventricular tachycardia) when they reach threshold voltage. *(From Haddad LM, Shannon MW, Winchester JF, et al: Clinical Management of Poisoning and Drug Overdose, 3rd ed. Philadelphia, 1998, WB Saunders Company.)*

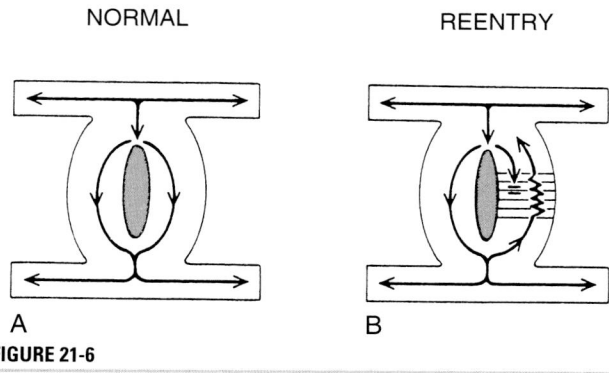

FIGURE 21-6

Reentry: Schema of Purkinje fibers or ventricular muscle through which impulse transmission occurs. **A**, Normal depolarization of a muscle segment. Impulses spread simultaneously down various conduction pathways to depolarize distal areas. Depolarization and repolarization proceed homogeneously. **B**, Reentry. The hatched area represents a local area with depressed conduction, which might be produced by a membrane-depressant drug or focal myocardial ischemia or necrosis. An impulse traveling antegradely in an area of depressed conduction is blocked *(dark horizontal lines)*; impulses traveling in adjacent pathways can pass through the area of conduction delay, however, in retrograde fashion. If tissue proximal to the depressed area is already repolarized and is now excitable, restimulation (reentry) occurs. *(From Haddad LM, Shannon MW, Winchester JF, et al: Clinical Management of Poisoning and Drug Overdose, 3rd ed. Philadelphia, 1998, WB Saunders Company.)*

TABLE 21-1 Fast Sodium Channel Inhibition

DRUGS AND TOXINS	ELECTROCARDIOGRAM FINDINGS
Antihistamines	Rightward deviation of QRS axis
Antiarrhythmics	R wave elevation lead AVR
Type Ia (quinidine, disopyramide, procainamide)	Prolonged QRS and interventricular conduction delay
Type Ic (flecainide, encainide, propafenone)	Ventricular tachycardia Ventricular fibrillation Ventricular bradycardia (severe poisoning)
Type II (propranolol*)	Asystole
Carbamazepine	
Chloroquine	
Cyclic antidepressants	
Cocaine	
Neuroleptics (thioridazine and mesoridazine)	
Propoxyphene	
Quinine	

*Propranolol and other membrane-depressant β-blockers may show fast sodium channel inhibition in poisoning. This is not a β-receptor mechanism.

gradient-dependent sodium-calcium pump (Fig. 21-8A).[14] This increase in intracellular calcium concentration has been associated with delayed ADs and certain digitalis-induced tachyarrhythmias (Fig. 21-8B).[15] Another result of the sodium-potassium pump blockade is a loss of intracellular potassium to the extracellular environment. Animal evidence suggests that potassium depletion results in modulation of sodium-potassium ATPase inhibition by digitalis, and persons with low serum potassium are more likely to develop digitalis-induced arrhythmias.[7,15]

Adrenergic Receptors

β-RECEPTORS

The β$_1$-adrenoceptor is the predominant subtype involved in drug-related cardiac poisoning. Activation of β$_1$-adrenoceptors results in increased cyclic adenosine monophosphate (cAMP) synthesis. cAMP leads to a cascade of events that culminates

in calcium entry into the myocardial cells and subsequent increased inotropic, chronotropic, and dromotropic effects (Fig. 21-9). Phosphodiesterase then hydrolyzes cAMP and terminates its activity. Poisonings from direct β-agonists are uncommon. More often, toxins (e.g., cocaine and amphetamines) increase release of or inhibit reuptake or degradation of catecholamines and cause diffuse activation of adrenoceptors. Typically, α$_1$ and β$_1$ effects predominate, resulting

TABLE 21-2 Selected Causes of Acquired Long QT Syndrome

Antiarrhythmic drugs
  Type Ia—quinidine, disopyramide, procainamide
  Type III—sotalol, amiodarone
Antibiotics
  Macrolides—erythromycin, clarithromycin
  Pentamidine
  Sparfloxacin, grepafloxacin*
Histamine receptor antagonists
  Terfenadine,* astemizole*
Psychiatric drugs
  Neuroleptics (thioridazine, mesoridazine, and other phenothiazines; haloperidol)
Cholinergic agonists
  Cisapride, organophosphates
Toxins
  Arsenic, fluoride
Plants and herbals
  Aconitine
Metabolic conditions
  Hypokalemia, hypomagnesemia, hypocalcemia

*Withdrawn from U.S. markets.
Modified from Viskin S: Long QT syndromes and torsades de pointes. Lancet 354:1629, 1999.

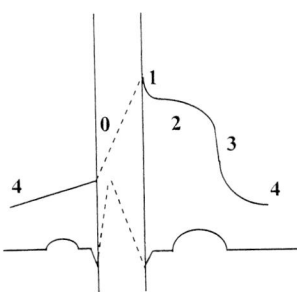

FIGURE 21-7

Cardiac action potential showing that when sodium channels are blocked, the rate or rise of phase 0 is decreased corresponding to a widening of the QRS complex on the electrocardiogram. *(From Haddad LM, Shannon MW, Winchester JF, et al: Clinical Management of Poisoning and Drug Overdose, 3rd ed. Philadelphia, 1998, WB Saunders Company.)*

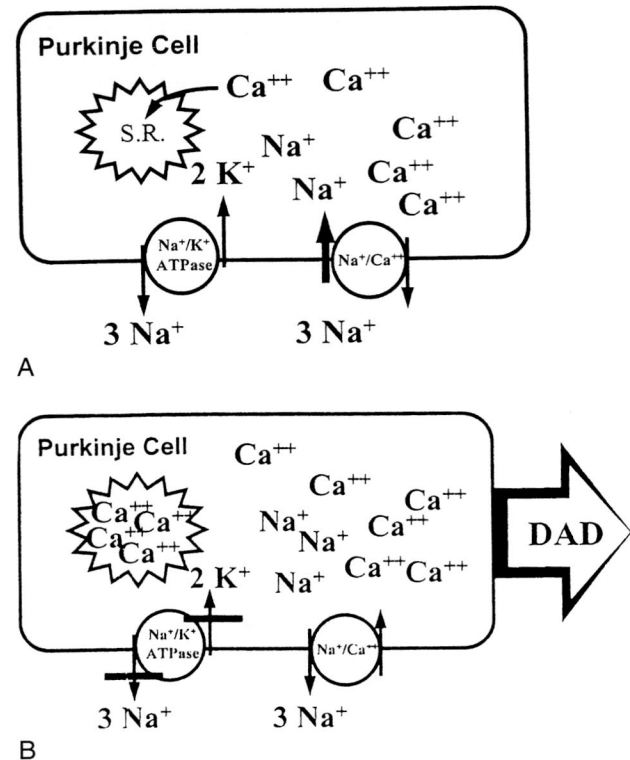

FIGURE 21-8

A, The inhibition of the Na^+,K^+-ATPase pump leads to an increase of intracellular Na^+, which leads to an exchange of Na^+ for Ca^+ via the Na^+-Ca^+ pump. The excess Ca^+ is sequestered in the sarcoplasmic reticulum (S.R.). **B**, With continuing Ca^+ overload of the cell, the S.R. is unable to compensate by sequestration, and the internal charge begins to increase, leading to delayed afterdepolarization (DAD) formation. *(From Haddad LM, Shannon MW, Winchester JF, et al: Clinical Management of Poisoning and Drug Overdose, 3rd ed. Philadelphia, 1998, WB Saunders Company.)*

β_2-adrenoceptors on the peripheral vasculature causes vasodilation, whereas activation of cardiac β_2-adrenoceptor increases ventricular contractility.[16]

α-ADRENOCEPTORS

In poisoning, clinically significant toxicity involves activation of the α_1-adrenoceptor subtype in arterial vasculature and α_2-adrenoceptor subtype activation in the brainstem. *α_1 activation* results in elevated intracellular calcium levels and subsequent arterial constriction with a rise in blood pressure. *Central α_2 agonism* decreases cAMP levels and inhibits sympathetic output, increases parasympathetic output, and produces sedation (see Fig. 21-3). *α_1-Antagonist activity* results in decreased intracellular calcium with subsequent arteriolar relaxation and hypotension (see Fig. 21-3).

Cholinergic Receptors

Acetylcholinesterase is the enzyme responsible for degradation of acetylcholine. Toxins (i.e., organophosphates) that inhibit acetylcholinesterase result in elevated acetylcholine concentrations at muscarinic and nicotinic receptors. A variety of sympathetic and parasympathetic signs and symptoms may be present after toxicity (see Fig. 21-3).

NICOTINIC RECEPTORS

Cardiovascular toxicity can occur from agonist activity at the ganglionic nicotinic receptor. Although these receptors are present on parasympathetic and sympathetic postganglionic fibers, toxicity is manifested initially by predominantly sympathetic stimulation. With higher doses, parasympathetic stimulation and neuromuscular blockade are seen. Aside from nicotine poisoning, overdose from direct nicotinic agonists or antagonists is unusual.

MUSCARINIC RECEPTORS

Stimulation of the muscarinic receptor on the myocardium causes decrease in SA node excitability and AV node conduction, resulting in sinus bradycardia and varying degrees of AV block (see Fig. 21-3). *Inhibition* of the cardiac muscarinic receptors prevents acetylcholine from binding to the

in hypertension and tachyarrhythmias (see Fig. 21-3). β_1-Adrenoceptor blockade decreases cAMP and subsequently blunts chronotropic, dromotropic, and inotropic effects of endogenous and exogenous catecholamines. Activation of

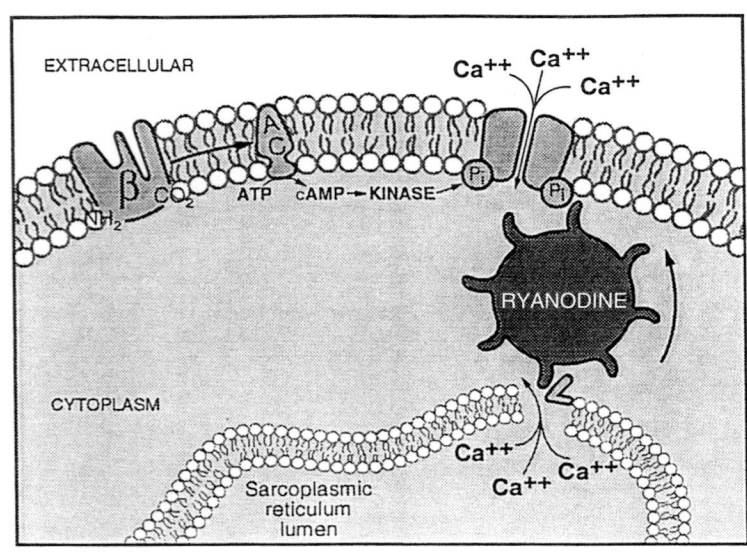

FIGURE 21-9

Schematic overview of Ca^{2+} homeostasis during myocardial contraction. The β-adrenergic receptor (β), when stimulated, increases adenylate cyclase activity (AC), leading to activation of kinases that phosphorylate the L-channel, increasing Ca^{2+} entry. Ryanodine is the receptor that couples plasmalemmal Ca^{2+} currents to the sarcoplasmic reticulum, allowing release of intracellular pools of Ca^{2+}.

receptors, reducing parasympathetic restraint of heart rate and resulting in unopposed sympathetic stimulation. This stimulation causes a modest sinus tachycardia with heart rate generally less than 150 beats/min and a modest rise in blood pressure due to increased cardiac output (see Fig. 21-3).

Altered Central Autonomic Nervous System Activity

Many toxins suppress or enhance ANS activity through the central nervous system (CNS) and subsequently result in peripheral cardiovascular effects. Poisoning from clonidine, a central α_2-agonist, often results in reduced CNS-mediated sympathetic activity and increased parasympathetic tone, causing a decrease in heart rate. Conversely, many CNS stimulants (e.g., cocaine and amphetamines) cause an increase in CNS-mediated sympathetic tone, resulting in tachycardia and hypertension. In a healthy heart, sympathetic stimulation can increase cardiac output twofold to threefold.

Systemic Influences

Many critically poisoned patients have coexisting systemic factors that further influence and exacerbate cardiotoxicity. Hemodynamic changes resulting from hypovolemia, fever, electrolyte abnormalities, acidosis, and hypoxia also must be taken into consideration and corrected.

CLINICAL MANIFESTATIONS OF TOXIC EFFECTS: CARDIAC ARRHYTHMIAS AND CONDUCTION ABNORMALITIES

This section discusses the recognition of cardiac arrhythmias, conduction abnormalities, and specific ECG findings that might help the clinician narrow the differential diagnosis in an unknown overdose. Because most conduction abnormalities are accompanied by abnormalities in heart rate, our clinical approach to a patient begins with categorizing them as having bradycardia or tachycardia. Some toxins cause conduction disturbances without rate alteration and are considered separately.

Bradycardia

As outlined in Figure 21-10, our approach to the diagnosis and management of bradycardia begins by classifying the patient into two broad categories, based on ECG findings and perfusion status. Similarly, we separate cardiodepressant drugs into two categories based on how they impair cardiovascular parameters. Drugs may have *indirect* effects on the cardiovascular system, such as altering autonomic output or causing reflex changes in heart rate (i.e., γ-hydroxybutyrate or phenylpropanolamine). Other drugs depress cardiovascular parameters by *directly* interacting with myocardial membranes and receptors (i.e., calcium channel blockers and β-blockers).

BRADYCARDIA WITH CONDUCTION ABNORMALITY OR HYPOPERFUSION

Agents (e.g., calcium channel blockers) that *directly* inhibit conduction and decrease contractility generally present with more profound ECG abnormalities and cardiovascular

instability than agents with *indirect toxicity*. Bradyarrhythmias and hypotension are the hallmark of these toxins. Mild sinus bradycardia may be the only ECG abnormality despite clinical findings of hypoperfusion (see Fig. 21-10). Hypotension in these cases is evidence for depressed contractility from a direct myocardial toxin or vasodilation as opposed to rate-related shock. High-degree heart block (Mobitz II or third-degree AV block), sinus arrest with AV junctional or ventricular escape rhythm, widening of QRS, and asystole also suggest the presence of a direct myocardial toxin. Some agents that cause these bradyarrhythmias (e.g., type IA antiarrhythmics, cardiac glycosides) predispose the patient to ventricular tachyarrhythmias through reentry mechanism or delayed ADs.

BRADYCARDIA WITHOUT CONDUCTION ABNORMALITIES OR HYPOPERFUSION

Patients who present with sinus bradycardia with first-degree or Wenckebach AV block may be manifesting signs of early poisoning from a direct myocardial toxin. More often, these findings suggest drugs and toxins with indirect toxicity that results in less myocardial depression and hemodynamic instability than direct effects on the conduction system. Most indirectly acting cardiodepressants either decrease sympathetic tone or increase parasympathetic tone, typically with heart rates of 40 to 60 beats/min, without causing severe hypoperfusion (see Fig. 21-10). Higher grades of AV block are seen infrequently.

TREATMENT

The goal of management in a patient with symptomatic bradycardia from an unknown poisoning is to improve perfusion by increasing cardiac output and reversing vasodilation. Treatment should focus on increasing heart rate if rate-related dysfunction is suspected or improving inotropy if myocardial contractility is impaired. Atropine and pacing should be initiated and generally are sufficient for indirectly acting cardiodepressants but may be ineffective in management of bradycardia associated with direct toxins. With severe intoxication, heart block or asystole sometimes is associated with an inability to generate an impulse even with high-voltage pacing.[17]

If hypotension is present despite normal or increased heart rate or in association with high-grade AV block, the clinician should assume contractile dysfunction and initiate treatment with crystalloid fluids and an inotropic agent. Epinephrine, dopamine, or norepinephrine should be started and titrated to a dose that restores perfusion. Glucagon has increased rate and contractility successfully in poisonings from β-blocker, calcium channel blocker, and severe tricyclic antidepressant (TCA) poisoning.[18] Isoproterenol also may be used for unresponsive sinus, junctional, or ventricular bradycardia. If the ECG reveals a wide QRS, sodium bicarbonate boluses should be considered to reverse the effects of cardiotoxins on fast sodium channels (see Table 21-1). If appropriate, toxin-specific therapy, such as calcium (for negative inotropic effects of calcium channel blockers) and digoxin antibodies, should be instituted. Electrolyte abnormalities, hypoxia, and acidosis should be corrected because they may contribute to failure of pacing stimulus to depolarize cardiac cells.

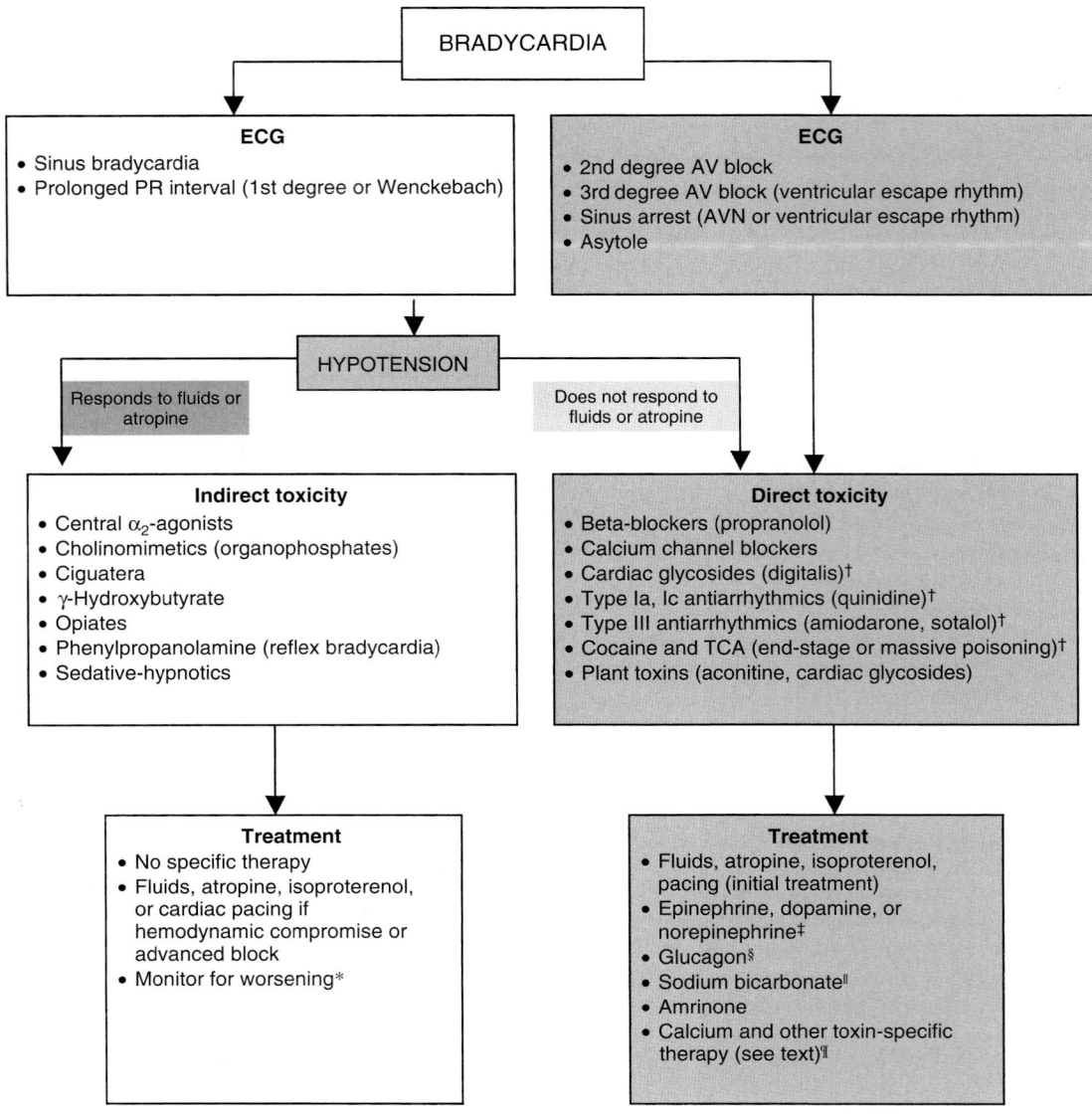

FIGURE 21-10

Algorithm for determining causes and management of bradycardia.

*Toxins with potential for direct toxicity may manifest only mild signs early in the course of poisoning.

†Agents also may cause tachyarrhythmias (see Table 21-4).

‡If low systemic vascular resistance.

§Glucagon is particularly helpful for β-blocker poisoning.

‖If signs of membrane depression.

¶Helpful in suspected calcium channel overdose; may be harmful in digoxin overdose.

Tachycardia

Our analysis of tachyarrhythmias in poisoned patients begins by classifying them into a wide-complex versus a narrow-complex rhythm. This distinction serves two primary purposes. First, it allows the clinician to narrow the differential diagnosis to a group of toxins responsible for the arrhythmia (Table 21-3). Second, the clinician can use the classification scheme to decide on initial therapy concomitant with an attempt to establish the diagnosis.

WIDE-COMPLEX TACHYCARDIA

Monomorphic tachycardia of uncertain origin, polymorphic ventricular tachycardia (PVT), and bidirectional ventricular tachycardia (VT) are three types of wide-complex tachycardia (WCT) that are encountered in poisoned patients. When the patient is hemodynamically stable, therapy varies for the three types of WCT. This discussion begins with ways to identify the WCT. Subsequently, we present treatment options for each of the WCTs.

Monomorphic Wide-Complex Tachycardia. When an ECG reveals a wide-complex QRS with a uniform morphology and a constant RR interval, the two common entities to consider are VT and supraventricular tachyarrhythmia (SVT) with intraventricular conduction delay. Although implementing the optimal therapy can be facilitated greatly if VT is distinguished from SVT (Fig. 21-11), previous studies in the general

TABLE 21-3 Differential Diagnosis of Drug-Induced or Toxin-Induced Tachyarrhythmias

NARROW-COMPLEX TACHYARRHYTHMIAS	WIDE-COMPLEX TACHYARRHYTHMIAS
Anticholinergic	Antiarrhythmics (type Ia, Ic, III)‡
Amantadine	Antihistamines‡
Antihistamines*	Arsenic‡
Atropine, belladonna, scopolamine	Carbamazepine
Cyclic antidepressants*	Cardiac glycosides
Mushrooms (e.g., *Amanita muscaria*)	Chloral hydrate
Neuroleptics (thioridazine* and mesoridazine*	Cocaine
also are membrane depressants)	Cyclic antidepressants
Plants (e.g., Jimson weed)	Sodium fluoride‡
	Freon (and other fluorocarbon aerosols)
Sympathomimetic	Hydrocarbon solvents
Amphetamines and their congeners (e.g., Ecstasy)	Neuroleptics (thioridazine, mesoridazine)‡
Caffeine	Propoxyphene
Chloral hydrate*	Quinine and related agents‡
Cocaine*	Theophylline
Ethanol	
Ephedrine and pseudoephedrine	**ECG**
Lysergic acid diethylamide (LSD) and other	VT (monomorphic or polymorphic)
hallucinogens	VF
Monoamine oxidase inhibitors	
Phencyclidine	*ECG Signs Preceding VF/VT*
Scorpion or spider envenomation	Supraventricular tachyarrhythmias
Sedative-hypnotic withdrawal	Intraventricular conduction delay (QRS
Selective serotonin reuptake inhibitors	prolongation)
Theophylline*	R wave elevation lead AVR
	Rightward deviation of QRS axis
Cholinomimetic	QT prolongation (see Table 21-2)
Organophosphates	
	Treatment
ECG	See treatment algorithm (Fig. 21-12)
Sinus tachycardia	
Supraventricular tachycardia (normal conduction)	
Treatment	
No specific therapy	
Correct hypotension, hypoxia, or electrolyte abnormalities	
If hemodynamic compromise and sympathomimetic	
poisoning: physostigmine†	

*Any supraventricular arrhythmia can deteriorate to a ventricular arrhythmia, but this occurs more frequently with these agents.
†Contraindicated if suspicion of membrane-depressant drug overdose.
‡Agents that can cause torsades de pointes and monomorphic VT.
ECG, electrocardiogram; VF, ventricular fibrillation; VT, ventricular tachycardia.

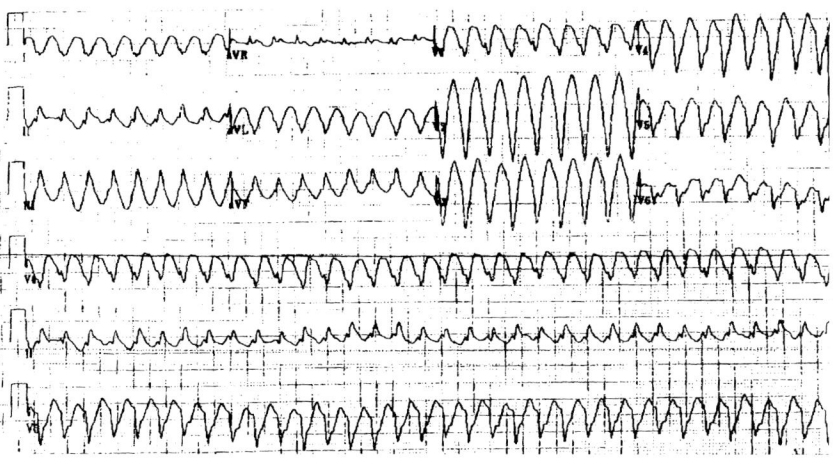

FIGURE 21-11

Electrocardiogram (ECG) from a 53-year-old woman who ingested unknown quantities of a tricyclic antidepressant. The patient had a sustained wide-complex tachycardia with a normal blood pressure despite receiving multiple ampules of sodium bicarbonate boluses and a lidocaine drip. After 17 hours in this rhythm, sinus tachycardia returned spontaneously, and the patient fully recovered without any specific interventions. This ECG was interpreted as ventricular tachycardia by two separate cardiologists.

population with WCT have shown that even experienced physicians have difficulty in differentiating VT from SVT.[19] Hemodynamic stability or instability cannot be used to determine between the two arrhythmias.[20] In poisoned patients with a monomorphic WCT, initially it is safer to assume and treat as if the arrhythmia is VT (see later). When initial treatment measures have been instituted and the patient is hemodynamically stable, attempts to differentiate between VT and SVT may be considered. In a hemodynamically stable patient, carotid sinus massage or another vagal maneuver can be applied and may indicate a supraventricular arrhythmia when it abolishes the rhythm or slows the rate. Certain key ECG features suggest VT, and these are listed in Table 21-4. These features have not been validated in poisoned patients. Adenosine may provide useful diagnostic information in patients with WCT of uncertain origin.[21] Table 21-3 lists toxic causes of WCT, and the later section on specific toxins discusses those that are commonly encountered in poisoning.

Treatment. Figure 21-12 is a modified advanced cardiac life support (ACLS) algorithm for managing a patient with a WCT secondary to poisoning. Because many overdoses resulting in a WCT are due to fast sodium channel inhibition, an important modification to the treatment algorithm involves the contraindication of type Ia and Ic antiarrhythmics (e.g., procainamide) and the introduction of sodium bicarbonate bolus therapy. The clinical status should dictate the initial method of treatment for the WCT. When associated with hemodynamic compromise, angina, or cerebral insufficiency, immediate termination of the arrhythmia should be attempted with direct current cardioversion and intravenous sodium bicarbonate. The patient who is clinically stable should be treated with sodium bicarbonate and antiarrhythmic therapy. Lidocaine is usually the antiarrhythmic of choice in this setting. Sodium bicarbonate has emerged to be the first line of treatment for membrane depression from TCA poisoning and other agents with fast sodium channel blockade activity (see Table 21-1).[22] Sodium bicarbonate is believed to be beneficial as a result of increasing extracellular sodium, increasing extracellular pH, and lowering extracellular potassium, all of which attenuate the effects of TCA and other fast sodium channel blockers.[23–25]

When these initial stabilizing measures have been implemented, further attempts to differentiate the cause of WCT should be undertaken so that toxin-specific therapy can be administered (e.g., digitalis antibodies for digitalis

overdose). Calcium channel blockers and β-blockers are contraindicated in WCTs of uncertain etiology because their vasodilatory or myocardial-depressant effects may cause sudden cardiovascular collapse. If pharmacologic therapy is unsuccessful, sustained WCT, especially with a rate greater than 150 beats/min, should be treated with electrical cardioversion.

ACLS guidelines recommend amiodarone before lidocaine for the treatment of stable WCT. Other than in two case reports and a case series, the use of amiodarone has not been studied in poisoned patients.[26–28] In a small case series in which 13 of 17 patients with aconite poisoning had ventricular tachyarrhythmias, amiodarone suppressed VT in the 5 patients in whom it was used.[28] Lidocaine was used in 11 patients and was ineffective in all cases. Another case report described the return of sinus rhythm after use of amiodarone in a 17-year-old patient who had cardiac arrest secondary to butane abuse. As part of the ACLS protocol, high doses of epinephrine, bicarbonate, lidocaine, and electrical cardioversion were tried unsuccessfully for 40 minutes before use of amiodarone. The patient subsequently made a full recovery.[27]

Because of the lack of experience with the use of amiodarone in poisoned patients, lidocaine should be tried first in arrhythmias related to drug overdose or poisoning. Amiodarone still may be considered for recalcitrant arrhythmias. Hypotension and bradycardia are the major adverse effects from amiodarone and are related to the rate of infusion. These adverse effects should be taken into consideration before its use in poisoned patients.

Polymorphic Ventricular Tachycardia. With PVT, the ECG reveals a WCT with beat-to-beat variation in the QRS morphology and RR interval (Fig. 21-13). The pathophysiology of PVT, as discussed earlier, is different from monomorphic VT, and consequently therapeutic options differ. PVT often occurs in the setting of a prolonged QT_c interval, in which case it is referred to as TdP.

Agents that cause TdP typically lengthen repolarization as evidenced by prolongation of QT_c interval and appearance of U waves on the ECG (see Fig. 21-13). These ECG changes represent early ADs. Although QT_c greater than 600 msec after drug exposure may place the patient at higher risk for TdP, the arrhythmia can occur at shorter QT_c intervals as well.[6] These arrhythmias often are associated with and precipitated by pauses due to sinus bradyarrhythmia or sinus arrest or a pause after a premature beat, because bradycardias enhance the ADs. Factors that are predictive of TdP in the setting of a prolonged QT_c interval are the presence of "warning signs," such as giant U waves, ventricular bigeminy, pause-dependent lengthening or enhancement of T-U wave, extrasystoles, and bradyarrhythmias.[6] Ventricular bigeminy with drug-induced prolonged QT_c interval has been called impending torsades.[6]

Treatment. If TdP is sustained and causes hemodynamic compromise, it should be treated primarily with electrical cardioversion. In general, treatment of TdP or prolonged QT_c with the above-mentioned warning signs is directed at suppression of early AD and acceleration of heart rate. Most often, the arrhythmia is not sustained and terminates spontaneously. The challenge lies, however, in prevention of its recurrence. TdP should be treated initially with a rapid bolus

---

TABLE 21-4 Electrocardiogram Features Strongly Suggestive of Ventricular Tachycardia*

Atrioventricular dissociation
QRS morphology
    Upgoing in V1: qR, RR' (R taller than R'), R
    Downgoing in V6: rS, QS
    5/6 or 6/6 V leads positively or negatively concordant
    Fusion beats or capture beats
    Frontal plan QRS axis −90 to −180 (northwest or right upper quadrant)
    Identical to previous PVC

*These criteria have not been validated in ventricular tachycardia associated with poisoning.
PVC, premature ventricular contraction.

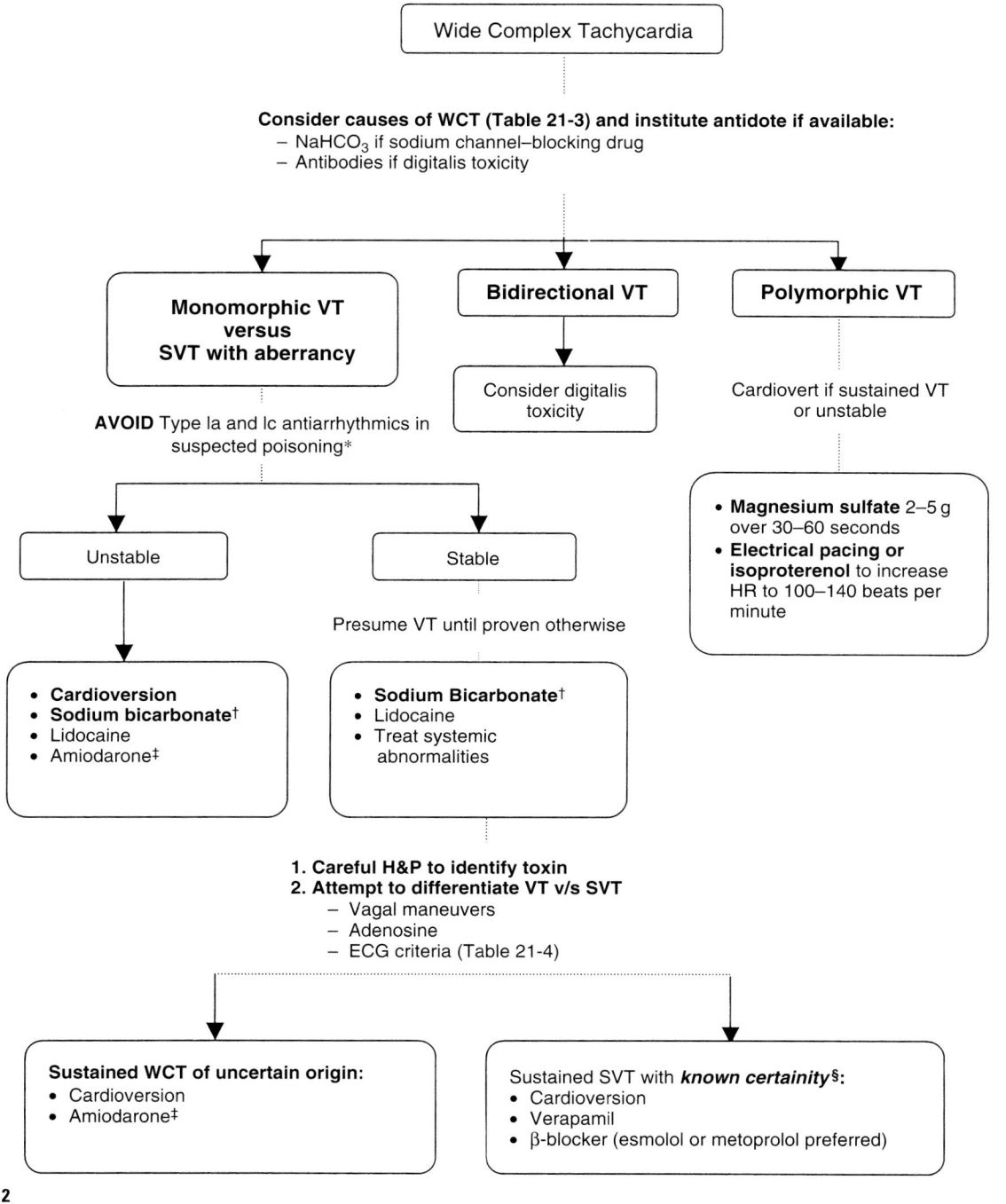

FIGURE 21-12

Algorithm for management of wide-complex tachycardia (WCT) of uncertain origin in poisoining and drug overdose.
*Quinidine, procainamide, disopyramide, flecainide, and propafenone.
†Unless contraindicated by pH greater than 7.55, cerebral edema, or severe hypokalemia.
‡Use for refractory ventricular arrhythmias, but may worsen hypotension in poisoned patients.
§Strongly recommend use of a cardiology consultant or esophageal lead confirmation of atrial rhythm before use of calcium channel blockers, β-blockers, or digitalis in WCT.
ECG, electrocardiogram; H & P, history and physical examination; HR, heart rate; NaHCO₃, sodium bicarbonate; SVT, supraventricular tachycardia; v/s, versus; VT, ventricular tachycardia.

of magnesium sulfate (2 to 5 g over 30 to 60 seconds), which decreases the amplitude of early AD and suppresses triggered rhythms. Treatment with a slower infusion of 2 g over 2 minutes should be considered in the presence of the warning signs (especially bigeminy) with a prolonged QT_c on ECG.[5,29] Recurrent warning signs or arrhythmias can be treated with a second bolus in 5 to 15 minutes and, if necessary, a maintenance infusion at 3 to 10 mg/min.

Bradycardia is associated with a more pronounced AD, and because toxin-induced TdP is pause dependent, increasing the heart rate generally suppresses the AD and the emergence of TdP. If magnesium sulfate is ineffective or

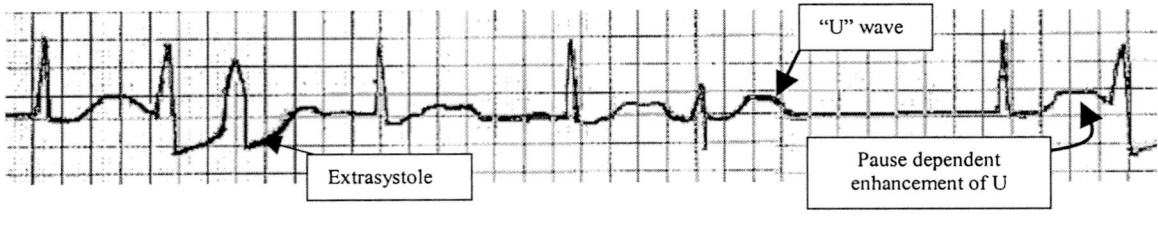

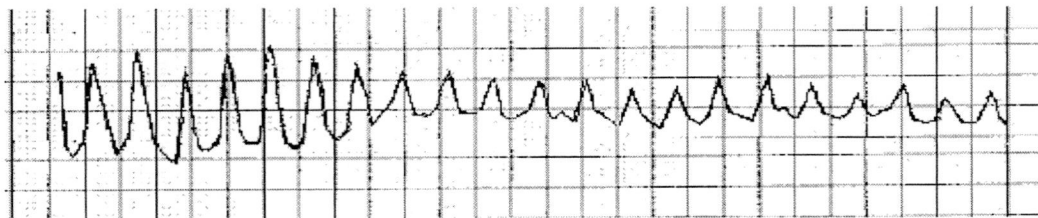

FIGURE 21-13

Electrocardiogram (ECG) from a 63-year-old woman who had ingested unknown amounts of thioridazine. She presented with sinus bradycardia at a rate of 20 to 50 beats/min and hypotension requiring atropine and dopamine. Six hours after ingestion, she developed several episodes of torsades de pointes (TdP) shown in the lower panel, which was preceded by the strip in the upper panel. (*Note the presence of "warning signs" of TdP discussed in the text*: giant U waves, bradycardia, extrasystoles, and pause-dependent enhancement of T-U wave). The patient was cardioverted and subsequently placed on an isoproterenol drip, and the ECG eventually became normal without any further episodes of TdP.

bradyarrhythmias occur, electrical pacing should be instituted to accelerate the heart rate or shorten the QT interval. If pacing is unavailable, isoproterenol (1 to 4 μg/min) may be used to accelerate the heart rate. A rate of 100 to 140 beats/min usually abolishes or prevents emergence of TdP, at which point the pacing rate should be decreased to the lowest rate that abolishes ventricular ectopy (usually 80 to 100 beats/min). Hypokalemia can exacerbate TdP, and potassium supplementation, even in normokalemic patients with drug-induced prolonged QT_c, has been shown to normalize repolarization abnormalities.[29,30] Serum potassium should be checked and maintained in the high-normal range (4.5 mEq/L) in patients at risk for TdP.[30]

Bidirectional Ventricular Tachycardia. ECG findings reveal a tachycardia with a wide QRS morphology that usually is alternating in direction with a constant RR interval (Fig. 21-14). A rare arrhythmia, bidirectional VT is almost pathognomonic for digitalis toxicity and should be treated with digoxin-specific antibodies.[31]

NARROW-COMPLEX TACHYCARDIA

Narrow-complex sinus tachycardia is probably the most common arrhythmia seen in poisoned patients. Sympathomimetic and anticholinergic drugs are the most common causes of supraventricular arrhythmias in poisoning, although other indirect influences, such as fever, hypoxia, hypovolemia, and agitation, often contribute to toxicity. Toxin-induced SVTs generally resolve with supportive care. Some toxins that induce tachycardia also possess membrane-depressant properties with a potential to cause myocardial depression (Figs. 21-15 and 21-16). The clinician can risk stratify these patients by assessing the ECG for conduction abnormalities. Impaired conduction in the His-Purkinje system resulting in QRS widening greater than 100 msec or rightward deviation of the terminal 40-msec frontal plane QRS vector (130 to 270 degrees) suggests significant cardiotoxicity and is predictive of seizures from TCA poisoning (see Fig. 21-15).[32,33] A positive deflection greater than 3 mm of the terminal portion of lead aVR (R') also is a significant predictor of seizures or arrhythmias in TCA poisoning (Fig. 21-17).[34] Although these ECG findings in poisoning most commonly suggest TCA involvement, similar intraventricular conduction delay is evident with other toxins that impede fast sodium channels (see Table 21-1).[35] The clinician should suspect digitalis toxicity in any patient with an atrial tachycardia and AV block (usually 2:1 AV block). Digitalis is well known to increase automaticity and cause AV nodal conduction blockade.

Treatment. Supportive therapy and cardiac monitoring usually are sufficient for a patient with narrow-complex tachycardia, because tachycardia frequently subsides when the offending agent is eliminated. Hypovolemia, fever, and hypoxia can exacerbate tachyarrhythmias in poisoned patients and should be corrected. Pharmacologic therapy or electrical cardioversion usually is reserved for SVTs or tachyarrhythmias associated with hemodynamic compromise, angina, or cerebrovascular insufficiency. When treatment is warranted for a narrow-complex supraventricular arrhythmia and the toxin is unknown, one option is to use a relatively specific and

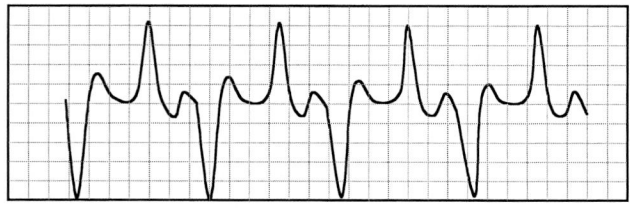

FIGURE 21-14

Bidirectional ventricular tachycardia suggestive of digitalis toxicity.

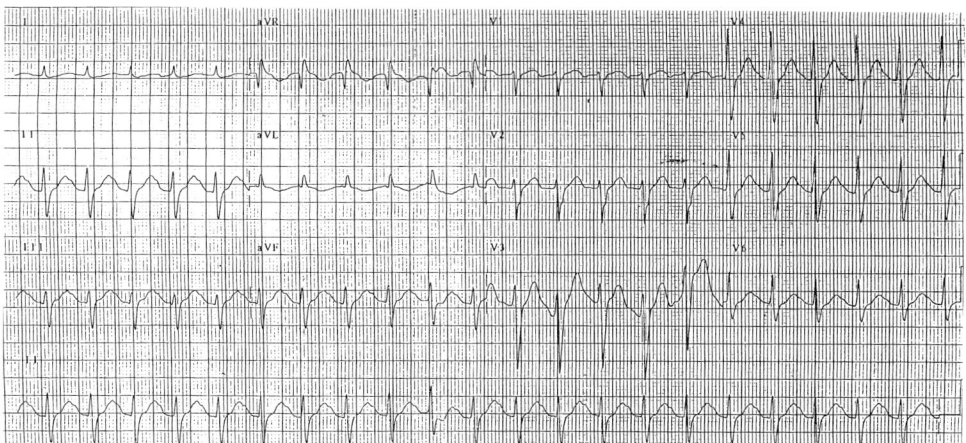

FIGURE 21-15

Electrocardiogram (ECG) from a 39-year-old man after a tricyclic antidepressant overdose. The ECG shows signs of impaired conduction in the His-Purkinje system: QRS widening greater than 100 msec and rightward deviation of the terminal 40-msec frontal plane QRS vector (aVR). In the presence of tricyclic antidepressant overdose, these ECG findings suggest significant cardiotoxicity.

short-acting β_1-selective blocker, such as esmolol, because many arrhythmias are a result of excess sympathetic activity. Arrhythmias from stimulant abuse (i.e., cocaine, amphetamines) are predominantly β-adrenergic receptor mediated, and a β-blocking agent is preferred. A nonselective β-blocking drug (i.e., propranolol) could worsen vasoconstriction, however, by antagonizing β_2-mediated vasodilation, resulting in unopposed α effects and aggravation of hypertension.[36] The use of esmolol or metoprolol may help avoid these deleterious effects owing to their β_1-receptor selectivity.[37] β-Blocking agents also are preferred for treating tachyarrhythmias from theophylline toxicity, but they may worsen airway obstruction. Esmolol and metoprolol are safer in such situations. If anticholinergic poisoning is suspected and is associated with hemodynamic instability, β-blockers or physostigmine may be used. Physostigmine, a cholinesterase inhibitor, increases acetylcholine at the neuronal junction, reversing anticholiner-

gic toxicity. Physostigmine and β-blockers should be used only in the absence of any AV conduction inhibition because they may result in worsening AV block, bradycardia, and asystole. Evidence of fast sodium channel blockade on the ECG should be treated with sodium bicarbonate bolus therapy as discussed earlier in the section on WCT and TCA poisoning.

SPECIFIC TOXINS

Poisonings may result in cardiotoxicity by a variety of mechanisms. To facilitate diagnosis, we categorize the toxins based on manifestations of cardiotoxicity, specifically bradyarrhythmias, tachyarrhythmias, or both. Some poisoned patients also may have abnormalities in conduction without any abnormalities in rate, but the principles of treatment remain the same.

Drugs Causing Bradyarrhythmias

β-ADRENERGIC RECEPTOR BLOCKERS

β-Adrenergic receptor blockers, with the exception of pindolol, cause cardiac disturbances as a result of β-receptor blockade and typically present with sinus bradycardia and varying degrees of AV block in patients with healthy hearts. Junctional and slow ventricular escape rhythms (heart rate 20 to

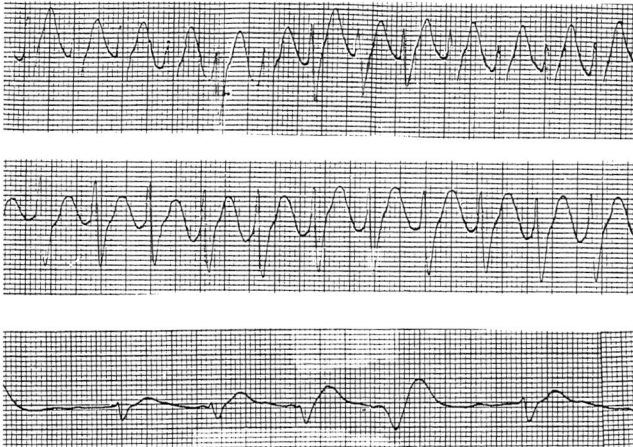

FIGURE 21-16

Electrocardiogram (ECG) from a 39-year-old man after a tricyclic antidepressant overdose (Fig. 21-15 was the presenting ECG). ECG changes associated with progressively impaired conduction in the setting of an untreated tricyclic antidepressant overdose are shown. QRS width was 120 msec in the upper strip, which was recorded after the patient had his first seizure. The middle strip reveals a QRS of 160 msec and was recorded 134 minutes later, immediately after the second seizure. The lower strip was recorded 60 minutes later, after the fourth seizure, in the radiology suite where the patient was undergoing a cranial computed tomography scan. Subsequently the patient experienced a cardiac arrest, and efforts at resuscitation were unsuccessful.

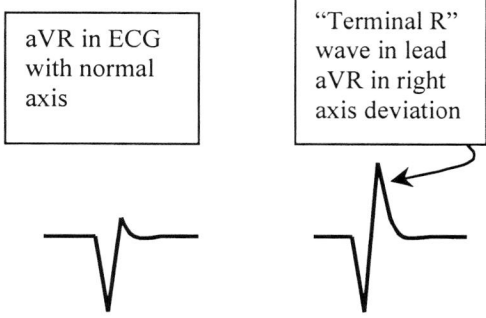

FIGURE 21-17

A positive deflection greater than 3 mm of the terminal portion of lead aVR (R'), frequently called a *terminal R*, is a significant predictor of seizures or arrhythmias in tricyclic antidepressant poisoning. Similar intraventricular conduction delay suggests presence of a fast sodium channel blocker in a poisoned patient.

40 beats/min) are seen in patients with underlying conduction disease or with massive overdose. Hypotension, shock, and pulmonary edema resulting from myocardial depression can be seen in any severe β-blocker poisoning, but they are more likely in patients with diseased myocardium that depends on sympathetic activity for contractility. Certain β-receptor–blocking drugs have membrane-depressant (acebutolol, pindolol, and propranolol) or sympathomimetic activity (acebutolol and pindolol) that contributes to toxicity.[38] β-Receptor–blocking agents with membrane-depressant effects can cause myocardial depression and conduction system abnormalities resulting in widening of QRS and hypotension.[39] Sotalol, which has type III antiarrhythmic activity, prolongs the QT interval in a dose-dependent manner and may cause TdP and ventricular fibrillation.

Crystalloid fluids, atropine, and cardiac pacing should be administered initially to patients with bradycardia and hypotension. Glucagon has been the most consistently useful agent in treating severe β-blocker poisonings (Fig. 21-18).[18,40] Glucagon activates adenylate cyclase by a non–β-receptor mechanism, enhancing heart rate and myocardial contractility. Epinephrine, dopamine, and isoproterenol also have been used successfully in β-blocker poisoning.[17,41]

CALCIUM CHANNEL BLOCKERS

The hallmark of poisoning by verapamil and diltiazem is myocardial depression and hypotension.[11] Sinus bradycardia, varying degrees of AV block, sinus arrest with AV junctional rhythm, and asystole may be seen (see Fig. 21-18).[42,43] Nifedipine and other dihydropyridines predominantly cause a reflex tachycardia, but with severe poisoning they also may reduce myocardial contractility and produce bradycardia.[44]

No single treatment consistently reverses calcium channel blocker cardiotoxicity. Atropine, cardiac pacing, and crystalloids should be tried but are often ineffective.[45] Calcium chloride and calcium gluconate reverse the negative inotropic effects of calcium channel blocker toxicity but not AV blockade or peripheral vasodilation.[46,47] Even high doses of calcium may not be successful in reversing toxicity.[17,48,49] Glucagon and epinephrine have produced favorable results in some cases.[18,38] Evidence from animal studies and case series suggests that high doses of insulin with euglycemia may be a superior antidote to calcium, glucagon, and epinephrine and should be considered in recalcitrant or severe cases of calcium

channel blocker poisoning.[49,50] The source of energy for the myocardium is altered from free fatty acids to carbohydrates in calcium channel blocker poisoning. Calcium channel blockers also inhibit insulin release, leading to inadequate carbohydrate use by the myocardium, hyperglycemia, and acidosis. High doses of insulin with euglycemia enhances carbohydrate use and the clearance of lactate, improving myocardial contractility in calcium channel blocker poisoning.[50]

SEVERE COCAINE AND TRICYCLIC ANTIDEPRESSANT POISONING

Although cocaine and TCAs primarily cause tachyarrhythmias, severe toxicity may result in ventricular bradycardia with reduced cardiac output and hypotension (see Figs. 21-16 and 21-19). In addition to sodium bicarbonate, treatment should include cardiac pacing or isoproterenol in conjunction with pressors such as norepinephrine or dopamine.

Drugs Causing Tachyarrhythmias

AMPHETAMINES AND COCAINE

Amphetamine and many of its analogues release catecholamines from the presynaptic terminals, producing symptoms through direct stimulation of postsynaptic adrenergic receptors. Cocaine is a potent inhibitor of catecholamine reuptake, which results in increased levels and longer persistence of catecholamines at the adrenergic receptors. Sympathetic overactivity causing sinus or atrial tachycardia and hypertension are common cardiac findings after cocaine or amphetamine use. Compared with amphetamines, cocaine is associated more commonly with cardiovascular complications, such as acute myocardial infarction, myocardial necrosis, and dissecting aortic aneurysm.[51] Increased myocardial work in the presence of fixed coronary artery disease, vasospasm, or thrombosis may be responsible for myocardial infarction.[52–54] Patchy myocardial necrosis and contraction band necrosis as a result of intense catecholamine stimulation has been described with acute and chronic use of cocaine.[53,54] The focal areas of necrosis may form a substrate for arrhythmias, which may lead to sudden cardiac death. Myocarditis and cardiomyopathy also have been reported after acute and chronic use of amphetamines and cocaine. Additionally, high doses of cocaine may impede fast sodium channels, resulting in widening QRS, myocardial depression, and hypotension (Fig. 21-19).[25]

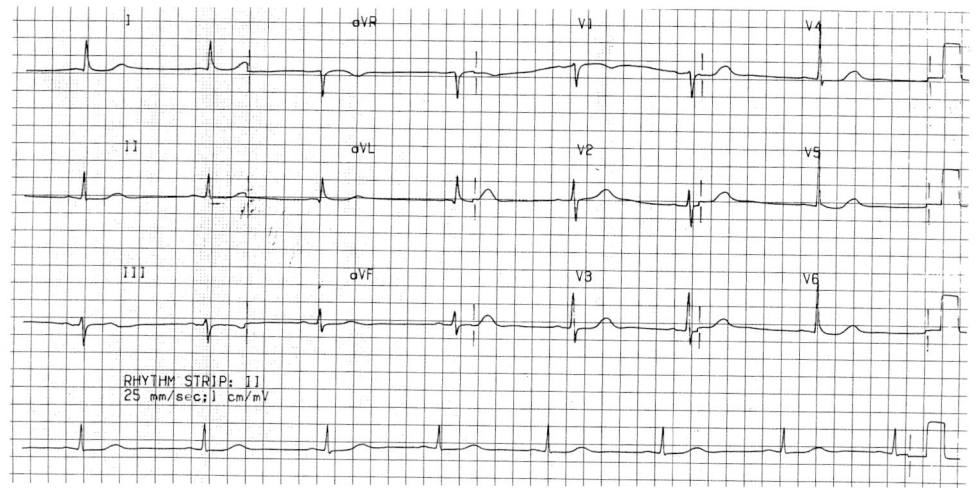

FIGURE 21-18

A 73-year-old woman presented with syncope and hypotension after accidentally ingesting three times her normal dose of atenolol. Her initial sinus bradycardia of 36 beats/min did not respond to atropine, and there was no capture with transcutaneous pacing. Glucagon, 3 mg intravenously followed by a 3 mg/hr drip, increased heart rate and blood pressure. Bradycardia and hypotension recurred over the next 8 hours with weaning of the glucagon infusion.

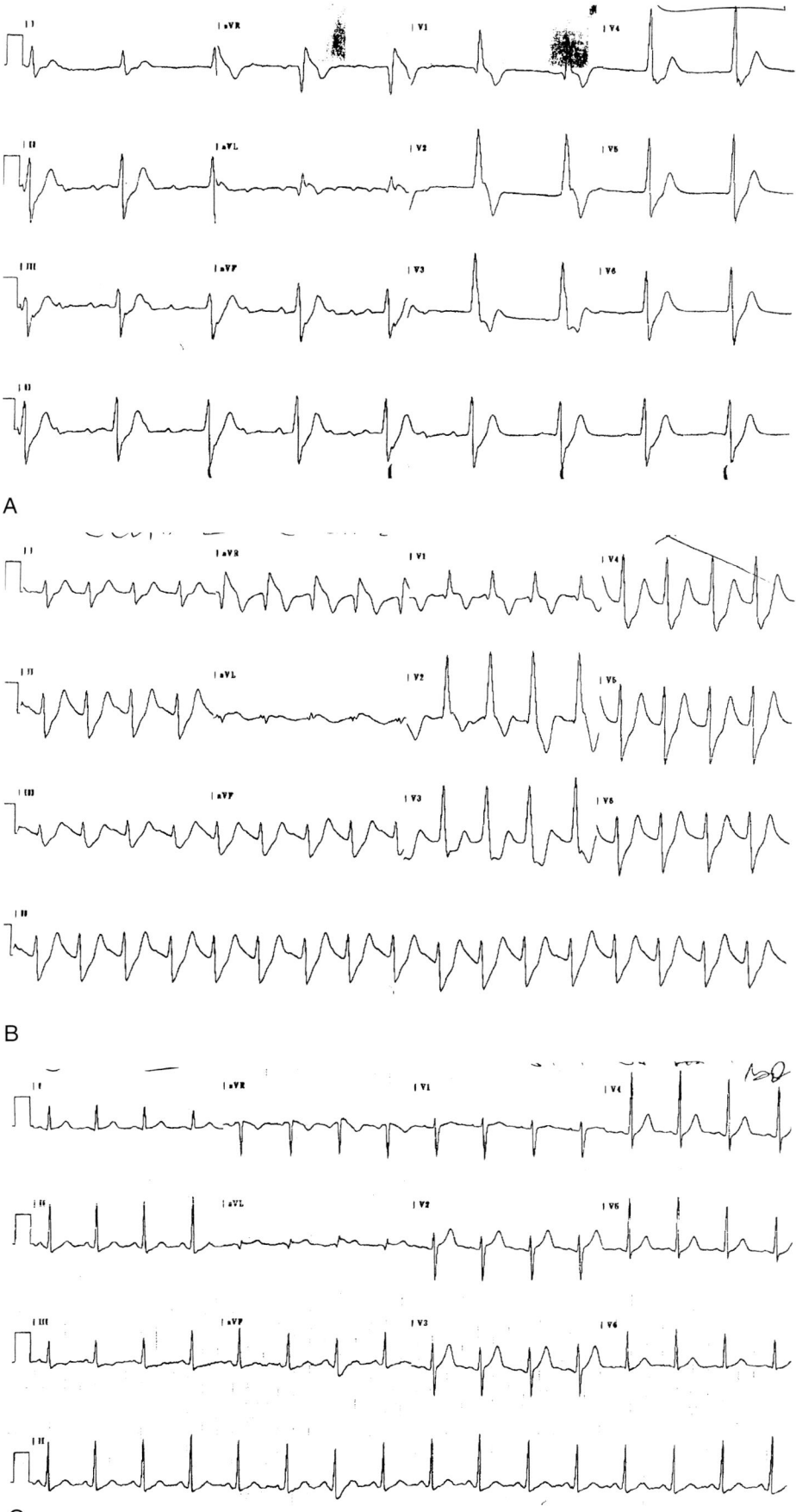

A

B

C

FIGURE 21-19

A 28-year-old man had a seizure in jail 1 hour after ingesting crack cocaine. The patient was asystolic when the medic arrived. **A**, The first electrocardiogram (ECG) was taken on presentation to the emergency department and showed atrioventricular dissociation. **B**, The second ECG revealed a QRS of 160 msec and a terminal R greater than 3 mm in lead aVR after intravenous fluids and 2 ampules of sodium bicarbonate. **C**, The third ECG showed sinus tachycardia with resolution of the conduction disturbances. It was recorded after 8 ampules of sodium bicarbonate over 3 hours with an improvement of arterial pH from 6.39 to 7.30. The patient recovered fully and was discharged after 5 days of hospitalization.

Management of cocaine and amphetamine intoxication should be directed toward specific cardiovascular manifestations.[37] Animal studies have shown benzodiazepines to reduce mortality from psychomotor agitation as a result of cocaine toxicity.[55] Benzodiazepines should be first-line therapy for treatment of agitation, tachycardia, and hypertension in these patients. Persistent severe hypertension or hypertension with end-organ damage can be treated with vasodilators, such as sodium nitroprusside or α- and β-blocking drugs. Treatment for arrhythmias has been discussed in a prior section.

ANTICHOLINERGICS

Anticholinergics competitively inhibit acetylcholine at its muscarinic receptor sites and produce the well-described anticholinergic syndrome. By blocking the cholinergic effects on the heart, these drugs cause sinus tachycardia with mild hypertension. Serious arrhythmias from anticholinergic agents are rare, unless patients have underlying cardiac disease (i.e., severe coronary artery disease with tachycardia-induced ischemia), or the ingested compound has other cardiotoxic properties in addition to muscarinic blockade. Common medications with anticholinergic effects that also cause conduction abnormalities in overdose include TCAs, phenothiazines, and antihistamines, all of which are discussed individually elsewhere in this book. Management of tachyarrhythmias from anticholinergic toxicity has been discussed previously.

ANTIHISTAMINES

Most antihistamines have some degree of anticholinergic activity and produce varying degrees of the anticholinergic syndrome after overdose. Additionally, other properties of these agents can cause primary cardiac disturbances. Fast sodium channel blockade may result in slowing of conduction and wide QRS, which should be treated similar to TCA poisoning. This condition has been reported most commonly with diphenhydramine. Two antihistaminic agents, terfenadine and astemizole, inhibit outward potassium currents, causing QT interval prolongation and occasionally TdP. This condition can occur if the parent compound builds up as a result of impaired metabolism secondary to hepatic dysfunction or drug interaction or in overdose. Although terfenadine and astemizole have been withdrawn from U.S. markets, they still are available in other countries. Management of prolonged QT interval and TdP is described elsewhere in this chapter.

TRICYCLIC ANTIDEPRESSANTS

Hypotension, tachyarrhythmias, and seizures are the most frequently encountered signs of toxicity from TCA poisoning.[56] Manifestations of toxicity are a result of various mechanisms, including anticholinergic properties, catecholamine reuptake inhibition, fast sodium channel blockade, and peripheral α_1-blockade.[57,58] Early in overdose, patients usually manifest sinus tachycardia as a result of anticholinergic effects and increased circulating catecholamines. With more severe poisoning, patients manifest signs of fast sodium channel blockade with impairment of conduction and myocardial depression. Peripheral α_1-blockade, depressed inotropy, and catecholamine depletion all may contribute to hypotension.

ECG changes often precede cardiovascular deterioration, and the ECG is used widely as a bedside tool in assessment and risk stratification of patients with possible TCA poisoning.[34] Aside from anticholinergic effects causing sinus tachycardia, most other ECG findings in TCA poisoning (e.g., wide QRS) result from fast sodium channel blockade and have been discussed in a prior section. Bundle-branch block, AV block, ventricular bradycardia, and asystole also may be seen with severe toxicity (see Fig. 21-16).[32] The absence of conduction inhibition does not rule out TCA poisoning because hypotension can occur with or without conduction inhibition.[59]

WCTs and intractable hypotension are the two most common reasons for death after TCA poisoning.[58] As described previously, manifestations of membrane depression that benefit from sodium bicarbonate include QRS widening greater than 100 to 120 msec, hypotension, and ventricular arrhythmias (see Fig. 21-16). Hyperventilation may be beneficial, but only transiently and only in cases in which sodium bicarbonate is not readily available or contraindicated (i.e., pulmonary edema).

Hypotension without evidence of conduction inhibition often can be treated with isotonic crystalloids.[58] If pressors are required, norepinephrine and dopamine are the recommended α-agonist agents. Profound cardiogenic shock with intractable hypotension is encountered occasionally in TCA poisoning and is associated with a high mortality. Intraaortic balloon pump or cardiopulmonary bypass may be the only means to stabilize these patients until their bodies can metabolize the TCA.[60]

In addition to TCAs, several other drugs possess "quinidine-like," membrane-depressant properties (see Table 21-1). Many of these other agents do not possess anticholinergic or sympathomimetic properties and do not manifest sinus tachycardia as with TCAs, cocaine, or antihistamines.

THEOPHYLLINE

Theophylline poisoning causes nonselective β-adrenergic stimulation through systemic and local catecholamine release. Additionally, at high concentrations, it inhibits phosphodiesterase, an enzyme that degrades cAMP, synergistically enhancing β-adrenergic stimulation. Cardiovascular manifestations of theophylline intoxication commonly include SVTs and VTs in addition to hypotension. Early in the course of poisoning, hypotension may be due to direct vasodilation, but prolonged catecholamine stimulation resulting in myocarditis and impaired contractility can occur later. Additionally, older patients with ischemic heart disease can have myocardial depression as a result of ischemia aggravated by tachycardia and hypotension. Convulsions and metabolic abnormalities (hypokalemia, acidosis) also contribute to arrhythmias and hypotension.

Management is often difficult because patients are generally older and have chronic lung disease. Management of tachyarrhythmias has been discussed. Hypotension may resolve with judicious use of fluids, treatment of arrhythmias, and correction of metabolic abnormalities. Pressors may be required for recalcitrant hypotension. Nonselective β-blockers, such as propranolol, can reverse hypotension by blocking β_2-mediated vasodilation. β_1-Selective blockers, such as esmolol and metoprolol, are preferred in the presence of bronchospastic lung disease.

Drugs Causing either Tachyarrhythmias or Bradyarrhythmias

CARDIAC GLYCOSIDES

Digitalis has a variety of pharmacologic properties that result in protean manifestations of toxicity. In overdose, morbidity and mortality may result from arrhythmias, heart block, and hyperkalemia. Disruption of sodium and potassium transport, with the associated hyperkalemia, depresses conduction velocity.[14] Increased rate of diastolic depolarization and delayed ADs may cause ventricular ectopy or tachyarrhythmias. Additionally, digitalis may enhance sympathetic activity, causing increased automaticity while decreasing parasympathetic activity and consequently accelerating conduction velocity. Resultant arrhythmias in overdose often are characterized by increased automaticity and depressed intracardiac conduction. The development of an atrial tachycardia with 2:1 or higher-degree AV conduction block suggests digitalis toxicity. AV junctional tachycardia and ventricular ectopy, tachycardia, or fibrillation may be more common in patients with diseased hearts.[15] Bradyarrhythmias, including sinus bradycardia, second-degree and complete AV block, atrial fibrillation with slow ventricular response, idioventricular rhythm, and asystole, also can occur with digitalis poisoning. Hyperkalemia, resulting from inhibition of sodium-potassium exchange, can contribute to AV block and depressed excitability and is an indicator of poor prognosis.

First-line treatment for arrhythmias or hyperkalemia in digitalis poisoning is administration of digoxin-specific antibodies.[61] If the antibodies are not immediately available, temporizing measures should be directed at the specific arrhythmia and normalization of serum potassium levels. Insulin, glucose, and bicarbonate are preferred treatment for digitalis-induced hyperkalemia. Use of calcium chloride for hyperkalemia may worsen toxicity because intracellular calcium levels are elevated in the presence of digitalis. Lidocaine and phenytoin may ameliorate tachyarrhythmias by increasing AV conduction and depressing automaticity.[15] Cardiac pacing should be reserved for high-grade AV blocks and bradyarrhythmias with hemodynamic compromise because some evidence suggests that pacing may enhance triggered rhythms due to delayed ADs.[8,9] Although esmolol can be used for tachyarrhythmias, other β-blockers, calcium channel blockers, and type Ia antiarrhythmics should be avoided because they can worsen conduction disturbances.[15]

QUINIDINE AND OTHER TYPE I ANTIARRHYTHMICS

In overdose, type Ia antiarrhythmic drugs block fast sodium channels, impede slow inward calcium and outward potassium channels, and reduce the rate of spontaneous depolarization.[62] ECG findings may include QRS widening, bundle-branch block, SA or AV block, and marked QT prolongation. Patients may present with bradycardia resulting from conduction delay and block.[35] Monomorphic VT from reentry as a result of membrane depression and PVT as a result of prolonged repolarization can occur with quinidine poisoning (overdose and sometimes with therapeutic doses). Hypotension also is a common manifestation secondary to depressant actions on the heart. Similarly, type Ic antiarrhythmics (flecainide, propafenone) cause bradyarrhythmias with conduction delays, depressed inotropy, and shock and monomorphic VT in overdose. The effects of these agents on cardiac conduction are rate dependent, so the extent of QRS widening is greater at faster heart rates. Recognition and management of conduction inhibition and hypotension are similar to that discussed in the previous section on TCAs. Treatment of PVT also is described elsewhere in this chapter.

NEUROLEPTICS

Cardiovascular manifestations of neuroleptics in overdose result from a combination of α-adrenergic blockade, anticholinergic activity, and "quinidine-like," membrane-depressant effects. Although these properties appear to be similar to TCAs, individual neuroleptics have varying potencies and different degrees of concentration in the myocardium. Most neuroleptics predominantly possess α-adrenergic and anticholinergic properties, the cardiovascular toxicity of which generally is not difficult to control. Thioridazine and mesoridazine are the most cardiotoxic neuroleptics and are responsible for most deaths from this group.[63] Their membrane-depressant effects and ECG manifestations are similar to those described for type Ia antiarrhythmics. Bradycardia with SA or AV block, prolonged QT interval, QRS widening, and bundle-branch blocks may occur in overdose.[64] Sinus tachycardia due to anticholinergic properties also may be seen with thioridazine and mesoridazine but not as predictably as with TCAs or with some of the other neuroleptics. Monomorphic VT and PVT have been reported with these neuroleptics.[65] TdP is reported more commonly with neuroleptics than with TCA overdose.[63] A likely explanation is that TCA-poisoned patients are frequently tachycardic because of the anticholinergic effects, which may be less prominent in thioridazine or mesoridazine overdose and are absent in quinidine poisoning. Because TdP is "pause dependent," and repolarization time is inversely proportional to heart rate, patients with bradyarrhythmias in the presence of these neuroleptics may be more likely to develop PVT (see Fig. 21-13). Treatment for PVT is described elsewhere. Conduction abnormalities and hypotension should be treated as with type Ia antiarrhythmics and TCA poisoning.

SUMMARY

Central to the treatment of critically poisoned patients is initial stabilization using the clinical approach outlined in this chapter followed by a thorough history, physical examination, and evaluation of the ECG. Autonomic disturbances, membrane-depressant effects, triggered rhythms, and systemic metabolic influences may contribute to cardiac conduction and rate disturbances in poisoned patients. Recognition of these disturbances facilitates further management of patients manifesting signs and symptoms of cardiotoxicity from an unknown drug or a poison.

REFERENCES

1. Rosen MR, Wit AL, Hoffman BF: Electrophysiology and pharmacology of cardiac arrhythmias: I. Cellular electrophysiology of the mammalian heart. Am Heart J 88:380–385, 1974.
2. Antman EM, Stone PH, Muller JE, et al: Calcium channel blocking agents in the treatment of cardiovascular disorders: Part I. Basic and clinical electrophysiologic effects. Ann Intern Med 93:875–885, 1980.

3. Aubert AE, Ramaekers D: Neurocardiology: The benefits of irregularity: The basics of methodology, physiology and current clinical applications. Acta Cardiol 54:107–120, 1999.

4. Waldo AL, Wit AL: Mechanisms of cardiac arrhythmias. Lancet 341:1189–1193, 1993.

5. Antzelevitch C, Sicouri S: Clinical relevance of cardiac arrhythmias generated by afterdepolarizations: Role of M cells in the generation of U waves, triggered activity and torsade de pointes. J Am Coll Cardiol 23:259–277, 1994.

6. Viskin S: Long QT syndromes and torsade de pointes. Lancet 354:1625–1633, 1999.

7. Rosen MR, Wit AL, Hoffman BF: Electrophysiology and pharmacology of cardiac arrhythmias: IV. Cardiac antiarrhythmic and toxic effects of digitalis. Am Heart J 89:391–399, 1975.

8. Taboulet P, Baud FJ, Bismuth C, et al: Acute digitalis intoxication—is pacing still appropriate? J Toxicol Clin Toxicol 31:261–273, 1993.

9. Bismuth C, Motte G, Conso F, et al: Acute digitoxin intoxication treated by intracardiac pacemaker: Experience in sixty-eight patients. Clin Toxicol 10:443–456, 1977.

10. Brennan FJ: Electrophysiologic effects of imipramine and doxepin on normal and depressed cardiac Purkinje fibers. Am J Cardiol 46:599–606, 1980.

11. Pearigen PD, Benowitz NL: Poisoning due to calcium antagonists: Experience with verapamil, diltiazem and nifedipine. Drug Saf 6:408–430, 1991.

12. Kunkel F, Rowland M, Scheinman MM: The electrophysiologic effects of lidocaine in patients with intraventricular conduction defects. Circulation 49:894–899, 1974.

13. Smith TW, Antman EM, Friedman PL, et al: Digitalis glycosides: mechanisms and manifestations of toxicity: Part I. Prog Cardiovasc Dis 26:413–458, 1984.

14. Smith TW, Antman EM, Friedman PL, et al: Digitalis glycosides: Mechanisms and manifestations of toxicity: Part II. Prog Cardiovasc Dis 26:495–540, 1984.

15. Smith TW, Antman EM, Friedman PL, et al: Digitalis glycosides: Mechanisms and manifestations of toxicity: Part III. Prog Cardiovasc Dis 27:21–56, 1984.

16. Newton GE, Azevedo ER, Parker JD: Inotropic and sympathetic responses to the intracoronary infusion of a β2-receptor agonist: A human in vivo study. Circulation 99:2402–2407, 1999.

17. Agura ED, Wexler LF, Witzburg RA: Massive propranolol overdose: Successful treatment with high-dose isoproterenol and glucagon. Am J Med 80:755–757, 1986.

18. White CM: A review of potential cardiovascular uses of intravenous glucagon administration. J Clin Pharmacol 39:442–447, 1999.

19. Akhtar M, Shenasa M, Jazayeri M, et al: Wide QRS complex tachycardia: Reappraisal of a common clinical problem. Ann Intern Med 109:905–912, 1988.

20. Morady F, Baerman JM, DiCarlo LA, et al: A prevalent misconception regarding wide-complex tachycardias. JAMA 254:2790–2792, 1985.

21. Sharma AD, Klein GJ, Yee R: Intravenous adenosine triphosphate during wide QRS complex tachycardia: Safety, therapeutic efficacy, and diagnostic utility. Am J Med 88:337–343, 1990.

22. Hoffman JR, Votey SR, Bayer M, et al: Effect of hypertonic sodium bicarbonate in the treatment of moderate-to-severe cyclic antidepressant overdose. Am J Emerg Med 11:336–341, 1993.

23. Nattel S, Mittleman M: Treatment of ventricular tachyarrhythmias resulting from amitriptyline toxicity in dogs. J Pharmacol Exp Ther 231:430–435, 1984.

24. Sasyniok BI, Jhamandas V: Mechanism of reversal of toxic effects of amitriptyline on cardiac Purkinje fibers by sodium bicarbonate. J Pharmacol Exp Ther 231:387–394, 1984.

25. Beckman KJ, Parker RB, Hariman RJ, et al: Hemodynamic and electrophysiological actions of cocaine: Effects of sodium bicarbonate as an antidote in dogs. Circulation 83:1799–1807, 1991.

26. Yeih DF, Chiang FT, Huang SK: Successful treatment of aconitine induced life threatening ventricular tachyarrhythmia with amiodarone. Heart 84:E8, 2000.

27. Edwards KE, Wenstone R: Successful resuscitation from recurrent ventricular fibrillation secondary to butane inhalation. Br J Anaesth 84:803–805, 2000.

28. Tai YT, But PP, Young K, et al: Cardiotoxity after accidental herb-induced aconite poisoning. Lancet 340:1254–1256, 1992.

29. Davidenko JM, Cohen L, Goodrow R, et al: Quinidine-induced action potential prolongation, early afterdepolarizations, and triggered activity in canine Purkinje fibers: Effects of stimulation rate, potassium, and magnesium. Circulation 79:674–686, 1989.

30. Choy AM, Lang CC, Chomsky DM, et al: Normalization of acquired QT prolongation in humans by intravenous potassium. Circulation 96:2149–2154, 1997.

31. Cohen SI, Deisseroth A, Hecht HS: Infra-His bundle origin of bidirectional tachycardia. Circulation 47:1260–1266, 1973.

32. Harrigan RA, Brady WJ: ECG abnormalities in tricyclic antidepressant ingestion. Am J Emerg Med 17:387–393, 1999.

33. Niemann JT, Bessen HA, Rothstein RJ, et al: Electrocardiographic criteria for tricyclic antidepressant cardiotoxicity. Am J Cardiol 57:1154–1159, 1986.

34. Liebelt EL, Francis PD, Wolf AD: ECG lead aVr versus QRS complex interval in predicting seizures and arrhythmias in acute tricyclic antidepressant toxicity. Ann Emerg Med 26:195–201, 1995.

35. Kim SY, Benowitz NL: Poisoning due to class IA antiarrhythmic drugs: Quinidine, procainamide and disopyramide. Drug Saf 5:393–420, 1990.

36. Lange RA, Cigarroa RG, Flores ED, et al: Potentiation of cocaine-induced coronary vasoconstriction by beta-adrenergic blockade. Ann Intern Med 112:897–903, 1990.

37. Sand IC, Brody SL, Wrenn KD, et al: Experience with esmolol for the treatment of cocaine-associated cardiovascular complications. Am J Emerg Med 9:161–163, 1991.

38. Kerns W, Kline J, Ford MD: Beta-blocker and calcium channel blocker toxicity. Emerg Med Clin North Am 12:365–390, 1994.

39. Frishman W, Jacob H, Eisenberg E, et al: Clinical pharmacology of the new beta-adrenergic blocking drugs: Part 8. Self-poisoning with beta-adrenoceptor blocking agents: Recognition and management. Am Heart J 98:798–811, 1979.

40. Love JN, Leasure JA, Mundt DJ, et al: A comparison of amrinone and glucagon therapy for cardiovascular depression associated with propranolol toxicity in a canine model. J Toxicol Clin Toxicol 30:399–412, 1992.

41. Weinstein RS: Recognition and management of poisoning with beta-adrenergic blocking agents. Ann Emerg Med 13:1123–1131, 1984.

42. Thomas SH, Stone CK, Koury SI: Cardiac dysrhythmias in severe verapamil overdose: Characterization with a canine model. Eur J Emerg Med 3:9–13, 1996.

43. Ashraf M, Chaudhary K, Nelson J, et al: Massive overdose of sustained-release verapamil: A case report and review of literature. Am J Med Sci 310:258–263, 1995.

44. Herrington DM, Insley BM, Weinmann GG: Nifedipine overdose. Am J Med 81:344–346, 1986.

45. Ramoska EA, Spiller HA, Winter M, et al: A one-year evaluation of calcium channel blocker overdoses: Toxicity and treatment. Ann Emerg Med 22:196–200, 1993.

46. Gay R, Algeo S, Lee R, et al: Treatment of verapamil toxicity in intact dogs. J Clin Invest 77:1805–1811, 1986.

47. Morris DL, Goldschlager N: Calcium infusion for reversal of adverse effects of intravenous verapamil. JAMA 249:3212–3213, 1983.

48. Crump BJ, Holt DW, Vale JA: Lack of response to intravenous calcium in severe verapamil poisoning. Lancet 2:939–940, 1982.

49. Yuan TH, Kerns WP, Tomaszewski CA, et al: Insulin-glucose as adjunctive therapy for severe calcium channel antagonist poisoning. J Toxicol Clin Toxicol 37:463–474, 1999.

50. Kline JA, Raymond RM, Leonova ED, et al: Insulin improves heart function and metabolism during non-ischemic cardiogenic shock in awake canines. Cardiovasc Res 34:289–298, 1997.

51. Levine SR, Brust JC, Futrell N, et al: Cerebrovascular complications of the use of the "crack" form of alkaloidal cocaine. N Engl J Med 323:699–704, 1990.

52. Lange RA, Cigarroa RG, Yancy CW, et al: Cocaine-induced coronary-artery vasoconstriction. N Engl J Med 321:1557–1562, 1989.

53. Kloner RA, Hale S, Alker K, et al: The effects of acute and chronic cocaine use on the heart. Circulation 85:407–419, 1992.

54. Karch SB, Billingham ME: The pathology and etiology of cocaine-induced heart disease. Arch Pathol Lab Med 112:225–230, 1988.

55. Derlet RW, Albertson TE: Diazepam in the prevention of seizures and death in cocaine-intoxicated rats. Ann Emerg Med 18:542–546, 1989.

56. Langou RA, Van Dyke C, Tahan SR, et al: Cardiovascular manifestations of tricyclic antidepressant overdose. Am Heart J 100:458–464, 1980.

57. Pentel PR, Benowitz NL: Tricyclic antidepressant poisoning: Management of arrhythmias. Med Toxicol 1:101–121, 1986.

58. Frommer DA, Kulig KW, Marx JA, et al: Tricyclic antidepressant overdose: A review. JAMA 257:521–526, 1987.

59. Shannon M, Merola J, Lovejoy FH: Hypotension in severe tricyclic antidepressant overdose. Am J Emerg Med 6:439–442, 1988.

60. Noble J, Kennedy DJ, Latimer RD, et al: Massive lignocaine overdose during cardiopulmonary bypass: Successful treatment with cardiac pacing. Br J Anaesth 56:1439–1441, 1984.

61. Antman EM, Wenger TL, Butler VP, et al: Treatment of 150 cases of life-threatening digitalis intoxication with digoxin-specific Fab antibody fragments: Final report of a multicenter study. Circulation 81:1744–1752, 1990.

62. Hoffman BF, Rosen MR, Wit AL: Electrophysiology and pharmacology of cardiac arrhythmias: VII. Cardiac effects of quinidine and procaine amide. Am Heart J 89:804–808, 1975.

63. Buckley NA, Whyte IM, Dawson AH: Cardiotoxicity more common in thioridazine overdose than with other neuroleptics. J Toxicol Clin Toxicol 33:199–204, 1995.

64. Le Blaye I, Donatini B, Hall M, et al: Acute overdosage with thioridazine: A review of the available clinical exposure. Vet Hum Toxicol 35:147–150, 1993.

65. Hulisz DT, Dasa SL, Black LD, et al: Complete heart block and torsade de pointes associated with thioridazine poisoning. Pharmacotherapy 14:239–245, 1994.

CHAPTER 22

Anticholinergic Syndrome

Thomas G. Martin

The anticholinergic syndrome is common and may result from exposures to many drugs or natural substances (Table 22-1). Anticholinergic effects are desired or intended effects for certain drugs (i.e., antispasmodics, mydriatics, and belladonna alkaloids) and are undesired or side effects for other drugs (i.e., antihistamines, antidepressants, antipsychotics, and antiparkinsonians). Both prescription and over-the-counter drugs may have anticholinergic effects. Combined use of more than one drug with anticholinergic effects increases the risk of anticholinergic toxicity. The anticholinergic syndrome, also called the *anticholinergic toxidrome*, has peripheral and central manifestations. The more serious adverse effects associated with large exposures to these agents are often a result of other physiologic properties of these agents rather than the anticholinergic effects.

Granacher and Baldessarini[1] and Hall and colleagues[2] were among the first to describe the central anticholinergic syndrome (CAS), a sometimes dramatic form of anticholinergic toxicity. CAS may result from abuse, intentional or unintentional overdoses, or adverse drug reactions. A moderate stage of CAS with euphoria and hallucinations is the desired end point of certain forms of substance abuse, but achieving the desired stage of intoxication and avoiding toxicity is difficult.

OVERVIEW AND INCIDENCE

Data from the American Association of Poison Control Centers Toxicological Exposure Surveillance System indicate that anticholinergic exposures are common but usually not severe or fatal (Table 22-2).[3] Of the more than 120,000 exposures reported in the United States in 2002, however, almost half were treated in health care facilities (Table 22-3). Use of drugs with anticholinergic activity is the most common cause of drug-induced delirium.[4] Differences in clinical effects result from not only the dose but also variability in the degree of muscarinic receptor blocking among agents.[5,6] Large intentional ingestions of sleeping pills (antihistamine type) and tricyclic antidepressants (TCAs) are common causes of serious toxicity within these groups. More anticholinergic exposures are due to intentional exposures to mushrooms, TCAs, and phenothiazines than to exposure to plants, gastrointestinal anticholinergics, antihistamines, and anticholinergic drugs.[3] Many anticholinergic-type adverse drug reactions and abuse are not reported to poison centers or adverse drug reaction programs, and their true incidence is unknown. In one study, 60% of elderly nursing home patients were taking at least one anticholinergic agent, and 13% of patients on anticholinergic drugs in one geriatric unit had significant adverse effects.[4]

HISTORY

Natural substances with anticholinergic properties, such as nightshade plants, have long been used for their mind-altering properties by different cultures.[7] The Solanaceae alkaloids, primarily atropine and scopolamine, have been the active ingredients of ancient witches' brews and ointments (Pharmaka diabolics), love potions, intoxicants, hallucinogens, knockout agents, and poisons. British soldiers were described as "natural fools" for 11 days after consuming a salad containing leaves of *Datura stramonium* (Jimson weed) (see Chapter 126).[8]

PATHOPHYSIOLOGY

Acetylcholine is the neurotransmitter for all preganglionic autonomic neurons and postganglionic parasympathetic neurons and some postganglionic sympathetic neurons. Acetylcholine stimulates muscarinic, nicotinic, and central nervous system cholinergic receptors. Nicotinic receptors are located primarily on the autonomic ganglion and neuromuscular end plates. There are 12 types of nicotinic receptors: α_2 through α_9 and β_2 through β_5. Nicotinic receptors are ligand-gated (ionotropic receptors) sodium (Na^+) and calcium (Ca^{2+}) channels whose activation leads to rapid depolarization and excitation. Muscarinic receptors are located primarily on the postganglionic parasympathetic neurons and less so on autonomic ganglions and the adrenal medulla.[9,10] There are five types of cloned muscarinic receptors (M_1 through M_5), whose effects are mediated more slowly by guanosine triphosphate–binding proteins (G proteins), or so-called metabotropic receptors. The primary intracellular messengers affected by muscarinic stimulation are calcium and cyclic adenosine monophosphate (cAMP). The intracellular effects of muscarinic receptor stimulation are summarized in Figure 22-1.[11] Odd-numbered receptors (M_1, M_3, M_5) activate a G protein that leads to the release of intracellular calcium, resulting in smooth muscle contraction and gland secretion. Even-numbered receptors (M_2, M_4) activate a G protein that inhibits adenylyl cyclase, leading to reduced levels of cAMP. The intracellular effects of muscarinic stimulation may lead to stimulatory (depolarizing) or inhibitory (hyperpolarizing) effects on membrane potentials.

TABLE 22-1 Anticholinergic Drugs and Natural Substances

Belladonna Alkaloids
Atropine sulfate
Belladonna extract
Belladonna tincture
Levo alkaloids of belladonna (Bellafoline)
Clidinium (Quarzan)
Homatropine hydrobromide
Hyoscine N-butylbromide
Hyoscyamine sulfate
Hyoscyamine
Scopolamine hydrobromide

Gastrointestinal Antispasmodics
Anisotropine methylbromide (Valpin)
Butylscopolamine bromide (Buscopan)
Clidinium bromide (Librax)
Dicyclomine hydrochloride (Bentyl)
Glycopyrrolate (Robinul)
Hexocyclium methylsulfate (Tral)
Isopropamide iodide (Darbid)
Mepenzolate bromide (Cantil)
Methantheline bromide (Banthine)
Atropine/diphenoxylate (Lomotil)
Methscopolamine bromide (Pamine)
Oxyphencyclimine hydrochloride (Daricon)
Oxyphenonium bromide (Antrenyl)
Propantheline bromide (Pro-Banthine)

Genitourinary Antispasmodics
Flavoxate hydrochloride (Urispas)
Oxybutynin chloride (Ditropan)
Tolterodine tartrate (Detrol)

Cycloplegics
Cyclopentolate (Cyclogyl)
Tropicamide (Mydriacyl)

Other Drugs
Cyclobenzaprine (Flexeril)
Mefloquine
Diphenidol (Vontrol)
Ipratropium bromide (Atrovent)

Antihistamines
Acrivastine
Antazoline
Azatadine
Bromodiphenhydramine
Brompheniramine
Buclizine
Carbinoxamine
Cetirizine
Chlorcyclizine
Chlorpheniramine
Clemastine
Cyclizine
Cyproheptadine
Dexbrompheniramine
Dexchlorpheniramine
Dimenhydrinate
Dimethindene
Diphenhydramine
Diphenylpyraline
Doxylamine
Fexofenadine
Hydroxyzine
Loratadine
Meclizine
Methapyrilene
Phenindamine
Pheniramine
Phenyltoloxamine
Promethazine

Pyrilamine
Pyrrobutamine
Tripelennamine
Triprolidine

Antiulcer Drugs
Cimetidine
Famotidine
Propantheline
Ranitidine

Antiparkinson Drugs
Benztropine mesylate (Cogentin)
Biperiden (Akineton)
Orphenadrine hydrochloride (Disipal)
Orphenadrine citrate (Norflex)
Procyclidine (Kemadrin)
Trihexyphenidyl hydrochloride (Artane)

Neuroleptics[6]
Chlorpromazine (Thorazine)
Prochlorperazine
Fluphenazine
Clozapine (Clozaril)
Prochlorperazine
Olanzapine (Zyprexa)
Thioridazine
Thiothixene

Tricyclic Antidepressants[5]
Amitriptyline (Elavil)
Clomipramine (Anafranil)
Imipramine (Tofranil)
Desipramine (Norpramin)
Doxepin (Sinequan)
Nortriptyline (Pamelor)

Protriptyline (Vivactil)
Trimipramine (Surmontil)

Plants
Atropa belladonna (deadly nightshade)
Brugmansia arborea (angel's trumpet)
Brugmansia suaveolens (angel's trumpet)
Cestrum diurnum (day jessamine)
Cestrum nocturnum (night jessamine)
Cestrum parqui (willow-leaved jessamine)
Datura metel (Hindu datura)
Datura stramonium (Jimson weed, thorn apple, locoweed)
Duboisra spp.
Hyoscyamus niger (black henbane)
Lantana camara (yellow sage)
Lycium halimifolium (matrimony vine)
Mandragora officinarum (mandrake)
Scopolia atropoides (crazy plant)
Solandra spp. (trumpet flower)
Solanum dulcamara (woody nightshade)
Solanum nigrum (black nightshade)

Mushrooms
Amanita cothurnata
Amanita gemmata
Amanita muscaria
Amanita pantherina
Amanita smithiana

TABLE 22-2 Anticholinergic Reported Exposures and Intent

AGENTS	EXPOSURES	UNINTENTIONAL	INTENTIONAL	OTHER
Natural substances				
Mushroom*	31	8	21	1
Plant†	1072	523	523	9
Medications				
Anticholinergic	5780	3539	1778	4
Antihistamine‡	69,107	48,210	18,345	56
Gastrointestinal antispasmodics†	1109	612	420	1
Cyclic antidepressants	13,198	4333	8189	20
Phenothiazine	5224	2282	2423	10
Atypical antipsychotics	25,252	7655	16,374	27
Total	120,773	67,162	48,073	128

*Ibotenic acid group.
†Anticholinergic type.
‡Not including H_2 receptor antagonists.
From Watson WA, Litovitz TL, Rodgers GC Jr, et al: 2002 annual report of the American Association of Poison Control Centers Toxic Exposure Surveillance System. Am J Emerg Med 21:353–421, 2003.

TABLE 22-3 Anticholinergic Health Care Facility Exposures and Outcomes

AGENTS	HEALTH CARE FACILITY EXPOSURES	OUTCOME				
		None	*Minor*	*Moderate*	*Severe*	*Death*
Natural substances						
Mushroom*	19	2	8	11	3	0
Plant†	613	179	124	358	34	1
Medications						
Anticholinergic	2926	1390	1046	811	194	10
Antihistamine‡	24,119	16,935	10,547	5559	904	71
Gastrointestinal antispasmodics†	611	294	213	172	27	1
Cyclic antidepressants	9967	1988	3029	3277	1418	119
Phenothiazine	3441	985	1168	1094	254	11
Atypical antipsychotics	19,291	4173	7228	5710	1448	78
Total	60,987	25,946	23,363	16,992	4282	291

*Ibotenic acid group.
†Anticholinergic type.
‡Not including H_2 receptor antagonists.
From Watson WA, Litovitz TL, Rodgers GC Jr, et al: 2002 annual report of the American Association of Poison Control Centers Toxic Exposure Surveillance System. Am J Emerg Med 21:353–421, 2003.

Toxic Mechanism

Anticholinergic agents antagonize the effects of acetylcholine by competitively blocking its binding to acetylcholine receptor sites. Muscarinic receptor antagonists (e.g., atropine) are generally ineffective at blocking binding to the nicotinic sites except at high doses. Some drugs, such as quaternary ammonium analogues of atropine (e.g., propantheline), may exhibit a greater degree of nicotinic receptor blockade, however. Although cholinergic receptors in the brain include muscarinic and nicotinic types, quaternary compounds do not cross the blood-brain barrier readily. Clinical cases of anticholinergic syndrome are due to predominantly muscarinic receptor antagonism. Muscarinic receptors differ in their sensitivity to muscarinic antagonists. Low levels of muscarinic antagonism result in decreased salivary and bronchial secretions and sweating. Higher levels of muscarinic antagonism result in mydriasis, loss of visual accommodation, and tachycardia. Even higher levels of antagonism are required for urinary, intestinal, and gastric atony.[10]

The anticholinergic syndrome may be divided into peripheral and central effects (Table 22-4). Patients may present with

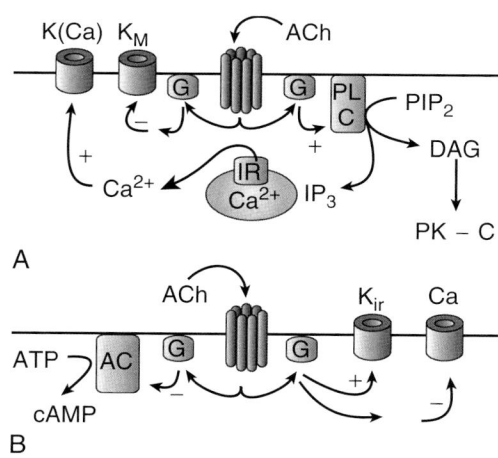

FIGURE 22-1

Intracellular effects of muscarinic receptor stimulation. **A,** Stimulation of odd-numbered muscarinic receptors leads to stimulation of two types of G proteins. One of these types of G proteins activates phospholipase C (PL-C), leading to the breakdown of phosphatidylinositol 4,5-biphosphate (PIP$_2$) into inositol trisphosphate (IP$_3$) and diacylglycerol (DAG). IP$_3$ stimulates its own receptor (IR), which releases internal stores of calcium (Ca^{2+}), which activate certain types of potassium channels (K[Ca]). DAG stimulates protein kinase C (PK-C). The other type of G protein stimulated inhibits certain other types of potassium channels (K$_M$). **B,** Stimulation of even-numbered muscarinic receptors leads to stimulation of two types of G proteins. One of these types of G proteins inhibits adenylyl cyclase (AC), which decreases production of cyclic adenosine monophosphate (cAMP). The other type of stimulated G protein inhibits an N-type of calcium channel and in cardiac tissue opens a K$_{ir}$ channel. *(Adapted from Durieux ME: Muscarinic signaling in the central nervous system. Anesthesiology 84:173–198, 1996.)*

TABLE 22-4 Anticholinergic Toxicity

Peripheral Anticholinergic Signs
Dry skin, mouth, and axilla
Flushing
Hyperthermia
Urinary retention
Diminished bowel signs
Mydriasis
Loss of accommodation
Myoclonus
Tachycardia
Hypertension
Peripheral vasodilation
Dysrhythmias
Cardiogenic shock

Central Anticholinergic Signs
Agitation
Altered mental status
Amnesia

Anxiety
Ataxia
Cardiorespiratory arrest
Choreoathetosis
Coma
Delirium
Disorientation
Dysarthria
Extrapyramidal reactions
Auditory and visual
  hallucinations
Incoherent speech
Lethargy
Paranoia
Psychosis
Seizures
Stereotypy*

*Repetitive gesturing or movements.

predominantly one form or both forms. Tertiary agents more readily cross the blood-brain barrier and are more likely to result in central anticholinergic toxicity, whereas the converse is true of quaternary agents. Tertiary and quaternary anticholinergic agents are listed in Table 22-5. Atropine typically causes predominantly peripheral anticholinergic effects at low doses and additional central anticholinergic effects at higher doses. Still higher doses of atropine may result in shock, coma, and respiratory failure.

Toxic Effects

The anticholinergic syndrome is a constellation of signs and symptoms potentially involving many different organ systems (see Table 22-4). Signs of peripheral anticholinergic toxicity characteristically, but not always, accompany CAS. The authors of a carefully controlled clinical study meticulously described the onset and course of iatrogenic CAS and its reversal by the cholinergic agent physostigmine.[12] They described three phases of CAS—induction, stupor, and delirium. In the induction phase, peripheral anticholinergic effects predominated. The stupor phase overlapped the induction phase and was characterized by somnolence, restlessness, ataxia, hyperthermia, and hypertension. The third phase, delirium, overlapped the second phase and was characterized by amnesia, confusion, incoherent speech, and hallucinations. The delirium phase often outlasted the first two phases. These phases may not apply to CAS from anticholinergic agents other than the three studied.[12]

The characteristic general appearance of the anticholinergic syndrome is a restless, delirious patient who is picking at the bed sheets, clothing, and imaginary objects in the air. Speech is characteristically rapid, mumbling, and incomprehensible.[13] Hallucinations are usually visual but sometimes may be auditory. Dilated pupils and tachycardia are often present, but neither is essential to the diagnosis. Public disrobing is a common feature, possibly due to the delirious uninhibited patient's sensation of flushing and hot skin.[13]

SEIZURES

Anticholinergic poisoning is a common cause of drug-induced seizures. Seizures were not observed, however, in a

series of 20 cases of severe atropinization secondary to mostly unintentional autoinjector discharge during the Persian Gulf War.[14] In TCA overdose, the prevalence of seizures has been reported to be 3 to 30%.[15–17] In nine children hospitalized after ingesting *Amanita pantherina* or *Amanita muscaria* mushrooms, seizures or myoclonic twitching occurred in 44%.[18] Abnormal muscle activity (e.g., jerks, twitches, rigidity) secondary to anticholinergic toxicity sometimes is confused with seizures by laypersons and less experienced health care providers. Because seizures are considered to be a relative contraindication to physostigmine use, the reported observation of seizures by less experienced or trained personnel must be evaluated carefully.

CARDIOVASCULAR EFFECTS

Mild to moderately severe anticholinergic syndrome is associated with sinus tachycardia and hypertension. The tachycardia may result primarily from blocking of the M_2-receptors on the sinoatrial node. Anticholinergic agents can enhance conduction in the atrioventricular node and increase ventricular rate. Hypertension results from antagonism of the acetylcholine-induced peripheral vasodilation. Poisoning with large amounts of anticholinergic agents possessing sodium channel–blocking or α-adrenergic receptor–blocking properties may lead to severe cardiovascular toxicity, including ventricular dysrhythmias, advanced heart block, vasodilation, and refractory shock. Moderate anticholinergic exposure in a susceptible host also may lead to severe toxicity.[19]

GASTROINTESTINAL EFFECTS

Anticholinergic agents may decrease intestinal peristalsis and delay gastric emptying.[20] For antispasmodic drugs, this is a desired effect and leads to decreased intestinal spasms. When undesired or excessive, these effects may lead to constipation or drug-induced ileus. This effect also may lead to delayed peak absorption and prolonged toxicity in anticholinergic overdose.

SKELETAL MUSCLE EFFECTS

Severe forms of the anticholinergic syndrome may be associated with rhabdomyolysis resulting in release of myoglobin into the blood and nephrotoxicity.[21–25] Rhabdomyolysis in this setting may be a result of hyperthermia, excess motor activity or muscle tone, or dependent-type pressure injury secondary to deep coma.

TEMPERATURE EFFECTS

Anticholinergic agents inhibit sweating, which reduces one's ability to dissipate excess body heat. Excess motor activity or muscle tone increases body heat. Hyperthermia can result from increased heat generation and impaired cooling secondary to sweating inhibition. This is especially true in environments with high ambient temperatures.

URINARY TRACT EFFECTS

Anticholinergic agents reduce bladder tone and may lead to urinary retention. This is especially a problem for an elderly man with prostatic hypertrophy and increases the risk of urinary tract infections. Urinary retention also necessitates the use of bladder catheterization in many patients with the anticholinergic syndrome.

TABLE 22-5 Belladonna Alkaloids

TERTIARY AMINES	QUATERNARY AMMONIUM
Naturally Occurring Alkaloids	
Atropine	
Belladonna	
Hyoscyamine	
Scopolamine	
Semisynthetic Derivatives	
Homatropine	Homatropine methylbromide
Methscopolamine	
Synthetic Amine Compounds	
Dicyclomine	Clidinium
Oxybutynin	Glycopyrrolate
Pirenzepine	Ipratropium
Tolterodine	Mepenzolate
	Propantheline

Laboratory Tests

Many toxicologic screens are immunoassays designed to detect common drugs of abuse at levels above the U.S. Substance Abuse and Mental Health Services Administration thresholds. This type of drug of abuse screen does not detect any of the anticholinergic agents listed in Table 22-1. Some immunoassay screens provide qualitative or semi-quantitative detection of TCAs. Gas chromatography combined with mass spectroscopy is a commonly employed technique in comprehensive drug and substance screening that can detect many but not all of these agents.[26,27] Although quantitative assays probably are available for all of the anticholinergic agents, they are usually unnecessary in the clinical management of patients with anticholinergic syndrome. In certain cases (e.g., in fatalities or atypical presentations), other laboratory techniques (e.g., gas-liquid chromatography, high-pressure liquid chromatography, or high-pressure thin-layer chromatography) may be required to identify the anticholinergic agent.

Toxicity

Toxicity varies greatly among the various substances with anticholinergic properties. Toxicity is greatest for the TCAs primarily because of their α-adrenergic receptor–blocking and sodium channel–blocking effects rather than their anticholinergic properties. In a pediatric series of autoinjector atropine exposures, lower injected doses resulted mainly in mild peripheral effects, whereas higher doses resulted in hyperthermia and central effects.[14] In adults, atropine doses of 0.032 mg/kg caused peripheral effects, and doses of 0.13 to 0.17 mg/kg caused central effects.[12] These studies suggest that peripheral effects occur at lower doses than do central effects. As little as 4 to 5 eye drops (probably less in children) containing 4% atropine or 0.25% scopolamine has been reported to cause the anticholinergic syndrome.[28,29]

DIFFERENTIAL DIAGNOSIS

The differential diagnosis includes many conditions that resemble the anticholinergic syndrome (Table 22-6). Many of these diagnoses can be eliminated by a careful history and physical examination combined with routine laboratory tests. A history of anticholinergic exposure, typical manifestations of peripheral and central anticholinergic toxicity, and a typical time course for resolution of symptoms are adequate for most clinical diagnoses of anticholinergic syndrome. In some cases, little to no peripheral anticholinergic findings are noted.[2] Although several physical findings, such as dry skin and decreased bowel sounds, are said to be useful in distinguishing anticholinergic syndrome from other causes of agitated delirium, the sensitivity and specificity of these findings are not well documented. Hall and colleagues[2] stated that fever was seen in only 20% of adults and 25% of children and that fewer than 10% of patients with CAS manifest constipation, ileus, urinary retention, and convulsions. These percentages appear to be estimates, and the number of cases on which they were based was not provided. This report also stated that the most reliable signs of the anticholinergic syndrome were dilated and sluggishly reactive pupils, confusion, disorientation, incoher-

TABLE 22-6 Differential Diagnoses of Anticholinergic Syndrome

Intoxications	
Caffeine	Hypercapnia
Dextromethorphan	Hyperthyroidism
Ketamine	Hypoglycemia
Lithium	Hyponatremia
Lysergic acid diethylamide (LSD)	Hypoxia
Monoamine oxidase inhibitors (MAOI)	Pheochromocytoma
Phencyclidine (PCP)	Uremia
Salicylates	Wernicke's syndrome
Selective serotonin reuptake inhibitors	**Infections**
Sympathomimetics (e.g., cocaine,	Encephalitis
amphetamines, methamphetamines)	Meningitis
Theophylline	Sepsis
Withdrawal Syndromes	**Psychiatric Illnesses**
Ethanol	Schizophrenia
Barbiturates	Dementia
Sedative-hypnotics	
Dysautonomia	**Other Causes**
Malignant hyperthermia	Cerebral vasculitis
Neuroleptic malignant syndrome	Cerebrovascular accident
Serotonin syndrome	Cerebral contusion
Metabolic Diseases	Postictal state
Disulfiram (Antabuse) reactions	Postconcussive syndrome
Hepatic failure	Partial complex seizures

ence, memory impairment, facial flushing, dry mucous membranes, tachycardia, agitation, picking or grasping movements, ataxia, motor incoordination, and visual and auditory hallucinations.[2] In eight victims of surreptitious scopolamine use, dry mouth and skin were noted in 100%, and decreased bowel sounds were noted in 25%.[30] In a review of stramonium intoxication, dry skin and mucous membranes were reported in only 25 of 54 (46%) cases.[31] In Jimson weed intoxications, dry mucous membranes were reported in 16 of 17 cases.[32] In unknown cases, comprehensive laboratory testing can be used to detect some of the more commonly used drugs and abused substances.

ROUTES OF EXPOSURE

The anticholinergic syndrome may result from oral, pulmonary (smoking), ocular, dermal, buccal, rectal, or vaginal routes of exposure to anticholinergic agents. Oral exposures are most common in reported cases and include intentional ingestion of pills, seeds, or teas. Pulmonary or inhalational exposures usually are associated with substance abuse, although nebulized atropine treatment of asthma is an exception.[33,34] Ocular and dermal exposures more commonly are unintentional exposures and are difficult to recognize. Witches' ointments were applied intentionally to the whole body, including the axillae, rectum, and vagina.[7] Horse traders rolled *Datura* leaves together and inserted them into the rectums of old nags to make them appear to be as fiery as thoroughbreds.[7] Exposure to ophthalmologic drops has resulted in the anticholinergic syndrome as an adverse effect of therapeutic use and has been an agent of drug-facilitated assault or robbery. Dermal exposures to topical diphenhydramine and scopolamine patches are well-known causes of systemic anticholinergic effects.[35–38]

INTENTION OR CAUSE OF EXPOSURES

Adverse Drug Reactions

Many authors have stated empirically that anticholinergic syndrome occurs frequently as an adverse drug reaction, but few data have been published to support this. Anticholinergic adverse drug reactions occur most frequently as a result of increased sensitivity to a therapeutic dose or as a result of combinations of anticholinergic agents. Very young and very old individuals and patients with underlying organic brain syndromes are said to be more susceptible to CAS.[2,39,40] For unknown reasons, some patients have developed the anticholinergic syndrome from exposures to anticholinergic skin patches that most patients tolerate without problems.[41]

Unintentional Overdose

Toddlers and mentally infirm people are common victims of unintentional or accidental overdose. Use of combinations of prescribed or over-the-counter anticholinergic agents is a common cause of unintentional overdose.

Intentional or Suicidal Overdose

Suicidal ingestions of over-the-counter sleeping pills usually involve anticholinergic antihistaminic agents. Although these exposures are common and usually mild to moderate in severity, severe outcomes or death occasionally results.[42,43]

Recreational Abuse

Self-administration of anticholinergic agents to induce CAS and the desired euphoria, stupor, and hallucinations is well described.[44,45] Abuse of anticholinergic drugs or natural substances is a particular problem of adolescents who are too young to buy alcoholic beverages legally.[32,46,47] In the 14th and 15th centuries, henbane often was added to beer for its hallucinogenic and mind-altering properties.[7] Anticholinergic agents prescribed to prevent or treat extrapyramidal or dystonic reaction due to neuroleptics have been abused by schizophrenics and individuals without psychiatric illnesses. In one study of schizophrenic patients, careful scrutiny revealed that 6.5% of 214 consecutively admitted schizophrenic patients abused trihexyphenidyl.[48] Emergency department physicians in the 1980s often gave a placebo saline injection to patients with suspected dystonic reactions in hopes of discovering individuals with feigned dystonia who were seeking intravenous anticholinergic drugs.[49–51] The delayed absorption associated with these agents plus the biologic variability in natural substances make it particularly difficult for users to titrate the dose of these agents to reach the desired end point of hallucinations while avoiding more severe toxicity.

Malicious Use

The addition of anticholinergic agents such as scopolamine to other substances of abuse may lead to unusual or serious toxicity. Substitution of scopolamine for cocaine[52] and addition of scopolamine to heroin[53] have been reported. Surreptitious addition of scopolamine to beverages is a well-known method of drug-facilitated sexual assault or crime.[30,54,55] The German term *Altsitzerkraut*, meaning "old sitter herb," refers to the use of henbane to induce a lethal form of anticholinergic toxicity to murder an inactive old person.[7] Because there is no history of exposure in these cases and the usual simple toxicologic screens are negative, misdiagnosis is common.

Toxic Causes or Sources

Many types of prescription and over-the-counter medications and natural substances have anticholinergic properties (see Table 22-1). The anticholinergic syndrome may result from intentional or unintentional exposure to toxic amounts of these individual agents or in combinations. Many members of the plant family Solanaceae contain tropane or belladonna alkaloids. Plants that can cause the anticholinergic syndrome contain variable amounts of the following toxic alkaloids: solanine, atropine, and scopolamine. Anticholinergic plant toxicity is discussed in detail in Chapter 126. Scopolamine is the primary tropane in Jimson weed. Toxin concentrations of specific types of plants and mushrooms are well known to vary with location, climate, and season. Natural brews, such as teas or wines made from these plants, are notorious for their intoxicating abilities.[56–59] Mushrooms containing muscimol/ibotenic acid are capable of causing hallucinations and a syndrome with features that resemble the anticholinergic syndrome. Intentional (recreational) and unintentional (toddler ingestions) exposures to these types of mushrooms only rarely produce severe anticholinergic-like syndrome.[18]

DIAGNOSTIC STUDIES

Toxicologic Analyses

Most of the common causes of the anticholinergic syndrome are not detected on routine toxicologic screens, which usually consist of immunoassays to detect drugs of abuse. An exception is the qualitative immunoassay for TCAs, which also can yield false-positive results in the presence of other anticholinergic drugs, such as diphenhydramine and certain phenothiazines. Although quantitative levels of most of the drugs and anticholinergic alkaloids in Table 22-1 are available from reference laboratories, they are rarely necessary. Because of variable susceptibility to these agents, quantitative levels for diagnostic confirmation may not be reliable.[60] Quantitative levels of other agents may be useful in ruling out the anticholinergic syndrome.

Abnormal Routine Laboratory Test Findings

Many standard laboratory tests may be abnormal in patients with the anticholinergic syndrome. Patients who are agitated or delirious may have a mild increase in white blood cell counts secondary to demargination. Increases in serum sodium, urine osmolarity, blood urea nitrogen, and creatinine may occur as a result of prerenal azotemia secondary to poor fluid intake and increased insensible losses associated with agitation and hyperthermia. Increased creatinine also may occur with rhabdomyolysis-induced acute renal failure. Hyperthermia and agitation may lead to rhabdomyolysis, which is associated with increased amounts of myoglobin in the serum and the urine. Urine with excess myoglobin appears brown or pink and tests positive on a urine ortho-tolidine test for blood, but no red blood cells are seen in the microscopic urinalysis. Quantitative serum levels of skeletal muscle enzymes and urinary myoglobin levels can confirm the diagnosis of rhabdomyolysis. Rhabdomyolysis also may increase the serum potassium and phosphate and decrease the serum calcium levels. Marked agitation may be associated with an increased anion gap metabolic (lactic) acidosis and decreased serum bicarbonate. Sustained or severe hyperthermia may result in disseminated intravascular coagulation syndrome, characterized by increased coagulation times, increased D dimer and fibrin split products, and decreased platelets and fibrinogen levels.

Differential Features

The anticholinergic syndrome is characterized by the mnemonic *Mad as a hatter, red as a beet, dry as a bone, blind as a bat, hot as a hare.* The syndrome is usually, but not always, a combination of peripheral and central anticholinergic toxicity (see Table 22-4). When it occurs without signs of peripheral anticholinergic toxicity, the syndrome may be misdiagnosed as a primary psychiatric disease, especially without a history of excess anticholinergic exposure and with a negative toxicologic screen.[61] Misdiagnoses are more common in very young and very old patients.[35,62,63] Many other toxicities and medical problems may resemble the anticholinergic syndrome and may be difficult to distinguish clinically (see Table 22-6). Although it is said that dry skin and absent bowel sounds distinguish anticholinergic syndrome from stimulant poisoning, there are few published data to evaluate the sensitivity or specificity of these findings. Ophthalmologic preparations are particularly problematic because many patients do not include them when listing their current medications.[40] In suspected cases of anticholinergic syndrome, a diagnostic challenge with carefully titrated physostigmine doses may be attempted as long as contraindications (see Chapter 153) are not present.[64]

TREATMENT

Most cases of the anticholinergic syndrome are not life-threatening and require little more than observation and general supportive care. Because these patients are at risk of hurting themselves or others and of sudden deterioration due to seizures or respiratory distress, they should be observed carefully until major signs of toxicity have dissipated. Less commonly encountered severe cases may require complicated and expert supportive care.[65,66] More severe cases of the anticholinergic syndrome usually are seen with agents that have other important, potentially toxic properties, such as sodium channel or α-adrenergic receptor blockade (e.g., TCAs, neuroleptics, diphenhydramine). Delayed gastric emptying and drug absorption are major concerns. In a reported case of severe benztropine toxicity, severe anti-

cholinergic poisoning persisted for 9 days after a large single ingestion.[67] Anecdotally, one author reported recovery of Jimson weed seeds 23 hours after ingestion.[68] A review of 15 cases of anticholinergic plant poisoning reported a mean latency to onset of symptoms of 2.7 hours.[69] Based on these reports, gastrointestinal decontamination may be useful for a longer time after ingestion of these agents than for the usual types of acute overdose. Patients with severe toxicity and patients who are unable to protect their airway should undergo rapid-sequence intubation.

Patients who are significantly agitated must be protected from hurting themselves or others. Significant agitation associated with the anticholinergic syndrome usually is treated by reversal with either an anticholinesterase (i.e., physostigmine) or a sedating agent (chemical restraint). The use of physical restraints alone may result in significant rhabdomyolysis if the patient fights vigorously or persistently against them. Physical restraint should be used only as an adjunct to chemical restraints, in case the latter wear off unexpectedly. Large amounts of sedatives may be required to achieve adequate chemical restraint or sedation in anticholinergic syndrome cases. In a comparative study of physostigmine versus benzodiazepines for the anticholinergic syndrome, the mean total benzodiazepine doses were diazepam, 53.1 mg; lorazepam, 35.5 mg; and midazolam, 31.7 mg.[70] Haloperidol can be used to calm delirious patients, but concerns about QT_c interval prolongation and proarrhythmias may warrant QT_c monitoring during its use.[71,72] Because haloperidol has anticholinergic properties, many medical toxicologists believe it should be avoided in patients with the anticholinergic syndrome.

Seizures may be seen in severe cases of anticholinergic toxicity. Although apparent successful terminations of anticholinergic-associated seizures with physostigmine have been reported,[73,74] seizures believed to be secondary to physostigmine use also have been reported.[75–77] Animal studies suggest that physostigmine has limited efficacy against seizures secondary to anticholinergic toxicity.[78–81] Because of concerns over limited efficacy and even enhancing propensity to seizures, physostigmine should not be used as a first-line anticonvulsant therapy, but instead benzodiazepine and other anticonvulsants should be tried.

Severe hyperthermia (temperature >40°C) may result in direct tissue injury and should be treated aggressively. Methods of rapid core cooling include cold water immersion; wet sheets and fans; ice packs in the groin or axilla; and ice water irrigation of the stomach, rectum, or peritoneum. If rigidity is present, dantrolene, a skeletal muscle relaxer, may be used.[82–84] Continued heat production from rigidity resistant to dantrolene may be treated with neuromuscular paralysis.

Rhabdomyolysis may occur secondary to marked agitation, increased muscle tone, or severe hyperthermia. In the absence of renal failure, rhabdomyolysis treatment includes intravenous fluids, mannitol, and sodium bicarbonate. Myoglobin is less likely to precipitate in the renal tubules and cause nephrotoxicity when the urine is dilute and alkaline.[85,86]

Specific Treatment

Some physicians prefer to treat the anticholinergic syndrome primarily with supportive care, carefully titrated sedation, and intubation and artificial ventilation if necessary.[87] If choosing sedation, one must avoid agents with known anticholinergic properties, such as chlorpromazine. Other physicians prefer to use physostigmine for cases of severe anticholinergic poisoning presenting without significant cardiovascular toxicity, in hopes of avoiding the need for excess sedation, intubation, and artificial ventilation.[63] Physostigmine is a short-acting, nonselective cholinesterase inhibitor that is a tertiary amine capable of crossing the blood-brain barrier. It has been reported to be effective in reversing anticholinergic toxicity from drugs[70,88–90] and natural substances (see Chapter 153).[91,92] Although physostigmine was popular in the 1970s and early 1980s, its use diminished after reports of serious adverse effects in TCA overdoses.[93–95] Currently the use of physostigmine to reverse CAS is controversial in medical toxicology and emergency medicine.[96] As discussed in Chapter 153, however, many of these perceived risks seem to be unfounded. Appropriate indications and doses of physostigmine are given in Chapter 153. Neostigmine is a quaternary amine, unable to cross the blood-brain barrier. It has been reported to be more efficacious than physostigmine in the treatment of paralytic ileus and other peripheral anticholinergic effects, but most physicians prefer supportive care and observation for these effects.[83]

REFERENCES

1. Granacher RP, Baldessarini RJ: Physostigmine: Its use in acute anticholinergic syndrome with antidepressant and antiparkinson drugs. Arch Gen Psychiatry 32:375–380, 1975.
2. Hall RCW, Fox J, Stickney SK, et al: Anticholinergic delirium: Etiology, presentation, diagnosis and management. J Psychedelic Drugs 10:237–241, 1978.
3. Watson WA, Litovitz TL, Rodgers GC Jr, et al: 2002 annual report of the American Association of Poison Control Centers Toxic Exposure Surveillance System. Am J Emerg Med 21:353–421, 2003.
4. Mintzer J, Burns A: Anticholinergic side effects of drugs in elderly people. J R Soc Med 93:457–462, 2000.
5. Frazer A: Pharmacology of antidepressants. J Clin Psychopharmacol 17(Suppl 1):2S-18S, 1997.
6. Richelson E: Receptor pharmacology of neuroleptics: Relation to clinical effects. J Clin Psychiatry 60(Suppl 10):5–14, 1999.
7. Muller JL: Love potions and the ointment of witches: Historical aspects of the nightshade alkaloids. J Toxicol Clin Toxicol 36:617–627, 1998.
8. Labianca DA, Reeves WJ: Scopolamine: A potent chemical weapon. J Chem Educ 61:678–680, 1984.
9. Lefkowitz RJ, Hoffman BB, Taylor P: The autonomic and somatic motor nervous systems. In Hardman JG, Limberd LE, Molinoff PB, et al (eds): Goodman and Gilman's the Pharmacological Basis of Therapeutics, 9th ed. New York, McGraw-Hill, 1996, 105–140.
10. Brown JH, Taylor P: Muscarinic receptors: Agonists and antagonists. In Hardman JG, Limberd LE, Molinoff PB, et al (eds): Goodman and Gilman's the Pharmacological Basis of Therapeutics, 9th ed. New York, McGraw-Hill, 1996, 141–160.
11. Durieux ME: Muscarinic signaling in the central nervous system. Anesthesiology 84:173–198, 1996.
12. Ketchum JS, Sidell FR, Crowell EB Jr, et al: Atropine, scopolamine, and ditran: Comparative pharmacology and antagonists in man. Psychopharmacologia 28:121–145, 1973.
13. Furbee B, Wermuth M: Life-threatening plant poisoning. Crit Care Clin 13:849–888, 1997.
14. Amitai Y, Almog S, Singer R, et al: Atropine poisoning in children during the Persian Gulf crisis: A national survey in Israel. JAMA 268:630–632, 1992.
15. Lavoie FW, Gansert GG, Weiss RE: Value of initial ECG findings and plasma drug levels in cyclic antidepressant overdose. Ann Emerg Med 19:696–700, 1990.
16. Boehnert MT, Lovejoy FH: Value of the QRS duration versus the serum drug level in predicting seizures and ventricular arrhythmias after an acute overdose of tricyclic antidepressants. N Engl J Med 313:474–497, 1985.
17. Pall H, Czech K, Kotzaurek R, et al: Experiences with physostigmine salicylate in tricyclic antidepressant poisoning. Acta Pharmacol Toxicol 14(Suppl 2):171–178, 1977.
18. Benjamin DR: Mushroom poisoning in infants and children: The Amanita pantherina/muscaria group. J Toxicol Clin Toxicol 30:13–22, 1992.
19. Brunner GA, Fleck S, Pieber TR, et al: Near fatal anticholinergic intoxication after routine funduscopy. Intensive Care Med 24:730–731, 1998.
20. Parkman HP, Trate DM, Knight LC, et al: Cholinergic effects on human gastric motility. Gut 45:346–354, 1999.
21. Mendoza FS, Atiba JO, Krensky AM, et al: Rhabdomyolysis complicating doxylamine overdose. Clin Pediatr 26:595–597, 1987.
22. Frankel D, Dolgin J, Murray BM: Non-traumatic rhabdomyolysis complicating antihistamine overdose. J Toxicol Clin Toxicol 31:493–496, 1993.
23. Emadian SM, Caravati EM, Herr RD: Rhabdomyolysis: A rare adverse effect of diphenhydramine overdose. Am J Emerg Med 14:574–576, 1996.
24. Yang CC, Deng JF: Anticholinergic syndrome with severe rhabdomyolysis—an unusual feature of amantadine toxicity. Intensive Care Med 23:355–356, 1997.
25. Leybishkis B, Fasseas P, Ryan KF: Doxylamine overdose as a potential cause of rhabdomyolysis. Am J Med Sci 322:48–49, 2001.
26. Nogue S, Pujol L, Sanz P, et al: Datura stramonium poisoning: Identification of tropane alkaloids in urine by gas chromatography-mass spectrometry. J Int Med Res 23:132–137, 1995.
27. Perrone J, Shaw L, De Roos F: Laboratory confirmation of scopolamine co-intoxication in patients using tainted heroin. J Toxicol Clin Toxicol 37:491–496, 1999.
28. Palmer EA: How safe are ocular drugs in pediatrics? Ophthalmology 93:1038–1040, 1986.
29. Barker DB, Solomon DA: The potential for mental status changes associated with systemic absorption of anticholinergic ophthalmic medications: Concerns in the elderly. DICP: The Annals of Pharmacotherapy 24:847–850, 1990.
30. Lauwers LF, Daelemans R, Baute L, et al: Scopolamine intoxications. Intensive Care Med 9:283–285, 1983.
31. Gowdy JM: Stramonium intoxication: Review of symptomatology in 212 cases. JAMA 221:585–587, 1972.
32. Shervette RE 3rd, Schydlower M, Lampe RM, et al: Jimson "loco" weed abuse in adolescents. Pediatrics 63:520–523, 1979.
33. Guharoy SR, Barajas M: Atropine intoxication from the ingestion and smoking of jimson weed (Datura stramonium). Vet Hum Toxicol 33:588–589, 1991.
34. Bergman KR, Pearson C, Waltz GW, et al: Atropine-induced psychosis: An unusual complication of therapy with atropine sulfate. Chest 78:891–893, 1980.
35. Filloux F: Toxic encephalopathy caused by topically applied diphenhydramine. J Pediatr 108:1018–1020, 1986.
36. Woodward GA, Baldassano RN: Topical diphenhydramine toxicity in a five year old with varicella. Pediatr Emerg Care 4:18–20, 1988.
37. Osterholm RK, Camoriano JK: Transdermal scopolamine psychosis. JAMA 247:3081, 1982.
38. Rubner O, Kummerhoff PW, Haase H: An unusual case of psychosis caused by long-term administration of a scopolamine membrane patch: Paranoid hallucinogenic and delusional symptoms. Nervenarzt 68:77–79, 1997.
39. Hall RCW, Feinsilver DL, Holt RE: Anticholinergic psychosis: Differential diagnosis and management. Psychosomatics 22:581–587, 1981.
40. Barker DB, Solomon DA: The potential for mental status changes associated with systemic absorption of anticholinergic ophthalmic medications: Concerns in the elderly. DICP: The Annals of Pharmacotherapy 24:847–850, 1990.
41. Parrott AC, Jones R: Effects of transdermal scopolamine upon psychological test performance at sea. Eur J Clin Pharmacol 28:419–423, 1985.
42. Hooper RG, Conner CS, Rumack BH: Acute poisoning from over-the-counter sleep preparations. J Am Coll Emerg Physicians 8:98–100, 1979.
43. Allen MD, Greenblatt DJ, Noel BJ: Self-poisoning with over-the-counter hypnotics. J Toxicol Clin Toxicol 15:151–158, 1979.
44. Smith JM: Abuse of the antiparkinson drugs: A review of the literature. J Clin Psychiatry 41:351–354, 1980.
45. Pullen GP, Best NR, Maguire J: Anticholinergic drug abuse: A common problem. BMJ 289:612–613, 1984.
46. Harrison G: The abuse of anti-cholinergic drugs in adolescents. Br J Psychiatry 137:495, 1980.

47. Klein-Schwartz W, Oderda GM: Jimsonweed intoxication in adolescents and young adults. Am J Dis Child 138:737–739, 1984.
48. Zemishlany Z, Aizenberg D, Weiner Z, et al: Trihexyphenidyl (Artane) abuse in schizophrenic patients. Int Clin Psychopharmacol 11:199–202, 1996.
49. Rubinstein JS: Abuse of antiparkinsonism drugs: Feigning of extrapyramidal symptoms to obtain trihexyphenidyl. JAMA 239:2365–2366, 1978.
50. Shipko S, Mancini JL: Simulated dystonia. Ann Emerg Med 9:279, 1980.
51. Dooris B, Reid C: Feigning dystonia to feed an unusual drug addiction. J Accid Emerg Med 17:311, 2000.
52. Nogue S, Sanz P, Munne P, et al: Acute scopolamine poisoning after sniffing adulterated cocaine. Drug Alcohol Depend 27:115–116, 1991.
53. Scopolamine poisoning among heroin users—New York City, Newark, Philadelphia, and Baltimore, 1995 and 1996. MMWR Morb Mortal Wkly Rep 45:457–460, 1996.
54. Brizer DA, Manning DW: Delirium induced by poisoning with anticholinergic agents. Am J Psychiatry 139:1343–1344, 1982.
55. Goldfrank L, Flomenbaum N, Lewin N, et al: Anticholinergic poisoning. J Toxicol Clin Toxicol 19:17–25, 1982.
56. Smith EA, Meloan CE, Pickell JA, et al: Scopolamine poisoning from homemade 'moon flower' wine. J Anal Toxicol 15:216–219, 1991.
57. Coremans P, Lambrecht G, Schepens P, et al: Anticholinergic intoxication with commercially available thorn apple tea. J Toxicol Clin Toxicol 32:589–592, 1994.
58. Anticholinergic poisoning associated with an herbal tea—New York City, 1994. MMWR Morb Mortal Wkly Rep 44:193–195, 1995.
59. Hassell LH, MacMillan MW: Acute anticholinergic syndrome following ingestion of Angel's Trumpet tea. Hawaii Med J 54:669–670, 1995.
60. Tune LE, Damlouji NF, Holland A, et al: Association of postoperative delirium with raised serum levels of anticholinergic drugs. Lancet 2:651–652, 1981.
61. Blaustein BS, Gaeta TJ, Balentine JR, et al: Cyproheptadine-induced central anticholinergic syndrome in a child: A case report. Pediatr Emerg Care 11:235–237, 1995.
62. Feinberg M: The problems of anticholinergic adverse effects in older patients. Drugs Aging 3:335–348, 1993.
63. Moreau A, Jones BD, Banno V: Chronic central anticholinergic toxicity in manic depressive illness mimicking dementia. Can J Psychiatry 31:339–341, 1986.
64. Heindl S, Binder C, Desel H, et al: Etiology of initially unexplained confusion of excitability in deadly nightshade poisoning with suicidal intent: Symptoms, differential diagnosis, toxicology and physostigmine therapy of anticholinergic syndrome. Dtsch Med Wochenschr 125:1361–1365, 2000.
65. Freedberg RS, Friedman GR, Palu RN, et al: Cardiogenic shock due to antihistamine overdose: Reversal with intra-aortic balloon counterpulsation. JAMA 257:660–661, 1987.
66. Rinder CS, D'Amato SL, Rinder HM, et al: Survival in complicated diphenhydramine overdose. Crit Care Med 16:1161–1162, 1988.
67. Fahy P, Arnold P, Curry SC, et al: Serial serum drug concentrations and prolonged anticholinergic toxicity after benztropine (Cogentin) overdose. Am J Emerg Med 7:199–202, 1989.
68. Levy R: Jimson seed poisoning—a new hallucinogen on the horizon. J Am Coll Emerg Physicians 6:58–61, 1977.
69. Jimenez-Mejias ME, Montano-Diaz M, Lopez Pardo F, et al: Atropine poisoning by *Mandragora autumnalis*: a report of 15 cases. Med Clin (Barc) 95:689–692, 1990.
70. Burns MJ, Linden CH, Graudins A, et al: A comparison of physostigmine and benzodiazepines for the treatment of anticholinergic poisoning. Ann Emerg Med 35:374–381, 2000.
71. Lawrence KR, Nasraway SA: Conduction disturbances associated with administration of butyrophenone antipsychotics in the critically ill: A review of the literature. Pharmacotherapy 17:531–537, 1997.
72. Sharma ND, Rosman HS, Padhi ID, et al: Torsades de pointes associated with intravenous haloperidol in critically ill patients. Am J Cardiol 81:238–240, 1998.
73. Gillick JS: Atropine toxicity in a neonate. Br J Anaesth 46:793–794, 1974.
74. Magera BE, Betlach CJ, Sweatt AP, et al: Hydroxyzine intoxication in a 13-month-old child. Pediatrics 67:280–283, 1981.
75. Newton RW: Physostigmine salicylate in the treatment of tricyclic antidepressant overdosage. JAMA 231:941–943, 1975.
76. Aquilonius SM, Hedstrand U: The use of physostigmine as an antidote in tricyclic anti-depressant intoxication. Acta Anaesth Scand 22:40–45, 1978.
77. Ordiway MV: Treating tricyclic overdose with physostigmine. Am J Psychiatry 135:1114, 1978.
78. Enginar N, Nurten A, Yamanturk P, et al: Scopolamine-induced convulsions in food given fasted mice: Effects of physostigmine and MK-801. Epilepsy Res 28:137–142, 1997.
79. Kamei C, Ohuchi M, Sugimoto Y, et al: Mechanism responsible for epileptogenic activity by first-generation H1-antagonists in rats. Brain Res 887:183–186, 2000.
80. Tanii H, Taniguchi N, Niigawa H, et al: Development of an animal model for neuroleptic malignant syndrome: heat-exposed rabbits with haloperidol and atropine administration exhibit increased muscle activity, hyperthermia, and high serum creatine phosphokinase level. Brain Res 743:263–270, 1996.
81. Holger JS, Harris CR, Engebretsen KM: Physostigmine, sodium bicarbonate, or hypertonic saline to treat diphenhydramine toxicity. Vet Hum Toxicol 44:1–4, 2002.
82. Pinder RM, Brogden RN, Speight TM, et al: Dantrolene sodium: A review of its pharmacological properties and therapeutic efficacy in spasticity. Drugs 13:3–23, 1977.
83. Ward A, Chaffman MO, Sorkin EM: Dantrolene: A review of its pharmacodynamic and pharmacokinetic properties and therapeutic use in malignant hyperthermia, the neuroleptic malignant syndrome and an update of its use in muscle spasticity. Drugs 32:130–168, 1986.
84. Gerbershagen MU, Fiege M, Krause T, et al: Dantrolene: pharmacological and therapeutic aspects. Anaesthesist 52:238–245, 2003.
85. Koppel C: Clinical features, pathogenesis and management of drug-induced rhabdomyolysis. Med Toxicol Adverse Drug Exp 4:108–126, 1989.
86. Curry SC, Chang D, Connor D: Drug- and toxin-induced rhabdomyolysis. Ann Emerg Med 18:1068–1084, 1989.
87. Rodgers GC Jr, Von Kanel RL: Conservative treatment of jimsonweed ingestion. Vet Hum Toxicol 35:32–33, 1993.
88. Crowell EB, Ketchum JS: The treatment of scopolamine-induced delirium. Clin Pharmacol Ther 8:409–414, 1967.
89. Duvoisin RC: Cholinergic-anticholinergic antagonism in parkinsonism. Arch Neurol 17:124–136, 1967.
90. Beaver KM, Gavin TJ: Treatment of acute anticholinergic poisoning with physostigmine. Am J Emerg Med 16:505–507, 1998.
91. Shenoy RS: Pitfalls in the treatment of Jimsonweed intoxication. Am J Psychiatry 151:1396–1397, 1994.
92. Orr R: Reversal of *Datura stramonium* delirium with physostigmine: Report of three cases. Anesth Analg 54:158, 1975.
93. Tong TG, Benowitz NL, Becker CE: Tricyclic antidepressant overdose. Drug Int Clin Pharm 10:711–713, 1976.
94. Pentel P, Peterson CK: Asystole complicating physostigmine treatment of tricyclic antidepressant overdose. Ann Emerg Med 9:588–590, 1980.
95. Shannon M: Toxicology reviews: Physostigmine. Pediatr Emerg Care 14:224–226, 1998.
96. Sivilotti MLA, Burns MJ, Linden CH: The attitudes of US regional poison centers toward physostigmine for anticholinergic delirium (Abstract). J Toxicol Clin Toxicol 35:653, 1999.

CHAPTER 23

Cholinergic Syndromes

D. Nicholas Bateman

Acetylcholine is a neurotransmitter that is distributed widely throughout the central nervous system (CNS) and peripheral nervous system. Functionally, it is responsible for transmitting impulses to a variety of specific receptor sites, including sites in the brain, within the autonomic nervous system, and the nerve endings of motor nerves acting on skeletal and smooth muscle. In addition to these neurologic sites of action, acetylcholine receptors have been identified in many other cells, including white blood cells. There is a wide distribution of potential acetylcholine-mediated effects at different organ sites: The effects of drugs that increase the activity of acetylcholine in the body and cause a "cholinergic syndrome" depend on the way in which the potential toxic agent interacts with the cholinergic components of the organism.

Historically, the investigation of compounds that affect the breakdown of acetylcholine predates the understanding of its pharmacology. In the 19th century, Scottish pharmacologists began to explore the pharmacologic effects of an extract of the Calabar bean, which had been brought back from West Africa. At that time, the bean was found to be in use by local West African tribesmen in various ceremonies, in which its CNS effects were noted by explorers. The active ingredient of the Calabar bean eventually was identified as physostigmine, which is an acetylcholinesterase inhibitor.

Full understanding of the significance of acetylcholine followed important discoveries in pharmacology that were made at the end of the 19th and beginning of the 20th centuries. These discoveries involved the use of naturally occurring compounds, two of which still are used to name the principal receptor groups of acetylcholine: the muscarinic receptors, named after muscarine, an extract of the fungus *Amanita muscarina*; and nicotinic receptors, named after nicotine, from tobacco.

As is discussed later in this chapter, acetylcholine itself acts on different subtypes of receptors, and drugs may mimic these agonist actions of acetylcholine. The consequences of these drugs depend on their specific receptor selectivity. These drugs sometimes are structural analogues of acetylcholine itself (e.g., bethanechol). Alternatively, they may be compounds that have been used traditionally to categorize the different acetylcholine receptor systems (e.g., nicotine). When acetylcholine has been released into a nerve ending, its clinical effect relates to its local concentration, which normally is limited by the activity of the enzyme acetylcholinesterase. The latter is present locally within nerve endings and metabolizes acetylcholine to acetic acid and choline, terminating its action (Fig. 23-1).

Clinically, although drugs such as carbachol and bethanechol were synthesized with structural resemblance to acetylcholine, there are now few clinical indications for the use of such agents, and their availability to patients is limited. In contrast, the use of anticholinesterase compounds in the management of myasthenia gravis and related abnormalities of skeletal nerve end plate function is an area in which systemic use of drugs that alter acetylcholine function is important. Myasthenia is managed by peripherally acting carbamate anticholinesterases, such as pyridostigmine and neostigmine. New developments in the use of anticholinesterases in dementia therapy seem likely to change the availability of anticholinesterases in the community. Rivastigmine, tacrine, galantamine, and donepezil have been approved in the United States for the treatment of senile dementia and Alzheimer's disease.

Acetylcholine is an important neurotransmitter in insects; chemicals that interfere with the enzyme acetylcholinesterase have a widespread use in agriculture as insecticides. The intensivist or medical toxicologist is most likely to see features of overactivity of acetylcholine in association with poisoning with such anticholinesterase compounds. Anticholinesterases also are used as nerve agents in chemical warfare and have been released intentionally for this purpose by terrorist groups (see Chapters 130 and 131). The need to develop effective therapies against these agents has been responsible for stimulating research into the management of patients who manifest symptoms of excess cholinergic activity.

The number of cases in which cholinergic features are prominent seen by individual clinicians to a large extent reflects their clinical environment. In developed countries, agricultural uses of pesticides are generally closely controlled, and engineering precautions are taken to avoid operator exposure. Exposures to spray drift occur, but in general these are unlikely to produce significant clinical poisoning. In developing countries, control of pesticide availability may be less stringent, and pest problems may be more common, making more widespread the use and availability of pesticides, particularly carbamate and organophosphate anticholinesterase compounds. Their availability for use as a means of self-harm and suicide is more likely. Epidemiologic data from such use and abuse in developing nations are more difficult to obtain because of the lack of detailed public health statistics. Published data require cautious interpretation because data acquisition methods and sources vary.

Some indication of the relative burden of these agents on the community in a developed country can be obtained

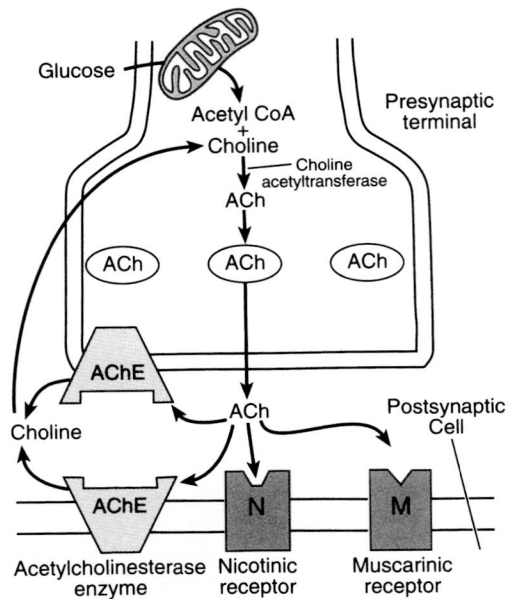

FIGURE 23-1

Cholinergic neurotransmission. Acetylcholine (ACh) is synthesized from choline and acetate via choline acetyltransferase. When released into the synaptic cleft, ACh binds to nicotinic and muscarinic receptors or is hydrolyzed by acetylcholinesterase (AChE) to choline and acetate. *(From Rhoades RA, Tanner GA [eds]: Medical Physiology. Boston, 1995, Little, Brown, p 46.)*

from publications of the American Association of Poison Control Centers; for example, in 1999, there were 15,000 inquiries involving pesticides that had an anticholinesterase action (carbamates and organophosphates). The total num-

ber of inquiries regarding potential human poisonings in that year was 2,201,000. In incidents involving only carbamates or organophosphates, there were 74 major poisonings and 5 deaths reported (Table 23-1).[1]

In Scotland (population approximately 5.1 million), pesticide use is less frequent, and severe accidental poisoning is extremely rare; poisoning usually is due to intentional ingestion.[2] In Spain, a case series of 187 organophosphate pesticide poisonings collected in the province of Almeria between 1981 and 1986 indicated that 62% of cases presenting were accidental and 38% were attempted suicide. Of patients, 86% were male, and the mean age was 31 years. The in-hospital mortality in this series was low, and the global mortality was 4%.[3] In Costa Rica in 1996, of 1274 pesticide exposures reported to the poison control center, 38.5% were occupational, 33.8% were accidental, and 22.5% were suicidal. Organophosphates accounted for 21.1% of the cases and carbamates for 13.2%.[4]

A report from Japan in 1997 indicated that of 130 cases of organophosphate poisoning, 25% resulted in death.[5] A high proportion of patients with significant depression of serum cholinesterase required ventilation. These investigators indicated that ventilatory support was in their view a crucial aspect of early care, and this is an area in which developing countries may have inadequate resources. In Sri Lanka, organophosphate insecticides are the most common cause of poisoning.[6]

The wide availability of organophosphate compounds has resulted in many patients presenting with illnesses that initially were ascribed to other causes. Fang and colleagues[7] and Greenaway and Orr[8] reported illnesses in developing countries that initially were attributed to food poisoning but subsequently were identified as being secondary to pesticide contamination of food.

TABLE 23-1   Epidemiology of Anticholinesterase Poisoning in the United States, 1999

SUBSTANCES IMPLICATED IN EXPOSURE	NO. EXPOSURES	AGE (YR)			REASON				TREATED IN HEALTH CARE FACILITY	OUTCOME				
		<6	6–19	>19	Unint	Int	Other	AdvRxn		None	Minor	Moderate	Major	Death
Carbamate only	3231	1377	336	1321	3094	84	23	26	657	717	474	140	9	0
Carbamate with other pesticide	963	309	101	503	915	25	11	12	166	149	191	31	1	0
Organophosphate only	11,193	3420	929	6003	10,725	258	40	140	2943	2350	1972	567	72	5
Organophosphate with carbamate	530	199	61	254	508	10	8	4	70	125	78	16	0	0
Organophosphate with chlorinated hydrocarbon	176	50	13	100	167	7	1	1	46	27	31	9	2	0
Organophosphate with other pesticide	1398	378	152	779	1348	28	7	13	279	291	359	71	9	0
Organophosphate with carbamate and chlorinated hydrocarbon	51	9	7	28	50	0	0	1	11	9	14	2	0	0

AdvRxn, adverse reaction; Int, intentional; Unint, unintentional.
Data from Litovitz TL, Klein-Schwatrz W, White S, et al: 1999 annual report of the American Association of Poison Control Centers Toxic Exposure Surveillance System. Am J Emerg Med 18:517–574, 2000.

In addition to anticholinesterase insecticides, other agents can cause the cholinergic syndrome. In North America, berries of the pokeweed plant (*Phytolacca americana*) produce peripheral and central cholinergic stimulation.[9] Some types of the *Amanita* species of mushroom contain muscarine and possibly other cholinomimetic compounds. Nerve gases, such as sarin, are anticholinesterases and produce features of cholinergic poisoning.[10]

PATHOPHYSIOLOGY

Acetylcholine is a transmitter in a wide range of nerves. It is convenient to divide the sites of action physiologically and anatomically and to examine the individual nerve ending responses pharmacologically.

Within the autonomic nervous system, acetylcholine is the agent responsible for transmission from preganglionic to postganglionic neurons in the parasympathetic and sympathetic systems. In the parasympathetic system, the postganglionic neuron uses acetylcholine as its transmitter. In the sympathetic nervous system, sweat gland innervation is also via acetylcholine. Motor nerves to smooth muscle in a variety of organs, including the lung and the gut, are postganglionic parasympathetic nerves with acetylcholine as their transmitter.

The anatomic divisions of the parasympathetic and sympathetic nerve supplies are shown in Table 23-2. The specific biologic effects that the stimulation of these nerves produces are shown in Table 23-3. Toxicologic effects can be predicted from Table 23-3. Separate from the autonomic nervous system, acetylcholine is a transmitter at two other sites: motor nerve endings on skeletal muscle and nerve endings within the CNS.

There has been a tremendous increase in understanding of the more basic aspects of the pharmacology of the receptor systems involved in acetylcholine transmission. Originally the separation of receptors into different subtypes was based on the differential activity of agonists and antagonists within in vitro systems. Subsequent cloning of putative receptors has led to the need for a more formal system of classification, such as is provided by the International Union of Pharmacology.

Nicotinic receptors, named because the compound nicotine generally can mimic their effects, are responsible for transmission at skeletal muscle sites and at autonomic ganglia. They also have been identified within the CNS, but their role here is uncertain. There is increasing evidence that the nicotinic acetylcholine receptor exists in a variety of subtypes. This type of receptor is a member of the multisubunit, neurotransmitter-gated family of ion channels.[11] Analysis of subunits within the receptor has suggested subtle differences in structure between the receptors appearing in fetal and adult skeletal muscle and these muscle receptors and the receptors in autonomic ganglia and the CNS. These small differences in structure suggest that it might be possible to synthesize more specific agonists and antagonists for the different receptor subtypes. The toxicologic significance of these differences is unclear.

The muscarinic receptor is part of a different functional group of receptors, in that it generally is linked to a G protein–coupled receptor. More work has been done on the cloning and typing of muscarinic than nicotinic receptors, and at present it is believed there are five separate types of muscarinic receptors (M_1 through M_5) present in humans.[12] The different muscarinic receptor groups are thought to have different functional properties. It seems likely that M_3 receptors are responsible for smooth muscle contraction and the stimulation of glandular secretion. M_2 receptors inhibit adenyl cyclase and inhibit voltage-gated calcium channels in the heart.[12] Table 23-4 shows some of these differences in receptor subtype function.

TOXICOLOGIC MECHANISMS

Present knowledge of receptors is well ahead of understanding of the toxicologic mechanisms of drug and toxin action in humans. In theory, increased activity of acetylcholine at any of the receptor sites identified could be caused by an increase in their stimulation. Potential toxic mechanisms include the following:

1. An increase in the quantity of acetylcholine released
2. A direct effect of a compound on the specific receptor site (agonist action)
3. An interaction with the systems responsible for the removal of acetylcholine (anticholinesterases)
4. Enhancement of second messenger systems and interactions with ion channels that increase the effects of released acetylcholine
5. Interaction with other neurotransmitter systems (e.g., D_2 antagonism leading to enhanced acetylcholine action in the basal ganglia and parkinsonian effects)

TABLE 23-2 Anatomy, Physiology, and Pharmacology of the Autonomic Nervous System		
	PARASYMPATHETIC	**SYMPATHETIC**
Location of cell body of		
Preganglionic fiber	Brainstem and sacral cord (S2–4)	Cord (T1-L2)
Postganglionic fiber	Ganglia associated with cranial nerves III, VII, and IX and in or near organs innervated by cranial nerves X and XI and the pelvic nerve	
Chemical mediation of transmission from		
Preganglionic fiber	Acetylcholine	Acetylcholine
Postganglionic fiber	Acetylcholine (relaxation of cardiac sphincter due to adrenergic fibers)	Norepinephrine (sweat glands innervated by acetylcholine)

TABLE 23-3 Effect of Stimulation of Autonomic Nerves on Organs and Tissues of Humans

ORGAN OR TISSUE	PARASYMPATHETIC	SYMPATHETIC
Eye		
Radial muscle of iris	–	Contraction
Circular muscle of iris	Contraction	–
Ciliary muscle	Contraction	–
Glands		
Sweat	–	Secretion*
Salivary	Secretion	Secretion
Lacrimal	Secretion	–
Respiratory tract	Secretion	–
Gastrointestinal tract	Secretion	–
Adrenal medulla	–	Secretion†
Heart		
Sinus nodal rhythm	Slowing	Acceleration
Refractory period, AV node	Increased	Reduced
Atrial conduction rate	Increased	Increased
Atrial contraction force	Decreased	Increased
Ventricular contraction force	Unknown	Increased
Blood vessels to		
Muscles	–	Dilation
Heart	Constriction	Dilation
Skin	–	Constriction
Viscera	–	Constriction
Salivary glands	Dilation	Constriction
Erectile tissue	Dilation	Constriction
Muscles of		
Hair	–	Contraction
Intestinal wall	Contraction	Relaxation
Cardiac sphincter	Relaxation‡	–
Spleen	–	Contraction
Fundus of urinary bladder	Contraction	Relaxation
Trigone and sphincter of bladder	Relaxation	Contraction
Uterus	–	Contraction

*The nicotinic action of acetylcholine results in the sympathetic effects indicated in the second column. Sweating is mediated by postsynaptic acetylcholine receptors in the sympathetic nervous system.
†The stimulation is preganglionic; the adrenal medulla is analogous to a ganglion.
‡Relaxation of the cardiac sphincter is via adrenergic nerves.
AV, atrioventricular.

Although animals and humans have been fed the acetylcholine precursor choline in an attempt to improve the functional activity of acetylcholine receptor systems, there is little evidence that this has much clinical benefit, and toxicologically it seems of no significance. Similarly the few compounds that increase acetylcholine release experimentally are not encountered normally in overdose.

There are many compounds that act at postsynaptic sites producing a spectrum of clinical responses due to selective receptor activity. This selectivity can be at muscarinic or nicotinic or both receptor systems. A more selective action at a subtype level within these broader classification groups (e.g., pure M_3 agonist action) is theoretically possible, but as yet no clinical examples are documented. There are rare instances in which second messenger enhancement or ion channel effects could be relevant to toxic effects in humans, an example being baclofen, but these have not been studied properly. Baclofen is an agonist at GABA B receptors, and these modulate acetylcholine release. Withdrawal symptoms have been reported after baclofen overdose that may be due to this phenomenon.[13]

SPECIFIC CHOLINERGIC POISONING SYNDROMES

The clinical manifestations of drugs that increase acetylcholine effects in theory can be divided into three distinct categories—pure muscarinic actions, pure nicotinic actions, and a combination of both of these effects. The last-mentioned syndrome is associated primarily with agents that prevent the breakdown of acetylcholine, principally organophosphates and carbamates. It is possible to predict the likely clinical consequences of poisoning with compounds that act on the cholinergic system by reference to Table 23-3. Bradycardia, excess salivation, sweating, increased gut motility, small pupils, and atrial stimulation occur with muscarinic agonists. Nicotinic effects include increased sympathetic activity, and clinical features are an unpredictable combination of muscarinic effects, cardiovascular effects, and fasciculation of skeletal muscle. The clinical effects of muscarinic and nicotinic stimulation are shown in Table 23-5. The clinical features seen depend on the pharmacology of the poison, its dose, and in some instances, its lipid solubility and ability to enter the brain.

Muscarinic Syndrome

Acetylcholine is not normally available itself as a pharmacologic preparation for use in humans. Bethanechol is a muscarinic agonist that was used in the treatment of gut and bladder disorders. The textbook *Therapeutic Drugs*[14] documents what is believed to be the only example of bethanechol poisoning, in which a paraplegic patient ingested 900 mg approximately 13 hours before presenting to the hospital. This patient developed hypotension, with a systolic blood pressure of around 50 mm Hg, which responded to atropine.

Pilocarpine is a quaternary compound that has muscarinic properties and is used primarily in eye drops. Pilocarpine eye drops have been implicated in poisoning in unexpected ways. Cordner and colleagues[15] reported deaths of two hospital patients who were in a female psychogeriatric ward. Most of the 24 patients in the ward developed coughing, salivation, and some degree of cyanosis after a meal. Five of the patients became more dyspneic, although two recovered quickly, but three deteriorated and were transferred to an acute medical facility. There two of the patients died. Following a police investigation, it was concluded that the patients' food had been contaminated with pilocarpine. More recently, Pfliegler and Palatka[16] reported an 18-year-old patient who attempted suicide by consuming pilocarpine orally and self-injecting the same compound. He vomited excessively, probably reducing the absorption of the compound orally. He was treated rapidly with atropine, which effectively reversed the cholinergic actions peripherally.

TABLE 23-4 Muscarinic Receptors: G-Protein Coupling, Transduction Pathways, Localization, and Functional Responses

	RECEPTOR TYPE				
	M_1	M_2	M_3	M_4	M_5
Preferred G-protein	q/11	i/o	q/11	i/o	q/11
Second messengers*	PLC IP$_3$/DAG Ca^{2+}/PKC	AC (–)	PLC IP$_3$/DAG Ca^{2+}/PKC	AC (–)	PLC IP$_3$/DAG Ca^{2+}/PKC
Locations	Brain (cortex, hippocampus) Glands Sympathetic ganglia	Heart Hindbrain Smooth muscle	Smooth muscle Glands Brain	Basal forebrain Striatum	Substantia nigra
Functional responses†	M-current inhibition	K$^+$ channels (βγ activates) Inhibit Ca^{2+} channels Decrease heart rate and force Decrease neurotransmitter release (presynaptic)	Smooth muscle contraction Gland secretion Decrease neurotransmitter release (presynaptic)	Inhibit Ca^{2+} channels	

*AC, acetylcholine; DAG, diacylglycerol; IP$_3$, inositol, 1,4,5-triphosphate; PKC, protein kinase C; PLC, phospholipase C.
†Main responses; several other responses have been suggested to be elicited by defined subtype.
From Caulfield MP, Birdsall NJM: International Union of Pharmacology XVII: Classification of muscarinic acetylcholine receptors. Pharmacol Rev 50:279–290, 1998.

TABLE 23-5 Cholinergic Toxicologic Syndromes

MUSCARINIC	NICOTINIC
Lung	Skeletal muscle
Wheeze and cough	Fasciculation
Bronchorrhea	Twitching
Dyspnea	Muscle weakness (including respiratory muscles)
Gastrointestinal	Nicotinic effects at sympathetic ganglia (e.g., in anticholinesterase poisoning)
Excess salivation	Hyperglycemia
Nausea	
Vomiting	
Abdominal cramp	
Diarrhea	
Cardiovascular system	Nicotinic effects at sympathetic ganglia (e.g., in anticholinesterase poisoning)
Bradycardia	Hypertension
Hypotension	
Ventricular tachycardia (rare)	
Eyes	
Lacrimation	
Miosis	
Blurred vision	
Bladder	
Urinary frequency	
Incontinence	
Skin	Nicotinic effects at sympathetic ganglia (e.g., in anticholinesterase poisoning) Skin pallor (vasoconstriction)
Sweating	
Central nervous system	Nicotinic effects at sympathetic ganglia (e.g., in anticholinesterase poisoning)
Confusion	Hypertonia
Agitation	
Convulsions	

Benjamin[17] reported a case series of nine children who had been exposed to mushrooms of the *Amanita* species, eight exposed to *Amanita pantherina* and one to *Amanita muscaria*. Because these mushrooms contain a range of toxins, it is by no means certain that all features are directly attributable to muscarinic effects. Most of these ingestions were in young children, and the author reported that symptoms occurred 30 to 180 minutes after ingestion, with variable CNS depression, ataxia, hallucinations, agitation, and hyperkinetic behavior being features. Seizures or myoclonic twitching were reported in four of the nine patients. In this case series, recovery was reported to be rapid and complete. Treatment of the symptoms principally consisted of anticonvulsant therapy with diazepam or barbiturates. Elonen and colleagues[18] reported three patients who appeared to have eaten the European northern mushroom *Amanita regalis*, mistaking it for an alternative edible mushroom, *Macrolepiota procera*. Symptoms began 1 to 2 hours after ingestion and included marked gastrointestinal symptoms of nausea and vomiting, and in two patients central cholinergic effects included hallucinations, confusion, loss of consciousness, excess salivation, and sweating. Patients recovered within 4 to 24 hours and developed no other organ toxicity.

An unusual potential cause of increased cholinergic activity was reported by Chen and colleagues[19] in a case series of patients with severely impaired renal function who were treated with baclofen. The most common presenting feature of excess baclofen therapy was sedation. The authors noted with interest, however, that in this case series five of the nine patients developed abdominal pain. They postulated that the effects of baclofen on γ-aminobutyric acid increased cholinergic activity in the gut and as a result produced abdominal symptoms. This suggestion requires further elucidation but illustrates the potential interaction between various neurotransmitters within the autonomic system and may represent an ion channel effect manifesting as an increased cholinergic response.

With rapid withdrawal of anticholinergic psychotropic medications, a cholinergic syndrome may develop. Symptoms include bradykinesis, motor retardation, slowed thinking and speech, lassitude, irritability, dysphoria, nausea, vomiting, and diarrhea. Tandon and colleagues[20] reported the onset of cholinergic symptoms after withdrawal of anticholinergic therapy in a schizophrenic patient who also was abusing marijuana. Initially thought to be an increase in psychotic symptoms, the syndrome resolved after institution of appropriate anticholinergic medication. These withdrawal syndromes are unusual, although syndromes were seen in patients with Parkinson's disease in whom sudden cessation of anticholinergic therapy resulted in acute akinesia. These withdrawal syndromes suggest that up-regulation of muscarinic cholinergic receptor expression may occur in humans.

Nicotinic Syndrome

It is likely that clinical toxicologists will see increasing numbers of patients experiencing the clinical effects of ingested nicotine as it becomes more widely used as a treatment for tobacco addiction. Nicotine is an alkaloid, and poisoning can occur after ingestion of cigarettes, snuff, and nicotine gum or patches. Clinical features of poisoning are more likely in children, owing to the lower doses required, and children are unlikely to be habituated to the effects of the drug. Tolerance to nicotine is well documented. Nicotine is available as an insecticide and has been ingested in this formulation.

Classic signs of nicotine poisoning develop about 15 minutes after ingestion, although features may be more rapid after ingestion of a liquid formulation of insecticide. Deaths have been reported within 5 minutes of liquid ingestions. Malizia and coworkers[21] reported that 4 to 8 mg of nicotine by mouth would produce serious symptoms in nonhabituated children. Initial features were gastrointestinal, including burning in the mouth and throat followed by salivation, nausea, vomiting, abdominal pain, and occasionally diarrhea. In children ingesting smaller amounts (less than two cigarettes),[22] vomiting occurred in about 20 minutes. In this series, seizures were not reported, and the investigators noted that the absence of vomiting predicted a favorable outcome. Cigarette ingestion in children rarely requires specific treatment.[23] In more severe poisoning, CNS features are seen, including headache, confusion, dizziness, agitation, restlessness, and incoordination, followed later by convulsions and coma. Other cholinergic features may be observed, probably resulting from stimulation of the autonomic ganglia, and include sweating, salivation, lacrimation, early miosis, and later mydriasis. Neuromuscular symptoms include hypotonia, decreased tendon reflexes, weakness, fasciculation, and paralysis of muscles, which if it includes the respiratory muscles is life-threatening.

In Malizia and coworkers' case series,[21] four children who ingested two cigarettes each developed salivation, vomiting, diarrhea, tachypnea, tachycardia, and hypertension within 30 minutes. Subsequently, cardiac arrhythmias and respiratory depression occurred. About 1 hour after ingestion, convulsions occurred. It is possible to develop

tolerance to nicotine, and prediction of dosage required to produce symptoms depends on previous ingestions. The industrial condition "green tobacco sickness" occurs in young workers who do not smoke and have been exposed to the wet, uncured tobacco leaf. Usually they experience nausea, vomiting, and faintness.[24]

The effects of nicotine reflect effects at the classic sites seen in basic pharmacology. CNS stimulation results in vomiting, then excitation. Autonomic ganglia stimulation results in increased effects at the sympathetic and parasympathetic systems manifesting as cardiovascular disturbances. Actions on the neuromuscular junction typically result in muscle weakness.

Combined Muscarinic and Nicotinic Syndrome

The compound carbachol is a combined muscarinic/nicotinic agonist that has been used therapeutically. This therapeutic use has been relatively uncommon, particularly in more recent years, and the numbers of cases reported in the literature are low.

Sangster and associates[25] reported two cases, a father and son, who developed attacks of sweating, intestinal cramps, defecation, temperature disturbance, hypotension, and bradycardia. The older patient was the 36-year-old father of the 10-year-old son, who had died from identical symptoms before the more detailed investigations of the father's case. Initially, this condition was thought to be "familial disease," but subsequent investigation showed the father had been taking carbachol prescribed for his wife for micturition disturbances. The clinical features of the father on presentation when the diagnosis was made are noteworthy. About 1 hour after eating chicken soup thought to contain carbachol, the patient became sick, developing abdominal cramps and explosive defecation. He was sweating excessively and had excess salivation. By the time he reached the hospital, he was somnolent, his heart rate was 10 to 25 beats/min, his blood pressure was 100/35 mm Hg, and his body temperature was 35°C. The electrocardiogram showed extreme sinus bradycardia with an atrial rate of 30 beats/min with atrial ventricular block and a subsequent ventricular response of 10 to 15 beats/min. The patient's cardiovascular problems responded to isoprenaline. Further symptoms occurred in the same patient after visits from his wife, and it was in this way the diagnosis was made. These symptoms suggest a predominantly muscarinic range of effects.

Sangster and associates[25] referred to deaths occurring in the 1940s after use of carbachol by accidental administration of 400 times the recommended dose. These investigators concluded that a dose of around 1 mg/kg could be considered potentially lethal.

A far more common cause of this syndrome is exposure to anticholinesterase compounds, of which there are three main types—tertiary and quaternary ammonium compounds, carbamates, and organophosphates. Figure 23-2 shows the general chemical structure of carbamate and organophosphate insecticides and of quaternary and tertiary ammonium compounds used clinically. Clinical features reflect the increase in activity of acetylcholine within the peripheral nervous system and CNS on autonomic and skeletal targets. Some compounds (e.g., neostigmine) penetrate the blood-brain barrier less well, and as a result overdose with this compound is less likely

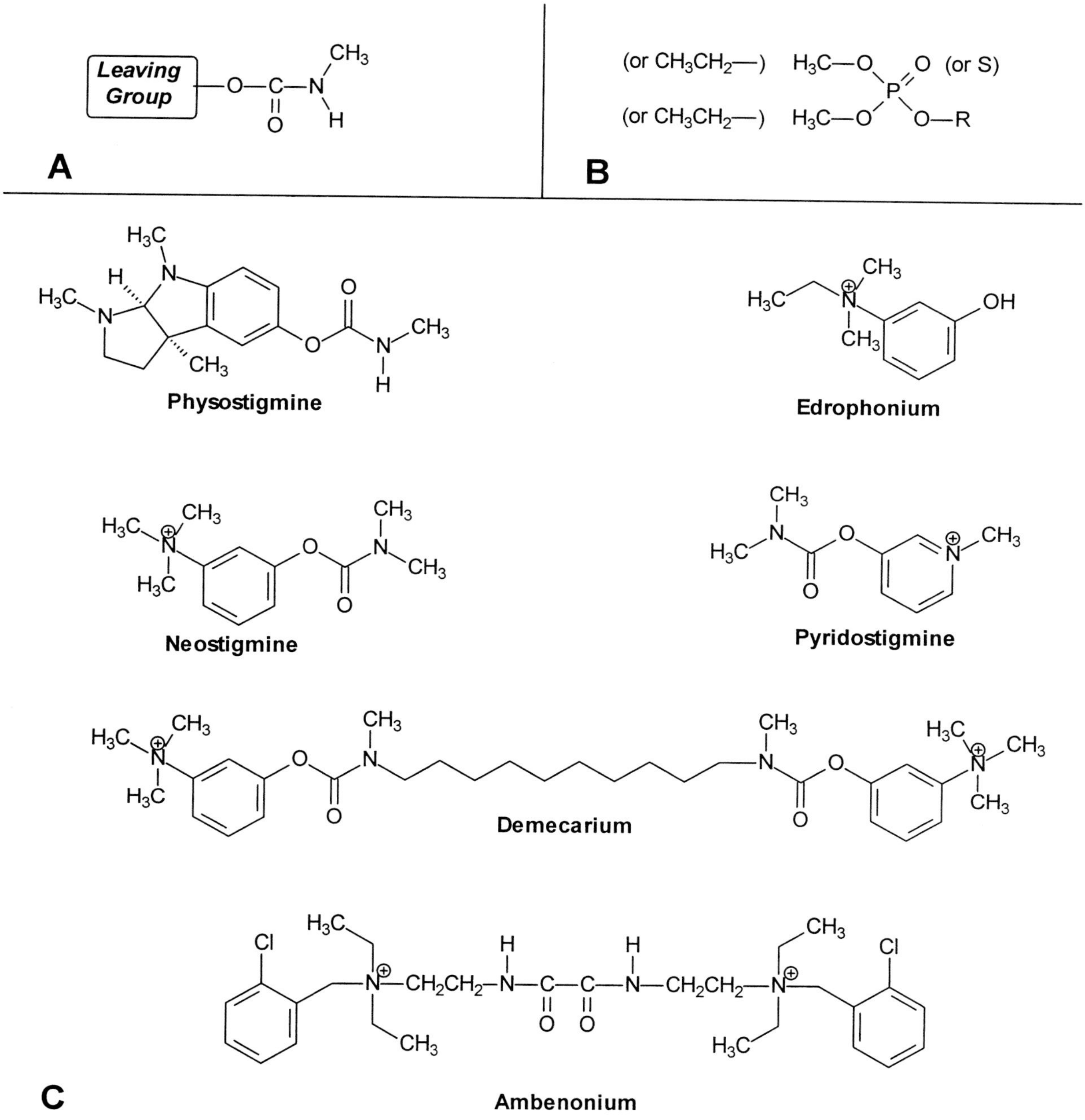

FIGURE 23-2

Chemical structures of anticholinesterase compounds. **A**, Basic structure of carbamate insecticides. **B**, Basic structure of organophosphate agents. **C**, Structures of various quaternary and tertiary ammonium compounds.

to cause CNS effects than the related physostigmine. The increasing use of agents that inhibit acetylcholinesterase as treatments for dementia[26] may alter the epidemiology of poisoning with this type of agent. The availability of these possibly toxic compounds to elderly, potentially confused patients is a potential risk. A dramatic clinical effect of rivastigmine has been a case of esophageal rupture.[27] The availability of nerve agents to terrorist groups poses another cause for concern[10] (this is discussed in further detail in Chapter 130).

An unusual presentation with cholinergic poisoning was that of a case reported from Belgium in which the carbamate aldicarb was used in an attempted murder case. The

individuals involved developed marked cholinergic effects after drinking coffee. The ingestion was confirmed by measurement of serum aldicarb concentration, but the patients recovered after 12 days in the hospital and required treatment principally with atropine and toxigonin. The investigators attributed the recovery, despite high serum aldicarb concentrations, to the reversibility of the action of carbamates on acetylcholinesterase.[28]

One well-documented report of the effects of a peripherally acting quaternary ammonium, pyridostigmine, in overdose was produced after the consumption of this agent as a potential antidote to organophosphorus nerve gases during the Gulf War. Many individuals overdosed with pyridostigmine in doses of 300 to 900 mg by injection.[29] Although pyridostigmine caused no CNS manifestations in this group, its ingestion resulted in mild-to-moderate peripheral cholinergic symptoms, including abdominal cramps, diarrhea, nausea and vomiting, hypersalivation, urinary incontinence, and muscle fasciculation. Some individuals also noted muscle weakness and blurred vision. The investigators noted that serum cholinesterase measurement was a useful indicator of pyridostigmine poisoning, although they could not show a clear relationship between the extent of serum cholinesterase inhibition and the incidence and severity of the cholinergic signs. Atropine was required for reversal of the clinical syndrome in only three of the patients, and the authors concluded that at the doses administered pyridostigmine was relatively well tolerated by normal young adults.

Manoguerra and colleagues[30] reported an unusual case in which echothiophate iodide ophthalmic drops were absorbed in sufficient quantities to produce symptoms thought to be due to myasthenia gravis. Clinical evaluation showed extreme depression of red blood cell and serum cholinesterase levels. The patient's symptoms reversed after cessation of therapy.

Some drugs have unexpected adverse effects on the cholinergic system, producing a cholinergic syndrome. The new cytotoxic agent irinotecan has been found to cause severe gastrointestinal adverse effects, particularly diarrhea. This effect seems to be due to two separate mechanisms. The first, the direct effect of irinotecan itself, can be reversed with atropine. A second syndrome of late-onset diarrhea also occurs in most patients, and this has been thought to be due to the effects of the active metabolite of irinotecan, a compound that undergoes biliary excretion. The precise mechanisms of this late-onset diarrhea were not identified by Hecht[31] at the time of writing the review and may not have been cholinergic in origin.

Many organophosphate compounds are in use as pesticides; common examples include diazinon, malathion, methylparathion, parathion, chlorpyrifos, and dichlorvos (Table 23-6). These compounds act by irreversibly inhibiting acetylcholinesterase. The binding of the organophosphate compounds to the enzyme may result in an irreversible change in its structure (aging), which means that the enzyme no longer can be reactivated to break down acetylcholine.[32] If this change occurs, the effects of the toxic ingestion last until new enzyme has been synthesized by the body. This process may take several days to weeks. It is possible to displace organophosphate from acetylcholinesterase by the use of oximes, such as pralidoxime and obidoxime. Poisoning by organophosphate and the related carbamate pesticides is discussed in detail in Chapter 91. The clinical pharmacology of oximes is discussed in Chapter 145.

Atropine competitively antagonizes the muscarinic peripheral and CNS effects of organophosphate poisoning. It alleviates the symptoms shown in Table 23-5 that result from action on the muscarinic system. Atropine has no effect, however, on the nicotinic receptors responsible for muscle weakness or respiratory failure, which occurs in more severe poisoning. These effects require ventilatory support. Because atropine is a pure competitive antagonist and the duration of effect of organophosphate compounds may be long, large doses of atropine may be required for considerable periods. In one case of parathion ingestion, a patient required 20 g of atropine over a 24-day period.[33] Le Blanc and associates[34] reported the use of atropine by intravenous infusion for more than 6 weeks. The major hazard of organophosphate poisoning on the muscarinic system is bronchosecretions.

TABLE 23-6 Examples of Compounds that Potentially Cause Toxic Effects in Cholinergic Mechanisms

Agents that increase acetylcholine release
   Guanidine, linopiridin
Pure muscarinic agonists
   Acetylcholine, bethanecol, methacholine, muscarine, pilocarpine, mushrooms
Nicotinic agonists
   Nicotine (tobacco)
Muscarinic-nicotinic agonists
   Carbachol
Anticholinesterases
   Quaternary ammonium compounds
   Demecarium, distigmine/neostigmine, physostigmine, pyridostigmine, ecothiopate, eduphonium, galantamine
   Carbamates
      Aldicarb, 4-benzothienyl-*N*-methyl carbamate, bufencarb (BUX), carbaryl, carbofuran, isolan,
      2-isopropyl phenyl-*N*-methyl carbamate, 3-isopropyl phenylmethyl carbamate, propoxur, Zectran
   Organophosphates
      Azinphos methyl, carbophenothion, chlorpyrifos, demeton-*O*-methyl, demeton-methyl, diazinon, dichlorvos,
      dicrotophos, dimethoate, endothion, fensulfothion, fenthion, malathion, methyl demeton, methyl parathion,
      mevinphos, mipafox, mononcrotophos, naled, paraoxon, parathion, phorate, phosphamidon, tetraethyl
      pyrophosphate (TEPP), thiometon, tichlorofon
Nerve agents (normally organophosphate derivatives)
   Sarin, tabun, VX
Anticholinesterases used in Alzheimer's disease
   Tacrine, rivastigmine, donepezil, galantamine

This particular effect of anticholinesterases, rather than pupillary size or heart rate, is used as the end point of treatment. In symptomatic patients, atropine may be lifesaving and should be used on clinical suspicion before the result of cholinesterase estimations become available. Atropine is of no use as a prophylactic agent in asymptomatic patients. The diagnostic doses of atropine usually advised are 1 mg in an adult or 0.015 mg/kg in a child. Atropinization should occur within 10 minutes of administration. In significantly symptomatic patients, most toxicologists recommend initial doses of 4 mg in an adult every 15 minutes. The duration of atropinization depends on the clinical scenario, and as can be seen from the above-mentioned case reports, atropinization may need to be continued for a significant period. Far larger doses than normally used in standard clinical practice may be required. For nicotinic effects on the CNS and circulatory system, appropriate sedative and cardiac supportive therapies are indicated.

LABORATORY INVESTIGATIONS

Few specific laboratory tests are applicable to the management of agents that cause cholinergic symptoms. Confirmation of an ingested agent by appropriate laboratory assay may be possible, particularly with modern gas chromatography–mass spectrometry techniques. Urinary assays may confirm the presence of metabolites of organophosphates. The most useful laboratory tests are those involved in the management of patients with organophosphate and carbamate poisoning, in which estimations of red blood cell cholinesterase confirm the diagnosis. One problem with the use of red blood cell cholinesterase is the lack of a "normal" value in patients who present acutely. There is interindividual variability in baseline levels, and in mild cases of poisoning acute measurements are difficult to interpret. Serial estimations often are needed to show a return of a marginally depressed level to normal. Urinary metabolites of organophosphates also can be estimated, and these may be of use in confirming exposure, although they are less useful in determining the precise degree of intoxication. Other laboratory investigations depend on the clinical scenario being treated.

DIFFERENTIAL DIAGNOSIS

The full range of cholinergic symptoms as described in Table 23-5 is unlikely to be seen in other clinical situations. Each individual component of the syndrome could be mimicked by another drug, however. Effects on the eye causing miosis may be mimicked by opioids. Nausea and vomiting may be caused by infectious gastroenteritis and by many toxins, including ciguatera, heavy metals, plants such as rhododendrons, and drugs, including opioids and selective serotonin reuptake inhibitor antidepressants. Excessive sweating, nausea, and vomiting are seen in salicylate poisoning. Bronchospasm may be seen in β-blocker poisoning, as is bradycardia, but not the gastrointestinal effects. The overall picture, however, is unique to these types of agent. Table 23-7 lists some of the other drugs, toxins, and conditions that may mimic some of the symptoms and signs of the cholinergic syndrome.

TABLE 23-7 Differential Diagnosis of Cholinergic Syndrome	
ACUTE POISONING	**CHRONIC POISONING**
Overdose	
Opiates	Alcohol
Phenothiazines	Opiates
Nicotine	Arsenic
β-Blockers	Thallium
Salicylates	
SSRIs	
Bites	
Venomous arthropod bites	
Spider	
Scorpion	
Venomous snake bite	
Mushrooms	
Mushrooms containing muscarine	
Infective/Other Causes	
Pneumonia and aspiration	
Septicemia	Irritable bowel syndrome
Meningitis	Bronchitis/asthma
Encephalitis	Chronic fatigue syndrome
Leptospirosis, shigellosis	
Botulism	
Gastroenteritis	
Neurologic Causes	
Epilepsy	Depression
Subarachnoid bleeding	Guillain-Barré syndrome
Subdural hematoma	Other polyneuropathies
Cerebral vasculitis	Motor neuron disease
Metabolic Causes	
Uremia	Chronic renal failure
Hypoglycemia/hyperglycemia	Thyrotoxicosis
Myxedema coma	
Thyrotoxic crisis	
Reye's syndrome	
Serotonin syndrome	

SSRIs, selective serotonin reuptake inhibitors.
Modified from Bardin PG, Van Eden SF, Moolman JA, et al: Organophospate and carbamate poisoning. Arch Intern Med 154:1433–1441, 1994.

TREATMENT

The treatment of cholinergic poisoning depends on the severity in individual patients. Decontamination techniques are applicable and relevant to patients who have been exposed to organophosphates via the dermal route, and appropriate decontamination techniques in this situation are necessary. Removal of the individual subjects from exposure, without placing bystanders and rescuers at risk, may be a necessary technique when organophosphate nerve gas exposure has occurred. It is unlikely, however, that in practice sufficient warning will have been given to emergency services to enable this to be done optimally.

The specific pharmacologic treatments for individual muscarinic, nicotinic, and muscarinic/nicotinic poisoning have been discussed previously. Atropine remains the mainstay of treatment of muscarinic symptoms. Nicotinic effects on skeletal muscle are treated symptomatically, if necessary using respiratory support or ventilation. The reader is referred to specific chapters for further information regarding the treatment of specific classes of cholinergic agents. CNS agitation secondary to muscarinic effects may respond in part to atropine, but sedative agents, such as diazepam, may be required for convulsions. The nicotinic sympathetic effects of acetylcholine exerted on the sympathetic ganglia should be treated symptomatically. In patients who have taken organophosphate and carbamate insecticides, it is general clinical experience that the effects on respiratory muscles and on bronchorrhea are dominant. When cardiovascular effects occur, their profile is unpredictable because of the muscarinic actions that occur at the same time as the nicotinic-induced sympathetic stimulation. Case-by-case clinical care is necessary.

REFERENCES

1. Litovitz TL, Klein-Schwartz W, White S, et al: 1999 annual report of the American Association of Poison Control Centers Toxic Exposure Surveillance System. Am J Emerg Med 18:517–574, 2000.
2. Good AM, Bateman DN: The Scottish experience of pesticide poisoning since 1963. J Toxicol Clin Toxicol 38:259, 2000.
3. Yelamos F, Diez F, Martin C, et al: Acute organophosphate insecticide poisonings in the province of Almeria: A study of 187 cases. Med Clin 98:681–684, 1992.
4. Leveridge YR: Pesticide poisoning in Costa Rica during 1996. Vet Hum Toxicol 40:42–44, 1998.
5. Yamashita M, Yamashita M, Tanaka J, Ando Y: Human mortality of organophosphate poisonings. Vet Hum Toxicol 39:84–85, 1997.
6. Senanayake N: Organophosphorus insecticide poisoning. Ceylon Med J 43:22–29, 1998.
7. Fang T-C, Chen K-W, Wu M-H, et al: Coumaphos intoxications mimic food poisoning. Clin Toxicol 33:699–703, 1995.
8. Greenaway C, Orr P: A foodborne outbreak causing a cholinergic syndrome. J Emerg Med 14:339–344, 1996.
9. Jaeckle KA, Freemon FR: Pokeweed poisoning. South Med J 74:639–640, 1981.
10. Okumura T, Takasu N, Ishimatsu S, et al: Report on 640 victims of the Tokyo subway sarin attack. Ann Emerg Med 28:129–135, 1996.
11. Lukas RJ, Changeux J-P, Le Novère N, et al: Current status of the nomenclature for nicotinic acetylcholine receptors and their subunits. Pharmacol Rev 51:397–401, 1999.
12. Caulfield MP, Birdsall NJM: International Union of Pharmacology XVII: Classification of muscarinic acetylcholine receptors. Pharmacol Rev 50:279–290, 1998.
13. Peng C-T, Ger J, Yang C-C, et al: Prolonged severe withdrawal symptoms after acute-on-chronic baclofen overdose. Clin Toxicol 36:359–363, 1998.
14. Dollery C [ed]: Therapeutic Drugs. CD Rom database release 1.0. Edinburgh, Elsevier, 1999.
15. Cordner SM, Fysh RR, Gordon H, Whitaker SJ: Deaths of two hospital inpatients poisoned by pilocarpine. BMJ 293:1285–1287, 1986.
16. Pfliegler GP, Palatka K: Attempted suicide with pilocarpine eyedrops. Am J Ophthalmol 120:399–400, 1995.
17. Benjamin DR: Mushroom poisoning in infants and children: The *Amanita panetherina/muscaria* group. J Toxicol Clin Toxicol 30:13–22, 1992.
18. Elonen E, Tarssanen L, Harkonen M: Poisoning with brown fly agaric, *Amanita regalis*. Acta Med Scand 205:121–123, 1979.
19. Chen KS, Bullard MJ, Chien YY, Lee SY: Baclofen toxicity in patients with severely impaired renal function. Ann Pharmacother 31:1315–1320, 1997.
20. Tandon R, Dutchak D, Greden JF: Cholinergic syndrome following anticholinergic withdrawal in a schizophrenic patient abusing marijuana. Br J Psychiatry 154:712–714, 1989.
21. Malizia E, Andreucci G, Alfani F, et al: Acute intoxication with nicotine alkaloids and cannabinoids in children from ingestion of cigarettes. Hum Toxicol 2:315–316, 1983.
22. McGee D, Brabson T, McCarthy J, Picciotti M: Four-year review of cigarette ingestions in children. Pediatr Emerg Care 11:13–16, 1995.
23. Sisselman SG, Mofenson HC, Caraccio TR: Childhood poisonings from ingestion of cigarettes. Lancet 347:200–201, 1996.
24. Gehlbach SH, Williams WA, Freeman JI: Protective clothing as a means of reducing nicotine absorption in tobacco harvests. Arch Environ Health 34:111–114, 1979.
25. Sangster B, Savelkoul TJF, Nieuwenhuis MG, van der Sluys Veer J: Two cases of carbachol intoxication. Neth J Med 22:27–28, 1979.
26. Cummings JL: Cholinesterase inhibitors: A new class of psychotropic compounds. Am J Psychiatry 157:4–15, 2000.
27. Babic T, Banfic L, Papa J, et al: Spontaneous rupture of oesophagus (Boerhaave's syndrome) related to rivastigmine. Age Ageing 29:370–371, 2000.
28. Covaci A, Manirakiza P, Coucke V, et al: A case of aldicarb poisoning: A possible murder attempt. J Analyt Toxicol 23:290–293, 1999.
29. Almog S, Winkler E, Amitai Y, et al: Acute pyridostigmine overdose: A report of nine cases. Isr J Med Sci 27:659–663, 1991.
30. Manoguerra A, Whitney C, Clark RF, et al: Cholinergic toxicity resulting from ocular instillation of ecothiophate iodide drops. J Toxicol Clin Toxicol 33:463–465, 1995.
31. Hecht JR: Gastrointestinal toxicity of irinotecan. Oncology 12:72–78, 1998.
32. Marrs TC: Organophosphate poisoning. Pharmacol Ther 58:51–66, 1993.
33. Golsousidis H, Kokkas V: Use of 19,590 mg of atropine during 24 days of treatment after a case of unusually severe parathion poisoning. Hum Toxicol 4:339–340, 1985.
34. Le Blanc FN, Benson BE, Gilg AD: A severe organophosphate poisoning requiring the use of an atropine drip. J Toxicol Clin Toxicol 24:69–76, 1986.

CHAPTER 24

Serotonin Syndrome

Kirk C. Mills

Serotonin syndrome (SS) is a potentially life-threatening complication of psychopharmacologic drug therapy characterized by variable alterations in cognition and behavior, autonomic nervous system function, and neuromuscular activity. Any drug or combination of drugs that has the net effect of increasing brainstem serotoninergic neurotransmission theoretically can produce SS (Table 24-1). It most commonly occurs when two or more serotoninergic drugs are used concurrently, but it has been reported with single-drug therapy[1,2] or overdose.[3] Serotoninergic drugs are used most commonly to treat major depression, migraine headaches, Parkinson's disease, bipolar affective disorders, obsessive-compulsive disorders, anxiety disorders, eating disorders, and attention-deficit disorders.[4] SS often is misdiagnosed because of its nonspecific symptoms, variations in severity of illness, and lack of awareness by many health professionals. In its mildest form, SS often is attributed to an exacerbation of the underlying psychiatric or medical condition. In its most severe presentation, SS may be misdiagnosed as neuroleptic malignant syndrome (NMS) (see Chapter 26).

SS is an idiosyncratic and iatrogenic condition. There have been approximately 200 reported cases of SS (depending on diagnostic criteria) since the 1950s. This number assuredly underestimates its true incidence. A prospective study attempted to determine the incidence of SS using clomipramine as a single agent. Of patients, 25% developed mild symptoms suggesting SS, and one patient (2.5%) developed moderate symptoms. The fatality rate for SS is reported to be approximately 10%,[6] but this number probably is inflated as a consequence of publication bias. SS does not have a gender predilection and has been reported in pediatric[2,3] and geriatric patients.[1]

HISTORY OF SEROTONIN SYNDROME

The earliest published account of SS is attributed to a 1955 case report discussing toxic encephalitis.[7] In the late 1950s and early 1960s, physicians began reporting cases of significant and sometimes fatal drug reactions involving meperidine and monoamine oxidase (MAO) inhibitors.[8,9] Similar reports followed involving the combination of MAO inhibitors and tricyclic antidepressants.[10,11] Prospective human experiments showed that high-dose tryptophan alone or in combination with MAO inhibitors could produce neurologic symptoms explained by serotoninergic hyperactivity.[12,13] A rodent experimental model of SS was developed during the 1960s and 1970s and helped clarify its pathophysiology.[14] The first published case report including the words *serotonin syndrome* in its title was published in 1982.[9,15]

Criteria for the diagnosis of SS were proposed in 1991 after reviewing the first 38 cases of SS.[16] The original criteria excluded the most severe manifestations of SS, however, and should not be considered as absolute criteria. Modified criteria have been proposed but still have significant limitations.[17]

PATHOPHYSIOLOGY

A general review of serotonin physiology is necessary to understand the different pharmacologic mechanisms involved in producing SS and the basis for proposed drug therapy. Serotonin acts centrally as a modulator of excitatory neurotransmission. It helps regulate many functions, such as personality, sleep, appetite, temperature, sexual function, aggression, motor control, and pain perception.[18] Peripherally, serotonin stimulates smooth muscle contraction, which leads to vasoconstriction, bronchoconstriction, uterine contraction, platelet aggregation, and increased intestinal peristalsis. Serotonin also is the primary precursor to melatonin in the pineal gland.[19]

Serotonin does not cross the blood-brain barrier.[20] It is synthesized from the dietary neutral amino acid L-tryptophan, which is able to cross the blood-brain barrier via a nonspecific amino acid transporter.[20] Centrally, serotonin is produced in nine discrete nuclei located in the lower pons and upper brainstem. The axonal projections from these nuclei communicate with almost every area of the central nervous system. The brainstem nuclei can be simplified into two groups: a superior or rostral group, which sends ascending axonal projections to the thalamus and cortex (generally inhibitory), and an inferior or caudal group, which sends descending axonal projections to the medulla and spinal cord (generally excitatory) (Fig. 24-1).[19] When inside the neuronal cytoplasm, L-tryptophan undergoes hydroxylation (rate-limiting step) to form 5-hydroxytryptophan and subsequent decarboxylation to form 5-hydroxytryptamine (5-HT, serotonin) (Fig. 24-2). It is stored in protective vesicles and released into the synapse on neuronal depolarization. After its release, serotonin binds to presynaptic and postsynaptic receptors (Fig. 24-3). Stimulation of presynaptic receptors decreases further release of serotonin.[20] Stimulation of postsynaptic receptors produces varied responses depending on which receptor subtype is stimulated. Serotoninergic neurotransmission is terminated primarily by removal of

TABLE 24-1 Mechanism of Action of Serotoninergic Drugs*

Increase Serotonin Synthesis	Selegiline (Eldepryl)	Fluvoxamine (Luvox)	Sumatriptan (Imitrex)
L-Tryptophan	Tranylcypromine (Parnate)	Paroxetine (Paxil)	Zolmitriptan (Zomig)
	St. John's wort	Sertraline (Zoloft)	Phenylalkylamines
Increase Serotonin Release		Other serotonin uptake inhibitors	(mescaline) (?)
Amphetamines	**Inhibit Serotonin Uptake**	Amphetamines	
Cocaine	Tricyclic antidepressants	Cocaine	**Dopamine Agonists**
Dexfenfluramine (Redux)	Amitriptyline (Elavil)	Dextromethorphan	Amantadine (Symmetrel)
Fenfluramine (Pondimin)	Amoxapine (Asendin)	Meperidine (Demerol)	Bromocriptine (Parlodel)
Reserpine	Clomipramine (Anafranil)	Nefazodone (Serzone)	Bupropion (Wellbutrin)
Dextromethorphan (?)	Desipramine (Norpramin)	Sibutramine (Meridia)	Levodopa (L-dopa)
	Doxepin (Sinequan, Adapin)	Tramadol (Ultram)	Pergolide (Permax)
Decrease Metabolism	Imipramine (Tofranil)	Trazodone (Desyrel)	
Amphetamine metabolites	Maprotiline (Ludiomil)	Venlafaxine (Effexor)	**Nonspecific Serotoninergic**
Monoamine oxidase inhibitors	Nortriptyline (Pamelor)		**Agents**
Isocarboxazid (Marplan)	Protriptyline (Vivactil)	**Direct Serotonin Receptor**	Electroconvulsive therapy
Moclobemide (Auronex,	Selective serotonin reuptake	**Agonists**	Lithium (Lithobid, Eskalith)
Manerix)	inhibitors	Buspirone (Buspar)	
Pargyline	Citalopram (Celexa)	Lysergic acid diethylamide (LSD)	
Phenelzine (Nardil)	Fluoxetine (Prozac)	Rizatriptan (Maxalt)	

*Names in parentheses are examples of common proprietary names of these agents.

serotonin from the synapse via presynaptic reuptake pumps (protein transporters) (see Fig. 24-3). On reuptake into the presynaptic nerve terminal, serotonin can be either repackaged into the storage vesicles for future release or metabolized by MAO and eliminated as 5-hydroxyindoleacetic acid (Fig. 24-4; see Fig. 24-3).

MAO is a cytoplasmic enzyme located on the outer mitochondrial membrane, which catalyzes the deamination and inactivation of serotonin. There are two isoenzymes of MAO: MAO-A and MAO-B. These isoenzymes differ in their catalytic affinity for serotonin, with MAO-A having the greater ability to metabolize 5-HT. MAO-B seems to be

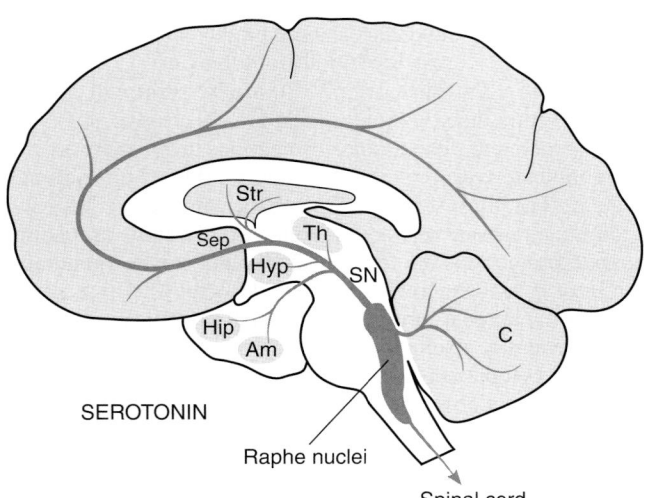

FIGURE 24-1

Serotoninergic pathways in the brain. Am, amygdaloid nucleus; C, cerebellum; Hip, hippocampus; Hyp, hypothalamus; Sep, septum; SN, substantia nigra; Str, corpus striatum. *(From Rang HP, Dale MM, Ritter JM, Gardner P (eds): Other transmitters and modulators. In Pharmacology, 4th ed. Philadelphia, Churchill-Livingstone, 2001, p 491.)*

the more prevalent isoenzyme in the human brain and serotoninergic neurons.[21] One explanation for this apparent paradox is that MAO-B probably functions to metabolize other biogenic amines and maximizes the percentage of 5-HT that gets recycled.

There currently are seven known classes of serotonin receptors, designated 5-HT$_1$ through 5-HT$_7$.[22] Some receptor classes contain separate subclasses of receptors. Only the first four classes have been studied extensively, allowing for any meaningful clinical correlations (Table 24-2). The 5-HT$_1$ class is the most studied of all the 5-HT receptors. It also has the most subclasses—5-HT$_{1A}$, 5-HT$_{1B}$, 5-HT$_{1D}$, 5-HT$_{1E}$, 5-HT$_{1F}$, 5-HT$_{1P}$, and 5-HT$_{1S}$. The 5-HT$_{1A}$ receptor subtype is predominantly a somatodendritic receptor located on serotonin nerve cell bodies in the brainstem.[21] The 5-HT$_{1A}$ receptors function as autoreceptors that inhibit subsequent serotonin release.[20] Postsynaptic 5-HT$_{1A}$ receptors are less common than 5-HT$_{1A}$ somatodendritic receptors, are found throughout the central nervous system, and are generally inhibitory. The 5-HT$_2$ receptors always are located postsynaptically, and there are three subclasses: 5-HT$_{2A}$, 5-HT$_{2B}$, and 5-HT$_{2C}$. The 5-HT$_{2A}$ receptor is found peripherally on smooth muscle cells (vasoconstriction) and platelets (aggregation). Centrally the 5-HT$_{2A}$ receptor is located predominately in the frontal cortex and produces excitation. Central 5-HT$_3$ receptors are located near the chemoreceptor trigger zone and when stimulated promote vomiting. Drugs that inhibit 5-HT$_3$ receptors are used as antiemetics. The 5-HT$_4$ receptor is associated with intestinal function and motility. Drugs that stimulate 5-HT$_4$ receptors promote gastric emptying (e.g., cisapride). Medications that act on 5-HT$_3$ and 5-HT$_4$ receptors do not produce SS.[19] The remaining serotonin receptors—5-HT$_5$, 5-HT$_6$, and 5-HT$_7$—have not been characterized fully to date.[22]

Animal models of SS suggest that it occurs primarily as a result of stimulation of brainstem postsynaptic 5-HT$_{1A}$ receptors.[23,24] Stimulation of postsynaptic 5-HT$_2$ receptors also

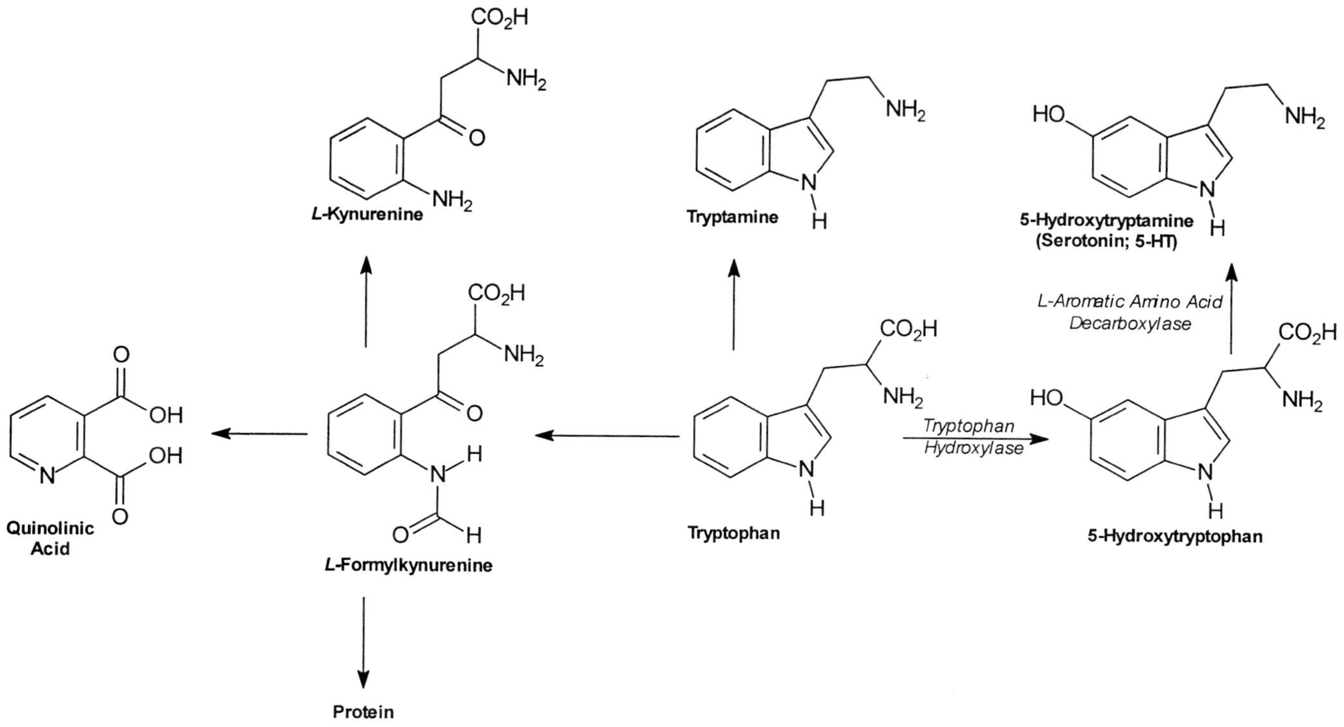

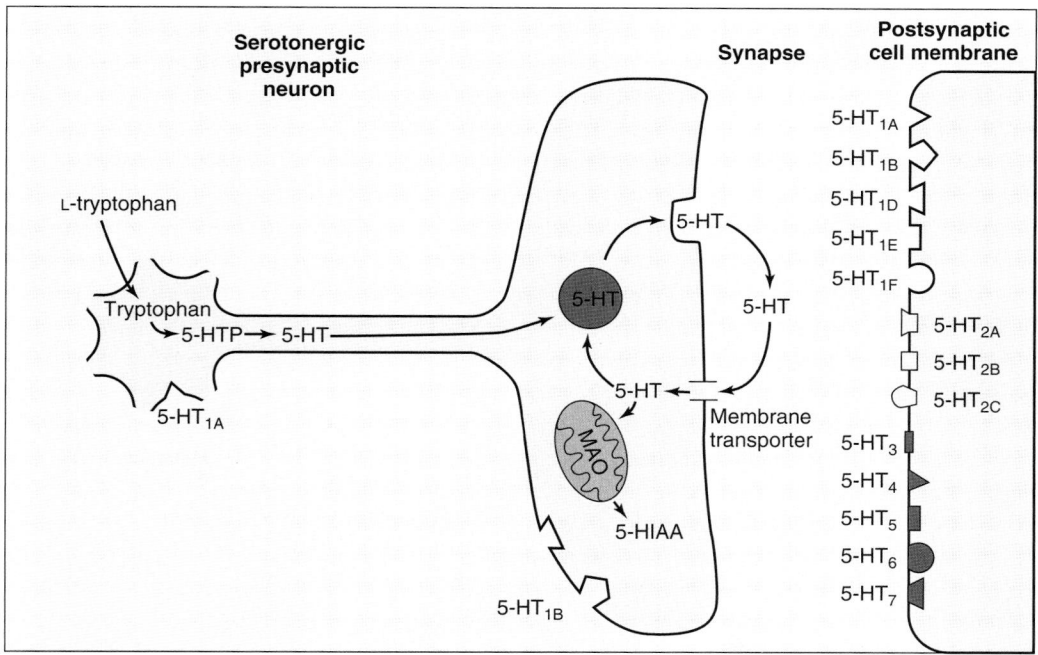

FIGURE 24-2

Biosynthesis of 5-hydroxytryptamine and alternative metabolic pathways for tryptophan.

FIGURE 24-3

A serotoninergic presynaptic neuron impinging on a postsynaptic cell. L-Tryptophan is accumulated into the cell body by an active process and converted to 5-hydroxytryptophan (5-HTP) and then to 5-hydroxytryptamine (5-HT), which is stored in granules. The stored 5-HT is released after depolarization then is available for reuptake by the membrane transporter back into the presynaptic terminal for further release or metabolism, for activation of presynaptic autoreceptors on cell bodies or nerve terminals modulating further transmitter release, or for interaction with receptors on the postsynaptic cell membrane. The postsynaptic cell membrane shown displays all known 5-HT receptor subtypes; however, several combinations of 5-HT receptors are present on different cells. MAO, monoamine oxidase. *(From Cohen ML, Brody TM: 5-Hydroxytryptamine (serotonin) and therapeutic agents that modulate serotonergic neurotransmission. In Brody TM, Larner J, Minneman KP [eds]: Human Pharmacology: Molecular to Clinical, 3rd ed. St Louis, 1998, Mosby, p 162.)*

seems to contribute to the full expression of the syndrome.[25,26] Data from animal dissection experiments indicate that stimulation of the descending serotonin pathways is an absolute requirement for SS expression.[27] The ascending pathways are also probably involved to a certain degree, however, because cognitive abnormalities commonly are seen in humans. Other neurotransmitters, such as dopamine and norepinephrine, also may contribute to the expression of SS as a result of complex interactions with serotoninergic systems.[26]

There are five basic pharmacologic mechanisms by which serotonin neurotransmission can be increased: (1) augmentation of serotonin synthesis, (2) increased release of 5-HT, (3) inhibition of 5-HT uptake, (4) inhibition of 5-HT metabolism, and (5) direct stimulation of postsynaptic 5-HT receptors (see Table 24-1). The mechanism by which some serotoninergic agents (e.g., lithium) work has yet to be elucidated, and some serotoninergic agents work by more than one mechanism. Cocaine and amphetamines primarily increase release of serotonin, but they also are capable of blocking its reuptake. Drugs that act indirectly (i.e., do not stimulate postsynaptic receptors directly) potentially can stimulate all subtypes of serotonin receptors and produce nonspecific receptor stimulation. The most common mechanism by which drugs increase serotonin activity is via inhibition of 5-HT reuptake. Drugs that have an extended half-life or an active metabolite, such as fluoxetine and its metabolite norfluoxetine, can produce SS weeks after the last dose. Drugs that irreversibly inhibit MAO require at least 2 weeks after discontinuation before the addition of another serotoninergic drug because it takes 2 weeks to produce enough new MAO to return enzyme activity to 50% of normal.[6]

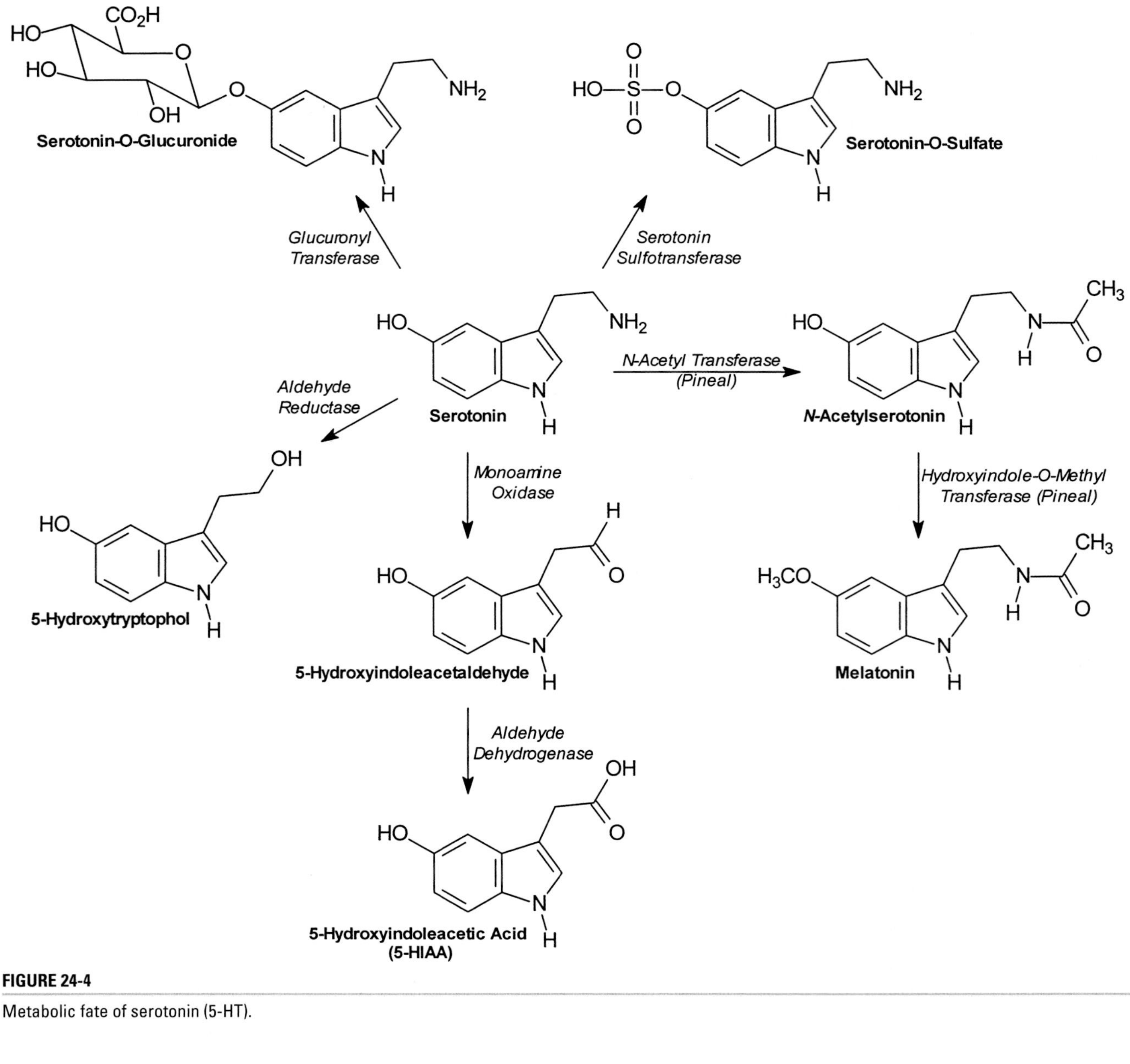

FIGURE 24-4

Metabolic fate of serotonin (5-HT).

TABLE 24-2 Classes of Serotonin Receptors*

RECEPTOR	ANATOMIC LOCATION	PHYSIOLOGIC FUNCTION	RESPONSE TO AGONIST	RESPONSE TO ANTAGONIST
5-HT$_{1A}$ presynaptic	Brainstem raphe nuclei Hippocampus	Limit release of serotonin	Decrease anxiety	Antidepressant
5-HT$_{1A}$ postsynaptic	Hippocampus Spinal cord	Hypothermia Increase prolactin Locomotion Appetite Sexual activity	Antidepressant Serotonin syndrome	Improves serotonin syndrome Depression
5-HT$_{1B}$ presynaptic	Substantia nigra Basal ganglia	Decrease release of 5-HT and other neurotransmitters	Prevents further release of serotonin	NA
5-HT$_{1B}$ postsynaptic	Extracranial blood vessels Diffuse CNS distribution	NA	Improves migraine headaches Myocardial ischemia	NA
5-HT$_{2A}$ postsynaptic	Frontal cortex Limbic area Platelets	Increase temperature Increase blood pressure Affect and alertness Platelet aggregation	Serotonin syndrome Anxiety Psychosis Drug hallucinations Hypertension	Improves serotonin syndrome Antidepressant actions Antipsychotic effect Blocks drug-induced hallucinations Antihypertensive
5-HT$_3$ postsynaptic	Intestinal tract Brainstem (area postrema) Limbic area	Promote emesis to noxious stimulation Modulates dopamine release	Nausea and vomiting	Antiemetic Mild antipsychotic effect
5-HT$_4$ postsynaptic	Intestinal tract Heart	Modulates intestinal activity	Increase intestinal motility Tachycardia	NA

*Note that most receptor information is derived from animal studies and may not apply directly to humans.
CNS, central nervous system; NA, not available (known).
Based on references 18, 22, and 41.

CLINICAL PRESENTATION

Patients with SS can present with abnormalities in cognition, behavior, autonomic nervous system, or neuromuscular function. SS is associated with many potentially severe complications, such as hyperthermia, seizures, coma, disseminated intravascular coagulation, hypotension, ventricular tachycardia, and metabolic acidosis.[6,28] It is not unusual for signs and symptoms from only one or two of these categories to predominate. The onset and intensity of clinical manifestations is extremely variable. In general, SS onset occurs soon after either an increase in dose of the primary drug or the addition of another serotoninergic drug. Information regarding the clinical characteristics of SS has come primarily from reviewing published case reports, which are difficult to interpret because of incomplete data, different drug combinations and doses, and uncontrolled treatment regimens. Nonetheless, case series based on individual reports still provide a general pattern of presentation. Five retrospective series are available for comparison (Table 24-3).[6,16,28–30] Each one of these series differs in scope, inclusion criteria, duration, number of cases, and interpretation, but each contributes to providing a consensus of the most common clinical characteristics of SS.

Disorders of neuromuscular function are the most frequently reported clinical manifestations of SS. Myoclonus and hyperreflexia occur in more than 50% of all reported cases. Their true incidence is probably higher because numerous case reports did not include neurologic examination results. Muscle rigidity, which serves as a specific yet insensitive marker for SS, is the third most commonly reported neuromuscular abnormality and often is limited to the lower extremities.[6] Ataxia may be the only presenting complaint; affected patients should be examined carefully for lower extremity hypertonia. Unilateral muscle rigidity has not been reported. Specific types of muscle rigidity, such as opisthotonos and trismus, also have been reported.[6] Rhabdomyolysis can result from prolonged or severe muscle rigidity. Generalized shivering occurs in approximately 25% of cases. Nystagmus and Babinski sign occur with equal frequency and are always bilateral. Less commonly reported neuromuscular abnormalities include teeth chattering, paresthesias, and head twitching.

Abnormalities of cognition and behavior, such as confusion and agitation, are common but risk being unrecognized

TABLE 24-3 Clinical Presentation of Serotonin Syndrome

	PERCENT OF TOTAL CASES REVIEWED				
	Mills[6] (N* = 127)	Hilton[29] (N = 105)	Sporer[28] (N = 79)	Mason[30] (N = 41)	Sternbach[16] (N = 38)
Cognitive-Behavioral					
Confusion/disorientation	54		57	41	42
Agitation	35	42		37	
Coma/unresponsiveness	28				
Anxiety	16				
Hypomania	15				21
Drowsy/lethargic	15			7	
Seizures	14		10	5	
Insomnia	10				
Hallucinations	6				
Dizziness	6	4			
Autonomic Dysfunction					
Hyperthermia	46	34	35	27	
Diaphoresis	46	39	39	49	26
Sinus tachycardia	41			18	
Hypertension	33			5	
Tachypnea	28				
Dilated pupils	26			8	
Unreactive pupils	18				
Flushed skin	14				
Hypotension	14				
Diarrhea	12	17	13		16
Abdominal cramps	5				
Salivation	5				
Neuromuscular Dysfunction					
Myoclonus	57	63	54	49	34
Hyperreflexia	55	44	60	41	29
Muscle rigidity	49	66		20	
Extremity tremor	49	61		17	26
Hyperactivity/restlessness	43			30	45
Ataxia/incoordination	38	40	48		13
Shivering/chills	25	30	27		26
Nystagmus	13				
Babinski (extensor response)	14			12	
Teeth chattering	6	3			
Opisthotonos	6				
Trismus	6			7	

*Number of patients.

due to subtle presentations. Coma is reported more often than less severe alterations of consciousness, which may reflect reporting bias more than true incidence. Changes in behavior such as anxiety and hypomania initially may be misinterpreted as an exacerbation of underlying psychiatric illness. Generalized tonic-clonic seizures have been reported in roughly 10% of cases. These are usually self-limiting, but treatment-resistant seizures also have been reported.[6] Focal seizures are extremely unusual and should prompt an evaluation for an alternative diagnosis.[31] Subjective symptoms, such as headache, insomnia, visual hallucinations, and dizziness, are reported less commonly.

Autonomic disturbances may represent a manifestation of SS. Numerically, autonomic disturbances occur less frequently than cognitive or neuromuscular abnormalities; however, numerous case reports fail to mention vital sign measurements or physical examination results. Their incidence most likely is underestimated. Diaphoresis is observed commonly, having been reported in approximately half of all cases. Hyperthermia is reported commonly and usually is moderate, but severe elevations have been reported. Hypertension also is usually moderate in severity but can achieve extreme levels. Patients frequently present with asymptomatic sinus tachycardia ranging from 100 to 180 beats/min. Ventricular tachycardia has been observed rarely.[22,10,57] Tachypnea is present in more than one third of cases. Hypotension occurs in 14% of cases and usually portends an unfavorable prognosis. Flushed skin, diarrhea, salivation, and abdominal pain occur relatively infrequently. Dilated pupils have been reported; they frequently are unreactive to light. A peculiar ocular finding described as "Ping-Pong" gaze has been observed with some cases of MAO inhibitor toxicity and refers to bilateral wandering horizontal eye movements.[32] The mechanism of this gaze disorder is unknown. In all cases, it gradually resolves as the patient improves.

DIAGNOSIS

Laboratory and Ancillary Tests

There are no confirmatory laboratory or ancillary tests for SS. Laboratory tests are used best to identify potential complications, rule out other diagnoses, and assist in supportive patient care. Serum electrolytes and glucose concentrations, hemoglobin, hematocrit, cerebrospinal fluid analysis, and computed tomography brain scans are almost always normal.[6] Leukocytosis is seen in approximately 13% of cases but rarely exceeds 20,000 cells/cm. Electroencephalography, when performed, either is normal or shows general slowing consistent with diffuse encephalopathy. Electrocardiograms most commonly show normal sinus rhythm or sinus tachycardia. Elevated noncardiac creatine phosphokinase levels are reported in 18% of cases and are more common in association with muscle rigidity. Complications such as disseminated intravascular coagulation, metabolic acidosis, and hypoxia are infrequent but have been reported in severe cases of SS.[6,28] In cases in which drug concentrations (including metabolites) have been determined, they have been either therapeutic or low in 80% to 90% of cases.[6] Therapeutic drug concentrations do not exclude the diagnosis.[33]

Differential Diagnosis

The best way to make the diagnosis of SS is a high clinical suspicion based on a history of serotoninergic drug exposure combined with signs and symptoms consistent with SS and the exclusion of other potential causes. Previous diagnostic criteria were vague and limited. They excluded many symptoms that are common, severe, and more specific to the diagnosis of SS. Retrospective studies have allowed for a greater understanding and appreciation of this syndrome since the original criteria[16] and subsequent attempt at modification.[17] This new information should be incorporated into the existing diagnostic criteria for greater accuracy (Table 24-4). Potential signs and symptoms should be expanded to include any of the signs and symptoms listed in Table 24-3. Diagnostic accuracy increases when patients have symptoms from each of the three main categories,

especially when symptoms either are commonly observed (e.g., hyperthermia) or are unique to SS (e.g., bilateral lower leg muscle rigidity). Neuromuscular symptoms are more specific for SS, and it is imperative to perform a complete neuromuscular examination to detect any of these abnormalities. A rapid and complete response to antiserotoninergic agents (e.g., cyproheptadine) is less likely among the other disorders listed in the differential diagnosis and strongly favors the diagnosis of SS (see Table 24-4).

The differential diagnosis of SS most commonly involves disorders capable of producing muscle rigidity and autonomic dysfunction. In its most severe presentation, SS frequently is confused with NMS (Table 24-5) (NMS is discussed in detail in Chapter 26). Differentiation between SS and NMS becomes especially difficult in patients having recently been exposed to serotoninergic and neuroleptic drugs. There may be a neurochemical explanation for the similarity between these two syndromes because serotonin tends to inhibit dopamine secretion,[34] as evidenced by increased prolactin levels.[22] Serotonin uptake inhibitors have been associated with extrapyramidal syndromes, such as dystonia, akathisia, and parkinsonism.[35] It may be speculated that SS and NMS may represent two different pathways with the same clinical end point. There also is some speculation that serotonin may be involved in producing malignant hyperthermia.[36]

There are numerous other possibilities in the differential diagnosis of SS, such as drug-related toxicity secondary to MAO inhibitors, phencyclidine, cocaine, amphetamine, methylphenidate, strychnine, nicotine, lithium, and antimuscarinic (anticholinergic) agents. Because of the similarities in presentation between SS and overdoses of MAO inhibitors, their differential diagnoses are the same (see Table 43-2). Special note should be made concerning 3,4-methylenedioxymethamphetamine (MDMA)-related toxicity especially because many of these cases resemble severe SS.[37,38]

TREATMENT

SS generally is associated with a favorable prognosis.[30] The management of SS encompasses five basic elements: (1) supportive care, (2) discontinuation of all serotoninergic agents, (3) anticipation of complications, (4) possible administration of antiserotoninergic agents, and (5) reassessment of the need for continuing serotoninergic drug therapy when SS has resolved. Despite the favorable prognosis, many patients with SS require admission to an intensive care unit, with 25% of these patients needing endotracheal intubation and ventilatory support. Most patients show some improvement within the first 24 hours with supportive care alone. Many patients experience complete resolution of SS within the first 12 to 24 hours.[6,28,30] Clinical manifestations occasionally last longer than 96 hours, but this usually occurs only in cases associated with medical complications (e.g., multiple organ failure) or drugs with prolonged duration of action. In cases of acute drug overdose, gastrointestinal decontamination (e.g., gastric lavage, activated charcoal) may be warranted if done early, but airway protection should be ensured first. The pharmacokinetics of the most commonly encountered serotoninergic agents is such that repeated doses of activated charcoal are unlikely to be of benefit. Lithium is the only serotoninergic agent for which extracorporeal removal may be indicated.

TABLE 24-4 Criteria for Diagnosis of Serotonin Syndrome	
Documented exposure to one or more serotoninergic agents	Absolute
Exclusion of other causes	Absolute
Presence of three or more symptoms consistent with diagnosis (see Table 24-3)	Absolute
No recent addition or dosage increase of antipsychotic medications	Absolute
No recent discontinuation of dopamine agonists	Relative
Rapid improvement with antiserotoninergic medications	Relative

TABLE 24-5 Comparison of Serotonin Syndrome versus Neuroleptic Malignant Syndrome		
	SEROTONIN SYNDROME	**NEUROLEPTIC MALIGNANT SYNDROME**
Etiology		
Dopamine antagonists (e.g., haloperidol)	No	Antagonism of dopamine receptors is believed to be the main pathophysiologic mechanism producing NMS
Withdrawal of dopamine agonists	No	It has been reported to produce NMS
Dopamine agonists (e.g., levodopa)	Dopamine agonist may increase CNS serotonin activity indirectly	No
Serotonin agonists (e.g., MAO inhibitors)	By definition, serotonin syndrome occurs only in the presence of serotoninergic drugs	No
Serotonin antagonists (e.g., cyproheptadine)	Drugs that block serotonin receptors are incapable of producing serotonin syndrome	No
Symptoms/Signs		
Onset of symptoms	Symptoms frequently begin within minutes to hours after addition of second drug or increase in dose of primary drug	Symptom development is usually more gradual, occurring over days to weeks
Resolution of symptoms	Often improve or resolve in <24 hr	Symptoms are slower to resolve (average 9 days)
Hyperthermia (>38°C)	46%	>90%
Altered level of consciousness	54%	>90%
Autonomic dysfunction	50–90%	>90%
Muscle rigidity	49%	>90%
Leukocytosis	13%	>90%
Increased creatinine phosphokinase level	18%	>90%
Liver transaminase enzyme levels	9%	>75%
Metabolic acidosis	9%	Very common
Hyperreflexia	55%	Rare
Myoclonus	57%	Rare
Treatments		
Dopamine agonists (e.g., bromocriptine)	No reason to believe they would be of benefit, and theoretically they may exacerbate condition	Are commonly believed to improve condition
Serotonin antagonists	May improve condition	No beneficial effect

CNS, central nervous system; MAO, monoamine oxidase; NMS, neuroleptic malignant syndrome.

Hyperthermia is the most significant complication of SS and is seen almost exclusively in the setting of muscle rigidity. Based on experience with drug-induced sympathomimetic syndromes, most clinical toxicologists believe that hyperthermia should be treated rapidly and aggressively.[28] Benzodiazepines generally are considered the initial agents of choice to relieve muscle rigidity, but nondepolarizing paralyzing agents may be needed as second-line agents. Dantrolene has been used empirically in some cases, especially when NMS was suspected initially.[6] Seizures generally respond to benzodiazepines or barbiturates.[6,28] Phenytoin is not expected to be effective (see Chapter 20). Metabolic acidosis typically is seen only in cases involving hyperthermia, seizures, muscle rigidity, or multiple organ failure.

There are no true antidotes for SS. Animal studies have shown that antagonists at the 5-HT$_{1A}$ and 5-HT$_2$ receptors, such as chlorpromazine, cyproheptadine, methysergide, and propranolol, are effective in preventing SS.[24,25] Isolated case reports have suggested that these same agents may be beneficial in treating SS in humans. Chlorpromazine has been used in more than a dozen cases with generally favorable results,[39] with a typical dose of 50 mg given intramuscularly and repeated every 6 hours up to four doses.

The main advantage of chlorpromazine is that it can be given to patients who are unable to take oral medications. The concerns of lowering the seizure threshold, producing hypotension, and predisposing to dystonic reactions have not been realized in case reports.[39] Benzodiazepines have been administered frequently but rarely have been effective as single agents, perhaps as a result of inadequate doses.[6] The potential benefit of benzodiazepines is most marked in patients with generalized muscle rigidity or significant agitation. There are no controlled human studies using any of these drugs, and any benefit attributed to their use is purely speculative and anecdotal.

Cyproheptadine seems to be the most consistently effective antiserotoninergic agent in humans.[40] It is a nonspecific antagonist of 5-HT$_{1A}$ and 5-HT$_2$ receptors. In addition, it has antimuscarinic and antihistaminic characteristics, which may be disadvantageous. Cyproheptadine is available as a 4-mg tablet with a typical adult dose of 0.5 mg/kg/day. A syrup (2 mg/5 mL) preparation is available for children with the usual pediatric dose of 0.25 mg/kg/day. Cyproheptadine is considered relatively safe in pregnancy. Initial adult cyproheptadine doses in SS can range from 4 to 8 mg and can be repeated every 1 to

4 hours until a therapeutic response is obtained, or a maximum daily dose of 32 mg in adults and 12 mg in children is achieved. Methysergide has been used in a few cases with mixed results.[6] Propranolol also has had mixed success.[6] Propranolol, benzodiazepines, and chlorpromazine have the potential advantage of being available in parenteral form.

When the patient recovers from SS, the next decision is to reevaluate the necessity of reinstituting serotoninergic medications. Controlled data on this topic are lacking, and it is best to proceed with caution. A few guidelines may be beneficial. First, if psychopharmacologic drug therapy is warranted, nonserotoninergic medications should be considered. Second, if serotoninergic agents are necessary, using single-drug therapy or drugs of lower potency is recommended. Third, a drug-free "washout" period lasting 6 weeks may be necessary in drugs with long half-lives or active metabolites, such as fluoxetine, before restarting serotoninergic medications.

Finally, it is important not to precipitate SS unknowingly in patients admitted to the hospital for other conditions. This situation is most likely to occur through the administration of meperidine or dextromethorphan to patients already taking other serotoninergic agents. Morphine, hydromorphone, aspirin, and acetaminophen are nonserotoninergic analgesic alternatives.

Key Points in Serotonin Syndrome

1. Serotonin syndrome is a clinical diagnosis. There are no confirmatory tests.
2. Most serotoninergic drugs are not identified on routine drug screens.
3. Most cases of serotonin syndrome involve two or more medications. Look for all possibilities, including prescription medications, over-the-counter dextromethorphan, herbal supplements such as St. John's wort or 5-hydroxytryptophan, and drugs of abuse (e.g., 3,4-methylenedioxymethamphetamine [MDMA], lysergic acid diethylamide [LSD]).
4. Most cases of serotonin syndrome involve medications within therapeutic limits.
5. When in doubt about whether the diagnosis is serotonin syndrome or neuroleptic malignant syndrome, give cyproheptadine and avoid dopamine agonists or chlorpromazine. If the patient responds, serotonin syndrome is the diagnosis.
6. Do not give meperidine, tramadol, or dextromethorphan to patients taking serotoninergic agents.
7. Patients can present with vague nonspecific complaints, which are mistaken for an exacerbation of their psychiatric condition.
8. Most physicians do not perform a complete neuromuscular examination and miss important findings.
9. Serotonin syndrome rarely produces focal physical findings.
10. Serotonin syndrome does not develop as a result of carcinoid syndrome.
11. Cyproheptadine and chlorpromazine may produce a false-positive tricyclic antidepressant serum drug screen result.
12. A urine amphetamine drug screen does not always detect MDMA.
13. Patients still are susceptible to serotonin syndrome 4 weeks after discontinuation of an irreversible monoamine oxidase inhibitor.
14. Hyperthermia is the main contributing factor to patient deaths from serotonin syndrome.

REFERENCES

1. Fischer P: Serotonin syndrome in the elderly after antidepressive monotherapy. J Clin Psychopharmacol 15:440–442, 1995.
2. Gill M, LoVecchio F, Selden B: Serotonin syndrome in a child after a single dose of fluvoxamine. Ann Emerg Med 33:457–459, 1999.
3. Kaminski C, Robbins M, Weibley R: Sertraline intoxication in a child. Ann Emerg Med 23:1371–1374, 1994.
4. Chojnacka-Wojcik E: 5-Hydroxytrptamine in the central nervous system. Pol J Pharmacol 47:219–235, 1995.
5. Lejoyeux M, Ades J, Rouillon F: Serotonin syndrome incidence, symptoms and treatment. CNS Drugs 2:132–143, 1994.
6. Mills KC: Serotonin syndrome, a clinical update. Med Toxicol 13:763–783, 1997.
7. Mitchell R: Fatal toxic encephalitis occurring during iproniazid therapy in pulmonary tuberculosis. Ann Intern Med 42:417–424, 1955.
8. Taylor D: Antidepressives in chronic schizophrenics. Lancet 2:401–402, 1962.
9. Reid N, Jones D: Pethidine and phenelizine. BMJ 1:408, 1962.
10. Brachfeld J, Wirtshafter A, Wolfe S, et al: Imipramine-tranylcypromine incompatibility. JAMA 186:1172–1173, 1963.
11. Rom W, Benner E: Toxicity by interaction of tricyclic antidepressant and monoamine oxidase inhibitor. Calif Med 117:65–66, 1972.
12. Oates J, Sjoerdsma A: Neurologic effects of tryptophan in patients receiving a monoamine oxidase inhibitor. Neurology 10:1076–1078, 1960.
13. Smith B, Prockop D: Central nervous system effects of ingestion of L-tryptophan by normal subjects. N Engl J Med 267:1338–1341, 1962.
14. Jacobs B: An animal behavior model for studying central serotonergic synapses. Life Sci 19:777–786, 1976.
15. Insel T, Roy B, Cohen R, et al: Possible development of the serotonin syndrome in man. Am J Psychiatry 139:954–955, 1982.
16. Sternbach H: The serotonin syndrome. Am J Psychiatry 148:705–713, 1991.
17. Hegerl U, Bottlender R, Gallinat J, et al: The serotonin syndrome scale: First results on validity. Eur Arch Psychiatry Clin Neurosci 248:96–103, 1998.
18. Leonard B: Serotonin receptors and their function in sleep, anxiety disorders and depression. Psychother Psychosom 65:66–75, 1996.
19. Mills KC: Serotonin toxicity: A comprehensive review for emergency medicine. Top Emerg Med 15:54–73, 1993.
20. Curry SC, Mills KC, Graeme KA: Neurotransmitters. In Goldfranks LR, Flomenbaum NE, Lewin NA, et al (eds): Goldfranks's Toxicologic Emergencies, 7th ed. New York, McGraw-Hill, 2002, pp 133–165.
21. Boulton A, Eisenhofer G: Catecholamine metabolism from molecular understanding to clinical diagnosis and treatment. Adv Pharmacol 42:273–292, 1998.
22. Barnes N, Sharp T: A review of central 5-HT receptors and their function. Neuropharmacology 38:1083–1152, 1999.
23. Goodwin G, De Souza R, Wood A, et al: The enhancement by lithium of the 5-HT1a mediated serotonin syndrome produced by 8-OH-DPAT in the rat: Evidence for a post-synaptic mechanism. Psychopharmacology 90:488–493, 1986.
24. Gerson S, Baldessarini R: Motor effects of serotonin in the central nervous system. Life Sci 27:1435–1451, 1980.
25. Glennon R, Darmani N, Martin B: Multiple populations of serotonin receptors may modulate the behavioral effects of serotonin agents. Life Sci 48:2493–2498, 1991.
26. Nisijima K, Yoshino T, Ishiguro T: Risperidone counteracts lethality in an animal model of the serotonin syndrome. Psychopharmacology 150:9–14, 2000.
27. Jacobs B, Klemfuss H: Brain stem and spinal cord mediation of a serotonergic behavioral syndrome. Brain Res 100:450–457, 1975.
28. Sporer KA: The serotonin syndrome: implicated drugs, pathophysiology and management. Drug Saf 13:94–104, 1995.
29. Hilton S, Maradit H, Moller H: Serotonin syndrome and drug combinations: Focus on MAOI and RIMA. Eur Arch Psychiatry Clin Neurosci 247:113–119, 1997.
30. Mason PJ, Morris VA, Balcezak TJ: Serotonin syndrome: Presentation of 2 cases and review of the literature. Medicine 79:201–209, 2000.
31. Pascual J, Combarros O, Berciano J: Partial status epilepticus following single low dose of clomipramine in a patient on MAO-inhibitor treatment. Clin Neuropharmacol 10:565–567, 1987.
32. Erich J, Shih R, O'Connor R: "Ping-Pong" gaze in severe monoamine oxidase inhibitor toxicity. J Emerg Med 13:653–655, 1995.

33. Goeringer K, Raymon L, Christian G, et al: Postmortem forensic toxicology of selective serotonin reuptake inhibitors: A review of pharmacology and report of 168 cases. J Forens Sci 45:633–648, 2000.

34. Leiberman J, Mailman R, Duncan G, et al: Serotonergic basis of antipsychotic drug effects in schizophrenia. Biol Psychiatry 44:1099–1117, 1998.

35. Gerber PE, Lynd LD: Selective serotonin reuptake inhibitor induced movement disorders. Ann Pharmacother 32:692–698, 1998.

36. Wappler F, Fiege M, Schulte am Esch J: Pathophysiologic role of the serotonin system in malignant hyperthermia. Br J Anaesth 87:794–798, 2001.

37. Demirkiran M, Jankovic J, Dean JM: Ecstasy intoxication: An overlap between serotonin syndrome and neuroleptic malignant syndrome. Clin Neuropharmacol 19:157–164, 1996.

38. Mueller PD, Korey WS: Death by "Ecstasy": The serotonin syndrome? Ann Emerg Med 32:377–380, 1999.

39. Gillman PK: The serotonin syndrome and its treatment. J Psychopharmacol 13:100–109, 1999.

40. Graudins A, Stearman A, Chan B: Treatment of the serotonin syndrome with cyproheptadine. J Emerg Med 16:615–619, 1998.

41. Gareri P, Falconi U, De Fazio P, et al: Conventional and new antidepressant drugs in the elderly. Prog Neurobiol 61:353–396, 2000.

CHAPTER 25

Malignant Hyperthermia

Henry Rosenberg ■ Jordan Miller

Malignant hyperthermia (MH) syndrome is an unusual disorder. Like a person who has an allergy, the MH-susceptible patient is unaware of his or her problem until exposed to the "triggering" agent. MH syndrome may not develop on all exposures. The resemblance to an allergy breaks down, however, on further analysis. MH is an inherited disorder.[1] Patients develop a hypermetabolic condition on exposure to drugs that are used to produce general anesthesia or skeletal muscle paralysis.[2,3] The pathophysiologic change relates to an uncontrolled increase of intracellular calcium in skeletal muscle that leads to hypermetabolism, depletion of energy sources, acidosis, and membrane breakdown.[1–4] Untreated, MH syndrome is fatal in most cases. With prompt discontinuation of trigger agents and administration of the drug dantrolene, mortality may be eliminated.[5] This chapter discusses clinical presentation, pathophysiology, molecular genetics, diagnosis, treatment, and sources of information for this unusual cause of anesthetic morbidity and mortality.

HISTORY

MH was recognized in the early 1960s by clinical anesthesiologists and a clinical geneticist in Melbourne, Australia.[6] The event that attracted their attention related to surgery for a young man who sustained a motor vehicle injury. The patient expressed great concern because many members of his family had died unexpectedly while under anesthesia. The anesthesiologists administered halothane anesthesia, and, warned by the patient's concern, stopped the anesthetic and the procedure when the patient developed hypertension, then hypotension, tachycardia, and sweating. Denborough, a consultant internist with an interest in inherited diseases, was called to investigate. He then described many salient features of the syndrome.

After Denborough and Lovell[6] described the syndrome, many others described similar cases throughout the world. By the end of the 1960s, the syndrome was called *malignant hyperthermia* or *malignant hyperpyrexia*. The reason for the appellation was the mortality of greater than 80% and the strikingly elevated body temperature that accompanied the disorder. Other peculiar features that were described included muscle rigidity, rhabdomyolysis, and in some cases, rigidity limited to the jaw muscles after the muscle relaxant succinylcholine was administered.

At the first international workshop on MH, held in 1971 in Toronto, Canada, clinicians and basic researchers began to exchange information about MH. Veterinarians and pig breeders reported that certain breeds of pigs developed what seemed to be MH on a regular basis when stressed.[7] The breeds were known for their muscle mass and included Pietrain, Poland-China, and others.

Although there was great concern initially that MH-susceptible humans would develop the syndrome with stress, that has not been shown to be the case.[2,3] There are many other differences between human and swine MH. The inheritance of the syndrome is autosomal recessive in pigs but autosomal dominant in humans. The pig has served as a useful model, however, for understanding the pathophysiology of MH, determining which drugs precipitate the syndrome, and determining the effective treatment of MH.

Since the early 1970s, there has been an enormous growth in knowledge and awareness of how to diagnose and treat MH syndrome. Landmark advances are outlined in Table 25-1. All of these findings and many others have led to the reduction of mortality from MH to less than 7% in developed countries.[11]

In a sense, the term *malignant hyperthermia* has become a misnomer. Fever is a late sign of MH and is often not manifest when the diagnosis is made, and the fatality rate of MH is low. The name of MH may be too firmly entrenched to be changed, however. Other names given to the syndrome include *anesthesia-induced myodystrophy* and *rhabdomyolysis of anesthesia*.

INCIDENCE

MH, being an inherited myopathy, should be amenable to epidemiologic investigation of incidence, prevalence, and perhaps penetrance. The data have been difficult to gather, however. The reason is that MH patients in general have no specific phenotypic sign, other than when exposed to anesthetic drugs; the signs of MH during anesthesia may be nonspecific and mimicked by other processes, such as fever, iatrogenic overheating, and myotonia. In addition, until late 1998, there was no specific ICD-9 (*International Classification of Diseases–ninth revision*) code for MH, and the syndrome did not appear in the diagnostic databases of diseases.

The incidence of fulminant cases of MH is approximately 1 in 200,000 instances of exposure to anesthesia, and the incidence of clinical signs that resemble MH but for which the diagnosis is not certain is 1 in 5000 instances of exposure to anesthesia.[12] In addition, the incidence of MH in children is about three times higher than in adults.[13] The incidence of clinical MH depends on the use of the trigger agents for MH and the gene prevalence in the population. In the

TABLE 25-1 Landmarks in Malignant Hyperthermia

Demonstration that biopsied muscle responds with abnormal contractures to halothane and to caffeine[8,9]

Recognition that all potent volatile anesthetic gases are triggers for MH, as is the depolarizing relaxant succinylcholine[2,3]

Demonstration that local anesthetics and intravenous anesthetics are not triggers of MH[2,3]

The finding, in 1975, that dantrolene sodium is a specific treatment for MH[5,10]

The routine use of capnography in anesthesia and the recognition that elevated end-tidal carbon dioxide is an early sensitive and specific sign of MH[2,3]

The creation of patient advocacy groups and hotlines throughout the world to assist anesthesia providers and others to recognize MH and guide treatment

Demonstration that mutations in a specific gene that elaborates a calcium channel in muscle, the ryanodine receptor, is responsible for almost all cases of pig MH and perhaps 50% of human MH[1]

MH, malignant hyperthermia.

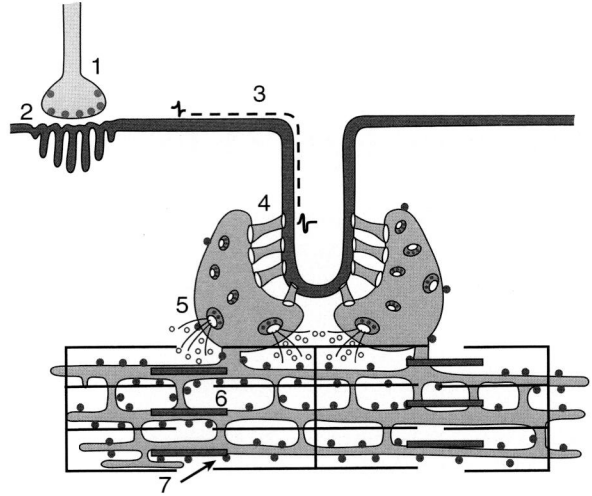

FIGURE 25-1

Schematic diagram of the steps involved in muscle activation and contraction. (1) Nerve endings showing acetylcholine stores. (2) Muscle end plate. (3) Propagation of action potential. (4) Ryanodine receptor calcium channel. (5) Terminal cisternae containing calcium release channels. (6) Thick and thin filaments mediating contraction. (7) Calcium-ATPase protein that pumps calcium back into the longitudinal elements of the sarcoplasmic reticulum. *(From Nelson TE, Sweo T: Calcium uptake and calcium release by skeletal muscle sarcoplasmic reticulum. Anesthesiology 69:572, 1988.)*

United States and Canada, a higher incidence of MH is found in Ontario, Wisconsin, Michigan, and West Virginia. MH has been identified in every country and ethnic group where it has been looked for.[11]

A study has determined that the incidence of susceptibility to MH in one province of Quebec is about 1 in 200 individuals.[14] The study was performed because many patients in the province had been tested for MH susceptibility with biopsy (see under Diagnostic Testing). The province was settled by a small number of families in the 19th century, and there had not been a large admixture of other families in the province. A few families with MH accounted for most of the cases. A more recent study using molecular genetic techniques estimated that the prevalence of MH mutations may be 1 in 2000 in the French population.[15]

A great deal of further investigation is needed to determine the epidemiologic characteristics of the disorder. To the best of our knowledge, there are fewer than five deaths from MH each year in the United States and several hundred nonfatal cases.

PATHOPHYSIOLOGY

MH is a disorder of skeletal muscle biochemistry and physiology (Fig. 25-1).[1–4] It is doubtful that other tissues are primarily responsible for the clinical manifestations of MH or are significantly altered during a case of MH. Based on the recognition that muscle rigidity was a dramatic part of most cases of MH, Kalow and colleagues[8] tested muscle biopsy specimens from susceptible pigs and humans for their response to caffeine, the agent known to produce muscle contracture secondary to calcium release from the sarcoplasmic reticulum. The response of biopsied skeletal muscle in vitro to caffeine was clearly abnormal. Contractures developed with concentrations of 0.5 mM in MH muscle but not in normal muscle. MH muscle showed significant (>0.5 g) contractures on exposure to clinical concentrations of halothane.[9,16–18] The same findings cannot be shown in smooth or cardiac muscle.

Further investigations using calcium-sensitive dyes and calcium ion electrode showed markedly increased levels of intracellular calcium in whole muscle or cultured muscle from MH-affected animals and humans on exposure to anesthetics.[19–21] The defect in MH is related to enhanced *release* of calcium from the terminal cisternae of the sarcoplasmic reticulum (Fig. 25-2).[4] Reuptake does not seem to be at fault in these tissues.[4,22] The consequence of enhanced release of calcium is muscle contraction/contracture resulting from release of inhibition of actin-myosin interaction. Adenosine triphosphate (ATP) levels decline as a result of activation of processes to resequester calcium, leading to anaerobic metabolism and acidosis. Presumably the declining levels of ATP lead to breakdown of membrane integrity and release of intracellular enzymes, such as creatine kinase (CK), along with potassium and hydrogen ions.

Evidence of abnormal calcium control in MH-susceptible patients, even without exposure to anesthetic agents, is suggested by nuclear magnetic resonance studies in exercising human muscle in vivo.[23–27] These studies show greater inorganic phosphate levels (owing to ATP breakdown) at rest and with exercise, exercise-induced acidosis, and slower recovery of ATP levels in MH-susceptible patients. These changes do not lead to clinical signs of MH.

Further refinement of understanding of the pathophysiology of MH has focused on the mechanisms responsible for calcium control in muscle.[4] Several proteins mediate calcium release and control intracellular calcium levels. Most attention has been focused on the ryanodine receptor, a calcium channel that mediates excitation contraction coupling in skeletal muscle (Fig. 25-3).[1–4] Molecular biologic studies

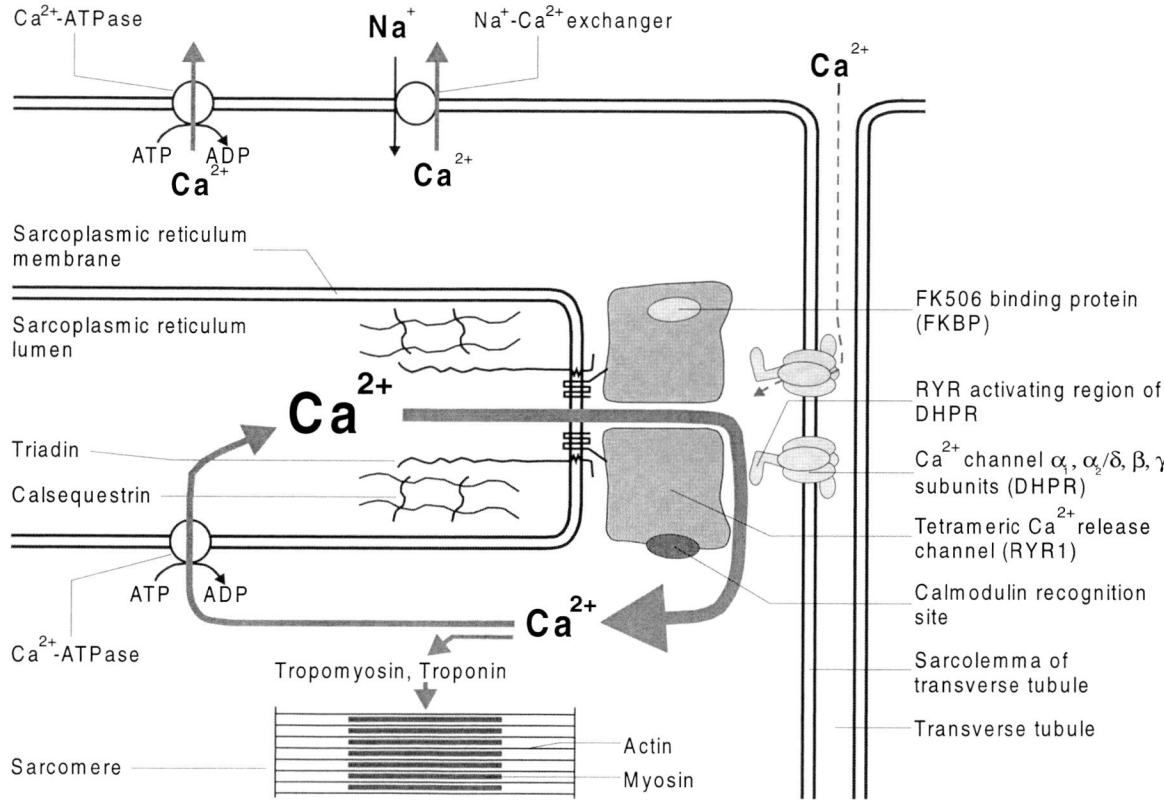

FIGURE 25-2

Diagram of structures involved in excitation-contraction coupling in skeletal muscles. *(From Schulte am Esch J, Wappler F: Malignant Hyperthermia. Vienna, Pabst Science, 2000.)*

have shown that 50% of families susceptible to MH harbor 1 of about 30 mutations in the gene that elaborates this protein.[1,28] At least six other genes have been implicated in MH,[1,29–32] however, including another protein that mediates excitation contraction, the dihydropyridine receptor,[33] the sodium channel,[34] and other genes whose function is not yet clarified in relation to MH syndrome.

Although mutations in the ryanodine receptor may be an important factor in the pathophysiology of MH, only about 50% of MH-susceptible families have been linked to ryanodine mutations.[1,28] The presence of a mutation does not explain the interindividual and intraindividual variability in the human MH syndrome in terms of clinical expression. In several families, there is discordance between the

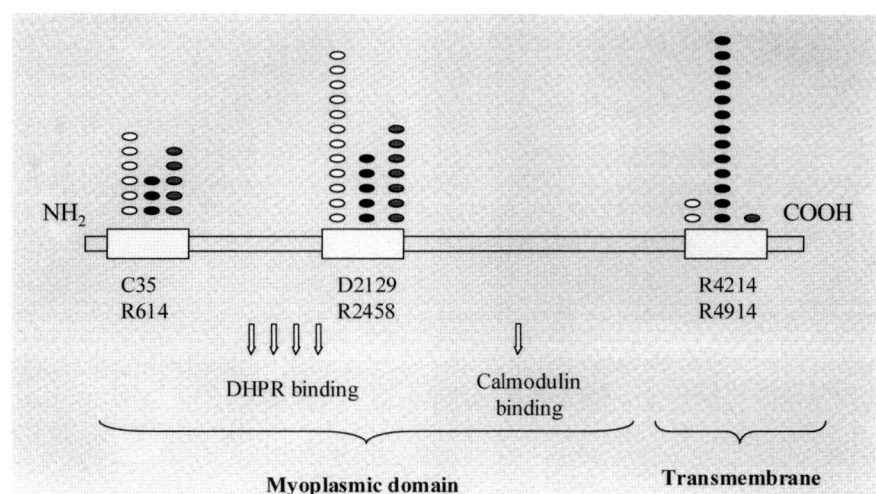

FIGURE 25-3

Diagram of the ryanodine receptor gene illustrating the regions of the most common mutations.

MH-ryanodine genotype and the phenotype as determined by the halothane-caffeine contracture test.[35–39]

We have proposed several modulators that influence the expression of the clinical syndrome. One modulator is fatty acids.[40] Skeletal muscle from MH-susceptible patients exhibits elevated fatty acid production.[41] These fatty acids have been shown to increase the sensitivity of halothane-induced calcium release in vitro.[40,42] In addition, in MH muscle, there is a shift of subtypes of sodium channels[43,44] leading to longer membrane depolarization[44] and an increased period of calcium release from the terminal cisternae. There also is evidence for linkage of MH to chromosome 17 at or near the locus encoding the sodium channel α subunit. In one family, a mutation in the sodium channel has been associated with an unusual form of myotonia and with MH susceptibility.[34] These changes in sodium channel function, either through sodium channel mutations or through effects of fatty acids on sodium channel and other proteins, may be essential for the phenotypic expression of certain aspects of the MH syndrome, such as muscle rigidity.[45]

Central core disease, a dominantly inherited neuromuscular weakness, is one of the myopathies associated with MH. Mutations in the ryanodine receptor gene have been shown to be causal for central core disease.[46,47] Hypokalemic periodic paralysis is another myopathy that has been associated with mutations in the dihydropyridine receptor in the same region as the mutations for MH.[33] Some patients with these disorders have displayed clinical MH reactions, but others have not.

The fine details of calcium control and its alteration in MH patients require further study and examination to characterize better the clinical presentations of MH. It is hoped that advances in molecular genetics will assist this effort. Nevertheless, the basic finding that MH results from a hypermetabolic response to increased levels of intracellular calcium in skeletal muscle in genetically predisposed patients exposed to potent inhalational agents and succinylcholine is an essential tenet of the pathophysiology of the disorder.

DIAGNOSTIC TESTING

After the demonstration that biopsied skeletal muscle behaved abnormally on exposure to caffeine[8] and to halothane[9] in vitro, a standardized testing protocol to diagnose MH was developed. There are three major testing protocols in common use throughout the world.[11] The protocols in Europe[48] and North America[49] are similar. The one in Japan is different.[50]

In protocols using muscle bundles (Europe and North America) weighing about 100 mg, the tissue is tested on the same day as harvest.[48,49] The muscle tested is either the vastus lateralis or the vastus medialis. Tests are conducted in duplicate or triplicate. The muscle is electrically stimulated to produce contractions of at least 0.5 g. Exposure to caffeine and to halothane results in contracture development (Figs. 25-4 and 25-5).

In the European protocol, exposure to halothane is done in increments of 0.5%, 1%, and 2%. A positive response is a contracture of at least 0.2 g on exposure to 2% or less of halothane (see Fig. 25-4). Other strips are exposed to incremental doses of caffeine (0.25 mM, 0.5 mM, 1 mM, 1.5 mM, 2 mM, 3 mM, and 4 mM), and a positive response is 0.2-g contracture to 2 mM of caffeine or less (see Fig. 25-5). If the response to both agents is positive, the patient is considered *MH susceptible*. If the test is positive to only one agent, the patient is designated as *MH equivocal* but for clinical purposes is considered as MH susceptible.

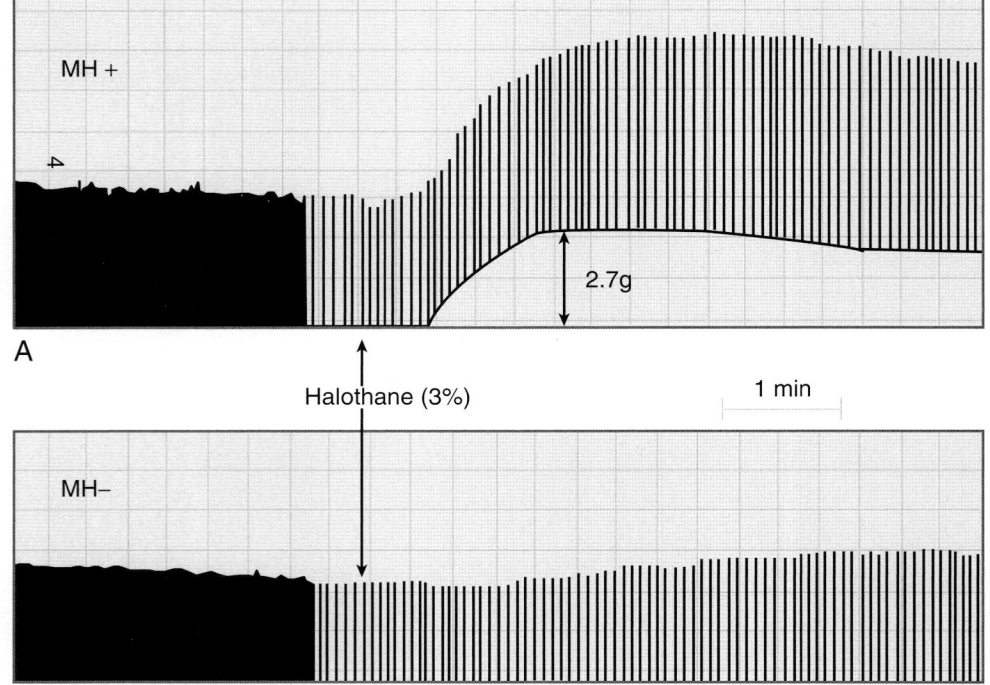

A

Halothane (3%) 1 min

B

FIGURE 25-4

In vitro contracture response. Cut muscle bundles from the vastus muscle weighing approximately 150 mg are mounted in a temperature-controlled bath. The muscle is stimulated at 0.1 Hz with a supramaximal stimulus. Halothane 3% in 95% oxygen and 5% carbon dioxide are introduced into the bath. **A**, 3 g contracture typical of malignant hyperthermia susceptibility. **B**, Normal response to halothane.

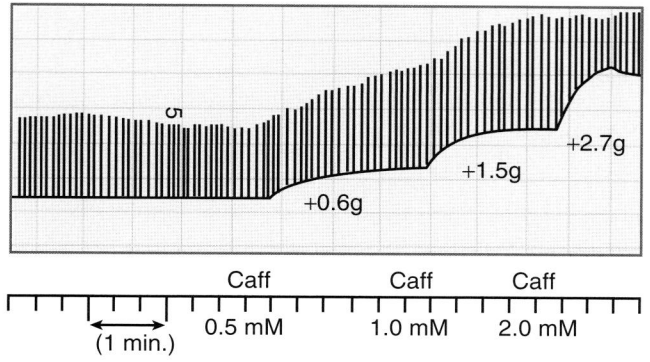

Abnormal caffeine dose response

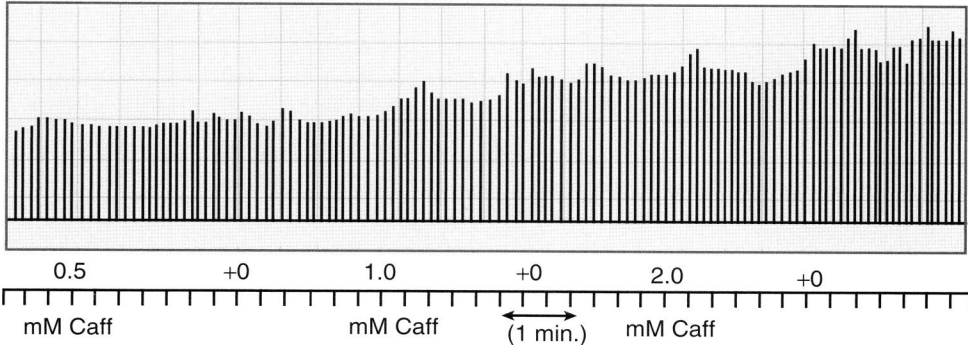

FIGURE 25-5

Responses to caffeine in vitro. Same preparation with different muscle bundles as in Figure 25-4 except the muscle bundle is exposed to incremental concentrations of caffeine for 4 minutes each. A positive response indicating malignant hyperthermia susceptibility is a contracture of 0.3 g or more to 2 mM of caffeine.

Normal caffeine dose response

In the North American protocol, the exposure is to 3% halothane, and a contracture of 0.5 g or greater is considered positive. Exposure to caffeine is essentially similar to that in Europe except that the concentrations are 0.5 mM, 1 mM, 2 mM, 4 mM, 8 mM, and 32 mM. A contracture of greater than or equal to 0.3 g at 2 mM of caffeine is considered positive. Patients are considered MH susceptible if the response to one of the agents is abnormal.

Multicenter studies have shown a sensitivity of close to 100%[16,17] but a specificity of about 82% to 93% in Europe[16,28] and 78% in North America.[17] In both tests, considerable interlaboratory variability is noted—not surprising, given that these are biologic tests. Because 5% to 15% of responses are considered equivocal by the European test, alternative agents have been used with some benefit. Responses to ryanodine[18,51] and to chlorocresol[52] have been shown to be abnormal in MH muscle.

There are about 12 biopsy centers for MH in North America (Table 25-2) and more than 20 in Europe. Other biopsy centers exist in other countries, including Australia, New Zealand, Brazil, and Israel. The test is time-consuming and expensive to perform. Despite the promise of other testing procedures, such as determination of high-energy phosphate depletion with exercise in vivo as measured by nuclear magnetic resonance spectroscopy,[23–27] the biopsy response to caffeine and halothane remains the gold standard diagnostic test.

In Japan, the diagnostic test also uses skeletal muscle, but muscle in which the sarcolemma has been chemically removed.[50] Such skinned muscle showed accentuated responses to calcium and to caffeine. Comparison between the skinned muscle test and biopsy contracture test using whole muscle bundles showed a discordance between the two tests, however.[53] As a result, biopsy centers in Europe and North America have decided not to employ this test.

Histologic examination of the biopsied muscle usually reveals nonspecific findings, such as type 1 atrophy, internal nuclei, and variation of fiber size. A few patients show changes consistent with central core or minicore disease, however.[54] Aside from this occasional finding, there is no distinctive pathologic change in MH muscle.[55]

TABLE 25-2 Biopsy Centers in the United States and Canada*

United States

Philadelphia, PA	Thomas Jefferson University
Los Angeles, CA	University of California, Los Angeles
Bethesda, MD	Uniformed Services University of Health Sciences (military only)
Winston-Salem, NC	Bowman Gray School of Medicine
Chicago, IL	Northwestern School of Medicine
Minneapolis, MN	University of Minnesota
Mayo Clinic, MN	Mayo School of Medicine
Sacramento, CA	University of California, Davis

Canada

Toronto, Ontario	Toronto General Hospital
Ottawa, Ontario	Ottawa Civic Hospital

*Further information may be obtained from the Malignant Hyperthermia Association of the United States (MHAUS) at 1-607-674-7901 or www.mhaus.org.

For diagnostic purposes, the patient must be sent to a biopsy center for testing.

With the demonstration of the association between *RYR1* mutations and MH susceptibility in certain families,[1,28] many believe that routine testing for ryanodine mutations has become essential.[56] Some investigators believe that if a known mutation in *RYR1* is found in a family member, other family members showing that mutation may be considered as MH susceptible. Further investigation is needed to rule out susceptibility if the mutation is not found in a family member. This is a promising and exciting prospect for simplified diagnosis of MH.[57] In Germany and in Australia, where several families have been identified and screened for *RYR1* mutations, 25% of families can be characterized by a *RYR1* mutation.[27] Family members may be evaluated by DNA testing for susceptibility to MH.

The virtue of molecular genetic testing is the high specificity and the fact that DNA may be harvested from white blood cells or buccal cells. Many other, less invasive tests are in development. These include measurement of carbon dioxide production after microinjection of caffeine into muscle[58] and calcium release measurement on exposure of cultured muscle cells to halothane. B lymphocytes also manifest activity of the ryanodine receptor, and the calcium flux changes that are found in muscle may be shown in isolated B lymphocytes.[59]

CLINICAL PRESENTATION

The clinical diagnosis of MH may be easy and straightforward or challenging. MH is precipitated on exposure to the potent inhalational anesthetic agents or succinylcholine. Other drugs used in anesthesia to produce insensibility or muscle paralysis are not triggers for MH (Table 25-3).

TABLE 25-3   Safe and Unsafe Pharmacologic Agents in Malignant Hyperthermia

Malignant Hyperthermia Triggers

Succinylcholine
All potent inhalational anesthetics
    Halothane
    Desflurane
    Sevoflurane
    Isoflurane
    Enflurane
    Methoxyflurane
    Cyclopropane
    Ethers
    Fluroxene

Agents That Do Not Trigger Malignant Hyperthermia

Nitrous oxide
All local anesthetics
Intravenous anesthetics (e.g., thiopental, etomidate, propofol, ketamine)
Nondepolarizing muscle relaxants (e.g., curare, rocuronium, vecuronium, atracurium, cisatracurium, mivacurium, pancuronium)
Opioids (e.g., morphine, fentanyl, sufentanil)
Anxiolytics and benzodiazepines
Reversal agents (e.g., naloxone, flumazenil, anticholinesterases, anticholinergics)
Mixed opioid agonists/antagonists (e.g., nalbuphine, butorphanol)
Droperidol/haloperidol

In the past, MH most often occurred shortly after induction of anesthesia and was marked by a paradoxical rigid response to succinylcholine, with tachycardia, hypertension, increase in end-tidal carbon dioxide, and fever.[1–3] As anesthetic practice has evolved and succinylcholine use has declined, the manifestations of MH also have changed. MH now occurs later in the course of anesthesia and even in the recovery room.[60–63]

The earliest, most sensitive and specific sign of MH is an increase in end-tidal carbon dioxide levels that requires large minute ventilation to control. Patients who require two or more times predicted minute ventilation to maintain normocarbia are hypermetabolic. End-tidal carbon dioxide may increase to 50 or 100 mm Hg during MH episodes. Besides MH, other causes of hypermetabolism include sepsis, iatrogenic overheating, faulty monitor function, and rarely thyrotoxicosis or pheochromocytoma (see later discussion of differential diagnosis of MH).

Despite the appellation, hyperthermia is a late sign of MH in almost all cases. If the patient's body temperature has increased to 40°C (104°F), early signs of MH have been missed. If core temperature exceeds 42°C, disseminated intravascular coagulation almost always supervenes, leading to a high fatality rate. It is vital to monitor a patient's core temperature during all general anesthesia exposures lasting longer than about 20 minutes. Hyperthermia is sometimes an important tip-off to the diagnosis of MH.

Muscle rigidity during anesthesia exposure is another important warning sign for MH.[64,65] One of the common forms of muscle rigidity that has been noted in MH is masseter muscle rigidity after the use of succinylcholine. Of children anesthetized with an inhalational agent followed by administered succinylcholine, 1% develop masseter muscle rigidity.[66,67] Clinical MH follows in about 20% of cases, but the onset may be delayed. It is not clear why some patients who are not MH susceptible also develop succinylcholine-induced muscle rigidity. When there is generalized muscle rigidity, MH is almost certain. Masseter rigidity along with generalized rigidity is virtually pathognomonic for MH.

Rhabdomyolysis is another characteristic feature of MH. CK elevation may be dramatic and extreme, whereas myoglobinuria may occur soon after the onset of the MH episode. Myoglobinuria and CK elevation peak at about 14 hours after the episode, however, and repeated determinations of CK are needed to diagnose MH or confirm the suspicion of MH. An easy screening test for myoglobin is urine dipstick for blood in the absence of red blood cells.

Hyperkalemia, hypercalcemia, and hypocalcemia are the typical electrolyte changes during an MH episode. Hyperkalemia may lead to arrhythmias. Hyperkalemia sufficient to cause ventricular fibrillation has been reported after the use of trigger agents in patients with a wide variety of myopathies, especially central core disease, muscular dystrophy, and various forms of myotonia.

Nonspecific signs of MH include tachycardia, tachyarrhythmias, tachypnea, sweating, hypertension, and hypotension. Coagulation abnormalities are more common in patients experiencing marked hyperthermia. Arterial blood gas analysis is essential in confirming the diagnosis of MH in many cases. Typically, respiratory and metabolic acidosis are found. Hypoxemia is not common during MH. Venous blood gas is

TABLE 25-4 Signs and Symptoms of Malignant Hyperthermia

SYMPTOM	INCIDENCE (FIRST 30 MIN)
Tachycardia	90%
Hypercarbia	80%
Rigidity	80%
Hypertension	75%
Hyperthermia	70%

a good substitute for arterial sampling. Elevation of venous carbon dioxide tension and marked acidosis are seen during MH crisis.

The presentation of MH may consist of a mixture of all of the above-mentioned signs or may be limited to only a few, making the diagnosis challenging. When MH is suspected but not easily confirmed, it is advisable to treat with dantrolene, control the metabolic signs, and investigate the patient later. Table 25-4 lists common signs and symptoms of MH and their incidence.

TIME OF ONSET

Most episodes of MH occur in the early part of the anesthesia exposure, certainly within the first few hours. Late-onset postoperative rhabdomyolysis is unlikely to be MH, but frequently there are not enough data to allow a true differential diagnosis.[60-63] Perioperative rhabdomyolysis or myoglobinuria may occur in patients who are not susceptible to MH.

Normal patients who are not susceptible to MH may have 10-fold to 100-fold increases in serum myoglobin[68,69] after succinylcholine; repeated administration (i.e., intermittent intravenous bolus) is associated with more prominent increases in myoglobin level. Other causes of perioperative rhabdomyolysis include (1) pressure-induced muscle ischemia from prolonged surgical positioning[70,71]; (2) muscle ischemia from prolonged tourniquet inflation[72-74]; (3) extensive soft tissue trauma; (4) electrical injury; and (5) underlying myopathy or metabolic disorder rendering muscle more susceptible to injury from ischemia, fever, or fasting. It is difficult to exclude MH from consideration with confidence unless the medical record clearly shows absence of hypermetabolism during anesthesia and in the early postoperative period. If the patient later undergoes a biopsy and is found to be MH susceptible by the in vitro halothane caffeine contracture test, there is a tendency to assume the episode was MH related. A patient after an uneventful triggering anesthetic of 8 hours' duration had the onset of flank pain and rhabdomyolysis starting more than 24 hours postoperatively. The biopsy specimen was abnormal 3 months after the event.[75] Whether this was an MH event is highly debatable, although based on the biopsy the patient should be treated as MH susceptible. In the absence of sepsis, patients who experience perioperative rhabdomyolysis should be referred for biopsy diagnosis of MH.

RELATED MALIGNANT HYPERTHERMIA CONDITIONS

Sudden Cardiac Arrest in Young Patients

In the early 1990s, a series of young, mostly male patients who developed unexpected cardiac arrest soon after induction of anesthesia or in the recovery room were reported to the MH hotline. Further investigation revealed that these patients were harboring a myopathy that had not produced clinical signs and symptoms. The cause of the cardiac arrest was related to hyperkalemia. Hyperthermia, tachycardia, and muscle rigidity were not constant features. Rhabdomyolysis was common, however. The younger patients were found to harbor classic muscular dystrophy.[76] The older patients were found to have Becker's muscular dystrophy.[76] It is now almost an axiom of anesthesia care that sudden cardiac arrest in an otherwise healthy boy should be considered as a hyperkalemic event and therapy should be directed to that cause.

Becker's muscular dystrophy is also an X-linked dystrophinopathy, but onset is in adolescence. Hyperkalemic cardiac arrest during anesthesia has been the presenting sign of Becker's dystrophy in a few instances. It is unclear why a myopathy related to abnormality of a structural protein, dystrophin, makes the muscle susceptible to marked disintegration of muscle membrane integrity.

As a result of such reports, the U.S. Food and Drug Administration ordered a change in the package insert for succinylcholine. At present, a black box warning states that succinylcholine should be administered only on indication in children or young adults, such as full stomach or airway problem. Most pediatric anesthesiologists have phased out the routine use of succinylcholine, replacing it with a rapid-onset nondepolarizing agent. The routine use of this drug for intubation in the emergency department also should be reconsidered.

Awake Malignant Hyperthermia

MH in the awake state is much harder to diagnose than MH in the operating room. A large increase in the production of carbon dioxide in an immobile and anesthetized patient is unusual. The cold operating room environment, depression of thermoregulation, and frequent use of neuromuscular blockade makes the classic signs and symptoms unusual except in an MH episode. Even patients who are febrile from bacteremia usually lose heat and reduce metabolic rate under anesthesia. Clinical signs frequently suggest the diagnosis of MH early in the disease process. Further confirmation using laboratory tests and, if necessary, muscle biopsy is helpful.

The patient who awakens from anesthesia shivering, who may or may not have been febrile preoperatively, is much more difficult to evaluate for MH susceptibility. Although most patients awaken with little to suggest hypermetabolism, many who are hypothermic in the operating room shiver on awakening. This shivering may be confused with evidence of MH[77] and is frequently treated with low-dose meperidine or acetaminophen. If this treatment results in lysis of fever, MH is ruled out. Some patients have an exaggerated response on emergence from anesthesia, with excitement and physical agitation, and may need physical restraint. There may be marked abnormal laboratory results (e.g., lactic acidosis, elevated CK levels). This response, although uncommon, is more frequent than the incidence of MH susceptibility in the population (1 in 10,000). Most such patients are not MH susceptible,[78,79] based on in vitro halothane and caffeine contracture tests (IVCT).

Nonanesthetic Drugs and Circumstances

It is even harder to diagnose MH in the patient who has not had an anesthetic or who is more than 24 hours post-anesthetic. Several cases of awake MH have been reported. It is unlikely that MH would have been considered if not for the presence of a history of MH in the patient or family. There are several cases of awake MH related to sports,[80–82] heat stress,[83–85] and sudden death.[86] Cases of infection[86,87] or emotional stress associated with cocaine and alcohol consumption triggering MH also have been suggested. Intrinsic myotoxicity or direct stimulation of muscle metabolism by cocaine does not seem to be a factor. Cocaine does not cause in vitro contracture of MH-susceptible muscle, and it does not change the response to low concentrations of halothane.[88] In vivo cocaine nonetheless might potentiate the effects of triggering agents via its many effects on catecholamines, central excitation, and temperature regulation.

Not everyone agrees that these cases are truly MH. Even if the IVCT is positive, given the 10% to 20% false-positive rate, the diagnosis of MH is uncertain. This issue will be clarified only when the biochemistry of MH is understood along with the molecular genetic underpinnings of the syndrome.

Because MH-susceptible muscle is known to be more sensitive to caffeine in vitro, one concern often raised is whether patients who are MH susceptible should avoid caffeine or the other methylxanthines such as theophylline. Sufficient evidence seems to have accumulated to indicate that both are safe at doses that are not toxic in normal individuals. Based on in vitro studies, it is possible that triggering agents will be more likely to cause an MH episode in patients who have high levels of these agents.[89]

Cardiac glycosides may increase myoplasmic calcium levels, but MH-susceptible swine do not respond abnormally to digoxin.[90] α-Adrenergic stimulation may aggravate the MH process by limiting transcutaneous heat loss; however, α-adrenergic agonists do not trigger MH in susceptible swine.[91]

Amide local anesthetics previously were thought to be harmful because lidocaine may enhance in vitro contracture by inhibition of calcium sequestration into the sarcoplasmic reticulum. Reexamination has shown, however, that lidocaine does not trigger MH in susceptible swine, even when given in doses above the convulsive threshold[92]; all local anesthetics including the amides are acceptable for anesthetic purposes.[93,94]

Other drugs and compounds have been suggested as triggers of MH. Chlorocresol, a preservative in many drugs, is a potent, specific trigger in the IVCT[95] and is a trigger of MH in vivo in susceptible pigs. Large doses need to be given over a short time. Such high blood levels are close to the

toxic dose in all animals and are not likely to occur from the use of drugs preserved with this agent[96] (>100 U/kg insulin would be the threshold dose to trigger MH). Agents discharged by fire extinguishers (bromochlorodifluoromethane),[97] other chlorofluorocarbons, and gasoline vapors[98,99] have been suggested as possible nonanesthetic triggers. Not all investigators agree, however, that human cases are related to exposure to these agents, given the phenotypic heterogeneity of MH.

Centrally acting agents, such as serotonin agonists and neuroleptic drugs, may produce a syndrome comprising fever, acidosis, and rhabdomyolysis that resembles MH. Caroff and associates[100] reported a high incidence of positive response to the IVCT in seven patients with previous neuroleptic malignant syndrome (NMS).[100] In contrast, Bello and coworkers[101] reported normal contracture tests in 29 of 32 patients with previous NMS (see Chapter 26).

To assume that any patient with NMS is MH susceptible is not reasonable and puts patients at risk. Many patients with NMS need electroconvulsive therapy, and the optimal anesthetic technique includes the triggering agent succinylcholine. The rare possibility of an MH episode does not warrant prohibiting the use of succinylcholine in patients with acute NMS. Similarly a patient with heatstroke or NMS who requires urgent intubation should not be excluded from receiving succinylcholine because of fear of MH.

INFECTION

Infection as a trigger for MH has been studied in susceptible pigs. Endotoxin injection and the febrile state that follows does not lead to MH. Outcome of septic, MH-susceptible pigs was worse, however, when they also were given a triggering agent. This finding is not surprising because both stresses are potentially lethal.[102] In humans, a study of patients and their families after a suspected MH episode associated with appendicitis showed that only 1 of 13 were MH susceptible, but 3 other patients died and were assumed to be MH susceptible.[103] Death occurred in two patients despite dantrolene. No criteria could distinguish the septic patients from the patients who were MH susceptible. One study did not find any MH susceptibility by IVCT in a group of 30 patients who developed postoperative fever.[78]

EXERCISE AND HEAT STRESS

In the pig model, hypothermia[104] is protective against development of MH, whereas hyperthermia per se has been shown to worsen MH. MH may be triggered in susceptible swine if body temperature is greater than 42°C (107.6°F).[105] Although it may be imprudent to extrapolate from the pig model, one might be concerned that MH-susceptible patients who became febrile might be triggered to develop MH. Although frequently combined with heat stress, there have been several deaths attributed to MH after or during exercise. Most deaths can be dismissed easily as cardiac arrhythmias; underlying cardiac abnormalities were frequently found. Against the association is the fact that many patients with the diagnosis of MH susceptibility have undergone strenuous exercise with little evidence for an unusual response. Some patients have been exposed to exercise in a controlled environment with no adverse effects.[106] Suspicious cases remain, however.[81,82,107] Wappler and colleagues[108] studied 12 young men who developed rhabdomyolysis after exertion. Nine were positive on the halothane-caffeine contracture test, and three of those displayed one of the typical causative MH mutations. Tobin and colleagues[109] reported a 12-year-old boy with a history of clinical MH who developed muscle rigidity after soccer practice and subsequently developed ventricular fibrillation and elevation of CK and died. The boy, his father, and other relatives were identified as harboring a typical MH causative mutation.

The major diagnostic criteria seem to be rigidity and postmortem fever[110] because some degree of rhabdomyolysis, acidosis, and hyperthermia may be attributed to exercise or resuscitation. One must be careful to order biopsy for patients after an adequate recovery period from rhabdomyolysis ($\geq$6 months), because abnormal IVCTs have been found with damaged muscle.

DIFFERENTIAL DIAGNOSIS

Given that the signs of MH consist of tachycardia, acidosis, hypercarbia, fever, and muscle destruction, either together or in various combinations, it is not surprising that other syndromes may resemble MH (Table 25-5). Sepsis probably is confused most often with MH. Patients undergoing urinary tract surgery; ear, nose, and throat surgery; or appendectomy for appendicitis develop fever and sometimes acidosis. Elevated CK also may occur during episodes of sepsis. In contrast to MH, muscle rigidity is uncommon, although rigors may be mistaken for rigidity. In addition, signs of sepsis are treated effectively with nonsteroidal antiinflammatory drugs and antibiotics. MH does not respond to such nonspecific therapy. Dantrolene often may be associated with acute reduction of fever. This finding is also nonspecific, however. Differentiating sepsis from MH is often not possible clinically.

Another syndrome that has been mistaken for MH is hypoxic encephalopathy or brain injury from a variety of causes.[111,112] Patients may become febrile owing to hypothalamic damage or blood in the cerebral ventricles and may become rigid owing to posturing. If adequate ventilation is not provided, patients also may become hypercarbic. Marked elevation of temperature ($\geq$42°C [107.6°F]) is often associated with muscle destruction. Seizures can produce a similar picture. In contrast to MH, neuromuscular blocking agents relax the muscles and prevent the acidosis.

Thyrotoxicosis and pheochromocytoma produce tachycardia, hypertension, and fever. Occasionally they have been misdiagnosed as MH. Pheochromocytoma is particularly difficult to diagnose because patients often do not provide a history suggesting episodic hypertension.[113]

Iatrogenic overheating has been misdiagnosed as MH. In these situations, the patient is usually completely draped, the patient is externally warmed, and the procedure is lengthy. The patient develops fever, hypercarbia, tachycardia, and tachypnea if unparalyzed. Simple undraping leads to lysis of the fever, especially in an unanesthetized patient.

NMS is an idiosyncratic adverse drug reaction associated with the use of neuroleptic drugs and the newer, atypical neuroleptics, such as olanzapine and clozapine. NMS typically occurs gradually over days to weeks after the onset of neuroleptic drug use, in contrast to the typically rapid onset of MH soon after use of inhalational anesthetics. MH-susceptible individuals tolerate neuroleptics, and individuals with NMS have tolerated general anesthetics and succinylcholine. Paralyzing agents cause muscle flaccidity in patients with NMS but do not resolve the rigidity of MH. NMS would be unusual in the perioperative setting, but a careful medication history is essential to the differential.

Drug toxicity also may clinically resemble MH, particularly from anticholinergics, sympathomimetics, cocaine, and amphetamines. In general, these agents cause myoclonus rather than the myotonia characteristic of MH and respond to antidotes such as physostigmine for anticholinergics and benzodiazepines for the sympathomimetics. Also, respiratory alkalosis, rather than hypercarbia, would be the norm with poisoning from the sympathomimetics and amphetamines. The clinical setting would be different in most cases, although record of their use should be reviewed during the diagnostic process.

The serotonin syndrome is another drug-related complication and is secondary to increased central nervous system serotonin neurotransmission. This syndrome can result from interactions of antidepressants; opiate analgesics such as meperidine, dextromethorphan, or fentanyl; lithium; or the hallucinogens lysergic acid diethylamide (LSD) or methylenedioxymethamphetamine (MDMA). It also can occur as the result of a single dose or an overdose of a serotonergic agent or the use of dopamine agonists. It is characterized by a constellation of neuromuscular, autonomic, and central nervous system manifestations that could resemble MH or NMS. The onset is usually rapid ($\leq$24 hours) after introduction or increased dose of a serotonergic drug, and it typically resolves within 24 to 36 hours. Severity of hyperthermia, rhabdomyolysis, and muscle rigidity typically is less than seen in NMS or MH, but these can be life-threatening. In the perioperative setting, the syndrome could appear after the use of meperidine or fentanyl in a patient who had been taking antidepressants or other serotonergic drugs.[114] A comprehensive medication history helps establish the diagnosis. Serotonin syndrome is usually self-limited with drug abstinence and responds to simple cooling measures and sedatives (see Chapters 24 and 26).

A unusual syndrome, but one that is characteristic in its presentation, is the syndrome of radiologic contrast agent–induced neurotoxicity. In this syndrome, a water-soluble contrast agent is inadvertently injected into the central nervous system, usually during the course of a myelogram.

TABLE 25-5 Differential Diagnosis of Malignant Hyperthermia	
Amphetamine toxicity	Intracranial bleed
Anticholinergic syndrome	Lethal catatonia
Brain injury	Meningitis
Cocaine toxicity	Neuroleptic malignant syndrome
Contrast-induced neurotoxicity	Pheochromocytoma
Drug/alcohol withdrawal	Salicylate toxicity
Extrapyramidal syndrome	Sepsis
Heatstroke	Serotonin syndrome
Hypoxic encephalopathy	Sympathomimetic toxicity
Iatrogenic overheating	Thyrotoxicosis

Within a few hours, the patient, who may be completely awake, begins to exhibit muscle jerking in the lower extremities. These myoclonic movements ascend to the upper extremities. Fever and acidosis may follow, particularly when seizure activity occurs. This syndrome is self-limiting, however. Nevertheless, the patient should be intubated and observed in a critical care unit. Myoglobinuria and hyperkalemia are the result of the muscle hyperactivity.[115] Other causes of misdiagnosis of MH include faulty temperature monitoring devices, faulty calibration of capnograph, absorption of carbon dioxide during laparoscopic procedures, underventilation of a septic patient, and a variety of causes of fever.

Although the only way to diagnose MH definitively is by means of the IVCT, the constellation of clinical signs may be helpful in determining the likelihood that a clinical event was related to MH. The so-called clinical grading scale employs a point system based on the presence of signs of MH to score an episode. The details of the scoring system may be found elsewhere.[116] The utility of the scoring system depends on the completeness of data that are collected in a given patient. At present, the scoring system is used as a research tool only.

Help in diagnosing and managing clinical cases of MH is available through a hotline service offered by the Malignant Hyperthermia Association of the United States (MHAUS) at no cost. Experts in MH share responsibility in answering questions regarding MH and its treatment 7 days a week, 24 hours per day. The hotline number is 1-800-MH-HYPER (1-800-644-9737). Outside the United States the number is 0011-315-464-7079. Further details about MHAUS are given subsequently. More than 1500 calls are handled by the hotline each year; only about 300 are related to actual MH cases.

MANAGEMENT OF PATIENTS WITH KNOWN MALIGNANT HYPERTHERMIA SUSCEPTIBILITY

Patients with MH susceptibility should have a preoperative evaluation. Safe anesthesia consists of either regional anesthesia with local anesthesia (all local anesthetics are safe) or general anesthesia using nitrous oxide and intravenous agents such as propofol, barbiturates, benzodiazepines, opioids, or ketamine. Nondepolarizing neuromuscular blocking agents also are safe. All potent inhalational agents and succinylcholine are MH triggers and must be avoided. Known triggers of MH are halothane, desflurane, sevoflurane, enflurane, methoxyflurane, cyclopropane, and ether. Dantrolene pretreatment is *not* necessary.

Preparation of the anesthesia machine consists of closing or disabling gas vaporizers, flowing 10 L/min of oxygen or air through the machine for at least 20 minutes, and changing the carbon dioxide absorbent. If a ventilator is to be used, the rebreathing bag should be affixed to the y piece and the ventilator cycled at 5 to 8/min during the 20-minute flushing.

TREATMENT

The success in controlling deaths from MH is due to early recognition of the syndrome and prompt treatment with dantrolene sodium intravenously. Dantrolene is a hydantoin derivative that inhibits calcium release from the sarcoplasmic

reticulum. It has no effect on cardiac or smooth muscle. Toxicity is limited when given over only a few days. Long-term administration is associated with hepatotoxicity. The elimination half-life is 7 to 12 hours.

Dantrolene is poorly soluble and is prepared in a lyophilized powder with 3 g of mannitol and sodium hydroxide to maintain pH of 9 to 10. The drug should be mixed with 60 mL of *sterile water* and shaken vigorously. Each vial contains 20 mg of dantrolene.

It is recommended that 36 vials be immediately available wherever general anesthesia with potent agents or succinylcholine is used. Short-term side effects include muscle weakness, phlebitis, nausea, and vomiting. The drug does not impair respiration except in patients with muscle disease and should be given carefully to those individuals. Any facility where general anesthesia is administered should be prepared to treat MH. A treatment protocol should be readily available, such as the one available from the MHAUS (Table 25-6). Table 25-7 lists suggested items to be kept in a treatment cart.

SOURCES OF INFORMATION CONCERNING MALIGNANT HYPERTHERMIA

Updated information may be obtained from the MHAUS (PO Box 1069, Sherburne, NY 13460), a not-for-profit patient advocacy organization. Formed in 1981 to provide information to practitioners and patients regarding MH, MHAUS sponsors a hotline and the North American MH Registry and produces pamphlets, a newsletter, a fax-on-demand service, and a website (www.mhaus.org), among other services.

TABLE 25-6 Malignant Hyperthermia Treatment Protocol

When MH is identified, all potent agents should be stopped.

Hyperventilation at a tidal volume of at least 10–15 mL/kg at 12–15 times/min should be instituted.

Dantrolene should be mixed and a dose of 2.5 mg/kg injected rapidly.

Additional dantrolene should be given titrated to heart rate, rigidity acidosis. Control of the syndrome usually occurs with doses <10 mg/kg. During this time, if the patient is decompensating, bicarbonate should be given, 1–2 mEq/kg.

Cooling should begin using surface cooling; nasogastric lavage with cold solution; and wound, bladder, or rectal irrigation as appropriate. In the case of cardiac arrest, potassium levels should be obtained immediately.

If elevated, treatment should begin with calcium chloride, glucose, and insulin along with hyperventilation. Epinephrine and other β-agonists may be lifesaving.

Arterial blood gases, electrolytes, creatine kinase, and coagulation studies should be obtained.

Arrhythmias should be treated with antiarrhythmics, with the exception of calcium channel blockers, because they may produce hyperkalemia in the presence of dantrolene.

When the initial crisis is under control, the patient should receive 1 mg/kg of dantrolene every 4–6 hr titrated to signs of MH for at least 36 hr. Creatine kinase should be assessed every 12–24 hr until stable.

If myoglobinuria occurs, vigorous diuresis should be instituted with furosemide, alkalinization, and fluids. Each vial of dantrolene contains 3 g of mannitol; 2.5 mg/kg of dantrolene gives the patient 0.4 g/kg of mannitol.

TABLE 25-7 Treatment Cart for Care of Malignant Hyperthermia: Suggested Supplies and Equipment

Dantrolene, 20 mg/vial, 36 vials
Bacteriostatic free sterile water, 2 L
Sodium bicarbonate, 8.4%, 3 ampules
Glucose 50%, 2 ampules
Furosemide, 10 mg/mL, 2 vials
Calcium chloride 10%, 2 vials
Lidocaine 1%, 10 mL, 2 vials
Regular insulin
Nasogastric tube
Blood collection tubes for CK, PT, PTT, fibrin-split products, electrolytes, platelets
Arterial and central venous pressure kits
Plastic bags for ice
Minispike or similar transfer pin to mix water with dantrolene
Urinary dip-stick for hemoglobin
Esophageal or tympanic temperature probes
Rectal or bladder and skin temperature probes

CK, creatine kinase; PT, prothrombin time; PTT, partial thromboplastin time.

The phone number is 1-607-674-7901. The board of directors of MHAUS consists of laypersons and professionals. Support for MHAUS is from a variety of sources, but mostly from voluntary contributions. In addition, MHAUS sponsors and supports the Neuroleptic Malignant Syndrome Information Service (www.nmsis.org) with goals similar to the goals described previously. Another useful resource is Genetests (www.genetests.org).

REFERENCES

1. MacLennan DH, Phillips MS: Malignant hyperthermia. Science 256: 789–794, 1992.
2. Gronert G: Malignant hyperthermia. In Engel AG, Franzini-Armstrong C (eds): Myology: Basic and Clinical, 2nd ed. New York, McGraw-Hill, 1994, pp 1661–1678.
3. Rosenberg H, Fletcher JE, Seitman D: Pharmacogenetics. In Barash PG, Cullen BF, Stoelting RK (eds): Clinical Anesthesia, 3rd ed. Philadelphia, Lippincott-Raven, 1997, pp 489–517.
4. Mickelson JR, Louis CF: Malignant hyperthermia: Excitation-contraction coupling, Ca^{2+} release channel, and cell Ca^{2+} regulation defects. Physiol Rev 76:537–592, 1996.
5. Kolb ME, Horne ML, Martz R: Dantrolene in human malignant hyperthermia. Anesthesiology 56:254–262, 1982.
6. Denborough MA, Lovell RRH: Anaesthetic deaths in a family. Lancet 2:45, 1960.
7. Harrison GG: Pale, soft exudative pork, porcine stress syndrome and malignant hyperpyrexia—an identity? J S Afr Vet Assoc 43:57–63, 1972.
8. Kalow W, Britt BA, Terreau ME, et al: Metabolic error of muscle metabolism after recovery from malignant hyperthermia. Lancet 2: 895–898, 1970.
9. Ellis FR, Harriman DG, Keaney NP, et al: Halothane-induced muscle contracture as a cause of hyperpyrexia. Br J Anaesth 43:721–722, 1971.
10. Harrison GG: Control of the malignant hyperpyrexic syndrome in MHS swine by dantrolene sodium. Br J Anaesth 47:62–65, 1975.
11. Rosenberg H, Fletcher JE: Report of a Scientific Meeting. International Malignant Hyperthermia Workshop and Symposium. Hiroshima, Japan, July 16–19, 1944. Anesthesiology 82:803–805, 1995.
12. Ording H: Incidence of malignant hyperthermia in Denmark. Anesth Analg 64:700–704, 1985.
13. Lunn JN, Farrow SC, Fowkes FG, et al: Epidemiology in anaesthesia: I. Anaesthetic practice over 20 years. Br J Anaesth 54:803–809, 1982.
14. Bachand M, Vachon N, Boisvert M, et al: Clinical reassessment of malignant hyperthermia in Abitibi-Temiscamingue. Can J Anaesth 44:696–701, 1997.
15. Monnier N, Krivosic-Horber R, Payen J-F, et al: Presence of two different genetic traits in malignant hyperthermia families: Implication for genetic analysis, diagnosis, and incidence of malignant hyperthermia susceptibility. Anesthesiology 97:1067–1074, 2002.
16. Ording H, Brancadoro V, Cozzolino S, et al: In vitro contracture test for diagnosis of malignant hyperthermia following the protocol of the European MH Group: Results of testing patients surviving fulminant MH and unrelated low-risk subjects. The European Malignant Hyperthermia Group. Acta Anaesthesiol Scand 41:955–966, 1997.
17. Allen GC, Larach MG, Kunselman AR: The sensitivity and specificity of the caffeine-halothane contracture test: A report from the North American Malignant Hyperthermia Registry. The North American Malignant Hyperthermia Registry of MHAUS. Anesthesiology 88:579–588, 1998.
18. Fletcher JE, Rosenberg H, Aggarwal M: Comparison of European and North American malignant hyperthermia diagnostic protocol outcomes for use in genetic studies. Anesthesiology 90:654–661, 1999.
19. Iaizzo PA, Klein W, Lehmann-Horn F: Fura-2 detected myoplasmic calcium and its correlation with contracture force in skeletal muscle from normal and malignant hyperthermia susceptible pigs. Pflugers Arch 411:648–653, 1988.
20. Lopez JR, Allen PD, Alamo L, et al: Myoplasmic free $[Ca^{2+}]$ during a malignant hyperthermia episode in swine. Muscle Nerve 11:82–88, 1988.
21. Censier K, Urwyler A, Zorzato F, et al: Intracellular calcium homeostasis in human primary muscle cells from malignant hyperthermia-susceptible and normal individuals: Effect of overexpression of recombinant wild-type and Arg163Cys mutated ryanodine receptors. J Clin Invest 101:1233–1242, 1998.
22. Louis CF, Zualkernan K, Roghair T, et al: The effects of volatile anesthetics on calcium regulation by malignant hyperthermia-susceptible sarcoplasmic reticulum. Anesthesiology 77:114–125, 1992.
23. Olgin J, Argov Z, Rosenberg H, et al: Non-invasive evaluation of malignant hyperthermia susceptibility with phosphorus nuclear magnetic resonance spectroscopy. Anesthesiology 68:507–513, 1988.
24. Webster DW, Thompson RT, Gravelle DR, et al: Metabolic response to exercise in malignant hyperthermia-sensitive patients measured by 31P magnetic resonance spectroscopy. Magn Reson Med 15:81–89, 1990.
25. Olgin J, Rosenberg H, Allen G, et al: A blinded comparison of noninvasive, in vivo phosphorus nuclear magnetic resonance spectroscopy and the in vitro halothane/caffeine contracture test in the evaluation of malignant hyperthermia susceptibility. Anesth Analg 72:36–47, 1991.
26. Payen JF, Fouilhe N, Sam-Lai E, et al: In vitro 31P-magnetic resonance spectroscopy of muscle extracts in malignant hyperthermia-susceptible patients. Anesthesiology 84:1077–1082, 1996.
27. Bendahan D, Kozak-Ribbens G, Rodet L, et al: 31Phosphorus magnetic resonance spectroscopy characterization of muscular metabolic anomalies in patients with malignant hyperthermia: Application to diagnosis. Anesthesiology 88:96–107, 1998.
28. Brandt A, Schleithoff L, Jurkat-Rott K, et al: Screening of the ryanodine receptor gene in 105 malignant hyperthermia families: Novel mutations and concordance with the in vitro contracture test. Hum Mol Genet 8:2055–2062, 1999.
29. Robinson RL, Monnier N, Wolz W, et al: A genome wide search for susceptibility loci in three European malignant hyperthermia pedigrees. Hum Mol Genet 6:953–961, 1997.
30. Sudbrak R, Procaccio V, Klausnitzer M, et al: Mapping of a further malignant hyperthermia susceptibility locus to chromosome 3q13.1. Am J Hum Genet 56:684–691, 1995.
31. Iles DE, Lehmann-Horn F, Scherer SW, et al: Localization of the gene encoding the alpha 2/delta-subunits of the L-type voltage-dependent calcium channel to chromosome 7q and analysis of the segregation of flanking markers in malignant hyperthermia susceptible families. Hum Mol Genet 3:969–975, 1994.
32. Levitt RC, Olckers A, Meyers S, et al: Evidence for the localization of a malignant hyperthermia susceptibility locus (MHS2) to human chromosome 17q. Genomics 14:562–566, 1992.
33. Monnier N, Procaccio V, Stieglitz P, et al: Malignant-hyperthermia susceptibility is associated with a mutation of the alpha 1-subunit of the human dihydropyridine-sensitive L-type voltage-dependent calcium-channel receptor in skeletal muscle. Am J Hum Genet 60:1316–1325, 1997.

34. Vita GM, Olckers A, Jedlicka AE, et al: Masseter muscle rigidity associated with glycine1306-to-alanine mutation in the adult muscle sodium channel alpha-subunit gene. Anesthesiology 82:1097–1103, 1995.

35. Deufel T, Sudbrak R, Feist Y, et al: Discordance, in a malignant hyperthermia pedigree, between in vitro contracture-test phenotypes and haplotypes for the MHS1 region on chromosome 19q12–13.2, comprising the C1840T transition in the RYR1 gene. Am J Hum Genet 56:1334–1342, 1995.

36. MacLennan DH: Discordance between phenotype and genotype in malignant hyperthermia. Curr Opin Neurol 8:397–401, 1995.

37. Serfas KD, Bose D, Patel L, et al: Comparison of the segregation of the RYR1 C1840T mutation with segregation of the caffeine/halothane contracture test results for malignant hyperthermia susceptibility in a large Manitoba Mennonite family. Anesthesiology 84:322–329, 1996.

38. Fagerlund TH, Ording H, Bendixen D, et al: Discordance between malignant hyperthermia susceptibility and RYR1 mutation C1840T in two Scandinavian MH families exhibiting this mutation. Clin Genet 52:416–421, 1997.

39. Fortunato G, Carsana A, Tinto N, et al: A case of discordance between genotype and phenotype in a malignant hyperthermia family. Eur J Hum Genet 7:415–420, 1999.

40. Fletcher JE, Mayerberger S, Tripolitis L, et al: Fatty acids markedly lower the threshold for halothane-induced calcium release from the terminal cisternae in human and porcine normal and malignant hyperthermia susceptible skeletal muscle. Life Sci 49:1651–1657, 1991.

41. Cheah KS, Cheah AM, Fletcher JE, et al: Skeletal muscle mitochondrial respiration of malignant hyperthermia-susceptible patients: Ca^{2+}-induced uncoupling and free fatty acids. Int J Biochem 21:913–920, 1989.

42. Fletcher JE, Tripolitis L, Rosenberg H, et al: Malignant hyperthermia: Halothane- and halothane-induced calcium release in skeletal muscle. Biochem Mol Biol Int 29:763–772, 1993.

43. Fletcher JE, Wieland SJ, Karan SM, et al: Sodium channel in human malignant hyperthermia. Anesthesiology 86:1023–1032, 1997.

44. Wieland SJ, Fletcher JE, Rosenberg H, et al: Malignant hyperthermia: Slow sodium current in cultured human muscle cells. Am J Physiol 257:C759–765, 1989.

45. Fletcher JE, Adnet PJ, Reyford H, et al: ATX II, a sodium channel toxin, sensitizes skeletal muscle to halothane, caffeine, and ryanodine. Anesthesiology 90:1294–1301, 1999.

46. Quane KA, Healy JM, Keating KE, et al: Mutations in the ryanodine receptor gene in central core disease and malignant hyperthermia. Nat Genet 5:51–55, 1993.

47. Zhang Y, Chen HS, Khanna VK, et al: A mutation in the human ryanodine receptor gene associated with central core disease. Nat Genet 5:46–50, 1993.

48. European Malignant Hyperpyrexia Group: A protocol for the investigation of malignant hyperpyrexia (MH) susceptibility. The European Malignant Hyperpyrexia Group. Br J Anaesth 56:1267–1269, 1984.

49. Larach MG: Standardization of the caffeine halothane muscle contracture test. North American Malignant Hyperthermia Group. Anesth Analg 69:511–515, 1989.

50. Maehara Y, Mukaida K, Hiyama E, et al: Genetic analysis with calcium-induced calcium release test in Japanese malignant hyperthermia susceptible (MHS) families. Hiroshima J Med Sci 48:9–15, 1999.

51. Hopkins PM, Hartung E, Wappler F: Multicentre evaluation of ryanodine contracture testing in malignant hyperthermia. The European Malignant Hyperthermia Group. Br J Anaesth 80:389–394, 1998.

52. Ording H, Glahn K, Gardi T, et al: 4-Chloro-m-cresol test—a possible supplementary test for diagnosis of malignant hyperthermia susceptibility. Acta Anaesthesiol Scand 41:967–972, 1997.

53. Adnet P, Bortlein ML, Tavernier B, et al: Caffeine skinned fiber tension test: application to the diagnosis of susceptibility to malignant hyperthermia. Ann Fr Anesth Reanim 18:624–630, 1999.

54. De Cauwer H, Heytens L, Lubke U, et al: Discordant light microscopic, electron microscopic, and in vitro contracture study findings in a family with central core disease. Clin Neuropathol 16:237–242, 1997.

55. Mezin P, Payen JF, Bosson JL, et al: Histological support for the difference between malignant hyperthermia susceptible (MHS), equivocal (MHE) and negative (MHN) muscle biopsies. Br J Anaesth 79:327–331, 1997.

56. Urwyler A, Deufel T, McCarthy T, West S: Guidelines for molecular genetic detection of susceptibility to malignant hyperthermia. Br J Anaesth 86:283–287, 2001.

57. Urwyler A, Deufel T, McCarthy T, West S: Guidelines for molecular genetic detection of susceptibility to malignant hyperthermia. Br J Anaesth 86:283–287, 2001.

58. Anetseder M, Hager M, Muller CR, et al: Diagnosis of susceptibility to malignant hyperthermia by use of a metabolic test. Lancet 359:1579–1580, 2002.

59. Sei Y, Brandom B, Bina S, et al: Patients with malignant hyperthermia demonstrate an altered calcium control mechanism in B lymphocytes. Anesthesiology 97:1052–1058, 2002.

60. Schulte-Sasse U, Hess W, Eberlein HJ: Postoperative malignant hyperthermia and dantrolene therapy. Can Anaesth Soc J 30:635–640, 1983.

61. Carr AS, Lerman J, Cunliffe M, et al: Incidence of malignant hyperthermia reactions in 2,214 patients undergoing muscle biopsy. Can J Anaesth 42:281–286, 1995.

62. Grinberg R, Edelist G, Gordon A: Postoperative malignant hyperthermia episodes in patients who received "safe" anaesthetics. Can Anaesth Soc J 30:273–276, 1983.

63. Souliere CR Jr, Weintraub SJ, Kirchner JC: Markedly delayed postoperative malignant hyperthermia. Arch Otolaryngol Head Neck Surg 112:564–566, 1986.

64. Relton JE, Creighton RE, Conn AW, et al: Generalized muscular hypertonicity associated with general anaesthesia: A suggested anaesthetic management. Can Anaesth Soc J 14:22–25, 1967.

65. Donlon JV, Newfield P, Sreter F, et al: Implications of masseter spasm after succinylcholine. Anesthesiology 49:298–301, 1978.

66. Schwartz L, Rockoff MA, Koka BV: Masseter spasm with anesthesia: Incidence and implications. Anesthesiology 61:772–775, 1984.

67. Lazzell VA, Carr AS, Lerman J, et al: The incidence of masseter muscle rigidity after succinylcholine in infants and children. Can J Anaesth 41:475–479, 1994.

68. Plotz J: Letter. Anesth Analg 67:798, 1988.

69. Airaksinen MM, Tammisto T: Myoglobinuria after intermittent administration of succinylcholine during halothane anesthesia. Clin Pharmacol Ther 7:583–587, 1966.

70. Ziser A, Friedhoff RJ, Rose SH: Prone position: Visceral hypoperfusion and rhabdomyolysis. Anesth Analg 82:412–415, 1996.

71. Targa L, Droghetti L, Caggese G, et al: Rhabdomyolysis and operating position. Anaesthesia 46:141–143, 1991.

72. Palmer SJ, Graham G: Tourniquet-induced rhabdomyolysis after total knee replacement. Ann R Coll Surg Eng 76:416, 1994.

73. Vold PL, Weiss PJ: Rhabdomyolysis from tourniquet trauma in a patient with hypothyroidism. West J Med 162:270–271, 1995.

74. Day RL, Zale BW: The effect of tourniquets on muscle enzymes during foot and ankle surgery. J Foot Ankle Surg 32:280–285, 1993.

75. Harwood TN, Nelson TE: Massive postoperative rhabdomyolysis after uneventful surgery: A case report of subclinical malignant hyperthermia. Anesthesiology 88:265–268, 1998.

76. Larach MG, Rosenberg H, Gronert GA, et al: Hyperkalemic cardiac arrest during anesthesia in infants and children with occult myopathies. Clin Pediatr (Phila) 36:9–16, 1997.

77. Ciofolo MJ, Clergue F, Devilliers C, et al: Changes in ventilation, oxygen uptake, and carbon dioxide output during recovery from isoflurane anesthesia. Anesthesiology 70:737–741, 1989.

78. Halsall PJ, Ellis FR: Does postoperative pyrexia indicate malignant hyperthermia susceptibility? Br J Anaesth 68:209–210, 1992.

79. Christiaens F, Gepts E, D'Haese J, et al: Malignant hyperthermia suggestive hypermetabolic syndrome at emergence from anesthesia. Acta Anaesthesiol Belg 46:93–97, 1995.

80. Ogletree JW, Antognini JF, Gronert GA: Postexercise muscle cramping associated with positive malignant hyperthermia contracture testing. Am J Sports Med 24:49–51, 1996.

81. Gronert GA, Thompson RL, Onofrio BM: Human malignant hyperthermia: Awake episodes and correction by dantrolene. Anesth Analg 59:377–378, 1980.

82. Hunter SL, Rosenberg H, Tuttle GH, et al: Malignant hyperthermia in a college football player. Physician Sportsmed 15:77–84, 1987.

83. Denborough MA: Heat stroke and malignant hyperpyrexia. Med J Aust 1:204–205, 1982.

84. Hopkins PM, Ellis FR, Halsall PJ: Evidence for related myopathies in exertional heat stroke and malignant hyperthermia. Lancet 338:1491–1492, 1991.

85. Kochling A, Wappler F, Winkler G, et al: Rhabdomyolysis following severe physical exercise in a patient with predisposition to malignant hyperthermia. Anaesth Intensive Care 26:315–318, 1998.

86. Britt BA: Combined anesthetic- and stress-induced malignant hyperthermia in two offspring of malignant hyperthermic-susceptible parents. Anesth Analg 67:393–399, 1988.

87. Denborough MA, Collins SP, Hopkinson KC: Rhabdomyolysis and malignant hyperpyrexia. BMJ (Clin Res Educ) 288:1878, 1984.

88. Sato N, Brum JM, Mitsumoto H, et al: Effect of cocaine on the contracture response to 1% halothane in patients undergoing diagnostic muscle biopsy for malignant hyperthermia. Can J Anaesth 42:158–162, 1995.

89. Flewellen EH, Nelson TE: Is theophylline, aminophylline, or caffeine (methylxanthines) contraindicated in malignant hyperthermia susceptible patients? Anesth Analg 62:115–118, 1983.

90. Gronert GA, Ahern CP, Milde JH, et al: Effect of CO_2, calcium, digoxin, and potassium on cardiac and skeletal muscle metabolism in malignant hyperthermia susceptible swine. Anesthesiology 64:24–28, 1986.

91. Maccani RM, Wedel DJ, Hofer RE: Norepinephrine does not potentiate porcine malignant hyperthermia. Anesth Analg 82:790–795, 1996.

92. Wingard DW, Bobko S: Failure of lidocaine to trigger porcine malignant hyperthermia. Anesth Analg 58:99–103, 1979.

93. Brownell AKW: Counseling of malignant hyperthermia susceptible individuals. In Britt BA (ed): Malignant Hyperthermia. Boston, Martinus Nijhoff, 1987, pp 309–323.

94. Berkowitz A, Rosenberg H: Femoral block with mepivacaine for muscle biopsy in malignant hyperthermia patients. Anesthesiology 62:651–652, 1985.

95. Wappler F, Scholz J, Fiege M, et al: 4-chloro-m-cresol is a trigger of malignant hyperthermia in susceptible swine. Anesthesiology 90:1733–1740, 1999.

96. Iaizzo PA, Johnson BA, Nagao K, et al: 4-chloro-m-cresol triggers malignant hyperthermia in susceptible swine at doses greatly exceeding those found in drug preparations. Anesthesiology 90:1723–1732, 1999.

97. Denborough MA, Hopkinson KC, Banney DG: Firefighting and malignant hyperthermia. BMJ (Clin Res Educ) 296:1442–1443, 1988.

98. Wingard DW, Gatz EE: Some observations on stress susceptible patients. In Aldrete JA, Britt BA (eds): Malignant Hyperthermia. New York, Grune & Stratton, 1978, pp 363–372.

99. Anetseder M, Hartung E, Klepper S, et al: Gasoline vapors induce severe rhabdomyolysis. Neurology 44:2393–2395, 1994.

100. Caroff SN, Rosenberg H, Fletcher JE, et al: Malignant hyperthermia susceptibility in neuroleptic malignant syndrome. Anesthesiology 67:20–25, 1987.

101. Bello N, Adnet P, Saulnier F, et al: Lack of sensitivity to per- anesthetic malignant hyperthermia in 32 patients who developed neuroleptic malignant syndrome. Ann Fr Anesth Reanim 13:663–668, 1994.

102. Musley SK, Beebe DS, Komanduri V, et al: Hemodynamic and metabolic manifestations of acute endotoxin infusion in pigs with and without the malignant hyperthermia mutation. Anesthesiology 91:833– 838, 1999.

103. Strecker G, Adnet P, Forget AP, et al: Malignant hyperthermia and appendicular sepsis: Can they be differentiated during surgical procedure? Ann Fr Anesth Reanim 16:234–238, 1997.

104. Nelson TE: Porcine malignant hyperthermia: Critical temperatures for in vivo and in vitro responses. Anesthesiology 73:449–454, 1990.

105. Denborough M, Hopkinson KC, O'Brien RO, et al: Overheating alone can trigger malignant hyperthermia in piglets. Anaesth Intensive Care 24:348–354, 1996.

106. Green JH, Ellis FR, Halsall PJ, et al: Thermoregulation, plasma catecholamine and metabolite levels during submaximal work in individuals susceptible to malignant hyperpyrexia. Acta Anaesthesiol Scand 31:122–126, 1987.

107. Hackl W, Winkler M, Mauritz W, et al: Muscle biopsy for diagnosis of malignant hyperthermia susceptibility in two patients with severe exercise-induced myolysis. Br J Anaesth 66:138–140, 1991.

108. Wappler F, Feige M, Steinfath M, et al: Evidence for susceptibility to malignant hyperthermia in patients with stress-induced rhabdomyolysis. Anesthesiology 94:95–100, 2001.

109. Tobin JR, Jason DR, Challa VR, et al: Malignant hyperthermia and apparent heat stroke. JAMA 286:168–169, 2001.

110. Ryan JF, Tedeschi LG: Sudden unexplained death in a patient with a family history of malignant hyperthermia. J Clin Anesth 9:66–68, 1997.

111. Francoise M, Francois C, Sandre D, et al: Hemorrhagic shock with encephalopathy syndrome or major hyperthermia syndrome? Pediatrie 48:792–795, 1993.

112. Itaya K, Takahata O, Mamiya K, et al: Anesthetic management of two patients with mitochondrial encephalopathy, lactic acidosis and stroke-like episodes (MELAS). Masui 44:710–712, 1995.

113. Allen GC, Rosenberg H: Phaeochromocytoma presenting as acute malignant hyperthermia—a diagnostic challenge. Can J Anaesth 37:593–595, 1990.

114. Giese SY, Neborsky R: Serotonin syndrome: Potential consequences of Meridia combined with Demerol or fentanyl. Plast Reconstr Surg 107:293–294, 2001.

115. Karl H, Talbott GA, Toberts TS: Intraoperative administaration of radiologic contrast agents: Potential neurotoxicity. Anesthesiology 81:1068–1071, 1994.

116. Larach MG, Localio AR, Allen GC, et al: A clinical grading scale to predict malignant hyperthermia susceptibility. Anesthesiology 80:771–779, 1994.

CHAPTER 26

Neuroleptic Malignant Syndrome

Michael J. Burns

Neuroleptic malignant syndrome (NMS) is an uncommon but potentially fatal idiosyncratic complication of neuroleptic drug therapy. It was first described in 1960 when Delay and colleagues[1] reported rigidity and fever associated with haloperidol therapy. The syndrome subsequently was named and classified as a drug-induced extrapyramidal syndrome (EPS) by Delay and Deniker in 1968.[2] The term *neuroleptic malignant syndrome* is derived from the French *syndrome malin des neuroleptiques*.[3] Although now infrequently fatal and not always associated with neuroleptic therapy, NMS remains the preferred term to describe this illness.

NMS is a heterogeneous disorder with a wide spectrum of clinical severity.[4,5] It commonly is characterized by the tetrad of altered consciousness, fever, muscular rigidity, and autonomic dysfunction.[6] NMS has been reported with all neuroleptic drugs.[7] It also has been reported with other drugs that antagonize dopaminergic neurotransmission in the central nervous system (CNS) (e.g., amoxapine, metoclopramide, lithium) and in patients with Parkinson's disease who abruptly discontinue dopamine agonist therapy.[5,8–20] Many drugs that are not known to antagonize dopamine neurotransmission rarely have been implicated as etiologic agents for NMS (Table 26-1).[21–37] These drugs produce movement disorders, muscular rigidity, and fever by a mechanism different from that of NMS and are better characterized as producing NMS-like syndromes rather than true NMS.

To date, more than 1000 cases of NMS have been reported in the literature, largely as individual case reports, case series, and reviews.[4,5,21,39–41] Collectively, these cases have heightened awareness of NMS, facilitated its early recognition, promoted a reduction of suspected risk factors, and allowed more timely treatment. As a result, the incidence and mortality from NMS have decreased since the 1980s.[5,7,41–44] However, the lack of animal models and controlled, prospective treatment studies for NMS has hampered a full understanding of its pathophysiology and optimal treatment. Further study is necessary to reduce the incidence, morbidity, and mortality from NMS.

EPIDEMIOLOGY

Incidence

NMS is uncommon. From retrospective studies, reported incidences have ranged from 0.02% to 3.2% of individuals exposed to neuroleptic drugs.[6,40] In two prospective studies, incidences were 0.07% and 0.9%.[44–46] Estimates of frequency are influenced by diagnostic criteria, patient populations studied, prevalence of risk factors, setting, and methods of data collection.[6] If NMS were recognized across a spectrum of severity, and widened diagnostic criteria were employed to diagnose it, the prevalence of this disorder would be higher. When data are pooled from many studies, NMS is estimated to occur in 2 of every 1000 patients treated with neuroleptics.[6]

Demographics

NMS occurs in all age groups. Most cases occur in patients between 20 and 50 years old with a mean age of 40.[5–7,40] This age distribution likely reflects the pattern of neuroleptic use in society rather than a true age predilection for the disease.[5,6] NMS occurs approximately twice as often in men compared with women.[5–7] This occurrence also likely reflects the pattern of neuroleptic use, with a higher frequency of use in men.

Risk Factors

Several potential risk factors for the development of NMS have been identified from case series and reviews; these include rapid initiation of antipsychotic therapy; use of high-potency agents and depot preparations; dehydration; severe agitation or catatonia; requirement of restraints or seclusion; preexisting organic brain disease, mental retardation, or affective disorder; previous treatment with electroconvulsive therapy (ECT); previous history of NMS; poorly controlled EPS; and concomitant use of predisposing drugs, such as lithium, anticholinergic agents, and antiparkinson agents.[5–7,40,42] In two similarly designed case-control studies in which 43 patients with NMS were compared with 75 matched neuroleptic-treated controls, risk factors were better delineated.[47,48] NMS was more likely to occur in patients who had been agitated, been dehydrated, required restraint or seclusion, received a larger number of intramuscular injections, and received larger doses of neuroleptic agents soon after hospital admission (rapid dose titration).

NMS has been associated with all neuroleptic agents. Most cases have been reported, however, with high-potency agents and depot preparations. NMS also has been reported with atypical antipsychotics, but it is not yet known whether the incidence of NMS is lower with use of these newer agents. In one review of 115 cases of NMS, 57% were attributed to haloperidol, 16% to fluphenazine, and 17% to a depot preparation.[5] The higher frequency of NMS associated with higher-potency neuroleptics may reflect their more frequent prescribing pattern or rates of administration, however, and

TABLE 26-6 Agents Reported to Cause Neuroleptic Malignant Syndrome

NEUROLEPTIC AGENTS		NONNEUROLEPTIC AGENTS	
Typical Agents	**Atypical Agents**	**Agents that Deplete Dopamine**	**Monoamine Oxidase Inhibitors**
Butyrophenone	Benzamides	α-Methylparatyrosine[10]	Phenelzine (Nardil)[25,35,*]
Droperidol (Inapsine)	Raclopride	Reserpine (Serpasil)	
Haloperidol (Haldol)	Remoxipride	Tetrabenazine[10,21]	**Psychotropic Agents**
Dihydroindolone	Sulpiride		Lithium[17,20]
Molindone (Moban)	Sultopride	**Antiepileptics**	
Diphenylbutylpiperidine	Benzisothiazoyl piperazine	Carbamazepine (Tegretol)[22,23,*]	**Skeletal Muscle Relaxants**
Pimozide (Orap)	(ziprasidone)	Phenytoin (Dilantin)[24,*]	Cyclobenzaprine (Flexeril)[36,*]
Phenothiazine	Benzisoxazole		Diazepam (Valium)[37,*]
Aliphatic	Risperidone (Risperdal)	**Cyclic Antidepressants**	Lorazepam (Ativan)[21,*]
Chlorpromazine (Thorazine)	Dibenzodiazepine	Amitriptyline (Elavil)[21,25,*]	
Promethazine (Phenergan)	Clozapine (Clozaril, Leponex)	Desipramine (Norpramin)[26,*]	**Withdrawal of Dopamine Agonists**
Piperazine	Dibenzothiazepine	Dothiepin[27,28,*]	Amantadine (Symmetrel)[9,10,12]
Fluphenazine (Prolixin)	Quetiapine (Seroquel)	Fluoxetine (Prozac)[29,*]	Bromocriptine (Parlodel)[9–11]
Perphenazine (Trilafon)	Dibenzoxazepine	Imipramine[30,*]	Levodopa/carbidopa (Sinemet)[11,13]
Prochlorperazine (Compazine)	Loxapine (Loxitane)	Maprotoline (Ludiomil)[31,*]	
Trifluoperazine (Stelazine)	Thienobenzodiazepine	Trimipramine (Surmontil)[32,*]	
Piperidine	Olanzapine (Zyprexa)*		
Mesoridazine (Serentil)		**Dopamine Receptor Antagonists**	
Thioridazine (Mellaril, Millazine)		Amoxapine (Asendin)[17,18]	
Thioxanthene		Metoclopramide (Reglan)[14–16]	
Chlorprothixene (Taractan)			
Clopenthixol		**Miscellaneous Agents**	
Flupenthixol		Cocaine[33,*]	
Thiothixene (Navane)		Estrogen[39,*]	
Zuclopenthixol (Clopixol)			

*Although these agents have been reported to cause neuroleptic malignant syndrome (NMS), evidence consists of one or two case reports for each agent, and the reported cases often have coingestants that may produce muscular rigidity and fever. For each case, the syndrome reported should be characterized as an NMS-like syndrome rather than true NMS.

not a true increased risk. In this same review, the low-potency agent chlorpromazine was implicated in 24% of cases of NMS; its overrepresentation in NMS cases probably reflects its frequent use at the time of the study.[5] Whether the incidence of NMS is truly higher with depot preparations is not clear either. In this same NMS case review, the depot preparation fluphenazine decanoate was implicated in 16% of cases compared with 5% for patients treated with oral fluphenazine. In contrast, oral haloperidol was implicated in 57% of NMS cases compared with 1% for its depot preparation.[5]

NMS is idiosyncratic; its occurrence is not correlated with dose, and it usually occurs with antipsychotic serum levels in the therapeutic range.[5–7,40,42] Although NMS may occur at any time during therapy, it usually appears in the first 1 to 2 weeks of treatment or soon after a change in dosage.[5–7,40] The rate of increase of neuroleptic dose correlates with the likelihood of developing NMS.[40,47] The decline in the incidence of NMS may reflect an appreciation of this risk factor and a significant decline in "rapid tranquilization" of agitated psychiatric patients.[44–46]

NMS occurs independent of race, geographic location, environmental temperature, and humidity.[5–7] There is no seasonal variation in incidence.[6] Although there have been rare reports of NMS occurring within the same family, there does not seem to be any significant genetic predisposition to its occurrence.[5–7,49] Although individuals with preexisting affective and organic brain disorders are at greater risk for developing NMS, the illness occurs across the neuropsychiatric disease spectrum and occurs in

patients without organic and functional brain disorders as well.[5–7,47,50]

PATHOPHYSIOLOGY

Although the pathophysiology of NMS is not fully understood, it primarily involves dopaminergic hypoactivity in the CNS.[6–8,51,52] Several lines of clinical evidence support this theory. First, all neuroleptic agents have been associated with NMS, and all share the ability to bind and antagonize D_2-dopamine receptors.[51,53,54] Second, other agents that block D_2-receptors (e.g., amoxapine, metoclopramide) or result in depletion of dopamine (e.g., reserpine, α-methylparatyrosine, tetrabenazine) have been reported to produce NMS.[5,8,10,14–18,55] Third, the abrupt discontinuation of dopamine agonists (e.g., amantadine, levodopa/carbidopa) in patients with Parkinson's disease has been reported to produce a syndrome identical to NMS.[8–13] Fourth, treatment with dopamine agonists (e.g., bromocriptine, amantadine) improves the signs and symptoms of NMS.[5,6,40,41,56–61] Fifth, if dopamine agonist therapy is withdrawn prematurely from patients with NMS who have been treated, signs and symptoms may return.[61] Sixth, a significant reduction of the dopamine metabolite homovanillic acid has been observed in the cerebrospinal fluid of some patients with NMS compared with control subjects.[62]

Functionally the signs and symptoms of NMS largely can be explained by neuroleptic blockade of D_2-dopamine receptors in the hypothalamus, striatum, mesocortical and mesolimbic areas, peripheral sympathetic nerve terminals, and vasculature.[8,51,63] Neuroleptic blockade of D_2-receptors in the nigrostriatum may produce muscle rigidity and parkinsonism.[51,63] Neuroleptic blockade of D_2-receptors in the thermoregulatory center (preoptic area) of the anterior hypothalamus may produce hyperthermia.[51,63] Injection of dopamine into the preoptic area of the hypothalamus of animals results in hypothermia, and this effect can be blocked by haloperidol.[64] Intraventricular injection of chlorpromazine causes a rise in core temperature.[65] The fever of NMS is the result of increased heat production from muscle rigidity, impaired heat dissipation, and possibly a higher set-point of core temperature in the hypothalamus. Neuroleptic blockade of mesocortical and mesolimbic D_2 pathways partly mediates the altered mentation of NMS.[51] Neuroleptic antagonism of dopamine receptors present on peripheral sympathetic nerve terminals and vascular smooth muscle cells may mediate the autonomic dysfunction associated with NMS.[66] Antagonism of presynaptic D_2-autoreceptors increases the release of norepinephrine, whereas antagonism of postsynaptic D_2-receptors results in vascular relaxation in select areas.[67] Supersensitivity of these receptors that results from repeated neuroleptic administration contributes to autonomic irregularity. Clinically, tachycardia, hypertension, blood pressure lability, diaphoresis, pallor, tachypnea, and incontinence may result.

The time delay between the administration of neuroleptics and the occurrence of NMS suggests that factors other than acute effects of neuroleptics are operative in the initiation of the syndrome. Centrally, nigrostriatal and mesolimbic regions have presynaptic D_2-autoreceptors, which diminish the release of dopamine when stimulated.[67] Peripherally, sympathetic ganglia and postganglionic sympathetic nerve terminals have presynaptic D_2-autoreceptors, which diminish the release of norepinephrine when stimulated.[68] Exposure to neuroleptics may initiate the development of supersensitivity at the presynaptic and the postsynaptic dopamine receptors. Autoreceptors are more sensitive to dopamine, however, than are postsynaptic receptors and are affected to a greater degree.[67] Supersensitivity at the presynaptic area results in decreased dopamine output and contributes to dopaminergic hypoactivity. Although supersensitivity of postsynaptic receptors occurs with repeated neuroleptic administration, the acute administration of rapidly escalating doses predominantly results in postsynaptic depolarization blockade.[67,69] When postsynaptic blockade is coupled with presynaptic downregulation (decreased dopamine production and release), marked dopaminergic hypoactivity results, and patients are at risk for NMS. Why NMS occurs in such a small minority of patients treated with neuroleptics is unknown.

NMS and EPS (e.g., acute dystonia, parkinsonism, akathisia) are closely related entities, both of which result from neuroleptic blockade of nigrostriatal D_2-receptors.[51,53,63,69] NMS is often considered a severe form of EPS with fever that has progressed from unrecognized or inadequately treated milder forms of EPS.[4,5,7,50,70,71] Despite its similarity to EPS, however, NMS has a unique pathophysiology that probably reflects complicated, time-dependent neuroreceptor effects yet to be elucidated. Anticholinergic agents are not efficacious for the treatment of NMS but are highly effective for acute dystonia and parkinsonism. Time-dependent changes in neuroreceptor function may be responsible for a lack of response to these agents in the setting of NMS.

The pathophysiology of NMS may involve iron. Iron is a positive modulator of dopamine receptor activity. Low serum iron levels often are found in patients with NMS and may lead to a decreased expression of dopamine receptors in the brain.[72,73] It is not known whether low serum iron levels are a primary cause of NMS or occur as a result of the illness.

Although dopaminergic blockade is central to the pathobiology of NMS, the alterations of other neurotransmitter systems are likely important as well. Neuroleptics may modulate the activity of a variety of other neurochemicals (e.g., γ-aminobutyric acid [GABA], acetylcholine, norepinephrine, serotonin, glutamate, aspartate, enkephalin, dynorphin, substance P, somatostatin, cholecystokinin, neurotensin, vasoactive intestinal peptide, and various prostaglandins) through specific receptor binding or indirectly as a result of altered dopamine neurotransmission.[8,52] Imbalance between dopaminergic activity and one or more of these neurochemicals may mediate the signs and symptoms of NMS. The interactions are complex, varied throughout the CNS, and not well understood. In addition to striatal D_2-receptor antagonism, the muscular rigidity and akinesia associated with NMS result from alterations in levels of substance P, dynorphin, enkephalin, glutamate, and GABA in various basal ganglial pathways.[8,52]

One provocative theory suggests that NMS results from disinhibition of glutamatergic and other excitatory amino acid pathways in the CNS.[52,74] Normally, excitatory amino acid activity in corticostriatal and subthalamic pathways is antagonized by nigrostriatal dopaminergic neurons. Blockade of dopamine receptors by neuroleptics disinhibits the N-methyl-D-aspartate (NMDA) glutamate receptor, resulting in an excess of glutamatergic neurotransmission and the rigidity of NMS.[52,74] There is evidence to support this theory. Amantadine, an NMDA-receptor antagonist, ameliorates the rigidity of NMS and induces hypothermia in animals.[52,75] GABA-receptor agonists (e.g., benzodiazepines) inhibit glutamate neurotransmission and are helpful in the treatment of NMS.[5,8,52]

Direct skeletal muscle effects from neuroleptics may mediate partly the rigidity, fever, and serum elevations of creatine kinase associated with NMS. In vitro, neuroleptics have been shown to inhibit calmodulin, increase ionized calcium, and result in skeletal muscle fiber contraction; this action may be inhibited by dantrolene.[76–78] A primary peripheral cause of NMS is unlikely, however, because dantrolene sometimes is ineffective for the treatment of this syndrome.[5,21,41,79]

CLINICAL FEATURES

NMS is most commonly characterized by fever, muscular rigidity, altered mental status, and autonomic dysfunction.[5,6] Fever and muscular rigidity usually are present but are not required for diagnosis. NMS is a heterogeneous syndrome that occurs across a spectrum of severity.[4] Signs and symptoms vary and are influenced by the timing of diagnosis and treatment. Fever (temperature $\geq 38°C$ [100.4°F]) occurs in 79% to 100% of patients, and temperatures exceed 40°C in approximately 40% of patients.[5,6,21,39–41] Muscular rigidity is present in 92% to 97% of patients and is usually parkinsonian or "lead pipe" in nature.[5,6,8,40,41,80] The rigidity of NMS typically is unresponsive to anticholinergic treatment.[5,6] Mental status alteration is reported in 97% of cases and may range from mild inattentiveness, lethargy, and confusion to severe unresponsive catatonia, stupor, and coma.[5,6,8,41,80] Agitation and delirium also have been described. Autonomic dysfunction has been reported in 100% of patients and includes fever, tachycardia, tachypnea, hypertension or hypotension, blood pressure lability, diaphoresis, sialorrhea, pallor, flushing, urinary incontinence, and cardiac dysrhythmias.[5–7,40,41,80]

Extrapyramidal movement disorders frequently are present in patients with NMS and include tremor, bradykinesia, akinesia, hypomimia, festinating gait, chorea, dystonias (e.g., opisthotonos, trismus, blepharospasm, buccofacial dyskinesia, and oculogyric crisis), nystagmus, opsoclonus, dysphagia, dysarthria, and aphonia.[5–7,41,80] These findings are expected if one accepts NMS as an extreme form of EPS. Other neurologic abnormalities include akinetic mutism, hyperreflexia, extensor plantar responses, ataxia, abnormal flexor or extensor posturing, ocular flutter, impaired upward gaze, and seizures.[5–7,40,41,80]

CLINICAL COURSE

Although NMS may occur at any time during neuroleptic therapy, most cases (66% to 89%) occur within 2 weeks of drug initiation, dose increase, or change to a different agent.[5,6,40,41] NMS peaks within 72 hours of symptom onset in most patients (79% to 90%).[5,6,40,41] In one review of 115 cases of NMS, however, it took 4 to 30 days for 18 patients (21%) to evolve into the full syndrome.[5] When neuroleptics are stopped, signs and symptoms of NMS resolve within 1 to 61 days.[5,6,40,41] In one study of 65 patients not treated with dantrolene or dopamine agonists, the mean duration of NMS was 9.6 ± 9.1 days.[79] The duration of illness is not different in pediatric patients.[41] The clinical course is nearly twice as long, however, for patients who have received intramuscular depot preparations.[5,6,40] In one study of 115 patients, the mean duration of NMS was 13 days for nondepot neuroleptics and 26 days for depot agents.[5]

Most cases of NMS seem to follow a sequence of development. Mental status changes or muscular rigidity precede autonomic dysfunction and hyperthermia in 82.3% of cases.[70] These findings support the theory that psychomotor agitation and muscular rigidity contribute to the development of fever. Early recognition of confusion, catatonia, or worsening EPS may facilitate prompt treatment and halt progression to a fulminant syndrome.[50,70]

LABORATORY FINDINGS

Although laboratory abnormalities frequently are present with NMS, none are specific to or pathognomonic for NMS. Elevation of serum creatine phosphokinase (CPK) (greater than three times normal) is the most frequent laboratory abnormality, present in 97% of patients.[5,6] Elevation of CPK reflects myonecrosis and often is associated with rhabdomyolysis, myoglobinuria, and acute renal failure from acute tubular necrosis. Myonecrosis results from muscular rigidity, fever, and psychomotor agitation. Leukocytosis (white blood cell count 10,000 to 40,000/mm³), with or without a left shift, is present in 70% to 98% of patients.[5–7,40,41] Other laboratory abnormalities that may occur include hypernatremia or hyponatremia, mild elevations of hepatic aminotransferases,

and low serum iron.[5–7] Patients with NMS may develop anion gap metabolic acidosis (due to increased lactic acid), hypoxemia, and elevations of creatinine and coagulation parameters.[5–7,40]

For patients with NMS, results of lumbar puncture, radionuclide brain scans, and computed tomography and magnetic resonance imaging of the head are usually normal or show nonspecific abnormalities.[5–7,40] Electroencephalograms are normal or suggest nonspecific encephalopathy.[5] In one review of 45 patients with NMS who had electroencephalograms, 21 (47%) had nonspecific slowing, and 20 (44%) had normal studies.[5] Electromyograms and muscle biopsy specimens are normal or show nonspecific changes.[5–7,40] Postmortem histopathologic examinations of the brain do not reveal specific structural abnormalities associated with NMS.[6,7]

COMPLICATIONS AND MORTALITY

Medical complications from NMS are more likely to occur in patients with a higher severity of illness (e.g., longer duration, higher fever) or preexisting comorbid conditions (e.g., organic brain syndrome, mental retardation).[5–7,21,39,40] Rhabdomyolysis is the most frequent complication.[5,6] Other complications include renal failure, aspiration pneumonia, pulmonary edema, pulmonary embolism, respiratory failure, sepsis, coagulopathy, disseminated intravascular coagulation, sepsis, seizures, myocardial infarction, peripheral neuropathy, periarticular ossification, necrotizing enterocolitis, cardiac arrhythmias, and cardiorespiratory arrest.[5–8]

NMS initially was characterized as "malignant" because of its fatal outcome in a significant percentage of patients. Before 1986 the mortality rates ranged from 17% to 28%, whereas since 1986 they have ranged from 0% to 11.6%.[5–8,39–44,81,82] In one review of 77 cases of NMS in adolescents and children, the mortality rate was 9%, and serious sequelae occurred in 20%.[41] As in adults, the mortality rate has declined since the mid-1980s; no fatalities in children have been reported since 1986.[41] Mortality is correlated closely with the severity of hyperthermia. In one review of 374 patients with NMS, survival was 100% for patients with peak temperature less than 38°C, 88% for patients with peak temperature between 39.0°C and 39.9°C, but only 44% for patients with peak temperature greater than 42°C.[39] The duration of hyperthermia likely also is associated with the incidence of secondary complications and lethality. In all patients with NMS, death usually is secondary to respiratory failure (e.g., aspiration pneumonia, hypoventilation), cardiovascular collapse, myoglobinuric renal failure, arrhythmias, thromboembolism (e.g., pulmonary embolism), and disseminated intravascular coagulation.[5–7,40] Renal failure is associated with a 50% mortality rate.[43] Most adult patients who recover from NMS recover fully and do not manifest persistent neurologic sequelae.[5–7]

DIAGNOSIS

Confirmatory laboratory tests do not exist for NMS, and diagnosis is based on history, suggestive physical findings, and a high level of suspicion in the appropriate clinical setting. It is unclear whether NMS is a qualitatively distinct entity with all-or-none clinical expression or an extrapyramidal complication that occurs at the end of a spectrum of neuroleptic-induced side effects. Some investigators believe that the diagnosis should not be made unless all four classic features (i.e., fever, muscular rigidity, altered mentation, and autonomic dysfunction) are present.[6,83,84] Other investigators believe that NMS is a heterogeneous disorder that may be diagnosed in its milder, atypical, and incipient forms.[4,5,50,70,71] To date, a lack of uniform diagnostic criteria in the literature has produced inconsistencies in diagnosis.[85] Adoption of a single set of standardized but flexible criteria to assist diagnosis is important to advance understanding of NMS and to differentiate it from other illnesses. The use of rigid diagnostic criteria may unnecessarily delay diagnosis and treatment, whereas flexible criteria may reduce morbidity by ensuring earlier recognition and prompt intervention.[4,50,70,71,85] Sets of clinical criteria that seem to allow for some flexibility in diagnosis are presented in Table 26-2.[86,87] Fever and muscle rigidity are required for diagnosis with these criteria.

DIFFERENTIAL DIAGNOSIS

The diagnosis of NMS should be considered whenever a patient develops fever and muscular rigidity while taking neuroleptics. Early signs of NMS also may include an unexpected deterioration of mental status, new catatonia, and the development of EPS refractory to anticholinergic therapy.[50,70] Because NMS is an uncommon syndrome, however, the diagnosis should not be made before other causes have been considered and ruled out. Studies have shown that patients initially suspected of having NMS often have other medical disorders that account for their signs and symptoms.[4,88] Alternative conditions that should be considered in the differential diagnosis of NMS are listed in Table 26-3.

One disorder that is difficult to differentiate from NMS is lethal catatonia. Lethal catatonia is a rapidly progressive, idiopathic psychiatric syndrome that is characterized by catalepsy, rigidity, waxy flexibility, stupor, mutism, fever, autonomic instability, and death.[6–8,89] In contrast to NMS, lethal catatonia begins with extreme agitation that, if unchecked, leads to exhaustion and mutism; rigidity is a late finding in lethal catatonia. Neuroleptics are ineffective in lethal catatonia.[89] Withdrawal of neuroleptics is recommended when either NMS or lethal catatonia is suspected.[89]

Although NMS and malignant hyperthermia (see Chapter 25) have similar clinical characteristics, they are differentiated easily on the basis of history, clinical setting, and rapidity of onset. The two illnesses are distinct clinical entities with different pathophysiology. Malignant hyperthermia is a rare genetically transmitted abnormality of skeletal muscle calcium metabolism. After exposure to certain anesthetic agents (e.g., succinylcholine, halothane) or stress, enhanced release and impaired reuptake of calcium occur from muscle cell sarcoplasmic reticulum. Excessive excitation-contraction coupling and a syndrome of muscle rigidity and fever that

TABLE 26-2 Two Sets of Diagnostic Criteria for Neuroleptic Malignant Syndrome

CAROFF ET AL[86]	AMERICAN PSYCHIATRIC ASSOCIATION[87]

1. Treatment with neuroleptics within 7 days of illness onset (2–4 wk for depot agents)
2. Hyperthermia (>38°C)
3. Muscle rigidity
4. Five of the following:
  Change in mental status
  Tachycardia
  Hypertension or hypotension
  Tachypnea or hypoxia
  Diaphoresis or sialorrhea
  Dysarthria or dysphagia
  Tremor
  Incontinence
  Increased CPK or myoglobinuria
  Leukocytosis
  Metabolic acidosis
5. Exclusion of other drug-induced, systemic, or neuropsychiatric illness
	A. Development of muscle rigidity and fever associated with the use of neuroleptics
	B. ≥Two of the following:
	  Change in level of consciousness
	  Mutism
	  Tachycardia
	  Hypertension or labile blood pressure
	  Diaphoresis
	  Dysphagia
	  Tremor
	  Incontinence
	  Leukocytosis
	  Laboratory evidence of muscle injury (e.g., elevated CPK)
	C. Symptoms in A and B are not due to another substance or to a neurologic or general medical condition
	D. Symptoms in A and B are not better accounted for by a mental disorder

CPK, creatine phosphokinase.

TABLE 26-3 Differential Diagnosis of Neuroleptic Malignant Syndrome

TOXIN-MEDIATED ALTERNATIVE DIAGNOSES	NON–TOXIN-MEDIATED ALTERNATIVE DIAGNOSES
Anticholinergic agents Central hallucinogens (e.g., ketamine, LSD, MDMA, MDEA, PCP) Cyclic antidepressants Drug-induced parkinsonism (e.g., amoxapine, carbon monoxide, carbon disulfide, cyanide, disulfiram, ethylene glycol, methanol, metoclopramide, MPTP, neuroleptics) Drug interactions (e.g., monoamine oxidase inhibitor tyramine reaction, serotonin syndrome) Drug withdrawal states (e.g., barbiturates, benzodiazepines, ethanol) Heavy metals (e.g., manganese, mercury, lead) Lithium Monoamine oxidase inhibitors Salicylates Strychnine Sympathomimetics (e.g., amphetamines, cocaine, designer drugs, methylxanthines)	Cerebrovascular accident (e.g, hemorrhagic stroke) CNS tumors Endocrinopathies (e.g., pheochromocytoma, thyrotoxicosis) Heatstroke Infections (e.g., brain abscess, CNS HIV infection, meningoencephalitis, postinfectious encephalomyelitis, pneumonia, sepsis, rabies, tetanus) Lethal catatonia Malignant hyperthermia Seizures Stiff-man syndrome Systemic lupus erythematosus Trauma

CNS, central nervous system; HIV, human immunodeficiency virus; LSD, lysergic acid diethylamide; MDEA, 3,4-methylenedioxyamphetamine; MDMA, 3,4-methylenedioxymethamphetamine; MPTP, 1-methyl-4-phenyl-1,2,3,6-tetrahydropyridine; PCP, phenylcyclohexyl piperidine (phencyclidine).

may appear clinically similar to NMS result. In contrast to NMS, however, malignant hyperthermia has a genetic predisposition, it is associated with general anesthesia and not neuroleptic therapy, it is characterized by rapid onset and high mortality, and its rigidity does not respond to nondepolarizing paralytic agents.[5–8,83] In addition, muscle fibers from patients with malignant hyperthermia have positive in vitro contracture responses to caffeine and halothane, whereas muscle fibers from patients with NMS do not contract.[90]

EVALUATION

The history should include the duration of neuroleptic treatment; identity, dosing pattern, and route of administration of the neuroleptic; concurrent medications; identity of any preexisting illness and NMS risk factors; and time of onset, nature, sequence, and progression of signs and symptoms. The ingestion of other substances should be documented. The initial physical examination should include a detailed assessment of vital signs, cardiopulmonary status, and neurologic function. There are no bioassays that can confirm the diagnosis of NMS. Laboratory and adjunctive diagnostic tests are used primarily to exclude alternative diagnoses and complications.[6,7] Typical laboratory evaluation may include a complete blood count; blood cultures; measurement of serum electrolytes, blood urea nitrogen, creatinine, glucose, calcium, magnesium, CPK, thyroid-stimulating hormone, and iron; a toxicologic screen of blood or urine or both; a urinalysis; and an electrocardiogram. Pregnancy testing is suggested for women of childbearing age. There is no known direct effect of NMS on pregnancy or the fetus. Sicker patients also require measurements of coagulation parameters and liver function tests, arterial blood gas analysis, and a chest radiograph. Quantitative serum concentrations of concurrent medications (e.g., lithium) should be obtained. Other studies that may be necessary to exclude alternative diagnoses include a lumbar puncture, electroencephalogram, and computed tomography or magnetic resonance imaging of the head. Serial evaluations of vital signs, neurologic function, and serum CPK are important to determine the course of the illness and the need for further testing and intervention.

TREATMENT

Prevention is the most important aspect of treatment.[50] Risk factors (e.g., dehydration, agitation) should be identified and modified when possible, and neuroleptics should be discontinued in instances in which the incipient phase of NMS (e.g., severe EPS) is suspected. Management of suspected or established cases of NMS requires immediate withdrawal of neuroleptics and NMS-potentiating drugs (e.g., anticholinergics, lithium), exclusion of other medical conditions that may simulate NMS, and aggressive supportive care. The role of adjunctive pharmacotherapies is less well established. Supportive care includes provision of adequate ventilation and oxygenation; rehydration; temperature reduction; nutritional support; low-dose heparin to prevent thromboembolic disease; and treatment of metabolic, renal, and cardiopulmonary complications.[7] Because NMS is an idiosyncratic complication that results from therapeutic dosing of neuroleptics, gastrointestinal decontamination is not indicated if the diag-

nosis of NMS is secure. Empirical antibiotic administration is recommended because of the initial difficulty in differentiating NMS from systemic infection. Prophylactic intubation should be considered for patients with excessive sialorrhea, swallowing dysfunction, coma, significant hypoxemia and acidosis, and rigidity with severe hyperthermia. Rehydration should be aggressive and rapid to achieve a minimum urine output of 50 to 100 mL/hr (1 mL/kg/hr) to avoid renal failure.

The effectiveness of specific treatments for NMS remains unclear; no individual therapy or combination of therapies has been shown to be universally effective or clearly superior to supportive care alone.[5–7,50,54] Evidence to support efficacy of individual agents is not based on controlled, prospective studies but largely on inferences from retrospective data and case reports. Selection bias, variation in the onset and severity of NMS, lack of standardized drug-dosing protocols, multiple simultaneous treatments, and the self-limited course of NMS make it difficult to establish the relative efficacy of any specific therapy compared with supportive care alone.[5–7,50,54] The possibility of a prospective, controlled study is unlikely because of the low incidence of NMS. Specific treatment measures include dantrolene, nondepolarizing neuromuscular paralysis, benzodiazepines, bromocriptine, amantadine, levodopa/carbidopa, nifedipine, nitroprusside, and ECT. All of these measures have been reported effective anecdotally in the management of NMS.

Most evidence does not support the use of anticholinergic agents for the treatment of NMS. Anticholinergic agents do not decrease the incidence of NMS when coadministered with neuroleptics, and they are usually ineffective at reducing symptoms or in shortening the duration of illness for established cases of NMS.[5,6,8,40,76] Anticholinergics may worsen hyperthermia by impairing heat dissipation. In one retrospective review of NMS in children and adolescents, however, anticholinergic therapy was associated with a shorter duration of illness.[41]

Dantrolene, a hydantoin derivative, inhibits ionized calcium release from the sarcoplasmic reticulum (see Chapter 156). It causes direct muscle relaxation by uncoupling excitation-contraction in skeletal muscle. It is used mainly to treat NMS-associated hyperthermia and rigidity. By reducing tonic contraction of skeletal muscles, dantrolene reduces thermogenesis and CPK release. It is given orally or by intravenous infusion. Initially, dantrolene should be administered at doses of 1 to 2.5 mg/kg every 6 hours.[5–8,83] Doses of up to 10 mg/kg/day are considered safe.[5–8,83] Dantrolene should be continued until the signs and symptoms of NMS resolve, typically after 5 to 10 days of therapy.[8,28,91] On symptom resolution, some authorities recommend that dantrolene be tapered over 3 to 10 days to avoid syndrome recrudescence.[50,71,91] Dantrolene may produce a variety of adverse effects, including muscle weakness, lethargy, nausea, vomiting, diarrhea, and urinary incontinence. Hepatotoxicity and seizures may occur with doses greater than 10 mg/kg/day and when treatment extends beyond 60 days.[6] In one review of 534 cases of NMS, a positive response was noted in 84% of 44 patients treated with dantrolene alone.[39]

Bromocriptine, amantadine, carbidopa-levodopa (Sinemet), and levodopa alone are dopamine agonists that are given to overcome neuroleptic-induced dopaminergic blockade. Dopamine agonists are given alone or in conjunction with dantrolene or other muscle relaxants. Bromocriptine, a dopamine receptor agonist, initially is administered in doses of 2.5 to 10 mg three to four times daily (see Chapter 146).[5–7,82] Doses of 20 mg four times daily have been used.[5–8,41] The appropriate dosing in children is not well established.[41] Bromocriptine is administered until the signs and symptoms of NMS resolve, typically after 5 to 10 days of therapy.[8,28,91] Duration of treatment has ranged from 2 to 56 days.[58,60,67] Abrupt discontinuation of bromocriptine has resulted in recrudescence of the signs and symptoms of NMS.[61,67] As with dantrolene, it is recommended that bromocriptine be tapered over 3 to 10 days on symptom resolution.[50,71,91] Amantadine, which enhances presynaptic dopamine release, is given orally two times daily (100 to 200 mg/dose).[6,40,83] The therapeutic actions of amantadine also are mediated by its noncompetitive antagonism at the NMDA-glutamate receptor.[52,74,75] Sinemet, which increases presynaptic dopamine stores, is given orally three to four times daily (25/250 to 75/300 mg dose).[40,80,92] In one review of 536 cases of NMS, bromocriptine was administered alone to 42 patients and was effective for 88%.[39] In this same review, amantadine and levodopa each were used in 16 cases; amantadine was effective in all, and levodopa was effective for 94% of patients.[39] These patients were treated concurrently with other pharmacotherapies, however, and the independent effects of amantadine and levodopa alone are unclear. In one study of adolescents and children with NMS, bromocriptine and levodopa were associated with a significantly shorter duration of illness.[41] In some cases of NMS, premature discontinuation of bromocriptine treatment has resulted in relapse of the syndrome; subsequent reinitiation of the drug has been effective.[8,61,67]

Studies that have examined the efficacy of dantrolene and dopamine agonists have been largely retrospective. In one retrospective analysis of 67 cases of NMS, dantrolene or bromocriptine reduced the time to clinical improvement and resolution compared with supportive care alone.[82] Mean response time to clinical improvement was 1.0 day for bromocriptine, 1.7 days for dantrolene, and 6.8 days for supportive care alone. Mean time to complete resolution was 9.0 days for dantrolene, 9.8 days for bromocriptine, and 15.8 days for supportive care alone. A prospective, open, nonrandomized study of 20 patients with NMS showed a more prolonged illness and greater complication rates with bromocriptine or dantrolene treatment, however, compared with supportive care alone.[92] The mean duration of illness was 9.9 days for patients treated with bromocriptine or dantrolene versus 6.8 days for patients treated supportively. The treatment groups in this study had a higher incidence of underlying medical illness, which may have biased results. In retrospective analyses, dopamine agonists have been reported to reduce NMS mortality rates significantly from 21% to 9.2%.[93,94] When used alone, bromocriptine reduces mortality to 7.8% and amantadine reduces mortality to less than 6%.[93,94] The combination of dantrolene with bromocriptine does not offer additional survival advantage over either drug alone.[93]

Benzodiazepines have shown efficacy as adjunctive therapy for NMS.[95–99] Benzodiazepines not only decrease neuromuscular agitation in a nonspecific manner but also inhibit glutamergic neurotransmission as GABA-receptor agonists.[5,8,10,40,76,95,99] Administration of benzodiazepines early in the course of illness may diminish psychomotor agitation and muscular rigidity and halt progression to the fulminant hyperthermic syndrome. Benzodiazepines also may hasten recovery from NMS.[98,99] In one retrospective study

of 16 patients with NMS, clinical improvement was noted within 24 to 72 hours of benzodiazepine treatment initiation (e.g., lorazepam)[99]; this compares favorably with the rates of recovery reported with other pharmacotherapies and with supportive care alone.[5,6,99] Initial intravenous doses of diazepam (0.1 to 0.2 mg/kg) or lorazepam (0.05 to 0.1 mg/kg) may be repeated at 10- to 30-minute intervals until the desirable effect is achieved or CNS or respiratory depression occurs. Although experience is limited, phenobarbital (5 to 10 mg/kg intravenously) may be used if psychomotor agitation is resistant to repeated benzodiazepine therapy.

ECT has been an effective treatment for NMS.[5–8,21,39] The beneficial effects are believed to result from an increased turnover of dopamine in the brain and increased receptor sensitivity to dopamine after ECT.[100] In one review of 29 cases of NMS treated with ECT, a positive response was noted in 83% of patients.[101] Some investigators suggest that the incidence of mortality for NMS patients treated with ECT is lower than for patients treated supportively.[101] Cardiac arrhythmias, cerebral edema, and death have occurred after ECT in a few patients, however.[6] ECT may be reserved more appropriately for patients who fail to respond to standard pharmacotherapies or have refractory catatonia.

Prompt reduction of NMS-associated muscle rigidity and hyperthermia can be expected to minimize the risk of rhabdomyolysis, renal failure, pneumonia, respiratory failure, disseminated intravascular coagulation, and cardiovascular collapse. These complications are responsible for most NMS-associated deaths, making their prevention paramount.[5–7,21,39–41,76,83] The severity of hyperthermia is correlated closely with the likelihood of death in patients with NMS.[39,41] Although hypothalamic thermoregulatory dysfunction may have a causal role in NMS-associated fever, thermogenesis ultimately is due to tonic skeletal muscle contraction.[5–8,76,79,83] Rapid muscle relaxation is the goal in patients who are severely ill. Bromocriptine and dantrolene often take 1 or more days to reduce fever and rigidity in patients with NMS.[82] In select instances, when patients are extremely rigid and have temperatures that exceed 40°C, it makes intuitive sense to use nondepolarizing neuromuscular paralysis (e.g., pancuronium) to achieve the most rapid, predictable, and effective reduction of rigidity and fever. Pancuronium has been used successfully to control rigidity and fever rapidly in two case reports; one of the patients had failed dantrolene therapy.[79,102] A reasonable first approach to manage the rigidity and fever associated with NMS includes intravenous benzodiazepines (diazepam, 0.1 to 0.4 mg/kg, or lorazepam, 0.05 to 0.1 mg/kg), antipyretics, evaporative cooling, ice packs, cooled intravenous fluids, and dopamine agonist therapy (e.g., bromocriptine). Adjunctive dantrolene therapy may be beneficial as well. If rigidity persists and patient temperature exceeds 40°C, timely neuromuscular paralysis is recommended. Immediate paralysis also is recommended for patients who have severe hyperthermia and rigidity on initial presentation. The sequence, type, and rapidity of intervention depend on the time course and severity of illness. In general, all patients suspected of having NMS should be admitted initially to an intensive care unit for aggressive supportive care. When the appropriate disposition or management of a patient is in question, consultation with a medical toxicologist is recommended.

To date, evidence suggests that patients with a history of NMS have a significantly greater risk for syndrome recurrence when a neuroleptic agent is reintroduced. In one review of 47 patients in whom neuroleptics were reintroduced, 14 (30%) developed recurrent episodes of NMS.[81] The risk is greater when high-potency (greater D_2-receptor binding affinity) and long-acting (depot) agents are reintroduced. Of 21 patients, 10 (48%) developed a recurrent episode when rechallenged with a high-potency agent compared with 4 (15%) of 26 patients rechallenged with a low-potency agent.[81] When reinitiation of neuroleptic therapy is necessary to treat severe psychotic illness in a patient with a history of NMS, steps should be taken to minimize the risk of syndrome recurrence. Potential risk factors, such as patient agitation and dehydration, should be minimized. The risk of recurrence is reduced significantly (8% versus 86% recurrence rate) if reintroduction of neuroleptic therapy is delayed by at least 2 weeks from an initial NMS episode.[76,103,104] When neuroleptics are reinitiated, low-potency or atypical agents (e.g., clozapine) should be used. In addition, low doses should be used initially, dose titration should be gradual, and patients should be monitored closely for incipient signs of NMS.[5,6,8,40,76]

Key Points in Neuroleptic Malignant Syndrome

1. When neuroleptic malignant syndrome (NMS) is first suspected, neuroleptic agents should be discontinued immediately.
2. The diagnosis of NMS should be considered whenever a patient develops fever and muscular rigidity while taking neuroleptics.
3. The diagnosis of NMS should not be made before other medical conditions have been considered and ruled out.
4. Timely and aggressive supportive care is the most important aspect of treatment.
5. Prompt reduction of muscle rigidity and fever minimizes medical complications and optimizes survival.
6. Because NMS is a life-threatening medical emergency, all patients suspected of having the illness should be managed initially in an intensive care unit.

REFERENCES

1. Delay J, Pichot P, Lemperiere T, et al: Un neuroleptique majeur non-phenothiazine et non-reserpinique, l'haloperidol, dans le traitement des psychoses. Ann Med Psychol 118:145–152, 1960.
2. Delay J, Deniker P: Drug-induced extrapyramidal syndromes. In Vinken PJ, Bruyn GW (eds): Handbook of Clinical Neurology: Diseases of the Basal Ganglia, vol 6. Amsterdam, 1968, North-Holland Publishing, pp 248–266.
3. Bourgeois M, Tignol J, deBouchard D: Le syndrome malin des neuroleptiques. Bourd Med 4:1115–1128, 1971.
4. Levinson DF, Simpson GM: Neuroleptic-induced extrapyramidal symptoms with fever: Heterogeneity of the "neuroleptic malignant syndrome." Arch Gen Psychiatry 43:839–848, 1986.
5. Addonizio G, Susman VL, Roth SD: Neuroleptic malignant syndrome: Review and analysis of 115 cases. Biol Psychiatry 22:1004–1020, 1987.
6. Caroff SN, Mann SC: Neuroleptic malignant syndrome. Med Clin North Am 77:185–202, 1993.
7. Pelonero AL, Levenson JL, Pandurangi AK: Neuroleptic malignant syndrome: A review. Psychiatr Serv 49:1163–1172, 1998.
8. Ebadi M, Pfeiffer RF, Murrin LC: Pathogenesis and treatment of neuroleptic malignant syndrome. Gen Pharmacol 21:367–386, 1990.
9. Toru M, Matsuda O, Makiguchi K, Sugano K: Neuroleptic malignant syndrome-like state following a withdrawal of antiparkinsonian drugs. J Nerv Ment Dis 169:324–327, 1981.
10. Burke RE, Fahn S, Mayeux R, et al: Neuroleptic malignant syndrome caused by dopamine depleting drugs in a patient with Huntington's chorea. Neurology 31:1022–1026, 1981.
11. Figa-Talamanca L, Gualandi C, DiMeo L, et al: Hyperthermia after discontinuance of levodopa and bromocriptine therapy: Impaired dopamine receptors a possible cause. Neurology 35:258–261, 1985.
12. Simpson DM, Davis GC: Case report of neuroleptic malignant syndrome following withdrawal from amantadine. Am J Psychiatry 141:796–797, 1984.
13. Sechi G, Tanda F, Mutani R: Fatal hyperpyrexia after withdrawal of levodopa. Neurology (Cleveland) 34:249–251, 1984.
14. Robinson MB, Kennett RP, Harding AE, Legg NJ: Neuroleptic malignant syndrome associated with metoclopramide. J Neurol Neurosurg Psychiatry 40:1305–1312, 1985.
15. Friedman LS, Weinrauch LA, D'Elia JA: Metoclopramide-induced neuroleptic malignant syndrome. Arch Intern Med 147:1495–1497, 1987.
16. Patterson JF: Neuroleptic malignant syndrome associated with metoclopramide. South Med J 81:674–675, 1988.
17. Madakasira S: Amoxapine-induced neuroleptic malignant syndrome. DICP Ann Pharmacother 23:50–51, 1989.
18. Taylor NE, Schwartz HI: Neuroleptic malignant syndrome following amoxapine overdose. J Nerv Ment Dis 176:249–251, 1988.
19. Rosenberg PB, Pearlman CA: NMS-like syndrome with a lithium/doxepin combination. J Clin Psychopharmacol 11:75–76, 1991.
20. Koehler PJ, Mirandolle JR: Neuroleptic malignant syndrome and lithium. Lancet 2:1499–1500, 1988.
21. Kellam AMP: The neuroleptic malignant syndrome, so-called: A survey of the world literature. Br J Psychiatry 150:752–759, 1987.
22. Keepers GA: Neuroleptic malignant syndrome associated with withdrawal from carbamazepine. Am J Psychiatry 147:1687, 1990.
23. O'Griofa FM, Voris JC: Neuroleptic malignant syndrome associated with carbamazepine. South Med J 84:1378–1380, 1991.
24. Woolf DCS: Neuroleptic malignant syndrome associated with phenytoin intoxication. S Afr Med J 73:620–621, 1988.
25. Heyland D, Sauvé M: Neuroleptic malignant syndrome without the use of neuroleptics. Can Med Assoc J 145:817–819, 1991.
26. Baca L, Martinelli L: Neuroleptic malignant syndrome: A unique association with a tricyclic antidepressant. Neurology 40:1797–1798, 1990.
27. Grant R: Neuroleptic malignant syndrome. BMJ 228:1960, 1984.
28. Lev R, Clark RF: Neuroleptic malignant syndrome presenting without fever: Case report and review of the literature. J Emerg Med 12:49–55, 1994.
29. Halman M, Goldbloom DS: Fluoxetine and neuroleptic malignant syndrome. Biol Psychiatry 28:518–521, 1990.
30. Merriam AE: Neuroleptic malignant syndrome after imipramine withdrawal. J Clin Psychopharmacol 7:53–54, 1987.
31. Kiyataka I, Yamaji K, Shirato I, et al: A case of neuroleptic malignant syndrome with acute renal failure after the discontinuation of sulpiride and maprotoline. Jpn J Med 30:387–391, 1991.
32. Langlow JR, Alarcon RD: Trimipramine-induced neuroleptic malignant syndrome after transient psychogenic polydipsia in one patient. J Clin Psychiatry 50:144–145, 1989.
33. Kosten TR, Kleber HD: Rapid death during cocaine abuse: A variant of neuroleptic malignant syndrome? Am J Drug Alcohol Abuse 14:355–346, 1988.
34. Rivera JM, Iriarte LM, Lozano F, et al: Possible estrogen-induced NMS. DICP Ann Pharmacother 23:811, 1989.
35. Brennan D, MacManus M, Howe J, McLoughlin J: 'Neuroleptic malignant syndrome' without neuroleptics. Br J Psychiatry 52:578–579, 1988.
36. Theoharides TC, Harris RS, Weckstein D: Neuroleptic-malignant-like syndrome due to cyclobenzaprine? J Clin Psychopharmacol 15:79–81, 1995.
37. Velamoor VR: NMS complicated by diazepam. Br J Psychiatry 160:324–327, 1992.
38. Davis JM, Janicak P, Sakkas P, et al: Neuroleptic malignant syndrome: The first 1000 cases (Abstract). Biol Psychiatry 27:132A, 1990.
39. Kellam AMP: The (frequently) neuroleptic (potentially) malignant syndrome. Br J Psychiatry 157:169–173, 1990.
40. Shalev A, Munitz H: The neuroleptic malignant syndrome: Agent and host interaction. Acta Psychiatr Scand 73:337–347, 1986.
41. Silva RR, Munoz DM, Alpert M, et al: Neuroleptic malignant syndrome in children and adolescents. J Am Acad Adolesc Psychiatry 38:187–194, 1999.
42. Pearlman CA: Neuroleptic malignant syndrome: A review of the literature. J Clin Psychopharmacol 6:257–273, 1986.

43. Shalev A, Hermesh H, Munitz H: Mortality from neuroleptic malignant syndrome. J Clin Psychiatry 50:18–29, 1989.

44. Keck PE, Pope HG, McElroy SL: Declining frequency of neuroleptic malignant syndrome in a hospital population. Am J Psychiatry 148:880–882, 1991.

45. Gelenberg AJ, Bellinghansen B, Wojcik JD, et al: A prospective survey of neuroleptic malignant syndrome in a short-term psychiatric hospital. Am J Psychiatry 145:517–518, 1988.

46. Keck PE, Sebastianelli J, Pope HG, et al: Frequency and presentation of neuroleptic malignant syndrome in a state psychiatric hospital. J Clin Psychiatry 50:352–355, 1989.

47. Keck PE, Pope HG, Cohen BM, et al: Risk factors for neuroleptic malignant syndrome: A case-control study. Arch Gen Psychiatry 46:914–918, 1989.

48. Sachdev P, Mason C, Hadzi-Pavlovic DH: Case-control study of neuroleptic malignant syndrome. Am J Psychiatry 154:1156–1158, 1997.

49. Otani K, Horiuchi M, Kondo T, et al: Is the predisposition to neuroleptic malignant syndrome genetically transmitted? Br J Psychiatry 158:850–853, 1991.

50. Velamoor VR, Swamy GN, Parmar Late-RS, et al: Management of suspected neuroleptic malignant syndrome. Can J Psychiatry 40:545–550, 1995.

51. Henderson VW, Wooten GF: Neuroleptic malignant syndrome: A pathophysiologic role for the dopamine receptor blockade? Neurology 1331:132–137, 1981.

52. Kornhuber J, Weller M: Neuroleptic malignant syndrome. Curr Opin Neurol 7:353–357, 1994.

53. Richelson E: Neuroleptic affinities for human brain receptors and their use in predicting adverse effects. J Clin Psychiatry 45:331, 1984.

54. Buckley PF, Hutchinson M: Neuroleptic malignant syndrome. J Neurol Neurosurg Psychiatry 58:271–273, 1995.

55. Haddad PM: Neuroleptic malignant syndrome may be caused by other drugs. BMJ 308:200, 1994.

56. McCarron MM, Boettger ML, Peck JJ: A case of neuroleptic malignant syndrome successfully treated with amantadine. J Clin Psychiatry 43:381–382, 1982.

57. Mueller PS, Vester JW, Fermaglich J: Neuroleptic malignant syndrome: Successful treatment with bromocriptine. JAMA 249:386–388, 1983.

58. Verhoeven WM, Elderson A, Westenberg HG: Neuroleptic malignant syndrome: Successful treatment with bromocriptine. Biol Psychiatry 20:680–684, 1985.

59. Zubenko G, Pope HG: Management of a case of neuroleptic malignant syndrome with bromocriptine. Am J Psychiatry 140:1619–1620, 1983.

60. Levenson JL: Neuroleptic malignant syndrome. Am J Psychiatry 142:1137–1145, 1985.

61. Dhib-Jalbut S, Hesselbrock R, Mouradian MM, et al: Bromocriptine treatment of neuroleptic malignant syndrome. J Clin Psychiatry 48:69–73, 1987.

62. Nisijima K, Ishiguro T: Neuroleptic malignant syndrome: A study of CSF monoamine metabolism. Biol Psychiatry 27:280–288, 1990.

63. Mann SC, Caroff SN, Lazarus A: Pathogenesis of neuroleptic malignant syndrome. Psychiatr Ann 21:175–180, 1991.

64. Cox B, Kerwin R, Lee TF: Dopamine receptors in the central thermoregulatory pathways of the rat. J Physiol 282:471–483, 1978.

65. Rewerski WJ, Jori A: Microinjection of chlorpromazine in different parts of rat brain. Int J Neuropharmacol 7:359–364, 1968.

66. Lindvall O, Bjorklung A, Skagerberg G: Dopamine-containing neurons in the spinal cord: Anatomy of some functional aspects. Ann Neurol 14:255–260, 1983.

67. Sitland-Marken PA, Wells BG, Froemming JH, et al: Psychiatric applications of bromocriptine therapy. J Clin Psychiatry 51:68–82, 1990.

68. Stoof JC, Kebabian JW: Two dopamine receptors: Biochemistry, physiology and pharmacology. Life Sci 34:2281–2286, 1984.

69. Baldessarini RJ: Drugs and the treatment of psychiatric disorders: Psychosis and anxiety. In Hardman JG, Limbird LE, Molinoff PB, et al (eds): Goodman and Gilman's the Pharmacological Basis of Therapeutics, 9th ed. New York, 1996, McGraw-Hill, pp 399–430.

70. Velamoor VR, Norman RMG, Caroff SN, et al: Progression of symptoms in neuroleptic malignant syndrome. J Nerv Ment Dis 182:168–173, 1994.

71. Nierenberg D, Disch M, Manheimer E, et al: Facilitating prompt diagnosis and treatment of the neuroleptic malignant syndrome. Clin Pharmacol Ther 50:580–586, 1991.

72. Rosebush PI, Mazurak MF: Serum iron and neuroleptic malignant syndrome. Lancet 338:149–151, 1991.

73. Garcia FM, Duarte J, Perez A, et al: Low serum iron and neuroleptic malignant syndrome. Ann Pharmacother 27:101–102, 1993.

74. Kornhuber J, Weller M, Riederer P: Glutamate receptor antagonists for neuroleptic malignant syndrome and akinetic hyperthermic parkinsonian crisis. J Neural Transm 6:63–72, 1993.

75. Weller M, Kornhuber J: A rationale for NMDA receptor antagonist therapy of the neuroleptic malignant syndrome. Med Hypotheses 38:329–333, 1992.

76. Dickey W: The neuroleptic malignant syndrome. Prog Neurobiol 36:425–436, 1991.

77. Takagi A: Chlorpromazine and skeletal muscle: A study of skinned single fibres of the guinea pig. Exp Neurol 73:477–486, 1981.

78. Lopez JR, Sanchez V, Lopez MJ: Sarcoplasmic ionic calcium concentration in neuroleptic malignant syndrome. Cell Calcium 10:223–233, 1989.

79. Sangai R, Dimitrijevic R: Neuroleptic malignant syndrome: Successful treatment with pancuronium. JAMA 254:2795–2796, 1985.

80. Kurlan R, Hamill TR, Shoulson I: Neuroleptic malignant syndrome. Clin Neuropharmacol 7:109–120, 1984.

81. Caroff SN, Mann SC: Neuroleptic malignant syndrome. Psychopharmacol Bull 24:25–29, 1988.

82. Rosenberg MR, Green M: Neuroleptic malignant syndrome: Review of response to therapy. Arch Intern Med 149:1927–1931, 1989.

83. Guze BH, Baxter LR: Neuroleptic malignant syndrome. N Engl J Med 313:163–166, 1985.

84. Adityan J, Sing S, Sing G, Ong S: Spectrum concept of neuroleptic malignant syndrome. Br J Psychiatry 153:107–111, 1988.

85. Gurrera RJ, Chang SS, Romero JA: A comparison of diagnostic criteria for neuroleptic malignant syndrome. J Clin Psychiatry 53:56–62, 1992.

86. Caroff SN, Mann SC, Lazarus A, et al: Neuroleptic malignant syndrome: Diagnostic issues. Psychiatr Ann 21:130–147, 1991.

87. American Psychiatric Association: Diagnostic and Statistical Manual for Mental Disorders, 4th ed (DSM-IV). Washington, DC, 1994, American Psychiatric Press, pp 739–742.

88. Sewell D, Jeste DV: Distinguishing neuroleptic malignant syndrome (NMS) from NMS-like acute medical illnesses: A study of 34 cases. J Neuropsychiatry 4:265–269, 1992.

89. Mann SC, Caroff SN, Bleier HR, et al: Lethal catatonia. Am J Psychiatry 143:1374–1381, 1986.

90. Adnet PJ, Krivosic-Horber RM, Adamantidis MM, et al: The association between neuroleptic malignant syndrome and malignant hyperthermia. Acta Anesthesiol Scand 33:676–680, 1989.

91. Olmsted TR: Neuroleptic malignant syndrome: Guidelines for treatment and reinstitution of neuroleptics. South Med J 81:888–891, 1988.

92. Knezevic W, Mastaglia FL, Lefroy RB, Fisher A: Neuroleptic malignant syndrome. Med J Aust 140:28–30, 1984.

92. Rosebush PI, Stewart TD, Marzurek MF: The treatment of neuroleptic malignant syndrome: Are dantrolene and bromocriptine useful adjuncts to supportive care? Br J Psychiatry 159:709–712, 1991.

93. Sakkas P, Davis JM, Hua J, et al: Pharmacotherapy of neuroleptic malignant syndrome. Psychiatr Ann 21:157–164, 1991.

94. Sakkas P, Davis JM, Janicak PG, et al: Drug treatment of the neuroleptic malignant syndrome. Psychopharmacol Bull 27:381–384, 1991.

95. Kumar V: A case of neuroleptic malignant syndrome treated with diazepam. Can J Psychiatry 32:815–816, 1987.

96. O'Brien P: Neuroleptic malignant syndrome treated with diazepam. Can J Psychiatry 33:780, 1988.

97. Fricchione GL, Cassem NH, Hoberman D, Hobson D: Intravenous lorazepam in neuroleptic-induced catatonia. J Clin Psychopharmacol 3:338–342, 1983.

98. Khaldarov V: Benzodiazepines for treatment of neuroleptic malignant syndrome. Hosp Physician 36:51–55, 2000.

99. Francis A, Koch M, Chandragiri S, et al: Is lorazepam a treatment for neuroleptic malignant syndrome? CNS Spectrum 5:54–57, 2000.

100. Lerer B, Belmaker RH: Receptors and the mechanism of action of ECT. Biol Psychiatry 17:497–511, 1982.

101. Davis JM, Janicak PG, Sakkas P, et al: Electroconvulsive therapy in the treatment of the neuroleptic malignant syndrome. Convulsive Therapy 7:111–120, 1991.

102. Mahmoodian S: Neuroleptic malignant syndrome. W Va Med J 82:435–439, 1986.

103. Rosebush P, Stewart T, Glenberg AJ: Twenty neuroleptic challenges after neuroleptic malignant syndrome in 15 patients. J Clin Psychiatry 50:295–298, 1989.

104. Susman VL, Addonizio G: Recurrence of neuroleptic malignant syndrome. J Nerv Ment Dis 176:234–241, 1987.

CHAPTER 27

Toxic Pulmonary Syndromes

Jefferey L. Burgess

The lung is a major target organ of inhaled toxicants and may be injured as a result of systemic toxicity from select ingestions. Similar to the liver, the lung has the capacity to metabolize xenobiotics. The lung is susceptible to oxidant injury from direct chemical exposure and from inflammatory cells located in the lung, including alveolar macrophages and neutrophils. The lung also may be injured through immune response mechanisms. Lung injury may present immediately after a toxic exposure or in a delayed fashion, particularly after exposure to gases with low water solubility or other toxicants affecting the lower respiratory tract.

Incidence data are not obtained easily for many acute toxic pulmonary syndromes, although some statistics are available. Occupational inhalation accidents sufficient to cause respiratory illness have been reported to occur at a rate of 1.1 patients per 100,000/yr.[1] Acute lung injury (ALI) and adult respiratory distress syndrome (ARDS) incidence varies by study. In a study of northern European countries, incidence was 17.9 and 13.5 patients per 100,000/yr for ALI and ARDS.[2] For inhalation fever, incidence rates vary markedly by exposure source and occupation. Among welders, approximately 20% have experienced symptoms consistent with metal fume fever[3]; among male farmers, approximately 60% have experienced symptoms consistent with grain fever.[4] Persistent asthma or reactive airways dysfunction syndrome (RADS) after occupational inhalation accidents is less common, with an estimated 0.1 cases per 1 million workers/yr.[1] Aspiration pneumonia rates are highest in compromised individuals, such as nursing home patients; in one study of nursing home patients, 22.9% of gastrostomy tube–fed patients aspirated.[5] Hypersensitivity pneumonitis rates vary by population. Rate of confirmed disease in farmers in one study was 44 patients per 100,000/yr.[6]

HISTORY

Lung injuries after occupational exposures have long been reported, although new recognition of various disease forms continues through the present. In the early 1700s, Ramazzini[7] described the adverse pulmonary effects of dust exposure in miners. Morbidity and mortality from lung injury was well documented after exposure to chlorine, phosgene, and mustard agents used in chemical warfare in World War I.[8] The German army killed several thousand Allied troops using chlorine in Ypres, Belgium, in 1915, and the Allies retaliated using the same gas later that year. More recently, inhalation exposure incidents such as the release of methyl isocyanate in Bhopal

have caused death and persistent respiratory compromise.[9] RADS and cryptogenic organizing pneumonia (COP) (also known as *bronchiolitis obliterans organizing pneumonia*) first were described in 1985,[10,11] and new causes of respiratory disease continue to be discovered.

The treatment of acute toxic pulmonary syndromes is a relatively more recent and evolving field. The danger of oxygen toxicity first was reported in studies in rabbits in 1916.[12] The Cocoanut Grove Fire in Boston in 1942 showed the importance of pulmonary injury in burns,[13] and the development of blood gas analysis, new respirators, and intensive care units in the 1950s and 1960s greatly advanced the clinical care of patients with pulmonary injuries. ARDS first was described in 1967, as was the beneficial effect of positive end-expiratory pressure in treating this condition.[14] ARDS was a frequent complication of battlefield injuries among American casualties in the Vietnam war. Controversy continues over the proper ventilation of patients with ARDS.[15,16] Other than improvements in ventilatory and other supportive care, however, relatively few advances have been made in the treatment of ALI.

PATHOPHYSIOLOGY

The two main functions of the lung are ventilation and gas exchange. To serve both of these functions, the lung is composed of conducting airways and gas exchange regions. The conducting airways start with the trachea and extend into the primary and secondary bronchi and terminal bronchioles. The loss of cartilage characterizes the transition from bronchi to bronchioles. The gas exchange region is composed of respiratory bronchioles and associated alveolar ducts and sacs. Cell types in the lung vary by region, with the conducting airways lined by ciliated epithelial cells, mucus-secreting goblet cells, and fluid-producing serous cells. The resulting mucus layer traps particles and is believed to have additional protective effects for the conducting airways. The ciliated cells beat synchronously, moving the mucus toward the pharynx, where it generally is swallowed. The alveolar epithelium is lined predominantly by flattened type I pneumocytes (covering 90% to 95% of the surface) and type II pneumocytes, which serve as progenitor cells for type I pneumocytes and as the source for pulmonary surfactant. Clara cells are prevalent in the bronchioles and contain P-450 metabolizing enzymes. Additional cells in the alveolar interstitium include fibroblasts, monocytes, and lymphocytes.

Ventilation of the lungs is driven during inhalation by reduced intrathoracic pressure created by contraction of the diaphragm and thoracic wall musculature and during exhalation by relaxation of these muscles. Although the total lung capacity in an adult usually exceeds 5 L, resting tidal volume is approximately 500 mL, and vital capacity, which is the volume exhaled after maximum inhalation and full exhalation, is approximately 4.5 L. After full exhalation, the remaining air constitutes the residual volume. Resting respiratory rate is 12 to 20 breaths/min in adults. Minute volume, which is the product of inhalation rate and tidal volume, increases with exercise.

Perfusion involves the flow of blood into the lungs. Blood supply to the lungs is provided through bronchial arteries, which parallel the airways and provide oxygenated blood, and the pulmonary artery, which carries blood with low oxygen content from the right ventricle. The alveolar septa are composed of the following layers: capillary endothelium, basement membrane, and alveolar epithelium. Diffusion across these septa occurs between the blood and air in the alveolar space. A variety of pathologic processes can affect air exchange, through loss or thickening of alveolar septa.

TOXIC MECHANISMS

Pulmonary toxicity may manifest in the conducting airways, alveolar region, or both. One of the major toxic mechanisms in the lung is the constellation of oxidative injury and inflammation. Free radicals may be inhaled or generated within the lung by tobacco smoke, ozone, nitrogen dioxide, and immune cells within the lung (predominantly macrophages and neutrophils). Important reactive oxygen species (ROS) include superoxide, hydrogen peroxide, and hydroxyl radicals. These free radicals damage cells through initiation of lipid peroxidation chain reactions.[17–19] ROS react with arachidonic acid, leading to the formation of inflammatory mediators, including prostaglandins and leukotrienes.[20] The release of inflammatory mediators increases the recruitment of neutrophils to the lung, neutrophil activation, and their migration into the alveolar space. Death of phagocytic cells during an inflammatory response releases proteolytic enzymes, with resultant lung tissue damage. Inflammation within the lung alters alveolar permeability, with resultant entry of water and blood proteins into the alveoli. With sufficient damage, pulmonary edema occurs. Certain drugs, such as opiates and salicylates, theoretically may alter lung permeability through neurogenic mechanisms, and other drugs, such as penicillamine and gold salts, may affect repair of lung injury through alteration of collagen metabolism.[21]

Water solubility of inhaled toxicants and particle size affect the location and extent of lung injury. Moderately to highly water-soluble gases, such as ammonia, chlorine, and sulfur dioxide, interact readily with the proximal respiratory tract. This reaction causes immediate symptoms but spares the lower lung from injury unless the exposure is to a high concentration or for a prolonged period. Low water-solubility toxicants, such as phosphine or nitrogen dioxide, react primarily at the alveolar level, where they have increased residence time. Initial warning symptoms may not occur, and symptomatic lung injury may be delayed for 8 or more hours.[22,23]

For exposure to particulate matter, particle size determines the location of deposition in the respiratory tract. Particles with median aerodynamic diameters less than 10 μm are considered respirable. Larger particles typically impact in the nasopharyngeal region. Particles 2.5 to 6 μm preferentially deposit in the bronchial tree, whereas particles less than 2.5 μm deposit predominantly in the alveoli.[24] Ultrafine particles less than 0.1 μm may deposit throughout the lungs and owing to their greater surface area may result in greater toxicity.[25] Approximately 60% of particles deposited in the conducting airways are cleared from the lung by the mucociliary escalator within 24 hours, whereas only 25% of particles deposited in the bronchiolar region are cleared within this time.[26] In patients without emphysema, smoking alters particle retention, resulting in decreased residence time of deposited particles within the lung and decrease in airway particle burden without altering parenchymal particle burden.[27,28] Particles deposited in the alveolar region may be phagocytized and carried to the regional lymph nodes.

Lung toxicity also may manifest through an immunologic mechanism. Asthma and hypersensitivity pneumonitis are classic examples. High-molecular-weight compounds, such as animal dander or excreta, may elicit a direct immune response, whereas low-molecular-weight compounds (molecular weight <100 d), such as phthalic anhydride and diisocyanates, can complex with proteins, which then elicit an immune response.[29] Exposure to some chemicals, including those in air pollution, may affect immune reactivity through alteration of the response to inhalation of other substances.[30] Certain pharmaceutical agents, such as bleomycin, β-sympathomimetics, amphotericin, and nitrofurantoin, also may induce lung toxicity through release of inflammatory mediators from macrophages,[31] complex activation, direct activation of neutrophils, or immune complex deposition.[21]

TOXIC EFFECTS

The lung may respond to toxic insults with a variety of clinical presentations, including ALI and its more severe form ARDS, inhalation fever, RADS and asthma, noncardiac pulmonary edema, COP, pulmonary vascular disease, pulmonary fibrosis, pleural effusions, and parenchymal hemorrhage. In addition, aspiration and smoke exposure may result in specific clinical presentations.

Acute Lung Injury

ALI is characterized by lung inflammation and increased alveolar-capillary permeability associated with a constellation of clinical, radiologic, and physiologic abnormalities not explained by cardiac dysfunction. ARDS is a more severe subset of ALI. Recommended criteria for ALI and ARDS are listed in Table 27-1. Development of ARDS is associated most often with sepsis, aspiration, primary pneumonia, and multiple trauma. Mortality from ARDS historically has been 10% to 90%.[32] Patients with sepsis or preexisting diseases, including chronic lung or liver disease, are at greater risk of death, as are patients developing multiple organ system failure.[33,34] In survivors, pulmonary function generally improves, although some patients continue to experience significant respiratory limitation.[35]

TABLE 27-1 Recommended Criteria for Acute Lung Injury and Adult Respiratory Distress Syndrome

Acute onset
Arterial partial pressure of oxygen/fraction of inspired oxygen (PaO_2/FiO_2)
    ratio
    ≤300 for ALI
    ≤200 for ARDS
Bilateral infiltrates seen on frontal chest radiograph
Pulmonary artery wedge pressure <18 mm Hg or absence of other
    evidence of left atrial hypertension

ALI, acute lung injury; ARDS, adult respiratory distress syndrome.
From Bernard GR, Artigas A, Brigham KL, et al: The American-European Consensus Conference on ARDS: Definitions, mechanisms, relevant outcomes, and clinical trial coordination. Am J Respir Crit Care Med 149:818–824, 1994.

In ALI and ARDS, lung permeability at the alveolar-capillary barrier increases, resulting in movement of fluid into the alveolar space. In addition, there is a reduction in surfactant production. A proinflammatory cytokine response results in migration of neutrophils into the alveolar space, with subsequent release of free radicals and proteolytic enzymes. Vascular injury within the lung may follow thrombus formation.[36,37] ALI and ARDS are common clinical end points to a variety of injurious exposures, including inhalation injury from chemical exposures, pneumonia, near-drowning, pulmonary contusion, and aspiration (Table 27-2). Lung injury also may occur as part of multisystem organ failure seen after sepsis, trauma, blood product transfusions, acute pancreatitis, and drug overdoses.[38] Pharmaceuticals such as tricyclic antidepressants causing severe cardiovascular toxicity are among the more common causes of overdose-induced ALI and ARDS.

Inhalation Fever

Exposure to a variety of agents, including metals, polymer combustion products, and bioaerosols (Table 27-3), may result in a clinical presentation characterized by fever and chills, often associated with chest discomfort, cough, myalgias, and headache. Common terms used to describe this condition include *metal fume fever, polymer fume fever*, and *humidifier fever*. The diagnosis is based on history and clinical findings. The condition is self-limiting, and tolerance may develop with repeated exposure, with the condition recurring after an exposure-free period; one common name of the illness is "Monday morning fever." Laboratory findings typically include a neutrophilic leukocytosis and airway neutrophilia.[39,40] Although the pathophysiology of inhalation fever is unclear, immunologic sensitization does not seem to play a role.[39] Increases in cytokines, including tumor necrosis factor-α, interleukin-6, and interleukin-8, may play a key role in modulating inflammation, including subsequent neutrophil migration and activation.[41–44]

During initial exposure, symptoms may not be present or may be limited to respiratory irritation and cough. The flulike symptoms occur 4 to 8 hours after exposure, with fever of 41°C. Symptoms typically resolve 24 to 48 hours after cessation of exposure. During the illness, pulmonary function, arterial blood gas, and chest radiograph findings usually are normal.[40] Inhalation fever generally does not require treatment other than termination of exposure and standard measures to reduce symptoms. Although inhalation fever usually is considered a benign, self-limited condition, at least one case report of progression to chronic obstructive pulmonary disease (COPD) with multiple episodes of inhalation fever after exposure to polytetrafluoroethylene has been published.[45]

In metal workers, exposure to welding, brazing, bronzing, or galvanizing may result in inhalation fever. These processes produce 0.1- to 1-μm particles that efficiently reach the alveoli. Exposure to zinc oxide is the most common cause of metal fume fever.[46] It is important to distinguish zinc oxide from zinc chloride, exposure to which may result in severe and persistent pulmonary damage.[47] For polymer fume fever, the most common exposure is to heated polytetrafluoroethylene (Teflon).[48] For bioaerosols, agents causing hypersensitivity pneumonitis also can cause inhalation fever. Exposure to molds, such as with moldy silage, are prominent examples.

TABLE 27-2 Agents Associated with Adult Respiratory Distress Syndrome

Drugs	Streptokinase[183]
Amiodarone[160,161]	Transretinoic acid[184]
Amitriptyline[162]	
Ampicillin[163]	**Chemicals**
Aprotinin[164]	Aluminum phosphide[185]
Aspirin[165]	Arsenic[186]
Bleomycin[166]	Carbofuran[187]
Cyclosporine[167]	Detergents[188]
Deferoxamine[168]	1,3-Dichloropropene[189]
Dextran 40[169]	Ethylene glycol (ingestion)[190,191]
Diphenhydramine[170]	Fluorocarbon resin[192]
Ethchlorvynol[171]	Hydrofluoric acid[193]
Gemcitabine[172]	Mercury vapor[194]
Heroin[173]	Nickel[195]
Ibuprofen[174]	Nitrogen dioxide[196]
Lidocaine[175]	Organophosphates[197]
Lithium[176]	Phenol-formaldehyde resin[198]
Methotrexate[177]	Phosgene (inhalation)[199]
3,4-Methylenedioxy-methamphthetamine (MDMA)[178]	Selenious acid[200]
	Sodium oleate[201]
Nitrofurantoin[179]	Sulfuric acid fume[202]
Propylthiouracil[180]	Toxic (denatured rapeseed) oil[203]
Quinine[181]	Welding on metal with a galvanized coating or containing zinc chloride or nickel[122]
Radiocontrast material (injectable)[182]	

TABLE 27-3 Agents Associated with Inhalation Fever

Metal Oxides	**Bioaerosol Mist/Organic Dusts**
Zinc[44]	Contaminated humidifiers[209–211]
Copper[204]	Textiles[212,213]
Magnesium[205]	Moldy silage, wood chips[214,215]
Other (antimony, cadmium, chromium, iron, mercury, tin)[206]	Animal confinement facilities[216]
Polymer Fume	Grain dust[4]
Polytetrafluoroethylene[207]	
Diisocyanates[208]	

TABLE 27-4 Original Diagnostic Criteria for Reactive Airways Dysfunction Syndrome

Absence of preexisting asthma
Onset of asthma-like symptoms within 24 hr after a single-exposure incident to an irritant gas, smoke, fume, or vapor present at high concentrations
Persistence of symptoms for at least 3 mo
A positive methacholine challenge test
Lack of other types of pulmonary disease that could explain the presentation

From Brooks SM, Weiss MA, Bernstein IL: Reactive airways dysfunction syndrome (RADS): Persistent asthma syndrome after high level irritant exposures. Chest 88:376–384, 1985.

Reactive Airways Dysfunction Syndrome

RADS is characterized by new-onset, nonspecific airway hyperresponsiveness after significant exposure to irritant compounds, such as ammonia, chlorine, sulfur dioxide, cleaning agents, smoke, and acid gases. The original diagnostic criteria for RADS are listed in Table 27-4. Subsequent suggested revisions of the definition of RADS include acceptance of more than one exposure and use of provocative tests other than methacholine challenge.[49]

The pathogenesis of RADS is not completely defined but is believed to include airway inflammation with epithelial cell damage, alterations in neuropeptides, microvascular leakage, and bronchial smooth muscle hyperresponsiveness.[50] Bronchial biopsy specimens of a patient with RADS after exposure to chlorine showed initial replacement of the respiratory epithelium by fibrohemorrhagic exudate, with gradual improvement in inflammation over 5 months.[51] Animal models of RADS have shown similar changes after

chlorine exposure.[52] Avoidance of exposure to chemicals at irritant concentrations is recommended. Because sensitization does not occur in RADS, subsequent low-dose exposures to these same chemicals may be tolerated. RADS may persist or resolve over time.

Noncardiogenic Pulmonary Edema

Noncardiogenic pulmonary edema is distinguished from cardiogenic pulmonary edema by measurement of pulmonary artery wedge pressure. Potential mechanisms include altered alveolar-capillary membrane permeability through direct toxic effect on respiratory epithelial or vascular endothelial cells, increased respiratory secretions such as after cholinergic poisoning, and altered neurogenic tone.[53,54] High-altitude pulmonary edema may occur through increased capillary pressure.[55] Although decreased vascular osmotic pressure secondary to hypoalbuminemic states theoretically could result in increased movement of fluid into the alveolar space, this potential mechanism does not seem to be an important clinical cause of pulmonary edema. Agents such as narcotics and tocolytics are some of the more common causes of this condition (Table 27-5), and complement activation may play a role in its pathophysiology.[56]

Typically, pulmonary edema occurs within a few hours of use of an agent in patients with depressed respiration. Cocaine use also can result in noncardiogenic pulmonary edema by any route of administration. "Crack lung" may result from smoking crack cocaine or freebase cocaine and is characterized by alveolar infiltrates, hemoptysis, fever, and respiratory failure.[57] Aspirin may cause noncardiogenic pulmonary edema at toxic levels.[58,59] Risk factors for salicylate-induced noncardiogenic pulmonary edema in adults include chronic ingestion, serum levels greater than 2.9 mmol/L (40 mg/dL),

TABLE 27-5 Agents Associated with Noncardiac Pulmonary Edema

Drugs		Other
Amphetamine[217]	Mitomycin C[241]	Organphosphates/carbamates[260]
Amphotericin B[218]	Naloxone[242]	Paraquat[261]
Antivenom[219]	Nitrofurantoin[243]	Phosgene[262]
Aspirin[220]	Nitrosoureas[31]	Phosphine[263]
Chlordiazepoxide[221]	Nonsteroidal antiinflammatory drugs[244]	Polytetrafluoroethylene[264]
Cocaine[222]	Phenothiazines[245]	Sodium azide[265]
Colchicine[223]	Propoxyphene[246]	Sulfur dioxide[266]
Contrast media[224]	Protamine[247]	Tear gas[267]
Cytosine arabinoside[225]	Sulfasalazine[248]	
Dextran 70[226]	Tocolytic agents[249]	**Other**
Diltiazem[227]	Transretinoic acid[225]	Aspiration[268]
Ethchlorvynol[228]	Tricyclic antidepressants[250]	Blood transfusion[269]
Gemcitabine[229]		Hepatic failure[270]
Haloperidol[230]	**Chemicals**	Infection[225]
Heroin[231,232]	Cadmium[251]	High altitude[271]
Hydrochlorothiazide[233,234]	Chlorine gas[252]	Meat tenderizer[272]
Interleukin-2[235]	Cyanide[253]	Near-drowning[273]
Ketamine[236]	Dimethyl sulfate[254]	Pregnancy[274]
Lidocaine[237]	Hydrocarbons[255]	Reexpansion pulmonary edema[275]
Methadone[238]	Hydrogen sulfide[256]	Scorpion venom[276]
Methamphetamine[239]	Nitric acid[257,258]	Shock[277]
Methotrexate[240]	Nitrogen dioxide[259]	Strenuous swimming/scuba diving[278]
		Tumor necrosis factor[279]

neurologic abnormalities, increased age, and smoking.[58] In advanced cases of pulmonary edema, hypoxia may result from the collection of fluid within the alveoli.

Cryptogenic Organizing Pneumonia

COP is predominantly a disease of the terminal and respiratory bronchioles. The term *cryptogenic organizing pneumonia* is synonymous with *bronchiolitis obliterans organizing pneumonia* and is used particularly for organizing pneumonias of idiopathic origin. In this disease, fibrinous connective tissue proliferates in the epithelial lining of the small conducting bronchioles and extends into the distal alveolar spaces. COP is contrasted with constrictive bronchiolitis that involves permanent constrictive narrowing or complete obstruction of the airway lumen. Although most cases of COP are idiopathic,[11] cases also are associated with acute inhalation exposures and drug or chemical reactions and may occur after viral and other respiratory infections.[60] COP is best diagnosed by obtaining high-resolution computed tomography (CT) scans of the chest. The lung typically shows bilateral areas of consolidation involving the subpleural and peribronchial regions, although findings in immunocompromised patients may vary (Fig. 27-1).[61]

COP may result from a variety of diseases and exposures (Table 27-6). The clinical presentation may include nonproductive cough, dyspnea, fever, sore throat, malaise, and weight loss.[11,62,63] Chest radiographic findings are variable and include unilateral or bilateral patchy consolidation in approximately 80% of patients and diffuse, small, linear or nodular opacities in less than 10% of patients (Fig. 27-2).[11] Histologic findings include granulation tissue filling the distal airspaces. The alveolar architecture is preserved, and extensive fibrosis or honeycombing is lacking (Fig. 27-3).[64] In bronchoalveolar lavage fluid, a neutrophilic infiltrate is common and may exceed 40% of inflammatory cells. Increased percentage of neutrophils may be associated with poor outcome.[63] Alveolar macrophages from patients with COP show increased gene expression of IL-8 and fibronectin

TABLE 27-6 Agents Associated with Cryptogenic Organizing Pneumonia	
Drugs	Methyl isocyanate[300]
Acebutolol[280]	Nitrogen dioxide[259]
Amiodarone[280]	Ozone[297,301]
Amphotericin B[281]	Phosgene[297,301]
Bleomycin[282]	Sulfur dioxide[297,301]
Carbamazepine[283]	Talc[302]
Cocaine[284]	Textile printing[303]
Cyclophosphamide[285]	Thionyl chloride[304]
Gold salts[286]	
Interferon beta-1a[287]	**Other**
L-tryptophan[288]	Bird droppings[63]
Methotrexate[289]	Connective tissue disorders
Minocycline[290]	Essential mixed cryoglobulinemia[305]
Nitrofurantoin[291]	Polymyositis and dermatomyositis[285,306]
Penicillamine[292]	Rheumatoid arthritis[307]
Phenytoin[293]	Sjögren's syndrome[306]
Sulfasalazine[294]	Systemic lupus erythematosus[308]
Sulfamethoxypyridazine[295]	Organ transplantation
Ticlopidine[296]	Chronic graft-versus-host disease[309]
	Heart-lung transplantation[310]
Chemicals	Infections
Ammonia[297]	Bacterial (e.g., *Legionella,*
Bromine[298]	*Mycoplasma*)[311]
Chlorine[297]	Viral (e.g., influenza, rhinovirus)[312]
Fly ash[299]	Radiation[313]
Hydrogen fluoride[299]	Idiopathic[142,314]
Hydrogen sulfide[297]	

compared with controls.[65] Generally, COP responds well to steroid therapy, with return to premorbid function,[64] although relapses may occur in more than 50% of patients.[66] The mortality rate from progressive disease for COP is in the range of 4%, although much higher rates have occurred with rapidly progressive disease.[11,63] Pulmonary fibrosis may occur in greater than 10% of affected individuals.[67]

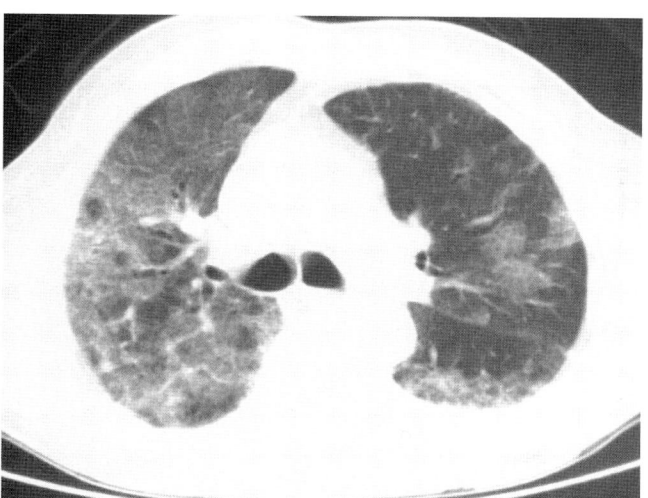

FIGURE 27-1

Cryptogenic organizing pneumonia (also known as *bronchiolitis obliterans–organizing pneumonia*). High-resolution computed tomography section through the midlung shows peripheral airspace consolidation.

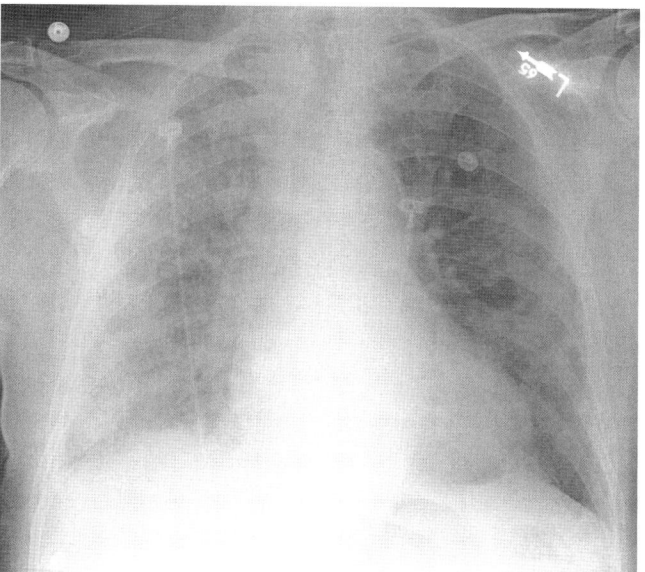

FIGURE 27-2

Cryptogenic organizing pneumonia. Frontal chest film shows extensive patchy consolidation, particularly in the right lung.

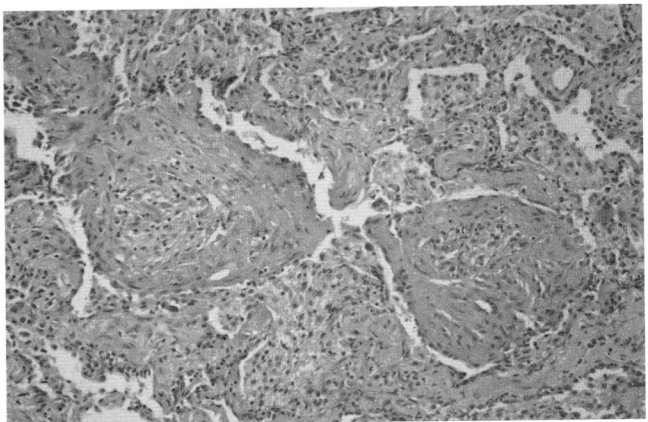

FIGURE 27-3

Cryptogenic organizing pneumonia. This high-power photomicrograph shows two nodules of young connective tissue (Masson bodies) in alveoli. Surrounding lung shows chronic inflammation. *(Courtesy of Richard Sobonya, MD, University of Arizona.)* See Color Fig. 27-3.

Vasculitis

Illicit drugs, or their diluents or contaminants, given intravenously may elicit an inflammatory response in the lung. Agents associated with pulmonary vascular disease are listed in Table 27-7. Drugs are associated with the development of systemic lupus erythematosus (SLE) in an estimated 5% to 12% of cases, and 80% of cases of drug-induced SLE involve the lungs and pleura.[68] This disease may present as pleural effusion, pleuritic chest pain, pneumonitis/alveolar infiltrates, or a combination of findings. Most cases of drug-induced SLE are caused by hydralazine and phenytoin.[69]

Forms of vasculitis in the lung also involving the kidney include Goodpasture's syndrome and Wegener's granulomatosis. Anti–glomerular basement membrane autoantibodies are generated in Goodpasture's syndrome, leading to pulmonary hemorrhage and glomerulonephritis. Goodpasture's syndrome may appear at any age, and symptoms typically include cough, shortness of breath, and hemoptysis. Pulmonary hemorrhage may vary from mild to life-threatening. Renal disease also may vary from mild to rapidly progressive renal failure.[70] Goodpasture's syndrome has been associated with D-penicillamine therapy and less frequently with a variety of inhaled and ingested solvents, hard metal dust, and crack cocaine.[71–78]

Wegener's granulomatosis commonly involves the upper and the lower respiratory tracts and the kidneys and may extend to other organs. Upper airway involvement may include the nose, sinuses, pharynx, and trachea, manifested as epistaxis, nasoseptal perforation, nasal congestion and pain, mucosal ulcers, and stenosis of the trachea. Endobronchial lesions commonly are present. Lower airway involvement occurs in approximately 85% of patients, and glomerulonephritis occurs in approximately 80%.[79] Histologically, Wegener's granulomatosis is characterized by a necrotizing vasculitis involving arterioles, venules, and capillaries (Fig. 27-4).[80] Symptoms may vary with the site of vasculitis and can include dyspnea and wheezing with stenosis of large airways. Parenchymal involvement can manifest with cough, dyspnea, and hemoptysis.[79] Wegener's granulomatosis has been associated with exposure to propylthiouracil, and renal carcinoma may trigger its development.[81,82] In addition, occupational exposure to pesticides and fumes or particulate materials and residential exposure to particulate materials from construction have been associated with development of Wegener's granulomatosis.[83,84]

Pulmonary Fibrosis

Pulmonary fibrosis predominantly involves the alveolar walls and interstitium and may occur as a result of many diseases and exposures (Table 27-8). Symptoms include progressive cough, dyspnea on exertion, fatigue, and malaise. There are a variety of forms of pulmonary fibrosis, including but not limited to acute interstitial pneumonitis, desquamative interstitial pneumonia, idiopathic pulmonary fibrosis (IPF), lymphoid interstitial pneumonia, nonspecific interstitial pneumonia, and usual interstitial pneumonia.[85] Drug-induced pulmonary fibrosis may occur over 1 to 2 months, or an accelerated form may occur over days.

TABLE 27-7 Agents Associated with Pulmonary Vascular Disease

Drugs	
Cocaine[315]	Procainamide[327]
Corticosteroids[316]	Isoniazid[328]
Cromoglycate[317]	Phenytoin[329]
Dexfenfluramine[136]	Penicillamine[330]
Estrogen[318]	Streptomycin[331]
Heroin[319]	Sulfonamides[332]
Methadone[320]	Tetracycline[333]
Methylphenidate[321]	Estrogens[334]
Propylthiouracil[322]	
Radiation[323]	**Chemicals**
Drug-induced SLE	Particulate exposure[84]
Hydralazine[324]	Pesticides[335]
Griseofulvin[325]	Silica[83]
Paraaminosalicylic acid[326]	**Other**
	Renal carcinoma[82]

SLE, systemic lupus erythematosus.

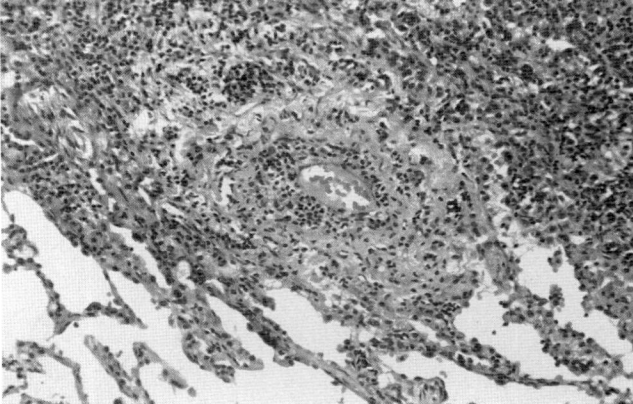

FIGURE 27-4

Wegener's granulomatosis. A small blood vessel shows infiltration by lymphocytes (vasculitis). Surrounding lung tissue shows chronic inflammation. *(Courtesy of Richard Sobonya, MD, University of Arizona.)* See Color Fig. 27-4.

TABLE 27-8 Agents Associated with Pulmonary Fibrosis

Drugs
Amiodarone[336]
Amphotericin B[337]
Azathioprine[338]
Bleomycin[339]
Busulfan[340]
Carbamazepine[86]
Chlorambucil[341]
Cocaine[342]
Cyclophosphamide[343]
Danazol[344]
Flecainide[345]
Gold[346]
Heroin[347]
Melphalan[348]
Mercaptopurine[349]
Methadone[350]
Methotrexate[351]
Methylphenidate[352]
Methysergide[353]
Mitomycin C[354]
Nitrofurantoin[355]
Nitrosoureas[356]
Penicillamine[357]
Peplomycin[358]
Phenytoin[359]
Sulfasalazine[294]
Tocainide[360]

Chemical
Aluminum dust[361]
Asbestosis[362]
Berylliosis[363]

Coal workers' pneumoconiosis[364]
Fiberglass[365]
Hard metal pneumoconiosis[366]
Hydrogen sulfide[367]
Mineral oil[368]
Mustard gas[369]
Oxygen toxicity[12]
Paraquat[370]
Radiation toxicity[371]
Radon[372]
Silicosis[373]

Other
Adult respiratory distress syndrome[374]
Ankylosing spondylitis[375]
Bronchiolitis obliterans organizing pneumonia[376]
Dermatomyositis/polymyositis[377]
Familial pulmonary fibrosis[378]
Fungal disease[379]
Hamman-Rich syndrome[380]
Hypersensitivity pneumonitis[381]
Idiopathic[382]
Mixed connective tissue disease[383]
Postviral[384]
Pulmonary hemosiderosis[385]
Rheumatoid arthritis[386]
Sarcoidosis[387]
Sjögren's syndrome[365]
Systemic lupus erythematosus[388]
Systemic sclerosis[389]
Thalassemia[390]

Bleomycin and amiodarone are common causes of drug-induced pulmonary fibrosis.[56] Acute interstitial pneumonitis may occur in children and adults and commonly may be associated with drug therapy.[86,87] IPF typically occurs in individuals 40 to 70 years old, and diagnostic criteria exclude known drug toxicity, collagen vascular disease, and environmental exposures. Potential risk factors for IPF include cigarette smoking; antidepressant drug ingestion; chronic aspiration; environmental exposures, including metal and wood dust; and various infectious agents, including Epstein-Barr virus.[85] In SLE, a fulminant, often fatal pneumonitis may develop with onset of tachypnea, dyspnea, fever, cough, and occasional hemoptysis.[88] A diffuse interstitial lung disease also may occur.[89] Patients with SLE who survive the acute pneumonitis often fail to return to their premorbid level of lung function.[88]

Crackles on chest auscultation and clubbing are common with IPF and other forms of pulmonary fibrosis. Pulmonary function studies typically show a restrictive pattern, and single-breath diffusion capacity of carbon monoxide is often one of the earliest abnormalities noted. Virtually all patients with IPF have abnormal chest radiographs. CT provides better definition of disease status. The erythrocyte sedimentation rate commonly is elevated in patients with IPF, and 10% to 20% have elevated antinuclear antibody or serum rheumatoid factor even without clearly established

rheumatologic disorders. Bronchoalveolar lavage and lung biopsy may help establish a specific diagnosis or prognosis, but their utility is limited. Neutrophil and eosinophil counts may be increased in bronchoalveolar lavage fluid of IPF patients, and elevations have been associated with more severe disease.[85]

Aspiration Syndromes

Aspiration may lead to either pneumonitis or pneumonia. Aspiration pneumonitis occurs from aspiration of sterile gastric contents and occurs most frequently in younger persons with a decreased level of consciousness, such as after drug overdose or with general anesthesia. Pulmonary injury occurs from the corrosive effects of stomach acids and the inflammatory effects of particulate material.[90] Risk factors for pneumonitis include large aspirate volume (>0.3 mL/kg body weight), particulate matter, bacterial contamination, and pH less than 2.5.[91] Initial lung injury due to the direct effects of low-pH media and particulate matter peaks at 1 hour after aspiration. This inflammation and cell death leads to the release of additional inflammatory mediators, including interleukin-8, cyclooxygenase and lipoxygenase products, and ROS.[92–94] Subsequent neutrophil response leads to release of proteolytic enzymes and exacerbated inflammatory response, peaking at 4 hours after aspiration.[95] Aspiration pneumonitis may resolve spontaneously or progress to infectious pneumonia or ALI including ARDS.

Aspiration pneumonia follows aspiration of oropharyngeal material, usually in elderly persons with dysphagia. Pulmonary injury occurs from infection with gram-positive cocci, gram-negative rods, and anaerobic bacteria.[90] Risk factors include anesthesia, decreased mental status, stroke, gastroesophageal reflux, dysphagia, feeding tube, diabetes, COPD, poor dentition, bacteria in saliva, and malnutrition.[5,90,96–99] Less acidic gastric contents may be more likely to lead to colonization of the upper gastrointestinal tract, although this has not been shown clearly to lead to pneumonia.[100,101] Patients with poor dental hygiene have higher concentrations of bacteria. In patients with chronic illness, bacteria may colonize the upper gastrointestinal tract. Topical antibiotic prophylaxis of oropharyngeal colonization has been shown to decrease the incidence of ventilator-associated pneumonia.[102] Aspiration pneumonia may progress without treatment or lead to lung abscess or emphysema.

Immunologic Pulmonary Syndromes

Idiosyncratic, hypersensitivity, or allergic reactions occur in approximately 5% of patients receiving any drug. Hypersensitivity reactions manifest with pulmonary infiltrates accompanied by cough, dyspnea, and fever, which resolve with withdrawal of the offending agent. Hypersensitivity reactions most typically occur with exposure to nitrofurantoin, ampicillin, bleomycin, carbamazepine, chlorpropamide, cromolyn, dantrolene, hydralazine, imipramine, isoniazid, methotrexate, methylphenidate, penicillin, phenytoin, procarbazine, sulfadimethoxine, and sulfasalazine, among others.[21,31] Pleural effusions also may occur as part of a hypersensitivity reaction, separately as a result of pleural hemorrhage, or associated with delayed hypersensitivity reactions or interstitial fibrosis. Pleural effusion may occur with exposure to dantrolene, busulfan, nitrofurantoin, and amiodarone, among others.[31] Methotrexate may cause a granulomatous pneumonitis.

Hypersensitivity pneumonitis results from repeat exposure and sensitization to a variety of antigens. A synonymous term is *extrinsic allergic alveolitis*; additional terms include *farmer's lung* and *bird fancier's lung*. A wide variety of exposures have been associated with development of hypersensitivity pneumonitis (Table 27-9). Microbial agents are the most common causes of hypersensitivity pneumonitis. Within bacterial causes, thermophilic actinomycetes are common, and exposure is associated with farmer's lung. Proteolytic enzymes from *Bacillus subtilis* may be found in detergent powders. Common fungal causes of hypersensitivity pneumonitis include *Aspergillus, Penicillium, Alternaria*, and *Cladosporium*. Within the diisocyanates, toluene diisocyanate, diphenylmethane diisocyanate, and hexamethylene diisocyanate have been identified as causing hypersensitivity pneumonitis.[103–105] Among pharmaceuticals, nitrofurantoin, phenytoin, carbamazepine, procarbazine, and methotrexate are well-known causes of hypersensitivity pneumonitis.[56]

Clinical presentation classically occurs 4 to 12 hours after exposure, with flulike symptoms similar to those following inhalation fever, including cough, dyspnea, fever, malaise, and myalgias. Wheezing also may be present. Physical examination findings may include tachycardia and rales.

TABLE 27-9 Agents Associated with Hypersensitivity Pneumonitis

Drugs
Acebutolol[391]
Bleomycin[392]
Carbamazepine[393]
Celiprolol[394]
Clozapine[395]
Cyclosporine[396]
Dextropropoxyphene[397]
Efavirenz[398]
Gold[399]
HMG-CoA reductase
 inhibitors[400]
Hydroxyurea[401]
Mesalamine[402]
Methotrexate[403]
Minocycline[404]
Nalidixic acid[405]
Nilutamide[406]
Nitrofurantoin[407]
Penicillamine[408]
Penicillin[409]
Perindopril[410]
Phenytoin[411]
Procarbazine[412]
Propranolol[413]
Sulfasalazine[414]
Trimethoprim[415]

Bacteria
Bacillus subtilis[416]
Contaminated hay[417]

Contaminated compost[418]
Mushroom compost[140]
Humidifiers/heated water
 reservoirs[419]
Metal working fluids[420]

Fungi
Moldy hay[417]
Humidifiers/heated water
 reservoirs[421]
Grain[39]
Cheese[422]
Moldy wood products[423]

Amebae

Animal Products
Bird droppings/feathers[424]
Mollusk shell[425]
Rodent urine[426]
Wheat weevil[427]

Chemicals
Cobalt[428]
Diisocyanates[103–105]
Pyrethrum[429]
Sodium diazobenzene sulfate[430]
Trimellitic anhydride[431]
Zinc[432]
Zirconium silicate[433]

HMG-CoA, 3-hydroxy-3-methylglutaryl-coenzyme A.

TABLE 27-10 Diagnostic Criteria for Hypersensitivity Pneumonitis

All of the following:
 History or documentation of exposure to offending antigens
 Symptoms of hypersensitivity pneumonitis occurring several hours after exposure
 Abnormal chest radiograph
 Exclusion of other diseases with similar clinical findings
At least two of the following:
 Basilar rales
 Decreased diffusion capacity
 Decreased oxygen saturation at rest or with exertion
 Histology consistent with hypersensitivity pneumonitis
 Reproducibility of symptoms with repeat exposure

From Terho EO: Work-related respiratory disorders among Finnish farmers. Am J Ind Med 18:269–272, 1990.

Diagnostic criteria for hypersensitivity pneumonitis are listed in Table 27-10. Hypersensitivity pneumonitis consists of a lymphocytic alveolitis and granulomatous pneumonitis (Fig. 27-5). Pulmonary macrophages in patients with hypersensitivity pneumonitis have been shown to produce greater concentrations of ROS and proinflammatory cytokines (macrophage inflammatory protein-1α and interleukin-8) than healthy controls.[106,107] Within 48 hours of exposure in a sensitized host, increased numbers of lung neutrophils can be shown by bronchoalveolar lavage,[108] with a change to 60% to 70% lymphocytes within several days.[109] T-cell lymphocytes predominate, and the CD4-to-CD8 ratio varies.[110] Bronchoalveolar lavage findings have not been shown to correlate with clinical disease, however. Viral infection may increase risk of hypersensitivity pneumonitis when there is a concomitant exposure to an offending antigen.[111]

Smoke Inhalation

Injury from smoke exposure varies with the source. Smoke may contain materials from pyrolysis, which is the thermal

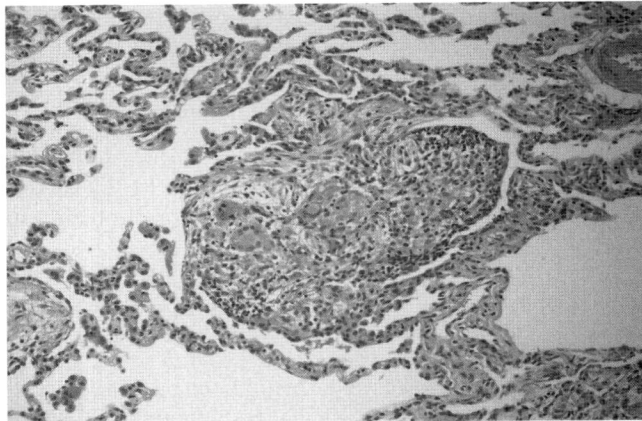

FIGURE 27-5

Hypersensitivity pneumonitis. A few poorly formed granulomas are present in the lung, associated with lymphocytic inflammation. *(Courtesy of Richard Sobonya, MD, University of Arizona.)* See Color Fig. 27-5.

degradation of a material, and combustion, which involves the oxidation of a material. Although thermal injury may occur, it is primarily a proximal finding and generally less important than chemical injury, secondary to the ability of the respiratory tract to remain at cooler temperatures through evaporation. Common toxic components of smoke, particularly wood smoke, include aldehydes, acid gases, particulates, and free radicals. Carbon monoxide and cyanide poisoning always must be considered in serious cases of smoke inhalation. Loss of consciousness from hypoxia, carbon monoxide, or cyanide or other volatile organics can lead to aspiration.[112]

The effects of smoke exposure depend on the dose, with large doses causing acute microvascular injury with pulmonary edema and slightly lower doses causing ARDS 48 to 96 hours after exposure.[113] The anatomic level of injury determines the time to clinical presentation. Upper airways injury occurs within a few hours and is often the result of thermal or chemical trauma. Tracheobronchial injury typically occurs within 12 hours and is most often the result of chemical exposure. Parenchymal injury usually is delayed ($\leq$24 hours) and is due primarily to chemical exposure. Within 3 days, asphyxia, upper airway obstruction, tracheobronchitis, pulmonary edema, pulmonary shunting, and atelectasis may occur. After approximately 3 days, pneumonia, ARDS, COPD, RADS, bronchiectasis, bronchiolitis obliterans, and pulmonary fibrosis may occur. Most individuals who survive smoke exposure make a full recovery, however.[112]

DIFFERENTIAL DIAGNOSIS

Nontoxic Causes

Infectious and autoimmune diseases are the most common causes of acute and chronic lung injury and must be considered in the differential diagnosis of any respiratory condition. Infectious pneumonias classically present with fever and leukocytosis, and history of exposure to toxicants is lacking. Autoimmune disorders often affect other organ systems as well. In certain instances, it may be difficult, however, to distinguish clinically between environmental and occupational lung diseases and diseases of nontoxic etiology. The granulomatous disease berylliosis commonly is misdiagnosed as sarcoidosis. These problems illustrate the necessity of obtaining a good occupational and environmental exposure history and a thorough medication history.

Toxic Causes

Several of the acute pulmonary syndromes described in this chapter may be difficult to distinguish. Although ALI and ARDS are diagnosed using specific criteria (see Table 27-1), these syndromes are common end points for a variety of pulmonary insults and could occur in combination with other acute toxic pulmonary syndromes. The differential diagnosis for inhalation fever includes hypersensitivity pneumonitis, chemical alveolitis, and viral syndrome. In contrast to patients with inhalation fever, patients with hypersensitivity pneumonitis and chemical alveolitis have abnormal chest radiographs, symptoms persist for weeks to months, and there is a risk of chronic respiratory

sequelae. The differential diagnosis for RADS includes occupational asthma, encompassing allergic response to agents such as the diisocyanates. Noncardiogenic pulmonary edema must be distinguished from cardiogenic pulmonary edema. The differential diagnosis for COP includes acute interstitial pneumonia and carcinoma of the lung.[114,115] Differential diagnoses for hypersensitivity pneumonitis include inhalation fever; granulomatous/immunologic diseases, including allergic bronchopulmonary aspergillosis, berylliosis, collagen vascular diseases, drug-induced pneumonitis, eosinophilic pneumonia, lymphomatoid granulomatosis, and sarcoidosis; infections, including viral pneumonias, mycoplasmal disease, fungal infections, and psittacosis; and fibrosing lung disease, including idiopathic pulmonary fibrosis, bronchiolitis obliterans, and pneumoconioses.

Medications

Within each of the toxic pulmonary syndromes, there is often little to diagnose toxic causes, other than the patient's history. Certain agents have particular characteristics, however, that may help to distinguish them. Nitrofurantoin is an antimicrobial agent with a high incidence of hypersensitivity reactions, which include hypersensitivity pneumonitis or pleural effusion or both. The pathophysiology may include development of autoantibodies to a nitrofurantoin-albumin complex and free radical production.[21,116] Although symptoms typically occur within 2 hours to 10 days after initiation of therapy, unusual cases may develop 1 year later. Typically, infiltrates resolve within 24 to 48 hours after cessation of therapy. Chronic reactions may occur, including interstitial fibrosis and desquamative interstitial pneumonitis. Amiodarone causes pulmonary toxicity in approximately 5% to 15% of patients, including interstitial and alveolar infiltrates, dyspnea, chest pain, and cough.[56] Although the exact mechanism of toxicity is not known, it causes phospholipidosis and associated vacuolization.[117] The relative susceptibility of the lung may be due to the preferential concentration of amiodarone in this organ.[118] Methysergide may cause pleural effusion acutely and may result in chronic pulmonary fibrosis.[119]

The pulmonary effects of antineoplastic drugs most commonly include interstitial pneumonitis and fibrosis (Fig. 27-6). Interstitial pneumonitis most often results from a hypersensitivity reaction and occurs sooner after drug initiation than does interstitial fibrosis. Clinical evaluation may reveal bibasilar fine crackles, infiltrates on chest x-ray or chest CT (Figs. 27-7 and 27-8), and reduced spirometry and diffusion capacity of carbon monoxide measurements. Definitive diagnosis may require lung biopsy to distinguish drug reaction from other causes, such as infection. Bleomycin produces ROS in association with iron in the lung.[120] Specific lung toxicity of bleomycin also is likely due to preferential distribution and decreased detoxification of bleomycin in the lung.[121]

Chemicals

Exposure to most metal fumes typically results in self-limited inhalation fever. Exposure to cadmium and mercury at high concentrations may cause more severe injury, however,

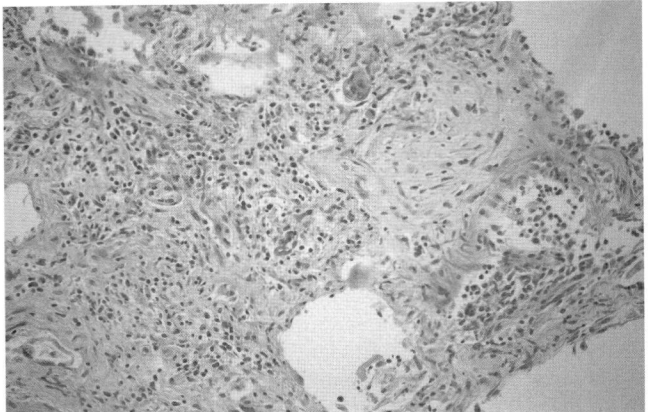

FIGURE 27-6

Interstitial fibrosis due to bleomycin. Nonspecific chronic inflammation and fibrosis with atypical reactive pneumocytes are present in the lung. *(Courtesy of Richard Sobonya, MD, University of Arizona.)* See Color Fig. 27-6.

including acute pneumonitis that can progress to ALI and ARDS.[122,123] Ingestion of paraquat, and in rare cases dermal exposure and potentially inhalation of paraquat, often causes progressive, fatal oxidative lung injury.[124] Hydrofluoric acid inhalation exposure can cause corrosive lung injury similar to other acids but also may cause systemic hypocalcemia.[125,126] Beryllium exposure at high concentrations can result in acute pneumonitis but more commonly causes berylliosis, a granulomatous lung disease. Along with history of exposure, a positive beryllium lymphocyte transformation test should help to establish the diagnosis.[127]

Toxic oil syndrome occurred in Spain in 1981 as a result of ingestion of rapeseed oil denatured with 2% aniline. Although initially imported for industrial use, the product was refined and mixed with other oils before being sold by street vendors as olive oil for human consumption. Individuals

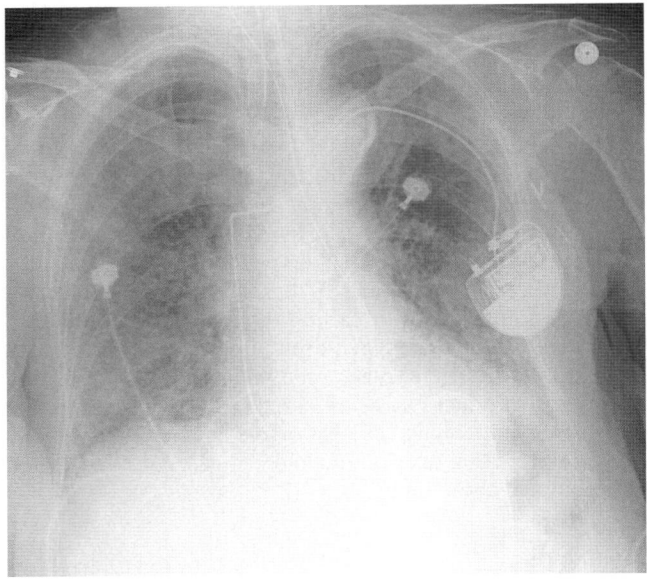

FIGURE 27-7

Pulmonary fibrosis. Frontal chest film of a patient treated with bleomycin shows reticular pattern, particularly at the lung bases.

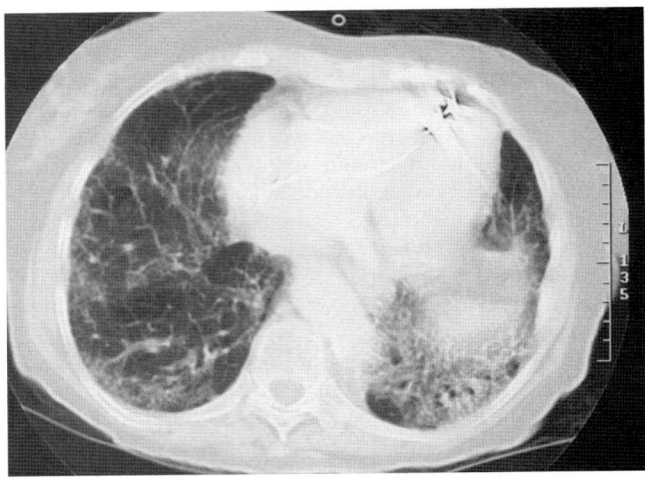

FIGURE 27-8

Pulmonary fibrosis. Computed tomography section through the lower lungs of a patient treated with bleomycin shows extensive reticular opacities, particularly in the periphery, typical of interstitial fibrosis.

having ingested the oil developed cough, pain, chest tightness, dyspnea, malaise, anorexia, headache, tissue edema, pruritus, and arthralgia. Deaths in the first 2 months after ingestion generally were due to respiratory failure from noncardiogenic edema.[128] The agents responsible were believed to be fatty acid anilides, in particular oleyl anilide.[129] The mechanism of toxicity was endothelial cell injury, most likely due to oxidative stress, with subsequent macrophage and T-cell activation.[130] This mechanism is believed to be similar to that present in eosinophilia-myalgia syndrome associated with L-tryptophan ingestion.[131]

Ingestion of toxic oil and L-tryptophan has been associated with development of pulmonary hypertension.[132,133] Although this disease has been associated with many pharmaceutical agents, including oral contraceptives,[134] it is best known for its association with appetite-suppressant agents, including fenfluramine, dexfenfluramine, and aminorex, all of which have been removed from the market in most countries. Pulmonary hypertension associated with use of these agents is indistinguishable clinically and histologically from primary pulmonary hypertension, including the findings of monoclonal pulmonary endothelial cell proliferation leading to plexiform pulmonary arteriopathy.[135] The clinical presentation of drug-induced pulmonary hypertension consistently includes fatigue and progressive dyspnea and may include syncope or near-syncope, chest pain, peripheral edema associated with right ventricular hypertrophy or failure, and tricuspid valve regurgitation or pulmonic insufficiency.[136,137] The rarity of this condition in exposed individuals suggests that there may be a strong component of genetic susceptibility in the development of this condition, possibly associated in part with nitric oxide deficiency.[137]

Biologics

Exposure to infectious agents is likely to cause pneumonia, in which case differential diagnosis is assisted by evaluation and culture of induced sputum. Inhaled toxins can elicit allergic reactions, such as in asthma or hypersensitivity pneumonitis, and antibody testing may help to confirm exposure. Direct toxic effects also may occur, such as with exposure to metal working fluids.

DIAGNOSIS

Assays

Arterial blood gas and oximetry measurements are essential guides to clinical care to optimize fraction of inspired oxygen and ventilator settings and oxygenate the patient adequately while minimizing oxygen toxicity. Sputum induction is used for collecting phlegm samples for identification of infectious organisms. Bronchoalveolar lavage may be used to diagnose infection and malignancies and to assess inflammatory conditions. Although the findings may not be pathognomonic, they are often helpful in supporting a diagnosis. White blood cell count and differential may help to distinguish infectious and toxicant-related pneumonias.

For hypersensitivity pneumonitis, hematology laboratory abnormalities may include leukocytosis with neutrophilia, mild elevation in erythrocyte sedimentation rate, and C-reactive protein. Serum precipitins may help to document immunologic response to an offending antigen, but sensitization may occur without disease, and false-negative tests also are problematic. Circulating antibodies directed against cytoplasmic components of neutrophils and monocytes (ANCA) typically are found in small vessel vasculitis, such as Wegener's granulomatosis. Specifically, antibodies with a cytoplasmic pattern on immunofluorescence (cANCA, specific for proteinase 3) are detected in approximately 90% of patients with untreated Wegener's granulomatosis and are detected in a few patients with microscopic polyangiitis and Churg-Strauss syndrome.[138,139] Antibodies with a perinuclear pattern (pANCA, specific for myeloperoxidase) also are present in most patients with microscopic polyangiitis, Churg-Strauss syndrome, and pauci-immune glomerulonephritis, but occur less commonly in Wegener's granulomatosis.[139]

Pulmonary Function Testing

Spirometry testing usually is normal in inhalation fever but may show a restrictive pattern in cases of hypersensitivity pneumonitis and fibrosis.[42,140,141] With RADS, spirometry testing may be normal or show reversible obstructive findings.[10] With bronchiolitis, obstructive, restrictive, or mixed patterns may be present.[62,142] Diffusion capacity testing likewise generally is normal in inhalation fever but decreased with hypersensitivity pneumonitis and fibrosis.[140,141]

Radiologic Imaging

The standard chest radiograph is the initial diagnostic test of choice for acute toxic pulmonary syndromes. Although the chest radiograph is abnormal in most of the lung diseases previously described with the exception of inhalation fever and RADS, there is often sufficient overlap in diagnostic findings to render differential diagnosis difficult. Toxic pneumonitis tends to have a diffuse pattern (Fig. 27-9). Chest radiographs often are normal in hypersensitivity pneumoni-

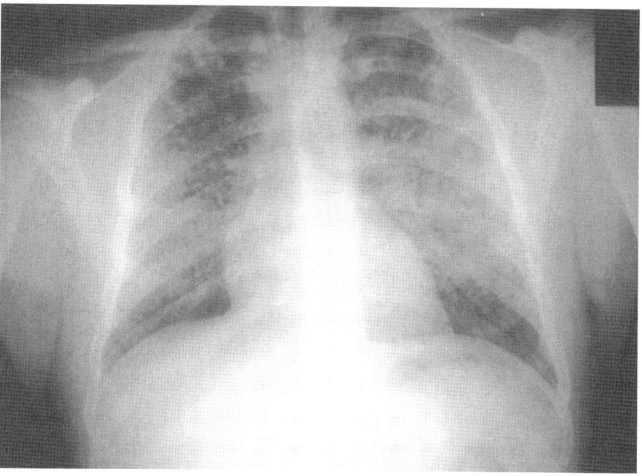

FIGURE 27-9

Toxic pneumonitis. Frontal chest film of a patient exposed to nitrogen dioxide shows extensive bilateral pulmonary consolidation in the periphery typical of capillary leak edema.

tis, although abnormalities can occur with acute or chronic disease (Fig. 27-10).[143,144]

Chest CT is indicated for further definition of abnormalities noted on chest radiographs. For diagnosis of disease not visible on chest radiograph, high-resolution chest CT is recommended, using 1.0- to 1.5-mm thin section cuts. High-resolution CT of the chest can provide more definitive information, particularly for the diagnosis of COP, pulmonary fibrosis, and hypersensitivity pneumonitis. On high-resolution chest CT of patients with hypersensitivity pneumonitis, a ground-glass appearance often is seen (Fig. 27-11).[145]

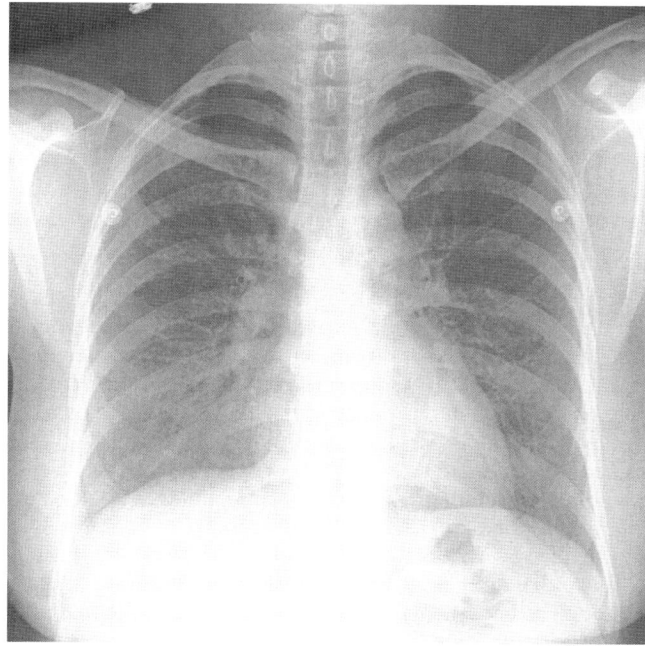

FIGURE 27-10

Hypersensitivity pneumonitis. Posteroanterior chest radiograph shows diffuse ground-glass density throughout both lungs.

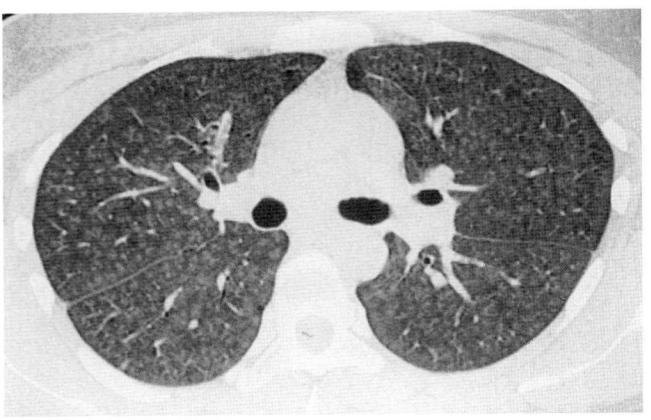

FIGURE 27-11

Hypersensitivity pneumonitis. High-resolution computed tomography of the midlungs shows diffuse nodular densities throughout in a centrilobular distribution.

More advanced imaging, such as with angiography, nuclear imaging, and ultrasonography, may be helpful for particular indications. CT angiography with rapid or spiral CT or ventilation (using ^{133}xenon gas) and perfusion (commonly using ^{99m}Tc) studies are indicated for evaluation of potential pulmonary embolus. Pulmonary angiography is used most commonly to confirm the diagnosis of pulmonary embolus and to evaluate arteriovenous malformations, aneurysms, and hemoptysis.

Biopsy

Biopsy may be necessary for establishing a definitive diagnosis, particularly in cases of bronchiolitis obliterans and pulmonary fibrosis. Transbronchial biopsy specimens often are of limited utility, whereas open-lung biopsy specimens or biopsy specimens using video-assisted thoracic surgery provide more definitive results. One exception may be COP; at least one report has been published of diagnostic results by transbronchial biopsy, whereas open-lung biopsy results were negative.[146]

TREATMENT

Treatment for ALI and ARDS is supportive. Studies have suggested that standard mechanical ventilation may worsen lung injury and that lowering tidal volume and increased positive end-expiratory pressure may decrease lung inflammation and lower mortality.[15,147] Steroid therapy has not proved beneficial early in the course of ARDS.[148] Later treatment with steroids has shown benefit, however, in reducing mortality in patients not responding to standard supportive therapy.[149] Inhaled bronchodilators can be used for acute exacerbations.

For inhalation fever, no specific treatment is necessary, although removal from exposure and symptomatic management are preferred. Treatment for RADS involves cessation of irritant exposures exacerbating the patient's clinical course and use of inhaled bronchodilators and steroids as necessary. Treatment for noncardiogenic pulmonary edema

is supportive. Most cases of COP respond to treatment with prednisone. Patients with consolidation may respond better to corticosteroid treatment than patients with reticulonodular infiltrates. A subset of patients with rapidly progressive COP may have much higher mortality despite treatment with prednisone or other immunosuppressive therapy.[150] Steroid therapy may be helpful in progressive pulmonary fibrosis, although response is not uniform.[141] For hypersensitivity pneumonitis, steroid treatment usually is reserved for cases not responding to the cessation of the inciting exposure.[151] Although the disease may progress to fibrosis with continued exposure, removal of the offending antigen usually leads to complete recovery. For smoke inhalation injury, systemic steroid therapy has not been shown to improve patient outcome.[152]

Wegener's granulomatosis usually responds to therapy with cyclophosphamide and glucocorticoids.[153] Maintenance therapy includes methotrexate, which seems superior to trimethoprim-sulfamethoxazole prophylaxis.[154,155] For Goodpasture's syndrome, oral cyclophosphamide and high-dose corticosteroids are used together with plasmapheresis.[156] Prednisone is generally the first choice for therapy of pulmonary fibrosis, although clear efficacy has not been proved, with other immunosuppressive therapy reserved for steroid failure.[141]

After witnessed aspiration, the upper airway should be suctioned, and endotracheal intubation should be considered for patients unable to maintain their airway. Prophylactic antibiotic treatment need not be administered, unless colonization of the gastric contents is suspected.[90] Antibiotics are not indicated routinely for infiltrates detected by chest radiograph, unless pneumonitis fails to improve within 48 hours. Antibiotic choice should be broad spectrum, such as levofloxacin or ceftriaxone. Culture of specimens obtained from the lower respiratory tract may help select more targeted antibiotic therapy.[90] In drug-overdose patients with aspiration pneumonitis, corticosteroid therapy improved blood gas measurements, infiltrates on chest radiographs improved more rapidly, and duration of ventilation and length of stay in the intensive care unit were reduced.[157] In addition, steroid therapy resulted in long-term improvement in pulmonary function tests compared with patients with aspiration pneumonitis not treated with steroids.[158] For aspiration pneumonia, coverage should be provided against gram-negative organisms. Suitable choices include third-generation cephalosporins, fluoroquinolones, and piperacillin.[90] Coverage for oral anaerobes is not indicated routinely.[159] If infection with *Pseudomonas aeruginosa* is suspected or documented, two antimicrobials active against *Pseudomonas* are recommended.

REFERENCES

1. Sallie B, McDonald C: Inhalation accidents reported to the SWORD surveillance project 1990–1993. Ann Occup Hyg 40:211–221, 1996.
2. Luhr OR, Antonsen K, Karlsson M, et al: Incidence and mortality after acute respiratory failure and acute respiratory distress syndrome in Sweden, Denmark, and Iceland. The ARF Study Group. Am J Respir Crit Care Med 159:1849–1861, 1999.
3. Ross DS: Welders' metal fume fever. J Soc Occup Med 24:125–129, 1974.
4. Manfreda J, Holford-Strevens V, Cheang M, Warren CP: Acute symptoms following exposure to grain dust in farming. Environ Health Perspect 66:73–80, 1986.

5. Cogen R, Weinryb J: Aspiration pneumonia in nursing home patients fed via gastrostomy tubes. Am J Gastroenterol 84:1509–1512, 1989.
6. Terho EO: Work-related respiratory disorders among Finnish farmers. Am J Ind Med 18:269–272, 1990.
7. Ramazzini B: Diseases of Workers. [Translated by Cave WC.] New York Academy of Medicine/History of Medicine Series, no. 23. New York, 1964, Hafner.
8. Smart JK: History of chemical and biological warfare: An American perspective. In Sidell FR, Takafuji ET, Franz DR (eds): Medical Aspects of Chemical and Biological Warfare. Office of the Surgeon General, United States Army, 1997, Washington, DC, pp 9–86.
9. Naik SR, Acharya VN, Bhalerao RA, et al: Medical survey of methyl isocyanate gas affected population of Bhopal: Part II. Pulmonary effects in Bhopal victims as seen 15 weeks after M.I.C. exposure. J Postgrad Med 32:185–191, 1986.
10. Brooks SM, Weiss MA, Bernstein IL: Reactive airways dysfunction syndrome (RADS): Persistent asthma syndrome after high level irritant exposures. Chest 88:376–384, 1985.
11. Epler GR, Colby TV, McLoud TC, et al: Bronchiolitis obliterans organizing pneumonia. N Engl J Med 312:152–158, 1985.
12. Karsner HT: The pathological effects of atmospheres rich in oxygen. J Exp Med 23:149, 1916.
13. Cope O: Care of the victims of the Cocoanut Grove fire at the Massachusetts General Hospital. N Engl J Med 229:138, 1943.
14. Ashbaugh DG, Bigelow DB, Petty TL, Levine BE: Acute respiratory distress in adults. Lancet 2:319–323, 1967.
15. Ventilation with lower tidal volumes as compared with traditional tidal volumes for acute lung injury and the acute respiratory distress syndrome. The Acute Respiratory Distress Syndrome Network. N Engl J Med 342:1301–1308, 2000.
16. Brochard L, Roudot-Thoraval F, Roupie E, et al: Tidal volume reduction for prevention of ventilator-induced lung injury in acute respiratory distress syndrome. The Multicenter Trial Group on Tidal Volume Reduction in ARDS. Am J Respir Crit Care Med 158:1831–1838, 1998.
17. Freeman BA, Crapo JD: Biology of disease: Free radicals and tissue injury. Lab Invest 47:412–426, 1982.
18. Chabot F, Mitchell JA, Gutteridge JM, Evans TW: Reactive oxygen species in acute lung injury. Eur Respir J 11:745–757, 1998.
19. Vallyathan V, Shi X: The role of oxygen free radicals in occupational and environmental lung diseases. Environ Health Perspect 105(Suppl 1):165–177, 1997.
20. Lewis RA, Austin KF: The biologically active leukotrienes: Biosynthesis, metabolism, receptors, functions and pharmacology. J Clin Invest 73:889–897, 1984.
21. Cooper JAD, White DA, Matthay RA: Drug-induced pulmonary disease: Part 2. Noncytotoxic drugs. Am Rev Respir Dis 133:488–505, 1986.
22. Jones AT, Jones RC, Longley EO: Environmental and clinical aspects of bulk wheat fumigation with aluminum phosphide. Am Ind Hyg Assoc J 25:376–379, 1964.
23. Schoonbroodt D, Guffens P, Jousten P, et al: Acute phosphine poisoning? A case report and review. Acta Clin Belg 47:280–284, 1992.
24. Pritchard JN: The influence of lung deposition on clinical response. J Aerosol Med 14:S19–26, 2001.
25. Churg A, Brauer M: Ambient atmospheric particles in the airways of human lungs. Ultrastruct Pathol 24:353–361, 2000.
26. Falk R, Philipson K, Svartengren M, et al: Assessment of long-term bronchiolar clearance of particles from measurements of lung retention and theoretical estimates of regional deposition. Exp Lung Res 25:495–516, 1999.
27. Agnew JE, Pavia D, Clarke SW: Factors affecting the 'alveolar deposition' of 5 microns inhaled particles in healthy subjects. Clin Phys Physiol Meas 6:27–36, 1985.
28. Churg A, Wright JL, Stevens B, Wiggs B: Mineral particles in the human bronchial mucosa and lung parenchyma: II. Cigarette smokers without emphysema. Exp Lung Res 18:687–714, 1992.
29. Chan-Yeung M: Occupational asthma. Chest 98:148–161, 1990.
30. D'Amato G: Outdoor air pollution in urban areas and allergic respiratory diseases. Monaldi Arch Chest Dis 54:470–474, 1999.
31. Cooper JAD, White DA, Matthay RA: Drug-induced pulmonary disease: Part 1. Cytotoxic drugs. Am Rev Respir Dis 133:321–340, 1986.
32. Bernard GR, Artigas A, Brigham KL, et al: The American-European Consensus Conference on ARDS: Definitions, mechanisms, relevant outcomes, and clinical trial coordination. Am J Respir Crit Care Med 149:818–824, 1994.
33. Fowler AA, Hamman RF, Good JT, et al: Adult respiratory distress syndrome: Risk with common predispositions. Ann Intern Med 98:593–597, 1983.
34. Montgomery AB, Stager MA, Carrico CJ, Hudson LD: Causes of mortality in patients with the adult respiratory distress syndrome. Am Rev Respir Dis 132:485–489, 1985.
35. Ghio AJ, Elliott CG, Crapo RO, et al: Impairment after adult respiratory distress syndrome: An evaluation based on American Thoracic Society recommendations. Am Rev Respir Dis 139:1158–1162, 1989.
36. Ware LB, Matthay MA: The acute respiratory distress syndrome. N Engl J Med 342:1334–1349, 2000.
37. Wyncoll DL, Evans TW: Acute respiratory distress syndrome. Lancet 354:497–501, 1999.
38. Baudouin SV, Howdle P, O'Grady JG, Webster NR: Acute lung injury in fulminant hepatic failure following paracetamol poisoning. Thorax 50:399–402, 1995.
39. Rask-Andersen A: Organic dust toxic syndrome among farmers. Br J Ind Med 46:233–238, 1989.
40. Blanc P, Boushey HA: The lung in metal fume fever. Semin Respir Med 14:212–225, 1993.
41. Fine JM, Gordon T, Chen LC, et al: Metal fume fever: Characterization of clinical and plasma IL-6 responses in controlled human exposures to zinc oxide fume at and below the threshold limit value. J Occup Environ Med 39:722–726, 1997.
42. Blanc P, Wong H, Bernstein MS, Boushey HA: An experimental human model of metal fume fever. Ann Intern Med 114:930–936, 1991.
43. Kuschner WG, D'Alessandro A, Wong H, Blanc PD: Early pulmonary cytokine responses to zinc oxide fume inhalation. Environ Res 75:7–11, 1997.
44. Kuschner WG, D'Alessandro A, Wintermeyer SF, et al: Pulmonary responses to purified zinc oxide fume. J Invest Med 43:371–378, 1995.
45. Kales SN, Christiani DC: Progression of chronic obstructive pulmonary disease after multiple episodes of an occupational inhalation fever. J Occup Med 36:75–78, 1994.
46. Mueller EJ, Seger DL: Metal fume fever: A review. J Emerg Med 2:271–274, 1985.
47. Pettila V, Takkunen O, Tukiainen P: Zinc chloride smoke inhalation: A rare cause of severe acute respiratory distress syndrome. Intensive Care Med 26:215–217, 2000.
48. Lewis CE, Kirby GR: An epidemic of polymer fume fever. JAMA 191:103–106, 1965.
49. Demeter SL, Cordasco EM, MacIntyre W, et al: Quantitation of abnormal 67Ga uptake in pulmonary interstitial vascular disease—a new test to detect diffuse lung disease. Angiology 41:1023–1028, 1990.
50. Alberts WM, Brooks SM: Reactive airways dysfunction syndrome. Curr Opin Pulm Med 2:104–110, 1996.
51. Lemiere C, Malo JL, Boutet M: Reactive airways dysfunction syndrome due to chlorine: Sequential bronchial biopsies and functional assessment. Eur Respir J 10:241–244, 1997.
52. Demnati R, Fraser R, Ghezzo H, et al: Time-course of functional and pathological changes after a single high acute inhalation of chlorine in rats. Eur Respir J 11:922–928, 1998.
53. Karliner JS: Noncardiogenic forms of pulmonary edema. Circulation 46:212–215, 1972.
54. Li C, Miller WT, Jiang J: Pulmonary edema due to ingestion of organophosphate insecticide. AJR Am J Roentgenol 152:265–266, 1989.
55. Scherrer U, Sartori C, Lepori M, et al: High-altitude pulmonary edema: From exaggerated pulmonary hypertension to a defect in transepithelial sodium transport. Adv Exp Med Biol 474:93–107, 1999.
56. Cooper JAD, Zitnik RJ, Matthay RA: Mechanisms of drug-induced pulmonary disease. Ann Rev Med 39:395–404, 1988.
57. Forrester JM, Steele AW, Waldron JA, Parsons PE: Crack lung: an acute pulmonary syndrome with a spectrum of clinical and histopathologic findings. Am Rev Respir Dis 142:462–467, 1990.
58. Heffner JE, Sahn SA: Salicylate-induced pulmonary edema: Clinical features and prognosis. Ann Intern Med 95:405–409, 1981.
59. Fisher CJ Jr, Albertson TE, Foulke GE: Salicylate-induced pulmonary edema: Clinical characteristics in children. Am J Emerg Med 3:33–37, 1985.
60. King TE Jr: Overview of bronchiolitis. Clin Chest Med 14:607–610, 1993.
61. Lee KS, Kullnig P, Hartman TE, Muller NL: Cryptogenic organizing pneumonia: CT findings in 43 patients. AJR Am J Roentgenol 162:543–546, 1994.

62. Alasaly K, Muller N, Ostrow DN, et al: Cryptogenic organizing pneumonia: A report of 25 cases and a review of the literature. Medicine 74:201–211, 1995.

63. Cohen AJ, King TE Jr, Downey GP: Rapidly progressive bronchiolitis obliterans with organizing pneumonia. Am J Respir Crit Care Med 149:1670–1675, 1994.

64. Epler GR: Bronchiolitis obliterans organizing pneumonia. Arch Intern Med 161:158–164, 2001.

65. Carre PC, King TE, Mortensen R, Riches DW: Cryptogenic organizing pneumonia: Increased expression of interleukin-8 and fibronectin genes by alveolar macrophages. Am J Respir Cell Mol Biol 10:100–105, 1994.

66. Lazor R, Vandevenne A, Pelletier A, et al: Cryptogenic organizing pneumonia: Characteristics of relapses in a series of 48 patients. Am J Respir Crit Care Med 162:571–577, 2000.

67. Yousem SA, Lohr RH, Colby TV: Idiopathic bronchiolitis obliterans organizing pneumonia/cryptogenic organizing pneumonia with unfavorable outcome: Pathologic predictors. Mod Pathol 10:864–871, 1997.

68. Dweik RA, Ahmad M, Demeter SL: Drug induced pulmonary disease. In Baum GL, Crapo BR, Karlinsky JB (eds): Textbook of Pulmonary Diseases. Philadelphia, 1998, Lippincott-Raven, pp 477–490.

69. Stratton MA: Drug-induced systemic lupus erythematosus. Clin Pharmacol 4:657–663, 1985.

70. Young KR Jr: Pulmonary-renal syndromes. Clin Chest Med 10:655–675, 1989.

71. Peces R, Riera JR, Arboleya LR, et al: Goodpasture's syndrome in a patient receiving penicillamine and carbimazole. Nephron 45:316–320, 1987.

72. Bernis P, Hamels J, Quoidbach A, et al: Remission of Goodpasture's syndrome after withdrawal of an unusual toxic. Clin Nephrol 23:312–317, 1985.

73. Carlier B, Schroeder E, Mahieu P: A rapidly and spontaneously reversible Goodpasture's syndrome after carbon tetrachloride inhalation. Acta Clin Belg 35:193–198, 1980.

74. Nathan AW, Toseland PA: Goodpasture's syndrome and trichloroethane intoxication. Br J Clin Pharmacol 8:28406, 1979.

75. Gaskin G, Thompson EM, Pusey CD: Goodpasture-like syndrome associated with anti-myeloperoxidase antibodies following penicillamine treatment. Nephrol Dial Transplant 10:1925–1928, 1995.

76. Garcia-Rostan y Perez GM, Garcia Bragado F, Puras Gil AM: Pulmonary hemorrhage and antiglomerular basement membrane antibody-mediated glomerulonephritis after exposure to smoked cocaine (crack): A case report and review of the literature. Pathol Int 47:692–697, 1997.

77. Lauwerys R, Bernard A, Viau C, Buchet JP: Kidney disorders and hematotoxicity from organic solvent exposure. Scand J Work Environ Health 11(Suppl 1):83–90, 1985.

78. Lechleitner P, Defregger M, Lhotta K, et al: Goodpasture's syndrome: Unusual presentation after exposure to hard metal dust. Chest 103:956–957, 1993.

79. Langford CA, Hoffman GS: Rare diseases: 3. Wegener's granulomatosis. Thorax 54:629–637, 1999.

80. Travis WD, Hoffman GS, Leavitt RY, et al: Surgical pathology of the lung in Wegener's granulomatosis: Review of 87 open lung biopsies from 67 patients. Am J Surg Pathol 15:315–333, 1991.

81. Pillinger M, Staud R: Wegener's granulomatosis in a patient receiving propylthiouracil for Graves' disease. Semin Arthritis Rheum 28:124–129, 1998.

82. Tatsis E, Reinhold-Keller E, Steindorf K, et al: Wegener's granulomatosis associated with renal cell carcinoma. Arthritis Rheum 42:751–756, 1999.

83. Nuyts GD, Van Vlem E, De Vos A, et al: Wegener granulomatosis is associated to exposure to silicon compounds: a case-control study. Nephrol Dial Transplant 10:1162–1165, 1995.

84. Duna GF, Cotch MF, Galperin C, et al: Wegener's granulomatosis: role of environmental exposures. Clin Exp Rheumatol 16:669–674, 1998.

85. American Thoracic Society: Idiopathic pulmonary fibrosis: Diagnosis and treatment. International consensus statement. American Thoracic Society (ATS), and the European Respiratory Society (ERS). Am J Respir Crit Care Med 161:646–664, 2000.

86. De Swert LF, Ceuppens JL, Teuwen D, et al: Acute interstitial pneumonitis and carbamazepine therapy. Acta Paediatr Scand 73:285–288, 1984.

87. Vourlekis JS, Brown KK, Cool CD, et al: Acute interstitial pneumonitis: Case series and review of the literature. Medicine 79:369–378, 2000.

88. Matthay RA, Schwarz MI, Petty TL, et al: Pulmonary manifestations of systemic lupus erythematosus: Review of twelve cases of acute lupus pneumonitis. Medicine 54:397–409, 1975.

89. Cheema GS, Quismorio FP: Interstitial lung disease in systemic lupus erythematosus. Curr Opin Pulm Med 6:424–429, 2000.

90. Marik PE: Aspiration pneumonitis and aspiration pneumonia. N Engl J Med 344:665–671, 2001.

91. James CF, Modell JH, Gibbs CP, et al: Pulmonary aspiration—effects of volume and pH in the rat. Anesth Analg 63:665–668, 1984.

92. Nader-Djalal N, Knight PR 3rd, Thusu K, et al: Reactive oxygen species contribute to oxygen-related lung injury after acid aspiration. Anesth Analg 87:127–133, 1998.

93. Folkesson HG, Matthay MA, Hebert CA, Broaddus VC: Acid aspiration-induced lung injury in rabbits is mediated by interleukin-8-dependent mechanisms. J Clin Invest 96:107–116, 1995.

94. Goldman G, Welbourn R, Kobzik L, et al: Synergism between leukotriene B4 and thromboxane A2 in mediating acid-aspiration injury. Surgery 111:55–61, 1992.

95. Kennedy TP, Johnson KJ, Kunkel RG, et al: Acute acid aspiration lung injury in the rat: Biphasic pathogenesis. Anesth Analg 69:87–92, 1989.

96. Wada H, Nakajoh K, Satoh-Nakagawa T, et al: Risk factors of aspiration pneumonia in Alzheimer's disease patients. Gerontology 47:271–276, 2001.

97. Leroy O, Vandenbussche C, Coffinier C, et al: Community-acquired aspiration pneumonia in intensive care units: Epidemiological and prognosis data. Am J Respir Crit Care Med 156:1922–1929, 1997.

98. Pick N, McDonald A, Bennett N, et al: Pulmonary aspiration in a long-term care setting: Clinical and laboratory observations and an analysis of risk factors. J Am Geriatr Soc 44:763–768, 1996.

99. Terpenning MS, Taylor GW, Lopatin DE, et al: Aspiration pneumonia: Dental and oral risk factors in an older veteran population. J Am Geriatr Soc 49:557–563, 2001.

100. Bonten MJ, Gaillard CA, van der Geest S, et al: The role of intragastric acidity and stress ulcer prophylaxis on colonization and infection in mechanically ventilated ICU patients: A stratified, randomized, double-blind study of sucralfate versus antacids. Am J Respir Crit Care Med 152:1825–1834, 1995.

101. Bonten MJ, Gaillard CA, de Leeuw PW, Stobberingh EE: Role of colonization of the upper intestinal tract in the pathogenesis of ventilator-associated pneumonia. Clin Infect Dis 24:309–319, 1997.

102. Bergmans DC, Bonten MJ, Gaillard CA, et al: Prevention of ventilator-associated pneumonia by oral decontamination: a prospective, randomized, double-blind, placebo-controlled study. Am J Respir Crit Care Med 164:382–388, 2001.

103. Fink JN, Schlueter DP: Bathtub refinisher's lung: An unusual response to toluene diisocyanate. Am Rev Respir Dis 118:955–959, 1978.

104. Walker CL, Grammer LC, Shaughnessy MA, et al: Diphenylmethane diisocyanate hypersensitivity pneumonitis: A serologic evaluation. J Occup Med 31:315–319, 1989.

105. Malo JL, Ouimet G, Cartier A, et al: Combined alveolitis and asthma due to hexamethylene diisocyanate (HDI), with demonstration of crossed respiratory and immunologic reactivities to diphenylmethane diisocyanate (MDI). J Allergy Clin Immunol 72:413–419, 1983.

106. Calhoun WJ: Enhanced reactive oxygen species metabolism of air space cells in hypersensitivity pneumonitis. J Lab Clin Med 117:443–452, 1991.

107. Denis M: Proinflammatory cytokines in hypersensitivity pneumonitis. Am J Respir Crit Care Med 151:164–169, 1995.

108. Fournier E, Tonnel AB, Gosset P, et al: Early neutrophil alveolitis after antigen inhalation in hypersensitivity pneumonitis. Chest 88:563–566, 1985.

109. Salvaggio JE, deShazo RD: Pathogenesis of hypersensitivity pneumonitis. Chest 89:190S–193S, 1986.

110. Cormier Y, Belanger J, Laviolette M: Prognostic significance of bronchoalveolar lymphocytosis in farmer's lung. Am Rev Respir Dis 135:692–695, 1987.

111. Cormier Y, Israel-Assayag E: The role of viruses in the pathogenesis of hypersensitivity pneumonitis. Curr Opin Pulm Med 6:420–423, 2000.

112. Haponik EF, Munster AM: Respiratory Injury: Smoke Inhalation and Burns. New York, 1990, McGraw-Hill.

113. Hales CA, Elsasser TH, Ocampo P, Efimova O: TNF-alpha in smoke inhalation lung injury. J Appl Physiol 82:1433–1437, 1997.

114. Ichikado K, Johkoh T, Ikezoe J, et al: A case of acute interstitial pneumonia indistinguishable from bronchiolitis obliterans organizing pneumonia/cryptogenic organizing pneumonia: High-resolution CT findings and pathologic correlation. Radiat Med 16:367–370, 1998.

115. Murphy J, Schnyder P, Herold C, Flower C: Bronchiolitis obliterans organising pneumonia simulating bronchial carcinoma. Eur Radiol 8: 1165–1169, 1998.

116. Teppo AM, Haltia K, Wager O: Immunoelectrophoretic "tailing" of albumin line due to albumin-IgG antibody complexes: A side effect of nitrofurantoin treatment? Scand J Immunol 5:249–261, 1976.

117. Heath MF, Costa-Jussa FR, Jacobs JM, Jacobson W: The induction of pulmonary phospholipoidosis and the inhibition of lysosomal phospholipases by amiodarone. Br J Exp Pathol 66:391–397, 1985.

118. Camus P, Mehendale HM: Pulmonary sequestration of amiodarone and desethylamiodarone. J Pharmacol Exp Ther 237:867–873, 1986.

119. Dunn JM, Sloan H: Pleural effusion and fibrosis secondary to Sansert administration. Ann Thorac Surg 15:295–298, 1973.

120. Sausville EA, Stein RW, Peisach J, Horowitz SB: Properties and products of the degradation of DNA by bleomycin and iron (II). Biochemistry 17:2746–2754, 1978.

121. Ohnuma T, Holland JF, Masuda H, et al: Microbiological assay of bleomycin: Inactivation, tissue distribution, and clearance. Cancer 33:1230–1238, 1974.

122. Barbee JY Jr, Prince TS: Acute respiratory distress syndrome in a welder exposed to metal fumes. South Med J 92:510–512, 1999.

123. Moromisato DY, Anas NG, Goodman G: Mercury inhalation poisoning and acute lung injury in a child: Use of high-frequency oscillatory ventilation. Chest 105:613–615, 1994.

124. Wesseling C, Hogstedt C, Picado A, Johansson L: Unintentional fatal paraquat poisonings among agricultural workers in Costa Rica: Report of 15 cases. Am J Ind Med 32:433–441, 1997.

125. Blodgett DW, Suruda AJ, Crouch BI: Fatal unintentional occupational poisonings by hydrofluoric acid in the U.S. Am J Ind Med 40: 215–220, 2001.

126. Kono K, Watanabe T, Dote T, et al: Successful treatments of lung injury and skin burn due to hydrofluoric acid exposure. Int Arch Occup Environ Health 73:S93–S97, 2000.

127. Kreiss K, Wasserman S, Mroz MM, Newman LS: Beryllium disease screening in the ceramics industry: Blood lymphocyte test performance and exposure-disease relations. J Occup Med 35:267–274, 1993.

128. Kilbourne EM, Rigau-Perez JG, Heath CW, et al: Clinical epidemiology of toxic-oil syndrome: Manifestations of a new illness. N Engl J Med 309:1408–1414, 1983.

129. Kilbourne EM, Bernert JT Jr, Posada de la Paz M, et al: Chemical correlates of pathogenicity of oils related to the toxic oil syndrome epidemic in Spain. Am J Epidemiol 127:1210–1227, 1988.

130. Yoshida SH, German JB, Fletcher MP, Gershwin ME: The toxic oil syndrome: A perspective on immunotoxicological mechanisms. Regul Toxicol Pharmacol 19:60–79, 1994.

131. del Pozo V, de Andres B, Gallardo S, et al: Cytokine mRNA expression in lung tissue from toxic oil syndrome patients: A TH2 immunological mechanism. Toxicology 118:61–70, 1997.

132. Tazelaar HD, Myers JL, Drage CW, et al: Pulmonary disease associated with L-tryptophan-induced eosinophilic myalgia syndrome: Clinical and pathologic features. Chest 97:1032–1036, 1990.

133. Mestre de Juan MJ, Martinez Tello FJ, Gomez Pajuelo C, et al: Severe pulmonary arterial hypertension due to toxic oil syndrome: A new cause of plexogenic arteriopathy. Cor Vasa 32:218–224, 1990.

134. Kleiger RE, Boxer M, Ingham RE, Harrison DC: Pulmonary hypertension in patients using oral contraceptives: A report of six cases. Chest 69:143–147, 1976.

135. Tuder RM, Radisavljevic Z, Shroyer KR, et al: Monoclonal endothelial cells in appetite suppressant-associated pulmonary hypertension. Am J Respir Crit Care Med 158:1999–2001, 1998.

136. Rashid A, Lehrman S, Romano P, et al: Primary pulmonary hypertension. Heart Dis 2:422–430, 2000.

137. Archer SL, Djaballah K, Humbert M, et al: Nitric oxide deficiency in fenfluramine- and dexfenfluramine-induced pulmonary hypertension. Am J Respir Crit Care Med 158:1061–1067, 1998.

138. van der Woude FJ, Rasmussen N, Lobatto S, et al: Autoantibodies against neutrophils and monocytes: Tool for diagnosis and marker of disease activity in Wegener's granulomatosis. Lancet 1:425–429, 1985.

139. Hewins P, Tervaert JW, Savage CO, Kallenberg CG: Is Wegener's granulomatosis an autoimmune disease? Curr Opin Rheumatol 12:3–10, 2000.

140. Sanderson W, Kullman G, Sastre J, et al: Outbreak of hypersensitivity pneumonitis among mushroom farm workers. Am J Ind Med 22:859–872, 1992.

141. Gay SE, Kazerooni EA, Toews GB, et al: Idiopathic pulmonary fibrosis: Predicting response to therapy and survival. Am J Respir Crit Care Med 157:1063–1072, 1998.

142. Cordier JF, Loire R, Brune J: Idiopathic bronchiolitis obliterans organizing pneumonia: Definition of characteristic clinical profiles in a series of 16 patients. Chest 96:999–1004, 1989.

143. Lynch DA, Rose CS, Way D, King TE: Hypersensitivity pneumonitis: sensitivity of high-resolution CT in a population-based study. AJR Am J Roentgenol 159:469–472, 1992.

144. Gurney JW: Hypersensitivity pneumonitis. Radiol Clin North Am 30:1219–1230, 1992.

145. Collins J: CT signs and patterns of lung disease. Radiol Clin North Am 39:1115–1135, 2001.

146. Dina R, Sheppard MN: The histological diagnosis of clinically documented cases of cryptogenic organizing pneumonia: Diagnostic features in transbronchial biopsies. Histopathology 23:541–545, 1993.

147. Ranieri VM, Suter PM, Tortorella C, et al: Effect of mechanical ventilation on inflammatory mediators in patients with acute respiratory distress syndrome: A randomized controlled trial. JAMA 282:54–61, 1999.

148. Bernard GR, Luce JM, Sprung CL, et al: High-dose corticosteroids in patients with the adult respiratory distress syndrome. N Engl J Med 317:1565–1570, 1987.

149. Meduri GU, Tolley EA, Chinn A, et al: Procollagen types I and III aminoterminal propeptide levels during acute respiratory distress syndrome and in response to methylprednisolone treatment. Am J Respir Crit Care Med 158:1432–1441, 1998.

150. King TE Jr, Mortenson RL: Cryptogenic organizing pneumonitis: The North American experience. Chest 102:8S–13S, 1992.

151. Fink JN: Hypersensitivity pneumonitis. Clin Chest Med 13:303–309, 1992.

152. Robinson NB, Hudson LD, Riem M, et al: Steroid therapy following isolated smoke inhalation injury. J Trauma 22:876–879, 1982.

153. Yi ES, Colby TV: Wegener's granulomatosis. Semin Diagn Pathol 18:34–46, 2001.

154. Langford CA, Talar-Williams C, Barron KS, Sneller MC: A staged approach to the treatment of Wegener's granulomatosis: Induction of remission with glucocorticoids and daily cyclophosphamide switching to methotrexate for remission maintenance. Arthritis Rheum 42:2666–2673, 1999.

155. de Groot K, Reinhold-Keller E, Tatsis E, et al: Therapy for the maintenance of remission in sixty-five patients with generalized Wegener's granulomatosis: Methotrexate versus trimethoprim/sulfamethoxazole. Arthritis Rheum 39:2052–2061, 1996.

156. Merkel F, Netzer KO, Gross O, et al: Therapeutic options for critically ill patients suffering from progressive lupus nephritis or Goodpasture's syndrome. Kidney Int 64(Suppl):S31–S38, 1998.

157. Sukumaran M, Granada MJ, Berger HW, et al: Evaluation of corticosteroid treatment in aspiration of gastric contents: A controlled clinical trial. Mt Sinai J Med 47:335–340, 1980.

158. Lee M, Sukumaran M, Berger HW, Reilly TA: Influence of corticosteroid treatment on pulmonary function after recovery from aspiration of gastric contents. Mt Sinai J Med 47:341–346, 1980.

159. Marik PE, Careau P: The role of anaerobes in patients with ventilator-associated pneumonia and aspiration pneumonia: A prospective study. Chest 115:178–183, 1999.

160. Ashrafian H, Davey P: Is amiodarone an underrecognized cause of acute respiratory failure in the ICU? Chest 120:275–282, 2001.

161. Greenspon AJ, Kidwell GA, Hurley W, Mannion J: Amiodarone-related postoperative adult respiratory distress syndrome. Circulation 84(5 Suppl 1):III407–III415, 1991.

162. Guharoy SR: Adult respiratory distress syndrome associated with amitriptyline overdose. Vet Hum Toxicol 36:316–317, 1994.

163. Poe RH, Condemi JJ, Weinstein SS, Schuster RJ: Adult respiratory distress syndrome related to ampicillin sensitivity. Chest 77:449–451, 1980.

164. Vucicevic Z, Suskovic T: Acute respiratory distress syndrome after aprotinin infusion. Ann Pharmacother 31:429–432, 1997.

165. Suarez M, Krieger BP: Bronchoalveolar lavage in recurrent aspirin-induced adult respiratory distress syndrome. Chest 90:452–453, 1986.

166. Luis M, Ayuso A, Martinez G, et al: Intraoperative respiratory failure in a patient after treatment with bleomycin: previous and current intraoperative exposure to 50% oxygen. Eur J Anaesthesiol 16:66–68, 1999.

167. Walsh RF, Springate JE, Spivack BS, et al: Cyclosporine and adult respiratory distress syndrome. Transplantation 46:776–777, 1988.

168. Tenenbein M, Kowalski S, Sienko A, et al: Pulmonary toxic effects of continuous desferrioxamine administration in acute iron poisoning. Lancet 339:699–701, 1992.

169. Taylor MA, DiBlasi SL, Bender RM, et al: Adult respiratory distress syndrome complicating intravenous infusion of low-molecular weight dextran. Cathet Cardiovasc Diagn 32:249–253, 1994.

170. Lindsay CA, Williams GD, Levin DL: Fatal adult respiratory distress syndrome after diphenhydramine toxicity in a child: a case report. Crit Care Med 23:777–781, 1995.

171. Burton WN, Vender J, Shapiro BA: Adult respiratory distress syndrome after Placidyl abuse. Crit Care Med 8:48–49, 1980.

172. Girard T, Mouthon L, Boaziz C, et al: Favorable outcome of gemcitabine-induced respiratory distress syndrome. Ann Med Int (Paris) 151:306–308, 2000.

173. McDonald CF, Thomson SA, Scott NC, et al: Benzodiazepine-opiate antagonism—a problem in intensive-care therapy. Intensive Care Med 12:39–42, 1996.

174. Le HT, Bosse GM, Tsai Y: Ibuprofen overdose complicated by renal failure, adult respiratory distress syndrome, and metabolic acidosis. J Toxicol Clin Toxicol 32:315–320, 1994.

175. Howard JJ, Mohsenifar Z, Simons SM: Adult respiratory distress syndrome following administration of lidocaine. Chest 81:644–645, 1982.

176. Friedman BC, Bekes CE, Scott WE, Bartter T: ARDS following acute lithium carbonate intoxication. Intensive Care Med 18:123–124, 1992.

177. Dai MS, Ho CL, Chen YC, et al: Acute respiratory distress syndrome following intrathecal methotrexate administration: A case report and review of literature. Ann Hematol 79:696–699, 2000.

178. Walubo A, Seger D: Fatal multi-organ failure after suicidal overdose with MDMA, 'ecstasy': Case report and review of the literature. Hum Exp Toxicol 18:119–125, 1999.

179. Israel RH, Gross RA, Bomba PA: Adult respiratory distress syndrome associated with acute nitrofurantoin toxicity: Successful treatment with continuous positive airway pressure. Respiration 39:318–322, 1980.

180. Chevrolet JC, Guelpa G, Schifferli JA: Recurrent adult respiratory distress-like syndrome associated with propylthiouracil therapy. Eur Respir J 4:899–901, 1991.

181. Wenstone R, Bell M, Mostafa SM: Fatal adult respiratory distress syndrome after quinine overdose. Lancet 1:1143–1144, 1989.

182. Machiels JP, Evrard P, Dive A, et al: Venovenous ECMO in life-threatening radiocontrast mediated-ARDS. Intensive Care Med 25:546, 1999.

183. Sandblom RL, Johnson RJ: Adult respiratory distress syndrome following thrombolytic therapy for pulmonary embolism. Chest 83:151–153, 1983.

184. Gruson D, Hilbert G, Boiron JM, et al: Acute respiratory distress syndrome due to all-trans retinoic acid. Intensive Care Med 24:642, 1998.

185. Chugh SN, Ram S, Mehta LK, et al: Adult respiratory distress syndrome following aluminium phosphide ingestion: Report of 4 cases. J Assoc Physicians India 37:271–272, 1989.

186. Bolliger CT, van Zijl P, Louw JA: Multiple organ failure with the adult respiratory distress syndrome in homicidal arsenic poisoning. Respiration 59:57–61, 1992.

187. Baban NK, Nunley DL, Borges AS Jr, Roy TM: Human sequelae of severe carbamate poisoning. Tenn Med 91:103–106, 1998.

188. Mapp CE, Pozzato V, Pavoni V, Gritti G: Severe asthma and ARDS triggered by acute short-term exposure to commonly used cleaning detergents. Eur Respir J 16:570–572, 2000.

189. Hernandez AF, Martin-Rubi JC, Ballesteros JL, et al: Clinical and pathological findings in fatal 1,3-dichloropropene intoxication. Hum Exp Toxicol 13:303–306, 1994.

190. Catchings TT, Beamer WC, Lundy L, Prough DS: Adult respiratory distress syndrome secondary to ethylene glycol ingestion. Ann Emerg Med 14:594–596, 1985.

191. Piagnerelli M, Carlier E, Lejeune P: Adult respiratory distress syndrome and medullary toxicity: Two unusual complications of ethylene glycol intoxication. Intensive Care Med 25:1200, 1999.

192. Bracco D, Favre JB: Pulmonary injury after ski wax inhalation exposure. Ann Emerg Med 32:616–619, 1998.

193. Bennion JR, Franzblau A: Chemical pneumonitis following household exposure to hydrofluoric acid. Am J Ind Med 31:474–478, 1997.

194. Lim HE, Shim JJ, Lee SY, et al: Mercury inhalation poisoning and acute lung injury. Korean J Intern Med 13:127–130, 1998.

195. Rendall RE, Phillips JI, Renton KA: Death following exposure to fine particulate nickel from a metal arc process. Ann Occup Hyg 38:921–930, 1994.

196. Yockey CC, Eden BM, Byrd RB: The McConnell missile accident: Clinical spectrum of nitrogen dioxide exposure. JAMA 244:1221–1223, 1980.

197. Kass R, Kochar G, Lippman M: Adult respiratory distress syndrome from organophosphate poisoning. Am J Emerg Med 9:32–33, 1991.

198. Cohen N, Modai D, Khahil A, Golik A: Acute resin phenol-formaldehyde intoxication: A life threatening occupational hazard. Hum Toxicol 8:247–250, 1989.

199. Borak J, Diller WF: Phosgene exposure: Mechanisms of injury and treatment strategies. J Occup Environ Med 43:110–119, 2001.

200. Pentel P, Fletcher D, Jentzen J: Fatal acute selenium toxicity. J Forensic Sci 30:556–562, 1985.

201. Okumura T, Suzuki K, Kumada K, et al: Severe respiratory distress following sodium oleate ingestion. J Toxicol Clin Toxicol 36:587–589, 1998.

202. Knapp MJ, Bunn WB, Stave GM: Adult respiratory distress syndrome from sulfuric acid fume inhalation. South Med J 84:1031–1033, 1991.

203. Esteban A, Guerra L, Ruiz-Santana S, et al: ARDS due to ingestion of denatured rapeseed oil. Chest 84:166–169, 1983.

204. Lyle WH, Payton JE, Hui M: Haemodialysis and copper fever. Lancet 1:1324–1325, 1976.

205. Hartmann AL, Hartmann W, Buhlmann AA: Schweizerische Medizinische Wochenschrift. [Magnesium oxide as cause of metal fume fever]. J Suisse Med 113:766–770, 1983.

206. Bluhm RE, Bobbitt RG, Welch LW, et al: Elemental mercury vapour toxicity, treatment, and prognosis after acute, intensive exposure in chloralkali plant workers: Part I. History, neuropsychological findings and chelator effects. Hum Exp Toxicol 11:201–210, 1992.

207. Shusterman DJ: Polymer fume fever and other fluorocarbon pyrolysis-related syndromes. Occup Med 8:519–531, 1993.

208. Nielsen J, Sango C, Winroth G, et al: Systemic reactions associated with polyisocyanate exposure. Scand J Work Environ Health 11:51–54, 1985.

209. Pal TM, de Monchy JG, Groothoff JW, Post D: The clinical spectrum of humidifier disease in synthetic fiber plants. Am J Ind Med 31:682–692, 1997.

210. Kateman E, Heederik D, Pal TM, et al: Relationship of airborne microorganisms with the lung function and leucocyte levels of workers with a history of humidifier fever. Scand J Work Environ Health 16:428–433, 1990.

211. Finnegan MJ, Pickering CA, Davies PS, et al: Amoebae and humidifier fever. Clin Allergy 17:235–242, 1987.

212. Rylander R: The role of endotoxin for reactions after exposure to cotton dust. Am J Ind Med 12:687–697, 1987.

213. Uragoda CG: An investigation into the health of kapok workers. Br J Ind Med 34:181–185, 1977.

214. Rask-Andersen A, Land CJ, Enlund K, Lundin A: Inhalation fever and respiratory symptoms in the trimming department of Swedish sawmills. Am J Ind Med 25:65–67, 1994.

215. Brinton WT, Vastbinder EE, Greene JW, et al: An outbreak of organic dust toxic syndrome in a college fraternity. JAMA 258:1210–1212, 1987.

216. Sprince NL, Lewis MQ, Whitten PS, et al: Respiratory symptoms: associations with pesticides, silos, and animal confinement in the Iowa Farm Family Health and Hazard Surveillance Project. Am J Ind Med 38:455–462, 2000.

217. Maury E, Darondel JM, Buisinne A, et al: Acute pulmonary edema following amphetamine ingestion. Intensive Care Med 25:332–333, 1999.

218. Boxer LA, Ingraham LM, Allen J, et al: Amphotericin-B promotes leukocyte aggregation of nylon-wool-fiber-treated polymorphonuclear leukocytes. Blood 58:518–523, 1981.

219. Singh A, Biswal N, Nalini P, et al: Acute pulmonary edema as a complication of anti-snake venom therapy. Indian J Pediatr 68:81–82, 2001.

220. Woolley RJ: Salicylate-induced pulmonary edema: a complication of chronic aspirin therapy. J Am Board Fam Pract 6:399–401, 1993.

221. Mountain R, Ferguson S, Fowler A, Hyers T: Noncardiac pulmonary edema following administration of parenteral paraldehyde. Chest 82:371–372, 1982.

222. Kline JN, Hirasuna JD: Pulmonary edema after freebase cocaine smoking—not due to an adulterant. Chest 97:1009–1010, 1990.

223. Zitnik RJ, Cooper JA Jr: Pulmonary disease due to antirheumatic agents. Clin Chest Med 11:139–150, 1990.

224. Greganti MA, Flowers WM Jr: Acute pulmonary edema after the intravenous administration of contrast media. Radiology 132: 583–585, 1979.

225. Briasoulis E, Pavlidis N: Noncardiogenic pulmonary edema: An unusual and serious complication of anticancer therapy. Oncologist 6:153–161, 2001.

226. Schinco MA, Hughes D, Santora TA: Complications of 32% dextran-70 in 10% dextrose: A case report. J Reprod Med 41:455–458, 1996.

227. Humbert VH Jr, Munn NJ, Hawkins RF: Noncardiogenic pulmonary edema complicating massive diltiazem overdose. Chest 99:258–259, 1991.

228. Conces DJ Jr, Kreipke DL, Tarver RD: Pulmonary edema induced by intravenous ethchlorvynol. Am J Emerg Med 4:549–551, 1986.

229. Briasoulis E, Pavlidis N: Noncardiogenic pulmonary edema: An unusual and serious complication of anticancer therapy. Oncologist 6:153–161, 2001.

230. Mahutte CK, Nakasato SK, Light RW: Haloperidol and sudden death due to pulmonary edema. Arch Intern Med 142:1951–1952, 1982.

231. Frand UI, Shim CS, Williams MH Jr: Heroin-induced pulmonary edema: Sequential studies of pulmonary function. Ann Intern Med 77:29–35, 1972.

232. Morrison WJ, Wetherill S, Zyroff J: The acute pulmonary edema of heroin intoxication. Radiology 97:347–351, 1970.

233. Mas A, Jordana R, Valles J, Cervantes M: Recurrent hydrochlorothiazide-induced pulmonary edema. Intensive Care Med 24:363–365, 1998.

234. Almoosa KF: Hydrochlorothiazide-induced pulmonary edema. South Med J 92:1100–1102, 1999.

235. Saxon RR, Klein JS, Bar MH, et al: Pathogenesis of pulmonary edema during interleukin-2 therapy: Correlation of chest radiographic and clinical findings in 54 patients. AJR Am J Roentgenol 156:281–285, 1991.

236. Pandey CK, Mathur N, Singh N, Chandola HC: Fulminant pulmonary edema after intramuscular ketamine. Can J Anaesth 47: 894–896, 2000.

237. Rooke NT, Milne B: Acute pulmonary edema after regional anesthesia with lidocaine and epinephrine in a patient with chronic renal failure. Anesth Analg 63:363–364, 1984.

238. Johnson BA, James AE Jr, Levey MS, Campbell HJ: Pulmonary edema caused by methadone. Va Med Mon 101:640–644, 1974.

239. Nestor TA, Tamamoto WI, Kam TH, Schultz T: Acute pulmonary edema caused by crystalline methamphetamine. Lancet 2:1277–1278, 1989.

240. Bernstein ML, Sobel DB, Wimmer RS: Noncardiogenic pulmonary edema following injection of methotrexate into the cerebrospinal fluid. Cancer 50:866–868, 1982.

241. Claycomb CL, Berkovic M: Microangiopathic hemolytic anemia, noncardiac pulmonary edema, and renal failure after treatment of metastatic adenocarcinoma of the colon with 5-fluorouracil and mitomycin-C: Report of a case. J Am Osteopath Assoc 86:499–503, 1986.

242. Schwartz JA, Koenigsberg MD: Naloxone-induced pulmonary edema. Ann Emerg Med 16:1294–1296, 1987.

243. Nicklaus TM, Snyder AB: Nitrofurantoin pulmonary reaction: A unique syndrome. Arch Intern Med 121:151–155, 1968.

244. Van den Ouweland FA, Gribnau FW: Nonsteroidal anti-inflammatory drugs as a prognostic factor in acute pulmonary edema. Arch Intern Med 147:176–179, 1987.

245. Li C, Gefter WB: Acute pulmonary edema induced by overdosage of phenothiazines. Chest 101:102–104, 1992.

246. Bogartz LJ, Miller WC: Pulmonary edema associated with propoxyphene intoxication. JAMA 15:259–262, 1971.

247. Urdaneta F, Lobato EB, Kirby RR, Horrow JC: Noncardiogenic pulmonary edema associated with protamine administration during coronary artery bypass graft surgery. J Clin Anesth 11:675–681, 1999.

248. Cooper JA Jr, Matthay RA: Drug-induced pulmonary disease. Dis Mon 33:61–120, 1987.

249. Alper M, Cohen WR: Pulmonary edema associated with ritodrine and dexamethasone treatment of threatened premature labor: A case report. J Reprod Med 28:349–352, 1983.

250. Shannon M, Lovejoy FH Jr: Pulmonary consequences of severe tricyclic antidepressant ingestion. J Toxicol Clin Toxicol 25:443–461, 1987.

251. Tibbits PA, Milroy WC: Pulmonary edema induced by exposure to cadmium oxide fume: Case report. Milit Med 145:435–437, 1980.

252. Pino F, Puerta H, D'Apollo R, et al: Effectiveness of morphine in non-cardiogenic pulmonary edema due to chlorine gas inhalation. Vet Hum Toxicol 35:36, 1993.

253. Graham DL, Laman D, Theodore J, Robin ED: Acute cyanide poisoning complicated by lactic acidosis and pulmonary edema. Arch Intern Med 137:1051–1055, 1977.

254. Ip M, Wong KL, Wong KF, So SY: Lung injury in dimethyl sulfate poisoning. J Occup Med 31:141–143, 1989.

255. Nierenberg DW, Horowitz MB, Harris KM, James DH: Mineral spirits inhalation associated with hemolysis, pulmonary edema, and ventricular fibrillation. Arch Intern Med 151:1437–1440, 1991.

256. Deng JF, Chang SC: Hydrogen sulfide poisonings in hot-spring reservoir cleaning: Two case reports. Am J Ind Med 11:447–451, 1987.

257. Hajela R, Janigan DT, Landrigan PL, et al: Fatal pulmonary edema due to nitric acid fume inhalation in three pulp-mill workers. Chest 97:487–489, 1990.

258. Bur A, Wagner A, Roggla M, et al: Fatal pulmonary edema after nitric acid inhalation. Resuscitation 35:33–36, 1997.

259. Horvath EP, doPico GA, Barbee RA, Dickie HA: Nitrogen dioxide-induced pulmonary disease: Five new cases and a review of the literature. J Occup Med 20:103–110, 1978.

260. Park CH, Kim KI, Park SK, Lee CH: Carbamate poisoning: high resolution CT and pathologic findings. J Comput Assist Tomogr 24:52–54, 2000.

261. Gardiner AJ: Pulmonary edema in paraguat poisoning. Thorax 27:132–135, 1972.

262. Misra NP, Manoria PC, Saxena K: Fatal pulmonary oedema with phosgene poisoning. J Assoc Physicians India 33:430–431, 1985.

263. Wilson R, Lovejoy FH, Jaeger RJ, Landrigan PL: Acute phosphine poisoning aboard a grain freighter: Epidemiologic, clinical, and pathological findings. JAMA 244:148–150, 1980.

264. Lee CH, Guo YL, Tsai PJ, et al: Fatal acute pulmonary edema after inhalation of fumes from polytetrafluoroethylene (PTFE). Eur Respir J 10:1408–1411, 1997.

265. Albertson TE, Reed S, Siefkin A: A case of fatal sodium azide ingestion. J Toxicol Clin Toxicol 24:339–351, 1986.

266. Woodford DM, Coutu RE, Gaensler EA: Obstructive lung disease from acute sulfur dioxide exposure. Respiration 38:238–245, 1979.

267. Vaca FE, Myers JH, Langdorf M: Delayed pulmonary edema and bronchospasm after accidental lacrimator exposure. Am J Emerg Med 14:402–405, 1996.

268. Pahade A, Green KM, de Carpentier JP: Non-cardiogenic pulmonary oedema due to foreign body aspiration. J Laryngol Otol 113:1119–1121, 1999.

269. Fitzgerald J, Chatwani A, Oyer R: Noncardiogenic pulmonary edema as a rare complication of blood transfusions: A case report. J Reprod Med 33:243–245, 1988.

270. Trewby PN, Warren R, Contini S, et al: Incidence and pathophysiology of pulmonary edema in fulminant hepatic failure. Gastroenterology 74:859–865, 1978.

271. Gibbs JS: Pulmonary hemodynamics: implications for high altitude pulmonary edema (HAPE): A review. Adv Exp Med Biol 474:81–91, 1999.

272. Hall ML, Huseby JS: Hemorrhagic pulmonary edema associated with meat tenderizer treatment for esophageal meat impaction. Chest 94:640–642, 1988.

273. Rumbak MJ: The etiology of pulmonary edema in fresh water near-drowning. Am J Emerg Med 14:176–179, 1996.

274. Davison JM: Edema in pregnancy. Kidney Int 59(Suppl):S90–S96, 1997.

275. Cinnella G, Dambrosio M, Brienza N, Ranieri VM: Reexpansion pulmonary edema with acute hypovolemia. Intensive Care Med 24:1117, 1998.

276. D'Suze G, Comellas A, Pesce L, et al: *Tityus discrepans* venom produces a respiratory distress syndrome in rabbits through an indirect mechanism. Toxicon 37:173–180, 1999.

277. Lee RP, Wang D, Kao SJ, Chen HI: The lung is the major site that produces nitric oxide to induce acute pulmonary oedema in endotoxin shock. Clin Exp Pharmacol Physiol 28:315–320, 2001.

278. Pons M, Blickenstorfer D, Oechslin E, et al: Pulmonary oedema in healthy persons during scuba-diving and swimming. Eur Respir J 8:762–767, 1995.

279. Ferro TJ, Hocking DC, Johnson A: Tumor necrosis factor-alpha alters pulmonary vasoreactivity via neutrophil-derived oxidants. Am J Physiol 265:L462–L471, 1993.

280. Camus P, Lombard JN, Perrichon M, et al: Bronchiolitis obliterans organising pneumonia in patients taking acebutolol or amiodarone. Thorax 44:711–715, 1989.

281. Roncoroni AJ, Corrado C, Besuschio S, et al: Bronchiolitis obliterans possibly associated with amphotericin B. J Infect Dis 161:589, 1990.

282. Santrach PJ, Askin FB, Wells RJ, et al: Nodular form of bleomycin-related pulmonary injury in patients with osteogenic sarcoma. Cancer 64:806–811, 1989.

283. Milesi-Lecat AM, Schmidt J, Aumaitre O, et al: Lupus and pulmonary nodules consistent with bronchiolitis obliterans organizing pneumonia induced by carbamazepine. Mayo Clin Proc 72:1145–1147, 1997.

284. Patel RC, Dutta D, Schonfeld SA: Free-base cocaine associated with bronchiolitis obliterans organizing pneumonia. Ann Intern Med 107:186–187, 1987.

285. Knoell KA, Hook M, Grice DP, Hendrix JD: Dermatomyositis associated with bronchiolitis obliterans organizing pueumonia (BOOP). J Am Acta Dermatol 40:328–330, 1999.

286. Blancas R, Moreno JL, Martin F, et al: Alveolar-interstitial pneumopathy after gold-salts compounds administration, requiring mechanical ventilation. Intensive Care Med 24:1110–1112, 1998.

287. Ferriby D, Stojkovic T: Clinical picture: Bronchiolitis obliterans with organising pneumonia during interferon beta-1a treatment. Lancet 357:751, 2001.

288. Mar KE, Sen P, Tan K, et al: Bronchiolitis obliterans organizing pneumonia associated with massive L-tryptophan ingestion. Chest 104:1924–1926, 1993.

289. Rossi SE, Erasmus JJ, McAdams HP, et al: Pulmonary drug toxicity: Radiologic and pathologic manifestations. Radiographics 20:1245–1259, 2000.

290. Piperno D, Donne C, Loire R, Cordier JF: Bronchiolitis obliterans organizing pneumonia associated with minocycline therapy: A possible cause. Eur Respir J 8:1018–1020, 1995.

291. Cameron RJ, Kolbe J, Wilsher ML, Lambie N: Bronchiolitis obliterans organising pneumonia associated with the use of nitrofurantoin. Thorax 55:249–251, 2000.

292. Boehler A, Vogt P, Speich R, et al: Bronchiolitis obliterans in a patient with localized scleroderma treated with D-penicillamine. Eur Respir J 9:1317–1319, 1996.

293. Angle P, Thomas P, Chiu B, Freedman J: Bronchiolitis obliterans with organizing pneumonia and cold agglutinin disease associated with phenytoin hypersensitivity syndrome. Chest 112:1697–1699, 1997.

294. Gabazza EC, Taguchi O, Yamakami T, et al: Pulmonary infiltrates and skin pigmentation associated with sulfasalazine. Clin Chest Med 87:1654–1657, 1992.

295. Godfrey KM, Wojnarowska F, Friedland JS: Obliterative bronchiolitis and alveolitis associated with sulphamethoxypyridazine (Lederkyn) therapy for linear IgA disease of adults. Br J Dermatol 123:125–126, 1990.

296. Alonso-Martinez JL, Elejalde-Guerra JI, Larrinaga-Linero D: Bronchiolitis obliterans-organizing pneumonia caused by ticlopidine. Ann Intern Med 129:71–72, 1998.

297. King TE Jr: Bronchiolitis obliterans. Lung 167:69–93, 1989.

298. Kraut A, Lilis R: Chemical pneumonitis due to exposure to bromine compounds. Chest 94:208–210, 1988.

299. Boswell RT, McCunney RJ: Bronchiolitis obliterans from exposure to incinerator fly ash. J Occup Environ Med 37:850–855, 1995.

300. Weill H: Disaster at Bhopal: The accident, early findings and respiratory health outlook in those injured. Bull Eur Physiopathol Respir 23:587–590, 1987.

301. McLoud TC, Epler GR, Colby TV, et al: Bronchiolitis obliterans. Radiology 159:1–8, 1986.

302. Reijula K, Paakko P, Kerttula R, et al: Bronchiolitis in a patient with talcosis. Br J Ind Med 48:140–142, 1991.

303. Romero S, Hernandez L, Gil J, et al: Organizing pneumonia in textile printing workers: A clinical description. Eur Respir J 11:265–271, 1998.

304. Konichezky S, Schattner A, Ezri T, et al: Thionyl-chloride-induced lung injury and bronchiolitis obliterans. Chest 104:971–973, 1993.

305. Zackrison LH, Katz P: Bronchiolitis obliterans organizing pneumonia associated with essential mixed cryoglobulinemia. Arthritis Rheum 36:1627–1630, 1993.

306. Imasaki T, Yoshi A, Tanaka S, et al: Polymyositis and Sjogren's syndrome associated with bronchiolitis obliterans organizing pneumonia. Intern Med 35:231–235, 1996.

307. Ippolito JA, Palmer L, Spector S, et al: Bronchiolitis obliterans organizing pneumonia and rheumatoid arthritis. Semin Arthritis Rheum 23:70–78, 1993.

308. Gammon RB, Bridges TA, al-Nezir H, et al: Bronchiolitis obliterans organizing pneumonia associated with systemic lupus erythematosus. Chest 102:1171–1174, 1992.

309. Kleinau I, Perez-Canto A, Schmid HJ, et al: Bronchiolitis obliterans organizing pneumonia and chronic graft-versus-host disease in a child after allogeneic bone marrow transplant. Bone Marrow Transplant 19:841–844, 1997.

310. Scott JP, Whitehead B, de Leval M, et al: Paediatric incidence of acute rejection and obliterative bronchiolitis: a comparison with adults. Transpl Int 7(Suppl 1):S404-S406, 1994.

311. Llibre JM, Urban A, Garcia E, et al: Bronchiolitis obliterans organizing pneumonia associated with acute *Mycoplasma pneumoniae* infection. Clin Infect Dis 25:1340–1342, 1997.

312. Staud R, Ramos LG: Influenza A-associated bronchiolitis obliterans organizing pneumonia mimicking Wegener's granulomatosis. Rheumatol Int 20:125–128, 2001.

313. Crestani B, Valeyre D, Roden S, et al: Bronchiolitis obliterans organizing pneumonia syndrome primed by radiation therapy to the breast. Am J Respir Crit Care Med 158:1929–1935, 1998.

314. Takehara H, Tada S, Kataoka M, et al: Intercellular adhesion molecule-1 in patients with idiopathic interstitial pneumonia. Acta Med Okayama 55:205–211, 2001.

315. Frazier SK: Diagnosing and treating primary pulmonary hypertension. Nurse Pract 24:18–26, 1999.

316. Palevsky HI, Fishman AP: Chronic cor pulmonale: Etiology and management. JAMA 263:2347–2353, 1990.

317. Burgher LW, Kass I, Schenken JR: Pulmonary allergic granulomatosis: A possible drug reaction in a patient receiving cromolyn sodium. Chest 66:84–86, 1974.

318. Shaul PW: Ontogeny of nitric oxide in the pulmonary vasculature. Semin Perinatol 21:381–392, 1997.

319. Antonelli Incalzi R, Ludovico Maini C, Giuliano Bonetti M, et al: Inapparent pulmonary vascular disease in an ex-heroin user. Clin Nucl Med 11:266–269, 1986.

320. Arnett EN, Battle WE, Russo JV, Roberts WC: Intravenous injection of talc-containing drugs intended for oral use: A cause of pulmonary granulomatosis and pulmonary hypertension. Am J Med 60:711–718, 1976.

321. Sherman CB, Hudson LD, Pierson DJ: Severe precocious emphysema in intravenous methylphenidate (Ritalin) abusers. Chest 92:1085–1087, 1987.

322. Ohtsuka M, Yamashita Y, Doi M, Hasegawa S: Propylthiouracil-induced alveolar haemorrhage associated with antineutrophil cytoplasmic antibody. Eur Respir J 10:1405–1407, 1997.

323. Seguchi M, Hirabayashi N, Fujii Y, et al: Pulmonary hypertension associated with pulmonary occlusive vasculopathy after allogeneic bone marrow transplantation. Transplantation 69:177–179, 2000.

324. Asherson RA, Benbow AG, Speirs CJ, et al: Pulmonary hypertension in hydralazine induced systemic lupus erythematosus: Association with C4 null allele. Ann Rheum Dis 45:771–773, 1986.

325. Bonilla-Felix M, Verani R, Vanasse LG, Hebert A: Nephrotic syndrome related to systemic lupus erythematosus after griseofulvin therapy. Pediatr Nephrol 9:478–479, 1995.

326. Jones FL, Spivey CG: Spread of pulmonary coccidioidomycosis associated with steroid therapy: Report of a case with a lupus-like reaction to antituberculosis chemotherapy. Lancet 86:226–230, 1966.

327. Goldberg SK, Lipschutz JB, Ricketts RM, Fein AM: Procainamide-induced lupus lung disease characterized by neutrophil alveolitis. Am J Med 76:146–150, 1984.

328. Guleria R, Behera D, Jindal SK: Systemic lupus erythematosus during isoniazid therapy. Ind J Chest Dis Allied Sci 32:55–58, 1990.

329. Muren C, Strandberg O: Cavitary pulmonary nodules in atypical collagen disease and lupoid drug reaction: Report of two cases. Acta Radiol 30:281–284, 1989.

330. Arroliga AC, Podell DN, Matthay RA: Pulmonary manifestations of scleroderma. J Thorac Imaging 7:30–45, 1992.

331. Agarwal MB, Anjaria PD, Mehta BC: Activation of systemic lupus erythematosus by antitubercular drugs. J Postgrad Med 26:263–266, 1980.

332. Cowan KN, Heilbut A, Humpl T, et al: Complete reversal of fatal pulmonary hypertension in rats by a serine elastase inhibitor. Nat Med 6:698–702, 2000.

333. Schlienger RG, Bircher AJ, Meier CR: Minocycline-induced lupus: A systematic review. Dermatology 200:223–231, 2000.

334. Mok CC, Lau CS, Wong RW: Use of exogenous estrogens in systemic lupus erythematosus. Semin Arthritis Rheum 30:426–435, 2001.

335. Balluz L, Philen R, Ortega L, et al: Investigation of systemic lupus erythematosus in Nogales, Arizona. Am J Epidemiol 154:1029–1036, 2001.

336. Iliopoulou A, Pagou H, Giannakopoulos G, Spiropoulos T: Amiodarone-induced pulmonary interstitial fibrosis. Intensive Care Med 26:1585, 2000.

337. Hadjiliadis D, Sporn TA, Perfect JR, et al: Outcome of lung transplantation in patients with mycetomas. Chest 121:128–134, 2002.

338. Panos RJ: Therapy and management of idiopathic pulmonary fibrosis. Compr Ther 20:289–293, 1994.

339. Oury TD, Thakker K, Menache M, et al: Attenuation of bleomycin-induced pulmonary fibrosis by a catalytic antioxidant metalloporphyrin. Am J Respir Cell Mol Biol 25:164–169, 2001.

340. Min KW, Gyorkey F: Interstitial pulmonary fibrosis, atypical epithelial changes and bronchiolar cell carcinoma following busulfan therapy. Cancer 22:1027–1032, 1968.

341. Refvem O: Fatal intraalveolar and interstitial lung fibrosis in chlorambucil-treated chronic lymphocytic leukemia. Mt Sinai J Med 44:847–851, 1977.

342. Bailey ME, Fraire AE, Greenberg SD, et al: Pulmonary histopathology in cocaine abusers. Hum Pathol 25:203–207, 1994.

343. Eliasson O, Cole SR, Degraff AC Jr: Adverse effects of cyclophosphamide in idiopathic pulmonary fibrosis. Conn Med 49:286–289, 1985.

344. Grange MJ, Dombret MC, Fantin B, Gougerot-Pocidalo MA: Fatal acute pulmonary fibrosis in a patient treated by danazol for thrombocytopenia. Am J Hematol 53:149, 1996.

345. Vigreux P, Lemozit JP, Delay M, et al: Antiarrhythmic drug-induced side effects: A prospective survey of 300 patients. Therapie 50:413–418, 1995.

346. Shaban MR, Golding DN, Letcher RG: Fatal intrahepatic cholestasis and interstitial lung fibrosis following gold therapy for rheumatoid arthritis. J R Soc Med 77:960–961, 1984.

347. Gottlieb LS, Boylen TC: Pulmonary complications of drug abuse. West J Med 120:8–16, 1974.

348. Mufti GJ, Hamblin TJ, Gordon J: Melphalan-induced pulmonary fibrosis in osteosclerotic myeloma. Acta Haematol 69:140–141, 1983.

349. Bruggers CS, Friedman HS, Phillips PC, et al: Leptomeningeal dissemination of optic pathway gliomas in three children. Am J Ophthalmol 111:719–723, 1991.

350. Pare JA, Fraser RG, Hogg JC, et al: Pulmonary 'mainline' granulomatosis: Talcosis of intravenous methadone abuse. Medicine 58:229–239, 1979.

351. van der Veen MJ, Dekker JJ, Dinant HJ, et al: Fatal pulmonary fibrosis complicating low dose methotrexate therapy for rheumatoid arthritis. J Rheumatol 22:1766–1768, 1995.

352. Stern EJ, Frank MS, Schmutz JF, et al: Panlobular pulmonary emphysema caused by i.v. injection of methylphenidate (Ritalin): Findings on chest radiographs and CT scans. AJR Am J Roentgenol 162:555–560, 1994.

353. Graham JR: Cardiac and pulmonary fibrosis during methysergide therapy for headache. Am J Med Sci 254:1–12, 1967.

354. Fielding JW, Crocker J, Stockley RA, Brookes VS: Interstitial fibrosis in a patient treated with 5-fluorouracil and mitomycin C. BMJ 2:551–552, 1979.

355. Robinson BW: Nitrofurantoin-induced interstitial pulmonary fibrosis: Presentation and outcome. Med J Aust 1:72–76, 1983.

356. Smith AC: The pulmonary toxicity of nitrosoureas. Pharmacol Ther 41:443–460, 1989.

357. de Clerck LS, Dequeker J, Francx L, Demedts M: D-penicillamine therapy and interstitial lung disease in scleroderma: A long-term followup study. Arthritis Rheum 30:643–650, 1987.

358. Ekimoto H, Aikawa M, Ohnuki T, et al: Immunological involvement in pulmonary fibrosis induced by peplomycin. J Antibiot 38:94–98, 1985.

359. Hostettler C, Amundson D, O'Connor S: Phenytoin hypersensitivity with pulmonary involvement in a hemophiliac patient with human immunodeficiency virus infection. Drug Intell Clin Pharm 21:875–876, 1987.

360. Feinberg L, Travis WD, Ferrans V, et al: Pulmonary fibrosis associated with tocainide: Report of a case with literature review. Am Rev Respir Dis 41:505–508, 1990.

361. Kraus T, Schaller KH, Angerer J, Letzel S: Aluminium dust-induced lung disease in the pyro-powder-producing industry: Detection by high-resolution computed tomography. Int Arch Occup Environ Health 73:61–64, 2000.

362. Nishimura SL, Broaddus VC: Asbestos-induced pleural disease. Clin Chest Med 19:311–329, 1998.

363. Chanana A, Sharma OP: Pulmonary involvement in unusual multisystem disorders. Curr Opin Pulm Med 3:384–390, 1997.

364. Gautrin D, Auburtin G, Alluin F, et al: Recognition and progression of coal workers' pneumoconiosis in the collieries of northern France. Exp Lung Res 20:395–410, 1994.

365. Takahashi T, Satoh M, Satoh H: Unilateral acute exacerbation of pulmonary fibrosis in association with Sjogren's syndrome. Intern Med 35:811–814, 1996.

366. Forrest ME, Skerker LB, Nemiroff MJ: Hard metal pneumoconiosis: another cause of diffuse interstitial fibrosis. Radiology 128:609–612, 1978.

367. Duong TX, Suruda AJ, Maier LA: Interstitial fibrosis following hydrogen sulfide exposure. Am J Ind Med 40:221–224, 2001.

368. Skyberg K, Ronneberg A, Christensen CC, et al: Lung function and radiographic signs of pulmonary fibrosis in oil exposed workers in a cable manufacturing company: A follow up study. Br J Ind Med 49:309–315, 1992.

369. Emad A, Rezaian GR: The diversity of the effects of sulfur mustard gas inhalation on respiratory system 10 years after a single, heavy exposure: Analysis of 197 cases. Chest 112:734–738, 1997.

370. Papiris SA, Maniati MA, Kyriakidis V, Constantopoulos SH: Pulmonary damage due to paraquat poisoning through skin absorption. Respiration 62:101–103, 1995.

371. Ringden O, Baryd I, Johansson B, et al: Increased mortality by septicemia, interstitial pneumonitis and pulmonary fibrosis among bone marrow transplant recipients receiving an increased mean dose rate of total irradiation. Acta Radiol Oncol 22:423–428, 1983.

372. Archer VE, Renzetti AD, Doggett RS, et al: Chronic diffuse interstitial fibrosis of the lung in uranium miners. J Occup Envron Med 40:460–474, 1998.

373. Bissonnette E, Rola-Pleszczynski M: Pulmonary inflammation and fibrosis in a murine model of asbestosis and silicosis: Possible role of tumor necrosis factor. Inflammation 13:329–339, 1989.

374. Martin C, Papazian L, Payan MJ, et al: Pulmonary fibrosis correlates with outcome in adult respiratory distress syndrome: A study in mechanically ventilated patients. Chest 107:196–200, 1995.

375. Davies D: Ankylosing spondylitis and lung fibrosis. QJM 41:395–417, 1972.

376. Nagai S, Kitaichi M, Itoh H, et al: Idiopathic nonspecific interstitial pneumonia/fibrosis: Comparison with idiopathic pulmonary fibrosis and BOOP. Eur Respir J 12:1010–1019, 1998.

377. Chow SK, Yeap SS: Amyopathic dermatomyositis and pulmonary fibrosis. Clin Rheumatol 19:484–485, 2000.

378. Davies BH, Tuddenham EG: Familial pulmonary fibrosis associated with oculocutaneous albinism and platelet function defect: A new syndrome. QJM 45:219–232, 1976.

379. O'Brien AA, Moore DP, Keogh JA: Pulmonary berylliosis on corticosteroid therapy, with cavitating lung lesions and aspergillomata—report on a fatal case. Postgrad Med J 63:797–799, 1987.

380. Parr LH: Hamman-Rich syndrome: Idiopathic pulmonary interstitial fibrosis of the lung. J Natl Med Assoc 61:8–12, 1969.

381. Murayama J, Yoshizawa Y, Ohtsuka M, Hasegawa S: Lung fibrosis in hypersensitivity pneumonitis: Association with CD4+ but not CD8+ cell dominant alveolitis and insidious onset. Chest 104:38–43, 1993.

382. Gross TJ, Hunninghake GW: Idiopathic pulmonary fibrosis. N Engl J Med 345:517–525, 2001.

383. Wiener-Kronish JP, Solinger AM, Warnock ML, et al: Severe pulmonary involvement in mixed connective tissue disease. Am Rev Respir Dis 124:499–503, 1981.

384. Lok SS, Egan JJ: Viruses and idiopathic pulmonary fibrosis. Monaldi Arch Chest Dis 55:146–150, 2000.

385. Buschman DL, Ballard R: Progressive massive fibrosis associated with idiopathic pulmonary hemosiderosis. Chest 104:293–295, 1993.

386. Gochuico BR: Potential pathogenesis and clinical aspects of pulmonary fibrosis associated with rheumatoid arthritis. Am J Med Sci 321:83–88, 2001.

387. Abehsera M, Valeyre D, Grenier P, et al: Sarcoidosis with pulmonary fibrosis: CT patterns and correlation with pulmonary function. AJR Am J Roentgenol 174:1751–1757, 2000.

388. Richards AJ, Talbot IC, Swinson DR, Hamilton EB: Diffuse pulmonary fibrosis and bilateral pneumothoraces in systemic lupus erythematosus. Postgrad Med J 51:851–855, 1975.

389. Bresser P, Jansen HM, Weller FR, et al: T-cell activation in the lungs of patients with systemic sclerosis and its relation with pulmonary fibrosis. Chest 120:66S–68S, 2001.

390. Freedman MH, Grisaru D, Olivieri N, et al: Pulmonary syndrome in patients with thalassemia major receiving intravenous deferoxamine infusions. Am J Dis Child 144:565–569, 1990.

391. Thompson RN, Grennan DM: Acebutolol induced hypersensitivity pneumonitis. BMJ 286:894, 1983.

392. Holoye PY, Luna MA, MacKay B, Bedrossian CW: Bleomycin hypersensitivity pneumonitis. Ann Intern Med 88:47–49, 1978.

393. Stephan WC, Parks RD, Tempest B: Acute hypersensitivity pneumonitis associated with carbamazepine therapy. Chest 74:463–464, 1978.

394. Lombard JN, Bonnotte B, Maynadie M, et al: Celiprolol pneumonitis. Eur Respir J 6:588–591, 1993.

395. Benning TB: Clozapine-induced extrinsic allergic alveolitis. Br J Psychiatry 173:440–441, 1998.

396. Roelofs PM, Klinkhamer PJ, Gooszen HC: Hypersensitivity pneumonitis probably caused by cyclosporine: A case report. Respir Med 92:1368–1370, 1998.

397. Matusiewicz SP, Wallace WA, Crompton GK: Hypersensitivity pneumonitis associated with co-proxamol (paracetamol + dextropropoxyphene) therapy. Postgrad Med J 75:475–476, 1999.

398. Behrens GM, Stoll M, Schmidt RE: Pulmonary hypersensitivity reaction induced by efavirenz. Lancet 357:1503–1504, 2001.

399. Agarwal R, Sharma SK, Malaviya AN: Gold-induced hypersensitivity pneumonitis in a patient with rheumatoid arthritis. Clin Exp Rheumatol 7:89–90, 1989.

400. Liebhaber MI, Wright RS, Gelberg HJ, et al: Polymyalgia, hypersensitivity pneumonitis and other reactions in patients receiving HMG-CoA reductase inhibitors: a report of ten cases. Chest 115:886–889, 1999.

401. Sandhu HS, Barnes PJ, Hernandez P: Hydroxyurea-induced hypersensitivity pneumonitis: A case report and literature review. Can Respir J 7:491–495, 2000.

402. Sviri S, Gafanovich I, Kramer MR, et al: Mesalamine-induced hypersensitivity pneumonitis: A case report and review of the literature. J Clin Gastroenterol 24:34–36, 1997.

403. Cron RQ, Sherry DD, Wallace CA: Methotrexate-induced hypersensitivity pneumonitis in a child with juvenile rheumatoid arthritis. J Pediatr 132:901–902, 1998.

404. Kloppenburg M, Dijkmans BA, Breedveld FC: Hypersensitivity pneumonitis during minocycline treatment. Neth J Med 44:210–213, 1994.

405. Dan M, Aderka D, Topilsky M, et al: Hypersensitivity pneumonitis induced by nalidixic acid. Arch Intern Med 146:1423–1424, 1986.

406. Akoun GM, Liote HA, Liote F, et al: Provocation test coupled with bronchoalveolar lavage in diagnosis of drug (nilutamide)-induced hypersensitivity pneumonitis. Chest 97:495–498, 1990.

407. Holmberg L, Boman G, Bottiger LE, et al: Adverse reactions to nitrofurantoin: Analysis of 921 reports. Am J Med 69:733–738, 1980.

408. Kumar A, Bhat A, Gupta DK, et al: D-penicillamine-induced acute hypersensitivity pneumonitis and cholestatic hepatitis in a patient with rheumatoid arthritis. Clin Exp Rheumatol 3:337–339, 1985.

409. de Hoyos A, Holness DL, Tarlo SM: Hypersensitivity pneumonitis and airways hyperreactivity induced by occupational exposure to penicillin. Chest 103:303–304, 1993.

410. Benard A, Melloni B, Gosselin B, et al: Perindopril-associated pneumonitis. Eur Respir J 9:1314–316, 1996.

411. Munn NJ, Baughman RP, Ploysongsang Y, et al: Bronchoalveolar lavage in acute drug-hypersensitivity pneumonitis probably caused by phenytoin. South Med J 77:1594–1596, 1984.

412. Brooks BJ, Hendler NB, Alvarez S, et al: Delayed life-threatening pneumonitis secondary to procarbazine. Am J Clin Oncol 13:244–246, 1990.

413. Akoun GM, Milleron BJ, Mayaud CM, Tholoniat D: Provocation test coupled with bronchoalveolar lavage in diagnosis of propranolol-induced hypersensitivity pneumonitis. Am Rev Respir Dis 139:247–249, 1989.

414. Leino R, Liippo K, Ekfors T: Sulphasalazine-induced reversible hypersensitivity pneumonitis and fatal fibrosing alveolitis: Report of two cases. J Intern Med 229:553–556, 1991.

415. Higgins T, Niklasson PM: Hypersensitivity pneumonitis induced by trimethoprim. BMJ 300:1344, 1990.

416. Johnson CL, Bernstein IL, Gallagher JS, et al: Familial hypersensitivity pneumonitis induced by *Bacillus subtilis*. Am Rev Respir Dis 122:339–348, 1980.

417. Baur X, Dexheimer E: Hypersensitivity pneumonitis concomitant with acute airway obstruction after exposure to hay dust. Respiration 46:354–361, 1984.

418. Vincken W, Roels P: Hypersensitivity pneumonitis due to *Aspergillus fumigatus* in compost. Thorax 39:74–75, 1984.

419. Suda T, Sato A, Ida M, et al: Hypersensitivity pneumonitis associated with home ultrasonic humidifiers. Chest 107:711–717, 1995.

420. Hodgson MJ, Bracker A, Yang C, et al: Hypersensitivity pneumonitis in a metal-working environment. Am J Ind Med 39:616–628, 2001.

421. Woodard ED, Friedlander B, Lesher RJ, et al: Outbreak of hypersensitivity pneumonitis in an industrial setting. JAMA 259:1965–1969, 1988.

422. Campbell JA, Kryda MJ, Treuhaft MW, et al: Cheese worker's hypersensitivity pneumonitis. Am Rev Respir Dis 127:495–496, 1983.

423. Dykewicz MS, Laufer P, Patterson R, et al: Woodman's disease: Hypersensitivity pneumonitis from cutting live trees. J Allergy Clin Immunol 81:455–460, 1988.

424. Nimkin K, Oates E: Gallium-67 lung uptake in extrinsic hypersensitivity pneumonitis. Clin Nucl Med 14:451–452, 1989.

425. Orriols R, Manresa JM, Aliaga JL, et al: Mollusk shell hypersensitivity pneumonitis. Ann Intern Med 113:80–81, 1990.

426. Carroll KB, Pepys J, Longbottom JL, et al: Extrinsic allergic alveolitis due to rat serum proteins. Clin Allergy 5:443–456, 1975.

427. Mitsuhashi M, Tamura H, Morikawa A, Kuroume T: A unique substance from the granary weevil: Nonspecific immunoglobulin binding substance. Int Arch Allergy Appl Immunol 72:310–315, 1983.

428. Migliori M, Mosconi G, Michetti G, et al: Hard metal disease: eight workers with interstitial lung fibrosis due to cobalt exposure. Sci Total Environ 150:187–196, 1994.

429. Carlson JE, Villaveces JW: Hypersensitivity pneumonitis due to pyrethrum: Report of a case. JAMA 237:1718–1719, 1977.

430. Evans WV, Seaton A: Hypersensitivity pneumonitis in a technician using Pauli's reagent. Thorax 34:767–770, 1979.

431. Tao Y, Sugiura T, Nakamura H, et al: Experimental lung injury induced by trimellitic anhydride inhalation on guinea pigs. Int Arch Allergy Appl Immunol 96:119–127, 1991.

432. Ameille J, Brechot JM, Brochard P, et al: Occupational hypersensitivity pneumonitis in a smelter exposed to zinc fumes. Chest 101:862–863, 1992.

433. Liippo KK, Anttila SL, Taikina-Aho O, et al: Hypersensitivity pneumonitis and exposure to zirconium silicate in a young ceramic tile worker. Am Rev Respir Dis 148:1089–1092, 1993.

CHAPTER 28

Hematologic Syndromes: Hemolysis, Methemoglobinemia, and Sulfhemoglobinemia

Steven C. Curry

Three main syndromes result from erythrocytic oxidant stress. Removal of electrons from the protein portion of hemoglobin and other erythrocytic macromolecules leads to *oxidant hemolytic anemia*, characterized by Heinz bodies and bite cells. Removal of electrons from ferrous iron in hemoglobin produces *methemoglobinemia*. Lastly, oxidation of hemoglobin's porphyrin ring by sulfur results in *sulfhemoglobinemia*. The etiology, pathophysiology, occurrence, diagnosis, and treatment of oxidant-induced hemolytic anemia, methemoglobinemia, and sulfhemoglobinemia are entangled (Fig. 28-1).[1–3]

Some chemical agents responsible for oxidant hemolysis, methemoglobinemia, or sulfhemoglobinemia frequently lack oxidizing potential in vitro. Their ability to produce oxidant stress is explained most commonly, however, by electrophiles produced from metabolism by cytochrome P-450 enzymes. For example, dapsone, benzocaine, and some sulfonamides are metabolized to hydroxylamines that are responsible for producing oxidant stress.

The circulating red blood cell lacks mitochondria and depends on glycolysis and the hexose monophosphate shunt for energy production (Fig. 28-2). Adenosine triphosphate produced in glycolysis meets energy requirements, whereas glycolytic production of reduced nicotine adenine dinucleotide (NADH) is essential in maintaining methemoglobin fractions within the normal range. The hexose monophosphate shunt produces reduced nicotine adenine dinucleotide phosphate (NADPH), which is used to protect against oxidant-induced hemolysis.[4]

HEMOLYSIS

Pathophysiology and Etiology

Erythrocytes constantly encounter oxidant stress from multiple sources, including food, infection, oxygen, drugs, and chemicals. Oxidation of the protein portion of hemoglobin (i.e., removal of an electron from globin) results in denaturation and attachment of damaged protein to the internal cell membrane, which is visible as Heinz bodies with special staining of blood smears. Erythrocytes filled with denatured hemoglobin are trapped in the microcirculation of the spleen, where pieces of plasma membrane are removed (resulting in bite cells) or where entire red blood cells undergo destruction, producing extravascular hemolysis (nonspherocytic).[3,5] Oxidant stress may produce hemolysis by several additional mechanisms as well, including depletion of intracellular glu-

tathione stores with direct damage to the erythrocytic membrane and oxidation of other proteins, such as enzymes needed for erythrocyte integrity. Tremendous oxidant stress (e.g., chlorates) can produce intravascular hemolysis as well.

The erythrocyte protects itself from oxidant-induced hemolysis by reducing (donating electrons) oxidants before protein denaturation occurs.[4] Reduced glutathione, nonenzymatically and enzymatically with glutathione peroxidase, is responsible for most reducing capacity in this regard. Catalase also reduces hydrogen peroxide; ascorbate is a mild reducing agent (Fig. 28-3).

Adequate stores of reduced glutathione are maintained within the erythrocyte through the conversion of NADPH to NADP (see Fig. 28-2). NADPH formation requires a properly functioning hexose monophosphate shunt. Patients who display congenital deficiency of glucose-6-phosphate dehydrogenase (G6PD), the first enzyme in the hexose monophosphate shunt, can be predisposed to hemolysis from sources of oxidant stress that would not affect normal phenotypes. The most common sources of oxidant stress producing hemolysis in these patients are infection, drugs, and food. Oxidant hemolysis can be produced in anyone, however, if oxidant stress is severe enough, such as after overdose with numerous drugs (e.g., phenazopyridine, dapsone) (Table 28-1).

Logically, substances producing oxidant hemolysis share the ability to produce methemoglobinemia and sulfhemoglobinemia. Some agents are known better for producing hemolysis than accompanying dyshemoglobinemias, however. Naphthalene, an aromatic hydrocarbon, produces hemolysis[6] and less commonly is associated with severe methemoglobinemia. Chlorates[7] produce hemolysis but also can cause marked methemoglobinemia.

Clinical Presentation and Diagnosis

Other than the expected effects of acute anemia, complications of hemolysis include hyperkalemia and pigment nephropathy. Jaundice may appear after a few days. Methemoglobinemia and occasionally sulfhemoglobinemia commonly accompany Heinz body hemolytic anemia, and evidence for this should be sought.

Hemolysis is diagnosed by showing decreases in blood hemoglobin and serum haptoglobin concentrations and a rise in plasma free hemoglobin concentration. Hemoglobinuria results when plasma concentrations of hemoglobin increase

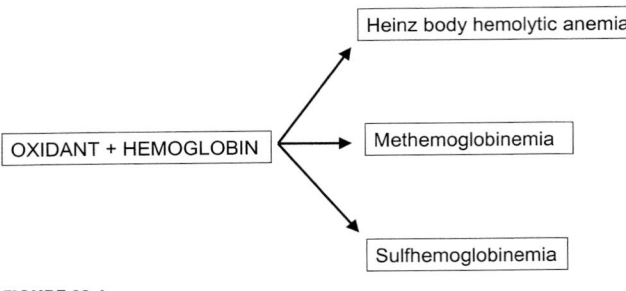

FIGURE 28-1

Consequences of erythrocytic oxidant stress.

high enough to saturate haptoglobin and turn plasma pink or red. In oxidant-induced disease, bite cells may be noted on routine Wright's stain of blood.[3] Heinz bodies can be detected with special staining, but they are not detectable with Wright's stain of blood. Spherocytes are typically absent or only mildly increased in number. Reticulocytosis is delayed for several days after onset of hemolysis.

Treatment

In general, treatment is supportive with blood transfusions, ensuring a brisk urine output, and monitoring for hyperkalemia. Specific therapies may be indicated with specific toxins (e.g., exchange transfusions for arsine; D-penicillamine for copper). Intravenous N-acetylcysteine prevented severe decreases in whole-blood glutathione concentration in cats with acetaminophen-induced methemoglobinemia,[8] and in vitro studies of human erythrocytes revealed that incubation in solutions containing N-acetylcysteine can prevent oxidant hemolysis produced by various agents.[9,10] No reports have shown N-acetylcysteine's effectiveness, however, at preventing or lessening oxidant hemolysis in humans with acute poisonings.

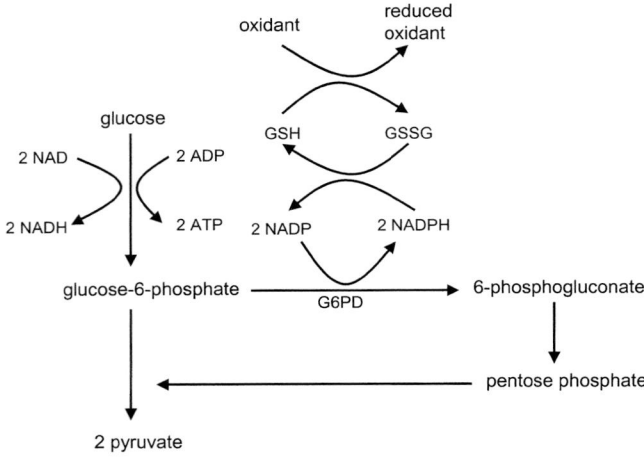

FIGURE 28-2

Erythrocytic energy production. ADP, adenosine diphosphate; ATP, adenosine triphosphate; G6PD, glucose-6-phosphate dehydrogenase; GSH, reduced glutathione; GSSG, oxidized glutathione; NAD, nicotinamide adenine dinucleotide; NADH, reduced nicotinamide adenine dinucleotide; NADP, nicotinamide adenine dinucleotide phosphate; NADPH, reduced nicotinamide adenine dinucleotide phosphate.

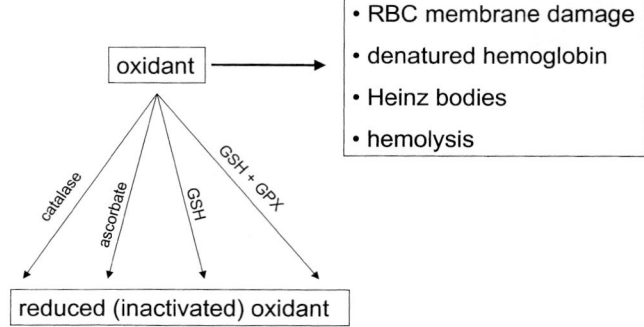

FIGURE 28-3

Protection against hemolysis by reduction of oxidants. GPX, glutathione peroxidase; GSH, reduced glutathione; RBC, red blood cell.

METHEMOGLOBINEMIA

Pathophysiology

Reduced hemoglobin (deoxyhemoglobin) contains four ferrous (Fe^{2+}) heme groups capable of binding and transporting oxygen. Oxidation to the ferric (Fe^{3+}) state produces methemoglobin. Oxidant stress produces denaturation of hemoglobin with hemolysis and methemoglobin, explaining the coexistence of both disorders in the same patient; (see Fig. 28-1).

Reduced (ferrous) hemoglobin continuously undergoes conversion to methemoglobin within erythrocytes, to a large extent from the oxidizing power of oxygen. Values for methemoglobin are reported most commonly in percentages (fractions). These fractions represent the percentage of all hemoglobin pigments present as methemoglobin. Methemoglobin fractions in whole blood normally are less than 1% to 2%. When fractions exceed this value, methemoglobinemia is said to be present. Hemoglobinemia refers to the presence of excess hemoglobin in plasma, whereas methemoglobinemia refers to elevated circulating fractions of methemoglobin within erythrocytes.

Methemoglobin does not transport oxygen. Ferric heme groups impair unloading of oxygen by ferrous heme on the same hemoglobin tetramer, shifting the oxygen-hemoglobin dissociation curve to the left.[4] Serious signs and symptoms from methemoglobinemia result from impaired oxygen delivery to tissues and from cyanosis, which can be seen before significant impairment of oxygenation.

Visible cyanosis is produced by 5 g of normal deoxyhemoglobin per 1 dL of capillary blood. Because methemoglobin is dark brown, however, only 1.5 g of methemoglobin/dL of blood is required to produce noticeable discoloration. In nonanemic patients, about 10% to 15% methemoglobinemia produces cyanosis without significant impairment of oxygen delivery. Progressive increases in methemoglobin fractions to 20% to 40% in nonanemic patients are accompanied by headache, dyspnea, tachypnea, tachycardia, and mild hypertension. Further increases in methemoglobin fractions into the 40% to 55% range (without anemia) may begin to produce confusion, lethargy, and metabolic acidosis. Additional increases result in coma, seizures, bradycardia, ventricular dysrhythmias, and hypotension; near 70% methemoglobinemia results in death. I have seen one nonanemic patient who

TABLE 28-1 Agents Producing Oxidant Stress*

Acetanilid	Dapsone	Monolinuron	Phenylhydroxylamine
Aminophenols	Diaminodiphenylsulfone	Mushrooms	Piperazine
p-Aminosalicylic acid	Dimethylamine	Naphthalene	Plasmoquine
Amyl nitrite	Dimethylaminophenol	Naphthylamine	Prilocaine‡
Aniline	Dimethylaniline	Nitrates	Primaquine
Anilinoethanol	Dimethyl sulfoxide	Nitric oxide	Propanil
Arsine†	Dimethyltoluidine	Nitrites	Pyridine
Benzocaine‡	Dinitrobenzene	Nitroalkanes	Pyrogallol
Bismuth subnitrate	Dinitrophenols	Nitroaniline	Quinones
Bromoaniline	Dinitrotoluene	Nitrobenzene	Resorcinol
Bupivacaine‡	Flutamide	Nitroethane	Riluzole
Chloramine	Hydrazines	Nitrofurans	Sodium nitrite‡
Chlorates†	Hydroquinone	Nitroglycerin	Sulfonamides
Chlorites	4′-Hydroxyacetanilid	Nitrophenol	Sulfones
Chloroanilines	Hydroxylamine	Pamaquine	Sulofenur
Chloroquine	Ifosfamide	Pendimethalin	Tetralin
Chromates†	Isobutyl nitrite	Phenacetin	Tetranitromethane tetronal
Clofazimine	Lidocaine‡	Phenazopyridine	Toluenediamine
Dichromates	Local anesthetics‡	Phenetidine	Toluidine
Cobalt preparations	Methylene blue	Phenols	Trichlorocarbanilide
Commercial inks	Metobromuron	p-Phenylenediamine	Trinitrotoluene
Copper sulfate†	Metoclopramide	Phenylhydrazine	Trional

*Poisoning (and sometimes therapeutic doses) by these agents variously produces combinations of Heinz body hemolytic anemia, methemoglobinemia, or sulfhemoglobinemia in individual patients. Why some patients develop methemoglobinemia, whereas others mainly develop sulfhemoglobinemia or hemolysis is not well understood.
†Known for producing extraordinarily severe hemolysis.
‡Hemolysis usually not significant after a single therapeutic dose, even when methemoglobinemia is present.

was awake with 73% methemoglobinemia who complained only of weakness and voices and noises sounding distant.

Anemic patients experience more severe impairment of oxygen delivery and more severe signs and symptoms at given methemoglobin fractions than nonanemic patients. Anemic patients exhibit less profound cyanosis, however, at given methemoglobin fractions.

Although inactivation of oxidants is the main mechanism by which oxidant hemolysis is prevented, oxidant inactivation remains relatively unimportant in maintaining methemoglobin fractions within the normal range. Patients with congenital glutathione deficiency, G6PD deficiency, catalase deficiency, and scurvy do not have elevated methemoglobin fractions. Rather, methemoglobin fractions are maintained at low levels by allowing methemoglobin to form, then immediately enzymatically reducing it back to ferrous hemoglobin.

Erythrocytic cytochrome-b_5 reductase accounts for virtually all normal methemoglobin reduction (Fig. 28-4).[11] In this process, electrons from NADH (produced in glycolysis) are used to reduce cytochrome b_5, which reduces methemoglobin to form ferrous hemoglobin. Normal enzymatic methemoglobin reduction requires an intact glycolytic pathway for NADH production, the presence of cytochrome b_5, and adequate activity of cytochrome-b_5 reductase. The normal rate of enzymatic methemoglobin reduction exceeds spontaneous background methemoglobin formation rate by several hundred–fold. Heterozygous erythrocytic cytochrome-b_5 reductase–deficient patients ordinarily

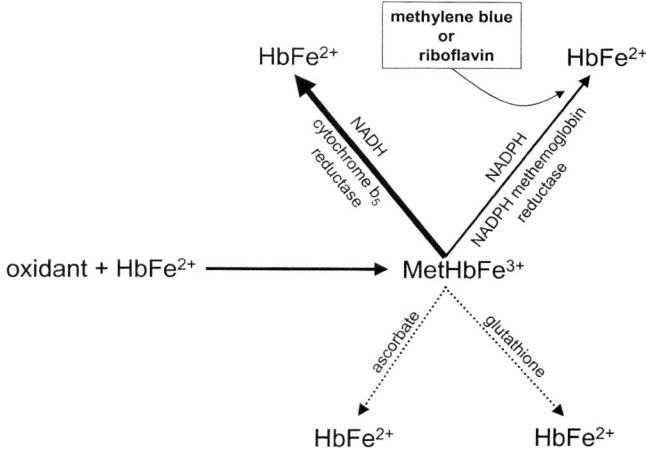

FIGURE 28-4

Mechanisms of maintaining low methemoglobin (MetHbFe^{3+}) fractions through MetHbFe^{3+} reduction. Significant MetHbFe^{3+} reduction in vivo occurs only through cytochrome-b_5 reductase, which uses reduced nicotine adenine dinucleotide (NADH) as a reducing agent. Methylene blue markedly enhances MetHbFe^{3+} reduction by acting as a cofactor for reduced nicotine adenine dinucleotide phosphate (NADPH) MetHbFe^{3+} reductase, an enzyme that normally plays no role in MetHbFe^{3+} reduction. Riboflavin can act like methylene blue and has been used in cases of congenital methemoglobinemia. Ascorbate and glutathione are responsible for a minority of MetHbFe^{3+} reduction in vitro but play an insignificant role in normal MetHbFe^{3+} reduction and are not known to be effective in treating methemoglobinemia. HbFe^{2+}, normal ferrous hemoglobin.

exhibit normal methemoglobin fractions but are predisposed to developing methemoglobinemia in response to oxidant stress. Patients homozygous for this deficiency have congenital methemoglobinemia.[11]

A second erythrocytic reducing enzyme, NADPH methemoglobin reductase, normally remains minimally active or completely inactive because of the absence of an electron transfer intermediate (e.g., cytochrome b_5) to serve as a cofactor for enzymatic methemoglobin reduction. Methylene blue is an acceptable electron acceptor/donor intermediate, however, and markedly accelerates NADPH methemoglobin reductase activity.[4] In this pathway (see Fig. 28-4), electrons are transferred from NADPH (produced in the hexose monophosphate shunt) to methylene blue to form leukomethylene blue. Leukomethylene blue donates an electron to methemoglobin to produce ferrous hemoglobin. Reduction of methemoglobin by this pathway requires an intact hexose monophosphate shunt; a cofactor, such as methylene blue; and normal activity of erythrocytic NADPH methemoglobin reductase. In vitro, some methemoglobin reduction can be shown by glutathione and ascorbate, but these are thought to be relatively minor in vivo. Ascorbate is not considered effective for treatment of acquired methemoglobinemia because of its slow action.

The predisposition of infants to methemoglobinemia is explained by normally low erythrocytic cytochrome-b_5 reductase activity and cytochrome b_5 concentrations. Oxidant stress resulting from gastroenteritis and other infections is the most common cause of acquired methemoglobinemia in this age group.[12,13]

Etiology

CONGENITAL CAUSES

Patients with homozygous deficiency for erythrocytic cytochrome-b_5 reductase have congenital methemoglobinemia and can be treated with oral methylene blue to lower methemoglobin fractions. In addition, several mutant hemoglobin species (hemoglobin M) in which the iron remains in the ferric form have been described. Most of these patients have congenital methemoglobinemia unresponsive to methylene blue. Rare mutant unstable hemoglobins undergo denaturation to produce congenital Heinz body hemolytic anemias; some of these also oxidize to form methemoglobin. These hemoglobins would be expected to produce disease before adulthood.[5,11]

ACQUIRED CAUSES

Most cases of methemoglobinemia in adults and nonneonates are acquired, resulting from exposure to chemical agents (see Table 28-1). One of the most common causes is benzocaine, which is metabolized to a methemoglobin-producing agent. Methemoglobinemia resulting from topical benzocaine spray used to perform transesophageal echocardiograms, endotracheal intubations, bronchoscopies, or other endoscopic procedures has been described repeatedly in the literature.[14,15] The use of benzocaine-containing teething ointments and hemorrhoidal creams also has produced methemoglobinemia in some patients, even after therapeutic doses. Prilocaine is the second local anesthetic most closely associated with methemoglobinemia, but methemoglobinemia has resulted from

many anesthetics, including lidocaine and bupivacaine.[16,17] Methemoglobinemia usually follows overdose of phenazopyridine (Pyridium) or dapsone and occasionally results from therapeutic use. A plethora of additional prescription drugs have been associated with methemoglobinemia; examples are valproate,[18] clofazimine,[19] flutamide,[20] and ifosfamide.[21] Oral overdoses with nitroglycerin and organic nitrates (which are esters of nitrite) and therapeutic doses of intravenous nitroglycerin are well known to produce methemoglobinemia.[22]

The conversion of nitrates to nitrites by bacteria in the upper gastrointestinal tract has produced fatal methemoglobinemia in infants who ingest well water high in nitrate concentrations—so-called well-water methemoglobinemia.[23] Nitrite contamination of public drinking water also explained a large outbreak of methemoglobinemia.[24] Methemoglobinemia results from the recreational use of inhalational nitrites (e.g., isobutyl nitrite) and from ingestion of meat containing excessive amounts of sodium nitrite as a preservative.[25] Topical contact with aniline dyes found in printing ink on diapers, leather dyes in new shoes, and commercial marking crayons has produced methemoglobinemia and death.[4] The ingestion of nitroethane, found in some over-the-counter fingernail products, produces methemoglobinemia.[26]

As expected, most agents producing methemoglobinemia also produce oxidant-induced hemolysis, and both disorders commonly coexist in the same patient. Hemolysis can be extraordinarily severe after poisonings by chlorates, arsine, stibine, and chromates. Methemoglobinemia resulting from local anesthetics usually is unaccompanied by serious hemolysis.

Diagnosis

The use of multiwavelength cooximetry allows for the diagnosis of methemoglobinemia. Modern cooximeters measure the absorption of multiple wavelengths of ultraviolet light by blood and calculate concentrations of oxyhemoglobin, reduced hemoglobin, methemoglobin, and carboxyhemoglobin. Because cooximetry determines methemoglobin concentrations by measuring absorption of light, substances that interfere with light absorption can produce false results on some cooximeters, depending on the model. Hyperlipemia, such as that seen after the infusion of lipid emulsions or in patients with diabetes mellitus, has resulted in reporting of falsely elevated methemoglobin fractions.[27] Cooximetry may be unreliable for several minutes immediately after a dose of methylene blue.[28] As discussed later, sulfhemoglobin is handled in various ways, depending on the specific instrument, but some cooximeters cannot differentiate between sulfhemoglobin and methemoglobin, reporting elevated methemoglobin fractions in both instances.

Other diagnostic clues commonly lead to the presumed diagnosis of methemoglobinemia before cooximetry is considered. Generalized cyanosis in the presence of a normal arterial PO_2 usually represents methemoglobinemia. As expected, cyanosis from methemoglobinemia persists despite oxygen therapy. Patients with significant methemoglobinemia may exhibit chocolate-colored or abnormally dark blood. When methemoglobin fractions exceed 10% to 15% in a nonanemic patient, a drop of blood allowed to dry on filter paper appears noticeably brown compared with venous blood from a normal person.[29] Many blood gas instruments do not measure percent hemoglobin saturation but report a calculated value derived from the PO_2 and pH. This calculated saturation represents what the saturation should be in the absence of abnormal hemoglobin pigments. In methemoglobinemia, the true percent saturation as determined by cooximetry is lower than the calculated percent saturation as reported by many blood gas instruments. The difference between the calculated and measured saturation is termed the *saturation gap* and normally is less than 3% to 5% in arterial blood. Large saturation gaps in arterial blood almost always result from methemoglobin or carboxyhemoglobin and less commonly result from sulfhemoglobin.

Pulse oximetry neither accurately nor reliably measures percent saturation in the presence of methemoglobinemia.[30] Depending on the true oxygen saturation, pulse oximetry may read falsely low or falsely high. The most common response to methemoglobinemia is that pulse oximeters read falsely high saturations, although reported saturations may decrease below the normal range. When the diagnosis of methemoglobinemia has been made, the pulse oximeter should be removed from the patient so that medical personnel cannot be misled by unreliable readings.

Methemoglobinemia does not change measurement of total blood hemoglobin concentration by the clinical laboratory. Methemoglobin fractions commonly increase after death. Postmortem methemoglobin concentrations do not reliably reflect antemortem methemoglobinemia.[31]

Differential Diagnosis

Arterial PO_2, in the absence of other causes of hypoxemia, is normal in methemoglobinemia, distinguishing abnormal coloration from hypoxia. The cyanosis from methemoglobinemia does not respond to oxygen therapy.

Patients with sulfide poisoning have been reported to exhibit an unusual, poorly characterized discoloration of skin and other organs, mainly as a postmortem finding. Rare cases of tellurium exposures have produced blue discoloration. Some patients with severe cyanide toxicity exhibit cyanosis, and many other signs and symptoms of cyanide poisoning would be similar to signs and symptoms of methemoglobinemia. Normal arterial PO_2 and increased saturation gaps also characterize carbon monoxide poisoning and sulfhemoglobinemia, and some cooximeters measure and report sulfhemoglobin as methemoglobin. Skin discoloration from dermal contact with new blue clothing or blue towels has been confused with methemoglobinemia, but this discoloration is removed with washing the skin. Excessive administration of methylene blue can produce skin discoloration that may be confused with continuing methemoglobinemia or cyanosis from other causes.

Treatment

Patients should receive oxygen to maximize oxygen carrying capacity of remaining normal hemoglobin. Blood should be drawn to screen for hemolysis (hemoglobin, blood smear, Heinz body stain, plasma free hemoglobin, serum haptoglobin), for arterial blood gases and cooximetry, and for routine laboratory studies. An electrocardiogram may help exclude myocardial ischemia.

ASYMPTOMATIC PATIENTS

Some patients with methemoglobinemia exhibit cyanosis but lack other signs and symptoms and do not require specific treatment. After exposure to the offending agent ends, methemoglobin levels usually return to normal within 36 hours with some exceptions (e.g., dapsone, nitroethane). Most of these patients require admission to the hospital, however, to follow them clinically for worsening signs and symptoms, to monitor for onset of hemolysis, and to follow serial methemoglobin fractions. Assuming normal hemoglobin concentrations, asymptomatic patients usually exhibit methemoglobin fractions between 10% and 15%.

SYMPTOMATIC PATIENTS

Patients who are symptomatic from methemoglobinemia (e.g., tachycardia, dyspnea, headache) should be considered for specific antidotal therapy with methylene blue, in the absence of a history of G6PD deficiency (see later). Parenteral methylene blue should be given intravenously over 3 to 5 minutes at an initial dose of 2 mg/kg (0.2 mL/kg of a 1% solution). Resolution of cyanosis usually occurs within 15 to 25 minutes. If the patient is seriously symptomatic and no response occurs within 15 minutes, or if the patient remains moderately symptomatic without any improvement for 30 to 60 minutes, repeat doses of 1 mg/kg (0.1 mL/kg of a 1% solution) should be given. If methemoglobin levels are readily available, repeat determinations of methemoglobin fractions should be performed before repeat dosing of methylene blue because large doses of methylene blue produce discoloration of skin. The total amount of methylene blue given during the first few hours generally should not exceed 5 to 7 mg/kg. Intraosseous infusion of methylene blue has been described when intravenous access cannot be obtained.[32]

Patients with methemoglobinemia always should be closely followed for evidence of hemolysis because the latter is common whether or not patients receive methylene blue. Hemolysis may be clinically apparent on presentation or, most commonly, appears 2 to 3 days after admission and after methemoglobin fractions have decreased.

Some toxins are known for producing methemoglobinemia that is refractory or only partially responsive to methylene blue therapy. In most instances, this situation results from the inability of methemoglobin reduction, even in the presence of methylene blue, to keep up with profound oxidant stress. Examples of these toxins include aniline, nitrobenzene, and chlorates.[7,33,34]

Some methemoglobin-producing toxins possess long half-lives and produce prolonged methemoglobinemia. Dapsone produces methemoglobinemia and hemolysis lasting for days.[35,36] In these cases, it may be necessary to administer methylene blue as a continuous infusion. Methylene blue is dissolved in the crystalloid of choice and, based only on case reports, started at 0.1 mg/kg/hr (0.01 mL/kg/hr of a 1% methylene blue solution),[35] although personal experience indicates that higher rates may be required at times. It is important to follow serial methemoglobin fractions and total hemoglobin concentrations.

Most methylene blue is excreted unchanged by the kidneys. Although patients with renal insufficiency do not require changes in initial methylene blue doses, they should receive lower continuous infusion doses of the drug based on creatinine clearance. No specific guidelines for dosing in renal failure patients have been developed.

Methylene blue should not be given to patients with *known* G6PD deficiency. These patients have low red blood cell NADPH concentrations, impairing augmentation of NADPH methemoglobin reductase by methylene blue.[37] Methylene blue triggers hemolysis in patients with G6PD deficiency, which would impair oxygen delivery further.[2,38] Methylene blue should never be withheld from symptomatic patients, however, simply because a history of G6PD deficiency cannot be excluded.

Large doses of methylene blue in normal volunteers have been associated with dysuria, substernal chest pain, nausea, tachycardia, hypertension, and anxiety. In my experience, however, patients with methemoglobinemia do not voice or experience these effects from methylene blue. Urine initially turns blue, then green. Although authors have cautioned that methylene blue paradoxically may increase methemoglobin fractions when given in large doses (e.g., 5 mg/kg over 35 to 70 minutes),[39] this has not been thought to be a significant problem in humans receiving recommended doses. This phenomenon has been attributed largely to results of in vitro studies during hypoxic conditions.[40,41] Worsening hemolysis also has been alleged after methylene blue therapy, even in patients with normal G6PD activity, but these allegations mainly arise from case reports in which hemolysis was expected from the agent producing methemoglobinemia,[42] making causal relationships unclear.

Fetuses and newborns seem to be sensitive to hemolytic actions of methylene blue. Intraamniotic injections of methylene blue, sometimes using large doses, have been associated with delivery of newborns with Heinz body hemolytic anemia. Hemolysis also has been reported in newborns receiving methylene blue through feeding tubes.[43,44] Reports of newborns with methemoglobinemia after intraamniotic injection of methylene blue[45] could reflect a peculiar susceptibility of neonates, the effects of a large relative dose of methylene blue, or in utero hypoxic conditions favoring methylene blue–induced oxidant stress in the fetus. Regardless of these concerns, the administration of methylene blue to a symptomatic patient with methemoglobinemia has never been proved to worsen methemoglobinemia.

Cimetidine has been used to help control methemoglobinemia from dapsone. Cimetidine inhibits cytochrome P-450 conversion of dapsone to the oxidizing metabolite responsible for methemoglobinemia, dapsone hydroxylamine. In patients receiving 1200 mg/day of cimetidine orally while taking therapeutic doses of dapsone, circulating methemoglobin fractions decreased by an average of 25%.[46] There are no studies describing the efficacy of cimetidine after dapsone overdose. Ascorbic acid works slowly and generally is considered ineffective for treatment of acute acquired methemoglobinemia.[4]

Riboflavin also can accept electrons from NADPH methemoglobin reductase and enhance methemoglobin reduction in a manner similar to that of methylene blue. Although endogenous riboflavin concentrations are not high enough to account for significant methemoglobin reduction, large oral doses (e.g., 60 to 100 mg/day) have been used successfully in patients with congenital methemoglobinemia.[47,48] The safety and efficacy of intravenous or oral riboflavin for the treatment of acquired acute methemoglobinemia has not been described.

Incubation of erythrocytes in high concentrations of *N*-acetylcysteine seems to enhance methemoglobin reduction.[49] These concentrations of *N*-acetylcysteine cannot be achieved safely in humans, however, and a randomized controlled trial found that conventional doses of intravenous *N*-acetylcysteine was ineffective in reducing nitrite-induced methemoglobin fractions in human volunteers.[50]

It is important always to monitor total oxygen carrying capacity by following total hemoglobin concentrations, methemoglobin fractions, and true percent saturation of oxyhemoglobin. A decrease in methemoglobin fraction from 25% to 15% would result in worsened oxygen delivery if accompanying hemolysis has resulted in a decrease of the hemoglobin concentration from 15 g/dL to 5 g/dL. In addition, the development of anemia alone may result in resolution of cyanosis despite worsening of oxygen delivery, without a decrease in methemoglobin fractions. In most persons, 15% methemoglobinemia with a hemoglobin concentration of 15 g/dL would produce visible cyanosis, whereas 20% methemoglobinemia in patients with a hemoglobin concentration of 5 g/dL produces no visible discoloration, yet may be lethal. Interpreting disappearance of cyanosis to mean that the patient has improved must be done with caution.

After initial signs and symptoms of methemoglobinemia have been addressed, routine gastrointestinal and skin decontamination should be performed as indicated. If the clinician chooses to use ascorbic acid in treating methemoglobinemia, a recommended dose has been 0.5 to 1 g of ascorbic acid given every 6 hours intravenously or orally.[4]

FAILURE TO RESPOND TO METHYLENE BLUE

When patients with methemoglobinemia do not improve with methylene blue therapy, several possibilities should be considered (Table 28-2). First, exposure to large amounts of drugs or chemicals can produce methemoglobin at rates greater than reducing capacity, even with methylene blue therapy. When methemoglobin fractions do not return to normal because of continued methemoglobin formation, methylene blue therapy almost always results in at least a transient decrease in methemoglobin fractions. As noted earlier, recurrent methemoglobinemia is common after exposure to etiologic agents with long half-lives. Second, patients who do not respond to methylene blue also may be suffering from unrecognized G6PD deficiency. Third, patients with congenital NADPH methemoglobin reductase

---

TABLE 28-2 Possible Explanations When Methemoglobinemia Fails to Respond to Methylene Blue

Overwhelming oxidant stress from ingestant or toxin
G6PD deficiency
NADPH methemoglobin reductase deficiency
Sulfhemoglobinemia
Blue skin discoloration from other sources
Hypoxemia (recheck arterial PO_2)

G6PD, glucose-6-phosphate dehydrogenase; NADPH, reduced nicotinamide adenine dinucleotide phosphate.

deficiency also fail to respond to methylene blue.[4] Fourth, sulfhemoglobinemia can be mistaken for methemoglobinemia (see later). Fifth, repeated doses or large doses of methylene blue produce blue skin coloration that may be mistaken for methemoglobinemia.[51]

For patients who cannot receive or fail to respond to methylene blue, treatment options are limited. Blood transfusions and exchange transfusions[34] have been used and suggested whenever refractory methemoglobin fractions approach 70% in nonanemic patients. Hyperbaric oxygen can be a temporizing measure that provides adequate oxygen delivery during preparation of blood transfusions. Oxygen toxicity limits the amount of time a patient can stay in a hyperbaric chamber, however. Oral riboflavin could be given (60 to 100 mg/day divided into three doses), but its efficacy is unknown in this setting, and it would not be expected to be effective in patients with G6PD deficiency. Intravenous ascorbic acid (500 mg) also can be given,[4] although it is stated that it works too slowly to be helpful for acquired methemoglobinemia.

SULFHEMOGLOBIN

Background and Characteristics

Sulfhemoglobin is a green molecule in which a sulfur atom has been incorporated into the porphyrin ring of hemoglobin.[52] Sulfhemoglobin cannot transport oxygen. No significant circulating sulfhemoglobin normally exists, but sulfhemoglobin fractions increase in some persons in response to oxidant stress. In contrast to methemoglobin, sulfhemoglobin persists for the life of the erythrocyte and does not undergo conversion back to hemoglobin. Only 0.5 g/dL of sulfhemoglobin produces slate-gray cyanosis (e.g., approximately 3% sulfhemoglobin in a patient with a total hemoglobin concentration of 16 g/L).

Although sulfhemoglobin cannot transport oxygen, additional factors usually prevent serious impairment of oxygen delivery in nonanemic patients. During sulfhemoglobinemia, hemoglobin tetramers usually contain only one or two sulfurated heme isomers, preventing extremely elevated sulfhemoglobin fractions. Sulfurated heme moieties in hemoglobin shift unaffected heme moieties toward the unliganded confirmation, reducing oxygen affinity of normal heme subunits and shifting the oxygen-hemoglobin dissociation curve to the right, which enhances oxygen delivery to tissues and partially ameliorates the effects of reduced oxygen binding capacity.[53] In contrast, methemoglobin and carboxyhemoglobin shift the dissociation curve to the left, compounding impaired oxygen delivery to tissues.

Sulfhemoglobin, methemoglobin, and hemoglobin M possess similar light absorption spectra. This fact prevented many early authors from distinguishing among these three pigments. Some multiwavelength cooximeters today report sulfhemoglobin as methemoglobin. In addition, early studies of "sulfhemoglobinemia" from hydrogen sulfide mixed with blood in vitro may have represented nothing more than a mixture of oxidized, denatured hemoglobin pigments that were unrelated to what is termed sulfhemoglobin today.[54] Readers must interpret cautiously confusing older medical literature on reports of sulfhemoglobinemia, which has been suggested to be better termed *pseudosulfhemoglobin*.[55] These articles might represent true reports of sulfhemoglobinemia, methemoglobinemia, hemoglobin M disease, various species of denatured hemoglobin from hydrogen sulfide mixed with blood in vitro, combinations of the aforementioned, or perhaps other chemical compounds.

Formation and Etiology

Agents that produce sulfhemoglobinemia (see Table 28-1) usually are known better for their ability to produce methemoglobinemia and hemolysis. Methemoglobinemia and sulfhemoglobinemia have followed exposures to metoclopramide,[56,57] flutamide,[20,58] dapsone,[59] and phenazopyridine.[60] Methemoglobinemia, sulfhemoglobinemia, and especially hemolysis may coexist in the same patient.[59] Why exposure to the same substance produces sulfhemoglobinemia in one person, methemoglobinemia in another, and both in another person remains unknown.

Sulfhemoglobin forms when elemental sulfur binds to the β-pyrrole ring of the heme moiety, where it persists for the life of the erythrocyte.[52] Although early authors suggested that the sulfur responsible for oxidizing hemoglobin was found in the etiologic chemical, many drugs that produce sulfhemoglobinemia do not contain sulfur. It also was an older belief that vague gastrointestinal dysfunction alone produced hemolytic anemia, sulfhemoglobinemia, and methemoglobinemia from the presumed absorption of endogenously produced nitrites and sulfides—so-called enterogenous cyanosis. Evidence indicates, however, that patients with enterogenous cyanosis were ingesting surreptitiously analgesics known to cause such disorders.[61]

Animal studies suggest that sulfur from intestinal bacterial metabolism in combination with oxidant stress from various agents might be responsible for sulfhemoglobin formation. Rats with jejunal pouches that received phenacetin were more likely to develop sulfhemoglobinemia than controls; neomycin prevented phenacetin-induced sulfhemoglobin formation.[62] Neomycin use for treatment of sulfhemoglobinemia in humans has been described in case reports.[63]

Diagnosis

In early attempts to clarify what was being measured when "sulfhemoglobin" was reported to be present, Micel and Harris[64] reported that the addition of cyanide or dithionite (hydrosulfite) to blood eliminated the spectral absorption of methemoglobin immediately, whereas the spectral absorption of sulfhemoglobin remained. This simple test did not exclude hemoglobin M (or perhaps other oxidation products of hemoglobin), however, which also remains after addition of these compounds. Carrico and colleagues[65] reported that carbon monoxide would bind to sulfhemoglobin to produce carbonmonoxysulfhemoglobin, a compound with a down-field shift, whereas neither methemoglobin nor hemoglobin M bound carbon monoxide. Light absorption in the presence of cyanide (or dithionite) and carbon monoxide served for several years as laboratory tools to measure "sulfhemoglobin" fractions and concentrations, although it is not known confidently exactly what species always was being measured. Park and Nagel[53] reported that electrophoresis with isoelectric focusing reliably delineates the three pigments, and isoelectric focusing generally serves as the gold standard today, although various methods of analysis (e.g., gas chromatography, manual spectrophotometry) are used at reference laboratories.

Results from isoelectric focusing, manual spectrophotometric analysis, or other reference methods do not return for hours to days, whereas multiwavelength cooximetry results are available within minutes in most intensive care units. Different brands of cooximeters and various models from the same manufacturer vary in how they handle sulfhemoglobin.[66] The IL 282 and IL 482 (Instrumentation Laboratory, Inc, Lexington, MA) do not distinguish between methemoglobin and sulfhemoglobin and report sulfhemoglobin as methemoglobin.[57,58,67] Zwart and colleagues[68] showed that a reported methemoglobin fraction greater than 10% in combination with a negative carboxyhemoglobin fraction on these instruments suggests that at least some sulfhemoglobin is present. Conversely the IL 682 is said to indicate sulfhemoglobin fractions greater than 1.5%.[67] The Chiron Rapidlab 865 (Bayer Diagnostics, Tarrytown, NY) reports a sulfhemoglobin fraction as being greater than 1.5% but does not quantify the concentration.[69] Wu and Kenny[70] noted that Radiometer's OSM3 cooximeter reports falsely elevated oxygen saturations in the presence of sulfhemoglobinemia, unless the blood specimen is analyzed with a service program configuration that can be activated only by a company representative. The intensivist must be familiar with how his or her particular cooximeter handles and reports sulfhemoglobin (if at all) and sometimes must remain skeptical of claims made by a manufacturer regarding ability to detect and quantify sulfhemoglobin accurately.

Few data exist on accuracy of pulse oximetry in the presence of sulfhemoglobinemia. I have seen one woman with slate-gray cyanosis and 18.6% sulfhemoglobin (total hemoglobin 9 g/dL) whose pulse oximeter read in the 60% range despite an elevated arterial PO_2 and absent methemoglobin (true saturation about 81%). Aravindhan and Chisholm[69] described a 48-year-old woman with an arterial PO_2 of 99 mm Hg, 28% sulfhemoglobinemia, and a pulse oximeter reading of 85% (true saturation about 72%). Langford and Sheikh[71] noted a pulse oximeter reading of 92% to 94% saturation with a sulfhemoglobin fraction of 16% (true saturation about 84%).

Clinical Presentation

The diagnosis of sulfhemoglobinemia usually is considered when confronted with a cyanotic or slate-gray patient who has a normal PO_2. Depending on the cooximeter being used, methemoglobin fractions may be reported as normal, or methemoglobin fractions may be reported as elevated and remain so after methylene blue therapy (other causes of this scenario were described previously). Except for discoloration, most patients with sulfhemoglobinemia remain asymptomatic, unless other abnormal hemoglobins are present (e.g., methemoglobin), or the typical accompanying oxidant hemolytic anemia is severe. Discoloration most often appears slate gray and lasts for weeks or months due to the

irreversible nature of sulfhemoglobin.[72] The coexistence of methemoglobinemia and anemia may alter the color of cyanosis and clinical symptoms.

Historically the most common drugs causing sulfhemoglobinemia were acetanilid, phenacetin, and sulfonamides. Bromo-Seltzer was the most common cause, but acetanilid, the offending ingredient, since has been removed as an ingredient. More recent reports describe sulfhemoglobinemia resulting from dapsone,[59] dimethyl sulfoxide,[73] flutamide,[58] metoclopramide,[57] and phenazopyridine.[60]

Treatment

There is no specific antidote for sulfhemoglobinemia. No beneficial effect results from therapy with methylene blue. Treatment centers on ensuring adequate oxygen delivery to tissues by correcting coexistent methemoglobinemia and anemia (from hemolysis) and ensuring maximal oxygen carrying capacity with administration of oxygen when the patient is symptomatic. Transfusions usually are required only in patients whose coexisting hemolytic anemia is severe, which increases the total hemoglobin concentration and decreases the sulfhemoglobin fraction. Patients need follow-up on an outpatient basis for several weeks because sulfhemoglobin concentrations decrease only as the red blood cell population is replaced in the absence of the offending agent.

Key Points in Hematologic Syndromes

1. Oxidant hemolysis, methemoglobinemia, and sulfhemoglobinemia share common etiologies and frequently coexist in the same patient.
2. Methemoglobinemia or sulfhemoglobinemia should be suspected when a cyanotic patient does not have a significantly depressed arterial PO_2 or when the history suggests toxic exposure to a known etiologic agent.
3. Methemoglobin impairs oxygen delivery by producing a functional anemia and by shifting the oxygen-hemoglobin dissociation curve to the left.
4. Oxygen carrying capacity can worsen while methemoglobin fractions decrease or cyanosis improves if accompanying hemolysis produces significant decreases in hemoglobin concentrations.
5. Methylene blue enhances enzymatic reduction of methemoglobin but is contraindicated in patients with glucose-6-phosphate dehydrogenase deficiency.
6. Pulse oximetry is unreliable in the presence of methemoglobinemia or sulfhemoglobinemia.
7. Cooximeters vary widely in their ability to detect, measure, and report sulfhemoglobinemia; some report sulfhemoglobin as methemoglobin.
8. Sulfhemoglobin cannot transport oxygen but shifts the oxygen-hemoglobin dissociation curve to the right; impaired oxygen delivery usually is not a problem unless accompanying hemolysis or methemoglobinemia is significant.
9. Methylene blue does not affect sulfhemoglobin. Sulfhemoglobin persists for the life of the erythrocyte.

**Common Errors in Management
of Hematologic Syndromes**

Failure to realize that arterial PO_2 is usually normal or at baseline values in patients with methemoglobinemia

Not recognizing that percent saturations reported by many blood gas machines are calculated, rather than measured, and can be reported as normal despite hemoglobinopathies such as methemoglobinemia

Forgetting to consider the total hemoglobin concentration when assessing impairment of oxygen carrying capacity from methemoglobinemia

Failure to seek evidence of hemolysis in patients with methemoglobinemia and vice versa

Believing that glucose-6-phosphate dehydrogenase deficiency predisposes to methemoglobinemia

Failure to understand whether a specific cooximeter being used in patient management detects or reports sulfhemoglobinemia

Not realizing that pulse oximetry does not provide reliable measurements of saturation in the presence of methemoglobinemia or sulfhemoglobinemia

Forgetting that known glucose-6-phosphate dehydrogenase deficiency is a contraindication to therapy with methylene blue

Failure to recognize that Heinz bodies cannot be seen on routine Wright's stain of blood

REFERENCES

1. Evans AS, Enzer N, Eder HA, et al: Hemolytic anemia with paroxysmal methemoglobinemia and sulfhemoglobinemia. Arch Intern Med 86:22–34, 1950.
2. Basset P, Bergerat JP, Lang JM, et al: Hemolytic anemia and sulfhemoglobinemia due to phenacetin abuse: A case with multivisceral adverse effects. Clin Toxicol 18:493–499, 1981.
3. Yoo D, Lessin LS: Drug-associated "bite cell" hemolytic anemia. Am J Med 92:243–238, 1992.
4. Curry S: Methemoglobinemia. Ann Emerg Med 11:214–221, 1982.
5. Weatherall DJ, Clegg JB, Higgs DR, et al: The hemoglobinopathies. In Scriver CR, Beaudet AL, Sly WS, et al (eds): The Metabolic and Molecular Bases of Inherited Disease, 7th ed. New York, 1995, McGraw-Hill, pp 3417–3484.
6. Melzer-Lange M, Walsh-Kelly C: Naphthalene-induced hemolysis in a black female toddler deficient in glucose-6-phosphate dehydrogenase. Pediatr Emerg Care 5:24–26, 1989.
7. Steffen C, Seitz R: Severe chlorate poisoning: Report of a case. Arch Toxicol 48:281–288, 1981.
8. Savides MC, Oehme FW, Leipold HW: Effects of various antidotal treatments on acetaminophen toxicosis and biotransformation in cats. Am J Vet Res 46:1485–1489, 1985.
9. Iciek M, Polak M, Wlodek L: Effect of thiol drugs on the oxidative hemolysis in human erythrocytes. Acta Pol Pharm 57:449–454, 2000.
10. Kondo H, Takahashi M, Niki E: Peroxynitrite-induced hemolysis of human erythrocytes and its inhibition by antioxidants. FEBS Lett 413:236–238, 1997.
11. Jaffe ER, Hultquist DE: Cytochrome b_5 reductase deficiency and enzymopenic hereditary methemoglobinemia. In Scriver CR, Beaudet AL, Sly WS, et al (eds): The Metabolic and Molecular Bases of Inherited Disease, 7th ed. New York, 1995, McGraw-Hill, pp 3399–3415.
12. Yano SS, Danish EH, Hsia YE: Transient methemoglobinemia with acidosis in infants. J Pediatr 100:415–418, 1982.
13. Luk G, Riggs D, Luque M: Severe methemoglobinemia in a 3-week-old infant with urinary tract infection. Crit Care Med 19:1325–1327, 1991.
14. Kern K, Langevin PB, Dunn BM: Methemoglobinemia after topical anesthesia with lidocaine and benzocaine for a difficult intubation. J Clin Anesth 12:167–172, 2000.
15. Stoiber TR: Toxic methemoglobinemia complicating transesophageal echocardiography. Echocardiography 16:383–385, 1999.
16. Karim A, Ahmed S, Siddiqui R, et al: Methemoglobinemia complicating topical lidocaine used during endoscopic procedures. Am J Med 111:150–153, 2001.
17. Schroeder TH, Dieterich HJ, Muhlbauer B: Methemoglobinemia after axillary block with bupivacaine and additional injection of lidocaine in the operative field. Acta Anaesthesiol Scand 43:480–482, 1999.
18. Lynch A, Tobias JD: Acute valproate ingestion induces symptomatic methemoglobinemia. Pediatr Emerg Care 14:205–207, 1998.
19. Methemoglobinemia secondary to clofazimine treatment of chronic graft-versus-host disease. Blood 92:4872–4873, 1998.
20. Khan AM, Singh NT, Bilgrami S: Flutamide induced methemoglobinemia. J Urol 157:1363, 1977.
21. Hadjiliadis D, Govbert JA: Methemoglobinemia after infusion of ifosfamide chemotherapy: First report of a potentially serious adverse reaction related to ifosfamide. Chest 118:1208–1210, 2000.
22. Curry SC, Arnold-Capell P: Toxic effects of drugs used in the ICU: Nitroprusside, nitroglycerin, and angiotensin-converting enzyme inhibitors. Crit Care Clin 7:555–581, 1991.
23. Lukens JN: The legacy of well-water methemoglobinemia. JAMA 257:2793–2795, 1987.
24. Methemoglobinemia attributable to nitrite contamination of potable water through boiler fluid additives—New Jersey, 1992 and 1996. MMWR Morb Mortal Wkly Rep 46:202–204, 1997.
25. Kennedy N, Smith CP, McWhinney P: Faulty sausage production causing methaemoglobinaemia. Arch Dis Child 76:367–368, 1997.
26. Sheperd G, Grover J, Klein-Schwartz W: Prolonged formation of methemoglobin following nitroethane ingestion. J Toxicol Clin Toxicol 36:613–616, 1998.
27. Spurzem JR, Bonekat HW, Shigeoka JW: Factitious methemoglobinemia caused by hyperlipemia. Chest 86:84–86, 1984.
28. Kirlangitis JJ, Middaugh RE, Zablocki A, et al: False indication of arterial oxygen desaturation and methemoglobinemia following injection of methylene blue in urological surgery. Mil Med 155:260–262, 1990.
29. Henretig FM, Gribetz B, Kearney T, et al: Interpretation of color change in blood with varying degree of methemoglobinemia. Clin Toxicol 26:293–301, 1988.
30. Ralston AC, Webb RK, Runciman WB: Potential errors in pulse oximetry: III. Effects of interference, dyes, dyshaemoglobins and other pigments. Anaesthesia 46:291–295, 1991.
31. Reay DT, Insalaco SJ, Eisele JW: Postmortem methemoglobin concentrations and their significance. J Forensic Sci 29:1160–1163, 1984.
32. Herman MI, Chyka PA, Butler AY, et al: Methylene blue by intraosseous infusion for methemoglobinemia. Ann Emerg Med 33:111–113, 1999.
33. Mier RJ: Treatment of aniline poisoning with exchange transfusion. J Toxicol Clin Toxicol 265:357–364, 1988.
34. Harrison MR: Toxic methaemoglobinaemia: A case of acute nitrobenzene and aniline poisoning treated by exchange transfusion. Anaesthesia 32:270–272, 1977.
35. Berlin G, Brodin B, Hilden J-O: Acute dapsone intoxication: A case treated with continuous infusion of methylene blue, forced diuresis, and plasma exchange. J Toxicol Clin Toxicol 22:537–548, 1985.
36. Southgate HJ, Masterson R: Lessons to be learned: A case study approach: Prolonged methaemoglobinaemia due to inadvertent dapsone poisoning; treatment with methylene blue and exchange transfusion. J R Soc Health 119:52–55, 1999.
37. Karadsheh NS, Shaker Q, Ratroat B: Metoclopramide-induced methemoglobinemia in a patient with co-existing deficiency of glucose-6-phosphate dehydrogenase and NADH-cytochrome b_5 reductase: Failure of methylene blue treatment. Haematologica 86:659–660, 2001.
38. Rosen PJ, Johnson C, McGehee WG, et al: Failure of methylene blue treatment in toxic methemoglobinemia: Association with glucose-6-phosphate dehydrogenase deficiency. Ann Intern Med 75:83–86, 1971.
39. Lamont AS, Roberts MS, Holdsworth DG, et al: Relationship between methaemoglobin production and methylene blue plasma concentrations under general anaesthesia. Anaesth Intensive Care 14:360–364, 1986.
40. Way JL, Leung P, Sylvester DM, et al: Methaemoglobin formation in the treatment of acute cyanide intoxication. In Ballantyne B, Marrs TC (eds): Clinical and Experimental Toxicology of Cyanides. Bristol, 1987, IOP Publishing Limited, pp 402–412.
41. Stossel TP, Jennings RB: Failure of methylene blue to produce methemoglobinemia in vivo. Am J Clin Pathol 45:600–604, 1966.
42. Liao Y-P, Hung D-Z, Yang D-Y: Hemolytic anemia after methylene blue therapy in aniline induced methemoglobinemia (Abstract). J Toxicol Clin Toxicol 39:292, 2001.

43. Kirsch IR, Cohen HJ: Heinz body hemolytic anemia from the use of methylene blue in neonates. J Pediatr 96:276–278, 1980.

44. Crooks J: Haemolytic jaundice in a neonate after intra-amniotic injection of methylene blue. Arch Dis Child 57:872–873, 1982.

45. McEnerney JK, McEnerney LN: Unfavorable neonatal outcome after intraamniotic injection of methylene blue. Obstet Gynecol 61(Suppl): 35S–37S, 1983.

46. Coleman MD, Rhodes LE, Scott AK, et al: The use of cimetidine to reduce dapsone-dependent methaemoglobinaemia in dermatitis herpetiformis patients. Br J Clin Pharmacol 34:244–249, 1992.

47. Hirano M, Matsuki T, Tanishima K, et al: Congenital methaemoglobinaemia due to NADH methaemoglobin reductase deficiency: Successful treatment with oral riboflavin. Br J Haematol 47:353–359, 1981.

48. Kaplan JC, Chirouze M: Therapy of recessive congenital methaemoglobinaemia by oral riboflavine. Lancet 2:1043–1044, 1978.

49. Wright RO, Woolf AD, Shannon MW, et al: N-acetylcysteine reduces methemoglobin in an in-vitro model of glucose-6-phosphate dehydrogenase deficiency. Acad Emerg Med 5:225–229, 1998.

50. Tanen DA, LoVecchio F, Curry SC: Failure of intravenous N-acetylcysteine to reduce methemoglobin produced by sodium nitrite in human volunteers: A randomized controlled trial. Ann Emerg Med 35:369–373, 2000.

51. Goluboff N, Wheaton R: Methylene-blue-induced cyanosis and acute hemolytic anemia complicating the treatment of methemoglobinemia. J Pediatr 58:86–89, 1961.

52. Chatfield MJ, La Mar GN: 1H Nuclear magnetic resonance study of the prosthetic group in sulfhemoglobin. Arch Biochem Biophys 295:289–296, 1992.

53. Park CM, Nagel RL: Sulfhemoglobinemia: Clinical and molecular aspects. N Engl J Med 310:1579–1584, 1984.

54. Curry SC, Gerkin RD: A patient with sulfhemoglobin? Ann Emerg Med 16:828–830, 1987.

55. Smith RP, Gosselin RE: Hydrogen sulfide poisoning. J Occup Med 21:93–97, 1979.

56. Mary AM, Bhupalam L: Metoclopramide-induced methemoglobinemia in an adult. J Ky Med Assoc 98:245–247, 2000.

57. Van Veldhuizen PJ, Wyatt A: Metoclopramide-induced sulfhemoglobinemia. Am J Gastroenterol 90:1010–1111, 1995.

58. Kouides PA, Abboud CN, Fairbanks VF: Flutamide-induced cyanosis refractory to methylene blue therapy. Br J Haematol 94:73–75, 1996.

59. Chawla R, Gurnani A, Bhattacharya A: Acute dapsone poisoning. Anaesth Intensive Care 21:349–351, 1993.

60. Halvorsen SM: Phenazopyridine-induced sulfhemoglobinemia: Inadvertent rechallenge. Am J Med 91:315–317, 1991.

61. Azen EA, Bryan GT, Shahidi NT, et al: Obscure hemolytic anemia due to analgesic abuse: Does enterogenous cyanosis exist? Am J Med 48:724–727, 1970.

62. Westphal RG, Azen EA: Experimental enterogenous cyanosis and anaemia. Br J Haematol 22:609–616, 1972.

63. Levine D, Brunton AT, Kruger A, Hersant M: Recurrent sulphaemoglobinaemia treated with neomycin. J R Soc Med 93:428, 2000.

64. Michel HO, Harris JS: The blood pigments: Properties and quantitative determination with special reference to spectrophotometric methods. J Lab Clin Med 25:445–463, 1940.

65. Carrico RJ, Peisach RJ, Peisach J, Alben JO: The preparation and some physical properties of sulfhemoglobin. J Biol Chem 253:2386–2391, 1978.

66. Zoppi F, Brenna S, Fumagalli C, et al: Discrimination among dyshemoglobins: Analytical approach to a toxicological query. Clin Chem 42:1300–1302, 1996.

67. Demedts P, Wauters A, Watelle M, et al: Pitfalls in discriminating sulfhemoglobin from methemoglobin. Clin Chem 43:1098–1099, 1977.

68. Zwart A, Buursma A, Oeseburg B, et al: Determination of hemoglobin derivatives with the IL 282 Co-oximeter as compared with a manual spectrophotometric five-wavelength method. Clin Chem 27:1903–1907, 1981.

69. Aravindhan N, Chisholm DG: Sulfhemoglobinemia presenting as pulse oximetry desaturation. Anesthesiology 93:833–834, 2000.

70. Wu C, Kenny MA: A case of sulfhemoglobinemia and emergency measurement of sulfhemoglobin with an OSM3 CO-oximeter. Clin Chem 43:162–166, 1997.

71. Langford SL, Sheikh S: An adolescent case of sulfhemoglobinemia associated with high-dose metoclopramide and N-acetylcysteine. Ann Emerg Med 34:538–541, 1999.

72. Finch CA: Methemoglobinemia and sulfhemoglobinemia. N Engl J Med 239:470–478, 1948.

73. Burgess JL, Hammer AP, Robertson WO: Sulfhemoglobinemia after dermal application of DMSO. Vet Hum Toxicol 40:87–89, 1998.

CHAPTER 29

Acid-Base Balance in the Poisoned Patient

Stephen W. Borron

It is what we think we know already that prevents us from learning.

Claude Bernard, 1813–1878

Acid-base disorders, a common feature of serious poisonings, may result from exogenously administered ions, metabolic production of organic acids, disruption of mitochondrial function, renal injury, hypoventilation, or inadequate tissue delivery of oxygen because of respiratory or circulatory insufficiency. In the intensive care setting, multiple additional sources of acid-base disturbances are encountered, including non–toxicant-induced acute or chronic renal insufficiency and pulmonary disease, side effects of therapy (diuretics, hyperalimentation, vasopressors), and secondary complications of poisoning such as sepsis. Combined, these factors render particularly challenging the evaluation of acid-base status in a critically ill patient with suspected or demonstrated poisoning. As such, critical care physicians caring for poisoned patients must be well versed in the evaluation and management of disorders of acid-base equilibrium.

A quiet revolution has come about in the evaluation of acid-base disorders in the last 20 years based on the work of Stewart,[1] who recognized that the Henderson-Hasselbalch equation alone cannot adequately explain complex acid-base disorders. His work calls to mind the admonition of Claude Bernard at the beginning of this chapter. We will thus explore the pitfalls in the "classic" approach to acid-base disorders, which depends on the base excess and/or the anion gap and summarize the concept of "strong ion," or quantitative acid-base chemistry, which has recently been demonstrated to be superior to standard methods in clinical trials.[2–4] The reader is referred to the seminal works of Stewart,[1] Fencl and colleagues,[2,5] and Kellum and associates[6,7] for a more complete understanding of the important underlying concepts.

RAPID REVIEW OF KEY FACTORS IN ACID-BASE EQUILIBRIUM

Acid-base balance under physiologic conditions is the simple sum of the production of organic acids occurring in metabolism and their elimination or neutralization by the body's buffer systems. The first line of defense is the respiratory buffer system. Carbon dioxide, produced by the metabolism of carbohydrates, forms carbonic acid (H_2CO_3) when combined with water:

Equation 1

$$H^+ + HCO_3^- \rightleftarrows H_2CO_3 \rightleftarrows CO_2 + H_2O$$
$$\downarrow$$
$$\text{Pulmonary clearance}$$

This buffer system is considered an "open system" because moderate increases in CO_2 are normally eliminated by a compensatory increase in minute volume. Acidosis stimulates respiratory chemoreceptors both centrally and peripherally to produce an increase in ventilation, hence shifting this equation to the right and thus reducing the acidosis. However, severe acidosis may actually impede ventilation and lead to a vicious cycle that may result in death unless rapidly corrected.

Plasma proteins and phosphate stores in bone serve as a second line of defense against acid-base abnormalities. The important role of these buffer systems will be developed further in the discussion of "strong ion" analysis of acidosis. A strong ion refers to one that generally exists in a dissociated or nearly dissociated form (Na^+, K^+, Cl^-, and others, to be discussed). The kidneys assist in the maintenance of physiologic acid-base conditions through their regulation of strong ions.

Both simple and mixed forms of alkalosis and acidosis may be observed in a poisoned patient. However, the most troublesome toxicant-induced acid-base disorder is metabolic acidosis, to which the majority of this chapter will be devoted.

Toxicant-Induced Respiratory Alkalosis and Acidosis

Respiratory alkalosis and acidosis are direct reflections of, respectively, increased and decreased ventilation. Ventilation may be altered through changes in tidal volume, the respiratory rate, and gas exchange across the alveoli or by combinations thereof. These disorders may be of central or peripheral origin. Stimulation of the central nervous system may result in tachypnea or hyperpnea and subsequent respiratory alkalosis. Salicylates,[8] nicotine,[9] and caffeine[10] are examples of agents that stimulate respiratory centers. Opiates tend to decrease the respiratory rate by depressing the central respiratory and brainstem regulatory centers,[11] but they may also reduce ventilation by induction of peripheral effects, such as noncardiogenic pulmonary edema and increases in thoracic muscle tone.[12] Benzodiazepines and barbiturates likewise have both central effects (γ-aminobutyric acid [GABA]-mediated depression in the medulla oblongata) and peripheral effects (muscle weakness resulting in upper airway obstruction and/or respiratory muscle inefficacy); however, the peripheral effects appear to be of greater clinical importance.[13] Inadequate ventilation may also result in inadequate oxygenation and thereby lead to anaerobic glycolysis and lactate production. Thus, combined respiratory and metabolic acidosis is not uncommon in poisoning by toxicants that interfere with ventilation. Clinical diagnosis of these disorders is rather straightforward and based on physical examination and arterial blood gases, particularly $PaCO_2$.

Toxicant-Induced Metabolic Alkalosis

Chemical-induced metabolic alkalosis is relatively rare. The milk-alkali syndrome, characterized by hypercalcemia, metabolic alkalosis, and renal failure, was more common when calcium-containing antacids were the primary treatment of peptic ulcer disease. Nowadays, it is seen in elderly women taking calcium supplements for osteoporosis.[14] It has also been reported in betel nut chewers who use calcium-rich oyster shell paste in its preparation.[15] Laxatives taken in excess may give rise to hypokalemia and metabolic alkalosis,[16] as can diuretics[17] and licorice.[18] A nonexhaustive list of toxicants responsible for metabolic alkalosis is found in Table 29-1.

Toxicant-Induced Metabolic Acidosis

Metabolic acidosis is induced by numerous drugs and chemicals through varying mechanisms. Ingested mineral acids (toilet bowl cleaners, battery acid) may serve as exogenous sources of metabolic acidosis. Toxic alcohols and glycols, including methanol and ethylene glycol, are notable causes of metabolic (endogenous) production of organic acids.

TABLE 29-1 Toxicants Reported to Cause Metabolic Alkalosis

AGENT	CLASSIFICATION	SELECTED REFERENCES
Calcium carbonate	Antacid	15, 19
Chlorthalidone	Diuretic	20
Corticosteroids	Corticosteroid	21
Ethacrynic acid	Diuretic	22
Furosemide	Diuretic	22
Gamma-hydroxybutyrate	Anesthetic	23
Gentamicin	Antibiotic	24
Laxative	Laxative	16, 25
Licorice	Candy	17, 26–29
Magnesium oxide	Electrolyte	30
Neo-Mull-Soy	Soy-based infant formula	31–33
Potassium sodium citrate	Antiurolithiasis agent	34
Sodium bicarbonate	Antacid	35
Sodium lactate	Antacid	36

Interference with mitochondrial function results in lactate production. Antiretroviral medications and cyanide are well known for their ability to induce lactic acidosis. Agents causing profound cardiovascular collapse, such as chloroquine and colchicine, may give rise to acidosis through diminished perfusion, as well as other mechanisms. In Table 29-2 the reader is provided with selected references for a nonexhaustive list of toxicants that may induce metabolic acidosis. A discussion of individual toxicants is beyond the scope of this chapter. Related chapters in this text pertaining to specific substances should be consulted.

CLINICAL SUSPICION OF ACID-BASE DISORDERS

Vigilance is required to promptly detect and treat acid-base disorders. The finding of altered mental status or abnormal vital signs should always invoke consideration of an acid-base disturbance. Clinical findings may be subtle early in the pathophysiologic process, so habits as elemental as truly counting the respiratory rate may make the difference in early recognition of these disorders. A thorough examination may detect sentinel breath odors (ketones, paraldehyde, cyanide), altered respiration (hyperpnea, Kussmaul respirations), cyanosis, pressure sores or bullae suggestive of rhabdomyolysis, or other clues to this diagnosis. Clinical signs and symptoms are insufficiently sensitive, however, so laboratory screening is necessary in all critically ill patients. Simple point-of-care monitoring devices such as pulse oximeters and end-tidal CO_2 detectors may also suggest the presence of an acid-base disturbance, although undue reliance on such devices is to be discouraged, given the possibility of both false-positive and false-negative readings.[167–174] Additionally, bedside testing for ketones, blood glucose, electrolytes, and lactate may assist in the early recognition of acid-base disorders. Notwithstanding the value of these bedside tools, definitive evaluation of acid-base disorders is based on carefully selected data provided by the chemistry and toxicology laboratories.

LABORATORY DIAGNOSTIC TOOLS IN ACID-BASE BALANCE

Gaps in Our Knowledge of Acid-Base Disturbances

This double entendre is not original[175] but reflects our incomplete comprehension of acid-base disorders in spite of more than 30 years of clinical studies and discussions in the literature regarding the use of various gaps—base excess, anion, delta, and osmolal. Each of these tools, their potential utility, and their shortcomings will be discussed, followed by a discussion of the quantitative approach to acid-base balance, which appears to overcome these gaps.

Given the ubiquity of its use in clinical medicine, the most frequently available laboratory indicator of acidosis is the serum electrolyte panel. For this reason, anion and delta gaps will be discussed before base excess and osmolal gaps.

TABLE 29-2 Toxicants Reported to Cause Metabolic Acidosis

AGENT	CLASSIFICATION	SELECTED REFERENCES
Acetaminophen (paracetamol)	Analgesic, antipyretic	37–43
Acetazolamide	Carbonic anhydrase inhibitor	44–46
Acetonitrile	Solvent, chemical intermediate	47–49
Acetylene	Welding gas	50
Aminocaproic acid	Hemostatic	51
Arginine	Amino acid	52
Aspirin (acetylsalicylic acid) and salicylates	Analgesic, antipyretic	53–58
Azide, sodium	Herbicide, fungicide, fumigant, bactericide, chemical intermediate, preservative, propellant	59–62
Boric acid	Insecticide	63
Carbon monoxide	Asphyxiant, chemical	64–67
Chlorine	Disinfectant, halide	68
Cocaine	Anesthetic, sympathomimetic, stimulant drug of abuse	69–71
Cyanide (HCN and salts)	Asphyxiant, chemical	72–77
Diazepam	Sedative hypnotic	78
Didanosine	Antiviral, nucleoside analogue	79
Diethylene glycol/ triethylene glycol	Glycol, solvent, brake fluid	80, 81
Endosulfan	Organochlorine insecticide	82
Ethanol	Alcohol	83–91
Ethylene glycol	Antifreeze, solvent	92–95
Ethylene glycol monobutyl ether (EGBE, butoxyethanol, butyl cellosolve)	Solvent, glass cleaner	96–100
Ethylene glycol monomethyl ether (EGME; methoxyethanol; methyl cellosolve)	Solvent, antifreeze	101
Etomidate	Anesthetic	102–104
Fialuridine	Antiviral, nucleoside analogue	105
Flumequine	Antimicrobial, fluoroquinolone	106
Formalin (40% formaldehyde in water)	Tissue fixative, embalming fluid	107, 108
Formic acid	Organic acid	109–114
Hydrogen sulfide	Petroleum production, decomposition of sulfur-containing organic matter	115
Iron	Mineral supplement	116
Isoniazid (INH)	Antimicrobial, antitubercular	117, 118
Lorazepam	Sedative-hypnotic	119–122
Methamphetamine	Sympathomimetic, appetite suppressant, stimulant drug of abuse	123
Methyl alcohol (methanol)	Solvent, antifreeze, chemical intermediate, paint remover	124, 125
Nalidixic acid	Antimicrobial, quinolone	126
Nitroprusside, sodium	Antihypertensive, vasodilator	127
Nortriptyline	Cyclic antidepressant	128
Parathion	Pesticide, organophosphate	129
Phenol	Disinfectant, aromatic organic solvent	130–132
Phosphoric acid	Metal cleaner, toilet bowl cleaner	133
Phosphorus, elemental	Pesticide, fireworks	134
Potassium chloroplatinate	Photographic toner solution	135
Propionitrile	Cyanogen	136
Propofol	Anesthetic	137–142
Propylene glycol	Solvent, pharmaceutical adjuvant	78, 102–104, 119–122, 143–148
Smoke, fire (see cyanide and carbon monoxide above)	Environmental toxicant	73, 149, 150
Sodium chloride	Electrolyte	151
Stavudine	Antiviral, nucleoside analogue	152
Teniposide	Anticancer chemotherapeutic agent	153
Theophylline	Thioxanthine bronchodilator	154–156
Thiamine deficiency	Vitamin	88
Toluene	Solvent, aromatic organic, paints, thinners, lacquers, adhesives	157–160
Topiramate	Anticonvulsant	161
Treosulfan (dihydroxybusulfan)	Anticancer chemotherapeutic agent	162
Trimethoprim/sulfamethoxazole	Antimicrobial, sulfonamide	163, 164
Valproic acid	Anticonvulsant	164a, 164b
Xylenol	Phenolic detergent	165
Zidovudine	Antiviral, nucleoside analogue	166

Anion Gap

The serum anion gap (AG) remains a useful but only moderately sensitive tool in the initial evaluation of potential acid-base disturbances. It suffers from numerous limitations, which will be discussed later. If the clinician is aware of these limitations and adjusts for them accordingly, the AG provides one of the most rapidly available tools in the evaluation of acid-base disorders.

In its most basic form,

$$AG = \text{Measured serum cations} - \text{Measured serum anions}$$

Because the most important anions after chloride and bicarbonate (protein, inorganic phosphate, and sulfate) are not routinely measured in a serum electrolyte panel, a "normal" AG exists. The presence of additional unmeasured anions (often organic acids) creates an "increased" AG. The most commonly used calculation for AG is

Equation 2
$$AG = Na^+ - (\{Cl^-\} + \{HCO_3^-\})$$

An alternative though less frequently used equation adds $[K^+]$ to the first term. Extremes of potassium may affect the AG and should be kept in mind; however, the discussion that follows will be based on Equation 2. Although its calculation is remarkably simple, its interpretation is not always straightforward.

Because of the body's requirement for electroneutrality, an increase in unmeasured anions (the AG) should be compensated by an equal decrease in serum bicarbonate.[176] Thus, the first evaluation of the calculated AG should be its relationship to serum bicarbonate. In the simplest case, AG increases in an amount equivalent to the fall in bicarbonate. However, this does not always occur. For example, in the case of diabetic ketoacidosis (DKA), a discordance is often found,[177] with AG being smaller than predicted based on the decrease in bicarbonate. This lower AG may be explained by the extensive tubular elimination of ketone bodies, along with concomitant retention of chloride, which results in a component of hyperchloremic metabolic acidosis (HCMA). Brivet and others[178] investigated this phenomenon and demonstrated that the hyperchloremic component of acidosis increases over the course of DKA. This increase is also probably due in part to the large amount of sodium chloride typically administered in DKA. Skellet and colleagues[151] have demonstrated that large-volume fluid resuscitation with isotonic saline can induce acidosis because the equimolar concentrations of sodium and chloride in normal saline (155 mmol/L) will increase plasma chloride to a greater extent than plasma sodium, thus lowering the strong ion difference (see discussion of strong ion difference later).

An HCMA component may also be observed in increased anion gap metabolic acidosis (AGMA) not caused by DKA.[178] This finding is of more than passing interest to the toxicologist. Brivet and coworkers[178] evaluated the ratio of AG/ΔAR (where ΔAR is the calculated serum bicarbonate −25 mmol/L). An AG/ΔAR ratio less than 0.8 suggests a hyperchloremic component to the metabolic acidosis. Among those with a ratio less than 0.8, the AG was significantly lower, chloride was higher, and plasma lactate tended toward lower values. Brivet and colleagues postulated that intracellular distribution of organic anions is followed by a compensatory extracellular increase in chloride, which causes a decrease in AG and thus a decrease in the AG/ΔAR ratio. As further evidence that this phenomenon occurs, they compared the ratio of Na^+/Cl^- and found that those with AG/ΔAR ratios less than 0.8 also had smaller Na^+/Cl^- ratios. This finding suggests that the presence of a component of HCMA may in fact belie an underlying intracellular organic anion acidosis (i.e., the calculated AG may be misleadingly low).

The limitations of the AG fall into two general categories: (1) analytic and (2) physiologic.

ANALYTIC LIMITATIONS

Early published normal ranges of AG values, 12 ± 4 mmol/L,[179] continue to be used by many clinicians. However, these values now represent, in many hospitals, a significant overestimate because of changes in technology that occurred in the 1980s. Ion-specific electrode methodology has led to an increase in normal values of chloride by 2 to 6 mmol/L, with a concomitant decrease in the AG. Winter and colleagues[180] demonstrated convincingly that the normal AG is probably closer to 6 mmol/L, with a rather small standard deviation. The 95% confidence intervals for AG in a group of 120 blood donors was 3 to 11 mmol/L. This difference from previous normal values may seem small, but as the authors point out, if the true normal AG is 6 mmol/L, a patient with 10 mmol/L of added organic acid and thus an AG of 16 mmol/L would, by generally accepted standards, have a normal AG. In a group of 222 patients with normal renal function and albumin, Sadjadi[181] found an AG of 6.6 ± 2 mmol/L, almost identical to that demonstrated in the study of Winter and coworkers. Referring to the study of Iberti and associates,[182] Sadjadi provides evidence that failure to take this change into account may result in failure to diagnose acidosis. Using the "normal" range of 12 ± 4 mmol/L, Iberti and colleagues found that 50% of critically ill patients with lactic acidemia in the range of 5 to 9.9 mmol/L and 79% of those with lactate concentrations between 2.5 and 5 mmol/L had AG values less than 16 mmol/L. Applying the current lower ranges of AG would clearly improve sensitivity. A further word of caution is in order, however. Other authors have reported that the normal range of AG values not only depends on the instrument being used (mean of 5.9 mmol/L for the Beckman Synchron versus 12.4 mmol/L for the Nova analyzer)[183] but also varies significantly according to the laboratory providing the measurements.[184] Finally, clinicians must also be aware that some laboratories have altered the calibration of the chloride-measuring instrument so that the normal ranges of chloride and AG in those institutions remain closer to "classic" published values. Given the changes in technology and interlaboratory variability, normal ranges based on the literature are patently unacceptable and may lead to false interpretation. Thus, it is imperative that clinicians discuss this issue with laboratory medicine specialists in their own institutions to ensure that the normal ranges provided by the laboratory have, in fact, been verified in that laboratory.

A closely related issue has to do with "pseudohyponatremia," which is most often associated with DKA but potentially of interest in intoxications that induce acidosis and hyperglycemia. In spite of continued references to this phenomenon in the literature, complete with formulas for correcting it, the move to ion-specific sodium electrodes has for all practical purposes eliminated "pseudohyponatremia" as an entity. Thus, sodium should not be corrected for an elevated glucose concentration before calculating the AG.[181]

PHYSIOLOGIC LIMITATIONS

Serum Albumin. Whereas the potential for abnormal proteins (such as cationic multiple myeloma proteins) to alter the AG is widely appreciated, the critical role of normal proteins such as albumin remains largely ignored. Albumin constitutes the largest component of unmeasured anions under normal physiologic conditions, with inorganic phosphate and sulfates representing most of the remainder. Calculation of the AG without consideration of serum albumin may be justifiable in normal healthy patients, but it is certainly not acceptable in the critically ill. Figge and coworkers studied 152 critically ill patients with documentation of 265 measurements. Marked hypoalbuminemia was found in 96% of the patients, and values less than 20 g/L (the normal range in nine healthy subjects was 44 ± 3 g/L) were found in 49%. The authors noted that each gram-per-liter decrease in serum albumin caused the observed AG to underestimate the total concentration of unmeasured anions by 0.25 mmol/L.[185] A severely malnourished patient may have a significant AG virtually obscured because of the influence of hypoalbuminemia.[2] Thus, in a malnourished patient a normal AG may be observed even in the presence of abnormal anions (poisoning). Correcting for protein abnormalities improves the reliability of the AG.[2,185] The AG may be corrected for hypoproteinemia as follows:

Equation 3
$$AG_{corrected} = Na^+ - (\{Cl^-\} + \{HCO_3\}) + 0.25 \times (\{Normal\ albumin\ g/L\} - \{Observed\ albumin\ g/L\})$$

If albumin values are reported in grams per deciliter, the factor is 2.5. Hyperalbuminemia from severe dehydration (cholera) may reach significant enough concentrations to contribute to metabolic acidosis.[186]

Water Excess/Deficit. Significant loss or gain of free water will alter serum sodium and chloride by the same percentage but not by the same absolute amount, which will clearly alter the AG.[175] The effect of hyponatremia (water excess) on the AG has been clinically documented.[175,187] Corrections for the effects of water excess/deficit are taken into account in calculation of the strong ion gap (to be discussed) but have not generally been applied to the AG. A prospective look at the value of such a correction in patients with metabolic acidosis is needed.

Assumptions Regarding Lactate in the Anion Gap. The presence of an AG acidosis not explained by the presence of ketoacids, renal failure, or historical and laboratory evidence of toxicant ingestion is often assumed to be due to lactate. However, Gabow and colleagues found that a measured increase in lactate of greater than 4 mmol/L was present in only 9 of 21 patients (43%) meeting these criteria, thus illustrating the potential for error in such an assumption.[188] Dorwart and Chalmers found normal AGs in 32 of 45 patients with plasma lactate levels between 2.5 and 9.9 mmol/L.[189] Schwartz-Goldstein and colleagues reported on a patient with

near-normal AG (measured AG of 11 to 16 mmol/L) and measured plasma lactate levels of 11.5 to 14.7 mmol/L.[190] Iberti and associates have also pointed out that the AG lacks sensitivity in detecting hyperlactatemia.[182] Thus, if lactic acidemia is in the differential diagnosis, lactate should be quantified in the laboratory or at the bedside. Such quantification is particularly important in poisoning, where measurement of exogenous anions such as oxalate or formate is not always readily available. Quantification of lactate may not only provide clues to the diagnosis but also increase or decrease the suspicion of the presence of another unmeasured anion and should thus be considered an integral part of the laboratory evaluation.

Role of Potassium in the Anion Gap. Serum potassium, as mentioned earlier, is often "discarded" in calculating the AG because the range of serum potassium in most patients is small enough that potassium variations cause only a minimal change in the calculated gap. Nonetheless, there are circumstances (digitalis and toluene poisoning, for example) in which extremes of serum potassium may occur and render its consideration in calculation of the AG more important. Furthermore, a reduction in "normal" mean AG (absent the potassium) from 12 to 6 mmol/L renders the variation in potassium of greater importance in terms of percent change in AG. (Regardless of whether potassium is included in the calculation used, it exerts an electrical force as a strong ion.)

Hyperphosphatemia. Because the contribution of inorganic phosphates to the normal AG is moderate and because normal phosphate concentrations are generally about 1.0 ± 0.2 mmol/L,[2] hypophosphatemia results in a negligible change in the AG. On the other hand, conditions that result in hyperphosphatemia, such as phosphate enema intoxication, may result in an increased AG.[191,192] Thus, hyperphosphatemia must be added to the differential diagnosis of an increased AG.

Delta Gap

Another method of evaluating acid-base disorders is to compare the change in AG with the change in alkaline reserve.[176] This relationship is expressed as the "delta gap," which is defined as

Equation 4
$$\Delta Gap = \Delta AG - \Delta HCO_3^-$$

where ΔAG is the observed AG minus the upper normal limit of the AG and ΔHCO_3^- is the lower normal HCO_3^- minus the observed HCO_3^-. The normal range for the delta gap is 0 ± 6. As mentioned previously, the body must maintain electroneutrality, so an increase in unmeasured anions (the AG) should be compensated by an equal decrease in serum bicarbonate.[176] Therefore, for a simple increased AG acidosis, the delta gap should be 0. A significantly positive (greater than +6) delta gap suggests the presence of metabolic alkalosis. A significantly negative (less than −6) delta gap suggests hyperchloremic acidosis. Because normal values for electrolytes (and AGs) vary among hospitals, depending on the methodologies used, it is imperative to calculate these values on the basis of local norms.[180] Wrenn demonstrated through a series of clinical cases that the delta gap can assist in the detection of mixed acid-base disorders that would go unsuspected on the basis of evaluation of the AG alone. It is not foolproof, however, as illustrated by one case in which a patient with a normal AG (4 mmol/L), a normal delta gap (−2 mmol/L), and a bicarbonate concentration of 19 mmol/L actually had a combination of AGMA, HCMA, and metabolic alkalosis from volume contraction.[176] Thus, one should not rely entirely on either the AG or the delta gap in the evaluation of potential acid-base disorders.[175]

Base Excess

Base excess (BE) was the first "gap" to be proposed as a useful approach to the evaluation of acid-base disturbances.[193] It is obtained as follows:

Equation 5
$$BE = 1.2 (\{HCO_3^-\} - 22.9)$$

The multiplier 1.2 takes into account the approximately 25% of buffer capacity not provided by the carbon dioxide/bicarbonate system. HCO_3^- is the "standard" bicarbonate, which is the concentration of bicarbonate in plasma when whole blood has been equilibrated at a $PaCO_2$ of 40 mm Hg, oxyhemoglobin saturation of 100%, and temperature of 38°C. Once the pH is measured, the standard bicarbonate can be obtained directly from Equation 6, the Henderson-Hasselbalch equation:

Equation 6
$$pH = 6.10 + \log \frac{HCO_3^-}{PaCO_2 \times 0.030}$$

The normal mean of standard bicarbonate is 22.9 mEq/L, so this value is subtracted in Equation 5 from the product to obtain the BE. A BE less than −5 mEq/L is thought to be consistent with metabolic acidosis. Salem and Majais[175] have warned against the use of this theoretical bicarbonate concentration when calculating the AG (in lieu of total CO_2) because rapidly changing conditions in apparent values of pK' may result in calculated errors in HCO_3^- as high as 50%.[175] Rosan and associates have likewise called attention to this problem.[194] Furthermore, excess heparin in blood gas samples may decrease $PaCO_2$ by up to 25%, which also falsifies the calculated bicarbonate value.[175] It then stands to reason that the BE, determined on the basis of calculated bicarbonate, also risks misinterpretation. In addition to the risk of analytic and calculated errors, the BE is dependent on a number of other factors "assumed" to be normal in this simple calculation: normal water content, electrolytes, and albumin. As pointed out by Balasubramanyan and colleagues, changes in these values will alter the calculated BE independent of changes in lactate, bicarbonate, or unmeasured anions.[3]

Quantitative Acid-Base Analysis: The Strong Ion Gap

The strong ion approach to acid-base management appears to be the most fundamentally sound from the perspective of physical chemistry.[6] This method, originally described by

Stewart[1] and refined by Fencl and Leith,[5] relies on the fact that systems operate under a number of restraints imposed by physical laws that must always and simultaneously be met:

1. Electroneutrality must always exist: the sum of all positive charges must always be equal to the sum of all negative charges.
2. Dissociation equilibria of all incompletely dissociated substances must always be satisfied.
3. Mass is conserved; that is, the total concentration of an incompletely dissociated substance can always be accounted for as the sum of the concentrations of its dissociated and undissociated forms.

The hydrogen ion concentration in blood is held within a very tight range, 36 to 43 nmol/L, because this range is critical to the maintenance of appropriate protein function (enzymes, pumps, etc.) and thus cellular function.[6] The source of hydrogen ions is the dissociation of water. Dissociation of water into hydrogen and hydroxyl ions is determined by three independent determinants (each can be changed independently of the others): the strong ion difference (SID), $PaCO_2$, and the total weak acid concentration (A_{TOT}).

The first independent variable is SID, or the net electrical charge of the strong electrolytes (i.e., those that are completely or nearly completely dissociated). This variable includes not only the electrolytes Na^+, K^+, Ca^{2+}, Mg^{2+}, and Cl^- but also other strong anions of low pK_a such as lactate and ketoacids, which are likewise almost completely dissociated at physiologic pH (Fig. 29-1). The second independent variable is $PaCO_2$, which, of course, varies with ventilation. The third independent variable is A_{TOT}, the sum of weak acids [HA] and their anions [A^-]. The weak acids

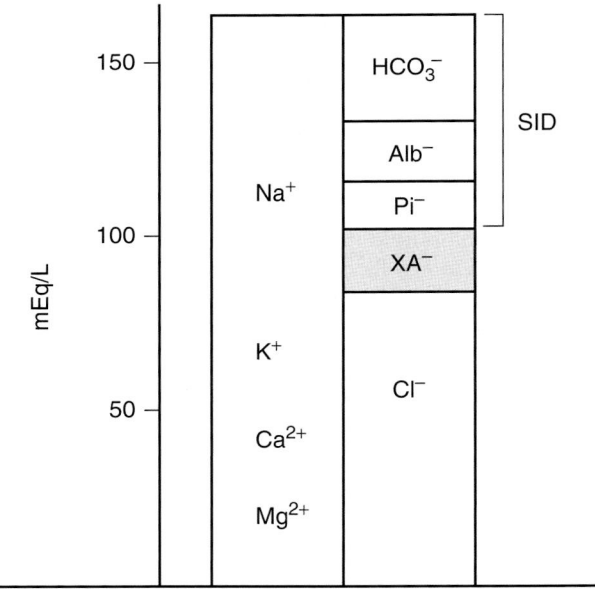

FIGURE 29-1

Electroneutrality must be maintained in blood plasma; thus, the sum of positive charges must equal the sum of negative charges. Hydroxyl, carbonate, and protons are not shown because their concentrations are in the nanomolar to micromolar range. XA^- represents unidentified strong anions (lactate, sulfate, ketoacids, others). SID, strong ion difference. *(Adapted from Fencl V, Jabor A, Kazda A, Figge J: Diagnosis of metabolic acid-base disturbances in critically ill patients. Am J Respir Crit Care Med 162:2246–2251, 2000.)*

are primarily composed of proteins (mainly albumin) and phosphates. Kellum and coworkers[7] point out that weak acids [HA] without their anions are not an independent variable because their equilibrium with A⁻ changes with alterations in SID and $PaCO_2$. *The central tenet of the strong ion approach is that neither [H⁺] nor HCO_3^- can change without a change in one or more of these three independent variables.* Neither H⁺ nor HCO_3^- is a strong ion. Strong ions cannot be created or destroyed to satisfy electrical neutrality, but hydrogen ions can be generated or consumed by changes in water dissociation.[7] Likewise, bicarbonate production or consumption is a result of changes in the three independent variables. Thus, the "classic" approach of looking at HCO_3^- is in a sense backward, in that we are examining the end result rather than the underlying cause of the disturbance. Acid-base disturbances may be classified according to the underlying change in these three independent variables (Table 29-3).

There are two basic approaches to using SID clinically. In the first approach, one calculates the strong ion gap (XA⁻), which, similar to the AG, identifies the presence of unmeasured anions. The second approach provides corrections to BE based on SID. Each approach has been shown to be more advantageous than use of the classic AG and BE.

Fencl and colleagues[2] recently used the first approach in a study involving 9 healthy subjects and 152 intensive care

unit patients and conclusively demonstrated that reliance on the AG (particularly if not corrected for albumin) or BE results in false interpretation of the acid-base status of critically ill patients. The strong ion approach, though requiring a few more direct laboratory measurements, is comprehensive and thus more sensitive. Figure 29-1 demonstrates that SID is equivalent to the following:

Equation 7
$$SID = \{HCO_3^-\} + 0.28 \times \{Alb, g/L\} + 1.8 \times \{Pi, mmol/L\}$$

$\{HCO_3^-\}$ is calculated from arterial blood gas measurements, and calculation of the effect of albumin (g/L) and inorganic phosphate (mmol/L) is based on their direct measurement in serum. This formula is a simplification and uses factors of 0.28 and 1.8 to correct for the actual charge (in mEq) provided by albumin and inorganic phosphates. If your laboratory provides {Pi} in mg/dL, the factor for {Pi} is 0.6 rather than 1.8.

The strong ion gap {XA⁻} is composed of strong ions other than Cl⁻ (lactate, ketoacids, and other organic anions such as toxic metabolites or sulfate), some of which are not readily measured in plasma. {XA⁻} is thus derived as

Equation 8
$$\{XA^-\} = \{Na^+\} + \{K^+\} + \{Ca^{2+}\} + \{Mg^{2+}\} - \{Cl^-\} - SID$$

where SID is obtained from Equation 7. Water excess or deficit, determined on the basis of an abnormal [Na⁺], will alter {Cl⁻} and {XA⁻}, both of which must be corrected:

Equation 9
$$\{Cl^-\}_{corrected} = \{Cl^-\}_{observed} \times (\{Na^+\}_{normal}/\{Na^+\}_{observed})$$

Correction of chloride allows one to determine the plasma excess or deficit in chloride.

Equation 10
$$\{XA^-\}_{corrected} = \{XA^-\}_{calculated} \times (\{Na^+\}_{normal}/\{Na^+\}_{observed})$$

Although this series of steps is a bit more demanding in time and cost than is calculation of AG, it allows recognition of complex acid-base disturbances that would be missed by simple examination of BE or AG.[2]

The second approach to using clinical quantitative acid-base chemistry is illustrated by Balasubramanyan and colleagues.[3] They used three equations of Fencl and Leith[5] to calculate a corrected BE that takes into account the fact that free water, changes in chloride concentration, and albumin all affect BE. First, the effect on BE caused by free water (BE_{fw}) is calculated as

Equation 11
$$BE_{fw} = 0.3 \times (\{Na^+\} - 140)$$

Changes in BE accounted for by chloride are calculated as

Equation 12
$$BE_{Cl} = 102 - Cl_{corr}$$

where Cl_{corr} is the corrected chloride: $Cl \times 140/Na$. Finally, the effect of albumin on BE (BE_{alb}) is calculated as

---

TABLE 29-3 Classification of Primary Acid-Base Disturbances

	ACIDOSIS	ALKALOSIS
I. Respiratory	↑ $PaCO_2$	↓ $PaCO_2$
II. Nonrespiratory (metabolic)		
1. Abnormal SID*		
a. Water excess/deficit†	↓ SID, ↓ {Na⁺}	↑ SID, ↑ {Na⁺}
b. Imbalance of strong ions		
i. Chloride excess/deficit	↓ SID, ↑ {Cl⁻}	↑ SID, ↓ {Cl⁻}
ii. Unidentified anion excess	↓ SID, ↑ {XA⁻}	—
2. Nonvolatile weak acids		
a. Serum albumin	↑ {Alb}	↓ {Alb}
b. Inorganic phosphate	↑ P_i	↓ P_i‡

*Changes in acid-base balance are controlled by changes in three independent variables—$PaCO_2$, the strong ion difference, and total weak acids. As such, these disorders may be classified on the basis of their underlying cause or causes. Assessment of these three variables can explain even complex acid-base disorders.

†Discerned by abnormal [Na⁺].

‡Because inorganic phosphate concentrations are normally low (≈1 mmol/L), hypophosphatemia has a negligible effect on acid-base balance.

{Alb}, plasma albumin concentration; {P_i}, plasma inorganic phosphate concentration; SID, difference between the sums of all the strong (fully dissociated, chemically nonreacting) cations (Na⁺, K⁺, Ca²⁺, Mg²⁺) and all the strong anions (Cl⁻ and other strong anions); {XA⁻}, plasma concentration of unidentified strong anions.

Adapted with permission from Fencl V, Leith DE: Stewart's quantitative acid-base chemistry: Applications in biology and medicine. Respir Physiol 91:1–16. 1993.

Equation 13

$$BE_{alb} = 3.4 \times (4.5 - albumin)$$

where albumin is reported in grams per deciliter.

The "classic" BE, as calculated from plasma bicarbonate, is really the sum of these three components plus a component attributable to unmeasured anions, BE_{ua}.

Equation 14

$$BE = BE_{fw} + BE_{Cl} + BE_{alb} + BE_{ua}$$

If one subtracts the first three from reported BE, one obtains BE_{ua}, or BE caused by unmeasured anions.

Equation 15

$$BE_{ua} = BE - (BE_{fw} + BE_{Cl} + BE_{alb})$$

In his study of 255 children in whom arterial blood gases, electrolytes, and albumin were measured simultaneously, Balasubramanyan demonstrated that BE_{ua} predicts increases in plasma lactate concentration better than BE does and, furthermore, that it is a better predictor of mortality than is BE or the lactate concentration.

Finally, Durward and colleagues recently showed that based on Stewart's principles, the chloride/sodium ratio can help identify acidotic patients with unmeasured anions. A ratio of less than 0.75 identified the presence of tissue acids (unmeasured anions + lactate) with a positive predictive value of 88%. A ratio over 0.79 excluded increased tissue acids with a positive predictive value of 81%.[195] The chloride-sodium ratio may thus be a useful initial parameter to establish in addition to the AG while awaiting the results of other elements for calculation of the strong ion gap. The studies of Balasubramanyan,[3] Fencl,[2] and their colleagues provide evidence that critical care patients warrant an aggressive evaluation of acid-base status. One of several examples offered by Fencl and coworkers demonstrates the value of quantitative acid-base analysis. A patient with head trauma, coma, and acute renal failure had the following laboratory findings: Na^+, 133 mEq/L; K^+, 3.9 mEq/L; Cl^-, 96 mEq/L; HCO_3^-, 25.5 mEq/L; AG (including K^+), 15 mEq/L; arterial pH, 7.36; and $PaCO_2$, 45 mm Hg. The AG is at the upper limit of normal, and analysis of BE reveals simple respiratory acidosis, with no metabolic disturbance. Adding the knowledge gained by measuring Ca^{2+} (4.2 mEq/L), Mg^{2+} (1.6 mEq/L), inorganic phosphates (0.4 mmol/L), and albumin (10 g/L) and calculating SID (29 mEq/L [normal, 39 ± 1]), we discover that a strong ion gap (XA^-) of 19 mEq/L exists (after correction for water excess) and represents unmeasured anions not detected by simple calculation of the AG. The corrected chloride is normal (no chloride deficit as suggested by the uncorrected chloride), and the AG corrected for severe hypoalbuminemia is 24 mEq/L. In summary, in this patient with plasma water excess, the presence of significant unmeasured anions causing acidosis, hypoalbuminemia masking that acidosis, and normal chloride, simple respiratory acidosis would be misdiagnosed on the basis of the classic AG-BE evaluation for acid-base disorders.[2]

Osmolal Gap

The utility of the osmolal gap in a poisoned patient, particularly one with suspected toxic alcohol ingestion, has been both lauded and lambasted in recent years. Osmolality is an expression of the number of particles in a given weight of solvent. Thus, each molecule of a substance, regardless of its molecular weight, contributes exactly the same as a molecule of another substance to osmolality. The vast majority of circulating osmoles consist of sodium (and its associated anions), glucose, and urea. The osmolar gap is calculated as

Equation 16

$$OG = MO - CO$$

where MO is the measured and CO the calculated (predicted) osmolality. There are normally a limited number of unmeasured osmoles, so a small gap is expected. In the context of a poisoned patient, the OG is most commonly measured in an attempt to determine whether substantial concentrations of circulating exogenous osmoles are present. Generally, the presence of excess measured, but not calculated, osmoles in a poisoned patient will be due to alcohols or glycols, such as ethanol, methanol, isopropanol, ethylene glycol, or propylene glycol, the last often present because of its widespread use in therapeutically administered medications. Since these molecules are volatile, MO should be determined by freezing point depression to ensure that they are not liberated during determination of osmolality. The relative contributions of these molecules to MO are indicated in Table 29-4. It should be

TABLE 29-4 Contributions of Some Solutes to Serum Osmolality

SUBSTANCE	MOLECULAR WEIGHT	1 mg/dL BLOOD OR PLASMA CONCENTRATION OF SUBSTANCE WILL INCREASE THE OSMOLAL GAP BY APPROXIMATELY (mOsm/kg)	1 mOsm/kg INCREASE IN THE OSMOLAL GAP CORRESPONDS TO AN ESTIMATED CONCENTRATION OF (mg/dL)
Acetone	58.1	0.17	5.8
Ethanol*	46.1	0.22	4.6
Ethylene glycol	62.1	0.16	6.2
Isopropanol	60.1	0.17	6.0
Methanol	32.1	0.31	3.2
Propylene glycol	76.1	0.13	7.6

Serum concentration (mg/dL) = (osmolal gap) × molecular weight/10. These calculated figures may be misleading and should be interpreted carefully.
*See the text for a revised calculation of ethanol concentration proposed by Purrsell and colleagues.[52]

emphasized that the figures in this table are theoretical and should be used only as a rough guide to expected changes in osmolality or, conversely, plasma concentration. Osmolality is measured in mOsm/kg H_2O. Numerous formulas have been used for calculation of this gap, and one such formula for the predicted serum osmolality follows:

Equation 17
$$\text{Calculated OG} = 2 \times \{Na^+\} + \{Glucose\} + \{BUN\}$$

where concentrations of sodium, glucose, and blood urea nitrogen (BUN) are expressed in mmol/L. Conversion of glucose and urea from mg/dL (mass units) to SI (standard international) molar units is accomplished by dividing glucose by 18 and urea by 2.8. An earlier formula used 1.86 as the multiplier of $\{Na^+\}$ and divided all solute concentrations by 0.93 because serum is normally only 93% water. Discerning mathematicians will quickly note that $1.86 \div 0.93 = 2$, so Smithline and Gardner proposed simply multiplying serum sodium by 2, as in Equation 17.[196] Others have abandoned the water correction and simply multiply by 1.86. Obviously, the choice of multiplying by 1.86 or 2 makes a great deal of difference if you consider that for a serum sodium value of 140, the product is either 280 or 260, thereby potentially "creating" (or destroying, depending on your point of view) 20 mOsm. To adjust for this difference, Dorwart and Chalmers proposed that a "correction factor" of 9 be added to the last term in the formula, with 1.86 used as the multiplier.[189]

The differences induced by these various and confusing formulas were studied by Osterloh and colleagues in a group of patients with ethanol concentrations varying from 0 to 561 mg/dL (median, 221 mg/dL).[83] They found that the osmolal gap calculated by using the formula of Smithline and Gardner ($\{2 \times Na\} + Glu/18 + BUN/2.8$) closely correlated with blood ethanol concentrations and had a much smaller bias than the Dorwart formula did. Osterloh and colleagues, like Smithline and Gardner, chose to ignore division of the molecular weights of glucose and urea by 0.93, and in fact, it is probably not important. For example, in a patient with a blood glucose concentration of 540 mg/dL (29.7 mmol/L), the calculated attributable osmoles are either 30 or 28, depending on this choice, and for a BUN concentration of 90 mg/dL (32.1 mmol/L), the attributable osmoles are calculated as 30 or 32. Thus, even in the presence of significant hyperglycemia and renal failure, the two calculations would alter the results of osmoles attributable to glucose and urea by only a small number.

In contrast to the conclusions of Osterloh and associates, Hoffman and colleagues found that using 2 as the multiplier for sodium routinely resulted in a markedly negative osmolal gap.[197] Instead, they found that using 1.86 as the multiplier for calculation of the osmolal gap (without addition of the "Dorwart factor" of 9) and correcting for the presence of ethanol yielded reliable results with mean values of −5 to 15 mOsm/kg, depending on whether they used the 0.93 (water content of serum) correction factor for ethanol only (thus introducing yet a new formula).[197]

More recently, this problem has been studied by Purssell and colleagues,[198] who derived a formula involving the use of linear regression for the osmolal gap, with the blood ethanol concentration taken into account, and then validated it in convenience samples from 128 patients. Their results agree with those of Osterloh and coworkers. They proposed a correction factor of 1.25 in SI units for the contribution to osmolality by ethanol. Given the frequency with which ethanol is found in poisoned patients, its presence should be confirmed and included in the calculation, although such inclusion may introduce a factor of bias. Thus, adding the Purssell ethanol correction factor, one arrives at a formula for CO, corrected for measured blood ethanol ($CO_{corrected}$):

Equation 18
$$CO_{corrected} = 2\,\{Na^+\} + \{Glucose\} + \{BUN\} - 1.25 \times \{Ethanol\}$$

If mass units (mg/dL) are used for the latter three, the following formula should be used:

Equation 19
$$CO_{corrected} = 2\,\{Na^+\} + \{Glucose\}/18 + \{BUN\}/2.8 - \{Ethanol\}/3.7$$

In fact, the choice of formula that one uses to calculate the osmolal gap is probably less important than knowing that the range of "normal" osmolal gaps will vary significantly, depending on the calculation chosen. Assuming that a "normal" osmolal gap is 0 to 10 mOsm/kg is arbitrary[196] and ill advised.[197] As astutely pointed out by Hoffman and associates,[197] large standard deviations in the normal range of osmolal gaps prevent the application of population norms to individual data. The osmolal gap appears to be most reliable when it exceeds 25 mOsm/kg, although it clearly diminishes in sensitivity at this cutoff.[199] Because of variations in the results (and normal values) obtained depending on the formula used, the relatively small number of milliosmoles produced by a toxic concentration of ethylene glycol (a blood concentration of 25 mg/dL {4 mmol/L} is equivalent to only ≈4 mOsm/kg; see Table 29-4), and the possibility of missing even *severe* very early or late manifestations of ethylene glycol or methanol toxicity, the osmolal gap should be viewed as helpful only if positive. Stated differently, the occurrence of severe metabolic acidosis, particularly if accompanied by a high AG and/or osmolal gap, in the absence of alcoholic or diabetic ketoacidosis or sepsis should strongly evoke the diagnosis of poisoning by a toxic alcohol or glycol. However, small or absent anion or osmolal gaps may be observed with severe toxic alcohol poisoning, depending on the extent of absorption and metabolism that have taken place since the ingestion. Therefore, both anion and osmolal gaps must be viewed as insensitive and do not rule out such poisonings. If any clinical suspicion exists, a direct measurement of the possible offending alcohols or glycols should be obtained. While these results are awaited, determination of the osmolal gap can be quite useful if its limitations are kept in mind. Jacobsen and colleagues have used the osmolal gap (minus the ethanol correction factor) in predicting blood concentrations of methanol and ethylene glycol in poisoned patients.[200] In six methanol-poisoned patients, the osmolal gap predicted the sum of ethanol and methanol concentrations with a coefficient of correlation of 0.95. Among six ethylene glycol–poisoned patients, none of whom had coingested ethanol, the correlation was 0.99.

An unvalidated algorithm in which the various gaps are used for evaluation of acid-base disorders is presented in Figure 29-2. Suggestions for use of the anion and delta gaps are found in Figures 29-3 and 29-4, respectively.

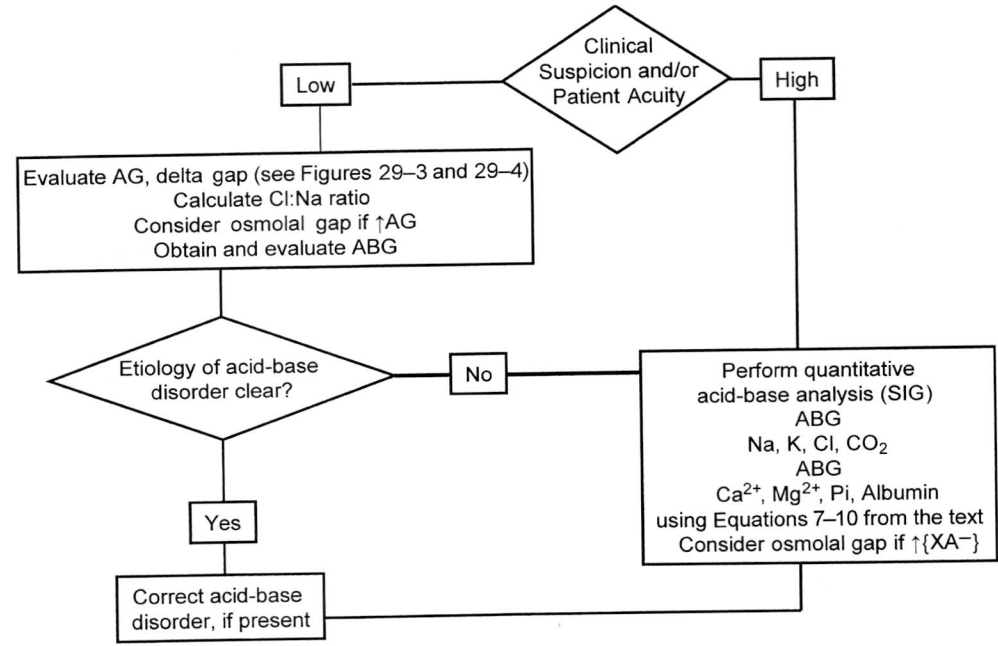

FIGURE 29-2

An unvalidated algorithm for the evaluation of acid-base disorders based on clinical suspicion of a disorder or patient acuity. While simple acid-base evaluation, using classic laboratory studies and calculation of "gaps," may suffice where suspicion of acid-base derangements and acuity is low, quantitative "strong ion" analysis is indicated where there is high suspicion of acid-base disorder or high acuity. Failure to clarify the etiology of the disorder with simple gaps and ABG analysis should also provoke quantitative acid-base analysis. SIG, strong anion gap. See text for details on calculation.

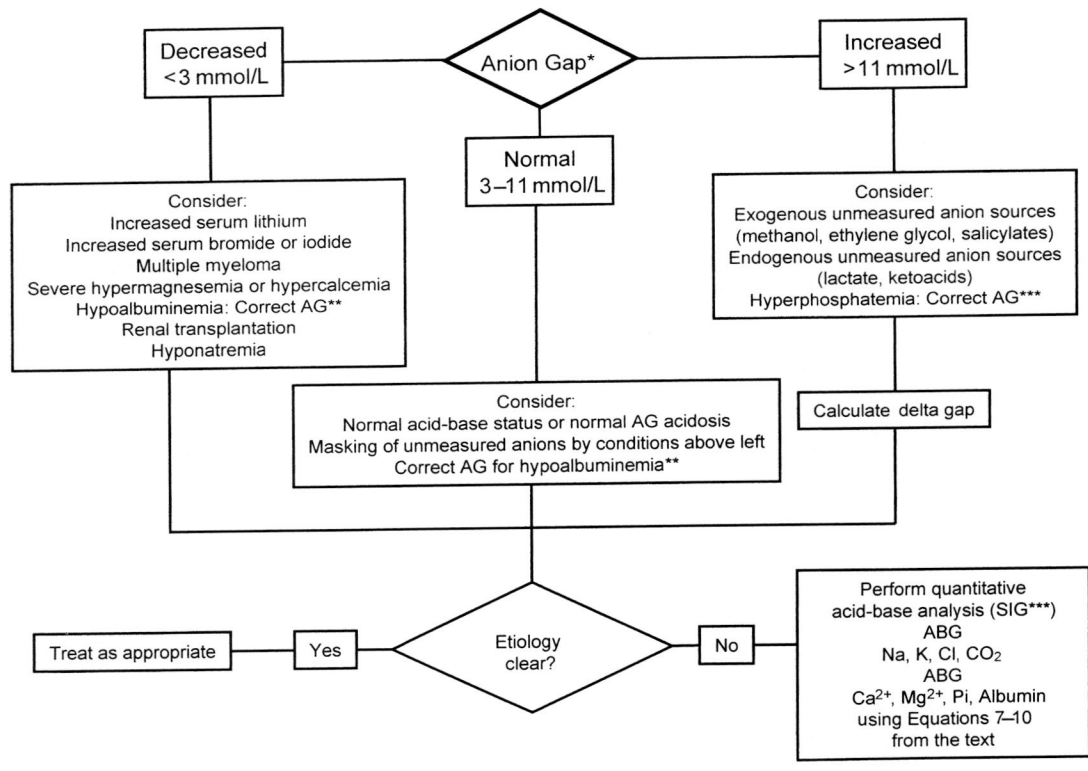

FIGURE 29-3

Evaluation of the anion gap (AG).
*AG is calculated as $Na^+ - (Cl^- + HCO_3^-)$. The normal range of AG is 3 to 11 mmol/L but will vary according to individual hospital laboratories.
**Correction for hypoalbuminemia: AG observed $+ 0.25 \times$ ([Albumin, nL] $-$ [Albumin observed]) = AG corrected, where normal albumin is considered to be 45 g/L.
***Correction for hyperphosphatemia: AG observed $- 0.32 \times$ ([Phosphate observed] $-$ [Phosphate, nL]) = AG corrected, where the upper normal phosphate level is considered to be 5 mg/dL.
If phosphate is reported in mmol/L, simply drop the multiplier of 0.32. ABG, arterial blood gases; SIG, strong ion gap.

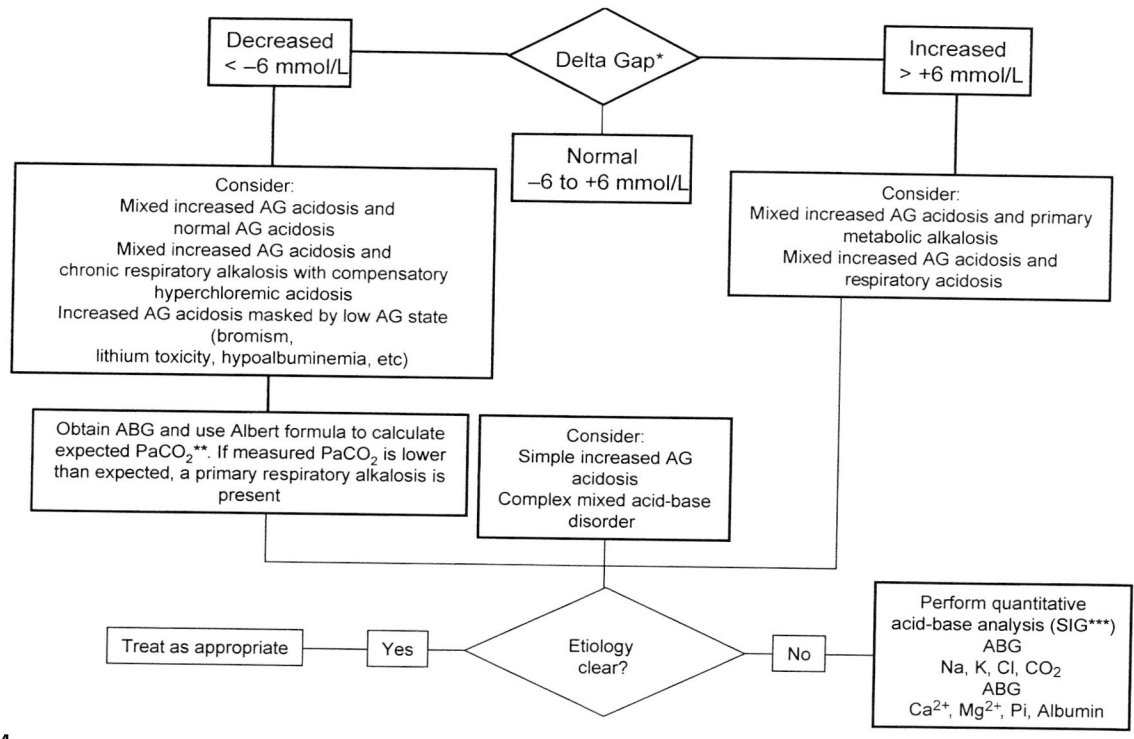

FIGURE 29-4

Evaluation of the delta gap.
*The delta gap is calculated as Δgap = ΔAG − ΔHCO$_3^-$, where ΔAG = observed AG − the upper normal limit of the AG and ΔHCO$_3^-$ = lower normal HCO$_3^-$ − observed HCO$_3^-$. The normal range for the delta gap is 0 ± 6.
**Albert formula: Expected PaCO$_2$ = 1.5 [HCO$_3^-$] + 8 + 2.
***See text and Figure 29-3 for calculation of SIG (XA$^-$).
(Adapted from Wrenn K: The delta (delta) gap: An approach to mixed acid-base disorders. Ann Emerg Med 19:1310–1313, 1990.)

Arterial Blood Gases

Interpretation of arterial blood gases in a poisoned patient does not differ significantly from that in other patients and is therefore not discussed in detail here. It is worthwhile, however, to note that according to the strong ion theory, the change in pH induced by a change in PaCO$_2$ will vary depending on SID and A$_{TOT}$, thus indicating that PaCO$_2$ is important not only in respiratory acidosis but also in metabolic acidosis, and reinforcing the importance of evaluation of all three independent variables (Fig. 29-5A and B). The compensation formulas for simple acid-base disorders proposed by Narins and Emmett[201] are provided in Table 29-5. The caveats discussed above with regard to "standard" bicarbonate hold.

TREATMENT OF ACID-BASE DISORDERS

The sine qua non of therapy for all acid-base disorders is correction of the underlying cause of the disorder. Attention to the patency of the airway and adequacy of ventilation and oxygenation cannot be overemphasized. In terms of metabolic derangements, the strong ion theory significantly simplifies the approach to the task of correction. A careful evaluation of strong ions will determine the need for electrolyte replacement, so reflexive administration of large volumes of solutions that alter SID, such as sodium chloride, is

avoided in the treatment of metabolic acidosis. Hypoperfusion persisting in spite of correction of vascular water and electrolyte deficits may require the use of vasoactive substances. It must be appreciated that their use may often worsen acidosis via the production of lactate, so careful attention to the risk-benefit ratio of their use is of utmost clinical interest.[202]

The specific (i.e., other than supportive) treatment of acid-base disorders remains controversial. Part of this controversy probably derives from the tendency of physicians to attempt to simplify approaches to "common" problems. For many years, the cornerstone of treatment of metabolic acidosis, with the exception of DKA, was the administration of bicarbonate, sometimes in very large quantities. Correction of abnormal pH (excess H$^+$) via administration of bicarbonate appears logical on the surface. However, Graf and colleagues[203] in 1985 pointed out that there is evidence that administration of bicarbonate may actually worsen intracellular acidosis, which led to proposals by some that we should "ban bicarbonate" in the treatment of acidosis.[204] Whether this rapid swing of the pendulum in the opposite direction is warranted depends on the belief that all metabolic acidosis is alike and should therefore be treated similarly. One might question, however, whether the "exogenous" acidosis produced by metabolic conversion of methanol is equivalent to the lactic acidosis produced in septic shock. Kellum has pointed out that when treatment is based on SID, the need for bicarbonate therapy becomes

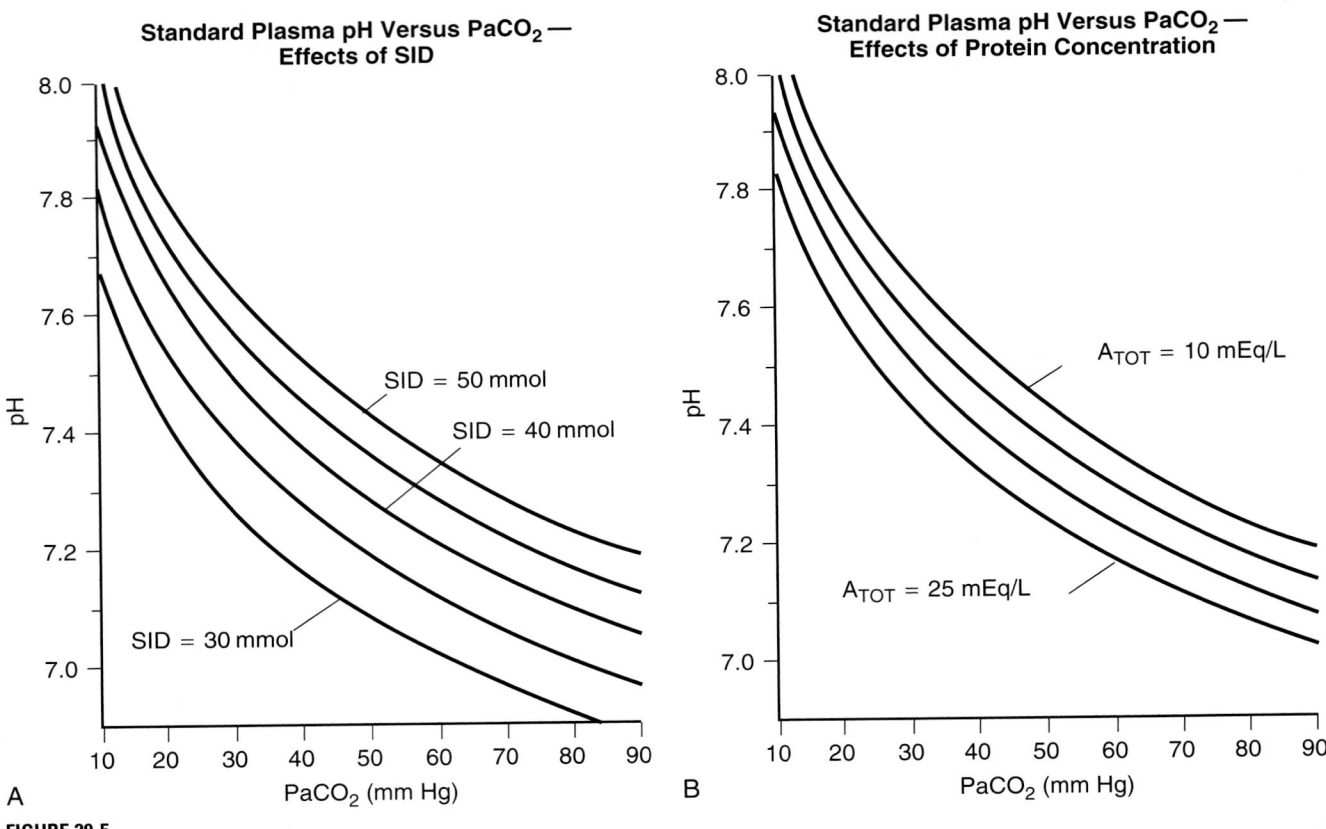

FIGURE 29-5

A, Interaction of the strong ion difference (SID) and $PaCO_2$ on pH. **B**, Interaction of the protein concentration and $PaCO_2$ on pH. *(From Stewart PA: Modern quantitative acid-base chemistry. Can J Physiol Pharmacol 61:1444–1461, 1983.)*

clear.[6] If the disorder involved is characterized by decreased or normal sodium, administration of sodium in the form of bicarbonate may in fact be warranted. However, it is in reality the sodium concentration (the strong ion) that is being treated. The bicarbonate will actually be determined by the three independent variables (strong ions, $PaCO_2$, and weak acids/salts). Only by increasing sodium relative to chloride can sodium bicarbonate "repair" metabolic acidosis. Thus, when sodium is already increased, there is no role for bicarbonate therapy.[6] Other considerations make the use of sodium bicarbonate potentially appropriate in metabolic acidosis of toxic origin. Alkalinization of the urine has a demonstrated beneficial effect on the distribution of salicylates and barbiturates by hastening elimination. Sodium administration (as bicarbonate or hypertonic saline) appears to be effective as well in the treatment of cyclic antidepressant–related dysrhythmias, which may be associated with metabolic acidosis.[205,206] In summary, although bicarbonate should no longer be viewed as the "universal antidote" for metabolic acidosis, its use should not be summarily abandoned in all cases of acidosis.

Use of the strong ion approach allows us to not only recognize the often multiple underlying causes of acid-base disorders but also correct them. Hypoalbuminemia contributing to severe metabolic alkalosis may warrant replacement therapy. Chloride excess leading to acidosis may be addressed by hemofiltration or the use of a weak base such as tris(hydroxymethyl)aminomethane (THAM,

TABLE 29-5 Formulas for Expected Compensation in Simple Acid-Base Disorders

DISORDER	FORMULA
Metabolic acidosis	Change in $PaCO_2$ = 1.2 × change in HCO_3^-
Metabolic alkalosis	Change in $PaCO_2$ = 0.6 × change in HCO_3^-
Acute respiratory acidosis	Change in HCO_3^- = 0.1 × change in $PaCO_2$
Acute respiratory alkalosis	Change in HCO_3^- = 0.2 × change in $PaCO_2$
Chronic respiratory acidosis	Change in HCO_3^- = 0.35 × change in $PaCO_2$
Chronic respiratory alkalosis	Change in HCO_3^- = 0.5 × change in $PaCO_2$

Changes represent differences from normal values for $PaCO_2$ (40 mm Hg) and HCO_3^- (24 mEq/L). See text for cautions regarding standard HCO_3^-.
Adapted from Narins RG, Emmett M: Simple and mixed acid-base disorders: A practical approach. Medicine (Baltimore) 59:161–187, 1980.

or tromethamine) (see later). The presence of a strong ion gap (excess unmeasured anions) calls for therapy to reduce their production or facilitate their removal.[6]

Three other pharmacologic methods of treatment of metabolic acidosis bear mention. Carbicarb is a mixture of 0.3 molar disodium carbonate and 0.3 molar sodium bicarbonate. This mixture has significant theoretical advantages over bicarbonate alone inasmuch as the carbon dioxide produced by the combination of bicarbonate and acids is buffered by the carbonate. This therapy has been demonstrated to be beneficial in the laboratory[207] and shown to be safe in a series of surgical patients,[208] but the drug is not currently commercialized in the United States.

THAM has also been proposed as an alternative to sodium bicarbonate. Several studies have shown promising results in selected patient populations,[209,210] but additional studies will be needed before its use can be generally recommended. Dichloroacetate (DCA) has been proposed as a treatment of lactic acidosis,[211] but like carbicarb, DCA is not currently available in many countries, including the United States. Finally, a treatment method of interest in acidosis of toxic etiology is peritoneal dialysis or hemodialysis.[212–214] Hemodialysis corrects not only the plasma bicarbonate (the result of the underlying disturbance in strong ion imbalance) but also some strong ion abnormalities (hyperkalemia). In addition, in contrast to parenterally administered bicarbonate, there is presumably little risk of worsening intracellular acidosis. Furthermore, it has the capacity to remove a number of endogenous (lactate, pyruvate) and exogenous (methanol and metabolites, ethylene glycol and metabolites) compounds of low molecular weight and limited volume of distribution. Although the number of cases treated precludes any definite conclusions regarding its efficacy, hemodialysis should perhaps be considered in the setting of grave poisoning with strong mineral acids (H_2SO_4, HCl), which may entirely overwhelm the capacity of physiologic buffer systems and supportive care.

SUMMARY

Acid-base disorders in poisoned patients may be of multiple toxic and nontoxic etiologies. A careful history and physical examination are necessary to suspect the disorder, and a thorough laboratory evaluation is required to distinguish the probable etiology. Reliance on simple calculations such as anion or osmolal gaps may result in errors, including missed diagnosis. A systematic approach using multiple diagnostic tools, including the quantitative (strong ion) method, will decrease the likelihood of errors. Treatment is largely supportive. Bicarbonate therapy is useful in selected cases but should be based on a quantitative analysis of acid-base derangements rather than being a rote response to abnormal laboratory values. Hemodialysis may also be of benefit in selected patients, again relying on the patient's clinical condition as a guide to therapy.

REFERENCES

1. Stewart PA: Modern quantitative acid-base chemistry. Can J Physiol Pharmacol 61:1444–1461, 1983.
2. Fencl V, Jabor A, Kazda A, Figge J: Diagnosis of metabolic acid-base disturbances in critically ill patients. Am J Respir Crit Care Med 162:2246–2251, 2000.
3. Balasubramanyan N, Havens PL, Hoffman GM: Unmeasured anions identified by the Fencl-Stewart method predict mortality better than base excess, anion gap, and lactate in patients in the pediatric intensive care unit. Crit Care Med 27:1577–1581, 1999.
4. Story DA, Morimatsu H, Bellomo R: Strong ions, weak acids and base excess: a simplified Fencl-Stewart approach to clinical acid-base disorders. Br J Anaesth 92:54–60, 2004.
5. Fencl V, Leith DE: Stewart's quantitative acid-base chemistry: Applications in biology and medicine. Respir Physiol 91:1–16. 1993.
6. Kellum JA: Metabolic acidosis in the critically ill: Lessons from physical chemistry. Kidney Int Suppl 66:S81–S86, 1998.
7. Kellum JA, Kramer DJ, Pinsky MR: Strong ion gap: A methodology for exploring unexplained anions. J Crit Care 10:51–55, 1995.
8. Meredith TJ, Vale JA: Non-narcotic analgesics. Problems of overdosage. Drugs 32(Suppl 4):177–205, 1986.
9. Fernandez R, Larrain C, Zapata P: Acute ventilatory and circulatory reactions evoked by nicotine: Are they excitatory or depressant? Respir Physiol Neurobiol 133:173–182, 2002.
10. Leson CL, McGuigan MA, Bryson SM: Caffeine overdose in an adolescent male. J Toxicol Clin Toxicol 26:407–415, 1988.
11. Kolarzyk E, Targosz D, Pach D, Misiolek L: Nervous regulation of breathing in opiate dependent patient. Part I. Respiratory system efficiency and breathing regulation in the first stage of controlled abstinence. Przegl Lek 57:531–535, 2000.
12. Campbell C, Weinger MB, Quinn M: Alterations in diaphragm EMG activity during opiate-induced respiratory depression. Respir Physiol 100:107–117, 1995.
13. Gueye PN, Lofaso F, Borron SW, et al: Mechanism of respiratory insufficiency in pure or mixed drug-induced coma involving benzodiazepines. J Toxicol Clin Toxicol 40:35–47, 2002.
14. Fiorino AS: Hypercalcemia and alkalosis due to the milk-alkali syndrome: A case report and review. Yale J Biol Med 69:517–523, 1996.
15. Wu KD, Chuang RB, Wu FL, et al: The milk-alkali syndrome caused by betelnuts in oyster shell paste. J Toxicol Clin Toxicol 34:741–745, 1996.
16. Muller-Lissner SA: Adverse effects of laxatives: Fact and fiction. Pharmacology 47(Suppl 1):138–145, 1993.
17. Rosenblum M, Simpson DP, Evenson M: Factitious Bartter's syndrome. Arch Intern Med 137:1244–1245, 1977.
18. Corsi FM, Galgani S, Gasparini C, et al: Acute hypokalemic myopathy due to chronic licorice ingestion: Report of a case. Ital J Neurol Sci 4:493–497, 1983.
19. Vanpee D, Delgrange E, Gillet JB, Donckier J: Ingestion of antacid tablets (Rennie) and acute confusion. J Emerg Med 19:169–171, 2000.
20. Olveira Fuster G, Mancha Doblas I, Vazquez San Miguel F, et al: [Surreptitious intake of diuretics as the cause of pseudo–Bartter's syndrome: Apropos of a case and differential diagnosis.] An Med Interna 13:496–499, 1996.
21. Fraley DS, Adler S, Bruns F: Life-threatening metabolic alkalosis in a comatose patient. South Med J 72:1024–1025, 1979.
22. Laudignon N, Ciampi A, Coupal L, et al: Furosemide and ethacrynic acid: Risk factors for the occurrence of serum electrolyte abnormalities and metabolic alkalosis in newborns and infants. Acta Paediatr Scand 78:133–135, 1989.
23. Entholzner E, Mielke L, Pichlmeier R, et al: [EEG changes during sedation with gamma-hydroxybutyric acid.] Anaesthetist 44:345–350, 1995.
24. Shetty AK, Rogers NL, Mannick EE, Aviles DH: Syndrome of hypokalemic metabolic alkalosis and hypomagnesemia associated with gentamicin therapy: Case reports. Clin Pediatr (Phila) 39:529–533, 2000.
25. Oster JR, Materson BJ, Rogers AI: Laxative abuse syndrome. Am J Gastroenterol 74:451–458, 1980.
26. Heikens J, Fliers E, Endert E, et al: Liquorice-induced hypertension—a new understanding of an old disease: Case report and brief review. Neth J Med 47:230–234, 1995.
27. Saito T, Tsuboi Y, Fujisawa G, et al: An autopsy case of licorice-induced hypokalemic rhabdomyolysis associated with acute renal failure: Special reference to profound calcium deposition in skeletal and cardiac muscle. Nippon Jinzo Gakkai Shi 36:1308–1314, 1994.
28. Fournier A, Lagrue G: [Hypertension caused by hypermineralocorticism.] Sem Hop 47:872–889, 1971.
29. Gautier J, Lamisse F, Lamagnere JP: [Quadriplegia with hypokalemia and metabolic alkalosis secondary to ingestion of licorice extract.] Cah Coll Med Hop Paris 10:461–466, 1969.
30. Bodanszky H, Leleiko N: Metabolic alkalosis with hypertonic dehydration in a patient with diarrhoea and magnesium oxide ingestion. Acta Paediatr Hung 26:241–246, 1985.
31. Garin EH, Geary D, Richard GA: Soybean formula (Neo-Mull-Soy) metabolic alkalosis in infancy. J Pediatr 95:985–987, 1979.
32. Hellerstein S, Duggan E, Grossman HM, et al: Metabolic alkalosis and Neo-Mull-Soy. J Pediatr 95:1083–1084, 1979.

33. Reznik VM, Griswold WR, Mendoza SA, McNeal RM: Neo-Mull-Soy metabolic alkalosis: A model of Bartter's syndrome? Pediatrics 66:784–786, 1980.

34. Herrmann U, Schwille PO, Schwarzlaender H, et al: Citrate and recurrent idiopathic calcium urolithiasis. A longitudinal pilot study on the metabolic effects of oral potassium sodium citrate administered as short-, medium- and long-term to male stone patients. Urol Res 20:347–353, 1992.

35. Acomb C, Hordon LD, Judd AT, Turney JH: Metabolic alkalosis induced by 'Panadol Soluble'. Lancet 2:614, 1985.

36. Chiolero R, Schneiter P, Cayeux C, et al: Metabolic and respiratory effects of sodium lactate during short i.v. nutrition in critically ill patients. JPEN J Parenter Enteral Nutr 20:257–263, 1996.

37. Pitt J: Association between paracetamol and pyroglutamic aciduria. Clin Chem 36:173–174, 1990.

38. Pitt JJ, Brown GK, Clift V, Christodoulou J: Atypical pyroglutamic aciduria: Possible role of paracetamol. J Inherit Metab Dis 13:755–756, 1990.

39. Pitt JJ, Hauser S: Transient 5-oxoprolinuria and high anion gap metabolic acidosis: Clinical and biochemical findings in eleven subjects. Clin Chem 44:1497–1503, 1998.

40. McClain CJ, Price S, Barve S, et al: Acetaminophen hepatotoxicity: An update. Curr Gastroenterol Rep 1:42–49, 1999.

41. Koulouris Z, Tierney MG, Jones G: Metabolic acidosis and coma following a severe acetaminophen overdose. Ann Pharmacother 33:1191–1194, 1999.

42. Dempsey GA, Lyall HJ, Corke CF, Scheinkestel CD: Pyroglutamic acidemia: A cause of high anion gap metabolic acidosis. Crit Care Med 28:1803–1807, 2000.

43. Yale SH, Mazza JJ: Anion gap acidosis associated with acetaminophen. Ann Intern Med 133:752–753, 2000.

44. Chapron DJ, Gomolin IH, Sweeney KR: Acetazolamide blood concentrations are excessive in the elderly: Propensity for acidosis and relationship to renal function. J Clin Pharmacol 29:348–353, 1989.

45. Heller I, Halevy J, Cohen S, Theodor E: Significant metabolic acidosis induced by acetazolamide. Not a rare complication. Arch Intern Med 145:1815–1817, 1985.

46. Watson WA, Garrelts JC, Zinn PD, et al: Chronic acetazolamide intoxication. J Toxicol Clin Toxicol 22:549–563, 1984.

47. Boggild MD, Peck RW, Tomson CR: Acetonitrile ingestion: Delayed onset of cyanide poisoning due to concurrent ingestion of acetone. Postgrad Med J 66:40–41, 1990.

48. Rainey PM, Roberts WL: Diagnosis and misdiagnosis of poisoning with the cyanide precursor acetonitrile: Nail polish remover or nail glue remover? Am J Emerg Med 11:104–108, 1993.

49. Turchen SG, Manoguerra AS, Whitney C: Severe cyanide poisoning from the ingestion of an acetonitrile-containing cosmetic. Am J Emerg Med 9:264–267, 1991.

50. Foley RJ: Inhaled industrial acetylene. A diabetic ketoacidosis mimic. JAMA 254:1066–1067, 1985.

51. Budris WA, Roxe DM, Duvel JM: High anion gap metabolic acidosis associated with aminocaproic acid. Ann Pharmacother 33:308–311, 1999.

52. Gerard JM, Luisiri A: A fatal overdose of arginine hydrochloride. J Toxicol Clin Toxicol 35:621–625, 1997.

53. Temple AR: Acute and chronic effects of aspirin toxicity and their treatment. Arch Intern Med 141(Spec No):364–369, 1981.

54. Cowan RA, Hartnell GG, Lowdell CP, et al: Metabolic acidosis induced by carbonic anhydrase inhibitors and salicylates in patients with normal renal function. Br Med J (Clin Res Ed) 289:347–348, 1984.

55. Bartels PD, Lund-Jacobsen H: Blood lactate and ketone body concentrations in salicylate intoxication. Hum Toxicol 5:363–366, 1986.

56. Germann R, Schindera I, Kuch M, et al: [Life-threatening salicylate poisoning caused by percutaneous absorption in severe ichthyosis vulgaris.] Hautarzt 47:624–627, 1996.

57. Pertoldi F, D'Orlando L, Mercante WP: [Acute salicylate intoxication after transcutaneous absorption.] Minerva Anestesiol 65:571–573, 1999.

58. Proudfoot AT, Brown SS: Acidaemia and salicylate poisoning in adults. BMJ 2:547–550, 1969.

59. Abrams J, el-Mallakh RS, Meyer R: Suicidal sodium azide ingestion. Ann Emerg Med 16:1378–1380, 1987.

60. Albertson TE, Reed S, Siefkin A: A case of fatal sodium azide ingestion. J Toxicol Clin Toxicol 24:339–351, 1986.

61. Emmett EA, Ricking JA: Fatal self-administration of sodium azide. Ann Intern Med 83:224–226, 1975.

62. Senda T, Nishio K, Hori Y, et al: [A case of fatal acute sodium azide poisoning.] Chudoku Kenkyu 14:339–342, 2001.

63. Restuccio A, Mortensen ME, Kelley MT: Fatal ingestion of boric acid in an adult. Am J Emerg Med 10:545–547, 1992.

64. Myers RA, Britten JS: Are arterial blood gases of value in treatment decisions for carbon monoxide poisoning? Crit Care Med 17:139–142, 1989.

65. Roshan M, Price DE: Carbon monoxide poisoning presenting as apparent ketoacidosis. Diabetes Care 16:956–957, 1993.

66. Sokal JA: The effect of exposure duration on the blood level of glucose, pyruvate and lactate in acute carbon monoxide intoxication in man. J Appl Toxicol 5:395–397, 1985.

67. Sokal JA, Kralkowska E: The relationship between exposure duration, carboxyhemoglobin, blood glucose, pyruvate and lactate and the severity of intoxication in 39 cases of acute carbon monoxide poisoning in man. Arch Toxicol 57:196–199, 1985.

68. Szerlip HM, Singer I: Hyperchloremic metabolic acidosis after chlorine inhalation. Am J Med 77:581–582, 1984.

69. Bethke RA, Gratton M, Watson WA: Severe hyperlactemia and metabolic acidosis following cocaine use and exertion. Am J Emerg Med 8:369–370, 1990.

70. Jonsson S, O'Meara M, Young JB: Acute cocaine poisoning. Importance of treating seizures and acidosis. Am J Med 75:1061–1064, 1983.

71. Stevens DC, Campbell JP, Carter JE, Watson WA: Acid-base abnormalities associated with cocaine toxicity in emergency department patients. J Toxicol Clin Toxicol 32:31–39, 1994.

72. Baud FJ, Borron SW, Megarbane B, et al: Value of lactic acidosis in the assessment of the severity of acute cyanide poisoning. Crit Care Med 30:2044–2050, 2002.

73. Baud FJ, Barriot P, Toffis V, et al: Elevated blood cyanide concentrations in victims of smoke inhalation. N Engl J Med 325:1761–1766, 1991.

74. Baud FJ, Borron SW, Bavoux E, et al: Relation between plasma lactate and blood cyanide concentrations in acute cyanide poisoning. BMJ 312:26–27, 1996.

75. Borron SW, Baud FJ: Acute cyanide poisoning: Clinical spectrum, diagnosis, and treatment. Arh Hig Rada Toksikol 47:307–322, 1996.

76. Benaissa ML, Hantson P, Bismuth C, Baud FJ: Mercury oxycyanide and mercuric cyanide poisoning: Two cases. Intensive Care Med 21:1051–1053, 1995.

77. Yen D, Tsai J, Wang LM, et al: The clinical experience of acute cyanide poisoning. Am J Emerg Med 13:524–528, 1995.

78. Wilson KC, Reardon C, Farber HW: Propylene glycol toxicity in a patient receiving intravenous diazepam. N Engl J Med 343:815, 2000.

79. Bissuel F, Bruneel F, Habersetzer F, et al: Fulminant hepatitis with severe lactate acidosis in HIV-infected patients on didanosine therapy. J Intern Med 235:367–371, 1994.

80. Borron SW, Baud FJ, Garnier R: Intravenous 4-methylpyrazole as an antidote for diethylene glycol and triethylene glycol poisoning: A case report. Vet Hum Toxicol 39:26–28, 1997.

81. Vassiliadis J, Graudins A, Dowsett RP: Triethylene glycol poisoning treated with intravenous ethanol infusion. J Toxicol Clin Toxicol 37:773–776, 1999.

82. Grimmett WG, Dzendolet I, Whyte I: Intravenous thiodan (30% endosulfan in xylene). J Toxicol Clin Toxicol 34:447–452, 1996.

83. Osterloh JD, Kelly TJ, Khayam-Bashi H, Romeo R: Discrepancies in osmolal gaps and calculated alcohol concentrations. Arch Pathol Lab Med 120:637–641, 1996.

84. Adams SL: Alcoholic ketoacidosis. Emerg Med Clin North Am 8:749–760, 1990.

85. Lamminpaa A, Vilska J: Acute alcohol intoxications in children treated in hospital. Acta Paediatr Scand 79:847–854, 1990.

86. Lamminpaa A, Vilska J, Korri UM, Riihimaki V: Alcohol intoxication in hospitalized young teenagers. Acta Paediatr 82:783–788, 1993.

87. Lien D, Mader TJ: Survival from profound alcohol-related lactic acidosis. J Emerg Med 17:841–846, 1999.

88. Mukunda BN: Lactic acidosis caused by thiamine deficiency in a pregnant alcoholic patient. Am J Med Sci 317:261–262, 1999.

89. Braden GL, Strayhorn CH, Germain MJ, et al: Increased osmolal gap in alcoholic acidosis. Arch Intern Med 153:2377–2380, 1993.

90. Schelling JR, Howard RL, Winter SD, Linas SL: Increased osmolal gap in alcoholic ketoacidosis and lactic acidosis. Ann Intern Med 113:580–582, 1990.

91. Wrenn KD, Slovis CM, Minion GE, Rutkowski R: The syndrome of alcoholic ketoacidosis. Am J Med 91:119–128, 1991.
92. Clay KL, Murphy RC: On the metabolic acidosis of ethylene glycol intoxication. Toxicol Appl Pharmacol 39:39–49, 1977.
93. Jacobsen D, Ovrebo S, Ostborg J, Sejersted OM: Glycolate causes the acidosis in ethylene glycol poisoning and is effectively removed by hemodialysis. Acta Med Scand 216:409–416, 1984.
94. Brent J: Current management of ethylene glycol poisoning. Drugs 61:979–988, 2001.
95. Ortuno Anderiz F, Rodriguez Palomares JR, Cabello Clotet N: [Survival in a case of ethylene glycol poisoning with extreme acidemia.] Rev Clin Esp 200:344–345, 2000.
96. Rambourg-Schepens MO, Buffet M, Bertault R, et al: Severe ethylene glycol butyl ether poisoning. Kinetics and metabolic pattern. Hum Toxicol 7:187–189, 1988.
97. Bauer P, Weber M, Mur JM, et al: Transient non-cardiogenic pulmonary edema following massive ingestion of ethylene glycol butyl ether. Intensive Care Med 18:250–251, 1992.
98. Dean BS, Krenzelok EP: Clinical evaluation of pediatric ethylene glycol monobutyl ether poisonings. J Toxicol Clin Toxicol 30:557–563, 1992.
99. Burkhart KK, Donovan JW: Hemodialysis following butoxyethanol ingestion. J Toxicol Clin Toxicol 36:723–725, 1998.
100. McKinney PE, Palmer RB, Blackwell W, Benson BE: Butoxyethanol ingestion with prolonged hyperchloremic metabolic acidosis treated with ethanol therapy. J Toxicol Clin Toxicol 38:787–793, 2000.
101. Nitter-Hauge S: Poisoning with ethylene glycol monomethyl ether. Report of two cases. Acta Med Scand 188:277–280, 1970.
102. Bedichek E, Kirschbaum B: A case of propylene glycol toxic reaction associated with etomidate infusion. Arch Intern Med 151:2297–2298, 1991.
103. McConnel JR, Ong CS, McAllister JL, Gross TG: Propylene glycol toxicity following continuous etomidate infusion for the control of refractory cerebral edema. Neurosurgery 38:232–233, 1996.
104. Van de Wiele B, Rubinstein E, Peacock W, Martin N: Propylene glycol toxicity caused by prolonged infusion of etomidate. J Neurosurg Anesthesiol 7:259–262, 1995.
105. McKenzie R, Fried MW, Sallie R, et al: Hepatic failure and lactic acidosis due to fialuridine (FIAU), an investigational nucleoside analogue for chronic hepatitis B. N Engl J Med 333:1099–1105, 1995.
106. Arnaudo JP, Maheut H, Martin B, Hesse JY: [Reversible ketoacidosis and hyperglycemia after absorption of flumequine. Effect of high doses in a non-diabetic adult.] Nouv Presse Med 9:636, 1980.
107. Koppel C, Baudisch H, Schneider V, Ibe K: Suicidal ingestion of formalin with fatal complications. Intensive Care Med 16:212–214, 1990.
108. Pandey CK, Agarwal A, Baronia A, Singh N: Toxicity of ingested formalin and its management. Hum Exp Toxicol 19:360–366, 2000.
109. Chan TC, Williams SR, Clark RF: Formic acid skin burns resulting in systemic toxicity. Ann Emerg Med 26:383–386, 1995.
110. Jefferys DB, Wiseman HM: Formic acid poisoning. Postgrad Med J 56:761–762, 1980.
111. Malizia E, Reale C, Pietropaoli P, De Ritis GC: Formic acid intoxications. Acta Pharmacol Toxicol (Copenh) 41(Suppl 2):342–347, 1977.
112. Rajan N, Rahim R, Krishna Kumar S: Formic acid poisoning with suicidal intent: A report of 53 cases. Postgrad Med J 61:35–36, 1985.
113. Rosewarne FA: Self poisoning with formic acid. Anaesthesia 38:1104–1105, 1983.
114. Verstraete AG, Vogelaers DP, van den Bogaerde JF, et al: Formic acid poisoning: Case report and in vitro study of the hemolytic activity. Am J Emerg Med 7:286–290, 1989.
115. Stine RJ, Slosberg B, Beacham BE: Hydrogen sulfide intoxication. A case report and discussion of treatment. Ann Intern Med 85:756–758, 1976.
116. McGuigan MA: Acute iron poisoning. Pediatr Ann 25:33–38, 1996.
117. Alvarez FG, Guntupalli KK: Isoniazid overdose: Four case reports and review of the literature. Intensive Care Med 21:641–644, 1995.
118. Romero JA, Kuczler FJ Jr: Isoniazid overdose: Recognition and management. Am Fam Physician 57:749–752, 1998.
119. Arbour RB: Propylene glycol toxicity related to high-dose lorazepam infusion: Case report and discussion. Am J Crit Care 8:499–506, 1999.
120. Arbour R, Esparis B: Osmolar gap metabolic acidosis in a 60-year-old man treated for hypoxemic respiratory failure. Chest 118:545–546, 2000.
121. Cawley MJ: Short-term lorazepam infusion and concern for propylene glycol toxicity: Case report and review. Pharmacotherapy 21:1140–1144, 2001.
122. Reynolds HN, Teiken P, Regan ME, et al: Hyperlactatemia, increased osmolar gap, and renal dysfunction during continuous lorazepam infusion. Crit Care Med 28:1631–1634, 2000.
123. Chan P, Chen JH, Lee MH, Deng JF: Fatal and nonfatal methamphetamine intoxication in the intensive care unit. J Toxicol Clin Toxicol 32:147–155, 1994.
124. Lanigan S: Final report on the safety assessment of methyl alcohol. Int J Toxicol 20(Suppl 1):57–85, 2001.
125. Liesivuori J, Savolainen H: Methanol and formic acid toxicity: Biochemical mechanisms. Pharmacol Toxicol 69:157–163, 1991.
126. Dash H, Mills J: Severe metabolic acidosis associated with nalidixic acid overdose [letter]. Ann Intern Med 84:570–571, 1976.
127. Humphrey SH, Nash DA Jr: Lactic acidosis complicating sodium nitroprusside therapy. Ann Intern Med 88:58–59, 1978.
128. Lipper B, Bell A, Gaynor B: Recurrent hypotension immediately after seizures in nortriptyline overdose. Am J Emerg Med 12:452–453, 1994.
129. Zadik Z, Blachar Y, Barak Y, Levin S: Organophosphate poisoning presenting as diabetic ketoacidosis. J Toxicol Clin Toxicol 20:381–385, 1983.
130. Haddad LM, Dimond KA, Schweistris JE: Phenol poisoning. JACEP 8:267–269, 1979.
131. Soares ER, Tift JP: Phenol poisoning: Three fatal cases. J Forensic Sci 27:729–731, 1982.
132. Stajduhar-Caric Z: Acute phenol poisoning. Singular findings in a lethal case. J Forensic Med 15:41–42, 1968.
133. Caravati EM: Metabolic abnormalities associated with phosphoric acid ingestion. Ann Emerg Med 16:904–906, 1987.
134. Fernandez OU, Canizares LL: Acute hepatotoxicity from ingestion of yellow phosphorus–containing fireworks. J Clin Gastroenterol 21:139–142, 1995.
135. Woolf AD, Ebert TH: Toxicity after self-poisoning by ingestion of potassium chloroplatinite. J Toxicol Clin Toxicol 29:467–472, 1991.
136. Bismuth C, Baud FJ, Djeghout H, et al: Cyanide poisoning from propionitrile exposure. J Emerg Med 5:191–195, 1987.
137. Cray SH, Robinson BH, Cox PN: Lactic acidemia and bradyarrhythmia in a child sedated with propofol. Crit Care Med 26:2087–2092, 1998.
138. Hanna JP, Ramundo ML: Rhabdomyolysis and hypoxia associated with prolonged propofol infusion in children. Neurology 50:301–303, 1998.
139. Martin PH, Murthy BV, Petros AJ: Metabolic, biochemical and haemodynamic effects of infusion of propofol for long-term sedation of children undergoing intensive care. Br J Anaesth 79:276–279, 1997.
140. Parke TJ, Stevens JE, Rice AS, et al: Metabolic acidosis and fatal myocardial failure after propofol infusion in children: Five case reports. BMJ 305:613–616, 1992.
141. Perrier ND, Baerga-Varela Y, Murray MJ: Death related to propofol use in an adult patient. Crit Care Med 28:3071–3074, 2000.
142. Strickland RA, Murray MJ: Fatal metabolic acidosis in a pediatric patient receiving an infusion of propofol in the intensive care unit: Is there a relationship? Crit Care Med 23:405–409, 1995.
143. Cate JC 4th, Hedrick R: Propylene glycol intoxication and lactic acidosis. N Engl J Med 303:1237, 1980.
144. Christopher MM, Eckfeldt JH, Eaton JW: Propylene glycol ingestion causes D-lactic acidosis. Lab Invest 62:114–118, 1990.
145. Demey HE, Daelemans RA, Verpooten GA, et al: Propylene glycol–induced side effects during intravenous nitroglycerin therapy. Intensive Care Med 14:221–226, 1988.
146. Glover ML, Reed MD: Propylene glycol: The safe diluent that continues to cause harm. Pharmacotherapy 16:690–693, 1996.
147. Kelner MJ, Bailey DN: Propylene glycol as a cause of lactic acidosis. J Anal Toxicol 9:40–42, 1985.
148. Lolin Y, Francis DA, Flanagan RJ, et al: Cerebral depression due to propylene glycol in a patient with chronic epilepsy—the value of the plasma osmolal gap in diagnosis. Postgrad Med J 64:610–613, 1988.
149. Buehler JH, Berns AS, Webster JR, et al: Lactic acidosis from carboxyhemoglobinemia after smoke inhalation. Ann Intern Med 82:803–805, 1975.
150. Taboulet P, Clemessy JL, Freminet A, Baud FJ: A case of life-threatening lactic acidosis after smoke inhalation—interference between

beta-adrenergic agents and ethanol? Intensive Care Med 21:1039–1041, 1995.

151. Skellett S, Mayer A, Durward A, et al: Chasing the base deficit: Hyperchloraemic acidosis following 0.9% saline fluid resuscitation. Arch Dis Child 83:514–516, 2000.

152. Miller KD, Cameron M, Wood LV, et al: Lactic acidosis and hepatic steatosis associated with use of stavudine: Report of four cases. Ann Intern Med 133:192–196, 2000.

153. McLeod HL, Baker DK Jr, Pui CH, Rodman JH: Somnolence, hypotension, and metabolic acidosis following high-dose teniposide treatment in children with leukemia. Cancer Chemother Pharmacol 29:150–154, 1991.

154. Bernard S: Severe lactic acidosis following theophylline overdose. Ann Emerg Med 20:1135–1137, 1991.

155. Hagley MT, Traeger SM, Schuckman H: Pronounced metabolic response to modest theophylline overdose. Ann Pharmacother 28:195–196, 1994.

156. Leventhal LJ, Kochar G, Feldman NH, et al: Lactic acidosis in theophylline overdose. Am J Emerg Med 7:417–418, 1989.

157. Caravati EM, Bjerk PJ: Acute toluene ingestion toxicity. Ann Emerg Med 30:838–839, 1997.

158. Gerkin RD Jr, LoVecchio F: Rapid reversal of life-threatening toluene-induced hypokalemia with hemodialysis. J Emerg Med 16:723–725, 1998.

159. Kamijima M, Nakazawa Y, Yamakawa M, et al: Metabolic acidosis and renal tubular injury due to pure toluene inhalation. Arch Environ Health 49:410–413, 1994.

160. Kamijo Y, Soma K, Hasegawa I, Ohwada T: Fatal bilateral adrenal hemorrhage following acute toluene poisoning: A case report. J Toxicol Clin Toxicol 36:365–368, 1998.

161. Wilner A, Raymond K, Pollard R: Topiramate and metabolic acidosis. Epilepsia 40:792–795, 1999.

162. Scheulen ME, Hilger RA, Oberhoff C, et al: Clinical phase I dose escalation and pharmacokinetic study of high-dose chemotherapy with treosulfan and autologous peripheral blood stem cell transplantation in patients with advanced malignancies. Clin Cancer Res 6:4209–4216, 2000.

163. Kaufman AM, Hellman G, Abramson RG: Renal salt wasting and metabolic acidosis with trimethoprim-sulfamethoxazole therapy. Mt Sinai J Med 50:238–239, 1983.

164. Porras MC, Lecumberri JN, Castrillon JL: Trimethoprim/sulfamethoxazole and metabolic acidosis in HIV-infected patients. Ann Pharmacother 32:185–189, 1998.

164a. Janssen F, Rambeck B, Schnabel R: Acute valproate intoxication with fatal outcome in an infant. Neuropediatrics 16:235–238, 1985.

164b. Isbister GK, Balit CR, Whyte IM, Dawson A: Valproate overdose: a comparative cohort study of self poisonings. Br J Clin Pharmacol 55:398–404, 2003.

165. Watson ID, McBride D, Paterson KR: Fatal xylenol self-poisoning. Postgrad Med J 62:411–412, 1986.

166. Aggarwal A, al-Talib K, Alabrash M: Type B lactic acidosis in an AIDS patient treated with zidovudine. Md Med J 45:929–931, 1996.

167. Costarino A, Davis D, Keon T: Falsely normal saturation reading with the pulse oximeter. Anesthesiology 67:830–831, 1987.

168. Grace R: Pulse oximetry. Gold standard or false sense of security? Med J Aust 160:638–644, 1994.

169. Kirlangitis J, Middaugh R, Zablocki A, Rodriquez F: False indication of arterial oxygen desaturation and methemoglobinemia following injection of methylene blue in urological surgery. Mil Med 155:260–262, 1990.

170. Lear J, Morgan M: False reassurance of pulse oximetry. Misunderstanding leads to dangerous practice. BMJ 307:733, 1993.

171. Maleck W, Koetter K: False-positive end-tidal CO2. Ann Emerg Med 30:116–117, 1997.

172. McCrory C, Ryan M, Doherty P: Falsely reassuring pulse oximetry in the presence of severe hypoxia. Can J Anaesth 44:1323–1324, 1997.

173. Montauk L, Michaels A, Barsotti M: False-positive end-tidal CO2. Ann Emerg Med 28:458–459, 1996.

174. O'Flaherty D, Adams A: False-positives with the end-tidal carbon dioxide detector. Anesth Analg 74:467–468, 1992.

175. Salem MM, Mujais SK: Gaps in the anion gap. Arch Intern Med 152:1625–1629, 1992.

176. Wrenn K: The delta (delta) gap: An approach to mixed acid-base disorders. Ann Emerg Med 19:1310–1313, 1990.

177. Adrogue HJ, Wilson H, Boyd AE 3rd, et al: Plasma acid-base patterns in diabetic ketoacidosis. N Engl J Med 307:1603–1610, 1982.

178. Brivet F, Bernardin M, Dormont J: [Hyperchloremic acidosis in metabolic acidosis with anion gap excess. Comparison with diabetic ketoacidosis.] Presse Med 20:413–417, 1991.

179. Gabow PA, Kaehny WD, Fennessey PV, et al: Diagnostic importance of an increased serum anion gap. N Engl J Med 303:854–858, 1980.

180. Winter SD, Pearson JR, Gabow PA, et al: The fall of the serum anion gap. Arch Intern Med 150:311–313, 1990.

181. Sadjadi SA: A new range for the anion gap. Ann Intern Med 123:807, 1995.

182. Iberti TJ, Leibowitz AB, Papadakos PJ, Fischer EP: Low sensitivity of the anion gap as a screen to detect hyperlactatemia in critically ill patients. Crit Care Med 18:275–277, 1990.

183. Roberts WL, Johnson RD: The serum anion gap. Has the reference interval really fallen? Arch Pathol Lab Med 121:568–572, 1997.

184. Paulson WD, Roberts WL, Lurie AA, et al: Wide variation in serum anion gap measurements by chemistry analyzers. Am J Clin Pathol 110:735–742, 1998.

185. Figge J, Jabor A, Kazda A, Fencl V: Anion gap and hypoalbuminemia. Crit Care Med 26:1807–1810, 1998.

186. Wang F, Butler T, Rabbani GH, Jones PK: The acidosis of cholera. Contributions of hyperproteinemia, lactic acidemia, and hyperphosphatemia to an increased serum anion gap. N Engl J Med 315:1591–1595, 1986.

187. Decaux G, Schlesser M, Coffernils M, et al: Uric acid, anion gap and urea concentration in the diagnostic approach to hyponatremia. Clin Nephrol 42:102–108, 1994.

188. Gabow PA, Kaehny WD, Fennessey PV, et al: Diagnostic importance of an increased anion gap. N Engl J Med 303:854–858, 1980.

189. Dorwart WV, Chalmers L: Comparison of methods for calculating serum osmolality from chemical concentrations, and the prognostic value of such calculations. Clin Chem 21:190–194, 1975.

190. Schwartz-Goldstein BH, Malik AR, Sarwar A, Brandstetter RD: Lactic acidosis associated with a deceptively normal anion gap. Heart Lung 25:79–80, 1996.

191. Kirschbaum B: The acidosis of exogenous phosphate intoxication. Arch Intern Med 158:405–408, 1998.

192. Oster JR, Singer I, Contreras GN, et al: Metabolic acidosis with extreme elevation of anion gap: Case report and literature review. Am J Med Sci 317:38–49, 1999.

193. Astrup P, Jorgensen K, Siggaard-Andersen O, et al: The acid-base metabolism—a new approach. Lancet 1:1035–1039, 1960.

194. Rosan RC, Enlander D, Ellis J: Unpredictable error in calculated bicarbonate homeostasis during pediatric intensive care: The delusion of fixed pK′. Clin Chem 29:69–73, 1983.

195. Durward A, Skellett S, Mayer A, et al: The value of the chloride:sodium ratio in differentiating the aetiology of metabolic acidosis. Intensive Care Med 27:828–835, 2001.

196. Smithline N, Gardner KD Jr: Gaps—anionic and osmolal. JAMA 236:1594–1597, 1976.

197. Hoffman RS, Smilkstein MJ, Howland MA, Goldfrank LR: Osmol gaps revisited: Normal values and limitations. J Toxicol Clin Toxicol 31:81–93, 1993.

198. Purssell RA, Pudek M, Brubacher J, Abu-Laban RB: Derivation and validation of a formula to calculate the contribution of ethanol to the osmolal gap. Ann Emerg Med 38:653–659, 2001.

199. Buckley N, Whyte I, Dawson A: Osmolal gap. J Toxicol Clin Toxicol 32:93–95, 1994.

200. Jacobsen D, Bredesen JE, Eide I, Ostborg J: Anion and osmolal gaps in the diagnosis of methanol and ethylene glycol poisoning. Acta Med Scand 212:17–20, 1982.

201. Narins RG, Emmett M: Simple and mixed acid-base disorders: A practical approach. Medicine (Baltimore) 59:161–187, 1980.

202. Kolendorf K, Moller BB: Lactic acidosis in epinephrine poisoning. Acta Med Scand 196:465–466, 1974.

203. Graf H, Leach W, Arieff AI: Evidence for a detrimental effect of bicarbonate therapy in hypoxic lactic acidosis. Science 227:754–756, 1985.

204. Forsythe SM, Schmidt GA: Sodium bicarbonate for the treatment of lactic acidosis. Chest 117:260–267, 2000.

205. Liebelt E: Targeted management strategies for cardiovascular toxicity from tricyclic antidepressant overdose: The pivotal role for alkalinization and sodium loading. Pediatr Emerg Care 14:293–298, 1998.
206. Mackway-Jones K: Towards evidence based emergency medicine: Best BETs from the Manchester Royal Infirmary. Alkalinisation in the management of tricyclic antidepressant overdose. J Accid Emerg Med 16:139–140, 1999.
207. Shapiro JI: Pathogenesis of cardiac dysfunction during metabolic acidosis: Therapeutic implications. Kidney Int (Suppl 61):S47-S51, 1997.
208. Leung JM, Landow L, Franks M, et al: Safety and efficacy of intravenous Carbicarb in patients undergoing surgery: Comparison with sodium bicarbonate in the treatment of mild metabolic acidosis. SPI Research Group. Study of Perioperative Ischemia. Crit Care Med 22:1540–1549, 1994.
209. Nahas GG, Sutin KM, Fermon C, et al: Guidelines for the treatment of acidaemia with THAM. Drugs 55:191–224, 1998.
210. Kallet RH, Jasmer RM, Luce JM, et al: The treatment of acidosis in acute lung injury with tris-hydroxymethyl aminomethane (THAM). Am J Respir Crit Care Med 161:1149–1153, 2000.
211. Preiser J, Vincent J: Specific therapies of biguanide-induced lactic acidosis. Anesthesiology 89:267–268, 1998.
212. Ledebo I: Acid-base correction and convective dialysis therapies. Nephrol Dial Transplant 15(Suppl 2):45–48, 2000.
213. Heaney D, Majid A, Junor B: Bicarbonate haemodialysis as a treatment of metformin overdose. Nephrol Dial Transplant 12:1046–1047, 1997.
214. Sabeel AI, Kurkus J, Lindholm T: Intensified dialysis treatment of ethylene glycol intoxication. Scand J Urol Nephrol 29:125–129, 1995.

CHAPTER 30

Withdrawal Syndromes

Adhi N. Sharma ▪ Robert S. Hoffman

Any discussion of withdrawal should begin with defining the following terms: *narcotic, tolerance, dependence, addiction, withdrawal,* and *cross-tolerance*. Defining these words not only allows for better understanding but also enables the appropriate application of these terms (Fig. 30-1). *Narcotic* literally means any drug that induces sleep, although it also has the sociolegal implication of an illegal substance. To maintain clarity, drugs should be referred to by clinical class (i.e., opioids, sedative-hypnotics, and stimulants [e.g., cocaine and amphetamines]). *Tolerance* is the physiologic process by which increasing drug concentrations are required to obtain a desired effect, which can be represented graphically by a shift in the dose-response curve to the right. This effect is exemplified best by heroin tolerance, in which one person's routine dose would be lethal to a naive user. Tolerance can be mediated via receptor modulation (opioids), induced metabolism (barbiturates), or both (ethanol). *Dependence* implies that cessation of the drug leads to withdrawal symptoms. *Withdrawal* can be physiologic (i.e., autonomic instability, nausea, vomiting, diarrhea, hyperactivity, or altered mentation), psychological (i.e., emotional symptoms and craving), or both. When continued use of a drug induces socially unacceptable behavior (theft) or results in unacceptable outcomes (a driving-while-intoxicated conviction), the user of the drug is considered *addicted*. Addiction does not require dependence, as in the case of crack cocaine. Crack addicts are not physiologically dependent on cocaine. Although they experience drug craving, overt physical withdrawal symptoms are lacking. Physiologic withdrawal is a response to lowered drug concentrations resulting in a predictable constellation of symptoms (i.e., psychological craving, tremors, hypertension, nausea, vomiting, diarrhea). These symptoms are reversible if the drug in question is reintroduced (herein lies the cocaine withdrawal debate because the symptoms of washout are not reversible). Not all withdrawal symptoms are negative or unpleasant. Piloerection, yawning, and lacrimation are associated with opioid withdrawal, but most patients do not perceive these symptoms as negative compared with their drug craving, nausea, and vomiting.

Understanding *cross-tolerance* is the key to treating certain withdrawal syndromes. The concept is that two different drugs share enough common receptor or metabolic activity that one drug can be substituted for the other to prevent withdrawal. This concept is most important for treatment of withdrawal from heroin, alcohol, benzodiazepine, barbiturates, and more recently γ-hydroxybutyrate (GHB) or its analogues γ-butyrolactone (GBL) and butanediol.

The nature of withdrawal and self-treatment behavior makes it impossible to describe its actual incidence. It would be expected that most dependent users go through mild withdrawal every day. The alcoholic who awakens in the morning and drinks an "eye-opener" may exemplify this concept best. Current estimates state that almost 19 million Americans are alcohol abusers or alcoholics, with a 2:1 male-to-female ratio.[1] There are 600,000 heroin addicts in the United States, 20% of whom are in methadone maintenance programs.[2] More recently, GHB and GBL abuse and dependence have been described, but this remains unquantified. Benzodiazepines are some of the most commonly prescribed drugs worldwide. Tolerance to any of these agents can lead to withdrawal, and in the case of alcohol and the sedative-hypnotics (including GHB/GBL), it can be life-threatening.

HISTORY

Spanish physicians described symptoms consistent with delirium tremens (DTs) in the first half of the 19th century.[3] Seven clinical cases were reported in the 1840s and were referred to as *alcoholic chorea* or *ataxis fever*. These patients received various treatments ranging from bleeding with leeches to tincture of opium. The differential diagnosis at that time included epilepsy and meningitis.

In North America, Osler[4] reportedly recognized DTs as a complication of alcoholism in the early part of the 20th century. His recommended treatment consisted of chloral hydrate, potassium bromide, hyoscine, opium, cessation of alcohol, and bed rest. Around 1919, Victor and Adams[5] credited Mellanby as being "among the first to become cognizant of the immediate adjustments of the nervous system to alcoholic intoxication." Alterations to Osler's treatment included the addition of restraints, paraldehyde, and strychnine or ergots to control tremor. Despite these innovations, mortality remained around 14%. It was not until the early 1950s with the work of Victor and Adams[5] and Isbell and colleagues[6] that DTs was recognized as a manifestation of abstinence. At the same time, treatment regimens began to focus on rehydration, substrate supplementation, and supportive care. By the early 1960s, mortality approached 5.4% at Philadelphia General Hospital.[7] Studies in the 1960s comparing paraldehyde and antipsychotics showed a 35% mortality rate with promazine versus a 4.5% mortality rate with paraldehyde.[8] In 1975, benzodiazepines were compared with paraldehyde, and a demonstrable benefit was recognized for this new class of drug in the treatment of

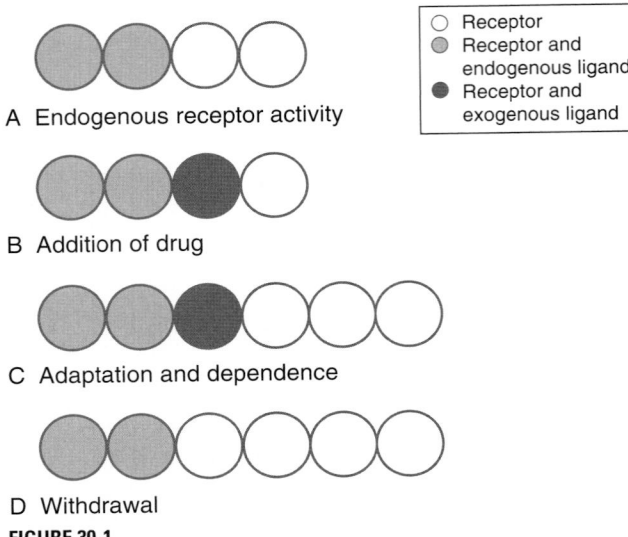

A Endogenous receptor activity

○ Receptor
◐ Receptor and endogenous ligand
● Receptor and exogenous ligand

B Addition of drug

C Adaptation and dependence

D Withdrawal

FIGURE 30-1

Schematic representation of receptor activity.

alcohol withdrawal. Since 1976, the mortality of alcohol withdrawal has been expected to be zero, unless insufficient therapy is provided.[9] Mortality still results from common medical conditions that force alcohol abstinence. Pancreatitis, pneumonia, head trauma, and ulcers commonly precede alcohol withdrawal.[10] A delay in diagnosis of these entities because of the obvious manifestations of withdrawal can result in significant morbidity and mortality.

The use of mind-altering substances predates written records. As new agents are developed, the potential for abuse, dependency, and withdrawal exists. GHB use has grown since the 1980s. Meanwhile, the use of cocaine in the United States has declined from its peak of 5.7 million users in 1985 to 1.5 million in 1998.[2] Since 1992, there has been an increasing trend in new heroin use, and in 1995, the U.S. National Institute for Drug Abuse estimated that there were 141,000 new heroin users, with an unusually high percentage of women from middle-class suburbs.[2] A basic understanding of the pathophysiology of withdrawal and its treatment has general applicability to any withdrawal syndrome, new or well known.

PATHOPHYSIOLOGY

Withdrawal is a phenomenon of altered neurochemistry with the central nervous system (CNS) as the most consequential target. Under normal conditions, the CNS maintains a balance between excitation and inhibition. Although there are several ways to achieve this balance, excitation is constant, and actions occur through removal of inhibitory tone.[11–13] The two major neurotransmitters in the CNS are glutamate and γ-aminobutyric acid (GABA). Glutamate's effects at the N-methyl-D-aspartate (NMDA) receptors increase intracellular calcium, resulting in excitation.[14] Stimulation of GABA receptors increases inhibitory tone via chloride (Cl^-) channel opening. This Cl^- channel is surrounded by receptors, which when activated exert various effects on the channel. The benzodiazepine receptor

increases the frequency of Cl^- channel opening, depolarizing the cell and inhibiting it (Fig. 30-2). This effect requires the presence of GABA.[15] The barbiturate receptor increases the duration of Cl^- channel opening, resulting in a similar effect.[15] Although this action is facilitated by the presence of GABA, the anesthetic barbiturates can depolarize the cell even in the relative absence of GABA. There is increasing evidence of a G protein–mediated GHB receptor, explaining the mechanism of action of GHB.[16] Although it previously was unclear how certain agents (alcohol, propofol, and inhaled anesthetics) interacted with the GABA receptor (subunit A), there is now mounting evidence that these drugs work via binding specific amino acid residues on ligand-gated ion channels to enhance receptor function.[17,18]

The most studied excitatory receptor in the CNS is the NMDA receptor. This receptor controls a voltage-gated and ligand-dependent Ca^{2+} channel.[19] Calcium and sodium influx result in cell depolarization, causing CNS stimulation. Many drugs act as NMDA receptor antagonists, including ethanol, ketamine, phencyclidine, and dextrorphan, the metabolite of dextromethorphan.[20–23]

Finally, opioids stimulate the opioid receptor subtypes μ, κ, and δ to varying extents. Although there are many different opioids available, the common pathway for the development of physical dependence is stimulation of the μ receptor. Stimulation of opioid receptors by opioids begins a cascade of events. These events are mediated via G proteins that alter the cell's conductance and decrease intracellular adenylyl cyclase.[24] Outward potassium channels are activated, decreasing intracellular potassium, hyperpolarizing the cell, and inhibiting its activation.[25,26] The decrease in adenylyl cyclase results in less cyclic adenosine monophosphate (cAMP), preventing protein kinase–mediated activation of Ca^{2+} influx (Fig. 30-3).[27] The net result is to hyperpolarize the cell and prevent neurotransmission of glutamate and substance P, which manifest clinically as CNS depression and analgesia.

Chronic receptor alteration by a drug results in changes in the receptors such that a constant concentration of that drug is needed to maintain baseline neuronal activity. When the drug is stopped abruptly or as the serum concentration drops below threshold, the patient manifests withdrawal symptoms specific to the class of drug used. For sedatives, the result is noradrenergic hyperactivity in the locus caeruleus. This hyperactivity may be produced by enhanced NMDA activity or decreased GABA tone. CNS excitation is the end result and leads to altered mental status, hyperactive muscular activity with resultant hyperthermia, and rhabdomyolysis.[28]

Chronic opioid use leads to cellular and synaptic adaptations. These adaptations include desensitization and internalization, or down-regulation, of receptors (removal of surface receptors), leading to tolerance.[29,30] In addition to these processes, counteradaptation occurs. Activation of the nuclear transcription factor CREB (cAMP responsive element-binding protein) increases the expression of adenylyl cyclase in the locus caeruleus, which may explain the autonomic hyperactivity that occurs in opioid withdrawal.[31] These compensatory changes also are a form of tolerance, increasing cellular excitability and requiring the presence of the drug to maintain basal activity. The best-studied adaptation is an increase in adenylyl cyclase (despite an initial

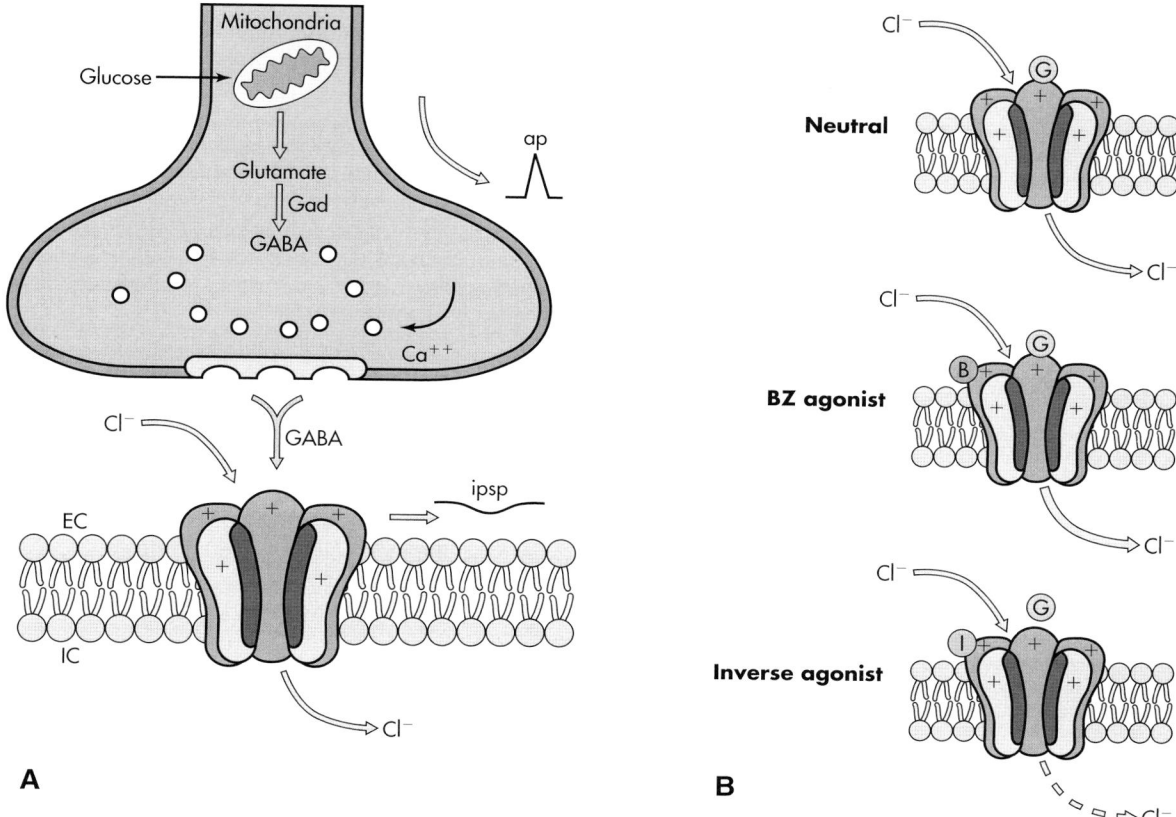

FIGURE 30-2

Idealized model of γ-aminobutyric acid (GABA)-benzodiazepine (BZ)-chloride (Cl⁻) channel at axosomatic (postsynaptic) inhibitory synapses. **A,** Presynaptic and postsynaptic elements. ap, action potential; Gad, glutamic acid decarboxylase; EC, extracellular; IC, intracellular; ipsp, inhibitory postsynaptic potential. **B,** GABA-BZ receptor interactions influencing permeability of chloride channels. Neutral: GABA receptor binds GABA (G) with moderate affinity in the absence of BZ ligand. BZ agonist: Direct BZ agonist (B) enhances GABA affinity for its receptor, resulting in maximal chloride permeability. Inverse agonist: Inverse agonists bound to BZ receptor result in poor GABA affinity and markedly reduced chloride permeability. *(From Rech RH: Drugs to treat anxieties and related disorders. In Brody TM, Larner J, Minneman KP: Human Pharmacology: Molecular to Clinical, 3rd ed. St. Louis, Mosby, 1998, p 367.)*

decrease), which results in Ca^{2+} influx and cellular depolarization. In this excitable state, the user goes through withdrawal when opioid use is discontinued or when an opioid antagonist, such as naloxone, is administered.

TOXIC EFFECTS: WITHDRAWAL SYNDROME

Although there is a great deal of overlap between different substances and their associated withdrawal syndromes, several drugs are discussed individually. These syndromes are alcohol, sedative-hypnotics (including GHB/GBL), opioids, and cocaine (Table 30-1). Finally, the unique aspects of neonatal withdrawal syndromes are discussed.

Alcohol Withdrawal

Alcohol withdrawal is one of the most common withdrawal syndromes, behind those of nicotine and caffeine. The alcohol withdrawal syndrome is multifaceted and should be considered a spectrum. The discrete aspects of alcohol withdrawal can follow a progression or occur independently. These aspects include alcoholic tremulousness, withdrawal seizures, hallucinosis, and DTs. These terms are preferred to the original terms described in the works of Victor and Adams[5] because they are less confusing. It may be more clinically relevant, however, to describe withdrawal as mild, moderate, or severe (life-threatening). Each aspect of alcohol withdrawal is discussed separately, with the understanding that they all are part of a single syndrome.

Alcohol withdrawal typically begins within a few hours after cessation of drinking, when serum ethanol concentrations fall below a threshold level. This level varies with the degree of tolerance the patient has developed. The initial features are usually mild, and tremor is a common symptom. Other accompanying features variably include tachycardia, hypertension, diaphoresis, and anxiety.[5,6] Intervention at this point may halt the progression or development of more significant symptoms and complications.

ALCOHOL WITHDRAWAL SEIZURES

Alcohol withdrawal seizures, previously called "rum fits," usually occur within 6 to 48 hours after cessation of drinking, although they may occur later. The syndrome is typified by a single brief, generalized seizure with a short postictal period. Occasionally the patient has multiple short seizures over a brief period, but status epilepticus occurs in less than 3% of cases.[5] Alcohol withdrawal seizures may be the initial manifestation of withdrawal and the sentinel event in approximately one third of untreated patients who develop DTs.[5]

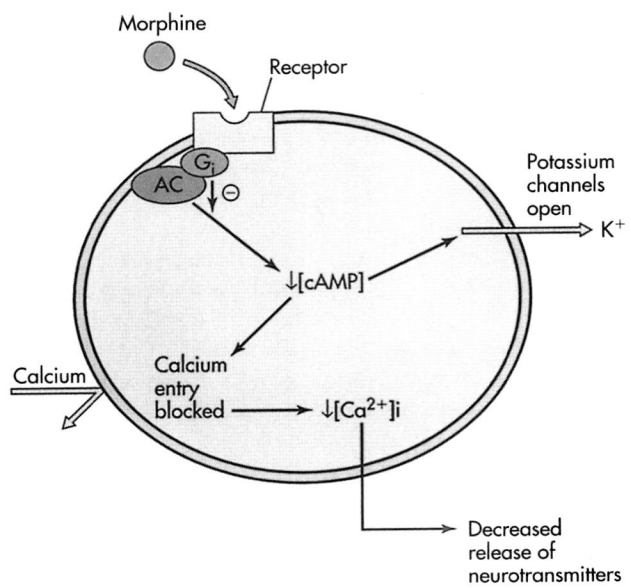

FIGURE 30-3

Mechanism of action of opioids on neurons. Opioid receptors μ, δ, and κ are coupled negatively to adenylyl cyclase by G proteins (G$_i$). Activation of an opioid receptor by an agonist decreases activity of adenylyl cyclase, resulting in a decrease in the production of cyclic adenosine monophosphate (cAMP). This leads to an increase in the efflux of K$^+$ (primarily with μ and δ opioid receptors), cellular hyperpolarization, a decrease in the influx of Ca^{2+} (primarily with κ opioid receptors), and lower intracellular concentrations of free calcium. The overall consequence is a decrease in the neuronal release of neurotransmitters. Opioid receptors also may be coupled by G proteins to intracellular second messengers other than cAMP. *(From Brody TM, Larner J, Minneman KP: Human Pharmacology: Molecular to Clinical, 3rd ed. St. Louis, Mosby, 1998.)*

ALCOHOLIC HALLUCINOSIS

In alcoholic hallucinosis, the hallucinations are typically visual or auditory and may have a persecutory tone. Onset is often within a few hours of abstinence. Alcoholic hallucinosis can occur independently of other signs or symptoms of withdrawal.[5] Although patients experience hallucinations, their mentation is otherwise clear. As such, the hallucinations often are disturbing to the oriented patient.

DELIRIUM TREMENS

DTs are the best studied of all the withdrawal syndromes. The term *delirium tremens* not only applies to alcohol withdrawal but also serves as a model for sedative-hypnotic withdrawal (including GHB/GBL). Symptoms develop 24 hours or more

after the last drink and usually last 3 to 5 days.[5] As the name implies, *delirium* is an important aspect of DTs. During mild withdrawal, or shortly after a rum fit, the patient's mental status generally is intact. An altered sensorium is one of the key distinguishing features of DTs. Patients may hallucinate, have seizures, and display extreme psychomotor agitation (tremens). Hallucinations can be visual or tactile (formication). Autonomic instability may manifest as hypertension, tachycardia, diaphoresis, miosis, and hyperthermia. Psychomotor agitation and autonomic instability associated with DTs represent the life-threatening aspects of alcohol withdrawal and should prompt aggressive therapy.

Sedative-Hypnotic Withdrawal

Sedative-hypnotic withdrawal (benzodiazepines, barbiturates, and GHB/GBL) may be indistinguishable from alcohol withdrawal. The chronology may offer a clue, however, as to the etiology of the withdrawal. Because of rapid metabolism and the lack of active metabolites, GHB/GBL withdrawal generally occurs within 2 to 3 hours of cessation of drug usage.[32] Seizures do not seem to be a part of GHB withdrawal. In a series of nine cases of presumed GHB withdrawal, only one had seizure-like activity, which was a preterminal event.[32] In contrast, diazepam has active metabolites, and withdrawal symptoms may not manifest for 1 week. Seizures are a common sign of benzodiazepine withdrawal. Regardless of the cause, the treatment is similar.

Opioid Withdrawal

Opioid withdrawal can be divided into physical signs and symptoms and psychological symptoms. Piloerection, yawning, and lacrimation are some of the physical signs; nausea, vomiting, and diarrhea are common symptoms. These patients also have intense opioid craving associated with the feeling of being unwell. In contrast to sedative-hypnotic withdrawal, opioid withdrawal is associated with minimal autonomic instability. Patients may be tachycardic and have minimal elevation in blood pressure, but this is partly in response to their physical and emotional symptoms. Opioid withdrawal always is associated with a normal mental status. Needle use in heroin abusers predisposes them to many infections, including CNS infections. Attributing fever and an altered mental status to opioid withdrawal could have catastrophic results. Opioid withdrawal, although thoroughly unpleasant, is unlikely to be life-threatening unless

TABLE 30-1 Vital Signs and Mental Status Changes in Withdrawal				
	OPIOIDS	**SEDATIVE-HYPNOTICS***	**ALCOHOL**	**COCAINE**
Heart rate	↑	↑ ↑	↑ ↑	↓
Blood pressure	↑	↑ ↑	↑ ↑	↓
Respiratory rate	↑	↑ ↑	↑ ↑	↓
Hyperthermia	−	+	+	−
Altered mental status	−	±	±	−

*Includes benzodiazepines, barbiturates, and γ-hydroxybutyrate/γ-butyrolactone.

complicated by aspiration or dehydration. The onset and duration of withdrawal secondary to opioid discontinuation depend on the agent in question. Heroin withdrawal can begin within 6 hours of the last dose, peak by 48 hours, and last 4 to 5 days. Although methadone withdrawal begins 2 to 3 days after the last dose and may last 2 weeks,[33] iatrogenic opioid withdrawal can occur immediately after naloxone administration. This type of opioid withdrawal is as short-lived as the duration of action of naloxone (approximately 40 to 60 minutes) and usually requires no intervention. With withdrawal induced by longer-acting antagonists or partial agonists, supportive therapy with benzodiazepines and antiemetics may be required.

Cocaine Withdrawal

Cocaine withdrawal is associated with an emotional component, whereas the existence of a physical component is debatable. The emotional component is associated with intense craving. This craving is the significant component of cocaine addiction and is the reason why detoxification from cocaine is more rehabilitation oriented. The "washed-out" syndrome that can occur after prolonged cocaine use may be interpreted as physical withdrawal symptoms.[34] Because this phenomenon is not prevented by continued cocaine use, defining it as withdrawal is debatable.[35] The chronic use of cocaine depletes presynaptic neurotransmitter stores, especially dopamine stores, leaving the user catecholamine depleted.[36,37] As a result, baseline adrenergic activity is diminished, and patients may appear lethargic or adynamic with depressed vital signs. This effect usually is self-limited and requires minimal if any supportive care.

Neonatal Withdrawal

Maternal addiction can lead to neonatal withdrawal. Time to symptom presentation after birth varies with the agent in question. Neonatal alcohol withdrawal typically begins within 3 days of parturition. Symptoms include opisthotonos, tremor, nystagmus, clonus, seizures, hypertonia, crying, hyperactive or asymmetric reflexes, excessive rooting, diarrhea, vomiting, startle, and inability to thermoregulate.[38,39] Opisthotonos and abdominal distention rarely occur in opioid withdrawal and can help differentiate the two when the mother has abused multiple substances. Although initially thought to occur only as a complication of fetal alcohol syndrome, neonatal alcohol withdrawal can occur independently of fetal alcohol syndrome.[39] Presentation of neonates withdrawing from sedative-hypnotics would be indistinguishable. Regardless of the etiology, treatment remains the same.

The development of neonatal opioid withdrawal symptoms depends on the agent used by the mother. Heroin withdrawal typically begins in the first few days, whereas methadone withdrawal may not be evident for 10 to 14 days.[40] Neonatal and adult opioid withdrawal are similar. In addition to vomiting, diarrhea, irritability, yawning, sleeplessness, diaphoresis, lacrimation, tremor, and hypertonicity, neonates can have seizures, a high-pitched cry, skin mottling, and excoriation. These latter signs and symptoms are more typical of opioid withdrawal and rarely occur with neonatal alcohol withdrawal.[38]

DIFFERENTIAL DIAGNOSIS

Most dependent users are skilled at treating their own withdrawal. While constructing a differential diagnosis for substance withdrawal, the clinician should try to elucidate the circumstances surrounding the patient's withdrawal. Although lack of finances and lack of availability are common reasons to develop withdrawal, patients often have an underlying illness that prevents "self-medication." An alcoholic may have pancreatitis, pneumonia, head trauma, CNS infections, or gastrointestinal hemorrhage.[41] Undiagnosed medical disorders may contribute significantly to mortality despite adequate withdrawal therapy. Additionally, complications of alcohol withdrawal can be catastrophic. Besides hyperthermia and a myriad of metabolic complications, myocardial infarction may occur secondary to the physical stress associated with withdrawal.

Many disorders may be mistaken for alcohol withdrawal. Among them are thyroid storm, hypoglycemia, encephalitis, and to a lesser extent serotonin syndrome and neuroleptic malignant syndrome (Table 30-2). Also, certain toxins can mimic withdrawal symptoms. Organophosphate poisoning can result in constricted pupils (dilated pupils can occur in organophosphate poisoning depending on how much autonomic stimulus there is), diaphoresis, vomiting, agitation, seizures, and an altered mental status. A combination of these symptoms could be confused easily for either opioid or sedative-hypnotic withdrawal. Sympathomimetic intoxication can present in a manner similar to sedative-hypnotic withdrawal, creating the same diagnostic dilemma. Additionally the anticholinergic patient may present with hallucinations, tachycardia, and hyperthermia. Symptomatic overdose of certain drugs may mimic substance withdrawal; these agents include lithium, aspirin, and theophylline (Table 30-3).

TABLE 30-2 Nontoxic Differential Diagnosis of Alcohol and Sedative-Hypnotic Withdrawal

Encephalitis
Hypomagnesemia
Meningitis
Neuroleptic malignant syndrome
Pneumonia
Serotonin syndrome
Thyrotoxicosis

TABLE 30-3 Toxins That May Mimic Alcohol and Sedative-Hypnotic Withdrawal

Amphetamines
Anticholinergics
Carbamates
Cocaine
Lithium
Organophosphates
Salicylates
Theophylline

DIAGNOSTIC STUDIES

The diagnosis of withdrawal cannot be established without first excluding the other life-threatening disorders in the differential diagnosis. All patients in withdrawal should have serum analysis performed for standard chemistries, including glucose, magnesium, and calcium. Patients may have underlying metabolic derangements stemming from poor nutritional status or from vomiting and diarrhea. A complete blood count should be performed to assess the status of all cell lines because bone marrow suppression and occult hemorrhage are common afflictions in alcoholic patients. An elevated white blood cell count does not necessarily indicate infection, as it may be a marker of a stress response. Liver function test and coagulation assays are important in alcoholics to determine metabolic and synthetic function. A serum ethanol concentration may be a helpful prognostic tool because patients in alcohol withdrawal with elevated ethanol levels tend to have more severe withdrawal and are less likely to be compliant with outpatient detoxification programs.[42]

A chest radiograph and computed tomography (CT) scan of the head are essential in the evaluation of the withdrawal patient with altered consciousness or seizures. A chest radiograph can help exclude pneumonia, whereas a CT scan of the brain can show subdural hematomas, cerebral edema, and other intracranial pathology that may be mistaken for delirium.[43] When symptoms are consistent with CNS infection, a lumbar puncture is necessary to exclude the diagnosis. A CT scan of the brain also should be part of the evaluation of anyone presenting with new-onset seizure before the diagnosis of a rum fit is established.[44] An abdominal CT scan can help identify other disorders in the differential diagnosis of withdrawal, including pancreatitis, cholecystitis, and intestinal obstruction.

TREATMENT

In the past, numerous agents were used to treat withdrawal. Mild withdrawal can be remedied by self-administration of the offending agent. When a patient is admitted for withdrawal or develops withdrawal as an inpatient, physicians must be aware of all treatment options. Logically, withdrawal responds best to reinstitution of the particular agent in question. Heroin and alcohol withdrawal present ethical dilemmas, however. Although some institutions may accept treatment of alcohol withdrawal with alcohol, most clinicians would find this treatment as enabling the underlying disorder, alcoholism.[45] Treatment with alcohol not only does not promote rehabilitation but also contributes to all the health risks associated with chronic alcohol use, including cirrhosis, bone marrow suppression, and gastritis. The principle of cross-tolerance may be applied in this instance. Benzodiazepines show therapeutic effect to varying extents for sedative-hypnotics, alcohol, and GHB/GBL. The safety and efficacy of benzodiazepine-based withdrawal therapy were borne out in studies performed in the mid-1970s.[46] Benzodiazepines are excellent anticonvulsants. Current practice guidelines for the treatment of alcohol withdrawal use benzodiazepines as first-line therapy.[47]

Ethanol Withdrawal

Mild-to-moderate ethanol withdrawal usually responds well to low-dose oral benzodiazepines. Treatment regimens vary, and fixed-schedule treatments are common. Studies show, however, that "front-loading" benzodiazepines relieves withdrawal symptoms faster.[48,49] In these studies, oral diazepam was given to patients in either a 10- or 20-mg dose at 1- to 2-hour intervals until patients were asymptomatic. In one study, patients used one third the amount of diazepam used under conventional therapy. More recently, as-needed chlordiazepoxide was compared with fixed-schedule dosing in a double-blind, placebo-controlled study.[50] Not only did the as-needed group require less chlordiazepoxide (100 mg versus 425 mg), but also total treatment time was reduced to 9 hours from 68 hours.

Moderate-to-severe withdrawal can be life-threatening and requires parenteral sedative-hypnotics or anesthetic agents. The use of the latter often necessitates intubation. Dosing regimens are not well established and are highly variable. Most patients respond to conventional doses of benzodiazepines. Occasionally, larger doses are required to treat the withdrawal symptoms. If more than 400 mg of diazepam or its equivalent is given to a patient without satisfactory effect, an alternative agent is often necessary. Historically the barbiturates have been the second-line agent of choice.[51] Physician familiarity and established history are the major benefits of barbiturate therapy. Phenobarbital has a lag time to response that can make titration difficult, and the kinetics of short-acting barbiturates may result in prolonged sedation when extended therapy is required (e.g., thiopental).[52] Barbiturate therapy often requires intubation.[53] Optimal therapy results in the patient's being sedated and arousable but not obtunded or comatose. Whether it uses benzodiazepines or barbiturates, prolonged therapy often leads to tolerance of the agent used. Tapering often is required to prevent withdrawal from the therapeutic agent. Agents with longer half-lives or active metabolites, such as diazepam or chlordiazepoxide, may facilitate tapering.

In Europe, GHB has been studied for the treatment of alcohol withdrawal.[54-56] The investigators concluded that although effective, the use of GHB could not be recommended for all alcohol withdrawal patients. Its use in the United States is restricted at this time. Propofol has been shown to have an increasing role in sedative-hypnotic withdrawal. It has been used for alcohol, barbiturate, and GHB withdrawal and has been studied for alcohol withdrawal.[57,58] The benefits of propofol include rapid onset of sedation, rapid emergence when discontinued, and anticonvulsant properties. In addition to being a GABA agonist, propofol has NMDA antagonist properties.[59] This dual activity is similar to that of alcohol and may explain why propofol works well for patients refractory to benzodiazepines. Propofol withdrawal is not well described. However, propofol is a costlier agent than the other options discussed. Other agents that have been used include antipsychotics, β-blockers, and clonidine.[8,60-62] These agents are able to treat psychosis and autonomic instability but fail to treat the underlying disorder and as such are not recommended. These agents also may mask some of the symptoms associated with withdrawal, resulting in suboptimal treatment. Finally, although the use of neuroleptics in patients with psychotic symptoms seems logical, they are not cross-tolerant with sedative-hypnotics, lower the seizure threshold, exacerbate tachycardia, and impair heat dissipation. In animal models and case reports, neuroleptics, such as haloperidol, exacerbate sedative-hypnotic withdrawal.[63,64]

Sedative-Hypnotic (and γ-Hydroxybutyrate) Withdrawal

Sedative-hypnotic and GHB withdrawal treatment is based on alcohol withdrawal treatment. Although specific regimens for GHB withdrawal have not been developed, the goal of therapy is the same: restoration of autonomic stability, reduction of psychomotor agitation, and mild-to-moderate sedation. Duration of withdrawal varies with the specific agent involved (Table 30-4).

Opioid Withdrawal

Heroin (and other opioids) withdrawal is treated best with a socially acceptable opioid alternative, methadone. Although methadone is available orally for maintenance therapy, acute withdrawal should be treated parenterally (10 mg of methadone intramuscularly). The intramuscular route is preferable because these patients may be vomiting, and this route guarantees delivery of methadone. When methadone is unavailable or unacceptable, morphine provides a suitable alternative in the acute setting. An initial dose of 0.1 mg/kg intravenously followed by titration to response can provide symptomatic relief. Many oral opioid agents are available and can be dosed similarly using morphine equivalents. Iatrogenic withdrawal induced by naloxone is treated best by supportive measures only. Although unpleasant, the withdrawal is not life-threatening in an awake patient and is self-limited, often lasting less than 1 hour. Other agents that have been used include clonidine, benzodiazepines, and antiemetics.[65–68] Although these agents treat some of the physiologic symptoms associated with heroin withdrawal, they do not relieve the intense craving, which may lead some patients to self-discharge. As such, these agents should be used as adjuncts to opioid therapy. Long-term therapy in this subgroup of patients has developed into methadone maintenance programs. These programs often combine counseling with high-dose oral methadone (>100 mg) to prevent heroin use in these patients.

SUMMARY

Familiarity with the terms *dependence, tolerance, cross-tolerance, addiction,* and *withdrawal,* coupled with an understanding of the pharmacology of the agents in question, not only facilitates the evaluation of patients in withdrawal but also enables appropriate management, decreasing morbidity and mortality in these patients. Substance abuse, which precedes withdrawal, is a multifaceted problem requiring a multidisciplinary approach. Although medical management of withdrawal may be sufficient initially, ultimately patients benefit from additional psychiatric and social counseling and support.

TABLE 30-4 Expected Onset and Duration of Withdrawal Symptoms by Agent

AGENT	SYMPTOM ONSET	DURATION
Alcohol	Hours	5–7 days
Alprazolam	24–48 hr	4–5 days
Diazepam	5–7 days	Weeks
Lorazepam	2–4 days	Weeks
Heroin/morphine	Hours	3–5 days
Methadone	1–2 days	5–7 days
Butalbital	4–6 days	3–5 days
Phenobarbital	7–10 days	3–5 days
GHB/GBL	Hours	3–5 days

GHB/GBL, γ-hydroxybutyrate/γ-butyrolactone.

REFERENCES

1. National Institute on Alcohol Abuse and Alcoholism. Available at: http://www.niallaa.nih.gov. Accessed March 27, 2001.
2. National Institute on Drug Abuse. Available at: http://www.nida.nih.gov. Accessed March 27, 2001.
3. Conde Lopez VJ, Plaza Nieto JF, Macias Fernandez JA, et al: [Historical study of seven cases of delirium tremens in Spain in the first half of the XIX century.] Actas Luso Esp Neurol Psiquiatr Cienc Afines 23:200–216, 1995.
4. Osler W: The Principles and Practice of Medicine, 8th ed. New York, Appleton, 1916, pp 398–400.
5. Victor M, Adams RD: The effect of alcohol on the nervous system. Res Publ Assoc Res Nerv Ment Dis 32:526–573, 1953.
6. Isbell H, Fraser HF, Wikler A, et al: An experimental study of the etiology of "rum fits" and delirium tremens. Q J Stud Alcohol 16:1–33, 1955.
7. Tavel ME: A new look at an old syndrome: Delirium tremens. Arch Intern Med 109:129–134, 1962.
8. Thomas DW, Freedman DX: Treatment of alcohol withdrawal syndrome: Comparison of promazine and paraldehyde. JAMA 188:316–318, 1964.
9. Sellers EM, Kalant H: Alcohol intoxication and withdrawal. N Engl J Med 294:757–769, 1976.
10. Liber CS: Medical disorders of alcoholism. N Engl J Med 333:1058–1065, 1995.
11. Krogsgaard-Larsen P, Scheel-Kruger J, Kofod H (eds): GABA-Neurotransmitters: Pharmacological, Biochemical and Pharmacological Aspects. New York, Academic Press, 1979, pp 102–103.
12. Squires RF (ed): GABA and Benzodiazepine Receptors, vol 1. Boca Raton, CRC Press, 1991, pp 2–10.
13. Tunniclif G, Raess BU: GABA Mechanism in Epilepsy. New York, Wiley, 1992, pp 54–55.
14. MacDermott AB, Mayer ML, Westbrook GL, et al: NMDA-receptor activation increases cytoplasmic calcium concentration in cultured spinal cord neurons. Nature 321:519–522, 1986.
15. Sivilotti L, Nistri A: GABA receptor mechanisms in the CNS. Prog Neurobiol 36:35–92, 1991.
16. Snead OC: Evidence for a G protein-coupled gamma-hydroxybutyric acid receptor. J Neurochem 75:1986–1996, 2000.
17. Wick MJ, Mihic SJ, Ueno S, et al: Mutations of gamma-aminobutyric acid and glycine receptors change alcohol cutoff: Evidence for an alcohol receptor? Proc Natl Acad Sci U S A 95:6504–6509, 1998.
18. Mascia MP, Trudell JR, Harris RA: Specific binding sites for alcohols and anesthetics on ligand-gated ion channels. Proc Natl Acad Sci U S A 97:9305–9310, 2000.
19. Thomas RJ: Excitatory amino acids in health and disease. J Am Geriatr Soc 43:1279–1289, 1995.

20. Steffensen SC, Nie Z, Criado JR, et al: Ethanol inhibition of N-methyl-D-aspartate responses involves presynaptic gamma-aminobutyric acid(B) receptors. J Pharmacol Exp Ther 294:637–647, 2000.

21. Martin D, Lodge D: Ketamine acts as a non-competitive N-methyl-D-aspartate antagonist on frog spinal cord in vitro. Neuropharmacology 24:999–1003, 1985.

22. Thornberg SA, Saklad SR: A review of NMDA receptors and the phencyclidine model of schizophrenia. Pharmacotherapy 16:82–93, 1996.

23. Tortella FC, Ferkany JW, Pontecorvo MJ: Anticonvulsant effects of dextrorphan in rats, possible involvement in dextromethorphan-induced seizure protection. Life Sci 42:2509–2514, 1988.

24. Minami MJ, Satoh M: Molecular biology of the opioid receptors: Structures, functions and distributions. Neurosci Res 23:121–145, 1995.

25. Grudt TJ, Williams JT: Kappa-opioid receptors also increase potassium conductance. Prod Natl Acad Sci U S A 90:11429–11432, 1993.

26. North RA, Williams JT, Surprenant A, et al: Mu and sigma receptors belong to a family of receptors that are coupled to potassium channels. Proc Natl Acad Sci U S A 84:5487–5491, 1987.

27. Piros E, Prather P, Law P, et al: Calcium channel and adenylyl cyclase modulation by cloned mu opioid receptors in GH$_3$ cells. Mol Pharmacol 47:1041–1049, 1995.

28. Glue P, Nutt D: Overexcitement and disinhibition: Dynamic neurotransmitter interactions in alcohol withdrawal. Br J Psychiatry 157:491–499, 1990.

29. Chirstie MJ, Williams JT, North RA: Cellular mechanism of opioid tolerance: Studies in single brain neurons. Mol Phamacol 32:633–638, 1987.

30. Crain SM, Shen KF: Modulatory effects of G$_s$-coupled excitatory opioid receptor functions on analgesia, tolerance and dependence. Neurochem Res 21:1347–1351, 1996.

31. Maldonado R, Blendy JA, Tzavar E, et al: Reduction of morphine abstinence in mice with mutation in the gene encoding CREB. Science 273:657–659, 1996.

32. Dyer JE, Roth B, Hyma BA: Gamma-hydroxybutyrate withdrawal syndrome. Ann Emerg Med 37:147–153, 2001.

33. Gossop M, Strang J: A comparison of the withdrawal responses of heroin and methadone addicts during detoxification. Br J Psychiatry 158:697–699, 1991.

34. Satel SL, Price LH, Palumbo JM, et al: Clinical phenomenology and neurobiology of cocaine abstinence: A prospective inpatient study. Am J Psychiatry 148:495–498, 1991.

35. Lago JA, Kosten TR: Stimulant withdrawal. Addiction 89:1477–1481, 1994.

36. Dackis CA, Gold MS: New concepts in cocaine addiction: The dopamine depletion hypothesis. Neurosci Biobehav Rev 9:469–477, 1985.

37. Pilotte NS, Sharpe LG, Roundtree SD, et al: Cocaine withdrawal reduces dopamine transporter binding in the shell of the nucleus accumbens. Synapse 1:87–92, 1996.

38. Robe LB, Gromisch DS, Iosub S: Symptoms of neonatal ethanol withdrawal. Curr Alcohol 8:485–493, 1981.

39. Coles CD, Smith IE, Fernhoff PM, et al: Neonatal ethanol withdrawal: Characteristics in clinically normal, nondysmorphic neonates. J Pediatr 105:445–451, 1984.

40. Zelson C, Lee SJ, Casalino M: Neonatal narcotic addiction: Comparative effects of maternal intake of heroin and methadone. N Engl J Med 289:1216–1220, 1973.

41. Lieber CS: Medical disorders of alcoholism. N Engl J Med 333:1058–1065, 1995.

42. Vinson DC, Menezes M: Admission alcohol level: A predictor of the course of alcohol withdrawal. J Fam Pract 33:161–167, 1991.

43. Feussner KR: Computed tomography brain scanning in alcohol withdrawal seizures. Ann Intern Med 94:519–524, 1981.

44. Earnest MP, Feldman H, Marx JA, et al: Intracranial lesions shown by CT scans in 259 cases of first alcohol-related seizures. Neurology 38:1561–1565, 1988.

45. DiPaula B, Tommasello A, Solounias B, et al: An evaluation of intravenous ethanol in hospitalized patients. J Subst Abuse Treat 15:437–442, 1998.

46. Thompson WL, Johnson AD, Maddrey WL, et al: Diazepam and paraldehyde for treatment of severe delirium tremens: A controlled trial. Ann Intern Med 82:175–180, 1975.

47. Mayo-Smith MF: Pharmacological management of alcohol withdrawal: A meta-analysis and evidence-based practice guideline. American Society of Addiction Medicine Working Group on Pharmacological Management of Alcohol Withdrawal. JAMA 278:144–151, 1997.

48. Manikant S, Tripathi BM, Chavan BS: Loading dose diazepam therapy for alcohol withdrawal state. Indian J Med Res 98:170–173, 1993.

49. Sellers EM: Clinical pharmacology and therapeutics of benzodiazepines. Can Med Assoc J 118:1533–1538, 1978.

50. Saitz R, Mayo-Smith MF, Roberts MS, et al: Individualized treatment for alcohol withdrawal: A randomized double blind controlled trial. JAMA 272:519–523, 1994.

51. Hemmingsen R, Kramp P, Rafaelsen OJ: Delirium tremens and related clinical states: Aetiology, pathophysiology and treatment. Acta Psychiatr Scand 59:337–369, 1979.

52. Ives TJ, Mooney AJ 3rd, Gwyther RE: Pharmacokinetic dosing of phenobarbital in the treatment of alcohol withdrawal syndrome. South Med J 84:18–21, 1991.

53. Cilip M, Chelluri L, Jastremski M, et al: Continuous intravenous infusion of sodium thiopental for managing drug withdrawal syndromes. Resuscitation 13:243–248, 1986.

54. Gallimberti L, Canton G, Gentile N, et al: Gamma-hydroxybutyric acid for treatment of alcohol withdrawal syndrome. Lancet 2:787–789, 1989.

55. Lenzenhuber E, Muller C, Rommelspacher H, Spies C: [Gamma-hydroxybutyrate for treatment of alcohol withdrawal syndrome in intensive care patients: A comparison between two symptom-oriented therapeutic concepts.] Anaesthetist 48:89–96, 1999.

56. Addolorato G, Balducci G, Capristo E, et al: Gamma-hydroxybutyric acid (GHB) in the treatment of alcohol withdrawal syndrome: A randomized comparative study versus benzodiazepine. Alcohol Clin Exp Res 23:1596–1604, 1999.

57. Coomes TR, Smith SW: Successful use of propofol in refractory delirium tremens. Ann Emerg Med 30:825–828, 1997.

58. McCowan C, Marik P: Refractory delirium tremens treated with propofol: A case series. Crit Care Med 28:1781–1784, 2000.

59. Orser BA, Bertlik M, Wang LY, et al: Inhibition by propofol (2,6 di-isopropylphenol) of the N-methyl-D-aspartate subtype of glutamate receptor in cultured hippocampal neurons. Br J Pharmacol 116:1761–1768, 1995.

60. Friedhoff AJ, Zitrin A: A comparison of the effects of paraldehyde and chlorpromazine in delirium tremens. N Y State J Med 59:1060–1063, 1959.

61. Adinoff B: Double-blind study of alprazolam, diazepam, clonidine and placebo in the alcohol withdrawal syndrome. Alcohol Clin Exp Res 18:873–878, 1994.

62. Horwitz RI, Gottlieb LD, Kraus ML: The efficacy of atenolol in the outpatient management of the alcohol withdrawal syndrome: Results of a randomized clinical trial. Arch Intern Med 149:1089–1093, 1989.

63. Blum K, Eubanks JD, Wallace JE, et al: Enhancement of alcohol withdrawal convulsions in mice by haloperidol. Clin Toxicol 9:427–434, 1976.

64. Greenblatt DJ, Gross PL, Harris J, et al: Fatal hyperthermia following haloperidol therapy of sedative-hypnotic withdrawal. J Clin Psychiatry 39:673–675, 1978.

65. Gold MS, Redmond ED, Kleber HD: Clonidine blocks acute opioid withdrawal symptoms. Lancet 2:599–602, 1978.

66. Uhde TW, Redmond DE Jr, Kleber HD: Clonidine suppresses the opioid abstinence syndrome without clonidine-withdrawal symptoms: A blind inpatient study. Psychiatry Res 2:37–47, 1980.

67. Gibert-Rahola J, Maldonado R, Mico JA, et al: Comparative study in mice of flunitrazepam vs diazepam on morphine withdrawal syndrome. Prog Neuropsychopharmacol Biol Psychiatry 12:927–933, 1988.

68. Pinelli A, Trivulzio S, Tomasoni L: Effects of ondansetron administration on opioid withdrawal syndrome observed in rats. Eur J Pharmacol 340:111–119, 1997.

CHAPTER 31

Immunologic Reactions

Stephen C. Dreskin

Drug reactions that lead to an intensive medical response are a significant medical problem. These reactions can be due to known pharmacologic activities of a drug, activation of the immune system, or other mechanisms. The reactions that involve the immune system account for only 10% of cases but can be dramatic and life-threatening.[1,2] Extrapolating from estimates of the cost for all drug reactions in the United States, the cost of drug reactions with an immunologic basis is approximately $3 to $13 billion/yr.[1,3] Reactions that involve immunologic mechanisms often are described as "allergic" or "pseudoallergic." The word *allergic* is used most often to describe reactions that are mediated through the IgE class of antibodies, although this term often is extended (as in this chapter) to include any immune reaction that involves specific recognition by the immune system (via antibodies or the T-cell receptor). The term *immunologic drug reaction* has been coined to include both of these mechanisms.[4] The term *pseudoallergic* often is used to refer to drug reactions that mimic allergic reactions (e.g., release of proinflammatory mediators). These reactions occur via activation of the immune system in a fashion that is independent of antibody or specific receptors.[4–7] The term *idiosyncratic*, as used in this chapter, refers to an uncharacteristic response to a drug that is qualitatively different from its pharmacologic activity and that is not immunologic in mechanism. These reactions may be genetically based and related to metabolic or enzyme deficiencies.[4,5] The terms *anaphylactic* and *anaphylactoid* refer to systemic reactions that have an allergic and pseudoallergic basis, respectively.[4,6]

HISTORY

At the end of the 19th century, there were dramatic advances in the use of inoculation of killed or attenuated organisms to prevent human infectious diseases, including smallpox, rabies, typhoid, cholera, and plague.[8] In this fertile intellectual environment, two other immunization strategies were undertaken that led to paradoxical reactions and inadvertently expanded our understanding of the immune system. In the first approach, animals were given injections of increasing doses of a toxin to protect them from subsequent exposure. The second approach was to protect or treat humans with sera from animals that had been injected previously with infectious agents or toxins.

The importance of these unexpected reactions first was appreciated by the Frenchman Richet, who immunized dogs with a toxin from the sea anemone with the objective of even-

tually treating Mediterranean Sea bathers who were stung by jellyfish.[9–11] Richet hypothesized that animals surviving a sublethal dose would be protected (prophylaxed) against subsequent injections. When given a subsequent dose of similar or smaller size, however, some of the dogs died within minutes. The symptoms of the reaction after the rechallenge were considerably different from the subacute toxic reaction progressing over 4 or 5 days seen after the initial injection. These reactions to rechallenge were characterized by the rapid (within minutes) onset of shortness of breath, lethargy, and diarrhea. Richet concluded that the first toxin injection had not prophylaxed the dogs but rather had changed the animals into a state of anaphylaxis (without protection).[10,12–14]

Reactions to heterologous (from another species) blood products were appreciated in 1667 after early attempts to use lamb's blood for transfusion.[15] The desire to treat human infectious diseases with sera from immune animals led to efforts to understand these reactions. In the early years of the 20th century, antiserum developed in horses, particularly anti–diphtheria antitoxin, came into general use and was associated with 38 reported fatal reactions and many more nonfatal reactions between 1895 and 1923. Some of these reactions occurred immediately and were similar to the reactions Richet observed in dogs, but most evolved more slowly with different manifestations. In 1905, Von Pirquet and Schick coined the term *serum sickness* to describe this latter reaction, characterized by fever, arthritis, and erythema multiforme occurring 7 to 10 days after exposure to heterologous serum.[15] During the next decade, the overlap between anaphylaxis and serum sickness became apparent, and the concept of different manifestations of "hypersensitivity" came to be appreciated. As medical care evolved during the 20th century, therapy with heterologous serum gave way to the use of antibiotics and recognition of allergic reactions to these agents. Antibiotics continue to be a substantial problem, and a plethora of drugs generated for a variety of illnesses also have become important sensitizing substances. On a positive note, the "humanization" of monoclonal antibodies offers the promise that novel biologics can be designed with minimal risk of sensitization.

PATHOPHYSIOLOGY

Reactions to drugs vary widely. Some reactions are limited to the skin or to specific internal organs; others are systemic. Although some agents are more prone to result in a specific type of reaction, almost any agent can cause any type of

TABLE 31-1 Immunopathologic Penicillin Reactions

GEL AND COOMBS TYPE	MECHANISM	EXAMPLES OF ADVERSE PENICILLIN REACTIONS
I	Anaphylactic (IgE-mediated injury)	Acute anaphylaxis; urticaria
II	C'-dependent cytolysis (IgG/IgM)	Hemolytic anemias Thrombocytopenia Interstitial nephritis
III	Immune complex damage	Serum sickness Drug fever Some cutaneous eruptions and vasculitis
IV	"Delayed" or cellular hypersensitivity	Contact dermatitis Morbilliform eruptions (?)

From Adkinson NF Jr: Drug allergy. In Middleton E Jr, Reed CE, Ellis EF, et al (eds): Allergy: Principles and Practice, Vol II, 5th ed. St Louis, Mosby, 1998, pp 1212–1224.

reaction. In the 1960s, Gel and Coombs characterized immunologic reactions by the major immunologic process operative in a reaction.[4] In this analysis, type 1 reactions are immediate hypersensitivity reactions involving cross-linkage of IgE bound to high-affinity receptors on mast cells or basophils. Type 2 reactions are due to cytotoxic antibodies. Type 3 reactions are due to immune complexes, and type 4 reactions are due to cell-mediated hypersensitivity. Adkinson[4] described this concept well for penicillin reactions (Table 31-1). Although this process is a useful method of discussing immunologic reactions to drugs, more recent data have shown that there is marked overlap among these arms of the immune system such that several of the Gel and Coombs–type reactions can be operative in a single reaction. A different approach that is more functional is to classify reactions to drugs based on the timing and predominant clinical manifestation.[2] This approach is outlined in Table 31-2.

Many drugs are small, immunologically inactive molecules, such as penicillin, that activate the immune system by virtue of their ability to "haptenate" naturally occurring plasma and cellular proteins. The process of forming haptens is fairly well understood for penicillin and probably is similar for other small molecules (Fig. 31-1). In this scenario, the drug itself is not recognized by the immune system because of its small size (molecular weight 100 to 1000 d). When the drug or its metabolic product is bound to a protein, however, it distorts the three-dimensional image of the protein so that the drug, now presented as part of a protein, is recognized as a novel structure leading to clonal expansion of T cells (not shown). T cells interact with B cells and produce cytokines that also drive the maturation of B cells. These maturing B cells express surface immunoglobulin for the drug, then form plasma cells that secrete immunoglobulins that recognize the drug with high affinity.[16] Susceptible patients

TABLE 31-2 Classification of Allergic Reactions Based on their Timing

REACTION TYPE	TIME OF ONSET (hr)	CLINICAL MANIFESTATION
Immediate	0–1	Anaphylaxis Angioedema Urticaria Bronchospasm
Accelerated	1–72	Angioedema Urticaria Bronchospasm
Late	>72	Morbilliform rash Interstitial nephritis Hemolytic anemia Thrombocytopenia Neutropenia Serum sickness Drug fever Stevens-Johnson syndrome Toxic epidermal necrolysis

Modified from Weiss ME: Drug allergy. Med Clin North Am 76:857–882, 1992.

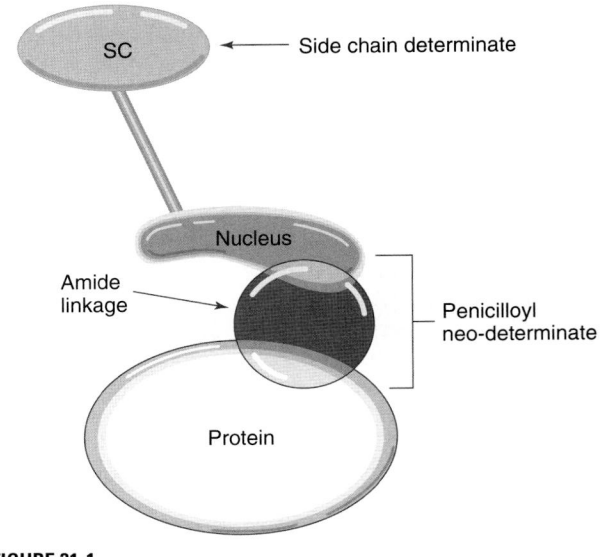

FIGURE 31-1

Generation of haptans. SC, side chain. *(From Adkinson NF Jr: Drug allergy. In Middleton E Jr, Reed CE, Ellis EF, et al [eds]: Allergy: Principles and Practice, Vol II, 5th ed. St Louis, Mosby-Year Book, 1998, pp 1212–1224.)*

undergo class switching from an IgG response to produce IgE that binds to the high-affinity receptor for IgE (FcεRI) on mast cells and basophils, sensitizing these patients. Subsequent exposure to the "haptenated" protein during a repeat course of therapy leads to cross-linking of the antigen-specific IgE bound to FcεRI, then to degranulation of mast cells and basophils.[1,4] This process also can occur during a single course of drug therapy in which either the first exposure was not appreciated (e.g., exposure to antibiotics in food) or the initial sensitization and the effects of sensitization occur in rapid sequence.[17]

The most limited reactions that are clearly IgE mediated are manifest as generalized urticaria (hives), but reactions can be generalized and include bronchospasm, allergic gastroenteritis, and vascular collapse. It is unknown why some but not all patients produce IgE and why the reactions are to certain agents and not to others. Patients with a history of allergic reactions to drugs are more prone to reactions with structurally unrelated medications.[2] This situation may be due to a genetic predisposition to recognize haptens.[1] A history of allergic disease, such as allergic rhinitis, does not predispose to allergic drug reactions, although these individuals may be at risk for serious reactions should they occur.[2] The lack of a history of previous allergic reactions to drugs or to other allergens is not helpful.

Foreign molecules (antigens) can activate the immune system in a highly specific fashion. The molecules of the immune system that recognize antigens are either soluble proteins called *antibodies* or receptors on the surface of T cells (T-cell receptors) and B cells (B-cell receptors). Antibodies fall into five distinct molecular groups (in order of predominance in the circulation): IgG, IgM, IgA, IgD, and IgE. Antigens that lead to an IgE response are called *allergens*. Antibody molecules have two critical regions—the Fab region, which binds avidly to unique structures (antigens), and the Fc region, which binds to Fc receptors on effector cells. The IgG antibodies (normal range, approximately 700 to 1500 mg/dL [7 to 15 mg/mL]) account for the greatest portion of the humoral (soluble) immune response to foreign proteins. They participate in immune reactions by forming immune complexes with antigen or by combining with specific receptors (Fc receptors) on effector cells. IgE antibodies (normal range, approximately 0 to 250 ng/mL) are present at the lowest concentration and participate in host defense against parasites. IgE is responsible for immediate hypersensitivity reactions. IgE antibodies sensitize mast cells and basophils by binding with high affinity to FcεRI receptors. The process of antigen presentation by antigen presenting cells (typically B cells, macrophages, and dendritic cells), immune recognition of T-cell epitopes by T cells via the T-cell receptor, T cell–mediated and antigen stimulation of B cells, maturation of B cells to become IgE-producing plasma cells, and sensitization of mast cells by IgE is illustrated in Figure 31-2.[18] IgE, bound to FcεRI and cross-linked by a specific antigen, causes degranulation of these cells with the rapid (0 to 30 minutes) release of potent vasoactive and proinflammatory mediators, such as histamine, leukotriene C_4, and prostaglandin D_2.[19] T cells recognize a specific antigen by virtue of their T-cell receptors that identify the unique specificity of a foreign peptide sequence in the context of the major histocompatibility loci.[18] A crucial precept of modern immunology is that the region of a foreign epitope recognized by the T-cell receptor (shown as rectangles in Fig. 31-2) is distinct from that recognized by the B-cell receptor and circulating antibodies (shown as ovals in Fig. 31-2).[18]

Examples of IgE-mediated reactions are generalized anaphylaxis and more limited reactions, such as some cases of acute asthma, hives, and allergic rhinitis (hay fever). IgG antibodies are responsible for more delayed adverse reactions, interacting with the immune system via Fcγ receptors (receptors for the Fc portion of IgG) and by forming soluble immune complexes. Immune complexes often activate the complement cascade, generating immunologically active

FIGURE 31-2

Production of IgE. Sensitization and activation of mast cells. **A,** Allergens contain specific sequences that define epitopes that are recognized by T cells (in the context of major histocompatibility complex [MHC] class 2) and different epitopes that are recognized by B cells. Activation of antigen-specific T cells by presentation of the T-cell epitopes leads to T:B cell interactions and the generation of specific cytokines. These cytokines, in the context of exposure of the maturing B cell to the B-cell epitopes of the allergen, cause B cells to proliferate and mature into antibody-producing plasma cells, some of which produce IgE. **B,** Allergen-specific IgE sensitizes mast cells by binding to the high-affinity receptor for IgE (FcεRI). These sensitized mast cells can be activated by exposure to a polyvalent allergen. LTC_4, leukotriene C_4; PGD_2, prostaglandin D_2.

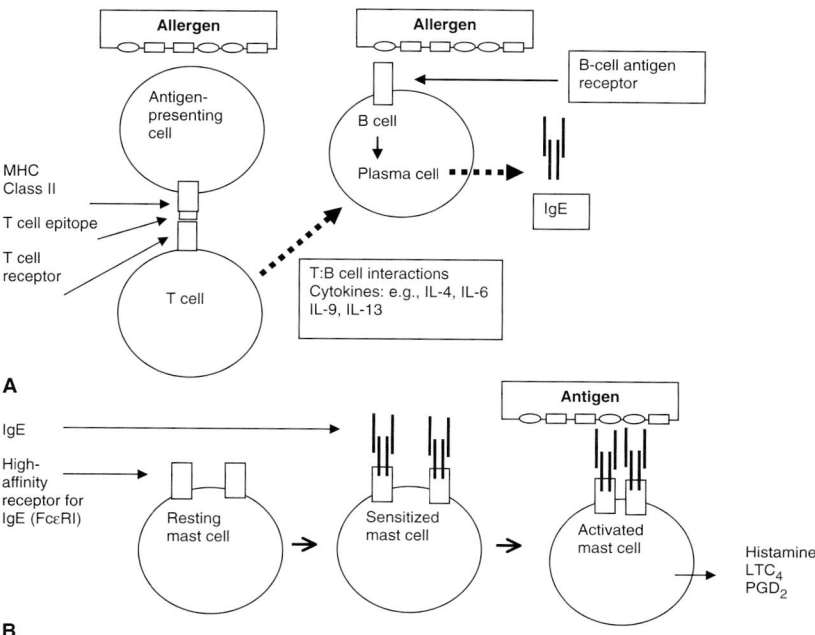

complement fragments. Examples of IgG-mediated immunologic reactions include serum sickness and immune complex glomerulonephritis. Specific antigen receptors on T cells (T-cell receptors) have the ability to recognize foreign material in much the same way as antibodies do. This recognition leads to expansion and activation of clones of T cells. These reactions generally are referred to as *delayed-type hypersensitivity* reactions. The most familiar example is the dermatitis seen secondary to poison ivy, but delayed-type hypersensitivity reactions also are seen with topical medications, such as neomycin, and can be seen in dermatologic reactions to systemically administered drugs.[1,20]

Although there are many reactions to drugs and chemicals that are mediated by the immune system, as discussed here, there are other reactions in which the immune system may be contributory but does not appear to be the entire cause. The Stevens-Johnson syndrome (SJS) is a prime example of the latter situation and is discussed subsequently.

SYSTEMIC REACTIONS

Systemic Anaphylaxis

The most terrifying reaction to an exogenous agent is systemic anaphylaxis. These reactions are observed most frequently within 1 to 30 minutes of parenteral administration of the offending agent but can occur minutes to hours after the ingestion of a food.[14,21] Typically the patient has a brief prodrome of anxiety and a sense of impending doom followed by cutaneous reactivity (diffuse erythema, hives, or angioedema), laryngeal edema, bronchospasm, hypotension, and vascular collapse. Not all of these signs and symptoms need be present. Even when anaphylaxis is observed contemporaneously by medical personnel who immediately administer epinephrine, antihistamines, corticosteroids, and pressor agents, resuscitation can fail. In the operating room, some of the above-mentioned warning signs and symptoms are not evident, and resistance to ventilation or vascular collapse may be the first sign of anaphylaxis. The patient usually already is intubated, however, so that patency of the airway is not an issue. In the hospital, a large array of agents can precipitate the clinical syndrome of anaphylaxis, including drugs, latex, blood transfusions, foods, and intravenous contrast material. In the outpatient setting, patients can have anaphylaxis as a result of drugs, latex, food, insect bites, or exercise; as a manifestation of systemic mastocytosis; and spontaneously (idiopathic anaphylaxis).[14,21]

Cross-linkage of IgE-FcεRI complexes on mast cells and basophils initiates the most common form of anaphylactic reaction—IgE-mediated anaphylaxis. For this reaction to occur, the patient generally has been exposed previously to the agent, and some time (weeks to months) has passed to allow for the production of sufficient IgE to sensitize mast cells and basophils. Systemic anaphylaxis can be caused by a wide variety of agents. Many drugs are of such small molecular weight that they by themselves are not recognized by the immune system. Penicillins are the best-studied example of this type of drug. In this case, it is the drug bound to a large-molecular-weight protein (i.e., albumin) that becomes antigenic. In this situation, the drug is called a *hapten*. Latex is an example of a complex material that has become a significant hazard in the hospital. Latex-sensitive patients are often medical personnel or patients who have had many surgeries or procedures. The most significant reactions occur when latex is introduced to a mucous membrane by inserting a catheter or when latex gloves are placed in the abdominal cavity at surgery. The most frequently used heterologous protein in current clinical practice is antithymocyte globulin. This is a rabbit IgG directed against human T cells. Patients can form an IgE and an IgG response, leading to anaphylaxis (IgE mediated) and serum sickness (IgG mediated).[14,21]

Anaphylactoid Reactions

Some agents cause a syndrome of anaphylaxis without involvement of IgE. These reactions, called *anaphylactoid reactions*, are caused by direct mast cell activation leading to hives, angioedema, and occasionally hypotension. Intravenous radiocontrast material is thought to cause activation and degranulation of mast cells by virtue of its hyperosmolality.[14] *N*-Acetylcysteine can cause a similar syndrome, although the mechanism is even more obscure.[22] In the perioperative period, neuromuscular relaxants, plasma substitutes, intravenous induction drugs, opioids, protamine, and ethylene oxide all have been implicated in anaphylactic reactions.[7,14] The extent to which any of these agents are acting by an IgE-mediated or non–IgE-mediated mechanism is controversial.

Other Systemic Reactions

The best-described nonanaphylactic systemic reaction is serum sickness. As mentioned earlier for horse serum, this reaction is characterized by fever, malaise, and a pruritic rash that is often urticarial but can be maculopapular or erythema multiforme–like. Associated findings include proteinuria (rarely with frank glomerulonephritis), gastrointestinal symptoms, adenopathy, vasculitis, and peripheral neuropathy.[23] Any heterologous protein can precipitate this type of reaction, which is thought to be due to circulating immune complexes. Heterologous proteins currently in clinical use include antivenin (Crotalidae) polyvalent (horse serum–derived antibody), Crotalidae polyvalent immune Fab (Fab fragments of sheep IgG), digoxin immune Fab antibody (Fab fragments of sheep IgG), and antithymocyte globulin (rabbit IgG).[24] The risk of serum sickness associated with the use of therapeutic IgG can be lessened greatly by production of "humanized" monoclonal antibodies. Serum sickness also can occur due to nonprotein drugs, such as β-lactam antibiotics and sulfonamides.

In susceptible individuals, nonsteroidal antiinflammatory drugs (NSAIDs) activate the immune system in a way distinct from that of radiocontrast dyes. Although specific NSAIDs, similar to almost any drug, can cause IgE-dependent anaphylaxis, this class of drugs also can activate the immune system in an IgE-independent fashion (pseudoallergic). Although the specifics still are largely unknown, the IgE-independent reactions to NSAIDs seem to involve macrophages, mast cells, and endothelial cells leading to excessive production of vasoactive lipid-derived molecules (e.g., leukotrienes and prostanoids).[25] Clinical manifestations include asthma, sinusitis, nasal polyps, and occasionally urticaria or angioedema or both. Vascular collapse is not typically part of this picture, but bronchospasm can be profound.[25]

The cause of drug fever is unknown, and it can be seen with many drugs. It may be associated with eosinophilia, leukocytosis, and an elevated erythrocyte sedimentation rate, but it is most frequently present as an isolated symptom and poses a diagnostic dilemma. Because drug fevers usually resolve within 48 to 72 hours of stopping the drug, this forms a useful diagnostic test.[1]

REACTIONS WITH A PREDOMINANT ORGAN INVOLVEMENT

Cutaneous reactions can occur with almost any drug taken systemically and vary from relatively benign to severe life-threatening lesions with morbidity similar to that seen with severe burns. Diffuse urticaria or angioedema is due to degranulation of cutaneous mast cells. Although usually this is a self-limited process, urticaria and angioedema are severely distressing to the patient. This should be considered to be a systemic (not local) reaction and may be a harbinger of a more severe generalized reaction that is developing over time. If compromise of the airway is present, it must be treated aggressively. Angiotensin-converting enzyme inhibitors cause angioedema by virtue of their ability to inhibit important esterases, leading to excessive levels of vasoactive kinins. The localization of this swelling to the upper airway is not understood but can cause significant diagnostic problems in patients who present with an isolated cough. Other agents that can activate cutaneous mast cells by non–IgE-mediated mechanisms include radiocontrast media; vancomycin; *N*-acetylcysteine; opiates; amphotericin; tubocurarine; and physical stimuli, such as sunlight, pressure, vibration, heat, and cold. By virtue of location or the presence of specific receptors, many of these agents most often activate only cutaneous mast cells, leading to a syndrome limited to erythema, pruritus, dermatitis, or hives, but more severe systemic reactions do occur.[1,4,6]

Erythema multiforme appears as raised erythematous lesions predominantly on the extremities with varied shapes, including target lesions, maculopapular rashes, urticaria, and vesicles.[1] In most patients, infection or exposure to drugs or both are thought to be responsible.[1,26] Erythema multiforme minor is an acute, self-limited mucocutaneous syndrome with a wide range of causes, including infections and drugs.[26] Erythema multiforme major includes SJS and toxic epidermal necrolysis (TEN). These are examples of a cutaneous disease that should be thought of as a systemic illness because of the extensive involvement of mucous membranes. The pathophysiology is largely unknown but does seem to have an immunologic component that is independent of IgE. TEN often is considered to be a more severe variant of SJS based on the percentage of skin detachment.[27,28]

Henoch-Schönlein purpura is predominantly a disease of children characterized by cutaneous vasculitis with the deposition of IgA. Although most often associated with a precedent infection, particularly group A β-hemolytic streptococcus, it occasionally is associated with the recent intake of a variety of drugs. Henoch-Schönlein purpura also can present as a systemic vasculitis and can be seen in adults.[29]

Drug-induced hepatitis most often is due to toxic effects of drugs (e.g., acetaminophen) but infrequently is due to immunologic activation. Immunologic reactivity within the liver can manifest as cholestasis, hepatocellular damage, and granulomatous reactions. Although many drugs can cause allergic hepatitis, halothane and anticonvulsants (phenobarbital, carbamazepine, phenytoin, and halothane) are most prominent.[1] Drug-induced, immunologically mediated hepatitis is characterized by a delay in presentation; a lack of dose dependence; the presence of drug-specific antibodies or drug-reactive T cells; an accelerated course on rechallenge; and hallmarks of hypersensitivity, such as fever, rash, and eosinophilia. Associated manifestations may include lymphadenopathy, hemolysis, and involvement of other organs.[1,30,31]

Drug-induced glomerulonephritis can occur secondary to immune complex formation (serum sickness) or because immunologic activation occurs primarily in the kidney. Interstitial nephritis resulting from drugs (e.g., β-lactam antibiotics, rifampin, NSAIDs, sulfonamides, captopril, and allopurinol) is characterized by eosinophils in the urinary sediment (a positive Hansel stain). Eosinophiluria is not always found in drug-induced renal damage, however, and a biopsy may be needed to make the diagnosis.[32]

Immune-mediated hematologic disorders, such as thrombocytopenia and hemolytic anemia, are well described.[33] Patients can present with eosinophilia, thrombocytopenia, hemolytic anemia, or leukopenia.[1] In most occurrences, drugs (e.g., penicillins) or their metabolic by-products bind to cellular membranes and initiate an immunologic reaction via the hapten mechanism by forming new antigenic determinants. IgG antibodies thus formed react with the blood elements, leading to sequestration by splenic macrophages. Cell lysis may occur if complement is activated. A less common mechanism has been documented with α-methyldopa, levodopa, and procainamide, in which autoantibodies (against red blood cells) are formed, generating a clinical picture that looks like autoimmune hemolytic anemia.[33]

Hypersensitivity pneumonitis can be seen with many drugs, including antimicrobial agents (nitrofurantoin, sulfonamides), anticonvulsants (phenytoin, carbamazepine), diuretics (hydrochlorothiazide), antiarrhythmics (amiodarone), narcotics (heroin, methadone, propoxyphene, cocaine), antirheumatics (gold, methotrexate, penicillamine, naproxen), and chemotherapeutics (bleomycin). The clinical picture is similar to that seen after inhalation of organic dusts from multiple sources, such as moldy hay (farmer's lung), bird proteins (pigeon breeder's disease), or contaminated humidifiers.[34,35] This syndrome is characterized by fever, nonproductive cough, and dyspnea associated with bilateral patchy infiltrates suggestive of a pulmonary infection. A separate pulmonary syndrome, drug-induced systemic lupus erythematosus, can be caused by hydralazine, procainamide, isoniazid, and chlorpromazine.[36]

IMMUNOLOGIC REACTIONS DUE TO SPECIFIC AGENTS

Antibiotics

Antibiotics are associated most commonly with immunologic drug reactions, probably due to their widespread and intermittent usage. Fatality from penicillin has been estimated to occur in 0.0001% of treatments, resulting in 400 to 800 deaths per year during the 1970s.[2] Parenteral administration is associated with more allergic reactions, but it is unclear whether this is related to the route of administration or to the dose administered.[2] The best-studied responses to penicillin are the IgE responses, although IgG and T-cell responses can be important. Although these are small molecules, penicillins and other β-lactam antibiotics (cephalosporins, carbapenems, and monobactams) present a range of antigenic determinants to the immune system.[37,38] Penicillins bind covalently to proteins by an amide linkage to the side chain ε-amino group on lysine residues, generating the "penicilloyl" residue (the major determinant) and less characterized "minor" determinants.[39] Antibodies to the penicilloyl group constitute up to 95% of the responses to penicillin.[16] IgE antibodies to the minor determinants (breakdown products) of penicillin, which account for less than 15% of the positive skin tests, are associated more frequently with anaphylaxis, however.[1,2] More delayed reactions, such as late-appearing hives, are usually associated with IgE against the major determinants.[2] Serum sickness is probably due to IgG antibodies against the major determinants.

In addition to patients who have developed sensitivity to the shared penicillin β-lactam ring or its metabolites, there are fewer patients who have sensitivity to a specific side chain and react only to a single agent. Because of this mechanism, IgE-mediated drug reactions require sufficient time for development of an antibody response. Allergic reactions can develop, however, during the course of a single treatment and can become manifest 2 weeks after termination of the treatment.[17] The typical maculopapular or morbilliform rash commonly seen with ampicillin in patients with infectious mononucleosis, other viral illnesses, chronic lymphocytic leukemia, or concomitant allopurinol therapy is not IgE mediated.[1]

CROSS-REACTIVITY OF β-LACTAMS

Early studies with first-generation cephalosporins suggested strong but incomplete cross-reactivity with penicillins. As newer drugs were analyzed, similar cross-reactivity with penicillin was seen with the carbapenems (e.g., imipenem), but minimal cross-reactivity was seen with the monobactams (e.g., aztreonam). Overall, deShazo and Kemp[1] estimated that there is approximately a 10% cross-reactivity between penicillins and first-generation cephalosporins, 1% to 3% cross-reactivity between penicillins and third-generation cephalosporins, and minimal cross-reactivity with aztreonam. For practical purposes, because the impact of a reaction is great, patients with generalized reactions to penicillins should be considered to be reactive to all other penicillins and to cephalosporins and carbapenems but are not likely to be sensitive to the monobactams. Patients with a maculopapular (not urticarial) rash associated with intake of a penicillin (most often amoxicillin), especially in the context of a viral infection (Epstein-Barr virus or cytomegalovirus), are unlikely to have systemic reactions to penicillin in the future and, in clinical practice, often are given a test dose of a cephalosporin in a controlled setting. Anaphylactoid reactions have been reported with procaine penicillin and may be related to inadvertent intravenous administration and resultant toxic and embolic effects.[2]

OTHER ANTIBIOTICS

Reactions to sulfa drugs may be immunologically mediated and manifest as hives or anaphylaxis or both. The major concern for sulfa drugs is development of SJS and TEN, however. The pathophysiology of these syndromes was discussed earlier. In a patient with a rash in the context of a sulfa drug, it is crucial to consider these severe cutaneous reactions early and to consider them often. Vancomycin can cause mast cell degranulation directly, leading to the "red man syndrome" and can induce an IgE response. The pseudoallergic activation of mast cells with vancomycin is functionally similar to the nonspecific degranulation of mast cells seen with radiocontrast material, although the red man syndrome is limited to the skin. It is unknown why this activation manifests as a diffuse erythema rather than hives and why is it limited to the skin.

Antiepileptics

Similar to other drugs, antiepileptic drugs can cause a maculopapular or morbilliform rash and more severe cutaneous reactions, including SJS and TEN.[40] The concomitant administration of valproate and lamotrigine seems to increase the risk. Valproate is known to increase the half-life of lamotrigine, and the dose should be adjusted accordingly.[41] Antiepileptic drugs also are associated with a specific pattern of hypersensitivity characterized by a maculopapular rash that can evolve into a severe exfoliative dermatitis, fever, tender lymphadenopathy, hepatitis, and eosinophilia, most often referred to as the *antiepileptic drug hypersensitivity syndrome* or the *anticonvulsant hypersensitivity syndrome*.[40,42] This is a potentially life-threatening, multiorgan syndrome beginning 1 week or more than 3 months after initiating therapy. It generally is defined as a triad of fever, skin rash, and internal organ involvement. Allergic hepatitis is prominent, but the kidneys and the lungs also can be involved.[42] Lymphadenopathy typically shows benign lymphoid hyperplasia or pseudolymphoma, which may be difficult to distinguish from malignant lymphoma. Hepatitis is usually anicteric, but it can be severe. Other organs that may be involved include the kidneys, heart, lungs, and thyroid gland.[40] This syndrome is relatively common (1:1000 to 1:10,000) and is distinguished from SJS by the rarity of mucosal involvement and by more severe organ involvement. It can be distinguished from TEN less easily but can be distinguished by the nature of the evolving rash and by the presence of eosinophilia. A similar syndrome can be caused by other, nonepileptic drugs, such as sulfonamides, azathioprine, and allopurinol.[42] Evidence that this syndrome has an immunologic basis includes the need for a sensitization period (reactions occur at least 7 days after the beginning of the drug therapy or after repeated exposure), no clear relationship to dose, the presence of blood and tissue eosinophilia, the presence of fever, positive rechallenges, and the presence of drug or drug-specific antibodies or drug-reactive T cells.[43]

Local Anesthetics

Bona fide reactions to local anesthetics are extremely rare, although there are many patients who profess that they have had reactions, mostly during dental procedures. The most generally accepted alternative explanations for these histories are that these either are vasovagal reactions or are due to the inadvertent intravenous injection of the local anesthetic agent with epinephrine. Some of these patients may be allergic to latex (see later). A simple approach to these patients is to perform skin testing to reassure the patient and to switch to a different class of local anesthetic agent (benzoic acid esters versus amide-type local anesthetics).[2,44]

General Anesthesia

The incidence of life-threatening immunologic reactions to drugs used in general anesthesia has been estimated to be 1 in 3500 to 1 in 6000.[45] These reactions typically occur with administration of multiple drugs. This situation obscures temporal relationships and complicates determination of the specific offending agent. The patient typically is unconscious and covered, delaying awareness that a systemic reaction is taking place. Increased ventilatory resistance or loss of blood pressure may be the earliest signs of anaphylaxis. Based on the demonstration of drug-specific IgE, 50% of these reactions may be IgE mediated; the remainder are thought to be pseudoallergic. Muscle relaxants, such as suxamethonium, are the cause in approximately 60% of the IgE-mediated reactions. Quaternary ammonium ions, which are present in many drugs and cosmetics, may be the active epitope.[46] Other agents, such as hypnotics and morphine derivatives, occasionally are identified as causal. Some agents, such as tubocurarine, may be able to release histamine from mast cells on a pseudoallergic basis (without the presence of drug-specific IgE), but the clinical importance of this is controversial.[2,45] Latex sensitivity may explain many episodes of intraoperative anaphylaxis.[14]

Latex

Latex reactivity is included in this chapter because sensitivity to latex proteins is an important consideration in patients presenting with immediate hypersensitivity reactions in the hospital. The early reports of anaphylaxis after exposure to latex were in patients undergoing barium enemas and in children with spina bifida.[47] In the 1990s, it became apparent that many individuals are sensitized to latex, and individuals at highest risk are patients who have undergone multiple surgeries or invasive procedures, health care professionals, and latex workers.[47] Prevalence of antilatex IgE in health care workers is 9% to 18% compared with about 6% in unselected blood donors.[48] This higher rate of sensitization has been attributed to the institution of universal precautions in 1987 with the concomitant increased use of rubber gloves.[49] Although many patients present with dermatitis, conjunctivitis, rhinitis, or asthma, life-threatening allergic reactions can be the initial presentation for latex allergy.[47] Gloves marked "hypoallergenic" likely contain significant latex allergen and are *not safe* for sensitized individuals. Powdered gloves are the most allergenic because the powder acts as a vehicle for the latex proteins.[47] The task force on Allergic Reactions to Latex of the American Academy of Allergy and Immunology recommends that medical procedures performed on latex-sensitive persons be conducted in a latex-free environment.[47]

Latex is a natural product manufactured from the sap of the rubber tree and contains many proteins, several of which are allergenic in susceptible individuals. An important corollary is that other plants, particularly those of tropical origin, such as the kiwi fruit, papaya, banana, and avocado, contain similar proteins and can be cross-reactive. Cross-reactivity between latex and chestnuts, grass pollen, and ragweed pollen also has been reported. Seasonal rhinitis and food allergies are often present in latex-sensitive patients, and inadvertent exposure to specific foods can cause anaphylactic reactions.[47,49]

Nonsteroidal Antiinflammatory Drugs

The most common immunologic reactions to NSAIDs involve either the respiratory tract or the skin, although other reactions, such as anaphylaxis, aseptic meningitis, and hypersensitivity pneumonitis, occur.[2,25] Aspirin-induced bronchospasm occurs in approximately 10% of asthmatics older than age 10 years and in 30% to 40% of asthmatics with nasal polyps. The clinical syndrome, triad asthma, refers to patients with aspirin sensitivity, asthma, and nasal polyps. These individuals typically have sinusitis and a predisposition to a variety of adverse responses to NSAIDs. These reactions are not IgE mediated and are due to exaggerated pharmacologic actions of these drugs on cells of the immune system in select individuals. NSAIDs share the pharmacologic property of inhibiting cyclooxygenases (cyclooxygenase type 1 and type 2), the proximal enzymes for the production of prostanoids from arachidonic acid. Although this effect is advantageous to most individuals, patients with triad asthma, after ingestion of less than or equal to 1% of a standard dose of an NSAID, may experience intense rhinorrhea, conjunctivitis, periorbital edema, laryngospasm, and prolonged bronchospasm.[25] Increased production of leukotriene E_4, the terminal metabolic product of cystinyl leukotriene production, has been shown in the urine of these patients. Increased levels of a key enzyme, leukotriene synthase, have been shown in lung tissue from some of these patients. This finding suggests that when the cyclooxygenase pathway is inhibited, these patients may overproduce proinflammatory leukotrienes.[50] Urticarial and anaphylactic reactions to aspirin and NSAIDs seem to be IgE mediated; this is based on observations that the reactivity is limited to agents of similar structure, the reactions generally are limited to the skin or are anaphylactic, and the reactions tend to occur within minutes of oral ingestion.[25]

Radiographic Contrast Material

Reactions to radiographic contrast material have been discussed previously as the best example of a pseudoallergic drug reaction. Understanding of these reactions and their management has been advanced by the studies of Greenberger and Paterson.[51,52] The most important approach to these reactions is to be prepared for them, to identify patients who have had previous reactions, and to premedicate or use low-ionic-strength contrast material in susceptible patients. One must be prepared because, even without a history of previous reactions, 1% to 2% of patients have a systemic reaction, which can include cutaneous hives, angioedema, asthma, and systemic anaphylaxis. Severe reactions were rare in a large-scale Japanese study, occurring in 0.04% to

0.22% of the reactions, and resulted in 1 death per 169,000 procedures.[53] History of a previous reaction to radiocontrast material is the best historical clue to predict a reaction. Of patients with a generalized reaction to a previous exposure, 17% to 35% react on a subsequent exposure at an increased risk of 8 to 35 times that of patients without a prior reaction.[51] Other less important risk factors that have been recognized include a history of asthma, a history of skin-test positivity to common allergens, and a history of allergy to penicillin.[53] A history of cutaneous reactivity to iodine-containing skin disinfectants, a history of parotid swelling after radiocontrast material administration, a positive cutaneous reaction to radiocontrast material, and a history of allergic reactions to seafood are not predictive.[51] Several caveats are important. Use of β-blockers interferes with the action of epinephrine and complicates resuscitation of patients from anaphylaxis. These agents should be stopped, if clinically possible, before radiocontrast material is administered.[53] Patients without the aforementioned risk factors but with personal concerns regarding reactions to radiocontrast material should be pretreated with prednisone and antihistamines because this does not entail a significant risk.[52] Pretreatment with diphenhydramine and prednisone (Table 31-3) reduces the frequency of repeat reactions to approximately 10% and reduces the reactions' severity. The addition of ephedrine further reduces the rate of reaction to approximately 3% but must be balanced by the risk of that drug. Ephedrine should not be used in patients with hypertension and heart disease. The combination of premedication and the use of low osmolar radiocontrast material in patients with a history of severe reactivity reduces the risk of systemic reaction to approximately 0.7%.[52] Table 31-3 lists recommendations for administration of radiocontrast material in susceptible patients.[53]

Biologics

As mentioned at the beginning of the chapter, horse serum was used extensively in the first half of the 20th century to treat a variety of infectious diseases and was associated with frequent immunologic reactions. More recently, purified polyclonal IgG, purified Fab fragments of polyclonal IgG, monoclonal IgG, and humanized monoclonal IgG have provided safer, biologically derived therapeutic agents. An example of a therapeutic material containing unfractionated horse globulins (not purified IgG) is black widow spider antivenin.[54] Examples of materials containing predominantly polyclonal horse IgG currently in use are antivenin (Crotalidae) polyvalent and antithymocyte globulin.[54] Crotalidae polyvalent immune Fab and digoxin immune Fab antibody (sheep IgG) (Digibind) are

---

TABLE 31-3 Management of Patients at Risk for Anaphylactoid Reactions to Radiographic Contrast Media

1. Remove any β-blockers if possible.
2. Have emergency therapy available.
3. Pretreat with prednisone 50 mg PO 13, 7, and 1 hr prior to the procedure and diphenhydramine 50 mg IM or PO 1 hr prior to the procedure.
4. For patients with a history of generalized anaphylaxis, pretreat and use a lower osmolar radiographic contrast medium.

---

produced from sheep by papain digestion of serum from immunized sheep and the subsequent isolation of the less immunogenic Fab portion of the antibody.[24]

Murine monoclonal antibodies also have been useful clinically. An example is anti-CD3 (Orthoclone OKT3), which binds to CD3 on T cells, leading to activation and subsequent blockade of T-cell function.[54] To decrease the immune response against the murine monoclonal antibodies, humanized monoclonal antibodies have been engineered that include only the essential murine sequences within the Fab region necessary to retain the immunologic activity. Agents designed in this way and in current clinical use include infliximab (Remicade; anti–tumor necrosis factor-α) and rituximab (Rituxan; anti CD20).[54] Another approach has been to engineer novel chimeric proteins consisting of sequences for soluble human receptors and the Fc region of human IgG. The Fc region of IgG imparts a long half-life to these agents. Because the sequences are all human, immunologic reactions are unlikely. An example is etanercept (Enbrel), a fusion protein containing the extracellular ligand-binding portion of the human tumor necrosis factor receptor linked to the Fc portion of human IgG_1.[54]

Allergic Reactions

Antithymocyte globulin is an effective treatment for severe, resistant aplastic anemia. Because this is purified equine IgG, there is ample opportunity for immune activation even in patients who have severely dysfunctional bone marrow and are leukopenic. In a prospective study of 35 patients treated for aplastic anemia, 86% developed serum sickness. Urticaria and anaphylaxis were rare, but one patient died.[55,56] In a study of 43 patients receiving multiple courses of treatment, serum sickness occurred in 66% of the patients.[57] A skin test has been developed to screen for anaphylactic sensitivity to antithymocyte globulin.[56]

Antivenin Crotalidae polyvalent also has been associated with numerous case reports of acute allergic reactions and a reported incidence rate ranging from 23% to 56%.[24] In a prospective study, the incidence of acute reactions to the potentially less immunogenic Crotalidae polyvalent immune Fab was 14%, and most of the events were of mild to moderate severity. Crotalidae polyvalent immune Fab has not been used as extensively as antivenin (Crotalidae) polyvalent, however, and these differences should be considered preliminary. Serum sickness also is seen with each of these agents, with reported rates between 15% and 86% of patients receiving antivenin Crotalidae polyvalent and 16% of patients receiving Crotalidae polyvalent immune Fab.[24]

A postmarketing survey of the efficacy and safety of Digibind included 717 patients with life-threatening digitalis intoxication treated in 487 hospitals. Six subjects had adverse reactions that probably or possibly were due to Digibind. These reactions included pruritic rashes, angioedema, chills, and thrombocytopenia and occurred more frequently in patients with a history of allergic reactions. None of the reactions were life-threatening, and all resolved with cessation of the infusion and appropriate medical treatment.[58]

Murine monoclonal antibodies also are heterologous proteins, and the production of a human antimouse antibody response is common. These antibodies generally do not produce as severe a reaction as the polyclonal equine antithymocyte globulin does, although anaphylactic reactions can occur.[59] Humanized monoclonal antibodies do not seem to cause significant immune responses.[60]

Cytokine Syndrome

Anti-CD3 is the prototypic biologic with the propensity to activate T cells. This agent has been used widely in clinical transplantation and has been associated with transient T-cell activation and the subsequent production of proinflammatory cytokines.[61]

DIFFERENTIAL DIAGNOSIS

In a hospitalized patient who has had a severe systemic reaction, the main considerations are allergic reactions to drugs, blood products, foods, or latex and distinguishing these anaphylactic reactions from septic shock. Cutaneous eruptions, such as hives (with or without angioedema) or angioedema (with or without hives), are typical manifestations of an acute allergic reaction. In the acute setting, the presence of hives is the best predictor that a reaction is allergic.[62] Angioedema (with or without hives; localized or diffuse) may be due to an allergic reaction or to a known pharmacologic activity of a drug in a sensitive patient (NSAIDs or angiotensin-converting enzyme inhibitors). Other causes of angioedema need to be considered, however, including hereditary angioedema and acquired angioedema. These latter diseases are caused by deficiencies in the quantity or function of a protein called *C1 esterase inhibitor* and should not be accompanied by urticaria. C1 esterase inhibitor exerts regulatory control on complement activation and activation of vasoactive peptides called *kinins*.

Severe cutaneous eruptions may be due to drugs, infections, or intercurrent disease. Infections associated with severe dermatitis include upper respiratory viruses, cytomegalovirus, human immunodeficiency virus, Epstein-Barr virus, viral hepatitis, staphylococcal scalded skin syndrome, and *Staphylococcus aureus*–induced toxic shock syndrome. Concomitant collagen vascular diseases, lymphoma, porphyria, and syphilis also can be the cause of severe cutaneous eruptions (Table 31-4).[40]

TABLE 31-4 Differential Diagnosis of Immunologic Reactions

Angioedema with or without urticaria	Human immunodeficiency virus
Pharmacologic response (NSAIDs or ACE inhibitors)	Epstein-Barr virus
	Viral hepatitis
	Scalded skin syndrome
Immediate hypersensitivity reaction	Toxic shock syndrome
	Collagen vascular diseases
Hereditary angioedema	Lymphoma
Severe cutaneous eruptions	Porphyria
Upper respiratory viruses	Syphilis
Cytomegalovirus	Septic shock

ACE, angiotensin-converting enzyme; NSAIDs, nonsteroidal antiinflammatory drugs.

Crucial diagnostic concerns are distinguishing sepsis from anaphylaxis and recognizing pseudoallergic reactions when they occur. The possibility of a pseudoallergic reaction should be considered if a patient becomes symptomatic in the context of administration of an agent known to cause this type of a reaction (see earlier under Systemic Reactions).

When one has determined that a specific reaction is an allergic or a pseudoallergic reaction, the work to determine the cause of the reaction begins. A decision regarding which of many suspects is the etiologic agent is not straightforward and often cannot be determined absolutely. As in all aspects of medicine, a detailed history is the beginning step. The history as it relates to a possible drug allergy must include a detailed analysis of all medications that have been used, including prescribed medications, over-the-counter medications, dietary supplements, and herbals. If the reactions occurred in the operating room, exposure to latex may be important. In the emergency department, inadvertent exposure to foods in a patient with a bona fide food allergy is a common cause of a systemic reaction. The temporal relationship between administration of a suspected agent and the onset of the reaction is crucial, but it is most helpful in the evaluation of patients who have had systemic anaphylactic reactions or hives. A history of a previous reaction to a suspected or chemically similar drug is useful, whereas a history of other allergies or a family history of a reaction to a given drug is not useful. Systemic allergic reactions tend to develop more abruptly and are often in the context of recent administration of an agent with the potential to produce an allergic reaction. For reactions with later onset, such as maculopapular rashes, other rashes, or serum sickness, the relationships may be much less clear.

The physical examination is useful because some manifestations are more typically "allergic" than others. In the acute setting, a patient with rapid onset of vascular collapse often can be recognized easily to be having an anaphylactic reaction because of associated urticaria. Other cutaneous presentations, such as maculopapular rashes, diffuse erythema, or the symptom of pruritus, are less specific, however, and there may be no cutaneous changes at all. Wheezing can be a prominent sign of anaphylaxis, although in the operating room this may be manifest only as increased resistance to ventilation. Fever typically is not part of an acute allergic reaction (but it can be a manifestation of more delayed reactions, such as a drug fever or serum sickness), and its presence should raise the likelihood of sepsis.

Laboratory Testing

IN VITRO TESTS

Results from general laboratory testing can be helpful. Elevated numbers of eosinophils generally indicate an allergic process. Antigen-specific IgE measurements (radioallergosorbent test [RAST]) are helpful if positive but have poor negative predictive value. Products from mast cells can be measured. Plasma levels of histamine increase rapidly (approximately 5 to 10 minutes) after an allergic reaction and return to baseline within 30 minutes. Plasma samples must be handled carefully and processed promptly. Determination of urinary histamine in a 4-hour collection beginning immediately after the onset of a reaction can be helpful if the values are quite elevated. Modest levels of elevation of urinary histamine are of limited usefulness. Levels of β-tryptase increase more slowly than serum histamine (peak at about 1 hour) and stay elevated longer (3 to 4 hours).[63] These laboratory tests are complementary, but normal values do not rule out an allergic reaction. There is no value in ordering a total IgE level.

The syndromes of hereditary angioedema and acquired angioedema are due to abnormal complement pathway activation and need to be considered in patients with angioedema. Typically, these syndromes have low levels of C4 between attacks and nearly absent C4 during attacks. The diagnostic test is to measure levels and function of C1 esterase inhibitor. Not all laboratories report C4 values in such a way that one can distinguish between low and absent levels of C4, and complement activation occurs in a variety of conditions seen in the hospital.

IN VIVO TESTING

Skin tests can be useful diagnostic tools to distinguish among various possible etiologic agents that may have precipitated an allergic reaction. When applied to drugs, these are not standardized tests, however, and they have many limitations. A critical limitation is that after a severe reaction, IgE may be depleted so that one should wait 4 to 6 weeks before conducting these tests. A second limitation is that for many drugs, the reactive species may be a metabolic product or a haptenated protein and not the original drug itself. The best-characterized skin tests are those for penicillins, but they are suboptimal because the minor determinant mix is not commercially available.

To perform skin tests, one first must determine if the patient can react appropriately to skin tests by placing a positive (histamine) and negative (saline) control. The main cause of lack of reactivity to the positive control is recent administration of an antihistamine, but conditions such as uremia also give a false-negative reaction to histamine. The most common cause of unexpected reactivity to the negative control is inappropriate activation of dermal mast cells by the physical stimulus of pricking the skin. This activation occurs in patients who have dermatographism. One cannot interpret skin tests in patients when the positive control is negative or the negative control is positive. For penicillin testing, it first should be established that the patient can mount a skin response to histamine that is substantially (>3 mm wheal with erythema) more than the control. Then skin tests should be performed to the penicillin in question, to a polymerized β-lactam product (benzylpenicilloyl polylysine [Pre-Pen]), and to a mixture of breakdown products of penicillin called a *minor determinant mix*. Many academic medical practices produce their own minor determinant mix for internal use. The lack of a standardized minor determinant mix is of significant concern because reactivity to the minor determinant mix is correlated best with systemic anaphylaxis from penicillins. The presence of a negative skin test to these penicillin reagents reduces the risk of anaphylaxis to nearly zero.[1] If the minor determinant mix reagent is not available, one may miss 7% of the allergic patients, and these seem to be at higher risk of anaphylaxis.[1,2] Skin tests and RAST for other drugs are useful if positive, but if negative they do not exclude the possibility of an allergy to the tested drug. These tests are for IgE-mediated processes and have no bearing on non–IgE-mediated immunologic reactions, such as serum sickness or dermatologic manifestations other than angioedema and/or hives.

A detailed allergy history should be taken, and percutaneous skin tests should be performed before infusing any animal-derived biologics, unless there is a specific experience that argues to the contrary.[64] Patients receiving Fab fragments should be questioned regarding a history or sensitivity to papaya, papain, chymopapain, and the pineapple enzyme bromelain. Patients with allergies to latex, other tropical fruits, and dust mites may be at risk.[54] As discussed earlier, skin tests to assess sensitivity to these agents always should be accompanied by appropriate negative (saline) and positive (histamine) controls.

TREATMENT

Treatment of anaphylaxis requires the immediate administration of epinephrine and the establishment of a large-bore intravenous catheter for infusion of intravenous fluids, colloids, and pressor agents.[21] Current advanced cardiac life-support guidelines should be followed. Epinephrine is the drug of choice for anaphylaxis; 0.3 mL of a 1:1000 dilution should be given intramuscularly (as opposed to subcutaneously) to maximize absorption. In extreme cases, intravenous administration of a more dilute solution (1:10,000) is appropriate. Nebulized epinephrine can be useful, especially in the case of severe bronchospasm. Antihistamines and corticosteroids should be given as soon as possible. Diphenhydramine (Benadryl), 0.5 to 1 mg/kg up to 50 mg intravenously, or hydroxyzine, 0.5 to 1 mg/kg intramuscularly, and methylprednisolone (Solu-Medrol), 1 mg/kg intravenously, should be given as soon as possible. The effects of epinephrine may give a false sense of security; close monitoring and support are necessary for 24 hours after the initiation of a reaction. The ameliorative effect of epinephrine in anaphylaxis is mediated predominantly through β2-receptors, and the concurrent treatment of a patient with nonselective and selective β-blockers either systemically or intraconjunctivally can interfere with its effect. Patients who have anaphylaxis while on a β-blocker are notoriously difficult to treat. In this setting, glucagon is given, 1 to 5 mg intravenously as a bolus followed by an infusion of 5 to 15 μg/min titrated to the clinical response.[14]

Compromise of the airway constitutes a medical emergency. A patient with angioedema due to either an allergic reaction or lack of C1 esterase inhibitor activity may experience closure of the larynx. Intubation in this situation is difficult and may be unsuccessful. The local trauma of an unsuccessful intubation may make angioedema worse. In this situation, it is essential to call for an anesthesiologist (or an emergency physician) as soon as the problem is recognized and to be ready to perform an emergency cricothyrotomy.

Avoidance of the offending agent is the simplest treatment, but for a variety of reasons this may not be possible because the offending agent may not be identified easily. This is often the case in intrasurgical anaphylaxis, in which multiple agents are suspect and percutaneous skin tests and RAST are of only limited usefulness. Alternatively, there are clinical settings in which administration of the offending drug is clearly indicated, and there is no acceptable alternative treatment. An example is treatment of a pregnant woman who is allergic to penicillin and has syphilis. The second-line drug is doxycycline, which is contraindicated in pregnancy. In this case, desensitization is an option but must be undertaken with caution.

Desensitization is a potentially life-threatening procedure that should be performed only by physicians with substantial experience and should be done in carefully controlled settings, such as an intensive care unit or an emergency department. The most extensive experience in desensitization to drugs is with β-lactam antibiotics, although this approach has been generalized to include many other agents. In general, patients with acute systemic reactions (urticaria or anaphylaxis) are good candidates for desensitization because there is good reason to think that their reactions are mediated by IgE. Patients with positive skin tests to the suspect drug are likely at greater risk than patients with negative skin tests. The presence of a negative skin test is not a guarantee, however, that the patient can tolerate the drug. The patient is placed in a setting that allows careful monitoring (e.g., intensive care unit). After informed consent is obtained, an initial dose of the drug that is approximately 10^5 less than the therapeutic dose is administered, and the patient is observed for 20 minutes. Incremental doses are administered every 20 minutes until the therapeutic dose is achieved. Desensitization is maintained only as long as the drug is administered on a frequent basis. Patients with atypical reactions (e.g., morbilliform rashes) to agents known to cause IgE-mediated reactions and negative skin tests often are given test doses in a controlled setting because the index of suspicion of an IgE-mediated allergic reaction is not high.

Certain drugs are associated with aggressive cutaneous reactions, and these agents are not good candidates for desensitization. Examples of agents for which desensitization is not used are antiepileptic drugs in patients who have had severe cutaneous reactions and sulfa drugs in patients who are not immunosuppressed. Although the cutaneous reactions to sulfa drugs are not thought to be immune mediated, patients who are immunosuppressed may have successful desensitization to sulfa drugs. Trimethoprim-sulfamethoxazole has been administered successfully (using a desensitization protocol) to patients with human immunodeficiency virus and to patients who are status post–lung transplantation.[65,66]

REFERENCES

1. deShazo RD, Kemp SF: Allergic reactions to drugs and biologic agents. JAMA 278:1895–1906, 1997.
2. Weiss ME: Drug allergy. Med Clin North Am 76:857–882, 1992.
3. White TJ, Arakelian A, Rho JP: Counting the costs of drug-related adverse events. Pharmacoeconomics 15:445–458, 1999.
4. Adkinson NF Jr: Drug allergy. In Middleton E Jr, Reed CE, Ellis EF, et al (eds): Allergy: Principles and Practice, Vol II, 5th ed. St Louis, 1998, Mosby-Year Book, pp 1212–1224.
5. Vervloet D, Durham S: Adverse reactions to drugs. BMJ 316:1511–1514, 1998.
6. DiPiro JT, Stafford CT, Schlesselman LS: Allergic and pseudoallergic drug reactions. In DiPiro JT, Talbert RL, Yee GC, et al (eds): Pharmacotherapy: A Pathophysiologic Approach, Vol 1. Stamford, CT, 1999, Appleton & Lange, pp 1393–1405.
7. Bircher AJ: Drug-induced urticaria and angioedema caused by non-IgE mediated pathomechanisms. Eur J Dermatol 9:657–663, 1999.
8. Plotkin SL, Plotkin SA: A short history of vaccination. In Plotkin SA, Orenstein WA (eds): Vaccines. Philadelphia, 1999, WB Saunders, pp 1–12.
9. Cohen SG: From immunity to autoimmune disease, a historic trail: Part III. Allergy Asthma Proc 21:177–183, 2000.
10. Cohen SG: From immunity to autoimmune disease, a historic trail: Part II. Allergy Asthma Proc 21:117–122, 2000.
11. Cohen SG: From immunity to autoimmune disease, a historic trail: Part I. Allergy Asthma Proc 21:63–68, 2000.
12. Ratner B: Allergy, Anaphylaxis, and Immunotherapy. Baltimore, 1943, Williams & Wilkins.
13. May CD: The ancestry of allergy: Being an account of the original experimental induction of hypersensitivity recognizing the contribution of Paul Portier. J Allergy Clin Immunol 75:485–495, 1985.
14. Lieberman P: Anaphylaxis and anaphylactoid reactions. In Middleton E Jr, Reed CE, Ellis EF, et al (eds): Allergy: Principles and Practice, Vol II, 5th ed. St Louis, 1998, Mosby-Year Book, pp 1079–1092.
15. Wilson SGS: The Hazards of Immunization. London, 1967, The Athlone Press.
16. Torres MJ, Mayorga C, Garcia JJ, et al: New aspects in betalactam recognition. Clin Exp Allergy 28(Suppl 4):25–28, 1998.
17. Sogn DD: Is it a penicillin allergy? Diagnosis. April, 36–44, 1984.
18. Abbas AK, Lichtman AH, Pober JS: Cellular and Molecular Immunology. Philadelphia, 2000, WB Saunders.
19. Holgate ST, Church MK. Allergy. London, 1993, Mosby.
20. Pichler WJ, Schnyder B, Zanni MP, et al: Role of T cells in drug allergies. Allergy 53:225–232, 1998.
21. Wyatt R: Anaphylaxis: How to recognize, treat and prevent potentially fatal attacks. Postgrad Med 100:87–90, 1996.
22. Bailey B, McGuigan MA: Management of anaphylactoid reactions to intravenous N-acetylcysteine. Ann Emerg Med 31:710–715, 1998.
23. Wintroub BU, Wasserman SI: Allergic reactions to drugs. In Frank MM, Austin KF, Claman HN, Unanue ER (eds): Samter's Immunologic Diseases, Vol 2. Boston, 1995, Little, Brown, pp 1207–1221.
24. Dart RC, McNally J: Efficacy, safety, and use of snake antivenoms in the United States. Ann Emerg Med 37:181–188, 2001.
25. Stevenson DD, Simon RA: Sensitivity to aspirin and nonsteroidal anti-inflammatory drugs. In Middleton E Jr, Reed CE, Ellis EF, et al (eds): Allergy: Principles and Practice, Vol II, 5th ed. St Louis, 1998, Mosby-Year Book, pp 1225–1234.
26. Martin Mateos MA, Roldan Ros A, Munoz-Lopez F: Erythema multiforme: A review of twenty cases. Allergol Immunopathol (Madr) 26:283–287, 1998.
27. Roujeau JC, Stern RS: Severe adverse cutaneous reactions to drugs. N Engl J Med 331:1272–1285, 1994.
28. Wolkenstein PE, Roujeau JC, Revuz J: Drug-induced toxic epidermal necrolysis. Clin Dermatol 16:399–408, 1998.
29. Saulsbury FT: Henoch-Schonlein purpura in children: Report of 100 patients and review of the literature. Medicine (Baltimore) 78:395–409, 1999.
30. Beaune PH, Lecoeur S: Immunotoxicology of the liver: Adverse reactions to drugs. J Hepatol 26:37–42, 1997.
31. Zimmerman H: Drug-induced liver disease. In Schiff ER, Sorrell MF, Maddrey WC (eds): Schiff's Diseases of the Liver. Philadelphia, 1999, Lippincott-Raven, pp 973–1064.
32. Kelly CJ, Neilson EG: Tubulointerstitial diseases. In Brenner BM (ed): The Kidney, Vol II. Philadelphia, 2000, WB Saunders, pp 1509–1538.
33. Thomas AT: Autoimmune hemolytic anemias. In Lee GR, Foerster J, Lukens J, et al (eds): Wintrobe's Clinical Hematology, Vol 1. Baltimore, 1999, Williams & Wilkins, pp 1233–1263.
34. Tanoue LT: Pulmonary toxicity associated with chemotherapeutic agents. In Fishman AP (ed): Fishman's Pulmonary Diseases and Disorders, Vol 2. New York, 1998, McGraw-Hill, pp 1003–1016.
35. Fink JN, Zacharisen MC: Hypersensitivity pneumonitis. In Middleton E Jr, Reed CE, Ellis EF, et al (eds): Allergy: Principles and Practice, Vol II, 5th ed. St Louis, 1998, Mosby-Year Book, pp 994–1004.
36. Swartz MN: Approach to the patient with pulmonary infections. In Fishman AP (ed): Fishman's Pulmonary Diseases and Disorders, Vol 2. New York, 1998, McGraw-Hill, pp 1905–1938.
37. Blanca M, Vega JM, Garcia J, et al: New aspects of allergic reactions to betalactams: Crossreactions and unique specificities. Clin Exp Allergy 24:407–415, 1994.
38. Adkinson NF Jr: Beta-lactam crossreactivity. Clin Exp Allergy 28(Suppl 4):37–40, 1998.
39. Coleman JW: Protein haptenation by drugs. Clin Exp Allergy 28(Suppl 4):79–82, 1998.
40. Hamer HM, Morris HH: Hypersensitivity syndrome to antiepileptic drugs: A review including new anticonvulsants. Cleve Clin J Med 66:239–245, 1999.

41. Faught E, Morris G, Jacobson M, et al: Adding lamotrigine to valproate: Incidence of rash and other adverse effects. Postmarketing Antiepileptic Drug Survey (PADS) Group. Epilepsia 40:1135–1140, 1999.

42. Schlienger RG, Shear NH: Antiepileptic drug hypersensitivity syndrome. Epilepsia 39:S3–7, 1998.

43. Leeder JS: Mechanisms of idiosyncratic hypersensitivity reactions to antiepileptic drugs. Epilepsia 39:S8–16, 1998.

44. Gall H, Kaufmann R, Kalveram CM: Adverse reactions to local anesthetics: Analysis of 197 cases. J Allergy Clin Immunol 97:933–937, 1996.

45. Gueant JL, Aimone-Gastin I, Namour F, et al: Diagnosis and pathogenesis of the anaphylactic and anaphylactoid reactions to anaesthetics. Clin Exp Allergy 28(Suppl 4):65–70, 1998.

46. Naguib M, Magboul MM: Adverse effects of neuromuscular blockers and their antagonists. Drug Saf 18:99–116, 1998.

47. Yunginger JW: Natural rubber latex allergy. In Middleton E Jr, Reed CE, Ellis EF, et al (eds): Allergy: Principles and Practice, Vol II, 5th ed. St Louis, 1998, Mosby-Year Book, pp 1073–1078.

48. Saxon A, Ownby D, Huard T, et al: Prevalence of IgE to natural rubber latex in unselected blood donors and performance characteristics of AlaSTAT testing. Ann Allergy Asthma Immunol 84:199–206, 2000.

49. Warshaw EM: Latex allergy. J Am Acad Dermatol 39:1–24, 1998.

50. Cowburn AS, Sladek K, Soja J, et al: Overexpression of leukotriene C4 synthase in bronchial biopsies from patients with aspirin-intolerant asthma. J Clin Invest 101:834–846, 1998.

51. Greenberger PA, Patterson R, Tapio CM: Prophylaxis against repeated radiocontrast media reactions in 857 cases: Adverse experience with cimetidine and safety of beta-adrenergic antagonists. Arch Intern Med 145:2197–2200, 1998.

52. Greenberger PA, Patterson R: The prevention of immediate generalized reactions to radiocontrast media in high-risk patients. J Allergy Clin Immunol 87:867–872, 1991.

53. Wittbrodt ET, Spinler SA: Prevention of anaphylactoid reactions in high-risk patients receiving radiographic contrast media. Ann Pharmacother 28:236–241, 1994.

54. Physicians' Desk Reference. Montvale, NJ, 2002, Medical Economics.

55. Bielory L, Gascon P, Lawley TJ, et al: Human serum sickness: A prospective analysis of 35 patients treated with equine anti-thymocyte globulin for bone marrow failure. Medicine (Baltimore) 67:40–57, 1988.

56. Bielory L, Wright R, Nienhuis AW, et al: Antithymocyte globulin hypersensitivity in bone marrow failure patients. JAMA 260:3164–3167, 1988.

57. Tichelli A, Passweg J, Nissen C, et al: Repeated treatment with horse antilymphocyte globulin for severe aplastic anaemia. Br J Haematol 100:393–400, 1998.

58. Kirkpatrick CH. Allergic histories and reactions of patients treated with digoxin immune Fab (ovine) antibody. The Digibind Study Advisory Panel. Am J Emerg Med 9:7–10, 1991.

59. Gruber R, van Haarlem LJ, Warnaar SO, et al: The human antimouse immunoglobulin response and the anti-idiotypic network have no influence on clinical outcome in patients with minimal residual colorectal cancer treated with monoclonal antibody CO17-1A. Cancer Res 60:1921–1926, 2000.

60. Milgrom H, Fick RB Jr, Su JQ, et al: Treatment of allergic asthma with monoclonal anti-IgE antibody. rhuMAb-E25 Study Group. N Engl J Med 341:1966–1973, 1999.

61. Sgro C: Side-effects of a monoclonal antibody, muromonab CD3/orthoclone OKT3: Bibliographic review. Toxicology 105:23–29, 1995.

62. Lin RY, Schwartz LB, Curry A, et al: Histamine and tryptase levels in patients with acute allergic reactions: An emergency department-based study. J Allergy Clin Immunol 106:65–71, 2000.

63. Schwartz LB, Huff TF: Biology of mast cells. In Middleton E Jr, Reed CE, Ellis EF, et al (eds): Allergy: Principles and Practice, Vol II, 5th ed. St Louis, 1998, Mosby-Year Book, pp 261–276.

64. Brooks CD, Karl KJ, Francom SF: ATGAM skin test standardization: Comparison of skin testing techniques in horse-sensitive and unselected human volunteers. Transplantation 58:1135–1137, 1994.

65. Absar N, Daneshvar H, Beall G: Desensitization to trimethoprim/sulfamethoxazole in HIV-infected patients. J Allergy Clin Immunol 93:1001–1005, 1994.

66. Mann R, Badesch D, Zamora M, Dreskin SC: Desensitization to trimethoprim-sulfamethoxazole following lung transplantation (Letter). Chest 111:1147, 1997.

CHAPTER 32

Sympathomimetic Syndrome

Cynthia K. Aaron ■ Kathleen Northrup

Sympathomimetics have been available as medicinal agents from antiquity. More than 5000 years ago, the ancient Chinese recognized ephedrine, the primary active ingredient from the ephedra plant Ma Huang, as an active ingredient to treat asthmatic conditions and to stanch bleeding. Pliny, in the 1st century AD, used ephedrine to treat bleeding.[1] Caffeine made from brewing the seeds of the cocoa plant was used in South America and brought back to Europe in the Middle Ages. In the 1960s, home chemists experimented with merging various combinations of mescaline and amphetamine derivatives to yield the alphabet soup of hallucinogenic amphetamines described in Chapter 73. Now in the 21st century, sympathomimetics are ubiquitous in daily life (Table 32-1). They are found in over-the-counter medications, alternative medicinal agents, and illicit drugs. Most cough and cold preparations contain a sympathomimetic. Caffeine can be found in beverages in latte bars, flavored waters advertised to teenagers (Table 32-2), cocaine, methamphetamine, and 3,4-methylene-dioxymethamphetamine (MDMA) found on the street or at "alcohol-free" rave parties.

SYMPATHOMIMETIC TOXIDROME

The sympathomimetic toxidrome comprises a broad constellation of signs and symptoms that are aggregated because of similarity in appearance. Although sympathomimetics are thought of as being interchangeable, there can be significant differences in physiologic effects. These effects are based on whether the agent has predominant effects on dopaminergic or adrenergic neurotransmission, whether the agent is a direct-acting or indirect-acting agent, and which receptors are involved. The effects of specific sympathomimetic agents are described in Chapter 41. In general, the classic picture of a sympathomimetic toxidrome is a patient who presents with signs of significant adrenergic excess. This presentation can include dilated pupils, tachycardia, tachypnea, hypertension, hyperthermia, and psychomotor agitation—the classic "fight-or-flight response." The patient may be agitated, confused, or having seizures. If the patient has been on a prolonged "speed run," he or she may show signs of catecholamine depletion with lethargy, unresponsiveness, and relatively normal vital signs. Because few illicit sympathomimetic agents are pure agonists at a single receptor, however, one may see signs of other neurotransmitter effects, such as dopamine and serotonin. These effects include tremor, myoclonus, hypotension, hallucinations, and parkinsonian activity. Dopamine and serotonin also may contribute to the confusion, mental status changes, and seizures that cannot be explained by central nervous system (CNS) hemorrhage.

PATHOPHYSIOLOGY

Sympathomimetics are defined as catecholamine-like substances that have physiologic actions similar to those engendered by activation of the autonomic sympathetic nervous system. These actions include an excitatory effect on some types of smooth muscle with an inhibitory effect on others, modulation of glycogenolysis in the liver and muscle, and alterations in free fatty acid metabolism in adipose tissues. In some cases, sympathomimetics alter the effects of insulin by affecting the islet α_2-receptors and β_2-receptors and pituitary hormone secretion (antidiuretic hormone) by stimulation of central β_1-receptors.[2] More commonly recognized are the effects on the heart and CNS. Sympathomimetics have an excitatory effect on the heart, enhancing inotropy and chronotropy. Agents that cross the blood-brain barrier stimulate the CNS to increase wakefulness and psychomotor activity. Most have an anorectant effect. Sympathomimetics affect presynaptic nerve terminals in the adrenergic system, leading to enhancement or inhibition of the release of neurotransmitters.[4]

Structurally, sympathomimetic amines are created from a β-phenylethylamine parent compound (Fig. 32-1). Sympathomimetics with adjacent dihydroxy (–OH) substitutions on the benzene ring are called *catecholamines*. By altering the location of the hydroxyl groups on the phenyl ring and the size and location of the alkyl substitutions on the ethylamine moiety, the molecule can assume variable α and β selectivity,[3,4] as described in Chapter 41.

Normal biosynthesis of catecholamines (dopamine, norepinephrine, and epinephrine) occurs in the neuronal tuberosities. Tyrosine diffuses into the neuron and is taken up into storage granules containing tyrosine hydroxylase. This enzyme converts the tyrosine to 3,4-dihydroxyphenylalanine. Further conversion by L-aromatic amino acid decarboxylase converts 3,4-dihydroxyphenylalanine to dopamine. Dopamine-β-hydroxylase converts dopamine to norepinephrine within synaptic storage vesicles. Epinephrine is created in the adrenal medulla by the same process except that norepinephrine diffuses out of the storage vesicle and is converted by phenethanolamine-N-methyltransferase to epinephrine. It is then transported back into vesicles for release (see Fig. 41-2).[5,6]

On stimulation of a sympathic postganglionic neuron, norepinephrine-containing vesicles are transported to the

TABLE 32-1 Selected Sympathomimetic Agents

Albuterol	Mitodrine
Amphetamine	Norepinephrine
Cocaine	Other hallucinogenic
Dextroamphetamine	amphetamines
Diethylpropion	Pemoline
Dopamine	Phendimetrazine
Ephedrine	Phenmetrazine
Epinephrine	Phentermine
Isoproterenol	Phenylephrine
Ketamine	Phenylpropanolamine
MDEA	Propylhexedrine
MDMA	Pseudoephedrine
Metaproterenol	Ritodrine
Methamphetamine	Terbutaline
Methylphenidate	Tyramine

MDEA, 3,4-methylenedioxyethamphetamine;
MDMA, 3,4-methylenedioxymethamphetamine.

TABLE 32-2 Caffeine Content of Certain Beverages and Drugs

SOURCE	APPROXIMATE AMOUNT OF CAFFEINE PER UNIT (5 OZ CUP OR TABLET) (mg)
Beverages	
Brewed coffee	80–150
Instant coffee	85–100
Decaffeinated coffee	2–4
Tea (bag or leaf)	30–75
Cocoa	5–40
Cola drinks	35–60*
Nonprescription (OTC) Drugs	
Analgesics	
Anacin, Bromo-Seltzer, Cope, Empirin compound	32
Excedrin	60
Stimulants	
No Doz	100
Vivarin	200
Caffedrine	250
Many cold preparations	32

*12 oz.
OTC, over-the-counter.
From Oakley R: Drugs, Society and Human Behavior. St Louis, 1978, CV Mosby, p 196.

nerve membrane, where they fuse and release norepinephrine into the synaptic cleft. Neurotransmission is halted by reuptake of norepinephrine back into the presynaptic terminal or diffusion away in the cleft. Reuptake occurs by way of the norepinephrine transporter. This transporter has a high affinity for norepinephrine but also transports dopamine, tyramine, monoamine oxidase (MAO), and other phenylethylamines such as amphetamine.[7] Although both the enzymes catechol O-methyltransferase and MAO are present, neurotransmission is halted mostly by reuptake and not by enzymatic degradation of the neurotransmitter (Fig. 32-2).[8,9] In addition to normal neurotransmission, the presence of other endogenous agents can alter neurotransmission by affecting prejunctional neuroreceptors (Fig. 32-3). These agents include adenosine triphosphate (ATP), opioids, and prostanoids. By altering ionic influx at the receptors, the nerve stimulation is affected (Table 32-3).[10]

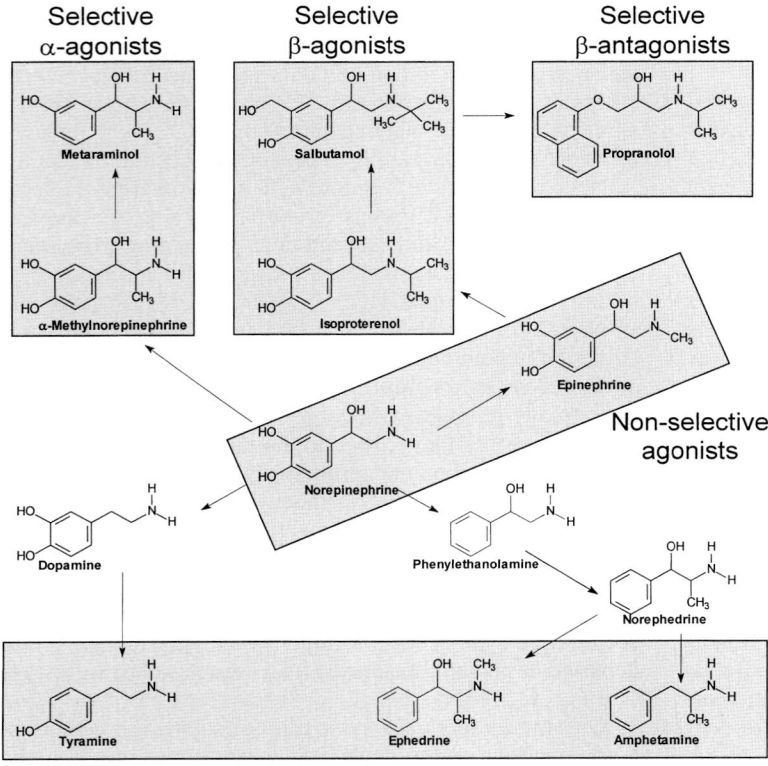

Indirectly Acting Sympathomimetic Amines

FIGURE 32-1

Graphic depiction of the structure-activity relationships among the catecholamines and related phenylethylamines.

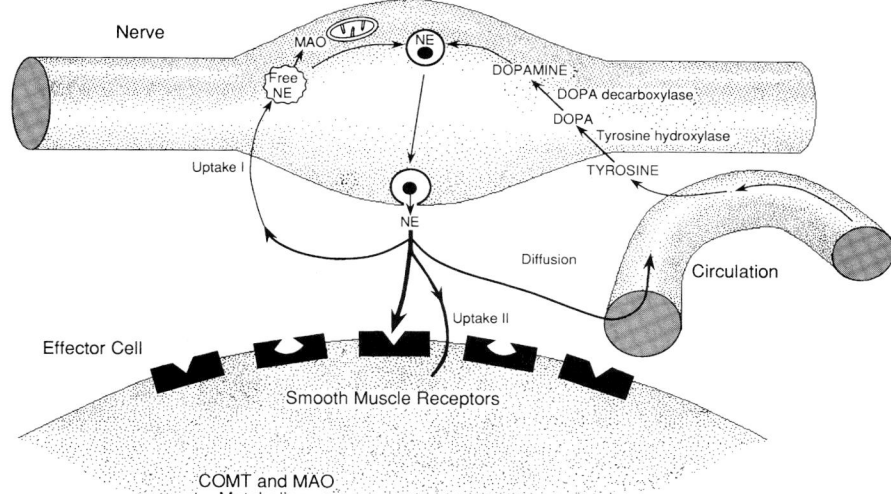

FIGURE 32-2

Adrenergic neuroeffector transmission; the termination of norepinephrine (NE) neurotransmission. MAO, monoamine oxidase; COMT, catechol *O*-methyltransferase. *(From Brown OM: Adrenergic drugs. In Smith CM, Reynard AM [eds]: Textbook of Human Pharmacology. Philadelphia, WB Saunders, 1992, p 144.)*

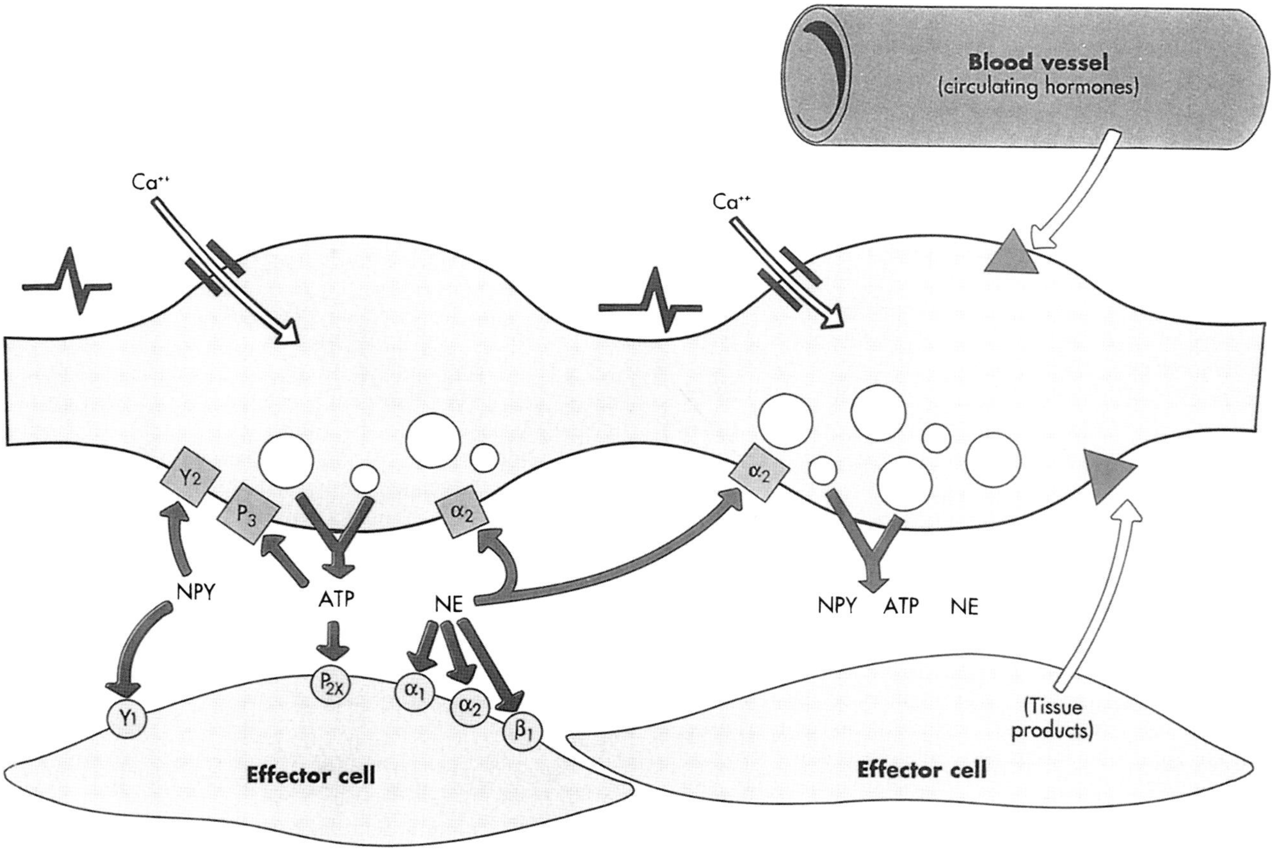

FIGURE 32-3

Prejunctional regulation at the sympathetic neuroeffector junction. The left varicosity illustrates autoinhibition of neurotransmitter release, including possible "lateral" inhibition (i.e., transmitter from one varicosity inhibiting release from an adjacent varicosity). The right varicosity illustrates prejunctional regulation of transmitter release by tissue and blood-borne chemicals. See Table 32-3 for a list of involved substances. Postjunctional receptors are shown as *circles*; prejunctional inhibitory autoreceptors are shown as *squares*; prejunctional heteroreceptors are shown as *triangles*. ATP, adenosine triphosphate; NE, norepinephrine; NPY, neuropeptide Y. *(From Fink GD: Regulation of blood pressure by the autonomic nervous system. In Brody TM, Larner J, Minneman KP [eds]: Human Pharmacology: Molecular to Clinical, 3rd ed. St. Louis, Mosby, 1998, p 177.)*

TABLE 32-3 Prejunctional Modulators of Sympathetic Neurotransmitter Release

CHEMICAL	SOURCE	RECEPTOR	MECHANISM	EFFECT
Norepinephrine	SNT	α_2	$\downarrow Ca^{2+}$	$\downarrow$
Neuropeptide Y	SNT	Y_2	$\downarrow Ca^{2+}$	$\downarrow$
ATP	SNT	P_3, P_{2x}	$\downarrow Ca^{2+}$	$\downarrow$
Epinephrine	Blood	β_2	$\uparrow cAMP$	$\uparrow$
Angiotensin II	Blood/PJT	AT_1	$\uparrow PLC$	$\uparrow$
Prostanoids	PJT	?	$\downarrow Ca^{2+}$	$\downarrow$
Adenosine	PJT	P_1	$\downarrow Ca^{2+}$	$\downarrow$
Opioids	Blood	μ, κ, δ	$\downarrow Ca^{2+}$	$\downarrow$
Acetylcholine	Nerve	M_2	$\uparrow cGMP$	$\downarrow$
Dopamine	SNT	D_2	$\uparrow K^+$	$\downarrow$
Atrial natriuretic peptide	Blood	?	$\uparrow cGMP$	$\downarrow$
Nitric oxide	EC	?	$\uparrow cGMP$	$\downarrow$

cAMP, cyclic adenosine monophosphate; cGMP, cyclic guanosine monophosphate; EC, endothelial cell; PJT, postjunctional tissue; PLC, phospholipase C; SNT, sympathetic nerve terminal.
From Fink GD: Regulation of blood pressure by the autonomic nervous system. In Brody TM, Larnes J, Minneman KP (eds): Human Pharmacology: Molecular to Clinical, 3rd ed. St. Louis, Mosby, 1998, p 176.

In the neurons, norepinephrine is stored in the synaptic vesicles in high concentration along with ATP, chromogranin, and dopamine-β-hydroxylase. When norepinephrine is released, all of these agents are released simultaneously. The effects of MAO, which is an intracellular enzyme, and the high-affinity norepinephrine transporter protein keep the concentration of cytosolic norepinephrine low. The enzyme dopamine-β-decarboxylase is not specific to dopamine and is involved in the synthesis of serotonin from 5-hydroxytryptamine (5-HT).[11]

Sympathomimetic actions are mediated through the effects of the adrenergic nervous system via neurotransmitters. Norepinephrine, epinephrine, and dopamine are the predominant adrenergic neurotransmitters. Although these neurotransmitters tend to be thought of in isolation, they are intricately interconnected in the CNS and can alter acetylcholine and serotonin release and uptake. The main noradrenergic nucleus is located in the cortical locus caeruleus. Its axons radiate into the cortex, cerebellum, and other structures. Norepinephrine released from the locus caeruleus into the hippocampal projections increases cortical neurologic activity through β-adrenergic receptor stimulation. Norepinephrine release into the outer cortical area has an inhibitory effect mediated by α-receptor agonism. If the locus caeruleus receives a nonspecific stimulus, there is widespread cortical activation with excitation. This activation may be part of the effect of nonspecific sympathomimetics resulting in hyperattentiveness and lack of fatigue.[12] Medullary cholinergic neurons, opioid peptide neurons, and central raphe serotonin neurons all penetrate into the locus caeruleus. Stimulation of the locus caeruleus may lead to norepinephrine release but also may affect serotonin, endogenous opioid, and acetylcholine neurotransmission.[12,13] Dopamine neurotransmission also is altered by endogenous opioids at the μ and κ receptors in the mesolimbic system.[14] This interplay gives the varied presentation of patients with a sympathomimetic syndrome. Although we speak mostly of the hyperadrenergic state, there can be overlap into other neurotransmitter systems creating unexpected toxicity.

Noradrenergic Receptors

Noradrenergic receptors (Table 32-4) act as the binding site for sympathomimetic agents. Receptors are divided into ligand-gated ion channel receptors and G protein receptors. When an agent binds to a ligand-gated ion channel, the pore undergoes a conformational change and allows entry of a specific ion, which triggers secondary effects. G-linked proteins are coupled to cyclic guanosine triphosphatase (GTPase). Activation of these receptors leads to phosphorylation of the cyclic GTPase and a cascade of activities eventually altering the ionic flow. A sympathomimetic agent may affect ligand-gated ion channels, G protein receptors, or both. All adrenergic receptors are of the G protein type. Noradrenergic receptors generally have been classified as α_1, α_2, β_1, β_2, and β_3,[15] and their receptor distribution is variable throughout the various organ systems. The ocular radial muscle is α_1, but the ciliary body is predominantly β_2. The heart contains β_1 and β_2 receptors. Arteries vary in their concentration of α_1, α_2, and β_2, whereas the CNS has α_1. The venous system has α_1, α_2, and β_2 receptors.[15] Bronchodilation occurs from stimulation of β_2 receptors in the bronchiole smooth muscle.[16]

Sympathomimetic agents mimic adrenergic nervous system effects. Sympathomimetic agents classified as direct agents bind directly to α and β receptors. For the most part, these agents do not cross the blood-brain barrier. Indirect sympathomimetic agents cause the release of cytoplasmic norepinephrine or dopamine without vesicular exocytosis. They do this by changing the free cytoplasmic norepinephrine or dopamine concentration, causing a mass action effect. The neuronal membrane bidirectional transporter facilitates the uptake of many polar sympathomimetics, such as amphetamine and ephedrine, which normally would have problems crossing the bilipid membrane (Fig. 32-4).[17] When the sympathomimetic has entered the cell, the agent is transported into a storage vesicle. Normal vesicular pH is 5.5, but indirectly acting sympathomimetics buffer the storage vesicle pH, reducing the pH gradient across the membrane, which causes the release of stored norepinephrine and dopamine into the cytoplasm. Because of the chemistry of norepinephrine

TABLE 32-4 Noradrenergic Receptors

RECEPTOR TYPE	EFFECTOR	RESPONSE TO STIMULATION
α_1	Arterioles (resistance vessels)	Constriction
	Veins	Constriction
	Uterus	Contraction
α_2	Presynaptic nerve ending	Inhibit NE release
		Vasodilation
	Postsynaptic CNS	Decreased sympathetic tone
	Pancreatic islets	Vasodilation
		Decreased secretion
β_1	Heart	Increased inotropy
		Increased chronotropy
β_2	Bronchioles	Dilation
	Arterioles	Dilation
	Metabolic sites	Enhanced metabolism (glycogenolysis and gluconeogenesis)
	Uterine smooth muscle	Relaxation
	Pancreatic islets	Increased secretion
Dopamine	Mesenteric arterioles	Dilation (low dose)
		Constriction (high dose)

CNS, central nervous system; NE, norepinephrine.
Data from references 9 and 54.

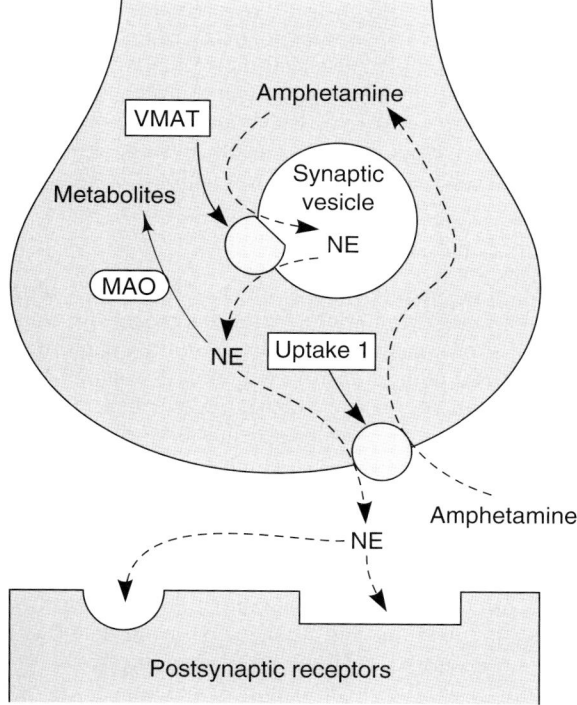

FIGURE 32-4

The mode of action of amphetamine, an indirectly acting sympathomimetic amine. Amphetamine enters the nerve terminal via the norepinephrine (NE) carrier (uptake 1) and enters synaptic vesicles via the vesicular monoamine transporter, in exchange for NE, which accumulates in the cytosol. Some of the NE is degraded by monoamine oxidase (MAO) within the nerve terminal, and some escapes, in exchange for amphetamine via uptake 1, to act on postsynaptic receptors. Amphetamine also reduces NE reuptake via uptake 1, enhancing the action of the released NE. VMAT, vesicular monamine transporter. *(From Rang HP, Dale MM, Ritter JM, Gardner P: Pharmacology, 4th ed. New York, Churchill-Livingstone, 2001, p 158.)*

formation, there is always some dopamine in the storage vesicle. Release of norepinephrine is accompanied by a small amount of dopamine. As the cytoplasmic concentration of catechol increases, norepinephrine and dopamine compete with sympathomimetic agents for the transport vesicle. The increased cytoplasmic catechol concentration facilitates exchange diffusion, via the transporter, to the extracellular synapse. Nonpolar agents do not require the transporter to enter the cell but diffuse across the lipid bilayer.[3] The release of norepinephrine has an inhibitory effect on its own release through the presynaptic α_2 receptor; this occurs by inhibiting adenylate cyclase (Fig. 32-5).[18] Inhibition of the transporter protein by tricyclic antidepressants abolishes amphetamine-induced norepinephrine release.[4]

PRESENTATION

Central Nervous System

The effects of sympathomimetics on the CNS are extensive, ranging from hyperpyrexia to mental status changes to seizures. Because the locus caeruleus innervates most of the CNS, including the cerebral cortex, cerebellum, and spinal cord, stimulation of this nucleus causes release of norepinephrine, leading to widespread cortical activation and excitation.[19] Indirect-acting sympathomimetics augment this excitation, increasing overall norepinephrine concentration; this explains the hyperattentiveness and lack of fatigue that accompany the use of amphetamines, Ecstasy (MDMA), and similar sympathomimetics.[20] At the extreme end of this spectrum is the psychosis and marked agitation that can be seen with overdoses of these agents.

In addition to behavioral effects, abuse of sympathomimetic agents can lead to hemorrhagic strokes. Subarachnoid

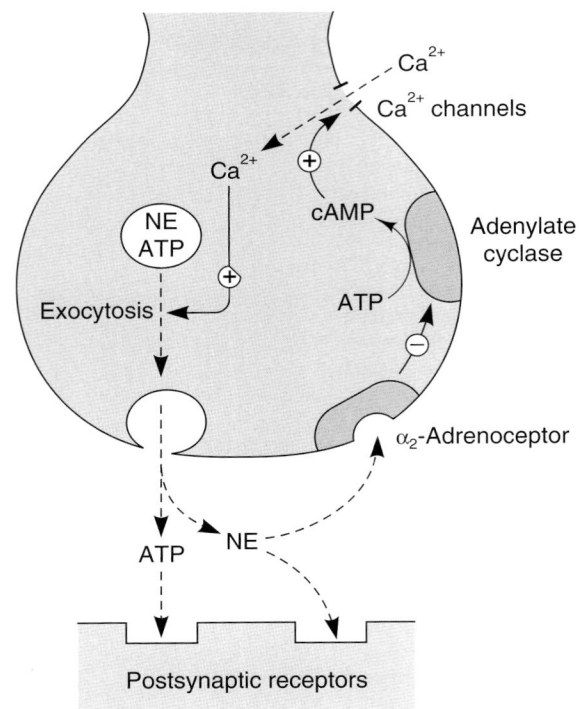

FIGURE 32-5

Feedback control of norepinephrine (NE) release. The presynaptic α_2-adreno-ceptor inhibits adenylate cyclase, reducing intracellular cyclic adenosine monophosphate (cAMP). cAMP acts to promote Ca^{2+} influx in response to membrane depolarization and to promote the release of norepinephrine and adenosine triphosphate (ATP). *(From Rang HP, Dale MM, Ritter JM, Gardner P: Pharmacology, 4th ed. New York, Churchill-Livingstone, 2001, p 144.)*

hemorrhage has been reported as a complication of cocaine use. This event is seen most frequently in individuals who have a preexisting cerebral aneurysm or arteriovenous malformation.[21] The transient but intense elevation in blood pressure that can be seen with cocaine use is enough to cause such defects to rupture.[21] Phenylpropanolamine (PPA) is an α-adrenergic sympathomimetic that formerly was available over the counter in the United States as a component of cold remedies and appetite suppressants.[22] In November 2000, the U.S. Food and Drug Administration issued a public health advisory concerning the risk of hemorrhagic stroke in users of PPA and urged drug manufacturers to remove products containing PPA from the market. This advisory was prompted by the findings of the Hemorrhagic Stroke Project, which reported that use of PPA is an independent risk factor for hemorrhagic stroke in women[22] using these products as diet aids. Ephedra alkaloids, frequently sold over the counter as dietary supplements for weight loss or improved energy, have been linked only anecdotally to adverse cerebrovascular events[23]; the link has not been shown in a controlled trial.

In addition to hemorrhagic strokes, thrombotic strokes have been reported in association with cocaine use. An increased risk of these ischemic strokes has not been shown, however, in a controlled trial. If stroke does occur, it has been hypothesized that α stimulation may cause vasoconstriction of large cerebral arteries, leading to thrombosis as a result of stasis and sympathomimetic-induced platelet activation.[24] This

hypothesis is questionable, however, because these vessels lack endothelial α receptors. Cocaine-induced vasospasm of coronary arteries also can lead to ischemia. Vasospasm may be secondary to the hypertension seen with cocaine use; however, the blockade of serotonin reuptake also may be a factor. Serotonin is a potent vasoconstrictor and may contribute to reduced blood flow to the brain.[25]

Seizures are an additional possible complication of sympathomimetic overdose. Massive cocaine overdose, such as that seen in body packers, can lead to generalized tonic-clonic activity and status epilepticus. Seizures are considered a major indicator of cocaine-related lethality in humans.[26] The long-term neurologic sequelae of cocaine-induced seizures also have been documented.[27] Seizures also may be seen in individuals who use relatively small amounts of cocaine.[28] Part of the difficulty in dealing with cocaine-related seizures is the refractory nature of the seizures to many standard anticonvulsants.[29] This refractoriness is related in part to the lack of knowledge of the precise mechanism by which cocaine causes seizures. Although seizures can result from a single high dose of cocaine, there is evidence that repetitive administration of subconvulsive doses of cocaine can lead to a decreased seizure threshold, a phenomenon known as *pharmacologic kindling*.[28,30] This feature, combined with the epileptogenic nature of cocaine, contributes to the significant neurologic impairment that can be associated with cocaine use.

On a neurophysiologic level, cocaine causes a threefold increase in D_3 binding sites in the locus accumbens and parts of the caudate and putamen, with up-regulation of κ_2 receptors in the amygdala. This activity can contribute to the hallucinations and aggressive and violent behavior seen in patients with cocaine overdoses.[7,14] The pathophysiology of cocaine intoxication is described in detail in Chapter 75.

Cardiovascular System

Cardiovascular manifestations are seen frequently with the sympathomimetic toxidrome. Because many of these agents have α-, β-, or mixed-receptor agonism, the effects also are varied. Agents with almost pure α effects, such as phenylpropanolamine, may cause isolated hypertension with reflex bradycardia. The hypertension is caused by the α effect on the vasculature, resulting in significant vasoconstriction. Other agents, depending on the amount of β_1 or β_2 predominance, can cause hypotension from β_2-induced vasodilation and β_1-enhanced tachycardia. Generally, with the exception of patients intoxicated with the mostly α agents, patients present with tachycardia, arrhythmias, and hypertension followed by, in the premorbid state, hypotension. The β stimulation and resulting calcium entry into the myocytes is arrhythmogenic. Tachydysrhythmias, including ventricular tachycardia and fibrillation, may occur.[31] There is a significant amount of literature linking sympathomimetics to myocardial necrosis with subsequent arrhythmogenesis and loss of inotropy.[32,33]

Renal System

The most significant renal-related side effect is acute renal failure associated with rhabdomyolysis, which has been reported mostly for cocaine and the amphetamines. Renal failure can occur via several mechanisms. Prolonged seizures can lead to rhabdomyoglobinuric renal failure. Overdose-related coma with associated muscle compression also can cause rhabdomyolysis.[34,35] Prolonged vasoconstriction of intramuscular arteries also may contribute; it also is hypothesized that cocaine may have some direct toxic effects on skeletal muscle.[34,36,37] Hyperthermia resulting from prolonged dancing at Ecstasy-driven rave parties is another well-documented cause of rhabdomyolysis.[38]

Renal failure also has been reported without associated rhabdomyolysis.[37] This renal failure is believed to be secondary to the vasoconstriction frequently seen with cocaine abuse. Renal artery vasoconstriction can lead to ischemia, and even infarction, of the kidney.[35] Additionally, chronic use of sympathomimetic drugs can lead to accelerated hypertension with associated renal failure.[38]

DIAGNOSTIC STUDIES

The laboratory diagnosis is nonspecific. Patients may show secondary evidence of adrenergic excess with hypokalemia, hypomagnesemia, hyperglycemia, and leukocytosis without left shift. If the patient has a significant sympathomimetic syndrome, is hyperpyrexic, or shows evidence of prolonged muscle activity, there is a lactic acidosis.[39] Ketonuria may be present if the patient has been using a sympathomimetic for a prolonged period without eating or if there is evidence of metabolic hyperactivity and lipolysis. The electrocardiogram most often shows sinus tachycardia, but paroxysmal supraventricular tachycardia or other tachydysrhythmias may be present. Routine radiographic studies are not helpful unless there is suspicion of body packing or body stuffing.

Differential Diagnosis

It may be difficult to distinguish between a true sympathomimetic syndrome and many other overdoses and conditions (Tables 32-5 and 32-6). In particular, ethanol and sedative-hypnotic withdrawal may present with all of the same signs and symptoms, including mental status changes and seizures. In many respects, this could be considered an endogenous sympathomimetic syndrome because withdrawal causes a large release of catecholamines and creates the same physiologic state.[39]

Anticholinergics tend to present with their own stereotypical syndrome that can be differentiated with careful observation and examination of the patient (see Table 32-6). In our experience, the anticholinergic toxidrome leads to mydriasis with cycloplegia, dry mucous membranes, tachycardia (but not usually as fast as seen with sympathomimetics), hypertension, hyperpyrexia, and tachypnea, usually in contrast to the extremes seen with sympathomimetics. Key differentiation points are loss of compensatory sweating, absence of bowel sounds, urinary retention, and red flushed skin in anticholinergic poisoning. The mental status change also is different. Patients with an anticholinergic toxidrome are nonfocally agitated, with picking motions of their hands. Their mouths appear cottony, and they answer with slurred, nearly incomprehensible speech. Many patients, when lying quietly, appear to be listening to internal voices. Treatment with haloperidol seems to make patients worse, and benzo-

TABLE 32-5 Differential Diagnosis of Sympathomimetic Syndrome

Toxic
Anticholinergics (antihistamines, scopolamine, atropine, hyoscyamine, hydroxyzine)
Serotonin syndrome
Neuroleptic malignant syndrome
MAO inhibitor intoxication
Strychnine poisoning
Drug interactions (MAO inhibitor plus meperidine, lithium, or haloperidol)
Salicylates
Pentachlorophenol
Cyclic antidepressants

Metabolic
Ethanol withdrawal
Sedative-hypnotic withdrawal

Thyrotoxicosis/thyroid storm
Status epilepticus
Heatstroke
Hypertensive encephalopathy
Hypoglycemia
Malignant hyperthermia

Infectious
Sepsis
Meningitis

Structural
Brain tumor
Pheochromocytoma

MAO, monoamine oxidase.

diazepines may not be effective until large doses are reached.[40] Physostigmine reorients the anticholinergic patient, restores vital signs toward normal, and confirms the diagnosis. The patient with a sympathomimetic syndrome also may be nonfocally agitated and restless but constantly in motion, requiring significant restraint. Benzodiazepines in appropriate dosing can be useful.[41,42]

The neuroleptic malignant syndrome (NMS) and serotonin syndrome are becoming more frequently recognized occurrences and result in a patient presenting in what appears to be similar to a sympathomimetic toxidrome. In NMS, there is evidence of dopamine depletion or a central D_2 receptor block with decrease in dopaminergic activity in the CNS striatum and hypothalamus. This situation leads to a disrupted core temperature regulation, enhanced centrally mediated muscle activity with rigidity, increased sympathetic tone and autonomic instability, and a change in mental status. To be diagnosed with NMS, patients currently must be taking or recently have been taking a neuroleptic or another antidopaminergic medication and satisfy several additional criteria, including increased core temperature, lead-pipe rigidity, autonomic instability, elevated creatine kinase, and change in mental status.[44] NMS is discussed in Chapter 26. By contrast, in the serotonin syndrome, there is an excess of 5-HT$_{1A}$ receptor stimulation, and this may involve 5-HT$_2$ receptor agonists, catecholamines, dopamine, and tryptamine. These patients have less remarkable extremity rigidity, but they should have the triad of altered mental status, autonomic dysfunction, and neuromuscular abnormalities. The neuromuscular findings are myoclonus, shivering, tremor, and hyperreflexia. In addition, patients may have fever, incoordination, diaphoresis, and diarrhea. The patient may be on a single serotonin agent, on a series of agents, or overdosed on a serotonin agent.[45,46] The serotonin syndrome is described in detail in Chapter 24.

Most serious MAO inhibitor overdoses involve agents that irreversibly inhibit MAO, the enzyme responsible for deaminating biogenic amines, leading to an increased availability

TABLE 32-6 Differential Diagnostic Features of Stimulant Syndromes

	BP	HR	TEMPERATURE	MS	SKIN	PUPILS	SPECIAL FEATURES
Sympathomimetic syndrome	↑	↑	↑	Altered	Diaphoretic	↑	Normal bowel sounds, reactive mydriasis
Alcohol/sedative-hypnotic withdrawal	↑	↑	Normal to ↑	Altered	Piloerection	↑	History of alcohol or sedative-hypnotic abuse, reactive mydriasis
Anticholinergic syndrome	↑↓	↑	↑	Altered	Dry	↑	Hypoactive bowel sounds, urinary retention, unreactive mydriasis
Complex status epilepticus	↓↑	Unreactive	Normal to ↑	Altered	Normal	Normal	Involuntary repetitive movements, unreactive pupils
Heatstroke	↓	↑	↑	Altered	Dry/hot	Normal	Core temperature >105°F, history of exposure
Hypertensive encephalopathy	↑	↑ or ↓	Normal	Altered	Normal	Normal	Visual changes, papilledema, headache
Hypoglycemia	Normal	↑	Normal or ↓	Altered	Diaphoretic	Normal to ↑	Resolves with glucose
Meningitis	Normal or ↓	↑	↑	Altered	Normal to hot	Normal	Meningismus, headache
Neuroleptic malignant syndrome	Labile	Labile	↑	Altered	Normal to diaphoretic	Normal to ↑	Skeletal muscular rigidity, history of neuroleptic use
Serotonin syndrome	Labile	↑	Normal to ↑	Altered	Diaphoretic	↑	History of serotonin agent, myoclonus, shivering, hyperreflexia
MAO inhibitor	Labile	↑↓	↑	Altered	Diaphoretic	↑	History of MAO inhibitor agent, wide swings in vital signs with use of pressors, tremor, myoclonus
Cyclic antidepressants	↓	↑	Normal to ↑	Altered	Dry/flushed	↑	Widened QRS, R wave in aVR and S wave in I, II
Pheochromocytoma	↑	↑	Normal	Normal to altered	Flushed	Normal	Paroxysms of hypertension and tachycardia
Sepsis	↓	↑	↑↓	Altered	Cool/clammy or hot/dry	Normal	Source of infection may be evident, low peripheral vascular resistance
Thyrotoxicosis	↑↓	↑	↑	Altered	Normal	Normal	Thyromegaly or tender thyroid, tachycardia disproportionate to fever

BP, blood pressure; HR, heart rate; MAO, monoamine oxidase; MS, mental status.

of these amines in the cytosol. The patient may present with an initial asymptomatic phase, possibly with headache, then develop neuromuscular excitation and evidence of enhanced sympathetic stimulation. The patient then becomes diaphoretic, agitated, hyperthermic, hyperreflexic, rigid, and tremulous and may develop myoclonus and seizures. CNS depression, cardiac dysrhythmias, and cardiovascular collapse may follow. These patients are sensitive to indirect-acting agents and may show wide autonomic instability if pressors are used. The MAO inhibitor overdose may mimic serotonin syndrome but with lead-pipe rigidity; the patient also develops evidence of profound autonomic collapse.[47,48] Overdoses of MAO inhibitors are discussed in Chapter 43.

Patients with heatstroke may present with a high core temperature, tachycardia, altered mental status, and tachypnea. Patients may have some muscular rigidity. Heatstroke is caused by loss of normal thermoregulation under some amount of heat stress. Patients may appear to be extremely toxic with sympathomimetic syndrome, and differentiation may not be possible initially. The heatstroke patient initially may be diaphoretic and hypertensive but eventually becomes hypovolemic and hypotensive, with dry skin. Multiple organ system failure then ensues. Treatment is the same as with the sympathomimetic syndrome, with supportive care and rapid cooling. Diagnosis may not be determined until after resolution of the acute event.[49]

Malignant hyperthermia occurs in patients with abnormalities in their muscular excitation-contraction mechanisms. These patients present with tachycardia and central hyperpyrexia. Differentiation from sympathomimetic syndrome is helped by a family history of similar events or temporally related exposure to general anesthesia or similar agents. The patients always have muscular rigidity and usually are sweating.[49] Malignant hyperthermia is discussed in Chapter 25.

Diagnostic Studies

Certain studies may help in the differential diagnosis. Although leukocytosis is present in most sympathomimetic states, septic patients should show a left shift with other

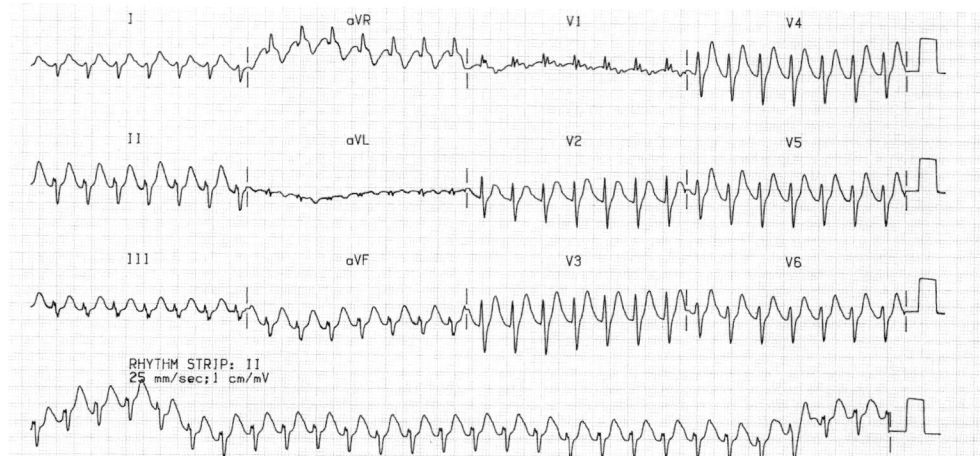

FIGURE 32-6

A classic electrocardiogram from a tricyclic antidepressant–poisoned patient, showing sinus tachycardia, QTc and QRS prolongation, elevated R wave in aVR, S waves in I, II. This ECG would be highly suggesive of any fast inward sodium channel blocker toxicity.

evidence of infection, such as toxic granules, Döhle's bodies, or leukopenia. In thyrotoxicosis, thyroid-stimulating hormone is markedly depressed. In hypoglycemic patients, serum glucose is less than 70 mg/dL (3.89 mmol/L). Urinary collection of vanillylmandelic acid helps differentiate pheochromocytoma.

The electrocardiogram may be useful in differentiating neuroleptic agents and cyclic antidepressants from other causes. Most neuroleptics cause a nonspecific widening of the QT_c. Classic cyclic antidepressants frequently show a rightward deviation of the terminal 40 msec of the frontal plane QRS (an R wave in aVR and an S wave in I, II) and QT_c and QRS prolongation (Fig. 32-6).

A computed tomography scan of the head is useful to rule out CNS bleeding or mass. In the case of pheochromocytoma, scanning of the abdomen and adrenals may elicit useful information.

Toxicologic screening may identify some of these agents. Specific testing for lithium and salicylates is available. The most common immunoassays for drugs of abuse for the most part are positive for amphetamine, methamphetamine, and cocaine. Because there is structural similarity to ephedrine and pseudoephedrine, the test also may show a false-positive result for amphetamine for these agents. These assays are not useful for anticholinergic agents and serotoninergic amphetamines such as MDMA. Some tests assay for tricyclic antidepressants, and these may be positive for the classic cyclics, which have a central seven-membered ring. β Agents, MAO inhibitors, and neuroleptics do not show on these immunoassays. Comprehensive thin-layer chromatography coupled with immuoassay, high-performance liquid chromatography, and gas chromatography–mass spectroscopy may identify many compounds. A negative toxicologic screen does not mean that the drug is not present and may represent only the fact that the test does not look for it or that it is present in insufficient quantity.

TREATMENT

Because sympathomimetic toxicity reflects a general increase in catechol effect, treatment is directed toward attenuating this pathway. The simplest and most efficient way is to depress the CNS release of catecholamines with benzodiazepine or barbiturate sedation[50,51]; this decreases norepinephrine release. We recommend that tachycardia and hypertension be treated cautiously with β blockade only in the presence of an α-receptor antagonist, such as phentolamine. β Blockade alone theoretically may lead to unopposed α effect and worsening hypertension. Hypertension unresponsive to α blockade and sedation may require nitroprusside infusion. Arrhythmias usually respond to sedation, but the patient may need a calcium channel blocker or other antiarrhythmic agent. Chest pain can be treated with the usual nitrates.[52] Because sympathomimetics can induce the serotoninergic response in platelets, aspirin therapy in the presence of cardiac-type chest pain also is suggested.[53] Hyperpyrexia must be treated aggressively with rapid cooling and prevention of muscle hyperactivity. Sedation may be helpful, but if the patient has rigidity, marked myoclonus, or prolonged seizure activity, paralysis with a nondepolarizing agent may be necessary to halt the continued lactic acidosis and heat production. Seizures generally are brief and should respond to benzodiazepines. If continued seizures develop, an anticonvulsant such as a barbiturate is suggested.

SPECIAL POPULATIONS

Patients who take β-blockers may not present with the tachycardia associated with the sympathomimetic syndrome. If there is a significant α component to the sympathomimetic agent, the patient may present with exaggerated hypertension from the unopposed α effect.

REFERENCES

1. Manjo G: The Healing Hand: Man and Wound in the Ancient World. Cambridge, MA, Harvard University Press, 1991, pp 349–352.
2. Hoffman B: Catecholamines, sympathomimetic drugs, and adrenergic receptor antagonists. In Hardman JG, Limbird LE, Goodman Gilman A (eds): Goodman and Gilman's The Pharmacologic Basis of Therapeutics, 10th ed. New York, McGraw-Hill, 2001, p 216.
3. Hoffman B, Taylor P: Neurotransmission. In Hardman JG, Limbird LE, Goodman Gilman A (eds): Goodman and Gilman's The Pharmacologic Basis of Therapeutics, 10th ed. New York, McGraw-Hill, 2001, pp 132–133.

4. Bylund DB: Physiology and biochemistry of the peripheral autonomic nervous system. In Brody TM, Larner J, Minneman KP (eds): Human Pharmacology: Molecular to Clinical, 3rd ed. St Louis, Mosby, 1998, p 92.
5. Moore KE: Drugs affecting the sympathetic nervous system. In Brody TM, Larner J, Minneman KP (eds): Human Pharmacology: Molecular to Clinical, 3rd ed. St Louis, Mosby, 1998, p 120.
6. Staley JE, Hearn WL, Ruttenberg J, et al: High affinity cocaine recognition sites on the dopamine transporter are elevated in fatal cocaine overdose victims. J Pharm Exp Ther 271:1678–1685, 1994.
7. Rang HP, Dale MM, Ritter JM, Gardner P: Pharmacology, 4th ed. New York, Churchill-Livingstone, 2001, pp 145–146.
8. Brown OM: Adrenergic drugs. In Smith CM, Reynard AM (eds): Textbook of Human Pharmacology. Philadelphia, WB Saunders, 1992, p 146.
9. Fink GD: Regulation of blood pressure by the autonomic nervous system. In Brody TM, Larner J, Minneman KP (eds): Human Pharmacology: Molecular to Clinical, 3rd ed. St Louis, Mosby, 1998, pp 176–177.
10. Hoffman B, Taylor P: Neurotransmission. In Hardman JG, Limbird LE, Goodman Gilman A, et al (eds): Goodman and Gilman's The Pharmacologic Basis of Therapeutics, 10th ed. New York, McGraw-Hill, 2001, pp 122–125.
11. Bloom F: Neurotransmission and the central nervous system. In Hardman JG, Limbird LE, Goodman Gilman A, et al (eds): Goodman and Gilman's The Pharmacologic Basis of Therapeutics, 10th ed. New York, McGraw-Hill, 2001, p 310.
12. Ordway GA, et al: Pharmacology and distribution of norepinephrine transporters in the human locus ceruleus. J Neurosci 17:1710–1716, 1997.
13. Mash DC, Staley JK: D3 dopamine and kappa opioid receptor alterations in human brain of cocaine-overdose victims. Ann N Y Acad Sci 877:507–522, 1999.
14. Gutstein HB, Akil H: Opioid analgesics. In Hardman JG, Limbird LE, Goodman Gilman A, et al (eds): Goodman and Gilman's The Pharmacologic Basis of Therapeutics, 10th ed. New York, McGraw-Hill, 2001, p 582.
15. Hoffman B, Taylor P: Neurotransmission. In Hardman JG, Limbird LE, Goodman Gilman A, et al (eds): Goodman and Gilman's The Pharmacologic Basis of Therapeutics, 10th ed. New York, McGraw-Hill, 2001, pp 119–120.
16. Rang HP, Dale MM, Ritter JM, Gardner P: Pharmacology, 4th ed. New York, Churchill-Livingstone, 2001, p 158.
17. Rang HP, Dale MM, Ritter JM, Gardner P: Pharmacology, 4th ed. New York, Churchill-Livingstone, 2001, p 144.
18. Nolte J: The Human Brain: An Introduction to Its Functional Anatomy. St. Louis, Mosby-Year Book, 1993, pp 165–166.
19. Katzung B: Basic and Clinical Pharmacology. Norwalk, CT, Appleton & Lange, 1995, p 124.
20. Fessler RD, Esshaki CM, Stankewitz RC, et al: The neurovascular complications of cocaine. Surg Neurol 47:339–345, 1997.
21. Jacobs IG, Roszler MH, Kelly JK, et al: Cocaine abuse: Neurovascular complications. Radiology 170:223–227, 1989.
22. Kernan WN, Viscoli CM, Brass LM, et al: Phenylpropanolamine and the risk of hemorrhagic stroke. N Engl J Med 343:1826–2000, 2000.
23. Haller CA, Benowitz NL: Adverse cardiovascular and central nervous system events associated with dietary supplements containing ephedra alkaloids. N Engl J Med 343:1833–1838, 2000.
24. Spivey WH, Euclic B: Neurologic complications of cocaine abuse. Ann Emerg Med 19:1422–1428, 1990.
25. Catravas JD, et al: Acute cocaine intoxication in the conscious dog: Pathophysiologic profile of acute lethality. Arch Int Pharmacodyn Ther 235:328–340, 1978.
26. Kunisaki TA, Augenstein WL: Drug and toxin-induced seizures. Emerg Med Clin North Am 12:1027–1056, 1994.
27. Kramer LD, Locke GE, Ogunyemi A, Nelson L: Cocaine-related seizures in adults. Am J Drug Alcohol Abuse 16:307–317, 1990.
28. Gasior M, Ungard JT, Witkin JM: Preclinical evaluation of newly approved and potential antiepileptic drugs against cocaine-induced seizures. J Pharmacol Exp Ther 290:1148–1156, 1999.
29. Miller KA, et al: Pharmacological and behavioral characterization of cocaine-kindled seizures in mice. Psychopharmacology 148:74–82, 2000.
30. Pentel PR: Toxicity of over-the-counter stimulants. JAMA 252:1898–1903, 1984.
31. Isner JM, Estes NA 3rd, Thompson PD, et al: Acute cardiac events temporally related to cocaine abuse. N Engl J Med 315:1438–1443, 1986.
32. Pentel P, Jentzen J, Sievert J: Myocardial necrosis due to interperitoneal administration of phenylpropanolamine. Fundam Appl Toxicol 9:167–172, 1987.
33. Rosenblum I, Wohl A, Stein A: Studies in cardiac necrosis: I. Production of cardiac lesions with sympathomimetic amines. Toxicol Appl Pharmacol 7:1–8, 1965.
34. Crowe AV, et al: Substance abuse and the kidney. QJM 93:147–152, 2000.
35. Roth D, et al: Acute rhabdomyolysis associated with cocaine intoxication. N Engl J Med 319:673–677, 1988.
36. Murthy BVS, Wilkes RG, Roberts NB: Creatine kinase isoform changes following Ecstasy overdose. Anaesth Intensive Care 25:156–159, 1997.
37. LeBlanc M, Hebert MJ, Mongeau JG: Cocaine-induced acute renal failure without rhabdomyolysis. Ann Intern Med 121:721–722, 1994.
38. Woodrow G, Harnden P, Turney JH: Acute renal failure due to accelerated hypertension following ingestion of 3,4-methylenedioxymethamphetamine (Ecstasy). Nephrol Dial Transplant 10:399–400, 1995.
39. Hoffman RJ, Hoffman RS, Freyberg CL: Clenbuterol ingestion causing prolonged tachycardia, hypokalemia, and hypomagnesemia with confirmation by quantitative levels. J Toxicol Clin Toxicol 39:339–344, 2001.
40. Burns MJ, Linden CH, Graudins A, et al: A comparison of physostigmine and benzodiazepines for the treatment of anticholinergic poisoning. Ann Emerg Med 35:374–381, 2000.
41. Guaza C, Borrell S: Effect of naloxone administration upon responses of adrenal hormones to withdrawal from ethanol. Psychopharmacologia 82:181–189, 1984.
42. Paine TA, Jackman SL, Olmstead MC: Cocaine-induced anxiety: Alleviation by diazepam, but not buspirone, dimenhydrinate, or diphenhydramine. Behav Pharmacol 13:511–523, 2002.
43. Aaron CK: Sympathomimetics. Emerg Med Clin North Am 8:513–526, 1990.
44. Nierenberg D, Disch M, Manheimer E, et al: Facilitating prompt diagnosis and treatment of the neuroleptic malignant syndrome. Clin Pharmacol Ther 50:580–586, 1991.
45. Martin TG: Serotonin syndrome. Ann Emerg Med 28:520–526, 1996.
46. Sternbach H: The serotonin syndrome. Am J Psychiatry 148:705–713, 1991.
47. Linden CH, Rumack BH, Strehlke C: Monoamine oxidase inhibitor overdose. Ann Emerg Med 13:1137–1144, 1984.
48. Robertson JC: Recovery after massive MAOI overdose complicated by malignant hyperpyrexia. Postgrad Med J 48:64–65, 1972.
49. Vassallo SU, Delaney KA: Pharmacologic effects on thermoregulation: Mechanisms of drug-related heatstroke. J Toxicol Clin Toxicol 27:199–224, 1989.
50. Richards JR, Derlet RW, Duncan DR: Chemical restraint for the agitated patient in the emergency department. J Emerg Med 16:567–573, 1998.
51. Derlet RW, Albertson TE: Anticonvulsant modification of cocaine-induced toxicity in the rat. Neuropharmacology 29:255–259, 1991.
52. Hollander JE, et al: Nitroglycerin in the treatment of cocaine associated chest pain: Clinical safety and efficacy. J Toxicol Clin Toxicol 32:243–256, 1994.
53. Wang RY: pH-dependent cocaine-induced cardiotoxicity. Am J Emerg Med 17:364–369, 1999.
54. Hoffman B, Taylor P: Neurotransmission. In Hardman JG, Limbird LE, Goodman Gilman A, et al (eds): Goodman and Gilman's The Pharmacologic Basis of Therapeutics, 10th ed. New York, McGraw-Hill, 2001, pp 119–120.

PART 3

Medications
CARDIOVASCULAR

CHAPTER **33**

Digitalis Glycosides

Frédéric Lapostolle ▪ Frédéric J. Baud ▪ Stephen W. Borron ▪ Bruno Mégarbane

The medical use of cardiac glycosides began in 1785 with the publication of Withering's monograph on the therapeutic efficacy and toxicity of the leaves of the common foxglove plant, *Digitalis purpurea*. Thereafter, various related glycosides, including digitoxin and ouabain, were extracted from plants. Cardiac glycosides have been widely prescribed for more than 2 centuries. A better understanding of the pathophysiology of cardiac diseases, particularly dysrhythmias, and the pharmacotoxicology of cardiac glycosides progressively has restricted their use, however, to the treatment of heart failure due to systolic dysfunction with or without supraventricular dysrhythmias or atrial fibrillation.

Digitalis may cause life-threatening toxicity. Digitalis poisoning most often results from chronic toxicity in patients with cardiac disease because many factors can alter patient sensitivity to digitalis glycosides. It also may be the result of acute overdose in patients with or without cardiac disease. In 1976, Smith and colleagues[1] reported the first case of acute human life-threatening digoxin poisoning treated with digoxin-specific Fab fragments, unveiling the modern era of treatment of cardiac glycoside toxicity.

BIOCHEMISTRY OF DIGITALIS GLYCOSIDES

Cardiac glycosides of therapeutic interest share a molecular motif common to these agents—a steroid nucleus and one or more glycosidic residues bound at C3 of this nucleus (Fig. 33-1). Removal of the glycoside moieties, resulting in the corresponding genin (or aglycone), only minimally affects their pharmacodynamic action. The potent and highly selective property of cardiac glycosides to bind and inhibit the membrane Na^+, K^+-ATPase is related to the presence of a β hydroxyl group at C14 and

an unsaturated lactone at the C17 position of the steroid nucleus. The genin part of digitoxin differs from that of digoxin only by the absence of a hydroxyl group at C12. In addition to foxglove (*Digitalis*), the most important sources of cardiac glycosides are dogbane (*Strophantus*) and red squill (*Urginea maritima*). Scilliroside and proscillaridin are glycosides derived from red squill. Related compounds also can be found in other plants, such as lily of the valley (*Convallaria majalis*), oleander (*Nerium oleander*), yellow oleander (*Theretia peruviana*), and henbane (*Helleborus niger*). Poisoning by cardiac glycoside–containing plants is discussed in Chapter 125. A ouabain-like compound (resibufogenin) found in the skin of the bufo toad (*Bufo* spp.) shares the characteristics of a cardiac glycoside.

Pharmacokinetics of Digoxin and Digitoxin

Digoxin

Volume of distribution: 5.6 L/kg
Protein binding: 25%
Mechanism of clearance: digoxigenin, digoxigenin mono-digitoxiside and bis-digitoxiside
*Active metabolites:** renal
Methods to enhance clearance: activated charcoal

Digitoxin

Volume of distribution: 0.56 L/kg
Protein binding: 95%
Mechanism of clearance: hepatic
*Active metabolites:** digoxin
Methods to enhance clearance: activated charcoal

*More than 10% of the relative activity compared with digoxin.

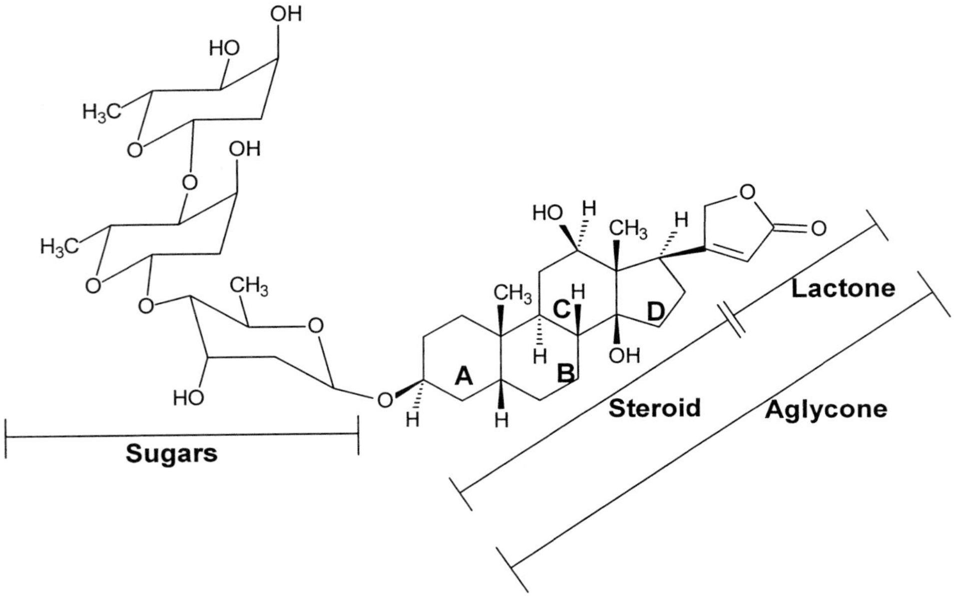

FIGURE 33-1

Chemical structure of digoxin. Digitoxin lacks a hydroxyl group on the C ring, resulting in greater lipophilicity.

PHARMACOLOGY OF THERAPEUTIC AND TOXIC EFFECTS

Cardiac glycosides have numerous sites of action, including the cardiac myocytes, vascular smooth muscle, and central nervous system.[2,3] The net effect on the cardiovascular system depends on the patient's cardiac status and the dose of cardiac glycoside. Therapeutic and toxic effects result from the same mechanism of action. Cardiac glycosides reversibly bind with high affinity to specific subunits of the Na^+, K^+-ATPase in cardiac, smooth, and skeletal muscles; lung; and kidney, resulting in its inhibition (see Fig. 125-5). This inhibition results in an increase in intracellular Na^+ and a decrease in intracellular K^+ concentrations with a corresponding increase in extracellular K^+ concentration. Through the resultant effects on Na^+ and Ca^{2+} membrane transporters, an increased intracellular Ca^{2+} concentration follows. Therapeutic actions of digitalis are based partially on this increase in intracellular Ca^{2+}, which is taken up by the sarcoplasmic reticulum, resulting in increased contractile force (Fig. 33-2).[3] Excessive increase in intracellular Ca^{2+} caused by excessive intracellular cardiac glycoside concentration results in transient late depolarization (delayed afterdepolarization) that may be accompanied by an aftercontraction often seen with digitalis toxicity.

Within the central nervous system, cardiac glycosides interact with the sympathetic and the parasympathetic systems. At therapeutic doses, digoxin increases vagal tone and decreases sympathetic activity, whereas at toxic doses, digoxin increases sympathetic activity. The vagal response is a toxic and a therapeutic effect, which involves increased coronary and carotid sinus cell Na^+ influx and the resultant Bezold-Jarisch reflex–mediated increase in vagal tone. Direct and indirect effects contribute to the complex electrophysiologic effects on the myocardial cells. At toxic doses, the simultaneous nonuniform increase in automaticity and a vagally mediated depression of conduction in His-Purkinje and ventricular myocytes may cause life-threatening dysrhythmias.

CLINICAL PRESENTATION AND LIFE-THREATENING COMPLICATIONS

Poisonings mainly result from pharmaceutical preparations of digitalis and more rarely from self-made preparations of cardiac glycoside–containing plants.

Chronic Toxicity

Because digitalis glycosides have a narrow therapeutic index, toxicity has been reported in 6% to 23% of treated patients, particularly in the elderly.[4-6] Many factors can alter a patient's sensitivity to cardiac glycosides (Table 33-1). Acute renal impairment may precipitate digoxin intoxication.[5,7,8] The gradual decrease in the glomerular filtration rate with age predisposes to digoxin accumulation. Most patients on long-term digitalis therapy are taking multiple medications, which may be responsible for drug-drug interactions through either pharmacodynamic or pharmacokinetic mechanisms. Although the possible interactions of digitalis glycosides with other drugs are too numerous to review in this chapter, a few cogent examples merit specific mention.[3,6] The concurrent administration of digoxin and quinidine may result in decreased clearance of the former, with resulting major increases in serum digoxin concentrations. Similarly, concomitant amiodarone and digoxin therapy may result in elevations of the serum concentration of the latter to toxic levels. Serum digoxin concentrations also may be increased by the simultaneous administration of calcium channel inhibitors (e.g., verapamil).

The noncardiac manifestations of digitalis toxicity are nonspecific but highly prevalent in patients with suspected digoxin toxicity.[9] Noncardiac signs and symptoms include gastrointestinal, neurologic, and visual manifestations. Gastrointestinal signs and symptoms include anorexia, nausea, vomiting, malaise, abdominal pain, and diarrhea. At times, symptoms may be severe enough that the patient is unable to eat or drink, contributing to dehydration and renal insufficiency. Other complications, such as mesenteric ischemia,

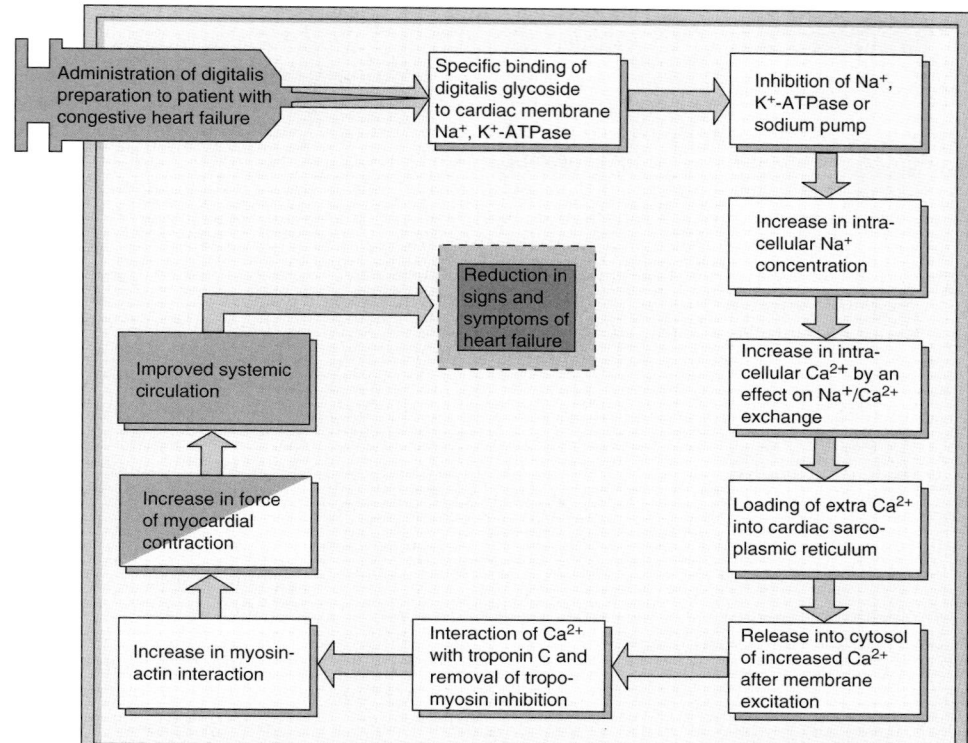

FIGURE 33-2

Molecular interaction of digitalis with cell constituents and the subsequent cascade of events resulting in pharmacologic response in the treatment of left ventricular dysfunction. *(From Brody TM: Introduction and definitions. In Brody TM, Larner J, Minneman KP [eds]: Human Pharmacology: Molecular to Clinical, 3rd ed. St. Louis, Mosby, 1998, p 5.)*

have been reported rarely. Neurologic manifestations include fatigue, lethargy, and weakness, and visual manifestations include scotoma, blurred vision, color aberration, and blindness. Mental status changes include confusion, hallucinations, delirium, and other psychiatric disorders. Any onset of gastrointestinal, neurologic, or visual manifestations in a patient treated with digitalis should raise the suspicion of toxicity and call for the measurement of serum digoxin concentration.

Digitalis cardiac toxicity results from the combination of conduction and rhythm disturbances.[7] A variety of electrocardiogram (ECG) abnormalities are characteristic of digitalis toxicity. The ECG may reveal premature contractions of junctional or ventricular origin, which are more frequent rhythm disturbances than atrial extrasystoles, and varying types and degrees of conduction disturbance,

including bradycardia, sinoatrial block, and all degrees of atrioventricular (AV) block. Rhythm disturbances, such as atrial fibrillation and conduction disturbances, may be seen in combination, resulting in an irregular bradycardia. Toxicity should be suspected when there is evidence of increased automaticity and depressed AV or myocardial conduction. The typical arrhythmias associated with digoxin toxicity include atrial tachycardia with variable AV conduction; accelerated junctional rhythms, especially associated with the sudden regularization of the ventricular response to atrial fibrillation; and fascicular tachycardia.[10] Life-threatening arrhythmias primarily consist of third-degree AV block, ventricular tachycardia, and ventricular fibrillation. The contribution of underlying cardiac disease, including cardiomyopathy and coronary artery disease, to digitalis toxicity is less clear.[5] In cases of long-term treatment, digitalis effect on the ST segment cannot be considered as a criterion of intoxication.

Acute Overdose

Acute digitalis poisoning may result from accidental or suicidal exposure to a single high dose of the glycoside in patients with or without antecedent digitalis therapy. Symptoms generally occur within 6 hours of ingestion, but life-threatening symptoms may occur later, reflecting the relatively slow tissue distribution of digoxin and digoxin-like cardiac glycosides. The onset of gastrointestinal disturbances (nausea and vomiting), slow heart rate, and dysrhythmias suggests the clinical diagnosis of acute digitalis poisoning. At presentation, bradycardia and conduction disturbances are the most frequent ECG abnormalities. Bradycardia is associated with

---

TABLE 33-1 Main Predisposing and Precipitating Factors for Digitalis Toxicity

Advanced age
Underlying cardiac disease
Respiratory disease
  Hypoxia, respiratory alkalosis or acidosis
Renal insufficiency
Hypothyroidism
Electrolytes disturbances
  Hypokalemia, hyperkalemia, hypercalcemia, hypomagnesemia
Drug-drug interactions
  Diuretics, quinidine, amiodarone, verapamil, β-adrenergic blockers,
    β-adrenergic agonists, amphotericin B, corticosteroids

ventricular dysrhythmias. Poor prognostic factors in acute digitalis glycoside poisonings include age older than 55 years, male sex, hyperkalemia, and any degree of AV block.[11] Mortality rate is increased significantly when serum potassium concentration is greater than 4.5 mmol/L (Table 33-2). A mortality rate of 35% was observed in digitoxin-poisoned patients who had a serum potassium greater than 5 mmol/L, reaching 100% when potassium was greater than 6.4 mmol/L.[12] Ventricular dysrhythmias were the leading cause of death (70%), followed by advanced AV block (20%) and pump failure secondary to negative inotropic effect (10%). Death also may result from mesenteric infarction.

DIAGNOSIS

The clinical and laboratory basis for diagnosis depends on whether the digitalis poisoning is chronic or acute.

Chronic Toxicity

The definitive diagnosis of chronic toxicity is difficult because noncardiac symptoms are nonspecific, whereas some of the ECG abnormalities also may result from the underlying cardiac disease itself.[7] The presence of rhythms such as junctional tachycardia that occur almost always secondary to digitalis intoxication simplifies the diagnosis, however. Serum digitalis glycoside concentration should be determined in every case of suspected digitalis

intoxication. Properly obtained and interpreted serum digoxin concentrations significantly aid in diagnosis and the management of digitalis poisoning. The range of therapeutic (steady-state) concentrations of digoxin and digitoxin are 0.5 to 2.0 ng/mL (0.6 to 2.6 nmol/L) and 10 to 30 ng/mL (13 to 39 nmol/L).[13] According to the numerous factors that may increase digoxin toxicity, however, no single serum digoxin concentration can establish the presence or absence of toxicity.[4] In a retrospective study dealing with 6133 levels measured in 5100 patients, Ordog and coworkers[4] showed that of 460 patients with serum digoxin concentration greater than 2 ng/mL (>2.6 nmol/L), only 13 were diagnosed by the examining physician as having digoxin toxicity before obtaining the digoxin level. Hospitalized patients with serum digoxin concentrations greater than 2.1 ng/mL (>2.7 nmol/L) spent a mean of 12.1 ± 17.1 days in hospital. The mean time to death for patients in this group who died was 5 ± 3.1 days.[4] Two thirds of the patients who died in the hospital had increasing digoxin levels before death. In this study, renal failure was not associated with a statistically significant increase in mortality compared with patients with similar digoxin levels and normal blood urea nitrogen.[4] The mortality rate in patients with elevated digoxin levels and pre-existing ECG abnormalities was 8% compared with 40% for patients with elevated digoxin levels and new ECG abnormalities.[4] There was a significant relationship between the serum digoxin concentration and the mortality rate in this series. A mortality rate of 50% was reported in patients with serum digoxin concentrations greater than 6 ng/mL (7.7 mmol/L).[4]

TABLE 33-2 Prognostic Factors of Acute Digitoxin Poisoning*

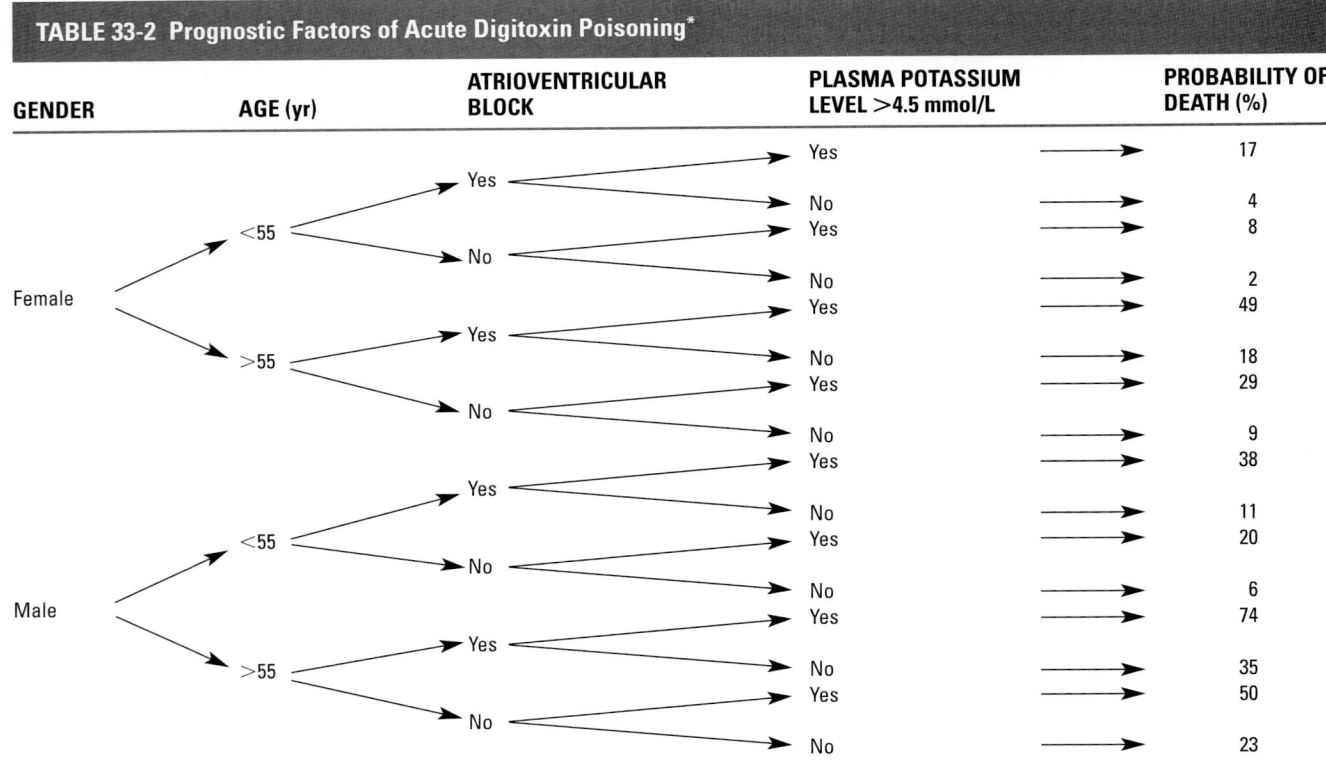

GENDER	AGE (yr)	ATRIOVENTRICULAR BLOCK	PLASMA POTASSIUM LEVEL >4.5 mmol/L	PROBABILITY OF DEATH (%)
Female	<55	Yes	Yes	17
			No	4
		No	Yes	8
			No	2
	>55	Yes	Yes	49
			No	18
		No	Yes	29
			No	9
Male	<55	Yes	Yes	38
			No	11
		No	Yes	20
			No	6
	>55	Yes	Yes	74
			No	35
		No	Yes	50
			No	23

*These data are based on 179 patients who had acutely ingested >2 mg of digitoxin. Adapted from Dally S, Alperovitch A, Lagier G, et al: [Prognostic factors in acute digitalis poisoning]. Nouv Presse Med 10:2257–2260, 1981.

Serum potassium concentration significantly influences the toxicity associated with a given digitalis concentration.[14] In contrast to acute poisoning, most of the more serious arrhythmias found in patients with chronic toxicity are associated with a serum potassium level less than 3.7 mmol/L.[15] An indication for transient pacemaker placement was present much more frequently when digitalis intoxication was accompanied by hypokalemia (72%) compared with normokalemia (37%).[15] In a group of patients with dysrhythmias typical of digitalis intoxication, normokalemic patients had a mean serum digoxin level of 6.68 ± 0.17 ng/mL (8.55 ± 0.22 mmol/L), whereas hypokalemic patients had a mean serum digoxin level of 1.13 ± 0.04 ng/mL (1.45 ± 0.05 mmol/L). Repletion of serum potassium sometimes corrected the dysrhythmia without a significant change in serum digoxin level. Hypomagnesemia likewise increases the toxicity of digitalis and may be a more frequent contributor to digoxin toxicity than hypokalemia.[15] Finally, prompt termination of the arrhythmias in temporal relationship to cessation of drug administration or after the administration of digoxin-specific Fab fragments supports the diagnosis of chronic toxicity.[7]

Acute Toxicity

The diagnosis of acute digitalis poisoning is typically straightforward. QT interval modifications are of diagnostic value only in patients not previously treated with digitalis. The diagnosis is confirmed by the measurement of the serum digitalis concentration. The plasma potassium concentration indicates the degree of inhibition of the Na^+, K^+-ATPase pump in patients without established causes of potassium depletion.[16]

Endogenous Digoxin-like Substance

Significant differences in measured digoxin concentrations in the serum of patients with impaired renal function (defined as a serum creatinine concentration ≥2.0 mg/dL [≥177 μmol/L]) have been reported when assayed by different commercially available ^{125}I-digoxin immunoassays, with differences as great as 2.9 ng/mL (3.7 nmol/L). The magnitude of the discrepancies was not related to the degree of renal impairment. More than 60% of patients with renal impairment not on digoxin therapy had false-positive digoxin values on immunoassay with apparent digoxin concentration of 1.0 ng/mL (1.3 nmol/L). Potentially cross-reactive substances, such as endogenous steroids, digitalis metabolites, and nonspecific binding, did not explain the false-positive digoxin values. Therapeutic monitoring of individuals with renal insufficiency may be confounded by endogenous digoxin-like immunoreactive substances. Endogenous digoxin-like immunoreactive substances also have been reported in the serum of premature or full-term neonates; children; pregnant women; and patients with hypertension, congestive heart failure, subarachnoid hemorrhage, acromegaly, insulin-dependent diabetes, and liver disease. Several methods, including immunoassays and the use of ultrafiltration, have been reported to minimize or eliminate confounding from these endogenous digoxin-like immunoreactive substances.[17–20] The chemical structure and physiologic role of the endogenous digoxin-like immunoreactive substances remain to be elucidated.[21–24]

Several other exogenous compounds may be detected by or may interfere with digoxin immunoassays, including a metabolite of spironolactone, a toad venom–containing Chinese medicine known as Kyushin, and some herbal teas. Hyperbilirubinemia similarly interferes with digoxin immunoassays.

TREATMENT

Most cases of chronic toxicity are minor, and the patient can be treated by temporary withdrawal or reduction in the dose of digoxin on an outpatient or inpatient basis. In the United States, several thousand patients each year require more aggressive hospital treatment, however.[25]

Gastrointestinal Decontamination

A single dose of activated charcoal may be administered if a patient has ingested a potentially toxic dose of cardiac glycoside within the previous 2 hours. Although activated charcoal may reduce peak serum digoxin concentrations, it is unknown whether this affects the patient's clinical course or outcome. Repeated doses of activated charcoal increase the elimination of digoxin and digitoxin. There are insufficient clinical data, however, to support or exclude the use of this therapy.[26] The usefulness of gastrointestinal decontamination in chronically poisoned patients also remains to be determined.

Extracorporeal Removal Techniques

There is no supporting outcome evidence or basis for assuming that extracorporeal removal techniques, such as hemodialysis, continuous arteriovenous hemofiltration, and activated charcoal hemoperfusion, have any role in the management of digoxin poisoning, given the large volume of distribution of digoxin, high degree of protein binding by digitoxin, and, once distributed, the high affinity for Na^+, K^+-ATPase pumps. Digoxin-specific Fab fragments (see later) are effective even in anephric patients.

Indications for ICU Admission in Digitalis Glycoside Poisoning

Clinically stable patients receiving digoxin who meet the following criteria:
  Mildly elevated serum digoxin concentrations
  Without signs and symptoms of digoxin toxicity
  With serum potassium >3.7 mmol/L and <4.5 mmol/L
  No history of severe cardiac disease
  Seem at low risk of developing serious digoxin toxicity and may not require treatment beyond the discontinuation of digoxin therapy
All symptomatic patients suspected of chronic or acute digitalis poisoning. Given the high mortality associated with digitalis poisoning, it is prudent to admit all patients with electrocardiogram or electrolyte abnormalities or other significant underlying pathology to an intensive care unit.

Electrolyte Disorders

Correction of hypokalemia, hypomagnesemia, and dehydration are important in the presence of chronic toxicity. Table 33-3 lists the indications for administration of potassium.[7] In chronically treated patients, hyperkalemia may result not only from the direct toxic effect of cardiac glycosides[4] but also from coadministered medications, including potassium-sparing diuretics, nonsteroidal antiinflammatory drugs, angiotensin-converting enzyme inhibitors, and nonselective β-blockers. Given that these drugs may have a role in electrolyte disorders, impaired digitalis clearance, or cardiovascular compromise, they should be withdrawn temporarily.

In acute poisoning, hyperkalemia (>4.5 mmol/L) is the hallmark of severe toxicity, and treatment with Fab fragments should be considered. Otherwise, conventional treatment of severe hyperkalemia (>5.6 mmol/L) consists of administering glucose, insulin, and bicarbonate and sodium polystyrene sulfonate enema.[27] If Fab fragments are administered simultaneously, however, severe hypokalemia may result. Although calcium salts are one treatment for hyperkalemia, they should be avoided in patients with digitalis poisoning because the pathophysiology of this condition is primarily calcium loading of the myocardium.

Nonantidotal Treatment

Atropine is the initial treatment of choice for digitalis-induced sinus bradycardia or AV conduction disturbance. Atropine should be administered in adults with severe AV block in doses of 0.5 mg, repeated to a total dose of 2 mg. Therapeutic success of atropine is unpredictable because at high doses the more direct nonvagotonic cardiac effects of digitalis may predominate. In the presence of refractory bradycardia, the use of a large cumulative dose of atropine may lead to anticholinergic encephalopathy.

Many antidysrhythmics, including phenytoin, lidocaine, procainamide, propranolol, and amiodarone, have been used to treat digitalis-induced arrhythmias. Propranolol and procainamide must be avoided because of their adverse effects on cardiac conduction and contractility. Quinidine should not be used because it may prolong digoxin toxicity as a result of drug-impaired clearance.[13] Lidocaine and phenytoin

---

TABLE 33-3 Acute Potassium Administration in Suspected Chronic Digitalis Poisoning

Indications

Serum potassium <4.0 mmol/L and ventricular premature complexes or ventricular tachycardia or supraventricular tachycardia with AV block

Serum potassium <3.0 mmol/L and (in addition to those listed above) first-degree AV block and second-degree AV block with Wenckebach's periodicity (Mobitz type I)

Contraindications

Mobitz type II or third-degree AV block if temporary electrical pacing unavailable

---

AV, atrioventricular.
From Kelly RA, Smith TW: Recognition and management of digitalis toxicity. Am J Cardiol 69:108G–119G, 1992.

---

should be considered antiarrhythmic drugs of choice to treat digitalis-induced dysrhythmias because they have little effect on the sinus node and on AV conduction.[7] The role of fosphenytoin has not been evaluated in this setting.

Intravenous magnesium sulfate has been reported to be effective in the treatment of digoxin-induced arrhythmias, even in patients with normal or slightly elevated serum magnesium concentrations.[28–31] Magnesium potentiates the activity of Na^+, K^+-ATPase without affecting the binding of digoxin. A decrease in serum potassium concentration after magnesium therapy has been reported in digitalis intoxication. Treatment with magnesium potentially could lead to adverse effects from hypermagnesemia, particularly in patients with impaired renal function. Hypermagnesemia is unlikely to occur with an initial bolus of 10 to 20 mmol of magnesium, but it may be a problem with continuous infusion or with repeat doses.[28,29] Fab therapy is the most effective and safe antidysrhythmic strategy, however, in digitalis-induced life-threatening arrhythmias.

Transvenous or transcutaneous cardiac pacing may be used to correct digitalis-induced bradycardia or conduction disturbances and to prevent ventricular dysrhythmias.[32] Cardiac pacing is not universally available, however, and may be associated with life-threatening ventricular dysrhythmias. Retrospective studies have suggested that pacing does not significantly decrease the mortality rate of acute digitalis intoxication.[32,33] Given the high rate of nonfatal and fatal complications associated with cardiac pacing in acute digitalis toxicity, Fab fragment therapy should be considered first-line treatment.[33] Electrical cardioversion is potentially hazardous in severe arrhythmias with advanced digitalis toxicity and should be avoided if other treatment, such as Fab fragments, is available.[7]

Digoxin-Specific Fab Fragments

The efficacy and safety of digoxin-specific Fab fragments have been reported consistently in adults[5,8,27,34,35] and children[36] and in acute and chronic poisonings. An analysis by Maushopf and Wenger[25] supported the cost-effectiveness of Fab fragments in the treatment of digoxin toxicity.

Digoxin-specific Fab fragments may be used for the treatment of digoxin and digitoxin toxicity. According to their cross-reactivity, Fab fragments also can effectively neutralize methyl-digoxin, β-acetyl-digoxin, lanatoside, ouabaine, proscillaridin, and scilliroside and cardiac glycosides contained in yellow oleander and in toad venom.[37–39]

Fab fragments are indicated for digitalis-induced life-threatening dysrhythmias or severe hyperkalemia (>5.5 mmol/L)[27] refractory to conventional treatment. Life-threatening dysrhythmias include progressive bradyarrhythmias resulting from severe sinus bradycardia, second-degree or third-degree heart block unresponsive to atropine, and ventricular tachycardia or fibrillation.[5,8,27,40] Fab fragments also may be considered in the treatment of noncardiovascular complications of digitalis intoxication, including recent onset of altered mental status and mesenteric infarction.[41,42]

The theoretical maximum dose is that required to neutralize the body burden of digitalis. This dose can be calculated using either the supposed ingested dose or the serum digitalis concentration (Table 33-4). When no data are available

TABLE 33-4 Calculation of Digoxin Body Load

Based on suspected ingested amount

Digoxin body load (mg) = 0.8* × suspected ingested amount (mg)

Digitoxin body load (mg) = 1* × suspected ingested amount (mg)

Based on serum concentration

Digoxin body load (mg) = [serum concentration (ng/mL)] × Vd × weight (kg)]/ 1000

Vd: 5.6 L/kg

Digitoxin body load (mg) = [serum concentration (ng/mL)] × Vd × weight (kg)]/ 1000

Vd: 0.56 L/kg

One vial of 40 mg of Fab fragments (Digibind) neutralizes 0.6 mg of digitalis (either digoxin or digitoxin)

One vial of 80 mg of Fab fragments (Digidote) neutralizes 1 mg of digitalis (digoxin or digitoxin)

---

*This represents the bioavailability of either digoxin or digitoxin in tablet form. This term increases to 0.95 for elixir and gel tablet forms.

Vd, volume of distribution.

---

regarding the supposed body load of digitalis, empirical dosing recommendations are to administer 400 to 800 mg of Fab (closely equivalent to 10 to 20 vials of Digibind, containing 38 mg digoxin immune Fab per vial) in acute toxicity and 120 to 240 mg of Fab (3 to 6 vials of Digibind) in chronic toxicity.

There are no clear differences regarding the indication and the dosage of Fab fragments in chronic and acute poisonings. Data suggest, however, that in acute digitalis poisonings resulting from the ingestion of a massive dose, the indication and the dose of Fab fragments could be refined. In this instance, the definitive diagnosis is established with relative ease and expediency. Because equimolar neutralization with Fab fragments is expensive and sometimes not available in small hospitals, Fab administration often is delayed or withheld until serious arrhythmias occur. Under these conditions, ventricular fibrillation and asystole often result in postanoxic brain damage or refractory cardiogenic shock.[5,8,27,33,34,40] With the exception of one series by Antman and colleagues[8] of 56 patients with digoxin-induced cardiac arrest among whom 54% survived hospitalization and an additional series reported by Smolarz and coworkers[34] in which 94% of 34 patients with severe digitalis poisoning survived, the mortality rates of patients with cardiac arrest or ventricular arrhythmias remain dramatically high in large series of digitalis poisonings treated with Fab fragments.[5,8,27,35] Considering the safety of Fab fragments, prophylactic administration of Fab fragments to prevent the occurrence of life-threatening arrhythmias was first proposed by Smolarz and coworkers in 1985.[34] This approach was refined further by Taboulet and colleagues,[33,35] who took into account (1) the prognostic factors of acute digitoxin poisoning,[11,16] (2) the lack of evidence for the efficacy of pacing, and (3) the frequency and severity of adverse effects of cardiac pacing. Taboulet and colleagues[33,35] suggested that Fab fragments should be employed as first-line therapy in acute digitalis poisoning. Two treatment strategies for two distinct situations of acute digitalis poisonings were proposed, as follows:[35]

In patients exhibiting life-threatening disturbances, an equimolar neutralizing dose of Fab (curative dose) must be administered rapidly.

In patients with mild bradycardia (<60 beats/min), regardless of the conduction disturbances, especially in patients with associated poor prognostic factors,[11] when atropine fails to accelerate the cardiac rhythm to greater than 60 beats/min, a half equimolar neutralizing dose should be administered ("prophylactic" dose). Particular attention should be paid to patients older than age 55 years, patients with cardiac disease, and patients with serum potassium concentration equal to or greater than 5.5 mmol/L. If the heart rate remains less than 60 beats/min, based on the experience of Taboulet and colleagues,[35] it is recommended that the remaining half-dose be administered. In their experience, a full dose of Fab was not always necessary. So-called prophylactic treatment requires close and prolonged monitoring of patients, however, necessitating a 72-hour minimal stay in the intensive care unit.

Several lines of evidence support the use of less than an equimolar initial dose of Fab. A series of 717 patients treated with Fab fragments showed that there was no clear relationship between initial response to treatment and percent of the estimated adequate dose of Fab.[5] Schaumann and associates[43] reported on 17 acute digoxin poisonings successfully treated with Fab fragments. Six of these patients, with serum digoxin concentrations before Fab fragments therapy ranging from 4.9 to 20 ng/mL (6.4 to 26 nmol/L), were treated with a standard dosage regimen including a loading dose of 160 mg of Fab followed by an infused dose of 160 mg without any adjustment of the serum digoxin concentration.[43] The calculation of the equimolar dose of Fab fragments based on either the estimated ingested dose or the serum digitalis concentration frequently overestimates the amount of digitalis in the body. The calculation based on the estimate of ingested dose uses only the theoretical bioavailability of cardiac glycosides, whereas during the time interval between ingestion of digitalis and Fab administration, a fraction of the dose of digitalis already has been eliminated.[34] The relationship between the serum digitalis concentration and the corresponding actual amount in the body should be considered accurate only during the drug elimination phase, not during the distribution phase, which may last 6 hours for digoxin.[13] After acute poisoning, patients frequently are admitted early during the course of the poisoning, and the accuracy of the relationship can be questioned. In the series of 717 patients, the lone factor associated with recrudescent toxicity was shown to be inadequacy of the Fab initial fragment dose. These data and the data from Schaumann and colleagues[43] strongly suggest that the minimal efficient dose of this therapy and the dosage regimen for optimal binding of Fab fragments to digitalis remain to be determined.

The sole contraindication to the use of Fab fragments is a reported history of anaphylaxis after prior treatment with this product. During and after Fab administration, vital signs, ECG, and serum potassium levels should be recorded frequently to assess the efficacy and safety of treatment. Improvement in cardiac and noncardiac signs and symptoms of digitalis toxicity occurs rapidly after specific Fab administration. Antman and colleagues[8] reported a median time to initial response of 19 minutes from termination of infusion, whereas the median time to complete response was 88 minutes. Treatment response was observed by 1 hour in 75% of patients, and reversal of glycoside effects was usually evident within 4 hours of administration.[8] Neither age nor concurrent cardiac disease was associated with any significant delay in initial response.[8] Among 56 patients whose digitalis toxicity culminated in cardiac arrest, 30 (54%) survived hospitalization after treatment with Fab fragments.[8,27,40]

Hypokalemia may occur after Fab administration as elevated serum potassium concentrations decline rapidly. In all patients who had elevated serum potassium concentrations, Fab therapy reversed the hyperkalemia.[8,40] Decline in serum potassium concentration often was noted within 1 hour and seemed complete within 4 hours.[8,27,40]

After the administration of Fab fragments, serum digoxin concentrations determined by conventional methods no longer are useful because they represent free plus bound digitalis, and many laboratories are not equipped to determine free serum digoxin concentrations. Detectable free digoxin concentrations may reappear 5 to 24 hours or longer after Fab administration.[44]

Partial response or even no response at all to the initial dose of Fab fragments has been reported in clinical trials. Partial or no response may result from (1) a moribund state at the time of infusion, (2) an inadequate dose of Fab, (3) concomitant toxicity from other drugs or treatments, (4) and underestimated severity of underlying cardiac disease.[5,8,27,40] No clear relationship was observed, however, between initial response to treatment and percent of the estimated adequate dose administered.[5] None of the patients without heart disease who ingested a single acute dose of digitalis were nonresponders to Fab.[5]

The administration of additional doses of Fab fragments should be considered in patients in whom life-threatening toxicity reappears or persists despite initial treatment. Recrudescent toxicity was reported in 20 of the 717 patients (2.8%) and was observed within 3 days of the initial Fab treatment in most of the patients, although as late as 4 to 11 days in a few patients.[5] Inadequacy of the initial dose was the only factor associated with recrudescent digitalis toxicity. This risk in patients receiving less than 50% of the estimated adequate dose was 5.8 times greater than the risk of patients receiving 100% of the adequate dose.[5] In cases of massive digitoxin poisoning, recurrent toxicity has been reported 1 to 4 days after Fab administration and when the initial dose was less than the estimated adequate dose.[35] Measurement of the free digoxin concentration may be of value to determine the need for additional doses of Fab. Reports have shown that when free serum digoxin concentration rebounds beyond 0.8 ng/mL (1.02 nmol/L), signs and symptoms of digoxin intoxication recurred in some patients.[44]

Adverse events in response to Fab fragments have been reported in 7%[5] and 9%[8] of treated patients. These untoward events include allergic responses and withdrawal of the therapeutic effect of digitalis. Allergic responses have been reported rarely. Some authors did not report adverse effects.[8,27,33,34] Wenger and coworkers[40] reported slight erythema at the site of skin testing. Of the 717 patients, 6 (0.8%) developed allergic reaction during treatment with Fab, including pruritic rash, facial swelling and flushing, urticaria, thrombocytopenia, episodes of shaking and chills

without fever, wheezing, and dyspnea.[5] Withdrawal of the therapeutic effects of digitalis may be associated with an onset of congestive heart failure or an increase in ventricular rate in previously ill patients. In the former group of patients, caution is advised in the use of catecholamines owing to the increased risk of digitalis-associated dysrhythmias. Worsening of cardiac dysfunction after Fab fragment infusion is reported rarely in clinical studies (<3%).[8] Reversal of the therapeutic effect of digoxin typically occurs within 24 to 48 hours of Fab administration.[44] Transient apnea has been reported in a several-hour-old neonate.[8] Data regarding the safety of Fab fragments in patients treated for more than one episode of digitalis toxicity are too limited to allow any conclusion.[5]

Therapeutic redigitalization of the patient, if necessary, should be delayed until elimination of Fab fragments from the body is complete. Digoxin therapy can be administered safely 48 to 72 hours after Fab administration in patients with normal renal function.[44]

SPECIAL POPULATIONS

Pediatric Patients

Digitalis poisoning has been reported in pediatric patients ranging from 1 day old to 17 years old.[36] Errors in the calculation or administration of the digitalizing and maintenance doses in smaller children are common and result in episodes of iatrogenic intoxication. Accidental poisonings also occur in young children who have access to adult medication. Less commonly, adolescents may ingest digitalis in a suicidal attempt. Children treated with digoxin also may be taking other medications that can result in drug-drug interactions. Acute digitalis intoxication in infants or young children is accompanied most often by few clinical effects and requires only close monitoring and nonspecific therapy. There are numerous reports of digoxin-poisoned children, however, who developed neurologic manifestations, life-threatening arrhythmias, conduction defects, and secondary hypotension requiring medical intervention and cardiopulmonary resuscitation. Hyperkalemia is uncommon in children. Fab therapy has been reported consistently to be effective and safe in pediatric patients. In children with digoxin poisoning, digoxin-specific Fab fragments are recommended based on the following criteria:[36]

Known digoxin intoxication
Strong historical evidence of an acute ingestion of greater than 0.1 mg/kg digoxin
Or an elevated (steady-state) serum digoxin concentration greater than 5 ng/mL (6.4 nmol/L)

And *signs and symptoms of digitalis toxicity*
Rapidly progressing symptoms and signs of digoxin toxicity
Or potentially life-threatening arrhythmias, including cardiac conduction disturbances
Or severe hyperkalemia (≥6.0 mmol/L).

Woolf and colleagues[36] proposed that although it is not recommended that Fab fragments be used prophylactically, it is desirable to institute Fab therapy early in the course of a severe poisoning to forestall progression to more refractory, malignant cardiac arrhythmias.

The dosage of Fab fragments in children, similar to in adults, is related to the calculated total body burden of digitalis, either from the known amount of drug ingested or from calculation using the serum digitalis concentration. In children, the dose of Fab is always equimolar to that of the calculated total body burden of digitalis. Particular attention should be paid to the dilution of Fab to avoid fluid overload in small children. When no data are available regarding the supposed body load of digitalis, our empirical dosing recommendation is to administer 400 to 800 mg of Fab in acute poisoning. Empirical dosing recommendations for chronic toxicity in children are 40 to 80 mg. In the package insert, digoxin immune Fab (Digibind) provides a table to determine the dose of Fab fragments according to the serum digoxin concentration and patient body weight. In treated children, conduction defects and ventricular or supraventricular ectopy typically resolve within 24 hours, and often within 4 hours, of the administration of Fab fragments. Increased serum potassium concentration usually returns to the normal range within 4 hours of administration.[36] To our knowledge, no cases of hypersensitivity to Fab fragments have been reported in children. Adverse effects include hypokalemia in one case and recurrence of cardiac conduction defects after treatment, which resolved on administration of a repeated dose of specific Fab fragments in three children.[36]

Pregnant Patients

During pregnancy, digitalis overdose may result in maternal and fetal digitalis poisoning. To our knowledge, there are no data regarding the efficacy or safety of Fab fragments in pregnant women.

Elderly Patients

Digoxin toxicity in the elderly is common, ranging from easily overlooked symptoms, such as nausea and anorexia, to life-threatening dysrhythmias. The elderly are at greater risk of toxicity for several reasons.[6] First, they frequently are taking multiple medications (e.g., quinidine, amiodarone, verapamil), which may interfere with digoxin elimination or otherwise increase its toxicity. The elderly have diminished creatinine clearance, which may be masked by their decreased muscle mass, giving the false impression of normal renal function. Finally, Alzheimer's or other forms of dementia may lead to unintentional repeated doses of digoxin. Mild-to-moderate digoxin toxicity in the elderly may be difficult to discern from other "signs of old age"—somnolence, decreased hearing, confusion, agitation, poor appetite, nausea, vomiting, and diarrhea. In elderly patients treated with cardiac glycosides, chronic toxicity should be suspected in the face of new-onset dysrhythmias, malaise, gastrointestinal disturbances, or mental status changes. Lethargy, depression, and confusion seem to occur almost exclusively in the elderly.[45] These signs and symptoms may be ignored or misdiagnosed by the physician.[46] Advanced age seems to be an independent poor prognostic factor.

Renal Dysfunction Patients

Patients with renal dysfunction are at risk of digoxin poisoning. Fab therapy is effective in patients with renal dysfunction.[5,8] Fab fragments should be given to patients with renal impairment at the same dose as for patients with normal renal function.[47] Elimination of digoxin-specific Fab complexes is prolonged in digoxin-poisoned patients with renal dysfunction. Total body clearance of Fab fragments is related linearly to creatinine clearance, whereas their apparent volume of distribution is not affected.[47] Free digoxin concentrations decrease rapidly after Fab therapy but rebound at about 77 ± 46 hours postinjection.[48] The magnitude by which free digoxin concentration rebounds is unaffected by the degree of renal dysfunction.[48] There is no evidence to support a dissociation of the Fab/digoxin complexes over extended periods.[44] In a patient with end-stage renal disease, plasmapheresis was effective in removing Fab and the digoxin/Fab complexes. Because there are rarely complications resulting from circulating digoxin/Fab complexes for a prolonged period, however, there is little evidence to recommend this procedure in patients with end-stage renal disease receiving Fab therapy.[44] Monitoring free serum digoxin concentrations with special methods after the administration of Fab may be of value in selected patients to guide additional Fab dosing, confirm possible rebound toxicity, or guide the reinitiation of digoxin therapy.[48]

Key Points in Digitalis Glycoside Poisoning

1. Digitalis poisoning may result from chronic toxicity in patients with cardiac disease because many factors can alter patient sensitivity to digoxin or from the exposure, either accidentally or with suicidal intent, to a single high dose of cardiac glycoside in patients on or not previously on digitalis treatment.
2. Acute and chronic digitalis poisonings may be life-threatening with sudden onset of fatal dysrhythmias.
3. Any suspicion of digitalis toxicity should result in the emergency determination of the serum digitalis concentration.
4. In acute digitalis poisoning, several prognostic factors (age >55 years, serum potassium >4.5 mmol/L, and atrioventricular block of any degree) have been identified that place the patient at high risk of fatal outcome.
5. Chronic digitalis toxicity is overlooked easily owing to symptoms that mimic common diseases.
6. Chronic toxicity may result from digitalis accumulation owing to renal insufficiency or pharmacokinetic drug-drug interactions; extrinsic factors, including hypokalemia, hypomagnesemia, and pharmacodynamic drug-drug interactions; progressive cardiac disease; or a combination of these factors.
7. Poor prognostic factors of chronic digitalis toxicity include serum digoxin concentration on admission, further increase of serum digoxin level during hospitalization, and onset of new electrocardiogram abnormalities.
8. Digitalis-specific Fab fragments constitute the treatment of choice when hyperkalemia, cardiac conduction disturbances, poor prognostic factors, or life-threatening arrhythmias are present.

REFERENCES

1. Smith TW, Haber E, Yeatman L, Butler VP Jr: Reversal of advanced digoxin intoxication with Fab fragments of digoxin-specific antibodies. N Engl J Med 294:797–800, 1976.
2. Smith TW: Digitalis: Mechanisms of action and clinical use. N Engl J Med 318:358–365, 1988.
3. Kelly R, Smith T: Pharmacological treatment of heart failure. In Hardman J, Limbrid L, Molinoff P (eds): Goodman and Gilman's The Pharmacological Basis of Therapeutics. New York, McGraw-Hill, 1996, pp 809–838.
4. Ordog G, Benaron S, Bhasin V: Serum digoxin levels and mortality in 5100 patients. Ann Emerg Med 16:32–39, 1987.
5. Hickey AR, Wenger TL, Carpenter VP, et al: Digoxin Immune Fab therapy in the management of digitalis intoxication: Safety and efficacy results of an observational surveillance study. J Am Coll Cardiol 17:590–598, 1991.
6. Borron S, Bismuth C, Muszynski J: Advances in the management of digoxin toxicity in the older patient. Drugs Aging 10:18–33, 1997.
7. Kelly RA, Smith TW: Recognition and management of digitalis toxicity. Am J Cardiol 69:108G–119G, 1992.
8. Antman EM, Wenger TL, Butler VP Jr, et al: Treatment of 150 cases of life-threatening digitalis intoxication with digoxin-specific Fab antibody fragments: Final report of a multicenter study. Circulation 81:1744–1752, 1990.
9. Mahdyoon H, Battilana G, Rosman H, et al: The evolving pattern of digoxin intoxication: Observations at a large urban hospital from 1980 to 1988. Am Heart J 120:1189–1194, 1990.
10. Marchlinski F, Hook B, Callans D: Which cardiac disturbances should be treated with digoxin immune Fab (ovine) antibody. Am J Emerg Med 9:24–28, 1991.
11. Dally S, Alperovitch A, Lagier G, et al: [Prognostic factors in acute digitalis poisoning]. Nouv Presse Med 10:2257–2260, 1981.
12. Gaultier M, Welti J, Bismuth C, et al: Intoxication digitalique grave: Facteurs pronostiques. Intérêt et limites de l'entrainement électrosystolique (à propos de 133 cas). Ann Med Int 127:761–766, 1976.
13. Mooradian A: Digitalis: An update of clinical pharmacokinetics, therapeutic monitoring techniques and treatment recommendations. Clin Pharmacokinet 15:165–179, 1988.
14. Shapiro W: Correlative studies of serum digitalis levels and the arrhythmias of digitalis intoxication. Am J Cardiol 41:852–859, 1978.
15. Lehmann HU, Witt E, Temmen L, Hochrein H: [Life-threatening digitalis intoxication with and without additional diuretic treatment]. Dtsch Med Wochenschr 103:1566–1571, 1978.
16. Bismuth C, Gaultier M, Conso F, Efthymiou ML: Hyperkalemia in acute digitalis poisoning: Prognostic significance and therapeutic implications. Clin Toxicol 6:153–162, 1973.
17. Pudek MR, Seccombe DW, Jacobson BE, Humphries K: Effect of assay conditions on cross reactivity of digoxin-like immunoreactive substance(s) with radioimmunoassay kits. Clin Chem 31:1806–1810, 1985.
18. Graves SW, Sharma K, Chandler AB: Methods for eliminating interferences in digoxin immunoassays caused by digoxin-like factors. Clin Chem 32:1506–1509, 1986.
19. Kulaots IA, Pudek MR, Seccombe DW: Endogenous digoxin-like immunoreactive substances eliminated from serum samples from patients with liver disease by the EMIT column digoxin assay. Clin Chem 33:1490–1491, 1987.
20. Seccombe DW, Pudek MR, Humphries KH: Minimizing analytical interferences from digoxin-like immunoreactive substances (DLIS) in cases of digoxin toxicity. J Forensic Sci 32:650–657, 1987.
21. Naomi S, Graves S, Lazarus M, et al: Variation in apparent serum digitalis-like factor levels with different digoxin antibodies: The immunochemical fingerprint. Am J Hypertens 4(10 Pt 1):795–801, 1991.
22. Hollenberg NK, Graves SW: Endogenous sodium pump inhibition: Current status and therapeutic opportunities. Prog Drug Res 46:9–42, 1996.
23. Tao QF, Hollenberg NK, Price DA, Graves SW: Sodium pump isoform specificity for the digitalis-like factor isolated from human peritoneal dialysate. Hypertension 29:815–821, 1997.
24. Tao QF, Hollenberg NK, Graves SW: Sodium pump inhibition and regional expression of sodium pump alpha-isoforms in lens. Hypertension 34:1168–1174, 1999.
25. Mauskopf J, Wenger T: Cost-effectiveness analysis of the use of digoxin immune Fab (ovine) for the treatment of digoxin toxicity. Am J Cardiol 68:1709–1714, 1991.
26. Position statement and practice guidelines on the use of multi-dose activated charcoal in the treatment of acute poisoning. American Academy of Clinical Toxicology; European Association of Poisons Centres and Clinical Toxicologists. J Toxicol Clin Toxicol 37:731–751, 1999.
27. Smith TW, Butler VP Jr, Haber E, et al: Treatment of life-threatening digitalis intoxication with digoxin-specific Fab antibody fragments: Experience in 26 cases. N Engl J Med 307:1357–1362, 1982.
28. Cohen L, Kitzes R: Magnesium sulfate and digitalis-toxic arrhythmias. JAMA 249:2808–2810, 1983.
29. French JH, Thomas RG, Siskind AP, et al: Magnesium therapy in massive digoxin intoxication. Ann Emerg Med 13:562–566, 1984.
30. Reisdorff EJ, Clark MR, Walters BL: Acute digitalis poisoning: The role of intravenous magnesium sulfate. J Emerg Med 4:463–469, 1986.
31. Kinlay S, Buckley NA: Magnesium sulfate in the treatment of ventricular arrhythmias due to digoxin toxicity. J Toxicol Clin Toxicol 33:55–59, 1995.
32. Bismuth C, Motte G, Conso F, et al: Acute digitoxin intoxication treated by intracardiac pacemaker: Experience in sixty-eight patients. J Toxicol Clin Toxicol 10:443–456, 1977.
33. Taboulet P, Baud FJ, Bismuth C, Vicaut E: Acute digitalis intoxication—is pacing still appropriate? J Toxicol Clin Toxicol 31:261–273, 1993.
34. Smolarz A, Roesch E, Lenz E, et al: Digoxin specific antibody (Fab) fragments in 34 cases of severe digitalis intoxication. J Toxicol Clin Toxicol 23:327–340, 1985.
35. Taboulet P, Baud FJ, Bismuth C: Clinical features and management of digitalis poisoning—rationale for immunotherapy. J Toxicol Clin Toxicol 31:247–260, 1993.
36. Woolf AD, Wenger TL, Smith TW, Lovejoy FHJ: Results of multicenter studies of digoxin-specific antibody fragments in managing digitalis intoxication in the pediatric population. Am J Emerg Med 9(2 Suppl 1):16–20, 33–34, 1991.
37. Cambridge D, Morgan C, Allen G: Digoxin and digoxin derivative induced arrhythmias: In vitro binding and in vivo abolition of arrhythmias by digoxin immune fragments (Digibind). Cardiovasc Res 26:906–911, 1992.
38. Sabouraud A, Urtizberea M, Cano N, et al: Specific anti-digoxin Fab fragments: An available antidote for proscillaridin and scilliroside poisoning. Hum Exp Toxicol 9:191–193, 1990.
39. Eddleston M, Rajapakse S, Rajakanthan K, et al. Anti-digoxin Fab fragments in cardiotoxicity induced by ingestion of yellow oleander: A randomised controlled trial. Lancet 355:967–972, 2000.
40. Wenger TL, Butler VP Jr, Haber E, Smith TW: Treatment of 63 severely digitalis-toxic patients with digoxin-specific antibody fragments. J Am Coll Cardiol 5(5 Suppl A):118A–123A, 1985.
41. Bourhis F, Riard P, Danel V, et al: [Digitalis poisoning with severe ischemic colitis: A favorable course after treatment with specific antibodies]. Gastroenterol Clin Biol 14:95, 1990.
42. Varriale P, Mossavi A: Rapid reversal of digitalis delirium using digoxin immune Fab therapy. Clin Cardiol 18:351–352, 1995.
43. Schaumann W, Kaufmann B, Neubert P, Smolarz A: Kinetics of the Fab fragments of digoxin antibodies and of bound digoxin in patients with severe digoxin intoxication. Eur J Clin Pharmacol 30:527–533, 1986.
44. Ujhelyi MR, Robert S: Pharmacokinetic aspects of digoxin-specific Fab therapy in the management of digitalis toxicity. Clin Pharmacokinet 28:483–493, 1995.
45. Portnoi V: Digitalis delirium in the elderly. J Clin Pharmacol 19:747–750, 1979.
46. Brunner G, Zweiker R, Krejs GJ: A toxicological surprise. Lancet 356:1406, 2000.
47. Renard C, Grene-Lerouge N, Beau N, et al: Pharmacokinetics of digoxin-specific Fab: Effects of decreased renal function and age. Br J Clin Pharmacol 44:135–138, 1997.
48. Ujhelyi MR, Robert S, Cummings DM, et al: Influence of digoxin immune Fab therapy and renal dysfunction on the disposition of total and free digoxin. Ann Intern Med 119:273–277, 1993.

β-Receptor Antagonists

Jeffrey Brent

β-receptor antagonists (β-blockers) are used therapeutically for their ability to attenuate the expression of functions mediated by β-adrenergic receptors. β-Blockers have found a prodigious number of uses in common therapy and are prescribed widely. Among the most frequent indications for their use are the treatment of hypertension, cardiac tachydysrhythmias, congestive heart failure, migraine headaches, and certain movement disorders.

Major toxicity from the use of β-receptor antagonists can occur with therapeutic doses, with overdoses, or as a result of drug interactions. Toxicity at therapeutic doses typically occurs as a result of an adverse effect deriving from the normal physiologic properties of the drug or from excessive systemic absorption after ocular installation. An example of the former would be the development of bronchospasm as a result of blockade of pulmonary β-receptors in susceptible patients. Drug interactions can cause serious toxicity with β-blockers, particularly bradycardias or heart block resulting from the simultaneous use of a β-blocker with a cardioactive calcium channel blocker, such as verapamil. Some of the most serious manifestations of β-receptor antagonist toxicity follow the intentional or unintentional ingestion or administration of excessive doses.

BIOCHEMISTRY AND CLINICAL PHARMACOLOGY

β-Receptor antagonists comprise a group of structurally related agents that act as antagonists at β_1-receptor, β_2-receptor, or both receptor subtypes. In addition, these drugs are thought to exert varying, although as yet uncharacterized, degrees of antagonism at β_3-receptors and β_4-receptors. Virtually all of these agents used clinically are either selective β_1-receptor antagonists or nonselective antagonists at β_1-receptors and β_2-receptors (Table 34-1). Figure 34-1 shows that these agents typically are ethers of an aromatic group and a propylamine moiety to which is bound, via the nitrogen terminus, an isopropyl or similar group. The aromatic component of these agents most often is a phenyl group. They have considerable structural similarity to phenylethylamine β-receptor agonists. The isopropyl or related group covalently bound to the amino nitrogen is an important structural feature for binding to the β-receptor.

Pharmacokinetics

There is some variation from agent to agent, but in general β-receptor antagonists are absorbed orally, have modest volumes of distribution (0.7 L/kg [sotalol] to 9.46 L/kg [labetalol]), are variably protein bound (0% [sotalol] to 93% [pindolol]), and are hepatically metabolized. Exceptions are noted in Table 34-1. Most hepatically cleared β-blockers are metabolized by cytochrome P-450 2D6, an enzyme well known for its genetic polymorphism, as originally was shown for its role in debrisoquine oxidation.[1,2] Although various 2D6 phenotypes have been described, they have not been reported to influence the clinical course of β-receptor antagonist intoxication.

β-Receptor antagonists may be absorbed and achieve clinically significant systemic concentrations after ophthalmic application.[3–5] Absorption after ocular administration is through the nasolacrimal duct and directly into the systemic circulation. Normal first-pass hepatic metabolism, a prominent feature of the oral administration of these agents, is thus bypassed.

Subtypes

As shown in Table 34-1, many β-receptor antagonists are used throughout the world. These agents vary as a function of many characteristics that potentially can affect their clinical presentation during poisoning. These individual characteristics are primarily β_2 selectivity, intrinsic sympathomimetic activity, and membrane-stabilizing activity (MSA). MSA often is referred to as local anesthetic effect or sodium channel blockade. Agents with intrinsic sympathomimetic activity, of which pindolol is the prototype, have the potential for producing sympathomimetic effects during poisoning. Agents with MSA, such as propranolol, may exhibit sodium channel–blocking effects on the myocardium similar to quinidine. Agents with relatively high lipid solubility, such as propranolol, readily penetrate the blood-brain barrier and may be associated with altered sensorium, coma, or seizures.

PATHOPHYSIOLOGY

β-Receptors

β-Adrenergic receptors comprise a group of interrelated guanine nucleotide binding protein (G protein)–linked ligand binding sites, of which there are three established

TABLE 34-1 β-Receptor Antagonists

AGENT	β₁ SELECTIVITY	ISA	MSA	COMMENTS
Acebutolol	Yes	Slight	Slight	Most activity attributed to its metabolite diacetolol
Alprenolol	No	Yes	Yes	Highly lipid soluble
Atenolol	Yes	No	No	Primarily renally excreted
Betaxolol	Yes	No	Slight	
Bevantolol	Yes	No	No	Weak α₁-receptor antagonist
Bisoprolol	Yes	No	No	
Bopindolol	No	Yes	No	
Bucindolol	No	Slight	No	α-Receptor antagonist
Carteolol	No	Moderate	No	
Carvedilol	No	No	No	α-Receptor antagonist and vasodilator; antioxidant
Celiprolol	Yes	Slight	No	Mild β₂-agonist, α₂-antagonist, and vasodilator
Esmolol	Yes	No	No	Short half-life (8 min)
Labetalol	No	No	No	α-Receptor antagonist
Levobunolol	No	No	No	Used mostly as a topical agent to treat glaucoma
Metipranolol	No	No	No	Used mostly as a topical agent to treat glaucoma
Metoprolol	Yes	No	No	Inverse β-agonist; stereoselective hepatic metabolism
Nadolol	No	No	No	Renally excreted; long plasma half-life (approximately 20 hr)
Nebivolol	Yes	No	No	Effects mediated through nitric oxide; bronchodilator
Oxyprenolol	No	Yes	Slight	
Penbutolol	No	Slight	Slight	
Pindolol	No	Strong	Slight	5-hydroxytryptamine₁ₐ somatodendritic autoreceptor antagonist that leads to serotonin release; intrinsic sympathomimetic activity
Practolol	Yes	Yes	No	Causes ocular and skin injury and sclerosing peritonitis
Propafenone	No	No	No	Type I antiarrhythmic
Propranolol	No	No	Moderate	Lipid soluble with high CNS penetration; inverse β-agonist
Sotalol	No	No	No	Additional antiarrhythmic activity
Timolol	No	Minimal	No	

CNS, central nervous system; ISA, intrinsic sympathomimetic activity; MSA, membrane-stabilizing activity.

subtypes known as the β₁₋₃. As described subsequently, there also is evidence for the existence of a β₄-receptor subtype. G protein–linked receptors represent a superfamily of similar ligand binding sites with different affinities for a variety of agonists and antagonists. All are membrane-spanning receptors with intracellular sites that regulate the activity of these receptors.

The β₁-receptor is found predominantly in the heart, where it is the most abundant type of adrenergic receptor. It is diffusely distributed throughout the heart, and agonist binding causes increased chronotropy, inotropy, automaticity, and action potential conduction velocity. Most of the significant effects from β-receptor antagonist intoxication occur as a result of cardiac β₁-receptor blockade. β₁-Receptors also are found in the bowel, kidney, and posterior pituitary and on adipocytes.

The β₂-receptor also is found in cardiac tissue, although at considerably lower density than receptors of the β₁ subtype; it too is cardiostimulatory by a mechanism similar to the β₁-receptor (see later). β₂-Receptors also are found on arterioles and veins, where they cause vasodilation, and on smooth muscles of airways, where they cause relaxation. Most of the relevant toxicologic effects of β₂-receptors are due to effects on the heart, arterioles, and airways. β₂-Receptors also can be found in the eye, uterus, skeletal muscle, pancreas, urinary bladder, spleen, liver, and intestines and throughout the gastrointestinal system.

The β₃-receptor is best known for its action on adipocytes, in which β₃-receptors stimulate lipolysis. This receptor also is important in modulating the mast cell degranulatory response to IgE-mediated and non–IgE-mediated immune system stimulation (i.e., anaphylactic and anaphylactoid reactions). The toxicologic significance of this receptor derives from its existence on the heart, however, where it may have cardioinhibitory properties. The effects of the β₃-receptor are most marked in patients with heart failure; however, as described subsequently, they may be important in the clinical manifestations of β-receptor antagonist intoxication and have a potentially significant influence on the response to therapy with adrenergic agents.[6] The β₄-receptor is postulated to exist based on cardiostimulatory affects of β-receptor agonists that can be shown when β₁-receptors, β₂-receptors, and β₃-receptors are blocked.[6]

The physiology of β-receptors is complex.[7,8] The β₁-receptor (Fig. 34-2) exists in two forms—the active (R*) and inactive (R) state, which exist in equilibrium. β-Agonists bind to and stabilize the R* state; by doing so, they shift the equilibrium to an increased proportion of R*. Agonist binding to R* activates the stimulatory guanine nucleotide-binding protein (G_s), which binds to and activates adenylyl

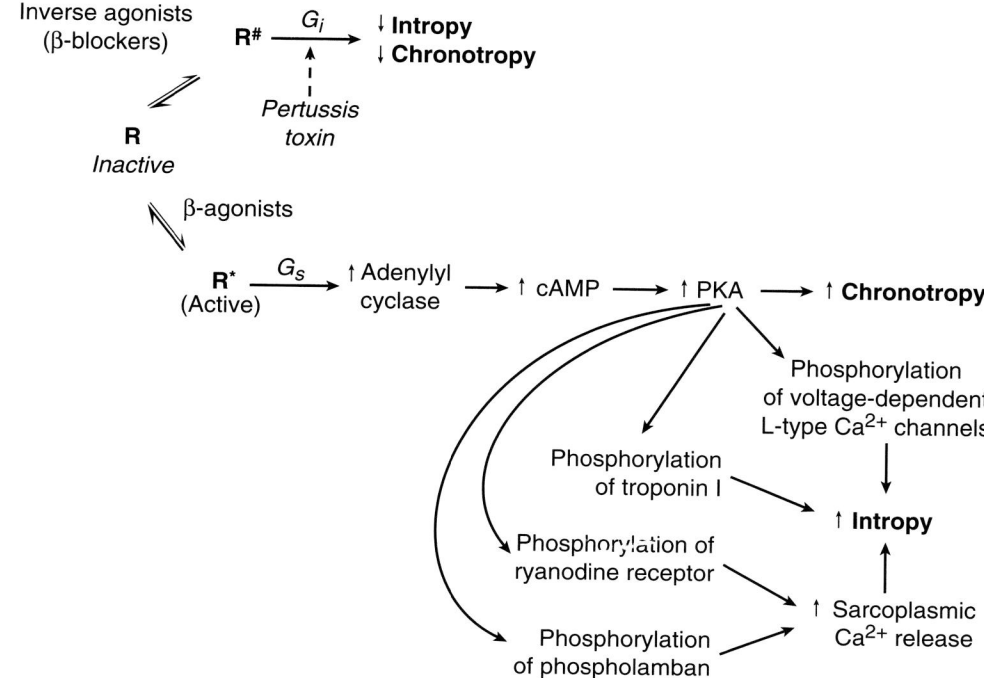

Esmolol

Atenolol

Propranolol

FIGURE 34-1

Chemical structures of some common β-adrenergic antagonists. Note that the side chain is widely conserved throughout this group.

cyclase, the enzyme responsible for the formation of cyclic adenosine monophosphate (cAMP), which activates protein kinase A. Protein kinase A is the mediator of stimulatory adrenergic effects on the myocardium, a feat accomplished

by its ability to phosphorylate many important proteins. Prominent among these is the voltage-dependent L-type calcium channel, which, when phosphorylated, allows calcium influx into the myocardium during phase II of the action potential. Phosphorylation of troponin I enhances muscle contraction by actinomyosin. Phosphorylation of the ryanodine receptor and phospholamban on the sarcoplasmic reticulum enhances calcium release, further stimulating excitation-contraction coupling. β-Antagonists bind to and stabilize the R form of the β_1-receptor and shift the equilibrium away from the activated receptor.

The β_2-receptor is stimulated by β-agonists in a manner similar to that of the β_1-receptor. The β_2-receptor also has the capability of mediating an important cardioinhibitory function, however. This receptor may exist in a third isoform ($R^\#$), which acts through an inhibitory protein G_i.[7] G_i is inhibited by pertussis toxin, which provides an important experimental tool by which the role of this protein has been elucidated; it is unclear whether G_i accomplishes this by the inhibition of adenylyl cyclase or through other mechanisms (see Fig. 34-2). Agents that bind to and stabilize $R^\#$ and mediate the β_2 receptor–induced cardioinhibitory effects are known as *inverse agonists*. Most β-receptor antagonists function, to various degrees, as inverse agonists at this receptor, explaining the potential effects of these agents beyond that which would be expected from simple removal of β_1 receptor–mediated adrenergic tone.

β_3-Adrenergic receptors constitute only a small fraction of the β-receptors on the heart and are cardioinhibitory, at least partially by a nitric oxide–mediated pathway, which seems to be independent of the above-described pathways for the β_2-receptor.[8,9] The β_3-receptor seems to be cardiostimulatory in the R^* state and may be cardioinhibitory in a G_i protein–linked manner via an $R^\#$ state analogous to that of the β_2-receptor.[6] It appears that all β-receptor antagonists

FIGURE 34-2

Isoforms of the β-adrenergic receptor and effects of their agonism. See text for further details. cAMP, cyclic adenosine monophosphate; PKA protein kinase A.

bind to the β_3-receptor,[6] although it is unclear which isoform of this receptor (R or R#) these agents stabilize.

When a β-receptor antagonist and a β-receptor agonist are pharmacologically present, there is competition between them for binding to the various isoforms of β-receptors. The end result is a much greater dose of agonist required for a pharmacologic effect. The avid binding of β-receptor antagonists to β-receptors means that the amount of agonist required to achieve its effect can be enormous. For example,[10] the avidity of propranolol for the β-receptor is shown by the striking magnitude of its binding constant, (K_B), 2×10^{-9}.

Effects of β-Receptor Blockade

CARDIAC

There are many mechanisms by which β-receptor antagonists may exert negative inotropic and chronotropic effects on the heart, including β_1-receptor antagonism, inverse agonism at β_2-receptor and β_3-receptors, membrane stabilization (i.e., sodium channel blockade), and metabolic derangements (e.g., relative hypoglycemia related to increased myocardial demands for glucose). Agents with MSA exert their effects via unique, non–β receptor–mediated mechanisms. There also are certain uniquely individual properties of individual agents, the most prominent of which is associated with sotalol, as described subsequently.

The mechanism of inverse agonism was described earlier. Germane to this consideration is the fact that although normal human hearts contain a large predominance of β_1-receptors,[11] the proportion of β_2-receptors increases dramatically in the setting of heart failure.[12] It is theoretically possible that the greater expression of inverse agonism that would occur with an increased proportion of β_2-receptors may make the failing heart hypersusceptible to poisoning with these agents.

There is a theory that β-receptor antagonists, by virtue of their modulation of ion channels, cause hyperpolarization of the cell membrane and decreased inotropy and chronotropy.[13] This idea is speculative, however, and it is unclear to what degree, if any, this occurs physiologically with poisoning by these agents.

Sotalol requires special mention. Sotalol is a Vaughn-Williams class III antiarrhythmic agent that increases the duration of the myocardial action potential and causes prolongation of the QT interval. Because the QT interval prolongation is due to an increase in the duration of phase 2 of the action potential and not increased duration of repolarization, it is unclear whether sotalol predisposes to torsades de pointes; however, cases of this arrhythmia have been reported after intoxication with sotalol.[14–16]

BLOOD VESSELS

β_2-Adrenergic stimulation of blood vessels causes vasodilation. It is anticipated that isolated β-receptor antagonist effects on vasculature allow for unopposed α receptor–mediated vasoconstriction. This vasoconstriction is rarely seen as an isolated event in poisonings, however, probably because of the clinical inability to separate cardiac from vascular effects without the assistance of invasive hemodynamic monitoring. In general, the theoretical vasoconstrictive effect of β-antagonists has little clinical implication in the absence of excess adrenergic stimulation (e.g., cocaine).

AIRWAYS

β_2 agonism is associated with relaxation of smooth muscles of the airways and bronchodilation. β_2 antagonism can result in clinically significant bronchoconstriction in susceptible individuals. It is not known to what degree, if any, inverse agonism at the β_2-receptor causes bronchoconstriction.

METABOLIC

Under therapeutic[17] or toxic[18] conditions, β-receptor antagonists cause a shift in substrate preference of the myocardium from free fatty acids to carbohydrates. Associated with this shift is a reduction in myocardial metabolic rate. This reduction may create an energy deficit for the heart and may explain further why insulin treatment, which increases myocardial glucose uptake, has had beneficial effects in an experimental model of propranolol intoxication.[19] It is unknown to what degree this observation can be generalized to other β-receptor antagonists.

MEMBRANE-STABILIZING ACTIVITY

Agents with MSA, of which the prototype is propranolol, exert not only β-receptor antagonism but also sodium channel–blocking antiarrhythmic effects characteristic of the Vaughn-Williams class I agents. In overdose, they cause QRS widening and other myocardial effects similar to quinidine.[20,21] These agents can be characterized as class IA antiarrhythmics in electrophysiologic action and toxicity. A further discussion of these antiarrhythmics is given in Chapter 36. Therapeutic approaches to MSA toxicity from β-receptor antagonists having this characteristic should address not only their β-blocking effects but also their sodium channel–blocking effects, as outlined in Chapter 36.

MAST CELL EFFECTS

β-Receptors exert a regulatory effect on reuptake by mast cells. This modulation influence can be lost in the presence of β-receptor antagonism, even at therapeutic doses.

CLINICAL PRESENTATION

Patients intoxicated with β-receptor antagonists present primarily with hypotension and cardiac bradydysrhythmias. In major intoxications, a variety of additional effects may become manifest, as described subsequently. The clinical picture depends on the dose ingested, the underlying physiologic status of the patient, and the particular agent involved. Propranolol is the most common agent implicated in cases in which toxicity is severe or fatal.[22,23]

Cardiac

The cardiovascular manifestations of β-blocker poisoning typically are bradydysrhythmias, cardiac conduction defects, pump failure, hypotension, and circulatory shock. Pindolol poisoning has been reported to cause hypertension, a likely consequence of its sympathomimetic actions.[24,25] Severe β-receptor antagonist poisoning may cause ventricular arrhythmias, including torsades de pointes and cardiac arrest; this is particularly true after sotalol intoxication.[14,16]

BRADYDYSRHYTHMIAS

Because the heart has an intrinsic rhythm, the removal of β_2 stimulation primarily prevents adrenergic stimulatory tone. This action by itself would not be expected to cause severe bradycardia in the absence of heightened vagal tone. Inverse agonism, as described earlier, theoretically can worsen bradydysrhythmias, however. β-Receptor antagonists with MSA, particularly propranolol, seem to be the primary cause of bradydysrhythmias,[10] although they have been reported with other β-receptor antagonists as well.[26–28]

Hemodynamically significant bradydysrhythmias may occur from the ocular administration of β-receptor antagonists, even at recommended therapeutic doses. Although bradydysrhythmias are unlikely to occur in otherwise healthy patients, those with compromised cardiovascular function seem to be at risk. These effects have been observed most frequently after the ocular application of timolol, which is the agent most commonly used to treat glaucoma.[4,5,29] The National Registry of Drug-Induced Ocular Side Effects in the United States contains multiple reports of cardiovascular adverse effects in patients receiving this agent.[4,5] Published case reports also have described significant bradydysrhythmias in patients being treated with timolol as an ophthalmic preparation.[30–32] One published series of patients receiving long-term treatment with ophthalmic timolol included two patients with asymptomatic, yet profound, bradydysrhythmias.[37]

The U.S. National Registry contains many reports of sudden death in patients receiving ocular timolol.[34] As in any spontaneous reporting system, however, a cause-and-effect relationship cannot be inferred from these anecdotal observations.

CARDIAC CONDUCTION DEFECTS

There have been many case reports of various degrees of heart block, atrioventricular dissociation, junctional escape rhythms, and bundle-branch blocks associated with poisoning by many different β-receptor antagonists.

PUMP FAILURE

Cardiac pump failure from β-receptor antagonist intoxication may be due to hemodynamically significant arrhythmias, to characteristic bradydysrhythmias, or to a decrease in inotropy. It is important to make this distinction because these three mechanisms have different therapeutic implications. Clinically documented decreases in dP/dT, a widely accepted measure of myocardial contractility, are sparse; however, this may be an artifact of the lack of determination of this parameter in many clinical case reports. If there is significant bradycardia, it should be corrected (see treatment section). Pump failure not attributable to bradydysrhythmias should be characterized further through measurement of hemodynamic parameters (cardiac index, pulmonary capillary wedge pressure, total peripheral resistance), unless it resolves with empirical treatment, such as a trial of dobutamine.

HYPOTENSION

Hypotension has been associated anecdotally with β-receptor antagonist intoxication in case reports involving almost all agents of this class. The relative frequency of this effect has not been determined in a large case series, and it has not been associated with any particular β-receptor antagonist or pharmacologic characteristic. A study comparing the lipophilic, membrane-stabilizing agent propranolol with atenolol, a β-blocker that does not possess these properties, showed no difference in the incidence of either systolic or diastolic hypotension after poisonings.[22] Hypotension also has been reported after the ocular administration of therapeutic doses of β-blockers.[5,29]

Pulmonary

Many pulmonary complications may be anticipated with poisonings by β-receptor antagonists. Patients with a depressed level of consciousness also may develop hypoventilatory respiratory failure and should be considered at increased risk for aspiration. The blockade of pulmonary β_2-receptors can result in increased airflow resistance and clinical bronchospasm. Patients with severe cardiovascular dysfunction may develop adult respiratory distress syndrome.

RESPIRATORY DEPRESSION

There have been multiple reports of respiratory depression after overdose with β-receptor antagonists. Respiratory failure seems to be secondary to cardiovascular or central nervous system depression and has not occurred independent of these effects. A clinical study comparing the propensity of propranolol and atenolol to cause bradypnea did not show a significant difference.[22]

BRONCHOCONSTRICTION

Bronchospasm may occur in susceptible individuals after either therapeutic or sympathomimetic doses of β-receptor antagonists. There have been multiple case reports, including fatalities, of bronchospasm associated with therapeutic use. Bronchospasm also has been reported after therapeutic ocular administration.[4,5] Similarly, several case reports, although no studies or series, have shown bronchospasm after β-receptor antagonist overdose.[35,36] Significant bronchospasm likely occurs only in individuals with hyperreactive airways. Most cases of β-receptor antagonist intoxication, including cases associated with high doses, do not manifest this effect.

Neurologic

The two primary neurologic manifestations of β-receptor antagonist intoxication are depressed sensorium and seizures. The former may be due primarily to cardiovascular depression and decreased cerebral perfusion. In addition, lipophilic agents, such as propranolol, would be expected to have a more direct effect on the central nervous system.

Seizures have been associated with a variety of β-receptor antagonists in overdose. Seizures are reported far more frequently, however, in patients who have ingested propranolol. Most patients have seizures in association with hemodynamic instability,[22] and it is possible that their convulsions are a result of cerebral hypoperfusion. One series, comparing propranolol poisonings with and without seizures, showed that the patients who had ictal events were more likely to be hypotensive, had a relatively wider QRS interval, and were more likely to have a respiratory rate less than 12 breaths/min. There was no association, however, between having seizures and presenting with a Glasgow Coma Scale score less than 15 or an abnormal QT_c interval.[22] The minimal dose of propranolol associated with seizures was 1.2 g, whereas at doses greater than 2 g, most patients had ictal events.[22]

Other

β-Receptor antagonist intoxication may be expected to cause many potential effects that can complicate therapy, including hypoglycemia, rhabdomyolysis, acute renal failure on the basis of decreased renal perfusion, and metabolic acidosis secondary to hypoperfusion.

DIAGNOSIS

The diagnosis of β-receptor antagonist poisoning is a clinical one that should be based on the history and clinical syndrome. Patients who present with hypotension, brady-dysrhythmias, or cardiac conduction defects should have these agents included in the differential diagnosis, including toxicity from the use of β-receptor antagonist eye drops. Routine drug screening tests may not detect this class of medications. If there is a possibility of intoxication by a β-receptor antagonist, however, the laboratory should be informed so that they may look specifically for them with more comprehensive assays. Quantitative serum concentrations of β-receptor antagonists generally are not available and are useful only for retrospective verification of the diagnosis and corroboration of the severity of intoxication. In rare cases it is necessary to obtain these determinations, however, to establish the diagnosis.

TREATMENT

As with all poisonings, the treatment of β-receptor antagonist intoxications often relies on appropriate supportive care, including airway support for standard indications and monitoring for complications.

Decontamination

In the past, one component of the treatment of serious poisonings was gastric emptying with either syrup of ipecac or gastric lavage. As described in detail in Chapter 5, however, syrup of ipecac no longer has an accepted, evidence-based role in the treatment of major poisonings. Similarly, gastric lavage is unlikely to have a significant effect and carries with it increased risk of iatrogenic morbidity (e.g., aspiration, mechanical injury). There are no studies suggesting that gastric lavage alters either the outcome or the clinical course in patients with β-blocker intoxication. The scientific data supporting these points are discussed further in Chapter 5. There also is the theoretical concern that gastric lavage may enhance vagal tone and worsen bradyrhythmias in β-receptor antagonist–poisoned patients.

The administration of activated charcoal may reduce blood concentrations of ingested β-receptor antagonists. In a study of volunteer subjects who ingested nadolol, the administration of 3 g of activated charcoal over 9 hours reduced the area under the curve (AUC) of the absorbed drug.[36] There have been no studies, however, validating the use of activated charcoal in patients poisoned by these agents. It is speculated that the administration of activated charcoal may decrease peak plasma concentrations and corresponding AUCs and possibly ameliorate the clinical course of β-receptor antagonist overdose. This theoretical benefit is less likely to be significant as time passes postingestion. I recommend the administration of activated charcoal only if it can be accomplished within the first few hours after ingestion. If the patient has a depressed sensorium, activated charcoal should be administered only with appropriate precautions to reduce the risk of aspiration. There is no supporting clinical or pharmacokinetic evidence for multidose activated charcoal after β-receptor antagonist ingestion, and its use is not recommended.

Whole-bowel irrigation with electrolyte-balanced polyethylene glycol solutions has been touted as an alternative to activated charcoal. There are no data supporting the use of this technique in the treatment of β-receptor antagonist intoxication, however, and its use is not recommended. There are no data to support the use of this technique for substances, such as β-receptor antagonists, that are well absorbed to activated charcoal; this includes sustained-release preparations (see Chapter 5).

Patients who have β-blocker intoxication secondary to ocular administration may benefit from aggressive eye irrigation, including the conjunctival recesses, possibly with concurrent nasolacrimal duct occlusion. This is a theoretical recommendation and has not been subjected to a controlled study.

Owing to their relatively high volumes of distribution, there is little role for extracorporeal techniques for enhancing the clearance of most β-receptor antagonists. Commonly used β-receptor antagonists that may be amenable to extracorporeal drug removal are listed in Table 34-2. Propranolol, the agent most commonly causing severe toxicity, has a moderately large volume of distribution (4 L/kg) and is greater than 90% protein bound; it is unlikely that it would be cleared to any significant degree by these techniques.

Indications for ICU Admission in β-Blocker Poisoning

Hemodynamic instability
Coma or seizures
Bronchoconstriction not responsive to initial bronchodilator therapy

---

TABLE 34-2 Common β-Receptor Antagonists Amenable to Extracorporeal Removal

AGENT	VOLUME OF DISTRIBUTION (L/kg)	PROTEIN BINDING (%)
Acebutolol	1.2	30–40
Atenolol	1.1	<5
Sotalol	0.7	0

Cardiovascular Effects

BRADYDYSRHYTHMIAS

The various treatment modalities available for β-receptor antagonist–induced bradydysrhythmias have not been studied in individual or comparative trials. There is published case experience with the use of atropine, glucagon, β-receptor agonists, phosphodiesterase inhibitors, insulin, electrical pacing, intraaortic balloon counterpulsation, and extracorporeal circulatory support for this indication.

Atropine increases heart rate by its muscarinic anticholinergic, a non–β receptor–mediated effect. Although atropine may provide a transient increase in cardiac rate and index, its effect is variable and short-lived. Repeated doses may induce anticholinergic delirium and other, more peripheral adverse effects (e.g., urinary retention). Its primary use is limited to the initial stabilization of a bradycardic, hemodynamically compromised patient.

Glucagon has been widely suggested as a means of producing a positive chronotropic effect, independent of the β-receptor. There have been multiple reports of its apparent beneficial effects, although these generally were in uncontrolled clinical cases involving several pharmacologic therapies.[37-42] Typically, when used for the treatment of poisonings, glucagon is administered as a 10-mg intravenous bolus in adults, followed by a continuous infusion generally at 10 mg/hr. The pediatric bolus dose is 50 to 150 μg/kg up to 10 mg. Some preparations of glucagon have been packaged with a phenol-containing diluent. Because the doses of glucagon used in the treatment of β-receptor antagonist intoxication are higher than doses for other purposes, patients may receive an excessive amount of phenol if this diluent is used. If the diluent is phenol, it should be replaced with any simple intravenous solution, such as normal saline or dextrose in water.

The use of β-receptor agonists, in an attempt to overcome receptor blockade competitively, may be attempted in cases of hemodynamically significant cardiac bradydysrhythmias. The options that may be considered are isoproterenol, dobutamine, epinephrine, and prenalterol. Prenalterol is not available in many countries, however, including the United States. There are few data to rely on for assessing the effects of β-agonists in the treatment of these bradycardias. For patients who are refractory to simple supportive therapy, an empirical trial with a dobutamine or isoproterenol infusion can be attempted. As described subsequently, isoproterenol may worsen hypotension or cause cardiac dysrhythmias and should be used cautiously and only in a well-monitored patient. The typical adult dose of isoproterenol for conditions not related to β-blocker poisoning is 2 to 10 μg/min. Because of the potential adverse effects of this therapy, the lowest effective dose should be used. The typical pediatric dose is 0.1 to 1.5 μg/kg/min, with the lowest effective dose suggested.[43] As described subsequently, however, it is unlikely that conventional doses of isoproterenol would be effective in a patient with serious β-blocker poisoning.

There are few published data on the use of dobutamine or epinephrine as a β-adrenergic agonist in patients poisoned by these agents. Because of the high binding affinity of β-antagonists to the β-receptor, it is likely that unusually high doses of receptor agonists would be required to over-come the blockade competitively. This likelihood may explain cases of failure of adrenergic agents. It has been calculated that a 10,000 times increase over standard isoproterenol dosing would be required to overcome the blockade induced by an overdose of propranolol.[10] For β-adrenergic agents that have any α-agonist properties, the administration of high doses may increase afterload to the point of causing adverse effects on cardiac hemodynamics or coronary perfusion or both, in part due to the unopposed α-adrenergic agonism that occurs as a consequence of β-receptor antagonist intoxication.

Cardiac pacing may be attempted for the treatment of bradyarrhythmias, although there is little clinical experience with this in the management of β-receptor antagonist intoxication. Successful use of the intraaortic balloon pump has been reported in select cases.[44,45] Similarly, in patients unresponsive to all other measures, extracorporeal cardiac support could be attempted. This approach was reported to be successful in a patient who was refractory to multiple other therapies after propranolol intoxication.[46]

Phosphodiesterase inhibitors, such as an inamrinone (formerly amrinone) or milrinone, theoretically should have a positive chronotropic effect on the myocardium because the β-receptor exerts its effect by increasing intracellular cAMP, a molecule that is metabolized by phosphodiesterase. The heart contains the isoform phosphodiesterase III, which is bound to the sarcoplasmic reticulum.[47] Inhibiting this enzyme enhances calcium release from the sarcoplasm.[8] There have been several case reports of increasing cardiac index with these agents,[44] although in a canine model of propranolol intoxication, inamrinone increased cardiac contractility but not rate.[50] In another canine study of propranolol intoxication, milrinone, in combination with glucagon, caused severe tachycardia.[51]

If inamrinone is elected, typical initial loading dose is 0.75 mg/kg as a bolus given over 2 to 3 minutes followed by an infusion of 5 to 40 μg/kg/min. Milrinone typically is administered in a loading dose of 50 μg/kg over 10 minutes, followed by an infusion of 0.375 to 1 μg/kg/min. These dosing protocols should be adjusted in patients with significant renal insufficiency.

CARDIAC CONDUCTION DEFECTS

As described earlier, various degrees of cardiac conduction defects have been observed after intoxication with β-receptor antagonists, including agents with and without MSA. There has been no systematic study of this phenomenon, and few data are available in the published literature on its treatment. Minor degrees of heart block in an otherwise hemodynamically stable patient can be managed expectantly. If the heart block is associated with significant bradycardia, it is possible that it may resolve with treatment of the latter, as described earlier. The fluid and electrolyte status of the patient also should be optimized. If the heart block is significant enough to cause pump failure, treatment should be initiated as described in the following section.

PUMP FAILURE

There have been no clinical trials to date addressing the optimal therapy of β-blocker–induced reduction in myocardial contractility. Pump failure due to hemodynamically significant bradycardias should be treated initially as described earlier. Pump failure that is not solely rate related can be managed, however, by the administration of inotropes, glucagon, or possibly phosphodiesterase inhibitors. So-called insulin-euglycemia therapy has been proposed, although there are few clinical data supporting its use for this condition.

Pump failure resistant to pharmacologic interventions and optimal management of fluid status may require the use of a left ventricular assist device or extracorporeal circulation. If pump failure is refractory to initial therapeutic approaches, it may be helpful to obtain precise hemodynamic parameters through invasive monitoring. The clinical benefits and risks of this intervention have not been studied, however.

Some inotropic agents (e.g., dobutamine) act by stimulating cardiac β_1-receptors and are expected to be antagonized competitively by the β-blocker. These agents may not be clinically effective, although a cautious empirical trial of this approach cannot be criticized. Theoretically, much higher doses of β-agonists may be necessary than doses typically used in the absence of β-receptor antagonist poisoning, but this has not been studied. Of the various options for β_1-specific inotropes, dobutamine is the most appropriate based on theoretical considerations, in my opinion. These effects may be magnified at higher doses. An emerging concern regarding the use of β-antagonists in the presence of a β-receptor antagonist relates to the cardioinhibitory β_3-receptor. It is possible that blockade of the cardiac β_1-receptor and β_2-receptor could cause adrenergic inotropes preferentially to agonize the β_3-receptor. In the presence of nadolol, isoproterenol exerts an inhibitory effect on dP/dt in the human myocardium.[6]

The use of glucagon in β-receptor antagonist poisoning was described earlier. Several case reports have described improvement in multiple hemodynamic parameters after the administration of glucagon in patients poisoned by these agents.[37–42] Most of these patients were receiving several treatments at the same time, however. Studies on propranolol intoxication in dog models have shown beneficial effects of glucagon on multiple hemodynamic parameters, including cardiac output, stroke volume, left ventricular end-diastolic pressure, and dP/dT.[50–52]

Phosphodiesterase inhibitors may be beneficial in the treatment of β-receptor antagonist–induced pump failure. Investigations using canine models showed hemodynamic improvement with inamrinone[50] and milrinone.[51,53] Similarly, in clinical cases, amrinone has been reported to be efficacious in treating β-receptor antagonist–induced pump failure.[49]

Insulin-euglycemia therapy has been touted as a potential treatment for β-receptor antagonist intoxication, based on a dog model of propranolol intoxication. In that model, an infusion of 4 U/min of insulin with supplemental 50% glucose to prevent hypoglycemia improved the dP/dT.[19] There is little experience with this therapy in humans with β-receptor antagonist poisoning. There is experimental animal and anecdotal human experience with insulin-euglycemia therapy in calcium channel antagonist poisoning. If this therapy is attempted in the treatment of β-receptor antagonist toxicity, reasonable starting doses would be those used in calcium channel antagonist toxicity, which are reviewed in Chapter 35.

HYPOTENSION

Hypotension from β-receptor antagonist intoxication may be secondary to vasodilation, myocardial depression, or cardiac dysrhythmias. Because of the potential vasodilatory nature of the hypotension, an initial crystalloid fluid trial generally is appropriate. At the same time, attention should be paid to optimizing cardiac output, as described subsequently.

Although it is intuitively appealing to treat β-receptor antagonist–induced hypotension with β-agonists, results with this approach generally have been disappointing. Attempts to antagonize competitively the effect of β-blocking agents at the β-receptor with the β-agonist isoproterenol theoretically may worsen the hypotension by inducing vasodilation, or it may induce cardiac arrhythmias. Case series of β-receptor antagonist–intoxicated patients have failed to support a beneficial effect of isoproterenol. A likely explanation is an insufficient dose to overcome the β blockade competitively.

Prenalterol, a β-receptor agonist that is not universally available, has been evaluated in a dog model of metoprolol toxicity in which it seemed to improve blood pressure, pulmonary capillary wedge pressure, cardiac output, central venous pressure, and stroke volume. It reduced peripheral vascular resistance, however.[54] There have been several case reports of clinical improvement in patients treated with prenalterol.[55,56] These patients were treated with multiple other therapies, however, and it is unclear to what extent, if any, the prenalterol was effective.

Vasopressors may be beneficial in the treatment of vasodilation secondary to β-receptor antagonist stimulation of β_2-receptors. Dopamine and norepinephrine are used commonly. Neither dopamine nor norepinephrine has been studied systematically in β-receptor antagonist intoxication, however. An appropriate approach to using vasopressors in these patients is to use them empirically, evaluating their efficacy in the particular patient by assessment of neurodynamic response. In a dog model of propranolol toxicity, glucose and insulin euglycemia therapy prevented hypotension.[19]

Noncardiovascular Effects

Respiratory depression, bronchoconstriction, depressed mentation, seizures, hypoglycemia, and secondary problems such as rhabdomyolysis or acute renal failure should be treated by standard measures for the approach to these complications in the intensive care unit. It should be anticipated, however, based on theoretical considerations, that attempts to treat bronchospasm with β-agonists may be unsuccessful due to the blockade of β-receptors. Similarly, because this bronchospasm is due to loss of β-adrenergic tone and not inflammation, it is unlikely that corticosteroids would offer significant therapeutic effects. Alternative bronchodilator approaches with greater potential efficacy include anticholinergic agents (e.g., ipratropium, glycopyrrolate), phosphodiesterase inhibitors (e.g., aminophylline), and possibly glucagon. Seizure secondary to β-receptor antagonist poisoning, seen most commonly with propranolol, should be treated in the same manner as other toxicant-induced convulsions (see Chapter 20).

Criteria for ICU Discharge in β-Blocker Poisoning

Hemodynamic stability
Normal sensorium
Pulmonary disorder requiring intensive care unit–level care

SPECIAL POPULATIONS

Pediatric Patients

There is little information concerning significant differences in the pathophysiology, presentation, or treatment of β-receptor antagonist intoxication in children compared with adults. Among more than 50,000 β-receptor antagonist intoxications reported to U.S. poison centers over an 11-year period, nearly 20,000 occurred in children younger than age 6, and there were no fatalities in this group.[23] A 7-year retrospective study of cases reported to a regional poison center in the United States evaluated children younger than 7 years old with β-receptor antagonist ingestions. As is typical for ingestions in children of this age, most involved either a small number of pills or only the suspicion of ingestion.[57] Only 8 of the 378 children evaluated developed any significant signs of toxicity. The toxicities that did occur were bradycardias, lethargy, and hypotension. These were manifest at a median of 3 hours postingestion, with a maximal time from ingestion of 3.5 hours. This study did not have enough cases with sustained-release preparations to reach any conclusions regarding ingestion of these formulations. From the limited information available, it seems that the clinical presentation of β-receptor antagonist intoxication in children is similar to that in adults, and with the exception of sustained-release preparations, children who will become symptomatic tend to do so within several hours. Patients who are asymptomatic but who have ingested sustained-release preparations should be observed for a longer time. Although there are no guidelines to follow in the latter case, a survey of poison centers in the United States found that most suggest that children who have ingested sustained-release preparations of these agents be observed for more than 8 hours.[57]

Pregnant Patients

Most of the adverse experiences associated with β-receptor antagonists in pregnancy involve propranolol, which seems to cross the placenta and may concentrate in the fetus.[58] Bradydysrhythmias, hypoglycemia, respiratory depression (and even neonatal apnea), and circulatory collapse have been described in women who received propranolol before delivery.[58-60]

A case of neonatal respiratory depression, hypotonia, and circulatory collapse was reported in a 33-week-gestation neonate delivered by cesarean section whose mother received intravenous labetalol before surgery.[59] A case report of a major overdose of metoprolol in a woman in her 20th week of pregnancy described cardiac arrest in the mother. Despite successful resuscitation, the event led to fetal demise.[61]

Breast-feeding Patients

Most β-receptor antagonists that have been studied in regard to breast-feeding are excreted in breast milk. A case report described an infant with β-receptor antagonist intoxication from breast-feeding by a mother who was treated with atenolol.[62]

Common Errors in β-Blocker Poisoning

Not realizing that therapeutic use of β-receptor antagonist–containing eye drops can cause significant toxicity
Induction of bronchospasm by these agents in susceptible individuals
Assuming that whole-bowel irrigation is superior to activated charcoal for gastrointestinal decontamination of sustained-release preparations

Key Points in β-Blocker Poisoning

β-Blockers may cause the following:
  Bradydysrhythmia
  Cardiac conduction disturbances
  Hypotension
  Central nervous system depression and seizures
  Bronchoconstriction
  Secondary complications deriving from the above
Therapeutic options beyond supportive care comprise
  Gastrointestinal decontamination
  Atropine
  Phosphodiesterase inhibitors
  Glucagon
  Insulin
  Cardiac pacing
  Left ventricular assist
  Extracorporeal circulation
  Extracorporeal drug removal for certain agents

REFERENCES

1. Meyer UA: The molecular basis of genetic polymorphisms of drug metabolism. J Pharm Pharmacol 46(Suppl 1):409–415, 1994.
2. Gonzalez FJ, Idle JR: Pharmacogenetic phenotyping and genotyping: Present status and future potential. Clin Pharmacokinet 26:59–70, 1994.
3. Korte J-M, Kaila T, Saari KM: Systemic bioavailability and cardiopulmonary effects of 0.5% timolol eyedrops. Graefe Arch Clin Exp Ophthalmol 240:430–435, 2002.
4. Fraunfelder FT, Meyer SM: Systemic reactions to ophthalmic drug preparations. Med Toxicol 2:287–293, 1987.
5. Fraunfelder FT: Ocular β-blockers and systemic effects. Arch Intern Med 146:1073–1074, 1986.
6. Schnabel P, Maack C, Mies F, et al: Binding properties of β-blockers at recombinant β1-, β2-, and β3-adrenoceptors. J Cardiovasc Pharmacol 36:466–471, 2000.
7. Gong H, Sun H, Koch WJ, et al: Specific β-AR blocker ICI 118,551 actively decreases contraction through a Gi-coupled form of the β2AR in myocytes from failing human heart. Circulation 105:2497–2503, 2002.
8. Zaugg M, Schaub MC, Pasch T, et al. Modulation of β-adrenergic receptor subtype activities in perioperative medicine: Mechanisms and sites of action. Br J Anaesth 88:101–123, 2002.

9. Varghese P, Harrison RW, Lofthouse RA, et al: β_3-adrenoceptor deficiency blocks nitric oxide-dependent inhibition of myocardial contractility. J Clin Invest 106:693–703, 2000.

10. Critchley, JAJH, Ungar A: The management of acute poisoning due to β-adrenoceptor antagonists. Med Toxicol 4:32–45, 1898.

11. White M, Roden R, Minobe W, et al: Age-related changes in β-adrenergic neuroeffector systems in the human heart. Circulation 90:1225–1238, 1994.

12. Bristow MR, Ginsburg R, Minobe W, et al: Decreased catecholamine sensitivity and β-adrenergic receptor density in failing human hearts. N Engl J Med 307:205–211, 1982.

13. Kerns W II, Ransom M, Tomaszewski C, et al: The effects of extracellular ions on β-blocker cardiotoxicity. Toxicol Applied Pharmacol 137:1–7, 1996.

14. Baliga BG: Beta blocker poisoning: Prolongation of Q-T interval and inversion of T wave. J Indian Med Assoc 83:165, 1985.

15. Beattie JM: Sotalol induced torsade de pointes. Scott Med J 29:240–244, 1984.

16. Totterman KJ, Turto H, Pellinen T: Overdrive pacing as treatment of sotalol-induced ventricular tachyarrhythmias (torsades de pointes). Acta Med Scand 668(Suppl):28–33, 1982.

17. Bravo EL: Metabolic factors and sympathetic nervous system. Am J Hypertens 2:339S–344S, 1989.

18. Masters TN, Glaviano W: Effects of D-L-propranolol on myocardial free fatty acid and carbohydrate metabolism. J Pharmacol Exp Ther 167:187–193, 1969.

19. Kerns W II, Schroeder D, Williams C, et al: Insulin improves survival in a canine model of acute β-blocker toxicity. Ann Emerg Med 29:748–757, 1997.

20. Hashimoto K, Hiroyasu S, Shoichi I: Effects of etafenone and antiarrhythmic drugs on Na and Ca channels of guinea pig atrial muscle. J Cardiovasc Pharmacol 1:561–570, 1979.

21. Nies AS, Shand DG: Clinical pharmacology of propranolol. Circulation 52:6–15, 1975.

22. Reith DM, Dawson AH, Epid D, et al: Relative toxicity of beta blockers in overdose. Clin Toxicol 34:273–278, 1996.

23. Love JN, Litovita TL, Howell JM, et al: Characterization of fatal beta blocker ingestion: A review of the American Association of Poison Control Centers data from 1985 to 1995. Clin Toxicol 35:353–359, 1997.

24. Thorpe P: Pindolol in hypertension. Med J Aust 58:1242, 1974.

25. Offenstadt G, Hericord P, Amstutz P: Voluntary poisoning with pindolol. Nouv Presse Med 5:1539, 1976.

26. Love JN, Elshami J: Cardiovascular depression resulting from atenolol intoxication. Eur J Emerg Med 9:111–114, 2002.

27. Eibs HG, Oberdisse U Brambach U: Intoxikation mit beta rezeptoren blockers. Dtsch Med Wochenschr 107:1139–1143, 1982.

28. Kulling P, Eleborg L, Persson H: β-adrenoceptor blocker intoxication: Epidemiological data: Prenalterol as an alternative in the treatment of cardiac dysfunction. Hum Toxicol 2:175–181, 1983.

29. Munroe WP, Rindone JP, Kershner RM: Systemic side effects associated with the ophthalmic administration of timolol. Drug Intell Clin Pharm 19:85–89, 1985.

30. Coppeto JR: Transient ischemic attacks and amaurosis fugax from timolol. Ann Ophthalmol 98:64–65, 1984.

31. McMahon CD, Shaffer RN, Hoskins HD, et al: Adverse effects experienced by patients taking timolol. Am J Ophthalmol 88:736–738, 1979.

32. Wilson RP, Spaeth GL, Poryzees E: The place of timolol in the practice of ophthalmology. Ophthalmology 87:451–454, 1980.

33. Boger WP, Puliafito CA, Steinert RF, et al: Long-term experience with timolol ophthalmic solution in patients with open-angle glaucoma. Ophthalmology 85:259–267, 1978.

34. Vanbuskirik EM: Adverse reactions from timolol administration. Ophthalmology 87:447–450, 1980.

35. Weinstein RS, Cole S, Knaster HB, et al: Beta-blocker overdose with propranolol and with atenolol. Ann Emerg Med 14:161–163, 1985.

36. duSouich P, Caille G, Larochelle P: Enhancement of nadolol elimination by activated charcoal and antibiotics. Clin Pharmacol Ther 33:585–590, 1983.

37. Illingsworth RW: Glucagon for beta-blocker poisoning. Practitioner 223:683–685, 1979.

38. Kosinski EJ: Glucagon and propranolol (Inderal) toxicity. N Engl J Med 285:1325, 1971.

39. O'Mahony D, O'Leary P, Molloy MG. Severe oxprenolol poisoning: The importance of glucagon infusion. Hum Exp Toxicol 9:101–103, 1990.

40. Ehgartner GR, Zelinka MA: Hemodynamic instability following intentional nadolol overdose. Arch Intern Med 148:801–802, 1988.

41. Peterson CD, Leeder JS, Sterner S: Glucagon therapy for β-blocker overdose. Drug Intell Clin Pharm 18:394–398, 1984.

42. Vadhera RB: Propranolol overdose. Anaesthesia 47:279–280, 1992.

43. Benitz WE, Tatro DS: The Pediatric Drug Handbook, 3rd ed. St Louis, Mosby-Year Book, 1995.

44. Lane AS, Woodward AC, Goldman MR, et al: Massive propranolol overdose poorly responsive to pharmacologic therapy: use of the intra-aortic balloon pump. Ann Emerg Med 16:1381–1383, 1987.

45. Koppel C, Winkler M, Preib H, et al: Extreme doses of catecholamines and intra-aortic balloon counterpulsation in serious atenolol overdose. Presented at EAPCCT XUI, International Congress, Vienna, Austria, 1994.

46. McVey FK, Corke CF: Extracorporeal circulation in the management of massive propranolol overdose. Anaesthesia 46:744–746, 1991.

47. Yang J, Drazba JA, Ferguson DG, et al: A-kinase anchoring protein 100 (AKAP100) is localized in multiple subcellular compartments in the adult rat heart. J Cell Biol 142:511–522, 1998.

48. Berridge MJ: Elementary and global aspects of calcium signaling. J Exp Biol 200:315–319, 1997.

49. Kollef MH: Labetalol overdose successfully treated with amrinone and alpha-adrenergic receptor agonists. Chest 105:626–627, 1994.

50. Love JN, Leasure JA, Mundt DJ, et al: A comparison of amrinone and glucagon therapy for cardiovascular depression associated with propranolol toxicity in a canine model. Clin Toxicol 30:399–412, 1992.

51. Sato S, Tsuji MH, Okubo N, et al: Combined use of glucagon and milrinone may not be preferable for severe propranolol poisoning in the canine model. Clin Toxicol 33:337–342, 1995.

52. Kosinski EJ, Malindzak GS: Glucagon and isoproterenol in reversing propranolol toxicity. Arch Intern Med 132:840–843, 1973.

53. Sato D, Tsuji MH, Okubo N, et al: Milrinone versus glucagon: Comparative hemodynamic effects in canine propranolol poisoning. Clin Toxicol 32:277–289, 1994.

54. Andersson T, Heath A, Mattson H: Prenalterol as an antidote to massive doses of metoprolol—a cardiovascular study in the dog. Acta Med Scand 659(Suppl):71–88, 1982.

55. Kulling P: Clinical experiences with prenalterol as an antidote to β-adrenoceptor blockade (Abstract). Acta Med Scand 212(Suppl 59):191–199, 1982.

56. Freestone S, Thomas HM, Bhamra RK, et al: Severe atenolol poisoning: Treatment with prenalterol. Hum Toxicol 5:343–345, 1986.

57. Belson MG, Sullivan K, Geller RJ: Beta-adrenergic antagonist exposures in children. Vet Hum Toxicol 43:361–365, 2001.

58. Cottril CM, McAllister RG, Guttes L, et al: Propranolol therapy during pregnancy, labor and delivery: Evidence for transplacental drug transfer in impaired neonatal drug disposition. J Pediatr 91:812–814, 1977.

59. Haraldsson A, Geven W: Severe adverse effects of maternal labetalol in a premature infant. Acta Paediatr Scand 78:956–958, 1989.

60. Habib A, McCarthy JS: Effects on the neonate of propranolol administered during pregnancy. J Pediatr 91:808–811, 1977.

61. Tai YT, Lo CW, Chow WH, et al. Successful resuscitation and survival following massive overdose of metoprolol. Br J Clin Pract 44:746–747, 1990.

62. Schmimmel MS, Eidelman AJ, Wilschanski MA, et al: Toxic effects of atenolol consumed during breast feeding. J Pediatr 114:476–478, 1989.

CHAPTER **35**

Calcium Channel–Blocking Agents

Jeffrey Brent

The role of calcium in physiologic processes has been long recognized. In approximately 1960, it was first noted that calcium channel antagonists being developed as vasodilators had negative inotropic and chronotropic effects. This observation gave rise to the concept that reducing calcium influx into myocardial cells and arterial vascular smooth muscle could negatively modulate excitation-contraction coupling, accounting for their vasodilating and negative inotropic effects. Subsequently, it was recognized that inhibiting the inward calcium flux decreased the rate of spontaneous depolarization of cardiac pacemaker cells. Because this inward calcium current is slow compared with the fast sodium channel of cardiac myocytes, the former has been called the *slow calcium channel*, frequently referred to as simply the *calcium channel*.

The vasodilating and negative chronotropic effects of calcium channel antagonists have led to their development for many important indications, such as the treatment of hypertension, cardiac tachyarrhythmias, arterial vasospasm, angina pectoris, hypertropic cardiomyopathy, congestive heart failure, premature labor, and pulmonary hypertension.

Several classes of calcium channel antagonists are in use. These classes vary in their effects on arterial smooth muscle and the heart. The pharmacologic actions of the various agents on these two end organs account for their major clinical effects when used therapeutically and when toxicity develops.

The major calcium channel antagonists in clinical use around the world are verapamil, nifedipine, diltiazem, and amlodipine. As described in this chapter, the first three of these drugs are prototypes of the three major distinct classes of calcium channel antagonists; most of the data concerning the toxicity of these respective classes come from observations on these three specific agents. To the extent that information is available on toxic effects of the other calcium channel antagonists, these are described as well.

CLINICAL PHARMACOLOGY

Five classes of calcium channel antagonists are in clinical use (Table 35-1), although verapamil, diltiazem, and members of the dihydropyridine class have been the most frequently employed clinically. Examples of the structures of these agents are shown in Figure 35-1. All share the common property of antagonizing the slow, or so-called L-type, calcium channel. Further discussion of calcium channels follows in the pathophysiology section. Most of these agents

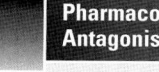

Pharmacokinetics of Calcium Channel Antagonists

Volume of distribution: generally large*
Protein binding: extensive
Removal by extracorporeal techniques: minimal*
Mode of clearance: hepatic metabolism
Active metabolites: generally none†

*See text for exceptions.

†Verapamil and diltiazem have active metabolites, norverapamil and desacetyldiltiazem. These metabolites are significantly less active than are the parent molecules.

have volumes of distribution greater than 2 L/kg, making clinically significant enhanced clearance of these drugs by extracorporeal techniques unfeasible. Exceptions are nicardipine (volume of distribution 0.64 to 1.4 L/kg) and possibly nifedipine (volume of distribution 0.6 to 2.21 L/kg) and nimodipine (volume of distribution 0.94 to 2.5 L/kg). Because these and all other calcium channel antagonists are highly protein bound, however, they are not cleared to any significant degree by hemodialysis. Theoretically the aforementioned agents with relatively low volumes of distribution may be eliminated by other techniques, such as charcoal hemoperfusion.

The pharmacokinetic features of these agents in overdose have not been well characterized. One well-conducted pharmacokinetic investigation of two cases of verapamil overdose found that despite markedly elevated plasma concentrations, the elimination of the parent drug and its primary metabolite norverapamil followed first-order kinetics, suggesting that their metabolism was not saturated in overdose.[1] At verapamil concentrations greater than 2000 ng/mL, the fraction of non–protein bound drug increased to 12% to 15%, which is two to six times the free fraction seen at lower levels.[1] Despite the apparent first-order kinetics, the half-life of elimination of verapamil was prolonged in these cases, an observation made in other cases of verapamil poisoning.[2,3]

PATHOPHYSIOLOGY

Although there are a prodigious number of effects of the calcium channel antagonists, the end organs of greatest importance to their clinical toxicity are the heart and the arterial vasculature. The effects of calcium channel antagonists on

413

TABLE 35-1 Calcium Channel Antagonists

CLASS	AGENT(S)	CLASS EFFECTS		
		Heart Rate	Peripheral Arterial Tone	Cardiac Contractility
Phenylalkylamine	Verapamil	↓	↓	↓↓
Dihydropyridine	Amlodipine	↑	↓↓↓	±
	Felodipine			
	Isradipine			
	Nicardipine			
	Nifedipine			
	Nimodipine			
	Nitrendipine			
	Nisoldipine			
Benzothiazepine	Diltiazem	−/↓	↓↓	↓↓
Diphenylpiperazine or tetralene	Mibefradil*	↓	↓↓	−/↓
Diarylaminopropylamine or diarylaminopropylether	Bepridil	↓	↓	↓

*Withdrawn from the market in many countries because of numerous severe cytochrome P-450–related drug interactions. Mibefradil was unique among calcium channel antagonists in that it blocked the T and the L calcium channel.

these two organs differ among the various classes of agents (see Table 35-1). The selectivity of the various agents, in terms of their clinical effects, may derive from their tissue-dependent differential binding to L-type channels.[4,5] Verapamil tends to bind nonselectively to vascular and cardiac tissue L-type calcium channels, whereas the dihydropyridine class binds primarily to tissue L-type calcium channels in vascular tissue.

There are five different types of voltage-gated calcium channels, designated *L, T, P, Q,* and *N.* The L-type (or long-lasting) channel is found primarily on the heart, arterial smooth muscle, and pancreatic beta cells, although it is present on a diverse group of other organs.[6] It is the largest channel and is the slowest to undergo inactivation when opened—hence the designation *slow* calcium channel. The T-type (or transient) calcium channel is the fastest to become inactivated and is found on cardiac nodal and conducting cells. The P-type channel is found on cerebellar Purkinje cells. Q-type channels are similar to P channels. The N-type (or neuronal) calcium channel is found on neurons. The calcium channel antagonists inhibit calcium influx through the L-type channel, of which there are at least five subclasses.

Normally, there is an enormous concentration gradient of calcium across cell membranes, with serum concentrations in the millimolar range and intracellular free calcium concentration of less than 10^{-7} M. The cell maintains this gradient by allowing calcium influx only through voltage-gated calcium channels, sequestering free calcium in the sarcoplasmic reticulum of muscle cells, and maintaining an adenosine triphosphate (ATP)–driven calcium export pump (Fig. 35-2). When activated by membrane depolarization, the opening of the L-type channel results in an increase in intracellular calcium concentrations to the micromolar, or higher, range.[7]

Pharmaceutical calcium channel antagonists act by binding to the dihydropyridine, or the α_{1c} receptor on the L-type calcium channel (Fig. 35-3). The exact binding site of the α_{1c} subunit for the various classes of calcium channel antagonists varies.[6]

In the cardiac myocyte, or smooth muscle cell, the resulting increased intracellular calcium concentration initiates a cascade that results in muscle concentration (see Fig. 35-2). This process is reversed by the active reuptake of calcium into the sarcoplasmic reticulum. In contrast to skeletal muscle, most of the calcium for cardiac myocyte or smooth muscle relaxation comes from influx through the L-type calcium channel.[8] Calcium channel antagonists have little effect on skeletal muscle.

The L-type calcium channel is activated when phosphorylated by intracellular protein kinases (Fig. 35-4; see Fig. 35-3), which are stimulated by cyclic adenosine monophosphate (cAMP), the mediator of effects caused by agonism at cardiac β-receptors (see Fig. 34-2). Phosphorylation of the calcium channel occurs with each depolarization. This site of phosphorylation is the regulatory subunit of the calcium channel, called *phospholamban.*[7]

In contrast to cardiac myocytes, the nodal cell's resting potential is due to a calcium gradient, not a sodium gradient. The spontaneous depolarization of the sinoatrial and atrioventricular nodes is due to slow calcium influx through L-type channels.[9]

Cardiac Effects

Calcium channel antagonists affect both the myocardium and cardiac pacemaker cells. These effects are seen primarily with the phenylalkylamine and benzothiazepine classes of agents and less commonly with toxicity from the dihydropyridines. The effects of the cardioactive calcium channel antagonists are exerted on the cardiac pacemaker cells and on the myocardium itself. As described earlier, cardiac pacemaker cells, such as those that make

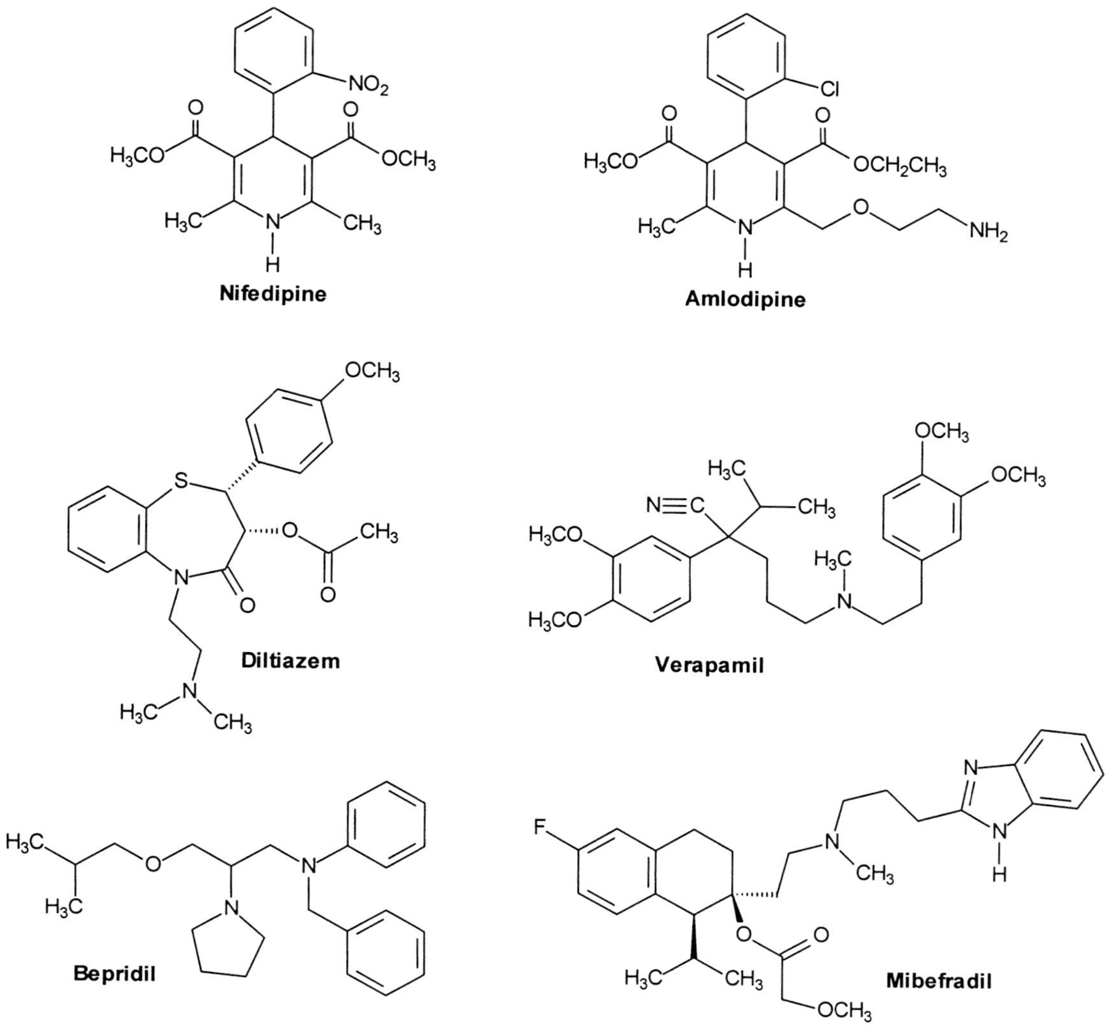

FIGURE 35-1

Chemical structures of representative calcium channel antagonists, including the dihydropyridines, nifedipine and amlodipine; the benzothiazepine, diltiazem; the phenylalkylamine, verapamil; the diarylaminopropylamine, bepridil; and the tetrate, mibefradil.

up the atrioventricular node, spontaneously depolarize as a result of a slow inward calcium flux. Inhibition of this calcium influx by calcium channel antagonists reduces the rate of pacemaker cell depolarization and, in cases of severe toxicity, can cause a complete arrest of this process.

The myocardium itself uses calcium through the action of voltage-dependent calcium channels that allow for calcium influx during phase II of the myocardial action potential, which is necessary for myocardial excitation-contraction coupling (see Fig. 35-2). The calcium influx that occurs at this time triggers further increases in intracellular free calcium concentrations by stimulating the sodium-calcium exchange pump on the myocardial cell membrane and by causing release of stored sarcolemmal calcium. The combined result is a sharp increase in intracellular calcium concentration, which leads to increased calcium binding to tropomyosin. Tropomysin, a negative modulator of excitation-contraction coupling, acts by inhibiting the interaction of actin and myosin filaments. After calcium-induced activation of tropomyosin, the actin and myosin filaments are free to interact, causing

muscle contraction. Inhibition of calcium influx results in decreased excitation-contraction coupling, manifested clinically by reduced cardiac inotropy.

Arterial Vasculature

In contrast to skeletal muscle and venous smooth muscle, arterial smooth muscle is highly dependent on external calcium for contraction. This calcium enters arterial myocytes by voltage-gated calcium channels, which, in a manner analogous to that in the heart, causes excitation-contraction coupling and increased arterial vascular tone. Inhibition of arterial smooth muscle calcium channels causes vasodilation. This effect is most marked with the dihydropyridine calcium channel antagonists (e.g., nifedipine).

Pancreatic Effects

Pancreatic insulin release is under the influence of the L-type calcium channel, which may become inhibited at

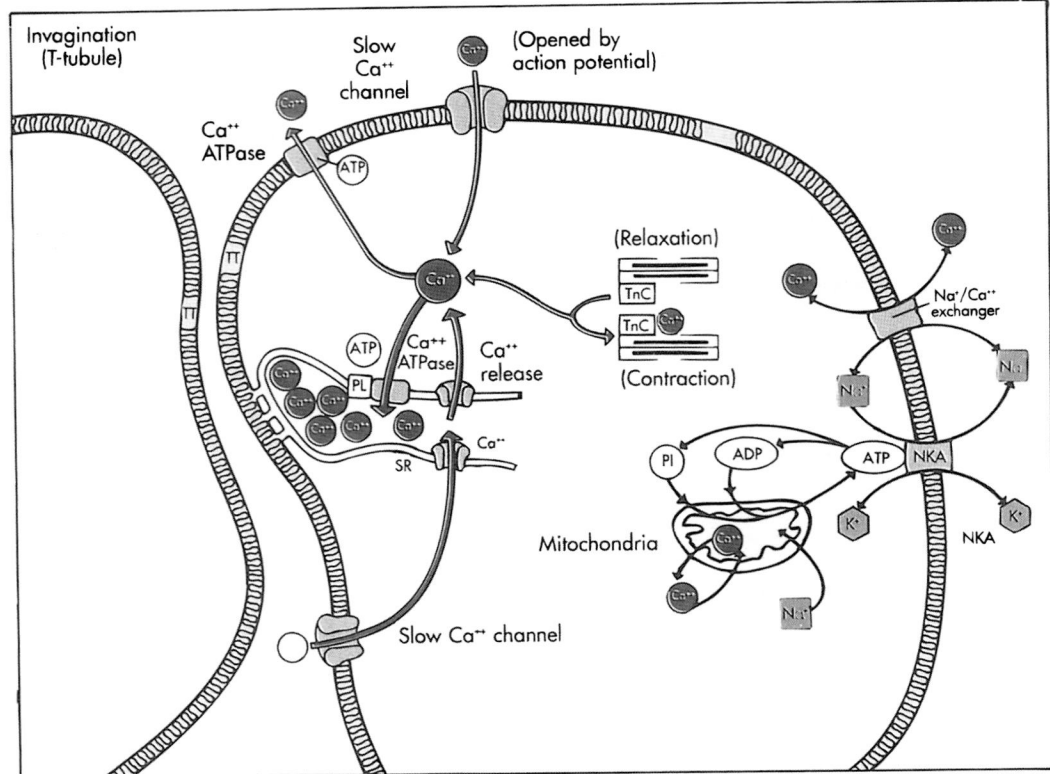

FIGURE 35-2

Ca^{2+} influx through the L-type (or slow) calcium channel results in excitation-contraction coupling in myocardial and arterial smooth muscle. NKA, Na$^+$,K$^+$-ATPase; PL, phospholamban; SR, sarcoplasmic reticulum; TT, T-tubule; TnC, troponin complex. *(From Brody TM, Larner J, Minneman KP [eds]: Human Pharmacology: Molecular to Clinical, 3rd ed. St Louis, Mosby, 1998, p 231.)*

high concentrations of channel blockers and lead to hyperglycemia. A theoretical concern regarding hypoinsulinemia in patients with calcium channel antagonist poisoning is that in shock states the myocardium shifts its substrate preference from free fatty acids to glucose.[10,11] Hypoinsulinemia adversely affects cardiac myocyte glucose uptake, which may be crucial to meeting its energy requirements under these conditions.[12]

Metabolic Effects

Calcium channel antagonism can cause a decrease in mitochondrial calcium intake,[11,13] resulting in a reduction in pyruvate dehydrogenase activity and lactate accumulation.[14] This enzyme is required for pyruvate oxidation and subsequent Krebs cycle metabolism. Inhibition of pyruvate dehydrogenase causes hyperlactatemia.

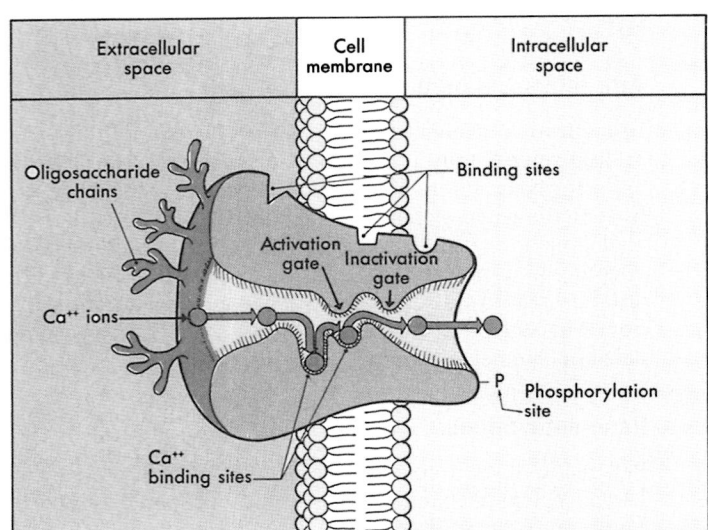

FIGURE 35-3

Schematic L-type Ca^{2+} channel spanning the sarcolemmal membrane. The activation and inactivation gates control the flux of calcium through this channel. Binding sites for calcium channel antagonists, which decrease Ca^{2+} flux through the pore, are depicted. The actions of these channels also are regulated by changes in electrochemical gradient across the sarcolemma. As shown in Figure 35-4, the calcium channel can exist in open, resting, or inactivated states. *(From Brody TM, Larner J, Minneman KP [eds]: Human Pharmacology: Molecular to Clinical, 3rd ed. St Louis, Mosby, 1998, p 229.)*

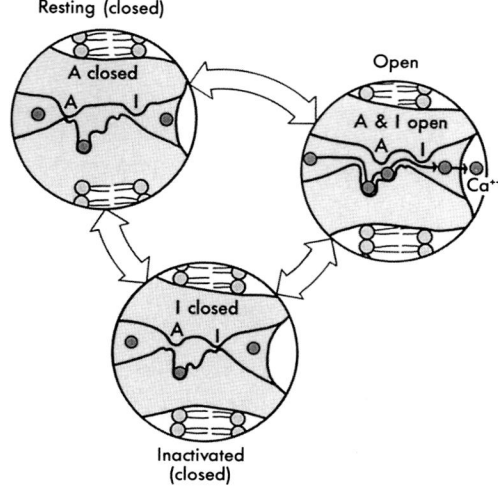

FIGURE 35-4

Depiction of the three states of the calcium channel. In the open state, the activation and inactivation sites (see Fig. 35-3) are open. If either of these two sites is closed, the channel does not permit Ca²⁺ flux. *(From Brody TM, Larner J, Minneman KP [eds]: Human Pharmacology: Molecular to Clinical, 3rd ed. St Louis, Mosby, 1998, p 229.)*

CLINICAL PRESENTATION

Although there are major differences in the effects of the different classes of calcium channel antagonists when used therapeutically, some of these distinctions may be lost in overdose, wherein various pharmacologic actions tend to become clinically amplified. In general, the clinical presentation of calcium channel antagonist toxicity is one of hypotension, sinus node and myocardial depression, atrioventricular block, cardiac arrhythmias, and mental status changes. Other effects that commonly have been described with these agents are respiratory arrest, seizures, gastroenteritis, hyperglycemia, noncardiogenic pulmonary edema, and lactic acidosis.[12,15-18] Of the various calcium channel antagonists, verapamil seems to be associated with the greatest incidence of adverse effects in overdose.[15-18] Effects of intoxication with these agents may be delayed (>6 hours) and prolonged (>24 hours) after the ingestion of sustained-release preparations.[18]

Hypotension

In a prospective case series of 113 hospitalized patients with calcium channel antagonist overdose, hypotension (defined as systolic blood pressure <100 mm Hg) was present in 43%. Systolic blood pressure less than 60 mm Hg was reported in 8% (nine patients).[16] Hypotension occurred in 53% of verapamil overdoses, 32% of nifedipine overdoses, and 38% of diltiazem overdoses.[16] These data are consistent with the plentiful case report data in which verapamil poisoning is relatively overrepresented among patients with hypotension compared with other calcium channel antagonists. Despite nifedipine's vasodilating properties, there were no cases of severe hypotension (systolic blood pressure <60 mm Hg) in the above-described series.[16] Hypotension, caused by either decreased peripheral resist-

ance or cardiac pump failure, should be considered to be a possibility, however, with poisoning by all calcium channel antagonists. The classic peripheral signs of shock (e.g., impaired capillary refill, skin pallor, and coolness on examination) may be absent in patients with significant calcium antagonist–induced hemodynamic instability, particularly when vasodilatory agents in the dihydropyridine class are involved. Other parameters of tissue-organ hypoperfusion (e.g., urine output, acid-base status) should be monitored closely in these patients.

Cardiac Conduction Deficits

Sinus node depression, all degrees of heart block, junctional rhythms, and QT interval prolongation have been reported after calcium channel antagonist intoxication, almost exclusively after verapamil or diltiazem overdoses. Most often, these conditions resolve within the first 24 hours, but they have been reported to persist for 7 days.[16,19]

Cardiac Dysrhythmias

In the major series addressing cardiac dysrhythmias, bradycardia has been reported to occur in 29% of verapamil and diltiazem overdoses and 14% of nifedipine overdoses. One half to two thirds of patients poisoned with the former two agents had heart rates less than 40 beats/min. There were no such cases reported in the same series in nifedipine-poisoned patients.[16]

Sinus tachycardia is a common feature of poisonings by vasodilating (primarily dihydropyridine) calcium channel antagonists, occurring in one series in 57% of nifedipine overdoses, 26% of diltiazem overdoses, and 18% of verapamil poisonings.[16] Tachycardia also has been reported in several case reports of amlodipine overdose,[20,21] possibly secondary to carotid sinus reflex stimulation. In patients with preexisting accessory pathways, such as occur in Wolff-Parkinson-White syndrome, verapamil may cause accelerated conduction through these pathways.[22]

Adult Respiratory Distress Syndrome

Although it is the impression of medical toxicologists that severe calcium channel antagonist poisoning may be accompanied by adult respiratory distress syndrome (ARDS), the true incidence of this complication has not been formally studied, and documentation of its occurrence exists primarily in the form of case reports.[18,20,21,23-30] Several of these cases probably represent cardiogenic pulmonary edema related to aggressive fluid resuscitation in patients who have calcium channel antagonist–induced pump failure. There has been little published documentation, however, of hemodynamic parameters, such as cardiac output, cardiac index, or pulmonary capillary wedge pressure, in these patients. Some of these cases represent true ARDS based on parameters obtained via invasive hemodynamic monitoring.[30] Dilation of prepulmonary capillary or a drug-induced change in alveolar membrane permeability may contribute to the ARDS.[25,31-33] This theory may explain the anecdotal observation that patients with calcium channel antagonist intoxication who have required mechanical ventilatory support, when extubated and subjected to the associated abrupt reduction in thoracic pressure, may have "flash" pulmonary edema.

The incidence of cardiac pump failure after overdoses by calcium channel antagonists has not been determined because it is a notable omission as an end point of series on this topic and is reported only anecdotally. On theoretical grounds, it is expected that pump failure primarily would be a characteristic of poisoning by verapamil and, to a lesser degree, diltiazem.

DIAGNOSIS

The determination of calcium channel antagonist toxicity generally starts with a history of ingestion of these substances. In the absence of such a history, suspicion of toxicity by these medications should arise in a patient who presents with hypotension and other signs of toxic effects of these agents as described earlier, which may be complicated by the diversity of presentation provoked by the different classes and pharmacokinetic formulations of agents. Routine drug screens typically do not detect calcium channel antagonists, and when they do, their interpretation is limited by their qualitative nature. Quantitative calcium channel antagonist determinations are generally available only from commercial reference laboratories and, when they can be obtained, have not been shown to correlate with clinical presentation. When calcium antagonists are present above therapeutic plasma or serum concentrations, however, this provides confirmatory support for the diagnosis of toxicity.

Calcium channel antagonists generally are not considered to be radiopaque, although one case report has suggested that sustained-release verapamil may be detected radiologically.[34] Another case report of fatal overdose with a sustained-released verapamil preparation found a large concretion of this material at autopsy, although it was not seen in abdominal radiographs obtained before death.[35]

TREATMENT

As with all serious poisonings, the initial approach to the treatment of patients with calcium channel antagonist toxicity should be focused on maintaining adequate airway, ventilation, oxygenation, and hemodynamic support. Because these patients may have depressed mentation or evolving ARDS, serious poisonings with these agents often warrant endotracheal intubation and mechanical ventilation. Close monitoring of cardiac rhythm, vital signs, respiratory status, and urine output is fundamental to intensive care unit management. Because some of the manifestations of calcium channel antagonist intoxication may be caused by different mechanisms, additional monitoring and diagnostic modalities may be indicated. Hypotension caused by these poisonings may be the result of decreased cardiac output, systemic vascular resistance (SVR), or both. For some patients, it may be necessary to employ invasive hemodynamic monitoring techniques to distinguish among these possibilities and choose the appropriate therapeutic modality and monitor the efficacy of these treatments.

For a patient who sustains a cardiac arrest, the pathophysiologic changes induced by calcium channel antagonists are potentially completely reversible despite prolonged resuscitations, as exemplified by one patient who was in cardiac arrest for 2.5 hours and recovered fully.[36,37] A patient in cardiac or circulatory arrest should be treated aggressively using the approaches to hypotension, conduction defects, and bradydysrhythmias that are described in this chapter.

If a patient with calcium channel antagonist poisoning presents after acute ingestion, administration of a single dose of oral activated charcoal may decrease peak serum concentrations.[38] In a human volunteer study of sustained-release verapamil ingestion, whole-bowel irrigation did not reduce drug absorption significantly.[38] The gastrointestinal decontamination modality of choice for calcium channel antagonist intoxication is a single dose of activated charcoal.

In a study of volunteers, activated charcoal was effective in reducing gastrointestinal absorption of non–sustained release verapamil if given immediately after ingestion, but not 2 hours later. Activated charcoal significantly reduced the absorption of sustained-release verapamil, however, 4 hours postingestion, the temporal end point of the study.[39] Based on available data, if a sustained-released preparation is ingested, a dose of activated charcoal is indicated, even if given more than 2 hours after ingestion. There are no data supporting the use of whole-bowel irrigation with or without activated charcoal, even for sustained-release calcium channel antagonist ingestions. Because these agents tend to be highly protein bound and have large volumes of distribution, there is no theoretical support for extracorporeal drug elimination in the treatment of their toxicity.

Many modalities typically are employed in the treatment of cardiovascular system impairment associated with these agents. Calcium, glucagon, sympathomimetics, insulin, inamrinone, pacing, and mechanical cardiac assist devices have been used. Empirical attempts to use these various therapeutic modalities are often successful and allow for the cardiovascular support of the patient until clinical toxicity resolves. Empirical treatments can be accomplished often without formal determinations of hemodynamic parameters beyond monitoring vital signs, heart rhythm, urine output, and acid-base status (e.g., base excess). For a patient who does not respond to empirical treatment, however, it is advisable to use invasive hemodynamic monitoring to tailor therapy to the specific pathophysiology of the individual patient. Following is a suggested approach to the therapy of cardiovascular system manifestations of calcium channel antagonist toxicity. These recommendations are the product of my synthesis of the reported pathophysiology of these poisonings, animal data, published anecdotal experience, and personal experience in caring for many patients poisoned by these agents. There are no prospective clinical trials on the treatment of calcium channel antagonist intoxication.

Although ARDS and other complications related to calcium channel antagonist poisoning may occur, their treatment is not discussed in this chapter. These effects usually are

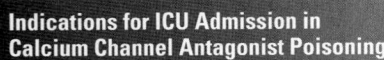

Indications for ICU Admission in Calcium Channel Antagonist Poisoning

Hemodynamic instability
Anticipatorily in cases of (even if minor):
    Decreasing blood pressure
    Decreasing heart rate
    Cardiac conduction disturbances

secondary to the cardiovascular dysfunction induced by these agents, and the clinical approach taken to these complications is not calcium channel antagonist specific. They should be treated by generally recommended supportive approaches (see Chapter 8).

Hypotension

Hypotension should be treated by intravascular volume support and empirical use of parenteral calcium and vasopressors. If there is clinically evident pump failure not responsive to calcium infusion, then insulin-glucose or high-dose glucagon therapy (dose discussed later) may be tried. For continued hypotension not responsive to these interventions, placement of a Swan-Ganz catheter is indicated to determine whether the patient's hemodynamic instability is due primarily to depressed inotropy, decreased SVR, or both. Pressor agents such as dobutamine, phosphodiesterase inhibitors, or left ventricular assist devices also may be used. In the extreme case in which the patient is refractory to all of these interventions, temporary cardiopulmonary bypass may be an effective stabilizing measure. For patients with depressed SVR unresponsive to calcium and an initial trial of sympathomimetics, further increase in the infusion rates of the latter also may be effective. A discussion of some of these therapeutic modalities follows. Figure 35-5 is a suggested algorithm for the treatment of calcium channel antagonist–induced hypotension.

CALCIUM

Given that the fundamental pathophysiology of calcium channel antagonist toxicity is an inhibition of calcium flux into target tissues, it seems intuitive that calcium supplementation would be effective treatment, and to a significant degree, relevant data bear this out. Most animal studies of calcium channel antagonist intoxication have shown the beneficial effect of calcium chloride administration on hypotension from these agents.[40–43]

Controlled studies with human subjects pretreated with intravenous calcium followed by verapamil showed that calcium prevented the development of hypotension.[44] The data on calcium administration in patients poisoned by these agents are uncontrolled and anecdotal, however. Several case reports have suggested that calcium administration had a positive effect on calcium channel antagonist–induced hypotension.[17,45,46] In a prospective observational poison control center–based study of 113 patients poisoned by calcium channel antagonists, 22 showed hypotension, of whom 16 (80%) reportedly responded to calcium treatment.[16] Not every patient predictably responds to calcium administration, however.[15–17,47] It is likely that patients who are severely poisoned and patients in whom therapy is started late constitute the population that may be refractory to calcium therapy of their hypotension.[47] Insufficient doses of calcium are another potential explanation for apparent nonresponders.[48]

Calcium concentrations typically are expressed in mg/dL or mmol/L; 1 mg/dL is equivalent to 0.25 mmol/L. Because calcium is a divalent cation, 1 mmol is equivalent to 2 mEq. The use of calcium chloride ($CaCl_2$) in the treatment of calcium channel antagonist toxicity is preferable to calcium gluconate because the former has approximately three times the molar calcium concentration of the latter. There are 13.6 mEq (or 270 mg) of calcium in 10 mL of 10% $CaCl_2$ compared with 4.6 mEq (90 mg) in an equivalent ampule of calcium gluconate; 10 mL of 10% $CaCl_2$ or calcium gluconate contains 1 g of the respective salt. The 13.6 mEq/L of $CaCl_2$ means that calcium constitutes 27% of the chloride versus 9% in the 4.6 mEq of calcium gluconate.

There are no uniformly accepted infusion protocols for calcium administration in this setting. I endorse an aggressive calcium administration protocol of 10% $CaCl_2$ administered at a rate of 10 mL over 2 to 3 minutes, repeated until an adequate clinical response is obtained, QT narrowing is observed, or more than doubling of ionized serum calcium occurs.[48] Patients receiving this regimen should be on a continuous cardiac monitor. If the patient stabilizes after this treatment, a maintenance infusion of 10% $CaCl_2$ at 10 mL/hr could be administered. Doses of 30 g of calcium preparation in less than 12 hours have resulted in only a transient rise in serum calcium concentrations and no evidence of clinical hypercalcemia.[18,46,49] Nevertheless, patients who are receiving calcium infusions should be monitored for hypotension, bradydysrhythmias, and conduction disturbances.[50] The pediatric dose is 0.2 mL/kg of 10% $CaCl_2$ or 1 mL/kg of calcium gluconate. Further calcium doses should be appropriately reduced in pediatric cases.

Animal studies have shown that the treatment of severe toxicity may require a doubling of serum calcium concentrations.[42,45] Lam and Lau[45] reported a case of a patient with severe refractory hypotension from a nifedipine overdose who responded to calcium administration when the patient's ionized serum calcium increased from 1.14 mmol/L to approximately 2 mmol/L. The accumulated human experience has not verified the need for this magnitude of increment in serum calcium, however. More marked increase in ionized serum calcium caused a decline in cardiac contractility and index in a swine model of diltiazem poisoning.[50] It may be imprudent to allow the ionized serum calcium to exceed 2 mmol/L. Because of the caustic nature of $CaCl_2$, it is preferable that it be administered through a large, and ideally central, line.

SYMPATHOMIMETICS

Vasopressors constitute a diverse group of agents, consisting primarily of dopamine, norepinephrine, epinephrine, dobutamine, isoproterenol, and phenylephrine (see Appendix B). Each has its unique physiologic properties, which render it potentially useful under various clinical circumstances. Ideally, it is advantageous to determine whether the hypotension after calcium channel–blocker intoxication is due to myocardial depression or vasodilation. An empirical trial of dopamine frequently increases blood pressure and cardiac output in patients poisoned by different members of this class,[16,51,52] however, and constitutes a reasonable first step in treatment of hemodynamic instability. Patients who do not respond to an initial trial of dopamine should have calcium therapy instituted as described in the prior section. Patients who do not respond to either of these interventions are best managed using invasive hemodynamic monitoring to determine cardiac index, filling pressure, and SVR. Patients with myocardial depression seem to benefit most from agents with β-adrenergic activity, such as intermediate-dose dopamine (see Appendix B) or dobutamine. Isoproterenol, the most potent β-agonist of this group, has been used successfully in animal models,[53]

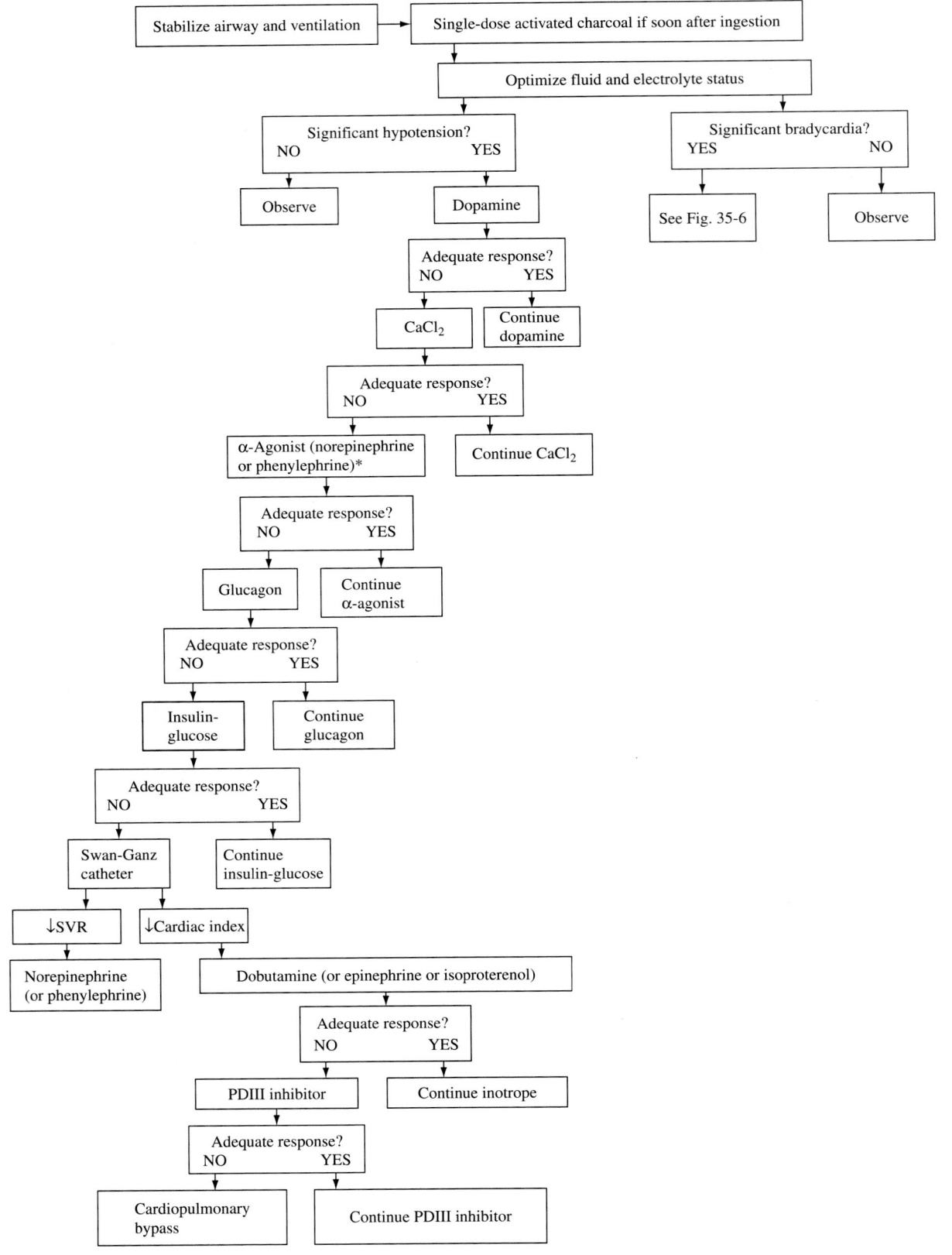

FIGURE 35-5

Recommended algorithm for treatment of calcium channel antagonist–induced hypotension. Use of this algorithm presumes that airway management and ventilatory support, if needed, have been initiated. This algorithm also presumes that a dose of activated charcoal has been administered, if warranted, and fluid and electrolyte status is being optimized. See text for details. $CaCl_2$, calcium chloride; Norepi, norepinephrine; PDIII, phosphodiesterase III; SVR, systemic vascular resistance.

*May also add a potent β-agonist (i.e., isoproterenol or epinephrine) at this stage for verapamil or diltiazem overdose.

although evidence for its efficacy in humans is only anecdotal. There is concern for the arrhythmogenic and myocardial ischemic effects of isoproterenol. Theoretically, dobutamine is a better inotropic support agent; however, there is little experience with it in the treatment of calcium channel–blocker intoxication, and patients treated with this agent should be monitored for vasodilation. Epinephrine has been shown to increase cardiovascular function in canine models of calcium channel–blocker intoxication.[53,54] Here, too, however, there is concern for its potential to cause vasodilation and a reduction in blood pressure at low doses. Theoretically, it is a useful agent in patients who do not have signs of vasodilation, unless relatively high, non-vasodilating doses are used. Appropriate epinephrine doses are given in Appendix B.

Patients with significantly reduced SVR may benefit from the α_1-agonist actions of norepinephrine or phenylephrine. However, in one animal study of calcium channel antagonist intoxication, increasing SVR with phenylephrine appeared to worsen myocardial depression by increasing afterload.[55] It is possible that some patients may require inotropic support and vasoconstriction; accomplishing this may require the simultaneous administration of two agents with different pharmacologic actions, such as phenylephrine for the latter effect and dobutamine for the former. The ideal approach is empirically based (i.e., directed by the individual patient's response).

GLUCAGON

Glucagon is a 29–amino acid polypeptide hormone secreted by pancreatic beta cells. It has a molecular weight of 3485 d, and its volume of distribution is 0.04 L/kg. Well known for its biologic actions of increasing blood glucose and glycogenolysis, glucagon is also a potentially powerful cardiac inotrope and chronotrope,[56,57] acting at specific cardiac G-protein coupled receptors.[58] When bound to its receptor, glucagon stimulates an increase in cAMP, which leads to an increase in myocardial calcium influx.[59,60]

A study in isolated rat hearts, using a Langendorff preparation poisoned with various calcium channel blockers, showed that glucagon can reverse the depression of dP/dt by these agents. A clinically achievable serum glucagon concentration of 0.5 mmol was required.[60]

Another study in rats showed that glucagon administration antagonizes verapamil-induced hypotension in these animals.[61] Four of five studies employing canine models of verapamil intoxication failed to show a beneficial effect of glucagon on mean arterial pressure.[54,55,62–64] Two of these studies assessed cardiac contractility, and both of these reported a beneficial effect[54,62]; however, in one study,[54] this increase was only transient. Three of these studies evaluated cardiac output, and all showed an increase in this parameter.[54,55,64]

In a canine model of diltiazem toxicity, glucagon was effective in increasing blood pressure.[50] Anecdotally, glucagon has been reported to be effective in the treatment of calcium channel antagonist–induced refractory hypotension.[65]

Dosing of glucagon in various reports has varied from single doses of 2 mg[66] to 17 mg.[16] I recommend a 10-mg (or 0.15 mg/kg) initial bolus. If there is a response to glucagon at this dose, it may be followed by a continuous infusion, given glucagon's half-life of 3 to 6 minutes.[67] A

recommended regimen for continuous infusion of glucagon in this setting is 1 to 5 mg/hr (or 0.05 to 0.1 mg/kg/hr).[68]

INAMRINONE

Inamrinone is an inhibitor of phosphodiesterase III, the phosphodiesterase isoenzyme that is found in vascular and cardiac muscle. Inhibition of phosphodiesterase III prevents the degradation of cAMP, theoretically resulting in enhanced flux of calcium into the cell. The inhibition of this enzyme may be insufficient, however, to increase cAMP concentrations above the threshold required for an inotropic myocardial response.[69] It is questionable whether simply increasing intracellular cAMP is sufficient to generate an inotropic effect.[70] There is the theoretical concern that because inamrinone may up-regulate the dihydropyridine receptor, the potential for antagonism of the calcium channel is increased.[71] This antagonism has not been shown to occur, however, during the short-term treatment relevant to the treatment of acute toxicity.

In a Langendorff preparation of verapamil-poisoned isolated rat hearts, inamrinone appeared to provide little reversal of depressed cardiac inotropy.[61] Several canine studies have shown a potentially beneficial effect of inamrinone on cardiac function, however, in the treatment of verapamil intoxication.[72–75] There is concern that inamrinone may worsen the vasodilation caused by one of these agents; in a canine study of verapamil intoxication, inamrinone increased cardiac index with concomitant reduction in SVR.[75] Based on this type of experimental evidence, inamrinone should be used cautiously, in particular, with the vasodilating dihydropyridine class of calcium channel antagonists.

Several human case reports have suggested that verapamil-induced shock may respond to inamrinone therapy.[76,77] The regimen used in these studies was a 1 mg/kg loading dose followed by an infusion of 3–6 μg/kg/min.

Typically, inamrinone is diluted to a concentration of 1 to 3 mg/mL in normal saline. The initial bolus should be given over 15 minutes. If there is a response, an infusion may be started and titrated to a maximal rate of administration of 15 μg/kg/min. Because inamrinone may cause hypotension, the hemodynamic response should be monitored closely.

INSULIN-GLUCOSE

Insulin is a potential inotrope, particularly when the myocardium is depressed.[54,78] In the setting of calcium channel antagonist intoxication, this effect may be due to the correction of drug-induced metabolic abnormalities of the myocardium. Normally, free fatty acids are the preferred myocardial energy substrate. In a canine model of verapamil toxicity,[10] the change in myocardial preference to carbohydrate as an energy substrate is accompanied by the development of relative insulin resistance.[79,80] After supplemental insulin infusion, the suppressed phosphodiesterase III activity was enhanced, preventing lactate formation and allowing for more efficient myocardial carbohydrate use to meet demands for ATP production.

Insulin also enhances the influx of potassium into the intracellular space, causing hypokalemia and prolonging phase II of the myocardial action potential. During phase II there is calcium influx, and the prolongation of this phase increases intracellular calcium concentrations, promoting increased contractility.[81] In this way, the hypokalemia associated with insulin administration may be beneficial, and it has been suggested that unless it is severe, it should not be treated.[12]

Several canine studies have shown that therapy with insulin and supplemental glucose is effective in the treatment of verapamil intoxication. In this model, animals developed cardiac conduction deficits, decreased dP/dt, and hypotension. Survival was markedly enhanced in animals treated with insulin-glucose compared with animals receiving sham treatment, epinephrine, or glucagon. The increase in survival in the insulin-glucose group was attributable to improved cardiac contractility.[54] In the same model, this enhanced survival was associated with insulin-glucose–induced improvement in carbohydrate uptake and metabolism.[10,80]

Several human case reports[82,83] and case series[12,84] have described patients who seemed to be refractory to other therapies yet showed significant improvements in blood pressure after euglycemic insulin treatment. Failure of this treatment also has been reported, however.[85]

I recommend that an initial insulin dose of 10 U of regular insulin intravenously be followed by infusion of 0.5 U/kg/hr, a rate that can be adjusted based on the patient's response to treatment (Table 35-2). The initial insulin bolus should be accompanied by 25 g of glucose, unless blood glucose is greater than 200 mg/dL (11 mmol/L), following which an infusion of 50% dextrose should be administered at a rate determined by serial blood glucose determinations, which can be accomplished by simple finger-stick methods. These determinations should be done hourly while the patient is receiving glucose treatment. In the series by Yuan and coworkers,[12] the mean maximal dextrose requirement was 28.4 g/hr (range 10 to 75 g/hr). A total of 100 mL of 50% dextrose solution contains 50 g of glucose. Because of its osmolar effects at this concentration, dextrose infusion in this setting should be administered through a central venous line. Given the hyperglycemia that may occur as an associated effect of calcium channel antagonist intoxication, not all patients receiving insulin therapy require dextrose supplementation.[82,84]

MECHANICAL CIRCULATORY SUPPORT

In addition to the pharmacologic measures described earlier, left ventricular assist devices, cardiac pacing, and cardiopulmonary bypass are options for severely poisoned patients. A series of patients[86] with various overdoses requiring pacing included three calcium channel antagonist–poisoned patients who were profoundly bradycardic and hypotensive on presentation, all having nodal bradycardia on electrocardiogram. The interpretation of these cases is complicated because none were pure calcium channel blocker overdoses. Two patients, and possibly the third, also overdosed on β-blockers, and two also ingested nitrates. Two of the three patients responded with an elevation of blood pressure when bradycardia was treated effectively with electrical pacing.

In a porcine model of verapamil intoxication, cardiopulmonary bypass was successful in reversing hypotension and allowed resuscitation when combined with high-dose calcium treatment. Combining cardiopulmonary bypass with epinephrine or glucagon was not demonstrably effective in this model, however.[87] There have been several reports in which cardiopulmonary bypass was attempted after severe verapamil overdoses, although in these cases it was not successful.[87,88] Holzer and colleagues[37] described a case of a 41-year-old man after a massive verapamil overdose who presented in cardiac arrest with pulseless electrical activity and was put on cardiopulmonary bypass 2.5 hours after unsuccessful closed chest compression attempts at resuscitation. After restoration of circulation on bypass, the patient was successfully weaned from this support modality and eventually had a total recovery.

Cardiac Conduction Defects

Most cardiac conduction deficits in calcium channel–blocker poisoning can be managed expectantly as long as adequate tissue perfusion is ensured. In the presence of cardiac conduction abnormalities, it is important to optimize electrolyte status, and in cases of significant bradycardia, improvement in heart rate may have beneficial effects on conduction. The treatment of significant bradycardia is described in the next section.

In one case series involving the use of euglycemic insulin treatment, two patients in third-degree heart block reverted to normal sinus rhythm when therapy was started.[12] It is unclear, however, whether it was the insulin treatment that was responsible for enhancing cardiac conduction.

One study of calcium channel antagonist–poisoned rats showed that in that model, sympathomimetic amines were superior to calcium in the treatment of cardiac conduction disturbances.[41] In the series by Ramoska and associates,[16] isoproterenol administration, although enhancing heart rate, did not seem to affect cardiac conduction. Of the sympathomimetic amines, dopamine, dobutamine, or perhaps even epinephrine might be more appropriate choices.

Several case reports have suggested the efficacy of $CaCl_2$ in the treatment of cardiac conduction disturbances after poisoning with calcium channel antagonists.[46,89,90] Failure of this treatment also has been reported, however.[91] Three studies using canine models of verapamil toxicity[54,55,64] have

---

TABLE 35-2 Suggested Regimen for Insulin-Glucose Therapy

Set up D_{50} IV* (D_{25} for small children*)
Treat initial hypokalemia, if present
Rapid beside capillary blood glucose determination. If <200 mg/dL (11 mmol/L):
    Adults: administer bolus of 25 g of glucose (50 mL D_{50})
    Small children: administer bolus of 0.25 g/kg of glucose (1 mL/kg)
Prepare 1 U/mL IV solution of regular insulin
Give initial insulin bolus of 10 U/mL insulin IV (1 U/mL/kg if <10 kg)
Followed by an infusion of 0.5 U/kg/hr
Adjust infusion rate based on clinical response
Rapid bedside capillary blood glucose determination at least after 0.5 hr and hourly thereafter
Infuse D_{50} (D_{25} for small children) at a rate such that blood glucose maintained in the 150–200 mg/dL range (5.5–11 mmol/L)
Determine serum potassium concentrations hourly for at least 4 hr, then every 2 hr if it has been stable

*Preferentially in a central line because of its high concentration.
D_{50}, 50% dextrose; D_{25}, 25% dextrose.

shown beneficial effects of glucagon on cardiac conduction, although these effects tended to be transient.

Bradydysrhythmias

The suggested approach to the treatment of bradydysrhythmias is given in Figures 35-5 and 35-6. In a canine model of vera-pamil toxicity, atropine was effective in causing a rate response,[53] suggesting that this may be a useful agent for initial stabilization. Repeated administration of atropine may induce an anticholinergic syndrome, however, and should be avoided.

CALCIUM

Animal studies have suggested that $CaCl_2$ administration may not affect heart rate in patients poisoned by calcium channel antagonists.[90] In many case reports, calcium administration was associated with increases in sinoatrial rate, however.[17,46] In one case series, calcium administration was reported to be beneficial in almost two thirds of patients with calcium channel antagonist–induced bradydysrhythmias.[16] Doses of calcium should be the same as those described in the section on the treatment of hypotension.

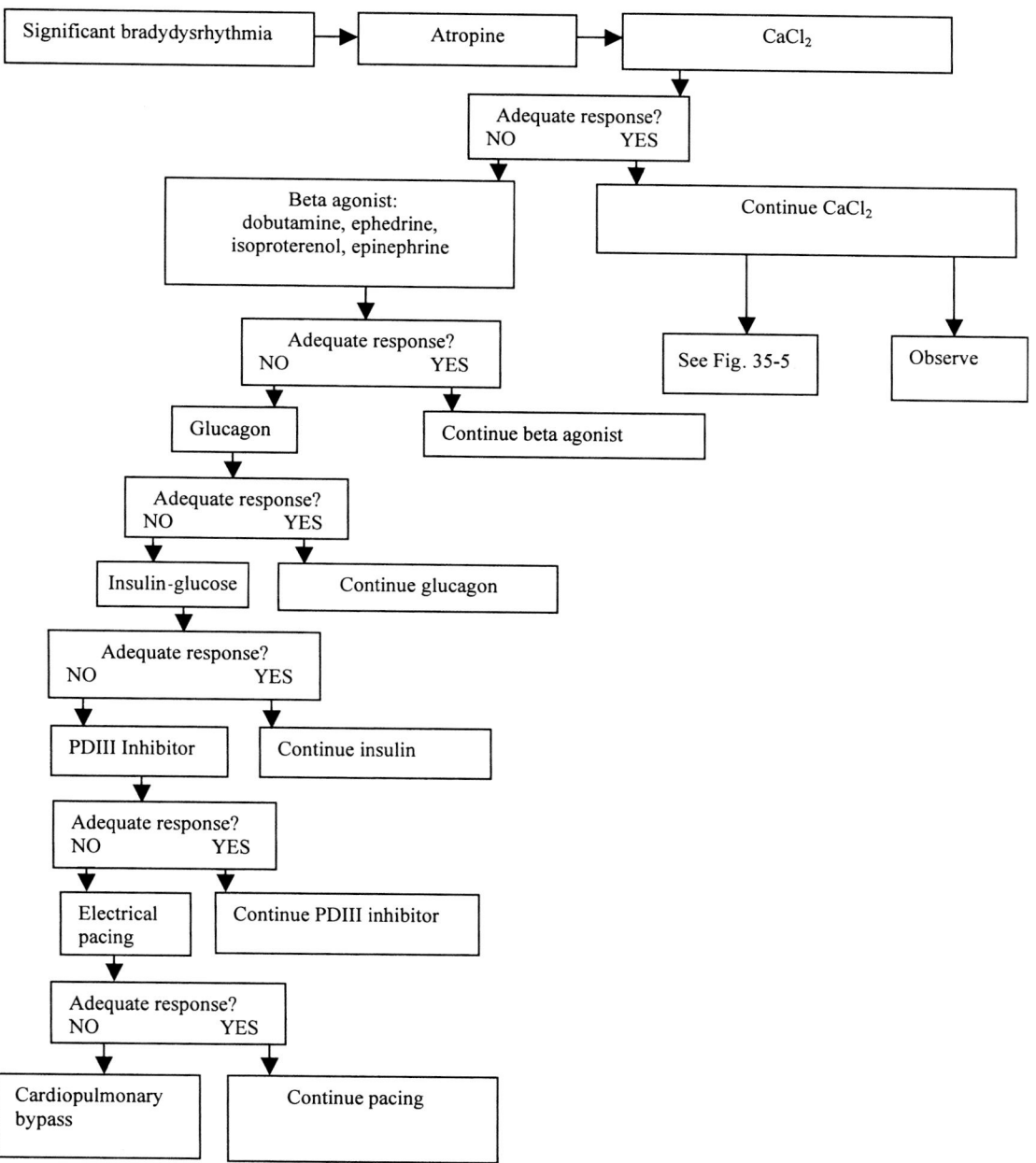

FIGURE 35-6

Recommended algorithm for treatment of calcium channel antagonist–induced bradydysrhythmias. Use of this algorithm presumes that airway manage-ment and ventilatory support, if needed, have been initiated. This algorithm also presumes that a dose of activated charcoal has been administered, if war-ranted, and fluid and electrolyte status is being optimized. $CaCl_2$, calcium chloride; PDIII, phosphodiesterase III.

SYMPATHOMIMETICS

Most of the available data regarding the use of sympathomimetic agents to increase heart rate in bradycardias induced by calcium channel antagonists are from the use of isoproterenol. In a canine model of verapamil intoxication, isoproterenol was effective in increasing heart rate.[53]

The clinical data are extremely limited. In the series of 113 calcium channel antagonist–poisoned patients by Ramoska and associates,[16] isoproterenol was used in only 3 patients, 2 of whom had a rate response. Dopamine was ineffective.

It is expected, based on pharmacodynamic considerations, that agents with β-adrenergic properties would increase heart rate, although because of their β2 effects, they also might cause vasodilation. There is no clinically useful, completely selective β1-adrenergic agonist. β-Adrenergic agents that are viable candidates for use in calcium channel antagonist poisoning are dobutamine, ephedrine, and isoproterenol. Because of the possibility of vasodilation with these agents, it is important to monitor blood pressure or SVR closely when these agents are used. If there is a good rate response but unacceptable vasodilation, it may be beneficial to add an α-adrenergic vasoconstricting agent, such as norepinephrine or phenylephrine, to the treatment regimen.

GLUCAGON

There is little published clinical experience with glucagon in the treatment of calcium channel antagonist–induced bradydysrhythmias. In a Langendorf preparation of a rat heart poisoned with verapamil, glucagon was effective in increasing heart rate.[92] Similarly, several animal studies with rodents[61,93] and dogs[54,55,63,64] reported that glucagon reverses verapamil-induced bradycardias. Anecdotal data suggest that glucagon may be effective in the treatment of bradydysrhythmias,[77] although there is little experience with its use as the sole agent.

INSULIN-EUGLYCEMIA

Several reports have described patients who have responded to insulin treatment for calcium channel antagonist–induced bradycardias.[12,82]

INAMRINONE

There is little experience with the use of phosphodiesterase III inhibitors in the treatment of bradydysrhythmias.

CARDIAC PACING

Cardiac pacing has been reported to be effective in patients with bradydysrhythmias induced by calcium channel antagonists.[16,86] It has been reported in some patients with high-degree atrioventricular nodal block, however, that pacemaker capture may not occur.[16]

Criteria for ICU Discharge in Calcium Channel Antagonist Poisoning

Stable hemodynamic status
Resolution of adult respiratory distress syndrome

SPECIAL POPULATIONS

Pediatric Patients

There have been two retrospective case series of pediatric calcium channel antagonist ingestions. One involved only 29 cases.[94] The second study comprised 283 patients of mean age 27 months (range 8 months to 6 years).[95] The first study called attention to the potential seriousness of sustained-release calcium channel antagonist ingestions in children. In the larger study, 61% of the cases involved this type of formulation. Even the larger study by Belson and colleagues[95] is limited, however, in the amount of information available because it was simply an analysis of data available to one poison control center over a 6-year period. Much about patient history, presentation, and clinical course is unknown. Little information can be gleaned about therapeutic options in children based on these studies, and in the absence of other data, they should be treated in the same fashion as adults. Because pediatric cases often involve relatively small doses or questionable exposures, younger pediatric patients frequently never develop clinical manifestations of toxicity, in contrast to older patients who have ingested substantial amounts as an intentional overdose. The Belson study data suggest that an observation period of 3 hours is sufficient for children with a history of ingestion of regular-release formulations. An observation period of 18 hours may be sufficient for children who may have ingested a sustained-release preparation formulation.

Common Errors in Calcium Channel Antagonist Poisoning

Resorting to whole-bowel irrigation despite its lack of documented efficacy for reducing calcium channel antagonist absorption

Resorting to whole-bowel irrigation despite its lack of documented efficacy for reducing sustained-release preparations of calcium channel antagonists

Failing to recognize when invasive hemodynamic monitoring is indicated

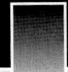

Key Points in Calcium Channel Antagonist Poisoning

1. Calcium channel antagonists induce a syndrome primarily characterized by
   Hypotension
   Bradydysrhythmia
   Cardiac conduction disturbances
2. The above triad may not be present in all patients.
3. Treatment options are the following:
   Administration of pressors, glucagon, calcium chloride, or insulin-glucose
   Phosphodiesterase inhibition
   Pacing
   Cardiopulmonary bypass
4. These agents are not removed effectively by hemodialysis.

REFERENCES

1. Kivisto KT, Neuvonen PJ, Tarssanen L: Pharmacokinetics of verapamil in overdose. Hum Exp Toxicol 16:35–37, 1997.
2. Buckley CD, Aronson JK: Prolonged half-life of verapamil in a case of overdose: Implications for therapy. Br J Clin Pharmacol 39:680–683, 1995.
3. Sauder P: Acute verapamil poisoning: Six cases. J Toxicol Clin Exp 10:261–270, 1990.
4. Morel N, Buryi V, Feron O, et al: The action of calcium channel blockers on recombinant L-type calcium channel alpha1-subunits. Br J Pharmacol 125:1005–1012, 1998.
5. Soldatov NM, Bouron A, Reuter H: Different voltage-dependent inhibition by dihydropyridines of human Ca^{2+} channel splice variants. J Biol Chem 270:10540–10543, 1995.
6. Abernathy DR, Schwartz JB: Calcium-antagonist drugs. N Engl J Med 341:1447–1457, 1999.
7. Morgan JP: Abnormal intracellular modulation of calcium as a major cause of cardiac contractile dysfunction. N Engl J Med 325:625–632, 1991.
8. Hope RR, Lazzora R: The clinical uses of calcium antagonists. Adv Intern Med 27:435–452, 1982.
9. Braunwald E: Mechanism of action of calcium-channel blocking agents. N Engl J Med 307:1618–1627, 1983.
10. Kline JS, Leonova E, Raymond RM: Beneficial myocardial metabolic effects of insulin during verapamil toxicity in the anesthetized canine. Crit Care Med 23:1251–1263, 1995.
11. Buss WC, Savage DD, Stepanek J, et al: Effect of calcium channel antagonists on calcium uptake and release by isolated rat cardiac mitochondria. Eur J Pharmacol 152:247–253, 1988.
12. Yuan TH, Kerns WP 2nd, Tomaszewski WP, et al: Insulin-glucose as adjunctive therapy for severe calcium channel antagonist poisoning. J Toxicol Clin Toxicol 37:463–474, 1999.
13. Rafael J, Patzelt J: Binding of diltiazem and verapamil to isolated rat heart mitochondria. Basic Res Cardiol 82:246–251, 1987.
14. McCormack JG, Cromptom M: The role and study of mammalian mitochondrial calcium transport and matrix calcium. In McCormack JG, Cobbold PH (eds): Cellular Calcium. New York, Oxford University Press, 1991, pp 345–382.
15. Ramoska EA, Spiller HA, Myers A: Calcium channel blocker toxicity. Ann Emerg Med 19:649–655, 1990.
16. Ramoska EA, Spiller HA, Winter M, et al: A one-year evaluation of calcium channel blocker overdoses: toxicity and treatment. Ann Emerg Med 22:196–200, 1993.
17. Pearigen PD, Benowitz NL: Poisoning due to calcium antagonists: Experience with verapamil, diltiazem and nifedipine. Drug Saf 6:408–430, 1991.
18. Howarth DM, Dawson AH, Smith AJ, et al: Calcium channel blocking drug overdose: An Australia series. Hum Exp Toxicol 13:161–166, 1994.
19. Quezado A, Lippmann M, Wertheimer J: Severe cardiac, respiratory, and metabolic complications of massive verapamil overdose. Crit Care Med 19:436–438, 1991.
20. Stanek EJ, Nelson CE, DeNofrio D: Amlodipine overdose. Ann Pharmacother 31:853–855, 1997.
21. Cosbey SH, Carson DJL: A fatal case of amlodipine poisoning. J Analyt Toxicol 21:221–222, 1997.
22. McGovern B, Garan H, Ruskin JN: Precipitation of cardiac arrest by verapamil in patients with Wolff-Parkinson-White syndrome. Ann Intern Med 104:791–794, 1986.
23. Snook CP, Sigvaldson K, Kristinsson J: Severe atenolol and diltiazem overdose. Clin Toxicol 38:661–665, 2000.
24. Satchithananda DK, Stone DL, Chauhan A, et al: Unrecognized accidental overdose with diltiazem. BMJ 321:160–161, 2000.
25. Humbert VH Jr, Munn JN, Hawkins RF: Noncardiogenic pulmonary edema complicating massive diltiazem overdose. Chest 99:258–259, 1991.
26. Spurlock BW, Virani NA, Henry CA: Verapamil overdose. West J Med 154:208–211, 1991.
27. Leesar MA, Martyn R, Talley JD, et al: Noncardiogenic pulmonary edema complicating massive verapamil overdose. Chest 105:606–607, 1994.
28. Ori Y, Korzets A, Caneti M, et al: Lymphocytic intracellular calcium in a patient with complicated verapamil overdose. Am J Med Sci 319:63–67, 2000.
29. Szekely LA, Thompson BT, Woolf A: Use of partial liquid ventilation to manage pulmonary complications of acute verapamil-sustained release poisoning. Clin Toxicol 37:475–479, 1999.
30. Harchelroad F: ARDS associated with calcium channel blocker overdose. Vet Hum Toxicol 34:328, 1992.
31. Low RI, Takeda P, Mason DT, et al: The effects of calcium channel blocking agents on cardiovascular function. Am J Cardiol 49:547–553, 1982.
32. Payne DK, Fuseler JW, Owens MW: Modulation of endothelial cell permeability by lung carcinoma cells: A potential mechanism of malignant pleural effusion formation. Inflammation 18:407–417, 1994.
33. Simon RP: Neurogenic pulmonary edema. Neurol Clin 11:309–323, 1993.
34. Linowiecki KA, Tillman DJ, Ruggles D, et al: Radiopacity of modified release cardiac medications: A case report and in vitro analysis (Abstract). Vet Hum Toxicol 34:350, 1992.
35. Sporer KA, Manning JJ: Massive ingestion of sustained-release verapamil with a concretion and bowel infarction. Ann Emerg Med 22:603–605, 1993.
36. Romano MJ, Gaylor A, Sang CH Jr: Life-threatening isradipine poisoning in a child. Pharmacotherapy 22:766–770, 2002.
37. Holzer M, Sterz F, Schoerkhuber W, et al: Successful resuscitation of a verapamil-intoxicated patient with percutaneous cardiopulmonary bypass. Crit Care Med 27:2818–2823, 1999.
38. Lapatto-Reiniluoto O, Kivisto KT, Neuvonen PJ: Efficacy of activated charcoal versus gastric lavage half an hour after ingestion of moclobemide, temazepam, and verapamil. Eur J Clin Pharmacol 56:285–288, 2000.
39. Laine K, Kivisto KT, Neuvonen PJ: Effect of delayed administration of activated charcoal on the absorption of conventional and slow-release verapamil. Clin Toxicol 37:263–268, 1997.
40. Bania TC, Blaufeux B, Hughes S, et al: Calcium and digoxin vs calcium alone for severe verapamil toxicity. Acad Emerg Med 7:1089–1096, 2000.
41. Strubelt O, Diederich KW: Experimental investigations on the antidotal treatment of nifedipine overdosage. J Toxicol Clin Toxicol 24:135–149, 1986.
42. Hariman RJ, Mangiardi LM, McAllister RG, et al: Reversal of the cardiovascular effects of verapamil by calcium and sodium: Differences between electrophysiologic and hemodynamic responses. Circulation 59:797–804, 1979.
43. Spivey WH, Schoffstall JM, Gambone L, et al: Effects of calcium channel blocker-induced hypotension on systemic hemodynamics in the conscious dog, with evaluation of antidotes (Abstract). Ann Emerg Med 18:915, 1989.
44. Jameson SJ, Hargarten SW: Calcium pretreatment to prevent verapamil-induced hypotension in patients with SVT. Ann Emerg Med 21:84, 1992.
45. Lam Y-M, Lau C: Continuous calcium chloride infusion for massive nifedipine overdose. Chest 119:1280–1282, 2001.
46. Luscher TF, Noll G, Sturmer T, et al: Calcium gluconate in severe verapamil intoxication. N Engl J Med 330:718–720, 1994.
47. Crump JD, Hold DW, Vale JA: Lack of response to intravenous calcium in severe verapamil poisoning. Lancet 939–940, 1982.
48. Buckley NA, Whyte IM, Dawson AH: Overdose with calcium channel blockers. BMJ 308:1639, 1994.
49. Haddad LM: Resuscitation after nifedipine overdose exclusively with intravenous calcium chloride. Am J Emerg Med 14:602–603, 1996.
50. Ross M, Sorenson E, Matyunas N: Treatment of experimental diltiazem poisoning with continuous infusion of calcium chloride and glucagon. J Toxicol Clin Toxicol 35:535, 1997.
51. Enyeart JJ, Price WA, Hoffman DA, et al: Profound hyperglycemia and metabolic acidosis after verapamil overdose. J Am Coll Cardiol 2:1228–1231, 1983.
52. Passal DB, Crespin FH: Verapamil poisoning in an infant. Pediatrics 73:543–544, 1984.
53. Gay RG, Alego S, Lee R, et al: Treatment of verapamil toxicity in intact dogs. J Clin Invest 77:1805–1811, 1986.
54. Kline JA, Tomaszewski CA, Schroeder JD, et al: Insulin is a superior antidote for cardiovascular toxicity induced by verapamil in the anesthetized canine. J Pharmacol Exp Ther 267:744–750, 1993.
55. Stone CB, Thomas SH, Koury SI, et al: Glucagon and phenylephrine combination vs glucagon alone in experimental verapamil overdose. Acad Emerg Med 3:120–125, 1996.
56. Hall-Boyer K, Zaloga GP, Chernow B: Glucagon: Hormone or therapeutic agent? Crit Care Med 12:584, 1984.
57. Glick G, Parmsley WW, Wechsler AS, et al: Glucagon: Its enhancement of cardiac performance in the cat and dog and persistence of its action despite beta-receptor blockade with propranolol. Circ Res 22:789–799, 1968.

58. Farah AE: Glucagon and the circulation. Pharmacol Rev 35:181, 1983.

59. Chernow B, Zaloga GP, Malcolm D, et al: Glucagon's chronotropic action is calcium-dependent. J Pharmacol Exp Ther 241:833, 1987.

60. Zaritsky AL, Horowitz M, Chernow B: Glucagon antagonism of calcium channel blocker-induced myocardial dysfunction. Crit Care Med 16:246–251, 1988.

61. Tuncok Y, Apaydin S, Kalkan S, et al: The effects of amrinone and glucagon on verapamil-induced cardiovascular toxicity in anesthetized rats. Int J Exp Pathol 77:207–212, 1996.

62. Jolly SR, Kipnis JN, Lucchesi BR: Cardiovascular depression by verapamil: Reversal by glucagon and interactions with propranolol. Pharmacology 35:249–255, 1987.

63. Sabatier J, Pouyet T, Shelvey G: Antagonistic effects of epinephrine, glucagon and methylatropine but not calcium chloride against atrioventricular conduction disturbances produced by high doses of diltiazem, in conscious dogs. Fundam Clin Pharmacol 5:93–106, 1991.

64. Stone CK, May WA, Carroll R: Treatment of verapamil overdose with glucagon in dogs. Ann Emerg Med 25:369–374, 1995.

65. Fant JS, James LP, Fiser RT, et al: The use of glucagon in nifedipine poisoning complicated by clonidine ingestion. Pediatr Emerg Care 13:417–419, 1997.

66. Anthony T, Jastremski M, Elliot W, et al: Charcoal hemoperfusion for the treatment of a combined diltiazem and metoprolol overdose. Ann Emerg Med 15:1344–1348, 1986.

67. Parmsley WW, Glick G, Sonnenblick EH: Cardiovascular effects of glucagon in man. N Engl J Med 279:12–17, 1968.

68. Bailey B: Glucagon in β-blocker and calcium channel blocker overdoses: A systematic review. J Toxicol Clin Toxicol 41:595–602, 2003.

69. Tenor H, Bartel S, Krause EG: Cyclic nucleotide phosphodiesterase activity in the rat myocardium: Evidence of four different PDE subtypes. Biomed Biochim Acta 46:S749–753, 1987.

70. Frangakis CJ, Lanni C, Lasher KP, et al: The role of cyclic AMP and the dihydropyridine-sensitive channels on the mechanism of action of milrinone (Corotrope). J Cardiovasc Pharmac 13:915–925, 1989.

71. Rump AFE, Acar D, Klaus W: A quantitative comparison of the phosphodiesterase-inhibitors, amrinone, milrinone and levosimendan in rabbit isolated hearts. Br J Pharmacol 112:757–762, 1994.

72. Alousi AA, Canter JM, Fort DJ: The beneficial effect of amrinone on acute drug-induced heart failure in the anaesthetized dog. Cardiovasc Res 19:483–494, 1985.

73. Koury SI, Stone CK, Thomas SH: Amrinone as an antidote in experimental verapamil overdose. Acad Emerg Med 3:762–767, 1996.

74. Mahr NC, Valdes A, Lamas G: Use of glucagon for acute intravenous diltiazem toxicity. Am J Cardiol 79:1570–1571, 1997.

75. Makela VHM, Kapur PA: Amrinone and verapamil-propranolol induced cardiac depression during isoflurane anesthesia in dogs. Anesthesiology 66:792–797, 1987.

76. Goenen M, Col J, Compere A, et al: Treatment of severe verapamil poisoning with combined amrinone-isoproterenol therapy. Am J Cardiol 58:1142–1143, 1986.

77. Wolf LR, Spadafora MP, Otten EJ: Use of amrinone and glucagon in a case of calcium channel blocker overdose. Ann Emerg Med 22:1225–1228, 1993.

78. Farah AE, Alousi AA: Minireview: The actions of insulin on cardiac contractility. Life Sci 29:975–1000, 1981.

79. Kline JA, Raymond RM, Leonova E, et al: Insulin improves heart function and metabolism during non-ischemic cardiogenic shock in awake canines. Cardiovasc Res 34:289–298, 1997.

80. Kline JA, Raymond RM, Schroeder JD, et al: The diabetogenic effects of acute verapamil poisoning. Toxicol Appl Pharmacol 145:357–362, 1997.

81. Thomas LJ: Increase in labeled calcium uptake in heart muscle during potassium lack. J Gen Physiol 43:1193–1206, 1960.

82. Boyer EW, Shannon M: Treatment of calcium-channel-blocker intoxication with insulin infusion. N Engl J Med 344:1721–1722, 2001.

83. Meyer M, Stremski E, Scanlon M: Verapamil-induced hypotension reversed with dextrose-insulin. J Toxicol Clin Toxicol 39:500, 2001.

84. Boyer EW, Duic PA, Evans A: Hyperinsulinemia/euglycemia therapy for calcium channel blocker poisoning. Pediatr Emerg Care 18:36–37, 2002.

85. Herbert JX, O'Malley C, Tracey JA, et al: Verapamil overdosage unresponsive to dextrose/insulin therapy. J Toxicol Clin Toxicol 39:293–294, 2001.

86. McGlinchey PG, McNeill AJ: Drug overdoses requiring temporary cardiac pacing: A study of six cases treated at Altnagelvin Hospital, Londonderry. Ulster Med J 67:13–18, 1998.

87. Martin TG, Tisherman SA, Stein K: Massive diltiazem OD unresponsive to cardiopulmonary bypass. EAPCCT XVI International Congress, Vienna, 1994.

88. Hendren WG, Schiebere RS, Garrettson LK: Extracorporeal bypass for the treatment of verapamil poisoning. Ann Emerg Med 18:984–987, 1989.

89. Harlman RJ, Manglardi LM, McAllister RG, et al: Reversal of the cardiovascular effects of verapamil by Ca and Na: Differences between electrophysiologic and hemodynamic responses. Circulation 59:797–804, 1979.

90. Vick JA, Kandil A, Herman EH, et al: Reversal of propranolol and verapamil toxicity by calcium. Vet Hum Toxicol 25:8–10, 1983.

91. Horowitz BZ, Rheo KJ: Massive verapamil ingestion: A report of two cases and a review of the literature. Am J Emerg Med 7:624–631, 1989.

92. Tuncok Y, Apaydin S, Gidener S, et al: The effects of amrinone and glucagon on verapamil-induced myocardial depression in a rat isolated heart model. Gen Pharmacol 28:773–776, 1997.

93. Zaloga GP, Malcolm D, Holaday J, et al: Glucagon reversed the hypotension and bradycardia of verapamil overdose in rats. Crit Care Med 13:273, 1985.

94. Brayer AF, Wax P: Accidental ingestion of sustained release calcium channel blockers in children. Vet Hum Toxicol 40:104–106, 1998.

95. Belson MG, Gorman SE, Sullivan K, et al: Calcium channel blocker ingestions in children. Am J Emerg Med 18:581–586, 2000.

CHAPTER 36

Sodium Channel–Blocking Antidysrhythmics

Paul Kolecki

Many antidysrhythmic agents block myocardial sodium channels as their main pharmacologic action. Class I antidysrhythmics are classic examples of agents that act in accordance with this pharmacologic mechanism.[1] However, other antidysrhythmics (e.g., propafenone and propranolol), as well as a variety of other drugs, including antidepressants (e.g., amitriptyline), antihistamines (e.g., diphenhydramine), anticonvulsants (e.g., carbamazepine), and narcotic analgesics (e.g., propoxyphene), also possess sodium channel–blocking properties.[2,3] Poisoning by any sodium channel–blocking antidysrhythmic agent is potentially life-threatening inasmuch as myocardial sodium channel blockade can lead to serious intraventricular conduction defects, ventricular arrhythmias, hypotension, and bradydysrhythmias.[4] Poisoning by these agents may also produce morbidity and mortality secondary to their other pharmacologic effects.

Important research into the toxicologic properties of sodium channel–blocking antidysrhythmics began in the 1950s, when molar sodium lactate was used to reverse the sodium-blocking effects of quinidine and procainamide.[5] Based on these initial studies, the ability of antidysrhythmic agents to block sodium channels has come to be described as a "quinidine-like" effect. The phrases "membrane-stabilizing effect" and "local anesthetic effect" are also commonly used synonymously with sodium channel blockade.

PHARMACOLOGY

The so-called type I antidysrhythmic agents block myocardial sodium channels (Table 36-1). These agents, as a group, produce similar cardiac manifestations when taken in overdose. In general, sodium channel–blocking antidysrhythmics all have high volumes of distribution and large molecular weights. These pharmacologic properties exclude hemodialysis as a method of treating poisoned patients.

Transmembrane sodium channels have been grouped into two functional classes. One such class is composed of ligand-gated sodium channels that are triggered (opened or closed) in response to the binding of a ligand (e.g., neurotransmitter substance). The second class of sodium channels is voltage gated, that is, they are triggered (opened) in response to depolarization of the cell membrane in which they reside (Fig. 36-1).[6] The antidysrhythmic agents discussed in this chapter block voltage-gated sodium channels (Fig. 36-2). At any given time, functioning voltage-gated sodium channels may exist in one of three possible states: resting, activated, and inactivated (see Fig 16-2). During the resting state, the

channel is closed and impermeable to sodium. Depolarization of the cell membrane activates (opens) the sodium channel, thus permitting the influx of sodium. After activation, the channel undergoes a conformational change (inactivation) that prevents further sodium influx. Inactivated channels must then conformationally revert to the resting state before opening again. This conformational change occurs during the repolarization phase of the action potential, as discussed in the next section.

PATHOPHYSIOLOGY OF CARDIAC ACTION POTENTIALS AND MYOCARDIAL TOXICITY RESULTING FROM SODIUM CHANNEL–BLOCKING ANTIDYSRHYTHMIC POISONING

An appreciation of mechanisms of action potential generation in nonpacemaker and pacemaker cells of the heart is essential to understanding the toxicity of sodium channel–blocking antidysrhythmics. In nonpacemaker cells, the action potential consists of five phases (see Fig. 39-4). Phase 4 refers to the resting state, during which voltage-gated sodium channels are closed until activated in response to the spread of electrical membrane depolarization from adjacent tissue or the opening of nearby ligand-gated excitatory ion channels. Once the voltage-gated sodium channels are activated, slow influx of sodium results in membrane depolarization. When the threshold potential (about −90 mV) is reached, voltage-gated sodium channels open, and a massive influx of sodium ensues and causes the onset of phase 0. The upslope of phase 0 is directly responsible for the normally rapid rate of conduction of the action potential through the ventricle, and such conduction results in the narrow QRS interval seen on the electrocardiogram. Phase 1 of the nonpacemaker cell action potential begins with inactivation of sodium channels at the peak of the action potential and is marked by a brief period of rapid electrical repolarization. Phase 2, or the plateau phase, results from a balance between calcium influx through voltage-gated calcium channels and potassium efflux. There is a relatively smaller and more gradual change in the membrane potential during phase 2 because the net ion conductance is minimal. Rapid repolarization (phase 3) results from further activation of transmembrane potassium channels and outward movement of potassium. The cell membrane and its sodium channels then return to the resting state (e.g., phase 4) and again are ready for depolarization and activation.

TABLE 36-1 Classification and Pharmacokinetics (Baselt, 2000) of Sodium Channel–Blocking Antidysrhythmic Drugs

DRUG CLASS	DRUG	VOLUME OF DISTRIBUTION (L/kg)	PROTEIN BINDING (%)	ELIMINATION HALF-LIFE (hr)
Class IA	Quinidine*†	1.8–3.0	74–88	5–12
	Procainamide*†	3.3–4.8	15	2–5
	Disopyramide*	0.6–1.5	25–40	5–8
Class IB	Lidocaine	1.3	55–79	0.7–1.8
	Mexiletine	6–12	70	8–17
	Phenytoin	0.5–0.8	87–93	8–60
	Tocainide	1.4	10–15	12–15
Class IC	Encainide	2.7–4.3	75–85	2.3 (slow: 11)
	Flecainide	9–10	40	12–27
	Propafenone	2.5–4.0	77–97	2–10 (slow: 10–32)
Class II	Propranolol‡	3–5	93	2–4
Class III	Amiodarone	18–148	94	3–80 (single dose) 35–68 days (chronic therapy)

*Anticholinergic.
†Extended-release preparations available.
‡Propranolol is one of the most potent sodium channel–blocking antidysrhythmics among β-blockers.

Unlike the five-phase action potential of nonpacemaker cells, the action potential of pacemaker cells is composed of three phases (see Fig. 21-2). In phase 4, which is relatively slow, spontaneous efflux of potassium and influx of sodium occur. Whether slow depolarization to threshold voltage in phase 4 results mainly from decreased potassium efflux or from increased sodium influx remains unknown. When the threshold potential is reached, phase 0 is initiated, and influx of calcium occurs. In contrast to nonpacemaker tissue, very little sodium influx occurs during phase 0. Phase 3 repolarization, as in nonpacemaker cells, is due almost entirely to potassium efflux.

Sodium channel–blocking antidysrhythmics can have four major cardiotoxic effects: intraventricular conduction defects,

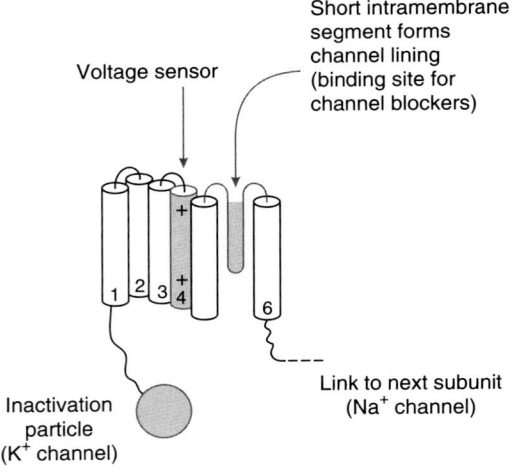

FIGURE 36-1

Structure of voltage-gated ion channels. The diagram shows one of the four domains of the channel. In sodium channels, the four domains are linked as a single chain; in potassium channels, they are separate subunits and may consist of fewer than six membrane-spanning helices. Movement of helix 4 (voltage sensor) is responsible for channel activation. Inactivation occurs when the intracellular inactivation particle blocks the channel. (In the sodium channel, the inactivating particle is formed from one of the intracellular loops; see the text.) The channel pore is formed from the short intramembrane segment plus adjacent helices; channel-blocking drugs bind in this region. *(From Rang HP, Dale MM, Ritter JM, Gardner P: Pharmacology, 4th ed. Philadelphia, Churchill-Livingstone, 2001, p 638.)*

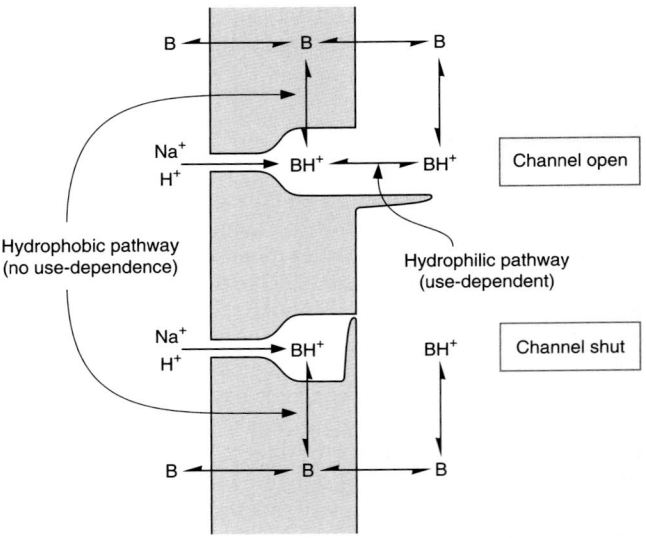

FIGURE 36-2

Interaction of local anesthetics with sodium channels. The blocking site within the channel can be reached via the open channel gate on the inner surface of the membrane by the charged species BH⁺ (hydrophobic pathway) or directly from the membrane by the uncharged species B (hydrophobic pathway). *(From Rang HP, Dale MM, Ritter JM, Gardner P: Pharmacology, 4th ed. Philadelphia, Churchill-Livingstone, 2001, p 641.)*

TABLE 36-2 Differences among Class I Antiarrhythmic Drugs			
CLASS	**PHASE 0 DEPRESSION**	**REPOLARIZATION**	**ACTION POTENTIAL DURATION**
IA	Moderate	Prolonged	Increased
IB	Weak	Shortened	Decreased
IC	Strong	No effect	No effect

From Hume JR, Woosley RL: Cardiac electrophysiology and antiarrhythmic agents. In Brody TM, Larner J, Minnerman KP (eds): Human Pharmacology: Molecular to Clinical, 3rd ed. St. Louis, CV Mosby, 1998.

ventricular dysrhythmias, hypotension, and bradydysrhythmias.[4] The effects of the various types of type I agents are presented in Table 36-2. Intraventricular conduction defects, which occur as a result of a sodium channel blockade–related reduction in the slope of phase 0 of the nonpacemaker cell action potential, are seen as decrements in the conduction velocity of the myocardial action potential (Fig. 36-3). Clinically, this decreased conduction velocity is represented by a widening of the QRS complex and/or the development of bundle-branch block morphology. An increase in the severity of the phase 0 conduction decrement is accompanied by progressive QRS widening to the point of sine wave morphology or asystole (Fig. 36-4).

Toxic exposure to sodium channel–blocking antidysrhythmics may also induce ventricular monomorphic tachycardia or fibrillation. These potentially lethal dysrhythmias are thought to occur by slowing intraventricular conduction to the point that unidirectional block and reentrant circuits develop.[7] These reentrant circuits can further degenerate into ventricular tachycardia and fibrillation.[8]

Rarely, poisoning by sodium channel–blocking antidysrhythmics may also produce polymorphic ventricular tachycardia (torsades de pointes). Torsades typically occurs with the class IA antidysrhythmics (e.g., quinidine, procainamide, disopyramide) and other drugs that inhibit potassium efflux during phase 3 of the nonpacemaker cell action potential.[1] Prolonged repolarization from impairment of outward potassium currents produces a lengthening of the QT interval (see Fig. 39-5) and predisposes the involved myocardium to the occurrence of polymorphic ventricular tachycardia (Fig. 36-5). The sinus tachycardia resulting from the anticholinergic properties of many drugs with sodium channel–blocking actions, including class IA antidysrhythmics (e.g., quinidine), is associated with a decrease in the QT interval and may help explain why polymorphic ventricular tachycardia, though possible, is relatively uncommon after an overdose of these antidysrhythmics.[4]

Hypotension after sodium channel–blocking antidysrhythmic poisoning probably results from decreased myocardial contractility because influx of sodium and calcium is coupled to the release of intracellular calcium stores.[9,10] Hypotension may also occur secondary to reduced vascular smooth muscle contractility and resultant vasodilation. The peripheral α-adrenergic antagonist actions of selected sodium channel–blocking antidysrhythmics (e.g., quinidine) may also contribute substantially to this clinical effect.

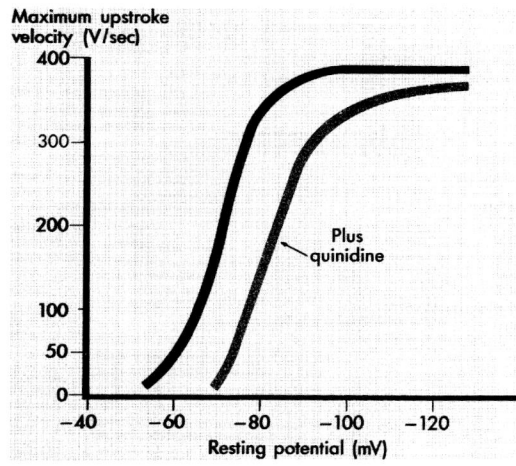

FIGURE 36-3

$\dot{V}_{max}$ of the action potential during phase 0, as influenced by the resting membrane potential. This relationship is called membrane responsiveness. The plot to the *left* is in the absence of drugs. The addition of many class I antiarrhythmic agents such as quinidine shifts the curve to more negative membrane potentials (hyperpolarizing direction). *(From Hume JR, Woosley RL: Cardiac electrophysiology and antiarrhythmic agents. In Brody TM, Larner J, Minneman KP [eds]: Human Pharmacology: Molecular to Clinical, 3rd ed. St. Louis, CV Mosby, 1998, p 204.)*

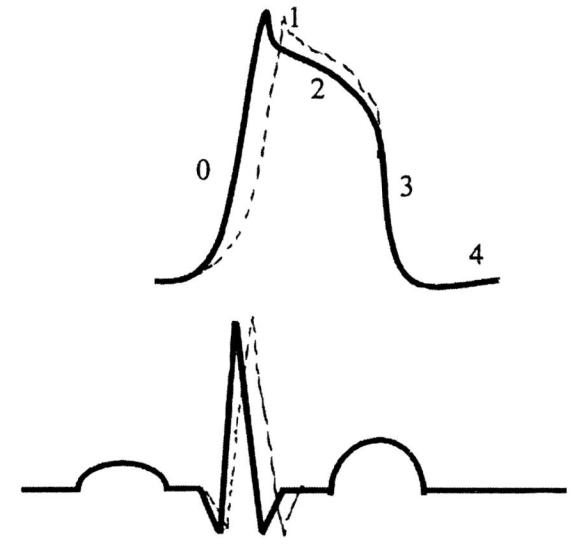

FIGURE 36-4

Pacemaker action potential.

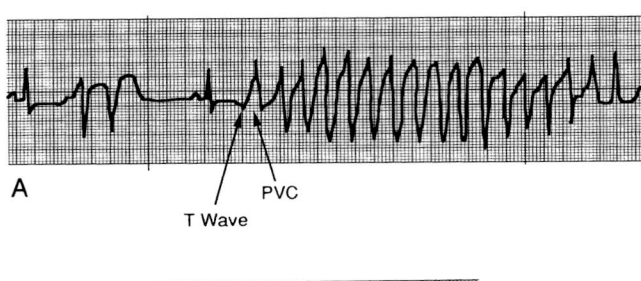

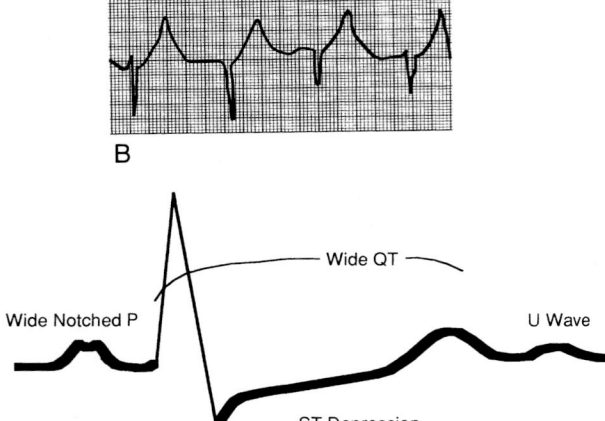

FIGURE 36-5

Quinidine toxicity and torsades de pointes. One of the effects of quinidine toxicity is a lengthening of the QT interval (**A**) and an arrhythmia known as torsades de pointes (**B**). Torsades de pointes is characterized by ventricular tachycardia with an electrocardiographic strip that looks as though the QRS peaks were undulating about an axis, a "roller coaster" pattern. This rhythm may terminate itself or may lead to ventricular fibrillation. (**C**) Schematic summary of the effects of quinidine. PVC, premature ventricular contraction. *(From Lathers CM, O'Rourke DK: Antiarrhythmic agents. In Smith CM, Reynard AM [eds]: Textbook of Pharmacology. Philadelphia, WB Saunders, 1992, p 515.)*

Many sodium channel–blocking antidysrhythmic agents (e.g., type IA agents) possess anticholinergic properties that cause sinus tachycardia after an overdose.[1] However, large overdoses of these antidysrhythmics may depress pacemaker cell automaticity, causing sinus bradycardia, junctional escape or other ventricular arrhythmias, and even asystole.[1] In sodium channel blocker poisoning by anticholinergic antidysrhythmics, the combination of a wide QRS complex and bradycardia is ominous because it indicates that the sodium channel blockade is so profound that the myocardium cannot mount a tachycardic response to muscarinic antagonism.

The mechanism of decreased automaticity in pacemaker cells during severe sodium channel blockade is unclear, in part because the exact ion currents responsible for spontaneous depolarization of pacemaker cells remain undefined. If sodium influx during phase 4 causes pacemaker cells to reach threshold, massive sodium channel blockade could explain slowed depolarization and the resulting bradycardia. An analogous situation has been studied in Purkinje fibers, in which high doses of imipramine, an anticholinergic sodium channel–blocking tricyclic antidepressant (TCA), depressed the slope of phase 4 of the pacemaker action potential to the point of asystole.[11]

CLINICAL PRESENTATION AND LIFE-THREATENING COMPLICATIONS

Patients exposed to toxic doses of non–sustained-release sodium channel–blocking antidysrhythmics can usually be expected to become symptomatic within 6 hours after oral ingestion and much sooner after parenteral overdoses. Patients who ingest sustained-release sodium channel–blocking antidysrhythmic preparations generally become symptomatic within 24 hours of ingestion. Intraventricular conduction defects (e.g., prolonged QRS, bundle-branch blocks), ventricular dysrhythmias (e.g., ventricular tachycardia, ventricular fibrillation), hypotension, and bradydysrhythmia (e.g., bradycardia, junctional escape, asystole) have been observed after an overdose of sodium channel–blocking antidysrhythmics. Lidocaine, a type IB antidysrhythmic, has minimal effect on phase 0 of the action potential in nondiseased myocardium at therapeutic doses and thus does not generally cause ventricular dysrhythmias.[12] Poisoning by type IA antidysrhythmics and other drugs that inhibit potassium efflux during phase 3 of the nonpacemaker cell action potential may result in the development of torsades de pointes. Poisoning by sodium channel–blocking antidysrhythmics can involve other adverse organ system manifestations in addition to the cardiotoxic effects. Overdose of anticholinergic antidysrhythmics (e.g., quinidine, disopyramide) may result in a rapid-onset anticholinergic syndrome manifested by agitation, coma, respiratory depression, urinary retention, tachycardia, anhidrosis, and depressed gastrointestinal motility. Seizures are common after an overdose of lidocaine, with some evidence suggesting that central nervous system sodium channel blockade by lidocaine and its metabolite monoethylglycine is the responsible proconvulsant mechanism.[12] Several type IA antidysrhythmics (e.g., quinidine, disopyramide) also block potassium efflux in pancreatic beta islet cells, thereby resulting in increased insulin release and hypoglycemia after an overdose.[13,14]

DIAGNOSIS

The diagnosis of sodium channel–blocking antidysrhythmic poisoning is primarily clinical and electrocardiographic (ECG). Intraventricular conduction defects frequently occur in poisoned patients. Clinically, these conduction defects are manifested by prolongation of the QRS interval beyond 100 milliseconds, and they typically develop within 6 hours of an overdose involving non–sustained-release drugs. Right axis deviation greater than 120 degrees of the terminal 40 milliseconds has been proposed as a reliable ECG criterion for TCA toxicity[15]; however, its predictive value for sodium channel–blocking antidysrhythmic toxicity has not been well studied.

Because hypoglycemia may occur, close monitoring of blood glucose levels is warranted for patients with type IA antidysrhythmic toxicity. Most of these drugs are not detected by standard hospital urine drug-screening methods; therefore, qualitative and/or quantitative analysis performed at a commercial reference laboratory may be required for confirmatory assessment.

TREATMENT

Securing an airway, as needed, and ensuring adequate ventilation are of top priority in the initial management of sodium channel–blocking antidysrhythmic toxicity. The patient should be placed on a cardiac monitor and intravenous access established. Hypotension should initially be treated with judicious crystalloid boluses, unless they are contraindicated (e.g., as in pulmonary edema). Because of the severe toxicity associated with overdose of these agents, gastrointestinal decontamination via gastric lavage, oral activated charcoal, or both may be considered if the patient is seen within 1 hour after ingestion. However, gastric lavage has not been shown to alter the clinical course of these patients and may rarely result in additional morbidity (see Chapter 5). Activated charcoal administered within the first few hours after ingestion may result in decreased peak drug levels, although this treatment has also not been demonstrated to alter the clinical course of poisoning with these agents. Once life-threatening clinical manifestations have occurred, the risks of gastrointestinal decontamination probably exceed the benefits. Because of the large volume of distribution of these agents, their clearance is not significantly enhanced by hemodialysis or hemoperfusion. It is beyond the scope of this chapter to discuss every nuance of treating sodium channel–blocking antidysrhythmic poisoning because of the numerous and diverse additional pharmacologic properties that these drugs possess. What follows is a synopsis of the treatment of the cardiotoxic manifestations of poisoning by these agents.

Hypertonic Sodium Bicarbonate Therapy

Hypertonic sodium bicarbonate is currently the initial treatment of choice for intraventricular conduction defects, ventricular dysrhythmias, and the negative inotropic effects of a sodium channel–blocking antidysrhythmic overdose. One of the first reports of its use as an antidote for antidysrhythmic poisoning was published in 1958 and involved the administration of hypertonic sodium lactate in a patient with quinidine poisoning, with apparent correction of hypotension and reversal of QRS complex prolongation.[16] This treatment was soon used successfully in the treatment of procainamide poisoning.[5] When TCAs were introduced, hypertonic sodium bicarbonate was used in the treatment of their toxicity.[17,18] Successful treatment with sodium bicarbonate has been reported in patients poisoned with many

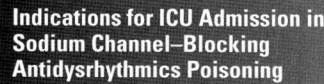

Indications for ICU Admission in Sodium Channel–Blocking Antidysrhythmics Poisoning

Bradydysrhythmias
Hypotension
Conduction defects (2nd-, 3rd-degree atrioventricular block; intraventricular delay)
Respiratory failure
Moderate to severe anticholinergic toxicity
Ventricular dysrhythmias

other sodium channel–blocking antidysrhythmics, including encainide, flecainide, and propafenone.[2,19–21]

Intravenous hypertonic sodium bicarbonate (one or more intravenous [IV] boluses of 1 mEq/kg or 1 mL/kg of an 8.4% injectable aqueous solution) produces a rise in both the serum sodium concentration and blood pH. Depending on the experimental species and drug or drugs studied, there is considerable variation with regard to the relative role of change in sodium concentration versus change in blood pH on pertinent hemodynamic and ECG parameters. Serum alkalization is thought to benefit sodium channel blockade inasmuch as acidosis has been shown to exacerbate quinidine toxicity in vitro.[22] Amitriptyline-induced ventricular tachyarrhythmias in dogs demonstrated a greater response to the administration of sodium bicarbonate than to an equimolar quantity of hypertonic sodium chloride.[23] Increasing the extracellular sodium concentration without a change in blood pH, however, has been shown to reverse quinidine-induced depression of phase 0 in atrial fibers.[24] An elegant study involving canine Purkinje fibers published in 1984 demonstrated that increases in serum sodium concentration and blood pH are additive in their reversal of amitriptyline-induced cardiotoxicity, thus indicating that both alkalization and a rise in serum sodium concentration are beneficial.[25] A more recent in vitro study demonstrated that the combination of increases in extracellular sodium to 160 mmol/L and pH to 7.6 reduced the depressant effects of flecainide, mexiletine, and imipramine.[26]

The molecular mechanism by which hypertonic sodium bicarbonate appears to reverse sodium channel blockade is unclear. Older studies suggested that alkalization increased protein binding of the sodium channel–blocking agent, thereby effectively reducing the free concentration of the drug.[27] This mechanism seems unimportant because hypertonic sodium bicarbonate has been reported to be effective in reversing amitriptyline-poisoned isolated Purkinje fibers in the absence of protein.[25] A more recent study of the sodium channel–blocking TCA imipramine demonstrated that dissociation from the sodium channel occurred secondary to alkalization.[28]

A 1993 study demonstrated that flecainide dissociates from the sodium channel when the local sodium concentration is raised.[29] This study suggests that the increase in serum sodium concentration lowers the binding affinity of the drug for the channel and thereby results in dissociation of the blocking agent. This and other studies have led to the suggested use of hypertonic saline as a therapeutic agent for the treatment of sodium channel blockade.[30–32] In 1998, a group of investigators reported the results of a swine study in which hypertonic saline (10 mL/kg of 7.5% NaCl) was compared with sodium bicarbonate (3 mEq/kg of 8.4% sodium bicarbonate) in the treatment of nortriptyline poisoning. They found that hypertonic saline was more effective than sodium bicarbonate in correcting hypotension and narrowing the QRS complex.[33] Thus, the preponderance of currently available data does not conclusively demonstrate the superiority of hypertonic sodium bicarbonate over hypertonic saline in this setting.

Intraventricular Conduction Delays

The administration of IV boluses of sodium bicarbonate has been widely observed to narrow widened QRS complexes resulting from exposure to toxic doses of various sodium channel–blocking antidysrhythmics. Much of the clinical experience with this therapy to date has been derived from hospitalized patients poisoned with TCAs. Based on the experience with TCAs, it has become common practice to administer sodium bicarbonate boluses when the duration of the QRS complex reaches or exceeds 120 milliseconds. Recommended treatment commonly consists of an initial 1- to 2-mEq/kg bolus of sodium bicarbonate (1 to 2 mL/kg of 8.4% $NaHCO_3$) and then further induction and maintenance of alkalemia until the arterial pH is in the range of 7.45 to 7.5. If life-threatening clinical manifestations are present (e.g., hypotension, ventricular arrhythmias), the targeted end point of such therapy may be further increased to an arterial pH of 7.55. It is advisable to refrain from higher elevations in pH because of the adverse effects of excessive alkalosis. With rapid administration of relatively large amounts of hypertonic sodium bicarbonate, hypernatremia may be reasonably anticipated. Theoretically, a modest rise in serum sodium concentration may be desirable, although this has not been well studied.

Sodium Bicarbonate versus Serum Alkalization by Induced Respiratory Alkalosis

Based on the discussion just presented, it can be concluded that both sodium supplementation and serum alkalization are important components of the treatment of poisoning with these agents if ECG manifestations of sodium channel blockade are present. Theoretically, this can be accomplished by the administration of sodium bicarbonate by repetitive boluses or infusion or by inducing respiratory alkalosis and infusing normal saline. The latter option can easily be accomplished because patients with toxicity to the point of ECG abnormalities almost invariably require mechanical ventilation. Using this option also prevents severe hypernatremia and fluid overload, which are undesirable because of the myocardial depressant qualities of sodium channel–blocking agents. However, no clinical trial has compared the primary administration of sodium bicarbonate with induced alkalization and saline. If the latter option is chosen, sodium bicarbonate boluses should be administered until an induced serum alkalization, to a pH of 7.45 to 7.55, is achieved.

Hypotension

The hypotension that accompanies sodium channel–blocking antidysrhythmic poisoning usually responds to judicious intravascular volume expansion with crystalloid solution (e.g., normal saline or lactated Ringer's solution). Persistent hypotension in the absence of dysrhythmia most commonly results from depression of myocardial contractility (i.e., negative inotropy) and peripheral vasodilation. If hypotension is unresponsive to fluid boluses, norepinephrine is generally recommended for its β-adrenergically mediated positive inotropic effect and relatively potent α-adrenergic vasoconstrictive properties. In patients who require more than minimal doses of norepinephrine or who remain in shock, pulmonary artery catheterization is of theoretical benefit. Intraaortic balloon counterpulsation or even cardiopulmonary bypass may be lifesaving for patients in extreme and/or refractory cardiogenic shock.[34]

Ventricular Dysrhythmias

The generally recommended, though clinically unproven, initial treatment of sodium channel antidysrhythmic–induced ventricular arrhythmia is sodium bicarbonate boluses. Lidocaine is usually recommended as the first-line antidysrhythmic drug for the treatment of ventricular dysrhythmias. Lidocaine administration has minimal effect on phase 0 of the action potential in nondiseased hearts at therapeutic doses and thus does not appear to add significantly to the cardiotoxic effects of other sodium channel–blocking drugs. In dogs, lidocaine has been demonstrated to halt ventricular dysrhythmias induced by amitriptyline.[23] However, these effects were transient and associated with a significant drop in blood pressure. Lidocaine should not be given to patients suffering toxicity from other type IB antidysrhythmics. Treatment options for ventricular dysrhythmia resistant to sodium bicarbonate and lidocaine include bretylium, transcutaneous and transvenous cardiac pacing, and cardiopulmonary bypass. Class IA and class IC antidysrhythmics, potent depressants of phase 0 of the action potential, are expected to only worsen myocardial toxicity in the setting of sodium channel blockade and are therefore contraindicated in the management of sodium channel blocker toxicity.

Bradydysrhythmias

Bradydysrhythmias are characteristic of severe sodium channel antidysrhythmic poisoning. In the presence of severe bradycardia, a wide QRS complex, and hypotension, it is recommended, based on anecdotal and theoretical considerations, that IV epinephrine be administered by continuous infusion if the administration of IV sodium bicarbonate does not elicit an immediate beneficial response. Intravenous epinephrine infusions for these indications should be started at 5 μg/min (0.1 μg/kg/min in pediatric patients) and titrated to effect. Transcutaneous or transvenous cardiac pacing should be initiated if the hemodynamically significant bradydysrhythmia persists despite drug therapy. Intraaortic balloon counterpulsation and cardiopulmonary bypass are of theoretical benefit in patients who do not respond to the aforementioned therapies. There is no compelling theoretical support or clinical evidence for the use of atropine in the treatment of sodium channel blockade–induced bradydysrhythmias.

Supraventricular Dysrhythmias

Sinus tachycardia accompanying sodium channel antidysrhythmic poisoning usually results from the anticholinergic effects of these agents and rarely requires treatment. Physostigmine, a short-acting anticholinesterase, has been reported to both slow the heart rate and subsequently narrow the QRS complex in patients poisoned with sodium channel blockers.[35,36] Slowing the heart rate by physostigmine allows greater sodium influx during phase 0 of the action potential. However, there are major potential complications associated with the use of physostigmine as an antidote for this poisoning. By reversing the anticholinergically induced sinus tachycardia, physostigmine may potentially unmask sodium channel blockade in pacemaker cells and predispose the patient to the development of bradydysrhythmia, heart block, and asystole.[37,38] It is also possible that slowing the heart rate may increase the QT interval, thus predisposing to torsades de pointes. These serious adverse effects are the reason why physostigmine should not be used in treating patients poisoned with sodium channel–blocking antidysrhythmics, TCAs, or any sodium channel–blocking agents, at least not during the early phases of poisoning when sodium channel blockade is clinically and/or electrocardiographically evident.

Hypertonic Saline

As mentioned previously, there are reports of successful treatment of sodium channel blockade poisoning–induced ventricular arrhythmias, QRS widening, or hypotension with hypertonic (3%) saline when initial hypertonic sodium bicarbonate therapy was unsuccessful.[31,32] The optimal human dose of hypertonic saline has not been established, and careful attention is necessary to prevent severe hypernatremia. Current data do not conclusively demonstrate the superiority of hypertonic saline over sodium bicarbonate for the treatment of sodium channel–blocking antidysrhythmic toxicity. In addition, the safety and efficacy of the use of hypertonic solution in the treatment of poisoning by these agents have not been demonstrated in controlled clinical studies. Pulmonary edema may occur if hypertonic solutions are used and cardiac output is depressed. Hypertonic saline may not reverse sodium channel blockade secondary to lidocaine poisoning.[39]

Disposition

Though not systematically studied, anecdotal experience strongly suggests that patients poisoned with non–sustained-release sodium channel–blocking antidysrhythmics can usually be expected to become symptomatic with 6 hours after ingestion and much sooner after parenteral overdoses. The vast majority of patients who show no signs of toxicity after 6 hours of monitored observation and have normal ECG findings are most likely safe for medical clearance. Documented ingestion of any of the sustained-release sodium channel–blocking antidysrhythmic formulations or uncertainty regarding the exact formulation ingested may warrant 24 hours of cardiac-monitored observation.

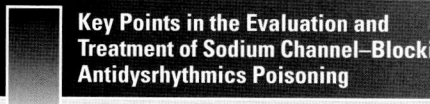

Key Points in the Evaluation and Treatment of Sodium Channel–Blocking Antidysrhythmics Poisoning

1. Clinical toxicity is usually evident within 6 hours of exposure to a non–sustained-release formulation; ingestion of a sustained-release formulation may result in delayed onset and/or prolonged toxicity
2. ECG evidence of sodium channel blockade–induced toxicity includes hypotension, bradydysrhythmias, atrioventricular and intraventricular conduction delays, and ventricular tachydysrhythmias.
3. Other cardiotoxic manifestations associated with sodium channel–blocking antidysrhythmics include prolonged QT/torsades de pointes (potassium efflux blockade) and sinus tachycardia (antimuscarinic effects, e.g., quinidine).
4. Noncardiovascular toxicity associated with sodium channel–blocking antidysrhythmic drugs includes central and peripheral anticholinergic syndrome, and hypoglycemia.

continued

Key Points in the Evaluation and Treatment of Sodium Channel–Blocking Antidysrhythmics Poisoning *continued*

5. Appropriate treatment of toxicity includes airway/ventilatory support, cautious IV volume expansion, hypertonic sodium bicarbonate (1-mEq/kg IV boluses to an arterial pH of 7.45 to 7.55), IV vasopressors (norepinephrine, epinephrine), IV lidocaine for ventricular tachydysrhythmias, and hypertonic (3%) saline for hemodynamic instability or dysrhythmia refractory to other treatments.
6. Consider intraaortic balloon pump or cardiopulmonary bypass for severe refractory cardiogenic shock.

REFERENCES

1. Kim SY, Benowitz NL: Poisoning due to class 1A antidysrhythmic drugs. Quinidine, procainamide, and disopyramide. Drug Saf 5:393, 1990.
2. Fonck K, Haenebalcke C, Hemeryck A, et al: ECG changes and plasma concentrations of propafenone and its metabolites in a case of severe poisoning. J Toxicol Clin Toxicol 36:247, 1998.
3. Taboulet P, Cariou A, Berdeaux A, et al: Pathophysiology and management of self-poisoning with β-blockers. J Toxicol Clin Toxicol 31:531, 1993.
4. Kolecki PF, Curry SC: Poisoning by sodium channel blocking agents. Crit Care Clin Med Toxicol 13:829, 1997.
5. Wasserman F, Brodsky L, Dick MM, et al: Successful treatment of quinidine and procainamide intoxication. Report of three cases. N Engl J Med 259:797, 1958.
6. Katz AM: Cardiac ion channels. N Engl J Med 328:1244, 1993.
7. Vohra J, Burrows G, Hunt D, et al: The effect of toxic and therapeutic doses of TCA drugs on intracardiac conduction. Eur J Cardiol 3:219, 1975.
8. Nattel S, Keable H, Sasynuik BI: Experimental amitriptyline intoxication: Electrophysiologic manifestations and management. J Cardiovasc Pharmacol 6:83, 1984.
9. Nawada T, Tanaka Y, Sirai S, et al: Evaluation of negative inotropic and antidysrhythmic effects of class I antidysrhythmic drugs. Int J Clin Pharmacol Ther 32:347, 1994.
10. Reiter M: Calcium mobilization and cardiac inotropic mechanisms. Pharmacol Rev 40:189, 1988.
11. Rodriguez S, Tamargo J: Electrophysiologic effects of imipramine (sic) on bovine ventricular muscle and Purkinje's fibres. Br J Pharmacol 70:15, 1980.
12. Denaro CP, Benowitz NL: Poisoning due to class 1B antidysrhythmic drugs. Lignocaine, mexiletine, and tocainide. Med Toxicol Adverse Drug Exp 4:412, 1989.
13. Cacoub P, Deray G, Baumelou A, et al: Disopyramide-induced hypoglycemia: Case report and review of the literature. Fundam Clin Pharmacol 3:527, 1989.
14. White NJ, Warrell DA, Chanthavanich P, et al: Severe hypoglycemia and hyperinsulinemia in falciparum malaria. N Engl J Med 309:61, 1983.
15. Wolfe TR, Caravati EM, Rollins DE: Terminal 40-ms frontal plane QRS axis as a marker for TCA overdose. Ann Emerg Med 18:348, 1989.
16. Bellet S, Hamden G, Somlyo A, Lara R: Reversal of the cardiotoxic effects of quinidine by molar sodium lactate. Clin Res 6:226, 1958.
17. Brown TCK: Sodium bicarbonate treatment for TCA arrhythmias in children. Med J Aust 2:380, 1976.
18. Hoffman JR, McElroy CR: Bicarbonate therapy for dysrhythmia and hypotension in TCA overdose. West J Med 134:60, 1981.
19. Mortensen ME, Bolon CE, Kelley MT, et al: Encainide overdose in an infant. Ann Emerg Med 21:998, 1992.
20. Lovecchio F, Berlin R, Brubacher JR, Sholar JB: Hypertonic sodium bicarbonate in an acute flecainide overdose. Am J Emerg Med 16:534, 1998.
21. Goldman MJ, Mowry JB, Kirk MA: Sodium bicarbonate to correct widened QRS in a case of flecainide overdose. J Emerg Med 15:183, 1997.
22. Nattel S, Elharrar V, Zipes DP, et al: pH-dependent electrophysiological effects of quinidine and lidocaine on canine cardiac Purkinje's fibers. Circ Res 48:55, 1981.

23. Nattel S, Mittleman M: Treatment of ventricular tachyarrhythmias resulting from amitriptyline toxicity in dogs. J Pharmacol Exp Ther 231:430, 1984.

24. Cox AR, West TC: Sodium lactate reversal of quinidine effect studied in rabbit atria by the microelectrode technique. J Pharmacol Exp Ther 131:212, 1961.

25. Sasyniuk BI, Jhamandas V: Mechanism of reversal of toxic effects of amitriptyline on cardiac Purkinje's fibers by sodium bicarbonate. J Pharmacol Exp Ther 231:387, 1984.

26. Bou-Abboud E, Nattel S: Relative role of alkalosis and sodium ions in reversal of class I antidysrhythmic drug–induced sodium channel blockade by sodium bicarbonate. Circulation 94:1954, 1996.

27. Levitt MA, Sullivan JB, Owens SM, et al: Amitriptyline plasma protein binding: Effects of plasma pH and relevance to clinical overdose. Am J Emerg Med 4:121, 1986.

28. Bou-Abboud E, Nattel S: Molecular mechanisms of the reversal of imipramine-induced sodium channel blockade by alkalinization in human cardiac myocytes. Cardiovas Res 38:395, 1998.

29. Ranger S, Sheldon R, Fermini B, et al: Modulation of flecainide's cardiac sodium channel blocking actions by extracellular sodium: A possible cellular mechanism for the action of sodium salts in flecainide cardiotoxicity. J Pharmacol Exp Ther 264:1160, 1993.

30. Scalabrini A, Simonetti Mdos P, Velasco IT, Rocha e Silva M: Hypertonic NaCl solution prevents bupivacaine-induced cardiovascular toxicity. Circ Shock 36:231, 1992.

31. Dolara P, Franconi F: Hypertonic sodium chloride and lidocaine in a case of imipramine intoxication. Clin Toxicol 10:395, 1977.

32. Hoegholm A, Clementsen P: Hypertonic sodium chloride in severe antidepressant overdosage [letter]. J Toxicol Clin Toxicol 29:297, 1991.

33. McCabe JL, Cobaugh DJ, Menegazzi JJ, Fata J: Experimental TCA toxicity: A randomized, controlled comparison of hypertonic saline solution, sodium bicarbonate, and hyperventilation. Ann Emerg Med 32:329, 1998.

34. Lane AS, Woodward AC, Goldman MR, et al: Massive propranolol overdose poorly responsive to pharmacologic therapy: Use of the intra-aortic balloon pump. Ann Emerg Med 16:1381, 1987.

35. Tobis J, Das BN: Cardiac complications in amitriptyline poisoning. Successful treatment with physostigmine. JAMA 235:1474, 1976.

36. Weisdorf D, Kramer J, Goldberg A, et al: Physostigmine for cardiac and neurologic manifestations of phenothiazine poisoning. Clin Pharmacol Ther 24:663, 1978.

37. Pentel P, Peterson C: Physostigmine and asystole. Ann Emerg Med 10:228, 1981.

38. Pentel P, Peterson CD: Asystole complicating physostigmine treatment of TCA overdose. Ann Emerg Med 9:588, 1980.

39. Ujhelyi MR, Schur M, Frede T, et al: Hypertonic saline does not reverse the sodium channel blocking actions of lidocaine: Evidence from electrophysiologic and defibrillation studies. J Cardiovasc Pharmacol 29:61, 1997.

CHAPTER 37

Sodium Nitroprusside

Steven C. Curry

Sodium nitroprusside (SNP) entered into clinical practice in 1955 and gained popularity as a vasodilator for hypertensive emergencies because of its rapid onset of action and short duration, which allowed for bedside titration to the desired effect.[1] The introduction of a freeze-dried preparation in 1974 was followed by an additional increase in popularity, and it continued to gain favor for producing controlled hypotension during anesthesia and afterload reduction during low cardiac output states.

SNP therapy can result in two major distinct toxic syndromes: cyanide toxicity and thiocyanate (SCN^-) toxicity.[2] Each of these two disorders differs in risk factors, pathophysiology, signs and symptoms, diagnostic strategies, methods of prevention, and treatment. Cyanide toxicity is described in greater detail in Chapter 95 and is covered more superficially here.

CYANIDE TOXICITY FROM SODIUM NITROPRUSSIDE

Chemistry and Pathophysiology

The structure of SNP explains why desired vasodilation and cyanide toxicity may result from its use (Fig. 37-1). SNP contains about 50% cyanide by weight. Early investigators attributed SNP's in vivo decomposition to hydrocyanic acid (HCN) to a reaction with oxyhemoglobin. It has been accepted for many years, however, that each SNP molecule decomposes when it reacts with sulfhydryl groups on endothelial cells,[3,4] releasing nitric oxide (producing vasodilation) and five cyanide moieties (Fig. 37-2).

When solutions of SNP are exposed to intense sunlight, they decompose relatively quickly to release cyanide. Solutions of SNP are relatively stable, however, when exposed to artificial light. When protected from light, acidic or neutral solutions of SNP remain stable for months to years. It is unnecessary to prepare fresh solutions of SNP every 4 hours if the solution has been protected from bright sunlight.[2] The infusion of SNP in the same line as intravenous solutions containing sulfhydryl groups (e.g., amino acid solutions, N-acetylcysteine) also would be expected to accelerate its breakdown to cyanide.[4,5]

At physiologic pH, all cyanide exists as HCN, and HCN has two main fates. First, HCN can be detoxified by being transsulfurated to SCN^-, probably through several mechanisms. SCN^- undergoes renal excretion with an elimination half-life of 2.7 days in patients with normal renal function

(see Fig. 37-2).[6] Second, HCN can move into tissue and mitochondria to bind to the binuclear copper-iron center of cytochrome oxidase, where it inhibits electron transport, oxygen consumption, and oxidative phosphorylation. Because oxidative phosphorylation is a major buffer of protons, inhibition of cytochrome oxidase by cyanide is accompanied by metabolic acidosis. Hyperlactatemia reflects increased glycolytic adenosine triphosphate production and a shift in the redox potential.

An important and probably the dominant sulfur donor for detoxification of HCN is thiosulfate ($S_2O_3^{2-}$) A healthy adult seems to possess enough thiosulfate to metabolize about 50 mg of SNP over the short term.[7] Patients coming off cardiac bypass or receiving diuretics may have lower plasma thiosulfate concentrations and might be predisposed to cyanide toxicity from a given dose of SNP, although this has never been proved. Short-term starvation, such as after other types of surgery, has been associated with increases in circulating thiosulfate levels,[7] probably as a result of mobilization of sulfur-containing amino acids from skeletal muscle catabolism. There are no data supporting the contention that hepatic insufficiency predisposes to SNP-induced cyanide poisoning. Animals with hepatic damage detoxify HCN without difficulty.[8] In dogs, renal insufficiency is associated with lower circulating cyanide levels for a given SNP infusion rate.

Pharmacokinetics

Absorption of SNP is instantaneous and complete with intravenous infusion.[4] In blood, SNP is found almost wholly in plasma, with little to none in blood cells. This fact suggests that the nitroprusside anion distributes mainly to the extracellular space. The rapid breakdown of nitroprusside through interactions with sulfhydryl groups results in an elimination half-life of about 2 minutes, explaining the requirement of a continuous infusion and the ease with which infusion rates may be titrated to clinical effects.

Clinical Findings and Toxic Doses

Cyanide poisoning has resulted from short-term and long-term infusions of SNP.[9–12] When used as *short-term* infusions, such as those used during anesthesia, circulating HCN concentrations begin to increase when the total dose (not infusion rate) of SNP exceeds 0.5 to 1.5 mg/kg.[13,14] For *long-term* infusions, such as those used in the intensive care unit, circulating

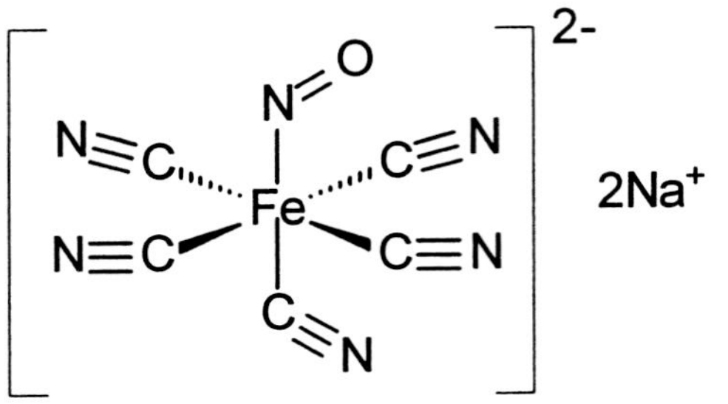

FIGURE 37-1

Chemical structure of sodium nitroprusside.

HCN concentrations begin to increase when SNP infusion rates exceed approximately 2 μg/kg/min.[2,4] Vesey and Cole[15] showed that on average, SNP infusion rates less than about 4 μg/kg/min would not be expected to produce toxic plasma cyanide concentrations. Toxic HCN concentrations may be reached within a few hours when infusion rates exceed 5 to 10 μg/kg/min, but this is not always the case. Cyanide toxicity also may not appear until several days after beginning a SNP infusion.

The signs and symptoms of cyanide poisoning are described in detail in Chapter 95. Briefly, cyanide toxicity is characterized by central nervous system and cardiovascular dysfunction and metabolic acidosis. All of these abnormalities are seen commonly in critically ill patients, making it sometimes difficult to discern whether cyanide toxicity accounts for a patient's declining course. Central nervous system dysfunction includes agitation, confusion, convulsions, coma, and cerebral death. Cardiovascular findings comprise tachycardia, bradycardia, hypotension, and, sometimes, early hypertension. SNP and HCN produce vasodila-

tion and a decline in systemic vascular resistance. Serial measurements of cardiovascular parameters with a pulmonary artery catheter reveal a decrease in oxygen consumption and, if cardiac output and hemoglobin concentrations remain unchanged, an increase in mixed venous oxygen content. There are no established values, however, for oxygen consumption or mixed venous oxygen content that provide reliable positive and negative predictive values for the presence of cyanide poisoning. A low systemic vascular resistance, anion gap metabolic acidosis, elevated arterial lactate concentrations, and depressed oxygen consumption are typical of SNP-induced cyanide poisoning, as are sepsis, hepatic failure, toxic shock syndrome, and systemic inflammatory response syndrome.

Diagnosis

The diagnosis of cyanide poisoning from SNP should be considered whenever central nervous system dysfunction, metabolic acidosis, and cardiovascular dysfunction accompany SNP infusion rates greater than about 4 μg/kg/min. Theoretically, however, infusion rates greater than 2.5 μg/kg/min over many hours might be capable of producing HCN toxicity in an exceptional patient. Serious cyanide poisoning always results in metabolic acidosis, unless the patient is receiving alkaline infusions (e.g., sodium bicarbonate) or has a significant baseline metabolic alkalosis. Arterial lactate concentrations are elevated. Most patients with cyanide toxicity do not have unusually pink or bright red skin or blood; many are cyanotic. The presence of bright red skin or unusually bright red venous blood or retinal veins suggests the possibility of cyanide poisoning, however. Hypothermia commonly is noted in comatose victims of cyanide toxicity. An abnormal odor, including that of bitter almonds, would not result from SNP-induced cyanide poisoning.

It has been noted anecdotally that the onset of cyanide poisoning is accompanied by an increase in blood pressure and what seems to be resistance to SNP-induced vasodilation. Whether this is true and serves as a useful clinical clue or whether simply the higher doses of SNP result in cyanide toxicity has not been clarified in controlled trials with serial measurements of red blood cell or plasma cyanide concentrations. Resistance to SNP certainly can occur in the absence of cyanide poisoning.

Whole-blood cyanide concentrations, as performed at most reference laboratories, commonly are elevated falsely in patients receiving long-term SNP infusions because of elevated plasma SCN⁻ concentrations (see Chapter 95),[16] and this has led to the misdiagnosis of cyanide poisoning from SNP in patients without evidence of cyanide toxicity.[17,18]

Plasma cyanide concentrations would be more helpful but are difficult to measure accurately. *Red blood cell* cyanide concentrations are easier to measure and correlate well with severity of cyanide poisoning. In general, metabolic disturbances from cyanide poisoning appear with red blood cell cyanide concentrations of about 1 mg/L (approximately 40 mmol/L). Obvious cyanide poisoning is evident with red blood cell HCN concentrations of 5 mg/L (approximately 200 mmol/L).[17]

Many laboratories do not offer this test, and results from any of these tests usually do not return for hours to days after

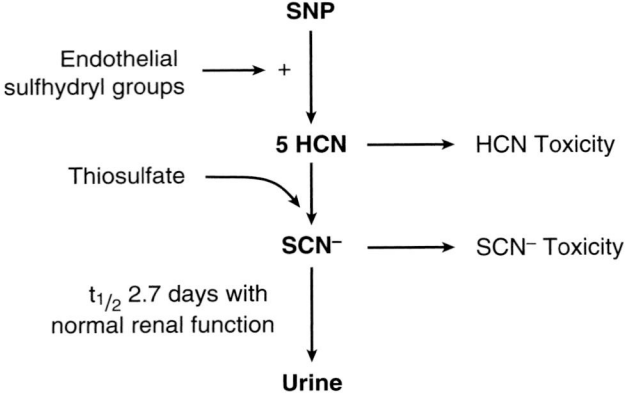

FIGURE 37-2

The fate of sodium nitroprusside (SNP). Nitroprusside reacts with endothelial sulfhydryl groups to release nitric oxide (producing vasodilation) and five cyanide moieties (HCN). In the presence of adequate stores of thiosulfate, HCN is transsulfurated to form thiocyanate (SCN⁻), which is excreted in the urine with a half-life of 2.7 days in patients with normal renal function. Inadequate thiosulfate stores lead to accumulation of HCN, which can move into tissue to produce cyanide toxicity. Large doses of nitroprusside, prolonged infusions, and renal insufficiency can cause the accumulation of SCN⁻, which produces a separate toxic syndrome. If SNP routinely is coinfused with sodium thiosulfate, HCN does not accumulate, and cyanide toxicity is prevented.

the specimen is obtained and sent. The delay in obtaining results, false elevation in whole-blood cyanide concentrations in many patients receiving SNP, and difficulty in obtaining red blood cell cyanide concentrations or accurately measured plasma cyanide concentrations limit the practical value of cyanide bioassay in establishing a timely diagnosis of cyanide toxicity.

Most patients with SNP-induced cyanide poisoning have nontoxic serum SCN$^-$ concentrations, although they may be elevated above the reference range. Serum SCN$^-$ levels are not helpful in establishing or excluding the diagnosis of cyanide toxicity.

Prevention

Numerous studies have shown that the coinfusion of sodium thiosulfate with SNP prevents increases in circulating HCN concentrations, even with SNP infusion rates approaching 20 μg/kg/min.[4,19] Each 100 mg of SNP should be mixed with 1 g of sodium thiosulfate.[2] These mixtures are stable for at least 7 days when protected from light.[19] Each 1 g of sodium thiosulfate contains 12.6 mmol of sodium.

Cyanide poisoning from SNP becomes virtually impossible if the correct dose of sodium thiosulfate has been coinfused. Patients receiving mixtures of thiosulfate and nitroprusside experience more rapid detoxification of HCN to SCN$^-$, however, and higher plasma SCN$^-$ levels. SCN$^-$ toxicity is rarely a problem, however, and can be monitored easily with measurement of serum or plasma SCN$^-$ concentrations.

Treatment

SNP should be discontinued in patients suspected of having cyanide toxicity. The SNP infusion can be restarted if SNP is mixed or coinfused with sodium thiosulfate as described earlier. Patients with serious cyanide poisoning (e.g., coma, hypotension, moderate-to-severe metabolic acidosis) should receive sodium nitrite and sodium thiosulfate from a cyanide antidote kit as described in Chapter 95 or whichever cyanide antidote is locally available. One should begin treating promptly on the basis of clinical suspicion, rather than waiting for results of blood cyanide concentrations. In a nonanemic adult, 300 mg of sodium nitrite intravenously should be infused, followed by 12.5 g intravenously of sodium thiosulfate if using the cyanide antidote kit. For doses of other cyanide antidotes, see Chapters 150 and 160. Patients who are only mildly symptomatic from cyanide toxicity and in whom induction of methemoglobinemia with sodium nitrite may be dangerous (e.g., those with severe anemia) are likely to improve with discontinuance of SNP and infusion of sodium thiosulfate alone.

Vesey and Cole[15] showed that accurately measured red blood cell and plasma HCN concentrations decrease with a half-life of about 30 minutes after SNP is halted and decrease with a half-life of about 10 minutes if thiosulfate (without nitrite) is also given. These HCN concentrations were not in the highly toxic range, however, and it is not known if this half-life can be extrapolated to much higher HCN levels.

THIOCYANATE TOXICITY FROM SODIUM NITROPRUSSIDE

Most of the HCN released from SNP undergoes transulfuration to form SCN$^-$, which is excreted in the urine with an elimination half-life of 2.7 days in patients with normal renal function and 9 days in patients with severe renal insufficiency.[6,15] Because of its long elimination half-life, SCN$^-$ can accumulate in patients receiving SNP infusions over several days.

Clinical Findings and Toxic Doses

Most knowledge concerning SCN$^-$ toxicity and the definition of toxic plasma concentrations has resulted from past extensive use of oral SCN$^-$ salts in the treatment of hypertension. This older literature describes SCN$^-$ toxicity as comprising abdominal colic, vomiting, weakness, rash, tinnitus, and hypothyroidism. More severe toxicity results in delusions, agitation, disorientation, tremor, convulsions, coma, and death.

The mechanism by which SCN$^-$ produces toxicity is unknown. The older literature described the enzymatic conversion of SCN$^-$ to HCN, but this now is known to have been an in vitro artifactual phenomenon. In contrast to cyanide poisoning, SCN$^-$ toxicity is not accompanied by a metabolic acidosis in the absence of other causes, such as convulsions or shock.

Diagnosis

Although serum or plasma SCN$^-$ concentrations do not assist in establishing or excluding the diagnosis of cyanide poisoning, they are of diagnostic utility with regard to SCN$^-$ toxicity. Normal plasma SCN$^-$ concentrations in nonsmokers are approximately less than 4 mg/L (<0.4 mg/dL [<0.07 mmol/L]), whereas smokers, who inhale HCN in cigarette smoke, have plasma SCN$^-$ levels of less than 8 mg/L (<0.8 mg/dL [<0.14 mmol/L]). Even serum or plasma SCN$^-$ concentrations of 100 mg/L (10 mg/dL [1.7 mmol/L]) are not accompanied by significant toxicity. Serious SCN$^-$ toxicity occurs when plasma SCN$^-$ concentrations are greater than 150 to 200 mg/L (>15 to 20 mg/dL [>2.6 to 3.4 mmol/L]).[15]

Prevention of and Monitoring for Toxicity

Patients receiving long-term infusions of SNP commonly have plasma SCN$^-$ concentrations above normal reference values.[15] Plasma concentrations only rarely reach a level associated with systemic toxicity, however. SCN$^-$ toxicity is not expected until the total SNP dose infused (not infusion rate) exceeds about 70 mg/kg.[15] In patients with normal renal function, SCN$^-$ toxicity could occur in 7 to 14 days, whereas in patients with renal insufficiency, SCN$^-$ toxicity can occur as early as 3 to 6 days.[4]

Patients receiving coinfusions of sodium thiosulfate with SNP form SCN$^-$ more readily and develop higher plasma SCN$^-$ concentrations for a given SNP infusion rate. SCN$^-$ toxicity remains uncommon, however, when SNP infusions are limited to 1 to 2 days in patients with renal failure or to 6 to 7 days in patients with normal renal function.

Treatment

Several authors have described effective removal of SCN⁻ with hemodialysis.[20,21] Hemodialysis is considered the treatment of choice for patients with severe SCN⁻ toxicity, especially in the presence of renal insufficiency.

Common Errors in the Management of Sodium Nitroprusside Toxicity

Using sodium nitroprusside without coinfusion of sodium thiosulfate

Failing to recognize falsely elevated whole-blood cyanide concentrations in many patients receiving sodium nitroprusside

Using serum or plasma thiocyanate levels to diagnose or exclude cyanide toxicity

Believing that most patients with cyanide poisoning have bright red skin or blood or exude a bitter almond odor

Believing it is necessary to mix a new bag of sodium nitroprusside every 4 hours when the solution is covered and protected from bright sunlight

SPECIAL POPULATIONS

Pregnant Patients

Case reports and series document successful use of SNP for short infusions (e.g., during aneurysm clipping), with low total doses (e.g., ≤60 mg) and with low infusion rates (e.g., <3 μg/kg/min) in pregnant women and gravid ewes.[22–25] Concern has been raised appropriately, however, with regard to the induction of fetal cyanide toxicity during maternal use of SNP. SNP infusions in gravid ewes can produce increases in maternal and fetal red blood cell cyanide concentrations.[26] Nitroprusside crosses the ovine placenta to produce equal concentrations in fetal and maternal blood.[27] Hydrogen cyanide, a small, lipophilic molecule, also crosses the placenta easily.

In gravid near-term ewes, the coinfusion of sodium thiosulfate with SNP prevents increases in maternal and fetal cyanide concentrations.[27] In this model, thiosulfate does not cross the placenta to enter the fetal circulation.[28] Maternally administered thiosulfate prevents ovine fetal cyanide toxicity by keeping maternal HCN concentrations low, allowing HCN to diffuse from the fetal circulation back into the maternal circulation for detoxification.[28] Fetal SCN⁻ concentrations do not increase during short-term infusions of maternal SCN⁻ in the ewe model.[27]

No studies examining fetal and maternal HCN concentrations in pregnant women receiving SNP compared with pregnant women receiving SNP mixed with thiosulfate have been conducted. Given the safety and lack of adverse effects associated with sodium thiosulfate combined with data from ewe studies, it is recommended that the use of SNP in pregnant women always be accompanied by coinfusion of sodium thiosulfate as described previously for nonpregnant patients.

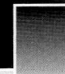

Key Points in Sodium Nitroprusside Toxicity

1. SNP therapy produces two toxic syndromes: cyanide poisoning and thiocyanate toxicity.
2. Doses of SNP for short-term administration (e.g., 1 to 2 hours) should not exceed 0.5 to 1.5 mg/kg to prevent cyanide toxicity.
3. Circulating cyanide concentrations begin to increase when long-term SNP infusions (>2 or 3 hours) exceed about 2 μg/kg/min. Cyanide toxicity may occur when infusion rates exceed about 4 μg/kg/min.
4. Cyanide toxicity may occur within minutes to hours with large doses or fast infusion rates or may be delayed for hours to days with lower infusion rates.
5. The clinical picture of SNP-induced cyanide poisoning is similar to that of septic shock, liver failure, and other disorders (e.g., low systemic vascular resistance, hypothermia, lactic acidosis, lethargy/coma, tachycardia and hypotension, decreased oxygen consumption).
6. SNP-induced cyanide poisoning is prevented completely with coinfusion of sodium thiosulfate; 1 g of sodium thiosulfate should be mixed with each 100 mg of SNP.
7. SNP-induced cyanide toxicity is treated in a nonanemic adult by stopping the SNP infusion and administering 300 mg of sodium nitrite and 12.5 g of sodium thiosulfate intravenously from a cyanide antidote kit or another cyanide antidote (see Chapters 150 and 160).
8. Whole-blood cyanide concentrations rarely return quickly enough to be helpful and commonly are falsely elevated in patients receiving SNP infusions.
9. Serum or plasma thiocyanate concentrations are nontoxic in most patients with cyanide toxicity and are not helpful in establishing or excluding the diagnosis of cyanide poisoning.
10. Thiocyanate accumulates over days to weeks to produce thiocyanate toxicity. Thiocyanate toxicity is prevented by limiting total SNP doses to <70 mg/kg and by monitoring serum or plasma thiocyanate concentrations.
11. Moderate-to-severe thiocyanate toxicity (e.g., confusion, coma, rash, abdominal pain, seizures) does not appear until serum or plasma thiocyanate concentrations exceed about 150 to 200 mg/L (15 to 20 mg/dL).
12. Severe thiocyanate toxicity is treated with hemodialysis, especially in patients with renal insufficiency.

SNP, sodium nitroprusside.

REFERENCES

1. Page IH, Corcoran AC, Dustan HP, et al: Cardiovascular actions of sodium nitroprusside in animals and hypertensive patients. Circulation 11:188–198, 1955.
2. Curry SC, Arnold-Capell P: Nitroprusside, nitroglycerin, and angiotensin-converting enzyme inhibitors. Crit Care Clin 7:555–581, 1991.
3. Kreye VAW, Reske SN: Possible site of the in vivo disposition of sodium nitroprusside in the rat. Arch Pharmacol 32:260–265, 1982.
4. Schulz V: Clinical pharmacokinetics of nitroprusside, cyanide, thiosulphate and thiocyanate. Clin Pharmacokinet 9:239–251, 1984.
5. Rodkey FL, Collison HA: Determination of cyanide and nitroprusside in blood and plasma. Clin Chem 23:1969–1975, 1977.
6. Schulz V, Bonn R, Kindler J: Kinetics of elimination of thiocyanate in seven healthy subjects and in eight subjects with renal failure. Klin Wochenschr 57:243–247, 1979.
7. Ivankovich AD, Braverman B, Stephens TS, et al: Sodium thiosulfate disposition in humans: Relation to sodium nitroprusside toxicity. Anesthesiology 58:11–17, 1983.

8. Rutkowski JV, Roebuck BD, Smith RP: Liver damage does not increase the sensitivity of mice to cyanide given acutely. Toxicology 38:305–314, 1986.
9. Jack RD: Toxicity of sodium nitroprusside (Letter). Br J Anaesth 46:952, 1974.
10. MacRae WR, Owen M: Severe metabolic acidosis following hypotension induced with sodium nitroprusside. Br J Anaesth 46:795–797, 1974.
11. Mellino M, Phillips DF: Severe lactic acidosis in a case of nitroprusside resistance. Cleve Clin Q 47:119–122, 1980.
12. Humphrey SH, Nash DA: Lactic acidosis complicating sodium nitroprusside therapy. Ann Intern Med 88:58–59, 1978.
13. Aitken D, West D, Smith F, et al: Cyanide toxicity following nitroprusside-induced hypotension. Can Anaesth Soc J 24:651–660, 1977.
14. Vesey CJ, Cole PV, Simpson PJ: Cyanide and thiocyanate concentrations following sodium nitroprusside infusion in man. Br J Anaesth 48:651–660, 1976.
15. Vesey CJ, Cole PV: Blood cyanide and thiocyanate concentrations produced by long-term therapy with sodium nitroprusside. Br J Anaesth 57:148–155, 1985.
16. Vesey CJ, Wilson J: Red cell cyanide. J Pharm Pharmacol 30:20–26, 1978.
17. Patel CB, Laboy V, Venus B, et al: Use of sodium nitroprusside in post-coronary bypass surgery: A plea for conservatism. Chest 89:663–667, 1986.
18. Cole PV, Vesey CJ: Sodium thiosulphate decreases blood cyanide concentration following sodium nitroprusside (Letter). Br J Anaesth 60:745, 1988.
19. Schulz V, Gross R, Pasch T, et al: Cyanide toxicity of sodium nitroprusside in therapeutic use with and without sodium thiosulphate. Klin Wochenschr 60:1393–1400, 1982.
20. Pahl MV, Vaziri ND: In-vivo and in-vitro hemodialysis studies of thiocyanate. J Toxicol Clin Toxicol 19:965–974, 1982.
21. Elberg AJ, Gorman HM, Baker R, et al: Prolonged nitroprusside and intermittent hemodialysis as therapy for intractable hypertension. Am J Dis Child 132:988–989, 1978.
22. Rigg D, McDonogh A: Use of sodium nitroprusside for deliberate hypotension during pregnancy. Br J Anaesth 53:985–987, 1981.
23. Donchin Y, Amirav G, Sahar A, et al: Sodium nitroprusside for aneurysm surgery in pregnancy. Br J Anaesth 50:849–851, 1978.
24. Stempel JE, O'Grady JP, Morton MJ, et al: Use of sodium nitroprusside in complications of gestational hypertension. Obstet Gynecol 60:533–538, 1982.
25. Ellis SC, Wheeler AS, James FM III, et al: Fetal and maternal effects of sodium nitroprusside used to counteract hypertension in gravid ewes. Am J Obstet Gynecol 143:766–770, 1982.
26. Curry SC, Carlton MW, Raschke RA: Prevention of fetal and maternal cyanide toxicity from nitroprusside with coinfusion of sodium thiosulfate in gravid ewes. Anesth Analg 84:1121–1126, 1997.
27. Naulty J, Cefalo RC, Lewis PE: Fetal toxicity of nitroprusside in the pregnant ewe. Am J Obstet Gynecol 139:708–711, 1981.
28. Graeme KA, Curry SC, Bikin DS, et al: The lack of transplacental movement of the cyanide antidote thiosulfate in gravid ewes. Anesth Analg 89:1448–1452, 1999.

CHAPTER **38**

Imidazoline, Guanidine, and Oxazoline Antihypertensives and Decongestants

Anthony J. Tomassoni ■ Kevin L. Wallace

Clonidine and other imidazoline derivatives have a variety of treatment indications, including hypertension and mucous membrane congestion. Clonidine is the most thoroughly studied of the centrally acting antihypertensive agents and is chemically and pharmacologically similar to other members of the imidazoline class, such as guanabenz and guanfacine. The development and clinical introduction of two newer oxazolines, moxonidine and rilmenidine, has led to better understanding of the mechanism of action of the imidazolines. These more recently developed agents are used primarily as antihypertensives. The introduction of clonidine initially as a mucous membrane decongestant was followed by the development and approval of several other imidazoline compounds for this indication, including naphazoline, oxymetazoline, tetrahydrozoline, and xylometazoline, which now are available over the counter or by prescription as decongestant solutions intended for nasal or ocular use. As expected, based on their chemical and pharmacologic similarity, these agents have similar toxicity. Most reported cases of severe imidazoline intoxication pertain to clonidine.

Clonidine initially was developed for use as a decongestant in 1962. Shortly thereafter, this compound's sympatholytic and hypotensive effects were noted,[1] leading to its clinical application as an antihypertensive[2,3] and subsequently to its use in the management of glaucoma[4–8]; migraine headache[9]; attention-deficit disorder with hyperactivity[10]; menopausal flushing[11]; and, in conjunction with opioids or local anesthetics (or both) in epidural infusion, intractable cancer pain, postsurgical pain, and labor.[12–15]

The existence of a central nonadrenergic binding site responsible for the antihypertensive effect of clonidine was advanced in the 1980s after the investigation of structurally similar compounds synthesized to have fewer adverse effects.[16] Subsequently the oxazoline compounds rilmenidine and moxonidine were approved for clinical application in several countries. These compounds have little α_2-agonist potency compared with clonidine but nonetheless exert marked hypotensive effects. The study of these drugs has led to improved understanding of the imidazoline receptor concept, further described in the pathophysiology section.

These compounds also possess antidysrhythmic activity.[17] Long-term use results in remodeling of the left ventricle. A hypoglycemic effect due to improved insulin sensitivity[18] without atherogenic effect also has been attributed to these agents.[19–21]

Tetrahydrozoline, naphazoline, oxymetazoline, and xylometazoline currently are used in nasal and ocular decongestants. These are available in a wide variety of sprays and drops available by prescription and over the counter. Ingestion of 2.5 mL of 0.05% tetrahydrozoline (1.25 mg) has resulted in respiratory depression. Drowsiness, sweating, marked hypotension, and shock resulting from the inadvertent ingestion of small amounts of these agents by children were recognized and reported by the mid-1960s.[22,23]

In general, the use of topical or systemic imidazolines in children younger than age 6 years has not been recommended in the Western English language literature for many years, but such indications still persist in the literature of other regions. Aside from the age of the patient, some factors suggested as contributors to the intoxication of young children with "therapeutic" use of imidazoline decongestants include the difficulty of administering drops to children and packaging inadequate for proper dosing of children.[24]

Despite numerous reports of imidazoline intoxication after ingestion of 2.5 mL of solution, availability of over-the-counter imidazoline-containing nasal and ocular decongestants remains widespread.[22] Poison-prevention efforts should focus on increasing public and professional awareness of the hazard posed by imidazolines and on the safe packaging, use, and storage of these agents.

CLINICAL PHARMACOLOGY

The chemical structures of clonidine and other imidazoline and oxazoline compounds is shown in Figure 38-1. Clonidine is absorbed completely and rapidly from the gastrointestinal tract with rapid onset of action in 30 to 60 minutes and essentially 100% bioavailability. Peak effects have been reported to occur at 2 to 3 hours with a

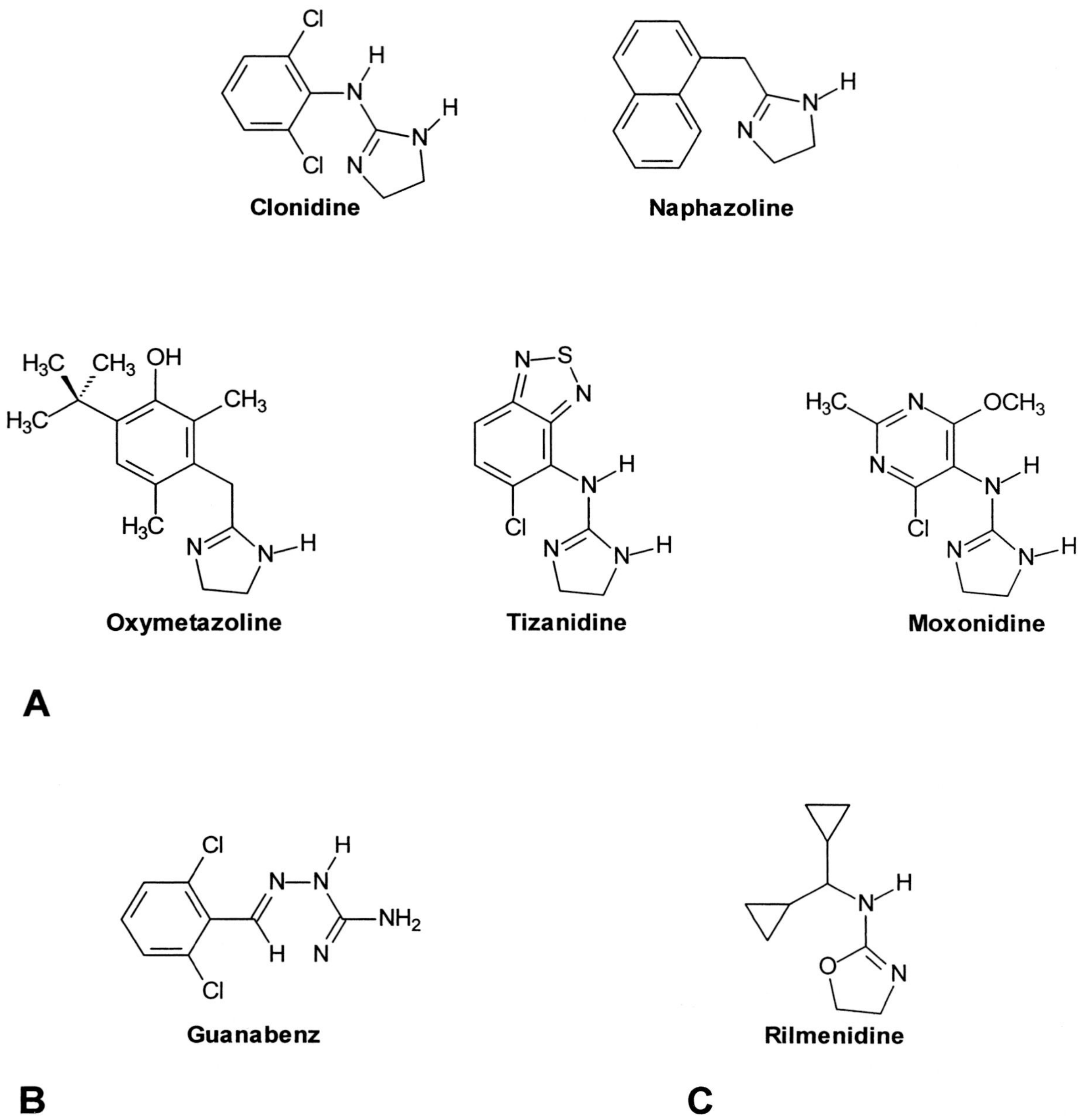

FIGURE 38-1

Chemical structures of imidazoline, guanidine, and oxazoline compounds. **A**, Imidazoline compounds. **B**, A guanidine compound. **C**, An oxazoline compound.

duration of 8 hours when administered in therapeutic amounts.[1] Topical imidazolines are well absorbed through ocular and nasal mucosa and the gastrointestinal tract. Although clonidine is excreted predominantly unchanged through the kidney, other imidazoline, guanidine, and oxazoline compounds vary in terms of their clearance mechanisms.[25–28]

As might be inferred from the diverse uses of clonidine mentioned earlier, the drug has been available in a variety of doses and formulations ranging from tablets to drops, solutions for injection, transdermal patches, and ophthalmic rods.[29] Systemic effects may result from the topical use of imidazolines. The use of clonidine 0.5% eye drops intended to treat open-angle glaucoma has been noted to lower substantially the systemic blood pressure.[30]

Transdermal delivery of imidazolines is effective, but the conversion from oral to transdermal dosing is not predictable, presumably because of interpatient variability in transdermal absorption. Transdermal dosing of clonidine always should begin with a patch designed to deliver 0.1 mg/24 hr applied once every 7 days to avoid accidental hypotension or intoxication.[31] The rate of drug absorption from patches also varies with the site of application on any given individual.[32] The use of transdermal delivery systems has resulted in unintentional drug transfer. Used transdermal patches of clonidine contain large residual amounts of medication. A 0.3 mg/24 hr clonidine patch (7.5 mg/10.5 cm²) might contain approximately 5.4 mg residual clonidine after being worn for 1 week.

Discarded patches may pose a particular hazard to toddlers, who might retrieve these after they are discarded and then wear the patch or, worse, swallow them or suck or chew on them, liberating toxic amounts of clonidine.[33] Inadvertent parent-to-child transfer of a transdermal clonidine patch resulting in toxic effects in the toddler also has been reported.[34] In addition, we have witnessed hypotension resulting from excess drug delivery when multiple transdermal patches were worn by a confused elderly patient who mistakenly placed new patches of medication without removing the old transparent patches, which she had difficulty locating once they were placed on her skin.

Pharmacokinetics of Selected Imidazoline and Guanidine Drugs

Clonidine

Volume of distribution: 3.2–5.6 L/kg; 0.96 L/kg in children[4]
Protein binding: 20–40%
Active metabolites: None reported
Mechanisms of clearance: 40–60% excreted unchanged via kidney
Elimination half-life: 12–16 hr

Guanabenz

Volume of distribution: 7.4–13.4 L/kg
Protein binding: 90%
Active metabolites: None reported
Mechanisms of clearance: Hepatic (<1% excreted unchanged via kidney)
Elimination half-life: 12–14 hr

Oxymetazoline

Volume of distribution: NA
Protein binding: NA
Active metabolites: None reported
Mechanisms of clearance: 30–72% renal; 10–22% fecal; 40–50% excreted unchanged
Elimination half-life: 5–8 hr

NA, no information available.

Data from references 25 through 28.

PATHOPHYSIOLOGY

Initial speculation regarding the mechanism of action attributed the sedation, oral hyposecretion, and antihypertensive effects of clonidine to its activation of brainstem α_2-adrenergic receptors.[35] Stimulation of these receptors results in inhibition of the nucleus tractus solitarius and ultimately in decreased norepinephrine release. This reduced sympathetic outflow from the thoracolumbar spinal tracts to the periphery has been thought to be the primary basis for the cardiovascular and neurobehavioral effects of these drugs.[36,37] Sedation is thought to result primarily from the α_2-agonist

actions of imidazolines and guanidines, such as clonidine and guanabenz, in the locus caeruleus. The peripheral sympathomimetic effects of clonidine and other α_2-agonists in this class (e.g., transient vasoconstriction and initial rise in blood pressure) have been explained on the basis of postsynaptic α_2-agonist actions in vascular smooth muscle.[38] The presynaptic α_2-receptor agonist actions of these drugs at central and peripheral adrenergic synapses, resulting in suppression of norepinephrine release, also may contribute to the antihypertensive effects of clonidine. Imidazolines and the other drugs in this treatment category have little effect on β-adrenergic receptors.

The development of more potent α_2-agonists did not yield compounds with improved antihypertensive properties, leading to the hypothesis that the central antihypertensive action of these agents may result in part from agonist actions at specific imidazoline receptors. As previously noted, investigations of structure-activity relationships of compounds synthesized in an effort to reduce or eliminate the adverse effects (e.g., sedation) of clonidine led to development of the oxazoline class of antihypertensives (e.g., rilmenidine).

Parallels between effects resulting from the stimulation of opiate receptors and central α_2-adrenergic receptors have led to speculation about a potential relationship between these receptors. This speculation is reinforced by the successful use of clonidine in detoxification regimens for opiate dependence[39,40] and as a spinal analgesic.[12–15] Current hypotheses regarding such a link between opiate receptors and central α_2-adrenergic receptors remain unproven.

CLINICAL PRESENTATION AND LIFE-THREATENING COMPLICATIONS

On the basis of numerous case reports and case series,[22,24,41–46] the life-threatening effects of acute imidazoline intoxication may be characterized by initial hypertension and reflex bradycardia, followed by hypotension with bradycardia and a cyclical pattern of agitation alternating with coma/respiratory depression (bradypnea or apnea) that typically responds to vigorous physical stimulation. Peripheral vasoconstriction may manifest as skin pallor. Pupillary miosis is common. Hypotonia, hyporeflexia, and hypothermia also may be present in severe intoxication. Bowel sounds may be reduced or absent, indicating gastrointestinal hypomotility.

Prominent α_2 effects associated with imidazolines include sedation and reduced salivation. These common adverse effects of clonidine and guanabenz (compounds that possess strong α_2-agonist properties) have limited their use at recommended doses by some patients. Although oral hyposecretion may be used to help characterize the toxidrome, this effect is less pronounced with oxazolines, such as moxonidine and rilmenidine, which have markedly reduced α_2-agonist potency.

Abrupt cessation of clonidine has been associated with a hyperadrenergic syndrome characterized by what commonly is referred to as *rebound hypertension*. This effect may be dose dependent and has not been observed so far with the newer oxazoline group of antihypertensives.[47,48]

DIAGNOSIS

A broad differential diagnosis should be considered in patients suspected of imidazoline, guanidine, or oxazoline drug toxicity, as for all patients presenting in coma (see Chapter 19). Systemic oxygenation status and blood glucose concentration should be monitored early in the diagnostic evaluation. Given the potential for inhibition of glycogenolysis secondary to sympatholytic actions, the clinician should consider these patients to be at increased risk for hypoglycemia.

The toxicologic differential diagnosis of imidazoline poisoning includes intoxication with opioids, β-blockers, calcium channel blockers, phenothiazines (e.g., chlorpromazine), acetylcholinesterase inhibitors (i.e., organophosphates or carbamates), barbiturates, and other sedative-hypnotic agents. Although routine toxicology immunoassay screens generally do not include imidazolines, these compounds can be identified in clinical specimens (e.g., urine) by gas chromatography/mass spectroscopy when clinically or forensically warranted.

TREATMENT

Because imidazoline compound–intoxicated or guanidine compound–intoxicated patients may develop light coma with or without apneic spells, special attention must be paid to airway and ventilatory status. Endotracheal intubation and mechanical ventilatory support are rarely required but may be warranted in severe intoxications. Successful management of imidazoline poisoning often has been limited to close observation with physical stimulation to terminate apneic episodes.[41]

Transient hypertension may be observed in patients who present early after overdose. This hypertension is generally of brief duration and often requires no therapy. Severe hypertension should be treated only with short-acting, readily controlled vasodilator treatment (e.g., nitroprusside or possibly phentolamine) because it is likely to be transient and followed by hypotension as central sympatholytic effects become predominant.

Intravenous administration of crystalloid should be considered as first-line therapy for hypotension in centrally acting antihypertensive overdose. The use of atropine for bradycardia in normotensive or hypertensive individuals may precipitate or prolong hypertensive crisis in individuals with a reflex increase in vagal tone secondary to peripheral vasoconstrictive effects. We recommend that atropine be avoided in imidazoline-poisoned patients except in the event of clinically significant bradycardia *and* hypotension. Intravenous dopamine, with or without atropine, is an appropriate choice of pressor in the treatment of hypotension associated with bradycardia.[49]

Hypothermia should be managed with active or passive rewarming as indicated. Given the potential for these drugs to cause central nervous system depression shortly after ingestion, gastric emptying procedures (e.g., administration of ipecac or gastric lavage) are not recommended. A single dose of activated charcoal may be administered to patients who are alert and present shortly after ingestion and is likely to be more effective after the ingestion of tablets than of imidazoline-containing solutions, given the rapid absorption of drugs in solution. In the event of clonidine patch ingestion, whole-bowel irrigation with polyethylene glycol/balanced electrolyte solution has been reported to be effective in enhancing clearance from the gastrointestinal tract.[33] Extracorporeal removal by hemodialysis has not been shown to be efficacious in enhancement of clonidine clearance.[25]

There is no generally accepted specific antidotal therapy for imidazoline poisoning. Imidazoline-induced coma, respiratory depression, and miosis have suggested a role for intravenous naloxone as a means of reversing life-threatening clinical manifestations of toxicity. Reports of the efficacy of this treatment are inconsistent and are confounded by the typically cyclical course of the central nervous system effects of untreated poisoning.[45,46,50–53] It is possible that physical stimulation associated with the administration of this medication may be responsible for some reports of the efficacy of naloxone in reversing apnea and lightening sedation in some cases of imidazoline intoxication. Administration of naloxone to clonidine-poisoned children also has been reported to result in hypertension.[54] In cases in which naloxone has been suggested to have reversed clonidine-induced coma, the "response" has been transient and consistent with the untreated, cyclical course of the intoxication. The case of a 3-year-old child treated with naloxone after ingestion of 30 mL of 0.05% tetrahydrozoline solution reported by Holmes and Berman[55] illustrated this transient response. Two hours after the ingestion, incontinence of urine, hypotonia, and lethargy were noted. Naloxone (1.5 mg) was administered intravenously, followed by improvement in sensorium and increased heart rate and blood pressure. The effect was short-lived, however, and 10 minutes later the child again became somnolent with decreased pulse and blood pressure. The child subsequently was awake and alert approximately 8 hours after ingestion without further administration of naloxone.

Despite the lack of convincing evidence that naloxone administration is beneficial in clonidine poisoning, its efficacy has not been excluded definitively by controlled clinical trials. If one is faced with the prospect of impending endotracheal intubation after the failure of vigorous stimulation to arouse an imidazoline-intoxicated patient in coma, it seems reasonable to proceed with an empirical trial of relatively high-dose naloxone (4 to 10 mg intravenously) as long as this intervention does not delay the institution of appropriate supportive care measures. Perhaps the most appropriate empirical use of naloxone is in the setting of

---

Indications for ICU Admission in Clonidine and Other Imidazoline Derivatives Poisoning

Coma/respiratory depression
Bradycardia/hypotension
Rebound (i.e., abrupt cessation–related) hypertension

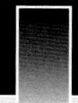

Criteria for ICU Discharge in Clonidine and Other Imidazoline Derivatives Poisoning

Intact sensorium
Stable hemodynamic status

suspected or confirmed imidazoline intoxication to address the possibility of unrecognized or concomitant opioid toxicity.

Tolazoline, also an imidazoline compound, is a mixed central and peripheral α_2-antagonist that has been used in the treatment of imidazoline intoxication, based on its theoretical potential for reversal of the central sympatholytic and peripheral sympathomimetic actions of imidazoline and guanidine drugs. Tolazoline generally is not recommended, however, given mixed clinical case experience and reported instances of hypertension, tachycardia, and arrhythmias after its administration.[56] Yohimbine, an indole derivative with central α_2-antagonist actions, and idazoxan, an imidazoline and α_2-adrenergic receptor antagonist, similarly lack sufficient supporting clinical evidence of efficacy and safety to recommend their use in the treatment of α_2-agonist toxicity.[57,58]

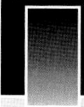

Key Points in the Evaluation and Management of Clonidine and Other Imidazoline Derivatives Poisoning

1. Severe toxicity, especially in young children, has resulted from the ingestion of small amounts (<15 mL) of over-the-counter topical and prescription imidazoline and guanidine preparations.
2. Clinical toxicity frequently presents as cyclical coma/respiratory depression alternating with agitation.
3. Appropriate treatment commonly is limited to routine supportive care and close observation, with physical stimulation as needed for episodes of apnea.
4. Although to date there is no convincing evidence that it reverses imidazoline-induced central nervous system depression, the empirical administration of high-dose intravenous naloxone in respiratory depression refractory to physical stimulation seems reasonable as long as it does not delay the provision of appropriately more aggressive supportive care (i.e., endotracheal intubation and mechanical ventilation).
5. Atropine use should be avoided in imidazoline-poisoned patients except in patients with clinically significant bradycardia *and* hypotension.
6. There is currently no antidote for centrally acting α_2-agonist poisoning that has proved safe and effective.

SPECIAL POPULATIONS

Pregnant Patients

The teratogenicity of common prescription and over-the-counter imidazolines has not been studied completely. Given the relatively high fetoplacental penetration of imidazolines, developing fetuses are at potential risk of toxicity.

Clonidine crosses the placenta readily with cord blood levels similar to maternal blood levels at delivery.[59] Maternal hypotension and hypoxia resulting from severe imidazoline intoxication also might result in reproductive toxicity. Fetal bradycardia is reported to occur with increased frequency in women who are administered epidural clonidine concomitantly with an epidural anesthetic in labor.[60,61] Infants born to women treated with oral clonidine late in pregnancy uncommonly may experience transient neonatal hypertension.[62,63] Although high-dose animal studies of clonidine revealed effects on uterine blood flow, intraamniotic pressure, and fetal oxygenation,[64,65] clonidine generally does not seem to be associated with significant adverse effects at doses that are nontoxic to the mother.[66–68] A case report of an infant with multiple severe birth defects (Roberts' syndrome) born to a mother treated with 0.3 mg/day of clonidine throughout pregnancy for hypertension suggests, however, the preferable use of an alternative agent for the treatment of hypertension during pregnancy,[69] with clonidine considered relatively contraindicated in this context. Clonidine is listed as a class C drug under the U.S. Food and Drug Administration Fetal Risk Summary classification (see Appendix A).[70]

Epidemiologic studies have not revealed definitive evidence of associations between the use of oxymetazoline and birth defects, despite one study in which maternal use of oxymetazoline, phenylpropanolamine, and pseudoephedrine revealed an association with gastroschisis. Pseudoephedrine and phenylpropanolamine apparently accounted for the major portion of this association.[71–74] A nonreactive nonstress test and late decelerations have been reported, however, in a patient presenting at 41 weeks' gestation. The fetus was delivered due to late decelerations and term pregnancy. The mother reportedly had overused an oxymetazoline-containing nasal spray before examination. Fetal heart rate changes were thought to result indirectly from decreased uterine perfusion or perhaps through a direct effect on the fetal central nervous system.[75] The safest policy is to advise against the use of imidazolines during pregnancy.

Pediatric Patients

Infants and young children are relatively susceptible to systemic effects from topical imidazoline use.[76] Pediatric patients also are at relatively high risk for poisoning due to their smaller body mass and greater likelihood of ingesting imidazolines intended for topical use from containers supplied with dropper-type or spray-type dispensers resembling baby bottle nipples. Abundant case experience suggests that younger children are at particularly high risk for imidazoline-induced central nervous system depression and respiratory failure.[22–24,43–46,76] Clonidine has been found in human breast milk at concentrations about twice those in maternal blood, but the significance of this finding to nursing infants is unknown.[59,77]

Geriatric Patients

The elderly seem to be at increased risk of systemic adverse effects from topical imidazoline use. Bradycardia and hypotension have been reported in an elderly patient.[78]

Some caution against the use of these drugs in the elderly seems appropriate.

Other Special Populations

Clonidine may be used to relieve symptoms in patients withdrawing from opioids, alcohol, or nicotine. Clonidine is used best in conjunction with other agents in the process of opioid or alcohol detoxification.[79,80] Monotherapy with clonidine is not recommended, and clonidine alone does not reduce the incidence of seizures or delirium. Alcohol-dependent patients also should receive benzodiazepines.[81] Care must be exercised in treating opioid-dependent patients with possible polysubstance abuse because clonidine may mask symptoms of life-threatening sedative-hypnotic or ethanol withdrawal.[82]

REFERENCES

1. Lowenstein J: Clonidine. Ann Intern Med 92:74–77, 1980.
2. Nayler WG, Rosenbaum M, McInnes I, et al: Effect of a new hypotensive drug, ST 155, on the systemic circulation. Am Heart J 72:764–770, 1966.
3. Smet G, Hoobler SW, Sanbar S, et al: Clinical observations on a new antihypertensive drug, 2-(2,6-dichlorophenylamine)-2-imidazoline hydrochloride. Am Heart J 77:473–478, 1969.
4. Harrison R, Kaufmann CS: Clonidine: Effects of a topically administered solution on intraocular pressure and blood pressure in open-angle glaucoma. Arch Ophthalmol 95:1368–1373, 1977.
5. Gold MS, Redmonde DE, Kleber HD: Clonidine blocks acute opiate-withdrawal symptoms. Lancet 2:599–602, 1978.
6. Gold MS, Pottash AC, Sweeney DR, et al: Opiate withdrawal using clonidine: A safe, effective and rapid non-opiate treatment. JAMA 243:343–346, 1980.
7. Glassman AH, Stetner F, Walsh BT, et al: Heavy smokers, smoking cessation, and clonidine. JAMA 259:2863–2866, 1988.
8. Cohen DJ, Young JG, Nathanson JA, et al: Clonidine in Tourette's syndrome. Lancet 2:551–553, 1979.
9. Shafer I, Tallett ER, Knowlson PA: Evaluation of clonidine in prophylaxis of migraine: Double-blind trial and follow-up. Lancet 1:403–407, 1972.
10. Hunt RD, Minderaa RB, Cohen DJ: Clonidine benefits children with attention deficit disorder and hyperactivity: A report of a double-blind placebo-crossover therapeutic trial. J Am Acad Child Psychiatry 24:617–629, 1985.
11. Clayden JR, Bell JW, Pellard P: Menopausal flushing: Double-blind trial of a non-hormonal medication. BMJ 9:409–412, 1974.
12. Milligan KR, Convery PN, Weir P, et al: The efficacy and safety of epidural infusions of levobupivacaine with and without clonidine for postoperative pain relief in patients undergoing total hip replacement. Anesth Analg 91:393–397, 2000.
13. Motsch J, Graber E, Ludwig K: Addition of clonidine enhances postoperative analgesia from epidural morphine: A double-blind study. Anesthesiology 73:1067–1073, 1990.
14. Naulty JS: Continuous infusions of local anesthetics and narcotics for epidural analgesia in the management of labor. Int Anesthesiol Clin 28:17–24, 1990.
15. Bonnet F, Boico O, Rostaing S, et al: Postoperative analgesia with extradural clonidine. Br J Anaesth 63:465–469, 1989.
16. Bousquet P, Feldman J, Schwartz J: Central cardiovascular effects of α-adrenergic drugs: Differences between catecholamines and imidazolines. J Pharmacol Exp Ther 230:230–236, 1984.
17. Bousquet P, Feldman J: Drugs acting on imidazoline receptors: A review of their pharmacology, their use in blood pressure control and their potential interest in cardioprotection. Drugs 58:799–812, 1999.
18. Lithell HO: Insulin resistance and diabetes in the context of treatment of hypertension. Blood Press 3(Suppl):28–31, 1998.
19. Laurent S, Safar M: Rilmenidine: A novel approach to first-line treatment of hypertension. Am J Hypertens 5(4 Pt 2):99S–105S, 1992.
20. Elliott HL: Moxonidine: Pharmacology, clinical pharmacology and clinical profile. Blood Press 7(Suppl 3):23–27, 1998.
21. Schachter M: Moxonidine: A review of safety and tolerability after seven years of clinical experience. J Hypertens 17(Suppl 3):37–39, 1999.
22. Higgins GL, Campbell B, Wallace K, et al: Pediatric poisoning from over-the-counter imidazoline-containing products. Ann Emerg Med 20:655–658, 1991.
23. Mindlin RL: Accidental poisoning from tetrahydrozoline eyedrops (Letter). N Engl J Med 275:112, 1966.
24. Vitezic D, Romanic V, Franulovic J, et al: Naphazoline nasal drops intoxication in children. Arh Hig Rada Toksikol 45:25–29, 1994.
25. Dollery SC (ed): Clonidine. In Therapeutic Drugs, vol 1. New York, Churchill Livingstone, 1991.
26. Lowenthal DT: Pharmacokinetics of clonidine. J Cardiovasc Pharmacol 2(Suppl):529–537, 1980.
27. Meacham RH, Emmett M, Kyriakopoulos AA, et al: Disposition of C-guanabenz in patients with essential hypertension. Clin Pharmacol Ther 27:44–52, 1980.
28. Covington TR, Pau AK: Oxymetazoline. Am Pharmacol NS25:21–26, 1985.
29. Alani SD, Hammerstein W: The ophthalmic rod—a new drug delivery system II. Graefes Arch Clin Exp Ophthalmol 228:302–304, 1990.
30. Petursson G, Cole R, Hanna C: Treatment of glaucoma using minidrops of clonidine. Arch Ophthalmol 102:1180–1181, 1984.
31. AHFS Drug Information 2000. Bethesda, MD, American Society of Health-System Pharmacists, 2000.
32. Ebihara A, Fujimura A, Ohashi K, et al: Influence of application site of a new transdermal clonidine, M5041T, on its pharmacokinetics and pharmacodynamics in healthy subjects. J Clin Pharmacol 33:1188–1191, 1993.
33. Henretig FM, Wiley J, Brown L: Clonidine patch toxicity: The proof's in the poop! (Abstract). J Toxicol Clin Toxicol 33:520, 1995.
34. Reed MT, Hamburg EL: Person-to-person transfer of transdermal drug delivery systems: A case report. N Engl J Med 314:1120–1121, 1986.
35. Timmermans PBMW, Van Zwieten PA: α2-Adrenoreceptors: Classification, localization, mechanisms and targets for drugs. J Med Chem 25:1389–1401, 1982.
36. Abrams WB: In summary: Satellite symposium on central α-adrenergic blood pressure regulating mechanisms. Hypertension 6(Suppl II):87–93, 1984.
37. Reid JL: Alpha-adrenergic receptors and blood pressure control. Am J Cardiol 19:19–24, 1981.
38. Kobinger W: Central α-adrenergic systems as targets for hypotensive drugs. Rev Physiol Biochem Pharmacol 81:39–100, 1978.
39. Franz DN, Hare BD, McCloskey KL: Spinal sympathetic neurons: Possible site of opiate-withdrawal suppression by clonidine. Science 215:1643–1645, 1982.
40. Aghajanian GK: Tolerance of locus coeruleus neurons to morphine and suppression of withdrawal response to clonidine. Nature 276:186–188, 1978.
41. Anderson FJ, Hart GR, Crumpler CP, et al: Clonidine overdose: Report of six cases and review of the literature. Ann Emerg Med 10:107–112, 1981.
42. Olsson JM, Pruitt AW: Management of clonidine ingestion in children. J Pediatr 103:646–650, 1983.
43. Knapp JF, Fowler MA, Wheeler CA, Wasserman GS: A two-year-old female with alteration of consciousness. Pediatr Emerg Care 11:62–65, 1995.
44. Heidemann SM, Sarnaik AP: Clonidine poisoning in children. Crit Care Med 18:618–620, 1990.
45. Fiser DH, Moss MM, Walker W: Critical care for clonidine poisoning in toddlers. Crit Care Med 18:1124–1128, 1990.
46. Wiley JF II, Wiley CC, Henretig FM: Clonidine poisoning in young children. J Pediatr 116:654–658, 1990.
47. Ram CV, Engelman K: Abrupt discontinuation of clonidine therapy. JAMA 242:2104–2105, 1979.
48. Sarlis NJ, Caticha O, Anderson JL, et al: Hyperadrenergic state following acute withdrawal from clonidine used at supratherapeutic doses. Clin Auton Res 6:115–117, 1996.
49. Maggi JC, Iskra MK, Nussbaum E: Severe clonidine overdose in children requiring critical care. Clin Paediatr 25:453–455, 1986.
50. Kulig K, Rumack BH: Efficacy of naloxone in clonidine poisoning. Am J Dis Child 137:807–808, 1983.
51. Banner W Jr, Lund ME, Clawson L: Failure of naloxone to reverse clonidine toxic effect. Am J Dis Child 137:1170–1171, 1983.
52. Nichols MH, King WD, James LP: Clonidine poisoning in Jefferson County, Alabama. Ann Emerg Med 29:511–517, 1997.
53. Wedin GP, Edwards LJ: Clonidine poisoning treated with naloxone. Am J Emerg Med 7:343–344, 1989.

54. Gremse DA, Artman M, Boerth RC: Hypertension associated with naloxone treatment for clonidine poisoning. J Pediatr 108(5 Pt 1):776–778, 1986.

55. Holmes JF, Berman DA: Use of naloxone to reverse symptomatic tetrahydrozoline overdose in a child. Pediatr Emerg Care 15:193–194, 1999.

56. Schieber RA, Kaufman ND: Use of tolazoline in massive clonidine poisoning. Am J Dis Child 135:77–78, 1981.

57. Roberge RJ, McGuire SP, Krenzelok EP: Yohimbine as an antidote for clonidine overdose. Am J Emerg Med 14:678–680, 1996.

58. Shannon M, Neuman MI: Yohimbine. Pediatr Emerg Care 16:49–50, 2000.

59. Hartikainen-Sorri AL, Heikkinen JE, Koivisto M, et al: Pharmacokinetics of clonidine during pregnancy and nursing. Obstet Gynecol 69:598–600, 1987.

60. Chassard D, Mathon L, Dailler F, et al: Extradural clonidine combined with sufentanil and 0.0625% bupivacaine for analgesia in labour. Br J Anaesth 77:458–462, 1996.

61. Cigarini I, Kaba A, Bonnet F, et al: Epidural clonidine combined with bupivacaine for analgesia in labor. Reg Anesth 20:113–120, 1995.

62. Boutroy MJ, Gisonna CR, Legagneur M: Clonidine: Placental transfer and neonatal adaption. Early Hum Dev 17:275–286, 1988.

63. Horvath JS, Phippard A, Korda A, et al: Clonidine hydrochloride: A safe and effective antihypertensive agent in pregnancy. Obstet Gynecol 66:634–638, 1985.

64. Eisenach JC, Castro MI, Dewan DM, et al: Intravenous clonidine hydrochloride toxicity in pregnant ewes. Am J Obstet Gynecol 160:471–478, 1988.

65. Bamford OS, Dawes GS, Hanson MA, et al: Effects of the alpha2-adrenergic agonist clonidine and its antagonist idazoxan on the fetal lamb. J Physiol 381:29–37, 1986.

66. Johnson CI, Aickin DR: The control of high blood pressure during labor with clonidine. Med J Aust 2:132–135, 1971.

67. Tuimala R, Punnonen R, Kauppila E, et al: Clonidine in the treatment of hypertension during pregnancy. Ann Chir Gynaecol 74(Suppl 197):47–50, 1985.

68. LeMoine PM, Coggins G: The use of clonidine, Catapres, in hypertensive and toxemic syndromes of pregnancy. Aust N Z J Med 3:432, 1973.

69. Stoll C, Levy JM, Beshara D: Roberts' syndrome and clonidine. J Med Genet 16:486–488, 1979.

70. Briggs GG, Freeman RK, Yaffe SJ (eds): Drugs in Pregnancy and Lactation, 6th ed. Philadelphia, Lippincott Williams & Wilkins, 2002.

71. Aselton P, Jick H, Milunsky A, et al: First-trimester drug use and congenital disorders. Obstet Gynecol 65:451–455, 1985.

72. Rayburn WF, Anderson JC, Smith CV, et al: Uterine and fetal Doppler flow changes from a single dose of a long-acting intranasal decongestant. Obstet Gynecol 76:180–182, 1990.

73. Jick H, Holmes LB, Hunter JR, et al: First-trimester drug use and congenital disorders. JAMA 246:343–346, 1981.

74. Torfs CP, Katz EA, Bateson TF, et al: Maternal medications and environmental exposures as risk factors for gastroschisis. Teratology 54:84–92, 1996.

75. Baxi LV, Gindoff PR, Pregenzer GJ, et al: Fetal heart rate changes following maternal administration of a nasal decongestant. Am J Obstet Gynecol 153:799–800, 1985.

76. Soderman P, Sahlberg J, Wilholm BE, et al: CNS reactions to nose drops in small children. Lancet 1:573, 1984.

77. Bunjes R, Schaefer C: Clonidine and breast-feeding. Clin Pharmacol 12:178–179, 1993.

78. Glazener F, Blake K, Gradman M: Bradycardia, hypotension, and near-syncope associated with Afrin (oxymetazoline) nasal spray. N Engl J Med 309:731, 1983.

79. O'Connor PG, Carroll KM, Shi JM, et al: Three methods of opioid detoxification in a primary care setting: a randomized trial. Ann Intern Med 127:526–530, 1997.

80. American Academy of Pediatrics Committee on Drugs: Neonatal drug withdrawal. Pediatrics 101:1079–1088, 1998.

81. Mayo-Smith MF: Pharmacological management of alcohol withdrawal: A meta-analysis and evidence-based practice guide. JAMA 278:144–151, 1997.

82. Hughes PL, Morse RM: Use of clonidine in a mixed-drug detoxification regimen: Possibility of masking of clinical signs of sedative withdrawal. Mayo Clin Proc 60:47–49, 1985.

CHAPTER 39

Antihistamines

Daniel E. Rusyniak ■ R. Brent Furbee

By the turn of the 20th century, interest in allergic response and particularly the phenomenon of anaphylaxis had become intense. In 1902, Portier and Richet[1] provided further focus for study by developing the concept of altered animal reactivity, which they termed *allergy*. Of the biologic amines released in the inflammatory process, histamine was the first described, originally termed β-*aminoethylimidazole*. Histamine's actions on the gut, bronchioles, and heart were reported in 1910.[2,3] Work on the receptor theory of drug action was well under way when the first articles on anaphylaxis were published. It was not until 1933, however, when Clark published *The Mode of Action of Drugs on Cells*,[4] that acceptance of that theory became sufficient to stimulate a search for compounds that might block histamine's effects. Many compounds with antihistaminic activity were produced, but their toxicity precluded use in humans. In 1941, a French patent was obtained for N_1N-dimethyl-N_1-benzyl-N-phenyl-ethylenediamine, the first antihistamine in human clinical use. Diphenhydramine followed in 1945. The designation *H_1 receptors* was proposed in 1966,[5] and by 1972, the existence of H_2 receptors had been confirmed.[6] Subsequently, use of H_1 and H_2 antagonists became widespread. Nonsedating second-generation antihistamines were developed in the 1980s when their inability to penetrate the central nervous system (CNS) was exploited. Adverse effects, particularly the occasional occurrence of torsades de pointes, was noted in the late 1980s. Emanuel[7] provides a detailed history of the understanding and development of antihistamines.

CLINICAL PHARMACOLOGY

Kinetics for Oral Exposure in Healthy Adults

Compound	Peak Effect (hr)	Half-life (hr)
H_1-Blockers		
Brompheniramine	3–9	12–34
Chlorpheniramine	2	12–43
Cyproheptadine	0.5 (dogs)	?
Dexchlorpheniramine	3	3–6 (duration)
Dimenhydrinate	0.25–0.5 (onset)	?
Diphenhydramine	1–3	2–8

continued

Kinetics for Oral Exposure in Healthy Adults *continued*

H_1-Blockers		
Hydroxyzine	0.25–0.5 (onset)	3–6 (duration)
Loratadine	8–12	12–15
Meclizine	1 (onset)	8–24 (duration)
Promethazine	0.3 (onset)	2–6 (duration)
Tripelennamine	0.25–0.5 (onset)	2–8 (duration)
H_2-Blockers		
Cimetidine	1–2	2–4
Famotidine	1 (onset)	10–12 (duration)
Nizatidine	0.5–3	1.3
Ranitidine hydrochloride	1–3	2.5

Antihistamines are classified based on their affinities for either H_1 or H_2 receptors. Antihistamines classified as H_1-receptor antagonists are divided further into first-generation agents (less H_1 receptor specificity and high blood-brain barrier penetration) and second-generation agents (more H_1 receptor specificity and low blood-brain barrier penetration) (Figs. 39-1 and 39-2).[8]

PATHOPHYSIOLOGY

The therapeutic effects of antihistamines are related to their ability to bind to and block histaminic receptors throughout the body (Fig. 39-3). The therapeutic effects of H_1-receptor antagonists result from the blockade of receptors in the vasculature, bronchioles, cardiac tissues, and sensory nerves and prevention of release of further histamine from mast cells and basophils.[9] This activity results clinically in decreasing the systemic effects of allergic reactions. H_2-receptor antagonists derive their benefit from inhibiting gastric acid secretion and subsequently treating and preventing gastric and duodenal ulcers. The toxic effects of antihistamines occur when either histaminic receptors in the CNS or nonhistaminic receptors in the CNS and peripheral nervous system are antagonized.

In the CNS, there are three classes of histamine receptors: H_1, H_2, and the more recently discovered H_3 receptors.[10,11] H_1 receptors are thought to have a modulatory role in

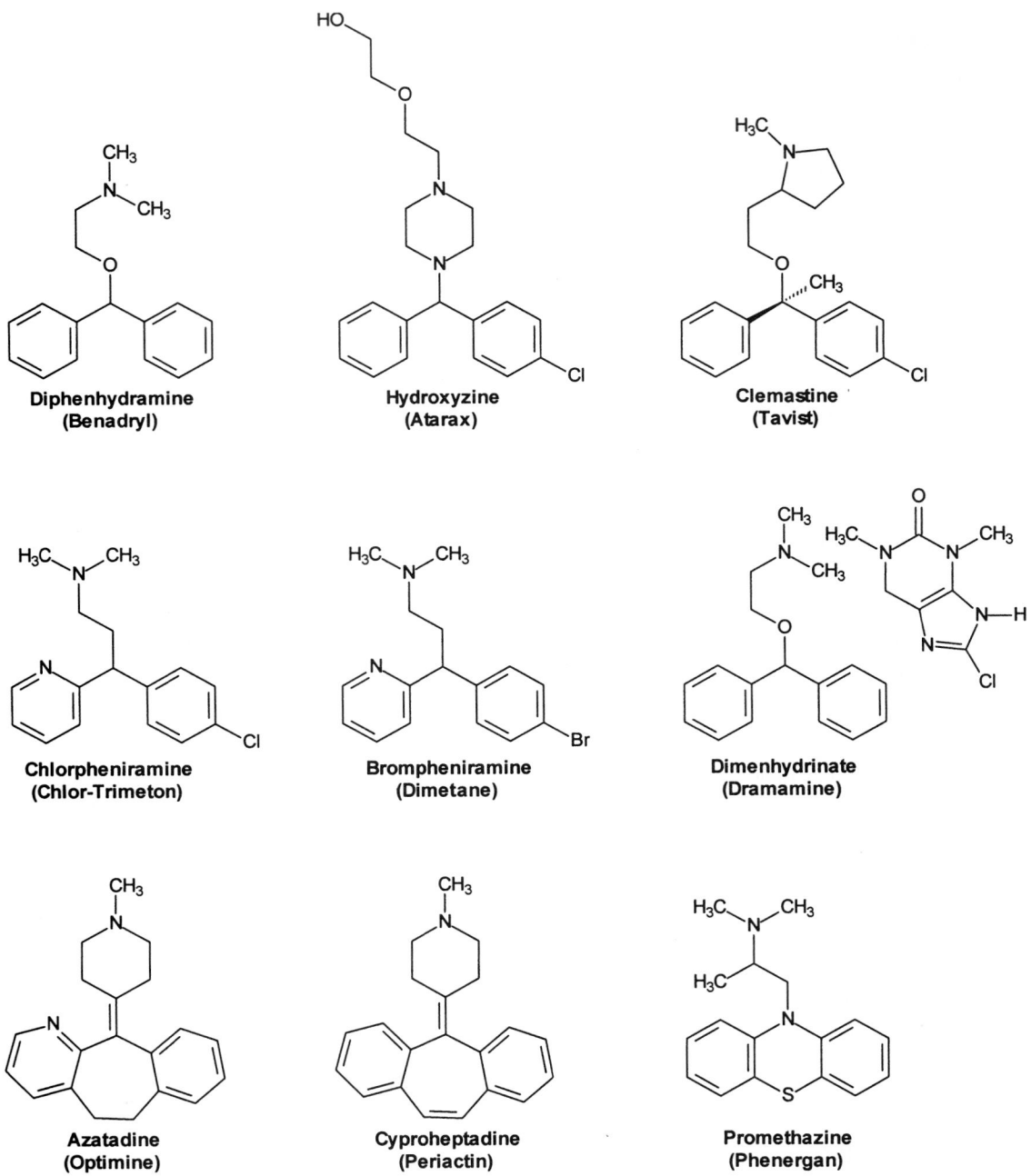

FIGURE 39-1

Chemical structures of first-generation antihistamines (sedating).

the CNS, affecting numerous functions, including sleep-wake cycles, thirst, thermoregulation, and prevention of seizures.[12,13] Antagonism of central H_1 receptors can result in somnolence[14] and seizures.[15]

The mechanism of sedation is believed to be the inhibition of central H_1 receptors.[16] In cultured human cortical neurons, histamine blocks background leakage of potassium, resulting in neuronal membrane depolarization and consequent generation of action potentials. This blockage, along with histamine's distribution in the CNS, is the basis of histamine's presumed role in arousal. Blockade of background potassium currents can be inhibited by selective H_1- but not H_2-receptor

antagonists, resulting in decreased neuronal firing and CNS depression.[14] Traditionally, antihistamine-induced seizures were thought to be due to either their local anesthetic effects or their anticholinergic effects. Antihistamines' ability to cause seizures does not correlate, however, with their affinity for muscarinic receptors and is not reversed by physostigmine.[15,17] Laboratory studies in mice and rats using histidine, a histamine precursor, and blockers of histamine metabolism have shown significant decreases in the incidence of experimentally induced seizures, suggesting that histamine may play a role in the CNS in seizure prevention. Administration of H_1 antagonists lowers the seizure threshold, resulting in epileptic

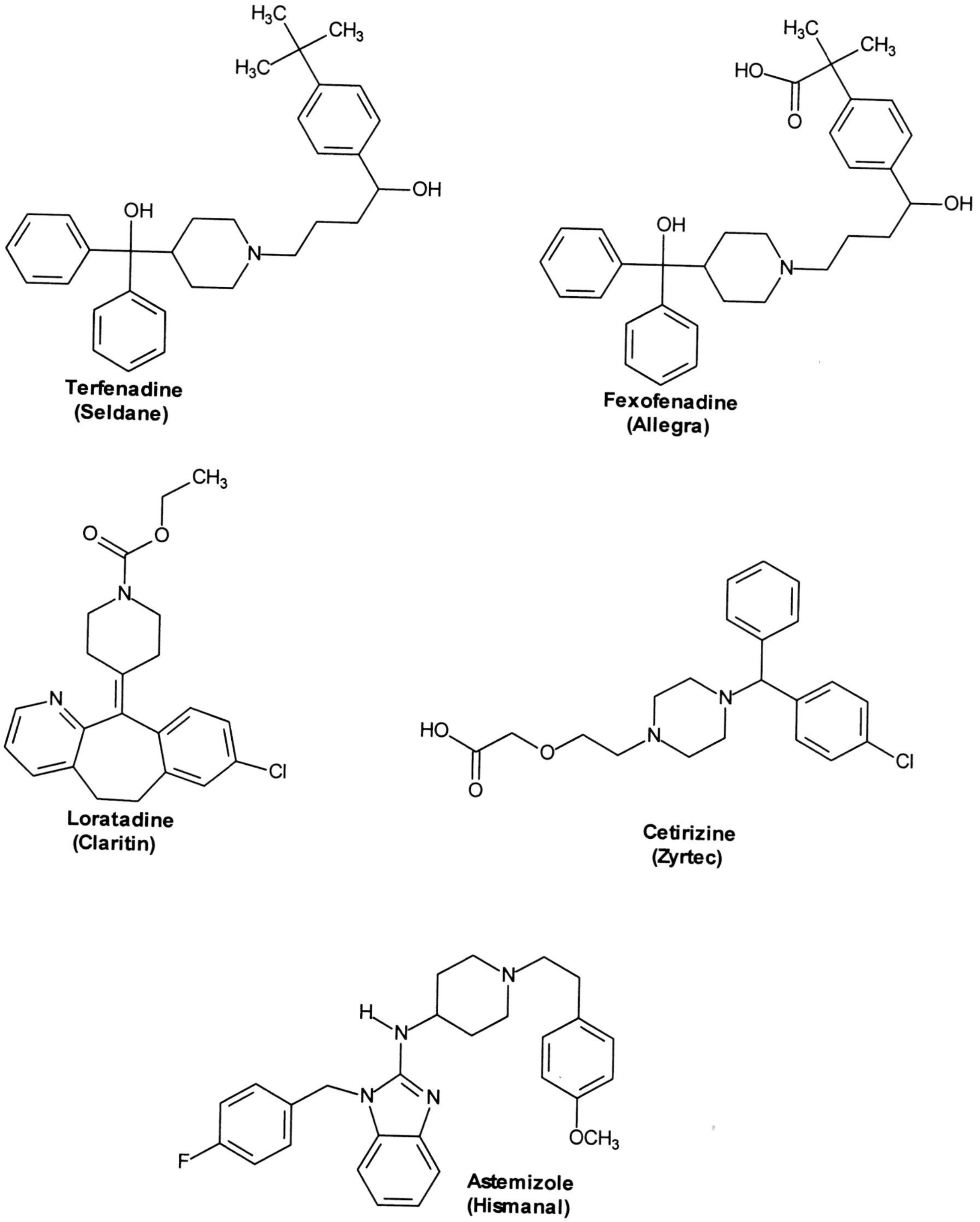

FIGURE 39-2

Chemical structures of second-generation antihistamines (nonsedating).

activity.[13,18–21] The role of central H_2 receptors is not well known, but when animals are given large doses of H_2 blockers, seizures may occur.[22] The presynaptic H_3 receptor works as an autoreceptor regulating the release and synthesis of histamine. Although experimental H_3-receptor antagonists are being investigated as possible anticonvulsants,[23] no clinically relevant agents currently are available.

In part as a result of the similarity in amino acid sequences between H_1 and muscarinic receptors,[24] first-generation H_1 antagonists cause CNS and peripheral nervous system anticholinergic effects. Some adverse effects of antihistamines are related to complications of overdosage (aspiration pneumonia, anoxia, and rhabdomyolysis) or are idiosyncratic (dystonia, thrombocytopenia, and leukopenia).

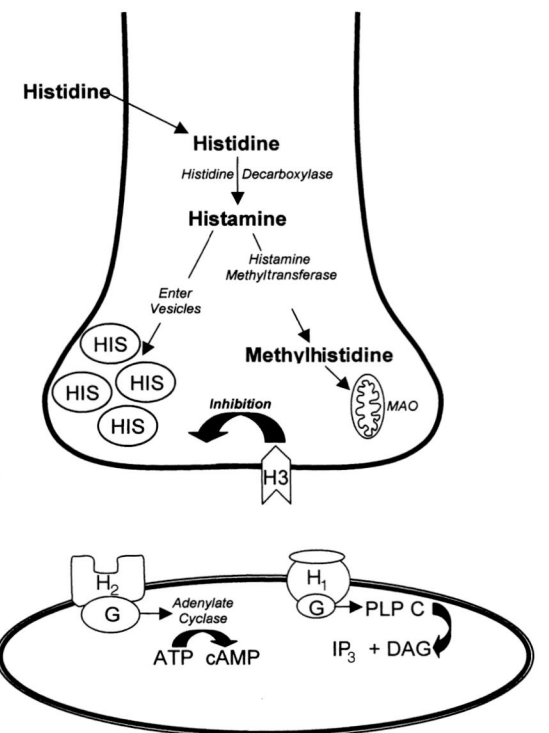

FIGURE 39-3

Schematic model of a central histaminergic neuron. Histidine crosses the blood-brain barrier and, when inside neurons, is converted to histamine (H) via the enzyme histidine decarboxylase. H is transported into vesicles, where it is stored before release. Free H can be metabolized by histamine methyltransferase with methylhistidine and then metabolized further through the monoamine oxidase (MAO) system. H binding to H_1 receptors stimulates phospholipase C (PLP C) with the liberation of inositol triphosphate (IP_3) and diacylglycerol (DAG) as second messengers. H binding to H_2 receptors stimulates adenylate cyclase with the generation of cyclic adenosine monophosphate (cAMP) as a second messenger. H binding to H_3 autoreceptors results in feedback inhibition and decreases release of H and numerous other neurotransmitters. ATP, adenosine triphosphate; G, G protein.

The cardiac effects of antihistamines include effects resulting from sodium channel blockade (e.g., ventricular tachycardia, potassium efflux blockade, and torsades de pointes). Serious cardiac effects of first-generation (sedating) antihistamines generally are thought to be secondary to sodium channel blockade. Numerous reports of diphenhydramine toxicity have shown QRS widening and hypotension. Some of these patients showed resolution of these effects after receiving doses of physostigmine and sodium bicarbonate,[25,26] whereas others responded to sodium bicarbonate alone, supporting the theory that sodium channel blockade was a major factor. Wang and colleagues[27] studied the effects of "conventional" antihistamines on cardiac conduction and found that cardiac repolarization was slowed in the following order: clemastine, hydroxyzine > brompheniramine, chlorpheniramine, diphenhydramine > cyproheptadine, chlorcyclizine, promethazine. They also showed the dose-dependent ability of these drugs to prolong the QT interval. Wang and colleagues[27] suggested that large doses of these medications might have adverse effects on cardiac conduction. Zareba and associates[28] reviewed 12-lead electrocardiograms of 126 consecutive patients with diphenhydramine overdoses reported to regional poison centers. Of patients, 25% had

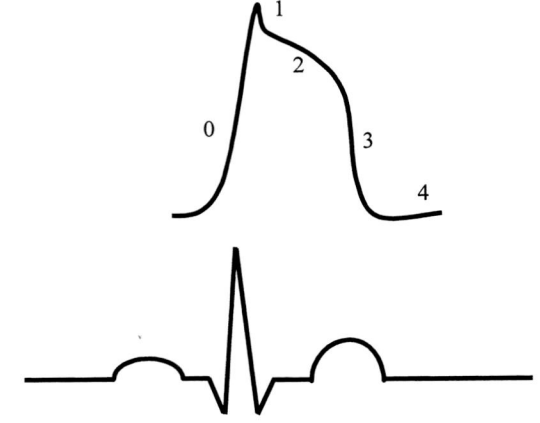

FIGURE 39-4

The relationship between the action potential and the QRS. Although changes in sodium influx during phase 0 leads to QRS prolongation, blockade of potassium channels in phase 2 and phase 3 lengthens the QT interval.

heart rates greater than 120 beats/min, probably owing to the anticholinergic effects of diphenhydramine. QT_c prolongation was common, with 50% of the patients having a QT_c interval of greater than 450 msec and 11% greater than 500 msec. Only one patient presented with monomorphic ventricular tachycardia, and no patients had torsades de pointes.

Second-generation antihistamines, such as astemizole, terfenadine, and ebastine, seem to cause torsades de pointes by inhibiting potassium efflux from cells in the cardiac conductive system. The blockade of the "delayed rectifier" potassium current in late phase 2 and early phase 3 of the action potential seems to be responsible for prolongation of the QT interval and a contributor to the development of torsades de pointes (Fig. 39-4).[29]

Blockade of potassium channels leads to an increase in membrane potential (i.e., toward zero) and allows Purkinje fibers to "refire." This event is termed an *afterdepolarization* because it must follow a normal cellular depolarization and cannot arise de novo. When an afterdepolarization occurs in late phase 2 or early phase 3, it is termed an *early afterdepolarization*. These early afterdepolarizations initiate "triggered" activity, such as torsades de pointes (Fig. 39-5).[30]

CLINICAL PRESENTATION

Neurologic Effects

Diphenhydramine and the older first-generation H_1-receptor antagonists commonly are used in over-the-counter sleep preparations, and one of the most common manifestations of H_1-receptor antagonist overdose is sedation. At therapeutic doses, H_1-receptor antagonists have been shown to decrease time to sleep, psychomotor function, and cognitive function.[16,31] In a well-designed simulated driving performance test, drivers who ingested 50 mg of diphenhydramine performed similarly to, and in some scenarios worse than, drivers ingesting ethanol (blood ethanol concentration 0.1%).[32] As a result of diminished CNS penetration, second-generation H_1 antagonists have a lower incidence of sedation.[31] In overdose, patients can present with a spectrum of CNS depression ranging from mild sedation to coma.

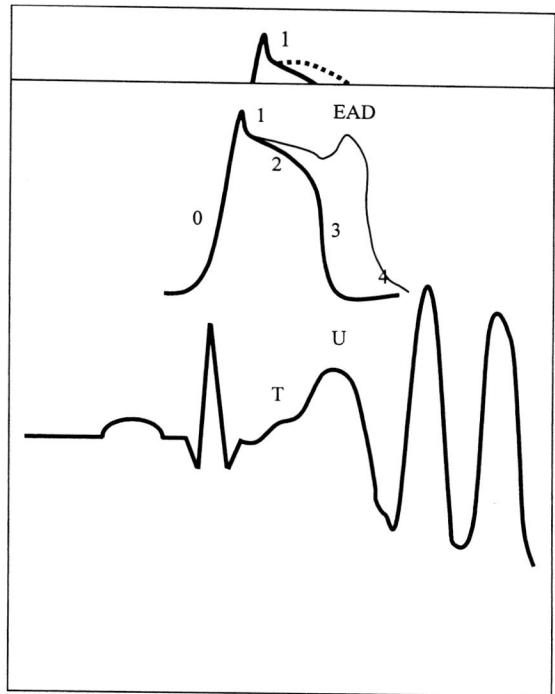

FIGURE 39-5

The production of early afterdepolarizations (EAD) and torsades de pointes. The retention of potassium ions within Purkinje cells leads to a refiring of the cell and the production of an EAD. This can lead to the onset of torsades de pointes, which is heralded by a slowing of the rate and a prominent U wave. T, T wave.

Antihistamines' association with seizures has been known since shortly after their initial clinical usage.[33] Focal and generalized seizures in overdoses, supratherapeutic doses, and therapeutic doses were reported.[33–35] In a 2-year retrospective poison center review of 191 cases of poisoning associated with seizure, Olson and colleagues[36] showed diphenhydramine to be the third leading cause. In fatal overdoses involving antihistamines, seizures often are premonitory to cardiac arrhythmias and death.[37–39]

All first-generation H_1-receptor antagonists have the potential to cause anticholinergic syndrome. There are many examples in the literature of anticholinergic poisoning with peripheral nervous system signs (dry mouth, dry skin, decreased bowel sounds, urinary retention, mydriasis, and tachycardia) and CNS anticholinergic signs (altered mental status, confusion, psychosis) in antihistamine overdoses. For further discussion on the presentation and treatment of anticholinergic poisonings, see Chapter 22.

Diphenhydramine often is used as a first-line treatment for extrapyramidal effects secondary to dopamine antagonists. Its mechanism of reversal may occur through either its central antimuscarinic effects[40] or its ability to inhibit dopamine uptake in neuronal cells.[41–43] Despite this, antihistamines also have been reported to be a cause of extrapyramidal symptoms. Cases of orofacial dyskinesias, acute dystonia, torticollis, trismus, tremors, and incoordination have been reported in patients with acute and long-term usage of antihistamines in therapeutic doses and overdoses.[44–53] Patients who develop antihistamine-associated extrapyramidal effects should be treated with either benzodi-

azepines or benztropine, a relatively potent inhibitor of central dopamine uptake (see Chapter 45).

Cardiac Effects

Tachycardia due to anticholinergic effects is the most common cardiac presentation[54] and seldom requires treatment. Wide QRS and ventricular tachycardia have been reported and may be treated with sodium bicarbonate in a fashion similar to that caused by tricyclic antidepressants.[55] Prolonged QT_c and torsades de pointes also have been reported, especially with nonsedating agents, such as terfenadine and astemizole. Hypertension[56] and hypotension[56] have been documented.

Nonsedating second-generation H_1 antagonists were introduced in the 1980s. In 1986, Craft[57] reported torsades de pointes in a 16-year-old who ingested an overdose of astemizole. By 1990, reports of an association between second-generation antihistamines (terfenadine, ebastine, and astemizole and its metabolite desmethylastemizole)[58] and torsades de pointes began to appear in the medical literature.[59,60] In 1988, Snook and colleagues[61] reported torsades de pointes associated with astemizole use. Monahan and coworkers[62] reported 25 cases of terfenadine toxicity resulting in torsades de pointes. The cardiac effects of these drugs seem to be independent of their antihistaminic properties and better associated with substitutions at the nitrogen atom (see Fig. 39-2).[63]

Other Effects

Rhabdomyolysis in uncomplicated antihistamine overdose is a rare event without complicating factors. As with other serious intoxications, however, antihistamine overdose can result in rhabdomyolysis. Severe cases of rhabdomyolysis typically are associated with seizures and hyperthermia.[64–66] Other features of antihistamine overdose that may contribute to the development of rhabdomyolysis include prolonged periods of inactivity with the development of compartment syndromes and agitation in patients fighting against restraints.

Therapeutic use of H_2 antagonists has been associated idiosyncratically (i.e., in a non–dose-related fashion) with thrombocytopenia and granulocytopenia. Numerous case reports have been published of thrombocytopenia isolated[67–79] or in combination with anemia or leukopenia or both.[80–87] The data behind most of these case reports are confused, however, by complicating factors and other medications not taken into account. In a systematic review of published case reports of drug-induced thrombocytopenia, only cimetidine had data considered level I evidence (definite), and ranitidine had level II evidence (probable).[88] The cause of thrombocytopenia with H_2 antagonists generally is thought to be immune mediated with the development of IgE[75,88,89] or IgG and IgM antibodies[73,74,79] against an H_2 antagonist–platelet complex. Although some authors have suggested cross-reactivity between different H_2 antagonists,[79,89] others have shown no recurrence of thrombocytopenia when a different H_2 antagonist was used.[77,90] Similarly, numerous case reports of granulocytopenia have been associated with therapeutic administration of cimetidine[81–86,91–94] and famotidine.[87] In most of these cases, patients either were critically ill or were using other medications with suspected bone marrow toxicity. The causes of leukopenia have been thought to be either H_2

blockade on bone marrow cells[95] or peripheral destruction of leukocytes secondary to antibodies to cimetidine.[86]

DIAGNOSIS

There are no specific laboratory or physical examination findings that indicate a diagnosis of antihistamine poisoning. Rather, a combination of CNS depression, anticholinergic findings, and electrocardiogram findings would put antihistamines on the list of differential diagnoses. Anticholinergic findings typically predominate. More important is the ability of the critical care physician to recognize and treat the features of antihistamine overdoses that are potentially life-threatening, including a loss of airway protection, widened QRS, prolonged QT_c, torsades de pointes, rhabdomyolysis, and seizures.

TREATMENT

Treatment of antihistamine poisoning focuses on the prevention and treatment of life-threatening complications. Although antihistamines are effectively bound to charcoal, there are no specific decontamination recommendations for antihistamines because none have been validated empirically. For a general review of gastrointestinal decontamination, see Chapter 5.

Secondary to the relatively high volume of distribution and protein binding of most antihistamines, extracorporeal removal is not effective in antihistamine poisoning. The management of CNS sedation with H_1-receptor antagonists rests largely on supportive care, including airway management in a patient who is unable to protect the airway. The anticholinergic effects of antihistamines can be reversed with physostigmine.[96] Because of the remote risk of seizures and arrhythmias, the empirical use of physostigmine should be reserved for patients with major anticholinergic manifestations (see Chapter 153).[97-99]

Benzodiazepines (e.g., diazepam and lorazepam) should be considered the first-line treatment for seizures associated with antihistamine overdosage, followed by barbiturates (e.g., phenobarbital and pentobarbital) or propofol (see Chapter 20). Phenytoin is not recommended in most cases of toxin-induced seizures because numerous animal studies have suggested that it is inferior to benzodiazepines or barbiturates and, in some overdoses, may lower the seizure threshold.[100]

Indications for ICU Admission in Antihistamine Toxicity
Central nervous system depression or coma
Seizures
Anticholinergic delirium
New-onset QRS widening beyond 110 msec
New-onset QT_c interval widening
Ventricular tachycardia
Hypotension

Tachycardia associated with anticholinergic effects seldom requires treatment. Ventricular tachycardia may respond to boluses of sodium bicarbonate.[55] Dosage is variable, with a starting point of 1 to 2 mEq/kg. Sodium bicarbonate infusions of 100 to 150 mL in 1000 mL of 5% dextrose in water (with potassium chloride added) often have been used after conversion of ventricular tachycardia, although the scientific basis for this practice is marginal (see Chapter 36). Lidocaine is a second-line drug for ventricular tachycardia. Intravenous magnesium sulfate may be effective in the treatment of torsades de pointes. Although there are no clear guidelines for magnesium sulfate dosage, adults may be treated with 2 g (16 mEq) mixed in 50 to 100 mL of 5% dextrose in water intravenously over 5 minutes and repeated if no improvement is noted; infusion of 3 to 50 mg/min also may be administered. Other treatment modalities for torsades de pointes include intravenous administration of isoproterenol and use of electrical cardiac pacing. Both modalities have had some success in torsades de pointes treatment. Isoproterenol may be used in patients who are bradycardic but should be avoided in patients with poor left ventricular function or severe coronary artery disease.[101] Other drugs that have been used include verapamil[102,103] and drugs that facilitate potassium channel opening, such as pinacidil[104,105]; however, their roles in treatment remain to be determined. Torsades de pointes is discussed further in Chapter 21.

SPECIAL POPULATIONS

Pediatric Patients

In one reported case series of antihistamine poisonings, it was suggested that children are more prone to seizures than adults.[34] This association has not been validated prospectively. Antihistamines are used widely in children and carry risks similar to those in adults. Patients with long QT syndrome due to congenital alteration in cardiac ion channels (Jervell and Lange-Nielsen and Romano-Ward syndromes) may be at increased risk for drug-induced torsades de pointes.

Female Patients

Women seem to be at a greater risk of developing torsades de pointes because of genetic differences in the number of potassium channels.[106] In a review of 332 cases of torsades de pointes, Makkar and associates[107] found a female predominance among all of the drug-induced cases except procainamide.

Elderly Patients

Elderly patients may be more prone to develop altered mental status in association with H_1- and H_2-receptor antagonists. A prospective cohort study showed that patients older than 70 years of age who received a dose of antihistamines during hospitalization had a relative risk of 1.7 for delirium symptoms.[108] Other articles have suggested a similar trend with H_2 antagonists in the elderly, particularly if concomitant renal impairment is present.[109]

Patients Taking Other Medications

As a result of its ability to inhibit cytochromes 1A2, 2C18, 2D6, and 3A4, cimetidine can increase serum concentrations of numerous drugs, including theophylline, opioids, antihypertensives, antibiotics, and antidepressants. H_2 antagonists can reduce the bioavailability and effectiveness of the antifungal medications ketoconazole and itraconazole because these medications require an acidic medium in the gut for absorption.

Coingestion of cytochrome 3A4 inhibitors, such as ketoconazole, itraconazole, cyclosporine, erythromycin, nifedipine, verapamil, and grapefruit juice, may lead to a buildup of the cardiotoxic second-generation antihistamine (i.e., terfenadine and astemizole) parent compounds, which can induce torsades de pointes. Terfenadine and astemizole have been removed from the market in many countries.

Pregnant Patients

Safety ratings for use in pregnancy vary with specific agents, but antihistamines often are rated category C (see Appendix A). In a meta-analysis of 24 articles involving 200,000 enrolled participants, Seto and colleagues[110] concluded: "H_1 blockers used mainly for morning sickness during the first trimester do not increase the teratogenic risk in humans and may, in fact, be associated with a protective effect."

REFERENCES

1. Portier P, Richet C: De l'action anaphylactique de certains venins. C R Soc Biol 54:170–172, 1902.
2. Barger G, Dale H: The presence in ergot and physiological activity of β-iminazoylethylamine. J Physiol 30:38–40, 1910.
3. Dale H, Laidlaw P: The physiological action of β-iminazoylethylamine. J Physiol 41:341–344, 1910.
4. Clark AJ: The Mode of Action of Drugs on Cells. London, Arnold, 1933.
5. Ash A, Schild H: Receptors mediating some actions of histamine. Br J Pharmacol 27:427–429, 1966.
6. Black J: Definition and antagonism of histamine H2 receptors. Nature 236:385–390, 1972.
7. Emanuel M: Histamine and the antiallergic antihistamines: A history of their discoveries. Clin Exp Allergy 29(Suppl 3):1–11, 1999.
8. Slater JW, Zechnich AD, Haxby DG: Second-generation antihistamines: A comparative review. Drugs 57:31–47, 1999.
9. Simons FE, Simons KJ: The pharmacology and use of H1-receptor-antagonist drugs. N Engl J Med 330:1663–1670, 1994.
10. Leurs R, Smit MJ, Timmerman H: Molecular pharmacological aspects of histamine receptors. Pharmacol Ther 66:413–463, 1995.
11. Hill SJ: Multiple histamine receptors: Properties and functional characteristics. Biochem Soc Trans 20:122–125, 1992.
12. Wada H, Inagaki N, Itowi N, et al: Histaminergic neuron system: Morphological features and possible functions. Agents Actions 33:11–27, 1991.
13. Scherkl R, Hashem A, Frey HH: Histamine in brain—its role in regulation of seizure susceptibility. Epilepsy Res 10:111–118, 1991.
14. Reiner PB, Kamondi A: Mechanisms of antihistamine-induced sedation in the human brain: H1 receptor activation reduces a background leakage of potassium current. Neuroscience 59:579–588, 1994.
15. Kamei C, Ohuchi M, Sugimoto Y, et al: Mechanism responsible for epileptogenic activity by first-generation H1-antagonists in rats. Brain Res 887:183–186, 2000.
16. Simons FER: Non-cardiac adverse effects of antihistamines (H1-receptor antagonists). Clin Exp Allergy 29:125–132, 1999.
17. Sangalli BC: Role of the central histaminergic neuronal system in the CNS toxicity of first generation H1-antagonists. Prog Neurobiol 52:145–157, 1997.
18. Yokoyama H, Onodera K, Iinuma K, et al: Proconvulsive effects of histamine H1-antagonists on electrically-induced seizure in developing mice. Psychopharmacology (Berl) 112:199–203, 1993.
19. Yokoyama H, Sato M, Iinuma K, et al: Centrally acting H_1 antagonists promote the development of amygdala kindling in rats. Neurosci Lett 217:194–196, 1996.
20. Kamei C, Ishizawa K, Kakinoki H, et al: Histaminergic mechanisms in amygdaloid-kindled seizures in rats. Epilepsy Res 30:187–194, 1998.
21. Scherkl R, Hashem A, Frey HH: Importance of histamine for seizure susceptibility. Agents Actions 33:85–89, 1991.
22. Amabeoku GJ, Chikuni O: Cimetidine-induced seizures in mice. Biochem Pharmacol 46:2171–2175, 1993.
23. Kakinoki H, Ishizawa K, Fukunaga M, et al: The effects of histamine H3-receptor antagonists on amygdaloid kindled seizures in rats. Brain Res Bull 46:461–465, 1998.
24. Smit MJ, Hoffmann M, Timmerman H, et al: Molecular properties and signalling pathways of the histamine H1 receptor. Clin Exp Allergy 29:19–28, 1999.
25. Kukovetz WR: [Effect of ortho-(beta-diethylaminoethoxy)phenylpropiophenone × HCl (etafenone) on the dynamics, metabolism, O2-utilization and coronary flow of heart]. Arzneimittelforschung 19:1672–1677, 1969.
26. Rinder CS, D'Amato SL, Rinder HM, et al: Survival in complicated diphenhydramine overdose. Crit Care Med 16:1161–1162, 1988.
27. Wang WX, Ebert SN, Liu XK, et al: "Conventional" antihistamines slow cardiac repolarization in isolated perfused (Langendorff) feline hearts. J Cardiovasc Pharmacol 32:123–128, 1998.
28. Zareba W, Moss AJ, Rosero SZ, et al: Electrocardiographic findings in patients with diphenhydramine overdose. Am J Cardiol 80:1168–1173, 1997.
29. Barbey JT, Anderson M, Ciprandi G, et al: Cardiovascular safety of second-generation antihistamines. Am J Rhinol 13:235–243, 1999.
30. Jackman W, Friday K, Anderson J, et al: The long QT syndromes: A critical review on new clinical observations and a unifying hypothesis. Prog Cardiovasc Dis 31:115–172, 1988.
31. Adelsberg BR: Sedation and performance issues in the treatment of allergic conditions. Arch Intern Med 157:494–500, 1997.
32. Weiler JM, Bloomfield JR, Woodworth GG, et al: Effects of fexofenadine, diphenhydramine, and alcohol on driving performance: A randomized, placebo-controlled trial in the Iowa driving simulator. Ann Intern Med 132:354–363, 2000.
33. Churchill JA, Gammon GD: The effect of antihistaminic drugs on convulsive seizures. JAMA 141:18–21, 1949.
34. Wyngaarden JB, Seevers MH: The toxic effects of antihistaminic drugs. JAMA 145:277–282, 1951.
35. Yasuhara A, Ochi A, Harada Y, et al: Infantile spasms associated with histamine H1 antagonist. Neuropediatrics 29:320–321, 1998.
36. Olson KR, Kearney TE, Dyer JE, et al: Seizures associated with poisoning and drug overdose. Am J Emerg Med 11:565–568, 1993.
37. Goetz CM, Lopez G, Dean BS, et al: Accidental childhood death from diphenhydramine overdosage. Am J Emerg Med 8:321–322, 1990.
38. Krenzelok EP, Anderson GM, Mirick M: Massive diphenhydramine overdose resulting in death. Ann Emerg Med 11:212–213, 1982.
39. Winn RE, McDonnell KP: Fatality secondary to massive overdose of dimenhydrinate. Ann Emerg Med 22:1481–1484, 1993.
40. Miyawaki E, Tarsy D: Tardive dyskinesia and other drug-related movement disorders. In Samuels MA (ed): Office Practice of Neurology. New York, Churchill Livingstone, 1996, pp 666–667.
41. Coyle JT, Snyder SH: Antiparkinsonian drugs: Inhibition of dopamine uptake in the corpus striatum as a possible mechanism of action. Science 166:899–901, 1969.
42. Symchowicz S, Korduba CA, Veals J: Inhibition of dopamine uptake into synaptosomes of rat corpus striatum by chlorpheniramine and its structural analogs. Life Sci Physiol Pharmacol 10:35–42, 1971.
43. Shishido S, Oishi R, Saeki K: In vivo effects of some histamine H1-receptor antagonists on monoamine metabolism in the mouse brain. Naunyn Schmiedebergs Arch Pharmacol 343:185–189, 1991.
44. Thach BT, Chase TN, Bosma JF: Oral facial dyskinesia associated with prolonged use of antihistaminic decongestants. N Engl J Med 293:486–487, 1975.
45. Sovner RD: Dyskinesia associated with chronic antihistamine use (Letter). N Engl J Med 294:113, 1976.
46. Favis GR: Facial dyskinesia related to antihistamine (Letter)? N Engl J Med 294:730, 1976.
47. Brait KA, Zagerman AJ: Dyskinesias after antihistamine use. N Engl J Med 296:111, 1977.
48. Lavenstein BL, Cantor FK: Acute dystonia: An unusual reaction to diphenhydramine. JAMA 236:291, 1976.

49. Granacher Jr RP: Facial dyskinesia after antihistamines (Letter). N Engl J Med 296:516, 1977.

50. Barone DA, Raniolo J: Facial dyskinesia from overdose of an antihistamine (Letter). N Engl J Med 303:107, 1980.

51. Roila F, Donati D, Basurto C, et al: Diphenhydramine and acute dystonia (Letter). Ann Intern Med 111:92–93, 1989.

52. Etzel JV: Diphenhydramine-induced acute dystonia. Pharmacotherapy 14:492–496, 1994.

53. Joseph MM, King WD: Dystonic reaction following recommended use of a cold syrup. Ann Emerg Med 26:749–751, 1995.

54. Zavitz M, Lindsay C, McGuigan M: Acute diphenhydramine ingestion in children (Abstract). Vet Hum Toxicol 31:349, 1989.

55. Clark R, Vance M: Massive diphenhydramine poisoning resulting in a wide-complex tachycardia: Successful treatment with sodium bicarbonate. Ann Emerg Med 21:318–321, 1992.

56. Mullins M, Pinnick R, Terhes J: Life-threatening diphenhydramine overdose treated with charcoal hemoperfusion and hemodialysis. Ann Emerg Med 22:104–107, 1999.

57. Craft T: Torsades de pointes after astemizole overdose. BMJ 292:660, 1986.

58. Valen G, Kaszaki J, Szabo I, et al: Histamine release and its effects in ischaemia-reperfusion injury of the isolated rat heart. Acta Physiol Scand 150:413–424, 1994.

59. Simons FE, Keselman MS, Giddins NG, et al: Astemizole-induced torsades de pointes. Lancet 2:624, 1988.

60. Davies AJ, Harindra V, McEwan A, et al: Cardiotoxic effect with convulsions in terfenadine overdose. BMJ 298:325, 1989.

61. Snook J, Boothman-Burrell D, Watkins J, et al: Torsades de pointes ventricular tachycardia associated with astemizole overdose. Br J Clin Pract 42:257–259, 1988.

62. Monahan B, Ferguson C, Killeavy E, et al: Torsades de pointes occurring in association with terfenadine use. JAMA 264:2788–2790, 1990.

63. Taglialatela M, Castaldo P, Pannaccione A, et al: Cardiac ion channels and antihistamines: Possible mechanisms of cardiotoxicity. Clin Exp Allergy 29:182–189, 1999.

64. Mendoza FS, Atiba JO, Krensky AM, et al: Rhabdomyolysis complicating doxylamine overdose. Clin Pediatr (Phila) 26:595–597, 1987.

65. Frankel D, Dolgin J, Murray BM: Non-traumatic rhabdomyolysis complicating antihistamine overdose. J Toxicol Clin Toxicol 31:493–496, 1993.

66. Soto LF, Miller CH, Ognibere AJ: Severe rhabdomyolysis after doxylamine overdose. Postgrad Med 93:227–229, 232, 1993.

67. Isaacs AJ: Cimetidine and thrombocytopenia. BMJ 280:294, 1980.

68. Yates VM, Kerr RE: Cimetidine and thrombocytopenia (Letter). BMJ 280:1453, 1980.

69. Reddy J, Bailey RR: Cimetidine and thrombocytopenia (Letter). N Z Med J 91:232, 1980.

70. Glotzbach RE: Cimetidine-induced thrombocytopenia. South Med J 75:232–234, 1982.

71. Mann HJ, Schneider JR, Miller JB, et al: Cimetidine-associated thrombocytopenia. Drug Intell Clin Pharm 17:126–128, 1983.

72. Wong YY, Lichtor T, Brown FD: Severe thrombocytopenia associated with phenytoin and cimetidine therapy. Surg Neurol 23:169–172, 1985.

73. Spychal RT, Wickham NW: Thrombocytopenia associated with ranitidine. BMJ 291:1687, 1985.

74. Gibson PR, Pidcock ME: Immune-mediated thrombocytopenia associated with ranitidine therapy (Letter). Med J Aust 145:661–662, 1986.

75. Gafter U, Komlos L, Weinstein T, et al: Thrombocytopenia, eosinophilia, and ranitidine. Ann Intern Med 106:477, 1987.

76. Yue CP, Mann KS, Chan KH: Severe thrombocytopenia due to combined cimetidine and phenytoin therapy. Neurosurgery 20:963–965, 1987.

77. Shalev O, Seror D: Cimetidine and ranitidine may not cross-react to cause thrombocytopenia. J Intern Med 230:87–88, 1991.

78. Arbiser JL, Goldstein AM, Gordon D: Thrombocytopenia following administration of phenytoin, dexamethasone and cimetidine: A case report and a potential mechanism. J Intern Med 234:91–94, 1993.

79. Gentilini G, Curtis BR, Aster RH: An antibody from a patient with ranitidine-induced thrombocytopenia recognizes a site on glycoprotein IX that is a favored target for drug-induced antibodies. Blood 92:2359–2365, 1998.

80. Pixley JS, MacKintosh FR, Sahr EA, et al: Mechanism of ranitidine associated anemia. Am J Med Sci 297:369–371, 1989.

81. James C, Prout BJ: Marrow suppression and intravenous cimetidine. Lancet 1:987, 1978.

82. Chang HK, Morrison SL: Bone-marrow suppression associated with cimetidine. Ann Intern Med 91:580, 1979.

83. Rate R, Bonnell M, Chervenak C, et al: Cimetidine and hematologic effects (Letter). Ann Intern Med 91:795, 1979.

84. Collen MJ: Cimetidine-associated thrombocytopenia and leukopenia. West J Med 132:257–258, 1980.

85. Chandrasekhara KL, Iyer SK, Macchia RJ: Leucopenia and thrombocytopenia with cimetidine (Letter). J Natl Med Assoc 73:92, 98, 1981.

86. Mar DD, Brandstetter RD, Miskovitz PF, et al: Cimetidine-induced, immune-mediated leukopenia and thrombocytopenia. South Med J 75:1283–1285, 1982.

87. Oymak O, Akpolat T, Arik N, et al: Reversible neutropenia and thrombocytopenia during famotidine treatment (Letter). Ann Pharmacother 28:406–407, 1994.

88. George JN, Raskob GE, Shah SR, et al: Drug-induced thrombocytopenia: A systematic review of published case reports. Ann Intern Med 129:886–890, 1998.

89. Gafter U, Zevin D, Komlos L, et al: Thrombocytopenia associated with hypersensitivity to ranitidine: Possible cross-reactivity with cimetidine. Am J Gastroenterol 84:560–562, 1989.

90. Burnakis TG: Inaccurate assessment of drug-induced thrombocytopenia: Reason for concern. Ann Pharmacother 28:726–729, 1994.

91. Lopez-Luque A, Rodriguez-Cuartero A, Perez-Galvez N, et al: Cimetidine and bone-marrow toxicity. Lancet 1:444, 1978.

92. Johnson NM, Black AE, Hughes ASB, et al: Leucopenia with cimetidine. Lancet 2:1226–1227, 1977.

93. Iyer SK, Chandrasekhara KL: Leukopenia with cimetidine. J Natl Med Assoc 72:805–806, 1980.

94. Khokhar N, Akavaram NR: Cimetidine-induced leukopenia: Case reports. Milit Med 145:853–855, 1980.

95. Byron JW: Pharmacodynamic basis for the interaction of cimetidine with bone marrow stem cell (CFU-5). Exp Hematol 8:256–263, 1980.

96. Cowen PJ: Toxic psychosis with antihistamines reversed by physostigmine. Postgrad Med J 55:556–557, 1979.

97. Newton RW: Physostigmine salicylate in the treatment of tricyclic antidepressant overdosage. JAMA 231:941–943, 1975.

98. Pentel P, Peterson CD: Asystole complicating physostigmine treatment of tricyclic antidepressant overdose. Ann Emerg Med 9:588–590, 1980.

99. Walker WE, Levy RC, Haneson IB: Physostigmine—its use and abuse. J Am Coll Emerg Physicians 5:436–439, 1976.

100. Blake KV, Massey KL, Hendeles L, et al: Relative efficacy of phenytoin and phenobarbital for the prevention of theophylline-induced seizures in mice. Ann Emerg Med 17:1024–1028, 1988.

101. Haverkamp W, Shenasa M, Borggrefe M, et al: Torsades de pointes. In Zipes D, Jalife J (eds): Cardiac Physiology: From Cell to Bedside, 3rd ed. Philadelphia, WB Saunders, 1999, pp 885–899.

102. Liao WB, Bullard MJ, Kuo CT, et al: Anticholinergic overdose induced torsades de pointes successfully treated with verapamil. Jpn Heart J 37:925–931, 1996.

103. Cosio FG, Goicolea A, Lopez Gil M, et al: Suppression of torsades de pointes with verapamil in patients with atrio-ventricular block. Eur Heart J 12:635–638, 1991.

104. Brosch SF, Studenik C, Heistracher P: Abolition of drug-induced early afterdepolarizations by potassium channel activators in guinea-pig Purkinje fibres. Clin Exp Pharmacol Physiol 25:225–230, 1998.

105. Carlsson L, Abrahamsson C, Drews L, et al: Antiarrhythmic effects of potassium channel openers in rhythm abnormalities related to delayed repolarization. Circulation 85:1491–1500, 1992.

106. Ebert SN, Liu XK, Woosley RL: Female gender as a risk factor for drug-induced cardiac arrhythmias: Evaluation of clinical and experimental evidence. J Womens Health 7:547–557, 1998.

107. Makkar R, Fromm B, Steinman R, et al: Female gender as a risk factor for torsades de pointes associated with cardiovascular drugs. JAMA 270:2590–2597, 1993.

108. Agostini JV, Leo-Summers LS, Inouye SK: Cognitive and other adverse effects of diphenhydramine use in hospitalized older patients. Arch Intern Med 161:2091–2097, 2001.

109. Slugg PH, Haug MT, Pippenger CE: Ranitidine pharmacokinetics and adverse central nervous system reactions. Arch Intern Med 152:2325–2329, 1992.

110. Seto A, Einarson T, Koren G: Pregnancy outcome following first trimester exposure to antihistamines: Meta-analysis. Am J Perinatol 14:119–124, 1997.

CHAPTER 40

Theophylline and Other Methyl Xanthines

Holly E. Perry ■ Michael Shannon

Theophylline is a bronchodilator and respiratory stimulant that has been used since the 1950s to treat asthma, chronic obstructive pulmonary disease, and apnea and bradycardia of prematurity. It is used less frequently today because new pharmacologic agents have been introduced to treat these diseases and because of concerns about its toxicity. Theophylline can cause either acute intentional or chronic unintentional intoxication. Severe intoxication may result in life-threatening arrhythmias and seizures and has a mortality of at least 10%. Acute caffeine intoxication has pathophysiology, symptoms, and management similar to those of theophylline intoxication.

BIOCHEMISTRY AND PHARMACOLOGY

Theophylline, caffeine, and pentoxifylline are all xanthine derivatives. Their structures closely resemble that of purines, such as adenosine (Fig. 40-1).

Theophylline is absorbed completely after oral therapeutic doses. For each 1 mg/kg ingested, a peak serum level of 2 μg/mL is expected to result. Oral forms are available as either immediate-release or sustained-release preparations; the sustained-release preparations have been prescribed more frequently. In therapeutic use, peak levels occur 1 to 2 hours after ingestion of an immediate-release formulation and 6 to 8 hours after ingestion of a sustained-release preparation. In the setting of overdose, sustained-release tablets may have prolonged and erratic absorption, possibly because of bezoar formation.[1,2] Peak levels may be delayed for 24 hours,[3] and levels may continue to rise despite repeated doses of activated charcoal.[4]

Theophylline has a relatively small volume of distribution, although patients at extremes of age have a larger volume of distribution. It is distributed rapidly to all tissues.[5] Theophylline is metabolized by cytochrome P-450 isoenzymes 1A2, 2E1, and 3A3. In older children and adults, 90% is metabolized, and 10% is excreted unchanged in the urine. In neonates and young children, 50% is metabolized in the liver, with the remainder excreted unchanged in the urine.[5]

Theophylline has a prolonged half-life in patients at extremes of age. The half-life in neonates is 25 hours, and the half-life in adults older than age 60 years is 10 hours. The half-life for patients 16 to 60 years old is 8 hours.[5] Across the therapeutic range, theophylline elimination follows first-order kinetics. With an elimination pattern best described as Michaelis-Menten kinetics, however, first-order kinetics changes to zero-order elimination as higher theophylline concentrations are attained. In the setting of

an acute overdose, elimination initially follows zero-order, unpredictable kinetics.[3]

Patients taking theophylline therapeutically are at risk for developing chronic theophylline toxicity for two reasons. First, because theophylline elimination follows Michaelis-Menten (i.e., saturable) kinetics, a small increase in dose (e.g., when a patient takes doses additional to those prescribed) may result in a disproportionately large increase in serum concentration. Second, the rate of theophylline metabolism depends on underlying disease processes, intercurrent illness, and ingestion of substances that interfere with specific cytochrome P-450 isoenzymes. Patients with liver disease, chronic obstructive pulmonary disease, or congestive heart failure have a 50% decrease in metabolism that can produce elevated serum concentrations quickly.[5] Acute febrile illness in children, regardless of cause, has been shown to decrease metabolism; the magnitude of effect is proportional to height of fever.[6] Many commonly prescribed medications can reduce theophylline clearance through inhibition of cytochrome P-450 isoenzymes (1A2, 3A4). Examples of important inhibitors include ciprofloxacin,[7] cimetidine, erythromycin, clarithromycin, interferon, disulfiram, verapamil,[8] and zafirlukast.[9] Cigarette smoking increases theophylline metabolism.[8] As a result, patients may become toxic if they cease smoking and the theophylline dose has not been decreased. This effect, the result of cytochrome P-450 induction followed by reversion to normal activity, appears 4 to 8 days after cessation of smoking.

Pharmacokinetics of Theophylline

Volume of distribution: 0.45 L/kg (0.3–0.7 L/kg)
Protein binding: 40–65%
Mechanism of clearance:
  Children <1 yr: hepatic 50%; renal 50%
  Adults: hepatic 90%; renal 10%
Half-life:
  Neonates: 25 hr
  Adults 16–60 yr: 8 hr
  Adults >60 yr: 10 hr
Active metabolites: caffeine (neonates only)
Methods to enhance clearance:
  MDAC
  Hemodialysis
  Hemoperfusion

Pharmacokinetics of Caffeine

Volume of distribution: 0.61 L/kg (0.4–0.8 L/kg)
Protein binding: 30–45%
Mechanism of clearance: hepatic
Half-life:
 Preterm neonates: 52 hr
 Neonates: 20 hr
 Adults: 5 hr
Active metabolites: none
Methods of enhance clearance:
 Hemoperfusion
 MDAC (theoretical)
 Hemodialysis (theoretical)

MDAC, multiple-dose activated charcoal.

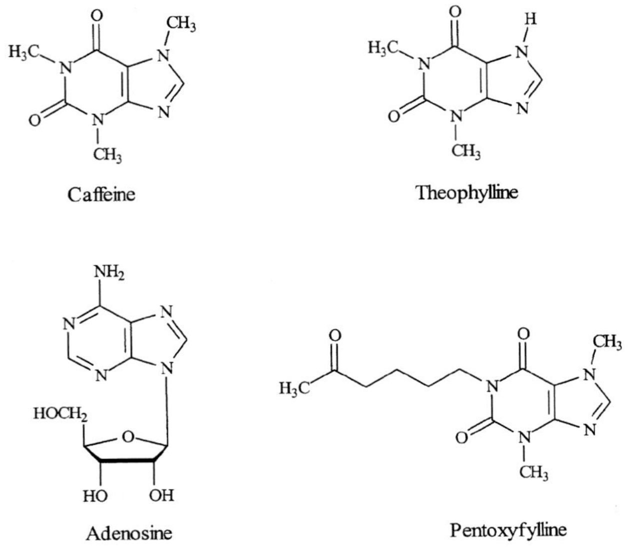

FIGURE 40-1

Chemical structures of selected xanthines (modification I).

PATHOPHYSIOLOGY OF THERAPEUTIC AND TOXIC EFFECTS

Toxic effects are mediated primarily through activity at adenosine and adrenergic receptors. Theophylline is a potent adenosine antagonist. Its beneficial effect is due primarily to antagonism of adenosine A_1 receptors in the lungs, which produce bronchodilation. Adenosine antagonism is also a major factor in producing toxicity. In the central nervous system, antagonism of A_1 receptors can result in sustained, unmodulated discharge of neurotransmitters—including glutamate, a major excitatory neurotransmitter—resulting in seizure activity. In the heart, A_1-receptor antagonism leads to an increase in the rate of discharge of cardiac pacemaker cells and increased arrhythmogenesis. Antagonism of A_2 receptors, present throughout the vascular system, results in vasoconstriction.[10] Vasoconstrictive effects have been shown to be important in the central nervous system[11] and are presumed to be important in the myocardium as well.[12]

In addition to being a potent adenosine antagonist, methyl xanthines have powerful indirect adrenergic activity. Theophylline intoxication has been shown to produce increased plasma catecholamines (epinephrine and norepinephrine) in animal models[13,14] and in case series of human victims of theophylline intoxication.[15,16] The magnitude of catecholamine elevation and the specific catecholamine released seem to vary depending on the type of intoxication. Acute intoxication has been shown to be associated with epinephrine concentrations elevated 4-fold to 8-fold greater than controls and norepinephrine levels 4-fold to 10-fold normal.[15,16] In the few patients with chronic overdose who have been studied, norepinephrine and dopamine levels were elevated compared with normal controls and patients with an acute theophylline overdose.[15]

Theophylline and caffeine are phosphodiesterase inhibitors at toxic concentrations. Inhibition of phosphodiesterase results in increased levels of cyclic adenosine monophosphate and augmentation of adrenergic effects. Alterations in intracellular calcium transport have also been postulated to be important in theophylline and caffeine toxicity, although this has not been well studied.[17]

CLINICAL PRESENTATION AND LIFE-THREATENING COMPLICATIONS

Theophylline toxicity primarily affects the gastrointestinal, cardiovascular, and central nervous systems. Characteristic metabolic disturbances, including hypokalemia and hyperglycemia, are noted frequently. Severe lactic acidosis and rhabdomyolysis have been reported. Caffeine intoxication has similar clinical features and so is not discussed separately.

Gastrointestinal Manifestations

Nausea and vomiting are the predominant gastrointestinal system manifestations. Vomiting is an almost universal feature of severe, acute intoxication; it is less common after chronic intoxication.[18–21] Vomiting results from gastric acid hyperstimulation[22] and central stimulation of the chemoreceptor trigger zone. Vomiting may be difficult to control and may make it impossible for the patient to tolerate activated charcoal, an initial therapeutic intervention.[19,23] Hematemesis may occur as a consequence of a Mallory-Weiss tear.[20,23]

Cardiovascular Manifestations

Theophylline predisposes the heart to develop arrhythmias even at therapeutic serum concentrations.[24] At toxic serum concentrations, tachyarrhythmias and hypotension are common findings. Any type of atrial (e.g., multifocal atrial tachycardia) or ventricular tachyarrhythmias may be seen after theophylline intoxication. Death frequently results from an intractable ventricular arrhythmia.[4,18,21] Theophylline predisposes to arrhythmias by reducing the ventricular fibrillation threshold and by nonuniformly increasing cardiac conduction, favoring reentrant arrhythmias. Other factors contributing to arrhythmias include coronary ischemia due to A_2 antagonism, increases in circulating catecholamines, hypokalemia, and acidosis.[12]

The hypotension associated with theophylline intoxication is multifactorial. Vasodilation occurs as a result of β$_2$-adrenoceptor stimulation from catecholamines, the release of which is stimulated by theophylline. Cardiac output may be impaired by tachyarrhythmias resulting in reduced filling time. Hypovolemia secondary to gastrointestinal losses and theophylline-induced diuresis also contribute to hypotension.

Central Nervous System Manifestations

Central nervous system manifestations of theophylline toxicity include agitation, tremor, and seizures. Seizures may occur without warning, particularly in victims of chronic theophylline intoxication[18]; these may be either focal or generalized. Some,[25,26] but not all,[18] studies have found seizures to occur more frequently in patients with underlying neurologic disorders, such as cerebrovascular accident or seizure disorder. When seizures begin, they are frequently difficult to control.[25,27]

Theophylline-induced seizures have a high morbidity and mortality. In most studies, mortality has been reported to be 10%, although 50% mortality has been reported.[27] Higher mortality and morbidity are associated with prolonged seizures.[28] In a study of children with status epilepticus from diverse causes, there was a 50% morbidity and mortality in children with status epilepticus associated with supratherapeutic theophylline concentrations compared with a 23% rate in children with status epilepticus from other causes.[29] Theophylline-induced seizures may be associated with poor neurologic outcome ranging from profound memory deficit to persistent vegetative state. Morbidity has been reported even when status epilepticus has not occurred.[28,30,31]

The origin of xanthine-induced seizures is incompletely understood, although it is most likely that they are due in part to inhibition of adenosine-mediated autoregulation of glutamate release (i.e., excitation-suppression).[32] In an animal model of theophylline-induced seizures, administration of adenosine directly into the cerebral ventricles delayed the onset of seizures.[33] Injury may be compounded by antagonism at A$_2$ receptors, which leads to vasoconstriction[11,34] and less oxygen and glucose delivery at a time when the brain has an increased need for these substrates.

Metabolic Manifestations

Theophylline toxicity also is associated with hypokalemia, hyperglycemia, mild hypomagnesemia,[35] and acidosis. In general, these manifestations have no physiologic significance, but they may have some diagnostic value. Hypokalemia and hyperglycemia are more common in acute than in chronic intoxication[15,18,20,36] and may be helpful in determining the type of intoxication if not clear by history. Significant alterations in pH are uncommon, although severe lactic acidosis has been reported with pH as low as 6.63.[37] Rhabdomyolysis and compartment syndrome have been reported after acute theophylline intoxication.[18,20,38]

Type of Intoxication: Acute, Chronic, or Acute on Chronic

Acute intoxication is defined as development of signs and symptoms of toxicity after an ingestion of a single dose of theophylline, usually at least 10 mg/kg. Chronic intoxication occurs in patients who have been receiving theophylline therapy for at least 72 hours. It may result from impaired drug metabolism due to addition of a cytochrome P-450 inhibitor to a drug regimen, cessation of a P-450 inducer (e.g., smoking), or an intercurrent illness. Patients also can develop chronic intoxication if they have been prescribed or take excessive doses of theophylline. Acute-on-chronic intoxication is considered to occur when a patient who has been receiving theophylline therapy for at least 72 hours ingests a single dose of theophylline large enough to produce signs and symptoms of toxicity.

Determining the type of intoxication is essential in caring for patients with theophylline toxicity because the incidence of and predictors for life-threatening events (LTEs), such as ventricular arrhythmias and seizures, differ substantially between acute and chronic intoxication. Patients with chronic intoxication have been reported to have as high or higher incidence of LTEs compared with patients with acute intoxication. They are less likely to have minor symptoms, such as vomiting, hypokalemia, or hyperglycemia.[18,20,21] Patients with acute intoxication superimposed on long-term theophylline therapy have not been studied as closely but seem to behave more like patients with chronic intoxication.

In acute intoxication, serum theophylline concentrations correlate with the risk for major complications, although no serum concentration has been shown to have an acceptable degree of sensitivity and specificity. In a series of 98 patients who were reported to a regional poison center, a serum theophylline concentration of 60 μg/mL (333 μmol/L) had a sensitivity of 90% and a specificity of 75% for identifying patients who developed major toxicity. In contrast, a serum theophylline concentration of 80 μg/mL (444 μmol/L) had a specificity of 97% but a sensitivity of only 67%.[39] Similarly, Paloucek and Rodvold,[18] in a review of cases of theophylline intoxication published between 1975 and 1985, found that seizures occurred only when the serum concentration was greater than 50 to 60 μg/mL (278 to 333 μmol/L).[18] In a series of 14 patients who presented to an emergency department after acute ingestion, LTEs were seen only in patients with serum concentrations greater than 80 μg/mL (444 μmol/L).[20] A serum theophylline concentration of 43 μg/mL (239 μmol/L) has been associated with seizures after acute overdose, however.[4]

For patients with chronic intoxication, age rather than serum theophylline concentration is the most important prognostic factor. In a prospective poison center–based study of 92 patients with chronic intoxication, patients older than age 60 had a 50% probability (confidence interval 38% to 63%) of developing LTEs. Using the criterion of age greater than 60 for predicting major toxicity had a sensitivity of 80% and specificity of 62%.[39] Other case series support the correlation of advanced age with occurrence of LTEs.[18,20,28,29] In the only study of children, LTEs were associated with younger age, with infants younger than 1 year being at greatest risk.[36] Serum theophylline concentrations have poor predictive value in chronic intoxication. In the only study designed to study risk factors systematically, there was no correlation between serum concentration and occurrence of LTEs.[39] There are reports of LTEs occurring with serum concentrations in the therapeutic range of 10 to 20 μg/mL (56 to 111 μmol/L).[18,40] Most case series have not reported LTEs, however, unless the serum theophylline concentration is greater than 30 μg/mL (167 μmol/L).[20,21,27,36]

DIAGNOSTIC CONSIDERATIONS

Theophylline intoxication should be considered in any patient presenting with seizures, agitation, tachyarrhythmias, hypotension, or persistent vomiting, particularly if there is hyperglycemia and hypokalemia. Patients with chronic intoxication may present relatively asymptomatically.

When theophylline intoxication is in the differential diagnosis, a serum theophylline concentration should be obtained on presentation. If a sustained-release preparation has been ingested, serial serum concentrations should be obtained every 2 hours until serum concentration begins to decline. Laboratory evaluation also should include electrolytes, calcium, magnesium, and venous or arterial blood gas analysis. Serial electrolytes should be obtained if the patient has significant metabolic abnormalities. Clinical indicators of respiratory abnormalities or decreased serum bicarbonate concentrations should prompt the evaluation of blood gas analyses. Important historical factors to consider include (1) type of intoxication (acute versus chronic); (2) type of preparation ingested (immediate or sustained release); (3) coingestants associated with arrhythmias, seizures, or hypotension; and (4) comorbid conditions, such as asthma, coronary artery disease, and seizure disorder.

TREATMENT

There are four components of treatment for xanthine poisoning: (1) supportive care, (2) gastrointestinal decontamination, (3) pharmacologic treatment of manifestations, and (4) enhancement of elimination.

Supportive Care

Supportive care is paramount. Crystalloid should be given to replace losses from diuresis and emesis. Hypokalemia should be treated cautiously with potassium supplementation because total body potassium is not depleted; rather, hypokalemia results from intracellular sequestration secondary to β2-receptor stimulation. Hyperkalemia may occur as the serum theophylline concentration decreases in a patient who is receiving potassium supplementation[41] or if a patient is being treated with propranolol.[42] Administration of magnesium and sodium bicarbonate should be considered for clinically significant hypomagnesemia and acidosis.

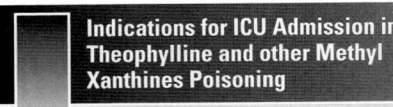

Indications for ICU Admission in Theophylline and other Methyl Xanthines Poisoning

Seizure
Ventricular arrhythmia
Hypotension
Rising theophylline concentration despite decontamination

Continuous electrocardiographic monitoring to assess for myocardial irritability should be instituted. Isolated premature ventricular contractions that are not associated with hemodynamic compromise require no treatment. More significant signs of myocardial irritability should be treated with appropriate doses of lidocaine. Although the proconvulsant actions of lidocaine pose a theoretical risk, there is no evidence suggesting that lidocaine is detrimental when used in appropriate doses.

Gastrointestinal Decontamination

Victims of acute theophylline intoxication may benefit from gastrointestinal decontamination. A single dose of activated charcoal always should be given. The American Academy of Clinical Toxicologists and the European Association of Poison Control Centres and Clinical Toxicologists recommended that whole-bowel irrigation be considered in an acute overdose with a sustained-release preparation,[43] although an animal model of acute theophylline overdose did not show that whole-bowel irrigation significantly reduces absorption of theophylline.[44,45] A bezoar should be suspected in patients who continue to have rising serum concentrations despite tolerating activated charcoal. Rarely, endoscopy has been used to remove a bezoar.[2]

Pharmacologic Management

Recommendations for pharmacologic treatment of theophylline overdose (Table 40-1) are based on an understanding of pathophysiology and anecdotal experience. No large series or randomized clinical trials have studied the efficacy of specific pharmacologic interventions for theophylline intoxication.

Clinically significant cardiac arrhythmias should be treated according to advanced cardiac life support algorithms. Atrial tachyarrhythmias have been shown to be reversed by β-blockers.[13,16,42,46] Nonspecific β-blockers, such as propranolol, should be administered cautiously to patients with asthma because they may precipitate bronchospasm. Additionally, use of nonspecific β-receptor antagonists may lead to unopposed α-adrenergic activity, resulting in coronary vasoconstriction and left ventricular dysfunction. Esmolol, a selective β1-adrenoreceptor antagonist, seems to be safe to use in patients with asthma; however, their respiratory status should be monitored closely. Some authors have recommended intensive hemodynamic monitoring when esmolol is used in theophylline intoxication because it has been shown to increase left ventricular stroke work index.[47] Adenosine has been reported to reverse theophylline-induced paroxysmal supraventricular tachycardia at typical adult doses of 6 mg,[48] although much higher doses may be required. Adenosine is likely to be of minimal clinical usefulness, however, because of its ultrashort half-life, and continuous infusions of adenosine can lead to bronchoconstriction and atrioventricular block.[49] Verapamil has been used to treat multifocal atrial tachycardia[50] but has failed in the treatment of supraventricular tachycardia.[4] Verapamil should be used cautiously because it may lead to heart block and hypotension.

Hypotension that persists despite fluid resuscitation and treatment of clinically significant arrhythmias should be treated initially with an α-receptor agonist, such as

TABLE 40-1 Pharmacologic Treatment in Theophylline Overdose*			
SYMPTOM	**AGENT**	**DOSE**	**COMMENT**
Emesis	Ondansetron	8 mg IV (0.15 mg/kg IV)	Cimetidine should not be used, as it inhibits metabolism of theophylline
	Ranitidine	50 mg IV (2 mg/kg)	
Seizure	Lorazepam	4 mg IV (0.1 mg/kg IV)	Other benzodiazepines may be used
	Phenobarbital	300–800 mg (20 mg/kg IV)	May augment respiratory depression
Hypotension	Propranolol	1–3 mg slow IV push (0.02 mg/kg IV)	May precipitate bronchospasm in asthmatic patients; if effective, consider infusion 5–10 mg/hr
	Esmolol	500 μg/kg over 1 min, then 50 μg/kg/min	May increase left ventricular stroke work index
			May be effective if hypotension is due to tachycardia

*Numbers in parentheses indicate pediatric dose.
IV, intravenous.

phenylephrine. Hypotension also has been successfully with propranolol, which antagonizes β$_2$-mediated vasodilation.[16,42] Invasive cardiovascular monitoring should be instituted for patients who are persistently hypotensive.

Seizures are frequently difficult to control in patients with theophylline intoxication. The initial choice of anticonvulsants should be a benzodiazepine, large doses of which may be required. Phenobarbital or other barbiturates may be used as adjunctive anticonvulsants. Barbiturates have the disadvantage of delayed onset and potentially adding to the respiratory depressant effects of benzodiazepines. Phenytoin should be considered to be contraindicated based on the empirical observation that it is ineffective in the termination of theophylline-induced seizures and based on animal data suggesting increased mortality.[51] If anticonvulsants are ineffective in terminating seizures, neuromuscular blockade may be indicated. In this circumstance, continuous electroencephalographic monitoring is needed to ensure that electrical seizure activity is not occurring.

Prophylactic administration of an anticonvulsant, either a benzodiazepine or a barbiturate, should be considered in patients at high risk for theophylline-induced seizures. High-risk patients include patients with acute overdose and with a serum theophylline concentration greater than or equal to 80 μg/mL (444 μmol/L), patients with chronic intoxication who are older than age 60 and with a serum theophylline concentration greater than or equal to 30 μg/mL (167 μmol/L), and patients with evidence of neuromuscular excitability. Although there is no reported experience in humans to support this practice, pretreatment with anticonvulsants in animal models of acute theophylline intoxication is beneficial.[51–53] The use of prophylactic anticonvulsants is not a substitute for and should not result in delay of institution of extracorporeal elimination in cases in which the latter is indicated.

Emesis must be controlled to administer activated charcoal effectively and to prevent further fluid loss. Control of emesis may be difficult to achieve for most patients with theophylline intoxication.[4,20,23] Standard antiemetics, such as phenothiazines, are frequently ineffective.[4,23] Additionally, phenothiazines may lower the seizure threshold significantly. Ondansetron, a 5-hydroxytryptamine antagonist that acts at the chemoreceptor trigger zone, has been shown to

reduce theophylline-associated vomiting when other anti-emetics have failed.[54,55] Ranitidine is an important adjunct because it decreases theophylline-induced gastric hyper-secretion[22] and does not inhibit cytochrome P-450 enzymes. Ranitidine has been shown to be effective in controlling emesis when used alone.[56]

Enhancement of Elimination

Multiple-dose activated charcoal (MDAC) (Fig. 40-2) has been shown to reduce theophylline's apparent half-life in a case series of intoxicated patients and in human experimental models of theophylline intoxication. In one series of five infants, MDAC reduced the expected half-life of theophylline from 25 hours to between 6.5 and 12.6 hours.[57] Similarly, in a human volunteer trial, the half-life of theophylline was reduced from 6.4 hours to 3.3 hours when MDAC was administered.[58]

The optimal regimen for MDAC has been studied in human volunteers who received 6 mg/kg of aminophylline intravenously. Frequency of administration was found to be more important than the total amount of charcoal given.

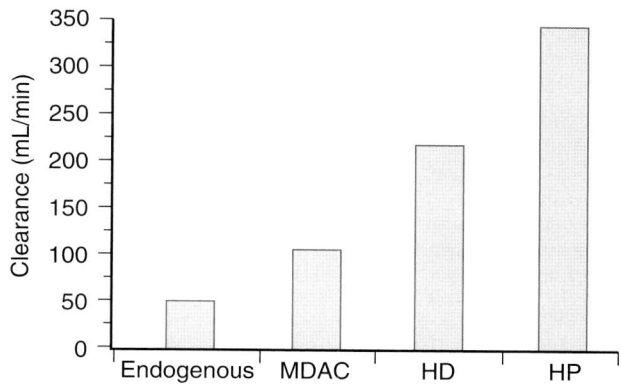

FIGURE 40-2

Clearance rate of theophylline using multiple-dose activated charcoal (MDAC), hemodialysis (HD), and hemoperfusion (HP) compared with endogenous clearance.

Administering activated charcoal every 2 hours maximally increased clearance of theophylline.[59] The recommended regimen is 25 g of activated charcoal administered every 2 hours until the serum theophylline concentration has declined to an acceptable level.[60] It is safe for most patients but must be administered cautiously to premature infants and to paralyzed patients. Activated charcoal should not be used if the patient has an ileus. MDAC is discussed in Chapter 6. When MDAC is administered, it is crucial to avoid using cathartics with each dose because these may lead to life-threatening volume depletion and electrolyte abnormalities. The activated charcoal should be administered as an aqueous suspension. Suggested indications for enhanced elimination are given in Table 40-2.

Extracorporeal drug removal (ECR) may be beneficial for selected patients. Acceptable ECR modalities include hemodialysis and charcoal hemoperfusion.[61] Triple-volume exchange transfusion was used successfully in a premature infant.[62] Peritoneal dialysis removes theophylline but too slowly to have a role in the treatment of theophylline intoxication.[63] Ideally, ECR should begin before LTEs are present because numerous case series and case reports have shown that ECR does not reliably terminate LTEs when they begin.[4,18,20,33,61,62] Patients have died or experienced significant neurologic disability despite the institution of ECR.[4,18,20,64]

Important differences exist between hemodialysis and hemoperfusion. Hemoperfusion effects a higher rate of clearance than does hemodialysis. Hemoperfusion has been shown to decrease the elimination half-life of theophylline to 1.23 ± 0.31 hours versus 2.39 ± 1.14 hours for hemodialysis.[61] Hemoperfusion has many disadvantages, however. It is not available in all centers, and it is associated with complications such as bleeding, thrombocytopenia, and hypocalcemia in 40% to 60% of patients undergoing the procedure. In contrast, hemodialysis is readily available at most centers and has a lower complication rate.[62] ECR is discussed in more detail in Chapter 7.

ECR should be considered for any patient who is at high risk for LTEs (see Table 40-2). As previously discussed, in an acute ingestion, high-risk patients include patients with a theophylline serum concentration of 80 to 100 µg/mL (444 to 555 µmol/L). In chronic intoxication, patients who are older than age 60 to 65 or younger than 1 year and who have supratherapeutic levels are at risk. Most patients do not experience LTEs until levels exceed 30 to 40 µg/mL (167 to 222 µmol/L), so most authorities do not recommend ECR unless these patients have levels greater than 40 µg/mL (222 µmol/L).

Although hemoperfusion is more efficient than hemodialysis at removing theophylline, it has not been shown to be better at improving clinical outcome. In the only study to compare clinical outcomes of theophylline-poisoned patients treated with either hemoperfusion or hemodialysis, there was no significant difference in the numbers of patients who had major toxicity during or after the procedure.[61] This study must be interpreted with some caution because patients were not assigned randomly to treatment groups, and it had limited power.

It seems reasonable to perform prophylactic hemodialysis for high-risk patients given the risks of hemoperfusion, the poor specificity of risk factors, and the lack of demonstrable benefit between hemodialysis and hemoperfusion. For patients who are already manifesting LTEs, however, hemoperfusion is the best choice given its higher clearance. If hemoperfusion is not immediately available, hemodialysis should be instituted promptly.

Common Errors in the Treatment of Methyl Xanthine Poisoning

Not instituting hemodialysis in a patient experiencing a life-threatening event if hemoperfusion is unavailable
Not monitoring serum concentrations closely (every 2 hours)
Not monitoring serum concentrations for 24 hours after an overdose of a sustained-release preparation

Key Points in the Evaluation and Management of Methyl Xanthine Poisoning

1. In acute intoxication, serum concentration is the most important prognostic indicator of life-threatening events.
2. In chronic intoxication, age is the most important prognostic indicator of life-threatening events.
3. Extracorporeal drug removal should be considered in any patient who is at high risk for a life-threatening event. When a life-threatening event occurs, there may be significant morbidity and mortality despite extracorporeal drug removal.

TABLE 40-2 Indications for Enhanced Elimination

MDAC
Acute intoxication
    After ingestion of >10 mg/kg; continue until concentration has peaked
Chronic intoxication
    Serum concentration >20 µg/mL in a patients who is symptomatic

Hemodialysis
Acute intoxication
    Serum concentration >80–100 µg/mL (or anticipated despite MDAC)
Chronic intoxication
    Age >60 yr and serum concentration >40 µg/mL
    Age <1 yr and serum concentration >40 µg/mL
Hemoperfusion not available and patient experiencing an LTE

Hemoperfusion*
Seizure
Ventricular arrhythmia
Persistent hypotension

---

*If hemoperfusion is unavailable, hemodialysis may be substituted.
LTE, life-threatening event; MDAC, multiple-dose activated charcoal.

OTHER METHYL XANTHINES: CAFFEINE AND PENTOXIFYLLINE

Caffeine is found in numerous prescription and nonprescription products. Chronic ingestion may produce caffeinism, a symptom complex consisting of irritability, insomnia, anxiety, and chronic abdominal pain. In contrast to theophylline, life-threatening toxicity has not been reported after chronic ingestion of caffeine. Symptoms after acute overdose of caffeine however, are similar, to symptoms of acute theophylline toxicity. Metabolic acidosis,[65] seizures,[65,66] and ventricular arrhythmias[65,67] all have been reported. Caffeine poisoning also has been associated with excessive catecholamine release similar to that seen with theophylline poisoning.[68] Fatal oral doses of caffeine have ranged from 5 to 50 g[69–71]; the lethal dose is estimated to be 100 to 200 mg/kg. Fatalities have been associated with serum caffeine concentrations ranging from 80 to 1560 μg/mL,[72] although concentrations of 297 μg/mL have been associated with survival after hemoperfusion.[67]

Treatment of acute caffeine overdose is similar to that for theophylline intoxication. Several case reports have shown that caffeine is removed effectively by hemoperfusion.[67,72] A serum concentration level greater than or equal to 120 μg/mL has been cited as a criterion for hemoperfusion.

Pentoxifylline is a xanthine derivative used in the treatment of peripheral vascular disease. Experience in overdose is limited. Acute overdose has been associated with hypokalemia, hyperglycemia, atrioventricular block, and hypotension.[73–76] Death has occurred after massive overdose.[77] Toxicity from chronic use has not been reported. Treatment is primarily supportive. Hypotension may be treated with crystalloid and seizures treated with benzodiazepines or phenobarbital.

CONCLUSION

Theophylline intoxication is associated with significant morbidity and mortality. Preventing the occurrence of arrhythmias and seizures by aggressive decontamination and ECR in selected patients is essential to prevent untoward outcomes after theophylline poisoning.

REFERENCES

1. Bernstein G, Jehle D, Bernaski E, et al: Failure of gastric emptying and charcoal administration in fatal sustained release theophylline overdose: Pharmacobezoar formation. Ann Emerg Med 21:1388–1390, 1992.
2. Cereda JM, Scott J, Quigley EM: Endoscopic removal of pharmacobezoar of slow release theophylline. BMJ Res Ed 293:1143, 1986.
3. Gaudreault P, Guay J: Theophylline poisoning: Pharmacological considerations and clinical management. Med Toxicol 1:169–191, 1986.
4. Henderson A, Wright DM, Pond SM: Management of theophylline overdose patients in the intensive care unit. Anaesth Intensive Care 20:56–62, 1992.
5. Hendeles L, Jenkins J, Temple R: Revised FDA labeling guidelines for theophylline oral dosage forms. Pharmacotherapy 15:409–427, 1995.
6. Weinberger M, Hendeles L: Theophylline use: An overview. J Allergy Clin Immunol 76:277–284, 1985.
7. Mizuki Y, Fujiwara I, Yamaguchi T: Pharmacokinetic interaction related to the chemical structures of the fluoroquinolones. J Antimicrob Chemother 37(Suppl A):41–45, 1996.
8. Cupp MJ, Tracy TS: Cytochrome p450: New nomenclature and clinical implications. Am Fam Physician 57:107–116, 1998.
9. Katial RK, Stelzle RC, Bonner MW, et al: A drug interaction between zafirlukast and theophylline. Arch Intern Med 158:1713–1715, 1998.
10. Pelleg A, Porter S: The pharmacology of adenosine. Pharmacotherapy 10:157–174, 1990.
11. Pinard E, Riche D, Puiroud S, et al: Theophylline reduces cerebral hyperaemia and enhances brain damage induced by seizures. Brain Res 511:303–309, 1990.
12. Minton NA, Henry JA: Acute and chronic human toxicity of theophylline. Hum Exp Toxicol 15:471–481, 1996.
13. Kearney TE, Manoguerra AS, Curtis GP, et al: Theophylline toxicity and the beta adrenergic system. Ann Intern Med 102:485–490, 1985.
14. Curry SC, Vance MV, Requa R, et al: Effects of toxic concentrations of theophylline on oxygen consumption, ventricular work, acid-base balance and plasma catecholamine levels in the dog. Ann Emerg Med 14:554–561, 1985.
15. Shannon M: Hypokalemia, hyperglycemia and plasma catecholamine after severe theophylline intoxication. Clin Toxicol 32:41–47, 1994.
16. Biberstein MP, Ziegler MG, Ward DM: Use of beta-blockade and hemoperfusion for acute theophylline poisoning. West J Med 141:485–490, 1984.
17. Whitehurst VE, Joseph X, Vick JA, et al: Reversal of acute theophylline toxicity by calcium channel blockers in dogs and rats. Toxicology 110:113–121, 1996.
18. Paloucek FP, Rodvold KA: Evaluation of theophylline overdose and toxicities. Ann Emerg Med 17:135–144, 1988.
19. Sessler CN: Poor tolerance of activated charcoal with theophylline overdose. Am J Emerg Med 5:492–495, 1987.
20. Sessler CN: Theophylline toxicity: Clinical features of 116 cases. Am J Med 88:567–576, 1990.
21. Shannon M: Life-threatening events after theophylline overdose: A 10-year prospective analysis. Arch Intern Med 159:989–994, 1999.
22. Cano R, Isenberg JI, Grossman MI: Cimetidine inhibits caffeine-stimulated gastric acid secretion in man. Gastroenterology 70:1055–1057, 1976.
23. Amitai Y, Lovejoy FH Jr: Characteristics of vomiting associated with acute sustained release theophylline poisoning: Implications for management with oral activated charcoal. Clin Toxicol 25:539–554, 1987.
24. Bittar G, Friedman HS: The arrhythmogenicity of theophylline: A multivariate analysis of clinical determinants. Chest 99:1415–1420, 1991.
25. Bahls F, Ma KK, Bird TD: Theophylline associated seizures with "therapeutic" or low serum concentrations: Risk factors for serious outcomes in adults. Neurology 41:1309–1312, 1991.
26. Covelli HD, Knodel AR, Heppner BT: Predisposing factors to apparent theophylline-induced seizures. Ann Allergy 54:411–415, 1985.
27. Zwillich CW, Sutton FD, Neff TA, et al: Theophylline-induced seizures in adults: Correlation with serum concentrations. Ann Intern Med 82:784–787, 1975.
28. Aitkin ML, Martin TR: Life-threatening theophylline toxicity is not predictable by serum levels. Chest 91:10–14, 1987.
29. Dunn DW, Parekh HU: Theophylline and status epilepticus in children. Neuropediatrics 22:24–26, 1991.
30. O'Riordan JI, Hutchinson J, FitzGerald MX, et al: Amnesic syndrome after theophylline associated seizures: Iatrogenic brain injury. J Neurol Neurosurg Psychiatry 57:643–645, 1994.
31. Bigler ED: Theophylline neurotoxicity resulting in diffuse brain damage. Dev Med Child Neurol 33:179–183, 1991.
32. Eldridge FL, Paydarfar D, Scott SC, et al: Role of endogenous adenosine in recurrent generalized seizures. Exp Neurol 103:179–185, 1989.
33. Shannon M, Maher T: Anticonvulsant effects of intracerebroventricular adenocard in theophylline-induced seizures. Ann Emerg Med 26:65–68, 1995.
34. Puiroud S, Pinard E, Seylaz J: Dynamic cerebral and systemic circulatory effects of adenosine, theophylline and dipyridamole. Brain Res 453:287–298, 1988.
35. Parr MJ, Anaes FC, Day AC: Theophylline poisoning—a review of 64 cases. Intensive Care Med 16:394–398, 1990.
36. Shannon M, Lovejoy FH: Effect of acute versus chronic intoxication on clinical features of theophylline poisoning in children. J Pediatr 121:125–130, 1992.
37. Bernard S: Severe lactic acidosis following theophylline overdose. Ann Emerg Med 20:1135–1137, 1991.
38. Titley OG, Williams N: Theophylline toxicity causing rhabdomyolysis and acute compartment syndrome. Intensive Care Med 18:129–130, 1992.
39. Shannon M: Predictors of major toxicity after theophylline overdose. Ann Intern Med 119:1161–1167, 1993.
40. Bertino JS Jr, Walker JW: Reassessment of theophylline toxicity: Serum concentrations, clinical course, and treatment. Arch Intern Med 147:757–760, 1987.
41. D'Angio R, Sabatelli F: Management considerations in treating metabolic abnormalities associated with theophylline overdose. Arch Intern Med 147:1837–1838, 1987.

42. Amin DN, Henry JA: Propranolol administration in theophylline overdose. Lancet 1:520–521, 1985.
43. Tenenbein M: Position statement: Whole bowel irrigation, American Academy of Clinical Toxicology; European Association of Poison Centres and Clinical Toxicologists. J Toxicol Clin Toxicol 35:753–762, 1997.
44. Burkhart KK, Wuerz RC, Donovan JW: Whole-bowel irrigation as adjunctive treatment for sustained-release theophylline overdose. Ann Emerg Med 21:1316–1320, 1992.
45. Minton NA, Henry JA: Prevention of drug absorption in a stimulated theophylline overdose. Clin Toxicol 33:43–49, 1995.
46. Seneff M, Scott J, Friedman B, et al: Acute theophylline toxicity and the use of esmolol to reverse cardiovascular instability. Ann Emerg Med 19:671–673, 1990.
47. Kempf J, Rusterholtz T, Ber C, et al: Haemodynamic study as guideline for the use of beta blockers in acute theophylline poisoning. Intensive Care Med 22:585–587, 1996.
48. Cairns CB, Niemann JT: Intravenous adenosine in the emergency department management of paroxysmal supraventricular tachycardia. Ann Emerg Med 20:717–721, 1991.
49. Biery JC, Kauflin MJ, Mauro VF: Adenosine in acute theophylline intoxication. Ann Pharmacother 29:1285–1287, 1995.
50. Levine JH, Michael JR, Guarnierit T: Treatment of multi-focal atrial tachycardia with verapamil. N Engl J Med 312:21–25, 1985.
51. Blake KV, Massey KL, Hendeles L, et al: Relative efficacy of phenytoin and phenobarbital for the prevention of theophylline-induced seizures in mice. Ann Emerg Med 17:1024–1028, 1988.
52. Hoffman A, Ointo E, Gilhar D: Effect of pretreatment with anticonvulsants on theophylline-induced seizures in the rat. J Crit Care 8:198–202, 1993.
53. Goldberg MJ, Spector R, Miller G: Phenobarbital improves survival in theophylline-intoxicated rabbits. Clin Toxicol 24:203–211, 1986.
54. Roberts JR, Carney S, Boyle SM, et al: Ondansetron quells drug-resistant emesis in theophylline poisoning. Am J Emerg Med 6:609–610, 1993.
55. Sage TA, Jones WN, Clark RF: Ondansetron in the treatment of intractable nausea associated with theophylline toxicity. Ann Pharmacother 27:584–585, 1993.
56. Amitai Y, Yeung AC, Moye J, et al: Repetitive oral actvated charcoal and control of emesis in severe theophylline toxicity. Ann Intern Med 105:386–387, 1986.
57. Shannon M, Amitai Y, Lovejoy FH Jr: Multiple dose activated charcoal for theophylline poisoning in young infants. Pediatrics 80:368–370, 1987.
58. Berlinger WG, Spector R, Goldberg MJ, et al: Enhancement of theophylline clearance by oral activated charcoal. Clin Pharmacol Ther 33:351–354, 1983.
59. Park GD, Radomski L, Goldberg MJ, et al: Effects of size and frequency of oral doses of charcoal on theophylline clearance. Clin Pharmacol Ther 34:663–666, 1983.
60. Position statement and practice guidelines on the use of multi-dose activated charcoal in the treatment of acute poisoning. American Academy of Clinical Toxiciology; European Association of Poison Centers and Clinical Toxicologists. J Toxicol Clin Toxicol 37:731–751, 1999.
61. Shannon M: Comparative efficacy of hemodialysis and hemoperfusion in severe theophylline intoxication. Acad Emerg Med 4:674–678, 1997.
62. Shannon M, Wernovsky G, Morris C, et al: Exchange transfusion in the treatment of severe theophylline poisoning. Pediatrics 89:145–147, 1992.
63. Colonna F, Trappan A, de Vonderweid U, et al: Peritoneal dialysis in a 6-weeks old pre-term infant with severe theophylline intoxication. Minerva Pediatr 48:383–385, 1996.
64. Park GD, Spector R, Roberts R, et al: Use of hemoperfusion for treatment of theophylline intoxication. Am J Med 74:961–966, 1983.
65. Dietrich AM, Mortensen ME: Presentation and management of an acute caffeine overdose. Pediatr Emerg Care 6:296–298, 1990.
66. Banner W, Czajka PA: Acute caffeine overdose in the neonate. Am J Dis Child 134:495–498, 1980.
67. Nagesh RV, Murphy KA: Caffeine poisoning treated by hemoperfusion. Am J Kidney Dis 12:316–318, 1988.
68. Benowitz NL, Osterloh J, Goldschlager N, et al: Massive cathecholamine release from caffeine poisoning. JAMA 248:1097–1098, 1982.
69. Dirmacio VJM, Garriot JC: Lethal caffeine poisoning in a child. Forensic Sci Int 3:275–278, 1974.
70. Sullivan JL: Caffeine poisoning in an infant. J Pediatr 90:1022–1023, 1977.
71. Turner JE, Cravey RH: A fatal ingestion of caffeine. Clin Toxicol 10:341–344, 1977.
72. Mrvos R, Reilly P, Dean B, et al: Massive caffeine ingestion resulting in death. Vet Hum Toxicol 31:571–572, 1989.
73. Zimmerman PM, Pulliam J, Schwengels J, et al: Caffeine intoxication: A near fatality. Ann Emerg Med 14:1227–1229, 1985.
74. Dolgin J, Abrams B, Tucker J: Survival with massive pentoxifylline overdose and high serum levels. Vet Hum Toxicol 36:369, 1994.
75. Garnier R, Riboulet-Delmas G, Chatenet T, et al: Acute pentoxifylline poisoning in children. Ann Pediatr 33:62–63, 1986.
76. Sznajder I, Bentur Y, Taitelman U: First and second degree atrioventricular block in oxpentifylline overdose. BMJ (Clin Res) 288:26, 1984.
77. Suarez-Penarranda JM, Rico-Boquete R, Lopez-Rivadulla M, et al: A fatal case of suicidal pentoxifylline intoxication. Int J Legal Med 111:151–153, 1998.

CHAPTER 41

Sympathomimetic Agents

Robert J. Hoffman ■ Lewis S. Nelson

Sympathomimetics constitute a large group of drugs with a spectrum of uses that range from over-the-counter cold preparations to critical care medications. Their clinical effects are similar and theoretically should be predictable based on an understanding of the specific pharmacology of the drugs. Because of the complexity of the autonomic nervous system and its responses to physiologic changes within the body, however, the actual clinical effects of these drugs vary and may be unpredictable.

CHEMISTRY AND BIOCHEMISTRY OF SYMPATHOMIMETIC AGENTS

β-Phenylethylamine, the parent compound of the sympathomimetic amines, consists of a benzene ring and ethylamide side chain (Fig. 41-1). Substitutions are possible on the aliphatic ring, the α and β carbon, or the terminal amino group to yield a variety of compounds with sympathomimetic activity. The particular groups substituted on the parent molecule impart the unique properties of each sympathomimetic amine. Its substituted groups often determine polarity or nonpolarity of a sympathomimetic amine. Less polar molecules are more lipophilic and possess a greater tendency to cross the blood-brain barrier, resulting in central effects. Examples of such sympathomimetic amines are ephedrine and amphetamines. The more polar compounds (e.g., epinephrine, norepinephrine, and isoproterenol) cross the blood-brain barrier poorly, and their effects are peripheral (see Fig. 41-1).

PATHOPHYSIOLOGY

The sympathomimetic toxidrome, addressed in detail in Chapter 32, is technically a misnomer. Excess autonomic stimulation and agents that mimic this process produce the clinical syndrome typically described as "sympathomimetic." Selective or receptor-specific adrenergic agonists produce clinical findings, however, that may be distinctly different. Prediction of the clinical effects of particular adrenergic agonists is possible based on their preferred adrenergic binding activity; their ability to cross the blood-brain barrier; and their direct, indirect, or mixed activity. After significant overdose, the receptor specificity may be diminished, however. The clinical effects of the various agents may become less predictable after overdose. The

sequelae of sympathomimetic overdose are generally related to the neurologic and cardiovascular systems and include psychomotor agitation–induced hyperthermia, cardiac dysrhythmia, hypertension and end-organ damage, myocardial ischemia and infarction, stroke, seizure, hypotension and vascular collapse, and hypokalemia.

The endogenous catecholamines include epinephrine, norepinephrine, and dopamine. These neurotransmitters, released from adrenergic and dopaminergic nerve endings, from the adrenal medulla, and locally within the sympathetic nervous system, are involved in numerous physiologic functions, including homeostasis and response to stressors. The actions of catecholamines are terminated rapidly by reuptake into nerve terminals with metabolic degradation by monoamine oxidase (MAO) or by repackaging in vesicles (Fig. 41-2). Alternatively, termination of catecholamine activity may result after diffusion from the synaptic cleft with subsequent degradation at extraneuronal sites by catechol *O*-methyltransferase (COMT).

Synthetic sympathetic amines are structural analogues of the endogenous catecholamines. They lack several crucial hydroxyl groups, a property that increases their oral bioavailability by reducing their hepatic metabolism by COMT. In some cases, substitutions on the phenyl group (see Fig. 41-1) confer MAO resistance to these agents.

Adrenergic Receptors

Adrenergic receptors are broadly classed as α and β, but numerous subtypes exist. The clinically relevant types addressed here are α_1, α_2, β_1, and β_2 (Table 41-1). α_1-Adrenergic receptors are postsynaptic and cause contraction of smooth muscle with various clinical effects. α_2-Receptors are primarily presynaptic and function in an autoregulatory capacity. Synaptic norepinephrine inhibits further release of norepinephrine by feedback inhibition. Postsynaptic α_2-receptors share many of the properties of α_1-receptors but also mediate a few unique effects (see Table 41-1).

β_1-Receptors are located primarily on the myocardium and are involved in cardiovascular stimulation. β_2-Receptors mediate numerous clinical effects, but the most important are related to smooth muscle relaxation (see Table 41-1).

The endogenous catecholamines are nonspecific adrenergic agonists; they stimulate α-adrenergic and β-adrenergic receptors. When administered exogenously, all are predominantly peripherally acting and do not exert significant central nervous system (CNS) effects. Epinephrine

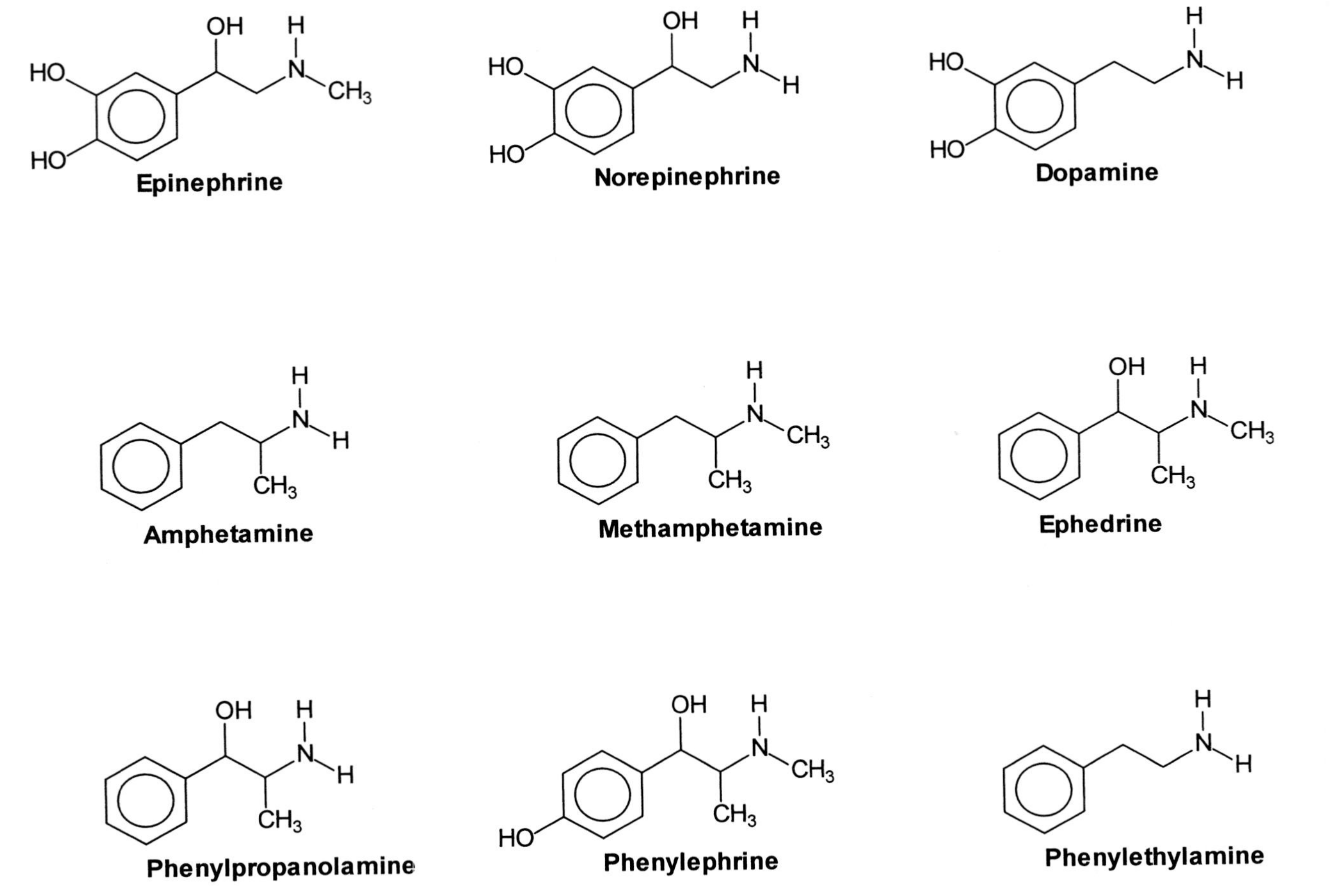

FIGURE 41-1

Chemical structure of phenylethylamine and related sympathomimetics.

and norepinephrine are direct-acting sympathomimetics, implying that they bind to and stimulate adrenergic receptors. They differ slightly, however, in their receptor selectivity. Most significantly, epinephrine is a potent β-adrenergic agonist, whereas norepinephrine is in all practicality a pure α-adrenergic agonist. Clinically, epinephrine has potent chronotropic and inotropic activity, and norepinephrine has less effect on cardiac contractility or rate. The β$_2$-adrenergic effects of therapeutic doses of epinephrine result in vasodilation and decrease in peripheral vascular resistance; in therapeutic doses, norepinephrine causes an increase in peripheral vascular resistance. Epinephrine also exerts many metabolic effects and hormone-like effects on secretory glands that norepinephrine does not (Table 41-2). Dopamine acts indirectly by effecting increased release of norepinephrine from the presynaptic neuron. At increased serum concentrations, dopamine may exert mixed, direct, and indirect activity. Several distinct types of dopamine receptors mediate the peripheral effects of dopamine. At low concentrations, dopamine's primary effect is stimulation of D$_1$ receptors. This stimulation results in vasodilation, particularly in the renal, mesenteric, and coronary vasculature. This unique property makes dopamine a valuable pressor agent because the typical effects of other pressors, such as norepinephrine and epi-

nephrine, include vasoconstriction of the aforementioned vascular beds. At increasing concentrations, dopamine stimulates β$_1$-adrenergic receptors, with resulting increase in cardiac chronotropy and inotropy, and stimulates α$_1$-receptors, resulting in vasoconstriction.

The synthetic sympathetic amines are a large group of agents each with a unique combination of pharmacologic effects. Their mechanism of action is similar to the endogenous catecholamines, but because of unique structural and chemical qualities, they have unique pharmacologic and clinical properties. As a group, these agents have much greater CNS penetration than the catecholamines, although there are tremendous variations within the group. Methamphetamine is a better CNS stimulant than other amphetamine congeners, such as ephedrine, owing to its enhanced CNS penetration and to receptor binding potency.

Specific agents can be classified by their activities at α-receptors and β-receptors and their subtypes or alternatively classified according to their direct, indirect, or mixed action as adrenergic agents. Because the clinical effects of these agents vary based on their receptor selectivity, this is the framework used for discussion. These effects from amphetamines and their derivatives are discussed in Chapter 73.

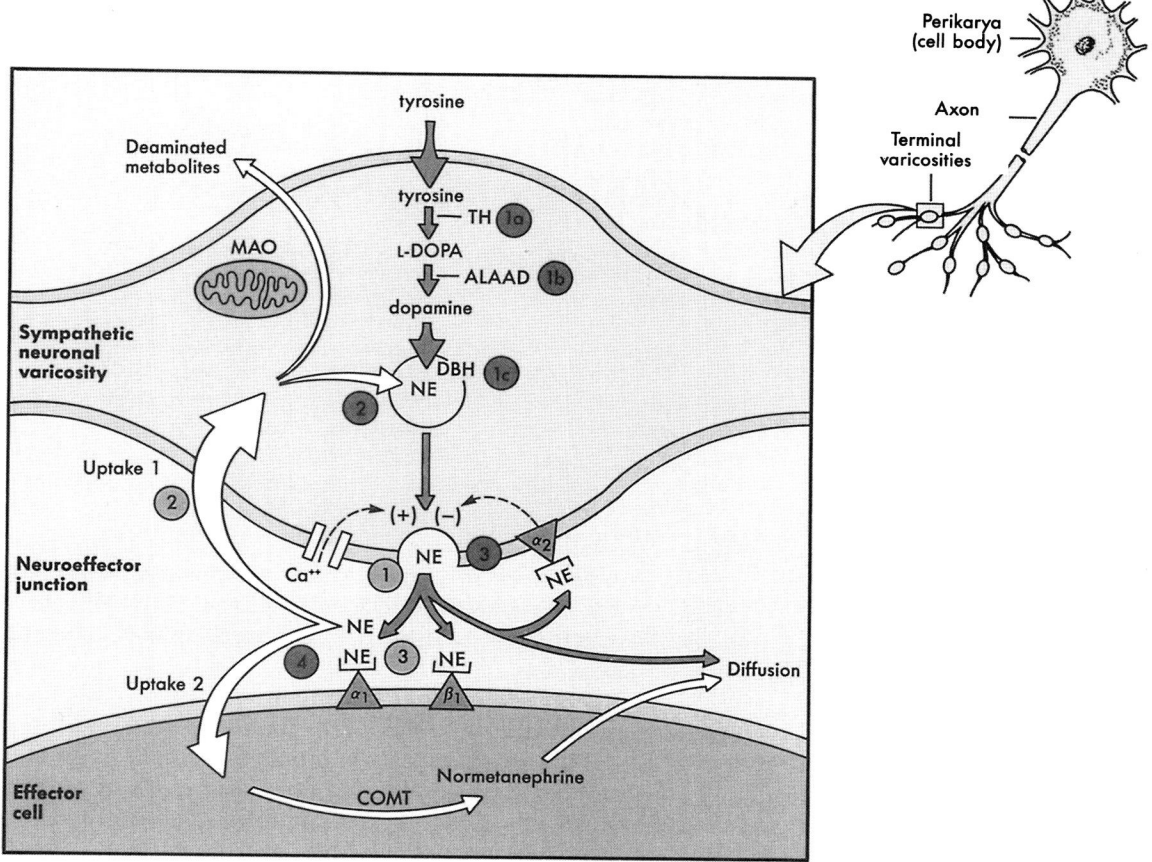

FIGURE 41-2

Prejunctional and postjunctional sites of action of drugs that modify noradrenergic transmission at a sympathetic neuroeffector junction. L-Tyrosine is actively transported into the axoplasm of the neuron, where it is converted first to L-dopa by tyrosine hydroxylase (TH) and then to dopamine by aromatic L-amino acid decarboxylase (ALAAD). Dopamine is actively transported into synaptic vesicles, where it is converted by dopamine β-hydroxylase (DBH) to norepinephrine (NE). The arrival of a nerve action potential at the varicosity causes the influx of calcium ions, which promotes the exocytotic release of NE into the neuroeffector junction, where NE can activate receptors on postjunctional smooth muscle or glandular cells (α_1 or α_2) or cardiac cells (β_1) or on the prejunctional neuronal membrane (α_2). Activation of the α_2-receptor inhibits the further release of NE. The action of NE is terminated by transport back into the varicosity, uptake 1. In the varicosity, NE can be stored in the synaptic vesicle or metabolized by monoamine oxidase (MAO) to inactive deaminated products. NE also is lost from the neuroeffector junction by diffusion and by transport into the postjunctional cell, uptake 2, where it is metabolized to normetanephrine by catechol *O*-methyltransferase (COMT). Drugs that enhance or mimic noradrenergic transmission (1) facilitate release (e.g., amphetamine), (2) block reuptake (e.g., cocaine), and (3) are receptor agonists (e.g., phenylephrine). Drugs that reduce noradrenergic transmission (1) inhibit synthesis (e.g., 1a, α-methyltyrosine; 1b, carbidopa; 1c, disulfiram), (2) disrupt vesicular storage (e.g., reserpine), (3) inhibit release (e.g., guanethidine), and (4) are receptor antagonists (e.g., phentolamine). *(From Brody TM, Larner J, Minneman KP [eds]: Human Pharmacology: Molecular to Clinical, 3rd ed. St. Louis, Mosby, 1998.)*

Agents with Combined α-Adrenergic and β-Adrenergic Activity

EPINEPHRINE, NOREPINEPHRINE, AND DOPAMINE

Poisoning from epinephrine, norepinephrine, and dopamine may result from inhalational, intravenous, or subcutaneous administration. Iatrogenic injury or death from administration of parenteral catecholamines is a common occurrence and may relate to improper preparation of an infusion, inappropriate infusion rate, or infusion pump malfunction. Administration of subcutaneous or intravenous epinephrine at inappropriate doses or to inappropriate locations also is common. Administration to inappropriate locations may occur as a result of inadvertent administration of topical anesthetic containing epinephrine into end organs, particularly digits, or similarly by release of an epinephrine autoinjector into the digit.[1]

Epinephrine and norepinephrine have direct α-adrenergic and β-adrenergic activity. Both are metabolized by COMT and MAO and are not bioavailable when taken orally. Similarly, because of this efficient metabolism, they have brief durations of action.

Dopamine, a mixed acting agent, produces principally α-adrenergic and β-adrenergic effects at low parenteral doses. As the dose escalates, the α-adrenergic effects predominate. Although the clinical effects of epinephrine, norepinephrine, and dopamine are qualitatively similar, there are important differences (Table 41-2).

EPHEDRINE AND PSEUDOEPHEDRINE

Ephedrine has been commonly available in its herbal form, *Ephedra* or Ma Huang, and its use at least has kept pace with, if not exceeded, the current trend of increased dietary

TABLE 41-1 Adrenoreceptor Subtypes

ADRENORECEPTOR TYPE	TISSUE	RESPONSE
α_1	Most smooth muscle	Contraction
	Hepatic	Glycogenolysis, gluconeogenesis
	Intestinal smooth muscle	Relaxation
	Pupillary dilator muscle	Contraction (dilates pupil)
α_2	Vascular smooth muscle	Contraction
	CNS adrenoreceptors	Multiple effects, including lowering blood pressure
	Nerve terminals	Inhibits norepinephrine release
	Fat cells	Inhibits lipolysis
	Pancreatic β cells	Decreases insulin secretion
β_1	Cardiac	Increases inotropy and chronotropy
β_2	Smooth muscle	Relaxation
	Skeletal muscle	Glycogenolysis
	Hepatic	Glycogenolysis, gluconeogenesis

CNS, central nervous system.

TABLE 41-2 Method of Action and Adrenoreceptor Effects of Sympathomimetics

DRUG	DIRECT, INDIRECT, OR MIXED ACTIVITY	PREDOMINANT ADRENORECEPTOR EFFECT	COMMENTS
Dopamine	Mixed	β_1	Dopaminergic activity as well
Dobutamine	Direct	β_1	
Epinephrine	Direct	$\alpha_1, \alpha_2, \beta_1, \beta_2$	
Norepinephrine	Direct	α_1, α_2	
Ephedrine	Mixed	$\alpha_1, \alpha_2, \beta_1, \beta_2$	
Pseudoephedrine			
Phenylpropanolamine	Mixed	α_1	β_1, β_2 effect in therapeutic dose
Phenylephrine	Direct	α_1	
Methoxamine			
Metaraminol	Mixed	$\alpha_1, \alpha_2, \beta_1, \beta_2$	Only α_1 effects at low dose
Mephentermine			
Mitodrine			
Isoproterenol	Direct	β_1, β_2	
Metaproterenol	Direct	$\beta_2 > \beta_1$	β_1, β_2 equivalent when used intravenously
Albuterol	Direct	β_2	
Bitolterol			
Formoterol			
Levalbuterol			
Pirbuterol			
Ritodrine			
Salmeterol			
Terbutaline			

supplement consumption. The surge in the use of Ma Huang has been particularly prevalent in products used for weight loss, athletics, bodybuilding, mood elevation, and euphoria (e.g., "herbal ecstasy").[2,3] Before this trend, ephedrine use was most widespread among college students and workers, such as truck drivers, seeking heightened alertness and wakefulness.[4]

Ephedrine and pseudoephedrine, optical isomers, are extremely similar to each other in pharmacologic properties and clinical use. Poisonings due to ephedrine or pseudoephedrine cause identical syndromes and require similar treatments. Ephedrine and pseudoephedrine are mixed-acting sympathomimetics, meaning that they have direct- and indirect-acting properties at adrenergic receptors. Similar to dopamine, they cause the release of norepinephrine. α-Adrenergic and β-adrenergic stimulation occur in cases of ephedrine or pseudoephedrine poisoning. The half-life of ephedrine and pseudoephedrine is approximately 5 hours.

α-Adrenergic Agonists

α-Adrenergic agents can be classified according to their relative affinity for α_1-adrenergic or α_2-adrenergic receptors. The primary effect of α_1-adrenergic agonists is vasoconstriction resulting in increased peripheral vascular resistance, increased blood pressure, and often reflex brady-cardia. Examples of α_1-agonists include phenylephrine and phenylpropanolamine. α_2-Receptors are found in the peripheral nervous system and CNS. Peripherally, α_2-receptors function similarly to the α_1 subtype and mediate smooth muscle contraction, causing vasoconstriction. At central adrenergic sites, α_2-adrenergic agonism results in feedback inhibition and a decreased release of cate-cholamines. The most prominent clinical effects include a centrally mediated reduction in blood pressure and heart rate. Common α_2-agonists are guanfacine; guanabenz; methyldopa; and the imidazoline agents clonidine, apra-clonidine, oxymetazoline, naphazoline, tetrahydrolazine, and xylometazoline. α_2-Adrenergic agonists are discussed in detail in Chapter 38.

CLINICAL PRESENTATION

Epinephrine, Norepinephrine, and Dopamine

The predominant clinical effects of epinephrine, norepi-nephrine, and dopamine are cardiovascular and include vasoconstriction and cardiac stimulation. The sequelae of poisoning with these agents include hypertension, tachycar-dia, dysrhythmia, acute coronary syndromes, pulmonary edema, and cerebrovascular injury.[5–12] In addition, patients often complain of anxiety, a sense of impending doom, apprehension, and headache. Catecholamines, which cross the blood-brain barrier only at high doses, produce minimal direct CNS symptoms. The psychological and cerebrovascu-lar effects likely are secondary to cardiovascular simulation.

Tissue necrosis secondary to localized vasoconstriction is the potential result of end-organ administration; this most typically occurs as a result of α-adrenergic vasoconstriction, usually due to locally applied epinephrine. The performance of "bloodless field" surgery, particularly hand and cosmetic surgery, demonstrates that epinephrine administration to dig-its or end organs is not an indication for mandatory therapy.

Ephedrine and Pseudoephedrine

The adverse effects of ephedrine and pseudoephedrine are the result of excessive cardiovascular stimulation by the auto-nomic nervous system. The expected complications of their use are qualitatively similar to the complications that occur with catecholamine use. Relative to amphetamine or metham-phetamine, ephedrine and pseudoephedrine have poor CNS penetration and cause much more profound peripheral sympa-thomimetic effects. Patients attempting to achieve the degree of CNS stimulation produced by methamphetamine may take massive doses of ephedrine or pseudoephedrine, resulting in profound cardiovascular stimulation and its sequelae.

β-Adrenergic Agonists

NONSELECTIVE β-ADRENERGIC AGONISTS

Nonselective adrenergic agonists, such as isoproterenol, typically are used in the intensive care setting. Isopro-terenol is a potent β_1-receptor and β_2-receptor agonist;

causes decreased peripheral vascular resistance in skeletal muscle, renal vasculature, and mesenteric vasculature; and has a positive chronotropic and inotropic effect on the heart. As a result, isoproterenol typically causes an increase in systolic blood pressure and a decrease in diastolic blood pressure. Isoproterenol is metabolized by COMT and has a half-life of 2 to 5 minutes.

SELECTIVE β₂-AGONISTS

The selective β_2-agonists stimulate receptors located in bronchial, uterine, and vascular smooth muscle and are used to treat bronchoconstriction and preterm labor. They have come into use more recently for the treatment of hyperkalemia because of their β-receptor–mediated ability to cause an intracellular influx of potassium. Although these agents primarily stimulate β_2-receptors, they may produce some β_1-agonist effects, particularly at high doses.

The β_2-agonists have nearly identical clinical effects, and the principal differences among the various agents derive from their pharmacokinetics. As such, this chapter does not examine each β_2-agonist individually; rather, they are discussed as a class. The β_2-agonists include albuterol, bitolterol, formoterol, pirbuterol, salmeterol, clenbuterol, terbutaline, and ritodrine.

Use of β_2-agonists is widespread, which presents several problems to the clinician treating potential toxicity. Exces-sive use of β_2-agonists such as those contained in metered-dose asthma inhalers or oral preparations can result in tachyphylaxis, a phenomenon in which down-regulation of receptors occurs, and the effects from this drug diminish as a result of excessive use.[13–15] Consequently, patients may require higher doses to achieve the same clinical effect they previously experienced at lower doses, resulting in more profound systemic side effects.

ADVERSE EFFECTS OF β-ADRENERGIC AGONISTS

The toxic effects of isoproterenol poisoning are related to its cardiostimulatory and vasodilatory properties and include tachycardia, hypotension, tachydysrhythmias, myocardial ischemia, and flushing. Commonly, CNS effects of anxiety, fear, and headache occur. Excess selective β_2-adrenergic agonism is associated with fewer clinically significant effects than combined β_1 and β_2 agonism; this probably relates to the vasodilatory properties of the β_2-agonists and the lack of vasoconstrictive and hyperten-sive effects after their overdose.

Severe hypokalemia can result from β_2-adrenergic stim-ulation.[16] This condition results from influx of extracellular potassium into the intracellular compartment despite nor-mal total-body potassium content. Electrocardiographic and neuromuscular complications of hypokalemia may develop. Although β_2-agonists cause hyperglycemia, prolonged poi-soning can result in hypoglycemia from depleted glucose and glycogen stores. Other effects of β_2-adrenergic poison-ing include tremor, agitation, vomiting, hypomagnesemia, and hypophosphatemia.[17–19]

Elevations of creatine phosphokinase muscle (CPK-MM) and cardiac (CPK-MB) fractions after large doses of β_2-agonists, particularly terbutaline infusions and continu-ous albuterol nebulization, are well described.[20–22] The clinical significance of increased CPK-MB is unclear, and it has not been shown to correlate with clinically adverse effects. Cardiac troponins may be elevated as a result of terbutaline infusion. Cardiac dysrhythmia, although described with β2-agonist poisoning, is most frequently supraventricular in origin and clinically inconsequential. Dysrhythmias other than sinus tachycardia should not be attributed routinely to β2-agonist toxicity until other causes have been excluded.

Ingestion of β2-agonists, which occurs predominantly in young children treated with oral albuterol preparations, can cause significant gastrointestinal symptoms and tachycardia.[23] Nevertheless, these unintentional poisonings are extremely well tolerated in children and rarely require more than supportive treatment. For oral albuterol poisoning, 1 mg/kg seems to be the dose threshold for developing significant toxicity.[24] Ritodrine, used in pregnant women for tocolysis, is associated with pulmonary edema, neutropenia, and agranulocytosis. In most reported cases, these effects resolve rapidly after discontinuation of ritodrine.[25–29]

α1-Selective Agonists

Direct-acting α1-selective agonists include phenylephrine and methoxamine, and mixed-acting α1-selective agonists include mephentermine, metaraminol, and mitodrine. All of these agents are used clinically for their vasoconstrictive effects. After overdose, hypertension and reflex bradycardia typically occur. The reflex bradycardia is a protective mechanism to keep cerebral blood flow in a physiologically acceptable range in the presence of a severely elevated blood pressure.

PHENYLEPHRINE

Phenylephrine is a direct-acting α1-adrenergic agonist used topically as a nasal decongestant and mydriatic and intravenously as a pressor. Toxicity from topical application is described, particularly in infants and geriatric patients. Phenylephrine undergoes extensive metabolism by MAO in the intestinal wall, resulting in poor oral bioavailability. Its duration of action is usually less than 60 minutes, so its primary effects typically are self-limited. Complications, including psychosis, seizure, myocardial infarction, and intracerebral hemorrhage, may persist beyond this time, however.[30]

PHENYLPROPANOLAMINE

Phenylpropanolamine, commonly used as an appetite suppressant, is an indirect-acting α-adrenergic and β-adrenergic agonist. After overdose, it acts almost exclusively as an α1-adrenergic agonist. Phenylpropanolamine crosses the blood-brain barrier much less readily than does amphetamine. The half-life of phenylpropanolamine is typically 2.5 hours in children and 5 to 6 hours in adults. Sustained-release preparations exist, and their duration of action may be two to three times longer than non–sustained-release preparations.

Although there is tremendous individual variability in blood pressure response to therapeutic doses of phenylpropanolamine,[31] severe hypertension and reflex bradycardia are typical after overdose. In addition, attempts to achieve psychoactive effects involve taking large doses and may result in hypertension and associated complications.[32] Cardiac dysrhythmias, myocardial injury, cardiomyopathy, and intracra-

nial hemorrhage also have been reported in association with greater than recommended doses of phenylpropanolamine.

METHOXAMINE, METARAMINOL, AND MIDODRINE

Methoxamine is a relatively selective direct-acting α1-adrenergic receptor agonist. Metaraminol and mephentermine have direct vasoconstrictive effects and cause release of endogenous norepinephrine. All of these agents result in typical complications of α-adrenergic agonist poisoning, including hypertension, tachydysrhythmias or bradydysrhythmias, and CNS stimulation.

DIAGNOSIS

Sympathomimetic overdose is a clinical diagnosis. Some laboratory findings, such as hypokalemia and hyperglycemia, may be present, but they play little role in diagnosis. Although sympathomimetic drugs and the endogenous catecholamines can be selectively assayed, the results typically are not available in a clinically relevant period of time. Urine drug screens, which can detect the structurally similar amphetamine derivatives by immunoassay, are neither sufficiently sensitive nor sufficiently specific to be clinically useful during the acute management of sympathomimetic drug toxicity. The differential diagnosis of sympathomimetic poisoning is listed in Table 41-3.

TREATMENT

The mainstay of therapy for adrenoreceptor overstimulation is correction and maintenance of vital signs to within acceptable limits. Because of the increased myocardial oxygen demand, supplemental oxygen should be administered unless specifically contraindicated. For agents that produce predominantly psychomotor agitation and increased autonomic activity, sedation is generally sufficient.

Patients poisoned by peripherally acting agents occasionally require the judicious use of specific α or β antagonists (Table 41-4). This therapy should not be initiated prematurely or indiscriminately because inappropriate use of these antagonists can result in unpredictable effects and potentially dire consequences. In a patient with a nonspecific

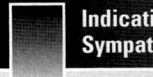
Indications for ICU Admission in Sympathomimetic Agent Poisoning

Manifestations of vital end-organ injury (e.g., myocardial ischemia or infarction, cerebrovascular accident, cerebral hemorrhage, liver function abnormality)
Cardiac dysrhythmias other than sinus tachycardia
Hypokalemia requiring cardiac monitoring or potassium supplementation
Cardiovascular effects requiring ongoing therapy with cardiovascular agents (e.g., nitroprusside infusion)
Ongoing morbidity requiring monitoring and treatment (e.g., hyperthermia, rhabdomyolysis, or renal insufficiency)

TABLE 41-3 Differential Diagnosis of Sympathomimetic Syndrome

Hyperthyroidism
Thyroid storm
Anticholinergic syndrome
Pheochromocytoma
Withdrawal syndromes
Mania
Subarachnoid hemorrhage
Serotonin syndrome
Neuroleptic malignant syndrome
Poisoning by illicit agents with adrenergic activity (e.g., cocaine or amphetamine derivatives)
Other situations of increased endogenous catecholamine release

adrenergic agonist overdose, such as ephedrine poisoning, the unopposed α-adrenergic stimulation that remains after β-adrenergic blockade may be associated with acute deterioration of the patient's vital signs.[31]

Treatment of Toxicity from Combined α-Adrenergic and β-Adrenergic Agents

Because of the short duration of action of epinephrine, norepinephrine, and dopamine, treatment of systemic toxicity, beyond supportive care, is typically unnecessary, unless complications arise. Discontinuation of the infused or administered drug is followed by fairly prompt cessation of signs and symptoms.

Treatment of systemic toxicity resulting from longer acting sympathomimetic agents should focus on correcting the vital sign abnormalities to within acceptable limits, including aggressive management of hyperthermia and control of neuro-

behavorial effects. Vasoconstrictive effects may be managed safely with phentolamine, a dihydropyridine calcium channel blocker, or sodium nitroprusside, but the chronotropic and inotropic effects are abated only by the administration of diltiazem, verapamil, or a β-adrenergic antagonist. β-Adrenergic antagonists are not advised routinely, however, unless a vasorelaxant agent is coadministered. The concern over the use of a β-blocker in such a situation is that it may result in unopposed α-adrenergic activity and hypertension. The danger of administering a β-blocker in the presence of an agent with combined α-adrenergic and β-adrenergic activity may be overstated, and β-blockers have been administered successfully in these situations.[32,33] At this time, there is insufficient evidence to support the safety or efficacy of β-blocker use to treat patients exposed to adrenergic agonists, such as cocaine, amphetamines, or ephedrine.

Psychomotor agitation should be treated with benzodiazepines, such as lorazepam or diazepam. Consideration for gastrointestinal decontamination in patients who ingest the sympathomimetic agents is discussed in detail in Chapter 5.

Although there are not sufficient published data to make broad-based recommendations about treatment for digital administration of epinephrine, it generally is accepted that in the absence of comorbidities, such as diabetic vasculopathy, pallor in a digit or end organ lasting only a few hours is usually safe. If deemed necessary, treatment for end-organ epinephrine administration is directed at increasing blood flow to the affected area; this can be accomplished by warming the area or by vasodilation achieved by application of topical nitroglycerin paste. Alternatively an appropriate amount of phentolamine may be injected into the affected area, directly into the initial puncture wound if possible, to antagonize epinephrine's α$_1$-adrenergic vasoconstrictive effect.[34-36] Many clinicians have limited experience with phentolamine, and because this agent is not used frequently, it is possible that obtaining it for use in

TABLE 41-4 Drugs Used in Treatment of Sympathomimetic Toxicity

DRUG	INDICATION	ACTION	DOSE
Nitroprusside	Hypertension	Vasodilation	0.3–10 μg/kg/min IV, titrated to effect
Phentolamine	Hypertension	α antagonism	Child: 0.1 mg/kg/dose (up to 5 mg/dose) IV repeated every 10 min PRN Adult: 5 mg IV repeated every 5 min PRN
	Extravasation of catecholamine	α antagonism	5–10 mg in 10 mL of normal saline infiltrated SC in appropriate quantity
Terbutaline	Extravasation of catecholamine	β$_2$ agonism	Child: 0.01 mg/kg/dose SC every 15 min to maximum of 0.4 mg/2 hr* Adult: 0.1 mg SC every 15 min to maximum of 0.4 mg/2 hr*
Esmolol	Hypertension	β antagonism	500 μg/kg/min IV bolus followed by infusion 50 μg/kg/min titrated to effect up to 500 μg/kg/min
Metoprolol	Hypertension	β antagonism	Child: Pediatric dose not established Adult: 2.5–5 mg IV every 5 min to a maximum of 15 mg
Propranolol	Hypertension	β antagonism	Child: 0.05–0.1 mg/kg slow IV (up to 1 mg/dose), repeated every 15 min to maximum of 5 mg total dose Adult: 0.5–1 mg slow IV, repeated every 15 min to maximum of 5 mg total dose
Labetalol	Hypertension	β antagonism, some α antagonism	Child: 0.2–0.5 mg/kg/dose IV, maximal dose 20 mg, followed by infusion of 0.25–1 mg/kg/hr Adult: 20 mg slow IV, may repeated every 10 min PRN *or* 2 mg/kg/min infusion titrated to effect

*These doses are based on 1 mg/mL solution.
IV, intravenously; PRN, as needed; SC, subcutaneously.

such situations may be difficult. Another therapy that may be effective is injection of terbutaline into the affected tissues. The β_2-adrenergic activity of terbutaline allows this agent to be used as a local vasodilator. In cases of inadvertent digital administration of epinephrine, terbutaline can be injected into the site of pallor in a manner similar to that described earlier.[37] Terbutaline offers the advantage of being much more readily available, and more clinicians have experience administering this agent. Terbutaline typically is available in a concentration of 1 mg/mL, and in such cases use of a dose similar to that used for bronchospasm is appropriate. In adults, an injection of 0.1 mg is an appropriate initial dose; this dose can be repeated in 15 minutes if necessary. If the epinephrine injection occurred in a fleshy area, such as the thenar eminence or pad of the distal phalanx, the dose of terbutaline can be diluted in 1 mL of normal saline to allow greater tissue distribution.

Treatment of β-Adrenergic Agonist Poisoning

Supportive care with elimination of the drug is the mainstay of treatment. Most patients with β-adrenergic agonist–mediated hypotension and tachycardia respond to intravascular volume expansion with intravenous saline. Administration of vasopressors generally is unnecessary but may be required in patients with refractory, symptomatic, vasodilatory hypotension.

Conceptually the use of a β-blocker would be the ideal therapy for hypotensive patients with β-adrenergic agonist poisoning. Although use of a β-blocker to treat hypotension may seem counterintuitive, reversal of the β_2-mediated vasodilation would be expected to cause a rise in the hypotensive patient's blood pressure. This use should be approached cautiously, however, and after other therapies have failed, particularly because there are currently no short-acting selective β_2-blockers. Patients with hemodynamically consequential tachydysrhythmias may be treated with β-blockers. In this situation, it is prudent to use a short-acting agent, such as esmolol. Although they are typically considered contraindicated in asthmatic patients, there is evidence that the judicious use of short-acting β-blockers such as esmolol may be acceptable in such patients.[38]

Treatment of clinically significant hypokalemia consists of cautious small boluses of potassium. This use must be distinguished from the higher doses used in total-body potassium repletion, however, because efflux of potassium from the extracellular compartment follows resolution of the β_2-agonist effect. Aggressive administration of potassium during the period of symptomatic hypokalemia potentially can result in hyperkalemia.

Treatment of α-Adrenergic Agonist Toxicity

General principles of normalization of vital signs within acceptable limits should be employed. Gastrointestinal decontamination can be considered for any intoxication or overdose with oral agents (see Chapter 5). Many agents are concentrated liquid preparations used parenterally, topically on mucous membranes, or as inhalational agents, so the ability to perform gastrointestinal decontamination may be limited.

Treatment of hypertension should be administered based solely on measured, not anticipative, elevations in blood pressure. This recommendation is particularly important in healthy patients whose normal blood pressures are far lower than the blood pressures used to define hypertensive urgency or emergency. A rise in mean arterial pressure of 30 mm Hg is associated with an increased risk of intracranial hemorrhage, even in asymptomatic patients.

Hypertension resulting from α_1-adrenergic stimulation can be treated with numerous drugs. The most specific therapy is phentolamine, an α_1-adrenergic antagonist. Less specific but still effective therapy more familiar to most clinicians includes direct-acting vasodilators, such as nitroprusside, nitroglycerin, or the dihydropyridine class of calcium channel blockers that includes nifedipine. Treatment of reflex bradycardia is rarely necessary and should resolve with improvement in the patient's blood pressure.

SPECIAL SITUATIONS

Several unique issues relevant to sympathomimetic toxicity warrant mention. MAO inhibitor use can result in exaggerated pressor response to indirect-acting sympathomimetics because of increased presynaptic stores of catecholamines. The concomitant use of inhalational or halogenated anesthetics can sensitize the myocardium to β-adrenergic agonism, resulting in dysrhythmia on release of endogenous or exposure to exogenous catecholamines. Patients requiring pressors after poisoning by catecholamine reuptake inhibitors, such as tricyclic antidepressants, may not respond to administration of dopamine or other indirect-acting pressors. These patients may respond, however, to a direct-acting adrenergic agonist. Similarly, patients with catecholamine depletion, such as patients who have been using large amounts of a sympathomimetic agent, may not respond to indirect-acting agents but do respond to direct-acting agents.

REFERENCES

1. Hinterberger JW, Kintzi HE: Phentolamine reversal of epinephrine-induced digital vasospasm: How to save an ischemic finger. Arch Fam Med 3:193–195, 1994.
2. Zahn KA, Li RL, Purssell RA: Cardiovascular toxicity after ingestion of "herbal ecstasy." J Emerg Med 17:289–291, 1999.
3. Gruber AJ, Pope HG Jr: Ephedrine abuse among 36 female weightlifters. Am J Addict 7:256–261, 1998.
4. Crouch DJ, Birky MM, Gust SW, et al: The prevalence of drugs and alcohol in fatally injured truck drivers. J Forensic Sci 38:1342–1353, 1993.
5. Karch SB: Coronary artery spasm induced by intravenous epinephrine overdose. Am J Emerg Med 7:485–488, 1989.
6. Saff R, Nahhas A, Fink JN: Myocardial infarction induced by coronary vasospasm after self-administration of epinephrine. Ann Allergy 70:396–398, 1993.
7. Woodard ML, Brent LD: Acute renal failure, anterior myocardial infarction, and atrial fibrillation complicating epinephrine abuse. Pharmacotherapy 18:656–658, 1998.
8. Davis CO, Wax PM: Prehospital epinephrine in a child resulting in ventricular dysrhythmias and myocardial ischemia. Pediatr Emerg Care 15:116–118, 1999.
9. Butte MJ, Nguyen BX, Hutchinson TJ, et al: Pediatric myocardial infarction after racemic epinephrine administration. Pediatrics 104:e9, 1999.
10. Tajima K, Sato S, Miyabe M: A case of pulmonary edema and bulbar paralysis after local epinephrine infiltration. J Clin Anesth 9:236–238, 1997.
11. Levine DH, Levkoff AH, Pappu LD, Purohit DM: Renal failure and other serious sequelae of epinephrine toxicity in neonates. South Med J 78:874–877, 1985.

12. Horowitz BZ, Jadallah S, Derlet RW: Fatal intracranial bleeding associated with prehospital use of epinephrine. Ann Emerg Med 28:725–727, 1996.
13. January B, Seibold A, Whaley B, et al: Beta 2-adrenergic receptor desensitization, internalization, and phosphorylation in response to full and partial agonists. J Biol Chem 272:23871–23879, 1997.
14. Conolly ME, Tashkin DP, Hui KK, et al: Selective subsenitization of beta-adrenergic receptors in central airways of asthmatics and normal subjects during long-term therapy with inhaled salbutamol. J Allergy Clin Immunol 70:423–431, 1982.
15. Hoffman BB, Lefkowitz RL, Taylor P: Neurotransmission. In Hardman JG, Limburb LE, Molinoff PB, et al (eds): Goodman and Gilman's the Pharmacologic Basis of Therapeutics, 9th ed. New York, McGraw-Hill, 1996, pp 129–130.
16. Udezue E, D'Souza L, Manajan M: Hypokalemia after normal doses of nebulized albuterol (salbutamol). Am J Emerg Med 13:168–171, 1995.
17. Wasserman D, Amitai Y: Hypoglycemia following albuterol overdose in a child. Am J Emerg Med 10:556, 1992.
18. King WD, Holloway M, Palmisano PA: Albuterol overdose: A case report and differential diagnosis. Pediatr Emerg Care 8:268–271, 1992.
19. Bodenhamer J, Bergstrom R, Brown D, et al: Frequently nebulized beta-agonists for asthma: Effects on serum electrolytes. Ann Emerg Med 21:1337–1342, 1992.
20. Craig VL, Bigos D, Brilli RJ: Efficacy and safety of continuous albuterol nebulization in children with severe status asthmaticus. Pediatr Emerg Care 12:1–5, 1996.
21. Craig TJ, Smits W, Soontornniyomiu V: Elevation of creatinine kinase from skeletal muscle with inhaled albuterol. Ann Allergy Asthma Immunol 77:488–490, 1996.
22. Sykes AP, Lawson N, Finnegan JA, Ayres JG: Creatine kinase activity in patients with brittle asthma treated with long term subcutaneous terbutaline. Thorax 46:580–583, 1991.
23. King WD, Holloway M, Palmisano PA: Albuterol overdose: A case report and differential diagnosis. Pediatr Emerg Care 8:268, 1992.
24. Wiley JF 2nd, Spiller HA, Krenzelok EP, Borys DJ: Unintentional albuterol ingestion in children. Pediatr Emerg Care 10:193–196, 1994.
25. Bloss JD, Hankins GD, Gilstrap LC 3d, Hauth JC: Pulmonary edema as a delayed complication of ritodrine therapy: A case report. J Reprod Med 32:469–471, 1987.
26. Muro M, Shono H, Oga M, et al: Ritodrine-induced agranulocytosis. Int J Gynaecol Obstet 36:329–331, 1991.
27. Wang-Cheng R, Davidson BJ: Ritodrine-induced neutropenia. Am J Obstet Gynecol 154:924–925, 1986.
28. Gupta RC, Foster S, Romano PM, Thomas HM 3d: Acute pulmonary edema associated with the use of oral ritodrine for premanture labor. Chest 95:479–481, 1989.
29. Crosby ET, Elliott RD: Anaesthesia for caesarean section in a parturient with quintuplet gestation, pulmonary oedema and thrombocytopenia. Can J Anaesth 35:417–421, 1988.
30. Fraunfelder FT, Meyer SM: Possible adverse effects from topical ocular 10% phenylephrine. Am J Ophthalmol 85:447–453, 1985.
31. Ramoska E, Sacchetti AD: Propranolol-induced hypertension in treatment of cocaine intoxication. Ann Emerg Med 14:1112–1113, 1985.
32. Pentel PR, Asinger RW, Benowitz NL: Propranolol antagonism of phenylpropanolamine-induced hypertension. Clin Pharmacol Ther 37:488–494, 1985.
33. Burkhart KK: Intravenous propranolol reverses hypertension after sympathomimetic overdose: Two case reports. J Toxicol Clin Toxicol 30:109–114, 1992.
34. Hardy SJ, Agostini DE: Accidental epinephrine auto-injector-induced digital ischemia reversed by phentolamine digital block. J Am Osteopath Assoc 95:377–378, 1995.
35. McCauley WA, Gerace RV, Scilley C: Treatment of accidental digital injection of epinephrine. Ann Emerg Med 20:665–668, 1991.
36. Maguire WM, Reisdorff EJ, Smith D, Wiegenstein JG: Epinephrine-induced vasospasm reversed by phentolamine digitial block. Am J Emerg Med 8:46–47, 1990.
37. Stier P, Bogner M, Webster K, et al: Subcutaneous terbutaline to reverse peripheral ischemia. J Toxicol Clin Toxicol 35:543, 1997.
38. Ramoska EA, Henretig F, Joffe M, Spiller HA: Propranolol treatment of albuterol poisoning in two asthmatic patients. Ann Emerg Med 22:1474–1476, 1993.

CHAPTER **42**

Cyclic Antidepressants

Kirk C. Mills

The popularity of tricyclic antidepressants (TCAs) in the treatment of major depression has decreased significantly as newer and safer antidepressants have become available (see Chapter 44). TCAs are associated with a low therapeutic index, severe cardiotoxicity in overdose, and a high incidence of adverse effects secondary to their nonspecific pharmacologic actions. TCAs are the most frequently implicated single class of prescription drugs resulting in overdose fatalities[1,2] and are responsible for more intensive care unit admissions than any other type of medication.[3] Three fourths of all TCA exposures occur in patients older than age 19 years, and 60% of all exposures are reported as intentional.[1] Only 12% of all exposures occur in children younger than 6 years old.[1] TCAs are used primarily to treat major depression, but they also are prescribed frequently for other psychiatric and medical conditions, such as chronic pain syndromes; peripheral neuropathies; nocturnal enuresis; migraine headache; selected drug withdrawal syndromes; and obsessive-compulsive, attention-deficit, panic and phobia, anxiety, and eating disorders.[4]

Currently available TCAs are listed in Table 42-1. The five most commonly reported TCAs involved in drug exposures in the United States are amitriptyline (63%), doxepin (14%), imipramine (10%), nortriptyline (10%), and desipramine (3%).[1,5] Worldwide, the order of TCA exposure is similar except that dothiepin and clomipramine are seen more commonly in overdose.[6–9] Two other cyclic antidepressants, maprotiline and amoxapine, have minor structural differences compared with traditional TCAs but have similar toxicity in overdose and are included in this chapter.

The most severe type of drug toxicity produced by TCAs is related to intentional overdose. There are seven ways, however, by which TCAs may produce mild-to-moderate clinical toxicity when administered in therapeutic doses (Table 42-2). First, the average therapeutic dose of TCAs is highly variable. Lower doses are used initially, followed by gradual increases until the desired therapeutic response is achieved, allowing for patients to become acclimated to the adverse effects. Patients started immediately at higher doses develop adverse effects more acutely. Second, toxicity can result when TCAs are combined with other medications having similar pharmacologic actions (e.g., antihistamines, antipsychotics).[10] Third, a subset of the population consists of slow metabolizers of TCAs, and these individuals

develop higher plasma TCA concentrations at any given dose.[11] Fourth, many drugs have the potential to inhibit the metabolism of TCAs, resulting in elevated TCA plasma concentrations.[11] Fifth, some TCAs are available as mixed-drug formulations combined with either benzodiazepines or antipsychotic agents, having the potential for additional drug toxicity. Sixth, patients with certain medical conditions, such as underlying cardiac problems or seizure disorders, are more susceptible to TCA toxicity at therapeutic doses.[11] Finally, TCAs have the potential to produce serotonin syndrome, especially in combination with other serotonergic medications (see Chapter 24).

BIOCHEMISTRY

TCAs have a distinct chemical structure comprising three aromatic rings: a central seven-member ring, two outer benzene rings, and an aminopropyl side chain connected to the central ring (Fig. 42-1).[4] There are only minor structural differences among the TCAs, usually on the central aromatic ring or aminopropyl side chain. Amoxapine is unique in that it has an aromatic substituent. Maprotiline has an ethylene bridge across a six-member center ring, giving it a tetracyclic chemical structure. Other chemicals that share the same basic tricyclic chemical structure as the TCAs produce similar toxicity in overdose and may trigger a false-positive TCA plasma or urine drug screen (Table 42-3).[12–15]

PHARMACOKINETICS

All TCAs share similar pharmacokinetic properties.[11] They are highly lipophilic and cross the blood-brain barrier. Peak plasma levels occur between 2 and 6 hours after ingestion at therapeutic doses. Gastrointestinal absorption may be prolonged because of their antimuscarinic effect on gut motility. Bioavailability is only 30% to 70% because of extensive first-pass hepatic metabolism. They are highly protein bound to α_1 acid glycoproteins. Their apparent volume of distribution is extremely large (range 10 to 50 L/kg). Tissue TCA levels are commonly 10 to 100 times greater than plasma levels.[11] Only 1% to 2% of the total body burden of TCAs is found in the blood.[16] These pharmacokinetic properties

TABLE 42-1 Tricyclic Antidepressants

GENERIC NAME	TRADE NAME	AVAILABLE IN U.S.	ACTIVE METABOLITE
Amitriptyline	Elavil	Yes	Nortriptyline
Amoxapine	Asendin	Yes	Hydroxyamoxapine
Clomipramine	Anafranil	Yes	Desmethylclomipramine
Desipramine	Norpramin, Pertofrane	Yes	None
Dothiepin	Prothiaden	No	Nesmethyldothiepin
Doxepin	Adapin, Sinequan	Yes	Desmethyldoxepin
Imipramine	Tofranil	Yes	Desipramine
Lofepramine	Tymelyt	No	Desipramine
Maprotiline	Ludiomil	Yes	Desmethylmaprotiline
Nortriptyline	Pamelor, Aventyl	Yes	None
Opipramol	Insidon	No	None
Protriptyline	Vivactil	Yes	None
Trimipramine	Surmontil	Yes	Desmethyltrimipramine

Pharmacokinetics of Tricyclic Antidepressants

Volume of distribution: large
Gastrointestinal absorption: rapid
Bioavailability: 30–70%
Peak blood levels: 2–6 hr after ingestion
Protein binding: highly protein bound
Half-life: ranges from 24–48 hr
Method of elimination: eliminated by hepatic metabolism using P-450 system
Active metabolites: some tricyclic antidepressants have active metabolites

explain why attempts at removing TCAs by hemodialysis, hemoperfusion, peritoneal dialysis, or forced diuresis are generally unproductive.[16]

TCAs are eliminated almost entirely by hepatic oxidation, which consists of *N*-demethylation of the amine side-chain groups and hydroxylation of ring structures (Fig. 42-2). The

TABLE 42-2 Mechanisms for Tricyclic Antidepressant Drug Toxicity at Therapeutic Doses

Combination medications containing other active ingredients (e.g., antipsychotics)
Development of serotonin syndrome
Elevated plasma concentrations of TCAs due to genetically based slow hepatic metabolism
Exacerbation of preexisting cardiovascular or CNS disease
Pharmacokinetic drug interactions with medications that inhibit hepatic metabolism
Pharmacodynamic drug interactions with medications sharing similar pharmacologic actions
Unacclimated (i.e., TCA-naive) individuals starting on high therapeutic doses

TCA, tricyclic antidepressant.

removal of a methyl group from the tertiary amine side chain usually produces an active metabolite designated by the *desmethyl-* (or *nor-*) prefix. These active metabolites often have different pharmacologic activities compared with the parent compounds. Amoxapine and maprotiline have active metabolites. Although secondary amines, such as desipramine, nortriptyline, and protriptyline, are effective antidepressants, their metabolites are generally considered inactive. Clinical toxicity from tertiary TCAs usually lasts longer than toxicity from secondary TCAs alone because of the production of active metabolites. Some TCAs undergo enterohepatic circulation before their eventual oxidation, conjugation, and renal elimination, but this does not contribute significantly to their toxicity. The average elimination half-life of TCAs is approximately 24 hours (range 6 to 36 hours) at therapeutic doses, which can increase to 72 hours after overdose. As previously noted, inhibition of TCA metabolism by other drugs that use the same hepatic enzymes can prolong the half-life of TCAs; this carries the risk of elevating TCA plasma concentrations and producing clinical TCA toxicity at therapeutic doses.

PATHOPHYSIOLOGY

TCAs are nonselective agents that exhibit a multitude of pharmacologic effects (Table 42-4). There are subtle and potentially clinically significant pharmacologic differences among the TCAs at therapeutic plasma concentrations. These differences become less important, however, at the higher plasma levels typically associated with overdose. Only a few of the pharmacologic actions of the TCAs are believed to have a direct therapeutic effect, among them inhibition of amine reuptake (norepinephrine, serotonin [5-hydroxytryptamine (HT)]) and antagonism of postsynaptic serotonin receptors (5-HT$_2$).[8,16] The remaining pharmacologic actions essentially have no therapeutic benefit but contribute significantly to TCA-related adverse effects and overdose toxicity. Most clinical findings seen in TCA overdose can be explained by the following pharmacologic actions.

Dibenzazepines

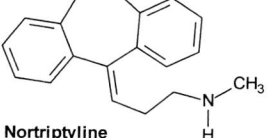

Imipramine

Desipramine

Clomipramine

Dibenzocycloheptenes

FIGURE 42-1

Chemical structures of some tricyclic antidepressants.

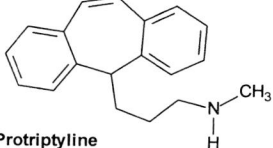

Amitriptyline

Nortriptyline

Protriptyline

Antihistaminic Effects

TCAs are potent inhibitors of peripheral and central post-synaptic histamine receptors.[8] Doxepin is a particularly potent antihistamine, but its nonspecific pharmacologic activity makes it impractical to use for treatment of seasonal allergies or other allergic conditions. Antagonism of central histamine receptors primarily leads to central nervous system (CNS) sedation and may contribute significantly to the development of coma frequently seen in TCA overdose.

Antimuscarinic Effects

TCAs frequently produce antimuscarinic effects.[8] They are competitive inhibitors of acetylcholine at central and peripheral muscarinic receptors. This action is commonly referred to by the term *anticholinergic*. *Antimuscarinic* is a more precise term, however, because TCAs do not antagonize acetylcholine at nicotinic receptors, which would produce muscle weakness or paralysis. Central antimuscarinic signs and symptoms vary from agitation to delirium, confusion, amnesia, hallucinations, slurred speech, ataxia, sedation, and coma. Peripheral antimuscarinic manifestations primarily comprise dilated pupils, blurred vision, tachycardia, hyperthermia, hypertension, decreased oral and bronchial secretions, dry skin, ileus, urinary retention, increased muscle tone, and tremor. Antimuscarinic signs and symptoms are especially common when TCAs are

TABLE 42-3 Agents That May Cause a False-Positive Tricyclic Antidepressant Qualitative Drug Screen

Carbamazepine
Cyclobenzaprine
Cyproheptadine
Dimenhydrinate
Diphenhydramine/Phenothiazines

combined with other medications that also have antimuscarinic activity. Examples of such medications include antihistamines, antipsychotics, antiparkinsonian drugs, antispasmodics, and some muscle relaxants.

Physostigmine is an inhibitor of acetylcholinesterase and can reverse antimuscarinic effects. Historically, physostigmine was used to reverse TCA-induced antimuscarinic effects, but it has been associated with life-threatening complications. Although antimuscarinic clinical manifestations are a common occurrence in TCA overdose, they are not directly responsible for TCA-related major toxicity or deaths. Antimuscarinic effects are an important clinical marker of TCA toxicity, but they do not require specific therapy other than supportive care. Physostigmine no longer is recommended in the current management of TCA overdose.[17]

Antagonism of α-Adrenergic Receptors

Inhibition of postsynaptic central and peripheral α-adrenergic receptors, but not β-adrenergic receptors, is characteristic of most TCAs.[8] TCAs have a much greater affinity for α₁-adrenergic than α₂-adrenergic receptors.[8] Inhibition of α₁-receptors results in CNS sedation, orthostatic hypotension, reflex tachycardia, and pupillary constriction. This action frequently offsets antimuscarinic-induced pupillary dilation. Patients with TCA toxicity can present with constricted, dilated, or midpoint-sized pupils.

Inhibition of Amine Reuptake

Inhibition of amine reuptake is believed to be the most important mechanism by which TCAs are efficacious in the treatment of depression. TCAs are potent inhibitors of norepinephrine and 5-HT reuptake, but they have little affinity for inhibition of dopamine reuptake.[8] Inhibition of neurotransmitter reuptake leads to an increase in synaptic concentrations and subsequent augmentation of the neurotransmitter response. Inhibition of norepinephrine reuptake is thought to produce the early sympathomimetic effects occasionally

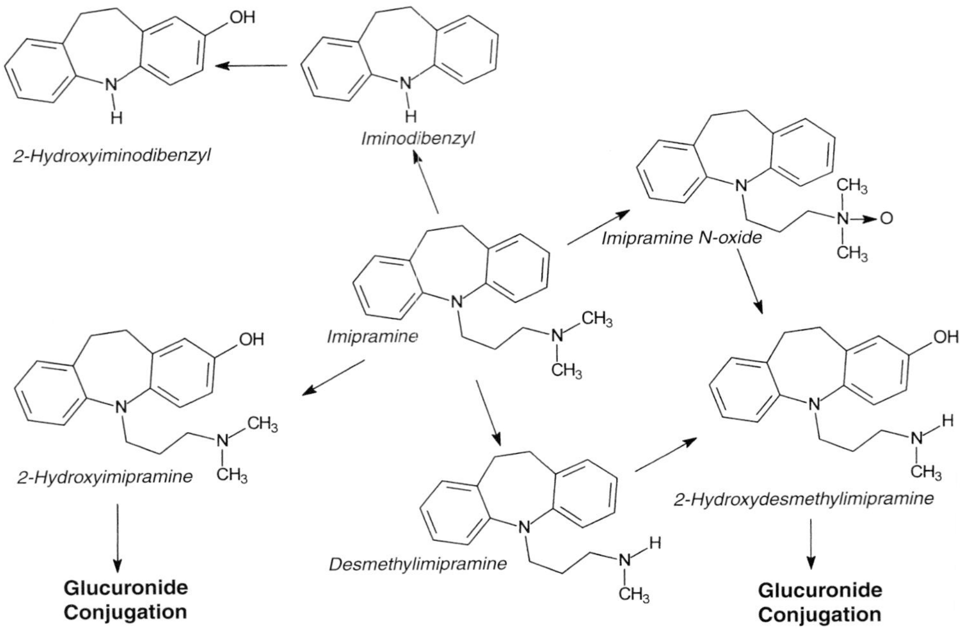

FIGURE 42-2

Structural depiction of the metabolic pathways of imipramine. These metabolic transformations are also typical of other tricyclic antidepressants.

seen in some TCA overdoses and may contribute to the development of cardiac dysrhythmias.[16] Serotonin syndrome results from increased 5-HT brainstem activity and has been produced by TCAs that are particularly potent 5-HT reuptake inhibitors, such as clomipramine and amitriptyline.[4] In general, TCAs must be used in combination with other serotonergic agents to produce serotonin syndrome. Myoclonus and hyperreflexia are often attributed to increased serotonin activity.

Sodium Channel Blockade

TCA-induced cardiotoxicity is the most important factor contributing to patient mortality.[7] Life-threatening cardiotoxicity results from TCA-induced inhibition of sodium influx through voltage-gated sodium channels. Inhibition of fast sodium channels in His-Purkinje cells leads to delayed depolarization and conduction abnormalities. Impaired sodium entry into myocardial tissue leads to decreased contractility. Sodium channel blockade, often referred to as a *membrane-stabilizing, quinidine-like*, or *local anesthetic effect*, results in a prolongation of phase 0 of the action potential. These effects become more pronounced with rapid heart rates, hyponatremia, and acidosis. Sodium channel blockade is expressed on the electrocardiogram (ECG) as prolongation of PR and QRS intervals and right-axis deviation (RAD) of the terminal 40 msec.[18] The RAD is most pronounced in the terminal 40 msec of limb leads, as shown on the ECG by a terminal R wave in lead aVR and an S wave in lead I (see Figs. 21-15, 21-16, and 21-17). Rapid influx of sodium is necessary for the release of intracellular calcium stores and subsequent myocardial contractility. Some of the negative chronotropic effects of sodium channel blockade can be attenuated by sinus tachycardia secondary to antimuscarinic activity.[18] Local changes in electrical conduction can predispose to ventricular dysrhythmias by establishing reentry loops. Severe sodium channel blockade culminates in depressed myocardial contractility, various types of heart block, hypotension, cardiac ectopy, and widening and RAD of the terminal 40 msec of the QRS complex.

Sodium channel blockade can be overcome in part by serum alkalization (pH 7.45 to 7.55) and increasing the serum sodium concentration. In humans, intravenous sodium bicarbonate ($NaHCO_3$) is thought by some to be more effective than either hyperventilation (serum alkalization) or intravenous sodium chloride in treating TCA cardiotoxicity.[19] One theoretical explanation for the postulated greater effectiveness of $NaHCO_3$ is that it produces plasma alkalization and increased serum sodium concentration.[19] The mechanism by which serum alkalization partially reverses sodium channel blockade is unknown but currently is not believed to be related to enhancement of plasma TCA serum protein binding, although it may involve reduced

---

TABLE 42-4 Pharmacologic Actions of Tricyclic Antidepressants*

Antagonism of histamine receptors
Antagonism of muscarinic receptors
Antagonism of α-adrenergic receptors
Antagonism of norepinephrine or serotonin reuptake
Antagonism of sodium channel conduction (influx)
Antagonism of potassium channel conduction (efflux)
Antagonism of GABA$_A$ receptors

---

*Listed in descending order of potency.
GABA$_A$, γ-aminobutyric acid A.

TCA binding to the sodium channel.[20] Serum alkalization is likely to result in a decrease in the overall inhibition of sodium ion influx. Animal data suggest that hypertonic saline (7.5% sodium chloride) may be as efficacious as NaHCO₃ in reversing TCA cardiotoxicity.[20] Whether this finding also would be applicable to humans is currently unknown. Hypertonic saline is believed to act primarily by increasing the extracellular sodium concentration gradient, favoring the inward movement of sodium ions.

Potassium Channel Antagonism

TCAs block myocardial potassium channels and inhibit potassium efflux during repolarization.[18] This effect is seen on the ECG as QT interval prolongation, which is more pronounced at slower heart rates.[20] Many TCA overdose patients develop sinus tachycardia, which is partially protective against severe QT_c interval prolongation. Torsades de pointes (see Chapter 21) is a life-threatening complication of severe QT interval prolongation that is seen more commonly with therapeutic doses than with TCA overdoses.[21] It is possible that the antimuscarinic-induced sinus tachycardia causes a relative narrowing of the QT interval and protection against torsades de pointes.

γ-Aminobutyric Acid A Receptor Antagonism

Generalized seizures occur in approximately 10% of TCA overdoses.[22] Possible mechanisms for these seizures include TCA-induced γ-aminobutyric acid A (GABA_A) receptor antagonism, neuronal sodium channel blockade, central anticholinergic activity, and effects on biogenic amines. Benzodiazepines and barbiturates are potent GABA_A agonists and are considered the anticonvulsants of choice in treating TCA-induced seizures.[22] Propofol (Diprivan) is a short-acting intravenous anesthetic with anticonvulsant activity. It should be considered for patients with refractory seizures, especially in the setting of hypotension.[23]

CLINICAL PRESENTATION

Therapeutic doses for TCAs are highly variable and are determined by many factors but generally range between 1 and 5 mg/kg/day. Doses greater than this have the potential to produce clinical toxicity, although some patients tolerate higher doses without adverse effects. Life-threatening toxicity usually occurs with ingestions of greater than 10 mg/kg in adults.[24] Some patients are at greater risk for TCA-related toxicity, including patients who have coingested cardiotoxic or CNS-depressive medications, geriatric patients, pediatric patients, and patients with heart disease. TCA-related fatalities commonly are associated with ingestions of greater than 1 g.[24] Most TCA overdose fatalities occur within the initial hours after ingestion, often before the patient reaches the hospital.[25] Fatalities are unusual for patients who are alive when they arrive at the hospital and receive appropriate care.[3] The mortality rate for hospitalized TCA overdose patients is approximately 2%.[3,26] The amount of TCA ingested in most overdose cases is unknown. The diagnosis of TCA

toxicity should be suspected from a history of TCA ingestion, clinical presentation consistent with TCA toxicity, characteristic ECG abnormalities, or positive plasma TCA drug screen.

Qualitative urine or plasma TCA drug screens have a low false-positive rate. This aspect makes them extremely helpful in confirming the presence of TCAs; their low cost and rapid turnaround time also are beneficial. Positive qualitative screens do not differentiate between therapeutic and toxic levels, however. Also, false-positive results have been reported with medications that structurally resemble TCAs (see Table 42-3).[12–15]

In contrast, quantitative determinations of plasma concentrations are specific for individual TCAs, with false-positive rates of essentially zero; however, these tests are costly and time-consuming. Quantitative assays allow for a certain degree of differentiation between therapeutic and toxic levels, but their greatest utility is in the monitoring of long-term drug therapy (e.g., compliance, metabolism). Quantitative levels have limited application to acute overdose patients.[27,28] The results of quantitative assays are rarely available at the time of patient evaluation and during initial treatment and have a negligible impact on patient care.

Some studies have shown that patients with a combined plasma concentration of parent TCA and metabolite of greater than 1000 ng/mL are at greater risk for developing seizures and cardiotoxicity.[27,28] The severity of clinical toxicity does not always correlate, however, with the extent of plasma TCA elevation. Patients can develop severe toxicity at plasma levels less than 1000 ng/mL.[27,28] Conversely, patients with plasma TCA concentrations much greater than 1000 ng/mL may not develop seizures or ventricular dysrhythmias.[27] Serious toxicity rarely develops at therapeutic concentrations (<300 ng/mL). For patients with plasma concentrations in this range, other causes should be considered to explain the patient's condition. As always, the primary focus should be on treating the patient, not the drug concentrations.

A confounding characteristic of TCAs is their ability to undergo significant postmortem drug redistribution.[29,30] Plasma concentrations can increase by 10-fold to 50-fold after death as tissue binding sites release TCAs, with resultant back diffusion into the blood as a time-dependent process. Theoretically, the accuracy of postmortem TCA levels as a reflection of immediate antemortem levels is related inversely to the time interval between death and subsequent specimen collection. Elevated TCA concentrations that are obtained long after death may be assigned inappropriately as the cause of death, when they simply reflect therapeutic body burdens that have undergone redistribution. Unless this possibility is recognized, it may raise false concerns about the care provided to the patient during his or her hospitalization or a misassignment of the cause of death to drug toxicity or overdose.

Clinical Manifestations of Acute Overdose

Signs and symptoms typically develop within the first few hours after ingestion.[31] The clinical presentation of TCA toxicity varies tremendously from mild antimuscarinic symptoms to coma and severe cardiotoxicity. Another consideration is that TCA ingestions often involve coingestion of other drugs, which can produce additional toxicity. Patients who do not manifest major toxicity (Table 42-5) by 6 hours postingestion are considered at low risk for life-threatening complications. The most frequently reported effects are CNS sedation and sinus tachycardia. Along with other antimuscarinic effects these effects serve as clinical markers of TCA toxicity, but alone they are rarely responsible for fatalities. Antimuscarinic symptoms are not uniformly present in TCA toxicity.[24] Antimuscarinic syndrome classically is associated with diminished bowel sounds and ileus. Gut function is fairly resistant to this effect, however, and active bowel sounds can be present even in seriously ill patients. The presence of normal bowel sounds does not rule out the possibility of antimuscarinic syndrome.

Mild-to-moderate TCA toxicity may present as drowsiness, confusion, slurred speech, ataxia, dry mucous membranes and axillae, sinus tachycardia, urinary retention, myoclonus, and hyperreflexia. CNS depression is often associated with respiratory depression leading to hypoxia or aspiration or both. Many TCA overdose patients require endotracheal intubation to manage their respiratory depression and loss of airway protection. Mild hypertension is observed occasionally and rarely requires treatment. Nontolerant individuals (e.g., young children) frequently develop coma and respiratory depression after relatively small overdoses without obvious peripheral antimuscarinic effects and without QRS widening.[32] Overflow urinary incontinence may be mistaken for normal micturition in pediatric (diaper-dependent) patients.

Serious toxicity almost always is seen within 6 hours of major TCA ingestion and consists of coma, cardiac conduction delays, wide-complex supraventricular tachycardia, hypotension, respiratory depression, premature ventricular beats, ventricular tachycardia, and seizures.[5,24,26,31,32] Secondary complications from serious toxicity include aspiration pneumonia, anoxic encephalopathy, hyperthermia, and rhabdomyolysis.[24] Pulmonary edema is a well-recognized complication of TCA overdose.[33] Seizures usually are generalized and brief and occur in roughly 10% of patients.[22] The risk of seizures increases as the QRS complex exceeds 100 msec. The exception to this rule is seen in amoxapine and maprotiline overdoses, which have been reported to cause status epilepticus.[7] Amoxapine-induced seizures commonly occur without corresponding QRS widening.[7]

ECG abnormalities are seen commonly with TCA toxicity and generally are useful in identifying patients at increased risk for seizures and ventricular dysrhythmias.[34] The "classic" TCA ECG, shown in Figures 21-15, 21-16, and 21-17, consists of sinus tachycardia; RAD of the terminal 40 msec (best seen as a terminal R wave in lead aVR); and prolongation of the PR, QRS, and QT intervals (Table 42-6). This classic ECG pattern is seen frequently in moderate-to-severe TCA toxicity,[34] but its absence does not eliminate the possibility of TCA toxicity during the first 6 hours after ingestion.[27,28] Moderate prolongation of the QT interval is noted frequently, even at therapeutic TCA doses. Nonspecific ST-segment and T-wave abnormalities are observed commonly in TCA overdose. Less commonly reported ECG abnormalities include right bundle-branch block and high-degree atrioventricular blocks.[34] These reports probably reflect the ECG similarities between TCA effects and right bundle-branch block.[35]

Life-threatening complications can occur in the absence of significant ECG abnormalities.[28] These complications are more likely, however, in the presence of a QRS interval greater than 100 msec or RAD of the terminal 40 msec greater than 120 degrees.[27,28,34] Ventricular dysrhythmias are more likely if QRS prolongation exceeds 160 msec. Widening of the QRS complex and positive deflection of the terminal QRS complex in lead aVR are equally helpful in identifying patients at risk for serious toxicity.[34] They usually occur together but may occur in the absence of each other. The development of RAD of the terminal 40 msec or QRS widening seems to be less predictive of TCA-induced cardiotoxicity in young children.[34] Pediatric ECGs tend to have a wider range of acceptable variant features, and this complicates the ECG identification of TCA toxicity.[34]

ECG abnormalities, if they are to occur, universally develop within 6 hours of ingestion and typically resolve over 24 to 48 hours.[36] The identification of either QRS widening greater than 100 msec or terminal RAD greater than 120 degrees warrants mechanical ventilation–induced respiratory alkalosis or $NaHCO_3$ therapy and admission to a monitored hospital bed.[30] A subset of the normal population has a QRS of more than 100 msec or terminal RAD, however, without exposure to sodium channel–blocking drugs; this includes individuals with right bundle-branch block. These ECG abnormalities in isolation are not specific for TCA toxicity. Many patients receiving TCA therapy do not have prior ECGs available for comparison. Any observed ECG abnormalities initially must be assumed attributable to TCA exposure until proven otherwise.

TABLE 42-5 Major Toxicity Criteria

Altered mental status
Cardiac dysrhythmias or conduction defects
Hypotension
Respiratory depression
Right-axis deviation of the terminal 40 msec of QRS in limb leads
Seizures
Widened QRS complex >100 msec

TABLE 42-6 Classic Electrocardiographic Abnormalities in Tricyclic Antidepressant Toxicity

Sinus tachycardia
Prolonged PR interval
Prolonged QT interval
Widened QRS complex >100 msec
Right-axis deviation (positive deflection) of terminal QRS complex in lead aVR >3 mm

DIAGNOSIS

TCA toxicity should be suspected in all patients with a positive serum or urine TCA drug screen in conjunction with corresponding clinical toxicity or characteristic ECG abnormalities or both (see Table 42-6). The differential diagnosis of TCA toxicity encompasses drugs that can mimic any one of the three criteria used in making the diagnosis. False-negative serum TCA drug tests are extremely unusual. They should be repeated with a new specimen if there is a high clinical suspicion of TCA exposure. The quintessential point, however, is that treatment should not be delayed while awaiting drug test results. A rapid screen for TCA toxicity is the ECG because most TCA-poisoned patients manifest major toxicity within 2 hours of ingestion or not at all. The combination of characteristic ECG changes and typical manifestations of toxicity is a sensitive and a specific approach to the diagnosis of poisoning by these agents.

TREATMENT

All patients should be evaluated immediately for alterations of consciousness, hemodynamic instability, and respiratory impairment. Every patient requires prompt placement of an intravenous line, continuous cardiac monitoring, and a 12-lead ECG. Serial ECGs may be required in patients manifesting any signs of toxicity. Suggested laboratory studies include determinations of serum electrolyte, creatinine, and glucose concentrations. A quantitative serum acetaminophen level is recommended in all overdose patients. Patients with antimuscarinic symptoms may require a urinary catheter to prevent urinary retention and a nasogastric tube if bowel sounds are absent. Patients who are initially asymptomatic may deteriorate rapidly and should be monitored closely for several hours.[21,22]

Gastrointestinal Decontamination. Although the best method of gastrointestinal decontamination in TCA ingestions is undefined, a few generalizations are supported by available evidence.[37] The risks associated with using ipecac syrup outweigh any beneficial effects, and its use cannot be recommended. Activated charcoal has been shown to bind TCAs effectively and reduce their absorption. All presenting patients who have ingested a TCA within the previous few hours should receive 1 g/kg of activated charcoal. Care should be taken, however, to ensure that the airway is adequately protected before activated charcoal administration. If activated charcoal is given, it should be administered as a single dose.

Common practice is to give activated charcoal, possibly in association with gastric lavage, to patients who present relatively early after intentional TCA ingestions. Whether gastric lavage in combination with activated charcoal is of greater clinical benefit than activated charcoal alone or no gastrointestinal decontamination is unproven. Gastric lavage is most likely to be effective when it is performed within the first hour after ingestion.[37]

Serum Alkalization and Sodium Bicarbonate Therapy. As described earlier, a theoretical rationale and empirical data support serum alkalization and the administration of sodium. This treatment can be achieved either by ventilator-driven hyperventilation with intravenous saline or by the administration of $NaHCO_3$. Although both approaches have their proponents, they have not been subjected to clinical comparison. The pros and cons of these two therapies are discussed in detail in Chapter 21.

Indications for ventilator-driven serum alkalization/saline or $NaHCO_3$ therapy include QRS complex widening greater than 100 msec and ventricular dysrhythmias (Table 42-7).[16,17,19] Intravenous $NaHCO_3$ and an increase in serum pH have been shown to improve conduction, increase contractility, and suppress ventricular ectopy.[19] If $NaHCO_3$ infusion is selected, it is given as an initial bolus of 1 to 2 mEq/kg, which can be repeated until clinical or ECG improvement is noted or until blood pH is between 7.50 and 7.55. Alkalization beyond this point can be deleterious and is discouraged. Continuous infusions of $NaHCO_3$ usually are administered as 3 ampules (50 mEq/50 mL) placed in 1 L of 5% dextrose in water or 2 ampules added to 5% dextrose/0.45 normal saline (slightly hypertonic with $NaHCO_3$ added) solution and infused initially at a rate of 2 to 3 mL/kg/hr. Adjustments in the intravenous rate are made based on blood pH measurements, serum sodium level, and clinical response to therapy. Because of the potential for cardiogenic and noncardiogenic pulmonary edema in TCA-toxic patients, it is important to reduce the rate of fluid administration when the patient is stabilized. Hypokalemia is an expected complication of $NaHCO_3$ therapy. Intravenous potassium supplementation usually is required, and serum potassium levels should be measured frequently. Induced hyperventilation, if that option is chosen, is accomplished by inducing a respiratory alkalosis, with the targeted end point being a pH range similar to that described earlier.

Altered Level of Consciousness

Patients with altered level of consciousness require a trial of intravenous dextrose, thiamine, naloxone, and oxygen to rule out reversible causes of CNS depression. Antagonism of postsynaptic muscarinic, histaminic, and α-adrenergic receptors may contribute to the development of altered mentation in TCA overdoses. It is possible that other direct CNS effects unrelated to these mechanisms may occur. Coma from TCA toxicity typically is of rapid onset. Unresponsive patients may have unrecognized head or neck trauma. Flumazenil should not be given to patients suspected of TCA overdose because this may precipitate generalized seizures.[38] Agitation may be

---

TABLE 42-7 Indications for Serum Alkalization in Tricyclic Antidepressant Toxicity*

Terminal right-axis deviation (positive deflection) in lead aVR >3 mm
Ventricular dysrhythmias
Widened QRS complex >100 msec

---

*With induced hyperventilation or sodium bicarbonate administration. See text for details.

observed before the onset of coma and in previously comatose patients as they awaken. Agitation is best controlled with reassurance, decreased environmental stimulation, and benzodiazepines. As mentioned previously, physostigmine probably is best avoided in TCA-toxic patients.

Seizures

Most seizures occur within the first 2 hours after TCA ingestion. Typically, but not always, these seizures are generalized, are brief, and commonly do not require anticonvulsant therapy.[22] Multiple seizures are reported in less than 10% of TCA overdoses.[17,22] Focal seizures are atypical and require further neurologic evaluation. Seizures are more common with maprotiline and amoxapine ingestions and require aggressive management because status epilepticus is associated more frequently with these two particular antidepressants.[23] Benzodiazepines (e.g., diazepam, lorazepam) are the anticonvulsants of choice for ongoing seizure activity.[22] Barbiturates (e.g., phenobarbital) are indicated in the treatment of recurrent seizures or seizures resistant to benzodiazepine therapy. The initial intravenous dose of phenobarbital is 15 mg/kg given in 5-mg/kg increments, but this can be increased safely in patients with continued seizure activity who are not hemodynamically compromised. Because of the potential for inducing hypotension, the initial phenobarbital loading dose should be given in 5-mg/kg increments. Propofol also may be employed as second-line or third-line anticonvulsant therapy, but there is limited clinical experience with this approach. If not already employed for TCA-induced respiratory failure, endotracheal intubation and respiratory support are required when benzodiazepines are combined with barbiturates or propofol or when high doses of either of the latter are used.[23]

If seizures continue despite adequate dosing with benzodiazepines, phenobarbital, and possibly propofol, consideration should be given to paralyzing the patient with a neuromuscular blocking agent. This paralysis stops the physical manifestations of the seizure and its secondary effects, which include metabolic acidosis, hyperthermia, rhabdomyolysis, and renal failure. It does not stop brain seizure activity, however. After induction of muscle paralysis, these patients require electroencephalographic monitoring and further anticonvulsant therapy. (Toxicant-induced seizures are discussed in detail in Chapter 20.)

Hypotension

Hypotension should be treated initially with isotonic crystalloid in increments of 10 mL/kg. In the setting of impaired cardiac contractility, pulmonary edema may develop if excessive fluids or NaHCO$_3$ is administered. Vasopressors should be used when hypotension is unresponsive to fluid therapy. Norepinephrine is believed to be the vasopressor of choice in the setting of TCA-induced α-adrenergic blockade, but dopamine and epinephrine also have been shown to be effective.[36,39,40] A pulmonary artery catheter should be placed in patients whose hypotension is refractory to fluid volume replacement and vasopressor therapy; this should be done cautiously, however, because mechanical irritation of the heart during pulmonary artery catheter placement may precipitate life-threatening conduction abnormalities and ventricular dysrhythmias. Severe TCA-induced hypotension represents a potentially reversible cause of cardiovascular collapse. Mechanical support of the circulation with cardiopulmonary bypass, overdrive pacing, or aortic balloon pump assistance may be warranted in patients with refractory hypotension, although no studies adequately document their effectiveness.[41,42]

Dysrhythmias

TCAs frequently alter cardiac rate, conduction, and contractility. Otherwise asymptomatic patients with sinus tachycardia, isolated PR and QT prolongation, or first-degree atrioventricular block do not require specific pharmacologic therapy. Conduction blocks greater than first-degree blocks can progress rapidly to complete heart block secondary to impaired infranodal conduction. Patients with isolated QRS duration greater than 100 msec may benefit from treatment with serum alkalization and NaHCO$_3$ therapy replacement, although this is controversial.[19] This recommendation is made despite the absence of randomized, controlled human trials showing NaHCO$_3$ therapy–related benefits in otherwise asymptomatic patients with QRS prolongation.[19] Nonetheless, the early use of serum alkalization with NaHCO$_3$ or induced hyperventilation in the setting of sodium channel blockade has become a common practice for treating QRS widening.[16]

Ventricular dysrhythmias should be treated immediately with NaHCO$_3$ bolus administration.[16] Lidocaine is the second agent of choice in treating ventricular dysrhythmias,[16] although excessive lidocaine administration is capable of producing seizures. Bretylium generally is considered a third-line drug for ventricular dysrhythmias. Synchronized cardioversion is appropriate in patients with unstable dysrhythmias. Torsades de pointes should be treated initially with at least 2 g of intravenous magnesium sulfate. Efforts should be made to rule out other causes of torsades de pointes. Overdrive pacing frequently is required to prevent recurrence of this dysrhythmia. Intravenous isoproterenol may be beneficial in treating recurrent torsades de pointes when overdrive pacing is not available. Treatment of torsades de pointes is discussed in Chapter 21. The medications in Table 42-8 should be considered contraindicated in the treatment of torsades de pointes–induced dysrhythmias.

TABLE 42-8 Medications Contraindicated in Tricyclic Antidepressant Overdose

Class Ia antidysrhythmics
Class Ic antidysrhythmics
Class III antidysrhythmics
β-Blockers
Calcium channel blockers
Flumazenil
Physostigmine

DISPOSITION

Patients who remain asymptomatic for at least 6 hours after ingestion do not require hospital admission for toxicologic reasons. They still may require hospital admission because of coexisting medical or psychiatric conditions. Psychiatric evaluation is warranted for intentional drug ingestions. All symptomatic patients require hospital admission to a monitored bed. Patients showing signs of moderate-to-severe toxicity should be admitted to an intensive care unit.

Indications for Emergency Department or ICU Admission in Cyclic Antidepressant Poisoning

All patients with evidence of moderate-to-severe TCA toxicity require ICU admission.
Patients with mild toxicity can be admitted to a monitored bed.

Criteria for Emergency Department or ICU Discharge in Cyclic Antidepressant Poisoning

Appropriate gastrointestinal decontamination completed if the patient presented within the first 1 to 2 hours of ingestion
No clinical manifestation of toxicity after at least 6 hours of observation, including normal vital signs
Normal or baseline electrocardiogram after 6 hours of observation
Psychiatric evaluation completed in cases of intentional overdose
Nontoxic serum acetaminophen concentration (intentional overdoses)
Neurologic and pulmonary stability
Absence of antimuscarinic signs

REFERENCES

1. Litovitz TL, Klein-Schwartz W, Rodgers GC, et al: 2001 Annual report of the American Association of Poison Control Centers Toxic Exposure Surveillance System. Am J Emerg Med 20:391–401, 2002.
2. Coleridge J, Cameron PA, Drummer OH, et al: Survey of drug-related deaths in Victoria. Med J Aust 157:459–461, 1992.
3. Henderson A, Wright M, Pond SM: Experience with 732 acute overdose patients admitted to an intensive care unit over six years. Med J Aust 158:28–30, 1993.
4. Braithwaite RA: The tricyclic antidepressants. Contemp Issues Clin Biochem 3:211–239, 1985.
5. Foulke GE: Identifying toxicity risk early after antidepressant overdose. Am J Emerg Med 13:123–126, 1995.
6. Battersby MW, O'Mahoney JJ, Beckwith AR, et al: Antidepressant deaths by overdose. Aust N Z J Psychiatry 30:223–228, 1996.
7. Cassidy S, Henry J: Fatal toxicity of antidepressant drugs in overdose. BMJ 295:1021–1024, 1987.
8. Buckley NA, McManus PR: Can the fatal toxicity of antidepressant drugs be predicted with pharmacological and toxicological data? Drug Saf 18:369–381, 1998.
9. Mason J, Freemantle N, Eccles M: Fatal toxicity associated with antidepressant use in primary care. Br J Gen Pract 50:366–370, 2000.
10. Jarvis MR: Clinical pharmacokinetics of tricyclic antidepressant overdose. Psychopharmacol Bull 27:541–550, 1991.
11. Preskorn SH: Pharmacokinetics of antidepressants: Why and how they are relevant to treatment. J Clin Psychiatry 54:14–34, 1993.
12. Spiller HA, Winter ML, Mann KV, et al: Five-year multicenter retrospective review of cyclobenzaprine. J Emerg Med 13:781–785, 1995.
13. Fleischman A, Chaing VW: Carbamazepine overdose recognized by a tricyclic antidepressant assay. Pediatrics 107:176–177, 2001.
14. Yuan CM, Spanorfer PR, Miller SC, et al: Evaluation of tricyclic antidepressant false positivity in a pediatric case of cyproheptadine overdose. Ther Drug Monit 25:299–304, 2003.
15. Matos ME, Burns MM, Shannon MW: False positive tricyclic antidepressant drug screen leading to the diagnosis of CBZ intoxication. Pediatrics 105:E66, 2000.
16. Glauser J: Tricyclic antidepressant poisoning. Cleve Clin J Med 67:704–719, 2000.
17. Newton EH, Shih RD, Hoffman RS: Cyclic antidepressant overdose: A review of current management strategies. Am J Emerg Med 12:376–379, 1994.
18. Kolecki PF, Curry SC: Poisoning by sodium channel blocking agents. Med Toxicol 13:829–845, 1997.
19. Hoffman JR, Votey SR, Bayer MB, et al: Effect of hypertonic sodium bicarbonate in the treatment of moderate-to-severe cyclic antidepressant overdose. Am J Emerg Med 11:336–341, 1993.
20. McCabe JL, Cobaugh DJ, Menegazzi JJ, et al: Experimental tricyclic antidepressant toxicity: A randomized, controlled comparison of hypertonic saline solution, sodium bicarbonate, and hyperventilation. Ann Emerg Med 32:329–333, 1998.
21. Phillips S, Brent J, Kulig K, et al: Fluoxetine versus tricyclic antidepressants: A perspective multicenter study of antidepressant drug overdoses. J Emerg Med 15:439–445, 1997.
22. Ellison DW, Pentel PR: Clinical features and consequences of seizures due to cyclic antidepressant overdose. Am J Emerg Med 7:5–10, 1989.
23. Merigian KS, Browning RG, Leeper KV: Successful treatment of amoxapine-induced refractory status epilepticus with propofol (Diprovan). Acad Emerg Med 2:128–133, 1995.
24. Crome P: Poisoning due to tricyclic antidepressant overdosage: Clinical presentation and treatment. Med Toxicol 1:261–285, 1985.
25. Bolster M, Curran J, Busuttil A: A five year review of fatal self-ingested overdoses involving amitriptyline in Edinburgh, 1983–87. Hum Exp Toxicol 13:29–31, 1994.
26. Foulke GE, Albertson TE, Walby WF: Tricyclic antidepressant overdose: Emergency department findings as predictors of clinical course. Am J Emerg Med 4:496–500, 1986.
27. Caravati EM, Bossart PJ: Demographic and electrocardiographic factors associated with severe tricyclic antidepressant toxicity. Clin Toxicol 29:31–34, 1991.
28. Hulten BA, Adams, R, Askenasi R, et al: Predicting severity of tricyclic antidepressant overdose. Clin Toxicol 30:161–170, 1992.
29. Pounder DJ, Owen V, Quigley C: Postmortem changes in blood amitriptyline concentration. Am J Forensic Med Pathol 15:224–230, 1994.
30. Hilberg T, Bugge A, Beylich KM, et al: An animal model of postmortem amitriptyline redistribution. J Forensic Sci 38:81–90, 1993.
31. Tokarski GF, Young MJ: Criteria for admitting patients with tricyclic antidepressant overdose. J Emerg Med 6:121–124, 1988.
32. Shannon M, Merola J, Lovejoy FH: Hypotension in severe tricyclic antidepressant overdose. Am J Emerg Med 6:439–441, 1988.
33. Flaherty JJ, Cerva D, Graff J: ARDS associated with massive imipramine overdose. Am J Emerg Med 4:195–196, 1986.
34. Liebelt EL, Francis PD, Woolf AD: ECG lead aVR versus QRS interval in predicting seizures and arrhythmias in acute tricyclic antidepressant toxicity. Ann Emerg Med 26:195–201, 1995.
35. Niemann JT, Bessen HA, Rothstein RJ, et al: Electrocardiographic criteria for tricyclic antidepressant cardiotoxicity. Am J Cardiol 57:1154–1159, 1986.
36. Vernon DD, Banner W, Garrett JS, et al: Efficacy of dopamine and norepinephrine for treatment of hemodynamic compromise in amitriptyline intoxication. Crit Care Med 19:544–549, 1991.
37. Bosse GM, Barefoot JA, Pfeifer MP, et al: Comparison of three methods of gut decontamination in tricyclic antidepressant overdose. J Emerg Med 13:203–209, 1995.
38. Mordel A, Winkler E, Almog S, et al: Seizures after flumazenil administration in a case of combined benzodiazepine and tricyclic antidepressant overdose. Crit Care Med 20:1733–1734, 1992.

39. Teba L, Schiebel F, Dedhia H, et al: Beneficial effect of norepinephrine in the treatment of circulatory shock caused by tricyclic antidepressant overdose. Am J Emerg Med 6:266–268, 1988.

40. Tran TP, Panacek EA, Rhee KJ, et al: Response to dopamine vs norepinephrine in tricyclic antidepressant-induced hypotension. Acad Emerg Med 4:864–868, 1997.

41. Williams JM, Hollingshed MJ, Vasilakis A, et al: Extracorporeal circulation in the management of severe tricyclic antidepressant overdose. Am J Emerg Med 12:456–458, 1994.

42. Goodwin DA, Lally KP, Null DM: Extracorporeal membrane oxygenation support for cardiac dysfunction from tricyclic antidepressant overdose. Crit Care Med 21:625–627, 1993.

CHAPTER 43

Monoamine Oxidase Inhibitors

Kirk C. Mills

Monoamine oxidase (MAO) inhibitors were the first effective agents in the treatment of major depression and have been in clinical use since the 1960s. Their use has been supplanted more recently, however, by newer antidepressants that have fewer serious adverse effects and are less hazardous in overdose. Despite their waning popularity, MAO inhibitors still are problematic because of their complex pharmacology and potential for fatality when taken in overdose. This chapter focuses on the traditional nonselective and irreversible MAO inhibitors, which are associated with a low therapeutic index and the potential for food (e.g., tyramine reaction) and drug (e.g., serotonin syndrome) interactions and manifest severe toxicity in overdose. There have been some major advances in developing less toxic MAO inhibitors, which are reversible and selective in their MAO activity (Table 43-1). These agents are discussed separately in this chapter because their toxicity seems to be less severe than that of irreversible MAO inhibitors. The MAO inhibitors used as antidepressants in the United States include phenelzine (Nardil), tranylcypromine (Parnate), and isocarboxazid (Marplan). In 2002, there were slightly more than 200,000 prescriptions filled for MAO inhibitors in the United States (personal communications with manufacturers), with phenelzine representing 55%, tranylcypromine representing 40%, and isocarboxazid representing 5% of these prescriptions.

Monoamine Oxidase Inhibitors Available in the United States

Isocarboxazid (Marplan)—used as an antidepressant
Phenelzine (Nardil)—used as an antidepressant
Selegiline (Eldepryl)—used to treat Parkinson's disease
Tranylcypromine (Parnate)—used as an antidepressant

For the period from 1989 to 2000, the American Association of Poison Control Centers Toxic Exposure Surveillance System recorded 6076 total exposures to MAO inhibitors with 58 fatalities.[1,2] Of these exposures, 75% occurred in adults, 40% were intentional ingestions, and 80% of patients developed symptoms.[2] On average, one death resulted from every 100 exposures to MAO inhibitors. In contrast, trazodone (an atypical antidepressant) averages one death for every 1200 drug exposures.[1] This striking difference in mortality between MAO inhibitors and newer antidepressants underscores the greater toxicity of MAO inhibitors. The mortality rate from MAO inhibitor overdose is one of the highest among all pharmaceutical agents. In one case series consisting of 12 MAO inhibitor overdose cases, the mortality rate was 33%. The true mortality rate from MAO inhibitor overdose is unknown because only isolated case reports and a few case series exist in the literature. These reports undoubtedly create reporting bias toward the more severe cases.

MAO inhibitors are used primarily to treat cases of atypical or refractory depression, but they also have produced positive responses in many other conditions, such as social phobia disorders, panic disorders, posttraumatic stress syndrome, obsessive-compulsive disorder, bulimia, and narcolepsy.[4] MAO inhibitors should be avoided during pregnancy. In the United States, they are not approved for use in children younger than 16 years of age.

Selegiline (Eldepryl) is an MAO inhibitor that is devoid of antidepressant activity but is used as an adjunct in the treatment of Parkinson's disease.[5] At higher doses, selegiline resembles the activity of traditional MAO inhibitor antidepressants.[5] Some drugs have been discovered to have MAO inhibitor activity as an unrelated pharmacologic action. Examples include procarbazine (Matulane), a chemotherapeutic agent for severe Hodgkin's lymphoma, and furazolidone (Furoxone), a synthetic nitrofuran with antimicrobial and antiprotozoan activity. Pargyline (Eutonyl) use has been discontinued since the 1990s in many parts of the world; this was an antihypertensive agent whose primary mechanism of action was MAO inhibition. St. John's wort (*Hypericum perforatum*) is a popular over-the-counter herbal treatment for depression and has been reported to show slight MAO inhibitor activity.[6] St. John's wort seems to function more like a nonselective neurotransmitter reuptake inhibitor, however, than like an MAO inhibitor.[6] Most patients taking St. John's wort do not consider it a drug and often omit the herbal product when being asked about medications. Harmaline alkaloids found in the plant *Peganum harmala* inhibit MAO activity but have limited popularity.[7,8]

BIOCHEMISTRY, PATHOPHYSIOLOGY, AND CLINICAL PHARMACOLOGY

MAO is an intracellular enzyme bound to the outer mitochondrial membrane. It can be found in most human cells, with the exception of erythrocytes, which lack mitochondria.

TABLE 43-1 Monoamine Oxidase Inhibitors

GENERIC NAME	TRADE NAME	AVAILABLE IN UNITED STATES	INHIBITS MAO-A	INHIBITS MAO-B	IRREVERSIBLE	REVERSIBLE
Brofaromine			X			X
Cimoxatone			X			X
Clorgyline			X		X	
Isocarboxazid	Marplan	X	X	X	X	
Moclobemide	Aurorix, Manerix		X			X
Pargyline	Eutonyl			X	X	
Phenelzine	Nardil	X	X	X	X	
Selegiline	Eldepryl	X		X	X	
Toloxatone			X			X
Tranylcypromine	Parnate	X	X	X	X	

*Data from references 7, 8, and 9.

MAO removes amine groups from endogenous and exogenous biogenic amines. This oxidative deamination process is the primary mechanism by which endogenous biogenic amines, such as norepinephrine, dopamine, and 5-hydroxytryptamine (serotonin),[9] become inactivated. An equally important function of MAO is the reduction in systemic bioavailability of absorbed dietary biogenic amines, such as tyramine, via hepatic and intestinal metabolism. Inhibition of MAO leads to the accumulation of neurotransmitters in central and peripheral presynaptic nerve terminals and allows for increased systemic availability of dietary amines.[9] MAO does not metabolize circulating catecholamines, which either are secreted endogenously (e.g., adrenal gland, sympathetic nerve terminals) or are administered intravenously (e.g., epinephrine). This metabolism is accomplished by catechol O-methyltransferase, an extraneuronally located enzyme that is not affected by MAO inhibitors.[9]

MAO is two separate isoenzymes, designated *MAO-A* and *MAO-B*. Each isoenzyme has a unique affinity profile for different neurotransmitters, dietary amines, and MAO inhibitors.[7–9] These substrate preferences are dose dependent, however, and become less relevant at higher substrate concentrations or MAO inhibitor doses. Norepinephrine and serotonin are metabolized primarily by MAO-A, whereas MAO-A and MAO-B have equal ability to metabolize dopamine and tyramine.[7–9] MAO-B is the exclusive isoenzyme found in serotoninergic neurons.[6] This paradox may be explained by simple conservation of energy, in which the MAO-B isoenzyme has a lower affinity for 5-HT and allows for more 5-HT to become recycled. It also allows for increased metabolism of nonserotonin bioamines, keeping the neuron free of false neurotransmitters.

The human brain contains more MAO-B than MAO-A, with MAO-B predominance increasing with advancing age. Dopamine neurons seem to lack MAO-B activity and have limited MAO-A activity.[7,9] Significant MAO-B activity has been detected in surrounding astrocytes and glial cells. Dopamine inactivation may depend on astrocyte and glial cell metabolism.[7,9] MAO-A constitutes approximately 75% of the MAO activity in the intestine, whereas approximately equal proportions of both isoenzymes are found in the liver. When only one isoenzyme is inhibited, such as in the presence of moclobemide, which selectively inhibits MAO-A, this dual representation of both isoenzymes in the intestines and liver affords greater protection against the hypertensive reaction to tyramine-containing foods. Similarities in chemical structure between MAO inhibitors and endogenous amines, such as norepinephrine, serotonin, and dopamine, make them eligible as potential substrates for MAO and cause inhibition of amine metabolism (Fig. 43-1).[8] The antidepressant activity of phenelzine, tranylcypromine, and isocarboxazid generally is attributed to their ability to increase norepinephrine and serotonin neurotransmission by increasing presynaptic concentrations of serotonin and norepinephrine.[7] The actual mechanism by which they exert their therapeutic action is unproven but more likely is related to delayed postsynaptic receptor modifications (e.g., downregulation). Other potential mechanisms of action include indirect release of neurotransmitters and inhibition of neurotransmitter reuptake. MAO inhibitors also inhibit other enzyme systems (e.g., pyridoxal phosphokinase, diamine oxidase), but this is of uncertain clinical significance. Selegiline has limited effects on norepinephrine and serotonin metabolism at therapeutic doses (typically 10 mg/day). At doses greater than 30 mg/day, however, selegiline is capable of increasing presynaptic norepinephrine and serotonin concentrations and has the potential to produce similar drug-related toxicity to that of nonselective MAO inhibitors, such as phenelzine and tranylcypromine.[5] Selegiline's therapeutic benefit in Parkinson's disease is thought to be related to increasing striatal dopamine neurotransmission and protection against neuronal damage from oxidative stress.[5]

All of the currently available MAO inhibitor antidepressants in the United States are irreversible and nonselective (MAO-A, MAO-B) in their enzyme inhibition. Irreversible MAO inhibitors form covalent bonds with the MAO enzymes, which renders the enzyme permanently inactive.[7] When an irreversible MAO inhibitor has been discontinued, it takes approximately 2 weeks before new enzyme synthesis returns MAO activity to 50% of normal.[6,7] This is the basis for the recommendation of waiting 2 weeks after the discontinuation of an irreversible MAO inhibitor before starting any new antidepressant therapy. MAO inhibitors do

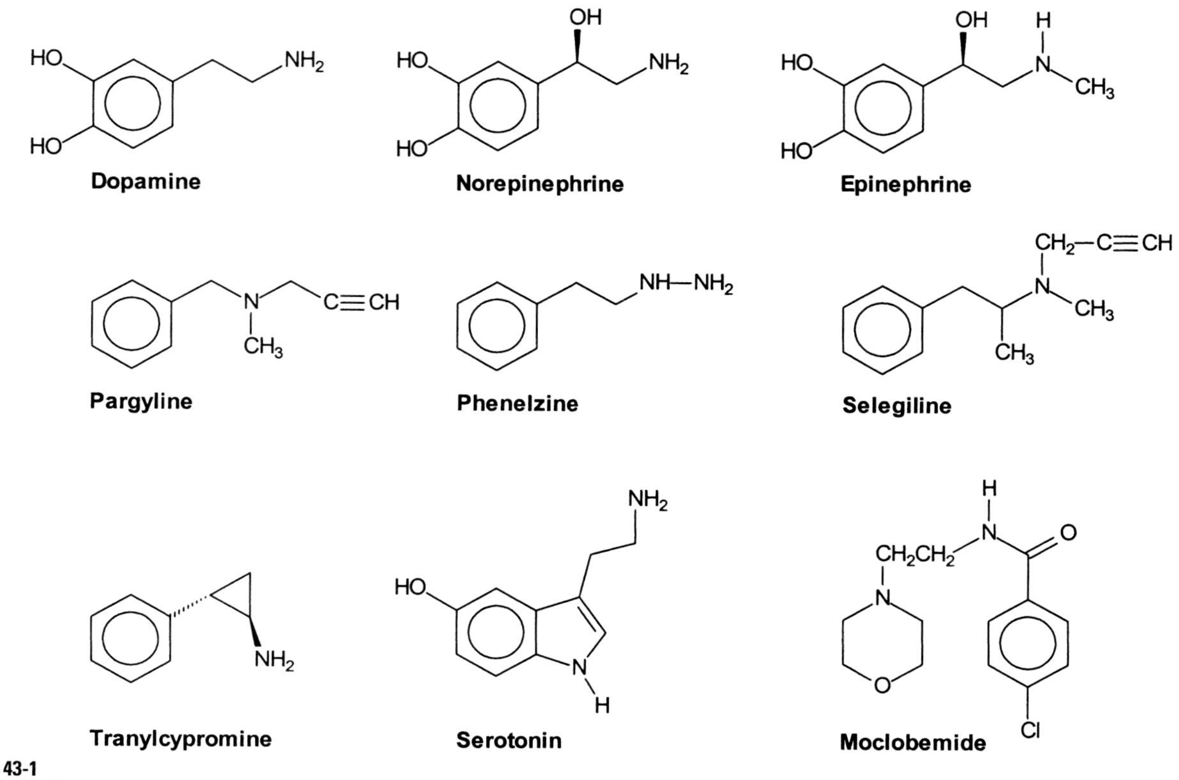

FIGURE 43-1

Chemical structures of monoamine oxidase inhibitors and pertinent neurotransmitters.

not affect enzyme production. Reversible MAO inhibitors do not form irreversible covalent bonds with MAO. New enzyme synthesis is not necessary to restore MAO, and MAO activity gradually returns to normal over a period of hours as the drug-enzyme complex spontaneously dissociates.[10] Examples of reversible MAO inhibitors include moclobemide, toloxatone, brofaromine, and cimoxatone.

PHARMACOKINETICS

Although MAO inhibitors have been used since the 1960s, there is a scarcity of information regarding their pharmacokinetics.[9,10] In general, they are absorbed rapidly and completely from the gastrointestinal tract but undergo significant first-pass hepatic metabolism, limiting their bioavailability. Their dependence on hepatic metabolism predisposes MAO inhibitors to potential drug interactions with other drugs requiring hepatic oxidation. Peak drug levels usually occur 1 to 4 hours after ingestion. Their volumes of distribution are relatively small (1 to 3 L/kg) compared with other antidepressants. Their degree of plasma protein binding is unknown, and their elimination half-life averages 2 to 3 hours.[11]

Selegiline has many active metabolites, such as desmethylselegiline, amphetamine, and methamphetamine. Tranylcypromine has long been suspected as having amphetamine as a metabolite, but this rarely has been detected.[12] Phenelzine metabolism results in multiple active metabolites, such as B-phenylethylamine, which also serves as a substrate for MAO-B.[11]

Clinical toxicity usually is delayed until well after most of the MAO inhibitor already has been metabolized. Blood MAO inhibitor concentrations do not correlate with clinical toxicity. The pharmacokinetic profile of most MAO inhibitors suggests that attempts at extracorporeal removal (e.g., hemodialysis) or administering repeat-dose activated charcoal would be unsuccessful in significantly reducing MAO inhibitor plasma concentrations.

Biphasic postmortem changes have been reported with tranylcypromine and moclobemide in fatal overdose cases.[13,14] Initially, MAO inhibitor blood levels increase in a similar, but less dramatic, fashion as other antidepressants. After 24 hours, drug concentrations show a rapid decline, however, suggesting bacterial degradation.

Pharmacokinetics of Monoamine Oxidase Inhibitors

Volume of distribution: 1–3 L/kg
Absorption rate: rapidly absorbed in 1–2 hr
Bioavailability: 50%
Peak levels: 2–4 hr after ingestion
Protein binding: 50%
Metabolism: hepatic metabolism (P-450 system)
Plasma half-life: 2–4 hr
Active metabolites: no significant active metabolites (except for selegiline)

CLINICAL PRESENTATION OF ACUTE OVERDOSE

Acute MAO inhibitor overdoses have two distinct characteristics. First, the lethal dose in relation to the therapeutic dose is relatively smaller than with other antidepressants. Second, the clinical manifestations of toxicity typically are delayed well beyond the usual observation period of other antidepressants.[15,16] These two characteristics distinguish MAO inhibitors from the other antidepressants, which have a much higher therapeutic index and usually develop toxicity within 6 hours after ingestion.

The usual therapeutic dose for most MAO inhibitors ranges from 0.25 to 1.0 mg/kg. Mild-to-moderate toxicity typically is seen with ingestions of less than 2 mg/kg. Severe toxicity often results from ingestions of 2 to 3 mg/kg. The lethal dose of irreversible MAO inhibitors is reported to be 4 to 6 mg/kg.[15] Deaths have been reported in adults with 170 mg of tranylcypromine and 375 mg of phenelzine. Selegiline overdoses have not been reported but should be assumed to produce similar toxicity as the traditional MAO inhibitor antidepressants until determined otherwise. The average therapeutic dose of tranylcypromine is 20 to 40 mg/day, with a maximum daily dose of 60 mg/day. Phenelzine therapeutic dose is 45 to 75 mg/day, with a maximum of 90 mg/day. Isocarboxazid has a therapeutic dose range of 10 to 30 mg/day. Selegiline usually is administered in a standard dose of 10 mg/day. An important clinical aspect of MAO inhibitor overdoses is that symptoms characteristically are delayed 6 to 12 hours after ingestion but can be delayed 24 hours.[15,16] The delayed onset of toxicity is believed to be secondary to the gradual accumulation of norepinephrine and serotonin in the brain and peripheral sympathetic neurons, which leads to excessive sympathetic receptor stimulation resulting in a hyperadrenergic state. Excess serotonin contributes to MAO inhibitor toxicity but is less prominent than adrenergic symptoms. Patients on long-term MAO inhibitor therapy may show earlier signs of toxicity owing to preexisting enzyme inhibition. In severe cases, the hyperadrenergic state can be followed rapidly by hypotension and central nervous system depression, a sympatholytic-like stage thought to reflect catecholamine depletion.[15] Toxicity usually persists 1 to 4 days after ingestion.[16]

The signs and symptoms of MAO inhibitor toxicity are often nonspecific. Even in its most severe form, it can resemble numerous other conditions (see discussion of differential diagnosis later). Information regarding MAO inhibitor overdoses primarily comes from limited case series[3,11,17] and isolated case reports.[18–27] These reports have tremendous variation in presentation, treatment, and outcome. There is no "typical" presentation to MAO inhibitor toxicity, and there is not an orderly progression of symptoms. After an initial latent period, the rapid development of life-threatening symptoms in all patients with MAO inhibitor overdose should be anticipated. The initial symptoms of MAO inhibitor overdose include headache, agitation, irritability, tremor, nausea, and palpitations. The earliest signs of MAO inhibitor toxicity include sinus tachycardia, hyperreflexia, drowsiness, hyperactivity, mydriasis, fasciculations, hyperventilation, nystagmus, and generalized flushing.[15]

In cases of moderate toxicity, opisthotonos, muscle rigidity, diaphoresis, hypertension, chest pain, diarrhea, hallucinations, combativeness, confusion, marked hyperthermia, and trismus may become evident.[16] A peculiar ocular finding has been observed with some cases of MAO inhibitor toxicity and is described as a "Ping-Pong" gaze because of the bilateral wandering horizontal eye movements.[19,27] The mechanism of this gaze disorder is unknown. In all cases, it resolved gradually with patient improvement.

Severe toxicity generally is manifested by bradycardia, cardiac arrest, hypoxia, hypotension, papilledema, seizures, coma, and worsening hyperthermia. Hypotension is an ominous finding that commonly remains resistant to therapeutic attempts at correction.[19,22] Fetal demise, cerebral edema, pulmonary edema, and intracranial hemorrhage all have been reported in association with MAO inhibitor overdoses.[15] The most common electrocardiographic abnormality seen in MAO inhibitor toxicity is sinus tachycardia, but T-wave abnormalities also are common.[15] Deaths usually are secondary to multiple organ failure.[16]

The newer reversible and selective MAO inhibitors seem to be less toxic in overdose than traditional MAO inhibitors. Most of these cases of newer MAO inhibitor overdose involve moclobemide,[28–30] although one large case series involved toloxatone.[31] The toxicity of both of these antidepressants is similar in overdose and probably can be generalized to other selective and reversible MAO inhibitors. Most adult patients with ingestions of less than 2000 mg are expected to remain asymptomatic or develop only minimal symptoms after a single drug overdose. Toxicity can become severe, however, when combined with other antidepressants or in large doses; when this occurs, the clinical manifestations are similar to those described previously with irreversible agents and can be just as severe. The toxicity from reversible MAO inhibitors resolves sooner than with the irreversible agents, and the mortality rate is believed to be less.

MAO inhibitors can produce hypertension by several mechanisms. It may result from spontaneous hypertensive crisis, tyramine reactions (see later), drug interactions, serotonin syndrome, or high-dose toxicity. Determining the cause of the hypertension depends largely on obtaining an accurate history of the preceding events. Spontaneous hypertensive crisis is a rare condition usually occurring in relation to recent MAO inhibitor dosing.[32] Hypertension can result from exposure to indirect-acting sympathomimetics commonly found in over-the-counter cold and sinus medications.[33] Serotonin syndrome most commonly occurs shortly after exposure to other serotoninergic agents and usually is associated with significant cognitive-behavioral and neuromuscular abnormalities.[34] The clinical presentation of the serotonin syndrome is discussed in Chapter 24.

TYRAMINE REACTION

Tyramine is a dietary amine that normally is metabolized by intestinal and hepatic MAO enzymes (Fig. 43-2), limiting its bioavailability. Nonselective MAO inhibitors interfere with this process, allowing for a greater amount of tyramine to reach the systemic circulation. Tranylcypromine is associated more frequently with tyramine reactions than phenelzine or isocarboxazid.[16,35,36] Selegiline is unlikely to produce a

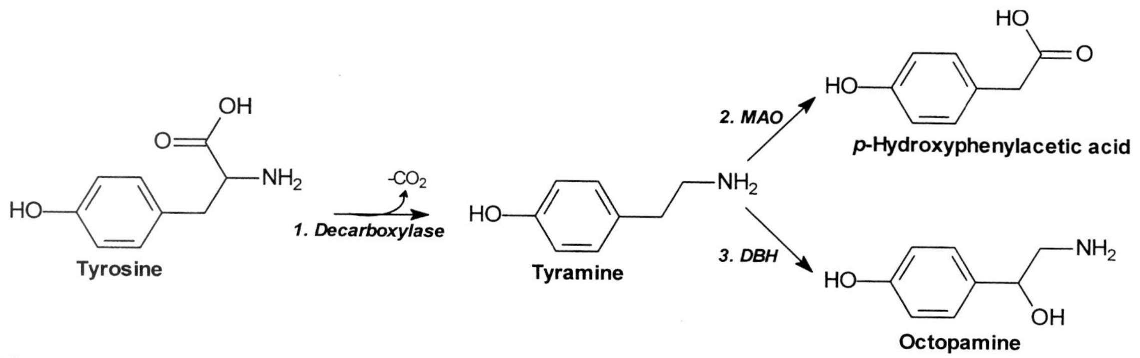

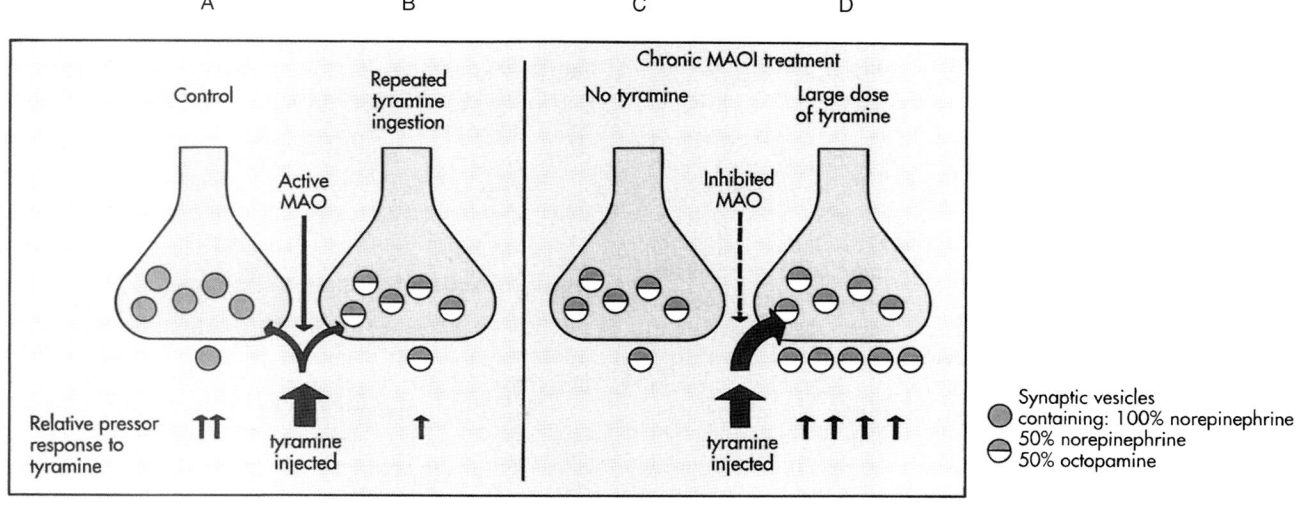

FIGURE 43-2

Synthesis and metabolism of tyramine. Reaction 1: decarboxylation of tyrosine in liver and gastrointestinal tract. Reaction 2: oxidative deamination of tyramine by monamine oxidase (MAO) in liver, kidney, and other tissues. Reaction 3: β-oxidation of tyramine by dopamine β-hydroxylase (DBH) located in synaptic vesicles within terminal of sympathetic neurons. *(Redrawn from Moore KE: Drugs affecting the sympathetic nervous system. In Brody TM, Larner J, Minneman KP [eds]: Human Pharmacology: Molecular to Clinical, 3rd ed. St. Louis, Mosby, 1998, p 132.)*

tyramine reaction if taken at therapeutic doses because of its selective inhibition of MAO-B. Tyramine is an indirect sympathomimetic and is structurally similar to amphetamine. As with most indirect sympathomimetics, tyramine enters the presynaptic neuron through amine uptake pumps.[35] When inside the neuron, tyramine is capable of releasing presynaptic stores of norepinephrine and to a lesser degree serotonin and dopamine (Fig. 43-3).[16] Tyramine also can displace epinephrine from the adrenal gland.[16]

Tyramine is found in more than 70 foods and beverages. Any one of these sources may trigger a reaction.[36] Tyramine is the basis for the so-called cheese reaction because aged cheese contains a large amount of tyramine. In similar fashion, broad (fava) beans contain large quantities of dopamine, a mixed-activity sympathomimetic compound. Patient compliance to an MAO inhibitor–restrictive diet has been reported to be less than 30% of patients.[35] In addition, approximately 4% to 8% of compliant patients experience a tyramine reaction during their therapy.[16] Nonetheless, newer MAO inhibitor

treatment guidelines call for avoiding only a few high-risk food groups, such as nonfresh meat or fish, sauerkraut, aged meats and cheeses, Chianti wine, vermouth, pickled herring, concentrated yeast extracts, and broad beans.[36]

The tyramine reaction characteristically occurs within 15 to 90 minutes after ingesting the dietary amine.[16] The severity of this reaction is highly variable and partially related to the total amount of tyramine ingested.[35,36] The hallmark symptom of tyramine reactions is a severe occipital or temporal headache.[16,33] Other associated symptoms include hypertension, palpitations, diaphoresis, mydriasis, neck stiffness, pallor, neuromuscular excitation, and chest pain.[16,33] Most symptoms gradually resolve over 6 hours without specific therapy.[16] Fatalities have been reported rarely, usually due to intracranial hemorrhage or myocardial infarction. An electrocardiogram should be obtained for all patients with tyramine-associated chest pain. Focal neurologic findings or a persistent severe headache warrants investigation with a computed tomography scan of the head.

FIGURE 43-3

Acute response to ingestion of tyramine (**A**); tolerance to repeated ingestions of tyramine (**B**); long-term treatment with a monoamine oxidase inhibitor (MAOI) (**C**); effects of tyramine after long-term MAOI pretreatment (**D**). The relative increase in blood pressure is denoted by the number of arrows. *(From Moore KE: Drugs affecting the sympathetic nervous system. In Brody TM, Larner J, Minneman KP [eds]: Human Pharmacology: Molecular to Clinical, 3rd ed. St. Louis, Mosby, 1998, p 132.)*

Tyramine Reaction

Diagnosed by rapid onset of headache and hypertension after tyramine ingestion

Can occur with other indirect sympathomimetics (e.g., levodopa)

Phentolamine is antihypertensive of choice

Avoid β-blockers because they may worsen hypertension

Persistent headaches should be evaluated for intracranial hemorrhage

Chest pain should be evaluated for myocardial ischemia

Most tyramine reactions rapidly resolve with appropriate treatment

Asymptomatic patients can be discharged after 4 hr of observation

Admit all patients symptomatic for >6 hr

DIAGNOSIS

MAO inhibitor toxicity is a clinical diagnosis based solely on the history of MAO inhibitor ingestion and hyperadrenergic symptoms. There are no readily available confirmatory tests. Routine drug screens do not detect MAO inhibitors but may be helpful in narrowing the differential diagnosis. A positive urine drug screen for amphetamine might be expected with selegiline ingestions because amphetamine is one of its major metabolites. Special toxicologic testing would be of little value in detecting MAO inhibitors because most of the parent compounds have a short half-life in relation to their duration of action and may not be detectable when symptoms develop. The best use of laboratory tests is to assist in the differential diagnosis of MAO inhibitor toxicity and to identify possible complications of MAO inhibitor overdose, which include hypoxia, rhab-

domyolysis, renal failure, hyperkalemia, metabolic acidosis, hemolysis, and disseminated intravascular coagulation. Leukocytosis[22,23] and thrombocytopenia[19,24] are seen commonly with MAO inhibitor toxicity.

The differential diagnosis of an unknown MAO inhibitor ingestion is extremely challenging and includes all drugs and medical conditions capable of producing a hyperadrenergic state, altered mental status, hyperthermia, or muscle rigidity (Table 43-2). MAO inhibitor toxicity also could be associated with a sympatholytic presentation, broadening the differential possibilities further. In reality, without a history of exposure, a conclusive diagnosis of MAO inhibitor poisoning cannot be made because no confirmatory tests are available.

TREATMENT

All patients with MAO inhibitor overdose require immediate physician evaluation, establishment of at least one peripheral intravenous line, intensive clinical and cardiac monitoring, and possibly gastric decontamination. There are no known antidotes for MAO inhibitor toxicity. There are no controlled

Indications for ICU Admission in Monoamine Oxidase Inhibitor Poisoning

1. Admit all patients who ingested >1 mg/kg to an ICU (except reversible MAO inhibitors).
2. Admit all symptomatic patients <24 hr since ingestion.
3. Consider ICU admission for most patients with serotonin syndrome.

TABLE 43-2 Differential Diagnosis of Monoamine Oxidase Inhibitor Overdose

	HYPERADRENERGIC	HYPERTHERMIA	ALTERED MENTATION	MUSCLE RIGIDITY
Amphetamine toxicity	XXX	X	X	X
Antimuscarinic toxicity	X	X	XX	0
Benzodiazepine withdrawal	X	X	XX	0
Cocaine toxicity	XX	X	X	0
Delirium tremens	XX	X	XX	0
Dystonic reaction	0	0	0	XX
Heat stroke	XX	XXX	XXX	X
Hyperthyroidism	X	X	X	0
Hypoglycemia	X	0	XX	0
Malignant hyperthermia	XXX	XXX	XXX	XXX
Meningitis	X	XX	XXX	X
Neuroleptic malignant syndrome	XXX	XXX	XXX	XXX
Phencyclidine toxicity	XX	X	XX	X
Serotonin syndrome	XX	XX	XX	XX
Strychnine toxicity	0	X	0	XXX
Tetanus	X	X	0	XXX
Tyramine reaction	XX	X	X	0

0, not expected to be present; X, expected in the minority of cases; XX, expected to be commonly present; XXX, expected to be present in almost all cases.

human studies on MAO inhibitor overdose treatment on which to base patient management recommendations. Medical management is based on providing excellent supportive care, avoiding potential drug interactions, and treating medical complications early. Onset of toxicity is usually gradual and delayed, sometimes 24 hours after ingestion. The abrupt development of seizures, coma, respiratory insufficiency, and cardiovascular collapse is possible, however. Certain patient groups, such as patients with underlying medical problems, children, and the elderly, may manifest greater toxicity at a given dose of an MAO inhibitor.

The best method of gastrointestinal decontamination in MAO inhibitor overdose has never been studied. The following recommendations are general guidelines based on the pharmacokinetic profile of MAO inhibitors and human case reports. Syrup of ipecac is contraindicated in MAO inhibitor overdose because of the significant potential for cardiovascular collapse and loss of consciousness. Activated charcoal should be administered as a single dose of 1 g/kg as soon as is safely possible, particularly if it can be given shortly after ingestion. The efficacy of activated charcoal treatment, if any, is expected to decrease as time passes postingestion (see Chapter 6). Multiple-dose activated charcoal administration is not expected to be advantageous. Some medical toxicologists recommend gastric lavage for all significant ingestions because it may be of benefit if it can be performed within 1 hour after ingestion. It is unknown, however, whether this intervention alters the clinical course or outcome after MAO inhibitor overdose (see Chapter 5). Because MAO inhibitors are absorbed rapidly, delayed gastric lavage or whole-bowel irrigation is unlikely to be of any clinical benefit. Urinary acidification is not recommended because it is ineffective at enhancing MAO inhibitor elimination, and it predisposes to acute renal failure secondary to myoglobin precipitation within renal tubules. Routine laboratory tests should be performed on all patients, with particular emphasis on identifying early hyperkalemia, metabolic acidosis, and rhabdomyolysis.

Hypertension

Acutely hypertensive patients should be treated with short-acting intravenous antihypertensive agents because of the potential to develop precipitous hypotension. In most cases, an intraarterial catheter is required for accurate blood pressure monitoring. Traditionally the antihypertensive agents of choice are phentolamine and nitroprusside. Phentolamine is a nonspecific α-adrenergic receptor antagonist, usually administered in 2.5- to 5.0-mg boluses every 10 to 15 minutes until blood pressure elevation is controlled. It also can be given as a continuous infusion (1 to 5 mg/hr) for maintenance therapy. Phentolamine use commonly is associated with reflex tachycardia. Nitroprusside is given as a continuous infusion with an initial rate of 1 μg/kg/min, then titrated according to blood pressure response. Prolonged high doses of nitroprusside can predispose to cyanide toxicity (see Chapter 37). The addition of thiosulfate to nitroprusside infusions eliminates the possibility of cyanide toxicity and is done routinely in many intensive care units (ICUs). Nitroglycerin can be used for the relief of cardiac-related chest pain. Fenoldopam is a new short-acting parenteral antihyper-

tensive agent.[17] Its mechanism of action is secondary to peripheral dopamine (D_1) receptor agonism.[37] Fenoldopam reportedly does not cross the blood-brain barrier. There are no known contraindications for its use in MAO inhibitor–induced hypertension. Fenoldopam is administered as a titratable infusion with a suggested starting dose of 0.05 to 0.1 μg/kg/min. Intravenous diltiazem is expected to be an effective antihypertensive agent, but its long duration of action makes it less desirable than the shorter acting agents. β-Blockers pose a theoretical risk of increasing the blood pressure through unopposed α-adrenergic receptor–mediated vasoconstriction and should be considered contraindicated. Labetalol is a β-blocker with slight α-receptor blocking ability. The theoretical benefit of its α-blocking capacity must be balanced against its much greater β-blocking activity. Because patients with MAO inhibitor toxicity may change rapidly from being hypertensive to being hypotensive, short-acting antihypertensive agents theoretically are preferable.

Hypotension

Hypotension carries a poor prognosis in MAO inhibitor overdose.[15,18,22] Isotonic intravenous fluid boluses of 10 to 20 mL/kg are the initial treatment of hypotension. When vasopressors are required, it is important to avoid all agents with indirect sympathomimetic actions (e.g., dopamine) and choose from available direct-acting sympathomimetics instead (Table 43-3). Norepinephrine is the vasopressor of choice, with epinephrine as the second drug of choice. Patients with MAO inhibitor toxicity may have increased sensitivity to vasopressors, and lower starting doses are recommended.

Dysrhythmias

Sinus tachycardia rarely requires specific drug therapy, unless it is producing myocardial ischemia. Lidocaine, procainamide, and phenytoin are the most effective antiarrhythmics in treating MAO inhibitor–induced dysrhythmias.[15] Bradycardia may degrade quickly into asystole in the later stages of the overdose[18] and require pacemaker placement. Pharmacologic treatment of bradycardia includes atropine, isoproterenol, and dobutamine. Bretylium should be avoided because of its indirect sympathomimetic activity.

Seizures

Benzodiazepines are the anticonvulsants of choice in treating MAO inhibitor–induced seizures.[15,16,26] Barbiturates also are effective[15,16,26] but may cause hypotension, especially at higher doses. Phenytoin theoretically is ineffective in stopping drug-induced seizures (see Chapter 20). General anesthesia with muscle paralysis may be necessary in cases of status epilepticus to prevent the metabolic acidosis, hyperthermia, and rhabdomyolysis commonly seen with persistent seizure activity. Muscle paralysis is accomplished best using nondepolarizing neuromuscular blocking agents (e.g., vecuronium). Pancuronium theoretically is less desirable than other nondepolarizing agents because of its propensity to produce elevations in heart rate and blood

TABLE 43-3 Drugs Contraindicated with Monoamine Oxidase Inhibitors

INDIRECT-ACTIVITY AND MIXED-ACTIVITY SYMPATHOMIMETICS	ANTIDEPRESSANTS	MISCELLANEOUS DRUGS
Benzphetamine	Amoxapine	β-Blockers
Bretylium	Amitriptyline	Buspirone
Caffeine	Bupropion	Carbamazepine
Cocaine	Citalopram	Clonidine
Dexfenfluramine	Clomipramine	Cyclobenzaprine
Dextroamphetamine	Desipramine	Dextromethorphan
Diethylpropion	Doxepin	Disulfiram
Dopamine	Fluoxetine	Ergot alkaloids
Ephedrine	Fluvoxamine	Fentanyl
Fenfluramine	Imipramine	Furazolidone
Guanethidine	Maprotiline	Ginseng
Isometheptene	Mirtazapine	Ketamine
Mephentermine	Nefazodone	Levodopa
Metaraminol	Paroxetine	Lithium
Methamphetamine	Sertraline	Meperidine
3,4-Methylenedioxymethamphetamine (MDMA)	St. John's wort	Oral hypoglycemic agents
Methyldopa	Trazodone	Phenothiazines
Methylphenidate	Venlafaxine	Procarbazine
Pemoline		Rizatriptan
Phentermine		Sumatriptan
Phencyclidine		Tramadol
Phenylpropanolamine		Tryptophan
Propylhexedrine		Zolmitriptan
Pseudoephedrine		
Reserpine		
Ritodrine		
Theophylline		
Tyramine		

pressure. Phenelzine may enhance the action of succinylcholine because it lowers pseudocholinesterase activity.[39] When muscle paralysis is used to control the peripheral manifestations of seizure activity, electroencephalographic monitoring is necessary to assess for the presence of central nervous system seizures.

Hyperthermia

Antipyretics generally are insufficient to reduce drug-induced hyperthermia, and other temperature reduction methods often are necessary. Benzodiazepines generally are considered to be useful first-line agents through centrally mediated reduction in muscle hyperactivity and decrease in heat production. Increasing evaporative and conductive heat loss is essential for the successful treatment of hyperthermia. Increasing heat loss is accomplished best by using cool mist spray, fans, and ice baths. Hyperthermia often is resistant to these measures in the setting of persistent muscle rigidity.[16] Muscle paralysis with nondepolarizing agents should be considered when diffuse rigidity is refractory to benzodiazepine therapy. Dantrolene has been used with apparent success as a muscle relaxant in resistant cases of muscle rigidity.[15,24] The intravenous dose of dantrolene is 0.5 to 2.5 mg/kg every 6 hours. Phenothiazines theoretically should be avoided because of their potential to impair

sweating (and evaporative heat loss), lower the seizure threshold, worsen hypotension, and produce extrapyramidal reactions.

Admission Criteria

All intentional MAO inhibitor overdoses and accidental exposures of greater than 1.0 mg/kg require admission to an ICU. Accidental exposures of less than 1.0 mg/kg still require hospital admission to a monitored bed; however, these patients are unlikely to develop life-threatening complications. Reversible MAO inhibitors are less toxic than traditional MAO inhibitors, and ingestions of less than 2000 mg in adults are unlikely to produce significant toxicity. Asymptomatic patients can be admitted to a monitored bed for 24-hour observation. Even a single MAO inhibitor tablet may produce life-threatening drug interactions, such as the serotonin syndrome, or other drug interactions under certain circumstances. Asymptomatic patients should be monitored for at least 24 hours before medical clearance. Vital sign abnormalities should be recognized early and treated appropriately. Dietary and medication restrictions should be followed meticulously during hospitalization. All patients should be instructed to avoid contraindicated foods and medications for a minimum of 2 weeks. Consultation with a medical toxicologist or a poison center is recommended. Patients requiring transfer to hospitals with ICU capabilities should be transferred as soon as possible to avoid the problems anticipated with delayed onset of toxicity. Medical personnel capable of performing advanced cardiac life support and endotracheal intubation should accompany all patients being transferred.

Extracorporeal Removal Techniques

Hemodialysis, hemoperfusion, and peritoneal dialysis have no established role in the treatment of MAO inhibitor poisoning.

Tyramine Reaction

In cases of severe hypertension, the drug of choice is phentolamine, which typically is given intravenously in 2.5- to 5-mg doses every 5 to 15 minutes until the blood pressure is controlled. The half-life of phentolamine is approximately 20 minutes, and its duration of action is less than 1 hour.[16] Nitroprusside is another rapidly acting direct vasodilator and is administered as a continuous infusion (1 to 4 μg/kg/min). In cases of moderate hypertension, nifedipine and prazosin have been reported to be effective.[16,33] Newer recommendations for the treatment of accelerated chronic hypertension discourage the use of nifedipine owing to concerns of excessive blood pressure reduction. These concerns may not apply to the acute hypertension seen in tyramine reactions. β-Adrenergic blocking drugs generally are considered to be contraindicated because of the risk of unopposed α-receptor stimulation. Hospital admission should be strongly considered for patients whose hypertension does not resolve completely within 6 hours after onset. Gastrointestinal decontamination is unlikely to offer any significant benefit because the onset of toxicity is so rapid after tyramine exposure. Tyramine reactions are immediate, without delayed sequelae. Asymptomatic patients require only 6 hours of observation.

Criterion for ICU Discharge in Monoamine Oxidase Inhibitor Poisoning

Stable patient who is at least 24 hr postingestion

DRUG INTERACTIONS

Long-term MAO inhibitor drug therapy predisposes to many potentially significant drug interactions (see Table 43-3). Documentation of human MAO inhibitor drug interactions often is limited to single case reports or case series. Controlled human studies are impractical owing to the life-threatening nature of these reactions. Animal studies often have limited applicability to human toxicity. Patients taking MAO inhibitors should not receive other prescription or nonprescription medications unless strongly warranted and only after drug compatibility with MAO inhibitors has been confirmed (Table 43-4).

Drug interactions involving MAO inhibitors can be grouped into three categories—pharmacodynamic, pharma-

TABLE 43-4 Drugs Considered Safe with Monoamine Oxidase Inhibitors*

DIRECT-ACTIVITY SYMPATHOMIMETICS	MISCELLANEOUS DRUGS
Albuterol	Acetaminophen
Dobutamine	Aspirin
Epinephrine	Barbiturates
Fenoldopam	Benzodiazepines
Isoproterenol	Calcium channel blockers
Norepinephrine	Cephalosporins
Terbutaline	Corticosteroids
	Inhalational anesthetics
	Lidocaine
	Morphine
	Nitroglycerin
	Nitroprusside
	Nitrous oxide
	Nonsteroidal antiinflammatory drugs
	Penicillin
	Phentolamine
	Procainamide
	Succinylcholine

*Always use the lowest effective dose.

cokinetic, and idiosyncratic. The most common pharmacodynamic reaction involves drugs with indirect sympathomimetic actions,[33,38] such as pseudoephedrine and possibly ephedrine. These drugs have the potential to produce a hyperadrenergic condition similar to the tyramine reaction and can be found in over-the-counter preparations, drugs of abuse, and some prescription products. Pharmacokinetic drug interactions have been noted with MAO inhibitors because they are metabolized through the cytochrome oxidase enzyme system and can inhibit the hepatic metabolism of other drugs. The potentiation of opiate and sedative-hypnotic drugs is an example of this type of enzyme inhibition.[33] Tranylcypromine and phenelzine have been shown to increase insulin release and predispose to hypoglycemia, especially in patients taking oral sulfonylurea agents.[40] Insulin dosage also may warrant reduction.

Serotonin syndrome is a rare, potentially life-threatening idiosyncratic reaction. It most commonly occurs when MAO inhibitors are combined with other serotoninergic agents. A complete description of serotonin syndrome and a listing of serotoninergic medications can be found in Chapter 24.[33] Given the relatively high frequency of their use, however, special mention is made to avoid administration of meperidine[16,21] and dextromethorphan, which are capable of producing serotonin syndrome in combination with MAO inhibitors.[39] All of these medications are contraindicated for 2 weeks after discontinuation of an irreversible MAO inhibitor. This recommendation is particularly important to prevent the development of serotonin syndrome.

Equally important is the recognition that certain medications are generally compatible with MAO inhibitors (see Table 43-4). Aspirin,[16] acetaminophen,[33] ibuprofen,[16] and morphine[40] have been used in combination with MAO inhibitors without complications. Morphine should be given in decreased doses because of MAO inhibitor–induced impaired morphine metabolism and enhanced opiate effects.[40] Direct-acting sympathomimetic agents, such as norepinephrine, can be used with caution, using lowest possible effective dose. Direct sympathomimetics do not rely on the release of neurotransmitters for their activity and are inactivated by catechol *O*-methyltransferase, which is unaffected by MAO inhibitors.[33]

Key Points in Monoamine Oxidase Inhibitor Poisoning

1. Clinical toxicity often is delayed 6–24 hr after ingestion.
2. MAO inhibitors are not detected by common drug tests.
3. Drug concentrations are not useful to managing overdosed patients.
4. Reversible MAO inhibitors are less toxic than irreversible MAO inhibitors.
5. MAO inhibitors have little effect on the electrocardiogram except for sinus tachycardia.
6. Consider serotonin syndrome in patients taking two or more serotoninergic agents.
7. Admit all patients who ingested >1 mg/kg for 24 hr of observation.
8. Do not use syrup of ipecac for gastrointestinal decontamination.
9. Do not use β-blockers to treat tachycardia or hypertension.
10. Do not give meperidine, tramadol, or dextromethorphan to patients taking MAO inhibitors.
11. Avoid combining serotoninergic agents.
12. Do not use indirect sympathomimetics.
13. Extracorporeal removal is an unproven modality in MAO inhibitor overdose.
14. Tranylcypromine rarely, if ever, produces amphetamine in the urine.
15. Selegiline is metabolized to methamphetamine.

REFERENCES

1. Litovitz TI, Bailey KM, Schmitz BF, et al: 1990 Annual report of the American Association of Poison Control Centers National Data Collection System. Am J Emerg Med 9:461–509, 1991.
2. Litovitz TI, Klein-Schwartz W, White SW, et al: 2000 Annual report of the American Association of Poison Control Centers Toxic Exposure Surveillance System. Am J Emerg Med 19:337–395, 2001.
3. Meredith T, Vale J: Poisoning due to psychotropic agents. Adverse Drug React Acute Poisoning Rev 4:313–329, 1985.
4. McDaniel K: Clinical pharmacology of monoamine oxidase inhibitors. Clin Neuropharmacol 9:207–234, 1986.
5. Youdim M, Finberg J: Pharmacological actions of l-deprenyl (selegiline) and other selective monoamine oxidase B inhibitors. Clin Pharmacol Ther 56(Part 2):725–730, 1994.
6. Muller WE, Singer A, Wonnermann M, et al: Hyperforin represents the neurotransmitter reuptake inhibiting constituent of hypericum extract. Pharmacopsychiatry 31:16–21, 1998.
7. Cesura A, Pletscher A: The new generation of monoamine oxidase inhibitors. Prog Drug Res 38:171–297, 1992.
8. Youdim M, Finberg J: New directions in monoamine oxidase A and B selective inhibitors and substrates. Biochem Pharmacol 41:155–162, 1991.
9. Boulton A, Eisenhofer G: Catecholamine metabolism from molecular understanding to clinical diagnosis and treatment. Adv Pharmacol 42:273–292, 1998.
10. Nair NPV, Ahmed SK, Ng Ying Kim NMK: Biochemistry and pharmacology of reversible inhibitors of MAO-A agents: Focus on moclobemide. J Psychiatr Neurosci 18:214–222, 1993.
11. Mallinger A, Smith E: Pharmacokinetics of monoamine oxidase inhibitors. Psychopharmacol Bull 27:493–502, 1991.
12. Iwersen S, Schmoldt A: One fatal and one nonfatal intoxication with tranylcypromine: Absence of amphetamines as metabolites. J Anal Toxicol 20:301–304, 1996.
13. Yonemitsu K, Pounder D: Postmortem changes in blood tranylcypromine concentration: Competing redistribution and degrading effects. Forensic Sci Int 59:177–184, 1993.
14. Rodge S, Hilberg T, Teige B: Fatal combined intoxication with new antidepressants: Human cases and an experimental study of postmortem moclobemide redistribution. Forensic Sci Int 100:109–116, 1999.
15. Linden C, Rumack B, Strehlke C: Monoamine oxidase inhibitor overdose. Ann Emerg Med 13:1137–1144, 1984.
16. Mills K: Monoamine oxidase inhibitor toxicity. Top Emerg Med 15:58–71, 1993.
17. Ciocatto E, Fagiano G, Bava G: Clinical features and treatment of overdosage of monoamine oxidase inhibitors and their interaction with other psychotropic drugs. Resuscitation 1:69–72, 1972.
18. Breheny F, Dobb G, Clarke G: Phenelzine poisoning. Anaesthesia 41:53–56, 1986.
19. Erich J, Shih R, O'Connor R: "Ping-Pong" gaze in severe monoamine oxidase inhibitor toxicity. J Emerg Med 13:653–655, 1995.
20. Lipkin D, Kushnick T: Pargyline hydrochloride poisoning in a child. JAMA 201:135–136, 1967.
21. Mallampalli A, Pentel P, Anderson D: Nonreactive pupils due to monoamine oxidase inhibitor overdose. Med Care Medicine 15:536–537, 1987.
22. Marra J, Minter D, Hobins T: Suicide by ingestion of tranylcypromine. JAMA 192:162–163, 1965.
23. Matter B, Donat P, Brill M, et al: Tranylcypromine sulfate poisoning. Arch Intern Med 116:18–20, 1965.
24. Pennings E, Verkes R, Koning J, et al: Tranylcypromine intoxication with malignant hyperthermia, delirium, and thrombocytopenia. J Clin Psychopharmacol 17:430–432, 1997.
25. Solberg C, Norway B: Phenelzine intoxication. JAMA 177:572–573, 1961.
26. Thorp M, Toombs D, Harmon B: Monoamine oxidase inhibitor overdose. WMJ 166:275–277, 1997.
27. Watkins H, Ellis C: Ping Pong gaze in reversible coma due to overdose of monoamine oxidase inhibitor. J Neurol Neurosurg Psychiatry 52:539, 1989.
28. Myrenfors PG, Eriksson T, Sandstedt CS: Moclobemide overdose. J Intern Med 233:113–115, 1993.
29. Iwersen S, Schmoldt A: Three suicide attempts with moclobemide. Clin Toxicol 34:223–225, 1996.
30. Hetzel W: Saftey of moclobemide taken in overdose for attempted suicide. Psychopharmacology 106:S127-S129, 1992.
31. Azoyan Ph, Garnier R, Baud FJ, et al: Intoxication aigue par la toloxatone: A propos de 122 observations. Therapie 45:139–144, 1990.
32. Lavin M, Mendelowitz A, Kronig M: Spontaneous hypertensive reactions with monoamine oxidase inhibitors. Soc Biol Psychiatry 34:146–151, 1993.
33. Lippman S, Nash K: Monoamine oxidase inhibitor update potential adverse food and drug interactions. Drug Saf 5:195–204, 1990.
34. Mills KC: Serotonin syndrome: A clinical update. Crit Care Clin 13:763–783, 1997.
35. Brown C, Taniguchi G, Yip K: The monoamine oxidase inhibitor-tyramine reaction. J Clin Pharmacol 29:529–532, 1989.
36. Shulman K, Walker S, MacKenzie S, et al: Dietary restriction, tyramine, and the use of monoamine oxidase inhibitors. J Clin Pharmacol 9:397–402, 1989.
37. Post J, Frishman W: Fenoldopam: A new dopamine agonist for the treatment of hypertensive urgencies and emergencies. J Clin Pharmacol 38:2–13, 1998.
38. Hunter K, Boakes A, Laurence D: Monoamine oxidase inhibitors and L-dopa. BMJ 3:388, 1970.
39. Stack C, Rogers P, Linter S: Momoamine oxidase inhibitors and anaesthesia. Br J Anaesth 60:222–227, 1988.
40. Cooper A, Ashcroft G: Potentiation of insulin hypoglycemia by M.A.O.I. antidepressant drugs. Lancet 1:407–409, 1966.

CHAPTER 44

Serotonergic Antidepressants

Kirk C. Mills

The amine hypothesis of depression has been generally accepted and popularized during the past 50 years, although the true mechanism by which antidepressants exert their therapeutic effects is currently unknown.[1] The serotonin neurotransmitter system has become the most common target for newly developed antidepressants in an effort to enhance serotonin (5-hydroxytryptamine [5-HT]) neurotransmission selectively without the unwanted and potentially toxic adverse effects of affecting other neurotransmitter systems.[2] The newer antidepressants commonly are referred to as *atypical, heterocyclic,* or *second-generation antidepressants.* For the purpose of this chapter, they are referred to as *serotonergic antidepressants,* which emphasizes their common effect on enhancing serotonin neurotransmission. These different terms distinguish this group of antidepressants from the more traditional selective monoamine oxidase (MAO) inhibitors and tricyclic antidepressants (TCAs). This distinction is important because newer antidepressants are more selective in their pharmacologic activity and have markedly different toxicologic behavior than MAO inhibitors and TCAs.[1]

Serotonergic antidepressants are the most popular form of psychopharmacologic therapy for the treatment of major depression. They are also commonly prescribed in the treatment of many other psychiatric disorders, such as obsessive-compulsive, panic, and eating disorders.[2] Serotonergic antidepressants increasingly are being used in older children and adolescents despite varying degrees of proven safety in these populations. The American Association of Poison Control Centers Toxic Exposure Surveillance System consistently has reported annual increases in drug exposures to serotonergic antidepressants since the 1990s.[3] The newer antidepressants produce less severe toxicity in overdose and are associated with fewer fatalities than either MAO inhibitors or TCAs.[3] This chapter discusses the expected clinical toxicity and general management of serotonergic antidepressant poisoning. The antidepressants discussed in this chapter include trazodone (Desyrel), nefazodone (Serzone), bupropion (Wellbutrin), mirtazapine (Remeron), and venlafaxine (Effexor). The selective serotonin reuptake inhibitors (SSRIs) also are discussed, including fluoxetine (Prozac), sertraline (Zoloft), paroxetine (Paxil), fluvoxamine (Luvox), citalopram (Celexa), and escitalopram (Lexapro).

GENERAL CHARACTERISTICS OF SEROTONERGIC ANTIDEPRESSANT POISONING

Serotonergic antidepressants are a heterogeneous group of drugs that differ significantly in chemical structure, mechanism of action, pharmacokinetic characteristics, and side-effect profile. Despite these differences, they share many important similarities that are summarized in the following nine points (Table 44-1). For brevity within this chapter, most of these points are not repeated for each individual drug.

1. Most serotonergic antidepressants are far less cardiotoxic than TCAs.[4] In general, these newer agents have a low affinity for cardiac sodium, calcium, or potassium ion channels. They typically do not show the same cardiotoxicity or electrocardiogram (.00ECG) conduction abnormalities as those seen with TCAs. Exceptions to this rule occur in large overdoses or mixed-drug ingestions. Citalopram, fluoxetine, trazodone, and venlafaxine are the most likely serotonergic antidepressants to show cardiotoxicity in large overdoses.
2. These agents do not inhibit MAO and are not associated with tyramine-like reactions. Unlike with the MAO inhibitors, the use of indirect sympathomimetics with the serotonergic antidepressants is not contraindicated.[1]
3. These agents have negligible affinity for acetylcholine, dopamine, γ-aminobutyric acid, glutamate, or β-adrenergic receptors.[1] Although the exact mechanism of action is poorly understood, it traditionally is attributed to inhibition of neurotransmitter reuptake (except mirtazapine). Some atypical antidepressants may act through postsynaptic serotonin receptor inhibition.[5]
4. Serotonergic antidepressants (except bupropion) have a much higher therapeutic index than MAO inhibitors and TCAs.[3] Nonetheless, they still can cause fatalities, especially at high doses or when combined with other drugs. For many of these agents, there are limited human data on poisoning presentation or optimal patient management. Current management recommendations may require modification as more information becomes available. Treating physicians should contact a medical toxicologist or a regional poison control center if there are any questions regarding the hazards of overdoses with newer antidepressants.
5. Based on their pharmacokinetic profiles,[6] attempts to enhance the elimination of serotonergic antidepressants via hemodialysis, hemoperfusion, forced diuresis,

TABLE 44-1 General Characteristics of Serotonergic Antidepressants

Capable of contributing to development of serotonin syndrome
Combination with MAO inhibitors contraindicated
Little ability to inhibit cardiac sodium, calcium, and potassium channels
Likely to undergo postmortem drug redistribution
Act primarily by inhibition of amine uptake (except mirtazapine)
Quantitative blood concentrations do not alter patient management
All U.S. FDA category C in pregnancy except bupropion (category B) (see Appendix A)
Do not inhibit MAO
Not associated with tyramine reactions
Do not block muscarinic receptors significantly
High therapeutic index (except bupropion)
Unlikely to be removed significantly by extracorporeal mechanisms
May interfere with metabolism of other drugs due to hepatic enzyme inhibition
Not detected by standard drug screening tests

FDA, Food and Drug Administration; MAO, monoamine oxidase.

---

multiple-dose activated charcoal, or whole-bowel irrigation are unlikely to offer any advantage over single-dose activated charcoal in the gastrointestinal decontamination of patients exposed to newer antidepressants.

6. The newer antidepressants are not detected by most routine hospital serum and urine drug screens. Comprehensive urine drug screens detect some of the newer antidepressants but cannot distinguish between therapeutic and toxic exposures. Some laboratories can measure plasma parent drug and metabolite levels, but obtaining this information is costly and time-consuming, and the multiple-dose activated charcoal does not affect patient management.

7. Postmortem drug redistribution is likely to occur with serotonergic agents because the newer antidepressants generally have large volumes of distribution. Interpretation of postmortem blood concentrations of these drugs must take this factor into consideration.[7–10]

8. The newer antidepressants are metabolized primarily by hepatic P-450 pathways. Drug interactions are possible when two medications that share the same metabolic pathway are given together.[6,11] In addition, hepatic dysfunction may lead to elevated plasma drug concentrations and theoretically to toxicity.

9. All antidepressants, especially MAO inhibitors and SSRIs, have the potential to produce the serotonin syndrome (see Chapter 24).[11] Although the manufacturers' contraindications do not encompass all serotonergic medications, significant caution should be exercised before combining two or more serotonergic agents in a patient's treatment.

TRAZODONE

Trazodone hydrochloride (Desyrel) was released in the United States in 1982 for the treatment of endogenous depression. During the 1990s, the frequency of reported trazodone exposures consistently increased.[12] The reported fatality rate is approximately 1 in 1000 exposures, which is 7 to 10 times less than the fatality rate for MAO inhibitor or TCA exposures.[3] The average daily therapeutic dose for trazodone is 150 to 400 mg (Table 44-2), with a maximal dose of 600 mg restricted to psychiatric inpatients. Trazodone is available as 50-mg, 100-mg, and 150-mg tablets. There is a low potential for trazodone abuse, and a distinct withdrawal syndrome has not been observed with its abrupt discontinuation.[13] Trazodone carries a U.S. Food and Drug Administration (FDA) pregnancy category C designation (see Appendix A).

Trazodone is a triazolopyridine derivative that, with the exception of trazodone, is structurally unrelated to other antidepressants.[12] Its antidepressant action is believed to be due to a combination of serotonin reuptake inhibition and antagonism of postsynaptic 5-HT$_2$ receptors.[12] Trazodone is a moderately potent nonselective α-adrenergic receptor blocker with at least five times greater affinity for α$_1$-adrenergic receptors than for α$_2$-adrenergic receptors. Consequently, trazodone frequently is associated with orthostatic hypotension, which is maximal within the first 6 hours of use and can be minimized by taking the medication at bedtime.[13] Sedation, which is a common side effect of trazodone therapy, is believed to be secondary to inhibition of central α-adrenergic and histamine receptors.

Clinical Pharmacology

Trazodone is absorbed rapidly and completely, with peak plasma levels occurring 1 to 2 hours after oral administration. It is highly protein bound and has an intermediate volume of distribution (1.2 L/kg).[12] Most trazodone undergoes hepatic oxidation by the cytochrome P-450 isoenzyme system. It has one active metabolite, m-chlorophenylpiperazine (m-CPP), which has a complex pharmacologic profile, including inhibition of 5-HT uptake, stimulation and inhibition of multiple postsynaptic serotonin receptors, and interactions with other neurotransmitter systems. The overall contribution of m-CPP to the therapeutic and toxic effects of trazodone is currently under investigation. The apparent half-life of trazodone is 5 to 9 hours at therapeutic doses but can increase to 13 hours in overdose.[12]

The most frequently reported dose-related adverse effects are drowsiness, dizziness, dry mouth, nausea and vomiting, and orthostatic hypotension.[12] There have been

TABLE 44-2 Trazodone Overdose

Typical therapeutic dose 150 to 400 mg/day
Risk of priapism in 1/1000 to 1/10,000 patients
Commonly produces orthostatic hypotension
Low incidence of cardiac toxicity but may cause QT interval prolongation
May produce CNS sedation in overdose
Serious toxicity most likely with ingestions of >2 g in adults
Adult ingestions of <2 g managed with activated charcoal and supportive care
Adult ingestions of >2 g may require gastric lavage and supportive care
Asymptomatic patients can be discharged after 6 hr of observation
Symptomatic patients after 6 hr of observation require hospital admission

CNS, central nervous system.

rare case reports of patients experiencing reversible liver enzyme elevation, jaundice, and abnormal liver histology in association with trazodone therapy.[13]

Acute Toxicity

There is no established toxic dose for trazodone. As a general guideline, serious toxicity in an average adult is not expected with ingestions of less than 2 g.[13] The safety margin is reduced significantly when other medications are coingested with trazodone.[14]

The most common sign of acute trazodone poisoning is central nervous system (CNS) depression.[14,15] Other CNS-related effects include ataxia, dizziness, coma, and seizures. Trazodone rarely produces coma or seizures when it is the only drug ingested.[14] Pupils are usually of normal size but can become dilated.[16] Trazodone-induced CNS effects show marked improvement within 6 to 12 hours after ingestion and almost always are resolved within 24 hours.[14]

Orthostatic hypotension is the most frequently reported cardiovascular abnormality noted in trazodone overdose and usually responds to fluid administration.[15] Therapeutic use of trazodone has been reported occasionally to be arrhythmogenic, especially in patients with underlying cardiac risk factors such as conduction abnormalities or ischemic heart disease. This arrhythmogenic potential is increased at higher concentrations, and various dysrhythmias have been attributed to trazodone toxicity, including sinus arrest, sinus bradycardia, atrioventricular blocks, complete heart block, atrial fibrillation, and ventricular dysrhythmias (premature ventricular beats or torsades de pointes).[13] The most common ECG abnormality is moderate prolongation of the QT_c interval.[16,17] Polymorphic ventricular tachycardia (torsades de pointes) has been reported in rare cases.[16,17]

Commonly reported gastrointestinal complaints include nausea, vomiting, and nonspecific abdominal pain. Respiratory depression is observed infrequently with pure trazodone overdoses.[14,15] Priapism has been reported after an acute overdose of 3.5 g.[18] The estimated incidence of priapism ranges from 1 in 1000 to 1 in 10,000 patients at therapeutic doses. Hyponatremia has been reported in association with trazodone toxicity.[19]

Treatment

Intravenous access should be obtained and cardiac monitoring initiated on all patients. Hypotension should be treated initially with isotonic intravenous fluid administration before initiating vasopressors.

Gastrointestinal decontamination with activated charcoal theoretically is useful for patients with large overdoses presenting within the first few hours after ingestion. It is not known whether this therapy alters the patients' outcome or clinical course. Ingestion of 2000 mg or less of trazodone in adults carries a low risk of toxicity, as long as trazodone is ingested as a single agent and the patient does not have any underlying cardiac or neurologic risk factors. Ingestions of more than 2000 mg of trazodone pose a greater risk for CNS and cardiovascular toxicity.[13]

Patients who have coingested other drugs or ethanol or both have a higher incidence of coma, seizures, and respira-

tory arrest.[14] Gastric decontamination in these patients possibly may be achieved by early gastric lavage followed by administration of activated charcoal. This intervention has not been shown to be beneficial, however.

NEFAZODONE

Nefazodone (Serzone) was approved in the United States in 1995 for the treatment of depression. It is related structurally and functionally to trazodone.[20] Nefazodone inhibits serotonin reuptake and antagonizes postsynaptic 5-HT$_2$ receptors.[20] It has little affinity for other receptors except slight antagonism of postsynaptic α_1-receptors.[20] Nefazodone is available in 50-mg, 100-mg, 150-mg, 200-mg, and 250-mg tablets. The recommended effective dose for nefazodone is 300 to 600 mg/day (Table 44-3).

Clinical Pharmacology

Nefazodone is absorbed rapidly but has a bioavailability of only 20% due to extensive first-pass hepatic metabolism. Peak serum concentrations occur within 1 hour, and its apparent elimination half-life ranges from 2 to 6 hours. Nefazodone is 99% protein bound, with a relatively small volume of distribution. It has three active metabolites: hydroxynefazodone, desethylhydroxynefazodone, and *m*-CPP.[20] The activity of the hydroxynefazodone metabolite is pharmacologically equivalent to that of the parent compound. The *m*-CPP metabolite is noteworthy only because it is also a metabolite of trazodone.

Nefazodone can inhibit the metabolism of terfenadine, astemizole, and pimozide, which can lead to prolongation of the QT interval and torsades de pointes.[20] Certain benzodiazepines, such as alprazolam and triazolam, have markedly increased CNS effects in the presence of nefazodone. Carbamazepine inhibits the metabolism of nefazodone by 75%. Overall, nefazodone has a favorable side-effect profile. Compared with placebo, nefazodone has a higher incidence of headache, dizziness, drowsiness, asthenia, tremor, dry mouth, nausea, constipation, and blurred vision. It also predisposes patients to postural hypotension and priapism but not to the same degree as trazodone. Nefazodone has a U.S. FDA pregnancy category C rating (see Appendix A).

Acute Toxicity

A prospective study collected data on 1004 acute nefazodone exposures from 1995 through 1996.[21] Of all exposures, 25% of patients remained asymptomatic and another 50%

TABLE 44-3 Nefazodone Overdose
Typical therapeutic dose 300–600 mg/day
Side-effect profile similar to trazodone's but less risk of priapism
Important drug interactions that may produce significant QT interval prolongation
Limited human overdose data available but considered relatively safe
Asymptomatic patients can be discharged after 6 hr of observation

were believed to develop only minor symptoms.[21] The maximal ingested asymptomatic dose was 13,500 mg. The lowest symptomatic dose was 300 mg. The most common symptoms reported were drowsiness (17%), nausea (10%), dizziness (10%), and vomiting (8%). Hypotension was reported in 1.6% of patients. There was only one major outcome: A patient developed premature ventricular contractions, bradycardia, and hypotension. No fatalities were reported. The onset of clinical effects ranged from 1 to 4 hours.

Treatment

Nefazodone is relatively safe in overdose. Supportive care alone is sufficient in most cases.[21] Gastrointestinal decontamination with activated charcoal theoretically is warranted for all large ingestions if they present within 1 or 2 hours of overdose. Cardiac toxicity is extremely unlikely. Symptomatic patients typically return to normal after 8 to 24 hours. Asymptomatic patients can be discharged after 6 hours of observation.

BUPROPION

Bupropion (Wellbutrin) has been available in the United States since 1989 for the treatment of major depression. It also has been approved for use in smoking cessation (Zyban). Approximately 7300 bupropion exposures were reported to the American Association of Poison Control Centers Toxic Exposure Surveillance System from 1998 through 1999, accounting for 5% of all antidepressant drug exposures.[22] For smoking cessation, Zyban (150 mg) is administered either once or twice daily for no more than 12 consecutive weeks. The maximum daily dose of Zyban is 300 mg (Table 44-4). Wellbutrin comes in a variety of doses and formulations, including sustained-release tablets (100 and 150 mg) and regular-release tablets (75 and 100 mg). The recommended starting dose of Wellbutrin is 100 mg given twice daily, gradually increasing to 300 mg/day. The incidence of seizures drastically increases at doses greater than 450 mg/day, and higher doses are prohibited.[23] The combination of the two bupropion preparations, Wellbutrin and Zyban, is contraindicated due to concern for bupropion toxicity. Bupropion also is contraindicated in patients with bulimia, anorexia nervosa, and epilepsy and patients taking MAO inhibitors.[22] Bupropion has a U.S. FDA pregnancy category B designation (see Appendix A). Most toxicologic information regarding bupropion is derived from exposures to the Wellbutrin formulation. It is assumed that this information is equally applicable to Zyban exposures, and no further distinction is made in this chapter between these two bupropion products.

Clinical Pharmacology

Bupropion has a monocyclic phenylaminoketone chemical structure that resembles the structures of the phenylethylamines (e.g., amphetamine). Bupropion does not produce stimulant effects or drug-addictive behavior at therapeutic doses, however.[24] The therapeutic mechanism of action for bupropion is poorly understood but currently attributed to a weak ability to inhibit neuronal reuptake of dopamine and to a lesser extent norepinephrine and serotonin.[25,26] It does not stimulate postsynaptic receptors directly.

Bupropion is absorbed rapidly after oral administration and undergoes extensive first-pass hepatic metabolism.[26] It is highly protein bound, has an extremely large volume of distribution, and readily crosses the blood-brain barrier. Peak plasma concentrations occur within 2 hours for regular-release tablets and 3 hours for sustained-release preparations. The elimination half-life ranges from 14 to 20 hours.[26] Bupropion has one important metabolite, hydroxybupropion, which is less potent than bupropion; preferentially inhibits norepinephrine reuptake; and may contribute to seizure development.

Bupropion antidepressant therapy is well tolerated. It does not produce CNS depression, orthostatic hypotension, or cardiovascular changes or impair sexual function at therapeutic doses.[24] The most commonly reported adverse effects are of mild severity and include dry mouth, dizziness, agitation, nausea, headache, constipation, tremor, anxiety, confusion, blurred vision, and increased motor activity. Bupropion has been reported infrequently to produce catatonia, hallucinations, psychosis, and paranoia, which probably are related to its dopaminergic activity.[24]

Theoretically, abrupt discontinuation of bupropion may pose a slight risk of precipitating neuroleptic malignant syndrome because bupropion is considered a dopamine agonist. Bupropion is relatively free of significant drug interactions.[26] In general, bupropion should not be combined with SSRIs, lithium, MAO inhibitors, TCAs, dopaminergic drugs (e.g., levodopa), or drugs that are known to lower patient seizure threshold (e.g., phenothiazines).

Acute Toxicity

Bupropion has a low therapeutic index, with toxicity occurring at doses equal to or slightly greater than the maximal therapeutic dose of 450 mg/day.[27] As a general rule, significant toxicity is not expected in pure bupropion overdose with adult ingestions of less than 450 mg. The largest case series of bupropion overdoses reported that symptomatic patients ingested a mean of 2310 mg, and the smallest symptomatic dose was 200 mg.[27] Patients who remained asymptomatic ingested a mean of 1325 mg, and the largest asymptomatic dose was 4000 mg. Another study reviewed

---

TABLE 44-4 Bupropion Overdose

Maximal therapeutic dose 300 mg/day
Wellbutrin (depression) and Zyban (smoking cessation) contain bupropion
Low therapeutic index
Considered dopamine agonist (may worsen some psychiatric disorders)
Adult overdoses of <450 mg not associated with significant toxicity
Overdose commonly associated with generalized seizures and sinus tachycardia
Observe overdoses of regular-release bupropion for 8 hr
Contact poison control center or medical toxicologist for management of extended-release overdoses
Cross-reacts on amphetamine immunoassays
Admit all patients with clinical manifestations of toxicity to monitored bed

symptoms after bupropion exposures and found similar symptoms, although drug doses were not available for comparison.[22] The most commonly reported symptoms in both studies included sinus tachycardia (34% to 43%), lethargy (25% to 41%), tremor (10% to 24%), generalized seizures (19% to 21%), confusion (6% to 14%), and vomiting (13% to 14%).[22,27]

Mild hyperthermia is reported occasionally.[25] Sinus tachycardia is the most common ECG abnormality. An isolated case of moderate QT interval prolongation has been reported in conjunction with a massive bupropion overdose. Otherwise, bupropion does not produce myocardial conduction abnormalities.[25] Hypotension is unexpected in pure bupropion overdoses but has been reported in mixed-drug overdoses.[22,27] Hypertension is usually of only mild-to-moderate severity. Coma and cardiac arrest have been reported in severe bupropion overdoses.[28,29]

The hallmark of bupropion toxicity is generalized seizures. The actual incidence of seizures is unknown but approximates 20% of intentional ingestions.[22,27] There is no correlation between the development of seizures and the presence of other signs, such as sinus tachycardia. Seizures can develop in otherwise asymptomatic patients. Seizures usually occur within the first 1 to 4 hours after ingestion of regular-release bupropion. The average time of seizure onset is 3.7 hours, but they may be delayed for 8 hours.[27] Case reports suggest that sustained-release preparations may predispose patients to seizures 14 hours after exposure.[29]

Laboratory study findings usually are normal except for rare cases of mild hypokalemia.[27] As a likely consequence of its phenylethylamine-like structure, bupropion cross-reacts with amphetamines on some screening immunoassays.[30]

Treatment

A peripheral intravenous line should be established and cardiac monitoring initiated in all patients. Supportive care alone is sufficient for most patients after bupropion exposure. The possible early onset of generalized seizures should be anticipated, however. Rapid gastrointestinal decontamination with activated charcoal is theoretically beneficial for large bupropion overdoses.

Significant cardiotoxicity is not expected except in mixed-drug overdoses. Sinus tachycardia is rarely of hemodynamic significance. Most seizures are short-lived and resolve without specific treatment.[22,27] Benzodiazepines generally have been effective in stopping bupropion seizures.[27] Diphenylhydantoin (phenytoin) reportedly was effective in stopping seizure activity in a single case of bupropion-induced status epilepticus.[27]

Hospital admission to a monitored setting is recommended for all patients with seizures, sinus tachycardia, or lethargy. Asymptomatic patients who have ingested only regular-release bupropion can be medically cleared after 8 hours of observation. Similar guidelines for sustained-release bupropion preparations have not been established. Patients who have ingested more than 450 mg of sustained-release bupropion probably require longer periods of monitoring before medical clearance. Consultation with a medical toxicologist or poison control center is recommended in all bupropion overdoses, especially with sustained-release preparations.

MIRTAZAPINE

Mirtazapine (Remeron) is a tetracyclic compound structurally unrelated to other currently available antidepressants. It has been available in the United States since 1996. Mirtazapine does not inhibit neuronal amine uptake, in contrast to the other serotonergic antidepressants.[31] Instead, it blocks central presynaptic α_2-adrenergic receptors and postsynaptic serotonin receptor, subtypes 5-HT$_2$ and 5-HT$_3$ (Table 44-5).[31] This activity has the net therapeutic effect of increasing central norepinephrine and serotonin (5-HT$_1$) neurotransmission. Mirtazapine has a high inhibitory affinity for H$_1$-receptors. This explains most adverse symptoms reported at therapeutic doses, such as somnolence, dry mouth, increased appetite, and weight gain.[31,32] Mirtazapine has a low affinity for cholinergic muscarinic receptors.[32] It is supplied as 15-mg, 30-mg, and 45-mg tablets, with an average daily dose range of 15 to 45 mg. It has a U.S. FDA pregnancy category C rating (see Appendix A). Postmarketing surveillance indicated a rare incidence of agranulocytosis associated with mirtazapine.[32]

Clinical Pharmacology

Mirtazapine has a pharmacokinetic profile similar to other serotonergic antidepressants. It is absorbed rapidly and completely after oral administration. Bioavailability is approximately 50% due to significant first-pass hepatic metabolism. Peak plasma concentrations occur within 2 hours of ingestion. Mirtazapine is metabolized by the hepatic oxidase enzyme system (P-450), with only minor active metabolites. The elimination half-life for mirtazapine averages 26 hours for men and 37 hours for women. The difference in mirtazapine half-life between men and women is attributed to decreased P-450 metabolism in women. Mirtazapine is highly protein bound (85%) and has a large volume of distribution (5 L/kg).[31,32] Plasma concentrations are unlikely to be affected by attempts at extracorporeal removal.

Acute Toxicity

Mirtazapine seems to be associated with minimal toxicity in overdose. There are only two published case series[33,34] and a few isolated case reports of mirtazapine overdoses.[35,36] The most common presentation includes sedation, confusion, sinus tachycardia, and mild hypertension. Doses of 1350 mg have been tolerated without significant sequelae.[33] The risk

---

TABLE 44-5 Mirtazapine Overdose

Antagonizes α_2-receptors and postsynaptic 5-HT$_2$ and 5-HT$_3$ receptors

Net effect of increasing norepinephrine and serotonin 5-HT$_1$ receptor activity

Therapeutic dose 15–45 mg/day

Expect CNS sedation, sinus tachycardia, and mild hypertension in overdose

Symptoms typically resolve within 24 hr

Consult poison control center or medical toxicologist for management recommendations

Asymptomatic patients can be discharged after 8 hr of observation

---

CNS, central nervous system; 5-HT, 5-hydroxytryptamine.

of coma and respiratory depression is greatest at larger doses or when it is combined with other CNS-depressant drugs. Vital sign abnormalities are rarely of clinical significance and have not required specific treatment. Mirtazapine does not seem to produce ECG abnormalities other than sinus tachycardia.[33–35]

Treatment

Treatment guidelines have not been established for mirtazapine overdoses. Based on the currently available data, the following recommendations seem logical but may require modification as experience with mirtazapine increases. For this reason, medical toxicology or poison control center consultation is encouraged for most cases involving the use of mirtazapine. Mirtazapine toxicity usually resolves over 24 hours with supportive care alone.[33,34] Single-dose activated charcoal is theoretically useful after large ingestions in patients who present within the first 1 or 2 hours. Whole-bowel lavage or multiple-dose activated charcoal is unnecessary and not validated with regard to efficacy and safety. Clinically affected patients should be admitted to a monitored bed, but significant cardiac toxicity is unlikely. Asymptomatic patients can be medically cleared after 8 hours of observation.

VENLAFAXINE

Venlafaxine (Effexor) is a bicyclic compound that is structurally different from other antidepressants. It was released in the United States in 1994 for treatment of depression. In contrast to the SSRIs, venlafaxine is a nonselective inhibitor of serotonin, norepinephrine, and dopamine reuptake (Table 44-6).[37] Whether this lack of selectivity offers any advantage over SSRIs, bupropion, trazodone, nefazodone, or mirtazapine is currently unknown. Venlafaxine has no significant direct effect on presynaptic or postsynaptic neurotransmitter receptors and does not inhibit MAO.[37] It is available in 25-mg, 37.5-mg, 50-mg, 75-mg, and 100-mg tablets. The recommended starting dose is 75 mg/day, which can be increased gradually to a maximal daily dose of 225 mg. It has a U.S. FDA pregnancy category C rating (see Appendix A).

Clinical Pharmacology

When taken therapeutically, venlafaxine serum concentrations peak approximately 2 hours after ingestion. It is poorly

---

TABLE 44-6 Venlafaxine Overdose

Maximal therapeutic dose 225 mg/day
Nonspecific inhibitor of serotonin, norepinephrine, and dopamine reuptake
Has an active metabolite
May produce mild-to-moderate hypertension even at therapeutic doses
Overdoses associated with CNS depression, seizures, and sinus tachycardia
May have electrocardiogram abnormalities with QRS widening
Asymptomatic patients can be discharged after 8 hr of observation
Admit all symptomatic patients to monitored bed

CNS, central nervous system.

---

protein bound (27%), and it has a volume of distribution of 6 to 7 L/kg and a half-life of approximately 5 hours. Most of an ingested dose of venlafaxine undergoes hepatic P-450 oxidation; however, it is also a weak inhibitor of P-450 enzyme activity.[10] To date, no significant pharmacokinetic drug interactions have been reported. It has one active metabolite, *O*-desmethylvenlafaxine, which is pharmacologically similar to its parent drug except for an apparently longer half-life (11 hours). The side-effect profile for venlafaxine is similar to that for the SSRIs. The only notable exception is the occurrence of mild-to-moderate hypertension when doses exceed 225 mg/day, which is probably secondary to inhibition of norepinephrine reuptake.[37]

Acute Toxicity

There is limited clinical experience with venlafaxine toxicity. A prospective case series reported that approximately 50% of venlafaxine exposures remain asymptomatic.[38] The most common symptom reported was drowsiness, seen in one third of cases. CNS sedation occasionally progressed to coma requiring endotracheal intubation and ventilatory support.[39–42] Sympathetic nervous system stimulation, via inhibition of norepinephrine reuptake, predisposes patients to tachycardia, hypertension, diaphoresis, tremor, and mydriasis, effects frequently seen in venlafaxine overdoses.[39–42] Severe hypotension, requiring vasopressors, has been reported in a few cases.[39,43] Otherwise, most vital sign abnormalities are of moderate severity and do not require specific pharmacologic therapy. Generalized seizures are reported frequently and tend to occur early after ingestion.[44] ECG abnormalities and cardiac rhythm disturbances may include QRS and QT$_c$ interval prolongation, sinus tachycardia, and ventricular tachycardia.[39,40,44] In most cases, symptoms completely resolve gradually over 36 hours with supportive care alone.

Treatment

There are no established guidelines for treating venlafaxine overdose. All patients require at least 8 hours of observation. Venlafaxine toxicity is often precipitous[40–42] and should be anticipated in all overdoses. These patients require immediate evaluation, establishment of a peripheral intravenous line, and cardiac monitoring. Venlafaxine seems to have greater toxicity in overdose than SSRIs and probably warrants more aggressive gastrointestinal decontamination with activated charcoal. Charcoal should be given as a single dose in patients presenting within the first 1 or 2 hours after ingestion. Benzodiazepines are the anticonvulsants of choice.[40] Hypertension and sinus tachycardia rarely require specific pharmacologic therapy. Sodium bicarbonate therapy should be considered in venlafaxine overdoses associated with QRS widening greater than 100 msec.[39] All symptomatic patients should be admitted to monitored acute care units.

SELECTIVE SEROTONIN REUPTAKE INHIBITORS

SSRIs represent a structurally heterogeneous group of drugs that share a selective affinity to inhibit presynaptic serotonin reuptake without significantly affecting norepinephrine or dopamine reuptake.[2] The increase in synaptic serotonin concentrations may not explain entirely their therapeutic effects. Cellular and receptor compensatory mechanisms currently are believed to play an important role in their mechanism of action.[1] SSRIs are essentially devoid of direct presynaptic or postsynaptic receptor interactions (Table 44-7). They are associated with few unwanted pharmacologic actions, in stark contrast to TCAs.

SSRIs represent the most common form of pharmacotherapy for depression in the United States. They also are the most frequent class of antidepressants reported in drug overdoses.[3] Fatalities involving SSRIs alone are extremely rare.[45-47] There are currently six SSRIs available in the United States: fluoxetine (Prozac, released in 1988), sertraline (Zoloft, released in 1991), paroxetine (Paxil, released in 1993), fluvoxamine (Luvox, released in 1994), citalopram (Celexa, released in 1998), and escitalopram (Lexapro, released 2002). There are slight potency differences between SSRIs, but their clinical efficacies seem to be comparable. The suggested average daily doses and maximal daily doses for SSRIs are as follows: fluoxetine, average 20 to 80 mg, maximal 80 mg; paroxetine, average 20 to 50 mg, maximal 50 mg; citalopram, average 20 to 40 mg, maximal 60 mg; escitalopram, average 10 to 20 mg; sertraline, average 50 to 200 mg, maximal 200 mg; and fluvoxamine, average 50 to 300 mg, maximal 300 mg. In pregnancy, all SSRIs have a U.S. FDA category C rating (see Appendix A).

The SSRIs have similar pharmacokinetic profiles, including rapid and complete oral absorption, peak plasma levels occurring 4 to 8 hours after ingestion (citalopram, 2 to 4 hours), significant first-pass hepatic metabolism, high degree of protein binding (except citalopram), and large volume of distribution. Fluoxetine is the only SSRI with a clinically significant active metabolite, norfluoxetine, which is equal in potency to fluoxetine.[48] The apparent half-lives of fluoxetine and norfluoxetine are 2 to 4 days and 7 to 14 days, respectively. The effects of fluoxetine may last 5 weeks because of the prolonged period necessary to allow for norfluoxetine metabolism. Sertraline and paroxetine have similar apparent half-lives of approximately 24 hours. The apparent half-life of citalopram is estimated at 33 hours, whereas fluvoxamine has the shortest half-life at 15 hours.[48] The SSRIs are metabolized almost entirely by the hepatic cytochrome P-450 isoenzyme system. It increasingly is recognized that SSRIs can inhibit

TABLE 44-7 Selective Serotonin Reuptake Inhibitor Overdose

Have little ability to inhibit other amine reuptake except serotonin
Hyponatremia a well-recognized complication of SSRI drug therapy
Fluoxetine (Prozac) has a long half-life and an active metabolite
Metabolized by hepatic enzymes and may produce drug interactions
Most likely class of antidepressants to produce serotonin syndrome
High therapeutic index and relatively safe in overdose
Electrocardiogram abnormalities unexpected except with citalopram and fluoxetine
Asymptomatic patients can be discharged after 6 hr of observation

SSRI, selective serotonin reuptake inhibitor.

the metabolism of other drugs dependent on the cytochrome P-450 isoenzyme system.[2,6,48] Clinically significant drug interactions are most likely to occur with drugs that have a low therapeutic index, such as TCAs, antipsychotics, anticonvulsants, benzodiazepines, opiates, theophylline, warfarin, terfenadine, astemizole, and pimozide.[2,6,48]

Serotonin has varying effects on the dopaminergic system. In many cases, extrapyramidal symptoms, such as dystonic reactions, akathisia, dyskinesia, hypokinesia, and parkinsonian symptoms, have been reported in association with SSRI therapy.[49] Consequently, SSRIs should be used cautiously with antipsychotic agents because SSRIs can potentiate antidopaminergic activity. A withdrawal syndrome consisting of nonspecific neurologic, psychiatric, and gastrointestinal symptoms has been described in conjunction with abrupt SSRI discontinuation.[50] It is less likely to occur with fluoxetine because it has a long-acting metabolite.

Acute Toxicity

The greatest amount of SSRI overdose experience has been with fluoxetine.[45-47] Information obtained involving the other SSRIs is consistent with the information accumulated on fluoxetine.[51-55] For the most part, all SSRIs produce similar toxicity in overdose. All of the SSRIs are characterized by a high toxic-to-therapeutic ratio, and fatalities are uncommon with pure SSRI overdoses. Approximately 25% to 50% of all patients and 75% to 90% of pediatric patients remain asymptomatic after SSRI overdose.[3,45,51,52] The most common effects seen in SSRI overdose include nausea, vomiting, sedation, tremor, and sinus tachycardia.[45-47,51-55] These are almost identical to the side-effect profile of SSRIs except for sinus tachycardia, which is more common in overdose and rarely reported as an adverse effect.[47] Less frequently observed effects include mydriasis, seizures, diarrhea, agitation, hallucinations, hypertension, and hypotension. Sertraline may produce mild CNS stimulation in pediatric patients.[53] Sinus bradycardia was observed more frequently in fluvoxamine overdoses than with other SSRIs.[54] Citalopram produced QRS widening in approximately one third of cases when more than 600 mg was ingested.[55] In another case series, prolongation of the QT interval has been reported in association with significant citalopram ingestions.[56] Other SSRIs rarely have been reported to produce similar ECG abnormalities.[57] In most cases, the ECG abnormalities gradually resolve over 24 hours. Tachycardia, mild hypotension, and lethargy are seen more commonly when SSRIs are combined with ethanol. Mixed-drug ingestions can produce a wide variety of additional symptoms, depending on the coingestant toxicity. Serotonin syndrome can occur as a consequence of acute SSRI overdose.[58] Routine laboratory studies usually are normal in SSRI overdoses. SSRI therapy has been associated with a drug-induced syndrome of inappropriate antidiuretic hormone secretion, which may result in symptomatic hyponatremia.[59,60]

Treatment

Patients who intentionally overdose with SSRIs require establishment of a peripheral intravenous line and cardiac monitoring. The value of gastrointestinal decontamination in

SSRI poisoning, if any, is not established. Based on the high therapeutic index and low likelihood of serious toxicity, single-dose activated charcoal (1 g/kg) is rational only for large ingestions, particularly if this can be administered within 1 hour after overdose. All patients should be observed for at least 6 hours, during which time supportive care generally is all that is required.[4,8,51–55] Psychiatric evaluation is warranted for intentional ingestions. Hospital admission is recommended for all patients who remain tachycardic or lethargic 6 hours after ingestion. Patients at higher risk for complications include patients with underlying seizure disorders, symptoms of serotonin syndrome, or mixed-drug overdoses that have the potential for additional or delayed toxicity. The use of sodium bicarbonate therapy has been reported in cases of SSRI-induced QRS prolongation[57]; however, the benefit of this intervention has not been established. If used, sodium bicarbonate should be administered in a manner identical to that described in Chapter 42 for TCAs. Benzodiazepines are recommended as initial anticonvulsant therapy. Barbiturates probably are equally effective compared with benzodiazepines but are more sedating. Delayed onset of serotonin syndrome and extrapyramidal reactions are theoretical possibilities that should be considered in all patients.[58]

REFERENCES

1. Gareri P, Falconi U, De Fazio P, et al: Conventional and new antidepressant drugs in the elderly. Prog Neurobiol 61:353–396, 2000.
2. Mourille P, Stokes PE: Risks and benefits of selective serotonin reuptake inhibitors in the treatment of depression. Drug Saf 18:57–82, 1998.
3. Litovitz TI, Klein-Schwartz W, Rodgers GC, et al: 2001 Annual Report of the American Association of Poison Control Centers Toxic Exposure Surveillance System. Am J Emerg Med 20:391–401, 2002.
4. Phillips S, Brent J, Kulig K, et al: Fluoxetine versus tricyclic antidepressants: Prospective multicenter study of antidepressant drug overdoses. J Emerg Med 15:439–445, 1997.
5. Caccia S: Metabolism of newer antidepressants: An overview of the pharmacological and pharmacokinetic implications. Clin Pharmacokinet 34:281–302, 1998.
6. DeVane CL: Pharmacokinetics of the newer antidepressants: Clinical relevance. Am J Med 97(Suppl 6A):13S-23S, 1994.
7. Anderson DT, Fritz KL, Muto JJ: Distribution of mirtazapine in thirteen postmortem cases. J Anal Toxicol 23:544–548, 1999.
8. Rohrig TP, Prouty RW: Fluoxetine overdose: A case report. J Anal Toxicol 13:305–307, 1989.
9. Martin A, Pounder DJ: Post-mortem toxico-kinetics of trazodone. Forensic Sci Int 56:201–207, 1992.
10. Jaffe PD, Batziris HP, van der Hoeven P, et al: A study involving venlafaxine overdoses: Comparison of fatal and therapeutic concentrations in postmortem specimens. J Forensic Sci 44:193–196, 1999.
11. Mitchell PB: Drug interactions of clinical significance with selective serotonin reuptake inhibitors. Drug Saf 17:390–406, 1997.
12. Haria M, Fitton A, McTavish D: Trazodone: A review of its pharmacology, therapeutic use in depression and therapeutic potential in other disorders. Drugs Aging 4:331–355, 1994.
13. Mills KC: Trazodone toxicity: Current concepts. Top Emerg Med 15:37–46, 1993.
14. Henry JA, Ali CJ: Trazodone overdosage: Experience from a poisons information service. Hum Toxicol 2:353–356, 1983.
15. Wedin GP, Oderda GM, Kelin-Schwartz W, et al: Relative toxicity of cyclic antidepressants. Ann Emerg Med 15:797–804, 1986.
16. de Meester A, Carbutti G, Gabriel L, et al: Fatal overdose with trazodone: Case report and literature review. Acta Clin Belg 56:258–261, 2001.
17. Tibbles PM, Burns MJ, Spencer FA, et al: Trazodone cardiotoxicity following overdose. J Toxicol Clin Toxicol 35:499, 1997.
18. Gamble DE, Peterson LG: Trazodone overdose: Four years of experience from voluntary reports. J Clin Psychiatry 47:544–546, 1986.
19. Vanpee D, Laloyaux P, Gillet JB: Seizure and hyponatremia after overdose of trazodone. Am J Emerg Med 17:430–431, 1999.
20. Cyr M, Brown CS: Nefazodone: Its place among antidepressants. Ann Pharmacother 30:1006–1012, 1996.
21. Benson BE, Mathiason M, Dahl B, et al: Toxicities and outcomes associated with nefazodone poisoning: An analysis of 1,338 exposures, Am J Emerg Med 18:587–592, 2000.
22. Belson MG, Kelley TR: Bupropion exposures: Clinical manifestations and medical outcome. J Emerg Med 23:223–230, 2002.
23. Davidson J: Seizures and bupropion. J Clin Psychiatry 50:256–261, 1989.
24. Shopson B: Bupropion: A new clinical profile in the psychobiology of depression. J Clin Psychiatry 44:140–142, 1983.
25. Storrow AB: Bupropion overdose and seizure. Am J Emerg Med 12:183–184, 1994.
26. Goodnick PJ: Pharmacokinetics of second generation antidepressants: Bupropion. Psychopharmacol Bull 27:513–519, 1991.
27. Spiller HA, Ramoska EA, Krenzelok EP, et al: Bupropion overdose: A 3-year multicenter retrospective analysis. Am J Emerg Med 12:43–45, 1994.
28. Harris CR, Gualtieri J, Stark G: Fatal bupropion overdose. J Toxicol Clin Toxicol 35:321–324, 1997.
29. Bergman F, Bleich S, Wischer S, et al: Seizure and cardiac arrest during bupropion SR treatment. J Clin Psychopharmacol 22:630–631, 2002.
30. Weintraub D, Linder MW: Amphetamine-positive toxicology screen secondary to bupropion. Depress Anxiety 12:53–54, 2000.
31. Stimmel GL, Dopheide JA, Stahl SM: Mirtazapine: An antidepressant with noradrenergic and specific serotonergic effects. Pharmacotherapy 17:10–21, 1997.
32. Kasper S, Praschak-Rieder N, Tauscher J, et al: A risk-benefit assessment of mirtazapine in the treatment of depression. Drug Saf 17:251–264, 1997.
33. Valazquez C, Carlson A, Stokes KA, et al: Relative safety of mirtazapine overdose. Vet Hum Toxicol 43:342–344, 2001.
34. Bremmer JD, Wingard P, Walshe TA: Safety of mirtazepine in overdose. J Clin Psychiatry 59:233–235, 1998.
35. Gerristen AW: Safety in overdose of mirtazapine: A case report. J Clin Psychiatry 58:271, 1997.
36. Hoes MJAJM, Zeijpveld JHB: First report of mirtazapine overdose. Int Clin Psychopharmacol 11:147, 1996.
37. Rudolph RL, Derivan AT: The safety and tolerability of venlafaxine hydrochloride: Analysis of the clinical trials database. J Clin Pharmacol 16(Suppl 2):54S–61S, 1996.
38. Setzer SC, Anderson DA, Lawler RJ, et al: Acute venlafaxine overdose: A multicenter study. J Toxicol Clin Toxicol 33:496–497, 1995.
39. Combes A, Peytavin G, Theron D: Conduction disturbances associated with venlafaxine. Ann Intern Med 134:166–167, 2001.
40. Leaf EV: Comment: Venlafaxine overdose and seizures. Ann Pharmacother 32:135–136, 1998.
41. Coorey AN, Wenck DJ: Venlafaxine overdose. Med J Aust 168:523, 1998.
42. Fantaskey A, Burkhart KK: A case report of venlafaxine toxicity. Clin Toxicol 33:359–361, 1995.
43. Banham NDG: Fatal venlafaxine overdose. Med J Aust 169:445–448, 1998.
44. Peano C, Leiken JB, Hanashiro PK: Seizures, ventricular tachycardia, and rhabdomyolysis as a result of ingestion of venlafaxine and lamotrigine. Ann Emerg Med 30:704–708, 1997.
45. Borys DJ, Setzer SC, Ling LJ: Acute fluoxetine overdose: A report of 234 cases. Am J Emerg Med 10:115–120, 1992.
46. Peretti S, Judge R, Hindmarch I: Safety and tolerability considerations: Tricyclic antidepressants vs. selective serotonin reuptake inhibitors. Acta Psychiatr Scand 101(Suppl 403):17–25, 2000.
47. Barbey JT, Roose SP: SSRI safety in overdose. J Clin Psychiatry 59(Suppl 15):42–48, 1998.
48. Catterson ML, Preskorn SH: Pharmacokinetics of selective serotonin reuptake inhibitors: Clinical relevance. Pharmacol Toxicol 78:203–208, 1996.
49. Caley CF: Extrapyramidal reactions and the selective serotonin reuptake inhibitors. Ann Pharmacother 31:1481–1489, 1997.
50. Coupland NJ, Bell CJ, Potokar JP: Serotonin reuptake inhibitor withdrawal. J Clin Psychopharmacol 16:356–362, 1996.
51. Myers LB, Krenzelok EP: Paroxetine (Paxil) overdose: A pediatric focus. Vet Hum Toxicol 39:86–88, 1997.
52. Lau GT, Horowitz BZ: Sertraline overdose. Acad Emerg Med 3:132–136, 1996.
53. Klein-Schwartz W, Anderson B: Analysis of sertraline-only overdoses. Am J Emerg Med 14:456–458, 1996.
54. Garner R, Azoyan P, Chataigner D, et al: Acute fluvoxamine poisoning. J Int Med Res 21:197–208, 1993.

55. Personne M, Sjoberg G, Person H: Citalopram overdose—review of cases treated in Swedish hospitals. Clin Toxicol 35:237–240, 1997.

56. Catalano G, Catalano MC, Epstein MA, et al: QTc interval prolongation associated with citalopram overdose: A case report and literature review. Clin Neuropharmacol 24:158–162, 2001.

57. Graudins A, Vossler C, Wang R: Fluoxetine-induced cardiotoxicity with response to bicarbonate therapy. Am J Emerg Med 15:501–503, 1997.

58. Brendel DH, Bodkin JA, Yang JM: Massive sertraline overdose. Ann Emerg Med 36:524–526, 2000.

59. Bradley ME, Foote EF, Lee EN, et al: Sertraline-associated syndrome of inappropriate antidiuretic hormone: Case report and review of the literature. Pharmacotherapy 16:680–683, 1996.

60. Johnson CR, Hoejlyng N: Hyponatremia following acute overdose with paroxetine. Int J Clin Pharmacol Ther 36:333–335, 1998.

CHAPTER 45

Neuroleptic Agents

Michael J. Burns

The discovery of chlorpromazine and other traditional antipsychotic agents in the early 1950s revolutionized the management of schizophrenia and led to a dramatic reduction in the number of hospitalizations necessary for patients with psychosis. Shortly after their introduction, however, it was noted that these agents often produced disabling neurologic side effects (e.g., sedation, extrapyramidal side effects [EPS], tardive dyskinesia [TD]) and were ineffective against the negative symptoms (e.g., anhedonia, apathy, inactivity, poverty of thought, social withdrawal) and neurocognitive deficits of schizophrenia. Initially, it was thought that EPS were linked inextricably to antipsychotic drug action. The introduction of clozapine in 1990 and other so-called atypical agents shortly thereafter has further revolutionized the management of schizophrenia. Compared with traditional antipsychotics, atypical agents produce minimal EPS at clinically effective antipsychotic doses and seem to be more effective for the negative symptoms and neurocognitive deficits of schizophrenia. This chapter describes in detail the pharmacology and toxicology of traditional and atypical antipsychotic agents.

The antipsychotics commonly are referred to either as *neuroleptics*, owing to their propensity to cause EPS, or as *major tranquilizers*, owing to their ability to cause sedation. These terms are misleading, however, because they refer to nonessential features of these agents. The newer atypical agents separate therapeutic from adverse effects; they are more likely to produce antipsychotic effects without producing EPS or sedation. The term *antipsychotic* is preferred by some experts but also is misleading.[1] Although these agents are used primarily to treat schizophrenia and other psychotic disorders, they also are used to facilitate induction of general anesthesia and to treat the manic phase of bipolar illness, agitated behavior, drug-associated hallucinations and delirium, migraine and tension headaches, nausea and vomiting, intractable hiccoughs, pruritus, and many extrapyramidal movement disorders (e.g., tics, chorea). Currently the terms *neuroleptic* and *antipsychotic* may be used interchangeably to classify these agents.

Poisoning by neuroleptic agents may occur after therapeutic doses or accidental or intentional overdose. Toxicity often results from an extension of pharmacologic actions and primarily manifests as neurologic and cardiovascular abnormalities. Neuroleptic agents have a wide therapeutic index; death after overdose is rare, particularly if medical care is initiated in a timely manner. Death most commonly occurs when neuroleptics have been coingested with other agents or after the ingestion of chlorpromazine, loxapine, mesoridazine, or thioridazine.[2,3] It has been estimated that the most toxic neuroleptic agents cause 1 death from poisoning for every 1000 patient-years of use.[2] In 1998, 8364 neuroleptic exposures were reported to U.S. poison centers, of which 294 (3.5%) resulted in major toxicity and 13 (0.2%) resulted in death.[4]

CLASSIFICATION

Currently, more than 40 neuroleptics are clinically available worldwide, and numerous others are in various stages of development. Neuroleptics are classified most commonly by structure, pharmacologic profile, and whether they are typical (traditional, conventional) or atypical (novel, second-generation). Neuroleptics are a structurally diverse group of heterocyclic compounds; 13 different chemical classes are available for clinical use worldwide, including benzamide, benzisothiazole, benzisoxazole, butyrophenone, dibenzodiazepine, dibenzoxazepine, dibenzothiazepine, diphenylbutylpiperidine, dihydroindolone, phenothiazine, quinolinone, rauwolfia alkaloid, and thioxanthene derivatives (Table 45-1). The phenothiazine and thioxanthene agents are subdivided further into three groups (aliphatic, piperidine, and piperazine) based on side-chain substitution of the central ring (Fig. 45-1). The nature of the substitution influences pharmacologic activity. Compared with the piperazine subclass, aliphatic (e.g., chlorpromazine) and piperidine (e.g., thioridazine) phenothiazines have lower antipsychotic potency and a lower incidence of EPS but have a higher incidence of sedation, hypotension, and anticholinergic effects.[5] Aside from the phenothiazine class, structure-activity relationships have not been elucidated for most neuroleptics. Neuroleptic classification based on chemical structure has little clinical utility.

It is more useful to classify neuroleptics based on relative receptor binding profiles (Table 45-2). Because clinical toxicity is often the result of exaggerated pharmacologic activity, knowledge of a neuroleptic's relative receptor binding can be used to predict adverse effects that will occur after therapeutic doses and overdose.[6-8] Clinically, agents are considered atypical if they

Produce minimal EPS at clinically effective antipsychotic doses

Have a low propensity to cause TD with long-term treatment

Are effective for treating the positive (delusions, disorganized behavior, hallucinations) and negative symptoms of schizophrenia[1,6-10]

TABLE 45-1 Neuroleptic Agents

STRUCTURAL CLASS	GENERIC NAME (TRADE NAME)	AFFINITY OF NEUROLEPTIC AGENT FOR D_2-DOPAMINE RECEPTOR (POTENCY)*	DAILY DOSE RANGE (mg)
Typical Agents			
Butyrophenone	Droperidol (Inapsine)	3+	1.25–30
	Haloperidol (Haldol)	2+	1–30
Dihydroindolone	Molindone (Moban)	1+	15–225
	Oxypertine[†]		
Diphenylbutylpiperidine	Pimozide (Orap)	2+	1–20
	Fluspirilene[†]		
Phenothiazine			
Aliphatic	Chlorpromazine (Thorazine)	2+	25–2000
	Promazine (Sparine)		50–1000
	Promethazine (Phenergan)	2+	25–150
	Levomepromazine[†]	2+	
	Triflupromazine (Vesprin)		5–90
Piperazine	Acetophenazine (Tindal)		40–400
	Fluphenazine (Prolixin)	3+	0.5–30
	Perphenazine (Trilafon)	3+	4–64
	Prochlorperazine (Compazine)	2+	10–150
	Trifluoperazine (Stelazine)	3+	2–40
	Thiethylperazine (Torecan)		10–30
Piperidine	Mesoridazine (Serentil)	2+	30–400
	Thioridazine (Mellaril, Millazine)	2+	20–800
Thioxanthene	Chlorprothixene (Taractan)	2+	30–600
	Clopenthixol[†]	3+	
	Flupentixol[†]	3+	
	Thiothixene (Navane)	3+	6–60
	Zuclopenthixol (Clopixol)[†]	3+	
Atypical Agents			
Benzamides	Amisulpride	2+	100–1200
	Raclopride	3+	5–8
	Remoxipride	1+	150–600
	Sulpiride	2+	100–1600
	Sultopride		
Benzisothiazole	Ziprasidone (Zeldox)[†]	3+	40–160
Benzisoxazole	Risperidone (Risperdal)	3+	2–16
	Iloperidone[†]		
Dibenzodiazepine	Clothiapine[†]		
	Clozapine (Clozaril, Leponex)	1+	150–900
Dibenzoxazepine	Loxapine (Loxitane)	1+	20–250
	Savoxepin[†]		
Dibenzothiazepine	Quetiapine (Seroquel)	1+	300–600
	Zotepine[†]	2+	150–300
Imidazolidinone	Sertindole (Serlect)[†]	3+	12–24
Quinolinone	Aripiprazole (Abilify)	2+	10–30
Thienobenzodiazepine	Olanzapine (Zyprexa)	2+	5–20

*A higher numerical value indicates greater binding affinity (greater antagonism) at D_2-receptor. Binding affinity (potency) at D_2-receptor correlates with daily dose range. 0 = minimal to none; 1+ = low; 2+ = moderate; 3+ = high to very high.
[†]Not currently available for clinical use in the United States.

CLINICAL PHARMACOLOGY

D_2-dopaminergic receptor antagonism (Fig. 45-2) seems to be necessary for antipsychotic effects; currently, there is no effective antipsychotic devoid of this property.[1,5–7] Neuroleptics bind to and antagonize presynaptic (autoreceptor) and postsynaptic D_2-receptors.[5] Initially, this antagonism stimulates dopamine neurons to synthesize and release more dopamine. With continued neuroleptic treatment, however, depolarization inactivation occurs, and decreased production and release of dopamine occur along with continued postsynaptic D_2-receptor antagonism.[5,10]

For most neuroleptics, the affinity (potency) for the D_2-receptor correlates with the daily dose used to treat schizophrenia and the likelihood of producing EPS.[1,7,11] Antagonism of mesolimbic D_2-receptors is believed to

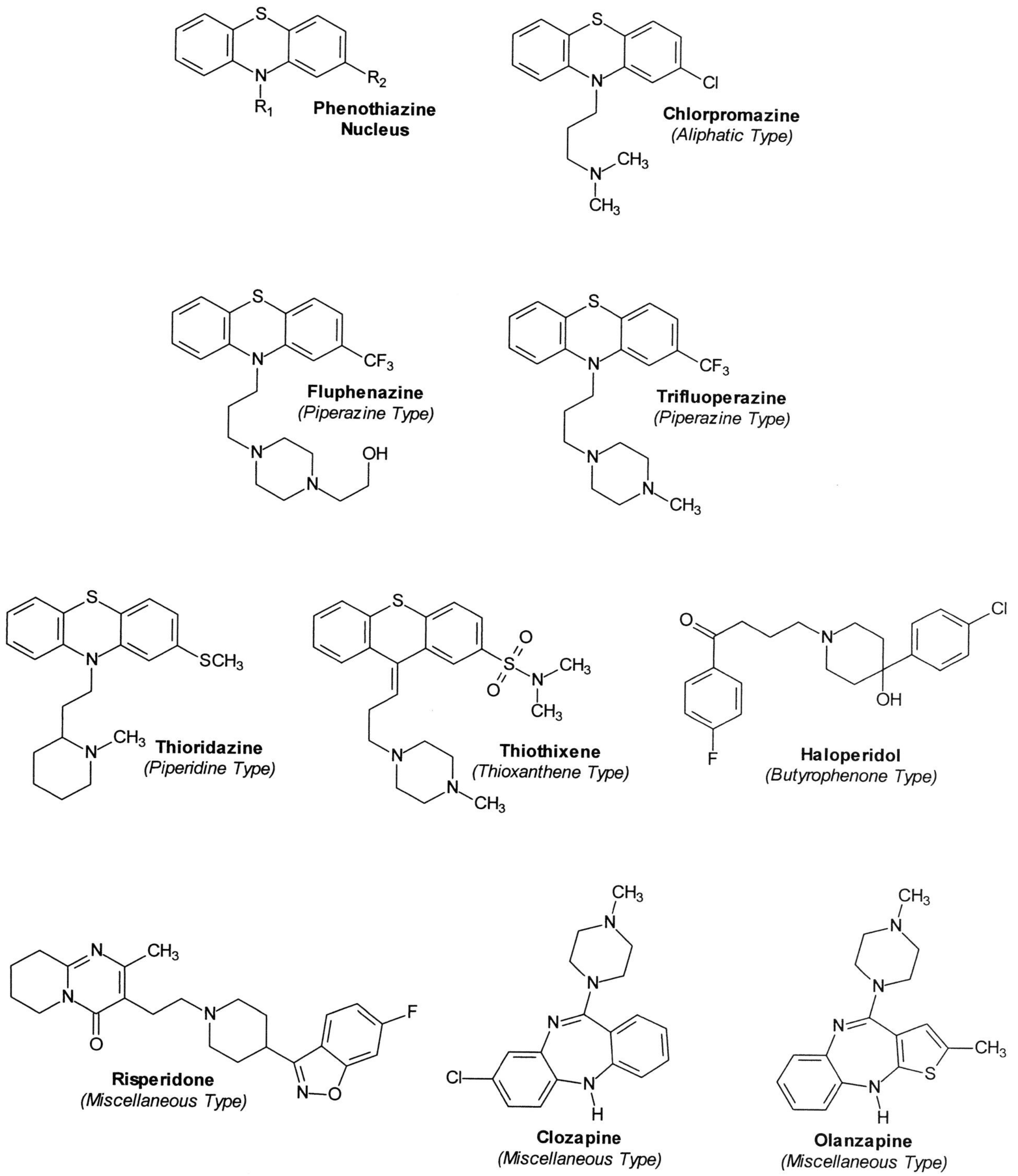

FIGURE 45-1

Chemical structures of various antipsychotic agents.

mediate antipsychotic effects (positive symptom amelioration). Based on in vivo radioligand binding studies with positron emission tomography (PET), the therapeutic effects of neuroleptics correlate with 70% or greater mesolimbic D_2-receptor occupancy.[6,12] Simultaneous antagonism of mesocortical D_2-receptors, however, is believed to exacerbate cognitive impairment and the negative symptoms of schizophrenia.[13] Blockade of nigrostriatal D_2-receptors produces EPS (e.g., acute dystonia, parkinsonism, akathisia). Agents with high affinity for D_2-receptors (e.g., fluphenazine,

TABLE 45-2 Relative Neuroreceptor Affinities for Neuroleptics*

NEUROLEPTIC AGENT	H_1	α_1	α_2	M_1	$5\text{-}HT_{2A}$	Other Receptor Binding	EPS RISK†
Typical Agents							
Chlorpromazine	2+	3+	0	1+	3+	D_1, D_3, D_4	1+
Fluphenazine	0	0	0	0	0		3+
Haloperidol	0	1+	0	0	1+	D_1, D_4, σ	3+
Loxapine	3+	3+	0	2+	3+	D_4, blocks NE reuptake	1+
Mesoridazine	3+	3+		1+			1+
Molindone	0	0	1+	0	0		3+
Perphenazine	1+	1+		0			3+
Pimozide	0	1+		0	1+		3+
Prochlorperazine	1+	1+		0	0		3+
Thioridazine	2+	3+	0	3+	2+		1+
Thiothixene	0	0	0	0	0		3+
Trifluoperazine	0	1+		0	1+		3+
Atypical Agents							
Amisulpride	0	0	0	0	0	D_3	1+
Aripiprazole	1+	1+	0	0	3+	D_3, 5-HT$_{2C}$, 5-HT$_7$	0
Clozapine	3+	3+	3+	3+	3+	D_1, D_4, M$_2$, M$_3$, M$_4$, M$_5$, 5-HT$_{2C}$, 5-HT$_{2D}$, 5-HT$_3$, 5-HT$_6$, 5-HT$_7$; blocks NE reuptake	0
Olanzapine	2+	2+	0	3+	3+	D_1, D_3, D_4, M$_2$, M$_3$, M$_4$, M$_5$, 5-HT$_{1C}$, 5-HT$_3$, 5-HT$_6$	0
Quetiapine	3+	3+	0	3+	1+	5-HT$_{1A}$, D_1	0
Remoxipride	0	0		0	0	σ	1+
Risperidone	0	2+	1+	0	3+	D_1, D_4	1+
Sertindole	0	1+	0	0	3+	5-HT$_{1C}$, 5-HT$_{2C}$	
Ziprasidone	0	3+	0	0	3+	5-HT$_{1A}$, 5-HT$_{1C}$, 5-HT$_{1D}$, 5-HT$_{2C}$, D_1; blocks NE, 5-HT reuptake	0
Zotepine	2+	0	2+	0	3+	D_1, D_3, D_4, 5-HT$_{2C}$; blocks NE reuptake	1+

*Relative neuroreceptor affinity (neuroreceptor affinity at receptor X/dopamine D_2-receptor affinity) indicates relative receptor antagonism at therapeutic (D_2-blocking) antipsychotic doses. 0 = minimal to none; 1+ = low; 2+ = moderate; 3+ = high; 4+ = very high.
†A higher M_1 and $5\text{-}HT_2$ relative neuroreceptor affinity confers a lower EPS risk.
EPS, extrapyramidal side effects; NE, norepinephrine.
Adapted from references 6 through 8, 108, and 132 through 137.

thiothixene, haloperidol) have a high likelihood of producing EPS.[6] Agents with low D_2-receptor affinity (e.g., clozapine, quetiapine) or agents that selectively antagonize limbic D_2-receptors over receptors in the nigrostriatum (e.g., sulpiride, remoxipride, raclopride) are less likely to produce EPS.[1,7–10] Data from PET studies show that EPS are seen with nigrostriatal D_2-receptor occupancy at 80% or greater.[6,12] At therapeutic doses of most conventional neuroleptics, there is minimal separation of D_2-receptor occupancies in the mesolimbic and nigrostriatal areas.[12]

Blockade of D_2-receptors in the area postrema (chemoreceptor trigger zone) of the medulla oblongata mediates the antiemetic action of neuroleptics. Antagonism of D_2-receptors in the anterior pituitary (tuberoinfundibular pathway) stimulates prolactin secretion and may result in galactorrhea, gynecomastia, menstrual changes, and sexual dysfunction.[6] D_2-receptor blockade in the anterior hypothalamus impairs temperature regulation and may result in hypothermia or hyperthermia, depending on ambient temperature.[5] D_2-receptor antagonism in the hypothalamus and nigrostriatum mediates the neuroleptic malignant syndrome (see Chapter 26), a rare hyperthermic condition associated with neuroleptic therapy.

A novel class of antipsychotic agents, called dopamine system stabilizers, has recently emerged. These agents (e.g., aripiprazole) function as partial agonists of the D_2-receptor; they reduce dopaminergic neurotransmission when such activity is excessive and enhance dopaminergic activity when such activity is deficient. These agents work to restore dopamine neurotransmission to the normal range and provide antipsychotic effects while

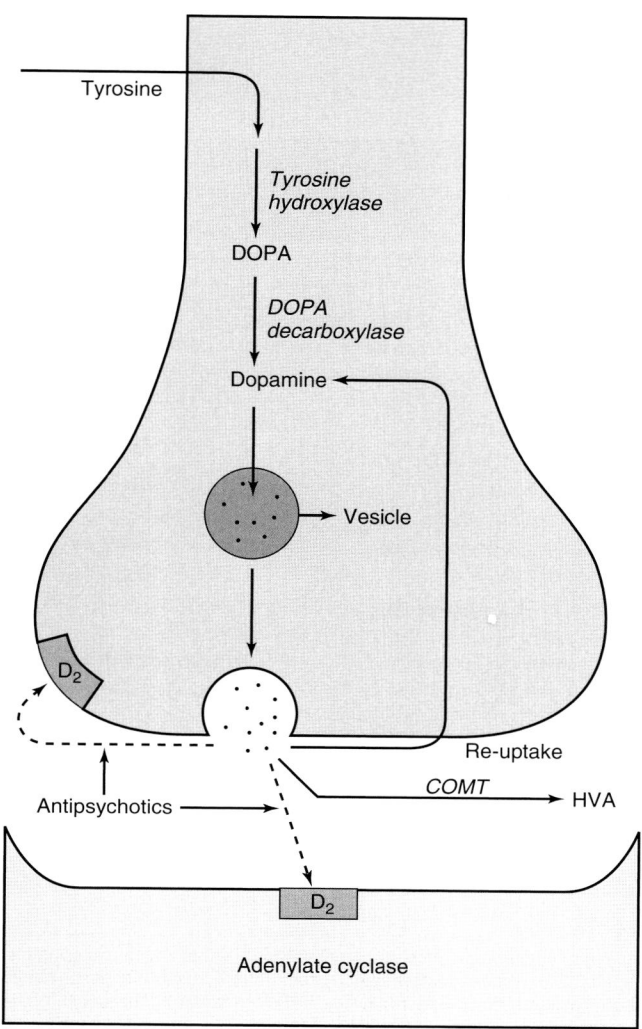

FIGURE 45-2

The release and inactivation of dopamine and blockade of the D_2-receptor by antipsychotics. COMT, catechol *O*-methyltransferase; HVA, hydroxy-vanillic acid. *(From Brody TM, Larner J, Minneman KP [eds]: Human Pharmacology: Molecular to Clinical, 3rd ed. St. Louis, Mosby, 1998, p 342.)*

minimizing adverse effects from excessive D_2-receptor antagonism.

Neuroleptics are competitive antagonists at a wide variety of neuroreceptors; each agent has a unique pharmacologic profile that determines its clinical profile. Because D_2-receptor potency closely correlates with the dose used to treat psychosis, the likelihood of an individual's developing effects from other neuroreceptors depends on the relative binding affinity at these receptor sites compared with that at the D_2-receptor (see Table 45-2).[6,14] Relative binding affinity data can be used to predict adverse effects at therapeutic doses and overdose. Agents with high relative α_1-adrenergic antagonism (e.g., aliphatic and piperidine phenothiazines, clozapine, olanzapine, risperidone, ziprasidone, sertindole) are likely to produce orthostatic hypotension, reflex tachycardia, miosis, and nasal congestion. High relative α_2-adrenergic receptor antagonism

(e.g., clozapine, risperidone) may result in sympathomimetic effects (i.e., tachycardia). High relative H_1-histamine receptor binding (e.g., aliphatic and piperidine phenothiazines, clozapine, loxapine, olanzapine, quetiapine) produces central nervous system (CNS) depression, appetite stimulation, and hypotension. Agents with high relative M_1-muscarinic receptor binding (e.g., aliphatic and piperidine phenothiazines, clozapine, olanzapine) produce central and peripheral anticholinergic stigmata (e.g., agitation, blurred vision, delirium, dry skin and mucous membranes, hallucinations, hypertension, ileus, mydriasis, tachycardia, urinary retention). Sialorrhea, a feature unique to clozapine, likely is mediated by its partial agonism at M_1- and M_4-receptors.[6] High relative potencies at M_1-receptors and 5-HT_{1A}- and 5-HT_{2A}-serotonin receptors are inversely related to the likelihood of EPS (Fig. 45-3; see Table 45-2).[6,10,15-17] The ability to block norepinephrine reuptake and antagonize the $GABA_A$ receptor may mediate partly the high incidence of seizures with certain agents (e.g., clozapine, loxapine). The clinical effects that result from neuroleptic binding at other neuroreceptor subtypes (see Table 45-2) are not well understood.

One or more of several different pharmacologic mechanisms define drug atypia. Although these mechanisms are incompletely understood, atypical agents have been subdivided into four functional groups as follows:

1. D_2-receptor, D_3-receptor antagonists (e.g., amisulpride, remoxipride, raclopride, sulpiride)
2. D_2-receptor, α_1-receptor, 5-HT_{2A}-receptor antagonists (e.g., risperidone, sertindole, ziprasidone), also called *serotonin-dopamine antagonists*
3. D_2-receptor, 5-HT_{1A}-receptor partial agonists, 5-HT_{2A}-receptor antagonists (e.g., aripiprazole), also called *serotonin-dopamine system stabilizers*
4. Broad-spectrum, multireceptor antagonists (e.g., clozapine, olanzapine, quetiapine)[8,18]

Characteristics Associated with Atypical Behavior of Neuroleptics

Low D_2-receptor potency (high milligram drug dosing)
Low D_2-receptor occupancy (<70%) by positron emission tomography in mesolimbic and nigrostriatal areas at therapeutic drug doses
High affinities for M_1-, D_1-, 5-HT_{1A}-, and 5-HT_{2A}-receptors relative to D_2-receptors
Selective mesolimbic D_2-receptor antagonism
Broad multireceptor antagonism
Partial agonist activity at D_2- and 5-HT_{1A}-receptors
Minimal propensity to elevate serum prolactin concentrations

Adapted from references 6 through 10, 12, 15, and 16.

Neuroleptics with a high relative 5-HT_{2A} binding affinity (5-HT_{2A}-to-D_2 receptor binding ratio >1) have a lower likelihood of producing EPS and mitigate the negative symptoms of schizophrenia by disinhibiting the dopamine system in the striatum and prefrontal cortex (see Fig. 45-3).[15,16,19] Normally, dopamine neurons in the nigrostriatum and

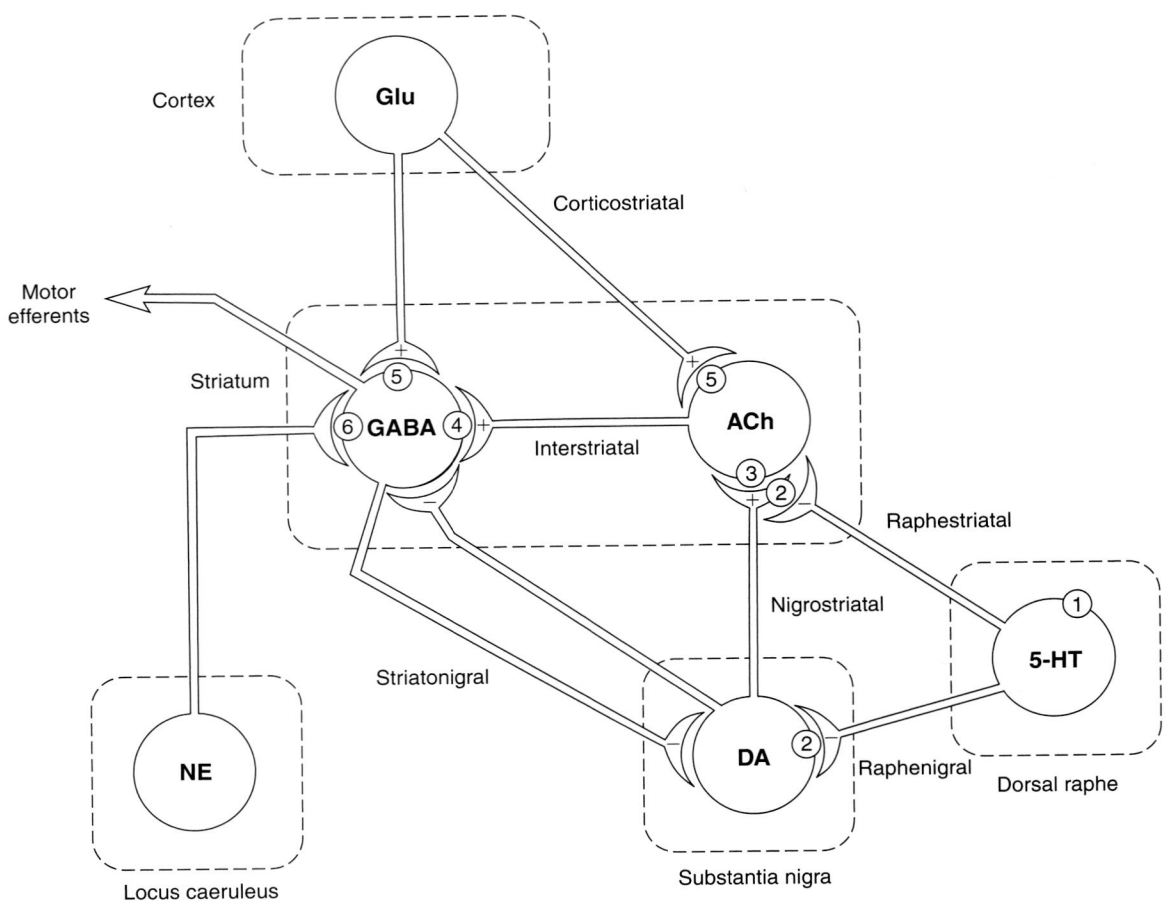

FIGURE 45-3

Schematic diagram of the complex neurotransmitter interactions that influence the appearance of extrapyramidal side effects with neuroleptics. 1, Inhibitory 5-HT$_{1A}$-somatodendritic autoreceptors; 2, inhibitory 5-HT$_2$-heteroreceptors; 3, excitatory postsynaptic D$_2$-receptors; 4, excitatory postsynaptic M$_1$-receptors; 5, excitatory postsynaptic NMDA-glutaminergic receptors; 6, inhibitory postsynaptic GABA$_A$-receptors. 5-HT$_{1A}$-receptor agonists and 5-HT$_2$-receptor antagonists release the nigrostriatal dopamine system from inhibition and decrease extrapyramidal side effects. GABA$_A$-receptor agonists and M$_1$-receptor antagonists decrease extrapyramidal side effects, whereas NMDA-receptor antagonists exacerbate extrapyramidal side effects. ACh, acetylcholine; GABA, γ-aminobutyric acid; Glu, glutamic acid; 5-HT, 5-hydroxytryptamine; NE, norepinephrine. (Adapted from references 10, 15, 16, 19, and 31.)

prefrontal cortex are inhibited by serotonin heteroreceptors. 5-HT$_2$-Receptor antagonism releases dopamine neurons from this inhibition (disinhibition) and ameliorates the effects of D$_2$-receptor blockade. 5-HT$_{1A}$-Autoreceptor agonism produced by certain atypical neuroleptics (e.g., aripiprazole, clozapine, ziprasidone) or stabilizers (e.g., aripiprazole) additionally releases dopamine neurons from this inhibition and mitigates EPS (see Fig. 45-3).[10,15,16] 5-HT$_{2A}$-Receptor antagonism in the limbic system seems to have an independent antipsychotic effect.[10,13] Serotonin-dopamine antagonists (e.g., amperozide, clozapine, olanzapine, risperidone, sertindole, ziprasidone) may be given at smaller doses and produce a lower incidence of EPS while maintaining clinical effectiveness.

PATHOPHYSIOLOGY OF THERAPEUTIC AND TOXIC EFFECTS

The aliphatic and piperidine phenothiazines (e.g., chlorpromazine, thioridazine, mesoridazine) have a direct negative inotropic action and quinidine-like (type IA) antiarrhythmic

effect on the heart.[5] These agents bind to inactivated fast-sodium channels responsible for membrane depolarization and potassium channels responsible for membrane repolarization.[20–22] This sodium channel blockade is voltage and rate dependent; block is enhanced greatly at less negative membrane potentials and faster heart rates.[20] Conduction disturbances are more apparent for drugs that also produce a tachycardia (e.g., drugs with anticholinergic properties). Potassium channel blockade is concentration, voltage, and reverse frequency dependent; block is enhanced at higher concentrations, at less negative membrane potentials, and at slower heart rates.[21,22] As elucidated for sertindole and thioridazine, these drugs specifically antagonize delayed rectifier, voltage-gated potassium channels encoded by the *HERG* gene.[21,22] Certain neuroleptics (e.g., haloperidol, mesoridazine, pimozide, and thioridazine) also are calcium channel antagonists.[23,24] Pimozide is known to antagonize calmodulin and T-type calcium channels.[25] Electrophysiologic effects variably include a depressed rate of phase 0 depolarization, depressed amplitude and duration of phase 2, and prolongation of phase 3 repolarization. Early afterdepolarizations that result from blockade of rectifying potassium channels may trigger ventricular arrhythmias, particularly torsades de pointes.

Neuroleptics produce hypotension from depressed peripheral vasomotor tone (from α_1-adrenergic blockade), central vasomotor reflex depression, and direct myocardial depression. Hypotension is most commonly orthostatic and occurs during initial therapeutic dosing or shortly after acute overdose with certain agents.

Neuroleptics produce dose-related electroencephalographic (EEG) changes and are believed to lower the threshold for new-onset seizures and recurrent seizures in epileptic patients.[26-29] The seizures are dose related.[27-29] For most neuroleptics, however, the risk of seizures is low, even after overdose.[3] Clozapine, loxapine, and chlorpromazine are the neuroleptics most commonly associated with seizures after therapeutic doses and overdose.[26-30] Clozapine and chlorpromazine also induce the most striking EEG alterations when schizophrenic patients are given neuroleptics in therapeutic doses.[26-29] The mechanisms by which neuroleptics lower the seizure threshold are not well understood. $GABA_A$-receptor antagonism, norepinephrine reuptake inhibition, and membrane-destabilizing activity (altered ionic flow through channels) may mediate seizures for certain agents. The $GABA_A$ antagonists clozapine and loxapine (the latter from its active metabolites, amoxapine and hydroxyamoxapine) also produce dose-related inhibition of norepinephrine reuptake, which may account partly for the high incidence of seizures with high doses of these agents.

Normal extrapyramidal motor function requires a balance among the excitatory nigrostriatal dopaminergic neurons and inhibitory intrastriatal cholinergic neurons, raphestriatal and raphenigral serotoninergic neurons, and GABAergic striatonigral neurons (see Fig. 45-3).[10,15,16,19,31] Numerous other neurotransmitter pathways (e.g., noradrenergic, σ, D_1-dopaminergic, and N-methyl-D-aspartate [NMDA] glutamatergic) converge on various basal ganglia nuclei to modulate extrapyramidal movement further.[10,31] All neuroleptics seem to produce EPS by nigrostriatal D_2-receptor blockade.[6] This blockade leads to striatal cholinergic excess and signs and symptoms of EPS.[32,33] Any agent that prevents cholinergic excess by balancing D_2-receptor blockade with M_1-receptor blockade at therapeutic doses is less likely to induce EPS (less relative dopamine antagonism in the nigrostriatum).[6] Similarly, agents with high relative 5-HT_2 antagonism or 5-HT_{1A} agonism release the nigrostriatal dopamine system from inhibition, prevent cholinergic excess, and ameliorate EPS.[10,15,16,19] Agents with low D_2-receptor potency in the nigrostriatum are unlikely to result in depolarization inactivation, receptor alterations, and signs of acute and chronic EPS.[10] σ- and NMDA-receptor antagonism modulates the dopaminergic-cholinergic balance to increase the likelihood of acute dystonia, whereas α-adrenergic and D_1 antagonism seems to protect against the development of acute dystonia.[10,31,34]

Although parkinsonism is known to result from decreased nigrostriatal dopaminergic activity, the pathophysiology of other extrapyramidal syndromes has not been elucidated fully.[35] Akathisia is possibly the manifestation of mesocortical D_2-receptor blockade.[35] Similar to parkinsonism, acute dystonic reactions (DRs) may result from decreased dorsal striatal dopaminergic activity. Paradoxi-

cally, acute DRs alternatively may result from increased nigrostriatal dopaminergic activity that occurs as a compensatory response to neuroleptics.[35,36] Acutely, postsynaptic D_2-receptor blockade produced by neuroleptics is matched by increased presynaptic dopamine synthesis and release (see Fig. 45-2). As midbrain concentrations of the neuroleptic decline hours to days after a dose, a state of dopamine excess develops, and sustained muscular contraction (dystonia) occurs.[35,36] TD is likely a compensatory response to prolonged D_2-receptor antagonism by neuroleptics. Up-regulated postsynaptic processes create a state of dopamine supersensitivity and an exaggerated response despite smaller quantal releases of dopamine.[5,35,36] An alternative theory postulates that TD results from the neurotoxic effects of free radicals, which are produced by increased dopamine metabolism associated with chronic neuroleptic D_2-receptor blockade.[37]

PHARMACOKINETICS

The pharmacokinetics of neuroleptics is complex. Although the pharmacokinetic parameters are similar for most classes of agents, there is substantial interindividual variability. Absorption is nearly complete after oral administration, but bioavailability is erratic and unpredictable (range, 10% to 70%) as a result of extensive first-pass hepatic and intestinal metabolism.[38,39] Bioavailability is increased 4 to 10 times after intramuscular administration. Plasma concentrations peak 1 to 6 hours after oral therapeutic dosing, 0.5 to 1 hour after immediate-release intramuscular administration, and within 24 hours of intramuscular administration of sustained-release preparations.[38,39] Sustained-release (depot) preparations are made by esterifying the hydroxyl group of a neuroleptic (e.g., fluphenazine, haloperidol) with a long-chain fatty acid (e.g., enanthate or decanoate). After oral overdose, absorption occurs more rapidly, but peak plasma concentrations are delayed; clinical effects occur sooner and last longer.

Most neuroleptics are highly lipophilic, are highly protein bound (75% to 99%), and accumulate in the brain and other tissues.[5,38,39] Volumes of distribution are large, and plasma concentrations after therapeutic doses are low (less than one to several hundred nanograms per milliliter). These pharmacokinetic characteristics make significant extracorporeal removal by hemodialysis and hemoperfusion impossible. Most neuroleptics readily cross the placenta to enter the fetal circulation and are secreted into breast milk. All neuroleptics are eliminated predominantly by hepatic metabolism. The main routes of metabolism are oxidation by cytochrome P-450 mixed-function oxidases (CYP) or flavin-containing monooxygenase (FMO), hydroxylation, sulfoxidation, N-dealkylation, and conjugation.[39,40] Metabolites commonly are active and metabolized further in the liver or excreted in the urine or bile. Large interindividual variation in the biotransformation of neuroleptics results in substantial differences in steady-state plasma concentrations with fixed therapeutic dosing.[5,38-41] In addition, many neuroleptics have metabolites that are not readily measured but are pharmacologically active. There is often little correlation among neuroleptic dose, serum concentrations, and

Pharmacokinetics of Commonly Used Neuroleptics

Neuroleptic Agent	t_{max} (hr)	$t_{1/2}$ (hr) (mean)	Protein Binding (%)	V_d (L/kg)	Route of Metabolism	Active Metabolite
Typical Agents						
Chlorpromazine	2–4	8–35	90–95	7–20	CYP2D6	Yes (7-hydroxychlor-promazine, others)
Haloperidol	1–6	17–36	92	10–35	CYP2D6, CYP3A4	Yes (reduced haloperidol, others)
Fluphenazine	2–5	5–27 (13)	90–95	220	Hepatic	Yes (7-hydroxy-fluphenazine, others)
Flupenthixol	2–6	22–36	90–93	12–24	Hepatic	No
Loxapine	1–6	2–8 (3.4)	—	—	CYP1A2, CYP2D6, CYP3A4	Yes (amoxapine, 7-hydroxyloxapine, others)
Perphenazine	2–6	8–21	90–95	10–35	CYP2D6	No
Pimozide	6–8	28–214	99	11–62	CYP3A4, CYP1A2	Yes
Thioridazine	2–4	9–36	99	18	CYP2D6	Yes (mesoridazine, sulforidazine, ring sulfoxide)
Thiothixene	1–3	12–36	90–95	—	Hepatic	No
Atypical Agents						
Aripiprazole	3–5	31–146 (75)	>99	4.9	CYP2D6, CYP3A4	Yes (dehydroaripiprazole)s
Clozapine	1–4	10–105 (16)	92–95	2–5	CYP1A2, CYP3A4	Yes (norclozapine)
Olanzapine	5–6	20–70 (30)	93	10–20	CYP1A2, CYP2D6	No
Quetiapine	1–2	4–10 (7)	83	10	CYP3A4	Yes (7-hydroxyquetiapine)
Remoxipride	1–2	4–7	80	0.7	Hepatic, renal	No
Risperidone	1–1.5	3–24 (3.6)	90	1–1.5	CYP2D6	Yes (9-hydroxyrisperidone)
Sertindole	10	24–200 (55–90)	>99	20–40	CYP3A4, CYP2D6	Yes (dehydrosertindole)
Sulpiride	3–6	5–14 (6.8)	40	2.7	Hepatic, renal	No
Ziprasidone	5	4–10 (NA)	>99	2	CYP3A4	No

NA, data not available; $t_{1/2}$, half-life; t_{max}, time to peak plasma concentration; V_d, volume of distribution.

Pharmacokinetic data obtained from references 5, 7, 9, 39, 40, 132, and 133.

clinical effects.[38–41] Elimination half-lives typically range from 18 to 40 hours and allow for once-daily dosing for many neuroleptics. Depot preparations have elimination half-lives of 7 to 21 days.[38]

DRUG INTERACTIONS

When neuroleptics are coadministered with other drugs, clinically significant interactions may occur.[42] Interactions may be additive or antagonistic and pharmacodynamic or pharmacokinetic. These interactions are most likely to be of clinical concern when therapy is begun or discontinued. The CNS and respiratory depressant effects of neuroleptics may be potentiated by alcohols, antihistamines, antidepressants, opiates, and sedative-hypnotics. Fatal cardiorespiratory arrest has been reported to occur when therapeutic doses of clozapine have been taken with diazepam and lorazepam.[43,44] Exaggerated anticholinergic effects may occur when certain neuroleptics are coadministered with tricyclic antidepressants, antihistamines, antiparkinsonian agents, and certain skeletal muscle relaxants (e.g., cyclobenzaprine). The hypotensive effects of neuroleptics with α_1-antagonist properties may be potentiated when coadministered with antihypertensives (e.g., prazosin) with similar pharmacologic properties. The dopamine receptor–blocking effects of neuroleptics antagonize the effects of levodopa and dopamine agonists used to treat patients with Parkin-

son's disease. Mesoridazine or thioridazine may potentiate the cardiotoxicity of other type IA antiarrhythmic agents (e.g., quinidine, tricyclic antidepressants) and vice versa. Certain neuroleptics (e.g., haloperidol, sertindole, thioridazine) may potentiate the QT prolongation produced by other cardioactive agents. The addition of selective serotonin reuptake inhibitors (e.g., fluoxetine) to patients taking neuroleptics may precipitate EPS. When combined with neuroleptics, lithium may precipitate a toxic syndrome that resembles neuroleptic malignant syndrome.[42]

The principal pharmacokinetic interactions that occur between neuroleptics and other drugs result from hepatic CYP P-450 enzyme induction and inhibition (Table 45-3).[39,40,42,45] Because many neuroleptics are metabolized by CYP2D6 and CYP1A2 enzymes, their clearance may be decreased significantly when coadministered with inhibitors of these enzymes, such as fluoxetine or paroxetine. Although these interactions occur frequently and often go unnoticed, they occasionally may result in clinically significant effects. Clozapine toxicity has been reported after coadministration with the CYP1A2 inhibitors cimetidine, erythromycin, and fluvoxamine.[46–49] Clarithromycin, a CYP3A4 and CYP1A2 inhibitor, can increase plasma concentrations of pimozide and can result in significant increases in the QT_c interval in human volunteers given a single dose of pimozide.[50] Selective serotonin reuptake inhibitors block CYP2D6 and may precipitate aripiprazole, chlorpromazine, clozapine, haloperidol, olanzapine, perphenazine, risperidone, quetiapine, and thioridazine toxicity.[39,40,42,45,51] In particular, selective serotonin reuptake inhibitors may precipitate thioridazine cardiotoxicity by increasing plasma concentrations of the unchanged parent drug and shunting metabolism to the cardioactive ring–sulfoxide metabolite. Conversely, the clearance of many neuroleptics may be increased significantly when coadministered with certain CYP isoenzyme inducers. Anticonvulsants (e.g., carbamazepine, phenytoin, phenobarbital) stimulate CYP3A4 and may decrease plasma concentrations of clozapine, olanzapine, and quetiapine. Cigarette smoking induces CYP1A2 and increases clearance of chlorpromazine, clozapine, fluphenazine, haloperidol, olanzapine, and numerous other neuroleptics.[42] Knowledge of the receptor profile and pharmacokinetic parameters of a drug facilitates recognition and treatment of clinically significant drug interactions.

CLINICAL PRESENTATION

Overdose

After accidental or intentional overdose, most patients remain asymptomatic or develop only mild toxicity.[4] Toxic effects are commonly an exaggeration of pharmacologic effects. Clinical effects begin within 30 to 90 minutes of ingestion and include CNS and consequent respiratory depression, miosis or mydriasis, hypertension or orthostatic hypotension, sinus tachycardia, agitation, confusion, delirium, anticholinergic stigmata, myoclonic jerking, seizures, hyperthermia or hypothermia, cardiac conduction disturbances, and atrial and ventricular arrhythmias. Rarely, pulmonary edema may occur.[52,53] Peak toxic effects are usually evident within 2 to 6 hours, and resolution of serious toxicity usually occurs by 24 to 48 hours. CNS depression is the most frequent clinical finding in overdose.[3,54–58] CNS effects may range from lethargy, slurred speech, ataxia, and confusion in mild poisoning to deep coma with apnea and loss of brainstem and deep tendon reflexes in severe poisoning. Anticholinergic manifestations are frequent after overdoses with chlorpromazine, clozapine, mesoridazine, olanzapine, and thioridazine. Sinus tachycardia is a frequent finding with chlorpromazine, clozapine, mesoridazine, olanzapine, quetiapine, risperidone, and thioridazine. Miosis is more likely to occur in severely poisoned patients; it has been described in greater than 70% of patients poisoned with phenothiazines and has been noted frequently in patients poisoned with clozapine, olanzapine, and quetiapine.[55,56,58,59] Although acute EPS are often idiosyncratic reactions that follow therapeutic neuroleptic doses, these effects also may be dose related and have occurred after overdose with many neuroleptics.[54,60,61] EPS may be the presenting manifestation in a child after accidental neuroleptic poisoning.[60–62] Sialorrhea, a feature unique to clozapine, has been observed in 13% of patients poisoned with this agent.[55,60] Acute pulmonary edema has been described after overdose of chlorpromazine, clozapine, haloperidol, and perphenazine.[52,53] Rhabdomyolysis, myoglobinuria, and acute renal failure have occurred in patients with repetitive seizures after loxapine overdose.[30,63]

Neuroleptics have a relatively high therapeutic index, particularly when compared with certain other psychotropic medications, such as tricyclic antidepressants. Overdoses of neuroleptics are rarely fatal.[4] Death most frequently results from respiratory arrest (before medical intervention), arrhythmias, or aspiration-induced respiratory failure.[5] The toxic and lethal doses are highly variable and depend largely on agent identity, the presence of coingestants, age and habituation of the patient, and time to treatment. Children and nonhabituated adults are more sensitive to the toxic effects of these agents than individuals who have taken the agents on a long-term basis before an acute overdose. Higher potency neuroleptics (e.g., fluphenazine, thiothixene, haloperidol) are safer after overdose than low-potency, multireceptor agents (e.g., chlorpromazine, thioridazine, clozapine). These latter agents are more likely to produce respiratory depression, seizures, and cardiovascular toxicity. The ingestion of a single tablet of chlorpromazine, clozapine, loxapine, mesoridazine, olanzapine, or thioridazine may cause serious toxicity in a toddler. Coma and respiratory arrest have been reported after the ingestion of 100 mg and 200 mg of clozapine, respectively, in toddlers.[60] Pronounced CNS sedation and anticholinergic delirium have occurred after the ingestion of 7.5 to 15 mg of olanzapine in children.[64,65] Death of an infant was reported after the ingestion of 350 mg of chlorpromazine.[66] Adult fatalities have been reported after the ingestions of 2 g of chlorpromazine and clozapine, 2.5 g of loxapine and mesoridazine, 600 mg of olanzapine, and 1.5 g of thioridazine.[66–69] Other patients have survived much larger ingestions.

Cardiovascular Toxicity

Orthostatic hypotension and sinus tachycardia are frequent clinical manifestations.[3,54,55,57,58,60,61,64–66] Electrocardiogram (ECG) abnormalities include prolongation of the PR, QRS, and QT intervals; T-wave and U-wave abnormalities (blunting, notching, inversion); ST-segment depression; rightward axis of the terminal 40 msec of the QRS; atrioventricular, bundle-branch, fascicular, and intraventricular conduction disturbances; and supraventricular and ventricular tachyarrhythmias.[3,70–76] These cardiac effects are observed most commonly with aliphatic and piperidine phenothiazines. Thioridazine is perhaps the most cardiotoxic agent. In one study of 299 patients with neuroleptic overdose, thioridazine had a significantly greater incidence of prolonged QT_c interval (60%), prolonged QRS interval (23%), and arrhythmia (5%) than chlorpromazine (34%, 15%, and 0%, respectively) and other neuroleptics (19%, 6%, and 0%, respectively).[3] ECG changes and arrhythmias occasionally have been described after overdose of the newer atypical neuroleptics.[54,55,77–82]

Repolarization abnormalities are the earliest and most common abnormalities noted on the ECG of patients with neuroleptic poisoning.[70–72,75] Although observed with therapeutic doses, repolarization abnormalities are dose and concentration dependent and more prevalent in overdose. Prolongation of the QT interval has been observed with aliphatic and piperidine phenothiazines, droperidol, haloperidol, loxapine, pimozide, quetiapine, sertindole, risperidone, and ziprasidone.[3,30,78,80–88] Therapeutic doses of sertindole have been associated with a mean QT_c interval increase of 21 msec in one premarketing trial and a QT_c interval greater than 500 msec in 50% of patients in another trial.[77,89] The manufacturer withdrew its new drug application in the

TABLE 45-3 Pharmacokinetic Drug Interactions of Neuroleptics

NEUROLEPTIC		INTERACTING DRUG(S)	DRUG EFFECT
Atypical	*Typical*		
Clozapine Olanzapine Quetiapine Ziprasidone	Loxapine Pimozide	Cimetidine Clarithromycin Erythromycin Fluvoxamine Fluoroquinolones Isoniazid Paroxetine	Elevated plasma neuroleptic concentrations from CYP1A2 inhibition
Clozapine Olanzapine Quetiapine Risperidone Sertindole	Chlorpromazine Fluphenazine Haloperidol Loxapine Perphenazine Thioridazine	Amiodarone Chloroquine Cimetidine Fluoxetine Paroxetine Propafenone Propoxyphene Propranolol Quinidine Risperidone Sertraline Tricyclic antidepressants	Elevated plasma neuroleptic concentrations from CYP2D6 inhibition
Clozapine Olanzapine Quetiapine Sertindole Ziprasidone	Haloperidol Pimozide	Amiodarone Antifungals (azoles) Cimetidine Clarithromycin Cyclosporine Erythromycin Fluoxetine Nefazodone Protease inhibitors Zafirlukast	Elevated plasma neuroleptic concentrations from CYP3A4 inhibition
Clozapine Olanzapine Quetiapine Sertindole Ziprasidone	Haloperidol Pimozide	Carbamazepine Dexamethasone Phenytoin Phenobarbital Primidone Rifampin	Decreased plasma neuroleptic concentrations from CYP3A4 stimulation
Clozapine Olanzapine Quetiapine Ziprasidone	Loxapine Pimozide	Carbamazepine Cigarettes Phenobarbital Phenytoin Rifampin Ritonavir Omeprazole	Decreased plasma neuroleptic concentrations from CYP1A2 stimulation
Clozapine Olanzapine Quetiapine Risperidone Sertindole	Chlorpromazine Fluphenazine Haloperidol Loxapine Perphenazine Thioridazine	Carbamazepine Phenobarbital Phenytoin Rifampin Ritonavir	Decreased plasma neuroleptic concentrations from CYP2D6 stimulation
	Chlorpromazine Haloperidol Fluphenazine	Cigarettes	Decreased plasma neuroleptic concentrations
	Haloperidol	Fluvoxamine	Elevated plasma neuroleptic concentrations
Quetiapine		Thioridazine	Decreased plasma neuroleptic concentrations

United States due to fear of polymorphic ventricular tachycardia from this agent. Torsades de pointes has been described after overdose with droperidol, haloperidol, mesoridazine, pimozide, and thioridazine.[86-88,90-92] This complication is particularly important to the intensivist who uses haloperidol to sedate agitated patients in the intensive care unit. In one study, torsades de pointes occurred in 3.6% of hospitalized critically ill patients who received intravenous haloperidol for sedation.[92] The incidence of torsades de pointes was increased significantly when greater than 35 mg of haloperidol was administered in less than 6 hours (64%) and when the QT_c interval was greater than 500 msec (84%). No patient who had a QT_c interval less than 500 msec developed torsades de pointes.

Ventricular tachyarrhythmias may underlie sudden death that has been associated with therapeutic doses of phenothiazines.[93-95] Thioridazine is likely the most dangerous. In one case series of 49 deaths associated with therapeutic doses of neuroleptics, more than half of the cases were associated with thioridazine.[94]

Seizures

Although all neuroleptics are considered to lower the seizure threshold and produce dose-related EEG abnormalities, seizures occur uncommonly.[3,26,27] Generalized and partial seizures have been reported, but generalized major motor seizures predominate. Seizures are most likely to occur in patients with one or more risk factors, at higher therapeutic doses, and after overdose with certain agents (e.g., chlorpromazine, clozapine, loxapine).[26-30] Risk factors for seizures include organic brain disease, epilepsy, a history of electroconvulsive therapy, abnormal baseline EEG, polypharmacy, large drug doses, and initiation or rapid dose escalation of neuroleptics.[26,29] Seizures have been reported to occur in 2.4% of patients taking clozapine and 1.2% of patients taking phenothiazines.[26,96] The incidence of seizures rises, however, to 4.4% for patients taking greater than 600 mg of clozapine daily and 9% for patients taking greater than 1 g of chlorpromazine daily.[27,28] Seizures are unlikely to occur when certain traditional agents (e.g., fluphenazine, haloperidol, molindone, pimozide) and newer atypical agents are used; these agents have a seizure incidence comparable to placebo (<1%) during therapeutic dosing.[26] Overall the incidence of seizures is low after neuroleptic overdose. In one study of 299 patients with neuroleptic overdose, the incidence of seizure was only 1%.[3] For clozapine and loxapine, however, the risk is much higher. To date, seizures have occurred in 10% of clozapine overdoses reported in the literature.[55] In one series of 10 patients with loxapine overdose, seizures occurred in 6 (60%) and were often multiple.[30]

Hepatotoxicity

Asymptomatic elevations of hepatic transaminases have occurred during treatment with most neuroleptics.[97,98] These abnormalities commonly are noted during the first 3 months of therapy and are self-limiting. The incidence is variable according to agent; incidences of 37%, 20%, and 16% have been described for clozapine, chlorpromazine, and haloperidol, respectively.[97,98] Clinically significant hepatotoxicity occurs in a small proportion of patients.

Hepatotoxic reactions are idiosyncratic and not observed with acute neuroleptic overdose. Chlorpromazine carries an incidence of overt liver disease of 0.1% to 1%.[97,99] Cholestatic jaundice is the characteristic pattern of injury. In support of a hypersensitivity mechanism, the injury most often occurs within 1 month of therapy onset, is characterized by a rash and eosinophilia in most cases, and is not dose related.[97,100] Cholestatic jaundice also has been associated rarely with haloperidol and risperidone therapy. Chlorpromazine and clozapine also may cause direct hepatocyte cytotoxicity.[97]

Blood Dyscrasias

Agranulocytosis (absolute neutrophil count $<500/mm^3$) is a life-threatening idiosyncratic reaction that rarely may occur with phenothiazine and clozapine therapy. It occurs in approximately 1 in 10,000 patients receiving chlorpromazine, usually within the first 8 to 12 weeks of treatment.[101,102] The incidence is higher with clozapine (1% to 2%) and, as for chlorpromazine, usually occurs within the first 3 months of therapy.[103,104] Mortality rates range from 30% to 85% when agranulocytosis occurs.[104] The risk of clozapine-associated agranulocytosis is minimized by weekly white blood cell count monitoring. With regular monitoring, the incidence (cumulative risk 0.8% at 1 year) of and mortality (4%) from agranulocytosis have been reduced.[103,104] The mechanism of clozapine-associated agranulocytosis has not been determined but is likely to result from immune-mediated and direct drug-induced myelotoxicity.[105] Granulocyte colony-stimulating factor has shortened recovery time significantly when administered to patients with neuroleptic-associated granulocytopenia.[106]

Extrapyramidal Syndromes

EPS are a group of sustained-movement disorders that occur in approximately 30% of patients treated with neuroleptics and often lead to medication noncompliance, inadequate treatment, and an exacerbation of the symptoms of schizophrenia.[107] New-generation atypical neuroleptics are associated with a significantly lower incidence and severity of EPS; rates not significantly different from placebo have been found with clozapine, olanzapine, quetiapine, and sertindole.[89,108,109] EPS may occur within hours to days (e.g., acute DRs, akathisia), days to months (e.g., akathisia, parkinsonism), or months to years (e.g., TD) from the initiation of therapy and may be reversible or irreversible. The neuroleptic malignant syndrome, a severe EPS, rarely may occur during treatment and is discussed in Chapter 26.

Acute DRs are reversible motor disturbances that occur soon after initiation of neuroleptic therapy or after an increase in dose. Of acute DRs, 50% occur within 48 hours, and 90% occur within 5 days of neuroleptic treatment.[110,111] Peak incidence occurs when neuroleptic concentrations are declining in the serum. Acute DRs are characterized by sustained muscle contractions resulting in abnormal posturing of the eyes, face, tongue, jaw, neck, back, abdomen, and pelvis. Clinical manifestations include facial grimacing, trismus, oculogyric crisis, blepharospasm, tongue protrusion, buccolingual dyskinesias, dysarthria, swallowing difficulties, retrocollis, torticollis, opisthotonos, tortipelvis, gait disturbance, and, rarely, stridor from laryngospasm. Impaired respiration caused by dystonia of laryngeal and pharyngeal muscles rarely may result in death.[112] Acute DRs are characterized by a patient who is awake and alert. The overall prevalence of acute DRs is approximately 2%, but the incidence varies according to individual susceptibility (presence of risk factors), agent identity, dose, and duration of therapy.[107] Patient-related risk factors include male sex, young age (5 to 45 years old), a personal or family history of acute dystonia, and recent alcohol or cocaine use.[111,113–115] High-potency D_2-receptor antagonists cause acute DRs more frequently than do low-potency agents. Acute DRs have been reported to occur in 25% of patients treated with intramuscular fluphenazine, 16% of patients treated with haloperidol, 8% of patients taking thiothixene, 3.5% of patients taking chlorpromazine, and 1% or less of patients treated with atypical agents.[32,108–111] Clozapine is the only known atypical neuroleptic that does not induce acute dystonia. Although previously considered an idiosyncratic reaction, acute DRs are more likely to occur with larger drug doses and frequently have been described after acute neuroleptic overdose.[54,60–62]

Akathisia is the subjective sensation of motor restlessness that occurs within hours to days of the initiation of neuroleptic therapy.[108,109] Akathisia is characterized by a compelling need to move and the inability to maintain a stable position or posture for several minutes. Patients may be irritable and anxious; have difficulty concentrating; and often constantly move their legs, rock, pace, or shift their weight from foot to foot. Vital signs are normal. Akathisia occurs in approximately 30% of patients taking neuroleptics.[108,109] In one study, akathisia developed in 44% of patients within 1 hour after taking a single 10-mg intravenous dose of prochlorperazine.[116] Akathisia occurs more commonly in women and is more prevalent with high-potency neuroleptics.

Parkinsonism is a reversible, intermediate-stage extrapyramidal syndrome that often occurs 5 to 30 days after starting neuroleptic therapy.[108,109] In a study of 1559 patients treated with neuroleptics, parkinsonism was noted in 66% of patients.[107] Parkinsonism is characterized by bradykinesia (slow movement) or akinesia, masked facies, muscular rigidity (e.g., cogwheeling), tremor (e.g., pill rolling), gait and postural instability, bradyphrenia (slow thinking), and cognitive impairment. The risk of drug-induced parkinsonism is greatest in the elderly, patients with organic brain injury, patients taking high-potency agents, and patients receiving long-term neuroleptic therapy.[107]

TD is a late-appearing, potentially irreversible movement disorder that occurs in approximately 20% of patients who receive long-term neuroleptic treatment and 50% of high-risk individuals (e.g., the elderly).[108,109] With conventional neuroleptic therapy, an annual incidence of 3% to 5% for TD has been reported. Atypical neuroleptics have a lower propensity to cause TD, with an annual incidence of less than 2%.[108,109] It has been associated with all neuroleptics except clozapine. TD is characterized by stereotyped, involuntary, repetitive, painless movements of the face, eyelids, mouth, tongue, extremities, or trunk. Clinically, patients show chewing, tongue protrusion, lip smacking and puckering, rapid eye blinking, facial grimacing, grunting, and, occasionally, slow choreoathetosis of the arms and legs. Orofacial movements are the earliest and most frequent clinical manifestations. The risk of developing TD is greatest in the elderly, patients with organic brain injury, patients taking high-potency agents, and patients receiving long-term neuroleptic therapy.[117]

DIAGNOSIS

The diagnosis of neuroleptic poisoning is based on a history of ingestion; suggestive physical findings; and corroborating evidence from ECG, laboratory, and other adjunctive tests. A history that suggests poisoning includes report of neuroleptic exposure by the patient or an acquaintance, a medication list that includes a neuroleptic, known history of psychosis or treatment with a neuroleptic, and the discovery of a neuroleptic near the patient before or on hospital arrival. The presence of CNS or respiratory depression, anticholinergic stigmata (see Chapter 22), miosis, sinus tachycardia, hypotension, and EPS on physical examination suggests neuroleptic poisoning. An ECG that shows repolarization abnormalities (e.g., nonspecific ST-T changes, QT interval prolongation) with or without sinus tachycardia is consistent with neuroleptic exposure. An abdominal radiograph may show radiopaque densities with phenothiazine and butyrophenone poisoning. The absence of this finding, however, does not rule out poisoning with these agents. The Forrest, ferric chloride, or Phenistix colorimetric urine test may be positive with phenothiazine ingestions.[118] These tests are insensitive and nonspecific, however, and cannot be used to rule in or out the presence of phenothiazines. Chlorpromazine, mesoridazine, quetiapine, and thioridazine often produce false-positive results for tricyclic antidepressants on immunoassay screens. When necessary, comprehensive urine toxicologic screening may be used to confirm the presence of most neuroleptics. Quantitative drug concentrations may be obtained but are not helpful in guiding therapy; they generally are not available in a timely manner and do not correlate well with clinical toxicity.[38–40]

Differential Diagnosis

Poisoning by neuroleptics may mimic the neurologic and cardiovascular effects produced by alcohols, antiarrhythmics, anticholinergics, antiepileptics, antihistamines, barbiturates, cyclic antidepressants, opiates, and sedative-hypnotics. Specifically, mesoridazine and thioridazine toxicity may be clinically indistinguishable from that produced by tricyclic antidepressants. CNS infection, occult trauma, cerebrovascular accident, and metabolic abnormalities always should be considered in the differential diagnosis and ruled out by appropriate testing. Acute dystonic reactions must be differentiated from alkalosis; anticholinergic, antiepileptic, and strychnine poisoning; cerebrovascular accident; CNS and oropharyngeal infections; conversion disorder; hypocalcemia; hypomagnesemia; and joint dislocations. In addition, numerous drugs other than neuroleptics may produce acute DRs. Akathisia often may be misinterpreted as acute anxiety or agitation. Parkinsonism produced by neuroleptics may be indistinguishable from that produced by cerebrovascular accidents; CNS infection and trauma; and poisoning by carbon disulfide, carbon monoxide, cyanide, manganese, methanol, metoclopramide, 1-methyl-4-phenyl-1,2,3,6-tetrahydropyridine (MPTP), and reserpine.

TREATMENT

Overdose

Treatment for neuroleptic overdose is primarily supportive. Endotracheal intubation and assisted ventilation should be instituted for patients with significant CNS or respiratory depression. All patients should have an intravenous line established, an ECG performed, and continuous monitoring of cardiac and respiratory function. Intravenous dextrose (or Dextrostix determination), naloxone, oxygen, and thiamine administration should be considered for patients with altered mental status, particularly patients with coma or seizures. Patients with mild-to-moderate CNS depression who do not initially require endotracheal intubation should be placed in the lateral decubitus, head-down position to minimize the risk of aspiration. Arterial blood gas; urinalysis; and measurements of serum creatine phosphokinase, calcium, and magnesium additionally should be obtained for patients with seizures, hyperthermia, or severe toxicity. A complete blood count should be obtained for any patient who presents with fever while taking clozapine or chlorpromazine. Serial evaluations of mental status and vital signs are important to determine the course of poisoning and the need for further testing and intervention.

Hypotension should be treated initially with Trendelenburg's position and rapid intravenous crystalloid infusion (i.e., 10 to 40 mL/kg normal saline or lactated Ringer's solution). Refractory hypotension should be treated with catecholamine pressors. Although dopamine may be effective, a direct α-agonist, such as norepinephrine or phenylephrine, may be necessary because many neuroleptics are α-adrenergic antagonists. Central venous, peripheral arte-

rial, and pulmonary arterial catheter monitoring is recommended for patients who require significant doses of pressors to maintain satisfactory blood pressure.

Sinus tachycardia does not require specific treatment. Supraventricular tachycardias may be treated according to standard advanced cardiac life-support guidelines. Ventricular tachyarrhythmias may be treated with standard doses of lidocaine and electrical cardioversion, depending on the hemodynamic stability of the patient. Sodium bicarbonate (1 to 2 mEq/L intravenous boluses) is indicated as first-line therapy for ventricular or wide-complex tachycardias associated with mesoridazine, thioridazine, and, rarely, other agents. Type IA (e.g., procainamide), type IC (e.g., propafenone), and type III (e.g., amiodarone) antiarrhythmic agents are not recommended and are potentially dangerous; these agents may impair cardiac conduction further. Torsades de pointes should be treated by standard methods (see Chapter 21).[119-122]

Seizures generally are treated best with benzodiazepines (e.g., diazepam, lorazepam) followed by barbiturates (e.g., phenobarbital), as necessary. The efficacy and safety of phenytoin have not been established for neuroleptic-associated seizures. Patients with recurrent seizures (e.g., loxapine poisoning) rarely may require neuromuscular paralysis and endotracheal intubation to prevent rhabdomyolysis and myoglobinuric renal failure. Continuous EEG monitoring is required for these patients to determine the efficacy of antiepileptic therapy (see Chapter 20).

Physostigmine may be used to control agitation and reverse delirium in patients who have significant anticholinergic stigmata from certain neuroleptics. Its duration of action is less than 1 hour, however, so repeat dosing may be necessary. Physostigmine is safe, provided that the ECG does not show cardiac conduction disturbances.[123] It has been used successfully to reverse the anticholinergic syndrome associated with chlorpromazine, clozapine, olanzapine, and thioridazine.[123,124] Physostigmine should be given slowly intravenously (0.02 mg/kg in children or 2 mg in adults) over 3 minutes (see Chapter 22). Physostigmine-treated patients should be observed closely for at least 15 minutes for evidence of cholinergic excess. Alternatively, agitated behavior associated with the anticholinergic effects of neuroleptics may be treated with benzodiazepines.

After patient stabilization, gastrointestinal decontamination should be initiated as soon as possible. Activated charcoal adsorbs these agents effectively and, for most patients, is the only decontamination intervention that is necessary. Gastric lavage is not routinely recommended for these patients (see Chapter 5). Because of slowed gut motility produced by the anticholinergic effects of many neuroleptics, it is reasonable to administer activated charcoal even several hours after overdose. The clinical utility of this recommendation is unknown, however.

Multiple-dose activated charcoal has no proven clinical benefit for neuroleptic poisoning and is not recommended. Because neuroleptics have large volumes of distribution, have high protein binding, and are metabolized predominantly in the liver, their elimination is not enhanced by hemodialysis, hemoperfusion, forced diuresis, or urinary alkalinization techniques.[125-127] Urinary alkalinization is reserved for patients with rhabdomyolysis that may result from neuroleptic-associated seizures or hyperthermia.

Indications for ICU Admission in Neuroleptics Poisoning

Significant central nervous system depression (unresponsive to verbal stimuli)
Significant central nervous system agitation (requiring chemical or physical restraint)
Respiratory depression ($PCO_2 > 45$ mm Hg)
Hypoxia or respiratory failure (adult respiratory distress syndrome)
Need for endotracheal intubation
Hypotension (systolic blood pressure ≤80 mm Hg) not immediately responsive to crystalloid
Multiple seizures with altered mental status
Nonsinus cardiac rhythm
Acute overdose with QRS > 120 msec or QT_c > 500 msec
Second-degree or third-degree atrioventricular block associated with poisoning
Need for invasive hemodynamic monitoring (e.g., pulmonary artery catheter, arterial line)
Extremes of temperature (e.g., ≥40°C or ≤32°C)
Significant acid-base or metabolic disturbances requiring close monitoring or aggressive correction
Initial diagnosis of neuroleptic malignant syndrome

Adapted from Brett AS, Rothschild N, Gray R, Perry M: Predicting the clinical course in intentional drug overdose: Implications for use of the intensive care unit. Arch Intern Med 147:133–137, 1987.

Acute Dystonic Reactions

Treatment of acute DRs rarely may require supplemental oxygen and assisted ventilation for patients with respiratory distress from laryngeal and pharyngeal dystonia. Pharmacologic therapy with a parenteral anticholinergic dopaminergic (antiparkinsonian) agent is highly effective and usually provides relief within 10 minutes of administration. Benztropine, which is a potent inhibitor of dopamine uptake (0.02 to 0.05 mg/kg) or diphenhydramine (1 mg/kg), may be given intramuscularly or slowly intravenously over 2 minutes. Repeat dosing may be necessary for complete resolution of acute DRs. Resistant cases may respond to diazepam (0.1 mg/kg intravenously) or lorazepam (0.05 to 0.1 mg/kg intravenously). A search for other underlying illnesses should be sought whenever acute DRs are resistant to antiparkinsonian treatment. After parenteral therapy, an oral antiparkinsonian agent should be administered for 48 to 72 hours to prevent acute DR recurrence.[128] When continued neuroleptic therapy is necessary, patients also should be maintained on an antiparkinsonian agent or switched to a neuroleptic with lower EPS liability.[109]

Akathisia

Although recommended as initial therapy, anticholinergic/antiparkinsonian agents often are ineffective for the treatment of akathisia.[109] These agents seem to be effective, however, when administered prophylactically. Pretreatment with diphenhydramine significantly decreases the incidence of akathisia that follows a single therapeutic dose of prochlorperazine.[129] Treatment with a benzodiazepine, propranolol (20 mg orally twice daily), or clonidine (0.1 mg orally three times daily) may be beneficial.[130,131] When continued neuroleptic therapy is necessary, akathisia may be minimized by reducing the neuroleptic dose, adding an anticholinergic agent, or switching to a neuroleptic with lower EPS liability.[109]

Parkinsonism

Parkinsonism effects may be minimized by using low doses of traditional neuroleptics, switching to an atypical agent, or adding an anticholinergic/antiparkinsonian agent (e.g., benztropine, biperiden, diphenhydramine, or trihexyphenidyl) or an agent that enhances dopaminergic activity (e.g., amantadine).[109]

Tardive Dyskinesia

TD is often irreversible and has no consistently effective treatment. The best treatment for TD is to minimize its risk of occurrence. The best preventive practice is to use the minimal effective dose of a neuroleptic for long-term therapy and to discontinue treatment when it is no longer medically necessary.[109] An alternative option is to treat patients with atypical agents, which have a lower propensity to induce TD with long-term treatment. Some atypical agents are antidyskinetic (e.g., clozapine, olanzapine, quetiapine, risperidone); the severity of TD is reduced after a change in regimen to these agents from a traditional neuroleptic.[109]

Disposition

For all neuroleptics, signs and symptoms develop rapidly (within 4 hours) after acute ingestion. After an initial treatment and observation period in the emergency department, clinical reassessment can reliably identify patients who are at high risk for complications and require intensive care and patients who may be medically discharged. Most patients with pure neuroleptic overdose develop only mild toxicity and are medically safe for psychiatric evaluation and disposition after an observation period of 4 to 6 hours in the emergency department. Patients who manifest persistent mild toxicity (e.g., ataxia, lethargy, sinus tachycardia, repolarization abnormalities on ECG) should be admitted to a monitored bed for continued observation. Patients with moderate to severe toxicity (e.g., moderate-to-severe CNS or respiratory depression, hypotension, seizures, marked agitation, acid-base disturbances, arrhythmias other than mild sinus tachycardia, and cardiac conduction disturbances) should be admitted to an intensive care unit for aggressive supportive care. Admission to a monitored bed also is recommended for patients who take phenothiazines on a long-term basis and have incidental ECG abnormalities (e.g., prolonged QRS or QT$_c$ intervals); these patients are considered at risk for sudden phenothiazine death. When the appropriate disposition of a patient is in question, consultation with a medical toxicologist or poison control center is recommended.

SPECIAL POPULATIONS

Patients with Renal Impairment

Because most neuroleptics are metabolized extensively in the liver before excretion, they are not affected significantly by changes in renal function. Normally, small amounts (1% to 3%) of a parent drug are excreted unchanged by the kidney.[38] Aside from the benzamide derivatives (e.g., remoxipride, sulpiride, and risperidone), these drugs commonly do not require dose alteration for patients with renal impairment.[39] Even when clearance is prolonged due to renal dysfunction, clinical toxicity is unlikely to be lengthened appreciably after overdose in this patient population.

Patients with Hepatic Impairment

Most patients with hepatic disease (e.g., cirrhosis, hepatitis) and conditions that decrease hepatic blood flow (e.g., congestive heart failure) have decreased neuroleptic clearance from plasma and require dose adjustment with long-term therapy.[39] After acute overdose, neuroleptic clearance may be prolonged but is unlikely to delay clinical recovery significantly.

Infants, Children, and Elderly Patients

Compared with normal adults, fetuses, infants, and elderly patients have a diminished capacity to metabolize and eliminate neuroleptics.[5] Children commonly metabolize these drugs more rapidly than adults. Compared with normal adults, plasma clearances of neuroleptics are reduced by 30% to 50% (elimination half-lives doubled) in the elderly.[38,39] In general, elderly individuals are more sensitive than young adults to the effects of neuroleptics; they have decreased CNS, hepatic, renal, and cardiac function and have a greater tendency to develop anticholinergic stigmata, EPS (e.g., parkinsonism, TD), sedation, confusion, and postural hypotension from these agents. The safety and efficacy of most neuroleptics have not been established in pediatric patients. Similar to elderly patients, children are more sensitive than normal adults to the CNS and respiratory depressant effects of these drugs. In addition, children are more likely to develop an acute DR than other age groups.

Patients of Different Races and Ethnic Groups

Genetic polymorphisms of hepatic CYP isoenzymes often are associated with race or ethnic group variations. These polymorphisms result in large interindividual differences in neuroleptic steady-state plasma concentrations and clearance.[40] CYP isoenzyme differences become clinically important with long-term dosing or when other CYP isoenzyme substrates are ingested concomitantly. Genetic polymorphisms of CYP2D6 may result in different concentrations of aripiprazole and thioridazine despite similar therapeutic doses in otherwise similar individuals.[40] Poor metabolizers at CYP2D6 are at greater risk for cardiovascular side effects from thioridazine and its metabolite mesoridazine. These individuals attain much higher plasma concentrations of unchanged thioridazine and the cardioactive ring sulfoxide metabolite.[41] The latter metabolite is CYP2D6 independent and preferentially formed when CYP2D6 activity is low.

Pregnant and Breast-feeding Patients

There are no adequate, well-controlled studies in pregnant women that establish the safety of neuroleptics for the developing fetus. Most neuroleptics are considered pregnancy category C and should be used during pregnancy only if the potential benefit justifies the potential risk to the fetus. Because most neuroleptics are secreted in breast milk and their safety to infants is not established, breast-feeding is not recommended for women taking neuroleptics.

Key Points in Neuroleptics Poisoning

1. Toxic effects are often an exaggeration of pharmacologic effects.
2. For all neuroleptics, clinical effects occur rapidly (within a few hours) of acute ingestion.
3. The presence of central nervous system and respiratory depression, anticholinergic stigmata, miosis, sinus tachycardia, hypotension, and extrapyramidal side effects on physical examination should suggest neuroleptic poisoning.
4. Timely supportive care should prevent death in most patients with neuroleptic poisoning.
5. An electrocardiogram should be obtained for all symptomatic patients with neuroleptic poisoning.
6. After an acute neuroleptic overdose, patients may be medically discharged if they remain asymptomatic after an observation period of 4 to 6 hours; symptomatic patients should be observed until they are alert and electrocardiogram abnormalities resolve.

REFERENCES

1. Tandon R, Milner K, Jibson MD: Antipsychotics from theory to practice: Integrating clinical and basic data. J Clin Psychiatry 60(Suppl 8):21–28, 1999.
2. Buckley N, McManus P: Fatal toxicity of drugs used in the treatment of psychotic illnesses. Br J Psychiatry 172:461–464, 1998.
3. Buckley NA, Whyte IM, Dawson AH: Thioridazine has greater cardiotoxicity in overdose than other neuroleptics. J Toxicol Clin Toxicol 33:199–204, 1995.
4. Litovitz TL, Klein-Schwartz W, Caravati EM, et al: 1998 annual report of the American Association of Poison Control Centers Toxic Exposure Surveillance System. Am J Emerg Med 17:435–487, 1999.
5. Baldessarini RJ: Drugs and the treatment of psychiatric disorders: Psychosis and anxiety. In Hardman JG, Limbird LE, Molinoff PB, et al (eds): Goodman and Gilman's The Pharmacological Basis of Therapeutics, 9th ed. New York, McGraw-Hill, 1996, pp 399–430.
6. Richelson E: Receptor pharmacology of neuroleptics: Relation to clinical effects. J Clin Psychiatry 60(Suppl 10):5–14, 1999.
7. Jibson MD, Tandon R: New atypical antipsychotic medications. J Psychiatr Res 32:215–228, 1998.
8. Blin O: A comparative review of new antipsychotics. Can J Psychiatry 44:235–244, 1999.
9. Borison RL: Recent advances in the pharmacotherapy of schizophrenia. Harv Rev Psychiatry 4:255–271, 1997.
10. Kinon BJ, Lieberman JA: Mechanisms of action of atypical antipsychotic drugs: A critical analysis. Psychopharmacology 124:2–34, 1996.
11. Seeman P, Lee T, Chau-Wong M, Wong K: Antipsychotic drug doses and neuroleptic dopamine receptors. Nature 261:717–719, 1976.
12. Farde L, Nordstrom AL, Wiesel GA, et al: Positron emission tomographic analysis of central D_1 and D_2 dopamine receptor occupancy in patients treated with classical neuroleptics and clozapine: Relation to extrapyramidal side effects., Arch Gen Psychiatry 49:538–544, 1992.
13. Risch SC: Pathophysiology of schizophrenia and the role of newer antipsychotics. Pharmacotherapy 16(suppl):11–14, 1996.
14. Black JL, Richelson E: Antipsychotic drugs: Prediction of side effect profiles based on neuroreceptor data derived from human brain tissue. Mayo Clin Proc 62:369–372, 1987.
15. Kapur S, Remington G: Serotonin-dopamine interaction and its relevance to schizophrenia. Am J Psychiatry 153:466–476, 1996.
16. Lieberman JA, Mailman RB, Duncan G, et al: Serotonergic basis of antipsychotic drug effects in schizophrenia. Biol Psychiatry 44:1099–1117, 1998.
17. Snyder S, Greenberg D, Yamamura JI: Antischizophrenic drugs and brain cholinergic receptors: Affinity for muscarinic sites predicts extrapyramidal effects. Arch Gen Psychiatry 31:58–61, 1974.
18. Gerlach J, Peacock L: New antipsychotics: The present status. Int Clin Psychopharmacol 10(Suppl 3):39–48, 1995.
19. Huttunen M: The evolution of the serotonin-dopamine antagonist concept. J Clin Psychopharmacol 15(Suppl 1):4S-10S, 1995.
20. Ogata N, Narahashi T: Block of sodium channels by psychotropic drugs in single guinea-pig cardiac myocytes. Br J Pharmacol 97:905–913, 1989.
21. Drolet B, Vincent F, Rail J, et al: Thioridazine lengthens repolarization of cardiac ventricular myocytes by blocking the delayed rectifier potassium current. J Pharm Exp Ther 288:1261–1268, 1999.
22. Rampe D, Murawsky K, Grau J, Lewis EW: The antipsychotic agent sertindole is a high affinity antagonist of the human cardiac potassium channel HERG. J Pharm Exp Ther 286:788–793, 1998.
23. Gould RJ, Murphy KMM, Reynolds IJ, et al: Antischizophrenic drugs of the diphenylbutylpiperidine type act as calcium channel antagonists. Proc Natl Acad Sci U S A 86:5122–5125, 1983.
24. Gould RJ, Murphy KMM, Reynolds IJ, et al: Calcium channel blockade: Possible explanation for thioridazine's peripheral side effects. Am J Psychiatry 141:352–357, 1984.
25. Arnoult C, Cardullo RA, Lemos JR, Florman HM: Activation of mouse sperm T-type Ca^{2+} channels by adhesion to the egg zona pellucida. Proc Natl Acad Sci U S A 93:13004–13009, 1996.
26. Cold JA, Wells BG, Froemming JH: Seizure activity associated with antipsychotic therapy. Drug Intell Clin Pharm 24:601–606, 1990.
27. Logothetis J: Spontaneous epileptic seizures and electroencephalographic changes in the course of phenothiazine therapy. Neurology 17:869–877, 1967.
28. Devinsky D, Honigfeld G, Patin J: Clozapine-related seizures. Neurology 41:369–371, 1991.

29. Alldredge BK: Seizure risk associated with psychotropic drugs: Clinical and pharmacokinetic considerations. Neurology 53(Suppl 2):S68–S75, 1999.
30. Peterson C: Seizures induced by acute loxapine overdose. Am J Psychiatry 138:1089–1091, 1981.
31. Carlsson A, Walters N, Carlsson ML: Neurotransmitter interactions in schizophrenia—therapeutic implications. Biol Psychiatry 46:1388–1395, 1999.
32. Rupniak NMJ, Jenner P, Marsden CD: Acute dystonia induced by neuroleptic drugs. Psychopharmacology 88:403–419, 1986.
33. Baldessarini RJ, Tarsy D: Dopamine and the pathophysiology of dyskinesia induced by antipsychotic drugs. Ann Rev Neurosci 3:23–41, 1980.
34. Jeanjean AP, Laterre C, Maloteaux J-M: Neuroleptic binding to sigma receptors: Possible involvement in neuroleptic-induced dystonia. Biol Pyschiatry 41:1010–1019, 1997.
35. Marsden CD, Jenner P: The pathophysiology of extrapyramidal side-effects of neuroleptic drugs. Psychol Med 10:55–72, 1980.
36. Kolbe H, Clow A, Jenner P, et al: Neuroleptic-induced acute dystonic reactions may be due to enhanced dopamine release or to supersensitive postsynaptic receptors. Neurology 31:434–439, 1981.
37. Cadet JL, Lohr JB: Possible involvement of free radicals in neuroleptic-induced movement disorders. Ann N Y Acad Sci 570:176–185, 1989.
38. Javaid JI: Clinical pharmacokinetics of antipsychotics. J Pharmacol 34:286–295, 1994.
39. Ereshefsky L: Pharmacokinetics and drug interactions: Update for new antipsychotics. J Clin Psychiatry 57(Suppl 11):12–25, 1996.
40. Fang J, Gorrod JW: Metabolism, pharmacogenetics, and metabolic drug-drug interactions of antipsychotic drugs. Cell Mol Neurobiol 19:491–510, 1999.
41. Dahl ML, Bertilsson L: Genetically variable metabolism of antidepressants and neuroleptics. Pharmacogenetics 3:61–70, 1993.
42. Goff DC, Baldessarini RJ: Drug interactions with antipsychotic agents. J Clin Psychopharmacol 13:57–67, 1993.
43. Edge SC, Markowitz JS, DeVane CL: Clozapine drug interactions: A review of the literature. Hum Psychopharmacol 12:5–20, 1997.
44. Klimke A, Klieser E: Sudden death after intravenous application of lorazepam in a patient treated with clozapine (Letter). Am J Psychiatry 151:780, 1994.
45. Tanaka E, Hisawa S: Clinically significant pharmacokinetic drug interactions with psychoactive drugs: Antidepressants and antipsychotics and the cytochrome P450 system. J Clin Pharm Ther 24:7–16, 1999.
46. Taylor D: Pharmacokinetic interactions involving clozapine. Br J Psychiatry 171:109–112, 1997.
47. Cohen LG, Chesley S, Eugenio L, et al: Erythromycin-induced clozapine toxic reaction. Arch Intern Med 156:675–677, 1996.
48. Funderburg LG, Vertrees JE, True JE, Miller AL: Seizure following addition of erythromycin to clozapine treatment. Am J Psychiatry 151:1840–1841, 1994.
49. Stevens I, Gaertner HJ: Plasma level measurement in a patient with clozapine intoxication. J Clin Psychopharmacol 16:86–87, 1996.
50. Desta Z, Kerbusch T, Glockhart DA: Effect of clarithromycin on the pharmacokinetics and pharmacodynamics of pimozide in healthy poor and extensive metabolizers of cytochrome P450 2D6 (CYP2D6). Clin Pharmacol Ther 65:10–20, 1999.
51. Lee HS, Tan CH, Au LSY: Serum and urine risperidone concentrations in acute overdose. J Clin Psychopharmacol 17:325–326, 1997.
52. Mahutte CK, Nakassuto SK, Light RW: Haloperidol and sudden death due to pulmonary edema. Arch Intern Med 142:1951–1952, 1982.
53. Li C, Gefter WB: Acute pulmonary edema induced by overdosage of phenothiazines. Chest 101:102–104, 1992.
54. Acri AA, Henretig FM: Effects of risperidone in overdose. Am J Emerg Med 16:498–501, 1998.
55. LeBlaye I, Donatini B, Hall M, Krupp P: Acute overdosage with clozapine: A review of the available clinical experience. Pharm Med 6:169–178, 1992.
56. O'Malley GF, Seifert S, Heard K, et al: Olanzapine overdose mimicking opioid intoxication. Ann Emerg Med 34:279–281, 1999.
57. Harmon TJ, Benitez JG, Krenzelok EP, Cortes-Belen E: Loss of consciousness from acute quetiapine overdosage. J Toxicol Clin Toxicol 36:599–602, 1998.
58. Barry D, Meyskens FL, Becker CE: Phenothiazine poisoning: A review of 48 cases. Calif Med 118:1–5, 1973.
59. Mitchell AA, Lovejoy FH, Goldman P: Drug ingestions associated with miosis in comatose children. J Pediatr 89:303–305, 1976.
60. Mady S, Wax P, Wang D, et al: Pediatric clozapine intoxication. Am J Emerg Med 14:462–463, 1996.
61. Bonin MM, Burkhart KK: Olanzapine overdose in a 1-year old male. Pediatr Emerg Care 15:266–267, 1999.
62. Cheslik TA, Erramouspe J: Extrapyramidal symptoms following accidental ingestion of risperidone in a child. Ann Pharmacother 30:360–363, 1996.
63. Tam CW, Olin BR, Ruiz AE: Loxapine-associated rhabdomyolysis and acute renal failure. Arch Intern Med 140:975–976, 1980.
64. Yip L, Dart RC, Graham K: Olanzapine toxicity in a toddler (Letter). Pediatrics 102:1494, 1998.
65. Bond GR, Thompson JD: Olanzapine pediatric overdose (Letter). Ann Emerg Med 34:292–293, 1999.
66. McGuigan MA: Phenothiazines. Clin Toxicol Review 3, 1981.
67. Meeker JE, Herrmann PW, Som SW, Reynolds PC: Clozapine tissue concentrations following an apparent suicidal overdose of Clozaril. J Anal Toxicol 16:54–56, 1992.
68. Elian AA: Fatal overdose of olanzepine. Forensic Sci Int 91:231–235, 1998.
69. Meeker JE, Herrmann PW, Som SW: Clozapine tissue concentrations following an apparent suicidal overdose of Clozaril. J Anal Toxicol 16:54–56, 1992.
70. Elkayam U, Frishman W: Cardiovascular effects of phenothiazines. Am Heart J 100:397–401, 1980.
71. Fowler ND, McCall D, Chou T, et al: Electrocardiographic changes and cardiac arrhythmias in patients receiving psychotropic drugs. Am J Cardiol 37:223–230, 1981.
72. Fletcher GF, Kazamias TM, Wenger NK: Cardiotoxic effects of Mellaril: Conduction disturbances and supraventricular arrhythmias. Am Heart J 78:135–138, 1961.
73. Fulop G, Phillips RA, Shapiro AK, et al: ECG changes during haloperidol and pimozide treatment of Tourette's disorder. Am J Psychiatry 144:673–675, 1987.
74. Marris-Simon P, Zell-Kanter M, Kendzlerski D, et al: Cardiotoxic manifestations of mesoridazine overdose. Ann Emerg Med 17:1074–1078, 1988.
75. Thornton CC, Wendkos MH: EKG T-wave distortions among thioridazine-treated psychiatric inpatients. Dis Nerv Syst 32:320–323, 1971.
76. Neimann JT, Stapczynski JS, Rothstein RJ, et al: Cardiac conduction and rhythm disturbances following suicidal ingestion of mesoridazine. Ann Emerg Med 10:585–588, 1981.
77. Lee AM, Knoll JL, Suppes R: The atypical antipsychotic sertindole: A case series. J Clin Psychiatry 58:410–416, 1997.
78. Brown K, Levy H, Brenner C, et al: Overdose of risperidone. Ann Emerg Med 22:1908–1910, 1993.
79. Lynch S, Fill S, Hoffman RS: Intentional quetiapine (Seroquel) overdose (Abstract). J Toxicol Clin Toxicol 37:631, 1999.
80. Hustey FM: Acute quetiapine poisoning. J Emerg Med 17:995–997, 1999.
81. Kopala LC, Day C, Dillman B, Gardner D: A case of risperidone overdose in early schizophrenia: A review of potential complications. J Psychiatry Neurosci 23:305–308, 1998.
82. Palatnick W, Meatherall R, Tenenbein M: Ventricular tachycardia associated with remoxipride overdose (Abstract). J Toxicol Clin Toxicol 33:492, 1995.
83. Flugelman MY, Tal A, Pollack S, et al: Psychotropic drugs and long QT syndromes: Case reports. J Clin Psychiatry 46:290–291, 1985.
84. Aunsholt NA: Prolonged QT interval and hypokalemia caused by haloperidol. Acta Psychiatr Scand 79:411–412, 1989.
85. Lawrence KR, Nasraway SA: Conduction disturbances associated with administration of butyrophenone antipsychotics in the critically ill: A review of the literature. Pharmacotherapy 17:531–537, 1997.
86. Frye MA, Coudreaut MF, Hakeman SM, et al: Continuous droperidol infusion for management of agitated delirium in an intensive care unit. Psychosomatics 36:301–305, 1995.
87. Riker RR, Fraser GL, Cox PM: Continuous infusion of haloperidol controls agitation in critically ill patients. Crit Care Med 22:433–440, 1994.
88. Krahenbuhl SI, Sauter B, Kupferschmidt H, et al: Reversible QT prolongation with torsades de pointes in a patient with pimozide intoxication. Am J Med Sci 309:315–316, 1995.
89. Tamminga CA: The promise of new drugs for schizophrenia treatment. Can J Psychiatry 42:265–273, 1997.
90. Hulisz DT, Dasa SL, Black LD, et al: Complete heart block and torsades de pointes associated with thioridazine poisoning. Pharmacotherapy 14:239–245, 1994.

91. Wilt JL, Minnema AM, Johnson RF, et al: Torsades de pointes associated with the use of intravenous haloperidol. Ann Intern Med 119:391–394, 1993.

92. Sharma ND, Rosman HS, Padhi D, Tisdale JE: Torsades de pointes associated with intravenous haloperidol in critically ill patients. Am J Cardiol 81:238–240, 1998.

93. Ravin DS, Levenson JW: Fatal cardiac event following initiation of risperidone therapy. Ann Pharmacother 31:867–870, 1997.

94. Mehtonen OP, Aranko K, Malkonen L, et al: A survey of sudden death associated with the use of antipsychotic or antidepressant drugs: 49 cases in Finland. Acta Psychiatr Scand 84:58–64, 1991.

95. Hollister LE, Kosek JV: Sudden death during treatment with phenothiazine derivatives. JAMA 192:1035–1038, 1965.

96. Marks RC, Luchins DJ: Antipsychotic medications and seizures. Psychiatr Med 9:37–52, 1991.

97. Selim K, Kaplowitz N: Hepatotoxicity of psychotropic drugs. Hepatology 29:1347–1351, 1999.

98. Hummer M, Kurz M, Kurzthalaer I, et al: Hepatotoxicity of clozapine. J Clin Psychopharmacol 17:314–317, 1997.

99. Ishak K, Irey N: Hepatic injury associated with the phenothiazines. Arch Pathol 93:283–304, 1972.

100. Derby L, Gutthann SP, Jick H, Dean A: Liver disorders in patients receiving chlorpromazine or isoniazid. Pharmacotherapy 13:354–358, 1993.

101. Litvak R, Kaelbling R: Agranulocytosis, leukopenia and psychotropic drugs. Arch Gen Psychiatry 24:265–267, 1971.

102. Trayle WH: Phenothiazine-induced agranulocytosis (Letter). JAMA 256:1957, 1986.

103. Alvir J, Lieberman J, Safferman A, et al: Clozapine-induced agranulocytosis: Incidence and risk factors in the United States. N Engl J Med 329:162–167, 1993.

104. Safferman A, Lieberman JA, Kane JM, et al: Update on the clinical efficacy and side effects of clozapine. Schizophr Bull 17:247–261, 1991.

105. Lorenz M, Evering WE, Provencher A, et al: Atypical antipsychotic-induced neutropenia in dogs. Toxicol Appl Pharmacol 155:227–236, 1999.

106. Geibig CB, Marks LW: Treatment of clozapine- and molindone-induced agranulocytosis with granulocyte colony-stimulating factor. Ann Pharmacother 27:1190–1194, 1993.

107. Muscettola G, Barbato G, Pampallona D, et al: Extrapyramidal syndromes in neuroleptic-treated patients: Prevalence, risk factors, and association with tardive dyskinesia. J Clin Psychopharmacol 19:203–208, 1999.

108. Casey D: The relationship of pharmacology to side effects. J Clin Psychiatry 58(Suppl 10):55–62, 1997.

109. Cortese L, Pourcher-Bouchard E, Williams R: Assessment and management of antipsychotic-induced adverse events. Can J Psychiatry 43(Suppl 1):15S-20S, 1998.

110. Swett C: Drug-induced dystonia. Am J Psychiatry 132:532–534, 1982.

111. Ayd FJ: A survey of drug-induced extrapyramidal reactions. JAMA 175:1054–1060, 1961.

112. Koek RJ, Edmond HP: Acute laryngeal dystonic reactions to neuroleptics. Psychosomatics 30:359–364, 1989.

113. Hegarty AM, Lipton RB, Merriam AE, et al: Cocaine as a risk factor for acute dystonic reactions. Neurology 41:1670–1672, 1991.

114. Lee AS: Treatment of drug-induced dystonic reactions. J Am Coll Emerg Physicians 8:453–457, 1979.

115. Freed E: Alcohol-triggered neuroleptic-induced tremor, rigidity and dystonia. Med J Aust 2:44–45, 1981.

116. Drotts DL, Vinson DR: Prochlorperazine induces akathisia in emergency patients. Ann Emerg Med 34:469–475, 1999.

117. Yassa R, Ananth J, Cordozo S, et al: Tardive dyskinesia in an outpatient population: Prevalence and predisposing factors. Can J Psychiatry 28:391–394, 1983.

118. Forrest FM, Forrest IS, Mason AS: Review of rapid urine tests for phenothiazine and related drugs. Am J Psychiatry 118:300–307, 1961.

119. Tranum BL, Murphy ML: Successful treatment of ventricular tachycardia associated with thioridazine (Mellaril). South Med J 62:357–358, 1969.

120. Lumpkin J, Watanabe AS, Rumack BH, et al: Phenothiazine-induced ventricular tachycardia following acute overdose. J Am Coll Emerg Physicians 8:476–478, 1979.

121. Pietro DA: Thioridazine-associated ventricular tachycardia and isoproterenol (Letter). Ann Intern Med 94:411, 1981.

122. Kemper A, Dunlop R, Pietro D: Thioridazine-induced torsades de pointes successful therapy with isoproterenol. JAMA 249:2931–2934, 1983.

123. Burns MJ, Linden CH, Graudins A, et al: A comparison of physostigmine and benzodiazepines for the treatment of anticholinergic poisoning. Ann Emerg Med 35:374–381, 2000.

124. Schuster P, Gabriel E, Luefferie B, et al: Reversal by physostigmine of clozapine-induced delirium. Clin Toxicol 10:437–441, 1977.

125. Koppel C, Schirop T, Ibe K, et al: Hemoperfusion in chlorprothixene overdose. Intensive Care Med 13:358–360, 1987.

126. Donlon PT, Tupin JP: Successful suicides with thioridazine and mesoridazine. Arch Gen Psychiatry 34:955–957, 1977.

127. Hals PA, Jacobsen D: Resin hemoperfusion in levomepromazine poisoning: Evaluation of effect on plasma drug and metabolite levels. Hum Toxicol 3:497–503, 1984.

128. Corre K, Neimann J, Bessen H: Extended therapy for acute dystonic reactions. Ann Emerg Med 13:194–197, 1984.

129. Vinson DR, Drotts DL: Diphenhydramine prevents akathisia induced by intravenous prochlorperazine: A randomized controlled trial (Abstract). Acad Emerg Med 6:533, 1999.

130. Adler L, Angrist B, Peselow E, et al: A controlled assessment of propranolol in the treatment of neuroleptic-induced akathisia. Br J Psychiatry 149:42–45, 1983.

131. Zubenko GS, Cohen BM, Lipinski JF, et al: Use of clonidine in treating neuroleptic-induced akathisia (Letter). Psychiatry Res 13:253, 1985.

132. Goren JL, Levin GM: Quetiapine, an atypical antipsychotic. Pharmacotherapy 18:1183–1194, 1998.

133. Markowitz JS, Brown CS, Moore TR: Atypical antipsychotics: Part I. Pharmacology, pharmacokinetics, and efficacy. Ann Pharmacother 33:73–85, 1999.

134. Pickar D: Prospects for pharmacotherapy of schizophrenia. Lancet 345:557–562, 1995.

135. Seeger TF, Seymour PA, Schmidt AW, et al: Ziprasidone (CP-88,059): A new antipsychotic with combined dopamine and serotonin receptor antagonist activity. J Pharmacol Exp Ther 275:101–113, 1995.

136. Bymaster FP, Perry KW, Nelson DL, et al: Olanzapine: A basic science update. Br J Psychiatry 174(Suppl 37):36–40, 1999.

137. Meltzer HY, Matsubara S, Lee JC: Classification of typical and atypical antipsychotic drugs on the basis of dopamine D-1, D-2 and serotonin$_2$ pK$_i$ values. J Pharmacol Exp Ther 251:238–246, 1989.

CHAPTER 46

Lithium

Jeffrey Brent ▪ Laura J. Klein

Lithium salts have found many therapeutic uses over the years. The major currently accepted indication is to treat bipolar disorders. Most commonly, lithium is used in the form of the carbonate salt.

The earliest attempted medicinal use of lithium was in 1841, when it was advanced as a potential therapy for gout, a condition for which it soon was recognized to be ineffective.[1] Several years later, lithium was proposed as a treatment of rheumatic nodes and bladder stones. Most literature cites the seminal article by the Australian psychiatrist Cade[2] as the initial study promulgating the efficacy of lithium salts in the treatment of mania. Many earlier publications recognized its potential utility in the treatment of mood disorders, however. The Cade article, showing an attenuation of mania, followed his observation of a sedating effect of lithium on pigs. In a book by Hammond[3] published in 1871, lithium was recommended for the treatment of mania and depression. Similarly a publication by Lange in 1897, as described by Hanson and Amdisen,[4] is reported to have promoted lithium's efficacy of the treatment of depression.

After the publication of the article by Cade,[2] lithium's use in the treatment of mood disorders became commonplace. Further studies on the use of lithium for bipolar disease were conducted in Europe, resulting in earlier widespread use of these salts there than in the United States.[5] The use of lithium salts in the United States lagged behind Europe because of many reports in the American literature in which the use of lithium as a salt substitute resulted in several deaths.

Along with the widespread use of lithium salts as a therapeutic agent, case reports were published describing significant toxic manifestations from this therapy associated with elevated serum lithium concentrations. El-Mallakh[6] described case reports of lithium toxicity dating back to 1948. In 1978, Hanson and Amdisen[4] described 100 case reports of lithium intoxication from the published literature dating back to 1949. There is little question that unmonitored lithium therapy, particularly in a susceptible patient, may result in toxicity.

BIOCHEMISTRY AND CLINICAL PHARMACOLOGY

Chemistry

Lithium, from the Greek *lithos* meaning "stone," is in group 1A of the periodic table, situated immediately above sodium, providing an explanation for the similarity in behavior of these two ions. Lithium's atomic number of 3 means that it contains three electrons with a single unpaired one in its outermost shell. This outermost electron is ionized easily, creating the Li^+ ion. Lithium has an atomic weight of 6.9.

Because of the chemical similarities between lithium and sodium, lithium chloride has a salty taste. Starting in the late 1940s, lithium chloride was available in the United States as a salt substitute (West Sal). Ingestion of lithium chloride led to virtually immediate adverse effects,[7,8] some fatal, resulting in the regulatory actions taken in regard to lithium salts by the U.S. Food and Drug Administration.[9,10]

Pharmacokinetics

Pharmacokinetics of Lithium

Volume of distribution: 0.7–1.4 L/kg
Therapeutic plasma concentration: 0.3–1.6 mmol/L
Protein binding: negligible
Plasma elimination half-life: 12–27 hr*
Mode of elimination: renal
Method to enhance elimination: hemodialysis

*The half-lives given are for volunteers. Many factors, primarily therapeutic use (as opposed to overdose in a lithium-naive patient), advanced age, and any decrease in renal clearance, may increase half-life.

Peak plasma lithium concentrations occur 30 minutes to 4 hours after a dose, although this can be prolonged further in delayed-release preparations.[5,6,11] Liquid preparations are absorbed most rapidly. For standard lithium preparations, absorption is usually complete within 8 hours.[11] When lithium is used therapeutically, target plasma concentrations vary from 0.3 to 1.6 mmol/L, depending on the indication. Lithium circulates as free Li^+ ion in plasma without significant protein binding. Plasma elimination half-life in volunteers ranges from 12 to 27 hours.[12–14] The elimination half-life is longer in patients with long-term lithium treatment, related to tissue stores of the Li^+ ion in this population. This same phenomenon probably explains the slow excretion of lithium after its therapeutic use has been discontinued.[15] The half-lives in patients with lithium toxicity range from 12.9 to 50.1 hours in different published series.[16]

Lithium elimination can be reduced dramatically in the elderly, and this population should be considered to be at particular risk for toxicity during therapeutic use. Lithium's serum half-life with therapeutic use has been reported to be 36 hours in elderly patients, increasing with reductions in creatinine clearance.[17,18] Similarly, any patient, regardless of age, with subnormal creatinine clearance should be considered to have at least a relative contraindication to lithium therapy.

When absorbed, lithium distributes to multiple tissues, with the most consequences in the brain, kidney, and thyroid.[19,20] Tissue concentrations of lithium may continue to increase for hours after plasma levels have peaked, with its distribution through the blood-brain barrier into the brain being slower than into other organs.[21] This slow distribution phase probably accounts for the delayed onset of action and the delayed resolution of lithium-induced central nervous system manifestations after toxic exposure. Its volume of distribution is reported variously to be between 0.7 and 1.4 L/kg.[22–24] Lithium is found in the cerebrospinal fluid, although only at approximately 40% of plasma concentrations[25] because of its active transport out of the cerebrospinal fluid.[26]

Virtually all of an ingested lithium dose is excreted renally, with only trace amounts found in sweat, saliva, or breast milk. When filtered through the glomerulus, lithium and sodium are reabsorbed in the proximal tubule. Approximately 80% of the filtered lithium undergoes active reabsorption against an electrical and a chemical gradient in this segment of the nephron.[5,15,27,29] Lithium is reabsorbed further in the loop of Henle.[5] In contrast to sodium, lithium is not reabsorbed in the distal tubule.[30] It has a reported renal clearance of 13 to 56 mL/minute,[12,13,27,31] and its fractional clearance (lithium clearance/creatinine clearance) has been reported to be 0.17 to 0.29.[13,27,32] The renal clearance and fractional excretion of lithium decrease during hemodialysis.[4] In volunteer studies, lithium clearance can be increased by the administration of sodium chloride or bicarbonate, acetazolamide, urea, or aminophylline.[27] Neither water loading nor loop diuretics affect lithium clearance.[27] The small amount of lithium that is not eliminated renally is excreted in the feces and perspiration. Lithium exhibits a high clearance by conventional hemodialysis (100 to 150 mL/min).[4,33] However, Hemodialysis effectively removes only plasma Li+, and there is often a posthemodialysis "rebound" increase in serum lithium concentration as a consequence of its diffusional flux down its concentration gradient from tissues into the vascular compartment.[4,31,34]

PATHOPHYSIOLOGY

Central Nervous System Effects

The mechanism of lithium's mood-stabilizing effect is unknown and a matter of considerable debate. Lithium causes a variety of effects on neurons, although the exact contribution, if any, of these neuropharmacologic actions to its therapeutic effects is uncertain.

It is tempting to speculate that the chemical similarity between lithium and sodium causes the former to modulate the action of the latter on neuronal function. Lithium, similar to sodium, can enter the neuron via the fast sodium channel and stimulate an action potential. In contrast to sodium, however, it is a poor substrate for the Na+-K+ pump, and no lithium-related electrochemical gradient across the cell

membrane can be maintained. It is further tempting to theorize that lithium entry by the fast sodium channel, coupled with its relative inability to be pumped out of the cell, causes intraneuronal lithium loading. How this loading might relate to the mood-stabilizing effects of lithium is unclear, however.

Lithium affects many enzymes and other proteins involved in neuronal and nonneuronal function and may modulate neurotransmission and central nervous system excitability. Neurons have many regulatory guanosine triphosphate–binding proteins, and lithium is known to inhibit their activities.[35]

Research focusing on the molecular mechanism underlying the therapeutic effect of lithium has revealed that it induces changes in the activities of cellular signal transduction systems, especially the phosphatidylinositol and cyclic adenosine monophosphate (cAMP) second messenger systems. Extracellular signal-related kinase pathways may mediate lithium's antimanic effects.[36] Lithium also may modulate phosphatases that have been implicated in the cause of bipolar disease.[37]

Cardiac Effects

Increase in myocardial lithium may lower intracellular potassium concentrations, causing T-wave flattening and ST-segment abnormalities.[39,40]

Thyroid Effects

Li+ ion concentrates in the thyroid gland, achieving concentrations four to five times those occurring simultaneously in the plasma. Normally the thyroidal response to thyroid-stimulating hormone is mediated by cAMP. The formation and the action of the latter may be inhibited by lithium, however. Additionally, in rodent models, lithium has been shown to reduce organification of iodine and colloid formation.[41–43]

Renal Effects

In 1970, the unresponsiveness of the kidney to antidiuretic hormone (ADH) was reported in patients being treated with lithium.[44] The result is loss of renal urine-concentrating ability. This effect is reflected further in the increased excretion of ADH during lithium treatment.[45] ADH acts by stimulating renal adenylyl cyclase to produce cAMP, a reaction inhibited by lithium.[46] ADH regulates the renal water channel (aquaporin). Lithium treatment causes a downregulation of this channel.[42] The end result of this loss of renal concentration ability is diabetes insipidus, characterized by excessive free water loss with resulting hypernatremia. Because of its nonresponsiveness to ADH, this effect is called *nephrogenic diabetes insipidus* (NDI). Lithium also may cause an alkaline urine and renal tubular acidosis.[5]

CLINICAL PRESENTATION

Lithium intoxication is characterized primarily by neuromuscular hyperexcitability and, in more severe cases, central nervous system dysfunction. Many renal abnormalities may occur, most prominently NDI. Although NDI may be seen with long-term therapy, it frequently becomes manifest after episodes of toxicity. Lithium may have adverse effects on the thyroid gland and may have adverse cardiac effects therapeutically and during periods of toxicity. Acute lithium toxicity is often associated with gastrointestinal symptoms. A modification of the grading scheme for lithium intoxication, promulgated by Hansen and Amdisen,[4,16,48] is presented in Table 46-1.

A dominant theme that must accompany all considerations of patients with lithium toxicity is the profound difference in clinical presentation between a lithium-naive patient who takes an acute overdose and an individual who presents with inadvertent toxicity after therapeutic use. The latter group shows markedly more profound manifestations of toxicity at much lower serum lithium concentrations.[49] This difference is due to the tissue lithium stores present in a patient taking lithium long-term. Lithium in the end organs, not the blood, is responsible for its toxic manifestations.

In the classic analysis of 123 cases of lithium intoxication by Hansen and Amdisen,[4] aside from the obvious acute overdose, intravascular volume depletion in association with negative water balance was found to be the major predisposing factor for lithium intoxication. Volume loss from decreased intake, excessive perspiration, gastrointestinal fluid loss, or diuretics can predispose to lithium toxicity.[50–53] Similarly, drugs that decrease renal glomerular blood flow, most notably angiotensin-converting enzyme inhibitors, may cause lithium toxicity. Although nonsteroidal antiinflammatory drugs decrease glomerular filtration rate, their propensity to induce lithium toxicity seems to be minimal.[11] Lithium-induced NDI and polyuria[11] can contribute to a vicious cycle of intravascular volume depletion and worsening toxicity. Because thiazide diuretics selectively act to decrease sodium (and increase lithium) reabsorption in the proximal tubule, this class of diuretics is most prone to cause lithium toxicity.[54]

TABLE 46-1 Grading System for Lithium Intoxication[4]

GRADE	FEATURES
0	Asymptomatic
1	Any of the following
	Nausea
	Vomiting
	Tremor
	Hyperreflexia
	Agitation
	Muscle weakness
	Ataxia
	Drowsiness
2	Any of the following
	Stupor
	Rigidity
	Hypotension
3	Any of the following
	Coma
	Seizures
	Myoclonia
	Cardiovascular instability

Data from references 4, 24, and 48.

Neurologic Effects

For reasons described earlier, there is overall a poor correlation between serum lithium concentration and clinical presentation. Patients with lithium intoxication present with a clinical picture predominantly characterized by hyperreflexia, tremor, motor hyperactivity, increased tone and rigidity, drowsiness, apathy, sluggishness, ataxia, fasciculations, and stupor, in approximately that order of decreasing frequency.[4,49]

Most patients with lithium toxicity have abnormal electroencephalograms (EEGs).[4,55] Some authors have suggested that EEG changes correlate better with lithium toxicity than do serum concentrations,[56] although this has not been studied systematically. EEG changes are typically polymorphic, with rhythmic slowing of theta and delta waves of moderate-to-high voltage. These can be continuous or paroxysmal and diffuse or focal. Epileptiform changes may occur and can even mimic status epilepticus.[56] In the series by Hansen and Amdisen,[4] 83% of patients had EEGs on admission, all of which were severely abnormal, mostly with 2 to 5 Hz spikes and sharp waves. All of these EEGs showed improvement over time as the lithium toxicity resolved, and most of them normalized.

Although in most patients lithium-induced neurotoxicity is transient, there have been many reports of permanent neurologic sequelae in patients with lithium intoxication.[4,11,56–61] Interpretation of these reports is limited, however, by the frequent lack of baseline information and other possible confounding factors, such as neuroleptic drug use, preexisting diagnoses, alcoholism, or brain damage due to other factors.

Renal Effects

Many lithium-induced renal abnormalities have been described with therapeutic use and intoxication. Various reports have described decreases in creatinine clearance,[62,63] oliguria[5,62,63] or polyuria,[5,49,61–63] renal tubular acidosis,[5,49,61–64] decreased urinary concentrating ability,[5,49,61–64] and nephrotic syndrome.[5,6,63] Acute renal failure after lithium intoxication is unusual, occurring in 7% of patients in one series.[49]

Diabetes insipidus and hypernatremia have been reported to occur in 20% of patients during therapeutic use or episodes of lithium intoxication.[49,65,66] Many more patients have polyuria, polydipsia, decreased urinary concentrating ability, and increased thirst.[67] This diabetes insipidus is not usually responsive to vasopressin (Pitressin) and is nephrogenic in origin.

Thyroid Effects

Hypothyroidism, even to the point of myxedema, or possibly with goiter, occasionally is related to lithium therapy.[68,69] The incidence of hypothyroidism associated with lithium therapy has been reported to be 1% to 20%.[69,71] Risk factors for developing lithium-induced hypothyroidism include female gender, a family history of thyroid disease, and age older than 60.[68–71] Because hypothyroidism and depression can appear clinically similar, it is possible for the former to be overlooked. Because of the inhibitory effect of lithium on the thyroid, hyperthyroidism can be suppressed by lithium therapy.[72] An illustrative case

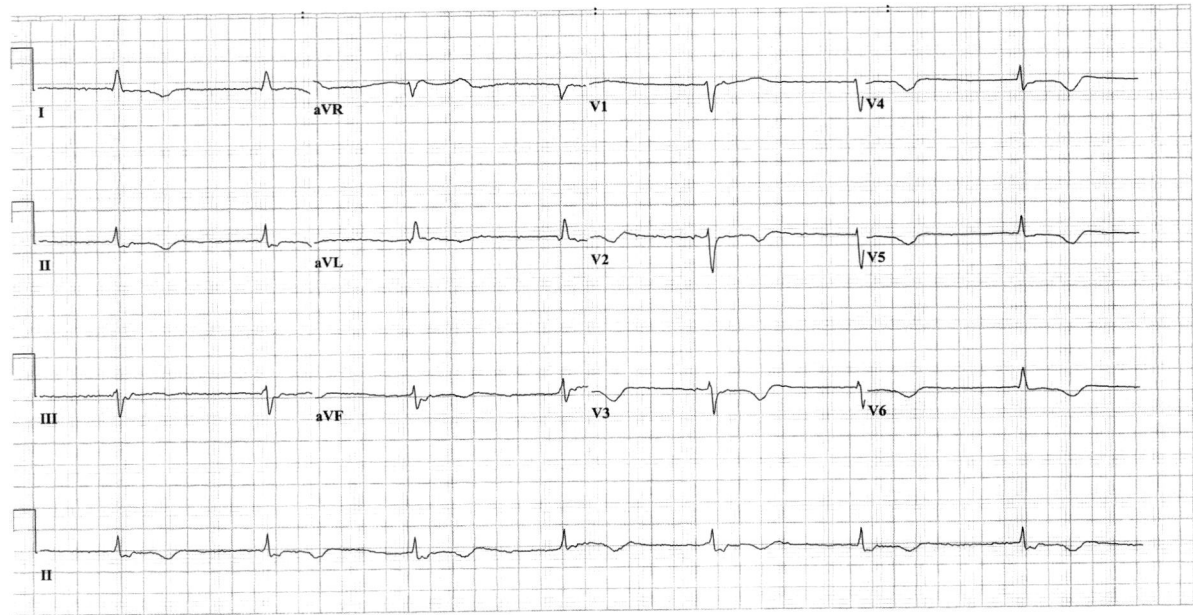

FIGURE 46-1

ECG of a 53-year-old woman with chronic lithium toxicity (level 2.4 mEq/L) and acute delirium. She presented with junctional bradycardia and underwent emergent hemodialysis on day 1 and had spontaneous conversion to normal sinus rhythm on hospital day 4. Note the diffuse T-wave inversion. *(Courtesy of J. Ward Donovan, MD, PinnacleHealth Toxicology Center, Harrisburgh, PA.)*

report described a patient with lithium toxicity and no prior diagnosis of hyperthyroidism who developed thyroid storm after hemodialysis.[72]

Cardiac Effects

Many electrocardiogram changes have been associated with therapeutic lithium use and toxicity, including nonspecific ST-T wave changes, bradycardia, conduction blocks, and junctional rhythms.[1,42] The most common effects seen with therapeutic use are T-wave flattening or inversion and depressed ST segments in the lateral leads (Fig. 46-1)[1,42]

DIAGNOSIS

The diagnosis of lithium toxicity usually is made on the basis of the clinical history, determination of serum or plasma lithium concentration, and clinical suspicion. In the absence of a history of lithium ingestion, patients who present with the various clinical features described in the preceding section, such as altered mental status, hyperreflexia, tremor, increased tone, and diabetes insipidus, should be suspected of having lithium toxicity. If a patient has a history of psychiatric disorder or access to lithium in the environment, this should heighten the suspicion.

Lithium typically is assayed in the plasma using emission photometry, atomic absorption spectroscopy, or an Li+ ion–specific electrode. In most instances, serum or plasma lithium concentrations are measured, and most clinical experience is with these analyses. Some authors have suggested that a better correlate of tissue lithium concentrations is provided by

measurement of red blood cell lithium concentrations; however, there is little clinical experience with the interpretation of these latter values.

A clue to unrecognized elevated plasma lithium concentrations may occur in the form of an abnormally low, or even negative, anion gap; this occurs because lithium is an unmeasured cation. Given the propensity of lithium to induce hypothyroidism, a thyroid-stimulating hormone determination is appropriate.

The blood lithium concentration must be interpreted in the context of whether the patient may have had an acute overdose, has been on long-term lithium therapy, or both. Patients who are on long-term lithium therapy and who overdose on this medication may present with a clinical picture that is intermediate between acute and chronic toxicity.[4]

Acute Toxicity

Acute lithium toxicity generally presents with markedly elevated plasma or serum lithium concentrations and a relative paucity of clinical signs, particularly if presentation is early after overdose. This represents the phase during which lithium is primarily in the plasma and has not distributed yet into tissues. If plasma lithium concentration remains elevated for a prolonged time, however, it may distribute into various tissue compartments, and clinical manifestations may become evident thereafter. Because lithium exerts its neurologic effects while resident in the brain, and because distribution of lithium into and out of the brain is slow, the development and resolution of these clinical manifestations lag behind the initial rise and subsequent fall in plasma concentrations.

Chronic Toxicity

The diagnosis of chronic lithium toxicity can be much more challenging than the diagnosis of acute lithium overdose. These patients may have significant tissue lithium stores yet have modest plasma lithium concentrations.[4,49,83] Lithium concentrations in the plasma may decrease to low or undetectable levels despite significant ongoing end-organ manifestations of toxicity.

TREATMENT

As with all poisonings, the treatment of lithium intoxication may require aggressive management of the patient's airway and ventilation and circulatory support, depending on clinical severity. Patients who are lithium intoxicated may be hypermetabolic, may be diaphoretic, may have decreased fluid intake or frank emesis, and are likely to be intravascularly volume depleted. Because lithium clearance depends on glomerular filtration rate, fluid resuscitation to normalize the patient's intravascular volume and establish normal urine flow is paramount. Because lithium clearance increases with sodium loading,[27] resuscitation with isotonic saline to the point of normal intravascular volume clinically with attainment or maintenance of eunatremia may enhance lithium's renal clearance. Because many of these patients have NDI, however, aggressive fluid management with normal saline may lead to hypernatremia. When the goal of eunatremia and volume resuscitation is achieved, it is advisable to change the intravenous fluid to half-normal saline.

Patients who have severe lithium toxicity may have many secondary complications, including seizures, acute renal failure, severe rhabdomyolysis, and adult respiratory distress syndrome. These complications should be treated by standard supportive measures, with no specific treatment indicated as a result of their occurrence in the context of lithium toxicity.

Gastrointestinal Decontamination

Lithium does not bind to activated charcoal.[74] Gastric lavage has not been shown to alter the outcome or clinical course of patients who have overdosed on lithium and is unlikely to be beneficial. Based on the current state of knowledge, however, the use of lavage in a patient who presents less than 1 hour after an acute ingestion cannot be discouraged completely because of the theoretical possibility of efficacy (see Chapter 5). Because the likelihood of gastric lavage having a major effect is small, its use should be considered optional at best.

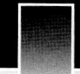

Indications for ICU Admission in Lithium Poisoning

Supratherapeutic and rising serum lithium concentrations
Significant manifestations of toxicity (e.g., altered mental status, rigidity, hyperreflexia)
Cardiovascular or other instability

WHOLE-BOWEL IRRIGATION

Because it is not bound to activated charcoal, lithium often is cited as a common example of a toxin for which whole-bowel irrigation (see Chapter 5) may be a useful technique after an acute overdose of a large amount of this substance. Although there is no question that whole-bowel irrigation is done on occasion, there is a striking lack of reported clinical experience with this technique in lithium overdose. In addition to the theoretical basis of this technique, its utility in the reduction of lithium absorption has been documented in a randomized crossover study using healthy volunteers.[75] In this study, there was a significant reduction of lithium absorption after whole-bowel irrigation was initiated 1 hour postingestion. Irrigation was accomplished by the administration of 2 L/hr of polyethylene glycol over 5 hours. The applicability of this approach to clinical practice is unknown, however, because it is difficult to administer whole-bowel irrigation solutions at rates greater than 1 L/hr, and in these volunteer studies the amount ingested was by necessity small. There are no controlled data relating to the effect, if any, of whole-bowel irrigation on either outcome or clinical course of patients who have lithium toxicity. Whole-bowel irrigation is a relatively benign procedure, however, and a reasonable, although untested, approach for patients who have large lithium ingestions is to administer polyethylene glycol solutions via a nasogastric tube at rates of up to 2 L/hr until it can be documented that either serum lithium concentrations are declining or there is radiologic evidence of gastrointestinal decontamination. The latter would apply if radiopaque tablets were visualized in the bowel on abdominal flat films. Some lithium preparations are radiopaque, but this is not universally true. In the event that a radiopaque preparation is ingested, whole-bowel irrigation could be administered until most of the tablets are shown to have been cleared from the gastrointestinal tract. There is no compelling reason to continue this procedure until every last one is removed.

SODIUM POLYSTYRENE SULFONATE

The cation exchange resin sodium polystyrene sulfonate (SPS) has been shown to bind lithium in vitro.[76,77] Many animal studies, reviewed in detail by Scharman,[78] have shown that SPS administration can reduce measured serum lithium concentrations after either single or multiple doses of the latter. This reduction has been shown to occur when SPS is given after a significant delay following oral administration[79] even when the lithium was administered intravenously.[80] These two studies show that SPS in the gastrointestinal tract has the capability of decreasing the absorption of lithium and enhancing its clearance. The latter probably is the result of enteral-enteral lithium recirculation. These animal data used larger doses of SPS (2.5 to 5 g/kg) than typically are used to treat hypokalemia in humans.[78,81] In a murine model of chronic lithium intoxication, oral administration of SPS reduced serum lithium concentrations. The SPS dose was 5 g/kg, repeated for a total of five doses over 60 minutes.[82] As described subsequently, however, this dose is greater than may be practical or safe in humans.

Two human volunteer studies showed that doses of SPS of less than 1 g/kg can reduce the absorption of small amounts of lithium.[83,84] A case report of a patient with lithium overdose described treatment with 150 g of SPS over a 24-hour period without significant adverse effects. The authors of this report cited the patient's elimination half-life of lithium of 12 hours as evidence of SPS's efficacy.[85]

The optimal dose of SPS is unknown. It seems that a single dose of 1 g/kg may be efficacious without significantly affecting either serum sodium or potassium concentrations.[84] Rather than administering repetitive doses of SPS, however, which may cause hypernatremia and hypokalemia, it may be prudent to use whole-bowel irrigation if serum lithium concentrations continue to increase. Because of the possibility of potassium loss during SPS treatment, it may be advantageous to administer supplemental potassium to patients with serum concentrations of this ion in the low normal range. In patients who are frankly hypokalemic, SPS should be avoided. If supplemental potassium is administered, it is theoretically best to give it intravenously to prevent loss of SPS binding capacity. Potassium supplementation may decrease lithium's binding to SPS. It is unknown if intravenous potassium administration affects the ability of SPS to bind lithium. In a volunteer study comparing the effects of a single oral dose of SPS (857 mg/kg) with that of 250 mL of polyethylene glycol every 10 minutes for a total dose of 4 L, with both treatments starting 1 hour after ingestion, there was an equivalent reduction in lithium absorption associated with both interventions compared with untreated controls.[86]

Enhancement of Elimination

A fundamental goal in the treatment of lithium toxicity is the enhancement of its elimination. Generally, studies aimed at evaluating the utility of this approach have focused on clearance of lithium from the vascular compartment. This clearance usually is accomplished easily and quickly, particularly in patients with normal renal function. Physiologically, it is most important, however, to remove the lithium from target tissue compartments. Because this removal cannot be done directly, the indirect approach of clearing the plasma of lithium and encouraging a flux of the Li^+ ion down its concentration gradient from the tissue to the blood is the theoretical rationale for enhancing its plasma clearance.

As noted earlier, there are data in a rodent model of lithium toxicity suggesting that SPS may be effective in enhancing the clearance of already absorbed Li^+ ion. Whether there is any clinical utility to this approach is unknown.

Renal elimination of lithium constitutes the exclusive means by which it is cleared from the body. Because renal lithium clearance is a direct function of glomerular filtration rate, it is important to maintain intravascular volume and renal perfusion. Conventional wisdom has held that because lithium and sodium are reabsorbed primarily in the proximal convoluted tubule, a sodium load would enhance lithium absorption. Normal saline treatment has been shown to enhance lithium and creatinine clearance in a group of lithium-intoxicated patients.[4,49,87] Hospitalized psychiatric patients with bipolar disorder who are opposed to their lithium therapy have been known to reduce their lithium levels by consumption of large amounts of table salt. Whether normal saline is efficacious because of the competitive effect of the sodium ion on proximal tubular cation uptake or simply by virtue of its utility in reconstituting glomerular filtration is unknown. As noted earlier, overzealous treat-

ment with normal saline can result in hypernatremia in patients with clinical or subclinical NDI. There does not seem to be any role for forced diuresis.[4,27,49]

Extracorporeal Techniques

Lithium is well cleared by hemodialysis, with reported clearances of 63 to 170 mL/min[4,31,34,88]; this compares favorably with an endogenous clearance of 13 to 56 mL/min.[88] Similarly, half-lives of lithium have ranged from 2.3 to 12.9 hours on hemodialysis.[16,31,88] Most of these studies were done with older generation dialysis membranes. High-flux hemodialysis membranes are likely to enhance lithium elimination markedly. In one report, lithium half-life during hemodialysis with a high-flux system was 1.36 to 1.91 hours.[89]

A rebound in plasma lithium concentration is seen frequently after the termination of hemodialysis.[31,88] This rebound undoubtedly represents the slow rate of flux from peripheral tissues to the vascular compartment. It also may reflect continued gastrointestinal absorption. It is possible that acetate hemodialysis is more efficient than hemodialysis performed with bicarbonate-containing dialysate for the removal of intracellular lithium.[90] It has been hypothesized that acetate, being a weak acid, moves into the cell along with protons via the Na^+/H^+ transporter, with resultant net lithium efflux rather than sodium efflux.[90]

There are no generally accepted indications for hemodialysis. The indications that are in the literature rely on serum lithium concentration, renal function, and clinical status.[4,24,87,88,91] The one indication that is unambiguously supported is compromised renal function because this would impair the elimination of lithium in the absence of an extracorporeal removal intervention. Because many patients are volume depleted at presentation, however, it is appropriate to resuscitate the patient rapidly and aggressively in support of the recovery of age-appropriate normal renal function. Beyond that, most experienced clinicians probably would agree that patients with Hansen and Amdisen grade III toxicity I (see Table 46-1) represent the population most likely to benefit from hemodialysis and that grade 0 patients are unlikely to achieve any improvement in prognosis. Unequivocal recommendations cannot be made regarding patients with grade I or grade II toxicity other than to rehydrate them, follow their clinical course, and contemplate hemodialysis for worsening clinical toxicity in the presence of slowly decreasing, stable, or increasing serum lithium concentrations. Even so, hemodialysis has not been shown, under any circumstances, to alter patient outcome after lithium intoxication. The one study that attempted to evaluate the efficacy of hemodialysis in a controlled fashion did not show any beneficial effect of this intervention.[16] This was a nonrandomized study of only 17 patients, however, only 1 of whom had grade III toxicity. No firm conclusions regarding the clinical efficacy of hemodialysis can be gleaned from this study. It seems unlikely that patients with grade 0 through grade II toxicity would gain significant benefit from hemodialysis, even if it is helpful for patients with more severe toxicity. It also seems unlikely that hemodialysis would be of appreciable benefit to patients with low serum lithium concentrations.

Peritoneal Dialysis

Peritoneal dialysis has been reported anecdotally for the enhancement of lithium clearance.[4,92,93] It is typically done with 2 L/hr fluid volume exchanges; however, the clearances reported were only 9 to 15 mL/min. It is not expected that peritoneal dialysis would be advantageous in enhancing lithium clearance, particularly in a patient with normal renal function.

Other Extracorporeal Techniques

Clearances reported with continuous extracorporeal removal techniques tend to be less than clearances achievable with hemodialysis. Continuous techniques have the advantage of being simpler than hemodialysis, however, and often can be used when the latter is unavailable or the patient is too unstable hemodynamically to undergo effective hemodialysis. Lithium clearances with continuous arterial-venous hemodiafiltration have been reported to be 20.5 to 55.6 mL/min.[94,95] Clearances with continuous venovenous hemodiafiltration have been reported to range from 27.68 to 61.9 mL/min.[95,96] Clearances with continuous venovenous hemodialysis have been reported to be 15.66 to 23 mL/min.[95,97] None of the continuous techniques provide clearances that approach those attainable with hemodialysis. In a patient who cannot tolerate hemodialysis because of hemodynamic instability, however, or if these facilities are unavailable, continuous arterial-venous hemodiafiltration or continuous venovenous hemodiafiltration seems to be preferable to continuous venovenous hemodialysis.

Other Therapies

Because theophylline, like aminophylline (the intravenous form of theophylline), has been reported to increase renal clearance, there is potential for these agents to be used adjunctively in the treatment of lithium toxicity.[27] This potential has been studied only in volunteers, however, in whom the effect of theophylline on lithium clearance has been highly variable. Because of the potential toxicity associated with aminophylline and the lack of clinical experience with this technique, we do not recommend this approach.

There is a case report describing the attempt to enhance glomerular filtration with so-called renal doses of dopamine (2 μg/kg/min) to enhance lithium excretion.[98] Other than this case report, there is little clinical experience with this approach.

Treatment of Nephrogenic Diabetes Insipidus

NDI may be an overt clinical consequence of lithium therapy or may be subclinical and only manifested with the institution of normal saline therapy in an attempt to treat lithium toxicity. The fundamental deficit in NDI is loss of free water. Treatment primarily should involve administration of intravenous hypotonic fluids, such as half-normal saline or 5% dextrose in water or enteral administration of water. Antidiuretic hormone therapy is typically ineffective. The reconstitution of intracellular and extracellular fluid volume using these fluids should be done cautiously. Although the fluid deficits can be large, the administration

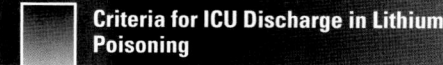

Criteria for ICU Discharge in Lithium Poisoning

Falling or nondetectable serum lithium concentrations
Resolving clinical signs of toxicity

of half-normal saline too rapidly may result in relative overexpansion of the extracellular compartment. The administration of 5% dextrose too rapidly may exacerbate hyperglycemia in a patient with glucose intolerance and on the basis of concomitant osmotic diuresis may aggravate the fluid volume loss. In either instance, the fluid volume deficit should be corrected gradually, with enteral sterile water supplementation in a patient with a functioning gut.

The goal of therapy is to gradually correct fluid volume deficits comprising the sum of the intracellular and extracellular volume losses. Normal intracellular fluid (ICF) volume is approximately 0.4 L/kg. A reliable estimate of the patient's actual ICF may be obtained using the following equation:

$$ICF = \frac{(normal\ ICF \times [2 \times normal\ serum\ Na^+]) \times weight}{2 \times measured\ Na^+}$$

In this equation, normal ICF is 0.4 L/kg, and normal serum sodium is 140 mmol/L. In a 70-kg patient, the normal ICF would be (0.4 L/kg × 70 kg), or 28 L. If with lithium-induced NDI the serum Na^+ is 150 mmol/L, the actual ICF would be approximately 26 L, representing a 2-L ICF deficit. The calculation of the extracellular fluid (ECF) volume cannot be done simply based on the measured serum Na^+ but rather must be estimated on clinical grounds. The normal ECF is approximately 0.2 L/kg, or 14 L/70 kg. It reasonably can be assumed that hypernatremic patients with NDI and relatively normal physical examinations have an approximately 10% decrease in ECF, although if signs of volume depletion are present, this can be 20%. If ECF volume decreases to 30% of normal, the patient is in frank circulatory shock. The total fluid volume deficit in need of replacement is the sum of the calculated ICF and estimated ECF deficits. An alternative, and in some cases simpler, approach to estimating the total fee water deficit (FWD) is to use the following formula and make empirical adjustments in replacement therapy:

$$FWD = \frac{(measured\ serum\ [Na^+] - 140) \times 0.66 \times wt\ (kg)}{140}$$

SPECIAL POPULATIONS

Pregnant Patients

Concern for the teratogenic potential of lithium has arisen from the demonstration, in several animal experiments, of adverse fetal outcomes occurring in treated pregnant dams.[99,100] These abnormalities occurred, however, only when animals were given overt maternally toxic amounts of lithium, were markedly dissimilar in various species, and did not occur in lithium-treated primates.[101]

In response to the possible teratogenic risk of lithium, a registry of treated patients was initiated in Denmark in 1969.[102] Similar registries were formed in other countries, leading ultimately to the International Register of Lithium Babies.[99,102,103] Based on the results of these registries, concern about potential adverse effects, particularly Ebstein's anomaly, surfaced. These registry data are uncontrolled, however, and prone to ascertainment bias. In contrast, there have been eight epidemiologic studies of offspring outcome among women treated with lithium during pregnancy: two cohort trials broadly dealing with teratogenicity and six case-control studies.[99] Collectively the data from these studies indicate that the initial concern for fetal risk raised by registry data was not verified. Risk has not been ruled out completely, however, and it may be prudent to avoid lithium therapy, particularly during the first trimester of pregnancy. In patients in whom lithium treatment is strongly indicated, it has been suggested that pregnancy be monitored by fetal echocardiography and ultrasound evaluation during the mid–second trimester.[99] Consistent with the demonstration that lithium crosses the placenta, a case has been published suggesting transient neonatal lithium toxicity after birth from a lithium-toxic mother.[104]

Because of the high glomerular filtration rate in pregnancy, renal lithium clearance is high. Given the rapid postpartum decline and normalization of glomerular filtration rate, it is important to reduce the maternal lithium dose and monitor plasma concentrations closely after parturition.

Although some lithium is excreted in breast milk, breast-feeding infants of treated mothers tend to have low circulating lithium concentrations.[100,105] As would be expected with older individuals, however, should the infant become volume depleted, serum lithium concentrations might rise.

Other Patients

Because lithium clearance depends completely on renal excretion, patients with decreased renal function are at particular risk for lithium toxicity. The presence of renal insufficiency should be considered at least a relative contraindication for treatment. Even in the absence of frank overt elevations in serum creatinine, normal decline in renal function with age suggests that the elderly are particularly vulnerable to lithium toxicity.

Common Errors in Lithium Poisoning

Thinking that diuresis beyond adequate urine production enhances lithium excretion

Failure to recognize significant lithium toxicity in the presence of normal or undetectable plasma concentrations

---

Key Points in Lithium Poisoning

1. Any factor that causes a decrease in lithium's renal clearance may predispose to toxicity.
2. Lithium toxicity is caused by its concentration in tissues (e.g., brain, kidney, thyroid), and its plasma levels may not reflect accurately the degree of intoxication.
3. Lithium is cleared renally. Its clearance may be enhanced further by hemodialysis.
4. Nephrogenic diabetes insipidus is a potential complication of its therapeutic use and toxic exposure.

REFERENCES

1. Tilkian AG, Schroeder JS, Kao JJ, et al: The cardiovascular effects of lithium in man: A review of the literature. Am J Med 61:665–670, 1976.
2. Cade JF: Lithium salts in the treatment of psychotic excitement. Med J Aust 2:349, 1949.
3. Hammond WA: A treatise on diseases of the nervous system. New York, D. Appleton & Company, 1871, p. 381.
4. Hansen HE, Amdisen A: Lithium intoxication. QJM 186:123–144, 1978.
5. Chan W-Y, Mosca P, Rennert OM: Lithium nephrotoxicity: A review. Ann Clin Lab Sci 11:343–349, 1981.
6. El-Mallakh RS: Acute lithium neurotoxicity. Psychiatr Dev 4:311–328, 1986.
7. Corcoran AC, Taylor RD, Page IH: Lithium poisoning from the use of salt substitutes. JAMA 139:685–688, 1949.
8. Hanlon LW, Romaine M, Gilroy FJ, et al: Lithium chloride as a substitute for sodium chloride in the diet. JAMA 139:688–692, 1949.
9. Bazilinski N, Mathew J: Lithium intoxication. Int J Artif Organs 9:5–6, 1986.
10. Editorial: Case of the substitute salt. Time 53:27, 1949.
11. Okusa MD, Jovita L, Crystal MD: Clinical manifestations and management of acute lithium intoxication. Am J Med 97:383–389, 1994.
12. Amdisen A: Monitoring of lithium treatment through determination of lithium concentration. Dan Med Bull 22:277–291, 1975.
13. Groth U, Prellwitz W, Jahnchen E: Estimation of pharmacokinetic parameters of lithium from saliva and urine. Clin Pharmacol Ther 16:490–498, 1974.
14. Thornhill DP: Pharmacokinetics of ordinary and sustained-release lithium carbonate in manic patients after acute dosage. Eur J Clin Pharmacol 14:267–271, 1978.
15. Singer I, Rotenberg D: Mechanisms of lithium action. N Engl J Med 289:254–260, 1973.
16. Bailey B, McGuigan M: Comparison of patients hemodialyzed for lithium poisoning and those for whom dialysis was recommended by PCC but not done: What lesson can we learn? Clin Nephrol 54:388–392, 2000.
17. Hicks R, Dysken MW, Davis JM, et al: The pharmacokinetics of psychotropic medication in the elderly: A review. J Clin Psychol 42:374–385, 1981.
18. Baldessarini RJ: Lithium salts: 1970–1975. Ann Intern Med 83:527–533, 1975.
19. Schou M: Lithium studies: Distribution between serum and tissues. Acta Pharmacol 15:115–124, 1958.
20. Berens SC, Wolff J, Murphy DL: Lithium concentration by the thyroid. Endocrinology 87:1085–1087, 1970.
21. Anderson RJ: Clinical Use of Drugs in Renal Failure. Springfield, IL, Charles C Thomas, 1976.
22. Lee C-F, Yang Y-Y, Hu OY-P: Single dose pharmacokinetic study of lithium in Taiwanese/Chinese bipolar patients. Aust N Z J Psychiatry 32:133–136, 1998.
23. Lehmann K, Merten K: Elimination of lithium in correlation with age in normal subjects and in renal insufficiency. Int J Clin Pharmacol Ther Toxicol 10:292–298, 1974.
24. Amdisen A: Clinical features and management of lithium poisoning. Med Toxicol 3:18–32, 1988.

25. Terhaag B, Scherber A, Schaps P, et al: The distribution of lithium into cerebrospinal fluid, brain tissue and bile in man. Int J Clin Pharmacol Biopharm 16:333–335, 1978.

26. Erlich BE, Diamond JM: Lithium, membranes and manic-depressive illness. J Membr Biol 52:187–200, 1980.

27. Thomsen K, Schou M: Renal lithium excretion in man. Am J Physiol 215:823–827, 1968.

28. Thomsen K, Schou M, Steiness I, et al: Lithium as an indicator of proximal sodium reabsorption. Pfluger Arch 308:180–184, 1969.

29. Singer I, Franko EA: Lithium-induced ADH resistance in toad urinary bladder. Kidney Int 3:151–159, 1973.

30. Amdisen A: Lithium. In Widdop B (ed): Therapeutic Drug Monitoring. Edinburgh, Churchill Livingstone, 1985, pp 302–329.

31. Jacobsen D, Aasen G, Frederichsen P, et al: Lithium intoxication pharmacokinetics during and after terminated hemodialysis in acute intoxications. Clin Toxicol 25:81–94, 1987.

32. Weder AB: Red-cell lithium-sodium countertransport and renal lithium clearance in hypertension. N Engl J Med 314:198–201, 1986.

33. Jacobsen D, Aasen G, Frederichsen P: Pharmacokinetics of lithium during and after terminated hemodialysis in intoxicated patients. Vet Hum Toxicol 26:475, 1987.

34. Jaeger A, Sauder P, Konferschmitt J, et al: Toxicokinetics of lithium intoxication created by hemodialysis. J Toxicol Clin Toxicol 23:501–507, 1986.

35. Manji HK, Chen G, Shimon H, et al: Guanine nucleotide-binding proteins in bipolar affective disorder. Arch Gen Psychiatry 52:135–144, 1995.

36. Gollub RL, Hyman SE: G proteins and second messengers in psychiatry. Harv Rev Psychiatry 3:41–44, 1995.

37. Agam G, Shaltiel G: Possible role of 3′(2′)-phosphoadenosine-5′ phosphate phosphatase in the etiology and therapy of bipolar disorder. Prog Neuropsychopharmacol Biol Psychiatry 27:723–727, 2003.

38. McKusick VA: The effects of lithium on the electrocardiogram of animals and the relation of these effects to the ratio of intracellular and extracellular concentrations of potassium. J Clin Invest 33:598–610, 1954.

39. Carmeliet EE: Influence of lithium ion on transmembrane potential and cation contents of cardiac cells. J Gen Physiol 47:501–530, 1964.

40. Ricciutti MA, Lis KR, Damato AN: A metabolic basis for the electrophysiologic effects of lithium. Circulation 44:217, 1971.

41. Kleiner J, Altshuler L, Hendrick V, et al: Lithium-induced subclinical hypothyroidism: Review of the literature and guidelines for treatment. J Clin Psychiatry 60:249–255, 1999.

42. Brady HR, Horgan JH: Lithium and the heart: Unanswered questions. Chest 93:166–169, 1988.

43. Capen CC: Pathophysiology of chemical injury of the thyroid gland. Toxicol Lett 64/65:381–388, 1992.

44. Angrist BM, Gershon S, Levitan SJ, et al: Lithium-induced diabetes insipidus-like syndrome. Comp Psychiatry 11:141–146, 1970.

45. MacNeil S, Jennings G, Eastwood PR, et al: Lithium and the antidiuretic hormone. Br J Clin Pharmacol 3:305–313, 1976.

46. Dousa TP: Interaction of lithium with vasopressin-sensitive cAMP system of human renal medulla. Endocrinology 95:1359, 1974.

47. Marples D, Christensen S, Christensen EI, et al: Lithium-induced downregulation of aquaporin-2 water channel expression in rat kidney medulla. J Clin Invest 95:1838–1845, 1995.

48. Amdisen A, Schou M: Lithium. In Dukes MNG (ed): Meyler's Side Effects of Drugs: An Encyclopedia of Adverse Reactions and Interactions. Amsterdam, Excerpta Medica, 1980, pp 43–50.

49. Dyson EH, Simpson D, Prescott LF, et al: Self-poisoning and therapeutic intoxication with lithium. Hum Toxicol 6:325–329, 1987.

50. Peterson V, Hvidt S, Thomsen K, et al: Effect of prolonged thiazide treatment on renal lithium clearance. BMJ 3:143–145, 1974.

51. Hurtig H, Pyson W: Lithium toxicity enhanced by diuresis. N Engl J Med 290:748–749, 1974.

52. Himmelhoch JM, Poust RI, Mallinger AG, et al: Adjustment of lithium dose during lithium-chlorothiazide therapy. Clin Pharmacol Ther 22:225–227, 1977.

53. Solomon K: Combined use of lithium and diuretics. South Med J 71:1098–1104, 1978.

54. Harvey NS, Merriman S: Review of clinically important drug interactions with lithium. Drug Saf 10:455–463, 1994.

55. Smith SJHM, Kocen RS: A Creutzfeldt-Jakob like syndrome due to lithium toxicity. J Neurol Neurosurg Psychiatry 51:120–123, 1988.

56. Gansaeuer M, Alsaadi TM: Lithium intoxication mimicking clinical and electrographic features of status epilepticus: A case report and review of the literature. Clin Electroencephalogr 34:28–31, 2003.

57. Bartha L, Marksteiner J, Bauer G, et al: Persistent cognitive deficits associated with lithium intoxication: A neuropsychological case description. Cortex 38:743–752, 2002.

58. Schou M: Long-lasting neurological sequelae after lithium intoxication. Acta Psychiatr Scand 70:594–602, 1984.

59. Saxena S, Mallikarjuna P: Severe memory impairment with acute overdose lithium toxicity: A case report. Br J Psychiatry 152:853–854, 1988.

60. Juul-Jensen P: Permanent brain damage after lithium intoxication. BMJ 4:673.

61. von Hartitzsch B, Hoenich NA, Leigh RJ, et al: Permanent neurological sequelae despite haemodialysis for lithium intoxication. BMJ 4:757–759, 1972.

62. Jorasky DK, Amsterdam JD, Oler J, et al: Lithium-induced renal disease: A prospective study. Clin Nephrol 30:293–302, 1988.

63. Markowitz GS, Radhakrishnan J, Kambham N, et al: Lithium nephrotoxicity: A progressive combined glomerular and tubulointerstitial nephropathy. J Am Soc Nephrol 11:1439–1448, 2000.

64. Rose SR, Klein-Schwartz W, Oderda GM, et al: Lithium intoxication with acute renal failure and death. Drug Intell Clin Pharm 22:691–694, 1988.

65. Paragas MG: Lithium adverse reactions in psychiatric patients. Pharmacol Biochem Behav 21:65–69, 1984.

66. Bendz H: Kidney function in lithium-treated patients. Acta Psychiatr Scand 68:303–324, 1983.

67. Simard M, Gumbiner B, Alexander L, et al: Lithium carbonate intoxication. Arch Intern Med 149:36–46, 1989.

68. Johnson AM, Eagles JM: Lithium-associated clinical hypothyroidism: Prevalence and risk factors. Br J Psychiatry 175:336–339, 1999.

69. Santiago R, Rashkin MC: Lithium toxicity and myxedema coma in an elderly woman. J Emerg Med 8:63–66, 1990.

70. Lindstedt G, Nilsson L, Walinder J, et al: On the prevalence, diagnosis and management of lithium-induced hypothyroidism in psychiatric patients. Br J Psychiatry 130:452–458, 1977.

71. Villeneuve A, Gautier J, Jus A, et al: Effect of lithium on thyroid in man. Lancet 1:502, 1973.

72. Oakley PW, Dawson AH, Whyte IM: Lithium: Thyroid effects and altered renal handling. J Toxicol Clin Toxicol 38:333–337, 2000.

73. Lewis DA: Unrecognized chronic lithium neurotoxic reactions. JAMA 250:2029–2030, 1983.

74. Favin FD, Klein-Schwartz W, Oderda GM, et al: In vitro study of lithium carbonate adsorption by activated charcoal. Clin Toxicol 26:443–450, 1988.

75. Smith SW, Ling LJ, Halstenson CE: Whole-bowel irrigation as a treatment for acute lithium overdose. Ann Emerg Med 20:536–539, 1991.

76. Watling SM, Gehrke JC, Gehrke CW, et al: In vitro binding of lithium using the cation exchange resin sodium polystyrene sulfonate. Am J Emerg Med 13:294–296, 1995.

77. Welch D, Driscoll J, Lewander W, et al: In vitro lithium binding with sodium polystyrene sulfonate. Vet Hum Toxicol 29:472, 1987.

78. Scharman EJ: Methods used to decrease lithium absorption or enhance elimination. Clin Toxicol 35:601–608, 1997.

79. Linakis JG, Hull KM, Lee CM, et al: Effect of delayed treatment with sodium polystyrene sulfonate on serum lithium concentrations in mice. Acad Emerg Med 3:333–337, 1996.

80. Linakis JG, Hull KM, Lacouture PG, et al: Enhancement of lithium elimination by multiple-dose sodium polystyrene sulfonate. Acad Emerg Med 4:175–178, 1997.

81. Linakis JG, Eisenberg MS, Lacouture PG, et al: Multiple-dose sodium polystyrene sulfonate in lithium intoxication: An animal model. Pharmacol Toxicol 70:38–40, 1992.

82. Linakis JG, Savitt DL, Wu T-Y, et al: Use of sodium polystyrene sulfonate for reduction of plasma lithium concentrations after chronic lithium dosing in mice. Clin Toxicol 36:309–313, 1998.

83. Belanger DR, Tierney MG, Dickinson G: Effect of sodium polystyrene sulfonate on lithium bioavailability. Ann Emerg Med 21:1312–1315, 1992.

84. Tomaszewski C, Musso C, Pearson JR, et al: Lithium absorption prevented by sodium polystyrene sulfonate in volunteers. Ann Emerg Med 21:1308–1311, 1992.

85. Roberge RJ, Martin TG, Schneider SM: Use of sodium polystyrene sulfonate in a lithium overdose. Ann Emerg Med 22:1911–1915, 1993.

86. Tilman DJ, Poddis BE, Watanabe MD, et al: Comparison of sodium polystyrene sulfonate (SPS) and polyethylene glycol solution (PEG) in decreasing area under the curve (AUC) of lithium carbonate. Vet Hum Toxicol 36:351, 1994.

87. Dyson EH, Freestone S, Simpson D, et al: Factors affecting renal lithium clearance. Kidney Int 28:278, 1985.

88. Jaeger A, Sauder P, Kopferschmitt J, et al: When should dialysis be performed in lithium poisoning? A kinetic study of 14 cases of lithium poisoning. J Toxicol Clin Toxicol 31:429–447, 1993.

89. Peces R, Pobes A: Effectiveness of haemodialysis with high-flux membranes in the extracorporeal therapy of life-threatening acute lithium intoxication. Nephrol Dial Transplant 16:1301–1303, 2001.

90. Szerlip H, Heeger P, Feldman GM: Comparison between acetate and bicarbonate dialysis for the treatment of lithium intoxication. Am J Nephrol 12:116–120, 1992.

91. Jaeger A, Sauder P, Kopferschmitt J, et al: Toxicokinetics of lithium intoxication treated by hemodialysis. J Toxicol Clin Toxicol 23:501–517, 1985.

92. Wilson JH, Donker AJ, van der Hem GK, et al: Peritoneal dialysis for lithium poisoning. BMJ 2:749–750, 1971.

93. O'Connor J, Gleeson J: Acute lithium intoxication: Peritoneal dialysis or forced diuresis. N Z Med J 95:790–791, 1982.

94. Bellomo R, Kealy Y, Parkin G, et al: Treatment of life-threatening lithium toxicity with continuous arterio-venous hemodiafiltration. Crit Care Med 19:836–839, 1991.

95. Leblanc M, Raymond M, Bonnardeaux A, et al: Lithium poisoning treated by high-performance continuous arteriovenous and venovenous hemodiafiltration. Am J Kidney Dis 27:365–372, 1996.

96. Hazouard E, Ferrandiere M, Rateau H, et al: Continuous veno-venous haemofiltration versus continuous veno-venous haemodialysis in severe lithium self-poisoning: A toxicokinetics study in an intensive care unit. Nephrol Dial Transplant 14:1605–1606, 1999.

97. Beckman U, Oakley PW, Dawson AH, et al: Efficacy of continuous venovenous hemodialysis in the treatment of severe lithium toxicity. J Toxicol Clin Toxicol 39:393–397, 2001.

98. MacDonald TM, Cotton M, Prescott LF: Low dose dopamine in lithium poisoning. Br J Clin Pharmacol 26:195–197, 1988.

99. Cohen LS, Friedman JM, Jefferson JW, et al: A re-evaluation of risk of in utero exposure to lithium. JAMA 271:146–150, 1994.

100. Weinstein MR, Goldfield MD: Administration of lithium during pregnancy. In Johnson FN (ed): Lithium Research and Therapy. New York, Academic Press, 1975, pp 237–264.

101. Gralla EJ, McIlhenny HM: Studies in pregnant rats, rabbits and monkeys with lithium carbonate. Toxicol Appl Pharmacol 21:428–433, 1972.

102. Weinstein MR: The International Register of Lithium Babies. Drug Info J 10:94–100, 1976.

103. Schou M, Goldfield MD, Weinstein MR, et al: Lithium and pregnancy: I. Report from the Register of Lithium Babies. BMJ 2:135–136, 1973.

104. Flaherty B, Dean BS, Krenzelok EP: Neonatal lithium toxicity as a result of maternal toxicity. Presented at NACCT 1995. Vet Hum Toxicol 39:92–93, 1997.

105. Linden S, Rich CL: The use of lithium during pregnancy and lactation. J Clin Psychiatry 44:358–360, 1983.

CHAPTER 47

Anxiolytic/Sedative-Hypnotics

Kevin L. Wallace ■ Daniel E. Brooks

Prescription sedative-hypnotic drug toxicity and withdrawal are commonly encountered clinical management challenges in the critical care arena. Although the chemical, pharmacokinetic, epidemiologic, and social characteristics of specific agents involved have changed dramatically over several decades, the essential features of sedative-hypnotic poisoning and withdrawal remain unchanged since the introduction of chloral hydrate (CH) in the mid-19th century. Over the ensuing decades, pharmaceutical research and development have led to a relative profusion of drugs prescribed for relief of anxiety and use as sleep aids.

By definition, sedative-hypnotic drugs exert a calming or anxiolytic effect, with associated drowsiness and induction of sleep. These pharmacologic agents include a variety of barbiturate, nonbarbiturate, and nonprescription (e.g., antihistamine) compounds. Prescription sedative-hypnotics that have been abused commonly since the 1980s primarily consist of benzodiazepine (e.g., diazepam) and benzodiazepine-like (e.g., zolpidem), barbiturate (e.g., butalbital), and barbiturate-like (e.g., meprobamate) drugs. The toxic effects of barbiturates are discussed in detail in Chapter 48.

Many prescription drugs with sedative-hypnotic activity exhibit significant abuse potential. The objectives of such misuse include achievement of a relaxed, euphoric state of intoxication; attenuation of undesirable effects of illicit drugs, such as cocaine and amphetamines; relief of withdrawal from other drugs (e.g., heroin); and the performance of criminal acts (e.g., robbery or sexual assault) against other individuals after surreptitious drug administration. As a result of the development of pharmacodynamic tolerance, chronic abuse of prescription sedative-hypnotic agents promotes a characteristic withdrawal syndrome after abrupt discontinuation, varying from agent to agent only with respect to intensity and timing (e.g., onset) and closely similar to the withdrawal syndrome associated with ethanol (see also Chapters 14, 30, and 48).

Benzodiazepines have been the most widely prescribed class of drugs worldwide since the market introduction of chlordiazepoxide in 1955. Many other prescription sedative-hypnotics, including glutethimide (Doriden), ethchlorvynol (Placidyl), chloral hydrate (Beta-Chlor, "Mickey Finn"), methaqualone (Quaalude), and methyprylon (Noludar), have been historically important sources of sedative-hypnotic abuse and poisoning. A marked decline in relative incidence of reported toxic exposures to these agents in the United States from 7.5% to less than 1% of the sedative-hypnotic category total over nearly two decades[1,2] suggests, however, that their role in more recent sedative-hypnotic abuse, acute

poisoning, and withdrawal has become relatively minor, although some are still marketed in the United States and elsewhere. The toxicology of these older, less prescribed, and less used agents is summarized briefly later in this chapter.

BENZODIAZEPINES AND BENZODIAZEPINE-LIKE DRUGS

The widespread clinical application of benzodiazepine sedative-hypnotics attests to their efficacy and safety. Unless it occurs in combination with other central nervous system (CNS) depressant agents (e.g., ethanol, tricyclic antidepressants, opioids, barbiturates, or antihistamines), benzodiazepine overdose, even in large amounts, rarely results in acute, life-threatening respiratory or hemodynamic manifestations. The wide margin of safety of benzodiazepines has made them appealing for the inpatient and outpatient management of anxiety disorders, agitation, and substance abuse and withdrawal.

It has been suggested that the newer, higher potency benzodiazepines (e.g., flunitrazepam) are more likely than the older, lower potency drugs (e.g., diazepam) to be associated with life-threatening CNS depression and ventilatory failure. A published forensic series in Australia involving eight deaths in which flunitrazepam was concluded to play either a causative or a significant contributory role in outcome has been cited in support of this agent-specific risk[3]; however, the presence of ethanol and other drugs confounded this interpretation in four of these cases. The facts that none of the deaths were witnessed and that the deaths were estimated to have occurred as long as 4 days before discovery further weaken support for the notion that flunitrazepam overdose has greater potential for lethality than overdose with other benzodiazepine drugs.

Flunitrazepam also has become known for its illicit use as a "date rape" drug.[4,5] Known to recreational and criminal users as "roofies," "rophies," and "forget me pill," flunitrazepam's rapid onset and induction of disinhibition and amnesia and the frequent failure to detect it on an immunoassay-based drug screen or by chromatographic assay enhance its criminal applications. Although not approved for use in the United States and banned from import into this country, flunitrazepam can be obtained elsewhere (e.g., Mexico), where it is sold legally and with fewer restrictions, in general, on prescription and distribution of substances than those that fall under regulatory control in the United States.

Zolpidem is a relatively recent addition to the sedative-hypnotic class of drugs. Despite its nonbenzodiazepine chemical classification, zolpidem mediates its effects through CNS benzodiazepine receptors. Its clinical pharmacology and toxicology are similar to those of benzodiazepine drugs.

Chemistry and Pharmacokinetics

The structures of representative benzodiazepine and benzodiazepine-like sedative-hypnotic drugs are shown in Figure 47-1. Except for clorazepate, whose bioavailability requires gastric decarboxylation to nordiazepam, benzodiazepines generally are absorbed completely after oral administration.[6] Another pharmacokinetic property that applies to benzodiazepines as a class is a relatively high degree of plasma protein binding (60% to 95%). Other relevant pharmacokinetic properties are summarized in Table 47-1. The interrelated pathways involved in the metabolism of selected benzodiazepines are shown schematically in Figure 47-2.

Particular attention should be directed to the fact that benzodiazepine elimination is primarily hepatic and that active metabolites result from phase I metabolism of selected drugs, such as chlordiazepoxide, diazepam, flurazepam, and alprazolam, the elimination of which may be significantly slower than that of the parent compound (see also Chapter 30). In addition, as is described in greater detail

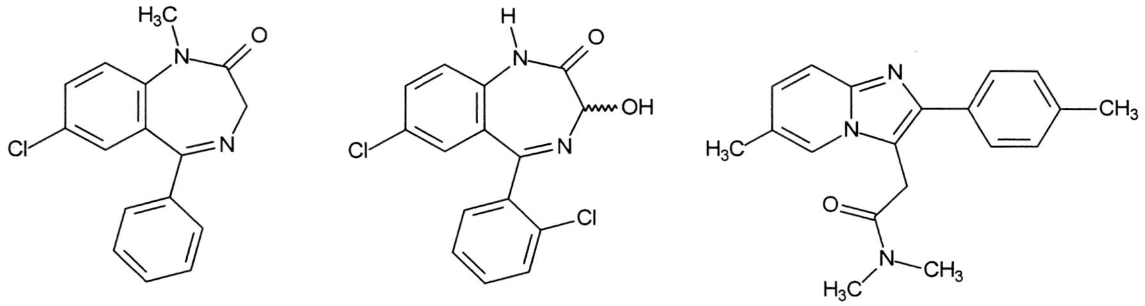

Diazepam   **Lorazepam**   **Zolpidem**

FIGURE 47-1

Chemical structures of representative benzodiazepine and benzodiazepine-like drugs.

TABLE 47-1   Benzodiazepines and Benzodiazepine-like Drugs

GENERIC DRUG (TRADE NAME)	ESTIMATED EQUIVALENCY (mg)	HALF-LIFE PARENT COMPOUND (hr)	ESTIMATED DURATION (hr)[†]
Onset: 2–3 hr			
Halazepam (Paxipam)	20	14–15	Long[‡]
Oxazepam (Serax*)	20	3–25	Intermediate
Prazepam (Centrax*)	20	Prodrug	Long[‡]
Temazepam (Restoril*)	15	5–20	Intermediate
Zolpidem (Ambien)	10	1.4–4.5	Short
Onset: 1–2 hr			
Alprazolam (Xanax*)	0.75	6.3–26.9	Intermediate
Chlordiazepoxide (Librium*)	25	5–48	Long[‡]
Clonazepam (Klonopin)	2	18–50	Long[‡]
Estazolam (ProSom)	2	10–34.6	Intermediate
Flurazepam (Dalmane*)	15	Prodrug	Long[‡]
Lorazepam (Ativan*)	1	10–20	Intermediate
Quazepam (Doral)	15	25–53	Long[‡]
Triazolam (Halcion*)	0.375	1.5–5.5	Short
Onset: <1 hr			
Clorazepate (Tranxene*)	15	Prodrug	Long[‡]
Diazepam (Valium*)	10	20–80	Long[‡]
Midazolam (Versed)	0.035	1.5–12	Intermediate
Flunitrazepam (Rohypnol)	1	10–30	Intermediate

*Generic available in United States.
[†]Arbitrarily based on mean half-life of parent compound: half-life <4 hr = short; half-life ≤24 hr = intermediate; half-life >24 hr = long duration.
[‡]Due to presence of active metabolite with a long half-life.

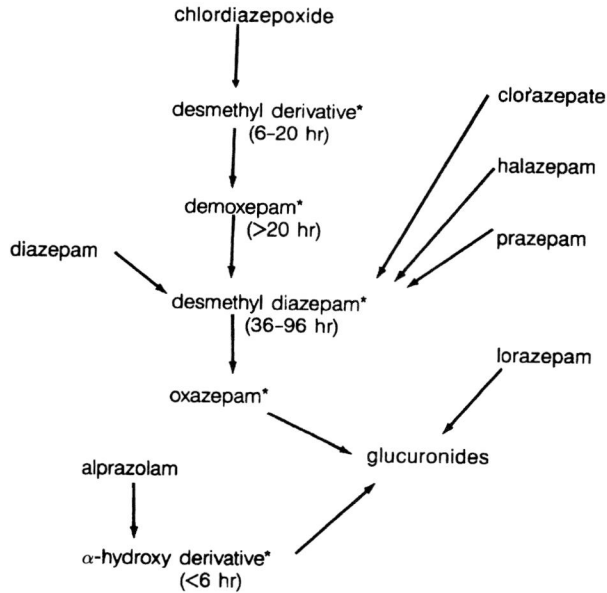

FIGURE 47-2

Metabolism of selected benzodiazepines. *(From Rech RH: Drugs to treat anxieties and related disorders. In Brody TM, Larner J, Minneman KP [eds]: Human Pharmacology: Molecular to Clinical, 3rd ed. St. Louis, Mosby, 1998, p 369.)*

elsewhere in this book, age (see Chapter 12), liver disease, and the coadministration of agents that inhibit hepatic metabolism (e.g., CYP3A4 inhibitors, such as selected macrolide antibiotics and imidazole antifungal agents) are important considerations in the individual who may have relatively pronounced or prolonged clinical effects of benzodiazepine administration.

Pathophysiology

The sedative-hypnotic and the anticonvulsant effects of benzodiazepine and benzodiazepine-like (e.g., zolpidem) drugs result from the drugs' effects on the activity of two CNS inhibitory neurotransmitters (see Chapter 20). In addition to their indirect γ-aminobutyric acid (GABA) agonist actions, enhancing the binding of GABA to postsynaptic neuronal Cl⁻ (GABA$_A$) (Fig. 47-3) channels, benzodiazepine compounds inhibit the presynaptic uptake of adenosine.[7] The latter neurotransmitter exerts a negative modulatory effect on the presynaptic release of glutamate, the principal excitatory neurotransmitter in the CNS. The consequences of these actions are (1) increased postsynaptic influx of negatively charged ions (Cl⁻) and (2) decreased glutamate-stimulated postsynaptic influx of positively charged ions (Na⁺ and Ca²⁺), resulting in widespread postsynaptic neuronal hyperpolarization and suppression of electrical impulse propagation.

Clinical Presentation and Life-Threatening Complications

The clinical manifestations of acute and chronic benzodiazepine overdose range from mildly depressed sensorium to coma. Impaired psychomotor skill, somnolence, dysarthria, nystagmus, ataxia, hyporeflexia, and, usually, non–life-threatening respiratory depression are common features of benzodiazepine intoxication.[6,8] In general, the incidence, severity, and duration of these effects increase with age, which is explained on the basis of age-related changes in drug disposition and neuropharmacologic actions (see Chapter 12). Hypoventilatory respiratory failure is an unusual complication of benzodiazepine overdose, even when ingested in massive amounts. If respiratory failure occurs, it should suggest the presence of another CNS depressant agent or existence of significant underlying disease (e.g., chronic obstructive pulmonary disease).

Retrograde and antegrade amnesia occur after therapeutic and supratherapeutic doses of benzodiazepines, which may be advantageous during the performance of medical or surgical procedures that produce discomfort. Benefit from acute ingestion of benzodiazepines may extend to their prophylactic anticonvulsant effects, particularly when overdose also involves ingestion of a proconvulsant agent, such as a cyclical antidepressant drug. Toxic delirium, transient global amnesia, and psychosis have been reported in association with the use of triazolam (Halcion),[9] although controlled studies have failed to support hypotheses that such untoward behavioral effects result with greater frequency after use of any one benzodiazepine than with others in the class.[10,11]

Diagnosis

The laboratory detection and identification of benzodiazepines in blood and urine have been major analytic challenges. The relatively low sensitivity[12] and low specificity[13,14] of immunoassay methods (e.g., enzyme multiplied immunoassay technique) and limited ability to detect benzodiazepines in biologic matrices by more specific methods (e.g., gas chromatography/mass spectrometry) are explained by the low concentrations of some benzodiazepine drugs in urine and their loss during gas chromatography.[14] A false-positive urine immunoassay for benzodiazepines was reported to occur after use of the nonsteroidal antiinflammatory drug oxaprozin (Daypro).[15] Although their value to forensic case investigation occasionally may be shown, there is little or no utility in obtaining quantitative or qualitative assays for benzodiazepine compounds in the clinical setting. The toxic differential diagnosis for acute benzodiazepine poisoning is extremely broad, including a variety of other agents with CNS depressant effects that are mediated by indirect GABA-agonist actions (e.g., ethanol, barbiturates, and meprobamate).

Treatment

 Indications for ICU Admission in Benzodiazepine Toxicity

Established or impending respiratory failure
Prolonged or profound level of obtundation
Withdrawal syndrome, refractory to initial treatment

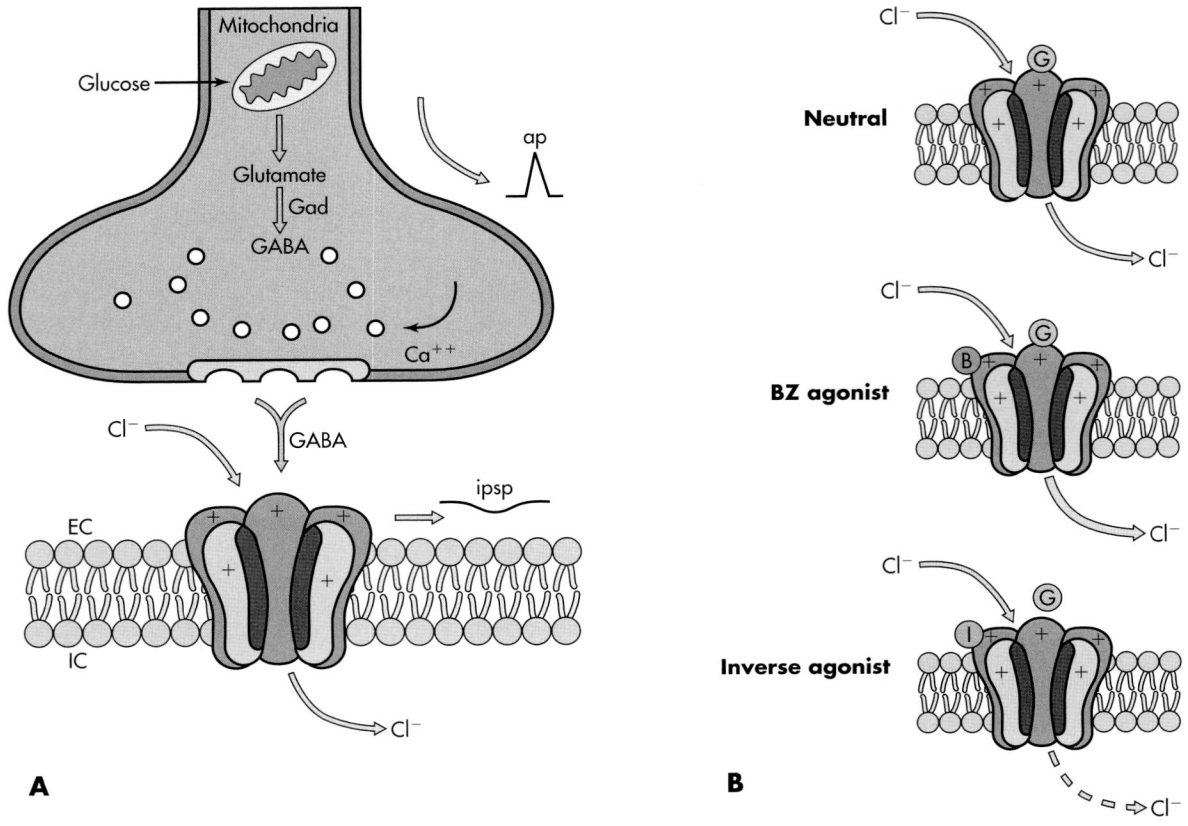

FIGURE 47-3

Idealized model of γ-aminobutyric acid (GABA)-benzodiazepine (BZ)-chloride (Cl⁻) channel at axosomatic (postsynaptic) inhibitory synapses. **A**, Presynaptic and postsynaptic elements. ap, action potential; Gad, glutamic acid decarboxylase; EC, extracellular; IC, intracellular; ipsp, inhibitory postsynaptic potential. **B**, GABA-BZ receptor interactions influencing permeability of chloride channels. Neutral: GABA receptor binds GABA (G) with moderate affinity in the absence of BZ ligand. BZ agonist: Direct BZ agonist (B) enhances GABA affinity for its receptor, resulting in maximal chloride permeability. Inverse agonist: Inverse agonist bound to BZ receptor results in poor GABA affinity and markedly reduced chloride permeability. *(From Rech RH: Drugs to treat anxieties and related disorders. In Brody TM, Larner J, Minneman KP [eds]: Human Pharmacology: Molecular to Clinical, 3rd ed. St. Louis, Mosby, 1998, p 367.)*

The management of acute and chronic benzodiazepine poisoning is mainly supportive (see Chapter 3). Appropriate initial intervention may include supplemental oxygen, dextrose, or thiamine, particularly if indicated on the basis of hypoxemia, altered mental status, documented hypoglycemia, or suspected malnutrition. Naloxone administration should be considered if hypoventilatory failure develops because benzodiazepines, in general, are less likely than μ-opioid receptor agonists to produce this degree of CNS depressant effect. The potential for significant aspiration should remain a concern in the stuporous and more obtunded individual, for whom care should include an appropriately intensive degree of clinical, laboratory, and radiographic monitoring. If clinical presentation occurs within 1 to 2 hours of ingestion, oral or nasogastric administration of a single dose of activated charcoal may be given, after appropriate airway protective measures are taken, to limit further drug absorption (see Chapter 5).

Flumazenil (Romazicon) is a drug with antagonist activity at the benzodiazepine binding site of the GABA$_A$ chloride complex that reverses the CNS depressant effects of benzodiazepines and benzodiazepine-like drugs (e.g., zolpidem).

The amplitude and duration of effect of flumazenil on benzodiazepine-induced respiratory depression may be limited, however. Given the demonstrated risks of flumazenil-induced benzodiazepine withdrawal in patients with established pharmacodynamic tolerance and convulsions in the setting of coingested proconvulsants (e.g., cyclic antidepressants), the risks of flumazenil administration seem to outweigh its benefits in many instances.[16,17]

The safe use of flumazenil seems limited to isolated acute benzodiazepine toxicity (e.g., in young children after acute overdose or after the controlled use of benzodiazepines for conscious sedation). An important caveat remains, however, that successful reversal of CNS depression in these instances does not obviate the need for further close monitoring because profound sedation may recur.[18] Chapter 138 provides a more detailed discussion regarding the mechanism of action, indications, contraindications, and administration of flumazenil.

Because uneventful recovery from acute benzodiazepine toxicity usually occurs within 12 to 36 hours and after routine and relatively conservative supportive care, extracorporeal enhancement of drug elimination is not indicated. Hemodialysis would not be expected to be efficacious due to the high degree of plasma protein binding of benzodiazepines.

Clinically significant benzodiazepine withdrawal may occur within hours of apparent recovery from the acute sedative effects of benzodiazepines, depending on the underlying degree of pharmacodynamic tolerance and the elimination kinetics of the specific drug or its active metabolites (see Chapter 30). Resumption of maintenance therapy with the benzodiazepine drug or an equivalent dose of another drug within the class is advisable when recovery of the sensorium has occurred.

Special Populations

PEDIATRIC PATIENTS

Children who have received oral and parenteral benzodiazepines for conscious sedation have been reported to have paradoxical behavioral reactions consisting of dysphoria, restlessness, disorientation, inconsolable crying, agitation, and combativeness.[8,19] These adverse reactions have been observed to occur at relatively low (0.6% to 1.4%) frequencies, although greater frequencies than in young and middle-aged adults. Case experience has shown, in addition, that flumazenil may be effective in reversing these paradoxical reactions and the excessive sedation that occurs as an iatrogenic effect of benzodiazepine administration.[19,20]

PREGNANT AND BREAST-FEEDING PATIENTS

Most benzodiazepines, including alprazolam, clonazepam, diazepam, and lorazepam, have been classified by the U.S. Food and Drug Administration (FDA) as teratogenicity category D drugs (see Appendix), on the basis that "there is positive evidence of human fetal risk, but the benefits from use in pregnant women may be acceptable despite the risk (e.g., if the drug is needed in a life-threatening situation or for a serious disease for which safer drugs cannot be used or are ineffective)."[21] Exceptions to this generalization are triazolam, temazepam, quazepam, and flurazepam, which are classified as category X drugs (i.e., drugs for which "studies in animals and human beings have demonstrated fetal abnormalities or there is evidence of fetal risk based on human experience or both, and the risk of the use of the drug in pregnant women clearly outweighs any possible benefit. The drug is contraindicated in women who are or may become pregnant."[21]). Zolpidem also has been classified under the same system as a category B agent (i.e., one for which "either animal-reproduction studies have not demonstrated a fetal risk but there are no controlled studies in pregnant women or animal-reproduction studies have shown an adverse effect [other than a decrease in fertility] that was not confirmed in controlled studies in women in the first trimester [and there is no evidence of a risk in later trimesters]").[21]

Two neonatal syndromes that have been described after relatively high-dose (>30 to 40 mg) or prolonged maternal diazepam administration during labor are floppy infant syndrome (lethargy, hypotonia, sucking difficulties) and withdrawal (tremors, irritability, hypertonicity, vomiting, diarrhea, vigorous sucking).[21] On the basis of their known excretion into human breast milk and reports of clinical withdrawal

and excessive sedation in some breast-feeding infants after maternal administration of benzodiazepine sedative-hypnotics, it is recommended that caution or avoidance be observed with regard to their administration in lactating women.[21]

ELDERLY PATIENTS

As stated previously in this chapter and elsewhere in this book (see Chapter 12), elderly individuals are at greater risk for more severe or prolonged toxicity as a result of age-dependent differences in pharmacokinetic and pharmacodynamic responses to the administration of benzodiazepines.

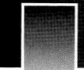

> **Key Points in the Diagnosis and Treatment of Benzodiazepine Toxicity**
>
> 1. Depressed sensorium without serious respiratory, cardiovascular, or other neurologic manifestations represents the typical clinical presentation of acute or chronic benzodiazepine or benzodiazepine-like drug (e.g., zolpidem) toxicity.
> 2. Paradoxical neuropsychiatric reactions (e.g., restlessness, agitation) occur uncommonly but with apparently greater frequency in children and elderly individuals.
> 3. The mainstay of treatment for benzodiazepine toxicity is supportive care.
> 4. Flumazenil, a benzodiazepine receptor antagonist, should be used selectively and with caution in the management of acute or chronic benzodiazepine and benzodiazepine-like drug toxicity, particularly when pharmacodynamic tolerance to the effects of benzodiazepine receptor agonists or concomitant proconvulsant (e.g., tricyclic antidepressant) intoxication is considered likely.
> 5. Reinstitution of maintenance regimen doses of benzodiazepine or benzodiazepine-like drugs, particularly drugs with relatively rapid elimination kinetics, should be implemented during the early convalescent phase of acute or chronic poisoning.

CHLORAL HYDRATE

CH was synthesized in 1832 by von Liebeg and introduced into clinical medicine by Liebreich in 1869. It originally was used intravenously, but this practice ended after prolonged sedation was an observed outcome. In 1890, Bornträger provided limited descriptions of 44 CH-related casualties, and in 1910 it was described as the most dangerous of all hypnotics.[22] Despite this dubious initial distinction, CH continues to be used in adults and extensively in children for procedural sedation in many clinical settings.[23] A review article described CH as the most common initial selection of pediatric sedative and discussed safe, effective CH dosing protocols.[24] The American Association of Pediatrics (AAP) acknowledges numerous reported postsedation complications with CH use but does not recommend its abandonment.[25]

Beginning in the 19th century, CH was used with malicious intent by adding it to alcoholic drinks before they were consumed by unsuspecting victims. Referred to as

"Mickey Finns" or "knockout drops," this practice was conducted by criminals with the objective of "rendering a person unconscious or stupefied . . . in order to rob him."[26] The pharmacologic interactions of ethanol and CH administered in this manner are discussed later.

CH is available as a liquid, capsule, or rectal suppository. The recommended and most commonly reported doses used for pediatric outpatient sedation range from 25 to 100 mg/kg.[24]

Chemistry and Pharmacokinetics

CH is the hydrated form of an aldehyde, chloral (2,2,2-trichloroacetaldehyde), and results from the condensation of each molecule of chloral with one molecule of water (Fig. 47-4). It is also a synthetic precursor in the production and an in vivo metabolite of trichloroethylene.[27,28] After complete absorption from the gastrointestinal (GI) tract, CH is metabolized rapidly in the liver, brain, and red blood cells to trichloroethanol (TCE*) and trichloroacetic acid (TCA).*,[29–31] The relative amounts of TCE and TCA produced depend on the amount of CH ingested.[27]

Rapid nicotinamide adenine dinucleotide (NADH)–dependent enzymatic reduction of CH by alcohol dehydrogenase (ADH) produces the active metabolite TCE,[32] which has two fates: hepatic glucuronidation to urochloralic acid with subsequent renal (major) and bile (minor) excretion, or oxidation to TCA (Fig. 47-5).[33,34] Animal research has shown ex vivo that metabolism of CH to TCE also occurs via reduced nicotinamide adenine dinucleotide (NADPH)–dependent aldehyde reductase.[30,35] Depending on the redox environment, CH also may be

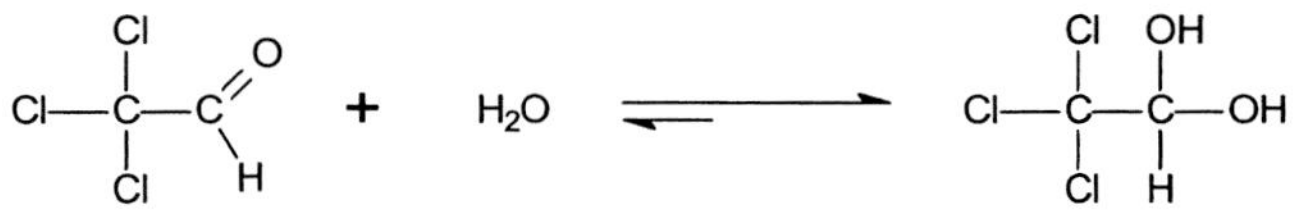

Chloral   **Chloral Hydrate**

FIGURE 47-4

Chemical structure of chloral hydrate shown in its equilibrium with chloral.

Pharmacokinetics of Chloral Hydrate

Volume of distribution: 0.6 L/kg (CH)
Protein binding: TCE, 40%; TCA, 85%
Mechanisms of elimination: CH, <10% excreted unchanged in urine; TCE, renal excretion as urochloralic acid or oxidation to TCA; TCA, renal excretion
Plasma half-life: CH, approximately 4 min; TCE, 10 hr (can be longer in overdose); TCA, 67 hr (can be longer in overdose)
Metabolites: chloral hydrate (CH) undergoes rapid conversion to two metabolites: trichloroethanol (TCE) (active) and trichloroacetic acid (TCA) (inactive).

---

*The acronyms TCE and TCA have been used in the scientific literature to denote trichloroethylene and trichloroethane and trichloroethanol and trichloroacetic acid. In this chapter, TCE and TCA refer only to the latter compounds.

oxidized directly via CH dehydrogenase to TCA, with nicotinamide adenine dinucleotide (NAD) as a cofactor.[34,36,37]

The coadministration of CH and ethanol leads to the formation of chloral alcoholate. Originally, it was thought that this compound was responsible for a "Mickey Finn" effect of prolonged, profound sedation. In aqueous solution, however, chloral alcoholate freely dissociates into CH and ethanol, which has been presumed to occur after ingestion of the mixture,[38,39] and it has been shown that there is no significant difference in the sedative potency of CH and chloral alcoholate.[40] The effects of chloral alcoholate are indistinguishable from equivalent doses of CH and ethanol.[38]

In addition to a competitive inhibitory effect on TCE metabolism, coadministration of ethanol, via its metabolism by ADH, results in a change in the redox potential and an associated net increase in the NADH-to-NAD ratio, which effectively drives primary CH metabolism to TCE (Fig. 47-6).[27,31,41] Simultaneous reduction in metabolism and an increase in production of TCE result in more rapidly developing and higher peak plasma concentrations of TCE, which, combined with TCE-mediated inhibition of ethanol metabolism through ADH, are thought to be the basis for the rapid onset and potency of CNS depressant effects that are characteristic of the "Mickey Finn" combination of CH and ethanol.

Because the hepatic enzymatic elimination of CH in normal healthy adults and older children is rapid (half-life 4 minutes), the rate of detection of the parent compound in urine in most clinical situations is low, limiting the utility of toxicologic assay for the parent compound itself.[37,42] The relatively more prolonged hypnotic effects of CH are attributed to the active metabolite TCE (half-life >6 hours).[37,42,43] With concurrent ethanol administration or after CH overdose, the elimination half-life of TCE reportedly has increased to greater than 30 hours.[44]

Pathophysiology

The precise mechanism of the sedative-hypnotic action of CH is unknown. Several lines of evidence, including the demonstration of CH's rapid bioconversion, suggest that the dose-dependent hypnotic and sedating effects of CH are due in large part to its active metabolite, TCE.[37,39,42,43] In addition, there is evidence to support TCE's indirect agonist actions at $GABA_A$ chloride channels in a manner similar to that of barbiturates.[45,46] TCA seems to have no direct physiologic effects, but as a strong organic acid, it may displace other xenobiotics from protein-binding sites.[22,37,47]

Several mechanisms of CH-induced myocardial toxicity have been postulated, including sensitization of the myocardium to the dysrhythmogenic effects of endogenous and exogenous catecholamines, similar to that associated with intense exposure to other halogenated hydrocarbons; reduction in myocardial contractility; and shortening of the refractory period of the myocardial action potential.[33] The subcellular and molecular bases for these physiologic effects remain undetermined.

Mild sedation (drowsiness) occurs at low doses (250 mg in adults and 8 mg/kg in children), with hypnotic responses seen at moderate doses (500 to 1000 mg in adults and 25 to

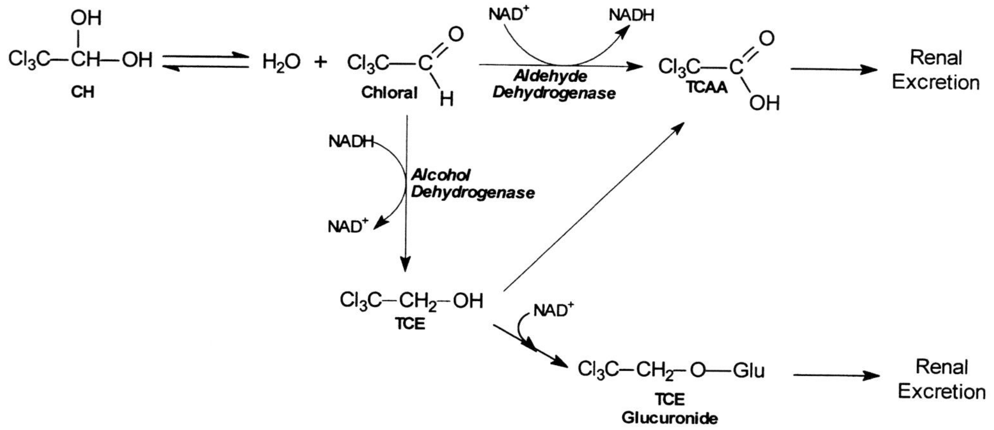

FIGURE 47-5

Metabolism of chloral hydrate (CH). TCAA, trichloroacetic acid; TCE, trichloroethanol.

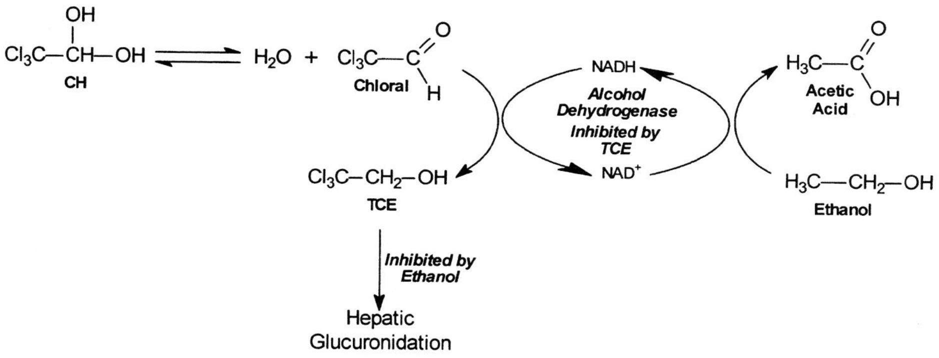

FIGURE 47-6

Metabolic interaction of ethanol and chloral hydrate. NAD, nicotinamide adenine dinucleotide; NADH, nicotinamide adenine dinucleotide, reduced form; TCE, trichloroethanol.

50 mg/kg in children). At therapeutic doses of CH, there is minimal depression of cardiovascular and respiratory function with maintenance of intact airway reflexes. Higher doses (>50 mg/kg in children) may produce more profound depression of respiratory and vasomotor functions. These effects typically occur within 1 hour of oral or rectal administration of a therapeutic dose. Although the occurrence of post-sedation "hangover" after therapeutic CH administration is less frequent or severe than that associated with other sedative-hypnotics, this cannot be generalized to the overdose setting.

Physiologic tolerance after long-term administration of CH has been reported, with CH-induced chemical dependence suggested by a single case report.[48] A withdrawal syndrome, mentioned in numerous sources but without references, seems biologically plausible based on experimental evidence that supports an indirect GABA agonist mechanism of action similar to that of barbiturates. Clinical and experimental evidence for the occurrence of a withdrawal syndrome after short-term or even relatively prolonged administration of CH is lacking, however; this supports the notion that when CH use is occasional and limited to the medical or surgical procedural setting, withdrawal is unlikely to be clinically significant.[49]

Clinical Presentation of Toxicity and Life-Threatening Complications

ACUTE TOXICITY

The acute lethal dose of CH is variable, with death reported after ingestion of 4 g in one case and survival reported after ingestion of 30 g in another.[50] Although excessive depression in level of consciousness and attendant respiratory compromise are the most commonly occurring and anticipated toxic effects of CH overdose, most deaths reported after CH overdose usually occurred after development of malignant cardiac dysrhythmias.[22,51–53]

Cardiovascular collapse and malignant ventricular tachy-dysrhythmias after acute CH overdose have been well documented.[22,54–66] Reported dysrhythmias include premature ventricular beats, ventricular tachycardia, ventricular fibrillation, bigeminy, accelerated junctional rhythm, torsades de pointes, and asystole. Cardiac dysrhythmias also have been associated with therapeutic doses of CH in children with congenital cardiac disease.[67]

Severe gastrointestinal irritant injury has been reported after oral overdose, including upper gastrointestinal hemorrhage, gastric necrosis and perforation, and esophagitis with subsequent stricture formation.[22,66,68–70] The dermal and soft tissue effects of direct exposure to CH were illustrated in a case series involving accidental intravenous administration of CH, in which skin sloughing and cyanosis were described.[64] Less life-threatening adverse reactions associated with the therapeutic use of CH include nausea and vomiting (5% to 7%), paradoxical hyperactivity (1% to 5%), and mild respiratory depression (≤9%).[71–74]

CHRONIC TOXICITY—CARCINOGENESIS

There has been extensive scientific investigation into the cancer risks of chronic CH exposure, in part owing to its metabolic relationship to trichloroethylene, a compound that has been shown to have carcinogenicity in laboratory animals.[50] CH is an intermediate metabolite of trichloroethylene in rodents and humans but is not thought to be responsible for trichloroethylene's carcinogenic effects.[75] Reviews of research findings more specifically pertinent to chloral and CH can be found in many sources, including the International Agency for Research on Cancer monograph series.[50,76] Chloral and CH are classified by the International Agency for Research on Cancer as group 3 substances (i.e., "not classifiable as to their carcinogenicity") based on inadequate human and limited animal evidence. The safety of CH, from a chronic effects standpoint, is supported further in a published report of the AAP.[23]

DRUG INTERACTIONS

At one time, CH was thought to induce a significant increase in the hypoprothrombinemic effects of warfarin.[77,78] The interaction was thought to involve displacement of warfarin from albumin by TCA, with a resultant increase in half-life and biologic activity.[47] Subsequent investigation revealed that the administration of CH during the induction of warfarin therapy produced a transient, clinically insignificant potentiation of warfarin's effect. This interaction is dose related and does not occur if CH administration is initiated after attainment of steady-state warfarin kinetics.[79–82]

The coadministration of CH and furosemide has been associated with adverse events in some patients, including hot flashes, diaphoresis, nausea, tachycardia, and alterations in blood pressure (hypertension and hypotension).[83,84] Typically, these clinical manifestations have been encountered shortly after intravenous furosemide administration in patients who had previously received CH. A toxicologic mechanism for these occurrences has not been established. Case reports suggest that these effects do not occur when furosemide is administered more than 24 hours after the last dose of CH. A retrospective study documented the occurrence of flushing-type reactions in 3 of 43 patients (7%) who received intravenous furosemide after CH.[85] This apparent adverse CH-furosemide interaction has had a documented clinical duration of 10 to 20 minutes, has not required specific intervention, and has not been considered life-threatening in patients without significant cardiovascular comorbidity.

Theoretically, CH should be used with caution in patients taking sympathomimetic medications (e.g., methylphenidate), based on theoretical concerns that the combination imposes an elevated risk of catecholamine-induced cardiac dysrhythmia. There is, however, no published clinical experience to support these concerns.

With regard to the "Mickey Finn" effects of CH and ethanol previously discussed, it seems that the interaction is synergistic if ethanol is given first and in a molar ratio of nearly 1:1.[39] Otherwise, the interaction between the two compounds seems to be only additive.

Diagnosis

CH use is associated with a pearlike odor, which, if present, may alert the clinician to the diagnosis. In addition, CH tablets are radiopaque and may be detected on an abdominal x-ray. Aside from these external clues and the increased risk of ventricular dysrhythmia associated with CH overdose, there are few clinical characteristics to distinguish CH toxicity from that caused by other sedative-hypnotics, including barbiturates and benzodiazepines. Because CH is metabolized rapidly to a relatively long-lived active metabolite, TCE, which is detected more readily in blood and urine, toxicologic analysis of biologic fluids for this compound may be useful in confirming and assessing the severity of exposure in the clinical or forensic setting.

Treatment

All CH overdose patients should be observed closely on a cardiac monitor for at least 3 hours after ingestion. Appropriate supportive measures, including endotracheal intubation, mechanical ventilation, and intravenous fluid volume replacement, should be provided as they are clinically indicated.

Tachydysrhythmias induced by CH poisoning should be treated with a β-adrenergic receptor antagonist. Numerous case reports document the successful use of propranolol (1 mg intravenous bolus followed by an infusion of 3 mg/hr) or other β-blocker, such as metoprolol (5 mg intravenous bolus), in the treatment of CH-induced dysrhythmias.[55,62,64–67] β-Blocker use often has been reported to be successful after failure to control the dysrhythmia with other drugs, such as lidocaine, procainamide, sodium bicarbonate, or magnesium. Because the duration of cardiotoxic action of TCE after overdose may be significantly longer than that of antidysrhythmic treatment, continuous cardiac monitoring is warranted, and repeated dosing of the β-blocker may be required. Cardioversion or defibrillation also has been employed to terminate dysrhythmias associated with CH poisoning.[65]

The administration of nonselective adrenergic agonists (e.g., dopamine, norepinephrine) to CH-poisoned individuals has been associated with an increase in dysrhythmias.[33,58,65]

Indications for ICU Admission in Chloral Hydrate Toxicity
Neurologic instability (coma, seizures)
Respiratory failure
Cardiac dysrhythmias
Significant effects (e.g., respiratory failure, hypotension) of chloral hydrate–drug (e.g., ethanol, furosemide) interactions

These agents should be used with caution or avoided in favor of α-selective agonists (e.g., phenylephrine) in the treatment of CH-induced hypotension.

There is no evidence to suggest that naloxone administration reverses CH-induced CNS depression.[86,87] Case reports suggest, however, that the use of flumazenil in CH overdose may reverse CH-induced sedation and may precipitate ventricular dysrhythmias.[86,88] It has been suggested that the induction of acute withdrawal states by naloxone or flumazenil administration increases the risk of TCE-induced dysrhythmias by increasing the release of endogenous catecholamines.[64] Naloxone and flumazenil should not be used routinely in the management of CNS depression associated with CH overdose.

The potential for effective enhancement of TCE clearance by hemodialysis is suggested by the compound's relatively long elimination half-life and its low molecular weight, volume of distribution, and degree of protein binding. Several reports show favorable outcomes after the use of hemodialysis in severe CH-induced toxicity, including a pregnant patient with malignant cardiac dysrhythmias.[22,44,54,65,89] In one case, the elimination half-life of TCE was shown to decline from 35 hours to 6 hours after hemodialysis was instituted.[44] Although there is no published clinical trial evidence to support outcome benefit, it seems reasonable to recommend that hemodialysis be considered when the CH poisoning is severe, prolonged, or refractory to other therapeutic interventions.

Key Points in the Management of Chloral Hydrate Toxicity

1. Monitor closely for signs or symptoms of toxicity for at least 3 hours after ingestion.
2. Provide supportive care, including intubation, oxygenation, and ventilation, when clinically indicated.
3. Use β-adrenergic blocker (e.g., propranolol) for tachydysrhythmias.

Special Populations

The use of CH has been associated with higher rates of adverse effects, including inadequate sedation, excessive sedation in patients with obstructive sleep apnea, wheezing, mental retardation, and diseases of cerebral white matter or the brainstem.[73,90]

PREGNANT AND BREAST-FEEDING PATIENTS

A study of 52 pregnant women who received CH while in active labor did not report any adverse maternal or fetal effects.[91] Analysis of fetal (cord) blood revealed significant concentrations of CH, TCE, and TCA. The FDA has classified CH as a category C (see Appendix) drug, or one for which "either studies in animals have revealed adverse effects on the fetus (teratogenic or embryocidal or other) and there are no controlled studies in women or studies in women and animals are not available" and one that "should be given only if the potential benefit justifies the potential risk to the fetus."[21] CH is found in breast milk but typically at concentrations too low to produce neonatal effects[91,92]; it is considered compatible with breast-feeding by the AAP.[93]

NEONATAL PATIENTS

Data suggest that neonates and preterm infants have impaired abilities to metabolize and excrete CH and its metabolites. Reports have documented significant increases in the half-life of TCE to 40 hours in neonates and critically ill children.[94,95] A similar report exists for a premature infant who received a supratherapeutic dose.[96] A study in neonates suggested that CH-induced sedation seems to correlate with plasma CH rather than TCE concentrations.[97] This finding corroborated earlier animal studies and may represent impaired metabolic capability of neonates to transform CH to TCE.

Published reports indicate the potential for increases in serum bilirubin (direct and indirect) in infants receiving CH.[98,99] This apparent dose-related phenomenon may reflect competition between CH and CH metabolites and bilirubin for conjugation in the immature liver.

ACUTE TOXICITY OF OLDER, LESS USED SEDATIVE-HYPNOTICS

Glutethimide, ethchlorvynol, meprobamate (Miltown, Equanil), and methaqualone (Fig. 47-7) are sedative-hypnotic drugs that have fallen out of common use, having been replaced largely by benzodiazepine and benzodiazepine-like drugs. Only one of these, meprobamate, is still available on the FDA-regulated pharmaceutical market[100] and only as a U.S. Drug Enforcement Agency (DEA) schedule III drug (i.e., a drug with a potential for abuse, although less so than drugs classified as schedule I or II, with a currently accepted medical use and for which abuse may lead to moderate or low physical dependence or high psychological dependence). Meprobamate is also the major active metabolite, however, of a relatively widely prescribed, non–DEA-scheduled, centrally acting muscle relaxant, carisoprodol (see Chapter 53).

A marked decline in the availability, prevalence, and therapeutic use of these older sedative-hypnotics is reflected in the marginal incidence of poisonings attributed to their continued use. The American Association of Poison Control Centers reported a 2001 annual combined total of less than 50 exposures and no deaths attributable to glutethimide, ethchlorvynol, and methaqualone out of a sedative-hypnotics/antipsychotics category total of greater than 100,000 exposures and 266 deaths.[101] Because these drugs continue to exhibit persistent availability, at least to a minor degree, it is appropriate to mention them briefly here.

Glutethimide

Glutethimide is a piperidine derivative that was introduced in the mid-1950s and became widely known in the 1970s and 1980s for its abuse potential, especially when combined with opioid drugs, such as codeine. Glutethimide is a

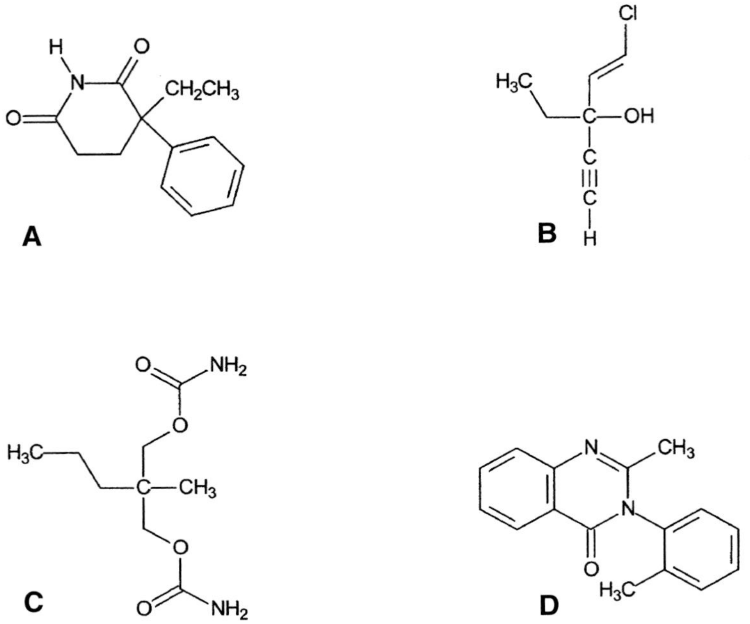

FIGURE 47-7

Chemical structures of older sedative-hypnotic agents. **A**, Glutethimide. **B**, Ethchlorvynol. **C**, Meprobamate. **D**, Methaqualone.

compound of relatively low water solubility that exhibits slow, erratic gastrointestinal absorption; is distributed relatively broadly (volume of distribution 2.7 L/kg); and undergoes inducible biotransformation and elimination through cytochrome P-450 pathways to active metabolites (e.g., 4-hydroxyglutethimide and 2-phenylglutarimide) (with an elimination half-life that ranges typically from 4 to >20 hours).[102]

Structurally similar to phenobarbital, glutethimide has sedative-hypnotic effects that are similar to the effects of barbiturates, but it lacks anticonvulsant properties. It also possesses relatively potent antimuscarinic activity, which accounts for the central and peripheral anticholinergic manifestations (see Chapter 22), including anhidrosis and pupillary mydriasis, which are perhaps the most distinctive clinical features of acute glutethimide poisoning. Reported clinical toxicity after acute glutethimide overdose characteristically has been prolonged and, consistent with its slow, erratic absorption and redistribution out of tissues, tends to assume a cyclical or fluctuating pattern of coma, convulsions, hypotension, and respiratory failure; pulmonary edema and renal failure also have been reported after glutethimide overdose.[103–105] The close structural similarity of glutethimide to phenobarbital also explains the occurrence of false-positive results on urine immunoassays for barbiturates after glutethimide administration.

Aggressive life support is the essence of the intensive care management after glutethimide overdose. Initial enteral administration of activated charcoal to prevent further absorption also is appropriate, given the potential for delayed gastric emptying associated with a drug that possesses anticholinergic and barbiturate-like depressant properties. There is no apparent clinical benefit from the use of extracorpo-

real clearance modalities (e.g., hemodialysis) in the management of glutethimide poisoning.[104,106]

Ethchlorvynol

Ethchlorvynol initially was marketed in the early to mid-1950s as a hypnotic agent; it was formulated in a gelatin capsule containing a liquid form of ethchlorvynol and a polyethylene glycol diluent that has been particularly noted for the characteristic vinyl plastic–like odor it has been reported to impart on the breath of the overdose victim. A highly lipophilic and volatile compound, ethchlorvynol has a rapid absorption and onset of action with the latter typically occurring before peak postabsorption serum concentrations are reached (1 to 1.5 hours). Consistent with its absorption kinetics and its relatively large volume of distribution (2.4 to 3.2 L/kg), distribution typically assumes a biphasic pattern over time, with a second, postredistribution peak seen at 7 to 14 hours.[102,107] Hepatic metabolism is extensive, with less than 1% urinary excretion occurring as the parent compound; elimination half-life ranges from 10 to 25 hours at therapeutic doses to greater than 100 hours after overdose.

The pharmacologic properties of ethchlorvynol are similar to those of barbiturates, including the capability for anticonvulsant and sedative-hypnotic actions. Prolonged (>10 days in some reports[107]) coma, respiratory failure, bradycardia, hypotension, hyporeflexia, and hypothermia are characteristic of the clinical presentation and course after oral overdose. Pulmonary edema has been documented to occur more frequently after parenteral overdose and is thought to result from an increase in pulmonary alveolar membrane permeability as an effect of the drug itself, rather than the coformulate excipient.[108,109] Bullous skin lesions and rhabdomyolysis are relatively common, although nonspecific, peripheral organ system complications of ethchlorvynol overdose, particularly in cases in which initial clinical discovery is delayed.[107]

Appropriate treatment, as for glutethimide and most other drugs in the sedative-hypnotic category, is entirely supportive. Given the potential for an extended period of severe intoxication after ethchlorvynol overdose, aggressive supportive care in an intensive care unit setting may be required for a prolonged time.

Meprobamate

Meprobamate was introduced in the 1950s and used widely for sedation and anxiolysis until it was recognized to be highly addictive and relatively lethal in overdose. Cariso-prodol, its metabolic precursor that has been marketed as a muscle relaxant (Soma) since the late 1950s, more recently has become an object of psychosocial and regulatory concern, given the barbiturate-like actions and risks of toxicity, abuse, tolerance, and withdrawal it shares with meproba-mate (see Chapter 53 for further details on carisoprodol, its metabolism to meprobamate, and their pharmacologic mechanisms).[110–112] Features of acute meprobamate poisoning that, in our opinion, are highly relevant to intensive care unit management and merit further emphasis are summarized here.

Meprobamate absorption, similar to that of carisoprodol, has been characterized in some cases of overdose as erratic or prolonged or both, which chiefly may reflect its apparent propensity to form gastric concretions.[113,114] Although there is no outcome evidence to support its benefit, there is limited clinical case experience with repeat administration of enteral activated charcoal beyond an initial dose at presentation to suggest that it may prevent further absorption or enhance elimination of meprobamate.[115,116] In addition, there is an attendant risk of delayed or recurrent clinical deterioration after acute meprobamate overdose, warranting cautious weaning of supportive care and monitoring measures in moderate-to-severe acute overdose.

Coma, clonus, seizures, profound and protracted hypotension, pulmonary edema, and cardiac dysrhythmias all have been reported after massive meprobamate overdose.[114] In cases in which hemodynamic compromise does not respond to aggressive supportive measures, including intravenous pressors, there may be clinical benefit from the use of extracorporeal enhancement of clearance (e.g., by hemodialysis or charcoal hemoperfusion), although support for this is limited to a few cases.[117] Theoretical support for the use of hemodialysis to enhance meprobamate elimination includes its known low molecular weight (218 d), volume of distribution (0.7 L/kg), and degree of protein binding (20%).[102]

Methaqualone

Methaqualone was withdrawn from the regulated U.S. market in 1983 after it was found to be relatively ineffective as a long-term maintenance drug in the treatment of anxiety and sleep disorders and instead developed widespread notoriety as a substance of abuse. It is pharmacologically and toxicologically similar to glutethimide and ethchlorvynol, with its slow biphasic pattern of elimination and associated prolonged duration of CNS depressant toxicity after moderate-to-severe acute overdose. As a result of the characteristically selective inhibition of polysynaptic spinal reflexes associated with methaqualone toxicity, clinical presentation and course have been notable, although not unique among CNS depressant drugs (see Chapter 53), for coma plus hyperactive motor dysfunction, seen clinically as increased muscle tone, hyperreflexia, clonus, and myoclonus.[118–120] In addition, it has been suggested that case reports of retinal and gastrointestinal hemorrhage occurring after methaqualone overdose may be explained on the basis of drug-induced effects on platelet dysfunction and coagulation factors.[121,122]

Aggressive supportive care of severe methaqualone toxicity should be directed at control of motor hyperreactivity (e.g., intravenous benzodiazepines or neuromuscular blockade or both). If paralytic agents are used, appropriate measures must be in place to monitor CNS status (e.g., electroencephalogram to monitor for seizures). Other aspects of the care of methaqualone-poisoned patients include the prevention of complications, such as rhabdomyolysis, renal failure, and aspiration pneumonitis. No clear evidence supports clinical benefit from extracorporeal enhancement of clearance after methaqualone overdose.

SEDATIVE-HYPNOTIC DRUG WITHDRAWAL

Available clinical and experimental evidence suggests that long-term administration of any of the sedative-hypnotics discussed in this chapter may result in pharmacodynamic tolerance to the degree that its abrupt discontinuation may result in life-threatening clinical effects. The dose-related tolerance to the sedative-hypnotic effects of these drugs, when administered on a prolonged and regular basis, is thought to occur predominantly as a result of down-regulation of neuroinhibitory cell membrane receptor expression or functional activity. The abrupt cessation of drug administration in the setting of established sedative-hypnotic tolerance triggers a sudden marked imbalance in central neurochemical tone in favor of excitatory neurotransmission. The clinical result of this imbalance is a syndrome of central sympathetic hyperactivity that, except for variations in time course and intensity, presents similarly after acute withdrawal from most, if not all, of the prescription drugs (e.g., benzodiazepines, barbiturates, CH, meprobamate) in this category.

The temporal course of sedative-hypnotic withdrawal depends on the elimination rate of the parent drug involved and whether it is metabolized to active compounds, the latter of which may have even longer half-lives (e.g., desmethyldiazepam, half-life 40 to 200 hours, compared with diazepam, half-life 30 to 60 hours). Withdrawal symptoms begin more rapidly with compounds having characteristically shorter elimination rates and can occur after cessation of administration, 12 to 24 hours for short-acting benzodiazepines, 24 to 36 hours for carisoprodol/meprobamate, and 4 to 8 days for long-acting benzodiazepine compounds.

In contrast to the relatively more benign clinical effects of opioid withdrawal, acute withdrawal from sedative-hypnotic agents—prescription (e.g., diazepam) and nonprescription (e.g., ethanol)—can be life-threatening. Depending on the dose and duration of use, symptoms and signs of withdrawal range from relatively minor, including restlessness, insomnia, anxiety, tremor, and gastrointestinal distress, to more severe, including agitation, delirium, psychosis, hyperthermia, tachyarrhythmias, and seizures. Hypertension, tachypnea, pupillary mydriasis, and diaphoresis commonly accompany, but are not specific for, sedative-hypnotic withdrawal.

A complete differential diagnosis for sedative-hypnotic withdrawal includes toxic and nontoxic diseases that may be indistinguishable from one another on the basis of presenting clinical features. Acute toxicity from sympathomimetic (e.g., amphetamines, cocaine) and methylxanthine (e.g., theophylline, caffeine) compounds, including thyrotoxicosis, hypoglycemia, thiamine deficiency, and neurosepsis, to name a few of these entities, shares clinical features with sedative-hypnotic withdrawal. Anticholinergic poisoning, with the exception of anhidrosis and neurobehavioral features (e.g., mumbling speech and carphologia) (see Chapter 22), also presents with clinical features similar to those of sedative-hypnotic drug withdrawal.

The diagnosis of sedative-hypnotic withdrawal is supported by minimal or absent sedative response to the administration of relatively large doses of rapidly acting sedative-hypnotic agents and may be supported further by the presence of sedative-hypnotic parent compounds or their metabolites on routine or comprehensive toxicologic analysis of biologic specimens (e.g., urine, blood, meconium).

Appropriate management of acute sedative-hypnotic withdrawal in the intensive care unit capitalizes on the broad cross-tolerance observed among drugs in this category. Rational choices of treatment are based on the relative safety and reliability of systemic administration, speed of therapeutic onset, and adequacy of effect duration. The optimal end point of pharmacotherapeutic titration with an intravenous benzodiazepine (e.g., diazepam) is resolution of sympathetic hyperactivity to the point of mild, rather than profound, sedation. The dose required to achieve this is highly variable and should be based on the closely monitored clinical response to incremental enteral or parenteral administration.

The failure of benzodiazepine therapy to reverse sedative-hypnotic withdrawal manifestations may reflect inadequate dosing, inadequate cross-tolerance secondary to differences in GABA$_A$-receptor subtype affinity (e.g., triazolobenzodiazepine versus non-triazolobenzodiazepine compounds), or some other toxic or nontoxic etiology. Long-term treatment of sedative-hypnotic dependence, including detoxification and discontinuation of therapy, can be accomplished safely and reliably using one or a combination of tapering regimens employing the same drug or a long-acting substitute (e.g., phenobarbital), as has been well described previously.[123-125] Optimal management of acute sedative-hypnotic withdrawal usually requires a health care facility capable of addressing the medical complications associated with acute or chronic underlying illness (e.g., sepsis, malnutrition) and treatment of substance withdrawal (e.g., excessive sedation and loss of airway protective reflexes) and, ultimately, referral for long-term behavioral treatment. See Chapter 30 for a more complete and general discussion of drug withdrawal and its management.

REFERENCES

1. Veltri JC, Litovitz TL: 1983 annual report of the American Association of Poison Control Centers National Data Collection System. Am J Emerg Med 2:420–423, 1984.
2. Litovitz TL, Klein-Schwartz W, White S, et al: 2000 annual report of the American Association of Poison Control Centers Toxic Exposure Surveillance System. Am J Emerg Med 19:337–395, 2001.
3. Drummer OH, Syrjanen ML, Cordner SM: Deaths involving the benzodiazepine flunitrazepam. Am J Forensic Med Pathol 14:238–243, 1993.
4. Ledray LE: Date rape drug alert. J Emerg Nurs 22:80, 1996.
5. Greenberg ML: Rohypnol (a.k.a. "rophies") draws national attention as "date rape" drug. Emerg Med News January:18–42, 1997.
6. Charney DS, Mihic SJ, Harris R: Hypnotics and sedatives. In Hardman JG, Limbird LE, Gilman AG (eds): Goodman and Gilman's the Pharmacological Basis of Therapeutics, 10th ed. New York, McGraw-Hill, 2001, pp 399–427.
7. Phillis JW, O'Regan MH: The role of adenosine in the central actions of the benzodiazepines. Prog Neuropsychopharmacol Biol Psychiatry 12:389–404, 1988.
8. Pena BM, Krauss B: Adverse events of procedural sedation and analgesia in a pediatric emergency department. Ann Emerg Med 34:483–491, 1999.
9. Wysowski DK, Barash D: Adverse behavioral reactions attributed to triazolam in the Food and Drug Administration's Spontaneous Reporting System. Arch Intern Med 151:2003–2008, 1991.
10. Jonas JM, Coleman BS, Sheridan AQ, Kalinske RW: Comparative clinical profiles of triazolam versus other shorter acting hypnotics. J Clin Psychiatry 53(Suppl):19–31, 1992.
11. Rothschild AJ: Disinhibition, amnestic reactions, and other adverse reactions secondary to triazolam: A review of the literature. J Clin Psychiatry 53(Suppl):69–79, 1992.
12. Boussairi A, Dupeyron J-P, Hernandez B, et al: Urine benzodiazepines screening of involuntarily drugged and robbed or raped patients. Clin Toxicol 34:721–724, 1996.
13. Raphan H: In reply to Pulini M: False-positive benzodiazepine urine test due to oxaprozin. JAMA 273:1905–1906, 1995.
14. Valentine JL, Middleton R, Sparks C: Identification of urinary benzodiazepines and their metabolites: Comparison of automated HPLC and GC-MS after immunoassay screening of clinical specimens. J Analyt Toxicol 20:416–424, 1996.
15. Pulini M: False-positive benzodiazepine urine test due to oxaprozin. JAMA 273:1905–1906, 1995.
16. Gueye PN, Hoffman JR, Taboulet P, et al: Empiric use of flumazenil in comatose patients: Limited applicability of criteria to define low risk. Ann Emerg Med 27:730–735, 1996.
17. Spivey WH, Roberts JR, Derlet RW: A clinical trial of escalating doses of flumazenil for reversal of suspected benzodiazepine overdose in the emergency department. Ann Emerg Med 22:1813–1821, 1993.
18. Hoffman RS, Goldfrank LR: The poisoned patient with altered consciousness—controversies in the use of a "coma cocktail." JAMA 274:562–569, 1995.
19. Massanari M, Novitsky J, Reinstein LJ: Paradoxical reactions in children associated with midazolam use during endoscopy. Clin Pediatr 36:681–684, 1997.
20. Weinbroum AA, Scold O, Ogorek D, Flashon R: The midazolam-induced paradox phenomenon is reversible by flumazenil. Epidemiology, patient characteristics and review of the literature. Eur J Anaesth 18:789–797, 2001.
21. Briggs GG, Freeman RK, Yaffe SJ (eds): Drugs in Pregnancy and Lactation, 6th ed. Philadelphia, Lippincott Williams & Wilkins, 2002.
22. Gerretsen M, de Groot G, van Heijst ANP, et al: Chloral hydrate poisoning: Its mechanism and therapy. Vet Hum Toxicol 21(Suppl):53–56, 1979.
23. American Academy of Pediatrics: Use of chloral hydrate for sedation in children. Pediatrics 92:471–473, 1993.
24. Malis DJ, Burton DM: Safe pediatric outpatient sedation: The chloral hydrate debate revisited. Otolaryngol Head Neck Surg 116:53–57, 1997.
25. American Academy of Pediatrics: Adverse sedation in pediatrics: Analysis of medications used for sedation. Pediatrics 106:633–644, 2000.
26. Wax P: Response to "a century of mickey finn—but who was he." Clin Toxicol 38:685, 2000.
27. Kawamoto T, Hobara T, Kobayashi H, et al: The metabolite ratio as a function of chloral hydrate dose and intracellular redox state in the perfused rat liver. Pharmacol Toxicol 60:325–329, 1987.
28. Ikeda M, Miyake Y, Ogata M, et al: Metabolism of trichloroethylene. Biochem Pharmacol 29:2983–2992, 1980.
29. Limpscomb JC, Mahle DA, Brashear WT, et al: A species comparison of chloral hydrate metabolism in blood and liver. Biochem Biophys Res Commun 277:340–350, 1996.

30. Tabakoff C, Vugrinic R, Anderson R, et al: Reduction of chloral hydrate to trichloroethanol in brain extracts. Biochem Pharmacol 23:455–460, 1974.

31. Sellers EM, Lang M, Koch-Weser J, et al: Interaction of chloral hydrate and ethanol in man: I. Metabolism. Clin Pharmacol Ther 13:37–49, 1972.

32. Hardman JG, Limbird LE (eds): Goodman and Gilman's the Pharmacological Basis of Therapeutics, 9th ed. New York, McGraw-Hill, 1996.

33. Graham SR, Day RO, Lee R, et al: Overdose with chloral hydrate: A pharmacological and therapeutic review. Med J Aust 149:686–688, 1988.

34. Silverman J, Muir WW III: A review of laboratory animal anesthesia with chloral hydrate and chloralose. Lab Anim Sci 43:210–216, 1993.

35. Ikeda M, Ezaki M, Kokeguchi S, et al: Studies on NADPH-dependent chloral hydrate reducing enzymes in rat liver cytosol. Biochem Pharmacol 30:1931–1939, 1981.

36. Cooper JR, Friedman PJ: The enzymatic oxidation of chloral hydrate to trichloroacetic acid. Biochem Pharmacol 1:76–82, 1958.

37. Marshall EK Jr, Owens AH Jr: Absorption, excretion and metabolic fate of chloral hydrate and trichloroethanol. Johns Hopkins Hosp Bull 95:1–18, 1954.

38. Gessner PK, Cabana BE: Chloral alcoholate: Reevaluation of its role in the interaction between the hypnotic effects of chloral hydrate and ethanol. J Pharmacol Exp Ther 156:602–605, 1967.

39. Gessner PK, Cabana BE: A study of the interaction of the hypnotic effects and of the toxic effects of chloral hydrate and ethanol. J Pharmacol Exp Ther 74:247–259, 1970.

40. Adams WL: The comparative toxicity of chloral alcoholate and chloral hydrate. J Pharmacol Exp Ther 78:340–345, 1943.

41. Kaplan HL, Forney RB, Hughes FW, et al: Chloral hydrate and alcohol metabolism in human subjects. J Forensic Sci 12:295–304, 1967.

42. Butler TC: The metabolic fate of chloral hydrate. J Pharmacol Exp Ther 92:49–58, 1948.

43. Mackay FJ, Cooper JR: A study in the hypnotic activity of chloral hydrate. J Pharmacol Exp Ther 135:271–274, 1961.

44. Stalker NE, Gambertoglio JG, Fukumitsu CJ, et al: Acute massive chloral hydrate intoxication treated with hemodialysis: A clinical pharmacokinetic analysis. J Clin Pharmacol 18:136–142, 1978.

45. Lovinger DM, Zimmerman SA, Levitin M, et al: Trichloroethanol potentiates synaptic transmission mediated by gamma-aminobutyric acid$_A$ receptors in hippocampal neurons. J Pharmacol Exp Ther 264:1097–1103, 1993.

46. Whiting PJ, McKernan RM, Wafford KA: Structure and pharmacology of vertebrate GABA$_A$ receptor subtypes. Int Rev Neurobiol 38:95–138, 1995.

47. Sellers EM, Koch-Weser J: Potentiation of warfarin-induced hypoprothrombinemia by chloral hydrate. N Engl J Med 283:827–831, 1970.

48. Stone CB: Chloral hydrate dependence: Report of a case. Clin Toxicol 12:377–380, 1978.

49. Leuschner J, Zimmermann T: Examination of the dependence potential of chloral hydrate by oral administration to normal monkeys. Arzneimittelforschung 46:751–754, 1996.

50. International Agency for Research on Cancer (IARC) website. Available at: http://193.51.164.11/monoeval/grlist.html.

51. Engelhart DA, Lavins ES, Hazenstab CB, et al: Unusual death attributed to the combined effects of chloral hydrate, lidocaine, and nitrous oxide. J Anal Toxicol 22:246–247, 1998.

52. Jastak JT, Pallasch T: Death after chloral hydrate sedation: Report of case. J Am Dent Assoc 116:345–348, 1988.

53. Levine B, Park J, Smith TD, et al: Chloral hydrate: Unusually high concentrations in a fatal overdose. J Anal Toxicol 9:232–233, 1985.

54. Vaziri ND, Kumar KP, Mirahmadi K, et al: Hemodialysis in treatment of acute chloral hydrate poisoning. South Med J 70:377–378, 1977.

55. Zahedi A, Grant MH, Wong DT: Successful treatment of chloral hydrate cardiac toxicity with propranolol. Am J Emerg Med 17:490–491, 1999.

56. Marshall AJ: Cardiac arrhythmias caused by chloral hydrate. BMJ 2:994, 1977.

57. Gustafson A, Svensson SE, Ugander L: Cardiac arrhythmias in chloral hydrate poisoning. Acta Med Scand 201:227–230, 1977.

58. Young JB, Vandermolen LA, Pratt CM: Torsades de pointes: An unusual manifestation of chloral hydrate poisoning. Am Heart J 112:181–183, 1986.

59. Seger D, Schwartz G: Chloral hydrate: A dangerous sedative for overdose patients. Pediatr Emerg Care 10:349–350, 1994.

60. Muller SA, Fisch C: Cardiac arrhythmias due to use of chloral hydrate. J Indiana Med Assoc 49:38–40, 1956.

61. Nordenberg A, Delisle G, Izukawa T: Cardiac arrhythmia in a child due to chloral hydrate ingestion. Pediatrics 47:134–135, 1971.

62. Bower K, Glasser SP: Chloral hydrate overdose and cardiac arrhythmias. Chest 77:232–235, 1980.

63. Bloom RA: Cardiopulmonary resuscitation. Lancet 16:164, 1966.

64. Sing K, Erickson T, Amitai Y, et al: Chloral hydrate toxicity from oral and intravenous administration. Clin Toxicol 34:101–106, 1996.

65. Ludwigs U, Divino Filho JC, Magnusson A, et al: Suicidal chloral hydrate poisoning. Clin Toxicol 34:97–99, 1996.

66. DiGiovanni AJ: Reversal of chloral hydrate-associated cardiac arrhythmia by a beta-adrenergic blocking agent. Anesthesiology 31:93–97, 1969.

67. Hirsch IA, Zauder HI: Chloral hydrate: A potential cause of arrhythmias. Anesth Analg 65:691–692, 1986.

68. Lee DC, Vassalluzzo C: Acute gastric perforation in a chloral hydrate overdose. Am J Emerg Med 16:545–546, 1998.

69. Vellar IDA, Richardson JP, Doyle JC, et al: Gastric necrosis: A rare complication of chloral hydrate intoxication. Br J Surg 59:317–319, 1972.

70. Gleich GJ, Mongan ES, Vaules DW: Esophageal stricture following chloral hydrate poisoning. JAMA 201:120–121, 1967.

71. Greenberg BS, Faerber EN, Aspinall CL, et al: High-dose chloral hydrate sedation for children undergoing MR imaging: Safety and efficacy in relation to age. AJR Am J Roentgenol 161:639–641, 1993.

72. Frush DP, Bisset GS III, Hall SC: Pediatric sedation in radiology. AJR Am J Roentgenol 167:1381–1387, 1996.

73. Vade A, Sukhani R, Dolenga M, et al: Chloral hydrate sedation of children undergoing CT and MRI imaging: Safety as judged by American Academy of Pediatrics guidelines. AJR Am J Roentgenol 165:905–909, 1995.

74. Rochera-Oms CL, Casillas C, Marti-Bonmati L, et al: Oral chloral hydrate provides effective and safe sedation in pediatric magnetic resonance imaging. J Clin Pharm Ther 19:239–243, 1994.

75. Keller DA, Heck HD: Mechanistic studies on chloral toxicity: Relationship to trichloroethylene carcinogenesis. Toxicol Lett 42:183–191, 1988.

76. Salmon AG, Phil D, Kizer KW, et al: Potential carcinogenicity of chloral hydrate—a review. J Toxicol Clin Toxicol 33:115–121, 1995.

77. Chloral hydrate and oral anticoagulants. Lancet 1:524, 1972.

78. Cucinell SA, Odessky L, Weiss M, et al: The effects of chloral hydrate on bishydroxycoumarin metabolism. JAMA 197:144–146, 1966.

79. Udall JA: Clinical implications of warfarin interactions with five sedatives. Am J Cardiol 35:67–71, 1975.

80. Udall JA: Warfarin-chloral hydrate interaction. Ann Intern Med 81:341–344, 1974.

81. Udall JA: Warfarin interactions with chloral hydrate and glutethimide. Curr Ther Res Clin Exp 17:67–74, 1975.

82. Griner PF, Raisz LG, Rickles FR, et al: Chloral hydrate and warfarin interaction: Clinical significance. Ann Intern Med 75:540–543, 1971.

83. Malach M, Berman N: Furosemide and chloral hydrate. JAMA 232:638–639, 1975.

84. Dean RP, Rudinsky BF, Kelleher MD: Interactions of chloral hydrate and intravenous furosemide in a child. Clin Pharm 10:385–387, 1991.

85. Pevonka MP, Yost RL, Marks RG, et al: Interaction of chloral hydrate and furosemide. Drug Intell Clin Pharm 11:332–335, 1977.

86. Donovan KL, Fisher DJ: Reversal of chloral hydrate overdose with flumazenil. BMJ 298:1253, 1989.

87. Chan MY: Naloxone interaction with some CNS depressant. Pharmacology 31:294–297, 1985.

88. Short TG, Maling T, Galletly DC: Ventricular arrhythmias precipitated by flumazenil. BMJ 296:1070–1071, 1988.

89. Buur T, Larsson R, Norlander B: Pharmacokinetics of chloral hydrate poisoning treated with hemodialysis and hemoperfusion. Acta Med Scand 223:269–274, 1988.

90. Biban P, Baraldi E, Pettenazzo A, et al: Adverse effects of chloral hydrate in two young children with obstructive sleep apnea. Pediatrics 92:461–463, 1993.

91. Bernstine JB, Meyer AE, Haymen HB: Maternal and foetal blood estimation following the administration of chloral hydrate during labour. J Obstet Gynaecol Br Emp 63:228–231, 1956.

92. Wilson JT: Drugs in Breast Milk. Lancaster, MTP, 1981.
93. Committee on Drugs, American Academy of Pediatrics: The transfer of drugs and other chemicals into human milk. Pediatrics 93:137–150, 1994.
94. Mayers DJ, Hindmarsh KW, Sankaran K, et al: Chloral hydrate disposition following single-dose administration to critically ill neonates and children. Dev Pharmacol Ther 16:71–77, 1991.
95. Gershanik J, Boecler B, Lertora JJL, et al: Monitoring levels of trichloroethanol (TCE) during chloral hydrate (CH) administration to sick neonates. Clin Res 29:895a, 1981.
96. Laptook AR, Rosenfeld CR: Chloral hydrate toxicity in a preterm infant. Pediatr Pharmacol 4:161–165, 1984.
97. Mayers DJ, Hindmarsh KW, Gorecki DKJ, et al: Sedative/hypnotic effects of chloral hydrate in the neonate: Trichloroethanol or parent drug. Dev Pharmacol Ther 19:141–146, 1992.
98. Reimche LD, Sankaran K, Hindmarsh KW, et al: Chloral hydrate sedation in neonates and infants—clinical and pharmacologic considerations. Dev Pharmacol Ther 12:57–64, 1989.
99. Lambert GH, Muraskas J, Anderson CL, et al: Direct hyperbilirubinemia associated with chloral hydrate administration in the newborn. Pediatrics 86:277–280, 1990.
100. Food and Drug Administration Center for Drug Evaluation and Research: Electronic Orange Book. October 2002. Available at: http://www.fda.gov/cder/ob/default.htm.
101. Litovitz TL, Klein-Schwartz W, Rodgers GC, et al: 2001 Annual Report of the American Association of Poison Control Centers Toxic Exposure. Am J Emerg Med 20:391–452, 2002.
102. Baselt RC: Disposition of Toxic Drugs and Chemicals in Man, 5th ed. Foster City, CA, 2000, Chemical Toxicology Institute.
103. Maher JF, Schreiner GE, Westervelt FB: Acute glutethimide intoxication: Clinical experience compared to acute barbiturate intoxication. Am J Med 33:70–82, 1962.
104. Chazen JA, Garella S: Glutethimide intoxication: A prospective study of 70 patients treated conservatively without hemodialysis. Arch Intern Med 128:215–219, 1971.
105. Wright N, Roscoe P: Acute glutethimide poisoning: Conservative management of 31 patients. JAMA 214:1704–1706, 1970.
106. Chazen JA, Cohen JJ: Clinical spectrum of glutethimide intoxication: Hemodialysis revisited. JAMA 208:837–839, 1969.
107. Yell RP: Ethchlorvynol overdose. Am J Emerg Med 8:246–250, 1990.
108. Glauser FL, Smith WR, Caldwell A, et al: Ethchlorvynol (Placidyl)-induced pulmonary edema. Ann Intern Med 84:46–48, 1976.
109. Fisher P, Glauser FL, Millen JE, et al: The effects of ethchlorvynol on pulmonary alveolar membrane permeability. Am Rev Respir Dis 116:901–906, 1977.
110. Rho JM, Donevan SD, Rogawski MA: Barbiturate-like actions of the propanediol dicarbamates felbamate and meprobamate. J Pharmacol Exp Ther 280:1383–1391, 1997.
111. Littrell RA, Hayes LR, Stillner V: Carisoprodol (Soma): A new and cautious perspective on an old agent. South Med J 86:753–756, 1993.
112. Elder NC: Abuse of skeletal muscle relaxants. Am Fam Pract 44:1223–1226, 1991.
113. Jenis EH, Payne AR, Goldbaum LR: Acute meprobamate poisoning. JAMA 207:361–365, 1969.
114. Schwartz HS: Acute meprobamate poisoning with gastrostomy and removal of a drug containing mass. N Engl J Med 295:1177–1178, 1976.
115. Hassan E: Treatment of meprobamate overdose with repeated oral doses of activated charcoal. Ann Emerg Med 15:73–76, 1986.
116. Linden CH, Rumack BH: Enhanced elimination of meprobamate by multiple doses of activated charcoal. Vet Hum Toxicol 26(Suppl 2):47, 1984.
117. Lin JL, Lim PS, Sai BC, Lin WL: Continuous arteriovenous hemoperfusion in meprobamate poisoning. J Toxicol Clin Toxicol 31:645–652, 1993.
118. Pascarelli EF: Methaqualone abuse, the quiet epidemic. JAMA 224:1512–1514, 1973.
119. Lawson AHH, Brown SS: Acute methaqualone (Mandrax) poisoning. Scott Med J 12:63–68, 1967.
120. Matthew H, Proudfoot AT, Brown SS, et al: Mandrax poisoning: Conservative management of 116 patients. BMJ 2:101–102, 1968.
121. Mills DG: Effects of methaqualone on blood platelet function. Clin Pharmacol Ther 23:685–691, 1978.
122. Trese M: Retinal hemorrhage caused by overdose of methaqualone (Quaalude). Am J Ophthalmol 91:201–203, 1981.
123. Smith DE, Wesson DR: Benzodiazepine dependency syndromes. J Psychoactive Drugs 15:85–95, 1983.
124. Marks J: Techniques of benzodiazepine withdrawal in clinical practice. Med Toxicol 3:324–333, 1988.
125. Benzer DG, Smith DE, Miller NS: Detoxification from benzodiazepine use: Strategies and schedules for clinical practice. Psychiatr Ann 25:180–185, 1995.

CHAPTER 48

Barbiturates

Kenneth D. Katz ■ Anne-Michelle Ruha

Barbiturates originally were introduced as sedative-hypnotics and anticonvulsants in the early 1900s. As a result of the frequency of prescription, intentional overdoses and the ensuing toxicities became commonplace. Barbiturates are hazardous and have the highest risk of morbidity and mortality among all sedative-hypnotics.[1] The use of newer, relatively less toxic medications, such as benzodiazepines, has largely supplanted the routine use of barbiturates. As a result, the incidence of serious toxicity related to barbiturate use has declined. Nevertheless, barbiturates still are used occasionally. Examples include phenobarbital and butalbital (Fiorinal), which currently are prescribed for seizure disorders and migraine headaches, respectively.[2] Primidone, used as an anticonvulsant, is metabolized to phenobarbital.[3] Barbiturates such as methohexital are used for induction of anesthesia, and pentobarbital is commonly relied on for control of intracranial hypertension and status epilepticus in intensive care units.[4,5] Barbiturates sometimes are used as adjunctive therapy for neonatal hyperbilirubinemia.[6] Illicit drug use also may involve barbiturates because of their potential for abuse. Consequently,

clinicians must be aware of the potential toxicities due to accidental or intentional ingestions of barbiturates and remain astute as to the potential addictive properties of barbiturates, with the attendant risk for tolerance and abstinence-induced withdrawal.

BIOCHEMICAL AND PHARMACOKINETIC PROPERTIES

All barbiturates are barbituric acid (2,4,6-trioxohexahydropyrimidine) derivatives (Fig. 48-1).[7] Barbiturates traditionally have been classified as short acting, intermediate acting, and long acting based on their duration of action and hepatic metabolism. These characteristics are influenced primarily by the lipid solubility and consequent distribution into tissues, rather than the actual elimination half-life. Lipid solubility, potency, and onset and duration of action are functions of various substitutions made at different positions on the common barbituric acid structure (see Fig. 48-1). Agents with long side chains, such as thiopental, have a high degree of lipid

Pharmacokinetics of Barbiturates					
Barbiturate	Duration of Action (hr)	pKa	Protein Binding (%)	Elimination Route	V_d (L/kg)
Ultra-short-Acting					
Thiopental (Penthothal)	0.3	7.60	80	Hepatic	1.4–6.7
Methohexital (Brevital)	0.3	7.90	73	Hepatic	1.1–2.6
Short-Acting					
Pentobarbital (Nembutal)	3	7.96	45–70	Hepatic	0.65–1.0
Secobarbital (Seconal)	3	7.90	52–57	Hepatic	1.5
Butalbutal (Fiorinal)	3–4	7.6	NA	Hepatic	NA
Intermediate-Acting					
Amobarbital (Amytal)	3–6	7.75	60	Hepatic	1.0–1.27
Aprobarbital (Alurate)	3–6	NA	NA	Hepatic	NA
Butabarbital (Butisol)	3–6	7.74	NA	Hepatic	0.78
Long-Acting					
Phenobaribital (Luminal)	6–12	7.24	51	Renal (25–30%)	0.5–0.7
Mephobarbital (Mebaral)	6–12	7.8	40–60	Renal (35–40%)	2.6
Primidone (Mysoline)	6–12	13.0	19	Renal (15%)	1.0

NA, not available; V_d, volume of distribution.

Numerical quantities from Baselt RC: Disposition of Toxic Drugs and Chemicals in Man, 5th ed. Foster City, CA, California Chemical Toxicology Institute, 2000.

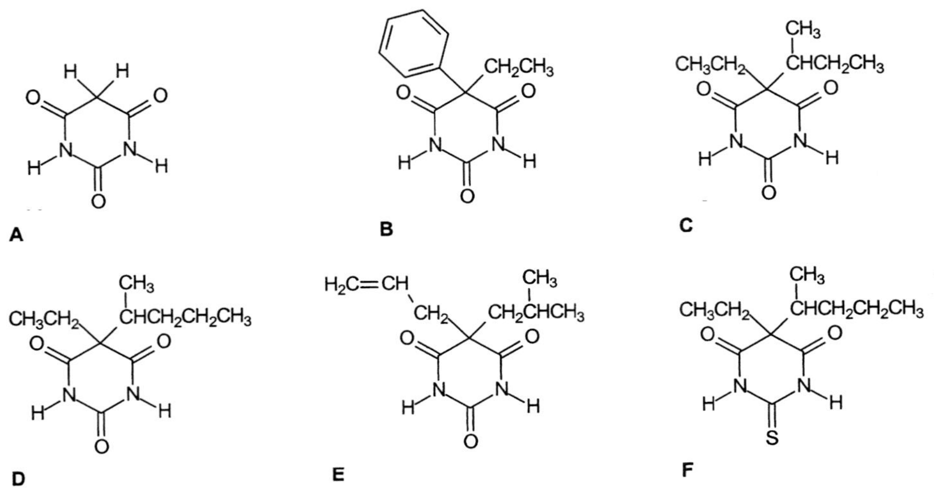

FIGURE 48-1

Chemical structures of barbituric acid (**A**), phenobarbital (**B**), butabarbital (**C**), pentobarbital (**D**), butalbital (**E**), and thiopental (**F**).

solubility and potency, with a rapid onset and short duration of action. In contrast, phenobarbital has a shorter side chain, which confers a relatively lower lipid solubility, lower potency, slower onset, and longer duration of action. Substitution of a phenyl group at the C5 position results in anticonvulsant activity, as observed with phenobarbital and mephobarbital. In general, the more lipid soluble the barbiturate compound, the more protein bound it is in the plasma[8]; this is shown by the relatively high protein binding of thiopental and the relatively lower amount of protein binding observed with phenobarbital. Protein binding plays an important role in the ability to remove a barbiturate effectively from the plasma using hemodialysis.

Barbiturates generally are well absorbed after oral administration and distribute widely to most body tissues, including the placenta and breast milk. Most barbiturates undergo nearly complete hepatic metabolism through cytochrome P-450 systems to inactive compounds, which then are renally excreted.[9] Two barbiturates, mephobarbital and metharbital, are endogenously converted to phenobarbital and barbital.[1] Renal excretion is more important for long-acting barbiturates, with nearly 25% of phenobarbital being excreted unchanged in the urine. Elimination of barbiturates is slower in neonates, elderly patients, and patients with liver and renal dysfunction; pregnancy may increase the half-life of a barbiturate, partly owing to an expanded volume of distribution.

Several noteworthy drug interactions occur with barbiturate administration. The sedative-hypnotic effects of barbiturates may be enhanced with concomitant administration of drugs such as ethanol or benzodiazepines. Repeated administration of barbiturates may induce hepatic CYP4503A4 microsomal enzymes, enhancing the metabolism of oral contraceptives, warfarin, vitamin D, tricyclic antidepressants, sulfonamides, doxycycline, corticosteroids, phenytoin, and barbiturates themselves.[3]

PATHOPHYSIOLOGY OF THERAPEUTIC AND TOXIC EFFECTS

Barbiturates generate their sedative-hypnotic effects in the central nervous system via several different mechanisms. They promote γ-aminobutyric acid (GABA) binding to the GABA$_A$ chloride channel complex, increasing the duration of chloride channel opening. At high concentrations they may open the GABA$_A$ chloride channel directly.[9,10] The result of these actions is increased chloride content in the nerve cell, hyperpolarizing the membrane and depressing neuronal electrical activity.[11] Barbiturates also can reduce excitatory α-amino-3-hydroxy-5-methyl-4-isoxazole propionate glutamate–induced depolarization.[9]

Barbiturates may inhibit nicotinic neurotransmission in autonomic ganglia. Other effects of barbiturates include depression of the medullary respiratory center, inhibition of myocardial contractility and conduction as a result of their "membrane-stabilizing" actions (i.e., fast Na$^+$ channel blockade), and suppression of gastrointestinal motility.[9]

Long-term barbiturate use may produce tolerance to its sedative-hypnotic effects. This phenomenon is related partially to barbiturate induction of hepatic microsomal enzymes (pharmacokinetic tolerance). It also is related to GABA$_A$ receptor down-regulation, which increases progressively as the drug dose increases (pharmacodynamic tolerance).[12]

CLINICAL PRESENTATION AND LIFE-THREATENING COMPLICATIONS

The clinical presentation of the acutely barbiturate-poisoned patient may vary depending on the patient's age and duration of use of the drug. A given dose of barbiturate may cause severe toxicity in a first-time user but only minor impairment in the long-term user because of the latter's pharmacodynamic tolerance to the drug. Barbiturate overdose management decisions should be based primarily on the clinical status of the patient in addition to the serum barbiturate concentration.

In general, acute intoxication with barbiturates may be clinically indistinguishable from that caused by other central nervous system depressant and sedative-hypnotic compounds, such as ethanol or benzodiazepines. These clinical manifestations include drowsiness, lethargy, sedation, ataxia, slurred speech, and incoordination. Vital sign stability and deep tendon reflexes may be preserved in mild barbiturate poisoning. Moderately severe poisoning frequently progresses, however, to the point of depressed levels of consciousness, slowed respirations, and diminished deep tendon reflexes.[13]

People with severe barbiturate intoxication present with coma, hypothermia, and circulatory collapse. Neurologic findings may include nonreactive pupils, loss of other brainstem reflexes (corneal, oculovestibular), absent deep tendon reflexes, and presence of the pathologic reflexes (i.e., Babinski's sign).[13] These manifestations mimic clinical brain death, which can be shown further by isoelectric electroencephalogram tracings. Skin bullae may be present but are nonspecific findings and occasionally are observed as a complication of other central nervous system depressant poisonings. Deleterious effects from other ingested toxins, anoxia, trauma, and rhabdomyolysis all may compound the initial insult and cloud the clinical picture.

Patients who chronically use or abuse barbiturates may experience withdrawal symptoms during the recovery phase of an acute poisoning episode or during other periods of medication abstinence. The severity of the withdrawal syndrome is a function of the daily dose of barbiturate and the degree of dependence.[12] This clinical syndrome is usually manifest within 24 hours and peaks depending on the elimination half-life and duration of effect of the barbiturate used. Withdrawal from other sedative-hypnotic drugs, such as benzodiazepines, presents similarly. Early signs and symptoms may include restlessness, anxiety, tremor, nausea, abdominal cramps, tachycardia, and diaphoresis. Progression to more severe signs and symptoms may occur and can include increased muscular tone, delirium, and seizures. In addition, progressive autonomic dysfunction and cardiovascular collapse may occur with severe withdrawal syndromes. Short-acting barbiturates, such as secobarbital, are associated with onset of withdrawal symptoms within the first 48 to 72 hours of their discontinuation, and withdrawal from long-acting barbiturates, such as phenobarbital, peaks in approximately 1 week. The abstinence syndrome usually clears within 14 days.[1] This syndrome may be seen in the intensive care unit in patients receiving continuous barbiturate administration for sedation.[14]

Chronic adverse effects of the barbiturates include induction of several enzyme systems, including hepatic microsomal CYP4503A4, the mitochondrial enzyme aminolevulinic acid synthetase, and the cytosolic enzyme aldehyde dehydrogenase.[9] Induction of aminolevulinic acid synthetase may precipitate exacerbations of porphyria because of enhanced porphyrin synthesis.[9]

Anticonvulsant hypersensitivity syndrome is a well-recognized pharmacogenetic and idiosyncratic reaction to aromatic anticonvulsant therapy with phenobarbital, phenytoin, primidone, and carbamazepine. The pathogenesis of this syndrome is thought to stem from formation of reactive metabolic intermediates, arene oxides, through the actions of hepatic microsomal enzymes. If these intermediates are not sufficiently detoxified by epoxide hydrolase, they may bind covalently to cell membrane constituents to form neoantigens that trigger hypersensitivity reactions. The clinical manifestations of anticonvulsant hypersensitivity syndrome arise most frequently on first exposure to the drug and occur usually within 1 to several weeks of initiation, earlier in previously sensitized patients. Fever, malaise, pharyngitis, cervical lymphadenopathy, atypical lymphocytosis, eosinophilia, and cutaneous eruption are part of the usual initial clinical presentation of the hypersensitivity syndrome. The rash may range from an exanthemous eruption to Stevens-Johnson syndrome or toxic epidermal necrolysis. Additional visceral organ involvement may include hepatitis, myocarditis, pericarditis, nephritis, pneumonitis, and thyroiditis.[15]

DIAGNOSIS

Laboratory tests obtained for a patient with suspected barbiturate intoxication should include a finger-stick blood glucose, electrolyte panel, serum creatine phosphokinase, and an electrocardiogram or rhythm strip. If there is concern for the possibility of acute overdose, it is advisable also to screen for acetaminophen and possibly salicylate poisoning. Urine immunoassay tests, such as enzyme magnified immunoassay technique, readily detect barbiturates at plasma concentrations associated with toxicity. Drugs such as glutethimide, a nonbarbiturate sedative-hypnotic, may cause false-positive results.[3] In addition, barbiturates other than phenobarbital cross-react with the latter compound in some immunoassays.[24] Gross crystalluria has been reported to occur as a clinical feature of toxicity with primidone, an anticonvulsant drug that undergoes biotransformation to phenobarbital and involves renal tubular precipitation of the parent compound.[3]

Serum barbiturate concentrations do not correlate with toxicity, particularly in the barbiturate-dependent patient. Prognostic or forensic information may be provided by serum drug concentrations, however, in barbiturate-poisoned patients; values greater than 35 mg/L of short-acting barbiturates, such as secobarbital, and greater than 80 mg/L of long-acting barbiturates, such as phenobarbital, are considered lethal.[1] In addition, serial serum barbiturate concentrations may assist in determining the need for continuing medical treatment or in the declaration of brain death after initial biologic detection of barbiturates.

TREATMENT

Standard treatment of acute barbiturate poisoning begins with aggressive airway management and ventilatory support as clinically indicated. Careful attention to hemodynamic monitoring is crucial. If hypotension occurs and persists despite aggressive fluid volume resuscitation, the addition of intravenous vasopressors, such as dopamine or norepinephrine, may be required to achieve hemodynamic stability. Forced diuresis is not recommended because of the attendant risks of sodium and fluid overload and probable lack of efficacy. Severe hypothermia should be treated by vigorous rewarming measures.

If a patient presents early after acute oral overdose, administration of a single dose of activated charcoal is recommended. Multiple doses of activated charcoal may reduce the duration of coma in an acutely intoxicated patient.[25,26] Caution is advised with this intervention because bowel motility may be compromised in a barbiturate-toxic patient. Administration of charcoal must be performed prudently to minimize the risk

Indications for ICU Admission in Barbiturate Poisoning

Hemodynamic instability
Requirement for mechanical ventilation
Coma
Severe hypothermia
Presence of comorbid medical conditions that may complicate therapy (e.g., severe coronary artery disease, congestive heart failure, renal failure)
Requirement for hemodialysis
Severe electrolyte disturbances or acidemia
Actively suicidal patient requiring close observation beyond general hospital floor capability
Increasing barbiturate level despite aggressive therapy
Significant withdrawal syndrome

Key Points in the Treatment of Barbiturate Poisoning

1. Give aggressive airway and ventilatory support.
2. Administer intravenous fluid (1–2 L) if hypotension is present; if no response, initiate vasopressors (e.g., dopamine or norepinephrine) to maintain systolic blood pressure <90 mm Hg and maintain adequate urine output.
3. Perform vigorous rewarming measures for severe hypothermia.
4. Consider administration of more than one enteral dose of activated charcoal.
5. Consider urinary alkalization (target urine pH 8) for moderate-to-severe phenobarbital overdose.
6. Consider serial barbiturate levels.
7. If the patient is clinically unstable or has rising serum barbiturate levels despite above measures, hemodialysis or hemoperfusion should be instituted.
8. The presence of rhabdomyolysis should be determined.
9. Skin bullae require local wound care; consider tetanus immunization.
10. Consider lower extremity compressive garments and gastric stress ulcer prophylaxis in critically ill patients.

of aspiration, which generally requires airway-protective measures and oronasogastric tube placement in comatose patients.

Alkalization of the urine has been shown to enhance clearance of phenobarbital, which has a pK_a of 7.2. The clearance of barbiturates with higher pK_a values has not been shown to increase in this manner.[12] Administration of sodium bicarbonate intravenously at dosages of 50 to 100 mmol of sodium bicarbonate in 1 L of 5% dextrose in water infused at 150 to 250 mL/hr may promote effectively formation of the ionized form of phenobarbital.[1] The rationale behind alkalization is that because ionized molecules are poorly reabsorbed in the kidney, phenobarbital is ion-trapped under alkaline conditions in the renal tubule and can undergo enhanced elimination. The goal of urinary alkalization is to maintain a urine pH of 7 to 8.[12] An additional benefit of urinary alkalization may be protection or treatment of accompanying rhabdomyolysis.[3]

Hemodialysis and hemoperfusion also can be employed to enhance elimination of long-acting barbiturates. These drugs are less protein bound and less lipid soluble than short-acting barbiturates and can be cleared effectively from the plasma by extracorporeal removal techniques. Indications include severely poisoned patients who are not responding adequately to the aforementioned supportive measures and patients who cannot excrete the barbiturate effectively because of renal failure. Several case reports have shown apparent clinical effectiveness of extracorporeal removal of phenobarbital in patients not responding to other supportive measures.[27] Exchange transfusion has been reported as an effective intervention for phenobarbital intoxication in neonates being treated for hyperbilirubinemia.[6]

Criteria for ICU Discharge in Barbiturate Poisoning

Mechanical ventilation no longer required
Vasopressors discontinued
Hemodynamic stability
Resolution of coma
Normothermia
Resolution of metabolic disturbances
Decreasing serum barbiturate concentrations

BARBITURATE WITHDRAWAL

The prevention and management of the barbiturate withdrawal syndrome primarily include gradual tapering of the previously administered medication regimen and institution of the same or a cross-tolerated sedative-hypnotic. In the critical care setting, discontinuation of a short-acting barbiturate such as pentobarbital may be accomplished safely and effectively after initiation of a long-acting barbiturate such as phenobarbital.[14] Withdrawal symptoms also may be managed by the administration of a benzodiazepine, such as diazepam or lorazepam, to control the sympathetic hyperactivity to the point of mild sedation, with care taken not to cause respiratory compromise. Gentle, incremental dose titration may be required at the patient's bedside. When control of withdrawal signs and symptoms is attained, further treatment may entail reintroduction of the barbiturate, depending on the clinical situation.[3]

SPECIAL POPULATIONS

Pediatric Patients

Neonatal exposure to barbiturates can occur in a variety of clinical scenarios, including administration during delivery or in the intensive care unit and maternal use during pregnancy. Pharmacologic effects of barbiturates in neonates are similar to those in adults, but strict adherence to drug doses and dosing intervals must be maintained because of relatively low levels of phase I enzyme activity in neonates.[16] In addition, phenobarbital has been associated with neonatal hemorrhage owing to a decrease in vitamin K–dependent clotting factors II, VII, IX, and X.[16]

Because barbiturates cross the placenta freely, neonatal withdrawal may be encountered. Symptoms of withdrawal in neonates usually begin 4 to 7 days after birth and may include overactivity, restlessness, insomnia, hyperphagia, tremor, and vasomotor instability. These symptoms may persist for weeks to months.[12]

Fetal abnormalities also have been reported with use of barbiturates during pregnancy, in a manner similar to that associated with use of phenytoin, trimethadione, and valproic acid. The name *fetal hydantoin syndrome* may be a misnomer because the etiologies of this syndrome also seem to include barbiturates. Clinical manifestations of this syndrome may include facial dysmorphism, prenatal and postnatal growth deficiency, and developmental delay. More recently, the notion of drug-specific syndromes has been supplanted by the term *fetal antiepileptic drug syndrome*.[17,18]

Pregnant and Breast-feeding Patients

Pregnancy is a multifaceted clinical arena because barbiturate use during this time may affect the mother and the fetus. Barbiturate toxicity in pregnant women may be associated with deleterious effects in the developing fetus, secondary to impaired maternal physiology (e.g., hypotension or hypoxemia). Resuscitation of the mother is the primary goal of the critical care provider.

Barbiturates may be employed in the treatment of pregnant women with epilepsy. One third of pregnant women with seizure disorders experience more frequent seizures; generalized motor seizures during pregnancy generate fetal bradycardia, decelerations, decreased variability, and intracranial hemorrhage.[18] As a result, optimal seizure control in a pregnant patient is essential to maintenance of fetal health. Although phenobarbital is considered a U.S. Food and Drug Administration pregnancy category D drug (see Appendix A), the risk to the mother and fetus may be greater if seizure control is lost. The lowest amount of drug required to control seizures should be used, and frequent monitoring of drug levels should be maintained.[19,20]

Phenobarbital is excreted in breast milk, and reports of infant sedation and withdrawal have been described. Breast-feeding women prescribed phenobarbital should be instructed to watch for sedation, and infant phenobarbital levels should be monitored if toxicity is suspected.[19]

Elderly Patients

Elderly patients present another set of special considerations with respect to barbiturates. Adverse drug reactions are commonplace in the elderly, who take an average of four or five prescribed medications and two over-the-counter medications.[21] In addition, alterations in the GABA–benzodiazepine receptor complex associated with aging may make older patients more sensitive to barbiturates.[22] Elderly patients also may have significant comorbid medical conditions that not only can lead to serious problems with medication compliance (e.g., excessive administration of sedative-hypnotics) but also may confound clinical presentation. Not only may the toxicity of the barbiturates be compounded in an elderly patient already taking other sedative-hypnotics or antihistamine medication, but also the diagnosis may be delayed or missed in patients with other medical illnesses clouding the clinical picture.

No specific data are available regarding the absorption, volume of distribution, protein binding, half-life, or changes in metabolism of phenobarbital in the geriatric patient. It has been shown, however, that phenobarbital clearance was reduced in older (>40 years old) patients compared with younger patients, and a reduction in maintenance dose was required in the older patients to maintain the same plasma phenobarbital concentration.[23] Decline in renal clearance associated with aging might lead to increased plasma phenobarbital concentrations at the same dose.[23]

Key Points in Barbiturate Poisoning

1. Assessment and treatment should be based primarily on the patient's clinical status, not just serum drug concentrations.
2. Barbiturates can cause isoelectric electroencephalogram (EEG) patterns; the diagnosis of brain death should not be made based on the EEG when these patterns are present.
3. Patients who are taking barbiturates on a long-term basis may develop a severe withdrawal syndrome if they are stopped abruptly.
4. There is no role for forced diuresis.

REFERENCES

1. Baltarowich L: Barbiturates. Top Emerg Med 7:46–53, 1985.
2. Mclean W, Boucher EA, Brennan M, et al: Is there an indication for the use of barbiturate-containing analgesic agents in the treatment of pain? Guidelines for their safe use and withdrawal management. Can J Clin Pharmacol 7:91–96, 2000.
3. Wallace KL, Morkunas AR: Commonly abused prescription sedative-hypnotic drugs. Top Emerg Med 19:27–33, 1997.
4. Lund N, Papadakos P: Barbiturates, neuroleptics, and propofol for sedation. Crit Care Clin 11:876–878, 1995.
5. Lerman B, Yoshida D, Levitt MA: A prospective evaluation of the safety and efficacy of methohexital in the emergency department. Am J Emerg Med 14:351–354, 1996.
6. Sancak R, Kucukoduk S, Tasdemir HA, Belet N: Exchange transfusion treatment in newborn with phenobarbital intoxication. Pediatr Emerg Care 15:268–269, 1999.
7. Osborn HH: Sedative-hypnotic agents. In Goldfrank LR, Flomenbaum N, Lewin N, et al (eds): Goldfrank's Toxicologic Emergencies, 6th ed. Stamford, CT, Appleton & Lange, 1998, pp 1001–1014.
8. Haddad LM, Winchester JF: Barbiturates. In Haddad LM, Shannon MW, Winchester JF (eds): Clinical Management of Poisoning and Drug Overdose, 3rd ed. Philadelphia, WB Saunders, 1998, pp 521–527.
9. Hobbs WR, Rall TW, Verdoon TA: Hypnotics and sedatives: Barbiturates. In Hardman JG, Limbird LE, et al (eds): Goodman and Gilman's the Pharmacological Basis of Therapeutics, 9th ed. San Francisco, McGraw-Hill, 1996, pp 373–380.
10. Mehta AK, Ticku MK: An update on GABA-A receptors. Brain Res Rev 29:204–205, 1999.
11. Curry SC, Mills KC, Graeme KA: Neurotransmitters. In Goldfrank LR, Flomenbaum N, Lewin N, et al (eds): Goldfrank's Toxicologic Emergencies, 6th ed. Stamford, CT, Appleton & Lange, 1998, pp 155–157.
12. Coupey SM: Barbiturates. Pediatr Rev 18:260–264, 1997.
13. Lindberg MC, Cunningham A, Lindberg NH: Acute phenobarbital intoxication. South Med J 85:803–806, 1992.
14. Tobias JD: Tolerance, withdrawal, and physical dependency after long-term sedation and analgesia of children in the pediatric intensive care unit. Crit Care Med 28:2130–2131, 2000.
15. Knowles SR, Shapiro LE, Shear NH: Anticonvulsant hypersensitivity syndrome. Drug Saf 21:489–499, 1999.
16. Gupta A, Waldhauser LK: Adverse drug reactions from birth to early childhood. Pediatr Clin North Am 44:79–82, 1997.

17. Seip M: Growth retardation, dysmorphic facies and minor malformations following massive exposure to phenobarbitone in utero. Acta Paediatr Scand 65:617–621, 1976.
18. Foldvary N: Treatment issues for women with epilepsy. Neurol Clin 19:409–425, 2001.
19. Briggs GG, Freeman RK, Yaffe SJ: Drugs in Pregnancy and Lactation, 6th ed. Philadelphia, Lippincott Williams & Wilkins, 2002, pp 1097–1105.
20. Zahn CA, Morrell MJ, Collins SD, et al: Management issues for women with epilepsy: A review of the literature. Neurology 51:949–956, 1998.
21. Kirk M, Pace S: Pearls, pitfalls and updates in toxicology. Emerg Med Clin North Am 15:427–449, 1997.
22. Kompoliti K, Goetz CG: Neuropharmacology in the elderly. Neurol Clin 16:599–610, 1998.
23. Bernus I, Dickinson RG, Hooper WD, Eadie MJ: Anticonvulsant therapy in the aged patient: Clinical pharmacokinetic considerations. Drugs Aging 10:278–289, 1997.
24. Nordt SP: Butalbital cross-reactivity to an Emit assay for phenobarbital. Ann Pharmacother 31:254–255, 1997.
25. Goldberg MJ, Berlinger WG: Treatment of phenobarbital overdose with activated charcoal. JAMA 247:2400–2401, 1982.
26. Amitai Y, Degani Y: Treatment of phenobarbital poisoning with multiple dose activated charcoal in an infant. J Emerg Med 8:449–450, 1989.
27. Palmer BF: Effectiveness of hemodialysis in the extracorporeal therapy of phenobarbital overdose. Am J Kidney Dis 36:640–643, 2000.

CHAPTER **49**

Phenytoin

Frank LoVecchio

Greater than 2 million Americans suffer from epilepsy, and 10% of the population have at least one convulsion in their lifetime. Phenytoin has been commercially available in the United States since 1938 and is a first-step anticonvulsant for all types of epilepsy, with the exception of absence seizures. In conjunction with benzodiazepines, phenytoin is efficacious in the acute treatment of status epilepticus[1] and has been used prophylactically after head injury.[2] Historically, it was used as a class 1B antidysrhythmic agent, particularly in the setting of digoxin toxicity, but it no longer is considered a first-line agent for that indication.

Significant morbidity or mortality is infrequent after intentional oral phenytoin overdose.[3] Hypersensitivity reactions, falls, rapid intravenous administration, and extravasation of the drug into soft tissues are responsible for most phenytoin-related deaths and morbidity. The latter two adverse effects are related directly to the propylene glycol–containing alkaline diluent in the available injectable form of the drug.[4] This diluent has been eliminated from the newer phenytoin prodrug preparation fosphenytoin.

In 1997, the American Association of Poison Control Centers reported 4630 phenytoin exposures, of which 13% were deemed to be of moderate severity, and less than 2% involved major effects. Two deaths were reported,[5] with none reported in the 2001 database.[6] Although poison center data are limited, these data at least suggest that significant morbidity and mortality are rare after acute phenytoin exposure.

BIOCHEMISTRY AND CLINICAL PHARMACOLOGY

Phenytoin, or 5,5-diphenyl-2,4-imidazolidinedione, is similar in chemical structure to the barbiturates but has a five-membered ring (Fig. 49-1). It is a weak acid with a pK_a of 8.3. To maintain parenteral phenytoin in solution, it is adjusted to a pH of 12.

PHARMACOKINETICS

Given phenytoin's relatively high pK_a, its solubility is limited at physiologic pH and in gastric acid. Absorption of oral phenytoin is slow and imperfect, particularly after an over-dose. Peak serum concentrations occur 3 to 12 hours after a single oral dose. Many factors influence kinetics in overdose (e.g., quantity, coingestions, long-term therapy). Intramuscular phenytoin administration results in local precipitation of the drug with sporadic absorption and is not recommended.

After absorption, phenytoin is distributed with a volume of distribution of 0.6 L/kg, approximating body water. Central nervous system concentrations equilibrate with concentrations in plasma within 10 minutes of intravenous infusion and correlate with therapeutic efficacy, whereas myocardial concentrations reach equilibrium with plasma within 30 to 60 minutes. Within the central nervous system, concentrations are higher in the brainstem and cerebellum than in the cerebral cortex.[7]

Phenytoin is 90% bound to plasma proteins, principally albumin. The free or unbound form is responsible for the drug's clinical effects. The free phenytoin fraction ordinarily constitutes 10% of the plasma level. The unbound fraction of the drug is greater in patients at extremes of age, pregnant women, patients with renal failure, patients with hypoalbuminemia, patients with hyperbilirubinemia, and individuals taking drugs that compete for phenytoin binding sites (e.g., salicylates, valproate, phenylbutazone, tolbutamide, and sulfisoxazole).[8]

Pharmacokinetics of Phenytoin
Therapeutic range: 10–20 µg/mL (20–40 µmol/L)
Free phenytoin concentration: 1–2 µg/mL (2–4 µmol/L)
Peak after therapeutic oral dose: 3–12 hr
Plasma half-life: 6–60 hr

Less than 5% of phenytoin is excreted unchanged in the urine. Most is metabolized by hepatic microsomal enzymes, primarily by CYP4502C9 and secondarily by CYP4502C19. Its major (60% to 70%) metabolite, the parahydroxyphenyl derivative, is generated by CYP4502C9. Inhibitors of CYP2C9 such as amiodarone, fluconazole, fluoxetine, metronidazole, or zafirlukast increase phenytoin serum concentrations. Although CYP4502C9 inducers such as phenobarbital and rifampin decrease in phenytoin concentrations, inhibitors of

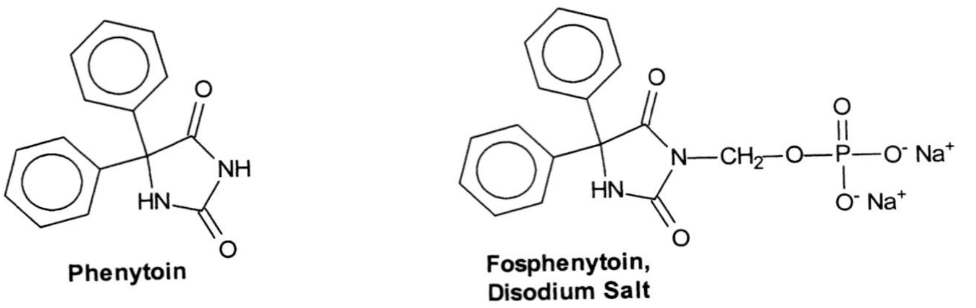

Phenytoin

Fosphenytoin, Disodium Salt

FIGURE 49-1

Chemical structures of anticonvulsant medications.

CYP4502C19 such as cimetidine, felbamate, fluvoxamine, ketoconazole, lansoprazole, omeprazole, paroxetine, and ticlopidine increase phenytoin levels. Finally, inducers of CYP2C19 such as carbamazepine and rifampin may lower serum phenytoin concentrations.[9]

Phenytoin is metabolized further by means of glucuronidation, then is secreted in the bile, reabsorbed, and subsequently excreted in the urine as the glucuronide. The metabolism of phenytoin is highly dose dependent at low concentrations. At plasma concentrations less than 10 μg/mL (40 μmol/L), its elimination is first order, with a constant percentage of drug being metabolized per unit of time. At higher concentrations, including concentrations in the therapeutic range (10 to 20 μg/mL [40 to 80 μmol/L]), its metabolism becomes saturated, however, and elimination changes to zero order (i.e., a fixed amount of drug metabolized per unit of time) (Fig. 49-2). This change in kinetics can markedly prolong the elimination rate of phenytoin, which has an apparent half-life during therapeutic use of 6 to 24 hours. When used therapeutically at the high therapeutic range, a modest increase in the daily dose may result in a disproportionate increase in the plasma concentration and subsequent toxicity. Individual variation occurs with regard to the serum or plasma concentration at which this transformation from first-order to zero-order kinetics occurs. Incremental increases in dose should be limited to the lowest increase

possible, and patients should be monitored carefully, particularly when it is necessary to increase phenytoin doses to greater than 300 mg/day (or approximately 5 mg/kg/day).[8]

PATHOPHYSIOLOGY

The precise mechanism by which phenytoin exerts its anticonvulsant action is unknown. The two presumed mechanisms of phenytoin's anticonvulsant effect are prolongation of neuronal sodium channel inactivation (Fig. 49-3) and the resulting inhibition of excitatory neurotransmitter release (see Chapter 20).

High frequency of neuronal action potential generation is responsible for seizure development. Suppression of this high-frequency firing may occur as a result of voltage-dependent sodium channel inactivation or prolongation of the recovery from inactivation. Phenytoin inhibits sodium channels by reducing their capacity for recovery from inactivation. Phenytoin stabilizes sodium channels in an inactive state and limits the ability of neurons to depolarize at high frequency.[9] Phenytoin does not affect low-frequency neuronal firing. At higher concentrations in vivo, phenytoin delays activation of outward potassium currents in neurons and prolongs the neuronal refractory period.[10]

Phenytoin also may exert some anticonvulsant effect by acting through adenosine receptors. Adenosine is an endogenous anticonvulsant that suppresses seizure propagation[11,12] by inhibiting excitatory neurotransmitter (e.g., glutamate) release. Phenytoin may inhibit adenosine reuptake, resulting in a net increase in extracellular synaptic adenosine and enhancement of its effect on neurotransmitter release.[12,13] Phenytoin has no clinically significant action at γ-aminobutyric acid receptors or known effects on calcium channel conductance.

At toxic levels in the brain, phenytoin suppresses memory and balance by inhibiting the only areas of the brain that exhibit spontaneous neuronal burst discharge: the hippocampus and the cerebellum. Cerebellar stimulation and alteration in dopaminergic and serotoninergic activity may be responsible for the acute dystonias and movement disorders such as opisthotonos and choreoathetosis that infrequently accompany phenytoin toxicity. Seizures after toxic phenytoin ingestion are extremely rare, and their mechanism is not understood.[11-14]

Phenytoin also may inhibit myocardial sodium channels; however, cardiac disturbances and negative inotropy attributed to this effect of phenytoin are reported infrequently. Similar to other class 1B antidysrhythmics, such as lidocaine, phenytoin blocks cardiac sodium channels and has a minimal effect on potassium efflux. At therapeutic doses,

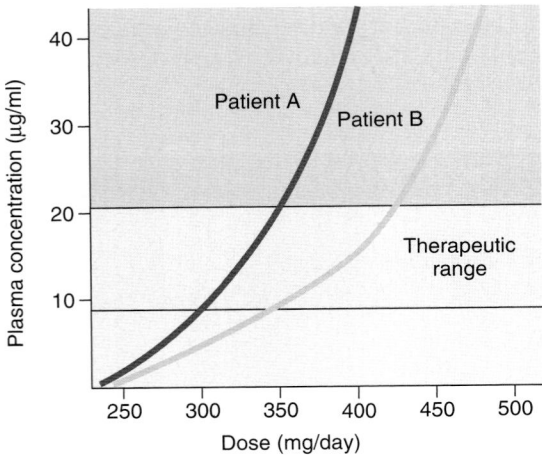

FIGURE 49-2

The relationship between the dose and steady-state plasma concentration of phenytoin is illustrated for two patients. In both patients, there is a linear relationship between the dose and the plasma concentration at low doses. As the dose increases, there is a transition to a nonlinear relationship. This transition occurs at different doses in each patient. *(From Stringer JL: Drugs for seizure disorders [epilepsies]. In Brody TM, Larner J, Minneman KP [eds]: Human Pharmacology: Molecular to Clinical, 3rd ed. St. Louis, Mosby, 1998, p 378.)*

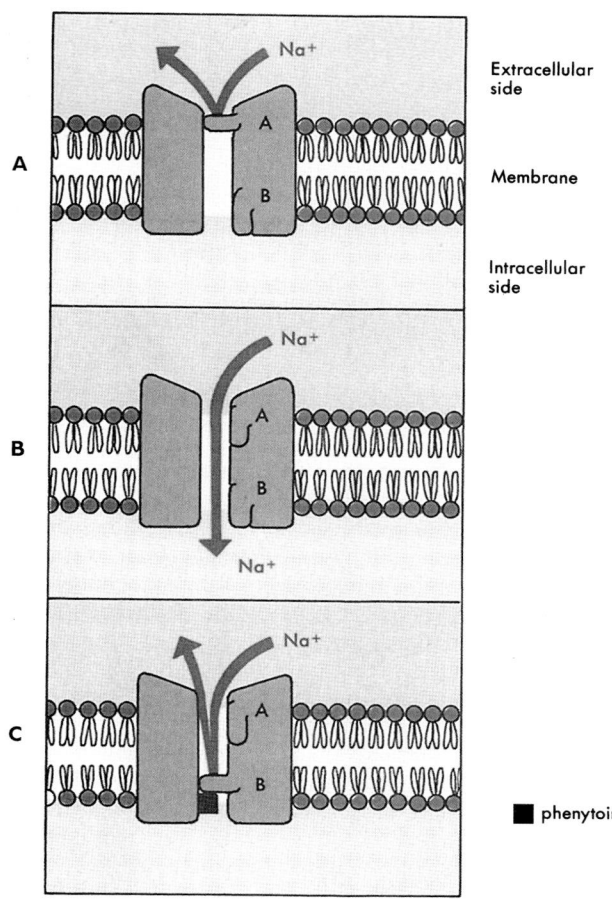

FIGURE 49-3

Action of phenytoin on sodium channel. **A,** Resting state in which sodium channel activation gate (A) is closed. **B,** Arrival of an action potential causes depolarization and opening of activation gate (A), and Na+ flows into the cell. **C,** When depolarization continues, an activation gate (B) moves into the channel. Phenytoin prolongs the inactivated state of the sodium channel, presumably by preventing reopening of the inactivation gate (B). *(From Stringer JL: Drugs for seizure disorders [epilepsies]. In Brody TM, Larner J, Minneman KP [eds]: Human Pharmacology: Molecular to Clinical, 3rd ed. St. Louis, Mosby, 1998, p 376.)*

no effects are noted on electrocardiogram, and at toxic doses, the effects are typically insignificant.[15–17]

Diluent Effects

The acute-onset cardiovascular toxicity seen with intravenously administered phenytoin has been attributed to its diluent. Older parenteral formulations of phenytoin contain 40% propylene glycol and 10% ethanol, adjusted to a pH of 12 with sodium hydroxide. The propylene glycol component seems to be responsible for the reported coma, seizures, circulatory collapse, and ventricular dysrhythmias[13] after rapid intravenous administration of phenytoin. Propylene glycol is a strong myocardial depressant with vasodilatory and vagal effects.[15,16] In animals, phenytoin partially reverses the toxic effects that occur when propylene glycol is given alone.[17] Noncardiovascular effects of propylene glycol include hyperosmolality, hemolysis, and lactic acidosis.[15] In addition, the ethanol diluent fraction of phenytoin may

precipitate a reaction in patients ingesting disulfiram or disulfiram-like medications.

CLINICAL PRESENTATION

The clinical toxicity of phenytoin varies as a function of dose, duration, route, and rate of administration. The latter two parameters are paramount. The rapid intravenous administration of phenytoin carries the greatest risk of life-threatening toxicity occurring as a result of the propylene glycol diluent. The gravest consequences occurring after intravenous administration of phenytoin are cardiovascular (bradycardia, hypotension, and asystole).[18–20] Toxicity from acute or chronic oral overdose may be manifested by nystagmus, nausea and vomiting, ataxia, dysarthria, choreoathetosis, opisthotonos, and central nervous system depression or excitation.[21] Deaths associated with oral ingestion of phenytoin are extremely rare and typically involve a coingestion.[21,22] Major cardiac toxicity after oral overdose has never been reported.[21,22] Tissue necrosis and sloughing after extravasation of intravenous phenytoin also have been described.[19,21,22]

Relationship between Plasma Concentration and Toxicity

Therapeutic plasma phenytoin concentrations are 10 to 20 µg/mL (20 to 40 µmol/L), with a free phenytoin concentration of 1 to 2 µg/mL (2 to 4 µmol/L). Some patients require plasma concentrations greater than 20 µg/mL (40 µmol/L) for adequate seizure control.[23] The therapeutic range for phenytoin is narrow, and some patients have a greater predisposition for toxicity than others. Individual variation in toxicity is a function of baseline neurologic status, individual response to the drug, and free drug fraction. Patients with underlying brain disease are predisposed to toxicity and may become toxic at lower plasma concentrations.[24] In general, toxicity correlates with increasing plasma concentration, but this is not a universal tenet. Some patients tolerate concentrations greater than 40 µg/mL (80 µmol/L) well.[24] Nystagmus typically appears first at phenytoin concentrations equal to or greater than 20 µg/mL (40 µmol/L) but may occur at lower or higher levels. Almost all patients with phenytoin-induced seizures have concentrations greater than 30 µg/mL (60 µmol/L). Signs of toxicity typically occur at free phenytoin concentrations equal to or greater than 2 µg/mL (4 µmol/L) and are consistently severe at greater than 5 µg/mL (10 µmol/L).[25,26]

Central Nervous System Toxicity

Central nervous system toxicity after acute or chronic phenytoin overdose is manifested by nystagmus, dysequilibrium, and cerebellar ataxia. Central nervous system depression and cognitive defects (confusion, dizziness, and memory impairment) may occur.[23,24] Paradoxically, high concentrations of phenytoin have been reported to be associated with seizures.[23–26]

When phenytoin concentrations in the brain increase beyond therapeutic values, inhibitory cortical and excitatory cerebellar/vestibular effects occur. The usual initial sign of toxicity is nystagmus, which is seen first on forced lateral gaze and subsequently becomes spontaneous. A decreased level of consciousness is common with initial sedation, lethargy, ataxic gait, and dysarthria. Progression to confusion, coma, and apnea can occur in massive ingestions.[29] Acute dystonias and movement disorders such as opisthotonos and choreoathetosis have been described.[30] Depressed or hyperactive deep tendon reflexes, clonus, and extensor toe responses also may be elicited.[30–32] Phenytoin-induced seizures are rare, universally preceded by other signs of toxicity, and usually brief and generalized.[33,34] Some signs of neurologic toxicity may outlast the presence of measurable drug levels by months, especially mild peripheral neuropathy or acute, typically reversible cerebellar ataxia.[35]

Vertical, bidirectional, or alternating nystagmus may occur with severe intoxication or be absent at levels high enough to cause coma, complete ophthalmoplegia, and loss of corneal reflexes. Absence of nystagmus does not exclude severe phenytoin toxicity. Nystagmus often returns as serum phenytoin concentrations decrease and coma lightens.[25–27]

Cardiovascular Toxicity

Cardiac toxicity after oral phenytoin overdose in an otherwise healthy patient has not been reported and if observed warrants aggressive assessment for other etiologies. Acute cardiovascular toxicity has been limited almost entirely to cases involving intravenous administration at rates greater than 50 mg/min and is manifested by hypotension, decreased peripheral vascular resistance, bradycardia, conduction delays that may progress to complete atrioventricular nodal block, asystole, ventricular tachycardia, or ventricular fibrillation.[15,17]

Electrocardiographic changes reported are increased PR interval, widened QRS interval, and ST-T wave changes. Most of these effects can be attributed to rapid intravenous administration of the preparation containing propylene glycol and typically are avoidable with slower administration (approximately 50 μg/min of phenytoin). In six healthy volunteers taking approximately 1 g of phenytoin in a simulated oral overdose, sinus bradycardia and a shortened PR interval were noted in two patients but did not correlate with peak plasma phenytoin concentration.[36]

Vascular and Soft Tissue Injury

Intramuscular injection of phenytoin may result in hematoma, sterile abscess, and myonecrosis[37] at the injection site. Reported complications after extravasation following intended intravenous infusion have included skin and soft tissue necrosis requiring skin grafting and compartment syndrome, gangrene, amputation, and death. Rhabdomyolysis is a potential complication. A syndrome of delayed bluish discoloration of the affected extremity, followed by erythema, edema, vesicles, bullae, and local tissue ischemia, also has been described.[38]

Non–Dose-Related Adverse Effects

Some adverse effects of long-term phenytoin administration are dose dependent and duration dependent, as noted earlier,

whereas others seem to be non–dose related (i.e., idiosyncratic), such as gingival hypertrophy[35] and anticonvulsant hypersensitivity syndrome.[33] Hypersensitivity reactions to phenytoin usually occur within the first few months of therapy and include fever, skin rashes, blood dyscrasia, and hepatitis. Phenytoin, phenobarbital, carbamazepine, and perhaps felbamate all are causes of anticonvulsant hypersensitivity syndrome, which is related causally to the generation of toxic arene oxide metabolites in some individuals receiving these drugs. Treatment is generally supportive with removal of the offending agent and avoidance of other anticonvulsants that are metabolized to arene oxide compounds.[30]

DIAGNOSIS

Determination of a plasma phenytoin concentration is the most commonly used method of diagnosing dose-dependent toxicity. Use of this metric is not infallible, however. The idiosyncratic phenytoin hypersensitivity syndrome is not dose dependent and is independent of the magnitude of the plasma concentrations. Patients with decreased plasma albumin concentrations generally have higher levels of free phenytoin (i.e., increased free fraction) and greater biologic effects. These patients may exhibit phenytoin toxicity despite total phenytoin levels in the usual therapeutic range. Patients who manifest toxic signs despite phenytoin levels in the therapeutic range, particularly if they may be hypoalbuminemic, should have free phenytoin concentrations measured, if available.[36]

Toxicity from other anticonvulsants such as carbamazepine or phenobarbital, sedative-hypnotics, ethanol, or phencyclidine and nontoxicologic causes constitute the major differential diagnosis of a patient presenting with altered mental status, ataxia, and nystagmus. Most of these toxicologic diagnoses can be excluded by history and determination of drug concentrations.

 Common Errors in the Assessment of Phenytoin Toxicity

Missing the diagnosis of phenytoin toxicity in hypoalbuminemic patients with normal blood phenytoin concentration
Failing to recognize that at toxic levels plasma phenytoin concentrations may decrease slowly owing to saturation of its metabolic enzymes

TREATMENT

Supportive treatment is the cornerstone of medical management for phenytoin toxicity. Appropriate initial management of acute oral phenytoin overdose includes intravenous access; airway and ventilatory support as clinically warranted; and, if presentation is early (within the first hour) after ingestion, possibly oral or orogastric activated charcoal administration. The administration of activated charcoal may reduce peak plasma phenytoin concentrations. Because virtually all patients with phenytoin toxicity as their sole acute medical diagnosis recover

Indications for ICU Admission in Phenytoin Poisoning

Rising serial plasma phenytoin concentrations
Coingestions
Coma
Poor reliability in caring for patient with regard to ataxia (fall prevention)

completely, it is unlikely that the administration of activated charcoal would alter their outcome. Whether activated charcoal administration shortens the clinical course of these patients is unknown.

In human volunteer studies, multiple doses of oral activated charcoal decreases the area under the curve and phenytoin half-life.[37,38] Multiple-dose activated charcoal is associated with possible aspiration in patients with depressed airway protective reflexes, however, and has never been of proven benefit to clinical outcome in any overdose patient population.[37,38]

Because phenytoin is extensively protein bound, it is not appreciably removed by hemodialysis or hemoperfusion, and these two modalities are not useful in phenytoin toxicity. Seizures should be treated with intravenous benzodiazepines (e.g., diazepam) or barbiturates or both, and their occurrence should prompt a search for other causes, given the low likelihood of their causation by phenytoin.

Cardiovascular toxicity is unexpected after oral phenytoin overdose and should suggest other causes. Prolonged cardiac monitoring after oral ingestion is unnecessary. Hypotension that occurs during intravenous administration of phenytoin usually responds to discontinuation of the infusion and the administration of isotonic crystalloid. Atropine and temporary cardiac pacing may be used for symptomatic bradydysrhythmias.

Patients with serious complications after acute oral ingestion (e.g., seizures, coma, altered mental status, ataxia) should be admitted for further evaluation and treatment. Others with only mild symptoms may be treated in the emergency department and discharged after their levels have returned to normal, provided that they are not actively suicidal and no coingestions warrant admission. Otherwise stable patients can be discharged even with supratherapeutic plasma phenytoin concentrations, provided that appropriate precautions against falling due to ataxia are taken (e.g., patient minimally ataxic, has caregiver at home, not anticoagulated).

Individuals with continuing signs and symptoms of phenytoin toxicity may need to be admitted or followed in an observation unit. Given the long, erratic absorption phase of phenytoin after oral overdose, the decision to discharge or clear a patient medically for psychiatric evaluation cannot be based on a single physical examination and serum level. Patients with symptomatic chronic intoxication should be admitted for observation and discharged when symptoms have resolved or minimized and consecutive serum levels are decreasing. Phenytoin therapy should be stopped in all cases, and if toxicity continues to resolve, a serum level may be reassessed in 2 to 3 days to guide resumption of therapy.

Patients with significant or persistent complications after intravenous administration of phenytoin should be admitted and managed by appropriate supportive and diagnostic means. Orthopedic or plastic surgical consultation should be obtained for patients with significant extravasation of intravenous phenytoin or other signs of local vascular or tissue toxicity after infusion.

To prevent complications due to intravenous infusion of phenytoin, it should be administered under close observation, with constant cardiac and blood pressure monitoring. The infused solution should be given slowly (no faster than 50 mg/min if under direct physician observation and intensive cardiovascular monitoring or 25 mg/min under less closely monitored conditions) through a large, well-positioned catheter. Proportionately slower administration (e.g., 0.5 to 1 mg/kg/min up to adult infusion rates) should be given to pediatric patients.

Criteria for ICU Discharge in Phenytoin Poisoning

Plasma phenytoin concentrations
No coma
Patient able to ambulate without danger to self (or appropriate assistance is available)

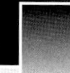

Key Points in the Management of Phenytoin Poisoning

1. Supportive care usually is all that is needed.
2. Charcoal (one dose, possibly a second dose) can be considered for increasing levels and normal bowel function).
3. Rule out coingestions.
4. Give benzodiazapine for seizures, which are rare.

FOSPHENYTOIN

The limiting properties of the parenteral form of phenytoin (incomplete aqueous solubility, toxic nature of the vehicle, and tendency to precipitate in intravenous solutions) have been addressed in the development of a prodrug of phenytoin (fosphenytoin) (see Fig. 49-1). With a pH of 8, fosphenytoin is less irritating to the tissues than is phenytoin. Fosphenytoin is the disodium phosphate ester of phenytoin and is converted to phenytoin by phosphatases in the blood and various organs, principally liver. The concentration and dose of fosphenytoin are expressed in phenytoin equivalents. The conversion half-life is 10 to 15 minutes. Fosphenytoin is tolerated intravenously and intramuscularly, and most patients can be loaded successfully within 30 minutes without significant side effects.[16–18] Given intravenously, fosphenytoin can cause pruritus and, much less commonly than with intravenous phenytoin, hypotension. Blood pressure and cardiac monitoring are recommended when loading with fosphenytoin intravenously but not intramuscularly. With intravenous infusion pumps set at lower rates of phenytoin administration (e.g., <30 mg/min), however, adverse effects are not reported as commonly, suggesting a continued role for the traditional form of the drug as a cost-effective alternative to fosphenytoin.

REFERENCES

1. Working Group on Status Epilepticus: Treatment of convulsive status. JAMA 270:854–859, 1993.
2. Brain Trauma Foundation: Role of antiseizure prophylaxis following head injury. J Neurotrauma 17:549–553, 2000.
3. Larsen JR, Larsen LS: Clinical features and management of poisoning due to phenytoin. Med Toxicol Adverse Drug Exp 4:229–245, 1989.
4. Golightly LK, Smolinske SS, Bennett ML, et al: Pharmaceutical excipients: Adverse effects associated with inactive ingredients in drug products (Part 1). Med Toxicol Adverse Drug Exp 3:128–165, 1988.
5. Litovitz TL, Klein-Schwarz W, Dyer KS, et al: 1997 Annual report of the American Association of Poison Control Centers Toxic Exposure Surveillance System. Am J Emerg Med 16:443, 1998.
6. Litovitz TL, Klein-Schwartz W, Rodgers GC Jr, et al: 2001 Annual report of the American Association of Poison Control Centers Toxic Exposure Surveillance System. Am J Emerg Med 20:391–452, 2002.
7. Barre J, Didey F, Delion F, Tillement JP: Problems in therapeutic drug monitoring: Free drug level monitoring. Ther Drug Monit 10:133–143, 1988.
8. Bachmann KA, Belloto RJ Jr: Differential kinetics of phenytoin in elderly patients. Drugs Aging 15:235–250, 1999.
9. Cuttle L, Munns AJ, Hogg NA, et al: Phenytoin metabolism by human cytochrome P450: Involvement of P450 3A and 2C forms in secondary metabolism and drug-protein adduct formation. Drug Metab Dispos 28:945–950, 2000.
10. Pisciotta M, Prestipino G: Anticonvulsant phenytoin affects voltage-gated potassium currents in cerebellar granule cells. Brain Res 941(1–2):53–61, 2002.
11. Ragsdale DS, Scheuer T, Catterall WA: Frequency and voltage-dependent inhibition of type IIA Na$^+$ channels, expressed in a mammalian cell line, by local anesthetic, antiarrhythmic, and anticonvulsant drugs. Mol Pharmacol 40:756–765, 1991.
12. Eldridge FL, Paydarfar D, Scott SC, et al: Role of endogenous adenosine in recurrent generalized seizures. Exp Neurol 103:179–185, 1989.
13. Weir RL, Padgett W, Daly JW, Anderson SM: Interaction of anticonvulsant drugs with adenosine receptors in the central nervous system. Epilepsia 25:492–498, 1984.
14. Osorio I, Burnstine TH, Remler B, et al: Phenytoin-induced seizures: A paradoxical effect at toxic concentrations in epileptic patients. Epilepsia 30:230–234, 1989.
15. Gross DR, Kitzman JV, Adams HR: Cardiovascular effects of intravenous administration of propylene glycol in calves. Am J Vet Res 40:783, 1979.
16. American Academy of Pediatrics Committee on Drugs: "Inactive" ingredients in pharmaceutical products: update (subject review). Pediatrics 99:268–278, 1997.
17. Louis S, Kutt H: The cardiocirculatory changes caused by intravenous Dilantin and its solvent. Am Heart J 74:523, 1967.
18. DeToledo JC, Ramsay RE: Fosphenytoin and phenytoin in patients with status epilepticus: Improved tolerability versus increased cost. Drug Saf 22:459–466, 2000.
19. Dean JC, Smith KR: Safety, tolerance, and pharmacokinetics of intramuscular fosphenytoin in neurosurgery patients. Epilepsia 34 (Suppl 6):111, 1993.
20. Earnest MP, Mark JA, Drury LR: Complications of intravenous phenytoin for acute treatment of seizures. JAMA 249:762, 1983.
21. Wyte CD, Berk WA: Severe oral phenytoin overdose does not cause cardiovascular morbidity. Ann Emerg Med 20:508, 1991.
22. Wheless JW: Pediatric use of intravenous and intramuscular phenytoin: Lessons learned. J Child Neurol 13(Suppl 1):S11-S14, 1998.
23. Mellick LB, Morgan JA, Mellick GA: Presentations of acute phenytoin overdose. Am J Emerg Med 7:61, 1989.
24. Curtis DL, Piibe R, Ellenhorn MJ, et al: Phenytoin toxicity: A review of 94 cases. Vet Hum Toxicol 31:164–165, 1989.
25. Berry DJ, Wiseman HM, Volans GN: A survey of non-barbiturate anticonvulsant drug overdose. Hum Toxicol 2:357, 1983.
26. Privitera M, Welty TE: Acute phenytoin toxicity followed by seizure breakthrough from a ticlopidine-phenytoin interaction. Arch Neurol 53:1191–1192, 1996.
27. Chua HC, Venketasubramanian N, Tan CB, et al: Paradoxical seizures in phenytoin toxicity. Singapore Med J 40:276–277, 1999.
28. De Diego JI, Prim MP, Marcos S, et al: Vestibular and hearing manifestations of phenytoin toxicity: A retrospective series. Ear Nose Throat J 80:404–409, 2001.
29. Moss W, Ojukwu C, Chiriboga CA: Phenytoin-induced movement disorder: Unilateral presentation in a child and response to diphenhydramine. Clin Pediatr (Phila) 33:634–638, 1994.
30. Corey A, Koller W: Phenytoin-induced dystonia. Ann Neurol 14:92–93, 1983.
31. Krupp E, Loscher W: Anticonvulsant drug effects in the direct cortical ramp-stimulation model in rats: Comparison with conventional seizure models. J Pharmacol Exp Ther 285:1137–1149, 1998.
32. Stark RJ: Spasticity due to phenytoin toxicity. Med J Aust 1:156, 1979.
33. Morkunas AR, Miller MB: Anticonvulsant hypersensitivity syndrome. Crit Care Clin 13:727–739, 1997.
34. Osorio I, Burnstein TH, Pemler B: Phenytoin induced seizures: A paradoxical effect at toxic concentrations in phenytoin patients. Epilepsia 30:230, 1989.
35. Luef G: Magnetic resonance volumetry of the cerebellum in epileptic patients after phenytoin overdoses. Eur Neurol 36:273–277, 1996.
36. Evens RP, Fraser DG, Ludden TM, et al: Phenytoin toxicity and blood levels after a large oral dose. Am J Hosp Pharm 37:232–235, 1980.
37. Asconape JJ: Some common issues in the use of antiepileptic drugs. Semin Neurol 22:27–39, 2002.
38. Hanna DR: Purple glove syndrome: A complication of intravenous phenytoin. J Neurosci Nurs 24:340, 1992.
39. Meraw SJ, Sheridan PJ: Medically induced gingival hyperplasia. Mayo Clin Proc 73:1196–1199, 1998.
40. Jack L, Cunningham C, Watson ID, et al: Micro-scale ultracentrifugation as an alternative to ultrafiltration for the determination of the unbound fraction of phenytoin in human serum. Ann Clin Biochem 23 (Pt 5):603–607, 1986.
41. Howard CE, Roberts S, Ely DS: Use of multiple-dose activated charcoal in phenytoin toxicity. Ann Pharmacother 28:201, 1994.
42. Rowden AM, Spoor JE, Bertino JS: The effect of activated charcoal on phenytoin pharmacokinetics. Ann Emerg Med 19:1144–1147, 1990.
43. Position statement and practice guidelines on the use of multi-dose activated charcoal in the treatment of acute poisoning. American Academy of Clinical Toxicology; European Association of Poisons Centres and Clinical Toxicologists. J Toxicol Clin Toxicol 37:731–751, 1999.

CHAPTER **50**

Carbamazepine

George Braitberg

Carbamazepine (CBZ) is as an antiepileptic agent that has been shown to be effective in the treatment of partial seizures (simple and complex) with and without secondary generalization, generalized tonic-clonic seizures (grand mal), and combinations of these seizure types.[1] CBZ is a carbamylated derivative of iminostilbene and is related structurally to the cyclical antidepressants.[2] In addition to its primary role as an anticonvulsant, CBZ has been used to treat many other medical conditions (Table 50-1).

CBZ has been reported as a substance of abuse.[9,10] Because of its widespread use, the occurrence of CBZ poisoning is relatively common. According to the American Association of Poison Control Centers, 6839 cases of CBZ overdose were recorded in 1996; of these, 4395 required treatment (283 in an intensive care unit) and 11 resulted in death.[11]

PATHOPHYSIOLOGY

The mechanism of action of CBZ has been elucidated partially. Through its inhibitory actions at voltage-gated sodium channels, CBZ stabilizes hyperexcited neurons, suppressing neuronal propagation of excitatory impulses.[2] It also inhibits presynaptic reuptake of adenosine, enhancing presynaptic inhibitory modulation of excitatory neurotransmitter (e.g., glutamate) release. Stabilization of neuronal membranes and inhibition of glutamate release from excitatory presynaptic nerve terminals also may contribute to the anticonvulsant actions of CBZ. It is speculated that an inhibitory effect on central dopaminergic and noradrenergic neurotransmission is responsible for the antimanic effects of CBZ.[1] In addition to its therapeutic actions, CBZ exerts central and peripheral antimuscarinic effects and antagonizes adenosine receptors of the A_1 subtype, providing an explanation for its reported "paradoxical" proconvulsant effects after therapeutic and supratherapeutic doses.[12]

CLINICAL PHARMACOLOGY

The chemical structure and molecular formula of CBZ are shown in Figure 50-1. Absorption from the gastrointestinal tract is relatively slow yet almost complete with the conventional tablet formulation.[2] When taken as a single oral dose, the conventional tablet yields a peak concentration of unchanged CBZ within 4 to 24 hours (most within 12 hours).[2,13] Liquid formulations are absorbed more quickly, and the controlled-release or extended-release tablet forms are absorbed more slowly and less completely than the conventional tablet.[1] An earlier peak is obtained with the suspension. Steady-state plasma concentrations of CBZ are attained within about 3 to 4 days.[13] When controlled-release tablets are administered singly and repeatedly, they yield about 25% lower peak concentrations of the parent compound in plasma than the conventional tablets do; the peaks are attained within 24 hours. Although controlled-release tablets provide a statistically significant decrease in the fluctuation index at steady state, the bioavailability of the conventional tablet approaches 100%, whereas it is about 15% lower for the controlled-release tablets.[1]

The apparent volume of distribution of CBZ is 0.8 to 1.9 L/kg.[1] Plasma protein binding is 70% to 80%.[13] The concentration of unchanged substance in saliva and cerebrospinal fluid reflects the non–protein-bound fraction present in plasma and is approximately 20% to 30% of that attained in plasma.[1,2] It is found in breast milk in concentrations ranging from 25% to 60% of that in plasma. CBZ readily crosses the placenta.[14]

CBZ is metabolized in the liver via the epoxide-diol pathway, the main metabolite (CBZ-10,11-epoxide) being pharmacologically active. Cytochrome P-450 3A4 has been identified as the major isoform responsible for the formation of CBZ-10,11-epoxide. A reactive arene oxide compound, distinct from the 10,11-epoxide metabolite, also is formed as a result of phase I oxidative metabolism of CBZ and is thought to be the toxic principal responsible for the hypersensitivity reactions and teratogenic effects associated with CBZ administration.[15] CBZ induces its own oxidative metabolism and that of other drugs, and given the gradual onset of this effect on drug clearance over the first few weeks of administration, it has been considered prototypical of drugs with time-dependent kinetics.[1,13]

The elimination half-life of unchanged CBZ after a single oral dose averages 36 hours. After repeated administration, however, it averaged 16 to 24 hours depending on the duration of treatment. In patients receiving concomitant treatment with other cytochrome P-450 enzyme–inducing drugs, half-life values averaging 9 to 10 hours have been shown. The mean elimination half-life of the 10,11-epoxide metabolite in the plasma is about 6 hours after single oral doses of the epoxide itself, which also is approved for clinical anticonvulsant use. After a single 400-mg dose, 72% was excreted in the urine mainly in the form of epoxide, hydroxylated, and conjugated metabolites, with 28% of the

TABLE 50-1 Medical Conditions for Which Carbamazepine Is Used

Trigeminal neuralgia*[,3,4]
Agitation and aggression[5,6]
Psychosis[7]
Bipolar disorder
Cocaine abuse[8]

*First used in the early 1960s and received U.S. Food and Drug Administration approval in 1968.

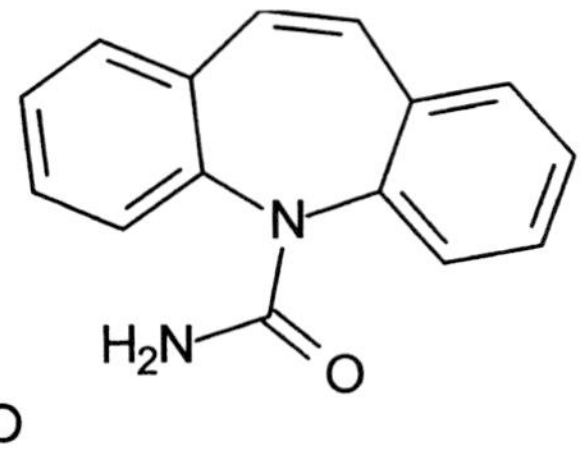

$C_{15}H_{12}N_2O$

FIGURE 50-1

Chemical structure and molecular formula of carbamazepine.

dose excreted in the feces.[1,13] Estimates of breast milk excretion range from 25% to 60% of the administered dose.[1] Clinically important pharmacokinetic interactions with other drugs that may result in elevated or reduced plasma concentrations of CBZ are listed in Table 50-2.[13,16]

CLINICAL PRESENTATION AND LIFE-THREATENING COMPLICATIONS

The presenting clinical manifestations of toxicity develop within 1 to 3 hours of overdose and usually involve the central nervous, cardiovascular, and respiratory systems. Symptoms may be prolonged or delayed in onset, depending on the form and amount of CBZ ingested; this is thought to be due to delayed or prolonged absorption owing to ingestion of an extended-release formulation or production of a gastric concretion of tablets, but there is limited clinical experience to support this.[17]

In reviewing published case reports and case series of patients with significant CBZ overdose, there is mixed evidence with regard to whether the CBZ peak serum concentrations correlate with the severity of clinical effects. Spiller and colleagues,[18] in a prospective study of 25 CBZ exposures, showed poor correlation between serious clinical signs and serum CBZ concentrations. Tibballs'[19] review of 82 pediatric patients found a statistically significant correlation, however, between the peak serum CBZ concentration and the depth of coma, convulsions, hypotension, and the requirement for mechanical ventilation.

In a retrospective chart review of accidental ingestion in 14 children age 2 to 5 years, Lifshitz and colleagues[20] reported the most prevalent sign to be nystagmus (12 of 14), followed by drowsiness (10 of 14), ataxia (4 of 14), and tachycardia (2 of 14). Peak serum concentrations did not distinguish among symptom groups. Other signs of poisoning included anticholinergic manifestations and abnormal electrocardiogram findings. More serious effects, such as seizure and coma, did not occur, with a documented maximal serum CBZ concentration of 32 μg/mL (130 μmol/L).

None of these studies measured the concentration of the pharmacologically active 10,11-epoxide metabolite. Potter and Donnelly[21] identified a subgroup of patients with normal CBZ levels who developed significant clinical toxicity secondary to a rise in CBZ epoxide levels, also reflected in a decrease in the CBZ-to-epoxide ratio. These findings suggest an indication for assaying the concentration of the CBZ epoxide; however, the clinical utility of this assay has not been studied.

Neurologic Toxicity

The most predominant neurologic signs (in descending order of incidence) are drowsiness, ataxia, nystagmus, and dystonia.[19] The central and peripheral anticholinergic toxidrome also is a relatively commonly occurring feature of CBZ poisoning (see Chapter 22).[19]

The frequency of seizures after CBZ overdose increases with a Glasgow Coma Scale score less than 8. Since the development of the first antiepileptic drugs, clinical observation of paradoxical drug-induced worsening of seizures involving a variety of antiepileptic drugs has been reported. CBZ, in particular, has been reported to cause seizures in overdose and to potentiate generalized seizures at therapeutic

TABLE 50-2 Examples of Pharmacokinetic Drug-Drug Interactions with Carbamazepine

MECHANISM	EFFECT	DRUG CAUSES
CYP3A4 inhibition	Reduced clearance/increased plasma concentration	Propoxyphene, fluconazole, itraconazole, ketoconazole, isoniazid, erythromycin, clarithromycin, cimetidine, verapamil, diltiazem, fluoxetine, fluvoxamine, nefazodone
CYP3A4 induction	Increased clearance/reduced plasma concentration	Phenytoin, phenobarbital, valproate, rifampin

levels.[17] Aggravation of other seizure types has been reported more rarely. CBZ has been reported to precipitate or exacerbate a variety of seizures, most notably absence, atonic, and myoclonic, in patients with generalized epilepsies. This exacerbation has been characterized by bursts of diffuse and bilaterally synchronous spike and wave electroencephalogram activity in epileptic patients while taking CBZ.[22–24] The mean time of electroencephalogram activity worsening was 1 to 2 days after introduction of CBZ. After CBZ withdrawal, electroencephalogram activity improved within a few days.[22,23]

It has been suggested that the concentration of the epoxide metabolite may play an important causative role in CBZ-induced seizures.[25,26] Other investigators have suggested that the precipitation of seizures may be facilitated by hyponatremia secondary to the antidiuretic actions of the drug.[27] Status epilepticus after CBZ overdose also has been described.[28,29]

Abnormal movements, including choreoathetosis, dyskinesia, and dystonia, have been described in patients taking CBZ and may be related to a central anticholinergic effect.[30–32] Zaidat and coworkers[33] described two children who presented in coma with diffuse hypotonia and areflexia after CBZ overdose. Repetitive nerve stimulation showed a decremental response only at high-frequency stimulation. Both patients made an uneventful recovery.

Deep coma has been described after CBZ overdose. Cordova and Lee[34] reported a 41-year-old man who presented with fixed, dilated pupils for 48 hours after an overdose of CBZ combined with an unknown quantity of venlafaxine. CBZ peaked at 69.9 μg/mL (295 μmol/L). The patient recovered with no neurologic sequelae. Similarly, Salcman and Pippenger[35] reported a 16-year-old boy with severe encephalopathy resulting from massive overdose of CBZ (5.8 g). He exhibited disconjugate gaze and absent oculovestibular reflexes. On the second hospital day the patient emerged from stupor, and by the fourth hospital day he was fully alert and oriented. Gary and associates[36] described a patient with absent doll's eye reflex and absent response to caloric testing who made an uneventful recovery.

Cardiovascular Toxicity

Although CBZ is structurally and, in some respects, pharmacologically similar to tricyclic antidepressants,[2] particularly with respect to its effects on myocardial sodium channel conductance and phase 0 of the cardiac action potential, CBZ poisoning results in serious cardiotoxicity much less frequently than does tricyclic antidepressant poisoning. Reports of heart block and bradycardia have been documented, however, even at therapeutic levels of CBZ.[37] Mordel and colleagues[38] reported the case of a 27-year-old man who developed CBZ-induced fatal rapid atrial fibrillation and an irregular wide-complex tachycardia. Life-threatening CBZ toxicity in adults has been reported to include significant cardiac dysfunction other than arrhythmia, including cardiogenic shock.[39]

Doyon and Zorc[40] retrospectively reviewed 56 pediatric patients with the discharge diagnosis of CBZ poisoning and noted that QRS prolongation occurred in 35% of cases. In another pediatric case series, Tibballs[19] described a group of patients with a mean peak serum CBZ concentration of 50.4 μg/mL (213 μmol/L), in whom cardiovascular instability was manifested by low cardiac output and poor myocardial contractility; two deaths occurred in this group.

Pulmonary Toxicity

Given the proconvulsant and profound central nervous system depressant effects of CBZ, hypoventilatory respiratory failure and aspiration are anticipated effects of acute overdose. Wilschut and coworkers[41] reported such an outcome in a 36-year-old woman who developed respiratory failure after overdose with CBZ. Analysis of bronchial washings and a lung tissue biopsy specimen showed diffuse alveolar damage. In addition, acute pulmonary edema is a potential complication of aggressive fluid volume replacement in the patient with CBZ-induced myocardial dysfunction.

Other Organ System Manifestations of Acute Carbamazepine Overdose

Rhabdomyolysis and myoglobinuric acute tubular nephropathy should be anticipated after CBZ overdose, particularly in patients who present after prolonged periods of unconsciousness or generalized seizure activity.

ADVERSE EFFECTS OF LONG-TERM CARBAMAZEPINE ADMINISTRATION

Anticonvulsant Hypersensitivity Syndrome

Anticonvulsant hypersensitivity syndrome is an uncommon but potentially fatal multisystem disorder that occurs after exposure to CBZ, phenytoin, and phenobarbital.[15,42] It is thought to be related to the benzene ring structure of these drugs and their oxidative metabolism to a toxic arene oxide metabolite. The first reported case of CBZ sensitivity was described by Coombes in 1965.[43] The hypersensitivity reaction that develops involves all organ systems, including the lung, liver, kidney, skin, and bone marrow.

Sudden Unexplained Death in Epilepsy

The phenomenon of sudden unexplained death in epilepsy (SUDEP) has been described,[44] although the data to support a causal association are not convincing at this time. A review of Cardiff Epilepsy Unit clinical data revealed that CBZ was disproportionately represented in patients experiencing SUDEP; 11 of 14 patients were taking CBZ at the time of death.[44] The CBZ subgroup represented 78% of SUDEP patients compared with a 38% prevalence of CBZ use among all patients on the same clinical unit. Proposed proarrhythmic mechanisms include those reflected in effects on QRS and QT interval (especially QT prolongation). It is speculated that such direct drug-induced arrhythmogenic effects, combined with the proarrhythmic effect of the epileptic seizure discharges, postictal hypercarbia, and hypoxia, may result in fatal cardiac rhythm disturbance.

Other Effects

Other adverse effects of CBZ therapy include the syndrome of inappropriate antidiuretic hormone secretion and hepatic and hematologic toxicity. Although aplastic anemia has occurred relatively uncommonly in association with CBZ therapy (1 in 200,000 patients treated), transient leukopenia and hepatic enzyme elevation have occurred in 10% and 5% to 10% of patients, respectively, during the initial few months of treatment.[2]

DIAGNOSIS

In addition to the investigations required for the general care and management of poisoned patients, quantitative serum analysis for CBZ should be performed. The accepted steady-state therapeutic concentration range for CBZ is 4 to 12 μg/mL (17 to 50 μmol/L).[1,2,13] CBZ-induced central nervous system toxicity has been reported, however, at levels of 9 μg/mL (38 μmol/L).[2] The main metabolite, CBZ-10,11-epoxide, possesses anticonvulsant activity and reaches concentrations in the brain and plasma of approximately 30% to 50% of that of the parent compound. The pharmacologic activity of unmeasured metabolite provides an explanation for the limited correlation observed between serum concentrations of the parent compound and clinical toxicity.[18]

The role of broad-spectrum toxicologic screening as a crucial adjunct to clinical diagnosis in suspected drug overdose is generally not well supported. Immunoassay has the advantage of being automated and rapid, inexpensive, and largely independent of operator skill. Interpretation of the results of this type of analysis is limited, however, by its use of polyvalent antibodies that may cross-react with a variety of other chemical compounds. False-positive results due to cross-reacting compounds in drug assays may have serious consequences.[45] CBZ is known to cross-react with tricyclic antidepressants in immunoassays developed to detect the latter group of compounds.[46,47] This cross-reaction occurred in two cases of CBZ overdose in which serum tested positive for tricyclic antidepressants despite the immunoassay's reported cross-sensitivity for CBZ of only 0.03%.[47]

TREATMENT

The mainstay of treatment of life-threatening clinical manifestations of CBZ poisoning is timely and appropriately aggressive provision of supportive care. Patients with large ingestions of CBZ need to be treated in an environment where they can be monitored closely and potential complications can be treated expeditiously. Tibballs[19] suggested a form of risk stratification based on the peak CBZ level in a pediatric population. He suggested that in patients with serum CBZ concentrations of equal to or greater than approximately 23.6 μg/mL (100 μmol/L), "close" monitoring and treatment with gastric lavage or activated charcoal or both are required. In patients with serum concentrations equal to or greater than 35.4 μg/mL (150 μmol/L), intensive life-support measures may be required; invasive methods to enhance drug clearance may be warranted if life-threatening manifestations are refractory to supportive treatment.

Endotracheal intubation and mechanical ventilation commonly are indicated in severe CBZ poisoning. Fluid volume resuscitation should be undertaken with caution in severely CBZ-poisoned patients because fluid volume over-

> ### Key Points in the Evaluation and Treatment of Carbamazepine Poisoning
>
> 1. Carbamazepine is used widely in the management of a variety of neurobehavioral disorders, including trigeminal neuralgia, bipolar affective disorder, and epilepsy.
> 2. The major clinical manifestations of acute toxicity are encephalopathy, coma, respiratory failure, seizures, tachycardia, cardiac conduction disturbance (prolonged QRS), and hypotension.
> 3. Treatment of acute carbamazepine poisoning is largely supportive and may include aggressive airway and ventilatory management, intravenous pressor or hypertonic sodium bicarbonate therapy, and seizure control with γ-aminobutyric acid agonist drugs (e.g., benzodiazepines, barbiturates).
> 4. Drug clearance has been shown to be enhanced by repeat-dose activated charcoal and by charcoal hemoperfusion; however, clinical benefit from these interventions has not been shown convincingly.
> 5. Carbamazepine is an established cause of anticonvulsant hypersensitivity syndrome and has been associated with birth defects. Its use is contraindicated in individuals with a previous history of anticonvulsant hypersensitivity syndrome. Caution is advised with regard to its use in pregnancy.

load may be accompanied more readily by pulmonary edema in patients with CBZ-induced myocardial dysfunction. Significant QRS interval prolongation, other acute cardiac conduction disorders, or hypotension should prompt reasonable consideration for intravenous hypertonic sodium bicarbonate (see Chapter 36) or intravenous pressor (e.g., dopamine) therapy. The goals of fluid volume therapy should include maintenance of adequate urine output, particularly in light of the increased risk of myoglobinuric renal tubular insult associated with severe poisoning. Because they generally are indicated for toxicant-induced convulsions (see Chapter 20), drugs with γ-aminobutyric acid (GABA)$_A$ agonist actions, such as benzodiazepines (e.g., diazepam, lorazepam) and barbiturates (e.g., phenobarbital), constitute the preferred anticonvulsant treatment options for CBZ-induced seizures.

Administration of enteral activated charcoal seems indicated as a means of gastrointestinal decontamination after CBZ overdose. Multiple-dose activated charcoal has been recommended as a method of enhancing drug clearance after CBZ overdose and after overdose of many other drugs, including dapsone, phenobarbital, quinine, and theophylline, although clinical benefit from this intervention has not been shown adequately.[48] In a review of 77 patients with CBZ overdose, Stremski and associates[32] reported that multiple doses of charcoal (0.5 g/kg every 4 hours until levels decreased to <12 μg/mL [<50 μmol/L]) significantly shortened serum CBZ half-life compared with single-dose charcoal (P = 0.008). Although generally a safe treatment, use of multiple-dose charcoal has been associated with adverse effects. Aspiration of charcoal; bowel obstruction (potentiated by the anticholinergic effects of CBZ); and fluid, electrolyte, and acid-base abnormalities (when mixed with cathartics) have been documented.[49] The influence of whole-bowel irrigation on the outcome of patients poisoned with slow-release preparations of CBZ has not been shown but may be considered theoretical after the ingestion of a potentially toxic amount of slow-release CBZ.[49] There is little evidence to support its superiority over activated charcoal therapy, however.

EXTRACORPOREAL REMOVAL OF CARBAMAZEPINE

Extracorporeal removal of CBZ should be considered in patients with life-threatening poisoning with deterioration despite adequate supportive care. Peritoneal dialysis has been found to be ineffective in the removal of CBZ, which can be explained by its relatively high degree of plasma protein binding and large volume of distribution. Many case reports show the effectiveness of charcoal hemoperfusion techniques, however, in the treatment of acute CBZ poisoning. The importance of charcoal hemoperfusion may lie in its ability to clear effectively the metabolically active epoxide metabolite in addition to the parent drug.[50]

Gary and colleagues[36] described a 48-year-old patient who presented after a multiple-drug ingestion that included CBZ. The patient's condition deteriorated despite supportive care, and the CBZ level continued to increase over the first 14 hours of admission. After 4 hours of charcoal hemoperfusion, the plasma CBZ concentration declined by 25% of its peak value, and the patient exhibited neurologic recovery. Chan and coworkers[51] reported a case of CBZ overdose treated with 2 hours of charcoal hemoperfusion, wherein a significant difference was shown between the half-life of CBZ elimination while undergoing hemoperfusion (almost 2 hours) and the half-life reported without extracorporeal treatment (39 hours). Anticipated complications of the procedure, including hypocalcemia, hypophosphatemia, and thrombocytopenia, were also observed in this patient.

Other modes of extracorporeal elimination, such as high-flux hemodialysis, also are worthy of consideration. Schuerer and coworkers[52] reported an elimination half-life of 2.7 hours using high-efficiency hemodialysis on an 18-month-old infant after life-threatening poisoning with a sustained-release CBZ preparation.

CARBAMAZEPINE TOXICITY AND PREGNANCY

Teratogenicity occurs at a rate of 9.7% with the use of anticonvulsant medication.[53] It is believed that the fetal abnormalities induced by aromatic anticonvulsants are due to a fetal deficiency of the epoxide hydrolase enzyme necessary to break down the arene oxide.[54] Although there are mixed reports of fetal adverse effects associated with CBZ use in pregnancy, it has been classified by the U.S. Food and Drug Administration as a teratogenicity category D drug (see Appendix).[55]

REFERENCES

1. Carbamazepine. In Caswell A (ed): MIMS Online. Version 1.1. August 1-October 31, 2000.
2. McNamara JO: Drugs effective in the therapy of the epilepsies. In Hardman JG, Limbird LE, Gilman AG (eds): Goodman and Gilman's the Pharmacologic Basis of Therapeutics, 10th ed. New York, McGraw-Hill, 2001, pp 521–547.
3. Lindsay B: Trigeminal neuralgia: A new approach. Med J Aust 1:8–13, 1969.
4. Burke WJ, Selby G: Trigeminal neuralgia: A therapeutic trial of tegretol. Proc Aust Assoc Neurol 3:89–96, 1965.
5. Azovi P, Jokic C, Attal N, et al: Carbamazepine in agitation and aggressive behaviour following severe closed head injury: Result of an open trial. Brain Inj 13:797–804, 1999.
6. Grossman F: A review of anticonvulsants in treating agitated demented elderly patients. Pharmacotherapy 18:600–606, 1998.
7. Gutierrez K, Walter H, Bankier B: Valproic acid and carbamazepine: A successful antipsychotic medication? The problem of diagnosis and its relevance for therapy. Psychopathology 32:235–241, 1999.
8. Hikas JA, Crosby RD, Pearson VL, Graves NM: A randomised double blind study of carbamazepine in the treatment of cocaine abuse. Clin Pharm Ther 62:89–105, 1997.
9. Crawford PJ, Fisher BM: Recreational overdosage of carbamazepine in Paisley drug abusers. Scott Med J 42:44–45, 1997.
10. Ramsay SG, Clee MD: Comment on recreational overdosage of carbamazepine in Paisley drug abusers. Scott Med J 42:95, 1997.
11. Litovitz TL, Smilkstein M, Felberg L, et al: 1996 annual report of the American Association of Poison Control Centers toxic exposure surveillance. Am J Emerg Med 15:447–492, 1997.
12. Clark M, Post RM: Carbamazepine, but not caffeine, is highly selective for adenosine A_1 binding sites. Eur J Pharmacol 164:399–401, 1989.
13. Brown TR: Pharmacokinetics of antiepileptic drugs. Neurology 51(Suppl 4):S2-S7, 1998.
14. Pienimaki P, Hartikainen AL, Arvela P, et al: Carbamazepine and its metabolites in human perfused placenta and in maternal and cord blood. Epilepsia 36:241–248, 1995.
15. Morkunas AR, Miller MB: Anticonvulsant hypersensitivity syndrome. Crit Care Clin 13:727–739, 1997.
16. Hansten PD, Horn JR: The Top 100 Drug Interactions. Edmonds, WA, H&H Publications, 2002, pp 38–41.
17. Sullivan JB Jr, Rumack BH, Peterson RG: Acute carbamazepine toxicity resulting from overdose. Neurology 31:621–624, 1981.
18. Spiller HA, Krenzelok EP, Cookson E: Carbamazepine overdose: A prospective study of serum levels and toxicity. J Toxicol Clin Toxicol 28:445–458, 1990.
19. Tibballs J: Acute toxic reaction to carbamazepine: Clinical effects and serum concentrations. J Pediatr 121:295–299, 1992.
20. Lifshitz M, Gavrilov V, Sofer S: Signs and symptoms of CBZ toxicity. Pediatr Emerg Care 16:26–27, 2000.
21. Potter JM, Donnelly A: Carbamazepine-10,11-epoxide in therapeutic drug monitoring. Ther Drug Monit 20:652–657, 1998.
22. Perucca E, Gram L, Avanzini G, Dulac O: Antiepileptic drugs as a cause of worsening seizures. Epilepsia 39:5–17, 1998.
23. Parmeggiani A, Fraticelli E, Rossi PG: Exacerbation of epileptic seizures by carbamazepine: Report of 10 cases. Seizure 7:479–483, 1998.
24. Dhuna A, Pascual-Leone A, Talwar D: Exacerbation of partial seizures and onset of nonepileptic myoclonus with carbamazepine. Epilepsia 31:275–278, 1991.
25. Pryse WEM, Jeavons PM: Effect of carbamazepine (Tegretol) on the electroencephalogram and ward behavior of patients with chronic epilepsy. Epilepsia 11:263–273, 1970.
26. So EL, Ruggles KH, Cascino GD, et al: Seizure exacerbation and status epilepticus related to carbamazepine-10,11-epoxide. Ann Neurol 35:743–746, 1994.
27. Van Amelsvoort T, Bakshi R, Devaux CB, Schwabe S: Hyponatraemia associated with carbamazepine and oxcarbamazepine therapy: A review. Epilepsia 35:181–188, 1994.
28. Spiller HA, Carlyle R: Status epilepticus after carbamazepine overdose. Abstract 109, 1998 North American Congress of Clinical Toxicology Annual Meeting. J Toxicol Clin Toxicol 36:472–473, 1998.
29. Sharma P, Gupta RC, Bharwaja B, et al: Status epilepticus and death following acute carbamazepine poisoning (Letter). J Assoc Physicians India 40:561–562, 1992.
30. Weaver DF, Camfield P, Fraser A: Massive carbamazepine overdose: Clinical and pharmacologic observations in five episodes. Neurology 38:755–759, 1988.
31. Drenck NE, Risbo A: Carbamazepine poisoning, a surprisingly severe case. Anaesth Intensive Care 8:203–205, 1980.
32. Stremski ES, Brady WB, Prasad K, et al: Pediatric carbamazepine intoxication. Ann Emerg Med 25:624–630, 1995.
33. Zaidat OO, Kaminski HJ, Berenson F, Katirji B: Neuromuscular transmission defect caused by carbamazepine. Muscle Nerve 22:1293–1296, 1999.

34. Cordova S, Lee R: Fixed dilated pupils in the ICU: Another recoverable cause. Anaesth Intensive Care 28:91–93, 2000.
35. Salcman M, Pippenger CE: Acute carbamazepine encephalopathy. JAMA 231:915, 1975.
36. Gary NE, Byra WM, Eisinger RP: Carbamazepine poisoning: Treatment by hemoperfusion. Nephron 27:202–220, 1981.
37. Hamilton DV: Carbamazepine and heart block (Letter). Lancet 1(8078):1365, 1978.
38. Mordel A, Sivlotti MLA, Linden CH: Fatal TCA-like cardiotoxicity following carbamazepine overdose. Abstract 108, 1998 North American Congress of Clinical Toxicology Annual Meeting. J Toxicol Clin Toxicol 36:472, 1998.
39. Cameron RJ, Hungerford P, Dawson AH: Efficacy of charcoal hemoperfusion in massive carbamazepine poisoning. J Toxicol Clin Toxicol 40:507–512, 2002.
40. Doyon S, Zorc J: Electrocardiographic changes associated with carbamazepine toxicity in the pediatric population. Abstract 130, 1999 North American Congress of Clinical Toxicology Annual Meeting. J Toxicol Clin Toxicol 37:635–636, 1999.
41. Wilschut FA, Cobben NA, Thunnissen FB, et al: Recurrent respiratory distress associated with carbamazepine overdose. Eur Respir J 10:2163–2165, 1997.
42. Braitberg G, Miller MB, Curry SC: Anticonvulsant hypersensitivity syndrome. Emerg Med 7:170–173, 1995.
43. Coombes BW: Stevens-Johnson syndrome associated with carbamazepine ("Tegretol"). Med J Aust 1:895–896, 1965.
44. Timmings PL: Sudden unexplained death in epilepsy: Is carbamazepine implicated? Seizure 7:289–291, 1998.
45. Fisher J: Immunoassay drug screen results: Easy to get, hard to interpret (Editorial). J Toxicol Clin Toxicol 36:115–116, 1998.
46. Matos ME, Burns MM, Shannon MW: False positive tricyclic antidepressant drug screen results leading to the diagnosis of carbamazepine intoxication. Paediatrics 105:E66, 2000.
47. Chattergoon DS, Verjee Z, Anderson M, et al: Carbamazepine interference with an immune assay for tricyclic antidepressants in plasma. J Toxicol Clin Toxicol 36:109–113, 1998.
48. Position statement and practice guidelines on the use of multi-dose activated charcoal in the treatment of acute poisoning. American Academy of Clinical Toxicology; European Association of Poison Centres and Clinical Toxicologists. J Toxicol Clin Toxicol 37:731–751, 1999.
49. Manoguerra AS: Gastrointestinal decontamination after poisoning: Where is the science? Crit Care Clin 13:709–729, 1997.
50. Deshpande G, Meerkt KL, Valenti RP: Repeat charcoal haemoperfusion treatments. Pediatr Nephrol 13:775–777, 1999.
51. Chan KM, Agnanno JJ, Jansen R, et al: Charcoal hemoperfusion for treatment of carbamazepine poisoning. Clin Chem 27:1300–1302, 1981.
52. Schuerer DJ, Brophy PD, Maxvold NJ, et al: High efficiency dialysis for carbamazepine overdose. J Toxicol Clin Toxicol 38:321–323, 2000.
53. Canger R, Battino D, Canevini MP, et al: Malformations in offspring with epilepsy: A prospective study. Epilepsia 40:1231–1236, 1999.
54. Buehler BA, Delmont BS, Van Wae MS, et al: Prenatal prediction of risk of the foetal hydantoin syndrome. N Engl J Med 322:1567–1572, 1990.
55. Briggs GG, Freeman RK, Yaffe SJ (eds): Drugs in Pregnancy and Lactation, 6th ed. Philadelphia, Lippincott Williams & Wilkins, 2002.

CHAPTER 51

Valproic Acid

Wayne R. Snodgrass

Valproic acid (VPA) was discovered by chance to have anti-convulsant activity when it was used as the vehicle for administration of other compounds that were being screened for antiepileptic activity. VPA now is used widely not only as an anticonvulsant but also in psychiatry as a mood stabilizer for patients with bipolar disorders. VPA was approved for use in the United States in 1978 after more than 10 years of use in Europe. In 2000 in the United States, the poison center data showed 9514 exposures, of which 5204 were intentional; there were 6 deaths.[1] There are various dosage forms: intravenous, 100 mg/mL (Depacon); oral VPA capsules USP, 250 mg (Depakene and generics); VPA syrup, 250 mg/5 mL (Depakene and generics); divalproex (a stable coordination compound of VPA and sodium valproate in a 1:1 molar ratio) (Depakote sprinkle capsules, 125 mg; Depakote delayed-release tablets, 125 mg, 250 mg, 500 mg; Depakote ER extended-release tablets).

BIOCHEMISTRY AND PHARMACOLOGY

VPA (n-dipropylacetic acid) is a branched-chain carboxylic acid. Its chemical structure is shown in Figure 51-1. VPA is metabolized in humans to multiple metabolites (Fig. 51-2). A major portion of a daily dose is conjugated and excreted as glucuronides in urine. β-Oxidation results in metabolites 2-en-VPA (2-propyl-2-pentenoic acid) and 3-keto-VPA (2-propyl-3-keto-pentanoic acid); both are major human plasma metabolites.[2] β-Oxidation metabolites are the major metabolites found in urine (about 70%); ω-oxidation and ω-1-oxidation metabolites (3-hydroxy, 4-hydroxy, 5-hydroxy, mostly as glucuronides) are found in lesser amounts in the urine (about 30%).[3] The hepatotoxic metabolite, 4-en-VPA, results from cytochrome P-450 enzyme activity, presumably mostly in the liver. Studies with human liver microsomes indicate that the cytochrome P-450 isozymes CYP2C9 and CYP2A6 are responsible for 4-en-VPA formation.[4] Additional in vitro studies with human hepatoblastoma cells showed that the P-450 isozyme CYP2E1 is responsible for further metabolism of 4-en-VPA to a reactive intermediate.[5] A carbon-centered free radical at the C-4 position in the VPA molecule probably serves as at least one key intermediate.[6] The 3-en-VPA is formed reversibly from 2-en-VPA by isomerization. In plasma, 2-en-VPA (less toxic than VPA or 4-en-VPA) is one of the major circulating metabolites of VPA. VPA therapy (assessed after 3 weeks) results in a small (1.5 to 2 times) autoinduction of its own metabolism by β-oxidation but not glucuronidation or 4-hydroxylation.[7]

VPA is highly (85% to 95%), but not tightly, bound to serum albumin.[8,9] Human brain-to-plasma ratios of VPA range approximately from 0.07 to 0.28. It is thought that an active transport process, the monocarboxylic acid transporter, regulates VPA distribution between plasma and brain.[2,10]

Cerebrospinal fluid concentrations of γ-aminobutyric acid (GABA), the major inhibitory neurotransmitter, are increased with VPA treatment, with values of approximately 120 pmol/mL in untreated children compared with approximately 250 pmol/mL in treated children.[11] VPA enters the human cerebrospinal fluid relatively rapidly after dosing. The time to maximum human subdural cerebrospinal fluid VPA concentration is 3.5 to 5.5 hours.[12]

Pharmacokinetics of Valproic Acid

Volume of distribution: 0.22 L/kg
Protein binding: 93%
Mechanism of clearance: 0.0066 L/kg/hr, liver
Plasma half-life: approximately 10 hr
pK$_a$: 4.6
Active metabolites: present but in small concentrations
Methods to enhance clearance: high-flux hemodialysis, multiple-dose activated charcoal; may consider hemoperfusion

---

PATHOPHYSIOLOGY

The mechanism of anticonvulsant action of VPA seems to be elevation of brain GABA (see Fig. 51-2). VPA-induced elevation of brain GABA in the substantia nigra is thought to be important because this area of the brain is involved in seizure control and propagation.[13] Laboratory animal data showed that VPA increases the apoenzyme of glutamic acid decarboxylase, the enzyme that synthesizes GABA. Some laboratory animal data showed that 2-en-VPA is more potent than VPA in potentiating brain GABA-mediated postsynaptic inhibitory responses[13]; 2-en-VPA may contribute significantly to the anticonvulsant effect of VPA in vivo. It is likely that the coma that characterizes VPA overdose also is due to elevation in brain GABA and possibly 2-en-VPA's postsynaptic inhibitory effects.

Hepatotoxicity

Most fatalities from VPA poisoning are due to hepatotoxicity, although cerebral edema with deep coma, which may

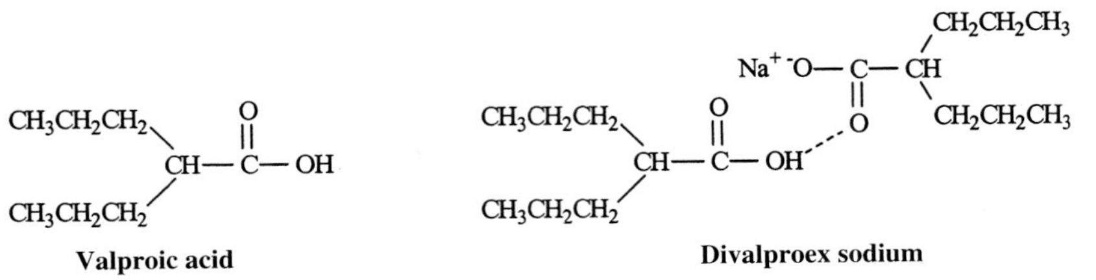

FIGURE 51-1

Chemical structures of valproic acid (VPA) and the dimeric congener valproex sodium.

occur in acute toxicity or as a consequence of hepatic encephalopathy, also poses risk for death. VPA hepatotoxicity may be dose dependent or idiosyncratic. Dose-dependent hepatotoxicity is more frequent, reproducible, and reversible, whereas idiosyncratic hepatotoxicity is unpredictable, is life-threatening, has a long latent period, and is rare (a frequency of <1 in 10,000). Risk estimates show 37 cases of the fulminant fatal form of VPA hepatotoxicity reported to the manufacturer for the 6-year period of 1978 through 1984. An estimated 400,000 patients were treated with this drug during this period. Of the 37 patients, 27 (73%) were between the ages of 5 months and 11 years. At highest risk for death were children 2 years of age or younger who were treated with multiple anticonvulsants and had significant disease beyond seizures, such as congenital defects and mental retardation.[14] The fatality rate due to hepatotoxicity in these children was 1 in 500, whereas the fatality rate in the entire group was 1 in 10,000. Use of multiple anticonvulsant drugs in young children increased the fatality rate to 1 in 500 compared with 1 in 7000 seen in children on monotherapy. Seventeen of the 37 patients with fatal VPA hepatotoxicity also were receiving phenobarbital.[14] Liver

histology typically shows steatosis and necrosis. Liver ultrastructure findings include enlarged mitochondria with distorted matrix and fragmented cristae.[15] Three risk factors for VPA hepatotoxicity are young age, multiple antiepileptic drug therapy, and high VPA plasma concentrations.[16] An immediately preceding febrile illness is present in about half of children who develop VPA hepatotoxicity.[14] Decreased caloric intake often is associated with a febrile illness. This decreased intake results in increased levels of endogenous fatty acids, which may compete with VPA for β-oxidation. Currently, it seems that the combination of factors of young age, polytherapy, status epilepticus, and febrile illness may result in mitochondrial dysfunction. Some epileptic children develop status epilepticus just before the onset of VPA hepatotoxicity[14] with implications for energy depletion in mitochondria.

The pathogenesis of VPA hepatotoxicity is uncertain. Hypotheses for the biochemical basis of VPA hepatotoxicity include hyperammonemia, carnitine deficiency, preexisting inborn errors of metabolism, diminished free radical scavenger activity, and toxicity caused by unsaturated VPA metabolites.

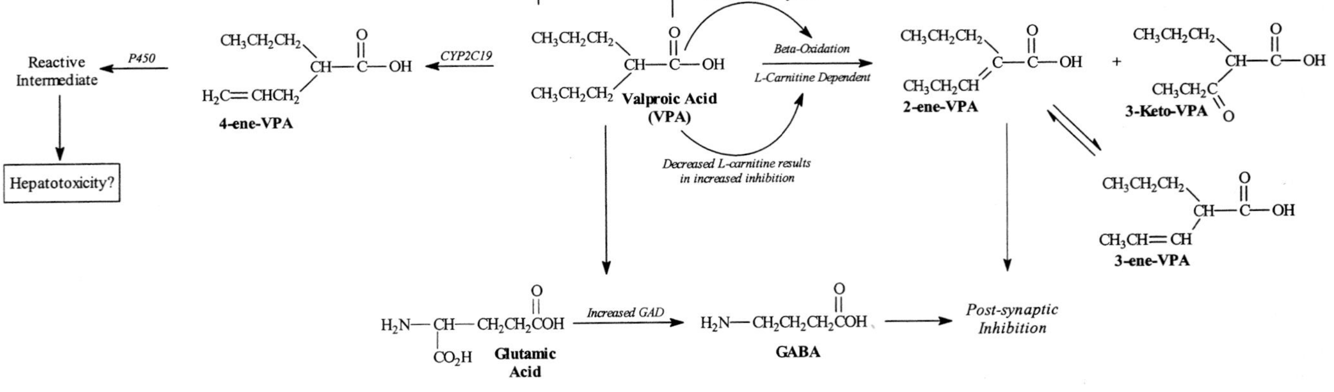

FIGURE 51-2

Metabolism of valproic acid (VPA) in humans. GABA, γ-aminobutyric acid; GAD, glutamic acid decarboxylase.

L-Carnitine increases fatty acyl group transport into mitochondria and helps maintain the ratio of acyl to free coenzyme A (CoA). Patients receiving VPA therapy have an ongoing biochemical process that uses L-carnitine to maintain mitochondrial metabolism.[15] Mitochondrial metabolic stress induced by increased catabolism brought on by seizures or infection increases the risk of development of hepatic failure due to an insufficient reserve of L-carnitine, needed for mitochondrial metabolism, including VPA detoxification (see Fig 51-2).

The 4-en-VPA metabolite is thought to be at least in part mechanistically related to dose-dependent VPA hepatotoxicity. This metabolite, 4-en-VPA, has structural similarity to other known liver toxins, such as hypoglycin A (methylene cyclopropylacetic acid) and 4-pentenoic acid. These two compounds can produce microvesicular steatosis in the livers of laboratory animals, a characteristic feature of Reye's syndrome.[17] A large increase in VPA plasma concentration results in a large increase in 4-en-VPA. An extensive, detailed study of VPA metabolism in cases of VPA hepatotoxicity concluded, however, that 4-en-VPA is not the decisive hepatotoxin.[18] In laboratory rats, 4-en-VPA in liver is steatogenic but does not cause hepatocyte necrosis. In one study, younger patients had greater formation of 4-en-VPA than older patients.[16] In another study, children younger than 2 years of age with valproate hepatotoxicity had lower 4-en-VPA plasma concentrations than children older than 2 years of age (whose age averaged 9.5 years).[18] The ratio of human plasma 4-en-VPA to VPA increases as the total plasma VPA concentration also increases. By contrast, the human plasma ratios of 2-en-VPA to VPA and 3-en-VPA to VPA decrease at high plasma concentrations of VPA. This decreased metabolic conversion of VPA to 2-en-VPA and 3-en-VPA at high plasma concentrations of VPA is probably due to autoinhibition or saturation of mitochondrial β-oxidation of VPA because VPA is an inhibitor of mitochondrial fatty acid β-oxidation (see Fig. 51-2), with inhibition of 3-ketoacyl-CoA thiolase being most important. What follows is a limited capacity for mitochondrial β-oxidation, which may become exhausted, leading to unknown metabolic reactions resulting in hepatotoxicity.[19] A 1.0-g oral dose or 400-mg intravenous dose of VPA given to fasting human adults results in approximately a 75% decrease in plasma 3-hydroxybutyrate and an approximate 60% decrease in plasma total ketones, with increases of lactate, pyruvate, alanine, and glycerol.[20] VPA decreases β-oxidation of endogenous fatty acids. Clinically, VPA hepatotoxicity incidence is increased in patients who also are treated with other antiepileptic drugs, such as phenytoin, phenobarbital, and carbamazepine, which are known to induce cytochrome P-450. It is likely that cytochrome P-450 enzyme induction results in increased 4-en-VPA production from VPA and further metabolism of 4-en-VPA to a reactive intermediate. Patients treated with multiple P-450 enzyme–inducing antiepileptic drugs seem to have increased inhibition of β-oxidation VPA that may be due to reduced valproyl-CoA formation and greater depletion of carnitine.[21,22] This altered VPA metabolic profile of production of 4-en-VPA and decreased β-oxidation of VPA also is reported in patients with fatal VPA hepatic failure.[23,24]

Autoantibodies

Covalent plasma protein adducts of VPA and antibodies to these protein adducts are formed in humans (9 of 57 persons tested), but at low titers. This formation occurs because VPA acyl glucuronide nonenzymatically reacts with plasma protein. Epileptic patients taking VPA on a long-term basis have measurable VPA plasma protein adducts at concentrations of approximately 0.75 μg VPA equivalents/mL.[25]

Teratogenicity

Structure-activity studies in laboratory animals showed that other branched-chain carboxylic acid analogues also have anticonvulsant activity. Some of these do not have teratogenic activity, in contrast to VPA, which is a known human teratogen. It is associated with neural tube defects.[26]

CLINICAL PRESENTATION AND LIFE-THREATENING COMPLICATIONS

After an acute large overdose, drowsiness progressing to coma usually occurs relatively rapidly but may progress more gradually, particularly with the divalproate form. Metabolic acidosis, hypoglycemia, hypocalcemia, hypophosphatemia, and hypernatremia may become severe and potentially life-threatening. Hyperammonemia and elevated serum liver enzymes may occur after either acute overdose or long-term therapy[27,28] and typically are not life-threatening in most patients. Occasionally, severe life-threatening hepatotoxicity may occur, especially in patients on long-term therapy. Thrombocytopenia, occasionally requiring platelet transfusion, and leukopenia are potential risks. Delayed, life-threatening cerebral edema appearing in a few to several days may occur in severely poisoned patients. In 133 VPA overdose patients with peak measured serum VPA concentrations averaging 380 mg/L (2660 μmol/L) and ranging from 110 to 1840 mg/L (770 to 12,880 μmol/L) (therapeutic range 50 to 100 mg/L [350 to 700 μmol/L]), findings included lethargy in 94, coma in 19, tachycardia in 24, aspiration in 8, metabolic acidosis in 8, and hypotension in 4.[29] Peak measured serum VPA concentrations greater than 850 mg/L (>5950 μmol/L) are more likely to be associated with coma; peak serum VPA levels greater than 450 mg/L (>3150 μmol/L) are more likely to be associated with moderate or major adverse outcome. Eleven of 133 patients with transient thrombocytopenia had peak measured serum VPA concentrations greater than 450 mg/L (>3150 μmol/L).[29] One of the highest reported serum VPA concentrations was 2700 mg/L (18,900 μmol/L) in an adult patient with a fatal outcome.[30]

DIAGNOSIS

The diagnosis of VPA poisoning, similar to many drug poisonings, is helped enormously by an available and accurate history of ingestion. When a patient presents with an unknown ingestion and laboratory data are pending, differential diagnosis is difficult. In this scenario, coma with or without a metabolic acidosis is typically present, and identification of VPA in urine or blood specimens is required to support the diagnosis. This identification should be followed by quantitative plasma concentrations for confirmation. Plasma concentrations of VPA greater than 100 mg/L (700 μmol/L) are of concern. Concentrations greater than 450 mg/L (3150 μmol/L) and 850 mg/L (5950 μmol/L) are of increasingly serious concern, although it is recognized that a close correlation between plasma concentrations and clinical severity does not exist.[29]

TREATMENT

Treatment considerations include general supportive care, gastrointestinal decontamination with activated charcoal, selective high-flux hemodialysis, and possibly L-carnitine and N-acetylcysteine administration. Some authors recommend the use of naloxone. All patients with VPA toxicity should be monitored closely for depression of mental status and need for airway protection. Patients with an altered mental status should have their arterial ammonia concentration determined. Glucose should be monitored because of the possibility of hypoglycemia.

Gastrointestinal Decontamination

Activated charcoal given 5 minutes after an oral dose of 300 mg of VPA to six healthy human volunteers reduced absorption of VPA by 65%.[31] When multiple-dose activated charcoal was started 4 hours after an oral dose of 300 mg of VPA (4 to 32 hours after VPA, repeated doses of activated charcoal, total of 80 g, were given), there was no significant difference in the area under the time-concentration curve or plasma half-life (20 hours versus 22 hours).[32] Single-dose activated charcoal given relatively soon after ingestion, but perhaps not multiple-dose activated charcoal, may be of benefit in patients with VPA overdoses. One patient with a fatal overdose of VPA had VPA levels in bile of 3000 mg/L (21,000 μmol/L),[30] however, suggesting the possibility that multiple-dose activated charcoal in poisoned patients might provide some benefit in interrupting enterohepatic circulation. There are no clinical prospective studies from which to assess the efficacy of multiple-dose activated charcoal in patients with large acute ingestions or patients who have ingested

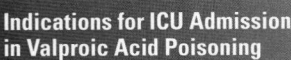

Indications for ICU Admission in Valproic Acid Poisoning

History of large-dose, symptomatic acute ingestion
Rapidly decreasing level of consciousness or coma
Cerebral edema
Markedly abnormal liver function tests, including serum elevated ammonia
Hypoglycemia
Metabolic acidosis

Common Errors in the Treatment of Valproic Acid Poisoning

Failure to use L-carnitine therapy
Unawareness of potential use of N-acetylcysteine
Unawareness of efficacy of high-flux hemodialysis

an overdose of a delayed-release preparation. Cholestyramine does not clinically decrease VPA absorption significantly in humans.[33]

Hemodialysis

Despite the high percentage of VPA bound to plasma proteins at therapeutic concentrations, hemodialysis may have a role in VPA poisoning. High-flux hemodialysis alone without hemoperfusion was effective in one patient with coma, hypotension, lactic acidosis, and a serum VPA level of greater than 1200 mg/L.[34] At high serum levels of VPA, its protein-binding fraction decreases owing to saturation of albumin binding sites. For example, 32% is bound at 1400 mg/L (9800 μmol/L),[35] resulting in the potential for greater effectiveness of hemodialysis than in patients with VPA concentrations in the therapeutic range when it is 85% to 95% bound to serum proteins. In one patient, high-flux hemodialysis of 6 hours' duration reduced serum VPA levels from 940 to 165 mg/L (6580 to 1155 μmol/L).[36] Case reports of extracorporeal methods indicate that this approach rapidly decreases elevated VPA serum levels.[37–40] Peritoneal dialysis does not seem to be effective, however.[41] Although hemodialysis is effective in reducing plasma VPA concentrations, it is unlikely to affect outcome because most patients survive with supportive care, generally consisting of airway support and mechanical ventilation. In patients with extremely high VPA concentrations, hemodialysis theoretically would decrease the duration of coma, and perhaps reduce complications, by enhancing drug clearance.

Naloxone

Anecdotal case report experience suggests that naloxone may be useful in some patients with VPA-induced coma and decreased ventilatory function.[42] Naloxone is relatively safe; its benefit-to-risk ratio is favorable for use in most patients with coma or ventilatory depression. Whether naloxone is truly effective in VPA poisoning is unknown.

L-Carnitine

VPA therapy and overdose may result in decreased plasma carnitine levels, which decreases β-oxidation.[17,43–47] In patients with VPA-induced hepatotoxicity, L-carnitine treatment resulted in a 48% survival in 42 patients compared with 10% survival in 50 patients treated with aggressive supportive care.[48] There was greater survival with intravenous L-carnitine compared with enteral L-carnitine, which is likely due to the 15% enteral bioavailability of L-carnitine. The dose of L-carnitine was 50 to

100 mg/kg/day, usually for a few days until there was clear evidence of clinical improvement. The optimal dose has not been established. L-Carnitine administration lowered elevated plasma ammonia concentrations to normal in VPA-treated children.[49] L-carnitine treatment, which is considered relatively safe, is recommended for patients with VPA hepatotoxicity. D-Carnitine is not active, and D,L-carnitine has been suspected of causing a myasthenia-like syndrome.

Based on the metabolic considerations discussed previously, use of L-carnitine is now common in all patients with VPA poisoning. L-Carnitine supplementation may be considered for most patients with VPA poisoning because of the associated reduction in plasma concentrations of carnitine in these patients, which occurs even in some patients treated with therapeutic doses of VPA. Recommended oral doses of L-carnitine for carnitine deficiency are 50 to 100 mg/kg/day in children and 1 to 3 g/day in adults. L-Carnitine should be given intravenously in VPA-poisoned patients.[48] To my knowledge, no studies to establish optimal doses of intravenous L-carnitine for VPA poisoning are published at the current time.

N-Acetylcysteine

Because the liver toxic metabolite 4-en-VPA is produced by oxidant cytochrome P-450 mechanisms and 4-en-VPA seems to be metabolized further by a cytochrome P-450 (probably CYP2E1) to a reactive, and perhaps toxic, intermediate, use of *N*-acetylcysteine has been recommended. There are no published prospective, randomized clinical trial outcome data, however, supporting it as an efficacious treatment for VPA hepatotoxicity or VPA-induced cerebral edema.[50] *N*-Acetylcysteine is a theoretical therapy for VPA hepatotoxicity and for VPA-induced delayed cerebral edema because of cytochrome P-450 production of a toxic metabolite of VPA (i.e., 4-en-VPA) (see Fig. 51-2). There are no clinical trials, however, showing the efficacy of *N*-acetylcysteine in the treatment of VPA toxicity. *N*-Acetylcysteine is used increasingly for the treatment of liver failure from multiple causes. A reasonable, although untested for this purpose, dosing regimen would be that currently used for acetaminophen poisoning (see Chapter 55).

Criteria for ICU Discharge in Valproic Acid Poisoning

Patient is awake enough to protect the airway
Improving liver function

SPECIAL POPULATIONS

Children, pregnant women, and the elderly are treated similarly for VPA poisoning. There is some evidence that L-carnitine is transported across the human placenta.[51]

Key Points in Valproic Acid Poisoning

1. Early recognition of hepatotoxicity in patients on long-term therapeutic doses improves outcome.
2. Early use of L-carnitine improves survival in patients with valproic acid hepatotoxicity.
3. High-flux hemodialysis is efficacious in enhancing drug clearance. It is not known if it affects outcome.

REFERENCES

1. Litovitz TL, Klein-Schwartz W, White S, et al: 2000 Annual report of the American Association of Poison Control Centers Toxic Exposure Surveillance System. Am J Emerg Med 19:337–395, 2001.
2. Nau H, Loscher W: Valproic acid and metabolites: Pharmacological and toxicological studies. Epilepsia 15(Suppl 1):s14-s22, 1984.
3. Tatsuhara T, Muro H, Matsuda Y, Imai Y: Determination of valproic acid and its metabolites by gas chromatography–mass spectrometry with selected ion monitoring. J Chromatogr 399:183–195, 1987.
4. Sadeque AJ, Fisher MB, Korzekwa KR, et al: Human CYP2C9 and CYP2A6 mediate formation of the hepatotoxin 4-ene-valproic acid. J Pharmacol Exp Ther 293:698–703, 1997.
5. Neuman MG, Shear NH, Jacobson-Brown PM, et al: CYP2E1-mediated modulation of valproic acid-induced hepatotoxicity. Clin Biochem 34:211–218, 2001.
6. Rettie AE, Boberg M, Rettenmeier AW, Ballie TA: Cytochrome P-450-catalyzed desaturation of valproic acid in vitro: Species differences, induction effects, and mechanistic studies. J Biol Chem 263:13733–13738, 1988.
7. McLaughlin DB, Andrews JA, Hooper WD, et al: Apparent autoinduction of valproate beta-oxidation in humans. Br J Clin Pharmacol 49:409–415, 2000.
8. Albani F, Riva R, Coritin M, Baruzzi A: Valproic acid binding to human serum albumin and human plasma: Effects of pH variation and buffer composition in equilibrium dialysis. Ther Drug Monit 6:31–33, 1984.
9. Kodama Y, Kodama H, Kuranari M, et al: Gender- or age-related binding characteristics of valproic acid to serum proteins in adult patients with epilepsy. Eur J Pharmaceut Biopharmaceut 52:57–63, 2001.
10. Bolanos JP, Medina JM: Effect of valproate on the metabolism of the central nervous system. Life Sci 60:1933–1942, 1997.
11. Loscher W, Siemes H: Valproic acid increases gamma-aminobutyric acid in CSF of epileptic children. Lancet 2:225, 1984.
12. Lindberger M, Tomson T, Wallstedt L, Stahle L: Distribution of valproate to subdural cerebrospinal fluid, subcutaneous extracellular fluid, and plasma in humans: A microdialysis study. Epilepsia 43:256–261, 2001.
13. Loscher W: Valproate: A reappraisal of its pharmacodynamic properties and mechanisms of action. Progr Neurobiol 58:31–59, 1999.
14. Dreifuss FE, Santilli N, Langer DH, et al: Valproic acid hepatic fatalities: A retrospective review. Neurology 37:379–385, 1987.
15. Partin JS: Valproic acid therapy and mitochondrial alterations. J Pediatr Gastroenterol Nutr 8:5–7, 1989.
16. Kondo T, Kaneko S, Otani K, et al: Associations between risk factors for valproate hapatotoxicity and altered valproate metabolism. Epilepsia 33:172–177, 1992.
17. Ishikura H, Matsuo N, Matsubara M, et al: Valproic acid overdose and L-carnitine therapy. J Analyt Toxicol 20:55–58, 1996.
18. Siemes H, Nau H, Schultze K, et al: Valproate (VPA) metabolites in various clinical conditions of probable VPA-associated hepatotoxicity. Epilepsia 34:332–346, 1993.
19. Bryant AE, Dreifuss FE: Valproic acid hepatic fatalities: III. US experience since 1986. Neurology 46:465–469, 1996.
20. Turnbull DM, Dick DJ, Wilson L, et al: Valproate causes metabolic disturbance in normal man. J Neurol Neurosurg Psychiatry 49:405–410, 1986.
21. Abbott FS, Kassam J, Orr JM, Farrell K: The effect of aspirin on valproic acid metabolism. Clin Pharmacol Ther 40:94–100, 1986.
22. Laub MC, Paetzke-Brunner I, Jaeger G: Serum carnitine during valproic acid therapy. Epilepsia 27:559–562, 1986.

23. Kochen W, Schneider A, Ritz A: Abnormal metabolism of valproic acid in fatal hepatic failure. Eur J Pediatr 141:30–35, 1983.

24. Kuhara T, Inoue Y, Matsumoto M, et al: Marked increased omega-oxidation of valproate in fulminant hepatic failure. Epilepsia 31:214–217, 1990.

25. Williams AM, Worrall S, de Jersey J, Dickinson RG: Studies on the reactivity of acyl glucuronides: III. Glucuronide-derived adducts of valproic acid and plasma protein and anti-adduct antibodies in humans. Biochem Pharmacol 43:745–755, 1992.

26. Bojic U, Elmazar MM, Hauck RS, Nau H: Further branching of valproate-related carboxylic acids reduces the teratogenic activity, but not the anticonvulsant effect. Chem Res Toxicol 9:866–870, 1996.

27. Eze E, Workman M, Donley B: Hyperammonemia and coma developed by a woman treated with valproic acid for affective disorder. Psychiatr Serv 49:1358–1359, 1998.

28. Lee WL, Yang CC, Deng JF, et al: A case of severe hyperammonemia and unconsciousness following valproate intoxication. Vet Hum Toxicol 40:346–348, 1998.

29. Spiller HA, Krenzelok EP, Klein-Schwartz W, et al: Multicenter case series of valproic acid ingestion: serum concentrations and toxicity. J Toxicol Clin Toxicol 38:755–760, 2000.

30. Connacher AA, Macnab MS, Moody JP, Jung RT: Fatality due to massive overdose of valproate. Scot Med J 32:85–86, 1987.

31. Neuvonen PJ, Kannisto H, Hirvisalo EL, et al: Effect of activated charcoal on absorption of tolbutamide and valproate in man. Eur J Clin Pharamcol 24:243–246, 1983.

32. Al-Shareef A, Buss DC, Shetty HG, et al: The effect of repeated-dose activated charcoal on the pharmacokinetics of sodium valproate in healthy volunteers. Br J Clin Pharmacol 43:109–111, 1997.

33. Malloy MJ, Ravis WR, Pennell AT, Diskin CJ: Effect of cholestyramine resin on single dose valproate pharmacokinetics. Int J Clin Pharmacol Ther 34:208–211, 1996.

34. Kane SL, Constintiner M, Staubus AE, et al: High-flux hemodialysis without hemoperfusion is effective in acute valproic acid overdose. Ann Pharmacother 34:1146–1151, 2000.

35. Franssen EJ, van Essen GG, Portman AT, et al: Valproic acid toxicokinetics: Serial hemodialysis and hemoperfusion. Ther Drug Monit 21:289–292, 1999.

36. Johnson LZ, Martinez I, Fernandez MC, et al: Successful treatment of valproic acid overdose with hemodialysis. Am J Kidney Dis 33:786–789, 1999.

37. Tank JE, Palmer BF: Simultaneous "in series" hemodialysis and hemoperfusion in the management of valproic acid overdose. Am J Kidney Dis 22:341–344, 1993.

38. Matsumoto J, Ogawa H, Maeyama R, et al: Successful treatment by direct hemoperfusion of coma possibly resulting from mitochondrial dysfunction in acute valproate intoxication. Epilepsia 38:950–953, 1997.

39. Graudins A, Aaron CK: Delayed peak serum valproic acid in massive divalproex overdose: Treatment with charcoal hemoperfusion. J Toxicol Clin Toxicol 34:335–341, 1996.

40. Roodhooft AM, Van Dam K, Haentjens D, et al: Acute sodium valproate intoxication: Occurrence of renal failure and treatment with haemoperfusion-haemodialysis. Eur J Pediatr 149:363–364, 1990.

41. Orr JM, Farrell K, Abbot FS, et al: The effects of peritoneal dialysis on the single dose and steady state pharmacokinetics of valproic acid in a uremic epileptic child. Eur J Clin Pharmacol 24:387–390, 1983.

42. Espinoza O, Maradei I, Ramirez M, Pascuzzo-Lima C: An unusual presentation of opioid-like syndrome in pediatric valproic acid poisoning. Vet Hum Toxicol 43:178–179, 2001.

43. Coulter DL: Carnitine, valproate and toxicity. J Child Neurol 6:7–14, 1991.

44. Hiraoka A, Arato T, Tominaga I: Reduction in blood free carnitine levels in association with changes in valproate disposition in epileptic patients treated with valproic acid and other antiepileptic drugs. Biol Pharmaceut Bull 20:91–93, 1997.

45. Murakami K, Sugimoto T, Woo M, et al: Effect of L-carnitine supplementation on acute valproic intoxication. Epilepsia 37:687–699, 1996.

46. Sakemi K, Hayasaka K, Tahara M, et al: The effect of carnitine on the metabolism of valproic acid in epileptic patients. Tohoku J Exp Med 167:89–92, 1992.

47. Beghi E, Bizzi A, Codegoni AM, et al: Valproate, carnitine metabolism, and biochemical indicators of liver function. Epilepsia 31:346–352, 1990.

48. Bohan TP, Helton E, McDonald I, et al: Effect of L-carnitine treatment for valproate-induced hapatotoxicity. Neurology 56:1405–1409, 2001.

49. Ohtani Y, Endo F, Matsuda I: Carnitine deficiency and hyperammonemia associated with valproic acid therapy. J Pediatr 101:782–785, 1982.

50. Farrell K, et al: Successful treatment of valproate hepatotoxicity with N-acetylcysteine. Epilepsia 3:700, 1989.

51. Schmidt-Sommerfeld E, Penn D, Sodha RJ, et al: Transfer and metabolism of carnitine and carnitine esters in the in vitro perfused human placenta. Pediatr Res 19:700–706, 1985.

CHAPTER **52**

Baclofen

Kimberlie A. Graeme

In the central nervous system, γ-aminobutyric acid (GABA) is the main inhibitory neurotransmitter. Three major GABA receptors—$GABA_A$, $GABA_B$, and $GABA_C$—have been identified. Baclofen (β-(4-chlorophenol)-γ-aminobutyric acid), a specific $GABA_B$ agonist, has been used to treat spasticity of various etiologies (e.g., multiple sclerosis, paraplegia, quadriplegia, cerebral palsy), dystonia, jerking, restless legs, chorea, stiff-person syndrome, torticollis, tetanus, hiccups, and pain.[1–14]

BIOCHEMISTRY, PHARMACOLOGY, AND PATHOPHYSIOLOGY

Baclofen is a structural analogue of GABA (Fig. 52-1).[15]

Pharmacokinetics

Baclofen is absorbed rapidly and completely after oral administration, but its central nervous system penetration is limited. Relatively large oral doses are required to achieve therapeutic effects. Oral baclofen has a low therapeutic index, primarily because it is distributed evenly between spinal and supraspinal levels after oral administration. Peak blood concentrations occur 1 to 3.5 hours after therapeutic ingestion; however, after overdose, absorption is prolonged and incomplete. Although signs and symptoms of toxicity can begin shortly after overdose, resolution can be protracted. After intrathecal or oral overdose, it may take days for the patient to become fully alert. Elimination from nerve and brain tissue is much slower than from serum, explaining the persistence of symptoms despite undetectable serum baclofen concentrations. Baclofen is excreted primarily by glomerular filtration, and its clearance is proportional to creatinine clearance. Generally, 50% to 85% of an ingested dose is eliminated unchanged in urine

Pharmacokinetics of Baclofen Poisoning

Protein binding: 30–35%
Volume of distribution: 0.8–2.4 L/kg
Serum half-life: 2–6.8 hr (longer after overdose)
Mechanism of clearance: primarily renal

within 72 hours. The remaining 15% is deaminated to β-(*p*-chlorophenol)-γ-hydroxybutyric acid.[5,11,12,15–27]

$GABA_B$ Receptors

$GABA_B$ receptors are expressed widely in the brain and the spinal cord, including the brainstem and dorsal horn of the spinal cord. The $GABA_B$ receptor comprises two subunits and is coupled to G proteins. Activation of these receptors promotes a decline in calcium conductance and intracellular cyclic adenosine monophosphate production.

Baclofen binds to presynaptic and postsynaptic $GABA_B$ receptors (Fig. 52-2). Presynaptic receptor binding of GABA or baclofen hyperpolarizes presynaptic terminals and decreases neurotransmitter (e.g., catecholamines, glutamate, substance P) release from excitatory spinal pathways (see Fig. 52-2B), producing an inhibitory effect. Presynaptic binding also occurs at GABAergic autoreceptors, hyperpolarizing presynaptic terminals and decreasing GABA release (see Fig. 52-2A), producing an excitatory effect. Postsynaptic binding to the $GABA_B$ receptor hyperpolarizes the neuron and results in inhibition (see Fig. 52-2A). Inhibitory and excitatory effects may occur with the binding of baclofen to $GABA_B$ receptors. Generally, when used therapeutically, the inhibitory effects prevail. The dual inhibitory and excitatory actions provide an explanation for the significant overlap of clinical manifestations (e.g., seizures) seen with overdose and withdrawal from baclofen.

Baclofen depresses γ and α motor neurons and inhibits monosynaptic extensor and polysynaptic flexor spinal reflexes. This activity accounts for the decreased muscle tone and the efficacy of baclofen in treating spasticity. Baclofen affects afferent depolarization in the dorsal horn of the spinal cord and modulates nociceptive input from primary afferent fibers to neurons of the spinothalamic tract. This effect, along with the inhibition of substance P release, accounts for the efficacy of baclofen in the treatment of pain. Central and peripheral GABA receptors also are known to play a role in regulation of body temperature; this may account for the hypothermia generally seen after overdose and the hyperthermia generally seen in withdrawal from baclofen. Central nervous system depression secondary to baclofen may be attributed to stimulation of $GABA_B$ receptors in the hippocampus, whereas respiratory and cardiovascular depression may result from stimulation of $GABA_B$ receptors in the brainstem.[1,6,7,15–17,23,28–34]

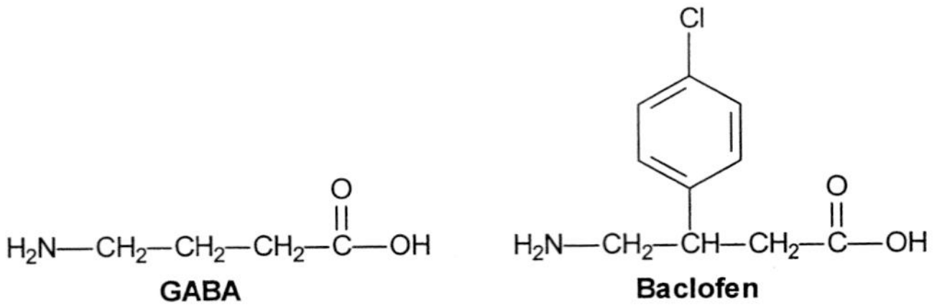

FIGURE 52-1

Chemical structures of γ-aminobutyric acid (GABA) and baclofen. Baclofen is a GABA analogue containing a *para*-chlorphenyl moiety in the β position relative to the carboxylate.

CLINICAL PRESENTATION

Routes of Exposure

ORAL

Acute ingestions of 300 to 970 mg in adults can be expected to produce serious intoxications, and doses of 1250 to 2500 mg have been fatal in adults.[11] Baclofen abuse has been reported in drug addicts and in adolescents seeking intoxication.[19,35]

INTRATHECAL

Intrathecal administration is accomplished by a pump with a reservoir that is implanted surgically in the subcutaneous tissue of the abdominal wall. A catheter is threaded into the intrathecal space, allowing direct delivery into the cerebrospinal fluid. Complications include mechanical problems (dislodgment, disconnection, kinking, blockage), pump failure, and infection.[15,36,37] In an 8-year study of 30 patients, the overall incidence of pump complications was 62%. The most frequent complication was catheter disconnection, followed by retraction of the intrathecal catheter.[36] Intrathecal overdose has occurred in continuous infusion and after bolus injection.[17]

Clinical Manifestations of Baclofen Poisoning

Lee and colleagues[28] attempted to differentiate between acute and chronic baclofen poisonings, suggesting that acutely poisoned patients are more likely to present with encephalopathy (disturbances of consciousness or seizure or both), respiratory depression, muscular hypotonia, and generalized hyporeflexia. Chronically poisoned patients are more likely to present with hallucinosis, impaired memory, catatonia, or acute mania.[28] The same authors also noted that the acute intoxication syndrome has a faster onset, a shorter duration, more severe clinical manifestations, and a higher incidence of seizures compared with the chronic intoxication syndrome.[28] There is significant overlap, however, in the clinical presentations of acute and chronic toxicity, and overlap with the presentation of withdrawal, as discussed later.

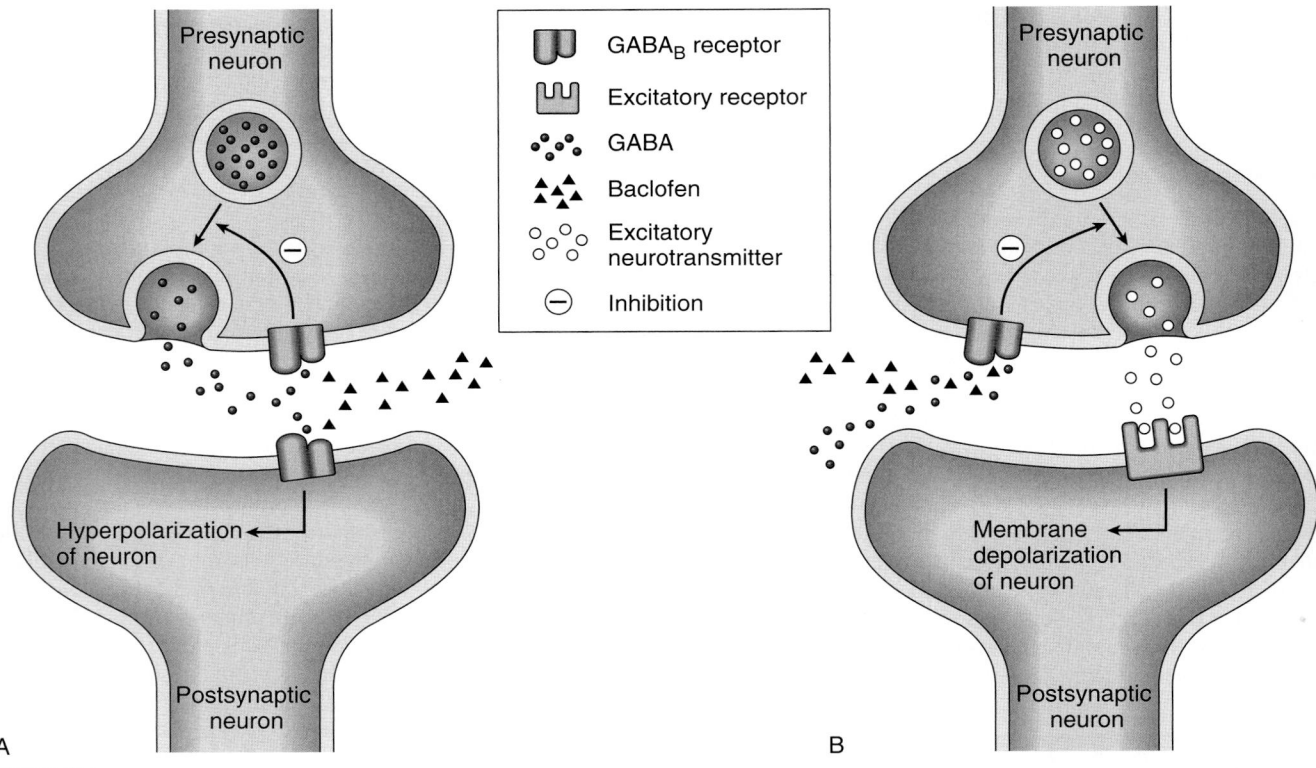

FIGURE 52-2

Binding of γ-aminobutyric acid (GABA) and baclofen to GABA_B receptors. **A**, GABA is released from presynaptic GABAminergic neurons and may bind to GABA_B receptors on postsynaptic neurons, resulting in hyperpolarization of postsynaptic neurons. This has an inhibitory effect on the nervous system. GABA released from presynaptic GABAminergic neurons also acts at GABA_B receptors on the presynaptic neurons, resulting in decreased release of GABA from the neuron, or autoregulation. This has an excitatory effect. **B**, GABA_B receptors also are located on presynaptic neurons that release excitatory neurotransmitters. When GABA binds to these receptors, the release of excitatory neurotransmitters is diminished. This has an inhibitory effect. Baclofen can bind at all of these GABA_B receptors and produces an effect similar to that of GABA binding.

ACUTE

Pulmonary. Respiratory depression and failure may occur.[11,12,17,19,22,27,38–42]

Cardiovascular. Hypertension or hypotension and tachycardia or bradycardia may occur. Tachycardia may alternate abruptly with bradycardia. Conduction abnormalities (including prolonged QT_c and first-degree heart block), premature atrial and ventricular contractions, supraventricular tachycardia, atrial flutter, and atrial fibrillation have been reported.[11,12,17–19,22,27,28,35,39–41]

Gastrointestinal. Nausea and vomiting can occur.[12,35,39,42]

Neurologic. Headache, dizziness, incoordination, ataxia, myoclonus, fatigue, weakness, areflexia, flaccid extremities, encephalopathy, coma, and seizures, including status epilepticus, may occur.[11,12,17–19,22,23,27,28,32,34,35,38,40–44] The clinician needs to be aware of the risk of nonconvulsive (akinetic) status epilepticus.[18,45] Although baclofen has antiepileptic properties at low concentrations, it is proepileptic at high concentrations.[17,32,43] Delayed psychosis and confusion with hallucinations have been reported during the recovery phase.[17,19,41]

Ocular. Blurred vision, horizontal or vertical nystagmus, unreactive pupils, absent corneal reflexes, and doll's eye reflexes may occur. Pupils may be small or large.[11,17,18,27,28,32,35,38,39,41,43]

Other. Hypothermia and hypersalivation may occur.[11,18,28,35,39] Hyperthermia is reported rarely.[28]

CHRONIC

Toxicity can occur gradually after long-term intrathecal or oral dosing, especially in patients with concomitant renal insufficiency. Chronic intoxication may present with impaired memory, acute mania or catatonia, and hallucinosis; this has been called *chronic baclofen intoxication syndrome*.[11,18,28] Respiratory depression, apnea, bradycardia, tachycardia, hypotension, hypertension, tremor, weakness, hypotonia, areflexia, urinary retention, sedation, coma, seizures, orofacial dyskinesia, and hypothermia also have been reported as manifestations of chronic baclofen toxicity.[4,5,24,25,28]

SIDE EFFECTS WITH LONG-TERM USE

Nausea, lightheadedness, vertigo, fatigue, drowsiness, confusion, and lethargy may occur as side effects of oral baclofen, owing to the narrow therapeutic margin.[12,24,28,46] Occasionally, hypotension also is seen.[24]

COMA AND THE DIAGNOSIS OF BRAIN DEATH

Deep coma and brainstem dysfunction may mimic brain death in patients with severe baclofen poisoning. Despite these findings, patients with baclofen poisoning may survive neurologically intact if aggressive supportive care is provided. The diagnosis of brain death should be made cautiously in patients with suspected baclofen toxicity. Several days of intensive care, serial neurologic examinations, and studies to determine brain death (e.g., cerebral blood flow studies) should be pursued before pronouncing brain death in these patients.[41]

Clinical Manifestations of Baclofen Withdrawal

Baclofen withdrawal may occur after diminished or discontinued oral administration or more commonly after intrathecal pump malfunction.[12,33] Withdrawal may occur shortly after recovery from baclofen toxicity when baclofen treatment is not reinitiated promptly in the long-term user.[27] The withdrawal syndrome occurs within 12 to 96 hours after cessation of use, and symptoms generally resolve within 24 to 72 hours of resumption of treatment, although some improvement may be seen sooner.[27,47]

Respiratory distress, tachypnea, hypotension or hypertension, bradycardia or tachycardia, dysrhythmias, heart block, sleeplessness, agitation, shaking, coma, areflexia, diplopia, dyskinesia, visual disturbances, loss of pupillary light and oculocephalic reflexes, hyperthermia, diaphoresis, and hypersalivation have been reported.[12,16,27,33,46–53] Rhabdomyolysis, disseminated intravascular coagulation, renal failure, hepatic failure, cerebral ischemia, and brain death may ensue.[16,48–50] Elevations in liver transaminase, creatinine, creatine phosphokinase, white blood cell count, and prothrombin time levels have been reported.[16,50] Acidosis may occur.[50] There is significant overlap in the clinical presentation of overdose and withdrawal (e.g., autonomic instability, coma, seizures, laboratory abnormalities), and differentiating between the two entities may be difficult.[27] One helpful clue is that spasticity and muscle spasms (likely unmasking an underlying condition) and hyperthermia are seen more commonly with withdrawal, whereas hypothermia is seen more commonly with overdose.

Baclofen withdrawal syndrome may appear clinically similar to neuroleptic malignant syndrome, infection, other febrile illnesses, or multiorgan system dysfunction of other etiology.[16,48,49] Infection of the pump pocket, meningitis, and sepsis must be considered in patients receiving intrathecal baclofen.[16,33,36] Modern pumps have bacterial filters that generally prevent overwhelming intrathecal infection; however, infection still may occur.[36,37,54] Pump function can be assessed using computer program systems and by aspirating and measuring the amount of drug remaining in the system.[16,36,48] These maneuvers may help differentiate among withdrawal, toxicity, and infection.[48]

DIAGNOSIS

Laboratory Studies

Baclofen can be detected by gas chromatography–mass spectrometry and high-performance liquid chromatography.[21,24,25,35] Plasma, rather than cerebrospinal fluid, concentrations generally are assessed.[25] Laboratory abnormalities may include elevated creatine phosphokinase, lactate dehydrogenase, glutamic oxaloacetic transaminase, alkaline phosphatase, amylase, blood glucose, and white blood cell count.[18,28] Analysis of cerebrospinal fluid should be considered to rule out other disease processes (e.g., meningitis).

Imaging Studies

Intrathecal pump systems are radiopaque. Radiographs may show loss of catheter integrity.[48,49] Imaging of the brain and spinal cord should be considered to rule out other disease processes (e.g., hemorrhage or infarction).

Special Studies

Electroencephalography often reveals reversible abnormalities. Typical electroencephalography findings are diffuse slowing of background activity and burst suppression.[17,28,32,35,44] In more severe cases, periodic delta and triphasic waves and generalized epileptiform discharges suggestive of seizures are seen.[17,23,28,43,44] Although some patients with severe baclofen toxicity may appear severely brain damaged by clinical and electroencephalography findings, these patients frequently recover fully with adequate supportive care.

TREATMENT

Generally, patients do well with aggressive supportive care. Fatalities have occurred, however, despite medical care.[19,21,55] Respiratory failure and deep coma should be managed promptly and aggressively with intubation and mechanical ventilation.

Gastrointestinal Decontamination

Because of the rapid onset of coma, induction of emesis is not recommended. The efficacy of gastric lavage followed by activated charcoal compared with activated charcoal alone has not been assessed. It is reasonable to administer oral activated charcoal without gastric lavage to patients with suspected ingestion of baclofen if an intact airway can be ensured.[19] The administration of activated charcoal has not been shown to alter the outcome of baclofen-poisoned patients, however. It is likely that any potential benefit of activated charcoal decreases as the time from ingestion increases (see Chapter 6).

Cerebrospinal Fluid Removal

If a large bolus of baclofen accidentally is injected intrathecally, some cerebrospinal fluid may be removed immediately in an attempt to limit toxicity.[17,43,56]

Extracorporeal Removal

Case series data indicate that duration of toxicity in patients with severe renal impairment may be shortened by hemodialysis.[4,57]

Specific Nonantidotal Treatments

CARDIOVASCULAR

Severe hypertension should be treated with short-acting agents because hypertension can deteriorate rapidly to hypotension.

Indications for ICU Admission in Baclofen Poisoning

Evidence of toxicity after acute ingestion
Evidence of toxicity after recent pump adjustment or filling of reservoir
Evidence of significant toxicity after chronic exposure
Evidence of withdrawal symptoms after cessation of baclofen
Evidence of withdrawal symptoms with suspected pump failure

Nitroprusside has been recommended.[19] If hypotension is unresponsive to intravenous fluid administration, vasopressor (e.g., norepinephrine) administration may be necessary.[17,27,49] Symptomatic bradycardia may respond to atropine.[19,27,39,58]

NEUROLOGIC

Seizures occur with baclofen toxicity and withdrawal. These seizures generally are brief and respond readily to treatment.[19] Benzodiazepines have been used to control seizures and other symptoms of toxicity and withdrawal (e.g., unmasked spasticity of withdrawal).[18,47,48,50] Paralytic agents may be used to limit spasticity and convulsions, but there is a risk of status epilepticus going unrecognized clinically in a chemically paralyzed patient.[48] Electroencephalography monitoring is recommended if these patients are chemically paralyzed.

Common Errors in Baclofen Poisoning

Failure to appreciate airway compromise
Failure to recognize the danger of succinylcholine administration in patients with neuromuscular disease
Failure to use short-acting agents when treating hypertension or hypotension and tachycardia
Failure to recognize nonconvulsive (akinetic) status epilepticus
Failure to diagnose baclofen toxicity, misdiagnosing patients as brain dead
Failure to differentiate between toxicity, withdrawal, and infection
Failure to resume baclofen treatment after acute or chronic toxicity resolves, precipitating withdrawal

Succinylcholine use should be limited; it should not be administered to patients who may have been comatose for prolonged periods, who have neuromuscular diseases, or who are suspected to be at risk of rhabdomyolysis or trauma. Patients with neuromuscular disease have altered muscle fiber receptors, resulting in hypersensitivity to the hyperkalemia that may follow succinylcholine administration. Cardiac arrest may occur in these patients after the administration of succinylcholine.[59,60]

Withdrawal from intrathecal baclofen may be resistant to various treatments and may require reinstitution of intrathecal baclofen.[49] Case reports suggest dantrolene may be helpful in treating baclofen withdrawal, but this is not well established.[61] It seems more sensible to resume baclofen promptly rather than initiate dantrolene therapy.[48,50]

INFECTIOUS

Pump infections may be treated by removal of the pump and intravenous antibiotic administration. Alternatively, antibiotics may be administered via the pump.[37,54]

Specific Antidotal Treatments

Although physostigmine and flumazenil have been given as antidotes by some, there is no convincing evidence that either agent is beneficial.[17,19,27,38,39,41,43,56,58,62,63] Risks of side effects from these treatments likely outweigh benefits.[38,63,64] Ondansetron also has been advocated as an antidote in a case report, but this agent has not been studied further.[42,65]

Criteria for ICU Discharge in Baclofen Poisoning

Resolution of altered mental status and seizures

Resolution of blood pressure, pulse, and temperature abnormalities

Resumption of baclofen initiated

SPECIAL POPULATIONS

Pediatric Patients

Respiratory arrest occurred in a 22-month-old infant who ingested 10.9 mg/kg of baclofen.[11] Six children, age 2 to 6 years, presented after oral baclofen overdose; two children required intubation, and one child experienced seizures. Signs and symptoms were similar to those reported in adults.[58] In a case series of adolescents ingesting baclofen, 9 of 14 required intubation; their symptoms were similar to the symptoms seen in adults.[19] Baclofen withdrawal syndrome also presents similarly in children and adults.[16]

Pregnant Patients

Pregnant women and nursing mothers generally are excluded from baclofen treatment.[12] If a pregnant woman presents with baclofen toxicity, she should be treated supportively, as recommended for nonpregnant patients.

Elderly Patients

Peak plasma concentrations occur later after ingestion in elderly patients.[25] This delay may prolong the clinical course in elderly patients.

Other Patients

Patients with impaired renal function are at risk for developing toxic symptoms soon after initiating even low-dose baclofen. Patients on stable regimens of baclofen may develop toxicity if creatinine clearance declines.[26,44,57] Serum creatinine levels may remain normal, despite diminished creatinine clearance.[26]

Key Points in Baclofen Poisoning

1. Patients who receive aggressive supportive care generally survive baclofen toxicity.
2. There is no clinically available antidote that reliably reverses baclofen toxicity.
3. Seizures, resulting from either toxicity or withdrawal, generally respond to benzodiazepines.
4. Differentiating between baclofen toxicity and withdrawal can be difficult.
5. Generally, hypothermia suggests toxicity, whereas hyperthermia suggests withdrawal or possibly infection.
6. Baclofen toxicity can mimic brain death clinically.
7. Prompt resumption of baclofen administration is often essential for the prevention and treatment of baclofen withdrawal.

REFERENCES

1. Van Hilten BJ, Van de Beek WJT, Hoff JI, et al: Intrathecal baclofen for the treatment of dystonia in patients with reflex sympathetic dystrophy. N Engl J Med 343:625–630, 2000.
2. Orsenes GB, Sorensen PS, Larsen TK, et al: Effect of baclofen on gait in spastic MS patients. Acta Neurol Scand 101:244–248, 2000.
3. VanSchaeybroeck P, Nuttin B, Lagae L, et al: Intrathecal baclofen for intractable cerebral spasticity: A prospective placebo-controlled, double-blind study. Neurosurgery 46:603–609, 2000.
4. Bassilios N, Launay-Vacher V, Mercadal L, Deray G: Baclofen neurotoxicity in a chronic haemodialysis patient. Nephrol Dial Transplant 15:715–716, 2000.
5. Peces R, Navascués RA, Baltar J, et al: Baclofen neurotoxicity in chronic haemodialysis patients with hiccups. Nephrol Dial Transplant 13:1896–1897, 1998.
6. Brauner-Osborne H, Krogsgaard-Larsen P: Functional pharmacology of cloned heterodimeric $GABA_B$ receptors expressed in mammalian cells. Br J Pharmacol 128:1370–1374, 1999.
7. Chebib M, Johnston GAR: The ABC of GABA receptors: A brief review. Clin Exp Pharmacol Physiol 26:937–940, 1999.
8. Taira T, Kawamura H, Tanikawa T, et al: A new approach to control central deafferentation pain: Spinal intrathecal baclofen. Stereotact Funct Neurosurg 65:101–105, 1995.
9. Seitz RJ, Blank B, Kiwit JC, et al: Stiff-person syndrome with anti-glutamic acid decarboxylase auto-antibodies: Complete remission of symptoms after intrathecal baclofen administration. J Neurol 242:618–622, 1995.
10. Gordon NC, Gear RW, Heller PH, et al: Enhancement of morphine analgesia by the $GABA_B$ agonist baclofen. Neuroscience 69:345–349, 1995.
11. Mack RB: Between a rock and a Charybdisian place: Baclofen (Lioresal) overdose. N C Med J 56:325–327, 1995.
12. Kamensek J: Continuous intrathecal baclofen infusions: An introduction and overview. Axone 20:93–98, 1999.
13. Nielsen JF, Anderson JB, Sinkjær T: Baclofen increases the soleus stretch reflex threshold in the early swing phase during walking in spastic multiple sclerosis patients. Mult Scler 6:105–114, 2000.
14. Dressnandt J, Konstanzer A, Weinzierl FX, et al: Intrathecal baclofen in tetanus: Four cases and a review of reported cases. Intensive Care Med 23:896–902, 1997.
15. Kita M, Goodkin DE: Drugs used to treat spasticity. Drugs 59:487–495, 2000.
16. Samson-Fang L, Gooch J, Norlin C: Intrathecal baclofen withdrawal simulating neuroleptic malignant syndrome in a child with cerebral palsy. Dev Med Child Neurol 42:561–565, 2000.
17. Fakhoury T, Abou-Khalil B, Blumenkopf B: EEG changes in intrathecal baclofen overdose: A case report and review of the literature. Electroencephalogr Clin Neurophysiol 107:339–342, 1998.
18. VanDierendonk DR, Dire DJ: Baclofen and ethanol ingestion: A case report. J Emerg Med 17:989–993, 1999.
19. Perry HE, Wright RO, Shannon MW, et al: Baclofen overdose: Drug experimentation in a group of adolescents. Pediatrics 101:1045–1048, 1998.
20. Gerkin R, Curry SC, Vance MV, et al: First-order elimination kinetics following baclofen overdose. Ann Emerg Med 15:843–846, 1986.
21. Fraser AD, MacNeil W, Isner AF: Toxicological analysis of a fatal baclofen (Lioresal) ingestion. J Forensic Sci 36:1596–1602, 1991.
22. Brodkey JA, Feler CA: Hypotension following a trial intrathecal dose of baclofen. J Tenn Med Assoc 86:297–298, 1993.
23. Lazzarino LG, Nicolai A, Valassi F: Acute transient cerebral intoxication induced by low doses of baclofen. Ital J Neurol Sci 12:323–325, 1991.
24. Aisen ML, Dietz MA, Rossi R, et al: Clinical and pharmacokinetic aspects of high dose oral baclofen therapy. J Am Paraplegia Soc 15:211–216, 1992.
25. Wuis EW, Dirks MJM, Vree TB, et al: Pharmacokinetics of baclofen in spastic patients receiving multiple oral doses. Pharm Week Sci 12:71–74, 1990.
26. Aisen ML, Dietz M, McDowell F, et al: Baclofen toxicity in a patient with subclinical renal insufficiency. Arch Phys Med Rehabil 75:109–111, 1994.
27. Peng CT, Ger J, Yang CC, et al: Prolonged severe withdrawal symptoms after acute-on-chronic baclofen overdose. J Toxicol Clin Toxicol 36:359–363, 1998.

28. Lee TH, Chen SS, Su SL, et al: Baclofen intoxication: Report of four cases and review of the literature. Clin Neuropharmacol 15:56–62, 1992.

29. Galvez T, Urwyler S, Prezeau L, et al: Ca^{2+} requirement for high-affinity γ-aminobutyric acid (GABA) binding at $GABA_B$ receptors: Involvement of serine 269 of the $GABA_BR1$ subunit. Mol Pharmacol 57:419–426, 2000.

30. Bonanno G, Carità F, Cavazzani P, et al: Selective block of rat and human neocortex $GABA_B$ receptors regulating somatostatin release by a $GABA_B$ antagonist endowed with cognition enhancing activity. Neuropharmacology 38:1789–1795, 1999.

31. Bonanno G, Fassio A, Schmid G, et al: Pharmacologically distinct $GABA_B$ receptors that mediate inhibition of GABA and glutamate release in human neocortex. Br J Pharmacol 120:60–64, 1997.

32. Kofler M, Kronenberg MF, Rifici C, et al: Epileptic seizures associated with intrathecal baclofen application. Neurology 44:25–27, 1994.

33. Naveira FA, Speight KL, Rauck RL, et al: Meningitis after injection of intrathecal baclofen. Anesth Analg 82:1297–1299, 1996.

34. Rush JM, Gibberd FB: Baclofen-induced epilepsy. J R Soc Med 83:115–116, 1990.

35. Weissenborn K, Wilkens H, Hausmann E, et al: Burst suppression EEG with baclofen overdose. Clin Neurol Neurosurg 93:77–80, 1991.

36. Levin AB, Sperling KB: Complications associated with infusion pumps implanted for spasticity. Stereotact Funct Neurosurg 65:147–151, 1995.

37. Zed PJ, Stiver G, Devonshire V: Continuous intrathecal pump infusion of baclofen with antibiotic drugs for treatment of pump-associated meningitis. J Neurosurg 92:347–349, 2000.

38. Byrnes SM, Watson GW, Hardy PA: Flumazenil: An unreliable antagonist in baclofen overdose. Anaesthesia 51:481–482, 1996.

39. Roberge R, Martin TG, Hodgman M, et al: Supraventricular tachyarrhythmia associated with baclofen overdose. J Toxicol Clin Toxicol 32:291–297, 1994.

40. Dressanandt J, Weinzieri FX, Konstanzer A, et al: Acute overdose of intrathecal baclofen. J Neurol 243:482–493, 1996.

41. Ostermann ME, Young B, Sibbald WJ, et al: Coma mimicking brain death following baclofen overdose. Int Care Med 26:1144–1146, 2000.

42. Broggi G, Dones I, Servello D, et al: A possible pharmacological treatment of baclofen overdose. Ital J Neurol Sci 17:179–180, 1996.

43. Saltuari L, Marosi MJ, Kofler M, et al: Status epilepticus complicating intrathecal baclofen overdose. Lancet 339:373–374, 1992.

44. Hormes JT, Benarroch EE, Rodriguez M, et al: Periodic sharp waves in baclofen-induced encephalopathy. Arch Neurol 45:814–815, 1988.

45. Zak R, Solomon G, Petito F, et al: Baclofen-induced generalized nonconvulsive status epilepticus. Ann Neurol 36:113–114, 1994.

46. Kofler M, Arturo LA: Prolonged seizure activity after baclofen withdrawal. Neurology 42:697–698, 1992.

47. Olmedo R, Hoffman RS: Withdrawal syndromes. Emerg Med Clin North Am 18:273–288, 2000.

48. Sampathkumar P, Scanlon PD, Plevak DJ: Baclofen withdrawal presenting as multiorgan system failure. Anesth Analg 87:562–563, 1998.

49. Reeves RK, Stolp-Smith DA, Christopherson MW: Hyperthermia, rhabdomyolysis, disseminated intravascular coagulation associated with baclofen pump catheter failure. Arch Phys Med Rehabil 79:353–356, 1998.

50. Green LB, Nelson VS: Death after acute withdrawal of intrathecal baclofen: Case report and literature review. Arch Phys Med Rehabil 80:1600–1604, 1999.

51. Mandac RR, Hurvitz EA, Nelson VS: Hyperthermia associated with baclofen withdrawal and increased spasticity. Arch Phys Med Rehabil 74:96–97, 1993.

52. Rivas DA, Chancellor MB, Hill K, et al: Neurological manifestations of baclofen withdrawal. J Urol 150:1903–1905, 1993.

53. Al-Khodairy AT, Vuagnat H, Uebelhart D: Symptoms of recurrent intrathecal baclofen withdrawal resulting from drug delivery failure: A case report. Am J Phys Med Rehabil 78:272–277, 1999.

54. Galloway A, Falope FZ: *Pseudomonas aeruginosa* infection in an intrathecal baclofen pump: Successful treatment with adjunct intra-reservoir gentamicin. Spinal Cord 38:126–128, 2000.

55. Stayer C, Tronnier V, Dressnandt J, et al: Intrathecal baclofen therapy for stiff-man syndrome and progressive encephalomyelopathy with rigidity and myoclonus. Neurology 49:1591–1597, 1997.

56. Rushman S, McLaren I: Management of intra-thecal baclofen overdose (Letter). Int Care Med 25:239, 1999.

57. Chen KS, Bullard MJ, Chien YY, et al: Baclofen toxicity in patients with severely impaired renal function. Ann Pharmacother 31:1315–1320, 1997.

58. Cooke DE, Glasstone MA: Baclofen poisoning in children. Vet Hum Toxicol 36:448–450, 1994.

59. Matthews JM: Succinylcholine-induced hyperkalemia and rhabdomyolysis in a patient with necrotizing pancreatitis. Anesth Analg 91:1552–1554, 2000.

60. Gronert GA, Theye RA: Pathophysiology of hyperkalemia induced by succinylcholine. Anesthesiology 43:89–99, 1975.

61. Knorasani A, Peruzzi WT: Dantrolene treatment for abrupt intrathecal baclofen withdrawal. Anesth Analg 30:1054–1056, 1995.

62. Sicignana A, Lorini FL: Does flumazenil antagonize baclofen? (Letter). Int Care Med 20:588, 1994.

63. Saltuari L, Baumgartner H, Kofler M, et al: Failure of physostigmine in treatment of acute severe intrathecal baclofen intoxication (Letter). N Engl J Med 322:1533–1534, 1990.

64. Chern TL, Kwan A: Flumazenil-induced seizure accompanying benzodiazepine and baclofen intoxication. Am J Emerg Med 14:231–232, 1996.

65. Broggi G, Dones I, Sevello D, et al: A possible pharmacological treatment of baclofen overdose. Ital J Neurol Sci 17:179–180, 1996.

CHAPTER 53

Centrally Acting Muscle Relaxants

Carl R. Baum

The centrally acting muscle relaxants are a group of drugs that act in the central nervous system (CNS) to mitigate tension and spasm of skeletal muscles. Drugs within this group are structurally heterogeneous and act at a variety of receptors in the CNS. Muscle relaxants that act at the level of the spinal cord, such as baclofen, or peripherally, such as dantrolene, are discussed in their respective chapters.

Many of the centrally acting muscle relaxants have been available for decades. Carisoprodol, for example, was licensed in 1956 as a prescription, noncontrolled, centrally acting skeletal muscle relaxant. It is metabolized to the anxiolytic meprobamate.[1,2] Others in the group may be compounded with analgesics: chlorzoxazone was first introduced in 1958 as the drug alone or in combination with salicylates or acetaminophen.[3,4] Methocarbamol was reported in 1960 to effectively relieve muscle spasm in a patient with black widow spider poisoning[5] and in a case series of 100 patients with a variety of acute and chronic orthopedic conditions.[6] Metaxalone was patented in 1962.[7] Diazepam, introduced in 1963, was the second benzodiazepine to be approved in the United States for humans and has been used as an anxiolytic and anticonvulsant, as well as a centrally acting muscle relaxant.[8,9] A 1964 double-blind investigation of 200 patients with low back pain and discomfort concluded that metaxalone diminished acute reflex skeletal muscle spasm.[10] Although a 1972 double-blind crossover trial of the tricyclic amine cyclobenzaprine demonstrated minimal improvement in patients with cerebral or spinal spasticity,[11] a 1975 study of several animal models suggested that the drug could be used to mitigate excessive tonic skeletal muscle activity in humans.[12] Cyclobenzaprine has been available as a centrally acting muscle relaxant since 1977.[9]

Meprobamate and diazepam may be habit forming. The United States, for example, officially lists them as controlled substances.[7] In overdose, the centrally acting muscle relaxants are relatively safe when not combined with other agents. For example, a 1-year retrospective review of pure skeletal muscle relaxant exposure, including the centrally acting agents carisoprodol, chlorzoxazone, and cyclobenzaprine, revealed that morbidity and mortality were low.[13]

Much of the clinical experience with muscle relaxants is limited to case reports and case series. Data reported in this chapter should therefore be interpreted cautiously.

BIOCHEMISTRY AND PHARMACOLOGY

The chemical structures of the agents discussed in this chapter are shown in Figure 53-1. Their pharmacokinetics and metabolism are summarized in the accompanying box.

Pharmacokinetics of Centrally Acting Muscle Relaxants

Carisoprodol
Volume of distribution: unknown
Protein binding: 58%
Mechanisms of clearance: hepatic to hydroxycarisoprodol, hydroxymeprobamate, and meprobamate
Active metabolites: meprobamate (4.7% of dose)

Chlorzoxazone
Volume of distribution: unknown
Protein binding: unknown
Mechanisms of clearance: unknown
Active metabolites: none

Cyclobenzaprine
Volume of distribution: unknown
Protein binding: 93%
Mechanisms of clearance: hepatic to norcyclobenzaprine; may undergo enterohepatic cycling; 50% renally as inactive metabolites; via bile in feces as unchanged drug
Active metabolites: none

Diazepam
Volume of distribution: 0.7–2.6 L/kg
Protein binding: 96–97%
Mechanisms of clearance: 4′-hydroxylation and conjugation; N-demethylation to nordiazepam
Active metabolites: nordiazepam

Meprobamate
Volume of distribution: 0.75 L/kg
Protein binding: 20%
Mechanisms of clearance: rapid hepatic; 8–20% in urine as unchanged drug; 10% as metabolites in feces
Active metabolites: none

Metaxalone
Volume of distribution: unknown
Protein binding: unknown
Mechanisms of clearance: unknown
Active metabolites: none

continued

Pharmacokinetics of Centrally Acting Muscle Relaxants *continued*

Methocarbamol

Volume of distribution: unknown
Protein binding: unknown
Mechanisms of clearance: O-demethylation and hydroxylation; conjugation; 99% excreted in 72-hour urine
Active metabolites: guaifenesin

Orphenadrine

Volume of distribution: 4.3–7.8 L/kg
Protein binding: 20%
Mechanisms of clearance: extensive hepatic; desmethylation; up to 30% may be eliminated unchanged in acidic urine; 60% excreted in 72-hour urine
Active metabolites: nororphenadrine

Data from references 7, 9, 15, 16.

Carisoprodol and Meprobamate

Carisoprodol is *N*-isopropyl-2-methyl-2-propyl-1,3-propanediol dicarbamate, or isopropyl meprobamate.[7] It is hepatically metabolized to hydroxycarisoprodol, hydroxymeprobamate, and the active form meprobamate.[2] Meprobamate is 2-methyl-2-propyl-1,3-propanediol dicarbamate.[7]

Chlorzoxazone

Chlorzoxazone is 5-chloro-2-benzoxazolinone and is derived from the more toxic zoxazolamine.[3]

Cyclobenzaprine

Cyclobenzaprine HCl is a tricyclic amine salt, 3-(5H-dibenzo [a,d]cyclohepten5-ylidene)-*N*,*N*-dimethyl-1-propanamine hydrochloride. It is structurally related to the tricyclic antidepressants; only a double bond on the central ring distinguishes it from amitriptyline.[9,14] Cyclobenzaprine, which may undergo enterohepatic cycling, is metabolized in the liver to norcyclobenzaprine.

Diazepam

Diazepam is a benzodiazepine that undergoes 4′-hydroxylation and conjugation as well as N-demethylation to the active metabolite nordiazepam; other metabolites are the active, but nonaccumulating 3-hydroxy derivatives temazepam and

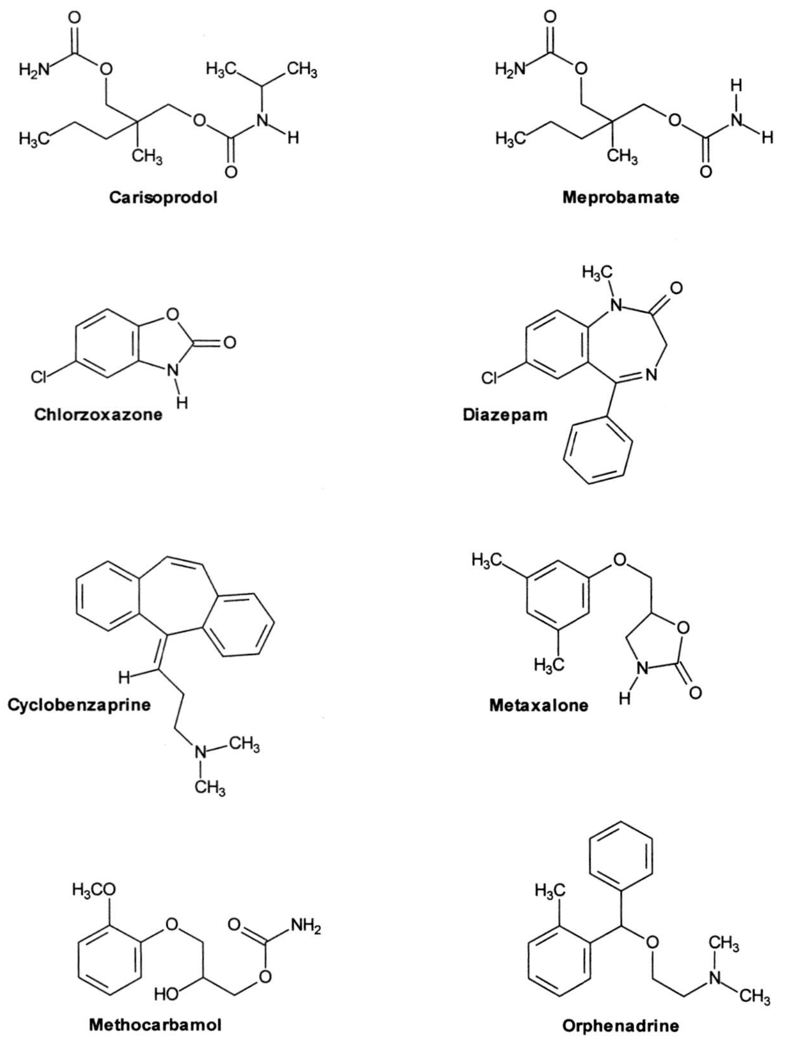

FIGURE 53-1.

Chemical structures of centrally acting muscle relaxants.

oxazepam.[9] The metabolism of diazepam is described in greater detail in Chapter 47.

Methocarbamol

Like carisoprodol and meprobamate, methocarbamol is a member of the carbamate class. Its formula is 3-(*o*-methoxyphenoxy)-2-hydroxypropyl-1-carbamate.[6] The phenyl ring undergoes O-demethylation and hydroxylation; conjugation of the parent drug and metabolites follows. Guaifenesin, an expectorant, is an active metabolite.[9]

Metaxalone

Metaxalone is 5-(3,5-dimethylphenoxymethyl)-2-oxazolidinone.[7]

Orphenadrine

Orphenadrine (*o*-methydiphenhydramine) is classified as a skeletal muscle relaxant, anticholinergic, and antihistaminic agent.[7] As a substrate for the cytochrome P-450 isoenzyme CYP3A4 and an inhibitor of CYP2D6, orphenadrine may have a number of unpredictable pharmacologic interactions.[15]

PATHOPHYSIOLOGY OF THERAPEUTIC AND TOXIC EFFECTS

Carisoprodol and Meprobamate

Carisoprodol is active in the descending reticular formation and spinal cord, where it inhibits interneuronal transmission. Both carisoprodol and its active metabolite meprobamate are indirect γ-aminobutyric acid GABA$_A$ receptor agonists that open the neuronal chloride channel and induce hyperpolarization. This mechanism is similar to that of the benzodiazepines (see Figs. 138-2 and 138-3).[1]

Chlorzoxazone

Chlorzoxazone inhibits polysynaptic reflex pathways that produce and maintain muscle tone in the subcortex and spinal cord, and it appears to relieve musculoskeletal spasm more effectively than neurogenic spasm.[3,4]

Cyclobenzaprine and Orphenadrine

Cyclobenzaprine relieves skeletal muscle spasm of local origin but does not exert its action directly on skeletal muscle, at the neuromuscular junction, or at the level of the spinal cord. Rather, it acts on the brainstem to reduce tonic somatic motor activity.[14] In overdose, its toxicity is related to its antagonism of muscarinic acetylcholine receptors and the resultant anticholinergic syndrome. A similar toxic profile is seen with the diphenhydramine analogue orphenadrine.[9] However, orphenadrine is a more potent fast voltage-gated sodium channel antagonist than cyclobenzaprine is, a property that may be important in the clinical manifestations of overdose.

Diazepam

The benzodiazepine diazepam has multiple therapeutic uses, one of which is skeletal muscle relaxation. It increases the action of the inhibitory neurotransmitter GABA in the limbic and reticular systems and in the CNS in general (see Figs. 138-2 and 138-3).[8,16] The pathophysiology of benzodiazepine effects is described in detail in Chapter 47.

Metaxalone

Metaxalone has an unknown mechanism of action, although no direct effects on striated muscle, the motor end plate, or the nerve fiber are reported.[17] As may largely be the case for several of the other agents discussed in this chapter, the drug's sedative properties are most likely to explain its therapeutic effects.[10]

Methocarbamol

This drug, which is believed to act primarily at the interneurons of the spinal cord, blocks multisynaptic reflexes.[6]

CLINICAL PRESENTATION AND LIFE-THREATENING COMPLICATIONS

The ingestion of pure centrally acting muscle relaxants is generally associated with low morbidity and mortality. The clinical manifestation of overdose is predominantly CNS depression. The available data on the clinical toxicology of these agents are relatively sparse, but several investigators have described their experience with certain members of this class. Logan and colleagues[18] compiled a series of 104 incidents of impaired driving in which the drugs carisoprodol and/or its metabolite meprobamate (used alone as an anxiolytic) were detected in the blood of drivers. Reports of erratic driving and symptoms consistent with CNS depression were common but may have been attributable to coingestion of ethanol. In 21 cases, however, such behavior was witnessed in the absence of drugs other than carisoprodol or meprobamate. A retrospective review of carisoprodol-related deaths in Jefferson County, Alabama, over a nearly 12-year period found that the skeletal muscle relaxant was present in 24 cases. Although the mechanism of death in 82% of these cases was respiratory depression, consistent with the action of carisoprodol, the drug was never the only one detected at autopsy and was never determined to be the sole cause of death. Of note, propoxyphene was present in a third of the cases.[19] Carisoprodol has been reported in three cases of illicit use in which it was combined with the nonopioid, nonsteroidal tramadol.[20] Carisoprodol has also been implicated in a case report of myoclonic encephalopathy. After the ingestion of 35 g of carisoprodol, agitation, tachycardia and myoclonus developed in a 39-year-old man. His plasma carisoprodol concentration was 71 mg/L, and the meprobamate concentration was 118 μmol/L (26 mg/L).[21]

In cases of cyclobenzaprine or orphenadrine overdose, an anticholinergic syndrome may be the predominant clinical manifestation (this syndrome is discussed in Chapter 22). In a 5-year review of cyclobenzaprine exposure,[22] toxicity appeared to be related primarily to anticholinergic effects, even if overdoses did not produce the neurologic and cardiovascular toxicity of the structurally related tricyclic antidepressants. Neurologic and cardiovascular complications may follow an overdose of orphenadrine. In a case report, a 3-year-old boy ingested an unknown quantity of orphenadrine and presented with tonic-clonic seizures and ventricular tachycardia.[23] A 2-year-old girl who ingested 400 mg also presented with seizures and an episode of ventricular tachycardia; her initial plasma orphenadrine concentration was 3.55 mg/L.[24]

In a case series of severe meprobamate poisoning, coma, hypotension, and hypothermia complicated the clinical course in four patients, and one required resuscitation after cardiac arrest. Peak plasma concentrations ranged from 800 to 923 μmol/L (176 to 203 mg/L) (therapeutic, 28 to 55 μmol/L [6 to 12 mg/L]). Three were treated with charcoal hemoperfusion (see later). All four survived without sequelae.[25]

Dependence and Withdrawal

Patients who are prescribed carisoprodol are at risk to become dependent on its metabolite meprobamate. In an uncontrolled Norwegian study of prisoners who had been taking carisoprodol for a minimum of 9 months, abstinence symptoms, including anxiety, insomnia, irritability, headache, and muscular pain, were observed when the drug was withdrawn over a 2-week period. No seizures or psychoses were noted.[26]

DIAGNOSIS

The diagnosis of skeletal muscle relaxant overdose depends primarily on the history and physical examination.

Some hospital laboratories may be able to detect or even measure concentrations, for example, of carisoprodol or meprobamate, but it is more likely, particularly in smaller hospitals, that outside reference laboratories must be contacted to arrange these assays. Furthermore, the screening immunoassays commonly used by hospital clinical laboratories may indicate false-positive results for tricyclic antidepressants if cyclobenzaprine is present. Cyclobenzaprine and its metabolite norcyclobenzaprine are among a number of polycyclic compounds that may cross-react with tricyclic antidepressants on immunoassay or high-performance liquid chromatography of blood, and cyclobenzaprine may have the same effect on a colloidal metal immunoassay of urine.[14,27] Although the cholinergic agent physostigmine may theoretically serve as a diagnostic tool in cases of cyclobenzaprine or orphenadrine overdose, it may cause seizures or asystole if given too rapidly.[16] With cautious administration, however, it is a relatively safe drug. The clinical pharmacology and cautions regarding its use are described in Chapter 153.

TREATMENT

The cornerstone of treatment of toxicity with these agents is supportive care.

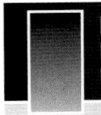

Gastrointestinal Decontamination

If a patient is seen shortly after ingestion, administration of activated charcoal may theoretically decrease drug absorption. However, there is no evidence that the administration of activated charcoal will affect either the clinical course or outcome. A complete discussion of gastrointestinal decontamination may be found in Chapter 5.

Extracorporeal Removal Techniques

Meprobamate has a small volume of distribution and limited protein binding; it is moderately dialyzable. In the case series of severe meprobamate poisoning noted earlier, charcoal hemoperfusion performed in three patients reduced the plasma half-life as much as threefold, from 8.3 to 2.6 hours.[25] Data concerning the efficacy of other centrally acting muscle relaxants are limited, although extracorporeal removal techniques would not be expected to significantly hasten the removal of agents with large volumes of distribution and/or extensive protein binding.

Flumazenil

Carisoprodol and its active metabolite meprobamate act as indirect GABA$_A$ agonists and, like the benzodiazepines, enhance GABA-mediated CNS neuronal chloride ion channel opening, thereby inducing hyperpolarization (see Figs. 138-2 and 138-3). Flumazenil was reported to reverse CNS depression in a woman who had a Glasgow Coma Scale score of 9 after carisoprodol ingestion. Her respirations were shallow at 18 breaths/min, and her pupils were reactive at 2 mm. She received two 2-mg naloxone doses without effect. Ten minutes later, she received flumazenil (0.2 mg intravenously over a period of 2 minutes), and within 2 minutes, she became more alert, with somewhat dysarthric speech. A second dose 5 minutes later normalized her mental status completely within 2 minutes.[2] Rarely reported in overdose, chlorzoxazone was cited in one case report of a patient who became comatose on two occasions after toxic ingestion of this skeletal muscle relaxant. Although the patient had only therapeutic to subtherapeutic benzodiazepine levels present, flumazenil was used and appeared to at least transiently reverse the CNS depression of chlorzoxazone.[4] The presence of an unrecognized benzodiazepine may explain the observed effect of flumazenil. Based on the aforementioned case reports, however, routine use of flumazenil is not recommended in the management of overdose, particularly if the patient has been taking any of these agents chronically. A complete discussion of the clinical pharmacology of flumazenil may be found in Chapter 138.

Physostigmine

Although case reports[23,24] of orphenadrine overdose attribute the resolution of ventricular tachycardia to physostigmine, the empirical use of this potentially toxic cholinergic agent should not precede the institution of standardized protocols for dysrhythmias.

Prevention and Treatment of Carisoprodol or Meprobamate Withdrawal

The authors of the Norwegian study noted earlier suggested that a gradual reduction in carisoprodol dosing may prevent withdrawal symptoms.[26] Similarly, if chronically administered carisoprodol or meprobamate is discontinued abruptly, prompt resumption of drug treatment may prevent withdrawal.

Criteria for ICU Discharge in Poisoning by Centrally Acting Muscle Relaxants

Patient awake with adequate airway protection
Patient otherwise stable

Key Points in Skeletal Muscle Relaxant Overdose

1. Consider skeletal muscle relaxant overdose in patients with anticholinergic signs such as hyperthermia, disorientation, hallucinations, delirium, seizures, sinus tachycardia, and mydriatic pupils.
2. Consider skeletal muscle relaxant overdose in patients with hypotension, bradycardia, depressed respirations, areflexia, hypotonia, myoclonic encephalopathy, or rapid onset of coma.
3. Most cases resolve with supportive care only.
4. Appropriate resumption of drug treatment may prevent carisoprodol/meprobamate withdrawal.

REFERENCES

1. Berger FM, Kletzkin M, Ludwig BJ, et al: Unusual muscle relaxant properties of *N*-isopropyl-2-methyl-2-propyl-1,3-propanediol dicarbamate (carisoprodol). J Pharmacol Exp Ther 127:66–74, 1959.
2. Roberge RJ, Lin E, Krenzelok EP: Flumazenil reversal of carisoprodol (Soma) intoxication. J Emerg Med 18:61–64, 2000.
3. Council on Drugs: New and non-official drugs: Chlorzoxazone (Paraflex). JAMA 170:195, 1959.
4. Roberge RJ, Atchley B, Ryan K, Krenzelok EP: Two chlorzoxazone (Parafon forte) overdoses and coma in one patient: Reversal with flumazenil. Am J Emerg Med 16:393–395, 1998.
5. Li JR: Methocarbamol in the treatment of black widow spider poisoning. JAMA 173:662, 1960.
6. Leventen EO, Vaccarino FP: Intravenous methocarbamol in 100 orthopaedic patients. Curr Ther Res 2:497–500, 1960.
7. O'Neil MJ, Smith A, Heckelman PE, Obenchain JR (eds): The Merck Index: An Encyclopedia of Chemicals, Drugs, and Biologicals, ed 13. Whitehouse Station, NJ, Merck & Co, 2001.
8. DiFrancesco A: Diazepam, a new tranquilizer. Am J Psychiatry 119: 989–990, 1963.
9. Baselt RC: Disposition of Toxic Drugs and Chemicals in Man, ed 5. Foster City, CA, Chemical Toxicology Institute, 2000.
10. Fathie K: A second look at a skeletal muscle relaxant: A double-blind study of metaxalone. Curr Ther Res 6:677–683, 1964.
11. Ashby P, Burke D, Rao S, Jones RF: Assessment of cyclobenzaprine in treatment of spasticity. J Neurol Neurosurg Psychiatry 35:599–605, 1972.
12. Share NN, McFarlane CS: Cyclobenzaprine: A novel centrally acting skeletal muscle relaxant. Neuropharmacology 14:675–684, 1975.
13. Lebby TI, Dugger K, Lipscomb JW, Leikin JB: Skeletal muscle relaxant ingestion. Vet Hum Toxicol 32:133–135, 1990.
14. Data on file, Flexeril (cyclobenzaprine). West Point, PA, Merck & Co, 1999.
15. Slordal L, Gjerden P: Orphenadrine [letter]. Br J Psychiatry 174: 275–276, 1999.
16. Leikin JB, Paloucek FP (eds): Poisoning & Toxicology Compendium. Hudson, OH, Lexi-Comp, 1998.
17. Data on file, Skelaxin (metaxalone). Cedar Knolls, NJ, Carnrick Laboratories, 1998.
18. Logan BK, Case GA, Gordon AM: Carisoprodol, meprobamate, and driving impairment. J Forensic Sci 45:619–623, 2000.
19. Davis GG, Alexander CB: A review of carisoprodol deaths in Jefferson County, Alabama. South Med J 91:726–730, 1998.
20. Reeves RR, Liberto V: Abuse of combinations of carisoprodol and tramadol. South Med J 94:512–514, 2001.
21. Roth BA, Vinson DR, Kim S: Carisoprodol-induced myoclonic encephalopathy. J Toxicol Clin Toxicol 36:609–612, 1998.
22. Spiller HA, Winter ML, Mann KV, et al: Five-year multicenter retrospective review of cyclobenzaprine toxicity. J Emerg Med 13:781–785, 1995.
23. Danze LK, Langdorf MI: Reversal of orphenadrine-induced ventricular tachycardia with physostigmine. J Emerg Med 9:453–457, 1991.
24. Van Herreweghe I, Mertens K, Maes V, Ramet J: Orphenadrine poisoning in a child: Clinical and analytical data. Intensive Care Med 25:1134–1136, 1999.
25. Jacobsen D, Wiik-Larsen E, Saltvedt E, Bredesen JE: Meprobamate kinetics during and after terminated hemoperfusion in acute intoxications, J Toxicol Clin Toxicol 25:317–331, 1987.
26. Wyller TB, Korsmo G, Gadeholt G: Dependence on carisoprodol (Somadril)? A prospective withdrawal study among prisoners. Tidsskr Nor Laegeforen 111:193–195, 1991.
27. Matos ME, Burns MM, Shannon MW: False-positive tricyclic antidepressant drug screen results leading to the diagnosis of carbamazepine intoxication. Pediatrics 105(5):E66, 2000.

CHAPTER 54

Anti-Parkinson's Medications

Kenneth D. Katz ■ Kevin L. Wallace

Parkinson's disease, named after James Parkinson, who first described the disorder in 1817, is a chronic, progressive neurologic disorder, clinically characterized by a combination of tremor, rigidity, and bradykinesia.[1,2] Estimates of the incidence of Parkinson's disease range from 5 to 20 new cases per 100,000 individuals per year, occurring with a slightly greater frequency in middle-aged and elderly men of European and North American descent.[1,3] The cause of Parkinson's disease is unknown, but it has been observed in humans and induced in primates by exposure to 1-methyl-4-phenylpyridine (MPP^+), a metabolite of 1-methyl-4-phenyl-1,2,3,6-tetrahydropyridine (MPTP), which poisons complex I of the mitochondrial electron transport chain (Fig. 54-1).[4] Other risk factors associated with the development of Parkinson's disease include oxidant stress, reduced glutathione stores, smoking (linked inversely to the development of Parkinson's disease), and caffeine consumption (correlated with reduced risk).[3,4] Current scientific evidence suggests that Parkinson's disease does not have a substantial genetic component.[3]

Pars compacta neurons located in the substantia nigra are responsible for dopaminergic input to the striatum, located within the basal ganglia (Figs. 54-2 and 54-3). Dopamine activates excitatory D_1-receptors in the striatum in a direct (monosynaptic) pathway and inhibits inhibitory striatal D_2-receptors in an indirect (polysynaptic) pathway (Table 54-1). With loss of dopaminergic nigral cells and subsequent striatal dopamine depletion, there is decreased activity of the direct pathway and increased activity of the indirect pathway. The net result of dopamine loss is reduced thalamic excitation of the motor cortex, resulting in the clinical manifestations of Parkinson's disease.[1,5]

The hallmark clinical features of Parkinson's disease are resting tremor, cogwheel rigidity, and bradykinesia. Patients with Parkinson's disease may manifest other motor signs and symptoms, including masked facies and gait abnormalities. Nonmotor signs and symptoms, such as sensory abnormalities, autonomic dysfunction, dementia, and depression, also are characteristic.[1]

Medical treatment of patients with Parkinson's disease can be categorized as either symptomatic or preventive. Symptomatic therapy involves administration of medications, including levodopa/carbidopa, anticholinergics/antihistamines, amantadine, dopamine agonists (e.g., bromocriptine), monoamine oxidase (MAO) B inhibitors (e.g., selegiline, rasagiline mesylate), catechol O-methyltransferase (COMT) inhibitors (e.g., entacapone), antidepressants, and atypical antipsychotics. Preventive treatment is targeted at slowing or halting the development and progression of the disease and includes medications such as MAO B inhibitors, dopamine agonists, antioxidants, antiinflammatories, and antiapoptotic agents. This chapter provides an overview of the various classes of medications commonly implemented to treat patients with Parkinson's disease and the tools with which to evaluate and treat toxicities associated with these medications in the critical care setting. Because patients who experience the toxic effects of anti-Parkinson's medications frequently are elderly, the clinical care provider is well advised to consider the toxicity risks associated with advanced age (see Chapter 12).

LEVODOPA/CARBIDOPA

Levodopa (L-3,4-dihydroxyphenylalanine) (Fig. 54-4), an amino acid, is the metabolic precursor of all catecholamines and normally is produced from tyrosine by the action of tyrosine hydroxylase (Fig. 54-5). It is decarboxylated to dopamine by dopa decarboxylase.[6] It has been stated: "Levodopa is the most reliable and effective symptomatic treatment for Parkinson's disease. Almost all patients with true idiopathic Lewy-body Parkinson's disease respond to levodopa treatment. Indeed, failure to respond suggests an alternative diagnosis."[4] Treatment of Parkinson's patients with levodopa is associated with decreased morbidity and mortality compared with treatment in the "pre-levodopa era."[2]

Pharmacokinetics

Levodopa is well absorbed from the gastrointestinal tract, but its bioavailability may be limited by many factors. Coingestion of other relatively large amino acids hinders levodopa absorption via saturation of the amino acid transport system in the proximal small intestine. Additionally, gut wall decarboxylase metabolizes 50% to 75% of orally administered levodopa before it reaches the systemic circulation. Delayed gastric emptying, which may occur with consumption of large meals or concomitantly administered anticholinergic medications, delays drug delivery to the small intestine and retards the onset of peak plasma concentrations.[6]

The volume of distribution of levodopa is approximately 0.9 to 1.6 mg/kg, with an apparent half-life of 0.78 to 1.74 hours. It is metabolized in the periphery by COMT to the inactive metabolite 3-O-methyldopa (3-OMD) and is excreted primarily in the urine as unchanged dopa and in the form of several metabolites, including homovanillic acid and dopamine.[6]

Levodopa penetrates the blood-brain barrier effectively. When given alone, however, levodopa is decarboxylated

Blood

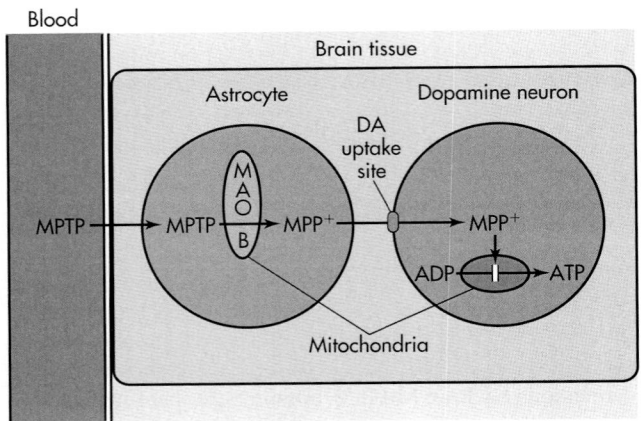

FIGURE 54-1

Mechanism of 1-methyl-4-phenyl-1,2,3,6-tetrahydropyridine (MPTP)–induced degeneration of nigrostriatal dopamine neurons. MPTP is converted by monoamine oxidase B (MAO-B) within astrocytes or other nondopaminergic neurons to the reactive intermediate 1-methyl-4-phenylpyridine (MPP⁺). MPP⁺ is taken up into the dopaminergic neuron by the dopamine (DA) transporter. Within the dopaminergic neuron, MPP⁺ acts on mitochondria to inhibit mitochondrial respiration, which results in cell death. ADP, adenosine diphosphate; ATP, adenosine triphosphate. *(From Gudelsky GA: Drugs for the treatment of Parkinson's disease. In Brody TM, Larner J, Minneman KP [eds]: Human Pharmacology: Molecular to Clinical, 3rd ed. St. Louis, Mosby, 1998, p 386.)*

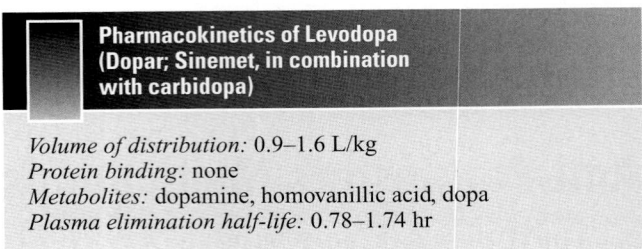

Pharmacokinetics of Levodopa (Dopar; Sinemet, in combination with carbidopa)

Volume of distribution: 0.9–1.6 L/kg
Protein binding: none
Metabolites: dopamine, homovanillic acid, dopa
Plasma elimination half-life: 0.78–1.74 hr

nearly completely in the peripheral circulation to dopamine, which does not penetrate the blood-brain barrier. In addition, common gastrointestinal side effects of levodopa, such as nausea and vomiting, occur secondary to the conversion of dopa to dopamine in the periphery and resultant dopamine-mediated stimulation of postrema areas not protected by the blood-brain barrier.[2] Coadministration of a dopa decarboxylase inhibitor, such as carbidopa or benserazide, minimizes peripheral conversion of levodopa to dopamine, promoting penetration of dopa to the brain and minimizing untoward gastrointestinal effects.[7] Another benefit gained from dopa decarboxylase inhibitor administration is the 70% to 80% reduction in daily levodopa dose needed for clinical efficacy.[6]

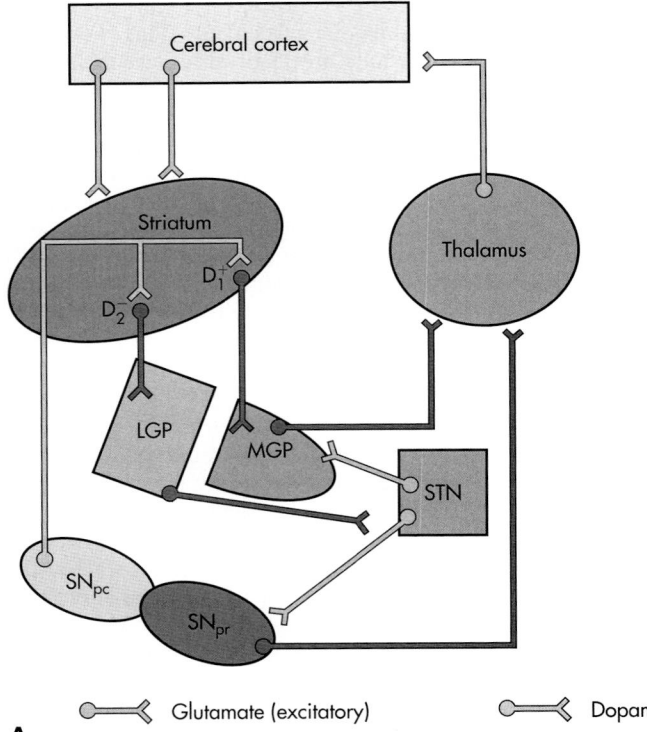

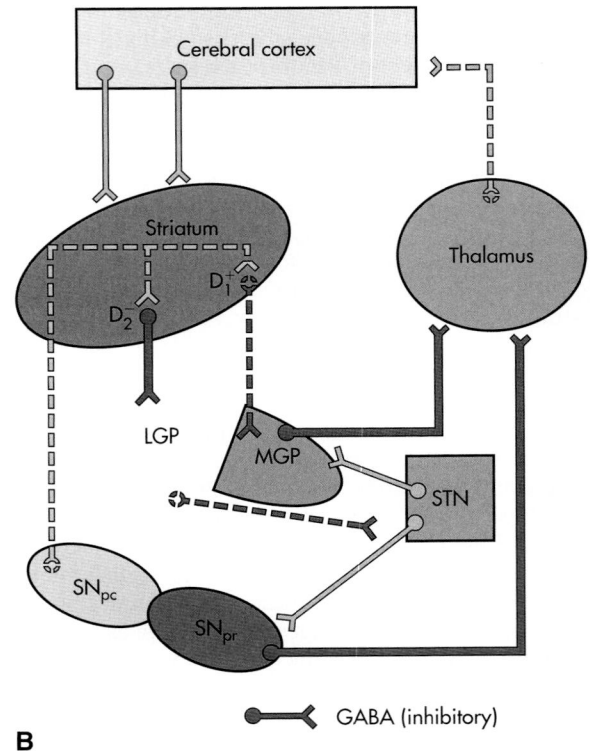

FIGURE 54-2

Parkinson's disease and the neural circuitry of the basal ganglia. **A**, The striatum is the principal input structure of the basal ganglia. Striatal D₁-receptors mediate an excitation of a direct-output pathway to the medial globus pallidus (MGP). Striatal D₂-receptors mediate an inhibition of an indirect-output pathway projecting through the lateral globus pallidus (LGP) and subthalamic nucleus (STN) to the substantia nigra pars reticulata (SNpr) and MGP. **B**, Loss of dopaminergic input to the striatum resulting from degeneration of nigrostriatal dopamine neurons results in a decrease in the activity of the direct-output pathway and an increased activity of the indirect-output pathway. The net effect is an increased inhibitory outflow from the SNpr and MGP to the thalamus. This outflow ultimately results in reduced excitatory input to the cerebral cortex. Thin lines, normal neuronal activity; dashed lines, reduced activity; thick lines, increased activity; SNpc, substantia nigra pars compacta. *(From Gudelsky GA: Drugs for the treatment of Parkinson's disease. In Brody TM, Larner J, Minneman KP [eds]: Human Pharmacology: Molecular to Clinical, 3rd ed. St. Louis, Mosby, 1998, p 390.)*

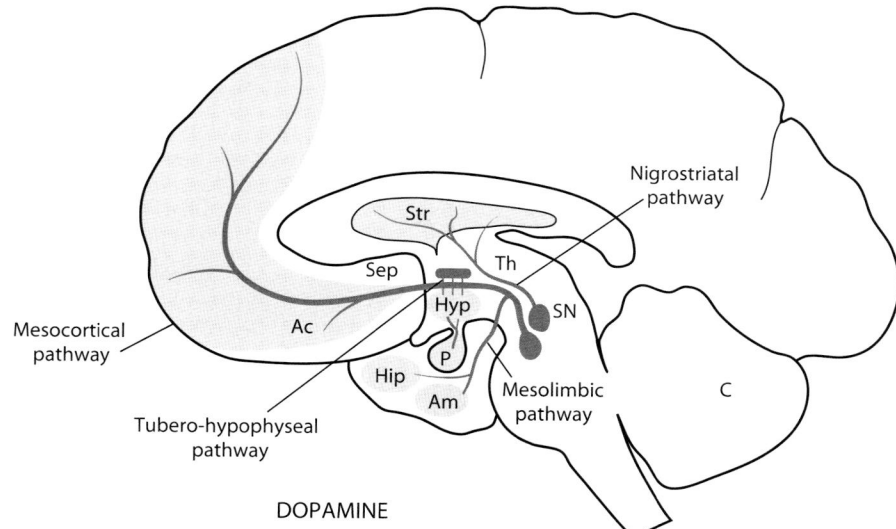

FIGURE 54-3

Dopamine pathways in the brain. Ac, nucleus accumbens; Am, amygdaloid nucleus; C, cerebellum; Hip, hippocampus; Hyp, hypothalamus; P, pituitary; Sep, septum; SN, substantia nigra; Str, corpus striatum; Th, thalamus. *(From Rang HP, Dale MM, Ritter JM, Gardner P: Other transmitters and modulators. In Pharmacology, 4th ed. Philadelphia, Churchill Livingstone, 2001, p 486.)*

Clinical Presentation

ADVERSE EFFECTS

Patients receiving therapeutic doses of levodopa commonly experience anorexia, nausea, and vomiting thought to be mediated by dopaminergic stimulation of the medullary emetic center.[8] Because dopamine is an active catecholamine possessing α-adrenergic and β-adrenergic agonist properties, administration of levodopa may cause tachycardia, cardiac dysrhythmia, hypertension, and, later, orthostatic hypotension.[8] Additionally, patients receiving levodopa may develop behavioral disturbances, including confusion, delirium, hallucinations, anxiety, and depression.[8] Long-standing use of levodopa may result in the development of dyskinesias, such as chorea, dystonia, and myoclonus. Levodopa-induced dyskinesia occurs in approximately 50% to 75% of Parkinson's patients after 5 to 10 years of therapy.[9] The mechanism of the dyskinesia has been suggested to be related to pulsatile stimulation of striatal dopamine receptors, with a resulting "down-flow supersensitivity."[10]

Levodopa is a phenylethamine compound and is structurally related to other central nervous system (CNS) stimulants and

TABLE 54-1 Dopamine Receptors

		D₁ TYPE		D₂ TYPE		
		D_1	D_5	D_2	D_3	D_4
Distribution	**Functional Role**					
Cortex	Arousal, mood	++	−	++	−	−
Limbic system	Emotion, stereotypical behavior	+++	−	+++	+	+
Basal ganglia	Motor control	++	+	+++	+	+
Hypothalamus	Autonomic and endocrine control	++	+	−	−	−
Pituitary gland	Endocrine control	−	−	+++	−	−
Agonists	Dopamine	+ (low potency)			+ (high potency)	
	Apomorphine	PA (low potency)			+ (high potency)	
	Bromocriptine	PA (low potency)			+ (high potency)	
Antagonists	Chlorpromazine	+	+	+++	+++	+
	Haloperidol	++	+	+++	+++	+++
	Spiperone	−	−	+++	+++	+++
	Sulpiride	−	−	+++	++	−
	Clozapine	+	+	+	+	++
Signal Transduction		Increase cyclic AMP		Decrease cyclic AMP and/or increase IP₃		
Effect		Mainly postsynaptic inhibition		Pre- and postsynaptic inhibition Stimulation/inhibition of hormone release		

AMP, adenosine monophosphate; IP₃, inositol 1,4,5-trisphosphate; PA, partial agonist.
From Rang HP, Dale MM, Ritter JM, Gardner P: Other transmitters and modulators. In Pharmacology, 4th ed. Philadelphia, Churchill Livingstone, 2001, p 486.

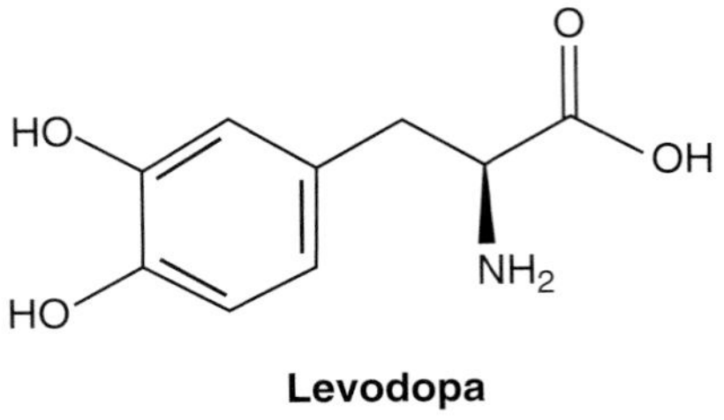

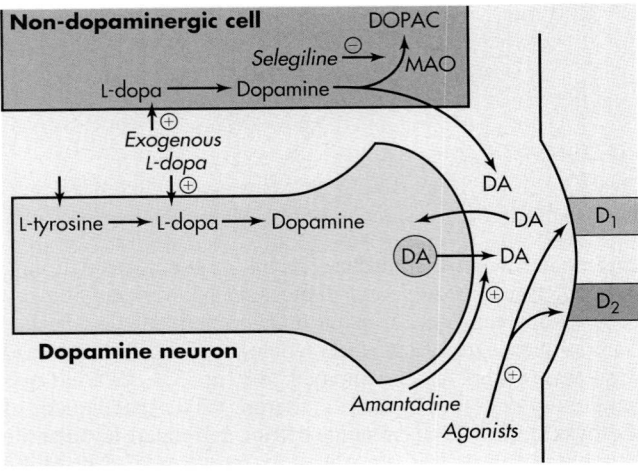

FIGURE 54-4

Chemical structure of levodopa.

FIGURE 54-5

Sites of action of antiparkinsonian agents to facilitate dopaminergic function. Levodopa (L-dopa) enhances the synthesis and ultimately the release of dopamine (DA). Amantadine facilitates the release of dopamine. Dopamine agonists directly activate dopamine receptors (D$_1$ and D$_2$) on the postsynaptic cell. Selegiline inhibits the metabolism of dopamine in nondopaminergic neurons or glia or both. *(From Gudelsky GA: Drugs for the treatment of Parkinson's disease. In Brody TM, Larner J, Minneman KP [eds]: Human Pharmacology: Molecular to Clinical, 3rd ed. St. Louis, Mosby, 1998, p 388.)*

sympathomimetic drugs (e.g., amphetamine). Similar to other drugs in this class, levodopa is subject to abuse, which is well described in Parkinson's patients who desire a particular psychological benefit from the medication.[11] Slow discontinuation and then reintroduction of levodopa to the desired clinical end point may prove successful in treating this problem.

Significant drug-drug interactions with levodopa are uncommon, but any substance or medication that alters gastric motility or emptying (e.g., presence of food, anticholinergic medications) may change levodopa absorption and plasma concentrations. Penicillamine increases plasma levodopa levels by greater than 50% by enhancing levodopa absorption.[12] Several other drugs have been shown to accentuate the clinical manifestations of Parkinson's disease and may interfere with levodopa therapy. Reserpine and tetrabenazine can reduce dopaminergic function by depleting presynaptic dopamine stores and may compromise and interfere with levodopa's efficacy. Methyldopa, after conversion to methyldopamine by dopa decarboxylase in presynaptic dopaminergic nerve terminals, can serve as a partial dopamine agonist and can competitively interfere with levodopa at the D$_2$ dopamine receptor. Additionally, coadministration of dopamine-blocking agents, such as high-potency neuroleptics or metoclopramide, can offset levodopa efficacy

and exacerbate manifestations of the underlying Parkinson's disease. Calcium channel–blocking agents (flunarizine, verapamil, diltiazem, amlodipine, manidipine) also may exacerbate parkinsonism due to interference with presynaptic striatal dopamine release.[12] Several other medications, including amiodarone, valproic acid, vigabatrin, cytosine, methotrexate, dacarbazine, cisapride, meperidine, isoniazid, and amoxapine, may cause or worsen parkinsonism.[12]

There is a hypothetical concern regarding levodopa neurotoxicity after long-term administration resulting from the propensity of the drug, once metabolized, to form oxygen free radicals. This potentially toxic phenomenon has been shown in vitro but has not been substantiated clinically.[2,13]

OVERDOSE AND TOXICITY

Although the adverse effects of levodopa therapy are well described, there is a relative paucity of literature describing acute levodopa overdose. Hoehn and Rutledge[14] described a 61-year-old Parkinson's patient who ingested approximately 100 g of levodopa and presented with marked confusion, agitation, some "jerking movements," restlessness, and initial hypertension followed by orthostatic hypotension. The effects of the acute overdose lasted nearly 1 week, and the patient did well with supportive care. A case report of a woman with no previous history of Parkinson's disease who ingested approximately 15 to 17 tablets of Sinemet (levodopa/carbidopa), ibuprofen, carisoprodol, and hydrocodone/acetaminophen described her as lethargic with choreiform movements. These choreiform movements were unaffected by administration of morphine sulfate and diazepam; pancuronium was administered intermittently for almost 60 hours until the patient's dyskinesias resolved. She was treated supportively and recovered without apparent sequelae.[15]

Additionally, Parkinson's patients can present not only after levodopa overdose but also with other levodopa-induced problems. Dyskinesias and motor fluctuations are common late complications of Parkinson's disease and may be related not only to progression of disease but also to fluctuations in serum levodopa concentrations.[16] Levodopa-induced dyskinesias may be ballistic, dystonic, myoclonic, or choreoathetotic and can affect any muscle group, including muscles involved with ventilatory function. Motor fluctuations range from "on," stable intervals, during which Parkinson's symptoms are controlled, to "off" periods, when the patient may experience disabling immobility, tremor, or postural instability. In addition, during the off periods, nonmotor features, such as autonomic instability, confusion, anxiety, and, rarely, neuroleptic malignant syndrome, from relative lack of central dopamine may be seen.[16] Several emergent complications may arise from these various disorders, including rhabdomyolysis and respiratory failure from aspiration or ineffective ventilation.

Acute dystonic reactions and neuroleptic malignant syndrome, thought to stem from D$_2$-receptor antagonism, can be seen in patients in whom levodopa is withdrawn abruptly. This syndrome generally responds to reinstitution of levodopa therapy.[17] Neuroleptic malignant syndrome is discussed in detail in Chapter 26.

Diagnosis

The initial diagnostic approach to a poisoned patient relies heavily on the history and physical examination. For a patient who has overdosed, it is recommended that several initial laboratory studies be obtained, including serum electrolytes, a serum acetaminophen assay level, and an electrocardiogram (ECG). Occasionally a blood salicylate determination or a urine toxicologic assay may be deemed necessary. The general diagnostic considerations in the evaluation of overdose patients are discussed in Chapter 2. The toxicologic differential diagnosis is broad and includes poisoning by sympathomimetic agents (e.g., amphetamine [see Chapter 73]), salicylates (see Chapter 57), or thyroid hormone.

In the case of acute ingestion of levodopa, the diagnosis is reached primarily by history and physical examination. Stuerenburg and Schoser[18] reported the value of measuring plasma concentrations of levodopa and 3-OMD (resulting from the ortho-methylation of levodopa) to the diagnosis and care of a patient who overdosed on levodopa/carbidopa.[18] Hoehn and Rutledge[14] reported the utility of measuring levodopa metabolites, such as dopamine dihydroxyphenylacetic acid, homovanillic acid, and norepinephrine, in urine to confirm levodopa exposure and to follow the eventual clearance of levodopa as it parallels clinical improvement. The availability of these assays in most clinical care settings is limited, however, and they are not essential to patient management, which is almost entirely supportive.

Parkinson's patients presenting with possible levodopa-induced clinical findings should be evaluated for other nontoxicologic diagnoses, such as sepsis. An infectious disorder, such as pneumonia or urinary tract infection, or another systemic disease process, such as congestive heart failure, can alter the patient's sensitivity to levodopa, triggering fluctuation in motor function.[16] Appropriate diagnostic and laboratory tests should be tailored to the individual clinical presentation and may include an ECG, chest radiograph (also needed for aspiration concerns), complete blood count, blood cultures, cardiac enzymes, and a urinalysis. Additionally, severe dyskinesia and neuroleptic malignant syndrome may promote rhabdomyolysis and myoglobinuric renal injury; serum creatine phosphokinase, electrolytes, blood urea nitrogen, and creatinine concentrations should be considered among the laboratory values obtained. Given the increased risk for thromboembolic disease in chronically immobilized patients, noninvasive vascular studies, such as lower extremity Doppler ultrasound, may be indicated.

Treatment

Treatment of the acutely levodopa-poisoned patient is largely supportive. The experience with levodopa overdose is extraordinarily limited, and suggestions regarding management of toxicity are based mainly on theoretical concerns. In the few instances of levodopa overdose that are documented in the medical literature, patients did well with supportive care alone.

As in all poisonings, attention initially should be focused on the patient's airway and circulatory status. If agitation is severe and uncontrollable, the airway should be secured by endotracheal intubation. A dose of oral activated charcoal may reduce further systemic drug absorption when administered within the first few hours of ingestion. It is unknown, however, whether the administration of activated charcoal alters the clinical course or outcome in these patients. There is no published evidence to support efficacy or clinical benefit of gastric lavage.

Hypertension has been described in the acute phase of levodopa overdose and generally has been transient.[14,15] If hypertension is persistent and severe, however, we prefer intravenous sodium nitroprusside over β-blockers because of the theoretical concern for unopposed α-adrenergic effects of levodopa poisoning. Hypotension should be treated initially with intravenous crystalloid; then, if hypotension is persistent, with intravenous vasopressor infusion. Catecholamines with relative α-adrenergic potency generally are preferred because dopamine-induced, β-adrenergically mediated vasodilation may occur in patients with hypotension refractory to volume resuscitation.

Agitation and dyskinesia may be managed initially with intravenous benzodiazepines, such as lorazepam or diazepam, titrated to mild sedation. If necessary, neuromuscular blockade may be implemented for control of extreme movement disorder or severe combativeness.

Treatment of other acute, subacute, or chronic manifestations of levodopa poisoning should be carried out on the basis of the specific presentation. Associated medical illness (e.g., infection) always must be considered and treated expeditiously. Another essential facet of therapy is directed at modification of the patient's anti-Parkinson's maintenance regimen, which may include discontinuation or reduction of levodopa dosage during periods of dyskinesia or increased levodopa administration during clinical off periods. Additionally, implementation of other anti-Parkinson's medications (see later), such as dopamine agonists or COMT inhibitors, may be indicated, depending on the clinical situation. Benzodiazepines, such as lorazepam, and atypical neuroleptics (e.g., clozapine) may be helpful in reducing the severity of dyskinesia. In the case of Parkinson's patients with acute psychosis, all anti-Parkinson's medications should be withheld, and benzodiazepines should be given for agitation.[16] Standard neuroleptics probably should be avoided because of their proparkinsonian effects. Consultation with a neurologist is recommended when adjustments are being made to the patient's medications.

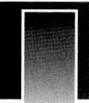

Indications for ICU Admission in Anti-Parkinson's Drug Toxicity

Levodopa/Carbidopa
Severe agitation
Autonomic instability
Altered level of consciousness
Uncontrollable movement disorder
Neuroleptic malignant syndrome

Key Points in the Evaluation and Treatment of Anti-Parkinson's Drug Toxicity

Levodopa/Carbidopa
1. Clinical toxicity is similar to that of sympathomimetic drugs (see Chapter 32), including delirium, dyskinesia, tachycardia, and hypertension.
2. Abrupt withdrawal after long-term administration may result in acute extrapyramidal manifestations.
3. Treatment of acute toxicity is mainly supportive.

ANTICHOLINERGIC AGENTS

Anticholinergic medications have been used in the treatment of Parkinson's disease dating to the mid-19th century and include trihexyphenidyl (Artane), procyclidine (Kemadrin), biperiden (Akineton), orphenadrine (Disipal, Norflex), and benztropine (Cogentin). The use of anticholinergic drugs in Parkinson's patients is directed at the imbalance between cholinergic and dopaminergic tone in their basal ganglia and is supported by their clinical efficacy. The anticholinergic agents employed are competitive antagonists at cholinergic muscarinic receptors throughout the body[19] and, in some cases, are inhibitors of dopamine reuptake, potentially exerting a dual action in restoring CNS neurotransmitter balance. The actual mechanism of action of anticholinergic medications in Parkinson's disease is uncertain, however.[2]

Pharmacokinetics

See Chapter 22 for a summary of the pharmacokinetics of anticholinergic agents. In general, anticholinergic anti-Parkinson's medications are well absorbed from the gastrointestinal tract, with peak plasma concentrations reached within 1 to 3 hours.[6] There are few published data regarding the distribution and metabolism of these drugs. Benz-hexol seems to follow a two-compartment model after ingestion with first-order terminal elimination kinetics.[6] Procyclidine may undergo "some first-pass metabolism, presumably in the liver, based on estimates of oral bioavailability."[6] Biperiden is eliminated via hepatic metabolism "with no unchanged drug being excreted in the urine."[6]

Some anticholinergic medications, such as benztropine and orphenadrine (Fig. 54-6), are structurally similar to the anti-

histamine diphenhydramine. Orphenadrine is the *O*-methyl analogue of diphenhydramine, allowing for prediction of additional toxicities (e.g., sodium channel blockade at high doses) based on shared structure-activity relationships.[6]

Clinical Presentation

ADVERSE EFFECTS

Adverse effects of anticholinergic medications are encountered commonly by patients and frequently limit their utility in clinical practice. This situation is particularly true in elderly patients, in whom side effects may be pronounced because of a myriad of concomitant physiologic perturbations (e.g., presence of dementia or autonomic insufficiency) and other prescribed medications. Central anticholinergic effects include confusion, memory difficulty, sedation, and hallucinations. Peripheral effects secondary to muscarinic inhibition include dry mouth, constipation, urinary retention, precipitation of glaucoma, blurry vision, anhidrosis, and tachycardia.[2,19]

With the exception of the potential effects of anticholinergic drug–induced gastrointestinal dysmotility on absorption of other drugs, pharmacokinetic drug-drug interactions generally are not clinically relevant to their use in Parkinson's patients. There are innumerable prescription and over-the-counter medications, however, that possess anticholinergic properties, adding to the adverse pharmacodynamic effects of these agents.

OVERDOSE AND TOXICITY

Intentional overdose and abuse of anticholinergic agents used to treat Parkinson's disease commonly are described in the medical literature. Drugs such as benztropine and

Procyclidine

Biperiden

Orphenadrine

Benztropine

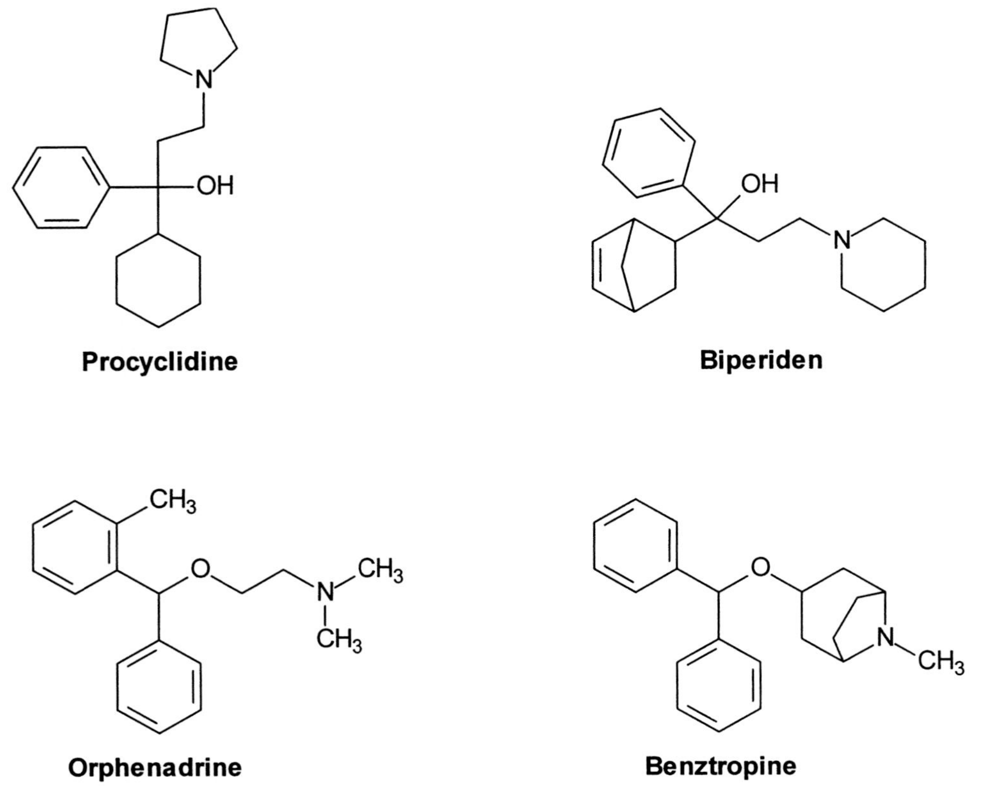

FIGURE 54-6

Chemical structures of procyclidine, biperiden, orphenadrine, and benztropine.

trihexyphenidyl are abused for their hallucinogenic and euphoric effects.[20]

The clinical presentation of anticholinergic toxicity results from blockade of central and peripheral muscarinic cholinergic receptors.[20,21] Confusion, hallucinations, incoherent speech, and agitation are hallmark central effects of anticholinergic drugs. The peripheral effects include hyperthermia, tachycardia, dry axillae, decreased bowel sounds, and urinary retention.[20,22] In addition, the antihistaminic properties of benztropine and orphenadrine may cause lethargy and sedation. Benztropine-induced dystonic and dyskinetic reactions, similar to those of antipsychotics, also have been reported.[23] The anticholinergic syndrome is described in detail in Chapter 22.

Special mention is warranted regarding orphenadrine poisoning. In addition to its antihistamine and anticholinergic properties, orphenadrine has relatively potent quinidine-like (i.e., sodium channel–blocking) effects on the cardiovascular system, with significant potential in overdose for producing cardiac conduction disturbances, depressed myocardial contractility, hypotension, and ventricular dysrhythmias.[24]

Diagnosis

The diagnosis of anticholinergic syndrome is based on a thorough history and careful physical examination, focusing on features that may distinguish acute antimuscarinic effects from features reflecting the presence of other toxidromes (e.g., hyperadrenergic states). In the case of acute overdose, measurement of serum electrolytes and acetaminophen concentrations is generally considered appropriate. Under some circumstances, additional diagnostic tests aimed at searching for coingestants may be indicated (see Chapter 22). An ECG should be performed to assess cardiac rhythm and the presence of significant interval (e.g., QRS or QT) prolongation, especially when dealing with orphenadrine poisoning.

Serum benztropine concentrations, although not readily obtainable in most clinical care settings, may be helpful in patients poisoned with this medication. Fahy and colleagues[22] reported following serial benztropine concentrations in a 38-year-old man who ingested a vial of 1-mg benztropine (Cogentin) tablets; levels peaked at 100 μg/L (325 μmol/mL), and anticholinergic symptoms persisted until the serum concentration reached 9 μg/L (29 μmol/mL).[22] A specific laboratory approach to anticholinergic poisoning may not only aid in the diagnosis of uncertain clinical presentations but also provide prognostic value.

Treatment

The treatment of anticholinergic syndrome is discussed in detail in Chapter 22. In general, meticulous supportive care, including maintenance of an airway, supplemental oxygen, intravenous fluids to correct intravascular volume deficits, cardiac monitoring, and bladder catheterization, is indicated in most patients with anticholinergic syndrome.[19,25] Particular attention should be focused on the detection of rhabdomyolysis secondary to agitation and impaired thermoregulation.[22]

Decontamination with activated charcoal theoretically is helpful because some anticholinergic medications, such as benztropine, undergo enterohepatic metabolism.[19] It is unknown, however, whether activated charcoal effectively

absorbs benztropine.[22] Physostigmine, a reversible inhibitor of central and peripheral cholinesterase activity, increases acetylcholine concentrations at nicotinic and muscarinic synapses.[19,21] This drug has been used not only as an aid in the diagnosis of anticholinergic syndrome but also in the control of its severe neuropsychiatric manifestations. Although most cases of anticholinergic syndrome can be treated successfully with supportive care alone, closely monitored, conservative administration of physostigmine may be beneficial in controlling severe anticholinergic agitation or convulsions or both.[22] Adverse effects of physostigmine include bronchospasm, seizures, and severe cardiac conduction abnormalities.[19,20] The clinical pharmacology of physostigmine is discussed in Chapter 153.

AMANTADINE

Amantadine (Fig. 54-7) is an antiviral drug that, by fortuitous discovery, was found to possess anti-Parkinson's efficacy. The mechanism of action of amantadine is unclear, but many actions have been suggested, including stimulation of catecholamine release, dopamine reuptake blockade, dopamine receptor stimulation, muscarinic antagonism, and *N*-methyl-D-aspartate receptor antagonism.[12] In clinical studies, amantadine administration has been found to alleviate akinesia, rigidity, and tremor in Parkinson's patients.[2]

Pharmacokinetics

Amantadine is well absorbed after oral administration.[26] The volume of distribution of amantadine is large, with estimates ranging from 6 to 10 L/kg, and it is believed to be highly protein bound.[6] The drug is not metabolized and is excreted unchanged in the urine through glomerular filtration and tubular secretion.[6] The plasma elimination half-life is approximately 12 to 18 hours in healthy adults. The half-life can increase twofold, however, in the elderly or in patients with renal insufficiency.[6,26]

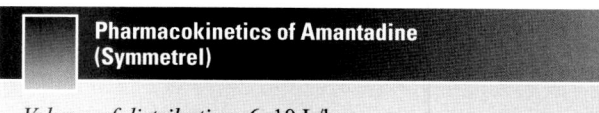

Pharmacokinetics of Amantadine (Symmetrel)

Volume of distribution: 6–10 L/kg
Protein binding: 0.67%
Metabolites: unchanged
Plasma elimination half-life: 12–18 hr

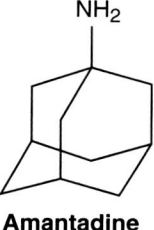

Amantadine

FIGURE 54-7

Chemical structure of amantadine.

Clinical Presentation

ADVERSE EFFECTS

The most common adverse effects experienced in patients taking amantadine are confusion, insomnia, hallucinations, and nightmares. Less troublesome side effects include ankle edema and livedo reticularis, which generally are well tolerated and do not limit treatment. Additionally, there may be acute worsening of Parkinson's disease when amantadine is withdrawn abruptly.[2] The adverse effects of long-term amantadine therapy may be exacerbated by coadministration of anticholinergics or drugs that reduce its renal clearance, such as hydrochlorothiazide/triamterene.[12]

OVERDOSE AND TOXICITY

The toxic effects of amantadine overdose principally involve the CNS and cardiovascular system. Patients typically present with agitation, psychosis, and restlessness, in addition to the other central and peripheral stigmata of anticholinergic poisoning (see Chapter 22).[27] Amantadine-induced coma has been reported.[28]

Cardiovascular effects of amantadine toxicity include hypotension, bradycardia, cardiac conduction defects, QT prolongation, malignant ventricular arrhythmias, and torsades de pointes. These findings may be explained by amantadine's tricyclic amine structure and similarity to tricyclic antidepressants.[29]

Diagnosis

Patients presenting with amantadine poisoning should be evaluated with routine laboratory tests and diagnostic studies previously mentioned for other anti-Parkinson's medications. Patients should be placed on a cardiac monitor and an ECG obtained to detect the initial presence or later development of significant QRS widening, QT prolongation, or dysrhythmia.

Serum amantadine concentrations have a confirmatory role in establishing the diagnosis of amantadine poisoning. Plasma concentrations greater than 1000 ng/mL (>6.6 nmol/mL) have been associated with CNS toxicity. The generally accepted therapeutic upper limit for this value is 300 ng/mL (2.0 nmol/mL).[26,30]

Treatment

Treatment of amantadine poisoning consists mainly of supportive care. Intravascular volume replacement should be initiated and maintained at a rate that supports adequate urine output. Amantadine-induced ventricular dysrhythmia should be managed pharmacologically, first with lidocaine in standard treatment doses; class IA antidysrhythmics should be

avoided because of their potential for exacerbation of cardiac conduction and repolarization abnormalities.[29] Torsades de pointes probably is managed best with parenteral magnesium sulfate or overdrive pacing. Isoproterenol should be avoided because it may worsen amantadine toxicity.[29] The onset of amantadine-induced cardiotoxicity may be delayed for 48 hours after ingestion; it is recommended that symptomatic patients undergo extended cardiac monitoring.[29]

Administration of oral activated charcoal may reduce systemic absorption of amantadine if given within the first few hours after ingestion. Multiple-dose activated charcoal treatment has been described anecdotally for amantadine toxicity 24 hours after ingestion[31]; however, it has not been subjected to further study in this setting and carries the risks associated with its use in anticholinergic poisoning (see Chapters 5 and 22). We do not recommend routine use of oral activated charcoal.

Physostigmine has been used successfully for control of severe amantadine-induced agitation.[32] The use of physostigmine may lead to cholinergic crisis, however. Because physostigmine has been associated with asystolic arrest in tricyclic antidepressant overdose, it should be avoided when significant cardiac conduction disturbance is evident.[31] A benzodiazepine, such as diazepam and lorazepam, would be the initial anticonvulsant of choice for amantadine-induced seizures.

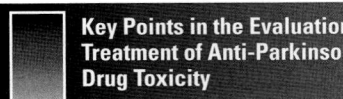

Key Points in the Evaluation and Treatment of Anti-Parkinson's Drug Toxicity

Amantadine
1. Major clinical manifestations of toxicity are anticholinergic syndrome, cardiac conduction disorder (e.g., QT prolongation), and ventricular dysrhythmia (e.g., torsades de pointes).
2. Administration of classes I and III antidysrhythmic drugs should be avoided.

SELEGILINE

MAO is responsible for the central (intraneuronal) and peripheral (intestinal and hepatic) degradation of dopamine (Fig. 54-8). The enzyme exists in two forms, A and B, and is found in the CNS and in peripheral tissue.[33] MAO A activity is found predominantly in the liver and intestine, and MAO B activity is found mainly in brain, liver, and platelets.[34] Irreversible and selective inhibition of MAO B by selegiline (Fig. 54-9) increases the duration of action of levodopa in Parkinson's patients and may increase the on time in advanced cases.[2] This action also may reduce levodopa dosing requirements.[2] Selective MAO B inhibition occurs at therapeutic doses (10 mg/day), but selectivity may be lost at higher doses.[12] Selegiline also is used as a potentially neuroprotective agent in Parkinson's patients based on its ability to block the MAO B–mediated oxidation of certain substrates (e.g., MPTP) to neurotoxic free radical species (e.g., MPP$^+$) (Fig. 54-10; see Fig. 54-1).[2] It has been speculated that administration of selegiline may retard striatal degeneration

Indications for ICU Admission in Anti-Parkinson's Drug Toxicity

Amantadine
Same as anticholinergic agents (see Chapter 22)
Cardiac dysrhythmia (especially QT prolongation, torsades de pointes)

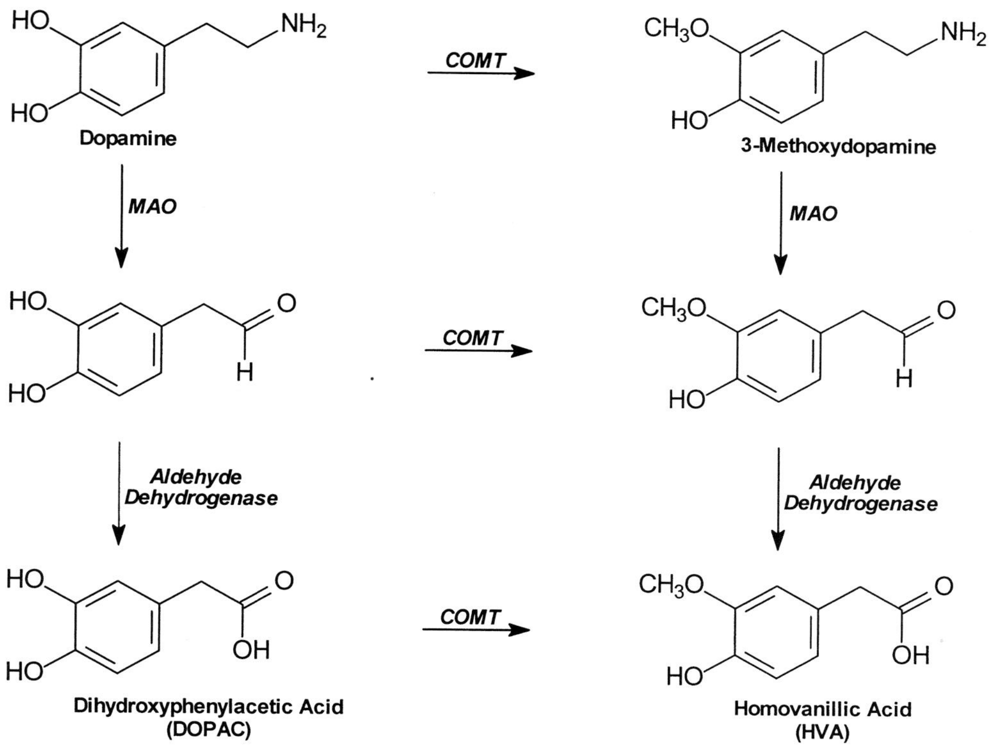

FIGURE 54-8

The main pathways for dopamine metabolism in the brain. COMT, catechol *O*-methyltransferase; MAO, monoamine oxidase.

Dopamine

3-Methoxydopamine

Dihydroxyphenylacetic Acid (DOPAC)

Homovanillic Acid (HVA)

in Parkinson's disease by inhibiting the formation of oxygen free radicals during CNS dopamine metabolism.[2]

Pharmacokinetics

Selegiline is absorbed rapidly after oral administration and attains peak serum concentration within 0.5 to 2 hours.[33] Selegiline has a volume of distribution of approximately 1.9 L/kg and exhibits an elimination half-life of approximately 2 hours.[35] The drug's major metabolites, L-methamphetamine and L-amphetamine, have longer half-lives of 29.5 and 17.7 hours, respectively.[36]

Pharmacokinetics of Selegiline (Eldepryl)

Volume of distribution: 1.9 L/kg
Protein binding: 94%
Metabolites: L-amphetamine, L-methamphetamine
Plasma elimination half-life: 2 hr

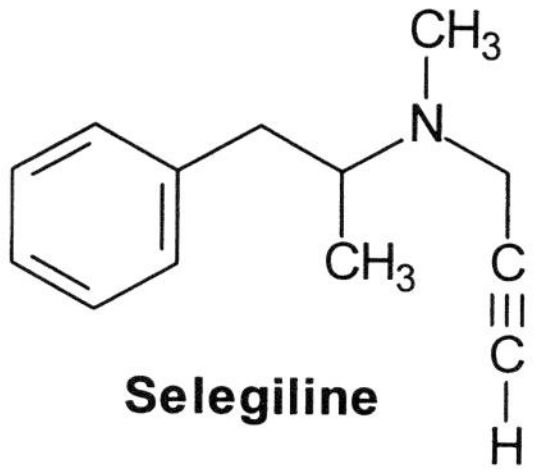

Selegiline

FIGURE 54-9

Chemical structure of selegiline.

Clinical Presentation

ADVERSE EFFECTS

Adverse effects of selegiline include CNS stimulation, insomnia, hallucinations, nausea, and vomiting. In addition, by inhibiting levodopa breakdown, selegiline may worsen levodopa-induced dyskinesia.[36] Orthostatic hypotension also has been reported with coadministration of selegiline and levodopa in Parkinson's patients.[37] Additionally, if taken at higher daily dosages, selegiline may inhibit MAO A and exhibit toxicities similar to those of the less selective antidepressant MAO inhibitors (see Chapter 43).

Case reports have described significant drug-drug interactions of selective serotonin reuptake inhibitors, tricyclic antidepressants, and selegiline, causing signs and symptoms resembling serotonin syndrome (see Chapter 24). The syndrome results from blockade of serotonin metabolism by MAO and excessive stimulation of brainstem and spinal cord 5-hydroxytryptamine ($5-HT_{1A}$ and $5-HT_2$) receptors.[38,39] This type of clinical presentation has been described with concomitant use of selegiline and meperidine, causing restlessness, agitation, delirium, and hyperthermia.[12]

OVERDOSE AND TOXICITY

An extensive literature review, including multiple case series of MAO inhibitor overdoses, failed to identify one published case of selegiline overdose. It is largely presumed and not supported by published clinical experience that selegiline overdose would inhibit MAO A and MAO B and produce a syndrome clinically similar to that of an antidepressant MAO inhibitor overdose (see Chapter 43).

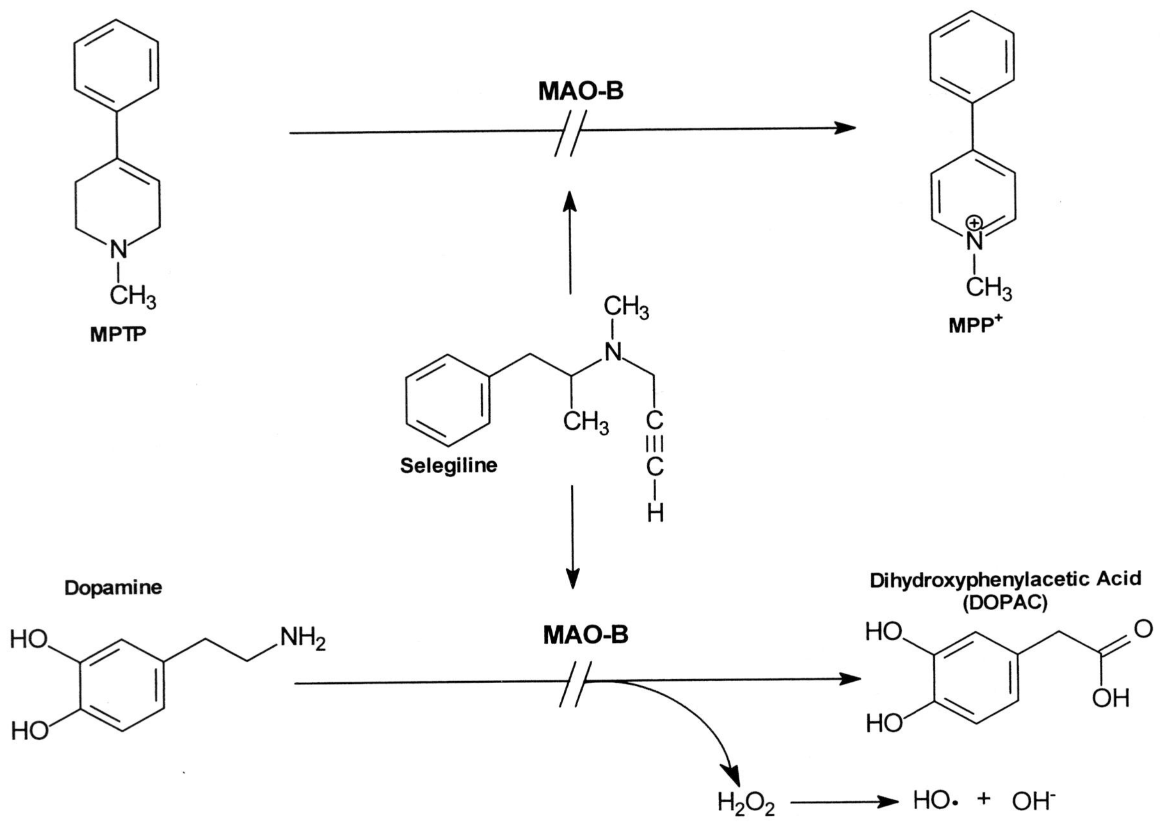

FIGURE 54-10

Mechanism of the potential neuroprotective effect of selegiline on the progressive neurodegeneration of 1-methyl-4-phenyl-1,2,3,6-tetrahydropyridine (MPTP)–induced toxicity and Parkinson's disease. Selegiline, an inhibitor of monoamine oxidase B (MAO-B), blocks the formation of the reactive intermediate 1-methyl-4-phenylpyridine (MPP^+) from MPTP and the formation of hydroxyl free radicals from the oxidation of dopamine.

Diagnosis and Treatment

Analysis of urine should detect the presence of methamphetamine and amphetamine after selegiline ingestion. So-called chiral assays that can distinguish the illicit D- from the L-isomeric form associated with selegiline use are commercially available. Appropriate therapeutic interventions for acute MAO inhibitor poisoning and serotonin syndrome are outlined in Chapters 24 and 43.

Indications for ICU Admission in Anti-Parkinson's Drug Toxicity

Selegiline
Monoamine oxidase inhibitor toxicity (see Chapter 43)

Key Points in the Evaluation and Treatment of Anti-Parkinson's Drug Toxicity

Selegiline
1. Interactions with other agents (e.g., sympathomimetic compounds, selective serotonin reuptake inhibitors) may result in excess adrenergic or serotoninergic tone, clinically manifested as a sympathomimetic toxidrome or serotonin syndrome.

continued

Key Points in the Evaluation and Treatment of Anti-Parkinson's Drug Toxicity *continued*

2. Overdose is characterized by toxicity similar to that of other MAO inhibitors (see Chapter 43).
3. Selegiline's major metabolites, L-methamphetamine and L-amphetamine, can be distinguished readily from the frequently illicit dextrorotatory forms of the same compounds by isomeric (chiral) determination.

DOPAMINE AGONISTS

Dopamine receptor agonists used in the treatment of parkinsonism are medications that, because of their dopamine-like molecular structure, directly stimulate striatal postsynaptic D_2-receptors. They are regarded as some of the most effective drugs to treat Parkinson's disease, second only to levodopa.[36] Traditionally, dopamine agonists have been used as adjuncts to levodopa in patients with Parkinson's disease. Initiation of dopamine agonists as first-line therapy may postpone the need for levodopa therapy, however, providing overall reduction of the risks of levodopa-induced dyskinesia.[2]

There are several advantages of dopamine agonists over levodopa: (1) They do not require conversion to an active metabolite to exert their pharmacologic effect, (2) circulating amino acids do not compete for their absorption and transport to the brain, (3) they have longer half-lives, (4) they do not undergo oxidative metabolism and do not produce potentially damaging oxygen free radicals, (5) they can target specific dopamine receptor subtypes, and (6) they offer a larger therapeutic window with decreased risk of dyskinesia.[2] Several dopamine agonists are currently available, including bromocriptine (Parlodel), pergolide (Permax), pramipexole (Mirapex), ropinirole (Requip), cabergoline (Cabaser, Dostinex), and lisuride (Dopergin).[40]

Pharmacokinetics

Bromocriptine (Fig. 54-11) is a potent D_2-receptor agonist, but it also possesses D_1 and 5-HT$_2$ agonist properties. It is absorbed rapidly after ingestion, is 90% metabolized by first-pass metabolism, and has a half-life of 3 to 8 hours.[40] Bromocriptine is largely protein bound and is excreted predominantly in the bile and feces.[6]

Pergolide is almost 10 times more potent than bromocriptine. It has a high affinity for D_2-receptors but also is a D_1-, D_3-, and α_2-receptor agonist.[40] Pergolide is well absorbed orally and has a half-life of approximately 3 to 7 hours.[7] It is also 90% protein bound.[40]

Pramipexole binds to D_2-receptors primarily but also possesses affinity for a myriad of other receptors, including D_1-, D_3-, D_4-, α_2-, acetylcholine-, and serotonin-receptors. Pramipexole has a half-life of about 8 to 12 hours and is 15% protein bound. Approximately 10% is metabolized, and the remainder is excreted unchanged in the urine.[40]

Ropinirole binds to the D_2-receptor and has relatively insignificant agonist activity to other brain receptors. It is absorbed quickly and completely from the stomach and has an elimination half-life of approximately 6 hours. Ropinirole is 40% protein bound, metabolized by CYP4501A2 to inactive metabolites, and excreted in the urine.[40]

Cabergoline is a D_2 agonist without effect on D_1-receptors. It has an elimination half-life of about 65 hours.[40]

Lisuride is a D_2 and 5-HT$_2$ agonist, but it has no D_1 activity. The onset of action is within 1 hour after intra-venous or subcutaneous administration. Lisuride possesses an elimination half-life of approximately 1 to 7 hours. There is no oral form because of minimal gastrointestinal absorption. Lisuride has effects comparable to those of dopa in treating Parkinson's patients. This drug is available in Europe but not in the United States.[40]

Significant drug-drug interactions may occur with the highly protein-bound dopamine agonists bromocriptine and pergolide. Coadministration of other highly protein-bound medications, such as warfarin or erythromycin, may result in elevation of dopamine agonist levels.[12]

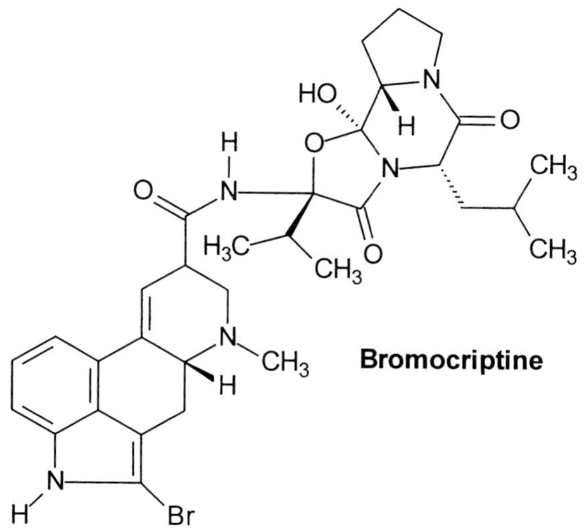

Pharmacokinetics of Dopamine Agonists

Bromocriptine (Parlodel)
Volume of distribution: 2 L/kg
Protein binding: 93%
Metabolites: –
Plasma elimination half-life: 3–8 hr

Pergolide
Volume of distribution: not available
Protein binding: >90%
Metabolites: extensive
Plasma elimination half-life: 27 hr

Pramipexole (Mirapex)
Volume of distribution: 5.6–9 L/kg
Protein binding: 15%
Metabolites: 10
Plasma elimination half-life: 8–12 hr

Ropinirole (Requip)
Volume of distribution: 7.5 L/kg
Protein binding: 40%
Metabolites: extensive
Plasma elimination half-life: 6 hr

Cabergoline (Dostinex)
Volume of distribution: not available
Protein binding: 40–42%
Metabolites: extensive
Plasma elimination half-life: 65 hr

Clinical Presentation

ADVERSE EFFECTS AND CHRONIC TOXICITY

The main side effects from dopamine agonists are similar to those of levodopa, including nausea, vomiting, orthostatic hypotension, hallucinations, psychosis, episodes of falling asleep ("sleep attacks"), and choreiform dyskinesias.[2] In addition, acute vasospastic crises (e.g., resulting in cerebral, coronary, or mesenteric ischemia), erythromelalgia, Raynaud's phenomenon, and retroperitoneal and pulmonary fibrosis have been reported with the ergot dopamine agonists (e.g., bromocriptine) but are uncommon with the newer nonergot medications.[2] Serotonin syndrome may occur theoretically as a result of dopaminergic-mediated increase in serotonin release.

FIGURE 54-11

Chemical structure of bromocriptine.

OVERDOSE AND ACUTE TOXICITY

Most reported cases of dopamine agonist overdose involve bromocriptine. Taken in overdose, bromocriptine produces nausea, vomiting, hypotension, lethargy, paranoia, aggressive behavior, and hallucinations. The neuropsychiatric manifestations most likely can be explained by the fact that bromocriptine is a lysergic acid derivative, similar to LSD.[41–43]

In a case report, a 17-month-old toddler who ingested her grandfather's pramipexole exhibited lethargy, which resolved within 24 hours.[44] Case reports of adult overdose printed in the manufacturer's package insert describe ataxia, drowsiness, tachycardia, and vomiting, which all spontaneously resolved.[44]

Diagnosis and Treatment

Indications for ICU Admission in Anti-Parkinson's Drug Toxicity

Dopamine Agonists
Uncontrolled agitation
Hypotension

Plasma bromocriptine concentrations vary widely among individuals on the same dose and do not correlate with clinical response or toxicity. Treatment of acute dopamine agonist overdose is largely supportive. The evaluation and management of ergotism are discussed in Chapter 69.

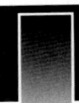

Key Points in the Evaluation and Treatment of Anti-Parkinson's Drug Toxicity

Dopamine Agonists
1. The presentation and treatment of acute and chronic bromocriptine toxicity is similar to that of other ergot alkaloids (see Chapter 69) and includes delirium, hallucinations, vasospastic crisis, and retroperitoneal fibrosis.

CATECHOL *O*-METHYLTRANSFERASE INHIBITORS

Because levodopa is metabolized in the periphery by COMT to the inactive metabolite 3-OMD, the addition of the reversible COMT inhibitors, tolcapone (Tasmar) or entacapone (Comtan), to Parkinson's disease treatment regimens has provided effective adjuncts to levodopa therapy.[2] These medications also decrease formation of 3-OMD, which, at least theoretically, competes with levodopa for transport to the brain.[2]

Pharmacokinetics

Tolcapone is absorbed rapidly from the gastrointestinal tract, with an elimination half-life of 2 to 3 hours, and is highly protein bound (>99.9%). It is metabolized nearly completely by the liver with little parent drug excreted in the urine.[45] Interaction between tolcapone and other highly protein-bound medications has not been shown.

Entacapone is readily absorbed and is predominantly protein bound (98%). The drug also nearly completely is hepatically metabolized, and small amounts of unchanged drug are found in the urine.[46] Similar to tolcapone, no significant interactions have been shown between entacapone and other protein-bound medications.

Catechol *O*-Methyltransferase Inhibitors

Tolcapone (Tasmar)
Volume of distribution: 0.10–0.14 L/kg
Protein binding: 99.9%
Metabolites: 3-*O*-methyl-tolcapone (>90)
Plasma elimination half-life: 2–3 hr

Etacapone (Comtan)
Volume of distribution: 0.24–0.56 L/kg
Protein binding: 98%
Metabolites: entacapone glucuronide (>90)
Plasma elimination half-life: 0.4–0.7 hr

Clinical Presentation

ADVERSE EFFECTS

Side effects of the COMT inhibitors are similar to those of levodopa and are related to increased levodopa availability. Severe and explosive diarrhea has been reported in approximately 5% to 10% of patients at therapeutic doses.[2] Harmless discoloration of urine also may occur. One potentially significant adverse effect of tolcapone is hepatotoxicity, an idiosyncratic effect found to occur in approximately 1% to 3% of patients on this drug.[2,47] The mechanism of liver injury seems to involve mitochondrial dysfunction.[48] Four cases of fulminant liver failure have occurred secondary to tolcapone, and, as a result, a "black box" warning has been issued in regard to this medication in the United States. Tolcapone is not available in Europe or Canada but can be obtained in the United States. Entacapone has not been associated with liver dysfunction.[2]

OVERDOSE AND TOXICITY

There are no reported human cases of overdose with either tolcapone or entacapone. Studies performed on healthy individuals taking larger-than-recommended daily amounts of both drugs resulted in minor symptoms that readily resolved on discontinuation of the medication. Theoretically, coadministration of a COMT inhibitor and MAO inhibitor could result in central and peripheral catecholamine excess, presenting clinically as a sympathomimetic poisoning syndrome.

Diagnosis and Treatment

Indications for ICU Admission in Anti-Parkinson's Drug Toxicity

Catechol *O*-Methyltransferase Inhibitors
Sympathomimetic toxicity (see Chapter 32)

No specific diagnostic tests are indicated in the setting of COMT inhibitor overdose. The emphasis of treatment should be on supportive care.

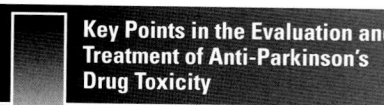

Key Points in the Evaluation and Treatment of Anti-Parkinson's Drug Toxicity

COMT Inhibitors

1. Chronic, dose-related adverse effects of COMT inhibitor treatment are similar to those of levodopa.
2. Hepatic toxicity is associated with tolcapone use.
3. Toxic interactions between COMT and MAO inhibitors are likely.

COMT, catechol *O*-methyltransferase; MAO, monoamine oxidase.

NEUROPROTECTIVE AGENTS

A broad variety of medications are aimed at protecting or preserving healthy striatal neurons in patients with Parkinson's disease. These neuroprotective agents include free radical scavengers, iron chelators (e.g., deferoxamine), nitric oxide synthesis inhibitors, calcium channel blockers, antiinflammatories, steroids, trophic factors, and antiapoptotic medicines. Many of these agents, such as calcium channel blockers and deferoxamine, are discussed elsewhere in this book (see Chapters 35 and 143).

REFERENCES

1. Aminoff MJ: Parkinson's disease. Neurol Clin 19:119–128, 2001.
2. Olanow CW, Watts RL, Koller WC: An algorithm (decision tree) for the management of Parkinson's disease (2001): Treatment guidelines. Neurology 56(11 Suppl 5):S1-S88, 2001.
3. Siderowf A: Parkinson's disease: Clinical features, epidemiology and genetics. Neurol Clin 19:565–578, 2001.
4. Marsden CD: Problems with long-term levodopa therapy for Parkinson's disease. Clin Neuropharmacol 17:32–34, 1994.
5. Amnioff MJ: Parkinson's disease and other extrapyramidal disorders. In Braunwald E, Fauci AS, Kasper DL, et al (eds): Harrison's Principles of Internal Medicine, 15th ed. New York, McGraw-Hill, 2001, pp 2356–2359.
6. Cedarbaum JM: Clinical pharmacokinetics of anti-parkinsonian drugs. Clin Pharmacokinet 13:141–178, 1987.
7. Standaert DG, Young AB: Treatment of central nervous system degenerative disorders. In Hardman JG, Limbird LE (eds): Goodman and Gilman's The Pharmacological Basis of Therapeutics, 9th ed. New York, McGraw-Hill, 1996, pp 552–560.
8. Sporer KA: Carbidopa-levodopa overdose. Am J Emerg Med 9:47–48, 1991.
9. Olanow CW: Preventing levodopa-induced dyskinesias. Ann Neurol 47:S167–178, 2000.
10. Rascol O: The pharmacological therapeutic management of levodopa-induced dyskinesias in patients with Parkinson's disease. J Neurol 247:51–57, 2000.
11. Nausieda PA: Sinemet "abusers." Clin Neuropharmacol 8:318–327, 1985.
12. Pfeiffer RF: Antiparkinsonian agents: Drug interactions of clinical significance. Drug Saf 14:343–354, 1996.
13. Murer MG, Raisman-Vozari R, Gershanik O: Levodopa in Parkinson's disease: Neurotoxicity issue laid to rest? Drug Saf 21:339–352, 1999.
14. Hoehn MM, Rutledge CO: Acute overdose with levodopa. Neurology 25:792–794, 1974.
15. Sporer KA: Carbidopa-levodopa overdose. Am J Emerg Med 9:47–48, 1991.
16. Factor SA, Molho ES: Emergency department presentations of patients with Parkinson's disease. Am J Emerg Med 18:209–215, 2000.
17. Chan TC, Evans SD, Clark R: Drug-induced hyperthermia. Crit Care Clin 13:785–808, 1997.
18. Stuerenburg HJ, Schoser BG: Acute overdosage and intoxication with carbidopa/levodopa can be detected in the subacute stage by measurement of 3-o-methyldopa. J Neurol Neurosurg Psychiatry 67:122–123, 1999.
19. Grace RF: Bentropine abuse and overdose: Case report and review. Adv Drug React Toxicol Rev 16:103–112, 1997.
20. Craig DH, Rosen P: Abuse of antiparkinsonian drugs. Ann Emerg Med 10:98–100, 1981.
21. Weiner M: Update on antiparkinsonian agents. Geriatrics 37:81–91, 1982.
22. Fahy P, Arnold P, Curry SC, Bond R: Serial serum drug concentrations and prolonged anticholinergic toxicity after benztropine (Cogentin) overdose. Am J Emerg Med 7:199–202, 1989.
23. Howrie DL, Rowley AH, Krenzelok EP: Bentropine-induced acute dystonic reaction. Ann Emerg Med 15:141–143, 1986.
24. Dilaveris P, Pantazis A, Vlasseros J, Gialafos J: Non-sustained ventricular tachycardia due to low-dose orphenadrine. Am J Med 111:418–419, 2001.
25. Catterson ML, Martin RL: Anticholinergic toxicity masquerading as neuroleptic malignant syndrome: A case report and review. Ann Clin Psychiatry 6:267–269, 1994.
26. Aoki FY, Sitar DS: Clinical pharmacokinetics of amantadine hydrochloride. Clin Pharmacokinet 14:35–51, 1988.
27. Snoey ER, Bessen HA: Acute psychosis after amantadine overdose. Ann Emerg Med 19:668–670, 1990.
28. Macchio GJ, Ito V, Sahgal V: Amantadine-induced coma. Arch Phys Med Rehabil 74:1119–1120, 1993.
29. Sartori M, Pratt CM, Young JB: Torsade de pointe malignant cardiac arrhythmia induced by amantadine poisoning. Am J Med 77:388–391, 1984.
30. Strong DK, Eisenstat DD, Bryson SM, et al: Amantadine neurotoxicity in a pediatric patient with renal insufficiency. Ann Pharmacother 25:1175–1177, 1991.
31. Pimentel L, Hughes B: Amantadine toxicity presenting with complex ventricular ectopy and hallucinations. Pediatr Emerg Care 7:89–92, 1991.
32. Berkowitz CD: Treatment of acute amantadine toxicity with physostigmine. J Pediatr 95:144–145, 1979.
33. Gerlach M, Youdim MBH, Riederer P: Pharmacology of selegiline. Neurology 47:S137–145, 1996.
34. Baldessarini RJ: Drugs and the treatment of psychiatric disorders. In Hardman JG, Limbird LE (eds): Goodman and Gilman's the Pharmacological Basis of Therapeutics, 9th ed. New York, McGraw-Hill, 1996, pp 447–483.
35. Heinomen EH, Anttila MI, Lammintansta RAS: Pharmacokinetic aspects of l-deprenyl (selegiline) and its metabolites. Clin Pharmacol Ther 56:742–749, 1994.
36. Lambert D, Waters CH: Comparative tolerability of the newer generation antiparkinsonian agents. Drugs Aging 16:55–65, 2000.
37. Churchyard A: Selegiline-induced postural hypotension in Parkinson's disease: A longitudinal study on the effects of drug withdrawal. Mov Disord 14:246–251, 1999.
38. Richard IH, Kurlan R, Tanner C, et al: Serotonin syndrome and the combined use of deprenyl and an antidepressant in Parkinson's disease. Neurology 48:1070–1077, 1997.
39. Hinds NP, Hillier CEM, Wiles CM: Possible serotonin syndrome arising from an interaction between nortriptiline and selegiline in a lady with parkinsonism. J Neurol 247:811, 2000.
40. Factor SA: Parkinson's disease and parkinsonian syndromes: Dopamine agonists. Med Clin North Am 83:415–443, 1999.
41. Mack RB: Mairzy doats and dozy doats and a kiddle eat almost anything. N C Med J 49:17–18, 1988.
42. Warren DE, Nakfoor E: Acute overdose of bromocriptine. Drug Intell Clin Pharm 17:374, 1983.
43. Vermunt SH, Goldstein RG, Romano AA, Atwood SJ: Accidental bromocriptine ingestion in childhood. J Pediatr 838–840, 1984.
44. Hack JB, Powell G, Nelson LS, et al: Acute pediatric exposure to pramipexole dihydrochloride (Mirapex). J Toxicol Clin Toxicol 37:891–892, 1999.
45. Jorga KM, Fotteler B, Heizmann P, Zurcher G: Pharmacokinetics and pharmacodynamics after oral and intravenous administration of tolcapone, a novel adjunct to Parkinson's disease therapy. Eur J Clin Pharmacol 54:443–447, 1998.
46. Keranen T, et al: Inhibition of soluble catechol *O*-methyltransferase and single dose pharmacokinetics after oral and intravenous administration of entacapone. Eur J Clin Pharmacol 46:151–157, 1994.
47. Watkins P: COMT inhibitors and liver toxicity. Neurology 55(11 Suppl 4):S51-S56, 2000.
48. Waters C: Catechol-*O*-methyltransferase (COMT) inhibitors in Parkinson's disease. J Am Geriatr Soc 48:692–698, 2000.

CHAPTER **55**

Acetaminophen (Paracetamol)

Holly E. Perry ■ Paul Wax

First developed in the 1890s, acetaminophen (paracetamol) was not marketed as an antipyretic and analgesic until the 1960s. Toxicity from acetaminophen overdose was initially recognized in 1966, when the first cases were reported in the British literature.[1,2] Since that time, morbidity and mortality from acetaminophen overdose have continued to climb steadily. Advertised for its therapeutic use as "strong," "proven stronger," and "easy to swallow," worldwide it is one of the most commonly used pharmaceutical agents for suicide.[3] Annually, more than 150 deaths in the United Kingdom[3] are attributable to acetaminophen overdose, with at least a similar number in the United States.[4] Acetaminophen-induced hepatotoxicity is the most common cause of acute liver failure (ALF) in both the United Kingdom[5] and the United States.[6] Additionally, toxicity from chronic ingestion of supratherapeutic amounts is increasingly being recognized. Antidote therapy is readily available and very effective when administered soon after an acute overdose.[7] The efficacy of antidote therapy after chronic ingestion of supratherapeutic amounts has not been well studied.

CLINICAL PHARMACOLOGY

Pharmacokinetics of Acetaminophen

Volume of distribution: 0.9 L/kg
Protein binding: 15–20%
Mechanisms of clearance: hepatic >90%, renal 4–7%
Active metabolites: N-acetyl-p-benzoquinoneimine
Methods to enhance clearance: dialysis (not clinically useful)

The kinetics and metabolism of acetaminophen are well understood. Gastric emptying is the rate-limiting step inasmuch as absorption of acetaminophen tablets occurs rapidly from the small intestine. Absorption is usually complete by 60 to 90 minutes after a therapeutic dose.[8] Liquid preparations are completely absorbed within 20 minutes.[8] With ingestion of excessive doses of standard-release preparations, absorption may be delayed but is invariably complete within 4 hours. Theoretically, acetaminophen absorption could be appreciably

delayed by coingestion of agents that slow gastric emptying. A peak serum acetaminophen concentration occurring later than 4 hours after overdose is rare but has been noted after coingestion of propoxyphene[9–11] and diphenhydramine.[12–14] Tylenol-ER, an extended-release acetaminophen preparation, has also been associated with peak levels delayed more than 4 hours after overdose.[15]

Acetaminophen elimination follows first-order kinetics. It has a half-life of 2.5 to 4 hours, which may be prolonged in patients with liver damage. Protein binding is 15% to 20%, and the volume of distribution is approximately 0.9 L/kg.[8]

PATHOPHYSIOLOGY

Metabolism of acetaminophen is the basis of its toxicity (Fig. 55-1). Acetaminophen is an example of a substance that undergoes hepatic toxification rather than detoxification; other examples include carbon tetrachloride, methanol, and ethylene glycol. More than 90% of acetaminophen is conjugated in the liver by a combination of sulfation and glucuronidation; approximately 4% to 7% is excreted unchanged in urine. The remainder (about 4%) is metabolized by the cytochrome P-450 mixed-function oxidase system (MFOS),[16] primarily by CYP2E1 with a smaller contribution by CYP1A2. The MFOS is distributed throughout the body, but the majority is found in the liver, with the highest concentration in the centrilobular region (zone 3), which is composed of hepatic acinar cells. A secondary area of increased concentration is in the kidneys. Neither acetaminophen nor its conjugated metabolites are harmful. However, the metabolite generated by CYP2E1 is potentially toxic.[17–19] This metabolite, N-acetyl-p-benzoquinoneimine (NAPQI), is short lived, with a half-life of nanoseconds. It binds to the hepatic cell membrane and injures the lipid bilayer if not neutralized by an antioxidant.[20] Hepatic glutathione appears to be the primary antioxidant that conjugates and detoxifies.[16,21–23] At therapeutic doses, acetaminophen is an extraordinarily safe drug with minimal side effects. However, in an animal model of acetaminophen overdose, NAPQI begins to bind to hepatocytes and causes arylation, cellular injury, and possibly death when hepatic glutathione stores have been depleted to less than 70% of normal values.[24]

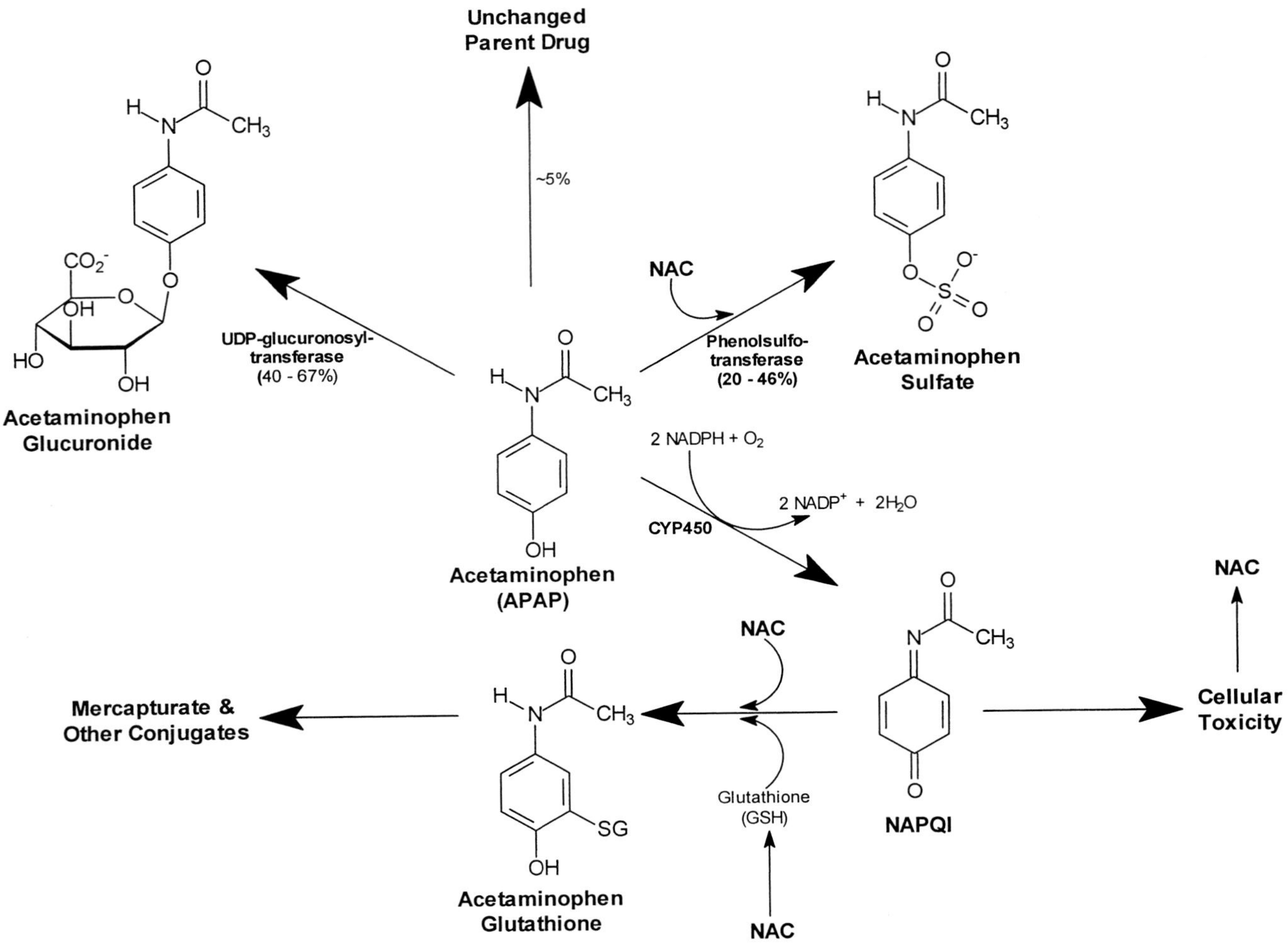

FIGURE 55-1

Metabolism of acetaminophen. APAP, acetyl-*para*-aminophenol; NADPH, reduced nicotinamide adenine dinucleotide phosphate; NAPQI, *N*-acetyl-*p*-benzoquinoneimine; UDP, uridine diphosphate.

In an adult, the minimum toxic dose of acetaminophen ingested as an acute overdose appears to be 10 g[25] or 150 mg/kg[26] (whichever is lowest). Children younger than 6 years appear to be more resistant to acetaminophen toxicity than adolescents and adults. Several large studies of young children have demonstrated that in this age group, a single ingestion of 200 mg/kg or less is highly unlikely to result in significant toxicity.[27–29]

Chronic supratherapeutic dosing of acetaminophen may also result in toxicity. The manufacturers' recommended daily amount is 4 g/day or less for adults and 75 mg/kg/day or less for children. Toxicity has been reported with ingestion of more than these recommended doses for a day or longer.[30–35] Retrospective case series in children have reported therapeutic doses (20 to 25 mg/kg/day) being associated with hepatotoxicity,[33,35] but the accuracy of these dose estimates is uncertain.

Modulators of Toxicity

Toxicity results when the amount of NAPQI produced from acetaminophen metabolism overwhelms the capacity for glutathione-mediated detoxification. Theoretically, any compound that induces CYP2E1 could increase the amount of NAPQI produced and thus increase the likelihood of toxicity. Inducers of CYP2E1 include ethanol, rifampin, isoniazid, and carbamazepine.[36] Clinical series suggest that patients who chronically ingest drugs that induce CYP2E1, such as certain anticonvulsants or ethanol, may have poorer outcomes than the general population after acetaminophen overdose.[37–41] Patients with depleted glutathione stores from malnutrition, such as chronic alcoholics, may also be at increased risk. However, concomitant ethanol and acetaminophen ingestion may decrease the effects of acetaminophen overdose because of competition for CYP2E1 activity. Phenytoin, which is not a CYP2E1 inducer, does not appear to increase the risk of acetaminophen-induced hepatotoxicity and, in fact, may offer hepatoprotection by increasing glucuronidation.[42]

Age is also a modulator of toxicity. Young children appear to be more resistant to the toxic effects of acute acetaminophen overdose. No fatalities have been documented after an acute, single overdose in any child younger than 7 despite reports of massive ingestion. Additionally, the incidence of hepatotoxicity is much lower than that observed in the general population.[43,44] However, severe hepatotoxicity has been reported. Young children are at risk for hepatotoxicity when supratherapeutic doses have been given chronically; numerous deaths have been reported in children in this context.[34,35]

CLINICAL PRESENTATION AND LIFE-THREATENING COMPLICATIONS

The clinical manifestations of acetaminophen toxicity can vary significantly, depending on the dose, time of presentation, and whether the toxicity results from acute or chronic ingestion. Patients who undergo medical evaluation within several hours after an acute ingestion may be asymptomatic or have only minor symptoms. Nausea, vomiting, and occasionally lethargy may occur early (typically within several hours of ingestion) in moderate to severe acetaminophen poisoning. In our experience, these symptoms usually decrease within 12 to 18 hours and may possibly reflect direct effects of the parent compound (because resolution occurs with declining acetaminophen levels). Depressed mental status, metabolic acidosis, and even coma within 4 to 6 hours of overdose have been reported after a massive overdose, but the pathophysiology of these complications is not understood.[45,46] Patients who first come to medical attention after the onset of signs of liver injury—generally at least 24 hours after acute ingestion—may initially present with encephalopathy, coagulopathy, and renal failure.

Hepatocytes are the primary target after an acetaminophen overdose. Given NAPQI's ultrashort half-life, its toxicity is limited to cells that elaborate it. Most of the life-threatening complications of acetaminophen poisoning are a direct result of acute liver injury and the systemic complications of liver failure. The clinical course most commonly observed with acute acetaminophen hepatotoxicity is hyperacute liver failure, which has been defined as the development of encephalopathy within 7 days of the onset of jaundice (although in some acetaminophen poisoning cases jaundice is never apparent).[47] Liver failure is the direct result of NAPQI-induced hepatocellular injury. The early histopathologic finding after acetaminophen overdose is centrilobular hepatic necrosis (zone 3) with periportal sparing.[48] The centrilobular region is chiefly composed of zone 3 hepatic acinar cells, the site of highest MFOS activity. Hepatic necrosis results in the release of a wide range of substances into serum and severe metabolic derangements (e.g., hypoglycemia and hyperammonemia) from the loss of functioning liver. Coagulopathy and renal failure usually accompany the encephalopathy, although the extent of different organ involvement may vary. Sepsis (both bacterial and fungal), cardiovascular collapse, and terminal ventricular dysrhythmias may also develop in patients with ALF. Nonetheless, given the injured liver's ability to regenerate, ALF is also potentially reversible, particularly in the case of acetaminophen poisoning, because hepatic regeneration occurs from cells situated in the periportal regions (zone 1), which tend to be unaffected by all but the most massive of acetaminophen overdoses.

Hepatic encephalopathy is the hallmark of ALF and develops in severe cases of acetaminophen-induced hepatotoxicity. In a series of 171 patients, grade II (Table 55-1) encephalopathy was noted at a median of 72 (range 38 to 120) hours after an acute acetaminophen overdose. Grade IV encephalopathy was noted within 89 (range 51 to 141) hours following an overdose occurring 12 (range 3 to 96) hours after grade

TABLE 55-1 Clinical Characteristics of Encephalopathy

Grade I	Slowed thought processes, slurred speech, untidy appearance, slight tremor
Grade II	Increased drowsiness, inappropriate behavior, easily elicited tremor
Grade III	Hypersomnolent, incoherent speech, marked confusion
Grade IV	Coma, no response to painful stimuli

II encephalopathy.[49] Patients with grade III encephalopathy are at significant risk for cerebral edema. Death is most likely to occur 72 to 96 hours after an overdose, although it may be delayed for up to 10 to 14 days. Death occurs most frequently as a complication of cerebral edema or sepsis. Patients who survive do not have permanent liver damage.[48]

Renal failure in the setting of acetaminophen poisoning may be due to a direct renal effect of NAPQI, prerenally mediated acute tubular necrosis, and/or hepatorenal syndrome. Because CYP2E1 is present in renal tubules, NAPQI is generated in the kidney. Renal injury manifested by hematuria, proteinuria, and modest elevations in blood urea nitrogen (BUN) and creatinine has been reported in as many as 8.9% of patients.[50] It typically develops within the first 24 to 48 hours, is transient, but may progress to anuric renal failure and require weeks of dialysis.[50,51] Oliguric renal failure necessitating dialysis has been reported to occur in 1% of patients.[52] Renal failure secondary to hepatorenal syndrome is typically delayed 48 to 72 hours after ingestion but seems to be more characteristic of non–acetaminophen-induced fulminant hepatic failure.[51] Clinically significant nephrotoxicity in the absence of hepatotoxicity has been reported but is rare.[53–55]

Other clinical manifestations associated with acetaminophen toxicity include pancreatitis and cardiotoxicity. Pancreatic inflammation, defined as serum lipase three times the upper limit of the normal laboratory value, may be found in 30% or more of patients with acetaminophen hepatotoxicity.[56] However, clinical pancreatitis is rare.[51] Cardiotoxicity, manifested by nonspecific electrocardiographic changes and alterations consistent with pericarditis, is also rare.[51,57] The mechanisms responsible for these less common findings are unclear.

Chronic Acetaminophen Overdose

The manufacturers' recommended maximum daily doses of acetaminophen are 4 g of acetaminophen in adults and 75 mg/kg in children. Ingestion of larger quantities constitutes chronic supratherapeutic doses and may result in hepatotoxicity. In young children, hepatotoxicity has developed after as little as 150 mg/kg/day.[33,58]

Chronic acetaminophen excess is usually a therapeutic misadventure. Common scenarios include those involving patients who increase their daily intake because they believe that it is safe, patients who use combination products such as acetaminophen and codeine along with acetaminophen, or caretakers who substitute adult for pediatric suppositories in a young child. The incidence of hepatotoxicity after chronic excess has not been extensively studied. The only study of this type examined 44 febrile children who had received more than 60 mg/kg/day and found small elevations in hepatic transaminases. There were no cases of severe liver injury.[59] Certain populations may be at risk, including patients who are fasting or who have ingested alcohol in the preceding 5 days.[32] Numerous cases of hepatotoxicity have been reported in alcoholics after chronic acetaminophen excess, although the apparent frequency may be due in part to ascertainment bias.[31] Indeed, in a randomized, double-blind, placebo-controlled trial of 201 long-term alcoholic patients, no liver injury was noted when recommended doses of acetaminophen were not exceeded.[60]

The clinical manifestations of chronic acetaminophen toxicity are highly variable. Some patients initially come to medical attention for other reasons such as acute or chronic pain disorders from low back pain, dental pain, or temporal mandibular joint pain. These patients may initially have few, if any, symptoms directly related to excessive acetaminophen use. Other cases of chronic acetaminophen poisoning may be manifested as altered mental status from incipient ALF.

DIAGNOSIS

Laboratory Evaluation

Within the first few hours after acute ingestion, the serum acetaminophen level is the only predictor of toxicity. The Rumack-Matthews nomogram, which plots the plasma acetaminophen concentration as a function of time since overdose, identifies patients who should receive antidote therapy after a single acute overdose (Fig. 55-2). According to this nomogram, which represents an acetaminophen poisoning treatment standard, two levels of risk for the development of severe hepatotoxicity after acetaminophen overdose are delineated: possible and probable. Patients are at "probable risk" if the serum acetaminophen concentration lies above the line beginning at 200 μg/mL (1323 μmol/L) at 4 hours and at "possible risk" if the serum acetaminophen concentration lies between the lines beginning at 150 to 200 μg/mL (992 to 1323 μmol/L) at 4 hours. The upper line reflects the actual

threshold for toxicity in the early studies; the so-called possible-risk level was added to the nomogram to give a 25% margin of safety to allow for variations in measurement of acetaminophen levels among laboratories, as well as uncertainty of the time of ingestion.[44] Although the probable-risk line is used widely as a threshold for treatment, in the United States the possible-risk line is often used. The nomogram is essential for determining which patients may benefit from N-acetylcysteine (NAC) after a single, acute ingestion. However, it may not be helpful if the patient is initially seen more than 20 hours after an overdose because the lower limit for detection of acetaminophen for many laboratories is 10 μg/mL (66 μmol/L) and this value represents a toxic level if obtained more than 20 hours after an overdose. The nomogram has not been validated for the assessment of patients with chronic acetaminophen ingestion.

Clinical and biochemical parameters are not usually helpful in a patient evaluated soon after ingestion. Hepatic transaminase levels should be normal unless the patient has preexisting liver disease. Initial laboratory evaluation should include a plasma acetaminophen concentration obtained 4 or more hours after ingestion; baseline aspartate aminotransferase (AST), alanine aminotransferase (ALT), prothrombin time (PT), and creatinine; a pregnancy test for women of childbearing age; and a salicylate level and toxicologic screen if coingestion is a concern. Aspirin is a frequent coingestant, and therefore a salicylate level should be considered in every patient who presents with an acetaminophen overdose. If Tylenol-ER has been ingested, some authors have suggested that two plasma acetaminophen concentrations be determined on blood samples drawn 4 hours apart. The value of a second acetaminophen concentration, however, has not been shown to predict toxicity. Consideration should be given to determining amylase and lipase levels, particularly in patients with protracted emesis, abdominal pain, or severe toxicity. For patients with signs of significant hepatotoxicity, ongoing evaluation should include at least daily PT, AST, ALT, and creatinine determinations. Arterial blood gas monitoring to evaluate acid-base disturbances should be performed for any patient with evidence of ALF.

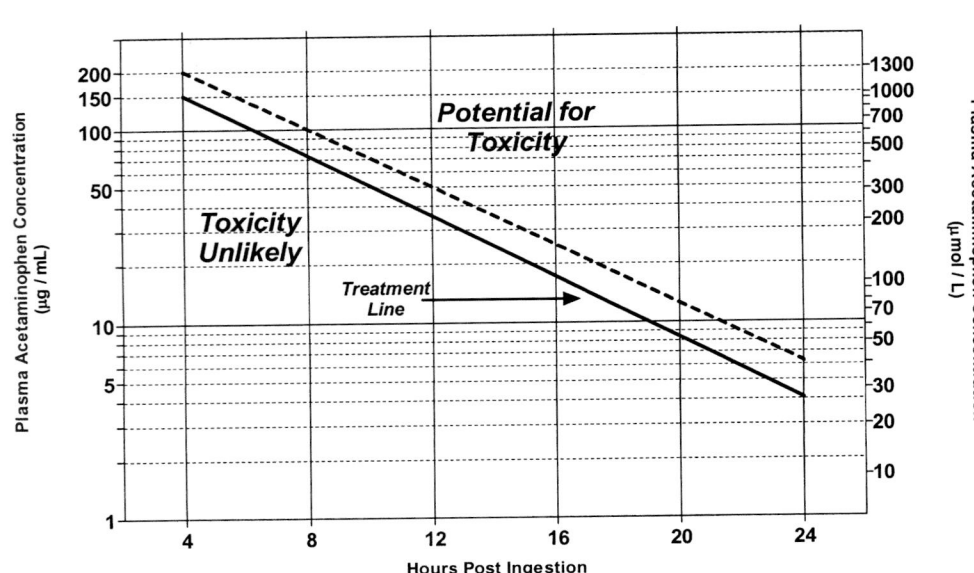

FIGURE 55-2

Acetaminophen treatment nomogram.

In more than half of all patients who ultimately manifest liver injury, some elevation in hepatic transaminases develops within 24 hours after an overdose.[61] In some cases, elevations in AST and ALT may appear as early as 8 hours after an overdose, but this finding is unusual, and a more remote time of ingestion or other cause of hepatic dysfunction should be considered. AST and/or ALT may rise to 10,000 IU/L or more, and in some cases, transaminase levels greater than 100,000 IU/L have been reported.[62] The degree of transaminase elevation by itself has little prognostic significance. In one large study of patients who died of acetaminophen overdose, the mean measured peak AST level was less than 3000 IU/L.[63] However, the possibility that these patients were initially evaluated after their transaminase levels peaked and were hence falling cannot be excluded.

In patients who recover, transaminases peak between 48 and 72 hours.[61] In a patient with significant hepatotoxicity, it may take up to 2 weeks before transaminases gradually return to normal. In our experience, the time to normalization of ALT is often much longer than that for AST, given the slower clearance of ALT. In some cases, AST may be elevated while ALT remains relatively normal. This transaminase profile suggests that the elevated AST may result from a nonhepatic source such as muscle breakdown. Rhabdomyolysis, either drug induced or from other causes, should be considered in this situation.

In a patient with alcoholic hepatitis, AST is minimally elevated (usually <300 IU/L), ALT is normal or slightly elevated, and the AST/ALT ratio is greater than 2. When acetaminophen toxicity is superimposed on alcoholic hepatitis, the transaminase profile differs in that both ALT and AST are markedly elevated, with ALT being less elevated than AST and the AST/ALT ratio remaining higher than 2.[64]

Patients with serum hepatic transaminase values over 1000 IU/L after a single acute acetaminophen overdose are at risk for progressive hepatic injury, development of ALF, and death. Patients with peak AST or ALT levels less than 1000 IU/L do not carry such a risk. However, decisions regarding prognosis or the need for transplantation should never be made on the basis of transaminase elevations alone. In two early British studies of 180 and 360 patients with acetaminophen overdose who did not receive an antidote, 16% had plasma acetaminophen concentrations above the probable-risk line on the acetaminophen nomogram.[65] In both series, 50% of patients with measured plasma acetaminophen concentrations above the probable-risk line had peak serum AST levels over 1000 IU/L. For those with AST levels higher than 1000 IU/L, mortality rates for each series were 50% and 11%, respectively. The much larger Rocky Mountain Poison Center study of 11,195 patients in which use of the antidote NAC was evaluated for acetaminophen overdose found that 18% of reported acetaminophen overdose cases had measured plasma acetaminophen concentrations above the possible-risk line and that 30% of those above the probable-risk line had AST levels higher than 1000 IU/L (n = 611), most of whom did not receive NAC until 10 hours or later after overdose because of delayed manifestations.[7] These 611 patients were treated with NAC, and only 11 (1.8%) died, a far different mortality rate than found in the earlier studies on untreated patients.

PT is one of the best readily available markers of functional hepatic damage. Whereas an increase in hepatic transaminase levels indicates hepatocyte injury and necrosis, PT determination provides information about hepatic synthetic function. A rise in PT is indicative of a decrease in hepatic synthesis of vitamin K–dependent clotting factors (factors II, VII, IX, X). A rising PT in the setting of falling transaminase levels is an ominous finding. Serum transaminase concentrations will invariably fall in both a patient who recovers from hepatic injury and one who develops ALF and massive hepatic necrosis. PT, however, will not usually improve if a patient has progressive liver injury, and it generally continues to rise in cases of ALF, especially in the absence of clotting factor replacement. The finding of a slightly elevated PT within hours after an acute overdose is common and usually the result of direct reversible inhibition by acetaminophen of vitamin K–dependent factor synthesis and not a marker of hepatic injury.[66]

Monitoring renal function by determination of serum creatinine is essential in the evaluation of acetaminophen toxicity. Unlike hepatic injury, which can be monitored by determination of transaminases and PT, comparable markers of renal injury do not exist. Renal injury will not be detected until functional impairment occurs as evidenced by an increasing serum creatinine concentration. Seventy-two to 96 hours may pass before an increase in serum creatinine is noted. BUN may be a misleading index of renal impairment in cases of ALF because hepatic production of BUN is reduced.

Some patients will have compensated or uncompensated metabolic acidosis shortly after ingesting a significant overdose.[67] This acidosis has been associated with increased lactate formation and has been postulated to occur as a consequence of impaired mitochondrial respiration at the level of ubiquinone by acetaminophen[68,69] or NAPQI.[70,71] This early-onset acidosis tends to resolve spontaneously within hours.[67] In patients whose clinical condition continues to deteriorate, however, acidosis often recurs and is highly predictive of lethality once ALF has developed.

Differential Diagnosis

Although acetaminophen is currently the primary cause of ALF, a number of other toxic and nontoxic etiologies must also be considered. Toxic causes include intrinsic, dose-related hepatotoxins such as carbon tetrachloride, chloroform, cyclopeptides (α-amanitine), copper sulfate, yellow phosphorus, and various herbal products. Botanicals that have been implicated as intrinsic hepatotoxins include pennyroyal oil from *Mentha pulegium*, chaparral, germander, Jin Bu Huan, and pyrrolizidine alkaloids from *Heliotropium, Senecio* (tansy ragwort), *Crotalaria*, and *Symphytum* (comfrey) species. ALF may also result from idiosyncratic hepatotoxins, including phenytoin, valproic acid, isoniazid, halothane, numerous nonsteroidal antiinflammatory agents, and troglitazone. Idiosyncratic hepatotoxicity is not dose related and may occur after therapeutic dosing. Liver failure from methylenedioxymethamphetamine (MDMA) has also been described and may occur in association with severe MDMA-induced heatstroke.[72] Other causes of fulminant liver failure include viral hepatitis, sepsis, hypovolemic shock, cardiogenic shock, heatstroke, and Reye's syndrome.[5] Serology, clinical history, and occasionally histopathology help differentiate these entities.

The time course and the clinical and biochemical characteristics of shock liver may appear remarkably similar to acetaminophen-induced hepatic failure. Shock liver generally results from hemorrhage, hypovolemia, and the resultant hypotension secondary to trauma and operative procedures. Differentiating between shock and acetaminophen as the primary hepatic insult may prove challenging, especially in situations in which hypotension may have occurred and the patient has been taking therapeutic amounts of acetaminophen.

In light of the increasing number of reports of hepatotoxicity associated with chronic supratherapeutic dosing,[30-35] acetaminophen should always be considered in cases that might otherwise be attributed to cryptogenic ALF. For any patient admitted to the critical care unit with ALF of unknown etiology, the earliest available blood specimen should be retrieved and tested for acetaminophen to assess whether it might be an etiologic factor.[73] However, depending on the timing of the last acetaminophen dose, the plasma concentration may be low or nondetectable and cannot reliably exclude acetaminophen as the cause. Furthermore, in the setting of severe hyperbilirubinemia ($\approx$25 mg/dL; 1.46 μmol/L), the conventional acetaminophen assay performed by enzyme assay (GDS Diagnostics, Elkhart, IN) may cross-react with the bilirubin and result in a falsely elevated or false-positive acetaminophen determination.[74] In the future, measurement of plasma levels of 3-(cystein-S-yl)-acetaminophen-protein adducts may be a useful diagnostic tool because it appears to be a relatively sensitive and specific marker of acetaminophen-associated hepatotoxicity.[75,76]

TREATMENT

Acetaminophen intoxication by itself does not typically produce cardiorespiratory compromise unless the patient is initially seen late and is in hepatic failure. Rare instances of patients presenting in coma and requiring endotracheal intubation shortly after an overdose have been reported.[45,46] Decontamination with a single dose of activated charcoal should be performed if the patient is seen within 1 hour of ingestion.[77,78] In the past, there was concern about activated charcoal and use of the oral antidote NAC, but the amount adsorbed is not considered clinically important.[79,80] Acetaminophen is removed by dialysis, but this modality has no role in overdose given the efficacy of NAC as an antidote and the rapid metabolism of the parent compound.

N-Acetylcysteine

NAC is a highly effective antidote when administered soon after an acetaminophen overdose. It acts as a glutathione substitute in addition to enhancing glutathione synthesis and

increasing the amount of acetaminophen that undergoes sulfation (see Fig. 55-1).[21] Its efficacy is primarily a function of time elapsed since the overdose. NAC is most effective when administered within the first 8 hours after an acetaminophen overdose, and its effectiveness decreases incrementally every hour thereafter.[7]

Three different NAC regimens have been studied (Table 55-2). In most of the world, NAC is administered as a continuous intravenous (IV) infusion. Prior to 2004, when IV NAC was approved by the FDA, the only approved protocol in the United States was 72 hours of oral NAC. Although this regimen is effective, successful administration is hindered by a high frequency of emesis. For this reason, an IV protocol has been devised that is a modification of the 72-hour oral protocol.[81] The results of clinical trials of these regimens are compared in Table 55-3.[7,81,82] Both the 20-hour IV protocol and the 72-hour oral protocol are efficacious when treatment is begun early. Previously, the 72-hour oral protocol was claimed to be superior to the 20-hour IV protocol when treatment was begun more than 15 hours after an overdose. However, a recent systematic review has shown that these protocols are essentially equivalent.[82] Efficacy is an inverse function of treatment delay. The 52-hour IV protocol appears to be equivalent to the 72-hour oral protocol, although results have been published on only 179 patients.[81]

Every patient with a plasma acetaminophen concentration that falls on or above the probable-risk line should receive NAC. In the United States, many recommend treatment for patients above the possible-risk line as well.[83] The earliest time after ingestion that can be plotted on the nomogram is 4 hours. However, it has been suggested that acetaminophen concentrations determined more than 1 hour after ingestion that are less than 100 μg/mL (661 μmol/L) are unlikely to be toxic at 4 hours.[84] Additionally, it has been suggested that in children younger than 5 years who have ingested a liquid preparation, a 2-hour acetaminophen level less than 225 μg/mL (1448 μmol/L) can be considered nontoxic.[85]

Treatment with either the oral or IV forms of NAC may be associated with adverse effects. A high incidence of nausea and vomiting is associated with the administration of oral NAC, but there is only a 2% to 3% incidence of anaphylactoid reactions.[81,86] In contrast, IV infusion of NAC has been associated with a 3% to 14% rate of adverse reactions, including erythema at the injection site, diffuse urticaria, bronchospasm, angioedema, and hypotension.[81,87-89] Most reactions are anaphylactoid in nature and are likely to be related to histamine release.[90] Fatal reactions to NAC are rare but

Indications for ICU Admission in Acetaminophen Poisoning

Significant acidosis
Any grade of encephalopathy
Coagulopathy requiring treatment
Significant renal failure

TABLE 55-2 N-Acetylcysteine Regimens

REGIMEN	LOADING DOSE	FOLLOWED BY	TOTAL DOSE
20 hr IV	150 mg/kg over 15 min	50 mg/kg over 4 hr 100 mg/kg over 20 hr	300 mg/kg
72 hr PO	140 mg/kg	70 mg/kg q4h for 17 doses	1330 mg/kg
52 hr IV	140 mg/kg over 60 min	70 mg/kg q4h for 12 doses	980 mg/kg

TABLE 55-3 Development of Hepatotoxicity as a Function of Protocol and Treatment Delay

TREATMENT DELAY (hr)	20 hr IV NAC (n = 205)	72 hr PO NAC (n = 2023)	48 hr IV NAC (n = 179)
0–10	3% (0–6)	6% (4–8)	8%
10–24	30% (5–55)	26% (24–29)	29%
16–24	46% (10–82)	41% (35–46)	58% (34–80)

Numbers in parenthesis represent 95% confidence intervals, where given. Hepatotoxicity is defined as aspartate or alanine transaminase levels higher than 1000 IU/L.
Data from references 7, 81, 82.
NAC, *N*-Acetylcysteine.

have been reported.[91] These reactions appear to be related to the rate of infusion because they are almost universally seen during the initial dose of 150 mg/kg over a 15-minute period and respond to decreasing the rate.[92] Many authorities recommend administration of the initial infusion over a period of 1 hour rather than 15 minutes to decrease the likelihood of this anaphylactoid reaction. Patients with a history of asthma are more likely to experience anaphylactoid reactions.[89] The anaphylactoid reactions typically respond to the administration of antihistamines and need not preclude further treatment with NAC.[86,88,89]

Effective administration of oral NAC may be hindered by emesis. The time to peak levels is approximately 1.4 hours. Acetaminophen overdose by itself is associated with emesis, and NAC, which is foul smelling and foul tasting, only adds to the nausea and vomiting triggers that may already be present. If the patient vomits within 1 hour of the initial dose, many toxicologists would recommend repeating that dose. Aggressive antiemetic therapy is often necessary for successful treatment when NAC is administered orally. High-dose metoclopramide (1 mg/kg; maximum of 50 mg IV) has been shown to relieve emesis in 78% of acetaminophen-poisoned patients.[93] If emesis persists, ondansetron (0.15 mg/kg IV) may be a useful adjunct.[94,95] If emesis is still persistent, a nasogastric or duodenal tube may be inserted and NAC dripped in over a 30-minute period. However, even for those who prefer the oral route, IV administration should be considered an important option in these circumstances.

In the United States, when an IV preparation was unavailable, clinical toxicologists gave the oral formulation of NAC intravenously. Traditionally, in the United States, IV NAC has been used in the following situations: inability to tolerate oral NAC despite aggressive antiemetic therapy, coingestant with the potential for morbidity and mortality necessitating ongoing gastrointestinal decontamination (e.g., whole-bowel irrigation), gastrointestinal bleeding or obstruction, medical or surgical conditions precluding oral NAC administration, acetaminophen toxicity manifested as encephalopathy severe enough to preclude oral administration of medication, and neonatal acetaminophen toxicity after maternal overdose.[96] Critically ill patients may have reduced absorption of oral NAC and thus may benefit from IV administration.

To prepare the oral preparation for IV use, the authors recommend that it be diluted to a 3% solution with 5% dextrose in water and administered through an in-line 0.2-μm Millipore filter. Each dose should be infused over a 1-hour period (140 mg/kg as a loading dose, followed by 70-mg/kg maintenance doses given over a 1-hour period every 4 hours for 12 doses) or administered as a continuous infusion after the loading dose is given. The incidence of adverse effects in 76 patients who were given the oral preparation intravenously was 5.3%. These events were classified as mild and did not interfere with subsequent IV NAC treatment.[96] Alternatively, the Prescott 20-hour protocol[97] could be considered (see Table 55-2).

Administration of NAC may also be of benefit to patients in whom ALF has already developed subsequent to acetaminophen overdose. Although NAC given to these patients does not change biochemical markers of liver function such as PT, it has been shown to improve survival and reduce the incidence of cerebral edema, as well as the incidence of hypotension requiring inotropic support.[98,99] In a prospective randomized study of patients who presented with signs of ALF, the survival rate was improved from 20% in patients who received intensive liver care to only 48% for those who were treated with NAC.[99] Groups were well matched for age, gender, and time to initial evaluation. Administration of NAC was continued until encephalopathy resolved or death ensued. The mechanism for the salutary effect of NAC is not completely understood but may be due in part to improvement in hepatic microcirculation and tissue oxygenation.[100]

The clinical pharmacology of NAC is discussed in detail in Chapter 136.

Role of Liver Transplantation and Management of Fulminant Hepatic Failure

In patients in whom ALF develops from acetaminophen toxicity, the most pressing question is whether orthotopic liver transplantation (OLT) is necessary for their survival. To make an informed recommendation with regard to OLT it is necessary to consider the natural history of patients who do not undergo transplantation, as well as the utility of prognostic indicators. Contrary to popular belief, most patients in whom ALF develops from acetaminophen toxicity survive and fully recover without transplantation. The King's College group reported their experience in 548 patients with ALF from acetaminophen toxicity treated at their center between 1990 and 1996.[101] The majority survived without OLT. Of the 424 patients (77% of the total) in this group who did not fulfill the transplantation criteria (Table 55-4), 93% survived.

TABLE 55-4 King's College Criteria for Transplantation

pH <7.25 24 hr after overdose despite fluid resuscitation and sodium bicarbonate

or

Concurrent presence of grade III-IV encephalopathy, creatinine >3.4 mg/dL (300 μmol/L), and prothrombin time >100 sec

Although 124 of 548 patients (23%) met the transplantation criteria, 56 of these 124 patients (45%) were not listed for transplantation mainly because of the rapid onset of multi-organ failure and cerebral edema. Rapid clinical deterioration also prevented transplantation in 24 of the 68 listed patients. Hence, only 44 patients (8% of the total) underwent OLT, and 33 survived to leave the hospital.

The search for highly sensitive and specific prognostic factors continues. Reliable indicators are critically important because patients may have sudden clinical deterioration and die before transplantation can take place. The window of opportunity for successful transplantation is often less than 24 hours. In contrast, transplantation should be avoided in patients expected to survive because liver function recovers completely and transplantation unnecessarily dooms the patient to a lifetime of immunosuppressive therapy.

AUXILIARY LIVER TRANSPLANTATION

Auxiliary liver transplantation is another alternative to OLT. In this procedure, the native liver is left in situ and a graft is implanted beside or below it. The aim of this procedure is to provide support while the patient's own liver regenerates. In a multicenter European study of 30 patients with hepatic failure of various etiology, 63% survived to 6 months and most had regained hepatic function and were able to stop immunosuppressive therapy.[102] Survival rates after auxiliary liver transplantation are similar to those after OLT.[103]

PROGNOSTIC INDICATORS

Several groups have studied prognostic indicators to develop criteria for transplantation. The most widely published transplant criteria were derived at the King's College Hospital liver unit in London. According to these criteria, patients should be considered for liver transplantation if their arterial pH is less than 7.25 at 24 hours or later after acetaminophen ingestion despite fluid resuscitation and treatment with sodium bicarbonate or if they have a combination of grade III or IV encephalopathy, serum creatinine level higher than 3.4 mg/dL (300 μmol/L), and PT longer than 100 seconds. These criteria were originally derived from 310 acetaminophen-poisoned patients studied between 1973 and 1985.[63] They were later validated by the same investigators in a group of 120 patients treated between 1990 and 1994. The positive predictive value of these criteria for a fatal outcome is 88%, and the negative predictive value is 65%.[104] However, other investigators have not found these criteria to be specific. For example, in a series of eight patients who met the criteria for transplantation, all but one recovered.[105]

Several groups have noted that mortality is low in the absence of encephalopathy. Makin and colleagues found that in 560 patients, mortality was a function of the grade of encephalopathy: 0% with grade I to II encephalopathy, 22% with grade III, 50% with grade IV, and 73% when cerebral edema was present.[106] In addition, Schiodt and associates were able to predict with 88% sensitivity (positive predictive value of 71%) and 90% specificity (negative predictive value of 96%) the occurrence of grade II or higher encephalopathy in a group of 32 acetaminophen-poisoned patients by using a combination of time to treatment, platelet count, and international normalized ratio (INR).[107] These results have not been subject to further investigation and validation. It is possible that in the future this model may prove useful for the prediction of who should undergo liver transplantation.

The utility of factor V as a prognostic indicator has also been studied. In a small series (n = 27) of patients, a finding of factor V levels less than 10% had a sensitivity of 91% but a specificity of only 55%. When both a factor V concentration less than 10% and grade III encephalopathy were present, the sensitivity was unchanged and the specificity rose to 91%.[108] A subsequent study, however, showed that the factor V level was much less useful than the King's College Hospital criteria in determining suitability for liver transplantation in acetaminophen-poisoned patients, although it may be useful when ALF is due to other causes.[109]

The utility of Acute Physiology and Chronic Health Evaluation (APACHE) III scores, which have been modified to include the grade of encephalopathy (grade I, 3 points; grade II, 8 points; grade III, 13 points; grade IV without cerebral edema, 24 points; grade IV with cerebral edema, 33 points), has also been studied. In 28 patients who did not fulfill either of the King's College Hospital criteria for transplantation and subsequently died, a cutoff score of over 60 had a sensitivity of 57%, a specificity of 84%, and a positive predictive value of 84%.[101] Further research is indicated before the decision to transplant can be reliably based on such disease severity indices.

Though not widely used, transjugular liver biopsy may also have a role in determining transplant suitability in patients with acetaminophen-induced ALF. Donaldson and coworkers showed in a group of 60 patients that only 2 of 19 survivors had greater than 70% hepatocellular necrosis.[110] Given some of the limitations of the King's College Hospital criteria, particularly its low negative predictive value for a poor outcome,[111] the addition of histologic data about the extent of hepatocellular necrosis may add important discriminatory prognostic information.

PSYCHIATRIC ASSESSMENT BEFORE ORTHOTOPIC LIVER TRANSPLANTATION

Psychiatric assessment for transplant feasibility is an essential aspect of the transplantation evaluation.[112] OLT is a major operative procedure, and its ultimate success is in part dependent on the transplant recipient's compliance with posttransplant care, including the need for lifelong immunosuppressive therapy. Although a suicide attempt or a history of ethanol or substance abuse by itself does not preclude transplant suitability, skilled assessment by a psychiatrist who has a close working relationship with the transplant team is essential to determine the likelihood of long-term posttransplant compliance. Ongoing substance abuse is a probable contraindication to this procedure.

THE BIOARTIFICIAL LIVER

Two artificial liver support systems that have been studied, the bioartificial liver (BAL) and the extracorporeal liver assist device (ELAD). These devices have been postulated to provide the critical time needed for hepatic recovery or serve as a "bridge" to liver transplantation. The BAL consists of porcine hepatocytes attached to microcarriers and an in-line charcoal hemoperfusion column. In an uncontrolled phase I clinical trial involving 18 patients with ALF of diverse etiology, 16 were bridged successfully to transplantation and 1 recovered.[113] In a series of eight patients with ALF from acetaminophen (three who subsequently underwent transplantation and five who recovered without transplantation), neurologic and metabolic improvement was noted in all after treatment with the BAL support system. Additionally, reductions in intracranial pressure (ICP) have been noted in patients with hepatic failure from acetaminophen who were treated with BAL.[114] The ELAD is a hollow-fiber membrane surrounded by immortalized human hepatocytes. A controlled clinical trial of patients with ALF (n = 24) did not demonstrate any difference in survival, although there were significant improvements in hemodynamic stability and the frequency of deterioration in mental status.[115]

Medical Management

Aggressive medical management is warranted for patients with ALF in an attempt to stabilize the patient and prevent further deterioration. Medical issues that arise include treatment of coagulopathy, renal failure, encephalopathy, cerebral edema, sepsis, cardiovascular collapse, metabolic derangements, and respiratory failure.

COAGULOPATHY

Coagulopathy will develop in many patients as demonstrated by an increased PT and INR. However, given the use of PT/INR as an indicator for the need for liver transplantation, many recommend that vitamin K and factor replacement with fresh frozen plasma be withheld unless the patient has frank bleeding or requires an invasive procedure such as an arterial line, central line, or ventriculostomy for monitoring of cerebrospinal fluid pressure. The efficacy of vitamin K therapy in patients with acetaminophen-induced hepatic synthetic dysfunction is of uncertain value. Active hemorrhage, most often upper gastrointestinal bleeding, necessitates treatment with fresh frozen plasma and red blood cell transfusion as needed. The use of H_2-blockers or sucralfate may reduce the risk of such bleeding.

RENAL FAILURE

Renal failure occurs in more than 75% of cases of ALF from acetaminophen overdose.[5] Decreased urine output may be the harbinger of acute renal failure, hepatorenal syndrome, and/or undertreated hypovolemia. Fluid resuscitation in these cases may inadvertently lead to fluid overload and pulmonary edema. Hemodialysis may be warranted, although the criteria for initiation are not well established. Venovenous hemofiltration is an alternative therapy but is more prone to clotting complications. Low-dose dopamine (2 to 4 μg/kg/hr) may improve renal perfusion and function. Nephrotoxic drugs should be avoided, and dosing of medications undergoing significant clearance by the kidney should be adjusted for renal insufficiency.

ENCEPHALOPATHY

Because the most common cause of death in patients with ALF is intracranial hypertension with resultant brain herniation, the onset of hepatic encephalopathy is an ominous finding. Blood ammonia concentrations are usually elevated, but the degree of ammonia elevation correlates poorly with the extent of encephalopathy. Computed tomography of the head should be performed if the patient's mental status deteriorates suddenly to evaluate for evidence of intracranial hemorrhage or cerebral edema. Neurosurgical placement of an ICP monitor may be useful to optimally control increased ICP. Extradural sensors may be preferable to intracerebral devices (e.g., ventricular catheters) because of the concomitant coagulation disorder and bleeding risk. Potentially effective interventions to lower ICP (target, <20 mm Hg) and thus maintain cerebral perfusion pressure (target, >50 mm Hg) include elevation of the patient's head 20 to 30 degrees to allow for jugular drainage; control of agitation (which may include neuromuscular blockage); hyperventilation to a $PaCO_2$ of 25 to 30 mm Hg; mannitol, 0.5 g/kg by IV bolus (which may be repeated if serum osmolality is less than 320 mm Hg); hypothermia (cooling blanket to a core temperature 33°C to 34°C); and pentobarbital coma.[5] Given the rapidly progressive time course of the encephalopathy in the setting of acetaminophen-induced liver failure, lactulose and bowel decontamination are not thought to be effective interventions.[116]

SEPSIS AND SHOCK

Patients with ALF who survive the first 4 to 5 days after an acute overdose remain at risk for complications of systemic inflammatory response syndrome (SIRS), sepsis, and hemodynamic collapse. SIRS is associated with worsening encephalopathy and a poorer prognosis.[117] Susceptibility to infection, both bacterial and fungal, appears to be as common in ALF secondary to acetaminophen overdose as in other etiologies. In a study of 39 patients with acetaminophen-induced ALF, documented bacterial infection developed in 82% and fungal infection in 34%.[118] Infections are thought to be the direct cause of death in 18% of patients with ALF.[5] The most common sites of infection are the respiratory tract, urinary tract, and blood. Bacteremia may be a direct result of seeding from a catheter or from decreased integrity of gastrointestinal mucosa. Endotoxemia, macrophage activation, and cytokine and tumor necrosis factor release may all occur and lead to a clinical condition resembling septic shock.[47] Because the only early sign of infection may be worsening encephalopathy or renal dysfunction, a high index of suspicion for infection, including daily cultures of blood, urine, and other fluids, has been recommended. The administration of broad-spectrum antibiotics is warranted if there is evidence of fever or other signs of infection. Antifungal agents may also need to be given to patients who do not respond rapidly to antibiotics. The use of prophylactic antibiotics and antifungals in these patients remains controversial.

Hemodynamic collapse and sudden death may also occur in patients with ALF secondary to acetaminophen overdose. Measurement of central venous pressure may prove useful to optimize fluid management. The insertion of a pulmonary artery catheter to frequently assess cardiac output, oxygen delivery and consumption, and systemic vascular resistance has also been recommended.[5] Continuous cardiac monitoring is essential. Norepinephrine or epinephrine infusions may be used to keep mean arterial pressure above 60 mm Hg.

HYPOGLYCEMIA

Hypoglycemia from impaired gluconeogenesis and decreased hepatic glycogen stores is one of the most significant metabolic derangements in patients with ALF. Hypoglycemia develops in more than 40% of these patients, and therefore frequent glucose monitoring is critical. Patients with hypoglycemia may require 10% dextrose infusions. The delivery of more concentrated glucose solutions through a central line may be necessary in patients with refractory hypoglycemia. Metabolic acidosis should be aggressively corrected with sodium bicarbonate infusion. Hypophosphatemia is also common and should be corrected.

SEDATION

Careful consideration must be given to which agents should be used for sedation in patients with ALF. No controlled studies have been conducted that address this issue. If benzodiazepines are used, an agent that does not have active metabolites, such as lorazepam, is preferable to diazepam. Recently, propofol infusions have been used in patients with ALF from acetaminophen overdose. Cessation of drug effect may be prolonged.

CHRONIC OVERDOSE

No treatment approach has been validated for patients who present with a history of chronic ingestion of supratherapeutic doses of acetaminophen. On initial evaluation, baseline plasma acetaminophen, AST, ALT, and bilirubin concentrations and PT/INR should be obtained. The nomogram has been validated only for patients who have taken a single overdose. No studies proving that NAC provides benefit in the setting of chronic excess have been performed. However, we recommend NAC therapy if either AST or ALT is abnormal. A more difficult treatment decision arises when the transaminases are normal but there is a detectable plasma acetaminophen concentration. Given the minimal side effect profile of NAC, we recommend the most conservative approach in this situation, which is to begin NAC therapy if the plasma acetaminophen concentration is higher than 10 μg/mL (66 μmol/L). NAC may be discontinued when the plasma acetaminophen concentration is nondetectable and transaminase levels begin to fall, unless the patient exhibits worsening coagulopathy or encephalopathy develops. In these cases, NAC should be continued until the patient shows improvement or dies.

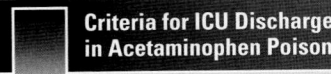

Criteria for ICU Discharge in Acetaminophen Poisoning
Resolution of major metabolic abnormalities
Improving coagulopathy
Resolving encephalopathy

SPECIAL POPULATIONS

Pregnant Patients

Acetaminophen is the preferred analgesic/antipyretic during pregnancy because it is safe at therapeutic doses and there is no evidence that it is teratogenic.[119] However, there is potential for fetal toxicity after a maternal overdose. Acetaminophen freely crosses the placenta, and the fetal liver is capable of elaborating detectable amounts of NAPQI by 14 weeks' gestation.[120] NAC also crosses the placenta; after a maternal overdose it was found in the cord blood of delivered infants (n = 4) at concentrations equivalent to those in maternal blood.[121] Despite the limited published experience about acetaminophen overdose in pregnancy, it has been reported to result in fetal morbidity[122] and mortality.[123] Treatment delay is significantly correlated with fetal wastage.[123] Therefore, we recommend that any pregnant woman who has ingested a potentially toxic amount of acetaminophen receive a loading dose of NAC on initial evaluation, regardless of the time after ingestion. If the acetaminophen concentration is then found to be in the nontoxic range, further doses of NAC are unnecessary. Other interventions such as emergency cesarean section are not usually warranted. However, cesarean section may be contemplated for near-term infants if the mother has substantial acetaminophen-induced hepatic necrosis.

Neonatal Patients

Neonates have been safely and effectively treated with IV NAC.[96,124] Care must be taken to not give excessive free

Key Points in Acetaminophen Poisoning
1. Nausea and vomiting must be treated aggressively if oral NAC is to be effective.
2. Oral NAC may be infused intravenously.
3. Unless clinically indicated, fresh frozen plasma and vitamin K should not be given if the patient has an elevated PT because the PT is an important prognostic indicator.
4. Most patients with significant hepatotoxicity (AST >1000 IU/L) and coagulopathy after acetaminophen overdose survive without liver transplantation.
5. Patients who survive an acetaminophen overdose have no residual liver damage.
6. NAC is a highly effective antidote when given shortly after an acute overdose.
7. Emesis must be controlled for oral NAC to be effective.
8. The oral formulation of NAC can be given intravenously.
9. NAC can decrease morbidity and mortality when administered to patients with fulminant hepatic failure after an acute acetaminophen overdose.
10. Selective use of liver transplantation as a treatment modality for patients with fulminant hepatic failure from acetaminophen toxicity, especially in the presence of acidemia, may prove beneficial.
11. Treatment decisions should not be overly reliant on the history (e.g., the timing and amount of ingestion) and should err on the side of prompt treatment with NAC, at least initially.

water, which can result in hyponatremia.[125] Neonatal acetaminophen poisoning has also been treated by exchange transfusion,[126] but such transfusion seems unnecessary given the proven efficacy of NAC in other populations.

REFERENCES

1. Davidson DGD, Eastham WN: Acute liver necrosis following overdose of paracetamol. BMJ 2:497, 1966.
2. Thomson JS, Prescott LF: Liver damage and impaired glucose tolerance after paracetamol overdosage. BMJ 2:506, 1966.
3. Gunnell D, Murray V, Hawton K: Use of paracetamol (acetaminophen) for suicide and nonfatal poisoning: Worldwide patterns of use and misuse. Suicide Life Threat Behav 30:313–326, 2000.
4. Litovitz TL, Klein-Schwartz W, White S, et al: 1999 annual report of the American Association of Poison Control Centers Toxic Exposure Surveillance System. Am J Emerg Med 18:517–580, 2000.
5. Mas A, Rodes J: Fulminant hepatic failure. Lancet 349:1081–1085, 1997.
6. Schiodt FV, Atillasoy E, Shakil AO, et al: Etiology and outcome for 285 patients with acute liver failure in the United States. Liver Transpl Surg 5:29–34, 1999.
7. Smilkstein MJ, Knapp GL, Kulig KW, et al: Efficacy of oral *N*-acetylcysteine in the treatment of acetaminophen overdose: Analysis of the National Multicenter Study (1976 to 1985). N Engl J Med 319:1557–1562, 1988.
8. Forrest JAH, Clements JA, Prescott LF: Clinical pharmacokinetics of paracetamol. Clin Pharmacokinet 7:93–107, 1982.
9. Augenstein WL, Kulig KW, Rumack BH: Delayed rise in serum drug levels in overdose patients despite multiple dose activated charcoal and after charcoal stools. Vet Hum Toxicol 29:491, 1987.
10. Bartle WR, Paradiso FL, Derry JE, et al: Delayed acetaminophen toxicity despite *N*-acetylcysteine use. Drug Intell Clin Pharmacol 23:509, 1989.
11. Tighe TV, Walter FG: Delayed toxic acetaminophen level after initial four hour non-toxic level. Clin Toxicol 32:431, 1994.
12. Gesell LB, Stephan M: Delayed acetaminophen peak and toxicity in combination products. J Toxicol Clin Toxicol 12:568–569, 1996.
13. Tsang WO, Nadroo AM: An unusual case of acetaminophen overdose. Pediatr Emerg Care 15:344–346, 1999.
14. Ho S, Arellano M, Zolkowski-Wynne J: Delayed increase in acetaminophen concentration after Tylenol PM overdose. Am J Emerg Med 17:315–317, 1999.
15. Cetaruk EW, Dart RC, Hurlburt KM, et al: Tylenol extended relief overdose. Ann Emerg Med 30:104–108, 1997.
16. Mitchell JR, Thorgiersson SS, Potter WZ, et al: Acetaminophen-induced hepatic injury: Protective role of glutathione in man and rationale for therapy. Clin Pharmacol Ther 16:676–684, 1974.
17. Mitchell JR, Jollow DJ, Gillette JR, et al: Drug metabolism as a cause of drug toxicity. Drug Metab Dispos 1:418–423, 1973.
18. Potter WZ, Davis DC, Mitchell JR, et al: Acetaminophen-induced hepatic necrosis. III. Cytochrome P-450–mediated covalent binding in vitro. J Pharmacol Exp Ther 187:203–210, 1973.
19. Corcoran GB, Mitchell JR, Vaishnav YN, et al: Evidence that acetaminophen and *N*-hydroxyacetaminophen form a common arylating intermediate, *N*-acetyl-*p*-benzoquinoneimine. Mol Pharmacol 18:536–542, 1980.
20. Jollow DJ, Mitchell JR, Potter WZ, et al: Acetaminophen-induced hepatic necrosis. II. Role of covalent binding in vivo. J Pharmacol Exp Ther 187:195–202, 1973.
21. Miners JO, Drew R, Birkett DJ: Mechanism of action of paracetamol protective agents in mice in vivo. Biochem Pharmacol 33:2995–3000, 1984.
22. Corcoran GB, Todd EL, Racz WJ, et al: Effects of *N*-acetylcysteine on the disposition and metabolism of acetaminophen in mice. J Pharmacol Exp Ther 232:857–863, 1985.
23. Buckpitt AR, Rollins DE, Mitchell JR: Varying effects of sulfhydryl nucleophiles on acetaminophen oxidation and sulfhydryl adduct formation. Biochem Pharmacol 28:2941–2946, 1979.
24. Mitchell JR, Jollow DJ, Potter WZ, et al: Acetaminophen-induced hepatic necrosis. IV. Protective role of glutathione. J Pharmacol Exp Ther 187:211–217, 1973.
25. Rumack BH, Peterson RG: Acetaminophen overdose: Incidence, diagnosis, and management in 416 patients. Pediatrics 62:898–903, 1978.
26. British Medical Association, Royal Pharmaceutical Society of Great Britain: Emergency treatment of poisoning. In British National Formulary, no 35. London, British Medical Association, 1998, pp 20–21.
27. Bond GR, Krenzelok EP, Normann SA, et al: Acetaminophen ingestion in childhood—cost and relative risk of alternative referral strategies. J Toxicol Clin Toxicol 32:513–525, 1994.
28. Anderson BJ, Holford NH, Armishaw JC, et al: Predicting concentrations in children presenting with an acetaminophen overdose. J Pediatr 135:290–295, 1999.
29. Caravati EM: Unintentional acetaminophen ingestion in children and the potential for hepatotoxicity. J Toxicol Clin Toxicol 38:291–296, 2000.
30. Leist MH, Gluskin LE, Payne JA: Enhanced toxicity of acetaminophen in alcoholics: Report of three cases. J Clin Gastroenterol 7:55–59, 1985.
31. Seeff LB, Cuccherini BA, Zimmerman HJ, et al: Acetaminophen hepatotoxicity in alcoholics: A therapeutic misadventure. Ann Intern Med 104:399–404, 1986.
32. Whitcomb DC, Block GD: Association of acetaminophen hepatotoxicity with fasting and ethanol use. JAMA 272:1845–1850, 1994.
33. Rivera-Penera T, Gugig R, Davi J, et al: Outcome of acetaminophen overdose in pediatric patients and factors contributing to hepatotoxicity. J Pediatr 130:300–304, 1997.
34. Heubi JE, Barbacci MB, Zimmerman HJ: Therapeutic misadventures with acetaminophen: Hepatotoxicity after multiple doses in children. J Pediatr 132:22–27, 1998.
35. Miles FK, Kamath R, Dorney SFA, et al: Accidental paracetamol overdosing and fulminant hepatic failure in children. Med J Aust 171:472–475, 1999.
36. Watkins PB: Drug metabolism by cytochromes P450 in the liver and small bowel. Gastroenterol Clin North Am 21:511–526, 1992.
37. Bray GP, Mowat CM, Muir DF, et al: The effect of chronic alcohol intake on prognosis and outcome in paracetamol overdose. Hum Exp Toxicol 10:435–438, 1991.
38. Bray GP, Harrison PM, O'Grady JG, et al: Long-term anticonvulsant therapy worsens outcome in paracetamol-induced fulminant hepatic failure. Hum Exp Toxicol 11:265–270, 1992.
39. Brotodihardjo AE, Batey RG, Farrell GC, et al: Hepatotoxicity from paracetamol self-poisoning in western Sydney: A continuing challenge. Med J Aust 157:382–385, 1992.
40. Wrights N, Prescott LF: Potentiation by previous drug therapy of hepatotoxicity following paracetamol overdosage. Scot Med J 18:56–58, 1973.
41. Scott CR, Stewart MF: Cysteamine treatment in paracetamol overdose. Lancet 1:452–453, 1975.
42. Rumack BH: Acetaminophen hepatotoxicity: The first 35 years. J Toxicol Clin Toxicol 40:3–20, 2002.
43. Rumack BH: Acetaminophen overdose in young children. Treatment and effects of alcohol and other additional ingestants in 417 cases. Am J Dis Child 138:428–433, 1984.
44. Peterson RG, Rumack BH: Age as a variable in acetaminophen overdose. Arch Intern Med 141:390–393, 1981.
45. Flanagan RJ, Mant TGK: Coma and metabolic acidosis early in severe acute paracetamol poisoning. Hum Toxicol 5:179–182, 1986.
46. Roth B, Woo O, Blanc P: Early metabolic acidosis and coma after acetaminophen ingestion. Ann Emerg Med 33:452–456, 1999.
47. Williams R: Classification, etiology, and considerations of outcome in acute liver failure. Semin Liver Dis 16:343–348, 1996.
48. Lesna M, Watson AJ, Douglas AP, et al: Evaluation of paracetamol-induced damage in liver biopsies. Acute changes and follow-up findings. Virchows Arch Pathol Anat 370:333–344, 1976.
49. Schiodt FV, Bondesen S, Tygstrup N, et al: Prediction of hepatic encephalopathy in paracetamol overdose: A prospective and validated study. Scand J Gastroenterol 34:723–728, 1999.
50. Boutis K, Shannon M: Nephrotoxicity after acute severe acetaminophen poisoning in adolescents. J Toxicol Clin Toxicol 39:441–445, 2001.
51. Jones AI, Prescott LF: Unusual complications of paracetamol poisoning. Q J Med 90:161–168, 1997.
52. Hamlyn AN, James O, Douglas AP: The spectrum of paracetamol (acetaminophen) overdose: Clinical and epidemiological studies. Postgrad Med J 54:400–404, 1978.
53. Curry RW, Robinson D, Sughrue MJ: Acute renal failure after acetaminophen ingestion. JAMA 247:1012–1014, 1982.

54. Kher K, Makker S: Acute renal failure due to acetaminophen ingestion without concurrent hepatotoxicity [letter]. Am J Med 82:1280–1281, 1987.

55. Campbell NR, Bayliss B: Renal impairment associated with an acute paracetamol overdose in the absence of hepatotoxicity. Postgrad Med J 68:116–118, 1992.

56. Yoo H, Witmer R, Wax P: Acute pancreatitis associated with acetaminophen hepatotoxicity [abstract]. J Toxicol Clin Toxicol 38:570, 2000.

57. Lip GYH, Vale JA: Does acetaminophen damage the heart? J Toxicol Clin Toxicol 34:145–147, 1996.

58. Henretig FM, Selbst SM, Forrest C, et al: Repeated acetaminophen overdosing causing hepatotoxicity in children. Clin Pediatr (Phila) 28:525–528, 1989.

59. Kozer E, Barr J, Evans S, et al: Potential hepatotoxicity of repeated acetaminophen administration in children [abstract]. J Toxicol Clin Toxicol 39:473, 2001.

60. Kuffner EK, Dart RC, Bogdan GM, et al: Effect of maximal daily doses of acetaminophen on the liver of alcoholic patients: A randomized, double-blind, placebo-controlled trial. Arch Intern Med 161:2247–2252, 2001.

61. Singer AJ, Carracio TR, Mofenson HC: The temporal profile of increased transaminase levels in patients with acetaminophen-induced liver dysfunction. Ann Emerg Med 26:49–53, 1995.

62. Ohtani N, Matsuzaki M, Anno Y, et al: A case of myocardial damage following acute paracetamol poisoning. Jpn Circ J 53:278–282, 1989.

63. O'Grady JG, Alexander GJM, Hayllar KM, et al: Early indicators of prognosis in fulminant hepatic failure. Gastroenterology 97:439–445, 1989.

64. Kumar S, Rex DK: Failure of physicians to recognize acetaminophen hepatotoxicity in alcoholics. Arch Intern Med 151:1189–1191, 1991.

65. Prescott LF: Paracetamol overdosage: Pharmacological considerations and clinical management. Drugs 25:290–314, 1983.

66. Whyte IM, Buckley NA, Reith DM, et al: Acetaminophen causes an increased international normalized ratio by reducing functional factor VII. Ther Drug Monit 22:742–748, 2000.

67. Gray TA, Buckley BM, Vale JA: Hyperlactataemia and metabolic acidosis following paracetamol overdose. Q J Med 65:811–821, 1987.

68. Porter KE, Dawson AG: Inhibition of respiration and gluconeogenesis by paracetamol in rat kidney preparations. Biochem Pharmacol 28:3057–3062, 1979.

69. Landin JS, Cohen SD, Khairallah EA: Identification of a 54-kDa mitochondrial acetaminophen-binding protein as aldehyde dehydrogenase. Toxicol Appl Pharmacol 141:299–307, 1996.

70. Esterline RL, Ray SD, Ji S: Reversible and irreversible inhibition of hepatic mitochondrial respiration by acetaminophen and its toxic metabolite, N-acetyl-p-benzoquinoneimine (NAPQI). Biochem Pharmacol 38:2387–2390, 1989.

71. Ramsey RR, Rashed MS, Nelson SD: In vitro effects of acetaminophen metabolites and analogs on the respiration of mouse liver mitochondria. Arch Biochem Biophys 273:449–457, 1989.

72. Carvalho M, Carvalho F, Bastos ML: Is hyperthermia the triggering factor for hepatotoxicity induced by 3,4-methylenedioxymethamphetamine (ecstasy)? An in vitro study using freshly isolated mouse hepatocytes. Arch Toxicol 74:789–793, 2001.

73. Wax P, Linden E: Fulminant hepatic failure after successful liver transplantation: Unmasking the culprit [abstract]. J Toxicol Clin Toxicol 37:665–666, 1999.

74. GDS Enzymatic Acetaminophen Reagent. Package insert. Elkhart, IN, GDS Diagnostics.

75. Webster PA, Roberts DW, Benson RW, et al: Acetaminophen toxicity in children: Diagnostic confirmation using a specific antigenic biomarker. J Clin Pharmacol 36:397–402, 1996.

76. Roberts DW, Bucci TJ, Benson W, et al: Immunohistochemical localization and quantification of the 3-(cystein-S-yl)-acetaminophen protein adduct in acetaminophen hepatotoxicity. Am J Pathol 138:359–371, 1991.

77. American Academy of Clinical Toxicology, European Association of Poisons Centres and Clinical Toxicologists: Single-dose activated charcoal. J Toxicol Clin Toxicol 35:721–741, 1997.

78. Green R, Grierson R, Sitar DS, et al: How long after drug ingestion is activated charcoal still effective? J Toxicol Clin Toxicol 39:601–606, 2001.

79. Smilkstein MJ: A new loading dose for N-acetylcysteine? The answer is NO. Ann Emerg Med 24:538, 1994.

80. Spiller HA, Krenzelok EP, Grande GA, et al: A prospective evaluation of the effect of activated charcoal before oral N-acetylcysteine in acetaminophen overdose. Ann Emerg Med 23:519–523, 1994.

81. Smilkstein MJ, Bronstein AC, Linden C, et al: Acetaminophen overdose: A 48-hour intravenous N-acetylcysteine treatment protocol. Ann Emerg Med 20:1058–1063, 1991.

82. Buckley NA, Whyte IM, O'Connell DL, et al: Oral or intravenous N-acetylcysteine: Which is the treatment of choice for acetaminophen (paracetamol) poisoning? J Toxicol Clin Toxicol 37:759–767, 1999.

83. Poisendex, Micromedex, vol 113, 2002.

84. Douglas DR, Smilkstein MJ, Rumack BH: APAP levels within 4 hours: Are they useful [abstract]? Vet Hum Toxicol 36:350, 1994.

85. Anderson BJ, Holford NHG, Armishaw JC, et al: Predicting concentration in children presenting with acetaminophen overdose. J Pediatr 135:290–295, 1999.

86. Tenenbein M: Hypersensitivity-like reactions to N-acetylcysteine. Vet Hum Toxicol 26(Suppl 2):3, 1984.

87. Miller LF, Rumack BH: Clinical safety of high oral doses of acetylcysteine. Semin Oncol 10(Suppl 1):76–85, 1983.

88. Chan TYK, Critchley JAJH: Adverse reactions to intravenous N-acetylcysteine in Chinese patients with paracetamol (acetaminophen) poisoning. Hum Exp Toxicol 13:542–544, 1994.

89. Schmidt LE, Dalhoff K: Risk factors in the development of adverse reactions to N-acetylcysteine in patients with paracetamol poisoning. Br J Clin Pharmacol 51:87–91, 2001.

90. Bateman DN, Woodhouse KW, Rawlins MD: Adverse reactions to N-acetylcysteine. Hum Toxicol 3:393–398, 1984.

91. Appelboam AV, Dargan PI, Knighton J: Fatal anaphylactoid reaction to NAC: Concern in asthmatics. Emerg Med J 19:594–595, 2002.

92. Dawson AH, Henry DA, McEwen J: Adverse reactions to N-acetylcysteine during treatment for paracetamol poisoning. Med J Aust 150:329–331, 1989.

93. Wright RO, Anderson AC, Lesko SL, et al: Effect of metoclopramide dosing on preventing emesis after oral administration of N-acetylcysteine for acetaminophen overdose. J Toxicol Clin Toxicol 37:35–42, 1999.

94. Clark RF, Chen R, Williams SR, et al: The use of ondansetron in the treatment of nausea and vomiting associated with acetaminophen poisoning. J Toxicol Clin Toxicol 34:163–167, 1996.

95. Scharman EJ: Use of ondansetron and other antiemetics in the management of toxic acetaminophen ingestions. J Toxicol Clin Toxicol 36:19–25, 1998.

96. Yip L, Dart RC, Hurlburt KM: Intravenous administration of oral N-acetylcysteine. Crit Care Med 26:40–43, 1998.

97. Prescott LF, Illingworth RN, Critchley JAJH, et al: Intravenous N-acetylcysteine: The treatment of choice for paracetamol poisoning. BMJ 2:1097–1100, 1979.

98. Harrison PM, Keays R, Bray GP, et al: Improved outcome of paracetamol-induced hepatic failure by late administration of acetylcysteine. Lancet 335:1572–1573, 1990.

99. Keays, R, Harrison PM, Wendon JA, et al: Intravenous acetylcysteine in paracetamol induced fulminant hepatic failure: A prospective controlled trial. BMJ 303:1026–1028, 1991.

100. Harrison PM, Wendon JA, Gimson AES, et al: Improvement by acetylcysteine of hemodynamics and oxygen transport in fulminant hepatic failure. N Engl J Med 324:1852–1857, 1991.

101. Bernal W, Wendon J, Rela M, et al: Use and outcome of liver transplantation in acetaminophen-induced acute liver failure. Hepatology 27:1050–1055, 1998.

102. Chenard-Neu M-P, Boudjema K, Bernuau J, et al: Auxiliary liver transplantation: Regeneration of the native liver and outcomes in 30 patients with fulminant hepatic failure—a multicenter European study. Hepatology 23:1119–1127, 1996.

103. van Hoek B, de Boer J, Boudjema K, et al: Auxiliary versus orthotopic liver transplantation for acute liver failure. J Hepatol 30:699–705, 1999.

104. Anand AC, Nightingale P, Neuberger JM: Early indicators of prognosis in fulminant hepatic failure: An assessment of the King's criteria. J Hepatol 26:62–68, 1997.

105. Gow PJ, Angus PW, Smallwood RA: Transplantation in patients with paracetamol-induced fulminant hepatic failure. Lancet 349:651–652, 1997.

106. Makin AJ, Wendon J, William R: A 7-year experience of severe acetaminophen-induced hepatotoxicity (1987–1993). Gastroenterology 109:1907–1916, 1995.

107. Schiodt FV, Bondesen S, Tygstrup N, Christensen E: Prediction of hepatic encephalopathy in paracetamol overdose: A prospective and validated study. Scand J Gastroenterol 7:723–728, 1999.
108. Pereira LMMB, Langley PG, Hayllar KM, et al: Coagulation factor V and VIII/V ratio as predictors of outcome in paracetamol induced fulminant hepatic failure: Relation to other prognostic indicators. Gut 33:98–102, 1992.
109. Izumi S, Langley PG, Wendon J: Coagulation factor V levels as a prognostic indicator in fulminant hepatic failure. Hepatology 23:1507–1511, 1996.
110. Donaldson BW, Gopinath R, Wanless IR, et al: The role of transjugular liver biopsy in fulminant liver failure: Relation to other prognostic indicators. Hepatology 18:1370–1376, 1993.
111. Shakil AO, Kramer D, Mazariegos GV, et al: Acute liver failure: Clinical features, outcome analysis, and applicability of prognostic criteria. Liver Transpl 6:163–169, 2000.
112. Forster J, Bartholome WG, Delcore R: Should a patient who attempted suicide receive a liver transplant? J Clin Ethics 7:257–267, 1996.
113. Watanbee FD, Mullon CJ-P, Hewitt WR, et al: Clinical experience with bioartificial liver in the treatment of severe liver failure: A phase I clinical trial. Ann Surg 225:484–494, 1997.
114. Detry O, Arkadopoulos N, Ting P, et al: Clinical use of a bioartificial liver in the treatment of acetaminophen-induced fulminant hepatic failure. Am Surg 65:934–938, 1999.
115. Hughes RD, Williams R: Use of bioartificial and artificial liver support devices. Semin Liver Dis 16:435–444, 1996.
116. O'Grady JG: Paracetamol-induced acute liver failure: Prevention and management. J Hepatol 26:41–46, 1997.
117. Rolando N, Wade J, Dabalos M, et al: Systemic inflammatory response syndrome in acute liver failure. Hepatology 32:734–739, 2000.
118. Rolando N, Harvey FAH, Brahm J, et al: Prospective study of bacterial infection in acute liver failure: An analysis of fifty patients. Hepatology 1:49–53, 1990.
119. McElhatton PR, Sullivan FM, Volans GN, Fitzpatrick R: Paracetamol poisoning in pregnancy: An analysis of the outcomes of cases referred to the Teratology Information Service of the National Poisons Information Service. Hum Exp Toxicol 9:147–153, 1990.
120. Yaffe SJ, Rane A, Sjoqvist F, et al: The presence of a monooxygenase system in human fetal liver microsomes. Life Sci 9:1189, 1970.
121. Horowitz RS, Dart RC, Jarvie DR, et al: Placental transfer of N-acetylcysteine following human maternal acetaminophen toxicity. J Toxicol Clin Toxicol 35:447–451, 1997.
122. Char VC, Fletcher AB, Avery GB: Polyhydramnios and neonatal renal failure—a possible association with maternal acetaminophen ingestion. J Pediatr 86:638, 1975.
123. Riggs BS, Bronstein AC, Kulig K, et al: Acute acetaminophen overdose during pregnancy. Obstet Gynecol 74:247–252, 1989.
124. Aw MM, Dhawan A, Baker A, et al: Neonatal paracetamol poisoning. Arch Dis Child Fetal Neonatal Ed 81:78F-81F, 1999.
125. Sung L, Simons JA, Dayneka NL: Dilution of intravenous N-acetylcysteine as a cause of hyponatremia. Pediatrics 100:389–390, 1997.
126. Lederman S, Fysh WJ, Tredger M, Gamsu HR: Neonatal paracetamol poisoning: Treatment by exchange transfusion. Arch Dis Child 58:631–633, 1983.

CHAPTER 56

Opioids

In-Hei Hahn ■ Lewis S. Nelson

Opium production dates back to the 4th millennium BC, and the first written documentation of its use dates to the writings of Theophrastus in the 3rd century BC.[1,2] Opium, which is the crude extract of the opium poppy plant, *Papaver somniferum*, was used for medicinal, recreational, and religious purposes. Morphine was isolated from opium in 1806 and was named after Morpheus, the Greek god of dreams. Diacetylmorphine, also called *heroin*, ironically was synthesized in the search for a safer, less addicting opioid. The endogenous opioid peptides, enkephalin, β-endorphin, and dynorphin, were isolated sequentially starting in 1975.[3] Although the medicinal benefits of opioids are undeniable, opioid use is fraught with tribulations for the patient and for society. This chapter focuses on the clinical issues concerning the acute and chronic effects of opioid use.

The term *opioid* refers to an agent that is capable of specific binding to an opioid receptor. This term is inclusive and alludes to all such agents, whether they are endogenous peptides, plant or animal derived, or synthetic, and does not specify whether the agent is an agonist or an antagonist at the receptor. *Opiates* are the subclass of drugs derived from the opium poppy plant. More than 20 naturally occurring opioid alkaloids can be extracted from this plant, including morphine, codeine, and thebaine. Semisynthetic opioids, such as heroin, oxycodone, and hydromorphone, are derived from structurally altering morphine's base structure with functional groups (Fig. 56-1). For example, heroin has acetyl functional groups added at the 3 and 6 positions to make diacetylmorphine.

Endogenous opioid peptides include three individual classes of peptides—enkephalins, dynorphins, and endorphins—that serve as innate agonists of the various human opioid receptors. The term *narcotic*, derived from the Greek word meaning "stupor" or "numbness," is used to refer to any drug that induces sleep. Although this use of the term encompasses one of the primary clinical roles of the opioid agonists, the term often is used to designate an illicit substance.

PHARMACOLOGY

Opioids interact with opioid receptors (Table 56-1) to modulate their various clinical effects. Opioid receptors may be categorized based either on location within the body or on the binding affinities for various endogenous or exogenous opioid agents. Similarly, opioids may be classified by their receptor preference or by pharmacologic characteristics. Because of this multiplicity of receptor and drug characteristics, most opioids produce a wide array of clinical effects. Opioid receptor families are identified in the central nervous system and are differentiated by anatomic location and function. The opioid receptor is stereospecific, and only the levorotatory (−) opioid isomers elicit clinical effects. The μ receptor, which exists in two subtypes, μ_1 and μ_2, is the binding site for the endogenous ligand β-endorphin.[4] When stimulated, the μ_1 receptor subtype produces supraspinal (e.g., brain) analgesia, euphoria, and peripheral antiinflammatory effects. Stimulation of the μ_2 receptor subtype mediates spinal-level analgesia and is the cause of most of the negative effects of opiate use, such as respiratory depression, miosis, constipation, pruritus, bradycardia, and physical dependence. These receptor subtypes are localized to the areas of the brain responsible for analgesia (periaqueductal gray matter, nucleus raphe magnus, medial thalamus), euphoria (limbic system), respiratory depression, and cough (medulla).[5,6] In the periphery, the μ_2 receptor is found in the gastrointestinal tract and peripheral terminals of nerve fibers in human synovia and immune cells, such as lymphocytes, macrophages, and mast cells.[7]

Although the κ receptors are named for their ability to bind ketocyclazocine, their endogenous ligand is dynorphin A.[8] κ receptors are found primarily in the spinal cord but also are found supraspinally in the antinociceptive regions of the brain, substantia nigra, cortex, and cerebellum. The functional opioid receptors in the cerebellum may be involved not only in motor control but also in motivational aspects of behavior and cognitive functions and in pain.[9–11] The κ_1 receptor subtypes produce primarily spinal analgesia and miosis. Agonism at the κ_2 receptor subtype is associated with dysphoria and psychotomimesis. The κ_3 receptor subtype, in contrast to the κ_1 receptor, provides supraspinal analgesia.[12] Dysfunction of the κ opioid receptor system may underlie some of the neurochemical mechanisms of drug abuse. Chronic administration of drugs with positive reinforcing properties, such as morphine, amphetamine, and cocaine, increases brain dynorphin levels,[13,14] which suggests that dynorphin may be part of homeostatic mechanisms to oppose the mood-enhancing and reinforcing effects of these drugs of abuse. Agonists at the κ receptor may increase the general dysphoric state, and the use of buprenorphine, a κ receptor antagonist/partial μ agonist, has been shown to be an effective treatment for opioid dependence by decreasing the imbalance of κ agonism. Buprenorphine also is reported to have antidepressant and antipsychotic effects.[15]

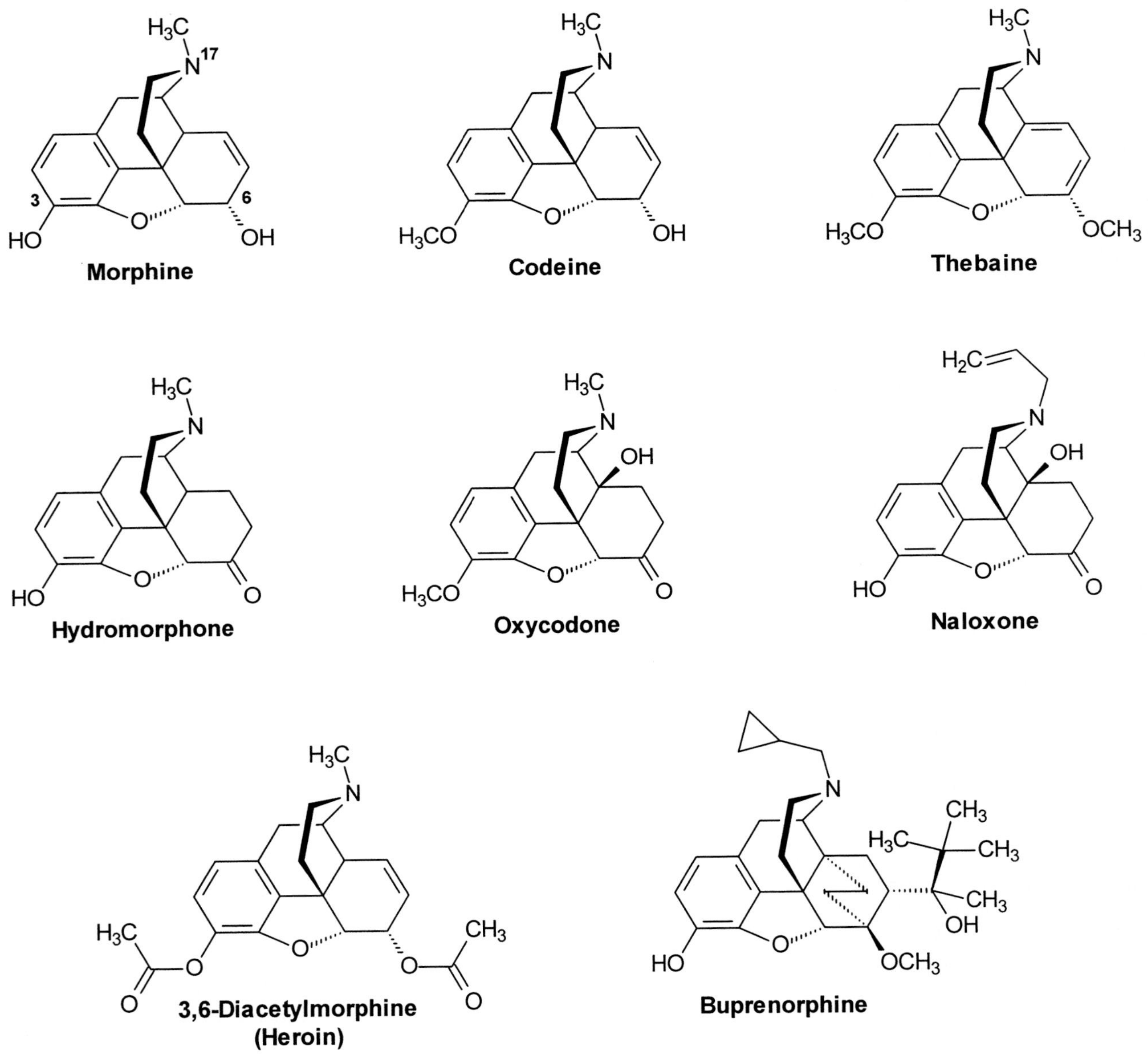

FIGURE 56-1

Chemical structures of opioids discussed in the text.

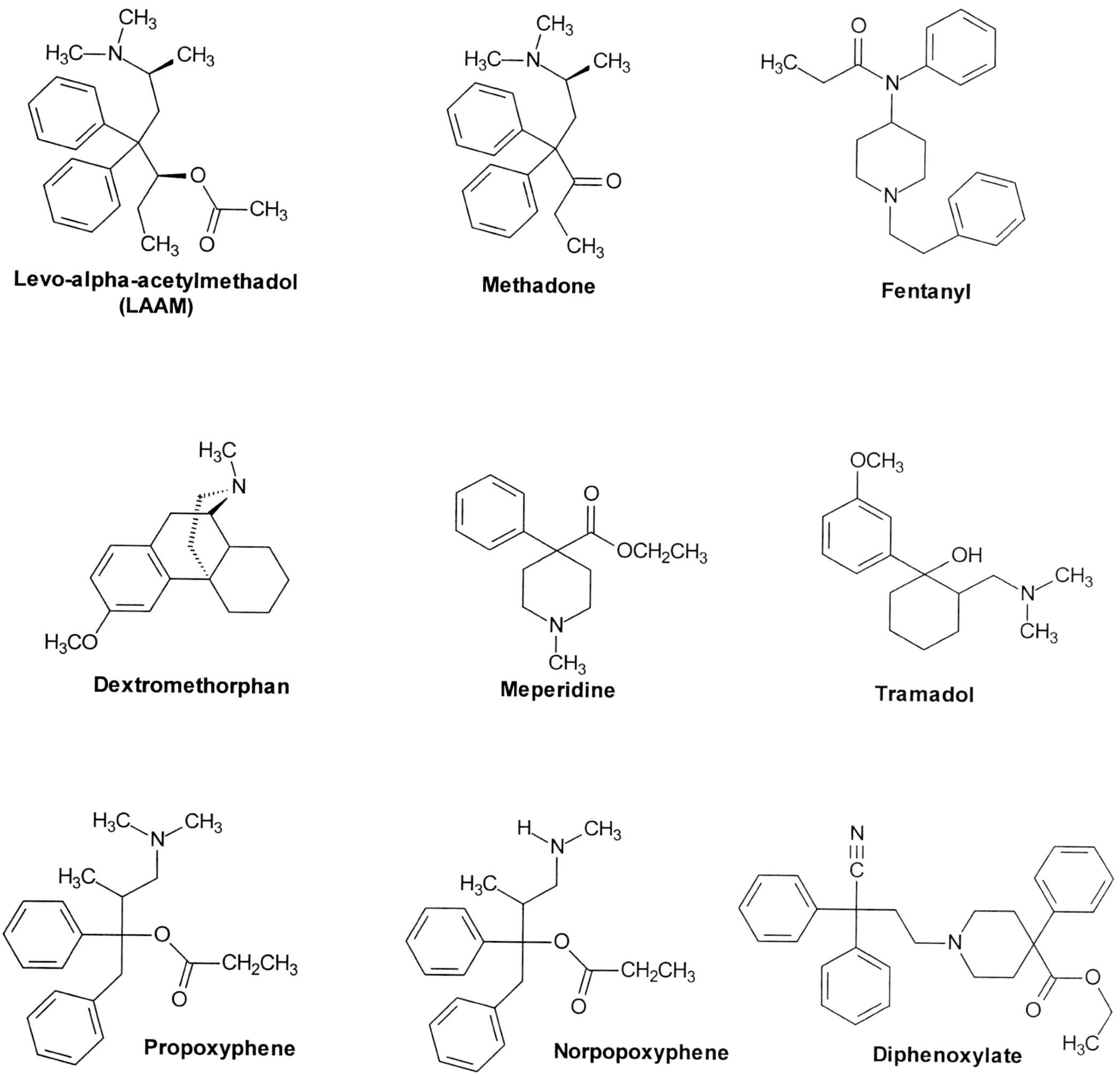

Levo-alpha-acetylmethadol (LAAM)

Methadone

Fentanyl

Dextromethorphan

Meperidine

Tramadol

Propoxyphene

Norpopoxyphene

Diphenoxylate

FIGURE 56-1 (*Continued*)

The δ receptor affects spinal analgesia. δ_1 and δ_2 receptor subtypes are established, and the enkephalins are their endogenous ligands.[16] Other δ receptor functions include alteration of nigrostriatal dopamine release, which modulates motor activity,[17] and inhibition of the cough reflex.[18]

A variety of opioid agonists are available for clinical use (Tables 56-2 and 56-3). Although useful for classification, whether the drug is natural, synthetic, or semisynthetic has little relevance to the clinical effects or pharmacology of the individual opioid agonists. Their predominant roles are in the management of acute and chronic pain syndromes or substitution therapy for illicit opioid use (e.g., methadone, buprenorphine). Their primary differences relate to their duration of effect, although most of the agents used for acute pain management are short acting, with duration of approximately 4 to 7 hours after a single dose.[2] Agents used for the other indications typically are longer acting. The ability to predict the duration of effect after chronic use and overdose is limited and is extended uniformly in this setting.[2]

A mixed opioid agonist-antagonist, such as pentazocine (κ agonist, μ antagonist), may act as an opioid agonist in an opioid-naive person but produce a withdrawal phenomenon

TABLE 56-1 Interaction of Opioids and Their Receptors in Modulating Various Clinical Effects

OPIOID RECEPTORS	AGONISTS	CLINICAL EFFECTS	LOCATION
μ_1, μ_2	Morphine	μ_1—supraspinal analgesia, peripheral analgesia, euphoria, prolactin release μ_2—spinal analgesia, respiratory depression, physical dependence, gastrointestinal dysmotility, miosis, pruritus, bradycardia	Periaqueductal gray matter, nucleus raphe magnus, medial thalamus, limbic system, medulla
κ_1, κ_2, κ_3	Ketocyclazocine—κ_1	κ_1—spinal analgesia, miosis	Spinal cord, antinociceptive regions of brain as listed above, substantia nigra
	Pentazocine—κ_2 Nalorphine—κ_3	κ_2—psychotomimesis, dysphoria κ_3—supraspinal analgesia	
σ (no longer considered opioid receptor)	Dextromethorphan, pentazocine	Spinal analgesia, psychotomimesis, movement disorders	Hypothalamus, limbic forebrain, midbrain, cerebellum, brainstem, hippocampus

in an opioid-dependent patient[2]; this is due to its ability to bind, but only incompletely stimulate, the μ opioid receptor. Similarly, butorphanol, another opioid agonist-antagonist, derives its beneficial clinical effects through κ receptor stimulation and antagonizes the μ opioid receptor. A partial agonist, such as buprenorphine, mediates its effects by μ agonism and κ antagonism. Partial agonists can be effective opioid analgesics in opioid-naive patients. In opioid-dependent patients, buprenorphine competes with the existing opioid for the μ receptor and can produce the opioid withdrawal

syndrome. Diphenoxylate is a congener of meperidine that is used as an agent to reduce gastrointestinal motility. Because of its insolubility, diphenoxylate acts locally within the gastrointestinal tract. Typically, diphenoxylate is combined with atropine (Lomotil) for the treatment of diarrhea. Opioid and anticholinergic effects may occur in an overdose. Delayed and recurrent presentation may be noted secondary to the delay in gastric emptying by both agents. Naloxone is effective in reversing recurrent central nervous system and respiratory depression. One patient was noted to present 18 hours

TABLE 56-2 Opioids Available for Clinical Use

AGENT	CLASS	COMMENTS
Agonists		
Codeine	Natural	Often combined with acetaminophen; used as antitussive
Morphine	Natural	Gold standard opioid
Buprenorphine (Buprenex)	Semisynthetic	Opioid substitution therapy requires 6–16 mg/day
Dextromethorphan (Robitussin DM)	Semisynthetic	Antitussive; abused for psychoactive effects
Heroin	Semisynthetic	Diacetylmorphine, more euphoric than morphine
Hydromorphone (Dilaudid)	Semisynthetic	Potent opioid for chronic pain therapy
Oxycodone (Percocet)	Semisynthetic	Sustained-release preparation (OxyContin)
Fentanyl (Sublimaze)	Synthetic	Very short acting, parenteral only
Meperidine (Demerol)	Synthetic	Seizures due to metabolite accumulation
Methadone (Dolophine)	Synthetic	Very long acting (approximately 24 hr)
Propoxyphene (Darvon)	Synthetic	Seizures, dysrhythmias in overdose
Tramadol (Ultram)	Synthetic	Seizures may occur
Antagonists		
Nalmefene (Revex)	Semisynthetic	Long acting (4–6 hr)
Naltrexone (Trexan)	Semisynthetic	Very long acting (24 hr)
Naloxone (Narcan)	Semisynthetic	Short acting (0.5 hr)
Mixed Agonists-Antagonists		
Pentazocine (Talwin)	Semisynthetic	
Butorphanol (Stadol)	Semisynthetic	
Nalbuphine (Nubain)	Semisynthetic	
Partial Agonist		
Buprenorphine (Buprenex)	Semisynthetic	Gaining wide acceptance in opioid-substitution therapy

TABLE 56-3 Comparison of Opioid Analgesics with Respect to Dosage and Duration of Action

DRUG	ROUTE	DOSE (mg)	PLASMA HALF-LIFE (hr)	DURATION OF EFFECT (hr)
Morphine	IM, SC	10	2	2–3
	PO	60		3–5
Heroin (diacetylmorphine)	IM, SC	5	0.5	2–3
	PO	60		
Hydromorphone (Dilaudid)	IM, SC	1.3	2–3	3–5
	PO	7.5		
Methadone (Dolophine)	IM	10	15–40	12–24
	PO	20		12–24
Meperidine (Demerol)	IM, SC	75	3–4	3–5
	PO	300		4–6
Fentanyl (Sublimaze)	IM	0.1	3–4	<1
Codeine	IM	130	2–4	3–5
	PO	200		
Oxycodone	PO	5–10		3–5

IM, intramuscular; PO, oral; SC, subcutaneous.

Data from Reisine T, Pasternak G: Opioid analgesics and antagonists. In Hardman J, Limbird L, Molinoff P, et al (eds): Goodman and Gilman's The Pharmacological Basis of Therapeutics, 9th ed. New York, McGraw-Hill, 1996, pp 521–555.

after ingestion with marked signs of atropinism, whereas other patients presented with delayed respiratory depression.[19] Because of the possibility of delayed and severe effects, all patients with significant ingestions of diphenoxylate-atropine should be admitted for monitored observation.

Certain agents with opioid activity also have additional pharmacologic effects mediated by nonopioid mechanisms. Dextromethorphan, an abused, nonanalgesic, opioid antitussive agent,[20,21] is a σ receptor agonist, through which it produces sedation and perhaps the dissociative state similar to that produced by phencyclidine.[22,23] It is also a noncompetitive antagonist at N-methyl-D-aspartate (NMDA) receptors with an active metabolite dextrorphan and binds to the phencyclidine site on the NMDA receptor, with subsequent inhibition of calcium influx through this receptor-linked ion channel, causing psychotomimesis.[24] Dextromethorphan has affinity for dextromethorphan and phencyclidine receptors and reduces K+-evoked and NMDA-evoked increases in $[Ca^{2+}]_i$ in a concentration-dependent manner. The results of an in vitro study suggested that dextromethorphan may exert anticonvulsant and neuroprotective effects by reducing Ca^{2+} influx through voltage-activated Ca^{2+} channels.[25]

Propoxyphene and its metabolite norpropoxyphene possess myocardial sodium channel–blocking effects analogous to those of class I antidysrhythmics. Only propoxyphene is a proconvulsant, however.[26] Normeperidine, the renally eliminated metabolite of meperidine, is a proconvulsant. Patients who use high doses of meperidine, especially patients who have renal insufficiency, are at risk for developing normeperidine toxicity.[27] In 1982, intravenous drug users developed severe parkinsonian symptoms and were labeled "frozen addicts" due to their extreme bradykinesia.[28] Intensive investigations led to the discovery of MPTP (1-methyl-4-phenyl-1,2,3,6- tetrahydropyridine), a by-product from the illicit synthesis of a meperidine analogue, MPPP (1-methyl-4-phenyl-4-propionoxy-piperidine). MPTP is metabolized to MPP+, which selectively destroys dopamine-containing cells in the substantia nigra through inhibition of oxidative phosphorylation.[29]

PATHOPHYSIOLOGY AND CLINICAL PRESENTATION

At sufficient doses, all opioid agonists produce the opioid toxidrome, a constellation of signs consisting of depression of mental status, ventilatory rate, and tidal volume; miosis; and reduced bowel motility. Many of these effects are due to a μ receptor–mediated reduction in sympathetic autonomic tone. Patients exposed to opioids, whether therapeutically or otherwise, typically present with bradycardia or hypotension, generally to a degree that is appropriate for their level of consciousness. Profound hemodynamic disturbances are unlikely to be the direct effect of an opioid agonist but represent an epiphenomenon secondary to hypoxia.

Most opioid-induced mortality relates directly to hypoxia, and patients rarely suffer significant discomfort from the other acute effects of opioids (e.g., gastrointestinal hypomotility, miosis). The opioid-induced reduction in ventilation occurs secondary to a reduced sensitivity of the medullary chemoreceptors to hypercapnia and hypoxia.[30] This effect is dose related, and agents with full agonist effect may produce apnea in sufficient dose. Opioid agonist-antagonists and partial agonists have ceilings on their ventilatory depressant effects.[31] After overdose with these agents, life-threatening hypoventilation is rare. The ventilatory effects may manifest as a decreased respiratory rate, decreased tidal volume, or both. The initial ventilatory effects of the opioids commonly include a reduction in tidal volume, which is difficult to assess and often overlooked.[32] Respiratory depression results predominantly through agonism at μ_2 receptors.[33] Because all currently available μ_1 agonists also exert effects at the μ_2 receptor, all opioids should be expected to produce respiratory depression.

Miosis is a relatively consistent finding among patients exposed to opioid agonists and likely results from a complex excitatory action on parasympathetic nerves.[34] Alternatively, patients using opioids occasionally may present with mydriasis, so this finding cannot be relied on diagnostically. Patients using heroin in combination with cocaine, called a *speedball*, may present with dilated pupils depending on the relative balance of the two agents. Patients with toxicity resulting from meperidine and propoxyphene have been reported to have normal pupil sizes.[35] Patients who have asphyxia or hypoxic brain damage also may have mydriasis.

Nausea and vomiting result from stimulation of dopamine-2 receptors at the chemoreceptor trigger zone. This effect has not been proved to be alleviated by low-dose naloxone.[36] Opioid agonists reduce gastrointestinal motility, producing constipation and bloating. These effects occur through increasing myenteric smooth muscle tone mediated through μ opioid receptors and can be reversed by low-dose oral naloxone, which is poorly bioavailable and rarely induces any opioid withdrawal symptoms.[37] Another agent that could be used to reverse constipation is methylnaltrexone, the first quaternary ammonium opioid receptor antagonist that does not cross the blood-brain barrier in humans. Methylnaltrexone reverses the unwanted peripheral opioid effects, such as constipation, without reversing the desired central effects, such as analgesia.[38] Although some gastrointestinal tolerance develops, patients who chronically take opioids generally remain constipated.[39]

Although the cardiovascular effects of opioids are mediated primarily by regulation of the autonomic nervous system, certain opioids, such as propoxyphene, may be directly cardiotoxic after overdose. Propoxyphene and its metabolite norpropoxyphene are sodium channel blockers and produce wide-complex dysrhythmias and negative inotropy after overdose. The clinical syndrome associated with sodium channel blockade is discussed in Chapter 36. Historically, quinine-adulterated heroin was associated with cardiac dysrhythmias and death.[40,41]

Acute lung injury, formerly called *noncardiogenic pulmonary edema*, is associated commonly with opioid overdose. Its cause is likely multifactorial, and its association with naloxone administration, although likely valid, is probably overestimated. Acute lung injury unmistakably is described in autopsy series in the 1880s, long before the introduction of naloxone. The association more probably relates to the improved auscultative ability of the examining physician after reinstitution of spontaneous ventilation with naloxone. Still, precipitation of a fulminant opioid withdrawal syndrome after naloxone may produce a catecholamine surge sufficient to impair myocardial relaxation and produce transitory congestive heart failure.[42] Canine models suggest that an elevated PCO_2 at the time of opioid-antagonist reversal of opioid-induced respiratory depression is associated with a more dramatic increase in systolic blood pressure and heart rate.[43]

Another mechanism implicated in opioid-associated acute lung injury involves inspiration against a closed airway glottis, the so-called Müller maneuver. Such a respiratory effort, occurring when the larynx is occluded due to pharyngeal laxity, creates negative intrathoracic pressure and may result in fluid's being drawn into alveoli through hydrostatic forces.[44] Alternatively, hypoxic damage producing an alveolar capillary leak syndrome may result in pulmonary edema.

Rapid administration or high doses of fentanyl can produce life-threatening chest wall rigidity. This effect occurs most commonly during anesthesia with high doses of fentanyl but also occurs in intravenous drug users who unknowingly inject fentanyl-adulterated heroin. Although incompletely characterized, it seems that the locus caeruleus and the caerulospinal noradrenergic pathways in the spinal cord are responsible.[45] Naloxone produces a variable, but generally beneficial, response.[2]

Although not part of the opioid toxidrome, seizures are another rare manifestation of therapeutic opioid use. After opioid overdose, patients may seize as a result of hypoxia or as a direct result of a drug or its metabolite. Accumulation of proconvulsant metabolites of certain opioids, such as meperidine, propoxyphene, and tramadol, causes seizures. Morphine injected into various regions of the brain of experimental animals causes epileptic activity not inhibited by naloxone.[46] In humans, only neonates have morphine-induced seizures, presumably due to the immaturity of the blood-brain barrier.[47] In mice, naloxone antagonizes the convulsant effects of propoxyphene but is not as effective in preventing seizures from meperidine or its metabolite normeperidine.[48]

DIAGNOSIS

Opioid poisoning is a clinical diagnosis, linking data from the patient's medical and situational history, physical examination, and, perhaps, response to naloxone therapy. Laboratory data (blood and urine testing) are not necessary for the management of opioid poisoning, other than to assess for concurrent medical conditions or to evaluate complications. The differential diagnosis of opioid poisoning includes other causes of depressed mental status, such as intracranial hemorrhage; postictal state; sepsis; postanoxic encephalopathy; hypoglycemia; hypothermia; and poisoning by various agents, including carbon monoxide, clonidine and other imidazolines, phenothiazines, and sedative-hypnotics (benzodiazepines and ethanol). Coingestants, such as ethanol and other opioid formulations containing acetaminophen and aspirin, also must be considered, and their presence may make the diagnosis more difficult. Drug screens are of mixed utility depending on the situation. In general, screens for recreational drugs are of little value in the acute setting but may be helpful for monitoring "detox" patients to ensure compliance with abstinence and methadone use. In an overdose, the serum drug screen may be helpful in detecting agents other than opioids that may alter therapy, such as acetaminophen.

TREATMENT

Proper airway management is crucial to managing opioid-poisoned patients. Patients experiencing ventilatory depression or hypoxia require either mechanical respiratory support or antidote administration. Use of nasopharyngeal or oral airway support can be considered in obtunded patients with non–life-threatening ventilatory depression and the absence of a gag reflex. Because both of these maneuvers can result in emesis, however, which can be life-threatening in a patient without an appropriate protective reflex, they should be used only with extreme caution. More appropriately, patients who are hypoventilating or hypoxic should be ventilated initially using a bag-valve-mask device with 100% oxygen supplementation. The decision to place an endotracheal tube depends on the patient's clinical condition, his or her response to less aggressive means of ventilation, and the environment in which care is delivered.

Patients experiencing inadequate ventilation, as defined by an inadequate respiratory rate or tidal volume, may benefit from the administration of an opioid antagonist, such as naloxone. In adult patients who are unconscious for undefined reasons, a respiratory rate of less than 12 breaths/min is most predictive of response to naloxone.[49] Although this finding is neither highly sensitive nor specific, opioid poisoning rarely is diagnosed in patients with respiratory rates at or above normal. Because unneeded treatment with naloxone, regardless of the dose delivered, is rarely detrimental in patients who are not opioid dependent, a therapeutic trial in patients with depressed respiration or mental status generally is warranted. Alternatively, in opioid-dependent patients, emesis due to precipitated opioid withdrawal in the setting of a non–naloxone-responsive etiology for mental status depression (e.g., ethanol intoxication) risks pulmonary aspiration. Regardless, if chronic opioid use cannot be determined, judicious administration of small doses of naloxone, with titration upward to effect, should allow the therapeutic trial to be aborted if signs of withdrawal develop. Depending on the population served and region of the United States (e.g., availability of methadone maintenance therapy), the prevalence of opioid dependence varies widely, so the empirical use of naloxone must be tailored to the clinical setting. The clinical pharmacology of naloxone is discussed in detail in Chapter 137.

Dysphoria due to dextromethorphan is treated with the administration of sedative-hypnotics such as benzodiazepines. Naloxone is not effective and may cause a withdrawal syndrome in chronic users. Naloxone at least partially reverses the respiratory and central nervous system depressant effects of dextromethorphan. The myocardial effects of propoxyphene should be treated with sodium bicarbonate and serum alkalinization in a fashion analogous to the tricyclic antidepressants (see Chapter 42).

The need for gastrointestinal decontamination depends on the circumstances surrounding the exposure, although administration of a single dose of oral activated charcoal generally is considered appropriate after an oral opioid overdose. The only opioid-exposed patients likely to benefit from more aggressive gastrointestinal decontamination are patients who are attempting to conceal large amounts of drug in their gastrointestinal tract to avoid detection by law enforcement. These patients are called *body packers*. The diagnosis usually can be confirmed with an abdominal radiograph, but occasionally false-negative radiographs occur even when patients carry large numbers of packets.[50] Patients suspected of carrying packets with a negative radiograph should receive either an abdominal computed tomography scan or a contrast-enhanced upper gastrointestinal series with bowel follow-through for full evaluation. In this patient population, whole-bowel irrigation (described in Chapter 5) may speed clearance of packets from the body. In our experience, in contrast to cocaine body packing patients, in whom symptoms mandate surgery, heroin body packers can be managed with activated charcoal, whole-bowel irrigation, and a continuous naloxone infusion until the packets pass. Intestinal perforation or obstruction generally requires surgical intervention.

Indications for ICU Admission in Opioid Poisoning

Requirement for mechanical ventilation
Symptomatic poisoning with methadone, levomethadyl acetate, or other long-acting opioid
Requirement for naloxone infusion
Acute lung injury or other hypoxic insult
Cardiovascular manifestations of hypotension or bradycardia requiring treatment
Neonatal withdrawal

Criteria for ICU Discharge in Opioid Poisoning

Resolution of ventilatory depression with adequate respirations
Resolution of acute lung injury or other hypoxic insult
Cessation of a naloxone infusion
Resolution of hypotension or bradycardia
Resolution of neonatal withdrawal

SPECIAL POPULATIONS

Pediatric Patients

Neonatal opioid withdrawal syndrome occurs in newborns of opioid-using mothers. Although it is similar to the adult opioid withdrawal syndrome in many respects, fever, myoclonic jerks, and life-threatening seizures are unique to

---

Dosing of Naloxone

Opioid dependence unlikely: 0.2–0.4 mg IV, escalating to 10 mg
Opioid dependence possible: 0.01–0.05 mg IV, additional doses every 1–2 min until response or signs of withdrawal
Positive response, short-acting opioid suspected: observe for resedation for 6 hr
Positive response, with resedation: rebolus as needed or continuous infusion starting at two thirds of the initial reversal dose hourly titrated to effect

IV, intravenously.

the neonatal syndrome. The withdrawal syndrome typically presents minutes after birth to 2 weeks later. The half-life of the particular opioid used by the mother directly correlates with the time at which opioid withdrawal symptoms manifest in the neonate.[51] Treatment of neonatal opioid withdrawal includes various regimens, such as paregoric, phenobarbital, diazepam, diluted opium tincture, and methadone. Further discussion of this withdrawal syndrome can be found in Chapter 30.

Pregnant Patients

For a pregnant opioid-tolerant patient acutely poisoned, reversal with naloxone may precipitate uterine contractions and possible induction of labor.[52] Slow titration of naloxone should reduce this effect.

Elderly Patients

Because of altered liver or kidney function in elderly patients, the pharmacokinetics of certain opioid agents may be unpredictable, and toxic effects may develop. Morphine is metabolized by the liver; any patients with cirrhosis or on medications that can interfere with liver function may be at risk for increased toxicity. In particular, elderly patients in the intensive care unit receiving ranitidine and morphine may have enhanced effects leading to confusion and hallucinations.[53,54] In one study in humans, ranitidine was found to inhibit morphine glucuronidation, decreasing the morphine- 3-glucuronide (M3G)-to-morphine-6-glucuronide (M6G) ratio and increasing the presence of morphine.[55] The active morphine metabolites, M3G and M6G, are renally excreted. M3G and M6G need to be considered when administering morphine because both metabolites can cause significant toxicity in elderly patients and patients with renal failure.[56] M6G has potent opioid agonist effects and is considered 4-fold to 20-fold more potent than morphine. M3G has no antinociceptic properties and has neuroexcitatory effects (allodynia, myoclonus, seizures).[57]

Acquired Immunodeficiency Syndrome Patients

Patients with acquired immunodeficiency syndrome (AIDS) who contracted the disease as a result of intravenous opioid use are susceptible to all the complications associated with intravenous drug use, including endocarditis, septic pulmonary emboli, tetanus, hepatitis, cellulitis, abscesses, osteomyelitis, and pneumothorax.

Key Points in Opioid Poisoning

1. Miosis is *not* present in all opioid users.
2. Miosis does not rule in opioid toxicity.
3. Naloxone should be administered in small amounts (starting with 0.05 mg) to avoid withdrawal. If opioid withdrawal results, do not attempt to reverse the withdrawal symptoms with another opioid. Allow naloxone's effect to wane spontaneously (typically 20–60 min).
4. Methadone and other semisynthetic or synthetic opioids do not cross-react with the standard urine opioid drug assay.

REFERENCES

1. Booth M: Opium: A History. New York, St. Martin's Press, 1996.
2. Reisine T, Pasternak G: Opioid analgesics and antagonists. In Hardman J, Limbird L, Molinoff P, et al (eds): Goodman and Gilman's The Pharmacological Basis of Therapeutics, 9th ed. New York, McGraw-Hill, 1996, pp 521–555.
3. Hughes J: Isolation of an endogenous compound from the brain with pharmacologic properties similar to morphine. Brain Res 88:295–308, 1975.
4. Pasternak GW: Pharmacological mechanisms of opioid analgesics. Clin Neuropharmacol 16:1–18, 1993.
5. Goodman RR, Snyder SH, Kuhar MJ, Young WS: Differentiation of δ and μ opiate receptor localization by light microscopic autoradiography. Proc Natl Acad Sci U S A 77:6239–6243, 1980.
6. Minami M, Satoh M: Molecular biology of the opioid receptors: Structures, functions and distributions. Neurosci Res 23:121–145, 1995.
7. Stein C, Pfluger M, Yassouuridis A, et al: No tolerance to peripheral morphine analgesia in presence of opioid expression in inflamed synovia. J Clin Invest 98:793–799, 1996.
8. Martin WR, Eades CG, Thompson JA, et al: The effects of morphine- and nalorphine-like drugs in the nondependent and morphine-dependent chronic spinal dog. J Pharmacol Exp Ther 197:517–532, 1976.
9. Derbyshire SWG, Jones AKP: Cerebral responses to a continual tonic pain stimulus measured using positron emission tomography. Pain 76:127–135, 1998.
10. Fiez JA: Cerebellar contribution to cognition. Neuron 16:13–15, 1996.
11. Grant S, et al: Activation of memory circuits during cue-elicited cocaine craving. Proc Natl Acad Sci U S A 93:12040–12045, 1996.
12. Martin WR, Sloan JW: Neuropharmacology and neurochemistry of subjective effects, analgesia, tolerance, and dependence produced by narcotic analgesics. In Martin WR (ed): Handbook of Experimental Pharmacology, Vol 45/I, Drug Addiction I: Morphine, Sedative/Hypnotic and Alcohol Dependence. Berlin, Springer-Verlag, 1977, pp 43–158.
13. Trujillo KA, Akil H: Changes in prodynorphin peptide content following treatment with morphine or amphetamine: Possible role in mechanisms of action of drugs of abuse. Natl Inst Drug Abuse Res Monogr 95:550–551, 1989.
14. Smile PL, Johnson M, Bush L, et al: Effects of cocaine on extrapyramidal and limbic dynorphin systems. J Pharmacol Exp Ther 253:938–943, 1990.
15. Rothman RB, et al: An open-label study of a functional opioid κ antagonist in the treatment of opioid dependence. J Subst Abuse Treat 18:277–281, 2000.
16. Portoghese PS, Larson DL, Sultana M, Takemori AE: Opioid agonist and antagonist activities of morphindoles related to naltrindole. J Med Chem 5:4325–4329, 1992.
17. Jones DNC, Holtzman SG: Interaction between opioid antagonists and amphetamine: Evidence for mediation by central delta opioid receptors. J Pharmacol Exp Ther 262:638–645, 1992.
18. Kotzer CJ, Hay DWP, Dondio G, et al: The antitussive activity of δ-opioid receptor stimulation in guinea pigs. J Pharmacol Exp Ther 292:803–809, 2000.
19. McCarron MM, Challoner KR, Thompson GA: Diphenoxylate-atropine (Lomotil) overdose in children: An update (report of eight cases and review of the literature). Pediatrics 87:694–700, 1991.
20. Schneider SM, Michelson EA, Boucek CD, Ilkhanipour K: Dextromethorphan poisoning reversed by naloxone. Am J Emerg Med 9:237–238, 1991.
21. Shaul WL, Wandell M, Robertson WO: Dextromethorphan toxicity: Reversal by naloxone. Pediatrics 59:117–118, 1977.
22. Klein M, Musacchio JM: High affinity dextromethorphan binding sites in guinea pig brain: Effect of sigma ligands and other agents. J Pharmacol Exp Ther 251:207–215, 1989.
23. Szekely JI, Sharpe LG, Jaffe JH: Induction of phencyclidine-like behavior in rats by dextrorphan but not dextromethorphan. Pharmacol Biochem Behav 40:381–384, 1991.
24. Church J: Neuromodulatory effects of dextromethorphan: Role of NMDA receptors in responses. Trends Pharmacol Sci 11:146–147, 1990.
25. Church J, Shacklock JA, Baimbridge KG: Dextromethorphan and phencyclidine receptor ligands: Differential effects on K$^+$ and NMDA-evoked increases in cytosolic free Ca^{2+} concentration. Neurosci Lett 124:232–234, 1991.
26. Lund-Jacobsen H: Cardio-respiratory toxicity of propoxyphene and norpropoxyphene in conscious rabbits. Acta Pharmacol Toxicol 42:171–178, 1978.

27. Kaiko RF, Foley KM, Grabinski PY, et al: Central nervous system excitatory effects of meperidine in cancer patients. Ann Neurol 13:180–185, 1983.

28. Langston JW, Ballard P, Tetrud JW, et al: Chronic parkinsonism in humans due to a product of meperidine-analog synthesis. Science 219:979–980, 1983.

29. Nicklas WJ, Youngster SK, Kindt MV, Heikkila RE: MPTP, MPP+ and mitochondrial function. Life Sci 40:721–729, 1987.

30. Weil JV, McCullough BS, Kline JS, Sodal IE: Diminished ventilatory response to hypoxia and hypercapnia after morphine in normal man. N Engl J Med 21:1103–1106, 1975.

31. Gal TJ, DiFazio CA, Moscicki J: Analgesic and respiratory depressant activity of nalbuphine: A comparison with morphine. Anesthesiology 57:367–374, 1982.

32. Shook JE, Watkins WD, Camporesi EM: Differential roles of opioid receptors in respiration, respiratory disease, and opiate-induced respiratory depression. Am Rev Respir Dis 142:895–909, 1990.

33. Ling GSF, Spiegel K, Lockhart SH, Pasternak GW: Separation of opioid analgesia from respiratory depression: Evidence for different receptor mechanisms. J Pharmacol Exp Ther 232:149–155, 1985.

34. Murray RB, Tallarida RJ: Pupillometric analysis of morphine action in the rabbit: Role of the autonomic nervous system. Eur J Pharmacol 80:197–202, 1982.

35. Ghoneim MM, Dhanaraj J, Choi WW: Comparison of four opioid analgesics as supplements to nitrous oxide anesthesia. Anesth Analg 63:405–412, 1984.

36. Cepeda MS, Gonzalez F, Granados V, et al: Incidence of nausea and vomiting in outpatients undergoing general anesthesia in relation to selection of intraoperative opioid. J Clin Anesth 8:324–328, 1996.

37. Meissner W, Schmidt U, Hartmann M, et al: Oral naloxone reverses opioid-associated constipation. Pain 84:105–109, 2000.

38. Yuan CS, Foss JF, O'Connor M, et al: Methylnaltrexone for reversal of constipation due to chronic methadone use: A randomized controlled trial. JAMA 283:367–372, 2000.

39. Manara L, Bianchetti A: The central and peripheral influences of opioids on gastrointestinal propulsion. Annu Rev Pharmacol Toxicol 25:249–273, 1985.

40. Lupovich P, Pilewski R, Sapira JD, Juselius R: Cardiotoxicity of quinine as adulterant of drugs. JAMA 212:1216, 1970.

41. Shesser R, Jotte R, Olshaker J: The contribution of impurities to the acute morbidity of illegal drugs of abuse. Am J Emerg Med 9:336–342, 1991.

42. Mills CA, Flacke JW, Flacke WE, et al: Narcotic reversal in hypercapnic dogs: Comparison of naloxone and nalbuphine. Can J Anaesth 37:238–244, 1990.

43. Mills CA, Flacke JW, Miller JD, et al: Cardiovascular effects of fentanyl reversal by naloxone at varying arterial carbon dioxide tensions in dogs. Anesth Analg 67:730–736, 1988.

44. Kollef MH, Pluss J: Noncardiogenic pulmonary edema following upper airway obstruction. Medicine 70:207–215, 1991.

45. Lui PW: Involvement of spinal adenosine A1 and A2 receptors in fentanyl-induced muscular rigidity in the rat. Neurosci Lett 224:189–192, 1997.

46. Turski WA, Czucawar SJ, Kleinrok Z, et al: Intraamygdaloid morphine produces seizures and brain damage in rats. Life Sci 33:615–618, 1983.

47. Koren G, Butt W, Pape K, Chinyanga H: Morphine-induced seizures in newborn infants. Vet Hum Toxicol 27:519–520, 1985.

48. Gilbert PE, Martin WR: Antagonism of the convulsant effects of heroin, d-propoxyphene, meperidine, normeperidine and thebaine by naloxone in mice. J Pharmacol Exp Ther 192:538–541, 1975.

49. Hoffman JR, Schriger DL, Luo JS: The empiric use of naloxone in patients with altered mental status: A reappraisal. Ann Emerg Med 20:246–252, 1991.

50. McCarron MM, Wood JD: The cocaine body packer syndrome: Diagnosis and treatment. JAMA 250:1417–1420, 1983.

51. Desmond MM, Wilson GS: Neonatal abstinence syndrome: Recognition and diagnosis. Addict Dis 2:113–121, 1975.

52. Flomenbaum NE, Goldfrank LR, Lewin NA, et al: Managing the patient with an unknown overdose. In Goldfrank LR, Flomenbaum NE, Lewin NA, et al (eds): Goldfrank's Toxicological Emergencies, 6th ed. Stamford, CT, Appleton & Lange, 1998, pp 515–522.

53. Martinez-Abad M, Gomis FD, Ferrer JM, Morales-Olivas FJ: Ranitidine-induced confusion with concomitant morphine. Drug Intell Clin Pharm 22:914–915, 1988.

54. Jellema JG: Hallucination during sustained-release morphine and methadone administration. Lancet 2:392, 1987.

55. Aamundstad TA, Storset P: Influence of raniditidine on the morphine-3-glucuronide to morphine-6-glucuronide ratio after oral administration of morphine in humans. Hum Exp Toxicol 17:347–352, 1998.

56. Ravenscroft P, Schneider J: Bedside perspectives on the use of opioids: Transferring results of clinical research into practice. Clin Exp Pharmacol Physiol 27:529–532, 2000.

57. Smith MT: Neuroexcitatory effects of morphine and hydromorphone: Evidence implicating the 3-glucuronide metabolites. Clin Exp Pharmacol Physiol 27:524–528, 2000.

CHAPTER 57

Salicylates

Steven C. Curry

Salicylate intoxication carries significant morbidity and mortality that are compounded when the seriousness of the situation is not recognized by the treating physician.[1] Progressive central nervous system (CNS) depression demands several immediate, aggressive actions, not just endotracheal intubation and ventilation. A small decrease in arterial pH to 7.3 may be of little consequence to most patients in a critical care unit, but in patients with salicylate intoxication, this decrease may result in rapid shifts of salicylate into the brain and heart, causing surprisingly swift deterioration and death. A decrease in serum drug concentrations is accompanied by clinical improvement in most other drug intoxications, but this frequently is not the case with serious salicylate poisoning. Patients may deteriorate and die as serum salicylate levels decrease.

A successful outcome for a patient with salicylate poisoning frequently requires prolonged physician time at the bedside with rapid responses to frequently changing laboratory and clinical parameters. The intensivist must become familiar with the pathophysiology, pharmacokinetics, potential pitfalls, and treatment options for salicylate intoxication in order to be successful in preventing death.

SOURCES OF SALICYLATE

Numerous forms of salicylate are available in over-the-counter and prescription preparations (Table 57-1). Regardless of the product, all of these formulations are converted to salicylate during or shortly after absorption.

Many keratolytic agents contain salicylic acid, and toxicity and death have followed dermal application.[2,3] Various liniments and some flavoring agents contain methyl salicylate (oil of wintergreen). Death has resulted from the ingestion of these liniments or from exposure to pure methyl salicylate.[4] Although salicylate is poorly absorbed after single ingestions of bismuth subsalicylate, the repeated use of large quantities of bismuth subsalicylate, such as those used in the treatment of diarrhea associated with acquired immunodeficiency syndrome, can result in serum salicylate concentrations in the toxic range.

PATHOPHYSIOLOGY

General and Metabolic Effects

Salicylate toxicity produces numerous metabolic derangements (Table 57-2), including respiratory alkalosis, metabolic acidosis, ketosis, hypokalemia, hypoglycemia, and hyperglycemia. Salicylate stimulates the respiratory center in the brainstem to produce tachypnea, hyperpnea, and respiratory alkalosis.[5] Most adults who present early with acute salicylate toxicity display alkalemia. As toxicity progresses, the onset of metabolic acidosis (described later) first normalizes pH and then produces acidemia as respiratory alkalosis is overwhelmed by acidosis or as respiratory depression ensues from worsening toxicity (e.g., coma, apnea). The coingestion or iatrogenic administration of CNS depressants (e.g., benzodiazepines, opiates) or neuromuscular blockade and controlled mechanical ventilation may blunt hyperventilation and respiratory alkalosis, allowing for clinical expression of only metabolic acidosis.[6]

Salicylate impairs adenosine triphosphate (ATP) synthesis through various mechanisms, and impaired ATP production from mitochondrial toxicity is the common denominator for much of salicylate's toxicity. A mitochondrion is surrounded by an external and an inner membrane. As electrons travel down the electron transport chain on the inner mitochondrial membrane (cristae), the released energy is used to pump H^+ ions out of the matrix into the mitochondrial intermembrane space, producing an electrical and pH gradient across the inner mitochondrial membrane. The electrons moving down the transport chain within the mitochondrion eventually combine with oxygen, the terminal electron acceptor, to form water. Meanwhile, hydrogen ions that have been concentrated within the intermembrane space reenter the mitochondrion through a pore in ATP synthase, a protein spanning the inner membrane, providing the energy needed to generate ATP from adenosine diphosphate (ADP) and phosphate inside the organelle. In mitochondria, ATP production via oxidative phosphorylation normally is "coupled" to oxygen consumption.

Salicylate uncouples oxidative phosphorylation through at least two mechanisms. First, similar to many weak organic acids, un-ionized salicylate crosses the inner mitochondrial membrane to release an H^+ into the matrix, where the pH is higher.[7] The remaining salicylate anion or other anions or both are transported out of the mitochondria. Second, salicylate may cause formation of pores in the inner mitochondrial membrane that are permeable to numerous substances, including H^+.[8] The end result of these two processes is a decrease in the H^+ gradient across the inner mitochondrial membrane, allowing H^+ ions to reenter the mitochondrial matrix without traveling through ATP synthase, decreasing ATP formation.[8] Electron transport and oxygen consumption continue and even accelerate in an effort to generate ATP uncoupling of oxidative phosphorylation. When uncoupling is severe, hyperthermia may develop as a consequence of heat production rather than ATP generation.

Impairment of ATP production also occurs within the mitochondrial matrix, where salicylate inhibits α-ketoglutarate dehydrogenase and succinic acid dehydrogenase of the tricarboxylic acid (Krebs) cycle.[9,10] This activity decreases formation of reduced nicotine adenine dinucleotide and reduced flavin adenine dinucleotide, the main electron donors for the respiratory chain.

The metabolic acidosis accompanying serious salicylate poisoning is poorly understood. Glycolysis (anaerobic conversion of glucose to lactate) is accelerated in salicylate poisoning in an attempt to meet ATP requirements in the presence of impaired oxidative phosphorylation. As emphasized by others,[11-13] however, the conversion of glucose to lactate does not result in the production of hydrogen ions, as illustrated in a balanced equation of glycolysis:

$$\text{Glucose} + 2\,ADP^{3-} + 2\,HPO_4^{2-} + 10\,H^+ \rightarrow 2\,\text{lactate}^- + 2\,ATP^{4-} + 2\,H_2O + 10\,H^+$$

Cellular pH and concentrations of substrates influence the amounts of ATP and H^+ produced during glycolysis, but glycolytic production of lactate and ATP is not acidifying, regardless of pH.[12,13] A large portion of the aci-

dosis of salicylate poisoning most likely results from hydrolysis of ATP:

$$ATP^{4-} + 4\,H^+ + H_2O \rightarrow ADP^{3-} + HPO_4^{2-} + 5\,H^+$$

Just as the hydrolysis of ATP always results in a net production of a H^+, the synthesis of ATP via oxidative phosphorylation in the inner mitochondrial membrane results in H^+ consumption by the reverse reaction:

$$ADP^{3-} + HPO_4^{2-} + 5\,H^+ \rightarrow ATP^{4-} + 4\,H^+ + H_2O$$

During normal metabolism, H^+ consumption via oxidative phosphorylation balances H^+ production from hydrolysis of ATP. Impaired oxidative phosphorylation (from uncoupling and inhibition of the tricarboxylic acid cycle) provides a state in which the hydrolysis of ATP produced in glycolysis generates H^+ faster than they can be buffered, excreted, or, most importantly, consumed via oxidative phosphorylation.

Circulating lactate concentrations are usually within the normal range or are slightly elevated in most patients with salicylate toxicity.[14] Occasionally lactate concentrations can be notably elevated.

The metabolic acidosis of salicylate toxicity is also in part a ketoacidosis.[5,14] Salicylate stimulates lipolysis and ketone formation. Most patients with salicylate toxicity excrete increased urine ketones that are detected easily by laboratory studies.

Elevated circulating cytokine concentrations have been described in patients with salicylate toxicity.[15] Their role in contributing to disease is undefined, however, because various cytokines are elevated in the blood of patients who are critically ill from many different causes.

Serum glucose concentrations vary during salicylate intoxication. During serious salicylate intoxication, glucose consumption is increased as glycolytic generation of ATP increases to compensate for impaired oxidative phosphorylation. Increased epinephrine and glucagon secretion results in mobilization of glycogen stores, commonly producing hyperglycemia early in the intoxication. Serum glucose concentrations commonly reach 200 to 300 mg/dL (11 to 17 mmol/L). As salicylate toxicity continues, glycogen stores become depleted, and increased glucose demands can be met only by a marked increase in gluconeogenesis. Salicylate is an inhibitor of alanine aminotransferase, preventing the conversion of alanine to pyruvate to fuel gluconeogenesis.[16] Serum glucose concentrations normalize and can reach the hypoglycemic range, especially in children[17,18] but also in adults.[19]

Hypoglycorrhachia and neuroglycopenia are noted in animal models of salicylate toxicity,[20] even without hypoglycemia. It has been suggested that some CNS toxicity from salicylate may reflect low CNS glucose concentrations and that this might occur without hypoglycemia.

Most patients with moderate-to-severe salicylate toxicity have hypokalemia, unless severe dehydration, impaired renal function, or rhabdomyolysis has resulted in hyperkalemia. Hypokalemia probably reflects gastrointestinal losses (vomiting) and obligate urinary excretion of potassium, with the salicylate anion or other organic acids or both resulting from toxicity.

A symptomatic adult patient with moderate-to-severe salicylate toxicity typically has a fluid deficit of at least 4 to 6 L on presentation. Water losses from hyperventilation, diaphoresis, third spacing of fluids in muscle from rhabdomyolysis, and vomiting are easily underestimated. Failing to rehydrate the patient adequately and maintain adequate intravascular volume is a common error made by treating physicians.

Gastrointestinal Tract and Liver Effects

Aspirin produces corrosive injury to the gastrointestinal tract. Patients with acute intoxications frequently have abdominal pain, vomiting, and hematemesis. Reports of gastric perforation after acute aspirin overdose appear in the literature.[21,22] Gastrointestinal toxicity contributes to dehydration and electrolyte losses, and occasionally anemia is severe enough to require transfusion. Salsalate produces less gastrointestinal injury than aspirin. Methyl salicylate can be very irritating, and salicylic acid keratolytic agents may produce oropharyngeal burns and more severe distal corrosive injury.[23]

Asymptomatic elevation in serum transaminases may be noted in patients with chronic ingestion of salicylates, most commonly in patients with connective tissue diseases.[62] A few of these patients have abdominal pain, nausea, and jaundice. Although clinical evidence of meaningful hepatotoxicity is not typical of acute salicylate toxicity, investigators have reported a high prevalence of hepatic microvesicular steatosis in children who died as a result of salicylate poisoning.[24] Microvesicular steatosis, as a reflection of impaired fatty acid oxidation, can be secondary to mitochondrial dysfunction from numerous causes. In the outer mitochondrial membrane, however, salicylate also sequesters extramitochondrial coenzyme A, preventing the activation of fatty acids and fatty acid β oxidation.

Pulmonary Effects

Adult respiratory distress syndrome occasionally complicates acute salicylate toxicity but is more common in chronic salicylate toxicity.[25,26]

Cardiovascular Effects

Impaired myocardial ATP production and, to a lesser extent, acid-base disorders produce sinus tachycardia, despite correction of hypovolemia. Heart failure and hypotension occur in seriously ill patients[27] but usually are not a problem until patients are near death. Ventricular arrhythmias, including sudden, unexpected ventricular fibrillation, are possible.

Effects on Coagulation and Platelets

Of all salicylate products, only aspirin significantly impairs platelet function. Salicylate (resulting from the ingestion of any product) inhibits the formation of vitamin K–dependent coagulation factors in a manner similar to that of warfarin

(Coumadin), mainly by preventing reduction of vitamin K quinone to the active hydroquinone.[28] Elevated prothrombin times usually occur 8 to 24 hours after acute overdose and respond promptly to the administration of vitamin K_1. Despite coagulopathies and potential platelet dysfunction, hemorrhage remains a rare cause of serious morbidity or mortality in patients with salicylate toxicity, with the exception of occasional gastrointestinal bleeding.

Central Nervous System Effects

Given the large energy requirements of the brain, it is not surprising that neurotoxicity from impaired ATP formation may accompany salicylate toxicity. Agitation, combativeness, disorientation, confusion, and hallucinations characterize severe toxicity. Even more severe cases progress (sometimes rapidly) to convulsions, coma, respiratory depression, cerebral edema, and brain death.[1,27–30]

Hill[31] showed in rats that elevated CNS salicylate concentration, leading to coma and seizures, was the most critical determinant of death, and this is consistent with clinical experience. Serious neurotoxicity, especially CNS depression or convulsions, carries a high mortality and commonly portends death in the next few minutes to hours. Even patients exhibiting shock and hypotension almost always develop CNS dysfunction before life-threatening cardiovascular toxicity. CNS depression, disorientation, agitation, or convulsions always should be interpreted as an ominous sign when due to salicylate toxicity.[27,30–32]

Miscellaneous Effects

Hypocalcemia and hypercalcemia have been described as a component of serious salicylate toxicity.[33,34] Rhabdomyolysis,[35] commonly seen in any metabolic poisoning, may produce the typical complications, including disseminated intravascular coagulation, compartment syndromes, renal failure, hyperkalemia, and hypocalcemia. Acute tubular necrosis has been reported in the absence of rhabdomyolysis.[36]

Tinnitus generally occurs when serum salicylate levels are greater than 20 mg/dL (>1.46 mmol/L). The patient may not complain of tinnitus, but instead simply may complain of difficulty in hearing. Auditory musical hallucinations also have been reported.[63]

Significant hyperthermia is seen in only a few cases and is seen more commonly in patients who die, reflecting more severe toxicity.[27] Even comatose patients may have a normal temperature.

Finally, I have encountered two cases of severe poisoning (leading to coma) in which the administration of succinylcholine was followed immediately by diffuse rigidity and hyperthermia resistant to neuromuscular blockade. That both patients could have had familial malignant hyperthermia seems extremely unlikely. Rather, because ATP also is required for muscle relaxation, presumably low muscle ATP levels prevented relaxation after initial depolarization by succinylcholine. As in any poisoning characterized by low ATP levels (e.g., nitrophenol, fluoroacetate), rigor mortis may develop within a few minutes after death. I have noticed similar rigidity as a near-terminal finding on one occasion in which no succinylcholine was given.

Pharmacokinetics

Pharmacokinetics of Salicylates

Volume of distribution: 0.15–0.35 L/kg or greater
Protein binding: 40–80%
Elimination: (1) mainly hepatic at low salicylate concentrations; (2) mainly renal at upper therapeutic and toxic serum salicylate concentrations
Active metabolites: none
Methods to enhance clearance: hemodialysis, alkaline diuresis

ABSORPTION

During and after ingestion, all salicylate products are converted rapidly to salicylate. Salicylate impairs gastric emptying, and gastric bezoars have formed in patients with chronic ingestion of enteric-coated aspirin tablets.[64] I have seen salicylate concentrations increase for more than 24 hours after large acute ingestions, although toxic levels commonly occur within 6 hours. Enteric-coated aspirin tablets may undergo delayed absorption, with nontoxic levels seen at 6 hours despite serious ingestions.[37] Liquid salicylate preparations (e.g., methyl salicylate, salicylic acid, pediatric aspirin products) undergo more rapid absorption than solid products. Toxic and fatal amounts of salicylate can be absorbed across skin after the use of salicylic acid–containing keratolytic agents.[2,3,38] Of topical salicylate, 60% is absorbed across psoriatic skin when covered with an occlusive dressing.[38]

DISTRIBUTION

About 40% to 80% of salicylate is bound to serum proteins, mainly albumin. As binding sites become saturated at high serum salicylate concentrations, the free, unbound fraction increases. Hypoalbuminemia, azotemia, and elevated serum salicylate levels all result in increased unbound serum salicylate concentrations.[39–41] The wide range of reported protein-bound fractions represents, to a large extent, variations in serum drug levels and albumin concentrations.

Salicylate exists in blood in an equilibrium between the ionized and un-ionized forms (Fig. 57-1). At physiologic pH, most salicylate resides in the ionized form. Only unbound, un-ionized salicylate readily crosses cell membranes. Any condition that increases the unbound fraction (e.g., high serum salicylate concentrations, hypoalbuminemia) or increases the un-ionized fraction of salicylate (e.g., decrease in pH) increases salicylate's apparent volume of distribution. A decrease in pH can result in a movement of salicylate from blood into tissue, raising the tissue levels of salicylate and worsening systemic toxicity, while serum salicylate concentrations decline. A drop in pH of only 0.25 (e.g., 7.45 to 7.2) almost doubles the amount of un-ionized drug capable of diffusing into tissue. In a healthy patient with low serum salicylate concentrations, the typical volume of distribution is about 0.16 L/kg. Salicylate's volume of distribution in the same patient with an elevated serum salicylate concentration and acidemia may reach 0.34 L/kg or greater.[42]

The changing volume of distribution of salicylate makes interpretation of serum salicylate concentrations potentially

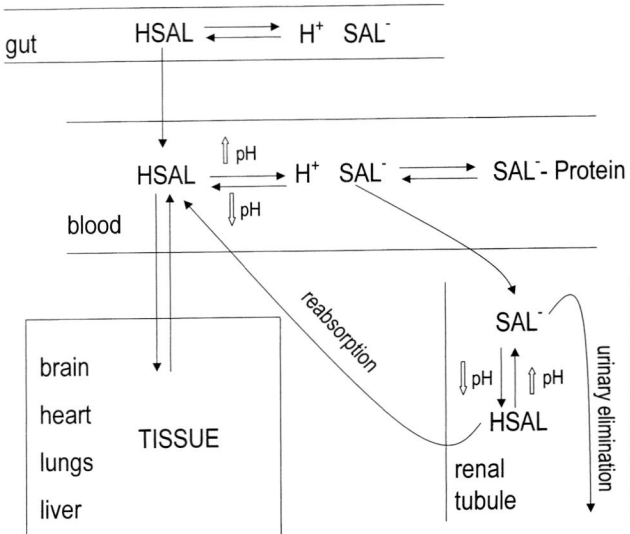

FIGURE 57-1

Salicylate exists in blood in an equilibrium between the ionized and un-ionized forms. HSAL, un-ionized salicylate; SAL−, ionized salicylate.

misleading. Two patients with identical serum salicylate concentrations may differ markedly in degree of toxicity because their tissue burden of salicylate may vary tremendously, depending on plasma albumin concentration, pH, and other factors that influence the volume of distribution for salicylate. Similarly, serum salicylate concentrations decline not only because of renal and hepatic elimination but also because a rise in the volume of distribution causes salicylate to leave blood and enter tissue, producing more severe toxicity. Patients may deteriorate and die as serum salicylate concentrations decrease.[27,29] Similarly, it is important to treat the patient and not simply the serum salicylate concentration. This point is especially important in patients with chronic salicylate toxicity, who characteristically have a large volume of distribution and more severe toxicity for a given serum salicylate concentration.

ELIMINATION

Salicylate undergoes hepatic metabolism, mainly by glucuronidation and by conjugation with glycine to form salicyluric acid (see Fig. 11-1).[43] Both of these pathways become saturated within the range of therapeutic serum salicylate concentrations, leading to zero-order elimination kinetics and an increasing role for renal elimination. During zero-order elimination kinetics, a set amount of drug is eliminated per unit time (not a set fraction of drug, as in first-order elimination), regardless of how much serum salicylate concentrations increase. The elimination "half-life" (a term that should not be used in zero-order kinetics) is changing constantly and increases as the serum salicylate concentration increases.

An increased fraction of unbound salicylate at high plasma concentrations also enhances renal clearance, making the kidneys the major route of elimination during salicylate toxicity.[44] Un-ionized salicylate undergoes reabsorption by renal tubules, prolonging elimination. Alkaline urine favors the formation of ionized salicylate, preventing reabsorption and enhancing secretion of un-ionized salicylate down its concentration gradient, both of which increase urinary elimination. Urinary clearance of salicylate can increase more than 500% by raising urine pH from 7.0 to 8.0.[65]

Saturable hepatic elimination kinetics, an increasing volume of distribution, dehydration, and aciduria act to prolong markedly the elimination of salicylate. In untreated or dehydrated patients with aciduria who have moderate-to-severe salicylate toxicity, more than 1 to 2 days may be required for serum salicylate concentrations to decrease by half, and prolonged absorption further attenuates decline in serum salicylate levels.

A shift to zero-order elimination also allows serum salicylate concentrations to increase out of proportion to the daily dose. Doubling a daily aspirin intake may result in a threefold or fourfold increase in serum salicylate concentrations; this explains why chronic salicylate toxicity is produced with relatively small increases in salicylate doses.

Toxic Doses

The acute ingestion of 150 mg/kg of aspirin or an equivalent amount of another salicylate-containing product mainly produces gastrointestinal irritation and vomiting. Ingestion of 150 to 300 mg/kg of aspirin results in mild-to-moderate toxicity with abdominal pain, vomiting, dehydration, hyperpnea, tinnitus, and acid-base disturbances. Ingestion of more than 300 mg/kg of aspirin produces moderate-to-severe toxicity and death. Patients with medical conditions that predispose them to a large volume of distribution (e.g., renal failure, hypoalbuminemia, acidemia) and patients who have ingested salicylate previously within the last 12 to 24 hours become more toxic for a given amount ingested.

Historically the Done nomogram[45] was suggested to assist in determining the degree of toxicity after salicylate ingestion. A serum salicylate level drawn 6 hours or more after ingestion could be plotted on the nomogram, and the patient could be placed at various degrees of toxicity. The Done nomogram can be misleading, however. The nomogram can overestimate and, most importantly, greatly underestimate the degree of toxicity. A person with a level in the "mild" range may still become severely ill hours later if acidemia or dehydration is not corrected or if salicylate levels continue to increase. Use of the Done nomogram is not recommended.[46] All symptomatic patients should be treated regardless of where their serum salicylate levels fall on the nomogram.

CLINICAL PRESENTATION

Acute Salicylate Toxicity

Presenting complaints and findings after acute ingestion of a salicylate product include vomiting (sometimes with hematemesis), abdominal pain, tinnitus, tachypnea, hyperpnea, diaphoresis, tachycardia, dehydration, leukocytosis, and ketonuria (Table 57-3). If rhabdomyolysis is not present or severe and if dehydration has not limited potassium excretion, laboratory analysis in most patients reveals hypokalemia. Adults usually present with respiratory alkalosis with or with-

TABLE 57-3 Clinical Findings of Salicylate Toxicity

Gastrointestinal
  Nausea, vomiting, abdominal pain
  Gastrointestinal bleeding
  Gastric perforation (rare)
Metabolic
  Respiratory alkalosis
  Metabolic acidosis
  Ketosis
  Hypokalemia
  Hyperglycemia, normoglycemia, or hypoglycemia
  Ketosis
Central nervous system
  Confusion, agitation, combativeness, hallucinations
  Seizures, coma, cerebral death
  Cerebral edema
  Low cerebrospinal fluid glucose (in animals)
Cardiovascular
  Sinus tachycardia
  Hypotension, ventricular arrhythmias
  Shock, asystole
Pulmonary
  Adult respiratory distress syndrome
Hematologic
  Leukocytosis
  Prolongation of prothrombin time
Miscellaneous
  Diaphoresis
  Hyperthermia
  Rhabdomyolysis
  Renal failure
  Tinnitus, auditory hallucinations (e.g., musical)

out a mild metabolic acidosis and with alkalemia. Young children commonly present with acidemia. Serum glucose concentrations usually are normal or elevated early in acute poisoning.

As the severity of poisoning progresses, worsening acidosis, worsening tachycardia, and diaphoresis appear, with progressive CNS dysfunction characterized by agitation, lethargy, confusion, combativeness, seizures, or coma. Although young children are more likely to develop hypoglycemia as glycogen stores are depleted, adults can develop hypoglycemia as well. Adult respiratory distress syndrome is more common in chronic salicylate poisoning but can occur in severe, acute poisonings. Elevated prothrombin times do not occur until hours after ingestion.

Patients who will die from acute salicylate poisoning usually exhibit CNS dysfunction and then die from refractory shock with terminal ventricular arrhythmias or asystole. Acidemia usually is present by this time, and the combination of tachycardia, diaphoresis, and CNS dysfunction, especially in the presence of acidemia, is an ominous indication of severe toxicity and great risk of deterioration and death if aggressive action is not taken immediately.[27,30-32] Clinical deterioration can be rapid; patients who are awake and alert may die within 6 hours.[1] Because of the increasing volume of distribution with higher salicylate concentrations and acidemia, patients may die while serum salicylate concentrations are declining.

CHRONIC SALICYLATE TOXICITY

Chronic salicylate toxicity is described best as a syndrome rather than as a specific dose over a particular time. A dehydrated and azotemic patient may develop chronic toxicity while taking doses that would not affect an otherwise healthy person.

Most patients with chronic salicylate toxicity are brought in by family members because of altered mental status characterized by lethargy, irritability, confusion, hallucinations (including auditory), seizures, or coma. Although dehydration is common, vomiting and abdominal pain usually are not major complaints. Tinnitus is common, and an elevated prothrombin time frequently is noted. Many patients are acidemic. Elevated hepatic transaminases are seen commonly in many patients using salicylate products regularly and are not specific for this syndrome. Tachypnea is common.

Leatherman and Schmitz[15] described invasive hemodynamic measurements in five selected hypotensive patients with chronic salicylate toxicity who exhibited low systemic vascular resistance and cardiac outputs ranging from 5.1 to 8.5 L/min. How representative these hemodynamic findings are of all patients with salicylate toxicity, including patients without hypotension, is unknown.

Because of a large volume of distribution, patients with chronic salicylate toxicity appear sicker than acutely toxic patients with the same serum salicylate level. Patients taking carbonic anhydrase inhibitors and salicylate may develop serious salicylate toxicity[47,48] at therapeutic or minimally elevated serum salicylate concentrations because carbonic anhydrase inhibitors alkalize cerebrospinal fluid while lowering blood pH,[49,50] both of which processes concentrate and trap salicylate within the CNS. Salicylate increases the unbound and active fraction of acetazolamide in blood,[48] enhancing acetazolamide's effect on salicylate distribution.

Differences between acute and chronic salicylate toxicity are not always clear, but rather represent a progression of signs and symptoms. The longer a patient presents after an acute ingestion, the more he or she behaves like a patient presenting with chronic toxicity. Altered CNS function, elevated prothrombin times, and acidemia that characterize chronic salicylate toxicity also are typical of an acute overdose patient hours after ingestion.

DIFFERENTIAL DIAGNOSIS

The differential diagnosis for salicylate toxicity is large and includes many disorders that produce metabolic acidosis (with an increased anion gap in more ill patients), respiratory alkalosis, gastroenteritis, and CNS dysfunction. Examples include sepsis, Reye's syndrome, diabetic ketoacidosis, hepatic failure, and alcoholic ketoacidosis. Poisonings by theophylline, caffeine, ethylene glycol, methanol, iron, ethylene glycol ethers, and heavy metals may produce acidemia, gastrointestinal symptoms, and coma and convulsions. A generalized seizure from any cause (e.g., isoniazid, cocaine, meningitis) usually produces transient metabolic acidosis that resolves over 20 to 60 minutes after the seizure is terminated. Direct or indirect β-adrenoceptor stimulation (e.g., bronchodilators, theophylline, sympathomimetics) produces tachycardia, metabolic acidosis, respiratory alkalosis, hypokalemia, hyperglycemia, leukocytosis, ketosis, and, depending on the agent (e.g., amphetamines, theophylline), convulsions. Diflunisal, a nonsteroidal anti-inflammatory drug, does not produce salicylate toxicity but causes falsely elevated serum salicylate concentrations by some colorimetric laboratory methods.[51]

EVALUATION AND TREATMENT

Special Airway and Ventilatory Considerations

Special considerations must be addressed when instituting sedation or mechanical ventilation. The administration of a sedative or narcotic to a patient poisoned with salicylate may decrease respirations, lessen respiratory alkalosis, and result in a prompt decrease in arterial pH from an unopposed metabolic acidosis. This situation may produce a prompt movement of salicylate into the brain with resultant clinical deterioration. A similar scenario occurs when a physician sedates or relaxes the patient for endotracheal intubation and then provides normal minute ventilation volumes with mechanical ventilation. Because of adverse hemodynamic effects and risks for barotrauma, aggressive mechanical hyperventilation should not be used to maintain pH in these settings, but rather the physician should recognize the probable consequences of sedation or controlled mechanical ventilation and should administer additional intravenous sodium bicarbonate to prevent dangerous decreases in arterial pH.

Decontamination and Initial Evaluation

Oral activated charcoal alone has been reported to be superior to induction of vomiting with ipecac syrup.[52,53] Activated charcoal (e.g., 100 g) should be given to patients who have ingested potentially toxic doses of a salicylate product. Although repeated-dose oral activated charcoal has been claimed to be effective in shortening elimination half-life in a retrospective study,[54] a prospective randomized study in human volunteers who ingested nontoxic doses of salicylate suggested that the routine use of repeated-dose charcoal might be without benefit.[55] If serum salicylate concentrations continue to increase after administration of activated charcoal, most toxicologists administer additional oral charcoal. Severe nausea and vomiting in an acutely poisoned patient may limit charcoal dosing.

In symptomatic patients, laboratory studies should include analysis of serum or plasma for electrolytes, blood urea nitrogen, glucose, creatine kinase, creatinine, prothrombin time, and salicylate concentration. Because of the ready availability of acetaminophen and frequency of acetaminophen overdose and because acetaminophen-containing products may have brand names that are similar to the names of products containing aspirin, serum acetaminophen concentration should be measured whenever salicylate toxicity is being considered. Urinalysis and complete blood count also should be obtained. Arterial blood gases should be measured to determine type and degree of acid-base imbalance. A chest radiograph should be obtained on all moderately to severely ill patients or any patient with respiratory distress or hypoxemia.

A patient who appears ill from salicylate toxicity should be treated regardless of serum salicylate concentration. Most symptomatic patients have serum salicylate concentrations greater than 20 mg/dL (>1.46 mmol/L). Severe toxicity commonly accompanies serum salicylate concentrations greater than 70 mg/dL (>5.1 mmol/L). Severe toxicity and death can be seen at lower levels, however. Because of variability in volume of distribution, serum salicylate concentrations in patients who die are, on average, similar to concentrations in patients who live. Chapman and Proudfoot[56] reported plasma salicylate concentrations ranging from 55 to 120 mg/dL (4.01 to 8.76 mmol/L) in fatal cases and ranging from 18 to 135 mg/dL (1.31 to 9.85 mmol/L) in survivors.

The acute ingestion of enteric-coated salicylate may result in nontoxic serum salicylate concentrations for the first few hours after ingestion but high serum salicylate concentrations and severe toxicity later.[37] Because of inaccurate histories provided from overdose victims or relatives and the delayed and prolonged absorption of enteric-coated products, anyone who may have ingested more than 150 mg/kg of enteric-coated aspirin should be admitted for observation and measurement of serial serum salicylate concentrations for 18 to 24 hours.

Moderately to severely ill patients belong in the intensive care unit. The purpose of admitting relatively asymptomatic patients or patients with only mild symptoms is usually concern for possible clinical deterioration that can be rapid. Patients who are awake and alert can die within 6 hours. This fact, along with the frequent need for vital signs and laboratory studies, means that almost all patients requiring admission for salicylate toxicity should be placed in an intensive care unit setting.

Supportive Treatment

All patients with an abnormal mental status or seizures should be presumed hypoglycemic and should receive appropriate doses of intravenous glucose, especially if bedside determinations of serum glucose levels are not immediately available. As with all drug-induced and toxin-induced seizures, benzodiazepines and barbiturates are the anticonvulsants of choice.

The average adult patient who presents several hours after an acute ingestion of salicylate with vomiting, perhaps tinnitus, and hyperventilation typically is dehydrated by 4 to 6 L or more. The insensible fluid losses from diaphoresis, hyperventilation, and third spacing into muscles undergoing rhabdomyolysis are frequently underestimated and limit initial attempts at rehydration and prevention of further negative fluid balances, which impairs salicylate elimination. Aggressive initial rehydration should be monitored carefully, and the treating intensivist must recognize that despite continuous intravenous infusions of 500 to 600 mL/hr, many patients continue to experience negative fluid balances with rising hematocrits and serum sodium concentrations that must be met with additional fluid boluses and increases in continuous infusion rates. These actions can be undertaken only with frequent bedside assessments and frequent laboratory studies. Frequent blood and urine collections are facilitated by indwelling arterial and urinary catheters.

After initial hydration, primary efforts should be directed at keeping arterial pH greater than 7.4 in symptomatic patients. A reasonable goal is an arterial pH of 7.5 to limit increases in volume of distribution and tissue (e.g., CNS) salicylate concentrations. A secondary goal of therapy is to alkalinize urine

to enhance urinary salicylate excretion. The more alkaline the urine (up to a pH of approximately 8.0), the greater the excretion of salicylate. Intensivists must recognize that the main reason for alkalization is to elevate blood pH. Alkaluria, although desirable, is of secondary concern. Alkaluria seems to be more important than diuresis with regard to enhancing salicylate excretion.[66]

Two important methods for sodium reabsorption in the renal distal and collecting tubules are tubular secretion of potassium ions and tubular secretion of hydrogen ions. Even during alkalemia and normokalemia, aciduria persists, impairing salicylate elimination, if the kidney is preferentially reabsorbing sodium by excreting hydrogen ions rather than potassium ions into the tubular lumen. Therefore, both bicarbonate and potassium supplementation are usually required to ensure alkaluria.

There are no randomized trials examining outcomes in patients treated with different infusion solutions. Based on experience, I initially rehydrate patients aggressively with either 0.9% sodium chloride or Ringer's lactate (if hyperkalemia is not present). In moderately to severely ill patients, I begin a continuous infusion of 1000 mL of 5% dextrose in water, to which is added 150 mEq of sodium bicarbonate and at least 50 mEq of potassium as potassium chloride at 250 to 300 mL/hr, assuming adequate urine output and the absence of hyperkalemia. Additional simultaneous infusions of crystalloid (e.g., 5% dextrose in 45% sodium chloride) usually are required to maintain adequate hydration, and total infusion rates greater than 500 mL/hr may be required in moderately to severely ill patients. A urinary output of 2 to 3 mL/kg/hr is desirable. Hemoglobin concentrations and hematocrits are followed to detect occult gastrointestinal bleeding. Arterial blood gases, serum electrolytes, serum salicylate concentrations, and urine pH are measured every 2 to 4 hours in moderately ill patients and at least every 1 to 2 hours in severely ill patients to ensure absence of acidemia and to detect disorders in serum potassium concentrations that may require adjustment in the electrolyte composition of the infusion solution. This monitoring also detects hypernatremia and hemoconcentration, which suggest insensible losses requiring further replacement. Serial (e.g., daily) serum creatine kinase activity is monitored to detect rhabdomyolysis.

Decreases in arterial pH from metabolic acidosis are treated with repeated intravenous boluses of 1 to 2 mEq/kg of sodium bicarbonate as needed. A decrease in urine pH less than 7.5 to 8 despite normokalemia is treated with additional potassium (intravenous or oral) as long as hyperkalemia is not present. After ensuring adequate hydration and urine flow, the potassium requirements in some patients with moderate-to-severe salicylate toxicity exceed 25 mEq/hr to ensure alkaluria. I administer 10 to 15 mg of vitamin K_1 intravenously to all patients with moderate-to-severe toxicity because prothrombin times usually are elevated within several hours without such therapy.

If objective evidence of hypervolemia develops and there is no appropriate increase in urine flow, intravenous furosemide can be given. However, the most common cause of oliguria is hypovolemia. Pulmonary edema usually represents adult respiratory distress syndrome, not fluid overload.

In patients with renal failure and oliguria who require less than 200 mL/hr to maintain good hydration, I commonly infuse crystalloid solutions containing 10% dextrose to prevent neuroglycopenia, which in animals may occur despite normoglycemia. Carbonic anhydrase inhibitors, such as acetazolamide, are best not given to alkalize urine because they also alkalize cerebrospinal fluid,[49,50] trapping salicylate in the CNS—opposing the aforementioned goals of therapy.

Severe neurotoxicity, characterized by lethargy, agitation, confusion, seizures, coma, or continued deterioration in level of consciousness despite supportive care, is an ominous sign and an indication for immediate hemodialysis, even if serum salicylate concentrations have been declining yet remain greater than 20 to 40 mg/dL (>1.46 to 2.91 mmol/L). Many toxicologists also administer intravenous mannitol (0.25 to 0.5 g/kg) in an effort to reduce or prevent further worsening of cerebral edema in these patients.

Hemodialysis

Salicylate's high water solubility, relatively low protein binding, small volume of distribution, and low molecular weight allow for effective removal by hemodialysis.[57] Hemodialysis is indicated for patients with one or more of the following: significant neurotoxicity (e.g., lethargy, agitation, coma, convulsions), renal failure, cardiovascular instability, and extremely elevated serum salicylate concentrations that are increasing despite hydration and attempts at alkaline diuresis. Others have recommended hemodialysis for pulmonary edema as well. On the one hand, previous recommendations that all patients with serum salicylate concentrations greater than 80 to 100 mg/dL (>5.84 to 7.3 mmol/L) must undergo hemodialysis immediately were too extreme because awake and alert patients with good blood pressure and urine output who have a serum salicylate concentration of 105 mg/dL (7.66 mmol/L) that is known to be falling can do well with intensive medical therapy. On the other hand, successful treatment of these patients requires a great deal of physician time, frequent bedside evaluations, frequent laboratory studies, and often 2 to 3 days in the intensive care unit. Most patients with serum salicylate concentrations greater than 100 mg/dL (>7.3 mmol/L) eventually meet the criteria for hemodialysis (e.g., CNS dysfunction), even while serum salicylate concentrations decrease. Failure to institute hemodialysis promptly in deteriorating patients leads to unnecessary deaths.[1,56] Mildly to moderately encephalopathic patients with chronic salicylate toxicity, in whom absorption has peaked, can do well with intensive medical therapy alone.

At our center, extraction ratios across the dialysis cartridge commonly range from 35% to 70% using double-lumen dialysis catheters and high-flux membranes with blood flow rates of 400 mL/min. In general, hemodialysis is performed until serum salicylate concentrations have decreased to less than 20 mg/dL (<1.46 mmol/L). Most patients with salicylate toxicity require 4 to 6 hours of hemodialysis to achieve this goal. Because of prolonged absorption, some patients require more than 6 hours of hemodialysis or require a repeat session of hemodialysis if salicylate levels increase again to produce serious toxicity.

Occult or minor gastrointestinal bleeding from the corrosive action of salicylate can become more severe and apparent when the patient is heparinized for hemodialysis, but this is uncommon. I routinely type and screen the patient for

transfusion, however, when arranging for hemodialysis and monitor hemoglobin concentrations and hematocrit values more closely during and shortly after dialysis. Because clinically significant gastrointestinal bleeding during hemodialysis is uncommon, concern for gastrointestinal bleeding from salicylate rarely should be considered a contraindication for heparinization and hemodialysis for life-threatening salicylate toxicity. Blood volume can be supported with transfusions, if needed, whereas death from salicylate is possible and often probable without hemodialysis.

Charcoal hemoperfusion also removes salicylate well; however, hemodialysis has the valuable added advantage of immediately correcting electrolyte and acid-base balance without the potential adverse effects associated with hemoperfusion (e.g., thrombocytopenia, hypocalcemia).[56,57] Peritoneal dialysis is relatively ineffective at removing salicylate compared with hemodialysis and should be used only when hemodialysis is not an option.

Intensive Care Unit Discharge

Criteria for ICU Discharge in Salicylate Poisoning

Awake, alert, and no clinical evidence of toxicity
Serum salicylate concentrations <20 mg/dL (1.46 mmol/L) and known to be declining

Patients can be discharged from the intensive care unit when they are awake and alert and metabolically stable and when serum salicylate concentrations are less than 20 mg/dL (<1.46 mmol/L) and known to be decreasing.

Common Errors in the Management of Salicylate Poisoning

Underestimating the seriousness of salicylate toxicity
Failing to consider the diagnosis of chronic salicylate toxicity in elderly patients with altered mental status
Failing to recognize potential for delayed and continued absorption of salicylate for >24 hours after overdose
Forgetting that coingestion of central nervous system depressants masks hyperventilation and respiratory alkalosis
Believing that most patients with salicylate poisoning are hyperthermic
Confusing units of measurement for serum salicylate concentrations, which vary among laboratories (10 mg/dL = 100 mg/L)
Using the Done nomogram
Failing to recognize potential for clinical deterioration and death despite decreasing salicylate serum concentrations
Underestimating insensible fluid losses and allowing patients to become hypovolemic despite what may seem like liberal fluid administration
Focusing on alkalizing urine rather than alkalizing blood
Not giving required potassium supplementation to alkalize urine successfully
Failing to obtain and review laboratory studies frequently
Failing to institute hemodialysis at the onset of neurotoxicity

continued

Key Points in the Management of Salicylate Poisoning

1. Salicylate absorption may continue for >24 hours and onset of absorption may be delayed with enteric-coated aspirin.
2. Patients with moderate-to-severe salicylate toxicity typically are 4–6 L dehydrated and may exhibit large maintenance fluid requirements because of insensible losses from hyperventilation, sweating, and vomiting.
3. Direct main efforts at correcting and maintaining euvolemia and keeping blood pH alkaline. Urinary alkalization usually requires sodium bicarbonate *and* potassium supplementation.
4. Bedside evaluations and laboratory studies (electrolytes, blood gases, salicylate concentrations, urine pH) every 1–2 hours are required for patients with serious salicylate toxicity.
5. Decreases in pH and elevated serum salicylate levels result in an increase in volume of distribution, with a movement of salicylate from blood into brain and other tissue. Patients can deteriorate and die while serum salicylate concentrations are decreasing. Awake and alert patients can die within 6 hours.
6. Monitor for and prevent decreases in arterial pH when giving sedatives/relaxants or controlling ventilation.
7. Hemodialysis should be instituted at the onset of neurotoxicity.
8. Pulmonary edema usually reflects adult respiratory distress syndrome.
9. Do not confuse units of measurement for serum salicylate concentrations, which vary among laboratories (10 mg/dL = 100 mg/L).

SPECIAL POPULATIONS

Pregnant Patients

Salicylate crosses the placenta and concentrate in the fetus at higher serum levels than in the mother.[58,59] The relative acidemia of the fetus also contributes to higher fetal *tissue* salicylate levels for already elevated fetal *serum* salicylate concentrations (large fetal volume of distribution). The fetus possesses less capacity to buffer acidemic stress imposed by salicylate and, compared with the mother, a reduced capacity to excrete the toxin. This situation collectively places the fetus at greater risk of death for a given maternal serum salicylate concentration than the mother.

Because the fetus has greater toxicity than the mother, it seems wise to institute hemodialysis for lesser degrees of maternal toxicity than those in nonpregnant patients.

Maternal hemodialysis can decrease placental blood flow. There are no studies to guide clinicians in deciding what maternal serum salicylate concentration crosses the threshold for hemodialysis. In a woman with a premature fetus, I institute hemodialysis for signs of fetal distress in the presence of maternal chronic salicylate toxicity or whenever maternal salicylate concentrations are greater than 40 mg/dL (>2.92 mmol/L).[60] In a woman with a mature fetus, immediate delivery might allow more intensive care for the infant.[61] Alternatively, maternal hemodialysis might remove salicylate more safely and effectively from the fetus (through redistribution) than fetal therapies after delivery. In general, I lean toward hemodialysis in the latter situation because it is much easier to perform hemodialysis on the mother than on a newborn.

REFERENCES

1. McGuigan MA: A two-year review of salicylate deaths in Ontario. Arch Intern Med 147:510–512, 1987.
2. von Weiss JF, Lever WF: Percutaneous salicylic acid intoxication in psoriasis. Arch Dermatol 90:614–619, 1964.
3. Brubacher JR, Hoffman RS: Salicylism from topical salicylates: Review of the literature. J Toxicol Clin Toxicol 34:431–436, 1996.
4. Howrie DL, Moriarty R, Breit R: Candy flavoring as a source of salicylate poisoning. Pediatrics 75:869–871, 1985.
5. Temple AR: Pathophysiology of aspirin overdosage toxicity, with implications for management. Pediatrics 62(Suppl):873–876, 1978.
6. Gabow PA, Anderson RJ, Potts DE, et al: Acid-base disturbances in the salicylate-intoxicated adult. Arch Intern Med 138:1481–1484, 1978.
7. Gutknecht J: Aspirin, acetaminophen and proton transport through phospholipid bilayers and mitochondrial membranes. Mol Cell Biochem 114:3–8, 1992.
8. Trost LC, Lemasters JJ: Role of the mitochondrial permeability transition in salicylate toxicity to cultured rat hepatocytes: Implications for the pathogenesis of Reye's syndrome. Toxicol Appl Pharmacol 147:431–441, 1997.
9. Kaplan E, Kennedy J, Davis J: Effects of salicylate and other benzoates on oxidative enzymes of the tricarboxylic acid cycle in rat tissue homogenates. Arch Biochem Biophys 51:47–61, 1954.
10. Dawkins P, Gould B, Sturman J, et al: The mechanism of the inhibition of dehydrogenases by salicylate. J Pharm Pharmacol 19:355–366, 1967.
11. Mizock BA: Lactic acidosis. Disease a Month 35:233–300, 1989.
12. Mizock BA: Controversies in lactic acidosis. JAMA 258:497–501, 1987.
13. Zilva JF: The origin of acidosis in hyperlactatemia. Ann Clin Biochem 15:40–43, 1978.
14. Bartels PD, Lund-Jacobsen H: Blood lactate and ketone body concentrations in salicylate intoxication. Hum Toxicol 5:363–366, 1986.
15. Leatherman JW, Schmitz PG: Fever, hyperdynamic shock, and multiple-system organ failure: A pseudo-sepsis syndrome associated with chronic salicylate intoxication. Chest 100:1391–1396, 1991.
16. Gould B, Dawkins P, Smith M, et al: The mechanism of the inhibition of aminotransferases by salicylate. Mol Pharmacol 2:525–533, 1966.
17. Limbeck GA, Ruvalcaba RHA, Samols E, et al: Salicylates and hypoglycemia. Am J Dis Child 109:165–167, 1965.
18. Snodgrass W, Rumack BH, Peterson RG, et al: Salicylate toxicity following therapeutic doses in young children. Clin Toxicol 18:247–259, 1981.
19. Raschke R, Arnold-Capell PA, Richeson R, et al: Refractory hypoglycemia secondary to topical salicylate intoxication. Arch Intern Med 151:591–593, 1991.
20. Thurston JH, Pollock PG, Warren S, et al: Reduced brain glucose with normal plasma glucose in salicylate poisoning. J Clin Invest 49:2139–2145, 1970.
21. Gumpel JM: Enteric-coated aspirin overdose and gastric perforation (Letter). BMJ 4:287, 1975.
22. Robins JB, Turnbull JA, Robertson C: Gastric perforation after acute aspirin overdose. Hum Toxicol 4:527–528, 1985.
23. Sacchetti A, Ramoska E: Ingestion of Compound W, an unusual caustic. Am J Emerg Med 4:554–555, 1986.

24. Starko K, Mullick FG: Hepatic and cerebral pathology findings in children with fatal salicylate intoxication: further evidence for a causal relation between salicylate and Reye's syndrome. Lancet 1:326–329, 1983.
25. Walters JS, Woodring JH, Stelling CB, et al: Salicylate-induced pulmonary edema. Radiology 146:289–293, 1983.
26. Heffner JE, Sahn SA: Salicylate-induced pulmonary edema: Clinical features and prognosis. Ann Intern Med 95:405–409, 1981.
27. Thisted B, Krantz T, Stroom J, et al: Acute salicylate self-poisoning in 177 consecutive patients treated in ICU. Acta Anaesthesiol Scand 31:312–316, 1987.
28. Hildebrandt EF, Suttie JW: The effects of salicylate on enzymes of vitamin K metabolism. J Pharm Pharmacol 35:421–426, 1983.
29. Dove DJ, Jones T: Delayed coma associated with salicylate intoxication. J Pediatr 100:493–496, 1982.
30. Proudfoot AT, Brown SS: Acidaemia and salicylate poisoning in adults. BMJ 2:547–550, 1969.
31. Hill JB: Salicylate intoxication. N Engl J Med 288:1110–1113, 1973.
32. Proudfoot AT: Toxicity of salicylates. Am J Med 75:99–103, 1983.
33. Fox GN: Hypocalcemia complicating bicarbonate therapy for salicylate poisoning. West J Med 141:108–109, 1984.
34. Reid IR: Transient hypercalcemia following overdoses of soluble aspirin tablets (Letter). Aust N Z J Med 15:364, 1985.
35. Skjoto J, Reikvam A: Hyperthermia and rhabdomyolysis in self-poisoning with paracetamol and salicylates. Acta Med Scand 205:473–476, 1979.
36. Rupp DJ, Seaton RD, Wiegmann TB: Acute polyuric renal failure after aspirin intoxication. Arch Intern Med 143:1237–1238, 1983.
37. Henry AF: Overdoses of Entrophen (Letter). Can Med Assoc J 128:1142, 1983.
38. Taylor J, Halprin K: Percutaneous absorption of salicylic acid. Arch Dermatol 111:740–743, 1975.
39. Alvan G, Bergman U, Gustafsson LL: High unbound fraction of salicylate in plasma during intoxication. Br J Clin Pharmacol 11:625–626, 1981.
40. Perez-Matao M, Erill S: Protein binding of salicylate and quinidine in plasma from patients with renal failure, chronic liver disease and chronic respiratory insufficiency. Eur J Clin Pharmacol 11:225–231, 1977.
41. Borga O, Cederlof IO, Ringberger VA, et al: Protein binding of salicylate in uremic and normal plasma. Clin Pharmacol Ther 20:464–475, 1976.
42. Levy G, Yaffe SJ: Relationship between dose and apparent volume of distribution of salicylate in children. Pediatrics 54:713–717, 1974.
43. Patel DK, Hesse A, Ogunbona A, et al: Metabolism of aspirin after therapeutic and toxic doses. Hum Exp Toxicol 9:131–136, 1990.
44. Needs CJ: Clinical pharmacokinetics of the salicylates. Clin Pharmacokinet 10:164–177, 1985.
45. Done AK: Salicylate intoxication: Significance of measurements of salicylate in blood in cases of acute ingestion. Pediatrics 26:800–807, 1960.
46. Kulig K: Salicylate intoxication: Is the Done nomogram reliable? AACT Update, American Academy of Clinical Toxicology 3:2–3, June 1990.
47. Anderson CJ, Kaufman PL, Sturm RJ: Toxicity of combined therapy with carbonic anhydrase inhibitors and aspirin. Am J Ophthalmol 86:516–519, 1978.
48. Sweeney KR, Chapron DJ, Brandt JL, et al: Toxic interaction between acetazolamide and salicylate: Case reports and a pharmacokinetic explanation. Clin Pharmacol Ther 40:518–524, 1986.
49. Rollins DE, Withrow CD, Woodbury DM: Tissue acid-base balance in acetazolamide-treated rats. J Pharmacol Exp Ther 174:535–540, 1970.
50. Javaheri S: Effects of acetazolamide on cerebrospinal fluid ions in metabolic alkalosis in dogs. J Appl Physiol 62:1582–1588, 1987.
51. Adelman HM, Wallach PM, Flannery MT: Inability to interpret toxic salicylate levels in patients taking aspirin and diflunisal. J Rheumatol 18:522–523, 1991.
52. Danel V, Henry JA, Glucksman E: Activated charcoal, emesis, and gastric lavage in aspirin overdose, BMJ 296:1507, 1988.
53. Curtis RA, Barone J, Giacona N: Efficacy of ipecac and activated charcoal/cathartic: Prevention of salicylate absorption in a simulated overdose. Arch Intern Med 144:48–52, 1984.
54. Hillman RJ, Prescott LF: Treatment of salicylate poisoning with repeated oral charcoal. BMJ 291:1472, 1985.
55. Kirshenbaum LA, Mathews SC, Sitar DS, et al: Does multiple-dose charcoal therapy enhance salicylate excretion? Arch Intern Med 150:1281–1283, 1990.
56. Chapman BJ, Proudfoot AT: Adult salicylate poisoning: Deaths and outcome in patients with high plasma salicylate concentrations. QJM 72:699–707, 1989.
57. Winchester JF, Gelfand MC, Helliwell M, et al: Extracorporeal treatment of salicylate or acetaminophen poisoning: Is there a role? Arch Intern Med 141:370–374, 1981.
58. Garrettson LK, Procknal JA, Levy G: Fetal acquisition and neonatal elimination of a large amount of salicylate. Clin Pharmacol Ther 17:98–103, 1975.
59. Levy G, Procknal JA, Garrettson LK: Distribution of salicylate between neonatal and maternal serum at diffusion equilibrium. Clin Pharmacol Ther 18:210–214, 1975.
60. Curry SC, Braitberg G: Poisoning in pregnancy. In Foley MR, Strong TH Jr (eds): Obstetric Intensive Care. Philadelphia, WB Saunders, 1997, pp 347–367.
61. Tenenbein M: Poisoning in pregnancy. In Koren G (ed): Maternal-Fetal Toxicology. New York, Marcel Dekker, 1994, pp 223–247.
62. Kanada SA, Kolling WM, Hindin BL: Aspirin hepatotoxicity. Am J Hosp Pharm 35:330–336, 1978.
63. Allen JR: Salicylate-induced musical perceptions. N Engl J Med 313:642–643, 1985.
64. Baum J: Enteric-coated aspirin and the problem of gastric retention. J Rheumatol 11:250–251, 1984.
65. Smith PK, Gleason HL, Stoll CG, Ogorzalek S: Studies on the pharmacology of salicylates. J Pharmacol Exp Ther 87:237–255, 1946.
66. Prescott LF, Balali-Bood M, Critchley JH, et al: Diuresis or urinary alkalinization for salicylate poisoning? BMJ 285:1383–1386, 1982.

CHAPTER 58

Nonsteroidal Antiinflammatory Drugs

Kimberlie A. Graeme ■ Anthony Morkunas

Nonsteroidal antiinflammatory drugs (NSAIDs) are a chemically diverse group of compounds that share antiinflammatory, analgesic, and antipyretic properties.

BIOCHEMISTRY AND CLINICAL PHARMACOLOGY

NSAIDs can be divided into different groupings (Table 58-1). One common method of classifying these agents uses the specific pharmacologic indicator of whether an agent is a specific or nonspecific inhibitor of the enzyme cyclooxygenase (COX). Recently, two isoenzymes of cyclooxygenase, COX-1 and COX-2, have been discovered.[1–5] Generally, COX-1 performs housekeeping functions, such as gastric mucosal protection, whereas COX-2 is involved in inflammatory responses.[3–6] Examples of selective COX inhibitors are celecoxib, rofecoxib, and valdecoxib. Celecoxib and rofecoxib have a 200- to 300-fold selectivity for inhibition of COX-2 relative to COX-1.[3] Some older NSAIDs are relatively selective for COX-2 at low doses.[3] Another method of classifying NSAIDs is by their chemical structure (Fig. 58-1).[7] This latter classification scheme is useful when discussing the adverse effects of these agents.

PATHOPHYSIOLOGY

Metabolism of phospholipids by the enzyme phospholipase A_2 results in the formation of arachidonic acid (Fig. 58-2). Arachidonic acid can be metabolized by either lipoxygenase to produce the leukotrienes or by COX to produce various prostaglandins and thromboxane. NSAIDs inhibit COX. In theory, highly selective COX-2 inhibitors should be antiinflammatory without the major adverse effects of NSAIDs.[3] However, although COX-2 expression is most evident at sites of inflammation and COX-1 accounts for the majority of prostaglandin synthesis in the normal gastrointestinal tract, there is clearly some overlap.[8] For instance, COX-2–derived prostaglandins play a role in maintenance of gastrointestinal mucosal integrity, especially ulcerated or inflamed mucosa.[8] In addition, animal models and clinical trials indicate that COX-1–derived prostaglandins contribute to the generation of inflammation.[8] Animal and human clinical trials also indicate that both COX-1 and COX-2 are important for maintaining renal function.[5,9]

COX-1 is a constitutive enzyme that is always expressed in most tissues.[4] It is found especially in gastrointestinal mucosal cells, platelets, vascular endothelial cells, and collecting tubule cells of the kidney.[1,3,4,10–14] Under normal circumstances, the action of COX on arachidonic acid produces the prostaglandins I_2, E_1 and E_2, $F_{2\alpha}$, and thromboxane A_2.[1] The function of these end products is gastrointestinal mucosal protection, maintenance of renal perfusion, and regulation of platelet aggregation.[1]

COX-2 is inducible, except where it is constitutively expressed in the brain and kidney.[3] Tissue concentrations under normal circumstances are low, but with induction, they can rise 10- to 80-fold.[1] Induction of COX-2 occurs primarily with inflammation. It can be induced in response to a variety of physiologic stimuli in cartilage, bone, gastric mucosa, colon, reproductive organs (ovary and uterus), and other tissues.[1,3,15–17]

Another functional difference is that COX-1 inhibitors are antithrombotic whereas COX-2 inhibitors are prothrombotic.[6] There is concern that COX-2–selective agents, when compared with traditional NSAIDs, may increase the risk of serious cardiovascular events, although this risk has not been clearly established.[6,18]

Inhibition of COX by NSAIDs can be irreversible or reversible. Aspirin irreversibly acetylates the COX enzyme. Once the use of aspirin is discontinued, new COX must be produced for normal enzymatic function to resume. All other NSAIDs reversibly inhibit the COX enzyme. It is important to note that "reversibility" is a function of the half-life of the drug used. Drugs with long half-lives (e.g., piroxicam, with a half-life of 30 to 86 hours) stay in plasma longer, thus continuing to affect COX, and therefore falsely appear to have irreversible effects.

Most older NSAIDs nonselectively inhibit both COX-1 and COX-2. Some older agents have a modest degree of COX-2 selectivity (etodolac, nabumetone, and meloxicam),[1–3,14,19–23] which may explain the low incidence of adverse gastrointestinal effects from these agents. The newer COX-2–selective NSAIDs (e.g., celecoxib, rofecoxib and valdecoxib) are expected to have less of an adverse gastrointestinal effect and fewer antiplatelet effects.

CLINICAL PRESENTATION

The various types of NSAIDs generally share similar toxicity therapeutically and after an overdose, with a few notable exceptions. Multiple organ systems can be involved. A description of effects on organ systems follows, with special note made of specific NSAIDs more likely than others to

TABLE 58-1 Classification of Nonsteroidal Antiinflammatory Drugs

Acetic Acids
Bromfenac (Duract)—off U.S. market, a benzene
  acetic acid
Diclofenac (Voltaren, Cataflam)—a phenylacetic acid
Etodolac (Lodine, Lodine XL)—an indole
  acetic acid
Indomethacin (Indocin)—an indole acetic acid
Sulindac (Clinoril)—an indene acetic acid
Tolmetin (Tolectin)

Butanones (a Ketone)
Nabumetone (Relafen)—nonactive prodrug; its metabolite is a
  naphthylacetic acid

Carboxylic Acids
Ketorolac (Toradol)

Fenamic Acids or Anthranilic Acids
Meclofenamic acid (Meclomen)—a benzoic acid
Mefenamic acid (Ponstel)—a benzoic acid

Furanones
Rofecoxib (Vioxx)—selective COX-2 inhibitor

Isoxazoles
Valdecoxib (Bextra)–a sulfonamide derivative and a selective COX-2
  inhibitor

Oxicams
Meloxicam (Mobic)
Piroxicam (Feldene)

Propionic Acids
Fenoprofen (Nalfon)
Flurbiprofen (Ansaid)
Ibuprofen (Motrin)
Ketoprofen (Orudis)
Naproxen (Naprosyn)
Oxaprozin (Daypro)
Suprofen (Suprol)—off U.S. market

Pyrazoles
Celecoxib (Celebrex)—a sulfonamide derivative and a selective COX-2
  inhibitor

Pyrazolidines or Pyrazolidinediones
Oxyphenbutazone
Phenylbutazone (Butazolidin)

Salicylic Acids
Acetylated Salicylates
Acetylsalicylic acid—commonly known as aspirin

Nonacetylated Salicylates
Choline salicylate (Arthropan)
Diflunisal (Dolobid)
Magnesium salicylate (Doan's Original, Magan, Mobidin)
Salicylamide
Salsalate (Disalcid)
Sodium salicylate
Sodium thiosalicylate (Rexolate Injection)
Trolamine salicylate (Aspercreme, Myoflex Creme, Mobisyl Creme)

Data from Brouwers JRBJ, deSmet PAGM: Pharmacokinetic-pharmacodynamic drug interactions with nonsteroidal
anti-inflammatory drugs. Clin Pharmacokinet 27:462–485, 1994.

produce certain types of toxicity. Major drug interactions associated with NSAIDs are presented in Table 58-2.

Neurologic Effects

Central nervous system depression, including coma, may occur after an overdose (e.g., >400 mg/kg of ibuprofen).[84–90] Agitation and irritability may precede the central nervous system depression.[87–89] Acute psychosis and auditory hallucinations have been seen after the ingestion of indomethacin, diclofenac, sulindac, and mefenamic acid.[91–93] Seizures, including status epilepticus, may occur, especially after an overdosage of mefenamic acid.[85,86,88,90,91,94,95] Patients commonly complain of dizziness, tinnitus, or headache.[89,96,97] Both transient and persistent sensorineural hearing loss have been reported to occur after therapeutic doses of ketorolac.[37,98] Nystagmus, diplopia, miosis, and blurred vision have also been reported.[93,96,97] Aseptic meningitis is an uncommon adverse effect of therapeutic doses of ibuprofen, naproxen, sulindac, and tolmetin.[99,100]

Respiratory Effects

Pulmonary edema and adult respiratory distress syndrome (ARDS) in conjunction with multiorgan failure have occurred after an overdose.[87,101,42] Respiratory failure as a result of respiratory depression, without evidence of ARDS or pulmonary edema, has likewise been reported.[86] At therapeutic

doses, angioedema, bronchospasm, and rarely, shock and death may occur in susceptible individuals.[37,103,104]

Cardiovascular Effects

Volume depletion, with secondary hypotension, and tachycardia are relatively common effects of NSAID overdose.[84,86,87] Less commonly, bradycardia, arrhythmias, or cardiogenic shock may occur.[85,96,105–108]

Gastrointestinal Effects

An overdose of NSAIDs often results in nausea, vomiting, diarrhea, abdominal pain, and rarely, gastrointestinal bleeding.[87–89,94,97,101,103,105] Gastric and duodenal ulceration and significant gastrointestinal bleeding may accompany chronic use. Selective COX-2 inhibitors have a lower incidence of ulcers, gastrointestinal bleeding, mucosal damage, and perforation, but these complications still occur.[3,17,18,109–113] Ketorolac is generally more gastrotoxic than other NSAIDs.[37] The mortality rate in patients who are hospitalized for NSAID-induced upper gastrointestinal bleeding is approximately 5% to 10%.[3]

Hepatic injury and right upper quadrant pain may be seen after an acute overdose, especially after the ingestion of phenylbutazone and conversion to its metabolite oxyphenbutazone.[85,87,93,114] Hepatic injury can include hepatocellular injury, cholestasis, granuloma formation, and steatosis.[87,115,116] Hepatitis may also occur on a more

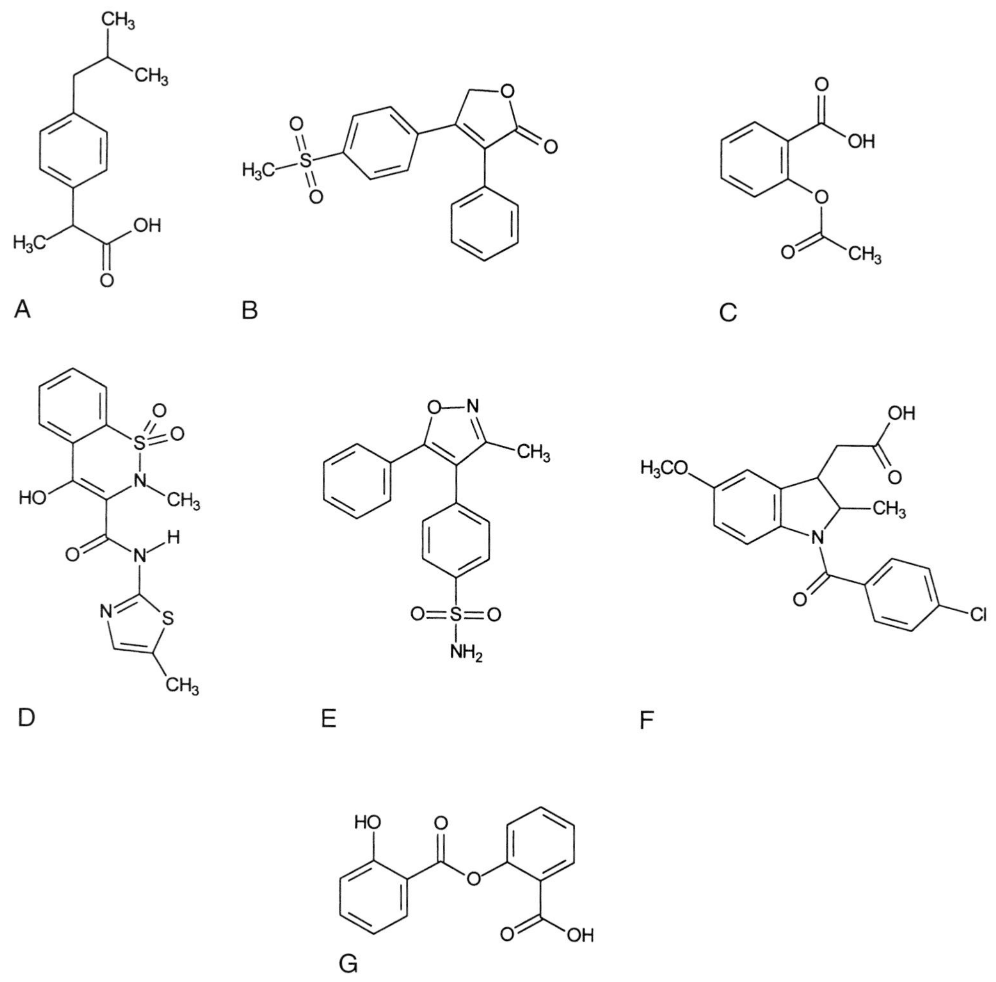

FIGURE 58-1

Chemical structures of various nonsteroidal antiinflammatory drugs. **A**, Ibuprofen, a propionic acid; **B**, rofecoxib, a furanone; **C**, acetylsalicylic acid, an acetylated salicylate; **D**, meloxicam, an oxicam or enolcarboxamide; **E**, valdecoxib, an isoxazole; **F**, indomethacin, an acetic acid; **G**, salsalate, a nonacetylated salicylate.

idiosyncratic basis, with hypersensitivity-like liver injury associated with fever and rash.[116] Fatal hepatitis is rare.[37,117,118] Resected liver from a patient with ibuprofen-induced subfulminant hepatitis revealed an atrophic liver with large areas of necrosis and confluent collapse of zone 3, with infiltration by mononuclear cells, leukocytes, and macrophages.[117] Pancreatitis has also been reported.[118,119]

Renal Effects

NSAID-induced renal disease may be manifested as sodium and water retention, acute renal failure, or nephrotic syndrome.[87,88] Patients with NSAID-induced renal failure may complain of lumbar pain.[105] Acute tubular necrosis and interstitial nephritis may occur at therapeutic doses of some NSAIDs such as ketorolac.[37,86,88] Inhibition of prostaglandin production is thought to be the cause of renal failure.[88,101] Normally, the afferent glomerular vasodilation caused by several prostaglandins helps maintain renal blood flow.[101,105,120] If the production of vasodilating prostaglandins is inhibited by an NSAID, afferent vasoconstriction occurs, and glomerular filtration and renal blood flow diminish.[120] Renal failure may

require hemodialysis for several weeks to months,[87,101,105,108] but it is generally reversible.[86,108]

The effects of COX-2 inhibition on renal function in humans are similar to those observed with nonselective NSAIDs.[3,8,109] Selective COX-2 inhibitors appear to have a renal safety profile similar to that of traditional NSAIDs because these agents alter renal blood flow, urine formation, and salt and water retention.[9,17,109] Rofecoxib appears to be more nephrotoxic than celecoxib.[5]

Musculoskeletal Effects

Hypotonia, muscle fasciculations, and myoclonic twitching have been reported after NSAID overdose.[93,96,115,121]

Hematopoietic Effects

Bone marrow suppression may occur, with bone marrow biopsy samples revealing granulomatous lesions.[105,122] Thrombocytopenia, leukopenia, aplastic anemia, hemolytic anemia, agranulocytosis, and pancytopenia have developed after therapeutic use as well as acute overdose.[87,102,122–125] The

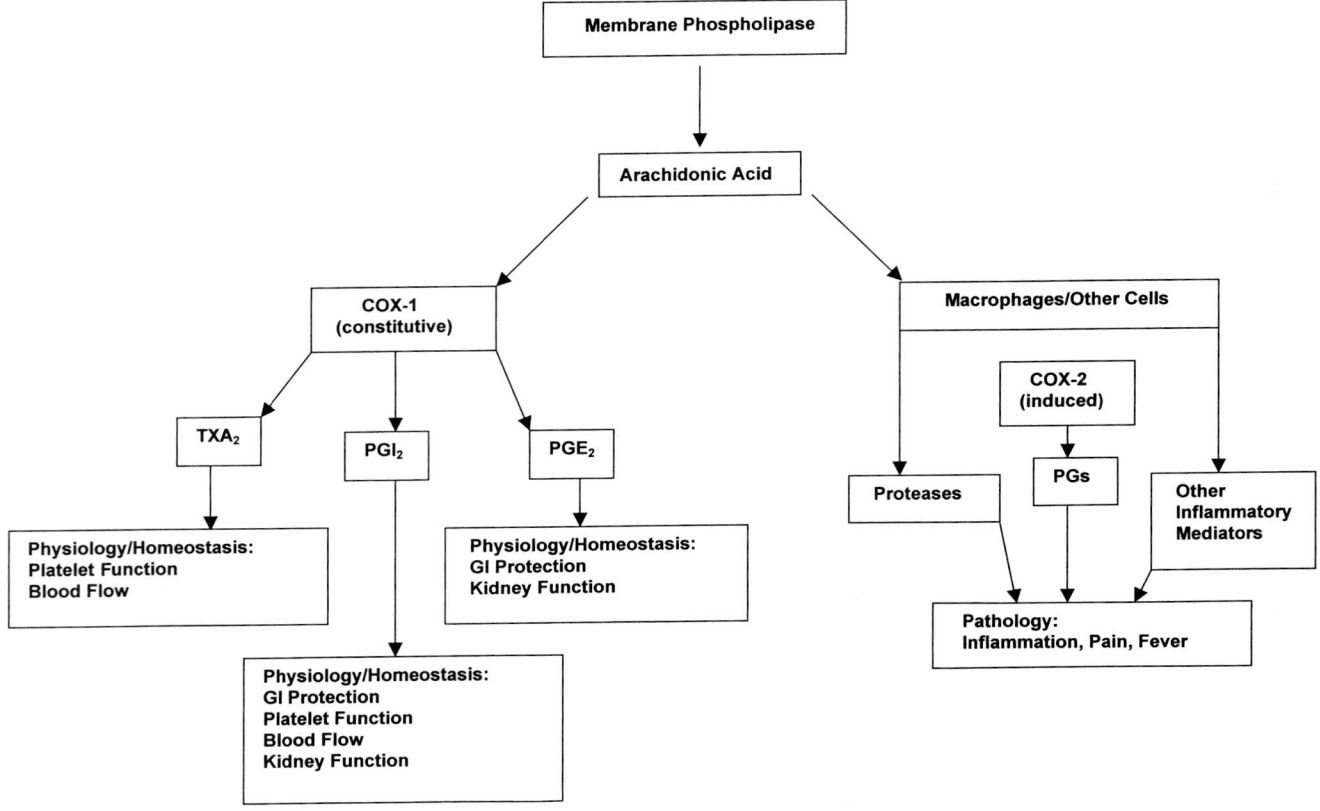

FIGURE 58-2

Mechanism of action of nonsteroidal antiinflammatory drugs (NSAIDs)—phospholipids are converted to arachidonic acid through the action of the enzyme phospholipase. NSAIDs inhibit the enzyme cyclooxygenase, which converts arachidonic acid to various prostaglandins and thromboxanes. The recent discovery of isoenzymes for cyclooxygenase (COX-1 and COX-2) has resulted in development of specific COX inhibitor NSAIDs. Selective COX-2 inhibitors primarily inhibit inflammation and pain. Nonspecific COX-1 and COX-2 inhibitors (e.g., older NSAIDs) also affect the homeostatic effects of prostaglandins and thromboxanes, thereby resulting in adverse systemic (e.g., renal, gastrointestinal) effects. PG, prostaglandin; TX, thromboxane.

TABLE 58-2 Drug Interactions

ACE Inhibitors
Several studies have shown that indomethacin inhibits the antihypertensive response of captopril. Other nonsteroidal antiinflammatory drugs (NSAIDs) probably have a similar effect. Sulindac is a possible exception in that it has been shown to have a small opposing effect on the antihypertensive efficacy of captopril and enalapril. The combination of angiotensin-converting enzyme (ACE) inhibitors (efferent vasodilation) and NSAIDs also occasionally results in an acute reduction in renal function that is reversible.

Acetazolamide
Salicylates displace acetazolamide from plasma protein binding sites and inhibit its renal excretion, thereby leading to accumulation of acetazolamide. Acetazolamide also enhances salicylate tissue penetration by producing a systemic acidosis while increasing renal elimination of salicylate through alkalinization of urine.

Anticoagulants, Oral
NSAIDs can result in hypoprothrombinemia, but the effect is highly variable and depends on the NSAID used. Most nonselective COX inhibitor NSAIDs also inhibit platelet function and are potentially ulcerogenic. Salicylate doses over 2 to 3 g/day may enhance the effect of warfarin through inhibition of vitamin K–dependent clotting factors. Aspirin also inhibits platelet function and is ulcerogenic. COX-2–selective agents may have platelet-aggregating effects and compete with warfarin for albumin binding sites. It is not known whether celecoxib (a sulfonamide) inhibits warfarin metabolism. Bleeding has been reported in patients receiving celecoxib and warfarin. When rofecoxib is used with warfarin, it can increase the prothrombin time by 10% and may increase the risk of bleeding.[24,25]

Antidiabetic Agents (Sulfonylureas and Insulin)
Phenylbutazone enhances the hypoglycemic response of antidiabetic agents. Fatalities have been reported. Tolmetin, naproxen, and sulindac do not interfere with the action of tolbutamide, but little is known regarding other combinations of sulfonylureas and NSAIDs. Salicylates in large doses have an intrinsic effect on carbohydrate metabolism through increased effects of insulin and inhibition of gluconeogenesis (see Salicylates, Chapter 57). The effect on chlorpropamide is seen at serum salicylate concentrations of 10 mg/dL (952 μmol/L). Cases have been reported in which aspirin appeared to have contributed to the hypoglycemic effect of sulfonylureas or insulin.[26]

TABLE 58-2 Drug Interactions—cont'd

β-Blockers

NSAIDs reduce the antihypertensive effects of β-blockers. It has been proposed that the antihypertensive effects of β-blockers may involve the production of prostaglandins. Attenuation of this antihypertensive effect has been reported with indomethacin, naproxen, and piroxicam in patients taking atenolol, labetalol, pindolol, and propranolol. Sulindac appears to be least likely to interfere with the antihypertensive effects of β-blockers. Using other antihypertensives may not circumvent the interaction because NSAIDs tend to inhibit the effects of antihypertensives in general.

Corticosteroids

Concurrent use of corticosteroids and NSAIDs results in an increased likelihood of gastrointestinal bleeding and ulceration.

Cyclosporine

It has been proposed that NSAIDs inhibit the formation of prostaglandins that are protective against cyclosporine-induced nephrotoxicity. Diclofenac can increase serum creatinine, potassium, and blood pressure without affecting cyclosporine levels. This effect may be seen within 48 hours of starting the NSAID.[27–29] Sulindac administration has resulted in a twofold to threefold increase in serum creatinine and cyclosporine concentration within 3 days.[30] In animal studies, indomethacin produced an increase in nephrotoxicity.[31] Mefenamic acid resulted in a rapid increase in serum creatinine and a twofold increase in cyclosporine concentration within 1 day.[32]

Ethanol

Both NSAIDs and ethanol damage the gastrointestinal mucosa, with the combination resulting in additive or synergistic effects. A twofold to threefold increase in the incidence of minor gastric bleeding can be seen.[33–35]

Heparin

NSAIDs can increase the incidence of bleeding in patients receiving heparin therapy.

Hydralazine

Indomethacin reportedly increases blood pressure through inhibition of prostaglandin synthesis.[36]

Lithium

NSAIDs increase serum lithium concentrations.[26] The magnitude of this effect varies considerably. Depending on which NSAID is used, serum lithium concentrations can be increased by 12% to 67%. The onset of this effect is delayed and has ranged anywhere from 3 to 10 days. It has been proposed that renal prostaglandins are involved in the excretion of lithium and that NSAIDs interfere with this mechanism.[37] Such interference has been reported with diclofenac, ibuprofen, indomethacin, ketorolac, mefenamic acid, naproxen, phenylbutazone, and piroxicam.[38–51] Sulindac has been reported to temporarily reduce lithium concentrations; however, other more recent studies also indicate elevated lithium levels.[52–54]

Methotrexate

NSAIDs may increase methotrexate levels, especially in patients taking high methotrexate doses.[25,26] Serious methotrexate toxicity has been reported with diclofenac given before high-dose methotrexate therapy.[55,56] Flurbiprofen has been reported to cause neutropenia, thrombocytopenia, and gastrointestinal bleeding in a patient with rheumatoid arthritis who was taking low-dose methotrexate.[57] Ibuprofen decreases the renal clearance of methotrexate by 50% and doubles the methotrexate area under the curve.[58] Deaths have been reported from concomitant use of methotrexate with indomethacin, ketoprofen, naproxen, and phenylbutazone.[55,59–62] Salicylates have produced a decrease in methotrexate renal clearance and an elevation in the methotrexate area under the curve.[63–67] Concomitant use of low-dose methotrexate (as used in the treatment of rheumatoid arthritis) and NSAIDs has been well tolerated. The risk of adverse effects from this interaction is more likely from patients receiving antineoplastic doses of methotrexate. However, an occasional patient may have reduced methotrexate clearance after NSAID administration, and some patients may experience clinically significant increases in methotrexate levels with concomitant NSAID administration.[68,69]

Potassium-Sparing Diuretics

Hyperkalemia has been reported with the concurrent use of indomethacin, diclofenac, and ibuprofen in patients taking triamterene.[70–74] Indomethacin may inhibit the formation of prostaglandins, which protect against drug-induced nephrotoxicity.[70–72]

Probenecid

Large doses of salicylates (those that produce salicylate levels greater than 5 mg/dL [476 μmol/L]) inhibit the uricosuric effect of probenecid.[75–78] Probenecid also inhibits uricosuria from large doses of salicylates.[75] However, a recent study demonstrated no adverse effect of aspirin, 325 mg/day, on serum urate concentrations or urinary urate clearance rates.[79]

Sulfinpyrazone

The amount of salicylate needed to inhibit sulfinpyrazone uricosuria is not well established. Sulfinpyrazone also inhibits the uricosuria from large doses of salicylates.

Valproic Acid

Salicylates displace valproic acid from plasma proteins.[80,81] In addition, salicylates may inhibit the hepatic metabolism of valproic acid by interfering with its beta oxidation and may also enhance valproic acid conjugation.[82,83]

---

prothrombin time may be prolonged.[87,89,102,118] Phenylbutazone, oxyphenbutazone, and indomethacin are the most hematotoxic NSAIDs.[87,102,122] Oxyphenbutazone, a metabolite of phenylbutazone, possesses toxicity similar to that of phenylbutazone and has a long half-life (50 to 80 hours).[87]

Metabolic Effects

Metabolic acidosis is occasionally seen after an overdose and may be associated with respiratory alkalosis.[86,87,101,107,108] Hyperkalemia and hyponatremia have been noted as well.[108,126] Hyperkalemic quadriparesis has occurred after chronic diclofenac use.[126] Hypokalemia and hypophosphatemia have also been reported.[3]

Skin Effects

Edema may occur at therapeutic doses.[122] Hepatotoxicity may be manifested as jaundice.[115,117] Mucocutaneous reactions have also occurred, with toxic epidermal necrolysis (Lyell's syndrome or Stevens-Johnson syndrome) being reported after therapeutic doses.[118,122,127–133] With chronic NSAID use, pseudoporphyria (bullous photosensitivity with similarities to porphyria cutanea tarda) has likewise been observed.[134–137]

Other Effects

Both hyperthermia and hypothermia have been described in the setting of NSAID toxicity.[85,93,122] A multisystem hypersensitivity syndrome characterized by fever, rash, hepatic injury, and lymphadenopathy is a reported effect of NSAID administration.[122]

DIAGNOSIS

Symptomatic patients should undergo the following blood studies: complete blood count, electrolytes, renal function tests (blood urea nitrogen, creatinine), and liver function tests (alanine transaminase and bilirubin).[87,117] Creatine phosphokinase levels may be elevated without myoglobin's being detected in the urine.[87,88,108] Serum concentrations of NSAIDs have no clinical utility and are rarely available.[84] In addition, the previously touted nomogram developed to assess the severity of illness based on ibuprofen levels is not helpful clinically.[84,96,97,101] It should be noted that diflunisal cross-reacts with some salicylate assays and may produce a falsely positive salicylate test.[93]

Urinalysis may reveal proteinuria and hematuria.[102,105] Red discoloration of urine, caused by a rubazonic acid metabolite, may be noted after phenylbutazone toxicity.[85]

Specialized studies may be indicated for evaluation of specific organ systems. Ultrasound of the kidneys may show general swelling of the parenchyma.[105] Bone marrow biopsy may reveal marrow aplasia.[102] Liver biopsy may reveal intrahepatic cholestasis and eosinophilia, consistent with a drug reaction.[116]

TREATMENT

Indications for ICU Admission in Antiinflammatory Drug Poisoning

Seizures
Coma or encephalopathy
Respiratory failure or potential for obstructive airway angioedema
Hemodynamic instability (hypotension, shock)
Cardiac arrhythmias
Gastrointestinal hemorrhage

Treatment is supportive. No antidotes are available for NSAID toxicity.

Decontamination

Activated charcoal is effective in adsorbing many NSAIDs[93] and may be administered, although it may also interfere with gastrointestinal endoscopy in cases of bleeding. Repeat-dose activated charcoal has been shown to decrease the absorption of phenylbutazone and reduce its half-life by 30%, as well as reduce the half-life of piroxicam in human volunteers.[87,93] The clinical significance of this effect is not known.

Neurologic Effects

Seizures should be treated with benzodiazepines and barbiturates.[93] Further discussion of the treatment of toxicant-induced seizures can be found in Chapter 20.

Respiratory Effects

Endotracheal intubation and mechanical ventilation may be required if respiratory failure, ARDS, or pulmonary edema develops.[101]

Cardiovascular Effects

Hypotension should be treated initially with intravenous fluids and, if persistent, with vasopressors.[86,87,93]

Gastrointestinal Effects

Endoscopy, proton-pump inhibitors, or H_2-antagonists and blood transfusions may be indicated for gastrointestinal bleeding.[93] Liver failure occasionally warrants liver transplantation, if available.[117]

Renal Effects

Hemodialysis may be needed if renal failure develops or to correct severe electrolyte abnormalities.[33,43,47]

Hematopoietic Effects

Blood transfusions may be necessary for acute gastrointestinal bleeding.[93] Platelet transfusions have been given for thrombocytopenia,[123,125] but thrombocytopenia may also resolve without transfusion.[124]

Metabolic Effects

Electrolyte and fluid imbalances should be monitored and abnormalities corrected.[93]

Skin Effects

Patient transfer to a burn center should be considered for those with toxic epidermal necrosis. It has not been established whether systemic corticosteroids are beneficial.[132]

Prevention and Prophylaxis

Patients at risk for gastrointestinal complications from NSAID use include those older than 65 years and those with a previous history of ulceration, perforation, or gastrointestinal bleeding. Other factors that may be associated with an increased risk for gastrointestinal complications include the dose and duration of NSAID use, smoking, the use of multiple NSAIDs, and concurrent use of corticosteroids. The use of either misoprostol, a proton-pump inhibitor, or high-dose H_2-antagonists has been proposed to reduce the risk of NSAID-induced gastrointestinal ulceration and damage in patients requiring continued NSAID use.[138–143]

Misoprostol in doses of 200 μg given four times a day has been shown to decrease the incidence of gastrointestinal ulcer perforation, gastric outlet obstruction, and bleeding in patients with rheumatoid arthritis who are taking NSAIDs. The protective effect was related to the misoprostol dose. Daily misoprostol doses of 400 μg provided the least protection, whereas daily doses of 800 μg offered the most benefit. Diarrhea and abdominal pain were also dose-related adverse effects of misoprostol.[138]

Lansoprazole, a proton-pump inhibitor, can be used for the treatment of NSAID-induced gastric ulceration in patients needing continued NSAID treatment and to reduce the risk of NSAID-induced gastric ulcers in patients with a previous history of ulcers in whom continued NSAID treatment is deemed beneficial. A dose of 15 mg daily is used to reduce risk whereas a 30-mg daily dose is indicated for healing of gastric ulceration.[139] Omeprazole in daily doses of 20 and 40 mg has shown similar results.[140,141]

Famotidine in oral doses of 40 mg twice daily has been shown to heal endoscopic ulcerations or lesions in patients continuing NSAID treatment. It has also prevented gastric and duodenal ulceration in patients without previous peptic ulcers who are taking chronic NSAIDs.[142,143]

An alternative approach to the therapy just presented would be to switch to a selective COX-2 agent.

SPECIAL POPULATIONS

Patients with heightened susceptibility to nephrotoxicity include the elderly and those with congestive heart failure, hepatic cirrhosis, hypovolemia (e.g., hypotensive or taking diuretics), or renal disease.[37,101,120]

Pediatric Patients

There may be an association of necrotizing enterocolitis and intestinal perforation in preterm infants treated with intravenous indomethacin, although such an association is controversial because preterm infants receiving 10 to 100 times the planned dose have done well, without the development of these complications.[144,145] Iatrogenic overdoses of intravenous indomethacin in these patients are rare and associated with elevated creatinine and decreased urine output.[144] In more severe iatrogenic overdosage, transient renal failure with oliguria, mild hyponatremia, and hyperkalemia have been reported.[145]

The clinical picture of acute ibuprofen ingestion is generally similar to that of adults.[146] Apnea has been reported in a 16-month-old child who acutely ingested 469 mg/kg of ibuprofen.[97]

The death of a 1-year-old was reported after the ingestion of 2 g of phenylbutazone.[87] A 2½-year-old acutely ingested phenylbutazone and presented with coma, recurrent convulsions, vomiting, diarrhea, and cholestatic jaundice with hepatomegaly that evolved over a period of 10 days.[115] Irreversible renal failure was observed in an adolescent treated with ketorolac.[120]

Pregnant Patients

A preterm infant born 8 hours after a maternal overdose of naproxen experienced hyponatremia, water retention, and hypoglycemia with associated lethargy and hypotonia; the infant recovered.[93,147] In infants exposed prenatally to maternal therapeutic doses of NSAIDs (ibuprofen, indomethacin, and nimesulide), both reversible and irreversible renal failure has developed.[120,148] Furthermore, prenatal exposure to NSAIDs may constrict the fetal ductus arteriosus and increase the incidence of intracranial hemorrhage and necrotizing enterocolitis.[120]

 Key Points in Antiinflammatory Drug Poisoning

1. Patients who have ingested less than 100 mg/kg of ibuprofen are not likely to become ill, and greater than 400 mg/kg is generally required to produce severe effects, including central nervous system depression, gastrointestinal disturbances, and less commonly, metabolic acidosis, renal failure, and seizures.[84,96,97,101] Other propionic acid derivatives produce similar effects.[86]
2. The toxicity of phenylbutazone is greater than that of most other NSAIDs. Phenylbutazone, also termed "bute," is occasionally abused by jockeys, grooms, and other racetrack workers.[87]
3. Acute overdose with mefenamic acid is characterized by convulsions,[90] and seizures develop in more than a third of all patients with confirmed mefenamic acid overdose.[93] Status epilepticus may ensue, and seizures may be resistant to standard treatment.[93]
4. Although COX-2–selective NSAIDs tend to have fewer adverse gastrointestinal effects than nonselective agents do, the selective agents have similar nephrotoxicity and may produce adverse effects related to their prothrombic acitivity.[3,4,6]

REFERENCES

1. Kaplan-Machlis B, Klostermeyer BS: The cyclooxygenase-2 inhibitors: Safety and effectiveness. Ann Pharmacother 33:979–988, 1999.
2. Meade EA, Smith WL, DeWitt DL: Differential inhibition of prostaglandin endoperoxide synthase (cyclooxygenase) isoenzymes by aspirin and non-steroidal anti-inflammatory drugs. J Biol Chem 268:6610–6614, 1993.
3. Oviedo JA, Wolfe M: Clinical potential of cyclo-oxygenase-2 inhibitors. Biodrugs 15:563–572, 2001.
4. Rajadhyaksha VD, Dahanukar SA: Rofecoxib: A new selective COX-2 inhibitor. J Postgrad Med 47:77–78, 2001.
5. Zhao SZ, Reynolds MW, Lefkowith J, et al: A comparison of renal-related adverse drug reactions between rofecoxib and celecoxib,

based on the World Heath Organization/Uppsala monitoring centre safety database. Clin Ther 23:1478–1491, 2001.

6. Mukherjee D, Nissen SE, Topol EJ: Risk of cardiovascular events associated with selective COX-2 inhibitors. JAMA 286:954–959, 2001.

7. Budavari S (ed): The Merck Index: An Encyclopedia of Chemicals, Drugs, and Biologicals, 12th ed. Whitehouse Station, NJ, Merck Research Laboratories, Division of Merck & Co, 1996.

8. Wallace JL: Selective COX-2 inhibitors: Is the water becoming muddy? Trends Pharmacol Sci 20:4–6, 1999.

9. Swan SK, Rudy DW, Lasseter KC, et al: Effect of cyclooxygenase-2 inhibition on renal function in elderly persons receiving a low-salt diet. Ann Intern Med 133:1–9, 2000.

10. Bjorkman DJ: The effect of aspirin and non-steroidal anti-inflammatory drugs on prostaglandins. Am J Med 105(1B):8S–12S, 1998.

11. Vane JR, Botting RM: Mechanism of action of non-steroidal anti-inflammatory drugs. Am J Med 104(3A):2S–8S, 1998.

12. Jouzeau JY, Terlain B, Abid A, et al: Cyclo-oxygenase isoenzymes: How recent findings affect thinking about nonsteroidal anti-inflammatory drugs. Drugs 53:563–582, 1997.

13. Emery P: Clinical implications of selective cyclooxygenase-2 inhibition. Scand J Rheumatol 25(Suppl 102):23–28, 1996.

14. Bolten WW: Scientific rationale for specific inhibition of COX-2. J Rheumatol 23(Suppl 51):2–7, 1998.

15. Wallace JL: Non-steroidal anti-inflammatory drugs and gastroenteropathy: The second hundred years. Gastroenterology 112:1000–1016, 1997.

16. Wolfe MM: Future trends in the development of safer non-steroidal anti-inflammatory drugs. Am J Med 105(5A):44S–52S, 1998.

17. Weaver AL: Rofecoxib: Clinical pharmacology and clinical experience. Clin Ther 23:1323–1338, 2001.

18. Silverstein FE, Faich G, Goldstein JL, et al: Gastrointestinal toxicity with celecoxib vs. nonsteroidal antiinflammatory drugs for osteoarthritis and rheumatoid arthritis: The CLASS study: A randomized controlled trial. JAMA 284:1247–1255, 2000.

19. Cryer B, Feldman M: Cyclooxygenase-1 and cyclooxygenase-2 selectivity of widely used non-steroidal anti-inflammatory drugs. Am J Med 104:413–421, 1998.

20. Glaser K, Sung ML, O'Neill K, et al: Etodolac selectively inhibits human prostaglandin G/H synthetase 2 (PGHS-2) versus human PGHS-1. Eur J Pharmacol 281:107–111, 1995.

21. Laneuville O, Breuer DK, DeWitt DL, et al: Differential inhibition of human prostaglandin endoperoxide H synthases-1 and -2 by non-steroidal anti-inflammatory drugs. J Pharmacol Exp Ther 27:927–934, 1994.

22. Mitchell JA, Akarasereenont P, Thiemermann, C, et al: Selectivity of nonsteroidal antiinflammatory drugs as inhibitors of constitutive and inducible cyclooxygenase. Proc Natl Acad Sci U S A 90:11693–11697, 1993.

23. Spangler RS: Cyclooxygenase 1 and 2 in rheumatic disease: Implications for non-steroidal anti-inflammatory drug therapy. Semin Arthritis Rheum 26:436–447, 1996.

24. Chan TYK: Adverse interactions between warfarin and nonsteroidal antiinflammatory drugs: Mechanisms, clinical significance, and avoidance. Ann Pharmacother 29:1274–1283, 1995.

25. Rofecoxib for osteoarthritis and pain. Med Lett Drugs Ther 41(1056):59–61, 1999.

26. Brouwers JRBJ, deSmet PAGM: Pharmacokinetic-pharmacodynamic drug interactions with nonsteroidal anti-inflammatory drugs. Clin Pharmacokinet 27:462–485, 1994.

27. Branthwaite JP, Nicholls A: Cyclosporine and diclofenac interaction in rheumatoid arthritis. Lancet 337:252, 1991.

28. Kovarik JM, Kurki P, Mueller E, et al: Diclofenac combined with cyclosporine in treatment of refractory rheumatoid arthritis: Longitudinal safety assessment and evidence of pharmacokinetic/dynamic interaction. J Rheumatol 23:2033–2038, 1996.

29. Deray G, Le Hoang P, Aupetit B, et al: Enhancement of cyclosporine A nephrotoxicity by diclofenac. Clin Nephrol 27:213–214, 1987.

30. Sesin GP, O'Keefe E, Roberto P: Sulindac induced elevation of serum cyclosporine concentration. Clin Pharm 8:445, 1989.

31. Whiting PH, Burke MD, Thompson AW: Drug interactions with cyclosporine: Implications from animal studies. Transplant Proc 18(6 Suppl 5):56, 1986.

32. Agar JW: Cyclosporine A and mefenamic acid in a renal transplant patient. Aust N Z J Med 21:784–785, 1991.

33. Goulston K, Cooke AR: Alcohol, aspirin, and gastrointestinal bleeding. BMJ 4:664, 1968.

34. Dobbing J: Fecal blood-loss after sodium acetyl salicylate taken with alcohol. Lancet 1:527, 1969.

35. Needham CD, Kyle J, Jones PF, et al: Aspirin and alcohol in gastrointestinal haemorrhage. Gut 12:819–821, 1971.

36. Cinquegrani MP, Liang CS: Indomethacin attenuates the hypotensive action of hydralazine. Clin Pharmacol Ther 39:564–570, 1986.

37. Reinhart D: Minimizing the adverse effects of ketorolac. Drug Saf 22:487–497, 2000.

38. Reimann JW, Frolich JC: Effects of diclofenac on lithium kinetics. Clin Pharmacol Ther 30:348–352, 1981.

39. Ragheb M, Ban TA, Buchanan D, et al: Interaction of indomethacin and ibuprofen with lithium in manic patients under a steady-state lithium level. J Clin Psychiatry 41:397–398, 1987.

40. Ragheb M: Ibuprofen can increase serum lithium levels in lithium-treated patients. J Clin Psychiatry 48:161–163, 1987.

41. Frolich JC, Leftwich R, Ragheb M, et al: Indomethacin increases plasma lithium. BMJ 1:1115–1116, 1979.

42. Reimann IW, Diener U, Frolich JC: Indomethacin but not aspirin increases plasma lithium ion levels. Arch Gen Psychiatry 40:283–286, 1983.

43. Langlois R, Paquette D: Increased serum lithium levels due to ketorolac therapy. Can Med Assoc J 150:1455–1456, 1994.

44. Iyer V: Ketorolac (Toradol) induced lithium toxicity. Headache 34:442–444, 1994.

45. Shelly RK: Lithium toxicity and mefenamic acid: A possible interaction and the role of prostaglandin inhibition. Br J Psychiatry 151:847, 1987.

46. MacDonald J, Nealt TJ: Toxic interaction of lithium carbonate and mefenamic acid. BMJ 297:1339, 1988.

47. Ragheb M, Powell AL: Lithium interaction with sulindac and naproxen. J Clin Psychopharmacol 6:150–154, 1986.

48. Ragheb M: The clinical significance of lithium–nonsteroidal anti-inflammatory drug interactions. J Clin Psychopharmacol 10:350–354, 1990.

49. Ragheb M: The interaction of lithium with phenylbutazone in bipolar affective patients. J Clin Psychopharmacol 10:149, 1990.

50. Walbridge DG, Bazier SR: An interaction between lithium carbonate and piroxicam presenting as lithium toxicity. Br J Psychiatry 145:206–207, 1985.

51. Kerry RJ, Owen G, Michaelson S: Possible toxic interaction between lithium and piroxicam. Lancet 1:418–419, 1983.

52. Ragheb MA, Powell AL: Failure of sulindac to increase serum lithium levels. J Clin Psychiatry 47:33–34, 1986.

53. Furnell MM, Davies J: The effect of sulindac on lithium therapy. Drug Intell Clin Pharm 190:374–376, 1985.

54. Jones M, Stoner S: Increased lithium concentrations reported in patients treated with sulindac. J Clin Psychiatry 61:7, 2000.

55. Thyss A, Milano G, Kubar J, et al: Clinical and pharmacokinetic evidence of a life-threatening interaction between methotrexate and ketoprofen. Lancet 1:256–258, 1986.

56. Todd PA, Sorkin EM: Diclofenac: A reappraisal. Drugs 35:244–285, 1988.

57. Frenia ML, Long KS: Methotrexate and nonsteroidal antiinflammatory drug interactions. Ann Pharmacother 26:234–237, 1992.

58. Tracy TS, Krolin K, Jones Dr, et al: The effects of a salicylate, ibuprofen, and naproxen on the disposition of methotrexate in patients with rheumatoid arthritis. Eur J Clin Pharmacol 42:121–125, 1992.

59. Ellison NM, Servi RJ: Acute renal failure and death following sequential intermediate-dose methotrexate and 5-FU: A possible adverse effect due to concomitant indomethacin administration. Cancer Treat Rep 69:342–343, 1985.

60. Maiche AG: Acute renal failure due to concomitant action of methotrexate and indomethacin. Lancet 1:1390, 1986.

61. Adams JD, Hunter GA: Drug interactions in psoriasis. Aust J Dermatol 17:39–40, 1976.

62. Singh RR, Malaviya AN, Pandey JN, et al: Fatal interaction between methotrexate and naproxen. Lancet 1:1390, 1986.

63. Liegler DG, Henderson ES, Hahn MA, Oliverio VT: The effect of organic acids on renal clearance of methotrexate in man. Clin Pharmacol Ther 10:849–857, 1969.

64. Mandel NA: The synergistic effect of salicylates on methotrexate toxicity. Plast Reconstr Surg 57:733, 1976.

65. Stewart CF, Fleming RA, Germain BF, et al: Aspirin alters methotrexate disposition in rheumatoid arthritis patients. Arthritis Rheum 34:1514–1520, 1991.

66. Baker H: Intermittent high dose oral methotrexate therapy in psoriasis. Br J Dermatol 82:65, 1970.

67. Furst DE: Clinically important interactions of nonsteroidal antiinflammatory drugs with other medications. J Rheumatol Suppl 17:58–62, 1988.

68. Aherne M, Booth J, Loxton A, et al: Methotrexate kinetics in rheumatoid arthritis: Is there an interaction with non-steroidal anti-inflammatory drugs? J Rheumatol 15:1356–1360, 1988.

69. Dupuis LL, Shore A, Silverman ED, et al: Methotrexate–nonsteroidal anti-inflammatory drug interaction in children with arthritis. J Rheumatol 17:1469–1473, 1990.

70. Mor R, Pitlik S, Rosenfeld JB: Indomethacin- and Moduretic-induced hyperkalemia. Isr J Med Sci 19:535–537, 1983.

71. Favre L, Glasson P, Riondel A, et al: Interaction of diuretics and non-steroidal anti-inflammatory drugs in man. Clin Sci 64:407–415, 1983.

72. Favre L, Glasson P, Vallotton MB: Reversible acute renal failure from combined triamterene and indomethacin. Ann Intern Med 96:317–320, 1982.

73. Harkonen M, Ekblom-Kullberg S: Reversible deterioration of renal function after diclofenac in a patient receiving triamterene. BMJ 293:698, 1986.

74. Gehr TWB, Sica MD, Steiger M, et al: Interaction of triamterene-hydrochlorothiazide and ibuprofen. Clin Pharmacol Ther 47:200, 1990.

75. Pascale L, Dubin A, Bronsky D, et al: Inhibition of the uricosuric action of Benemid by salicylate. J Lab Clin Med 45:771–777, 1955.

76. Brooks CD, Ulrich JE: Effect of ibuprofen or aspirin on probenecid-induced uricosuria. J Int Med Res 8:283–285, 1980.

77. Diamond HS, Meisel AD: Postsecretory reabsorption of urate in man. Arthritis Rheum 18:805–809, 1975.

78. Seegmiller JE, Grayzel AI: Use of newer uricosuric agents in the management of gout. JAMA 173:1076, 1960.

79. Harris M, Bryant L, Danaher P, et al: Effect of low dose daily aspirin on serum urate levels and urinary excretion in patients receiving probenecid for gouty arthritis. J Rheumatol 27:2873–2876, 2000.

80. Goulden KG, Dooley JM, Camfield PR, et al: Clinical valproate toxicity induced by acetylsalicylic acid. Neurology 37:1392–1394, 1987.

81. Farrell K, Orr JM, Abbott FS, et al: The effect of acetylsalicylic acid on serum free valproate concentrations and valproate clearance in children. J Pediatr 101:142–144, 1982.

82. Abbott FS, Kassam J, Orr JM, et al: The effect of aspirin on valproic acid metabolism. Clin Pharmacol Ther 40:94–100, 1986.

83. Orr JM, Abbott FS, Farrell K, et al: Interaction between valproic acid and aspirin in epileptic children: Serum protein binding and metabolic effects. Clin Pharmacol Ther 31:642–649, 1982.

84. McElwee NE, Veltri JC, Bradford DC, et al: A prospective, population-based study of acute ibuprofen overdose: Complications are rare and routine serum levels not warranted. Ann Emerg Med 19:657–662, 1990.

85. Okonek S, Reinecke HJ: Acute toxicity of pyrazolones. Am J Med 75(5A):94–98, 1983.

86. Kolodzik JM, Eilers MA, Angelos MG: Nonsteroidal anti-inflammatory drugs and coma: A case report of fenoprofen overdose. Ann Emerg Med 19:378–381, 1990.

87. Newton TA, Rose SR: Poisoning with equine phenylbutazone in a racetrack worker. Ann Emerg Med 20:204–207, 1991.

88. Turnbill AJ, Campbell P, Hughes JA: Mefenamic acid nephropathy—acute renal failure in overdose [letter]. BMJ 296:646, 1988.

89. Sheehan TMT, Boldy DAR, Vale JA: Indomethacin poisoning. J Toxicol Clin Toxicol 24:151–158, 1986.

90. Gossinger H, Hruby K, Haubenstock A, et al: Coma in mefenamic acid poisoning [letter]. Lancet 2:384, 1982.

91. Balali-Mood M, Proudfoot AT, Critchley JAJG, et al: Mefenamic acid overdosage. Lancet 1:1354, 1981.

92. Hoppmann RA, Peden JG, Ober SK: Central nervous system side effects of nonsteroidal anti-inflammatory drugs. Arch Intern Med 151:1309, 1991.

93. Smolinske SC, Hall AH, Vandenberg SA, et al: Toxic effects of nonsteroidal anti-inflammatory drugs in overdose: An overview of recent evidence on clinical effects and dose-response relationships. Drug Saf 5:252–274, 1990.

94. Court H, Volans GN: Poisoning after overdose with non-steroidal anti-inflammatory drugs. Adverse Drug React Toxicol Rev 3:1, 1984.

95. McKillop G, Canning GP: A case of intravenous and oral mefenamic acid poisoning. Scot Med J 32(3):81–82, 1987.

96. Hall AH, Smolinske SC, Stover B, et al: Ibuprofen overdose in adults. J Toxicol Clin Toxicol 30:23–37, 1992.

97. Hall AH, Smolinske SC, Conrad FL, et al: Ibuprofen overdose: 126 cases. Ann Emerg Med 15:1308–1313, 1986.

98. Schabb KC, Dickinson ET, Setzen G: Acute sensorineural hearing loss following intravenous ketorolac administration. J Emerg Med 13:509–513, 1995.

99. Neufeld MY, Korczyn AD: Encephalopathy associated with sulindac. Hum Toxicol 5:55, 1986.

100. Wong JG, Hathaway SC, Paat JJ, et al: Drug-induced meningitis. Postgrad Med 96:117–124, 1994.

101. Le HT, Bosse GM, Tsai Y: Ibuprofen overdose complicated by renal failure, adult respiratory distress syndrome, and metabolic acidosis. J Toxicol Clin Toxicol 32:315–320, 1994.

102. MacDougall LG, Taylor-Smith A, Rothberg AD, Thomson PD: Piroxicam poisoning in a 2 year old child. S Afr Med J 66:31–33, 1984.

103. Halpern SM, Fitzpatrick R, Volans GN: Ibuprofen toxicity: A review of adverse reactions and overdose. Adverse Drug React Toxicol Rev 12:107, 1993.

104. Szczeklik A: Antipyretic analgesics and the allergic patient. Am J Med 75(5A):82–84, 1983.

105. Kulling PEJ, Bechman EA, Skagius ASM: Renal impairment after acute diclofenac, naproxen, and sulindac overdoses. J Toxicol Clin Toxicol 33:173–177, 1995.

106. McCune KH, O'Brien CJ: Atrial fibrillation induced by ibuprofen overdose. Postgrad Med J 69:325–328, 1993.

107. Downie A, Ali A, Bell D: Severe metabolic acidosis complicating massive ibuprofen overdose. Postgrad Med J 69:575–577, 1993.

108. Mattana J, Perinbasekar S, Brod-Miller C: Near-fatal reversible acute renal failure after massive ibuprofen ingestion. Am J Med Sci 313:117–119, 1997.

109. Valdecoxib (Bextra)—a new COX-2 inhibitor. Med Lett Drugs Ther 44(1129):39–40, 2002.

110. Emery P, Zeidler H, Kvien TK, et al: Celecoxib versus diclofenac in long-term management of rheumatoid arthritis: Randomized double-blind comparison. Lancet 354:2106–2111, 1999.

111. Simon LS, Weaver AL, Graham DY, et al: Anti-inflammatory and upper gastrointestinal effects of celecoxib in rheumatoid arthritis: A randomized controlled trial. JAMA 282:1921–1928, 1999.

112. Goldstein JL, Silverstein FE, Agrawal NB, et al: Reduced risk of upper gastrointestinal ulcer complications with celecoxib, a novel COX-2 inhibitor. Am J Gastroenterol 95:1681–1690, 2000.

113. Feldman M, McMahon AT: Do cyclooxygenase-2 inhibitors provide benefits similar to those of traditional nonsteroidal anti-inflammatory drugs, with less gastrointestinal toxicity? Ann Intern Med 132:134–143, 2000.

114. Rodriguez LAG, Williams R, Derby LE, et al: Acute liver injury associated with nonsteroidal anti-inflammatory drugs and the role of risk factors. Arch Intern Med 154:311, 1994.

115. Bury RW, Mashford ML, Glaun BP, Saaroni G: Acute phenylbutazone poisoning in a child. Med J Aust 1:478–479, 1983.

116. Galan MV, Gordon SC, Silverman AL: Celecoxib-induced cholestatic hepatitis. Ann Intern Med 134:254, 2001.

117. Laurent S, Rahier J, Geubel AP, et al: Subfulminant hepatitis requiring liver transplantation following ibuprofen overdose [letter]. Liver 20:93–94, 2000.

118. Klein SM, Khan MA: Hepatitis, toxic epidermal necrolysis and pancreatitis in association with sulindac therapy. J Rheumatol 10:512–513, 1983.

119. Jick SS, Walker AM, Perera DR, et al: Non-steroidal anti-inflammatory drugs and hospital admission for perforated peptic ulcer. Lancet 2:380, 1987.

120. Cuzzolin L, Dal Cere M, Fanos V: NSAID-induced nephrotoxicity from the fetus to the child. Drug Saf 24:9–18, 2001.

121. Netter P, Lambert H, Larean A, et al: Diclofenac sodium–chlormezanone poisoning. Eur J Clin Pharmacol 26:535, 1984.

122. Andersson DEH, Langworth S, Newman HC, Ost A: Reversible bone marrow granuloma—adverse effect of oxyphenbutazone therapy. Acta Med Scand 207:131–133, 1980.

123. Kramer MR, Levene C, Hershko C: Severe reversible autoimmune haemolytic anaemia and thrombocytopenia associated with diclofenac therapy. Scand J Haematol 36:118–120, 1986.

124. Hunt PJ, Gibbons SS: Naproxen induced thrombocytopenia: A case report. N Z Med J 108:483–484, 1995.

125. Jain S: Ibuprofen-induced thrombocytopenia. Br J Clin Pract 48:51, 1994.

126. Patel P, Mandal B, Greenway MW: Hyperkalaemic quadriparesis secondary to chronic diclofenac treatment. Postgrad Med J 77:50–51, 2001.

127. Roujeau JC, Guillaume JC, Fabre JP, et al: Toxic epidermal necrolysis (Lyell syndrome). Arch Dermatol 126:37–42, 1990.

128. Stotts JS, Fang ML, Dannaker CJ, Steinman HK: Fenoprofen-induced toxic epidermal necrolysis. J Am Acad Dermatol 18:755–757, 1988.

129. Small RE, Garnett WR: Sulindac-induced toxic epidermal necrolysis. Clin Pharm 7:766–771, 1988.

130. Roujeau JC, Kelly JP, Naldi L, et al: Medication use and the risk of Stevens-Johnson syndrome or toxic epidermal necrolysis. N Engl J Med 333:1600–1607, 1995.

131. Ikeda N, Umetsu K, Suzuki T: A fatal case of sulindac-induced Lyell syndrome (toxic epidermal necrolysis). Z Rechtsmed 98:141–146, 1987.

132. Levitt L, Pearson RW: Sulindac-induced Stevens-Johnson toxic epidermal necrolysis syndrome. JAMA 243:1262–1263, 1980.

133. O'Sullivan M, Hanly JG, Molloy M: A case of toxic epidermal necrolysis secondary to indomethacin. Br J Rheumatol 22:47–49, 1983.

134. Ingrish G: Oxaprozin-induced pseudoporphyria. Arch Dermatol 132:1519–1520, 1996.

135. Al-Khenaizan S, Schechter JF, Sasseville D: Pseudoporphyria induced by propionic acid derivatives. J Cutan Med Surg 3:162–166, 1999.

136. Lang BI, Finlayson LA: Naproxen-induced pseudoporphyria in patients with juvenile rheumatoid arthritis. J Pediatr 124:639–642, 1994.

137. Magro CM, Crowson AN: Pseudoporphyria associated with Relafen therapy. J Cutan Pathol 26:42–47, 1999.

138. Silverstein FE, Graham DY, Senior JR, et al: Misoprostol reduces serious gastrointestinal complications in patients with rheumatoid arthritis receiving non-steroidal anti-inflammatory drugs: A randomized, double-blind, placebo-controlled trial. Ann Intern Med 123:241–249, 1995.

139. Agrawal NM, Campbell DR, Safdi MA, et al: Superiority of lansoprazole vs. ranitidine in healing non-steroidal anti-inflammatory drug–associated gastric ulcers. Arch Intern Med 160:1455–1461, 2000.

140. Yeomans ND, Tulassay Z, Juhasz L, et al (ASTRONAUT Study Group): A comparison of omeprazole with ranitidine for ulcers associated with non-steroidal anti-inflammatory drugs. N Engl J Med 338:719–726, 1998.

141. Hawkey DJ, Karrasch JA, Szczepanski L, et al (OMNIUM Study Group): Omeprazole compared with misoprostol for ulcers associated with non-steroidal anti-inflammatory drugs. N Engl J Med. 338:727–734, 1998.

142. Hudson N, Taha AS, Russell RI, et al: Famotidine for healing and maintenance in non-steroidal anti-inflammatory drug–associated gastroduodenal ulceration. Gastroenterology 112:1817–1822, 1997.

143. Taha AS, Hudson N, Hawkey CJ, et al: Famotidine for the prevention of gastric and duodenal ulcers caused by non-steroidal anti-inflammatory drugs. N Engl J Med 334:1435–1439, 1998.

144. Narayanana M, Sclueter M, Clyman RI: Incidence and outcome of a 10-fold indomethacin overdose in premature infants. J Pediatr 135:105–107, 1999.

145. Schuster V, von Stockhausen HB, Seyberth HW: Effects of highly overdosed indomethacin in a preterm infant with symptomatic patent ductus arteriosus. Eur J Pediatr 149:651–653, 1990.

146. Zukerman GB, Uy CC: Shock, metabolic acidosis, and coma following ibuprofen overdose in a child. Ann Pharmacother 29:869–871, 1995.

147. Alun-Jones E, Williams J: Hyponatremia and fluid retention in a neonate associated with maternal naproxen overdose. J Toxicol Clin Toxicol 24:257–260, 1986.

148. Peruzzi L, Gianoglio B, Porcellini MG, Coppo R: Neonatal end-stage renal failure associated with maternal ingestion of cyclo-oxygenase-type-1 selective inhibitor nimesulide as tocolytic. Lancet 354:1615, 1999.

CHAPTER 59

Gold Compounds

Jeffrey Brent ■ Michael Parra

Exposure to gold may occur by way of occupational exposure; contact with dental materials or gold-containing jewelry; or ingestion of gold-containing schnapps, liqueurs, or traditional remedies that may contain gold.[1-4] Gold reactions of medical significance are almost entirely due to the use of gold compounds in the treatment of autoimmune conditions, particularly rheumatoid arthritis (RA). A potential emerging context for possible gold toxicity is its use as a carrier for native DNA. Because the elemental form of gold is so nonreactive, it is well suited in microparticle form to be a carrier for DNA injected for gene therapy.[5]

The Chinese used elemental gold as a medicinal agent in 2500 B.C.[6] Since that time, gold in various forms has been advocated for the treatment of many different conditions. This enthusiasm for gold as a medicinal agent fueled the practice of alchemy. Even Paracelsus, often called the father of modern toxicology, an attribution deriving from his articulation of the cardinal dose-response principle ("the dose makes the poison"), advocated the use of gold as a universal remedy. More recently, gold was promoted as a treatment for tuberculosis.[7] Although used for this purpose even in Paracelsus' time, gold first was systematically studied for its tuberculostatic properties by Koch in the 19th century. Ultimately, gold turned out not to be an effective agent for treating tuberculosis. Its presumed antitubercular properties led to the early use of gold in the treatment of RA in the 1920s, however, because the latter condition was thought to be causally related to tuberculosis at that time.

Organic gold compounds initially were described as being therapeutic in the treatment of RA in 1927.[8] The term *chrysotherapy* (derived from the Greek *Chrysops*, meaning gold) has been generally adopted to describe therapy with gold compounds. In 1937, a series of 900 patients treated with chrysotherapy was reported, with the authors concluding that "gold is the best single form of treatment of RA."[9] In 1961, a controlled prospective trial of gold therapy in RA conclusively showed the efficacy of these compounds in the treatment of RA.[10] From nearly the beginning of the medicinal use of gold compounds, however, reports of significant adverse reactions to these compounds began to surface. A meta-analysis of the utility of gold compounds and other pharmaceuticals as second-line therapy for RA systematically reviewed 66 studies and found that auranofin, a commonly used oral gold compound, is the least effective and that injectable gold is the most toxic of the agents evaluated.[11] Since that time, there has been some tempering of enthusiasm for gold therapy of RA. Presently available gold compounds used therapeutically are summarized in Table 59-1.

Gold in its various forms has been associated with several different types of organ system toxicity. These are primarily mucocutaneous reactions, nephropathy, and blood dyscrasias—most commonly thrombocytopenia.

BIOCHEMISTRY AND PHARMACOLOGY

Gold has an atomic weight of 197 and is a member of the group IB elements on the periodic table. It exists in three forms: elemental, Au (I), and Au (III). Most of the gold compounds that have been used therapeutically are organic gold salts containing Au (I). The properties of the various medicinal organic gold compounds are presented in Table 59-1.

Gold, similar to platinum, rhodium, and palladium, is one of a group of elements that are referred to as *precious metals*. This designation describes metals that tend to be chemically stable in elemental form and are safe when in direct contact with skin. These metals are used for making jewelry. The more precious a metal is, the more resistant it is to ionization and subsequent release and reaction.

Gold compounds can be divided into those consisting of crystalline or colloidal gold. The latter are absorbed slowly after intramuscular administration. The crystalline gold compounds are divided into soluble forms, which are absorbed rapidly, and insoluble forms, which are absorbed at a rate intermediate between the soluble crystalline and the colloidal preparations (see Table 59-1).

During oral gold therapy, approximately 25% of an administered dose is absorbed.[12] After absorption and distribution, gold is found primarily in the reticuloendothelial system and the kidney.[7] The high renal gold concentration seems to be due to the excretion of gold in the kidney, rather than any selective concentration in that organ.[7]

During oral chrysotherapy, approximately two thirds of the total gold clearance is renal, and one third is fecal.[7,12,13] Colloidal gold (e.g., gold thioglucose in oil suspension) is cleared slowly and is excreted almost exclusively in feces.[7]

Normal whole-blood gold concentrations are usually less than or equal to 0.1 μg/mL, and serum concentrations are generally less than 0.5 ng/mL. Normal urine gold concentrations are less than 0.1 μg/24 hr. Although these values are markedly increased during chrysotherapy, there are no defined *therapeutic* or *toxic* gold concentrations. At concentrations greater than 3 μg/mL, albumin's gold-binding capacity may be exceeded. In a group of patients treated orally with aurothiomalate (gold sodium thiomalate [GSTM]), gold was found in the urine 10 months after therapy was

TABLE 59-1 Gold Compounds Used in Chrysotherapy

COMPOUND	GENERIC OR BRAND NAMES	ROUTE OF ADMINISTRATION	% GOLD	PROTEIN BINDING (%)	HALF-LIFE (DAYS)	AQUEOUS (A) OR OIL SUSPENSION (O)
Aurothioglucose or gold thioglucose	Solganal	IM	50	79	3–168	O
Gold sodium thiomalate, or aurothiomalate	Myocrisin	IM	50	79	1–5.5	A
SKF-D-3962	Auranofin	Oral	29	60–82	15–31	A
Gold sodium thiosulfate	Sanocrysin, Sanochrysine	IM or IV	37	79	Unknown	A

IM, intramuscular; IV, intravenous.

stopped.[14] The serum half-life of gold during oral auranofin therapy is 17 to 26 days.[12] The total body half-life has been estimated to be approximately 67 days.[15]

Peak serum gold levels range from 20 μg/dL during oral therapy to 1000 μg/mL when parenterally administered. Circulating gold is found primarily in the plasma, where it is bound to α-globulin.[16]

PATHOPHYSIOLOGY

Therapeutic Effects

The exact mechanism by which gold compounds exert their therapeutic effects is unknown. Gold therapy is known, however, to affect multiple aspects of humoral and cellular immunity and enzyme function. When inside phagocytes, the acidic pH, metallothionein, and oxygen radicals of the phagolysome cause gold to be oxidized from the Au (I) to the Au (III) form.[17] This oxidation may be important in some of the therapeutic and toxic effects of gold compounds. Au (III) is highly reactive and, similar to most reactive metals, binds to sulfhydryl groups on proteins, causing an oxidative cross-linking reaction.[18] Gold therapy also seems to decrease the gene transcription and production of proinflammatory cytokines.[19] There seems to be little correlation between serum gold concentration and therapeutic response.[19]

Toxic Reactions

The data are conflicting concerning whether the adverse affects of gold are dose dependent. Several studies have shown that there is no relationship between serum gold concentrations and the development of toxic reactions.[20,21] Other studies have yielded evidence, however, that such a relationship does exist.[22]

The immune system seems to be involved in some, and possibly all, of the adverse reactions related to gold therapy. In one study of 47 patients with RA treated with GSTM, it was found that serum IgE concentrations, which all were normal at baseline, increased in 22 patients. Patients with elevated IgE concentrations had a greater likelihood of an adverse affect.[23] It seems that serious adverse reactions occur in only a proportion of patients who are treated with gold salts and that if there is a dose dependency to these reactions, it is not easily demonstrable. The question of

dose dependency is best considered in light of the particular effect being considered. Non–dose-dependent reactions may characterize pathogenic mechanisms that are immunologic in nature.

Considerable support to the immunologic concept of gold toxicity derives from a 1978 report on 95 patients with rheumatoid disease treated with GSTM, showing that patients who were positive for HLA-DRw3 or HLA-DRw2 have an increased risk of certain adverse reactions.[24] Being positive for these HLA antigens also conferred an increased risk of adverse reaction to treatment with penicillamine. A striking component of this story followed the demonstration in 1994 by Bjorkner and colleagues[25] that 8.6% of patients skin tested with gold thiosulfate had positive tests. Several similar studies have reached similar conclusions.[5,26,27] There is considerable doubt, however, as to whether these positive skin tests in any way represent a phenomenon related to, or predictive of, adverse reactions to therapeutic gold salts. Patients who were positive to gold thiosulfate did not test positive to GSTM or metallic gold. It is not known whether patients who have an adverse reaction to gold salts are the same population who are skin test positive. As described subsequently, several of the gold-related adverse affects, particularly nephropathy, seem to be due to circulating immune complexes induced by gold treatment.[28] There also are data implicating non–HLA-linked slow sulfoxidation phenotype in an increased propensity to the adverse effects of gold therapy.[29]

The immunologic mechanisms associated with gold toxicity may be related to T-cell sensitization by gold salts. In animal models, Au (III), but not Au (I) is a T-cell sensitizer.[18,30] Au (III) is formed in vivo from the Au (I) in therapeutic agents. The use of Au (III) compounds (Krysolgan) for the treatment of tuberculosis in the early part of the 20th century was associated with a high incidence of adverse immunologic effects.

BLOOD DYSCRASIAS

Because thrombocytopenia has been the most commonly encountered hematologic complication, most of the data regarding gold-induced blood dyscrasias relates to this effect. Several studies have shown that patients with chrysotherapy-induced thrombocytopenia have normal-appearing bone marrow[31,32] and a decreased platelet life span.[31] It generally is assumed that the decreased platelet life span is immune mediated, although this has not been shown conclusively. In one of the early reports investigating this phenomenon, anti-platelet antibodies could not be shown in a patient with thrombocytopenia after GSTM therapy. Another study evaluated 23 patients with chrysotherapy-induced thrombocytopenia, of whom 6 were tested for antiplatelet antibodies. These antibodies were demonstrable in three of the six cases.[31,32]

Wooley and colleagues[33] reported the relationship between HLA type and adverse reactions in 91 RA patients treated with GSTM and reported that there was no demonstrable relationship between HLA subtype and incidence of hematologic complication. Coblyn and associates,[32] however, reported in a series of 23 patients with chrysotherapy-induced thrombocytopenia that possessing the HLA-DR3 phenotype conferred an 8.9-fold increased risk of thrombocytopenia. Contrary to the above-described immunologic data, Howell and coworkers[34] showed that colony formation in bone marrow is inhibited by GSTM in a dose-dependent fashion. Such in vitro studies are of questionable clinical relevance, however, because it is unknown whether bone marrow cells in vivo are exposed to GSTM in concentrations and under conditions comparable to those imposed experimentally in vitro.

It is presently unknown if there is a dose-dependent basis for chrysotherapy-induced blood dyscrasias. Lorber and colleagues[35] adjusted gold compound doses based on serum gold concentrations in 44 RA patients and reported no hematologic abnormalities despite 2500 cumulative weeks of observation. It is possible that if high peak gold concentrations are avoided, hematologic effects would be reduced.

Eosinophilia occurs in about 5% of gold salt–treated patients. Frequently, eosinophilia is of no significance and resolves despite continued chrysotherapy. It is unknown whether eosinophilia predicts future toxicity. Gold-related blood dyscrasias do not seem to be mediated by an autoimmune mechanism.[29]

GOLD NEPHROPATHY

Gold nephropathy does not seem to be dose related.[36] There is no relationship between serum or urine gold levels and the development of nephropathy.[36] In addition, gold nephropathy seems to be unrelated to T-cell sensitization by gold salts.[29] Although it remains unproven, most authors believe that the pathogenesis of gold nephropathy is due to immune complex formation. One report described the presence of elemental gold granules in renal proximal tubule cells in patients with gold nephropathy.[38]

There is a strong association for certain HLA types and the development of proteinuria. Patients who are positive for HLA-DRw3 or HLA-B8 have a 32 times increased risk for development of proteinuria.[33]

MUCOCUTANEOUS REACTIONS

The mucocutaneous reactions related to chrysotherapy are the most common side effects encountered, constituting 65% to 75% of all adverse reactions to gold therapy. These reactions to gold salts seem to be dose related and rarely occur with less than 250 mg of cumulative dose. Early studies have suggested that there is no causal relationship between serum gold levels and rashes[39,40]; however, in a series of 33 patients treated with GSTM, of whom 11 patients developed skin manifestations, the 5 patients who had the most severe skin reactions had serum gold levels that were significantly higher

than those of the patients without such reactions.[19] This study also found that the 5 patients with the most severe skin reactions all had eosinophilia, a relationship that was confirmed in another study of 43 patients in whom there was an increased likelihood of rash if the patients developed eosinophilia.[23] The latter study also found that there was an increased likelihood of rash if patients developed increased serum IgG levels during chrysotherapy.

In contrast to patients with blood dyscrasias or nephropathy, patients with gold dermatitis tend to exhibit T-cell sensitization to Au (III) salts.[29] Au (III) salts have been reported to be capable of inducing delayed hypersensitivity reactions.[39] Similar reactions have been reported in people chronically ingesting gold-containing schnapps. Lichen planus is generally thought to be a cellular immune reaction directed against epithelial cell antigens.[3] The mucocutaneous reactions associated with gold therapy are paradoxical in that they have features of classic dose-dependent toxicity and features of an immunologic reaction. The latter tend to be idiosyncratic and non–dose dependent. The mucocutaneous complications of gold therapy do not exhibit specific associations with HLA phenotypes, and they are not associated with bone marrow or nephrotoxicity.

CLINICAL PRESENTATION

The incidence of toxic reactions in patients treated with gold salts varies considerably from trial to trial. In the aggregate, they seem to occur in approximately one third of all treated patients. The most concerning reactions are the exfoliative dermatitides, blood dyscrasias, and nephropathy. Several cases of "pulmonary fibrosis" in patients receiving gold therapy have been described.[41] It is questionable, however, to what extent, if any, gold therapy can be implicated in causing this condition. Pulmonary fibrosis may occur secondary to the underlying RA. In several of the reported cases, the "pulmonary fibrosis" appeared to be reversible infiltrates.[40,41]

Mucocutaneous Reactions

The types of mucocutaneous reactions are prodigious and involve pruritus, stomatitis, lichenoid reactions, and rashes of all varieties. *Chrysiasis* denotes the gray-blue discoloration of the skin that has been described in patients receiving gold therapy for tuberculosis.[42] Skin discoloration is generally not seen in gold therapy of RA,[43] however, probably because of the lower doses used. Pathologically, in patients with gold-associated rashes there is an accumulation of CD4+ T cells.[44] Gold has been reported to be fixed in the dermis more than 20 years after the cessation of chrysotherapy.[45] These reactions are of concern to critical care providers only when they progress to exfoliative dermatitis, which is rare.

Blood Dyscrasias

Although a diverse variety of hematologic abnormalities has been associated with chrysotherapy, the most commonly encountered abnormality other than eosinophilia is thrombocytopenia, which occurs in 1% to 3% of gold salt–treated patients.[17] Other potential hematologic complications are neutropenia, anemia, pancytopenia, aplastic anemia, and agranulocytosis. Severe pancytopenia may be preceded by progressive thrombocytopenia as an early warning sign and may be prolonged for weeks or months. Severe pancytopenia or aplastic anemia may be seen with therapeutic doses of medicinal gold during and after therapy.

Nephropathy

Renal manifestations of gold therapy are frequent and consist primarily of proteinuria, hematuria, and nephrotic syndrome. The most common of these complications is proteinuria, which occurs in 2.6% to 17% of patients.[36] The most concerning is the nephrotic syndrome, which occurs in 0.1% to 2.6% of patients. Renal tubular lesions have been rarely described.[37,38,45,47] Gold-induced renal failure is uncommon. It is important that the proteinuria be distinguished from the increased urinary protein excretion that is seen occasionally as one component of RA. The latter is rare, however, occurring in approximately 3% of patients. Histologically, patients with gold nephropathy seem to have a membranous glomerulonephritis.[17] A similar lesion is seen in gold-treated animals.[17,48]

TREATMENT

The treatment of severe manifestations of gold toxicity should begin with the usual emergent stabilization that is done on any critically ill patient; this includes ensurance of the adequacy of an airway, appropriate intervenous access, and maintenance of ventilation and circulation. Most gold poisoning is oral, and the possibility of gastrointestinal decontamination therapy should be entertained. Because most gold therapy is associated with chronic oral use, however, as opposed to a single overdose, the likelihood of any beneficial effect from gastrointestinal decontamination is minimal. If a patient presents after an acute overdose, particularly within the first several hours of ingestion, it may be beneficial to administer a dose of activated charcoal. Gastrointestinal decontamination in a poisoned patient is described in detail in Chapter 5. As with most poisonings, usual supportive intensive care measures are crucial.

Chelation

DIMERCAPROL (BRITISH ANTILEWISITE)

Because gold is a heavy metal, it is natural to consider the possibility that chelating agents may provide a potential therapy for adverse reactions to chrysotherapy. Early and intense interest focused on the chelating agent British antilewisite, or dimercaprol, which had been developed during World War II by research groups in the United States

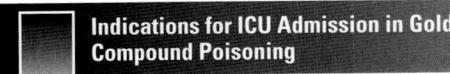

Indications for ICU Admission in Gold Compound Poisoning

Severe mucocutaneous reaction
Significant hemorrhage from thrombocytopenia

and the United Kingdom as a potential therapy for exposure to the arsenical chemical warfare agent lewisite. Although lewisite was not used in World War II, the anticipation of chemical warfare led to the development of this important antidote. Reports of its use in the treatment of adverse reactions to gold compounds were first published shortly after dimercaprol was made available for medicinal use.[49,50] The use of dimercaprol for poisoning by gold compounds also was supported by several animal studies showing that it protected against lethal doses of gold thiosulfate in mice and rats.[51,52] Dimercaprol given to gold thiosulfate–treated rabbits results in an approximately 10-fold increase in urinary gold excretion.[52] The administration of dimercaprol to patients receiving chrysotherapy also has been shown to increase urinary gold excretion.[53] Within 5 years of the introduction of dimercaprol, a report reviewed 50 cases of toxic reactions to chrysotherapy and concluded that dimercaprol is effective in greater than 90% of cases.[54] There are no data addressing the use of dimercaprol, or any other chelators, in acute gold overdoses. One case report described an individual who was given a chronic 10-fold dosing excess of Solganal who was treated with dimercaprol. The patient did well, and serial plasma and urine gold levels indicated a progressively decreasing gold concentration in both. No values before dimercaprol were reported, however.[55] The clinical pharmacology of dimercaprol is discussed in detail in Chapter 139.

PENICILLAMINE AND N-ACETYLCYSTEINE

Another potential chelating agent that may be of at least theoretical benefit in gold toxicity is penicillamine, an agent that also has therapeutic benefit in the treatment of RA. Penicillamine forms a strong complex with gold in vitro,[89] forming a more stable compound with the metal than is found by any other chelators.[57] In a series of nine patients being treated with GSTM, the amount of gold excreted after the administration of 1 g of penicillamine (500 mg administered intramuscularly in two doses separated by 12 hours) increased 12-fold. The significance of this result is questionable, however, because even then the patients' urinary gold excretion amounted to approximately 0.17% of their total dose. There was no adverse effect of the penicillamine treatment.[56] Use of penicillamine in the treatment of adverse effects of chrysotherapy has not been reported as extensively as has use of dimercaprol.

The sulfhydryl agent N-acetylcysteine complexes with several heavy metals to make a water-soluble complex that is excreted renally. In a series of 12 patients receiving intravenous chrysotherapy, N-acetylcysteine approximately doubled urine gold excretion.[58] There is little additional experience with the use of this agent in the treatment of gold compound toxicity.

CHELATION CONCLUSIONS

Although there are some theoretical data and early empirical observations that suggest that chelation therapy, particularly with dimercaprol, may benefit patients who are having adverse reactions to chrysotherapy, a diverse group of reactions may occur, and these have apparently distinct, although not always fully understood, pathogenic mechanisms. It is important to consider the potential beneficial effects, if any, of chelation therapy in the context of the specific adverse effect being treated.

Severe Skin Reactions

Although skin reactions are the most common adverse effects associated with chrysotherapy, rarely do they merit intensive care unit management. Severe exfoliative dermatitides may occur, however. By analogy to burn cases, if these affect more than 15% to 30% of total body surface area, management should be undertaken in an intensive care setting because of issues regarding fluid volume management, skin care, and the prevention and treatment of sepsis. Therapy for exfoliative dermatitides should be aimed at fluid management in a fashion similar to that used for burns; treatment of exfoliated areas, as for burns; and symptomatic treatment for pain and pruritus. Gold therapy should be halted. Patients who have mucocutaneous manifestations of chrysotherapy may frequently be restarted on gold compounds, however, usually at a lower dose, without recurrence of symptoms. There is no role for attempted extracorporeal drug removal for gold-induced dermatitis.

Shortly after the introduction of dimercaprol, several case series that suggested significant improvement in gold-induced dermatitides when dimercaprol was administered were published.[49,58] In one series of five patients, urinary gold excretion was found to increase markedly, reaching a maximum of approximately 1000 μg/day after initiation of dimercaprol.[58] Davis and Hughes[23] published a case report of a patient with apparent penicillamine-responsive, severe gold dermatitides that persisted for months after therapy was stopped. Urinary levels of gold increased from 158 μg to a peak of 618 μg during treatment with penicillamine. Fecal gold levels also increased approximately 2.5-fold. These were less than one tenth, however, of the urinary excretion levels. Plasma gold levels increased from approximately 45 μg/mL to approximately 90 μg/mL during penicillamine treatment.[23,40] This increase suggests that penicillamine was chelating free or bioavailable gold in the circulatory compartment and causing (a flux) redistribution of tissue gold into the plasma.

Although the anecdotal case reports on chelation therapy suggest that it has been useful for the treatment of gold dermatitides, the total number of cases reported is few, and these data may be subject to reporting bias or publication bias or both. Cases in which the patients apparently responded are more likely to have been reported or published than cases in which the patients did not respond. No patient-controlled study has been published to date. It can be concluded that the existing data, although of limited quantity and quality, suggest the possibility that chelation therapy with either dimercaprol or penicillamine may be useful in the treatment of gold-induced dermatitides. We suggest that it is reasonable, in a severe case, to employ an empirical trial of dimercaprol or penicillamine. In the absence of a clear-cut response, however, it does not seem that there would be any utility in continuing this treatment.

Blood Dyscrasias

Although multiple blood dyscrasias have been described in association with chrysotherapy, the hematopoietic disorders of greatest concern are aplastic anemia, pancytopenia, granulocytopenia, and thrombocytopenia. As with most poisonings, it is crucial to discontinue exposure by stopping chrysotherapy as soon as possible and to treat medical complications (e.g., septicemia) aggressively. For patients who have significant anemia or thrombocytopenia, blood component replacement may be necessary. In patients with significant granulocytopenia, the evaluation and treatment of infections and isolation may be warranted. For patients with severe pancytopenia or aplastic anemia, bone marrow transplantation may be necessary. There has been little published experience with this as a treatment for complications of chrysotherapy, however. Similarly, bone marrow–stimulating factors, such as granulocyte colony-stimulating factor, are of theoretical utility; however, there is little published experience with this approach. In our opinion, it would be reasonable or prudent to use colony-stimulating factors because they may promote hematopoietic recovery with little toxicity. For thrombocytopenia associated with gold therapy, megakaryocyte-stimulating factor also would be a reasonable treatment option.

CHELATION

Several case reports and case series have evaluated the potential role of chelation therapy for gold-induced blood dyscrasias. Most of these cases have focused on thrombocytopenia, largely because this is the most common of the hematologic abnormalities. These cases have been quite variable, with some reports describing a response to chelation[31,50,59,60] and others reporting no beneficial effect.[50,60–62] One report described a patient who had a dramatic increase in urinary gold excretion in response to dimercaprol; however, there was no effect on platelet count.[60]

One of the largest series retrospectively reviewed 55 patients who developed blood dyscrasias during the course of chrysotherapy with Myochrysine. Of the nine patients who received less than 200 mg, six had thrombocytopenia, which resolved spontaneously after withdrawal of the drug. The other three patients had neutropenia, which after cessation of chrysotherapy also resolved, although all the patients were additionally treated with dimercaprol. Of the patients who received greater than 400 mg, the 26 patients with thrombocytopenia alone recovered without specific treatment. Of the 20 patients with pancytopenia, however, 15 died despite therapy with corticosteroids and chelating agents. The investigators concluded that there is little apparent benefit to treatment with gold chelators.[63] No controlled studies have evaluated the efficacy of chelation therapy in the treatment of gold-related blood dyscrasias. The largest retrospective case series[63] suggested that patients with thrombocytopenia recover without the use of chelators. This series also suggested that pancytopenia does not tend to respond to chelators. It seems that there has been no demonstrable benefit to the use of chelation therapy for the treatment of gold-induced thrombocytopenia or pancytopenia. Because the data to support it are limited, it seems reasonable, however, to embark on an empirical course of treatment with one of these agents in treating blood dyscrasias.

CORTICOSTEROIDS

Several studies have reported a beneficial effect of corticosteroid treatment in the treatment of gold-induced thrombocytopenia.[31,61,64] Some of the outcomes were confounded, however, by simultaneous chelation therapy.[7,31,61]

Gold Nephropathy

Gold nephropathy, usually manifested by proteinuria, may produce a full-blown nephrotic syndrome. The most important single specific treatment for this condition is stopping chrysotherapy.[17,65,70] Although dimercaprol protects rats from gold-induced nephropathy,[71] there are few data on the utility of chelating agents in humans. Because gold nephropathy tends to resolve without specific treatment, there seems to be little reason to resort to chelation therapy. Corticosteroids for this indication do not seem to be beneficial.[65]

Criteria for ICU Discharge in Gold Compound Poisoning

Mucocutaneous Reaction

Nonseptic
Adequate post–intensive care unit nursing capabilities

Hemorrhage

No active hemodynamically significant bleeding
Stable hematocrit

Key Points in Gold Compound Poisoning

1. Gold therapy is associated with blood dyscrasias, nephropathy, and potentially serious dermatitides.
2. Adverse reactions may not be dose-dependent.
3. Stopping gold therapy and providing supportive care are the mainstays of treatment of adverse reactions.
4. The role of chelation therapy has not been established.

REFERENCES

1. Guenthner T, Stork CM, Cantor RM: Goldschlager allergy in a gold allergic patient. Vet Hum Toxicol 41:246, 1999.
2. Bajaj S, Vohora SB: Analgesic activity of gold preparations used in Ayurveda and Unani-tibb. Indian J Med Res 108:104–111, 1998.
3. Russell MA, Langley M, Truett AP III, et al: Lichenoid dermatitis after consumption of gold-containing liquor. J Am Acad Dermatol 36:841–844, 1997.
4. Burrows DD: Metals. Clin Dermatol 15:505–509, 1997.
5. Merchant B: Gold, the noble metal and the paradoxes of its toxicology. Biologicals 26:49–59, 1998.
6. Lewis AJ, Walz DT: Immunopharmacology of gold. Prog Med Chem 19:1–58, 1982.
7. Block WD, VanGoor K: Metabolism, Pharmacology and Therapeutic Uses of Gold Compounds. Publication 282, American Lecture Series, monograph in American Lectures in Dermatology. Springfield, IL, Charles C Thomas, 1956.
8. Lande K: Die gunstige beunflussung schleichender dauerinfehte durch Solganal. Munch Med Wochenschr 74:1132–1134, 1927.
9. Bluhm GB, Sigler JW, Ensign DC: D-penicillamine therapy of thrombocytopenia secondary to chrysotherapy: A case report. Arthritis Rheum 5:638, 1968.
10. Research Subcommittee of the Emire Rheumatism Council: Gold therapy in rheumatoid arthritis: Final report of a multicentered controlled trial. Ann Rheum Dis 20:315–333, 1961.
11. Felson DT, Anderson JJ, Meenan RF: The comparative efficacy and toxicity of second-line drugs in rheumatoid arthritis. Arthritis Rheum 33:1449–1461, 1990.
12. Bernhard GC: Auranofin therapy in rheumatoid arthritis. J Lab Clin Med 100:167–177, 1982.
13. Gottlieb NL, Smith PM, Smith EM: Gold excretion correlated with clinical course during chrysotherapy in rheumatoid arthritis. Arthritis Rheum 15:582–592, 1972.
14. Hartnung EF, Cotter J, Gannon C: The excretion of gold following the administration of gold sodium thiomalate in rheumatoid arthritis. J Lab Clin Med 26:1750–1755, 1941.
15. Blocka K, Furst DE, Landow E, et al: Single dose kinetics of auranofin in rheumatoid arthritis. Presented at Worldwide Auranofin Symposium, October 1981.
16. Freyberg RH: Gold therapy for rheumatoid arthritis. In Hollander JL (ed): Arthritis and Allied Conditions. Philadelphia, Lea & Febiger, 1972, pp 455–482.
17. Bigazzi PE: Metals and kidney autoimmunity. Environ Health Persp 107:753–765, 1999.
18. Shaw CF III: The mammalian biochemistry of gold: An inorganic perspective of chrysotherapy. Inorg Perspect Biol Med 2:287–355, 1979.
19. Jessop JD, Johns RGS: Serum gold determinations in patients with rheumatoid arthritis receiving sodium aurothiomalate. Ann Rheum Dis 32:228–232, 1973.
20. Freyberg RH: Gold therapy for rheumatoid arthritis. In Hollander JL (ed): Arthritis and Allied Conditions. Philadelphia, Lea & Febiger, 1966, pp 322–347.
21. Rothermich NO, Bergen W, Philips VK: The use of plasma gold levels in determining dose, frequency, type of gold salt, and impending toxicity in chrysotherapy for rheumatoid arthritis. Arthritis Rheum 19:308, 1967.
22. Krusius FE, Markkanen A, Peltola P: Plasma levels and urinary excretion of gold during routine treatment of rheumatoid arthritis. Ann Rheum Dis 29:232–235, 1970.
23. Davis P, Hughes GRV: Significance of eosinophilia during gold therapy. Arthritis Rheum 17:964–968, 1974.
24. Panayi GS, Wooley P, Batchelor JR: Genetic basis of rheumatoid disease: HLA antigens, disease manifestations, and toxic reactions to drugs. BMJ 2:1326–1328, 1978.
25. Bjorkner B, Bruze M, Moller H: High frequency of contact allergy to gold sodium thiosulfate: An indication of gold allergy? Contact Derm 30:144–151, 1994.
26. Ehrlich A, Belsito DV: Allergic contact dermatitis to gold. University of Kansas Medical Center 65:323–326, 2000.
27. Trattner A, David M: Gold sensitivity in Israel—consecutive patch test. Contact Derm 42:301–302, 2000.
28. Hostynek JJ: Gold: An allergen of growing significance. Food Chem Toxicol 35:839–844, 1997.
29. Verwilghen J, Kingsley GH, Gambling L, et al: Activation of gold-reactive T lymphocytes in rheumatoid arthritis patients treated with gold. Arthritis Rheum 35:1413–1418, 1992.
30. Bruze M, Andersen KE: Gold—a controversial sensitizer. Contact Derm 40:295–299, 1999.
31. Stavem P, Stromme J, Bull O: Immunological studies in a case of gold salt induced thrombocytopenia. Scand J Haematol 5:271–277, 1968.
32. Coblyn JS, Weinblatt M, Holdsworth D, et al: Gold-induced thrombocytopenia. Ann Intern Med 95:178–181, 1981.
33. Wooley PH, Griffin J, Panayi GS, et al: HLA-DR antigens and toxic reactions to sodium aurothiomalate and d-penicillamine in patients with rheumatoid arthritis. N Engl J Med 303:300–302, 1980.
34. Howell A, Gumpel JM, Watts RWE: Depression of bone marrow colony formation in gold-induced neutropenia. BMJ 1:432–434, 1975.
35. Lorber A, Simon TM, Leeb J, et al: Chrysotherapy: Pharmacological and clinical correlates. J Rheumatol 2:401–410, 1975.
36. Fillastre J-P, Godin M: Drug-induced neuropathies. In Davison AM, Cameron JW, Grunfeld J-P, et al (eds): Oxford Textbook of Clinical Nephrology, Vol III, 2nd ed. Oxford, Oxford University Press, 1998, pp 2645–2657.
37. Silverberg DS, Kidd EG, Shnitka TK, et al: Gold nephropathy: A clinical and pathologic study. Arthritis Rheum 13:812–825, 1970.
38. Watanabe I, Whittier FC, Moore J, et al: Gold nephropathy. Arch Pathol Lab Med 100:632–635, 1976.
39. Kligman AM: The identification of contact allergens by human assay: III. The maximization test: A procedure for screening and rating contact sensitizers. J Invest Dermatol 47:393–409, 1966.
40. Smith W, Ball GV: Lung injury due to gold treatment. Arthritis Rheum 23:351–354, 1980.
41. Davis P, Ezeoke A, Munro J, et al: Immunological studies on the mechanism of gold hypersensitivity reactions. BMJ 3:676–678, 1973.
42. Hansborg H: Chrysiasis: Ablagerung von gold in vivo. Acta Tuberc Scand 4:124–132, 1928.

43. Sundalin F: Die goldbehandlung der chronischen arthritis unter besondered berucksichtingung der komplikationen. Acta Med Scand 107:1–291, 1941.

44. Pennys NS, Ackerman AB, Gottlieb NL: Gold dermatitis: A clinical and histopathological study. Arch Dermatol 109:372–376, 1974.

45. Cox AJ, Marich KW: Gold in the dermis following gold therapy for rheumatoid arthritis. Arch Dermatol 108:655–657, 1973.

46. Strunk SW, Ziff M: Ultrastructural studies of the passage of gold thiomalate across the renal glomerular capillary wall. Arthritis Rheum 13:39–52, 1970.

47. Katz A, Little AH: Gold nephropathy: An immunopathologic study. Arch Pathol 96:133–136, 1973.

48. Nagi AH, Alexander F, Barabas AZ: Gold nephropathy in rats—light and electron microscopic studies. Exp Mol Pathol 15:354–362, 1971.

49. Cohen A, Goldman J, Dubbs AW: The treatment of acute gold and arsenic poisoning. JAMA 133:749–752, 1947.

50. Thompson M, Sinclair RJ, Duthie JJ: Thrombocytopenic purpura after administration of gold—comparison of treatment with dimercaprol, ACTH and cortisone. BMJ 4867:899–902, 1954.

51. Swanson R, Ney J, Smith PK: Influence of BAL on the acute toxicity of gold salts in mice. Fed Proc 6:375, 1947.

52. Kuzell WC, Pillsbury PL, Gellert SA: The effects of 2,3-dimercaptopropanol (BAL) on toxicity and excretion of gold. Stanford Medical Bulletin 5:197–202, 1947.

53. Honkapohja H: Treatment with BAL of a case of thrombocytopenic purpura. Ann Med Int Fenniae 38:33–37, 1949.

54. Straiss KF, Barrett RM, Rosenberg EF: BAL treatment of toxic reactions to gold: A review of the literature and report of two cases. Ann Intern Med 37:323–331, 1952.

55. Bunch TW: Gold overdose treated with BAL. Arthritis Rheum 19:123–125, 1976.

56. Eyring EJ, Engleman EP: Interaction of gold and penicillamine. Arthritis Rheum 6:216–223, 1963.

57. Rubin M, Sliwinski A, Photias M, et al: Influence of chelation on gold metabolism in rats. Proc Soc Exp Biol Med 124:290–296, 1967.

58. Godfrey NF, Peter A, Simon TM, et al: IV N-acetylcysteine treatment of hematologic reactions to chrysotherapy. J Rheumatol 9:519–526, 1982.

59. Lockie ML, Norcross BM, George CW: Treatment of two reactions due to gold: Response of thrombopenic purpura and granulocytopenia. JAMA 133:754–755, 1947.

60. Herbst KD, Stone WH, Flannery EP: Chronic thrombocytopenia following gold therapy. Arch Intern Med 135:1622, 1975.

61. Deren B, Masi R, Weksler M, et al: Gold-associated thrombocytopenia. Arch Intern Med 134:1012–1015, 1974.

62. Canada AT: Gold-induced thrombocytopenia. Am J Hosp Pharm 30:340–342, 1973.

63. Kay AG: Myelotoxicity of gold. BMJ 22:1266–1268, 1976.

64. Harth M, Hickey JP, Coulter WK, et al: Gold-induced thrombocytopenia. J Rheum 5:165–172, 1978.

65. Fillastre JP, Druet P, Mery JP: Proteinuric nephropathies associated with drugs and substances of abuse. In Cameron JS, Glassock RJ (eds): The Nephrotic Syndrome. New York, Marcel Dekker, 1988.

CHAPTER 60

Methotrexate

Mary Beth Hines

Previously reserved for the treatment of cancer, methotrexate (MTX) now is used for a variety of illnesses, ranging from immune disorders to asthma (Table 60-1). The dosage and route of administration vary and are based on the patient's diagnosis. Doses for the treatment of rheumatoid arthritis (RA) range from 7.5 to 20 mg weekly and may be given orally, intramuscularly, or intravenously. Dosing for the treatment of various cancers normally is expressed in terms of surface area rather than body weight and, depending on the diagnosis and specific treatment protocol, may be 15 g/m^2 (approximately 16.5 g for an average 70-kg human subject). Intrathecal administration of 15 mg may be given for the treatment of meningeal leukemia. The severity of symptoms associated with MTX toxicity makes it imperative to understand the potential for catastrophic outcomes after long-term therapeutic and short-term supratherapeutic exposure.

CLINICAL PHARMACOLOGY

Absorption of orally administered MTX is variable and saturable at doses greater than 80 mg/m^2. MTX is moderately (11% to 57%) protein bound; however, concerns about concomitant use of drugs that displace protein binding now are thought to have little clinical significance.[1] MTX is metabolized primarily via microsomal enzymes to 7-hydroxymethotrexate, which is 200-fold less active than its parent compound (Fig. 60-1). Greater than 80% is excreted renally unchanged within 48 hours; active tubular secretion and glomerular filtration occur. Elimination may be prolonged in the presence of ascites or pleural effusion because MTX may be "trapped" in third space fluids. Although elimination of the drug is primarily renal, enterohepatic circulation may occur.[1] The half-life of MTX is approximately 7 hours.[1] Toxicity is thought to

depend on the area under the concentration curve and not the specific dose.[1]

PATHOPHYSIOLOGY

An understanding of folate metabolism is crucial in explaining the pharmacology and toxicity of MTX (Fig. 60-2). Dietary folate must be reduced to N^5-methyl-tetrahydrofolate (N^5-methyl-FH$_4$) before it is transported actively into the cell; the enzyme required is dihydrofolate reductase (DHFR, no. 1 in Fig. 60-2). When inside the cell, N^5-methyl-FH$_4$ is converted to its polyglutamate form. When N^5-methyl-FH$_4$ is converted to tetrahydrofolate (FH$_4$), a single carbon moiety is transferred to homocysteine to form methionine. This reaction is reversible and requires vitamin B$_{12}$ as a cofactor. FH$_4$ may be converted to N^{5,10}-methylene-FH$_4$. This reaction, also reversible, involves the transfer of a single carbon group from serine to FH$_4$, resulting in the formation of glycine. N^{5,10}-methylene-FH$_4$ can be converted back to N^5-methyl-FH$_4$ or to dihydrofolate (FH$_2$), which is converted to FH$_4$ via DHFR. These reactions are essential to maintain normal protein synthesis.

N^{5,10}-methylene-FH$_4$ formation also is crucial in the process of nucleotide synthesis. During its conversion to FH$_2$, a single-carbon group is transferred to 2'-deoxyuridylate (dUMP) to form 2'-deoxythymidylate (dTMP), which is required for DNA synthesis. The enzyme responsible for this reaction is thymidylate synthase (TS, no. 2 in Fig. 60-2). N^{5,10}-methylene-FH$_4$ also can be converted to N^{5,10}-methenyl-FH$_4$ and then to N^{10}-formyl-FH$_4$. As N^{10}-formyl-FH$_4$ is converted back to FH$_4$, a carbon group is transferred in a series of reactions that create inosinate, which is used in DNA and RNA synthesis. One of the enzymes involved in this process is aminoimidazole carboxamide ribonucleotide transferase (AICRT, no. 3 in Fig. 60-2).

MTX gains entrance into the cell via the same active transport mechanism as dietary folate. It also may diffuse across the cell membrane when extracellular concentrations are greater than 20 μM. When inside the cell, it is converted to a polyglutamate form and has three important actions. First, it competitively inhibits DHFR. This leads to depletion of the intracellular FH$_4$ necessary for the one-carbon transfers required for protein synthesis and the reactions required in the synthesis of inosinic acid (purine precursor) and thymidylic acid (DNA-specific nucleotide). Second, it directly inhibits TS, further limiting nucleotide synthesis. Third, it inhibits AICRT, which affects DNA and

---

Pharmacokinetics of Methotrexate

Volume of distribution: 2.6 L/kg
Protein binding: 11–57%
Mechanism of clearance: >80% renal
Plasma half-life: 7 hr
pK$_a$: 4.3, 5.5
Active metabolites: 7-hydroxymethotrexate

TABLE 60-1   Clinical Uses of Methotrexate

Crohn's disease
Ectopic pregnancy
Graft-versus-host reactions
Lupus erythematosus
Neoplasm
    Breast carcinoma
    Choriocarcinoma
    Head and neck carcinomas
    Acute lymphocytic/nonlymphocytic leukemia
    Small cell lung carcinoma
    Diffuse histiocytic lymphoma
    Medulloblastoma
    Meningeal carcinomatosis
    Osteosarcoma
    Ovarian carcinoma
Psoriasis
Rheumatoid arthritis
Sarcoidosis
Systemic sclerosis
Wegener's granulomatosis

RNA synthesis. Evidence suggests that the inhibition of AICRT causes the release of adenosine, which may be responsible for the antiinflammatory effects of MTX.[2]

Folinic acid (leucovorin) is administered as rescue therapy during high-dose MTX treatment and as the antidote for toxicity caused by MTX overdose. It competes for entry into the cell at the same transport site as MTX, limiting cellular uptake. It also competes with MTX for the binding site on DHFR, limiting MTX's inhibitory effect on FH_4 synthesis. It can be converted directly to $N^{5,10}$-methenyl-FH_4 and in this manner bypasses the MTX-induced blockade of substrate formation needed for protein, RNA, and DNA synthesis.

Supplemental folate also is transported actively into the cell, but it does not share the same transport site as dietary folate. It is reduced in two steps to FH_4; the second step requires DHFR. It is converted to a polyglutamate form, then participates in the reactions described in Figure 60-2. Supplemental folate would not be expected to alleviate MTX toxicity because inhibition of DHFR would prevent its conversion to FH_4. As its entry site is not the same as MTX, supplemental folate does not provide competition for entry into the cell.

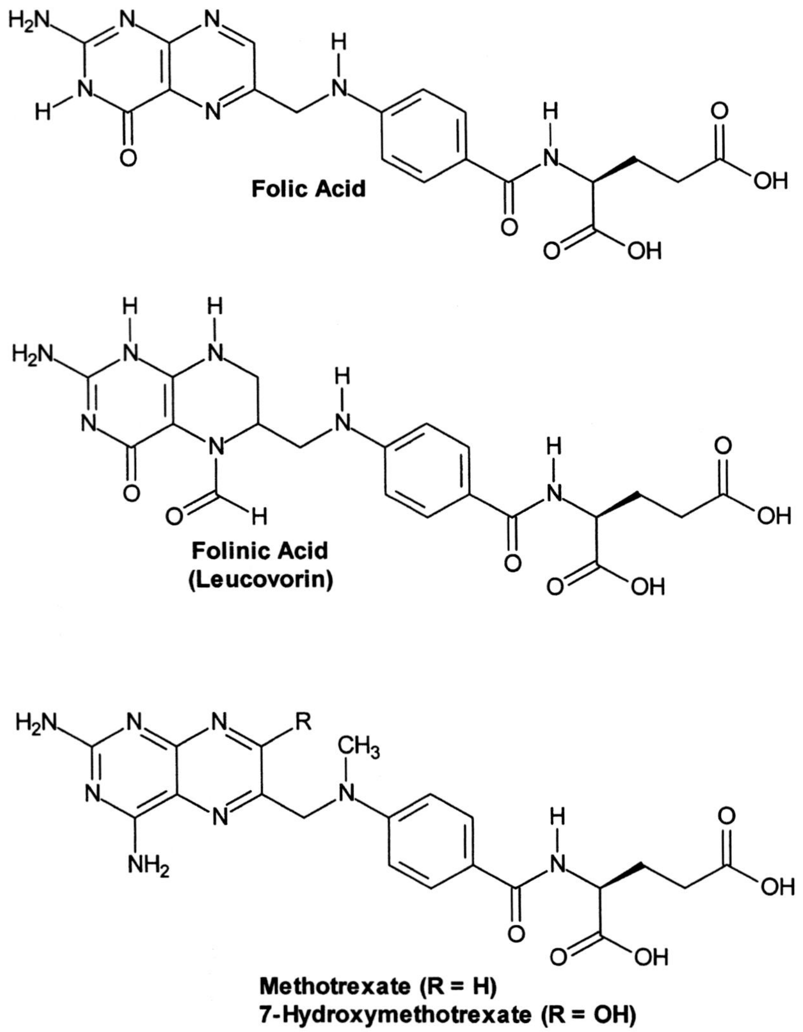

Folic Acid

**Folinic Acid
(Leucovorin)**

**Methotrexate (R = H)
7-Hydroxymethotrexate (R = OH)**

FIGURE 60-1

Chemical structures of folate-related and methotrexate-related compounds.

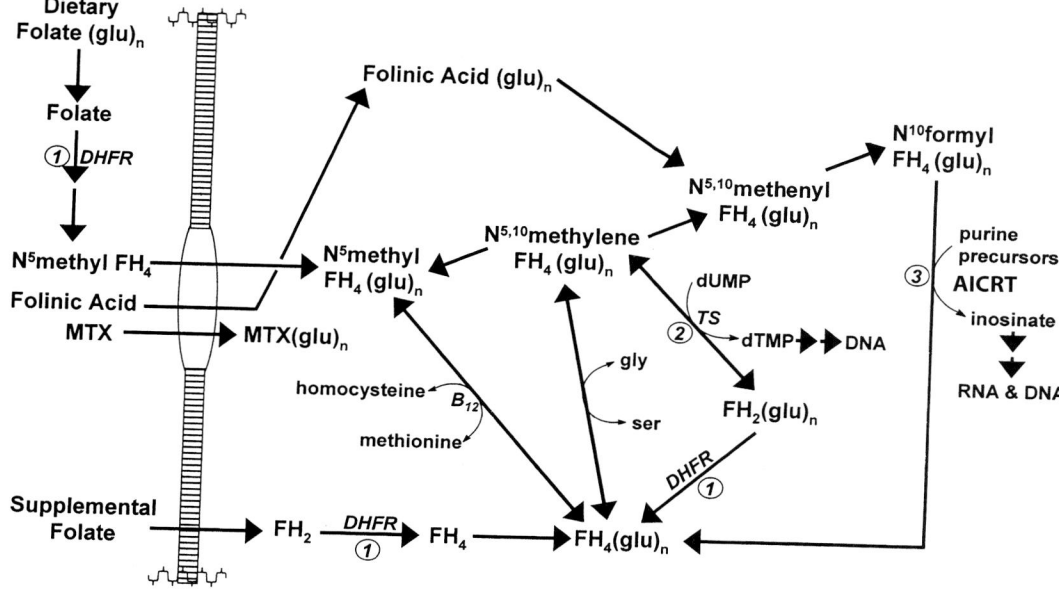

FIGURE 60-2

Folate metabolism. See text for explanation of abbreviations.

CLINICAL PRESENTATION

Much of the understanding regarding the toxic effects of MTX comes from the use of this drug in short-term, high-dose courses for cancer treatment and as long-term, low-dose maintenance therapy for dermatologic and rheumatic disorders. There are only five cases in the literature involving the acute ingestion of MTX by individuals not previously taking the drug. Three were children, and each was treated immediately with folinic acid. Two had mildly elevated liver function tests, and the third had an elevated lactate level. All three children were asymptomatic.[3,4] Two women ingested MTX in an attempt to induce an abortion. They presented with mucositis, pancytopenia, rash, and elevated hepatic enzymes. Both women were treated with leucovorin and survived.[5] Despite the paucity of published experience with acute intentional or unintentional overdose, it seems logical that the better-documented effects seen in long-term, low-dose treatment or high-dose MTX chemotherapy also might develop in the setting of an acute ingestion. The following sections describe some of these manifestations.

Gastrointestinal Effects

Anorexia, nausea, vomiting, diarrhea, weight loss, stomatitis, and abdominal pain are reported in 60% of patients treated with low-dose MTX.[6] Reports of gastrointestinal hemorrhage and toxic megacolon also exist.[7] These symptoms vary in severity and may respond to supplemental folate[8] but do not usually necessitate discontinuation of the drug.[9] Enteral products containing soy reduced weight loss and intestinal crypt necrosis compared with products containing other protein sources.[10] The use of intravenous glutamine has decreased enterocolitis in patients with breast cancer receiving high-dose MTX therapy.[11]

Hematopoietic Effects

Pancytopenia is a rare but potentially life-threatening complication. In one review, its incidence in RA patients receiving low-dose MTX was calculated at 1.4%, whereas the fatality rate was 12%. The most common risk factors in these cases were renal insufficiency and the use of nonsteroidal anti-inflammatory drugs.[12] Other potential predictors may be the presence of folate deficiency and an increase in mean corpuscular volume.[13] Trimethoprim, which also inhibits DHFR, should not be used in patients receiving MTX because of the increased risk of pancytopenia.[1]

Hepatobiliary Effects

Hepatic transaminase elevations have been reported after acute overdose and long-term therapeutic doses of MTX therapy. Fibrosis and cirrhosis may occur in oral low-dose therapy and are reported more often in patients with psoriasis than in patients with RA.[14] Risk factors include alcohol consumption, previous hepatic or renal disease, and the presence of obesity in a diabetic patient. Histologic progression does not always occur but is associated with increased alcohol use, psoriasis, and cumulative dose of MTX.[14] Serial transaminase determinations, liver biopsy, and drug withdrawal should be done in accordance with established guidelines.[15] Use of folinic acid supplementation (in weekly doses of 2.5 to 7.5 mg) has been shown to decrease the incidence of hepatotoxicity.[16]

Neurologic Effects

The incidence of neurologic complications in patients treated with low-dose MTX has been reported to range from 1% to 35% in various studies. Symptoms may be vague, such as dysphoria, depression, headache, or dizziness.[17] Acute complications resulting from high-dose MTX include encephalopathy and seizures; weekly treatments have been reported to cause transient neurologic deficits, which occur an average of 6 days after treatment. Intrathecal administration may cause aseptic meningitis in 40% of patients. Transverse myelopathy, focal neurologic deficits, and encephalopathy are rare.[18] Seizures have been described after intrathecal overdose of MTX.[19] Intrathecal and high-dose MTX may cause leukoencephalopathy.[18]

Pulmonary Effects

Five types of pulmonary pathology associated with the use of MTX have been reported. Interstitial pneumonitis is the most common, occurring in 50% of patients on low-dose therapy, with reported fatality rates of 17%.[20] Although it also has been called *hypersensitivity pneumonitis*, the etiology is not clearly immunologic. Interstitial fibrosis has occurred even in patients being treated for conditions other than RA whose diseases are not associated with this finding.[21] Noncardiogenic pulmonary edema and pleuritis, with and without pleural effusions, are rare and have been reported only in patients receiving intravenous and intrathecal MTX.[22,23] Rapidly progressing pulmonary nodules have been reported in a patient with RA receiving long-term MTX treatment. Discontinuation of MTX alleviated the patient's symptoms but did not lead to the resolution of the nodules.[24] Conflicting studies have not shown any clear risk factors for the development of pulmonary disease associated with MTX.

Laboratory and radiographic tests are useful in establishing other causes for respiratory symptoms temporally associated with MTX administration. Supportive care is the mainstay of treatment. Discontinuation of MTX is recommended in most cases, and rechallenge has been discouraged. Systemic corticosteroids have been shown to be helpful in the treatment of MTX-induced pneumonitis, with most reports using at least 60 mg/day of prednisone with a taper over 2 to 4 weeks.[20] The use of folinic acid has not been shown to reduce the risk or aid in treatment of pulmonary disease.[25]

Renal Effects

High-dose MTX (>100 mg/kg) has been reported to cause oliguria, azotemia, and renal failure.[26] At these doses, insoluble metabolites accumulate and precipitate in the renal tubule. The solubility of MTX itself is directly proportional to pH, with a tendency to form precipitates in acidic urine. Risk factors for nephrotoxicity include age; low glomerular filtration rate; and use of drugs that reduce renal blood flow (e.g., nonsteroidal antiinflammatory drugs), are themselves nephrotoxic (e.g., gentamicin), or are weak organic acids (e.g., aspirin).[27] Adequate hydration, urinary alkalinization, and folinic acid all have been used successfully to prevent these complications.[26,28,29]

Other Effects

Alopecia has been reported with low-dose MTX and is usually reversible with cessation of therapy. In addition to its teratogenicity (see later under Special Populations), low-dose MTX may induce oligospermia[30] and gynecomastia.[31] MTX inhibits human osteoblast proliferation, which may lead to diffuse osteopenia and associated stress fractures of the distal tibia and fibula or metatarsals. This condition, termed *MTX osteopathy*, has been reported in long-term treatment of pediatric leukemia, psoriasis, and RA.[32] It may be distinguished from advanced RA by the preferential loss of cortical bone (distal radius) compared with trabecular bone (spine). Toxic epidermal necrolysis also has been reported in a patient with psoriasis on low-dose MTX therapy.[33]

DIAGNOSIS

Serum MTX concentrations are obtained routinely during the course of chemotherapy and should be obtained after overdose. Some authors advocate the use of serial MTX levels at 12, 24, and 48 hours postexposure so that folinic acid therapy may be adjusted. MTX concentrations greater than 9×10^{-7} mol/L at 48 hours postexposure are considered a risk for bone marrow and gastrointestinal toxicity.[34] Care must be taken, however, with specific laboratory assays. Trimethoprim may interfere with radioenzymatic and enzyme inhibition assays for MTX, and folinic acid may be mistaken for MTX in spectrophotofluorometric assays, making results unreliable.[35–37] Inability to obtain serum MTX concentrations should prompt consideration of patient transfer to a facility that has this capability.

TREATMENT

Aggressive supportive care is essential to the treatment of MTX toxicity. A thorough history and physical examination should be performed to assess the risk of toxicity. A complete blood count and baseline liver and renal functions should be assessed. Serum MTX concentrations should be drawn, although they may not be immediately available to guide antidotal therapy. Intravenous access should be established and isotonic fluids given to ensure adequate hydration (urine output of 1 to 3 mL/kg/hr).[38] Urinary alkalinization is recommended to prevent precipitation of MTX in renal tubules and to decrease the incidence of nephrotoxicity.[29] Intravenous sodium bicarbonate should be administered with the goal of maintaining urine pH in the range of 7 to 8. Pancytopenia has been treated successfully with granulocyte colony-stimulating factor.[39] Use of granulocyte colony-stimulating factor should be considered in patients with severe neutropenia, evidence of infection, and undetectable MTX concentrations.

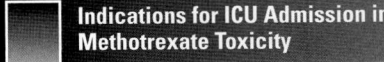
Indications for ICU Admission in Methotrexate Toxicity

Acute renal failure
Evidence of sepsis
Gastrointestinal bleeding
Need for ventilatory support
Severe neurologic dysfunction (seizure, coma)
Suicidal ideation (if adequate supervision is not available elsewhere)

There is no evidence to support the use of gastric lavage after MTX overdose. MTX is bound to activated charcoal,[40] and administration is advisable if performed early after ingestion. Multiple doses of activated charcoal are not currently recommended.[41] The clinical efficacy of these treatments in acute overdose is unknown.

Conflicting information exists in the literature regarding the use of hemodialysis and hemoperfusion in the treatment of MTX toxicity. Although animal data may suggest charcoal hemoperfusion to be the preferred technique,[42,43] anecdotal success has been reported for both modalities.[44–46] The experience of other authors and computer modeling show extracorporeal techniques to be of little value,[47,48] however, and many cases of toxicity have been treated successfully with the use of antidotal therapy alone.[49] There are no randomized clinical studies regarding the use of extracorporeal removal techniques in MTX toxicity, so it is difficult to recommend routine employment. Dialysis should be performed as indicated for the routine treatment of renal failure. Standard nonantidotal treatments are listed in Table 60-2.

Folinic acid (leucovorin), the reduced, active form of folate, is a widely accepted antidote for MTX toxicity. It competes with MTX for the binding site of DHFR and bypasses the blocked enzyme, allowing production of proteins, purines, and thymidylate through other pathways (see Fig. 60-2). Although it is used routinely in oncology as rescue therapy for a variety of cancers, straightforward guidelines for the administration of leucovorin in an acute overdose have not been established. In general, however, the dose of leucovorin given should be based on either the dose of MTX ingested or the plasma MTX concentration; this should allow adequate competitive inhibition of MTX to occur. When MTX levels are available, administration may be guided by the use of dosing regimens previously established for leucovorin rescue in chemotherapy (Table 60-3).[50] Although oral and intramuscular administration have been used, the preferred route of leucovorin administration is intravenous. Because leucovorin preparations contain calcium, the rate of infusion should be no faster than 160 mg/min. In general, the minimal recommended dose of leucovorin for the treatment of MTX toxicity is 15 mg/m^2. Leucovorin should be given within 1 hour of overdose for greatest efficacy. The dose should be repeated every 6 hours and continued for 2 to 3 days or until the serum MTX concentration is less than 5×10^{-8} mol/L.[3]

Other potential antidotes for MTX poisoning also have been studied. The use of thymidine is investigational; it has been used in combination with other therapies.[51,52] This treatment allows DNA synthesis to continue through the enzyme thymidine kinase, which is not inhibited by

MTX.[53] Carboxypeptidase G2 is a recombinant bacterial enzyme that hydrolyzes the terminal glutamate group of MTX, rendering it inactive. Its use has been documented only in several case reports, and it has been given intravenously and intrathecally.[54,55] Neither of these therapies currently is considered standard treatment for MTX poisoning.

Intrathecal MTX overdose merits particular mention because special measures may be needed. Patients in whom intrathecal overdose is detected soon after administration should be placed immediately in the upright position because this may delay the flow of MTX to the cisterna magna.[56] Cerebrospinal fluid drainage should be performed as soon as possible with the intention of removing *at least* 50% of the MTX injected. Guidelines for achieving this are in Table 60-4. When greater than 1 hour has elapsed since intrathecal overdose has occurred, cerebrospinal fluid exchange also is indicated. This exchange can be accomplished by lavaging the intrathecal space with lactated Ringer's solution.

When an intrathecal overdose is greater than 100 mg, ventriculolumbar perfusion generally is reccommended.[57] With this technique, a ventriculostomy is performed, and isotonic fluid is given via the cannula and drained from the lumbar site. MTX concentrations of effluent are used to guide cerebrospinal fluid exchange and perfusion therapies.[57] Standard leucovorin rescue is used in addition to these modalities but should not be given intrathecally because it may induce seizure activity.[58] Leucovorin also has been used without invasive measures to treat a child successfully with an intrathecal overdose of 300 mg of MTX.[59] The use of intravenous thymidine and intrathecal carboxypeptidase G2 also has been reported but again cannot be recommended as standard therapy.[51,55]

TABLE 60-3 Dosage of Leucovorin Based on Serum Methotrexate Concentrations

MTX CONCENTRATION (mol/L)	LEUCOVORIN DOSE (mg/m^2)*
5×10^{-7}	15
1×10^{-6}	100
2×10^{-6}	200

*Given every 6 hours.
MTX, methotrexate.
Adapted from Jolivet J, Cowan KH, Curt GA, et al: The pharmacology and clinical use of methotrexate. N Engl J Med 309:1094–1104, 1983.

TABLE 60-2 Nonantidotal Treatment of Methotrexate Toxicity

Charcoal
Intravenous fluid to maintain urine volume of 1–3 mL/kg/hr
Alkalinization of urine to achieve pH of 7–8
Hemodialysis as indicated for supportive treatment of renal failure

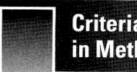

Criteria for ICU Discharge in Methotrexate Toxicity

Hemodynamic stability
No active bleeding
No requirement for ventilatory support
Psychiatric issues adequately addressed, if necessary

TABLE 60-4 Volume of Cerebrospinal Fluid Drainage Required to Reduce Methotrexate Concentrations*

TIME AFTER MTX INJECTION (min)	VOLUME TO REDUCE SPECIFIC CONCENTRATION (mL)		
	>50%	>70%	>90%
15	10	—	20
30	—	20	—
45	20	30	—
60	30	40	—

*Assumes 10 mL of MTX-containing fluid injected.
MTX, methotrexate.
Adapted from Addiego JE, Ridgeway D, Bleyer WA: The acute management of intrathecal methotrexate overdose: Pharmacologic rationale and guidelines. J Pediatr 98:825–828, 1981.

SPECIAL POPULATIONS

MTX has been used safely in the treatment of childhood leukemia, and dosage recommendations have been published for use in infants. Elderly patients receiving MTX should be watched closely because low glomerular filtration rates associated with advanced age would be expected to increase the risk of nephrotoxicity.[27] MTX is teratogenic and has been used in the treatment of ectopic pregnancy. Its misuse as an abortifacient has led to two reported cases of maternal toxicity and the birth of an infant with cranial, facial, and limb malformations.[5]

  Key Points in Methotrexate Toxicity

1. Methotrexate now is used to treat a variety of illnesses in the outpatient setting.
2. Methotrexate may be misused in attempts to induce abortion.
3. Methotrexate poisoning presentation may include gastrointestnal upset, mucositis, hepatitis, and renal toxicity.
4. Pancytopenia may be delayed.
5. Adequate urinary output and urinary alkalinization are important aspects of therapy.
6. Folinic acid should be started when the diagnosis is suspected, not when the results of methotrexate levels are obtained.
7. Inability to monitor methotrexate levels should be a consideration for transfer to another facility.
8. Intrathecal exposure requires cerebrospinal drainage and possible ventriculolumbar perfusion.

REFERENCES

1. Hillson JL, Furst DE: Pharmacology and pharmacokinetics of methotrexate in rheumatic disease. Rheum Dis Clin North Am 23:757–778, 1993.
2. Cronstein BN: The mechanism of action of methotrexate. Rheum Dis Clin North Am 23:739–755, 1993.
3. Gibbon BN, Manthey DE: Pediatric case of accidental overdose of oral methotrexate. Ann Emerg Med 34:98–100, 1999.
4. Pruitt AW, Kinkade JM, Patterson JH: Accidental ingestion of methotrexate. J Pediatr 85:686–688, 1974.
5. Alfaro J, Von Muhlenbrock R, Burgos N, et al: Intoxicacion aguda con methotrexate usado con fines abortivos: descripcion de 2 casos [Acute poisoning with methotrexate used as an abortifacient: description of 2 cases]. Rev Med Chil 128:315–318, 2000.
6. McKendry RJ: The remarkable spectrum of methotrexate toxicities. Rheum Dis Clin North Am 23:940–954, 1997.
7. Atherton LD, Leib ES, Kaye MD: Toxic megacolon associated with methotrexate therapy. Gastroenterology 86:1583–1585, 1984.
8. Morgan SL, Baggott JE, Refsum H, et al: Supplementation with folic acid during methotrexate therapy for rheumatoid arthritis: A double-blind, placebo-controlled trial. Ann Intern Med 121:833–841, 1994.
9. Zeiders RS: Oral methotrexate therapy in rheumatoid arthritis. Arthritis Rheum 25(Suppl):S65, 1982.
10. Chevreau N, Funk-Archuleta M: Effect of enteral formulas on methotrexate toxicity. Nutr Cancer 23:185–204, 1995.
11. Rubio IT, Yihong Cho MS, Hutchins LF, et al: Effect of glutamine on methotrexate efficacy and toxicity. Ann Surg 227:772–780, 1988.
12. Gutierrez-Urena S, Molina JF, Garcia CO, et al: Pancytopenia secondary to methotrexate in patients with rheumatoid arthritis. Arthritis Rheum 39:272–277, 1996.
13. Weinblatt ME: Mean corpuscular volume as a predictor of hematologic toxicity due to methotrexate therapy. Arthritis Rheum 32:1592–1596, 1989.
14. West SG: Methotrexate hepatotoxicity. Rheum Dis Clin North Am 23:883–915, 1997.
15. Roenigk HH Jr, Auerbach R, Maibach HI, et al: Methotrexate in psoriasis: Revised guidelines. J Am Acad Dermatol 19:145–156, 1988.
16. Ravelli A, Migliavacca D, Viola S, et al: Efficacy of folinic acid in reducing methotrexate toxicity in juvenile idiopathic arthritis. Clin Exp Rheum 17:625–627, 1999.
17. Kremer JM, Phelps CT: Long-term prospective study of the use of methotrexate in the treatment of rheumatoid arthritis. Arthritis Rheum 35:138–145, 1992.
18. Schiff D, Batchelor T, Wen PY: Neurologic emergencies in cancer patients. Neurol Clin 16:449–483, 1998.
19. Lee AC, Wong KW, Fong KW, et al: Intrathecal methotrexate overdose. Acta Paediatr 86:434–437, 1997.
20. Kremer JM, Alarcon GS, Weinblatt ME, et al: Clinical, laboratory, radiographic, and histopathologic features of methotrexate-associated lung injury in patients with rheumatoid arthritis: A multicenter study with literature review. Arthritis Rheum 40:1829–1837, 1997.
21. Kaplan RL, Waite DH: Progressive interstitial lung disease from prolonged methotrexate therapy. Arch Dermatol 114:1800–1802, 1978.
22. Bernstein ML, Sobel DB, Wimmer RS: Noncardiogenic pulmonary edema following injection of methotrexate into the cerebral spinal fluid. Cancer 50:866–868, 1982.
23. Walden PA, Mitchell-Heggs PF, Coppin C, et al: Pleurisy and methotrexate treatment. BMJ 2:867, 1977.
24. Alarcon GS, Koopman WJ: Nonperipheral accelerated nodulosis in a methotrexate-treated rheumatoid arthritis patient. Arthritis Rheum 36:132–133, 1993.

25. Pesce C, Mansi C, Bogliolo G, et al: Pulmonary toxicity in mice after high-dose methotrexate administration with and without leucovorin rescue. Eur J Cancer Clin Oncol 21:875–880, 1985.

26. Bleyer WA: The clinical pharmacology of methotrexate. Cancer 41:36–51, 1978.

27. Iven H, Brasch H: The effects of antibiotics and uricosuric drugs on the renal elimination of methotrexate and 7-hydroxy-methotrexate in rabbit. Cancer Chemother Pharmacol 21:337–342, 1988.

28. Isacoff WH, Eilber F, Block JB: Clinical pharmacology of high dose methotrexate. Proc Am Assoc Cancer Res 17:190, 1976.

29. Pitman SW, Frei E III: Weekly methotrexate-calcium leucovorin rescue: Effect of alkalinization on nephrotoxicity; pharmacokinetics in the CNS; and use in CNS non-Hodgkin's lymphoma. Cancer Treat Rep 61:695–701, 1977.

30. Sussman A, Leonard JM: Psoriasis, methotrexate and oligospermia. Arch Dermatol 116:215–217, 1980.

31. Del Paine DW, Leek JC, Jackle C, et al: Gynecomastia associated with low-dose methotrexate therapy. Arthritis Rheum 26:691–692, 1983.

32. Zonneveld IM, Bakker WK, Dijkstra PF, et al: Methotrexate osteopathy in long-term, low-dose methotrexate treatment for psoriasis and rheumatoid arthritis. Arch Dermatol 132:184–187, 1996.

33. Primka EJ, Camisa C: Methotrexate-induced toxic epidermal necrolysis in a patient with psoriasis. J Am Acad Dermatol 36:815–818, 1997.

34. Stoller RG, Hande KR, Jacobs SA, et al: The use of plasma pharmacokinetics to predict and prevent methotrexate toxicity. N Engl J Med 297:630–633, 1977.

35. Bock JL, Pierce R: Trimethoprim influence in methotrexate assays. Clin Chem 26:1510–1511, 1980.

36. Hande K, Gober J, Fletcher R: Trimethoprim interferes with serum methotrexate assay by the competitive protein binding technique. Clin Chem 26:1617–1619, 1980.

37. Kinkade JM, Volger WR, Dayton PG: Plasma levels of methotrexate in cancer patients as studied by an improved spectrophotofluorometric method. Biochem Med 10:337–350, 1974.

38. Christensen ML, Rivera GK, Crom WR, et al: Effect of hydration on methotrexate plasma concentrations in children with acute lymphocytic leukemia. J Clin Oncol 6:797–801, 1988.

39. Steger J, Mader RM, Gnant MFX, et al: GM-SCF in the treatment of a patient with severe methotrexate intoxication. J Intern Med 233:499–502, 1993.

40. Gadgil SD, Damle SR, Advani SH, et al: Effect of activated charcoal on the pharmacokinetics of high-dose methotrexate. Cancer Treat Rep 66:1169–1171, 1982.

41. American Academy of Clinical Toxicology, European Association of Poison Centres and Clinical Toxicologists: Position statement and practice guidelines on the use of multi-dose activated charcoal in the treatment of acute poisoning. J Toxicol Clin Toxicol 37:731–751, 1999.

42. Isacoff WH: Effects of extracorporeal charcoal hemoperfusion on plasma methotrexate. Proc Am Assoc Cancer Res 18:145, 1977.

43. Giardino R: Comparison of hemodialysis versus hemoperfusion in the clearance of high dose methotrexate in pigs. Artif Organs 19:362–365, 1995.

44. McIvor A: Charcoal hemoperfusion and methotrexate toxicity. Nephros 58:378, 1991.

45. Gauthier E, Gimonet JF, Piedbois P, et al: [Effectiveness of hemodialysis in a case of acute methotrexate poisoning]. Presse Med 19:2023–2025, 1990.

46. Frappaz D, Bouffet E, Cochat P, et al: [Hemoperfusion on charcoal and hemodialysis in acute poisoning by methotrexate]. Presse Med 17:1209–1213, 1988.

47. Winchester JF, Rahman A, Tilstone WJ, et al: Will hemoperfusion be useful for cancer chemotherapeutic drug removal? Clin Toxicol 17:557–569, 1980.

48. Pond SM: Extracorporeal techniques in the treatment of poisoned patients. Med J Aust 154:617–622, 1991.

49. Flombaum CD, Meyers PA: High-dose leucovorin as sole therapy for methotrexate toxicity. J Clin Oncol 17:1589–1594, 1999.

50. Jolivet J, Cowan KH, Curt GA, et al: The pharmacology and clinical use of methotrexate. N Engl J Med 309:1094–1104, 1983.

51. Spiegal RJ, Cooper PR, Blum RH, et al: Treatment of massive intrathecal methotrexate overdose by ventriculolumbar perfusion. N Engl J Med 311:386–388, 1984.

52. Howell SB, Ensminger WD, Krishnan A, et al: Thymidine rescue of high-dose methotrexate in humans. Cancer Res 38:325–330, 1978.

53. Tattersall MHN, Brown B, Frei E III: The reversal of methotrexate toxicity by thymidine with maintenance of antitumor effects. Nature 253:198–200, 1975.

54. Zoubek A, Zaunschirm HA, Lion T, et al: Successful carboxypeptidase G2 rescue in delayed methotrexate elimination due to renal failure. Pediatr Hematol Oncol 12:471–477, 1995.

55. O'Marcaigh AS, Johnson CM, Smithson WA, et al: Successful treatment of intrathecal methotrexate overdose by using ventriculolumbar perfusion and intrathecal instillation of carboxypeptidase G2. Mayo Clin Proc 71:161–165, 1996.

56. Echelberger CK, Riccardi R, Bleyer A, et al: Influence of body position on ventricular cerebral spinal fluid methotrexate concentration following intralumbar administration (Abstract C-131). Proc Am Assoc Cancer Res Am Soc Clin Oncol, March 1981, p 365.

57. Addiego JE, Ridgeway D, Bleyer WA: The acute management of intrathecal methotrexate overdose: Pharmacologic rationale and guidelines. J Pediatr 98:825–828, 1981.

58. Jardine LF, Ingram LC, Bleyer WA: Intrathecal leucovorin after intrathecal methotrexate overdose. J Pediatr Hematol Oncol 18:302–304, 1996.

59. Riva L, Conter V, Rizzari C, et al: Successful treatment of intrathecal methotrexate overdose with folinic acid rescue: A case report. Acta Pediatr 88:780–782, 1999.

CHAPTER **61**

Isoniazid and Related Hydrazines

K. Sophia Dyer ■ Michael Shannon

Isoniazid (isonicotinic acid hydrazide [INH]) was first released in 1952 as a drug to treat tuberculosis. Although tuberculosis was already on the decline in the United States and much of the Western world at the time of the release of INH, it is currently estimated that approximately one third of the world's population has been exposed to this disease. INH has remained the drug of choice for prophylactic treatment in individuals with a positive tuberculin skin test.[1] Because of the toxicity of the drug, even at standard doses, concern still exists regarding the use of INH for prophylaxis of latent tuberculosis infection.[2-5]

In the United States, there has been an increase in the incidence of tuberculosis infection since the late 1980s, as a consequence of the prevalence of human immunodeficiency virus (HIV). Although the incidence of tuberculosis has decreased in many subpopulations, its prevalence among foreign-born citizens has increased.[6] Other social and medical ills, such as homelessness, overcrowding, alcoholism, and intravenous drug use, have contributed to the rising rate of tuberculosis infection. The World Health Organization (WHO) proclaimed tuberculosis a *global emergency* in 1993.[7] With societal changes in the former Soviet Union and Eastern Europe, public health crises soon followed with a rise in new cases. The HIV epidemic in sub-Saharan Africa threatens attempts of tuberculosis control in Africa. It is estimated that there were 8 million newly diagnosed cases of tuberculosis in 1997.[8] According to the WHO, direct observed therapy of antituberculin drugs in the developing world would help curb the spread. If further public health measures are not instituted, such as direct observed therapy, the WHO estimated that a 41% increase in new cases would be seen, from 7.4 to 10.6 million cases.[9]

According to the American Association of Poison Control Centers, in 1997 and 1998, respectively, there were 480 and 452 recorded acute toxic exposures to INH by U.S. poison centers, resulting in 1 reported death each year.[10,11] Intentional exposures constituted 236 of the 480 and 196 of the 452.[10,11] Because these data depend on voluntary reporting of exposures, they undoubtedly underestimate the true incidence of INH poisonings.

INH belongs to a family of related chemicals called *hydrazines* (Fig. 61-1), and acute poisoning by these chemicals is similar to that seen with INH. INH is structurally related to isonicotinic acid. It is also referred to as *isonicotinylhydrazide*. Hydrazines are also found in the *Gyromitra* family of mushrooms, which contain the toxin gyromitrin (*N*-methyl-*N*-formyl hydrazone) (see Fig. 61-1), a substance that is eventually hydrolyzed to monomethylhydrazine in vivo. Species of this mushroom group include *G. esculenta, G. californica, G. brunnea,* and *G. infula.* All of these mushrooms are considered to have similar toxicity to that of INH. *Gyromitra* spp. mushrooms are discussed in Chapter 121.

BIOCHEMISTRY OF ISONIAZID AND HYDRAZINES

As chemicals, the hydrazines are used as rocket fuel and are powerful reducing agents. Hydrazine (see Fig. 61-1) is used in the manufacture of anticorrosive materials, pesticides, plastics, pharmaceuticals, dyes, and textile treatments. Hydrazine also may be called *diamine, anhydrous hydrazine,* and *hydrazine base.* Violent reactions occur when hydrazine is mixed with any oxidizing agent (e.g., peroxides or chlorates, metal oxides, and strong acids). As with any flammable liquid, its proximity to any source of ignition could be hazardous. The Chemical Abstract Service number of hydrazine is 302-01-2. Considered a flammable liquid, hydrazines can spontaneously ignite on contact with oxidizers or porous materials.[12] The American Conference of Governmental Industrial Hygienists gives a time-weighted average exposure limit of 0.01 ppm for hydrazine exposure.[13]

INH is produced initially as a white crystal; its injectable form is a clear to slightly greenish yellow liquid with a pH of 6 to 7 and a pK_a of 1.9.[14,15] It is available as an oral solution or tablets (usually 50 mg, 100 mg, or 300 mg). Various combination products are available, such as a capsule containing 150 mg of INH with 300 mg of rifampin (Rifamate) and a tablet preparation of 50 mg of INH, 300 mg of pyrazinamide, and 120 mg of rifampin (Rifater).[14]

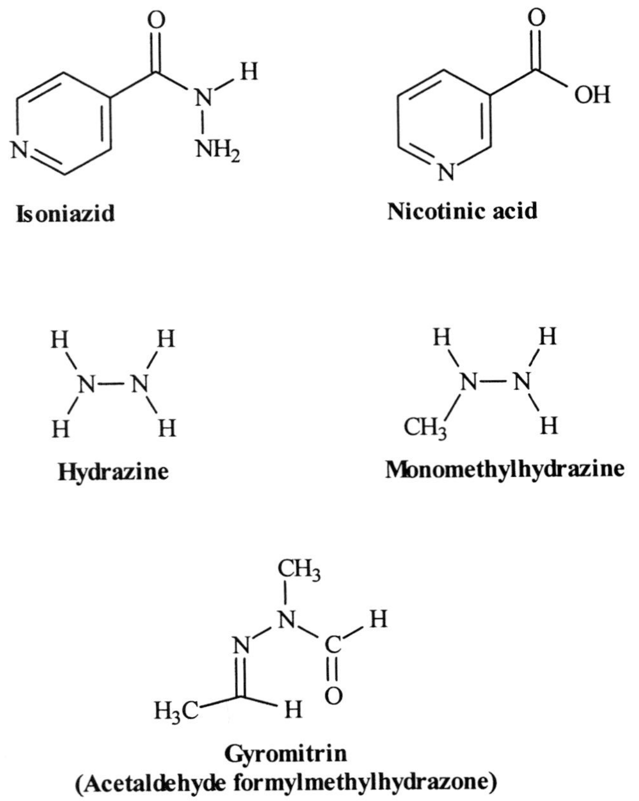

FIGURE 61-1

Chemical structures of isoniazid and related hydrazines.

Pharmacokinetics of Isoniazid and Related Hydrazines

Volume of distribution: 0.6–0.75 L/kg
Cerebrospinal fluid concentrations: 90–100% of plasma 3 to 4 hr after standard oral dose
Protein binding: 4–30%
Oral bioavailability: 90%
Metabolites: acetylisoniazid, isonicotinic acid, monoacetylhydrazine, diacetylhydrazine, isonicotinyl glycine, isonicotinyl hydrazones, methylisoniazid
Elimination: inactivated by liver acetylation* and dehydrazination, P-450 system hydrolysis, methylation; 75% to 96% of standard dose excreted in urine within 24 hours as parent drug or metabolites (assuming normal renal function)
Methods to enhance elimination: hemodialysis or peritoneal dialysis in specific populations

*Acetylation rate is genetically influenced; see text.

PATHOPHYSIOLOGY OF THERAPEUTIC AND TOXIC EFFECTS

The exact therapeutic mechanism of action of INH has not been elucidated. One commonly invoked mechanism is the drug's inhibition of mycolic acid synthesis during cell division, resulting in breaks in the mycobacterial cell wall (Fig. 61-2). Toxic effects in humans are better understood;

they seem to hinge on INH's effects on pyridoxine metabolism and the hepatotoxic effects of INH metabolites.

Ingestions of 1500 mg can cause minor toxicity in adults and major toxicity in children. Individuals with underlying seizure disorders may be more susceptible to INH-induced seizure activity. Ingestion of 6 to 10 g in an adult can produce severe metabolic acidosis, seizures, cardiovascular collapse, and death.

INH engages in critical interactions with pyridoxine (vitamin B_6). Pyridoxine is an essential cofactor in the production of γ-aminobutyric acid (GABA), the main inhibitory central nervous system neurotransmitter. Normally, pyridoxine is converted to pyridoxine 5′phosphate, which acts as a coenzyme for glutamic acid decarboxylase, the enzyme that catalyzes the conversion of glutamic acid to GABA (Fig. 61-3). INH inhibits pyridoxine kinase, the enzyme that catalyzes the production of pyridoxine 5′phosphate, and to a lesser extent INH directly inhibits glutamic acid decarboxylase. Hydrazines bind pyridoxine. The acute deficiency of pyridoxal phosphate resulting from INH overdose also is believed to inhibit catecholamine synthesis, contributing to cardiovascular instability and coma.[16]

CLINICAL PRESENTATION

The classic triad of acute INH poisoning consists of refractory seizures, coma, and metabolic acidosis.[16–18] The metabolic acidosis caused by INH is typically associated with a high anion gap. In one report, a 14-year-old child survived seizures, with a serum pH of 6.69, without sequelae.[19] Hankinns and colleagues reported a pH of 6.49 in a surviving INH overdose patient.[16] Excessive production of lactic acid and hydrolysis of adenosine triphosphate secondary to seizure activity are thought to be the major causes of this acidosis[20]; however, respiratory depression in the setting of intractable seizures also may contribute to profound acidosis. It is common for the pH to approach values of 6.8 in severe INH poisoning. Being structurally similar to nicotinic acid (vitamin B_3) (see Fig. 61-1), INH is believed to block nicotinamide-adenine dinucleotide activity, which is important for the conversion of lactate to pyruvate; this probably makes little, if any, contribution to INH-associated acidosis. If the patient has a seizure, however, the reduced metabolic clearance of lactate may cause the acidosis to be prolonged.

Persistent seizures are the toxic effect of INH most clearly resulting from pyridoxine deficiency. Other potential central nervous system effects of INH overdose include psychosis, ataxia, memory impairment, nystagmus, hyperreflexia, areflexia, light-headedness, and cerebellar syndrome.[21–25]

Peripheral neuropathy is a side effect of long-term INH therapy that is believed to result from pyridoxine deficiency. In a 1954 case report, therapy with pyridoxine relieved the peripheral neuropathy of a patient taking INH. The neuropathy recurred after pyridoxine therapy was discontinued.[26] Microscopic evaluation of patients with INH-associated peripheral neuropathy has shown wallerian degeneration.[27] Risk factors for INH-induced peripheral neuropathy include malnutrition, pregnancy, diabetes, alcoholism, and slow acetylator status. Because pyridoxal phosphate is removed by hemodialysis, patients receiving this therapy are theoretically at risk for neurotoxicity.[28] In a study of 38 children receiving INH,

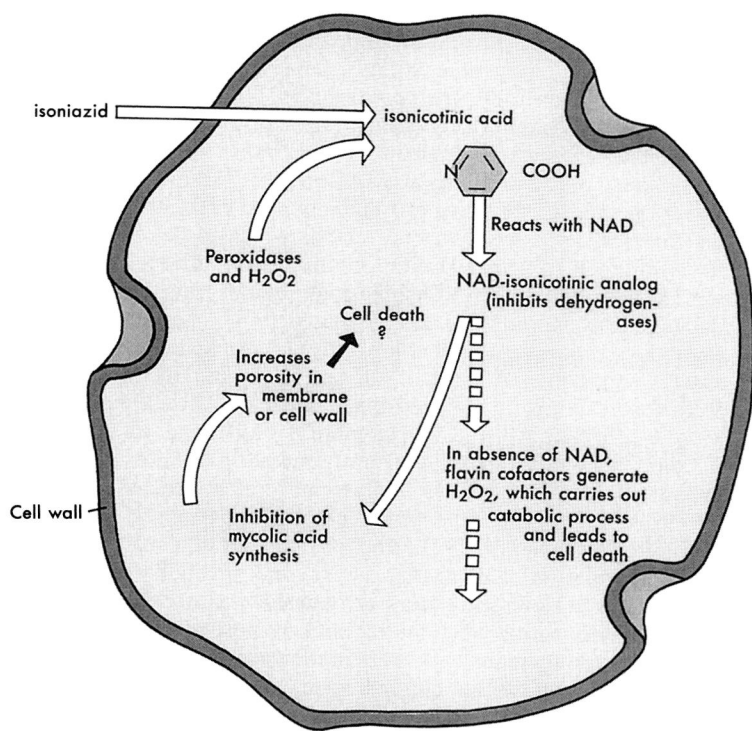

FIGURE 61-2

Postulated mechanism of action of isoniazid on *Mycobacterium tuberculosis. (From Brody TM, Larner J, Minneman KP: Human Pharmacology: Molecular to Clinical, 3rd ed. St. Louis, Mosby, 1998.)*

13% were found to be pyridoxine deficient, although none had definitive symptoms of the deficiency.[29] Doses of INH greater than 6 mg/kg/day also are considered to place the patient at risk for peripheral neuropathy. Pellagra also may result from deficiency of pyridoxal phosphate. Optic neuritis is another recognized adverse effect of INH therapy[30,31] and may be exacerbated by concomitant use of ethambutol, another antituberculous drug with established optic toxicity.

Although rhabdomyolysis has been reported in patients taking INH intermittently, it is primarily a consequence of seizure activity.[32] Other, less commonly reported adverse effects of INH include isolated fevers, rash, worsening of asthma symptoms, pancreatitis, red blood cell aplasia, and a

lupus-like syndrome.[33–41] One theory is that INH is oxidized by activated leukocytes to a reactive intermediate, which could induce the lupus-like syndrome.[42] Hyperglycemia, glycosuria, ketonemia, and ketonuria all have been reported in INH overdose.[17,24] This constellation may lead the clinician to believe the patient has diabetic ketoacidosis.

FOOD AND DRUG INTERACTIONS

Although reports of food and drug interactions with INH are infrequent, the potential for interactions does exist. INH weakly inhibits the enzyme monoamine oxidase (MAO)

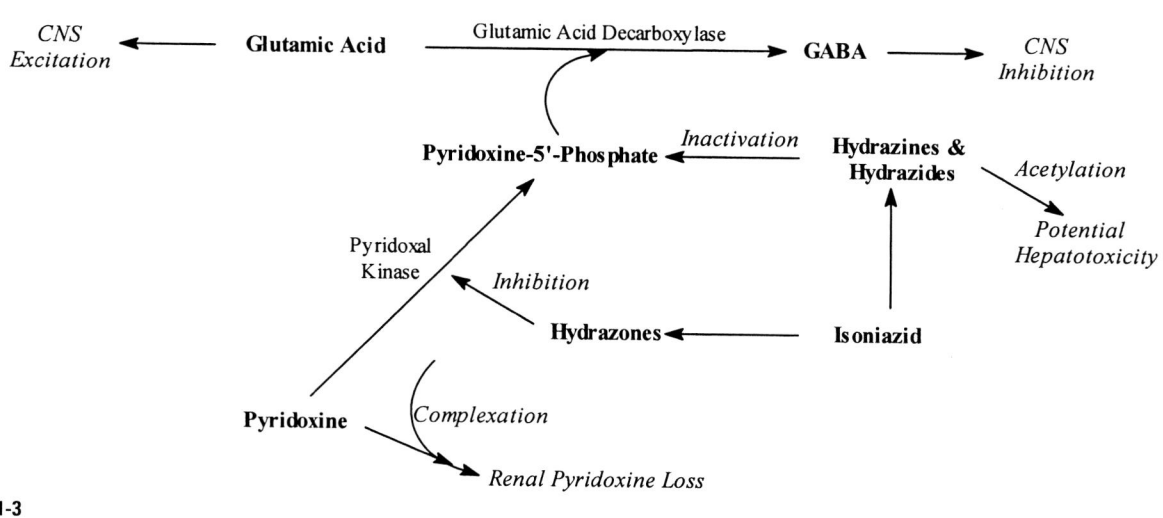

FIGURE 61-3

Inhibitory effect of isoniazid on pyridoxine-related metabolic processes. CNS, central nervous system; GABA, γ-aminobutyric acid.

and is a congener of isocarboxazid, an early MAO inhibitor used as an antidepressant and antituberculosis agent. The typical drug and dietary precautions given to patients on MAO inhibitors generally are not expanded, however, to include INH. It is likely that because INH is only a weak inhibitor of MAO, patients often appear to tolerate the drug without dietary precautions. As an MAO inhibitor, however, INH decreases the metabolism of tyramine, present in some wines, cheeses, and soy products. Increased sensitivity to dietary tyramine is associated with long-term INH administration and is manifested by flushing, palpitation, pruritus, headache, nausea, vomiting, and hypertension.[43]

Another notable MAO inhibitor drug-drug reaction is that with meperidine. A case of meperidine and INH in combination resulting in hypotension has been reported.[44] Caution has been advised when combining INH and tricyclic antidepressants.[45,46] Aside from the weak MAO inhibition attributed to INH, INH inhibits the metabolism of several benzodiazepines, phenytoin, carbamazepine, warfarin, and valproic acid.[47,48] Rifampin administration may induce the formation of hepatotoxic hydrazine metabolites. Patients who are slow acetylators are considered to be at greater risk for hepatitis when taking both of these drugs.[49] Some INH drug interactions are thought to result from INH-induced inhibition of the cytochrome isoenzyme CYP2E1.[50] Acetaminophen clearance has been shown to decrease by 15.2% when INH is given.[51] Paradoxically, INH not only inhibits but also induces CYP2E1. This is the basis of what seems to be an increased risk of hepatotoxicity in patients who take acetaminophen during INH therapy.[52,53] INH also inhibits the enzyme diamine oxidase, which metabolizes histamine.

Hepatotoxicity

One of the interesting properties of all hydrazines, most notably INH, is the ability to produce hepatotoxicity. The true incidence of hepatotoxicity during INH therapy is unclear. Even the definition of hepatotoxicity differs in much of the literature. It is estimated that 20% of patients receiving INH develop an elevation in liver function tests.[54,55] In contrast, one study of 921 patients found an incidence of only 0.4%.[56] Other studies have reported an incidence of hepatotoxicity ranging from 0.15% to 0.6%.[57,58] A trend toward higher rates of hepatotoxicity in women has been suggested.[58] In many of these studies of hepatotoxicity, serial serum transaminases were not performed, and toxicity was defined on the basis of clinical findings only. Elevations of liver function tests are typically transient and normalize despite continued therapy with the drug.

Elevations in liver function tests can appear within the first 2 weeks of therapy to 6 months after initiation; most cases develop within the first 3 months of therapy. Some authors have recommended discontinuing use of INH when transaminases exceed three times normal values. Clinically a patient with INH hepatotoxicity may voice vague digestive complaints (55%) or viral-like complaints (35%), according to one review comprising 114 patients.[59] A 1972 report described 2321 patients who required INH prophylaxis, 19 of whom (mean age 49.4 years) developed clinical symptoms of hepatic injury, occurring within the first 2 months in 9 patients. Two patients died.[60] This attracted the attention of the U.S. Public Health Service, which in 1972 undertook a surveillance study of 13,838 persons taking INH prophylaxis therapy and identified 8 deaths (0.06%). In the 21 cities examined, the rate of hepatotoxicity varied; 92 cases were determined to be probably related to INH, 82 cases were possibly related, and 22 cases had insufficient data.[61] These data also showed the higher incidence of hepatotoxicity in persons older than age 35 years and persons with daily alcohol intake. In 1983, the American Thoracic Society changed its recommendation for INH prophylaxis, recommending chemoprophylaxis for persons at increased risk of developing active tuberculosis and persons younger than 35 years. If patients are at high risk for developing tuberculosis and they are older than 35 years old, periodic liver function tests are recommended.[62]

Liver function tests are not always reported in case reports of acute INH overdose. In one series of eight overdoses, six had aspartate aminotransferase levels ranging from 40 to 1581 U/L, suggesting acute hepatotoxicity as a potential complication.[24] The fatality rate of patients with fulminant hepatitis has been reported to be 5%.[61,63] There seems to be a higher mortality in women, particularly during pregnancy and in the postpartum period.[64,65] Liver transplantation has provided rescue treatment in select cases of fulminant hepatitis.[66,67] A hepatitis B carrier state does not seem to be a risk factor for INH hepatitis.[68] A higher rate of hepatotoxicity is seen in patients receiving INH and rifampin.[57] Ethanol consumption is considered a significant factor by some authors; however, alcohol consumption is difficult to quantify in retrospective evaluations of the incidence.[61,69] Advancing age also is considered to be a risk factor for INH hepatotoxicity.

At one time, acetylator status was thought to be a major risk factor of INH-induced hepatotoxicity. Slow acetylation is found in 50% to 60% of American whites and blacks. Fast acetylator phenotype is found primarily in Japanese and Inuit populations. Acetylation status does not seem to change with age. Slow acetylators exhibit longer elimination half-life and higher plasma concentrations of INH and acetylhydrazine, particularly if they are taking high INH doses (>10 mg/kg/day). Both acetylhydrazine and the nonacetylated metabolite, hydrazine, yield hepatotoxic intermediates.[70,71] More recent studies have provided evidence, however, refuting a major role of acetylator status as a risk factor for INH-induced hepatotoxicity.

Industrial Hydrazines

Industrial hydrazines have toxic effects similar to those of INH, including seizures and hepatotoxicity. Additionally, they can produce direct tissue damage. Hydrazines are corrosive to the skin, resulting in manifestations ranging from simple itching to severe burns. Solutions with hydrazine concentrations greater than 25% are likely to produce significant dermal injury. High ambient concentrations can lead to hydrazine vapor exposure with irritation of mucous membranes and eyes. Similarly, concentrated vapor exposure can result in irritation of the respiratory tract, producing cough, shortness of breath, or pulmonary edema.[12] Combustion of hydrazines liberates nitrogen oxides, which can be toxic to the lung parenchyma. Methemoglobinemia (see Chapter 28) and hemolysis may occur after hydrazine exposures.

DIAGNOSIS OF HYDRAZINE POISONING

Toxic exposures associated with seizures or metabolic acidosis or both include cyanide, salicylates, tricyclic antidepressants, theophylline, iron, ibuprofen, cocaine, amphetamines, phencyclidine, ethylene glycol, and methanol. Ethanol/benzodiazepine withdrawal also should be considered in the differential diagnosis. Hyperglycemia and acetonuria should suggest the diagnosis of diabetic ketoacidosis, particularly if the history does not include seizure activity. INH overdose always should be considered in a patient with new onset of seizures of unknown etiology, particularly if the patient is from a tuberculosis-prone population. Generally the diagnosis is made clinically and based on the history of exposure. Laboratory testing usually cannot verify a diagnosis of INH poisoning within a clinically useful time frame. Serum transaminases at baseline and regular intervals are required to identify INH-induced hepatitis.

TREATMENT OF ISONIAZID AND HYDRAZINES POISONING

Skin and Eye Decontamination of Hydrazine Chemicals

Skin and eye decontamination for industrial hydrazine exposure is crucial because these agents are very corrosive. Skin decontamination focuses on administration of copious amounts of water and prompt removal of contaminated clothing, jewelry, watches, and shoes. If possible, decontamination should occur away from other patients if it is being performed in a hospital. The patient may be able to participate in decontamination by self-removal of clothing and self-washing of the skin. If minimal vapor exposure has occurred in an asymptomatic patient, removal of clothing may be all that is required. If doubt exists about the extent of exposure, water decontamination is advisable. The concentration of the chemical also determines the hazard, but for most hospital and prehospital medical providers that information may not be immediately available. Because hydrazine and monomethylhydrazine are flammable liquids, decontamination should take place away from any possible sources of ignition. Sources of ignition can include electrical switches, radios, and other electronics. Eye decontamination consists of irrigation with large amounts of water. A Morgan lens after topical anesthesia may facilitate eye decontamination. Because hydrazines are alkalis, the goal of ocular decontamination is to restore a constant pH of 7.0 to the conjunctival sac.

Medical Management

As with all overdoses, supportive care is crucial in the management of intoxication by INH or other hydrazine compounds, with close attention to vital signs, monitoring for early signs of cardiovascular collapse or airway compromise. Secure intravenous access is of particular importance because seizures may occur suddenly, although they are typically preceded by hyperreflexia or areflexia. Supple-

mental oxygen, fluid volume support, and maintenance of a patent airway are immediate priorities.

Ipecac syrup should never be administered to a patient who has ingested INH. Gastrointestinal decontamination is discussed further in Chapter 5. Activated charcoal has been shown to adsorb INH well and theoretically should be administered.[72] There are no data, however, indicating that the administration of activated charcoal alters outcome in INH-treated patients. If the patient presents to a health care facility soon after INH ingestion, the clinician may consider the use of orogastric lavage. Lavage is not without its hazards, however, and, as described in Chapter 5, is of questionable utility. The clinician should consider carefully the risks of the procedure versus its limited benefit.

In patients with profound metabolic acidosis, administration of intravenous sodium bicarbonate may be warranted. Sodium bicarbonate should not be used to correct metabolic acidosis in the absence of aggressive efforts to control seizure activity because most acidosis is related to seizure activity. Rhabdomyolysis should be assessed by following serum creatine phosphokinase or urine myoglobin. In cases of severe rhabdomyolysis, urine alkalization to pH greater than 6.5 may be beneficial.

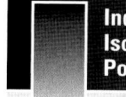

Indications for ICU Admission in Isoniazid and Related Hydrazines Poisoning

Prolonged or severe metabolic acidosis
Multiple seizures
Significant rhabdomyolysis
Depressed mental status
Hemodynamic instability
Seizures not easily controlled by pharmacologic intervention

Pyridoxine

Pyridoxine is the drug of choice for treating INH (or other hydrazine)-induced seizures. Because adequate doses of pyridoxine hydrochloride may not be available for immediate administration, other anticonvulsants are generally administered in the first few minutes. An anticonvulsant that works as an agonist at the GABA receptor, such as a benzodiazepine or barbiturate, is preferred. These agents alone rarely can provide full control of INH-induced seizures, however. Benzodiazepines and barbiturates are indirect agonists at the GABA receptor, requiring sufficient amounts of GABA to be effective. If there are insufficient amounts of pyridoxine in hospital stores, addition of a benzodiazepine, such as diazepam, can potentiate the pyridoxine.[73] Phenobarbital is a rational choice for adjunctive therapy if there is an insufficient supply of pyridoxine. Phenytoin, having a different mechanism of anticonvulsant action (working on sodium channels rather than GABA receptors), is theoretically ineffective in the treatment of INH-induced seizures. Although pyridoxine availability is crucial in the treatment of an INH-poisoned patient, one pediatric case series found that the average delay to its administration was 5.8 hours.[73] In a survey of U.S. hospitals with pediatric emergency medicine fellowships or emergency medicine residencies, immediate availability of the recommended 5-g dose was lacking for half of the institutions, and the dose was not kept in the emergency department in an even greater adult proportion of responding programs.[74] Areas where tuberculosis is relatively endemic should strongly consider keeping pyridoxine close at hand in the emergency department. If a patient presents shortly after a known INH overdose, pyridoxine administration may prevent seizures. In addition to therapy for seizure activity, pyridoxine may be useful in the treatment of INH-induced coma.[18,75]

Generally recommended pyridoxine dosing for an adult patient in whom the amount of INH ingested is unknown is 5 g (70 mg/kg in children); the dose is repeated if necessary.[17] When the amount ingested is known, pyridoxine should be administered in gram-for-gram equivalents.[17–19,22] Large doses of pyridoxine are not benign. Severe peripheral neuropathies, some permanent, have been reported in very high short-term and high long-term pyridoxine dosing (0.5 to 2 g/day).[76,77] The clinical pharmacology of pyridoxine is discussed in Chapter 147.

Other Hydrazines

Reports of severe hydrazine and monomethylhydrazine poisoning in the medical literature are few compared with reports involving INH. However, the use of pyridoxine is recommended on theoretical grounds for seizures and coma in victims of serious industrial exposure to hydrazine or major exposures to gyromitrin-containing mushrooms. Because gram-for-gram dosing of pyridoxine may not be calculable in an occupationally exposed patient, the generally accepted empirical adult dosing for seizure control is 5 g administered intravenously as a bolus.

Hemodialysis

Hemodialysis is theoretically likely to enhance INH clearance based on its low degree of protein binding and relatively small volume of distribution. Hemodialysis is generally unnecessary, however, if aggressive supportive care, pyridoxine, and sodium bicarbonate are provided, especially given INH's short elimination half-life and the typically short duration of severe symptoms after INH overdose. Patients without the ability to clear INH and its metabolites because of renal failure could be considered for peritoneal dialysis or hemodialysis.[22]

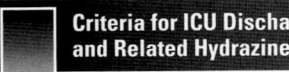

Criteria for ICU Discharge in Isoniazid and Related Hydrazines Poisoning

Resolution of metabolic acidosis and all seizure activity
Return to baseline mental status
Resolving rhabdomyolysis, if present

Common Errors in Isoniazid and Related Hydrazines Poisoning

Overaggressive pyridoxine therapy for prolonged periods
Failure to recognize coma as a toxic effect of overdose from isoniazid
Failure to recognize potential hazards of industrial hydrazines from a contaminated patient
Forgetting the usefulness of adjunctive benzodiazepine therapy in the treatment of seizures

Key Points in Isoniazid and Related Hydrazines Poisoning

1. Never use ipecac syrup.
2. Seizures are most likely to present within the first 3 hours of ingestion.
3. Pyridoxine is the drug of choice for seizures.
4. Benzodiazepines may be useful as adjunctive therapy until sufficient pyridoxine is available.
5. Monitor renal function and hydration status if the patient develops multiple or prolonged seizures.
6. Use sodium bicarbonate therapy for metabolic acidosis.

REFERENCES

1. Mandell GL, Petri WA: Drugs used in the chemotherapy of tuberculosis, mycobacterium avium complex disease, and leprosy. In Hardman JG, Limbird LE (eds): Goodman and Gilman's the Pharmacological Basis of Therapeutics, 9th ed. New York, McGraw-Hill, 1996, pp 1155–1167.
2. Colice GL: Decision analysis, public health policy, and isoniazid chemoprophylaxis for young adult tuberculin skin test reactors. Arch Intern Med 150:2517–2522, 1990.
3. Jordan TJ, Lewit EM, Reichman LB: Isoniazid preventive therapy for tuberculosis: Decision analysis. Am Rev Respir Dis 144:1357–1360, 1991.
4. Tsevat J, Taylor WC, Wong JB, Parker SG: Isoniazid for the tuberculin reactor: Take it or leave it. Am Rev Respir Dis 137:215–220, 1988.
5. Taylor WC, Aaronson MD, Delbanco TL: Should young adults with a positive tuberculin tests take isoniazid? Ann Intern Med 94:808–813, 1981.
6. McCray E, Weinbaum CM, Braden CR, Onorato IM: The epidemiology of tuberculosis in the United States. Clin Chest Med 18:99–113, 1997.
7. New report confirms global spread of drug-resistant tuberculosis. http://www.int/archives/inf-pe-1997/en/pr57–74.html. Accessed 9.21.01.
8. Dye C, Scheele S, Dolin P, et al: Consensus statement: Global burden of tuberculosis: Estimated incidence, prevalence, and mortality by country: WHO Global Surveillance and Monitoring Project. JAMA 282:677–686, 1999.
9. Dye C, Garnett GP, Sleeman K, Williams BG: Prospects for worldwide tuberculosis control under the WHO DOTS strategy. Lancet 352:1886–1191, 1998.
10. Litovitz TL, Klein-Schwartz W, Caravati EM, et al: 1998 Annual report of the American Association of Poison Control Centers Toxic Exposure Surveillance System. Am J Emerg Med 17:435–487, 1999.
11. Litovitz TL, Klein-Schwartz W, Dyer KS, et al: 1997 Annual report of the American Association of Poison Control Centers Toxic Exposure Surveillance System. Am J Emerg Med 16:443–497, 1998.
12. NIOSH Pocket Guide to Chemical Hazards. U.S. Department of Health and Human Services. Washington, DC, 1997, pp 166–167.
13. 1998 TLVs and BEIs. Cincinnati, American Congress of Governmental Industrial Hygienists, 1998, p 42.
14. McEvoy GK (ed): Drug Information 1999. Americal Society of Health System Pharmacists. Bethesda, MD, 1999, pp 481–487.

15. Weber WW, Hein DW: Clinical pharmacokinetics of isoniazid. Clin Pharmacol 4:401–422, 1979.
16. Hankinns DG, Saxena K, Faville RJ, et al: Profound acidosis caused by isoniazid ingestion. Am J Emerg Med 5:165–166, 1987.
17. Siever ML, Herrier RN: Treatment of acute isoniazid toxicity. Am J Hosp Pharm 32:202–206, 1975.
18. Brent J, Nguyen V, Kulig K, Rumack BH: Reversal of prolonged isoniazid-induced coma by pyridoxine. Arch Intern Med 150:1751–1753, 1990.
19. Black LE, Ros SP: Complete recovery from severe metabolic acidosis associated with isoniazid poisoning in a young boy. Pediatr Emerg Care 5:257–258, 1989.
20. Chin L, Sievers ML, Herrier RN, et al: Convulsions as the etiology of lactic acidosis in acute isoniazid toxicity in dogs. Toxicol Appl Pharmacol 49:377–384, 1979.
21. Alao AO, Yolles JC: Isoniazid-induced psychosis. Ann Pharmacother 32:889–891, 1998.
22. Asnis DS, Bhat JG, Melchert AF: Reversible seizures and mental status changes in a dialysis patient on isoniazid preventive therapy. Ann Pharmacother 27:444–446, 1993.
23. Pallone KA, Goldman MP, Fuller MA: Isoniazid-associated psychosis: Case report and review of the literature. Ann Pharmacother 27:167–170, 1993.
24. Blanchard PD, Yao JD, McAlpine DE, Hurt RD: Isoniazid overdose in the Cambodian population of Olmsted County Minnesota. JAMA 256:3131–3133, 1986.
25. Blumberg EA, Gill RA: Cerebellar syndrome caused by isoniazid. DICP 24:829–831, 1990.
26. Biehl JP, Vilter RW: Effects of isoniazid on pyridoxine metabolites. JAMA 156:1549–1552, 1954.
27. Ochoa J: Isoniazid neuropathy in man: Quantitative electron microscope study. Brain 93:831–850, 1970.
28. Siskind MS, Thienemann D, Kiklin L: Isoniazid-induced neurotoxicity in chronic dialysis patients: Reports of three cases and a review of the literature. Nephron 64:303–306, 1993.
29. Pellock JM, Howell J, Kendig EL, Baker H: Pyridoxine deficiency in children treated with isoniazid. Chest 87:658–661, 1985.
30. Holdiness MR: Neurological manifestations and toxicities of the antituberculosis drugs—a review. Med Toxicol 2:33–51, 1987.
31. Gonzalez-Gay MA, Sanchez-Andrade A, Aguerro JJ, et al: Optic neuritis following treatment with isoniazid in a hemodialysed patient (Letter). Nephron 63:360, 1993.
32. Cronkright PJ, Szymaniak G: Isoniazid and rhabdomyolysis (Letter). Ann Intern Med 110:945, 1989.
33. Henderson RP, Davis HL, Self TH: Spiking fevers induced by isoniazid. Drug Intell Clin Pharm 17:741–742, 1983.
34. Polasa R, Colombrita R, Prosperini G, Cacciola R: A case of acute deterioration in asthma symptoms induced by isoniazid prophylaxis. Respir Med 91:438–440, 1997.
35. Rabassa AA, Trey G, Shukla U, et al: Isoniazid-induced acute pancreatitis. Ann Intern Med 121:433–434, 1994.
36. Hoffman R, McPhedran P, Benz EJ, Duffy TP: Isoniazid-induced pure red cell aplasia. Am J Med Sci 286:2–9, 1983.
37. Salazar-Paramo M, Rubin RL, Garcia-De La Torre I: Systemic lupus erythematosus induced by isoniazid. Ann Rheum Dis 51:1085–1087, 1992.
38. Greenberg JH, Lutcher CL: Drug induced systemic lupus erythematosus: A case with life threatening pericardial tamponade. JAMA 22:191–193, 1972.
39. Gaultier, Griscelli C, Hayem F, et al: Lupus induced by isoniazid. Ann Pediatr (Paris) 19:459–468, 1972.
40. Hothersall TE, Mowat AG, Duthie JJ, et al: Drug induced lupus syndrome: A case report implicating isoniazid. Scot Med 18:245, 1968.
41. Grunwald M, David M, Feuerman EJ: Appearance of lupus erythematosus in a patient treated by isoniazid. Dermatologica 165:172–177, 1982.
42. Hofstra AH, Li-Muller SM, Uetrecht JP: Metabolism of isoniazid by activated leukocytes: Possible role in drug induced lupus. Drug Metab Dispos 20:205–210, 1992.
43. Hauser MJ, Baier H: Interactions of isoniazid with foods. Drug Intell Clin Pharm 16:617–618, 1982.
44. Gannon R, Pearsall W, Rowley R: Isoniazid, meperidine, and hypotension (Letter). Ann Intern Med 99:415, 1983.
45. DiMartini A: Isoniazid, tricyclics and the 'cheese reaction.' Int Clin Psychopharmacol 10:197–198, 1995.
46. Judd FK, Mijch AM, Cockram A, Norman TR: Isoniazid and antidepressants: Is there cause for concern? Int Clin Psychopharmacol 9:123–125, 1994.

47. Miller RR, Porter J, Greenblatt DJ: Clinical importance of the interaction of phenytoin and isoniazid: A report from the Boston Collaborative Drug Surveillance Program. Chest 75:356–358, 1979.
48. Block SH: Carbamazepine-isoniazid reaction. Pediatrics 69:494–495, 1982.
49. Sarma GR, Immanuel C, Kailasam S, et al: Rifampin-induced release of hydrazine from isoniazid: A possible cause of hepatitis during the treatment with regimens containing isoniazid and rifampin. Am Rev Respir Dis 133:1072–1075, 1986.
50. O'Shea D, Kim RB, Wilkinson GR: Modulation of CYP2E1 activity by isoniazid in rapid and slow N-actylators. Br J Clin Pharmacol 43:99–103, 1997.
51. Epstein MM, Nelson SD, Slattery JT, et al: Inhibition of the metabolism of paracetamol by isoniazid. Br J Clin Pharmacol 31:139–142, 1991.
52. Self TH, Chrisman CR, Baciewicz, AM, Bronze MS: Isoniazid drug and food interactions. Am J Med Sci 317:304–311, 1999.
53. Zand R, Nelson SD, Slattery JT, et al: Inhibition and induction of cytochrome P450 2E1-catalyzed oxidation by isoniazid in humans. Clin Pharmacol Ther 54:142–149, 1993.
54. Lee WM: Drug induced hepatotoxicity. N Engl J Med 333:1118–1127, 1995.
55. Mitchell JR, Zimmerman HJ, Ishak KG, et al: Isoniazid liver injury: Clinical spectrum, pathology and probable pathogenesis. Ann Intern Med 84:181–192, 1976.
56. Derby LE, Gutthann SP, Jick H, et al: Liver disorders in patients receiving chlorpromazine or isoniazid. Pharmacotherapy 13:353–358, 1993.
57. Steele MA, Burk RF, DesPrez RM: Toxic hepatitis with isoniazid and rifampin: A meta-analysis. Chest 99:465–471, 1991.
58. Nolan CM, Goldberg MD, Buskin SE: Hepatotoxicity associated with isoniazid preventive therapy. JAMA 281:1014–1018, 1999.
59. Black M, Mitchell JR, Zimmerman HJ, et al: Isoniazid-associated hepatitis in 114 patients. Gastroenterology 69:289–302, 1975.
60. Garbaldi RA, Drusin RE, Ferebee SH: Isoniazid-associated hepatitis. Am Rev Respir Dis 106:357–365, 1972.
61. Kopanoff DE, Snider DE, Caras GJ: Isoniazid-related hepatitis. Am Rev Respir Dis 117:991–1001, 1978.
62. American Thoracic Society: Treatment of tuberculosis and other mycobacterial diseases. Am Rev Respir Dis 127:790–796, 1983.
63. Snider DE, Caras GJ: Isoniazid-associated hepatitis deaths: A review of available information. Am Rev Respir Dis 145:494–497, 1992.
64. Franks AL, Binkin NJ, Snider DE, et al: Isoniazid hepatitis among pregnant and post-partum Hispanic patients. Public Health Rep 104:151–155, 1989.
65. Millard PS, Wilcosky TC, Reade-Christopher SJ, Weber DJ: Isoniazid-related fatal hepatitis. West J Med 164:486–491, 1996.
66. Farrell FJ, Keeffe EB, Man KM, et al: Treatment of hepatic failure secondary to isoniazid hepatitis with liver transplantation. Dig Dis Sci 39:2255–2259, 1994.
67. Hasagawa T, Reyes J, Nour B, et al: Successful liver transplantation for isoniazid-induced hepatic failure—a case report. Transplantation 57:1274–1277, 1994.
68. McGlynn KA, Lustbader ED, Sharrar RG, et al: Isoniazid prophylaxis in hepatitis B carriers. Am Rev Respir Dis 134:666–668, 1986.
69. Dickinson DS, Bailey WC, Hirschowitz BI, et al: Risk factors for isoniazid-induced liver dysfunction. J Clin Gastroenterol 3:271–279, 1981.
70. Lauterburg BH, Smith CV, Todd EL, Mitchell JR: Pharmacokinetics of the toxic hydrazino metabolite formed from isoniazid in humans. J Pharm Exp Ther 235:566–570, 1985.
71. Lauterberg BH, Smith CV, Todd EL, Mitchell JR: Oxidation of hydrazine metabolites formed from isoniazid. Clin Pharmacol Ther 38:566–571, 1985.
72. Siefer AD, Albertson TE, Corbett MG: Isoniazid overdose: Pharmacokinetics and effects of oral charcoal in treatment. Hum Toxicol 6:497–501, 1987.
73. Shah BR, Santucci K, Sinert R, Steiner P: Acute isonizid neurotoxicity in an urban hospital. Pediatrics 95:700–704, 1995.
74. Santucci KA, Shah BR, Linakis JG: Acute isoniazid exposures and antidote availability. Pediatr Emerg Care 2:99–101, 1999.
75. Brown A, Mallett M, Fiser D, Arnold WC: Acute isoniazid intoxication: Reversal of CNS symptoms with large doses of pyridoxine. Pediatr Pharmacol (New York) 4:199–202, 1984.
76. Albin RL, Albers JW, Greenberg HS, et al: Acute sensory neuropathy-neuronopathy from pyridoxine overdose. Neurology 37:1729–1732, 1987.
77. Schaumburg H, Kaplan J, Windebank A, et al: Sensory neuropathy from pyridoxine abuse. N Engl J Med 309:445–448, 1983.

CHAPTER 62

Rifampin, Dapsone, and Vancomycin

Cyrus Rangan ▪ Richard F. Clark

RIFAMPIN

Rifampin is a macrocyclic antimicrobial agent synthetically derived from many generations of rifamycin B, a virtually inactive metabolite of *Streptomyces mediterranei*. After laboratory manipulation, a new product, rifamycin SV, was conceived, which showed activity against gram-positive organisms.[1] Rifampin is used today in various settings as a broad-spectrum agent against gram-positive organisms (*Staphylococcus aureus, Staphylococcus epidermidis, Neisseria meningitidis, Haemophilus influenzae*) and gram-negative organisms (*Escherichia coli, Klebsiella, Proteus, Pseudomonas*).[2] More commonly, rifampin is used as a synergistic, bactericidal agent against tuberculous and nontuberculous mycobacteria.

Pharmacology and Pharmacokinetics

The structure of rifampin is shown in Figure 62-1.

Pharmacokinetics of Rifampin

Volume of distribution: 0.97–1.6 L/kg
Protein binding: 75–90%
Mechanism of clearance*: 7% renal
Active metabolites: 25-desacetylrifampin, 3-formylrifamycin
Methods to enhance clearance: multiple-dose activated charcoal

*Assumes normal renal function.

Pathophysiology

By binding to DNA-dependent RNA polymerase in bacteria, rifampin prevents initiation of messenger RNA synthesis (Fig. 62-2).[3] This binding does not occur in mammalian cells. Rifampin induces hepatic microsomal enzymes (CYP3A4), resulting in the increased metabolism of numerous drugs (Table 62-1). Of particular concern in the critical care setting is the increased metabolism (and decreased action) of anticoagulants and corticosteroids.

Clinical Presentation

Daily use of rifampin has few serious side effects. Red-orange discoloration of body fluids (e.g., urine, tears) is common with therapeutic and toxic doses, and its incidence

increases in a dose-dependent fashion.[4] Mild elevation of hepatic transaminases and cholestatic jaundice occur, especially when rifampin is used in combination with isoniazid, but symptomatic hepatitis or liver failure seems to be limited to elderly patients, undernourished patients, and patients with chronic liver disease.[5,6] When rifampin is administered on an intermittent basis (once-weekly or twice-weekly dosing) or when it is reintroduced after prolonged discontinuation, there is an increased incidence of a flulike syndrome, including fever and chills, headache, malaise, and weakness with colitis and eosinophilia.[7,8] Hemolytic anemia and thrombocytopenia also occur in these circumstances and may be antibody mediated. Acute renal failure has been reported, including rapidly progressive glomerulonephritis, acute interstitial nephritis, and light-chain proteinuria.[9] Although the mechanism for renal failure is unclear, it may be hemoglobinuric in association with intravascular hemolysis or mediated by rifampin-dependent IgG and IgM antibodies cross-reacting with the I-antigen on tubular epithelium.[10] Rifampin-induced lupus-like syndrome also has been reported when rifampin is used in combination with clarithromycin or ciprofloxacin and may involve autoantibody production.[11] Drowsiness and confusion have been observed in massive overdoses. Anaphylactoid reactions can occur with therapeutic use and overdosage and may require intensive care unit admission.

Diagnostic Considerations

Rifampin serum concentrations are available, but studies to correlate levels with occurrence or severity of toxicity are lacking. Determination of hepatic transaminases and fractionated bilirubin may be useful, especially when rifampin is used in combination with isoniazid or other potential hepatotoxins or used in the elderly. These laboratory parameters should be followed closely in symptomatic patients. There are no commercially available tests for the detection of rifampin-dependent antibodies.[12]

Treatment

Indications for ICU Admission in Rifampin Poisoning

Severe anaphylactoid reaction
Fulminant hepatic failure
Acute renal failure requiring dialysis

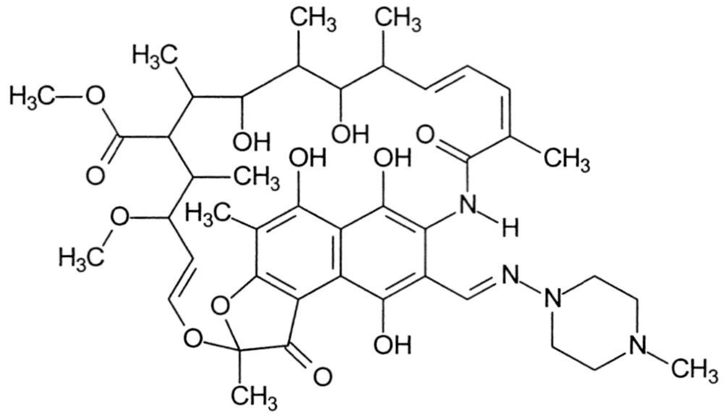

FIGURE 62-1

Chemical structure of rifampin.

TABLE 62-1 Agents with Increased Metabolism during Coadministration of Rifampin

Benzodiazepines	Phenobarbital
β-Blockers	Quinidine
Calcium channel blockers	Sulfonylureas
Clofibrate	Theophylline
Corticosteroids	Warfarin
Dapsone	Lamotrigine
Fungicidal agents	Reverse transcriptase inhibitors
Methadone	HMG-CoA reductase inhibitors
Oral contraceptives	

HMG-CoA, 3-Hydroxy-3-methylglutaryl–coenzyme A.

Discontinuation of rifampin usually is sufficient to correct mild elevations in hepatic transaminases and rifampin-induced renal failure.[5,10] There are no formally validated or accepted general criteria for discontinuation, however. The red-orange skin discoloration is treated with simple cleansing.[4] In cases of fulminant hepatic failure, liver transplantation may be considered.[13,14] For patients who experience a toxic effect of rifampin, standard supportive care is fundamental. There are no specific antidotes to rifampin toxicity. Several other specific therapeutic interventions are described subsequently.

ACTIVATED CHARCOAL

Single-dose activated charcoal generally is recommended for acute overdose of large amounts if this administration can be accomplished soon after ingestion (see Chapter 6). There are no data indicating whether activated charcoal alters the outcome or clinical course after rifampin ingestion. Multiple-dose activated charcoal (described in detail in Chapter 6) may increase rifampin clearance, but improvement in clinical outcome with this intervention has not been shown.[15]

EXTRACORPOREAL REMOVAL

Rifampin's high protein binding and large volume of distribution preclude the elimination of rifampin by extracorporeal removal.

Special Populations

PEDIATRIC PATIENTS

There are no special considerations regarding rifampin in pediatric patients.

PREGNANT PATIENTS

Rifampin is classified by the U.S. Food and Drug Administration (FDA) as Pregnancy Category C (see Appendix A). Rifampin has been shown to cause fetal malformations in mice, but this has not been shown in humans. Rifampin is recommended in cases of pregnant women with active tuberculosis.

ELDERLY PATIENTS

There is an increased incidence of hepatic and renal injury with rifampin in elderly patients.[6,9]

CHRONIC LIVER DISEASE PATIENTS

Patients with chronic liver disease are at increased risk for rifampin-induced hepatic failure.[14]

DAPSONE

Dapsone is a synthetic sulfone antimicrobial used for the prophylaxis of *Pneumocystis carinii* in immunocompromised patients with documented adverse reactions to trimethoprim-sulfamethoxazole.[16] Sulfones have experimental activity against many mycobacteria, and they are used clinically as a bacteriostatic agent in the treatment of *Mycobacterium leprae*, although drug resistance is increasing.[17] Occasionally, dapsone is used to treat chloroquine-resistant malaria, although resistance to dapsone therapy is increasing as well.[18] Dapsone is capable of suppressing neutrophil

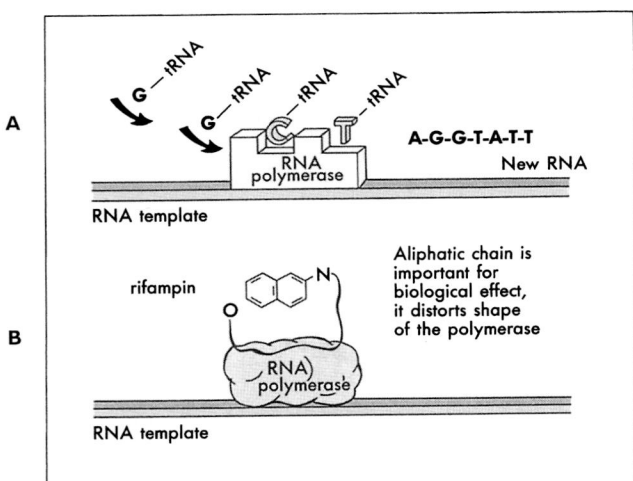

FIGURE 62-2

Mechanism of rifampin action. The drug binds to the β-subunit of DNA-dependent RNA polymerase and inhibits initiation of (but not ongoing) RNA synthesis. **A**, Drug is absent. **B**, Drug is bound to the polymerase and distorts the conformation of the enzyme so that it cannot initiate a new chain. *(From Brody H, Larner J, Minneman KP, et al: Human Pharmacology: Molecular to Clinical, 3rd ed. St. Louis, Mosby, 1998, p 725.)*

migration by blocking integrin-mediated adherence.[19] For this reason, it has been successful in the treatment of dermatologic disorders, such as dermatitis herpetiformis, pemphigus vulgaris, pyoderma gangrenosum, psoriasis, and systemic lupus erythematosus.[20] The often-touted use of dapsone as a treatment for the necrotic lesions caused by the brown recluse spider is not well supported.[21]

Pharmacology and Pharmacokinetics

The structure of dapsone is shown in Figure 62-3.

Pharmacokinetics of Dapsone

Volume of distribution: 1.0–1.5 L/kg
Protein binding: 70–90%
Mechanism of clearance*: 15% renal
Active metabolite: monoacetyldapsone
Methods to enhance clearance: multiple-dose activated charcoal, charcoal hemoperfusion

*Assumes normal renal function.

Pathophysiology

Dapsone is a bacteriostatic antimicrobial agent that binds to dihydropteroate synthase, which catalyzes the conversion of paraaminobenzoic acid and pteridine into dihydropteroic acid in the first step of folic acid synthesis. Folic acid is essential for the formation of methionine, which is necessary for nucleic acid synthesis. Bacteria that depend on intrinsic folic acid are affected by dapsone.[18]

Dapsone causes oxidant stress to the hematologic system. Hemolysis and methemoglobinemia may occur either separately or together. Dapsone-derived free radicals, formed by the biotransformation of dapsone into free arylamines and hydroxylamines, bind to the red blood cell membrane and to hemoglobin, leading to the formation of precipitated, denatured proteins (Heinz bodies). Heinz bodies attach to the red blood cell membrane, causing the affected erythrocytes to be destroyed by the reticuloendothelial system.[22] When oxidants, such as dapsone, are directed specifically toward the iron ion within hemoglobin, they act as electron acceptors, oxidizing divalent iron (Fe^{2+}) to trivalent iron (Fe^{3+}), forming methemoglobin, which is unable to transport oxygen. In addition, induction of methemoglobinemia shifts the oxygen-hemoglobin dissociation curve to the left, further impairing oxygen delivery to tissues. Although red blood cells have a natural defense (reduced glutathione) against oxidizing agents, these stores can be depleted rapidly in cases of drug-

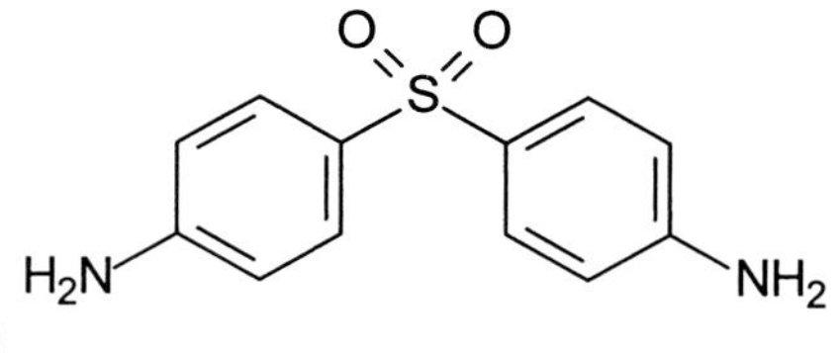

FIGURE 62-3

Chemical structure of dapsone.

induced hemolysis or methemoglobinemia, which may occur separately or together.[23] Oxidant effects on erythrocytes are discussed in greater detail in Chapter 28.

Sulfhemoglobinemia also can be induced by dapsone. Sulfhemoglobin also is incapable of carrying oxygen. It shifts the oxygen-hemoglobin dissociation curve to the right, however, which enhances overall oxygen delivery to tissues.[24]

Dapsone-induced maculopathy is presumed to occur secondary to the physical effects of red blood cell fragmentation in the vascular supply to the macular and perimacular regions of the eye, resulting in ischemic necrosis.[25] Dapsone-induced acute renal failure is thought to occur via a similar mechanism.[26] The "sulfone syndrome" may be induced by antibodies directed toward the free arylamine and hydroxylamine metabolites of dapsone.[26]

Clinical Presentation

Hemolysis and methemoglobinemia are the most widely known toxicities of dapsone. Although doses of greater than 200 mg/day are thought to be required to induce hemolysis in adults, the induction of methemoglobinemia seems to be a critical adverse therapeutic effect. Hemolytic anemia may manifest with tachycardia, pallor, jaundice, hypoxia, acidemia, and shock. Methemoglobinemia presents with cyanosis if blood methemoglobin concentration exceeds 1.5 g/dL. If hemolysis is excessive and hemoglobin concentrations decrease, the cyanosis may disappear (see Chapter 28).

The clinical presentation of dapsone-induced methemoglobinemia may be delayed (up to 3 days) and may be prolonged and recurrent, owing to the drug's delayed peak (up to 20 hours in overdose) and long half-life (30 hours in therapeutic settings; up to 77 hours in overdose).[27,28] Children younger than 4 years old may express much higher methemoglobin contents secondary to a relative deficiency in reduced nicotine adenine dinucleotide (NADH)–dependent methemoglobin reductase,[29] the enzyme responsible for reducing methemoglobin to hemoglobin.

The clinical presentation of sulfhemoglobinemia is generally similar to but less severe than that of methemoglobinemia. In both cases, patients may present with falsely low pulse oximetry readings yet with normal arterial blood gas PO_2. Patients with sulfhemoglobinemia rarely present with significant cyanosis because the amount of sulfhemoglobin generated in most cases is less than 5% of total hemoglobin.[24]

Other nonspecific effects include nausea, vomiting, rashes, and psychosis. There is controversial evidence that dapsone causes axonal degeneration, resulting in peripheral neuropathy.[27] Although dapsone is used as a treatment for leprosy, it also has been shown to exacerbate the condition.[17] Agranulocytosis is a rare effect of dapsone therapy.[30] Also reported is the "sulfone (hypersensitivity) syndrome," which can develop 2 months after starting long-term treatment with dapsone; methemoglobin and hemolytic anemia occur in addition to fever, exfoliative dermatitis, and fulminant hepatic necrosis with jaundice.[31]

Diagnostic Considerations

Any immunocompromised patient who presents with cyanosis or signs of hemodynamic instability should be suspected of dapsone poisoning. Serum concentrations of dapsone are available but do not correlate well with signs of toxicity.[23] Because of the long half-life of dapsone and the gradual cumulative process of injury to red blood cells, signs of toxicity may be delayed so that patients may be asymptomatic for hours before developing methemoglobinemia or hemolysis in overdose. In dapsone-induced hemolysis, hemoglobin concentrations may be low or normal, but the appearance of Heinz bodies on the peripheral blood smear may be an early indication of hemolysis. The reticulocyte count also may be elevated, although this typically is delayed for several days.[22] During hemolysis, testing for glucose-6-phosphate dehydrogenase (G6PD) activity may not be clinically useful because these patients have a predominance of young peripheral red blood cells with possibly normal G6PD activity.[23] In dapsone-induced methemoglobinemia, cooximetry can be used to measure methemoglobin concentrations but may read sulfhemoglobin falsely as methemoglobin. Most cooximeters are not designed to distinguish between methemoglobin and sulfhemoglobin.[24] Pulse oximetry is potentially misleading and should not be used alone as a diagnostic tool to assess tissue hypoxia; however, a low pulse oximetry reading that does not change with oxygen therapy should raise suspicion of methemoglobinemia.[32]

Treatment

Discontinuation of dapsone with subsequent observation usually is sufficient for most cases of mild dapsone-induced hemolytic anemia and methemoglobinemia. A normal bone marrow typically compensates for mild red blood cell loss. Exchange or conventional (packed red blood cell) transfusion may be required in severe cases. The reduction of methemoglobin in red blood cells normally occurs predominantly via the action of NADH cytochrome-b_5 reductase (see Fig. 28-4). This mechanism decreases methemoglobin content by approximately 15% per hour.[33] Slower endogenous detoxification rates may reflect intrinsic defects in cytochrome-b_5 reductase activity or ongoing production of methemoglobinemia. Pulse oximetry usually gives falsely low measurements in sulfhemoglobinemia and methemoglobinemia.[27] Management of oxidant-induced hemolysis and methemoglobinemia is discussed in detail in Chapter 28.

GASTROINTESTINAL DECONTAMINATION

Single-dose activated charcoal generally is recommended for acute overdose if it can be administered soon after ingestion (see Chapter 6). There are no data indicating, however, whether activated charcoal administration alters the outcome or clinical course after dapsone overdose.

Indications for ICU Admission in Dapsone Poisoning

Severe hemolysis or methemoglobinemia with secondary hypoxia, cardiovascular impairment, or shock
Renal failure requiring dialysis
Hepatic failure and/or presence of severe cutaneous involvement in the "sulfone syndrome"

EXTRACORPOREAL REMOVAL

Hemodialysis generally is not recommended because of dapsone's high protein binding and large volume of distribution (see Table 62-1). Charcoal hemoperfusion may be beneficial in severe cases that do not respond to conventional treatment because the long half-life of dapsone can be decreased significantly.[34] There are no studies documenting improvement, however, in clinical outcome or course after hemoperfusion.

METHYLENE BLUE

Methylene blue's antidotal actions reflect its function as a cofactor for reduced nicotine adenine dinucleotide phosphate (NADPH) methemoglobin reductase (see Fig. 28-4). This enzyme, normally a minor contributor to methemoglobin reduction, uses products from the hexose monophosphate shunt as a source of electrons for the reduction of methemoglobin. The conversion of glucose-6-phosphate to 6-phosphogluconate by G6PD in the first step of the pentose monophosphate shunt provides electrons for the conversion of NADP to NADPH. Methylene blue first is reduced to leukomethylene blue by electron donation from cellular NADPH stores. Leukomethylene blue, through the actions of NADPH methemoglobin reductase, donates these electrons to methemoglobin, reducing the Fe^{3+} in the heme group to the Fe^{2+} state and consequently reverting back to methylene blue (see Chapter 28). The usual dose of methylene blue is 1 to 2 mg/kg intravenously over 5 to 10 minutes.[35] Repeat dosing may be considered in 1 hour. If cyanosis persists, one must consider ongoing methemoglobin production, G6PD deficiency, or sulfhemoglobinemia. There is no antidote for sulfhemoglobinemia.

OTHER TREATMENTS

Multiple-dose activated charcoal may increase dapsone clearance, but improvement in clinical outcome has not been shown.[15] Severe methemoglobinemia and sulfhemoglobinemia unresponsive to conventional therapy can be treated with exchange transfusion.[32] Sulfone syndrome is best treated by the cessation of dapsone use. The administration of systemic corticosteroids is advocated in case studies, although controlled trials documenting their efficacy are lacking.[27,31]

Special Populations

PEDIATRIC PATIENTS

Dapsone doses of 100 mg (one tablet) in a child have been reported to cause hemolysis and methemoglobinemia.[32]

PREGNANT PATIENTS

Dapsone is a U.S. FDA Pregnancy Category C drug (see Appendix A). Studies documenting teratogenicity are lacking. Dapsone is theorized to be a potential cause of neural tube defects secondary to its effects on the folate synthesis pathway. Nursing mothers should avoid dapsone due to the potential for hemolysis and methemoglobinemia in the infant.

ELDERLY PATIENTS

There are no special considerations in elderly patients.

PATIENTS WITH GLUCOSE-6-PHOSPHATE DEHYDROGENASE DEFICIENCY

Patients with G6PD deficiency have a decreased capacity in the red blood cells to produce adequate levels of NADPH (see Fig. 28-2). NADPH is required to maintain appropriate stores of reduced glutathione, the red blood cell's primary defense against oxidants. These patients are more susceptible to developing hemolysis and methemoglobinemia after dapsone administration. There may be an increased risk of hemolysis or methemoglobinemia induced by methylene blue administration because the antidote itself is a mild oxidant that competes for the same NADPH required for maintenance of glutathione stores.[36] In a patient in whom methylene blue is contraindicated on the basis of G6PD deficiency, exchange transfusion can be beneficial.[32]

VANCOMYCIN

Vancomycin is a complex glycopeptide antimicrobial agent derived from *Streptomyces orientalis* bacteria found in the soil in the Far East. It is used primarily as a parenteral agent against gram-positive bacterial infections, particularly resistant strains of *S. epidermidis* and *S. aureus*, and as a synergistic agent with aminoglycosides against resistant *Enterococcus*, viridans streptococci, *Streptococcus pyogenes*, and *Streptococcus pneumoniae*.[37] Vancomycin also is used orally in patients with pseudomembranous colitis secondary to *Clostridium difficile*[38]

and in bone marrow transplant patients to maintain gastrointestinal sterility during transplantation.[39]

Pharmacology and Pharmacokinetics

The structure of vancomycin is shown in Figure 62-4.

Pharmacokinetics of Vancomycin

Volume of distribution: 0.11–0.39 L/kg
Protein binding: 30–55%
Mechanism of clearance*: 79% renal
Active metabolites: none
Methods to enhance clearance: hemodialysis, hemodiafiltration

*Assumes normal renal function

Pathophysiology of Therapeutic and Toxic Effects

Vancomycin inhibits cell wall synthesis in bacteria by binding to the D-alanyl-D-alanine moiety of cell wall precursors. Transpeptidase is unable to catalyze the linkage of D-alanine to glycine into the peptidoglycan chain, and cell wall synthesis subsequently stops.[40] Dividing cells are particularly susceptible to the actions of vancomycin, which is well known to cause hypersensitivity reactions, particularly "red man"

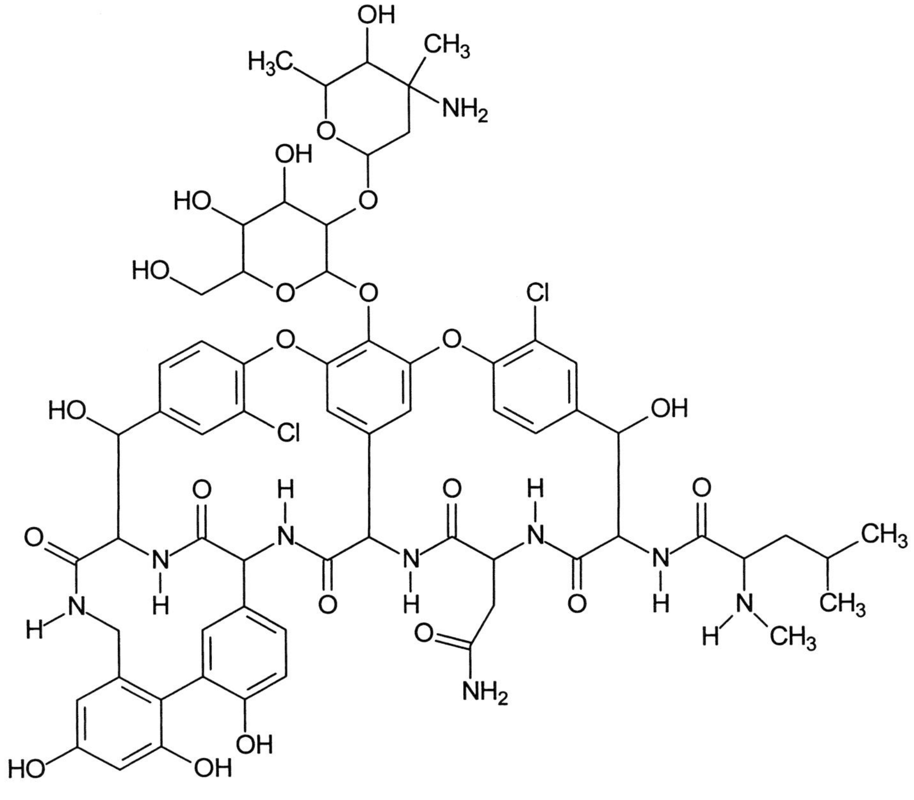

FIGURE 62-4

Chemical structure of vancomycin.

syndrome, thought to be a histamine-mediated anaphylactoid reaction.[41] The pathophysiologic mechanisms of ototoxicity and nephrotoxicity are unclear.

Clinical Presentation

Red man syndrome seems to be rate related and dose related. Symptoms usually are self-limited and commonly include urticaria and pruritus but also may include dyspnea, chest tightness, and hypotension. Tachyphylaxis is common, although reductions in dosages and dosing rates have improved cases.[42] Anaphylaxis also has been reported, suggesting that red man syndrome may represent true vancomycin allergy.[43] Transient and permanent hearing loss has occurred in patients with high peak plasma vancomycin concentrations (60 to 100 mg/L), but the mechanism of action is unclear.[44]

Nephrotoxicity has been reported in adults with high peak concentrations (>40 mg/L). A case-control study in newborns showed that no patients with measured serum peak concentrations greater than 40 mg/L developed nephrotoxicity (defined as a doubling of baseline creatinine or a creatinine level >0.6 mg/dL [>6.0 mg/L]), whereas 9 of 61 newborns with vancomycin peaks less than 40 mg/L did develop elevations in serum creatinine.[45] Conclusive evidence regarding the correlation between vancomycin drug levels and the appearance of ototoxicity and nephrotoxicity is lacking, and a mechanism of action has not been proved.[46] Although rare, vancomycin-dependent antiplatelet and antineutrophil antibodies can be induced by vancomycin administration.[47,48]

Diagnostic Considerations

Serum vancomycin concentration provides the most direct measure of potential vancomycin toxicity. Patients with end-stage renal disease are at particular risk for developing toxicity with conventional therapeutic dosing of vancomycin.[49] Pharmacokinetic evidence suggests that vancomycin fits a two-compartment profile in children, with a first-phase half-life ($t_{1/2\alpha}$) of 0.80 hours and a second-phase half-life ($t_{1/2\beta}$) of 5.63 hours. Serum vancomycin concentrations measured earlier than 4 hours after a dose may not reflect the postdistribution peak concentrations. Measured peak serum concentrations of vancomycin in children may not be predictive of toxicity.[50,51]

Treatment

Slowing the rate or diluting intravenous vancomycin infusions can prevent the occurrence of red man syndrome. Concomitant or prior administration of diphenhydramine also has been effective.[52] Ototoxicity and nephrotoxicity are generally reversible with dose readjustment or discontinuation.[53]

GASTROINTESTINAL DECONTAMINATION

Vancomycin is poorly absorbed orally, so gastrointestinal decontamination is not necessary.

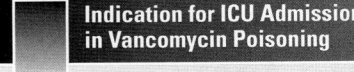

Indication for ICU Admission in Vancomycin Poisoning

Severe anaphylactoid reaction

EXTRACORPOREAL REMOVAL

Hemodialysis can remove vancomycin effectively in patients with impaired renal function.[50,53] Charcoal hemoperfusion also may be useful, but no studies have documented its superiority over dialysis.

Special Populations

PEDIATRIC PATIENTS

Dosing intervals may have to be adjusted in neonates, secondary to relatively decreased excretion of vancomycin by neonatal kidneys. High vancomycin trough levels in neonates may necessitate twice-daily or once-daily dosing.[50]

PREGNANT PATIENTS

Vancomycin is a U.S. FDA Pregnancy Category C drug (see Appendix A). Because vancomycin appears in cord blood, it is thought to pose risks of ototoxicity and nephrotoxicity to the fetus, but this effect has not been shown by controlled studies.

ELDERLY PATIENTS

Dosing intervals may have to be adjusted for hepatic or renal insufficiency.

REFERENCES

1. Sensi P: History of the development of rifampin. Rev Infect Dis 5(Suppl 3):S402-S406, 1983.
2. Loeffler AM: Uses of rifampin for infections other than tuberculosis. Pediatr Infect Dis J 18:631–632, 1999.
3. Campbell EA, Korzheva N, Mustaev A, et al: Structural mechanism for rifampicin inhibition of bacterial RNA polymerase. Cell 104:901–912, 2001.
4. Holdiness MR: A review of the redman syndrome and rifampicin overdosage. Med Toxicol Adverse Drug Exp 4:444–451, 1989.
5. Hong Kong Chest Service/Tuberculosis Research Centre, Madras/British Medical Research Council: A double-blind placebo-controlled clinical trial of three antituberculosis chemoprophylaxis regimens in patients with silicosis in Hong Kong. Am Rev Respir Dis 145:36–41, 1992.
6. Dossing M, Wilcke JT, Askgaard DS, et al: Liver injury during antituberculosis treatment: An 11-year study. Tuber Lung Dis 77:335–340, 1996.
7. Lange P, Oun H, Fuller S, et al: Eosinophilic colitis due to rifampicin. Lancet 344:1296–1297, 1994.
8. Dutt AK, Moers D, Stead WW: Undesirable side effects of isoniazid and rifampin in largely twice-weekly short-course chemotherapy for tuberculosis. Am Rev Respir Dis 128:419–424, 1983.
9. Covic A, Goldsmith DJ, Segall L, et al: Rifampicin-induced acute renal failure: A series of 60 patients. Nephrol Dial Transplant 13:924–929, 1998.
10. De Vriese AS, Robbrecht DL, Vanholder RC, et al: Rifampicin-associated acute renal failure: Pathophysiologic, immunologic, and clinical features. Am J Kidney Dis 31:108–115, 1998.
11. Patel GK, Anstey AV: Rifampicin-induced lupus erythematosus. Clin Exp Dermatol 26:260–262, 2001.
12. Burman WJ, Gallicano K, Peloquin C: Comparative pharmacokinetics and pharmacodynamics of the rifamycin antibacterials. Clin Pharmacokinet 40:327–341, 2001.
13. McKeon J, Patel AM: Antituberculous therapy and acute liver failure. Lancet 345:1170–1171, 1995.
14. Di Piazza S, Cottone M, Craxi A, et al: Severe rifampicin-associated liver failure in patients with compensated cirrhosis. Lancet 1:774, 1978.
15. Position statement and practice guidelines on the use of multi-dose activated charcoal in the treatment of acute poisoning. American Academy of Clinical Toxicology; European Association of Poisons Centres and Clinical Toxicologists. J Toxicol Clin Toxicol 37:731–751, 1999.
16. Blanchet KD: Current management practices in the treatment of Pneumocystis carinii pneumonia (PCP). AIDS Patient Care STDS 10:116–121, 1996.

17. Williams DL, Pittman TL, Gillis TP, et al: Simultaneous detection of *Mycobacterium leprae* and its susceptibility to dapsone using DNA heteroduplex analysis. J Clin Microbiol 39:2083–2088, 2001.

18. Triglia T, Menting JG, Wilson C, et al: Mutations in dihydropteroate synthase are responsible for sulfone and sulfonamide resistance in *Plasmodium falciparum*. Proc Natl Acad Sci U S A 94:13944–13949, 1997.

19. Booth SA, Moody CE, Dahl MV, et al: Dapsone suppresses integrin-mediated neutrophil adherence function. J Invest Dermatol 98:135–140, 1992.

20. Zhu YI, Stiller MJ: Dapsone and sulfones in dermatology: Overview and update. J Am Acad Dermatol 45(3 Pt 1):420–434, 2001.

21. Rees R, Campbell D, Rieger E, et al: The diagnosis and treatment of brown recluse spider bites. Ann Emerg Med 16:945–949, 1987.

22. Jollow DJ, Bradshaw TP, McMillan DC: Dapsone-induced hemolytic anemia. Drug Metab Rev 27:107–124, 1995.

23. Solheim L, Brun AC, Greibrokk TS, et al: Methemoglobinemia—causes, diagnosis, and treatment. Tidsskr Nor Laegeforen 120:1549–1551, 2000.

24. Lambert M, Sonnet J, Mahieu P, et al: Delayed sulfhemoglobinemia after acute dapsone intoxication. J Toxicol Clin Toxicol 19:45–60, 1982.

25. Kenner DJ, Holt K, Agnello R, et al: Permanent retinal damage following massive dapsone overdosage. Br J Ophthalmol 64:741–744, 1980.

26. Chugh KS, Singhal PC, Sharma BK, et al: Acute renal failure due to intravascular hemolysis in the North Indian patients. Am J Med Sci 274:139–146, 1977.

27. Woodhouse KW, Henderson DB, Charlton B, et al: Acute dapsone poisoning: Clinical features and pharmacokinetic studies. Hum Toxicol 2:507–510, 1983.

28. Elonen E, Neuvonen PJ, Halmekoski J, et al: Acute dapsone intoxication: A case with prolonged symptoms. Clin Toxicol 14:79–85, 1979.

29. Kugler W, Pekrun A, Laspe P, et al: Molecular basis of recessive congenital methemoglobinemia, types I and II: Exon skipping and three novel missense mutations in the NADH-cytochrome b_5 reductase (diaphorase 1) gene. Hum Mutat 17:348, 2001.

30. Coleman MD: Dapsone-mediated agranulocytosis: Risks, possible mechanisms and prevention. Toxicology 162:53–60, 2001.

31. Chalasani P, Baffoe-Bonnie H, Jurado RL: Dapsone therapy causing sulfone syndrome and lethal hepatic failure in an HIV-infected patient. South Med J 87:1145–1146, 1994.

32. Coleman MD, Coleman NA: Drug-induced methaemoglobinaemia: Treatment issues. Drug Saf 14:394–405, 1996.

33. Mansouri A, Lurie AA: Concise review: Methemoglobinemia. Am J Hematol 42:7–12, 1993.

34. Endre ZH, Charlesworth JA, Macdonald GJ, et al: Successful treatment of acute dapsone intoxication using charcoal hemoperfusion. Aust N Z J Med 13:509–512, 1983.

35. Dawson AH, Whyte IM: Management of dapsone poisoning complicated by methaemoglobinaemia. Med Toxicol Adverse Drug Exp 4:387–392, 1989.

36. Goldstein BD: Exacerbation of dapsone-induced Heinz body hemolytic anemia following treatment with methylene blue. Am J Med Sci 267:291–297, 1974.

37. Drori-Zeides T, Raveh D, Schlesinger Y, et al: Practical guidelines for vancomycin usage, with prospective drug-utilization evaluation. Infect Control Hosp Epidemiol 21:45–47, 2000.

38. Gerding DN: Treatment of *Clostridium difficile*-associated diarrhea and colitis. Curr Top Microbiol Immunol 250:127–139, 2000.

39. Arns da Cunha C, Weisdorf D, Shu XO, et al: Early gram-positive bacteremia in BMT recipients: Impact of three different approaches to antimicrobial prophylaxis. Bone Marrow Transplant 21:173–180, 1998.

40. Chiosis G, Boneca IG: Selective cleavage of D-Ala-D-Lac by small molecules: Re-sensitizing resistant bacteria to vancomycin. Science 293:1484–1487, 2001.

41. Veien M, Szlam F, Holden JT, et al: Mechanisms of nonimmunological histamine and tryptase release from human cutaneous mast cells. Anesthesiology 92:1074–1081, 2000.

42. Polk RE: Anaphylactoid reactions to glycopeptide antibiotics. J Antimicrob Chemother 27:17–29, 1991.

43. Hassaballa H, Mallick N, Orlowski J: Vancomycin anaphylaxis in a patient with vancomycin-induced red man syndrome. Am J Ther 7:319–320, 2000.

44. Brummett RE: Ototoxicity of vancomycin and analogues. Otolaryngol Clin North Am 26:821–828, 1993.

45. Bhatt-Mehta V, Schumacher RE, Faix RG, et al: Lack of vancomycin-associated nephrotoxicity in newborn infants: A case-control study. Pediatrics 103:E48, 1999.

46. Cantu TG, Yamanaka-Yuen NA, Lietman PS: Serum vancomycin concentrations: Reappraisal of their clinical value. Clin Infect Dis 18:533–543, 1994.

47. Christie DJ, Van Buren N, Lennon SS, et al: Vancomycin-dependent antibodies associated with thrombocytopenia and refractoriness to platelet transfusion in patients with leukemia. Blood 785:518–525, 1990.

48. Domen RE, Horowitz S: Vancomycin-induced neutropenia associated with anti-granulocyte antibodies. Immunohematology 6:41–43, 1990.

49. Somerville AL, Wright DH, Rotschafer JC: Implications of vancomycin degradation products on therapeutic drug monitoring in patients with end-stage renal disease. Pharmacotherapy 19:702–707, 1999.

50. Wrishko RE, Levine M, Khoo D, et al: Vancomycin pharmacokinetics and Bayesian estimation in pediatric patients. Ther Drug Monit 22:522–531, 2000.

51. Lamarre P, Lebel D, Ducharme MP: A population pharmacokinetic model for vancomycin in pediatric patients and its predictive value in a naive population. Antimicrob Agents Chemother 44:278–282, 2000.

52. Wallace MR, Mascola JR, Oldfield EC: Red man syndrome: Incidence, etiology, and prophylaxis. J Infect Dis 164:1180–1185, 1991.

53. Appel GB, Given DB, Levine LR, et al: Vancomycin and the kidney. Am J Kidney Dis 8:75–80, 1986.

CHAPTER 63

Chloroquine and Quinine

Alison L. Jones

CHLOROQUINE

Chloroquine is used to prevent and treat malaria and to manage systemic lupus erythematosus and rheumatoid arthritis. It is the most severe and frequent cause of poisoning by antimalarial drugs. Among 167 chloroquine poisoning cases admitted to a toxicology critical care unit, the mortality was less than 10%; these are the best survival figures quoted in the literature to date.[1] Chloroquine is a frequent method of suicide in Africa[2] and France.[3]

Chemistry and Pharmacology

The chemical name of chloroquine is 7-chloro-4-(4′-diethyl-amino-1′-methylbutylamino)-quinoline ($C_{18}H_{26}ClN_3$) (Fig. 63-1). Its molecular weight is 319.9, and it has pK_a values of 8.4 and 10.8. It is insoluble in water.

Chloroquine is absorbed readily from the gastrointestinal tract; the bioavailability is 78% for solution and 89% for tablets. Chloroquine accumulates in high concentrations in tissues such as kidneys, liver, lungs, and spleen. It is bound strongly in melanin-containing cells, such as those in the eyes and retina. It has a low toxic/therapeutic margin, and care must be taken in prescription to prevent unintentional intoxication.

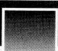

Pharmacokinetics of Chloroquine*

Apparent volume of distribution: 116–285 L/kg[28]
Protein binding: 50–65% in plasma
Mechanism of clearance: 61% urinary excretion
Active metabolite: desethylchloroquine
Terminal half-life:† 60 days
Methods to enhance clearance: none effective other than activated charcoal

*The half-life correlates well with peak plasma concentration; toxicokinetics is dose dependent.

†Terminal half-life of desethylchloroquine even longer.

Pathophysiology of Toxic Effects

Cardiovascular toxicity of chloroquine is due to its quinidine-like (class Ia) actions. It inhibits spontaneous depolarization, slows conduction, lengthens the refractory period, and raises the electrical depolarization threshold. These actions cause depressed contractility, impaired conductivity, and decreased excitability but heighten the possibility of reentrant arrhythmias.[4] The pathophysiology of the effect of these sodium channel–blocking agents is described in Chapter 36. Hypotension and shock are due to negative inotropic activity rather than peripheral vasodilation.[5] Neurologic symptoms of chloroquine are due to either direct central nervous system toxicity, which lowers the threshold for convulsions, or cerebral ischemia secondary to cardiovascular disturbances.

The mechanisms of hypokalemia have not been established, but its close temporal relationship with chloroquine toxicity suggests a potassium transport disturbance.[6,7] The data collected in the study by Clemessy and colleagues[7] do not favor the idea of hypokalemia as a result of potassium depletion. Hypokalemia cannot be attributable to gastrointestinal losses because diarrhea is not common, and vomiting occurs in only about 30% of cases and is not prolonged. Urinary potassium wasting is not responsible because potassium losses in urine are low. Alkalosis is not the cause because most patients are acidotic.[7] Hypokalemia by intracellular transport of potassium is the most likely scenario.[7]

Clinical Presentation and Life-Threatening Complications

Chloroquine overdoses usually have several characteristics in common. The interval between ingestion and onset of symptoms is short, and death, when it occurs, is often within 12 hours. At autopsy, common findings include cerebral and pulmonary edema. Tissue concentrations in a fatal overdose are shown in Table 63-1.[8] Therapeutic plasma concentration is 1 mg/L (3.1 μmol/L).[9] Plasma values reflect only a small proportion of total body chloroquine load because its apparent volume of distribution is high. The mortality rate in published studies is 12% to 35% and is among the highest in clinical toxicology.[10,11] Symptoms of chloroquine overdose usually start within 1 to 3 hours of ingestion and include nausea, vomiting, agitation, drowsiness, hypokalemia, headaches, and visual disturbances.[12] After large ingestions, rigidity, coma, convulsions, hypotension, and arrhythmias occur.

CARDIOVASCULAR

In severe poisoning, cardiovascular signs promptly follow the appearance of the initial symptoms.[2,11] Cardiac arrest can be the first sign of overdose, however.[5] Hypotension is one of the most frequent signs of chloroquine poisoning

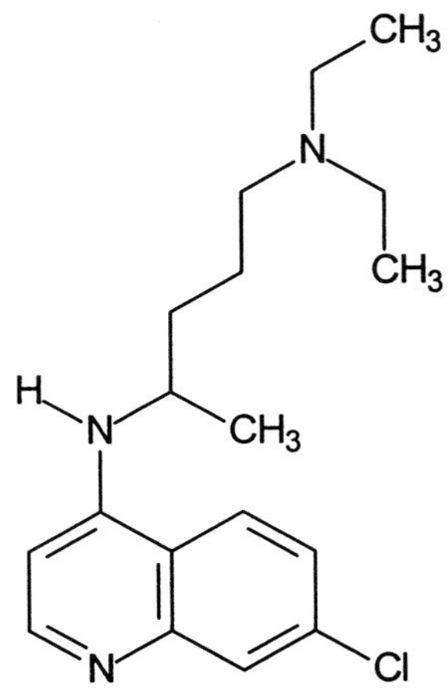

FIGURE 63-1

Chemical structure of chloroquine.

and without appropriate therapy may progress rapidly to cardiogenic shock with increased central venous pressure.

Electrocardiographic abnormalities include modifications of repolarization with prolonged QT_c or QRS interval, increased U waves, and depression of the ST-T segment and flattened or inverted T waves. Intraventricular conduction delay and QRS widening are common. Atrioventricular block is less common. Ventricular tachycardia or fibrillation is observed early in chloroquine poisoning, and cardiac arrests tend to occur during the first hours. Ventricular extrasystoles and torsades de pointes may occur after 8 hours. Delayed cardiac arrest (after 8 hours) has been reported secondary to ventricular arrhythmias.[13]

RESPIRATORY

Tachypnea is common in chloroquine poisoning. Apnea may occur suddenly, especially when convulsions start.[14]

CENTRAL NERVOUS SYSTEM

Neurologic effects appear rapidly after ingestion and include central nervous system depression and visual disturbances, such as blurred vision, diplopia, photophobia, and sometimes blindness. Blindness in acute chloroquine poisoning is transient and resolves without sequelae, in contrast to acute quinine poisoning or long-term chloroquine-induced retinopathy. Coma is less common and tends to be associated with circulatory failure.[15] Central nervous system excitation with agitation and seizures usually precedes cardiac arrest.

MYOPATHY AND NEUROPATHY

Chloroquine overdose can cause a painless proximal myopathy with normal or slight elevation of creatine kinase in plasma. It can also be associated with a peripheral neuropathy.[16]

HYPOKALEMIA

Hypokalemia in chloroquine poisoning has been recognized since the 1980s. It is almost always present in severe chloroquine intoxication[15] and tends to appear within 3 hours of ingestion. In one series stratified by severity, mild, moderate, and severe intoxications were associated with mean serum potassium concentrations of 3.5 mmol/L, 3.26 mmol/L, and 3 mmol/L, respectively.[12] Potassium administration may lead to sudden hyperkalemia as chloroquine is eliminated, and rapid rigorous correction of early hypokalemia is not recommended.[7]

Diagnosis

In the first 12 hours after overdose, serum chloroquine concentrations correlate well with severity of intoxication, with severe effects being seen when serum concentrations are greater than 5 mg/L (15.5 μmol/L).[12] Mild intoxication without clinical symptoms is associated with serum concentrations less than 2.5 mg/L (7.8 μmol/L). High serum chloroquine concentrations have been reported for 8 to 10 days, however, whereas clinical symptoms have resolved after 2 days.[15] In general, serum chloroquine concentrations are not needed to make the diagnosis or guide therapy.

Treatment

GENERAL CONSIDERATIONS

Activated charcoal should be given (and gastric lavage considered) in all patients who present within 1 hour of ingestion of more than 15 mg/kg of chloroquine.[17] Gastrointestinal decontamination in poisoned patients is discussed in detail in Chapter 5. The use of antiarrhythmic agents should be avoided if possible because this may precipitate further arrhythmias by additional negative chronotropic activity. Overdrive pacing is the treatment of choice for ventricular tachycardia or torsades de pointes.[15] Inotropic support with epinephrine may be required.[15,18] Plasma potassium must be monitored. Hypokalemia may have a protective effect and should not be corrected aggressively in the early stages of poisoning.[7] If hypokalemia persists longer than 8 hours, potassium should be replaced cautiously because rebound hyperkalemia often occurs during the recovery

TABLE 63-1 Chloroquine Concentrations in a Fatal Case	
SPECIMEN	**CONCENTRATION**
Blood	33 mg/L (103 μmol/L)
Kidney	110 mg/kg (344 μmol/kg)
Liver	169 mg/kg (528 μmol/kg)
Lung	73 mg/kg (228 μmol/kg)
Urine (antemortem)	367 mg/L (1147 μmol/kg)

From Weingarten HL, Cherry EJ: A chloroquine fatality. Clin Toxicol 18:959–963, 1981.

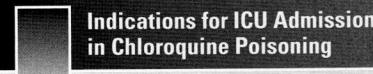

Indications for ICU Admission in Chloroquine Poisoning

Cerebral edema
Pulmonary edema
Coma
Persistent fits
Ventricular arrhythmias

phase.[7] High-dose diazepam (2 mg/kg intravenously over 30 minutes) may have a protective effect in chloroquine poisoning, but respiratory support should be present before it is given.[13,15] Early and continuous cardiorespiratory and neurologic support of these patients is crucial to their survival.

SPECIAL AIRWAY AND VENTILATORY CONSIDERATIONS

It is essential to intubate and ventilate patients early in chloroquine poisoning if arrhythmias or hypotension is present. Similarly, early intubation is advised if central nervous system features, such as recurrent seizures or coma, occur, especially if use of high-dose diazepam is contemplated.

ROLE OF DIAZEPAM IN CHLOROQUINE POISONING

Diazepam (0.1 to 0.3 mg/kg) given by slow intravenous injection, repeated as necessary, is effective at controlling convulsions.[18] In addition, diazepam at approximately 10 times higher doses has been reported to have a specific cardioprotective action in severe chloroquine poisoning.[13,15] In one series of severely chloroquine-intoxicated patients given diazepam, no clinical symptoms of chloroquine toxicity were seen in three patients who respectively had ingested 2.2 g, 2.6 g, and 5 g of chloroquine together with diazepam.[2] Crouzette and coworkers[19] subsequently reported that diazepam reduces mortality in rats acutely poisoned with chloroquine, whereas Riou and colleagues[20] showed cardioprotection and increased urinary chloroquine excretion in chloroquine-poisoned pigs after treatment with diazepam.

Diazepam (2 mg/kg intravenously over 30 minutes) together with early mechanical ventilation and intravenous epinephrine (0.25 μg/kg/min and increased until systolic blood pressure was >100 mm Hg) for 4 days was used to treat 11 patients with severe chloroquine poisoning. All of these patients would have been expected to die on the basis of historical control data. Ten of these 11 patients survived.[21] Mechanical ventilation was instituted in part because of the respiratory depressant effect of high-dose diazepam.

The mechanism of the cardioprotective effect of diazepam in acute chloroquine poisoning is unknown. Croes and coworkers[22] reported a patient with severe chloroquine poisoning who also had ingested clorazepate (initial whole-blood chloroquine and plasma nordiazepam [a clorazepate metabolite] concentrations 7.9 mg/L [24.7 μmol/L] and 2.3 mg/L [8.4 μmol/L], respectively) and in whom mechanical ventilation was instituted. The patient was treated successfully with diazepam (2 mg/kg over 30 minutes, followed by 1 to 2 mg/kg over 24 hours) and norepinephrine (0.25 μg/kg/min for 18 hours). Despite plasma diazepam and nordiazepam concentrations of equal to or greater than 3 mg/L (10 μmol/L) (therapeutic level is 2 mg/L), however, the patient required additional sedation with piritramide to facilitate mechanical ventilation.[22] Although it is possible that chloroquine antagonized the sedative effects of diazepam, the patient may have acquired tolerance to these effects because of prior use of clorazepate. A study in animals suggested that barbiturate anesthesia and isoprenaline (isoproterenol) infusion may be a more effective combination than diazepam and epinephrine in treating severe chloroquine poisoning.[23]

CARDIOTOXICITY

Studies in animals and humans suggested that early aggressive management of severe chloroquine intoxication has a cardioprotective effect and reduces the fatality rate.[1,21] Hypotension should be managed initially with intravenous fluids. Inotropes, such as epinephrine (1 to 5 μg/kg/min), may be necessary for hypotension that is nonresponsive to an intravenous fluid bolus. Sodium bicarbonate intravenously is considered the treatment of choice for arrhythmias and should be used in patients with widened QRS and QT_c intervals (1 to 2 mL/kg of 8.4% sodium bicarbonate repeated if necessary, aiming for a pH of 7.45 to 7.5). There are no randomized controlled trials of efficacy of sodium bicarbonate in chloroquine poisoning, but its use now is recommended widely.[1,24] Its use has rationale, given the quinidine-like action of the drug and the efficacy of sodium bicarbonate in reversing similarly induced cardiovascular effects in poisoning by tricyclic antidepressants.[1,24,25] It also may reverse the cardiotoxic effects of hyperkalemia.[26] The treatment of choice for ventricular tachycardia and torsades de pointes is overdrive pacing.[15] All antiarrhythmic drugs are potentially arrhythmogenic and should be avoided. Class I agents in particular are contraindicated, and lidocaine should not be used because it may precipitate convulsions.[1,24]

HYPOKALEMIA

Exogenously administered potassium has an effect on the heart similar to quinidine-like drugs in that it depresses excitability, slows the rate of depolarization, and decreases conduction.[26] The slowed depolarization and increased refractory period favors reentrant tachycardia. Mild hypokalemia protects dogs against conduction failure and increases the median lethal dose of quinidine.[27] It is recommended to avoid potassium replacement in the early hours of chloroquine intoxication, especially when cardiovascular effects are present.[15] In the second phase of poisoning, when ventricular extrasystoles and torsades de pointes are present, administration of potassium may be helpful, but it must be given cautiously to avoid sudden hyperkalemia. The best recommendation to date is to give patients with hypokalemia of less than 2 mmol/L no more than the equivalent of 160 mmol of K^+ per 24 hours for an adult.[7] Lesser degrees of hypokalemia may be treated with 80 mmol of K^+ per 24 hours for an adult.[7] The rationale for this relatively conservative therapy is that there is no total-body deficit of potassium, and because the hypokalemia is due to a transport problem, it is difficult to correct. Although there is a correlation between the degree of hypokalemia and death, in most cases hypokalemia is not the direct cause of death.[7] As the intoxication resolves, there is serious documented risk of hyperkalemia.[7]

EXTRACORPOREAL REMOVAL TECHNIQUES

Hemofiltration, hemodialysis, and hemoperfusion have no role in the management of chloroquine poisoning because of the large volume of distribution, relatively high protein binding, and long terminal elimination half-life (see Table 63-1).[28]

Criteria for ICU Discharge in Chloroquine Poisoning

Resolution of cerebral edema
Resolution of pulmonary edema
Resolution of coma
Resolution of persistent fits
Resolution of ventricular arrhythmias
Resolution of QRS prolongation

Special Populations

Elderly patients and patients with preexisting cardiovascular disease are likely to be more susceptible to the cardiotoxicity of chloroquine.

Key Points in the Management of Chloroquine Poisoning

1. The interval between ingestion and symptoms is usually short (1–3 hr).
2. The main risks are cardiovascular and central nervous system risks.
3. Early aggressive therapy is needed.
4. Use diazepam combined with epinephrine for severe chloroquine poisoning.
5. Chloroquine level in blood is not necessary for management—clinical features are more important.
6. Correcting hypokalemia early worsens cardiovascular toxicity.
7. Treating arrhythmias with antiarrhythmic drugs may result in negative inotropic and chronotropic effects, and cardiovascular status worsens.
8. Treating with high-dose diazepam without recognizing the need for ventilation may result in pulmonary aspiration.

QUININE

Quinine is an alkaloid extracted from the bark of various species of cinchona tree (*Rubiaceae*). It first was employed as an antipyretic, albeit not a very effective one, by the Portuguese in the first half of the 17th century.

Quinine salts are used in the treatment of chloroquine-resistant malaria.[29] It also commonly is employed for the treatment of nocturnal cramps, for which it has limited efficacy.[30] Quinine has been used as an illegal abortifacient.[31] Quinine also has been used to cut street heroin.[32] It is used widely in tonic water for its bitter taste, and there are several case reports of allergic reactions when it has been consumed this way.[33] Detailed review of overdoses in Scotland showed that 64% of overdoses occurred with prescriptions for other family members, and in only 36% of cases had patients taken their own quinine.[34]

Chemistry and Pharmacology

The chemical name of quinine is 6-methoxy-α-(5-vinyl-2-quinudidinyl)-4-quinoline-methanol ($C_{20}H_{24}N_2O_2 3H_2O$) (Fig. 63-2). It is the *d*-isomer of quinidine. Its molecular

weight is 378.5, pK_a values are 4.1 and 8.5, and it has low solubility in water. Quinine is absorbed rapidly and almost completely from the gastrointestinal tract when given orally, with peak plasma concentrations occurring 1 to 3 hours after ingestion.[15]

Pharmacokinetics of Quinine

Apparent volume of distribution: 2.1–3.1 L/kg
Protein binding: 70–89%
Mechanisms of clearance: 0.22–0.29 mL/min/kg*
Elimination half-life: 26.5 ± 5.8 hr at toxic levels
Active metabolites: liver, kidneys, and muscles metabolize 80% of ingested dose†
Methods to enhance clearance: multiple-dose activated charcoal effective

*20% is excreted unchanged in urine.

†Quinine is metabolized by P-450 CYP3A4; there is interindividual variance in expression of this.

Pathophysiology

Toxicity of quinine can be divided into effects that are immunologically induced, such as purpura and skin rashes, and effects that are direct toxic actions, such as cardiotoxicity and ocular toxicity. Quinine has sodium channel–blocking or local anesthetic actions but also is an irritant.[35] The latter effects may be responsible for nausea in clinical use. The actions on cardiac muscle are class IA antiarrhythmic. It produces sodium channel blockade with moderate phase 0 depression, resulting in slowed conduction and repolarization. The effects on cardiac muscle include an increased threshold in atrial, ventricular, and Purkinje fibers. As a result, the rate of Purkinje cell firing is decreased, and conduction velocity is decreased in ventricular muscle. The refractory period of cardiac muscle is increased. In the pacemaker cells of the sinoatrial node, spontaneous depolarization is inhibited, and this phenomenon extends particularly to the site of ectopic pacemaker activity. In larger doses, quinine causes atrioventricular beat generation (i.e., R-on-T phenomenon) because of its effects on ventricular refractory periods. When higher doses are used, ventricular fibrillation may supervene. The pathophysiology of sodium channel blockade effects on the myocardium is

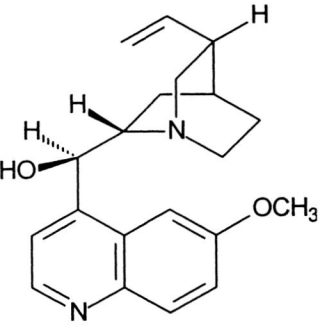

FIGURE 63-2

Chemical structure of quinine.

described in detail in Chapter 36. There is a direct myocardial depressant effect of quinine on cardiac muscle in addition to the sodium channel blockade. Quinine is a vasodilator, probably owing to α-blocking activity.[35]

Quinine has an oxytoxic action on the uterus, which becomes more pronounced as pregnancy progresses. The exact mechanisms for this action are poorly understood. In skeletal muscle, quinine has a curare-like effect, reducing end motor plate excitability. Its use is known to cause deterioration in patients with myasthenia gravis.[35] Quinine probably does not have an effect on gastric smooth muscle. The emetic effect is likely due to a central action on the chemoreceptor trigger zone.[35]

Quinine has been reported to stimulate insulin release in patients receiving treatment for falciparum malaria and causes hypoglycemia.[36] The mechanism of quinine-induced insulin release is a sulfonylurea-like suppression of potassium efflux, leading to β cell membrane depolarization and release of insulin and proinsulin from secretory granules in response to calcium influx via voltage-gated calcium channels.

Quinine has toxic effects that can result in blindness.[37,38] This effect was postulated to be due to retinal arteriole vasoconstriction, but quinine has a direct toxic effect on retinal photoreceptor cells.[37,39] There are no reports of retinal vascular changes being observed before the onset of severe peripheral field constriction or blindness.[40] Normal arteriolar caliber has been observed with fluorescein angiography in a blind patient, and electroretinographic and electrooculographic studies performed soon after patients became blind all showed that the primary disturbance was in retinal function rather than impaired blood flow.[38,40] Photoreceptor cells are affected first, followed by the ganglion layer and possibly the pigment epithelium.[38,40] Visual evoked responses show abnormal waveform and prolonged latency from 3 days after poisoning to several months later, implying some damage to the nerve fiber, the retina, or both.[41,42]

Quinine has direct toxicity on the auditory nerve. Audiometry reveals bilateral nerve deafness due to inhibition of the transducing outer hair cells of the organ of Corti.[43] The decreased acuity is not usually clinically apparent, although the patient recognizes tinnitus.[43]

Clinical Presentation and Life-Threatening Complications

Many clinical effects are common to an acute single overdose in self-poisoning and accumulation of quinine during therapy for malaria. These effects are known as *cinchonism* and include auditory symptoms, gastrointestinal disturbances, vasodilation, sweating, and headache.[35] As concentrations become greater, visual disturbance (plasma concentration >10 mg/L [31 μmol/L]) followed by cardiac and neurologic features (plasma concentration >15 mg/L [46 μmol/L]) occurs.[44] Similar levels in individuals who are ill with malaria do not result in toxicity owing to reduced free quinine present as a consequence of increased binding to α₁ acid glycoprotein. No clear fatal concentrations of quinine have been identified, however, and the patient with the highest plasma concentration of quinine at presentation in one series (20.4 mg/L [63 μmol/L]) survived with retinal damage. The fatal dose of quinine in an adult is approximately 8 g.[45]

CARDIOVASCULAR

Vasodilation[45] and sweating are common. Mild systemic hypotension can occur in the absence of disturbance of cardiac rhythm. Cardiotoxicity of quinine is the predominant cause of death in overdose patients and the ultimate predictor of outcome. These features usually occur within 8 hours of ingestion, although one case report claimed that torsades de pointes occurred 25 hours after ingestion.[46] Generalized myocardial depression is seen. Electrocardiographic changes include prolonged PR, QRS, and QT_c intervals; ST segment changes and T wave changes; and the appearance of U waves.[41] Atrial sinus node block or arrest, high-degree atrioventricular block, and complete atrioventricular dissociation also can occur. After large overdoses, broad-complex tachycardias, such as torsades de pointes, ventricular tachycardia, and ventricular fibrillation, may be seen.[15]

PULMONARY

A 17-year-old man took 5 g of quinine bisulfate and presented 3.5 hours later with deafness. He collapsed shortly after with broad-complex tachycardia. He had pulmonary edema and infection with *Pseudomonas* and *Staphylococcus*. His highest blood level of quinine was 17.8 mg/L (55 μmol/L). Autopsy revealed adult respiratory distress syndrome, but whether it was due to direct toxicity of quinine or due to severity of illness in the patient is unknown. Adult respiratory distress syndrome is not widely reported in patients seriously poisoned with quinine.[47]

GASTROINTESTINAL TRACT

Mild nausea may be the only symptom in therapeutic doses. Profuse vomiting, epigastric pain, and diarrhea characterize large overdoses, however.[35] These symptoms are due to direct irritant action on the gastrointestinal tract and central effects on the chemoreceptor trigger zone.[35]

HEMATOLOGIC

Quinine is a well-recognized cause of drug-induced thrombocytopenia and purpura.[48] The amounts needed are small, and these complications have been documented even after consumption of soft drinks containing quinine.[35] Agranulocytosis also has been reported.[49] In patients with malaria due to *Plasmodium falciparum*, anemia and intravascular hemolysis with renal failure are recognized complications. Attacks are reported to follow irregular quinine use.

RENAL

Intravascular hemolysis can precipitate oliguria and acute renal failure. Notelovitz[50] reported a case of a 21-year-old woman who ingested 90 g of quinine during her 8th week of pregnancy. The patient subsequently became drowsy with dark red urine, which was positive for blood and protein. The patient became oliguric, and urea levels increased to 2080 g/L. The patient was treated with blood transfusion and hemodialysis and was discharged within 72 hours.

AUDITORY

Tinnitus is common, and with large overdoses the patient may be deaf.[35] Vertigo also can occur.[35] The auditory symptoms nearly always resolve within a few days of the overdose. There have been no cases reported of permanent deafness as a result of quinine overdosage.

OCULAR

In quinine overdose, ocular toxicity depends on plasma concentration and often develops 6 to 15 hours after the overdose but may be delayed for 1 or more days.[41,44] The first symptoms are blurring of vision and disturbance of color perception; this can occur during quinine accumulation in malarial therapy. After acute overdose, however, more severe disturbances may occur with progressive constriction of the visual fields, reduced central acuity, and finally complete blindness. Many years after quinine-induced blindness, retinal pigment degeneration still may be apparent, giving the appearance of retinitis pigmentosa.

The fundus appears normal when visual symptoms begin. The pupils may be fixed and dilated some time before light perception is lost, particularly if the patient has marked tunnel vision. Thereafter there may be progressive constriction of retinal arterioles, a cherry-red macular spot, and macular edema; several days or weeks after the overdose, optic atrophy appears.[51,52] There are, however, reports of entirely normal funduscopic appearances after the onset of blindness and of normal retinal artery appearances after blindness has developed.[41,53] Many patients recover completely, although a significant number are rendered permanently blind. In general, the quicker the onset of recovery, the lower the degree of permanent impairment.[41] Of 30 overdose patients in a Scottish study, 8 had documented evidence of visual impairment, of whom 6 had visual problems at 32 months.[34] Fixed dilated pupils strongly suggest blindness due to quinine. Disk pallor does not indicate that permanent blindness will result.[54]

CENTRAL NERVOUS SYSTEM

Headache, confusion, and vertigo can occur.[15] Ataxia can occur after moderate overdose.[15] After massive overdoses, convulsions, coma, and respiratory depression occur and have high associated cardiovascular mortality.[15] A case of "myelopticoneuropathy" after quinine poisoning has been reported, but this case most likely represents vitamin B[12] deficiency and alcoholic neuropathy.[55]

HYPOGLYCEMIA

Hypoglycemia is thought to be due to quinine-stimulated insulin release and can be a severe problem.[56]

Diagnosis

All patients should have a 12-lead electrocardiogram, and plasma should be assayed for urea and electrolytes and glucose because quinine can cause hypokalemia and hypoglycemia. Quinine can be assayed in plasma by immunoassay, and there is a correlation between plasma concentration and clinical features. Usually levels less than 10 mg/L (31 μmol/L) are not associated with clinically significant poisoning.[57] Quinine concentrations are not performed routinely in the management of quinine-poisoned patients because knowledge of concentrations does not alter the patient's management.

Along with methanol, quinine should be considered in the differential diagnosis of patients presenting with acute bilateral blindness. The two can be differentiated easily because patients with methanol toxicity have a high anion gap acidosis and a positive methanol assay. Ergot derivatives, lead, and mercuric chloride are less common causes of blindness secondary to poisoning.

Treatment

GENERAL CONSIDERATIONS

Maintenance of the airway, breathing, and ventilation is crucial. If respiratory failure with or without pulmonary edema occurs, positive-pressure ventilation may be required. Intensive supportive therapy should be the mainstay of treatment, with meticulous correction of electrolyte abnormalities and hypoxia. As with chloroquine, it is theoretically likely that mild hypokalemia protects the myocardium from the effects of quinine, so zealous overcorrection of hypokalemia is not advised. The guidelines provided earlier for chloroquine reasonably may be applied to the management of hypokalemia in quinine poisoning as well. Blood glucose concentrations should be monitored.

Gastric lavage should be considered if a patient presents within 1 hour of ingestion of greater than 15 mg/kg of quinine. Firm recommendation concerning this technique cannot be made at present, however, because lavage has not been shown to affect outcome in poisoned patients but is known to have potential morbidity (albeit rarely). Gastrointestinal decontamination is reviewed in detail in Chapter 5. Multiple-dose activated charcoal (see Chapter 6) should be given to all patients who may have ingested greater than 15 mg/kg of quinine. The justification for this approach comes from the study of Prescott and colleagues,[57] which showed that after treatment with repeated oral charcoal, plasma quinine concentrations decreased rapidly with a mean half-life of 8.1 ± 1.1 hours compared with more than 24 hours in a report of similarly poisoned patients. The visual impairment, which was expected in a patient with cardiotoxicity and a plasma quinine concentration of 12.6 mg/L (39 μmol/L), did not occur. Repeated doses of oral charcoal have been shown to increase the rate of elimination of a therapeutic dose of quinine in healthy volunteers.[58] In another study,[41] the rate of spontaneous quinine elimination was much slower, pointing to a dose-dependent metabolism of quinine.[57] Activated charcoal remains the only practical means of enhancing removal of this drug after overdose. The effect is not due so much to interference with absorption as it is to concentration-dependent diffusion of drug from the circulation to the gastrointestinal lumen, where it is bound irreversibly by charcoal.[59] Activated charcoal usually is given in repeated doses until the patient improves clinically (i.e., cardiotoxicity has settled, ocular toxicity is improving). It is not possible to

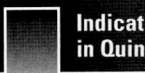
Indications for ICU Admission in Quinine Poisoning

Persistent hypotension
Ventricular arrhythmias
Intravascular hemolysis
Convulsions
Coma

show from the literature to date that treatment with charcoal enhanced the outcome of these patients.[57]

All patients with quinine overdoses should be placed on a cardiac monitor. Antiemetics may be given if vomiting is prolonged and severe, but theoretically agents with cardiotoxic or neurotoxic actions should be avoided (e.g., antihistamines). Intravenous fluids are necessary in cases with profuse vomiting or diarrhea.

CARDIOTOXICITY

Hypotension should be treated initially with intravenous fluids. If fluids do not correct the hypotension, inotropic agents may be necessary. Intravenous sodium bicarbonate is recommended to treat quinine-induced sodium channel blockade (e.g., QRS prolongation). The recommended initial dosing is 1 to 2 mL/kg of 8.4% sodium bicarbonate repeated if necessary, aiming for a pH of 7.45 to 7.5. Intravenous sodium bicarbonate is considered the treatment of choice for arrhythmias and should be used in patients with widened QRS and QT_c intervals (1 to 2 mL/kg of 8.4% sodium bicarbonate repeated if necessary, aiming for a pH of 7.45 to 7.5). There are no randomized controlled trials of efficacy of sodium bicarbonate in quinine poisoning, but its use is widely recommended.[24] Its use has rationale, given the class Ia action of the drug and the efficacy of sodium bicarbonate in reversing similarly induced cardiovascular effects in poisoning by tricyclic antidepressants.[25] The treatment of choice for ventricular tachycardia and torsades de pointes is overdrive pacing.[46] The threshold for pacing may have to be increased to above 1 V because the quinine-poisoned heart is relatively insensitive to pacing stimuli.[15,18]

All antiarrhythmic drugs are potentially arrhythmogenic and should be avoided. Class I agents specifically are contraindicated, and theoretically lidocaine in particular should not be used because it may precipitate convulsions and it potentiates the action of quinine on the heart.[24] Similarly, class III drugs (e.g., amrinone, sotalol, bretylium) are unsuitable.

Transvenous pacing may be indicated for complete heart block. If an inotropic agent is required, epinephrine, norepinephrine, or both are recommended. Epinephrine is the drug of first choice, unless vasodilation predominates, when a mixture of epinephrine and norepinephrine (vasoconstrictor action) is preferred.

OCULAR

Visual effects of quinine are largely untreatable because the mechanism of toxicity still is poorly understood. In the past, many measures were advocated, such as bilateral stellate ganglion block[51]; retrobulbar injections[60]; and vasodilators, including nitrates.[52] As with all rare conditions with some spontaneous recovery, it has been difficult to evaluate the outcome of these procedures. In my experience, however, these procedures make no difference to outcome, and I would not advocate their routine use. A report suggested efficacy for hyperbaric oxygen, but the same caveats of spontaneous recovery apply.[61]

CENTRAL NERVOUS SYSTEM

Quinine-induced convulsions are often short-lived, but if they persist, they should be treated with diazepam (0.1 to 0.3 mg/kg) or a similar benzodiazepine.[18] Coma should be managed conventionally.

EXTRACORPOREAL REMOVAL TECHNIQUES

Visual recovery has been taken by some workers to indicate the benefit of treatment. This improvement frequently is spontaneous and rapid. The actual amount of quinine cleared is limited, however, and cannot account for improvement.

Hemodialysis and hemoperfusion are ineffective in quinine poisoning because there is rapid tissue distribution, a relatively large volume of distribution, and extensive protein binding (see Table 63-3). Studies of the efficacy of hemodialysis showed that in 6 hours only 25 to 30 mg (77 to 93 μmol) of quinine were removed.[62] In other patients, only a few hundred milligrams of quinine were removed by hemoperfusion.[44,63] In one patient, charcoal hemoperfusion was complicated in one reported case by repeated clotting of the charcoal cartridge despite heparinization, thrombocytopenia, and hypoprothrombinemia. The patient died.[45] Resin hemoperfusion is equally ineffective because it removes toxicologically insignificant amounts.[64]

In one report, peritoneal dialysis was claimed to remove 640 mg (1970 μmol), but no analysis of plasma quinine concentrations was done to validate these findings.[65] Other authors recorded less than 60 mg (184 μmol) removed in 24 hours.[66] In another case report, plasmapheresis was similarly ineffective, removing only 8.5 mg (26 μmol) of quinine.[62] There currently is no evidence that any of the previously advocated extracorporeal elimination techniques for quinine are effective in practice.

Urinary acidification or forced diuresis is not advised. Although it may increase renal quinine excretion slightly, it would be expected to worsen cardiotoxicity. Quinine has two pK_a values (8.0 and 4.11), causing confusion in analysis of urine pH manipulation data.

ROLE OF OCTREOTIDE

The hyperinsulinemia and resultant hypoglycemia, which complicates quinine treatment of falciparum malaria, responds to octreotide. In Thai volunteers, octreotide (100 μg intramuscularly) suppressed quinine-induced hyperinsulinemia within 15 minutes.[67] The effect lasted for 6 hours. Octreotide (50 μg intravenously over 15 minutes followed by 50 μg/hr by intravenous infusion, increasing to 200 μg/hr or decreasing to 10 μg/hr as appropriate) together with intravenous glucagon or *d*-glucose or both was effective in treating hyperinsulinemia and hypoglycemia in five patients with falciparum malaria who were treated with quinine.[67] The clinical pharmacology of octreotide is described in detail in Chapter 159.

Criteria for ICU Discharge in Quinine Poisoning

Resolution of hypotension
Resolution of ventricular arrhythmias
Resolution of intravascular hemolysis
Resolution of convulsions
Resolution of coma

Special Populations

In children, quinine's volume of distribution is less and its elimination half-life is shorter than in adults, but a kinetic difference from adults in the overdose situation is unlikely.[15] In patients with malaria, there is increased protein binding, an increased elimination half-life, and a decreased volume of distribution.[15] The pharmacokinetics of therapeutic doses is altered in patients with chronic liver disease; the time to maximum plasma concentrations was prolonged and the terminal elimination half-life was prolonged to 23.4 hours versus 9.7 hours in healthy controls. No change in quinine clearance was seen, however.[68] The volume of distribution of quinine is decreased in the third trimester of pregnancy, but the clearance of therapeutic concentrations is similar, and toxicokinetics is not expected to be different from the nonpregnant state.[69]

Key Points in Quinine Poisoning

1. Toxicity can occur quickly (within 1–3 hr).
2. Cardiovascular toxicity is a bad prognostic sign.
3. No specific therapy works in ocular toxicity.
4. Extracorporeal elimination methods are of no value.
5. Multiple-dose activated charcoal is the best treatment modality available.
6. Correcting hypokalemia early worsens cardiovascular toxicity.
7. Treating arrhythmias with antiarrhythmic drugs worsens cardiovascular toxicity.

REFERENCES

1. Clemessy JL, Taboulet P, Hoffman JR, et al: Treatment of acute chloroquine poisoning: A 5 year experience. Crit Care Med 24:1189–1195, 1996.
2. Bondurand A, N'Dri K, Coffi S, Saracino E: L'intoxication à la chloroquine au CHU Abidjan. Afr Med 179:239–242, 1980.
3. Riou B, Barriot P, Rimailho A, Baud FJ: Treatment of severe chloroquine poisoning. N Engl J Med 318:1–6, 1988.
4. Cann HM, Verhulst HL: Fatal acute chloroquine poisoning in children. Pediatrics 27:95–101, 1961.
5. Britton WJ, Kevau JH: Intentional chloroquine overdosage. Med J Aust 21:407–410, 1978.
6. Lofaso F, Baud FJ, Halna du Fretay X, et al: Hypokalemia in massive chloroquine poisoning: 2 cases [in French]. Presse Med 16:22–24, 1987.
7. Clemessy JL, Favier C, Borron SW, et al: Hypokalaemia related to acute chloroquine ingestion. Lancet 346:877–880, 1995.
8. Weingarten HL, Cherry EJ: A chloroquine fatality. Clin Toxicol 18:959–963, 1981.
9. McChesney EW, Fasco MJ, Banks WF: The metabolism of chloroquine in man during and after repeated oral dosage. J Pharm Exp Ther 158:323–331, 1967.
10. Burg F: Intoxications volontaires par la chloroquine. These Medecine, Strasbourg, Universite Louis Pasteur, 1976.
11. Conso F: Death from acute poisoning in man. Vet Hum Toxicol 21:68–69, 1979.
12. Vitris M, Aubert M: Intoxications a la chloroquine: notre expérience a propos de 80 cas. Dakar Med 28:593–602, 1983.
13. Bouvier AM, Bertrand D, Timsit JF, Ricome JL: Intoxications massives et prolongées par la nivaquine: Effets du diazepam. Réanimation Soins Intensifs, Medecine d'Urgence 2:265–268, 1986.
14. Frija GA: Intoxications aigues a la chloroquine: A propos de 38 cas. Méd Trop 35:23–30, 1975.
15. Jaeger A, Sauder P, Kopferschmitt J, Flesch F: Clinical features and management of poisoning due to antimalarial drugs. Med Toxicol 2:242–273, 1987.
16. Havens PL, Splaingard ML, Bousounis D, Hoffman GM: Survival after chloroquine ingestion in a child. Clin Toxicol 26:381–388, 1988.
17. Neuvonen PJ, Kivisto KT, Laine K, Pyykko K: Prevention of chloroquine absorption by activated charcoal. Hum Exp Toxicol 11:117–120, 1992.
18. Jones AL, Dargan PI: Churchill's Pocketbook of Toxicology. Edinburgh, Churchill Livingstone, 2001.
19. Crouzette J, Vicaut E, Palumbo S, et al: Experimental assessment of the protective activity of diazepam on the acute toxicity of chloroquine. Clin Toxicol 20:271–279, 1983.
20. Riou B, Rimailho A, Galliot M, Bourdon R: Effets du diazepam dans l'intoxication expérimentale aigue par la chloroquine. Réanimation Soins Intensifs 2:236–238, 1986.
21. Riou B, Rimailho A, Galliot M, Baud F: Protective cardiovascular effects of diazepam in experimental acute chloroquine poisoning. Intensive Care Med 14:610–616, 1988.
22. Croes K, Augustinijs P, Sabbe M, et al: Diminished sedation during diazepam treatment for chloroquine intoxication. Pharm World Sci 15:83–85, 1993.
23. Buckley NA, Smith AJ, Dosen P, O'Connell DL: Effects of catecholamines and diazepam in chloroquine poisoning in barbiturate anaesthetized rats. Hum Exp Toxicol 15:909–914, 1996.
24. Jaeger A, Raguin O, Liegeon MN: Acute poisoning by Class I antiarrhythmic agents and by chloroquine [in French]. Rev Prat 47:748–753, 1997.
25. Bou-Abboud E, Nattel S: Relative role of alkalosis and sodium ions in reversal of Class I antiarrhythmic drug-induced sodium channel blockade by sodium bicarbonate. Circulation 94:1954–1961, 1996.
26. Bellet S, Wasserman F: The effects of molar sodium lactate in reversing the cardiotoxic effect of hyperpotassemia. Arch Intern Med 100:565–575, 1957.
27. Brandfonbrener M, Kronholm J, Jones HR: The effect of serum potassium concentration and quinidine toxicity. J Pharm Exp Ther 154:250–254, 1966.
28. Gustafsson LI, Walker O, Alvan G, et al: Disposition of chloroquine in man after single intravenous and oral doses. Br J Clin Pharmacol 15:471–479, 1983.
29. Wilairatana P, Looareesuwan S: Guidelines in management of severe malaria. J Indian Med Assoc 98:628–631, 2000.
30. Man-Son-Hing M, Wells G: Meta-analysis of efficacy of quinine for treatment of nocturnal leg cramps in elderly people. BMJ 310:13–17, 1995.
31. Dennenberg AL, Dorpman SF, Johnson J: Use of quinine for self-induced abortion. South Med J 76:846–849, 1983.
32. Levine LH, Hirsch CS, White LW: Quinine cardiotoxicity: A mechanism for sudden death in narcotic addicts. J Forensic Sci 18:167–172, 1973.
33. Belkin GA: Cocktail purpura: An unusual case of quinine sensitivity. Ann Intern Med 66:583–586, 1967.
34. Mackie MA, Davidson J, Clarke J: Quinine-acute self-poisoning and ocular toxicity. Scot Med J 42:8–9, 1997.
35. Bateman DN, Dyson EH: Quinine toxicity. Adv Drug React Ac Pois Rev 4:215–233, 1986.
36. White NJ, Warell DA, Chanthavich P, et al: Severe hypoglycaemia and hyperinsulinaemia in falciparum malaria. N Engl J Med 309:61–66, 1983.
37. Berggren L, Rendahl I: Quinine amblyopia: A report of four cases, two of them studied with electroretinography. Acta Ophthalmol 33:217–228, 1955.
38. Behrman J, Mushin A: Electrodiagnostic findings in quinine amblyopia. Br J Ophthalmol 52:925–928, 1968.
39. Cibis GW, Burian HM, Blodi FC: Electroretinogram changes in acute quinine poisoning. Arch Ophthalmol 90:307–309, 1973.
40. Brinton GS, Norton EWD, Zahn JR, Knighton RW: Ocular quinine toxicity. Am J Ophthalmol 90:403–410, 1980.
41. Dyson EH, Proudfoot AT, Prescott LF, Heyworth R: Death and blindness due to overdose of quinine. BMJ 291:31–33, 1985.
42. Gangitano JL, Keitner JL: Abnormalities of the pupil and visual-evoked potentials in quinine amblyopia. Am J Ophthalmol 89:425–430, 1980.
43. Roche RJ, Silamut K, Pukrittayakamee S, et al: Quinine induces reversible high-tone hearing loss. Br J Clin Pharmacol 29:780–782, 1990.
44. Bateman DN, Blain PG, Woodhouse KW, et al: Pharmacokinetics and clinical toxicity of quinine overdosage: Lack of efficacy of techniques intended to enhance elimination. QJM 54:125–131, 1985.

45. Goldenberg AM, Wexler LF: Quinine overdose: Review of toxicity and treatment. Clin Cardiol 11:716–718, 1988.
46. Bodenhamer JE, Smilkstein MJ: Delayed cardiotoxicity following quinine overdosage: A case report. J Emerg Med 11:279–285, 1993.
47. Wenstone R, Bell M, Mostafa SM: Fatal adult respiratory distress syndrome after quinine overdose. Lancet 1:1143–1144, 1989.
48. Helmly RB, Bergin JJ, Shulman NR: Quinine-induced purpura. Arch Intern Med 120:59–60, 1967.
49. Sutherland R, Vincent PC, Raik E, Burgess K: Quinine-induced agranulocytosis: Toxic effect of quinine bisulphate on bone marrow cultures in vitro. BMJ 1:605–607, 1977.
50. Notelovitz M: Acute renal failure following quinine poisoning. South Afr Med J 44:649, 1970.
51. Bankes JLK, Hayward JA, Jones MBS: Quinine amblyopia treated with stellate ganglion block. BMJ 4:85–88, 1972.
52. Pelner L, Saskin E: Toxic amaurosis due to quinine: Treatment with sodium nitrate administered intravenously. JAMA 119:1175–1176, 1942.
53. Francois J, de Rouck A, Cambie E: Retinal and optic evaluation in quinine poisoning. Ann Ophthalmol 4:177–185, 1972.
54. Hla KK, Leahy N, Henry JA: Accidental quinine poisoning in children under five. Vet Hum Toxicol 29:121–123, 1987.
55. Banerji NK, Martin VAF: Myelo-optico-neuropathy following quinine poisoning. J Irish Med Assoc 67:46–47, 1974.
56. Henquin J: Quinine and the stimulus secretion coupling in pancreatic beta-cells: Glucose-like effects on potassium permeability and insulin release. Endocrinology 110:1325–1332, 1992.
57. Prescott LF, Hamilton AR, Heyworth R: Treatment of quinine overdosage with repeated oral charcoal. Br J Clin Pharmacol 27:95–97, 1989.
58. Lockey D, Bateman DN: Effect of oral activated charcoal on quinine elimination. Br J Clin Pharmacol 27:92–94, 1989.
59. Boldy DAR, Vale JA, Prescott LF: Treatment of phenobarbitone poisoning with repeated oral administration of activated charcoal. QJM 61:997–1002, 1986.
60. Dyson EH, Proudfoot AT, Bateman DN: Quinine amblyopia: Is current management appropriate? J Toxicol 23:571–578, 1985–1986.
61. Wolff RS, Wirtshafter D, Adkinson C: Ocular quinine toxicity treated with hyperbaric oxygen. Undersea Hyperb Med Soc 24:131–134, 1997.
62. Sabto J, Pierce RM, West RH, Gurr FW: Haemodialysis, peritoneal dialysis, plasmapheresis and forced diuresis for the treatment of quinine overdose. Clin Nephrol 16:264–268, 1981.
63. Boereboom FT, Ververs FF, Meulenbelt J, van Dijk A: Hemoperfusion is ineffectual in severe chloroquine poisoning. Crit Care Med 28:3346–3350, 2000.
64. Heath A: Resin haemoperfusion for quinine poisoning. Lancet 1:1224, 1985.
65. Mckenzie IFC, Mathew TH, Baillie MJ: Peritoneal dialysis in the treatment of quinine overdose. Med J Aust 1:58–59, 1968.
66. Donadio JV, Whelton A, Gilliland PF, Cirksena WJ: Peritoneal dialysis in quinine intoxication. JAMA 204:274, 1968.
67. Phillips RE, Looareesuwan S, Molyneux ME, et al: Hypoglycaemia and counterregulatory hormone responses in severe falciparum malaria: Treatment with Sandostatin. QJM 86:233–240, 1993.
68. Auprayoon P, Sukontason K, Na-Bangchang K, et al: Pharmacokinetics of quinine in chronic liver disease. Br J Clin Pharmacol 40:494–497, 1995.
69. Krishna S, White N: Pharmacokinetics of quinine, chloroquine and amodiaquine. Clin Pharmacol 30:263–299, 1996.

CHAPTER 64

Lactic Acidosis and Nucleoside Analogue Reverse Transcriptase Inhibitors

Michael P. Dubé ■ George Mathew

The nucleoside analogue reverse transcriptase inhibitors (NRTIs)—zidovudine (ZDV), stavudine (D4T), didanosine (ddI), zalcitabine (ddC), abacavir (ABC), and lamivudine (3TC)—are used in the treatment of most human immunodeficiency virus type 1 (HIV-1)–infected patients who require antiretroviral therapy (Fig. 64-1). Among the adverse effects that have been associated with use of NRTIs, lactic acidosis now is being recognized as an important and more prevalent adverse event than was initially recognized. Many toxicities of the NRTI class of drugs are thought to be mediated by mitochondrial toxicity.[1–3] The association between ZDV and mitochondrial dysfunction first was noted in seven patients with ZDV-induced myopathy.[1] Several cases of severe lactic acidosis were described early in the 1990s.[4]

The normal blood lactate level in nonstressed patients is 1.0 ± 0.5 mmol/L, whereas in critically ill patients normal lactate levels are considered to be less than 2 mmol/L.[5] *Hyperlactatemia* or *lactic acidemia* is defined as a mild-to-moderate elevation of blood lactate (2 to 5 mmol /L) without metabolic acidosis, whereas *lactic acidosis* is defined as a elevated lactate level with metabolic acidosis.[5] Lactic acidosis is classified as either anaerobic (type A), seen in patients with tissue hypoxia, or aerobic (type B), examples of which include malignancies, glycogen storage disease, myopathies, or the lactic acidosis that occurs during NRTI treatment. This chapter discusses the lactic acidosis that occurs during NRTI treatment.

INCIDENCE

In a retrospective study of 1590 HIV-infected individuals taking NRTIs with 2220 person-years of follow-up, Fortgang and colleagues[6] found an incidence of 1.3 cases of lactic acidosis per 1000 person-years of NRTI use. Among 349 patients studied over 516 patient-years, 2 developed severe fulminant lactic acidosis and hepatic steatosis, whereas 5 patients developed symptomatic hyperlactatemia.[7] Lonergan and coworkers[8] estimated the incidence of hyperlactatemia associated with abdominal symptoms or hepatic abnormalities at 20.9 cases per 1000 person-years of NRTI treatment in patients receiving two or more NRTIs. Most early cases of severe lactic acidemia were reported in women, but there are no firm data regarding differences by gender, body mass index, race, or age.

PATHOPHYSIOLOGY

Elevated blood lactate is considered a good noninvasive marker for mitochondrial dysfunction. As long as other medical causes of hyperlactatemia are excluded (e.g., hypovolemia, cardiogenic causes, or septic shock), hyperlactatemia is considered more directly and primarily consistent with mitochondrial dysfunction.

NRTIs deplete mitochondrial DNA (mtDNA) in cell culture by inhibiting DNA polymerase gamma, the enzyme primarily responsible for the synthesis of mtDNA. The degree of DNA polymerase gamma inhibition, and subsequently of mtDNA depletion, depends on the type of nucleosides used, listed in order of decreasing inhibition: ddc > D4T > ddI > ZDV > 3TC > ABC.[2,3] In susceptible individuals, it is thought that NRTI-induced progressive loss of functional mtDNA results in loss of vital mitochondrial functions over time, including oxidative phosphorylation.[9,10] Ultimately a shift to anaerobic glycolysis leads to lactic acid production and lactic acidosis. A preliminary report documented marked increases in endogenous lactate production, without decrements in lactate clearance, in symptomatic NRTI-treated subjects with mild hyperlactatemia (lactate 2 to 4 mmol/L).[11] In patients with NRTI-induced hyperlactatemia, electron microscopic analysis of mitochondria revealed subsarcolemmal presence of increased number and size of mitochondria, abnormal lipid droplets in myocytes, and focal degeneration and loss of myofilamentous structure.[12]

CLINICAL FEATURES

The primary clinical features of severe lactic acidemia are fatigue, weight loss, nausea, abdominal complaints, dyspnea, and preterminal cardiac dysrhythmias. The onset can be acute or subacute. In the Swiss HIV Cohort Study, 33 of 42 (79%) patients who had hyperlactatemia presented with clinical symptoms, the most common being fatigue and diarrhea. Of 42 patients, 25 (26%) had additional laboratory abnormalities, the most frequent of which were elevated urate and hepatic abnormalities.[13]

Hepatic dysfunction is common and can include tender hepatomegaly, peripheral edema, ascites, and encephalopathy; jaundice is rare, however. Modest elevations in liver enzymes are common.[6,14] Evidence of hepatic steatosis is common on biopsy[6]; features of chronic liver disease, such

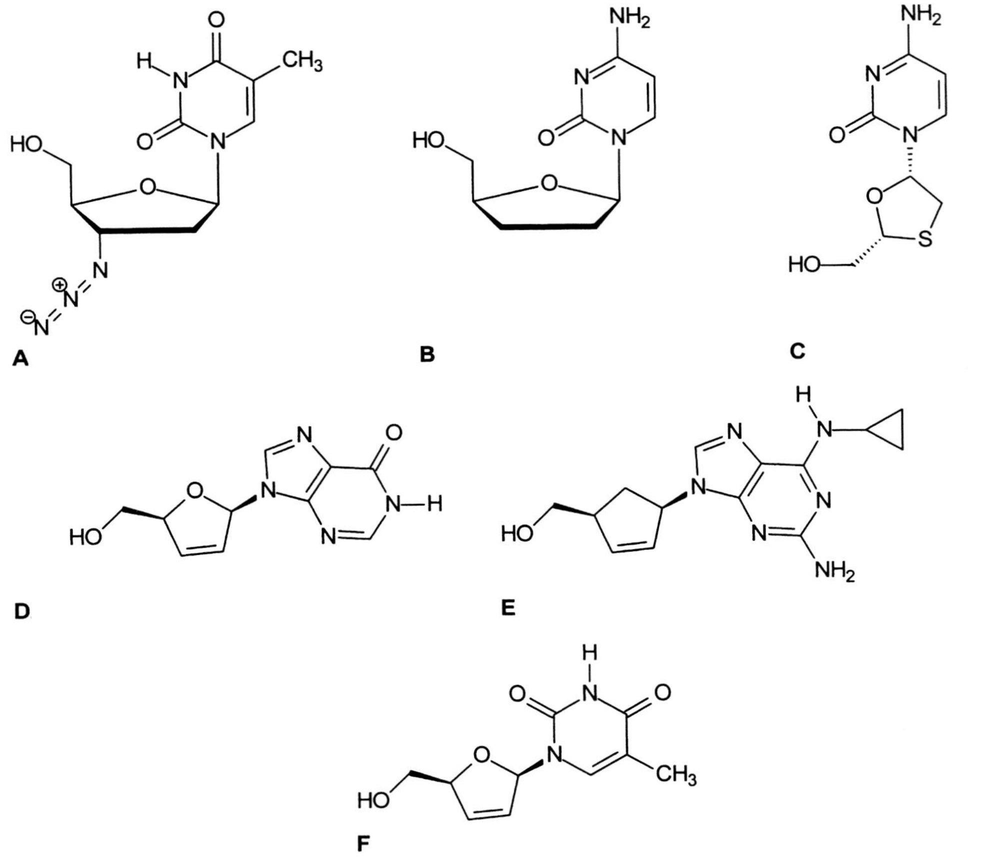

FIGURE 64-1

Chemical structures of the reverse transcriptase inhibitors. **A,** Zidovudine. **B,** Zalcitabine. **C,** Lamivudine. **D,** Didanosine. **E,** Abacavir. **F,** Stavudine.

as portal hypertension, have not been described. The presence of hypovolemia and sepsis should suggest other diagnoses. Patients with mild-to-moderate lactic acidemia (2 to 5 mmol/L) without acidosis may have milder systemic and hepatic abnormalities but often are asymptomatic.

In a report of four cases of NRTI-related fatal lactic acidosis, all the patients had gastrointestinal symptoms of nausea and vomiting followed by tachypnea, which preceded lactic acidosis.[15] Several studies suggested that there is a milder and earlier presentation of the lactic acidosis/hepatic steatosis syndrome characterized by abdominal pain and distention, nausea, and elevated alanine aminotransferase and lactate levels.[7,16] It is not clear how frequently milder syndromes precede severe lactic acidosis, but many, if not most, patients fail to develop more severe manifestations.

LABORATORY ABNORMALITIES

It is important that blood specimens be collected properly because improper collection techniques may result in falsely elevated lactate levels. In critically ill patients, arterial sampling yields the optimal specimen for testing, although venous collection also is acceptable.[17] When venous collection is done, it is crucial to instruct patients not to clench the fist before or during the procedure[18] and to relax the hand as much as possible. Although use of a tourniquet may not affect lactate concentrations,[18] it is

preferable if possible to avoid the use of a tourniquet. If immediate processing (within minutes) of the sample is not available, blood should be collected in a chilled gray-top (sodium fluoride–potassium oxalate) tube[19] and placed immediately on ice.

TREATMENT

The optimal management of NRTI-associated hyperlactatemia has not been established. Most clinical authorities at least transiently would discontinue the antiretroviral regimen if lactate levels are more than four times the upper limit of normal on repeat testing, or if lactate levels of more than two times the upper limit of normal occur in a

---

Indications for ICU Admission in Antiretroviral Toxicity

Hypotension
Severe acidosis
Lactic acidosis with diagnostic uncertainty (e.g., possible sepsis)
Evidence of major end organ dysfunction

symptomatic patient. Because of the prevalence of nonspecific systemic complaints in HIV-infected patients, it may be difficult to ascribe particular symptoms accurately to new-onset lactate acidosis. Occasionally, it is necessary to discontinue antiretroviral therapy to establish the link between symptoms and medications. The significance of milder elevation of blood lactate levels and the need to discontinue or change treatment in asymptomatic subjects are uncertain.

There are no established guidelines regarding the treatment protocol to be used in patients on NRTI therapy who develop lactic acidosis or severe hyperlactatemia. Brinkman and colleagues[20] suggested that in a case of lactic acidosis (serum lactate >5 mmol/L and serum bicarbonate <20 mmol/L), NRTI treatment be stopped; volume status be maintained with intravenous fluids if needed; and therapy be started with vitamin B complex twice a day and 1000 mg of L-carnitine twice daily, both given intravenously until lactate levels decrease to less than 3 mmol/L, after which oral therapy can be started. Using this protocol, Brinkman and colleagues treated six patients, all of whom survived.[20]

When an episode of serious hyperlactatemia or lactic acidosis is recognized in a patient receiving NRTIs, all antiretroviral therapy should be discontinued immediately. Antiretrovirals other than NRTI agents also must be stopped to prevent emergence of resistance during single-agent or dual-agent regimens, which are considered suboptimal. Patients not requiring hospitalization should be followed every 2 weeks until symptoms resolve. Patients requiring hospitalization should be followed in a closely monitored setting depending on the severity of illness. Supportive management with intravenous fluids, vasopressors, hyperventilation using mechanical ventilators, and judicious use of intravenous alkali bicarbonate should be employed when appropriate. In one instance of metabolic acidosis not responding to the aforementioned measures, hemodialysis was used with success.[21]

After the patient is stabilized, the clinician is faced with a difficult decision of which antiretrovirals to use. This decision is best left to an HIV care provider with experience with hyperlactatemia. Generally there is no acute need to rechallenge with the same antiretroviral drugs. Two strategies have been proposed: switch to a potentially less mitochondrial-damaging NRTI, such as from d4T to a non–d4T-containing regimen,[22] or switch to a regimen composed entirely of drugs other than NRTI agents, such as protease inhibitor agents plus a nonnucleoside reverse transcriptase inhibitor. The latter option may be safer, but many HIV-infected patients already have been exposed to all the available classes of antiretrovirals and may lack this option. For a patient whose virus already has developed resistance to the nonnucleoside reverse transcriptase inhibitor class of drugs, a virologically potent "NRTI-sparing regimen" would be difficult to construct with currently available antiretrovirals. The nucleotide reverse transcriptase inhibitor tenofovir, which has been newly improved in the United States, lacks mitochondrial toxicity in an in vitro model[23] and represents another option to NRTI-based regimens.

One mechanism for the tissue damage induced by NRTI-associated mitochondrial dysfunction is the accumulation of reactive oxygen free radicals, normally neutralized by functional mitochondria. Use of antioxidants in this dis-

order may be of value, as has been suggested in experimental models.[24,25] The safety and efficacy of vitamins B_1 (thiamine), B_2 (riboflavin), C, and E in the acute management of hyperlactatemia have not been assessed systematically. Case series suggest dramatic improvement of lactic acidosis after initiation of thiamine or riboflavin.[26–28] No data exist on the use of vitamins C and E in the acute management of hyperlactatemia. Thiamine and riboflavin are important for intact mitochondrial function. Deficiency of either or both B vitamins may play a role in NRTI-associated mitochondrial dysfunction.

Thiamine deficiency may be present in HIV-infected individuals and may predispose to lactic acidosis in patients receiving NRTIs. Anecdotal reports of the efficacy of 100 to 200 mg of thiamine in NRTI-induced mitochondrial dysfunction exist[20,26] without noted adverse events. A woman with acquired immunodeficiency syndrome on NRTI therapy with lactic acidosis was given 200 mg of thiamine intravenously as a single dose along with multivitamins, and within 12 hours pH and serum lactate normalized.[26]

Fouty and colleagues[28] found riboflavin deficiency in three patients with lactic acidosis and liver steatosis who subsequently recovered fully after riboflavin therapy at 50 mg/day. The authors hypothesized that impaired mtDNA replication owing to NRTI-mediated inhibition of DNA polymerase gamma, combined with riboflavin deficiency or decreased activity, led to lactic acidosis and that repletion of normal riboflavin levels helped mitochondrial function and lactic acid levels to return to normal. Riboflavin indirectly acts as a cofactor for respiratory chain complexes I and II. It is converted to flavin mononucleotide, which is converted to flavin adenine dinucleotide. These flavin coenzymes are cofactors for respiratory chain complexes I and II and are necessary for proper functioning of the electron-transport chain. Luzzati and associates[27] also reported a case of a pregnant woman with HIV on NRTI therapy who developed lactic acidosis, which responded to 50 mg/day of riboflavin.

L-Carnitine therapy also has been proposed as therapy for NRTI-induced lactic acidosis. ZDV therapy can cause L-carnitine deficiency, which may predispose to lactic acidosis,[29] presumably as a consequence of impaired β-oxidation of fatty acids. The dose commonly used is 50 mg/kg/day. One patient who received this dose of L-carnitine by infusion improved rapidly after a deterioration that occurred during routine supportive care plus hemodialysis.[30]

Key Points in the Diagnosis and Management of Antiretroviral Toxicity

1. Consider other causes of lactic acidosis to avoid delays in diagnosis.
2. Hyperlactatemia should be considered as a cause of abdominal complaints or abnormal liver enzymes.
3. *All* antiretroviral agents should be stopped simultaneously (if any are stopped).
4. Presence of mildly elevated plasma lactate (<2 times normal) in a patient who is receiving nucleoside analogue reverse transcriptase inhibitors seldom leads to severe lactic acidosis.

SPECIAL POPULATIONS

Pregnancy may increase the risk of NRTI-associated lactic acidosis. The manufacturer reported three pregnancy-related cases of fatal lactic acidosis with the combination of d4T and ddI (Letter to Healthcare Providers, A.C. Smyth, Bristol-Myers-Squibb Company, January 5, 2001). This combination, which is used commonly in the general HIV-infected population, has not been linked otherwise to increased incidence of severe lactic acidosis.

REFERENCES

1. Arnaudo E, Dalakas M, Shanske S, et al: Depletion of muscle mitochondrial DNA in AIDS patients with zidovudine-induced myopathy. Lancet 337:508–510, 1991.
2. Chen C, Vasquez-Padua M, Cheng Y-C: Effect of anti-human immunodeficiency virus nucleoside analogs on mitochondrial DNA and its implication for delayed toxicity. Mol Pharmacol 39:625–628, 1991.
3. Medina D, Tsai C, Hsuing D, Cheng Y: Comparison of mitochondrial morphology, mitochondrial DNA content and cell viability in cultured cells treated with three anti-human immunodeficiency virus dideoxynucleosides. Antimicrob Agents Chemother 38:1824–1828, 1994.
4. Chattha G, Arieff A, Cummings C, Tierny LM Jr: Lactic acidosis complicating the acquired immunodeficiency syndrome. Ann Intern Med 118:37–39, 1993.
5. Mizock B, Falk J: Lactic acidosis in critical illness. Crit Care Med 20:80–93, 1992.
6. Fortgang IS, Belitsos PC, Chaisson RE, Moore RD: Hepatomegaly and steatosis in HIV infected patients receiving nucleoside analog antiretroviral therapy. Am J Gastroenterol 90:1433–1436, 1995.
7. John M, Moore C, James I, et al: Chronic hyperlactatemia in HIV-infected patients taking antiretroviral therapy. AIDS 15:717–723, 2001.
8. Lonergan JT, Behling C, Pfander H, et al: Hyperlactatemia and hepatic abnormalities in 10 human immunodeficiency virus-infected patients receiving nucleoside analogue combination regimens. Clin Infect Dis 31:162–166, 2000.
9. Lewis W, Dalakas MC: Mitochondrial toxicity of antiviral drugs. Nat Med 1:417–422, 1995.
10. Brinkman K, Burger D, Smeitink J, et al: Adverse effects of reverse transcriptase inhibitors: Mitochondrial toxicity as common pathway. AIDS 12:1735–1744, 1998.
11. Leclerq P, Roth H, Bosseray A, et al: Investigating lactate metabolism to estimate mitochondrial status. Antiviral Ther 6(Suppl 4):16, 2001.
12. Zell S: Clinical features in HIV patients manifesting electron microscopic evidence of mitochondrial toxicity: A case series. First IAS Conference on Pathogenesis and Treatment. Buenos Aires, 2001.
13. Boubaker K, Sudre P, Flepp M, et al: Hyperlactatemia and antiretroviral therapy in the Swiss HIV Cohort Study (Abstract 57). Seventh Conference on Retroviruses and Opportunistic Infections, San Francisco, 2000.
14. Carr A, Miller J, Law M, et al: A syndrome of lipoatrophy, lactic acidaemia and liver dysfunction associated with HIV nucleoside analogue therapy: Contribution to protease inhibitor-related lipodystrophy syndrome. AIDS 14:F25–32, 2000.
15. Hofstede H, De Marie S, Foudraine S: Four cases of fatal lactic acidosis due to mitochondrial toxicity of NRTI treatment: analysis of clinical features and risk factors (Abstract 592). Seventh Conference on Retroviruses and Opportunistic Infections. San Francisco, 2000.
16. Gérard Y, Maulin L, Yazdanpanah Y, et al: Symptomatic hyperlactatemia: An emerging complication of antiretroviral therapy. AIDS 14:2723–2730, 2000.
17. Gallagher EJ, Rodriguez K, Touger M: Agreement between peripheral venous and arterial lactate levels. Ann Emerg Med 29:479–483, 1997.
18. Chen YD, Varasteh BB, Reaven GM: Plasma lactate concentration in obesity and type 2 diabetes. Diabete Metab 19:348–354, 1993.
19. Astles R, Williams CP, Sedor F: Stability of plasma lactate in vitro in the presence of antiglycolytic agents. Clin Chem 40:1327–1330, 1994.
20. Brinkman K, Vrouenraets S, Kauffmann R, et al: Treatment of nucleoside reverse transcriptase inhibitor-induced lactic acidosis. AIDS 14:2801–2802, 2000.
21. Chodock R, Mylonakis E, Shemin D, et al: Survival of a human immunodeficiency patient with nucleoside-induced lactic acidosis—role of haemodialysis treatment. Nephrol Dial Transplant 14:2484–2486, 1999.
22. Lonergan JT, Havlir D, Barber E, et al: Incidence and outcome of hyperlactatemia associated with clinical manifestations in HIV-infected adults receiving NRTI-containing regimens (Abstract 624). Eighth Conference on Retroviruses and Opportunistic Infections. Chicago, 2001.
23. Cihlar T, Chen MS: Incorporation of selected nucleoside phosphonates and anti-human immunodeficiency virus nucleotide analogues into DNA by human DNA polymerases alpha, beta, and gamma. Antiviral Chem Chemother 8:187–195, 1997.
24. Garcia de la Asuncion JdO, Millan M, Pellin A, et al: AZT treatment induces molecular and ultrastructural oxidative damage to muscle mitochondria. J Clin Invest 102:4–9, 1998.
25. Paulik M, Lancaster M, Croom D, et al: Anti-oxidants rescue NRTI-induced metabolic changes in AKR/J mice. Antiviral Ther 5(Suppl 5):6–7, 2000.
26. Schramm C, Wanitschke R, Galle PR: Thiamine for the treatment of nucleoside analogue-induced severe lactic acidosis. Eur J Anaesthesiol 16:733–735, 1999.
27. Luzzati RDB, Perrl P, Luzzani G, et al: Riboflavin and severe lactic acidosis. Lancet 353:901–902, 1999.
28. Fouty B, Frermon F, Reves R: Riboflavin to treat nucleoside analogue-induced lactic acidosis. Lancet 352:291–292, 1998.
29. Dalakas M, Leon-Monzon M, Bernardini I, et al: Zidovudine-induced mitochondrial myopathy is associated with muscle carnitine deficiency and lipid storage. Ann Neurol 35:482–487, 1994.
30. Claessens YE, Cariou A, Chiche JD, et al: L-Carnitine as a treatment of life-threatening lactic acidosis induced by nucleoside analogues. AIDS 14:472–473, 2000.

CHAPTER **65**

Iron

Sean M. Bryant ■ Jerrold B. Leikin

Iron poisoning historically has been a significant toxicologic problem and remains so at present. In the pediatric population, iron has been regarded as the most fatal of all toxic exposures.[1] Because of regulations on packaging in the United States, serious poisoning has declined in this country.[2] Visible warning labels and dispensing of tablets and capsules in blister packages have limited the dose a child might consume. Total reported exposures in children younger than 6 years old has declined from 3026 in 1995 to 2094 in 2001 in the United States.[3,4] The other patient population at risk is individuals older than age 19 years, most notably women of childbearing age with access to iron products. In 2001, 27% of exposures occurred in women of childbearing age.[4] Despite the significant toxic potential of iron, death and serious sequelae are uncommon because most exposures are unintentional and involve negligible amounts.

BIOCHEMISTRY AND PHARMACOKINETICS OF IRON

The primary functions of iron include participation in oxygen delivery as a constituent of hemoglobin and myoglobin and production of adenosine triphosphate via oxidative phosphorylation. It is a highly reactive ion and functions in many enzymatic biochemical processes. Iron is a transition metal (number 26 on the periodic table) with an atomic weight of 55.8. It is the second most prevalent metal and the fourth most abundant element in the earth's crust.

Iron has interesting and unique properties related to its absorption, distribution, and elimination. Intestinal iron absorption is a complex and active process that occurs mostly in the proximal small intestine.[5] Most dietary inorganic iron is in the ferric (Fe^{3+}) form. Iron in the gut lumen may form complexes with other constituents, forming insoluble nonbioavailable products. Mucin, at the cell surface of the enterocyte, binds iron, preparing it for integrin-mediated systemic absorption. Mobilferrin binds the iron within the enterocyte cytoplasm. Iron eventually is transferred to paraferritin and ferritin before entering the bloodstream complexed to transferrin. Because the proportion of iron absorbed decreases with increasing dose,[6] an overdose

patient absorbs disproportionately less of the dose ingested than the amount absorbed when iron is given therapeutically. In healthy adults, 2% to 10% of dietary iron eventually is absorbed. A canine model showed that only 14% of a fatal oral dose of ferrous sulfate was absorbed.[7] In contrast, people with iron deficiency may absorb 80% to 90% of an oral dose.[8]

After oral ingestion, iron either remains in the gut mucosa and eventually is excreted in the stool or is transported in the blood by transferrin primarily to the bone marrow for hemoglobin synthesis. The liver differs from the rest of the body, including the placenta, in that its capacity for iron uptake is unlimited.[9,10] This first-pass effect is chiefly responsible for the decrease in plasma iron concentration after ingestion. These concepts support early iron concentration determination—4 to 6 hours after ingestion—as being useful after overdose, followed by the use of clinical parameters to predict prognosis after 8 to 12 hours.

Pharmacokinetics of Iron

Volume of distribution: preparation dependent
Protein binding: 99%
Mechanisms of clearance: renal, fecal, skin desquamation
Active metabolites: none
Methods to enhance clearance: deferoxamine

Total iron body stores are approximately 3 to 4 g in adults, with 70% distributed in hemoglobin in the ferrous (Fe^{2+}) state. It also is present in ferritin and hemosiderin, which are stored in the liver, spleen, and bone marrow. About 1 to 2 mg of iron is eliminated daily through urinary and fecal excretion and skin desquamation. The usually recommended daily allowance of iron is 10 mg in men, 18 mg in women, and 30 to 60 mg in women during pregnancy and lactation.

The amount of elemental iron ingested is the key factor in predicting the severity of toxicity. Common preparations contain various percentages of elemental iron (Table 65-1). Although 20 mg/kg of elemental iron or less may result in gastric upset, potentially severe toxicity may follow

TABLE 65-1 Iron Content of Common Preparations

PREPARATION	ELEMENTAL IRON (%)
Ferrous gluconate	12
Ferrous sulfate*	20
Ferric chloride*	20
Ferrous chloride	28
Ferrous fumarate	33

*Hydrated.

ingestions of 40 to 60 mg/kg, and potentially lethal doses range from 200 to 250 mg/kg.[11] In toddlers, doses of 1.0 g of elemental iron have been reported to be fatal.[12,13]

PATHOPHYSIOLOGY

Iron, an essential element for bodily functions, must come from outside sources. It is a catalyst for the Haber-Weiss reaction resulting in free radical production:

$$O^-_2 \text{ (superoxide)} + H_2O_2 \text{ (hydrogen peroxide)} \rightarrow OH^- + OH^{\cdot} \text{ (hydroxyl radical)} + O_2$$

This iron-catalyzed reaction generates the highly reactive hydroxyl radical. Iron-induced lipid peroxidation, resulting from the production of these free radicals, is the primary mechanism of iron poisoning.[14,15] These free radicals induce local injury, most notably in locations of high iron concentrations, such as the intestine and liver. The primary intracellular target of toxicity is the mitochondria, resulting in destruction of cristae and loss of respiratory enzyme activity in a manner that is consistent with suppression of cellular respiration, without uncoupling oxidative phosphorylation.[16,17] Iron primarily affects the gastrointestinal (GI) tract, liver, cardiovascular system, and acid-base status of the poisoned patient. Because of the high metabolic activity of the heart, the myocardial mitochondria are particularly vulnerable to the toxic effects of iron poisoning.

Gastrointestinal

The initial GI symptoms after iron overdose are due to a direct local irritant effect. With large ingestions, free radical–induced lipid peroxidation causes secondary injury to the GI tract. There is a significant risk of hemorrhage and ulcerative damage from segmental gut infarction in children and adults.[18] Because of this damage, there is a concern for emerging GI bleeding during the first 48 to 72 hours after ingestion. Delayed effects, classically stricture formation, may occur weeks after exposure. Gastric outlet obstruction occurring 2 to 4 weeks after exposure is a consequence of healing and scarring of the gut. A high index of suspicion for gastric outlet obstruction exists in patients who have continual vomiting 2 to 3 weeks after the exposure incident or an onset of emesis after a symptom-free period.[19] Although pyloric injury is most common, lesions may occur at any location in the gut.[18]

Hepatic

Characteristic hemorrhagic hepatic periportal necrosis has been described in autopsy reports of patients who died from iron poisoning and in experimental animal models.[20] Other reports indicate similar damage in patients and animal models.[21] After absorption, iron is transported to the liver via the portal vein, where carrier-mediated uptake into zone 1 acinar cells eventually becomes overwhelmed. Microscopic observations indicate that hepatic mitochondrial injury within zone 1 is the primary mechanism of toxicity.[22] Because liver cell regeneration is a zone 1 function, injury to this region is of particular significance. After this injury, acute hepatic failure with elevated hepatic transaminases and serum ammonia concentrations, jaundice, steatosis, and hepatic coma may occur.[23]

Coagulopathy

Coagulopathy resulting from severe iron poisoning is characteristically biphasic.[24] A dose-related reversible coagulopathy has been shown in a canine model and in humans.[24] This condition results from a transient, early, dose-dependent depression of coagulation factors V, VII, IX, and X, causing a prolongation of the partial thromboplastin time.[24] An in vitro study showed that free iron may inhibit the formation of thrombin and subsequently thrombin's ability to form fibrin from fibrinogen.[25] This early coagulopathy may subside as iron levels decrease; however, severe poisoning may result in a second phase (2 to 7 days postingestion) of progressive dysfunction of coagulation secondary to hepatotoxicity.

Cardiovascular

Circulatory shock is the most common cause of death due to iron poisoning. In addition to hypovolemia resulting from GI volume loss and hemorrhage, an early distributive shock has been shown in animal models.[26,27] The myocardium has high metabolic activity, and acute iron-induced cardiotoxicity may be mediated by free radical generation.[28] In addition to interference with mitochondrial adenosine triphosphate production, membrane lipid peroxidation may interfere directly with slow-channel calcium exchange or the activity of the sarcoplasmic reticulum.[29] Diminished myocardial contractility is an important component of the pathogenesis of iron-induced shock.[30] Cardiac failure may occur 1 to several days after a major iron overdose.[31] The pathophysiology of shock resulting from iron overdose is multifactorial.

Metabolic

Metabolic acidosis is a prominent feature of iron poisoning. As discussed earlier, circulatory shock is one pathophysiologic mechanism responsible for this metabolic acidosis. Acidosis also may occur, however, in the absence of cardiovascular instability.[32] As described previously, iron poisoning suppresses cellular respiration. A principal mechanism by which iron causes a metabolic acidosis occurs, however, after absorption of a quantity of iron that exceeds the binding capacity of transferrin. When unbound iron is present, its hydrolysis liberates three unbuffered protons from each ferric ion:[33]

$$3H_2O + Fe^{3+} \rightarrow Fe(OH)_3 + 3H^+$$

Other Pathophysiologic Effects

Altered mental status may occur after large ingestions and is presumably multifactorial and related to the factors described earlier. Although no major direct toxicity is clinically apparent and relevant to the central nervous system, kidney, lung, and spleen, autopsy studies have revealed elevated iron concentrations in these organ systems and in the stomach, liver, and small intestine.[34]

CLINICAL PRESENTATION AND LIFE-THREATENING COMPLICATIONS

Classically, iron poisoning is described as occurring in five clinical stages (Table 65-2). Not all patients manifest this "textbook" presentation after overdose, however, and there is the potential for considerable temporal variability and overlap among these stages. The severity and stage of a particular patient's poisoning should be determined by his or her individual clinical evaluation, not simply by the number of hours since ingestion.

Stage I (the GI stage) of poisoning is encountered almost universally in all patients after significant iron ingestion. Epigastric pain, nausea, vomiting, and diarrhea typically occur immediately after ingestion in cases of overdose.[35] Hypotension, pallor, and lethargy often occur, resulting from vasodilation, intravascular volume loss, gastroenteritis, hematemesis, melena, or hematochezia secondary to the local effects of iron on the gut mucosa. Metabolic acidosis may occur at this stage. If acidosis is significant, blood volume loss occurs, resulting in circulatory shock, and the patient may progress directly into stage III.

Stage II is the time period associated with iron poisoning that is described as the *latent phase*. During this interval, which may begin several hours postingestion, the patient is in transition between the resolution of direct GI signs and symptoms and the appearance of overt systemic toxicity. This often-described quiescent phase may reflect failure to recognize ongoing clinical toxicity. The patient may have fewer overt GI manifestations during this time, lulling the clinician into an underestimation of the true seriousness of the ingestion.[36] During this apparently clinically benign period, however, patients may have a worsening metabolic acidosis if volume resuscitation is not sufficient to restore adequate tissue perfusion. Patients who progress through stage I with resolution of clinical manifestations and without development of a metabolic acidosis are unlikely to develop more serious systemic iron toxicity.

Stage III, the shock stage of iron toxicity, is defined by evidence of insufficient tissue perfusion and shock and typically

becomes manifest at least several hours after ingestion. Most deaths due to iron poisoning occur in this stage. Multiple organ dysfunction as a result of cellular toxicity and inadequate perfusion may result in hypotension, tachycardia, altered mental status, seizures, coma, worsening metabolic acidosis, renal failure, hepatic dysfunction, coagulopathy, myocardial depression, pulmonary edema, and mesenteric ischemia.[37] Hepatotoxicity often is evident during stage III; however, this may occur without concomitant shock.

Stage IV (hepatotoxicity) is not a universal finding in iron-poisoned patients.[38] The onset of this stage typically occurs 12 to 24 hours postingestion but may occur 2 to 3 days after overdose.[23] Hepatic dysfunction is a poor prognostic sign when present,[24] with hemorrhage secondary to coagulopathy often contributing to patient demise.[24]

The hallmark of stage V is gastric outlet obstruction; however, this stage rarely occurs.[11] Local mucosal injury may lead to development of stricture formation several weeks postingestion.[18] Although the classic site of obstruction is the pylorus, segmental injury may occur along the length of the gut.[18] The diagnosis of gastric outlet obstruction should be considered in patients with persistent vomiting, achlorhydria, abdominal pain, and distention more than 1 week postingestion.

Iron poisoning may present in any of the above-mentioned discrete stages, may skip specific stages, or may reflect overlap between or among different stages. The stages of toxicity are used as a guide to the conceptualization of the natural course of iron poisoning rather than as a consistently predictable sequence of events.

DIAGNOSIS

The diagnosis of iron toxicity may be evident based on a history of ingestion and corresponding signs of iron toxicity. GI symptoms are present in virtually all patients with significant iron ingestions.[39] If no history of iron ingestion is offered, however, the differential diagnosis includes other medical and surgical reasons for the varied manifestations of iron poisoning. Other poisonings to consider include those involving mercuric chloride, salicylates, pesticides, and colchicine.

All patients with known or suspected iron overdose should receive an x-ray of the abdomen to evaluate for radiopaque tablets.[40,41] Large overdoses of tablets can be visualized in the GI tract, helping to verify historical features and guide management with GI decontamination. If the patient ingested a liquid preparation, the abdominal film typically is unrevealing.[41] Pediatric multivitamins containing iron have such a low iron content that x-rays after ingestion of these also typically are negative.[42] Clinically significant poisoning after ingestion of iron-containing multivitamins is virtually nonexistent.[43] Negative abdominal plain films after iron ingestion also may be explained by dissolution of an ingested solid formulation; this is especially true in patients who present late after ingestion.

We recommend that a serum iron concentration be obtained on presentation and then every 1 to 2 hours to monitor the symptomatic patient further. When a clear downward trend of serum iron concentrations is established, it is no longer necessary to follow this parameter. Iron concentrations less than 500 μg/dL (<90 μmol/L)

TABLE 65-2 Stages of Iron Poisoning

STAGE	TYPICAL
I—Gastrointestinal	30 min–6 hr
II—Quiescent	2–8 hr
III—Shock	2–48 hr
IV—Hepatotoxicity	12–24 hr
V—Gut obstruction	1–7 wk

typically are not associated with significant systemic toxicity.[44,45] Systemic toxicity often is seen with iron concentrations of 500 to 1000 μg/dL (90 to 180 μmol/L), with levels greater than 1000 μg/dL (>180 μmol/L) being associated with severe life-threatening illness.

A high anion gap metabolic acidosis accompanying an elevated lactate concentration should be assumed to be an indication of serious toxicity from iron ingestion[37] and the need for chelation therapy. Because of the possibility of hemorrhage and multiple-organ toxicity, a complete blood count, hepatic and renal function tests, electrolytes, and coagulation profile should be obtained. The presence of hemorrhage or anemia should prompt preparation for possible blood product replacement.

Historically, other laboratory findings, such as leukocytosis (white blood cell count >15,000/mm³) and hyperglycemia (serum glucose >150 mg/dL [8.25 mmol/L]), were used as indices of severity of iron poisoning.[46] These parameters have not been shown to be sensitive predictors of toxicity, however.[44,47] Likewise, a serum iron concentration greater than the total iron-binding capacity, previously considered an indication for chelation therapy, has not been found to be a reliable index of toxicity and no longer is recommended.[44,48,49]

TREATMENT

Patients with significant iron ingestions or severe systemic toxicity warrant monitoring in the intensive care unit. Secure intravenous access, fluid volume replacement, oxygen supplementation, cardiac monitoring, and airway and ventilatory support are essential to the initial management of the critically iron-poisoned patient. Swan-Ganz catheter placement may be indicated for monitoring of hemodynamic parameters during treatment and to differentiate between cardiogenic and distributive shock.

Limiting the absorption of ingested iron should be considered during initial management. Administering syrup of ipecac is not supportable after presentation because of the lack of evidence of outcome benefit and concerns about aspiration risk.[50,51] Similarly, patients consistently develop GI symptoms after significant ingestion, and ipecac may obfuscate this marker of toxicity. Gastric lavage is an alternative form of gastric emptying. This procedure also has serious risks, has not proved to change outcome after iron ingestion, and should be considered only in life-threatening ingestions presenting within 1 hour.[50,52] Even in these circumstances, the efficacy of gastric lavage is questionable. Although activated charcoal is a standard method of GI

decontamination, it has not been shown to be effective in adsorbing iron.[53] Consideration of activated charcoal is appropriate when coingestion of noniron products has occurred.

The mainstay of GI decontamination for iron poisoning generally is considered to be whole-bowel irrigation.[54] This procedure has not been shown, however, to alter the clinical course or outcome of iron-poisoned patients.[55] Whole-bowel irrigation theoretically is important only in patients with abdominal radiographs revealing substantial numbers of radiopaque iron tablets. Whole-bowel irrigation is reviewed in Chapter 6. Although whole-bowel irrigation usually is limited to several hours of administration, one case report of multiple iron tablet persistence in the gut described a 5-day course of whole-bowel irrigation.[56] This case also may be taken as evidence, however, of the lack of efficacy of this technique. Subsequent abdominal x-rays can help guide the clearance of iron from the gut.

Gastroenterologic or surgical consultation should be considered in the event that a concretion or bezoar is shown or suspected; this is unusual, however. Concretions may be present when iron levels continue to rise. Usually there is a downward trend toward clearing by 6 to 24 hours postingestion. Several authors reported successful gastrotomy and removal of massive amounts of iron tablets not amenable to removal by less invasive measures.[57–61] Clinical evidence of bowel obstruction may indicate intestinal necrosis. Lifesaving small-bowel resection was performed 24 hours after presentation in a patient with a distended abdomen and signs of peritonitis.[62]

Other attempts at reducing iron absorption from the gut have been undertaken without success. Oral bicarbonate, phosphate, and magnesium hydroxide have been used with the idea that if they formed insoluble complexes with iron this would decrease absorption. Except for one canine study, data from in vitro and in vivo studies do not support bicarbonate or phosphate use, and these treatments may result in severe electrolyte imbalances.[63–66] Animal and human volunteer studies revealed a reduction in iron absorption after the administration of magnesium hydroxide; however, it does not affect absorption in humans after large overdoses of iron.[67–69] At present, there are insufficient data to support routine use of these modalities in human iron poisoning. Oral deferoxamine was shown in one prospective human study to reduce GI absorption of ferrous sulfate when mixed as a slurry with activated charcoal. Ferrioxamine, the deferoxamine-iron complex, has been shown to be lethal in animals after it is absorbed, but ferrioxamine absorption is reduced when activated charcoal is coadministered with deferoxamine.[70,71] Because of the concerns about the toxicity of ferrioxamine, oral deferoxamine is not recommended.

Iron-induced hepatotoxicity should be regarded as a marker of severe toxicity. Because the periportal area is most affected, iron-induced hepatotoxicity portends a much poorer overall prognosis than similar insults caused by other toxicants.[21] In light of this, hepatic monitoring and treatment of organ failure or coagulopathy should be pursued. Profound liver dysfunction warrants surgical consultation for possible transplantation. Correction of electrolyte and glucose abnormalities also may be crucial to patient outcome.

Hemodialysis should be used on a supportive basis for acute renal failure, usually developing in response to circulatory shock. Iron is not amenable to hemodialysis, even though the iron-deferoxamine complex can be cleared in this manner.[72]

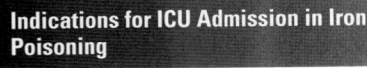

Indications for ICU Admission in Iron Poisoning

Significant acidemia (arterial pH <7.3)
Shock/neurodynamic compromise
Altered mental status
Serum iron concentration >500 μg/dL (90 μmol/L)
Radiologic evidence of a significant gastrointestinal burden of iron (>50 mg of elemental iron/kg)

Deferoxamine, derived from *Streptomyces pilosus*, is the specific chelator of choice for iron poisoning. After complexing with free iron (iron not found in hemoglobin, myoglobin, ferritin, or transferrin), it forms ferrioxamine, which is excreted in the urine. Deferoxamine also has been shown to promote clearance of intracellular iron effectively. Ferrioxamine produces a reddish brown or "vin rose" appearance to the urine. Deferoxamine challenge tests have been used in the past as a marker of iron excretion, as indicated by this urine color change. This test no longer is recommended; however, it is recommended to observe a urine sample before treatment and follow the course of color change during chelation. A total of 100 mg of deferoxamine mesylate chelates approximately 8.5 mg of ferric iron. Although the use of deferoxamine in severe iron poisoning is considered the standard of care, there are no published controlled studies that show a change in outcome with this treatment.

Deferoxamine treatment should be administered as early as possible after poisoning. Indications for deferoxamine are moderate to severe systemic toxicity, such as shock, GI bleeding, lethargy, and central nervous system depression. Metabolic acidosis is a reliable marker of cellular iron toxicity[37] and an indication for initiating treatment. Chelation should not be withheld while waiting for a serum iron concentration in significantly poisoned patients. An iron level 4 to 6 hours postingestion of equal to or greater than 500 μg/dL (≥90 μmol/L) also is considered to be an indication for treatment.[44,45] After 12 hours, the serum iron concentration is of no practical significance because the systemic burden has been distributed from the vascular compartment into tissues.

Recommendations for deferoxamine dosing are based primarily on case reports and have been established arbitrarily.[73] The intravenous route of administration is preferred. Intramuscular administration was used previously for less severe poisoning, but it is not considered to be reliable. Titration of the intravenous infusion to a rate of 15 mg/kg/hr should be initiated while the patient is carefully monitored for adverse effects, including rate-related hypotension.[74,75] Histamine release may underlie the hypotension and the flushing and urticaria that may be observed during deferoxamine infusion.[75] Administration of deferoxamine at even higher rates has been shown to be safe in ill patients and in patients on long-term hemodialysis.[76] There have been recommendations to administer less than 6 to 8 g/day even though 16 g/day has been given without concomitant side effects.[77] It is vital to maintain adequate intravenous fluid volume replacement during deferoxamine therapy to protect against the development of acute renal failure.[78] Finally, continuous infusions for greater than 24 hours have been reported to be associated with adult respiratory distress syndrome; however, this interpretation is confounded by the presence of adult respiratory distress syndrome in severe iron poisoning, even in untreated cases.[79–81] A reasonable end point of therapy is cessation of metabolic acidosis and resolution of systemic toxicity. Because the deferoxamine-iron complex acts as a siderophore for the growth of *Yersinia enterocolitica*, sepsis after chelation therapy is a risk, and appropriate antimicrobial therapy should be considered.[82–84] It is important to determine serum iron concentrations by atomic absorption spectroscopy in deferoxamine-treated patients because deferoxamine interferes with most other routine assays.

Criteria for ICU Discharge in Iron Poisoning

Absence of acidemia or other systemic disorders (e.g., coagulopathy)
Hemodynamic stability
Clear sensorium
Declining serum iron concentrations

SPECIAL POPULATIONS

Pregnant Patients

Iron overdose has occurred with relative frequency in pregnant patients.[85] There is no proven teratogenic risk of deferoxamine therapy during pregnancy, and fetal loss may occur as a result of severe maternal iron toxicity. Similar to trauma and many other diseases of pregnant women, the goals are to stabilize and treat the mother, which stabilizes and treats the fetus. The approach to a pregnant patient is no different from that for any other patient, other than that if the fetus is potentially viable it should be monitored for distress. Although spontaneous abortion, preterm delivery, and malformations are potential sequelae of treatment in severe iron poisoning, several cases reported successful use of deferoxamine in pregnancy.[86–89] One report described a postnatal fatality in a 30-year-old woman who was treated with deferoxamine 1 day after ingestion and successfully delivered a healthy infant 2 weeks before experiencing lethal multiple organ dysfunction.[90] The placenta serves as the fetus's barrier to systemic iron overload and associated toxicity. This concept is supported in an ovine model.[10] Deferoxamine may cross the placenta when the mother is treated for toxicity.[86] Harm to the fetus from deferoxamine use in pregnancy is referenced[10,88] yet not supported by the actual evidence. Cases describe first-trimester use of deferoxamine in women with chronic overload without subsequent fetal abnormalities.[91,92] Deferoxamine therapy should not be withheld out of concern for the fetus. Appropriately treating the mother is tantamount to treating the fetus.

Common Errors in Iron Poisoning

Withholding deferoxamine in an ill patient while waiting for a serum iron concentration
Withholding deferoxamine in a pregnant patient who meets criteria for treatment
Assessing a patient in stage II of toxicity as improved or fully recovered
Relying on leukocytosis and hyperglycemia to predict prognosis or guide therapy
Using total iron-binding capacity or a chelation challenge test to indicate need for deferoxamine
Administering deferoxamine to patients who exhibit only direct gastrointestinal toxicity from iron

Key Points in Iron Poisoning

1. Estimate total iron ingested based on the elemental dose and not the weight of the salt.
2. Serum iron concentrations beyond 12 hours after ingestion are of no benefit in managing the patient.
3. The end point of deferoxamine therapy is guided best by clinical stability of the patient and cessation of academia.
4. Fluid hydration is crucial during deferoxamine administration to help prevent acute renal failure.
5. Pregnant patients are approached in the same way and as aggressively as nonpregnant patients.

REFERENCES

1. Litovitz T, Manoguerra A: Comparison of pediatric poisoning hazards: An analysis of 3.8 million exposure incidents. Pediatrics 89:999–1006, 1992.
2. Nightingale SL: From the Food and Drug Administration. JAMA 277:1343, 1997.
3. Litovitz TL, Felberg L, White S, Klein-Schwartz W: 1995 annual report of the American Association of Poison Control Centers Toxic Exposure Surveillance System. Am J Emerg Med 14:487–537, 1996.
4. Litovitz TL, Klein-Shwartz W, Rodgers GC, et al: 2001 annual report of the American Association of Poison Control Centers Toxic Exposure Surveillance System. Am J Emerg Med 20:391–452, 2002.
5. Umbreit JN, Conrad ME, Moore EG, Latour LF: Iron absorption and cellular transport: The moriferrin/paraferritin paradigm. Semin Hematol 35:13–26, 1998.
6. Smith MD, Pannacciulli IM: Absorption of inorganic iron from gradient doses: Its significance in relation to iron absorption tests and the mucosal block theory. Br J Haematol 4:428–434, 1958.
7. Reissman KR, Coleman TJ, Budai BS, Moriarty LR: Acute intestinal iron intoxication: Iron absorption, serum iron and autopsy findings. Blood 10:35–45, 1955.
8. Harju E: Clinical pharmacokinetics of iron preparations. Clin Pharmacokinet 17:69–89, 1989.
9. Zimelman AP, Zimmerman HJ, McLean R, Weintraub LR: Effects of iron saturation of transferrin on hepatic iron uptake: An in vitro study. Gastroenterology 72:129–131, 1977.
10. Curry SC, Bond GR, Raschke R, et al: An ovine model of maternal iron poisoning in pregnancy. Ann Emerg Med 19:632–638, 1990.
11. Banner W Jr, Tong TG: Iron poisoning. Pediatr Clin North Am 33:393–409, 1986.
12. Spencer IOB: Ferrous sulphate poisoning in children. BMJ 2:1112–1117, 1951.
13. Thomson J: Two cases of ferrous sulfate poisoning. BMJ 1:640–641, 1947.
14. Halliwell B, Gutteridge JMC: Oxygen free radicals and iron in relation to biology and medicine: Some problems and concepts. Arch Biochem Biophys 246:501–514, 1986.
15. Bacon BR, Britton RS: The pathophysiology of hepatic iron overload: A free radical-mediated process? Hepatology 11:127–137, 1990.
16. Link G, Saada A, Pinson A, et al: Mitochondrial respiratory enzymes are a major target of iron toxicity in rat heart cells. J Lab Clin Med 131:466–474, 1998.
17. Witzleben CL: An electron microscopic study of ferrous sulfate induced liver damage. Am J Pathol 49:1053–1058, 1966.
18. Tenenbein M, Littman C, Stimpson RE: Gastrointestinal pathology in adult iron overdose. J Toxicol Clin Toxicol 28:311–320, 1990.
19. Gandhi RK, Robarts FH: Hour-glass stricture of the stomach and pyloric stenosis due to ferrous sulphate poisoning. Br J Surg 49:613–617, 1962.
20. Luongo MA, Bjornson SS: The liver in ferrous sulfate poisoning. N Engl J Med 251:995–999, 1954.
21. Tenenbein M: Hepatoxicity in acute iron poisoning. J Toxicol Clin Toxicol 39:721–726, 2001.
22. Ganote CE, Nahara G: Acute ferrous sulfate hepatotoxicity in rats: An electron microscopic and biochemical study. Lab Invest 28:426–436, 1973.
23. Gleason WA, deMello DE, deCastro FJ, Conners JJ: Acute hepatic failure in severe iron poisoning. J Pediatr 95:138–140, 1979.
24. Tenenbein M, Israels SJ: Early coagulopathy in severe iron poisoning. J Pediatr 113:695–697, 1988.
25. Rosenmund A, Haeberli A, Straub PW: Blood coagulation and acute iron toxicity. J Lab Clin Med 103:524–533, 1984.
26. Whitten CF, Chen YC, Gibson GW: Studies in acute iron poisoning: III. The hemodynamic alterations in acute experimental iron poisoning. Pediatr Res 2:479–485, 1968.
27. Vernon DD, Banner W, Dean JM: Hemodynamic effects of experimental iron poisoning. Ann Emerg Med 18:863–866, 1989.
28. Artman M, Olsen RD, Boucek RJ, Boerth RC: Depression of contractility in isolated rabbit myocardium following exposure to iron: role of free radicals. Toxicol Appl Pharmacol 72:324–332, 1984.
29. Pinson GL, Hershko C: Heart cells in culture: A model of myocardial iron overload and chelation. J Lab Clin Med 106:147–153, 1985.
30. Artman M, Olson RD, Boerth RC: Depression of myocardial contractility in acute iron toxicity in rabbits. Toxicol Appl Pharmacol 66:329–337, 1982.
31. Tenenbein M, Kopelow ML, deSa DJ: Myocardial failure and shock in iron poisoning. Hum Toxicol 7:281–284, 1988.
32. Tenenbein M: Toxicokinetics and toxicodynamics of iron poisoning. Toxicol Lett 102–103:653–656, 1998.
33. Reissman KR, Coleman TJ: Acute intestinal iron intoxication: II. Metabolic, respiratory, and circulatory effects of absorbed iron salts. Blood 10:46–51, 1955.
34. Pestaner JP, Ishak KG, Mullick FG, Centeno JA: Ferrous sulfate toxicity: A review of autopsy findings. Biol Trace Elem Res 69:191–198, 1999.
35. Robotham JL, Lietman PS: Acute iron poisoning: A review. Am J Dis Child 134:875–879, 1980.
36. Banner W, Tong TG: Iron poisoning. Pediatr Clin North Am 33:393–409, 1986.
37. Mills KC, Curry SC: Acute iron poisoning. Emerg Med Clin North Am 12:397–413, 1994.
38. Henretig FM, Karl SR, Weintraub WH: Severe iron poisoning treated with enteral and intravenous deferoxamine. Ann Emerg Med 12:306–309, 1983.
39. Knasel AL, Collins-Barrow MD: Applicability of early indicators of iron toxicity. J Natl Med Assoc 78:1037–1040, 1986.
40. Ng RC, Perry K, Martin DJ: Iron poisoning: Assessment of radiography in diagnosis and management. Clin Pediatr 18:614–616, 1979.
41. Staple TW, McAlister WH: Roentgenographic visualization of iron preparations in the gastrointestinal tract. Radiology 83:1051–1056, 1964.
42. Everson GW, Oudjhane K, Young LW, Krenzelok EP: Effectiveness of abdominal radiographs in visualizing chewable iron supplements following overdose. Am J Emerg Med 7:459–463, 1989.
43. Linakis JG, Lacouture PG, Woolf A: Iron absorption from chewable vitamins with iron versus iron tablets: Implications for toxicity. Pediatr Emerg Care 8:321–324, 1992.
44. Chyka PA, Bradyr AY: Assessment of acute iron poisoning by laboratory and clinical observations. Am J Emerg Med 11:99–103, 1993.
45. Bosse GM: Conservative management of patients with moderately elevated serum iron levels. J Toxicol Clin Toxicol 33:135–140, 1995.
46. Lacouture PG, Wason S, Temple AR, et al: Emergency assessment of severity in iron overdose by clinical and laboratory methods. J Pediatr 99:89–91, 1981.
47. Palatnick W, Tenenbein M: Leukocytosis, hyperglycemia, vomiting, and positive x-rays are not indicators of severity of iron overdose in adults. Am J Emerg Med 14:454–455, 1996.
48. Siff JE, Meldon SW, Tomassoni AJ: Usefulness of total iron binding capacity in the evaluation and treatment of acute iron overdose. Ann Emerg Med 33:73–76, 1999.
49. Tenenbein M, Yatscoff RW: The total iron-binding capacity in iron poisoning: Is it useful? Am J Dis Child 145:437–439, 1991.
50. Tenenbein M: Inefficacy of gastric emptying procedures. J Emerg Med 3:133–136, 1985.
51. American Association of Clinical Toxicology, European Association of Poisons Centres and Clinical Toxicologists: Position statement: Ipecac syrup. J Toxicol Clin Toxicol 35:699–709, 1997.
52. American Association of Clinical Toxicology, European Association of Poisons Centres and Clinical Toxicologists: Position statement: Gastric lavage. J Toxicol Clin Toxicol 35:711–719, 1997.
53. Decker WJ, Combs HF, Corby DG: Adsorption of drugs and poisons by activated charcoal. Toxicol Appl Pharmacol 13:454–460, 1968.
54. Tenenbein M: Whole bowel irrigation in iron poisoning. J Pediatr 111:142–145, 1987.

55. American Association of Clinical Toxicology, European Association of Poisons Centres and Clinical Toxicologists: Position statement: Whole bowel irrigation. J Toxicol Clin Toxicol 35:753–762, 1997.

56. Kaczorowski JM, Wax PM: Five days of whole-bowel irrigation in a case of pediatric iron ingestion. Ann Emerg Med 27:258–263, 1996.

57. Peterson CD, Fifield GC: Emergency gastrotomy for acute iron poisoning. Ann Emerg Med 9:262–264, 1980.

58. Venturelli J, Kwee Y, Morris N, Cameron G: Gastrotomy in the management of acute iron poisoning. J Pediatr 100:768–769, 1982.

59. Foxford R, Goldfrank L: Gastrotomy—a surgical approach to iron overdose. Ann Emerg Med 14:1223–1226, 1985.

60. Landsman I, Bricker JT, Reid BS, Bloss RS: Emergency gastrotomy: Treatment of choice for iron bezoar. J Pediatr Surg 22:184–185, 1987.

61. Tenenbein M, Wiseman N, Yatscoff RW: Gastrotomy and whole bowel irrigation in iron poisoning. Pediatr Emerg Care 7:286–288, 1991.

62. Roberts RJ, Nayfield S, Soper R, Kent TH: Acute iron intoxication with intestinal infarction managed in part by small bowel resection. Clin Toxicol 8:3–12, 1975.

63. Czajka PA, Konrad JD, Duffy JP: Iron poisoning: An in vitro comparison of bicarbonate and phosphate lavage solutions. J Pediatr 98:491–494, 1981.

64. Dean BS, Krenzelok EP: In vivo effectiveness of oral complexation agents in the management of iron poisoning. Clin Toxicol 25:221–230, 1987.

65. Bachrach L, Correa A, Levin R, Grossman M: Iron poisoning: Complications of hypertonic phosphate lavage therapy. J Pediatr 94:147–149, 1979.

66. Geffner ME, Opas LM: Phosphate poisoning complicating treatment for iron ingestion. Am J Dis Child 134:509–510, 1980.

67. Wallace KL, Curry SC, LoVecchio F, Raschke RA: Effect of magnesium hydroxide on iron absorption following simulated mild iron overdose in human subjects. Acad Emerg Med 5:961–965, 1998.

68. Corby DG, McCullen AH, Chadwick EW, Decker WJ: Effect of orally administered magnesium hydroxide in experimental iron intoxication. J Toxicol Clin Toxicol 23:489–499, 1985–86.

69. Snyder BK, Clark RF: Effect of magnesium hydroxide administration on iron absorption after a supratherapeutic dose of ferrous sulfate in human volunteers: A randomized controlled trial. Ann Emerg Med 33:400–405, 1999.

70. Gomez HF, McClafferty HH, Flory D, et al: Prevention of gastrointestinal iron absorption by chelation from an orally administered premixed deferoxamine/charcoal slurry. Ann Emerg Med 30:587–592, 1997.

71. Whitten CF, Chen Y, Gibson GW: Studies in acute iron poisoning: II. Further observation on desferrioxamine in the treatment of acute experimental iron poisoning. Pediatrics 38:102–110, 1966.

72. Richardson JR, Sugerman DL, Hulet WH: Extraction of iron by chelation and desferrioxamine and hemodialysis. Clin Res 15:368, 1967.

73. Westlin WF: Deferoxamine in the treatment of acute iron poisoning: Clinical experiences with 172 children. Clin Pediatr 5:531–535, 1966.

74. Leikin S, Vossough P, Mochis-Fatemi F: Chelation therapy in acute iron poisoning. J Pediatr 71:425–430, 1967.

75. Whitten CF, Gibson GW, Good MH, et al: Studies in acute iron poisoning: Desferrioxamine in the treatment of iron poisoning: Clinical observations, experimental studies and theoretical considerations. Pediatrics 36:322–325, 1965.

76. Berland Y, Carhon SA, Olmer M, Meunier PJ: Predictive value of desferrioxamine infusion test for bone aluminum deposit in hemodialyzed patients. Nephron 40:433–435, 1985.

77. Leikin JB, Paloucek FP (eds): Poisoning and Toxicology Handbook, 3rd ed. Hudson, OH, Lexi-Comp, 2002.

78. Koren G, Bentur Y, Strong D, et al: Acute changes in renal function associated with deferoxamine therapy. Am J Dis Child 143:1077–1080, 1989.

79. Tenenbein M, Kowalski S, Sienko A, et al. Pulmonary toxic effects of continuous desferrioxamine administration in acute iron poisoning. Lancet 339:699–701, 1992.

80. Anderson KJ, Rivers RPA: Desferrioxamine in acute iron poisoning. Lancet 339:1602, 1992.

81. Ioannides AS, Panisello JM: Acute respiratory distress syndrome in children with acute iron poisoning: The role of intravenous desferrioxamine. Eur J Pediatr 159:158–159, 2000.

82. Melby K, Skordahl S, Guttebert TJ, Nordbo SA: Septicaemia due to *Yersinia enterocolitica* after oral overdose of iron. BMJ 285:467–468, 1982.

83. Mofenson HC, Caraccio TR, Sharieff N: Iron sepsis: *Yersinia enterocolitica* septicemia possibly caused by an overdose of iron. N Engl J Med 316:1092–1093, 1987.

84. Milteer RM, Sarpong S, Poydras U: *Yersinia enterocolitica* septicemia after accidental oral iron overdose. Pediatr Infect Dis J 8:537–538, 1989.

85. Tran T, Wax JR, Philput C, et al: Intentional iron overdose in pregnancy—management and outcome. J Emerg Med 18:225–228, 2000.

86. Rayburn WF, Donn SM, Wulf ME: Iron overdose during pregnancy: Successful therapy with deferoxamine. Am J Obstet Gynecol 14:717–718, 1983.

87. Lacoste H, Goyert GL, Goldman LS, et al: Acute iron intoxication in pregnancy: Case report and review of the literature. Obstet Gynecol 80:500–501, 1992.

88. McElhatton PR, Roberts JC, Sullivan FM: The consequences of iron overdose and its treatment with desferrioxamine in pregnancy. Hum Exp Toxicol 10:251–259, 1991.

89. Turk J, Aks S, Ampuero F, Hryhorczuk DO: Successful therapy of iron intoxication in pregnancy with intravenous deferoxamine and whole bowel irrigation. Vet Hum Toxicol 35:441–444, 1993.

90. Olenmark M, Biber B, Dottori O, Rybo G: Fatal iron intoxication in late pregnancy. Clin Toxicol 25:347–359, 1987.

91. Thomas RM, Skalicka AE: Successful pregnancy in transfusion-dependent thalassaemia. Arch Dis Child 55:572–574, 1980.

92. Martin K: Successful pregnancy in β-thalassaemia major. Aust Paediatr J 19:182–183, 1983.

CHAPTER 66

Oral Anticoagulants

Jeffrey R. Suchard ▪ Steven C. Curry

In the 1920s, a hemorrhagic disorder of cattle feeding on spoiled clover silage was recognized. Studies of "sweet clover disease" led to the isolation in 1939 of dicumarol (bishydroxycoumarin), the first oral anticoagulant (OAC) drug. A more potent synthetic derivative, 3-(α-acetonylbenzyl)-4-hydroxycoumarin, was produced in 1948 and named warfarin, after the Wisconsin Alumni Research Foundation. Warfarin initially was used mostly as a rodenticide because of concerns of unacceptable toxicity. Then in 1951, an army inductee uneventfully survived a massive overdose of a warfarin rodenticide. Warfarin also was used to treat President Eisenhower after a heart attack in 1955, contributing to its general acceptance as a therapeutic drug. Many rat populations have become resistant to warfarin, leading to the use of "superwarfarins" (see Chapter 93) since the 1970s. These newer rodenticides have higher potencies and considerably longer half-lives than warfarin and the other therapeutic OACs.

Warfarin is the most commonly used OAC worldwide. Although not used in the United States, phenprocoumon (Fig. 66-1) and acenocoumarol are used in other parts of the world. These three drugs are 4-hydroxycoumarin derivatives with nonpolar carbon substituents at the 3 position. Indane-1,3-dione OACs are available but are used infrequently therapeutically.

PHARMACOKINETICS

Absorption is nearly complete when oral anticoagulants are ingested. Warfarin is detectable in plasma within 1 hour of ingestion, and concentrations of therapeutic doses peak in 2 to 8 hours. Warfarin is greater than 99% protein bound, principally to albumin, with a small volume of distribution of 0.14 L/kg. Fetal plasma warfarin concentrations approximate those of the mother.

S-Warfarin, the more potent enantiomer, undergoes metabolism by cytochrome P-450 2C9 (CYP2C9), with

an elimination half-life ranging from 0.5 to 3 days. CYP2C9 polymorphism explains the variation in half-life and individual sensitivities to warfarin doses required to reach therapeutic anticoagulation[1]

PATHOPHYSIOLOGY

The OACs interfere with the production of functional clotting factors. The vitamin K–dependent factors (factors II, VII, IX, and X and the anticoagulant factors protein C and protein S) undergo posttranslational γ-carboxylation at several glutamate residues, necessary for binding calcium ions involved in establishing a functional clotting cascade. This carboxylation step oxidizes the fully reduced, active vitamin K_1 (vitamin K hydroquinone) to vitamin K_1 2,3-epoxide (Fig. 66-2). Regenerating the active form of vitamin K occurs continuously in normal subjects. The epoxide first is reduced to a quinone, then to the hydroquinone; both of these reducing steps are inhibited by OAC drugs. Supplemental vitamin K_1 can be administered and is metabolized to the hydroquinone form in a reduced nicotinamide adenine dinucleotide phosphate–dependent step not inhibited by anticoagulants, resulting in active clotting factor synthesis. In the presence of OACs, however, the inactive, epoxide form of vitamin K accumulates and cannot be reduced to the active form.

CLINICAL PRESENTATION, DIAGNOSIS, AND TREATMENT

Chronic Toxicity

Most articles about OAC "overdose" actually refer to chronic, often asymptomatic, supratherapeutic dosing and not to acute, intentional ingestions. As expected, the worse the coagulopathy, the higher the risk. In all patients taking OACs for therapeutic purposes, the overall frequency of bleeding is 7.6 to 16.5 events per 100 patient-years, and frequency of major or life-threatening bleeds is 1.3 to 2.7 events per 100 patient years. The risk of an acute bleeding event within a 48-hour period increases from 1 in 4000, for an international normalized ratio (INR) between 2 and 2.9, to 1 in 100, for an INR of 7 or greater.[2] Gastrointestinal bleeding is the most common type, whereas intracranial bleeding carries the highest risk of mortality.

> ### Pharmacokinetics of Warfarin
>
> *Volume of distribution:* approximately 0.14 L/kg
> *Protein binding:* 99%
> *Mechanism of elimination:* S warfarin enantiomer metabolized by CYP2C9, with half-life ranging from 0.5 to 3 days

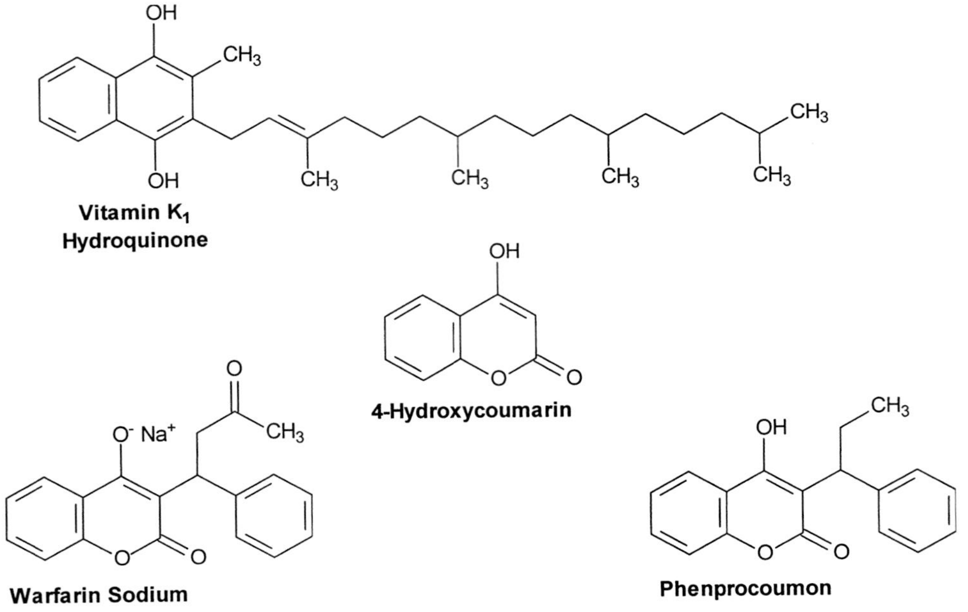

Vitamin K₁
Hydroquinone

4-Hydroxycoumarin

Warfarin Sodium

Phenprocoumon

FIGURE 66-1

Chemical structures of vitamin K active compounds.

Indications for ICU Admission in Oral Anticoagulant Poisoning

Oral anticoagulant–induced coagulopathy associated with
    Intracranial hemorrhage
    Gastrointestinal hemorrhage
    Other clinically significant bleeding
Intentional overdose of oral anticoagulant drugs

The ideal management of chronic OAC toxicity is unclear because most studies have been retrospective, have been of poor quality, and have had interstudy variance in treatment groups and doses. Notwithstanding these limitations, the American College of Chest Physicians has published consensus treatment guidelines.[3] Over the last several years, similar guidelines have recommended conservative treatment of overanticoagulated patients, with less reliance on active interventions in stable patients.[4]

In the absence of clinically significant bleeding, patients with an INR less than 5 should have warfarin withheld and resumed when a therapeutic INR is reached. For INR values of 5 to 9, warfarin is held for one or two doses and resumed when a therapeutic INR is achieved, or warfarin is held for one dose and 1 to 2.5 mg vitamin K₁ (phytonadione) is given orally. When an INR is greater than 9, warfarin is held, and the patient is given 3 to 5 mg of vitamin K₁ orally. Twenty-four hours after vitamin K₁ is given by any route to patients with asymptomatic coagulopathy after chronic, therapeutic dosing, the reduction in INR is comparable—47% to 86% for oral administration, 25% to 67% for subcutaneous administration, 40% to 75% for intravenous administration—versus only 21% to 42% for simply discontinuing warfarin.[5]

The American College of Chest Physicians recommendations are more aggressive when rapid reversal of coagulopathy is indicated. These recommendations specify that if surgery is planned and the INR is between 5 and 9, warfarin should be held and the patient given 2 to 4 mg of vitamin K₁ orally about 24 hours before the procedure. Additional vitamin K₁, 1 to 2 mg orally, may be given if necessary. If the INR is greater than 20 or the patient is experiencing serious bleeding, vitamin K₁, 10 mg, should be given by slow intravenous infusion and may be repeated every 12 hours as needed. If immediate reversal of coagulopathy is indicated (e.g., intracranial bleed, hemodynamically significant gastrointestinal hemorrhage), intravenous infusion of fresh frozen plasma or prothrombin complex concentrate is indicated. Warfarin resistance can be induced by administering excessive vitamin K₁, and patients may require heparinization temporarily if continued therapeutic anticoagulation is desired.

Criteria for ICU Discharge in Oral Anticoagulant Poisoning

Absence of clinically significant bleeding
Laboratory values stable for at least 12 (preferably 24) hours
    Prothrombin time/international normalized ratio
    Hemoglobin

Acute Overdose

Published experience of acute overdoses of OAC drugs intended for therapeutic use is limited. In the absence of a positive or suggestive history, evidence supporting the

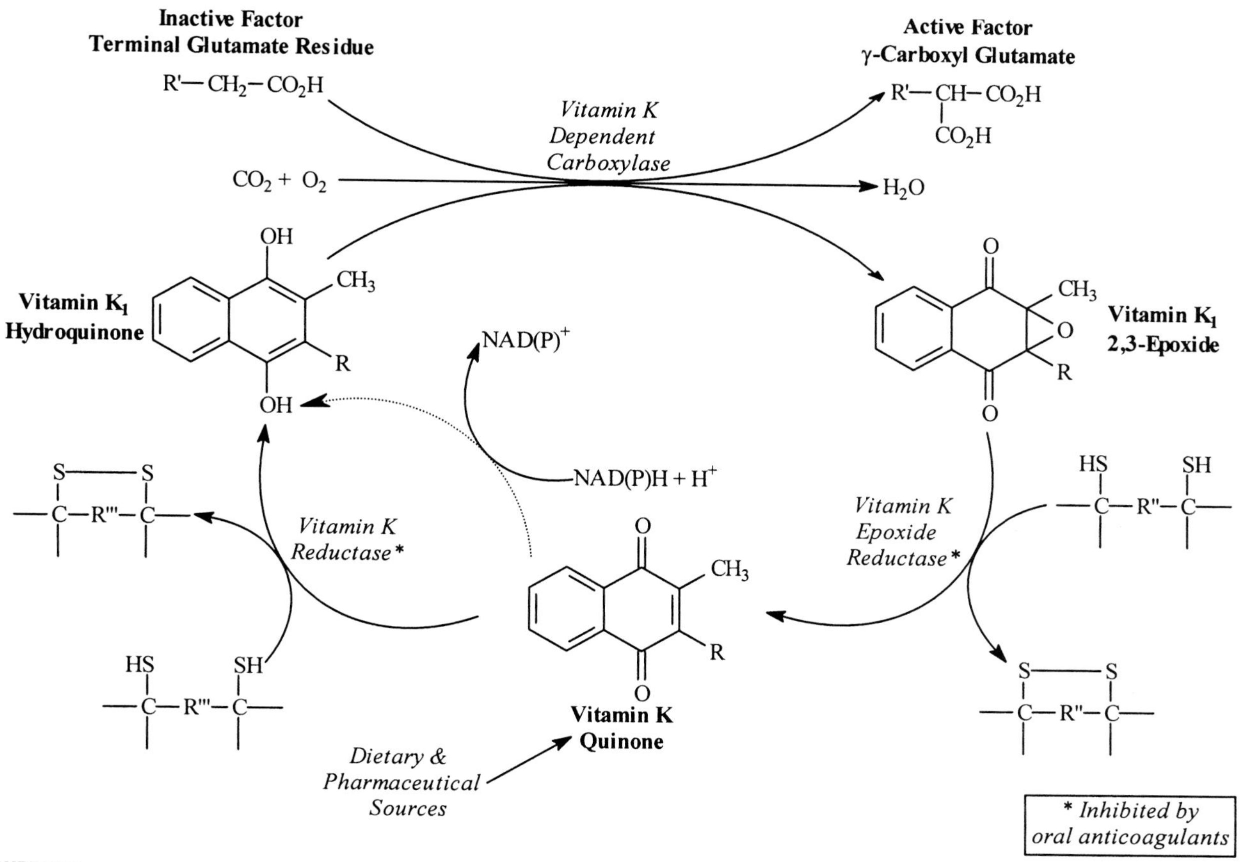

FIGURE 66-2

Mechanism of action of the oral anticoagulants.

diagnosis of OAC overdose is summarized in Table 66-1. OACs are not detected by most commonly used urine or plasma drug screens. Peak elevations in prothrombin times may not occur for a few days after overdose.[6] Treatment of OAC toxicity should be easier than for the anticoagulant rodenticides, mostly owing to their shorter half-lives. Superwarfarin toxicity may last many months, warranting long-term vitamin K_1 maintenance therapy and follow-up. In contrast, most patients with acute warfarin overdose require less than 1 week of therapy.[7]

Reported treatments for acute warfarin overdose have varied. An asymptomatic toddler who ingested 45 to 50 mg warfarin sodium 20 minutes earlier was treated with acti-

---

TABLE 66-1 Diagnostic Clues to Oral Anticoagulant Overdose

Prolongation of prothrombin time out of proportion to activated partial thromboplastin time (both may be unmeasurable in severe overdoses)

Coagulopathy that responds, at least temporarily, to vitamin K_1

Selective decreased activity of vitamin K–dependent factors—factors II, VII, IX, and X; protein C; and protein S (antigenic levels should be normal)

---

vated charcoal and daily prothrombin time monitoring.[6] When the prothrombin time increased from 11.8 seconds (baseline) to 18 seconds on day 3, the toddler was given 2.5 mg of intramuscular vitamin K_1 daily for 3 days. It is debatable whether this treatment was necessary, because no bleeding complications occurred. Adults with acute OAC overdoses typically present after coagulopathy has developed. A man presenting with bruising, gingival bleeding, and hematuria 1 day after ingesting 2000 mg of warfarin and injecting 250,000 units of heparin subcutaneously was treated successfully with intravenous prothrombin complex concentrate and several 20-mg intravenous doses of vitamin K.[8] Other cases of acute warfarin overdose have been managed with infusions of fresh frozen plasma, which seems especially helpful in cases in which maintaining therapeutic anticoagulation is desirable.[9]

Patients presenting within a few hours after an acute OAC ingestion should receive oral activated charcoal based on the theoretical possibility of reducing drug absorption. Acute gastrointestinal bleeding is a relative contraindication to charcoal because it may obscure endoscopic evaluation. Oral cholestyramine may increase clearance by interrupting enterohepatic circulation. Cholestyramine (4 g three times a day) reduced the half-life of single-dose intravenous warfarin from 1.98 ± 0.48 days to 1.34 ± 0.46 days ($P < 0.001$) in human volunteers.[10] In a case report of oral warfarin overdose, cholestyramine (4 g four times a day) decreased warfarin elimination half-life from 53 hours to 33 hours.[11]

Key Points in the Management of Acute Oral Anticoagulant Overdose

1. Prothrombin time peaks in 0.5 to 4.5 days—do not be falsely reassured by minimal prothrombin time prolongation early after ingestion.
2. Gastrointestinal decontamination with activated charcoal or cholestyramine may be beneficial.
3. Vitamin K orally or intravenously reverses coagulopathy; dosing every 4 to 8 hours may be required (in contrast to treating excessive coagulopathy after therapeutic doses).
4. Fresh frozen plasma (15 mL/kg) or prothrombin complex concentrates (50 IU/kg) should be used to treat potentially life-threatening bleeding—may need to be repeated.

VITAMIN K_1

Vitamin K_1 is an antidote for OAC toxicity, although it does not reverse enzyme inhibition in the vitamin K cycle (see Fig. 66-2). Rather, supplemental vitamin K_1 bypasses the inhibited enzymes, allowing for production of active clotting factors. Vitamin K_1 may be administered orally, subcutaneously, or intravenously. The optimal dose and route of vitamin K_1 has not been established.[5] The intravenous route is most predictable but occasionally is associated with anaphylactoid reactions; intravenous vitamin K_1 should be given at a rate not exceeding 5 mg/min, although some have suggested 1 mg/min.[12]

Regardless of route, vitamin K_1 does not have immediate effects, and significant bleeding should be treated with blood products. In massive acute warfarin overdose, three to five daily doses of vitamin K_1 may be necessary, owing to the latter's short plasma half-life.[13] With chronic OAC toxicity, a single dose often is sufficient.

Common Errors in the Management of Acute Oral Anticoagulant Overdose

Relying on negative urine drug screen to exclude ingestion
Failing to recognize that the coagulopathy may not peak for several days
Giving only a single dose of vitamin K_1 when some patients require vitamin K_1 doses several times daily

COAGULATION FACTORS

Patients with life-threatening bleeding require rapid reversal of coagulopathy. Fresh frozen plasma generally is administered at a dose of 15 mL/kg. Repeat dosing may be necessary because coagulation factor half-lives are in the range of several hours. Because many patients receiving OACs have underlying cardiopulmonary disease, fluid overload is a concern with repeat fresh frozen plasma dosing.

Coagulation factor concentrates also may be used. Prothrombin complex concentrate contains factors II, IX, and X, with dosage based on factor IX content. Doses of 12 IU/kg have been used in moderate coagulopathy, although 50 IU/kg should be given in the most serious cases, such as intracranial hemorrhage.[14] Some newer prothrombin complex concentrates are "four-factor" concentrates that also contain factor VII. If only the three-factor concentrate is used, an infusion of factor VII concentrate (25 to 30 IU/kg) or fresh frozen plasma should be added. Normal coagulation is achieved more rapidly with prothrombin complex concentrate infusion than with fresh frozen plasma. Maintenance therapy with supplemental vitamin K_1 still is necessary when using blood products because the effects are temporary.

DRUG INTERACTIONS WITH ORAL ANTICOAGULANTS

As a result of several unfavorable pharmacologic properties of the OACs, great potential exists for life-threatening interactions with other drugs and foods. First, the OACs possess a narrow therapeutic index; small changes in drug dosing, metabolism, or distribution can alter coagulability radically. The coumarins are highly bound to serum albumin, and drugs competing for binding to this protein cause an increased free fraction, resulting in enhanced coagulopathy. Coumarin metabolism depends on the activity of several CYP enzymes. Agents that inhibit this metabolism may induce hemorrhage, whereas metabolism inducers may result in loss of effective anticoagulation. The R and S stereoisomers of warfarin are metabolized by different, but overlapping, sets of CYP isoenzymes. The more potent S-warfarin is metabolized primarily by CYP2C9 and to a lesser degree by CYP3A4; R-warfarin is metabolized primarily by CYP1A2 and by CYP3A4 and CYP2C19. Even when the aforementioned issues are tightly controlled, dietary intake of vitamin K can vary, making therapeutic dosing difficult.

Systematic review of reported warfarin-drug interactions found that the drugs listed in Table 66-2 were considered

TABLE 66-2 Drugs Likely to Have Clinically Significant Interactions with Warfarin: Agents Likely to Cause Potentiation

Acetaminophen	Isoniazid
Amiodarone	Itraconazole
Anabolic steroids	Metronidazole
Aspirin	Miconazole
Chloral hydrate	Omeprazole
Cimetidine	Phenylbutazone
Ciprofloxacin	Phenytoin
Clofibrate	Piroxicam
Co-trimoxazole	Propafenone
Dextropropoxyphene	Propranolol
Disulfiram	Quinidine
Erythromycin	Simvastatin
Ethanol (if liver disease is present)	Sulfinpyrazone
Fluconazole	Tamoxifen
Influenza vaccines	Tetracycline

Table 66-3 Drugs Likely to Have Clinically Significant Interactions with Warfarin: Agents Likely to Cause Lessening of Warfarin's Effect

Barbiturates
Carbamazepine
Chlordiazepoxide
Cholestyramine
Diets or enteral feeds high in vitamin K content (including green leafy vegetables, avocados, and green tea)[13]
Griseofulvin
Nafcillin
Rifampin
Sucralfate

probable or highly probable to potentiate warfarin. Drugs considered probable or highly probable to reduce warfarin's action are listed in Table 66-3.

Acetaminophen's apparent potentiation of warfarin's effect has important potential clinical implications. Because of the antiplatelet effects of aspirin and other nonsteroidal antiinflammatory drugs, physicians often recommend acetaminophen for patients taking warfarin. A few patients taking both of these drugs develop prolonged prothrombin times unaccounted for by warfarin alone. A potential mechanism for this interaction is acetaminophen competitively inhibiting warfarin metabolism or vitamin K carboxylase.[1]

Several drugs impair vitamin K metabolism even in the absence of OACs. Drugs with such a warfarin-like effect include cephalosporin antibiotics with *N*-methyl-thiotetrazole side chains (cefamandole, moxalactam, cefoperazone, cefazolin, cefazedone) and salicylates. Aspirin may induce bleeding with an additive effect to that of warfarin and by a synergistic effect through platelet inhibition.

NONHEMORRHAGIC COMPLICATIONS OF ORAL ANTICOAGULANT THERAPY

OACs are associated with several adverse effects unrelated to their therapeutic effect. Nonhemorrhagic complications include warfarin skin necrosis, the "purple toes syndrome," hepatitis, and warfarin embryopathy.

Warfarin Skin Necrosis

Skin necrosis occurs in 0.01% to 0.10% of patients taking OACs. Most reported cases have occurred in association with warfarin, although it may occur with any of the coumarin-derived OACs. The usual presentation is the rapid development of painful, well-localized hemorrhagic or erythematous skin lesions 3 to 10 days after initiating OAC therapy. Occasionally, these lesions are heralded by paresthesias or a pressure-like sensation and poorly demarcated erythema. The lesions become edematous, producing a peau d'orange effect, and may develop petechiae and hemorrhagic bullae. The affected areas develop full-thickness skin necrosis, form eschars, and eventually slough. Small lesions can heal by granulation, but larger lesions usually

require surgical débridement, skin grafting, or amputation, depending on their extent.[15]

Warfarin skin necrosis occurs more commonly in obese, middle-aged women, with the preponderance of lesions found on the skin of the breast, buttock, and thigh.[15] Nearly all cases occur with OAC treatment for deep venous thrombosis or pulmonary embolism; necrosis does not occur with treatment for atrial fibrillation or cerebrovascular indications. Patients with protein C or protein S deficiencies and patients receiving large oral loading doses also are at higher risk.[15] These associations suggest that the high-risk population is already prone to thrombosis and that the early hypercoagulable state occurring with oral anticoagulants (due to decreased protein C and S activities) may precipitate localized thrombosis.

Although late treatment clearly consists of wound care and surgical intervention, early treatment before completed skin necrosis is not so obvious. Recommended strategies include intravenous vitamin K_1, substitution of heparin or low-molecular-weight heparins for anticoagulation, and prostacyclin infusions.[15] Patients with protein C deficiency may benefit from infusion of protein C concentrate. Even with optimal medical treatment, surgical intervention ultimately is required in about half of patients.[15]

Purple Toes Syndrome

The purple toes syndrome is a rare complication of OAC therapy. Patients can develop purplish discoloration of the plantar surfaces and sides of the toes, usually within 3 to 8 weeks of initiation of therapy. These lesions are painful and tender, blanch with pressure, and fade with leg elevation. Several cases with biopsy or autopsy specimens show an association with cholesterol microemboli. The purple toes syndrome may represent a sentinel event, presaging further emboli from atherosclerotic lesions, possibly from OAC interference with the healing of ulcerated atheromatous plaques. Other cases of warfarin-related cholesterol embolization (without purple toes) have responded to withdrawal of the offending drug. Consideration should be given to withdrawing OACs when the purple toes syndrome occurs.[16]

Hepatitis

Rare cases of drug-induced hepatitis have been reported with therapeutic dosing of warfarin, phenprocoumon, and acenocoumarol. Hepatocellular injury mimicking a viral hepatitis has been described, occurring within several months of initiating therapy; less commonly, a cholestatic pattern is evident. In some patients with phenprocoumon-induced hepatitis, the substitution of warfarin has resulted in recurrent hepatitis, suggesting cross-reactivity between these agents. This cross-reactivity is not the rule, because other patients with phenprocoumon-induced hepatitis have been treated successfully with either acenocoumarol or warfarin.[17]

SPECIAL POPULATIONS

Pregnant Patients

Pregnancy generally is considered a contraindication to warfarin therapy owing to teratogenic effects. The U.S. Food and Drug Administration has categorized warfarin as pregnancy class X (see Appendix A). Intrauterine exposure has resulted in the fetal warfarin syndrome, characterized by nasal/midface hypoplasia, bone stippling of the epiphyses (evident on plain radiographs), optic atrophy, and mental retardation.[18] Warfarin crosses the placenta, but its mechanism of teratogenesis is unclear. Hemorrhage into cartilage with subsequent scarring and calcification has been postulated as causing bone stippling, but this mechanism does not explain adequately the other observed abnormalities.[18] Roughly one sixth of pregnancies with warfarin exposure result in an infant with fetal warfarin syndrome, and another one sixth result in stillbirths or spontaneous abortions; the remaining two thirds result in apparently normal newborns.[19] Heparin usually is substituted for warfarin in pregnant women requiring anticoagulation, although one third of these cases still result in prematurity or stillbirth.[19]

REFERENCES

1. Shek KLA, Chan LN, Nutescu E: Warfarin-acetaminophen drug interaction revisited. Pharmacotherapy 19:1153–1158, 1999.
2. Baglin T: Management of warfarin (coumarin) overdose. Blood Rev 12:91–98, 1998.
3. Hirsch J, Dalen JE, Anderson DR, et al: Oral anticoagulants: Mechanism of action, clinical effectiveness, and optimal therapeutic range. Chest 114:445S–469S, 1998.
4. Glover JJ, Morrill GB: Conservative treatment of overanticoagulated patients. Chest 108:987–990, 1995.
5. Taylor CT, Chester EA, Byrd DC, et al: Vitamin K to reverse excessive anticoagulation: A review of the literature. Pharmacotherapy 19:1415–1425, 1999.
6. Montanio CD, Wruk KM, Kulig KW, et al: Acute pediatric warfarin (Coumadin) ingestion: Toxic effects despite early treatment. Am J Dis Child 147:609–610, 1993.
7. Bates D, Mintz M: Phytonadione therapy in a multiple-drug overdose involving warfarin. Pharmacotherapy 20:1208–1215, 2000.
8. Hackett LP, Ilett KF, Chester A: Plasma warfarin concentrations after a massive overdose. Med J Aust 142:642–643, 1985.
9. Toolis F, Robson RH, Critchley JAJH: Warfarin poisoning in patients with prosthetic heart valves. BMJ 283:581–582, 1981.
10. Jähnchen E, Meinertz T, Gilfrich HJ, et al: Enhanced elimination of warfarin during treatment with cholestryramine. Br J Clin Pharmacol 5:437–440, 1978.
11. Renowden S, Westmoreland D, White JP, et al: Oral cholestyramine increases elimination of warfarin after overdose. BMJ 291:513–514, 1985.
12. Rich EC, Drage CW: Severe complications of intravenous phytonadione therapy. Postgrad Med 72:303–306, 1982.
13. Bjornsson TD, Blaschke TF: Vitamin K1 disposition and therapy of massive warfarin overdose. Lancet 2:846–847, 1978.
14. Butler AC, Tait RC: Management of oral anticoagulant-induced intracranial hemorrhage. Blood Rev 12:35–44, 1998.
15. Chan YC, Valenti D, Mansfield AO, et al: Warfarin induced skin necrosis. Br J Surg 87:266–272, 2000.
16. Hyman BT, Landas SK, Ashman RF, et al: Warfarin-related purple toes syndrome and cholesterol microembolization. Am J Med 82:1233–1237, 1987.
17. Ehrenforth S, Schenk JF, Scharrer I: Liver damage induced by coumarin anticoagulants. Semin Thromb Hemost 25:79–83, 1999.
18. Harrod MJE, Sherrod PS: Warfarin embryopathy in siblings. Obstet Gynecol 57:673–676, 1981.
19. Pauli RM, Hall JG: Warfarin embryopathy. Lancet 2:144, 1979.

CHAPTER **67**

Thrombolytics, Heparin and Derivatives, and Antiplatelet Agents

Robert A. Raschke ■ Steven C. Curry

Toxicologic events related to therapeutic administration of heparins, antiplatelet drugs, and thrombolytic agents are far more common than accidental or intentional overdoses. This chapter focuses on the adverse effects of these agents most commonly encountered by intensivists—in particular, hemorrhage and hematologic dyscrasias.

THROMBOLYTIC THERAPY

Thrombolytic therapy is indicated in the treatment of acute myocardial infarction, hemodynamically significant pulmonary embolism, hyperacute stroke, and peripheral arterial occlusive disease. Agents in clinical use include streptokinase (SK), urokinase (UK), tissue plasminogen activator (t-Pa and rt-Pa), and anisoylated plasminogen streptokinase activator complex (APSAC).

Pathophysiology

The hematologic effects of thrombolytic agents may be divided into two phases. In the first phase, drug action results in the cleavage of the $arginine_{560}$-$valine_{561}$ bond of the inactive zymogen plasminogen; this produces a molecule of plasmin, which may be free in the plasma or fibrin-associated. Plasmin catalyzes proteolysis of cross-linked fibrin present in clots. This is the main therapeutic effect of thrombolytic agents and the main explanation for bleeding complications. Duration of plasminogen activation is relatively brief; the half-lives of thrombolytic agents are 6 minutes for t-Pa, 20 minutes for SK and UK, and 90 minutes for APSAC.[1,2] In general, circulating plasminogen activator is cleared from the circulation within 6 hours of discontinuation, regardless of the thrombolytic agent administered.[1,3,4]

Plasmin is a nonspecific serine protease. During the first phase of plasminogen activation, circulating fibrinogen, factor V, factor VIII, and other coagulation-related proteins also are cleaved and depleted. After plasminogen activation ceases, the resulting coagulopathy persists. Some have referred to this second phase as the *lytic state*, although lysis of fibrin occurs predominantly in the phase of plasminogen activation.[5] Complete hemostatic recovery from this phase may take 48 hours or longer.[3,5–7]

Hypofibrinogenemia is perhaps the most important characteristic of the second phase. Cleavage of fibrinogen into fibrin is the final common pathway by which clots form, and fibrinogen is essential to platelet aggregation. Fibrinogen concentrations less than 100 mg/dL are inadequate for normal hemostasis in patients with congenital hypofibrinogenemia and in surgical patients.[8,9] This degree of hypofibrinogenemia is common after thrombolytic therapy.[3,6,10] Fibrinogen proteolysis is agent specific and is more severe after administration of SK than after use of t-Pa.[4] Fibrinogen may remain at the nadir for hours and take 48 hours to normalize.[6] Fibrinogen degradation by plasmin results in the accumulation of fragments X, Y, and D. These have been shown to exhibit potent anticoagulant effects[11] and to weaken newly formed clot.[12] It is disquieting that fibrinogen levels in patients receiving thrombolytics have not been associated convincingly with bleeding complications.[4,13]

Factors V and VIII also reach levels that probably are inadequate for hemostasis in many patients receiving thrombolytic agents. Minimally acceptable levels for factor V and factor VIII ($<10\%$ to 30% activity) generally have been based on studies of patients with isolated factor deficiencies.[14] Because thrombolysis involves multiple additional hemostatic defects, it is possible that higher levels are necessary in these patients to control bleeding.

Plasmin activation also results in platelet dysfunction. Plasmin has been shown to inhibit platelet release of thromboxane B_2, which recruits other platelets to sites of vascular injury.[15] It also cleaves platelet glycoprotein Ib[16] and glycoprotein IIb/IIIa[17]—essential for platelet adherence and aggregation. In our experience, inhibition of platelet function commonly is overlooked by physicians treating patients with bleeding complications resulting from thrombolytic therapy.

Clinical Presentation and Life-Threatening Complications

The most common systemic adverse event associated with thrombolytic therapy is hemorrhage. The anatomic origin of hemorrhage is usually a site of previous vascular trauma, such as the site of an intravenous line.[4] We have seen a patient develop a forearm compartment syndrome from a hemorrhage originating at the site of a radial artery blood gas puncture. Hemothorax and hemomediastinum have been reported in patients receiving thrombolytic agents after undergoing cardiopulmonary resuscitation.[18]

The most devastating hemorrhagic complication is intracranial hemorrhage. The risk for intracranial hemorrhage is highest in patients receiving thrombolytics for stroke (6%

to 9%),[19–21] but the risk also is significant in patients with acute myocardial infarction (0.3% to 0.6%)[22–25] and pulmonary embolism (1.2%).[26] Intracranial hemorrhage is typically lobar and usually presents within 24 hours of the initiation of thrombolytic therapy. Presenting symptoms, in order of frequency, include decreased level of consciousness, focal neurologic deficits, vomiting, seizure, and headache.[27] Diffuse pulmonary hemorrhage[28] and localized hematoma of the airway[29] are thrombolytic complications that can be life-threatening in the absence of exsanguination.

Treatment

Bleeding complications of thrombolytic therapy can be minimized by excluding patients with contraindications; this is particularly important in the treatment of patients with hyperacute stroke. The administration of t-Pa to patients with mass effect or edema on brain computed tomography (CT) has been associated with a 31% rate of intracranial hemorrhage, and administration later than 6 hours after onset of stroke has been associated with a rate of 53%.[30,31] Bleeding also may be prevented by avoiding vascular procedures that are unnecessary or in locations that are difficult to compress adequately, such as the subclavian vein.

Treatment of bleeding complications can be divided into antifibrinolytic therapy and replacement of depleted coagulation factors. Although fibrin lysis is widely believed to be the major mechanism for bleeding complications,[2] antifibrinolytic therapy may result in life-threatening thrombotic complications and usually is held in reserve unless transfusion therapy fails. Randomized, controlled trials have not been performed to discern the best course of management; the following is a rational, opinion-based approach.[2]

Cryoprecipitate and fresh frozen plasma (FFP) are administered rapidly to replace clotting factors depleted by plasmin. The standard unit of cryoprecipitate provides a minimum of 150 mg and an average of 250 mg of fibrinogen. In addition, it contains 80 U of factor VIII. The volume of distribution is equal to the plasma volume—approximately 3200 mL in a 70-kg patient. Intravenous infusion of 10 U of cryoprecipitate increases the fibrinogen concentration by approximately 75 mg/dL and the factor VIII level by 30%.

FFP contains 180 to 300 U of factor V per unit. In a 70-kg patient, 6 U of FFP would be required to increase the factor V level by 30%. Often, lesser amounts result in clinical hemostasis. Laboratory assessment of fibrinogen and factors V and VIII levels can be helpful in guiding therapy if initial transfusions of cryoprecipitate and FFP are unsuccessful. Several factors complicate the interpretation of results, however. If blood is drawn during the phase of plasminogen activation, proteolysis may proceed in vitro, falsely diminishing levels of coagulation factors as measured in the laboratory.[32]

Platelet transfusion should be considered, especially if the bleeding time is abnormal or dilutional thrombocytopenia occurs as a complication of massive red blood cell transfusion. Theoretically, transfused platelets should function better than native platelets previously exposed to high levels of plasmin. In addition, platelet-bound factor V may help correct factor V deficiency. One unit of single-donor platelets usually provides adequate numbers of functioning platelets.

Antifibrinolytic agents (e.g., aminocaproic acid or tranexamic acid) may be considered early in treatment if transfusion therapy fails to control bleeding. Aminocaproic acid is a lysine analogue that binds to lysine binding sites on plasmin and plasminogen. It may be administered as a bolus of 0.1 g/kg over 30 minutes, followed by an infusion of 0.5 to 1 g/hr.[33] Administration of aminocaproic acid has been associated with life-threatening thrombotic complications, including stroke, myocardial infarction, limb gangrene, and renal cortical thrombosis. Antifibrinolytic agents would not be expected to be beneficial when the initial phase of plasminogen activation is over (>6 hours after infusion of a thrombolytic agent).

Life-threatening immunologic reactions have been reported in association with thrombolytic agents. SK is a bacterial protein and is an integral component of APSAC. Fever, angioedema, bronchospasm, and anaphylaxis have been associated with their use.[34] UK is derived from human embryonic kidney cells, and t-PA is a naturally occurring human protein. Allergic reactions to these agents are rare. Anaphylactoid reactions and oropharyngeal angioedema have been reported, however, in association with rt-PA.[35] Anaphylaxis and anaphylactoid reactions are treated with fluid resuscitation, epinephrine, H_1 and H_2 receptor antagonists, and corticosteroids. SK activates the kallikrein-bradykinin system. The administration of SK or APSAC may result in hypotension.[36]

Treatment of Clinically Significant Bleeding Due to Thrombolytic Agents

- Cryoprecipitate (approximately 10 U) *and*
- Fresh frozen plasma (approximately 2 U)
If bleeding continues:
- Platelets (1 U single donor or 10 U random donor)
If bleeding continues and thrombolytics were administered within last 6 hours:
- Consider aminocaproic acid (Amicar)

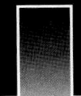

Common Errors in the Diagnosis and Treatment of Complications of Thrombolytic Therapy

Giving thrombolytics despite late presentations and contraindications

Failure to recognize platelet dysfunction in patients who are bleeding after thrombolytic therapy

UNFRACTIONATED AND LOW-MOLECULAR-WEIGHT HEPARINS

Unfractionated heparin (UH) acts by binding to antithrombin and catalyzing the inactivation of thrombin, factor Xa, and other clotting factors. Inactivation of thrombin requires a heparin chain length of at least 18 saccharides, and inactivation of factor Xa requires 5 saccharides. Low-molecular-weight heparins (LMWHs) have reduced antithrombin activity compared with UH. The antithrombotic activity of LMWH commonly is attributed to its anti–factor Xa activity. The anti-Xa assay is the laboratory test most often used in monitoring and adjusting LMWH.[37]

Heparins also have complicated effects on coagulation that are independent of interaction with antithrombin, and their relative importance is uncertain. Heparins (UH and LMWH) trigger endothelial cell release of tissue factor pathway inhibitor.[38–40] Tissue factor pathway inhibitor is a serine protease inhibitor that blocks tissue factor/factor VIIa–dependent coagulation. Tissue factor pathway inhibitor release seems to account for a significant fraction of heparin's antithrombotic activity and can be quantitated by the Heptest assay (Wako Chemicals USA Inc., Richmond, VA).[41] Heparins also interact with heparin cofactor II, which is a serine protease that is structurally similar to antithrombin but has specific antithrombin activity.[42] The antithrombin activity of LMWH might be clinically important, even though low antithrombin/anti-Xa activity previously was thought to be a theoretical advantage of LMWHs.[43,44] Antithrombin activity can be measured by anti-IIa assays.

Recognition of uncertainty concerning the mechanism of action of LMWH is important during attempts to use anti-Xa activity to guide clinical administration. Because LMWH does not produce isolated factor Xa inhibition, anti-Xa assays do not fully reflect clinical therapeutic or toxic effects.[37] In addition, the anti-Xa test has been reported to exhibit wide interassay variability.[45,46] Several studies have failed to show a significant relationship between anti-Xa results and the therapeutic or adverse effects of LMWHs.[47–49]

Clinical Presentation

The most common toxicologic effect of heparin seen in the intensive care unit (ICU) is bleeding. Rarely, bleeding occurs when single, inappropriately high doses of heparin are given in error. We saw a case in which a 25,000-U bag of heparin was given erroneously in response to an order for a hetastarch (Hespan) bolus. Pseudo–heparin resistance also has been reported, in which inappropriately high doses of heparin are given because of unrecognized suppression of activated partial thromboplastin time (APTT) by elevated factor VIII levels.[50]

Most often, hemorrhagic complications occur during appropriate administration of heparin. Although bleeding often is attributed to "overanticoagulation"—defined by supratherapeutic APTT results—several large studies showed no correlation between bleeding and the APTT.[51–54] The most important risk factors for bleeding are patient specific, such as underlying peptic ulcer disease or thrombocytopenia, and procedural trauma.

The gastrointestinal and urinary tracts are the most common sites for heparin-induced bleeding. Approximately 50% of these patients have an underlying pathologic lesion.[55] Appropriate workup should not be neglected with the logic that the heparin administration alone is a sufficient explanation.

Retroperitoneal hemorrhage often presents with nonspecific findings that commonly are misdiagnosed initially. Patients may complain of back, hip, or thigh pain, and the initial decline in hemoglobin may not be dramatic. Radiation of the pain to the thigh associated with decreased quadriceps strength indicates compression of the femoral nerve.[56] Rarely, findings such as Cullen's or Grey Turner's signs are present. CT should be considered in any patient receiving heparin who has unexplained back or flank pain. Surgical decompression or exploration generally is not recommended.[57]

Rectus sheath hematomas are usually caused by bleeding from the inferior epigastric artery. They present as a painful abdominal mass. Careful examination usually shows the mass to be external to the rectus muscle.[58] One case series showed, however, that delays in diagnosis of rectus sheath hematomas are common and seem to contribute to morbidity and mortality.[57] We have seen a rectus sheath hematoma misdiagnosed as a hernia and "reduced," with catastrophic results. Rectus sheath hematomas may require surgical intervention.

Bilateral adrenal hemorrhage may present with findings that are nonspecific in the ICU, including abdominal pain, nausea, fever, hypotension, tachycardia, hypoglycemia, and anemia. A cosyntropin stimulation test usually shows inability to produce serum cortisol levels greater than 18 μg/dL (>497 nmol/L). The hemorrhagic cause of the adrenal insufficiency can be shown by CT.[59]

Spinal epidural hematoma presents as severe, persistent back pain radiating in a dermatomal pattern. This condition can occur spontaneously or in association with lumbar puncture or epidural anesthesia. The concomitant use of prophylactic-dose LMWH and indwelling epidural analgesia has been recognized as a risk factor for this complication.[60] Neurologic findings, such as paraparesis, sensory loss, and urinary retention, are indications for urgent decompression.

The nonhemorrhagic toxicologic effects of heparin include hyperkalemia, skin necrosis, and osteoporosis.[55] These effects are not discussed in further detail here.

Treatment

The treatment of clinically severe bleeding related to heparin therapy includes heparin neutralization, supportive care, and transfusion. The effects of UH can be neutralized rapidly by an intravenous bolus of protamine sulfate. Protamine is a cationic protein derived from fish sperm, which strongly binds to (anionic) heparin. A dose of 1 mg of protamine sulfate neutralizes approximately 100 U of UH. A patient who bleeds immediately after an intravenous bolus of 5000 U of UH requires 50 mg of protamine sulfate. When UH is given as an intravenous infusion, only heparin given during the preceding several hours needs to be included in the dose calculation because the half-life of intravenous UH is short (approximately 90 minutes). A patient receiving a continuous intravenous infusion of 1250 U/hr requires approximately 20 mg of protamine sulfate. Neutralization of a subcutaneous dose of UH may require a prolonged infusion of protamine sulfate. The APTT can be used to confirm neutralization of UH.[61]

The risk of severe adverse reactions from protamine, such as hypotension and bradycardia, can be minimized by administering protamine slowly (over 1 to 3 minutes).[62] Development of antiprotamine antibodies and increased risk for allergic reactions, including anaphylaxis, are associated with (1) previous administration of protamine-containing insulin (e.g., neutral protamine Hagedorn [NPH] Insulin), (2) vasectomy, and (3) allergic sensitivity to fish.[61,63,64] Patients at risk for protamine allergy can be pretreated effectively with corticosteroids and antihistamines.

Many other methods have been used to neutralize the effects of UH, including hexadimethrine,[65] heparinase (Neutralase),[66] platelet factor 4 (PF4),[67] extracorporeal heparin removal devices,[68] and synthetic protamine variants.[69] These therapies are not widely available.

There is no proven method for neutralizing LMWH. Protamine neutralizes the antithrombin activity of LMWH but fails to neutralize completely the anti-Xa activity.[70–73] Protamine-heparin binding is related to the molecular weight of the heparin,[74] and it is theorized that failure of anti-Xa neutralization occurs because of reduced binding to low-molecular-weight components.[73,75] Others have suggested that plasma proteins inhibit protamine binding to LMWH.[76]

The clinical significance of incomplete anti-Xa neutralization by protamine is unclear. Animal studies have shown a hemostatic benefit of protamine in microvascular bleeding models despite persistent anti-Xa activity.[77–79] In a small case series, protamine failed to completely correct abnormal bleeding associated with LMWH in two of three patients.[71] There are no published clinical studies that show a beneficial effect of protamine on bleeding complications of LMWH; however, the package insert for enoxaparin suggests the following approach: If the LMWH heparin was given within 8 hours, protamine sulfate may be given in a dose of 1 mg per 100 anti-Xa U of LMWH (1 mg of enoxaparin equals approximately 100 anti-Xa U). A second dose of 0.5 mg of protamine sulfate per 100 anti-Xa U may be administered if bleeding continues.

In animal studies, synthetic protamine variants have been shown to be highly effective in neutralizing LMWH and seem to be less toxic than protamine.[80,81] Other reversing agents that have been or are being investigated include adenosine triphosphate, synthetic heparin binding peptide, heparinase 1, and lactoferrin.[82,83] These agents are not yet available for clinical use.

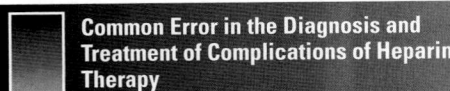

Common Error in the Diagnosis and Treatment of Complications of Heparin Therapy

Delay in recognition of occult bleeding, including retroperitoneal hemorrhage, rectus sheath hematomas, and adrenal hemorrhage

HEPARIN-INDUCED THROMBOCYTOPENIA

Heparin-induced thrombocytopenia (HIT) is a clinicopathologic syndrome characterized by a greater than 50% decrease in platelet count 5 days or more after the initiation of heparin therapy. Most authors include specific abnormalities in platelet function or antibodies to heparin/PF4 in the definition of HIT. The risk for venous and arterial thrombosis reaches 50% to 80% in patients with laboratory-confirmed HIT.[84–86] The syndrome of thrombocytopenia and thrombosis after heparin therapy also has been described in the absence of specific laboratory abnormalities typically associated with HIT.

Pathophysiology

IgG antibodies to the heparin/PF4 complex exhibit platelet-activating and endothelium-activating properties that are thought to be pathogenic in the platelet consumption and thrombotic complications of HIT. Seventeen percent of patients receiving UH and 8% of patients receiving LMWH develop detectable titers of these antibodies.[84,87] Most of these patients have stable platelet counts and no thromboembolism.[84,88] Approximately 25% of patients with heparin/PF4 antibodies develop clinical HIT.[89]

Clinical Presentation

HIT occurs in about 2% of patients receiving UH.[84] Bovine-derived UH is more likely than porcine-derived UH to be associated with HIT. Even small quantities of UH used to flush intravenous catheters have been reported to cause HIT.[90] LMWH is far less likely than UH to cause HIT.[84] When HIT occurs, however, LMWH consistently cross-reacts with existing heparin/platelet factor 4 antibodies. LMWH should not be used in therapy of HIT.[91] An increased risk for HIT sometimes can be recognized before thrombocytopenia occurs. The clinical clues include acute systemic reactions to heparin administration (chills, rigors, fever, tachycardia, and dyspnea)[92] and dermal plaques or necrosis at heparin injection sites.[93]

Thrombocytopenia typically becomes apparent 5 to 14 days after the onset of heparin therapy. The platelet nadir is usually less than 150×10^9/L, and the median platelet count in one large study was 60×10^9/L.[86] Approximately 10% of patients have thromboembolic events consistent with HIT, despite platelet counts greater than 150×10^9/L.[86] These patients typically have had significant decreases in platelet count, albeit to levels greater than 150×10^9/L. Bleeding complications are unusual, even when thrombocytopenia is severe.[94]

Venous thromboembolism occurs in approximately 50% of patients with HIT, with an incidence rate of 5% to 10% per day.[95,96] Progressive, recurrent, or bilateral lower extremity deep venous thromboses are seen in 50% of affected individuals, and pulmonary embolism is seen in 25%.[94] Deep venous thromboses often occur at the site of venous catheters. Rare forms of venous thromboembolism associated with HIT include bilateral adrenal hemorrhage and cerebral dural sinus thrombosis. HIT-associated deep venous thrombosis has progressed to venous limb gangrene in a subset of patients receiving warfarin. The gangrene apparently is triggered by warfarin-induced, acute protein C deficiency.[97]

Arterial thrombosis also occurs with increased frequency. Aortic or iliofemoral thrombosis resulting in acute limb ischemia occurs in 5% to 10% of patients with HIT. Stroke and myocardial infarction each occur in 3% to 5%, and spinal cord infarction has been reported.[94] Approximately 35% of patients with HIT who develop thromboembolic complications lose a limb or ultimately die.[95,96]

Diagnosis

Two general types of laboratory tests are useful in the diagnosis of HIT: platelet function assays and antibody tests (enzyme-linked immunosorbent assay [ELISA]). Platelet function tests include the platelet aggregation test and the serotonin release assay; the performance characteristics of these depend on technical aspects of laboratory method. The platelet aggregation test has a sensitivity of 26% to 91% and a specificity of 77%. The serotonin release assay has a sensitivity of 55% to 88% and a specificity of 96% to 100%. The ELISA platelet antibody test has a sensitivity of 64% to 97% and a specificity of 86%.[84,98–100] Sensitivity is enhanced for all tests when the diagnosis is confined to patients with thromboembolic complications.[100] Studies on the test performance characteristics are difficult to integrate because laboratory methods vary, and there is no relevant uniform independent gold standard. The ELISA test is the easiest and quickest to perform. The ELISA also seems to be the most sensitive test and would be expected to have a positive likelihood ratio of 5 to 6 and a negative likelihood ratio of 0.1 to 0.2. Because the sensitivity of the functional tests and the specificity of the ELISA assay are lacking, neither test by itself provides a conclusive answer in all patients. We have taken the following diagnostic approach: We order the platelet aggregation study and the ELISA in any patient with clinically suspected HIT. If either test yields a positive result, we consider the diagnosis of HIT confirmed.

Treatment

When HIT is suspected, all heparin (including heparin flushes) should be discontinued immediately, pending confirmatory laboratory testing. In patients with suspected HIT with thromboembolism, alternative antithrombotic therapy should be started immediately. It is likely that patients with laboratory-confirmed HIT who do not have overt thromboembolism also would benefit from antithrombotic therapy. Two therapeutic agents are approved by the U.S. Food and Drug Administration: lepirudin and argatroban.

Lepirudin is a recombinant form of hirudin—a direct thrombin inhibitor. Two historically controlled trials have shown reductions in thromboembolic events, limb gangrene, and death[95,96] in patients with HIT treated with lepirudin. Lepirudin is initiated as a bolus of 0.4 mg/kg body weight (up to 44 mg) over 20 seconds, followed by a continuous intravenous infusion at 0.15 mg/kg (up to 16.5 mg/hr). Monitoring with APTT is recommended, with adjustment of infusion made to achieve APTT values 1.5 to 2.5 times control values. Lepirudin is renally excreted, and patients with even mild renal insufficiency require dosage adjustment. Some patients receiving lepirudin develop anti-hirudin antibodies that have a paradoxical antithrombotic effect.[101] Warfarin therapy can be started cautiously when the platelet count is clearly recovering (i.e., >100 × 10⁹/L), but administration of warfarin during active HIT has been associated with venous limb gangrene.[97] This devastating syndrome may be heralded by an inordinate prolongation of the international normalized ratio (INR) after the first dose of warfarin. Lepirudin can be discontinued when concomitant warfarin therapy has resulted in prolongation of the INR to a value greater than 2 and when the platelet count is normalized.[102]

Argatroban is a synthetic direct thrombin inhibitor. A historically controlled trial showed a reduction in thromboembolic events in patients with HIT without thromboembolism who received argatroban,[103] but there was not a significant reduction in death or limb amputation. The initial infusion dose is 2 μg/kg/min, adjusted to attain an APTT value 1.5 to 3 times baseline. Argatroban significantly prolongs the prothrombin time, so during overlap therapy with warfarin, an INR greater than 4 usually is required before argatroban can be discontinued. Argatroban is metabolized in the liver, and it should not be used in patients with significant liver dysfunction.

We recommend lepirudin based on more convincing results of efficacy studies, although the published studies are not strictly comparable. In patients with renal insufficiency, argatroban is preferable. The optimal duration of warfarin anticoagulation in patients with HIT is unknown, but a 6-week duration seems reasonable.

Common Errors in the Diagnosis and Treatment of Heparin-Induced Thrombocytopenia

Failure to monitor for or consider the diagnosis
Failure to stop all heparin immediately while the diagnosis is being confirmed
Failure to recognize that the cross-reactivity between heparin and low-molecular-weight heparin is 100% in patients with heparin-induced thrombocytopenia

ANTIPLATELET DRUGS

Ticlopidine and Clopidogrel

Ticlopidine hydrochloride and clopidogrel are antiplatelet agents indicated for use in stroke, in peripheral arterial disease, in unstable angina, and after coronary stent placement. They are thienopyridine derivatives and act by irreversibly inhibiting the platelet membrane adenosine diphosphate receptor.[104] Stimulation of this receptor normally activates the glycoprotein IIb/IIIa complex, binding fibrinogen to the platelet membrane and allowing platelet aggregation. Patients who have received either of these agents within approximately 10 days of a bleeding episode should be considered to have potentially significant platelet dysfunction. If the bleeding is serious, this would warrant platelet transfusion despite normal platelet counts. We have seen several episodes of life-threatening bleeding associated with these agents in patients who had undergone high-risk procedures, such as gynecologic-oncologic surgery.

Thrombotic thrombocytopenic purpura (TTP) is one of the hematologic complications of this class of drugs that might present in the ICU. TTP is a life-threatening syndrome characterized by microangiopathic hemolytic anemia and thrombocytopenia in association with renal insufficiency, fever, and central nervous system abnormalities. Laboratory findings consistent with the diagnosis of TTP include elevated lactate dehydrogenase; schistocytes on blood smear; and normal prothrombin time, partial thromboplastin time, and fibrin split products. No cases of ticlopidine-associated TTP were reported during phase III trials,[105] but postmarketing surveillance has shown that TTP occurs in approximately 1/1600 to 1/5000 patients receiving ticlopidine. Mortality of TTP is 20% to 60%.[106,107,108]

Ticlopidine seems to induce the formation of autoantibodies to von Willebrand factor metalloproteinase in patients who subsequently develop TTP; this leads to reduced degradation of ultralarge von Willebrand factor multimers, increased binding of platelets to von Willebrand factor, and widespread microvascular thrombosis.[109] Most patients with ticlopidine-associated TTP develop it within 3 months of initiating therapy,[105,108] but a significant minority may develop delayed TTP. A nonrandomized study showed a reduction in mortality from 60% to 20% in patients with ticlopidine-associated TTP receiving plasma exchange.[108] Ticlopidine also has been associated with life-threatening neutropenia and aplastic anemia.

Clopidogrel is closely related chemically to ticlopidine. It has largely replaced ticlopidine in clinical application due to its relative lack of hematologic toxicity. TTP has been reported in association with its use, however.[110] Clopidogrel-associated TTP has occurred within the first 2 weeks of therapy and seems to respond to plasma exchange.

Glycoprotein IIb/IIIa Receptor Antagonists

The glycoprotein IIb/IIIa receptor plays a pivotal role in platelet aggregation. When activated by adhesion or agonist receptors, this integrin can bind soluble ligands, such as fibrinogen and von Willebrand factor, that mediate platelet cohesion. A detailed review of this process is referenced.[111] Platelet aggregation is particularly important in the formation of arterial clots. Antagonists of the glycoprotein IIb/IIIa integrin have been found to be efficacious in the therapy of acute coronary syndromes. The intravenous agents abciximab, eptifibatide, and tirofiban hydrochloride are in clinical use in the United States.

The pharmacokinetic properties of these agents are important in the management of hematologic complications. Abciximab has the highest affinity for platelet binding and the slowest rate of dissociation. Although the plasma half-life is 26 minutes, the "biologic" half-life (recovery of platelet aggregation) is approximately 8 hours. Platelet-associated abciximab can be detected for more than 14 days postinfusion.[112] Eptifibatide and tirofiban have lower platelet binding affinity and significantly faster dissociation kinetics. Their serum half-lives are approximately 2 hours and their biologic half-lives are less than 4 hours.[112] After a dose of any of these agents, the bleeding time corrects more rapidly than does platelet aggregation[113] and is of little utility in the evaluation of bleeding complications.[114]

Bleeding associated with glycoprotein IIb/IIIa antagonists occurs most commonly at the site of intravascular catheters in the groin. Although this bleeding is overt, the quantity of blood loss often is underestimated. We have seen several patients experience life-threatening hemodynamic compromise from groin hemorrhages that had been recognized previously but treated inadequately. Abciximab given within 12 hours of emergent cardiac surgery has been associated with a significant increase in perioperative bleeding.[115] The risk of intracranial hemorrhage with glycoprotein IIb/IIIa antagonists is 0.07%—equal to the risk with heparin.[116] Diffuse alveolar hemorrhage has been reported by several authors.[117,118]

Manual compression of enlarging groin hematomas is often sufficient treatment. Certain aspects of the treatment of bleeding complications are agent specific. The unbound fractions of eptifibatide and tirofiban typically are large enough to negate any benefit of platelet transfusion. Both of these agents undergo rapid renal clearance, with significant recovery of platelet function within 4 hours.[119] Treatment of bleeding associated with these agents is often supportive care. It is unclear whether either agent is dialyzable. In contrast, abciximab is almost entirely platelet bound in vivo, with little unbound drug to inhibit the function of transfused platelets. In addition, abciximab has a significantly prolonged antiplatelet effect. Platelet transfusion is much more likely to be of clinical benefit.[119]

Severe thrombocytopenia occurs in 1% to 2% of patients receiving abciximab. Although major bleeding seems to be infrequent in these patients,[120] mortality rates are higher in thrombocytopenic patients.[121] An immune mechanism has been suggested in which a ligand-induced antigen leads to a humoral immune response.[122] It has been recommended that glycoprotein IIb/IIIa inhibitors be discontinued when the platelet count decreases to less than 100×10^9 (along with other possible offending medications such as heparin).[122] Platelet transfusion should be considered if the platelet count decreases to less than 20×10^9. Thrombocytopenia related to abciximab administration has been shown to be readily correctable with platelet transfusion.[122]

REFERENCES

1. Nunn S, Esmail R, Fears H, et al: Pharmacokinetic properties of anisoylated plasminogen streptokinase activator complex and other thrombolytic agents in animals and in humans. Drugs 3(Suppl):88–92, 1987.
2. Sane DC, Califf RM, Topol RJ, et al: Bleeding during thrombolytic therapy for acute myocardial infarction: Mechanisms and management. Ann Intern Med 111:1010–1022, 1989.
3. Mentzer RL, Budzynski AZ, Sherry S: High dose, brief-duration intravenous infusion of streptokinase in acute myocardial infarction: description of effects in the circulation. Am J Cardiol 57:1220–1226, 1986.
4. Koneti Rao A, Pratee C, Berke A, et al, for the TIMI investigators: Thrombolysis in Myocardial Infarction (TIMI) trial—Phase I: Hemorrhagic manifestations and changes in plasma fibrinogen and the fibrinolytic system in patients treated with recombinant tissue plasminogen activator and streptokinase. J Am Coll Cardiol 11:1–11, 1988.
5. Owen J, Friedman KD, Grossman BA, et al: Quantitation of fragment X formation during thrombolytic therapy with streptokinase and tissue plasminogen activator. J Clin Invest 79:1642–1647, 1987.
6. Marder VJ: Comparison of thrombolytic agents: Selected hematologic, vascular and clinical events. Am J Cardiol 64:2A-7A, 1989.
7. Marder VJ, Tothbard RL, Fitzpatrick PG, Francis CW: Rapid lysis of coronary artery thrombi with anisoylated plasminogen streptokinase activator complex. Ann Intern Med 104:304–310, 1986.
8. Gralnick HR: Congenital disorders of fibrinogen. In Williams WJ, Beutler E, Ersley AJ, Lichtman MA (eds): Hematology. New York, McGraw-Hill, 1983, p 1400.
9. Salzman EW: Hemostatic problems in surgical patients. In Colman RW, Hirsh J, Marder VJ, Salzman EW (eds): Hemostasis and Thrombosis: Basic Principles and Clinical Practice. Philadelphia, JB Lippincott, 1987, p 922.

10. Verstraete M, Miller GAH, Bounameaux H, et al: Intravenous and intrapulmonary recombinant tissue-type plasminogen activator in the treatment of acute massive pulmonary embolism. Circulation 77:353–360, 1988.

11. Marder VJ, Shulman NR, Carroll WR: The importance of intermediate degradation products of fibrinogen in fibrinolytic hemorrhage. Trans Assoc Am Physicians 80:156–167, 1967.

12. Francis CW, Marder VJ: Increased resistance to plasmic degradation of fibrin with highly crosslinked alpha-polymer chains formed at high factor XIII concentrations. Blood 71:1361–1365, 1988.

13. Rao AK, Pratt C, Berke A, et al, for the TIMI Investigators: Thrombolysis in Myocardial Infarction (TIMI) trial—Phase 1: Hemorrhagic manifestations and changes in plasma fibrinogen and fibrinolytic system in patients treated with recombinant tissue plasminogen activator and streptokinase. J Am Coll Cardiol 11:1–11, 1988.

14. Rizza ER: Management of patients with inherited blood coagulation defects. In Bloom AL, Thomas DP (eds): Haemostasis and Thrombosis. London, Churchill Livingstone, 1981, p 371.

15. Schafer AI, Adelman B: Plasmin inhibition of platelet function and of arachidonic acid metabolism. J Clin Invest 75:456–461, 1985.

16. Adelman B, Michelson AD, Loscalzo J, et al: Plasmin effect on platelet glycoprotein Ib-von Willebrand factor interactions. Blood 65:32–40, 1985.

17. Stricker RB, Wong D, Shiu DT, et al: Activation of plasminogen by tissue plasminogen activator in normal and thrombasthenic platelets: Effect of surface proteins and platelet aggregation. Blood 68:275–280, 1986.

18. Cafri C, Gilutz H, Ilia R, et al: Unusual bleeding complications of thrombolytic therapy after cardiopulmonary resuscitation: Three case reports. Angiology 48:925–928, 1997.

19. The NINDS t-PA Stroke Study Group: Intracerebral hemorrhage after intravenous t-PA therapy for ischemic stroke. Stroke 28:2109–2118, 1997.

20. Hacke W, Kaste M, Fieschi C, et al: Randomized double-blind placebo controlled trial of thrombolytic therapy with intravenous alteplase in acute ischemic stroke (ECASS II). Lancet 352:1245–1251, 1998.

21. Trouillas P, Nighoghossian N, Derex L, et al: Thrombolysis with intravenous rt-PA in a series of 100 cases of acute carotid territory stroke. Stroke 29:2529–2540, 1998.

22. Gruppo Italiano per lo Studio della Sofravvivenza nell'Infarto Miocardio: GISSI 2: A factorial randomised trial of anistreplase versus streptokinase and heparin versus no heparin among 12,490 patients with acute myocardial infarction. Lancet 336:65–71, 1990.

23. ISIS-3 (Third International Study of Infarct Survival) Collaborative Group: ISIS-3: A randomized comparison of streptokinase versus tissue plasminogen activator versus anistreplase and of aspirin plus heparin versus aspirin alone among 41,299 cases of suspected acute myocardial infarction. Lancet 339:753–770, 1992.

24. ISIS-2 (Second International Study of Infarct Survival) Collaborative Group: ISIS-2: Randomised trial of IV streptokinase, oral aspirin, both or neither among 17,187 cases of suspected acute myocardial infarction. Lancet 2:349–360, 1988.

25. Wilcox RG, von der Lippe G, Olsson CG, et al: Trial of tissue plasminogen activator for mortality reduction in acute myocardial infarction. Anglo-Scandinavian Study of Early Thrombolysis (ASSET). Lancet 2:525–530, 1988.

26. Kanter DS, Mikkola KM, Patel SR, et al: Thrombolytic therapy for pulmonary embolism. Chest 111:1241–1245, 1997.

27. Sloan MA, Price TR, Petito CK, et al: Clinical features and pathogenesis of intracerebral hemorrhage after rt-PA and heparin therapy for acute myocardial infarction: The Thrombolysis in Myocardial Infarction (TIMI) II pilot and randomized clinical trial combined experience. Neurology 45:649–658, 1995.

28. Awadh N, Ronco JJ, Bernstein V, et al: Spontaneous pulmonary hemorrhage after thrombolytic therapy for acute myocardial infarction. Chest 106:1622–1624, 1994.

29. Klauser R, Roggla G, Pidlich J, et al: Massive upper airway bleeding after thrombolytic therapy: Successful airway management with the Combitube. Ann Emerg Med 21:431–433, 1992.

30. The NINDS t-PA Stroke Study Group: Generalized efficacy of t-PA for acute stroke: Subgroup analysis of the NINDS t-PA Stroke Trial. Stroke 28:2119–2125, 1997.

31. del Zoppo GJ, Poeck K, Pessin MS, et al: Recombinant tissue plasminogen activator in acute thrombotic and embolic stroke. Ann Neurol 32:78–86, 1992.

32. Topol EJ, Bell WR, Weisfeldt ML: Coronary thrombolysis with recombinant tissue-type plasminogen activator: A hematologic and pharmacologic study. Ann Intern Med 103:837–843, 1985.

33. Hillman RS: Anticoagulants, thrombolytic and antiplatelet drugs. In Hardman JG, Limbird LE, Molinoff PB, et al (eds): Goodman and Gilman's The Pharmacologic Basis of Therapeutics, 9th ed. New York, McGraw-Hill, 1996, p 1353.

34. Tisdale JE, Stringer KA, Antalek M, Matthews GE: Streptokinase-induced anaphylaxis. DICP 23:984–987, 1989.

35. Hill MD, Barber PA, Takahashi J, et al: Anaphylactoid reactions and angioedema during alteplase treatment of acute ischemic stroke. Can Med Assoc J 162:1281–1284, 2000.

36. Green J, Dupe RJ, Smith RAG, et al: Comparison of the hypotensive effects of streptokinase plasmin activator complex and BRL 26921 in the dog after high dose bolus administration. Thromb Res 36:29–36, 1984.

37. Cornelli U, Fareed J: Human pharmacokinetics of low molecular weight heparins. Semin Thromb Haemost 25:57–61, 1999.

38. Hansen JB, Sandset PM, Huseby KR, et al: Differential effect of unfractionated heparin and low molecular weight heparin on intravascular tissue factor pathway inhibitor: Evidence for a difference in antithrombotic action. Br J Haematol 101:638–646, 1998.

39. Altman R, Scazziota A, Rouvier J: Efficacy of unfractionated heparin, low molecular weight heparin and both combined for releasing total and free tissue factor pathway inhibitor. Haemostasis 28:229–235, 1998.

40. Hoppensteadt DAm, Jeske W, Fareed J, Bermes EW: The role of tissue factor pathway inhibitor in the mediation of the antithrombotic actions of heparin and low-molecular-weight heparin. Blood Coagul Fibrinolysis 6(Suppl 1):S57–64, 1995.

41. Hoppensteadt DAm, Walenga JM, Fasnella A, et al: TFPI antigen levels in normal human volunteers after intravenous and subcutaneous administration of unfractionated heparin and a low molecular weight heparin. Thromb Res 77:175–185, 1995.

42. Tollefsen DM, Sugimori T, Maimone MM: Effect of low molecular weight heparin preparations on the inhibition of thrombin by heparin cofactor II. Semin Thromb Hemost 16(Suppl):66–70, 1990.

43. Agnelli G: Pharmacological activities of heparin chains: Should our past knowledge be revised? Haemostasis 26(Suppl 2):2–9, 1996.

44. Padilla A, Gray E, Pepper DS, Barrowcliffe TW: Inhibition of thrombin generation by heparin and low molecular weight heparins in the absence and presence of platelet factor 4. Br J Haematol 82:406–413, 1992.

45. Kitchen S, Theaker J, Preston FE: Monitoring unfractionated heparin therapy: Relationship between eight anti-Xa assays and a protamine titration assay. Blood Coagul Fibrinolysis 11:137–144, 2000.

46. Sie P, Aillaud MF, de Prost D, et al: Measurement of low molecular weight heparin ex vivo activities in clinical laboratories using various anti-Xa assays: Interlaboratory variability and requirement for an agreed low molecular weight heparin standard. Thromb Haemost 58:879–883, 1987.

47. Bara L, Planes A, Samama MM: Occurrence of thrombosis and haemorrhage, relationship with anti-Xa, anti-IIa activities, and D-dimer plasma levels in patients receiving a low molecular weight heparin, enoxaparin or tinzaparin, to prevent deep vein thrombosis after hip surgery. Br J Haematol 104:230–240, 1999.

48. Leizorovicz A, Bara L, Samama MM, Haugh MC: Factor Xa inhibition: correlation between the plasma levels of anti-Xa activity and occurrence of thrombosis and haemorrhage. Haemostasis 23(Suppl 1):89–98, 1993.

49. Bara L, Leizorovicz A, Picolet H, Samama MM: Correlation between anti-Xa and occurrence of thrombosis and haemorrhage in post-surgical patients treated with either logiparin (LMWH) or unfractionated heparin. Post-surgery Logiparin Study Group. Thromb Res 65:641–650, 1992.

50. Raschke RA, Guidry JA, Foley MR: Apparent heparin resistance due to elevated factor VIII during pregnancy. Obstet Gynecol 96:804–806, 2000.

51. Hull RS, Raskob GE, Rosenbloom D, et al: Optimal therapeutic level of heparin therapy in patients with venous thrombosis. Arch Intern Med 152:1589–1595, 1992.

52. Basu D, Gallus A, Hirsh J, Cade J: A prospective study of the value of monitoring heparin treatment with the activated partial thromboplastin time. N Engl J Med 287:324–327, 1972.

53. Salzman EW, Deykin D, Shapiro RM, Rosenbert R: Management of heparin therapy: Controlled prospective trial. N Engl J Med 292: 1046–1053, 1975.
54. Doyle DJ, Turpie GG, Hirsh J, et al: Adjusted subcutaneous heparin or continuous intravenous heparin in patients with acute deep vein thrombosis. Ann Intern Med 107:441–445, 1987.
55. Guidry J, Raschke R, Morkunis A: Anticoagulants and thrombolytics: Risks and benefits. Crit Care Clin North Am 7:533–554, 1991.
56. Chui WS: The syndrome of retroperitoneal hemorrhage and lumbar plexus neuropathy during anticoagulant therapy. South Med J 69: 595–599, 1976.
57. Stanton PE, Wilson JP, Lamis PA, Letton AH: Acute abdominal conditions induced by anticoagulant therapy. Am Surg 40:1–14, 1974.
58. Babb RR, Spittell JA, Bartholomew LG: Hematoma of the rectus abdominus muscle complicating anticoagulant therapy. Mayo Clin Proc 40:760–768, 1965.
59. Scott WW, Fishman EK, Siegelman SS: Anticoagulants and abdominal pain: The role of computerized tomography. JAMA 252:2053–2056, 1984.
60. Wysowski DK, Talarico L, Bacsanyi J, Botstein P: Spinal and epidural hematoma and low-molecular-weight heparin. N Engl J Med 338: 1774–1775, 1998.
61. Protamine sulfate: Antiheparin agents 20:12.08. In McEvoy GK, Litvak K, Welsh OH, Snow EK (eds): AHFS Drug Information 1999. Bethesda, MD, American Society of Health-System Pharmacists, 1999, pp 1265–1267.
62. Horrow JC: Protamine: A review of its toxicity. Anesth Analg 64:348–361, 1985.
63. Caplan SN, Berkman EM: Protamine sulfate and fish allergy. N Engl J Med 295:172, 1976.
64. Stewart WJ, McSweeney SM, Kellett MR, et al: Increased risk of severe protamine reactions in NPH insulin-dependent diabetics undergoing cardiac catheterization. Circulation 70:788–792, 1984.
65. Kikura M, Lee MK, Levy JH: Heparin neutralization with methylene blue, hexadimethrine, or vancomycin after cardiopulmonary bypass. Anesth Analg 83:223–227, 1996.
66. Despotis GJ, Summerfield AL, Joist JH, et al: In vitro reversal of heparin effect with heparinase: Evaluation with whole blood prothrombin time and activated partial thromboplastin time in cardiac surgical patients. Anesth Analg 79:670–674, 1994.
67. Dehmer GJ, Fisher M, Tate DA, et al: Reversal of heparin anticoagulation by recombinant platelet factor 4 in humans. Circulation 91:2188–2194, 1995.
68. Tao W, Deyo DJ, Brunston RL Jr, et al: Extracorporeal heparin adsorption following cardiopulmonary bypass with a heparin removal device—an alternative to protamine. Crit Care Med 26:1096–1102, 1998.
69. Hulin MS, Wakefield TW, Andrews PC, et al: A novel protamine variant reversal of heparin anticoagulation in human blood in vitro. J Vasc Surg 26:1043–1048, 1997.
70. Lindblad B, Borgstrom A, Wakefield TW, et al: Protamine reversal of anticoagulation achieved with a low molecular weight heparin: The effects on eicosanoids, clotting and complement factors. Thromb Res 48:31–40, 1987.
71. Massonnet-Castel S, Pelissier E, Bara L, et al: Partial reversal of low molecular weight heparin (PK 10169) anti-Xa activity by protamine sulfate: In vitro and in vivo study during cardiac surgery with extracorporeal circulation. Haemostasis 16:139–146, 1986.
72. Woltz M, Weltermann A, Nieszpaur-Los M, et al: Studies on the neutralizing effects of protamine on unfractionated and low molecular weight heparin (Fragmin) at the site of activation of the coagulation system in man. Thromb Hemost 73:439–443, 1995.
73. Sugiyama T, Itoh M, Ohtawa M, Natsuga T: Study on neutralization of low molecular weight heparin by protamine sulfate and its neutralization characteristics. Thromb Res 68:119–129, 1992.
74. Ramamurthy N, Baliga N, Wakefield TW, et al: Determination of low-molecular-weight heparins and their binding to protamine and a protamine analog using polyion-sensitive membrane electrodes. Analyt Biochem 266:116–124, 1999.
75. Hirsh J, Levine MN: Low molecular weight heparin. Blood 79:1–17, 1992.
76. Hubbard AR, Jennings CA: Neutralization of heparan sulphate and low molecular weight heparin by protamine. Thromb Haemost 53:86–89, 1985.
77. Van Ryn-McKenna J, Cai L, Ofosu FA, et al: Neutralization of enoxaparine-induced bleeding by protamine sulfate. Thromb Haemost 63: 271–274, 1990.
78. Doutremepuich C, Bonini F, Toulemonde F, et al: In vivo neutralization of low-molecular weight heparin fraction CY 216 by protamine. Semin Thromb Hemost 11:318–322, 1985.
79. Bang CJ, Berstad A, Talstad I: Incomplete reversal of enoxaparin-induced bleeding by protamine sulfate. Haemostasis 21:155–160, 1991.
80. Wakefield TW, Andrews PC, Wrobleski SK, et al: Effective and less toxic reversal of low-molecular-weight heparin anticoagulation by a designer variant of protamine. J Vasc Surg 21:839–850, 1995.
81. Byun Y, Singh VK, Yang VC: Low molecular weight protamine: A potential nontoxic heparin antagonist. Thromb Res 94:53–61, 1999.
82. Dietrich CP, Shinjo SK, Fabio AM, et al: Structural features and bleeding activity of commercial low molecular weight heparins: Neutralization by ATP and protamine. Semin Thromb Hemost 25(Suppl 3):43–50, 1999.
83. Shenoy S, Sobel M, Harris RB: Development of heparin antagonists with focused biological activity. Curr Pharm Design 5:965–986, 1999.
84. Warkentin TE, Levine MN, Hirsh J, et al: Heparin-induced thrombocytopenia in patients treated with low-molecular-weight-heparin or unfractionated heparin. N Engl J Med 332:1330–1335, 1995.
85. Warkentin TE, Kelton JG: A 14-year study of heparin-induced thrombocytopenia. Am J Med 101:502–507, 1996.
86. Warkentin TE: Clinical presentation of heparin-induced thrombopenia. Semin Hematol 35(Suppl 4):9–16, 1998.
87. Amiral J: Diagnostic tests in heparin-induced thrombocytopenia. Platelets 8:68–72, 1997.
88. Amiral J, Peynaud-Debayle E, Wolf M, et al: Generation of antibodies to heparin-PF4 complexes without thrombocytopenia in patients treated with unfractionated or low molecular weight heparin. Am J Hematol 52:90–95, 1996.
89. Chong BH, Eisbacher M: Pathophysiology and laboratory testing of heparin-induced thrombocytopenia. Semin Hematol 35(4 Suppl 5): 3–8, 1998.
90. Kadidal VV, Mayo DJ, Horne MK: Heparin-induced thrombocytopenia (HIT) due to heparin flushes: A report of three cases. J Intern Med 246:325–329, 1999.
91. Greinacher A: Treatment of heparin-induced thrombocytopenia. Thromb Haemost 82:457–467, 1999.
92. Warkentin TE, Soutar RL, Panju A, Ginsberg JS: Acute systemic reactions to intravenous bolus heparin therapy: Characterization and relationship to heparin-induced thrombocytopenia (Abstract). Blood 80(Suppl 1):160a, 1992.
93. Warkentin TE: Heparin-induced thrombocytopenia, heparin-induced skin lesions, and arterial thrombosis. Thromb Haemost 77(Suppl):562, 1997.
94. Warkentin TE: Heparin-induced thrombocytopenia: A clinicopathologic syndrome. Thromb Haemost 82:439–447, 1999.
95. Breinacher A, Volpel H, Janssens U, et al: Recombinant hirudin (lepirudin) provides safe and effective anticoagulation in patients with the immunologic type of heparin-induced thrombocytopenia: A prospective study. Circulation 99:73–80, 1999.
96. Greinacher A: Leprirudin for the treatment of heparin-induced thrombocytopenia: A prospective study (Abstract). Blood 92:1490, 1998.
97. Warkentin TE, Elavathil LJ, Hayward CPM, et al: The pathogenesis of venous limb gangrene associated with heparin-induced thrombocytopenia. Ann Intern Med 127:804–812, 1997.
98. Pouplard C, Amiral J, Borg JY, et al: Decision analysis for use of platelet aggregation test, carbon 14-serotonin release assay, and heparin-platelet factor 4 enzyme-linked immunosorbent assay for diagnosis of heparin-induced thrombocytopenia. Am J Clin Pathol 111:700–706, 1999.
99. Walenga JM, Jeske WP, Wood JJ, et al: Laboratory tests for heparin-induced thrombocytopenia: A multicenter study. Semin Hematol 36(Suppl 1):22–28, 1999.
100. Sheridan D, Carter C, Kelton JG: A diagnostic test for heparin-induced thrombocytopenia. Blood 67:27–30, 1986.
101. Raskob GE, Hull RD, Pineo GF: Heparin, hirudin and related agents. In Beuller E, Coller BS, Lichtman MA, et al (eds): Williams Hematology, 6th ed. New York, McGraw-Hill, 2001, pp 1793–1801.
102. Warkentin TE: Current agents for the treatment of patients with heparin-induced thrombocytopenia. Curr Opin Pulm Med 8:405–412, 2002.
103. Lewis BE, Wallis DE, Berkowitz SD, et al: Argatroban anticoagulant therapy in patients with heparin-induced thrombocytopenia. Circulation 103:1838–1843, 2001.

104. Saltiel E, Ward A: Ticlopidine: A review of its pharmacodynamic and pharmacokinetic properties, and therapeutic efficacy in platelet-dependent disease states. Drugs 34:222–262, 1987.
105. Bennett CL, Davidson CJ, Raisch DW, et al: Thrombotic thrombocytopenic purpura associated with ticlopidine in the setting of coronary artery stents and stroke prevention. Arch Intern Med 159:2524–2528, 1999.
106. Bennett CL, Kiss JE, Weinberg PD, et al: Thrombotic thrombocytopenic purpura after stenting and ticlopidine. Lancet 352:1036–1037, 1998.
107. Steinhubl SR, Tan WA, Foody JM, et al: Incidence and clinical course of thrombotic thrombocytopenic purpura due to ticlopidine following coronary stenting. JAMA 281:806–810, 1999.
108. Bennett CL, Davidson CJ, Raisch DW, et al: Thrombotic thrombocytopenic purpura associated with ticlopidine in the setting of coronary artery stents and stroke prevention. Arch Intern Med 159:2524–2528, 1999.
109. Tsai HM, Rice L, Sarode R, et al: Antibody inhibitors to von Willebrand factor metalloproteinase and increased binding of von Willebrand factor to platelets in ticlopidine-associated thrombotic thrombocytopenic purpura. Ann Intern Med 132:794–799, 2000.
110. Bennett CL, Connors JM, Carwile JM, et al: Thrombotic thrombocytopenic purpura associated with clopidogrel. N Engl J Med 342:1773–1777, 2000.
111. Topol EJ, Byzova TV, Plow EF: Platelet GPIIb-IIIa blockers. Lancet 353:227–231, 1999.
112. Kleiman NS: Pharmacokinetics and pharmacodynamics of glycoprotein IIb/IIIa inhibitors. Am Heart J 138:s263–275, 1999.
113. Blankenship JC: Bleeding complications of glycoprotein IIb-IIIa receptor inhibitors. Am Heart J 138:s287–296, 1999.
114. Burns ER, Lawrence C: Bleeding time: A guide to its diagnostic and clinical utility. Arch Pathol Lab Med 113:1219–1224, 1989.
115. Gammie JS, Zenati M, Kormos RL, et al: Abciximab and excessive bleeding in patients undergoing emergency cardiac operations. Ann Thorac Surg 65:465–469, 1998.
116. Memon MA, Blankenship JC, Wood GC, et al: Incidence of intracranial hemorrhage complicating treatment with glycoprotein IIb/IIIa receptor inhibitors: A pooled analysis of major clinical trials. Am J Med 109:252–254, 2000.
117. Sitges M, Villa FP: Massive pulmonary hemorrhage in a patient treated with a platelet glycoprotein IIb/IIIa inhibitor. Int J Cardiol 62:269–271, 1997.
118. Ali A, Patil S, Grady KJ, Schreiber TL: Diffuse alveolar hemorrhage following administration of tirofiban or abciximab: A nemesis of platelet glycoprotein IIb/IIIa inhibitors. Catheter Cardiovasc Interv 49:181–184, 2000.
119. Tcheng JE: Clinical challenges of platelet glycoprotein IIb/IIIa receptor inhibitor therapy: Bleeding, reversal, thrombocytopenia, and retreatment. Am Heart J 139:s38–45, 2000.
120. Sasgupta H, Blankenship JC, Wood GC, et al: Thrombocytopenia complicating treatment with intravenous glycoprotein IIb/IIIa receptor inhibitors: A pooled analysis. Am Heart J 140:206–211, 2000.
121. Kereiakes DJ, Berkowitz SD, Lincoff AM, et al: Clinical correlates and course of thrombocytopenia during percutaneous coronary intervention in the era of abciximab platelet glycoprotein IIb/IIIa blockade. Am Heart J 140:74–80, 2000.
122. Madan M, Berkowitz SD: Understanding thrombocytopenia and antigenicity with glycoprotein IIb-IIIa inhibitors. Am Heart J 138:317–326, 1999.

CHAPTER 68

Antitubulin Agents: Colchicine, Vinca Alkaloids, and Podophyllin

Lisa K. Snyder ■ Louise W. Kao ■ R. Brent Furbee

Microtubules are present in all eukaryotic cells. They are responsible for movement of vesicles within cells, motion of cilia and flagella, and chromosome separation in mitosis. In neurons, microtubules serve as tracks for protein particles and organelles that move up and down the axon. They also can direct proteins for repair of cellular injury. Antitubulin agents, including colchicine, vincristine, vinblastine, and podophyllin, inhibit the construction of microtubules, which accounts for the therapeutic and the toxic actions of these agents.

COLCHICINE

Colchicine is an alkaloid derived from *Colchicum autumnale*, a member of the family Liliaceae,[1] and from *Gloriosa superba*.[2,3] *C. autumnale* is a perennial plant that is known commonly as *autumn crocus, wild saffron, meadow saffron, naked lady, naked boy*, and *son before the father*. This plant is indigenous to temperate areas of Europe, Asia, and America. It is unusual because it flowers after the long, lanceolate leaves wither back and fall off (hence the "son before the father"). All parts of the plant contain colchicine, but the highest concentration is in the bulb, which is rooted underground.[1]

Colchicine has been used since the 6th century A.D., when it was introduced by Alexander of Tralles as a treatment for gout. It is said that Benjamin Franklin also used colchicine as a remedy for his gouty arthritis and possibly introduced it into the United States.[1,4] Purified colchicine later was isolated from *C. autumnale* tubers in 1820 by Syng Dorsey and became widely known as a treatment for gouty arthritis.[2]

The currently approved indications for colchicine are treating gouty arthritis, preventing gout attacks, and managing familial Mediterranean fever.[5] It has also been advocated for pseudogout, sarcoidosis,[6] scleroderma,[7] amyloidosis,[8] Behçet's disease,[9,10] psoriasis,[11] systemic sclerosis,[12] Paget's disease, condyloma acuminatum,[13] brown recluse spider envenomation,[14] alcoholic cirrhosis,[15] primary biliary cirrhosis,[16] Sweet's syndrome,[17] and low back pain.[18,19]

Guidelines for intravenous colchicine use in the treatment of acute gout were outlined by Wallace and Singer.[20] Their recommendations are as follows: (1) A single intravenous dose should not exceed 2 to 3 mg, and cumulative doses for each attack should not exceed 4 to 5 mg; (2) after intravenous colchicine, no other form of the drug should be given by any route for at least 7 days; (3) doses of colchicine should be reduced in a patient with hepatic or renal insufficiency and in geriatric patients; (4) bolus dosing by intravenous route should be half the oral dose; (5) absolute contraindications include renal and hepatic disease, creatinine clearance of less than 10 mL/min, and extrahepatic biliary obstruction.[20]

Biochemistry and Pharmacokinetics

Colchicine has a complex structure (Fig. 68-1). Tropolones have a hydrogen ion, which resonates between an oxygen and methyl group. Wallace[21] identified five colchicine analogues. It was found that one analogue lacked a tropolone structure; that particular analogue failed to have antigout activity.

The kinetics of colchicine varies, but the most frequently cited observations regarding absorption from the gastrointestinal tract show the occurrence of a peak plasma concentration in 30 minutes to 2 hours. Approximately 50% of the drug is protein bound, and its volume of distribution is estimated to be 2.2 L/kg. This information allows for an understanding of the limited efficacy of hemodialysis as a means of enhancing drug clearance. The major route of elimination of colchicine is through hepatic metabolism and biliary excretion. It is believed that enterohepatic recirculation may prolong exposure of the intestinal mucosa to colchicine.[1] Twenty percent of unchanged drug is excreted in the urine.[31] In the setting of preexisting renal or hepatic impairment, these elimination percentages may change.

Colchicine has been reported to have a half-life of 10 to 16 hours and has been found in white blood cells and in urine 9 days after a single intravenous bolus.[4,29,33] Because colchicine is metabolized through cytochrome P-450 CYP3A4, its breakdown may be inhibited or induced. Inhibitors of CYP3A4, such as cimetidine, ketoconazole, erythromycin, diltiazem, and grapefruit juice, frequently produce increases in serum concentrations of colchicine. Inducers of CYP3A4 include rifampin, phenobarbital, and phenytoin, which tend to lower serum colchicine concentrations.

Pathophysiology

Microtubules are formed by polymerization of protein subunits, G actin and tubulin. Tubulin is present in α, β, and γ forms; α and β tubulin combine as dimers that serve as the building blocks of microtubules, and γ tubulin seems to

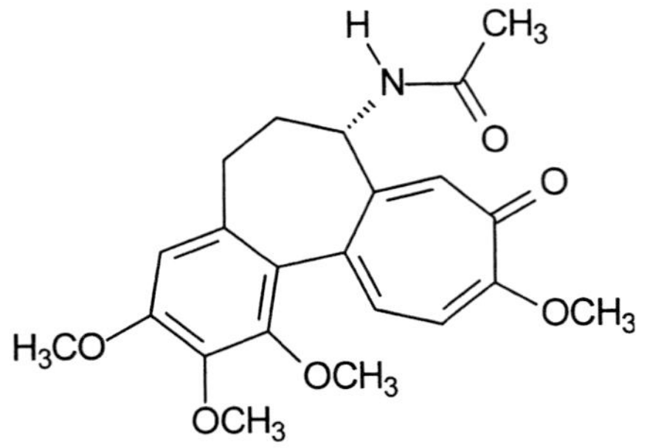

FIGURE 68-1

Chemical structure of colchicine.

play a role in the organization of these dimers during the assembly of a tubulin sheet. The sheet connects end to end to form the cylindrical origin of the microtubule.[22] The microtubule is composed of repeating α and β tubulin subunits in a helical array measuring 24 nm in diameter (Fig. 68-2).[23] The tubulin dimer has oppositely charged ends. Because the dimers are aligned repetitively, the microtubule they form has a positive end and a negative end. This alignment confers polarity to microtubules, which is crucial to their function. They are connected in elaborate networks depending on the function they serve within the cell. Microtubules form a diverse array of permanent (stable) and transient (unstable) structures. Stable microtubules are found when long-lived microtubules are needed, such as the axoneme in the flagellum of sperm and the marginal band of microtubules in most red blood cells and platelets or nerve cells. Unstable microtubules are found when cell structures composed of microtubules need to disassemble and assemble quickly. During mitosis, the cytosolic microtubule network that occurs in interphase disappears, and the tubulin from it is used to form the spindle-shaped apparatus that partitions chromosomes equally into daughter cells. Neurons must maintain long axons and do this with the aid of microtubules that continue to assemble (polymerize), and add to the chain. Disassembly of these stable structures has catastrophic effects, such as nonmobile sperm, nonpliable red blood cells, and retracting axons.[22]

Vinca alkaloids, colchicines, and podophyllin all inhibit the construction of microtubules that compose spindles in metaphase. This inhibition interrupts migration of the chromosomes toward the poles during mitosis but does not affect chromosome condensation. Because of this ability, colchicine is used in research to produce metaphase chromosomes for cytogenic study. Each dimer of tubulin has a single high-affinity binding site for colchicine. When one or two vinca alkaloid–bound, podophyllin-bound, or colchicine-bound tubulin dimers attach to the end of the developing microtubule, additional assembly stops. Although these compounds inhibit spindle formation, they do not cause their disassembly at lower doses. When assembly is halted at the positive end of the microtubule, naturally occurring disassembly at the negative end continues. At high doses, however, some of these compounds also may enhance disassembly.[24]

Microtubule formation is regulated by the number of tubulin dimers. As the number of "free" dimers within the cell increases, they bind to ribosomes and shut down the production of tubulin mRNA. The antitubulin compounds, via their inhibition of tubulin dimer polymerization, increase the number available to inhibit mRNA production. They do not seem to affect the more permanent microtubules because at therapeutic doses their impact is primarily on the *assembly* of the microtubule.

Vincristine and vinblastine also inhibit formation of mitotic spindles, interrupting cell division. They appear to crystallize free tubulin dimers. As a result of this action, they preferentially kill rapidly dividing cells, such as tumor cells. This effect also causes cell death in gut and hair cells because of their rapid division. Although the vinca alkaloids bind to tubulin, preventing polymerization in a fashion similar to that of colchicine and podophyllotoxin, they seem to have a different binding site.[23]

The mechanisms of action of colchicine have been studied extensively but remain unclear. Colchicine's action seems to depend on its rings, which are believed to bind microtubules, inhibiting the movement of intracellular granules. This inhibition disturbs the excretion of various components to the cell exterior. Colchicine inhibits multiple aspects of neutrophil activity, including adhesiveness, ameboid activity, mobilization, and degranulation of lysosomes, but the most studied is the inhibition chemotaxis.[25] Colchicine is thought

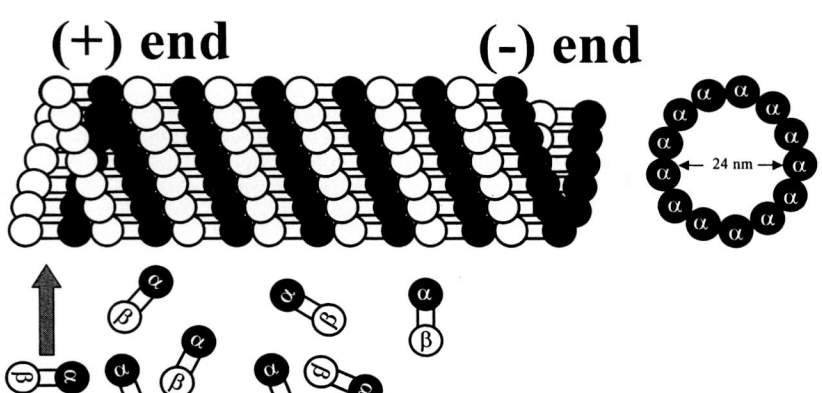

FIGURE 68-2

Microtubule assembly occurs at the positive end, whereas disassembly occurs at the negative end. Antitubulin compounds prevent the addition of tubulin at the positive end and stop assembly.

to work primarily through this inhibited chemotactic mechanism in the treatment of gout.[26,27]

Clinical Presentation

Cases of overdose of colchicine are not common but are associated with significant morbidity and mortality. Mortality overall is approximately 10% but approaches 100% for cases in which the ingestion is 0.8 mg /kg or greater.[3] A review by Baum and Meyerowitz[28] found that although about 90% of persons treated with colchicine for gout are men, the intentional use of this drug in overdose occurs more often in women.

Acute ingestion of colchicine is heralded by gastrointestinal symptoms for the first 24 hours. Profound nausea, vomiting, and diarrhea are common.[29] Abdominal cramping also is reported in several cases,[2,30] and melanotic stools have been seen.[31] These symptoms can cause circulatory collapse due to fluid losses and electrolyte abnormalities. Gastrointestinal symptoms are used as an end point of therapy in the treatment of gout. Typically, these symptoms ensue within minutes of ingestion. The cause is believed to be a direct toxic effect of colchicine on the gut epithelial cells.[1] Emesis may be centrally mediated as well, however, as suggested by an animal study by Ferguson[32] in which gastrectomized animals vomited anyway.

Beginning at 24 to 36 hours, the second stage consists of multiple organ failure. Hematopoietic changes begin with noticeable peripheral leukocytosis,[1,13,33] which reverses quickly and is followed by pancytopenia. Hemorrhage may develop secondary to hepatic dysfunction and thrombocytopenia. Hepatotoxicity and adult respiratory distress syndrome are described in multiple cases. Disseminated intravascular coagulation frequently is reported.[2,29,31,33,34]

Bradycardia and irregular rhythms have been seen with intravenous colchicine administration. Hemodynamic profiles of cardiac failure in acute ingestions have been described in several case reports.[3] Cardiac profiles obtained by Sauder and coworkers[35] in a study of eight patients revealed that four patients had declining cardiac index and rising systemic vascular resistance; these patients subsequently died. Asystole has been reported within 24 hours of ingestion. In one case, the ingestion of 0.4 mg/kg resulted in death. Eight of 12 deaths due to colchicine, according to poison center statistics from 1985 through 1997, indicated the cause of death to be cardiac.[36]

Oliguric renal failure is a common problem in severe colchicine poisoning. One likely cause of renal dysfunction is the profound hypovolemia from sensible gastrointestinal fluid losses and accumulation of fluids that results from paralytic ileus and marked gastrointestinal tract edema.[1,2] Volume depletion, combined with hypoxia and myoglobinuria secondary to colchicine-induced rhabdomyolysis, has resulted in azotemia, proteinuria, and hematuria.[1,29,31]

Reported electrolyte abnormalities include hypokalemia, hyponatremia, hypocalcemia, and hypophosphatemia.[31,33,35] Hypocalcemia may be due to a direct effect of colchicine on bone resorption. Animal studies have shown that colchicine inhibits the rise of serum calcium after injection of parathyroid hormone.[37]

Neurologic complications reflect central nervous system (CNS) and peripheral nervous system involvement. Mental status changes, including sedation, delirium, and coma, are the most common CNS manifestations. Seizures also have been reported. Peripheral nervous system involvement includes myoneuropathy and axonopathy as consequences of chronic and acute overdose.[38] Ascending paralysis and loss of deep tendon reflexes typically occur.[39] Myelin degeneration found on postmortem pathologic examination was thought to be the underlying peripheral manifestation in colchicine poisoning.[1,2]

Metabolic derangements also are well described in cases of colchicine intoxication. Lactic acidosis secondary to shock and tissue hypoxia is associated with colchicine toxicity; however, a more disruptive effect on cell metabolism also may contribute to the acid-base disturbance seen in many cases.[33] Rhabdomyolysis occurs fairly commonly in colchicine poisoning, manifested by myalgia, weakness, and marked elevation in serum creatine phosphokinase concentrations.

Alopecia marks the third stage of toxicity, which may be seen as early as day 6 and as late as day 14. Alopecia is due to the inhibition of mitotic activity in the hair follicles. Most commonly, alopecia begins on the scalp, then involves the axillae, trunk, extremities, and genital area. Regrowth generally occurs after several months, but failure of regrowth has been reported.[40–42] Rebound leukocytosis also occurs in phase III (Table 68-1).

Diagnosis

Intensive monitoring of vital physiologic parameters is imperative in a patient with colchicine intoxication. Systemic abnormalities may include pancytopenia; coagulopathy; hepatic transaminase elevation; acidemia; renal insufficiency; and electrolyte abnormalities, such as hypophosphatemia, hypomagnesemia, hypocalcemia, and hypokalemia. Serum creatine phosphokinase or urine myoglobin concentrations initially should be monitored serially. Septic workup, including blood cultures, is indicated for unexplained fever. Chest radiographs may show interstitial lung changes. Colchicine plasma concentration may confirm the presence of the drug but in many cases does not correlate with the patient's condition.[13] Without preexisting colchicine levels, interpretation of these values is limited. Hepatic and renal dysfunction may prolong drug metabolism and elimination.[33]

Treatment

After initial resuscitative measures, attempts may be made to delay absorption. If performed within 1 hour of ingestion, gastric lavage may be useful, but there is no outcome evidence to support clinical benefit. It generally is recommended that activated charcoal (1 g/kg) be administered. Owing to enterohepatic recirculation of colchicine, multidose activated charcoal may be beneficial; however, evidence of paralytic ileus is a contraindication to this intervention. Hemodialysis has not proved to be beneficial for colchicine poisoning. Any patient with a suspected toxic ingestion of colchicine should be observed for symptoms or signs of toxicity for a minimum of 12 hours. If symptoms develop, intensive care unit admission is warranted.

Supportive care is the mainstay of treatment. Intravascular volume and blood product replacement may be necessary, especially if coagulation parameters are abnormal or bleeding is noted. Ventilatory status should be monitored closely,

TABLE 68-1 Clinical Features of Antitubulin Agent Overdose

	COLCHICINE	VINCRISTINE	VINBLASTINE	PODOPHYLLIN	ETOPOSIDE/TENIPOSIDE
Peripheral neuropathy	Reported	Common	Rare	Common	With vincristine
Hypotension	Reported	Reported	Rare	Reported	With IV infusion
Nausea, vomiting	Common	Common	Common	Common	Common
Fever	Reported	Common	Reported	Common	NR
Leukocytosis	Common	Common	Rare	Reported	NR
Marrow suppression	Common	Reported	Common	Common	Common
Renal failure	Reported	Rare	Rare	In fatal cases	Rare
Liver function abnormalities	Common	Rare	Reported	Common	Reported
Alopecia	Common	Reported	Reported	NR	Reported
Seizures	Reported	Reported	Rare	Rare	With CNS tumors
Acidosis	Reported	Rare	Rare	Reported	NR

CNS, central nervous system; IV, intravenous; NR, not reported.

with intubation and mechanical ventilation provided as indicated. Hemodynamic monitoring also should be performed in a critical care setting initially and on a continuing basis as needed. Vasopressor support and electrolyte replacement may be necessary. Urine output should be followed closely and adjustments made accordingly. As clinical toxicity progresses, patients should be watched for signs of infection, as they become neutropenic and susceptible to opportunistic pathogens. Seizures should be treated with benzodiazepines or barbiturates, and the possibility of underlying acidosis, hypoxia, or electrolyte abnormalities should be considered and corrected aggressively.[2]

Injections of granulocyte colony-stimulating factor (G-CSF) have been used in several cases to treat bone marrow suppression. Dramatic increases have been reported in some but not all cases.[29,43,44]

The development of colchicine-specific antibodies is a promising but as yet unavailable therapy. These antibodies bind to colchicine and restore tubulin activity in vitro.[45] Studies performed in mice, using thermoregulation as an end point, showed a significant improvement in the group that received colchicines-specific IgG.[46] Anticolchicine antibodies were used successfully in a 25-year-old woman who presented 24 hours after ingesting 60 mg (0.96 mg/kg) of colchicine, phenobarbital, and opium extract. She was hemodynamically unstable and required vasopressor support. Colchicine-specific Fab fragments derived from goats were administered intravenously 40 hours after the ingestion. The patient's blood pressure began to increase 30 minutes after Fab administration. During the 6-hour infusion of the maintenance dose of Fab fragments, fluid replacement continued, and urine output improved.[47]

Special Populations

Intravenous colchicine administration is relatively contraindicated in elderly patients owing to their increased risk of underlying hepatic or renal dysfunction.[20] Patients with impaired hepatic or renal function have reduced colchicine clearance. Pediatric patients may be administered colchicine during therapy for conditions such as familial Mediterranean fever,[5,48] acne vulgaris,[49] renal amyloidosis,[50] or pericarditis,[51] to mention only a partial list. There are no published studies addressing colchicine toxicity in children.

VINCA ALKALOIDS

The vinca alkaloids are derived from the Madagascar periwinkle (*Catharanthus roseus*), a perennial evergreen herb found in most warm regions of the world. It grows throughout the southern United States. Interest in *C. roseus* among Western researchers began in 1949, when they studied its use in a tea made by Jamaicans for the treatment of diabetes mellitus. Although its use as a hypoglycemic agent did not evolve as a result of this investigation, bone marrow suppression was observed. Many alkaloids eventually were extracted from the plant, including vincristine, vinblastine, vindesine, and vinorelbine. Semisynthetic vinca alkaloids are also in use or under development. Although structurally similar (Fig. 68-3), these compounds vary in their clinical effects and application in the treatment of neoplastic diseases. The mechanism of action of these compounds is similar to that of colchicine and podophyllin, although with different binding sites on the tubulin dimer. Vincristine is used in the treatment of solid tumors, lymphoma, and leukemia. For normal patients (not children, older people, or people in renal failure), it is administered at 1.4 mg/m²/week. Individual doses should not exceed 2 mg.

Pharmacokinetics

The vinca alkaloids commonly are injected intravenously and seem to follow a three-compartment model (see Fig. 68-3). When ingested, vinca alkaloids' absorption is unpredictable,

Pharmacokinetics of Vinca Alkaloids

Compound	Renal Elimination (%)	Elimination Half-Life (hr)
Vincristine*	<1	24
Vinblastine	<1	24
Vinorelbine	>18	27.7–43.6

IV, intravenous.

*Clearance[81]
 Adults: 189 mL/min/m²
 Children: 482 mL/min/m²

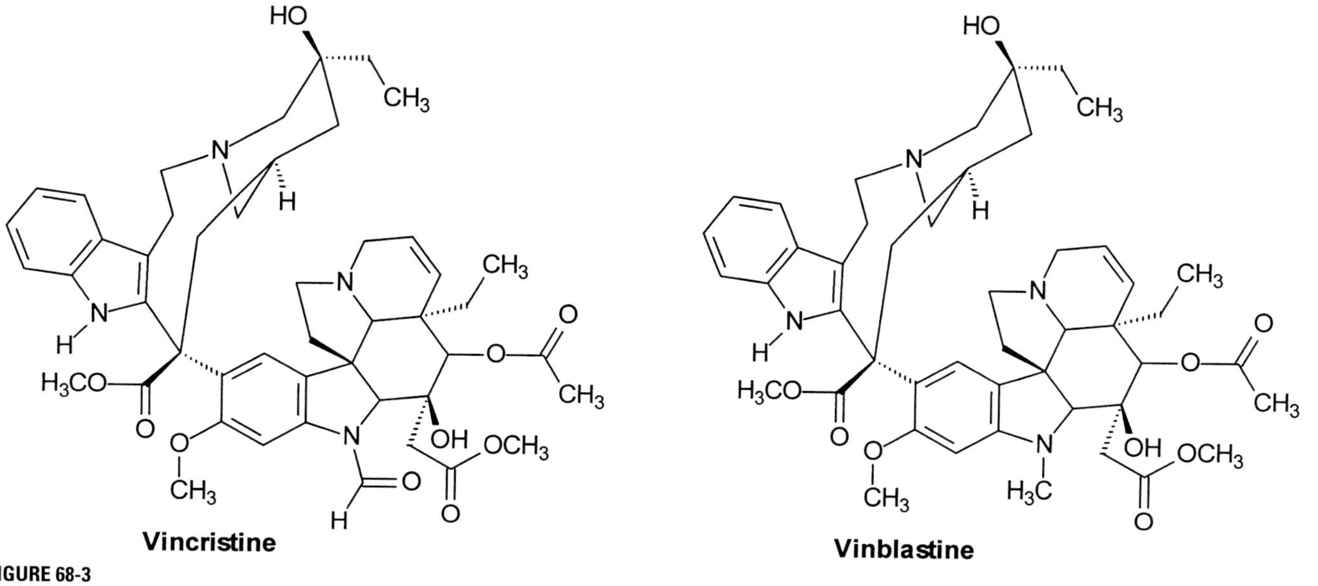

FIGURE 68-3

Chemical structures of vincristine and vinblastine.

although vinorelbine is frequently administered orally. When administered intravenously, vincristine rapidly distributes into tissue of the ileum, skeletal muscle, and kidney. It penetrates the blood-brain barrier poorly. Metabolism of these compounds is primarily hepatic. They are excreted in the bile, and less than 1% of vincristine and vinblastine are excreted in the urine. Renal elimination accounts for 18% of vinorelbine excretion.

Vincristine, and probably all the vinca alkaloids, inhibits the CYP3A subfamily. Troleandomycin, ketoconazole, nifedipine, erythromycin, cyclosporine, and vindesine all seem to increase serum concentrations of the vinca alkaloids. Calcium channel blockers, such as verapamil, seem to decrease protein binding of the vinca alkaloids, increasing the risk of neurotoxicity.[82]

Pathophysiology

The nervous system is the primary target organ of vincristine toxicity. Vincristine disrupts the normal process of microtubule formation, interfering with axoplasmic transport, which accounts for the prevalence of neural injury associated with its administration.[52,54] At therapeutic doses of vincristine of 1.5 mg/m^2 (0.06 mg/kg), the onset of peripheral neuropathies may begin within 2 weeks and occurs with a nearly 100% incidence.[53]

Vinblastine and vinorelbine seem to depolymerize microtubules at the negative terminus while stabilizing the positive terminus.[24] They cause less inhibition of microtubular polymerization and are less neurotoxic than vincristine. Their primary toxicity is bone marrow, which is often the dose-limiting factor during therapy with either drug.

Clinical Presentation

ACUTE TOXICITY

Vincristine. Paresthesias usually begin in the hands, followed by sensory loss in the feet. Loss of ankle-jerk reflex

occurs soon thereafter.[55] Although the sensory loss may progress, it seldom results in more proximal stocking-glove distribution deficits. Motor symptoms follow, with weakness of the extensors of the hands and feet being most pronounced. Cranial neuropathies are rare; however, ototoxicity with sudden transient hearing loss has been reported.[56] Sensory and motor symptoms usually abate within a few weeks of discontinuation of therapy, although mild distal sensory loss and absence of ankle-jerk reflexes may persist.

Although CNS penetration at therapeutic doses is relatively low, encephalopathy and seizures have been reported.[57,58] In rare cases they are the presenting sign of intravenous overdose and frequently occur a few days to a week after exposure. Initial signs and symptoms of overdose may include bone or muscle pain, abdominal pain, bleeding, or marrow depression.[59-61] Other adverse effects of vincristine use include autonomic dysfunction, mucositis, paralytic ileus, bladder atony, fever, bone marrow suppression, alopecia, and hypertension.[53,59] Trinkle and Wu[62] reviewed 18 cases of intravenous vincristine overdose in children (average age 10 years). There were four fatalities with a dose range of 0.2 to 0.6 mg/kg. The major lethal risk factors were hemorrhage due to thrombocytopenia and neutropenia-related infection. Paresthesias and loss of deep tendon reflexes occurred as early as 24 hours. Nausea, vomiting, diarrhea, and abdominal pain usually occurred within 48 hours. Paralytic ileus occurred in 66% of patients within a mean of 5 days. Thrombocytopenia and leukocytopenia occurred in most cases.[62] Syndrome of inappropriate secretion of antidiuretic hormone (SIADH) has been a relatively frequent occurrence after vincristine overdose.[59,60,63]

Accidental intrathecal injection accounts for a large portion of the fatalities, and survival from such exposures is rare regardless of therapy.[64] These therapeutic mishaps usually involve vincristine administration by personnel unfamiliar with the drug or confusion with other antineoplastic drugs that may be administered via that route. Dermal extravasation of vinca alkaloids has been associated with tissue loss.[65]

Vinblastine and Vinorelbine. These vinca alkaloids are less potent inhibitors of microtubular polymerization and are less neurotoxic than vincristine. Their primary toxicity is bone marrow suppression, which often is the dose-limiting factor during therapy with either drug and is the most common toxic effect of these drugs (see Table 68-1). Granulocytopenia occurs frequently. There are relatively few reports of overdose.[66–69] After overdose, onset of fever and diarrhea has been reported within a few hours. Pulmonary edema developed in one reported case at day 4.[66] Vinorelbine also has been associated with bronchospasm and respiratory failure, but concurrent disease may have played a significant role.[70]

CHRONIC ADVERSE EFFECTS

Myocardial ischemia has been reported after therapeutic doses of the vinca alkaloids[71–75]; however, this patient population tends to be at greater age-related cardiovascular risk. Delayed (24 hours) onset of epithelial keratopathy was reported after ocular exposure to vinblastine solution; it resolved over 2 weeks without treatment. Ototoxicity also has been reported (with vincristine and vinblastine). Tinnitus occurred in a 29-year-old man within hours of treatment with vinblastine, doxorubicin, bleomycin, and dacarbazine and lasted 7 to 10 days after each of multiple treatments; mild sensorineural hearing loss persisted in the high-decibel range.[76] Pancreatitis has been reported after therapeutic doses of vinorelbine.[77,78] As these cases show, predicting the toxicity of the vinca alkaloids frequently is confounded by coexistent disease and the presence of other chemotherapeutic agents. Similar to vincristine, vinblastine and vinorelbine also have been associated with SIADH.[79,80]

Treatment

INTRAVENOUS EXPOSURE

Supportive measures are the mainstay of care. Peripheral neuropathies usually resolve or improve on withdrawal of the drug. Seizures usually respond to benzodiazepines or barbiturates or both. A theoretical concern with the use of phenytoin is that it seems to potentiate the effects of vincristine and vinblastine by interfering with tubulin polymerization.[83] SIADH is managed most appropriately by fluid restriction. Vincristine has a large volume of distribution due to tissue uptake and is highly protein bound. Hemodialysis is of little benefit with regard to enhancement of drug clearance. Plasmapheresis has been performed with a favorable outcome,[84] but data supporting

its use are inadequate. Folinic acid has been used in humans[85] and studied in animals,[86] but its efficacy is controversial. Finally, glutamate also has been studied as a preventive intervention against neurotoxicity. In patients receiving therapeutic doses, neurotoxicity seemed to be reduced.[87] This particular intervention, too, is based on limited data.

INTRATHECAL EXPOSURE

With few exceptions, the accidental intrathecal or intraventricular injection of vincristine has resulted in death.[64,88,91] Autopsy results have shown evidence of an ascending chemical leptomeningitis; ventriculitis; and necrosis of the spinal cord, brainstem, and cerebellum.[89,90] Folinic acid and glutamic acid have been administered in many of these cases despite the relative paucity of supporting data and in response to the devastating and typically lethal nature of this injury. CNS washout involves removal of cerebrospinal fluid and replacement by Ringer's lactate. Ferayan and associates[92] reported significant motor and sensory impairment in a 7-year-old patient who ultimately survived. They employed a technique first described by Dyke.[93] During a routine admission for chemotherapy, 0.5 mg of vincristine accidentally was injected intrathecally. The error was recognized before the injection was complete, and 75 mL of cerebrospinal fluid was withdrawn immediately thereafter. That volume was replaced with Ringer's lactate via an additional lumbar puncture. In less than 2 hours, a catheter was placed in the right lateral ventricle by way of a bur hole; 1 L of Ringer's lactate was infused through the ventricular catheter at a rate of 100 mL/hr. Afterward, 15 mL of fresh frozen plasma was mixed with each liter of Ringer's lactate, and the rate was reduced to 55 mL/hr. That infusion was continued for 24 hours with the effluent passing through the lumbar catheter. Glutamic acid (250 mg every 8 hours) was administered via nasogastric tube, then continued orally for 1 month. The patient became symptomatic 7 days postexposure with urinary retention and sensorimotor impairment of the lower extremities. There was significant residual impairment at follow-up 34 months after exposure.[92] Aggressive replacement and lavage washout is not always successful,[64,89] but at present it seems to be the only viable therapy.

EXTRAVASATION

Subcutaneous injection of 250 U of hyaluronidase in 6 mL of normal saline circumferentially at the site has been recommended; this should be followed by the application of heat for 1 hour in the event of extravasation of vincristine or vinblastine. This procedure should be repeated four times daily for 3 to 5 days.

Special Populations

Children are the most common victims of accidental overdose or intrathecal injection. This is usually due to lack of familiarity with the drug or confusing it with another agent. It is imperative that stringent protocols for identification and administration of these compounds be followed because toxicologic treatment, particularly after intrathecal administration, is of limited efficacy.

Indications for ICU Admission in Vinca Alkaloid Overdose

1. The maximum tolerated doses of these drugs are not established. Patients who have received excessive amounts should be admitted for observation on a cardiac monitor.
2. The length of observation after intravenous overdose with one of the vinca alkaloids should be 3 to 4 days because the onset of symptoms may involve that degree of delay. This is dose dependent, with high-dose exposures reportedly causing onset of symptoms within only a few hours.[59,60]

PODOPHYLLIN AND PODOPHYLLIN DERIVATIVES

Podophyllotoxin (Fig. 68-4) is found in the rhizome and roots of *Podophyllum peltatum*, also known as *mandrake* or *May apple*. Native Americans used podophyllotoxin as an emetic, and the Chinese used it (*gui jiu*) as an abortifacient, as treatment for snakebites, and as an aid to purging intestinal parasites.[94–96] Podophyllin was included in the United States Pharmacopoeia in 1820.[97] Purification and isolation of podophyllotoxin first was accomplished in 1880.[94,95] Podophyllotoxin resin, or podophyllin, was used widely in the United States as a cathartic and an ingredient in proprietary medicines (e.g., Carter's Little Liver Pills) and topically in a 20% to 25% solution for condylomata until such uses were associated with reports of serious toxicity.[98–107]

Herbal remedies erroneously may contain podophyllin because *mandrake* also is used to refer to *Mandragora officinarum*, which has anticholinergic properties.[108] Poisoning also has been reported with herbal remedies obtained in countries outside the United States.[109–112]

In 1942, podophyllin was reported to treat venereal warts successfully, and in 1947 podophyllin-induced mitotic arrest was shown, leading to the investigation of its use for cancer treatment.[94,97] In response to the high toxicity and low water solubility of purified podophyllin, chemical modification of the compound was carried out, and many of the resulting compounds were studied. In the 1960s, synthesis and biologic testing of the podophyllin derivatives teniposide and etoposide was initiated. Currently, prescription ointment containing 0.5% podophyllin (podofilox [Condylox]) and physician-applied 25% podophyllin solution are used for the treatment of anogenital warts.[113,114] Podophyllin also is used topically to treat oral hairy leukoplakia.[115] Etoposide (VePesid, Etopophos) and teniposide (Vumon) are used in chemotherapy regimens for cancers, including testicular cancer, small cell lung cancer, lymphoma, and acute lymphoblastic leukemia.[23,94,97,116–118]

Pharmacokinetics of Podophyllin and Podophyllin Derivatives

Podophyllin[105,151,161]

Available in topical preparation from 0.5% to 25% in alcohol or benzoin tincture
Highly lipid soluble
Well absorbed across friable tissue
Dermal application of 0.1 to 1.5 mL of 0.5% topical preparation led to peak serum levels of 1 to 17 ng/mL 1 to 2 hours after application with an elimination half-life of 1 to 4.5 hours
Oral and intravenous pharmacokinetic data unavailable

Etoposide[114,116,128]

Oral formulation with polyethylene glycol, citrate, and glycerin
Intravenous formulation with polyethylene glycol, polysorbate 80, and 30% ethanol
Poor water solubility
Renal elimination (significant in children, 55% recovery in urine at 24 hours)
Oral bioavailability of 50%
No significant first-pass effect

continued

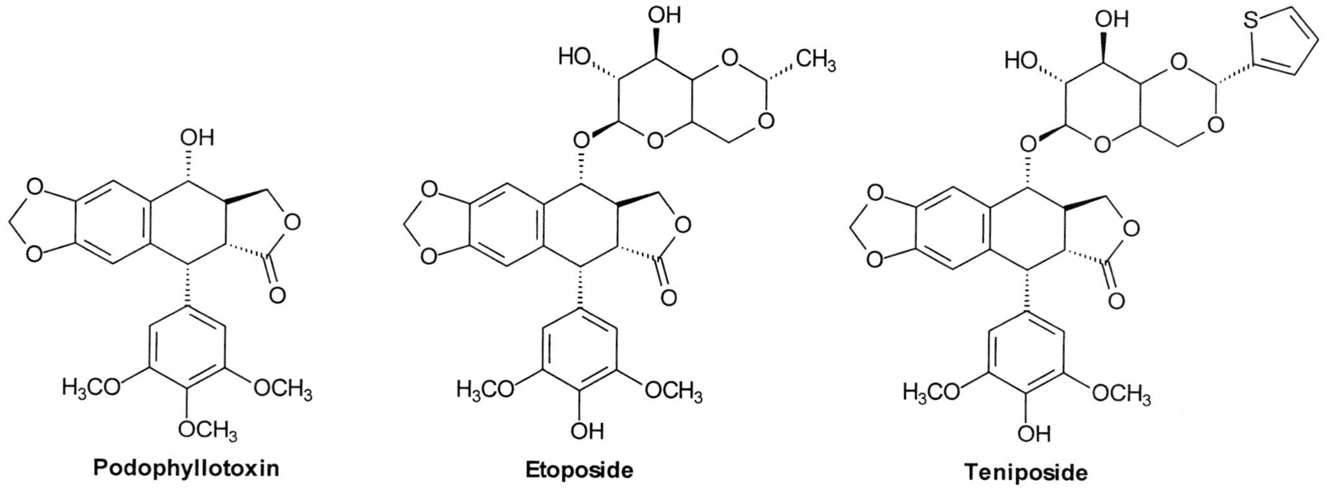

Podophyllotoxin   **Etoposide**   **Teniposide**

FIGURE 68-4

Chemical structures of podophyllotoxin, etoposide, and teniposide.

Pharmacokinetics of Podophyllin and Podophyllin Derivatives *continued*

97% protein bound
Volume of distribution highly variable between 7 and 17 L/m²
Terminal half-life 3 to 11 hours after intravenous infusion

Teniposide
Intravenous formulation with ethanol, which is reconstituted
   before infusion
Greater than 99% protein bound
Volume of distribution highly variable between 3 and 44 L/m²
Half-life variable between 6 and 48 hours, depending on the
   model
Biliary excretion 10% of elimination
Some central nervous system penetration

Pathophysiology

The cell cycle consists of four phases: G_1 (growth), S (DNA duplication), G_2 (preparation for cell division), and M (mitosis—cell division). Interphase consists of all phases except mitosis.[119] Although the spindle poisons, such as colchicine, podophyllin, and the vinca alkaloids, act in mitosis (specifically, causing metaphase arrest), podophyllin derivatives (etoposide and teniposide) act in interphase and prevent mitosis.

Podophyllin, similar to colchicine, binds reversibly to tubulin at the colchicine-binding site, resulting in mitotic arrest.[23,96] Microscopically, this activity results in metaphase arrest with clumped chromosomes because the mitotic spindle is unable to form without microtubules.[94] Disruption of microtubules also causes decreased cellular transport. Podophyllotoxin also inhibits the incorporation of labeled thymidine and uridine into cells by inhibiting nucleoside transport.[120] Neurotoxicity is thought to be related to microtubule binding and inhibition of axoplasmic flow.[121]

Podophyllotoxin derivatives have a mechanism of action distinct from that of the parent compound. Etoposide does not inhibit microtubule assembly compared with podophyllin.[120,122] Cells treated with etoposide, teniposide, and similar derivatives were found to have a low mitotic index, indicating that cells were inhibited from entering mitosis.[124] Time analyses indicated that the cells likely arrest in late S or early G_2 phase.[123,125] Later analyses showed that these derivatives may bind to tubulin, but this effect is seen at much higher and clinically impractical doses.[94]

Radiolabeled nucleoside (thymidine) incorporation into DNA is inhibited with etoposide and teniposide.[120,123] This mechanism of action is shared with podophyllin. Inhibition of cell proliferation is not linked to this mechanism, however.[123,124]

In 1974, DNA fragmentation by etoposide and teniposide was reported and represented a breakthrough in the understanding of the mechanism of action of podophyllin derivatives.[120] Podophyllin itself has no effect on DNA. Structure-activity studies indicated that derivatives with a hydroxyl group at the C-4′ position are required for this activity.[120,122] DNA breakage was found to correlate well with the cytotoxic effects of the drugs.[126] Subsequently, podophyllin derivative–induced DNA fragmentation has been correlated with inhibition of topoisomerase type II, which is essential for uncoiling of DNA before replica-

tion.[127] Topoisomerase II inhibition is now believed to represent the primary mechanism of action of these drugs, and they are classified today as topoisomerase interactive agents along with anthracyclines, such as doxorubicin.[94,97,116]

Clinical Presentation

During therapeutic administration of etoposide and teniposide, the most significant dose-limiting effect is bone marrow suppression (seen in 90% of patients), with granulocyte nadirs occurring in 7 to 14 days and platelet nadirs occurring in 9 to 16 days after administration. Marrow recovery usually occurs within 20 days.[97,118,128,129] Nausea, vomiting, anorexia, and diarrhea are reported but are milder than when caused by other chemotherapeutic agents.[97] At high doses, mucositis may be dose limiting. Anaphylaxis may occur. CNS depression and hypotension have been reported during intravenous infusion (see Table 68-1). Transient elevations in liver function tests have been reported. In children with acute lymphocytic leukemia, treatment has been associated with the development of secondary leukemias.[130,131] Hemolysis and renal failure have been reported in conjunction with teniposide-related antibody.[132] CNS depression, hypotension, and metabolic acidosis have been reported in children treated with teniposide; however, they also had clinically significant ethanol levels due to the high ethanol concentration in the infusion.[133] Neurologic manifestations, such as peripheral neuropathy, are less common after administration of the topoisomerase II inhibitors than with the spindle poisons, but they have been reported as well, often in high-dose use and in conjunction with drugs such as vincristine.[134,135] Neurologic symptoms, such as somnolence and increased seizure activity, have been reported after high-dose etoposide therapy for malignant glioma.[136] One case report of inadvertent supratherapeutic use of oral etoposide for 25 days detailed a reduction in T lymphocytes and blastic transformation that persisted at 57 months along with relapse-free remission.[137]

Podophyllin is far more toxic than its derivatives and has clinical effects similar to those of colchicine. Fatality has been reported after ingestion of 350 mg,[138] and survival has been reported after ingestion of 2.8 g.[98] Toxicity has occurred from ingestion,[101–103,110,118,138–141] cutaneous absorption,[94,105,107,121,142,143] subcutaneous injection,[144] and intramuscular injection.[145] Cases of toxicity from cutaneous absorption typically involved prolonged contact, large surface areas, or friable mucosa. Death has been reported after cutaneous application.[142,146]

The hallmarks of toxicity include nausea, vomiting, altered mental status progressing to coma, rapidly progressive peripheral neuropathy with paresis and areflexia, and delayed myelosuppression. Symptoms have been reported to be delayed 10 hours after ingestion[101] and 20 hours after topical application.[143] Review of the case reports indicates, however, that the patients initially developed gastrointestinal symptoms (one was given ipecac) and alteration in mental status (one also was ethanol intoxicated), followed by delayed and profound CNS depression and coma. Several reports of toxicity after cutaneous exposure detailed vomiting 12 to 13 hours postapplication followed by a coma within 30 hours of application.[107,142] Other reports included early gastrointestinal symptoms followed by delayed (24 hours) coma. Some patients may present primarily with peripheral neurologic symptoms, such as neuropathy and paresthesia.[106,109,112,145,147] Patients may recover fully from coma, which may last 10 days.[98,100,105,107,143] Electroencephalogram may show diffuse slowing, with cerebrospinal fluid findings typically normal but, at times, showing elevated protein.[98,148] Fever, seizure activity, and visual/auditory hallucinations also have been reported.

Patients often present with tachycardia and tachypnea. Hypotension has been reported. In fatal cases, renal failure and circulatory collapse may occur.[103,140,142,146] Noncardiogenic pulmonary edema and idioventricular bradycardia have been reported in a fatal case.[146] Necrotizing myopathy has been reported in a patient who died 9 weeks after podophyllin ingestion owing to sepsis.[140]

Survivors may have neurologic sequelae, such as persistent peripheral neuropathy lasting months to several years, that may manifest after the initial encephalopathy has resolved.[139,149] Some patients have developed persistent lower extremity paralysis and encephalopathy and radiologic findings of cerebral atrophy.[110,150] Dorsal radiculopathy, manifesting as profound loss of position sense, is reported.[139] Podophyllin has been proposed as an experimental model for deafferentation.[109] Absence of alopecia is notable in that it clinically differentiates podophyllin from acute colchicine or vinca alkaloid toxicity.

Diagnosis

Initially, leukocytosis may be seen (55,000/mm³).[105] Granulocytopenia and thrombocytopenia are delayed by 5 days and typically resolve over 2 to 3 weeks. Peripheral leukocytes may show enlarged nuclei with dense chromatin granules and cytoplasmic and nuclear vacuolization.[101] Bone marrow examination may reveal evidence of mitotic arrest[104,105,143] and vacuolization of erythroblasts and plasma cells.[151] Lactic acidosis has been described in a fatal case in a patient who had concomitant alcoholic cirrhosis.[101] Hypocalcemia has been reported,[102] along with elevated serum hepatic transaminase and uric acid concentrations.

Autopsy findings include mitotic arrest in granulocytes and intestinal mucosal cells; diffuse petechial hemorrhages; pulmonary, renal, and hepatic congestion; and cerebral edema.[101,103,142] The bone marrow is hypocellular with cytoplasmic vacuolization of myeloid precursors.[152]

Abnormalities on computed tomography or magnetic resonance imaging show cerebral atrophy in some survivors.[110,150] Some patients have developed persistent lower extremity paralysis; nerve biopsy specimens may reveal axonal degeneration and loss of large myelinated fibers, with gradual regeneration as recovery occurs.[110,112,149]

Because of its prominent early gastrointestinal effects, toxicity with podophyllin and derivatives may be confused with gastrointestinal disorders. In addition, podophyllin use may not be reported to the treating physician if it is applied as an ointment or applied by the patient's physician in the office. The common presentation of fever, lethargy, and leukocytosis mimics CNS infection. The presentation of hypotension, altered mental status, and fever mimics septic shock. Podophyllin toxicity may present with ascending paralysis and loss of reflexes similar to Guillain-Barré syndrome. Delayed bone marrow suppression leads to thrombocytopenia, granulocytopenia, and anemia, which may cause the treating physician to suspect other causes of bone marrow suppression, such as infection or malignancy.

Treatment

Gastrointestinal decontamination with activated charcoal may be beneficial after an acute suicidal podophyllin ingestion. Decontamination of skin should be performed if

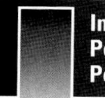

Indications for ICU Admission in Podophyllin or Podophyllin Derivatives Poisoning

1. Because of delayed and profound central nervous system effects, observation in an ICU setting for at least 24 hours should be considered for any patient with a significant exposure to podophyllin or podophyllin derivatives, particularly patients with evidence of altered mental status and rapidly progressive neuropathy.
2. Hemodynamic instability, intractable seizures, and respiratory distress also mandate ICU admission.

topical preparation has been applied. The mainstay of treatment is supportive care, including prevention of infection and screening for delayed bone marrow suppression. Blood products should be used if needed. Hemoperfusion has been used for podophyllin toxicity with variable results.[101,104,105,110,141,143,146] Because of the high lipid solubility, volume of distribution, and degree of protein binding (97% to 99%) of podophyllin and its derivatives, hemodialysis is not likely to be useful.

Although G-CSF has been used with some success to treat colchicine-induced neutropenia, its use has not been reported in podophyllin poisoning. G-CSF has been used in combination chemotherapy, including etoposide, for the prevention and treatment of hematopoietic toxicity and to facilitate more intensive chemotherapy regimens.[153–158] There is no specific antidotal therapy for podophyllin toxicity or that of its derivatives, etoposide and teniposide.

Special Populations

PREGNANT PATIENTS

These drugs are not intended for use in pregnancy. Podophyllin has been used to induce abortion. Reports link podophyllin to intrauterine fetal demise and birth defects.[106,159,160]

ONCOLOGY PATIENTS

In addition to increased risks of infection associated with immunosuppression and bone marrow suppression, after single-agent administration, concomitant cytotoxic medication use may lead to a synergistic increase in neurologic and hematologic toxicity.

REFERENCES

1. Hood RL: Colchicine poisoning. J Emerg Med 12:171–177, 1994.
2. Milne ST, Meek PD: Fatal colchicine overdose: Report of a case and review of the literature. Am J Emerg Med 16:603–608, 1998.
3. Borron S, Scherrmann J, Baud F: Markedly altered colchicine kinetics in a fatal intoxication: Examination of contributing factors. Hum Exp Toxicol 15:885–890, 1996.

4. Woodbury D, Fingl E: Analgesic-antipyretics, antiinflammatory agents, and drugs employed in the therapy of gout. In Goodman L, Gilman A (eds): The Pharmacologic Basis of Therapeutics, 5th ed. New York, MacMillan, 1975, pp 350–355.

5. Stahl N, Weinberger A, Benjamin D, et al: Fatal colchicine poisoning in a boy with familial Mediterranean fever. Am J Med Sci 278:77–81, 1979.

6. Kaplan H: Sarcoid arthritis with a response to colchicines. N Engl J Med 263:778–781, 1960.

7. Torres M, Furst D: Treatment of generalized systemic sclerosis. Rheum Dis Clin North Am 16:217–241, 1990.

8. Cohen A, Rubinow A, Anderson J: Colchicine treated cases from 1976 to 1983 compared with cases seen in previous years. Am J Med 82:1182–1190, 1987.

9. Sander H, Randal H: Use of colchicine in Behçet's syndrome. Cutis 37:344–348, 1986.

10. Anonymous: Criteria for diagnosis of Behçet's disease. International Study Group for Behçet's Disease. Lancet 335:1078–1080, 1990.

11. Seidman P, Fjellner B, Johannesson A: Psoriatic arthritis treated with oral colchicines. J Rheumatol 14:777–779, 1987.

12. Medsger Jr TA Jr: Treatment of systemic sclerosis. Ann Rheum Dis 50:877–886, 1991.

13. Naidus R, Rodviein R, Meikle H: Colchicine toxicity—a multisystem disease. Arch Intern Med 137:394–396, 1977.

14. Russell FE, Gertsch WJ: For those who treat spider or suspected spider bites (Letter). Toxicon 21:337–339, 1983.

15. Kershenobich D, Varga F, Garcia-Tsao G, et al: Colchicine in the treatment of cirrhosis of the liver. N Engl J Med 318:1709–1713, 1988.

16. Kaplan M, Alling DHJZ: A prospective trial for colchicine for primary biliary cirrhosis of the liver. N Engl J Med 315:1448–1454, 1986.

17. von den Driesch P: Sweet's syndrome (acute febrile neutrophilic dermatosis). J Am Acad Dermatol 31:535–560, 1994.

18. Simmons JW, Harris WP, Koulisis CW, et al: Intravenous colchicine for low-back pain: A double-blind study. Spine 15:716–117, 1990.

19. Schnebel BE, Simmons JW: The use of oral colchicine for low-back pain: A double-blind study. Spine 13:543–357, 1988.

20. Wallace S, Singer J: Review: Systemic toxicity associated with the intravenous administration of colchicine—guidelines for use. J Rheumatol 15:495–499, 1988.

21. Wallace S: Mechanism of action of colchicines. Arthritis Rheum 8:744–748, 1965.

22. Lodish H, Berk A, Zipursky SL, et al: Microtubules and cellular movement. In Molecular Cell Biology, 4th ed. New York: Freeman & Company, 1999, pp 795–847.

23. Jordan A, Hadfield J, Lawrence N, et al: Tubulin as a target for anticancer drugs: Agents which interact with the mitotic spindle. Med Res Rev 18:259–296, 1998.

24. Panda D, Jordan M, Chu K, et al: Differential effects of vinblastine on polymerization and dynamics at opposite microtubule ends. J Biol Chem 271:29807–29812, 1996.

25. Ben-Chetrit E, Levy M: Colchicine: 1998 update. Semin Arthritis Rheum 28:48–59, 1998.

26. Spilberg I, Mandell B, Mehta J, et al: Mechanism of action of colchicine in acute urate crystal-induced arthritis. J Clin Invest 64:775–780, 1979.

27. Chang Y: Mechanism of action of colchicines: III. Anti-inflammatory effect of colchicine compared with phenylbutazone and indomethacin. Arthritis Rheum 18:493–496, 1975.

28. Baum J, Meyerowitz S: Colchicine: Its use as a suicidal drug by females. J Rheumatol 7:124–127, 1980.

29. Folpini A, Furfori P: Colchicine toxicity—clinical features and treatment: Massive overdose case report. J Toxicol Clin Toxicol 33:71–77, 1995.

30. Wells S, Anderson D: Colchicine toxicity: A case report. Vet Hum Toxicol 32:313–316, 1989.

31. Murray SS, Dramlinger KG, McMichan JC, et al: Acute toxicity after excessive ingestion of colchicines. Mayo Clin Proc 58:528–532, 1983.

32. Ferguson F: Colchicine: I. General pharmacology. J Pharmacol Exp Ther 106:261–270, 1952.

33. Wallace SL, Omokoku B, Ertel NH: Colchicine plasma levels: Implications as to pharmacology and mechanism of action. Am J Med 48:443–448, 1970.

34. Hill R, Spragg R, Wedel M, et al: Adult respiratory distress syndrome associated with colchicine intoxication. Ann Intern Med 83:523–524, 1975.

35. Sauder P, Kopferschmitt J, Jaeger A, et al: Haemodynamic studies in eight cases of acute colchicine poisoning. Hum Toxicol 2:169–173, 1983.

36. Mullins M, Carrico E, Horowitz B: Fatal cardiovascular collapse following acute colchicine ingestion. Clin Toxicol 38:51–54, 2000.

37. Heath D, Palmer J, Aurbach G: The hypocalcemic action of colchicines. Endocrinology 90:1589–1593, 1972.

38. Kuncl R, Duncan G, Watson D, et al: Colchicine myopathy and neuropathy. N Engl J Med 316:1560–1561, 1987.

39. Neuss M, McCallum R, Brenckman WD, et al: Long-term colchicine administration leading to colchicine toxicity and death. Arthritis Rheum 29:448–449, 1986.

40. Stanley MW, Taurog JD, Snover DC: Fatal colchicine toxicity: Report of a case. Clin Exp Rheumatol 2:167–171, 1984.

41. Gooneratne BW: Massive generalized alopecia after poisoning by Gloriosa superba. BMJ 5494:1023–1024, 1966.

42. Ellwood MG, Robb GH: Self-poisoning with colchicines. Postgrad Med J 47:129–131, 1971.

43. Critchley J, Critchley L, Yeung E: Granulocyte colony stimulating factor in the treatment of colchicine poisoning. Hum Exp Toxicol 16:229–232, 1997.

44. Harris R, Marx G: Colchicine-induced bone marrow suppression: Treatment with granulocyte colony stimulating factor. J Emerg Med 18:435–440, 2000.

45. Wolff J, Capraro H: Colchicine binding to antibodies. J Biol Chem 255:7144–7148, 1980.

46. Terrien N, Urtizgerea M, Schermann J: Reversal of advanced colchicine toxicity in mice with goat colchicine-specific antibodies. Toxicol Appl Pharmacol 104:504–510, 1990.

47. Baud F, Sabourand A, Vicaut E, et al: Brief report: Treatment of severe colchicine overdose with colchicine specific Fab fragments. N Engl J Med 332:642–645, 1995.

48. Tutar HE, Imamoglu A, Atalay S: Recurrent pericarditis in familial Mediterranean fever (Letter). Acta Paediatr 88:1045–1046, 1999.

49. Sadjadi SJ, Moshir M: Treatment of acne vulgaris with colchicine (Letter). Acta Derm Venereol 78:388, 1998.

50. Paydas S: Report on 59 patients with renal amyloidosis. Int Urol Nephrol 31:619–631, 1999.

51. Yazigi A, Abou-Charaf LC: Colchicine for recurrent pericarditis in children. Acta Paediatr 87:603–604, 1998.

52. Sahenk Z, Brady S, Mendell J: Studies on the pathogenesis of vincristine-induced neuropathy. Muscle Nerve 10:80–84, 1987.

53. Chae L, Moon H, Kim S: Overdose of vincristine: Experience with a patient. J Korean Med Sci 13:334–338, 1998.

54. Schlaepfer W: Vincristine-induced axonal alteration in rat peripheral nerve. J Neuropathol Exp Neurol 30:448–505, 1971.

55. McLeod J, Penny R: Vincristine neuropathy: An electrophysiological and histological study. J Neurol Neurosurg Psychiatry 32:297–304, 1969.

56. Mahajan SL: Acute acoustic nerve palsy associated with vincristine therapy. Cancer 47:2404–2406, 1981.

57. Dallera F, Gamoletti R, Costa P: Unilateral seizures following vincristine intravenous injection. Tumori 70:243–244, 1984.

58. Hurwitz RL, Mahoney Jr DH, Armstrong DL, et al: Reversible encephalopathy and seizures as a result of conventional vincristine administration. Med Pediatr Oncol 16:216–219, 1988.

59. Kaufman I, Dung F, Koenig H, et al: Overdosage with vincristine. J Pediatr 89:671–674, 1976.

60. Casteels-Van Daele M, Beirinckx J, Baines P: Overdosage with vincristine. J Pediatr 90:1042–1043, 1977.

61. Johnson FL, Bernstein ID, Hartmann JR, et al: Seizures associated with vincristine sulfate therapy. J Pediatr 82:699–702, 1973.

62. Trinkle R, Wu JK: Errors involving pediatric patients receiving chemotherapy: A literature review. Med Pediatr Oncol 26:344–351, 1996.

63. Suskind R, Brusilow S, Zehr J: Syndrome of inappropriate secretion of antidiuretic hormone produced by vincristine toxicity (with bioassay of ADH level). J Pediatr 81:90–92, 1972.

64. Meggs W, Hoffman R: Fatality resulting from intraventricular vincristine administration. J Toxicol Clin Toxicol 36:243–246, 1998.

65. Dorr RT, Alberts DS: Vinca alkaloid skin toxicity: Antidote and drug disposition studies in the mouse. J Natl Cancer Inst 74:113–120, 1985.

66. Lotz JP, Chapiro J, Voinea A, et al: Overdosage of vinorelbine in a woman with metastatic non-small-cell lung carcinoma (Letter). Ann Oncol 8:714–715, 1997.

67. Gutowski MC, Fix DV, Corvalan JR, et al: Reduction of toxicity of a vinca alkaloid by an anti-vinca alkaloid antibody. Cancer Invest 13:370–374, 1995.

68. Conter V, Rabbone ML, Jankovic M, et al: Overdose vinblastine in a child with Langerhans' cell histiocytosis: toxicity and salvage therapy. Pediatr Hematol Oncol 8:165–169, 1991.

69. Fiorentino MV, Salvagno L, Chiarion Sileni V, et al: Vindesine overdose (Letter). Cancer Treat Rep 66:1247–1248, 1982.

70. Kouroukis C, Hing I: Respiratory failure following vinorelbine tartrate infusion in a patient with non-small cell lung cancer. Chest 112:846–848, 1997.

71. Subar M, Muggia F: Apparent myocardial ischemia associated with vinblastine administration. Cancer Treat Rep 70:690–691, 1986.

72. Yancey R, Talpaz M: Vindesine-associated angina and ECG changes. Cancer Treat Rep 66:587–589, 1982.

73. Lejonc J, Vernant J, MacWuin I, et al: Myocardial infarction following vinblastine treatment. Lancet 2:692, 1980.

74. Mandel E, Lewinski U, Djaldetti M: Vincristine induced myocardial infarction. Cancer 36:1979–1982, 1975.

75. Somers G, Abramow M, Witter M, et al: Myocardial infarction: A complication of vincristine treatment? Lancet 2:690, 1976.

76. McLendon B, Bron A: Corneal toxicity from vinblastine solution. Br J Ophthalmol 62:97–99, 1978.

77. Raderer M, Kornek G, Scheithauer W: Re: Vinorelbine-induced pancreatitis: A case report (Letter). J Natl Cancer Inst 90:329, 1998.

78. Tester W, Forbes W, Leighton J: Vinorelbine-induced pancreatitis: A case report (Letter). J Natl Cancer Inst 89:1631, 1997.

79. Winter S, Arbus G: Syndrome of inappropriate secretion of antidiuretic hormone secondary to vinblastine overdose. Can Med Assoc J 117:1134, 1977.

80. Garrett DA, Simpson Jr TA: Syndrome of inappropriate antidiuretic hormone associated with vinorelbine therapy. Ann Pharmacother 32:1306–1309, 1998.

81. Crom W, DeGraff S, Synold T, et al: Pharmacokinetics of vincristine in children and adolescents with acute lymphocytic leukemia. J Pediatr 125:642–649, 1994.

82. Chan JD: Pharmacokinetic drug interactions of vinca alkaloids: Summary of case reports. Pharmacotherapy 18:1304–1307, 1998.

83. Lobert S, Ingram J, Correia J: Additivity of dilantin and vinblastine inhibitory effects on microtubule assembly. Cancer Res 59:4816–4822, 1999.

84. Pierga J, Beuzeboc P, Dorval T, et al: Favourable outcome after plasmapheresis for vincristine overdose. Lancet 340:185, 1992.

85. Gale RP: Antineoplastic chemotherapy myelosuppression: Mechanisms and new approaches. Exp Hematol 13:3–7, 1985.

86. Thomas W, Bailony M, Lightsey A, et al: Folinic acid rescue in vincristine overdosage in mice. Am J Pediatr Hematol Oncol 8:266–268, 1986.

87. Jackson D, Wells H, Atkins J, et al: Amelioration of vincristine neurotoxicity by glutamic acid. Am J Med 84:1016–1022, 1988.

88. Williams M, Walker A, Bracikowski J, et al: Ascending myeloencephalopathy due to intrathecal vincristine sulfate: A fatal chemotherapeutic error. Cancer 51:2041–2047, 1983.

89. Gaidys W, Dickerman J, Walters C, et al: Intrathecal vincristine: Report of a fatal case despite CNS washout. Cancer 52:799–801, 1983.

90. Lau G: Accidental intraventricular vincristine administration: An avoidable iatrogenic death. Med Sci Law 36:263–265, 1996.

91. Manelis J, Freundlich E, Ezekiel E, et al: Accidental intrathecal vincristine administration. J Neurol 228:209–213, 1982.

92. Ferayan A, Russell N, Wohaibi M, et al: Cerebrospinal fluid lavage in the treatment of inadvertent intrathecal vincristine injection. Child Nerv Syst 15:87–89, 1999.

93. Dyke R: Treatment of inadvertent intrathecal injection of vincristine. N Engl J Med 321:1270–1271, 1989.

94. Stahelin HF, Von Wartburg A: The chemical and biological route from podophyllotoxin glucoside to etoposide. Ninth Cain Memorial Award Lecture. Cancer Res 51:5–15, 1991.

95. Vogelzang NJ, Raghavan D, Kennedy BJ: VP-16-213 (etoposide): The mandrake root from Issyk-Kul. Am J Med 72:136–144, 1982.

96. Chui FC: Podophyllotoxin and related compounds. In Herbert H, Schumburg PSS (eds): Experimental and Clinical Neurotoxicology, 2nd ed. New York, Oxford University Press, 2000, pp 1008–1010.

97. Stewart CF, Ratain MJ: Topoisomerase interactive agents. In Vincent TDJHS (ed): Cancer: Principles and Practice of Oncology, 5th ed. Philadelphia, Lippincott-Raven, 1997, pp 452–467.

98. Clark ANG, Parsonage MJ: A case of podophyllum poisoning with involvement of the central nervous system. BMJ 2:1155–1157, 1957.

99. Coruh M, Argun G: Podophyllin poisoning: A case report. Turk J Pediatr 7:100–103, 1965.

100. Campbell AN: Accidental poisoning with podophyllum. Lancet 1:206–207, 1980.

101. Cassidy DE, Drewry J, Fanning JP: Podophyllum toxicity: A report of a fatal case and a review of the literature. J Toxicol Clin Toxicol 19:35–44, 1982.

102. McFarland MFD, McFarland J: Accidental ingestion of podophyllum. Clin Toxicol 18:973–977, 1981.

103. West WM, Ridgeway NA, Morris AJ, et al: Fatal podophyllin ingestion. South Med J 75:1269–1270, 1982.

104. Rate RG, Leche J, Chervenak C: Podophyllin toxicity. Ann Intern Med 90:723, 1979.

105. Slater GE, Rumack BH, Peterson RG: Podophyllin poisoning: Systemic toxicity following cutaneous application. Obstet Gynecol 52:94–96, 1978.

106. Chamberlain MJ, Reynolds AL, Yeoman WB: Medical memoranda: Toxic effect of podophyllum application in pregnancy. BMJ 3:391–392, 1972.

107. Montaldi DH, Giambrone JP, Courey NG, et al: Podophyllin poisoning associated with the treatment of condylomata acuminatum: A case report. Am J Obstet Gynecol 119:1130–1131, 1974.

108. Frasca T, Brett AS, Yoo SD: Mandrake toxicity: A case of mistaken identity. Arch Intern Med 157:2007–2009, 1997.

109. Chang MH, Liao KK, Wu ZA, et al: Reversible myeloneuropathy resulting from podophyllin intoxication: An electrophysiological follow up. J Neurol Neurosurg Psychiatry 55:235–236, 1992.

110. Ng TH, Chan YW, Yu YL, et al: Encephalopathy and neuropathy following ingestion of a Chinese herbal broth containing podophyllin. J Neurol Sci 101:107–113, 1991.

111. Dobb GJ, Edis RH: Coma and neuropathy after ingestion of herbal laxative containing podophyllin. Med J Aust 140:495–496, 1984.

112. Chu CC, Huang EE, Chu NS: Sensory neuropathy due to Bajiaolian (podophyllotoxin) intoxication. Eur Neurol 44:121–123, 2000.

113. Bonnez W, Elswick Jr RK, Bailey-Farchione A, et al: Efficacy and safety of 0.5% podofilox solution in the treatment and suppression of anogenital warts. Am J Med 96:420–425, 1994.

114. Anonymous: Podofilox for genital warts. Med Lett Drugs Ther 33:117–118, 1991.

115. Gowdey G, Lee RK, Carpenter WM: Treatment of HIV-related hairy leukoplakia with podophyllum resin 25% solution. Oral Surg Oral Med Oral Pathol Oral Radiol Endod 79:64–67, 1995.

116. Donehower R, Rowinsky E: DNA topoisomerase II inhibitors. In Perry MC (ed): Chemotherapy Source Book, 2nd ed. Baltimore, William & Wilkins, 1996, pp 434–445.

117. Arnold AM, Whitehouse JM: Etoposide: A new anti-cancer agent. Lancet 2:912–915, 1981.

118. Anonymous: Podophyllotoxin derivatives. In Kastrup E (ed): Drug Facts and Comparisons. St Louis, Wolter & Kluwer, 2000, pp 1879–1881.

119. Hoffe PA: Cell cycle, mitosis, and meiosis. In Medical Molecular Genetics. Madison, CT, Fence Creek Publishing, 1998, pp 92–102.

120. Loike JD, Horowitz SB: Effects of podophyllotoxin and VP-16-213 on microtubule assembly in vitro and nucleoside transport in HeLa cells. Biochemistry 15:5434–5443, 1976.

121. Filley CM, Graff-Radford NR, Lacy JR, et al: Neurologic manifestations of podophyllin toxicity. Neurology 32:308–311, 1982.

122. Loike JD, Brewer CF, Sternlicht H, et al: Structure activity study of the inhibition of microtubule assembly in vitro by podophyllotoxin and its congeners. Cancer Res 38:2688–2693, 1978.

123. Grieder A, Maurer R, Stahelin H: Effect of an epipodophyllotoxin derivative (VP 16-213) on macromolecular synthesis and mitosis in mastocytoma cells in vitro. Cancer Res 34:1788–1793, 1974.

124. Grieder A, Maurer R, Stahelin H: Comparative study of early effects of epipodophyllotoxin derivatives and other cytostatic agents on mastocytoma cultures. Cancer Res 37:2998–3005, 1977.

125. Krishan A: Cytofluorimetric studies on the action of podophyllotoxin and epipodophyllotoxins (VM-26, VP-16-213) on the cell cycle traverse of human lymphoblasts. J Cell Biol 66:521–530, 1975.

126. Kalwinsky DK, Look AT, Ducore J, et al: Effects of the epipodophyllotoxin VP 16-213 on cell cycle traverse, DNA synthesis, and DNA

strand size in cultures of human leukemic lymphoblasts. Cancer Res 43:1592–1597, 1983.

127. Long BH, Minocha A: Inhibition of topoisomerase II by VP-16-213 (etoposide), VM-26 (teniposide), and structural congeners as an explanation for in vivo DNA breakage and cytotoxicity. Proc Am Assoc Cancer Res 24:321, 1983.

128. Anonymous: Cavinton, injection, tablet. Geographia Medica 14:361–363, 1984.

129. O'Dwyer PJ, Leyland-Jones B, Alonso MT, et al: Etoposide (VP-16-213): Current status of an active anticancer drug. N Engl J Med 312:692–700, 1985.

130. Hawkins MM: Secondary leukaemia after epipodophyllotoxins (Letter). Lancet 338:1408, 1991.

131. Kumar L: Epipodophyllotoxins and secondary leukaemia. Lancet 342:819–820, 1993.

132. Habibi B, Baumelou A, Seradaru M: Acute intravascular haemolysis and renal failure due to teniposide related antibody (Letter). Lancet 1:1423–1424, 1981.

133. McLeod HL, Baker DK, Pui C, et al: Somnolence, hypotension, and metabolic acidosis following high dose teniposide treatment in children with leukemia. Cancer Chemother Pharmacol 29:150–154, 1991.

134. Imrie KR, Couture F, Turner CC, et al: Peripheral neuropathy following high-dose etoposide and autologous bone marrow transplantation. Bone Marrow Transplant 13:77–79, 1994.

135. Thant M, Hawley RJ, Smith MT, et al: Possible enhancement of vincristine neuropathy by VP-16. Cancer 49:859–864, 1982.

136. Leff RS, Thompson JM, Daly MB, et al: Acute neurologic dysfunction after high dose etoposide therapy for malignant glioma. Cancer 62:32–35, 1988.

137. Pawlicki M, Zuchowska-Vogelgesang B, Sliz E: The case of VePesid overdosage in a patient with Hodgkin's disease. Cancer Chemother Pharmacol 25:387, 1990.

138. Dudley WH: Fatal podophyllin poisoning. Med Rec 37:409, 1890.

139. Gorin F, Kindall D, Seyal M: Dorsal radiculopathy resulting from podophyllin toxicity. Neurology 39:607–608, 1989.

140. Oliveira AS, Calia LC, Kiyomoto BH, et al: Acute necrotizing myopathy and podophyllin toxicity. Arq Neuropsiquiatr 54:288–292, 1996.

141. Heath A, Mellstrand T, Ahlmen J: Treatment of podophyllin poisoning with resin hemoperfusion. Hum Toxicol 1:373–378, 1982.

142. Ward JW, Clifford WS, Monaco AR, et al: Fatal systemic poisoning following podophyllin treatment of condyloma acuminatum. South Med J 47:1204–1206, 1954.

143. Moher LM, Maurer SA: Podophyllum toxicity: Case report and literature review. J Fam Pract 9:237–240, 1979.

144. Tomczak RL, Hake DH: Near fatal systemic toxicity from local injection of podophyllin for pedal verrucae treatment. J Foot Surg 31:36–42, 1992.

145. Freeman MC, Weimer LH, Arnaudo E, et al: Neuropathic and autonomic effects of intramuscular podophyllin. Ann Neurol 42:416, 1997.

146. Conard PF, Hanna N, Rosenblum M, et al: Delayed recognition of podophyllum toxicity in a patient receiving epidural morphine. Anesth Analg 71:191–193, 1990.

147. Chang MH, Lin KP, Wu ZA, et al: Acute ataxic sensory neuropathy resulting from podophyllin intoxication. Muscle Nerve 15:513–514, 1992.

148. Cabrera Rodriguez J, Munoz Garcia J: Acute pain due to vinorelbine. Rev Clin Espan 198:514–516, 1998.

149. O'Mahony S, Keohane C, Jacobs J, et al: Neuropathy due to podophyllin intoxication. J Neurol 237:110–112, 1990.

150. Chan YW: Magnetic resonance imaging in toxic encephalopathy due to podophyllin poisoning. Neuroradiology 33:372–373, 1991.

151. Stoehr GP, Peterson AL, Taylor WJ: Systemic complications of local podophyllin therapy. Ann Intern Med 89:362–363, 1978.

152. Leslie KO, Shitamoto B: The bone marrow in systemic podophyllin toxicity. Am J Clin Pathol 77:478–480, 1982.

153. Gianni AM, Bregni M, Siena S, et al: Granulocyte-macrophage colony-stimulating factor or granulocyte colony-stimulating factor infusion makes high-dose etoposide a safe outpatient regimen that is effective in lymphoma and myeloma patients. J Clin Oncol 10:1955–1962, 1992.

154. Maslak PG, Weiss MA, Berman E, et al: Granulocyte colony-stimulating factor following chemotherapy in elderly patients with newly diagnosed acute myelogenous leukemia. Leukemia 10:32–39, 1996.

155. Bernstein SH, Fay JP, Christiansen NP, et al: Sequential interleukin-3 and granulocyte-colony stimulating factor prior to and following high-dose etoposide and cyclophosphamide: A phase I/II trial. Clin Cancer Res 3:1519–1526, 1997.

156. Jakacki RI, Jamison C, Heifetz SA, et al: Feasibility of sequential high-dose chemotheraphy and peripheral blood stem cell support for pediatric central nervous system malignancies. Med Pediatr Oncol 29:553-559, 1997.

157. Neill HB, Miller AA, Clamon GH, et al: A phase II study evaluating the efficacy of carboplatin etoposide, and paclitaxel with granulocyte colony-stimulating factor in patients with stage IIIB and IV non-small cell lung cancer and extensive small cell lung cancer. Semin Oncol 24(4 Suppl 12);130–134, 1997.

158. Weaver CH, Schwartzberg LS, Birch R, et al: Collection of peripheral blood progenitor cells after the administration of cyclophosphamide, etoposide, and granulocyte-colony-stimulating factor: An analysis of 497 patients. Transfusion 37:896–903, 1997.

159. Rosenstein G, Rosenstein H, Freeman M, et al: Podophyllum—a dangerous laxative. Pediatrics 57:419–421, 1976.

160. Karol MD, Conner CS, Murphrey KJ: Podophyllum: Suspected teratogenicity from topical application. Clin Toxicol 16:283–286, 1980.

161. Anonymous: Condylox Gel 0.5%. In Murray L (ed): Physician's Desk Reference, 55th ed. Montvale, NJ, Medical Economics Company, 2001, pp 2248–2249.

CHAPTER 69

Ergot Alkaloids

Ken Kulig

The ergot alkaloids comprise a group of naturally occurring chemicals and semisynthetic pharmaceuticals with similar molecular structures and properties. They are of great historical interest, being responsible for massive epidemics of debilitating disease and deaths over the course of many centuries.[1] The first recorded epidemic was in Assyria, circa 600 BC. The most recent was in Africa in 1978.[2] Perhaps the largest and best-known epidemic occurred in the French village of Pont-St.-Espirit in 1951, where hundreds of residents became acutely psychotic, convulsed, and developed ischemic limbs, and an unknown number died.[3,4]

Numerous ergot alkaloids are produced by the fungus *Claviceps purpurea*, which grows under warm, wet conditions on the rye plant. Epidemic ergotism is a toxicologic syndrome caused by vasospasm, resulting in painful ischemia of the extremities or of vital organs, sometimes resulting in death. Epidemics occurred because bread made from rye contaminated with the *Claviceps* fungus was widely consumed.

Peripheral epidemic ergotism is characterized by extreme burning pain caused by the peripheral ischemia and gradual limb necrosis. It has been called *St. Anthony's fire* because it often disappeared when a pilgrimage was made to the shrine of St. Anthony, where bread made from rye was not available.[3,4] Many epidemics occurred with thousands of deaths, particularly in Europe, before the link between the clinical syndrome and the ingestion of bread made with contaminated rye was made in the late 1800s.

CHEMISTRY

The basic ergot nucleus is the four-ringed compound 6-methylergoline (Fig. 69-1). The naturally occurring ergots contain a double bond in the D ring and a variety of substitutions at the carbon 8 position, allowing for optical isomers to exist. Natural ergots are invariably a mixture, with the most prominent members being ergotamine, ergocornine, ergocristine, and ergocriptine, all potent vasoconstrictors.

Chemists manipulated the molecular structure of the naturally occurring ergots to create pharmaceuticals that are used primarily to treat migraine headache and to reduce postpartum hemorrhage. Although each may have different properties as a result of that manipulation, they are vasoconstrictors with similarities in their adverse reaction profiles. Lysergic acid diethylamide (LSD) is an ergot but is not discussed here (see Chapter 72). Ergonovine is used in the cardiac catheterization laboratory to induce coronary artery vasospasm to aid in the diagnosis of Prinzmetal's angina,[5–7] sometimes with disastrous consequences.[8] Figure 69-1 shows examples of semisynthetic ergots created from the ergot substrates found in nature. These ergots are divided into amines and amino acids; the latter have a peptide moiety attached to the carbon 8 position. The dihydrogenated derivatives (e.g., dihydroergotamine) are saturated at the D ring.

Bromocriptine (2-bromo-α-ergocriptine) has a bromine atom attached to the carbon 2 of the A ring, which gives it more potent dopaminergic properties. This structure makes bromocriptine useful in the treatment of parkinsonism and prolactin-secreting tumors. From 1980 until 1994, bromocriptine (Parlodel) was used to inhibit lactation in the postpartum period in women desiring not to breast-feed in the United States, Canada, Italy, and other countries. This indication was removed because of the risk of vasospastic phenomena, such as stroke, myocardial infarctions, seizures, and death.[9] Bromocriptine, similar to other ergots, is clearly a vasoconstrictor.[10,11]

Carbergoline is a newer, entirely synthetic ergot, which also has potent dopaminergic properties without the addition of a bromine atom to the A ring. Because dopamine inhibits the release of prolactin from the anterior pituitary, this drug, similar to bromocriptine, is useful in treating prolactinomas and other hyperprolactinemic disorders.[12]

PATHOPHYSIOLOGY AND PHARMACOKINETICS

The chief action of the ergots is vasoconstriction. Their therapeutic value usually is based on this property, as are the most common serious adverse drug events. Vasoconstriction may be systemic, resulting in hypertension, or focal, resulting in end-organ ischemia or necrosis. The latter is commonly termed *vasospasm*. The pathophysiologic consequences include stroke, myocardial infarction, seizures, gangrene of the extremities, or ischemia/infarction of other organs.[13–18] The treatment of ergotism in the intensive care unit is aimed primarily at reversing vasoconstriction or vasospasm and treating the end-organ damage it has caused.

Vasoconstriction or vasospasm from ergots can result from therapeutic use in normal doses. This condition may occur despite tolerance of similar doses by an individual in the past. Identical doses may result in life-threatening vasospasm in one individual but no clinically apparent vasoconstriction in another. Patients with a history of vascular phenomena, such as toxemia of pregnancy, Prinzmetal's angina, Raynaud's phenomenon, or migraine headache, may be more susceptible to ergot-induced vasospasm.

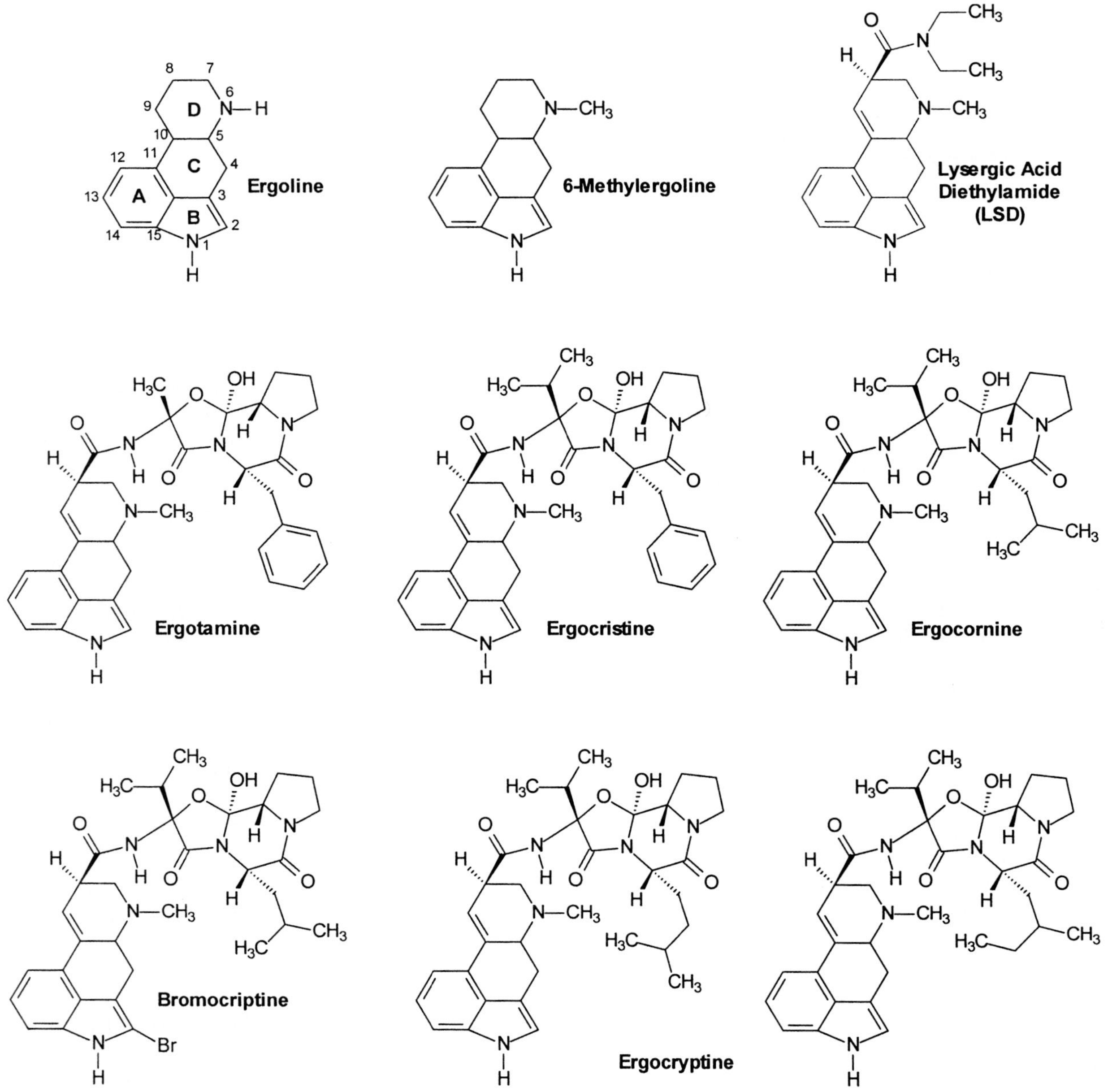

FIGURE 69-1

Chemical structures of ergoline, 6-methylergoline, lysergic acid diethylamide (LSD), ergotamine, ergocristine, ergocornine, bromocriptine, and the two structural isomers of ergocryptine. Ring designations and position numbers are shown on the structure of ergoline.

Although the physiologic mechanism for ergot disease is vasospasm, the receptor pharmacology causing this is less clear. Ergots interact at dopaminergic, serotonergic, and adrenergic receptors as either agonists or antagonists, in ways that may exert opposing effects. They show the curious property of being either vasodilators or vasoconstrictors, depending on the underlying vascular tone of the affected artery.[19,20] This is called the *amphoteric effect* of the ergots, and the degree of the underlying vascular tone at which a given ergot becomes a vasodilator (at higher tone) instead of a vasoconstrictor (at the lower underlying tone) is called the *inversion point*. The inversion points for some ergots in a canine model are shown in Table 69-1.

This intrinsic property of the ergots may help explain their unpredictable nature of inducing vasospasm in some patients and not others, in the same patient at certain times and not others, or in select arteries but not others at the same time. It also may help explain why the postpartum period, when vascular tone tends to be low, is one when patients seem unusually sensitive to the vasospastic effect of the ergots. Because of their adverse side-effect profile in the postpartum period (primarily vasospastic phenomena, such as hypertension, seizures, stroke, and myocardial infarction), ergots such as ergonovine, methyergonovine, and bromocriptine now are rarely used in postpartum women.[21–28]

TABLE 69-1 Inversion Points* for Some Ergots

	mm Hg/mL/min
Dihydroergotamine	4
1-Methylergotamine	2.3
Bromocriptine	3.8–4.2
Ergostine	4
Dihydroergostine	4
1-Methylergostine	2.3
Dihydroergocristine	2

*Initial resistance at which the test compound becomes a vasoconstrictor (at low vascular resistance) from a vasodilator (at higher vascular resistance).

The pharmacokinetic properties of the ergots as a class[29-40] may be less useful than for other drugs because hospital laboratories are unable to assay for ergots, and the pharmacologic and toxicologic effects of the ergots are well known to persist long after the drugs would be expected to be detectable in blood.

Pharmacokinetics of the Ergots

Absorption: oral absorption of the ergots is generally low and variable, ranging from less than 1% (e.g., ergotamine) to 28% (e.g., bromocriptine)

Distribution: widely distributed, with large volumes of distribution—5 L/kg

Metabolism: metabolized by the liver primarily by demethylation, hydroxylation, and ring cleavage. Not all metabolites are adequately identified or known; some are active. Most ergots have a large first-pass effect. Some ergots (e.g., bromocriptine) are metabolized in part by cytochrome P-450 CYP3A4. Drug-drug interactions with erythromycin, clarithromycin, ketoconazole, and troleandomycin and others may result in a more pronounced or prolonged ergot effect because of competitive binding of the CYP3A4 receptors

Elimination: most metabolites are eliminated via the bile into the feces. The α half-life of elimination of the parent compound may be significantly shorter than the β half-life, which is more biologically relevant. Ergots may show a prolonged pharmacologic effect, sometimes weeks after the last dose, much longer than the half-life might predict

Data from references 29 through 40.

CLINICAL PRESENTATION

Patients with ergotism may present with any of the clinical syndromes listed in Table 69-2. Commonly the chief complaint is referable to one organ system and not multiple systems at the same time. If the patient is unconscious (e.g., postictal or after a stroke), the history of ergot ingestion may not be obtainable. While obtaining a medication history, it is important to ask what medications the patient has taken in the last several weeks. Because the effects of ergots can persist long after the patient has stopped taking them, the patient might not mention an ergot preparation that was discontinued days ago, especially when being asked about "current" medications.

TABLE 69-2 Symptoms and Signs of Acute or Chronic Ergotism*

Seizures
Stroke (hemorrhagic or ischemic)
Headache (may be harbinger of stroke)
Chest pain/angina/myocardial infarction
Cardiac arrhythmias, sudden death
Limb paresthesias/pain/ischemia/gangrene
Vascular stasis/thrombosis
Nausea/vomiting/diarrhea
Hypertension or hypotension
Bradycardia or tachycardia
Psychosis/delirium/hallucinations
Lethargy/confusion/coma
Abdominal pain/bowel ischemia/pancreatitis/hepatitis
Pleuropulmonary fibrosis
Spontaneous abortion
Renal ischemia/flank pain/hematuria/oliguria/azotemia

*Clinical findings often involve only one organ system in a particular patient, with or without vital sign abnormalities.

Headache is a common side effect of ergot alkaloids.[28] Some ergot alkaloids (e.g., ergotamine, dihydroergotamine, methysergide) are used to treat migraine headaches. The clinical presentation may be similar in both cases. Some drugs used to treat migraines, such as sympathomimetics[41,42] or triptans, may acutely exacerbate ergot-induced vasospasm and cause a stroke.

Patients with ergotism who might require an intensive care unit admission are most likely to have chest pain/myocardial infarction, neurologic deficits/stroke, severe hypertension, seizures, limb ischemia/gangrene, or ischemia of other organs such as the kidney[43] or intestines[44] resulting in severe pain. It is important always to consider vasospasm in a patient taking an ergot alkaloid as a possible cause of the clinical picture and to rule it out using differential diagnosis and medical testing for conditions that may be unrelated to ergot ingestion.[45-48]

DIAGNOSTIC CONSIDERATIONS

Laboratory testing specifically looking for the presence of ergot alkaloids in the body is unavailable except in sophisticated research facilities. The physician must look for the residual of ergot-induced vasospasm in the organs affected. Angiography is often useful[48,49] but may not show vasospasm if there has been a delay in testing or if the vessel that had been in spasm has ruptured and is no longer seen radiographically.

Other causes of the syndrome seen (e.g., ruptured aneurysm or severe untreated hypertension in the case of hemorrhagic stroke or severe coronary artery disease in the case of myocardial infarction) should be pursued. Ergots can be administered in the cardiac catheterization laboratory to induce coronary artery spasm deliberately. When this is seen, the patient can be assumed to be susceptible to the vasospastic effects of ergots, which should then be avoided.

Migraine patients taking ergots therapeutically who then present with severe headache are problematic. The ergot preparation they are taking may be the cause rather than the treatment of the current headache they are experiencing.

Concurrent stroke also may have to be ruled out. A negative computed tomography scan does not rule out an early ischemic stroke. It may be prudent to take the patient off the ergot and use opiate analgesics and adjunctive treatment to manage the headache.

TREATMENT

The treatment of ergotism is basically the treatment of vasospasm and the organ damage it causes. A general treatment approach is outlined in Table 69-3. Supportive therapy along with specific treatment aimed at reversing vasospasm is the optimal approach. There are no effective means to enhance elimination of ergot alkaloids from the body. For headaches thought possibly related to ergots, it would be prudent to avoid sympathomimetics, triptans, and other ergots.

Aggressive monitoring, in some cases including serial angiograms, should be considered. Because ergot-induced vasospasm may be due primarily to serotonin agonism, cyproheptadine given orally as a serotonin antagonist is theoretically attractive. Cyproheptadine comes in 4-mg tablets; the optimal dose for this condition is unknown. Alprostadil (prostaglandin E_1) and epoprostenol (prostcyclin) also have been used to treat ergot-induced vasospasm, with some success. Calcium channel blockers also may be of theoretical benefit in the treatment of spasm, but clinical efficacy has not been tested in this setting.

Thrombosis at the site of vasospasm can occur. Treating the patient with aspirin, anticoagulants, glycoprotein IIb/IIIa inhibitors, or thrombolytics in select cases should be considered when thrombosis is diagnosed.

Ergot-induced hypertension may be severe and require a nitroprusside drip to normalize. Calcium channel blockers or angiotensin-converting enzyme inhibitors may be tried first if the hypertension is not immediately life-threatening. Bradycardia or tachycardia, if present, is unlikely to require any treatment. The other vital signs, respiratory rate and temperature, usually are unaffected by ergotism.

Indications for ICU Admission in Ergot Alkaloid Poisoning

Significant vital sign abnormalities, particularly hypertension
Chest pain, angina, or myocardial infarction
Neurologic symptoms and signs suggesting cerebrovascular accident (with or without CT evidence of stroke)
Severe headache suggesting new-onset vascular headache with or without positive CT (in part to rule out subarachnoid hemorrhage or ischemic stroke when CT negative)
Seizures
Evidence of limb ischemia
Evidence of other organ ischemia, particularly renal or intestinal

CT, computed tomography.

Criteria for ICU Discharge in Ergot Alkaloid Poisoning

1. Ergot-induced vasospasm has been adequately diagnosed and treated, with resolution of the symptoms and signs.
2. If angiograms have shown significant vasospasm, follow-up studies are done and show resolution.
3. Thrombosis at the site of vasospasm has been adequately addressed with anticoagulants, thrombolytics, or surgical procedures.
4. If the patient has had abnormal or unstable vital signs, they are now normal and stable without the necessity of vasodilators or pressors.

TABLE 69-3 Suggested Treatment of Ergot-Induced Vasospasm

The ergot medication must be discontinued immediately.
If patient has received an oral dose within the past several hours or has taken an acute overdose, 50 g of activated charcoal should be administered orally or via a nasogastric tube to help prevent further absorption. In a large overdose, the charcoal dose may be repeated several times.
If patient is severely hypertensive, start a nitroprusside drip, a nitroglycerin drip, or a phentolamine drip. Phentolamine may be preferable if significant peripheral ischemia is present.
If patient is hypertensive, but not severely so, consider the use of a calcium channel blocker or an angiotensin-converting enzyme inhibitor orally.
If patient has ergot-induced chest pain without hypertension, a nitroglycerin drip should be started and heparin should be considered. Aspirin also should be given. Because thrombosis can occur in the vessel that is in spasm, thrombolytics might be considered in patients who seem to have thrombosis on angiography. Glycoprotein IIb/IIIa inhibitors also might be useful, but efficacy in this setting is unproven.
If patient has had a stroke, it should be determined if it is hemorrhagic or ischemic. Cerebral angiography may help determine if there is an anatomic lesion.
If it appears that thrombosis at the site of vasospasm exists, anticoagulation or thrombolytics might be considered. Glycoprotein IIb/IIIa inhibitors also might be useful, but efficacy in this setting is unproven.
Ergot-induced headache should not be treated with an ergot, a tryptan, or a sympathomimetic. Opiates with or without a vasodilator are preferable in this setting.
Usual anticonvulsant therapy, including diazepam, lorazepam, dilantin, or phenobarbital, as needed may be required.
For severe peripheral ischemia, phentolamine infusions either systemically or intraarterially may reverse the vasospasm. Heparin should be administered and aspirin considered. If thrombosis is definitely present, thrombolytics also might be considered. Glycoprotein IIb/IIIa inhibitors also might be useful, but efficacy in this setting is unproven.
For any serious effects of ergots, including any of the above, consider oral cyproheptadine (Periactin), a nonspecific serotonin antagonist, which may reverse the serotonin agonist effects of the ergot causing the vasospasm.
Prostaglandin E_1 (alprostadil [Caverject]) and prostacyclin (epoprostenol [Flolan]) have been reported to reverse ergot-induced vasospasm in a few patients.[50–52]
Hyperbaric oxygen also has been used adjunctively in a case of peripheral ischemia with possible beneficial effects.[53] Especially when tissue oxygen concentrations can be measured to determine efficacy, this treatment is attractive but also should be considered experimental.

Common Errors in Ergot Alkaloid Poisoning

In general, not considering vasoconstriction/vasospasm as the cause of symptoms or signs in a patient taking an ergot derivative and not pursuing vascular insufficiency diagnostically

In taking a medication history, not recognizing that the patient may have recently stopped taking an ergot preparation (perhaps because of side effects) and not included it in the list of current medications, even though the effect of the ergot is still present

Not considering chest pain as being secondary to ergot-induced coronary artery vasospasm

Not considering neurologic deficits as being secondary to ergot-induced cerebral vasospasm and subsequent ischemic or hemorrhagic stroke

Not considering severe headache as being secondary to ergot-induced vasospasm and treating the headache with another ergot, a triptan, or a sympathomimetic

Not considering limb pain as being secondary to ergot-induced peripheral vasospasm and subsequent extremity ischemia

Not considering flank or abdominal pain in a patient taking an ergot as possibly being due to renal or intestinal ischemia

Not considering drug-drug interactions when prescribing a new drug (e.g., erythromycin, clarithromycin, ketoconazole, sympathomimetics, triptans, troleandomycin) to a patient taking an ergot derivative, resulting in ergotism

Key Points in Ergot Alkaoid Poisoning

1. The ergot alkaloids are not found on routine toxicologic screens, and their presence cannot be ruled out by a negative screen. Hospital laboratories in general are incapable of detecting ergots in biologic specimens. Because the vasospastic effects of the ergots persist long after the agent is no longer found in blood or urine above the detection limit, however, such testing would have limited usefulness.
2. Patients presenting with a clinical syndrome suggesting either central or peripheral vasospasm should have ingestion of ergots ruled out by extensive history taking, including from family members or friends when available. Medical records or prescriptions also may be valuable in documenting medication history.
3. Ergot-induced vasospasm can be present in some cases weeks after the last dose. Patients may not inform the physician that they are taking an ergot because they may consider themselves as not taking the drug at that time.
4. Angiograms are usually the best way to determine if vasospasm is present, but they may be negative at the time of testing if there has been a delay or if the vessel in spasm has ruptured.

REFERENCES

1. Thompson CJ (ed): Poisons and Poisoners with Historical Accounts of Some Famous Mysteries in Ancient and Modern Times. New York, Barnes & Noble Books, 1993.
2. Demeke T, Kidane Y, Wuhib E: Abstract, ergotism—a report on an epidemic 1977–1978. Ethiop Med J 17:107–112, 1978.
3. Fuller JG: The Day of St. Anthony's Fire. New York, Macmillan, 1968.
4. Weaver R, Phillips M, Vacek J: St. Anthony's fire: A medieval disease in modern times: Case history. Angiology 40:929–931, 1989.
5. Bory M, Joly P, Bonnet JL, et al: Methergin testing with angiographically normal coronary arteries. Am J Cardiol 61:298–302, 1988.
6. Frantz RP, Lerman A, Edwards BS, et al: Methylergonovine-induced diffuse coronary spasm in a patient with exercise-induced coronary spasm after heart transplantation. J Heart Lung Transplant 13:834–839, 1994.
7. Igarashi Y, Yamazoe M, Shibata A: Effect of direct intracoronary administration of methylergonovine in patients with and without variant angina. Am Med J 121:1094–1100, 1991.
8. Piatt J: Massive intracerebral hemorrhage complicating cardiac catheterization with ergonovine administration. Stroke 15:904–907, 1984.
9. Hardman JG, Limbird LE, Molinoff PB, Ruddon RW (eds): Goodman and Gilman's the Pharmacological Basis of Therapeutics, 9th ed. New York: McGraw-Hill, 1996.
10. Warlow CP, Dennis MS, van Gijn J, et al (eds): Stroke: A Practical Guide to Management, 2nd ed. Blackwell Science, 2001.
11. Parkes D: Bromocriptine. Adv Drug Res 12:247–344, 1977.
12. Rains CP, Bryson HM, Fitton A: Cabergoline—a review of its pharmacological properties and therapeutic potential in the treatment of hyperprolactinemia and inhibition of lactation. Drugs 49:255–279, 1995.
13. VanDenBrink A, Reekers M, Bax W, et al: Coronary side-effect potential of current and prospective antimigraine drugs. Circulation 98:25–30, 1998.
14. Senter H, Lieberman A, Pinto R: Cerebral manifestations of ergotism. Stroke 7:88–92, 1979.
15. Henry PY, Larre P, Aupy M: Reversible cerebral arteriopathy associated with the administration of ergot derivatives. Cephalalgia 4:171–178, 1984.
16. Ahlgren I, Haeger K, Nylander G: Imminent gangrene of the leg after ergot poisoning. Angiology 19:354–361, 1968.
17. Fujiwara Y, Yamanaka O, Nakamura T, et al: Acute myocardial infarction induced by ergonovine administration for artificially induced abortion. Jpn Heart J 34:803–808, 1993.
18. Galer B, Lipton R, Solomon S, et al: Myocardial ischemia related to ergot alkaloids: A case report and literature review. Headache 31:446–450, 1991.
19. Aellig WH: The effects on peripheral circulation by ergotamine, dihydroergotamine and l-methylergotamine in the innervated, perfused rear limb of the dog. Helv Physiol 25:374–396, 1967.
20. Bertholet A, Sutter R: Action of 15–754 on the innervated, perfused pelvic extremity of the dog. Internal Communique, Biomedical Research, Department of Experimental Therapy, Sandoz LTD, 1971.
21. Abouleish E: Postpartum hypertension and convulsion after oxytocic drugs. Anesth Analg 55:813–815, 1976.
22. Dutt S, Wong F, Spurway JH: Fatal myocardial infarction associated with bromocriptine for postpartum lactation suppression. Aust N Z J Obstet Gynaecol 38:116–117, 1998.
23. Comabella M, Alvarez-Sabin J, Rovira A: Bromocriptine and postpartum cerebral angiopathy: A causal relationship? Neurology 46:1754–1756, 1996.
24. Eickman FM: Recurrent myocardial infarction in a postpartum patient receiving bromocriptine. Clin Cardiol 15:781–783, 1992.
25. Katz M, Kroll D, Pak I, et al: Puerperal hypertension stroke and seizures after suppression of lactation with bromocriptine. Obstet Gynecol 66:822–824, 1985.
26. Ringrose D: The obstetrical use of ergot: A violation of the doctrine "Primum Non Nocere." Can Med Assoc J 87:712–714, 1962.
27. Simolke GA, Cox SM, Cunningham F: G1 cerebrovascular accidents complicating pregnancy and the puerperium. Obstet Gynecol 78:37–42, 1991.
28. Andersson PG: Ergotamine headache. Headache 15:118–121, 1975.
29. Berde B, Schild HO (eds): Ergot Alkaloids and Related Compounds. Berlin, Springer-Verlag, 1978.
30. Berde B: Pharmacology of ergot alkaloids in clinical use. Med J Aust (Special Suppl)2:3–13, 1978.
31. Aellig WH, Nuesche E: Comparative pharmacokinetic investigations with tritium-labeled ergot alkaloids after oral and intravenous administration in man. Int J Clin Pharmacol 15:106–112, 1977.
32. Kanto J: Clinical pharmacokinetics of ergotamine, dihydroergotamine, ergotoxine, bromocriptine, methysergide, and lergotrile. Int J Clin Pharmacol Ther Toxicol 21:135–142, 1983.
33. Mantyla R, Kanto J: Clinical pharmacokinetics of methylergometrine (methylergonovine). Int J Clin Pharmacol Ther Toxicol 19:386–391, 1981.
34. Mantyla R, Kleimola T, Kanto J: Pharmacokinetics of methylergometrine (methylergonovine) in the rabbit and man. Acta Pharmacol Toxicol 40:561–569, 1977.

35. Mantyla R, Kleimola T, Kanto J: Methylergometrine (methylergonovine) concentrations in the human plasma and urine. Int J Clin Pharmacol 16:254–257, 1978.
36. Muller-Schweinitzer E: Pharmacological actions of the main metabolites of dihydroergotamine. Eur J Pharmacol 26:699–705, 1984.
37. Peroutka S: The pharmacology of current anti-migraine drugs. Headache 30:5–11, 1990.
38. Ausband SC, Goodman PE: An unusual case of clarithromycin induced ergotism. J Emerg Med 21:411–413, 2001.
39. Horowitz R, Dart R, Gomez H: Clinical ergotism with lingual ischemia induced by clarithromycin-ergotamine interaction. Arch Intern Med 156:456–458, 1996.
40. Nelson M, Berchou R: Pharmacokinetic evaluation of erythromycin and caffeine administered with bromocriptine. Clin Pharmacol Ther 47:694–697, 1990.
41. Kulig K, Moore L, Kirk M, et al: Bromocriptine-associated headache: Possible life-threatening sympathomimetic interaction. Obstet Gynecol 78:941–943, 1991.
42. Chan J, Critchley JA, Cockram C: Postpartum hypertension, bromocriptine and phenylpropanolamine. Drug Invest 8:254–256, 1994.
43. Fedotin M, Hartman C: Ergotamine poisoning producing renal arterial spasm. N Engl J Med 283:518–519, 1970.
44. Buenger RE, Hunter JA: Reversible mesenteric artery stenoses due to methysergide maleate. JAMA 198:144–146, 1966.
45. Barinagarrementeria F: Postpartum cerebral angiopathy with cerebral infarction due to ergonovine use. Stroke 23:1364–1366, 1992.
46. Janssens E, Hommel M, Mounier-Vehier F, et al: Postpartum cerebral angiopathy possibly due to bromocriptine therapy. Stroke 26:128–130, 1995.
47. Larrazet F, Spaulding C, Lobreau H, et al: Possible bromocriptine-induced myocardial infarction. Ann Intern Med 118:199–200, 1993.
48. Richter AM, Banker VP: Carotid ergotism. Radiology 106:339–340, 1973.
49. Cutler D, Ghazzal Z, Deam G: Angiographic demonstration of inhibition of methyl-ergonovine-induced coronary vasospasm in a patient with sudden death. Cathet Cardiovasc Diag 39:181–184, 1996.
50. Levy JM, Ibrahim F, Ny Kamp PW, et al: Prostaglandin E for alleviating symptoms of ergot intoxication: A case report. Cardiovasc Intervent Radiol 7:28–30, 1984.
51. Zimran A, Ofek B, Hershko C: Treatment with captopril for peripheral ischemia induced by ergotamine. BMJ 288:364, 1984.
52. McKiernan TL, Bock K, Leya F, et al: Ergot-induced peripheral vascular insufficiency, noninterventional treatment. Cathet Cardiovasc Diag 31:311–314, 1994.
53. Merrick R, Gufler K, Jacobsen E: Ergotism treated with hyperbaric oxygen and continuous epidural analgesia. Acta Anesth Scand 67:87–90, 1978.

CHAPTER 70

Antidiabetic Agents

Christopher H. Linden

Antidiabetic agents include insulin and five classes of oral drugs: sulfonylureas, meglitinides, biguanides, glitazones, and α-glucosidase inhibitors. Although they may have other effects, antidiabetic agents are used primarily for the treatment of hyperglycemia, the cardinal feature of all forms of diabetes mellitus and the consequence of overproduction and underuse of glucose due to underlying insulin deficiency (low levels of circulating insulin) and insulin resistance (decreased tissue responsiveness to insulin). Insulin therapy provides exogenous hormone, sulfonylureas and meglitinides enhance endogenous insulin secretion, biguanides and glitazones enhance the tissue insulin activity, and α-glucosidase inhibitors reduce the intestinal absorption of carbohydrates. Insulin, sulfonylureas, and meglitinides can cause hypoglycemia and are classified as hypoglycemic agents. Biguanides, glitazones, and α-glucosidase inhibitors, when taken alone, do not cause hypoglycemia and are characterized as antihyperglycemic agents. However, they can potentiate the action of hypoglycemic agents and precipitate hypoglycemia when added to a therapeutic regimen that includes hypoglycemic agents. Biguanide exposure also has been associated with the development of lactic acidosis.

CHEMISTRY AND PHARMACOKINETICS

Insulin

Insulin is a protein hormone that is related structurally to the somatomedins or insulin-like growth factors, which act as paracrine modulators.[1,2] It consists of two chains of amino acids linked by disulfide bonds and is synthesized by β cells of pancreatic islets of Langerhans. These cells first produce a single long chain of amino acids known as *preproinsulin*. After entering the rough endoplasmic reticulum, an end portion of preproinsulin is cleaved off to form proinsulin (Fig. 70-1). Proinsulin then spontaneously folds on itself as disulfide bonds are established between the two ends. It subsequently is packaged in vesicles and transported to the Golgi complex. Here, proinsulin is repackaged in secretory granules, along with enzymes that convert it to a double-stranded insulin molecule by cleaving a connecting segment or C peptide from the fold or midportion of proinsulin. Insulin stored in granules complexes with zinc to produce insulin hexamers, a concentrated crystalline form of insulin. This process facilitates the conversion of proinsulin to insulin.

Although C peptide has no known biologic activity, equimolar amounts of insulin and C peptide are produced from the cleavage of proinsulin and released into the circulation from secretory granules (along with small quantities of proinsulin).

Insulin for therapeutic use originally was obtained by extracting it from pork or beef pancreas, with doses and concentrations expressed in units of insulin based on bioassay in rabbits. In 1921, Banting and Best were the first to use such an extract to treat a human patient successfully. Pork and beef insulins, which differ from human insulin by one (pork) and three (beef) amino acids, and mixtures of these insulins are still available. Human insulin, now more widely used, is prepared by enzymatic modification of pork insulin or produced by strains of *Escherichia coli* or *Saccharomyces cerevisiae* using recombinant DNA technology. Insulin lispro is a recombinant DNA–derived human insulin analogue. Insulin doses still are expressed in bioassay units, but solutions and suspensions now have been standardized to concentrations of 100 U/mL. This standardization is also true for fixed combinations, such as those containing 70/30 U/mL and 50/50 U/mL of regular and NPH (isophane) insulin (e.g., Humulin, Novolin). As with endogenously stored insulin, exogenous preparations often consist of hexameric insulin complexed with zinc.

Insulin must be given parenterally, usually by subcutaneous injection, although transdermal and inhalational delivery systems are under investigation.[1-3] Therapeutic subcutaneous doses range from 0.2 to 2.5 U/kg/day. After absorption (or secretion), hexameric insulin dissociates and circulates in the blood as the more biologically active free monomer. It is distributed in extracellular fluid, has a volume of distribution of about 0.4 L/kg, and is minimally bound to plasma proteins. Elimination occurs by liver, kidney, and muscle metabolism, with a half-life of 5 to 9 minutes after intravenous injection. The half-life is prolonged in patients with antiinsulin antibodies, patients with renal failure, and, to a lesser extent, patients with hepatic disease. The apparent half-life of insulin after subcutaneous administration is much longer (hours to days). More importantly, it depends on the insulin formulation. Differences in the duration of action after subcutaneous administration reflect differences in the rate of dissolution and absorption (not metabolism) of insulin preparations, and these differences affect times of onset and peak effect and apparent half-life. Regular insulin is the only preparation that can be given intravenously. By this route, its action begins in minutes, peaks within 0.5 hour, and lasts 2 to 3 hours.

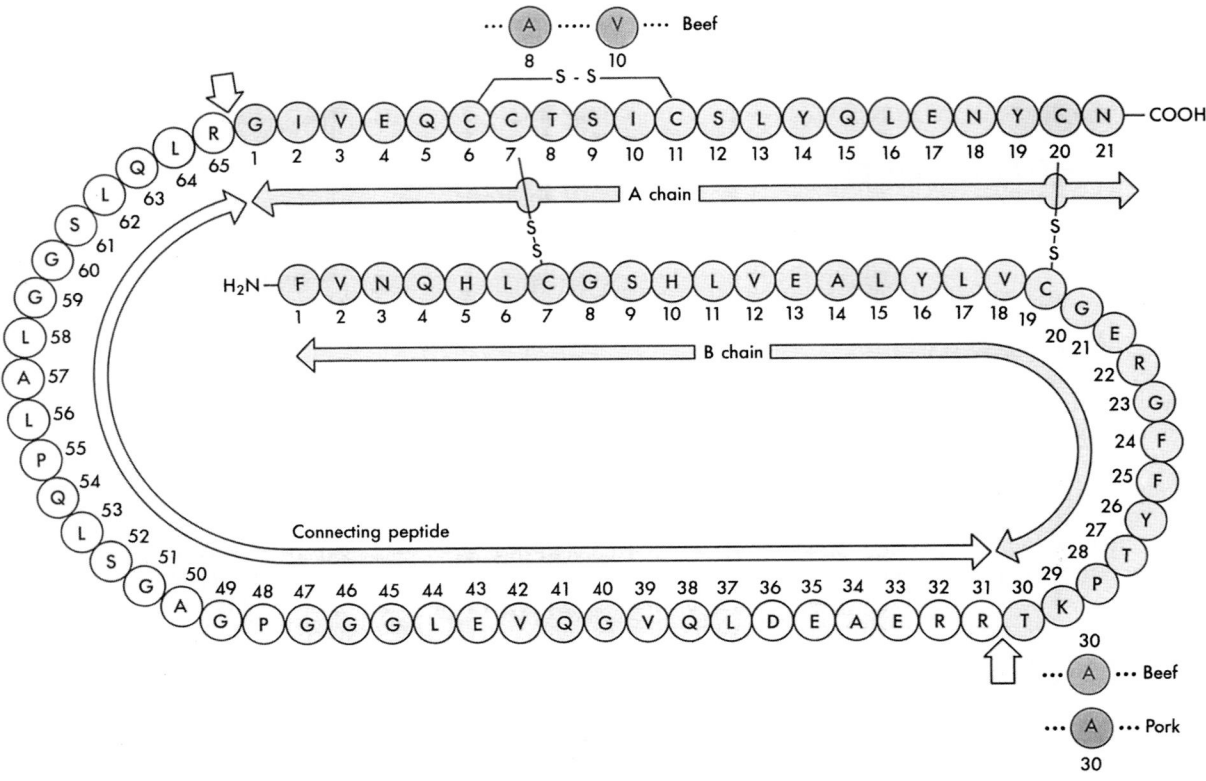

FIGURE 70-1

Amino acid sequence of human proinsulin. When the connecting peptide is removed (the portion between the arrows), the remaining primary structure is that of insulin. Amino acid substitutions in the sequence for pork insulin and beef insulin also are noted. *(From Lawrence JC: Insulin and oral hypoglycemic agents. In Brody TM, Larner J, Minneman KP [eds]: Human Pharmacology: Molecular to Clinical, 3rd ed. St. Louis, Mosby, 1998, p 549.)*

Under fasting conditions, the pancreas secretes about 1 U (40 μg [7 nmol]) of insulin per hour in nondiabetics, resulting in an average serum insulin level of about 12 μU/mL (0.5 ng/mL [84 pmol/L]) by radioimmunoassay. After ingestion of a meal, insulin levels in nondiabetics average about twice this amount. Normally, about 10% of the immunoreactive insulin level is due to the presence of proinsulin, with normal levels of the latter being 36 to 126 ng/mL (4 to 14 pmol/L). Because proinsulin has a longer half-life than insulin (about 17 minutes), a slightly higher fraction is seen in non–insulin-dependent diabetes. A much higher fraction of proinsulin (20% to 80%) is seen in patients with insulinomas because of abnormal processing of this peptide by these tumors. Also, because proinsulin has only about 1/50 the biologic activity of insulin, the effective insulin level is actually lower than that determined by radioimmunoassay. Similarly, because C peptide has a longer half-life than insulin (about 30 minutes), serum concentrations of this protein (also measured by radioimmunoassay) are higher than serum concentrations of insulin (1 to 4 ng/mL [500 to 2000 pmol/L]). Lower insulin and C peptide concentrations may be seen in untreated insulin-dependent diabetics who are insulin deficient, and higher concentrations may be seen in non–insulin-dependent diabetics (treated and untreated) who are insulin resistant. Serum insulin concentrations may be many times higher in insulin-dependent diabetics treated with nonhuman insulin because they rapidly develop antibodies capable of binding large amounts of exogenous insulin in the plasma, and radioimmunoassays measure total rather than free immunoreactive insulin (unless a preliminary separation step is employed).

Classification/Preparation	Onset (hr)	Peak (hr)	Duration of Action (hr)
Rapid-Acting			
Lispro	0.25–0.5	0.5–2.5	3–6
Regular (crystalline)	0.3–1	1–5	5–10
Intermediate-Acting			
Lente	1–3	6–14	16–24
NPH (isophane)	1–2	6–14	16–24
Long-Acting			
Ultralente	4–6	8–20	24–36

*After subcutaneous administration.

Sulfonylureas

The sulfonylureas (substituted arylsulfonylureas) are related structurally to sulfonamide antibiotics (Fig. 70-2).[1–3] Agents in current use differ in potency, with the newer or second-generation analogues being about 100 times more potent than the original or first-generation ones. They also differ in half-life and duration of action but are similar in terms of their high (>90%) plasma protein binding, primarily to albumin, and low (0.1 to 0.2 L/kg) volumes of distribution. Atypically and for unclear reasons, duration of action does not correlate with half-life.[4]

Sulfonylureas are well absorbed from the gastrointestinal tract with bioavailabilities of 80% or greater. Food can decrease their absorption and bioavailability. Antihyperglycemic effects typically begin within 1 hour and peak in 2 to 6 hours, with first-generation agents having a longer time to peak effect than second-generation agents. The

coadministration of other drugs that are highly protein bound (e.g., oral anticoagulants, phenytoin, salicylates and nonsteroidal antiinflammatory agents, sulfonamides) can displace sulfonylureas from binding sites and enhance their effects (and vice versa). These agents are eliminated by hepatic metabolism (to a variety of active and inactive metabolites) and renal excretion (along with their metabolites). Hepatic or renal insufficiency can prolong their half-lives. The renal elimination of chlorpropamide is increased in an alkaline urine and decreased in an acidic one. Because all sulfonylureas are weak acids with pK_a values of about 5, the urinary excretion of other agents also is likely to be dependent on urinary pH. Chlorpropamide, which has relatively greater renal elimination, and acetohexamide, glyburide, and tolazamide, which have active metabolites, are more likely than other agents to cause hypoglycemia in patients with renal failure.

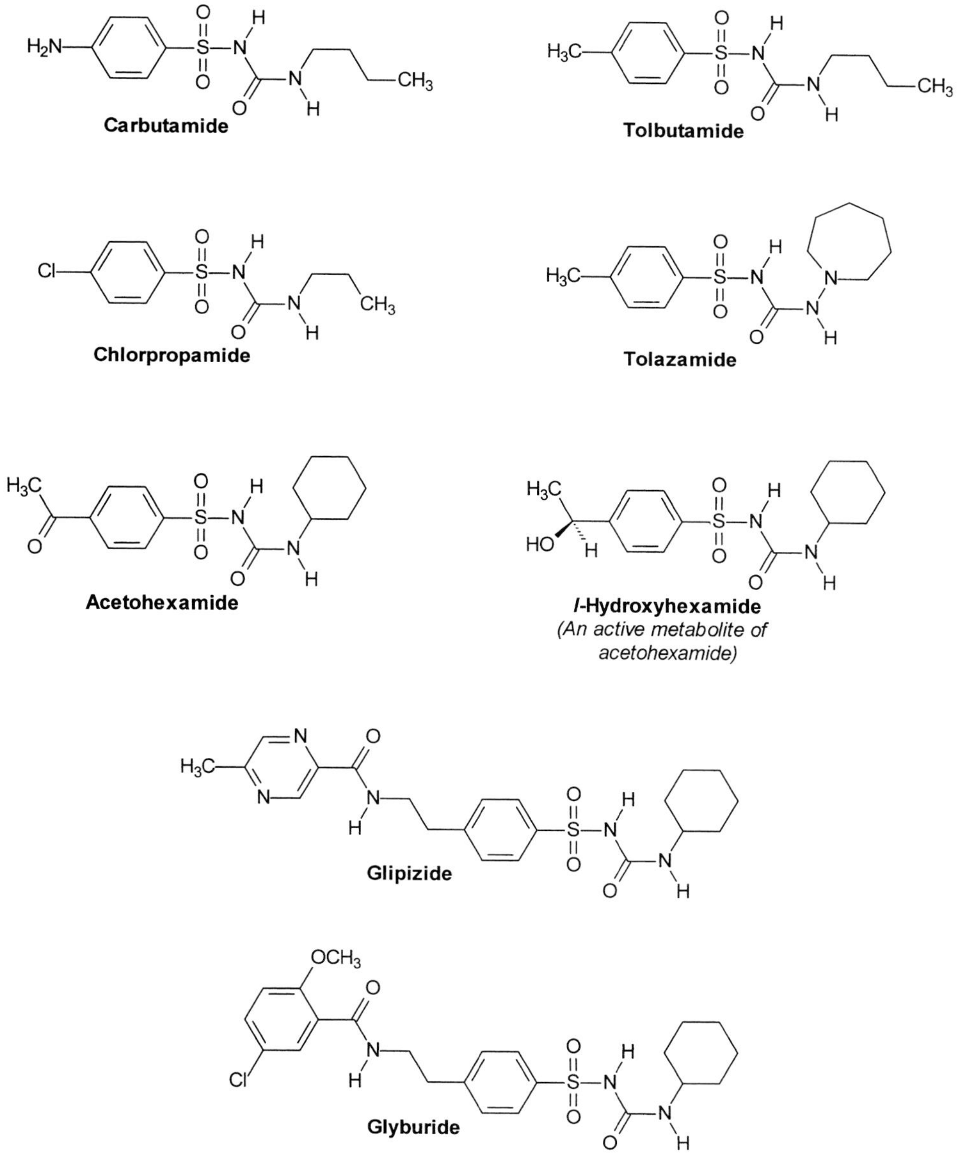

FIGURE 70-2

Chemical structures of sulfonylurea hypoglycemic agents.

Selected Pharmacokinetics and Pharmacodynamics of Sulfonylureas

	Usual Dose (mg/day)	Half-life (hr)	Duration of Action (hr)
First-Generation Agents			
Acetoheximide (Dymelor)	500–750*	1.4 (0.8–2.4)	12–24
Chlorpropamide (Diabinese)	250–375†	36 (25–60)	24–72
Tolazamide (Tolinase)	250–500*	7 (5–11)	14–16
Tolbutamide (Orinase)	1000–2000‡	7 (4–25)	6–12
Second-Generation Agents§			
Glimepiride (Amaryl)	1–4†	5 (2–8)	12–24
Glipizide (Glucotrol)¶	10–20*	2.8 (1.1–3.7)	12–24
Glyburide (Diaβeta, Glynase, Micronase)	3–20*	1.6 (0.7–3)	12–24

*Once a day or divided.

†Once a day.

‡Divided.

§Gliclazide, glimepiride, and gliquidone are additional agents in use outside the United States.

¶Also known as glibenclamide.

Meglitinides

Meglitinides are analogues of the nonsulfonylurea moiety of gliburide.[5,6] Repaglinide (Prandin) and nateglinide (Starlix) are the only agents in this class currently available in the United States. The recommended dose is 0.5 to 4 mg for repaglinide and 60 to 120 mg for nateglinide two to four times a day before or with meals. These agents are well absorbed orally and are highly (>98%) bound to plasma proteins, primarily albumin. They have relatively low volumes of distribution (about 0.4 L/kg) and are eliminated by hepatic metabolism, with renal excretion of inactive metabolites. Half-lives are about 1.5 hours. Elimination may be impaired in patients with hepatic or renal insufficiency. Because cytochrome P-450 enzymes, CYP3A4 in particular, are partly responsible for their metabolism, the coadministration of drugs that induce CYP3A4 (e.g., barbiturates, carbamazepine, rifampin, pioglitazone) or inhibit CYP3A4 (e.g., azole antifungals, calcium channel blockers, cimetidine, human immunodeficiency virus protease inhibitors, macrolide antibiotics, oral contraceptives) could potentially decrease or increase the effect of meglitinides, respectively.

Biguanides

Biguanides (diguanides) are derivatives of guanidine.[1–3,7] Above-ground parts of the flowering plant *Galega officinalis* (Goat's rue, French lilac, Italian fitch) contain the guanidine analogues galegine and 4-hydroxygalegine. This plant was used in medieval Europe for the treatment of diabetes and is still available as an herbal medicine, primarily used as a diuretic and secondarily as supportive therapy in diabetes. Metformin (Glucophage) is the only biguanide prescription medication currently available in the United States. It has been in clinical use in Europe since 1970 but was withdrawn from most markets in 1977 along with the related agent phenformin because use of the latter was associated with a low but unacceptable incidence of fatal lactic acidosis. Although this complication also can occur during metformin therapy, it is extremely rare and much less common than it is with phenformin. Metformin was reintroduced in Europe in the late 1980s and approved for use in the United States in 1995. Phenformin is still available in other areas of the world.[8,9]

Metformin is absorbed slowly and incompletely from the gastrointestinal tract. It does not bind to plasma proteins and has a volume of distribution of 3.7 L/kg. It is eliminated by urinary excretion and to a lesser extent in the feces as unchanged drug. The usual therapeutic dose is 500 or 850 mg, taken during or after meals; doses generally should not exceed 2550 mg/day. Sustained-release formulations (e.g., Glucophage XR) are also available for once- or twice-daily dosing (e.g., 2000 mg once a day or 1000 mg twice a day). Bioavailability is about 50%. Antihyperglycemic effects begin about 1 hour after ingestion and persist for 12 hours (longer with sustained-release formulations). The half-life averages 4 to 8 hours and is prolonged in patients with renal impairment. Renal insufficiency decreases the volume of distribution and increases peak plasma drug levels and the risk of toxicity. For these reasons, metformin is contraindicated in patients with renal disease or dysfunction and in patients who have conditions that predispose to renal impairment, such as congestive heart failure, dehydration, sepsis, and shock. It also is recommended that therapy be discontinued when performing radiographic imaging with intravenous iodinated contrast material, which can cause renal failure (particularly in diabetics), and not be resumed until post-procedure renal function is determined to be normal. Because metformin undergoes proximal tubular secretion and glomerular filtration, its renal clearance is about 3.5 times that of creatinine. Cimetidine and possibly other drugs that undergo renal tubular secretion, such as amiloride, digoxin, morphine, quinidine, procainamide, triamterene, trimethoprim, and vancomycin, can compete with metformin for proximal tubular transport and increase its plasma level.

Usual therapeutic doses of phenformin are 25 to 200 mg/day. It is well absorbed and has limited protein binding. Being more lipophilic than metformin, phenformin has a larger volume of distribution (5 to 10 L/kg). Also in contrast to metformin, it is eliminated by hepatic metabolism (hydroxylation to inactive metabolites) and by enzymes, which are saturable and subject to genetic polymorphism. Phenformin's half-life ranges from 7 to 15 hours.

Glitazones

Glitazones (thiazolidinediones) currently available in the United States include pioglitazone (Actos) and rosiglitazone (Avandia).[3] Troglitazone (Rezulin), the first widely used glitazone, was introduced in 1997 but removed from the market in March 2000 because of potentially fatal idiosyncratic liver toxicity associated with its use. The risk of this toxicity seems to be much less with pioglitazone and rosiglitazone.

Therapeutic doses are 15 to 45 mg/day for pioglitazone and 2 to 8 mg/day for rosiglitazone. Both drugs are well absorbed from the gastrointestinal tract, are highly (>99%) bound to plasma proteins (primarily albumin), have relatively small volumes of distribution (0.3 to 0.6 L/kg), and are eliminated by hepatic metabolism. Half-lives are approximately 3 hours, and there is renal excretion of active and inactive metabolites. Pioglitazone, but not rosiglitazone, is metabolized by CYP3A4 and could be subject to interactions with drugs that are metabolized by or inhibit this enzyme (see under Meglitinides).

α-Glucosidase Inhibitors

α-Glucosidase inhibitors currently available in the United States include acarbose (Precose) and miglitol (Glyset).[3] Voglibose, another α-glucosidase inhibitor, is awaiting U.S. Food and Drug Administration approval. Therapeutic doses of acarbose and miglitol are 25 to 100 mg three times a day given with meals. Acarbose, an oligosaccharide, has limited systemic absorption and is eliminated by metabolism within the gut, primarily by intestinal bacteria but also by digestive enzymes. Miglitol, a monosaccharide derivative, is well absorbed after oral administration. It has negligible protein binding, has a small volume of distribution (0.18 L/kg), and is eliminated by renal excretion of unchanged drug. Although its elimination may be impaired in patients with renal insufficiency, absorption does not contribute to its therapeutic effect (see later), and dosage adjustments are unnecessary in these patients.

PATHOPHYSIOLOGY

Insulin

Endogenous insulin secretion (i.e., the exocytosis of secretory granules from pancreatic β cells) depends primarily on and is inversely related to the blood glucose concentration.[1,2] It is influenced to a lesser degree by other nutrients, gastrointestinal hormones, and the autonomic nervous system. Increases in plasma glucose, amino acid, fatty acid, and ketone concentrations; the release of gastrointestinal inhibitory peptide, glucagon-like peptide-1, enteroglucagon, cholecystokinin, gastrin, gastrin-releasing peptide, secretin, and vasoactive intestinal peptide; and vagal stimulation, all of which occur after the ingestion of glucose or other foods, promote insulin secretion. β2-Adrenergic receptor stimulation enhances insulin secretion, whereas α2-adrenergic receptor stimulation inhibits it. Hormonal and vagal effects explain why oral glucose is a more potent stimulant of insulin secretion than intravenous glucose is.

Insulin secretion ultimately is triggered by a rise in the intracellular concentration of calcium in response to the generation of adenosine triphosphate (ATP), primarily by the oxidation of glucose but also by the metabolism of other nutrients. It is thought that ATP binds to and blocks the pore-forming unit of ATP-sensitive and voltage-sensitive potassium channels in β-cell membranes. This activity inhibits potassium efflux, with consequent membrane depolar-

ization leading to activation of voltage-sensitive calcium channels and the influx of calcium. Hormones and adrenergic receptors seem to potentiate or antagonize the action of glucose by stimulating or inhibiting adenylyl cyclase, increasing or decreasing intracellular cyclic adenosine monophosphate and calcium concentrations.

Insulin lowers the serum glucose concentration by facilitating glucose uptake by the liver, myocardium, skeletal muscle, and adipose tissue and by inhibiting hepatic gluconeogenesis and glycogenolysis. Glucose enters cells by diffusion that is facilitated by a family of at least six distinct membrane glycoproteins that are known as glucose transporters (GLUT). Insulin stimulates glucose uptake by promoting the translocation of intracellular vesicles that contain GLUT (subtypes 1 and 4) to the cell membrane and by enhancing the synthesis of GLUT4. It first binds to insulin receptors, membrane glycoproteins that are ligand-activated tyrosine kinases, with consequent enzyme activation. The intervening cascade of events is not well characterized. Other actions of insulin are mediated, at least in part, by its ability to bind and stimulate insulin-like growth factor (IGF) receptors, particularly IGF-1 (also called *somatomedin C receptors*).

In excessive doses, insulin can cause hypoglycemia. Hypoglycemia inhibits endogenous insulin secretion and stimulates the secretion of a variety of counterregulatory hormones, most notably glucagon but also cortisol, epinephrine, estrogens, growth hormone (somatotropin), norepinephrine, somatostatin, and thyroid hormones. Epinephrine and norepinephrine contribute to the autonomic (sympathetic nervous system) symptoms of hypoglycemia (see later), and glucagon may be responsible for the Somogyi phenomenon (morning hyperglycemia after an episode of nocturnal hypoglycemia). Other counterregulatory hormones seem to have only a permissive role during recovery from hypoglycemia. Central nervous system manifestations of hypoglycemia are due to decreased cellular metabolism resulting from the lack of glucose (neuroglycopenia), an essential, and nearly exclusive, energy substrate for brain tissue, which is unable to synthesize glucose.

Sulfonylureas

Sulfonylureas enhance the secretion of insulin in response to increases in blood glucose.[1–3] They bind to a distinct "sulfonylurea receptor" site associated with ATP-sensitive and voltage-sensitive potassium channels on the β-cell membrane with consequent blocking of these channels, inhibition of potassium efflux, membrane depolarization, calcium influx, and insulin secretion. It is unclear whether their extrapancreatic effects (e.g., decreased hepatic gluconeogenesis and insulin clearance, increased peripheral insulin sensitivity, stimulation of somatostatin secretion, and suppression of glucagon secretion) are clinically significant. Toxic effects are secondary to hyperinsulinemic hypoglycemia.

Meglitinides

Similar to the sulfonylureas, these agents bind to receptors on the β-cell membrane with consequent blocking of potassium channels, membrane depolarization, opening of calcium channels, and insulin secretion in response to increases in blood glucose.[5,6] Toxic effects are due primarily to hyperinsulinemia.

Biguanides

Antihyperglycemic effects are due to enhanced peripheral glucose uptake and inhibition of hepatic gluconeogenesis.[1-3,7] Other important effects include decreased plasma triglyceride concentrations, increased high-density lipoprotein cholesterol levels, and inhibition of platelet aggregation. Metformin promotes glucose uptake by increasing the binding of insulin to its receptor and by increasing the synthesis and intracellular translocation of GLUT1 and GLUT4 glucose transporters. It also enhances the tyrosine kinase activity of insulin receptors by inhibiting the activity of membrane glycoprotein PC-1, an inhibitor of tyrosine kinase whose increased activity seems to be responsible for the phenomenon of insulin resistance, with enhanced tyrosine kinase activity also promoting the uptake of glucose. Although insulin (endogenous or exogenous) is required for biguanides to be effective, insulin levels are not affected, and hypoglycemia does not occur with biguanide monotherapy or overdose.

Biguanide-induced lactic acidosis is due to inhibition of gluconeogenesis, the pathway for converting pyruvate to glucose.[10-14] Gluconeogenesis occurs primarily in the liver but also in the kidney. At supratherapeutic concentrations, biguanides inhibit the enzyme pyruvate carboxylase, which converts pyruvate to oxaloacetate, the first step of gluconeogenesis. Pyruvate is the end product of skeletal muscle glycolysis (which generates ATP). Most of it is reduced to lactate by lactate dehydrogenase before entering the circulation. Lactate is taken up by the liver, where it is converted back to pyruvate by lactate dehydrogenase, and is used for gluconeogenesis. Inhibition of pyruvate carboxylase seems to be secondary to lowering of the intracellular pH, an effect that also inhibits lactate uptake. Glucose produced by hepatic gluconeogenesis enters the bloodstream and is taken up by skeletal muscle, where it is used for glycolysis. This recycling process, known as the *Cori cycle*, shifts the burden of metabolism from skeletal muscle to the liver. Some amino acids (most notably alanine), derived from dietary proteins and from the catabolism of skeletal muscle during starvation, also are precursors of pyruvate. Hence, inhibition of pyruvate carboxylase can result in the accumulation of pyruvate and alanine as well as lactate.

Biguanides also have direct negative inotropic effects that can reduce hepatic blood flow and impair lactate clearance further. In addition, phenformin, but not metformin, inhibits glucose oxidation and oxidative phosphorylation. Ethanol, whose metabolism generates reduced nicotinamide adenine dinucleotide (NADH), can promote lactic acidosis because lactate dehydrogenase oxidizes NADH to NAD as it reduces pyruvate to lactate, and an increased NADH-to-NAD ratio inhibits the conversion of lactate to pyruvate. Severe acidosis results in depression of cardiovascular and central nervous system function.

Lactic acidosis can be divided into two types, aerobic and anaerobic. In the aerobic type, tissue hypoxia is not present, and biguanide accumulation resulting in impaired lactate metabolism is the predominant mechanism. Predisposing factors include advanced age, ethanol use, excessive dosing, liver disease (with impaired lactate and phenformin metabolism), and renal insufficiency (with impaired metformin elimination). Acute renal insufficiency may be precipitated by any condition that causes dehydration and by the administration of intravenous aminoglycoside antibiotics, dextran, or iodinated radiographic contrast material.

In anaerobic acidosis, enhanced lactate production is the primary cause, with conditions that reduce arterial oxygenation and tissue perfusion (e.g., congestive heart failure, myocardial infarction, respiratory failure, sepsis, severe dehydration) usually being responsible. Vigorous exercise also can increase lactate production.

Glitazones

Glitazones primarily act by decreasing insulin resistance in adipose tissue, the liver, and skeletal muscle, potentiating the effects of hypoglycemic agents.[3,15,16] They also decrease hepatic gluconeogenesis and have favorable effects on other risk factors for cardiovascular disease (e.g., blood pressure, fibrinolysis, lipid profile). Stimulation of peroxisome proliferator–activated receptors, primarily the gamma subtype, which enhances the transcription of insulin-responsive genes involved in the control of glucose transport, use, and production (and in the regulation of fatty acid metabolism), is the underlying mechanism. Because glitazones enhance the effects of insulin, insulin and C peptide plasma concentrations are reduced, and hypoglycemia does not occur with monotherapy or overdose.

α-Glucosidase Inhibitors

α-Glucosidase inhibitors competitively and reversibly inhibit membrane-bound α-glucosidase, glucoamylase, maltase, and sucrase, enzymes that hydrolyze oligosaccharides (dextrins, maltose, maltotriose, and sucrose) to glucose in the brush border of the small intestine. This activity delays and partially decreases the absorption of glucose.[3] Acarbose also inhibits pancreatic α-amylase, which hydrolyzes ingested polysaccharides, such as amylose and amylopectin, or starch, to oligosaccharides. Although neither agent significantly inhibits lactase, the resultant malabsorption of nonlactose carbohydrates can result in gastrointestinal symptoms that are identical to those of lactase deficiency. Taken alone, α-glucosidase inhibitors do not cause hypoglycemia.

CLINICAL PRESENTATION

Hypoglycemia

Hypoglycemia, the hallmark of poisoning by insulin, sulfonylureas, and meglitinides, may result from therapeutic doses of these agents in nondiabetics and excessive doses in diabetics.[17-20] Accidental poisoning may occur after therapeutic dosing in individuals with diabetes who miss a meal or eat at a time that does not correspond to that of peak drug effects; increase their dose of a hypoglycemic agent or physical activity; change agents, formulations, or brands; or have another antidiabetic drug added to their therapeutic regimen. Agents without intrinsic hypoglycemic activity also can precipitate hypoglycemia when added to existing antidiabetic therapy (Table 70-1). Predisposing factors include congestive heart failure; renal insufficiency; malignancy; sepsis; and conditions associated with limited glycogen reserves, such as extremes of age, malnutrition, and advanced liver disease.[21]

Accidental poisoning also may result from dispensing errors (wrong drug or wrong dose). Poor handwriting and sound-alike drug names (e.g., chlorpropamide/chloroquine/chlorpromazine, Diabinese/Diamox, Tolinase/Tolectin) are responsible for some medication errors. Neonatal hypoglycemia can result from maternal drug exposure. As for all other agents, poisoning can occur in young children as a consequence of accidental ingestion, an innocent exploratory behavior in this age group.

Nonaccidental self-poisoning usually occurs in depressed, suicidal individuals but also may be encountered in individuals with Munchausen syndrome. Surreptitious poisoning or factitious hypoglycemia can involve anyone who has access to hypoglycemic agents, such as diabetics, relatives of diabetics, and health care workers.[22] Difficult-to-diagnose but rare presentations of antidiabetic agent poisoning include attempted homicide and Munchausen syndrome by proxy.[23] A puncture wound, bogginess, skin discoloration, and tenderness may be noted at the site of an insulin injection.[24]

Autonomic manifestations of hypoglycemia include anxiety, diaphoresis, hunger, nausea and vomiting, palpitations and tachycardia, tachypnea, paresthesias, tremors, and peripheral vasoconstriction with pallor and widening of the pulse pressure.[17–20,25–29] The absence of autonomic findings does not preclude a diagnosis of hypoglycemia, however, particularly in patients who are taking medications with sympatholytic activity, such as β-blockers, clonidine, and prazosin, and in patients with long-standing diabetes who may have impaired autonomic function and counter-regulatory hormone responses.

Tachydysrhythmias, primarily atrial fibrillation and premature atrial and ventricular beats but also atrial flutter; supraventricular, junctional, and ventricular tachycardia (monomorphic and polymorphic); and ventricular fibrillation have been reported.[30,31] Electrocardiographic manifestations also include T-wave flattening and increases in the QT interval and QT dispersion.[32] ST segment depression also has been described.[33] Repolarization effects seem to be common yet subtle and often go unrecognized. These effects are thought to promote tachydysrhythmias and, similar to other autonomic effects, ultimately result from the action of counterregulatory hormones (primarily epinephrine).[34] Tachydysrhythmias may be responsible for many cases of sudden, unexplained death in diabetics, particularly patients with early autonomic neuropathy, which results in sympathetic hyperactivity.[35] Bradycardia and heart block also can occur, but bradydysrhythmias seem to be much less common than tachydysrhythmias.[36] Both fetal bradycardia and tachycardia have been attributed to maternal hypoglycemia.[25,37] Hypoglycemia also has been associated with congestive heart failure, worsening heart failure, and sudden death in patients with heart failure, but in most cases, it is not clear that a causal relationship exists.[21,38]

Prolonged (>1 hour) hypoglycemia may lead to hypothermia, particularly if it occurs in the morning.[39,40] Neonates and infants also seem to be particularly susceptible to hypothermia. Less commonly, sympathetic hyperactivity secondary to hypoglycemia may cause hyperthermia. Other complications include respiratory failure and adult respiratory distress syndrome.[41] Cyanosis and respiratory failure have been noted in newborns and infants. Metabolic abnormalities commonly associated with hypoglycemia include hypokalemia; hypomagnesemia; hypophosphatemia[42]; and, rarely, hyponatremia, hypocalcemia, and metabolic acidosis. Serum insulin concentrations are always inappropriately high.

Neuroglycopenia initially causes impaired cognitive function manifested as altered affect, perception, and personality; difficulty with calculations, concentration, memory, and speech; and delirium.[17–20,25–29] Ataxia, blurred vision, dizziness, fatigue, headache, generalized weakness, and malaise also may be noted. Neonates, infants, and young children may exhibit irritability and feeding problems. If neuroglycopenia persists, progressive deterioration in the level of consciousness occurs, with manifestations ranging from agitation and seizures to lethargy and coma, with or without focal findings.[43–46] Seizures may be single

TABLE 70-1 Agents That Can Cause Hypoglycemia*

AGENT	MECHANISM
Akee fruit (unripe)	Inhibition of gluconeogenesis by hypoglycin A toxin
Anabolic steroids	Enhanced peripheral insulin effect
ACE inhibitors	Inhibition of catecholamine release/effects
β2-Agonists	Enhanced insulin secretion
β-Blockers	Inhibition of catecholamine effects
Bromocriptine	Inhibition of growth hormone secretion/catecholamine effects
Calcium	Enhanced insulin secretion
Clofibrate	Enhanced peripheral insulin effect
Disopyramide	Unknown
Ethanol	Inhibition of gluconeogenesis
Lidocaine	Unknown
Lithium	Unknown
NSAIDs[†]	Unknown
Para-aminobenzoic acid	Unknown
Pentamidine	Destruction of pancreatic β cells with release of insulin
Propoxyphene	Unknown
PNU	Destruction of pancreatic β cells with release of insulin
Quinidine/quinine	Enhanced insulin secretion
Salicylates[†]	Enhanced insulin secretion and peripheral insulin effect
Streptozocin	Destruction of pancreatic β cells with release of insulin
Sulfonamides[†]	Unknown

*Other agents, implicated on the basis of isolated case reports, include chlorpromazine, cocaine, haloperidol, orphenadrine, para-aminosalicylic acid, sulfinpyrazone, and valproate.
†These and other highly protein-bound agents, such as warfarin and phenytoin, also can enhance the effect of sulfonylureas by decreasing the protein binding of sulfonylureas.
ACE, angiotensin-converting enzyme; NSAIDs, nonsteroidal antiinflammatory drugs; PNU, N-3-pyridylmethyl-N′-p-nitrophenylurea, Vacor.

or recurrent and focal or generalized. Both brief and prolonged postictal periods have been described. Coma may be associated with decerebrate posturing, but brainstem reflexes, such as oculocephalic, oculovestibular, and pupillary reflexes, are usually preserved. Hemiplegia, with or without coma, and choreoathetosis also can occur. With prompt treatment, complete recovery is expected, but prolonged neuroglycopenia may result in permanent neurologic damage (e.g., cognitive dysfunction, cranial nerve palsies, cerebral infarction, coma, recurrent seizures, or death).

The time of onset and duration of hypoglycemia depend on the agent and dose involved. They also depend on the baseline glucose and the presence or absence of insulin antibodies and insulin resistance, with insulin-dependent diabetics tending to be less susceptible than nondiabetics to a given dose. Hypoglycemia after usual or slightly greater doses of insulin would be expected to begin around the time of peak effect of a therapeutic dose (see Table 70-1).[42] Because insulin typically is administered in the morning and late afternoon or evening, hypoglycemia most commonly occurs between noon and suppertime (from the morning dose) and during the late night or early morning hours (from the afternoon/evening dose). Larger doses likely would result in an earlier onset. Delayed onset of hypoglycemia also has been reported (23 hours for regular insulin, 30 hours for NPH insulin, and 44 hours for Lente insulin).[47] The duration of action seems to be dose related, with persistent or recurrent hypoglycemia lasting up to 6 days after massive insulin overdose.[48] Although serum insulin concentrations do not seem to correlate with the severity of hypoglycemia, they do correlate with its duration, with hypoglycemia persisting until insulin concentrations return to normal.[48,49]

The incidence of hypoglycemia during sulfonylurea therapy seems to be related to the half-life of the agent involved, occurring more frequently with agents that have longer half-lives. In this setting, hypoglycemia most commonly occurs in the afternoon. In children with accidental sulfonylurea ingestions, the time of onset of hypoglycemia ranges from 0.5 to 16 hours, with 50% occurring within 2 hours and 96% occurring within 8 hours, and a single tablet is potentially toxic.[50,51] Data based on dispensing errors indicate that therapeutic doses also are potentially toxic in nondiabetic adults, but hypoglycemia sometimes may not occur until after the second or third dose. A single or extra therapeutic dose is unlikely to cause hypoglycemia in an adult diabetic. Although patients with intentional overdose often present with hypoglycemia long after ingestion (up to 48 hours),[52] the maximal interval between ingestion and symptom onset in these patients is unclear. The duration of hypoglycemia seems to be dose related and typically ranges from hours to several days, although a case lasting 27 days has been reported.[53]

Biguanide-Induced Lactic Acidosis

Biguanide-induced lactic acidosis may occur acutely after large intentional overdose in adults,[54–57] but it has not been described after the accidental ingestion of 1 or 2 tablets by young children.[58] More commonly, this complication occurs when a therapeutic dose is increased, or patients on long-term therapy develop conditions that decrease drug or lactate metabolism or increase lactate production (see under Pathophysiology).[8–14] In these settings, onset typically is

insidious. Symptoms are nonspecific and include anorexia, lethargy, nausea, vomiting, diarrhea, thirst, and abdominal pain. Hyperpnea and signs of dehydration, hypoxia, or shock may be present. Laboratory evaluation reveals an increased anion gap metabolic acidosis with elevated plasma lactate (>5 mEq [or mmol]/L) and, to a lesser extent, pyruvate and alanine levels.[59] In the aerobic form of acidosis, drug levels, blood urea nitrogen, and serum creatinine are increased, and anuria often is present.[60] In the anaerobic form, drug levels may be normal or mildly elevated, and blood urea nitrogen and serum creatinine tend to be elevated to a lesser degree. Ketosis (of unclear origin) may or may not be present.[12,61] Mortality is low with aerobic acidosis but may be as high as 50% in the anaerobic form, in which it is due primarily to predisposing conditions (see under Pathophysiology).[10,60]

Meglitinide, Glitazone, and α-Glucosidase Inhibitor Overdose

Few or no data are available regarding meglitinide, glitazone, and α-glucosidase inhibitor overdose. Meglitinides can be expected to have a toxicity profile similar to that of the sulfonylureas. Glitazones and α-glucosidase inhibitors could potentiate the hypoglycemic action of other antidiabetic agents, with an onset and duration of action that are likely to be similar to those of their therapeutic effects. Both agents can cause hepatitis during long-term therapy. α-Glucosidase inhibitor overdose also would be expected to result in nausea, abdominal cramps, bloating, flatulence, and diarrhea.

DIAGNOSTIC CONSIDERATIONS

Although a blood glucose concentration of less than 70 mg/dL (3.9 mmol/L) is considered low, clinical hypoglycemia requires the presence of symptoms. Whipple's triad[27–29,62] for the diagnosis of hypoglycemia consists of low blood glucose, symptoms of hypoglycemia, and improvement after glucose administration. There are situations of clinical hypoglycemia, however, in which these criteria are not met, including the empirical administration of glucose when a blood sample cannot be obtained and failure to respond to glucose because irreversible neurologic damage has occurred. Patients with serious sulfonylurea toxicity may also not respond to intravenous glucose therapy.[52]

Signs and symptoms of hypoglycemia usually occur when the serum glucose level decreases to 40 to 45 mg/dL (2.2 to 2.5 mmol/L), but there is substantial individual variation. Although autonomic manifestations typically precede manifestations of neuroglycopenia, diabetics with autonomic neuropathy may be asymptomatic until symptoms of neuroglycopenia develop. Women tend to be asymptomatic at lower blood glucose concentrations than men, and children tend to be asymptomatic at lower values than adults. Symptoms are more likely to occur when glucose concentrations decrease rapidly or by a large amount and depend on the baseline glucose value. Symptoms can occur in diabetics with normal or even elevated glucose levels if they are accustomed to a higher baseline level and experience a rapid decline in their glucose concentrations. Conversely, when glucose levels slowly decline, such as with prolonged fasting, symptoms may be absent despite glucose levels of 20 to 30 mg/dL (1.1 to 1.6 mmol/L)[63] because high levels of free fatty acids and ketone bodies provide alternative energy substrate.

The differential diagnosis of hypoglycemia includes nonantidiabetic drug exposure (see Table 70-1),[18–20] a variety of medical conditions (Table 70-2), and antidiabetic agent poisoning. Direct inspection of all prescribed pills and independent confirmation of their identity by imprint code may disclose a medication error. Failure of the blood glucose concentration to normalize after intravenous glucose administration is usually a consequence of severe sulfonylurea poisoning.[52] The presence of low birth weight and other metabolic abnormalities (e.g., high lactate acidemia or high free fatty acid levels, ketosis) in a neonate suggests an inborn error of metabolism.[64] Although virtually any neurologic manifestation, including focal findings, is consistent with a diagnosis of hypoglycemia, failure of the dysfunction to respond to normalization of the blood glucose concentration should prompt evaluation (e.g., computed tomography scan, lumbar puncture) for conditions such as central nervous system infarction, infection, or hemorrhage.

After clinical evaluation, if the cause of hypoglycemia is not apparent, measurement of serum insulin, C peptide, and proinsulin levels and toxicology testing may be helpful.[21] To interpret hormone levels properly, samples must be obtained at the time of hypoglycemia. Insulin secretion normally is suppressed and insulin and C peptide levels are low when hypoglycemia is present. When hypoglycemia is due to exogenous insulin or to oral hypoglycemics and other agents and conditions that enhance endogenous insulin secretion (see Tables 70-1 and 70-2), however, serum insulin concentrations are elevated. Except with exogenous

insulin exposure, C peptide also is elevated. An alternative, more sophisticated approach is to determine the molar ratio of insulin to C peptide.[65] Because C peptide has a longer half-life than insulin, this ratio is less than 1, unless exogenous insulin has been administered. This relationship seems to hold for patients with renal failure, who may have abnormally high baseline levels of insulin and C peptide, but not for diabetics who have insulin antibodies, which can elevate insulin levels falsely. Diabetics with insulin antibodies who have insulin-like activity (i.e., autoimmune hypoglycemia) have low C peptide levels, whereas diabetics with insulin antibodies who lack such activity (e.g., diabetics with insulin resistance) have elevated C peptide levels.[66]

Proinsulin levels also are elevated when hypoglycemia is due to enhanced endogenous insulin secretion.[67] Insulinomas can be differentiated from other causes by the presence of an increased ratio of proinsulin to insulin. Although sulfonylurea overdose also can produce these findings, proinsulin levels are not nearly as high as they are with insulinomas. An inappropriately low level of IGF-1 binding protein[68] and exaggerated insulin[69] and glycemic (>30 mg/dL increase in blood glucose level)[70] responses to glucagon also are seen in patients with endogenous hyperinsulinemia, with the latter being a potentially useful rapid bedside test.

Nonantidiabetic drugs often can be detected by routine, comprehensive urine toxicology screening. Detection of oral hypoglycemic agents and measurement of insulin concentration require more sophisticated laboratory methods that are not routinely available. For the laboratory investigation of potential antidiabetic agent poisoning, it is advisable to consult with laboratory personnel to determine the appropriate specimen (blood or urine) and test for detecting or measuring the suspected agent or agents involved.

TREATMENT

Hypoglycemia

Although standard life-support measures sometimes may be required, increasing the blood glucose level is often all that is necessary when hypoglycemia is the underlying cause of physiologic derangement. This is the rationale for performing a rapid bedside glucose determination or empirically administering glucose in patients with altered mental status, the hallmark of neuroglycopenia. It has even been suggested that *D* (dextrose) or *S* (sugar) be added to the well-known *ABC* (airway, breathing, circulation) resuscitation mnemonic (i.e., *ABCD* or *ABC'S*).[71] Supportive care also should include correction of fluid and electrolyte abnormalities.

The preferred treatment for hypoglycemia is dextrose (*d*-glucose). As discussed earlier, this diagnosis requires that symptoms be present. Giving dextrose to patients with a history of antidiabetic agent exposure (e.g., acute intentional or unintentional overdose) who have a low blood glucose level but are asymptomatic not only obscures the diagnosis but also may delay the onset of symptoms and necessitate monitoring for a longer period than otherwise might be necessary. The administration of glucose to asymptomatic patients with sulfonylurea overdose seems to be responsible for most cases in which the onset of hypoglycemia occurred more than 8 hours after ingestion.

TABLE 70-2 Medical Conditions That Can Cause Hypoglycemia

Decreased Glucose Availability

Decreased glucose absorption: diarrhea, malabsorption syndromes

Decreased glucose intake: fasting, acute or chronic malnutrition due to illness or starvation, vomiting

Inability to synthesize glucose: inborn errors of metabolism (gluconeogenic enzyme deficiency)

Inability to synthesize, store, or metabolize glycogen: inborn errors of metabolism (glycogen synthesis and glycogenolysis enzyme deficiency, glycogen storage diseases), liver disease (especially acute hepatic failure, Reye's syndrome), end-stage renal failure

Increased Glucose Utilization

Deficiency of counterregulatory hormones: adrenal, pancreatic, pituitary and thyroid disease

Increased insulin activity or secretion: insulin antibodies with insulin-like activity (pseudohyperinsulinemia), pancreatic β-cell adenoma (insulinoma) or ductal overgrowth (neonatal nesidioblastosis), reactive hypoglycemia (dumping syndrome, postprandial)

Increased metabolic demands: fever/sepsis, large tumor loads, pregnancy

Lack of alternative energy sources: decreased fat stores (malnutrition), inability to metabolize or mobilize fat (carnitine deficiency)

Indications for ICU Admission in Antidiabetic Agent Poisoning

Patients with unstable vital signs or unstable cardiac rhythm and evidence of myocardial ischemia or acute infarction associated with hypoglycemia

Patients with neurologic dysfunction that persists despite normalization of the blood glucose and for those with significant acidemia owing to biguanide poisoning

Note:

ICU admission is not routinely indicated for the monitoring of asymptomatic patients with a history of antidiabetic agent overdose and the monitoring and treatment of those with reversible hypoglycemia, but it may be necessary if continuous observation, frequent blood testing for glucose and other analytes, and therapy for hypoglycemia cannot be provided elsewhere.

Cardiac monitoring is not routinely necessary for patients who are asymptomatic or have reversible hypoglycemia, but it may be appropriate for those with underlying cardiovascular disease.

Dextrose can be given orally to patients who are awake and cooperative. Chewable 5-g tablets and 40% (w/w) gels containing 10 g of dextrose/25 g of gel are available. The usual adult dose is 10 to 20 g. Alternatively, candy or a cup of fruit juice with several teaspoons of added sugar can be given. Table sugar (sucrose) may not be effective, however, for patients taking α-glucosidase inhibitors. Oral glucose solutions should not be given to patients who lack adequate protective airway reflexes because aspiration can result in pulmonary edema.[72]

Intravenous dextrose is necessary for patients who cannot take it orally. Dextrose is available in a variety of formulations, with 50-mL ampules of 10%, 25%, and 50% solutions (i.e., D10, D25, and D50) containing 5 g, 12.5 g, and 25 g of dextrose, respectively, being the most common. The 50% solution can be used in adults and children, but lower concentrations are recommended for infants and neonates. The goal of therapy is to increase the serum glucose to normal levels (70 to 110 mg/dL [3.9 to 6.1 mmol/L]). Care should be taken not to overtreat because hyperglycemia stimulates endogenous insulin secretion and promotes recurrent hypoglycemia. This phenomenon of rebound hyperinsulinemia after glucose administration, which has been well documented in sulfonylurea poisoning,[52] also seems to occur after insulin overdose.[73] It can lead to a vicious cycle of alternating hyperglycemia and hypoglycemia, making treatment unduly complicated. In addition, there are wide individual variations in the magnitude of rise in serum glucose in response to a given dose of intravenous dextrose.[74,75] For these reasons, starting with a relatively low dose of dextrose (0.25 g/kg) and repeating it a few minutes later if the glucose level remains low are recommended. Except in prolonged neuroglycopenia resulting in permanent brain damage and in severe sulfonylurea poisoning, return to normal mental status can be expected to occur rapidly (within seconds to minutes of dextrose administration).

Proper functioning of the intravenous line should be confirmed before administering intravenous dextrose because these solutions are extremely hypertonic (2525 mOsm/L for D50) and can cause tissue necrosis if extravasation occurs. They also can cause vein irritation, with pain, phlebitis, and venous thrombosis. Rapid administration also can cause hyperosmolarity and consequent central nervous system dysfunction. For these reasons, slow injection (over several minutes) is recommended. Other potential complications include fluid overload, hypokalemia, hypophosphatemia, and hypomagnesemia. Because dextrose can precipitate Wernicke's encephalopathy in patients with thiamine deficiency, the coadministration of thiamine (100 mg orally, intramuscularly, or intravenously) is prudent for patients at risk for this condition (e.g., alcoholics and malnourished patients).

If an intravenous line cannot readily be established, intramuscular or subcutaneous glucagon, 1 mg for adults and children weighing more than 20 kg and 0.5 mg for children weighing less than 20 kg, can be given.[1-3] Glucagon increases serum glucose by enhancing glycogenolysis. Clinical effects are slower in onset than they are with intravenous dextrose, with return to normal mental status occurring in 5 to 20 minutes. Glucagon may be ineffective if hepatic stores of glycogen are diminished (e.g., in malnourished patients). Because effects may be transient, supplemental glucose should be given subsequently. Glucagon, like glucose, stimulates insulin secretion and can promote recurrent hypoglycemia.[76] Vomiting is a relatively common side effect.

Patients who respond to dextrose or glucagon then should be fed a meal. Diabetics with therapeutic misadventures involving insulin or an antihyperglycemic agent are unlikely to experience recurrent hypoglycemia and can be discharged, provided that they can monitor their blood glucose at home and have a responsible third party stay with them. Medication dosage adjustment also may be necessary. Patients with intentional insulin overdose and intentional or unintentional oral hypoglycemic agent exposure are at risk for delayed or recurrent hypoglycemia and require prolonged and frequent or continuous clinical monitoring with hourly blood glucose determinations, which generally can be accomplished only in an emergency, intermediate, or intensive care unit setting. A 6- to 12-hour period of observation (depending on the preparation involved) is prudent for patients with intentional insulin overdose who remain asymptomatic or become so after initial therapy. The optimal period of observation for patients with oral hypoglycemic agent exposures is controversial, with recommendations ranging from 6 to 8 hours[51,77,78] to 12 to 24 hours.[79-81] I prefer a conservative approach (i.e., longer observation).

Recurrent hypoglycemia, which is particularly common after sulfonylurea overdose, should be treated initially with an intravenous bolus of dextrose as described earlier. A continuous infusion of D10 also should be given, starting at a basal glucose requirement rate of about 0.1 g/kg/hr or 1 mL/kg/hr and adjusted upward as necessary.[82] This therapy may not be successful because it stimulates insulin secretion and may necessitate high doses, which often are prohibited by volume constraints and pain at the infusion site. Although giving higher concentrations of dextrose through a central venous line is one option, administration of an inhibitor of insulin secretion, such as diazoxide (Hyperstat) or octreotide (Sandostatin), makes more sense in terms of efficacy and safety. Adjunctive therapy with corticosteroids and glucagon has not been shown to be effective.[52] As noted earlier, glucagon can cause rebound hyperinsulinemia with subsequent hypoglycemia and may complicate therapy. Although the use of an artificial pancreas was reported to be beneficial in preventing fluctuations in blood glucose,[83] such aggressive, expensive, and technically difficult therapy seems unwarranted.

Diazoxide is a vasodilator antihypertensive agent that is related structurally to thiazide diuretics.[1,3] It also interacts with ATP-sensitive and voltage-sensitive potassium channels on the pancreatic β-cell membrane (possibly at the sulfonylurea receptor site) and prevents their closing or prolongs their opening, with consequent promotion of potassium efflux, membrane stabilization, and inhibition of calcium influx and insulin secretion, effects that are opposite to those of the sulfonylureas. When used for the treatment of sulfonylurea-induced hypoglycemia, diazoxide is given as an intravenous infusion rather than by rapid bolus injection (as for hypertension).[52] The initial dose, 3 mg/kg administered over 30 minutes, can be repeated every 4 hours or followed by an infusion of 1 mg/kg/hr. When used in this manner and setting, no significant side effects have been reported. Although tachycardia and orthostatic hypotension are common, the risk of clinically significant hypotension seems to be negligible. The other main side effect of diazoxide, sodium and water retention, could add to the free water effects of dextrose therapy. Patients receiving this therapy should be monitored for volume overload and have frequent blood pressure measurements.

Octreotide is a synthetic analogue of the naturally occurring pituitary gland hormone somatostatin.[1,3] Similar to somatostatin, it regulates the function of the pituitary gland, pancreas, and intestine by inhibiting the secretion of insulin, glucagon, and other hormones from these organs (see Chapter 159 for full details). To treat oral hypoglycemic poisoning, octreotide usually is given subcutaneously in a dose of 1 to 2 μg/kg every 8 hours.[84] Continuous infusions also have been used. When used in this setting, no significant side effects have been reported.

Presently, there are insufficient data to support either of these insulin secretion inhibitors as the superior antidote for sulfonylurea poisoning. Octreotide was found to be superior to diazoxide in preventing hypoglycemia in glipizide-poisoned volunteers.[85] It was so effective that some subjects did not even require supplemental glucose. There is more published experience with diazoxide in sulfonylurea overdose patients, however. Although no studies have directly compared octreotide and diazoxide in this population, I believe that availability, cost, drug familiarity, ease of administration, and side effect profile favor the octreotide. The fact that rebound hyperinsulinemia also may occur after insulin overdose suggests that either octreotide or diazoxide may be helpful in preventing recurrent hypoglycemia in this setting.

When a second episode of hypoglycemia occurs, more episodes are likely. Because the risk of recurrence and the duration of risk are variable and unpredictable, however, the optimal duration of insulin secretion inhibitor therapy is unknown. One approach is an initial treatment period of 24 hours followed by close monitoring for hypoglycemia for another 12 to 24 hours, because delayed recurrence of hypoglycemia has been reported after such therapy.[84,85] Should another episode of hypoglycemia occur, reinstitution of treatment for an additional 24 hours should be considered.

Measures to prevent drug absorption and enhance drug elimination also should be considered. Gastric decontamination measures may be appropriate for acute oral overdoses involving hypoglycemic agents and biguanides. Activated charcoal adsorbs sulfonylureas[86] and is the preferred modality. Surgical excision of tissue from the site of injection of insulin overdose has been reported,[87,88] but the efficacy of this intervention is anecdotal, and the necessity of performing it remains questionable. Multiple-dose activated charcoal therapy and urinary alkalization enhance the elimination of chlorpropamide[89] and probably other sulfonylureas. Although charcoal hemoperfusion also can enhance the elimination of chlorpropamide (and probably other sulfonylureas), this therapy should be considered only in patients with renal failure and intentional (i.e., large) overdoses.[90]

Biguanide-Induced Lactic Acidosis

The treatment of biguanide poisoning is supportive.[11,12,57] Intravenous saline should be given to correct dehydration, with caution not to cause fluid overload in patients with decreased urinary output. Intravenous saline also should enhance the elimination of metformin, but the efficacy of inducing diuresis for this purpose, although theoretically attractive, has not been proved. Severe acidosis (i.e., pH <7.1) should be treated with intravenous sodium bicarbonate. Insulin also may be effective.[11] Hemodialysis, using a high-bicarbonate bath, should be considered for refractory acidosis.[55,91] It also is effective in removing lactate, pyruvate, ketones, and metformin (but not phenformin) and as supportive therapy for uremia. Continuous venovenous hemofiltration, using lactate-free volume replacement fluid, also has been used to treat refractory acidosis.[57] Although not approved currently for human use, sodium dichloroacetate, a stimulant of pyruvate dehydrogenase, which catalyzes the decarboxylation of pyruvate to acetyl coenzyme A, thereby decreasing lactate production and increasing lactate disposal, has been shown to prevent and reverse lactic acidosis and to increase cardiac output directly in biguanide-poisoned animals.[92]

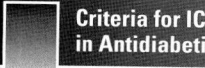

Criteria for ICU Discharge in Antidiabetic Agent Poisoning

Normal vital signs, normal cardiac rhythm, and no sign of hypoglycemia-induced cardiac ischemia

Resolution or stabilization of hypoglycemia-induced neurologic dysfunction

In the case of biguanides, resolution of the metabolic acidosis

Common Errors in Antidiabetic Agent Poisoning

Failure to consider the possibility of occult exposure to antidiabetic agents or their surreptitious use in patients with unexplained hypoglycemia, particularly those who are health care workers or relatives of diabetics

Failure to include exposure to nonantidiabetic drugs and potential drug interactions in the differential diagnosis of hypoglycemia

Failure to appreciate that a blood glucose level less than 70 mg/dl (3.9 mmol/L), while statistically abnormal, is not sufficient to make a diagnosis of hypoglycemia; that there is substantial individual variability in the glucose level at which signs and symptoms of hypoglycemia develop; that an abnormally low blood sugar be may seen in individuals who are asymptomatic, particularly women and children; that some individuals, especially diabetics, may exhibit signs and symptoms of hypoglycemia at normal or even elevated blood glucose levels; and that the administration of glucose solely on the basis of an abnormally low blood glucose level is unnecessary and will obscure the diagnosis of antidiabetic agent poisoning

Failure to appreciate that sulfonylurea-induced hypoglycemia may be delayed in onset and prolonged in duration and that an extended period of observation is required for patients with unintended or excessive exposure to such agents

Failure to appreciate that the oral administration of table sugar and complex carbohydrates may not be effective in treating hypoglycemia in patients taking alpha-glucosidase inhibitors

Failure to appreciate that overzealous treatment of hypoglycemia resulting in hyperglycemia will stimulate insulin secretion and can promote recurrent hypoglycemia, particularly in patients with sulfonylurea poisoning

Key Points in Antidiabetic Agent Poisoning

1. Hypoglycemia, the hallmark of antidiabetic agent poisoning, can result from exposure to hypoglycemic agents, which cause hyperinsulinemia either directly (exogenous insulin) or indirectly by enhancing endogenous insulin release (sulfonylureas and meglitinides), or to antihyperglycemic agents, which do not cause hypoglycemia when taken alone but which enhance the tissue action of insulin (biguanides and glitazones) or prevent the intestinal absorption of carbohydrates (alpha-glucosidase inhibitors) and thus potentiate the effect of hypoglycemic agents.

2. Signs and symptoms of hypoglycemia are due to central nervous system dysfunction resulting from the lack of essential energy substrate (neuroglycopenia) and autonomic dysfunction (sympathetic hyperactivity) caused by the effects of counter-regulatory hormones, primarily epinephrine.

3. The magnitude of increase in blood glucose that occurs in response to exogenous glucose administration, the preferred treatment for hypoglycemia, is variable and unpredictable, making it difficult to avoid causing hyperglycemia, a phenomenon that occurs most commonly, but not exclusively, in sulfonylurea poisoning.

Key Points in Antidiabetic Agent Poisoning   *continued*

4. The administration of octreotide, which inhibits endogenous insulin secretion, can prevent rebound hyperinsulinemia and decrease the incidence of recurrent hypoglycemia resulting from glucose therapy in patients with sulfonylurea-induced hypoglycemia.

5. Biguanides, by inhibiting gluconeogenesis and thus hepatic lactate uptake and utilization, can cause lactic acidosis following acute overdose and under conditions of reduced drug elimination or increased lactate production. Therapy is primarily supportive, with extracorporeal elimination being reserved for refractory acidosis.

REFERENCES

1. Davis SN, Granner DK: Insulin, oral hypoglycemic agents, and the pharmacology of the endocrine pancreas. In Hardman JG, Limbird LE, Molinoff PB, et al (eds): Goodman and Gilman's the Pharmacological Basis of Therapeutics, 9th ed. New York, McGraw-Hill, 1996, pp 1487–1517.
2. Sims EAH, Calles-Escandon J: Insulin, glucagon, and oral hypoglycemics in the treatment of diabetes mellitus. In Munson PL, Mueller RA, Breese GR (eds): Principles of Pharmacology: Basic Concepts and Clinical Applications, rev reprint. New York, Chapman & Hall, 1996, pp 697–723.
3. McEvoy GK, Litvak K, Welsh OH, et al (eds): AHFS Drug Information. Bethesda, 2000, American Society of Health-System Pharmacists.
4. Ferner RE, Chaplin S: The relationship between the pharmacokinetic and the pharmacodynamic effects of oral hypoglycemic drugs. Clin Pharmacokinet 12:397–401, 1987.
5. Malaisse WJ: Stimulation of insulin release by non-sulfonylurea hypoglycemic agents: The meglitinide family. Horm Metab Res 27:263–266, 1995.
6. Massi-Benedetti M, Damsbo P: Pharmacology and clinical experience with repaglinide. Expert Opin Invest Drugs 9:885–898, 2000.
7. Bailey CJ, Turner RC: Metformin. N Engl J Med 334:574–579, 1996.
8. McGuinness ME, Talbert RL: Phenformin-induced lactic acidosis: A forgotten adverse drug reaction. Ann Pharmacother 27:1183–1187, 1993.
9. Enia G, Garozzo M, Zoccali C: Lactic acidosis induced by phenformin is still a public health problem in Italy. BMJ 315:1466–1467, 1997.
10. Luft D, Schmulling RM, Eggstein M: Lactic acidosis in biguanide-treated diabetics: A review of 330 cases. Diabetologia 14:75–87, 1978.
11. Misbin RI: Phenformin-associated lactic acidosis: Pathogenesis and treatment. Ann Intern Med 87:591–595, 1984.
12. Gan SC, Barr J, Arieff AI, et al: Biguanide-associated lactic acidosis: Case report and review of the literature. Arch Intern Med 152:2333–2336, 1992.
13. Lalau JD, Race JM: Lactic acidosis in metformin therapy. Drugs 58(Suppl 1):55–60, 1999.
14. Wiholm BE, Myrhed M: Metformin-associated lactic acidosis in Sweden 1977–1991. Eur J Clin Pharmacol 44:589–591, 1993.
15. Horikoshi H, Hashimoto T, Fujiwara T: Troglitazone and emerging glitazones: New avenues for potential therapeutic benefits beyond glycemic control. Prog Drug Res 54:191–212, 2000.
16. Parulkar AA, Pendergrass ML, Granda-Ayala R, et al: Nonhypoglycemic effects of thiazolidinediones. Ann Intern Med 134:61–71, 2001.
17. Spiller HA: Management of antidiabetic agents in overdose. Drug Saf 19:411–424, 1998.
18. Seltzer HS: Drug-induced hypoglycemia: A review of 1418 cases. Endocrinol Metab Clin North Am 18:163–183, 1989.
19. Chan JC, Cockram CS, Critchley JA: Drug-induced disorders of glucose metabolism: Mechanisms and management. Drug Saf 15:135–157, 1999.
20. Marks V, Teale JD: Drug-induced hypoglycemia. Endocrinol Metab Clin North Am 28:555–577, 1999.
21. Shilo S, Berezovsky S, Friedlander Y, et al: Hypoglycemia in hospitalized nondiabetic older patients. J Am Geriatr Soc 46:978–982, 1998.

continued

22. Klonoff DC, Barrett BJ, Nolte MS, et al: Hypoglycemia following inadvertent and factitious sulfonylurea overdosages. Diabetes Care 18:563–567, 1995.

23. Owen L, Ellis M, Shield J: Deliberate sulphonylurea poisoning mimicking hyperinsulinaemia of infancy. Arch Dis Child 82:392–393, 2000.

24. Roberge RJ, Martin TG, Delbridge TR: Intentional massive insulin overdose: Recognition and management. Ann Emerg Med 22:228–234, 1993.

25. Haymond MW: Hypoglycemia in infants and children. Endocrinol Metab Clin North Am 18:211–252, 1989.

26. Moore DF, Wood DF, Volans GN: Features, prevention, and management of acute overdose due to antidiabetic drugs. Drug Saf 9:218–229, 1993.

27. Field JB: Hypoglycemia: Definition, clinical presentations, classification, and laboratory tests. Endocrinol Metab Clin North Am 18:27–43, 1989.

28. Service FJ: Hypoglycemia. Med Clin North Am 79:1–8, 1995.

29. Cryer PE: Hypoglycemia: pathophysiology, diagnosis, and treatment. Oxford, Oxford University Press, 1997.

30. Odeh M, Oliven A, Bassan H: Transient atrial fibrillation precipitated by hypoglycemia. Ann Emerg Med 19:565–567, 1990.

31. Chelliah YR: Ventricular arrhythmias associated with hypoglycaemia. Anaesth Intensive Care 28:698–700, 2000.

32. Marques JL, George E, Peacey SR, et al: Altered ventricular repolarization during hypoglycaemia in patients with diabetes. Diabet Med 14:648–654, 1997.

33. Lindstrom T, Jorfeldt L, Tegler L, et al: Hypoglycaemia and cardiac arrhythmias in patients with type 2 diabetes mellitus. Diabet Med 9:536–541, 1992.

34. Shimada R, Nakashima T, Nunoi K, et al: Arrhythmia during insulin-induced hypoglycemia in a diabetic patient. Arch Intern Med 144:1068–1069, 1984.

35. Weston PJ, Gill GV: Is undetected autonomic dysfunction responsible for sudden death in type 1 diabetes mellitus? The 'dead in bed' syndrome revisited. Diabet Med 16:626–631, 1999.

36. Pollock G, Brady WJ Jr, Hargarten S, et al: Hypoglycemia manifested by sinus bradycardia: A report of three cases. Ann Emerg Med 3:700–707, 1996.

37. Kramer DC, Fleischer FS, Marx GF: Fetal bradycardia resulting from maternal hypoglycemia: A report of two cases. J Reprod Med 40:394–396, 1995.

38. Luu M, Stevenson WG, Stevenson LW, et al: Diverse mechanisms of unexpected cardiac arrest in advanced heart failure. Circulation 80:1675–1680, 1989.

39. Kedes LH, Field JB: Hypothermia: A clue to the diagnosis of hypoglycemia. N Engl J Med 271:785–787, 1964.

40. Passias TC, Meneilly GS, Mekjavic IB: Effect of hypoglycemia on thermoregulatory responses. J Appl Physiol 80:1021–1032, 1996.

41. Matsumura M, Nakashima A, Tofuku Y: Electrolyte disorders following massive insulin overdose in a patient with type 2 diabetes. Intern Med 39:55–57, 2000.

42. Arem R, Zoghbi W: Insulin overdose in eight patients: Insulin pharmacokinetics and review of the literature. Medicine 64:323–332, 1985.

43. Plum S, Posner JB: The Diagnosis of Stupor and Coma, 3rd ed. Philadelphia, FA Davis, 1980, pp 219–222.

44. Luber SD, Brady WJ, Brand A, et al: Acute hypoglycemia masquerading as head trauma: A report of four cases. Am J Emerg Med 14:543–547, 1996.

45. Gold AE, Marshall SM: Cortical blindness and cerebral infarction associated with severe hypoglycemia. Diabetes Care 14:309–315, 1997.

46. Spiller HA, Schroeder S, Ching DSY: Hemiparesis and altered mental status in a child after glyburide ingestion. J Emerg Med 16:433–435, 1998.

47. Stapczynski JS, Haskell RJ: Duration of hypoglycemia and need for intravenous glucose following intentional overdoses of insulin. Ann Emerg Med 13:505–511, 1984.

48. Samuels MH, Eckel RH: Massive insulin overdose: Detailed studies of free insulin levels and glucose requirements. Clin Toxicol 27:157–168, 1989.

49. Shibutani Y, Ogawa C: Suicidal insulin overdose in a type 1 diabetic patient: Relationship of serum insulin concentrations to the duration of hypoglycemia. J Diabetes Complications 14:60–62, 2000.

50. Quadrani DA, Spiller HA, Widder P: Five year retrospective evaluation of sulfonylurea ingestion in children. J Toxicol Clin Toxicol 34:267–270, 1996.

51. Spiller HA, Villalobos D, Krenzelok EP, et al: Prospective multicenter study of sulfonylurea ingestion in children. J Pediatr 131:141–146, 1997.

52. Palatnick W, Meatherall RC, Tenenbein M: Clinical spectrum of sulfonylurea overdose and experience with diazoxide therapy. Arch Intern Med 151:1859–1862, 1991.

53. Cienchanowski K, Borowiak KS, Potocka BA, et al: Chlorpropamide toxicity with survival despite 27-day hypoglycemia. Clin Toxicol 37:869–871, 1999.

54. McLelland J: Recovery from metformin overdose. Diabet Med 2:410–411, 1985.

55. Heaney D, Majid A, Junor B: Bicarbonate haemodialysis as a treatment of metformin overdose. Nephrol Dial Transplant 12:1046–1047, 1997.

56. Brady WJ, Carter CT: Metformin overdose. Am J Emerg Med 15:107–108, 1997.

57. Teale KF, Devine A, Stewart H, Harper NJ: The management of metformin overdose. Anaesthesia 53:698–701, 1998.

58. Spiller HA, Weber JA, Winter ML, et al: Multicenter case series of pediatric metformin ingestion. Ann Pharmacother 34:1385–1388, 2000.

59. Lalau JD, Race JM: Lactic acidosis in metformin-treated patients: Prognostic value of arterial lactate levels and plasma metformin concentrations. Drug Saf 20:377–384, 1999.

60. Lalau JD, Lacroix C, Compagnon P, et al: Role of metformin accumulation in metformin-associated lactic acidosis. Diabetes Care 18:779–784, 1995.

61. Jurovich MR, Wooldridge JD, Force RW: Metformin-associated nonketotic metabolic acidosis. Ann Pharmacother 31:53–55, 1997.

62. Whipple AO: The surgical therapy of hyperinsulinism. J Int Chir 3:237–245, 1938.

63. Merimee TJ, Tyson JE: Stabilization of plasma glucose during fasting: normal variations in two separate studies. N Engl J Med 291:1275–1278, 1974.

64. Stanley CA: Hyperinsulinism in infants and children. Pediatr Clin North Am 44:363–374, 1997.

65. Lebowitz MR, Blumenthal SA: The molar ratio of insulin to C peptide: An aid to the diagnosis of hypoglycemia due to surreptitious (or inadvertent) insulin administration. Arch Intern Med 153:650–655, 1993.

66. Kim MR, Sheeler LR, Mansharamani N, et al: Insulin antibodies and hypoglycemia in diabetic patients. Endocrine 6:285–291, 1997.

67. Hampton SM, Beyzavi K, Teale D, et al: A direct assay for proinsulin and its applications in hypoglycemia. Clin Endocrinol 29:9–16, 1988.

68. Matchinsky FM, Sweet IR: Annotated questions and answers about glucose metabolism and insulin secretion of β-cells. Diabetes Rev 4:130–144, 1996.

69. Kumar D, Mehtalia S, Miller L: Diagnostic use of glucagon-induced insulin response: Studies in patients with insulinoma or other hypoglycemia conditions. Ann Intern Med 80:697–701, 1974.

70. Feingold DN, Stanley CA, Baker L: Glycemic response to glucagon during fasting hypoglycemia: An aid in the diagnosis of hyperinsulinism. J Pediatr 96:257–259, 1980.

71. Losek JD: Hypoglycemia and the ABC'S (Sugar) of pediatric resuscitation. Ann Emerg Med 35:43–46, 2000.

72. Kaneki T, Kubo K, Sone S, et al: Acute pulmonary edema caused by accidental aspiration of sweetened water in two cases of diabetes mellitus. Intern Med 37:969–972, 1998.

73. Bayly GR, Ferner RE: Persistent insulin secretion after insulin overdose in a non-diabetic patient. Lancet 341:370, 1993.

74. Adler PM: Serum glucose changes after administration of 50% dextrose solution: Pre- and in-hospital calculations. Am J Emerg Med 4:504–506, 1986.

75. Balentine JR, Gaeta TJ, Kessler D, et al: Effect of 50 milliliters of 50% dextrose in water administration on the blood sugar of euglycemic volunteers. Acad Emerg Med 5:691–694, 1998.

76. Thoma ME, Glauser J, Genuth S: Persistent hypoglycemia and hyperinsulinemia: Caution in using glucagon. Am J Emerg Med 14:99–101, 1996.

77. Erickson T, Arora A, Lebby TI, et al: Acute oral hypoglycemic ingestions. Vet Hum Toxicol 33:256–258, 1991.

78. Robertson WO: Sulfonylurea ingestions: Hospitalization not mandatory. J Toxicol Clin Toxicol 35:115–118, 1997.

79. Burkhart KK: When does hypoglycemia develop after sulfonylurea ingestion? Ann Emerg Med 31:771–772, 1998.

80. Borowski H, Caraccio T, Mofenson H: Sulfonylurea ingestion in children: Is an 8-hour observation period sufficient? J Pediatr 133:584–585, 1998.

81. Szlatenyi CS, Capes KF, Wang RY: Delayed hypoglycemia in a child after ingestion of a single glipizide tablet. Ann Emerg Med 31:773–776, 1998.

82. Fasching P, Roden M, Stuhlinger HG, et al: Estimated glucose requirement following massive insulin overdose in a patient with type 1 diabetes. Diabet Med 11:323–325, 1994.

83. Gin H, Larnaudie B, Aubertin J: Attempted suicide by insulin injection treated with artificial pancreas. BMJ (Clin Res Ed): 287:249–250, 1983.

84. McLaughlin SA, Crandall CS, McKinney PE: Octreotide: An antidote for sulfonylurea-induced hypoglycemia. Ann Emerg Med 36:133–138, 2000.

85. Boyle PJ, Justice K, Krentz AJ, et al: Octreotide reverses hyperinsulinemia and prevents hypoglycemia induced by sulfonylurea overdoses. J Clin Endocrinol Metab 76:752–756, 1993.

86. Kannisto H, Neuvonen PJ: Adsorption of sulfonylureas onto activated charcoal in vitro. J Pharm Sci 73:253–255, 1984.

87. Campbell IW, Ratcliffe JG: Suicidal insulin overdose managed by excision of insulin injection site. BMJ (Clin Res Ed) 285:408–409, 1982.

88. McIntyre AS, Woolf VJ, Burnham WR: Local excision of subcutaneous fat in the management of insulin overdose. Br J Surg 73:538, 1986.

89. Neuvonen PJ, Karkkainen S: Effects of charcoal, sodium bicarbonate, and ammonium chloride on chlorpropamide kinetics. Clin Pharmacol Ther 33:386–393, 1983.

90. Lalau JD, Andrejak M, Moriniere P, et al: Hemodialysis in the treatment of lactic acidosis in diabetics treated by metformin: A study of metformin elimination. Int J Clin Pharmacol Ther Toxicol 27:285–288, 1989.

91. Ludwig SM, McKenzie J, Faiman C: Chlorpropamide overdose in renal failure: Management with charcoal hemoperfusion. Am J Kidney Dis 6:457–460, 1987.

92. Stacpoole PW: The pharmacology of dichloroacetate. Metabolism 38:1124–1144, 1989.

PART 4

Drugs of Abuse

CHAPTER 71

Gamma Hydroxybutyrate and Its Congeners

Patrick E. McKinney* ■ Steven A. McLaughlin ■ Robert B. Palmer

Gamma hydroxybutyric acid was synthesized by Laborit[1] in 1960 as a γ-aminobutyric acid (GABA) analogue, gamma hydroxybutyrate (GHB), that could cross the blood-brain barrier. Initial clinical investigations showed it to be a sedative-hypnotic agent without significant cardiovascular effects. These properties led to its subsequent use as an anesthetic induction agent, primarily in Europe and Japan, in the 1960s and 1970s.[2] Its use as an anesthetic agent was limited by lack of analgesic and muscle relaxant properties and by side effects, including vomiting, emergence delirium, and apparent seizure activity. Currently, GHB is being evaluated as a potential therapeutic agent for narcolepsy, insomnia, intensive care unit (ICU) sedation, ethanol dependence, and ethanol and opioid withdrawal and as an obstetric anxiolytic. There also is evidence that GHB may protect tissue against hypoxic/ischemic insults. It has been investigated as an organoprotective agent after ischemic insults to the heart, brain, and other organs and as an adjunct in preserving function and integrity of transplant organs while awaiting replantation. GHB also has become a valuable tool for producing clinical and electroencephalogram (EEG) absence-type seizures in animals, although it does not seem to have these effects in humans.[3]

Much of the initial illicit use of GHB can be traced to a study from Japan in the late 1970s, which showed that GHB administration was associated with an increased release of growth hormone in normal volunteers.[4] Although this and subsequent studies provided no data suggesting that the increased release of growth hormone was associated with any change in soft tissue composition or muscle mass, GHB began to be used as a dietary supplement by bodybuilders in hopes of increasing lean muscle mass.[5,6] Primarily available at health food stores and gyms, GHB also was marketed as a sleep aid and a general nutritional supplement. The growing popularity and increasing availability of GHB was accompanied by increasingly broad but unsubstantiated claims of efficacy, and manufacturers promoted it for sexual enhancement, stress relief, combating depression, weight loss, hair restoration, increasing longevity, and enhancing cognition and as a euphoriant. In 1990, reports of the use of GHB as a recreational drug began to surface, especially in the club/bar and rave dance populations, and these soon were followed by reports of toxicity and eventually death.[7] Actions initiated by the San Francisco Poison Center, the California state health department, and the U.S. Food and Drug Administration led to legislation first restricting production and sale and later restricting possession.[7] Additional legislation has been prompted by the use of GHB as a "date rape drug." Because GHB is manufactured easily from many widely used and easily available precursors, there has been some attempt to regulate these precursors as "designer drugs." The widespread use of some of these agents (gamma-butyrolactone [GBL] and 1,4-butanediol) in industry and commercial products is likely to prevent scheduling of these substances, although restrictions may be placed on their sale and availability.

CHEMISTRY AND BIOCHEMISTRY

GHB is a four-carbon carboxylic acid (Fig. 71-1) that typically is distributed as the sodium or potassium salt, which is a white crystalline solid. These salts are freely soluble in water, ethanol, and methanol. GHB salt solutions typically are clear and colorless, although some may have a yellow tinge or other coloring agents added (blue food coloring has been suggested as a marker by some users). Technical grade GHB is available through chemical supply companies. Large amounts of GHB available illicitly are produced through saponification of GBL (see Fig. 71-1). GHB is available illicitly in liquid, tablet, capsule, or powder form. Liquid formulations often are sold in small (approximately 6 oz) plastic bottles with multiple doses per bottle. Concentrations of the solutions are reported to vary widely.

*Patrick E. McKinney, MD, 1962–2003. Clinician, educator, friend. You are missed.

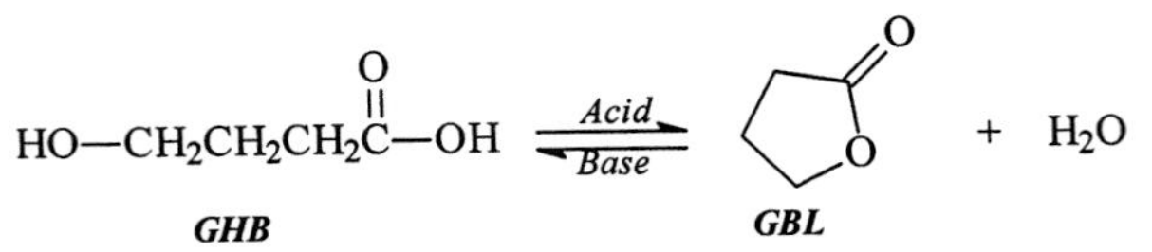

FIGURE 71-1

Saponification of gamma butyrolactone (GBL) to produce gamma hydroxybutyrate (GHB).

GBL is an oily solvent that exists in equilibrium with GHB in aqueous solution. Acid and base catalyzed methods of opening this lactone ring are known, but most recipes available on the Internet describe some variant of alkaline hydrolysis (saponification). GHB "kits" available over the Internet usually include premeasured (stoichiometrically correct) amounts of GBL and sodium hydroxide along with pH paper. Methods of preparation vary but usually involve dissolving sodium hydroxide in water with or without ethanol (an exothermic reaction), adding the lactone and heating. The reaction is continued for a recommended time or until a neutral pH has been reached. If the pH does not drop spontaneously to 7, an acid (vinegar, hydrochloric acid, or citric acid) is added. The resulting solution is reduced in volume through continued boiling and evaporation. The product, a concentrated aqueous solution of the sodium salt of GHB, is stored as a clear, slightly yellow liquid, or the salt may be precipitated and stored as a solid. Potential health risks of this procedure include caustic injury from dermal or ocular exposure to a boiling solution of sodium or potassium hydroxide and the risk of ingesting an incompletely reacted solution with alkaline pH. Residual sodium chloride or potassium chloride in the preparation is said to result in the characteristic salty taste. As legislative efforts restrict the availability of GBL, methods to synthesize this precursor from tetrahydrofuran or butyric acid derivatives may become more common. Structurally similar carboxylic acids or lactones, such as gamma valerolactone, may be substituted if GHB or GBL is not easily obtained. Gamma hydroxybutanol (1,4-butanediol) is a colorless oily liquid with a mild odor. It may be sold as a GHB prodrug. Structures of these agents are shown in Figure 71-2 and alternative names listed in Table 71-1.

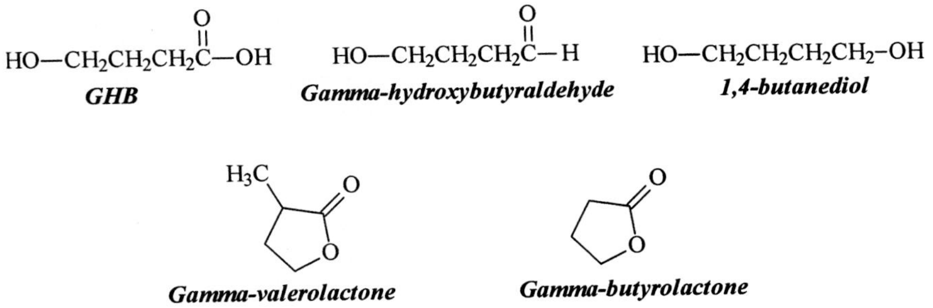

FIGURE 71-2

Gamma hydroxybutanol (1,4-butanediol) and structurally similar carboxylic acids and lactones. GHB, gamma hydroxybutyrate.

TABLE 71-1 Street and Chemical Names of Gamma Hydroxybutyrate and Its Congeners

Gamma Hydroxybutyrate

Street Names
GHB, γ-OH, Easy Lay, Everclear, Georgia Home Boy, Great Hormones at Bedtime, Grievous Bodily Harm, Goops, Liquid X, Liquid E, Natural Sleep-500, Oxy-sleep, Gamma-O, Liquid Ecstasy, Nature's Quaalude, Oxy-Sleep, Poor Man's Heroin, Salty Water, Scoop, Soap, Somatomax PM, Somsanit, Vita-D, Water, Wolfies, Zonked, Growth Hormone Booster, Cherry Meth, KGHB

Chemical Names
Butanoic acid, 4-hydroxy, monosodium salt, γ-hydroxybutyric acid, 4-hydroxybutanoic acid, sodium oxybate (product names: sodium oxybutyrate, 4-hydroxybutyrate, γ-hydrate), CAS 502-85-2

Gamma Butyrolactone

Street Names
Fire Water, RenewTrient, Blue Nitro, Blue Nitro Vitality, Revivarant, Revivarant G, GH Revitalizer, Remforce, Gamma-G

Chemical Names
Gamma butyrolactone, γ-hydroxybutyric acid lactone, 4-butyrolactone, 1,4-butanolide, 2(3)-furanone dihydro, dihydro-2(3)-furanone, 4-butanolide, 2(3H) furanone dihydro, tetrahydro-2-furanone, CAS 96-48-0

1,4-Butanediol

Street Names
Pine needle oil, Fubar, BlueRaine, Thunder, Dream on, SomatoPro

Chemical Names
1,4-Butanediol, 1,4-butylene glycol, 1,4-dihydroxybutane, 1,4-tetramethylene glycol CAS 110-63-4

Gamma Hydroxybutyraldehyde:
Fully reduced succinic semialdehyde (Revitalize Plus)

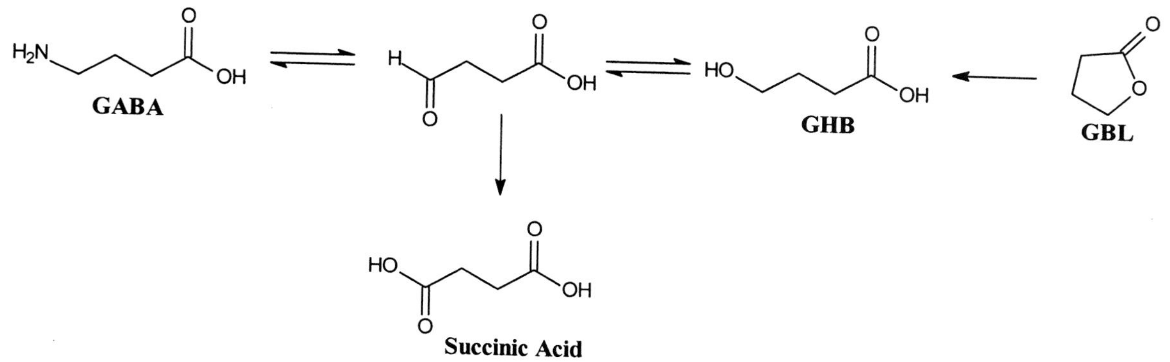

FIGURE 71-3

Metabolism of γ-aminobutyric acid (GABA), succinic acid, gamma hydroxybutyrate (GHB), and gamma butyrolactone (GBL).

PHARMACOKINETICS

GHB is an endogenous metabolite of the inhibitory neuro-transmitter, GABA (Fig. 71-3). GABA is transaminated to succinate semialdehyde, which is reduced to GHB. This reaction is reversible (i.e., GHB may be metabolized to GABA, or it may enter the tricarboxylic acid cycle to be metabolized to water and carbon dioxide).[8] GHB appears to show nonlinear absorption and distribution kinetics.[9] Related compounds, such as GBL and 1,4-butanediol, can be converted in vitro to GHB, or they can be ingested as prodrugs with in vivo conversion to GHB. GBL may undergo hydrolysis to GHB in the stomach. 1,4-Butanediol is metabolized in peripheral tissues by alcohol/aldehyde dehydrogenase to gamma hydroxybutyraldehyde and then to GHB in a manner similar to that of alcohols such as ethanol.[10] There is minimal aldehyde dehydrogenase activity in the brain, however, and 1,4-butanediol may be metabolized to GHB via enzymatic pathways independent of aldehyde dehydrogenase in the brain.[11] Ethanol and fomepizole may inhibit the in vivo conversion of 1,4-butanediol to GHB.[11,12]

Pharmacokinetics of Gamma Hydroxybutyrate and Its Congeners

Volume of distribution: 0.3 L/kg
Protein binding: <1%
Mechanism of clearance: hepatic
Half-life: 20–53 min
Active metabolites: gamma hydroxybutyrate (GHB), none; gamma butyrolactone (GBL), GHB; 1,4-butanediol, GBL, GHB
Methods to enhance clearance: none

PATHOPHYSIOLOGY OF TOXIC EFFECTS AND THERAPEUTIC POTENTIAL

Mechanism of Action

GHB is an endogenous neuromodulator whose exact mechanism of action has not been defined completely. It is found in the central nervous system (CNS) at micromolar concen-trations and at higher concentrations in peripheral tis-sues.[13,14] GHB administration is associated with changes in the synthesis and release of several neurotransmitters in animal models. Supratherapeutic doses of GHB seem to be associated with increased levels of acetylcholine in the CNS.[15] GHB also has been shown to increase serotonin and 5-hydroxyindolacetic acid (5-HIAA) in areas of rat brain.[16] Norepinephrine release in the hypothalamus may be inhibited by GHB, whereas endogenous opioid-like substances may be modulated in the striatum.[17] GHB does not seem to bind directly to opioid receptors.[18] Modulation of the dopaminer-gic system seems to be an important facet of GHB activity, as an endogenous compound and as an exogenously adminis-tered pharmaceutical agent. GHB seems to decrease dopamine release, leading to accumulation of dopamine within nerve terminals.[19] Data also suggest, however, that GHB may stimu-late dopamine release later. Other evidence suggests that lower doses inhibit and higher doses stimulate dopamine release.[20] A third line of evidence suggests that GHB inhibits dopamine release in awake animals but stimulates release in anesthetized models.[17,21] A variety of factors may modify the effect of GHB on dopamine synthesis and release, but it is difficult to extrapolate these data to clinical cases of human intoxication at this point.

In addition to modulating other neurotransmitters, GHB binds to at least two receptor types within the CNS. GHB binds with low affinity to the $GABA_B$ receptor, producing membrane hyperpolarization that can be antagonized by the $GABA_B$ antagonist CGP 35348.[22,23] An alternative expla-nation of the apparent GHB binding to the $GABA_B$ receptor suggests that GHB is metabolized first to GABA at loca-tions proximate to the $GABA_B$ receptor, and it is GABA derived from GHB that binds to this receptor.[24] GHB does not seem to bind to $GABA_A$ receptors.[25]

A GHB-specific receptor that is distinct from the $GABA_B$ binding site has been shown in the brain.[26] In the rat, the GHB binding sites are present in the highest concentrations in the cerebral cortex, hippocampus, and olfactory bulbs.[27] The pons, the medulla, most of the hypothalamus, and the peripheral tissues lack these high-affinity binding sites.[28] Evidence from rat brains suggests that these receptors are linked to G proteins and that receptor binding is mediated by calcium channels and is accompanied by an increase in cyclic guanosine monophosphate and inositol phosphate.[29–31] Mod-ulation of dopamine activity may be related to stimulation of the GHB receptor.[32] Other dopamine-modulating drugs, including prochlorperazine and (−)-sulpiride, also bind to the GHB receptor.

A variety of agents have been tested as antagonists or reversal agents for some or all of the properties of GHB. An experimental agent, NCS-382, is a selective GHB receptor antagonist, but it is not clinically available and may not reverse all of the effects of pharmacologic doses of GHB.[33] Animal models of GHB intoxication show EEG patterns suggestive of petit mal and grand mal seizure activity. These EEG patterns can be reversed with valproate, phenobarbital, clonazepam, and ethosuximide.[20,34] These EEG patterns are not seen in humans receiving GHB, however. Naloxone, flumazenil, and physostigmine have been investigated as reversal agents and are discussed in the treatment section.

Dose Response

The clinical effects of GHB at doses ranging from 10 to 100 mg/kg are well studied. Doses of 10 mg/kg produce short-term memory dysfunction and hypotonia. Drowsiness and sleep are induced at doses of 20 to 30 mg/kg. Doses of 50 mg/kg reliably produce sleep, and higher doses produce a state of general anesthesia with bradycardia, hypoventilation, and other effects generally associated with GHB toxicity.[35] The lethal dose has been estimated to be 5 to 15 times the dose required to produce unconsciousness.[36,37] GHB often is used in combination with other CNS depressant agents, which may produce synergistic CNS depression.[38] Serum GHB concentrations of greater than 260 mg/L (>2.5 mmol/L) have been associated with coma and loss of airway reflexes, and levels of less than 52 mg/L (<0.5 mmol/L) are found in spontaneously awakening patients.[39]

Place in Therapy

GHB has been used for a variety of therapeutic indications. Initial investigations focused on its use as a general anesthetic agent, a purpose for which it still is used in some pediatric populations. Lack of analgesic properties and the presence of myoclonus/seizures have limited its use in modern anesthesia practice, however. The sedative effects of GHB led to its use as a sleep aid, although most current research focuses on its use in narcolepsy. GHB seems to preserve normal sleep architecture, inducing rapid-eye-movement sleep followed by slow-wave sleep, with minimal "hangover" effect.[40,41] GHB has been shown to reduce frequency of cataplexy and sleep attacks, hypnagogic hallucinations, and subjective nocturnal arousals in patients with narcolepsy.[42] Sleep studies in narcoleptic patients used a split nighttime dosing schedule because of rapid drug metabolism and the propensity for patients to awaken abruptly in the middle of the night.

GHB also has been shown to have a protective effect against ischemia-induced organ injury.[43] The mechanism of this protective effect has not been determined precisely but may involve decreased glucose utilization, altered cerebrovascular reactivity, or indirect free radical scavenging effects.[41,44] Currently, most of this research centers on GHB-mediated reduction in ischemic damage after stroke or coronary artery occlusion, but studies also have shown protection from ischemia related to sepsis, hemorrhagic shock, bowel ischemia, hepatic ischemia, fetal hypoxia, and other conditions.[45–47] The addition of GHB to solutions used to preserve transplant organs seems to prolong organ viability before replantation.[45] It is not known whether these organoprotective effects may afford some margin of safety in overdose patients who have cardiac or respiratory insufficiency during use.

Because of its neuroinhibitory properties, GHB has been used to treat ethanol and opioid withdrawal.[48,49] In clinical trials, GHB decreases ethanol withdrawal symptoms, including tremor, diaphoresis, nausea, and anxiety. In a model examining cocaine self-administration in rats, GHB decreased the frequency and total dose of cocaine administration, suggesting a potential role in the treatment of cocaine addiction.[50]

CLINICAL PRESENTATION AND LIFE-THREATENING COMPLICATIONS

γ-Hydroxybutyric acid and related compounds are CNS depressants that are abused for their ability to induce euphoria, hypnosis, and amnesia. Their clinical toxicity largely reflects these depressant effects. The toxicity of GHB precursors (GBL and 1,4-butanediol) is similar to the toxicity seen with the parent compound. GHB often is abused in conjunction with other drugs, including ethanol, amphetamines, cocaine, benzodiazepines, and marijuana.[51–54] Approximately 59% to 86% of GHB-intoxicated patients are male, with a mean age of 28 to 30 years (reported range 16 to 51 years).[51,52,55] The typical patient with GHB intoxication presenting to a health care facility is a young man with CNS and respiratory depression, vomiting, and mild bradycardia.

Fatalities from isolated GHB and 1,4-butanediol overdoses have been reported,[55,56] but most patients with GHB poisoning recover without apparent complications.[7,52,53,55,57] Most reported fatalities from GHB have occurred in mixed intoxications with ethanol,[58] heroin,[59] or other drugs. The potentially life-threatening effects of GHB are CNS depression with loss of airway reflexes, vomiting with a potential for aspiration, respiratory depression, injury, and occasionally symptomatic bradycardia or other cardiac dysrhythmias. The CNS effects of GHB seem to be increased by ethanol and other CNS depressants. Chronic ethanol users may develop tolerance to the sedating effects of GHB.[60] Table 71-2 provides a summary of clinical effects.

γ-Hydroxybutyric acid can be used intravenously, but most illicit exposures are through ingestion of tablets, capsules, or liquid solutions. The onset of symptoms after oral overdose is rapid, typically occurring within 15 to 30 minutes.[37] The purity of powders sold as GHB is highly variable, making accurate dose calculation difficult and inadvertent overdose possible. High-purity GHB (97% to 99%) provides 2.9 g of GHB per level teaspoon.[53] The normal recreational dose of GHB ranges from 1.5 g to slightly more than 5 g.[7,53,61]

The primary neurologic effect of GHB is dose-related CNS depression with spontaneous awakening as GHB concentrations decline.[39] One series reported a Glasgow Coma Scale (GCS) score of 3 in 25% of patients, 4 to 8 in 32% of patients, and 14 to 15 in only 19% of patients.[52] Other common findings are myoclonus, tremor, amnesia, dizziness,

TABLE 71-2 Clinical Effects of Gamma Hydroxybutyrate*

CARDIOVASCULAR	RESPIRATORY	NEUROLOGIC	GASTROINTESTINAL	METABOLIC
Bradycardia	*Respiratory*	*CNS depression*	Nausea	*Respiratory*
Hypotension	*depression*	*Coma*	Vomiting	*acidosis*
Hypertension	*Apnea*	*Myoclonus*	Caustic burns	Metabolic
ECG changes	Aspiration	Seizures		acidosis
	Cheyne-Stokes	Miosis > mydriasis		Hypernatremia
		Headache		Hypokalemia
		Ataxia		Hyperglycemia
		Agitation		
		Incontinence		
		Euphoria		
		Amnesia		
		Dizziness		
		EPS		
		Withdrawal		

*Common effects in *italics*.
CNS, central nervous system; ECG, electrocardiogram; EPS, extrapyramidal side effects.

euphoria, disinhibition, incontinence, hypotonia, headache, and ataxia.[7,35,53,57,62,63] Pupillary abnormalities are common, with miosis being more common than mydriasis. Agitation may develop, especially during painful procedures, such as endotracheal intubation, lumbar puncture, or Foley catheter placement, and during awakening from coma.[54] The CNS depression typically lasts 1 to 3 hours with complete recovery by 6 to 8 hours.[52,53] Patients with more profound coma require longer to recover.[52] Other effects that have been noted occasionally include nystagmus,[64] extrapyramidal side effects[64] hallucinations, dystonias, and hypomania.[53,65]

Although seizures have been reported in 9% of patients with GHB intoxication,[53,66–69] most studies[52,54,55,57,63,70] have shown that generalized seizures do not occur commonly. This discrepancy may result from the misdiagnosis of myoclonus as generalized convulsive activity. Alternatively, generalized tonic-clonic seizures may occur secondary to hypoxia.

The cardiovascular effects of GHB include mild bradycardia, mild hypotension, and occasional electrocardiogram (ECG) abnormalities. Bradycardia is seen when GHB is used recreationally and for anesthesia.[52,63,71] It is usually mild, with an average decrease of 8 beats/min below baseline, and rarely causes hemodynamic compromise in the setting of anesthesia.[63,71] In a series of 88 GHB-intoxicated patients, 32 (36%) developed bradycardia, but only 1 patient required treatment with atropine.[52] Of the remaining patients in this series, 10 (11%) had an initial systolic blood pressure of less than 90 mm Hg, 6 (7%) were bradycardic, and all of these patients had a coingestion of alcohol or other drugs. It also was noted that patients with a lower GCS score were more likely to be bradycardic.[52] Mild hypertension also has been reported with therapeutic intravenous administration of GHB.[72] A variety of ECG abnormalities have been documented, which are discussed in the diagnosis section.

The respiratory effects of GHB include primarily dose-related respiratory depression, Cheyne-Stokes respirations, and apnea. Virtually all of the case series and case reports describe some degree of respiratory depression.[7,52,54,55,57,63,70,73–75] The respiratory depression is usually mild, with a mean increase in PCO_2 of 4 mm Hg in patients given 70 mg/kg of intravenous GHB.[63] In a series of 30 GHB-intoxicated patients, 21 had a PCO_2 of greater than 45 mm Hg with pH values ranging from 7.24 to 7.34.[52] Apnea has been reported in adults and children.[7,54,74,76] Despite the significant CNS and respiratory depression, many patients have been managed without endotracheal intubation, although more recent data suggest that the rate of endotracheal intubation is higher than previously estimated.[52–55,77] Endotracheal intubation may be difficult in these patients because of procedure-induced agitation, even in cases of near-apnea.[54]

Gastrointestinal toxicity includes nausea and vomiting, commonly seen after oral or intravenous GHB administration.[52,63] Emesis occurs in 22% to 30% of patients with GHB intoxication, and most patients with emesis have a lowered GCS score, increasing the risk of aspiration.[52,66]

Hypothermia has been reported in 25% to 31% patients in some series but has not been seen in other clinical settings.[52–54] In a rat model, GHB doses of 5 to 10 mg/kg produced hyperthermia, whereas doses of 300 to 500 mg/kg produced hypothermia.[78] In general, the hypothermia associated with GHB seems to be mild and may be treated easily by simple noninvasive warming techniques.[63]

Metabolic effects of GHB intoxication include metabolic acidosis, hypokalemia, hypernatremia, diaphoresis, hyperglycemia, and increased growth hormone and prolactin concentrations.[4,37,66] There is one reported case of Wernicke-Korsakoff syndrome occurring in a 24-year-old woman with a history of GHB use, anorexia, and remote ethanol abuse.[79]

Indirect toxicity secondary to adulterants or the persistence of alkaline reagents used in GBL saponification has been reported and includes reports of alkali burns to the mouth, esophagus, and airway from ingestion of illicitly manufactured GHB containing residual sodium hydroxide.[80] Tolerance to the effects of GHB and its precursors can occur with repeated dosing over time, and there seems to be cross-tolerance to the effects of ethanol and benzo-diazepines.[60,81,82] A GHB withdrawal syndrome including anxiety, tremors, diarrhea, tachycardia, diaphoresis, hyper-tension, insomnia, confusion, hallucinations, and paranoia also has been described and may occur within hours of a missed dose.[64,79,81–85] The GHB withdrawal syndrome occurred in 50% of patients in one small series and lasted 3 to 15 days.[81,82] Withdrawal symptoms can progress to severe delirium and autonomic instability similar to ethanol withdrawal. There are no controlled data to suggest an optimal treatment or prevention plan, but reported cases suggest that supportive care, with attention to electrolyte balance, vital signs, and treatment with benzodiazepines, produces optimal outcomes.[82,86]

Overall the clinical presentation of GBL or 1,4-butanediol toxicity is similar to that of GHB.[87–91] The reported cases describe CNS and respiratory depression, vomiting, bradycar-dia, and myoclonus. The duration of toxicity seems to be about 3 to 5 hours. Fatalities have been reported from isolated GBL and 1,4-butanediol ingestions.[91,92] GBL is rapidly hydrolyzed in the body to GHB, the active form, by peripheral lactonases. GBL is absorbed more rapidly from the gastro-intestinal tract, which may decrease the first-pass effect and result in increased plasma drug concentrations compared with equivalent doses of GHB.[93] GBL may be expected to be more potent on a volume basis, have a more rapid onset of toxicity, and have a longer duration of action.[13,93,94]

DIAGNOSIS

A patient with GHB intoxication typically presents with coma, respiratory depression, mild bradycardia, and vomit-ing. The pupils may be miotic, although midposition and mydriatic pupils have been reported. The patient may respond to painful stimuli with agitation before falling back into a coma. Occasionally, there may be myoclonic move-ments of the trunk and extremities. The physical exami-nation is otherwise largely unrevealing. This toxidrome does not provide many specific clues to separate GHB from other sedative-hypnotic exposures.

The history and description of the scene may be helpful in raising the suspicion of GHB poisoning. History of prior GHB use or the presence of bottles labeled as containing GHB, GBL, or 1,4-butanediol is helpful. Unlabeled GHB can appear as a clear or colored liquid or a white powder, which may be of limited diagnostic value. Because GHB often is used at parties, raves, and nightclubs and by weightlifters and bodybuilders, an increased suspicion is indicated in these situations. Emergency medical service providers, witnesses, and friends of the patient may be able to provide valuable information about recent events and the names of any ingested substances.

The differential diagnosis of GHB intoxication reflects the main symptom of depressed mental status and includes the following medical conditions: CNS infection, CNS mass, CNS trauma, cerebrovascular accident, intracranial hemor-rhage, hyperglycemia or hypoglycemia, thyroid disease,

seizures, uremia, electrolyte abnormalities, and hepatic encephalopathy. Possible toxicologic causes of the same pre-sentation include intoxication with opioids, benzodiazepines, barbiturates, carbon monoxide, cocaine, ethylene glycol, methanol, isopropyl alcohol, phenothiazines, phencyclidine, ketamine, other sedative-hypnotics, and ethanol.

No specific laboratory investigations are required in GHB-poisoned patients. A bedside capillary blood glucose measurement is indicated if the patient has an altered level of consciousness. An arterial blood gas evaluation is indi-cated in patients with signs of hypoventilation or hypoxia. Serum electrolytes and salicylate and acetaminophen levels may be indicated in certain patients, especially when diag-nosis is uncertain (see Chapter 2). A urine drug screen may be helpful to identify coingestants but rarely has any effect on treatment or disposition of GHB intoxication as a single-substance poisoning.

ECG findings in GHB poisoning are nonspecific. Reported ECG changes include bradycardia, transient P-wave inversions in lead II in 20% of cases,[63] U waves, right bundle-branch block, and first-degree atrioventricular block.[54,74] Transient atrial fibrillation also has been reported.[52] The most important role of the ECG may be to rule out ingestion of other cardiotoxic agents with similar clinical presentations (e.g., digoxin). There does not seem to be any role for routine radiography in the management of GHB toxicity or exposure. A chest radiograph may be indi-cated in patients with possible aspiration, with respiratory distress, and after endotracheal intubation.

GHB is not detected in routine urine and serum toxico-logic screens. Most common clinical laboratory techniques (e.g., immunoassay) are poorly suited for quantitative assess-ment of GHB and GBL concentrations. Although a qualita-tive screening test for GHB in urine has been reported,[95] it is not in widespread use in clinical laboratories. Most cases of GHB intoxication can be managed adequately without labora-tory determination of GHB concentrations.

In selected forensic cases, quantitation of GHB or ana-logues may be useful; however, accurate quantitation of these compounds in biologic matrices is a significant analytic challenge. The difficulty is due to its chemical structure and the presence of GHB as an endogenous substance. The sim-ple structure and small molecular size make development of an antibody with high specificity for immunoassay diffi-cult. The parent molecule also is suited poorly for gas chromatographic analysis owing to difficult extraction from biologic matrices and poor peak shape. Rapid elimination kinetics (a 100-mg/kg dose of GHB may be undetectable in the urine by 12 hours) and extensive hepatic metabolism to other compounds (<5% of an oral dose of GHB is elimi-nated unchanged in the urine) make prompt sample collec-tion vital to drug detection.[96]

Despite these challenges, many analytic methods have been reported for GHB and GBL quantitation. Among these are gas chromatography with flame ionization detec-tion, electron capture detection, mass spectral detection, and high-performance liquid chromatography methods using detection techniques such as ultraviolet-visible spec-trophotometry and thermospray mass spectrometry.[61,97] Treatment of GHB with acid drives the GHB-GBL equi-librium to the ring-closed lactone (GBL) (see Fig. 71-1), which is far more amenable to organic extraction and gas chromatography analysis.[98] Extraction recoveries vary by the specific method employed but range from approximately 63% to 83%.[97] The obvious disadvantage of converting GHB to GBL before analysis is that this method disallows simultaneous analysis of relative concentrations of GHB and GBL.

Simultaneous monitoring of relative concentrations of GHB and GBL has been accomplished through the use of high-performance liquid chromatography with ultraviolet-visible and thermospray mass spectrometry.[99] Techniques that can discriminate between GHB and GBL in the urine have been used in situations in which the direct detection of GHB is important,[61,100] although the accuracy of relative concentration measurements of these compounds in biologic samples has been questioned.[97]

Interpretation of postmortem GHB concentrations is problematic. Endogenously produced GHB usually is not detectable (levels <1 mg/L) in the blood or urine of living humans. Postmortem blood levels (refrigerated, fluoride treated) of GHB of 168 mg/L (typical range 12 to 25 mg/L) have been reported, however, in forensic cases without a history of exposure to GHB. Much higher concentrations (433 mg/L) are reported in nonrefrigerated blood in the absence of sodium fluoride.[101,102] Urine samples do not seem to be susceptible to the mechanisms that produce this artifactual rise in GHB concentrations in postmortem blood.[102]

TREATMENT

The treatment of GHB toxicity centers on protecting the airway with support of oxygenation and ventilation, while ruling out other ingestions or disease states that require specific therapy. The toxicity from acute GHB ingestions is short-lived, and patients generally do well with simple supportive measures. Clinicians should be vigilant for signs of airway compromise, respiratory failure, aspiration, and coingestants because these are the most likely contributors to poor patient outcomes.

Patients with probable GHB poisoning should be in a closely monitored environment with intravenous access, continuous cardiac and blood pressure monitoring, and pulse oximetry. Equipment and personnel for emergent airway management should be immediately available. Initial evaluation should include a bedside capillary blood glucose measurement and consideration of a trial of naloxone and empirical administration of thiamine, especially if the patient appears to be debilitated or suffering from alcoholism or malnutrition.

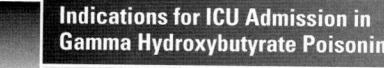

Indications for ICU Admission in Gamma Hydroxybutyrate Poisoning

Intubated patient
Uncertain diagnosis
Hemodynamic instability
Suicidal intent
Failure to arouse in the emergency department
Aspiration pneumonitis

Airway management of GHB-intoxicated patients is controversial. Some data suggest that selective intubation of deeply GHB-intoxicated comatose patients is safe and effective.[52,53] Despite coma and near-apnea, however, patients may respond violently to attempted intubation[70,103] and may require sedation or paralysis to facilitate the procedure. GHB-intoxicated patients with loss of airway protective reflexes, hypercarbia, or hypoxia not responsive to supplementary oxygen should be intubated. Especially in a mixed ingestion with GHB and another CNS depressant, the risk of vomiting and aspiration or apnea is high, and careful management of the airway either invasively or noninvasively is crucial to good patient outcomes.[52]

Gastrointestinal decontamination, if done, must be instituted rapidly because these agents are absorbed rapidly from the gastrointestinal tract, especially when consumed in a liquid form.[35] Because of the high incidence of altered mental status, airway compromise, and vomiting, induction of emesis is not recommended. Because GHB is absorbed rapidly and patients do well with supportive care, gastric lavage is not likely to be beneficial. Activated charcoal and cathartic can be considered in patients with large, recent (within 1 hour) ingestions and patients with coingestants in which gastrointestinal decontamination is an appropriate therapeutic intervention (see Chapter 5). Caution should be exercised when giving activated charcoal to patients who have altered mental status from GHB due to the high incidence of vomiting and airway compromise.

Most patients with GHB-induced bradycardia are asymptomatic and hemodynamically stable.[52,63] Adequate oxygenation and ventilation with continuous monitoring of vital signs are adequate in the asymptomatic bradycardic patient. Cases of bradycardia with hypotension have been reported,[52,75] and atropine has been used successfully to treat these patients.[52]

GHB is more likely to cause myoclonic movements than generalized seizures in acute overdose. Myoclonus can be managed with observation and supportive care (see earlier). Management of generalized seizure activity includes initial attention to the airway and breathing, then use of benzodiazepines or barbiturates to control persistent seizures. No other specific therapy is needed for seizures in GHB poisoning.

There are no specific antidotes for GHB poisoning in humans. The dopaminergic, EEG, and behavioral effects of GHB have been reversed by naloxone in two animal models.[104,105] A third study showed that high-dose naloxone failed to reverse GHB-induced narcosis in mice.[106] The relevance of these animal data to human clinical practice is uncertain. Naloxone seems to have no effect on GHB-poisoned or 1,4-butanediol-poisoned patients in a clinical setting.[54,70,73,74,80,103] Flumazenil reduces GHB-induced growth hormone release in humans[107] and antagonizes GHB intoxication in mice when given before GHB.[108] Flumazenil has failed to show any effect, however, in reversing clinical GHB toxicity.[70,75] Physostigmine effectively reversed the sedative effects of GHB in two patients with GHB overdose.[109] A second case series described three patients with GHB overdose treated with intravenous physostigmine, with equivocal results.[110] Some improvement in level of consciousness was noted, but it was not associated clearly with the administration of physostigmine and may have reflected

Criteria for ICU Discharge in Gamma Hydroxybutyrate Poisoning

Return of normal mental status (Glasgow Coma Scale score = 15)
Hemodynamically stable
Extubated and able to maintain patent airway

the natural course and rapid resolution of GHB intoxication. Physostigmine also has been used with some success as a reversal agent in patients undergoing GHB-induced anesthesia.[111,112] These studies were uncontrolled or confounded by the presence of neuromuscular blocking agents and a delay from physostigmine injection to possible response. At this time, there are no clear data to support physostigmine as an effective reversal agent. In addition to its limited proven benefit are the potential safety concerns of administering physostigmine to an overdose patient, including the development of seizures, bradycardia (including exacerbation of GHB-associated bradycardia), cholinergic syndrome, and death.

There are no data to suggest a role for extracorporeal removal of GHB from acutely intoxicated patients. Most patients with GHB intoxication awaken spontaneously within 4 to 6 hours, so it is appropriate to observe a stable, breathing patient in the emergency department.[53,63,68,70,103,113] Clinical experience to date suggests that patients who are asymptomatic after 6 hours can be discharged safely. Patients who are intubated, are unstable, show signs of aspiration, or have other significant coingestions should be admitted to the ICU. Reported rates of ICU admission for GHB-intoxicated patients range from 0% to 43%.[52,53,55] When the diagnosis is uncertain, there is suicidal ideation, or the patient does not improve within 6 hours, consideration of admission to an ICU or subacute floor should be renewed.

SPECIAL POPULATIONS

Pediatric Patients

Children may ingest GHB inadvertently, especially in its liquid form, because it often is stored in small plastic bottles or beverage containers.[74] Adolescents may encounter GHB as a recreational drug of abuse or in the underground athletic community, or they may be given the drug surreptitiously, sometimes with the intent of sexual assault.[114] The profile of GHB toxicity in children generally reflects what is seen in adults. Children who received intravenous GHB ($\geq$70 mg/kg intravenous) as part of a sedative protocol for a variety of procedures showed most of the expected clinical effects of sedation (bradycardia, vomiting, and mild respiratory insufficiency). Of 54 cases, 12 also developed transient P-wave inversion on the ECG.[63] Two cases of GHB toxicity have been reported in the pediatric population. The first was a 9-year-old boy who presented apneic and pulseless and recovered after 18 hours with supportive care.[74] The second case was a 12-year-old boy who presented with apnea, vomiting, and a GCS score of 6 unresponsive to naloxone. Although he required endotracheal intubation and gastrointestinal decontamination, he recovered within 4 hours. The ECG was notable for a transient right bundle-branch pattern.[74]

A 14-month-old boy had a decreased level of consciousness, flaccidity, and vomiting 1 hour after an accidental GBL ingestion. He recovered without treatment in 5 hours.[89]

An inborn error of metabolism caused by deficiency of succinic semialdehyde dehydrogenase results in the accumulation of GHB in the absence of ingestion.[115] Clinical findings in patients with this disorder are variable but may include delayed development, hypotonia, behavioral problems, and more serious manifestations. These patients have elevated concentrations of GHB in blood and urine.[115] Another autosomal dominant inherited disease, startle disease, has been postulated to be related to a defect in the GHB receptor.[116]

Pregnant Patients

No specific information exists regarding the treatment of GHB toxicity in pregnancy. It has been found to decrease uterine contractility and minimize hypoxic insult to the fetus in animal models. GHB is known to cross the placenta but has not been noted to cause fetal distress and increased uterine contractions.[36,37,72]

Elderly Patients

No specific information exists regarding the clinical syndrome or treatment of GHB toxicity in the elderly. It may be expected to have a longer half-life in patients with hepatic dysfunction or decreased hepatic blood flow from vascular or cardiac disease.

Other Special Populations

One case of GHB toxicity has been described in a patient with human immunodeficiency virus type 1 who took his usual dose of GHB after beginning ritonavir and saquinavir therapy. He became unresponsive and was intubated. The investigators hypothesized that these antiretroviral drugs inhibited GHB metabolism through their activity on the cytochrome P-450 system.[117] GHB dehydrogenase is inhibited by many anticonvulsant drugs, including barbiturates, valproate, ethosuximide, trimethadione, and salicylate.[118] Administration of these substances in rats results in increased CNS concentrations of GHB.[119] The clinical significance of these data is unclear.

Key Points in Gamma Hydroxybutyrate Poisoning

1. Gamma hydroxybutyrate, gamma butyrolactone, and 1,4-butanediol are commonly available chemicals that are used frequently as drugs of abuse.
2. The gamma hydroxybutyrate clinical syndrome most commonly consists of central nervous system depression, nystagmus, respiratory depression, and miosis. Myoclonus and vomiting also occur commonly.
3. Cardiovascular effects include electrocardiogram changes, bradycardia, and hypotension.
4. The clinical effects may be profound and may require cardiorespiratory support, but the toxicity is short-lived (patients usually awaken within 4 to 6 hours).
5. No specific antidote currently is available.
6. Laboratory confirmation is difficult and requires specialized assays that may not be available on a stat basis.

Common Misconceptions about Gamma Hydroxybutyrate Poisoning

1. There is a specific antidote for gamma hydroxybutyrate (GHB) intoxication.
2. GHB is detected on a urine drug screen.
3. GHB-intoxicated patients do not require aggressive airway management or intensive care unit admission.

REFERENCES

1. Laborit H: Sodium 4-hydroxybutyrate. Int J Neuropharmacol 3:433–452, 1964.
2. Laborit G, Larcan A, Kind A: Le gamma Hydroxybutyrate en anesthesie neuro-chirurgicale. Neurochirurgie 8:104–107, 1962.
3. Entholzner E, Mielke L, Pichlmeier R, et al: EEG changes during sedation with gamma-hydroxybutyric acid. Anaesthetist 44:345–350, 1995.
4. Takahara J, Yunoki S, Yakushiji W, et al: Stimulatory effects of gamma-hydroxybutyric acid on growth hormone and prolactin release in humans. J Clin Endocrinol Metab 44:1014–1017, 1977.
5. Racagni G, Apud JA, Cocchi D, et al: GABAergic control of anterior pituitary hormone secretion. Life Sci 31:823–838, 1982.
6. Gerra G, Marcato A, Fertonani Affini G, et al: Gamma-hydroxybutyric acid (GHB) and neuroendocrine function in humans. Neuroendocrinol Lett 7:55–63, 1994.
7. Dyer JE, Kreutzer R, Quattrone A, et al: Multistate outbreak of poisonings associated with illicit use of gamma hydroxy butyrate. MMWR Morb Mortal Wkly Rep 39:861–863, 1990.
8. Vayer P, Mandel P, Maitre M: Conversion of γ-hydroxybutyrate to γ-aminobutyrate in vitro. J Neurochem 45:810–814, 1985.
9. Palatini P, Tedeschi L, Frison G, et al: Dose dependent absorption and elimination of gamma-hydroxybutyric acid in healthy volunteers. Eur J Clin Pharmacol 45:353–356, 1993.
10. Barker SA, Snead OC III, Poldrugo F, et al: Identification and quantification of 1,4-butanediol in mammalian tissues: An alternative biosynthetic pathway for gamma hydroxybutyric acid. Biochem Pharmacol 34:1849–1852, 1985.
11. Poldrugo F, Snead OC: 1,4 Butanediol and ethanol compete for degradation in rat brain and liver in vitro. Alcohol 3:367–370, 1986.
12. Quang L, Maher T, Shannon M, et al: Pretreatment of CD-1 mice with 4-methylpyrazole (4-MP) blocks 1,4-butanediol (BD) toxicity (Abstract). J Toxicol Clin Toxicol 38:527, 2000.
13. Roth RH, Giarman NJ: Natural occurrence of gamma-hydroxybutyrate in mammalian brain. Biochem Pharmacol 19:1087–1093, 1970.
14. Nelson T, Kaufman EE, Kline E, et al: The extraneural distribution of gamma hydroxybutyrate. J Neurochem 37:1345–1348, 1981.
15. Giarman NJ, Schmidt KF: Some neurochemical aspects of the depressant action of γ-butyrolactone on the central nervous system. Br J Pharmacol 20:563–568, 1963.
16. Waldmeier PC, Fehr B: Effects of baclofen and gamma-hydroxybutyrate on rat striatal and mesolimbic 5-HT metabolism. Eur J Pharmacol 49:177–184, 1978.
17. Hechler V, Gobaille S, Bourguinon JJ, et al: Extracellular events induced by gamma-hydroxybutyrate in striatum: A microdialysis study. J Neurochem 56:938–944, 1991.
18. Feigenbaum JJ, Simantov R: Lack of effect of γ-hydroxybutyrate on μ, δ and κ opioid receptor binding. Neurosci Lett 212:5–8, 1996.
19. Walters JR, Rosh RH, Aghajanian GK: Dopaminergic neurons: Similar biochemical and histochemical effects of γ-hydroxybutyrate and acute lesions of the nigrostriatal pathways. J Pharmacol Exp Ther 186:630–639, 1973.
20. Tunnicliff G: Sites of action of gamma-hydroxybutyrate (GHB)—a neuroactive drug with abuse potential. J Toxicol Clin Toxicol 35: 581–590, 1997.
21. Howard SG, Feigenbaum JJ: Effect of γ-hydroxybutyrate on central dopamine release in vivo: a microdialysis study in awake and anesthetized animals. Biochem Pharmacol 53:103–110, 1997.
22. Nissbrandt H, Engberg G: The GABA$_B$-receptor antagonist, CGP 35348, antagonizes γ-hydroxybutyrate and baclofen induced alterations in locomotor activity and forebrain dopamine levels in mice. J Neural Transm 103:1255–1263, 1996.
23. Xie X, Smart TG: γ-Hydroxybutyrate hyperpolarizes hippocampal neurons by activating GABA$_B$ receptors. Eur J Pharmacol 212:291–294, 1992.
24. Hechler V, Ratomponirina C, Maitre M: γ-Hydroxybutyrate conversion into GABA induces displacement of GABA$_B$ binding that is blocked by valproate and ethosuximide. J Pharmacol Exp Ther 281:753–760, 1997.
25. Serra M, Sanna E, Foddi C, et al: Failure of gamma-hydroxybutyrate to alter the function of GABA$_A$ receptor complex in rat cerebral cortex. Psychopharmacology 104:351–355, 1991.
26. Benavides J, Rumigny JF, Bourguignon JJ, et al: A high-affinity, Na+-dependent uptake system for γ-hydroxybutyrate in membrane vesicles prepared from rat brain. J Neurochem 38:1570–1575, 1982.
27. Hechler V, Weissman D, Mach E, et al: Regional distribution of γ-[^{3}H]Hydroxybutyrate binding sites as determined by quantitative autoradiography. J Neurochem 49:1025–1032, 1987.
28. Hechler V, Gobaille S, Maitre M: Selective distribution pattern on γ-hydroxybutyrate receptors in the rat forebrain and midbrain as revealed by quantitative autoradiography. Brain Res 572:345–348, 1992.
29. Ratomponirina C, Hode Y, Hechler V, et al: γ-Hydroxybutyrate receptor binding in rat brain is inhibited by guanyl nucleotides and pertussis toxin. Neurosci Lett 189:51–53, 1995.
30. Cash CD, Gobaille S, Kemmel V, et al: γ-Hydroxybutyrate receptor function studied by the modulation of nitric oxide synthase activity in rat frontal cortex punches. Biochem Pharmacol 58:1815–1819, 1999.
31. Vayer P, Maitre M: γ-Hydroxybutyrate stimulation of the formation of cyclic GMP and inositol phosphates in rat hippocampal slices. J Neurochem 52:1382–1387, 1989.
32. Chrapusta SJ, Karoum F, Egan MF, et al: γ-Butyrolactone-sensitive and -insensitive dopamine release, and their relationship to dopamine metabolism in three rat brain regions. Eur J Pharmacol 222:129–135, 1992.
33. Schmidt C, Gobaille S, Hechler V, et al: Anti-sedative and anticataleptic properties of NCS-382, a gamma-hydroxybutyrate receptor antagonist. Eur J Pharmacol 203:393–397, 1991.
34. Vayer P, Gobaille S, Mandel P, et al: 3'-5' cyclic-guanosine monophosphate increase in rat brain hippocampus after gamma-hydroxybutyrate administration: Prevention by valproate and naloxone. Life Sci 41:605–610, 1987.
35. Kam PCA, Yoong FFY: Gamma-hydroxybutyric acid: An emerging recreational drug. Anaesthesia 53:1195–1198, 1998.
36. Vickers MD: Gamma hydroxybutyric acid. Proc R Soc Med 61:821–823, 1968.
37. Vickers MD: Gammahydroxybutyric acid. Int Anaesth Clin 7:75–89, 1969.
38. McCabe ER, Layne EC, Sayler DF, et al: Synergy of ethanol and a natural soporific—gamma hydroxybutyrate. Science 171:3441–3445, 1971.
39. Helric M, McAslan TC, Skolnik S, et al: Correlation of blood levels of 4-hydroxybutyrate with state of consciousness. Anesthesiology 25:771–775, 1964.
40. Mamelak M: Gamma hydroxybutyrate: An endogenous regulator of energy metabolism. Neurosci Biobehav Rev 13:187–198, 1989.
41. Mamelak M, Scharf MB, Woods M: Treatment of narcolepsy with γ-hydroxybutyrate: A review of clinical and sleep laboratory findings. Sleep 9:285–289, 1986.
42. Scrima L, Hartman PG, Johnson FH Jr, et al: Efficacy of gamma-hydroxybutyrate versus placebo in treating narcolepsy-cataplexy: Double-blind subjective measures. Biol Psychiatry 26:331–343, 1989.
43. Lavyne M, Hariri R, Tankosic T, et al: Effect of low dose gamma-butyrolactone therapy on forebrain neuronal ischemia in the unrestrained, awake rat. Neurosurgery 12:430–434, 1983.
44. Haller C, Mende M, Schuier F, et al: Effect of γ-hydroxybutyrate on local and global glucose metabolism in the anesthetized cat brain. J Cereb Blood Flow Metab 10:493–498, 1990.
45. Sherman IA, Saibil FG, Janossy TI: γ-Hydroxybutyrate mediated protection of liver function after long-term hypothermic storage. Transplantation 57:8–11, 1994.
46. Boyd AJ, Sherman IA, Saibal FG, et al: The protective effect of γ-hydroxybutyric acid in regional intestinal ischemia in the hamster. Gastroenterology 99:860–862, 1990.
47. Boyd AJ, Sherman IA, Saibil FG: The cardiovascular effects of gamma-hydroxybutyrate following hemorrhage. Circ Shock 38:115–121, 1992.

48. Gallimberti L, Cibin M, Pagnin P, et al: Gamma-hydroxybutyric acid for treatment of opiate withdrawal syndrome. Neuropsychopharmacology 9:77–81, 1993.

49. Gallimberti L, Canton G, Gentile N, et al: Gamma-hydroxybutyric acid for treatment of alcohol withdrawal syndrome. Lancet 30:787–789, 1989.

50. Martellotta MC, Balducci C, Fattore L, et al: Gamma-hydroxybutyric acid decreases intravenous cocaine self-administration in rats. Pharmacol Biochem Behav 59:697–702, 1998.

51. Luby S, Jones J, Zalewski A: GHB use in South Carolina. Am J Public Health 82:128, 1992.

52. Chin R, Sporer KA, Cullison B, et al: Clinical course of gamma-hydroxybutyrate overdose. Ann Emerg Med 31:716–722, 1998.

53. Dyer JE: Gamma-hydroxybutyrate: A health food producing coma and seizure like activity. Am J Emerg Med 9:321–324, 1991.

54. Li J, Stokes SA, Woeckener A: A tale of novel intoxication: Seven cases of gamma-hydroxybutyric acid overdose. Ann Emerg Med 31:723–728, 1998.

55. Carter J, Mofenson H, Caraccio T, et al: Gamma hydroxy-butyrate use—New York and Texas, 1995–1996. MMWR Morb Mortal Wkly Rep 46:281–283, 1997.

56. Smith SW, Zvosec DL: Death and central nervous system depression after ingestion of 1,4-butanediol, a γ hydroxybutyrate-related dietary supplement (Abstract). Ann Emerg Med 36:S85, 2000.

57. Gast JA, Frenia ML: Gamma hydroxybutyrate toxicity. Vet Hum Toxicol 36:348, 1994.

58. James C: Another case of gamma hydroxybutyrate (GHB) overdose. J Emerg Nurs 22:97, 1996.

59. Ferrara SD, Tedeschi L, Frison G, et al: Fatality due to gamma-hydoxybutyric acid (GHB) and heroin intoxication. J Forensic Sci 40:501–504, 1995.

60. Colombo G, Agabio R, Lobina C, et al: Cross-tolerance to ethanol and gamma-hydroxybutyric acid. Eur J Pharmacol 273:235–238, 1995.

61. Ropero-Miller JD, Goldberger BA: Recreational drugs: Current trends in the 90s. Clin Lab Med 18:727–745, 1998.

62. Louagie HK, Verstraete AG, De Soete CJ, et al: A sudden awakening from a near coma after combined intake of gamma hydroxybutyric acid and ethanol. J Toxicol Clin Toxicol 35:591–594, 1997.

63. Hunter AS, Long WJ, Ryrie CG: An evaluation of gamma-hydroxybutyric acid in paediatric practice. Br J Anaesth 43:620–628, 1971.

64. Price PA, Schachter M, Smith SJ, et al: Gamma hydroxybutyrate in narcolepsy. Ann Neurol 9:198, 1981.

65. Ferrara SD, Giorgetti R, Zancaner S, et al: Effects of single dose of gamma-hydroxybutyric acid and lorazepam on psychomotor performance and subjective feelings in healthy volunteers. Eur J Clin Pharmacol 54:821–827, 1999.

66. Garrison G, Mueller P: Clinical features and outcomes after unintentional gamma hydroxybutyrate (GHB) overdose. J Toxicol Clin Toxicol 36:503–504, 1998.

67. Adornato BT, Tse V: Another health food hazard: Gamma-hydroxybutyrate-induced seizures. West J Med 157:471, 1992.

68. Ryan JM, Stell I: Gamma hydroxybutyrate—a coma inducing recreational drug. J Accid Emerg Med 14:259–261, 1997.

69. Steele MT, Watson WA: Acute poisoning from gamma hydroxybutyrate (GHB). Mo Med 92:354–357, 1995.

70. Ross TM: Gamma hydroxybutyrate overdose: Two cases illustrate the unique aspects of this dangerous recreational drug. J Emerg Nurs 21:374–376, 1995.

71. Virtue RW, Lund LO, Beckwitt HJ, et al: Cardiovascular reactions to gammahydroxybutyrate in man. Can Anaesth Soc J 13:119–123, 1966.

72. Geldenhuys FG, Sonnedecker EW, DeKlerk MCC: Experience with sodium gamma-4-hydroxybutyric acid in obstetrics. J Obstet Gynaecol Br Commonwlth 75:405–413, 1968.

73. Libetta C: Gamma hydroxybutyrate poisoning. J Accid Emerg Med 14:411, 1997.

74. Suner S, Szlatenyi C, Wang R: Pediatric gamma hydroxybutyrate intoxication. Acad Emerg Med 4:1041–1045, 1997.

75. Thomas G, Bonner S, Gascoinge A: Coma induced by abuse of gamma-hydroxybutyrate (GBH or liquid ecstasy): A case report. BMJ 314:35–36, 1997.

76. Einsprunch BC: Near fatality results from health food store sleeping potion. Tex Med 88:10, 1992.

77. Harraway T, Stephenson L: Gamma hydroxybutyrate intoxication: The gold coast experience. Emerg Med 11:45–48, 1999.

78. Kaufman EE, Porrino LJ, Nelson T: Pyretic action of low doses of gamma-hydroxybutyrate in rats. Biochem Pharmacol 40:2637–2640, 1990.

79. Friedman J, Westlake R, Furman M: "Grievous bodily harm": Gamma hydroxybutyrate abuse leading to Wernicke-Korsakoff syndrome. Neurology 46:469–471, 1996.

80. Dyer JE, Reed JH: Alkali burns from illicit manufacture of GHB (Abstract). J Toxicol Clin Toxicol 35:553, 1997.

81. Galloway GP, Frederick SL, Staggers FE, et al: Gamma-hydroxybutyrate: An emerging drug of abuse that causes physical dependence. Addiction 92:89–96, 1997.

82. Dyer JE, Roth B, Hyma BA: Gamma-hydroxybutyrate withdrawal syndrome. Ann Emerg Med 37:147–153, 2001.

83. Hernandez M, McDaniel CH, Costanza CD, et al: GHB-induced delirium: A case report and review of the literature on gamma hydroxybutyric acid. Am J Drug Alcohol Abuse 24:179–183, 1998.

84. Sanguineti VR, Angelo A, Frank MR: GHB: A home brew. Am J Drug Alcohol Abuse 23:637–642, 1997.

85. Craig K, Gomez HF, McManus JL, et al: Severe gamma-hydroxybutyrate withdrawal: A case report and literature review. J Emerg Med 18:65–70, 2000.

86. Bowles TM, Sommi RW, Amiri M: Successful management of prolonged gamma-hydroxybutyrate and alcohol withdrawal. Pharmacotherapy 21:254–257, 2001.

87. Ingels M, Rangan C, Bellezzo J: Coma and respiratory depression following the ingestion of GHB and its precursors: three cases. J Emerg Med 19:47–50, 2000.

88. LoVecchio F, Curry SC, Bagnasco T: Butyrolactone-induced central nervous system depression after ingestion of RenewTrient a "dietary supplement," N Engl J Med 339:847–848, 1998.

89. Ramborg-Schepens M, Buffet M, Durak C, et al: Gamma butyrolactone poisoning and its similarities to gamma hydroxybutyric acid: Two case reports. Vet Hum Toxicol 39:234–235, 1997.

90. Higgins TF, Borron SW: Coma and respiratory arrest after exposure to butyrolactone. J Emerg Med 14:435–437, 1996.

91. Zvosec DL, Smith SW, McCutchear R, et al: Adverse events, including death, associated with the use of 1,4 butanediol. N Engl J Med 344:87–94, 2001.

92. Davis LG: Fatalities attributed to GHB and related compounds. South Med J 92:1037, 1999.

93. Lettieri J, Fung H: Improved pharmacological activity via pro-drug modification: Comparative pharmacokinetics of sodium gamma-hydroxybutyrate and gamma-butyrolactone. Res Commun Chem Pathol Pharmacol 22:107–118, 1978.

94. Kohrs FP, Porter WH: Gamma hydroxybutyric acid intoxication and overdose (Letter). Ann Emerg Med 33:475, 1999.

95. Badcock NR, Zotti R: Rapid screening test for gamma-hydroxybutyric acid (GHB, fantasy) in urine (Letter). Ther Drug Monit 21:376, 1999.

96. Hoes MJ, Vree TB, Guelen PJM: Gamma-hydroxybutyric acid as hypnotic. L'Encephale 6:93–99, 1980.

97. Lettieri JT, Fung H: Evaluation and development of gas chromatographic procedures for the determination of gamma-hydroxybutyric acid and gamma-butyrolactone in plasma. Biochem Med 20:70–80, 1978.

98. Ferrara SD, Tedeschi L, Frison G, et al: Therapeutic gamma-hydroxybutyric acid monitoring in plasma and urine by gas chromatography-mass spectrometry. J Pharm Biomed Anal 11:483–487, 1993.

99. Mesmer MZ, Satzger RD: Determination of gamma-hydroxybutyrate (GHB) and gamma-butyrolactone (GBL) by HPLC/UV-VIS spectrophotometry and HPLC/thermospray mass spectrometry. J Forensic Sci 43:489–492, 1998.

100. McCusker RR, Paget-Wilkes H, Chronister CW, et al: Analysis of gamma-hydroxybutyrate (GHB) in urine by gas chromatography-mass spectrometry. J Anal Toxicol 23:301–305, 1999.

101. Anderson DT, Kuwuhara T: Endogenous gamma-hydroxybutyrate (GHB) levels in postmortem specimens. Presented at the quarterly meeting of the California Association of Toxicologists, Las Vegas, NV, November 6, 1997.

102. Fieler EL, Coleman DE, Baselt RC: Gamma-hydroxybutyrate concentrations in pre- and postmortem blood and urine. Clin Chem 44:692, 1998.

103. Li J: Gamma hydroxybutyrate intoxication and overdose (Letter). Ann Emerg Med 33:475–476, 1999.

104. Snead OC III, Bearden LJ: Naloxone overcomes the dopaminergic, EEG, and behavioral effects of γ-hydroxybutyrate. Neurology 30:832–838, 1980.

105. Feigenbaum JJ, Howard SG: Naloxone reverses the inhibitory effects of gamma-hydroxybutyrate on central DA release in vivo in awake animals: A microdialysis study. Neurosci Lett 218:5–8, 1996.

106. Devoto P, Colombo G, Cappai F, et al: Naloxone antagonizes ethanol but not gamma-hydroxybutyrate-induced sleep in mice. Eur J Pharmacol 252:321–324, 1994.

107. Gerra G, Caccavari R, Fontanesi B, et al: Flumazenil effects on growth hormone response to gamma-hydroxybutyric acid. Int Clin Psychopharmacol 9:211–215, 1994.

108. Satz WA, Greene T, Dougherty T, et al: An investigation of flumazenil to antagonize gamma hydroxybutyrate intoxication in a murine model (Abstract). Acad Emerg Med 4:439, 1997

109. Yates SW, Viera AJ: Physostigmine in the treatment of γ-hydroxybutyric acid overdose. Mayo Clin Proc 75:401–402, 2000.

110. Caldicott DGE, Kuhn M: Gamma-hydroxybutyrate overdose and physostigmine: Teaching new tricks to an old drug? Ann Emerg Med 37:99–102, 2001.

111. Henderson RS, Holmes CM: Reversal of the anesthetic action of sodium gamma-hydroxybutyrate. Anaesth Intensive Care 4:351–354, 1976.

112. Holmes CM, Henderson RS: The elimination of pollution by a non inhalational technique. Anaesth Intensive Care 6:120–124, 1978.

113. Ryan JM, Stell I: Gamma hydroxbutyrate—a coma inducing recreational drug (Abstract). J Accid Emerg Med 14:259–261, 1997.

114. Bismuth C, Dally S, Borron SW: Chemical submission: GHB, benzodiazepines, and other knock out drops. J Toxicol Clin Toxicol 35:595–598, 1997.

115. Gibson KM, Hoffman GF, Hodson AK, et al: 4-Hydroxybutyric acid and the clinical phenotype of succinic semialdehyde dehydrogenase deficiency, an inborn error of GABA metabolism. Neuropediatrics 28:14–22, 1998.

116. Berthier M, Bonneau D, Desbordes J-M, et al: Possible involvement of a gamma-hydroxybutyric acid receptor in startle disease. Acta Paediatr 83:678–680, 1994.

117. Harrington RD, Woodward JA, Hooton TM, et al: Life threatening interactions between HIV-1 protease inhibitors and the illicit drugs MDMA and γ-hydroxybutyrate. Arch Intern Med 159:2221–2224, 1999.

118. Kaufman EE, Nelson T, Goochee C, et al: The purification and characterization of an NADP+-linked alcohol oxido-reductase which catalyzes the interconversion of γ-hydroxybutyrate and succinic semialdehyde. J Neurochem 32:699–712, 1979.

119. Snead OC III, Bearden LJ, Pegram V: Effect of acute and chronic anticonvulsant administration on endogenous gamma-hydroxybutyrate in rat brain. Neuropharmacology 19:47–52, 1980.

CHAPTER 72

Indole Hallucinogens

Curtis P. Snook

The hallucinogenic indolealkylamines include many natural substances, such as psilocin and psilocybin from mushrooms of the genus *Psilocybe*; ibogaine found in the African shrub *Tabernathe iboga*; harmine found in the South American plants *Peganum harmala* and *Banisteria caapi*; a tryptamine derivative found in the secretions of the Sonoran desert toad *Bufo alvarius*; and lysergic acid amide and isolysergic acid amide found in the American tropical morning glory species *Ipomoea violacea* and *Rivea corymbosa*. Hallucinogens of this class have been used in ritual for centuries. Ceremonial use of hallucinogenic mushrooms by native populations was documented in the 1500s after the Spanish conquest of Mexico.[1] Evidence suggests that bufotenine (5-hydroxydimethyltryptamine), a toxin found in many toad and plant species and reputed to be hallucinogenic, is not psychoactive in vivo owing to its poor penetration of the blood-brain barrier.[2,3]

Because of their similarity of structure, the synthetic hallucinogens lysergic acid diethylamide (LSD), dipropyltryptamine, α-methyltryptamine, diethyltryptamine, and 6-hydroxydimethyltryptamine, often are considered as belonging to this group. LSD is an ergot derivative and an especially potent hallucinogen that has had an enormous cultural impact since its discovery by the Swiss chemist Hofmann in 1938.[4] Additionally it has provided insight into the chemical and molecular bases of human psychosis.

Severe toxicity from indolealkylamine hallucinogens is uncommon, although abuse of these agents is prevalent. The exact prevalence of use is impossible to determine because of the inherent inaccuracies of self-reporting, the substitution of one substance for another by dealers, and the lack of laboratory confirmation in most cases. In one survey of 1500 American college students, 15% admitted to mushroom abuse and 5% admitted to misuse of LSD.[5]

Death from poisoning is rare and often related to secondary events, such as trauma while intoxicated. Many toxic sequelae of poisoning with the indole hallucinogens are potentially life-threatening, however, and could result in the necessity of intensive care unit admission.

BIOCHEMISTRY AND CLINICAL PHARMACOLOGY

The three main chemical groups of hallucinogens of clinical importance are the indolealkylamines (the subject of this chapter), phenylethylamines, and atypicals (arylcyclohexylamines). Representative chemical structures of indolealkylamines are illustrated in Figure 72-1. There is substantial chemical similarity between the indolealkylamine hallucinogens and the neurotransmitter serotonin (5-hydroxytryptamine [5-HT]). Although there is variety in structure among hallucinogens, which may account for differences in their clinical presentation overall, agonism at select cerebral serotonin receptors seems to be a necessary common denominator for their ability to produce hallucinations.[6–8] The commonly encountered indolealkylamines are psilocin (dimethyl-4-hydroxytryptamine); psilocybin, harmine, and ibogaine (all dimethyl-4-phosphoryltryptamine); 5-methoxydimethyltryptamine; LSD; lysergic acid amide; isolysergic acid amide; dimethyltryptamine; dipropyltryptamine; α-methyltryptamine; diethyltryptamine; and 6-hydroxymethyltryptamine.

Tryptamine (see Fig. 72-1) serves as the basic structural unit for serotonin and the indolealkylamine hallucinogens. Dialkyltryptamines, such as dimethyltryptamine, diethyltryptamine, and 5-methoxydimethyltryptamine, are not psychoactive if given orally, presumably owing to rapid hepatic metabolism, and generally are smoked or, in native cultures, inhaled as snuff.[9] Exceptions to this lack of oral activity are psilocin and psilocybin. The latter is converted by hydrolysis in vivo to the former, which is the active species.[10,11] Affinity of indolealkylamines for 5-HT$_2$ receptors seems to be influenced by the lipophilicity and electron-withdrawing properties of the four-position substituents.[12] The mechanism of hallucinogenesis seems to be sensitive to ring substitution. With the exception of 5-methoxy, 4-methoxy, or 4-phosphoryloxy (psilocybin) substituents, all other compounds with ring substitutions have not been found to be psychoactive in humans.[9]

Structural features on the aliphatic side chains also influence activity. An α-methyl group confers the ability to resist degradation by monoamine oxidase and to be orally bioavailable. α-Methyltryptamine is not degraded by monoamine oxidase, preventing the metabolism that so rapidly befalls other non–α-methylated tryptamine derivatives. The α-methylated compounds, such as α-methyltryptamine, have an increased duration of action.[13] Stereochemical considerations also are important. With α-methyltryptamine and 5-methoxy-α-methyltryptamine, the (+) enantiomer is the most active.[14,15]

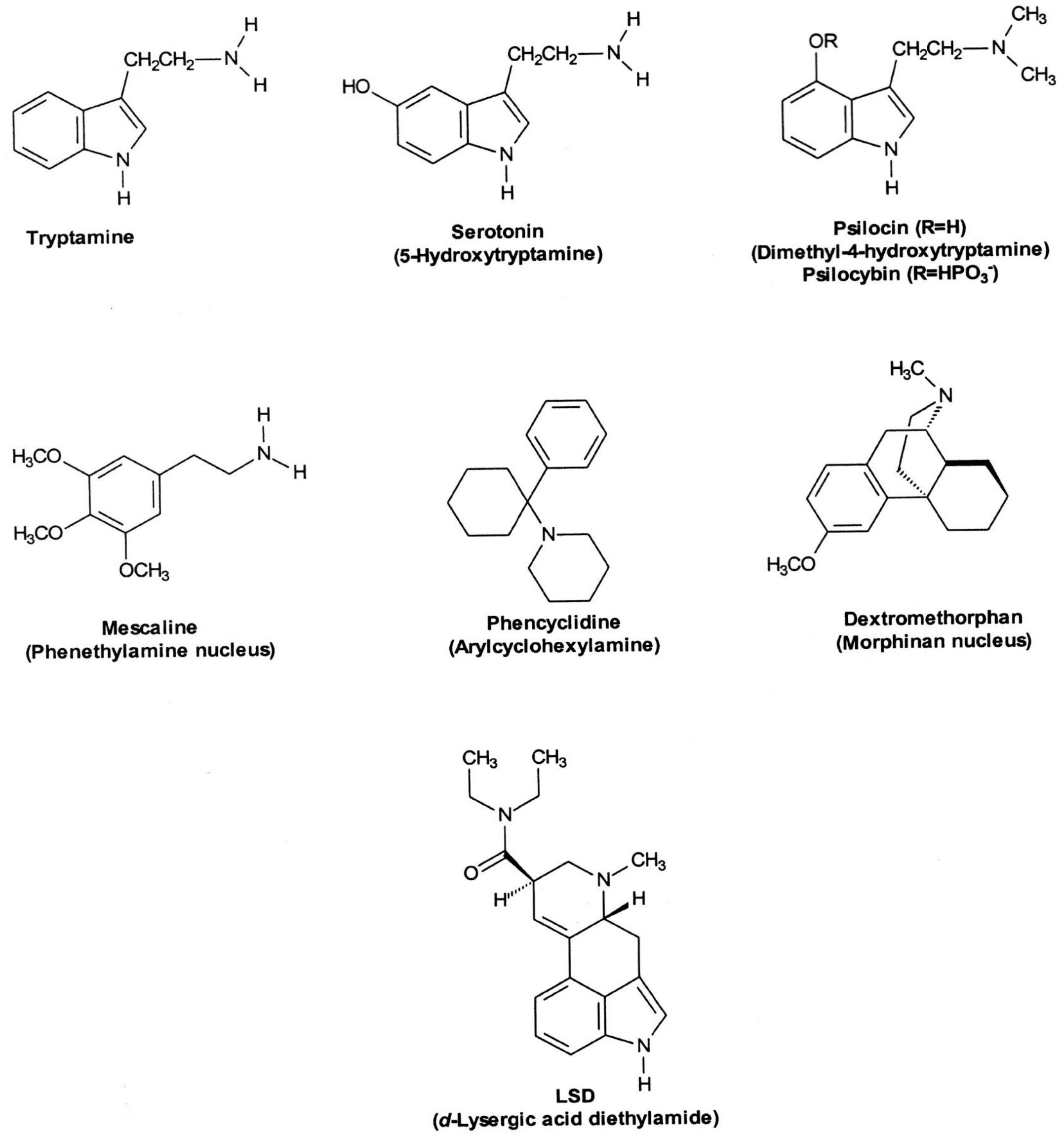

FIGURE 72-1

Chemical structures of the common indolealkylamine hallucinogens psilocin and lysergic acid diethylamide (LSD). These are tryptamines structurally similar to serotonin. For comparison, the structures of mescaline, dextromethorphan, and phencyclidine are included.

Pharmacokinetics of Indole Hallucinogens

Lysergic Acid Diethylamide (LSD)

Volume of distribution: 0.27 L/kg after 2 μg/kg intravenously, elimination half-life calculated at 103 min, hepatic elimination via hydroxylation, glucuronidation and excretion in bile, small amounts excreted unchanged in urine[52]

Absorption: well absorbed via gastrointestinal tract

Peak levels: 30–60 min after 2 μg/kg orally, reduced slightly and delayed by food[50]

Plasma protein binding: >80%

Elimination half-life: approximately 2.5 hr, approximately 0.01% crosses blood-brain barrier[51]

Psilocybin

Duration of action: briefer than LSD's, usually approximately 4 hours[53] (6–12 hr for LSD)

Dimethyltryptamine

Intense and shorter trip than LSD, lasting 30–60 min

Smoked, snorted, or injected[53]

Mechanism of clearance: dimethyltryptamine and 5-MeODMT eliminated:[54] (1) via monoamine oxidase by oxidative deamination (major route of metabolism in brain, liver, and kidney); (2) by *N*-oxidation (major metabolic route in peripheral tissues [e.g., liver and kidney], minor in brain); (3) only 8% of administered dose of either recovered as metabolites in urine

Bufotenines (5-Methoxydimethyltryptamine)

Single deep inhalations of vaporized venom powerfully psychoactive within 15 sec[34]

PATHOPHYSIOLOGY

The existence of cross-tolerance among hallucinogens suggests that they have a common site of action. Considerable evidence exists implicating 5-HT$_2$ receptors as that site. The affinity of substances for the 5-HT$_2$ receptor in rats and humans correlates well with hallucinogenic potency of these same agents in humans.[7,8] Risperidone, a potent 5-HT$_2$ receptor and dopamine-D$_2$ antagonist, completely blocks the discriminative stimulus properties of LSD in rats.[16] Antagonism of LSD's behavioral effects by 5-HT$_2$ antagonists, without change in the typical LSD-induced suppression of serotonin neuronal activity, suggests that these effects are mediated postsynaptically rather than presynaptically.[17] That 5-HT$_2$ agonism is the primary mode of action of LSD's behavioral effects is not firmly established, however. There is some evidence against a mechanism of direct pure 5-HT$_2$ agonism. LSD does not stimulate 5-HT$_2$-mediated phosphatidylinositol turnover in rat cortex, yet it inhibits serotonin's ability to produce these effects.[18]

More recent work with receptor subpopulations has determined that LSD and the phenylethylamine DOI (1-(2,5-dimethoxy-4-iodophenyl)-2-aminopropane) serve as potent partial agonists for cortical 5-HT$_{2A}$ receptors, inhibiting pyramidal cells in layer II, via stimulation of GABAergic interneurons in layer III, of the rat piriform cortex.[19] Indole hallucinogens initiate a 5-HT$_{2A}$ receptor–mediated enhancement of nonsynchronous, late components of glutaminergic excitatory postsynaptic potentials in layer V pyramidal cells, which may help explain the changes in higher level cognition, perception, and mood experienced from these drugs.[20]

It is clear in any case that the effects of the indolealkylamines are much more complex than can be explained by interaction with one receptor or binding site. LSD and dimethyltryptamine have been found to have high affinity for the DOB (a phenylalkylamine, 1-(2,5-dimethoxy-4-bromophenyl)-2-aminopropane) binding site and 5-HT$_{1A}$ and 5-HT$_{1D}$ receptors in addition to 5-HT$_2$ receptors. This high affinity for the DOB site may be crucial to the ability to produce hallucinations. It is believed that the DOB binding site represents 5-HT$_2$ receptors when they are in an agonist high-affinity state. The high affinity of indolealkylamines and other hallucinogens for this site may explain why they are hallucinogenic, whereas serotonin itself is not because the latter does not have high affinity for this site.[12] LSD is a potent partial agonist for 5-HT$_{2A}$ and a partial agonist for 5-HT$_{2C}$ receptors.[21] LSD also displays high affinity for α_2-adrenergic receptors and submicromolar affinity for α_1-adrenergic and β-adrenergic receptors.[18] It also has been suggested that hallucinogens are partial agonists at 5-HT$_2$ receptors because they occasionally seem to act as antagonists.[22]

Given their status as serotonergic agonists, the indolealkylamine hallucinogens have the potential to produce a serotonin syndrome. A report of eight patients with massive LSD overdose noted many clinical findings suggesting serotonin syndrome.[23] Interaction also has been noted between serotonergic and dopaminergic agonists with respect to hyperthermia.[24] Drug-induced hyperthermia is antagonized by serotonin receptor antagonists.[25] Psychoactive agents with dopaminergic effects, such as 3,4-methylenedioxymethamphetamine, are noted to be more potent in producing hyperthermia.[26]

A case report described what the authors called neuroleptic malignant syndrome after consumption of ethanol and LSD. This case had clinical features similar to those of serotonin syndrome.[27] It was the opinion of the authors of that report that the central nervous system effects of LSD resulted in continuous muscle contraction and hyperthermia, producing muscle damage and its sequelae. Symptoms from poisoning with the indolealkylamines are attributed primarily to their effects on serotonergic neurotransmission and the sympathetic nervous system.

CLINICAL PRESENTATION

Many life-threatening complications are possible with poisoning from indolealkylamine hallucinogens. Most commonly, trauma or self-harm may occur secondary to the mental and behavioral changes associated with the hallucinatory state and accompanying panic reactions or paranoia. Patients for whom little or no history is available should be assumed to have associated trauma until proved otherwise. Serotonergic excess may result in life-threatening hyperthermia, muscle rigidity, and rhabdomyolysis leading to myoglobinuric renal failure, hepatic necrosis, and disseminated intravascular coagulation. Elevation of blood pressure is common from these agents, and hypertensive crisis is theoretically possible, although it has not been reported to date.

True hallucinations are marked by changes in thought, perception, and mood without significant impairment of intellect or memory. Usual doses of hallucinogens typically are not associated with alterations in consciousness. In addition, there is not excessive stimulation or autonomic side effects at these doses. To the extent that they do occur, autonomic side effects tend to be mild and not disturbing to the patient. Addictive craving is minimal.[28]

Typical presentations for acute LSD toxicity include psychiatric and constitutional symptoms. Psychiatric manifestations include acute hyperanxiety, paranoia, panic reactions, dangerous or self-destructive behavior, hallucinations, sensory distortions (e.g., misperception of shape or color), acute psychosis, and major depressive or dysphoric reactions.[29] Constitutional symptoms include nausea, diaphoresis, mydriasis, severe headache, muscle weakness, fatigue, and impaired concentration. Cases of severe toxicity also have presented with coma, hyperactivity, seizures, marked visual and auditory hallucinations, respiratory depression requiring intubation, sinus tachycardia, fixed and dilated pupils, vomiting, vasodilation, and coagulopathy.[23] A single patient also was documented as presenting unconscious with severe extrapyramidal rigidity and hyperthermia.[27]

Ingestion of hallucinogenic mushrooms containing psilocin or psilocybin results in perceptual distortions or hallucinations, dysphoria, mydriasis, dry mouth, hyperreflexia, tachycardia, drowsiness, euphoria, nausea, cramping, abdominal pain, and distortions of body image.[30,31] One fatal mushroom poisoning was reported in a 6-year-old child who ingested *Psilocybe baeocystis* and developed hyperthermia and status epilepticus.[32]

As stated previously, because of its poor penetration of the blood-brain barrier, bufotenine (5-hydroxydimethyltryptamine), found in many toad and plant species, is not believed to be psychoactive if ingested. One species of toad, the Sonoran Desert (also known as Colorado River) toad, *Bufo alvarius*, is unique within its genus, however, in possessing the enzyme *O*-methyltransferase, which converts bufotenine to the potent hallucinogen 5-methoxydimethyltryptamine.[33] A 5-year-old boy was reported to have developed profuse salivation and status epilepticus within 15 minutes of licking a toad identified positively as *B. alvarius*.[34] He survived but remained symptomatic for 1 week. It has been shown that inhalation of the vaporized venom results in an intense but short-lived "trip" after 15 seconds, marked by auditory and visual hallucinations.[33] This mode of intake apparently denatures the venom's more toxic fractions, avoiding serious toxicity. Toad venoms contain many toxic substances in addition to indolealkylamines (bufotenines), including biogenic amines (epinephrine, norepinephrine), cardioactive steroids similar to digitalis (bufotalins or bufogenins), and conjugates of bufogenins (bufotoxins).[35] The clinical presentation of patients intoxicated with other indolealkylamine hallucinogens is similar to the presentations described earlier for LSD and psilocybin.

DIAGNOSIS

The differential diagnosis of severe poisoning with the indolealkylamines includes intoxication with the phenylalkylamine (e.g., amphetamine derivatives) or cycloarylhexyl (e.g., phencyclidine) hallucinogens, which present in a similar manner, with the exception that small fixed pupils and nystagmus can be prominent distinguishing features of phencyclidine (and congener) intoxication. Other toxicologic causes in the differential diagnosis include anticholinergic poisoning (e.g., jimsonweed, scopolamine), sympathomimetic poisoning (e.g., cocaine), the serotonin syndrome, malignant hyperthermia, and neuroleptic malignant syndrome. Possible nontoxicologic causes with similar symptoms include psychosis, central nervous system infections, and delirium from metabolic causes and withdrawal syndromes.

Diagnosis of indolealkylamine poisoning depends first on the acquisition of a thorough history if available. Smoking or licking of toad venom, use of blotter "acid," or ingestion of "psychedelic mushrooms" suggests the diagnosis. Adult patients with uncomplicated hallucinogenic experiences usually do not present to health care facilities. Adults who do present to health care facilities usually have presentations similar to those described in the prior section. Hallucinations, fixed and dilated pupils, muscle rigidity, and hyperthermia in the absence of other explanations should raise a high index of suspicion for this type of intoxication.

Standard drugs-of-abuse screening tests do not detect these agents. LSD and its major metabolite, 2-oxy-LSD, remain in the urine for 12 hours and can be detected by radioimmunoassay, requiring specific reagents.[29] LSD degrades on exposure to light, so specimens should be wrapped in opaque paper or aluminum foil and frozen. Identification of hallucinogenic mushrooms requires a proper specimen and the services of an experienced mycologist. Exposure to a toad in the area of the Sonoran Desert should raise suspicion of toad toxicity. The toad should be identified if available.

TREATMENT

Treatment of intoxication by indole hallucinogens includes gastrointestinal decontamination with activated charcoal if the patient presents soon after oral ingestion (see Chapter 5). Gastric lavage, considered to be of limited utility in the management of poisoned patients in general, should be avoided in patients intoxicated by indole hallucinogens. Similarly, use of activated charcoal should be limited in patients with panic reactions. These procedures are unlikely to be beneficial and could worsen the agitation of the patient. Extracorporeal removal techniques play no role in the treatment of poisoning with the indolealkylamines.

Specific treatments have proved helpful for various complications of indolealkylamine intoxication. Hyperanxiety states and panic attacks are helped by treatment with someone at bedside in a quiet room with a soothing, reassuring, nonjudgmental approach. Patients are "talked down" by repeated orientation to person and place, explaining that symptoms are drug related and they are not losing their sanity.[30] The use of phenothiazines should be avoided because two fatalities have resulted from their administration to patients with the phenylethylamine hallucinogen, DOM (4-methyl-25-dimethoxyamphetamine).[36] Haloperidol or phenothiazines are recommended, however, for prolonged drug-induced psychosis when the acute intoxication phase has passed.[36,37] Given the serotonin receptor agonism of indoles, serotonin reuptake inhibitors should not be used. Benzodiazepines are recommended if sedation is required[29] or if treatment is needed for sympathetic excess.

It is crucial that hyperthermia be managed quickly and aggressively by active external cooling, hydration, and paralysis with mechanical ventilation in severe cases.[38] As in nonexertional heatstroke, spraying a patient with tepid water and use of fans with adjunctive use of ice packs and ice water gastric lavage as needed is effective and prevents maladaptive shivering.[39] Although rapid cooling may help prevent rhabdomyolysis, treatment to minimize renal damage from deposition of myoglobin should be ongoing, with fluid administration to maintain urine output. Urine alkalinization, although controversial, may be beneficial in the prevention of myoglobinuric renal injury.[24]

It has been suggested that if hallucinogens are psychoactive because of their affinity for 5-HT$_2$ receptors, treatment of toxicity from these agents may benefit from the use of 5-HT$_2$ receptor antagonists.[8] Cyproheptadine, an agent sometimes used to treat serotonin syndrome, seems to be a partial 5-HT$_2$ agonist.[40] Although there are reported human cases of

Indications for ICU Admission in Indole Hallucinogen Poisoning

Respiratory depression requiring mechanical ventilation
Hyperthermia requiring external cooling
Muscle rigidity requiring neuromuscular blockade
Myoglobinuric renal failure
Hypertensive crisis
Malignant arrhythmia
Seizures/status epilepticus

Criteria for ICU Discharge in Indole Hallucinogen Poisoning

Adequate oxygenation and ventilation without ventilator support

Normalization of vital signs (tachycardia, hypertension) without pressor or inotropic support

Core temperature <39 °C with no evidence of life-threatening end-organ damage*:

No evidence of cerebral edema, hemorrhage or infarction, seizures

No evidence of pulmonary aspiration or edema

No evidence of cardiac failure or infarction

No evidence of hepatic or renal injury

No evidence of rhabdomyolysis

No evidence of disseminated intravascular coagulation

*Should end-organ damage occur, timing of intensive care unit discharge is situation dependent.

Common Errors in Indole Hallucinogen Poisoning

Exacerbating agitation in hallucinogen intoxication from over-aggressive gastrointestinal decontamination

Failure to recognize and treat hyperthermia aggressively

Overlooking therapy to limit renal effects of myoglobin in treating hyperthermia

Treatment-induced hypertension from use of β-blockers for psychostimulant-induced hypertensive crisis

Mistaken use of serotonin reuptake inhibitors or phenothiazines in indolealkylamine-induced hyperthermia

Key Points in Indole Hallucinogen Poisoning

1. Intoxication with indolealkylamines in most instances responds to reassurance and good supportive care.
2. Serotonergic excess from these drugs requires aggressive treatment: (a) Hyperthermia necessitates active external cooling, benzodiazepines, neuromuscular blockade, and possibly serotonin (5-HT$_2$) receptor antagonists; (b) muscle rigidity may benefit from the addition of dantrolene sodium.
3. Consultation with an experienced mycologist is necessary to confirm *Psilocybe* mushroom poisoning (and rule out hepatotoxic mushroom ingestion).

benefit from cyproheptadine in serotonin syndrome,[41–46] animal data suggest that a pure 5-HT$_2$ antagonist might be more effective. In a fatal rat model of serotonin syndrome, treatment with chlorpromazine and cyproheptadine prevented lethality only at high doses.[47] In this study, the potent 5-HT$_{2A}$ receptor antagonists ritanserin and pipamperone prevented lethality and increase in temperature while muting the associated rise of hypothalamic norepinephrine better than the other treatments. In cases in which muscle rigidity is prominent, dantrolene (see Chapter 156) may be beneficial. In a case of reported neuroleptic malignant syndrome associated with LSD intoxication, hyperpyrexia with muscle rigidity responded to the administration of dantrolene sodium, 25 mg three times daily.[27]

In the intensive care unit setting, if dantrolene therapy is desired for indolealkylamine-induced serotonin syndrome associated with muscle rigidity, the suggested dose would be the same as that used for malignant hyperthermia, that is, 1 to 2 mg/kg administered intravenously rapidly, repeated every 5 to 10 minutes as needed to a maximum total dose of 10 mg/kg.

SPECIAL POPULATIONS

Pediatric Patients

Given the reemergence of hallucinogen use among American teenagers and the availability of unsupervised access to information regarding synthesis and administration of these agents on the Internet,[48] heightened awareness of the presentation and knowledge of treatment of toxicity from these agents are needed.

Pregnant Patients

Available data concerning use of these agents in pregnancy are inconclusive. A review of the genetic toxicity of LSD found the available information on teratogenicity to be contradictory and inconclusive.[49]

REFERENCES

1. Schultes RE, Hofmann A: The Botany and Chemistry of Hallucinogens, 2nd ed. Springfield, IL, Charles C Thomas, 1980.
2. Lyttle T, Goldstein D, Gartz J: Bufo toads and bufotenine: Fact and fiction surrounding an alleged psychedelic. J Psychoact Drugs 28:267–290, 1996.
3. Gessner PK, Page IH: Behavioral effects of 5-methoxy-N,N-dimethyltryptamine, other tryptamines and LSD. Am J Physiol 203:167–172, 1962.
4. Hofmann AA: LSD: My Problem Child. Los Angeles, JP Tarcher, 1983.
5. Thompson JP, Anglin MD, Emboden W, et al: Mushroom use by college students. J Drug Educ 15:111–124, 1985.
6. Lyon RA, Titeler M, Seggel MR, et al: Indolealkylamine analogs share 5-HT$_2$ binding characteristics with phenylalkylamine hallucinogens. Eur J Pharm 145:291–297, 1988.
7. Glennon RA, Titeler M, McKenney JD: Evidence for 5-HT$_2$ involvement in the mechanism of action of hallucinogenic agents. Life Sci 35:2505–2511, 1984.
8. Sadzot B, Baraban JM, Glennon RA, et al: Hallucinogenic drug interactions at human brain 5-HT$_2$ receptors: Implications for treating LSD-induced hallucinogenesis. Psychopharmacology 98:495–499, 1989.
9. Nichols DE: Studies of the relationship between molecular structure and hallucinogenic activity. Pharm Biochem Behav 24:335–340, 1986.
10. Horita A, Weber LJ: The enzymatic dephosphorylation and oxidation of psilocybin and psilocin by mammalian tissue homogenates. Biochem Pharmacol 7:47–54, 1961.
11. Horita A, Weber LJ: Dephosphorylation of psilocybin in the intact mouse. Toxicol Appl Pharmacol 4:730–737, 1962.
12. Glennon RA, Teitler M, Sanders-Bush E: Hallucinogens and serotonergic mechanisms. NIDA Res Monogr 119:131–135, 1992.
13. Lessin AW, Long RF, Parkes MW: Central stimulant actions of α-alkyl substituted tryptamines in mice. Br J Pharmacol 24:49–67, 1965.
14. Glennon RA: The effect of chirality on serotonin receptor affinity. Life Sci 24:1487–1492, 1979.

15. Glennon RA, Young R, Jacyno M: Indolealkylamine and phenalkylamine hallucinogens: Effect of α-methyl and N-methyl substituents on behavioral activity. Biochem Pharmacol 32:1267–1273, 1983.

16. Meert TF, de Haes P, Janssen PA: Risperidone (R 64 766), a potent and complete LSD antagonist in drug discrimination by rats. Psychopharmacology 97:206–212, 1989.

17. Jacobs BL: How hallucinogenic drugs work. Amr Sci 75:386–392, 1987.

18. Pierce PA, Peroutka SJ: Hallucinogenic drug interactions with neurotransmitter receptor binding sites in human cortex. Psychopharmacology 97:118–122, 1989.

19. Marek GJ, Aghajanian GK: LSD and the phenylethylamine hallucinogen DOI are potent partial agonists at 5-HT$_{2A}$ receptors on interneurons in rat piriform cortex. J Pharmacol Exp Ther 278:1373–1382, 1996.

20. Aghajanian GK, Marek GJ: Serotonin and hallucinogens. Neuropsychopharmacology 21(2 Suppl):16S-23S, 1999.

21. Egan CT, Herrick-Davis K, Miller K, et al: Agonist activity of LSD and lisuride at cloned 5HT$_{2A}$ and 5HT$_{2C}$ receptors. Psychopharmacology 136:409–414, 1998.

22. Glennon RA: Do classical hallucinogens act as 5-HT$_2$ agonists or antagonists? Neuropsychopharmacology 3:509–517, 1990.

23. Klock JC, Boerner U, Becker CE: Coma, hyperthermia, and bleeding associated with massive LSD overdose, a report of eight cases. Clin Toxicol 8:191–203, 1975.

24. Callaway CW, Clark RF: Hyperthermia in psychostimulant overdose. Ann Emerg Med 24:68–76, 1994.

25. Yamawaki S, Lai H, Horita A: Dopaminergic and serotonergic mechanisms of thermoregulation: Mediation of thermal effects of apomorphine and dopamine. J Pharm Exp Ther 227:383–388, 1983.

26. Gordon CJ, Watkinson WP, O'Callahan JP, et al: Effects of 3,4-methylenedioxymethamphetamine on autonomic thermoregulatory responses of the rat. Pharmacol Biochem Behav 38:339–344, 1991.

27. Behan WM, Bakheit AM, Behan PO, et al: The muscle findings in the neuroleptic malignant syndrome associated with lysergic acid diethylamide. J Neurol Neurosurg Psychiatry 54:741–743, 1991.

28. Hollister LE: Effects of hallucinogens in humans. In Jacobs BL (ed): Hallucinogens: Neurochemical, Behavioral, and Clinical Perspectives. New York, Raven Press, 1986, pp 19–33.

29. Schwartz RH: LSD: Its rise, fall, and renewed popularity among high school students. Pediatr Clin North Am 42:403–413, 1995.

30. Leikin JB, Krantz AJ, Zell-Kanter M, et al: Clinical features and management of intoxication due to hallucinogenic drugs. Med Toxicol Adverse Drug Exp 4:324–350, 1989.

31. Schwartz RH, Smith DE: Hallucinogenic mushrooms. Clin Pediatr 27:70–73, 1988.

32. McCawley EL, Brummett RE, Dana GW: Convulsions from *Psilocybe* mushroom poisoning. Proc West Pharmacol Soc 5:27–33, 1962.

33. Weil AT, Davis W: *Bufo alvarius*: A potent hallucinogen of animal origin. J Ethnopharm 41:1–8, 1994.

34. Hitt M, Ettinger DD: Toad toxicity. N Eng J Med 314:1517, 1986.

35. Mebs D: Chemistry of animal venoms, poisons and toxins. Experientia 29:1328–1334, 1973.

36. Haddad LM: Management of hallucinogen abuse. Am Fam Physician 14:82–87, 1976.

37. Litovitz T: Hallucinogens. In Haddad LM, Winchester JF (eds): Clinical Management of Poisoning and Drug Overdose. Philadelphia, WB Saunders, 1983, pp 455–466.

38. Gay GR: Clinical management of acute and chronic cocaine poisoning. Ann Emerg Med 11:562–572, 1982.

39. Graham BS, Lichtenstein MJ, Hinson JM, et al: Nonexertional heatstroke: Physiologic management and cooling in 14 patients. Arch Intern Med 146:87–90, 1986.

40. Colpært FC, Niemegeers CJ, Janssen PA: In vivo evidence of partial agonist activity exerted by purported 5-hydroxytryptamine antagonists. Eur J Pharmacol 58:505–509, 1979.

41. Graudins A, Stearman A, Chan B: Treatment of the serotonin syndrome with cyproheptadine. J Emerg Med 16:615–619, 1998.

42. Horowitz BZ, Mullins ME: Cyproheptadine for serotonin syndrome in an accidental pediatric sertraline ingestion. Pediatr Emerg Care 15:325–327, 1999.

43. Lappin RI, Auchincloss EL: Treatment of the serotonin syndrome with cyproheptadine. N Engl J Med 331:1021–1022, 1994.

44. McDaniel WW: Serotonin syndrome: Early management with cyproheptadine. Ann Pharmacother 35:870–873, 2001.

45. Vandemergel X, Beukinga I, Neve P: [Serotonin syndrome secondary to the use of sertraline and metoclopramide]. Rev Med Brux 21:161–163, 2000.

46. Weiner AL, Tilden FF Jr, McKay CA Jr: Serotonin syndrome: Case report and review of the literature. Conn Med 61:717–721, 1997.

47. Nisijima K, Yoshino T, Yui K, et al: Potent serotonin (5-HT) (2A) receptor antagonists completely prevent the development of hyperthermia in an animal model of the 5-HT syndrome. Brain Res 890:23–31, 2001.

48. Halpern JH, Pope HG Jr: Hallucinogens on the Internet: A vast new source of underground drug information. Am J Psychiatry 158:481–483, 2001.

49. Cohen MM, Shiloh Y: Genetic toxicology of lysergic acid diethylamide (LSD-25). Mutat Res 47:183–209, 1977–1978.

50. Upshall DG, Wailling DG: The determination of LSD in human plasma following oral administration. Clin Chem Acta 36:67–73, 1972.

51. White FJ: Comparative effects of LSD and lisoride: Clues to specific hallucinogenic drug actions. Pharmacol Biochem Behav 24:365–379, 1986.

52. Wagner JG, Aghajanian GK, Bing OH: Correlation of performance test scores with "tissue concentrations" of lysergic acid diethylamide in human subjects. Clin Pharmacol Ther 9:635–638, 1968.

53. Cohen S: The hallucinogens and the inhalants. Psychiatr Clin North Am 7:681–688, 1984.

54. Sitoram BR, McLeod WR: Observations on the metabolism of the psychotomimetic indolealkylamines: Implications for future clinical studies. Biol Psychiatry 28:841–848, 1990.

CHAPTER 73

Amphetamines and Derivatives

Patrick E. McKinney* ■ Robert B. Palmer

This chapter addresses drugs that have the basic phenethylamine structure with various substitutions (Fig. 73-1). Amphetamine and methamphetamine, substituted amphetamines (3,4-methylenedioxymethamphetamine [MDMA or Ecstasy] and related compounds), and related anorexigens are discussed.

Although amphetamine was first synthesized more than 100 years ago, the first pharmacologic investigations of its properties and its clinical use began in the 1920s. Related plant-derived stimulants have been used by much of the world, however, for thousands of years. Ephedrine from *Ephedra (ma huang)* has been used in China for more than 5000 years, and cathine and cathinone from *Catha edulis* have been used in East Africa for more than 600 years. Both of these plants and their isolated active ingredients continue to be used today as medications, as drugs of abuse, and in social rituals.

Investigations into the pharmacologic properties of amphetamine began in the late 1920s and early 1930s, when these drugs were investigated as therapies for asthma and rhinitis.[1] In 1932, Smith, Kline, and French introduced an over-the-counter nasal inhaler containing *d/l*-amphetamine under the trade name Benzedrine. Although marketed for congestion, it was rapidly discovered that amphetamine had marked central nervous system (CNS) stimulant properties, and it rapidly became a source of abuse. Each Benzedrine inhaler contained a folded paper impregnated with 250 mg of amphetamine base together with other aromatic compounds. The papers were removed and portions of them were swallowed or soaked in beverages and consumed.[2] Benzedrine abuse within prisons and various American subpopulations (students, musicians, truck drivers) became problematic, and the medical problems now classically associated with amphetamines were well described in the medical literature of the 1930s and 1940s. In 1949, the inhaler was renamed Benzedrex and reformulated to contain propylhexedrine, a potent vasoconstricting agent with only approximately 8% of the CNS stimulant activity of amphetamine. Abuse of propylhexedrine soon was reported, however, and continues to be seen sporadically.[3]

Early claims of efficacy against fatigue and tiredness were reported in the lay press and the medical literature, and by the 1940s, amphetamines were prescribed widely for a variety of indications, including barbiturate overdose,

shock, coma, smooth muscle spasm of the genitourinary or gastrointestinal tract, chronic encephalitis, postural hypotension, and "fatigue or drowsiness of any cause whatsoever."[1-3] Experiences in World War II led to epidemics of use in the armed forces and civilian workforces in Japan and the United States. By 1970, legal production of amphetamine had risen to more than 100 tons, enough to make 5 billion 5-mg tablets.[1] Legitimate prescription of amphetamine in the 1960s and 1970s reflected its use as an anorexiant, but vast amounts of these drugs were diverted for illicit use. Federal regulation of prescribing patterns and restrictions on the approved indications for amphetamines and related drugs led to a decrease in the quantity manufactured by legitimate pharmaceutical companies. As legitimate production declined, illicit production of amphetamine and methamphetamine occurred, and it has become one of the largest problems related to clandestine drug synthesis and production in many parts of the world today.

The true incidence and prevalence of amphetamine and related drug use and resultant medical complications are difficult to gauge. Data from the 1998 U.S. National Household Survey of Drug Abuse suggested that 1.5% to 3.2% of respondents reported ever using an amphetamine-related drug.[4] Figures from the 1998 U.S. Drug Abuse Warning Network (DAWN) emergency department data indicated that methamphetamine-related emergency department visits leveled off from highs in the mid-1990s but showed that amphetamines remain a large problem, particularly in the western United States.[5] Of the 21 reporting DAWN metropolitan areas, 80% of methamphetamine cases came from six western U.S. metropolitan areas. DAWN medical examiner data also showed that methamphetamine accounted for a larger number of drug-related deaths in several western U.S. cities compared with the rest of the United States. Most of these deaths occurred in males, and in many cases they were secondary to external events (trauma) rather than direct drug toxicity.[6] Reports of amphetamine and amphetamine derivative use and adverse effects continue to accumulate from around the world, notably Southeast Asia, Europe, and Australia.[7] Law enforcement surveillance in the United States suggests that many illicit drug suppliers are diversifying from traditional cocaine and heroin trades to amphetamine derivatives.[8]

Available forms of amphetamines include pharmaceutical preparations and clandestinely synthesized preparations. Pharmaceutical preparations include amphetamine, methamphetamine, methylphenidate, and 3,4-methylenedioxymethamphetamine (see also Fig. 73-1). These preparations generally are approved only for short-term weight loss, narcolepsy, and

---

*Patrick E. McKinney, MD, 1962–2003. Clinician, educator, friend. You are missed.

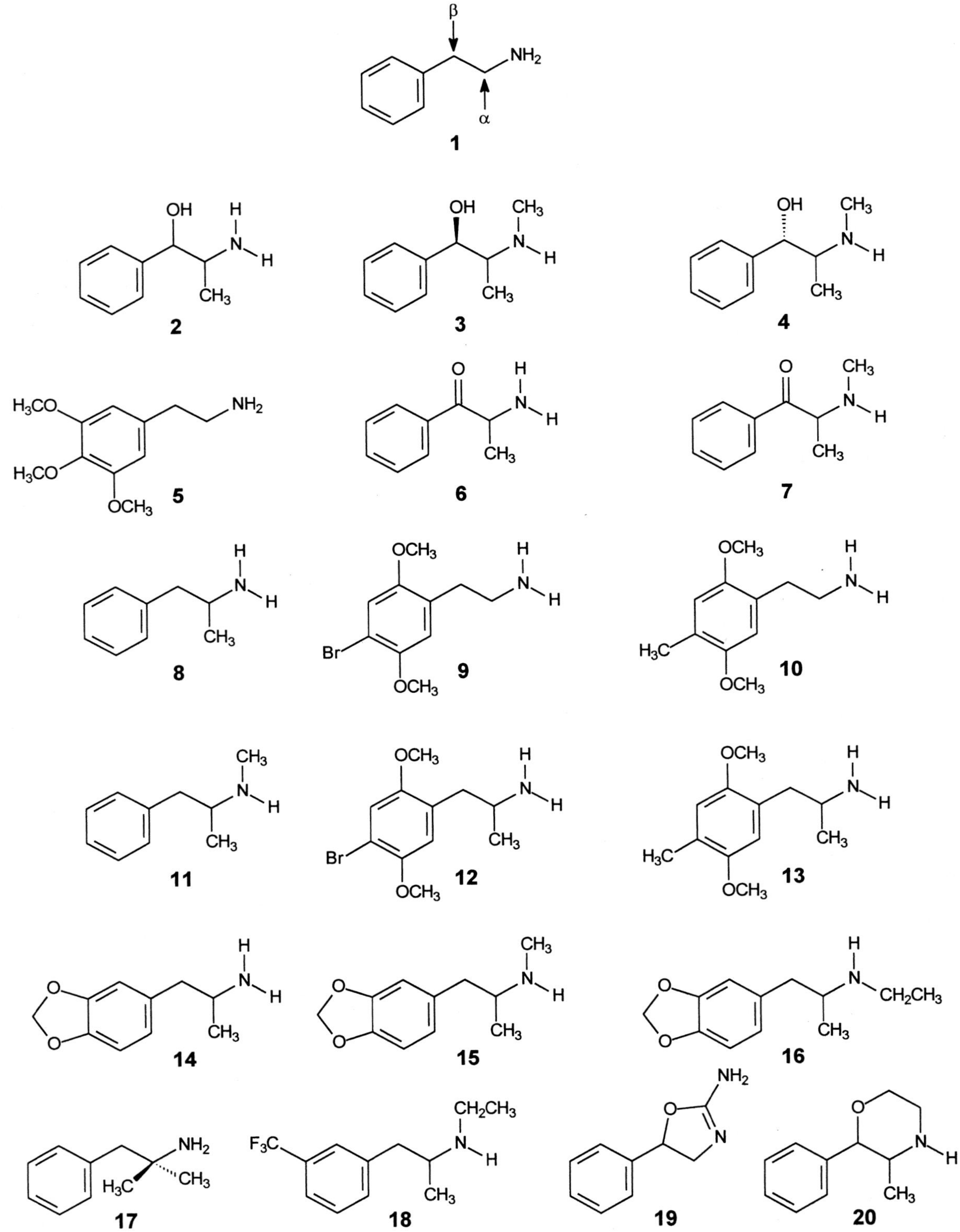

FIGURE 73-1

Chemical structures of phenethylamines: **1**, phenethylamine; **2**, phenylpropanolamine; **3**, ephedrine; **4**, pseudoephedrine; **5**, mescaline; **6**, cathinone; **7**, methcathinone; **8**, amphetamine; **9**, 4-bromo-2,5-dimethoxyphenethylamine; **10**, 4-methyl-2,5-dimethoxyphenethylamine (2-CD); **11**, methamphetamine; **12**, 2,5-dimethoxy-4-bromophenylisopropylamine (DOB); **13**, 2,5-dimethoxy-4-methylphenylisopropylamine (DOM); **14**, 3,4-methylenedioxyamphetamine (MDA); **15**, 3,4-methylenedioxymethamphetamine (MDMA); **16**, 3,4-methylenedioxyethamphetamine; **17**, phentermine; **18**, fenfluramine; **19**, aminorex; **20**, phenmetrazine.

attention-deficit disorder; however, they have been used clinically for a variety of conditions, including depression, Tourette's syndrome, closed head injury, pain, stroke, and depression. Paradoxically, they have been used for psychiatric conditions, including mania, schizophrenia, and obsessive-compulsive disorder, although these are symptoms of amphetamine toxicity as well. Available forms include tablets, capsules, sustained-release forms, and elixirs. Currently available clandestinely synthesized amphetamine and methamphetamine are often of high purity (98%); however, as with all street drugs, concentration of active ingredients may vary, and impurities, adulterants, and by-products of synthesis may contribute to toxicity. Amphetamine and methamphetamine often are called "speed" and "crank" (Table 73-1) and may be snorted, injected, or taken orally. A highly purified crystalline form of methamphetamine, known as "ice," has a relatively low melting point, allowing it to be smoked. Ice abuse first was reported in Asia in the early 1980s.[9] Concerns that ice might produce epidemic problems of a magnitude similar to that of problems seen with cocaine have been largely unfounded.

Designer drug is a term that originated in the United States in the early 1980s to describe compounds manufactured by "street" chemists that resembled various parent drugs of abuse with minor structural modifications.[10] Because of structural differences, these drugs were not illegal because they were not formally scheduled by the U.S. Drug Enforcement Administration. Because of this loophole in drug regulations, minor structural modifications of drugs resembling mescaline and amphetamine yielded compounds that had pharmacologic activity similar to that of these parent drugs but were legal to manufacture, possess, and use. The U.S. Controlled Substances Analogue Enforcement Act of 1986 largely closed the designer drug loophole. The synthesis of many of these compounds is relatively uncomplicated and inexpensive, however, and the lure of potentially large profits and the continued popularity of many of these substances make the designer drug phenomenon unlikely to be short-lived.

Contrary to popular belief, most designer amphetamines are not novel compounds developed by street chemists; rather, they are compounds that have been studied in the past by researchers and pharmaceutical companies, usually as part of the study of a series of related compounds. The description of the synthetic process and pharmacologic activity of these compounds (numbering in the hundreds) is easily accessible in the scientific literature and the popular press.[11] Many of these substances have never been formally tested for safety, efficacy, and side effects, however, and their pharmacokinetics and pharmacodynamics may be poorly characterized, if studied at all. The manufacture of these substances often occurs in conditions that are unsanitary; chemical reactions may be monitored poorly; and substitutions for unavailable reagents may occur.

The incidence and prevalence of designer drug use are difficult to estimate. Many of these substances are difficult to identify specifically using standard urine or blood toxicologic screens. A random, anonymous poll conducted among Stanford University students reported in 1987 indicated that of the 369 subjects interviewed, 149 (39%) indicated that they had used MDMA, a substituted amphetamine, at least once.[12] A similar study conducted at Tulane University in 1990 showed that 24.3% of the 1264 respondents indicated using MDMA at least once, an increase from 15.5% in 1986.[13] The popular press noted the worldwide phenomenon of MDMA use, especially at "rave parties," large dance gatherings where MDMA often is found.[14] Pharmaceutical companies currently do not produce the designer amphetamines; available street drugs in this class are produced by clandestine synthesis. MDMA and related compounds usually are taken orally and commonly are available as tablet, capsule, or powder. Injection of MDMA-like drugs is uncommon.

TABLE 73-1 Commonly Available Forms of Amphetamine Derivatives

Aminorex*
Amphetamine
Benzphetamine
Cathinone
Dexfenfluramine*
Dextroamphetamine
Diethylpropion
Fenfluramine*
Mephentermine
Mescaline
Methamphetamine
Methcathinone
p-Methoxyamphetamine
Methylphenidate
Pemoline
Phendimetrazine
Phenylpropanolamine
Pseudoephedrine
Sibutramine

*Withdrawn from the market in most countries.

CHEMISTRY AND PHARMACOLOGY OF AMPHETAMINES AND DERIVATIVES

The word *amphetamine* is an abbreviation for *a*lpha-*m*ethyl*ph*ene*t*hyl*amine*.[15] The class of CNS stimulant drugs to which amphetamine belongs is called the phenethylamines. The basic structural motif of this group of drugs is an aromatic ring (*phen* for phenyl) attached to a two-carbon chain (*ethyl*) bearing a basic nitrogen at the distal end of the carbon chain (*amine*) (see Fig. 73-1). Although primarily regarded as CNS stimulants, substitution of the fundamental phenethylamine nucleus can result in effects ranging from sedation to stimulation to hallucination induction.[15] The large number of phenethylamine derivatives that have been prepared allows detailed study of the structure-activity relationships of this series of compounds.[15,16] Based on structure-activity relationship investigations, some general inferences can be made about the pharmacologic effects of a given phenethylamine derivative based on its chemical structure. The specific chemical structure has significant effects on which neurotransmitter is principally affected. There are essentially four sites on the phenethylamine on which substitution would affect the overall pharmacology of the compound: the amino nitrogen, the α and β carbons of the ethyl chain, and the aromatic ring.

Substitution on the amino nitrogen with a single methyl group increases central activity, as is seen when comparing methamphetamine with amphetamine. Conversely, amphetamine causes more pronounced peripheral actions than methamphetamine. Mono-*N*-substituents larger than methyl cause a decrease in excitatory properties with retention of anorexiant effects. This observation has been exploited in the development of antiobesity agents, such as benzphetamine and diethylpropion, that have diminished abuse potential relative to the amphetamines. Di-substitution of the nitrogen to form a tertiary amine significantly reduces activity, frequently to the point of abolition.

Substitution of the α carbon (to the nitrogen) with lower alkyl groups causes the agent to have CNS stimulant and anorexiant effects. The lack of significant CNS effects in compounds without substitutions at the α-position (e.g., β-phenethylamine) apparently is due largely to their facile degradation by monoamine oxidase (MAO) into compounds that do not penetrate the CNS. Compounds with an alkyl α-substituent (e.g., amphetamine) are poor substrates for MAO and readily penetrate the CNS.

Several compounds oxidized at the β-carbon (e.g., cathinone, ephedrine, and pseudoephedrine) retain CNS activity. Hydroxylation at this position does result, however, in a less potent agent. This decreased potency is due largely to the diminished ability of the hydroxylated compound to cross the blood-brain barrier. Phenylpropanolamine has only about 1% of the ability to cross the blood-brain barrier as its nonhydroxylated congener, amphetamine.[17]

Substitution of the phenyl ring, particularly with alkoxy moieties, leads to agents with diminished central sympathetic activity but significant CNS effects ranging from altered perceptions to frank hallucinations. Hydroxylation of the aromatic ring also leads to diminished central activity presumably due to decreased blood-brain barrier penetration. These structure-activity relationship properties are shown in Figure 73-1.

The branching at the α-carbon induces a chiral center. With specific respect to the absolute configuration of amphetamine, two isomers exist (*dextro [d]* and *levo [l]*). The pharmacologic profiles of these two compounds are distinct. The alerting activity of the *levo* (R)-isomer is only about one tenth that of the *dextro* (S)-isomer and about half the strength as a psychotomimetic.[17] This stereospecificity also is apparent with methamphetamine. The *l*-isomer of methamphetamine (present in Vicks Inhalers as *l*-desoxyephedrine) is reported to have greater peripheral sympathomimetic and less CNS stimulant activity than the *d*-isomer. The *l*-isomer is also formed as a metabolite of the anti-Parkinson's drug selegiline (Fig. 73-2).[18]

The greater CNS stimulation induced by *d*-methamphetamine has made it the preferred agent not only as an illicit stimulant but also as a therapeutically useful antiobesity agent. The *d*-isomer of methamphetamine is a metabolite of the antiobesity agent benzphetamine.[19] The European over-the-counter analgesic/antipyretic famprofazone is metabolized to the *d*-isomer and *l*-isomer of methamphetamine, although the *l*-isomer predominates (see Fig. 73-2; Table 73-2).[20]

Pharmacokinetics of Amphetamine and Methamphetamine

Amphetamine
Volume of distribution: 3.2–6.1 L/kg
Half-life: 3.5–34 hr
Protein binding: 16%
pK_a: 9.9
Active metabolite: norephedrine
Method to enhance clearance: urinary acidification*

Methamphetamine
Volume of distribution: 3–7 L/kg
Half-life: 6–15 hr
Protein binding: 10–20%
pK_a: 9.9
Active metabolites: amphetamine, norephedrine
Method to enhance clearance: urinary acidification*

3,4-Methylenedioxymethamphetamine
Half-life: 7.6–8.7 hr
Active metabolite: 3,4-methylenedioxyamphetamine

*Half-life longer with alkaline urine.

ILLICIT SYNTHESIS OF METHAMPHETAMINE

The illicit synthesis of methamphetamine is not difficult and requires little or no formal education in synthetic chemistry. Although a wide variety of synthetic approaches are possible for the preparation of methamphetamine, only a handful are used with any regularity for illicit production of the drug. Other derivatives, such as MDMA, 3,4-methylenedioxyamphetamine (MDA), and 2,5-dimethoxy-4-bromomphetamine (DOB), tend to be more difficult to prepare and are prepared illegally less commonly, although this is changing rapidly. Methamphetamine street chemists or "cooks" learn synthetic procedures in a variety of ways, including word-of-mouth or apprenticeship with another cook; in jail; through a wide variety of books available through underground sources; through the Internet; and occasionally through the primary chemical literature. Poor training, technique, and facilities, combined with generalized chemical ignorance and misinformation from the training sources, can lead to relatively poor yields of methamphetamine and production of potentially toxic synthetic by-products.

Historically, illicit preparation of methamphetamine centered on derivatization of phenyl-2-propanone (P2P); typically, this involved condensation of the P2P with methyl amine to form the imine (Schiff base) followed by reduction to form the amine (methamphetamine) (scheme I in Fig. 73-3). The P2P method is not a stereospecific synthesis (i.e., it produces a 50:50 *d:l* mixture). Although popular for many years, use of methods involving P2P has declined substantially since the 1990s. The impetus for this decline is multifactorial. In the United States, P2P is now a Drug Enforcement Administration schedule II compound (restricted), and the detection of a "P2P lab" is easy because P2P has a pungent odor. Ephedrine and pseudoephedrine

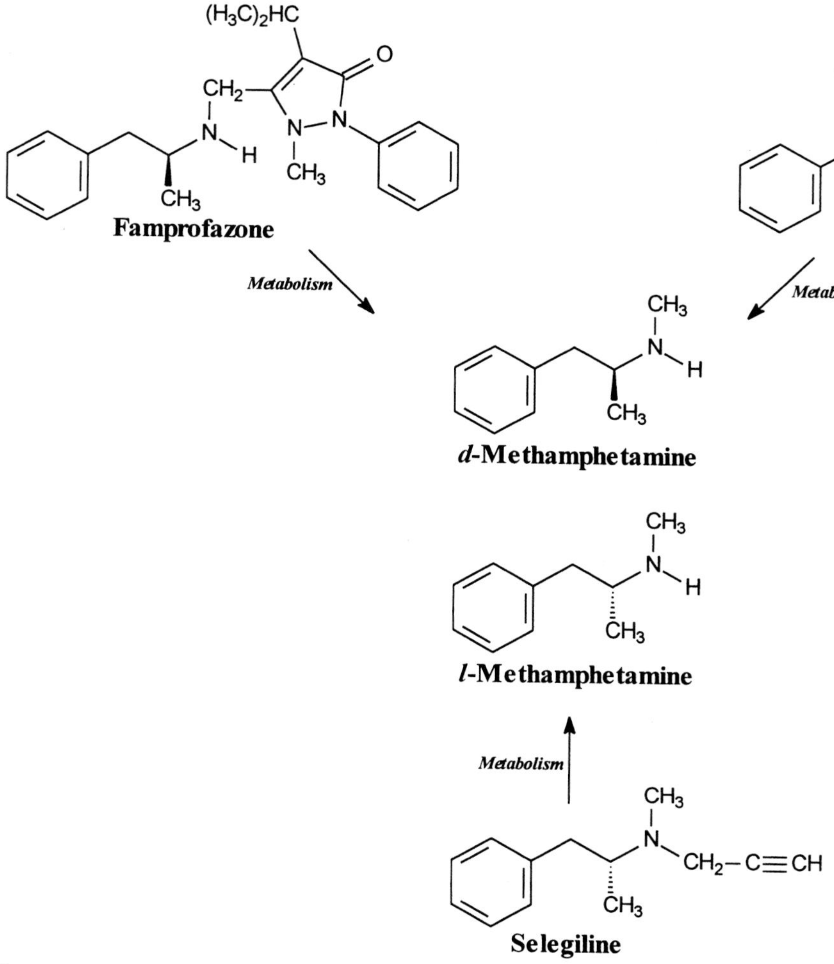

FIGURE 73-2

Metabolic transformations of prescription medications to both isomers of methamphetamine.

(starting materials for alternative reductive dehydroxylation methods) are readily available.

More recently, the reductive removal of the benzylic (β) hydroxy group of ephedrine or pseudoephedrine has become the preferred synthetic approach to methamphet-amine. One of the most common methods of reductive methamphetamine production from ephedrine or pseudoephedrine employs red phosphorus and hydriodic acid (scheme II in Fig. 73-3). In efforts to avoid detection, cooks often obtain the necessary chemicals from veiled sources. Red phosphorus

TABLE 73-2 Common Street Names of Amphetamine Derivatives

Amphetamine

amp, browns, hearts, fives, tens, white cross, beans, bam, black beauties, speed, bennies, cranks, crystal, dexies, greenies, lidpoppers, pep pills, pink and green amps, sparkle plenty's, uppers, whites

Methamphetamine

bambita, crystal, meth, speed, crank, ice, glass, shabu, peanut butter crank

3,4-Methylenedioxymethamphetamine

XTC, Ecstasy, Adam, X, E, clarity, essence

4-Bromo-2,5-dimethoxyphenethylamine

CBr, bromomescaline, nexus, Venus, N, Eve, synergy

3,4-Methylenedioxyamphetamine

love drug

Note: Street names are region specific and often overlap. The actual content of illicit drugs may be a function of drug substitutions, by-products of synthesis, and adulterating agents.

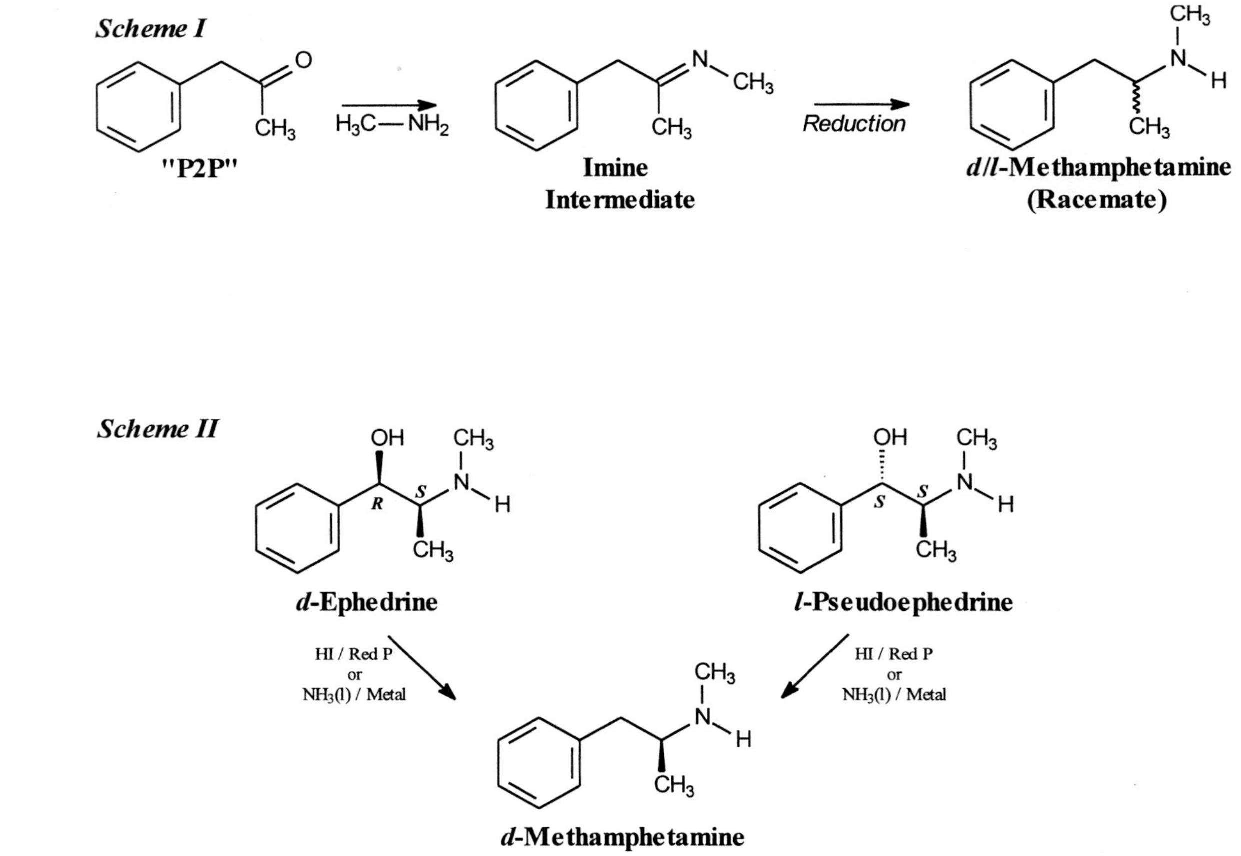

FIGURE 73-3

Methods of illicit preparation of methamphetamine.

is extracted from matchbook strikers or road flares, and hydriodic acid is produced in situ by mixing mineral acids with iodine crystals used for water purification.

Another common method employed by clandestine chemists for reductive dehydroxylation of ephedrine or pseudo-ephedrine involves the use of an alkali metal, such as lithium or sodium, in the presence of liquid ammonia (scheme II in Fig. 73-3). Although it is a misnomer, this method of illicit methamphetamine production often is referred to as the "Nazi" method. The metals typically are obtained from batteries, and the ammonia is obtained from agrochemical sources. Reduction of either *l*-ephedrine or *d*-pseudoephedrine via the red phosphorus/hydriodic acid or the "Nazi" method yields primarily *d*-methamphetamine—another reason cooks tend to favor these methods and starting materials.

Methamphetamine clandestine laboratories may be the source of significant toxic exposures. Mineral acids may cause serious burns, and metal/ammonia reduction has associated inhalational and dermal burn hazards due to residual ammonia or metal hydroxide left after production. Red phosphorus does not share the propensity to induce catastrophic liver damage possessed by yellow phosphorus (see Chapter 81). Residual unreacted sodium or lithium metals or hydride-reducing agents may present an explosive or corrosive hazard if they come in contact with atmospheric moisture or decontamination water. Additional concerns

associated with clandestine methamphetamine synthesis are exposure to a variety of organic solvents, such as diethyl ether, acetone, and dichloromethane, and burns and blast injuries from chemical explosions.

Because of impure starting materials, primitive facilities, and chemical ignorance, even when methamphetamine is actually synthesized, many synthetic by-products are produced concomitantly.[21,22] These by-products can be structurally diverse and may be present in highly variable amounts in a given mixture of methamphetamine. These by-products may contribute to the toxicity of a given batch of illicit methamphetamine, but few studies have examined this possibility. Drugs sold as amphetamines may contain nonprescription stimulants (e.g., caffeine, ephedrine, or phenylpropanolamine), other scheduled stimulants (e.g., cocaine or a variety of phenethylamine derivatives), or unrelated chemicals (e.g., strychnine, lead, solvents). Acute lead poisoning has been reported in association with the intravenous use of methamphetamine.[23]

PATHOPHYSIOLOGY OF PHENETHYLAMINE EFFECTS

Although the data are complex and sometimes conflicting, most data suggest that amphetamines cause their clinical effects indirectly, through increased release and decreased uptake of biogenic amines (dopamine, norepinephrine, serotonin) from presynaptic nerve terminals.[24] The degree to which any of these neurotransmitters is affected depends on the structure of the particular amphetamine derivative. Some evidence indicates that amphetamine may act directly on catecholamine receptors, but this is believed to be a minor mechanism. The effects of amphetamine on neurotransmitter systems have been studied most extensively on dopaminergic neurons. Examination of the data regarding the effect of amphetamine on dopamine neurophysiology provides a model to explain amphetamine-induced biogenic amine effect. Normally the dopamine uptake transporter system removes dopamine released from the synapse after cell firing. In the presence of amphetamines, the direction of this transport is reversed, however, resulting in movement of catecholamines out of the neuron. The uptake transporter system is Na^+ dependent, although evidence exists for Na^+-independent transporters as well.[25] Amphetamines act on the neuronal synapse at the dopamine uptake transporter system not only to block uptake but also to cause release of intracellular dopamine in a manner that is independent of depolarization and Ca^{++} flux. Amphetamines also may enter the nerve cell either by passive diffusion or by exchange diffusion through the uptake transporter, in which case amphetamine enters the cell concurrent with transport of dopamine out of the cell.[26] This intracellular amphetamine may enter dopamine storage vesicles and cause displacement of dopamine from these storage vesicles into the cytoplasm. The increased intracellular dopamine may contribute to the pool available for release from the cellular transporter uptake system.[27] At high doses, amphetamines also may have a weak inhibitory effect on MAO type A; however, this effect on neurotransmission is unlikely at commonly used doses.[28,29]

At low doses of amphetamine, increased central release of norepinephrine seems to induce appetite suppression and, in animal models, some forms of increased locomotor behavior. Amphetamines reduce appetite and food intake in humans and many animal models.[24,30,31] Higher doses are associated with an increased release of dopamine, which contributes to the anorexient effect and results in stereotypical behaviors and other forms of increased locomotor activity in animal models.[24,32] High doses of amphetamines (or lower doses of serotonin-selective forms, such as MDMA) may result in increased release of serotonin, which may result in altered perceptions and, together with dopamine increase, may result in a psychotic syndrome.

Amphetamine-induced psychosis and stereotypies have been used as a model for schizophrenia in animals, and there are many similarities between these conditions in humans. Both conditions result from dopaminergic overactivity, and both respond to typical antidopaminergic antipsychotic agents. In animal models, increased amphetamine-induced dopaminergic activity in the nucleus accumbens results in an increase in general locomotor activity, whereas a dopamine increase in the striatum results in species-specific stereotypical behaviors, such as rearing, licking, and gnawing. These behaviors also may be dose dependent; higher doses are required to induce the more characteristic individual stereotypies.[24] These stereotypical behaviors may be represented in humans as compulsive performance of repetitive tasks, such as assembling or disassembling mechanical objects, pacing, or foot tapping.

The designer amphetamines, notably MDMA, and some pharmaceutically developed preparations, such as fenfluramine, have prominent serotonergic actions that may account for some of their short-term and long-term effects. Much of the research regarding these compounds has centered on MDMA. Because of MDMA's importance as a drug of abuse, it is discussed in detail. It has been suggested that MDMA acts by several mechanisms (similar to the previous discussion of dopamine) to increase release of serotonin into the synaptic space.[33–35] MDMA and related drugs may act acutely to increase serotonin concentrations at the synapse and be implicated in the development of serotonergic effects, including a clinical serotonin syndrome. Animal models have shown, however, that MDMA, when given at excessive doses, also is associated with serotonergic neuronal injury, as evidenced by lasting decreases in the serotonin metabolite, 5-hydroxyindoleacetic acid, the serotonin synthetic enzyme tryptophan hydroxylase, and the serotonin uptake transporter.[36] The loss of serotonergic axons, as shown by histopathologic studies, has been shown in a variety of animal models.[37,38] Primate studies have documented serotonin neuronal loss lasting 7 years, suggesting that these changes are permanent.[39] Human data may support these findings. Controlled studies in MDMA users documented decreased levels of 5-hydroxyindoleacetic acid in cerebrospinal fluid, altered neuroendocrine responses to serotonin agonists, and decreased 5-HT transporter binding as shown by positron emission tomography.[40–42] These studies, when coupled with clinical investigations suggesting that MDMA users have impaired memory and cognitive performance and long-term psychiatric complaints, build a case for serotonergic neuronal toxicity, especially in cases of high dose or prolonged use.[42–45] All of these data are confounded, however, by the fact that the subjects studied had exposure to multiple other drugs as well. Similar data suggest that methamphetamine may cause persistent neurochemical deficits in dopaminergic and serotonergic neurons.[46]

CLINICAL PRESENTATION AND LIFE-THREATENING COMPLICATIONS

Systemic Effects

The most dramatic pattern of systemic toxicity after use of the amphetamine agents reflects a severe hyperadrenergic crisis. The relative contribution of norepinephrine and serotonin to the genesis of this clinical picture is unknown, and these patients may share features of serotonin syndrome and the sympathomimetic toxidrome (see Chapters 24 and 32). This clinical picture of an agitated delirium can occur with the traditional amphetamines and the substituted amphetamines and has been reported at therapeutic doses and in overdose.[47–49] Fulminant hyperpyrexia, tachycardia, hypertension, and agitation may occur, resulting in rhabdomyolysis; hepatorenal failure; disseminated intravascular coagulation; and ultimately, dysrhythmias, cardiovascular collapse, and death.[47,48] The features of the clinical presentation of phenethylamine toxicity are summarized in Table 73-3.

TABLE 73-3 Clinical Manifestations of Phenethylamine Toxicity						
CARDIOVASCULAR	**NEUROLOGIC**	**PULMONARY**	**GASTROINTESTINAL**	**METABOLIC**	**MUSCULAR**	**SKIN**
Hypertension	Euphoria	Pulmonary edema, cardiogenic and noncardiogenic	Nausea	Acidosis	Bruxism	Flushing
Sinus tachycardia	Agitation/violent behavior		Vomiting	Hyperpyrexia	Trismus	Diaphoresis
Ventricular tachydysrhythmias	Paranoia	Pulmonary hypertension	Hepatitis	Hyponatremia: SIADH or dilutional	Rhabdomyolysis	Excoriations
Vasculitis	Hallucinations		Diarrhea			
Valvulopathy	Seizures		Gut ischemia			
Cardiomyopathy	Coma					
Myocardial ischemia/ infarction	Intracranial bleed/ infarction					
Hypotension	Venous sinus thrombosis					
	Hyperreflexia					
	Mydriasis					
	Chorea					

SIADH, syndrome of inappropriate antidiuretic hormone.

Severe hyperthermia is associated with poor clinical outcome. The mechanism of amphetamine-mediated temperature elevation is unknown. In animal models, hyperthermia was not attenuated by decapitation, but it was improved with curare, suggesting that temperature elevation was secondary to muscular heat generation.[50,51] Other animal models suggest, however, that hyperthermia is centrally mediated and appears to be blunted by treatment with serotonin antagonists and dopamine antagonists.[52] Clinical reports describe cases of hyperthermia with and without excess agitation or muscular activity.[53] The data suggest that serotonin-mediated and dopamine-mediated central effects may be augmented by peripheral effects, which cause muscular heat generation in selected cases.[53]

Central Nervous System Effects

The CNS is one of the primary sites of action of the amphetamines, and consequently many of the clinical signs and symptoms of intoxication reflect CNS toxicity. Therapeutic use of amphetamines usually is accompanied by feelings of energy and well-being. Anorexia is common and often the desired effect. As toxicity progresses, energy turns to agitation and unpredictable behavior. Animal studies note frequent stereotypical species-specific behaviors.[24] This behavior may be seen in the clinical setting as repetitive ticlike movements or continued performance of certain tasks. Aggressive and paranoid behavior is common, and injuries and death due to violent behavior and excessive risk taking while amphetamine intoxicated are common.[6] Rodent studies show that aggressive behaviors (and mortality) are magnified under crowded conditions.[54,55] This magnification may account for the escalation of violent behavior that often occurs when the patient is confronted with the police or hospital security force. Larger doses may result in seizures that may be due to drug effect or may be secondary to intracranial hemorrhage.[56,57]

Chronic high-dose consumption of amphetamines and their derivatives may result in amphetamine psychosis.[58] Typically, users have paranoid ideation with ideas of reference.[43,44] Delusions may be well formed; individuals often believe they are under surveillance and may spend a great deal of time and effort to prove this. As the psychosis progresses, frank hallucinations may develop, and the paranoid delusions may provoke sudden violent responses. Symptoms usually abate or disappear with abstinence, but recovery may be delayed and occasionally incomplete.[43] A variety of other psychiatric illnesses, including depression, anxiety disorders, and panic attacks, also have been reported in conjunction with use of amphetamines.[43,59]

Intracerebral hemorrhage has been associated with amphetamines in hypertensive patients and in normotensive individuals.[60] Intraparenchymal and subarachnoid bleeding can occur, and patients with preexisting arteriovenous malformations may be at increased risk. Vasculitis has long been reported from oral and intravenous use of amphetamine. This small- and medium-vessel disease produces a beading pattern on radiologic imaging and can occur in the brain and other vascular beds.[56,57] Ischemic strokes also may occur.

Cardiovascular Effects

The acute cardiovascular effects of amphetamines largely reflect sympathomimetic effects. Lower doses typically are associated with sinus tachycardia and mild hypertension. Palpitations may occur. Larger doses may produce supraventricular and ventricular dysrhythmias.[59] Hypertension may be severe and result in end-organ damage. Occasionally, isolated constriction of vascular beds may result in localized organ ischemia.[61,62] In addition to vasospasm, necrotizing angiitis of smaller vessels may occur, which causes a beading pattern on radioangiography.[56] Myocardial ischemia, infarction, and global cardiomyopathy have been reported, although these complications seem to be less frequent compared with cocaine users.[63] Fenfluramine, dexfenfluramine, and aminorex fumarate, anorexigenic agents that are no longer sold in most countries, have been associated with pulmonary hypertension and valvulopathy.[64]

Gastrointestinal Effects

Gastrointestinal effects of amphetamines probably reflect the ability of these drugs to compromise vascular supply, either through systemic hypoperfusion or through localized vasculitis. Ischemic gut has been reported.[62] Many cases of hepatitis associated with amphetamine use have been reported, and these cases continue to accumulate with regard to the designer drugs.[65–67] The mechanism of liver injury is not clear; some cases are associated with hyperpyrexia, but other cases occur in the absence of fever.[67] Direct toxic effects (of the drug, contaminants, or by-products of synthesis), immune-mediated mechanisms, glutathione depletion, and vasculitis have been hypothesized as potential causes. Currently, no antidotal therapy seems to be successful. The mainstay of therapy is supportive care. The role of liver transplantation in cases of amphetamine-induced liver failure is unclear, and success rates are low.[67]

Dermatologic/Muscular Effects

Along with other stimulants, the amphetamines have been reported to cause rhabdomyolysis.[68] The mechanism of muscle damage is unclear but may include agitation, seizures, hyperthermia, coingestion of other toxins (e.g., cocaine, tobacco, ethanol), or a combination of these factors.[69] Patients present with an elevation of creatine phosphokinase and may or may not have a positive urine dip-stick orthotoluidine test for hemoglobin and myoglobin.[69] Chronic amphetamine use has been associated with alopecia, although the mechanism is unknown.[70] Self-inflicted excoriations may be seen when compulsive or repetitive behaviors cause the patient to scratch repeatedly. Delusions of parasitosis ("crank bugs") may be accompanied by disfiguring attempts to remove the perceived insects or worms from the skin. The poor nutritional status of many chronic amphetamine users may predispose them to nutritional deficiency dermatoses.

Pulmonary Effects

Amphetamines have been associated with cardiogenic and noncardiogenic pulmonary edema.[63] Pulmonary hypertension has been well described with fenfluramine, dexfenfluramine, and aminorex fumarate, but it also has been associated, in a case report, with illicit amphetamines.[71] Asthma may be exacerbated. Any pulmonary complication associated with injection drug use (e.g., infection, granulomas) also may be seen. Pneumothorax or pneumomediastinum may occur with inhalational drug use.

Genitourinary Effects

Urinary frequency and acute urinary retention have been associated with MDMA.[72] Although renal dysfunction may be seen in conjunction with amphetamine toxicity, it is believed to be secondary to rhabdomyolysis, volume depletion,

vasculitis, hyperpyrexia, or a combination of secondary factors rather than direct drug toxicity.

Clinical Presentation and Life-Threatening Complications Associated with Various Designer Drugs

The toxicity of the substituted amphetamines or designer drugs largely reflects the sympathomimetic syndrome seen with overdose of amphetamine and methamphetamine. The ring substitutions of the designer amphetamines convey serotonergic activity, however, that may be accompanied by specific clinical findings and toxicity (see Chapter 24). Data for some of the lesser used phenethylamines are sparse. There are considerable data, however, regarding MDMA, and some generalizations regarding the other amphetamine derivatives may be gleaned from the experience with this compound. Data regarding the clinical presentation of MDMA intoxication and toxic effects come from case reports and series describing side effects and toxicity in the psychotherapeutic setting, after pharmacokinetic/pharmacodynamic studies, or after recreational use. Typical recreational doses range from 50 to 175 mg.

Hayner and McKinney[73] divided adverse reactions to MDMA into three classes: (1) acute reactions with therapeutic doses, (2) overdose reactions, and (3) residual effects. Acute reactions at therapeutic doses commonly include tachycardia, tremor, tight jaw muscles, bruxism, nausea, headache, and sweating. Less commonly, numbness and tingling extremities, hallucinations, ataxia, blurry vision, and nystagmus have been reported. Mydriasis, hyperreflexia, and gait instability also may occur. Tachycardia and hypertension have been documented in healthy volunteers.[74] Ventricular dysrhythmias and cerebrovascular accidents have occurred after allegedly "therapeutic ingestions" of amphetamine and MDMA.[47] Users also report a variety of emotional and cognitive effects, including euphoria, increased energy, decreased appetite, positive changes in attitude or feelings, expanded mental perspective, and heightened sensual arousal.[75] Although MDMA often is referred to as the "love drug," its effect on sexual function is often detrimental.[76] Although most of MDMA's psychological effects are described as positive and relate to the perception of improved insight and interpersonal communication, undesirable symptoms, such as anxiety, nervousness, and depression, have been reported. Difficulty with cognition (multiplication) and judgment has been noted in volunteers.[74]

Overdose reactions consist of symptoms of sympathetic excess similar to amphetamine toxicity, including tachycardia, dysrhythmias, hypertension progressing to hypotension, hyperthermia, muscular rigidity, disseminated intravascular coagulation, rhabdomyolysis, and renal failure.[47,73,77] It is likely that patients with MDMA overdoses also have superimposed serotonin syndrome (see Chapter 24) caused by the serotoninergic effect of the drug. This clinical scenario has been described after ingestion of presumed therapeutic doses and overdose. Because these drugs are metabolized in part by CYP2D6, individuals who are deficient in this enzyme or are on medications that inhibit this enzyme may be at increased risk.[78,79] These signs and symptoms of toxicity have been associated with the use of MDMA at rave parties.[47] Rave parties typically are mass gatherings of young people where dance music is played and MDMA (along with a variety of other drugs) often is found.[80] It has been postulated that vigorous dancing coupled with inadequate fluid intake may predispose MDMA users to hyperthermic crisis and collapse.[47] Recommendations to keep hydrated have been taken to excess, however, and several cases of severe hyponatremia have been reported in rave participants.[81,82] Hyponatremia also has been attributed directly to inhibition of vasopressin in this setting.[83] Severe hypoglycemia also has been seen in MDMA-induced hyperthermia being treated with dantrolene.[84]

Cases of hepatitis have been reported after single doses and chronic use of MDMA.[47,65,66] Hepatitis usually resolves, but some cases have progressed to liver transplantation or death.[65] Aplastic anemia with recovery has been reported.[85,86] MDMA also modulates immune function in vitro, but the clinical correlates of this finding are uncertain.[87] Few data exist regarding the effect of phenethylamines in pregnancy; however, 2,5-dimethoxy-4-methyl-amphetamine (DOM) was found to cause significant uterine and umbilical artery vasoconstriction and evidence of fetal distress in sheep.[88] Diffuse vascular spasm responding to tolazoline hydrochloride and nitroprusside also has been reported after ingestion of DOB.[89]

The third category of reactions described by Hayner and McKinney[73] are attributable to residual effects. Mild residual reactions, such as exhaustion, fatigue, depression, nausea, numbness, and flashbacks, and more significant symptoms, such as anxiety attacks, persistent insomnia, rage reactions, and psychosis, were described. These residual symptoms persisted for hours to 2 weeks. Other authors have described a variety of psychiatric effects, primarily panic disorders, psychosis, flashbacks, and depression, which may be delayed in onset and may persist for months.[44,90,91] These cases seem to vary with respect to duration of symptoms and response to various psychotherapeutic agents, including haloperidol, amitriptyline, and fluoxetine. Because serotonin is implicated in several psychiatric disorders, including depression, psychosis, anxiety, panic, and eating disorders, it is hypothesized that MDMA disruption of serotonin homeostasis may be responsible for these symptoms.

The most concerning long-term potential adverse effect of MDMA is the possibility of CNS serotonergic neuron dysfunction or damage that may be long-lasting or permanent. As of yet, the clinical correlation of serotonergic dysfunction is uncertain. Serotonin dysfunction has been implicated, however, in MDMA's adverse effects on mood, sleep, and emotional and psychiatric state.[41,42]

3,4-METHYLENEDIOXYAMPHETAMINE

MDA is one of the original illicitly used substituted amphetamines. Initial investigations into the serotonergic toxicity of MDA were the catalyst that led to the scheduling of ring-substituted amphetamines.[92] Use is associated with stimulant effects and altered perceptions and hallucinations. Overdose cases may present with severe hyperthermia and subsequent multisystem organ failure.[93]

2,5-DIMETHOXY-4-METHYLAMPHETAMINE

DOM is a powerful hallucinogen with 100 times the potency of mescaline. Adrenergic effects, including tachycardia, elevated temperature, and elevated systolic blood pressure, occur at recreational doses.[94]

PARA-METHOXYAMPHETAMINE

Para-methoxyamphetamine has been involved in many deaths from hyperthermia or intracerebral hemorrhage, in which it was represented as "ecstasy."[49] *Para*-methoxyamphetamine has a reputation of being a dangerous drug, and most case reports indicate that it is a contaminant or substituted agent of specimens marketed as Ecstasy.

4-BROMO-2,5-DIMETHOXYPHENETHYLAMINE

There is little information regarding specific aspects of toxicity of 4-bromo-2,5-dimethoxyphenethylamine, a popular rave drug also known as "nexus." It typically is described as producing altered perception, intoxication, and euphoria, with hallucinations and agitation in higher doses.[95]

3,4-METHYLENEDIOXYETHAMPHETAMINE

The toxicity of 3,4-methylenedioxyethamphetamine appears to mirror that seen with MDMA.[96,97]

4-METHYLAMINOREX

4-Methylaminorex is a methylated derivative of the prescription drug aminorex fumarate. The latter was withdrawn from the European market after it was associated with an increased incidence of pulmonary hypertension.[64] It is not known whether this methylated derivative shares this toxicity.

N-METHYL-1-(3,4-METHYLENEDIOXYPHENYL)-2-BUTANAMINE

Specific human toxicologic data for *N*-methyl-1-(3,4-methylenedioxyphenyl)-2-butanamine are sparse. It commonly is detected in forensic specimens, however. Deaths have been reported.[98] Clinical effects appear to be similar to effects seen with MDMA, and consequently similar toxicologic effects might be expected.[99]

2,5-DIMETHOXY-4-BROMOAMPHETAMINE

One of the most potent hallucinogenic amphetamine derivatives is DOB. Usual oral doses range from 1 to 4 mg.[89,100] Use has been associated with prolonged and severe arterial spasm, resulting in amputation in one case.[89]

METHCATHINONE

Methcathinone is the methylated derivative of cathinone, one of the active constituents of the plant khat (*Catha edulis*). It is synthesized primarily through oxidation of ephedrine. Early reports of methcathinone use originated in Russia, followed by reports from the northern midwest United States. Existing case reports document sympathomimetic toxicity similar to that seen with methamphetamine.[101,102] Prominent psychiatric effects, including paranoia and hallucinations, can occur.[101]

DIAGNOSIS OF INTOXICATION BY PHENETHYLAMINES

The diagnosis of phenethylamine use and toxicity should be based primarily on the recognition of the clinical symptoms of sympathetic excess (see Chapter 32), hallucinations, and, in the case of ring-substituted derivatives such as MDMA, a serotonin syndrome (see Chapter 24). Any disease that results in the appearance of excess sympathetic tone, fever, or hallucinations should be considered. See Table 73-4 for a list of differential diagnoses. Some phenethylamines are associated with other toxicities that may not be secondary to this sympathetic excess, such as hepatotoxicity. Clinicians should be aware of these idiosyncratic toxicities as well.

Laboratory tests and radiographic studies serve primarily to identify medical or traumatic causes that may account for the patient's clinical condition or that may be present concurrently with phenethylamine use. During initial stabilization, a rapid blood glucose determination should be made, or the patient should be given 25 g of 50% dextrose in water by the intravenous route empirically. Empirical naloxone should be considered in unconscious patients. In patients with altered mental status, tachycardia, and fever with unclear history, infectious processes should be suspected, and an appropriate search for a source should be conducted, including chest x-ray, urinalysis, and lumbar puncture and blood cultures, as clinically indicated. These signs and symptoms also may reflect an intraparenchymal hemorrhage (unrelated or secondary to stimulant use), and a computed tomography scan of the head may be indicated. The complete blood count may show hemoconcentration if there has been decreased fluid intake or increased insensible fluid losses. The white blood cell count may be elevated with a leftward shift secondary to demargination from catecholamine excess. Electrolyte analysis may show hyponatremia, hypernatremia, or hyperkalemia. A metabolic acidosis may be present due to volume depletion, hypoperfusion, or seizure activity. Respiratory alkalosis may be seen as compensation for metabolic abnormalities, or it may occur primarily, as a result of anxiety or amphetamine

TABLE 73-4 Differential Diagnosis of Phenethylamine Intoxication

Toxicologic
Cocaine
PCP/ketamine
Anticholinergic agents
Salicylates
Lithium
MAO inhibitors
Theophylline/caffeine
Nitrophenols
LSD
Psilocybin
Isoniazid/monomethylhydrazine
Amoxapine
Tricyclic antidepressants
Scorpion envenomation (*Centruroides sculpturatus*)
Serotonin syndrome
Neuroleptic malignant syndrome
Ethanol/sedative-hypnotic withdrawal

Nontoxicologic
Sepsis/meningitis/encephalitis
Intracerebral hemorrhage or infarction
Pheochromocytoma
Thyrotoxicosis
Temporal lobe epilepsy
Heat-related illness
Psychosis
Hypoglycemia/hyperglycemia

LSD, lysergic acid diethylamide; MAO, monoamine oxidase; PCP, phencyclidine.

stimulation of the respiratory center. In cases of significant toxicity, creatine kinase and troponin-I may be measured to assess rhabdomyolysis and cardiac ischemia. Urinalysis may show a positive dip-stick ortho-toluidine test indicating blood, free hemoglobin, or myoglobin. Liver function tests may be indicated if amphetamine-induced hepatitis is suspected.

Measurement of serum salicylate, theophylline, and lithium concentrations also should be considered because these substances may show a similar clinical picture in overdose. Another medical illness that may mimic amphetamine intoxication is thyrotoxicosis, which may be assessed by measurement of thyroid hormone concentration. Amphetamine use may cause elevation of serum thyroxine concentrations, which resolves when drug use is stopped.[103] Withdrawal from ethanol or sedative-hypnotic drugs may present a similar clinical picture that may be deduced from historical details.

Laboratory Analysis for Amphetamine Compounds

It is often desirable to obtain a quick, inexpensive qualitative determination of drugs of abuse. The most common analytic technique for qualitative screening for amphetamine-like stimulants is the immunoassay. A variety of immunoassays have been developed to detect phenethylamines, including radioimmunoassay, kinetic interaction of microparticles in solution, cloned enzyme donor immunoassay, and enzyme-multiplied immunoassay technique, among others. Although there are differences among all of the techniques listed, they all share the common feature that the antibody used is "tuned" specifically to recognize the chemical structure of the analyte (e.g., amphetamine). The specificity of the antibody depends on the uniqueness of the chemical structure of the analyte. In the case of structurally unique compounds, such as cocaine, there are few substances that would interfere with the immunoassay and cause a false-positive result. As has been shown in this chapter, there are a wide variety of compounds containing the basic phenethylamine nucleus, some of which frequently are prepared illicitly and abused (e.g., methamphetamine) and others that are available over the counter and used therapeutically (e.g., pseudoephedrine). The possibility of a false-positive result from a structurally related compound is increased greatly. There is not a complete lack of specificity, however. The antibodies are designed specifically for interaction with amphetamine and methamphetamine. Although other compounds interact with the antibodies, it is typically only at drug concentrations greater than those required to give a positive result for amphetamine and methamphetamine. A positive result for an immunoassay is reported when a concentration greater than a predetermined cutoff value is detected. Levels less than this cutoff are considered negative because there exists a statistically significant chance that a level below the cutoff is the result of an interfering compound. One of the more commonly used immunoassays is the EMIT-II monoclonal amphetamine/methamphetamine assay (Syva Company, Deerfield, IL). This assay uses a cutoff of 1000 ng/mL for *d*-amphetamine and *d*-methamphetamine.[104] The package insert reports the concentrations of a series of other phenethylamine compounds that produce a positive result approximately equal to that of the 1000 ng/mL cutoff calibrator (Table 73-5). A few nonstimulant compounds do not possess the classic phenethylamine skeleton but may give a false-positive result for a phenethylamine immunoassay screen.

TABLE 73-5 Approximate Concentrations Producing a Positive Result Equivalent to the 1000 ng/mL Cutoff Calibrator in Syva's Emit II Monoclonal Amphetamine/Methamphetamine Assay

COMPOUND	CONCENTRATION (ng/mL) TESTING POSITIVE
d-Amphetamine	1000
d-Methamphetamine	1000
Phentermine	2000
MDA	3000
MDMA	6000
Fenfluramine	36,000
Tranylcypromine	65,000
Propranolol	160,000
l-Ephedrine	180,000
Tyramine	200,000
Phenylpropanolamine	290,000
Pseudoephedrine	670,000

MDA, 3,4-methylenedioxyamphetamine; MDMA, 3,4-methylenedioxymethamphetamine.
Data from Syva product insert.[104]

Two such compounds are ranitidine and chloroquine. The exact reasons for these interactions are not clear.

Forensic cases, such as those involving employment or litigation, may require confirmation of a positive immunoassay result. Confirmation is performed using an alternative methodology, typically gas chromatography with mass spectrometric detection. This method allows positive structural identification and quantitation of the analyte that produced the positive result in the immunoassay analysis. The lack of correlation between blood or urine levels of phenethylamine stimulants and clinical response makes such confirmation in clinical cases typically unnecessary.

Clinical and forensic interpretation of concentrations of methamphetamine in blood is an area fraught with difficulty. There does not seem to be a consistent link between measured concentration and level of intoxication or impairment. Similarly, deaths have been attributed to methamphetamine intoxication at levels well below those in individuals who have survived without deficit. Any detectable level of methamphetamine should be considered potentially toxic and correlated with the clinical circumstances.

TREATMENT OF PHENETHYLAMINE TOXICITY

Initial treatment of toxicity from amphetamine derivatives should be directed toward assessment and stabilization of the airway, breathing, circulation, and temperature. Agitation and combativeness may make the initial evaluation and treatment of these patients difficult. Rapid control of the situation is essential because significant hyperthermia or other vital sign or laboratory abnormalities may require emergent therapy. Benzodiazepines (e.g., diazepam or lorazepam) and butyrophenones (e.g., haloperidol or droperidol) have been recommended for agitation in these cases.[68,105] Benzodiazepines decreased tremor, piloerection, and seizures in rats but did not prevent death in a pretreatment model.[106] Conversely,

haloperidol and propranolol decreased fatality rates in the same study but did not prevent seizures. In amphetamine-intoxicated patients, droperidol may act more quickly than lorazepam and require fewer repeat doses.[107] The potential disadvantages of butyrophenones include dose-dependent QT_c interval prolongation, reduction of seizure threshold, impaired heat dissipation, and dystonias. Because of these potential complications, benzodiazepines should be considered to be the preferable first-line agents for sedation. Physical restraint of the patient also may be necessary. Intravenous access should be obtained in all cases of significant vital sign abnormalities or mental status changes. Patients should be placed on a cardiac monitor and be given oxygen as needed. Endotracheal intubation should be performed if hypoventilation is present or if airway protective reflexes are impaired.

Hyperthermia must be diagnosed rapidly and treated aggressively. Initial control of agitation must be obtained rapidly in these circumstances to prevent further heat generation. Vigorous use of benzodiazepines or butyrophenones should be followed by cooling with mist and fans or ice bath. If this approach is not successful, consider intubation and chemical paralysis to reduce muscular thermogenesis. Acetaminophen, aspirin, and cooling blankets have little value in these circumstances. The use of dantrolene (see Chapter 156) in this circumstance has not been studied, but it may be considered if the above-listed measures have failed.[108] In cases of significant temperature elevation, core temperature should be monitored with a continuous esophageal, rectal, or bladder probe, if available.

Gastrointestinal decontamination is not frequently an issue because many patients have used amphetamines by the intravenous or inhalational route. Nasal insufflation is not likely to be accompanied by a significant amount of drug in the gastrointestinal tract. In patients with a significant recent oral ingestion, ingestion of contraband drug packets, or ingestion of sustained-release products, gastrointestinal decontamination can be considered (see Chapter 5). Gastric lavage is unlikely to be of benefit. Activated charcoal has been shown to delay the onset to symptoms and reduce mortality when given after methamphetamine in a mouse model.[109] Oral activated charcoal should be considered if a patient presents within approximately 1 hour of ingestion of an amphetamine or has evidence of progressive toxicity. Charcoal should be administered cautiously in these patients because of the risk of seizures and loss of airway protective reflexes.

Seizures should be treated initially with a benzodiazepine. If seizure activity persists, phenobarbital or propofol should

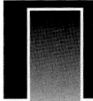

Indications for ICU Admission in Amphetamine and Amphetamine-Derivative Intoxication

Clinically significant cardiac dysrhythmia
Cardiac ischemia
Severe hypertension
Coma
Intracranial hemorrhage/infarction
Intractable seizures
Agitated delirium with fever
Multisystem organ failure

be added, with airway protection as needed. The role of phenytoin in toxin-induced seizures is likely to be minor. Continued seizure activity that is unresponsive to benzodiazepines and barbiturates, especially if it is contributing to significant hyperthermia, should be treated with chemical paralysis followed by electroencephalographic monitoring and consideration for general anesthesia. If focal neurologic deficits or persistent nonfocal findings such as coma are present, consideration should be given to the possibility of intracranial bleeding or infarction, and a computed tomography scan of the head should be obtained.

Amphetamines may cause a variety of dysrhythmias. Sinus tachycardia alone without hemodynamic compromise usually does not require treatment. Sinus tachycardia with hypertension may respond to a β-blocking agent, but a β-adrenergic blocking agent alone should be used with caution because of the possibility of unopposed α-adrenergic stimulation and worsening hypertension. An α-adrenergic blocking agent or a combination of an α-adrenergic blocking agent, such as phentolamine, with a β-adrenergic blocking agent or a β-blocker with α-blocking properties, such as labetalol, would be a rational choice in such cases. Likewise, titratable agents, such as nitroprusside or nitroglycerin, may be used for significant hypertension. Ventricular tachyarrhythmias should be treated by standard measures.

Hypotension, if present, should be treated first with normal saline or lactated Ringer's solution. Hypotension unresponsive to crystalloid infusion requires the use of standard vasopressor agents.

Vasospasm has been reported with amphetamine use.[89] Local vasospasm may be treated with vasodilators, such as nitroprusside, or α-adrenergic blocking agents, such as phentolamine. These agents may be administered by venous infusion or by local arterial infusion to the affected area. Vasospasm may be recurrent and require prolonged therapy.[89]

Rhabdomyolysis, if present, should be treated with adequate hydration and maintenance of urine output. Many clinicians recommend urinary alkalinization to prevent renal myoglobin deposition. To alkalinize the urine, 88 to 132 mEq/L of sodium bicarbonate can be added to 1 L of 5% dextrose in water. The rate can be adjusted to maintain adequate urine flow and urine pH of 7.5. Serum potassium concentrations should be monitored closely in this setting because rhabdomyolysis may be accompanied by hyperkalemia, and sodium bicarbonate administration may result in hypokalemia. Alkalinization of the urine may impair renal clearance of the amphetamines.

Elimination Enhancement

The enhanced renal elimination of amphetamines by urinary acidification is mentioned only to be condemned. The elimination half-life of amphetamine is 8 to 10.5 hours with acidic urine and 16 to 31 hours with alkaline urine.[110] Intoxication from amphetamines may be accompanied by rhabdomyolysis, however, and the risk of precipitating renal failure due to the precipitation of myoglobin in acidic urine is believed to outweigh any potential benefit from increased drug clearance. Hemodialysis, hemoperfusion, and hemofiltration play no role in increasing drug clearance in amphetamine toxicity.

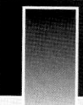

Criteria for ICU Discharge in Amphetamine and Amphetamine-Derivative Intoxication

Hemodynamic stability
Ability to protect airway
Resolution of hyperthermia and lack of evidence of hyperthermia-related multisystem organ failure
No requirement for continued intravenous medication infusion for hypertension, cardiac dysrhythmias, or seizures
No evidence of continued drug absorption in cases of oral exposure
Intracranial hemorrhage/infarction
Intractable seizures
Agitated delirium with fever
Multisystem organ failure

Pharmacologic Treatment Options for Amphetamine and Amphetamine-Derivative Intoxication

Lorazepam: 1–4 mg IV/IM
Diazepam: 2–10 mg IV
Midazolam: 1–4 mg IV/IM
Phenobarbital: 10–20 mg/kg IV
Propofol: 5–50 μg/kg/min IV
Haloperidol*,†: 2–10 mg IV/IM
Droperidol*,†: 1.25–10 mg IV/IM
Labetalol: 20 mg over 2 min IV‡
Phentolamine: 1–10 mg IV/IM
Nitroprusside: 0.3–10 μg/kg/min IV
Nitroglycerin: 5–100 μg/min IV

*May be used in combination with benzodiazepines.

†Use with caution in patients with elevated temperature.

‡May repeat at doses of 40 mg, then 80 mg, at 10-min intervals as needed.

IM, intramuscular; IV, intravenous.

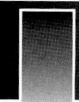

Key Points in the Treatment of Amphetamine and Amphetamine-Derivative Intoxication

1. Rapidly gain control of agitated patients, using physical and pharmacologic restraint as needed.
2. Rapidly assess all vital signs, including core temperature.
3. Treat hyperthermia aggressively with sedation, physical cooling measures, and paralysis, as clinically indicated.
4. Consider rhabdomyolysis as a complication of intoxication.

SPECIAL POPULATIONS

Pediatric Patients

Neonatal effects associated with maternal amphetamine use include tachycardia and bradycardia, which typically resolve as the drug is eliminated or as catecholamine homeostasis is restored.[111] Infants born to amphetamine-using mothers may lag behind their peers in various measures of intellectual performance and show abnormal growth and maturation patterns at puberty.[111] Children also may ingest amphetamines inadvertently, and these children may present a diagnostic dilemma to the clinician. In one series describing accidental methamphetamine ingestion, children commonly manifested tachycardia, irritability, inconsolable crying, agitation, and vomiting.[112] These symptoms can mimic many serious childhood diseases. A urine toxicologic screen for amphetamines may be a valuable diagnostic tool in these cases.

Pregnant Patients

Methamphetamine has been shown to cross the placenta rapidly in sheep and distribute rapidly into fetal tissues with a longer elimination half-life than in the mother.[113] Doses similar to those seen in recreational use caused maternal and fetal hypertension and a decrease in fetal oxyhemoglobin saturation and arterial pH in this model.[113] Amphetamine use during pregnancy has been associated with maternal hypertension, tachycardia, proteinuria, premature labor, and placental hemorrhage in humans.[111] Reported adverse pregnancy outcomes associated with maternal amphetamine use include cleft lip and palate, cardiac defects, growth retardation, cerebral hemorrhage, hyperbilirubinemia, biliary atresia, low birth weight, and reduced head circumference.[111] Preliminary data regarding prenatal exposure to MDMA indicate that there may be increased risk of cardiovascular and musculoskeletal abnormalities.[114]

Patients with Drug-Drug Interactions

Drug-drug interactions with amphetamines fall into two categories: interactions that result in increased amphetamine action and interactions that result from decreased renal excretion or hepatic metabolism of amphetamine. MAO inhibitors and possibly tricyclic antidepressants (catecholamine reuptake inhibitors) when taken together with amphetamines may result in an exaggerated release of catecholamines and sympathomimetic toxidrome or serotonin syndrome.[115] Similarly, antidepressants with serotonergic activity may increase clinical effects and toxicity seen with MDMA and related drugs. Any drug or dietary change that results in alkaline urine (acetazolamide, antacid therapy, sodium bicarbonate) results in a decrease in the urinary clearance of amphetamine, although this effect is of little significance because of the small urinary clearance of these drugs. The amphetamines are metabolized in part by the CYP2D6 enzyme. Users who are deficient in CYP2D6 activity (7% of whites) or who are taking medications that are CYP2D6 inhibitors (e.g., paroxetine and fluoxetine) may be susceptible to increased toxicity from these drugs. This susceptibility may account for reported cases of toxicity with therapeutic or usual recreational doses of amphetamines and derivatives.[49,79] In addition, the amphetamines may inhibit the metabolism of other drugs that are metabolized by this cytochrome isoform.[78]

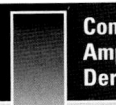

Common Errors in the Treatment of Amphetamine and Amphetamine-Derivative Intoxication

Failure to rapidly detect and aggressively treat hyperthermia or other significant vital sign abnormalities because of violent behavior on the part of the patient

Failure to consider primary or secondary intracranial hemorrhage as a cause of mental status changes

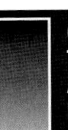

Common Misconceptions about the Treatment of Amphetamine and Amphetamine-Derivative Intoxication

1. Urinary alkalinization is useful in amphetamine toxicity.
2. All amphetamine compounds can be detected reliably by commonly available urine drug screens.

REFERENCES

1. Karch SB: Synthetic stimulants. In: The Pathology of Drug Abuse. Boca Raton, FL, CRC Press, 1993, pp 165–234.
2. Monroe RR, Drell HJ: Oral use of stimulants obtained from inhalers. JAMA 135:909–915, 1947.
3. Smith DE, Wesson DR, Sees KL, et al: An epidemiological and clinical analysis of propylhexedrine abuse in the United States. J Psychoact Drugs 20:441–442, 1988.
4. Office of Applied Statistics, Substance Abuse and Mental Health Services Administration, U.S. Department of Health and Human Services: Summary of Findings from the 1998 National Household Survey on Drug Abuse. Washington, DC, Department of Health and Human Services, 1999.
5. Office of Applied Statistics, Substance Abuse and Mental Health Services Administration: Year-end 1998 Emergency Department Data from the Drug Abuse Warning Network. Washington, DC, Department of Health and Human Services, 2000.
6. Office of Applied Statistics, Substance Abuse and Mental Health Services Administration: Drug Abuse Warning Network Annual Medical Examiner Data 1998. Washington, DC, Department of Health and Human Services, 1999.
7. Christophersen AS: Amphetamine designer drugs—an overview and epidemiology. Toxicol Lett 112–113:127–131, 2000.
8. Drug Enforcement Agency: 3,4-Methylenedioxymethamphetamine (MDMA, XTC, X, ECSTASY, ADAM). U.S. Department of Justice. Alexandria, Virginia, 1999. Available at: http://www.usdoj.gov/dea/concern/mdma/mdma.htm.
9. Cho AK: Ice: A new dosage form of an old drug. Science 249:631–634, 1990.
10. Henderson GL: Designer drugs: Past history and future prospects. J Forensic Sci 33:569–575, 1988.
11. Shulgin A, Shulgin A: Pihkal: A Chemical Love Story. Berkeley, CA, Transform Press, 1991.
12. Peroutka SJ: Incidence of recreational use of 3,4-methylene dimethoxymethamphetamine (MDMA, "ecstasy") on an undergraduate campus. N Engl J Med 317:1542–1543, 1987.
13. Cuomo MJ, Dyment PG, Gammino VM: Increasing use of "ecstasy" (MDMA) and other hallucinogens on a college campus. J Am Coll Health 42:271–274, 1994.
14. White JM, Bochner F, Irvine RJ: The agony of "ecstasy." Med J Aust 166:117–118, 1997.
15. Nichols DE: Medicinal chemistry and structure-activity relationships. In Cho AK, Segal DS (eds): Amphetamine and Its Analogs: Psychopharmacology, Toxicology and Abuse. San Diego, Academic Press, 1994, pp 3–41.

16. Jacob P 3rd, Shulgin AT: Structure-activity relationships of the classic hallucinogens and their analogs. In National Institute on Drug Abuse: Hallucinogens: An Update. NIDA Research Monograph 146. Rockville, MD, National Institute on Drug Abuse, 1994, pp 74–91.

17. Isaacson EI: Central nervous system stimulants. In Delgado JN, Remers WA (eds): Wilson and Gisvold's Textbook of Organic Medicinal and Pharmaceutical Chemistry, 10th ed. Philadelphia, Lippincott-Raven, 1998, pp 463–477.

18. Heinonen EH, Anttila MI, Lammintausta RA: Pharmacokinetic aspects of l-deprenyl (selegiline) and its metabolites. Clin Pharmacol Ther 56:742–749, 1994.

19. Cody JT, Valtier S: Detection of amphetamine and methamphetamine following administration of benzphetamine. J Anal Toxicol 22:299–309, 1998.

20. Cody JT: Enantiomeric composition of amphetamine and methamphetamine derived from the precursor compound famprofazone. Forensic Sci Int 80:189–199, 1996.

21. Soine WH: Clandestine drug synthesis. Med Res Rev 6:41–74, 1986.

22. Tanaka K, Ohmori T, Inoue T: Analysis of impurities in illicit methamphetamine. Forensic Sci Int 56:157–165, 1992.

23. Allcott JV III, Barnhart RA, Mooney LA: Acute lead poisoning in two users of illicit methamphetamine. JAMA 258:510–511, 1987.

24. Seiden LS, Sabol KE, Ricaurte GA: Amphetamine: Effects on catecholamine systems and behavior. Annu Rev Pharmacol Toxicol 32:639–677, 1993.

25. Kennedy LT, Hanbauer I: Sodium sensitive cocaine binding to rat striatal membrane: Possible relationship to dopamine uptake sites. J Neurochem 41:172–178, 1983.

26. Fischer JF, Cho AK: Chemical release of dopamine from striatal homogenates: Evidence for an exchange diffusion model. J Pharmacol Exp Ther 208:203–209, 1979.

27. Parker EM, Cubeddu LX: Comparative effects of amphetamine, phenylethylamine and related drugs on dopamine efflux, dopamine uptake and mazindol binding. J Pharmacol Exp Ther 245:199–210, 1988.

28. Miller HH, Shore PA, Clarke DE: In vivo monoamine oxidase inhibition by d-amphetamine. Biochem Pharmacol 29:1347–1354, 1980.

29. Mantle TJ, Tipton KF, Garrett NJ: Inhibition of monoamine oxidase by amphetamine and related compounds. Biochem Pharmacol 25:2073–2077, 1976.

30. Ersner JS: The treatment of obesity due to dietary indiscretion (overeating) with benzedrine sulfate. Endocrinology 27:776–780, 1940.

31. Spengler J, Waser PG: Influence of various pharmacologic agents on the food intake of albino rats in acute experiments. Arch Exp Pathol Pharmakol 237:171–185, 1959.

32. Sugrue MF: Neuropharmacology of drugs affecting food intake. Pharmacol Ther 32:145–182, 1987.

33. Berger UV, Gu XF, Azmitia EC: The substituted amphetamines 3,4-methylenedioxyamphetamine, methamphetamine, p-chloroamphetamine and fenfluramine induce 5-hydroxytryptamine release via a common mechanism blocked by fluoxetine and cocaine. Eur J Pharmacol 215:153–160, 1992.

34. Heckmatpanah CR, Peroutka SJ: 5-hydroxytryptamine uptake blockers attenuate the 5-hydroxytryptamine releasing effects of 3,4-methylenedioxymethamphetamine and related agents. Eur J Pharmacol 177:95–98, 1990.

35. Mørland J: Toxicity of drug abuse–amphetamine designer drugs (ecstasy): Mental effects and consequences of single dose use. Toxicol Lett 112–113:147–152, 2000.

36. Steele TD, McCann UD, Ricaurte GA: 3,4-Methylenedioxymethamphetamine (MDMA, "ecstasy"): Pharmacology and toxicology in animals and humans. Addiction 89:539–551, 1994.

37. Ricaurte GA, Forno LS, Wilson MA, et al: (±)3,4-Methylenedioxymethamphetamine selectively damages central serotonergic neurons in nonhuman primates. JAMA 260:51–55, 1988.

38. Ricaurte GA, Martello AL, Katz JL, et al: Lasting effects of (±)3,4-methylenedioxymethamphetamine on central serotonergic neurons in non-human primates: Neurochemical observations. J Pharmacol Exp Ther 261:616–622, 1992.

39. Hatzidimitriou G, McCann UD, Ricaurte GA: Altered serotonin innervation patterns in the forebrain of monkeys treated with (±) 3,4-methylenedioxymethamphetamine seven years previously: Factors influencing abnormal recovery. J Neurosci 19:5096–5107, 1999.

40. McCann UD, Szabo Z, Scheffel U, et al: Positron emission tomographic evidence of toxic effect of MDMA ("ecstasy") on brain serotonin neurons in human beings. Lancet 352:1433–1437, 1998.

41. McCann UD, Eligulashvili V, Mertl M, et al: Altered neuroendocrine and behavioral responses to m-chlorophenylpiperazine in 3,4-methylenedioxyamphetamine (MDMA) users. Psychopharmacology 147:56–65, 1999.

42. Reneman L, Booij J, Schmand B, et al: Memory disturbances in "ecstasy" users are correlated with an altered brain serotonin neurotransmission. Psychopharmocology 148:322–324, 2000.

43. McGuire PK, Cope H, Fahy TA: Diversity of psychopathology associated with use of 3,4-methylenedioxymethamphetamine ("ecstasy"). Br J Psychiatry 165:391–395, 1994.

44. McGuire P: Long term psychiatric and cognitive effects of MDMA use. Toxicol Lett 112–113:153–156, 2000.

45. O'Shea E, Granados R, Esteban B, et al: The relationship between the degree of neurodegeneration of rat brain 5-HT nerve terminals and the dose and frequency of administration of MDMA ("ecstasy"). Neuropharmacology 37:919–926, 1998.

46. Gibb JW, Johnson M, Elayan I, et al: Neurotoxicity of amphetamines and their metabolites. In Rapaka RS, Chiang N, Martin BR (eds): Pharmacokinetics, Metabolism and Pharmaceutics of Drugs of Abuse. Rockville, MD, National Institute on Drug Abuse, 1997, pp 128–145.

47. Henry JA, Jeffreys KJ, Dawling S: Toxicity and deaths from 3,4-methylenedioxymethamphetamine ("ecstasy"). Lancet 340:384–387, 1992.

48. Ginsberg MD, Hertzman M, Schmidt-Nowara WW: Amphetamine intoxication with coagulopathy, hyperthermia and reversible renal failure: A syndrome resembling heatstroke. Ann Intern Med 73:81–85, 1970.

49. Byard RW, Gilbert J, James R, et al: Amphetamine derivative fatalities in south Australia—is "ecstasy" the culprit? Am J Forensic Med Pathol 19:261–265, 1998.

50. Weis J: On the hyperthermic response to d-amphetamine in the decapitated rat. Life Sci 13:475–484, 1973.

51. Zalis EG, Kaplan G, Lundberg GD: Acute lethality of amphetamines in dogs and its antagonism by curare. Proc Soc Exp Biol Med 118:557–561, 1965.

52. Yamawaki S, Lai H, Horita A: Dopaminergic and serotonergic mechanisms of thermoregulation: Mediation of thermal effects of apomorphine and dopamine. J Pharmacol Exp Ther 227:383–388, 1983.

53. Calloway CW, Clark RF: Hyperthermia in psychostimulant overdose. Ann Emerg Med 24:68–76, 1994.

54. Kataoka Y, Gomita Y, Fukuda T, et al: Effects of aggregation on methamphetamine toxicity in mice. Acta Med Okayama 40:121–126, 1986.

55. Shintomi K: Effects of psychotropic drugs on methamphetamine-induced behavioral excitation in grouped mice. Eur J Pharmacol 31:195–206, 1975.

56. Citron BP, Halpern M, McCarron M, et al: Necrotizing angiitis associated with drug abuse. N Engl J Med 238:1003–1011, 1970.

57. Koff RS, Widrich WC, Robbins AH: Necrotizing angiitis in a methamphetamine user with hepatitis B—angiographic diagnosis, five-month follow-up results and localization of bleeding site. N Engl J Med 288:946–947, 1973.

58. McGuire P, Fahy T: Chronic paranoid psychosis after misuse of MDMA ("ecstasy"). BMJ 302:697, 1991.

59. McCann UD, Slate SO, Ricaurte GA: Adverse reactions with 3,4,methylenedioxymethamphetamine (MDMA; "ecstasy"). Drug Saf 15:107–115, 1996.

60. Weiss SR, Raskind R, Morganstern NL, et al: Intracerebral and subarachnoid hemorrhage following use of methamphetamine ("speed"). Int Surg 53:123–127, 1970.

61. Furst SR, Fallon SP, Reznik GN, et al: Myocardial infarction after inhalation of methamphetamine. N Engl J Med 323:1147–1148, 1990.

62. Herr RD, Caravati EM: Acute transient ischemic colitis after oral methamphetamine ingestion. Am J Emerg Med 9:406–409, 1991.

63. Hong R, Matsuyama E, Nur K: Cardiomyopathy associated with the smoking of crystal methamphetamine. JAMA 265:1152–1154, 1991.

64. McCann UD, Seiden LS, Rubin LJ, et al: Brain serotonin neurotoxicity and primary pulmonary hypertension from fenfluramine and dexfenfluramine, a systematic review of the literature. JAMA 278:666–672, 1997.

65. Andreu V, Mas A, Bruguera M, et al: Ecstasy: A common cause of severe acute hepatotoxicity. J Hepatol 29:394–397, 1998.

66. Dykhuizen RS, Brunt PW, Atkinson P, et al: Ecstasy induced hepatitis mimicking viral hepatitis. Gut 36:939–941, 1995.

67. Jones AL, Simpson KJ: Review article: Mechanisms and management of hepatoxicity in ecstasy (MDMA) and amphetamine intoxications. Aliment Pharmacol Ther 13:129–133, 1999.

68. Derlet RW, Rice P, Horowitz BZ, et al: Amphetamine toxicity: Experience with 127 cases. J Emerg Med 7:157–161, 1989.

69. Richards JR, Johnson EB, Stark RW, et al: Methamphetamine use and rhabdomyolysis in the ED: A 5-year study. Am J Emerg Med 17:681–685, 1999.

70. Eckert J, Church RE, Ebling FJ, et al: Hair loss in women. Br J Dermatol 79:543–548, 1967.

71. Schaiberger PH, Kennedy TC, Miller FC, et al: Pulmonary hypertension associated with long-term inhalation of "crank" methamphetamine. Chest 104:614–616, 1993.

72. Bryden AA, Rothwell PJN, O'Reilly PH: Urinary retention with misuse of "ecstasy." BMJ 310:504, 1995.

73. Hayner GN, McKinney H: MDMA the dark side of ecstasy. J Psychoactive Drugs 18:341–347, 1986.

74. Downing J: The psychological and physiological effects of MDMA on normal volunteers. J Psychoactive Drugs 18:335–340, 1986.

75. Greer G, Tolbert R: Subjective reports of the effects of MDMA in a clinical setting. J Psychoactive Drugs 18:319–327, 1986.

76. Buffum J, Moser C: MDMA and human sexual function. J Psychoactive Drugs 18:355–359, 1986.

77. Brown C, Osterloh J: Multiple severe complications from recreational ingestion of MDMA ("ecstasy"). JAMA 258:780–781, 1987.

78. Wu D, Otton SV, Inaba T: Interactions of amphetamine analogs with human liver CYP2D6. Biochem Pharmacol 53:1605–1612, 1997.

79. Henry JA, Hill IR: Fatal interaction between ritonavir and MDMA. Lancet 352:1751–1752, 1998.

80. Schwartz RH, Miller NS: MDMA (ecstasy) and the rave: A review. Pediatrics 100:705–708, 1997.

81. Matthai SM, Davidson DC, Sills JA, et al: Cerebral oedema after ingestion of MDMA ("ecstasy") and unrestricted intake of water. BMJ 312:1359, 1996.

82. Parr MJA, Low HM, Botterill P: Hyponatremia and death after "ecstasy" ingestion. Med J Aust 166:136–137, 1997.

83. Holden R, Jackson MA: Near-fatal hyponatraemic coma due to vasopressin over-secretion after "ecstasy" (3,4-MDMA). Lancet 347:1052, 1996.

84. Montgomery H, Myerson S: 3,4-Methylenedioxymethamphetamine (MDMA, or "ecstasy") and associated hypoglycemia. Am J Emerg Med 15:218, 1997.

85. Clark AD, Butt N: Ecstasy-induced very severe aplastic anaemia complicated by invasive pulmonary mucormycosis treated with allogenic peripheral blood progenitor cell transplant. Clin Lab Haematol 19:279–281, 1997.

86. Marsh JC, Abboudi ZH, Gibson FM, et al: Aplastic anemia following exposure to 3,4-methylenedioxymethamphetamine ("ecstasy"). Br J Haematol 88:281–285, 1994.

87. House RV, Thomas PT, Bhargava HN: Selective modulation of immune function resulting from in vitro exposure to methylenedioxymethamphetamine (ecstasy). Toxicology 96:59–69, 1995.

88. Zhang L, Dyer DC, Hembrough FB, et al: Effect of R(−) 2,5-dimethoxy-4-methylamphetamine on uterine and umbilical blood flow in conscious pregnant sheep. Eur J Pharmacol 199:179–184, 1991.

89. Bowen JS, Davis GB, Kearney TE, et al: Diffuse vascular spasm associated with 4-bromo-2,5-dimethoxyamphetamine ingestion. JAMA 249:1477–1479, 1983.

90. Creighton FJ, Black DL, Hyde CE: "Ecstasy" psychosis and flashbacks. Br J Psychiatry 159:713–715, 1991.

91. McCann UD, Ricaurte GA: Lasting neuropsychiatric sequelae of (3,4) methylenedioxymethamphetamine ("ecstasy") in recreational users. J Clin Psychopharmacol 11:302–305, 1991.

92. Ricaurte GA, Bryan G, Strauss L, et al: Hallucinogenic amphetamine selectively destroys brain serotonin nerve terminals. Science 229:986–988, 1985.

93. Simpson DL, Rumack BH: Methylenedioxyamphetamine: Clinical description of overdose, death and review of pharmacology. Arch Intern Med 141:1507–1509, 1981.

94. Snyder SH, Faillace L, Hollister L: 2,5-Dimethoxy-4-methylamphetamine (STP): A new hallucinogenic drug. Science 158:669–670, 1967.

95. De Boer D, Gijzels MJ, Bosman IJ, et al: More data about the new psychoactive drug 2C-B. J Anal Toxicol 23:227–228, 1999.

96. Dowling GP, McDonough ET III, Bost RO: "Eve" and "ecstasy": A report of five deaths associated with the use of MDEA and MDMA. JAMA 257:1615–1617, 1987.

97. Weinmann W, Bohnert M: Lethal monointoxication by overdosage of MDEA. Forensic Sci Int 91:91–101, 1998.

98. Carter N, Rutty GN, Milroy CM, et al: Deaths associated with MBDB misuse. Int J Legal Med 113:168–170, 2000.

99. Nichols DE: Differences between the mechanism of action of MDMA, MBDB, and the classic hallucinogens: Identification of a new therapeutic class: Entactogens. J Psychoactive Drugs 18:305–313, 1986.

100. Shulgin AT: Profiles of psychedelic drugs: DOB. J Psychedelic Drugs 13:99, 1981.

101. Emerson TS, Cisek JE: Methcathinone: A Russian designer amphetamine infiltrates rural Midwest. Ann Emerg Med 22:1897–1903, 1993.

102. Goldstone MS: "Cat": Methcathinone—a new drug of abuse. JAMA 269:2508, 1993.

103. Morley JE, Shafer RB, Elson MK, et al: Amphetamine-induced hyperthyroxinemia. Ann Intern Med 93:707–709, 1980.

104. Syva Company: EMIT-II monoclonal amphetamine/methamphetamine assay. Product Insert, 1992.

105. Solursh LP, Clement WR: Use of diazepam in hallucinogenic drug crises. JAMA 205:644–645, 1968.

106. Derlet RW, Albertson TE, Rice P: Protection against d-amphetamine toxicity. Am J Emerg Med 8:105–108, 1990.

107. Richards JR, Derlet RW, Duncan DR: Methamphetamine toxicity: Treatment with a benzodiazepine versus a butyrophenone. Eur J Emerg Med 4:130–135, 1997.

108. Denborough MA, Hopkinson KC: Dantrolene and "ecstasy." Med J Aust 166:165–166, 1997.

109. McKinney P, Tomaszewski C, Phillips S, et al: Prevention of methamphetamine toxicity by activated charcoal in mice. Ann Emerg Med 24:220–223, 1994.

110. Davis JM, Kopin IJ, Lemberger L, et al: Effects of urinary pH on amphetamine metabolism. Ann N Y Acad Sci 179:493–501, 1971.

111. Plessinger MA: Prenatal exposures to amphetamines. Obstet Gynecol Clin North Am 25:119–138, 1998.

112. Kolecki P: Inadvertent methamphetamine poisoning in pediatric patients. Pediatr Emerg Care 14:385–387, 1998.

113. Burchfield DJ, Lucas VW, Abrams RM, et al: Disposition and pharmacodynamics of methamphetamine in pregnant sheep. JAMA 265:1968–1973, 1991.

114. McElhatton PR, Bateman DN, Evans C: Congenital anomalies after prenatal ecstasy exposure. Lancet 354:1441–1442, 1999.

115. Smilkstein MJ, Smolinske SC, Rumack BH: A case of MAO inhibitor/MDMA interaction: Agony after ecstasy. Clin Toxicol J Toxicol 25:149–159, 1987.

CHAPTER 74

Phencyclidine and Its Congeners

Michael J. Pali ■ R. Steven Tharratt ■ Timothy E. Albertson

Phencyclidine (PCP) and its related compounds are drugs that were popular in the mid- to late 1970s. Currently the use of these drugs is highly regional, mostly concentrated in Los Angeles and Washington, D.C.[1] In other areas, use of PCP and its related compounds is sporadic enough that they are often forgotten. A recent Annual Report of the American Association of Poison Control Centers revealed 372 reported PCP exposures, with 2 deaths.[2] Most patients were older than 19 years of age (Table 74-1).[3] The toxidrome of these drugs, which can be highly variable, may not be readily identified in a critically ill patient. To make things more difficult, coingestion of PCP with other compounds is the rule rather than the exception.

CHEMISTRY

PCP was created in 1926 as reported by Kotz and Merkel from 1-piperidinocyclohexanecarbonitrile (PCC) with Grignard reagents (Fig. 74-1).[4] Thirty years later in 1958, PCP was used as an investigational anesthetic under the name Sernyl, manufactured by the pharmaceutical company Parke Davis. The original investigators searched for an anesthetic with dissociative qualities with minimal systemic effects. Studies on rhesus monkeys showed surgical anesthesia without respiratory depression or hypotension.[5] Side effects of PCP use, such as prolonged coma and bizarre behavior, occurred during emergence from anesthesia and led to its withdrawal from human clinical use in 1965, when safer derivatives, such as ketamine, (Fig. 74-2) were used. Afterward, PCP was marketed as Sernalyn for use in veterinary medicine as a dissociative anesthetic but was eventually discontinued for that purpose as well.

PCP has been used under a variety of street names, many with animal derivations ("hog," "elephant tranquilizer") arising from its use in veterinary anesthesia (Table 74-2). PCP use surged in the mid-1970s because the drug was easy to create in small laboratories from readily available reagents. The precursor, piperidine (Fig. 74-3), was readily available in large quantities. Several other "designer" variants of PCP, such as phenylcyclopentylpiperidine (PCPP), thienylcyclohexylpiperidine (TCP), cyclohexamine (PCE), and phenylcyclohexylpyrrolidine (PHP), that have effects similar to those of PCP have been manufactured (see Fig. 74-3).[4]

Route of Ingestion

PCP can be smoked, snorted, ingested orally, or injected intravenously and intramuscularly. The most common route is through inhalation (Table 74-3) in tobacco and marijuana cigarettes laced with PCP; for example, "Sherms" is slang for Sherman cigarettes that are laced with PCP (hence, the user would have the strength of a Sherman tank). Many other street drugs reported to be pure are in fact adulterated with the cheaper and relatively easier-to-create PCP. In most cases, marijuana joints and cigarettes are the most likely media; 25% of most street-obtained products contain PCP.[6] Exposure often is self-limited in many cases because the user must be awake and alert enough to smoke. Serum concentrations of greater than 300 mg/dL are less likely to be achieved through smoking as the user becomes more stuporous, dissociated, and unable to self-dose to the more toxic levels.

PATHOPHYSIOLOGY

PCP (see Fig. 74-1) is a three-ringed structured molecule that exists as either a free base or its hydrochloride salt. The pK_a is 8.5, volume of distribution is 5.3 to 7.5 L/kg, and it is highly lipophilic. Because most of the drug redistributes quickly to adipose tissue, the redistribution half-life is probably less than the elimination half-life; however, this may not be clinically relevant because the drug redistributes to central nervous system tissue as well. There are no controlled studies on the pharmacokinetics in human subjects, so this has not been quantified. Elimination half-life has been estimated to be 7 to 46 hours.[7] Oral bioavailability is around 70%,[8] and absorption may be erratic.

When smoked, the compound has its initial effects within 2 to 5 minutes. With oral ingestion, the onset is approximately 30 minutes. The drug tends to be absorbed in the small intestine because it is generally insoluble in the acid environment of the stomach. Toxicity lasts 4 to 6 hours in a moderate ingestion. The drug's effect may linger for longer periods; some users report that they feel "normal" 1 to 2 days after the time of exposure.

The drug displays enterogastric recycling because it is mostly insoluble in the stomach. PCP concentrations found in the gastric fluid are 50 times higher than concentrations in the plasma.[9] When the drug moves into the duodenum and is in an alkaline environment, it is readily absorbed. Cerebrospinal fluid is slightly more acidic than plasma, and the same concentrating phenomenon applies. Experimentally the drug has been found in higher concentrations in brain tissue than blood samples in postmortem specimens.[10]

TABLE 74-1 Demographic Profile of PCP Exposures by Age

AGE (yr)	EXPOSURES (%)
<6	4.6
6–19	34
>19	56

From Litovitz TL, et al: 1998 Annual report of the American Association of Poison Control Centers Toxic Exposure Surveillance System. Ann Emerg Med 17:435–487, 1998.

PCP's mode of action is linked most closely to the *N*-methyl-D-aspartate (NMDA) receptor and has been studied extensively. PCP binds to a site within the L-type calcium channel, preventing influx of that ion when excitatory neurotransmitters bind to the receptor (Fig. 74-4).[11] PCP also prevents norepinephrine, dopamine, and serotonin reuptake and stimulates the σ receptor, explaining some of its catecholinergic and anesthetic properties.[12] Experimentally, calcium channel blockers, such as diltiazem, have been documented to potentiate the inhibitory effect of PCP on the NMDA calcium channel. Verapamil seems to displace PCP within the ion channel, however, and to block the effects of PCP at the NMDA receptor.[13]

Pharmacokinetics of PCP and Its Congeners

Volume of distribution: 5.3–7.5 L/kg
Protein binding: 70%
Mechanisms of clearance: primarily hepatic, 10% renal clearance
Active metabolites: none
Methods to enhance clearance: (1) continuous nasogastric suction—no significant clearance in literature; (2) forced acid diuresis—not recommended; (3) dialysis—not effective

CLINICAL PRESENTATION AND COMPLICATIONS

PCP-intoxicated patients usually present clinically to the intensivist as agitated with severely altered mental status of unknown etiology. The typical user is a man 18 to 25 years old who usually has ingested more than one substance.[14] Because a combination of sedatives and stimulants may be coingested with PCP, the overall picture of intoxication can be difficult to discern. PCP intoxication itself can be truly bizarre in presentation, often taking the inexperienced clinician by surprise.

Studies on monkeys under the influence of PCP yielded several stages of anesthesia and many symptoms and side effects with differing levels.[4] One of the many reasons PCP use is undesirable in humans is that each individual reacts to PCP in a different way. Given that the drug has a redistribution half-life of less than 60 minutes and a terminal half-life of days, the initial symptoms and duration of the most concerning symptoms are over within hours. The patient may have effects from the drug for 48 hours or more.[15] As early as its inception, PCP was noted to have several unwanted side effects, including emergence phenomena and prolonged coma.

The largest database of signs and symptoms of PCP intoxication was published in 1981 by McCarron and coworkers.[16] A total of 1000 patients who had known PCP ingestion (most from the Los Angeles County Prison Ward) were observed for patterns of toxicity. In this study, the most common findings in PCP ingestion were hypertension (57%) and nystagmus (57%) (Table 74-4).[16] Nystagmus seen in PCP patients can be vertical and horizontal. The hypertension from PCP is systolic and diastolic and tends to last less than 4 hours. Some patients may present without nystagmus or hypertension, and the lack of these hallmark traits does not rule out intoxication with PCP. Table 74-4 contains the most commonly seen findings in order of incidence.

The concept of *major* and *minor* clinical patterns of PCP intoxication was introduced by McCarron and coworkers (Table 74-5).[16] Although not prospectively validated, these patterns may serve as a predictor of severe sequelae of PCP use. These 11 patterns also serve as a guideline to understanding the myriad symptoms with which patients can present.

Major Patterns

Major patterns are usually associated with a more grim presentation. These patterns have significantly higher incidences of cardiac arrest, seizures including status epilepticus, hyperthermia, severe respiratory depression, and rhabdomyolysis. The four major patterns are *coma, catatonic syndrome, toxic psychosis,* and *acute brain syndrome* and are mutually exclusive of each other.

COMA

Patients may present with coma in approximately 10% of cases. Coma may be divided into three categories. *Mild coma,* which lasts less than 2 hours, occurs in 43%. *Moderate*

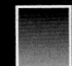

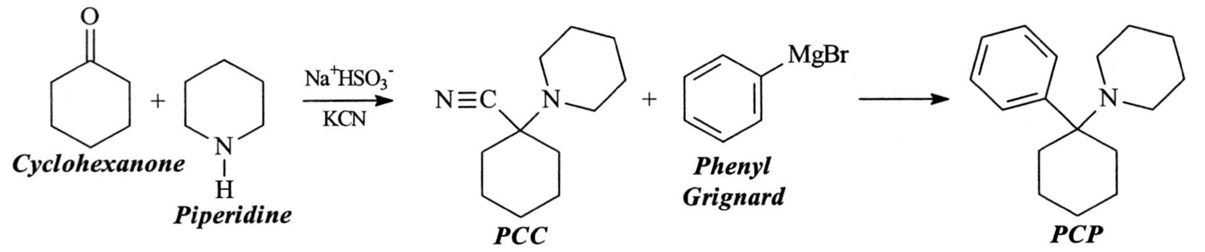

FIGURE 74-1

Synthesis of PCP from 1-piperidinylcyclohexanecarbonitrile (PCC) and phenyl grignard.

Cyclohexanone + Piperidine → (Na⁺HSO₃⁻ / KCN) → PCC + Phenyl Grignard → PCP

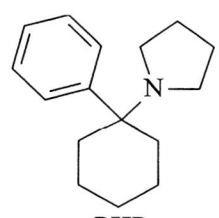

FIGURE 74-2

Chemical structure of the PCP analogue ketamine.

TABLE 74-2 PCP Aliases
Angel dust
Mist
Hog
PeaCe pill
Krystal joint (crystal joint)
Elephant tranquilizer
Super weed
Rocket fuel
Sheets
Cyclones
Snorts
Horse franks

coma lasts 2 to 24 hours and occurs in 38% of cases. Moderate coma is associated with more complications, such as aspiration pneumonitis and rhabdomyolysis. *Severe coma* occurs in 19% of cases, with a duration of 6 days. Complications from severe coma include those of persistent moderate coma and death. Emergence from severe coma can also be associated with acute brain syndrome, catatonic syndrome, and psychosis. Generally, as in most cases of coma, the longer the course, the more severe complications may be expected.

CATATONIC SYNDROME

Catatonic syndrome occurs in 12% of all cases and is diagnosed from the following criteria:

Motor signs (posturing, catalepsy, rigidity)
Psychosocial withdrawal (mutism, staring, negativism)
Excitement (nudism, impulsiveness, agitation, violence)
Stupor

A patient with catatonic syndrome is found motionless, with a blank stare and unresponsive to painful stimuli. The

syndrome usually lasts 4 to 6 hours, and 85% of patients are improved in less than 24 hours.

TOXIC PSYCHOSIS

Toxic psychosis is seen in 10% of PCP-intoxicated patients. In the absence of coma or catatonic syndrome, a patient with toxic psychosis presents as delusional or hallucinating. Delusions are usually religious in origin, and hallucinations are visual (brilliantly colored objects) and auditory.

ACUTE BRAIN SYNDROME

Acute brain syndrome constitutes the most common pattern of PCP intoxication. Patients present disoriented with any combination of confusion, lack of judgment, inappropriate affect, or loss of recent memory. This pattern is most confused with alcohol intoxication because patients usually are found wandering around (often into oncoming traffic) with ataxia and slurred speech. In contrast to individuals with alcohol intoxication, these patients present acutely ill with autonomic dysregulation, and many have traumatic injuries.

RHABDOMYOLYSIS

Rhabdomyolysis is a major complication of PCP intoxication. The overall incidence is 2.5% in patients presenting with PCP intoxication.[17] The incidence of rhabdomyolysis may be much higher for patients admitted the intensive care unit. Renal failure occurs in 40% of patients with clinically evident rhabdomyolysis (defined as myoglobinuria on urinalysis or a creatine phosphokinase >16,000 U/L). Most of these patients present catatonic, in a coma, or with acute brain syndrome. The cause for rhabdomyolysis cannot be attributed to the use of restraints because most cases occur in comatose patients with no need for restraints.

Minor Patterns

Minor patterns are found in patients with lower acuity intoxication. These patterns include *lethargy* or *stupor*, *bizarre* or *violent behavior*, *agitation*, *euphoria*, and *asymptomatic patterns*. Usually these patients are more likely to be detained by law enforcement or family members for behavioral disturbances. Patients who present with symptoms in these categories usually do not require hospitalization and are mostly alert and oriented. Medical complications still can occur in these minor categories, however. In contrast to the major patterns, these patterns often overlap.

LETHARGY OR STUPOR

Lethargy or stupor is defined as marked sedation with blunted response to verbal or tactile stimuli.

FIGURE 74-3

Synthetic analogues of PCP. PHP, 1-(1-phenyl-cyclohexyl) pyrrolidine; TCP, 1-(1-thiophenecyclo-hexyl) piperidine; PCE, 1-(1-phenylcyclohexyl) ethylamine.

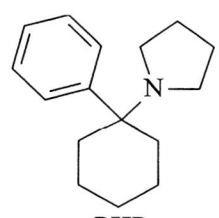
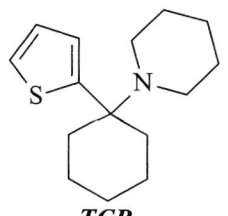
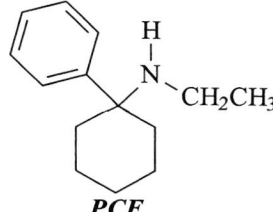

PHP   *TCP*   *PCE*

TABLE 74-3 Route of Exposure in PCP-Intoxicated Patients

ROUTE	PATIENTS (%)
Smoked	72
Snorted or sniffed	13
Oral ingestion	12
Intravenous	1.6

From McCarron MM, Schulze BW, Thompson GA, et al: Phencyclidine intoxication: Incidence of clinical findings in 1,000 cases. Ann Emerg Med 10:237–242, 1981.

BIZARRE BEHAVIOR

Bizarre behavior is described as strange or inappropriate behavior. Most patients in this category are alert and oriented without hallucinations or delusions. They may remove all of their clothing (20%) and may be agitated or violent.

VIOLENT BEHAVIOR

Violent behavior presents as threatening or combative behavior in an alert and oriented patient. Injuries are common in this pattern (41%), and about 75% of these patients are admitted to the hospital because of their behavior. Most of these patients need physical and pharmacologic restraints.

AGITATION

Agitation is seen in an alert and oriented patient who is restless with increased motor activity; the patient cannot keep still.

EUPHORIA

A patient with euphoria presents with elation, conveying a sense of well-being. Most of these patients are treated and released within hours.

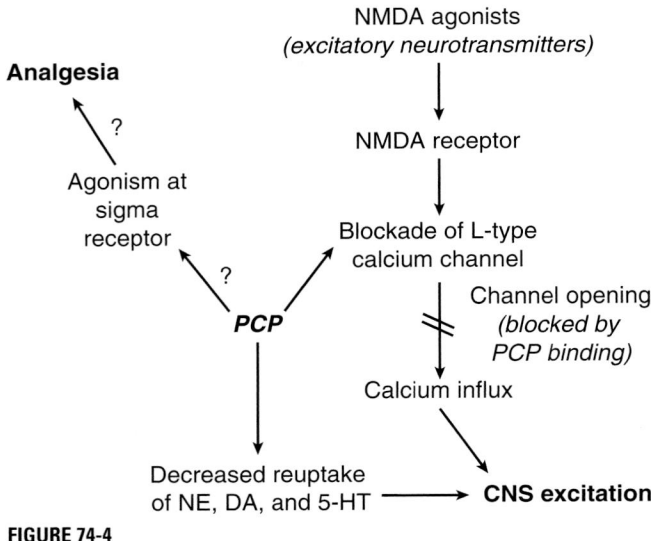

FIGURE 74-4

Mechanism of action and pharmacologic effects (in **boldface**) of PCP.

TABLE 74-4 PCP Findings in Order of Incidence

FINDING	%
Hallmarks	
Nystagmus	57.4
Hypertension	57.0
Sensorium	
Alert and oriented	45.9
Acute brain syndrome	36.9
Unconscious	10.6
Lethargy/stupor	6.6
Behavior	
Violent	35.4
Agitated	34.0
Bizarre	28.8
Hallucinating/delusional	18.5
Mute and staring	11.7
Nudism	3.3
No behavioral effects	3.5
Motor Signs	
Generalized rigidity	5.2
Grand mal seizures	3.1
Localized dystonias	2.4
Facial grimacing	1.7
Bronchorrhea	0.6
Anticholinergic Signs	
Pupils >4 mm	6.2
Urinary retention	2.4
Effects on Vital Signs	
Tachycardia	30.0
Hypothermia	6.4
Apnea/respiratory arrest	2.8
Hyperthermia	2.6
Cardiac arrest	0.3

From McCarron MM, Schulze BW, Thompson GA, et al: Phencyclidine intoxication: Incidence of clinical findings in 1,000 cases. Ann Emerg Med 10:237–242, 1981.

TABLE 74-5 McCarron Classification of Symptoms Related to PCP

MAJOR SYMPTOMS	MINOR SYMPTOMS
Coma	Lethargy
Catatonic syndrome	Stupor
Toxic psychosis	Bizarre behavior
Acute brain syndrome	Violent behavior
	Agitation
	Euphoria
	Asymptomatic patterns

From McCarron MM, Schulze BW, Thompson GA, et al: Acute phencyclidine intoxication: Clinical patterns, complications, and treatment. Ann Emerg Med 10:290–297, 1981.

DIAGNOSIS

In general, the diagnosis of PCP intoxication is based on clinical presentation. Serum levels of PCP formerly were frequently obtained, but many toxicology laboratories no

TABLE 74-6 Laboratory Abnormalities Associated with PCP Intoxication

LABORATORY TEST	% ABNORMAL
Hypoglycemia	22
Elevated CPK (>300 U)	70
Elevated AST/ALT	50
Hyperuricemia	24

AST/ALT, aspartate aminotransferase/alanine aminotransferase; CPK, creatine phosphokinase.
From McCarron MM, Schulze BW, Thompson GA, et al: Phencyclidine intoxication: Incidence of clinical findings in 1,000 cases. Ann Emerg Med 10:237–242, 1981.

longer test routinely for PCP. Because PCP has a higher affinity for lipid-based body tissue and because drug levels may be higher in the brain than in serum, the serum level may betray an inaccurate toxic picture. Clinical symptoms and degree of toxicity may not correlate with serum or urine PCP levels.[18]

The most sensitive method of detecting PCP is by gas chromatography using a nitrogen detector; this is superior to gas chromatography with flame ionization detection. Nitrogen-sensitive gas chromatography meets U.S. National Institute on Drug Abuse guidelines for ability to detect 2.5×10^{-4} mg/dL of PCP in urine for screening and confirmatory testing.[19] Enzyme-linked immunoassays exist for detecting PCP in urine at concentrations of 0.0015 mg/dL. Elimination and detection of PCP in urine are highly dependent on the acidity of urine. A urine pH should be obtained at the same collection time because alkaline urine may cause a false-negative result. Because of PCP's high volume of distribution, it may appear positive in the urine for 4 weeks with sensitive assays.

Most patients with PCP intoxication should have a creatine phosphokinase level determined because 70% have been shown to have levels greater than 300 U/L. A blood glucose test or finger-stick blood glucose level always should be obtained because hypoglycemia has been reported in 22% of patients.[15] Other laboratory abnormalities are shown in Table 74-6.

False-positive tests for PCP can occur with diphenhydramine,[20] dextromethorphan, and ketamine in high doses on screening assays. Confirmatory testing by gas chromatography can identify PCP conclusively, however.

TREATMENT

Indications for ICU Admission in PCP Intoxication

Rhabdomyolysis
Severe, refractory hypertension
Severe hyperthermia
Prolonged coma
Status epilepticus

Because the route of exposure for most PCP users is through inhalation, the typical user does not attain blood levels of greater than 3 mg/dL, self-limiting the toxicity of the agent. Intensivists should be aware, however, that when the drug is in the system of the patient, it is difficult to enhance its elimination owing to PCP's large volume of distribution. Patients with greater levels of toxicity need adjunctive therapy, as explained subsequently.

Decontamination

Because most patients with PCP ingestions survive with good supportive care measures, there is little use for aggressive decontamination measures. Activated charcoal may be appropriate if the patient presents early after oral ingestion and may bind other ingested materials as well. Multiple-dose activated charcoal has been shown in animal studies to be effective,[21] but its use must be weighed against the risk of aspiration from repeated doses. The use of multiple-dose activated charcoal in PCP ingestions has not been validated clinically.

Whole-bowel irrigation, in addition to activated charcoal, is possibly beneficial if the patient is a body packer or stuffer, potentially harboring a lethal or morbid amount of PCP within a bag or other container. General guidelines for the use of activated charcoal and whole-bowel irrigation are given in Chapter 5.

Nasogastric suction theoretically is ideal in that it may remove PCP in the concentrated environment of the stomach. Nasogastric suctioning does not remove a significant amount of the drug, however, because it is metabolized mostly through the hepatic route. Nasogastric suction has never been shown to be clinically beneficial in PCP exposures. Electrolytes should be monitored closely if continuous nasogastric suctioning is employed because chloride ions and protons are removed from the patient with this technique. The technique is difficult to apply in an agitated patient.

Enhanced Elimination Through Urinary Acidification—A Practice to Be Avoided

Forced acid diuresis was common practice in the treatment of PCP intoxication many years ago. Many detoxification centers and drug clinics recommended that patients drink cranberry juice to acidify their urine in hopes of eliminating PCP after casual use of the drug.[22] This technique has fallen out of favor for several reasons. The first is that most PCP patients survive even the most severe of ingestions with good supportive care. Second, acid diuresis may worsen rhabdomyolysis-induced renal injury. Third, elimination via the kidneys represents only 10% of the elimination route in a PCP-intoxicated patient. Most of the PCP is cleared through the liver. Finally, there are concerns about acidifying a patient's serum in the presence of lactic or other forms of acidosis. Forced acid diuresis is a potentially dangerous treatment that should not be used in PCP intoxication. The original data from Aranow and Done[23] that triggered the use of acidification for enhanced elimination was based on only three patients (Table 74-7). That study showed that a furosemide-stimulated urine pH of 5.5 comparatively had 25 times the elimination of PCP as a urine pH of 6.5 or

TABLE 74-7 Mean PCP Clearance Rate in Three Patients with Severe PCP Poisoning

PATIENT	SERUM pH	CLEARANCE RATE (mL serum/min)
Patient 1	6–6.5	4
Patient 2	5–6.5	20
Patient 3	5.0	53
Patient 3 with furosemide diuresis	4.5–5	100

From Aranow R, Done AK: Phencyclidine overdose: An emerging concept of management. J Am Coll Emerg Physicians 7:56–59, 1978.

greater. The limiting factor was acidifying the urine, however. Ascorbic acid has been used previously, but this has been shown to decrease urine pH by only 0.24 pH unit.[24] Because only a small fraction of the drug is eliminated in the urine, significant increases of the amount excreted still have little impact on total body PCP clearance.

Hemodialysis

Dialysis is not likely to be effective in removing clinically significant amounts of PCP because of the drug's large volume of distribution.

Hypertension

Management of hypertension rarely requires direct pharmacologic intervention. Most cases of hypertension resolve with sedation. Severe cases of hypertension are usually the cause of uncontrolled underlying hypertension exacerbated by PCP. These cases need specific treatments tailored to the patient's underlying disease states. If necessary, when severe hypertension is not responding to sedation, clonidine or a short-acting agent, such as nitroprusside or nitroglycerin, may be used (Table 74-8).

Electroencephalogram Monitoring

If available, continuous electroencephalogram (EEG) monitoring may predict patient improvement before there is

TABLE 74-8 Duration of Hypertension in PCP Patients

DURATION (hr)	PATIENTS (%)
≤4	62
5–12	19
13–24	8
>24	11

From McCarron MM, Schulze BW, Thompson GA, et al: Phencyclidine intoxication: Incidence of clinical findings in 1,000 cases. Ann Emerg Med 10:237–242, 1981.

clinical evidence. The EEG findings in PCP overdoses show slow delta rhythms during coma with more rhythmic theta activity as the patient becomes more alert.[25] Given that patients using PCP may have prolonged coma, with variable length, continuous EEG monitoring is not helpful. Most patients eventually awaken; the rest remain in a coma.

Sedation

Traditionally, haloperidol and other butyrophenones, such as droperidol, have been the mainstay of treating PCP patients who are combative and agitated. Although PCP does not interact directly with dopamine receptors, it prevents the reuptake of catecholamines and potentiates their action (see Fig. 74-4). Central dopamine antagonists have a definite role in the combative PCP-intoxicated patient. Characteristically, PCP users are dissociated from sensations of pain and often seem to possess superhuman strength. Intoxicated patients have been known to throw an enucleated eye or eviscerated testicle at staff and often break conventional restraints with ease.

In our experience, restraining a patient usually requires five or more people, regardless of the patient's size or estimated strength. A concerted effort in which each person is responsible for restraining a limb or the head followed by soft/hard or pharmaceutical restraints is the best approach for a takedown. A short-acting benzodiazepine, such as midazolam or lorazepam, or a butyrophenone may be given intramuscularly to control the patient temporarily in the absence of intravenous access. Care must be taken in a patient who presents with neuroleptic malignant syndrome (see Chapter 26) under the guise of PCP intoxication because use of butyrophenones may worsen the situation.

Experimental Therapies

VERAPAMIL AND FLUNARIZINE

Experimentally, verapamil has been shown to attenuate the action of PCP on the NMDA calcium channel (see Fig. 74-4). Two case reports of the success of verapamil on PCP-intoxicated patients have been published.[26,27] Each case showed a positive effect using verapamil, but with weak cause-and-effect relationships. There are no trials or case series on verapamil treatment to justify using it solely for reversing PCP toxicity. Because many PCP-intoxicated patients have hypertension and tachycardia, it may be efficacious to use such a drug in acute intoxication in select patients who do not respond to first-line therapies. It is uncommon, however, that PCP-induced hypertension requires direct pharmacologic intervention because the effects are seldom malignant. Most severe cases of PCP hypertension are exacerbations of the underlying essential type. In the rare instance when antihypertensive treatment is indicated, it should be based on the patient's prior medications.

In rats, verapamil potentiates PCP toxicity.[28] In the absence of clinical outcome–based data, verapamil use should be reserved for treatment of tachycardia and hypertension that is best suited for the patient and not for the treatment of PCP.

FAB FRAGMENTS

As yet, PCP-specific Fab fragments are not available for clinical use. The results of the initial experiments in dogs are promising.[29] No definitive human studies exist, however.[30]

SPECIAL POPULATIONS

Pregnant and Breast-feeding Patients

PCP crosses the placental barrier and has been associated with irritability, poor feeding, and hypertonicity in neonates.[31] The drug also is excreted into breast milk and may be present 40 days after last use.[32] In mice, PCP reaches concentrations 10 times that of plasma in breast milk; also there is a tenfold increase of PCP in fetal tissue compared with maternal blood concentrations.[33]

REFERENCES

1. Thombs DL: A review of PCP abuse trends and perceptions. Public Health Rep 104:325–328, 1989.
2. Litovitz TL: 1998 Annual report of the American Association of Poison Control Centers Toxic Exposure Surveillance System. Ann Emerg Med 17:435–487, 1998.
3. McCarron MM, Schulze BW, Thompson GA, et al: Acute phencyclidine intoxication: Clinical patterns, complications, and treatment. Ann Emerg Med 10:290–297, 1981.
4. Wong LK, Biemann K: Metabolites of phencyclidine. Clin Toxicol 9:583–591, 1976.
5. Chen GM, Weston JK: The analgesic and anesthetic effect of 1-(1-phenylcyclohexyl) piperidine on the monkey. Anesth Anesth Curr Res 39:132–137, 1964.
6. Sramek JJ, Baumgartner WA, Talos JA, et al: Hair analysis for detection of phencyclidine in newly admitted psychiatric patients. Am J Psychiatry 142:950–953, 1985.
7. Baselt RC: Disposition of Toxic Drugs and Chemicals in Man, 5th ed. Foster City, CA, Chemical Toxicology Institute, 2000.
8. Cook CE, Brome DR, Jeffcoat AR, et al: Phencyclidine disposition after intravenous and oral doses. Clin Pharm Ther 31:625–634, 1982.
9. Done AK, Aranow R, Miceli JN: The pharmacokinetics of phencyclidine in overdosage and its treatment. NIDA Res Monogr 21:210–217, 1978.
10. Anderson WH, Prouty RW: Postmortem redistribution of drugs. In Baselt RH: : Advances in Analytical Toxicology, Vol 2. Chicago, Year Book Medical Publishers, 1989, pp 70–102.
11. Johnson KM, Snell LD, Sacaan AI, et al: Pharmacologic regulation of the NMDA receptor ionophore complex. NIDA Res Monogr 133:14–40, 1993.
12. Javitt DC, Zukin SR: Recent advances in the phencyclidine model of schizophrenia. Am J Psychiatry 148:1301–1308, 1991.
13. Popoli P, Peezzola A, Benedetti M, Scotti de Carolis A: Verapamil and flunarizine inhibit phencyclidine-induced effects. Neuropharmacology 31:1185–1191, 1992.
14. McCarron MM, Schulze BW, Thompson GA, et al: Phencyclidine intoxication: Incidence of clinical findings in 1,000 cases. Ann Emerg Med 10:237–242, 1981.
15. Burns RS, Lerner SE: Perspectives: Acute phencyclidine intoxication. Clin Toxicol 9:477–501, 1976.
16. McCarron MM, Schulze BW, Thompson GA, et al: Acute phencyclidine intoxication: Clinical patterns, complications, and treatment. Ann Emerg Med 10:290–297, 1981.
17. Akmal M, Valdin JR, McCarron MM, et al: Rhabdomyolysis with and without acute renal failure in patients with phencyclidine intoxication. Am J Nephrol 1:91–96, 1981.
18. Bailey DN: Phencyclidine abuse. Am J Clin Pathol 72:795–799, 1979.
19. Bailey DN, Guba JJ: Gas chromatographic analysis for phencyclidine in plasma, with use of a nitrogen detector. Clin Chem 26:437–440, 1980.
20. Levine BS, Smith ML: Effects of diphenhydramine on immunoassay of phencyclidine in urine. Clin Chem 36:1258, 1990.
21. Picchioni AL, Consroe PF: Activated charcoal—a phencyclidine antidote, or hog in dogs. N Engl J Med 300:202, 1979.
22. Aranow R, Miceli JN, Done AK: A therapeutic approach to the acutely overdosed PCP patient. J Psychedelic Drugs 12:259–266, 1980.
23. Aranow R, Done AK: Phencyclidine overdose: An emerging concept of management. J Am Coll Emerg Physicians 7:56–59, 1978.
24. Nahata MC, Shimp L, Lampman T, et al: Effect of ascorbic acid on urine pH in man. Am J Hosp Pharm 34:1234–1237, 1977.
25. Rodin EA, Luby ED, Meyer JS: Electroencephalographic findings associated with Sernyl infusion. Electroencephalogr Clin Neurophysiol 11:796–798, 1959.
26. Price WA, Giannini AJ, Krishen A: Management of acute PCP intoxication with verapamil. Clin Toxicol 24:85–87, 1986.
27. Montgomery PT, Mueller ME: Treatment of PCP intoxication with verapamil. Am J Psychiatry 142:882, 1985.
28. McCann DJ, Smith CM, Winter JC: A caution against use of verapamil in phencyclidine intoxication. Am J Psychiatry 143:679, 1986.
29. Owens SM, Mayersohn M: Phencyclidine-specific Fab fragments alter phencyclidine disposition in dogs. Drug Metab Dispos 14:52–58, 1986.
30. MacDonald DI: New treatment for PCP? JAMA 257:3188, 1987.
31. Briggs GG: Drugs in Pregnancy and Lactation, 5th ed. Baltimore, Lippincott, Williams & Wilkins, 1998, pp 841–842.
32. Kauffman K, Petrucha RA, Pitts FN, et al: PCP in amniotic fluid and breast milk. J Clin Psychiatry 44:269–270, 1983.
33. Nicholas JM, Lipshitz J, Schreiber EC: Phencyclidine transfers across the placenta as well as into breast milk. Am J Obstet Gynecol 143:143–146, 1982.

CHAPTER 75

Cocaine

Ruben Olmedo ■ Robert S. Hoffman

Cocaine has been used for thousands of years for its recognized medicinal properties and for its personally gratifying qualities. The first archeological findings of human use of coca leaves date back to 3000 B.C. among pre-Colombian Andean societies.[1] The leaves were chewed by chasquis (on-foot mail carriers of the Incan empire) to decrease fatigue and enhance endurance as they delivered their royal messages by running from town to town.

Chewing the coca leaf was the preferred method of use until Niemann isolated cocaine in 1859. In the late 1800s, Freud advocated the use of cocaine for many ailments, including for the treatment of opioid addiction. During this same period, the renowned John Hopkins' surgeon Halsted reported the local anesthetic effects of cocaine. By the end of the 19th century, cocaine became widely used in various medicinal pastes and remedies. It was the main active ingredient in the soft drink Coca-Cola until 1903.[1] As accounts of addiction multiplied, legislation was enacted that curtailed its use.

Although resurgence of cocaine use in the United States occurred in the 1970s, use leveled off until 1983, when "crack" appeared, providing a fast and inexpensive method of self-administration. By 1985, the National Household Survey on Drug Abuse from the National Institute of Drug Abuse estimated that 25 to 40 million Americans had used cocaine at some time in their lives.[2] Cocaine use reached epidemic proportions in the mid-1980s, when it was reported to be the most frequent cause of illicit drug–related visits to emergency departments.[3] In the last 15 years of the 20th century, the use of the crystallized freebase form of cocaine became widespread, resulting in many cocaine-related hospitalizations and deaths.[4] Results from the National Institute of Drug Abuse indicate that cocaine use has been declining since 1992 to a plateau of 1.8 million regular users in 1998 (5.7 million in 1985).[5,6] Despite the decline in more recent years, the incidence of cocaine-related deaths increased by 14% from 1992 to 1995.[4,7]

Cocaine toxicity involves all of the body's organ systems. Its use brings patients to the hospital with a variety of medical symptoms. Complications include medical, psychiatric, and surgical emergencies. The estimated health care cost of patients with myocardial ischemia alone secondary to cocaine is greater than $80 million per year.[8] A retrospective study reported 1.1% incidence of positive urine screens for cocaine among all hospitalized nonnewborn patients during a 12-month period. These patients were predominantly young (average age 31.8 years) crack users and required admission to the intensive care unit 20% of the time.[9] An understanding of cocaine's pharmacology and its pathophysiology is beneficial in identifying and treating patients with the highest risks of complications.

COCAINE CHEMISTRY

The natural tropane alkaloid cocaine is extracted from the leaves of the plant *Erythroxylon coca*. First, coca paste is obtained after the leaves are processed with organic solvents and ammonia. The hydrophilic cocaine hydrochloride (HCl) salt is obtained after the latter undergoes treatment with hydrochloric acid. This form of cocaine (Fig. 75-1) is used intranasally and intravenously. The HCl salt cannot be smoked, however, because it undergoes pyrolysis at the higher temperatures required for vaporization.[10]

Cocaine HCl is converted back to its base form, by removing the HCl moiety, to obtain crack or freebase cocaine, which are chemically identical. Heating cocaine HCl in sodium bicarbonate or ammonia makes the hard crystallized cocaine base called *crack*. This crystallized base of cocaine received its name because when it is smoked a popping sound typically is heard. Another process called *freebasing* also gives rise to alkaloidal cocaine that can be smoked. First, cocaine HCl is dissolved in water and an alkaline substance. Then the base is extracted into ether or another organic solvent. The final product is obtained after evaporation of the organic phase. This final extraction with ether may be hazardous because these solvents are volatile and flammable. Facial and tracheal burn injuries are reported in freebase cocaine users, and fires in clandestine laboratories during the production process have been reported.[11]

PATHOPHYSIOLOGY OF COCAINE EFFECTS

Pharmacokinetics

Cocaine is absorbed rapidly from all mucous membranes, including the respiratory, gastrointestinal, and genitourinary tracts, giving rise to multiple potential routes of abuse.[12] Its onset of action is almost immediate from the intravenous or inhalational route (0.5 to 2 minutes) and is delayed 20 to 30 minutes after intranasal insufflation.[13,14] Gastrointestinal absorption is delayed further by a minimum of 90 minutes. The duration of effect is related closely to the onset of action, with intravenous and inhalational exposure lasting

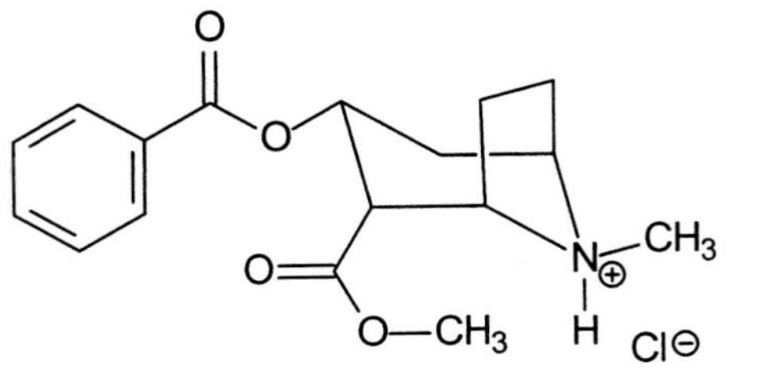

FIGURE 75-1

Chemical structure of the salt cocaine hydrochloride (HCl). When the hydrochloride salt is treated with base, the hydrochloride is removed, leaving cocaine in the alkaloid ("free base") form.

approximately 30 minutes, nasal insufflation lasting about 1 hour, and gastrointestinal use lasting at least 2 to 3 hours (Table 75-1).

The physiologic effect of cocaine is a sum of the effects of the parent compound, its metabolites, and their respective pharmacodynamics. More than 11 metabolites of cocaine have been described, and some deserve mention. Once absorbed, less than 5% of the parent compound is cleared in the urine.[15]

Cocaine is metabolized rapidly by a combination of enzymatic and nonenzymatic hydrolysis.[16] Enzymatic hydrolysis by plasma and liver esterases yields ecgonine methyl ester. Ecgonine methyl ester has mild vasodilating properties and has a plasma half-life of approximately 5 hours.[17–20] Decreased plasma cholinesterase activity enhances cocaine toxicity in mice.[21] Similarly, patients with relative plasma cholinesterase deficiency seem to be at increased risk of adverse consequences from cocaine toxicity.[22]

Another metabolite, benzoylecgonine, is formed mostly via nonenzymatic hydrolysis. Although an enzymatic hydrolysis pathway producing benzoylecgonine has been described, it probably accounts for only a small percentage of this metabolism.[16] Benzoylecgonine has potent vasoconstrictive properties, although less than the parent compound. It has a plasma half-life of approximately 8 hours.[19,20,23] One important fact about benzoylecgonine is that this metabolite is tested in most urine immunoassays. It is detected for 48 to 72 hours after infrequent cocaine use or 3 weeks in high-dose chronic cocaine users.[24,25]

Together, ecgonine methyl ester and benzoylecgonine constitute approximately 85% of cocaine's metabolism.[26] Less than 10% of cocaine is metabolized by N-demethylation in the liver, forming norcocaine. This metabolite is highly

vasoconstrictive and in animal models produces clinical effects similar to those of the parent compound.[19]

Additionally, in the presence of ethanol, cocaine is transesterified by a liver esterase to ethylcocaine or cocaethylene.[27] Cocaethylene has a longer half-life than cocaine. In humans, coadministration of cocaine and ethanol produces prolonged euphoria.[28] This metabolite has pharmacologically significant central and peripheral effects that are similar to those of cocaine.[29–32] Additionally, animal studies with cocaethylene show a dose-dependent myocardial depression effect and more potent Na^+ channel blockade than cocaine.[32,33]

Mechanism of Action

Cocaine's effects derive from its Na^+ channel blockade and its central and peripheral inhibition of monoamine reuptake. The first mechanism is responsible for cocaine's local anesthetic effects by inhibiting nerve conduction.[34] The effect is illustrated best in the myocardial conduction system, where it produces quinidine-like (Na^+ channel–blocking), membrane-stabilizing properties that result in QRS widening and decreased contractility.[35–37] In large doses, sodium channel blockade in the medullary centers produces respiratory depression and sudden death (Table 75-2).

Cocaine's second mechanism of action increases the concentrations of norepinephrine, dopamine, serotonin, and excitatory neurotransmitters in the synaptic space.[36,38,39] This mechanism is responsible for many of the stimulatory effects on the sympathetic nervous system. Some of the centrally mediated effects are euphoria, psychomotor agitation, and respiratory stimulation.

The increase in synaptic and circulating concentrations of catecholamines stimulates adrenergic nerve terminals, resulting in an increase in sympathetic activity.[38] Typically, sympathetic nervous system stimulation manifests as hypertension, tachycardia, diaphoresis, mydriasis, and hyperthermia. Pressor

TABLE 75-1 Toxicokinetic Parameters of Cocaine

METHOD OF USE	PEAK ONSET OF SYMPTOMS (min)	DURATION OF EFFECT (hr)
Oral (cocaine HCl)	60–90	>3
Intranasal (cocaine HCl)	30	1–2
Smoking (freebasing, crack, alkaline cocaine)	0.5–1.0	0.25–0.5
Intravenous (cocaine HCl)	0.5–2.0	0.25–0.5

HCl, hydrochloride.

TABLE 75-2 Mechanism of Action and Clinical Manifestations of Cocaine Poisoning

MECHANISM	CLINICAL MANIFESTATION
Na^+ channel blockade	Local anesthesia QRS widening on ECG Decreased cardiac muscle contractility Respiratory depression
Monoamine reuptake inhibition Epinephrine Norepinephrine Dopamine	 Tachycardia Hypertension Psychomotor agitation with attendant elevation in temperature. Reward leading to dependence. Movement disorders
Serotonin Excitatory amino acids	Various effects on mood and behavior Seizures
Platelet activation and alterations in plasma thrombogenic constituents	Thrombogenesis

ECG, electrocardiogram.

effects are mediated by norepinephrine of sympathetic neural origin, whereas tachycardic effects are secondary to epinephrine of adrenal medullary origin.[38]

Other effects of cocaine are secondary to its dopamine reuptake inhibition. Dopamine D_1/D_5 antagonists attenuate the euphoric effects of cocaine.[40] Administration of cocaine directly into motor centers produces an increase in locomotion that is reversed by coadministration of dopamine antagonists.[41] Restlessness, agitation, and seizures can occur from motor center stimulation after cocaine administration. This psychomotor stimulation after cocaine administration is absent in mice lacking the dopamine transporter.[42] Chronic cocaine use also depletes dopamine from reward centers in the brain. This mechanism is thought to be the basis for its reinforcement and addictive properties.[43]

The serotonergic effects of cocaine are unclear. Serotonin regulates certain biologic processes, such as mood, personality, temperature regulation, affect, appetite, motor function, sexual activity, sleep induction, hallucinations, and vasospasm. All of these processes may be affected during chronic cocaine abuse and withdrawal.[44]

Cocaine increases excitatory amino acid levels in the nucleus accumbens by enhancing dopamine stimulation of the *N*-methyl-D-aspartate receptor.[38] In animal models, *N*-methyl-D-aspartate antagonists attenuate cocaine's effect on the nucleus accumbens[45] and prevent cocaine-induced seizures and death.[46]

Cocaine has several hematologic actions, which may promote thrombogenesis. Tonga and colleagues[47] noted an increase in rabbit platelet aggregation and thromboxane production in vitro. Similar results of platelet activation are reported in in vitro human volunteer studies[48,49] and in an in vivo canine model.[50] Cocaine also alters plasma constituents (increases tissue plasminogen activator type I activity, increases von Willebrand factor) that regulate thrombus formation.[51,52] An additional direct effect of cocaine on the vascular endothelium causes release of endothelin-1, a potent endogenous vasoconstrictor.[53] Lastly, cocaine induces a transient erythrocytosis, further restricting blood flow. This latter effect is well described in patients chewing coca leaf during exercise.[54–56] As a result, intravascular thrombosis after cocaine use occurs in a variety of vascular beds[57–62] in diseased and nondiseased vessels.

CLINICAL PRESENTATION OF COCAINE TOXICITY

Cocaine toxicity may involve multiple organ systems. Although most patients with acute cocaine-associated symptoms may be managed in the emergency department, some require hospitalization because catastrophic complications occur. Most complaints are cardiopulmonary (56.2%), neurologic (39.1%), and psychiatric (36.8%), although multiple symptoms often are involved (57.5%).[63] In one study that evaluated the characteristics of cocaine users admitted to the hospital, a high admission rate to the intensive care unit was found among patients with a positive cocaine urine screen.[9]

The effects of cocaine on the different organ systems are a combination of the cocaine's overall intrinsic effect on the vascular tone and thrombogenicity and the specific physio-

logic response of that organ system. Arterial vasoconstriction and spasm and intravascular thrombosis after cocaine use occur in vascular beds throughout the body.[57–62,64–66] Some of the clinical manifestations of cocaine-induced vasospasm include cerebral infarction, myocardial infarction, blindness, central retinal artery occlusion, mesenteric ischemia, and renal infarction.[18,60,61,67–70] Secondary effects of cocaine that affect multiple organ systems are hypertension and tachycardia. Acutely, both of these initial effects increase tissue oxygen demand and further impair organ performance.

Hyperthermia

Cocaine use can result in serious toxic effects and death in part because of hyperthermia. Even relatively low doses of cocaine can elevate core temperature and hamper cardiac reserve.[71] High ambient temperature is associated with a significant increase in mortality from cocaine overdose.[72]

Cocaine causes hyperthermia in several ways. It increases psychomotor agitation, which results in increased heat production. As a vasoconstrictor of the peripheral vasculature, cocaine impairs the body's ability to dissipate heat. Additionally, because the heat-regulatory centers in the hypothalamus are dopamine modulated, cocaine has direct effects on temperature control.[73] Several case reports describe fatal hyperthermia without rhabdomyolysis in cocaine users.[74,75] Fatal elevations of core temperature have been documented in cocaine-poisoned dogs.[76] When ambient temperature increased from $-5°C$ to $5°C$ ($23°F$ to $41°F$) in this animal model, the survival rate decreased from 100% to 57%.[76] Of all vital sign abnormalities, hyperthermia seems to correlate most with fatality.

Neurologic Manifestations

Cocaine is a popular illicit drug of abuse because of its stimulatory effects on the central nervous system (CNS). Its use also generates a variety of untoward effects on the CNS. These CNS complications occur with all forms of cocaine administration and include cerebrovascular ischemia and infarction, transient ischemic attacks, subarachnoid hemorrhage, intraparenchymal hemorrhage, seizures, cerebrovascular thrombosis, cerebral vasculitis, migraine headache, anterior spinal artery syndrome, and movement disorders (Table 75-3).[65,66,69,77–85]

CEREBROVASCULAR ACCIDENTS

Cocaine-related strokes were first reported in the literature in 1977.[78] Strokes are ischemic and hemorrhagic. The incidence of ischemic and hemorrhagic strokes secondary to the alkaloidal form of cocaine is approximately the same,[65] whereas 80% of cocaine HCl–induced strokes are hemorrhagic.[66]

Patients with cerebrovascular ischemia or infarction may present with focal lateralizing neurologic deficits. Physical examination in these patients is typical of patients with cerebrovascular accidents, showing aphasia, hemiplegia, dysarthria, or paresthesias.

Cocaine-induced cerebral hemorrhage may be intraparenchymal or subarachnoid. The incidence of neurovascular

TABLE 75-3 Cocaine-Induced Central Nervous System Complications		
CNS COMPLICATIONS	**ETIOLOGY**	**REFERENCES**
Ischemic strokes	Vasospasm, thrombosis	65,66,69,78,80,82,87,94
Hemorrhagic stroke	Hypertension, vasospasm, thrombosis	65,66,69,78,80,82,83,87,91,94
Seizures	Reuptake inhibition of excitatory amino acids, CNS hemorrhage or infarction	86,87,92–98
Cerebral vasculitis	Direct effects	77
Migraine headaches	Dopamine reuptake inhibition, vasospasm	85
Movement disorders	Dopamine reuptake inhibition	79

CNS, central nervous system.

complications among cocaine-related hospital admissions is low (0.35% to 3%).[86,87] Autopsy studies of fatal nontraumatic intracranial hemorrhage reported an incidence of cocaine abuse to be 7% to 59%, however.[88,89] Headache is the most common symptom on presentation. Other presenting signs include meningismus, altered mental status, seizures, and focal neurologic deficits.[82]

The mechanisms of cocaine-related ischemic strokes are multiple and overlapping and have been related to focal vascular disease. Proposed causes include vasospasm (either pharmacologically induced or secondary to hypertension), thrombosis, and vasculitis. Cerebral vasoconstriction, documented by magnetic resonance angiography, occurs within 15 minutes of cocaine administration to asymptomatic human volunteers.[90] In head computed tomography (CT)–proven cerebral infarctions, angiography revealed evidence of vasospasm and thrombosis.[69] Biopsy-proven cerebral vasculitis as a cause of ischemic stroke also is rarely reported.[77]

Alternatively, acute systemic hypertension as a result of cocaine's sympathomimetic effects is the proposed mechanism for cocaine-related hemorrhagic strokes. The sudden increase in blood pressure may precipitate the rupture of a preexisting vascular malformation or aneurysms.[65] Arteriography has shown both of these vascular abnormalities in many cases of cocaine-induced subarachnoid hemorrhage and in some cases of intraparenchymal hemorrhage.[82,86,87,91]

Although most strokes occur either immediately or within the first 3 hours after cocaine use, Levine and associates[65] reported that 18% of strokes occur after an abstinence period of at least 2 days following a period of heavy crack use. Possible explanations for these delayed events are the prolonged half-life of cocaine's metabolites (benzoylecgonine) and cocaine's intrinsic thrombogenic effect.

SEIZURES

Although cocaine-related seizures are well associated with cocaine use, they are a rare presenting feature of emergency department visits and hospitalizations in patients with cocaine-related toxicity (2.8% to 8.4%).[92–94] Most cocaine-induced seizures occur as the only manifestation of cocaine toxicity. They are predominantly single, generalized, and tonic-clonic. Approximately 20% are focal in onset. Seizures that are focal or multiple often are associated with acute intracerebral complications.[95] Although some cocaine-induced

seizures occur secondary to a large CNS bleed or infarction, most are not associated with any lasting neurologic deficits.[94,96]

Most cocaine-induced seizures occur within 90 minutes of use.[96] Similar to cocaine-induced strokes, this corresponds temporally to peak plasma cocaine levels.[81,95,96] Delayed seizures may be caused by benzoylecgonine because this metabolite is also a potent CNS vasoconstrictor.[97]

OTHER NEUROLOGIC EFFECTS

Cocaine lowers the seizure threshold and precipitates seizures in patients with known seizure disorders.[98] Patients with a prior history of epilepsy have a higher frequency of cocaine-induced seizures than patients without a history of seizures.[95] Partial or multiple seizures occur more often in patients with prior history of epilepsy.[98] Additionally, animal studies and human case reports suggest cocaine's ability to "kindle" seizures after habitual use.[95,96] This process increases the sensitivity of the brain after repeated doses.

Cocaine induces a variety of movement disorders, which are presumed dopaminergic in origin. These movement disorders include dystonia, choreoathetosis (commonly known as *crack dancing*), akathisia, buccolingual dyskinesia (risus sardonicus), and Tourette's syndrome exacerbation. The high incidence of acute dystonic reactions in cocaine-addicted patients treated with antipsychotic medications suggests a dysfunctional dopamine-mediated basal ganglia effect.[79]

In addition to the kindling effect, chronic use of cocaine is associated with an increase in cerebral atrophy.[99] Because reward centers in the brain are under control of dopaminergic tone, depletion of dopaminergic transmission in these brain areas after repeated administration of cocaine produces a craving for the drug.

Cardiac Manifestations

Cardiac manifestations of cocaine poisoning are the most common and have been well recognized for years. Most symptoms relating to acute cocaine use suggest a cardiovascular etiology, with 40% of cocaine-related visits to the hospital having chest pain as the leading single presenting symptom.[63] Other frequently occurring cardiac symptoms at presentation are cardiac diaphoresis, palpitations, and dyspnea.[63,100] Because of cocaine's multiple effects on the coronary vasculature, evaluation of patients for myocardial ischemia or infarction is important.

The first myocardial infarction as a complication of cocaine abuse was reported in 1982.[101] It is now well recognized that myocardial infarction occurs with intranasal, intravenous, and inhalational use of cocaine.[102] Retrospective studies of cocaine-associated chest pain reported an incidence of myocardial infarction ranging from 0% to 31%. Subsequent prospective studies indicated that the frequency of infarction defined by creatine phosphokinase (CPK)-MB criteria more likely approximates 6%.[102–105]

The typical patient with cocaine-induced myocardial infarction is a man 18 to 52 years old (median age 33 years old). The typical patient has a history of regular tobacco smoking and frequent cocaine use. The quality of the chest pain is usually atypical of ischemia, and the location of the pain does not predict myocardial infarction.[102]

Two thirds of patients have symptoms of chest pain within 3 hours of cocaine use, and 93% have symptoms of chest pain within 24 hours of cocaine use.[68,102,106] A greater delay in the onset of symptoms is experienced rarely but has been documented.[107] Myocardial infarction 3 days after cocaine use was reported by Del Aguila and Rosman.[108] Additionally, Holter monitoring detected electrocardiogram (ECG) changes after 6 weeks in cocaine-addicted patients during an inpatient detoxification admission.[107]

Cocaine causes myocardial infarction by several mechanisms. Acutely, cocaine use leads to hypertension, tachycardia, and vasoconstriction, all of which increase myocardial demand. First, an elevation in heart rate and blood pressure increases myocardial workload. More dramatic elevations in blood pressure may intensify the shearing forces in the major vessels, causing aortic dissection and rupture.[109–114] Dissection of coronary arteries has occurred.[115,116] Second, cocaine causes local vasoconstriction of the coronary vasculature. In human volunteers, this effect occurs within 15 minutes of cocaine administration, as is well documented by angiography.[65] This arterial vasoconstriction is markedly worse in coronary artery segments previously narrowed by atherosclerosis.[117] In the presence of cocaine and its increased sympathetic activity, the normal coronary vasodilating response to a diminished oxygen supply is overwhelmed.

The vasoconstrictive effects of cocaine are established to be an α-adrenergically mediated function. Propranolol, a β-adrenergic antagonist, exacerbates coronary narrowing after cocaine infusion, whereas phentolamine, an α-adrenergic antagonist, reverses this effect.[118,119]

Acute and chronic effects of cocaine are associated with its thrombogenicity and ability to accelerate atherosclerosis. Coronary angiography performed in patients after cocaine-associated myocardial infarction often shows intracoronary thrombus and atherosclerotic lesions at different stages of stenosis in any of the coronaries.[106,120,121] Autopsy and coronary catheterization reports of chronic cocaine abusers show advanced atherosclerosis despite a young age.[68,114,122–125] Additionally, rabbits fed a 0.5% cholesterol diet and injected with cocaine develop atherosclerotic lesions in the aorta.[125] In humans, chronic cocaine use increases the prevalence of aortic atherosclerotic lesions independent of traditional cardiac risk factors.[127]

Cocaine use also has global cardiac effects that may produce ischemia. Echocardiography and catheterization data reveal that cocaine use depresses myocardial function. Dilated cardiomyopathy is reported with normal coronaries in patients with habitual cocaine use.[128,129] Ventricular angiography showed myocardial dysfunction as measured by worsening hemodynamic parameters in patients infused with cocaine.[130] Left ventricular systolic dysfunction, secondary to cocaine's myocardial depressant effect, presents as congestive heart failure and cardiomyopathy.[120,129] These cardiovascular hemodynamic changes alter the genetic expression of contractile proteins in cocaine-treated rats.[131] Inflammatory lymphocytic and eosinophilic infiltrates consistent with myocarditis are found in myocardial tissue from patients with cocaine-related deaths.[132,133] These anatomic alterations may provide a substrate for reentrant dysrhythmias and other conduction abnormalities.

Cocaine may produce cardiac dysrhythmias in several ways. It affects the conduction system directly or its release of endogenous catecholamines. In low doses, cocaine may result in bradycardia. Higher doses cause all types of tachydysrhythmias, with sinus tachycardia being the most common. Other rhythm disturbances frequently associated with cocaine use are atrial fibrillation, narrow-complex and wide-complex supraventricular tachycardia, ventricular tachycardia and fibrillation, and torsades de pointes.[35,37,106,134–136] Animal models and case reports of wide-complex supraventricular tachycardias suggest that these dysrhythmias resemble those following type I antidysrhythmic or tricyclic antidepressant poisonings. Slowing of phase 0 of the action potential in cocaine intoxication is secondary to the direct Na^+ channel–blocking effects of cocaine.[137] Additionally, ventricular dysrhythmias may develop secondary to cocaine-induced ischemia or infarction.

Pulmonary Manifestations

The pulmonary complications secondary to cocaine use arise from its pharmacologic effects on the pulmonary physiology and from the various methods of administering the drug. As a result of cocaine-induced vasoconstriction and platelet aggregation, pulmonary hemorrhage and pulmonary thrombus can occur. Hemoptysis is reported to occur in 5.7% of habitual smokers of freebase cocaine.[138] Histopathology of fiberoptic bronchoscopic lavage and autopsy reports of acutely cocaine-intoxicated patients reveal diffuse interstitial and alveolar hemorrhage, bronchial arterial constriction, and ischemic damage.[139,140] Pulmonary infarction is encountered less often,[141] mainly because of the dual blood supply to the lungs from the pulmonary and bronchial arteries.

Since the 1990s, habitual smoking of alkaloidal cocaine has replaced nasal insufflation of cocaine HCl as the most common method of use because of the faster onset and greater intensity of intoxication achievable with smoking. Each of these routes of administration is associated with unique pulmonary complications. Thermal burns of the upper airway, including the tongue, epiglottis, vocal cords, and subglottic area, occur after smoking cocaine[142]; this is from inhalation of either hot cocaine or ether used to prepare the alkaline form of cocaine. Acute respiratory symptoms (cough, black sputum, chest pain, shortness of breath, asthma)[143] occur with high frequency in temporal association with smoking the alkaloid form of cocaine.

Functional disorders of the lungs, gas exchange abnormalities, and reactive airway disease also occur commonly.[144] Subsequent pulmonary artery medial hypertrophy occurs in 20% of individuals who chronically abuse cocaine. This condition occurs in the absence of foreign particle embolization and is independent of the dose, frequency, or route of administration.[145]

The classic condition "crack lung" from inhalation of cocaine is described as pulmonary infiltrates, fever, and bronchospasm. An immunologic etiology of these symptoms is supported by the findings of eosinophilia, elevated IgE levels, and pruritus, all of which resolve with abstinence of drug use.[146–148] These findings suggest that heavy crack smoking produces respiratory tract injury manifested by acute respiratory symptoms and evidence of chronic airflow obstruction in large airways.

Acute pulmonary edema secondary to cocaine use is also encountered. It is due to cardiogenic and noncardiogenic causes. Noncardiogenic pulmonary edema results from cocaine's direct effect or from the impurities in cocaine on the pulmonary alveoli and endothelium by increasing their permeability.[149]

Barotrauma is often seen in individuals who use a Valsalva-type maneuver for rapid absorption of cocaine. There are numerous case reports of patients presenting to the emergency department with pneumomediastinum or pneumothorax or both and pneumopericardium. These abnormalities occur secondary to the mechanics of drug administration rather than directly related to cocaine itself.[150–157] A retrospective study that evaluated patients presenting with spontaneous pneumomediastinum found that 76% of the cases were associated with illicit inhalational drug use. Of these cases, 53% were secondary to cocaine use. Evaluation of the presenting clinical symptoms revealed that 82% of the patients had a complaint of chest pain or shortness of breath or both. The absence of an abnormal physical finding was uncommon: Most patients (88%) had subcutaneous emphysema, Hamman's crunch, or both.[155]

Chronic cocaine smokers show an abnormality in diffusion of gas at the alveolar-capillary level.[138] The cause of the diffusion defect is consistent with increased lung epithelial permeability secondary to damage to the alveolar-capillary membrane. This crack-related lung injury, reflected by abnormally rapid ^{99m}Tc-DTPA (diethylenetriamine pentaacetate aerosol) lung clearance, is at least partially reversible after a 3-month period of abstinence from smoking crack.[158]

Gastrointestinal Manifestations

Gastric and mesenteric arteries are abundant with α-adrenergic receptors, which constrict in response to cocaine. The intensity and location of vasoconstriction determine the extent of injury. Acute gastrointestinal ischemia occurs with all routes of cocaine administration. The most catastrophic outcomes are in patients who smuggle cocaine in the gastrointestinal tract in plastic-wrapped packets that have perforated.

Pathophysiologically, cocaine's decrease in mesenteric blood flow results in bowel edema, ulceration, and ultimately necrosis. Perforation of the duodenum, jejunum, ileum, and colon all are well described.[159–163] Large intestinal ischemia from localized vasoconstriction may present as colitis.[60,61]

Kram and colleagues[161] compared patients with cocaine-induced gastroduodenal ulceration and perforations with patients with perforations and ulcerations secondary to peptic gastroduodenal ulcer disease. These investigators reported the former patients to be younger, to have no prior history of peptic ulcer disease, and to differ in the location of their lesion. In cocaine users, the ulcerations occur in the first portion of the duodenum, the prepyloric region of the stomach, the pyloric canal, or the greater curvature of the stomach. In contrast, in patients with peptic ulcer disease, ulcers primarily develop in the duodenal bulb.[164]

Cocaine also has been associated with splenic infarction[165] and with abnormal spleen hemodynamics.[166] Cocaine administered intravenously to volunteers caused a 25% reduction in spleen volume and altered hematologic parameters (increase in hemoglobin levels, hematocrit values, and red blood cell counts).[167]

Renal Manifestations

The renal effects of cocaine are related primarily to its vasoconstrictive effect on the renal vasculature and secondarily to the effects subsequent to hyperthermia, seizures, and skeletal muscle breakdown. Additionally, cocaine-induced acute renal infarction is reported rarely.[70] In this setting, patients may present with flank or upper abdominal pain, nausea, vomiting, microscopic or gross hematuria, and proteinuria. The mechanism may be a combination of spasm of the renal vasculature and thrombogenesis from cocaine's direct effect on platelets and prostaglandins.

Rhabdomyolysis

Cocaine also produces atraumatic and traumatic rhabdomyolysis that may lead to acute renal failure.[168,169] In large doses, cocaine has a direct toxic effect on skeletal muscle, causing myofibrillar degeneration. Also, muscle ischemia from vasoconstriction may predispose further to rhabdomyolysis. Traumatic rhabdomyolysis occurs as cocaine impairs behavioral responses to the environment, causes agitation, and induces seizures.

A prospective case series of patients presenting to the emergency department with complaints related to cocaine use showed a high incidence of cocaine-associated rhabdomyolysis. Of all cocaine users, 24% had rhabdomyolysis, defined by an elevation of creatine kinase (CK) of more than fivefold that of the mean level (>1000 U/L). The same study found that only 13% of the patients presenting with rhabdomyolysis experienced any of the classic signs or symptoms (nausea, vomiting, myalgias, muscle swelling and tenderness, weakness).[170] Other causes of rhabdomyolysis also present without any signs and symptoms, which emphasizes the need for laboratory evaluation when establishing this diagnosis.

Patients at highest risk for complications from rhabdomyolysis are patients presenting with severe signs of cocaine toxicity. A retrospective study showed that patients with acute cocaine intoxication who had admission serum CK levels of less than 1000 U/L, a normal serum creatinine level, a normal WBC count, and no more than one additional risk factor for rhabdomyolysis (i.e., increased muscular activity, other mind-altering drugs, seizures) had little chance of developing complications.[171]

In severe cases, laboratory values are consistent with values associated with profound rhabdomyolysis. Serum CK values have been reported in the range of 100,000 U/L. Hyperkalemia, hyperphosphatemia, hyperuricemia, metabolic acidosis, and elevations of liver function tests may occur. Disseminated intravascular coagulation, usually fatal, may develop as a terminal event.

Uteroplacental Complications

The complications of cocaine use in pregnancy generally are thought to be secondary to its local vasoconstrictive effects on uterine blood flow.[172,173] Maternal complications include spontaneous abortion, abruptio placentae, and premature labor.[174,175] Fetal cocaine exposure results in developmental problems, including small head circumference, low birth weight, neurologic abnormalities, and uterogenital abnormalities.[176–182] The studies on the effects of cocaine on neonates are controversial because their results are limited and include other confounding factors.[183,184]

DIAGNOSIS

The diagnosis of acute cocaine toxicity is based on the patient's history and physical examination. Many patients present with symptoms of mild intoxication, and the physical examination reveals findings consistent with a sympathomimetic toxidrome. Most important clues to deciphering the etiology of the agitated patient are found in the vital signs. Hypertension, tachycardia, and hyperthermia are customary. An elevated body temperature (41.1°C [>106°F]) of any etiology is more ominous, however, than an elevated pulse or blood pressure. This information should be obtained early in the management. Because the differential diagnosis for agitated delirium is extensive, other immediate causes, including hypoxia, hypoglycemia, and infection, should be considered and treated promptly.

Unless a patient presents with a severe complication from cocaine, most laboratory tests are not helpful. Electrolyte abnormalities and acid-base abnormalities generally are secondary to seizures or agitated delirium and subsequent rhabdomyolysis. Patients should be monitored for hypokalemia, hyperkalemia, and hypocalcemia because subsequent dysrhythmias may be a cause of mortality in patients with rhabdomyolysis. Elevated liver enzymes are late findings in the severely hyperthermic patient.[185]

The clinical status should guide the use of adjunct diagnostic tools. A chest radiograph is helpful in clarifying the existence of pulmonary pathology or of a large vessel injury. Extrapulmonary air in the thoracic cavity or a widened mediastinum may be visible.

Similarly, patients with chest pain should have an ECG and CPK-MB or cardiac troponin I determination to help exclude cardiac ischemia and infarction. Although these parameters are not perfect tools in diagnosing cocaine-associated myocardial infarction, they are beneficial when definitively abnormal or evolving.

The ECG has a low predictive value for detection of an acute myocardial infarction in patients presenting with cocaine-related chest pain. The sensitivity of the ECG is 36%, and specificity is 90%.[102]

ECG abnormalities in patients with cocaine-associated chest pain are a common manifestation. ECGs of many patients with cocaine-induced myocardial infarctions are normal or nondiagnostic.[68,102,105] The typical ECG abnormalities include ST-segment elevations or depressions, T-wave inversions, QRS prolongation and Q waves, and J-point elevation due to early repolarization.[102,104,105,186,187] J-point elevation on the ECG of patients with cocaine-associated chest pain appeared with a mean frequency of 35%. These elevations in the precordial leads are misinterpreted easily as acute myocardial infarction. In one study, 43% of patients presenting with cocaine-associated chest pain had ST-segment elevations in the precordial leads, meeting ECG criteria for the use of thrombolytic therapy, with none of them meeting CPK criteria for infarction.[104] The high frequency of abnormal ECGs in this group of patients was attributed to early repolarization.

This subject is confounded further by the fact that similar ECG abnormalities are often found in asymptomatic chronic cocaine abusers.[107,188] Cocaine-addicted patients admitted for inpatient detoxification who wore ambulatory ECG monitors had frequent ST-segment elevations; 87% of the episodes for ST-segment elevations were silent. These ECG changes continued to occur in 25% of patients after 2 weeks of drug abstinence. None of the patients had ECG abnormalities after 6 weeks of ECG monitoring.[107]

Similarly, the value of CPK and CPK-MB measurements in cocaine-associated chest pain may be inadequate. These laboratory values may be elevated in patients with cocaine-associated chest pain with subsequent negative troponin I levels.[189] A study found that the specificities of CPK-MB for myocardial infarction in patients with and without cocaine use were only 75% versus 88%. In contrast, the specificities of troponin I were 94% versus 94%.[190] Troponin I may be a better serologic marker for acute myocardial infarction secondary to cocaine than a positive CK-MB concentration.[191]

In cocaine-associated chest pain, cardiac imaging studies may be useful in determining whether the chest pain is of cardiac origin. A prospective evaluation by myocardial perfusion imaging with ^{99m}Tc-sestamibi showed that only 5 of 216 (2%) patients presenting with cocaine-associated chest pain had a positive test, with 2 of the 5 patients ruling in for infarction by cardiac enzymes.[187] Results from studies of patients with chest pain indicate that this imaging modality may be sensitive for coronary artery disease.[192–195]

Cardiac catheterization may be able to localize an existing coronary lesion in cocaine-associated myocardial infarction. Of patients with cocaine-associated myocardial infarction who underwent angiography, 67% had significant coronary disease.[106] This high incidence of disease is found mainly because of selection bias, with angiography being performed preferentially in patients who were considered high risk.[68,120] An accurate incidence of coronary artery disease in all patients with cocaine-associated chest pain is unknown because patients in whom myocardial infarction is excluded rarely undergo further testing.

Numerous reports exist of sudden cardiac arrest secondary to cocaine use in the prehospital setting.[114,121,133] In patients who arrive at the hospital with a cocaine-associated myocardial infarction, incidence of complications ranges from 19.7% to 28%.[68,106] These complications consist of congestive heart failure, nonsustained ventricular tachycardia, sustained ventricular tachycardia, supraventricular tachycardia, and bradydysrhythmias. Despite this high frequency of occurrence, the mortality during acute hospital stay in one study was 0% (95% confidence interval 0% to 2%).[106] More importantly, patients who developed complications tended to do so within the first 12 hours of arrival to the emergency department. More than half of the complications already have manifested by arrival.[106]

The long-term outcome of patients who present to the emergency department with cocaine-associated chest pain also seems favorable. These patients have a 1-year survival of 98% and an incidence of late myocardial infarction of only 1%.[196]

Although the mortality from complications secondary to cocaine-induced myocardial infarction is low, certain patients need close monitoring. We recommend the following criteria for identifying patients who are at greatest risk:

Complications such as hypotension, dysrhythmias, or congestive heart failure at presentation or during a 12-hour observation period
Persistent chest pain despite standard therapy
An ECG that is classic for myocardial infarction or one that is evolving
A positive CPK-MB or troponin

When available, helical chest CT or angiography may be performed if an aortic dissection or a pulmonary infarction is suspected. Otherwise, a chest CT scan or a ventilation/perfusion scan may help exclude these two complications. Patients who present with global or focal neurologic symptoms should have a head CT scan or magnetic resonance imaging/magnetic resonance angiography. Similarly, in patients presenting with complaints of headache in which a subarachnoid hemorrhage is in question, a lumbar puncture should be performed if an initial head CT scan is normal.

TREATMENT

The peripheral complications of cocaine intoxication are likely the result of an increased central excitatory state secondary to an increased sympathomimetic outflow. Treatment is directed primarily at restoring this central imbalance, which by itself treats many of the peripheral manifestations providing specific treatment to the particular organ complications. Because the major cause of mortality from cocaine toxicity is secondary to the exceedingly severe psychomotor agitation and subsequent hyperthermia, primary attention is given to obtaining control of this agitated state.

Unless there is evidence of a catastrophic CNS or cardiovascular event, most patients with cocaine toxicity present to the hospital verbal and fully active and without the need of emergent airway management with endotracheal intubation. In an agitated delirious patient, hypoxia and hypoglycemia should be eliminated immediately by obtaining bedside pulse oximetry and a rapid reagent glucose.

Hyperthermia should be recognized early and treated immediately because of the increased mortality that it causes. Body temperatures greater than 41.1°C (106°F) place the patient at great risk for end-organ injury. Any temperature greater than 43.3°C (110°F) suggests a poor prognosis.[185]

Indications for ICU Admission in Cocaine Poisoning

Chest pain with ischemic changes on ECG, evolving ECG, persistent chest pain despite therapy, myocardial infarction, thrombolysis, symptomatic dysrhythmias
Focality on physical examination; prolonged or focal seizures, coma, subarachnoid hemorrhage, intraparenchymal hemorrhage, delirium
Aortic dissection, rupture; uncontrolled hypertension, hypotension
Hemorrhage, embolism, hypoxia, pneumothorax, pneumomediastinum
Rhabdomyolysis with signs of renal failure, renal infarction
Abruptio placentae, spontaneous abortion with prolonged bleeding
Mesenteric ischemia and infarction, splenic infarction, gastrointestinal perforation
Hyperthermia with change in mental status, metabolic acidosis
Evidence of disseminated intravascular coagulation (complication of hyperthermia)

ECG, electrocardiogram.

Management of hyperthermia consists of rapid immersion in an ice water bath while maintaining control over agitation. Adequate sedation controls the motor activity and prevents further temperature elevation.

Although agents such as haloperidol, chlorpromazine, pimozide, and propranolol may normalize some of the vital signs, they do not protect against the centrally mediated motor activity and lethality in most experimental models.[93,197–199] When comparing different therapeutic strategies in cocaine-toxic dogs, survival correlated best with therapies that corrected body temperature.[76] Benzodiazepines decrease mortality by controlling the agitation and lowering the body temperature.

Despite an elevated blood pressure, hyperthermic patients ordinarily are volume depleted secondary to the increased fluid loss from sweat.[200] Hydration status, electrolytes, and substrates should be replenished. When restrained, the patient should not be covered completely without adequate heat dissipation. Although effective for malignant hyperthermia, dantrolene is not effective for cocaine toxicity.[201–203]

Violent activity should be controlled with temporary physical restraint, if necessary, until sedation is achieved chemically. Continuous motor activity while in restraints may worsen hyperthermia from the increased muscle activity. Wrist and ankle bands instead of blankets should be used for physical restraints because blankets impair heat dissipation and worsen rhabdomyolysis and lactic acidosis.

Benzodiazepines are the pharmacologic agents of choice for sedation of cocaine-induced agitation. These agents control cocaine-induced agitation, hypertension, tachycardia, and hyperthermia in animal models.[76,204,205] Similarly, benzodiazepines resolve cardiac performance and symptoms of chest pain in patients with cocaine-associated coronary syndromes.[206] Additionally, they effectively treat agitation secondary to increased sympathomimetic activity from alcohol or sedative-hypnotic withdrawal. Benzodiazepines also are safe in controlling the CNS agitation from other potential causes, such as an infection. We recommend incremental doses of 5 to 10 mg of diazepam (or equivalent doses of lorazepam or midazolam) be given to adults until the desired level of sedation is achieved. As the mental status becomes controllable with treatment, the peripheral manifestations of cocaine toxicity also are alleviated (hypertension, tachycardia, hyperthermia, diaphoresis).

An elevated blood pressure that fails to respond to sedation may be controlled with sodium nitroprusside (0.5 to 10 μg/kg/min), nitroglycerin (starting dose 10 μg/min), or phentolamine (5 to 20 mg) with titration to a normal blood pressure. These drugs may be given without risk of cerebral hypoperfusion in patients without long-standing hypertension.

Additionally, benzodiazepines (e.g., lorazepam and diazepam) also control seizures that may occur early at presentation from acute cocaine intoxication or afterward as a manifestation of a CNS or cardiovascular complication. In a canine model of cocaine toxicity, only diazepam and induced hypothermia were able to reduce the incidence of seizures, control tachycardia and hypertension, and improve outcome.[76] Ultimately, barbiturate-induced coma also is effective in terminating seizure activity. Because of cardiovascular and respiratory depression caused by these agents, cardiac monitoring and ventilatory support must be provided.[207]

If a neuromuscular blocker is used, electroencephalogram monitoring is necessary because motor activity from a seizure otherwise may be overlooked. A nondepolarizing neuromuscular blocker is preferable because of the potential for exacerbating hyperkalemia and rhabdomyolysis from a depolarizing agent. Also, succinylcholine is degraded rapidly by plasma cholinesterase, the same enzyme that metabolizes cocaine. Theoretically, use of these agents simultaneously may extend the clinical effects of either or both.

Because most exposures to cocaine are from nasal insufflation or from inhalation, decontamination generally is not an issue. Ingestion may be lethal because this type of exposure occurs in the setting of smuggling large amounts of cocaine. Decontamination may require the administration of activated charcoal and, if packets were ingested, whole-bowel irrigation (see Chapter 5). Any symptomatic patient in whom there is confirmed packet ingestion should undergo a laparotomy to remove the cocaine packets.

Treatment of the cardiac manifestations of cocaine toxicity is directed at reversing its physiologic effects that cause ischemia or dysrhythmias. As stated earlier, benzodiazepines assist in normalizing the blood pressure and heart rate and diminish myocardial oxygen demand. If the physical examination denotes catecholamine excess, benzodiazepines should be the initial treatment modality in patients with cocaine-associated chest pain. Theoretically, aspirin may prevent cocaine's thrombogenic effects. Aspirin has an extensive beneficial record in the treatment of patients with ischemic heart disease. It should be administered in patients with cocaine-associated ischemic symptoms unless there is also a suspicion of cerebral hemorrhage.

Clinical and angiographic data support the use of nitroglycerin to relieve cocaine-associated chest pain caused by coronary artery vasoconstriction.[208,209] Cocaine-induced vasoconstriction was abolished in patients given sublingual nitroglycerin in a dose sufficient to reduce mean arterial pressure by 10% to 15%.[208] As in patients with classic ischemic chest pain, nitroglycerin should be the principal treatment for patients with cocaine-associated chest pain as well.

Because cocaine's vasoconstrictive effects are mediated by an α-adrenergic mechanism, the use of β-adrenergic antagonists for the treatment of cocaine-associated cardiac toxicity has resulted in deleterious consequences in human and animal studies.[44,76,117,197,205,210,211] In volunteers given 2 mg of cocaine intranasally or intravenously, the administration of the β-adrenergic antagonist propranolol caused further coronary artery constriction.[117–119,208] Similarly the use of mixed β-adrenergic antagonists, including labetalol, is contraindicated.[210,211]

Phentolamine, an α-adrenergic antagonist, reverses cocaine-induced ischemia.[119,212] A low starting dose (1 mg) of phentolamine is recommended to avoid hypotensive effects, while maintaining antiischemic effects.[8] This dose may be repeated in 5 minutes and be titrated to symptoms and blood pressure. This vasodilating agent with rapid-onset and short-lived pharmacodynamics is preferred because of its simple, dependable control.

Large multicenter clinical trials found calcium channel antagonists not to be beneficial in the treatment of myocardial ischemia unrelated to cocaine, whereas in cocaine intoxication, smaller animal and human studies yielded conflicting results.[119,213–221] In some animal studies, calcium channel antagonists decreased the incidence of seizures and cardiac dysrhythmias and increased survival[119,213,214,219,221]; others reported opposite results.[215–217] Verapamil reversed cocaine-induced coronary artery vasoconstriction in a human model[220] and is recommended for the treatment of refractory ischemia by some authors.[8] Because of these equivocal results, calcium channel antagonists should be used with caution and only when other therapies have failed.

Although the clinical safety of the use of thrombolytic therapy for cocaine-associated myocardial infarction has been documented,[222] this treatment modality has significant complications,[223,224] and the risk/benefit analysis in this setting is not yet conclusive. The poor predictive value of the ECG in cocaine-induced acute myocardial infarction and the low incidence of complications after such an event should discourage the routine use of thrombolytic therapy in this setting. In addition, because many patients with cocaine-induced myocardial infarction do not have a thrombus, cardiac catheterization may provide a definitive diagnosis and the ultimate reperfusion strategy when available. If invasive reperfusion facilities are unavailable and the patient has clear ECG evidence of myocardial infarction and no contraindications, thrombolytics may be used.

Most benign dysrhythmias secondary to cocaine toxicity respond to sedation, fluid administration, and cooling. Supraventricular dysrhythmias and atrial fibrillation that do not respond to this initial treatment may be treated with diltiazem or verapamil. Wide-complex supraventricular tachycardia occurring in an acutely cocaine-intoxicated patient is most likely secondary to cocaine's Na^+ channel–blocking effects on the conduction system of the heart. As such, this effect is similar to that of class I antidysrhythmic drugs.[135] Animal and human data report the reversal of the subsequent QRS prolonging effect on the ECG with treatment with sodium bicarbonate.[37,225–227]

Ventricular tachycardia may be treated with lidocaine. The effects of lidocaine on cocaine-poisoned animals are contradictory.[227–229] Concern of administering another class I antidysrhythmic agent with definitive CNS toxicity in cocaine toxicity exists. Evaluation of patients having cocaine-induced myocardial infarction who received lidocaine for various indications showed, however, clear absence of fatality, seizures, or cardiac complications in the emergency department or during subsequent hospitalization.[136]

REFERENCES

1. Kleber HD: Cocaine abuse: Historical, epidemiological, and psychological perspectives. J Clin Psychiatry 49(2Suppl):3–6, 1988.
2. National Institute of Drug Abuse: National Household Survey on Drug Abuse: Population Estimates, 1993. DHHS No. (ADM) 94–3017. Rockville, MD, 1994, USDHHS.
3. MacDonald DI: Cocaine leads emergency department drug visits. JAMA 258:2029, 1987.
4. Substance Abuse and Mental Health Services Administration: Drug Abuse Warning Network Medical Examiner: 1995; Annual Data, Series D1. (SMA)97–3126. Washington, DC, 1997, USDHHS.
5. National Institute of Drug Abuse: National Household Survey on Drug Abuse: Population Estimates, 1995. No. ADM (96–3095). Rockville, MD, 1996, USDHHS.
6. Substance Abuse and Mental Health Services Administration: National Household Survey on Drug Abuse. 1998. Available at: USDHHS. http://www.samhsa.gov.
7. Kandel D, Chen K, Warner LA, et al: Prevalence and demographic correlates of symptoms of last year dependence on alcohol, nicotine, marijuana and cocaine in the US population. Drug Alcohol Depend 44:11–29, 1997.
8. Hollander JD: The management of cocaine-associated myocardial ischemia. N Engl J Med 333:1267–1272, 1995.
9. Warner EA, Flores RM, Robinson BE: A profile of hospitalized cocaine users: Patient characteristics, diagnoses, and physical responses. Substance Abuse 16:205–212, 1995.
10. Goldfrank LR, Hoffman RS: The cardiovascular effects of cocaine. Ann Emerg Med 20:165–175, 1991.
11. Khalsa ME, Tashkin DP, Perrochet B: Smoked cocaine: Patterns of use and pulmonary consequences. J Psychoactive Drugs 24:265–272, 1992.
12. Mahler JC, Perry S, Sutton B: Intraurethral cocaine administration. JAMA 259:3126, 1988.
13. Javaid JI, Fischman MW, Schuster CR, et al: Cocaine plasma concentration: Relation to physiological and subjective effects in humans. Science 202:227–228, 1978.
14. Javaid JI, Musa MN, Fischman M, et al: Kinetics of cocaine in humans after intravenous and intranasal administration. Biopharm Drug Dispos 4:9–18, 1983.
15. Zhang JY, Foltz RL: Cocaine metabolism in man: Identification of four previously unreported cocaine metabolites in human urine. J Anal Toxicol 14:201–205, 1990.
16. Stewart DJ, Inaba T, Lucassen M, et al: Cocaine metabolism: Cocaine and norcocaine hydrolysis by liver and serum esterases. Clin Pharmacol Ther 6:464–468, 1979.
17. Borne RF, Bedford JA, Buelke JL, et al: Biological effects of cocaine, derivatives: I. Improved synthesis and pharmacologic evaluation of norcocaine. J Pharm Sci 66:119–129, 1977.
18. Devenyi P, Schneiderman JF, Devenyi RG, et al: Cocaine-induced central retinal artery occlusion. Can Med Assoc J 138:129–130, 1988.
19. Madden JA, Powers RH: Effect of cocaine and cocaine metabolites on cerebral arteries in vitro. Life Sci 47:1109–1114, 1990.
20. Schreiber MD, Madden JA, Covert RF, et al: Effects of cocaine, benzoylecgonine, and cocaine metabolites on cannulated pressurized fetal sheep cerebral arteries. J Appl Physiol 77:834–839, 1994.
21. Hoffman RS, Henry GC, Wax PM, et al: Decreased plasma cholinesterase activity enhances cocaine toxicity in mice. J Pharm Exp Ther 263:698–702, 1992.
22. Hoffman RS, Henry GL, Weisman RS, et al: Association between life-threatening cocaine toxicity and plasma cholinesterase activity. Am J Emerg Med 21:247–253, 1991.
23. Covert RF, Schreiber MD, Tebbett IR, et al: Hemodynamic and cerebral flow effects of cocaine, cocaethylene and benzoylecgonine in conscious and anesthetized fetal lambs. J Pharmacol Exp Ther 270:188–196, 1994.
24. Ambre J: The urinary excretion of cocaine and metabolites in humans: A kinetic analysis of published data. J Anal Toxicol 9:241–245, 1985.
25. Weiss RD: Protracted elimination of cocaine metabolites in long term high dose cocaine abuse. Am J Med 85:879–880, 1988.
26. Jatlow PI: Drug of abuse profile: Cocaine. Clin Chem 33:66b–71b, 1987.
27. Dean RA, Christian CD, Sample RH, et al: Human liver cocaine esterases: Ethanol-mediated formation of ethylcocaine. FASEB J 5:2735–2739, 1991.
28. McCance EF, Price LH, Kosten TR, et al: Cocaethylene: Pharmacology, physiology and behavioral effects in humans. J Pharmacol Exp Ther 274:215–223, 1995.
29. Elsworth JD, Bradberry CW, Taylor JR, et al: Cocaethylene is a pharmacologically active metabolite of cocaine formed after combined intake of cocaine and ethanol. Neurosci Abs 16:310–311, 1990.
30. Erzouki HK, Baum I, Goldberg SR, et al: Comparison of the effects of cocaine and its metabolites on cardiovascular function in anesthetized rats. J Cardiovasc Pharmacol 22:557–563, 1993.
31. McCance-Katz EF, Kosten TR, Jatlow P: Concurrent use of cocaine and alcohol is more potent and potentially more toxic than use of either alone—a multiple-dose study. Biol Psychiatry 44:250–259, 1998.
32. Wilson LD, Henning RJ, Suttheimer C, et al: Cocaethylene causes dose-dependent reduction in cardiac function in anesthetized dogs. J Cardiovasc Pharmacol 26:965–973, 1995.
33. Xu Y, Crumb WJ, Clarkson CW: Cocaethylene, a metabolite of cocaine and ethanol, is a potent blocker of cardiac sodium channels. J Pharm Exp Ther 271:319–325, 1994.
34. Billman GG: Mechanisms responsible for the cardiotoxic effects of cocaine. FASEB J 4:2469–2475, 1990.
35. Kerns II W, Garvey L, Owens J: Cocaine-induced wide complex dysrhythmia. J Emerg Med 15:321–329, 1997.
36. Kloner RA, Hale S, Alker K, et al: The effects of acute and chronic cocaine use on the heart. Circulation 85:407–421, 1992.
37. Wang RY: pH-Dependent cocaine-induced cardiotoxicity. Am J Emerg Med 17:364–369, 1999.
38. Smith JA, Mo Q, Guo H, et al: Cocaine increases extraneuronal levels of aspartate and glutamate in the nucleus accumbens. Brain Res Bull 683:264–269, 1995.
39. Tella SR, Schindler CW, Goldberg SR: Cocaine: Cardiovascular effects in relation to inhibition of peripheral neuronal monoamine uptake and central stimulation of the sympathoadrenal system. J Pharmacol Exp Ther 267:153–162, 1993.
40. Romach MK, Glue P, Kampman K, et al: Attenuation of euphoric effects of cocaine by the dopamine D_1/D_5 antagonist ecopipam (SCH 39166). Arch Gen Psychiatry 56:1101–1106, 1999.
41. Neisewander JL, O'Dell LE, Redmond JC: Localization of dopamine receptor subtypes occupied by intra-accumbens antagonists that reverse cocaine-induced locomotion. Brain Res 671:210–212, 1995.
42. Giros B, Jaber M, Jones S, et al: Hyperlocomotion and indifference to cocaine and amphetamine in mice lacking the dopamine transporter. Nature 379:606–612, 1996.
43. Volkow ND, Fowler JS, Wang GJ: Imaging studies on the role of dopamine in cocaine reinforcement and addiction in humans. J Psychopharmacol 13:337–345, 1999.
44. Spivey WH, Euerle B: Neurologic complications of cocaine abuse. Ann Emerg Med 19:1422–1428, 1990.
45. Pap A, Bradberry CW: Excitatory amino acid antagonists attenuate the effects of cocaine on extracellular dopamine in the nucleus accumbens. J Pharmacol Exp Ther 274:127–133, 1995.
46. Rockhold RW, Oden G, Ho IK, et al: Glutamate receptor antagonists block cocaine induced convulsions and death. Brain Res Bull 27:721–723, 1991.
47. Tonga G, Tempesta E, Tonga AR, et al: Platelet responsiveness and biosynthesis of thromboxane and prostacyclin in response to in vitro cocaine treatment. Haemostasis 15:100–107, 1985.
48. Heesch CM, Steiner M, Hernandez JA, et al: Effects of cocaine on human platelet aggregation in vivo. J Toxicol Clin Toxicol 34:673–684, 1996.
49. Rezkalla SH, Mazza JJ, Kloner RA, et al: The effects of cocaine on human platelets. Am J Cardiol 72:243–246, 1993.
50. Kuggelmass AD, Shannon RP, Yeo EL, et al: Intravenous cocaine induces platelet activation in the conscious dog. Circulation 91:1336–1340, 1995.
51. Moliterno DJ, Lange RA, Gerard RD, et al: Influence of intranasal cocaine on plasma constituents associated with endogenous thrombosis and thrombolysis. Am J Med 96:492–496, 1994.
52. Siegel AJ, Sholar MB, Mendelson JH, et al: Cocaine-induced erythrocytosis and increase in von Willebrand factor. Arch Intern Med 159:1925–1930, 1999.
53. Wilbert-Lampen U, Seliger C, Zilker T, Arendt RM: Cocaine increases the endothelial release of immunoreactive endothelin and its

concentrations in human plasma and urine: Reversal by co-incubation with σ-receptor antagonists. Circulation 98:385–390, 1998.

54. Casoni I, Ricci G, Ballarin E, et al: Hematological indices of erythropoietin administration in athletes. Int J Sports Med 14:307–311, 1993.
55. Favier R, Caceres E, Koubi H, et al: Effects of coca chewing on hormonal and metabolic responses during prolonged submaximal exercise. J Appl Physiol 80:650–655, 1996.
56. Sawka MN, Young AJ, Muza SR, et al: Erythrocyte reinfusion and maximal aerobic power. JAMA 257:1496–1498, 1987.
57. Ford PV, Parker HG: Unsuspected deep venous thrombophlebitis detected by gallium-67 imaging. Clin Nucl Med 12:556–557, 1987.
58. Galbe LI, Merkin MD: Cerebral infarction in a user of free base cocaine (crack). Neurology 36:1602–1604, 1986.
59. Mirzayan R, Hanks SE, Weaver FA: Cocaine-induced thrombosis of common iliac and popliteal arteries. Ann Vasc Surg 12:476–481, 1998.
60. Mizrahi S, Laor D, Stamler B: Intestinal ischemia induced by cocaine ingestion: Report of two cases. Surgery 97:374–376, 1985.
61. Mizrahi S, Loar D, Stamler B, et al: Intestinal ischemia induced by cocaine abuse. Arch Surg 123:394, 1988.
62. Wohlman RA: Renal artery thrombosis and embolization associated with intravenous cocaine injection. South Med J 80:928–930, 1987.
63. Brody SL, Slovis CM, Wrenn KD: Cocaine-related medical problems: Consecutive series of 233 patients. Am J Med 88:325–331, 1990.
64. Ascher EK, Stauffer JCE, Gaasch WH: Coronary artery spasm, cardiac arrest, transient electrocardiographic Q waves and stunned myocardium in cocaine-associated acute myocardial infarction. Am J Cardiol 61:939–941, 1988.
65. Levine SR, Brust JCM, Futrell N, et al: Cerebrovascular complications of the use of the "crack" form of alkaloidal cocaine. N Engl J Med 323:699–704, 1990.
66. Levine SR, Brust JCM, Futrell N, et al: A comparative study of the cerebrovascular complications of cocaine: Alkaloidal versus hydrochloride—a review. Neurology 41:1173–1177, 1991.
67. Hoffman RS, Reimer BI: "Crack" cocaine-induced bilateral amblyopia. Am J Emerg Med 11:35–37, 1993.
68. Hollander JE, Hoffman RS: Cocaine-induced myocardial infarction: An analysis and review of the literature. J Emerg Med 10:169–177, 1992.
69. Konzen K, Levine SR, Garcia JH: Vasospasm and thrombus formation as possible mechanisms of stroke related to alkaloidal cocaine. Stroke 26:1114–1118, 1995.
70. Sharff JA: Renal infarction associated with intravenous cocaine use. Ann Emerg Med 13:1145–1147, 1984.
71. Wetli CV, Fishbain DA: Cocaine-induced psychosis and sudden death in recreational cocaine users. J Forensic Sci 30:873–880, 1985.
72. Marzuk PM, Tardiff K, Leon AC, et al: Ambient temperature and mortality from unintentional cocaine overdose. JAMA 279:1795–1800, 1998.
73. Cox B, Kerwin R, Lee TF: Dopamine receptors in the central thermoregulatory pathways of the rat. J Physiol 282:471–483, 1978.
74. Daras M, Kakkouras L, Tuchman AJ, et al: Rhabdomyolysis and hyperthermia after cocaine abuse: A variant of the neuroleptic malignant syndrome. Acta Neurol Scand 92:161–165, 1995.
75. Roth D, Alarcon FJ, Fernandez JA, et al: Acute rhabdomyolysis associated with cocaine intoxication. N Engl J Med 319:673–677, 1988.
76. Catravas JD, Waters IW: Acute cocaine intoxication in the conscious dog: Studies on the mechanism of lethality. J Pharmacol Exp Ther 217:350–356, 1981.
77. Brust JC: Vasculitis owing to substance abuse. Neurol Clin 15:945–957, 1997.
78. Brust JCM, Richter RW: Stroke associated with cocaine abuse? N Y State J Med 77:1473–1475, 1977.
79. Daras M, Koppel BS, Atos-Radzion E: Cocaine-induced choreoathetoid movements ('crack dancing'). Neurology 44:751–752, 1994.
80. Daras M, Tuchman AJ, Koppel BS: Neurovascular complications of cocaine. Acta Neurol Scand 90:124–129, 1994.
81. Dhuna A, Pascual-Leone A, Langendorf F, et al: Epileptogenic properties of cocaine in humans. Neurotoxicology 12:621–626, 1991.
82. Fessler RD, Esshaki CM, Stankewitz RC, et al: The neurovascular complications of cocaine. Surg Neurol 47:339–345, 1997.
83. Kibayashi K, Mastri AR, Hirsh CS: Cocaine induced intracerebral hemorrhage: Analysis of predisposing factors and mechanisms causing hemorrhagic strokes. Hum Pathol 26:659–663, 1995.
84. Mody CK, Miller BL, McIntyre HB, et al: Neurologic complications of cocaine abuse. Neurology 38:1189–1193, 1988.
85. Satel SL, Gawin FH: Migraine-like headache and cocaine use. JAMA 261:2995–2996, 1989.

86. Jacobs IG, Roszler MH, Kelly JK, et al: Cocaine abuse: Neurovascular complications. Radiology 170:223–227, 1989.
87. Peterson PL, Rozzler M, Jacobs I, et al: Neurovascular complications of cocaine abuse. J Neuropsychiatry Clin Neurosci 3:143–149, 1991.
88. Davis GG, Swalwell CI: The incidence of acute cocaine or methamphetamine in deaths due to ruptured cerebral (berry) aneurysms. J Forensic Sci 441:626–628, 1996.
89. Nolte KB, Brass LM, Fletterick CF: Intracranial hemorrhage associated with cocaine abuse: A prospective autopsy study. Neurology 46:1291–1296, 1996.
90. Kaufman M, Levin JM, Ross MH, et al: Cocaine-induced cerebral vasoconstriction detected in humans with magnetic resonance angiography. JAMA 279:376–380, 1998.
91. Oyesiku NM, Colohan ART, Barrow DL, et al: Cocaine-induced aneurismal rupture: An emergent negative factor in the natural history of intracranial aneurysms? Neurosurgery 32:518–526, 1993.
92. Choy-Kwong M, Lipton RB: Seizures in hospitalized cocaine users. Neurology 39:425–427, 1989.
93. Derlet RW, Albertson TE, Rice P: The effect of haloperidol in cocaine and amphetamine intoxication. J Emerg Med 7:633–637, 1989.
94. Lowenstein DH, Massa SM, Rowbotham SD, et al: Acute neurological and psychiatric complications associated with cocaine abuse. Am J Med 83:841–846, 1987.
95. Pascual-Leone A, Dhuna A, Altafullah I, et al: Cocaine-induced seizures. Neurology 40:404–407, 1990.
96. Earnest MP: Seizures. Neurol Clin 11:563–575, 1993.
97. Konkol RJ, Erickson BA, Doerr JK, et al: Seizure induced by cocaine metabolite benzoylecgonine in rats. Epilepsia 33:420–427, 1992.
98. Koppel BS, Samkoff L, Daras M, et al: Relation of cocaine use to seizures and epilepsy. Epilepsia 37:875–878, 1996.
99. Pascual-Leone A, Dhuna A, Anderson DC: Cerebral atrophy in habitual cocaine abusers: A planimetric CT study. Neurology 41:34–38, 1991.
100. Rich JA, Singer DE: Cocaine-related symptoms in patients presenting to an urban emergency department. Ann Emerg Med 20:616–621, 1991.
101. Coleman DL, Ross TF, Naughton JI: Myocardial ischemia and infarction related to recreational cocaine use. West J Med 136:444–446, 1982.
102. Hollander JE, Hoffman RS, Gennis P, et al: Prospective multicenter evaluation of cocaine-associated chest pain. Acad Emerg Med 1:330–339, 1994.
103. Amin M, Gabelman G, Karpel J, et al: Acute myocardial infarction and chest pain syndromes after cocaine use. Am J Cardiol 66:1434–1437, 1990.
104. Gitter MJ, Goldsmith SR, Dunbar DN, et al: Cocaine and chest pain: Clinical features and outcome of patients hospitalized to rule out myocardial infarction. Ann Intern Med 115:277–282, 1991.
105. Tokarski GF, Paganussi P, Urbanski R, et al: An evaluation of cocaine induced chest pain. Ann Emerg Med 19:1088–1092, 1990.
106. Hollander JE, Hoffman RS, Burstein JL, et al: Cocaine-associated myocardial infarction: Mortality and complications. Arch Intern Med 155:1081–1086, 1995.
107. Nademanee K, Gorelick DA, Josephson AM, et al: Myocardial ischemia during cocaine withdrawal. Ann Intern Med 111:876–880, 1989.
108. Del Aguila C, Rosman H: Myocardial infarction during cocaine withdrawal (Letter). Ann Intern Med 112:712, 1990.
109. Adkins MS, Gaines WE, Anderson WA, et al: Chronic type A aortic dissection: An unusual complication of cocaine inhalation. Ann Thorac Surg 56:977–979, 1993.
110. Barth CW, Bray M, Roberts WC, et al: Rupture of the ascending aorta during cocaine intoxication. Am J Cardiol 57:496–497, 1986.
111. Chang RA, Rossi NF: Intermittent cocaine use associated with recurrent dissection of the thoracic and abdominal aorta. Chest 108:1758–1762, 1995.
112. Grannis FW Jr, Bryant C, Caffaratti JD, et al: Acute aortic dissection associated with cocaine abuse. Clin Cardiol 11:572–574, 1988.
113. Om A, Porter T, Mohanty PK: Transesophageal echocardiographic diagnosis of acute aortic dissection complicating cocaine abuse. Am Heart J 123:532–534, 1992.
114. Tardiff K, Gross E, Wu J, et al: Analysis of cocaine positive fatalities. J Forensic Sci 34:53–63, 1989.
115. Cohle SD, Lie JT: Dissection of the aorta and coronary arteries associated with acute cocaine intoxication. Arch Pathol Lab Med 116:1239–1241, 1992.
116. Jaffe BD, Broderick TM, Leier CV: Cocaine-induced coronary artery dissection (Letter). N Engl J Med 330:510–511, 1994.

117. Flores ED, Lange RA, Cigarroa RG, et al: Effects of cocaine on coronary artery dimensions in atherosclerotic coronary artery disease: Enhanced vasoconstriction at sites of significant stenosis. J Am Coll Cardiol 16:74–79, 1990.

118. Lange RA, Cigarroa RG, Flores ED, et al: Potentiation of cocaine induced coronary vasoconstriction by beta-adrenergic blockade. Ann Intern Med 112:897–903, 1990.

119. Lange RA, Cigarroa RG, Yancy CW, et al: Cocaine induced coronary artery vasoconstriction. N Engl J Med 321:1557–1562, 1989.

120. Om A, Warner M, Sabri N, et al: Frequency of coronary artery disease and left ventricle dysfunction in cocaine users. Am J Cardiol 69:1549–1552, 1992.

121. Smith HWB, Liberman HA, Brody SL, et al: Acute myocardial infarction temporally related to cocaine use: Clinical, angiographic, and pathophysiologic observations. Ann Intern Med 107:13–18, 1987.

122. Dressler FA, Malekzadeh S, Roberts WC: Quantitative analysis of amounts of coronary arterial narrowing in cocaine addicts. Am J Cardiol 65:303–308, 1990.

123. Majid PA, Patel B, Kim HS, et al: An angiographic and histologic study of cocaine-induced chest pain. Am J Cardiol 65:812–814, 1990.

124. Mittleman RE, Wetli CV: Cocaine and sudden "natural" death. J Forensic Sci 32:11–19, 1987.

125. Zimmerman JL, Dellinger RP, Majid PA: Cocaine associated chest pain. Ann Emerg Med 20:611–615, 1991.

126. Langner RO, Bernent CL: Cocaine-induced changes in the biochemistry and morphology of rabbit aorta. NIDA Res Monogr 108:154–166, 1991.

127. Kolodgie FD, Virmani R, Cornhill JF, et al: Cocaine: An independent risk factor for aortic sudanophilia: A preliminary report. Atherosclerosis 97:53–62, 1992.

128. Chokshi SK, Moore R, Pandian NG, et al: Reversible cardiomyopathy associated with cocaine intoxication. Ann Intern Med 111:1039–1040, 1989.

129. Weiner RS, Lockhart JT, Schwartz RG: Dilated cardiomyopathy and cocaine abuse. Am J Med 81:699–701, 1986.

130. Pitts WR, Vongpatanasin W, Cigarroa JE, et al: Effects of the intracoronary infusion of cocaine on left ventricular systolic and diastolic function in humans. Circulation 97:1270–1273, 1998.

131. Besse S, Assayag P, Latour C, et al: Molecular characteristics of cocaine-induced cardiomyopathy in rats. Eur J Pharmacol 338:123–129, 1997.

132. Karch SB, Billingham ME: The pathology and etiology of cocaine-induced heart disease. Arch Pathol Lab Med 112:225–230, 1988.

133. Virmani R, Robinowitz M, Smipek JE, et al: Cardiovascular effects of cocaine: An autopsy study of 40 patients. Am Heart J 115:1068–1076, 1988.

134. Monticciolo R, Sirop PA: Atrial fibrillation after the use of intranasal cocaine. Hosp Physician 24:48–49, 1988.

135. Schrem SS, Belsky P, Schwartzman D, et al: Cocaine-induced torsades de pointes in a patient with idiopathic long QT syndrome. Am Heart J 120:980–984, 1990.

136. Shih RD, Hollander JE, Burstein JL, et al: Clinical safety of lidocaine in patients with cocaine-associated myocardial infarction. Ann Emerg Med 26:702–706, 1995.

137. Schwartz AB, Janzen D, Jones RT, et al: Electrocardiographic and hemodynamic effects of intravenous cocaine in the awake and anesthetized dogs. J Electrocardiol 22:159–166, 1989.

138. Tashkin DP, Khalsa ME, Gorelick D, et al: Pulmonary status of habitual cocaine smokers. Am Rev Respir Dis 145:92–100, 1992.

139. Bailey ME, Fraire AE, Greenberg SD, et al: Pulmonary histopathology in cocaine abusers. Hum Pathol 25:203–207, 1994.

140. Murray RJ, Albin RJ, Mergner W, et al: Diffuse alveolar hemorrhage temporally related to cocaine smoking. Chest 93:427–429, 1988.

141. Delaney K, Hoffman RS: Pulmonary infarction associated with crack cocaine use in a previously healthy 23-year-old woman. Am J Med 91:92–94, 1991.

142. Dagget RB, Hahighi P, Terkeltaub RA: Nasal cocaine abuse causing an aggressive midline intranasal and pharyngeal destructive process mimicking midline reticulosis and limited Wegener's granulomatosis. J Rheumatol 17:838–840, 1990.

143. Rubin RB, Neugarten J: Cocaine-associated asthma. Am J Med 88:428–439, 1990.

144. Taylor RF, Bernard GR: Airway complications from freebasing cocaine. Chest 95:476–477, 1989.

145. Murray RJ, Smialek JE, Golle M, et al: Pulmonary artery medial hypertrophy in cocaine users without foreign particle microembolization. Chest 96:1050–1053, 1989.

146. Kissner AG, Lawrence D, Selis JE, et al: Crack lung: Pulmonary disease caused by cocaine abuse. Am Rev Respir Dis 136:1250–1252, 1987.

147. Rao AN, Polos PG, Walther FA: Crack abuse and asthma: A fatal combination. N Y State J Med 90:511–512, 1990.

148. Thadani PV: NIDA Conference report on cardiopulmonary complications of "crack" cocaine use: Clinical manifestations and pathophysiology. Chest 110:1072–1076, 1996.

149. Allred RJ, Ewer S: Fatal pulmonary edema following intravenous "freebase" cocaine use. Ann Emerg Med 10:441–442, 1981.

150. Barbera Mir JA, Vallejo Gavete J, Velo Plaza M, et al: Spontaneous pneumomediastinum after cocaine inhalation. Respiration 50:230–232, 1986.

151. Brody SL, Anderson AV, Gutman JBL: Pneumomediastinum as a complication of "crack" smoking. Am J Emerg Med 6:241–243, 1988.

152. Bush M, Rubenstein R, Hoffman I: Spontaneous pneumomediastinum as a consequence of cocaine use. N Y State J Med 84:618–619, 1984.

153. Birrer R, Calderon J: Pneumothorax, pneumomediastinum, and pneumopericardium following Valsalva's maneuver during marijuana smoking. N Y State J Med 84:619–620, 1984.

154. Palat D, Denson M, Sherman M, et al: Pneumomediastinum induced by inhalation of alkaloid cocaine. N Y State J Med 8:438–439, 1988.

155. Panacek EA, Singer AJ, Sherman BW, et al: Spontaneous pneumomediastinum: Clinical and natural history. Ann Emerg Med 21:10:1222–1227, 1992.

156. Shesser R, Davis C, Edelstein S: Pneumomediastinum and pneumothorax after inhaling alkaloidal cocaine. Ann Emerg Med 10:213–215, 1981.

157. Torre M, Barberis M: Spontaneous pneumothorax in cocaine sniffers. Am J Emerg Med 16:546–549, 1998.

158. Susskind H, Weber DH, Atkins HL: Does detoxification reverse the acute lung injury of crack smokers? Nucl Med Commun 17:963–970, 1996.

159. Dehesa AS, Cebrian JM: Ischemic colitis induced by cocaine abuse. Br J Surg 82:138, 1995.

160. Endress C, Gray DG, Wollschlaeger G: Bowel ischemia and perforation after cocaine use. AJR Am J Roentgenol 159:73–75, 1992.

161. Kram HB, Hardin E, Clark SR, et al: Perforated ulcers related to smoking "crack" cocaine. Am Surg 58:293–294, 1992.

162. Lee HS, LaMaute HR, Pizzi WF, et al: Acute gastroduodenal perforations associated with the use of crack. Ann Surg 211:15–17, 1990.

163. Nalbandian H, Sheth N, Dietrich R, et al: Intestinal ischemia caused by cocaine ingestion: Report of two cases. Surgery 97:374–376, 1985.

164. Abramson DL, Gertler JP, Lewis T, et al: Crack-related perforated gastropyloric ulcer. J Clin Gastroenterol 13:17–19, 1991.

165. Novielli KD, Chambers CV: Splenic infarction after cocaine use. Ann Intern Med 114:251–252, 1991.

166. Sarper R, Faraj BA, Tarcan DB, et al: Assessment of splanchnic blood flow in alcohol and drug abuse using radionuclide angiography. J Subst Abuse 5:295–303, 1993.

167. Kaufman MJ, Siegel AJ, Mendelson JH, et al: Cocaine administration induces human splenic constriction and altered hematologic parameters. J Appl Physiol 85:1877–1883, 1998.

168. Pogue VA, Nurse HM: Cocaine-associated acute myoglobinuric renal failure. Am J Med 86:183–186, 1989.

169. Rubin RB, Neugarten J: Cocaine-induced rhabdomyolysis masquerading as myocardial ischemia. Am J Med 86:551–553, 1989.

170. Welch RD, Todd K, Krause GS, et al: Incidence of cocaine-associated rhabdomyolysis. Ann Emerg Med 20:154–157, 1991.

171. Brody SL, Wrenn KD, Wilber MM, et al: Predicting the severity of cocaine-associated rhabdomyolysis. Ann Emerg Med 19:1137–1143, 1990.

172. Moore TR, Sorg J, Miller L, et al: Hemodynamic effects of intravenous cocaine on the pregnant ewe and fetus. Am J Obstet Gynecol 155:883–888, 1986.

173. Woods JR, Plessinger MA, Clark KE: Effect of cocaine on uterine blood flow and fetal oxygenation. JAMA 257:957–961, 1987.

174. Acker D, Sachs BP, Tracey KJ, et al: Abruptio placentae associated with cocaine use. Am J Obstet Gynecol 146:220–221, 1983.

175. Chasnoff IJ, Griffith DR, MacGregor S, et al: Temporal patterns of cocaine use in pregnancy: Perinatal outcome. JAMA 261:1741–1744, 1989.

176. Chasnoff IJ, Burns KA, Burns WJ: Cocaine use in pregnancy: Perinatal morbidity and mortality. Neurobehav Toxicol Teratol 9:291–293, 1989.

177. Chasnoff IJ, Griffith DR, Freier C, et al: Cocaine/polydrug use in pregnancy: Two-year follow-up. Pediatrics 89:284–289, 1992.
178. Chiriboga CA, Brust JCM, Bateman D, et al: Dose-response effect of fetal cocaine exposure on newborn neurologic function. Pediatrics 103:79–85, 1999.
179. Frank DA, McCarten KM, Robson CD, et al: Level of in utero cocaine exposure and neonatal ultrasound findings. Pediatrics 104:1101–1105, 1999.
180. Weathers WT, Crane MM, Sauvain KJ, et al: Cocaine use in women from a defined population: Prevalence at delivery and effects on growth in infants. Pediatrics 91:350–354, 1993.
181. Young LS, Heather JV, Phillips SA: Cocaine: Its effects on maternal and child health. Pharmacotherapy 12:2–17, 1992.
182. Zuckerman B, Frank DA, Hingson R, et al: Effects of maternal marijuana and cocaine use on fetal growth. N Engl J Med 320:762–768, 1989.
183. Richardson GA, Day NL: Maternal and neonatal effects of moderate cocaine use during pregnancy. Neurotoxicol Teratol 13:455–460, 1991.
184. Yawn RA, Thompson LR, Lupo VR, et al: Prenatal drug use in Minneapolis-St. Paul, Minn: A 4-year trend. Arch Fam Med 3:520–527, 1994.
185. Clowes GHA, O'Donnell TF Jr: Heat stroke. N Engl J Med 291:564–567, 1974.
186. Hollander JE, Lozano M, Fairweather P, et al: "Abnormal" electrocardiograms in patients with cocaine-associated chest pain are due to "normal" variants. J Emerg Med 12:199–205, 1994.
187. Kontos MC, Schmidt KL, Nicholson CS, et al: Myocardial perfusion imaging with technetium-99m sestamibi in patients with cocaine-associated chest pain. Ann Emerg Med 33:639–645, 1999.
188. Chakko S, Sepulveda S, Kessler KM, et al: Frequency and type of electrocardiographic abnormalities in cocaine abusers (electrocardiogram in cocaine abuse). Am J Cardiol 74:710–713, 1994.
189. MacLaurin M, Apple FS, Henry TD, et al: Cardiac troponin I and T concentrations in patients with cocaine-associated chest pain. Ann Clin Biochem 33:183–186, 1996.
190. Hollander JE, Levitt A, Young GP, et al: The effects of cocaine on specificity of cardiac markers (Abstract 242). Acad Emerg Med 4:422, 1997.
191. D'Amore J, Gallahue F, Shetty S, et al: A comparison of CK-MB and troponin I in the initial evaluation of cocaine induced chest pain (Abstract 42). Acad Emerg Med 7:442, 2000.
192. Hilton TC, Thompson RC, Williams HJ, et al: Technetium-99m sestamibi myocardial perfusion imaging in the emergency room evaluation of chest pain. J Am Coll Cardiol 23:1016–1022, 1994.
193. Kosnik JW, Zalenski RJ, Shamsa F, et al: Resting sestamibi imaging for the prognosis of low-risk chest pain. Acad Emerg Med 6:998–1004, 1999.
194. Tatum JL, Jesse RL, Kontos MC, et al: Comprehensive strategy for the evaluation and triage of the chest pain patient. Ann Emerg Med 29:116–125, 1997.
195. Varetto T, Cantalupi D, Altieri A, et al: Emergency room technetium 99m sestamibi imaging to rule out acute myocardial ischemia events in patients with nondiagnostic electrocardiograms. J Am Coll Cardiol 22:1804–1808, 1993.
196. Hollander JE, Hoffman RS, Gennis P, et al: Cocaine-associated chest pain: One year follow-up. Acad Emerg Med 2:179–184, 1995.
197. Spivey WH, Schoffstall JM, Kirkpatrick R, et al: Comparison of labetalol, diazepam, and haloperidol for the treatment of cocaine toxicity in a swine model. Ann Emerg Med 19:467–468, 1990.
198. Spivey WH, Schoffstall JM, Kirkpatrick R, et al: Comparison of labetalol, diazepam, and haloperidol for the treatment of cocaine-associated cardiovascular complications. Am J Emerg Med 9:161–163, 1991.
199. Witkin JM, Goldberg SR, Katz JL: Lethal effects of cocaine are reduced by the dopamine-1 receptor antagonists SCH 23390 but not by haloperidol. Life Sci 44:1285–1291, 1989.
200. O'Donnell TF Jr, Clowes GHA Jr: The circulatory abnormalities of heat stroke. N Engl J Med 287:734–737, 1972.
201. Amsterdam JT, Syverud SA, Barker WJ, et al: Dantrolene sodium for the treatment of heatstroke victims: Lack of efficacy in a canine model. Am J Emerg Med 4:399–405, 1986.
202. Bouchama A, Cafege A, Devol EB, et al: Ineffectiveness of peripheral sodium in the treatment of heatstroke. Crit Care Med 19:176–180, 1991.
203. Fox AW: More on rhabdomyolysis associated with cocaine intoxication (Letter). N Engl J Med 321:1271, 1989.
204. Derlet RW, Albertson TE: Diazepam in the prevention of seizures and death in cocaine-intoxicated rats. Ann Emerg Med 18:542–546, 1989.
205. Guinn MM, Bedford JA, Wilson MC: Antagonism of intravenous cocaine lethality in nonhuman primates. Clin Toxicol 16:499–508, 1980.
206. Baumann BM, Perrone JM, Shofer FS, et al: Randomized, double blind, placebo-controlled trial of diazepam, nitroglycerin or both for the treatment of cocaine associated acute coronary syndrome. Acad Emerg Med 7:878–885, 2000.
207. Lowenstein DH, Aldredge BK: Status epilepticus. N Engl J Med 338:970–976, 1998.
208. Brogan WC, Lange RA, Kim AS, et al: Alleviation of cocaine-induced coronary vasoconstriction by nitroglycerin. J Am Coll Cardiol 18:581–586, 1991.
209. Hollander JE, Hoffman RS, Gennis P, et al: Nitroglycerin in the treatment of cocaine associated chest pain—clinical safety and efficacy. J Toxicol Clin Toxicol 32:243–256, 1994.
210. Boehrer JD, Moliterno DJ, Willard JE, et al: Influence of labetalol on cocaine-induced coronary vasoconstriction in humans. Am J Med 94:608–610, 1993.
211. Sand IC, Brody SL, Wrenn KD, et al: Experience with esmolol for the treatment of cocaine-associated cardiovascular complications. Am J Emerg Med 9:161–163, 1991.
212. Hollander JE, Carter WA, Hoffman RS: Use of phentolamine for cocaine-induced myocardial ischemia. N Engl J Med 327:361, 1992.
213. Billman GE, Hoskins RS: Cocaine-induced ventricular fibrillation: Protection afforded by the calcium-induced coronary vasoconstriction in humans. Am J Med 94:608–610, 1993.
214. Billman GE: Effect of calcium channel antagonists on cocaine-induced malignant arrhythmias: Protection against ventricular fibrillation. J Pharmacol Exp Ther 266:407–416, 1993.
215. Derlet RW, Albertson TE: Potentiation of cocaine toxicity with calcium channel blockers. Am J Emerg Med 7:464–468, 1989.
216. Derlet RW, Tseng C-C, Albertson TE: Cocaine toxicity and the calcium channel blockers nifedipine and nimodipine in rats. J Emerg Med 12:1–4, 1994.
217. Hale SL, Alker KJ, Reskalla SH, et al: Nifedipine protects the heart from the acute deleterious effects of cocaine if administered before but not after cocaine. Circulation 83:1437–1443, 1991.
218. Knuepfer MM, Branch CA: Calcium channel antagonists reduce the cocaine-induced decrease in cardiac output in a subset of rats. J Cardiovasc Pharmacol 21:390–396, 1993.
219. Nahas G, Trouve R, Demus JF, et al: A calcium channel blocker as antidote to the cardiac effects of cocaine intoxication (Letter). N Engl J Med 313:519, 1985.
220. Negus BH, Willard JE, Hillis LD, et al: Alleviation of cocaine induced coronary vasoconstriction with intravenous verapamil. Am J Cardiol 73:510–513, 1994.
221. Trouve R, Nahas GG: Antidotes to lethal cocaine toxicity in the rat. Arch Int Pharmacodyn Ther 305:197–207, 1990.
222. Hollander JE, Burstein JL, Hoffman RS, et al: Cocaine-associated myocardial infarction: Clinical safety of thrombolytic therapy. Chest 107:1237–1241, 1995.
223. Bush HS: Cocaine-associated myocardial infarction: A word of caution about thrombolytic therapy. Chest 94:878, 1988.
224. LoVecchio F, Nelson L: Intraventricular bleeding after the use of thrombolytics in a cocaine user. Am J Emerg Med 14:663–664, 1996.
225. Beckman K, Parker RB, Hariman RJ, et al: Hemodynamic and electrophysiological actions of cocaine: Effects of sodium bicarbonate as an antidote in dogs. Circulation 83:1799–1807, 1991.
226. Grawe JJ, Hariman RJ, Winecoff AP, et al: Reversal of the electrocardiographic effects of cocaine by lidocaine: 2. Concentration effect relationships. Pharmacotherapy 14:704–711, 1994.
227. Winecoff AP, Hariman RJ, Grawe JJ, et al: Reversal of the electrocardiographic effects of cocaine by lidocaine: Part 1. Comparison with sodium bicarbonate and quinidine. Pharmacotherapy 14:698–703, 1994.
228. Derlet RW, Albertson TE, Tharratt RS: Lidocaine potentiation of cocaine toxicity. Ann Emerg Med 20:135–138, 1991.
229. Heit J, Hoffman RS, Goldfrank LR: The effects of lidocaine pretreatment on cocaine neurotoxicity and lethality in mice. Acad Emerg Med 1:438–442, 1994.

PART 5

Chemical Agents

METALS AND RELATED SUBSTANCES

CHAPTER **76**

Arsenic

Michael J. Kosnett

Arsenic has captured the attention of the medical community for more than 2 millennia as a cause of disease and as a cure. Hippocrates and other ancient Greek physicians described the use of arsenic sulfides such as realgar (As_2S_2) or orpiment (As_2S_3) as a topical treatment for ulcers. During the first millennium AD, the roasting of realgar led to the discovery of so-called white arsenic, or arsenic trioxide. Odorless, tasteless, and soluble in solution, it became a tool of deliberate poisoning and gained particular notoriety as a homicidal agent in Europe in the 15th through 17th centuries. In the late 18th century, Fowler[1] described the medical use of a 1% solution of potassium arsenite as an oral treatment for fever and chorea. Known as *liquor arsenicalis* or *Fowler's solution*, it was used extensively until the mid-20th century as a remedy for asthma and psoriasis. In the 19th century, arsenic compounds were used widely in commerce as pigments (e.g., copper arsenite or "Scheele's green"). Several arsenic compounds were used through most of the 20th century as pesticides (e.g., lead arsenate, calcium arsenate) or herbicides (e.g., sodium arsenite). Until recently, the wood preservative chromated copper arsenate represented the largest commercial use of arsenic, although use in new residential products has now been discontinued. Organic arsenic antibiotics were used extensively in humans in the first half of the 20th century in the treatment of protozoan and spirochetal diseases, and certain phenylarsenic agents still are used as feed additives for poultry and swine. The link between environmental and occupational arsenic exposure and chronic nonmalignant and malignant disease became well established in the latter half of the 20th century, leading to a reduction in many commercial applications and recent regulatory efforts to reduce permissible exposure levels in drinking water, where arsenic of geologic origin may occur as a natural contaminant.

Semiconductor manufacturing is one industrial sector that has seen expanded use of arsenic-containing compounds in recent decades. Hydride forms of arsenic, such as arsine gas, have been used as a source of arsenic dopants for silicon chips, and gallium arsenide has been used increasingly as a substrate for semiconductors. Inorganic arsenic has reemerged as a medicinal agent for the treatment of acute promyelocytic leukemia, and its potential utility in the therapy of other selected malignancies is under investigation. Arsenic trioxide was approved by the U.S. Food and Drug Administration as an orphan drug for the secondary treatment of acute promyelocytic leukemia in September 2000.

BIOCHEMISTRY

Arsenic

Elemental arsenic (atomic weight 74.92) is a naturally occurring silver-gray solid metalloid. The elemental (zero valence) form, which rarely exists in nature and has low solubility, is seldom a cause of human toxicity. Rather, human exposure may occur predominantly to a variety of inorganic arsenic salts and natural and synthetic organoarsenic compounds, whose toxicity varies considerably depending on the molecular form, valence state, solubility, and exposure circumstances.

The principal inorganic forms of arsenic of toxicologic concern are the soluble crystalline solids and salts of trivalent (As^{+3}) arsenite and pentavalent (As^{+5}) arsenate. Trivalent arsenic compounds generally have greater acute toxicity than the pentavalent forms, but in vivo interconversion occurs, and the two forms are capable of producing a similar pattern of acute and chronic intoxication. In the approach to a poisoned patient, there is seldom a clinical reason to distinguish whether the exposure has been to arsenite or arsenate. Arsenic trioxide (As_2O_3) is a commercially important crystalline solid that usually is produced from the smelting of copper or lead ores containing arsenic sulfides, such as arsenopyrite (FeAsS). Arsenic

Pharmacokinetics and Metabolism of Arsenic Compounds

Volume of Distribution

Experimentally derived human data on arsenic pharmacokinetics are sparse. In humans given an intravenous bolus of radiolabeled arsenite in a clinical study, the initial volume of distribution was calculated to be 0.2 L/kg.[2] Because initial plasma clearance was rapid (half-life approximately 0.45 hour), however, the volume of distribution after 2 to 3 hours appeared to increase to approximately 6 L/kg.

Protein Binding

At low background levels, arsenic in the blood follows a red blood cell-to-plasma ratio of approximately 1:1, but this ratio increases at higher levels of arsenic exposure in humans and animals.[3] Studies in patients undergoing peritoneal dialysis indicated that approximately 5% to 6% of the inorganic arsenic in serum is bound to protein, predominantly to transferrin.[4] The total serum arsenic in these patients (mean 4.7 μg/L) was higher than that of a reference population (0.96 ± 1.52 μg/L)[5] and was much lower than levels encountered in the early phases of acute arsenic intoxication.

Mechanisms of Clearance

In humans, inorganic arsenic and its methylated metabolites are excreted overwhelmingly (>95%) via the urine. Minor to trace amounts are eliminated via the feces, sweat, skin, and appendages (hair and nails).[2,6,7] In a study involving ingestion of radiolabeled arsenate, elimination was characterized by a three-component exponential function, with 66% of the arsenic eliminated with a half-life of 2.1 days, 30% with a half-life of 9.5 days, and 4% with a half-life of 38.4 days.[7] In other human ingestion studies, the half-life of urinary arsenic excretion after ingestion of 500 to 1000 μg arsenite was 2 to 3 days.[8,9] The elimination of arsenic is prolonged, however, after high-dose exposure.[3] In acutely poisoned humans, elevated urinary arsenic levels still may be detectable several weeks after termination of exposure.[10–12] Some data suggest that arsenic may undergo enterohepatic or enteroenteric circulation in humans, but the extent of this process has not been well characterized.

Active Metabolites

Inorganic arsenic undergoes in vivo biomethylation to form monomethylated and dimethylated metabolites. The principal metabolites are the pentavalent species, monomethylarsonic acid (MMA^V) and dimethylarsinic acid (DMA^V), which are less acutely toxic than inorganic arsenic by an order of magnitude.[13] After chronic low-dose exposure to inorganic arsenic, the methylated metabolites account for approximately 70% to 90% of arsenic excreted in the urine.[14] The biomethylation process also produces small amounts of the trivalent methylated species, monomethylarsonous acid (MMA^{III}) and dimethylarsinous acid (DMA^{III}), however, which have been found to be more acutely toxic than inorganic arsenic (arsenate or arsenite).[15–17] Methylation cannot be viewed exclusively as a detoxification process.

Methods to Enhance Clearance

Because arsenic is excreted via the kidney, intravenous hydration and other supportive care that maintains adequate urine output help to optimize clearance. Chelation may accelerate arsenic excretion. Arsenic is cleared rapidly from the blood, and hemodialysis contributes little to clearance in patients with intact renal function.

---

trioxide is moderately soluble in water (37 g/L at 20°C), and arsenic pentoxide (As$_2$O$_5$) is very soluble in water (1500 g/L at 16°C).[13] Commonly encountered soluble arsenic salts include sodium arsenite (NaAsO$_2$) and sodium arsenate (Na$_2$HAsO$_4$). Inorganic arsenic of geologic origin occurs in natural waters, particularly groundwater in the vicinity of arsenic-bearing soils or sediments, where local redox conditions influence the relative preponderance of arsenite or arsenate species. Inorganic compounds of low solubility seldom have been associated with overt acute toxicity because of poor absorption and limited systemic distribution. These compounds include the former pesticide and herbicide calcium arsenate, which still may be encountered as a natural contaminant of some coal fly ash, and gallium arsenide (GaAs), which is used in semiconductors.

Noteworthy organoarsenicals include synthetic and natural products. In humans, inorganic arsenate or arsenite undergoes in vivo biomethylation in certain tissues to monomethyl and dimethyl forms that ultimately are excreted in the urine. The main biomethylation products are the pentavalent species monomethylarsonic acid (MMA^V) and dimethylarsinic acid (DMA^V), which have lower acute toxicity than inorganic arsenic. More recent studies have shown that trivalent methylated forms, monomethylarsonous acid (MMA^{III}) and dimethylarsinous acid (DMA^{III}), which exist in small but stable amounts in vivo, have acute toxicities greater than the toxicity of arsenite. Synthetic MMA^V and DMA^V (also known as *cacodylic acid*) or their sodium salts formerly were used as agricultural chemicals, and cacodylic acid is still used as a laboratory buffer. Many marine organisms and a few terrestrial biota (principally fungi) biosynthesize the trimethylated arsenic compounds arsenocholine and arsenobetaine [(CH$_3$)$_3$As$^+$CH$_2$CO$_2^-$]. The latter, an amino acid analogue, exists in dietary seafood at concentrations ranging from approximately 1 to 100 ppm but appears not to be metabolized after ingestion and exerts no known toxicity. Arsenosugars and arsenolipids occur in edible marine organisms and certain plants; although arsenosugars are partially metabolized to DMA, they are not associated with acute human toxicity. The occurrence and chemistry of organoarsenicals in the diet have been reviewed.[18]

Trivalent and pentavalent arylarsenical antibiotics (e.g., arsphenamine and carbarsone) were used widely to treat spirochetal and protozoal infections in the first half of the 20th century. Today the only organoarsenical manufactured as a human pharmaceutical is melarsoprol, reserved for treatment of the meningoencephalitic stage of African trypanosomiasis. Other arylarsenical pharmaceuticals continue to be produced for veterinary applications. Pentavalent arylarsenicals, such as roxarsone (4-hydroxy-3-nitrophenylarsonic acid) and sodium arsanilate, are used as growth-promoting feed additives for poultry and swine. They are withheld from the feed 1 week before slaughter, which greatly reduces arsenic residues in the consumable meat. In general, arylarsenicals have lower acute toxicity than inorganic arsenite, and in the absence of accidental industrial exposure or misuse they are not a source of acute arsenic poisoning.

Arsine

Arsine (AsH_3) is an extremely toxic colorless gas with a density heavier than air. In contrast to the other arsenicals, which principally result in acute toxicity after ingestion of a sufficiently large dose, arsine gas is an acute inhalational hazard. Arsine gas is liberated when any inorganic arsenic–containing material comes in contact with nascent hydrogen. Severe accidental poisonings have occurred when metal ores, alloys, or metallic objects (particularly objects made of aluminum or zinc) have come in contact with acidic (or occasionally alkaline) solutions, producing arsine gas from arsenic impurities in the metal or the solution or both.[19] As discussed subsequently, arsine poisoning is distinguished from other forms of arsenic intoxication by its characteristic production of intravascular hemolysis.

Lewisite

The chemical warfare agent lewisite (dichloro [2-chlorovinyl] arsine $ClCH:CHAsCl_2$), named after Lewis, its American inventor, a chemist, is a volatile vesicant liquid that causes immediate severe irritation and necrosis to the eyes, skin, and airways. The median lethal dosage by inhalation is 1200 to 1500 mg-min/m3; eye injury occurs at dosages less than 300 mg-min/m3.[20] In recent decades, rare but significant accidental exposure to lewisite from old munitions has occurred. A current review of the acute and chronic effects of lewisite is available.[21]

PATHOPHYSIOLOGY

Arsenic

The acute and chronic noncancer toxicity of arsenic is a consequence of a multitude of interactions with cellular proteins, cofactors, and nucleic acids. Arsenite combines with the sulfhydryl groups of enzymes and cofactors, such as the vicinal dithiol lipoate component of the α-keto acid oxidation systems, that are vital to the main oxidative pathways of the tricarboxylic acid cycle.[22] In particular, arsenite has long been known to inhibit strongly pyruvate dehydrogenase,[23] and more recently MMA[III] has been shown to be even more potent in this regard.[16] Arsenite and to a greater extent MMA[III] are potent inhibitors of enzymes necessary for cellular protection against oxidative stress, such as glutathione reductase and thioredoxin reductase.[24,25] Arsenite exposure in vitro is associated with oxyradical production, mutagenesis, and cell death.[26] Arsenate and pentavalent methylarsenicals are reduced in vivo to trivalent species,[18] which subsequently may bind proteins, interfere with enzymatic function, or increase oxidative stress. Arsenate also may impair cellular energy production through unstable substitution for phosphate in

phosphorylation reactions, resulting in cellular depletion of adenosine triphosphate.[27] Inorganic arsenic may interfere with heme biosynthesis, reflected in part by elevated excretion of urinary porphyrins.[28]

In addition to the aforementioned effects, inorganic arsenic or its methylated metabolites are associated with numerous other cellular perturbations, such as alterations in gene expression, cell-cycle regulation, signal transduction, and apoptosis, that may contribute to acute and chronic cancer and noncancer effects.[29] Arsenite induces DNA-protein cross-links[30] and interferes with microtubule assembly.[31] Arsenic has been associated with chromosomal aberrations in multiple in vitro and in vivo studies, and one investigation has suggested that trivalent methylated arsenicals may damage DNA directly.[17] The numerous cellular effects induced by arsenic in experimental studies often depend on the intensity and duration of arsenic exposure, and the precise mode of action responsible for the spectrum of clinical effects of arsenic has not been elucidated. The fact that the biochemical targets of arsenic are ubiquitous in cells throughout the body is consistent, however, with the fundamental clinical observation that the effects of arsenic typically are multisystemic in their presentation.

Humans seem to be more susceptible than experimental animals to the toxic effects of inorganic arsenic. The median lethal dose of arsenite in hamsters is 8.5 mg/kg[16] and ranges from 15 to 75 mg/kg in mice and rats.[13] By comparison, potentially lethal complications have been observed in adult humans after the acute ingestion of approximately 200 to 300 mg (3 to 4 mg/kg) of a soluble form of inorganic arsenic. Although epidemiologic studies have shown unequivocally that arsenic is a human carcinogen, there is no well-established animal model of inorganic arsenic carcinogenicity.

Arsine

Arsine gas is a potent hemolytic agent. In vitro studies with human erythrocytes suggest that a large increase in intracellular calcium associated with an alteration in membrane sulfhydryl groups is a key feature of the hemolytic process.[32] In these experiments, arsine-induced changes in transmembrane ion flux appeared within 5 minutes of exposure, followed by significant hemolysis at 1 hour. The strong susceptibility of erythrocytes to the toxic effects of arsine, but not arsenite, suggests that the hemolysis might be induced by a reaction product of arsine formed in the presence of heme, which is highly abundant in these cells.[33] The pathophysiology of the adverse effects that follow arsine inhalation is multifactorial. The intrarenal deposition of hemoglobin and other cellular debris from lysed erythrocytes may produce acute tubular damage and oliguric renal failure. Severe hemolysis diminishes peripheral oxygen delivery and creates generalized hypoxic stress. Before hemolysis, some arsine is transported via the bloodstream to other tissues,[34] which may be damaged by the direct action of arsine or its reaction products. The kidney and possibly other organs convert arsine to arsenite, which further contributes to adverse effects.[33,35]

CLINICAL PRESENTATION AND LIFE-THREATENING COMPLICATIONS

Arsenic

ACUTE ARSENIC INTOXICATION

The clinical presentation of arsenic intoxication after a single acute ingestion is characterized by multisystemic findings that appear in stages over the course of hours to weeks (Table 76-1). The most common scenario results from the deliberate or accidental ingestion of several hundred milligrams or more of a soluble arsenic salt. The first stage typically begins 30 minutes to several hours postingestion, with prominent gastrointestinal distress consisting of nausea, vomiting, abdominal pain, and watery or mucoid diarrhea. There is often abdominal tenderness to palpation. The slightly delayed onset of these gastrointestinal symptoms and their appearance after parenteral arsenic overdose[12] are consistent with an acute mode of action dependent on acute cytotoxicity and increased vascular permeability rather than direct mucosal irritation.

During the initial stage of acute arsenic intoxication, diffuse capillary leak, alone or in combination with gastrointestinal fluid loss, produces cardiovascular signs and symptoms within a matter of hours. In mild-to-moderate cases, there may be thirst, tachycardia, or decreased urine output. More severe cases may result in hypotension, shock, malignant ventricular arrhythmias, and death.[36-42] The oliguria or anuria that occurs during the first 1 to 2 days after acute arsenic intoxication is most likely a consequence of decreased renal blood flow due to hypotension or diffuse extravascular fluid accumulation, rather than a consequence of acute tubular necrosis. The initial neurologic features of acute arsenic poisoning are highly variable and nonspecific. The mental status may be intact, or there may be lethargy, agitation, or delirium. Generalized convulsions have been reported but are relatively rare.[38,43] Low-grade fever may be present but is not an invariable finding.

Commonly the initial phase of gastrointestinal symptoms and hypotension stabilizes or improves within 24 to 48 hours but is followed within 1 to 7 days by a second phase of cardiovascular compromise characterized by mild congestive heart failure, noncardiogenic pulmonary edema, or both. The severity is variable, ranging from mild cardiomegaly or pleural effusions to full-blown adult respiratory distress syndrome.[39,44] In some cases, the peak manifestations of adult respiratory distress syndrome may be delayed 8 to 10 days postingestion.[45] The delayed appearance of isolated or recurrent malignant cardiac arrhythmias up to 10 days after an initial high-dose arsenic ingestion merits

---

TABLE 76-1 Clinical and Laboratory Findings in Acute Arsenic Poisoning*

Phase 1: Immediate (within hours postingestion)
Gastrointestinal
  Nausea, vomiting, diarrhea, abdominal pain
Cardiovascular
  Hypotension (shock), tachycardia, diminished urine output, malignant cardiac arrhythmias
Metabolic acidosis
Rhabdomyolysis
Neurologic
  Altered mental status (lethargy or agitation), seizures

Phase 2 (1 day to 1 week postingestion)
Cardiovascular
  Prolonged QT$_c$ interval, cardiac arrhythmias (torsades de pointes), **congestive cardiomyopathy, noncardiogenic pulmonary edema**
Neurologic
  Encephalopathy (agitation, delirium, stupor, coma)
Renal
  Low-grade proteinuria
Hepatic
  Elevated hepatic transaminases (slight to moderate), hyperbilirubinemia (slight)
Dermatologic
  Desquamation (especially palmar or plantar), macular-papular rash, periorbital edema

Phase 3 (1 to 4 weeks postingestion)
Hematologic
  Anemia, leukopenia, thrombocytopenia, relative eosinophilia, basophilic stippling of erythrocytes, disseminated intravascular coagulation
Neurologic
  Sensorimotor peripheral neuropathy, autonomic instability (hypertension, diaphoresis)
Dermatologic
  Transverse striate leukonychia (Mees' lines), herpetic lesions (zoster and/or simplex)

*More common findings are in **bold** type.

particular concern and clinical vigilance. A relatively specific feature is the development of the polymorphic ventricular tachycardia, torsades de pointes. Torsades de pointes frequently is preceded by the common arsenic-associated finding of prolongation of the QT interval, with the QT_c interval frequently greater than 500 msec.[46–50] Sudden cardiac arrest in the absence of QT prolongation or torsades de pointes also may occur within a few days of the initial onset of gastrointestinal symptoms.[51]

Patients may exhibit a decline in mental status, characterized by delirium or obtundation, 2 to 6 days after the onset of acute arsenic poisoning.[52–54] This delayed encephalopathy often resolves spontaneously within a week, but on rare occasions it may persist for a prolonged period.[55,56]

A third phase of acute intoxication, generally appearing 1 to 4 weeks after the initial high-dose ingestion, is heralded by hematologic abnormalities and peripheral neuropathy. The classic hematologic finding is pancytopenia, with the suppression of erythrocytes, leukocytes, and platelets usually reaching a nadir within 1 to 3 weeks. Complete recovery of all cell lines usually follows within weeks to months. The salient laboratory features are discussed further in the section on diagnosis.

In many but not all cases of acute arsenic intoxication, a symmetric distal sensorimotor axonal peripheral neuropathy evolves 1 to 5 weeks after the ingestion. Initial findings consist of dysesthesias in the distal extremities in a stocking-glove distribution. Dysesthesias often rapidly progress to "burning" paresthesias, with hyperpathia to mild stimuli, such as bed sheets rubbing against the feet.[52,57] Other sensory modalities (e.g., proprioception) also are affected, and within days to a week patients experience the onset of motor weakness. The lower extremities may be more affected than the upper extremities in the initial stages. Depending on the severity of the poisoning, sensory and motor deficits ascend symmetrically to involve the proximal musculature, and a marked quadriplegia can occur. In the most severe cases, neuromuscular respiratory failure requires mechanical ventilation, sometimes for several weeks.[44,58] Autonomic instability, characterized by episodic diaphoresis, temperature instability, and hypertension, may appear during the peak stages of neuropathy.[56] Although there have been rare reports of visual disturbances[36,59] and facial nerve paralysis,[60] cranial nerve function almost always is well preserved. Signs of slow improvement in the peripheral neuropathy begin to appear within a few weeks after deficits have reached their maximum. The extent of recovery depends on the severity of the peak insult. Patients with mild-to-moderate insults, such as cases with predominantly sensory involvement, have recovered completely, but in patients with severe motor and sensory deficits, distal weakness, wasting, and diminished sensation may persist for years.[53,54,61]

Several dermatologic signs variably appear after a delay of approximately 1 to 6 weeks following acute arsenic ingestion. A diffuse maculopapular rash, sometimes with areas of vesiculation, may be noted.[45,62] Mild-to-moderate desquamation of the skin, mainly in the hands and feet but occasionally in a more diffuse pattern, is common.[62–64] In many cases, the cutaneous reactions have appeared before treatment with chelating agents, which may induce allergic dermal manifestations. Patients may exhibit periorbital edema. Herpetic vesicular lesions, secondary to herpes simplex or herpes zoster, often erupt on the face or trunk days to weeks after substantial arsenic ingestion. This eruption may be triggered

by arsenic-related suppression of leukocytes and immune function. Transverse white striae (white bands 1 or 2 mm in width) classically appear on the emerging nail beds of the fingers and toes after 4 to 6 weeks. Although frequently referred to as *Mees' lines* after the report of Mees,[65] this finding of transverse striate leukonychia was described earlier by Aldrich[66] and by Reynolds[67] in arsenic-poisoned patients. The bands, which are thought to reflect an abrupt disruption of keratinization, are not pathognomonic for arsenic poisoning and may occur after other toxic insults, such as thallium poisoning.[68] Multiple bands on the nail beds may be visible in patients who have had multiple discrete episodes of acute poisoning in the preceding months.

SUBACUTE AND CHRONIC ARSENIC POISONING

Subacute arsenic poisoning shares many of the features of acute arsenic intoxication but is less often life-threatening. The magnitude of the recurrent dose influences the severity and time course of the presentation. A 2- to 4-month period of consumption of drinking water delivering arsenic doses that were probably on the order of 10 to 50 mg/day resulted in peripheral neuropathy, sometimes with antecedent gastrointestinal symptoms[69] and sometimes without gastrointestinal symptoms.[12] In a subset of 220 adult patients studied by Mizuta and colleagues,[70] 2 to 3 weeks of ingesting an estimated 3 mg of arsenite per day in contaminated soy sauce resulted in periorbital edema, gastrointestinal symptoms, decreased hematocrit, and mild peripheral neuropathy. During the Manchester beer epidemic of 1900, daily consumption for weeks to months of 1 to 5 mg of arsenic per day in contaminated beer caused a large outbreak of mild-to-moderate peripheral neuropathy. Hyperpigmentation and periorbital edema commonly were noted. Deaths from congestive heart failure were reported, but the contributory role of alcoholic cardiomyopathy in those cases remains uncertain.[67,71]

Experimental trials employing intravenous arsenite in the treatment of refractory or relapsed acute promyelocytic leukemia have provided new insights into the subacute toxicity of inorganic arsenic. The therapeutic mode of action of arsenic in treatment of this malignancy may involve a selective induction of apoptosis in the leukemic cells, possibly through degradation of a specific oncoprotein[72] or through interaction with the tubulin that is abundant in leukemic cells.[31] Experimental protocols generally have administered 10 to 20 mg of As_2O_3 intravenously daily for 2 months per course of treatment. Although many subjects have tolerated this regimen, some severe arsenic-related adverse effects have been reported, including arrhythmias, peripheral neuropathy, and hepatotoxicity. Ohnishi and coworkers[73] observed QT prolongation in eight of eight patients receiving daily infusions of 0.15 mg/kg As_2O_3 administered over 2 hours, and four of eight patients exhibited nonsustained monomorphic ventricular tachycardia, generally after 3 or more weeks of treatment. Unnikrishnan and associates[74] observed torsades de pointes in 3 of 19 patients, after 42, 16, and 12 days of treatment, respectively. In two of the three cases, the arrhythmia was refractory to treatment, and the patient died. Niu and coworkers[75] observed hepatic transaminase elevation in 7 of 11 newly diagnosed patients entering an arsenite treatment protocol. In five of the patients, hepatic dysfunction was reversible on cessation of treatment, but in two cases it seemed to be progressive. Sensorimotor peripheral neuropathy has occurred 6 to 8 weeks after initiation of treatment, and nausea, vomiting, and abdominal pain have been common.[76]

Chronic arsenic poisoning has been characterized extensively through studies of populations exposed to elevated levels of naturally occurring arsenic in drinking water and through historical accounts of the use of medicinal arsenic (e.g., Fowler's solution) for the treatment of asthma, psoriasis, and other maladies. The adverse effects of chronic arsenic ingestion have been reviewed in detail.[18,29] Noncancer chronic effects include a distinctive pattern of spotted hyperpigmentation and palmar-plantar hyperkeratosis, hematologic findings of anemia and leukopenia, a sensory predominant axonal peripheral neuropathy, vascular disease, and noncirrhotic periportal hepatic fibrosis and portal hypertension. Nonspecific gastrointestinal complaints, such as diarrhea and cramping, may also occur, but in many instances the cutaneous, neurologic, vascular, or hematologic effects of chronic arsenic poisoning develop without a history of antecedent gastrointestinal symptoms.[77] Epidemiologic studies have suggested a link between chronic arsenic ingestion and diabetes mellitus, hypertension, and increased cardiovascular disease mortality.[18,29] In the short term (days to months), gastrointestinal, hematologic, and neurologic symptoms may emerge with arsenic doses of 0.05 mg/kg/day. When exposure occurs over several years, noncancer symptoms may emerge at doses of approximately 0.01 mg/kg/day. Arsenic ingestion is associated with an increased risk of lung cancer, bladder cancer, and skin cancer, and occupational studies have identified arsenic inhalation as a cause of lung cancer.[18,29] Limited evidence suggests that the latency period for arsenic-induced cancers may be one or more decades.

Arsine

Although exposure to arsine occurs by inhalation, the gas is nonirritating, and there generally are *no immediate symptoms*. Although a garlic-like odor has sometimes but not invariably been reported, the reported odor threshold of 0.5 to 1.0 ppm does not provide sufficient warning properties.[89] Most arsine intoxications are associated with acute occupational exposure occurring over 30 minutes to a few hours. After a typical delay of 2 to 24 hours, patients often report nonspecific constitutional symptoms that may include malaise; headache; fever or chills; and gastrointestinal disturbance, particularly nausea, vomiting, and crampy abdominal pain.[78] In some cases, the pain has occurred predominantly in the low back or flank, rather than the abdomen.[79] Patients also may complain of numbness or coldness of the extremities. In severe exposures, sudden cardiovascular collapse and death may ensue within 1 or 2 hours.[80] The clinical features of acute arsine poisoning are summarized in Table 76-2.

In the absence of rapid fatality, a characteristic finding in the first 2 to 24 hours is the passage of dark, reddish urine, usually followed by oliguria and sometimes anuria.[81,82] There is often a concomitant appearance of a copper, bronze, or jaundiced discoloration to the skin.[83,84] The urine discoloration is attributable to hemoglobinuria, and the skin discoloration possibly is due to elevated plasma hemoglobin; both of these effects follow the significant intravascular hemolysis. Oliguria and anuria, which may last days to several weeks, are the hallmark of acute tubular necrosis. Within the first 1 to 2 days after presentation, a few patients with acute arsine poisoning may develop an altered mental status, ranging from agitation to frank hallucinosis.[84,85] Electrocardiogram changes during this time may include nonspecific T-wave changes or occasionally peaked T waves,[86] but in contrast to the picture in acute inorganic arsenic poisoning (see earlier), significant conduction abnormalities or malignant arrhythmias are uncommon. The delayed appearance (within weeks) of a mild-to-moderate sensorimotor peripheral neuropathy has been reported after acute arsine poisoning.[84,87] Transverse white striae of the fingernails, known as *Aldrich-Mees lines*, also may emerge during that time interval.

Chronic arsine poisoning has been described only rarely. Bulmer and colleagues[88] reported chronic arsine poisoning in 14 workers engaged in the cyanide extraction of gold. Five workers with the longest exposures (5 to 9 months) complained of persistent headache, weakness, shortness of breath, and nausea and vomiting and were noted to have severe anemia. Among the 14 subjects, the degree of anemia was proportional to the length of exposure, but specific exposure levels were not determined. In experimental models, subacute and subchronic exposure of rodents to arsine in the range of 0.025 to 5 ppm has been associated with reversible hematopoietic effects.[89]

TABLE 76-2 Clinical and Laboratory Features in Acute Arsine Poisoning*

Constitutional
  Malaise, fever or chills, acute sensation of numbness or cold in extremities
Gastrointestinal
  Nausea and vomiting, crampy abdominal pain, low back/flank pain, **hyperbilirubinemia (slight to moderate)**
Hematologic
  Hemolysis, elevated plasma hemoglobin
Renal
  Hemoglobinuria (dark red urine), oliguria or anuria (active urine sediment [cells and casts; may be delayed], increasing serum creatinine and BUN)
Dermatologic
  Bronze discoloration of skin
Neurologic
  Headache, altered sensorium (delirium or agitation), delayed sensorimotor peripheral neuropathy

---

*More common findings are in **bold** type.

DIAGNOSIS

Poisoning by Inorganic Arsenic

The diagnostic approach to arsenic poisoning should integrate (1) characteristic signs and symptoms, (2) a history consistent with sufficient exposure, (3) confirmatory laboratory findings, and (4) the relative exclusion of other factors in the differential diagnosis. Acute arsenic poisoning should be suspected in a patient with the abrupt onset of nausea, vomiting, watery diarrhea, abdominal pain, and hypotension, possibly in association with the evolving pattern of cardiovascular, hematologic, and neurologic findings discussed earlier. In symptomatic subacute and chronic poisoning, clinical or laboratory evidence of *multisystemic* adverse effects almost always is present.

Laboratory findings in the initial stage of acute arsenic poisoning often reveal evidence of an elevated anion-gap metabolic acidosis. The initial complete blood count (CBC) may be normal or may reveal an elevated hematocrit due to extravascular fluid loss and hemoconcentration. Rhabdomyolysis may be evidenced by increasing levels of creatinine phosphokinase.[90,91] The urinalysis may be normal or may reveal low levels of protein or heme. Microscopic examination of the urine usually lacks the prominent cellularity and sediment of acute tubular necrosis, however. Initially, blood urea nitrogen and serum creatinine may be normal or slightly elevated. These parameters of renal function often increase in the presence of diminishing urine output and shock, sometimes with a disproportionate rise in serum creatinine associated with rhabdomyolysis. The electrocardiogram commonly exhibits sinus tachycardia, sometimes with a prolonged QT_c interval, and nonspecific S-wave and T-wave changes.[46,49]

The chest x-ray in the initial phase of acute arsenic intoxication is generally unremarkable, but over the next several days the chest x-ray may exhibit mild cardiomegaly, pleural effusions, or both. The presence of radiopaque material in the gastrointestinal tract, detected incidentally in the region of the stomach on chest x-ray or in the stomach or small intestine on abdominal x-ray, sometimes may provide a clue to acute arsenic ingestion.[41,92,93] The presence of a radiopacity, owing to poorly dissolved arsenic compounds, is neither a sensitive nor a specific diagnostic finding, however.

Liver function tests in acute arsenic poisoning typically reveal slight-to-moderate increases in hepatic transaminases (alanine aminotransferase and aspartate aminotransferase), which may reach several hundred international units per liter within the first days to a week. Moderate hyperbilirubinemia (e.g., 1 to 3 mg/dL [17 to 51 μmol/L]) may be present initially or after a delay of several days. More severe elevations in bilirubin have been noted rarely,[90] and in two such cases, liver biopsy revealed slight cholestasis and a marked pattern of hepatocellular mitotic figures.[94]

Several abnormal hematologic test results usually are present in the second phase of acute arsenic poisoning and in subacute or chronic intoxication. Pancytopenia, particularly anemia and leukopenia, characteristically is evident on the CBC within 1 to 2 weeks after acute ingestion. The anemia is usually normochromic and normocytic, but megaloblastic changes also have been reported, with the peripheral smear showing regenerative macrocytes.[95]

Basophilic stippling of erythrocytes may be visible on the peripheral smear,[96,97] as may be nucleated red blood cells with karyorrhexis (irregular pyknotic nuclei). Leukopenia is evident as lymphocytopenia and neutropenia, and the differential white blood cell count often reveals a relative eosinophilia. Bone marrow examination typically reveals erythroid karyorrhexis and megaloblastoid dyserythropoiesis in the context of a hypercellular background. Hemostatic disorders have included a prolonged partial thromboplastin time and disseminated intravascular coagulation.[12,37,45,98]

The cerebrospinal fluid in the second or third phase of acute arsenic intoxication may be normal, or there may be mild-to-moderate elevations in protein, usually in the range of 50 to 100 mg/dL. Only rarely does the cerebrospinal fluid protein reach a few hundred milligrams per deciliter.[52,58,59] Cerebrospinal fluid cellularity classically is absent or scant. Electrodiagnostic studies and nerve biopsies performed to assess arsenic-induced peripheral neuropathy usually reveal distal axonal degeneration, although some investigators have reported that the early stages of acute arsenical polyneuropathy may exhibit features of a segmental demyelinating process.[54,58,61,99]

Measurement of urinary arsenic should be obtained for confirmatory diagnosis. Although a 24-hour urine collection sometimes yields information of forensic, toxicokinetic, or research interest, a spot urine collection that measures arsenic concentration is usually sufficient for diagnostic purposes. Most clinical laboratories report the result in terms of *total urinary arsenic*. Diagnostic interpretation sometimes requires a more specific assessment of the chemical forms or "species" of arsenic detected, however. Absorption of inorganic arsenate or arsenite by humans results in excretion of arsenate and arsenite, plus the products of in vivo biomethylation, principally MMA and DMA. Certain foods of marine origin, including many finfish, shellfish, and algal products, may contain large amounts of nontoxic organoarsenicals, such as arsenobetaine and arsenosugars. After a seafood meal, arsenobetaine may be excreted unchanged in the urine in concentrations of several hundred to several thousand micrograms (as arsenic) per liter over the next several days. Arsenosugars, abundant in bivalve mollusks, are metabolized at least partially to DMA.[100] After ingestion of clams or mussels, the DMA concentration of the urine may be increased to several hundred micrograms per liter. The arsenobetaine and DMA excreted after seafood ingestion is included in the laboratory measurement of total urine arsenic. By comparison, in North Americans and Europeans with average, "background" exposure to arsenic and no recent seafood consumption, the sum of inorganic arsenic (arsenate and arsenite), MMA, and DMA in the urine is generally less than 20 μg/L.[18]

Because of the potential presence of large amounts of seafood-derived arsenic in a patient's diet, the following approach is recommended when ordering urinary arsenic measurement on a potentially poisoned patient. If readily available, a speciated urine arsenic result that reports the concentration of inorganic arsenic (arsenite plus arsenate), MMA, and DMA should be requested. (It may be technically difficult, and not clinically necessary, for the laboratory to differentiate between arsenite and arsenate.) If only a total urinary arsenic measurement is readily available, this should be obtained, but a separate aliquot of the urine should be stored at $-4°F$ ($-20°C$). If the total urine arsenic concentration is elevated significantly above background values, (e.g., >50 μg/L), the retained aliquot should be sent to a toxicologic laboratory that can report the amount of inorganic arsenic, MMA, and DMA present. This practice reduces the potential for a total urine arsenic concentration that is elevated on the basis of recent arsenobetaine ingestion in seafood to be misinterpreted as evidence of recent overexposure to inorganic arsenic. Because DMA derived from seafood ingestion still may appear in the urine in large amounts for 3 days,[100,101] however, it nonetheless is important to obtain and consider a careful history of any recent seafood ingestion. If relevant, a follow-up urine specimen obtained after 3 or 4 days of strict abstinence from any seafood should be submitted for speciated arsenic analysis. Urine collected for speciated analysis should not be treated with dilute acids to prevent adsorption onto the sample container because this may alter the speciation profile.[102]

In the first 2 to 3 days after acute, symptomatic arsenic intoxication, the urinary arsenic concentration usually is greater than 1000 μg/L, and the urinary arsenic excretion in 24 hours is typically greater than several thousand micrograms. Depending on the severity of the poisoning, the urine arsenic concentration may not return to background levels (total urine arsenic concentration <50 μg/L) for several weeks.

Blood arsenic values are seldom of clinical utility in diagnosis or management for several reasons. Arsenic is cleared rapidly from the blood, and the relationship between symptomatic arsenic intoxication and blood arsenic levels is highly variable and time dependent. Blood values may decline to what some laboratories define as the "normal" range when the urine still contains hundreds of micrograms of arsenic per liter and the patient remains symptomatic. Blood arsenic also is technically more difficult to measure accurately, and speciation is seldom, if ever, available. Measurement of blood arsenic concentration should be reserved for cases when a urine arsenic measurement cannot be obtained, such as an anuric patient. Background levels of arsenic in whole blood usually are less than 5 μg/L.[18] In acutely poisoned patients, values greater than 100 μg/L (serum or whole blood) have been reported.[36,98]

Arsenic is incorporated from the circulation into fingernails, toenails, and the growing hair shaft at the root. As the hair and nails grow outward, portions that were formed during the time of increased circulating arsenic contain elevated arsenic concentrations. Scalp hair grows at the approximate rate of 1 cm/mo,[103,104] fingernails grow at the approximate rate of 4 to 5 mm/mo,[6] and toenails grow at the approximate rate of 1.1 mm/mo.[105] As a consequence, segmental analysis of hair shafts (e.g., analysis of longitudinally aligned hairs cut into centimeter or subcentimeter sections) or analysis of distal toenail or fingernail clippings may reveal evidence of increased arsenic exposure that occurred months earlier. Because arsenic levels in the urine generally return to baseline levels within a matter of weeks, the elevated arsenic levels remaining in hair or nails may yield important forensic evidence of past exposure. Arsenic can bind to hair and nails from external contamination, however, in a manner that is indistinguishable from that present as a result of

internal incorporation. Some data also suggest that arsenic extruded in the sweat during acute poisoning may contaminate distal segments of the hair and nail that were formed long before the arsenic exposure occurred.[6,106] Thus, the information obtained from analysis of the arsenic content of the hair and nails should be interpreted cautiously.[107] Background levels of arsenic in hair and nails are less than 1 ppm.

The differential diagnosis of acute arsenic intoxication includes other causes of multisystemic illness and organ dysfunction. Many clinical illnesses and poisonings can manifest with the severe gastrointestinal symptoms, hypotension, and metabolic acidosis that are typical of the initial stage of acute arsenic intoxication; examples include bacterial and viral gastroenteritis, naturally occurring food toxins (e.g., bacterial food poisoning), salicylate overdose, and iron overdose. Acute colchicine overdose may result in acute gastrointestinal distress and hypotension, followed within days by cardiovascular disturbances, altered mental status, and delayed bone marrow depression.

When the early symptoms of acute arsenic poisoning are followed by delayed peripheral neuropathy, the differential diagnosis shifts to several other entities. Guillain-Barré syndrome often occurs as an ascending polyradiculopathy in a patient with a history of an antecedent gastrointestinal illness. In contrast to Guillain-Barré syndrome, arsenical polyneuropathy features prominent early sensory deficits, absence of cranial nerve involvement, and generally lower cerebrospinal fluid protein levels. Noting that some of the early electrodiagnostic features of Guillain-Barré syndrome and arsenic polyneuropathy may be difficult to distinguish, Goddard and associates[108] recommended examination of the proximal F-loop latency, which is prolonged in Guillain-Barré syndrome but not in arsenic poisoning.

Thallium poisoning shares many of the features of arsenic poisoning, including marked initial gastroenteritis, central nervous system dysfunction, and cardiac toxicity, followed by painful peripheral neuropathy and Mees' lines on the nails. In contrast to arsenic poisoning, thallium poisoning does not cause prominent hematologic abnormalities, and it is more likely than arsenic poisoning to produce alopecia.

Patients presenting with alcoholic peripheral neuropathy can have histories of antecedent gastrointestinal distress, anemia, cardiac abnormalities, and liver dysfunction. Compared with arsenic peripheral neuropathy, alcoholic peripheral neuropathy has a slower tempo and may have less prominent motor involvement.

Patients with acute intermittent porphyria may present with a history of abdominal pain, central nervous system disturbance, and peripheral neuropathy, but the condition lacks the prominent sensory involvement of arsenic poisoning. Because acute intermittent porphyria is a genetic disease, it often is associated with a past history of recurrent attacks in adults. Certain nutritional deficiency syndromes, such as pellagra (dermatologic changes, gastrointestinal symptoms, peripheral neuropathy) and beriberi (mental status changes, cardiac failure, peripheral neuropathy), may share some features of arsenic intoxication.

The following two case summaries (of patients for whom the author provided consultation later in their courses) illustrate some classic clinical features of acute arsenic poisoning.

A 39-year-old woman presented to the emergency department complaining of 3 days of nausea, vomiting, diarrhea, and intermittent abdominal pain. Aside from her anxious and bizarre affect, physical examination was unremarkable. On laboratory testing, CBC and electrolytes were remarkable only for a hematocrit of 34% and a serum potassium of 2.8 mEq/L. She was administered 500 mL of intravenous fluids, given a prescription for prochlorperazine, and discharged with a presumptive diagnosis of viral gastroenteritis. She returned the next day with identical complaints. Physical examination remained unremarkable with the exception of a mild postural tachycardia. Laboratory testing revealed electrolytes (in mEq/L) of sodium 134, potassium 3, chloride 107, and bicarbonate 21; serum chemistry panel was remarkable for abnormal liver function tests, with total bilirubin of 1.9 mg/dL [32.5 μmol/L] (direct 0.3 mg/dL [5.1 μmol/L]) (reference range for total bilirubin 0.2 to 1.2 mg/dL [3.4 to 20.5 μmol/L], aspartate aminotransferase of 194 IU/L (reference range 5 to 35 IU/L), and alanine aminotransferase of 225 IU/L (reference range 5 to 35 IU/L). Serum β-human chorionic gonadotropin was negative. The diagnostic impression remained viral gastroenteritis, with inadequate oral intake at home. The patient was admitted to the medical ward for hydration. Past medical history was unremarkable.

During the first 3 hospital days, intermittent crampy abdominal pain, nausea, vomiting, and diarrhea continued. The patient remained afebrile. On hospital day 4, hematocrit was 28.7%, and white blood cell (WBC) count was 4900/mm³. Urinalysis revealed 2+ proteinuria. Stool cultures and ova and parasite examination were negative. Slowly progressive periorbital and pedal edema, unresponsive to furosemide, were noted. The patient complained of a dry mouth, and a faint malar rash was observed. On hospital day 7, the patient complained of lightheadedness, and an electrocardiogram revealed supraventricular tachycardia. She was transferred to the cardiac care unit, where additional monitoring over the next 2 days revealed frequent runs of nonsustained polymorphic ventricular tachycardia, including an episode of torsades de pointes. Chest x-ray revealed slight cardiomegaly and small bilateral pleural effusions.

Gastrointestinal complaints resolved by the second week of hospitalization. Aspartate aminotransferase peaked at 542 IU/L on day 7. CBC revealed slowly progressive pancytopenia, reaching a nadir on day 10 with hematocrit 22% and WBC count 1100/mm³. A bone marrow biopsy specimen showed erythroid hyperplasia and karyorrhexis; later, basophilic stippling and reticulocytosis appeared in the peripheral blood smear. A prodigious number of additional tests recommended by multiple consultants were essentially negative; the diagnosis of arsenic poisoning came to light with a blood arsenic level of 160 μg/L on hospital day 11. Repeat testing on day 16 yielded a blood arsenic level of 3 μg/L, and on day 17, a 24-hour urine arsenic collection contained 2279 μg (urine arsenic concentration was 426 μg/L).

Palmar desquamation was observed on day 23. A progressive sensorimotor peripheral neuropathy first became evident on day 30. Weakness progressed proximally, and on day 46, neuromuscular respiratory failure necessitated intubation and mechanical ventilation. Cranial nerves were intact. Head computed tomography scan and electroencephalogram were normal. Lumbar puncture revealed acellular fluid with a protein of 121 mg/dL. Seven to 10 days of autonomic instability, characterized by transient episodes of hypertension (systolic blood pressure 140 to 210 mm Hg), tachycardia (140 beats/min), and diaphoresis, appeared to respond to metoprolol. By day 62, motor strength began to return in a proximal-to-distal direction, and on day 73,

the patient was weaned successfully from the ventilator. Gross voluntary limb movement returned on day 83. Six months after the acute poisoning incident, the patient had recovered most motor strength in the upper extremities and proximal lower extremities, but residual weakness remained in the toes.

Comment: The source of the arsenic poisoning was never detected, but foul play was suspected. Because the initial attempt to investigate heavy metal poisoning was performed with a blood arsenic measurement, the diagnosis was almost missed. Although the blood arsenic level still was elevated on day 11, it had returned to normal range by day 16, a day before the preferred test, urine arsenic concentration, remained markedly elevated. The patient received 3 days of chelation with intramuscular dimercaprol (British antilewisite [BAL]) from day 17 to day 19, which did not avert the subsequent development of peripheral neuropathy (see later under Treatment).

A 27-year-old man self-injected approximately 0.6 mL of an arsenic-containing herbicide (arsenite dose 330 mg) in a suicide gesture. He presented to the emergency department 30 to 60 minutes later with an alert mental status and profuse vomiting. Vital signs included blood pressure 104/50 mm Hg, pulse 103 beats/min, temperature 98°F (37°C), and respiratory rate 40 breaths/min. Physical examination was normal except for slight diffuse erythema. Initial laboratory tests revealed an anion gap acidosis with serum electrolytes (mEq/L) of sodium 141, potassium 2.8, chloride 106, and bicarbonate 14 and an arterial blood gas on 6 L/min oxygen of pH 7.57, PCO₂ 14 mm Hg, and PO₂ 156 mm Hg. CBC included hematocrit 45.2%, WBC count 6000/mm³, and platelets 257,000/mm³. Prothrombin time was 11.7 seconds. Prompt chelation with dimercaprol, 300 mg intramuscularly every 4 hours (approximately 4 mg/kg every 4 hours), was begun 10 minutes after presentation. The patient became transiently delirious over the next 12 hours. A spot urine arsenic concentration on admission was 13,100 μg/L, and a 24-hour urine collected between the second and third day contained 11,396 μg of arsenic. Vomiting subsided within 36 hours. Transient oliguria that developed 24 to 48 hours postadmission was accompanied by a rise in serum creatinine from 1.6 mg/dL [141.4 μmol/L] to 2.1 mg/dL [185.6 μmol/L]. Urine output increased, however, with vigorous fluid hydration, and serum creatinine decreased to 1.0 mg/dL [88.4 μmol/L] on day 4.

A progressive thrombocytopenia developed during the first 6 days, with platelet count declining to 66,000/mm³. Fibrinogen was 175 mg/dL (reference range 200 to 400 mg/dL), and fibrin split products were increased slightly, leading to an impression of low-level disseminated intravascular coagulation. The patient developed episodic disorientation and hallucinations on day 6 and became markedly tachypneic. Dimercaprol was discontinued. Urine arsenic excretion on day 7 was 9623 μg/24 hr. Chelation with oral succimer, 800 mg every 8 hours (10 mg/kg three times a day), was begun on day 8, and the platelet count subsequently increased over the next 2 days to 137,000/mm³. The hematocrit decreased to 28%, however, and the WBC count reached a nadir of 3700/mm³. On day 10, there was an episode of ventricular tachycardia, and the chest x-ray after intubation revealed patchy bilateral infiltrates consistent with adult respiratory distress syndrome. Invasive hemodynamic monitoring revealed high-output congestive heart failure. Succimer was continued via a nasogastric tube. On day 14, cardiopulmonary and mental status improved, and the patient was extubated. On day 17, there was abrupt onset of a progressive sensorimotor peripheral neuropathy. Succimer dose was decreased to 250 mg three times a day on day 20 (when urine arsenic excretion was 992 μg/24 hr) and was continued through day 48 (when urine arsenic excretion was 129 μg/24 hr). The peripheral neuropathy advanced to quadriparesis by day 59. Slow improvement in limb strength began on day 64, and the patient was able to stand with the assistance of ankle braces by day 96.

Comment: In this rare case of intravenous arsenic overdose, the patient developed initial vomiting and intravascular volume depletion, followed more than 1 week later by life-threatening cardiopulmonary complications and delirium. These complications occurred despite the prompt initiation of chelation with intramuscular dimercaprol. Thrombocytopenia and low-level disseminated intravascular coagulation, which necessitated discontinuation of dimercaprol, coincidentally resolved when the chelation regimen was changed to oral succimer. A delayed sensorimotor peripheral neuropathy still ensued.

Poisoning by Arsine

Arsine poisoning should be suspected strongly in a patient with a history of premonitory constitutional complaints and gastrointestinal disturbance, notably cramping abdominal pain, which is followed within hours by passage of declining volumes of reddish urine and the development of a coppery or jaundiced discoloration to the skin. A history of recent work in which acidic solutions have come in contact with metallic ores or slag is highly suggestive of exposure but is neither specific nor essential.

Common laboratory tests almost always reveal a pattern of evolving, severe hemolysis. The urine is usually heme positive on dip-stick, but microscopic examination may be devoid of formed red blood cells in the initial hours. As oliguria develops, the scant urine usually is strongly dip-stick positive for heme and positive for protein, and microscopic examination reveals an active sediment with red blood cells, red blood cell casts, or granular casts. The urine hemoglobin level should be assessed quantitatively: It may be approach 3 g/L with significant hemolysis, and values ultimately may exceed 10 g/L.[83,109]

In the first few hours after acute overexposure, the CBC may reveal a hematocrit or hemoglobin that is normal or only moderately decreased, but within approximately 12 to 36 hours these values may decline dramatically, with hematocrits in the 20s and hemoglobin values in the range of 5 to 10 g/dL (50 to 100 g/L). Measurement of plasma or serum hemoglobin should be obtained because elevations greater than 1.5 g/dL (>15 g/L) are common in clinically significant arsine poisonings and may have prognostic significance. Plasma or serum hemoglobin initially rises, then remains elevated during the course of active hemolysis, which may persist for several days in the absence of treatment by exchange transfusion (see later). Erythrocyte morphology may include characteristic "ghost cells," which appear as an enlarged membrane enclosing a pale or vacant interior.[79,80,84] Erythrocyte fragmentation, spherocytes, and acanthocytes variably may be found. Leukocytosis is common, and reticulocytosis may appear within a few days. Coombs' test is negative.

Serum chemistries often reveal mild-to-moderate elevations in total bilirubin (e.g., 2 to 5 mg/dL [34.2 to 85.5 μmol/L]) within the initial 48 hours. Although the skin discoloration of arsine-poisoned patients sometimes has been described as "jaundiced," the typical elevation in serum bilirubin is inadequate to account for the dermal appearance. Plasma hemoglobin or degenerated heme products instead may be responsible. Serum transaminases may be slightly elevated, but lactate dehydrogenase typically is markedly elevated, consistent with the hemolytic state. Blood urea nitrogen and serum creatinine increase as acute tubular necrosis proceeds and renal output declines. As with most cases of acute tubular necrosis, the acute renal insufficiency of arsine poisoning generally is reversible after days to weeks of supportive care, although some residual insufficiency may persist.

Blood and urine arsenic concentrations are elevated in symptomatic arsine poisoning, but the range of values reported in the literature for similarly affected patients is extremely variable. This variability may reflect differences in the timing of collections, renal function, the impact of treatment, and laboratory precision. The total arsenic concentration in whole blood in severely affected patients has been reported to range from a few hundred to a few thousand micrograms per liter, and total urinary arsenic has ranged from a few hundred micrograms per liter to several thousand micrograms per liter. In one of the only reports of speciated urine arsenic measurements after acute arsine poisoning, marked elevations of inorganic arsenic and its methylated metabolites were detected, with the latter increasing in preponderance over 5 days.[110] Although total (and potentially speciated) urine arsenic levels and total whole-blood arsenic levels should be ordered for confirmatory or forensic purposes, the diagnosis usually can be established by the history, the clinical picture, and the pattern of common laboratory tests (urinalysis, CBC, and serum chemistries). In any case, the prompt and often intensive supportive care (Table 76-3) required in acute arsine poisoning should not be delayed pending the return of arsenic analyses. If industrial hygiene data on the patient's actual or estimated arsine exposure are available, this may help to confirm the diagnosis. The acute exposure guideline levels (AEGL) for arsine developed by the U.S. National Research Council[89] reported that disabling effects (AEGL-2) might result from 30 minutes of exposure to equal to or greater than 0.21 ppm, 1 hour of exposure to equal to or greater than 0.17 ppm, or 8 hours of exposure to equal to or greater than 0.02 ppm. Life-threatening or lethal effects (AEGL-3) could result from 30 minutes of exposure to equal to or greater than 0.63 ppm, 4 hours of exposure to equal to or greater than 0.13 ppm, or 8 hours of exposure to equal to or greater than 0.06 ppm.

An important element in the differential diagnosis of arsine poisoning is poisoning by stibine (SbH_3), the hydride gas of antimony. Stibine, a potent hemolytic agent that may cause signs and symptoms similar to those of arsine, also is liberated under similar occupational circumstances, such as contact of antimony-containing alloys or compounds with acidic solutions. Acute high-dose exposure to lead may result in a constellation of signs and symptoms that overlap with arsine poisoning, including acute central nervous system effects (headache or encephalopathy or both); abdominal pain; acute hemolysis; mild-to-moderate elevations in

TABLE 76-3 Treatment of Acute Arsine Poisoning

Supportive Care

In patients with evidence of hemolysis (especially plasma hemoglobin $\geq$1.5 g/dL [$\geq$15 g/L]), perform exchange transfusion with whole blood
Maintain vigorous urine output with intravenous fluids and mannitol (osmotic diuresis)
Perform hemodialysis as needed for progressive renal insufficiency

Chelation

Currently available chelating agents are of uncertain benefit in arsine poisoning (see text)
In first 24 hours, consider dimercaprol (BAL, British antilewisite): 3.0–5.0 mg/kg intramuscularly every 4–6 hr
Beyond first 24 hr, consider DMPS (oral or parenteral) or DMSA (oral) in patients with evidence of severe intoxication

DMPS, dimercaptopropanesulfonic acid; DMSA, dimercaptosuccinic acid.

liver function tests; and short-term, mild-to-moderate renal insufficiency. The tempo of severe acute lead intoxication is seldom as rapid as that seen with acute arsine intoxication, however. The hemolysis associated with severe acute lead intoxication is not as extensive as that due to arsine, and the acute renal insufficiency is not a consequence of hemoglobin deposition or acute tubular necrosis. Certain stages of malaria due to infection with *Plasmodium falciparum* may resemble clinically arsine poisoning, with patients displaying hemolysis ("blackwater fever"), renal failure, gastrointestinal symptoms, and occasionally central nervous system symptoms. Patients with paroxysmal nocturnal hemoglobinuria may present with hemolysis and abdominal pain.

TREATMENT

Arsenic

The treatment of acute arsenic poisoning is summarized in Table 76-4.

SUPPORTIVE CARE AND DECONTAMINATION

Treatment of acute arsenic poisoning requires supportive care (usually in the intensive care unit), decontamination, and prompt use of specific chelating agents. Immediate supportive care should address the hypotension or incipient shock that often accompanies the increased vascular permeability and the gastrointestinal fluid loss from vomiting and diarrhea that is common in acute arsenic poisoning. Large volumes of intravenous fluids may be needed to support blood pressure and maintain urine output. Moderate to high levels of urine output (1 mL/kg/hr) are desirable because the kidney is the major route of arsenic excretion. Because arsenic may result in congestive heart failure or noncardiogenic pulmonary edema, however, typically after several hours to days, determination of optimal fluid requirements ultimately may require invasive hemodynamic monitoring. Support with vasopressor agents, such as dopamine, or treatment of acidosis with bicarbonate may be indicated in severe cases. It may be prudent to avoid the use of phenothiazines as antiemetics or antipsychotics in these patients because these drugs may lower the seizure threshold or prolong the QT interval.

The potential development of malignant arrhythmias merits continuous cardiac monitoring for at least the first 24 to 48 hours in arsenic-poisoned patients who present with

 Indications for ICU Admission in Arsenic or Arsine Poisoning

Intensive care unit (ICU) admission is indicated for any patient with a history of acute ingestion of milligram quantities of inorganic arsenic or any patient with suspected arsenic ingestion who presents with overt signs of gastrointestinal, cardiovascular, or neurologic disturbance. Gastrointestinal manifestations, such as vomiting, diarrhea, or abdominal pain; cardiovascular findings, such as tachycardia or hypotension; or alterations in mental status, such as lethargy or agitation, may be followed abruptly by life-threatening shock, arrhythmias, or seizures.

Because of the potential for delayed cardiovascular or neurologic deterioration (congestive heart failure, noncardiogenic pulmonary edema, malignant arrhythmias, encephalopathy) continued ICU monitoring may be necessary for several days to a week after acute gastrointestinal symptoms or hypotension has been stabilized. Careful ongoing monitoring is indicated particularly in patients whose urinary arsenic concentration has been elevated markedly (e.g., >5000 μg/L) or in patients who exhibit prolongation of the QT_c interval on an electrocardiogram. Patients with arsenical peripheral neuropathy who display progressive signs of ascending motor weakness should be observed carefully for the abrupt appearance of neuromuscular respiratory failure.

Patients with known or suspected arsine intoxication should be admitted to the ICU, treated expectantly with vigorous intravenous hydration, and monitored carefully for progressive hemolysis and any compromise in cardiovascular, renal, or neurologic function. Because arsine-induced hemolysis may be associated with a latent interval of 2 to 24 hours, patients who initially are asymptomatic still may merit careful overnight observation.

any initial electrocardiogram abnormality or whose other presenting symptoms or signs (e.g., gastrointestinal distress, hypotension, metabolic acidosis, or altered mental status) indicate significant acute intoxication. Monitoring beyond 48 hours is indicated in patients with persistent symptoms or evidence of new (i.e., not preexisting) cardiovascular disturbances. These symptoms may include electrocardiogram abnormalities (e.g., tachycardia, ectopy, prolonged QT_c interval, U waves) or evidence of congestive heart failure, even to a mild degree. Antiarrhythmic drugs such as procainamide and other type Ia agents, which may exacerbate arsenic-related prolongation of the QT interval, should be avoided.

TABLE 76-4 Treatment of Acute Poisoning by Inorganic Arsenic

Supportive Care and Decontamination

Intravenous rehydration with crystalloid solutions

Vasopressor drugs

    In patients with gastrointestinal fluid loss and hypotension, use as needed to support blood pressure and
        optimize urine output (≥1 mL/kg/hr)

Sodium bicarbonate (as needed for severe metabolic acidosis)

Consider gastric lavage or whole-bowel irrigation for gut decontamination

Avoid phenothiazines and type 1a antiarrhythmics

Chelation*

Agent of first choice: DMPS (2,3-dimercaptopropanesulfonic acid, unithiol, Dimaval)

    Administer intravenously 3–5 mg/kg every 4 hr by slow infusion over 20 min

Agent of second choice if DMPS not immediately available: dimercaprol (BAL, British antilewisite)

    Administer intramuscularly 3–5 mg/kg every 4–6 hr

When patient stable and able to absorb an oral medication, consider change to oral chelation with either

    DMPS: 4–8 mg/kg orally every 6 hr

    DMSA (2,3-dimercaptosuccinic acid, succimer): 7.5 mg/kg orally every 6 hr, or 10 mg/kg every 8 hr

*DMPS and DMSA are not officially approved in all countries for chelation treatment of acute arsenic poisoning. Indications and dosages are the author's suggestion based on best available data.

Gastrointestinal decontamination of retained arsenic should be considered, but in practice the profuse vomiting that often accompanies acute arsenic poisoning obviates the need for gastric lavage. If ingestion has occurred recently (within approximately 1 hour) and no emesis has been noted, gastric lavage may be indicated. There are no data, however, that gastric lavage alters the course or clinical outcome in arsenic-poisoned patients. Gastric lavage is described in Chapter 5. As noted previously, abdominal x-rays (and occasionally chest x-rays) may reveal the presence of radiopacities consistent with gastrointestinal retention of poorly dissolved arsenic. In these cases, it may be prudent to perform gastric lavage or whole-bowel irrigation to hasten removal of this unabsorbed material.[93,111] Administration of oral activated charcoal often has been recommended, but because the binding affinity of activated charcoal for inorganic arsenic is extremely low in vitro, the clinical utility of this intervention is doubtful.[112] The detection of arsenic in human gastric aspirates 1 week after the last known ingestion raises the possibility that arsenic may undergo a degree of enterohepatic or enteroenteric circulation,[10,70] but the extent of this process has not been quantified, and a potential approach to interdict it with alternative binding agents has not been studied in humans.

Hemodialysis may increase arsenic elimination in patients with marked oliguria or anuria secondary to arsenic-induced acute renal failure, but because of the rapid distribution of arsenic to extravascular compartments, the total amount removed by this route (on the order of a few milligrams) is miniscule compared with the amount responsible for the intoxication or the amount eliminated via the urine in nonoliguric patients.[10,39,113–115] Because the oliguria associated with acute arsenic intoxication is generally due to hypotension and decreased renal blood flow rather than to acute tubular necrosis, fluid resuscitation to support blood pressure and maintain urine flow rates should be the focus of therapy. Hemodialysis should be considered only for patients with renal failure from another cause or patients whose oliguria or anuria is otherwise unresponsive.

Patients who develop delayed peripheral neuropathy should be monitored carefully for progressive involvement of the proximal musculature. There is a risk that neuromuscular respiratory failure might ensue abruptly when there is evidence of proximal limb weakness. Patients with this level of ascending motor involvement should undergo serial measurements of inspiratory muscle effort, and the possible requirement for mechanical ventilation on an emergent basis should be anticipated. Physical therapy is an important adjunctive measure in the recovery from arsenical neuropathy. Tricyclic antidepressants, such as amitriptyline, may be of value in treating the painful dysesthesias that often occur.[116]

CHELATION

The prompt use of dimercapto chelating drugs in the treatment of acute arsenic poisoning is recommended. The value of this treatment is based on the results of animal experimentation, however, and the therapeutic efficacy of chelation has not been established through carefully controlled human clinical trials.[117] The first chelating agent, dimercaprol (2,3-dimercaptopropanol), was developed by British scientists during World War II as a specific antidote for acute poisoning by the vesicant organoarsenical warfare agent lewisite.[23,118] Dimercaprol often has been referred to as *British antilewisite* or *BAL*. Water-soluble analogues of dimercaprol, dimercaptopropanesulfonic acid (DMPS, Unithiol, Dimaval), and dimercaptosuccinic acid (DMSA, succimer, Chemet) were developed as heavy metal chelators in the 1950s[119,120] and offer the advantage of higher therapeutic index and delivery by oral and intravenous routes.[121] Animal experiments have shown that dimercaprol, DMPS, and DMSA increase survival in experimental animals administered lethal doses of arsenite.[122,123] The effectiveness of chelation on survival declined, however, in proportion to the length of time after arsenic exposure that treatment was begun.[122,123] In an early study of the effectiveness of chelation against poisoning by organoarsenicals in rabbits, a single dose of dimercaprol given within 5 minutes of the arsenical resulted in survival of all the test animals, compared with a zero survival rate when treatment was delayed for 6 hours.[124] In humans exposed experimentally to low doses of diphenylcyanoarsine smoke, the percent increase in urinary arsenic excretion after dimercaprol was higher the sooner after exposure it was administered.[125] These experimental studies and limited clinical experience[52] suggest that chelation treatment begun within a few hours after acute arsenic ingestion offers an improved chance of a positive therapeutic outcome. Nevertheless, in many cases, death or delayed peripheral neuropathy has occurred despite prompt chelation treatment.[10,38,40,42,56,98,126] The clinical course of an incipient or established arsenical neuropathy, usually characterized by slow improvement over several months to years, generally is not influenced by chelation therapy.[44,52,54,59] Isolated case reports have associated chelation with more rapid resolution of arsenical neuropathy,[127,128] but because improvement would have been anticipated from the natural history of the illness, the added therapeutic role of chelation in these cases cannot be determined.

Of the chelating agents currently available, DMPS has the most favorable profile for the treatment of acute poisoning by inorganic arsenic. Although available as a pharmaceutical agent (Unithiol; Oktyabr) in the Soviet Union since the 1960s and in Germany since the 1970s (Dimaval; Heyl), DMPS has become available only more recently in the United States. Since 1999, DMPS has been sold legally in the United States as a bulk drug substance available for use by compounding pharmacists.[129]

DMPS offers several advantages over BAL, the chelating agent traditionally used for the treatment of arsenic poisoning in the United States and the United Kingdom, since its introduction in the 1940s.[130] DMPS has a higher therapeutic index and potency ratio in the treatment of experimental acute arsenic poisoning in animals.[121,123,131] DMPS was more effective than dimercaprol in mobilizing and decreasing the arsenic content of numerous tissues in animal models. This increased effectiveness was particularly noteworthy in the brain, where dimercaprol resulted in an *increase* in arsenic content compared with a significant decrease after use of DMPS.[121,123,132] The water-soluble nature of DMPS enables it to be given intravenously, in contrast to BAL, which is supplied dissolved in oil for administration by deep intramuscular injection only. The intravenous dosing available for DMPS allows more rapid delivery to the target tissues, especially in arsenic-poisoned patients who are hypotensive or in shock. In the therapeutic doses used to treat heavy metal poisoning, DMPS seems to be tolerated better than dimercaprol and in particular avoids the pain and discomfort associated with repeated intramuscular injections. The clinical pharmacology of these chelating agents is discussed in detail elsewhere.

For patients in the initial stages of acute inorganic arsenic poisoning, DMPS can be administered intravenously at total daily doses of 20 to 30 mg/kg/day. One sixth of the total daily dose can be given every 4 hours by slow intravenous infusion over 20 minutes.[133,134] Moore and associates[51] reported an initial intravenous dose of 5 mg/kg

every 4 hours, and Wax and Thorton[128] administered DMPS, 250 mg intravenously every 4 hours, to an arsenic-poisoned adult. Because it is important that chelation be started as soon as possible after arsenic ingestion, BAL should be used if DMPS is not immediately available. Dimercaprol is administered at doses of 3 to 5 mg/kg intramuscularly every 4 to 6 hours. A switch from parenteral to oral chelation is appropriate when the patient has no signs of adverse gastrointestinal effects (e.g., nausea, vomiting, diarrhea, abdominal pain) and no signs of cardiovascular compromise (e.g., hypotension or decreased urine output), which might be associated with decreased absorption of medication administered through the oral route. Chelation can be continued with oral preparations of DMPS. An adult daily dose of 1.2 to 2.4 g administered in 12 divided increments has been recommended (i.e., 100 to 200 mg every 2 hours),[135] but considering the elimination kinetics of DMPS,[136] a dose interval of every 6 hours seems satisfactory.

The dimercapto chelating agent DMSA also can be used for treatment of arsenic poisoning when an oral agent is appropriate. DMSA has exhibited clinical efficacy and pharmacodynamic properties similar to those of DMPS in animal studies of acute arsenic intoxication.[121,123] It can be administered at a total daily dose of 30 mg/kg/day. Although a dosing interval of every 8 hours has been recommended for chronic lead intoxication, more frequent dose intervals (e.g., every 6 hours) may be more appropriate for acute arsenic poisoning. The possibility that oral chelation with DMPS or DMSA might increase absorption of arsenic retained in the intestinal tract has not been studied directly, but negative studies with other metals and these chelators suggest that enhanced absorption of arsenic is not likely to be a problem.[137,138] D-Penicillamine has been shown to be ineffective in experimental arsenic intoxication,[121,139] and its use in human arsenic poisoning is not recommended. The clinical pharmacology of DMSA is discussed in Chapter 141.

The optimal duration of chelation treatment for acute or subacute arsenic intoxication is not well established. In cases in which the intoxication is not rapidly lethal, hemodynamic stabilization and resolution of gastrointestinal symptoms may enable parenteral chelation to be switched to oral chelation after 2 or 3 days. It may then be appropriate to continue oral chelation at least until urine arsenic excretion decreases to less than 500 μg/24 hr, or 400 μg/L, urinary values that are lower than values associated with overt symptoms in acutely exposed individuals. Alternatively, oral chelation might be continued until urinary arsenic excretion decreases to background levels (<50 μg/L), although the therapeutic benefit of extending chelation to this point is undetermined. A randomized, placebo-controlled clinical trial found no benefit of DMSA in the treatment of chronic arsenic poisoning in patients who already had been removed from ongoing exposure and whose urine arsenic levels were less than 50 μg/L.[140]

Arsine

Prompt exchange transfusion of whole blood is a key therapeutic intervention in acute severe arsine poisoning. The value of exchange transfusion is supported by clinical reports[80,109,141,142] and by mechanistic studies suggesting that a reaction of arsine with a hemoprotein, such as oxyhemoglobin, is an important step in the toxic effects of the gas.[32,35] Beneficial effects of exchange transfusion include (1) clearance from the blood of a toxic by-product or complex formed by arsine's reaction with hemoglobin; (2) removal of plasma hemoglobin or hemoglobin degradation products released by hemolysis, which then may precipitate in the renal tubules and cause acute tubular damage; and (3) restoration of a sufficient supply of intact erythrocytes to provide adequate oxygen delivery to the kidney and other tissues. A relatively simple technique of exchange transfusion in which whole donor blood is infused through a central line at the same rate of blood removal via a peripheral vein using a blood donor set has been described.[143] Other approaches have used modifications of hemodialysis circuits.[144] Exchange transfusion is recommended in any patient with suspected arsine poisoning exhibiting evidence of significant hemolysis. A plasma or serum hemoglobin level of 1.5 g/dL or greater has been suggested as a level that merits this therapy,[109] but given the delay inherent in securing the necessary donor blood, it would be prudent to plan for implementation of exchange transfusion in patients with lesser but rapidly escalating plasma hemoglobin levels. Evidence of renal insufficiency or incipient acute tubular necrosis also is an indication for exchange transfusion in arsine-poisoned subjects. Prompt exchange transfusion in patients with arsine hemolysis may avert significant renal failure in some, albeit not all, cases.[85,109]

Maintenance of vigorous renal output with intravenous fluids and mannitol-induced osmotic diuresis also may be protective against hemoglobinuric renal failure and should be started promptly in all patients with evidence of hemolysis or significant arsine exposure. Hemodialysis is indicated in cases of progressive oliguria and anuria. The toxic complexes or by-products formed by the action of arsine on hemoglobin and other proteins in the blood may not be removed adequately by hemodialysis,[145] however, and hemodialysis should not be considered a substitute for exchange transfusion.

The value of chelating agents in the treatment of arsine poisoning is uncertain. In experimental arsine poisoning, 1 mM of BAL added to human blood in vitro 5 minutes after exposure to arsine (2000 ppm) reduced observed hemolysis to 17% compared with 33.3% in controls (i.e., a 50% decline in hemolysis).[146] Although experiments with arsine-poisoned rabbits treated with dimercaprol within 30 minutes yielded a decline in observed lethality, the dose of BAL used was high, and the authors considered the observed results to be erratic.[146] A derivative of dimercaprol, 2,3-dimercaptopropyl ethyl ether, was more effective than dimercaprol in experimental studies of arsine poisoning, but further drug development was not pursued.[146] Soviet researchers reported that a highly lipid-soluble aryl thioether analogue of dimercaprol, 2,3-dimercaptopropyl-p-tolylsulfide (Mercaptide), was effective in experimental acute arsine poisoning in rats, whereas water-soluble DMPS (Unithiol) was completely ineffective.[147] Rael and colleagues[32] found that preincubation of human erythrocytes with high concentrations of DMSA or DMPS in vitro diminished hemolysis after subsequent exposure to arsine. In human case reports of arsine poisoning, the administration of dimercaprol has not yielded clinical impressions of therapeutic efficacy,[80,148] but because clinical

circumstances of poisoning and treatment are variable, little can be concluded from reports of this nature. It seems reasonable to initiate treatment with dimercaprol, a relatively lipid-soluble chelator, in patients who present in the early stages of acute arsine poisoning (i.e., within 24 hours). Later in the course of poisoning, treatment with oral DMSA or DMPS may exert some benefit in countering the adverse effects of arsenite, which eventually is produced in vivo after arsine poisoning.[110] The treatment of acute arsine poisoning is summarized in Table 76-3.

SPECIAL POPULATIONS

Pregnant Patients

Transport of arsenic across the placenta has been documented in animal models[149] and confirmed in studies of pregnant women exposed to elevated concentrations of arsenic in drinking water.[150] The developmental toxicity of arsenic has been reviewed.[18,29,151] Animal studies indicate that inorganic arsenic can cause malformations, prenatal fatality, and decreased fetal weight, usually at maternal exposures greater than 1 mg/kg/day.[18] Arsine exposure of pregnant rats and mice at concentrations of 0.025 ppm, 0.5 ppm, and 2.5 ppm resulted in increases in maternal spleen weight at the highest dose, but fetotoxicity was not observed.[152] Some human epidemiologic studies suggest an adverse reproductive effect of environmental arsenic exposure,[29,153] but the evidence is inconclusive, and further research is needed.

Two reports of pregnant women acutely poisoned with inorganic arsenic showed transplacental transport resulting in fetal or neonatal death. A 17-year-old woman who was 30 weeks pregnant developed abdominal pain, vomiting, hypotension, and acidosis shortly after ingestion of approximately 400 mg of arsenic trioxide.[154] A single dose of BAL was given 24 hours postingestion. The patient developed renal insufficiency and disorientation but subsequently recovered. A premature infant born 4 days after the arsenic ingestion had an Apgar score of 4 and hyaline membrane disease and died 11 hours after delivery. Autopsy revealed elevated levels of arsenic in the infant's organs. A 39-year-old woman who was 28 weeks pregnant developed the acute onset of slight abdominal pain and hypotension after eating chocolate later found to contain a large amount of arsenic trioxide.[45] The mother survived after a stormy course that included cardiopulmonary failure and moderately severe peripheral neuropathy. Intrauterine fetal death was confirmed on day 5, and 3 days later a maternal urine arsenic concentration of 5800 µg/L was reported. Examination of the organs of the aborted fetus revealed markedly elevated levels of arsenic.

The chelating agents DMPS and DMSA reduced, but did not eliminate, embryotoxic and teratogenic effects of sodium arsenite (12 mg/kg) in pregnant mice.[155,156] The protective effects occurred only with high doses of the chelating agents (≥150 mg/kg), administered within 1 hour of the arsenite. Nevertheless, these beneficial effects, combined with the apparent lack of adverse reproductive effects of the chelators given alone at therapeutic doses, suggest that pregnancy should not be considered a contraindication to chelation with DMPS or DMSA in a patient with acute arsenic poisoning.[157,158]

REFERENCES

1. Fowler T: Medical Reports of the Effects of Arsenic in the Cure of Agues, Remitting Fevers, and Periodic Headaches. London, Johnson & Brown, 1786.
2. Mealey J, Brownell GL, Sweet WH: Radioarsenic in plasma, urine, normal tissues and intracranial neoplasms. Arch Neurol Psychiatry 81:310–320, 1959.
3. Vahter M, Norin H: Metabolism of [74]As-labeled trivalent and pentavalent inorganic arsenic in mice. Environ Res 21:446–457, 1980.
4. Zhang X, Cornelis R, De Kimpe J, et al: Study of arsenic-protein binding in serum of patients on continuous ambulatory peritoneal dialysis. Clin Chem 44:141–147, 1998.
5. Zhang X, Cornelis R, De Kimpe J, et al: Speciation of arsenic in serum, urine, and dialysate of patients on continuous ambulatory peritoneal dialysis. Clin Chem 43:406–408, 1997.
6. Pounds CA, Pearson EF, Turner TD: Arsenic in fingernails. J Forensic Sci Soc 19:165–173, 1979.
7. Pomroy C, Charbonneau SM, McCullough RS, et al: Human retention studies with [74]As. Toxicol Appl Pharmacol 53:550–556, 1980.
8. Mappes R: Versuche zur Ausscheidung von Arsen im Urin [Experiments on excretion of arsenic in urine]. Int Arch Occup Environ Health 40:267–272, 1977.
9. Buchet JP, Lauwerys R, Roels H: Urinary excretion of inorganic arsenic and its metabolites after repeated ingestion of sodium meta arsenite by volunteers. Int Arch Occup Environ Health 48:111–118, 1981.
10. Mahieu P, Buchet JP, Roels HA, et al: The metabolism of arsenic in humans acutely intoxicated by As_2O_3: Its significance for the duration of BAL therapy. Clin Toxicol 18:1067–1075, 1981.
11. Foa V, Colombi A, Maroni M, et al: The speciation of the chemical forms of arsenic in the biological monitoring of exposure to inorganic arsenic. Sci Tot Environ 34:241–259, 1984.
12. Kosnett MJ, Becker CE: Dimercaptosuccinic acid: Utility in acute and chronic arsenic poisoning. Vet Hum Toxicol 30:369, 1988.
13. Agency for Toxic Substances and Disease Registry: Toxicological Profile for Arsenic (Update). Atlanta, ATSDR, 2000.
14. Vahter M: Variation in human metabolism of arsenic. In Chappell WR, Abernathy CO, Calderon RL (eds): Arsenic Exposure and Health Effects. Oxford, Elsevier, 1999, pp 267–279.
15. Petrick JS, Ayala-Fierro F, Cullen WR, et al: Monomethylarsonous acid (MMA[III]) is more toxic than arsenite in Chang human hepatocytes. Toxicol Appl Pharmacol 163:203–207, 2000.
16. Petrick JS, Jagadish B, Mash EA, et al: Monomethylarsonous acid (MMA[III]) and arsenite: LD50 in hamsters and in vitro inhibition of pyruvate dehydrogenase. Chem Res Toxicol 14:651–656, 2001.
17. Mass MJ, Tennant A, Roop BC, et al: Methylated trivalent arsenic species are genotoxic. Chem Res Toxicol 14:355–361, 2001.
18. National Research Council: Arsenic in Drinking Water. Washington, DC, National Academy Press, 1999.
19. Klimecki WT, Carter DE: Arsine toxicity: Chemical and mechanistic implications. J Environ Health 46:399–409, 1995.
20. Departments of the Army and the Air Force: Military Chemistry and Chemical Agents. Technical Manual No. 3–215, Air Force Manual No. 355–7. Washington, DC, Departments of the Army and the Air Force, 1956.
21. Institute of Medicine: Veterans at Risk: The Health Effects of Mustard Gas and Lewisite. Washington, DC, National Academy Press, 1993.
22. Webb JL: Enzyme and Metabolic Inhibitors, Vol III. Iodoacetate, Maleate, N-ethylmaleimide, Alloxan, Quinones, Arsenicals. New York, Academic Press, 1966.
23. Peters RA, Stocken LA, Thompson RHS: British anti-lewisite. Nature 156:616–619, 1945.
24. Lin S, Cullen WR, Thomas DJ: Methylarsenicals and arsinothiols are potent inhibitors of mouse liver thioredoxin reductase. Chem Res Toxicol 12:924–930, 1999.
25. Lin S, Del Razo LM, Styblo M, et al: Arsenicals inhibit thioredoxin reductase in cultured rat hepatocytes. Chem Res Toxicol 14:305–311, 2001.
26. Liu SX, Athar M, Lippai I, et al: Induction of oxyradicals by arsenic: Implication for mechanism of genotoxicity. Proc Natl Acad Sci USA 98:1643–1648, 2001.
27. Winski SL, Carter DE: Arsenate toxicity in human erythrocytes: Characterization of morphologic changes and determination of the mechanism of damage. J Toxicol Environ Health 53:345–355, 1998.
28. Garcia-Vargas GG, Del Razo LM, Cebrian ME: Altered urinary porphyrin excretion in a human population chronically exposed to arsenic in Mexico. Hum Exp Toxicol 13:839–847, 1994.
29. National Research Council: Arsenic in Drinking Water: 2001 Update. Washington, DC, National Academy Press, 2001.
30. Ramirez P, Del Razo LM, Gonsebatt ME: Arsenite induces DNA-protein crosslinks and cytokeratin expression in the WRL-68 human hepatic cell line. Carcinogenesis 21:701–706, 2000.
31. Li YM, Broome JD: Arsenic targets tubulins to induce apoptosis in myeloid leukemia cells. Cancer Res 59:776–780, 1999.
32. Rael LT, Ayala-Fierro F, Carter DE: The effects of sulfur, thiol, and thiol inhibitor compounds on arsine-induced toxicity in the human erythrocyte membrane. Toxicol Sci 55:468–477, 2000.
33. Ayala-Fierro F, Barber DS, Rael LT, et al: In vitro tissue specificity for arsine and arsenite toxicity in the rat. Toxicol Sci 52:122–129, 1999.
34. Levvy GA: A study of arsine poisoning. J Exp Physiol 34:47–67, 1947.
35. Ayala-Fierro F, Carter DE: LLC-PK1 cells as a model for renal toxicity caused by arsine exposure. J Toxicol Environ Health 60:67–79, 2000.
36. Kamijo Y, Soma K, Asari Y, et al: Survival after massive arsenic poisoning self-treated by high fluid intake. Clin Toxicol 36:27–29, 1998.
37. Fréjaville J-P, Bescol J, Leclerc L, et al: Intoxication aiguë par les dérivés arsenicaux; (à propos de 4 observations personnelles); troubles de l'hémostase; étude ultramicroscopique de foie et du rein. Ann Med Int 123:713–722, 1972.
38. Gillies AJD, Taylor AJ: Acute arsenical poisoning in Dunedin. N Z Med J 89:379–381, 1979.
39. Levin-Scherz JK, Patrick JD, Weber FH, et al: Acute arsenic ingestion. Ann Emerg Med 16:702–704, 1987.
40. Gerhardsson L, Dahlgren E, Eriksson A, et al: Fatal arsenic poisoning—a case report. Scand J Work Environ Health 14:130–133, 1988.
41. Jolliffe DM, Budd AJ, Gwilt DJ: Massive acute arsenic poisoning. Anaesthesiology 40:288–290, 1991.
42. Civantos DP, Rodriguez AL, Aguado-Borruey JM, et al: Fulminant malignant arrhythmia and multiorgan failure in acute arsenic poisoning. Chest 108:1774–1775, 1995.
43. Peterson RG, Rumack BH: D-Penicillamine therapy of acute arsenic poisoning. J Pediatr 91:661–666, 1977.
44. Greenberg C, Davies S, McGowan T, et al: Acute respiratory failure following severe arsenic poisoning. Chest 76:596–598, 1979.
45. Bollinger CT, van Zijl P, Louw JA: Multiple organ failure with the adult respiratory distress syndrome in homicidal arsenic poisoning. Respiration 59:57–61, 1992.
46. Glazener FS, Ellis JG, Johnson PK: Electrocardiographic findings with arsenic poisoning. Calif Med 109:158–162, 1968.
47. St. Petery J, Gross C, Victorica BE: Ventricular fibrillation caused by arsenic poisoning. Am J Dis Child 120:367–371, 1970.
48. Goldsmith S, From AHL: Arsenic-induced atypical ventricular tachycardia. N Engl J Med 303:1096–1097, 1980.
49. Fennell JS, Stacy WK: Brief report: Electrocardiographic changes in acute arsenic poisoning. Irish J Med Sci 150:338–339, 1981.
50. Little RE, Kay GN, Cavender JB, et al: Torsade de pointes and T-U wave alternans associated with arsenic poisoning. Pacing Clin Electrophysiol 13:164–170, 1990.
51. Moore DF, O'Callaghan CA, Berlyne G, et al: Acute arsenic poisoning: Absence of polyneuropathy after treatment with 2,3-dimercaptopropanesulphonate (DMPS). J Neurol Neurosurg Psych 57:1133–1135, 1994.
52. Jenkins RB: Inorganic arsenic and the nervous system. Brain 89:479–498, 1966.
53. O'Shaughnessy E, Kraft GH: Arsenic poisoning: Long-term follow-up of a nonfatal case. Arch Phys Med Rehabil 57:403–406, 1976.
54. LeQuesne PM, McLeod JG: Peripheral neuropathy following a single exposure to arsenic. J Neurol Sci 32:437–451, 1977.
55. Freeman JW, Couch JR: Prolonged encephalopathy with arsenic poisoning. Neurology 28:853–855, 1978.
56. Fincher R-ME, Koerker RM: Long-term survival in acute arsenic encephalopathy: Follow-up using newer measures of electrophysiologic parameters. Am J Med 82:549–552, 1987.
57. Murphy MJ, Lyon LW, Taylor JW: Subacute arsenic neuropathy: Clinical and electrophysiological observations. J Neurol Neurosurg Psychiatry 44:896–900, 1981.
58. Donofrio PD, Wilbourn J, Albers JW, et al: Acute arsenic intoxication presenting as Guillain-Barré-like syndrome. Muscle Nerve 10:114–120, 1987.

59. Heyman A, Pfeiffer JB, Willett RW, et al: Peripheral neuropathy caused by arsenical intoxication. N Engl J Med 254:402–409, 1956.

60. Zaloga GP, Deal J, Spurling T, et al: Unusual manifestations of arsenic intoxication. Am J Med Sci 289:210–214, 1985.

61. Goebel HH, Schmidt PF, Bohl J, et al: Polyneuropathy due to acute arsenic intoxication: Biopsy studies. J Neuropathol Exp Neurol 49:137–149, 1990.

62. Bartolome B, Cordoba S, Nieto S, et al: Acute arsenic poisoning: Clinical and histopathological features. Br J Dermatol 141:1106–1109, 1999.

63. Lawson GB, Jackson WP, Cattanach GS: Arsenic poisoning: Report of twenty-eight cases. JAMA 35:24–26, 1925.

64. Garner H: Arsenical polyneuritis. Arch Neurol Psychiatry 59:842, 1948.

65. Mees RA: The nails with arsenical polyneuritis (Abstract). JAMA 72:1337, 1919.

66. Aldrich CJ: Leuconychia striata arsenicalis transverses. Am J Med Sci 127:702–709, 1904.

67. Reynolds ES: An account of the epidemic outbreak of arsenical poisoning occurring in beer-drinkers in the north of England and the midland counties in 1900. Lancet 166–170, 1901.

68. Jenkins RB: Reynolds, Aldrich or Mees? A consideration of transverse striate leukonychia. Am J Med Sci 246:707–709, 1963.

69. Feinglass EJ: Arsenic intoxication from well water in the United States. N Engl J Med 288:828–830, 1973.

70. Mizuta N, Mizuta M, Fukashi I, et al: An outbreak of acute arsenic poisoning caused by arsenic contaminated soy-sauce (shuyu): A clinical report of 220 cases. Yamaguchi Med School 4:131–149, 1956.

71. Kelynack TN, Kirkby W, Delépine S, et al: Arsenical poisoning from beer-drinking. Lancet 1600–1603, 1900.

72. Chen Z, Chen G-Q, Shen Z-X, et al: Treatment of acute promyelocytic leukemia with arsenic compounds: In vitro and in vivo studies. Semin Hematol 38:26–36, 2001.

73. Ohnishi K, Yoshida H, Shigeno K, et al: Prolongation of the QT interval and ventricular tachycardia in patients treated with arsenic trioxide for acute promyelocytic leukemia. Ann Intern Med 133:881–885, 2000.

74. Unnikrishnan D, Dutcher JP, Varshneya N, et al: Torsades de pointes in 3 patients with leukemia treated with arsenic trioxide. Blood 97:1514–1516, 2001.

75. Niu C, Yan H, Yu T, et al: Studies on treatment of acute promyelocytic leukemia with arsenic trioxide: Remission induction, follow-up, and molecular monitoring in 11 newly diagnosed and 47 relapsed acute promyelocytic leukemia patients. Blood 94:3315–3324, 1999.

76. Huang S-Y, Chang C-S, Tang J-L, et al: Acute and chronic arsenic poisoning associated with treatment of acute promyelocytic leukaemia. Br J Haematol 103:1092–1095, 1998.

77. Goldstein NP, McCall JT, Dyck PJ: Metal neuropathy. In Dyck PJ, Thomas PK, Lambert EH (eds): Peripheral Neuropathy, Vol II. Philadelphia, WB Saunders, 1975.

78. Anthonisen P, Nielsen B, Pedersen K, et al: 3. Clinical picture and treatment in arsine poisoning. Acta Med Scand 496(Suppl):12–22, 1968.

79. Jones NB: Arseniuretted hydrogen poisoning: With report of five cases. JAMA 48:1099–1105, 1907.

80. Teitelbaum DT, Kier LC: Arsine poisoning, report of five cases in the petroleum industry and a discussion of the indications for exchange transfusion and hemodialysis. Arch Environ Health 19:133–143, 1969.

81. Muehrake RC, Pirani CL: Arsine-induced anemia: A correlative clinopathological study with electron microscope observations. Ann Intern Med 68:853–866, 1968.

82. Pedersen F, Ladefoged J, Winkler K, et al: The renal circulation in acute arsine poisoning. Acta Med Scand 496(Suppl):27–31, 1968.

83. Jenkins GC, Kazantzis G, Owen R: Massive haemolysis with minimal impairment of renal function. BMJ 2:78–80, 1965.

84. Levinsky WJ, Smalley RV, Hillyer PN, et al: Arsine hemolysis. Arch Environ Health 20:436–440, 1970.

85. Parish GC, Glass R, Kimbrough R: Acute arsine poisoning in two workers cleaning a clogged drain. Arch Environ Health 34:224–227, 1979.

86. Josephson CJ, Pinto SS, Petronella SJ: Arsine: electrocardiographic changes produced in acute human poisoning. Arch Ind Hyg Occup Med 4:43–52, 1951.

87. Phoon WH, Chan MO, Goh CH, et al: Five cases of arsine poisoning. Ann Acad Med Sing 13(2 Suppl):394–398, 1984.

88. Bulmer FMR, Rothwell HE, Polack SS, et al: Chronic arsine poisoning among workers employed in the cyanide extraction of gold: A report of 14 cases. J Ind Hyg Toxicol 22:111–124, 1940.

89. National Research Council: Arsine: Acute exposure guideline levels. In: Acute Exposure Guideline Levels for Selected Airborne Chemicals, Vol 1. Washington, DC, National Academy Press, 2000, pp 65–112.

90. Sanz P, Corbella J, Nogué S, et al: Rhabdomyolysis in fatal arsenic trioxide poisoning. JAMA 262:3271, 1989.

91. Fanton L, Duperret S, Guillaumée F, et al: Case report: Fatal rhabdomyolysis in arsenic trioxide poisoning. Hum Exp Toxicol 18:640–641, 1999.

92. Hilfer RJ, Mandel A: Acute arsenic intoxication diagnosed by roentgenograms: Report of a case with survival. N Engl J Med 266:663–664, 1962.

93. Michaux I, Haufroid V, Dive A, et al: Repetitive endoscopy and continuous alkaline gastric irrigation in a case of arsenic poisoning. Clin Toxicol 38:471–476, 2000.

94. Brenard R, Laterre P-F, Reynaert M, et al: Increased hepatocytic mitotic activity as a diagnostic marker of acute arsenic intoxication: A report of two cases. J Hepatol 25:218–230, 1996.

95. Westhoff DD, Samaha RJ, Barnes A Jr: Arsenic intoxication as a cause of megaloblastic anemia. Blood 45:241–246, 1975.

96. Kyle RA, Pease GL: Hematologic aspects of arsenic intoxication. N Engl J Med 273:18–23, 1965.

97. Eichner ER: Erythroid karyorrhexis in the peripheral blood smear in severe arsenic poisoning: A comparison with lead poisoning. Med J Clin Pathol 81:533–537, 1984.

98. Fesmire FM, Schauben JL, Roberge RJ: Survival following massive arsenic ingestion. Am J Emerg Med 6:602–606, 1988.

99. Ohta M: Ultrastructure of sural nerve in a case of arsenical neuropathy. Acta Neuropathol (Berl) 16:233–242, 1970.

100. Le XC, Ma M: Short-column liquid chromatography with hydride generation atomic fluorescence detection for the speciation of arsenic. Anal Chem 70:1926–1933, 1998.

101. Le X-C, Cullen WR, Reimer KJ: Human urinary arsenic excretion after one-time ingestion of seaweed, crab, and shrimp. Clin Chem 40:617–624, 1994.

102. Le XC, Ma M, Yalcin S, et al: Stability of arsenic species in urine. Paper presented at the Third International Conference on Arsenic Exposure and Health Effects, San Diego, CA, July 12–15, 1998.

103. Smith H: The interpretation of the arsenic content of human hair. J Forensic Sci Soc 4:192–199, 1964.

104. Pearson EF, Pounds CA: A case involving the administration of known amounts of arsenic and its analysis in hair. J Forensic Sci Soc 11:229–234, 1971.

105. Henke G, Nucci A, Queiroz LS: Detection of repeated arsenical poisoning by neutron activation analysis of foot nail segments. Arch Toxicol 50:125–131, 1982.

106. Lander H, Hodge PR, Crisp CS: Arsenic in hair and nails—its significance in acute arsenical poisoning. J Forensic Med 12:52–67, 1965.

107. Agency for Toxic Substances and Disease Registry: Hair Analysis Panel Discussion: Exploring the State of the Science. Summary Report. Atlanta, ATSDR, 2001.

108. Goddard MJ, Tanhehco JL, Dau PC: Chronic arsenic poisoning masquerading as Landry-Guillian-Barré syndrome. Electromyogr Clin Neurophysiol 32:419–423, 1992.

109. Pinto SS: Arsine poisoning: Evaluation of the acute phase. J Occup Med 18:633–635, 1976.

110. Apostoli P, Alessio L, Romeo L, et al: Metabolism of arsenic after acute occupational arsine poisoning. J Toxicol Environ Health 52:331–342, 1997.

111. Lee DC, Roberts JR, Kelly JJ, et al: Whole-bowel irrigation as an adjunct in the treatment of radiopaque arsenic. Am J Emerg Med 13:244–245, 1995.

112. Reichl FX, Hunder G, Liebl B, et al: Effect of DMPS and various adsorbents on the arsenic excretion in guinea-pigs after injection with As_2O_3. Arch Toxicol 69:712–717, 1995.

113. Vazari ND, Upham T, Barton CH: Hemodialysis clearance of arsenic. Clin Toxicol 17:451–456, 1980.

114. Smith SB, Wombolt DG, Venkatesan R: Results of hemodialysis and hemoperfusion in the treatment of acute arsenic ingestion. Clin Exp Dial Apher 5:399–404, 1981.

115. Mathieu D, Mathieu-Nolf M, Germain-Alonso M, et al: Massive arsenic poisoning—effect of hemodialysis and dimercaprol on arsenic kinetics. Intensive Care Med 18:47–50, 1992.

116. Wilner C, Low PA: Pharmacological approaches to neuropathic pain. In Dyck PJ (ed): Peripheral Neuropathy. Philadelphia, WB Saunders, 1993, pp 1709–1720.

117. Kosnett MJ: Unanswered questions in metal chelation. Clin Toxicol 30:529–547, 1992.

118. Stocken LA, Thompson RHS: British anti-lewisite: 2. Dithiol compounds as antidotes for arsenic. Biochem J 40:535–548, 1946.
119. Petrunkin VE: Synthesis and properties of dimercapto derivatives of alkylsulfonic acids: 1. Synthesis of sodium 2,3-dimercaptopropylsulfonate (unithiol) and sodium 2-mercaptoethyl-sulfonate. Ukr Khim Zhur 22:603–607, 1956.
120. Liang Y, Chu C, Tsen Y, et al: Studies on antibilharzial drugs: VI. The antidotal effects of sodium dimercaptosuccinate and BAL-glucoside against tartar emetic. Acta Physiol Sin 21:24–32, 1957.
121. Aposhian HV, Carter DE, Hoover TD, et al: DMSA, DMPS, and DMPA—as arsenic antidotes. Fundam Appl Toxicol 4:S58-S70, 1984.
122. Tadlock CH, Aposhian HV: Protection of mice against the lethal effects of sodium arsenite by 2,3 dimercapto-1-propane-sulfonic acid and dimercaptosuccinic acid. Biochem Biophys Res Commun 94:501–507, 1980.
123. Kreppel H, Reichl FX, Szinicz L, et al: Efficacy of various dithiol compounds in acute As$_2$O$_3$ poisoning in mice. Arch Toxicol 64:387–392, 1990.
124. Eagle H, Magnuson HJ, Fleischman R: Clinical uses of 2,3 dimercaptopropanol (BAL): I. The systemic treatment of experimental arsenic poisoning (marphasen, lewisite, phenyl arsenoxide) with BAL. J Clin Invest 25:451–466, 1946.
125. Wexler J, Eagle H, Tatum HJ, et al: Clinical uses of 2,3-dimercaptopropanol (BAL): II. The effect of BAL on the excretion of arsenic in normal subjects and after minimal exposure to arsenical smoke. J Clin Invest 25:467–473, 1946.
126. Jacobziner H, Raybin H: Accidental arsenic poisoning. N Y State J Med 58:1510–1513, 1958.
127. Dawson MA: Arsenic polyneuropathy. Ky Med Assoc 65:761–762, 1967.
128. Wax PM, Thornton CA: Recovery from severe arsenic-induced peripheral neuropathy with 2,3-dimercapto-1-propanesulphonic acid. Clin Toxicol 38:777–780, 2000.
129. Food and Drug Administration: List of drug substances that may be used in pharmacy compounding. Fed Reg 64:996–1003, 1999.
130. Randall RV, Seeler AO: BAL. N Engl J Med 239:1040–1046, 1948.
131. Aposhian HV, Tadlock CH, Moon TE: Protection of mice against the lethal effects of sodium arsenite: A quantitative comparison of a number of chelating agents. Toxicol Appl Pharmacol 61:385–392, 1981.
132. Hoover TD, Aposhian HV: BAL increases the arsenic-74 content of rabbit brain. Toxicol Appl Pharmacol 70:160–162, 1983.
133. Ruprecht J: Dimaval (DMPS): DMPS-Heyl. Scientific Monograph. Berlin, Heyl, 1997.
134. Federal Office for Environmental Protection (Germany): Einsatz von Chelatbildnern in der Umweltmedizin? [Use of chelating agents in environmental medicine?] Bundesgesundheitsbl-Gesundheitsforsch-Gesundheitsschutz 42:823–824, 1999.
135. Kommission B5: Preparatory monographs: Dimercaptopropanesulfonsäure (DMPS). Bundesanzeiger [Germany] Nv. 3, S. 59 v. 5.1, 1991.
136. Maiorino RM, Dart RC, Carter DE, et al: Determination and metabolism of dithiol chelating agents: XII. Metabolism and pharmacokinetics of sodium 2,3-dimercaptopropane-1-sulfonate in humans. J Pharmacol Exp Ther 259:808–814, 1991.
137. Nielsen JB, Andersen O: Effect of four thiol-containing chelators on disposition of orally administered mercuric chloride. Hum Exp Toxicol 10:423–430, 1991.
138. Cremin JD, Luck ML, Laughlin NK, et al: Oral succimer decreases the gastrointestinal absorption of lead in juvenile monkeys. Environ Health Perspect 109:613–619, 2001.
139. Kreppel H, Reichl FX, Forth W, et al: Lack of effectiveness of D-penicillamine in experimental arsenic poisoning. Vet Hum Toxicol 31:1–5, 1989.
140. Guha Mazumder DN, Ghoshal UC, Saha J, et al: Randomized placebo-controlled trial of 2,3-dimercaptosuccinic acid in therapy of chronic arsenicosis due to drinking arsenic-contaminated subsoil water. Clin Toxicol 36:683–690, 1998.
141. Hesdorffer CS, Milne FJ, Terblanche J, et al: Arsine gas poisoning: The importance of exchange transfusion in severe cases. Br J Ind Med 43:353–355, 1986.
142. Romeo L, Apostoli P, Kovacic M, et al: Acute arsine intoxication as a consequence of metal burnishing operations. Am J Ind Med 32:211–216, 1997.
143. Hoontrakoon S, Suputtamongkol Y: Exchange transfusion as an adjunct to the treatment of severe falciparum malaria. Trop Med Intern Health 3:156–161, 1998.
144. Weir EG, King KE, Ness PM, et al: Automated RBC exchange transfusion: Treatment for cerebral malaria. Transfusion 40:702–707, 2000.
145. Graham AF, Crawford TBB, Marrian GF: The action of arsine on blood: Observations on the nature of the fixed arsenic. Biochem J 40:256–260, 1946.
146. Kensler CJ, Abels JC, Rhoads CP: Arsine poisoning, mode of action and treatment. J Pharmacol Exp Ther 88:99–108, 1946.
147. Mizyukova IG, Pretunkin VE, Lysenko NM: Zavisimost' antidotnoi aktivnosti ryada tiolovykh soedinenii ot ikh stroeniya [The relation of antidotal potency of a series of thiol compounds to their structure]. Farmicol I toksikol 1:70–74, 1971.
148. Pinto SS, Petronella SJ, Johns DR, et al: Arsine poisoning: A study of thirteen cases. Arch Ind Hyg Occup Med 1:437–451, 1950.
149. Hood RD, Vedel-Macrander GC, Zaworotko MJ, et al: Distribution, metabolism and fetal uptake of pentavalent arsenic in pregnant mice following oral or intraperitoneal administration. Teratology 35:19–25, 1987.
150. Concha GC, Vogler D, Lezeano D, et al: Exposure to inorganic arsenic metabolites during early human development. Toxicol Sci 44:185–190, 1998.
151. Golub MS, Macintosh MS, Baumrind N: Developmental and reproductive toxicity of inorganic arsenic: Animal studies and human concerns. J Toxicol Environ Health B Crit Rev 1:199–241, 1998.
152. Morrisey RE, Fowler BA, Harris MW, et al: Arsine: Absence of developmental toxicity in rats and mice. Fundam Appl Toxicol 15:350–356, 1990.
153. Hopenhayn-Rich C, Browning SR, Hertz-Picciotto I, et al: Chronic arsenic exposure and risk of infant mortality in two areas of Chile. Environ Health Perspect 108:667–673, 2000.
154. Lugo G, Cassady G, Palmisano P: Acute maternal arsenic intoxication with neonatal death. Am J Dis Child 117:328–330, 1969.
155. Domingo JL, Bosque MA, Piera V: Meso-2,3-dimercaptosuccinic acid and prevention of arsenite embryotoxicity and teratogenicity in the mouse. Fundam Appl Toxicol 17:314–320, 1991.
156. Domingo JL, Bosque MA, Llobet JM, et al: Amelioration by BAL (2,3-dimercapto-1-propanol) and DMPS (sodium 2,3-dimercaptopropanesulfonic acid) of arsenite developmental toxicity in mice. Ecotox Environ Safety 23:274–281, 1992.
157. Domingo JL: Prevention by chelating agents of metal-induced developmental toxicity. Reprod Toxicol 9:105–113, 1995.
158. Domingo JL: Developmental toxicity of metal chelating agents. Reprod Toxicol 12:499–510, 1998.

CHAPTER 77

Cadmium

Jan Meulenbelt

Together with zinc and mercury, cadmium belongs to group IIb of the periodic table. It can be found in rocks, soil, water, coal, zinc ore, lead ore, and copper ore. In the environment, cadmium is present predominantly as the oxide or as the chloride, sulfide or sulfate salt. It has no recognizable taste or odor. The cadmium sulfide, carbonate, and oxide salts are practically insoluble in water, whereas the sulfate, nitrate, and halides are soluble in water.

Cadmium is consumed widely in industry. It is used for the production of glass and metal alloys and many consumer products, such as batteries or pigments in plastics. Exposure to relatively high cadmium concentrations occurs predominantly in the workplace. Workers also can be exposed during welding and soldering. Cadmium oxide is the compound most frequently inhaled.

BIOCHEMISTRY: KINETICS

The major route of cadmium exposure for the nonoccupational setting and nonsmoking persons is via food (e.g., leafy vegetables or potatoes). Normal daily exposure is approximately 30 μg/day, of which about 1 to 3 μg/day is absorbed. In smokers, 2 to 6 μg/day can be absorbed. The smoke of one cigarette contains about 1 to 2 μg of cadmium.

In water, the insoluble salts can be solubilized with changes in pH. Consequently, insoluble cadmium compounds, such as cadmium oxide and carbonate, can dissolve at gastric pH. Iron deficiency increases cadmium absorption, whereas oral zinc supplements decrease its absorption.[1] Approximately 25% of cadmium administered with food is still retained after 3 to 5 days. Retention decreases to approximately 6% after about 20 days.[2,3] Whole-body retention ranges from 1.2% to 7.6% (mean 2.7%).[4]

Depending on the kind of cadmium compound and particle size, 50% of inhaled cadmium can be absorbed. Some authors stated that exposure to relatively more soluble compounds in biologic fluids seems to be relatively more harmful,[5,6] but this was not confirmed by others.[7] The initial lung burden declines slowly after exposure.[6,8,9] Most inhaled or ingested cadmium is excreted in the feces.

Cadmium (+2) ion binds to anionic groups (especially sulfhydryl groups) in proteins (notably albumin and metallothionein).[10] It is absorbed by the intestinal mucosa, after which a cadmium-metallothionein complex is transported to the target organs. Cadmium does not undergo any direct metabolic conversion, such as oxidation, reduction, or alkylation. The cadmium concentrations in most tissues increase with age, especially in the kidneys and liver. Spleen, pancreas, and testis also contain relatively high concentrations after chronic cadmium exposure. After reviewing the literature, Kjellström and Nordberg[11] concluded that cadmium half-life in the kidney is 6 to 38 years (mean approximately 12 years) and in the liver is 4 to 19 years (mean approximately 7.5 years). Placental transfer of cadmium is slow and incomplete.[12]

CLINICAL PRESENTATION

Symptoms After Acute Exposure

Acute intoxication by inhalation of air with high cadmium levels rarely occurs except in cadmium welding, when exposure to high concentrations may cause severe pulmonary damage. During exposure, the symptoms are generally mild (comparable to symptoms seen in metal fume fever, such as cough, dyspnea, chest pain, and fever), but within a few days severe pulmonary edema and pneumonitis can develop, leading to respiratory failure, which can be fatal.[13] The lowest observed adverse effect level necessary in acute exposure to cause serious effects in humans seems to be 10 mg/m³. If a patient recovers from acute cadmium poisoning, the improvement seems to be rapid and complete. Limited data on follow-up after acute exposure are available.

Acute intoxication by ingestion may cause retrosternal pain (caused by esophageal irritation), nausea, vomiting, abdominal cramps, and diarrhea. Shock may be observed, which can be caused by fluid loss or cardiovascular depression or both. Ingestion of more than 150 g should be considered life-threatening.[14,15]

Chronic Exposure

Cortona and colleagues[16] measured respiratory function parameters (forced expiratory volume, forced vital capacity, residual volume, and carbon monoxide diffusion) in 69 smoking and nonsmoking male subjects exposed for years to concentrations of 0.008 to 1.53 mg/m³ of cadmium fumes in a factory producing cadmium alloys. In exposed workers, residual volume was more than 8% higher than in unexposed workers. In severely exposed workers, residual volume was increased by more than 10%.

Lung cancer risk also may be increased after long-term inhalational cadmium exposure. Stayner and coworkers[17] calculated that chronic exposure to 0.10 mg/m^3 cadmium oxide dust or fume 7 days/wk and 8 hr/day may cause 50 to 111 excess lung cancer deaths per 1000 workers.

Eating or inhaling lower levels of cadmium for a long period may cause a high cadmium body burden, which may result in renal damage. The kidney is the main target organ of cadmium toxicity, particularly the proximal tubules. Although intracellular metallothionein is induced by cadmium, offering partial protection, nephrotoxicity may occur at times when this protection is insufficient. Cadmium not bound to metallothionein presumably is responsible for the cadmium-related tissue injury. The mechanism of kidney damage is not fully understood. The lowest observed adverse effect level for chronic inhalational exposure causing renal effects in humans has been reported to be 0.05 to 0.1 mg/m^3, and the no-effect level is 0.02 to 0.05 mg/m^3.[18–21] Proteinuria has been reported at inhalational exposure levels of 0.067 or 0.0379 mg/m^3.[22,23]

There is no convincing evidence that cadmium causes hypertension. There is weak support that increased cadmium body burden may alter central nervous system function as evaluated by neuropsychologic tests.[24] A modest difference was found between cadmium-exposed and nonexposed workers in attention, psychomotor speed, and memory tests.

Cadmium exposure has been shown to alter zinc, iron, and copper metabolism, causing deficiencies of these trace elements.[25] Cadmium also influences selenium metabolism, inducing reduction in the activity of the selenoenzyme glutathione peroxidase.[26]

Cadmium affects calcium metabolism. Painful bone disorders, including osteomalacia, osteoporosis, and spontaneous bone fractures, have been reported in persons chronically exposed to cadmium in food (e.g., itai-itai disease).[27,28] Dietary deficiencies of calcium, protein, and vitamin D are likely to account for increased susceptibility to bone effects after cadmium exposure.[29] Cadmium-exposed people exhibit a progressive disturbance in renal metabolism of vitamin D to its biologically active form.[30–32] Cadmium exposure is associated with risk of renal stones.[33,34] Mason and associates[35] reported decreased renal reabsorption of calcium among cadmium alloy workers. This decreased calcium reabsorption is presumably responsible for the higher risk of renal stones in cadmium-exposed persons.

DIAGNOSIS

Cadmium can be measured in blood, urine, hair, and nails. The blood concentration of cadmium is the best indicator of recent exposure.[36,37] Urinary excretion of cadmium correlates with body burden and renal damage and less to recent exposure.[36,37] Cadmium-exposed persons with proteinuria generally have increased cadmium excretion. The urine cadmium excretion may decrease, however, if renal damage is severe.[12] Hair and nails are less reliable because they can be contaminated easily. Within 1 day after exposure, the cadmium in blood is contained mainly in the red blood cells, and the plasma concentration may be low.[38] Whole-blood cadmium concentrations normally range from 0.4 to 1 μg/L (approximately 4 to 9 nmol/L) for nonsmokers and

1.4 to 4 μg/L (approximately 13 to 36 nmol/L) for smokers.[10] Blood cadmium concentrations of 10 μg/L (approximately 89 nmol/L) are considered acceptable for occupational exposures.[39] The urine concentration is normally less than 1 μg/g of creatinine (approximately 1 nmol/mmol of creatinine).[10] The average urine cadmium concentration is 0.35 μg/g of creatinine (approximately 0.35 nmol/mmol of creatinine) in nonsmokers; levels greater than 2 μg/g of creatinine (approximately 2 nmol/mmol of creatinine) are rare.

Proximal renal tubular damage can be diagnosed by increased concentrations of low-molecular-weight proteins in the urine. The leakage of these proteins is not specific for cadmium toxicity but is a marker of proximal tubular damage. These proteins, such as β$_2$-microglobulin, light-chain immunoglobulins, retinol-binding protein, lysosomal enzyme N-acetyl-β-D-glucosaminidase (NAG), and ribonuclease, are filtered by the glomerulus and normally reabsorbed in the proximal tubules of the kidney. NAG and β$_2$-microglobulin are the most commonly used biomarkers of cadmium-induced proximal tubule injury. Of these, NAG is more sensitive. In severe kidney damage, high-molecular-weight proteins, such as albumin, also can be detected in urine. Decreased reabsorption of amino acids or glucose may be more sensitive for tubular dysfunction than the leakage of low-molecular-weight proteins.

TREATMENT

Acute Exposure

Therapy should begin by removal of the subject from the exposure. There is inadequate documentation on the usefulness of gastrointestinal decontamination in the case of ingestion of cadmium. Activated charcoal has no proven benefit after cadmium exposure. Hemodialysis and hemoperfusion are not useful in the treatment of cadmium intoxication. In cases of severe renal damage, hemodialysis is useful to replace kidney function.

In acute cadmium poisoning, chelating agents, such as ethylenediaminetetraacetic acid, penicillamine, and British antilewisite, have been used, but these seem to be of limited value and may increase kidney burden and damage.[40] Andersen[41,42] reported that 2,3-dimercaptosuccinic acid (DMSA) was effective in acute cadmium poisoning in mice. DMSA and 2,3-dimercapto-1-propane sulfonate (DMPS) were effective in reducing mortality and reducing cadmium burden in liver and kidneys in cadmium-intoxicated mice.[43,44] DMPS is also active intracellularly; DMSA is not. Chelation therapy for acute cadmium exposure may be useful, but this needs to be confirmed in human clinical

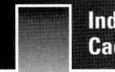

Indications for ICU Admission in Cadmium Poisoning

Acute inhalational exposure—respiratory failure due to pneumonitis or lung edema or both
Chronic exposure—severe metabolic disturbances due to renal failure

practice. Doses of DMSA or DMPS normally used during the chelation of other heavy metals should be used (see Chapters 141 and 142).

Chronic Exposure

The treatment of chronic cadmium poisonings is complicated by the difficulty in evaluating the body burden and the lack of data regarding chelating agents in this setting.[45] At present, chelation generally is not advised for chronic cadmium exposure. DMPS and DMSA may decrease cadmium body burden effectively. It has not been established, however, whether this therapy would decrease cadmium-induced end-organ toxicity.

In chronic cadmium exposure, removal from exposure is of fundamental importance. Adequate occupational hygiene, environmental monitoring, and worker surveillance are important to limit occupational vapor exposure. The American Conference of Governmental Industrial Hygienists time-weighted averaged permissible concentration for cadmium dust in air is 10 μ/m^3 with the respirable fraction limited to 2 μ/m^3.[46] The permissible exposure limits for cadmium, 10 μ/m^3 and 5 μ/m^3, have been established by the U.S. Occupational Safety and Health Administration.[47]

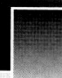

Criteria for ICU Discharge in Cadmium Poisoning

Patient weaned from the mechanical ventilator
Metabolic disorder mainly corrected

Key Points in Cadmium Poisoning

1. Cadmium accumulates in the body.
2. The kidney is the main target organ.
3. Measure whole-blood cadmium concentration to validate acute exposure.
4. Measure urine cadmium concentration to validate chronic exposure and increased body burden.
5. Treatment is primarily supportive.
6. The efficacy of chelation therapy is not proven.
7. In chronic cadmium exposure, be aware of osteomalacia and osteoporosis (itai-itai disease).
8. Chronic cadmium exposure is associated with risk of renal stones.

REFERENCES

1. Flanagan PR, McLellan JS, Haist J, et al: Increased dietary cadmium absorption in mice and human subjects with iron deficiency. Gastroenterology 74:841–846, 1978.
2. Rahola T, Aaran RK, Miettinen JK: Half-time studies of mercury and cadmium by whole-body counting. In: Assessment of Radioactive Contamination in Man. New York, 1972, International Atomic Energy Agency Unipublishers, pp 553–562.
3. Rahola T, Aaran RK, Miettinen JK: Retention and elimination of ^{115m}Cd in man. In: Health Physics Problems of Internal Contamination. Budapest, 1973, Akademia, pp 213–218.
4. Newton D, Johnson P, Lally AE, et al: The uptake by man of cadmium ingested in crab meat. Hum Toxicol 3:23–28, 1984.
5. Klimisch HJ: Lung deposition, lung clearance and renal accumulation of inhaled cadmium chloride and cadmium sulphide in rats. Toxicology 84:103–124, 1993.
6. Rusch GM, O'Grodnick JS, Rinehart WE: Acute inhalation study in rats of comparative uptake, distribution, and excretion for different cadmium containing materials. Am Ind Hyg Assoc 47:754–763, 1986.
7. Glaser U, Kloppel H, Hochrainer D: Bioavailability indicators of inhaled cadmium compounds. Ecotoxicol Environ Saf 11:261–271, 1986.
8. Henderson RF, Rebar AH, Pickrell JA, et al: Early damage indicators in the lung: III. Biochemical and cytological response of the lung to inhaled metal salts. Toxical Appl Pharmacol 50:123–136, 1979.
9. Moore W, Stara JF, Crocker WC, et al: Comparison of ^{115m}Cd retention in rats following different routes of administration. Environ Res 6:473–478, 1973.
10. Friberg L, Elinder CG, Kjellström T, Nordberg GF (eds): Cadmium and Health: A Toxicological and Epidemiological Appraisal, Vol I: Exposure, Dose, and Metabolism. Boca Raton, FL, CRC Press, 1985.
11. Kjellström T, Nordberg GF: A kinetic model of cadmium metabolism in the human being. Environ Res 16:248–269, 1978.
12. IPCS Environmental Health Criteria 134. Geneva, World Health Organization, 1992.
13. Beton DC, Andrews GS, Davies HJ, et al: Acute cadmium fume poisoning: Five cases with one death from renal necrosis. Br J Ind Med 23:292–301, 1966.
14. Bernard AM, Lauwerys R: Cadmium in human population. Experimenta 40:143–152, 1984.
15. Buckler HM, Smith WD, Rees WD: Self poisoning with oral cadmium chloride. BMJ 292:1559–1560, 1986.
16. Cortona G, Apostoli P, Toffoletto F, et al: Occupational exposure to cadmium and lung function. IARC Sci Publ 118:205–210, 1992.
17. Stayner L, Smith R, Thun M, et al: A dose-response analysis and quantitative assessment of lung cancer risk and occupational cadmium exposure. Ann Epidemiol 2:177–194, 1992.
18. EPA: 40 CFR261.31: Hazardous Wastes from Non-specific Sources. Washington, DC, Environmental Protection Agency, 1999.
19. EPA: 40 CFR261.32: Hazardous Wastes from Specific Sources. Washington, DC, Environmental Protection Agency, 1999.
20. EPA: 40 CFR261.33: Discarded Commercial Chemical Products, Off-Specification Species, Container Residues, and Spill Residues Thereof. Washington, DC, Environmental Protection Agency, 1999.
21. EPA: 40 CFR302.4: Designation, Reportable Quantities, and Notification: List of Hazardous Substances and Reportable Quantities. Washington, DC, Environmental Protection Agency, 1999.
22. Elinder CG, Edling C, Lindberg E, et al: β_2-Microglobulinuria among workers previously exposed to cadmium: Follow-up and dose-response analyses. Am J Ind Med 8:553–564, 1985.
23. Falck FY, Fine LJ, Smith RG, et al: Occupational cadmium exposure and renal status. Am J Ind Med 4:541–549, 1983.
24. Hart RP, Rose CS, Hamer RM: Neuropsychological effects of occupational exposure to cadmium. J Clin Exp Neuropsychol 11:933–943, 1989.
25. Petering HG, Choudhury H, Stemmer KL: Some effects of oral ingestion of cadmium on zinc, copper, and iron metabolism. Environ Health Perspect 28:97–106, 1979.
26. Jamall IS, Smith JC: Effects of cadmium treatment on selenium-dependent and selenium-independent glutathione peroxidase activities and lipid peroxidation in the kidney and liver of rats maintained on various levels of dietary selenium. Arch Toxicol 58:102–105, 1985.
27. Shigematsu I: The epidemiological approach to cadmium pollution in Japan. Ann Acad Med Singapore 13:231–236, 1984.
28. Kido T, Nogawa K, Yamada Y, et al: Osteopenia in inhabitants with renal dysfunction induced by exposure to environmental cadmium. Int Arch Occup Environ Health 61:271–276, 1989.
29. Kjellström T: Effects on bone, on vitamin D, and calcium metabolism. In Friberg L, Elinder CG, Kjellström T, Nordberg GF (eds): Cadmium and Health: A Toxicological and Epidemiological Appraisal, Vol II: Effects and Response. Boca Raton, FL, CRC Press, 1986, pp 111–158.
30. Nogawa K, Tsuritani I, Kido T, et al: Mechanism for bone disease found in inhabitants environmentally exposed to cadmium: Decreased serum α_1,25-dihydroxyvitamin D level. Int Arch Occup Environ Health 59:21–30, 1987.

31. Nogawa K, Tsuritani I, Kido T, et al: Serum vitamin D metabolites in cadmium-exposed persons with renal damage. Int Arch Occup Environ Health 62:189–193, 1990.

32. Buchet JP, Lauwerys R, Roels H, et al: Renal effects of cadmium body burden of the general population. Lancet 336:699–702, 1990.

33. Adams RG, Harrison JF, Scott P: The development of cadmium-induced proteinuria, impaired renal function, and osteomalacia in alkaline battery workers. QJM 38:425–443, 1969.

34. Thun MJ, Osorio AM, Schober S, et al: Nephropathy in cadmium workers—assessment of risk from airborne occupational cadmium exposure. Br J Ind Med 46:689–697, 1989.

35. Mason HJ, Davison HG, Wright AL, et al: Relations between liver cadmium, cumulative exposure, and renal function in cadmium alloy workers. Br J Ind Med 45:793–802, 1988.

36. Lauwerys R, Roels H, Regniers M, et al: Significance of cadmium concentration in blood and in urine in workers exposed to cadmium. Environ Res 20:375–391, 1979.

37. Lauwerys RR, Bernard AM, Roels HA, et al: Cadmium: Exposure markers as predictors of nephrotoxic effects. Clin Chem 40:1391–1394, 1994.

38. Nordberg GF, Kjellström T, Nordberg M: Kinetics and metabolism. In Friberg L, Elinder CG, Kjellström T, Nordberg GF (eds): Cadmium and Health: A Toxicological and Epidemiological Appraisal, Vol I: Exposure, Dose, and Metabolism. Boca Raton, FL, CRC Press, 1985, pp 103–178.

39. WHO: Recommended Health-Based Limits in Occupational Exposure to Heavy Metals. Technical Report Series No. 647. Geneva, World Health Organization, 1980.

40. Klaassen CD, Waalkes MP, Cantilena LR: Alteration of tissue disposition of cadmium by chelating agents. Environ Health Perspect 54:233–242, 1984.

41. Andersen O: Oral cadmium exposure in mice: Toxicokinetics and efficiency of chelating agents. Crit Rev Toxicol 20:83–112, 1989.

42. Andersen O: Choice of chelating antidotes for acute cadmium intoxication. Toxicol Environ Chem 23:105–120, 1989.

43. Basinger MA, Jones MM, Holscher MA, et al: Antagonists for acute oral cadmium chloride intoxication. J Toxicol Environ Health 23:77–89, 1988.

44. Srivastava RC, Gupta S, Ahmad N, et al: Comparative evaluation of chelating agents on the mobilization of cadmium: A mechanistic approach. Toxicol Environ Health 47:173–182, 1996.

45. Jones MM, Cherian MG: The search for chelate antagonist for chronic cadmium intoxication. Toxicology 62:1–25, 1990.

46. American Conference of Governmental and Industrial Hygiene (ACGIH): Threshold Limit Values for Chemical Substances and Physical Agents, Biological Exposure Indices. Cincinnati, ACGIH, 2000.

47. Occupational Safety and Health Administration: 29 CFR 1910.1027(c), 1992.

CHAPTER 78

Lead

Michael J. Kosnett

Lead poisoning is one of the oldest intoxications known to medicine. The ancient Greek physician Galen warned that consumption of water transported through lead pipes rendered individuals "subject to disorders in the intestines."[1] In 200 BC, Nikander of Colophon wrote that exposure to the lead oxide litharge could cause "deadly disturbances of the bowels, which, attacking with pains unexpected, overpower mankind."[2] More than 2 millennia later, lead poisoning continues to be a major issue in environmental and occupational health. Although reductions in high-dose exposure have shifted the focus of public health concern to the effects of chronic low-dose exposure, overt, symptomatic lead intoxication continues to arise in a diversity of settings. In industry, it occurs predominantly in tasks associated with high-level exposure to lead dust or fume, such as welding or torch cutting of painted metal during construction or demolition, grinding or sandblasting of lead-coated surfaces, smelting or refining of lead ores or scrap metal, repair of automotive radiators, use of powdered lead additives in fabrication of plastic, and manufacturing or recycling of lead storage batteries.[3] In environmental settings, high-dose lead exposure may result from use of oral folk remedies or tonics that contain large amounts of lead (e.g., azarcon, greta, paylooah), consumption of illicitly distilled alcohol (moonshine), pica ingestion by children of lead-contaminated paint chips or lead objects, and consumption of food or beverages prepared or stored in lead-glazed ceramics or lead-containing vessels. Fatal lead encephalopathy has resulted from the partial dissolution of retained lead bullets or shotgun pellets.[4] This process occurs primarily when the bullet, pellet, or lead fragment has lodged in or migrated to or is adjacent to a joint space or pseudocyst.

CHEMISTRY AND PHARMACOKINETICS

Lead is a soft, ductile, heavy metal that is obtained from the primary smelting of lead-containing ores, such as galena (lead sulfide) or cerusite ($PbCO_3$), or from the secondary smelting of recycled lead scrap. The potential for lead intoxication is highest after inhalation or ingestion of lead that is in a soluble and readily absorbable form. These forms include fume, particulate, and glaze composed of lead oxides (litharge, red lead [Pb_3O_4]); dust or particulate composed of basic lead carbonate (white lead [$Pb(OH)_2 \cdot 2PbCO_3$]), lead sulfate, or lead acetate; and solutions containing dissolved lead cations. Lead products of lower solubility, such as elemental lead, lead chromate, or lead sulfide, pose less acute risk but still may result in toxicity if the absorbed dose is high or if factors such as fine particle size, prolonged gut retention, or intraarticular contact promote in vivo dissolution. Organolead compounds, such as the oily liquid tetraethyl lead used as a fuel additive, are slightly soluble in water but are well absorbed by dermal, oral, and inhalational routes.

Pharmacokinetics of Inorganic Lead

Volume of Distribution

Because of the affinity of lead for proteins in the erythrocyte, the initial volume of distribution of lead is low. After intravenous injection of a lead isotope to human volunteers, approximately 70% to 80% of the dose is present in whole blood at 7 hours, and approximately 24% remains in whole blood at 20 days.[5–7] This time-dependent intravascular retention corresponds to a volume of distribution of 0.1 to 0.2 L/kg. With the passage of time, lead that is not excreted is redistributed predominantly to bone. Toxicokinetic studies in humans consuming stable lead isotopes over a period of months indicated that approximately 1% of lead is found in blood,[8] which is consistent with a final volume of distribution of approximately 7 L/kg.

Protein Binding

At low-to-moderate concentrations of lead in whole blood, >99% of the lead is associated with the erythrocyte. The fraction of lead in the plasma increases nonlinearly with dose and may reach a few percentage points as whole-blood lead concentrations become >80 to 100 μg/dL (>3.9 to 4.8 μmol/L).[9,10] The polymorphic enzyme δ-aminolevulinic acid dehydratase is the principal binding site for erythrocyte lead,[10] and genetic polymorphisms in δ-aminolevulinic acid dehydratase seem to influence the toxicokinetics of lead and susceptibility to its toxic effects.[11,12] Most plasma lead is protein bound, and only approximately 15% of the plasma lead is ultrafilterable.[13]

Mechanisms of Clearance

Approximately 70% of total lead clearance occurs through the urine, with the balance excreted mostly in the feces and to a minor extent in sweat, hair, and nails.[8,13,14] Clearance from the blood is greater after acute exposure than with chronic exposure; in both cases, clearance increases exponentially with increasing blood lead concentration. After chronic exposure, urinary clearance of lead from the blood of adults has ranged

continued

Pharmacokinetics of Inorganic Lead *continued*

from approximately 0.08 L/day at low blood lead concentrations to 0.3 L/day at high blood lead concentrations.[13] The overall temporal pattern of decline in blood lead concentration after removal from chronic lead exposure may be characterized by a multicompartment kinetic model, composed predominantly of a fast compartment in the blood and soft tissues (half-time 1 to 2 months) and slower compartments in the skeleton (half-times of years to decades).

Active Metabolites

There are no known active metabolites.

Methods to Enhance Clearance

In lead-poisoned patients, chelation initially may increase the rate of daily urinary lead excretion by 20-fold to 50-fold. There is no role for enhancement of clearance by extracorporeal methods in patients with intact renal function. In patients with severe renal insufficiency, clearance may be increased by calcium EDTA chelation combined with hemofiltration or dialysis (see text).

PATHOPHYSIOLOGY

Lead exerts a wide range of toxic effects involving multiple organ systems. The expression of lead toxicity is influenced by several factors, including the tempo and magnitude of the dose; the target organ; and the nutritional, genetic, and developmental characteristics of the host. On a biochemical level, many of the key effects of lead are mediated by interference with essential cations, particularly calcium, and interaction with enzymes and other proteins. Lead mimics or inhibits multiple cellular actions of calcium and alters calcium flux across membranes, ultimately increasing levels of cytoplasmic calcium in many cell types.[15,16] Increases in intracellular calcium in cerebrovascular endothelium may disturb microfilaments or other cellular components responsible for the integrity of tight junctions and contribute to cerebral edema.[17] Damage to brain capillaries and interstitial edema of white matter, particularly in the cerebellum, are a histopathologic feature of lead encephalopathy.[18,19] The increased susceptibility of juvenile animals to lead encephalopathy may be in part a consequence of the diminished ability of immature brain astrocytes to sequester lead.[20]

Lead's interaction with calcium flux seems partly responsible for its myriad effects on central and peripheral neurotransmission.[15] Alterations in synaptic transmission at the neuromuscular junction of visceral smooth muscle may underlie the disordered intestinal motility and tone that occurs during lead colic.[21,22] At low concentrations, lead can substitute for calcium in the activation of protein kinase C, which contributes to lead's amplification of glutamate-induced oxidative stress in the brain and other tissues.[23] In some neuronal cells, lead interacts with calcium-sensitive mitochondrial permeability transition pores, which results in mitochondrial depolarization and the initiation of the cytochrome-*c*–caspase cascade of apoptosis.[24]

Lead's disruption of mitochondrial membranes also may contribute to the diminished incorporation of iron into protoporphyrin IX, which is a feature of lead-induced anemia. Lead interferes with the action of enzymes and other proteins through its affinity for diverse biochemical ligands, including sulfhydryl, phosphate, and carboxyl groups. It may alter the conformation of the zinc finger motifs that are integral to the function of many DNA binding proteins, enzymes, and receptors.[25] Lead avidly binds to and inhibits the heme synthesis enzyme δ-aminolevulinic acid dehydratase. This action not only contributes to deficits in heme synthesis but also results in accumulation of heme precursors, such as aminolevulinic acid, that may have direct or indirect neurotoxic properties.[26] Lead's ability to be a potent agonist of calcium in its activation of calmodulin and protein kinase C affects multiple aspects of signal transduction. The potential for numerous additional biochemical modes of action has been documented and is the subject of ongoing research investigations. The complex interplay of these effects, which range from subtle alterations in cell signaling to overt cytotoxicity, are paralleled by the diverse manifestations of human lead intoxication.

CLINICAL PRESENTATION AND LIFE-THREATENING COMPLICATIONS

The adverse health effects of lead include a broad spectrum of multisystemic effects, ranging from subclinical impacts on cognitive and cardiovascular function to overt, life-threatening clinical presentations. This chapter focuses on the manifestations of lead poisoning that always require acute, inpatient medical care: *lead encephalopathy* and *lead colic*. These conditions are associated with high-dose lead exposure and blood lead concentrations that usually are greater than 80 to 100 μg/L (>3.9 to 4.8 μmol/L). As a result of preventive public health measures, these severe effects are now a relatively rare presentation of lead intoxication.

Lead Encephalopathy

Lead encephalopathy is a potentially life-threatening disturbance of central nervous system function associated with an altered sensorium, ataxia or incoordination, seizures, and coma. Because lead encephalopathy usually occurs in the context of recurrent lead exposure and a progressive increase in blood lead concentration, it often is preceded by several weeks or more of prodromal neurologic and constitutional symptoms, including severe headache, fatigue, sleep disturbance, anorexia, irritability, or loss of libido. Although rare, lead encephalopathy may occur after a single high-dose lead exposure.[27] An altered level of consciousness, which is expressed variably as delirium, hallucinations, lethargy, or stupor, may follow abruptly the prodromal symptoms. Isolated or recurrent seizures are common, affecting three quarters of the subjects in one survey.[28] Generalized seizures are most typical, but focal motor seizures also may occur. In some cases, convulsions may precede any evidence of an altered sensorium. Delirium, when it occurs, may persist or intensify over days to a week, even after the patient has been removed from lead exposure. Rarely the encephalopathic patient may lapse into a coma, and death may occur in the setting of progressive cerebral edema and increased intracranial pressure.

In children exposed acutely or recurrently to large doses of lead, the appearance of lead encephalopathy usually is preceded by 1 or more weeks of antecedent symptoms, which may include headache, lethargy, anorexia, vomiting, clumsiness, ataxia, and gait disturbance. In incipient cases, there may be evidence of a recent decline in visual acuity, and rarely reversible blindness has occurred in children and adults.[29,30] In all age groups, the classic lead-related gastrointestinal effects of colic (see later) and constipation do not always precede or accompany the emergence of even florid encephalopathy.[31,32]

The neurologic examination in lead encephalopathy is variable. Despite presentation with an altered sensorium or a history of recent convulsions, the patient may have no apparent neurologic deficits at the time of examination. In other cases, a wide variety of positive findings may be present. Reports have noted hyporeflexia and flaccidity[33,34] and hyperreflexia and hypertonia.[35-37] When present, ataxia frequently has been characterized as central or truncal, and an unsteady gait occasionally may be a prominent feature.[38,39] In a few cases, there may be lateralizing findings, such as hemiparesis.[28,40-43] There may be recent-onset strabismus, and cranial nerve palsies affecting the third or sixth cranial nerves have been noted, usually in conjunction with evidence of increased intracranial pressure.[32,33,35,42,44] Facial nerve (cranial nerve VII) palsy also may occur.[33,43,45] Papilledema, with or without retinal hemorrhages, was a rare finding in a series of adults with lead encephalopathy, most of whom survived.[28] Papilledema was more common with fatal lead encephalopathy in children,[40] but overall it is a finding with low sensitivity and negative predictive value. Bulging and tense anterior fontanelles may be present on physical examination of infants with lead-induced cerebral edema and elevated intracranial pressure.

Lead Colic

Although lead colic is not life-threatening, it causes severe abdominal pain and usually warrants intensive care for prompt parenteral chelation, pain control, and monitoring for the possible development of lead encephalopathy. Painful lead colic generally emerges in patients with blood lead concentrations greater than 80 μg/dL (>3.9 μmol/L). Milder, nonspecific gastrointestinal discomfort and constipation may appear at blood lead concentrations greater than 60 μg/dL (>2.9 μmol/L) in some individuals. The clinical presentation of lead colic was described extensively by Tanquerel des Planches and Dana,[46] who attended to 1217 cases of this disorder over 8 years. More than a century and half since its publication, Tanquerel des Planches' classic treatise on lead diseases remains unparalleled for the detail of its bedside observations and the extent of the case material. Tanquerel des Planches[46] observed the following:

This colic pain generally consists of a violent twisting sensation. In other cases less numerous it is an acute feeling of dilacerations, tearing out, pricking, burning, boring. Sometimes this increase of sensibility is compared by the patient to a simple constriction, or rather compression, produced by a weight upon the abdomen. In this last case the abdominal pains are generally obtuse, and their progress continues to be nearly uniform. In all other cases the pain is so intense that it throws the patient into the greatest agitation,

but then it is not always the same; it becomes more severe by fits, either by day or by night.

As noted further by Tanquerel des Planches[46] and other experienced observers,[47] the paroxysms of pain last minutes to hours and may recur at widely variable intervals, ranging from minutes to days. The pain typically is midline but may shift superiorly or inferiorly between bouts. Obstinate constipation almost always is present (>90% of cases), often resulting in a cessation of bowel movements for several days. Rarely a patient either may maintain a normal bowel pattern or may experience diarrhea. As observed by Tanquerel des Planches,[46] the abdomen is retracted in approximately half of cases of active colic, and in approximately two thirds of affected patients the pain is diminished by application of external pressure or palpation. Patients frequently press on their abdomens with both hands or shift to a prone position in a restless attempt to obtain relief. Abdominal tenderness to palpation occurs but is rare. Borborygmus was noted in three fourths of Tanquerel des Planches' cases, and vomiting occurred in one third. Despite the pain, the pulse is notably slow. The heart rate ranged from 30 to 60 beats/min in approximately 55% of the painful episodes observed by Tanquerel des Planches.[46] Blood pressure may be increased. Fever usually is absent. Although patients may be distraught and distracted by the intense pain, their sensorium usually is intact.

Other Clinical Features in Overt Lead Intoxication

Additional lead-induced medical problems may complicate the clinical presentation of lead encephalopathy or lead colic but seldom are the sole basis for inpatient medical attention. High-dose lead exposure that is chronic, but occasionally acute, may result in a predominantly *motor* polyneuropathy. Overtly affected individuals usually have blood lead concentrations greater than 80 to 100 μg/dL (>3.9 to 4.8 μmol/L). The classic presentation begins with weakness of the extensors of the fingers and wrists (wristdrop), but variants that primarily involve the extensors of the toes and feet or the shoulder girdle also may occur.[47,48] In chronic cases, there may be antecedent tremor. Patients with advanced neuropathy may note decreased sensation, but painful dysesthesias are absent. Patients with months to years of blood lead concentrations greater than 80 to 100 μg/dL (>3.9 to 4.8 μmol/L) may become emaciated and cachectic.

Rarely, jaundice may develop after acute or subacute high-dose exposure,[47,49-51] usually in association with hemolysis and indirect hyperbilirubinemia. Tanquerel des Planches[46] described the jaundice caused by heavy lead exposure to be an "earthy yellow" that was less green and bright than "common jaundice," which he presumably associated with infectious hepatitis.

In patients with poor oral hygiene, hydrogen sulfide released by the action of oral microbes present in the gingival sulcus may react with lead in the gingival circulation to form lead sulfide.[52] This precipitate may appear as a darkly pigmented blue-gray line a few millimeters wide at the gingival margins. Although the presence of a gingival "lead line" sometimes may provide a useful clue to the presence of lead poisoning, it has low sensitivity as a diagnostic finding.

Patients with chronic elevation of blood lead concentrations greater than 40 to 50 μg/dL (>1.9 to 2.4 μmol/L) may complain of prominent arthralgias and myalgias without evidence of localized synovitis or tenderness.[53,54] Lead-induced chronic renal insufficiency is associated with an increased risk of gout and gouty arthritis, a consequence of decreased renal clearance of uric acid.[55–57] As noted further subsequently, laboratory tests in a patient with overt lead poisoning frequently reveal hematologic abnormalities and less commonly renal dysfunction. Problems associated with lower-dose lead exposure, such as a history of hypertension, neuropsychologic dysfunction, developmental delay, and adverse reproductive outcome, also may be present in a patient who presents with lead colic or lead encephalopathy.

DIAGNOSIS

Rapid, Nonspecific Diagnostic Tests

Several readily available laboratory and radiographic tests can assist in the diagnosis of overt lead intoxication. Patients with lead encephalopathy or lead colic usually have evidence of anemia on the complete blood count. The anemia may be a consequence of hemolysis associated with acute or subacute high-dose exposure,[49,51] but more commonly there is the gradual onset of a hypochromic anemia with normocytic or microcytic indices. The microcytosis often may be related to coexistent iron deficiency.[58] Iron deficiency acts synergistically with lead in depressing heme synthesis,[59] and it may increase the risk of lead intoxication by enhancing gastrointestinal lead absorption.[60] Examination of the peripheral blood smear may reveal erythrocytes with basophilic stippling. The stippling is due to aggregation of ribosomal fragments in the maturing erythrocyte, possibly as a consequence of lead-induced inhibition of ribonuclease activity.[61] Basophilic stippling has been found within 3 to 4 days of acute, high-dose lead exposure,[62,63] and it may precede the appearance of anemia.[27,64] The number of stippled cells sometimes increases steeply within 1 to 3 days after the onset of lead colic.[64] Although basophilic stippling of erythrocytes may serve as an important diagnostic clue to the presence of lead intoxication, it is neither a sensitive nor a specific finding. It also can occur in other illnesses associated with hematologic effects, including arsenic poisoning, benzene exposure, thalassemia, and certain types of cancer.

Reticulocytosis is another hematologic finding that frequently but not invariably is present in patients with lead-induced anemia. Bone marrow examination may reveal either erythroid hyperplasia or hypoplasia, depending on whether the predominant hematologic impact has been hemolysis or suppression of erythropoiesis.[65] An increase in marrow ringed sideroblasts also may be observed. In adults, anemia due to lead exposure generally emerges at blood lead concentrations greater than 50 to 60 µg/dL (>2.4 to 2.9 µmol/L), but in children an increased prevalence of anemia has been found with blood lead concentrations greater than 25 µg/dL (>1.2 µmol/L).[66,67]

Other common, rapidly available laboratory tests are affected less consistently by overt lead intoxication. Transitory azotemia, possibly a consequence of intrarenal vasoconstriction, may accompany lead colic.[51,68] This condition causes moderate increases in blood urea nitrogen and serum

creatinine that typically resolve within 1 month or less. The urine transiently might reveal increased cellularity on urinalysis,[62,68] but it is often entirely normal.[69] Children with high-dose lead exposure may develop a reversible Fanconi syndrome characterized by aminoaciduria, glycosuria, and hypophosphatemia with relative hyperphosphaturia.[70] This tubular effect usually is not accompanied, however, by diminished glomerular filtration rate or overt renal insufficiency. The reversible renal abnormalities of acute or subacute lead intoxication should be distinguished from the irreversible interstitial and peritubular fibrosis of chronic lead nephropathy, a relatively rare condition that may appear after years of high-dose lead exposure (i.e., blood lead concentrations >80 µg/dL [>3.9 µmol/L]).[71]

Liver function tests in severe lead intoxication may be notable for mild-to-moderate elevations in serum transaminases.[51,61] The rare elevation in total bilirubin is usually a result of hemolysis, in which case the indirect (unconjugated) bilirubin fraction predominates.

The characteristic features of lumbar puncture in patients with lead encephalopathy are an elevated opening pressure, often greater than 300 mm H_2O, and an increased cerebrospinal fluid (CSF) protein count.[28,44] The CSF white blood cell count may be normal or slightly elevated (usually <30 white blood cells/high-power field), resulting in a mild albuminocytologic dissociation.

Several radiologic studies may be helpful in the diagnosis and management of overt lead intoxication. In patients with lead encephalopathy, computed tomography or magnetic resonance imaging of the brain frequently shows evidence of diffuse cerebral edema (e.g., effacement of the cerebral gyri or symmetrically narrowed ventricles). Other, less common findings include focal cerebellar edema,[34] which may cause compression of the fourth ventricle, and obstructive hydrocephalus.[35,37] Asymmetric compression of a lateral ventricle has also been shown.[72]

In children with a history of severe lead intoxication, plain radiographs of the skeleton may reveal dense, thick, transverse opacities at the metaphyseal ends of the bones. Commonly referred to as *radiographic lead lines*, these usually are best visualized at the ends of long bones, such as the tibia, fibula, femur, humerus, radius, or ulna. Lead lines also may be apparent at the iliac crests or the tips of the scapulae.[73] The opacities are not collections of "lead," but rather are bands of increased calcium deposition associated with lead-induced inhibition of calcified cartilage resorption. Although predominantly observed in children 2 to 6 years old,[74] radiographic lead lines also may be visible in neonates and infants.[37,75] Discrete lead lines migrate toward the diaphysis and eventually disappear as the child grows. They are not useful as markers of lead exposure in older children or adults. In one survey of 104 lead-poisoned children and 18 age-matched controls, the mean blood lead concentration of the children with lead lines was 49 ± 17.3 µg/dL (2.4 ± 0.8 µmol/L).[76] The authors of the survey suggested that the presence of a dense opacity in the proximal fibula may be helpful in distinguishing lead lines from bands that occur in physiologic sclerosis, particularly in children older than 3 years of age. Lead lines may be absent in patients with severe childhood lead intoxication, particularly in the setting of recent, acute exposure. In addition, lead lines do not form at low levels of lead exposure that nonetheless may be of public health concern. Accordingly, radiographic lead lines should not be used to screen for or rule out childhood lead poisoning. Lead lines should increase the index of suspicion for lead poisoning, however, in a child with consistent signs and symptoms and should prompt an investigation for potential lead exposure whenever they are observed as an incidental finding.

Plain radiographs of the abdomen may reveal flecks of a radiopaque substance, or discrete lead-containing foreign bodies (e.g., fishing weights), in the gastrointestinal tract of children or adults who recently have ingested substantial amounts of lead.[63,73,77] Because finely suspended or highly soluble lead formulations may be poorly visualized, however, or because the nonabsorbed portion of the ingested lead may have been evacuated by the time of the examination, the absence of suspicious radiopacities on abdominal radiographs does not rule out a significant recent ingestion. In patients with acute lead colic, abdominal x-rays may reveal focal intestinal dilation.[22,78]

Blood Lead Concentration

The blood lead concentration is the most specific and useful diagnostic test for lead intoxication. Because greater than 95% of the lead in blood occurs in the erythrocyte, the measurement is conducted on whole blood rather than serum or plasma. Blood intended for clinical evaluation of potential lead intoxication should be collected in a special trace metal evacuated tube (e.g., royal blue top in the United States) containing a small amount of ethylenediaminetetraacetic acid (EDTA) or heparin as an anticoagulant. In situations in which such a tube is unavailable, blood collected in a standard complete blood count tube (e.g., lavender top in the United States) still may yield useful information. In adults, the blood lead concentration in lead encephalopathy almost always is greater than 100 μg/dL (>4.8 μmol/L), and it is common for such cases to present first with levels greater than 150 μg/dL (>7.2 μmol/L). Children are more vulnerable to the central nervous system toxicity of lead, and blood lead concentrations greater than 70 μg/dL (>3.3 μmol/L) are considered to pose a risk of encephalopathy.[79] The mean blood lead concentration was 330 μg/dL (15.9 μmol/L) among a large series of children treated for lead encephalopathy in Baltimore between 1931 and 1970 (approximate range 90 to 800 μg/dL [4.3 to 38.6 μmol/L]).[80,81] The mean blood lead concentration of children who died as a result of lead poisoning in that series was nearly the same (327 μg/dL [15.6 μmol/L]). Lead colic in adults usually occurs at blood lead concentrations greater than 80 μg/dL (>3.9 μmol/L).

The time interval between the acquisition of an elevated blood lead concentration and the manifestation of overt symptoms is highly variable and depends in part on the tempo and intensity of the exposure and individual host factors. Exposure to massive doses of lead, which may occur with intentional oral overdose[62,82] or parenteral injection,[83] may produce overt gastrointestinal or neurologic symptoms in a few hours. Individuals with acute, high-dose inhalational exposure to lead fume or dust have developed symptoms within a few days to a week.[27,49] In one individual who ingested multiple metallic objects, there was a documented lag time of at least 8 days between a blood lead concentration of 436 μg/dL (21.1 μmol/L) and the development of

lead encephalopathy.[48] In most cases, a patient with severe lead intoxication has been exposed to lead repeatedly over weeks to months or longer. Accordingly, most of the data linking a given blood lead concentration to a particular constellation of signs and symptoms have been derived from studies or cases in which the presumed exposure occurred in a chronic, subacute, or acute-on-chronic pattern.

The geometric mean blood lead concentration in the United States from 1999 to 2000 was estimated to be 1.66 μg/dL (0.08 μmol/L) (95% confidence interval 1.58 to 1.73 μg/dL).[84] This represents an approximately 87% decline from the late 1970s, when the corresponding value was 12.8 μg/dL (0.6 μmol/L).[85] In 1991, the U.S. Centers for Disease Control and Prevention recommended that a blood lead concentration of 10 μg/dL (0.5 μmol/L) be considered a level of concern for children, based on the risk of adverse neurocognitive or neurobehavioral effects. A more recent study found subclinical neurocognitive effects in children at lower blood lead concentrations,[86] however, prompting a call for downward revision of the 1991 Centers for Disease Control recommendation.

In all age groups, the magnitude of lead exposure and the concentration of lead in blood associated with the onset of symptomatic lead intoxication are characterized by a wide range of interindividual variability. The clinical presentation of a symptomatic patient with a high blood lead concentration is highly variable; some patients exhibit severe lead colic without any evidence of encephalopathy, whereas others with comparable blood lead levels may present with delirium and seizures without any history of gastrointestinal symptoms. A rare adult or pediatric patient may be asymptomatic despite blood lead concentrations greater than 100 μg/dL (>4.8 μmol/L).[81] This wide interindividual variability applies to the entire scope of lead-related pathology, including constitutional, neuropsychologic, and cardiovascular effects that may occur at lower exposure levels. The biologic basis for the variability in response is poorly understood but might relate in part to polymorphisms in endogenous lead binding proteins and other genetic factors.[11]

Zinc Protoporphyrin and Other Indices of Lead Exposure

Lead inhibits the formation of heme by several mechanisms, including interference in the incorporation of reduced (ferrous) iron into protoporphyrin IX.[87] Zinc becomes incorporated into this precursor molecule instead, resulting in an accumulation of zinc protoporphyrin (ZPP) in developing erythrocytes. As erythrocytes with a normal concentration of heme disappear through senescence or hemolysis, there is a progressive increase in the blood concentration of ZPP, or the ratio of ZPP to erythrocyte heme. In general, an elevation in ZPP greater than background levels becomes detectable within 2 to 6 weeks after the blood lead concentration becomes greater than 30 μg/dL (>1.4 μmol/L). This lag time may provide information on the likely time course of a patient's lead exposure. A high blood lead concentration in the presence of a normal ZPP suggests that the lead exposure began recently. Conversely, a high blood lead concentration with an elevated ZPP suggests that the lead exposure began more than 2 weeks ago, provided that the patient does not have another medical condition (e.g., iron deficiency or anemia of chronic disease) that also can elevate ZPP.

Measurement of the amount of lead excreted in the urine in the first 24 hours after initiation of chelation (see later) may provide reassurance that a significant amount of lead has been mobilized, but as a practical matter, diagnostic and management decisions should be guided primarily by the blood lead concentration. A qualitative urine "heavy metal screen" offered by some laboratories frequently is subject to false-negative results and should never be relied on to rule out lead poisoning.[4] Chelation challenge or provocation tests that measure the urinary excretion of lead after a single dose of a chelating agent, such as calcium EDTA, do not reliably reflect the major body burden of lead found in the skeleton or a patient's long-term cumulative lead exposure.[88–90] At present, chelation challenge tests have not been validated as a means to identify patients who might derive therapeutic benefit from chelation. Measurement of lead in bone by noninvasive x-ray fluorescence may be a useful biomarker of a patient's long-term lead exposure, but it is not a tool for acute assessment.

Key Diagnostic Features and Differential Diagnosis

Lead encephalopathy should be considered in the differential diagnosis of patients who present with delirium or seizures and anemia. The coexistence of abdominal pain, constipation, and anemia should suggest the potential presence of lead colic. For both conditions, a history of antecedent constitutional or neurobehavioral symptoms (e.g., fatigue, lethargy, anorexia, irritability, myalgias, or headache) increases the index of suspicion. Less commonly, there may be a concurrent history of ataxia, motor neuropathy, developmental delay (in children), or renal insufficiency or gout (in adults). Basophilic stippling of erythrocytes, a gingival lead line, and (in children) the presence of radiographic lead lines on the long bones are relatively specific clues; however, they are insensitive findings and often are absent. Obtaining a careful environmental and occupational history is always indicated because it is likely to identify a potential source of lead exposure in many, albeit not all, cases. The ultimate diagnosis of lead poisoning should be confirmed by a sufficient elevation in blood lead concentration, but treatment for severe intoxication (see later) should not be withheld pending return of blood lead test results, which may take one or more days in many locations.

The differential diagnosis of lead encephalopathy includes a variety of infections of the central nervous system, particularly encephalitis, but also subacute meningitis and intracranial abscess. Similar to lead encephalopathy, these conditions can present with a history of headache, delirium, and seizures and can be accompanied by signs of increased intracranial pressure. Fever often is prominent in central nervous system infections but is relatively rare in lead encephalopathy. Lead encephalopathy is not associated with the CSF pleocytosis that is a feature of many central nervous system infections. Although some viral processes that cause encephalitis also may cause bone marrow depression, anemia is apt to be more common in patients with lead encephalopathy.

Patients in alcohol withdrawal can present with delirium and seizures and may have laboratory evidence of anemia

and elevations in transaminases and serum bilirubin. Alcohol withdrawal generally does not cause cerebral edema, however, and patients in withdrawal usually display a hyperadrenergic state that is not a feature of lead encephalopathy. In contrast to the normocytic or microcytic anemia of lead poisoning, the anemia common in chronic alcoholism tends to be macrocytic. In certain cases, prominent cerebellar edema in lead encephalopathy can mimic a midline cerebellar tumor, and both conditions can present with signs of altered mental status and obstructive hydrocephalus. Lead encephalopathy sometimes causes lateralizing neurologic signs that resemble presentations of subdural hematoma or focal brain edema from intracranial masses. These central nervous system lesions are not likely, however, to be accompanied by the anemia that often is found in patients with lead encephalopathy. Reye's syndrome is an encephalopathic process associated with vomiting, cerebral edema, and an acellular CSF. With rare exceptions,[91] the hyperammonemia and severe liver dysfunction of Reye's syndrome are not features of lead encephalopathy, however. In contrast to Reye's syndrome, laboratory findings in lead encephalopathy include elevated CSF protein and anemia. Carbon monoxide poisoning can present with a history of headache, nausea, and vomiting progressing to altered mental status and convulsions, but the cerebral edema and anemia common to patients with lead encephalopathy are absent.

The differential diagnosis of lead colic includes other causes of severe abdominal pain, including appendicitis, pelvic inflammatory disease, biliary colic, renal colic, intestinal obstruction, pancreatitis, and peptic ulcer. Gastrointestinal neoplasms can be associated with anemia, weight loss, and abdominal pain, although the pain generally is less severe and paroxysmal than that associated with lead colic. Attacks of acute intermittent porphyria and an even rarer condition, δ-aminolevulinic acid dehydratase deficiency porphyria, can share many of the features of severe acute lead intoxication, including colicky abdominal pain, constipation, nausea, and vomiting. In some cases, the gastrointestinal symptoms of porphyria are accompanied by neurologic derangements, including altered mental status, seizures, and motor neuropathy. Severe lead intoxication is usually associated with a more profound anemia, however. The attacks of abdominal pain in lead colic often are accompanied by a slowing of the pulse rate, in contrast to the tachycardia of acute intermittent porphyria.

TREATMENT

Effective treatment of lead intoxication requires attention to decontamination, supportive care, and use of specific chelating drugs.

Decontamination

Ingestion of lead-containing material (e.g., paint chips, small lead weights or pellets, or lead-contaminated folk remedies or food) has been a common cause of severe lead poisoning in children and occasionally is the source of lead poisoning in adults. What visibly might appear to be a small quantity (e.g., a single paint chip, a sip of a lead-containing glaze, or a small lead fishing weight) may contain hundreds of milligrams of lead. Ingestion of lead pellets[92] and lead-based ceramic glaze[63,93] has been associated with substantial increases in blood lead concentration within several hours. Partial dissolution of solid lead objects retained in the gastrointestinal tract has resulted in death within weeks.[77,94] As noted earlier, radiopacities on abdominal x-rays may suggest the presence of retained gastrointestinal lead, but a negative radiograph does not rule it out. The possible presence of lead in the gastrointestinal tract should be considered in all children and many adults who present with symptomatic lead intoxication, and an aggressive approach to decontamination is indicated when there are positive radiographs or when recent ingestion is otherwise suspected.

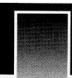 **Indications for ICU Admission in Lead Poisoning**

Suspected or Confirmed Lead Encephalopathy

History of potential lead exposure

Altered level of consciousness (delirium, hallucinations, lethargy, stupor, coma)

Seizure—focal or generalized

Ataxia or gait disturbance (often absent)

Prodromal symptoms of increasing headaches, lethargy, anorexia, vomiting, clumsiness, irritability, sleep disturbance; fever is uncommon

Neurologic examination findings consistent with increased intracranial pressure (often absent)—papilledema, cranial nerve palsies (especially cranial nerves III and VI), recent-onset strabismus, or decrease in visual acuity

Gingival lead line (helpful but often absent)

Neuroimaging consistent with increased intracranial pressure

Laboratory findings—anemia (common), basophilic stippling, indirect hyperbilirubinemia (rare), radiographic lead line (children only; helpful but insensitive), cerebrospinal fluid with elevated protein and relative acellularity

Blood lead concentration (whole blood)—usually >100 μg/dL (>4.8 μmol/L) in adults, >70 μg/dL (>3.4 μmol/L) in children

Lead Colic (Predominantly in Adults)

Severe, paroxysmal abdominal pain, often diminished by palpation, often with retraction of abdominal wall

History of severe constipation (common) or diarrhea (rare); nausea or vomiting

Slow or normal heart rate during episodes of abdominal pain

Blood concentration (whole blood)—usually >80 μg/dL (>3.9 μmol/L)

Patients with lead encephalopathy or lead colic may present with other features of lead poisoning. In adults, these features may include motor predominant peripheral neuropathy, tremor, gout, hypertension, acute or chronic renal insufficiency, neuropsychologic dysfunction (cognitive and behavioral), and history of adverse reproductive outcomes. In children, this may include developmental delay (neurocognitive, physical growth) and Fanconi-like renal syndrome. Because of the risk of incipient lead encephalopathy, intensive care unit admission should be considered for asymptomatic patients with extremely high blood lead concentrations (>150 μg/dL [>7.2 μmol/L]).

Activated charcoal has relatively low affinity for many metal ions, and its potential value in reducing gastrointestinal absorption of inorganic lead is doubtful but unknown. Case reports suggest that whole-bowel irrigation may accelerate the elimination of gastrointestinal lead and diminish further absorption.[95–97] This process requires the administration of commercially available solutions of polyethylene glycol and electrolytes by mouth or per nasogastric tube at a rate of 20 to 30 mL/kg/hr until a clear rectal effluent is achieved. Alternative approaches in cases of lead ingestion have included gastric lavage and cathartics.[63] Gastrointestinal decontamination techniques are discussed in Chapter 5.

Although gastrointestinal decontamination may be desirable, many patients with symptomatic lead poisoning, particularly lead colic, have severe constipation that may limit the potential effectiveness of whole-bowel irrigation or cathartics. Suspected lead foreign bodies that exhibit prolonged radiographic retention in the gastrointestinal tract (i.e., >48 hours), such as large intragastric objects or pellets lodged in the appendix, may require endoscopic or surgical removal.[98–100]

Retention of lead-containing bullets, shotgun pellets, or other metallic projectiles poses a well-documented risk of severe lead poisoning when the location of the foreign body results in dissolution and systemic distribution of lead.[4,101] The risk is greatest when the foreign body lodges or migrates into a joint space, where synovial fluid and mechanical factors accelerate breakdown of the object and dissolution of the lead.[102,103] Severe lead poisoning also has been reported when lead fragments have come in direct contact with bone or with fluid-filled spaces, such as paravertebral pseudocysts or a subscapular bursa.[4,104] An isolated lead bullet fragment embedded in muscle or other soft tissue often becomes encased in fibrous tissue that permanently minimizes systemic lead exposure. Patients with retained lead bullets or projectiles who present with symptomatic lead poisoning or with high blood lead levels in the absence of symptoms should receive prompt supportive care and chelation to stabilize their condition and lower blood concentrations (see later). If radiographic evaluation determines that the retained objects are in or adjacent to a joint space, bursa, or pseudocyst or in direct contact with bone, surgical removal should be strongly considered. Successful arthroscopic extraction of a lead shotgun pellet from the knee joint has been reported.[105] Patients with retained lead foreign bodies who are currently asymptomatic and who have negligible or mild elevations in blood lead require periodic monitoring for particle migration and blood lead elevation for at least the first year and possibly longer. Patient education and lifetime vigilance are warranted in all such cases because lead intoxication often insidiously or abruptly has emerged years to decades after the initial injury.

Supportive Care

Lead encephalopathy is a medical emergency that requires management in an intensive care unit. Supportive care is targeted to three key objectives: (1) diminution or normalization of increased intracranial pressure, (2) maintenance of a urine output that permits adequate urinary lead excretion, and (3) control of seizures with anticonvulsants. Critical elevations in intracranial pressure may be signaled on examination by a progressive decline in level of consciousness, papilledema, cranial nerve dysfunction, abnormal pupillary responses, or focal neurologic deficits. Elevated intracranial pressure may be confirmed by neuroimaging or direct intracranial pressure measurement. Emergent treatment should include intravenous administration of mannitol (0.25 to 1.0 g/kg as a 20% to 25% solution) and intubation and short-term hyperventilation initially targeted to a $PaCO_2$ of 30 to 35 mm Hg. Because the pathophysiology of cerebral edema in lead encephalopathy involves altered permeability of the brain microvasculature, there is theoretical benefit to the use of glucocorticoids, such as dexamethasone. If seizures occur, benzodiazepines, such as diazepam or lorazepam, are the anticonvulsants of choice, with recourse to supplemental phenobarbital or general anesthesia in recalcitrant cases. The use of phenothiazines for sedation or treatment of delirium should be avoided because they may lower the seizure threshold.

Lead is excreted predominantly through the kidney, and elimination is optimized when urine output is maintained at 1 to 2 mL/kg/hr. Patients with lead encephalopathy often may be volume depleted due to vomiting or decreased oral intake and require intravenous fluid to achieve this goal. Fluid supplementation must be managed carefully, however, to avoid volume overload and exacerbation of cerebral edema. In critically ill encephalopathic patients, optimization of fluid status may require invasive hemodynamic monitoring and intracranial pressure monitoring. In patients without intravascular volume depletion, fluids should be minimized, and urine output should be augmented as needed with loop diuretics or by the secondary diuretic effects of mannitol administered for treatment of cerebral edema.

Transfusion of packed red blood cells may be of potential therapeutic benefit in the severely symptomatic patient with a hematocrit less than 30 and a blood lead concentration greater than 100 μg/dL (>4.8 μmol/L). The fraction of blood lead found in plasma (normally <1%) increases at a supralinear rate in the presence of high blood lead concentrations or low hematocrits.[9,106] Plasma lead may have a greater capacity than erythrocyte-associated lead to cross endothelial barriers or cell membranes and partition into critical target organs, such as the brain. A high blood lead concentration in the presence of severe anemia is of even greater toxicologic concern than the same level in the presence of a normal hematocrit. Transfusion of packed red blood cells in an anemic, encephalopathic patient with a high blood lead level may be of benefit by lowering the plasma fraction of lead in the blood. Anecdotal experience suggests that this intervention is of clinical value, but it has not undergone systematic study.

Before the more widespread use of chelating agents in the 1960s, adults with acute lead colic frequently were treated with intravenous injection of calcium salts, which was observed to provide rapid, dramatic relief from the abdominal pain. Hunter[107] noted, "In severe cases, it is possible, by the slow intravenous injection of 15 mL of a 20% solution of calcium gluconate, or of 10 mL of a 5% solution of calcium chloride, to relieve the pain by the time the injection is over." Hamilton and Hardy[47] commented, "So dramatic is the effect of calcium that there is no need to use morphine or atropine." Soon after the introduction of the chelating agent calcium EDTA in the early 1950s, Belknap

and Perry[108] described the sequential use of calcium gluconate and calcium edetate in patients with acute lead colic, a regimen they believe combined the rapid pain relief of the former with the lead-mobilizing effect of the latter. These investigators noted the following:

Intravenous treatment with edathamil calcium disodium ($CaNa_2$-EDTA) does not give the prompt relief of lead colic which we expect within one-half hour with intravenously administered calcium gluconate. Therefore, a combination of intravenously administered calcium gluconate in alternate doses with intravenously administered edathamil calcium disodium is calculated to give immediate pain relief, combined with a sharp reduction of circulating, and therefore potentially dangerous lead.

By the mid-1960s, chelation alone supplanted the use of calcium salts in the treatment of the progressively rarer adult patient with acute lead colic. Aside from the observations of Belknap and Perry,[108] there seems to be scant discussion in the literature regarding clinical experience with calcium salts or opioids as adjuncts to chelation in the treatment of this condition.

Chelation

Several pharmaceuticals, known as *chelating agents* or *chelators*, are available for the treatment of lead intoxication. The principal agents are calcium edetate (calcium EDTA) and the three dimercapto compounds—dimercaprol (dimercaptopropanol, British antilewisite), succimer (dimercaptosuccinic acid [Chemet]), and unithiol (dimercaptopropanesulfonic acid [Dimaval]). Calcium EDTA and, in the case of the dimercapto agents, either the parent compound or the biotransformation products are thought to form relatively stable complexes with the lead atoms in vivo, enhancing lead mobilization and diminishing interaction with cellular proteins. Administration of each of the chelating agents results in reductions in blood lead concentrations and large increases in urinary lead excretion. There are no randomized clinical trials, however, that establish the ability of chelation to improve clinical outcome in lead-poisoned patients. There was no apparent benefit of chelation on survival in one of the few controlled animal studies that examined chelation treatment of acute high-dose lead poisoning.[109] A randomized, placebo-controlled, double-blind study of chelation with succimer in children with blood lead concentrations of 25 to 44 μg/dL (1.2 to 2.1 μmol/L) found no benefit in neuropsychologic outcome or long-term blood lead reduction.[110] For children with lead encephalopathy, the benefit of chelation has been suggested by the sharp decline in the case mortality rate since this treatment was introduced. In the 1940s, before the availability of chelating drugs, the case mortality rate for severe pediatric lead encephalopathy was approximately 65%, but it decreased to less than 5% among similar cases treated with chelation in the 1960s.[44,111,112] In nonencephalopathic patients with high blood lead concentrations, chelation has been advocated as a means to decrease blood lead concentration rapidly and avert possible progression to encephalopathy, a condition that potentially can result in death or permanent neurologic sequelae.[38]

Various chelation regimens have been proposed over the years. Dimercaprol was investigated as a chelating agent for lead intoxication soon after its introduction as an arsenic antidote in the mid-1940s. In contrast to its beneficial effect in acute arsenic poisoning, dimercaprol did not prolong survival in animals challenged with lethal doses of lead acetate, despite increasing urinary lead excretion.[113,114] In these animal experiments, dimercaprol actually increased the toxicity of lead. In early human case series, dimercaprol was thought to be of possible value in severe pediatric lead encephalopathy,[111] but it was considered to be less useful in adult cases, particularly patients with lead colic.[115,116] Calcium EDTA, introduced in the early 1950s, generated far more enthusiasm for its perceived therapeutic benefit.[117,118] Calcium EDTA replaced dimercaprol as a single agent in the treatment of lead intoxication after several pediatric case series associated it with better neurologic outcome among survivors and a higher therapeutic index.[40,119]

In a small randomized clinical trial conducted in the 1960s, Chisolm[112] observed that a two-drug regimen consisting of dimercaprol and calcium EDTA resulted in a more rapid decline in blood lead concentration and greater urinary lead excretion than those achieved with calcium EDTA alone. By administering the highest tolerable dose of two distinct types of agents, it was thought that the overall delivery of chelating moieties could be maximized. It also was suggested that the relatively higher lipophilicity of dimercaprol mobilized lead from intracellular sites and then shifted it extracellularly, where a more stable lead-EDTA chelate could be formed.[120] In a common two-drug regimen developed for pediatric lead encephalopathy,[121] treatment is begun with a priming dose of dimercaprol, 75 mg/m^2 intramuscularly, which is repeated every 4 hours for a total daily dose of 450 mg/m^2/day. Four hours after the initial dimercaprol dose, calcium EDTA, 1500 mg/m^2/day, is begun by slow, continuous intravenous infusion. Calcium EDTA (Calcium Disodium Versenate) is supplied in 5-mL ampules (200 mg/mL), which should be diluted to 2 to 4 mg/mL in saline or 5% dextrose for intravenous infusion. Although intramuscular injection of undiluted calcium EDTA (combined with lidocaine for local analgesia) sometimes has been advocated to minimize fluid load in encephalopathic patients with cerebral edema, the small amount of fluid required for intravenous infusion carries minimal risk and ensures efficient systemic delivery. The combined regimen of dimercaprol and calcium EDTA is continued for 5 days, although in some cases dimercaprol is discontinued after 3 days if the blood lead concentration has decreased to less than 50 μg/dL (<2.4 μmol/L). Other two-drug regimens have used a dimercaprol dose of 4 mg/kg intramuscularly every 4 hours (slightly higher than 5 mg/m^2 in an average-size child).[112] Alternative calcium EDTA doses have included 1000 mg/m^2/day (approximately 40 mg/kg/day in an average-size child)[122] or 50 mg/kg/day. [123]

Dimercaprol is supplied dissolved in peanut oil in 3-mL ampules (100 mg/mL) for deep intramuscular injection. Dimercaprol is associated with a high incidence of adverse side effects, including nausea and vomiting, hypertension, prolongation of the partial thromboplastin time, fever (particularly in children), and pain at the injection site. Sterile or pyogenic abscesses at the injection sites also may occur. Because it is supplied in a peanut oil vehicle, it should not be used in patients who have an allergy to peanuts. Although combined therapy with dimercaprol and calcium EDTA

accelerated the decline in blood lead concentration, there is little evidence that the addition of dimercaprol to calcium EDTA monotherapy measurably improved clinical outcome.[73,112] In 1992, a retrospective study of the treatment of hospitalized, nonencephalopathic children with blood lead concentrations of 50 to 60 μg/dL (2.4 to 2.9 μmol/L) found that treatment with calcium EDTA alone produced a greater short-term reduction in blood lead than did combined treatment with dimercaprol and calcium EDTA.[124] Patients not treated with dimercaprol displayed fewer adverse side effects. Because of dimercaprol's side-effect profile and the limited nature of the data supporting its added value, some clinicians omit it from chelation regimens of severely lead-poisoned patients, particularly adults. In encephalopathic adults with massively elevated blood lead concentrations (>400 μg/dL [>19.3 μmol/L]), treatment has been initiated with calcium EDTA alone without complications.[48,125,126] The dosage of calcium EDTA used in adults with lead encephalopathy or lead colic is usually 2 to 4 g/24 hr, or approximately 30 to 50 mg/kg/day, administered as a continuous intravenous infusion. Although formal dose-response studies have not been conducted, limited evidence suggests that higher doses are not associated with substantive increases in urinary lead excretion.[127]

Courses of treatment with calcium EDTA are limited to 5 consecutive days to diminish the risk of nephrotoxicity reported with prolonged high doses.[128–130] In patients with acute lead intoxication who receive chelation therapy soon after their lead exposure ends, the peak urinary lead excretion usually occurs within the first 2 days.[40,112,127] A report that an initial dose of calcium EDTA redistributed lead to the brain of rats[131] was not replicated in a more recent investigation conducted with sensitive measurement of a stable lead isotope tracer.[132]

Based on clinical trials conducted in nonencephalopathic patients with blood lead concentrations less than 100 μg/dL (<4.8 μmol/L), oral succimer, a water-soluble analogue of dimercaprol, seems equivalent or slightly more effective than parenteral calcium EDTA in lowering blood lead concentrations.[133–136] Oral succimer is nearly comparable to parenteral calcium EDTA in mobilizing lead into the urine.[136,137] Succimer is an acceptable alternative to calcium EDTA, or dimercaprol/calcium EDTA combination therapy, in nonencephalopathic lead-poisoned patients who are able to tolerate an oral medication. There is scant clinical experience with succimer as a single agent in the initial treatment of patients with lead encephalopathy or extremely high blood lead concentrations (e.g., >150 μg/dL [>7.2 μmol/L]). The initial use of an oral medication may be problematic in encephalopathic patients, who may have nausea and vomiting, or in patients with severe lead colic, in whom gastrointestinal motility often is compromised. There is some evidence that the chelating effect of succimer in humans requires in vivo biotransformation to form succimer-cysteine adducts.[138,139] The possible impact of very high blood lead concentrations on this biotransformation is unknown. In a case report, oral succimer was added to a regimen that included calcium EDTA and dimercaprol for treatment of an encephalopathic child with a blood lead concentration of 550 μg/dL (26.6 μmol/L).[96] In that case, blood lead concentrations rebounded upward when the parenteral chelators were stopped, even though succimer was continued. A controlled retrospective study in nonencephalopathic pediatric patients with mean blood lead concentrations of 50 to 60 μg/dL (2.4 to 2.9 μmol/L) found that two-drug therapy with succimer and calcium EDTA was equivalent to two-drug therapy with dimercaprol and calcium EDTA in lowering blood lead concentration but resulted in fewer adverse side effects.[140] A direct comparison of two-drug therapy with monotherapy was not conducted.

In North America and Europe, succimer is supplied as 100-mg capsules for oral administration. The small size of the capsules reflects the drug's U.S. Food and Drug Administration–approved indication as a treatment for lead poisoning in children. The medication is equally effective in adults, however. A commonly used treatment regimen consists of 10 mg/kg orally (in children, 350 mg/m²) every 8 hours for 5 days, decreasing to every 12 hours for the next 14 days.[141] Succimer generally is well tolerated, although adverse effects, including gastrointestinal distress, allergic skin rashes, mild reversible elevations in liver transaminases, and mild-to-moderate neutropenia, occasionally have been noted. A study conducted in primates found that oral treatment with succimer does not increase absorption of lead that may be present in the gastrointestinal tract.[142] Nonetheless, the gastrointestinal decontamination that is indicated in cases of recent lead ingestion (see earlier) prevents initiation of oral chelation until the decontamination process is completed. The clinical pharmacology of succimer is discussed in Chapter 141.

The sodium salt of succimer, sodium dimercaptosuccinate, has been used in the intravenous treatment of lead poisoning in the People's Republic of China, but at present this formulation is not available elsewhere. At a dose of 1 to 2 g/day, intravenous succimer was found to be equivalent to intravenous calcium EDTA in increasing urinary lead excretion in adults.[143,144]

Unithiol, another water-soluble analogue of dimercaprol, is similar to succimer in its capacity to decrease tissue levels of lead in experimental animals.[145] Treatment with oral unithiol has resulted in a decline in blood lead concentration and an increase in renal lead excretion in the relatively few reports of its use in the treatment of human lead intoxication.[146,147] No published reports are available regarding the use of unithiol in the treatment of patients with lead encephalopathy or patients with extremely high blood lead concentrations (>150 μg/dL [>7.2 μmol/L]). Unithiol is available in oral and parenteral formulations. It has been sold as a registered pharmaceutical in Germany and Russia for many years, but it only more recently became available in the United States for dispensation through compounding pharmacies.[148] Unithiol generally is well tolerated, although rare allergic cutaneous reactions and isolated cases of mild reversible transaminase elevation or leukopenia have been observed.[149] D-Penicillamine has been used for oral lead chelation but is inferior to succimer in lead mobilization[150] and is associated with a higher incidence of serious adverse effects.

The selection of a chelation regimen in a patient with symptomatic lead intoxication is influenced by the nature and severity of the clinical presentation. In patients with lead encephalopathy or severe lead colic, intravenous calcium EDTA is the current treatment of choice. As discussed earlier, some clinicians have advocated a combined regimen of dimercaprol and calcium EDTA, particularly in children. After 5 days, or possibly sooner if the patient is alert and able to tolerate an oral medication, the parenteral chelation agent may be replaced by an oral chelation agent, such as succimer or possibly unithiol. Measurement of blood lead concentration immediately before initiation or alteration of any chelation regimen and repeat measurements 24 to 48 hours later are indicated to confirm that blood lead levels are declining. Measurement of urinary lead during the first 24 hours of chelation therapy may provide further assurance of substantive lead excretion, which can exceed several milligrams in the initial days of therapy. If blood lead concentration increases after replacement of calcium EDTA with an oral chelator or if it remains greater than 100 μg/dL (>4.8 μmol/L), a second course of calcium EDTA is indicated. Each 5-day course of calcium EDTA should be separated, however, by a 2-day interval in which that drug is withheld. Further research is warranted to assess the clinical value of regimens that combine calcium EDTA with succimer or unithiol.

In adults who have symptomatic lead intoxication without evidence of encephalopathy or lead colic (usually at blood lead concentrations >60 to 80 μg/dL [>2.9 to 3.9 μmol/L]) and in children with blood lead concentrations greater than 45 μg/dL (>2.2 μmol/L) who likewise do not have encephalopathy or colic, chelation treatment may be initiated with oral succimer. Oral unithiol also may be appropriate in this setting. Because of limited experience regarding the use of succimer or unithiol as the sole chelating agent in patients with extremely high blood lead concentrations (>150 μg/dL [>7.2 μmol/L]), it is prudent to monitor the initial clinical progress and blood lead trend of such patients in an inpatient setting.

To avert potential progression to encephalopathy, which sometimes evolves abruptly after a symptom-free latent period,[48] chelation is warranted for asymptomatic adults with blood lead concentrations greater than 100 μg/dL (>4.8 μmol/L). Similarly, chelation has been recommended for all children with blood lead concentrations greater than 45 μg/dL (>2.2 μmol/L), even in the absence of symptoms.[79,123] Recent studies observed that the urinary excretion of lead after succimer administration is influenced by at least two genetic polymorphisms.[12] Occasionally, some individuals who excrete large quantities of lead after calcium EDTA excrete considerably lesser amounts after succimer.[151] A small study of the pharmacokinetics of succimer found that clearance of the drug and its metabolites may be prolonged in lead-poisoned children relative to lead-poisoned adults.[152] Although further study of these factors is necessary, the clinician should be alert to the possibility that an occasional patient may not respond to chelating agents with a substantial increase in urinary lead excretion or decline in blood lead concentration (≥20% by 48 to 96 hours). Although genetic or medical factors in the patient may be responsible, the possibility of noncompliance, ongoing occult exposure, or retention of lead in the gastrointestinal tract or in a synovial cavity also should be considered.

After termination of lead exposure, the pattern of decline in blood lead concentration is approximated by a two-compartment model: a fast, initial decline reflecting clearance of lead in the soft tissues, followed by a slow, second phase representing the major body burden of lead present in bone.[153] Chelating agents, which predominantly mobilize lead from the soft tissues, accelerate the initial rate of decline associated with the first compartment but exert a relatively modest impact on the second (skeletal) compartment. The ability of chelation to clear even the soft tissues of lead has limitations. In a study of juvenile primates, 77% of an injected lead isotope was retained in the body after 5 days of oral succimer, even though chelation was begun 15 minutes after the injection.[154] The amount of lead excreted in the urine during a course of chelation, often on the order of 10 mg within 1 week in a symptomatic individual, is small relative to the hundreds of milligrams that may be present in the skeleton after chronic or recurrent high-dose exposure.

In patients with a pattern of chronic or acute-on-chronic, high-dose lead exposure, cessation of chelation typically is followed by an upward "rebound" in blood lead concentration over the next few weeks as lead in the skeleton reequilibrates with the circulation. In general, the first one or two courses of chelation have an appreciable and enduring capacity to reduce blood lead concentrations below the high values associated with major, overt symptoms. Because of postchelation rebound from bone lead stores, however, subsequent courses of chelation may have only a modest impact on the long-term pattern of decline in blood lead concentration (Fig. 78-1).[155] The benefit of repeated courses of chelation in these settings has not been established.[156] A key component of successful clinical management is assurance that the patient is not discharged to an environment where hazardous lead exposure will continue.

PROGNOSIS

The long-term prognosis for complete recovery from severe lead intoxication in children is guarded. In a series of 425 children treated for lead intoxication published in 1966,

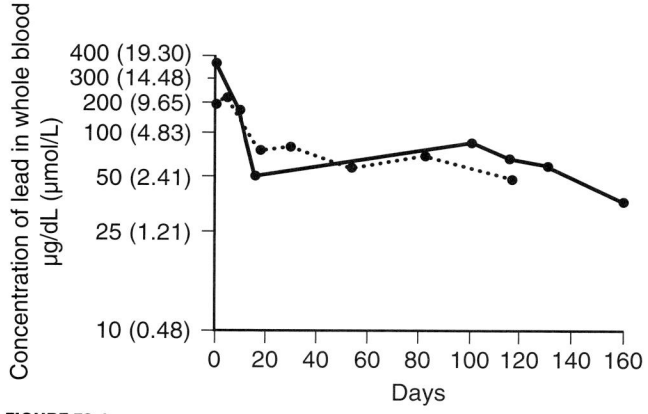

FIGURE 78-1

Response of blood lead concentrations to brief courses of chelation therapy. Data were obtained in two patients. Solid-line segments show decrease in blood lead concentrations during and after therapy with calcium disodium edetate (or dimercaprol and calcium disodium edetate), and dashed-line segments show trend in blood lead concentration without chelation therapy. *(From Moel DI, Sachs HK, Drayton MA: Slow, natural reduction in blood lead level after chelation therapy for lead poisoning in childhood. Am J Dis Child 140:905–908, 1986.)*

Perlstein and Attala[38] observed neurologic sequelae in 168 cases (39%). Among a subset of 59 patients who survived lead encephalopathy, 54% were noted to have a persistent seizure disorder; 38% were described as having mental retardation ("generally of a profound type"); and 13% were said to have cerebral palsy, usually characterized by spastic hemiplegia. Although 18% were believed to have no sequelae, this and other early studies did not assess the long-term effects of childhood plumbism on subclinical neurocognitive or neurobehavioral outcome. More recent long-term prospective studies of asymptomatic children with mild-to-moderate elevations in lead exposure have found evidence of enduring subclinical deficits in cognitive function or educational performance.[157–159]

The long-term outcome of adults with overt lead poisoning, including encephalopathy, has not been subject to formal prospective study, but in general these patients experience considerable improvement in symptoms after removal from exposure and decline in blood lead concentration. Most patients experience complete recovery from gastrointestinal symptoms and anemia. Peripheral neuropathy also improves, although patients who sustained severe insults may have residual deficits. The prospect for recovery of clinical neurocognitive and neurobehavioral function is favorable, although the rate of improvement may lag behind the decline in blood lead concentration. Reduction in brain lead occurs more slowly than reduction in blood lead, particularly during chelation.[19,154] A program of physical therapy and cognitive rehabilitation may foster improvement in neurologic function. Depending on the severity of intoxication, complete functional recovery in some patients may require 1 year or more, and occasional patients, particularly the elderly, may have persistent cognitive deficits. A study that used noninvasive x-ray fluorescence to measure lead in bone in former organolead workers found an association between past adult lead exposure and longitudinal decline in cognitive function.[160]

SPECIAL POPULATIONS

Patients with Renal Insufficiency

Lead excretion in humans occurs predominantly via the kidney. In patients with lead poisoning, chelating agents initially can increase daily urinary lead excretion by 20-fold to 50-fold.[133,147,161,162] The effect of chelation on lead elimination in the presence of renal failure has been best characterized for calcium EDTA. In patients with moderate renal insufficiency but preserved urine output, calcium EDTA results in large increases in urinary lead excretion, but at a slower rate than what occurs in patients with normal renal function.[163,164] When treating these patients for symptomatic lead intoxication, it is advisable to decrease the administered dose of calcium EDTA by half (e.g., 1 g/24 hr in an adult instead of 2 g/24 hr). A few case reports suggest that calcium EDTA can be combined with extracorporeal techniques to increase lead elimination in patients with severe renal failure. A patient with chronic lead poisoning and end-stage renal failure received calcium EDTA, 500 mg intravenously, before peritoneal dialysis. The amount of lead removed in the dialysate increased 4.5-fold, resulting in elimination of 16.8 mg of lead in 20 hours.[165] In another patient with chronic renal failure, calcium EDTA, 1.0 g intravenously, increased the amount of lead removed by peritoneal dialysis from a baseline of 16 μg/day to 1932 μg over 4 days.[166] Kessler and colleagues[167] used calcium EDTA, 1.0 g intravenously, 1 hour before hemofiltration to increase lead removal in patients with end-stage renal failure. Because effective lead mobilization by succimer may require biotransformation in the kidney to form a 1:2 dimercapto-succinic acid–cysteine adduct,[139,168] there is reason to doubt its potential ability to increase lead elimination in patients with end-stage renal failure. In limited unpublished reports, succimer did not seem to increase lead clearance by hemodialysis.[141]

Pregnant Patients

Lead undergoes transplacental transport, and at low-to-moderate blood lead concentrations, umbilical cord blood lead levels at delivery are approximately 85% to 90% of the maternal blood lead.[169] Factors that elevate the plasma fraction of maternal blood lead (e.g., high blood lead concentrations, anemia, or high maternal bone lead burden)[170] are likely to increase fetal lead exposure. High-dose lead exposure during pregnancy has been associated with an increased risk of spontaneous abortion and stillbirth. Lead has been used illicitly as an abortifacient,[171] and studies of reproductive outcome among women with relatively high occupational lead exposure in the late 19th and early 20th centuries noted a high incidence of miscarriage and stillbirth.[172] Contemporary epidemiologic studies generally have not detected an association between maternal blood lead concentrations less than 30 μg/dL (<1.4 μmol/L) and an increased risk of spontaneous abortion, although a nested case-control study found an odds ratio for spontaneous abortion of 1.8 (95% confidence interval 1.1 to 3.1) for every 5-μg/dL (0.24-μmol/L) increase in maternal blood lead over an approximate range of 5 to 20 μg/dL (0.24 to 1.0 μmol/L).[173]

Epidemiologic studies have yielded mixed results regarding a possible link between low-level lead exposure and preterm delivery or low birth weight.[174–176] Most long-term prospective studies have found postnatal but not prenatal low-level lead exposure to be associated with subclinical decrements in cognitive function.[177] A long-term prospective study in Yugoslavia observed prenatal and early postnatal exposure to have an enduring impact, however.[178] Although high-dose lead exposure has been teratogenic in animal studies, there is no established link between in utero lead exposure and structural deformities in humans.[80,177]

Animal studies found that chelating agents may reduce the fetotoxic and teratogenic effects of lead. When administered to pregnant rats simultaneously with lead, equimolar doses of calcium EDTA greatly diminished lead-induced resorptions and malformations.[179] Although the calcium EDTA transiently increased transplacental lead transfer during a 64-minute infusion, maternal lead clearance was enhanced, and fetal lead content was reduced greatly at 24 and 48 hours after injection.[180] Oral succimer administered to lead-exposed pregnant rats prevented lead-induced decrements in the body weight of the offspring assessed at the time of weaning and at 13 weeks of age.[181] Despite these beneficial effects, the use of chelating agents during pregnancy is tempered by the findings in animal studies that calcium EDTA was teratogenic at therapeutic doses[182] and that succimer was fetotoxic when administered at three times the standard therapeutic dose.[183] These findings may have been mediated by impacts on trace mineral metabolism, particularly zinc in the case of calcium EDTA[182] and copper in the case of succimer.[184,185] Judicious trace mineral supplementation conceivably might mitigate adverse effects on the fetus in the event of chelation for maternal lead poisoning. Reports of lead chelation during pregnancy in humans are sparse. In two cases, calcium EDTA treatment of lead poisoning during the third trimester was followed soon by delivery of a normal infant.[186,187]

Common Misconceptions about Lead Poisoning

1. The clinical presentation of *lead encephalopathy* sometimes is mistaken for a central nervous system infection or mass lesion.
2. The clinical presentation of *lead colic* sometimes is mistaken for appendicitis, pelvic inflammatory disease, biliary colic, renal colic, intestinal obstruction, pancreatitis, or peptic ulcer disease. Although useful, an occupational and environmental history often is omitted.
3. Basophilic stippling of erythrocytes, gastrointestinal radio-opacities, gingival lead lines, and radiographic skeletal lead lines (in children) occasionally provide useful clues, but the absence of these insensitive findings should not exclude the diagnosis.
4. An elevation in blood lead concentration ultimately should confirm the diagnosis, but treatment for clinically suspected severe lead intoxication should not be withheld pending a laboratory delay of one or more days.

Key Points in Lead Poisoning

1. Lead encephalopathy should be suspected in patients with delirium or seizures and laboratory evidence of anemia.
2. Lead colic should be suspected in patients with abdominal pain, constipation, and anemia.
3. Blood lead concentration usually is >100 μg/dL (>4.8 μmol/L) in adults with lead encephalopathy (>70 μg/dL [>3.4 μmol/L] in children). In lead colic, blood lead concentration usually is >80 μg/dL (>3.9 μmol/L).
4. Lead encephalopathy and lead colic may occur independently of each other, but other antecedent multisystemic findings almost always are present.
5. Effective treatment requires attention to decontamination, supportive care, and use of specific chelating agents. Intensive supportive care for lead encephalopathy may require mannitol, hyperventilation, corticosteroids for cerebral edema, and anticonvulsants for seizures.

REFERENCES

1. Nriagu JO: Lead and Lead Poisoning in Antiquity. New York, John Wiley & Sons, 1983.
2. Wedeen RP: Poison in the Pot. Carbondale, IL, Southern Illinois University Press, 1984.
3. Hipkins KL, Materna BL, Kosnett MJ, et al: Medical guidelines for the lead-exposed worker. Am Assoc Occup Health Nurs 46:330–339, 1998.
4. Linden MA, Manton WI, Stewart RM, et al: Lead poisoning from retained bullets: Pathogenesis, diagnosis, and management. Ann Surg 195:305–313, 1982.
5. Booker DV, Chamberlain AC, Newton D, et al: Uptake of radioactive lead following inhalation and injection. Br J Radiol 42:457–466, 1969.
6. Hursh JB, Mercer TT: Measurement of 212Pb loss rate from human lungs. J Appl Physiol 28:268–274, 1970.
7. Heard MJ, Chamberlain AC: Uptake of Pb by human skeleton and comparative metabolism of Pb and alkaline earth elements. Health Phys 47:857–865, 1984.
8. Rabinowitz MB, Wetherill GW, Kopple JD: Kinetic analysis of lead metabolism in healthy humans. J Clin Invest 58:260–270, 1976.
9. Manton WI, Cook JD: High accuracy (stable isotope dilution) measurements of lead in serum and cerebrospinal fluid. Br J Ind Med 41:313–319, 1984.
10. Bergdahl IA, Sheveleva M, Schutz A, et al: Plasma and blood lead in humans: Capacity-limited binding to δ-aminolevulinic acid dehydratase and other lead-binding components. Toxicol Sci 46:247–253, 1998.
11. Kelada SN, Shelton E, Kaufmann RB, Khoury MJ: δ-Aminolevulinic acid dehydratase genotype and lead toxicity: A HuGE review. Am J Epidemiol 54:1–13, 2001.
12. Schwartz BS, Lee BK, Lee GS, et al: Associations of blood lead, dimercaptosuccinic-chelatable lead, and tibia lead with polymorphisms in vitamin D receptor and δ-aminolevulinic acid dehydratase genes. Environ Health Perspect 108:949–954, 2000.
13. Leggett RW: An age-specific kinetic model of lead metabolism in humans. Environ Health Perspect 101:598–616, 1993.
14. O'Flaherty EJ: Physiologically based models for bone-seeking elements: IV. Kinetics of lead disposition in humans. Toxicol Appl Pharmacol 118:16–29, 1993.
15. Bressler JP, Goldstein GW: Mechanisms of lead neurotoxicity. Biochem Pharmacol 41:479–484, 1991.
16. Simons TJB: Lead-calcium interactions in cellular lead toxicity. Neurotoxicology 14:77–86, 1993.
17. Hariri RJ: Cerebral edema. Neurosurg Clin North Am 5:687–706, 1994.
18. Pentschew A: Morphology and morphogenesis of lead encephalopathy. Acta Neuropathol 5:133–160, 1965.
19. Goldstein GW, Asbury AK, Diamond I: Pathogenesis of lead encephalopathy: Uptake of lead and reaction with brain capillaries. Arch Neurol 31:382–389, 1974.
20. Tiffany-Castiglioni E, Sierra EM, Wu JN, et al: Lead toxicity in neuroglia. Neurotoxicology 10:417–443, 1989.
21. Silbergeld E, Fales JT, Goldberg AM: Evidence for a junctional effect of lead on neuromuscular function. Nature 247:49–50, 1974.
22. Janin Y, Couinaud C, Stone A, et al: The "lead-induced colic" syndrome in lead intoxication. Surg Ann 17:287–307, 1985.
23. Naarala JT, Loikkanen JJ, Ruotsalainen M, et al: Lead amplifies glutamate-induced oxidative stress. Free Rad Biol Med 19:689–693, 1995.
24. He L, Poblenz AT, Medrano CJ, et al: Lead and calcium produce rod photoreceptor cell apoptosis by opening the mitochondrial permeability transition pore. J Biol Chem 275:12175–12184, 2000.
25. Zawia NH, Crumpton T, Brydie M, et al: Disruption of the zinc finger domain: A common target that underlies many of the effects of lead. Neurotoxicology 21:1069–1080, 2000.
26. Goering PL: Lead-protein interactions as a basis for lead toxicity. Neurotoxicology 14:45–60, 1993.
27. Schneitzer L, Osborn HH, Bierman A, et al: Lead poisoning in adults from renovation of an older home. Ann Emerg Med 19:415–420, 1990.
28. Whitfield CL, Chien LT, Whitehead JD: Lead encephalopathy in adults. Am J Med 52:289–298, 1972.
29. Karpinski FE, Rieders F, Girsh LS: Calcium disodium versenate in the therapy of lead encephalopathy. J Pediatr 42:687–699, 1953.
30. Baghdassarian SA: Optic neuropathy due to lead poisoning. Arch Ophthalmol 180:721–723, 1968.
31. Nye LJJ: An investigation of the extraordinary incidence of chronic nephritis in young people in Queensland. Med J Aust 2:145–159, 1929.
32. Mirando EH, Ranasinghe L: Lead encephalopathy in children: Uncommon clinical aspects. Med J Aust 2:966–968, 1970.
33. Bucy PC, Buchanan DN: The simulation of intracranial tumor by lead encephalopathy in children, with remarks concerning the surgical treatment of the latter. JAMA 105:244–250, 1935.
34. Perelman S, Hertz-Pannier L, Hassan M, Bourrillon A: Lead encephalopathy mimicking a cerebellar tumor. Acta Paediatr 82:423–425, 1993.
35. Pappas CL, Quisling RG, Ballinger WE, et al: Lead encephalopathy: Symptoms of a cerebellar mass lesion and obstructive hydrocephalus. Surg Neurol 26:391–394, 1986.
36. Harrington JF, Mapstone TB, Selman WR, et al: Lead encephalopathy presenting as a posterior fossa mass. J Neurosurg 65:713–715, 1986.
37. Sharma RR, Chandy MJ, Lad SD: Transient hydrocephalus and acute lead encephalopathy in neonates and infants: Report of two cases. Br J Neurosurg 4:141–145, 1990.
38. Perlstein MA, Attala R: Neurological sequelae of plumbism in children. Clin Pediatr 5:292–298, 1966.
39. Mani J, Chaudhary N, Kanjalkar M, et al: Cerebellar ataxia due to lead encephalopathy in an adult. J Neurol Neurosurg Psychiatry 65:797–798, 1998.
40. Chisolm JJ, Harrison HE: The treatment of acute lead encephalopathy in children. Pediatrics 19:2–20, 1957.
41. Hess JW: Lead encephalopathy simulating subdural hematoma in an adult: Report of a case. N Engl J Med 264:382–384, 1961.
42. Segal I, Saffer D, Segal F: Diverse neurological manifestations of lead encephalopathy. S Afr Med J 48:1721–1722, 1974.
43. Powers JM, Rawe SE, Earlywine GR: Lead encephalopathy simulating a cerebral neoplasm in an adult. J Neurosurg 46:816–819, 1977.
44. Coffin R, Phillips JL, Staples WI, et al: Treatment of lead encephalopathy in children. J Pediatr 69:198–206, 1966.
45. Schirmer J, Anderson HA: Fatal pediatric poisoning from leaded paint—Wisconsin, 1990. MMWR Morbid Mortal Wkly Rep 40:193–195, 1991.
46. Tanquerel des Planches L, Dana SL: Lead Diseases: A Treatise from the French of L. Tanquerel des Planches, with Notes and Additions on the Use of Lead Pipe and Its Substitutes. Lowell, Bixby and Co, 1848.
47. Hamilton A, Hardy HL: Industrial Toxicology, 3rd ed. Acton, MA, Publishing Sciences, 1974.
48. Kosnett M, Rubens R, Goldman B: Delayed encephalopathy and proximal motor weakness in a patient with a blood lead level of 436 μg/dl (Abstract). Clin Toxicol 35:524, 1997.
49. Henderson LL: Jaundice due to lead poisoning. Arch Intern Med 89:967–969, 1952.
50. Beattie AD, Mullin PJ, Baxter RH, et al: Acute lead poisoning: An unusual cause of hepatitis. Scott Med J 24:318–321, 1979.
51. Carton JA, Maradona JA, Arribas JM: Acute-subacute lead poisoning: Clinical findings and comparative study of diagnostic tests. Arch Intern Med 147:697–703, 1987.
52. Bruggenkate CM, Cardozo EL, Maaskant P, et al: Lead poisoning with pigmentation of the oral mucosa. Oral Surg 39:747–753, 1975.
53. Cullen M, Robins JM, Eskenazi B: Adult lead intoxication: Presentation of 31 new cases and a review of recent advances in the literature. Medicine 62:221–247, 1983.
54. Gittleman JL, Engelgau MM, Shaw J, et al: Lead poisoning among battery reclamation workers in Alabama. J Occup Med 36:526–532, 1994.
55. Wyngaarden JB, Kelley WN: Saturnine gout. In Gout and Hyperuricemia. New York, Grune & Stratton, 1976, pp 360–366.
56. Batuman V, Maesaka JK, Haddad B, et al: The role of lead in gout nephropathy. N Engl J Med 304:520–523, 1981.
57. Craswell PW, Price JP, Boyle PD, et al: Chronic renal failure with gout: A marker of chronic lead poisoning. Kidney Int 26:319–323, 1984.
58. Clark M, Royal J, Seeler R: Interaction of iron deficiency and lead and the hematologic findings in children with severe lead poisoning. Pediatrics 81:247–254, 1988.

59. Marcus AH, Schwartz J: Dose-response curves for erythrocyte protoporphyrin vs blood lead: Effects of iron status. Environ Res 44:221–227, 1987.

60. Watson WS, Hume R, Moore MR: Oral absorption of lead and iron. Lancet 2:236–237, 1980.

61. Pagliucca A, Mufti GJ, Baldwin D, et al: Lead poisoning: Clinical, biochemical, and haematological aspects of a recent outbreak. J Clin Pathol 43:277–281, 1990.

62. Karpatkin S: Lead poisoning after taking Pb acetate with suicidal intent. Arch Environ Health 2:79–84, 1961.

63. Vance MV, Curry SC, Bradley JM, et al: Acute lead poisoning in nursing home and psychiatric patients from the ingestion of lead-based ceramic glazes. Arch Intern Med 150:2085–2092, 1990.

64. Belknap EL: Lead poisoning: Criteria for a diagnosis. Ind Med 9:505–509, 1940.

65. Leiken S, Eng G: Erythrokinetic studies of the anemia of lead poisoning. Pediatrics 31:996–1002, 1963.

66. Lilis R, Fischbein A, Diamond S, et al: Lead effects among secondary smelter workers with blood lead levels below 80 μg/100 ml. Arch Environ Health 32:256–266, 1977.

67. Schwartz J, Landrigan PJ, Baker KL, et al: Lead induced anemia: Dose-response relationships and evidence for a threshold. Am J Public Health 80:165–168, 1990.

68. Lilis R, Gavrilescu B, Nestorescu B, et al: Nephropathy in chronic lead poisoning. Br J Ind Med 25:196–202, 1968.

69. Radosevic Z, Saric M, Beritic T, et al: The kidney in lead poisoning. Br J Ind Med 18:222–230, 1961.

70. Chisolm JJ: Aminoaciduria as a manifestation of renal tubular injury in lead intoxication and a comparison with patterns of aminoaciduria seen in other diseases. J Pediatr 60:1–17, 1962.

71. Cramer K, Goyer RA, Jagenburg R, et al: Renal ultrastructure, renal function, and parameters of lead toxicity in workers with different periods of lead exposure. Br J Ind Med 31:113–127, 1974.

72. Hungerford GD, Ross P, Robertson HJF: Computerized tomography in lead encephalopathy: A case report. Radiology 123:91–92, 1977.

73. Greengard J: Lead poisoning in childhood: Signs, symptoms, current therapy, clinical expressions. Clin Pediatr 5:269–276, 1966.

74. Sachs HK: Evolution of the radiologic lead line. Radiology 139:81–85, 1981.

75. Veerula GR, Noah PK: Clinical manifestations of childhood lead poisoning. J Trop Med Hyg 93:170–177, 1990.

76. Blickman JG, Wilkinson RH, Graef JW: The radiologic "lead band" revisited. AJR Am J Roentgenol 146:245–247, 1985.

77. Hugelmeyer CD, Moorhead JC, Horenblas L, et al: Fatal lead encephalopathy following foreign body ingestion: Case report. J Emerg Med 6:397–400, 1988.

78. Esham RH, Sugg JH: Lead colic masquerading as intestinal obstruction. South Med J 66:959–960, 1973.

79. Centers for Disease Control and Prevention: Preventing lead poisoning in young children: A statement by the Centers for Disease Control—October, 1991. Atlanta, CDC, 1991.

80. Agency for Toxic Substances and Disease Registry: Toxicological Profile for Lead (Update). Atlanta, DHHS, 1999.

81. Davoli C, Serwint J, Chisolm JJ: Asymptomatic children with venous lead levels >100 microgram/dL. Pediatrics 98:965–968, 1996.

82. Karlog O, Moller KO: Three cases of acute lead poisoning: Analyses of organs for lead, and observations on polarographic lead determinations. Acta Pharmacol Toxicol 15:8–16, 1958.

83. Allcott JV, Barnhart RA, Mooney LA: Acute lead poisoning in two users of illicit methamphetamine. JAMA 258:510–511, 1987.

84. Centers for Disease Control and Prevention: Second National Report on Human Exposure to Environmental Chemicals. Atlanta, CDC, 2003.

85. Pirkle JL, Brody DJ, Gunter EW, et al: The decline in blood lead levels in the United States: The National Health and Nutrition Examination Surveys (NHANES). JAMA 272:284–291, 1994.

86. Lanphear BP, Dietrich K, Auinger P, et al: Cognitive deficits associated with blood lead concentrations <10 μg/dL in US children and adolescents. Public Health Rep 115:521–529, 2000.

87. Labbe RF: Lead poisoning mechanisms. Clin Chem 36:1870, 1990.

88. Schutz A, Skerfving S, Christoffersson JO, et al: Chelatable lead versus lead in human trabecular and compact bone. Sci Tot Environ 61:201–209, 1987.

89. Tell I, Somervaille LJ, Nilsson U, et al: Chelated lead and bone lead. Scand J Work Environ Health 18:113–119, 1992.

90. Kosnett MJ, Regan LS, Kelly TJ, et al: Interrelationships of urinary lead after DMSA challenge, bone lead burden, and blood lead in lead exposed workers (Abstract). Vet Hum Toxicol 36:363, 1994.

91. Magnus PD, Powers RJ, Leong A: Pb encephalopathy mimicking Reye syndrome. J Pediatr 95:495, 1979.

92. McKinney PE: Acute elevation of blood lead levels within hours of ingestion of large quantities of lead shot. Clin Toxicol 38:435–440, 2000.

93. Roberge RJ, Martin TG, Dean BS, et al: Ceramic lead glaze ingestions in nursing home residents with dementia. Am J Emerg Med 12:77–81, 1994.

94. Forsby N, Fristedt B, Kjellman B: Acute, lethal poisoning after ingestion of metallic lead. Acta Paediatr Scand 177(Suppl):107, 1967.

95. Roberge RJ, Martin TG: Whole bowel irrigation in an acute oral lead intoxication. Am J Emerg Med 10:577–583, 1992.

96. Gordon RA, Roberts G, Amin Z, et al: Aggressive approach in the treatment of acute lead encephalopathy with an extraordinarily high concentration of lead. Arch Pediatr Adolesc Med 152:1100–1104, 1998.

97. McNutt TK, Dethlefsen M, Shah R, et al: Bite the bullet: Lead poisoning after ingestion of 206 lead bullets (Abstract). Clin Toxicol 38:549, 2000.

98. Hillman FE: A rare case of chronic lead poisoning: Polyneuropathy traced to lead shot in the appendix. Ind Med Surg 36:488–492, 1967.

99. Lyons JD, Filston HC: Lead intoxication from a pellet entrapped in the appendix of a child: Treatment considerations. J Pediatr Surg 29:1618–1620, 1994.

100. Esernio-Jensen D, Donatelli-Guagenti RN, Mofenson HC: Severe lead poisoning from an imported clothing accessory: "Watch" out for lead. Clin Toxicol 34:329–333, 1996.

101. Dillman RO, Crumb CK, Lidsky MJ: Lead poisoning from a gunshot wound: Report of a case and review of the literature. Am J Med 66:509–514, 1979.

102. Leonard MH: The solution of lead by synovial fluid. Clin Orthop 64:255–261, 1969.

103. Manton WI, Thal ER: Lead poisoning from retained missiles: An experimental study. Ann Surg 204:594–599, 1986.

104. Stromberg BV: Symptomatic lead toxicity secondary to retained shotgun pellets: Case report. J Trauma 30:356–357, 1990.

105. Bolanos AO, Demizio JP, Vigorita VJ, et al: Lead poisoning from an intra-articular shotgun pellet in the knee treated with arthroscopic extraction and chelation therapy. J Bone Joint Surg Am 78:422–426, 1996.

106. deSilva PE: Determination of lead in plasma and studies on its relationship to lead in erythrocytes. Br J Ind Med 38:209–217, 1981.

107. Hunter D: The Diseases of Occupations, 3rd ed. London, English Universities Press, 1964.

108. Belknap EL, Perry MC: Treatment of inorganic lead poisoning with edathamil calcium-disodium. Arch Ind Hyg Occup Med 10:530–547, 1954.

109. Hofmann U, Segewitz G: Influence of chelation therapy on acute lead intoxication in rats. Arch Toxicol 34:213–225, 1975.

110. Rogan WJ, Dietrich KN, Ware JH, et al: The effect of chelation therapy with succimer on neuropsychological development in children exposed to lead. N Engl J Med 344:1421–1426, 2001.

111. Ennis JM, Harrison HE: Treatment of lead encephalopathy with BAL (2,3-dimercaptopropanol). Pediatrics 5:853–868, 1950.

112. Chisolm JJ: The use of chelating agents in the treatment of acute and chronic lead intoxication in childhood. J Pediatr 73:1–38, 1968.

113. Germuth FG, Eagle H: The efficacy of BAL (2,3 dimercaptopropanol) in the treatment of experimental lead poisoning in rabbits. J Pharm Exp Ther 92:397–410, 1948.

114. Graham JDP, Hood J: Actions of British Anti-Lewisite (2,3-dimercaptopropanol). Br J Pharmacol 3:84–90, 1948.

115. Stocken LA, Thompson RHS: Reactions of British Anti-Lewisite with arsenic and other metals in living systems. Physiol Rev 29:168–194, 1949.

116. Badstrup-Madsen P: Dimercaprol in acute lead poisoning. Lancet 2:171–172, 1950.

117. Sidbury JB: Lead poisoning: Treatment with disodium calcium ethylenediamine-tetra-acetate. Am J Med 18:932–946, 1955.

118. Foreman H: Use of chelating agents in treatment of metal poisoning (with special emphasis on lead). Fed Proc 20:191–196, 1961.

119. Bradley JE, Baumgartner RJ: Subsequent mental development of children with encephalopathy, as related to type of treatment. J Pediatr 53:311–315, 1956.

120. Haust HL, Ali H, Haines DSM, et al: Short-term administration of dimercaptopropanol (BAL) and calcium disodium edetate (EDTA) for diagnostic and therapeutic lead mobilization. Int J Biochem 12:897–904, 1980.

121. Piomelli S, Rosen JF, Chisolm JJ, et al: Management of childhood lead poisoning. J Pediatr 105:523–532, 1984.

122. 3M Pharmaceuticals: Product information on calcium disodium versenate. St. Paul, 3M, 2000.

123. Committee on Drugs, American Academy of Pediatrics: Treatment guidelines for lead exposure in children. Pediatrics 96:155–160, 1995.

124. O'Connor ME: CaEDTA vs CaEDTA plus BAL to treat children with elevated blood lead levels. Clin Pediatr 31:386–390, 1992.

125. Martinez Vea A, Soriano Marin E, Segura Porta F, et al: Encefalopatia plumbica en el adulto: Una forma inhabitual de intoxicacion. Rev Clin Espan 155:467–469, 1979.

126. Dubi J, Schneider PH, Regli F: L'intoxication saturnine: A propos d'un cas d'encephalopathie aigue chez un adulte. Schweiz Med Wochenschr 109:123–127, 1979.

127. Leckie WJH, Tompsett SL: The diagnostic and therapeutic use of edathamil calcium disodium (EDTA, Versene) in excessive inorganic lead absorption. QJM 27:65–82, 1958.

128. Foreman H, Finnegan C, Lushbaugh CC: Nephrotoxic hazard from uncontrolled edathamil calcium-disodium therapy. JAMA 160:1042–1046, 1956.

129. Rueber MD, Bradley JE: Acute versenate nephrosis occurring as the result of treatment for lead intoxication. JAMA 174:263–269, 1960.

130. Moel DI, Kumar K: Reversible nephrotoxic reactions to a combined 2,3-dimercapto-1-propanol and calcium disodium ethylenediaminetetraacetic acid regimen in asymptomatic children with elevated blood lead levels. Pediatrics 70:259–262, 1982.

131. Cory-Slechta DA, Weiss B, Cox C: Mobilization and redistribution of lead over the course of calcium disodium ethylenediamine tetraacetate chelation therapy. J Pharmacol Exp Ther 243:804–813, 1987.

132. Seaton CI, Lasman J, Smith DR: The effects of CaNa2EDTA on brain lead mobilization in rodents determined using a stable lead isotope tracer. Toxicol Appl Pharmacol 159:153–160, 1999.

133. Graziano JH, Siris ES, LoIacono N, et al: 2,3-dimercaptosuccinic acid as an antidote for lead intoxication. Clin Pharmacol Ther 37:431–438, 1985.

134. Graziano JH: Role of 2,3-dimercaptosuccinic acid in the treatment of heavy metal poisoning. Med Toxicol 1:155–162, 1986.

135. Graziano JH, LoIacono NJ, Meyer P: Dose-response study of oral 2,3-dimercaptosuccinic acid in children with elevated blood lead concentrations. J Pediatr 113:751–757, 1988.

136. Graziano JH, LoIacono NJ, Moulton T, et al: Controlled study of meso-2,3-dimercaptosuccinic acid for the management of childhood lead intoxication. J Pediatr 120:133–139, 1992.

137. Chisolm JJ: Evaluation of the potential role of chelation therapy in treatment of low to moderate lead exposures. Environ Health Perspect 89:67–74, 1990.

138. Maiorino RM, Akins JM, Blaha K, et al: Determination and metabolism of dithiol chelating agents: X. In humans, meso-2,3 dimercaptosuccinic acid is bound to plasma proteins via mixed disulfide formation. J Pharmacol Exp Ther 254:570–577, 1990.

139. Aposhian HV, Maiorino RM, Rivera M, et al: Human studies with the chelating agents, DMPS and DMSA. Clin Toxicol 30:505–528, 1992.

140. Besunder JB, Super DM, Anderson RL: Comparison of dimercaptosuccinic acid and calcium disodium ethylenediaminetetraacetic acid versus dimercaptopropanol and ethylenediaminetetraacetic acid in children with lead poisoning. J Pediatr 130:966–971, 1997.

141. Sanofi Pharmaceuticals: Chemet product information. New York, Sanofi Pharmaceuticals, 1999.

142. Cremin JD, Luck ML, Laughlin NK, et al: Oral succimer decreases the gastrointestinal absorption of lead in juvenile monkeys. Environ Health Perspect 109:613–619, 2001.

143. Wang S, Ting K, Wu C: Chelating therapy with Na-DMS in occupational lead and mercury intoxications. Chin Med J 84:437–439, 1965.

144. Wang S, Liu J, Shi Z: Chelating therapy in occupational metal intoxications in China. Plzen lek Sborn Suppl 56:111–113, 1988.

145. Xu Z, Jones M: Comparative mobilization of lead by chelating agents. Toxicology 53:277–288, 1988.

146. Chisolm JJ, Thomas DJ: Use of 2,3-dimercaptopropane-1-sulfonate in treatment of lead poisoning in children. J Pharmacol Exp Ther 235:665–669, 1985.

147. Bialonczyk C, Partsch H, Donner A: Bleivergiftung durch Langzeitanwendung von Diachylonsalbe [Lead poisoning following long-term application of diachylon ointment]. Z Hautkr 64:1118–1120, 1989.

148. Food and Drug Administration: List of drug substances that may be used in pharmacy compounding. Fed Reg 64:996–1003, 1999.

149. Ruprecht J: Dimaval (DMPS). DMPS-Heyl. Scientific Monograph. Berlin, Heyl, 1997.

150. Kapoor SC, Wielopolski L, Graziano JH, et al: Influence of 2,3-dimercaptosuccinic acid on gastrointestinal lead absorption and whole-body lead retention. Toxicol Appl Pharmacol 97:525–529, 1989.

151. Lee BK, Schwartz BS, Stewart W, et al: Provocative chelation with DMSA and EDTA: Evidence for differential access to lead storage sites. Occup Environ Med 52:13–19, 1995.

152. Dart RC, Hurlbut KM, Maiorino RM, et al: Pharmacokinetics of meso-2,3-dimercaptosuccinic acid in patients with lead poisoning and in healthy adults. J Pediatr 125:309–316, 1994.

153. Schutz A, Skerfving S, Ranstam J, et al: Kinetics of lead in blood after the end of occupational exposure. Scand J Work Environ Health 13:221–231, 1987.

154. Cremin JD, Luck ML, Laughlin NK, et al: Efficacy of succimer chelation for reducing brain lead in a primate model of human lead exposure. Toxicol Appl Pharmacol 161:283–293, 1999.

155. Moel DI, Sachs HK, Drayton MA: Slow, natural reduction in blood lead level after chelation therapy for lead poisoning in childhood. Am J Dis Child 140:905–908, 1986.

156. Kosnett MJ: Unanswered questions in metal chelation. Clin Toxicol 30:529–547, 1992.

157. Needleman HL, Schell A, Bellinger D, et al: The long-term effects of exposure to low doses of lead in childhood: An 11-year follow-up report. N Engl J Med 322:83–88, 1990.

158. Fergusson DM, Horwood LJ, Lynskey MT: Early dentine lead levels and educational outcomes at 18 years. J Child Psychol Psychiatr All Discip 38:471–478, 1997.

159. Tong S, Baghurst PA, Sawyer MG, et al: Declining blood lead levels and changes in cognitive function during childhood: The Port Pirie cohort study. JAMA 280:1915–1919, 1998.

160. Schwartz BS, Stewart WF, Bolla KI, et al: Past adult lead exposure is associated with longitudinal decline in cognitive function. Neurology 55:1144–1150, 2000.

161. Reiders F, Dunnington WG, Breiger H: The efficacy of edathamil calcium disodium in the treatment of occupational lead poisoning. Ind Med Surg 24:195–202, 1955.

162. Thomas DJ, Chisolm JJ: Lead, zinc, copper decorporation during calcium disodium ethylenediamine tetraacetate treatment of lead-poisoned children. J Pharmacol Exp Ther 239:829–835, 1986.

163. Emmerson BT: Chronic lead nephropathy: The diagnostic use of calcium EDTA and the association with gout. Aust Ann Med 12:310–324, 1963.

164. Osterloh J, Becker CE: Pharmacokinetics of CaNa2EDTA and chelation of lead in renal failure. Clin Pharmacol Ther 40:686–693, 1986.

165. Mehbod H: Treatment of lead intoxication: Combined use of peritoneal dialysis and edetate calcium disodium. JAMA 201:152–154, 1967.

166. Roger SD, Yiannikas C, Crimmins D, et al: Lead intoxication in an anuric patient: Management by intraperitoneal EDTA. Aust N Z J Med 20:814–817, 1990.

167. Kessler M, Durand PY, Huu TC, et al: Mobilization of lead from bone in end-stage renal failure patients with secondary hyperparathyroidism. Nephrol Dial Transplant 14:2731–2733, 1999.

168. Asiedu P, Moulton T, Blum CB, et al: Metabolism of meso-2,3-dimercaptosuccinic acid in lead-poisoned children and normal adults. Environ Health Perspect 103:734–739, 1995.

169. Graziano JH, Popovac D, Factor-Litvak P, et al: Determinants of elevated blood lead during pregnancy in a population surrounding a lead smelter in Kosovo, Yugoslavia. Environ Health Perspect 89:95–100, 1990.

170. Chaung HY, Schwartz J, Gonzalez-Cossio T, et al: Interrelations of lead levels in bone, venous blood, and umbilical cord blood with exogenous lead exposure through maternal plasma lead in peripartum women. Environ Health Perspect 109:527–532, 2001.

171. Hall A: The increasing use of lead as an abortifacient: A series of thirty cases of plumbism. BMJ 1:582–587, 1905.

172. Hertz-Picciotto I: The evidence that lead increases the risk for spontaneous abortion. Am J Ind Med 38:300–309, 2000.

173. Borja-Aburto VH, Hertz-Picciotto I, Lopez MR, et al: Blood lead levels measured prospectively and risk of spontaneous abortion. Am J Epidemiol 150:590–597, 1999.

174. Andrews KW, Savitz DA, Hertz-Picciotto I: Prenatal lead exposure in relation to gestational age and birth weight: A review of epidemiological studies. Am J Ind Med 26:13–32, 1994.

175. Gonzalez-Cossio T, Peterson KE, Sanin LH, et al: Decrease in birth weight in relation to maternal bone-lead burden. Pediatrics 100:856–862, 1997.

176. Torres-Sanchez LE, Berkowitz G, Lopez-Carrillo L, et al: Intrauterine lead exposure and preterm birth. Environ Res (A) 81:297–301, 1999.

177. Bellinger D: Teratogen update: Lead. Teratology 50:367–373, 1994.

178. Wasserman GA, Liu X, Popovac D: The Yugoslavia prospective lead study: Contributions of prenatal and postnatal lead exposure to early intelligence. Neurotoxicol Teratol 22:811–818, 2000.

179. McClain RM, Siekierka JJ: The effects of various chelating agents on the teratogenicity of lead nitrates in rats. Toxicol Appl Pharmacol 31:434–442, 1975.

180. McClain RM, Siekierka JJ: The placental transfer of lead-chelate complexes in the rat. Toxicol Appl Pharmacol 31:443–451, 1975.

181. Chen S, Golemboski KA, Sanders FS, et al: Persistent effect of in utero meso-2,3-dimercaptosuccinic acid (DMSA) on immune function and lead-induced immunotoxicity. Toxicology 132:67–79, 1999.

182. Brownie CF, Brownie C, Noden D, et al: Teratogenic effect of calcium edetate (CaEDTA) in rats and the protective effect of zinc. Toxicol Appl Pharmacol 82:426–443, 1986.

183. Domingo JL, Ortega A, Paternain JL, et al: Oral meso-2,3-dimercaptosuccinic acid in pregnant Sprague-Dawley rats: Teratogenicity and alterations in mineral metabolism: I. Teratological evaluation. J Toxicol Environ Health 30:181–190, 1990.

184. Taubeneck MW, Domingo JL, Llobet JM, et al: Meso-2,3-dimercaptosuccinic acid (DMSA) affects maternal and fetal copper metabolism in Swiss mice. Toxicology 72:27–40, 1992.

185. Domingo JL: Prevention by chelating agents of metal-induced developmental toxicity. Reprod Toxicol 9:105–113, 1995.

186. Angle CR, McIntire MS: Lead poisoning during pregnancy: Fetal tolerance of calcium disodium edetate. Am J Dis Child 108:436–439, 1964.

187. Timpo AE, Amin JS, Casalino MB, et al: Congenital lead intoxication. J Pediatr 94:765–767, 1979.

CHAPTER **79**

Mercury

Irma de Vries

Mercury is a naturally occurring metal that exists in several physical and chemical forms. *Inorganic mercury* refers to compounds formed after the combining of mercury with elements such as chlorine, sulfur, or oxygen. After combining with carbon by covalent linkage, the compounds formed are called *organic mercury compounds* or *organomercurials*. The most common forms of mercury in the environment are elemental mercury, mercuric sulfide (cinnabar ore, from which elemental mercury is refined by heating), mercuric chloride, and the organic mercury compound methylmercury. In the environment, methylmercury is produced by the methylation of inorganic mercury by microorganisms. This form of mercury may enter and accumulate in the aquatic food chain.[1] Major methylmercury poisonings occurred in Minamata Bay, Japan, in the 1950s after the consumption of contaminated seafood following severe industrial mercury discharge into the bay. Another mass tragedy occurred in Iraq in 1971–1972 after consumption of bread contaminated with methylmercury used as a fungicide on seed grain.[2]

All forms of mercury have specific toxicity profiles to consider on exposure. The routes of exposure, toxicokinetics, target organs, and treatments differ to a great extent. Acute toxicity usually is seen after inhalational exposure to elemental mercury vapors and ingestion of inorganic mercury compounds. Exposure to organic mercury most commonly occurs as a result of ingestion of seafood or other contaminated food products.[3]

Exposures to elemental mercury without appreciable clinical relevance are the following. A frequently occurring exposure, especially in children, is the ingestion of small amounts of elemental mercury from a broken oral thermometer. After ingestion, elemental mercury is absorbed poorly from a normally functioning gastrointestinal tract. Because of this limited absorption and the small volume typically ingested, these elemental mercury exposures are considered nontoxic. If gastrointestinal function or anatomy is abnormal, however, elemental mercury may be absorbed into the blood or extravasate into the peritoneal space. The same is true of elemental mercury in the rectum from a broken thermometer. Dermal exposure to elemental mercury vapor or liquid poses a minor occupational hazard compared with inhalational exposure because skin absorption is minimal.[4] Although there has been some concern about whether mercury vapors released from dental amalgam fillings pose health risks, there is no scientific evidence of toxic effects from these exposures.[5]

MERCURY COMPOUNDS AND SOURCES

Elemental Mercury

Synonyms for elemental mercury are metallic mercury (Hg^0), quicksilver, liquid silver, and hydrargyrum. Elemental mercury is a silvery, shining liquid at room temperature. It is a heavy metal with a high vapor pressure of 0.002 mm Hg at 25°C. Consequently, at room temperature, some mercury evaporates. These vapors are colorless and odorless; vaporization increases significantly when mercury is heated. After accidental spills, metallic mercury and its vapors are difficult to remove. Especially in enclosed rooms, significant concentrations may be reached. If decontamination is not carried out properly, this can result in prolonged exposure. Most intoxications arise from occupational exposures, mainly in mining and extracting processes; in industrial plants as chloralkali plants; in dental amalgam preparation; and in the manufacture and repair of instruments such as mercury thermometers, barometers, sphygmomanometers, batteries, and electrical switches. Elemental and inorganic mercury can be present in herbal preparations and used in religious and spiritual remedies.

Inorganic Mercury Salts

Synonyms for and examples of inorganic mercury salts are mercurous ion (Hg^+), mercuric ion (Hg^{2+}), mercurous chloride (HgCl, calomel), mercuric chloride ($HgCl_2$, corrosive sublimate), and mercuric oxide (HgO). Inorganic mercury exists primarily as a salt of monovalent (mercurous) or divalent (mercuric) forms. Ingestion of inorganic mercuric salts in concentrations exceeding 10% produces severe corrosive damage. Mercuric chloride is a common salt. Inorganic mercury compounds have had many uses (e.g., as antibacterials, topical antiseptics, components of skin-lightening products, paints, tattoo dyes [red mercuric sulfide], diuretics, and cathartics). Currently, mercuric oxide still is used in batteries and in fluorescent light bulbs.

Organic Mercury

Organic mercury exists in three major forms: aryl, short-chain alkyl, and long-chain alkyl compounds. Methylmercury, a short-chain alkyl compound, is the predominant form of organic mercury found in the environment. In the short-chain alkyl compounds, there is a stable carbon mercury bond. In the long-chain alkyl and aryl compounds, such as phenylmercury salts, the carbon mercury bond is less stable, and the toxicity of these compounds may be due to the divalent mercury released after the carbon mercury bond has been ruptured.[2] Organic mercury compounds have been used as biocides, as fungicides, as pesticides, as seed dressings, as antiseptics, as medicinal preservatives (thimerosal), and in paints.

TOXICOKINETICS

Elemental Mercury

The most important route of exposure is inhalation of mercury vapors. After inhalation, the lipid-soluble vapor rapidly diffuses across alveolar membranes, enters the blood, and partitions between plasma and red blood cells. Because of its high lipophilicity, mercury vapors are distributed throughout the body, including the central nervous system and fetus, if present. After absorption and distribution, most of the elemental mercury is oxidized intracellularly to inorganic mercurous ions (Hg^+) and subsequently to mercuric ions (Hg^{2+}) through the catalase-hydrogen peroxidase pathway. Mercuric mercury has a lower lipophilicity than unoxidized elemental mercury, which causes retention and accumulation of mercuric mercury in the brain, probably because of its presence as an insoluble selenium compound.[6] The further pattern of distribution changes toward that seen with inorganic mercury compounds, with accumulation primarily in the kidneys.[2] The overall retention of inhaled mercury vapor in human tissues is approximately 70% to 80%. Elimination of elemental mercury occurs through expired air, urine, and feces. Approximately 10% of an absorbed dose is exhaled in the first few days after exposure.[7] Urine and feces are the main excretory routes of mercury. In the first few days after acute exposure to high levels of mercury vapor, a large fraction of mercury can be found in the urine. In blood, there is an initial half-life of mercury of 2 to 16 days, followed by a half-life comparable to that observed in the kidneys of more than 1 month.[8,9] The whole-body half-life of elemental mercury is about 60 days (range 35 to 90 days).[2]

Inorganic Mercury Salts

Approximately 10% of ingested mercuric chloride is absorbed. Disruption of the gastrointestinal mucosa may enhance mercury absorption. The monovalent mercurous salts are less soluble, and absorption is thought to depend on their oxidation to the divalent form.[10] Some mercuric compounds (HgS, HgSe) have such low solubility that they are regarded as nontoxic. Cutaneous absorption of inorganic mercurials is possible, depending on the solubility of the vehicle. Although the mercuric ion's lipid solubility is low, with consequent poor penetration of the blood-brain barrier, chronic exposure, slow elimination, and the presence of a small amount of unoxidized elemental mercury (after reduction of inorganic mercuric ions) gradually result in accumulation of mercuric ions in the cerebellar and cerebral cortices of the brain.[11] Mercuric ions do not readily cross the placenta. In plasma, mercury is bound to protein. Most of the absorbed dose is accumulated in the kidneys. Excretion of the circulating mercuric ion is mainly via the

feces and urine. Elimination occurs by tubular secretion into the urine and by exfoliation of renal tubular cells. Because renal excretion is inefficient, however, the mercury continues to accumulate in the kidney. Inorganic mercury can be secreted into bile. Small amounts of mercuric ions are reduced to elemental mercury vapor by reductase enzymes and oxygen dismutase and exhaled. The half-life of inorganic mercury is 30 to 60 days, with an average of approximately 40 days.[2]

Organic Mercury

Most organic mercury compounds are absorbed readily after ingestion. Gastrointestinal absorption of methylmercury (a short-chain alkyl compound) is about 90%. The absorption of aryl and long-chain alkyl compounds is less, but greater than 50% has been reported.[12] Dermal and inhalational absorption occur, although the extent is not known exactly. The exception is phenylmercury, which is not well absorbed after ingestion or dermal contact. After absorption, intracellular cleavage of the labile carbon-mercury bond of the aryl and long-chain organic mercurials causes rapid conversion to inorganic forms, resulting in kinetics and toxicity similar to those in inorganic mercury. The short-chain alkyl mercurials are stable, and only a minor part is converted to inorganic forms. Because of their high lipophilicity, these short-chain alkyl compounds rapidly distribute throughout the body, with penetration of the blood-brain and placental barriers. The brain-to-blood concentration ratio after completion of the initial distribution of methylmercury is about 10:1.[2] Over the course of years, conversion of methylmercury to inorganic mercury in the brain has been reported.[13] Accumulation of methylmercury in red blood cells results in a large red blood cell–to–plasma ratio (10:1).[12] Accumulation of methylmercury is mainly in the kidneys and liver and to a lesser extent in brain tissues (although toxicity is expressed mostly in the brain) and hair. Slow conversion of methylmercury to inorganic mercury also takes place in the kidneys. Elimination of methylmercury is predominantly fecal. Methylmercury binds to reduced glutathione and is secreted in bile.[14] The methylmercury-glutathione complex is degraded to cysteine complexes that are subject to reabsorption. The N-acetyl-homocysteine-methylmercury metabolite undergoes enterohepatic recirculation. In the intestinal tract, a fraction of the methylmercury is converted to inorganic mercury and excreted in the feces. The whole-body half-life of methylmercury is about 70 days. The half-life in blood is approximately 44 days. After the intravenous administration of methylmercury in volunteers, however, the half-lives were 44 days for blood and whole body.[15]

PATHOPHYSIOLOGY OF TOXIC EFFECTS

Elemental Mercury

Damage to the airways by elemental mercury vapor may be by direct-contact effects or may be indirect due to binding to sulfhydryl groups of enzymes and proteins. The vapor may cause an exudative alveolar and interstitial edema, with desquamation of the bronchiolar epithelium. The ensuing partial obstruction may result in alveolar dilation and the complications discussed subsequently in the section on clinical presentation.[16] After absorption and distribution, elemental mercury vapor is subject to oxidation to mercuric ions (Hg^{2+}) by the catalase-hydrogen peroxidase pathway. The oxidation process depends on the amounts of catalase and hydrogen peroxide in the cell, and inhibitors of catalase or competitive substrates can slow down the oxidation. Mercuric cation can be reduced to elemental mercury by processes involving reductase enzymes and oxygen dismutase.[2] At steady state, the oxidation-reduction reaction of absorbed elemental mercury favors the mercuric cation, however.[17] This conversion to inorganic mercury is responsible for mercury's toxicity. Differences in the patterns of toxicity between inhaled mercury vapors and inorganic compounds are attributed to differences in lipophilicity and primary distribution and to specific characteristics of the inorganic compounds involved (e.g., corrosive features).

Inorganic Mercury Salts

The major mechanism of biologic activity of inorganic mercury in vivo is its reaction with sulfhydryl groups. The covalent binding to sulfur replaces the hydrogen ion in the sulfhydryl group. This is an almost instantaneous reaction, causing a high-affinity binding of the divalent mercuric ion to thiol-containing molecules as proteins, cysteine, and glutathione. Binding also occurs with phosphoryl, carboxyl, and amide groups. Because of the binding to glutathione, inorganic mercury is secreted from liver cells into bile. The accumulation of the divalent cation in the kidneys induces the thiol-containing protein metallothionein. This protein may play an important role in detoxification by forming a nontoxic Hg^{2+}-metallothionein compound. The divalent mercury cation also can give rise to oxidant free radicals that attack not only proteins but also DNA. Through alterations in intracellular thiol status, mercury can promote oxidative stress, lipid peroxidation, and mitochondrial dysfunction. Widespread dysfunction of enzymes, transport mechanisms, membranes, and structural proteins results, leading to multiple organ dysfunction. Mercuric ions may directly injure the epithelial cells of the proximal renal tubules, causing renal tubular necrosis.[18] After the ingestion of corrosive mercuric salts, renal hypoperfusion due to shock also may cause renal tubular necrosis. An immune mechanism is attributed to the development of membranous glomerulonephritis. Type IV hypersensitivity reactions, which develop over 21 to 28 days after the exposure to mercury, underlie the formation of granulomas. Granulomatous interstitial nephritis,[19] granulomas forming after intravenous injection, and cutaneous mercury granulomas have resulted. Also, an idiosyncratic hypersensitivity reaction is thought to be the underlying pathophysiologic etiology for acrodynia, or "pink disease," in children exposed to inorganic mercury.

The neuropathologic changes with elemental or inorganic mercury poisoning are different from the changes seen with organic mercury poisoning. Autopsy findings in patients who died after exposure to elemental mercury vapor reveal a well-preserved neuronal architecture, with the exception of decreased numbers of Purkinje and granular cells in the cerebellum[20] and prominent ischemic changes in the cerebellum in one patient and recent infarcts in the occipital lobe and the putamen in another.[11]

Organic Mercury

The biochemistry of the methylmercury cation (CH_3Hg^+), the prototype of organic mercury poisoning, is similar to the inorganic cation. There also is a high affinity for sulfhydryl groups. Methylmercury does not induce metallothionein.[2] In high doses, methylmercury can cause severe damage to the adult brain and the developing brain. Methylmercury is toxic to the cerebral and cerebellar cortex, causing neuronal loss and reactive proliferation of the glial cells, microcavitation, vascular congestion, petechial hemorrhage, and edema.[11] The visual cortex (calcarine cortex), the auditory center in the temporal cortex, the cortical motor and sensory centers, and the cerebellar cortex are especially affected. In the fetal brain and developing brain, damage is diffuse because neuronal cell division and migration are inhibited by blockage of the assembly process of microtubules in the neuronal cell.[2] Children can experience severe brain damage from prenatal exposure, even when the mother is much less affected.[21]

CLINICAL PRESENTATION

Elemental Mercury

After acute inhalation of vaporized elemental mercury, within hours of exposure, cough, chills, fever, headache, and shortness of breath can occur (metal fume fever). In addition, metallic taste; gastrointestinal complaints of nausea, vomiting, and diarrhea; salivation; excessive sweating; weakness; and visual disturbances can occur. Immune thrombocytopenia has been described in the acute phase.[22] At high concentrations, major pulmonary manifestations may develop, including necrotizing bronchitis, bronchiolitis, and pneumonitis, which can progress to pulmonary edema, respiratory failure, and death. Complications include multiple pneumothoraces, pneumomediastinum, and subcutaneous emphysema. Survivors of severe pulmonary manifestations may develop pulmonary fibrosis, granuloma formation, and residual restrictive pulmonary disease. Children may be particularly susceptible to the pulmonary toxicity of mercury vapors.[23]

The oxidation of elemental mercury to mercuric ions leads to features of inorganic mercury poisoning (described in the next section), characterized by renal toxicity, gingivostomatitis, and neurologic symptoms. In acute exposures to high levels, besides the lungs, the kidneys are the critical organs, with necrosis of the proximal tubuli and acute renal failure. Long-term, low-level exposure affects the neurologic system, with intention tremor and erethism (a condition characterized by increased irritability, excitability, anxiety, and shyness) as prominent features.[24]

There are several case reports of other routes of exposure to elemental mercury. Aspiration of metallic mercury into the tracheobronchial tree has resulted in endobronchial hemorrhage and death.[25] Aspiration usually does not lead to acute or chronic mercury poisoning. Intravenous injection of mercury can cause not only acute pulmonary embolus with respiratory failure but also pulmonary and systemic microembolisms. After oxidation to the mercuric cation, systemic inorganic mercury poisoning may occur. Subcutaneous injections or wounds contaminated with metallic mercury may cause local abscesses or granuloma formations. Systemic effects, including pulmonary embolization, have been reported but are unusual.[26]

Inorganic Mercury Salts

After acute ingestion of mercury salts, the immediate features observed are related to the direct caustic effects of these salts, with mercuric ions being more toxic than mercurous ions. After ingestion of mercuric chloride, symptoms can vary from severe irritation of the gastrointestinal tract to ulceration, necrosis, perforation, and acute hemorrhage, subsequently followed by hypovolemia, shock, electrolyte disturbances, and acute renal tubular necrosis with renal failure. Immediately after ingestion, grayish discoloration of mucous membranes, metallic taste, nausea, vomiting, diarrhea, and severe abdominal pain occur. With the disruption of the gastrointestinal mucosa, mercury absorption can be extensive, and the direct toxicity of the mercuric cation on the proximal tubules further increases renal toxicity. Deterioration of renal function starts within hours after exposure.

If the patient survives these acute initial effects, systemic toxicity develops, as also is observed in subacute or chronic poisoning. Systemic toxicity includes renal dysfunction, gastrointestinal symptoms, neurologic toxicity, and cutaneous symptoms. Chronic inorganic mercury poisoning also occurs after prolonged inhalation of elemental mercury vapor (owing to oxidation of elemental mercury) or after the in vivo dissociation of carbon-sulfur bonds of organic mercurial compounds, especially the aryl and long-chain alkyl mercurials. The primary target organ is the kidney, with proximal tubular dysfunction. This dysfunction can range from asymptomatic, reversible proteinuria to tubular necrosis and anuria. An immune glomerulonephritis may develop, which can lead to a full-blown nephrotic syndrome. Interstitial granulomatous nephritis has been described.[19] Oral symptoms of mercury intoxication include a metallic taste and burning sensation in the mouth, a blue lining of the gums, loose dentition, gingivitis, stomatitis, hypersalivation, and nausea. Neurologic toxicity is expressed by tremor and syndromes such as neurasthenia and erethism, which include headache, irritability, excitability, delirium, anxiety, shyness, emotional lability, depression, loss of concentration and memory, fatigue, weakness, anorexia, and insomnia. Other neurologic manifestations include a mixed sensorimotor peripheral neuropathy, ataxia, constriction of visual fields, and anosmia.[24]

Acrodynia (painful extremities), also known as *pink disease*, was described primarily in children exposed to inorganic mercury. Acrodynia is characterized by a pink maculopapular skin rash, particularly on the hands and feet, and hyperkeratotic induration also of the hands, feet, and face. In addition, excessive sweating, tachycardia, hypertension, photophobia, and neurologic symptoms, as mentioned previously, can occur.[27] Cutaneous manifestations of mercury toxicity may be a systemically induced allergic contact dermatitis, toxic contact dermatitis, or the formation of cutaneous granulomas, usually after injection of mercury.[28]

Organic Mercury

Features of poisonings by long-chain alkyl and aryl organic compounds have some similarities to inorganic mercury

toxicity but tend to be more subacute or chronic. Central nervous system toxicity is the hallmark of the short-chain alkyl compounds, particularly methylmercury. Clinical effects can be delayed for days to months after ingestion, depending on the amount ingested and the rate of enzymatic dysfunction. Neurologic symptoms start with paresthesias (facial and distal extremities) and headaches and progress to ataxia, dysarthria, visual field constriction, blindness, hearing disturbances, deafness, tremors, movement disorders, psychomotor retardation, and dementia. In severe cases, death ensues.[1,24] Dimethylmercury poisoning has been reported in only a few cases of human poisoning, each proving fatal.[29] After ingestion of ethylmercury, gastrointestinal symptoms, such as nausea, vomiting, abdominal pain, and diarrhea, can occur. High exposures to ethylmercury in the form of thimerosal have been reported to be associated with acrodynia, renal failure, and neuropathy, consistent with chronic inorganic mercury toxicity.[24] Dermal exposure may cause dermatitis.

DIAGNOSIS

In measuring mercury concentrations in blood and urine, it is essential to use mercury-free collection materials; generally, it is best to obtain blood and urine containers from the performing laboratories. There is not a good correlation between blood and urinary mercury concentrations and clinical manifestations. There is considerable overlap among concentrations of mercury found in the normal population, asymptomatic exposed individuals, and patients with clinical evidence of poisoning.

Urine Mercury Concentrations

Elemental and inorganic mercury exposure can be measured by determining urinary mercury concentration, preferably using a 24-hour urine collection rather than a spot urine level. Urine mercury concentrations correlate poorly, however, with exposure severity, symptoms, and total body burden.[11] Correlation is even less if the mercury exposure has been intermittent or variable in intensity.[24] In long-term exposures, the urinary excretion rate reflects the kidney content of mercury.[2] Urine mercury values have their greatest utility in confirming exposure and monitoring the efficacy of chelation therapy. Because methylmercury is hardly excreted in urine, urine mercury concentrations are not useful in evaluating methylmercury intoxication. The same is true for other alkylmercury compounds. Urine mercury concentrations less than 20 to 25 μg/L (<100 to 125 nmol/L) are considered normal, although in occupationally unexposed persons, levels greater than 10 μg/L (>50 nmol/L) (approximately 5 nmol/mmol creatinine) are seldom found.[30] Urine mercury concentrations greater than 100 μg/L (>500 nmol/L) have been associated with minor neurologic signs,[24] whereas levels greater than 300 μg/L (>1500 nmol/L) usually are associated with overt symptoms.[30]

Blood Mercury Concentrations

Soon after exposure to elemental and inorganic mercury, mercury concentrations in the blood may reflect mercury exposure accurately. As soon as redistribution takes place, these levels become less reliable in predicting toxicity. As a result of the relatively high concentration of methylmercury in red blood cells, whole-blood levels are relatively accurate in determining the acute/total body burden of methylmercury.[31] Whole-blood mercury concentrations are usually less than 10 μg/L (<50 nmol/L), but levels less than 20 μg/L (<100 nmol/L) still are considered to be in the normal range.[24] After long-term exposure to mercury vapor, whole-blood mercury concentrations of 35 μg/L (175 nmol/L) may be associated with nonspecific symptoms.[32]

Additional Laboratory Tests

Relevant laboratory tests, depending on the clinical scenario, may include arterial blood gas analysis, serum chemistry assessments including renal and liver functions, complete blood count, type and crossmatch of blood if exposed to caustic inorganic mercury, and screening for urinary markers of glomerular or proximal tubular damage (proteinuria, glucosuria, amino aciduria, enzymes such as α-*N*-acetylglucosaminidase, β$_2$-microglobulin, leucine aminopeptidase, retinol binding protein, γ-glutamyltranspeptidase, glutathione-*S*-transferases).

Radiographs and Other Diagnostic Procedures

With acute inhalation of elemental mercury vapor, chest radiographs initially may show interstitial or alveolar abnormalities (e.g., "bronchial thickening," diffuse alveolar infiltrates, and edema).[33] Thereafter, the radiologic features of adult respiratory distress syndrome may be apparent, as may be signs of complications (e.g., pneumothorax, pneumomediastinum, and subcutaneous emphysema). Elemental mercury is radiopaque and can be seen on radiographs after ingestion, intravenous exposure, or subcutaneous exposure. Reported pulmonary computed tomography findings in acute mercury vapor exposure are centrilobular nodules, ground-glass opacification, and alveolar consolidation, corresponding to acute interstitial pneumonitis.[34] Depending on the mercury compound involved, the circumstances of exposure, and the clinical features, other diagnostic procedures may be done, including endoscopic procedures, electrocardiogram, cardiovascular monitoring, pulmonary function tests, electroneuromyography, and neuropsychologic tests.

TREATMENT

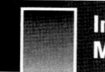

Indications for ICU Admission in Mercury Poisoning

Pulmonary symptoms after inhalation of mercury vapor
Corrosive damage to the oropharyngeal and gastrointestinal mucosa with risk of airway obstruction and hypovolemic shock

Immediate Considerations

Assessment and management of the patient's respiratory function, circulation, and urinary output are primary. Acute inhalational exposure to elemental mercury vapors requires monitoring for respiratory failure. Supplemental oxygen or endotracheal intubation and mechanical ventilation may be necessary. There are no known aerosolized antidotes for acute inhalational exposures. Ingestion of corrosive inorganic mercury requires the establishment of rapid vascular access and treatment to prevent serious fluid losses and shock. Caustic injury to the oropharyngeal mucosa may cause severe local edema, and endotracheal intubation or tracheostomy may be required to overcome obstruction of the airway.

Decontamination

Initial decontamination measures after skin or eye exposure are removal of contaminated clothing and copious flushing of contaminated skin and eyes. After ingestion of corrosive inorganic mercury, as with any caustic ingestion, the induction of emesis or gastric lavage is contraindicated.[35] If perforation is suspected or radiopaque objects remain present, direct endoscopic evaluation and removal should be performed. Activated charcoal hardly binds metallic compounds. In the absence of caustic injury, whole-bowel irrigation with polyethylene glycol may be considered until the rectal effluent is clear and the radiopaque material is absent.[36] After subcutaneous injection of elemental mercury, excision of mercury deposits in affected tissues is the most important treatment.

Role of Extracorporeal Removal Techniques

Extracorporeal removal techniques lack efficacy in removing mercury from the body. Hemodialysis may be necessary if renal failure ensues. Although plasma exchange therapy was reported to decrease plasma mercury in a 26-year-old woman with severe inorganic mercury poisoning,[37] prompt institution of chelation therapy is preferable.

Specific Treatment

NONANTIDOTAL

Corticosteroids have been administered in the case of interstitial granulomatous nephritis due to mercury poisoning. Their efficacy has not been shown in a controlled trial, however. In mercury vapor poisonings, corticosteroids do not seem to have a clear effect on the eventual outcome.[33]

ANTIDOTAL

Chelating agents effective in the treatment of mercury poisoning contain thiol groups, which are thought to compete with endogenous sulfhydryl groups for the binding of mercury. For years, elemental and inorganic mercury poisonings have been treated with dimercaprol and penicillamine. Dimercaprol was the primary chelating agent because it mobilizes mercury from the kidneys and protects against kidney damage. Dimercaprol cannot be used for the treatment of alkyl organic mercury poisoning because it might worsen neurotoxicity after redistribution of mercury into the brain.[10]

More recently, 2,3-dimercaptopropane-1-sulfonate (DMPS) and 2,3-dimercaptosuccinic acid (DMSA) have been shown to be effective agents in reducing the body burden of mercury and protecting against renal damage.[38] DMPS and DMSA are water-soluble analogues of dimercaprol and have the advantages that they can be administered intravenously and orally and they have better side-effect profiles. In animal studies comparing the various chelators, the highest efficacy for mobilizing mercury from exposed renal tissue was seen with DMPS.[39] In a patient treated with DMPS and hemodialysis because of anuric renal failure, after ingestion of mercuric chloride, mercury's half-life in the initial phase of elimination was estimated at 2.5 days. In the subsequent terminal phase, it was approximately 8.1 days. In this case, the nonrenal clearance of mercury through the biliary and gastrointestinal tract accounted for more than 80% of total elimination.[40] Chelation therapy with DMPS and DMSA in a patient with severe organic mercury poisoning resulted in complete recovery except for minor sensory deficits. Mercury elimination was biphasic, with blood mercury half-lives of 2.2 and 40.5 days.[41] Prompt institution of chelation therapy is important, however. Aggressive chelation therapy with DMSA was futile in a patient with rapid neurologic deterioration 3 months after exposure to dimethylmercury. From this case presentation, it was suggested that DMSA may have a limited capacity to distribute to and chelate organic mercury when this has been deposited in neuronal tissue or that DMSA cannot reverse tissue damage.[42,43]

Some studies have investigated a possible role for *N*-acetylcysteine in the chelation therapy for methylmercury poisoning.[24] A striking increase in urinary excretion of methylmercury has been reported in animal studies. In mice that received *N*-acetylcysteine (10 mg/mL) in the drinking water starting at 48 hours after methylmercury administration, the excretion of mercury in urine over the subsequent 48 hours was 47% to 54% compared with 4% to 10% in control animals. In mice, *N*-acetylcysteine was able to mobilize methylmercury from tissues, including the brain. Clearance of inorganic mercury was not accelerated by *N*-acetylcysteine.[44] Most methylmercury poisonings have a chronic course, however, and the efficacy of *N*-acetylcysteine in these situations is not yet established.

DMPS. At present, the chelator of choice in elemental and inorganic mercury poisoning is DMPS. In the case of organic mercury poisoning, there are conflicting results regarding the efficacy of DMPS and DMSA, possibly depending on the timing of chelation therapy. DMPS has been used safely for years in Europe. DMSA and dimercaprol are alternatives. Indications for chelation therapy after mercury intoxication are not firmly established. Chelation therapy should be started early after significant exposure in patients with features of severe poisoning and in patients with evidence of a large mercury burden shown by biologic monitoring.[24]

DMPS can be administered intravenously, dissolved in saline 0.9%, or orally. In a case of severe mercuric chloride poisoning in an adult, an adequate dosage regimen was 250 mg intravenously every 4 hours for the first 48 hours, then 250 mg intravenously every 6 hours for the second 48-hour period, followed by 250 mg intravenously every 8 hours afterward. The intravenous regimen was followed by oral treatment: 300 mg of DMPS three times a day for 7 weeks.[40] The duration of therapy depends on concentrations of mercury in blood and urine. Although not observed frequently, adverse reactions to DMPS include rash, nausea, and leukopenia.

DMSA. DMSA can be administered intravenously, dissolved in saline 0.9%, or orally. In adults, the dosage is

10 mg/kg three times a day for the first 5 days, followed by 10 mg/kg twice a day for the next 14 days. This same dosage schedule has been used in children, although a dosage based on body surface area may be a better choice because it prevents underdosing. In children, DMSA is administered at a dose of 350 mg/m² three times a day for the first 5 days, followed by 350 mg/m² twice a day for the next 14 days. Repeated administration may be necessary, with a 2-week interval between treatments. Adverse effects usually are limited to a mild, transient elevation of hepatic transaminase levels and mild gastrointestinal discomfort.

Dimercaprol. Dimercaprol must be administered intramuscularly. It can be administered at a dose of 2.5 to 5 mg/kg every 4 to 12 hours.[30] A decreasing dosing schedule for 10 days has been used, starting with 5 mg/kg intramuscularly once, 2.5 mg/kg intramuscularly every 8 to 12 hours for 1 day, and then 2.5 mg/kg intramuscularly every 12 to 24 hours thereafter. The dimercaprol-mercury chelate is excreted into bile and urine. Common side effects of dimercaprol include hypertension, tachycardia, pain at the injection site, nausea, vomiting, headache, and diaphoresis. Convulsions have been reported. Hemolysis may be induced if the patient is glucose-6-phosphate dehydrogenase deficient.[10]

SPECIAL POPULATIONS

Pregnant Patients

Methylmercury is of major concern in pregnant women because of its profound fetotoxicity.[21] Maternal exposure can lead to spontaneous abortion or severe developmental delay, deformities, mental retardation, and the clinical features described earlier.[21]

REFERENCES

1. Agency for Toxic Substances and Disease Registry (ATSDR): Toxicological Profile for Mercury. Atlanta, Department of Health and Human Services, 1999.
2. Clarkson TW: The toxicology of mercury. Crit Rev Clin Lab Sci 34:369–403, 1997.
3. Baum CR: Treatment of mercury intoxication. Curr Opin Pediatr 11:265–268, 1999.
4. Hursh JB, Clarkson TW, Miles EF, et al: Percutaneous absorption of mercury vapor by man. Arch Environ Health 44:120–127, 1989.
5. U.S. Public Health Service, Committee to Coordinate Environmental Health and Related Programs, Subcommittee on Risk Management: Dental Amalgam: A Scientific Review and Recommended Public Health Service Strategy for Research, Education, and Regulation. Washington, D.C., U.S. Public Health Service, 1993.
6. WHO: Environmental Health Criteria 118: Inorganic Mercury. Geneva, WHO, 1991.
7. Sandborgh-Englund G, Elinder CG, Johanson G, et al: The absorption, blood levels, and excretion of mercury after a single dose of mercury vapor in humans. Toxicol Appl Pharmacol 150:146–153, 1998.
8. Hursh JB, Cherian MG, Clarkson TW, et al: Clearance of mercury vapor (Hg-197, Hg-203) inhaled by human subjects. Arch Environ Health 31:302–309, 1976.
9. Barregard L, Quelquejeu G, Sallsten G, et al: Dose-dependent elimination kinetics for mercury in urine: Observations of subjects with brief but high-level exposure. Int Arch Occup Environ Health 68:345–348, 1996.
10. Klaassen C: Heavy metals and heavy-metal antagonists. In Hardman JG, Limbird LE (eds): Goodman and Gilman's The Pharmacological Basis of Therapeutics, 9th ed. New York, McGraw-Hill, 1996, pp 1649–1671.
11. Eto K, Takizawa Y, Akagi H, et al: Differential diagnosis between organic and inorganic mercury poisoning in human cases—the pathologic point of view. Toxicol Pathol 27:664–671, 1999.
12. Nordberg GF, Skerfving S: Metabolism. In Friberg L, Vostal J (eds): Mercury in the Environment: An Epidemiological and Toxicological Appraisal. Cleveland, CRC Press, 1972, pp 29–92.
13. Davis LE, Kornfeld M, Mooney HS, et al: Methylmercury poisoning: Long-term clinical, radiological, toxicological, and pathological studies of an affected family. Ann Neurol 35:680–688, 1994.
14. Ballatori N, Clarkson TW: Biliary transport of glutathione and methylmercury. Am J Physiol 244:G435-G441, 1983.
15. Smith JC, Allen P, Turner MD, et al: The kinetics of intravenously administered methylmercury in man. Toxicol Appl Pharmacol 128:251–256, 1994.
16. Jaffe KM, Shurtleff DB, Robertson WO: Survival after acute mercury vapor poisoning: Role of intensive supportive care. Am J Dis Child 137:749–751, 1983.
17. Magos L: Physiology and toxicology of mercury. In Sigel A, Sigel H (eds): Metal Ions in Biological Systems, Vol 34. New York, Marcel Dekker, Inc., 1997, pp 321–370.
18. Zalups RK, Lash LH: Advance in understanding the renal transport and toxicity of mercury. J Toxicol Environ Health 42:1–44, 1994.
19. Franco A, Antolin A, Trigueros M, et al: Two consecutive episodes of acute renal failure following mercury poisoning. Nephrol Dial Transplant 12:328–330, 1997.
20. Asano S, Eto K, Kurisaki E, et al: Acute inorganic mercury vapor inhalation poisoning. Pathol Int 50:169–174, 2000.
21. Harada M: Minamata disease: Methylmercury poisoning in Japan caused by environmental pollution. Crit Rev Toxicol 25:1–24, 1995.
22. Fuortes LJ, Weismann DN, Graeff ML, et al: Immune thrombocytopenia and elemental mercury poisoning. J Toxicol Clin Toxicol 33:449–455, 1995.
23. Moutinho ME, Tompkins AL, Rowland TW, et al: Acute mercury vapor poisoning. Am J Dis Child 135:42–44, 1981.
24. Goldman LR, Shannon MW, and the Committee on Environmental Health: Technical report: Mercury in the environment: Implications for pediatricians. Pediatrics 108:197–205, 2001.
25. Zimmerman JE: Fatality following metallic mercury aspiration during removal of a long intestinal tube. JAMA 208:2158–2160, 1969.
26. Smith SR, Jaffe DM, Skinner MA: Case report of metallic mercury injury. Pediatr Emerg Care 13:114–116, 1997.
27. Torres AD, Rai AN, Hardiek ML: Mercury intoxication and arterial hypertension: Report of two patients and review of the literature. Pediatrics 105:341–344, 2000.
28. Boyd AS, Seger D, Vannucci S, et al: Mercury exposure and cutaneous disease. J Am Acad Dermatol 43:81–90, 2000.
29. Siegler RW, Nierenberg DW, Hickey WF: Fatal poisoning from liquid dimethylmercury: A neuropathologic study. Hum Pathol 30:720–723, 1999.
30. Bates BA: Mercury. In Haddad LM, Shannon MW, Winchester JF (eds): Clinical Management of Poisoning and Drug Overdose, 3rd ed. Philadelphia, WB Saunders, 1998, pp 750–756.
31. Dales LG: The neurotoxicity of alkyl mercury compounds. Am J Med 53:219–232, 1972.
32. WHO: Environmental Health Criteria 1: Mercury. Geneva, WHO, 1976.
33. Solis MT, Yuen E, Cortez PS, et al: Family poisoned by mercury vapor inhalation. Am J Emerg Med 18:599–602, 2000.
34. Hashimoto M, Sato K, Heianna J, et al: Pulmonary CT findings in acute mercury vapour exposure. Clin Radiol 56:17–21, 2001.
35. AACT, EAPCCT: Position statement: Gastric lavage. J Toxicol Clin Toxicol 35:711–719, 1997.
36. AACT, EAPCCT: Position statement: Whole bowel irrigation. J Toxicol Clin Toxicol 35:753–762, 1997.
37. Yoshida M, Satoh H, Igarashi M, et al: Acute mercury poisoning by intentional ingestion of mercuric chloride. J Exp Med 182:347–352, 1997.
38. Aaseth J, Jacobsen D, Anderson O, Wickstrom E: Treatment of mercury and lead poisonings with dimercaptosuccinic acid and sodium dimercaptopropanesulphonate: A review. Analyst 120:853–854, 1994.
39. Keith RL, Setiarahardjo I, Fernando Q, et al: Utilization of renal slices to evaluate the efficacy of chelating agents for removing mercury from the kidney. Toxicology 116:67–75, 1997.
40. Toet AE, van Dijk A, Savelkoul TJF, Meulenbelt J: Mercury kinetics in a case of severe mercuric chloride poisoning treated with dimercapto-1-propane sulphonate (DMPS). Hum Exp Toxicol 13:11–16, 1994.
41. Pfab R, Muckter H, Roider G, Zilker Th: Clinical course of severe poisoning with thiomersal. J Toxicol Clin Toxicol 34:453–460, 1996.
42. Nierenberg DW, Nordgren RE, Chang MB, et al: Delayed cerebellar disease and death after accidental exposure to dimethylmercury. N Engl J Med 338:1672–1676, 1998.
43. Kulig K: A tragic reminder about organic mercury. N Engl J Med 338:1692–1693, 1998.
44. Ballatori N, Lieberman MW, Wang W: N-Acetylcysteine as an antidote in methylmercury poisoning. Environ Health Perspect 106:267–271, 1998.

CHAPTER 80

Antimony and Nickel

Javier Waksman ■ Scott D. Phillips

ANTIMONY

Antimony (stibium [Sb]) is a brittle, crystalline, silver-white metal found in nature in several ores. Stibnite (SbS_3) is the predominant ore; the others are mostly oxides. Antimony commonly is alloyed with other metals, such as lead, copper, and silver, to increase their hardness, mechanical strength, and corrosion resistance and to decrease their coefficient of friction. The common forms of antimony found in industry are antimony trioxide, pentoxide, trisulfide, oxysulfide, pentasulfide, and trichloride.

A significant amount of the consumption of antimony is for its use as a fire retardant (antimony trioxide) for plastics, textiles, rubber, building materials, adhesives, pigments, and papers.[1] It also is used in the manufacture of lead batteries, type metal, paints, ceramics, glass, solders, explosives, bearing metals, and semiconductors.[2] Antimony may be found in a gaseous state as stibine (SbH_3, hydrogen antimonide, antimony hydride), which is formed when antimony alloys are treated with acids and subjected to electrolytic action, as, for instance, during the charging of certain lead-containing batteries.

The ancient Romans used antimony compounds as emetic drugs (*calices vomitorum*) and expectorants.[3] Antimony potassium tartrate ("tartar emetic") historically was used in the treatment of schistosomiasis. Two pentavalent antimony-containing drugs—sodium stibogluconate (Pentostam) and meglumine antimoniate (Glucantime)—constitute the mainstays for contemporary treatment of visceral, mucosal, and cutaneous leishmaniasis.[4]

Biochemistry

Antimony has an atomic number of 51 and is found in group VA of the periodic table of elements directly below arsenic. Its atomic weight is 121.76, and it has four oxidation states: 0, +3, +5, and −3. The important toxicologic properties of antimony and common antimony-containing compounds are presented in Table 80-1.

Clinical Toxicology

The human data available regarding the pharmacokinetics and pharmacodynamics of antimony compounds are sparse and are derived mainly from animal studies, occupational exposures, and patients treated with antimony potassium tartrate, sodium stibogluconate, and meglumine antimoniate. Elevated antimony concentrations were found in the lungs of smelter workers 20 years after retirement,[5] and these concentrations seemed to increase with time of exposure.[6] The absorption of antimony from the respiratory tract depends on particle size,[7] whereas after oral ingestion less than 10% of antimony tartrate and 1% of all other forms of antimony are absorbed.[8] Cooper and colleagues[20] examined 28 smelter workers who had been exposed to antimony ore and antimony trioxide dust for 1 to 15 years. Antimony concentrations in area samples ranged from 0.08 to 138 mg/m³, but particle size was not specified. Pulmonary function studies carried out on 14 of these workers showed no consistent pattern of abnormalities. Three of the 13 workers who underwent radiographic examination were found, however, to have antimony pneumoconiosis, and 5 more were suspected of having this condition.

Valence states determine the distribution of antimony in blood and tissues; after inhalation, the trivalent and pentavalent forms concentrate in the erythrocytes and plasma. Antimony has been reported to accumulate in the liver when absorbed in the trivalent form and in the skeleton when given in the pentavalent form.[7] Other authors[9,10] found different distribution patterns, however, which also were related to oxidation state. Similar to the distribution pattern after inhalation, the distribution of antimony after gastrointestinal absorption also seems to depend on valence state.[11] Pentavalent antimony is excreted preferentially in urine; the trivalent forms are excreted in the feces.[12,13]

Biologic Half-Lives

A two-compartment pharmacokinetic model has been proposed by Chulay and coworkers[14] to describe the fate of antimony after being administered intramuscularly in the pentavalent form, consisting of a fast phase and a slow phase with elimination half-lives of 2.02 ± 0.25 hours and 76 ± 28 hours, respectively.

Pathophysiology

Being chemically, physically, and physiologically similar to arsenic, antimony toxicity is similar to arsenic toxicity.[15] Pentavalent compounds are considered less toxic than trivalent compounds. As with other metals, antimony interacts with sulfhydryl groups of enzymes and other proteins. In vitro antimony inhibits succinic oxidase, pyruvate oxidase,[16] and phosphofructokinase,[3] suggesting interference with cellular respiration.

TABLE 80-1 Properties of Antimony and Common Antimony Compounds[a]

PROPERTY	ANTIMONY	ANTIMONY PENTASULFIDE	ANTIMONY PENTOXIDE	ANTIMONY POTASSIUM TARTRATE
Atomic/molecular weight	121.75	403.80	323.5 (anhydrous)	333.93
Color	Silvery white	Yellow	Yellow	Colorless
Physical state	Solid	Solid	Solid	Solid
Valance state	0	+5	+5	+3
Melting point	630.5°C	75°C decomposes	380°C decomposes[f]	100°C ($-1/2H_2O$)
Boiling point	1750; 1325[b]; 1635[d]	No data	No data	No data
Density (g/cm3)	6684 (25°C); 6688 (20°C)[b]	4.12	3.78	2.6
Odor	No data	Odorless[d]	No data	Odorless[c]
Odor threshold				
Water	No data	No data	No data	No data
Air	No data	No data	No data	No data
Taste	No data	No data	No data	Sweetish, metallic[d]
Taste threshold	No data	No data	No data	No data
Solubility				
Water	Insoluble	Insoluble	Very slightly soluble	83 g/L (cold)
Organic solvents	No data	Insoluble in alcohol	No data	Insoluble in alcohol Soluble in glycerine
Partition coefficients				
Log K_{ow}	No data	No data	No data	No data
Log K_{oc}	No data	No data	No data	No data
Vapor pressure, mm Hg	1 (886°C)[e]	No data	No data	No data
Henry's law constant	No data	No data	No data	No data
Autoignition temperature	No data	No data	No data	No data
Flash point	No data	No data	No data	No data
Flammability limits	No data	No data	No data	No data
Conversion factors, ppm to mg/m3	None[g]	None[g]	None[g]	None[g]
Explosive limits	No data	No data	No data	No data

[a]All information obtained from Weast, 1988, except where noted.
[b]Herbst et al, 1985.
[c]Freedman et al, 1978.
[d]Windholz, 1983.
[e]HSDB, 1989, 1991.
[f]SAX, 1984.
[g]Because these substances exist in the atmosphere in the particulate state, the concentration is expressed as mg/m3.
From ATSDR: Toxicological Profile for Antimony. Report TP-92/14. Atlanta, GA, U.S. Public Health Service, Agency for Toxic Substances and Disease Registry, 1992.

Clinical Presentation

Antimony poisoning may occur in the industrial and occupational setting primarily with exposures to trivalent forms (antimony trioxide, trisulfide, and trichloride) and in patients treated with pentavalent antimony compounds for leishmaniasis. In the past, antimony toxicity commonly was reported in patients treated with antimony potassium tartrate for schistosomiasis.[17]

Acute poisoning after ingestion of antimony salts affects primarily the gastrointestinal tract, with manifestations of nausea, vomiting, watery diarrhea, abdominal pain, melena, and hematemesis.[18] These effects may lead to volume depletion and hypovolemic shock. Cardiac manifestations include premature ventricular beats, ventricular tachycardia, and fibrillation. The electrocardiogram may show T-wave changes with prominent U waves. Stokes-Adams syndrome, responsive to atropine, has been described with acute and long-term administration (orally or intravenously) of antimony potassium tartrate.[17] Hepatitis also may occur.[19]

Several organ systems are involved in chronic antimony toxicity. Organ system involvement may vary with the route of exposure (inhalation versus ingestion). With *inhalational exposure*, pneumoconiosis, bronchospasm,[20] chronic bronchitis with upper airway irritation,[21] abdominal pain, diarrhea, and vomiting[22] have been reported. After long-term *oral ingestion* of trivalent and pentavalent antimony compounds, cardiovascular and gastrointestinal systems are the most commonly involved, as previously described.

The cardiac toxicity associated with sodium stibogluconate and meglumine antimoniate treatment may occur at the recommended dose of 20 mg/kg/day and after prolonged therapy.[4] The manifestations of antimony cardiotoxicity are ventricular premature beats, first-degree atrioventricular block, T-wave and ST-T changes, and prolonged QT_c interval.[4,23–25] These changes are reversible with cessation of treatment.

Other reported affected systems (reported only with sodium stibogluconate and meglumine antimoniate) are as follows:

Hematologic
Thrombocytopenia
Leukopenia[26]

Hepatobiliary
Elevation of transaminases[25,27,28] (fulminant hepatic failure is seldom reported)
Acute pancreatitis with elevation of lipase and amylase (subsides when therapy is stopped[29,30]; three fatalities have been reported[27])
Acute renal tubular acidosis and necrosis have been described.[31]

Diagnosis

Antimony toxicity should be considered in patients who are treated for leishmaniasis or who work with antimony compounds if they present with gastrointestinal or pulmonary symptoms or both or have electrocardiogram changes as previously described. The diagnosis of antimony poisoning is made by measuring antimony concentrations via atomic absorption spectroscopy in blood or urine or both.[32]

Treatment

The ability of activated charcoal to reduce antimony absorption from the gastrointestinal tract in acute antimony poisoning has not been studied. Theoretically, activated charcoal may be efficacious in reducing absorption if it is administered within the first 1 to 2 hours after oral ingestion.

Aggressive intravenous administration of crystalloids with central venous pressure monitoring may be necessary to replace volume loss. Vasopressors, such as dopamine and norepinephrine, may be necessary to treat shock not responsive to fluid volume replacement.

Because QT_c prolongation may lead to the development of torsades de pointes, continuous cardiac monitoring should be implemented if there are electrocardiogram changes or other significant manifestations of antimony poisoning. The treatment of tachydysrhythmias is outlined in Chapter 21.

CHELATING AGENTS

In an attempt to enhance antimony elimination, the use of chelating agents has been proposed. Dimercaprol (British antilewisite [BAL]) was reported to decrease the toxicity of antimony potassium tartrate in animals[33] and to be effective in ameliorating the toxicity and adverse reactions during treatment with other trivalent antimonial drugs.[34,35] Dimercaptosuccinic acid (DMSA) and 2,3-dimercaptopropane-1-sulfonate, two BAL derivatives, have been shown to decrease mortality in mice given antimony tartrate in a dose twice the median lethal dose.

Penicillamine also reduced mortality in a mouse model, although less effectively than BAL or DMSA. BAL did not decrease mortality in this model.[36] In four patients who accidentally overdosed with antimony tartrate, BAL did not seem to change the course of their toxicity,[18] and DMSA did not increase antimony excretion in a patient who accidentally received an overdose with sodium stibogluconate.[37] Although the data are limited, we recom-

mend the use of DMSA, 10 mg/kg orally every 8 hours for 5 days followed by 10 mg/kg every 12 hours for 14 days, to be considered only in trivalent antimony compound poisoning. The current available data do not support chelation for pentavalent antimony toxicity. The duration of therapy should be guided by the clinical response. Penicillamine (250 mg in adults and 20 to 30 mg/kg in children four times a day) may serve as an alternative to DMSA. Penicillamine is not the preferred drug, however, because of its adverse effects.

Stibine

Stibine is a colorless gas formed when antimony alloys are treated with acid. In animals, stibine was shown to be lethal and to cause pulmonary edema[38] and hemolysis in a dose-dependent manner.[1] Several cases of poisoning from a mixture of gases including stibine (others being arsine and hydrogen sulfide) have been reported.[1] The affected patients had headache, nausea, weakness, abdominal and back pain, and severe hemolysis. The treatment for acute stibine poisoning is supportive. Fluid hydration and maintenance of urine output are important to prevent renal injury secondary to hemolysis. Erythrocyte transfusions may be required if the hemolytic anemia is severe or if the patient has compromised cardiopulmonary function. It is unknown whether chelating agents have any role in the management of this poisoning.

NICKEL

Nickel is the fifth most common metal in the earth's crust and is distributed widely in soils and sediment. It is found in many different industries, including mining, electroplating, and ceramics, and is used as yellow pigment in paint. Nickel ores are of two general types: magmatic sulfide ores, which are mined underground, and lateritic hydrous nickel silicates or garnierites, which are surface mined.[39,40]

Chemistry

Nickel's physical properties allow for its broad use in industry. Pure nickel is a hard, silvery-white metal that is combined with other metals to form alloys. It is a hard, yet malleable metal that is relatively resistant to corrosion. Nickel and its compounds have no characteristic odor or taste. The most familiar nickel-ferrous alloys are stainless steel and coinage metal. Nickel may be found in the metallic, inorganic, and organic forms. Although nickel can exist in oxidation states -1, 0, $+2$, $+3$, and $+4$, its only medically important oxidation state is $+2$.

Metallic nickel is a hard, lustrous, silvery-white metal, which in its bulk form is resistant to attack by air and water at ordinary temperatures. Powdered nickel is reactive in air, however, and may ignite spontaneously.

Nickel has typical metallic properties; it can be readily rolled, drawn into wire, forged, and polished. It also is ferromagnetic and a good conductor of heat and electricity. Nickel is positioned after hydrogen in the electrochemical series and slowly displaces hydrogen ions from dilute hydrochloric and sulfuric acids. It reacts more rapidly with nitric acid. Nickel is highly resistant to attack by strong alkali.[41] Black nickel oxide readily yields nickel salts on contact with mineral acids, whereas green nickel oxide is more refractory to solubilization.[42] The divalent state of nickel forms an extensive series of compounds and is the only important oxidation state in aqueous systems. Other oxidation states occur in special complexes and oxides. In alkaline solutions, nickel (+2) hydroxide can be oxidized to a hydrated nickel (+4) oxide, a reaction used in the Edison storage battery.

Nickel commonly forms complexes with a coordination number of six. These complexes have an octahedral configuration and generally are green. In aqueous solutions, nickel occurs as the octahedral hexahydrate ion $[Ni(H_2O)_6]$,[43] which is poorly absorbed by most living organisms.[42]

Nickel subsulfide is formed during the roasting and smelting of nickel ore and may be shipped as the matte for further processing, but it does not have any other significant commercial uses.[44] Data on the chemical properties of nickel and some important nickel compounds are presented in Table 80-2.

Pathophysiology

Nickel may be absorbed via inhalation or ingestion. Absorption by the respiratory route with secondary gastrointestinal absorption (insoluble and soluble) is the major pathway of exposure during occupational exposures. Similar to many inhaled particles, significant quantities may be swallowed after mucociliary clearance from the respiratory tract. The soluble nickel ion (Ni^{2+}) may be absorbed through the gastrointestinal tract, or less soluble compounds may be phagocytized in the lung. Percutaneous absorption is negligible for most nickel compounds, but for some forms, such as nickel chloride and nickel sulfate, 77% of an applied dose may be absorbed.[45] Nickel in many forms is a common cause of allergic dermatitis.

The organonickel compounds, such as nickel carbonyl, have the greatest propensity for absorption. It has been reported that 35% of inhaled nickel is absorbed into the blood.[46] Inhalation of nickel carbonyl may result in significant absorption.[47,48] Ingestion of nickel results in absorption of variable amounts. Bioavailability of nickel is altered by the presence of food in the gastrointestinal tract.[46] When nickel sulfate is given with water, 27% is absorbed, whereas only 0.75% is absorbed with food.[46]

After absorption, nickel enters the vascular compartment, where it is bound principally to albumin (34%) and nickeloplasmin (26%), with none as an unbound ultrafiltrable fraction.[49] Nickel carbonyl is distributed into the central nervous system to a greater extent than its other forms.

Metallic nickel is not metabolized; however, nickel carbonyl has been shown to be oxidized to nickel and carbon monoxide.[50] In a study of five subjects with nickel carbonyl poisoning, none developed elevated carboxyhemoglobin levels.[50] This finding was confirmed in a series of 25 cases.[51,52] Biomonitoring after nickel carbonyl exposure should focus

TABLE 80-2 Physical and Chemical Properties of Nickel and Compounds[a]

PROPERTY	NICKEL	NICKEL OXIDE	NICKEL SULFATE	NICKEL CHLORIDE
Molecular weight	58.69	74.69	154.75	129.60
Color	Silvery	Green	Greenish yellow	Golden yellow bronze
Physical state	Solid	Solid	Solid	Solid
Melting point	1455°C	1984°C	840°C	1001°C
Boiling point	2730°C	No data	No data	Sublimes at 973°C
Density	8.90 g/cm^3	6.67 g/cm^3	3.68 g/cm^3	3.55 g/cm^3
Odor	No data	No data	Odorless	None
Odor threshold				
Water	No data	No data	No data	No data
Air	No data	No data	No data	No data
Solubility				
Water	1.1 mg/L at 37°C[b]	1.1 mg/L at 20°C	293 g/L at 0°C	642 g/L at 20°C
Organic solvent(s)	No data	No data	Insoluble in ether and acetone; 0.2 g/L at 35°C in ethanol; 1.1 g/L at 35°C in methanol	Soluble in ethanol
Partition coefficients				
Log K$_{ow}$	No data	No data	No data	No data
Log K$_{oc}$	No data	No data	No data	No data
Vapor pressure	1 mm Hg at 1810°C	No data	No data	1 mm Hg at 671°C
Henry's law constant	No data	No data	No data	No data
Autoignition temperature	No data	No data	Nonflammable	Nonflammable
Flash point	No data	No data	Nonflammable	Nonflammable
Flammability limits	No data	No data	Nonflammable	Nonflammable
Conversion factors	No data	No data	No data	No data
Explosive limits	No data	No data	No data	No data

[a]All information obtained from HSDB 1996 except where noted.
[b]Ishimatsu et al, 1995.
From ATSDR: Toxicological Profile for Nickel. Report TP-92/14. Atlanta, GA, U.S. Public Health Service, Agency for Toxic Substances and Disease Registry, 1997.

on the detection of nickel in blood or urine samples.[53] In a rat model, 35% of nickel carbonyl was eliminated via the kidney.[50] Parenteral nickel is eliminated almost exclusively in the urine, where it is cleared rapidly from the body.[54] Nonabsorbed nickel (approximately 90%) is eliminated in the feces.[55]

Clinical Presentation

Nickel's toxicity may be related to its interference with physiologic processes involving other metal cations, such as manganese, zinc, calcium, and magnesium.

RESPIRATORY

Few nickel exposures result in a critical care admission. The exception is nickel carbonyl, which may cause pulmonary edema occurring within hours after significant inhalational exposure. The typical onset has been reported to be delayed,[56,57] following initial flulike symptoms.[56,58] Other investigators have reported pneumonitis and pulmonary irritation occurring immediately or with a delay, with infiltrations on chest x-ray that may persist for 4 weeks.[52]

Allergic contact dermatitis to nickel is common. More significant allergic reactions, including asthma, have been reported.[59,60] Transient pulmonary infiltrates and eosinophilia (Löffler's syndrome) have been reported after low-dose inhalational exposure to nickel carbonyl.[42]

RENAL

Nephrotoxic effects, such as renal edema with hyperemia and parenchymatous degeneration, have been reported in 32 cases of electroplaters who accidentally drank water contaminated with nickel sulfate and nickel chloride.[61] The workers developed signs and symptoms (e.g., nausea, vomiting, abdominal discomfort, diarrhea, giddiness, lassitude, headache, cough, shortness of breath) that were transient in most but persisted 1 to 2 days in seven cases. The nickel doses in workers with symptoms were estimated to range from 0.5 to 2.5 g. In 15 exposed workers who were tested on day 1 postexposure, serum nickel concentrations ranged from 13 to 1340 μg/L, and urine nickel concentrations ranged from 0.15 to 12 mg/g creatinine. Ten of the workers with initial urine nickel concentrations greater than 0.8 mg/g creatinine were hospitalized and treated with intravenous fluids. This treatment resulted in a mean elimination half-life for serum nickel of 27 ($\pm$7) hours, which was significantly shorter than the mean half-life of 60 ($\pm$11) hours in 11 subjects who did not receive intravenous fluids. All subjects recovered rapidly, without evident sequelae, and returned to work by the 8th day after exposure.

Treatment

The most important intervention after nickel exposure is the interruption of any potential ongoing absorption. Removal from exposure and decontamination are of primary importance. With nickel or nickel carbonyl poisoning, it is important to remove any contaminated clothing. Few specific therapeutic measures are available. Most traditional chelating agents are not of value. Sodium diethyldithiocarbamate (DDC) and disulfiram (Antabuse) have been proposed as effective nickel chelators, however. Two studies have

addressed the efficacy of these agents in animal models. In a rat model, DDC given parenterally at a dose of 50 to 100 mg/kg immediately after nickel carbonyl administration resulted in reduction of mortality from 73% to 8%.[62] In another animal study, mice were given 50 to 100 mg/kg of DDC, which was protective when given 8 hours after exposure. The efficacy declined at 24 hours. The 100-mg/kg dose was more efficacious than a lower dose.[63]

Disulfiram or bis (diethylthiocarbamoyl) disulfide is a metabolite of DDC. Given at a dose of 1000 mg/kg to rats, disulfiram offered complete protection against nickel carbonyl–induced toxicity when administered after exposure; however, 500 mg/kg offered no protection. Doses greater than 1500 mg/kg seemed to enhance mortality.[64] Patients have been treated with disulfiram with anecdotal results. In one case report, disulfiram was administered after inhalational exposure to nickel carbonyl for the first 2 days until sodium DDC was obtained. The patient gradually improved over 10 days.[58]

There are no adequately controlled clinical studies of the use of disulfiram or DDC in acute nickel carbonyl poisoning. Disulfiram or DDC may be considered as a possible therapeutic measure in seriously ill patients, however.

Special Populations

People with an increased susceptibility to nickel compounds are individuals with preexisting pulmonary disease, such as emphysema, asthma, interstitial lung disease, or possibly pulmonary hypertension. Nickel carbonyl may cause pulmonary edema, and individuals with preexisting atherosclerotic vascular disease may develop ischemia of end organs because of impaired oxygen diffusion. The fetus may be at increased risk should hypoxemia occur. Another group would be individuals who have topical allergies to nickel compounds. However, such an allergy is unlikely to result in admission to a critical care unit.

REFERENCES

1. U.S Bureau of Mines: Antimony in the first quarter of 1989. Mineral Industry Series. Pittsburgh, PA, U.S. Bureau of Mines, 1989.
2. Herbst KA, Rose G, Hanusch K: Antimony and antimony compounds. In Arpe HJ (ed): Ullman's Encyclopedia of Industrial Chemistry, Vol A3, 5th ed. Hoboken, NJ, Wiley, 1985, pp 55–76.
3. Browning E: Antimony. In Toxicity of Industrial Metals, 2nd ed. London, Butterworth & Co, 1969, pp 23–28.
4. Herwaldt BL, Berman JD: Recommendations for treating leishmaniasis with sodium stibogluconate (pentosam) and review or pertinent studies. Am J Trop Med Hyg 46:296–306, 1992.
5. Gerhardson L, Brune D, Nordberg CF, Webster CO: Antimony in the lung, liver, and kidney tissue from deceased smelter workers. Scand J Environ Health 8:201–209, 1982.
6. McCallum RI, Day MJ, Underhill J, Aird EGA: Measurement of antimony oxide dust in human lungs in vivo by x-ray spectrometry. In Walton WH (ed): Inhaled Particles. Oxford, England, Urwin Brothers Limited, The Gresham Press, Old Working, 1971, pp 611–618.
7. Felicetti SA, Thomas RG, McClellan RO: Metabolism of two valence states on inhaled antimony in hamster. Am Ind Hyg Assoc J 35:292–300, 1974.
8. International Commission on Radiological Protection: Limits of intakes of radionuclides by workers: Metabolic data for antimony. Annals of the ICRP. ICRP publication 30, part 3, 1981.

9. Djuric D, Thomas RG, Lie R: The distribution and excretion of trivalent antimony in the rat following inhalation. Arch Gewerbepatch Gewerbehyg 19:529–545, 1962.
10. Felicetti SA, Thomas RG, McClellan RO: Retention of inhaled antimony-124 in the beagle dog as a function of temperature of aerosol formation. Health Physics 26:515–531, 1974.
11. Sunagawa S: Experimental studies on antimony poisoning. Igaku Kenkyu 51:129–142, 1981.
12. Goodwin LG: The toxicity and trypanocidal activity of some organic antimonial. J Pharmacol 81:224, 1944.
13. Page JE: A study of the excretion of organic antimonials. Biochem J 37:198, 1943.
14. Chulay JD, Fleckenstein L, Smith DH: Pharmacokinetics of antimony during treatment of visceral leishmaniasis with sodium stibogluconate or meglumine antimonite. Trans R Soc Trop Med 82:69–72, 1988.
15. Norseth T, Martinsen I: Biological monitoring of antimony. In Clarkson TW, Friberg L, Nordberg G, Sager P (eds): Biological Monitoring of Toxic Metals. New York, Plenum Press, 1988.
16. Venugopal B, Luckey TD: Antimony. In Metal Toxicity in Mammals. New York, Plenum Press, 1978, pp 213–216.
17. Ming-Hsin H, Shao-Chi C, Ju-Sun P, et al: Mechanism and treatment of cardiac arrhythmias in tartar emetic intoxication. Chin Med J 76:103–115, 1958.
18. Lauwers LF, Roelants A, Roseel PM, et al: Oral antimony intoxication in man. Crit Care Med 18:324–326, 1990.
19. Chopra RN: Experimental investigation into the action of organic compounds of antimony. Indian J Med Res 15:41, 1927.
20. Cooper DA, Pendergrass EP, Vorwald AJ: Pneumoconiosis among workers in an antimony industry. Am J Roentgenol Rad Ther Nucl Med 103:495–508, 1968.
21. Potkonjak V, Pavlovich M: Antimoniosis: A particular form of pneumoconiosis: I. Etiology, clinical and x-ray findings. Int Arch Occup Environ Health 51:199–207, 1983.
22. Taylor PJ: Acute intoxication from antimony trichloride. Br J Ind Med 23:318–321, 1966.
23. Aronson NE, Wortmann GW, Johnson SC, et al: Safety and efficacy of intravenous sodium stibogluconate in the treatment of leishmaniasis: Recent U.S military experience. Clin Infect Dis 27:1457–1464, 1988.
24. Franke ED, Wignall S, Cruz ME, et al: Efficacy and toxicity of sodium stibogluconate for mucosal leishmaniasis. Ann Intern Med 113:934–940, 1990.
25. Bryceson ADM, ChulaYJD, Mugambi JD, et al: Visceral leishmaniasis unresponsive to antimonial drugs: II. Response to high dosage sodium stibogluconate or prolonged treatment with pentamidine. Trans R Soc Trop Med 79:705–714, 1985.
26. Braconier JH, Miorner H: Recurrent episodes of thrombocytopenia during treatment with sodium stibogluconate. J Antimicrob Chemother 31:187–188, 1993.
27. Saenz RE, Rodriguez CG, Johnson CM, Berman JD: Efficacy and toxicity of pentosam against Panamanian mucosal leishmaniasis. Am J Trop Med Hyg 44:394–398, 1991.
28. Herwaldt BL, Kaye ET, Lepore TJ, et al: Sodium stibogluconate (pentosam) overdose during treatment of American cutaneous leishmaniasis. J Infect Dis 165:968–971, 1992.
29. Delgado J, Macias J, Pineda JA, et al: High frequency of serious side effects from meglumine antimoniate given without an upper limit dose for the treatment of visceral leishmaniasis in human immunodeficiency virus type-1–infected patients. Am J Trop Med Hyg 61:766–769, 1999.
30. Gasser RA, Magill AJ, Oster CN, et al: Pancreatitis induced by pentavalent antimonial agents during treatment of leishmaniasis. Clin Infect Dis 18:83–90, 1994.
31. Horber FF, Lerut J, Jaeger PH: Renal tubular acidosis, a side effect of treatment with pentavalent antimony. Clin Nephrol 36:213, 1991.
32. Ludersdorf R, Fuchs A, Mayer P: Biological assessment of exposure to antimony and lead in the glass-producing industry. Int Arch Occup Environ Health 59:469–474, 1987.
33. Braun HA, Lusky LM, Calvery HO: The efficacy of 2,3-dimercaptopropanol (BAL) in the therapy of poisoning by compounds of antimony, bismuth, chromium, mercury and nickel. J Pharm Exp Ther 87(Suppl): 119–125, 1946.
34. Eagle H, Germuth FG, Magnuson HJ, Fleischman R: The protective action of BAL in experimental antimony poisoning. J Pharm Exp Ther 89:196–204, 1947.
35. Stevenson DS, Suarez RM, Marchand EJ: The use of BAL in heavy metal poisoning with particular reference to antimonial intoxication. Puerto Rico J Public Health Trop Med 23:535–553, 1948.
36. Basinger MA, Jones MM: Structural requirements for chelate antidotal efficacy in acute antimony (III) intoxication. Res Commun Chem Pathol Pharmacol 32:355–363, 1981.
37. Reymond JM, Desmeules J: Sodium stibogluconate (pentosan) overdose in a patient with acquired immunodeficiency syndrome. Ther Drug Monit 20:714–716, 1998.
38. Price NH, Yates WG, Allen SD: Toxicity evaluation for establishing IDLH values. PB87–229498. Cincinnati, OH, National Institute for Occupational Safety and Health, 1979.
39. Duke JM: Nickel in rocks and ores. In Nriagu JO (ed): Nickel in the Environment. New York, John Wiley & Sons, 1980, pp 27–50.
40. Warner JS: Occupation exposure to airborne nickel in producing and using primary nickel products. In Sunderman FW Jr, Aitio A, Berlin A (eds): Nickel in the Human Environment. IARC scientific publication no. 53. Lyon, France, International Agency for Research on Cancer, 1984, pp 419–437.
41. Hawley GG: Condensed Chemical Dictionary, 10th ed. New York, Van Nostrand Reinhold, 1981, pp 724–725.
42. Sunderman FW Jr, Oskarsson A: Nickel. In Merian E (ed): Metals and Their Compounds in the Environment. New York, VCH Verlagsgesellschaft, 1991, pp 1101–1126.
43. Windholz M: The Merck Index, 10th ed. Rahway, NJ, Merck & Co, 1983, pp 932–933, 1171.
44. Tien JK, Howson TE: Nickel and nickel alloys. In Grayson M, Eckroth D (eds): Kirk-Othmer Encyclopedia of Chemical Technology, Vol 15, 3rd ed. New York, John Wiley & Sons, 1981, pp 787–801.
45. ATSDR: Toxicological Profile for Nickel. Report TP-92/14. Atlanta, GA, U.S. Public Health Service, Agency for Toxic Substances and Disease Registry, 1993.
46. ATSDR: Toxicological Profile for Nickel. Report TP-92/14. Atlanta, GA, U.S. Public Health Service, Agency for Toxic Substances and Disease Registry, 1997.
47. Friberg L, Nordberg GF, Kessler E, et al (eds): Handbook of the Toxicology of Metals, 2nd ed. Amsterdam, Elsevier Science, 1986.
48. Sunderman FW: A pilgrimage into the archives of nickel toxicology. Ann Clin Lab Sci 19:1–16, 1989.
49. Webster JD, Parker TF, Alfrey AC, et al: Acute nickel intoxication by dialysis. Ann Intern Med 92:631–633, 1980.
50. National Academy of Sciences Committee on Medical and Biological Effects of Environmental Pollutants: Nickel. Washington, DC, National Academy of Sciences, 1975.
51. Sunderman FW, Kincaid JF: Nickel poisoning: II. Studies on patients suffering from acute exposure to vapors of nickel carbonyl. JAMA 155:889–890, 1954.
52. Vuopala U, Huhti E, Takkunen J, et al: Nickel carbonyl poisoning: Report of 25 cases. Ann Clin Res 2:214–222, 1970.
53. Baselt RC, Cravey RH: Disposition of Toxic Drugs and Chemicals in Man, 4th ed. Chicago, Year Book Medical Publishers, 1995.
54. HSDB: Hazardous Substances Data Bank. Bethesda, MD, National Institutes of Health, National Library of Medicine, 2002.
55. Baselt RC: Disposition of Toxic Drugs and Chemicals in Man, 6th ed. Foster City, CA, Chemical Toxicology Institute, 2002.
56. Jones CC: Nickel carbonyl poisoning: Report of a fatal case. Arch Environ Health 26:245–248, 1973.
57. Sunderman FW: Use of sodium diethyldithiocarbamate in the treatment of nickel carbonyl poisoning. Ann Clin Lab Sci 20:12–21, 1990.
58. Kurta DL, Dean BS, Krenzelok EP: Acute nickel carbonyl poisoning. Am J Emerg Med 11:64–66, 1993.
59. McConnell LH, Fink JN, Schlueter DP, Schmidt MG Jr: Asthma caused by nickel sensitivity. Ann Intern Med 78:888–890, 1973.
60. Goyer RA: Toxic effects of metals. In Amdur MO, Doull J, Klaassen C (eds): Casarett and Doull's Toxicology: The Basic Science of Poisons, 4th ed. New York, Pergamon Press, 1991, pp 651–652.
61. Sunderman FW Jr, Dingle B, Hopfer SM, Swift T: Acute nickel toxicity in electroplating workers who accidentally ingested a solution of nickel sulfate and nickel chloride. Am J Ind Med 14:257–266, 1988.
62. Bradberry SM, Vale JA: Therapeutic review: Do diethyldithiocarbamate and disulfiram have a role in acute nickel carbonyl poisoning? Clin Toxicol 37:259–264, 1999.
63. West B, Sunderman FW: Nickel poisoning: VII. The therapeutic effectiveness of alkyl dithiocarbamates in experimental animals exposed to nickel carbonyl. Am J Med Sci 236:15–25, 1958.
64. Basalt RC, Hanson VW: Efficacy of orally-administered chelating agents for nickel carbonyl toxicity in rats. Res Commun Chem Pathol Pharmacol 38:113–124, 1982.

CHAPTER 81

Phosphorus

Andrew Erdman

The element phosphorus exists in three common allotropic forms: red, black, and white. White phosphorus sometimes is called *yellow phosphorus* because of impurities. The forms differ in molecular structure (Fig. 81-1) and display unique chemical and biologic activities.

Black phosphorus consists of atoms arranged in a double-sheet crystalline structure. This form is stable and inert and has not been reported to cause toxicity in humans. Red phosphorus consists of linear chains of tetramers. Similar to black phosphorus, the red form is relatively stable and poorly soluble. It is not absorbed to a significant degree by the human body and exhibits minimal toxicity when ingested. Smoke from burning red phosphorus has been reported, however, to cause mild irritation to the respiratory tract and mucous membranes when inhaled.[1] White phosphorus, which is composed of isolated free tetramers, is extremely reactive owing to the instability of its interatomic bonds (see Fig. 81-1). White phosphorus is the primary form of medical concern.

Acute ingestions of white phosphorus can cause local gastrointestinal irritation and, if significant amounts are absorbed, cardiovascular collapse, hepatic and renal failure, and death.[2–4] Dermal contact with white phosphorus can cause chemical burns and, rarely, systemic toxicity or sudden death.[5–7] Inhalational exposures to smoke or unburned particles of white phosphorus can cause respiratory irritation. Chronic exposures to white phosphorus fumes can lead to oral tissue and mandibular necrosis, an occupationally related condition classically referred to as *phossy jaw*.[8]

Elemental phosphorus in any allotropic form does not occur freely in nature. Instead, it exists in combination with other minerals, for example, as calcium phosphate and fluoroapatite. To obtain elemental phosphorus, the base ore is processed and refined.[9] White phosphorus is used in a wide variety of industries, particularly in the manufacture of matches, munitions, fireworks, and roach or rodent poisons.[10] In addition, it is used to make phosphoric acid, fertilizers, food and beverage additives, cleansers, and many other products. In the past, most significant exposures and deaths from white phosphorus were related to ingestions of fireworks, rodenticide pastes, or matches.[3,11–14] Over the last century, however, the availability of white phosphorus has decreased as a result of legislation and international trade agreements that restrict its use, the development of safer rodenticides, and the advent of manufacturing techniques and munitions that use less toxic forms of phosphorus. As a result, acute poisonings seem to be far less common, and phossy jaw has all but been eliminated in Western society.[15]

In addition to its elemental forms, phosphorus may be present in many inorganic compounds, each of which has its own toxicity. Phosphoric acid can cause caustic injuries. Chloro compounds of phosphorus, such as phosphorus trichloride or pentachloride, can cause airway or mucous membrane irritation and pulmonary edema.[16] Sulfide compounds, such as phosphorus pentasulfide, have the potential to react with water, releasing phosphoric acid and hydrogen sulfide.

Phosphine gas (PH_3) is a phosphorus-containing molecule (Fig. 81-2) with the potential to cause significant toxicity or death if inhaled.[17–22] It is typically formed from the reaction of metal phosphide compounds with water or acids. Phosphine gas is used or produced in several industries, including the manufacture of organophosphate pesticides, semiconductors, and acetylene. Phosphine is employed extensively as a fumigant to kill insects and fungi during grain storage.[17] In this context, sachets of aluminum phosphide are stored along with the grain, and atmospheric moisture reacts with the aluminum phosphide to produce phosphine gas. The liberated gas permeates through the grain, killing any pests.[22] Metal phosphides, such as zinc or aluminum phosphide, are also used as rodenticides in some countries, either in powder or tablet form, and intentional ingestions of these products are a relatively common method of suicide in such countries.[23–25] After coming into contact with gastric acid or moisture from the oral mucosa, the metal phosphides release phosphine gas, which is inhaled or otherwise absorbed and can lead to systemic toxicity.[17–20] Fumigants are discussed in detail in Chapter 88.

The toxic gas phosphine sounds similar to phosgene, an unrelated non–phosphorus-containing gas. These two toxins often are confused, and care must be taken to ensure that the correct term is specified.

There is no specific antidote for poisoning by phosphorus in any of its forms. Treatment centers on decontamination and supportive care.

CHEMISTRY

Phosphorus

White phosphorus is a white-to-pale yellow, waxy solid with a distinctive garlic-like odor. It is oxidized easily and may ignite at room temperature (around 30°C), so it must be stored under water, depriving it of the oxygen necessary

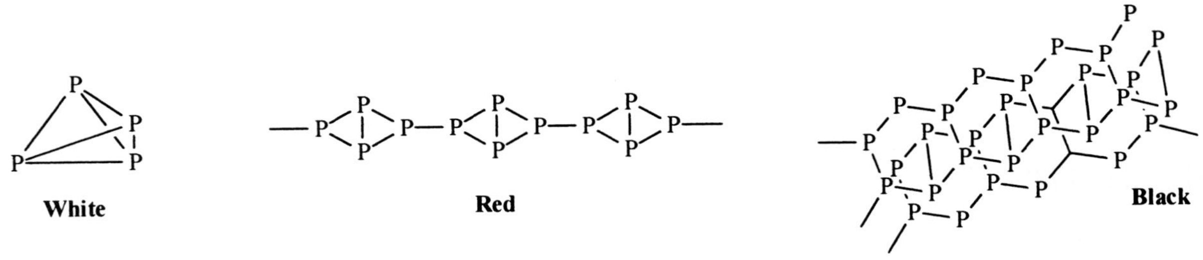

FIGURE 81-1

Structural diagrams of the allotropic forms of elemental phosphorus. The interatomic bonds of white phosphorus are highly strained, accounting for its reactivity.

for combustion. The oxidation of white phosphorus results in a smoke that consists of various phosphorus oxide compounds (primarily phosphorus pentoxide) and unburned phosphorus particles. This smoke has made phosphorus valuable in munitions and as an obscurant for military purposes. In the presence of oxygen, phosphorus may give off a faint greenish glow—hence the term *phosphorescence*. White phosphorus combines with various metals, such as copper, to form inactive, less toxic phosphorus salts.

White phosphorus is minimally soluble in water but dissolves readily in bile, fats, and oils. It may be absorbed across the gastrointestinal tract, respiratory tract, dermis, and mucous membranes. Its precise toxicokinetics after absorption is poorly understood but based on studies using radiolabeled phosphorus and postmortem tissue concentrations, it appears to be distributed widely and incorporated into a variety of body tissues, particularly the liver.[26-29] The metabolism of phosphorus is unclear, but its clearance has been suggested by some authors to occur via renal elimination in the form of various phosphates.[30]

Phosphine

Phosphine is a colorless, flammable gas, often with a fishy or garlic odor (owing to impurities). It is heavier than air and tends to settle in low-lying areas. Phosphine is liberated when metal phosphides, such as zinc, magnesium, or aluminum phosphide, react with water or acids or when phosphoric acid is heated. Phosphine is readily absorbed through the lungs after inhalational exposures. Poisonings are rare and generally the result of industrial or occupational exposures (e.g., grain storage elevators on ships, semiconductor industry, and methamphetamine manufacture). Occasionally phosphine poisoning occurs after ingestions of metal phosphide pesticides.[22] Toxicity after metal phosphide ingestion is believed to be due to liberation of phosphine in the acidic milieu of the stomach. The gas is either absorbed through the gastrointestinal tract or regurgitated and inhaled into the lungs. Based on the variety of organ systems affected, phos-

phine is believed to have a wide distribution throughout the body.[31] Its fate from there is unclear, but studies suggest that it may be exhaled unchanged through the lungs or converted to phosphite (PO_3) and hypophosphite (H_2PO_2), both of which may be excreted renally.[31]

PATHOPHYSIOLOGY

Phosphorus

SYSTEMIC EFFECTS

Significant systemic toxicity or death from white phosphorus may occur after inhalation or ingestion. Chronic inhalation or dermal exposure occasionally leads to phossy jaw and mild leukopenia or anemia.[8,10] Systemic toxicity has been noted after large dermal exposures in humans and animals.[7] It is not clear, however, whether these effects were the result of systemically absorbed phosphorus or merely an indirect result of massive burns. Most of the information on systemic phosphorus poisoning comes from case reports and case series of intentional ingestions of phosphorus-containing products (e.g., matches, fireworks, and rodenticides).

White phosphorus often is described as a "general protoplasmic poison."[4,11] Although it is true that most of the effects of phosphorus appear to take place in the cellular cytoplasm rather than the nucleus, this description is vague and does not describe adequately the variety of mechanisms involved.[32] The effects of these mechanisms on specific organ systems are described.

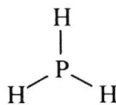

FIGURE 81-2

Chemical structure of phosphine.

Mechanisms of Phosphorus Poisoning
Inhibition of Krebs cycle reactions[33,34]
Altered ribosomal function and impaired protein synthesis[35-37]
Impairment of glycogen storage and blood glucose regulation[38,39]
Possible free radical injury and lipid peroxidation of membranes[40,41]
Impairment of lipoprotein synthesis and cellular triglyceride secretion, resulting in intracellular lipid accumulation and fatty degeneration of multiple organs (primarily liver, heart, brain, and kidneys)[28,36,37,41,42]

Cardiovascular Effects. Shock is a prominent feature in patients with significant phosphorus toxicity. Shock may begin within hours of ingestion, presumably as the result of hypovolemia from vomiting, diarrhea, and intestinal fluid or blood loss.[4,11,14,29,43,44] As phosphorus is absorbed systemically over the ensuing hours to days, direct cardiac or vascular toxicity may supervene, resulting in decreased cardiac contractility and vasodilation.[45] Clinically, these effects are manifested by hypotension, tachycardia, cyanosis, and other sequelae of shock. The hypotension may be poorly responsive to fluids and pressors. A variety of electrocardiogram (ECG) changes (particularly T-wave changes, ST-segment changes, and QT prolongation) and dysrhythmias may develop.[46,47] Torsades de pointes has not been reported.

The early onset of cardiovascular effects portends a poor prognosis. Cardiovascular collapse or dysrhythmias leading to cardiac arrest are the cause of most deaths occurring within the first 5 days after ingestion.[4,11,29] Deaths occurring later usually are the result of hepatic or renal failure.[11]

Hepatic Effects. White phosphorus is a well-known cause of hepatic injury.[2–4,11,12,14,28,32,44,48] Although the precise mechanism is uncertain, the histopathology of phosphorus-induced hepatic injury has been well characterized in humans and animals. Typically, within hours of ingestion, hydropic changes and fatty infiltration of hepatocytes occur.[2,13,14,28,38,41,49] This may be followed over the ensuing days by acute inflammatory infiltration and evidence of cellular necrosis.[3,28,44,50,51] Finally, over the course of months, fibrosis, scarring, and cirrhosis can develop. In most patients, however, the initial injury resolves without permanent sequelae.[3,13,14,28,50–53] The specific lobular location of hepatocellular injury has been the cause of some debate, but most authors suggest that injury first occurs in the periportal areas, then progresses to involve other areas of the lobule in more severe cases.[3,13,28,38,41,50,51] In a few patients, centrilobular or panlobular involvement predominates.[28,38,54] The primary event causing steatosis of the liver is believed to be a decrease in protein synthesis, resulting in impaired lipoprotein release. As a result, lipids and triglycerides accumulate, which impairs hepatocyte function (causing coagulopathy and hypoglycemia), and ultimately leads to necrosis.[35–37,41,45,55,56] Clinically, hepatic injury is manifested by abdominal pain, hepatomegaly, jaundice, and evidence of bleeding or coagulopathy. Laboratory abnormalities may include elevated serum transaminases and bilirubin, prolonged coagulation times, and hypoglycemia.[2,3,11,12,14,29,44,48] These clinical manifestations can last for weeks, but transaminases and bilirubin levels typically peak at 2 to 6 days before improving. Resolution of laboratory abnormalities seems to be the rule in survivors. The sooner after ingestion that hepatic injury develops, the worse the prognosis.[11,12] In the most severely poisoned patients, death occurs before evidence of liver injury develops.

Central Nervous System Effects. Nonspecific abnormalities of the central nervous system (CNS) are common with phosphorus toxicity and may be the initial presenting sign.[44] They also may become manifest later in the clinical course of poisoning. Mental status changes, such as delirium or obtundation, are generally a harbinger of severe toxicity.[11] The mechanism behind CNS dysfunction is unclear, but it may be due to neuronal fatty infiltration, particularly in the inferior olives. Presumably, the mechanism is similar to the development of hepatic steatosis.[57] Hypoglycemia, metabolic abnormalities, hypotension, ischemia, cerebral edema, and intracerebral hemorrhages secondary to coagulopathy may also contribute. The effects of any coingestants or underlying psychiatric illness should also be considered. Clinical CNS symptoms of phosphorus poisoning include restlessness, irritability, drowsiness, stupor, coma, hallucinations, psychosis, and delirium.[11,14,39,44,58]

Metabolic Effects. Several metabolic derangements have been described in patients with phosphorus poisoning. Metabolic acidosis may occur with significant toxicity.[12,59] The mechanisms have not been well studied but likely include inhibition of the Krebs cycle and hypotension, resulting in lactate accumulation.[44] Hypoglycemia or impaired regulation of blood glucose may occur, presumably due to alterations in energy production, depletion of glycogen stores, or liver failure.[12,38,39,48] With white phosphorus burns, animals and humans have been reported to develop significant hyperphosphatemia, hypocalcemia, or both, leading to a reversal in the normal serum calcium-to-phosphorus ratio.[60–62] One study suggests that these abnormalities may cause dysrhythmias and sudden death after otherwise minimal phosphorus burns.[62] After ingestions of white phosphorus, serum phosphorus levels seem to show no consistent pattern; they may be elevated, depressed, or within the normal range.[3,11,39,44,58] Hypocalcemia is common, however.[44] As would be expected, patients with more severe toxicity are more likely to exhibit metabolic derangements, and the presence of hypoglycemia or severe acidosis carries a poor prognosis.[12] Fever and chills can be seen in some patients.[39,44,58,63] Cyanosis has also been reported.[4,11,14]

Renal Effects. Renal toxicity is common with significant phosphorus ingestions.[3,11,44,48] Evidence of renal impairment typically manifests within days of initial exposure. Clinical features include oliguria, urinary changes (e.g., hematuria, proteinuria), and laboratory evidence of impaired renal function (e.g., elevated serum creatinine uremia).[3,11,44,48] Biopsy specimens may show tubular necrosis, cortical necrosis, or fatty infiltration.[3,28,64] Mechanisms underlying the renal injury have not been studied but may include direct toxicity of phosphorus on renal cells (e.g., via impaired metabolism, fatty infiltration, or oxidative stress), renal hypoperfusion from concomitant hypotension/hypovolemia, or hepatorenal syndrome.

LOCAL EFFECTS

White phosphorus is extremely reactive and can cause local tissue injury on contact with skin, mucous membranes, or the gastrointestinal and respiratory tracts.

Dermal Effects. White phosphorus causes chemical burns on contact with skin.[65,77,78,93] These burns occur most often in persons working with munitions or incendiary devices. Phosphorus burns tend to be more severe than simple thermal burns alone.[6,65,66] When exposed to the air, white phosphorus undergoes oxidation, an exothermic reaction causing thermal injury. Any phosphorus particles embedded in a wound may continue to oxidize and lead to ongoing tissue injury even after the initial exposure has ended.[65] In addition, the phosphorus oxides produced by this combustion reaction (particularly phosphorus pentoxide) are hygroscopic, leading to local tissue dehydration. The phosphorus oxides react with the water to form phosphoric acid, further damaging adjacent cells. The result is a potentially severe combination of chemical and thermal injury. Several authors have noted increased hospital stays and slower wound healing in patients with white phosphorus burns compared with patients with simple thermal burns.[6,65] Rarely, systemic effects may develop after dermal exposures to white phosphorus. These effects include liver and renal damage, metabolic abnormalities, dysrhythmias, and sudden death.[60–62,67] They have been well characterized in animals, but only a few human cases have been reported.[62] Whether these effects represent the sequelae of the burn or of systemically absorbed phosphorus is unclear.

Gastrointestinal Effects. Ingestion of white phosphorus generally causes significant gastrointestinal irritation as a result of its direct corrosive action on the local gastric mucosa. Mechanisms similar to the dermal injury are likely involved. Within hours of ingestion, most patients develop nausea, vomiting, and abdominal pain or cramping.[4,11,14,44] Gastrointestinal bleeding also has been reported.[11,14,29] Endoscopy findings include erythema, inflammation, erosions, and frank necrosis.[14,44,68] Occasionally, patients present without any significant gastrointestinal effects, so their absence does not rule out a significant ingestion.[11,44]

Inhalational Effects. Phosphorus smoke primarily comprises a mixture of phosphorus oxides and unburned phosphorus particles. Inhalation of these substances may cause irritation of the mucous membranes and respiratory tract, leading to cough, hoarseness, wheezing, and laryngeal edema or inflammation.[10] The mechanism of injury is likely due to a combination of heat formation from the oxidation of phosphorus, and hygroscopic or caustic injury caused by the products of this reaction. Animals exposed to high concentrations of phosphorus smoke have developed severe respiratory tract lesions, and some have died.[10]

Chronic inhalational exposure to phosphorus fumes, especially in the match manufacturing industry, used to be a common cause of phossy jaw.[8] Chronic inhalational exposures can also lead to anemia, leukopenia, and chronic cough.[10]

Phosphine

Phosphine poisoning causes severe systemic toxicity with a wide range of end-organ effects. A single tablet of metal phosphide may be enough to kill an adult.[24] Little is known, however, about the mechanisms of phosphine toxicity. A few studies have suggested that phosphine interacts with the heme moiety on cytochrome, inhibiting oxidative phosphorylation.[69] Phosphine also may alter hemoglobin's ability to carry oxygen to the tissues.[70] Regardless, the end result is cellular asphyxia.[71] Phosphine can also cause oxidative injury and lipid peroxidation.[72–74] Patients with phosphine toxicity may display clinical and echocardiographic evidence of myocardial depression. This myocardial depression

may exacerbate preexisting hypovolemia and lead to intractable shock.[22,75–77] Histologic evidence also suggests the possibility of direct myocardial toxicity.

CLINICAL PRESENTATION AND LIFE-THREATENING COMPLICATIONS

Phosphorus

Classically, acute white phosphorus poisoning has been described as occurring in three distinct stages. In practice, these stages tend not to be so well defined. The stages often overlap or vary in severity, and they may or may not be present in any given patient.[11,44] Factors such as amount of phosphorus ingested, time to medical treatment, adequacy of decontamination measures, individual differences in physiology or metabolism, underlying medical conditions, and presence of various coingestants may alter the development, timing, or presentation of these stages. The stages are presented here only to provide a general idea of how symptoms tend to progress. This information is intended to help the clinician anticipate the various complications of phosphorus poisoning.

STAGE I

Gastrointestinal effects are the hallmark of stage I. They generally begin within minutes to hours after ingestion but may be delayed several hours or more in some patients.[11,44] Occasionally, gastrointestinal effects do not develop.[44] As noted previously, these effects are the result of local corrosive injury. Symptoms include nausea, vomiting, diarrhea, abdominal pain and cramping, and gastrointestinal bleeding. The patient's stools, vomitus, or eructations may appear to smoke or phosphoresce, as intact particles of phosphorus continue to oxidize on contact with air. Occasionally a garlic-like odor is detectable.[3,4,11,14,29,44] In patients with massive ingestions, cardiovascular and CNS toxicity may develop rapidly during stage I, as a result of systemically absorbed phosphorus.[11] Death usually is caused by irreversible cardiovascular collapse or dysrhythmias.[11,29] In most patients, stage I lasts for many hours.

STAGE II

Survivors generally progress to stage II. This often is referred to as the *quiescent stage* because early authors described the appearance of almost complete recovery in patients who initially had exhibited significant toxicity.[2,14,43,59,79] Careful analysis of more recent literature suggests that this stage is almost never truly quiescent.[11] Patients invariably continue to experience some degree of anorexia, nausea, vomiting, diarrhea, or abdominal discomfort.[11] Nevertheless, many patients do appear to improve clinically as the initial corrosive effects of phosphorus subside but before clinical manifestations of systemic absorption and toxicity become apparent. This period of transient improvement may last 1 to 3 days.

STAGE III

Stage III is marked by clinical deterioration, coinciding with the systemic absorption of phosphorus and the evolution of its end-organ toxicity. The onset of stage III is classically heralded by the recurrence of nausea, vomiting, and abdominal discomfort several days after ingestion. Evidence of liver injury (e.g., jaundice, elevated serum transaminases, coagulopathy, and hypoglycemia), renal impairment (e.g., oliguria and elevated serum creatinine), CNS toxicity (e.g., delirium, obtundation, and restlessness), and cardiac dysfunction (e.g., ECG changes, shock, and dysrhythmias) may develop. Metabolic consequences (e.g., acidosis, hypocalcemia, and hypoglycemia) are common in this stage.[3,4,11,12,14,44,46–48] Death is usually the result of multiple organ failure, metabolic derangements, or irreversible cardiac impairment. A rapid onset of stage III implies a poor prognosis.[11,44] In survivors of this stage, recovery usually occurs over 1 to 3 weeks, but in some patients, laboratory abnormalities (e.g., elevated transaminases) may persist for months. Permanent sequelae are rare, but scattered reports of hepatic fibrosis and cirrhosis exist.[3,13,50,51,53]

Mortality rates in patients admitted to the hospital with white phosphorus poisoning range from 20% to 50%.[3,11,14,44] Mortality probably has decreased in more recent years with the advent of intensive care units and improvements in supportive care. Overall mortality seems to be directly related to the amount of phosphorus absorbed.[11,13,48] Although death has been reported in children ingesting only one to four firecrackers, most studies suggest that patients who ingest more than 1 mg/kg body weight of phosphorus are at risk for severe toxicity.[11,13,28] In one case series, all patients who ingested more than 1 g died.[11,48] Early gastric decontamination thus seems to be crucial in reducing systemic absorption.[3,11,13]

Besides a large ingestion, other historical features that suggest a poor prognosis include a long delay to decontamination and ingestions of phosphorus in a liquid vehicle. Clinical features portending a poor prognosis include the early onset of shock or CNS manifestations, the rapid development of hepatic injury, and the development of hypoglycemia or significant acidosis.[11,12,44]

Phosphine

Signs and symptoms of phosphine poisoning vary depending on the route of exposure. After ingestions of zinc or aluminum phosphide, symptoms of severe abdominal pain or burning, nausea, vomiting, and restlessness are common. These symptoms typically begin within minutes of ingestion. Cardiovascular shock may rapidly ensue and is often poorly responsive to most conservative measures. Evidence of pulmonary edema and acidosis are common. Other effects may include ECG changes, dysrhythmias, liver or renal injury, CNS depression, hemolysis, and electrolyte abnormalities (particularly hypokalemia and hypocalcemia). Unique characteristics include black vomitus (from zinc phosphide) or an unusual fishy odor.[18–20,25,80,81] Death occurs within hours to days of ingestion and is typically the result of intractable shock. The mortality in hospitalized patients has ranged from 25% to 71% depending on the study.[19,20,25,80] Recovery in survivors occurs over days to weeks.[18]

Inhalation of phosphine gas generally presents with milder gastrointestinal effects and more symptoms referable to the respiratory system. Initial effects include headache, weakness, paresthesias, ataxia, cough, respiratory irritation, chest discomfort, dyspnea, tachycardia, and occasionally

vomiting. Progression to pulmonary edema is common. Shock and renal or liver injury are rare.[22,80,82]

Phosphorus Burns

Dermal exposures to white phosphorus may result in chemical burns.[5–7,62,83] These are typically severe (e.g., second or third degree) and painful. The wounds may have a yellowish color or a garlic odor, and smoke may emanate from them due to the continued combustion of embedded phosphorus particles.[5,83] As noted previously, white phosphorus burns tend to heal more slowly than thermal burns. Contractures and prolonged hospitalizations are common.[6,65,66]

Complications unique to phosphorus burns may include systemic hypocalcemia and, rarely, dysrhythmias or sudden death.[62,83] Other complications include those seen with any burn, such as cellulitis, osteomyelitis, sepsis, fluid shifts and hypovolemia, renal injury, and associated trauma.[6,60]

DIAGNOSIS

Phosphorus

Because white phosphorus ingestions are now rare, particularly in developed countries, and because symptoms of toxicity are so nonspecific, the diagnosis is likely to be overlooked. There are no specific laboratory findings that definitively establish the diagnosis. Serum phosphorus concentrations may be low, normal, or high after ingestions.[11] Theoretically, samples of gastric fluid could be measured for phosphorus content or evaluated for fluorescence under ultraviolet light, but these cannot be relied on.[28] Consequently, making the diagnosis of phosphorus poisoning depends heavily on clinical suspicion and obtaining a history of access to products containing white phosphorus (e.g., fireworks or rodenticide pastes). Special efforts should be made to identify the exact product consumed or to locate containers or labels with specific ingredients. Histories are often inaccurate, so corroboration with information from with family or friends should be sought.

The classic three-stage progression of symptoms may help clue the clinician into the diagnosis, but other poisonings can present with similar symptoms (e.g., iron), and coingestants may confuse the picture. Specific clinical features that point to phosphorus ingestion include a characteristic garlic-like odor, smoking or luminescent stools or vomitus, and the presence of chemical burns. These features are relatively uncommon, however, and their absence does not exclude the diagnosis. A liver biopsy with periportal changes, such as steatosis or necrosis, may suggest phosphorus toxicity, but this pattern is neither specific nor sensitive. As with all poisonings, every effort should be made to rule out other medical and toxicologic diagnoses.

Phosphine

The diagnosis of phosphine poisoning can be difficult because clinical signs and symptoms are nonspecific. Phosphine levels have been measured in the blood and seem to correlate with the severity of clinical toxicity.[84] Blood levels are not readily available at most hospitals, however, and are of little utility in the acute management of most patients. Nonetheless, they may help confirm the diagnosis retrospectively. Poisoning should be suspected in patients with a history of exposure to areas that may have been fumigated, (e.g., railroad cars or structures used for grain storage) methamphetamine laboratories, or other industries where phosphine is commonly used. Access to older or foreign rodenticides can also be a clue. A fishy or garlic odor suggests the diagnosis but cannot be relied on. Some authors have measured aluminum or zinc concentrations in the serum or gastric aspirate as a surrogate marker for metal phosphide ingestion.[77,82] It is unlikely, however, that these results would be available soon enough to influence clinical decision making. Testing a patient's gastric aspirate or breath with silver nitrate–impregnated paper also has been suggested as a confirmatory bedside maneuver.[81,85] A small amount of gastric aspirate (about 5 mL) is mixed with water (about 15 mL) in a flask, which is then covered by silver nitrate–impregnated paper. The flask is heated gently until fumes develop and impregnate the paper for about 20 minutes. The paper is set aside to dry, and if phosphine is present, it turns black. Alternatively, the paper can be impregnated with the patient's breath for 20 minutes.

Phosphorus Burns

The diagnosis of phosphorus burns is usually readily apparent. Most exposures occur in military personnel or persons working in industries where white phosphorus is used regularly (e.g., munitions manufacturing and the fertilizer industry). As a result, patients often know the identity of the offending substance. Obtaining product composition information from the company may assist with the identification of specific chemicals or ingredients.

Clinical features that suggest phosphorus burns include smoking wounds, a garlic odor, and visualization of particles embedded in the tissue. Using an ultraviolet light may help with visualization.[6] Irrigation with a dilute copper sulfate solution can be useful because it combines with phosphorus to form black, easily recognizable particles of copper phosphate.[83] Unfortunately, these solutions have caused significant toxicity in some patients and should be used only with extreme caution.[65,86,87]

TREATMENT

Indications for ICU Admission in Phosphorus Poisoning

Significant exposure to phosphorus, phosphine, or metal phosphide suspected
Large phosphorus burn (>10%)
Evidence of shock
Respiratory compromise
Mental status changes
Patients with significant symptoms after exposure (due to risk of deterioration)

Phosphorus

There is no specific antidote for white phosphorus. Treatment should focus on aggressive decontamination and good supportive care. After ingestion, the most common cause of death in these patients is cardiovascular collapse or dysrhythmias. Liver failure, renal failure, and metabolic abnormalities may be the cause of death in later stages. Treatment and monitoring should focus on these areas in particular. A variety of specific decontamination and therapeutic modalities have been proposed, but little evidence exists in the literature to support or refute their use. Most of the recommendations are based on anecdotal reports, case series, animal data, or chemical principles alone.

GASTROINTESTINAL DECONTAMINATION

Because mortality seems to be closely related to the amount of phosphorus systemically absorbed, aggressive decontamination measures are important, especially if the ingestion is greater than 1 mg/kg body weight.[3,11,13,48] At least one case series indicated an improvement in survival with early decontamination, but others have suggested that benefits may be limited because most patients tend to self-decontaminate as a result of persistent emesis.[3,88] No controlled clinical study has established a benefit to aggressive gastrointestinal decontamination, however. Given the lack of other effective treatments, gastrointestinal decontamination seems prudent and should be performed as early as possible.

Charcoal is unlikely to adsorb phosphorus to a significant degree, so unless coingestants are suspected, it should not be administered. Gastric lavage is a reasonable option for decontamination because many phosphorus-containing products are in either paste or powder form and could be expected to pass through most lavage tubes. Phosphorus ingestions may result in corrosive injury to the esophagus and stomach, making the passage of a lavage tube risky. In general, the potential systemic toxicity of large phosphorus ingestions outweighs the risk for gastric injury or perforation from lavage, but this decision should be made on an individual basis. The smallest and most pliable tube should be used for the procedure, and it should be passed with care. Ordinary saline or tap water is adequate as a lavage fluid. Other types of fluid have been proposed but have not been studied formally. Potassium permanganate solution (1:5000 or 1:1000) has been suggested by multiple authors, primarily based on its ability to convert phosphorus in the stomach to less harmful phosphorus oxides.[3,4,11,44] Although this idea makes sense chemically, the use of potassium permanganate solution has not been evaluated for clinical efficacy or safety. Most physicians are unlikely to have experience with potassium permanganate solution or to find it readily available. Solutions of copper sulfate have also been proposed as lavage solutions, because copper binds with phosphorus to form insoluble, inactive salts.[14,43] Severe adverse sequelae, such as massive hemolysis and death, have been reported with their use, however, as a result of excessive systemic copper absorption.[89] Given these risks, the use of copper sulfate solution is strongly discouraged.

After lavage, many authors recommend giving a dose of mineral oil orally.[4,11,14,44] Theoretically, because phosphorus is fat soluble, it preferentially would dissolve in the mineral oil and be passed from the body (mineral oil is minimally absorbed through the gastrointestinal tract). Although there are no human trials investigating its use, one study in dogs suggested a benefit.[88] Another study in rats found no benefit.[32] Given the lack of significant side effects, however, in an awake patient, the use of mineral oil seems reasonable. Another potential method for enhancing the elimination of phosphorus from the gastrointestinal tract is whole-bowel irrigation. A polyethylene glycol solution for this purpose is safe and easy to administer through a nasogastric tube. It may help cleanse the gastrointestinal tract of unabsorbed phosphorus, but its use has not been reported, and it remains untested. Hemodialysis as a method of enhanced elimination has not been evaluated for patients with phosphorus poisoning. It should be considered when severe metabolic abnormalities or renal failure intervenes during the course of the illness.

Late decontamination procedures should be considered because many patients present hours or days after their ingestion. Case reports have shown that phosphorus can be recovered in vomitus or feces 2 to 3 days after ingestion.[88] As a result, even delayed institution of decontamination measures, such as lavage or whole-bowel irrigation, may be of potential benefit.

Dietary changes have been suggested to reduce the amount of phosphorus absorbed. If the patient is taking food orally, absorbable fats and oils should be avoided as much as possible. Absorbable fats and oils readily dissolve phosphorus and may increase its absorption systemically.[11,14,44,88]

As with many toxins, great care should be taken among medical personnel during decontamination procedures. Phosphorus in the patient's vomitus or feces potentially can cause burns on dermal contact. Personal protective equipment and universal precautions are essential.

SUPPORTIVE MEASURES

Serial measurements of vital signs and fluid status are essential for patients with phosphorus poisoning. In symptomatic patients or patients with potentially significant ingestions, it is important to monitor serum electrolytes (particularly phosphorus and calcium), acid-base status, renal function, liver function, and coagulation parameters regularly. Blood glucose measurements should be checked regularly in patients with significant toxicity. Patients should be examined for evidence of gastrointestinal bleeding; serial measurements of hematocrit may be helpful in this regard. Continuous ECG monitoring is important to detect any dysrhythmias or conduction abnormalities. Endoscopy may be indicated if significant gastrointestinal corrosive injury or life-threatening bleeding is suspected.

Given that phosphorus poisoning may lead to CNS depression, attention to the patient's airway and respirations should be paramount. If a patient is unable to maintain the airway, endotracheal intubation should be performed and ventilation assisted as necessary. Patients with significant ingestions should be observed closely, for rapid changes in mental status, airway protective reflexes, or respiratory drive. Continuous pulse oximetry is advised. Patients with altered mental status should also have rapid bedside measurement of serum glucose performed to rule out hypoglycemia.

If present, hypoglycemia should be treated with intravenous dextrose. Administration of naloxone, oxygen, and thiamine may be considered to rule out other causes for altered mentation.

Hypotension is common in patients with significant phosphorus toxicity, during the initial and later stages of illness, and the patients' blood pressure should be followed closely. If evidence of hypotension or poor perfusion develops, initial treatment should begin with intravenous fluids. In an adult, a bolus of 1 to 2 L is an adequate initial dose; however, more fluid may be necessary. Care should be taken to avoid hypervolemia, especially in patients with an underlying predisposition to fluid overload. Assessment of urine output may be helpful in guiding therapy. In patients who do not respond to fluids alone, intravenous pressors should be added. In ambiguous cases, invasive hemodynamic measurements may be helpful. Pressors may be particularly useful during the later stages of phosphorus poisoning, when vasodilation and myocardial depression can develop. No single pressor agent has been shown to be more effective than others in phosphorus-induced hypotension. The optimal choice is the pressor to which the patient responds best and with which the medical staff is most familiar. The dose should be titrated to clinical response, and more than one pressor may be necessary. α-Adrenergic agonists may be helpful in patients with low peripheral vascular resistance. Frequent vital signs and assessment of urine output, mentation, and acid-base status are good monitors of perfusion. All patients with suspected phosphorus poisoning should have intravenous access and be observed in a monitored setting, because conduction abnormalities and dysrhythmias may develop.

Supportive measures if liver failure develops include standard dietary restrictions and lactulose for encephalopathy. Various drugs to prevent or ameliorate phosphorus-induced hepatic injury are discussed in the following section. Coagulopathy may be treated with vitamin K supplementation. If significant bleeding develops, coagulation factor or blood replacement may be necessary.

Renal failure may necessitate hemodialysis if significant fluid or electrolyte abnormalities intervene. The indications for hemodialysis are similar to the indications for other medical conditions. A return to normal renal function over time is expected in survivors.

Electrolyte, acid-base, and metabolic abnormalities should be monitored and corrected. Hypoglycemia may develop with the advent of liver injury and needs to be addressed with intravenous dextrose.

SPECIFIC TREATMENTS

A variety of specific therapeutic and pharmacologic measures have been proposed for phosphorus poisoning, but human data are scant. The use of corticosteroids has been suggested, and temporal improvement in one patient was reported after their use.[63] A controlled, prospective trial of cortisone in 49 patients showed no benefit, however, and in one subgroup there was a trend toward increased mortality, although this was not statistically significant.[13] N-Acetylcysteine also has been tried in humans, but the case series investigating its use found no improvement.[12] Finally, exchange transfusions were attempted in a small group of patients with phosphorus poisoning and hepatic encephalopathy.[13] This nonrandomized trial seemed to show an improved mortality rate in the treated group versus controls, but the number of subjects was too small for statistical comparison.

There are more studies on therapeutic modalities for phosphorus poisoning in animals than there are in humans, yet no clear treatment has emerged from these models. In a Spanish study of rats poisoned with phosphorus, treatment with interferon alfa-2b improved survival and decreased hepatic injury.[90] Pentoxifylline reduced the incidence of scarring after liver injury in phosphorus-poisoned pigs.[53] Antioxidants such as glutathione, hexahydrocoenzyme Q_4, and propyl gallate all have been shown to be hepatoprotective in rats.[36,40] Adenine, an adenosine triphosphate precursor, also seemed to be beneficial in preventing hepatic steatosis in one study.[91] These studies are all isolated animal experiments, and the therapies described should be considered investigational.

Phosphine

As with white phosphorus, there is no specific antidote for phosphine, and treatment depends on decontamination and supportive care. Decontamination after phosphine gas exposures means simply moving them to a well-ventilated area. In the case of metal phosphide ingestions, after which phosphine gas may continue to be released for some time while the metal phosphide remains in contact with intestinal fluids, a more aggressive approach is necessary. Because some studies have correlated mortality to the amount of phosphide ingested, removal of even a portion could be beneficial.[19,92] This recommendation is supported by evidence that patients who spontaneously vomit after phosphide ingestions have improved survival.[92] Patients who have not self-decontaminated adequately by vomiting should undergo gastric lavage. Some authors recommend using a potassium permanganate or bicarbonate (2%) solution for gastric irrigation.[20,77,81] The theory behind bicarbonate is that by neutralizing the stomach acid one can reduce the hydrolysis of phosphides into phosphine.[81] Although these solutions probably are not harmful, there are no data to support their use. Unless they are readily available, these solutions should not be employed. Adequate personal protective equipment should be used during decontamination, and the procedure should be performed in a well-ventilated area. Gastric aspirate should be kept in a sealed container because any metal phosphide remaining continues to produce phosphine that may pose a potential hazard.

Supportive care is similar to that for patients with phosphorus poisoning. Blood pressure should be monitored, and shock should be corrected aggressively with fluids and pressors as needed. Pulmonary edema should be managed with mechanical ventilation, if necessary, and positive end-expiratory pressure should be employed. Care must be taken to avoid fluid overload. Continuous cardiac monitoring is important for the first 1 to 2 days to watch for dysrhythmias, and the patient's electrolytes should be monitored and replaced if necessary. Renal function, liver function, and acid-base status should be followed.

Intravenous magnesium has been employed in many patients with phosphine poisoning. Despite initially conflicting data, the evidence supporting its use is mounting. Several studies from India have shown an improvement in mortality, and many authors now advocate the use of intravenous magnesium.[93-96] The optimal dose has not been established. One author has recommended 2 g intravenously over 30 minutes followed by 5 g intravenously over the next 12 hours as an infusion, but other regimens have also been suggested.[81] Magnesium seems to be safe, but theoretically it may exacerbate hypotension. Until further studies are done, magnesium should be given, provided that there are no overriding contraindications. Corticosteroids also have been proposed based on a study that found evidence of adrenal suppression with phosphine poisoning.[97] Despite the lack of further evidence, corticosteroids should be considered in patients with refractory hypotension who do not respond to conservative measures. The recommended dose for dexamethasone is 4 mg intravenously every 4 hours.[81] Calcium supplementation also has been suggested as a "membrane stabilizer," but no benefit has been reported.[20,81] Newer research is evaluating the role of various antioxidants.[73]

Phosphorus Burns

Treatment of phosphorus burns primarily involves rapid decontamination and supportive measures. Immediate decontamination in the prehospital setting has been shown to improve outcome.[66] Decontamination should be instituted as quickly as possible after exposure. Particles of phosphorus that remain in contact with the skin can continue to oxidize in the presence of air, causing further tissue damage. Removing these particles or at least preventing their combustion by keeping them cool and moist is essential. Large particles should be brushed off immediately after exposure, but care must be taken not to push the phosphorus deeper into any wounds. Subsequently, wounds should be irrigated thoroughly. Irrigation helps wash away any remaining phosphorus and quenches any ongoing combustion.[5,98,99]

The optimal fluid for irrigation is the cause of some debate. Some authors have recommended using copper sulfate solutions (1% to 5%) or suspensions because copper combines with phosphorus to form a black inactive salt; theoretically this reduces the risk of ongoing injury and improves particle visualization and removal. A few animal studies have even suggested a benefit to irrigating with such solutions.[5,83,100] However, several patients have developed massive hemolysis due to systemic absorption of copper after prolonged dermal contact.[86,87] Another study in rats showed that irrigation with copper sulfate resulted in a higher mortality than irrigation with water alone.[98] Therefore, the use of copper sulfate should be discouraged. Other authors have suggested using silver nitrate solutions (1% to 3%) for similar reasons. In contrast to copper, silver does not seem to pose any significant systemic risks. Anecdotal reports suggest it may be beneficial, but no formal study has been published. Unless silver nitrate solutions are immediately available, plain water or saline should be used for irrigation. Any particles remaining should be débrided or removed manually with forceps. Ultraviolet light (i.e., Wood's lamp) may help with visualization of particles. Surgical excision is an option for tissues with significant amounts of phosphorus that cannot be removed by other measures. During transport, wounds should be kept covered with moist dressings. Using oil-impregnated or petrolatum-impregnated gauze should be avoided because the lipids may enhance phosphorus uptake through the dermis.[5]

Supportive care is similar to that recommended for other burn patients, including daily dressing changes, tetanus prophylaxis, observation for signs of infection, and evaluation for associated injuries (i.e., trauma). Consultation with a burn surgeon is advised because patients may require grafting, excision, escharotomy, or further measures. Close monitoring of fluid and electrolyte status is important, given the risk of hypocalcemia and hyperphosphatemia. Fluid requirements secondary to phosphorus burns may not be as great as the requirements for the treatment of comparable thermal injuries. Continuous cardiac monitoring should be performed for 1 to 2 days to watch for dysrhythmias.

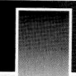

Criteria for ICU Discharge in Phosphorus Poisoning

Patients who have been monitored for an adequate period after suspected ingestions and have shown no signs of developing systemic toxicity (e.g., physical examination, electrolytes, liver function tests, and electrocardiogram show no significant abnormalities); the adequate observation period is not known and may vary based on the circumstances of exposure, but 24 to 48 hours should be adequate

Patients who had initial signs of poisoning (e.g., stage I toxicity) but who have shown no signs of developing systemic toxicity thereafter, despite an adequate observation period

Improving stage III systemic toxicity (e.g., improving mental or cardiovascular status, resolution of metabolic or electrolyte derangements, improving liver function)

SPECIAL POPULATIONS

Pediatric Patients

In the past, children were at increased risk of exposure to phosphorus because of its use as a rodenticide. The paste commonly would be spread on food to entice pests and was often eaten by children as well. These rodenticides are not used commonly any longer in most developed countries. Children are more susceptible to phosphine gas because of their increased minute ventilation compared with adults. The clinical course of phosphorus and phosphine poisoning is no different than in adults, and treatment should be the same.

Pregnant Patients

Phosphorus has been used as an abortifacient. It is known to cross the placenta, but no cases of fetotoxicity or teratogenicity have been reported.[101] Phosphine showed no evidence of teratogenicity in a rat study, and no reports of human fetotoxicity or teratogenicity have been published.[102] Pregnant patients should be managed similar to other patients, with aggressive decontamination and supportive care.

Military Personnel

Military personnel are at risk for phosphorus burns and inhalational exposures given the widespread use of phosphorus compounds in obscurants, incendiary devices, and munitions.

Common Errors in Phosphorus Poisoning

Not considering the diagnosis, which requires a high degree of suspicion and a detailed history

Relying on unusual signs, such as a garlic odor or smoking stools, to make the diagnosis; although relatively specific, these signs are insensitive and may not be present

Failing to monitor a patient with phosphorus ingestion after apparent initial improvement; later deterioration and end-organ toxicity may develop (i.e., stage III toxicity)

Key Points in Phosphorus Poisoning

1. Ingestions of white phosphorus can cause corrosive gastrointestinal injury followed hours to days later by systemic toxicity with multiple organ dysfunction, particularly hepatic damage.
2. Dermal contact with white phosphorus can cause severe burns and, potentially, systemic toxicity.
3. Inhalation of phosphine gas can cause pulmonary edema and systemic effects; ingestion of metal phosphides liberates phosphine gas, which can cause rapid, severe systemic toxicity with cardiovascular collapse.
4. Diagnosis may be difficult and depends heavily on a history of exposure.
5. Treatment is supportive; there are no specific antidotes for phosphorus or phosphine.
6. Early, aggressive decontamination may help prevent systemic toxicity from developing.

REFERENCES

1. Marrs TC: Histological changes produced by exposure of rabbits and rats to smokes produced from red phosphorus. Toxicol Lett 21:141–146, 1984.
2. Hann RG, Veale RA: A fatal case of poisoning by phosphorus with unusual subcutaneous hemorrhages. Lancet 1:163–164, 1910.
3. La Due JS, Schenken JR, Kuker LH: Phosphorus poisoning: A report of 16 cases with repeated liver biopsies in a recovered case. Am J Med Sci 208:223–234, 1944.
4. Simon FA, Pickering LK: Acute yellow phosphorus poisoning: "Smoking stool syndrome." JAMA 235:1343–1344, 1976.
5. Konjoyan TR: White phosphorus burns: Case report and literature review. Milit Med 148:881–884, 1983.
6. Mozingo DW, Smith AA, McManus WF, et al: Chemical burns. J Trauma Inj Inf Crit Care 28:642–647, 1988.
7. Obermer E: Phosphorus burns. Lancet 1:202, 1943.
8. Hughs JP, Baron R, Buckland DH, et al: Phosphorus necrosis of the jaw: A present day study. Br J Ind Med 19:83–99, 1962.
9. Llewellyn TO: Minerals Yearbook. U.S. Department of the Interior, Bureau of Mines, Washington, DC, 1993.
10. Duerkson-Hughs P, Richter P, Ingerman L, Thampi S: Toxicologic profile for white phosphorus. Agency for Toxic Substances and Disease Registry, Atlanta, GA, 1997.
11. Diaz-Rivera RS, Collazo PJ, Pons ER, Torregrosa MV: Acute phosphorus poisoning in man: A study of 56 cases. Medicine 29:269–298, 1950.

12. Fernandez OU, Canizares LL: Acute hepatotoxicity from ingestion of yellow phosphorus–containing fireworks. J Clin Gastroenterol 21:139–142, 1995.

13. Marin GA, Montoya CA, Sierra JL, Senior JR: Evaluation of corticosteroid and exchange-transfusion treatment of acute yellow-phosphorus intoxication. N Engl J Med 284:125–128, 1971.

14. Rubitsky HJ, Myerson RM: Acute phosphorus poisoning. Arch Int Med 83:164–178, 1949.

15. Phosphorus necrosis under control. Br Dent J 76:343, 1944.

16. Wason S, Gomolin I, Gross P, et al: Phosphorus trichloride toxicity: Preliminary report. Am J Med 77:1039–1042, 1984.

17. Anonymous: Deaths associated with exposure to fumigants in railroad cars—United States. MMWR Morb Mortal Wkly Rep 43:489–491, 1994.

18. Chopra JS, Kalra OP, Malik VS, et al: Aluminium phosphide poisoning: A prospective study of 16 cases in one year. Postgrad Med J 62:1113–1115, 1986.

19. Chugh SN, Aggarwal HK, Mahajan SK: Zinc phosphide intoxication symptoms: Analysis of 20 cases. Int J Clin Pharm Ther 36:406–407, 1998.

20. Khosla SN, Nand N, Khosla P: Aluminium phosphide poisoning. J Trop Med Hyg 91:196–198, 1988.

21. Willers-Russo LJ: Three fatalities involving phosphine gas, produced as a result of methamphetamine manufacturing. J Forens Sci 44:647–652, 1999.

22. Wilson R, Lovejoy FH, Jaeger RJ, Landrigan PL: Acute phosphine poisoning aboard a grain freighter: Epidemiologic, clinical, and pathological findings. JAMA 244:148–150, 1980.

23. Banjaj R, Wasir HS: Epidemic aluminium phosphide poisoning in Northern India. Lancet 1:820–821, 1988.

24. Jayaraman KS: Death pills from pesticide. Nature 353:377, 1991.

25. Sharma A, Gathwala G: Oral aluminium phosphide poisoning in Indian children. J Trop Med Hyg 95:221–222, 1992.

26. Cameron JM, Patrick RS: Acute phosphorus poisoning—the distribution of toxic doses of yellow phosphorus in the tissues of experimental animals. Med Sci Law 6:209–214, 1966.

27. Ghoshal AK, Porta EA, Hartroft WS: Isotopic studies on the absorption and tissue distribution of white phosphorus in rats. Exp Mol Pathol 14:212–219, 1971.

28. Salfelder K, Doehnert HR, Doehnert G, et al: Fatal phosphorus poisoning: A study of forty-five autopsy cases. Beitr Pathol 147:321–340, 1972.

29. Winek CL, Collom WD, Fusia EP: Yellow phosphorus ingestion—three fatal poisonings. Clin Toxicol 6:541–545, 1973.

30. Brewer E, Haggerty RJ: Toxic hazards: Rat poisons—phosphorus. N Engl J Med 258:147–148, 1958.

31. Bababunmi EA, Badaeva L, Jackson JR, et al: Environmental Health Criteria 73: Phosphine and Metal Phosphides. Geneva, World Health Organization International Programme on Chemical Safety, 1988.

32. Ganote CE, Otis JB: Characteristic lesions of yellow phosphorus–induced liver damage. Lab Invest 21:207–213, 1969.

33. Beloskurskaia GI: [The pathogenesis of toxic liver lesions in workers in phosphorus production] [Russian]. Vrachebnoe Delo July 7:104–106, 1989.

34. Kulkybaev GA, Merkusheva NV: [Dynamics of NAD-dependent isocitrate dehydrogenase activity in homogenized rat liver exposed to toxic products of the phosphorus industry] [Russian]. Gig Truda i Prof Zabol (1):21–23, 1992.

35. Barker EA, Smuckler EA, Benditt EP: Effects of thioacetamide and yellow phosphorus poisoning on protein synthesis. Lab Invest 12:955–960, 1963.

36. Pani P, Gravela E, Mazzarino C, Burdino E: On the mechanism of fatty liver in white phosphorus–poisoned rats. Exp Mol Pathol 16:201–209, 1972.

37. Seakins A, Robinson DS: Changes associated with the production of fatty livers by white phosphorus and by ethanol in the rat. Biochem J 92:308–312, 1964.

38. Althausen TL, Thoenes E: Influence on carbohydrate metabolism of experimentally induced hepatic changes. Arch Intern Med 50:58–75, 1932.

39. McIntosh R: Acute phosphorus poisoning. Am J Dis Child 34:595–602, 1927.

40. DiLuzio NR: Influence of intravenously administered hexahydrocoenzyme Q4 on liver injury. Life Sci 5:1467–1478, 1966.

41. Ghoshal AK, Porta EA, Hartroft WS: The role of lipoperoxidation in the pathogenesis of fatty livers induced by phosphorus poisoning in rats. Am J Pathol 54:275–291, 1969.

42. Foulerton AG: Acute yellow atrophy of the liver and the fatty infiltration of liver and kidney which results from the action of certain poisons on the liver. J Pathol Bacteriol 24:257–270, 1921.

43. Chretien TE: Acute phosphorus poisoning: Report of a case with recovery. N Engl J Med 232:247–249, 1945.

44. McCarron MM, Gaddis GP, Trotter AT: Acute yellow phosphorus poisoning from pesticide pastes. Clin Toxicol 18:693–711, 1981.

45. Talley RC, Linhart JW, Trevino AJ, et al: Acute elemental phosphorus poisoning in man: Cardiovascular toxicity. Am Heart J 84:139–140, 1972.

46. Diaz-Rivera RS, Morales FR, Garcia-Palmieri MR, Ramirez EA: The electrocardiographic changes in acute phosphorus poisoning in man. Am J Med Sci 241:758–765, 1961.

47. Pietras RJ, Stavrakos C, Gunnar RM, Tobin JR: Phosphorus poisoning simulating acute myocardial infarction. Arch Intern Med 122:430–434, 1968.

48. Fahim FA, El-Sabbagh M, Saleh NA, Sallam US: Biochemical changes associated with acute phosphorus poisoning (in humans). Gen Pharm 21:899–904, 1990.

49. Barone C, Cittadini A, Galeotti T, Terranova T: The effect of intoxication induced in rat liver by carbon tetrachloride, ethionine and white phosphorus on the level of microsomal cytochromes b5 and p-450. Experientia 29:73–74, 1973.

50. Fletcher GF, Galambos JT: Phosphorus poisoning in humans. Arch Intern Med 112:846–852, 1963.

51. Greenberger NJ, Robinson WL, Isselbacher KJ: Toxic hepatitis after the ingestion of phosphorus with subsequent recovery. Gastroenterology 47:179–183, 1964.

52. Mallory FB: Phosphorus and alcoholic cirrhosis. Am J Pathol 9:557–567, 1933.

53. Peterson TC, Neumeister M: Effect of pentoxifylline in rat and swine models of hepatic fibrosis: Role of fibroproliferation in its mechanism. Immunopharmacology 31:183–193, 1996.

54. Burnell JM, Dennis MB, Clayson KJ, et al: Evaluation in dogs of cross-circulation in the treatment of acute hepatic necrosis induced by yellow phosphorus. Gastroenterology 71:827–831, 1976.

55. Dianzani MU: Toxic liver injury by protein synthesis inhibitors. Prog Liver Dis 5:232–245, 1976.

56. Lombardi B, Recknagel RO: Interference with secretion of triglycerides by the liver as a common factor in toxic liver injury: With some observations on choline deficiency fatty liver. Am J Pathol 40:571–586, 1962.

57. Wertham F: Central nervous system in acute phosphorus poisoning. Arch Neuropsychiatry 28:320–330, 1932.

58. Blumenthal S, Lesser A: Acute phosphorus poisoning. Am J Dis Child 55:1280–1287, 1938.

59. Jacobinzer H, Raybin HW: Phosphorus poisoning including two fatal case reports. Arch Pediatr 396–402, 1961.

60. Appelbaum J, Ben-Hur N, Shani J: Subcellular morphological changes in the rat kidney after phosphorus burn. Pathol Eur 10:145–154, 1975.

61. Ben-Hur N, Appelbaum J: Biochemistry, histopathology and treatment of phosphorus burns: An experimental study. Isr J Med Sci 9:40–48, 1973.

62. Bowen TE, Whelan TJ, Nelson TG: Sudden death after phosphorus burns: Experimental observations of hypocalcemia, hyperphosphatemia and electrocardiographic abnormalities following production of a standard white phosphorus burn. Ann Surg 174:779–784, 1971.

63. Bayne JRD, Beck JC, Lowenstein L, Browne JSL: Cortisone acetate in the treatment of acute phosphorus poisoning. Can Med Assoc J 67:465–467, 1952.

64. Perry JW: Phosphorus poisoning with cortical necrosis of kidney: Report of 2 fatal cases. Australasia Ann Med 2:94–98, 1953.

65. Curreri PW, Asch MJ, Pruitt BA: The treatment of chemical burns: Specialized diagnostic, therapeutic, and prognostic considerations. J Trauma Inj Infect Crit Care 10:634–642, 1970.

66. Leonard LG, Scheulen JJ, Munster AM: Chemical burns: Effect of prompt first aid. J Trauma 22:420–423, 1982.

67. Ben-Hur N, Appelbaum J: The phosphorus burn and its specific treatment (a biochemical, histological, electron microscopy and radioactive study). Burns 1:222–232, 1975.

68. Wechsler L, Wechsler RL: Phosphorus poisoning: The latent period and unusual gastrointestinal lesions. Gastroenterology 17:279–283, 1951.

69. Kashi KP, Chefurka W: The effect of phosphine on the absorption and circular dichronine spectra of cytochrome-C and cytochrome oxidase. Pesticides Biochem Physiol 6:350–362, 1976.

70. Chin KL, Mai X, Meaklim J, et al: The interaction of phosphine with haemoglobin and erythrocytes. Xenobiotica 22:599–607, 1992.

71. Arora B, Punia RS, Kalra R, et al: Histopathological changes in aluminium phosphide poisoning. J Indian Med Assoc 93:380–381, 1995.

72. Chugh SN, Mittal A, Seth S, Chugh K: Lipid peroxidation in acute aluminium phosphide poisoning. J Assoc Physicians India 43:265–266, 1995.

73. Hsu C, Han B, Liu M, et al: Phosphine-induced oxidative damage in rats: Attenuation by melatonin. Free Rad Bio Med 28:636–642, 2000.

74. Hsu CH, Quistad GB, Casida JE: Phosphine-induced oxidative stress in hepa 1c1c7 cells. Toxicol Sci 46:204–210, 1998.

75. Bhasin P, Mittal HS, Mitra A: An echocardiographic study in aluminum phosphide poisoning. J Assoc Physicians India 39:851, 1991.

76. Kalra GS, Anand IS, Jit I, et al: Aluminium phosphide poisoning: Haemodynamic observations. Ind Heart J 43:175–178, 1991.

77. Stephenson JB: Zinc phosphide poisoning. Arch Environ Health 15:83–88, 1967.

78. Bajaj R, Wasir HS: Epidemiology of aluminium phosphide poisoning: Need for a survey. J Assoc Physicians India 38:197–198, 1990.

79. Swinton CF: Acute phosphorus poisoning. BMJ 2:1080, 1927.

80. Chugh SN, Malhotra KC: Acute pericarditis in aluminium phosphide poisoning. J Assoc Physicians India 40:564, 1992.

81. Gupta S, Ahlawat SK: Aluminum phosphide poisoning—a review. J Toxicol Clin Toxicol 33:19–24, 1995.

82. Garry VF, Good PF, Manivel JC, Perl DP: Investigation of a fatality from nonoccupational aluminum phosphide exposure: Measurement of aluminum in tissue and body fluids as a marker of exposure. J Lab Clin Med 122:739–747, 1993.

83. Chou TD, Lee TW, Chen SL, et al: The management of white phosphorus burns. Burns 27:492–497, 2001.

84. Chugh SN, Pal R, Singh V, Seth S: Serial blood phosphine levels in acute aluminum phosphide poisoning. J Assoc Physicians India 44:184–185, 1996.

85. Chugh SN, Ram S, Chugh K, Malhotra KC: Spot diagnosis of aluminium phosphide ingestion: An application of a simple test. J Assoc Physicians India 37:219–220, 1989.

86. Mendelson JA: Some principles of protection against burns from flame and incendiary munitions. J Trauma Inj Inf Crit Care 11:286–294, 1971.

87. Summerlin WT, Walder AI, Moncrief JA: White phosphorus burns and massive hemolysis. J Trauma Inj Inf Crit Care 7:476–484, 1967.

88. Atkinson HV: The treatment of acute phosphorus poisoning. J Lab Clin Med 7:148–150, 1921.

89. Stein RS, Jenkins D, Korns ME: Death after use of cupric sulfate as emetic. JAMA 235:801, 1976.

90. Gomez N, Andrade R, Roldos F, et al: [Use of interferon in hepatic necrosis produced by paraquat and yellow phosphorus: Experimental evaluation] [Spanish]. Acta Gastroent Latinoam 28:189–192, 1998.

91. Farber E, McConomy JM: Selective effect of adenine in preventing fatty liver. Lab Invest 15:1490–1491, 1966.

92. Singh S, Singh D, Wig N, et al: Aluminum phosphide ingestion—a clinico-pathologic study. J Toxicol Clin Toxicol 34:703–706, 1996.

93. Chugh SN, Kolley T, Kakkar R, et al: A critical evaluation of anti-peroxidant effect of intravenous magnesium in acute aluminium phosphide poisoning. Magnes Res 10:225–230, 1997.

94. Chugh SN, Ram S, Sharma A, et al: Adrenocortical involvement in aluminium phosphide poisoning. Indian J Med Res 90:289–294, 1989.

95. Katira R, Elhence GP, Mehrotra ML, et al: A study of aluminum phosphide (alp) poisoning with special reference to electrocardiographic changes. J Assoc Physicians India 38:471–473, 1990.

96. Siwach SB, Gupta S, Ahlawat S: A critical evaluation of magnesium sulfate therapy in aluminum phosphide poisoning. J Assoc Physicians India 39:850, 1991.

97. Chugh SN, Ram S, Sharma A, et al: Adrenocortical involvement in aluminium phosphide poisoning. Indian J Med Res 90:289–294, 1989.

98. Eldad A, Simon GA: The phosphorus burn—a preliminary comparative experimental study of various forms of treatment. Burns 17:198–200, 1991.

99. Eldad A, Wisoki M, Cohen H, et al: Phosphorous burns: Evaluation of various modalities for primary treatment. J Burn Care Rehabil 16:49–55, 1995.

100. Ben-Hur N, Giladi A, Applebaum J, Neuman Z: Phosphorus burns: The antidote: A new approach. Br J Plast Surg 25:245–249, 1972.

101. Gosselin RE, Smith RP, Hodge HC: Clinical Toxicology of Commercial Products, 5th ed. Baltimore, Williams & Wilkins, 1984.

102. Schroeder RE, Newton PE, Sullivan JD: An inhalation developmental toxicity study of phosphine in rats. Toxicologist 12:122, 1992.

CHAPTER 82

Thallium

Youngsoo Cho ■ Richard Y. Wang

Thallium, which is derived from the Greek word *thallos* or "young shoot," was discovered in 1861 by Sir William Crookes during his search for tellurium. An odorless, colorless, and tasteless heavy metal, thallium has a molecular weight between that of mercury and lead. It is highly reactive and is found mainly in the sulfate salt form, but it also exists in at least 18 different compounds. It can be found in the earth's crust in the form of minerals such as crooksite and ores such as sulfite ores and potassium minerals.[1]

Historically, thallium has been used as a treatment for syphilis, gonorrhea, gout, dysentery, and night sweats in tuberculosis patients. It also has been used as a depilatory agent for ringworm of the scalp.[2] Its use was limited, however, by toxic side effects. Thallium was first introduced as a rodenticide in the 1920s in Germany and since has been responsible for many occupational, accidental, and suicidal poisonings. It has been used as a homicidal agent in maliciously contaminated food, found in a Chinese herbal medication, and mistaken for cocaine.[3–5] The first reported outbreak of thallium poisoning in the United States occurred in 1932.[6] Thallium's use as a rodenticide and pesticide in the United States was banned in 1965, but it continues to be used in the manufacture of semiconductors, scintillation counters, fireworks, optical lenses, imitation jewelry, and industrial thermometers. Environmental contamination occurs from cement factories, coal-burning power plants, and smelters (of copper, zinc, cadmium, and lead).[7,8] Thallium[201] currently is used in myocardial imaging. Since thallium was restricted in the United States, thallium poisonings have fallen precipitously in this country. In some developing countries, use of thallium is unrestricted.[9] This chapter discusses the clinical toxicology and sequelae of thallium intoxication with a focus on an evidenced-based evaluation of various treatment protocols.

CLINICAL PHARMACOLOGY

Thallium is absorbed by the gastrointestinal tract after oral ingestion, by intact skin, and by the lungs after inhalation.[3,10,11] It distributes mostly intracellularly, accounting for its relatively large volume of distribution, estimated at 3.6 to 5.6 L/kg in humans.[10,11] Thallium distributes via the circulatory system, so organs that are well perfused, such as the heart, spleen, kidney, pancreas, and lungs, have the highest levels in humans.[10,11] Thallium's toxicity may be cumulative or manifest after a single dose. Lethal doses have been estimated at 1 g in humans, or 10 mg/kg, but

deaths have been reported with ingestions of 200 mg.[12,13] One hour after administration of thallium, it can be found in the urine and feces.[11] A three-compartment model has been described by de Groot and colleagues,[10] who proposed that in the first 4 hours, thallium is distributed over a central or fast exchange compartment, consisting of well-perfused organs, such as the kidney, liver, and muscle. During a second phase (4 to 24 hours), thallium is distributed to a slow exchange compartment consisting of the brain, causing thallium's neurotoxicity. A third compartment exists, consisting of the intestine, where there is extensive enteroenteral cycling between absorption and secretion.[14] After 24 hours, distribution is complete, and first-order elimination begins.[15] In animal experiments, thallium is secreted in all parts of the intestine. Approximately two thirds is excreted in the feces and one third in the urine.[11] The half-life for thallium in humans is estimated at 1.9 days, but it has been reported to be 15 days[16] depending on the amount of ingestion and individual variability.[10,15,17]

PATHOPHYSIOLOGY

The pathophysiology of thallium toxicity is not fully understood. Thallium behaves similarly to potassium physiologically and has chemical characteristics similar to those of that ion. Thallium is similar in size to potassium (ionic radii 1.44 Å for thallium and 1.33 Å for potassium) but has 10 times potassium's affinity for the Na^+, K^+-ATPase transporter.[7,18] Because potassium is distributed mainly intracellularly, it is not surprising that thallium is found in the intracellular compartment, explaining its volume of distribution. Thallium's ability to substitute for potassium has been used to advantage as an isotope in nuclear imaging of the heart.

Thallium, similar to other heavy metals, has an affinity for sulfhydryl groups and interferes with the function of sulfhydryl-containing enzymes.[7,18] It has been postulated that the alopecia and Mees' lines seen in thallium poisoning are due to thallium's binding to the sulfhydryl group on cysteine moieties.[7,19] Thallium combines with riboflavin and decreases the bioavailability of this vitamin; this decreases activity of flavin adenine dinucleotide–dependent processes because riboflavin is a vitamin precursor for flavin adenine dinucleotide.[7,20] Patients with thallium poisoning and riboflavin deficiency have similar presentations (i.e., peripheral neuropathy, alopecia, cheilosis).

CLINICAL PRESENTATION

Because thallium is distributed widely throughout the body, the signs and symptoms of its toxicity can be varied. The manifestations of thallium toxicity depend on dose, patient age, and time of presentation after ingestion. The classic triad of thallium toxicity is as follows:

Acute gastroenteritis
Polyneuropathy
Alopecia

Alopecia is considered the hallmark of thallium poisoning. After ingestion, there is a time course of the evolution of these signs and symptoms that can be classified as *early*, *intermediate*, *late*, and *chronic* manifestations (Table 82-1). There may be considerable overlap, however, in the timing and appearance of these effects.

In the early phase (within hours), gastrointestinal disturbances, such as nausea, vomiting, abdominal pain, hemorrhagic gastroenteritis, constipation, and diarrhea, predominate.[2,12,13]

In the intermediate phase (hours to weeks), cardiac and neurologic manifestations are most apparent. Cardiac signs, such as sinus tachycardia, hypertension, and chest pain,[2,13] are the most common, although bradycardia, ventricular arrhythmias, and atrial fibrillation, in the absence of structural heart disease, have been described.[21] The cause of thallium's effects on the heart is probably multifactorial; some authors hypothesize a component of vagal nerve involvement.[1,21]

Neurologic manifestations also are apparent in the intermediate phase. The initial neurologic symptoms are painful paresthesias, especially in the limbs. The pain in the feet and soles is often intense and can be accompanied by numbness in the fingers and toes, with loss of sensation. Motor weakness typically is more pronounced in the distal muscle distribution, with lower limbs affected more than the upper limbs.[22] Muscle wasting becomes noticeable weeks after ingestion of thallium. Reflexes are preserved in the early course of poisoning, enabling one to distinguish thallium poisoning from Gullain-Barre syndrome.[22] Plantar reflexes also usually are flexor. All of the cranial nerves can be involved, with the exception of cranial nerves I and VIII.[22] Ptosis, secondary to cranial nerve III dysfunction, is the most common cranial nerve finding and can be asymmetric. Cranial nerves IV and VI, leading to nystagmus, and cranial nerve VII also commonly are involved. Autonomic dysfunction has been reported, but clear clinical evidence of this is lacking.[22,23] The initial paresthesias can progress to severe peripheral neuropathy with weakness and atrophy of the musculature that can progress to death from respiratory failure. Many clinical findings point to involvement of the central nervous system. Ataxia, tremor, and change in mental state (i.e., psychosis, dementia) are common with extreme cases of poisoning, leading to convulsions and coma. Pathologic examination of the peripheral nervous system has revealed primary axonal damage with secondary loss of myelin.[22,24–26] In addition to cardiac and neurologic findings, proteinuria can occur. Studies in rats have revealed the damage to be localized to the thick ascending loop of Henle in the medulla. Renal damage is reversible by the 10th day after ingestion.[18]

In the late phase (2 to 4 weeks) of thallium poisoning, dermatologic manifestations predominate, with acne-like features being the first cutaneous sign. Sudden alopecia is the outstanding feature of thallium intoxication, however. The alopecia almost uniformly involves the scalp but also can include the axillae, pubic area, and lateral part of the eyebrows. If the patient survives, the alopecia usually resolves. Sweat and sebaceous glands are destroyed, and acne may be severe. Growth of fingernails is impaired, and Mees' lines develop.[19,27] Other dermatologic signs that have been described include eczema, anhidrosis, painful glossitis, stomatitis, and malar rash. The malar rash has been confused with systemic lupus erythematosus.[19,28]

Chronic thallium toxicity (>4 weeks) includes ophthalmologic features and residual neurologic deficits. Ophthalmoplegia, noninflammatory keratitis, lens opacities, optic atrophy, and optic neuropathy have been described. Functional changes due to optic nerve damage include abnormal color vision, impaired visual acuity, and central scotomas.[29] Mental abnormalities, dementia, memory loss, and muscle atrophy are some of the persisting neurologic impairments.[2,22,30,31]

TABLE 82-1 Time Course of Thallium Toxicity

Early Phase (within hours)
Gastrointestinal
  Nausea
  Vomiting
  Abdominal pain
  Gastroenteritis
  Diarrhea
  Constipation

Intermediate Phase (hours to weeks)
Cardiac
  Sinus tachycardia
  Hypertension
  Chest pain
Neurologic
  Painful paresthesias
  Distal motor weakness
  Ptosis
  Ataxia
  Mental status change
Renal
  Reversible proteinuria

Late Phase (2–4 weeks)
Dermatologic
  Alopecia
  Acne
  Mees' lines

Chronic Toxicity (>4 weeks)
Neurologic
  Memory loss
  Dementia
  Muscle atrophy
Ophthalmologic
  Ophthalmoplegia
  Optic neuropathy

DIAGNOSIS

Thallium toxicity should be considered in patients who present with gastrointestinal complaints, ascending polyneuropathy, and alopecia. Alopecia is a late finding, however (see Table 82-1).

The definitive diagnosis of thallium poisoning is made by measurement of thallium via atomic absorption assay of bodily fluids, typically in a 24-hour urine specimen.[13] Other clinical laboratory tests, electrocardiogram, and radiographic studies are not useful because findings are nonspecific and typically normal even in cases of large ingestions of thallium. Microscopic examination of hair roots by polarized light show distinctive tapered, distorted black anagen roots, but the specificity of this is poor.[19] The key to diagnosis is to have an index of suspicion for thallium toxicity. Because thallium toxicity is life-threatening, one should have a low threshold to obtain a urinary thallium measurement if any suspicion exists. The differential diagnosis should include Guillain-Barré syndrome, systemic lupus erythematosus, botulism, poisoning by other heavy metals (arsenic, lead, selenium), other toxic exposures (chronic alcoholism, organophosphates), thiamine or riboflavin deficiency, and, rarely, porphyria.

Common Error in the Diagnosis of Thallium Poisoning

Not considering thallium poisoning in patients who present with gastrointestinal symptoms, peripheral neuropathy, and alopecia

TREATMENT

Many therapeutic modalities have been tried to enhance the excretion of thallium via its two major routes of elimination—feces and urine. Many agents, such as British antilewisite, ethylenediaminetetraacetic acid, penicillamine, sodium iodide, sodium thiosulfate, and *N*-acetyl cysteine, have been tried in the past, but their use was limited due to low efficacy or unacceptable side effects. The data on various therapies rely almost exclusively on case reports. To our knowledge, no prospective or controlled study in humans has been performed.

Fecal Elimination

Many treatments focused on enhancement of fecal elimination of thallium have been tried. Lund[11] found that acti-

Indications for ICU Admission in Thallium Toxicity

Depressed neurologic respiratory status
Signs of cardiotoxicity

vated charcoal use in rats increased fecal elimination of thallium by 82%. Multiple-dose activated charcoal also enhanced fecal excretion of thallium in vitro[32] and in humans.[4] Activated charcoal acts as an adsorbent material for thallium and increases fecal elimination. Sodium polystyrene sulfonate also has been reported to increase fecal excretion in some studies. Holooggitas and colleagues[15] reported that sodium polystyrene sulfonate is of no benefit. Hoffman and colleagues[32] found that sodium polystyrene sulfonate strongly bound thallium in vitro, provided that no physiologic amount of potassium was present. Given the ubiquitous presence of potassium in biologic fluids, sodium polystyrene sulfonate does not seem to be promising. Based on the worldwide availability of activated charcoal and its limited side effects, we recommend a multiple-dose regimen.

The most reported method of enhancement of fecal elimination of thallium has been the use of Prussian blue (PB). PB is a crystal lattice of potassium ferric-cyanoferrate (II), which is not absorbed in the gut and which acts as an ion exchanger for univalent metal ions.[33,34] Thallium exchanges for potassium and attaches at the surface of the crystal lattice of PB. By binding to PB, thallium in the gut is not reabsorbed, interrupting enterohepatic cycling.[35] Heydlauf[33] first studied the effects of PB in 1969 in rats and found markedly increased fecal elimination and decreased body burden of thallium. This finding was corroborated by further studies in animals.[26,37,38] Meggs and colleagues,[39] Rios and Monroy-Noyola,[38] and Kravzov and coworkers[34] found decreased mortality in thallium-poisoned rats with administration of PB. Kamerbeek and associates[35] reported increased excretion of thallium when PB was given to humans. Subsequently, many case reports in humans reported apparent benefit of PB and increased fecal excretion.[40–44] In the series by Stevens and colleagues[43] of 11 cases, reporting treatment with PB, 250 mg/kg/24 hr in 50 mL of 15% mannitol as a laxative, variable amounts of thallium were recovered in the feces with no side effects noted. Fecal elimination largely exceeded urinary elimination. PB has no known side effects, and the numerous case reports cited support its use. Animal data show a decrease in mortality with the use of PB.[39] PB should be used in any case of serious thallium ingestion. Kamerbeek and coworkers[35] found a greater absorptive capacity of PB for thallium versus charcoal. In vitro studies found, however, that charcoal and PB adsorption of thallium are similar.[32,45]

Enhancement of Urinary Elimination

Chelating agents have been used in an attempt to enhance urinary excretion of thallium. Two chelating agents of note are diethyldithiocarbamate (dithiocarb) and diphenylthiocarbazone (dithizone). Dithiocarb initially was used in rats with increased excretion of thallium[46] and later was used with reported success in humans.[47,3] Enthusiasm for dithiocarb has waned because of potentially dangerous redistribution of thallium into the brain, with worsening of neurologic effects.[31,48] Dithizone increases urine excretion of thallium in rats[46,49] and humans.[50,51] Its use was abandoned, however, when concerns arose over its diabetogenic and goitrogenic properties.[49,50] Although these two agents can be used to increase thallium's urinary clearance, they should not be used in thallium poisoning.

The use of potassium chloride to enhance urine excretion of thallium has been attempted. That potassium chloride enhances thallium excretion has been shown by Lund[11,49] in rats and by Papp and associates[17] in humans. Lund[11,49] initially found potassium chloride to be useful in rats, and subsequently Papp and associates[17] found it useful in humans because it enhanced urinary clearance of thallium. Meggs and colleagues[52] and Koshy and Lovejoy[16] found, however, that potassium causes worsening of mental status in thallium-poisoned humans and animals. Given the concerning results of potassium and worsening of mental status, its use, beyond simple correction of hypokalemia, is not advocated.

Forced diuresis has been used with reported success in humans and animals.[40,53–56] It is safe and has been reported to eliminate 30% of thallium ingested, although this is probably a high estimate. Diuresis probably is most effective in the acute situation before redistribution occurs. Many of the case reports supporting forced diuresis used other treatment modalities as well, however. No human data exist strongly validating forced diuresis. It is a safe and potentially effective technique in the treatment of thallium toxicity, however, and diuresis is our recommendation.

Hemodialysis and hemoperfusion have been used with varying results. Pedersen and coworkers[56] found 143 mg of thallium was eliminated during the first 120 hours of hemodialysis after 1.6 g of thallium had been ingested. De Backer and coworkers[57] found that after 100 mg of ingested thallium, hemodialysis removed 1.2 mg, whereas hemoperfusion with a charcoal column eliminated 12 mg. These investigators concluded that hemoperfusion was superior to hemodialysis. De Groot and associates[10,58] found a 10-fold increase in thallium elimination with hemoperfusion and hemodialysis combined (12 to 25 mg/hr) versus renal excretion alone. It also has been suggested that hemoperfusion with charcoal is more efficacious at lower blood thallium concentrations.[58] Wainwright and colleagues[31] reported that hemodialysis and hemoperfusion were valuable in the early stages of thallium poisoning because the amount extracted was proportional to the serum concentration. Hemofiltration was found to be ineffective. Malbrain and associates[41] found hemodialysis to be effective when started early, with some rebound in thallium in serum after each hemodialysis session was finished. Paulson and colleagues[51] did not recommend hemodialysis, however, because only 13 mg of thallium was removed after 8 hours, and this value was not increased compared with dithizone, potassium chloride, and British antilewisite. Peritoneal dialysis also has been tried but without success.[16]

The data on extracorporeal elimination techniques are conflicting. Hemodialysis and hemoperfusion seem to be effective, however, in enhancing the clearance of thallium in cases of large ingestions, when used for a prolonged time, and when used in the early stages (within 48 hours). Extracorporeal techniques have side effects, are invasive, and are advocated only if a patient is in renal failure or has ingested large amounts of thallium. Extracorporeal techniques are most effective when initiated immediately after ingestion.

Criteria for ICU Discharge in Thallium Toxicity

Particular attention should be paid to stability of the following systems:

Central nervous
Cardiovascular
Respiratory

SPECIAL POPULATIONS

Pregnant Patients

Thallium has been shown to be teratogenic in animals,[59,60] but most evidence suggests that it has little mutagenic or carcinogenic potential.[61] It crosses the placenta; however, in cases in which the mother has severe thallium toxicity, some infants have been born grossly normal or with limited manifestations of thallium toxicity.[61–63] Thallium toxicity has been reported to cause premature birth and low birth weight. These data are limited, however, because there are too few cases reported to make any conclusions confidently.[61] PB is listed as a pregnancy category C drug by the FDA and is recommended for use in pregnant patients with thallium toxicity.

Women with thallium toxicity should not breastfeed until further consultation with a medical toxicologist is obtained because thallium can enter into breast milk.

CONCLUSION

Diagnosis is made on clinical grounds and urinary level of thallium. If patients present within hours of ingestion, forced diuresis should be initiated immediately. Multiple-dose activated charcoal at 0.5 g/kg twice a day and PB (if available) at 250 mg/kg/day in 15% mannitol for two or four divided doses should be started. In general, the dose of PB is 3 g orally three times a day for adolescents and adults, and 1 g orally three times a day for children (ages 2 through 12). If the patient presents early (within 24 to 48 hours) and has ingested a large amount of thallium, hemodialysis and hemoperfusion can be considered. If the patient is in renal failure, extracorporeal techniques should be initiated. PB should be used in all cases of thallium ingestion, but lack of Food and Drug Administration approval and limited availability in the United States make activated charcoal a much more feasible choice. All patients should be admitted to the intensive care unit for monitoring because the clinical course is variable and thallium toxicity is life-threatening.

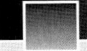

Key Points in Thallium Toxicity

1. The diagnosis of thallium toxicity is made on clinical grounds and urine thallium determinations.
2. The three hallmarks of thallium poisoning are gastrointestinal symptoms, peripheral neuropathy, and alopecia.
3. Therapy consists of Prussian blue, activated charcoal, diuresis, and extracorporeal thallium removal.

REFERENCES

1. Prick JJG: Thallium poisoning. In Vinkrn PJ, Bruyn GW (eds): Intoxication of the Nervous System: Handbook of Clinical Neurology. vol 36. New York, North-Holland, 1979, pp 239–278.
2. Reed D, Crawley J, Faro SN, et al: Thallotoxicosis. JAMA 183:516–522, 1963.
3. Insley BM, Grufferman S, Ayliffe E: Thallium poisoning in cocaine abusers. Am J Emerg Med 4:545–548, 1986.
4. Meggs WJ, Hoffman RS, Shih RD, et al: Thallium poisoning from maliciously contaminated food. Clin Toxicol 32:723–730, 1994.
5. Schaumberg: Alopecia and Chinese herbal medication. JAMA 268:2430–2431, 1992.
6. Munch J, Ginsberg H, Nixon C: Thallotoxicosis outbreak in California. JAMA 100:1315, 1933.
7. Saddique A: Thallium poisoning: A review. Vet Hum Toxicol 25:16–22, 1983.
8. Sullivan JB: Thallium. In Sullivan JB, Krieger GR (eds): Clinical Environmental Health and Toxic Exposures, 2nd ed. Philadelphia, Lippincott Williams & Wilkins, 2001, pp 954–958.
9. Anonymous. Thallium poisoning in Guyana—a national crisis. Lancet 1:604, 1987.
10. de Groot G, van Leusen R, van Heijst ANP: Thallium concentrations in body fluids and tissues in a fatal case of thallium poisoning. Vet Hum Toxicol 27:115–119, 1985.
11. Lund A: Distribution of thallium in the organism and its elimination. Acta Pharmacol Toxicol 12:251–259, 1954.
12. Grunfeld O, Hinostroza G: Thallium poisoning. Arch Intern Med 114:132–138, 1964.
13. Moeschlin S: Thallium poisoning. Clin Toxicol 17:133–145, 1980.
14. Rauws AG. Thallium pharmacokinetics and its modification by Prussian blue. Arch Pharmacol 284:295–306, 1974.
15. Holooggitas J, Ullucci P, Driscoll J: Thallium elimination kinetics in acute thallotoxicosis. J Analyt Toxicol 4:68–73, 1980.
16. Koshy KM, Lovejoy FH: Thallium ingestion with survival: Ineffectiveness of peritoneal dialysis and potassium chloride diuresis. Clin Toxicol 18:521–525, 1981.
17. Papp JP, Gay PC, Dodson VN, Pollard HM: Potassium chloride treatment in thallotoxicosis. Ann Intern Med 71:119–123, 1969.
18. Appenroth D, Gambaryan S, Winnefeld K, et al: Functional and morphological aspects of thallium-induced nephrotoxicity in rats. Toxicology 96:203–215, 1995.
19. Tromme I, Van Neste D, Dobbelaere F, et al: Skin signs in the diagnosis of thallium poisoning. Br J Dermatol 138:321–325, 1998.
20. Cavanagh JB: What have we learned from Graham Frederick Young? Reflections on the mechanism of thallium neurotoxicity. Neuropathol Appl Neurobiol 17:3–9, 1991.
21. Roby DS, Fein AM, Bennett RH, et al: Cardiopulmonary effect of acute thallium poisoning. Chest 85:236–240, 1984.
22. Cavanagh JB, Fuller NH, Johnson HRM, Rudge P: The effects of thallium salts, with particular reference to the nervous system changes. QJM 170:293–319, 1974.
23. Norfentoft T, Andersen EB, Mogensen PH: Initial sensorimotor and delayed autonomic neuropathy in acute thallium poisoning. Neurotoxicology 19:421–426, 1998.
24. Davis LE, Standefer JC, Kornfeld M, et al: Acute thallium poisoning: Toxicological and morphological studies of the nervous system. Ann Neurol 10:38–44, 1981.
25. Dumitru D, Kalantri A: Electrophysiologic investigation of thallium poisoning. Muscle Nerve 13:433–437, 1990.
26. Yokoyama K, Araki S, Abe H: Distribution of nerve conduction velocities in acute thallium poisoning. Muscle Nerve 13:117–120, 1990.
27. Heyl T, Barlow RJ: Thallium poisoning: A dermatological perspective. Br J Dermatol 121:787–792, 1989.
28. Alarcon-Segovia D, Amigo M, Reyes PA: Connective tissue disease features after thallium poisoning. J Rheumatol 16:171–174, 1989.
29. Tabandeh H, Crowston JG, Thompson GM: Ophthalmologic features of thallium poisoning. Am J Ophthalmol 117:243–245, 1994.
30. Gefel A, Liron M, Hirsch W: Chronic thallium poisoning. Israel J Med Sci 6:380–382, 1970.
31. Wainwright AP, Kox WJ, House IM, et al: Clinical features and therapy of acute thallium poisoning. QJM 258:939–944, 1988.
32. Hoffman RS, Stringer JA, Feinberg RS, et al: Comparative efficacy of thallium adsorption by activated charcoal, Prussian blue, and sodium polystrene sulfonate. Clin Toxicol 37:833–837, 1999.
33. Heydlauf H: Ferric-cyanoferrate (II): An effective antidote in thallium poisoning. Eur J Pharmacol 6:340–344, 1969.
34. Kravzov J, Rios C, Altagracia M, et al: Relationship between physio-chemical properties of Prussian blue and its efficacyas antidote against thallium poisoning. J Appl Toxicol 13:213–216, 1993.
35. Kamerbeek HH, Rauws AG, Ham M, Van Heijst ANP: Prussian blue in therapy of thallotoxicosis. Acta Med Scand 189:321–324, 1971.
36. Barroso-Moguel R, Villeda-Hernandez J, Mendez-Armenta M, et al: Combined D-penicillamine and Prussian blue as antidotal treatment against thallotoxicosis in rats: Evaluation of cerebellar lesions. Toxicology 89:15–24, 1994.
37. Mulkey JP, Oehme FW: Are 2,3-dimercapto-1-propanesulfonic acid or Prussian blue beneficial in acute thallotoxicosis in rats? Vet Hum Toxicol 42:325–329, 2000.
38. Rios C, Monroy-Noyola A: D-penicillamine and Prussian blue as antidotes against thallium intoxication in rats. Toxicology 74:69–76, 1992.
39. Meggs WJ, Cahill-Morasco R, Shih RD, et al: Effects of Prussian blue and N-acetylcysteine on thallium toxicity in mice. Clin Toxicol 35:163–166, 1997.
40. Ghezzi R, Marrubini B: Prussian blue in the treatment of thallium intoxication. Vet Hum Toxicol 21(Suppl):64–66, 1979.
41. Malbrain MLNG, Lambrecht GLY, Zandijk E, et al: Treatment of severe thallium intoxication. Clin Toxicol 35:97–100, 1997.
42. Pai V: Acute thallium poisoning: Prussian blue therapy in 9 cases. West Ind Med J 36:256–258, 1987.
43. Stevens W, van Peteghem C, Heyndrickx A, Barbier F: Eleven cases of thallium intoxication treated with Prussian blue. Int J Clin Pharmacol 10:1–22, 1974.
44. Van Der Merwe CF: The treatment of thallium poisoning. S Afr Med J 46:960–961, 1972.
45. Lehmann PA, Favari L: Parameters for the adsorption of thallium ions by activated charcoal and Prussian blue. Clin Toxicol 22:331–339, 1984.
46. Schwetz BA, O'Neil PV, Voelker FA, Jacobs DW: Effects of diphenylthiocarbazone and diethyldithiocarbamate on the excretion of thallium by rats. Toxicol Appl Pharmacol 10:79–88, 1967.
47. Sunderman FW: Diethyldithiocarbamate therapy of thallotoxicosis. Am J Med Sci 109:107–118, 1967.
48. Kamerbeek HH, Rauws AG, Ham M, Van Heijst ANP: Dangerous redistribution of thallium by treatment with sodium diethyldithiocarbamate. Acta Med Scand 189:149–154, 1971.
49. Lund A: The effect of various substances on the excretion and the toxicity of thallium in the rat. Acta Pharmacol Toxicol 12:260–268, 1956.
50. Bendl BJ: Thallium poisoning. Arch Dermatol 100:443–446, 1969.
51. Paulson G, Vergara G, Young J, Bird M: Thallium intoxication treated with dithizone and hemodialysis. Arch Intern Med 129:100–103, 1972.
52. Meggs WJ, Goldfrank LR, Hoffman RS: Effects of potassium in a murine model of thallium poisoning (Abstract). J Toxicol Clin Toxicol 33:558, 1995.
53. de Groot G, Van Heijst ANP: Toxicokinetic aspects of thallium poisoning: Methods of treatment by toxin elimination. Sci Total Environ 71:411–418, 1988.
54. Heath A, Ahlmen J, Branegard B, et al: Thallium poisoning: Toxin elimination and therapy in three cases. J Toxicol Clin Toxicol 20:451–463, 1983.
55. Nogue S, Mas A, Pares A, et al: Acute thallium poisoning: An evaluation of different forms of treatment. J Toxicol Clin Toxicol 19:1015–1021, 1982.
56. Pedersen RS, Olesen AS, Freund LG, et al: Thallium intoxication treated with long-term hemdialysis, forced diuresis, and Prussian blue. Acta Med Scand 204:429–432, 1978.
57. de Backer W, Zachee P, Verpooten GA, et al: Thallium intoxication treated with combined hemoperfusion-hemodialysis. J Toxicol Clin Toxicol 19:259–264, 1982.
58. de Groot G, van Heijst ANP, Kesteren RG, et al: An evaluation of the efficacy of charcoal haemoperfusion in the treatment of three cases of acute thallium poisoning. Arch Toxicol 57:61–66, 1985.
59. Gibson JE, Becker BA: Placental transfer, embryotoxicity, and teratogenicity of thallium sulfate in normal and potassium-deficient rats. Toxicol Appl Pharmacol 16:120–132, 1970.
60. Hall BK: Critical periods during development as assessed by thallium-induced inhibition of growth of embryonic chick tibiae in vitro. Teratology 31:353–361, 1985.
61. Hoffman RS: Thallium poisoning during pregnancy: A case report and comprehensive literature review. Clin Toxicol 38:767–775, 2000.
62. English JC: A case of thallium poisoning complicating pregnancy. Med J Aust 1:780–782, 1954.
63. Johnson W: A case of thallium poisoning during pregnancy. Med J Aust 47:540–542, 1960.

CHAPTER **83**

Ethylene Glycol and Other Glycols

Dag Jacobsen

ETHYLENE GLYCOL

Ethylene glycol is a colorless, almost nonvolatile liquid with an aromatic odor that is recognizable on the breath of some victims. It is used widely as antifreeze in internal combustion engines, and it is used as a solvent in various manufacturing processes.

There are many similarities between the pathophysiologies of ethylene glycol and methanol poisoning (see Chapter 86). Although few comparable epidemiologic data exist, ethylene glycol poisoning seems to be more frequent than methanol intoxication. Besides being the "poor man's" substitute for ethanol, ethylene glycol also has been used as a suicidal agent.

Clinical Pharmacology

Ethylene glycol is absorbed rapidly and probably completely after oral administration. The volume of distribution of ethylene glycol is approximately 0.7 L/kg based on studies in two male patients,[1] although values of 0.54 L/kg[2] and 0.83 L/kg[3] also have been reported in men.

The elimination kinetics of ethylene glycol has not been clarified completely. There is evidence for a saturable elimination with linear (first-order) elimination for low-to-moderate plasma concentrations (<40 mmol/L [<250 mg/dL]) with a half-life of 6 hours.[2] For higher plasma concentrations, the elimination seems to approach nonlinear (zero-order) kinetics.

In one male patient, the volume of distribution of glycolate, the major circulating ethylene glycol metabolite, was calculated to be 0.6 L/kg, with an estimated intrinsic half-life of 6 hours over the concentration range studied.[2] In four

---

Pharmacokinetics of Ethylene Glycol

Volume of distribution: 0.7 L/kg
Protein binding: none
Mechanisms of clearance: hepatic and renal
Active metabolites: glycolic acid and oxalic acid far more toxic than the mother compound
Methods to enhance clearance: hemodialysis

---

other patients, ethylene glycol elimination was slower, with a mean endogenous half-life of 10 hours and a mean elimination rate of 1.1 mmol/L/hr, whereas its metabolism was inhibited by fomepizole.[4]

Pathophysiology

The lethal dose of ethylene glycol in untreated patients is not well established, but 100 mL is the most frequently cited approximation. A value of 1 to 2 mL/kg seems reasonable.[5]

The primary enzyme in ethylene glycol metabolism is alcohol dehydrogenase (ADH) (Fig. 83-1). Similar to methanol, the toxicity of ethylene glycol is mediated through its metabolites. In contrast to methanol, ethylene glycol causes central nervous system (CNS) depression and inebriation in a manner similar to ethanol.

The mechanisms for the toxicity of ethylene glycol are not resolved completely. It was originally postulated that the formation of oxalate (see Fig. 83-1) was the main reason for ethylene glycol toxicity. This explanation was probably based on the visualization of oxalate-like crystals in the urine and the development of acute renal failure. Later, it was suggested that the aldehydes formed—mainly glycolaldehyde—were responsible for the toxic syndrome. It has been shown experimentally that these aldehydes were able to inhibit oxidative phosphorylation, glucose metabolism, protein synthesis, DNA replication, and RNA synthesis; these aldehydes may also be able to oxidize intracellular sulfhydryl groups.[6]

The mechanism for the renal toxicity of ethylene glycol is unresolved. Some human case studies[7] and controlled studies in animals[8] have shown tubular necrosis without the appearance of crystals. Two reports in humans—a controlled trial of ethylene glycol treatment with fomepizole[9] and an extensive case series[10]—found a strong correlation between increased plasma glycolate levels and the presence or development of acute renal failure. These results suggest that metabolites other than oxalate may play a significant role in the renal toxicity. Initial studies of the cellular toxicity of oxalate, glycolate, and glyoxylate in normal human proximal tubule cells showed, however, that the oxalate ion per se induced renal cell death at relevant concentrations,[11] whereas neither glyoxylate nor glycolate had an effect on cellular viability. Studies in

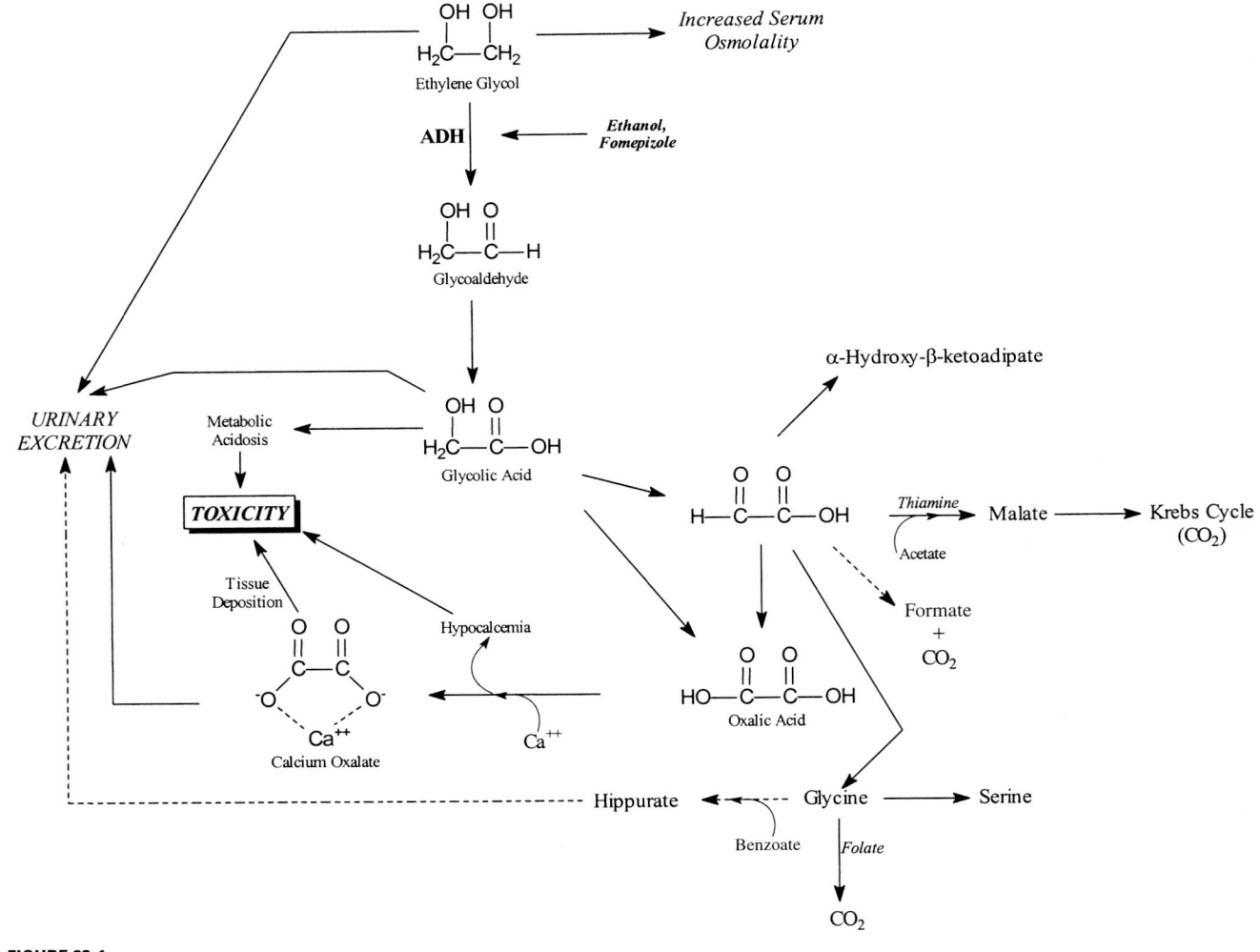

FIGURE 83-1

The complex metabolism of ethylene glycol. Solid arrows represent major routes or pathways. Dotted arrows are theoretical or less important routes. Direct renal excretion of ethylene glycol is a major pathway of elimination, provided that normal renal function is present. ADH, alcohol dehydrogenase.

transformed cell lines in culture also indicated that oxalate can induce cytotoxicity and may be the responsible agent for the tubular necrosis.[12,13]

As judged from experimental studies, there may be no major differences in the way rodents and humans handle ethylene glycol. This idea is based on the fact that both species become acidotic after exposure. The relative toxicities of the ethylene glycol metabolites (glyoxylate > glycolaldehyde > glycolate) established in rodents also may have some validity in humans.[14] In experimental studies with ethylene glycol–intoxicated rats, dogs, and monkeys, neither circulating glycolaldehyde nor glyoxylate was detected using gas chromatography–mass spectrometry techniques.[14–16] In addition, in six patients poisoned with ethylene glycol, plasma glyoxylate levels were less than 1.2 mg/dL (<0.2 mmol/L), and the glycolate concentrations ranged from 100 to 175 mg/dL (17 to 29 mmol/L).[17] Of the relevant metabolites, only glycolic acid seems to be present in the blood in amounts significant to produce the metabolic acidosis seen in ethylene glycol poisoning.

The toxicity of ethylene glycol probably is due to a combination of the severe metabolic acidosis caused by glycolic acid and the precipitation of calcium oxalate crystals resulting in impaired organ function, especially in the kidneys (see Fig. 83-1). The toxicity of the anion glycolate is probably less than that of formate, the major toxic metabolite in methanol poisoning.[5] Hypocalcemia and the resulting tetany and seizures probably are infrequent mechanisms of toxicity (see Fig. 83-1).

Clinical Presentation and Life-Threatening Complications

Many authors describe the clinical syndrome of ethylene glycol poisoning in three stages: (1) CNS depression, (2) cardiopulmonary complications, and (3) renal failure. Although there is some support for this classification, especially for the understanding of the pathophysiology, there is considerable clinical overlap between stages.

Ethylene glycol poisoning is characterized by an initial CNS depression phase associated with inebriation progressing to coma. After 4 to 12 hours, signs and symptoms resulting from the metabolites appear. The increasing accumulation of glycolic acid leads to metabolic acidosis, which may be severe, and to compensatory hyperventilation. In my clinical experience, in contrast to methanol poisoning, these patients usually are in coma when hyperventilation is pronounced, so there is no subjective feeling of dyspnea. Also in my experience, for unknown reasons, elevated blood pressure and tachycardia usually are prominent features.

For the first 12 to 18 hours postingestion, urine output generally is still adequate, and if proper treatment is started at this stage, full recovery is usually seen, although the patient may have some degree of acute kidney impairment. Another complication of calcium oxalate precipitation, such as hypocalcemia-induced tetanic contractions, also may occur. The prognosis of acute renal failure is good, although the plasma creatinine may not return to normal for months.[5,18]

Without adequate treatment, seriously poisoned patients rapidly deteriorate. In addition to CNS depression possibly associated with cerebral edema, convulsions, oliguric renal failure, and respiratory problems may develop. Pulmonary infiltrates may be observed radiologically, but these changes are thought to be noninfectious in origin. I have observed precipitated calcium oxalate crystals in the lungs of patients who have died from ethylene glycol poisoning. Given this observation, one could postulate that these changes may be an inflammatory reaction related to this precipitation. Although "cardiogenic pulmonary edema" is claimed to occur frequently in ethylene glycol poisoning, this is not frequent in my experience. Although the cardiac ejection fraction may be lowered (to about 40% in severely poisoned patients), this is not the major cause of the pulmonary infiltrations seen in these cases. The pulmonary capillary wedge pressure often is normal in this situation; as such, the diagnostic criteria for adult respiratory distress syndrome are fulfilled. The concomitant ingestion of ethanol may inhibit the metabolism of ethylene glycol to its toxic metabolites and may prolong the initial CNS phase of inebriation and delay the onset of the other clinical features of toxicity.

Patients admitted in extremis may survive the first days, provided that adequate treatment is given. These patients should undergo computed tomography or magnetic resonance imaging of the head to evaluate the degree of brain damage. Some of these patients develop (large) cerebral infarcts or cerebral edema resulting in brain death.[1,5] There are a few reports of ocular manifestations and methemoglobinemia associated with ethylene glycol poisoning.[19,20] No analytic investigations were performed, however, to rule out methanol contamination of the liquid ingested. I have seen one ethylene glycol–intoxicated patient with visual dyspraxia as a result of cerebral infarcts.[1] No objective ocular complications were observed.

Diagnosis

Ethylene glycol in biologic fluids can be determined easily by gas chromatography.[21] A method for simultaneous deter-

mination of ethylene glycol and glycolate has been developed more recently.[10]

If specific analysis is not available, the use of the anion and osmolal gaps may suggest the diagnosis (see Chapter 86).[18,22,23] An ethylene glycol concentration of 100 mg/dL (16 mmol/L) increases the osmolal gap by 16/0.93, or 17 mOsm/kg H_2O. Osmometry uses osmolality, which is expressed as milliosmoles per kilogram of water. Osmolarity is expressed as milliosmoles per liter. Because serum consists of 93% water, one has to divide by 0.93. Theoretically the sensitivity of the osmolal gap should be low at ethylene glycol concentrations less than 0.5 g/L (8 mmol/L), but in my experience, for unknown reasons, the osmolal gap tends to be higher than expected from molar contribution of ethylene glycol at such low levels. One possibility is that bicarbonate replacement by glycolate may increase the dissociation coefficient of sodium chloride.

To diagnose ethylene glycol poisoning, serum osmolality must be performed by the freezing point depression method, not by the vapor pressure method. If ethanol is coingested, there may be no metabolic acidosis, or anion gap, before the ethanol is metabolized. The details of the calculation of the osmolal gap are given in Chapter 29. In such circumstances, calculation of the osmolal and anion gaps must be repeated periodically. In late stages of ethylene glycol poisoning, most of the glycol is metabolized to glycolic acid. In this situation, the anion gap may be increased considerably, but the osmolal gap may be close to normal. A small or normal osmolal gap does not eliminate the possibility of toxic alcohol ingestion.[18]

Urine microscopy may reveal envelope-shaped or needle-shaped oxalate crystals (Fig. 83-2). These findings may be delayed, and a negative microscopy should be repeated if diagnosis still is unclear. About half of patients present with crystalluria on admission, and most develop this sign later. The crystalluria may be massive and easy to detect even by an inexperienced microscopist. In addition, there usually are erythrocytes, leukocytes, and different casts in the urine sediment.[18,24]

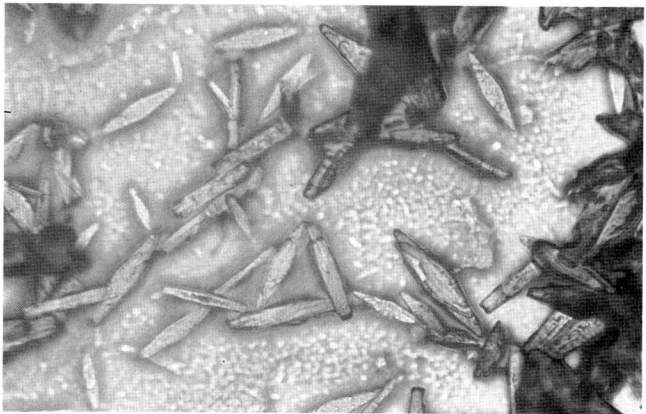

FIGURE 83-2

Typical needle-shaped calcium oxalate monohydrate crystals in the urine during ethylene glycol poisoning. Envelope-shaped calcium oxalate dehydrate crystals are less frequent but may occur in early stages of poisoning.[2]

Treatment

Treatment of ethylene glycol poisoning should follow the well-established principles of supportive care. If the patient is seen within 1 hour, gastric aspiration and lavage may be considered. Activated charcoal is of no value, unless coingestants are suspected.

METABOLIC ACIDOSIS

Although not studied in a formal clinical trial, it is generally accepted that the metabolic acidosis associated with ethylene glycol poisoning, particularly if severe, should be treated aggressively by infusion of sodium bicarbonate. In the first few hours, 600 to 800 mmol (milliequivalents) of bicarbonate may be needed, especially if antidotal therapy has not been initiated. Because ethylene glycol is metabolized faster than methanol, the acidosis develops more rapidly if an ADH inhibitor (ethanol or fomepizole) is not given, which can result in so-called bicarbonate-resistant metabolic acidosis. The rapid correction of acidosis in these patients may provoke tetanic signs, especially when hypocalcemia already is present.

INHIBITION OF ALCOHOL DEHYDROGENASE

For ethylene glycol–poisoned patients, it is critical that ethanol or fomepizole be given to inhibit the generation of toxic metabolites by ADH. The major advantage of fomepizole compared with ethanol is its documented effectiveness, lack of CNS depression, ease of administration, and ability to reduce the need for hemodialysis.[9] If fomepizole is given to a patient with ethylene glycol poisoning before renal failure develops, hemodialysis may not be necessary.[9,25] Fomepizole (molecular weight 82) is also removed by hemodialysis with a dialysance close to that of urea.[26] No drug monitoring is necessary, however, during this procedure. There is no clear evidence for when to start antidotal therapy, but I believe that in healthy patients without acidosis the treatment level should be 40 mg/dL (6.5 mmol/L). The conventional threshold for initiating ADH inhibitor therapy is 20 mg/dL (3.2 mmol/L), despite the lack of empirical data supporting this practice. In conventional acidotic patients or patients with renal impairment, 20 mg/dL (3 mmol/L) seems appropriate. If no ethylene glycol concentration is available, the degree of metabolic acidosis should be considered. ADH inhibition should be undertaken if the base deficit is greater than 10 mM. In borderline situations, one loading dose of ethanol (e.g., healthy adult with a serum ethylene glycol

concentration <40 mg/dL and base deficit <10 mM) may be better than fomepizole, which is more expensive.[27] For serious ethylene glycol poisoning, however, fomepizole is the preferred antidote.

 Dosing of Fomepizole

A loading dose of 15 mg/kg should be administered, followed by doses of 10 mg/kg every 12 hours for four doses, then 15 mg/kg every 12 hours thereafter until ethylene glycol levels have been reduced to <20 mg/dL (3 mmol/L). All doses should be given as a slow intravenous infusion over 30 minutes (dissolved in, e.g., 100 mL of isotonic saline or dextrose). During hemodialysis, the frequency of dosing should be increased to every 4 hours.

A therapeutic blood ethanol level of 100 mg/dL (22 mmol/L) may be achieved by giving a bolus dose of 0.6 g/kg (13 mmol/kg), followed by 66 to 154 mg/kg/hr (1.4 to 3.3 mmol/kg/hr) intravenously or orally, with the higher maintenance dose for heavy drinkers. Mixing 50 mL of absolute ethanol with 500 mL of isotonic glucose yields a 10% solution if a 10% ethanol solution for intravenous use is unavailable. With this solution, a bolus of 8 mL/kg (over 0.5 hour) followed by 1.5 mL/kg/hr should produce approximately the desired ethanol concentration. The maintenance infusion should be increased or decreased according to measured ethanol concentrations.

If ethanol is used as an antidote, it should be given as in methanol poisoning (see Chapter 86). The serum ethylene glycol concentration threshold for stopping antidotal therapy has been set arbitrarily at less than 20 mg/dL (<3.2 mmol/L). If an ethylene glycol concentration is not readily available, an osmolal gap less than 20 mOsm/kg H_2O may be a substitute value for stopping therapy. Although the affinity of ADH for ethylene glycol is lower than that for methanol,[28,29] this makes little practical difference in therapeutic dosing.

Several studies have indicated that ethanol can inhibit ethylene glycol elimination significantly.[2,3,27,30] An apparent half-life of ethylene glycol elimination of 14 to 17 hours during ethanol therapy has been shown in patients without renal failure[3,27]; this should be compared with a half-life of 6 hours without ethanol administration.[2] A similar half-life of 12 hours was observed by Baud and colleagues[31] using fomepizole instead of ethanol in a patient also without kidney failure; the elimination of ethylene glycol was due to its renal excretion, as also shown by others.[27] The apparent half-life of ethylene glycol during antidotal therapy depends on the diuresis and the degree of renal impairment. Although fomepizole gradually is replacing ethanol as the antidote of choice in ethylene glycol poisoning,[9,25,32] ethanol still may be used in some hospitals. Patients with CNS depression must be monitored closely if ethanol is given because this administration has been associated with respiratory arrest.[27] The American Academy of Clinical Toxicology has published practice guidelines indicating that fomepizole should be the first-line ADH

 Indications for ICU Admission in Ethylene Glycol Poisoning

There should be a low threshold for patients with pronounced metabolic acidosis >20 mM base deficit. Patients may deteriorate rapidly, and early treatment with "many nurse hands" is *essential* for outcome. Treatment is complicated (bicarbonate, antidote, seizures); patients without "normal admission criteria" also should be considered for the intensive care unit in cases of significant poisoning.

inhibitor in the treatment of serious ethylene glycol poisoning. Ethanol should be reserved for cases in which fomepizole is not available or the patient is allergic to fomepizole.[33]

HEMODIALYSIS

The dialysance of ethylene glycol has been well documented.[1,3,9] As should be expected from its higher molecular weight than that of methanol (62 d versus 32 d), ethylene glycol is less dialyzable than the latter (160 mL/min versus 130 mL/min, using a 1.6 m² dialyzer at blood flow of 200 mL/min). The dialysance of the major toxic metabolite glycolate also has been documented.[4,17] Because ethylene glycol has no significant pulmonary elimination, hemodialysis becomes the major route of its elimination if renal failure is present. Hemodialysis offers the additional possibility of correcting the metabolic and electrolyte disturbances seen in these patients.

If the patient is seen at an early stage (i.e., before severe metabolic acidosis and renal impairment have developed), hemodialysis may not be necessary, especially if fomepizole is the antidote used.[9,25,30,34] Under such circumstances, further metabolism of the glycol to its toxic metabolites is inhibited, and the glycol is excreted through the kidneys with an apparent plasma half-life of 12 to 17 hours. The onset of acute renal failure may require hemodialysis, hemodiafiltration, or peritoneal dialysis. In hypotensive patients, hemodiafiltration should be the treatment of choice for renal failure.

Although the anion glycolate may have a moderate toxicity by itself, it is a precursor for the probable nephrotoxic anion oxalate. The degree of metabolic acidosis is an important indicator of the need for dialysis.

As is evident from this discussion, it is not possible to establish strict indications for hemodialysis in ethylene glycol poisoning. This decision is difficult, and an experienced clinical toxicologist should be consulted. Hemodialysis may not be easily available in rural areas, and transport complications associated with critically ill patients must be taken into consideration, especially if ethanol is the antidote given. The introduction of fomepizole also limits the need for hemodialysis. Because hemodialysis also removes glycolate, the degree of metabolic acidosis and the renal status of the patient are more important than the serum ethylene glycol concentration. Most patients with normal renal function and moderate metabolic acidosis (base deficit <20 mM) are treated best with bicarbonate and fomepizole, even in patients with high serum ethylene glycol concentrations. The renal function of these patients must be monitored closely, however, because hemodialysis may be necessary later if oliguric or nonoliguric renal impairment develops. I have seen patients with serum ethylene glycol levels of 558 mg/dL (90 mmol/L) and moderate metabolic acidosis treated with bicarbonate and fomepizole alone.[35]

When initiated, hemodialysis generally is continued until the serum ethylene glycol concentration is less than 20 mg/dL (<3.2 mmol/L) and there are no acid-base disturbances. If blood concentrations are not available, hemodialysis should be continued for at least 8 hours and longer if the acidosis is not corrected. If ethanol is used as an anti-

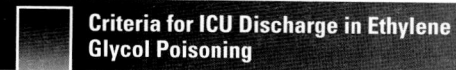

Criteria for ICU Discharge in Ethylene Glycol Poisoning

Resolution of metabolic acidosis
Hemodynamic stability
If ethanol treated, that treatment must be stopped, and the patient should be not inebriated

dote, persisting acidosis indicates that too little ethanol is being given during hemodialysis. If hemodialysis is not available, peritoneal dialysis also removes ethylene glycol,[35] although less efficiently. Hemoperfusion has no role in this poisoning.

The effectiveness of fomepizole and hemodialysis in two ethylene glycol–poisoned patients is shown in Figure 83-3. The effectiveness of fomepizole and selective hemodialysis is shown in Figure 83-4.

HYPOCALCEMIA AND SEIZURES

The hypocalcemia associated with ethylene glycol poisoning may cause tetany and seizures, which should be treated with intravenous calcium gluconate (or chloride). Calcium should not be given for hypocalcemia per se, however, because this may increase precipitation of calcium oxalate crystals in the tissues. If calcium therapy is not effective, convulsions should be treated conventionally with benzodiazepines, possibly phenytoin, or barbiturates in the most severe cases.

PYRIDOXINE AND THIAMINE

Pyridoxine and thiamine are thought to promote the alternative metabolism of glyoxylic acid to nontoxic metabolites (see Fig. 83-1). Data supporting this antidotal effect are sparse, however, and their use is not routinely recommended.

Prognosis

Outcomes are excellent for ethylene glycol–poisoned patients if they are diagnosed early and treated aggressively. If acute oliguric or nonoliguric renal failure develops, the prognosis for the renal function is always good with normalization of serum creatinine within 2 to 3 weeks (rarely months). In severe cases, patients with late diagnosis and treatment may experience cerebral infarcts.[5,18]

Special Populations

The toxicity of ethylene glycol in pediatric patients generally should be treated similar to toxicity in adults. The experience with fomepizole in children is limited, but cases have been published, and ethanol[30] and fomepizole seem to be effective antidotes in children.[36–39] Use of new drugs such as fomepizole generally is discouraged in the first trimester of pregnancy. The alternative antidote ethanol has documented ability to cause fetal harm, however. For use as an antidote for a couple of days, however, ethanol may be a more attractive antidote than fomepizole in the first trimester of pregnancy.

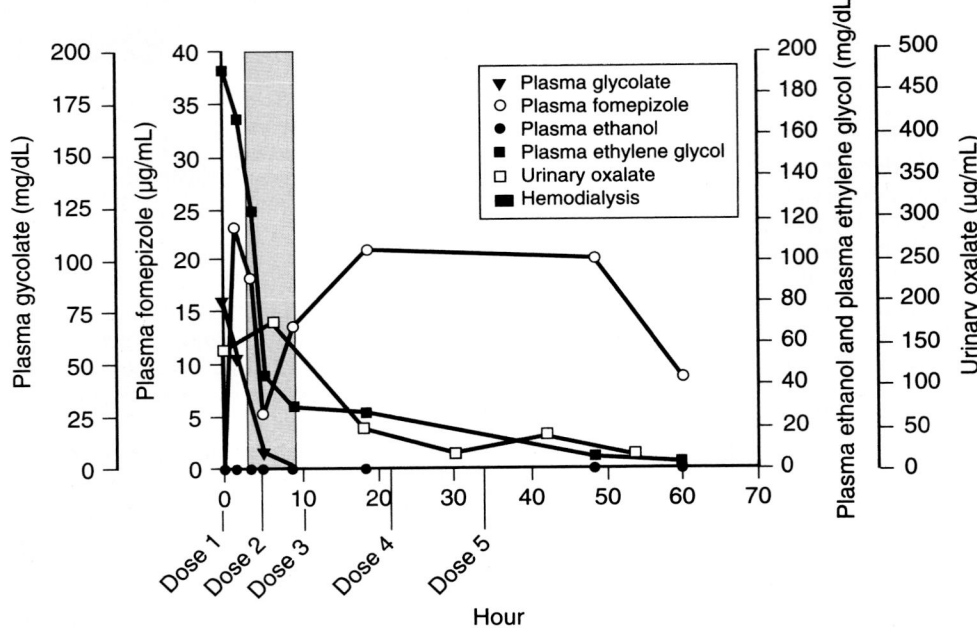

A

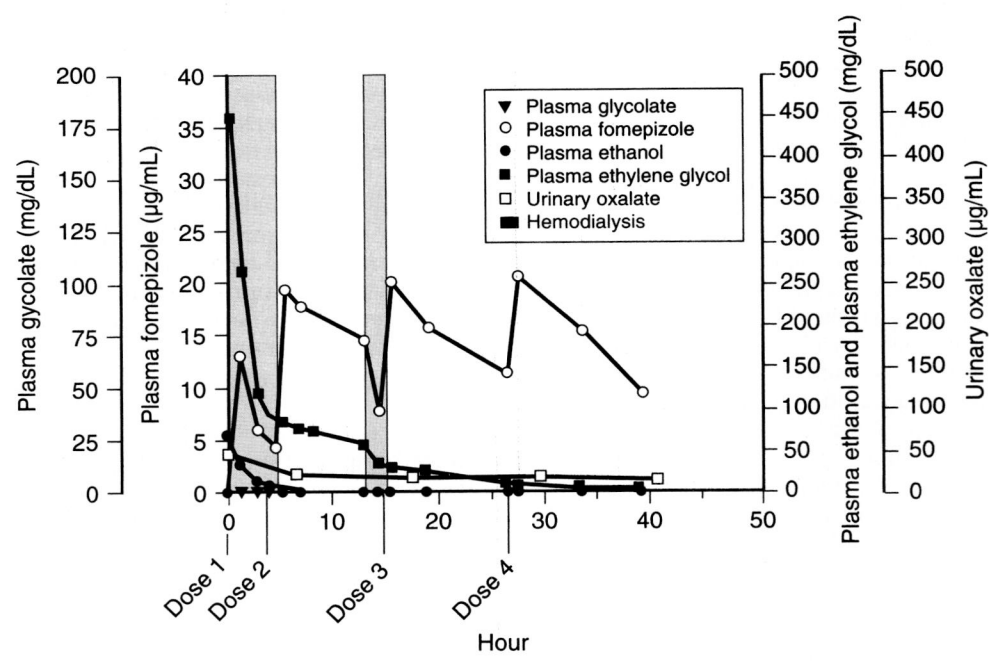

B

FIGURE 83-3

Serial plasma glycolate, fomepizole, ethanol, and ethylene glycol concentrations and urinary oxalate excretion in two patients with ethylene glycol poisoning. **A,** Values in a 73-year-old man who presented 7 hours after ingesting antifreeze in an attempt at suicide. His initial arterial pH was 7.22. He was treated with fomepizole, underwent hemodialysis for 6 hours, and recovered uneventfully. **B,** Values in a 35-year-old woman who presented 6 hours after ingesting antifreeze in an attempt at suicide. Her initial arterial pH was 7.42. She was treated with fomepizole, underwent hemodialysis twice (initially for 4 hours and subsequently for 2 hours), and recovered uneventfully. To convert the values for plasma ethylene glycol to millimoles per liter, multiply by 0.161. To convert the values for plasma glycolate to millimoles per liter, multiply by 0.132. To convert the values for serum creatinine to micromoles per liter, multiply by 88.4. To convert the values for plasma ethanol to millimoles per liter, multiply by 0.217. *(From Brent J, McMartin KE, Phillips S, et al: Fomepizole for the treatment of ethylene glycol poisoning. N Engl J Med 340:832–839, 1999.)*

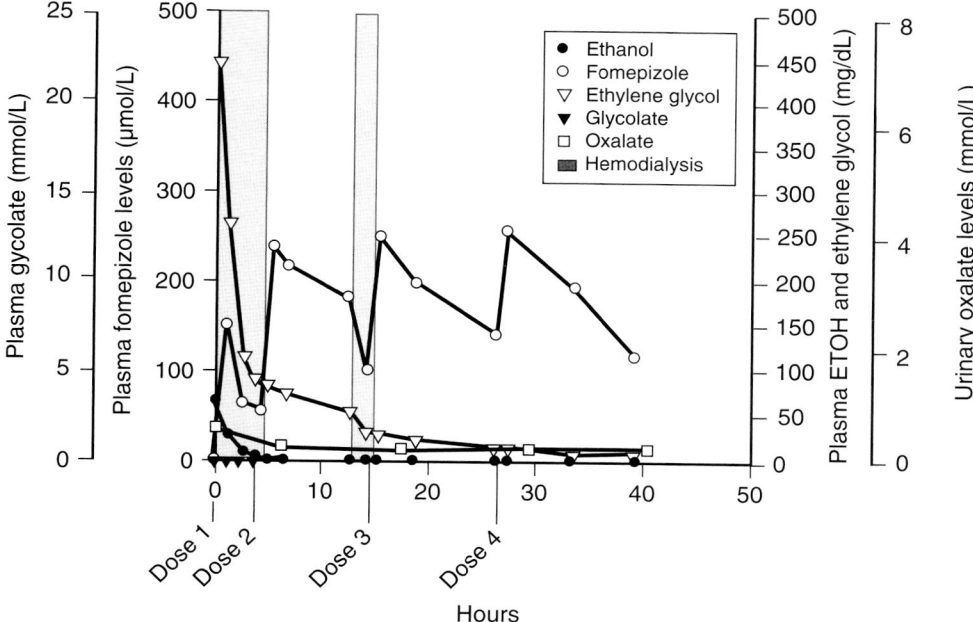

FIGURE 83-4

Clinical course of a patient with severe ethylene glycol poisoning treated with fomepizole and hemodialysis. The patient was treated as part of the multicenter clinical trial establishing the safety and efficacy of fomepizole in the treatment of ethylene glycol poisoning.[9] Although this patient was treated with adjunctive hemodialysis as per the study protocol, because she was nonacidotic, she would not be considered to require hemodialysis today, despite her high ethylene glycol level. Current clinical guidelines[33] support the nonuse of hemodialysis in patients treated with fomepizole who have high ethylene glycol levels but are nonacidotic and have normal renal function. *(From Brent J, McMartin KE, Phillips S, et al: Fomepizole for the treatment of ethylene glycol poisoning. N Engl J Med 340:832–839, 1999.)*

 Common Errors in Ethylene Glycol Poisoning

Delayed diagnosis because of failing to consider ethylene glycol poisoning in the differential diagnosis of metabolic acidosis of unknown origin

Failure to appreciate that the absence of early clinical features and the presence of normal anion or osmolal gaps do not exclude a potentially toxic ethylene glycol ingestion

Failure to give enough ethanol, if this is the antidote chosen, during hemodialysis

Failure to monitor closely blood ethanol concentrations, if this antidote is used

Failure to appreciate that prognosis may be good even in critically ill patients if correct treatment is given

Failure to stay at the bedside until bicarbonate and antidotal therapy have been initiated because time is critical in severely poisoned patients

Key Points in Ethylene Glycol Poisoning

1. Ethylene glycol toxicity is caused by its metabolites.
2. The initial step in ethylene glycol metabolism is catalysis by alcohol dehydrogenase.
3. Treatment is based on inhibition of alcohol dehydrogenase and correction of metabolic acidosis.

DIETHYLENE GLYCOL

The clinical course and the pathologic features of poisoning with diethylene glycol (Fig. 83-5) have been described in some reports, among which "the sulfanilamide Massengill disaster" probably is best known.[40] In that instance, diethylene glycol (73%) was used as a vehicle for the preparation of 10% sulfanilamide used to treat infections. A total of 105 deaths due to renal failure were related to this sulfonamide formulation. No oxalate crystals were reported found in the kidneys or other organs of these victims, but the variety of the oxalate crystals (not only the envelope form) was probably not known for most clinicians before 1980.[41] Except for the lack of oxalate crystals, the pathologic findings in the various organs of these victims were similar to those found in ethylene glycol–poisoned victims.

In the more recent Haitian acetaminophen episode, diethylene glycol–contaminated acetaminophen syrup caused renal failure in more than 100 children with a high mortality rate.[42] A similar episode also occurred in India.[43] The clinical features were renal failure, hepatitis, pancreatitis, and coma before death. Because of the acute renal failure, it is difficult to relate the metabolic acidosis reported in some cases[44] to possible acidic metabolites of diethylene glycol metabolism by ADH. In one case report, there is an indication of a positive effect from hemodialysis for the removal of diethylene glycol.[38] In another case report, the use of fomepizole was associated with correction of the metabolic acidosis.[45] Topical application of silver sulfadiazine contaminated with diethylene glycol to patients with burns resulted

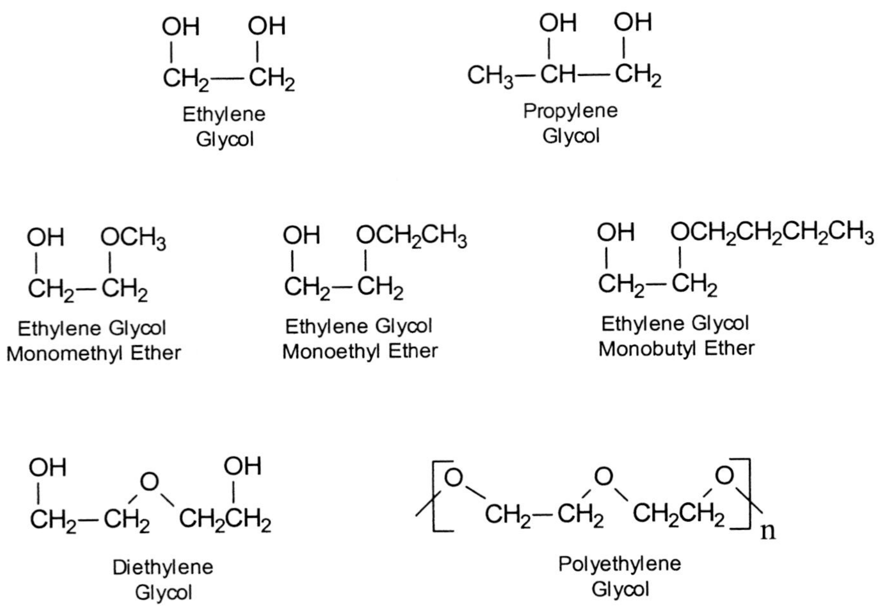

FIGURE 83-5

Chemical structures of common glycols and glycol ethers.

in increased anion gap metabolic acidosis and acute renal failure. All five patients reported died despite supportive treatment and bicarbonate replacement.[46] Autopsy was performed in one patient and showed no evidence of oxalate crystals.

Pathophysiology

Experimental studies in rats exposed to diethylene glycol showed similarities to ethylene glycol toxicity.[47,48] The animals developed metabolic acidosis as in ethylene glycol toxicity. Mortality was reduced if the animals were treated with bicarbonate or ethanol. The administration of the latter reduced mortality to nil and prevented acidosis. The untreated animals developed acute tubular necrosis with renal deposits of oxalate crystals. An experimental study in rats aimed at comparing some aspects of ethylene glycol and diethylene glycol toxicity indicated that the blood and kidney oxalate concentrations were higher when the former glycol was given.[49] Whether oxalate deposition actually occurs is questionable, however, because the ether bond generally is resistant to metabolic degradation.

Clinical Presentation

In humans exposed to diethylene glycol, the presence of acidosis has been questioned, but this may be due to the fact that these fatal cases were reported by pathologists with less emphasis on the clinical and metabolic features.[50] There is at least one clinical report in children supporting the rat data of metabolic acidosis in these poisonings.

Diagnosis

If there is no history of ingestion of diethylene glycol, diagnosing this condition is difficult. There are no clinical features or general laboratory analysis pointing to this diagnosis except for specific analysis, which is rarely available in hospital laboratories. These patients should be

observed for the development of metabolic acidosis, which should trigger treatment.

Treatment

As is evident from the foregoing discussion, the toxicities of ethylene glycol and diethylene glycol have similarities but are not identical. At present, treatment of diethylene glycol poisoning should be as for ethylene glycol poisonings: Bicarbonate and ADH inhibition should be given if metabolic acidosis is moderate or severe; hemodialysis should be considered in acidotic patients with an elevated osmolal gap. Because no strict treatment recommendations can be given, physicians dealing with these patients should consult a medical toxicologist or a poison center.

POLYETHYLENE GLYCOL

The polyethylene glycols (see Fig. 83-5) (molecular weight approximately 400 to 4000) are liquids but turn solid when the molecular weight is greater than 1000. The toxicity decreases with increasing molecular weight, probably as a result of poor absorption of the solid forms. In general, the toxicity is low but may be significant for the glycols with low molecular weight. The polyethylene glycols are used as solvents or excipients for different purposes. They also are used, and well tolerated, in the electrolyte solution (PEG-ES) recommended for whole-bowel irrigation.

Little is known about the clinical features of these poisonings. The reported CNS depression, metabolic acidosis, and renal failure may point to some similarities with ethylene glycol poisoning.[51]

A 2.5-year-old girl experienced severe toxicity with metabolic acidosis and renal impairment when polyethylene glycol was used as an excipient for the ointment applied on her severely burned skin (80% third-degree burns).[52] Treatment with ethanol, bicarbonate, and hemodialysis was associated with correction of acidosis and renal impairment. She died later as a result of the severe burns. No autopsy was performed, and no oxalate crystals were reported in the urine.

Treatment

The standard measures of gastric decontamination and supportive care are probably the mainstay of therapy in these rare poisonings if the patient is seen early. The efficacy of hemodialysis is hampered by the relatively high molecular weight of this group, but hemodialysis should be considered if low-molecular-weight glycols are ingested (molecular weight <600). If severe metabolic acidosis develops, fomepizole or ethanol treatment may be administered as in ethylene glycol poisoning, but the efficacy of this treatment has not been documented. Sodium bicarbonate should be given to correct severe acidosis.

PROPYLENE GLYCOL

The use of propylene glycol (1,2-propanediol) (see Fig. 83-5) in various cosmetics has little toxicologic significance. Its use as a solvent for intravenous drug formulations has shown that this compound is not completely inert from a toxicologic point of view. Renal failure may result in retention of the glycol, causing CNS depression, as about 50% is excreted in unchanged form by the kidneys, whereas the rest is metabolized mainly to lactate, acetate, and pyruvate.[53] Metabolic acidosis may be pronounced because of its metabolism to lactate (≤24 mmol/L).[54] The elimination half-life is about 19 hours.[55] In two children, CNS depression and seizures were observed after propylene glycol intoxication.[56,57]

Propylene glycol (molecular weight 76) also may raise the osmolal gap. If lactic acid acidosis develops, this rare poisoning may raise the osmolal and the anion gaps. Propylene glycol concentrations of 760 mg/dL (100 mM) did not cause CNS depression,[58] whereas stupor and metabolic acidosis were present in a patient with serum propylene glycol concentrations of 70 mg/dL (9 mM).[59] In these two cases, the osmolal gap theoretically would be elevated by about 108 mOsm/kg H_2O (100/0.93) and 10 mOsm/kg H_2O (9/0.93). From these few cases, there does not seem to be any correlation between serum propylene glycol levels and toxicity.

Treatment

Treatment is supportive. The effect of activated charcoal has not been documented.

ALKYL ETHERS OF ETHYLENE GLYCOL (CELLOSOLVES)

The group of alkyl ethers of ethylene glycol consists of the mono alkyl ethers of ethylene glycol—ethylene glycol butyl ether (butyl glycol, butyl Cellosolve), ethylene glycol monomethyl ether (methyl Cellosolve), and ethylene glycol monoethyl ether (Cellosolve) (see Fig. 83-5). These compounds are used mainly as solvents in hydraulic fluids and in household cleaning compounds. Few cases of toxicity from these compounds have been published, and the mech-

anisms of toxicity are not completely understood. Coma, hypotension, and metabolic acidosis with hyperventilation seem to be typical clinical signs of intoxication. The abnormal blood picture, including erythropenia, granulocytosis, hemolysis, and hemoglobinuria, seen in animals[60,61] also may be seen in the clinical situation.[62] Until more data are available, the treatment is considered to be uniform within this group.

Butyl glycol poisoning has been reported after the suicidal ingestion of a window-cleaning agent containing butyl glycol and ethanol.[62] Coma and hypotension were present on admission with blood levels of ethylene glycol butyl ether and ethanol being 432 mg/L and 36 mg/L, respectively. Metabolic acidosis developed and was confirmed by the presence of the butyl glycol metabolite butoxy acetic acid and lactate. No increase in urine oxalate content was observed. The patient was treated with forced diuresis, bicarbonate, and hemodialysis. There was a suggestion of ethanol-induced inhibition of butyl glycol metabolism and a beneficial effect of hemodialysis in this patient.

In another case without concomitant ethanol ingestion, metabolic acidosis was accompanied by coma, hypokalemia, hemoglobinuria, oxaluria, and a transitory rise in the serum creatinine level in a patient who survived on supportive therapy alone.[63] The measured increased urinary excretion of oxalate and butoxyacetic acid in this case gives an indication of different metabolic pathways, one of which includes degradation of ethylene glycol butyl ether to ethylene glycol.

Felgenhauer and colleagues[64] reported coma, metabolic acidosis, and mild renal impairment in a 27-year-old woman after the ingestion of 1 L of an ethylene glycol butyl ether–containing window cleaner. Hemolysis parameters were normal, no abnormal oxaluria was observed, and the osmolal gap was slightly elevated. Supportive therapy and hemodialysis were associated with an uneventful recovery.

Two patients with methyl Cellosolve ingestion developed metabolic acidosis and coma.[65] The patient with the more severe metabolic acidosis developed slight acute renal failure, and urine oxalate crystals were observed. The other patient had no evidence of renal effect or oxalate crystals in the urine. Both patients had an uneventful recovery after treatment with bicarbonate and ethanol.

Treatment

Based on these case reports and overall theoretical considerations, it seems reasonable to treat these poisonings with supportive therapy, including possibly gastric decontamination if the patient is seen early, and bicarbonate to correct significant metabolic acidosis. Hemodialysis also seems justified if large doses are ingested and the patient is acidotic. The role of hemodialysis in these poisonings is theoretical, however. It has not been validated empirically. The role of ADH inhibitors is controversial. Until more data are available, ADH inhibitors should be considered mostly in rare cases in which metabolic acidosis develops, to prevent an assumed formation of toxic metabolites by oxidation of the alcohol groups.

Because the role of ADH in the metabolism of these compounds is not clear, and fomepizole is expensive, some clinicians may prefer to use ethanol. If ethanol is used, however, patients must be placed in an intensive care unit and monitored closely as described previously.

REFERENCES

1. Jacobsen D, Ostby N, Bredesen JE: Studies on ethylene glycol poisoning. Acta Med Scand 212:11–15, 1982.
2. Jacobsen D, Hewlett TP, Webb R, et al: Ethylene glycol intoxication: Evaluation of kinetics and crystalluria. Am J Med 84:145–182, 1988.
3. Peterson CD, Collins AJ, Himes JM, et al: Ethylene glycol poisoning. N Engl J Med 304:21–23, 1981.
4. Moreau CL, Kerns W, Tomaszewski CA, et al: Glycolate kinetics and hemodialysis clearance in ethylene glycol poisoning. Clin Toxicol 36:659–666, 1998.
5. Jacobsen D, McMartin KE: Methanol and ethylene glycol poisonings: Mechanism of toxicity, clinical course, diagnosis and management. Med Toxicol 1:309–334, 1986.
6. Parry MF, Wallach R: Ethylene glycol poisoning. Am J Med 57:143–150, 1974.
7. Berman LB, Schreiner GE, Feys J: The nephrotoxic lesion of ethylene glycol. Ann Intern Med 46:611–619, 1957.
8. Smith BJ, Anderson BG, Smith SA, Chew DJ: Early effects of ethylene glycol on the ultrastructure of the renal cortex in dogs. Am J Vet Res 51:89–96, 1990.
9. Brent J, McMartin KE, Phillips S, et al: Fomepizole for the treatment of ethylene glycol poisoning. N Engl J Med 340:832–839, 1999.
10. Porter WH, Rutter PW, Bush BA, et al: Ethylene glycol toxicity: The role of serum glycolic acid in hemodialysis. J Toxicol Clin Toxicol 39:607–615, 2001.
11. McMartin KE, Cenac TA: Toxicity of ethylene glycol metabolites in normal human kidney cells. Ann N Y Acad Sci 919:315–317, 2000.
12. Scheid C, Koul H, Hill WA, et al: Oxalate toxicity in LLC-PK1 cells, a line of renal epithelial cells. J Urol 155:1112–1116, 1996.
13. Hackett RL, Shevock PN, Khan SR: Alterations in MDCK and LLC-PK1 cells exposed to oxalate and calcium oxalate monohydrate crystals. Scann Microscopy 9:587–596, 1995.
14. Laborit H, Baron C, London A, Olympie J: Activite nerveuse centrale et pharmacologie generale comparee du glyoxylate du glycolate et du glycolaldehyde. Aggressologie 12:187–212, 1971.
15. Chou JY, Richardson KE: The effect of pyrazole on ethylene glycol toxicity and metabolism in the rat. Toxicol Appl Pharmacol 43:33–44, 1978.
16. Clay KL, Murphy RC: On the metabolic acidosis of ethylene glycol intoxication. Toxicol Appl Pharmacol 39:39–49, 1977.
17. Jacobsen D, Ovrebo S, Ostborg J, Sejersted OM: Glycolate causes the acidosis in ethylene glycol poisoning and is effectively removed by haemodialysis. Acta Med Scand 216:409–416, 1984.
18. Jacobsen D, McMartin KE: Antidotes for methanol and ethylene glycol poisoning. Clin Toxicol 35:127–143, 1997.
19. Ahmed MM: Ocular effects of antifreeze poisoning. Br J Ophthalmol 55:854–855, 1971.
20. Friedman EA, Greenberg JB, Merril JP, Dammin GJ: Consequences of ethylene glycol poisoning. Am J Med 32:891–901, 1962.
21. Aarstad K, Dale O, Aakervik O, et al: A rapid gas chromatographic method for determination of ethylene glycol in serum and urine. J Analyt Toxicol 17:218–221, 1993.
22. Aabakken L, Johansen KS, Rydningen EB, et al: Osmolal and anion gaps in patients admitted to an emergency medical department. Exp Hum Toxicol 13:131–134, 1994.
23. Hoffman RS, Smilkstein MJ, Howland MA, Goldfrank LR: Osmolal gaps revisited: Normal values and limitations. J Toxicol Clin Toxicol 31:81–93, 1993.
24. Jacobsen D, Akesson I, Shefter E: Urinary calcium oxalate monohydrate crystals in ethylene glycol poisoning. Scand J Clin Lab Invest 42:321–324, 1982.
25. Borron SW, Megarbane B, Baud FJ: Fomepizole in treatment of uncomplicated ethylene glycol poisoning. Lancet 354:831, 1999.
26. Jacobsen D, Ostensen J, Bredesen L, et al: 4-methylpyrazole is effectively removed by hemodialysis in the pig model. Hum Exp Toxicol 15:494–496, 1996.
27. Kowalczyk M, Halvorsen S, Ovrebo S, Jacobsen D: Ethanol therapy in ethylene glycol poisoned patients. Vet Hum Toxicol 40:225–228, 1998.
28. Jakoby WB (ed): Enzymatic Basis of Detoxification, Vol. 1. New York, Academic Press, 1980.
29. Pietruszko R, Crawford K, Lester D: Comparision of substrate specificity of alcohol dehydrogenase from human liver, horse liver and yeast towards saturated and 2 enoic alcohols and aldehydes. Arch Biochem Biophys 159:50–60, 1973.
30. Hewlett TP, McMartin KE, Lauro AJ, Ragan FA: Ethylene glycol poisoning: The value of glycolic acid determination for diagnosis and treatment. J Toxicol Clin Toxicol 24:389–402, 1986.
31. Baud FJ, Galliot M, Astier A, et al: Treatment of ethylene glycol poisoning with intravenous 4-methylpyrazole. N Engl J Med 319:97–100, 1988.
32. Jacobsen D: New treatment for ethylene glycol poisoning. N Engl J Med 340:879–881, 1999.
33. Barceloux DG, Krenzelok EP, Olson K, Watson W: American Academy of Clinical Toxicology practice guidelines on the treatment of ethylene glycol poisoning. J Toxicol Clin Toxicol 37:537–560, 1999.
34. Baud FJ, Bismuth C, Garnier R, et al: 4-Methylpyrazole may be an alternative to ethanol therapy for ethylene glycol intoxication in man. J Toxicol Clin Toxicol 24:463–483, 1986–1987.
35. Aakervik O, Svendsen J, Jacobsen D: Ethylene glycol poisoning treated with fomepizole. Tidsskr Nor Laegeforen 122:2444–2446, 2002.
36. Baum CR, Langman CB, Oker EE, et al: Fomepizole treatment of ethylene glycol poisoning in an infant. Pediatrics 106:1489–1491, 2000.
37. Benitez JG, Swanson-Biearman B, Krenzelok EA: Nystagmus secondary to fomepizole administration in a pediatric patient. J Toxicol Clin Toxicol 38:795–798, 2000.
38. Brophy PD, Tenenbein M, Gardner J, et al: Childhood diethylene glycol poisoning treated with alcohol dehydrogenase inhibitor fomepizole and hemodialysis. Am J Kidney Dis 35:958–962, 2000.
39. Harry P, Jobard E, Briand M, et al: Ethylene glycol poisoning in a child treated with 4-methylpyrazole. Pediatrics 102:E21, 1998.
40. Geiling EMK, Cannon PR: Pathologic effects of elixir sulfanilamide (diethylene glycol) poisoning. JAMA 111:919–926, 1938.
41. Godolphin W, Meagher EP, Sanders HD, Frolich J: Unusual calcium oxalate crystals in ethylene glycol poisoning. J Toxicol Clin Toxicol 16:479–486, 1980.
42. O'Brien KL, Selanikio JD, Hecdivert C, et al: Epidemic of pediatric deaths from acute renal failure caused by diethylene glycol poisoning. Acute Renal Failure Investigation Team. JAMA 15:1175–1180, 1998.
43. Singh S, Dutta AK, Khare S, et al: Diethylene glycol poisoning in Gurgaon, India, 1998. Bull World Health Organ 79:88–89, 2001.
44. Bowie MD, McKenzie D: Diethylene glycol poisoning in children. South Afr Med J 46:931–934, 1972.
45. Borron SW, Baud FJ, Garnier R: Intravenous 4-methylpyrazole as an antidote for diethylene glycol and triethylene glycol poisoning: A case report. Vet Hum Toxicol 39:26–28, 1997.
46. Cantarell MC, Fort J, Camps J, et al: Acute intoxication due to topical application of diethylene glycol. Ann Intern Med 106:478–479, 1987.
47. Durand A, Auzepy P, Hebert JL, Trieu TC: A study of mortality and urinary excretion of oxalate in male rats following acute experimental intoxication with diethylene glycol. Eur J Intensive Care Med 2:143–146, 1976.
48. Hebert JL, Fabre M, Auzepy P, Paillas J: Acute experimental poisoning by diethylene glycol: Acid base balance and histological data in male rats. Toxicol Eur Res 1:289–294, 1978.
49. Winek CL, Shingleton DP, Shanor SP: Ethylene and diethylene glycol toxicity. J Toxicol Clin Toxicol 13:297–324, 1978.
50. Wordley E: Diethylene glycol poisoning: Report on two cases. J Clin Pathol 1:44–46, 1947.
51. Smyth HE, Carpenter CP, Weil CS: The toxicology of the polyethylene glycols. Am Pharm Assoc J 39:349–354, 1950.
52. Rodriguez EM, Gutierrez JCL, Jimenez JMT, Mar ZR: Metabolic acidosis: Intoxication caused by polyethylene glycol. Abstract No 5 at the Scientific Meeting of the European Association of Poison Centres and Clinical Toxicologists, Birmingham, UK, May 26–28, 1993.
53. Ruddick JA: Toxicology, metabolism and biochemistry of 1,2-propanediol. Toxicol Appl Pharmacol 21:102–111, 1972.
54. Kelner MJ, Bailey DN: Propylene glycol as a cause of lactic acidosis. J Analyt Toxicol 9:40–42, 1985.
55. Glasgow AM, Boeck RL, Miller MK, et al: Hyperosmolality in small infants due to propylene glycol. Pediatrics 72:353–355, 1983.
56. Arulanantham K, Genel M: Central nervous toxicity associated with ingestion of propylene glycol. J Pediatr 93:515–516, 1978.
57. Martin G, Finberg L: Propylene glycol: A potentially toxic vehicle in liquid dosage. J Pediatr 77:877–878, 1970.
58. Kulick MI, Lewis NS, Bansal V, et al: Hyperosmolality in the burn patient: Analysis of an osmolal discrepancy. J Trauma 20:223–228, 1980.

59. Cate JC, Hendricks R: Propylene glycol intoxication and lactic acidosis. N Engl J Med 303:1237, 1980.
60. Rowe VK, Wolf MA: Derivatives of glycols. In Clayton GA, Clayton FE (eds): Patty's Industrial Hygiene and Toxicology, 3rd ed. New York, Wiley, 1982.
61. Carpenter CP, Pozzani UC, Weil CS, et al: The toxicity of butyl cellosolve solvent. AMA Arch Ind Health 14:114–131, 1956.
62. Gijsenbergh FP, Jenco M, Veulemans H, et al: Acute butylglycol intoxication: A case report. Hum Toxicol 8:243–245, 1989.
63. Rambourg-Schepens MO, Buffet M, Bertault R, et al: Severe ethylene glycol butyl ether poisoning: Kinetics and metabolic pattern. Hum Toxicol 7:187–189, 1988.
64. Felgenhauer N, Zilker T, von Clarmann M: A case of severe ethylene glycol monobutyl ether poisoning. Abstract No 3 at The Scientific Meeting of the European Association of Poisons Centres and Clinical Toxicologists, Birmingham, UK, May 26–28, 1993.
65. Nitter-Hauge S: Poisoning with ethylene glycol monomethyl ether. Acta Med Scand 188:277–280, 1970.

CHAPTER 84

Hydrocarbon and Halogenated Hydrocarbons

Christopher S. Amato ■ Anthony Santilli ■ Richard Y. Wang

Hydrocarbon exposure is common, with more than 62,000 exposures reported in 1999 alone in the United States. Most of these exposures were unintentional. More than 24,000 of these exposures occurred in children younger than age 6 years. Although most of these exposures did not result in death, hydrocarbons were responsible for 21 of the 873 reported deaths from toxicologic exposures in 1999.[1] Accidental hydrocarbon ingestion usually occurs in the very old and the very young. Hydrocarbons are not packaged in child-resistant containers, and the fluid is attractive in color, odor, and taste.[2] These substances also are prone to abuse, however. They can produce a sense of euphoria, are easy to conceal, and are inexpensive. Of the 21 reported deaths in the United States in 1999, 9 were attributed to intentional inhalation of hydrocarbons. Seven of these occurred in children age 14 to 18.[1] A 20-year review of poisoning in adolescents found that abuse of inhalants was popular among teenage boys, and serious effects can result even after one use.[2]

Hydrocarbons traditionally are divided into two groups: aliphatic and aromatic. Aliphatic hydrocarbons are mostly compounds that result from the distillation of petroleum. If they have a halogen substituted for one or more of the hydrogen atoms, they are referred to as *halogenated aliphatic hydrocarbons*, an important and toxicologically distinct subgroup. Aromatic hydrocarbons are compounds that contain resonating ringed structures. Hydrocarbons of all varieties are present in many household and industrial chemicals. Kerosene, pine oil, and gasoline are hydrocarbons (Table 84-1).

PHARMACOKINETICS AND BIOCHEMISTRY

The ability to be absorbed by any route depends on the physical properties of the hydrocarbon involved. Aliphatic hydrocarbons' physical properties change depending on the number of carbon atoms in the chain. As the number increases, the compound is more likely to exist as a liquid than as a gas.

The four most important physical properties of aliphatic hydrocarbons are volatility, viscosity, solubility, and surface tension. *Volatility* is the ability of a substance to vaporize. *Viscosity* measures resistance to flow. *Surface tension* is the ability of liquid to move across a surface. Gaseous aliphatic hydrocarbons are highly volatile with low viscosity and low surface tension. They may be absorbed via the skin, gastrointestinal tract, and lung.[3,4] As the substances increase in molecular size and carbon chain length,

they become relatively less well absorbed through the gastrointestinal tract.[5] A major concern of hydrocarbons is that they may cause pulmonary aspiration. Viscosity is a crucial factor in the risk of aspiration. Viscosity usually is measured in Saybolt Seconds Universal (SSU) units. There is a high risk of aspiration when viscosity is less than 45 SSU at 100°F (37.8°C); this includes compounds such as gasoline, kerosene, and lighter fluid. When the viscosity is greater than 100 SSU at 100°F, there is a low risk of aspiration. Examples of low-viscosity substances are mothballs, petroleum jelly, and paraffin wax.[6]

Aromatic hydrocarbons, the most common of which are toluene and benzene, are absorbed through the gastrointestinal tract more readily than aliphatic hydrocarbons.[7] They are prone to cause pulmonary aspiration similar to aliphatic hydrocarbons because they tend to have a low viscosity.[6] These compounds also are potentially systemically absorbed through dermal exposure. Viscosity affects absorption by the dermal route as well. Highly viscous compounds have less dermal bioavailability.[8] The aromatic compound toluene is prone to abuse because it can produce a "high" when sniffed. Many serious complications have occurred when individuals were exposed via this route.[9]

Many halogenated hydrocarbons are volatile and exist as a gas at room temperature. They are easily absorbed via the lung. There have been many reports of clinically significant exposures after inhalation of these substances.[10–13] In one case, methyl bromide was detected in peripheral blood and other various organs after death from inhalation.[14] For the halogenated hydrocarbons that exist in nongaseous states at room temperature, there have been reports of disease from other modes of exposure. Extensive skin contact may result in absorption with systemic concentrations high enough to produce clinical effects.[15] Toxic effects of halogenated hydrocarbons have been reported in individuals who have ingested these compounds.[16]

CLINICAL MANIFESTATIONS

Table 84-2 lists clinical manifestations according to body system.

Pulmonary

Aspiration of low-viscosity hydrocarbons is the major cause of morbidity and mortality in acute ingestions. Pulmonary aspiration is typically clinically evident within 6 to

TABLE 84-1 Common Hydrocarbons and Substances Containing Hydrocarbons

Gasoline	Sterno fuel
Automotive products	Waxes
Pine oils	Furniture polish
Paint products	Solvents
Mineral oils and spirits	Disinfectants
Lighter fluid	Adhesives

8 hours after ingestion.[17] Clinical manifestations may range from dyspnea to respiratory failure (Fig. 84-1).

In a clinical series of hydrocarbon exposure, there was no statistical increase in patients who vomited or had gastric lavage, suggesting that chemical pneumonitis more likely was related to aspiration of hydrocarbons than to gastric contents.[17,18] Chemical pneumonitis can progress to pneumonia. Bacterial pneumonia has been described in studies of hydrocarbon aspiration.[17,19,20] Fever may occur, however, without clinical evidence of bacterial pneumonia.[17] Lipoid pneumonia has been cited as another consequence of hydrocarbon aspiration.[21] Other reported pulmonary complications include adult respiratory distress syndrome, pneumomediastinum, pneumothorax, pleural effusions, and pneumatocele formation.[17,21–23] Pulmonary function testing in these patients may show a restrictive pattern, which may resolve over time.[21] Aromatic and aliphatic hydrocarbons have been

TABLE 84-2 Clinical Effects of Hydrocarbon Exposure

Pulmonary	Nausea
ARDS	Vomiting
Bronchospasm	
Chemical pneumonitis	**Renal**
Pleural effusions	Acute renal failure
Pneumomediastinum	Acute tubular
Pneumonia	necrosis
Pneumatocele	Glomerulonephritis
	Type I RTA
Cardiac	
Arrhythmias	**Dermatologic**
Decreased inotropy	Chemical burns
Myocardial infarction	Compartment
	syndrome
Neurologic	Frostbite
Cerebellar dysfunction	Tissue necrosis
CNS depression	
Cranial nerve abnormalities	**Pregnancy**
Euphoria	Cardiotocographic
Myoclonus	Fetal malformations
Peripheral neuropathy	Oligohydramnios
Polyneuropathy	Restricted fetal growth
Psychiatric disorders	
Seizures	**Other**
	Adrenal hemorrhage
Gastrointestinal	Hemolysis
Abdominal pain	Methemoglobinemia
Hepatotoxicity	Primary ovarian failure

ARDS, adult respiratory distress syndrome; CNS, central nervous system; RTA, renal tubular acidosis.

implicated as causing pulmonary effects.[24,25] Decreased mentation, which may occur with hydrocarbon exposure, heightens the risk of pulmonary aspiration.[26] If present in high concentrations, hydrocarbons can displace alveolar oxygen, causing hypoxia. Hydrocarbons can cause pulmonary edema with intraalveolar hemorrhage.[14]

Cardiac

Hydrocarbons have been reported to cause various cardiac effects. In one case, a man developed atrial fibrillation after injection of gasoline.[27] Toluene has been associated with acute myocardial infarction in two cases of young men who intentionally inhaled the substance. One of the patients developed ventricular fibrillation.[9] Other studies have confirmed toluene's association with ventricular arrhythmias.[9,28,29] Bradycardia has been cited in one case report.[30] Multiple animal studies have shown effects of halogenated hydrocarbons on cardiac tissue. In an isolated ferret ventricular papillary muscle experiment, halothane and isoflurane were shown to decrease cardiac contractility.[31] The mechanism was decreasing Ca^{2+} release from the sarcoplasmic reticulum and transsarcolemmal Ca^{2+} influx. These were accomplished by a conformational change in a voltage-dependent Ca^{2+} channel,[32] an effect that was confirmed in a trial on human atria. Halogenated hydrocarbons can depress atrial conduction, prolong atrial refractory periods, and prolong atrioventricular node conduction time.[33] These compounds also were found to cause prolonged arrhythmias in rat hearts.[34] Hydrocarbon-induced vasospasm has been implicated in a patient with atherosclerosis who developed an asymptomatic myocardial infarction after inhalation of a trichloroethane.[35] In the same report, a second patient developed symptomatic myocardial ischemia that resolved after 4 hours.

Neurologic

Multiple neurologic complications can occur in patients exposed to hydrocarbons. These compounds can cross the blood-brain barrier and act as general anesthetics at high concentrations.[11,17,18] They may cause central nervous system depression secondary to hypoxia as a result of aspiration pneumonitis.[3] In the peripheral nervous system, n-hexane and methyl N-butyl ketone have been shown to cause a primary sensory peripheral polyneuropathy. In chronic solvent abuse, multiple central nervous system side effects can be seen. One study showed cognitive impairment in 60% of the subjects followed.[36] Abnormalities also were seen in the pyramidal, cerebellar, and cranial nerve tracts. Acute exposure to aromatic compounds has been shown to produce electroencephalogram alterations and resting tremors and seizures.[37,38] In the peripheral nervous system, polyneuropathy and quadriparesis have been reported.[24,39,40] Central nervous system depression with memory impairment, weakness, and numbness commonly is observed.[41–43] Centrally, cerebellar lesions and cranial nerve abnormalities resulting in problems walking, facial numbness, and blurry vision have been reported with trichloroethylene inhalation.[44] Other reported findings include spinal cord lesions producing motor and sensory disorders, myoclonus, and seizures.[14,42,45–47]

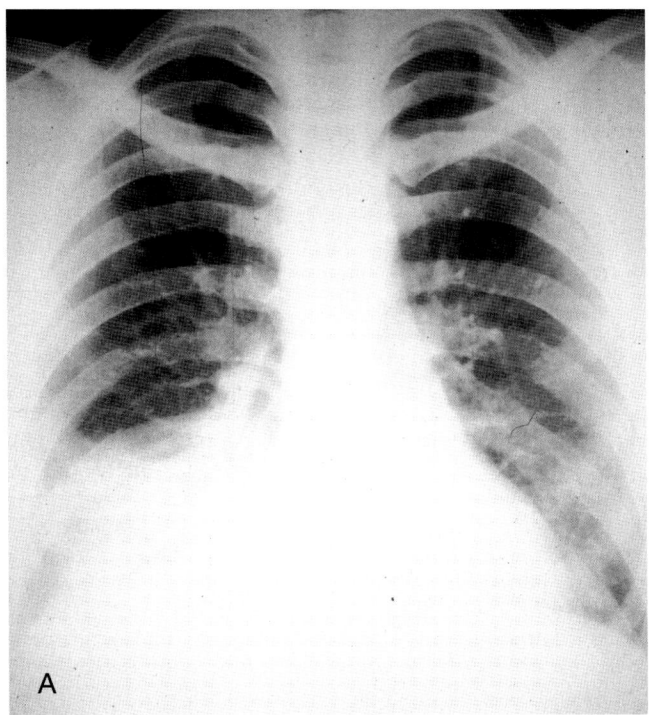

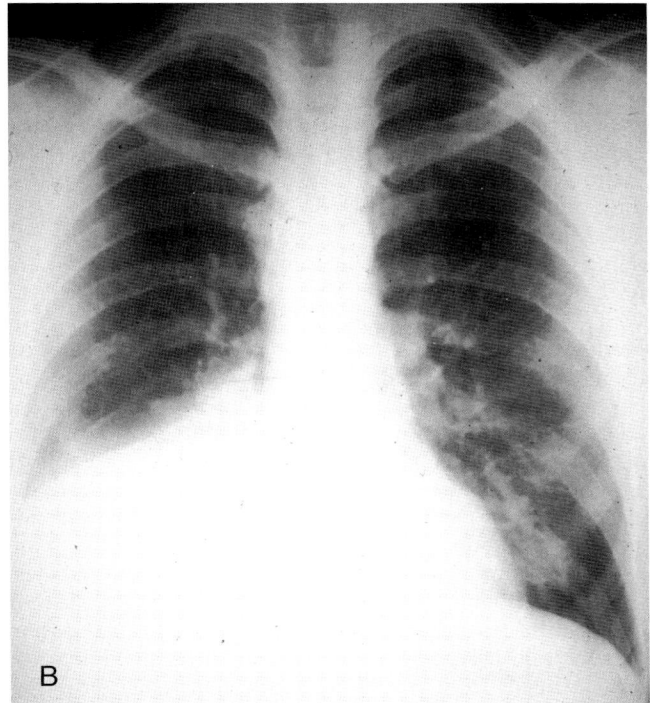

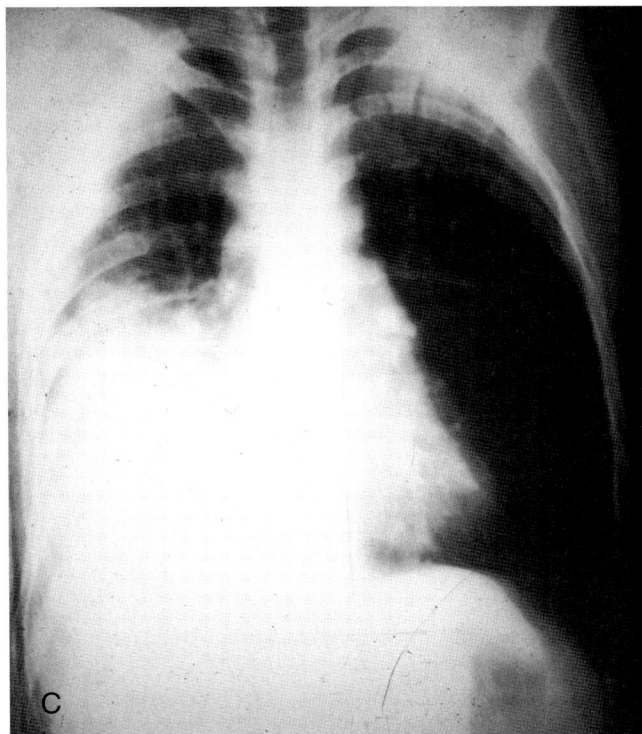

FIGURE 84-1

Serial chest radiographs taken during the inpatient evaluation and management of a 57-year-old man who ingested and aspirated gasoline during an attempt to siphon it from an automobile fuel tank. The plain film studies demonstrate right middle lobe infiltrate with possible right basilar effusion within 24 hours of the incident (**A**) and progression to diffuse and persistent right middle and lower lung field opacification on days 3 (**B**) and 5 (**C**). An ultrasound-guided tube thoracostomy was performed, yielding 60 mL of turbid, hemorrhagic fluid. The patient subsequently improved clinically and was discharged on hospital day 6.

Gastrointestinal

Hydrocarbon compounds tend to cause local irritation in the gastrointestinal tract, which results in abdominal pain, nausea, and vomiting.[17,42] There have been a few isolated reports, however, of abnormal liver function tests, including prolongation of prothrombin time with ingestion of these substances.[4,10,48] Aromatic hydrocarbons have the same gastrointestinal toxic profile as aliphatic hydrocarbons. Hepatic failure has been reported in one case confirmed by hepatocellular necrosis at autopsy.[49] Halogenated hydrocarbons (e.g., carbon tetrachloride) can cause a chemical hepatitis with abnormal liver function tests and progress rapidly to fulminant hepatic failure.[12,50,51]

Renal

Acute renal failure has been associated with exposure to hydrocarbons, usually occurring within the spectrum of multiorgan system failure.[20,41,52] There has been a report of isolated acute renal failure, however, and a report of acute tubular necrosis.[53,54] Chronic hydrocarbon exposure has been associated with rapidly progressive glomerulonephritis. The mechanism is thought to be a combination of immune complex–mediated injury and direct toxic effect on the kidney.[11] Aromatic hydrocarbons, particularly toluene, have been implicated in the development of type I renal tubular acidosis and reversible renal failure.[55,56] The renal effects of hydrocarbon exposure seem to be the exception, however, rather than the rule. Halogenated hydrocarbons have only minor nephrotoxic effects, thought to be secondary to a by-product of their degradation. These effects are on the glomerulus and the proximal and distal tubules. Clinically, albuminuria and glucosuria result.[12] A case of acute renal failure after a dermal application of carbon tetrachloride has been reported.[15] Acute renal failure also has resulted from rhabdomyolysis that occurred after inhalation of hydrocarbon vapors.[4]

Integument

Liquid aromatic and aliphatic hydrocarbons have been associated with contact dermatitis that can progress to a burn formation.[52,57] Inhalation of halogenated hydrocarbons has been associated with frostbite injury, with massive edema of the oral cavity and upper airway,[58] and with severe burns of the oral cavity.[59] Thermal burns may result from the accidental ignition of the hydrocarbon when being inhaled (e.g., sniffing, "bagging," or huffing). Injection of hydrocarbons has resulted in necrosis of subcutaneous fat tissue and the development of thrombosis.[60]

Other

Hematologic abnormalities have been described, including development of intravascular hemolysis[42] and methemoglobinemia with aniline exposure.[61] Carbon monoxide poisoning has been described in patients with methylene iodine and methylene chloride ingestion, as these substances are converted to carbon monoxide by the liver.[51,62]

DIAGNOSIS

Routine laboratory studies in any patient in whom there is concern for hydrocarbon poisoning should include the following: serum electrolytes, blood urea nitrogen, creatinine, complete blood count with differential, liver function tests, coagulation times, urinalysis with examination of sediment, and possibly an arterial blood gas. An electrocardiogram should be obtained, and patients should be monitored on telemetry, especially if halogenated hydrocarbons are involved. Echocardiography to evaluate for decreased cardiac ejection fraction and possibly pulmonary artery monitoring

should be obtained according to standard indications.[21,63] Hypotension can result from sepsis or cardiac dysfunction.[19,21,63] It is prudent to check a coagulation screen (i.e., for disseminated intravascular coagulopathy) and laboratory studies for intravascular hemolysis if the patient is significantly affected.[42]

In addition to the previously mentioned tests, an exposure to certain specific agents should prompt specific laboratory tests. If aniline exposure is suspected, a methemoglobin determination should be obtained; in methylene iodine and methylene chloride poisoning, one should measure blood carboxyhemoglobin.[51,62] Some hydrocarbons can be part of a mixture that contains other toxins. It is important to determine the composition of the material to which the patient has been exposed. For example, Sterno fuel contains methanol and certain gasolines, and ceramic glazes contain lead. A blood methanol or lead concentration should be obtained in these specific instances.[64,65]

Chest radiographs should be obtained at the time of admission and 6 hours later if the initial study was normal but the patient is symptomatic. Abnormalities on chest radiographs range from fine perihilar densities to lobar consolidation, pleural effusions, pneumothoraces, or pneumatoceles.[17,21,23,66] A computed tomography scan of the brain should be obtained in any patient with an altered sensorium, especially patients who have had chronic toluene exposure, because this produces a characteristic diffuse atrophy of the cortex.[38] Electroencephalography and electromyography may be useful, particularly if there has been chronic exposure, and there is a clinical suspicion of peripheral neuropathy.[38,43] Bronchoscopy has been used in the past, but its usefulness is uncertain.[21]

TREATMENT

The general approach toward the management of hydrocarbon poisoning is primarily supportive. Most severe poisonings can be managed in consultation with either a poison control center or a medical toxicologist. In 1999, the American Association of Poison Control Centers (AAPCC) reported 14,541 poisoned patients from hydrocarbon exposure that necessitated medical intervention.[67] Of these, 3200 exposures were deemed moderate to severe, with 18 fatal cases.

As in all emergent situations, a primary survey looking for life-threatening injuries is the best initial approach.

 Indications for ICU Admission in Hydrocarbon Poisoning

Hydrocarbon exposures involving toxic effects from coconstituents (e.g., organophosphate or heavy metals)
Intubated patients
Signs of respiratory failure—increasing alveolar-arterial gradient, hypoxia, increasing oxygen requirement, hypercarbia despite tachypnea, and respiratory acidemia
Altered sensorium
Seizures
Cardiac dysrhythmias that are either progressive or difficult to manage

Remembering the "A, B, C, D, and E's" can assist in this part of the patient assessment; this includes the *a*irway, *b*reathing, and *c*irculatory systems and *e*xposing the patient. In the care of a patient exposed to hydrocarbons, the "D" represents *d*ermal decontamination in addition to assessing neurologic *d*isability. The patient must be stripped of all involved clothing, especially contaminated leather goods, which can be a source of repeat exposure.[68] In addition, hospital personnel must wear the proper protective equipment to prevent secondary exposure until they are assured that adequate decontamination has occurred. Thorough irrigation with soapy water should be done to cleanse the patient of contaminants, except in the case of an organophosphate, which should be irrigated with a 0.5% hypochlorite solution. If there has been ocular involvement, copious eye irrigation should be initiated.

Mental status abnormalities, cyanosis, tachypnea, hypoxia, and other signs of respiratory distress are guides to airway stability. Nebulized bronchodilators and secretion control via suction help to maintain the airway.

Cardiopulmonary monitoring, pulse oximetry, and repeat physical examinations are essential to follow the clinical course and response to treatment of symptomatic patients. Cardiopulmonary monitoring helps to alert to cardiac dysrhythmias, which may be due to cardiac injury, heightened excitability, or hypoxia. Chest radiograph may or may not aid in determining the severity of illness of the patient because the findings often lag behind the clinical picture or may not correlate with symptoms.[69]

The decision to decontaminate the gastrointestinal tract is controversial. If an oral ingestion is large enough, the patient often vomits spontaneously. In common pediatric household ingestions, decontamination is not warranted because large quantities are rarely taken. The exception is when the ingested material contains toxic additives (e.g., camphor; halogenated, heavy metals; or pesticides). The primary morbidity associated with hydrocarbon poisoning is aspiration pneumonitis, and gastrointestinal decontamination may cause or worsen this complication. Activated charcoal may be indicated in the mixed overdose, but it does not adsorb hydrocarbons well. It may be useful for halogenated hydrocarbons, particularly if administered shortly after ingestion. Hemodialysis and hemoperfusion have no role in a hydrocarbon-poisoned patient. A critically poisoned patient can be difficult to identify because manifestations of hydrocarbon poisoning may not peak until 12 to 24 hours after exposure.[70]

The mainstay of treatment for hydrocarbon pneumonitis is predominantly supportive care. This may mean maintenance of the airway and respiratory system via ventilatory management and may require a large amount of positive end-expiratory pressure (PEEP).

Ventilator Management

Intubation is warranted in all patients who are critically ill from hydrocarbon exposure. In some exposures, it may be necessary to protect the patient's airway because he or she may have an altered sensorium. Other exposures may require ventilation because of hypoxia from chemical pneumonitis. In the latter group, increased PEEP may be required to maintain oxygenation. In one report, when a PEEP of 20 with 100%

oxygen was insufficient to maintain the patient's oxygenation, high-frequency jet ventilation seemed to be helpful.[23] Experimental models using rats showed a worsened outcome with partial liquid ventilation after the intratracheal instillation of perfluorocarbons.[71] In patients with carbon monoxide toxicity from either methyl iodine or methylene chloride exposure, oxygen therapy is indicated.[51,72] Carbon monoxide poisoning is discussed in detail in Chapter 94.

Ventilation is important when treating a patient exposed to halogenated hydrocarbons because increased minute ventilation may enhance the pulmonary clearance.[73] In mechanically ventilated patients who do not respond adequately to supplemental PEEP and high-frequency jet ventilation, extracorporeal membrane oxygenation (ECMO) may be considered as a last resort to maintain adequate oxygenation.

Extracorporeal Membrane Oxygenation

ECMO has been attempted as a possible alternative therapy for patients critically ill from hydrocarbon pneumonitis. In this technique, typically the circuit is run from a cannula inserted in the right atria via the right internal jugular to the ECMO apparatus then back to the patient's aortic arch via the right common carotid artery. The difficulty in using this procedure is knowing which patient warrants this invasive approach because most patients have a good outcome without ECMO. Patients who would benefit should be prepared early enough so that it may be effective. One finding in long-term trials of ECMO for a variety of diseases is that delay in starting ECMO decreases survival.[74] It also has been noted that younger children fare better than older children, and adults show no improved outcome on ECMO.[75] There are only 83 active ECMO centers in the United States and 21 more worldwide. The access to ECMO technology is another limiting step. In the U.S. AAPCC data for 1998, only four patients were treated with ECMO.

The criteria generally used for patient selection include lack of response to current therapy, signs of barotrauma, and increasing alveolar-arterial gradient. The decision to start ECMO should not be made lightly because there are significant risks involved, including altered cerebral circulatory flow, anticoagulation, and air emboli. Evidence indicates that ECMO is a useful resource if the patient has cardiac toxicity due to hydrocarbon poisoning without significant pulmonary involvement.[75]

Pharmacologic Therapy

Currently the only generally accepted pharmacologic therapy to aid a hydrocarbon-poisoned patient is nebulized bronchodilators. Steroids have not been shown to offer any improvement[76,77] despite the fact that the pathologic changes in the type II cells are inflammatory and similar to an adult respiratory distress syndrome reaction. The use of surfactant is being investigated. Prophylactic antibiotics are not considered beneficial. (Because there are no studies to show conclusively a lack of value of prophylactic antibiotics, some clinicians choose to start them in patients with significant pulmonary effects or patients with prior lung disease.) Sympathomimetic agents (e.g., epinephrine) should be avoided, if possible, because they could cause cardiac dysrhythmias. There have been reports of sudden death associated with

Criteria for ICU Discharge in Hydrocarbon Poisoning

Stabilized and improving cardiac status without requiring constant infusion of an antidysrhythmic or vasopressor agent

Improving mental status

Extubated patients and with improving respiratory function

Key Points in Hydrocarbon Poisoning

1. Significant exposures to hydrocarbons can affect multiple organs (e.g., central nervous system, cardiac, gastrointestinal, dermal, and respiratory).
2. Hydrocarbons are lipophilic and readily stored in adipose tissues, which can be a source of continued and delayed toxicity.

chlorinated and fluorinated hydrocarbons,[78] and it has been postulated that the myocardium is sensitized by the catecholamines.[79] The patient should be closely monitored for dysrhythmias if he or she requires vasopressor support. Treatment of methemoglobinemia with methylene blue may be necessary in exposures to aniline-containing or nitrobenzene-containing substances (see Chapter 28).

SPECIAL POPULATIONS

Pediatric Patients

Most pediatric ingestions do not require admission to the intensive care unit because children rarely ingest a large amount of toxin. Most are asymptomatic from the time of ingestion until after an observation period of 6 to 8 hours postingestion. Children who require admission often present with symptoms or develop symptoms during the observation period. An abnormal chest radiograph does not automatically necessitate admission unless it correlates with a symptomatic patient.[69] The risk of long-term complications in children is low.

Pregnant Patients

The acute ingestion of gasoline by a woman at 38 weeks' gestation was associated with respiratory distress in the mother and decelerations in fetal heart rate in the fetus.[80] The newborn was delivered by an immediate cesarean section and had Apgar scores at 1 minute of 4/10 and at 5 minutes of 8/10. The newborn was briefly intubated and did well otherwise. Retarded fetal growth occurred with third-trimester exposure to trihalomethane,[81] and fetal malformations developed after first-trimester exposure to organic solvents at the worksite.[82] Some of the chemicals in this latter category included aliphatic and aromatic hydrocarbons, phenols, trichloroethylene, xylene, vinyl chloride, and acetone.

Common Errors in Hydrocarbon Poisoning

Not considering chemical additives in hydrocarbon mixtures

Not considering additional chemical properties of certain hydrocarbons

Not considering delayed pulmonary or cardiac manifestations after hydrocarbon exposure

Not considering cardiac dysrhythmia as a cause of syncope after hydrocarbon exposure

REFERENCES

1. Shepherd G, Klein-Schwartz W: Accidental and suicidal adolescent poisoning deaths in the United States. Arch Pediatr Adolesc Med 152:1181–1185, 1998.
2. Burda AM, Leikin JB, Fischbein C, et al: Poisoning hazards of glass candle lamps. JAMA 277:885, 1997.
3. Gerarde HW: Toxicological studies on hydrocarbons: The aspiration hazard of hydrocarbons and hydrocarbon mixtures. Arch Environ Health 6:329–341, 1963.
4. Betrosian A: Rhabdomyolysis and suicidal hydrocarbon inhalation. Ann Emerg Med 29:301–303, 1997.
5. Mann MD, Pirie DJ, Wolfsdorf J: Kerosene absorption in primates. J Pediatr 91:495–498, 1977.
6. Michalodimitrakis MN, Tsatsakis AM, Christakis-Hampsas MG, et al: Death following intentional methyl bromide poisoning: Toxicology data and literature review. Vet Hum Toxicol 39:30–34, 1997.
7. Wolfsdorf J: Kerosene intoxication: An experimental approach to the etiology of the CNS manifestations in primates. J Pediatr 88:1037–1040, 1976.
8. Swan SH, Waller K: Disinfection by-products and adverse pregnancy outcomes: What is the agent and how should it be measured? Epidemiology 9:479–481, 1998.
9. Cunningham SR, Dalzell GW, McGirr P, Khan MM: Myocardial infarction and primary ventricular fibrillation after glue sniffing. BMJ 294:739–740, 1987.
10. Pyatt JR, Gilmore I, Mullins PA: Abnormal liver function tests following inadvertent inhalation of volatile hydrocarbons. Postgrad Med J 74:747–748, 1998.
11. Sesso R, Stolley PD, Salgado N, et al: Exposure to hydrocarbons and rapidly progressive glomerulonephritis. Braz J Med Biol Res 23:225–233, 1990.
12. Eger EL 2nd, Koblin DD, Bowland T, et al: Nephrotoxicity of sevoflurane versus desflurane anesthesia in volunteers. Anesth Analg 84:160–168, 1997.
13. Hanouz JL, Massetti M, Guesne G, et al: In vitro effects of desflurane, isoflurane, and halothane in isolated human right atria. Anesthesiology 92:116–124, 2000.
14. Potter D, Booth ED, Brandt HC, et al: Studies on the dermal and systemic bioavailability of polycyclic aromatic compounds in high viscosity oil products. Arch Toxicol 73:129–140, 1999.
15. Chang YC: An electrophysiological follow up of patients with n-hexane polyneuropathy. Br J Ind Med 48:12–17, 1991.
16. Javier PA, Courel M, Sobrado J, Gonzalez L: Acute renal failure after topical application of carbon tetrachloride (Letter). Lancet 1:515, 1987.
17. Anas N, Namasonthi V, Ginsburg C: Criteria for hospitalizing children who have ingested products containing hydrocarbons. JAMA 246:840–843, 1981.
18. Brook MP, McCarron MM, Mueller JA: Pine oil cleaner ingestion. Ann Emerg Med 18:391–395, 1989.
19. Welker JA, Zaloga GP: Pine oil ingestion: A common cause of poisoning. Chest 116:1822–1826, 1999.
20. Banner W Jr, Walson PD: Systemic toxicity following gasoline aspiration. Am J Emerg Med 3:292–294, 1983.
21. Segev D, Szold O, Fireman E, et al: Kerosene-induced severe acute respiratory failure in near drowning: Reports on four cases and review of the literature. Crit Care Med 27:1437–1440, 1999.
22. Rodriguez de la Vega A, Casaco A, Garcia M, et al: Kerosene-induced asthma. Ann Allergy 64:362–363, 1990.
23. Burns MJ, Dickson EW, Sivilotti AL, et al: Enhanced mortality from perfluorocarbon administration in a rat model of kerosene aspiration. J Toxicol Clin Toxicol 37:855–859, 1999.

24. Tan WP, Seow E: Case reports on acute toluene poisoning during parquet flooring. Ann Acad Med Singapore 26:138–140, 1997.
25. Nierenberg DW, Horowitz MB, Harris KM, James DH: Mineral spirits inhalation associated with hemolysis pulmonary edema and ventricular fibrillation. Arch Intern Med 151:1437–1440, 1991.
26. Bysani GK, Rucoba RJ, Noah ZL: Treatment of hydrocarbon pneumonitis. Chest 106:300–303, 1994.
27. Greenberg MD, Robinson T, Birner L: Atrial fibrillation after intravenous administration of gasoline. Am Heart J 125:1438–1439, 1993.
28. Carder JR, Fuerst RS: Myocardial Infarction after toluene inhalation. Pediatr Emerg Care 13:117–119, 1997.
29. Gerkin RD Jr, LoVecchio F: Rapid reversal of life-threatening toluene-induced hypokalemia with hemodialysis. J Emerg Med 16:723–725, 1998.
30. Einav S, Amitai Y, Reichman J, Geber D: Bradycardia in toluene poisoning. J Toxicol Clin Toxicol 35:295–298, 1997.
31. Housmans PR, Wanck LA, Carton EG, Bartunek AE: Effects of halothane and isoflurane on the intracellular Ca^{2+} transient in ferret cardiac muscle. Anesthesiology 93:189–201, 2000.
32. Lee DL, Zhang J, Blank TJ: The effects of halothane on voltage-dependent calcium channels in isolated Langendoff-perfused rat heart. Anesthesiology 81:1212–1219, 1994.
33. Raatikainen MJ, Trankina MF, Morey TE, Dennis DM: Effects of volatile anesthetics on atrial and AV nodal electrophysiological properties in guinea pig isolated perfused heart. Anesthesiology 89:434–442, 1999.
34. Goes S, Freire-Maia L, Almeida AP: Effects of anesthetics on the incidence and duration of reprofusion arrhythmias in isolated rat heart. Braz J Med Biol Res 26:1091–1095, 1993.
35. Baliey B, Loebstein R, Lai C, McGuigan MA: Two cases of chlorinated hydrocarbons–associated myocardial ischemia. Vet Hum Toxicol 39:298–301, 1997.
36. Hormes JT, Filley CM, Rosenberg NL: Neurologic sequelae of chronic solvent vapor abuse. Neurology 36:698–702, 1986.
37. Ottelio C, Giagheddu M, Marrosu F: Altered EEG pattern in aromatic hydrocarbon intoxication: A case report. Acta Neurol 15:357–362, 1993.
38. Litovitz TL, Klein-Schwartz W, White S, et al: 1999 Annual Report of the America Association of Poison Control Centers Toxic Exposure Surveillance System. Am J Emerg Med 18:517–574, 2000.
39. Kamijo Y, Soma K, Hasegawa I, Ohwada T: Fatal bilateral adrenal hemorrhage following acute toluene poisoning: A case report. J Toxicol Clin Toxicol 36:365–368, 1998.
40. Akisu M, Mir S, Genc B, Cura A: Severe acute thinner intoxication. Turk J Pediatr 38:223–225, 1996.
41. Garnier R, Rambourg-Schepens MO, Muller A, Hallier E: Glutathione transferase activity and formation of macromolecular adducts in two cases of acute methyl bromide poisoning. Occup Environ Med 53:211–215, 1996.
42. Algren JT, Rodgers GC Jr: Intravascular hemolysis associated with hydrocarbon poisoning. Pediatr Emerg Care 8:34–36, 1992.
43. Sclar G: Encephalomyeloradiculoneuropathy following exposure to industrial solvent. Clin Neurol Neurosurg 101:199–202, 1999.
44. Szlatenyi CS, Wang RY: Encephalopathy and cranial nerve palsies caused by intentional trichloroethylene inhalation. Am J Emerg Med 14:464–466, 1996.
45. Mazzini L, Galente M, Rezzonico M, Kokodoko A: Methylbromide intoxication: A case report. Schweiz Arch Neurol Psychiatr 143:75–80, 1992.
46. Uncini A, Basciani M, DiMuzio A, et al: Methyl bromide myoclonus: An electrophysiologic study. Acta Neurol Scand 81:159–164, 1990.
47. Horowitz BZ, Albertson TE, O'Malley M, Swenson EJ: An unusual exposure to methyl bromide leading to fatality. J Toxicol Clin Toxicol 36:353–357, 1998.
48. Garcia EB Jr, Makalinao IR, How CH: Kerosene-induced hepatotoxicity in children: A three-year retrospective study at Philippines General Hospital. Ann Emerg Med 26:718, 1995.
49. McIntyre AS, Long RG: Fatal fulminant hepatic failure in a 'solvent abuser.' Postgrad Med J 68:29–30, 1992.
50. Chittasobhaktra T, Wannanukul W, Wattanakrai P, et al: Fever, skin rash, jaundice and lymphadenopathy after trichloroethylene exposure: A case report. J Med Assoc Thailand 1:S144–S148, 1997.
51. Weimerskirich PJ, Burkhart KK, Bono MJ, et al: Methyl iodine poisoning. Ann Emerg Med 19:1171–1176, 1990.
52. Walsh WA, Scarpa FJ, Brown RS, et al: Gasoline immersion burn. N Engl J Med 291:830, 1974.
53. Li FK, Yip PS, Chan KW, et al: Acute renal failure after immersion in seawater polluted by diesel oil. Am J Kidney Dis 34:E26, 1999.
54. Jandry JF, Langlois S: Acute exposure to aliphatic hydrocarbons: An unusual cause of acute tubular necrosis. Arch Intern Med 158:1821–1823, 1998.
55. Taher SM, Anderson RK, McCartney R, et al: Renal tubular acidosis associated with toluene "sniffing." N Engl J Med 290:765–768, 1974.
56. Will AM, McLaren EH: Reversible renal damage due to glue sniffing. BMJ 283:525–526, 1981.
57. Schnetz E, Diepgen TL, Elsner P, et al: Multicentre study for the development of an in vivo model to evaluate the influence of topical formulation on irritation. Contact Derm 42:336–343, 2000.
58. Albright JT, Lebovitz BL, Lipson R, Luft J: Upper aerodigestive tract frostbite complicated volatile substance abuse. Int J Pediatr Otorhinolaryngol 49:63–67, 1999.
59. Kuspis DA, Krenzelok EP: Oral frostbite injury from intentional abuse of a fluorinated hydrocarbon. J Toxicol Clin Toxicol 37:873–875, 1999.
60. Rush MD, Schoenfeld CN, Watson WA: Skin necrosis and venous thrombosis from subcutaneous injection of charcoal lighter fluid (naphtha). Am J Emerg Med 16:509–512, 1998.
61. Phillips DM, Gradkek A, Hegselman DE: Methemoglobinemia secondary to aniline exposure. Ann Emerg Med 19:425–429, 1990.
62. Pamies RJ, Sugar D, Rives L, Herold AH: Methanol intoxication: Case report. J Fla Med Assoc 80:465–467, 1993.
63. Anene O, Castello FV: Myocardial dysfunction after hydrocarbon ingestion. Crit Care Med 22:528–530, 1994.
64. Matte TD, Proops D, Palazuelos E, et al: Acute high dose lead exposure from beverage contaminated by traditional Mexican pottery. Lancet 344:1064–1065, 1994.
65. Koppel C, Arndt I, Arendt U, Koeppe P: Acute tetrachloroethylene poisoning—blood elimination kinetics during hyperventilation therapy. J Clin Toxicol 23:103–105, 1985.
66. Franquet T, Gomez-Santos D, Gimenez A, et al: Fire eater's pneumonia: Radiographic and CT finding. J Comput Assist Tomogr 24:448–450, 2000.
67. Litovitz TL, Klein-Schwartz W, Martin Caravati E, et al: 1998 Annual Report of the America Association of Poison Control Centers Toxic Exposure Surveillance System. Am J Emerg Med 17:435–487, 1999.
68. Clifford NJ, Nies AS: Organophosphate poisoning from wearing a laundered uniform previously contaminated with parathion. JAMA 262:3035–3036, 1989.
69. Anas N, Namasonthi V, Ginsburg CM: Criteria for hospitalizing children who have ingested products containing hydrocarbons. JAMA 246:840–843, 1981.
70. Henretig FM: Special considerations in the poisoned pediatric patient. Emerg Med Clin North Am 12:549–567, 1994.
71. Dice WH, Ward G, Kelley J, Kilpatrick WR: Pulmonary toxicity following gastrointestinal ingestion of kerosene. Ann Emerg Med 11:138–142, 1982.
72. Watson WA, Chyka PA: Introduction: Clinical Controversies Symposium: ECMO American Board of Applied Toxicology. Clin Toxicol 34:355–371, 1996.
73. Parranga M, West J: Hydrocarbons. In Viccellio P: Emergency Toxicology, 2nd ed. Philadelphia, Lippincott-Raven, 1998, pp 299–312.
74. Green TP, Moler FW, Goodman DM: Probability of survival after prolonged extracorporeal membrane oxygenation in pediatric patients with acute respiratory failure. Crit Care Med 23:1132–1139, 1995.
75. Banner W: Risks of extracorporeal membrane oxygenation: Is there a role for the use in the management of the acutely poisoned patient? Clin Toxicol 34:365–371, 1996.
76. Wolfsdorf J, Kundig H: Dexamethasone in the management of kerosene pneumonia. Pediatrics 53:86–89, 1974.
77. Steele RW, Conklin RH, Mark HM: Corticosteroids and antibiotics for the treatment of fulminant hydrocarbon aspiration. JAMA 219:1434–1437, 1972.
78. Taylor GJ, Harris WS: Cardiac toxicity of aerosol propellants. JAMA 214:81–85, 1970.
79. Bass M: Sudden sniffing death. JAMA 212:2075–2079, 1970.
80. Fracas M, Wabersich J: Petrol ingestion poisoning in a pregnant women. Clin Exp Obstet Gynecol 24:223–225, 1997.
81. Gallagher MD, Nuckols JR, Stallones L, Savitz DA: Exposure to trihalomethanes and adverse pregnancy outcomes. Epidemiology 9:484–489, 1998.
82. Khattak S, Moghtader K, McMartin K, et al: Pregnancy outcome following gestational exposure to organic solvents. JAMA 281:1106–1109, 1999.

CHAPTER 85

Isopropyl Alcohol

Heath A. Jolliff

Isopropyl alcohol (isopropanol or 2-propanol) (IPA) is a clear, colorless, and volatile liquid that has an odor similar to that of acetone and a bitter taste.[1–3] Most commonly, it is found in rubbing alcohol as a 70% volume/volume solution. IPA also is found in solvents, inks, drug preparations, beauty products, and deicing agents.[4,5] Toxic effects of IPA are seen commonly in alcoholics,[6–8] who abuse it as a cheap, readily available substitute for ethanol. Toxicity also has been reported in small children who have ingested IPA or had long or repeated exposures to IPA through dermal or inhalational exposure.[9–14] Occupational exposure may occur by the dermal and inhalational routes. The primary effects of IPA toxicity are central nervous system (CNS) depression, gastrointestinal irritation, and ketosis. Treatment is symptomatic and supportive.

BIOCHEMISTRY AND PHARMACOKINETICS

IPA is highly volatile. It has a volume of distribution of 0.6 to 0.7 L/kg[9,15,16] and is metabolized to acetone via alcohol dehydrogenase (ADH) (Fig. 85-1). In contrast to ethylene glycol or methanol, IPA is not metabolized further to an acid (see Fig. 85-1).

Pharmacokinetics of Isopropyl Alcohol

Volume of distribution: 0.6–0.7 L/kg
Protein binding: negligible
Mechanism of clearance: hepatic alcohol dehydrogenase metabolism, first-order kinetics
Half-life: Isopropyl alcohol—2–8 hr; Acetone—22 hr
Solubility: miscible in water
Vapor pressure: 33 mm Hg

Data from references 9, 15, and 20.

PATHOPHYSIOLOGY

Central Nervous System Depression

CNS depression may occur rapidly after ingestion of IPA.[8–10,17,18] Peak serum levels of IPA occur 30 to 60 minutes after ingestion due to its rapid absorption from the gastrointestinal tract.[19–21] IPA seems to be the primary chemical responsible for CNS depression because the onset of these manifestations clinically correlates with the time to peak serum IPA levels.[22,23] Patients also tend to improve with declining serum IPA levels.[8,15,18,21,22,24] In clinical practice, patients commonly have prolonged coma, however, despite declining serum IPA levels. Most of these cases show rising serum acetone levels, which has led to the theory that acetone may be responsible for CNS depression. Acetone is known to cause CNS depression.[25–29] The literature also reports cases of patients with initial CNS depression whose mental status improved despite increasing acetone levels.[8,30] It seems that both compounds are responsible for the CNS depression seen with IPA toxicity.

Based on animal studies, IPA seems to have twice the intoxicating effect of ethanol at similar serum concentrations.[31] This effect may be due to the higher molecular weight of IPA compared with ethanol[9] or perhaps the additive effect of the acetone metabolite.

Respiratory depression and hypotension may accompany coma resulting from IPA intoxication.[9,13,20,22,23,32] These effects are most likely the result of depression of the brainstem and peripheral vasodilation.[8,9,14,15,18,20,22,24] Tachycardia is common and may be a compensatory response to the hypotension.[33]

Common CNS effects of ethanol ingestion, such as ataxia, nystagmus, and dysarthria, occur but are not as common in IPA toxicity.[33,34] Diminished reflexes commonly are seen in comatose patients with IPA toxicity.[20,30,33] Seizures are rare but have been reported in infants.[14]

Gastrointestinal Effects

IPA may cause gastritis, mucosal irritation, and, in severe cases, hemorrhagic gastritis. Patients who ingested IPA may present with vomiting and abdominal pain. It often is reported that hemorrhagic gastritis commonly is caused by IPA.[35,36] It is not clear, however, that hemorrhagic gastritis is any more common than the upper gastrointestinal bleeding seen with ethanol abuse. Most abusers of IPA also are alcoholics, and there is considerable overlap between these two groups. Systemic toxicity has been reported after rectal administration of IPA.[37–39] In these cases, serum IPA levels were comparable to serum levels attained after oral ingestion. Elevation of hepatic enzymes also has been reported after IPA ingestion.[40]

Metabolic Effects

Acetone is the major end product of IPA metabolism (see Fig. 85-1). Because no acidic product is generated, the metabolic

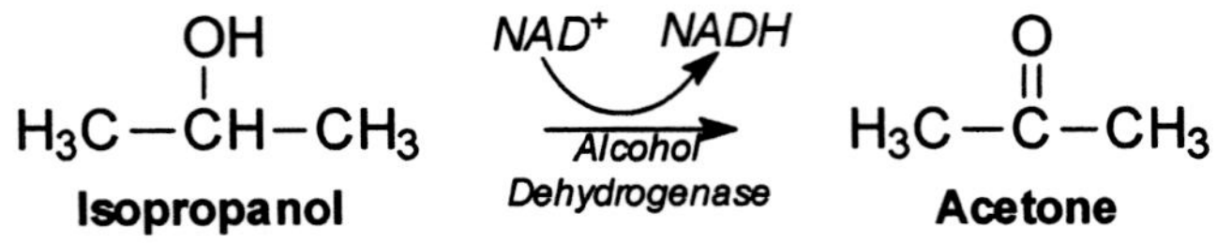

FIGURE 85-1

Conversion of isopropanol to its chief metabolite, acetone. Smaller amounts of isopropanol also are excreted unchanged in the urine and expired air.

acidosis associated with toxic alcohols such as methanol or ethylene glycol does not occur with IPA toxicity. Ketones or, more specifically, acetone can be measured in the serum and urine of patients with IPA toxicity. Acetone can be measured in the serum within 30 to 60 minutes of IPA ingestion but may not be measurable in the urine until after approximately 180 minutes.[8,19] Patients poisoned with IPA often have a ketotic or sweet smell to their breath secondary to the acetone metabolite.[8,18,41,42]

Other Manifestations

Hypothermia has been reported after IPA ingestion and is thought to be secondary to the CNS depression and peripheral vasodilation that can accompany IPA toxicity.[15,32,43] Hypothermia also should be ruled out in all patients with decreased mental status, especially if they are found outdoors. Hypothermia may be secondary to the toxic effects of IPA, the environment itself, or a combination of the two.

Miosis and mydriasis have been reported in patients poisoned with IPA.[9,11,14,30,32,33] Nystagmus has also been reported but is not a specific finding with IPA toxicity.[30]

Mild hyperglycemia has occurred in adults who ingested IPA. Hypoglycemia is rare but may be anticipated to occur in children with IPA toxicity.[7,9,17,44] Any patient with CNS depression always should be suspected to be hypoglycemic until proved otherwise.

Renal insufficiency and renal failure have occurred secondary to hypotension and rhabdomyolysis in IPA-toxic patients.[32,40,45,46] Rhabdomyolysis always should be ruled out in patients who are found comatose, especially when the duration of the coma is unknown. Coingestants always should be considered when patients present with altered mental status.

CLINICAL PRESENTATION AND LIFE-THREATENING COMPLICATIONS

Patients most commonly develop CNS depression, ketosis, fruity breath odor but not metabolic acidosis.[7] They also may present with abdominal pain, emesis, or gastritis. Patients with IPA toxicity should be monitored closely for rapid changes in their mental and cardiopulmonary status. Hypotension and respiratory failure have occurred after large ingestions of IPA.[14,15,20,22,32,43,46] If not monitored closely and treated, these conditions may lead to death.

IPA exposures occur primarily by ingestion; however, dermal, inhalational, and rectal exposures resulting in toxicity also have occurred.[9–13,23,37,43,47] A common exposure pathway in children is by bathing or sponge bathing with IPA to lower a fever.[10–12,14,30,35,43,47] Dermal and inhala-

tional exposures in adults may occur in the occupational setting.

DIAGNOSIS

IPA toxicity should be considered in the differential diagnosis of CNS depression. It also should be considered in an intoxicated patient who does not smell of ethanol or who has an unexplained ketosis. Ketosis without acidosis should make the physician think of IPA or acetone ingestion. IPA also should be a consideration in patients with an unexplained osmolar gap.

Serum IPA concentrations may not be readily available in many hospitals. If possible, however, they should be obtained in patients who are suspected to have been exposed. Serum concentrations can be used to document IPA exposure. The patient's overall clinical condition, not the IPA level, should be used to judge toxicity. Levels should be drawn at least 30 to 60 minutes after the exposure to identify peak IPA levels.[19–21] The best method for measuring serum IPA levels is gas chromatography or proton nuclear magnetic resonance imaging. If IPA levels are determined by ADH enzymatic assays, the assay may interpret IPA as ethanol and give a falsely low IPA level.[42] Although IPA may be detected with Breathalyzers used to measure ethanol, these levels are unreliable.[48]

A possible erroneous diagnosis of IPA poisoning may occur in patients with diabetic ketoacidosis. Cases of measurable IPA in these patients have been reported, although no exposure to IPA was known.[49] It has been theorized that the acetone produced with diabetic ketoacidosis might be converted to IPA via ADH. It is also possible that in these cases there was an unrecognized IPA exposure or that a laboratory error occurred.

Serum IPA levels greater than 120 mg/dL (>20 mmol/L) have been associated with deep coma.[12,15,17,46] An ingestion of 90 mL (3 oz) of 70% IPA theoretically can produce a serum IPA level of 100 mg/dL (16.6 mmol/L) in a 70-kg patient. As with ethanol, chronic alcoholics may tolerate higher IPA levels.[7,50]

Serum ketone or acetone levels may be helpful in the diagnosis of IPA toxicity. Acetone usually is not detected in the serum until 30 to 60 minutes postingestion.[8,19,41] Detection in the urine is usually delayed for at least 3 hours postingestion.[19] An initial nondetectable urine IPA level should be repeated in patients if there is a high index of suspicion for IPA ingestion. Acetone levels increase as ADH metabolizes IPA. Acetone should be measurable even after IPA levels are undetectable.

Laboratory tests useful for the management of IPA-poisoned patients are serum electrolytes, creatinine, glucose, and creatine phosphokinase. If a significant metabolic acidosis is present, other causes must be considered (see Chapter 29). Acetone interferes with certain colorimetric assays used to determine serum creatinine levels[51,52]; this has led to reports of falsely elevated serum creatinine levels in patients with acetone in their serum.[51] Serum osmolality and an osmolar gap may be determined. Caution must be used, however, because acetone and IPA are osmotically active compounds,[53,54] as are other substances, such as methanol and ethylene glycol. The absence of an osmolar gap does not rule out the presence of either compound and in clinical practice is not useful.[55,56]

TREATMENT

As with all toxic ingestions, treatment should be focused on the overall clinical condition of the patient. The primary treatment centers on supportive care. Because IPA is a CNS depressant, attention should be focused on the patient's ability to maintain the airway. If the patient is unable to maintain the airway, endotracheal intubation should be performed and assisted ventilation maintained. These patients warrant continuous cardiac monitoring and pulse oximetry. In patients who initially are able to maintain their airway, close monitoring for respiratory compromise is advised.

Any patient with altered mental status should have a rapid bedside assessment of the serum glucose to rule out hypoglycemia. Hypoglycemia should be treated with intravenous dextrose. Intravenous access should be established and normal saline administered to maintain blood pressure and ensure adequate hydration and urine output. At least 100 mg of thiamine should be administered intravenously or intramuscularly to any patient in whom nutritional status is uncertain and who may be at risk for the development of Wernicke-Korsakoff syndrome.

Hypotension should be treated initially with intravenous fluids. In adults, normal saline can be bolused in doses of 250 to 500 mL each. When the total amount of intravenous fluids has reached approximately 2000 mL, one should be cautious not to fluid overload the patient. If the hypotension does not respond to intravenous normal saline, an intravenous pressor should be the next step. No one pressor agent has been shown to be more efficacious than others in toxin-induced hypotension. Dopamine is often the pressor of first choice because of its relative ease of use and its availability as a premixed intravenous preparation. The dose administered should be based on clinical response. Hypotension that does not respond to the initial pressor of choice should be reassessed and may require additional pressors.

Gastrointestinal decontamination is not likely to be of benefit in IPA ingestions because IPA is absorbed from the gastrointestinal tract within 30 to 60 minutes.[23] Gastric lavage is not likely to influence this absorption. In a patient who presents within 30 minutes of a large IPA ingestion, nasogastric emptying with a standard nasogastric tube may decrease the total amount of IPA absorbed. Nasogastric emptying is theoretical and has not been tested. Activated charcoal also is of questionable benefit, especially when used in the standard dose of 1 g/kg. An in vitro model showed that a 20:1 ratio of charcoal to IPA was needed to adsorb 87% to 92% of the IPA.[57] It would require a large amount of charcoal to adsorb even small amounts of IPA. Using such large amounts of charcoal becomes impractical for the treating

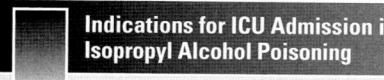
Indications for ICU Admission in Isopropyl Alcohol Poisoning

Coma
Hypotension
Respiratory failure
Patients needing hemodialysis

Criteria for ICU Discharge in Isopropyl Alcohol Poisoning

Mental status returned to baseline *and*
Normotensive without pressors *and*
Patient maintains own airway *and*
Oxygenation maintained without supplemental oxygen *and*
No further need for hemodialysis

physician and dangerous for the patient. It also is of questionable efficacy considering how rapidly IPA is absorbed from the gastrointestinal tract. If a coingestion is possible, the standard dose of charcoal might be appropriate (see Chapter 5).

IPA can be absorbed through the skin with resulting toxicity.[9–11,14] If dermal contact is suspected, washing the skin with a mild soap and water solution is appropriate for dermal decontamination.

Because of its small volume of distribution and negligible protein binding, IPA is easily dialyzable.[9] The clearance of IPA with hemodialysis has been reported as 137 mL/min.[18,58] The acetone metabolite of IPA also is amenable to dialysis. Hemodialysis is rarely indicated in these patients, however. It has been suggested that patients who are hypotensive due to IPA toxicity may benefit from dialysis.[58] Another suggested indication for dialysis is for patients who have serum IPA concentrations greater than 400 mg/dL (>66.6 mmol/L).[58] Most patients do well with supportive care alone, however, even if the patient presents with hypotension or an initially high serum IPA concentration. There are risks associated with hemodialysis, and the overall clinical picture of the patient should be considered. Peritoneal dialysis has been attempted in several reported cases, but the clearance of IPA with this method was only slightly better than the patients' endogenous clearance.[59] For patients who do not respond to aggressive supportive care or who are unstable due to high levels of IPA, hemodialysis should be considered in consultation with a medical toxicologist or poison control center.

There are no antidotes for IPA toxicity. Inhibiting ADH with ethanol or fomepizole would only prolong the time for the metabolism of IPA. Because acetone itself neither is life-threatening nor causes significant end-organ damage, treatment with ADH inhibition is unnecessary.

SPECIAL POPULATIONS

Pediatric Patients

Children may have a different susceptibility to dermal IPA absorption than adults owing to their larger body surface ratio and thin dermis. IPA has been applied dermally to reduce fever in children, with resultant significant toxicity.[11,12,43,47] It is unclear if the toxicity is due solely to the dermal absorption or possibly to a combination of dermal and inhalational absorption. Infants have become toxic when IPA was applied chronically to the umbilicus for cleaning.[14] Coma, hypotension, and seizures all have been reported in children with IPA toxicity.[13,14] Children also have been noted to experience dermal irritation and chemical burns when IPA was applied to the skin.[60] Hypoglycemia has not been reported to occur in children intoxicated with IPA.[61–63]

Pregnant Patients

Based on the size of the molecule, its solubility, and its similarity to ethanol, IPA is expected to cross the placenta. Hypotension in the mother is a concern for the overall status of the fetus. Supportive care for the mother is paramount for protecting the fetus. IPA is not considered a human carcinogen,[64] and its teratogenicity to humans is unknown.

Common Errors in Isopropyl Alcohol Poisoning

Not considering isopropyl alcohol as a potential cause in an intoxicated patient

Ruling out the diagnosis of isopropyl alcohol intoxication based on a normal osmolality and osmolar gap

Attributing an anion gap metabolic acidosis to isopropyl alcohol

Using hemodialysis instead of good supportive care as a cornerstone of treatment

Key Points in Isopropyl Alcohol Poisoning

1. Toxicity may occur after oral, inhalational, rectal, or dermal exposure.
2. Isopropyl alcohol can be a potent central nervous system depressant.
3. Hallmark of toxicity is ketosis without metabolic acidosis.
4. Isopropyl alcohol toxicity may cause gastritis as with other alcohols.
5. Treatment should focus on supportive care.

REFERENCES

1. Lewis R: Sax's Dangerous Properties of Industrial Chemicals, 9th ed. New York, Van Nostrand Reinhold, 1996.
2. O'Neil MJ, Smith A, Heckelman P, Obenchain J, et al: The Merck Index, 13th ed. Whitehouse Station, NJ, Merck & Co, 2002.
3. Ashford R: Ashford's Dictionary of Industrial Chemicals. London, Wavelength Publications, 1994.
4. Gosselin RE, Smith RP, Hodge HC (eds): Methyl alcohol. In Clinical Toxicology of Commercial Products. Baltimore, Williams & Wilkins, 1984, pp 111–275.
5. Leikin JB, Paloucek FP: Poisoning and Toxicology Compendium. Cleveland, Lexi-Comp, 1998.
6. Ford MD: Clinical Toxicology. Philadelphia, WB Saunders, 2001.
7. Alexander CB, McBay AJ, Hudson RP: Isopropanol and isopropanol deaths—ten years experience. J Forensic Sci 27:541–548, 1982.
8. Gaudet M, Fraser G: Isopropanol ingestion: Case report with pharmacokinetic analysis. Am J Emerg Med 7:297–299, 1989.
9. Lacouture PG, Wason S, Abrams A, Lovejoy FH Jr: Acute isopropyl alcohol intoxication: Diagnosis and management. Am J Med 75:680–686, 1983.
10. Lewin G, Oppenheimer P, Wingert W: Coma from alcohol sponging. J Am Coll Emerg Physicians 6:165–167, 1977.
11. McFadden S, Haddow J: Coma produced by topical application of isopropanol. Pediatrics 13:622–623, 1969.
12. Senz E, Goldfarb D: Coma in a child following use of isopropyl alcohol in sponging. J Pediatr 53:322–323, 1958.
13. Vicas IM, Beck R: Fatal inhalational isopropyl alcohol poisoning in a neonate. J Toxicol Clin Toxicol 31:473–481, 1993.
14. Vivier PM, Lewander WJ, Martin HF, Linakis JG: Isopropyl alcohol intoxication in a neonate through chronic dermal exposure: A complication of a culturally-based umbilical care practice. Pediatr Emerg Care 10:91–93, 1994.
15. Natowicz M, Donahue J, Gorman L: Pharmacokinetic analysis of a case of isopropanol intoxication. Clin Chem 31:326–328, 1985.
16. Baselt R: Disposition of Toxic Drugs and Chemicals in Man, 3rd ed. Chicago, Year Book Medical Publishers, 1995.
17. McCord W, Switzer P, Brill H: Isopropyl alcohol intoxication. South Med J 41:639–642, 1948.
18. Rosansky S: Isopropyl alcohol poisoning treated with hemodialysis: Kinetics of isopropyl alcohol and acetone removal. J Toxicol Clin Toxicol 19:265–271, 1982.
19. Lacouture PG, Heldreth DD, Shannon M, Lovejoy FH Jr: The generation of acetonemia/acetonuria following ingestion of a subtoxic dose of isopropyl alcohol. Am J Emerg Med 7:38–40, 1989.
20. Pappas A, Ackerman B, Olsen K: Isopropanol ingestion: A report of six episodes with isopropanol and acetone serum concentration time data. J Toxicol Clin Toxicol 29:11–21, 1991.
21. Parker K, Lere T: Acute isopropanol ingestion: Pharmacokinetic parameters in an infant. Am J Emerg Med 10:542–544, 1992.
22. King LH Jr, Bradley KP, Shires DL Jr: Hemodialysis for isopropyl alcohol poisoning. JAMA 211:1855, 1970.
23. Martinez TT, Jaeger RW, deCastro FJ, et al: A comparison of the absorption and metabolism of isopropyl alcohol by oral, dermal and inhalation routes. Vet Hum Toxicol 28:233–236, 1986.
24. Freireich A, Clinque T, Xanthaky G: Hemodialysis for isopropanol poisoning. N Engl J Med 277:699–700, 1967.
25. Ross D: Acute acetone intoxication. Occup Health 27:120–129, 1975.
26. Gamis A, Wasserman G: Acute acetone intoxication in a pediatric patient. Pediatr Emerg Care 4:24–26, 1988.
27. Gitelson S, Werczberger A, Herman J: Coma and hyperglycemia following drinking of acetone. Diabetes 15:810–811, 1966.
28. Ramu A, Rosenbaum J, Blaschke T: Disposition of acetone following acute acetone intoxication. West J Med 129:429, 1978.
29. Oliver J, Watson J: Abuse of solvents "for kicks": A review of 50 cases. Lancet 1:84, 1977.
30. Mydler TT, Wasserman GS, Watson WA, Knapp JF: Two-week-old infant with isopropanol intoxication. Pediatr Emerg Care 9:146–148, 1993.
31. Wallgren H: Relative intoxicating effects on rats of ethyl, propyl, and butyl alcohols. Acta Pharmacol Toxicol 16:217–222, 1960.
32. Alderson L: Fatal intoxication with isopropyl alcohol (rubbing alcohol). Am J Clin Pathol 38:144–151, 1962.
33. Kelner M, Bailey D: Isopropanol ingestion: Interpretation of blood concentrations and clinical findings. J Toxicol Clin Toxicol 20:497–507, 1983.
34. Rich J, Scheife RT, Katz N, Caplan LR: Isopropyl alcohol intoxication. Arch Neurol 47:322–324, 1990.
35. Lehmann A, Chase H: The acute and chronic toxicity of isopropyl alcohol. J Lab Clin Med 29:61–69, 1944.
36. Chan TYK, Sung JJY, Critchley AJH: Chemical gastro-oesophagitis, upper gastrointestinal haemorrhage and gastroscopic findings following Dettol poisoning. Hum Exp Toxicol 14:18–19, 1995.
37. Barnett JM, Plotnick M, Fine KC: Intoxication after an isopropyl alcohol enema. Ann Intern Med 113:638–639, 1990.
38. Corbett J, Meier G: Suicide attempted by rectal administration of drug. JAMA 206:2320–2321, 1968.
39. Haviv YS, Sadafi R, Osin P: Accidental isopropyl alcohol enema leading to coma and death. Am J Gastroenterol 93:850–851, 1998.
40. Chapin M: Isopropyl alcohol poisoning with acute renal insufficiency. J Maine Med Assoc 40:288–290, 1949.
41. Ashkar FS, Miller R: Hospital ketosis in the alcoholic diabetic: A syndrome due to isopropyl alcohol intoxication. South Med J 64:1409–1411, 1971.
42. Vasiliades J, Pollock J, Robinson C: Pitfalls of the alcohol dehydrogenase procedure for the emergency assay of alcohol: A case study of isopropanol overdose. Clin Chem 24:383–385, 1978.
43. Visudhiphan P, Kaufman H: Increased cerebrospinal fluid protein following isopropyl alcohol intoxication. N Y State J Med 71:887–888, 1971.
44. Trummel J, Ford M, Austin P: Ingestion of an unknown alcohol. Ann Emerg Med 27:368–374, 1996.

45. Juncos L, Taguchi JT: Isopropyl alcohol intoxication: Report of a case associated with myopathy renal failure, and hemolytic anemia. JAMA 203:732–734, 1968.

46. Manring E, Meggs W, Pape G: Toxicity of an intravenous infusion of isopropyl alcohol. J Toxicol Clin Toxicol 35:503, 1997.

47. Garrison R: Acute poisoning from use of isopropyl alcohol in tepid sponging. JAMA 152:317–318, 1953.

48. Logan BK, Gullberg RG, Elenbaas JK: Isopropanol interference with breath alcohol analysis. J Forensic Sci 39:1107–1111, 1994.

49. Bailey D: Detection of isopropanol in acetonemic patients not exposed to isopropanol. J Toxicol Clin Toxicol 28:459–466, 1990.

50. Mendelson J, Wexler D, Leiderman PH: A study of addiction to nonethyl alcohols and other poisonous compounds. Q J Stud Alcohol 18:561–580, 1957.

51. Hawley PC, Falko JM: "Pseudo" renal failure after isopropyl alcohol intoxication. South Med J 75:630–631, 1982.

52. Watkins F: The effect of ketone bodies on the determination of creatinine. Clin Chim Acta 18:191–196, 1967.

53. Chan K, Wong ET, Matthews WS: Severe isopropanolemia without acetonemia or clinical manifestations of isopropanol intoxication. Clin Chem 39:1922–1925, 1993.

54. Monaghan MS, Ackerman BH, Olsen KM: The use of delta osmolality to predict serum isopropanol and acetone concentrations. Pharmacotherapy 13:60–63, 1993.

55. Glaser D: Utility of the serum osmolar gap in the diagnosis of methanol or ethylene glycol ingestion. Ann Emerg Med 27:343–346, 1996.

56. Hoffman RS, Smilkstein MJ, Howland MA, et al: Osmolar gaps revisited: Normal values and limitations. J Toxicol Clin Toxicol 31:81–93, 1993.

57. Burkhart KK, Martinez MA: The adsorption of isopropanol and acetone by activated charcoal. Clin Toxicol 30:371–375, 1992.

58. Goldfrank LR, Flomenbaum NE: Toxic Alcohols. In Goldfrank L (ed): Goldfrank's Toxicologic Emergencies, 6th ed. Stamford, CT, Appleton & Lange, 1998, pp 1049–1060.

59. Mecikalski MB, Depner TA: Peritoneal dialysis for isopropanol poisoning. West J Med 137:322–325, 1982.

60. Schick JB, Milstein JM: Burn hazard of isopropyl alcohol in the neonate. Pediatrics 68:587–588, 1981.

61. Cummins L: Hypoglycemia and convulsions in children following alcohol ingestion. J Pediatr 58:23–26, 1961.

62. Hornfeldt CS: A report of acute ethanol poisoning in a child: Mouthwash versus cologne, perfume, and aftershave. Clin Toxicol 30:115–121, 1992.

63. Ricci LR, Hoffman SA: Ethanol-induced hypoglycemic coma in a child. Ann Emerg Med 11:202–204, 1982.

64. IARC Monographs on the Evaluation of Carcinogenic Risks to Humans: Overall Evaluations of Carcinogenicity: An Updating of IARC Monographs, Vol Supplement 7. Lyon, France, International Agency for Research on Cancer, 1987.

CHAPTER 86

Methanol and Formaldehyde Poisoning

Dag Jacobsen ▪ Kenneth McMartin

METHANOL

Methanol (methyl alcohol, "colonial spirit," "wood alcohol," "solvent alcohol") is a highly toxic alcohol that is widely used industrially as a solvent and in the production of formaldehyde and methylated compounds. It is found in commercial products such as gasoline, antifreeze, gasohol, windshield washer fluid, copy machine fluid, canned heat (Sterno), paint, shellac, and solvents for removing wood finishes. There also is a continuous discussion on the possible use of methanol as an alternative energy source in combustion engines.

Most cases of methanol poisoning are isolated episodes caused by accidental or intentional ingestion. Epidemics of methanol poisoning may occur when it is mistakenly substituted for ethanol by alcoholics or when methanol contaminants are used to ferment (e.g., wine) or illicitly distill (e.g., moonshine whisky) alcoholic beverages. In such circumstances, hundreds of victims have been reported.

Chemical Properties

The chemical structure of methanol is CH_3OH. It is a colorless, volatile, highly flammable liquid with a density of 0.81 g/mL and a weak smell that resembles that of ethanol.

Pathophysiology

Pharmacokinetics of Methanol

Volume of distribution: 0.6 L/kg
Protein binding: none
Mechanisms of clearance: hepatic, renal (minimal), pulmonary (minimal)
Active (toxic) metabolite: formic acid
Methods to enhance clearance: hemodialysis

The lethal dose of methanol is variably given as 30 to 240 mL, with 1 g/kg (1.2 mL/kg) as the best estimate.[1,2] The minimal dose that can cause permanent visual defects is unknown, but most probably ingestion of more than 30 mL (adults) is necessary.

Methanol is absorbed rapidly from the gut, skin, and lungs. It distributes in the total body water compartment of approximately 0.6 L/kg.[3] It is slowly metabolized first to formaldehyde and then to formic acid, which is responsible for the toxic effects in methanol intoxication (Fig. 86-1).[1] The oxidation of formaldehyde occurs rapidly; little formaldehyde accumulates in the serum. The metabolism of methanol by alcohol dehydrogenase, which accounts for about 90% of its elimination, is zero order, with a rate of 2.7 mmol/L/hr (8.5 mg/dL/hr) (half of that of ethanol) in one case.[4] Only small amounts are excreted in expired air and urine. The metabolism of formate depends on the folate pool.[1] Primates have a small folate reserve and are the only species that accumulates formate and experiences methanol toxicity.[5]

Similar to ethylene glycol, the toxicity of methanol is mediated through its metabolites. In contrast to ethylene glycol, however, methanol does not cause significant central nervous system (CNS) depression and ethanol-like inebriation. In the early stage of methanol poisoning, the toxic effects are due to the increasing metabolic acidosis caused by the accumulation of formic acid. Why the eye is the primary target organ for methanol's toxic effects is unknown.[1,6,7]

Formate inhibits cytochrome oxidase, the final enzyme in the mitochondrial electron transport chain, by binding to the ferric iron in the heme moiety of that enzyme. This inhibition occurs in the 5 to 30 mmol/L range,[8] which is similar to the formate concentrations associated with retinal toxicity in humans[1] and other primates.[9,10] Inhibition of mitochondrial energy metabolism markedly increases the production of reactive oxidative molecules and the likelihood of oxidative injury.[11] Formate also seems to increase retinal vulnerability to oxidative injury by causing a depletion of glutathione, which is the major endogenous molecule protecting against oxidative stress in the retina.[12] The retina is exposed to several sources of oxidative stress by virtue of its high intrinsic metabolic rate and its exposure to ambient radiation. Normally, retinal glutathione concentrations are relatively high compared with other organs.[13] Glutathione synthesis is highly dependent on mitochondrial respiration.[14] Studies using a folinic acid–dysfunctional rat model suggest that cones may be more sensitive than rods to long-term damage from methanol poisoning, possibly because of the greater number of mitochondria in cones than in rods.[12]

In late stages, as formate accumulates, the toxicity is caused mainly by the histotoxic effects of formate, which inhibits mitochondrial respiration. The resulting lactate production increases the metabolic acidemia and toxicity of formate, as more formate is protonated and able to

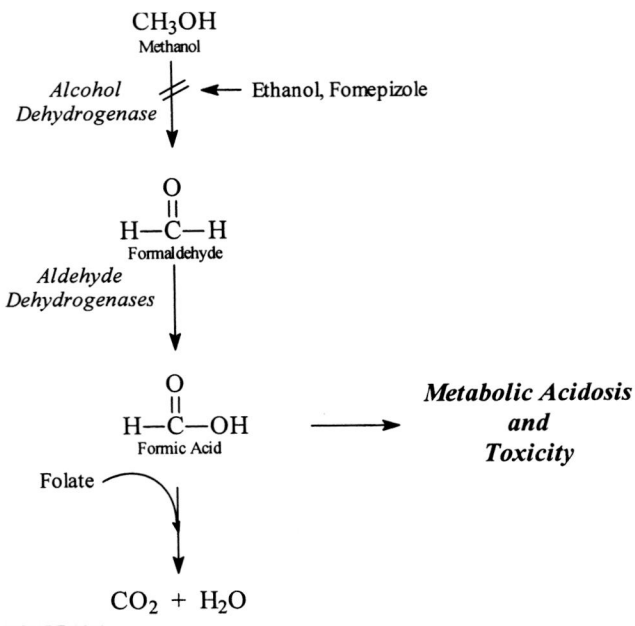

FIGURE 86-1

Methanol metabolism. Ethanol and fomepizole inhibit metabolism by alcohol dehydrogenase. As a result of the small folate pool in primates, little formic acid is metabolized further.

penetrate the blood-brain barrier.[15] A vicious hypoxic cycle is initiated.[16] In the late stages, specific lesions of the putamen may develop. It is not known why this structure is particularly vulnerable in late stages of methanol toxicity. Although the mechanism of these lesions is not known, it is reasonable to believe that the histotoxic effect of formate in late stages, causing a so-called circulus hypoxicus, is a contributing factor (Fig. 86-2).

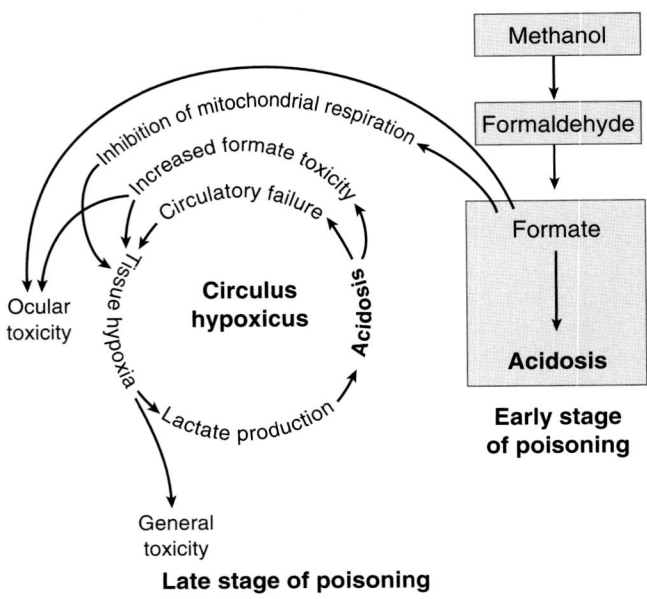

FIGURE 86-2

The "circulus hypoxicus" resulting from methanol ingestion. *(From Jacobsen D: Studies in methanol and ethylene glycol poisonings: Acidosis-kinetics-management. Thesis, University of Oslo, 1985.)*

Clinical Presentation and Life-Threatening Complications

The classic pattern of methanol toxicity includes a latent period of approximately 12 to 24 hours from the time of ingestion to the occurrence of signs and symptoms. It takes this much time for sufficient amounts of formic acid to be produced by methanol metabolism. This latent period may be longer if ethanol is coingested because the latter competitively inhibits methanol metabolism by alcohol dehydrogenase. A latent period of 90 hours has been reported when ethanol is coingested.[3] Methanol itself has few direct effects. Mild CNS depression and ethanol-like intoxication have been reported,[1] but patients with high methanol concentrations (137 mmol/L [438 mg/dL]) also have been sober.[3] With concentrated methanol solutions, nausea, vomiting, and abdominal pain may develop shortly after ingestion. A few cases also may present as acute abdomen, probably because of pancreatitis.[1,4]

The first clinical features of systemic toxicity are usually a feeling of weakness, anorexia, headache, nausea, and vomiting, accompanied or followed by increasing hyperventilation as metabolic acidosis progresses.[1,2,17,18] The first complaint may often be shortness of breath because of hyperventilation. Visual symptoms (blurred vision, decreased acuity, halo vision, tunnel vision, photophobia, and "snow fields") may appear first or with the above-mentioned symptoms. Usually ocular symptoms precede objective signs, such as dilated pupils that are partially reactive or nonreactive to light and funduscopy showing optic disk hyperemia with blurring of the margins.[1,2,18]

If treatment is not initiated at this early stage of poisoning, the patient may develop coma and respiratory and circulatory failure. A few patients also may develop methemoglobinemia with cyanosis, probably because of an interaction between formate and the ferric moiety of hemoglobin.[1]

The toxic effect on the putamen does not lead to detectable signs and symptoms in the acute stage because it is concealed by pronounced CNS depression. Survivors may manifest a Parkinson-like syndrome when they recover from the acute condition, usually after several days to a week.[19,20]

Diagnosis

Methanol poisoning can be difficult to diagnose in the absence of a history, especially if ethanol is coingested and the latency period is prolonged. Methanol usually is detected by gas chromatography or radioimmunoassay. Formate analyses usually are not available in the clinical setting. Laboratory evaluation of suspected methanol poisoning also should include arterial blood gas analysis; complete blood count; measurement of electrolytes, blood urea nitrogen, creatinine, glucose, and amylase; and urinalysis. The history should include the amount, concentration, and time of methanol ingestion; the nature and onset of symptoms; and whether ethanol was coingested. Patients also should be carefully questioned about the presence or absence of visual complaints, gastrointestinal symptoms, and feelings of intoxication.

The physical examination should focus on vital signs (especially respiratory rate) and the neurologic, visual, and cardiopulmonary status. Visual acuity and funduscopic examinations should be performed. The objective signs of ocular toxicity of methanol include dilated pupils, which are partially reactive or nonreactive to light, and optic disk hyperemia with blurring of the disk margins, and later pallor. This blurring of disk margin may look like papillary edema, but there is no diopter difference between the fundus and the disk.

The clinical diagnosis of methanol poisoning is difficult in the absence of a history of ingestion. Methanol poisoning should be considered in every patient presenting with a metabolic acidosis of unknown origin. The general evaluation of a patient with a metabolic acidosis of unknown etiology is described in detail in Chapters 2 and 29.

If methanol assay results are not immediately available, the anion and osmolal gaps should be calculated as a clue to the diagnosis. The accumulation of formate causes a metabolic acidosis, generally with an increased anion gap.[21] The "normal" range for the anion gap ($[Na + K] - [Cl + HCO_3]$) in unselected, acutely hospitalized patients is 13 ± 4 mmol/L; the reference range is 5 to 21 mmol.[22] Because of its low molecular weight (32 d) and the high concentrations associated with toxicity, methanol also increases the serum osmolality, as do other alcohols. This effect can be detected by calculating the difference between the measured osmolality (om) and the calculated osmolality (oc):

$$oc = [2 \times sodium] + blood\ urea\ nitrogen/3 + [glucose/18]$$

$$oc = (1.86 \times Na + blood\ urea\ nitrogen + glucose)/0.93\ (SI\ units)$$

The normal range for the osmolal gap in unselected patients is 5 ± 7 mOsm/kg H_2O (mean $\pm$ SD).[22] An osmolal gap greater than 19 (5 + 2 SD) strongly indicates exogenous osmoles of some kind.[1,21] A methanol concentration of 32 mmol/L (100 mg/dL) increases the osmolal gap by 32/0.93 = 34 mOsm/kg H_2O. The denominator of 0.93 accounts for serum's being 93% water. The osmolal contribution of methanol is so significant that interference from other causes should occur only at methanol levels less than 16 mmol/L (50 mg/dL). The presence of ethanol also influences the osmolal gap; 22 mmol/L (100 mg/dL) theoretically increases the osmolal gap by 22/0.93 = 24 mOsm/kg H_2O.

In late stages of methanol poisoning, all of the methanol is metabolized to formate. At this stage, the anion gap is elevated, but the osmolal gap is normal; formate detection is the only way to confirm the diagnosis. In early stages, or if ethanol is coingested, only the osmolal gap is elevated because the metabolism of methanol to formate has not yet begun.

If the diagnosis is based on the osmolal and anion gaps, osmometry must be performed by the freezing point depression technique and not by the vapor pressure technique because the latter does not detect the increased osmolality caused by volatile alcohols.[18] Computed tomography or magnetic resonance imaging of the brain may show necrosis of the putaminal areas, a finding seen late in the course of methanol poisoning.[18–20]

Increased anion and osmolal gaps also occur in ethylene glycol intoxication. Figure 86-3 enumerates various other causes of increased osmolar or anion gaps. Differentiating the two may be difficult, but the treatments are essentially the same. Hypocalcemia, seizures, and urine oxalate crys-

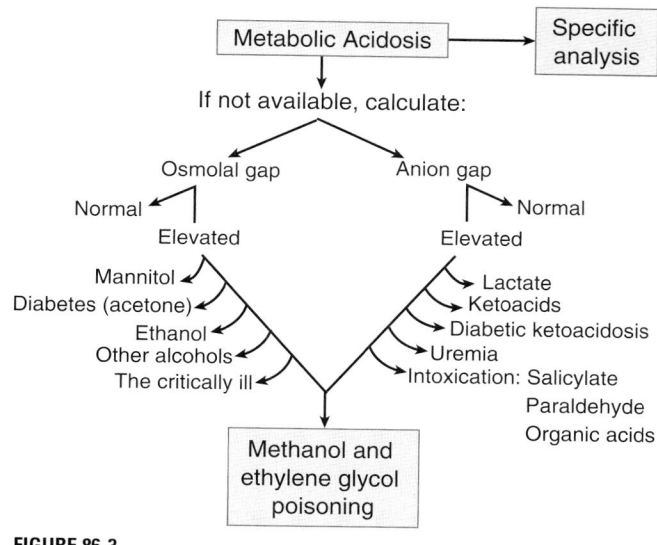

FIGURE 86-3

Causes of an increased anion gap and osmolal gap. Elevations in both gaps strongly indicate methanol or ethylene glycol intoxication. Per 100 mg/dL of alcohol concentration, the osmolal gap is increased by 32/0.93 = 34 for methanol, 22/0.93 = 24 for ethanol, and 16/0.93 = 17 for ethylene glycol.

tals indicate ethylene glycol poisoning; optic disk hyperemia indicates methanol poisoning.[1]

Treatment

Gastric decontamination is unlikely to be beneficial because methanol is rapidly and completely absorbed, and most patients do not present before onset of clinical features. Supportive treatment follows the established principles of intensive supportive care.

The specific treatment of methanol poisoning includes bicarbonate to counteract the metabolic acidosis, ethanol or fomepizole to inhibit methanol metabolism to formate, and selective hemodialysis to remove methanol and formate. Folic acid or folinic acid (leucovorin) is of theoretical value in increasing the metabolism of formate (see Fig. 86-1), but the clinical utility of this effect has not been proven.[23] The standard dose of folinic acid is 50 mg intravenously four times a day. Folic and folinic acids are discussed in Chapter 157.

CORRECTION OF METABOLIC ACIDOSIS

Although not prospectively studied, most clinical toxicologists recommend that the metabolic acidosis be treated aggressively by infusing sodium bicarbonate; 500 to 800 mEq (mmol) may be required during the first few hours. The goal should be full correction of the acidosis. Bicarbonate

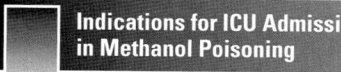

Indications for ICU Admission in Methanol Poisoning

Severe metabolic acidosis (manifested by a base deficit >20 mM)
Need for hemodialysis
General symptomatic indications

treatment decreases the amount of undissociated formic acid, resulting in less access of formate to the CNS.[2,15] In contrast to other types of metabolic acidosis, metabolic acidosis resulting from methanol poisoning should always be treated aggressively with bicarbonate. For acidotic methanol-poisoned patients, alkali treatment must be accompanied by ethanol or fomepizole; otherwise, the acidosis becomes bicarbonate resistant, as more formic acid is produced from the metabolism of methanol.

INHIBITION OF FORMATION OF TOXIC METABOLITES

Fomepizole. Central to the treatment of methanol poisoning is the inhibition of its metabolism to toxic metabolites (see Fig. 86-1). Fomepizole (4-methylpyrazole; Antizol), the frequently used antidote for the treatment of ethylene glycol poisoning,[24,25] is now also documented for use in methanol poisoning.[26–28] As in ethylene glycol poisoning, the major advantage of fomepizole is its documented effectiveness, lack of CNS depression, ease of administration, few side effects, and ability to reduce the need for hemodialysis. The lack of pancreatitis, a well-known side effect of ethanol, also makes fomepizole a more attractive antidote because pancreatitis is reported frequently in methanol-poisoned patients.[29] Fomepizole should be diluted in isotonic saline or dextrose and infused over 30 minutes. The initial loading dose should be 15 mg/kg, followed by 10 mg/kg every 12 hours for four doses, then 15 mg/kg every 12 hours, if necessary. During hemodialysis, the frequency of dosing should be increased to every 4 hours. Current guidelines suggest treatment until the blood level of methanol is less than 6 mmol/L (20 mg/dL) and the patient is without symptoms.

Ethanol. If ethanol is used to inhibit methanol metabolism, most authors recommend a therapeutic blood ethanol level of about 22 mmol/L (100 mg/dL). The amount of ethanol necessary to block methanol metabolism depends on the concomitant methanol level, however, because there is a dynamic competition for the enzyme alcohol dehydrogenase. If the blood methanol level is known, the molar ethanol concentration should be at least a quarter of the molar methanol concentration.[1,5]

A blood ethanol level of 22 mmol/L (100 mg/dL) may be achieved by giving a bolus dose of 0.6 g/kg (13 mmol/kg), followed by 66 to 154 mg/kg/hr (1.4 to 3.3 mmol/kg/hr) intravenously or orally, with the higher maintenance dose for heavy drinkers. Mixing 50 mL of absolute ethanol with 500 mL of isotonic glucose yields a 10% solution if a 10% ethanol solution for intravenous use is unavailable. With this solution, a bolus of 8 mL/kg (over 0.5 hour) followed by 1.5 mL/kg/hr should produce approximately the desired ethanol concentration. The maintenance infusion should be increased or decreased according to measured ethanol concentrations.

Monitoring the blood ethanol concentration is crucial. The blood ethanol concentration should be measured every 1 to 2 hours. Hemodialysis removes ethanol. As a rule of thumb, the maintenance dose of ethanol should at least be doubled during hemodialysis.

HEMODIALYSIS

If a blood methanol concentration cannot readily be obtained, fomepizole or ethanol therapy should be started in any suspected methanol-intoxicated patient with metabolic acidosis, clinical features (dyspnea, visual disturbances), or a history of a potentially toxic ingestion. By consensus, fomepizole or ethanol treatment should be discontinued when the methanol level decreases to less than 6 mmol/L (20 mg/dL). The use of this value has not been empirically validated, however. The lack of reported adverse effects associated with the practice of using the 6 mmol/L (20 mg/dL) value suggests that this practice is safe. It is likely, but unproven, that stopping therapy at higher blood methanol concentrations is also safe. This is particularly true of patients treated with fomepizole, because the inhibition of alcohol dehydrogenase caused by this agent is likely to be effective for more than 12 hours after the last dose.

Hemodialysis effectively removes methanol and formate and can be used to treat a metabolic acidosis.[1] It is difficult to establish strict indications for hemodialysis in methanol poisoning. The only generally accepted absolute indication for hemodialysis is a new visual impairment of any degree in a patient with metabolic acidosis or a detectable methanol level. Relative indications include severe metabolic acidosis (particularly if unresponsive to bicarbonate and ethanol or fomepizole therapy), a blood methanol concentration greater than 16 mmol/L (50 mg/dL), and ingestion of more than 1 g/kg of methanol. The slow elimination of methanol during ethanol/fomepizole treatment (plasma half-life of 45 to 50 hours[1]) must always be considered when the indication for hemodialysis is discussed. From a practical point of view (drunk patient for days in the intensive care unit), this means that ethanol therapy alone is not acceptable in patients with moderate methanol levels, even if they are admitted early or for some other reason (concomitant ethanol ingestion) have little metabolic acidosis. In some of these patients (e.g., blood methanol 32 mmol/L [100 mg/dL], no visual complaints, and almost normal acid-base status), fomepizole treatment should be considered to obviate the need for hemodialysis. If fomepizole is the antidote given, the need for hemodialysis is far less.

Hemodialysis is best continued until the blood methanol level is less than 6 mmol/L (20 mg/dL) and the acidosis is corrected. If methanol analyses are unavailable, we recommend that hemodialysis should be continued for at least 8 hours. Peritoneal dialysis also may remove methanol but not as effectively as hemodialysis.[30] Hemoperfusion is most probably ineffective.

OTHER

Consultation with a poison center or clinical toxicologist is strongly recommended if the treating physician is unfamiliar with the management of methanol poisoning. In addition, physicians who do not know how to obtain either methanol or formate levels may be able to obtain such information from these sources. When the diagnosis of methanol poisoning is made or suspected and hemodialysis is contemplated, a nephrologist should be consulted, especially when the patient is admitted in a late stage or after large ingestions.

All patients with suspected methanol poisoning for whom a methanol level is unavailable should be observed for continued clinical and laboratory evaluation. Every patient with a definite diagnosis of methanol intoxication should be admitted and have an initial and follow-up examination by an ophthalmologist.

If hemodialysis is unavailable, the patient who needs it, or will probably need it, should be transferred to a facility with this capability, and fomepizole or ethanol should be given immediately. Alkali treatment should be provided if any indication of a metabolic acidosis is present. These treatments should be continued during transport. Because plasma ethanol concentrations must be monitored during every 1 to 2 hours, fomepizole is the preferred agent for transfers that may last more than 1 hour. Alternatively, ethanol concentrations may be determined during transport by the use of an alcohol breath analyzer. The use of this kind of instrument requires an awake and cooperative patient, however.

Special Populations

When treating a methanol-poisoned patient, it always must be borne in mind that other people may also have ingested the illicit spirit (containing methanol), believing it was ethanol. If so, these victims must be traced and evaluated in an emergency department.

Common Errors in Methanol Poisoning

Delayed diagnosis because of failure to consider methanol poisoning in the differential diagnosis of metabolic acidosis of unknown origin

Failure to consider that there may be multiple victims when the source of methanol is unknown or is known to be contaminated ethanol

Failure to appreciate that the absence of early symptoms and the presence of normal anion or osmolal gaps do not exclude a potentially toxic methanol ingestion

Failure to observe all patients with known or suspected methanol ingestion until a methanol level can be obtained

Failure to give enough ethanol during hemodialysis because ethanol is removed as well

Failure to have visual function formally assessed by an ophthalmologist in patients with methanol poisoning

---

FORMALDEHYDE

Formaldehyde, the one-carbon aldehyde (HCHO), exists in the gaseous state as a reactive chemical with a distinctive disagreeable odor. The odor is sufficient to provoke flight responses in that humans cannot remain in intolerable atmospheres.[31] The most common liquid form of formaldehyde is formalin, which usually contains 37% formaldehyde in water by weight, along with methanol in concentrations of 15% as a stabilizing agent (preventing polymerization). Cases of oral ingestion of formaldehyde (mostly formalin solutions) have been reported,[32–37] albeit rarely because of the disagreeable nature of the solution.

Formalin is used as a disinfectant, tissue preservative, and embalming solution; occupational exposure generally involves inhalation or skin contact. Formaldehyde vapor is irritating to mucosal membranes and has caused problems in occupational settings where the concentrations reach levels of 1 ppm.[38] Formaldehyde also is present in resins, insu-

lation, plywood, and textiles, such that it also has been found in the indoor air of residential and business areas, particularly where urea-formaldehyde resins are used in insulation or furnishings. Regarding such vapor exposures, a major controversy exists as to whether formaldehyde is carcinogenic. The U.S. Environmental Protection Agency and the International Agency for Research on Cancer have classified formaldehyde as a probable human carcinogen.[31]

Pathophysiology

Formaldehyde reacts readily and covalently with amine groups such as are found in proteins and nucleic acids. Animal studies have confirmed that formaldehyde produces protein-DNA cross-links.[39] Such covalent adducts or cross-links would produce a loss of protein or nucleic acid function, which is a potential mechanism by which toxicity could be produced.

Formaldehyde is highly irritating to mucosal tissues, such as the eyes, nose, and respiratory tract, either by direct caustic reaction or through covalent interactions. These reactions include tearing, coughing, sneezing, and sometimes bronchospasm. Formaldehyde also reduces mucociliary clearance activity[31] and may affect lower respiratory tissue if attached to particulates. Formaldehyde may provoke allergic responses, including contact dermatitis and asthmatic reactions.[40]

Ingested formaldehyde is apparently absorbed rapidly into the bloodstream.[32] It is then rapidly degraded in the tissues by metabolism to formic acid, primarily through the enzyme formaldehyde dehydrogenase.[41] This enzyme catalyzes the reaction of glutathione, formaldehyde, and nicotinamide-adenine dinucleotide to yield S-formylglutathionine, which is hydrolyzed to formate and reduced glutathione by S-formylglutathionine hydrolase. These activities are widely expressed in all human tissues, although the highest activity is in the liver. Formaldehyde also can be oxidized to formate by a nonspecific aldehyde dehydrogenase and by the folate-dependent, one-carbon metabolic system.[38]

Because of the widespread metabolism, formaldehyde is eliminated extremely rapidly from the blood, with a half-life of 1 to 2 minutes.[42] Several studies in animals and one case report have indicated that systemic formaldehyde is completely converted to formic acid within a relatively short time.[32,43,44] Disposition of HCHO goes eventually to carbon dioxide (via oxidation of formate), although a small amount is incorporated into macromolecules via folate-dependent pathways or direct interaction of HCHO with amine groups. The systemic toxicity of formaldehyde primarily results from the accumulation of formic acid and the ensuing metabolic acidosis.[32]

Clinical Presentation

Several case reports of formalin ingestion have provided a general clinical picture. Ingestion of 45 mL of the typical 37% solution[34] has produced gastrointestinal ulceration with little systemic toxicity, whereas massive systemic toxicity and lethality were observed after consumption of 120 mL.[32] Ingestion of formalin often produces immediate vomiting and severe abdominal pain. Ulceration of the oropharynx, esophagus, and stomach is widespread. The duodenum appears less affected and often normal. In one patient who survived, these lesions did regress over 4 weeks, although there was some residual scarring of the distal body and antrum.[34]

Respiration becomes labored, with shortness of breath. Metabolic acidosis, with pH of 6.9, is reported.[32,36] Chest radiographs show pleural effusions and infiltrates. Muscles spasm, and the body may become stiff and rigid. There is laboratory evidence of rhabdomyolysis.[36]

The CNS becomes depressed, with weakness leading to stupor and coma. Hypotension and shock follow as the gastrointestinal damage and acidosis worsen. Ventricular tachycardia has been reported. Eventually anuria ensues, indicating development of renal failure. Death due to the failure of multiple organ systems can occur within 24 hours.[32]

Dialysis systems contaminated with formaldehyde have been associated with the occurrence of hemolysis[44] in patients. Chronic exposure to formaldehyde may therefore cause hemolytic anemia. Although significant formate accumulation seems to occur in patients with formaldehyde exposure, minimal ocular toxicity seems to be present. A patient with formaldehyde poisoning and metabolic acidosis should have vision checked, however, as noted earlier under methanol poisoning.

Diagnostic Considerations

A positive exposure history is the initial key to diagnosis. In a patient without confirmed ingestion, several features aid in the diagnosis. First, the odor of formaldehyde should be observed on the breath. On lavage in one patient, this odor was noted strongly in the gastric contents.[32,36] Two indicators of potential formaldehyde exposure are the presence of severe lesions of the gastrointestinal tract, especially in the oropharynx, and a severe, systemic metabolic acidosis (a decreased arterial blood pH, an increased anion gap, or a decreased serum bicarbonate concentration). Because these indicators are not definitive, an accompanying increase in blood formate concentrations would suggest that there had been an ingestion of formic acid or formaldehyde. Although the laboratory measurement of blood formate concentrations is rarely available, the treatment for either ingestion should be the same.

Treatment

Because of the potential for massive multiorgan damage, aggressive supportive care needs to be instituted rapidly.[32,36] Rapid intubation and ventilatory support should be instituted for standard indications. Gastric lavage with saline or bicarbonate solutions, even if applied within 1 to 3 hours of ingestion, is probably of questionable value because of the potential for further corrosive damage. If there is little corrosive damage to the esophagus, the benefit of decontamination must be weighed against the risk. The possibility of corrosive injury and the unlikely efficacy of the procedure suggest, however, that lavage should not be performed. Intravenous fluids help maintain cardiovascular and renal function. If necessary, vasopressors should be given to maintain blood pressure.

The mainstay of treatment beyond supportive care should be to aggressively counteract the systemic accumulation of formic acid. Initially, this counteraction should include intravenous administration of sodium bicarbonate to combat the acidosis.[32,36] Although never attempted in previous cases, administration of folate or folinic acid, as detailed earlier, should increase the metabolic elimination of formate. Hemodialysis should be initiated as soon as possible. The indications for hemodialysis are similar to those enumerated for methanol. In one patient who had consumed a lethal amount of formaldehyde and was nearly moribund, hemodialysis was started within 6 hours of ingestion.[36] The patient improved rapidly, the acidosis was reversed by the end of dialysis, and the patient recovered completely.

REFERENCES

1. Jacobsen D, McMartin KE: Methanol and ethylene glycol poisonings: Mechanism of toxicity, clinical course, diagnosis and treatment. Med Toxicol 1:309–334, 1986.
2. Roe O: Species differences in methanol poisonings. Crit Rev Toxicol 10:275–286, 1982.
3. Jacobsen D, Jansen H, Wiik-Larsen E, et al: Studies on methanol poisoning. Acta Med Scand 212:5–10, 1982.
4. Jacobsen D, Webb R, Collins TD, et al: Methanol and formate kinetics in late diagnosed methanol intoxication. Med Toxicol 3:418–423, 1988.
5. Makar AB, Tephly TR, Mannering GJ: Methanol metabolism in the monkey. Mol Pharmacol 4:471–483, 1968.
6. Martinasevic MK, Green MD, Baron J, Tephly TR: Folate and 10-formyltetrahydrofolate dehydrogenase in human and rat retina: Relation to methanol toxicity. Toxicol Appl Pharmacol 141:373–381, 1996.
7. McKellar MJ, Hidajat RR, Elder MJ: Acute ocular methanol toxicity: Clinical and electrophysiological features. Aust N Z J Ophthalmol 25:225–230, 1997.
8. Nicholls P: The effects of formate on cytochrome aa3 and on electron transport in the intact respiratory chain. Biochim Biophys Acta 430:13–29, 1976.
9. Hayreh MM, Hayreh SS, Baumbach GL, et al: Ocular toxicity of methanol: An experimental study. In Merigan W, Weiss B (eds): Neurotoxicity of the Visual System. New York, Raven Press, 1980, pp 35–53.
10. Hayreh MS, Hayreh SS, Baumbach P, et al: Methyl alcohol poisoning: III. Ocular toxicity of methanol: An experimental study. Arch Ophthalmol 95:1851–1858, 1977.
11. Erecinska M, Wilson DF: Inhibitors of cytochrome c oxidase. Pharmacol Ther 8:1–20, 1980.
12. Seme MT, Summerfelt P, Neitz J, et al: Differential recovery of retinal function after mitochondrial inhibition by methanol intoxication. Invest Ophthalmol Vis Sci 42:834–841, 2001.
13. Schutte M, Werner P: Redistribution of glutathione in the ischemic rat retina. Neurosci Lett 246:53–56, 1998.
14. Meister A: Mitochondrial changes associated with glutathione deficiency. Biochim Biophys Acta 127:35–42, 1995.
15. Herken W, Rietbrock N, Henschler D: Zum mechanismus der methanol-vergiftung: Toxisches Agens und Einfluss der Sure-Basenstatus auf die Giftwirkung. Arch Toxicol 24:214–238, 1969.
16. Jacobsen D: Studies in Methanol and Ethylene Glycol Poisonings: Acidosis-Kinetics-Management. Thesis, University of Oslo, 1985.
17. Roe O: The metabolism and toxicity of methanol. Pharmacol Rev 7:399–412, 1955.
18. Jacobsen D, McMartin KE: Antidotes for methanol and ethylene glycol poisoning. Clin Toxicol 35:127–143, 1997.
19. Aquilonius SM, Bergstrom K, Enoksson P, et al: Cerebral computed tomography in methanol intoxication. J Comput Assist Tomogr 4:425–428, 1980.
20. Kuteifan K, Oesterle H, Tajahmady T, et al: Necrosis and haemorrhage of the putamen in methanol poisoning shown on MRI. Neuroradiology 40:158–160, 1998.
21. Enger E: Acidosis, gaps and poisonings. Acta Med Scand 212:1–3, 1982.

22. Aabakken L, Johansen KS, Rydningen EB, et al: Osmolal and anion gaps in patients admitted to an emergency medical department. Hum Exp Toxicol 13:131–134, 1994.

23. Osterloh JD, Pond SM, Grady S, et al: Serum formate concentrations in methanol intoxication as criterion for hemodialysis. Ann Intern Med 104:200–203, 1986.

24. Baud FJ, Galliot M, Astier A, et al: Treatment of ethylene glycol poisoning with intravenous 4-methylpyrazole. N Engl J Med 319:97–100, 1988.

25. Jacobsen D: New treatment for ethylene glycol poisoning. N Engl J Med 340:879–881, 1999.

26. Brent J, McMartin KE, Phillips S, Aaron C, Kulig K: Fomepizole (4-methylpyrazole) treatment of methanol poisoning. N Engl J Med 344:424–429, 2001.

27. Hantson P, Wallemacq P, Brau M, et al: Two cases of acute methanol poisoning partially treated by oral 4-methylpyrazole. Intensive Care Med 25:528–531, 1999.

28. Burns MJ, Graudins A, Aaron CK, et al: Treatment of methanol poisoning with intravenous 4-methylpyrazole. Ann Emerg Med 30:829–832, 1997.

29. Hantson P, Mahieu P: Pancreatic injury following acute methanol poisoning. Clin Toxicol 38:297–303, 2000.

30. Keyvan-Larijani H, Tannenberg AM: Methanol intoxication. Arch Intern Med 134:293–296, 1974.

31. Council on Scientific Affairs: Formaldehyde. JAMA 261:1183–1187, 1989.

32. Eells JT, McMartin KE, Black K, et al: Formaldehyde poisoning: Rapid metabolism to formic acid. JAMA 246:1237–1238, 1981.

33. Kline BS: Formaldehyde poisoning. Ann Intern Med 36:220–228, 1925.

34. Kochhar R, Nanada V, Nagi B, Mehta SK: Formaldehyde-induced corrosive gastric cicatrization: Case report. Hum Toxicol 5:381–382, 1986.

35. Roy M Jr, Calonje MA, Mouton R: Corrosive gastritis after formaldehyde ingestion. N Engl J Med 266:1248–1250, 1962.

36. Spellman GG: Formaldehyde poisoning successfully treated with hemodialysis. J Iowa Med Soc 73:175–176, 1983.

37. Vinson PP, Harrington SW: Cicatricial stricture of the stomach without involvement of the esophagus following ingestion of formaldehyde. JAMA 93:917–918, 1929.

38. Ulsamer AG, Beall JR, Kang HK, Frazier JA: Overview of health effects of formaldehyde. In Saxena J (ed): Hazard Assessment of Chemicals: Current Developments, Vol 3. New York, Academic Press, 1984, pp 337–400.

39. Restani P, Galli CL: Oral toxicity of formaldehyde and its derivatives. Crit Rev Toxicol 21:315–328, 1991.

40. Imbus HR: Clinical evaluation of patients with complaints related to formaldehyde exposure. J Allergy Clin Immunol 76:831–840, 1985.

41. Uotila L, Koivusalo M: Formaldehyde dehydrogenase from human liver: Purification, properties and evidence for the formation of glutathione thiol esters by the enzyme. J Biol Chem 249:7653–7663, 1974.

42. McMartin KE, Martin-Amat G, Noker PE, Tephly TR: Lack of a role for formaldehyde in methanol poisoning in the monkey. Biochem Pharmacol 28:645–649, 1979.

43. Malorny G, Rietbrock N, Schneider M: Die oxydation des formaldehyds zu ameisensaure im blut, ein beitrag zum stoffwechsel des formaldehyds. N-S Arch Exp Path Pharmak 250:419–436, 1965.

44. Orringer EP, Mattern WD: Formaldehyde-induced hemolysis during chronic hemodialysis. N Engl J Med 294:1416–1420, 1976.

CHAPTER **87**

Chlorophenoxy Herbicides

Sally M. Bradberry ■ J. Allister Vale ■ Barbara E. Watt ■ Alex T. Proudfoot

Chlorophenoxy herbicides are weed killers that act as synthetic auxins (plant "hormones") and cause plant death by disrupting nutrient transport and growth. They are used widely for the control of broad-leaved weeds in pastures and cereal crops and along public rights of way. Chlorophenoxy herbicides are of limited persistence in the environment. These herbicides occasionally are coformulated with ioxynil or bromoxynil or both, which generally are more toxic than chlorophenoxy herbicides and have been shown experimentally to uncouple oxidative phosphorylation.

CHEMISTRY

Structurally, chlorophenoxy herbicides comprise an aliphatic carboxylic acid moiety attached to a chlorine-substituted or methyl-substituted aromatic ring. The most common herbicide of this class is 2,4-dichlorophenoxyacetic acid (2,4-D); its structural formula and that of related compounds are shown in Figure 87-1. Chlorophenoxy herbicides typically are formulated as salts or esters.

PATHOPHYSIOLOGY

Although not elucidated fully, experimental studies indicate the potential involvement of the following mechanisms in chlorophenoxy herbicide toxicity:

1. Dose-dependent cell membrane damage.[1] This mechanism is likely to be important in the mediation of central nervous system toxicity by damaging the blood-brain barrier[2] and disrupting neuronal membrane transport mechanisms.[3]
2. Interference in cellular metabolic pathways involving acetyl coenzyme A. Chlorophenoxy herbicides are related structurally to acetic acid and are able to form analogues of acetyl coenzyme A, such as 2,4-D-CoA. Also, chlorophenoxy herbicides can enter the acetylcholine synthetic pathway with the subsequent formation of choline esters (e.g., 2,4-D-ACh), which may act as false cholinergic messengers at muscarinic and nicotinic synapses.[4,5]

3. Uncoupling of oxidative phosphorylation due to the above-listed second mechanism or due to damage to intracellular membranes.[6] A variety of cellular activities may be compromised by subsequent adenosine triphosphate (ATP) depletion, including ATP-dependent ion pumps, DNA and protein synthesis, and processes involved in the maintenance of cell shape.

TOXICOKINETICS

Chlorophenoxy compounds are absorbed rapidly after oral administration in humans,[7,8] but dermal[9,8] and inhalational[10] absorption is limited. When absorbed, the salts or esters of these herbicides dissociate or hydrolyze rapidly. The free acid binds to serum albumin; increased length of the acid chain and increased substitution of the aromatic ring favor binding. Chlorophenoxy herbicides have relatively high volumes of distribution (approximately 0.1 L/kg for 2,4-D in humans).[11] However, bioavailability is affected not only by the extent of protein binding, which is saturable, but also by the extent of herbicide ionization. Because chlorophenoxy herbicides are acids (the pK_a of 2,4-D is 2.73), at physiologic pH only a small percentage is in the nonionized form and available to penetrate lipid membranes. 2,4-D undergoes little metabolic transformation in humans; the free acid is excreted predominately unchanged in urine[7] with small amounts as a 2,4-D conjugate. Limited experimental data suggest a similar process for other chlorophenoxy herbicides.[8] Active renal tubular secretion has been shown as a primary mechanism of renal clearance in animals.[8] The elimination half-life of 2,4-D in humans is of the order of 20 to 30 hours.[7,8]

CLINICAL PRESENTATION AND LIFE-THREATENING COMPLICATIONS

Chlorophenoxy herbicide poisoning is uncommon but may produce severe sequelae. Most cases of serious poisoning involve deliberate ingestion of 2,4-D alone, in combination with other chlorophenoxy herbicides, or in combination with

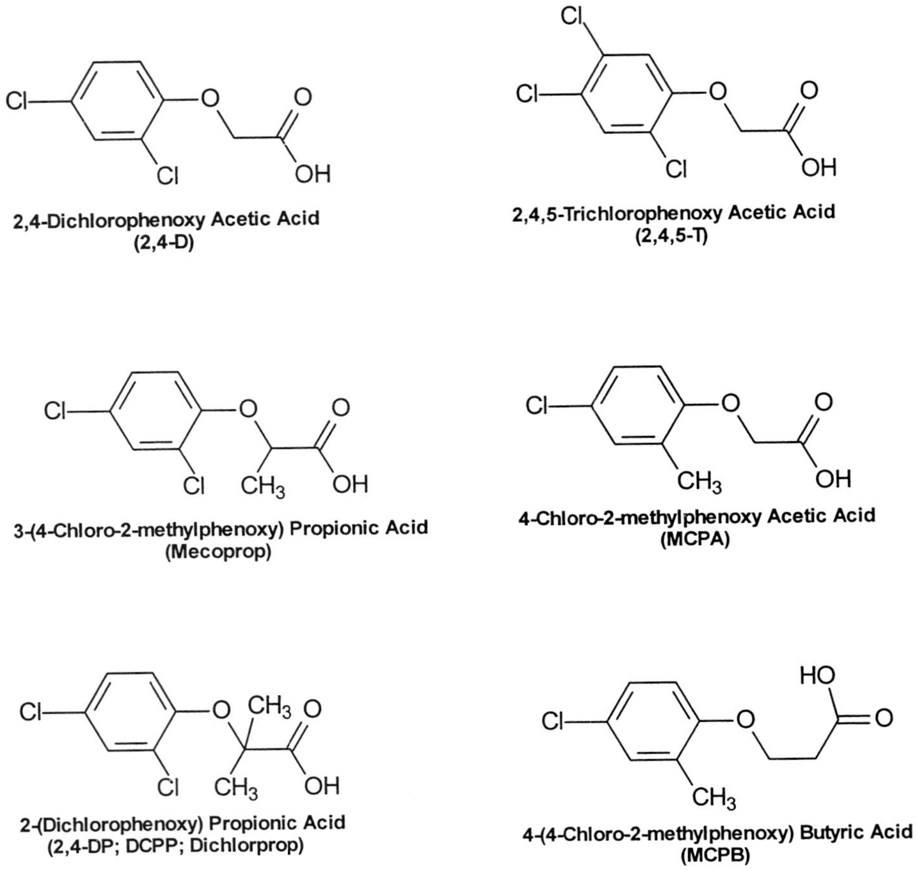

2,4-Dichlorophenoxy Acetic Acid
(2,4-D)

2,4,5-Trichlorophenoxy Acetic Acid
(2,4,5-T)

3-(4-Chloro-2-methylphenoxy) Propionic Acid
(Mecoprop)

4-Chloro-2-methylphenoxy Acetic Acid
(MCPA)

2-(Dichlorophenoxy) Propionic Acid
(2,4-DP; DCPP; Dichlorprop)

4-(4-Chloro-2-methylphenoxy) Butyric Acid
(MCPB)

FIGURE 87-1

Chemical structures of the chlorophenoxy herbicides.

ioxynil or bromoxynil. It is difficult to draw any conclusions regarding the relative toxicities of the different herbicides in this class.

Ingestion

Vomiting is a prominent early feature of chlorophenoxy herbicide ingestion and may be accompanied by burning in the mouth, abdominal pain, and diarrhea. Severe corrosive effects, including gastrointestinal hemorrhage, are rare and probably due predominantly to surfactants and solvents in the formulation. Gastrointestinal fluid loss, vasodilation, and direct myocardial toxicity contribute to hypotension, which may precipitate renal failure.

Rapid onset of coma is common in severe cases and may be preceded by a period of agitation and confusion. Coma is almost invariable in patients who die and often lasts several days in patients who survive. The incidence of other neurologic features varies widely. Hypertonia, hyperreflexia, clonus, and occasionally extensor plantar responses suggest upper motor neuron involvement.[12] Miosis, nystagmus, ataxia, hallucinations, and convulsions also have been reported.

Coma is associated frequently with inadequate ventilation. Aspiration of gastric contents may contribute to pulmonary complications. Hemoptysis and pulmonary edema may occur. Hypoventilation secondary to central nervous system depression is the primary cause of hypoxia, although respiratory

muscle weakness also may occur as part of a generalized myopathy. In such cases, there may be limb weakness or reduced or absent tendon reflexes and increased creatine kinase activity.

Some degree of peripheral neuromuscular involvement is common, as evidenced by loss of tendon reflexes, muscle twitching, fasciculation, weakness, or myotonia. Electromyography evidence of a peripheral neuropathy has been reported rarely.[13,14] Neuromuscular effects may persist for several weeks.

Metabolic complications include acidosis, hyperthermia in the absence of infection (possibly reflecting uncoupling of oxidative phosphorylation), and rhabdomyolysis. The latter may contribute to increased aspartate and alanine aminotransferase activities. Thrombocytopenia, hemolytic anemia, and hypocalcemia are recognized rarely.

Inhalational or Dermal Exposure

Because dermal and inhalational absorption of chlorophenoxy herbicides is poor, acute poisoning via these routes is uncommon. Local irritation to the skin and mucous membranes may occur, but there are few reports of systemic toxicity after such exposures. Interpretation of cases in which systemic effects are described is complicated, and the etiologic role of chlorophenoxy herbicides in many has been challenged.[15] Reported features include mild-to-moderate gastrointestinal symptoms followed by variable manifestations of peripheral neuropathy or myopathy.[16–22] Despite widespread use, there have been no published reports of systemic chlorophenoxy herbicide poisoning after dermal or inhalational exposure since at least the 1980s and no reported fatalities from such exposures.

DIAGNOSIS

There should be no diagnostic difficulty when a history of deliberate chlorophenoxy herbicide ingestion is forthcoming, but familiarity with the clinical presentation may hasten diagnosis when self-harm is suspected but no history is available. In cases of poisoning by an unknown substance, the toxicologic differential diagnosis most prominently includes poisoning by salicylates or psychotropic drugs. Measurement of plasma chlorophenoxy herbicide concentrations may be undertaken for diagnostic confirmation, although these assays are not widely available. There is no definite relationship between total plasma chlorophenoxy herbicide concentrations and severity of poisoning, although Flanagan and colleagues[23] suggested that a total plasma chlorophenoxy herbicide concentration greater than 500 mg/L is associated with severe toxicity.

TREATMENT

Initial assessment and treatment of patients exposed to chlorophenoxy herbicides should follow generally accepted guidelines of current practice for external and gastrointestinal decontamination and supportive care. In vitro studies showed that chlorophenoxy herbicides are adsorbed to activated charcoal.[24] The administration of oral activated charcoal, 50 to 100 g in an adult, may be considered reasonable in patients who have ingested a potentially toxic amount of a chlorophenoxy herbicide within 1 hour. Activated charcoal therapy has not been shown, however, to affect the outcome of chlorophenoxy herbicide–poisoned patients. Gastrointestinal decontamination is discussed in Chapter 5. Although most patients can be managed with symptomatic and supportive care alone, controversy surrounds the use of urine alkalization, hemodialysis, and hemoperfusion in enhancing herbicide elimination in severely poisoned patients.

Indications for ICU Admission in Pesticide Poisoning

Severe vomiting and diarrhea
Hypotension
Central neurologic or neuromuscular symptoms or signs

Urine Alkalization

No controlled trials of urine alkalization have been carried out in chlorophenoxy herbicide poisoning. Despite several case reports claiming enhanced elimination with urine alkalization,[23,25] there are sufficient data to examine this claim only

for one patient.[13,26] The patient, a 39-year-old man, developed features of severe poisoning after the ingestion of a calculated 6.8 g of 2,4-D and 13.6 g of mecoprop. The admission urine pH was 6.4, and the plasma 2,4-D concentration was 400 mg/L. An "alkaline diuresis" comprising 14 L of fluid containing 69.3 g of sodium bicarbonate (825 mmol) over 48 hours[13] was instituted approximately 42 hours postingestion, but a urine pH greater than 7.5 was not achieved until 70 to 75 hours postingestion.

The renal 2,4-D clearance corrected to a urine flow of 1 mL/min was related directly to urine pH ($r = 0.99$) and was estimated to increase almost fivefold for each unit increase in urine pH. The mean corrected 2,4-D renal clearance was 0.28 mL/min over the urine pH range 5.1 to 6.5 and 9.6 mL/min over the urine pH range 7.55 to 8.8 (Table 87-1).[26] At pH 5.1 and 8.3, the *uncorrected* 2,4-D renal clearances were 0.14 mL/min and 63 mL/min. The plasma half-life of 2,4-D decreased from approximately 219 hours before alkaline diuresis to 3.7 hours at 96 to 112 hours postingestion when the urine pH exceeded 8.0,[13] and the amount recovered in the urine was 6.66 g.

Similarly the renal mecoprop clearance corrected for urine flow the same as for 2,4-D was related directly to urine pH ($r = 0.94$). It was estimated to double for each unit increase in urine pH,[13] was 0.38 mL/min over the urine pH range 5.1 to 6.5, and was 2.08 mL/min over the urine pH range 7.55 to 8.8 (see Table 87-1). The plasma half-life of mecoprop was shortened from 39 to 14 hours, and the amount recovered in the urine was 7.64 g.[13] Clinical improvement paralleled the decrease in 2,4-D and mecoprop concentrations, and consciousness was regained on the fourth day after ingestion, when the plasma 2,4-D and mecoprop concentrations were approximately 100 mg/L.

The uncorrected renal 2,4-D clearance (0.14 mL/min at urine pH 5.1) determined by Prescott and coworkers[13] was similar to that found previously (0.17 to 1.4 mL/min).[27] A high 2,4-D renal clearance was achieved, however, only when the urine pH was greater than 7.5 and urine flow was greater than 200 mL/hr. The maximum uncorrected 2,4-D renal clearance of 63 mL/min at pH 8.3[13] would have required a urine flow rate of approximately 600 mL/hr and compared favorably with that achieved with hemodialysis (56.3 to 72.9 mL/min).[28] The corrected renal clearance data show, however, that urine alkalization without high urine flow is markedly less efficient than hemodialysis as a means of removing 2,4-D.

The less beneficial effect of alkaline diuresis on mecoprop clearance compared with 2,4-D clearance may be explained by the much greater clearance of mecoprop by metabolism and the fact that mecoprop is a weaker organic acid (pK_a of 3.78 and 2.73). Renal mecoprop clearance would be less affected by changes in urine pH.

Hemoperfusion and Hemodialysis

Durakovic and associates[28] treated four patients with 2,4-D poisoning by hemodialysis. In two cases, resin hemoperfusion also was instituted. The dialysis clearance in one patient was 68.7 mL/min, and in the two patients receiving combined therapy, the clearances were 56.3 mL/min and 72.9 mL/min, suggesting that hemodialysis with or without hemoperfusion is more efficient than urine alkalization, although urine alkalization combined with a high urine

TABLE 87-1 Effect of Urine Alkalization on Plasma Half-Life and Mean Corrected (to 1 mL/min Urine Flow) Renal Clearance of 2,4-Dichlorophenoxyacetic Acid (2,4-D) and Mecoprop

URINE pH (RANGE)	2,4-D		MECOPROP	
	Clearance (mL/min)	Half-Life (hr)	Clearance (mL/min)	Half-Life (hr)
5.10–6.5	0.28	219	0.38	39
6.55–7.5	1.14	42	0.65	22
7.55–8.8	9.60	4.7	2.08	14

Adapted from Park J, Darrien I, Prescott LF: Pharmacokinetic studies in severe intoxication with 2,4-D and mecoprop. Proc Eur Soc Toxicol 18:154–155, 1977.

flow (600 mL/hr) produced similar clearance values.[13,26] Nonetheless, in all severe cases, hemodialysis is the preferred elimination treatment because it greatly enhances clearance without the need for urine pH manipulation and the administration of substantial amounts of intravenous fluid to compromised patients.

Criteria for ICU Discharge in Pesticide Poisoning

Resolution of severe vomiting and diarrhea without new features
Resolution of hypotension, without new features
Resolution of, or substantial improvement in, central neurologic or neuromuscular symptoms or signs

Common Errors in Management of Pesticide Poisoning

Failure to consider the potential contribution to the clinical picture of solvents and adjuvants in the formulation
Inadequate monitoring and clinical review in first few hours after a substantial ingestion
Assumption that pyrexia must be due to infection when other metabolic explanations are possible

Key Points in Pesticide Poisoning

1. Severe poisoning is likely only after ingestion.
2. The level of consciousness may deteriorate rapidly after substantial ingestion.
3. Neuromuscular effects may persist for several weeks.

REFERENCES

1. Suwalsky M, Benites M, Villena F, et al: Interaction of 2,4-dichlorophenoxyacetic acid (2,4-D) with cell and model membranes. Biochim Biophys Acta 1285:267–276, 1996.
2. Hervonen H, Elo HA, Ylitalo P: Blood-brain barrier damage by 2-methyl-4-chlorophenoxyacetic acid herbicide in rats. Toxicol Appl Pharmacol 65:23–31, 1982.
3. Kim CS, Keizer RF, Ambrose WW, et al: Effects of 2,4,5-trichlorophenoxyacetic acid and quinolinic acid on 5-hydroxy-3-indoleacetic acid transport by the rabbit choroid plexus: Pharmacology and electron microscopic cytochemistry. Toxicol Appl Pharmacol 90:436–444, 1987.
4. Sastry BVR, Clark CP, Janson VE: Formation of 2:4-dichlorophenoxyacetylcholine (2:4-D-ACh) in human placenta and fetal growth retardation. Neurotoxicology 16:763, 1995.
5. Sastry BVR, Janson VE, Clark CP, et al: Cellular toxicity of 2,4,5-trichlorophenoxyacetic acid: Formation of 2,4,5-trichlorophenoxyacetylcholine. Cell Mol Biol 43:549–557, 1997.
6. Zychlinski L, Zolnierowicz S: Comparison of uncoupling activities of chlorophenoxy herbicides in rat liver mitochondria. Toxicol Lett 52:25–34, 1990.
7. Sauerhoff MW, Braun WH, Blau GE, et al: The fate of 2,4-dichlorophenoxyacetic acid (2,4-D) following oral administration to man. Toxicology 8:3–11, 1977.
8. Arnold EK, Beasley VR: The pharmacokinetics of chlorinated phenoxy acid herbicides: A literature review. Vet Hum Toxicol 31:121–125, 1989.
9. Feldmann RJ, Maibach HI: Percutaneous penetration of some pesticides and herbicides in man. Toxicol Appl Pharmacol 28:126–132, 1974.
10. Grover R, Cessna AJ, Muir NI, et al: Factors affecting the exposure of ground-rig applicators to 2,4-D dimethylamine salt. Arch Environ Contam Toxicol 15:677–686, 1986.
11. Baselt RC: Disposition of Toxic Drugs and Chemicals in Man, 5th ed. Foster City, CA, Chemical Toxicology Institute, 2000.
12. Dudley AW Jr, Thapar NT: Fatal human ingestion of 2,4-D, a common herbicide. Arch Pathol 94:270–275, 1972.
13. Prescott LF, Park J, Darrien I: Treatment of severe 2,4-D and mecoprop intoxication with alkaline diuresis. Br J Clin Pharmacol 7:111–116, 1979.
14. Lankosz-Lauterbach J, Kaczor Z, Kacinski M, et al: Severe polyneuropathy in a 3-year-old child after dichlorophenoxyacetic herbicide—Chwastox—intoxication, treated successfully with plasmapheresis (PF). Przegl Lek 54:750–752, 1997.
15. Mattsson JL, Eisenbrandt DL: The improbable association between the herbicide 2,4-D and polyneuropathy. Biomed Environ Sci 3:43–51, 1990.
16. Berkley MC, Magee KR: Neuropathy following exposure to a dimethylamine salt of 2,4-D. Arch Intern Med 111:351–352, 1963.
17. Goldstein NP, Jones PH, Brown JR: Peripheral neuropathy after exposure to an ester of dichlorophenoxyacetic acid. JAMA 171:1306–1309, 1959.
18. Todd RL: A case of 2,4-D intoxication. J Iowa Med Soc 52:663–664, 1962.
19. Tsapko VG: [On the probable harmful action of the herbicide 2,4-D on agricultural workers]. Gig Sanit 31:79–80, 1966.
20. Kolny H, Kita K: Zatrucie Aminopielikiem D. Med Pr 29:61–63, 1978.
21. Paggiaro PL, Martino E, Mariotti S: Su un caso di intossicazione da acido 2,4-diclorofenossiacetico. Med Lav 65:128–135, 1974.
22. Bezuglyi VP, Fokina KV, Komarova LI, et al: [Clinical manifestations of long-term sequels of acute poisoning with 2,4-dichlorophenoxyacetic acid]. Gig Tr Prof Zabol 3:47–48, 1979.

23. Flanagan RJ, Meredith TJ, Ruprah M, et al: Alkaline diuresis for acute poisoning with chlorophenoxy herbicides and ioxynil. Lancet 335:454–458, 1990.

24. Grover R, Smith AE: Adsorption studies with the acid and dimethylamine forms of 2,4-D and dicamba. Can J Soil Sci 54:179–186, 1974.

25. Schmoldt A, Iwersen S, Schlüter W: Massive ingestion of the herbicide 2-methyl-4-chlorophenoxyacetic acid (MCPA). J Toxicol Clin Toxicol 35:405–408, 1997.

26. Park J, Darrien I, Prescott LF: Pharmacokinetic studies in severe intoxication with 2,4-D and mecoprop. Proc Eur Soc Toxicol 18:154–155, 1977.

27. Wells WDE, Wright N, Yeoman WB: Clinical features and management of poisoning with 2,4-D and mecoprop. J Toxicol Clin Toxicol 18:273–276, 1981.

28. Durakovic Z, Durakovic A, Durakovic S, et al: Poisoning with 2,4-dichlorophenoxyacetic acid treated by hemodialysis. Arch Toxicol 66:518–521, 1992.

CHAPTER **88**

Fumigants

Scott D. Phillips

Fumigants are nonspecific pesticides that exist as gases or vapors or are capable of being changed to one of these states. They represent a diverse group of compounds (Table 88-1) that are dissimilar in their chemical structures, physical properties (Table 88-2), and mechanisms of injury. This broad category of substances includes liquids (ethylene dibromide, dibromochloropropane, formaldehyde) that can vaporize, solids that may release toxic gases when mixed with water (zinc phosphide, aluminum phosphide), cyanide salts (sodium or calcium cyanide) that liberate hydrogen cyanide gas when acidified, and gases (methyl bromide, hydrogen cyanide, ethylene oxide). Fumigants are used to control pests in confined, enclosed, or sealed environments. Examples of typical fumigant targets are rodents or insects in stored grain products, wood-destroying insects such as dry-wood termites or wood beetles, and nematodes and fungi in the soil that adversely affect crop production. Examples of specific confined areas are railroad hopper-cars, silos, and storage areas. Cyanide is discussed in Chapter 95 and is not addressed in this chapter.

Fumigant gases or vapors are intended to dissipate after the enclosed space has been opened and ventilated. For organisms living within that enclosed space, the fumigants are indiscriminate poisons. They affect targeted pests and other organisms that may not be an intended target, including workers that may enter the treated area unknowingly. Treated areas should have warning signs (placarding) indicating the date and time of safe entry.

Methyl bromide and sulfuryl fluoride are prototypic fumigants. They are gases at room temperature and 1 atmosphere pressure, are poorly water soluble, are odorless, and are not significantly irritating to the mucous membranes. Because many fumigants have poor warning properties, chloropicrin (CCl_3NO_2) often is added as a warning agent. Chloropicrin is intensely irritating to all mucous membranes and has been used as an incapacitating lacrimator in military poison gases.

The specific mechanisms of action, including specific molecular targets, have not been elucidated in detail for many of the fumigants. The clinical signs and symptoms of poisoning by these compounds are well known, but for many their effects at the cellular and molecular levels still are being explored.

PHOSPHIDES

Aluminum phosphide (AlP) and zinc phosphide (Zn_2P_3) are solids and usually formulated as pellets or encased in packets. When either phosphide reacts with water or acid,

phosphine gas (PH_3) is liberated, which acts as the fumigant. All typical routes of exposure may occur with fumigants, although inhalation is the most likely in the Untied States. In India, ingestion of fumigant pellets has become an important source of morbidity and mortality.[1]

There is experimental evidence that phosphine noncompetitively inhibits mitochondrial cytochrome oxidase,[2] interfering with cellular respiration and adenosine triphosphate formation. Myocardial cells are particularly sensitive to this noncompetitive inhibition of cytochrome oxidase.[3] Phosphine interferes with incorporation of amino acids into myocardial proteins,[3] which can result in heart failure. In the lung, phosphine directly damages the alveolar-capillary membrane, potentially resulting in noncardiogenic pulmonary edema and hypoxemia. Phosphine is a small peripheral arteriole vasodilator that may cause decreased systemic vascular resistance, with possible hypotension, and distributive shock.[4]

In a series of grain storage workers, acute inhalational exposure to aluminum phosphide was reported to cause cough, dyspnea, chest tightness, headache, numbness, lethargy, and epigastric pain.[5] In a report of eight intentional aluminum phosphide ingestions, the same investigators reported gastritis, altered sensorium, distributive shock, renal failure, and cardiac arrhythmias. Six patients died. Postmortem findings included pulmonary edema, intestinal edema, petechial hemorrhages on the liver and brain, and desquamation of the epithelial lining of the bronchioles.[6]

METHYL BROMIDE

Methyl bromide (CH_3Br) is colorless, odorless, and three times as heavy as air. The last-mentioned attribute is an important physical property in that this gas and others that are heavier than air collect in low-lying places. This property is beneficial for fumigation but is potentially responsible for unintended exposures. By cooperative agreement, methyl bromide is to be phased out of use by 2005 in industrialized nations.

Methyl bromide typically is used as a soil fumigant. It also has been used to treat stored fruit in ship holds or in special fumigation chambers in aircraft. Nonfumigant uses of methyl bromide include use as a methylating agent, refrigerant, and fire retardant. The main routes of exposure to humans are inhalation and skin contact.

Methyl bromide is a potent alkylating agent with high affinity for sulfhydryl and amino groups. It binds to amine groups in amino acids, interfering with protein synthesis

TABLE 88-1 Names and Common Uses of Selected Fumigants

COMMON NAME	SYNONYMS	USES
Methyl bromide	Bromomethane, monobromomethane, embafume	Pesticide fumigant for soil, mills, warehouses, vaults, ships, freight cars, etc. Wool degreaser
Sulfuryl fluoride	Sulfur difluoride dioxide, vikane	Pesticidal fumigant, especially for structures with dry-wood termites or wood beetles
Chloropicrin	Trichloronitromethane, nitrochloroform, larvacide, picfume	Pesticidal fumigant for soil, cereals, and grains; chemical synthesis; military "tear gas"
Aluminum phosphide	Celphos, detia, phostoxin	Pesticidal fumigant, especially for animal feed, bulk grain, cottonseed, leaf tobacco, and flour mills; phosphine source, semiconductor industry
Zinc phosphide	ZP	Rodenticidal fumigant
Carbon disulfide	Serafume, vertifume	Pesticide, manufacturing
Chlorine dioxide	Alcide, doxcide 50	Fumigant, algicide
Acrylonitrile	Acrylon, carbacryl, acrulofume	Pesticides, semiconductor industry

and function.[7] Sulfhydryl-containing amino acids and proteins can be damaged at their amino and sulfhydryl sites. Because methyl bromide is an alkylating agent, it may methylate many other cellular components, including glutathione, proteins, DNA, and RNA.[7]

Because of methyl bromide's lack of warning properties,[8] the unwary worker may come into contact with dangerous concentrations of this gas unknowingly. Symptoms may evolve over hours. Initially, mild symptoms, such as headache and eye, nose, and sinus irritation, may be reported.[9] At higher concentrations, central nervous system (CNS) and respiratory complaints predominate.[10] CNS complaints may include coma and convulsions.[11] Respiratory tract irritation, burns, and ultimately ventilatory failure may occur.[12] Skin irritation and burns may occur after large exposures.[13] The typical lesions are blisters with surrounding erythema.[14] Eye injuries may occur, with severe inflammation leading to temporary blindness.[15] Patients should have prompt skin and eye irrigation if indicated.

SULFURYL FLUORIDE

Sulfuryl fluoride (SO_2F_2) is odorless and colorless. The exact mechanism of action of sulfuryl fluoride is unknown. Its vapor pressure is similar to water. The respiratory system, CNS, and cardiovascular system are the primary target organ systems.[16] Free fluoride anion is released soon after contact.[16] At autopsy, markedly elevated fluoride concentrations have been found in the heart blood of one of two sulfuryl fluoride poisoning victims. The blood fluoride concentration obtained 6 days after exposure was 0.5 mg/L.[17] When sulfuryl fluoride is combusted in the presence of water vapor, it may form acidic vapors, such as hydrofluoric acid (see Chapter 100 for additional information concerning hydrofluoric acid).

Fluoride combines with divalent cations, primarily calcium and magnesium, potentially resulting in hypocalcemia, hypomagnesemia, and hyperkalemia from cellular destruction.[18] This constellation of electrolyte abnormalities can manifest as CNS irritability with agitation, tetany, or seizures.[18] These electrolyte abnormalities also may cause prolongation of the QT interval, torsades de pointes, bradydysrhythmias, wide QRS complexes, or asystole.[19] Acute bronchospasm has been reported after sulfuryl fluoride inhalation.[20] Limited exposures may cause nausea, vomiting, and diarrhea.[20] In one case report, a worker exposed to sulfuryl fluoride containing 1% chloropicrin developed nausea, vomiting, abdominal pain, pleuritis, and diffuse rhonchi after an inhalational exposure, all of which resolved promptly with supportive care.[20]

TABLE 88-2 Properties of Selected Fumigants

CHEMICAL	STATE	COLOR	ODOR/IRRITATION	WATER SOLUBILITY (% g/dL)	BOILING POINT (°F)	VAPOR PRESSURE (mm Hg)	IDLH (ppm)
Methyl bromide	Gas	Colorless	Odorless	2%	38	1.9	250
Sulfuryl fluoride	Gas	Colorless	Odorless	0.2%	−68	15.8	200
Chlorine dioxide	Gas	Yellow	Acidic	3%	51.8	760	5
Carbon disulfide	Liquid	Colorless to yellow	Sweet aromatic	0.08%	114.8	359	500
Chloropicrin	Liquid	Colorless to yellow	Intensely irritating	0.2%	234	18	2
Aluminum phosphide	Solid	Dark gray or yellow	Fishy	NA	NR	NR	NR
Zinc phosphide	Solid	Dark gray	Phosphorus-like	NA	2012	NR	NR
Acrylonitrile	Liquid	Pale yellow	Slight peach	7.2%	171.1	100	85
Ethylene dibromide	Liquid	Colorless	Sweet chloroform	0.4%	267.8	11.25	100

NR, not reported; NA, not applicable; IDLH, immediately dangerous to life and health.

CHLOROPICRIN

Chloropicrin is a lacrimator and a pulmonary irritant. It is a colorless-to-yellow liquid with a sweet, slightly aromatic odor. It is one of the more volatile fumigants. Chloropicrin is highly irritating to all mucous membranes and was used in World War I as a tear gas because of its strong lacrimating properties.[20,21] Chloropicrin's exact cellular mechanism of action has not been elucidated fully. It is slightly water soluble.[22] Its water solubility is intermediate between chlorine gas and phosgene gas, and its effects are similar to these gases. Chloropicrin is a corrosive toxicant with local toxic effects on exposed mucous membranes,[23] the respiratory tract including the alveolar-capillary membrane, and the eyes. Common clinical findings in patients after exposure to chloropicrin vapors include cough, erythema, tearing, rhinorrhea, headache, and irritation.[9,24] After ingestion, irritation of the gastrointestinal tract would be expected due to the corrosive nature of this substance.

ETHYLENE DIBROMIDE

Ethylene dibromide (CH_2BrCH_2Br) is a colorless substance, also referred to as *1,2-dibromoethane*. Ethylene dibromide first found use in 1948; its biocidal properties led to its use as a soil sterilant. In addition to its use as a fumigant, it has been used as an antiknocking agent in gasoline. In contrast to many other fumigants, ethylene dibromide is a dense liquid, and it has a sweet odor. The vapor pressure is approximately that of water, and poisoning typically occurs from direct contact. One chemical feature is its ability to penetrate protective clothing, including neoprene and rubber.[25]

Patients exposed to ethylene dibromide may have mucous membrane irritation,[26] skin irritation and blistering, and possibly respiratory distress.[27,28] Cardiac bundle-branch blocks, supraventricular tachycardia, ventricular fibrillation, and asystole have been described.[26-28] In cases of severe intoxication, hypotension and shock have been described.[27-29] Hepatic failure and renal insufficiency have been reported after significant exposure to ethylene dibromide.[30] Pathology of ethylene dibromide–related liver injury is characterized as centrolobular necrosis.[31] Ethylene dibromide has weak anesthetic properties that may result in CNS depression and ultimately coma if the dose is sufficient.[26,27,32]

Ethylene dibromide is converted by hepatic microsomal cytochrome P-450 isozymes (CYP2E1, CYP2A6, CYP2B6) and cytosolic glutathione-*S*-transferase isozymes (A1-1, A2-2, M1a-1a, P1-1) in vitro to bromoacetaldehyde, bromoacetic acid, thiodiacetic acid, *S*-2-bromoethylglutathione, and *S*-(2-hydroxyethyl) mercapturic acid.[33-37] The principal mechanism associated with carcinogenicity and mutagenicity is conjugation of ethylene dibromide catalyzed by glutathione-S transferases.[37,38] The conjugate rapidly rearranges to an episulfonium ion, which reacts with DNA.[37,39]

In a rat model, pretreatment with alcohol potentiated the hepatotoxicity of ethylene dibromide secondary to a reduction in ethylene dibromide conjugation, with a shift to the formation of reactive oxidative intermediates. The hepatotoxicity was blocked by the alcohol dehydrogenase inhibitor methylpyrazole.[40] In the rare case of concomitant ethylene dibromide and alcohol ingestion, there is a theoretical benefit to the use of fomepizole. This antidote is discussed in detail in Chapter 152.

ETHYLENE OXIDE

Ethylene oxide is one of the most common medical sterilants in use today. In addition to its use in the sterilization of medical devices, ethylene oxide has found use as a fumigant, a fungicide, and an intermediate in the production of plastics. Although it often is discussed in terms of its mutagenic potential, it also possesses the acute toxicologic properties of being a potent skin irritant and CNS depressant.

Ethylene oxide is a colorless gas at room temperature with an odor threshold of 250 to 690 ppm.[41] Levels of 200 ppm may cause mucous membrane irritation, however. Direct skin contact with liquid ethylene oxide may cause significant cutaneous burns resembling toxic epidermal necrolysis.[42] Concentrations approaching 1000 ppm may cause chest pain, dyspnea, gastrointestinal disturbances, weakness, and ataxia.[43] Uncommon but life-threatening acute reactions include hemolysis and anaphylactoid reactions[44] reported after exposure to ethylene oxide–treated cardiopulmonary bypass machines.

ACRYLONITRILE

Acrylonitrile (CH_2CHCN; vinyl cyanide) is a colorless–to–pale yellow liquid with an unpleasant odor. It is highly flammable and when combusted or ingested may form cyanide gas. The vapor pressure of acrylonitrile is 100 mm Hg (water is 25 mm Hg), and its vapor density is 1.9 (air is 1). Acrylonitrile easily volatilizes but remains low to the ground unless disturbed by air currents. In addition to its use in the plastics industry, it may be used as a fumigant. Exposure to acrylonitrile may occur by the dermal, inhalational, or oral routes. In human volunteers inhaling 2.3 or 4.6 ppm of acrylonitrile, 52% of the administered dose was retained.[45] It is absorbed through the forearm skin at a rate of 0.6 mg/cm²/hr.[46]

Acrylonitrile is metabolized less efficiently in humans than in rodents, which may explain partially why the cyanide-like toxicity plays a lesser role in humans than in rodents.[47] Its proposed metabolic pathways are shown in Figure 88-1. The typical half-life of acrylonitrile is approximately 3 to 6 hours in rodents.[48] Four main metabolic products have been detected: glucuronides; glutathione adducts, which form cyanoethyl mercapturic acid; protein thiol group adducts; and 2-cyanoethylene oxide, which is formed by epoxidation. The latter two pathways are considered to be responsible for acrylonitrile's toxicity.[30] The toxic mechanism of nitriles is via the liberation of cyanide in vivo and in vitro.[49]

Acrylonitrile may cause mucous membrane irritation, chest discomfort, dyspnea, and nausea at low doses. More significant exposure may cause loss of consciousness, seizures, respiratory arrest, and cardiovascular collapse[50] if the dose is sufficient. The acute systemic toxicity resembles cyanide poisoning, with the formation of lactic acidosis.[51] Liver and kidney injury may follow large exposures.[52] When acrylonitrile is ingested, the signs and symptoms may be slower in onset than after inhalation.[53]

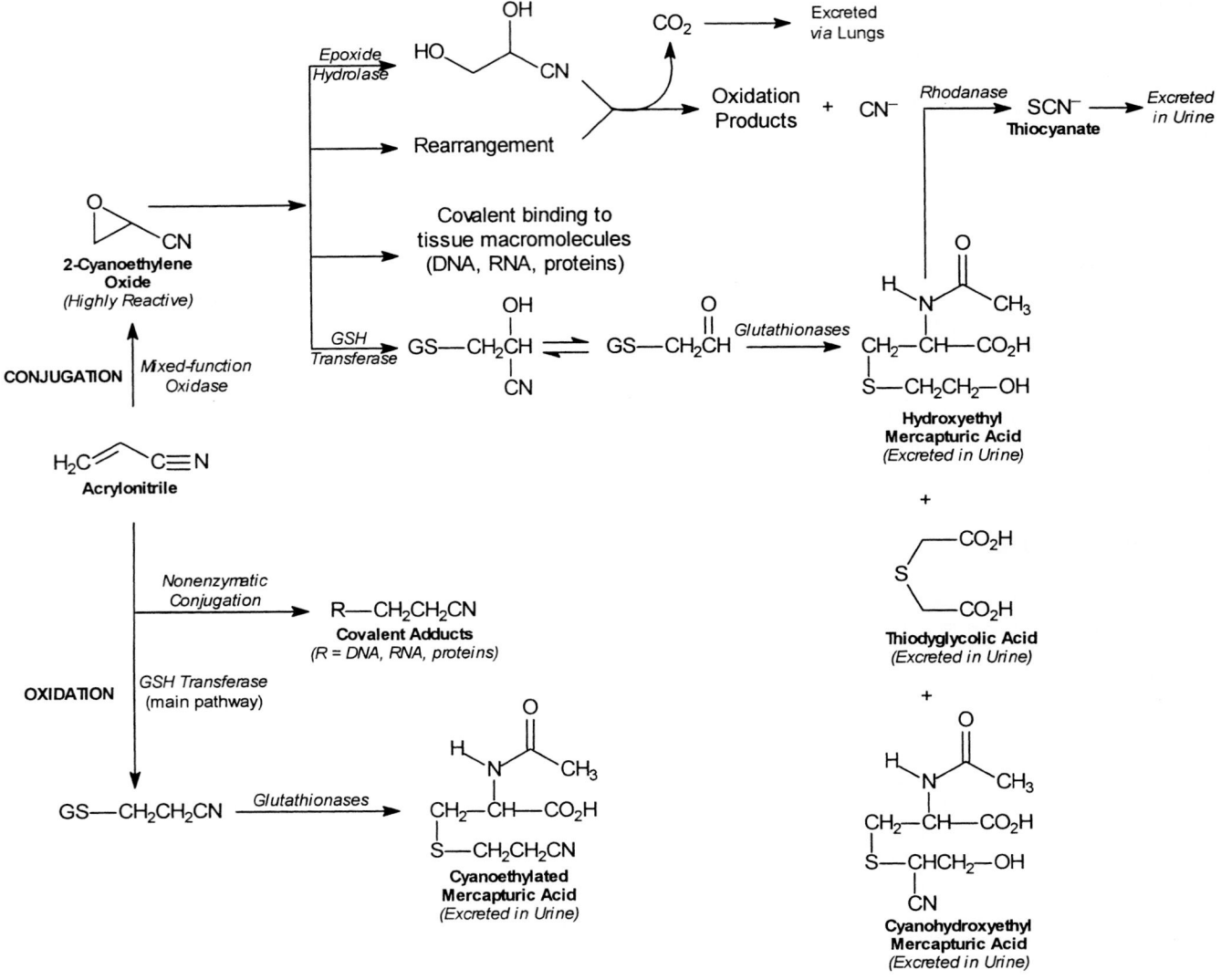

FIGURE 88-1

Proposed metabolic pathways of acrylonitrile metabolism. Note specifically the glutathione and rhodanase pathways.

CARBON DISULFIDE

Carbon disulfide (CS_2) is a colorless but volatile liquid. With proper engineering controls in the workplace, exposures are rare. Its vapor pressure is approximately 300 mm Hg (water is 25 mm Hg), so it is volatile. Carbon disulfide has been used principally in the manufacture of rayon, in the manufacture of cellophane, and in the semiconductor industry. It also has found use as a fumigant when mixed with carbon tetrachloride in a 20:80 ratio. This mixture has been used to fumigate boxcars of grains.[54,55] The major target organs are the CNS, eyes, skin, cardiovascular system, liver, and reproductive organs.

Acute effects of carbon disulfide are rare and generally are due to inhalation or dermal contact. An early effect of sufficient concentrations is irritation of the mucous membranes. After major skin contact, full-thickness corrosive burns may occur with erythema and blistering. Agitation, delirium, lethargy, blurred vision, hallucinations, and seizures have been described after carbon disulfide exposures.[56,57] Ingestion of carbon disulfide has been reported

rarely, with catastrophic features, including muscle spasms, Cheyne-Stokes respirations, hypotension, coma, and death.[58]

CHLORINE DIOXIDE

Chlorine dioxide (ClO_2) is a fumigant that also has found use in the bleaching of cellulose, flour, leather, and textiles. It is a yellow-to-red gas at room temperature, with an acrid odor; it is heavier than air; and it has a high vapor pressure (760 mm Hg). This compound typically is not used in routine fumigation processes. In 2001, anthrax spores were disseminated via the U.S. Postal Service. One site where anthrax spores were found was the Hart Senate Office Building in Washington, D.C. In this case, chlorine dioxide was pumped into the sealed building to soften and kill the spores. Because of chlorine dioxide's strong oxidizing properties, it was thought that it would be the most effective fumigant, based on the size of the job and risk to the building's inhabitants and adjacent urban population. After the fumigation process, the air was filtered through a scrubber containing the antioxidant ascorbic acid, which reacts with chlorine dioxide to inactivate the biocide.

Chlorine dioxide is an irritant gas that affects the mucous membranes and other moist tissue owing to its relatively high water solubility.[59] Expected clinical features are irritation of the eyes, nose, and throat.[60] Larger exposures may affect the tracheobronchial tree with the possibility of pulmonary irritation from very large exposures. Ingestion of this oxidizing agent would be expected to cause a corrosive injury to the gastrointestinal tract if the dose is sufficient. Chlorine dioxide is absorbed rapidly after ingestion or inhalation, with peak concentration occurring within 1 hour.[61]

TREATMENT

In all cases of fumigant exposure, it is important to remove the patient from further exposure. Rescuers must wear proper personal protective equipment. In many instances, removing the patient from the source is all that is necessary if these fumigants are in their gaseous states. For significant exposures with signs and symptoms that do not resolve, prompt evaluation at a medical facility is indicated.

During decontamination procedures, care should be taken to prevent secondary contamination of rescue workers; this is especially true for methyl bromide and sulfuryl fluoride in their liquid states. Secondary contamination may occur because a victim's skin temperature usually exceeds the boiling points of these substances, which may result in their volatilization.

Decontamination procedures should begin with the physical separation of the offending agent and the victim. If the product was in a liquid or solid state and skin contact has occurred, it is necessary to remove all clothing and personal items from the patient because these may contain residual fumigant. The patient should be decontaminated with mild soap and water for at least 15 minutes. A mild liquid detergent is necessary because these substances have low water solubilities (Table 88-2). Attention to exposed skin in skinfolds, the axillae, the genital area, feet, and hair is important. The patient's contaminated possessions should be disposed of as hazardous waste. It is not recommended to wash clothing because further exposure may occur during the intervals before washing the clothing.

Specific ocular decontamination may not be needed for patients exposed to these fumigants in their gaseous states; however, if there is irritation or if significant chloropicrin exposure has occurred, eye decontamination should be considered. If it is necessary, large quantities of water or sterile saline solution are preferred. Use of irrigation lenses with ophthalmic local anesthetics, such as proparacaine, can make decontaminating the eyes more comfortable for the patient.

Patients with significant fumigant exposures should be placed on a cardiac monitor and observed for dysrhythmias. If dysrhythmias occur, American Heart Association advanced cardiac life support guidelines generally are sufficient, with the exception of the use of calcium as a specific antidote in sulfuryl fluoride poisoning. Specific details of the treatment of fluoride poisoning may be found in Chapter 100.

The patient's level of consciousness should be assessed continually. If seizures develop despite adequate supportive care and blood glucose, the patient should be treated with intravenous diazepam or lorazepam. Status epilepticus can occur, necessitating high doses of intravenous diazepam or lorazepam and possibly the addition of a barbiturate. Tetany or seizures due to sulfuryl fluoride poisoning should be treated with intravenous calcium in addition to intravenous diazepam or lorazepam. Monitoring of liver and renal laboratory markers on a daily basis is indicated if there have been major exposures to these agents.

Ethylene Dibromide

There are no specific antidotes for ethylene dibromide poisoning, and supportive care is the mainstay of treatment. Although not studied, *N*-acetylcysteine is a theoretically beneficial sulfhydryl donor in these patients. *N*-Acetylcysteine is discussed in detail in Chapter 136. Hemodialysis has been used; its use should be considered for the management of renal insufficiency.[62] No data are available regarding clearance of ethylene dibromide with dialysis. Although the molecular weight is favorable (187.9), it has poor water solubility (4 g/L), which does not favor hemodialysis. The fumigants discussed in this chapter all have poor water solubility that would diminish the efficacy of hemodialysis (see Table 88-2), with the possible exception of methyl bromide.

Methyl Bromide

In a series of three patients occupationally exposed to methyl bromide, hemodialysis and, in the case of a child, peritoneal lavage were performed. The initially high bromide levels (67.8 to 91.5 μg/mL) returned to normal ranges with clinical improvement.[63]

Methyl bromide is known to form methylcysteine adducts in albumin and globulin.[64] Some authors have noted that glutathione may be protective of the alkylating effect of methyl bromide, so *N*-acetylcysteine may be useful. Some data, however, suggest a different metabolic mechanism that may lead to the formation of methanethiol and formaldehyde, which the authors suggest may be responsible for the neurotoxicity of methyl bromide.[64]

Acrylonitrile

If exposure to acrylonitrile has occurred, use of a cyanide antidote kit may be considered when the patient has altered consciousness or metabolic acidosis. Acrylonitrile is oxidized by the mixed-function oxidase pathway to an oxide (see Fig. 88-1). This oxide is metabolized further by epoxide hydrase, which releases cyanide. The latter is converted by rhodanase, in the presence of thiosulfate, to thiocyanate, which is excreted in the urine. Most cases involve minor exposure, however, which resolves with supportive care. Limited experience using the traditional cyanide antidotes generally has proved ineffective because conjugation via glutathione transferase is the dominant pathway of metabolism.[65] In addition to supportive measures and cyanide antidotes, it has been suggested that the treatment of acrylonitrile toxicity should include intravenous *N*-acetylcysteine.[66] In a rat model, Bondarev and associates[67] found that a combination of thiosulfate and cysteine had a pronounced prophylactic effect when looking at mortality as an end point. Because thiosulfate and *N*-acetylcysteine are safe when administered properly, their use should be considered in patients with significant acrylonitrile poisoning.

REFERENCES

1. Kabra SG, Narayanan R: Aluminum phosphide: Worse than Bhopal. Lancet 11:1333, 1988.
2. Chefurka W, Kashi KP, Bond EJ: The effect of phosphine on electron transport in mitochondria. Pestic Biochem Physiol 6:65–81, 1976.
3. Nakakita H: The inhibitory site of phosphine. J Pestic Sci (Nihon Noyakugaky Kaishi) 1:235–238, 1976.
4. Chugh SN, Aggarwal HK, Mahajan SK: Zinc phosphide intoxication symptoms: Analysis of 20 cases. Int J Clin Pharmacol Ther 36:406–407, 1998.
5. Misra UK, Bhargava SK, Nag D, et al: Occupational phosphine exposure in Indian workers. Toxicol Lett 42:257–263, 1988.
6. Misra UK, Tripathi AK, Pandey R, Bhargwa B: Acute phosphine poisoning following ingestion of aluminum phosphide. Hum Toxicol 7:343–345, 1988.
7. Starratt AN, Bond EJ: In vitro methylation of DNA by the fumigant methyl bromide. J Environ Sci Health B 23:513–525, 1988.
8. Lenhart SW, Gagnon YT: NIOSH Health Hazard Evaluation Report HETA 93-0012-2711, U.S. Department of Agriculture, Animal and Plant Health Inspection Service, Raleigh, NC. Government Reports, Announcements, and Index (GRA&I), Issue 20, 1999.
9. Goldman LR, Mengle D, Epstein DM, et al: Acute symptoms in persons residing near a field treated with the soil fumigants methyl bromide and chloropicrin. West J Med 147:95–98, 1987.
10. De Haro L, Gastaut J-L, Jouglard J, Renacco E: Central and peripheral neurotoxic effects of chronic methyl bromide intoxication. J Toxicol Clin Toxicol 35:29–34, 1997.
11. Deschamps FJ, Turpin JC: Methyl bromide intoxication during grain store fumigation. Occup Med 46:89–90, 1996.
12. Herzstein J, Cullen MR: Methyl bromide intoxication in four field-workers during removal of soil fumigation sheets. Am J Ind Med 17:321–326, 1990.
13. Zwaveling JH, de Kort WLAM, Meulenbelt J, et al: Exposure of the skin to methyl bromide: A study of six cases occupationally exposed to high concentrations during fumigation. Hum Toxicol 6:491–495, 1987.
14. Jarowenko DG, Mancusi-Ungaro HR Jr: The care of burns from methyl bromide (case report). J Burn Care Rehabil 6:119–123, 1985.
15. Chavez CT, Hepler RS, Straatsma BR: Methyl bromide optic atrophy. Am J Ophthalmol 99:715–719, 1985.
16. Eisenbrandt DL, Nitschke KD: Inhalation toxicity of sulfuryl fluoride in rats and rabbits. Fundam Appl Toxicol 12:540–557, 1989.
17. Fatalities resulting from sulfuryl fluoride exposure after home fumigation—Virginia. MMWR Morb Mortal Wkly Rep 36:602–604, 609–611, 1987.
18. Heard K, Hill RE, Cairns CB, Dart RC: Calcium neutralizes fluoride bioavailability in a lethal model of fluoride poisoning. J Toxicol Clin Toxicol 39:349–353, 2001.
19. Schuerman EH: Suicide by exposure to sulfuryl fluoride. J Forensic Sci 31:1154–1158, 1986.
20. Taxay EP: Vikane inhalation. J Occup Med 8:425–426, 1966.
21. Gonmori K, Muto H, Yamamoto T, et al: A case of homicidal intoxication by chloropicrin. Am J Forensic Med Pathol 8:135–138, 1987.
22. Budavari S (ed): The Merck Index Encyclopedia of Chemicals, Drugs and Biologicals. Rahway, NJ, Merck & Co, 1989.
23. American Conference of Governmental Industrial Hygienists, Inc: Documentation of the Threshold Limit Values and Biological Exposure Indices, Vols I-III, 6th ed. Cincinnati, ACGIH, 1991.
24. TeSlaa G, Kaiser M, Biederman L, et al: Chloropicrin toxicity involving animal and human exposure. Vet Hum Toxicol 28:323–324, 1986.
25. Zwavling JH, deKort WLAM, Meulenbelt J, et al: Exposure of the skin to methyl bromide: A study of six cases occupationally exposed to high concentrations during fumigation. Hum Toxicol 6:491–495, 1987.
26. Lentz GA, Pond SA, Osterloh JD, et al: Two fatalities after acute occupational exposure to ethylene dibromide. JAMA 252:2428–2431, 1984.
27. Nouchi T, Miuri H, Kanayama M, et al: Fatal intoxication by 1,2-dichloroethane—a case report. Int Arch Occup Environ Health 54:111–113, 1984.
28. Yodaiken RE, Babcock JR: 1,2-dichloroethane poisoning. Arch Environ Health 26:281–284, 1973.
29. Olmstead KV: Pathological changes in ethylene dibromide poisoning. Arch Ind Health 21:525–529, 1960.
30. Singh S, Gupta A, Sharma S, et al: Case report: Non-fatal ethylene dibromide ingestion. Hum Exp Toxicol 19:152–153, 2000.
31. Letz GA, Pond SM, Osterloh JD, et al: Two fatalities after acute occupational exposure to ethylene dibromide. JAMA 252:2428–2431, 1984.
32. Aneja EK, Mitra A, Mital HS, Mehrotra TN: Ethylene dibromide (EDB) poisoning. J Assoc Physicians India 36:672–673, 1988.
33. Edwards K, Jackson H: Studies with alkylating esters: II. A chemical interpretation through metabolic studies of the antifertility effects of ethylene dimethanesulphonate and ethylene dibromide. Biochem Pharmacol 19:1783–1789, 1970.
34. van Bladeren PJ, Hoogeterp JJ, Breimer DD, et al: The influence of disulfiram and other inhibitors of oxidative metabolism on the formation of 2-hydroxyethyl-mercapturic acid from 1,2-dibromoethane by the rat. Biochem Pharmacol 30:2983–2987, 1981.
35. van Bladeren PJ, Breimer DD, van Huijgevoort JA, et al: The metabolic formation of N-acetyl-S-2-hydroxyethyl-L-cysteine from tetradeutero-1,2-dibromoethane: Relative importance of oxidation and glutathione conjugation in vivo. Biochem Pharmacol 30:2499–2502, 1981.
36. Hayes WJ: Pesticides Studied in Man. Baltimore, Williams & Wilkins, 1982.
37. Ploemen J-P, Wormhoudt LW, Haenen GR, et al: The use of human in vitro metabolic parameters to explore the risk assessment of hazardous compounds: The case of ethylene dibromide. Toxicol Appl Pharmacol 143:56–69, 1997.
38. Fossett NG, Byrne BJ, Tucker AB, et al: Mutation spectrum of 2-chloroethyl methanesulfonate in Drosophila melanogaster premeiotic germ cells. Mutat Res 331:213–224, 1995.
39. Graves RJ, Green T: Mouse liver glutathione S-transferase mediated metabolism of methylene chloride to a mutagen in the CHO/HPRT assay. Mutat Res 367:143–150, 1996.
40. Aragno M, Tamagno E, Danni O, et al: In vivo potentiation of 1,2-dichloroethane hepatotoxicity by ethanol through inactivation of glutathione-s-transferase. Chem Biol Interact 5:277–288, 1996.
41. American Industrial Hygiene Association: Odor thresholds for chemicals with established occupational health standards. Fairfax, VA, AIHA Press, 1998.
42. Biro L, Fisher AA, Price E: Ethylene oxide burns—a hospital outbreak involving 19 women. Arch Dermatol 110:924–925, 1974.
43. Salinas E, Sasic L, Hall DH, et al: Acute ethylene oxide intoxication. Drug Intell Clin Pharm 15:384–385, 1981.
44. Poothullil J, Shimizu A, Day RP, et al: Anaphylaxis from products and ethylene oxide gas. Ann Intern Med 82:58–60, 1975.
45. Jakubowski M, Linhart I, Pielas G, et al: 2-Cyanoethylmercapturic acid (CEMA) in the urine as a possible indicator of exposure to acrylonitrile. Br J Ind Med 44:834–840, 1987.
46. Hazardous Substance Data Bank. Bethesda, MD, National Library of Medicine. Available at: http://toxnet.nlm.nig.gov/cgi-bin/sis/search/f?./temp/-BAARfaOpH:1.
47. Muller G, Verkoyen C, Soton N, et al. Urinary excretion of acrylonitrile and its metabolites in rats. Arch Toxicol 60:464–466, 1987.
48. Hazardous Substances Data Bank. Bethesda, MD, National Library of Medicine. Hazardous Substances Databank Number: 176, Last Revision Date: 2002-11-08.
49. Zhang H, Kamendulis LM, Klaunig JE: Mechanisms for the induction of oxidative stress in Syrian hamster embryo cells by acrylonitrile. Toxicol Sci 67:247–255, 2002.
50. Plunkett ER: Handbook of Industrial Toxicology. New York, Chemical Publishing Company, 1976.
51. Hathaway GJ, Proctor NH, Hughes JP, et al: Chemical Hazards of the Workplace. New York, Van Nostrand Reinhold Company, 1996.
52. Buchter A, Peter H: Clinical toxicology of acrylonitrile. G Ital J Med Lav 6:83–86, 1984.
53. Sakurai H, Onodera M, Utsunomiya T, et al: Health effects of acrylonitrile in acrylic fibre factories. Br J Ind Med 35:219–222, 1980.
54. Peters HA, Levine RL, Matthews CG, et al: Synergistic neurotoxicity of carbon tetrachloride/carbon disulfide (80/20 fumigants) and other pesticides in grain storage workers. Acta Pharmacol Toxicol (Copenh) 59(Suppl 7):535–546, 1986.
55. Peters H: Extrapyramidal and other neurological manifestations associated with carbon disulfide fumigant exposure. Arch Neurol 45:537–540, 1988.
56. VanHoorne M, DeBacquer D, Barbier F: Epidemiological study of gastrointestinal and liver effects of carbon disulfide. Int Arch Occup Environ Health 63:517–523, 1992.
57. Spyker DA, Gallanosa AG, Suratt PM: Health effects of acute carbon disulfide exposure. J Toxicol Clin Toxicol 19:87–93, 1982.

58. Foreman W: Notes of fatal case of poisoning by bisulfide of carbon. Lancet 2:118–122, 1986.

59. American Conference of Governmental Industrial Hygienists: TLVs and other occupational exposure values (CD-ROM). Boulder, Colorado, NexData Solutions, Inc., 2002.

60. Couri D, Mohamed S, Abdel-Rahman MS, Bull RJ: Toxicological effects of chlorine dioxide, chlorite and chlorate. Environ Health Perspect 46:13–17, 1982.

61. Yogendra P, Wong D: Toxicological review of chlorine dioxide and chlorite (CAS Nos. 10049-04-4 and 7758-19-2) in support of summary information on the Integrated Risk Information System (IRIS). Government Reports, Announcements, and Index (GRA&I), Issue 02, 2001.

62. Agarwal SK, Tiwari SC, Dash SC: Spectrum of poisoning requiring haemodiaylsis in a tertiary care hospital in India. Int J Artif Organs 16:20–22, 1993.

63. Yamano Y, Kagawa J, Ishizu S, Harayama O: Three cases of acute methyl bromide poisoning in a seedling farm family. Ind Health 39:353–358, 2001.

64. Garnier R, Rambourg-Schepens MO, Muller A, Hallier E: Glutathione transferase activity and formation of macromolecular adducts in two cases of acute methyl bromide poisoning. Occup Environ Med 53:211–215, 1996.

65. Agency for Toxic Substances Disease Registry: Toxicological Profile: Cyanide. Atlanta, U.S. Department of Health and Human Services, Public Health Service, Centers for Disease Control and Prevention, 1997.

66. Buchter A, Peter H: Clinical toxicology of acrylonitrile. G Ital Med Lav 6:83–86, 1984.

67. Bondarev GI, Stasenkova KP, Vissarionova VI: Protective action of sulfur-containing compounds in acrylonitrile poisoning. Vopr Pitan Jul-Aug:55–58, 1976.

CHAPTER 89

Fungicides

Daniel Sudakin

The fungicides are a diverse group of structurally unrelated chemicals that are used widely in agricultural, industrial, and domestic settings. As a group, fungicides are responsible for a small proportion of human exposures leading to acute morbidity and mortality. In 1999, fungicides accounted for 1054 cases reported to regional poison control centers in the United States, of which there were no deaths and only three life-threatening or disabling outcomes.[1] Despite these findings, fungicides are important from historical and international health perspectives. Some of the most serious poisoning epidemics in the 20th century have been attributed to accidental fungicide exposures. The lessons learned from these epidemics have led to the severe restriction or discontinued use of several classes of fungicides, such as methylmercury and hexachlorobenzene (HCB), in many parts of the world. Even with these restrictions, the acute and chronic effects after exposure to some of these compounds continue to pose diagnostic and therapeutic challenges to treating physicians.

This chapter is divided into six subsections, corresponding to the different chemical classifications of fungicides that are relevant to the critical care physician (Table 89-1). Several of the modern organic fungicides (Table 89-2) are not discussed in detail. In general, many of these modern organic fungicides can have irritant effects on the skin and mucous membranes, although systemic effects and acute poisonings have not been reported. The manufacturer of benomyl (Benlate) announced that it would discontinue worldwide sales and production of this widely used fungicide, citing difficulties encountered in defending the product from claims of human health and environmental impact. Although benomyl has been suggested to be a weak dermal sensitizer,[2] reports of reproductive toxicity (anophthalmia and microphthalmia) do not seem to be supported by the weight of the scientific evidence.[3,4]

ORGANOMERCURY COMPOUNDS

The organomercury compounds are a class of fungicides formulated as dusts and aqueous solutions, used primarily as seed protectants. Although their use has been banned or restricted severely in many countries, they are of historical importance because of their severe toxicity in humans. In 1971, a poisoning epidemic occurred in rural Iraq as a result of the ingestion of bread prepared with wheat that was treated with methylmercury as a fungicide, resulting in 50,000 exposures and at least 439 deaths.[5] The scientific study of this tragedy has provided further insight into the toxic effects of methylmercury on the central nervous system (CNS).

Biochemistry and Pharmacokinetics

> **Pharmacokinetics of Methylmercury**
>
> *Volume of distribution:* >1 L/kg
> *Protein binding:* >90%
> *Mechanisms of clearance:* 90% biliary, 10% renal
> *Active metabolite:* inorganic mercury
> *Methods to enhance clearance:* DMPS (?), DMSA (?)

Organomercury fungicides (Fig. 89-1) can be divided into short-chain alkyl (e.g., methylmercury) and aryl (e.g., phenylmercuric acetate) compounds. Their absorption, distribution, and metabolic fate vary depending on the chemical structure.[6] Ingestion is the predominant route of human exposure to methylmercury. Absorption is nearly complete across the gastrointestinal tract. Methylmercury has a high volume of distribution and is transferred readily across the blood-brain and placental barriers. When absorbed, more than 90% of methylmercury detected in blood is bound to hemoglobin in red blood cells. About 10% of the body burden of methylmercury is found in the brain, where it undergoes a slow metabolic transformation into inorganic mercury and becomes relatively fixed in neural tissue.[6] It is unclear whether the CNS injury is due to methylmercury, inorganic mercury, or the biotransformation process between the two forms. The major route of excretion of methylmercury in humans is through biliary and fecal elimination,[6] with a whole-body half-life of approximately 70 to 80 days.[6] Approximately 10% of a given dose of methylmercury is excreted in urine.[6]

In contrast to short-chain alkyl compounds, phenylmercuric acetate is not as well absorbed from the gastrointestinal tract and undergoes more rapid transformation into inorganic mercury.[6] Dermal absorption and inhalation may be important routes of exposure to phenylmercuric acetate. A case of acrodynia was reported in a child whose house was painted with latex paint containing phenylmercuric acetate.[7] An epidemiologic study conducted in follow-up to this case report found higher levels of mercury in the urine of individuals whose houses had been painted recently with products containing phenylmercuric acetate as a preservative.[7]

TABLE 89-1 Major Classifications of Clinically Relevant Fungicides

Organomercury compounds (methylmercury, phenylmercuric acetate)
Chlorinated phenols (pentachlorophenol)
Substituted benzenes (hexachlorobenzene)
Dithiocarbamates (metam-sodium, thiram, ethylene bisdithiocarbamate [EBDC] compounds)
Copper compounds (copper sulfate)
Organotin compounds (triphenyltin, tributyltin oxide)

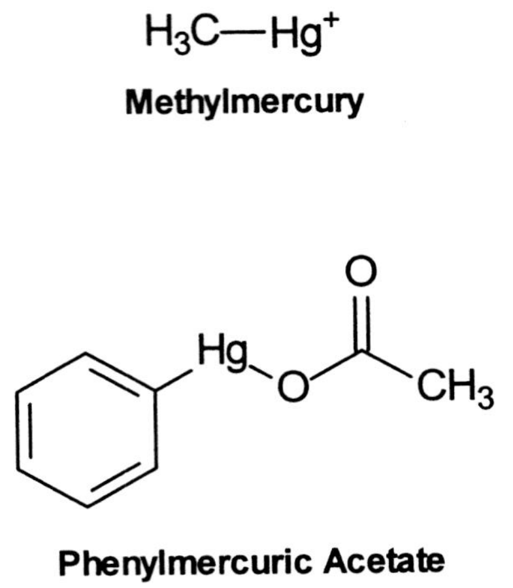

Pathophysiology

The pathophysiology of inorganic mercury exposure is believed to relate to its ability to form covalent bonds to sulfhydryl groups, resulting in enzyme dysfunction and cellular toxicity.[8] The biochemical mechanism of toxicity from methylmercury exposure is complex and not well understood.[9] Inhibition of protein synthesis, induction of lipid peroxidation, mitochondrial changes, and microtubule dysfunction have been proposed as mechanisms of cellular toxicity, although no single common pathway has been identified.

Clinical Presentation

The clinical course of methylmercury poisoning is most remarkable for its effects on the CNS.[10] The cardiovascular, renal, and gastrointestinal systems are not usually affected.[11] A latent period of 2 to 8 weeks between the time of exposure and the onset of symptoms has been described. Initial signs and symptoms include peripheral and perioral paresthesias, followed by prominent cerebellar findings, including incoordination, ataxic gait, and dysarthria.[11] Visual disturbances frequently are present, consisting of constriction of the visual field, reduced acuity, abnormal funduscopic examination, and blindness.[10] Audiologic impairment and dysequilibrium also frequently are reported.[10] Emotional lability, confusion, and delirium develop in severe cases. Most fatalities have been attributed to respiratory failure.[11]

Diagnosis

Mercury can be measured in whole blood and urine using atomic absorption spectrometry. Blood generally is considered the most appropriate biomarker of acute methylmercury exposure.[12] There are conflicting data on the correlation between blood mercury levels and clinical findings after

TABLE 89-2 Miscellaneous Organic Fungicides (Trade Names)

Benomyl (Benex, Benlate, Tersan 1991)
Dodine (Carpene, Curitan, Melprex, Venturol)
Etridiazole (Aaterra, Ethazol, Koban, Pansoil, Terrazole, Truban)
Iprodione (Glycophene, Rovral)
Metalaxyl (Ridomil, Subdue)
Thiabendazole (Apl-Luster, Arbotect, Meretect, Tecto, Thibendazole)
Triadimefon (Amiral, Bayleton)
Triforine (Denarin, Funginex, Saprol)

$$H_3C-Hg^+$$

Methylmercury

Phenylmercuric Acetate

FIGURE 89-1

Chemical structures of organomercurials.

methylmercury poisoning,[10,13] an observation that might be attributed to differences in the timing of clinical presentation and specimen collection. If blood mercury measurements are obtained after distribution to the CNS and other tissues is complete, the blood level may underestimate the total-body mercury burden. A relatively small proportion of methylmercury undergoes renal excretion (10%)[6]; urine mercury concentrations are less useful than concentrations in blood in the diagnosis of methylmercury poisoning. Urine mercury concentrations are useful, however, in monitoring response to chelation therapy. Compared with whole-blood mercury measurements, urine mercury concentrations are a more valid biomarker of exposure to phenylmercuric acetate, which is converted rapidly to inorganic mercury after absorption.[7]

Methylmercury incorporated into hair is stable, and hair analysis has been used to document timing of exposure in epidemiologic studies[14] using a variety of methods of analysis. Hair analysis may be useful in the diagnosis of methylmercury exposure occurring in the weeks or months before presentation. An important source of error in hair analysis for mercury is the presence of inorganic mercury from environmental contamination, an error that may be reduced by washing the sample before analysis.[15] All of the methods of measuring mercury in biologic specimens are subject to considerable variation as a result of contamination during preparation and analysis. Only an experienced laboratory should perform the collection and analysis of specimens.

Treatment

The clinical management of organomercury intoxication begins with the identification of and removal from the source of exposure. In most cases of methylmercury ingestion, the

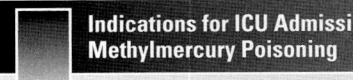

Indications for ICU Admission in Methylmercury Poisoning

Cerebellar signs
Visual impairment
Delirium

development of symptoms occurs after a considerable latent period,[10,11] which limits the potential benefit of gastrointestinal decontamination. Owing to the extensive enterohepatic recirculation of methylmercury,[6] orally administered thiolated resin has been investigated as a means to enhance elimination. In one study,[13] thiolated resin was found to significantly decrease the blood half-life of methylmercury-exposed adults and children, although there was no observed improvement in clinical signs and symptoms. In one of the cases treated with thiolated resin, an individual with an initial blood mercury concentration of 3622 ppb and mild neurologic signs at presentation had no further deterioration in neurologic status on longitudinal follow-up. In the same study, other treatment groups received sodium 2,3-dimercaptopropane-1-sulfonate (DMPS), penicillamine, and N-acetyl-D,L-penicillamine (an experimental analogue of penicillamine). Treatment with each of these agents resulted in a significant decrease in the blood half-life compared with untreated controls. DMPS was reported to have the best efficacy. Although no adverse effects were noted, none of these therapies resulted in observable clinical improvement. This finding is consistent with more recent reports of poisoning with organomercury compounds, in which the therapeutic benefit of chelating agents has been questionable.[16]

Although dimercaprol (British antilewisite) is considered the chelator of choice in the treatment of acute inorganic mercury poisoning, it is not recommended as a therapeutic option in the treatment of methylmercury or phenylmercury toxicity. Experimental animal data suggest that organomercurials may be redistributed to the brain after the administration of dimercaprol.[17] The role of dimercaptosuccinic acid (DMSA) has not been defined in methylmercury toxicity. DMSA has been used effectively to enhance the urinary elimination of mercury in a case report of dimethylmercury poisoning, although no clinical improvement was observed.[16] The limited available human data suggest that the initiation of chelation therapy after serious neurotoxicity has developed provides little to no clinical benefit.[16] In the absence of data supporting the safety and clinical efficacy of chelating agents in this scenario, their use for methylmercury poisoning should not be recommended routinely. The large volume of distribution and extensive protein binding of methylmercury predict that extracorporeal removal techniques would not be successful in enhancing the elimination of the compound.

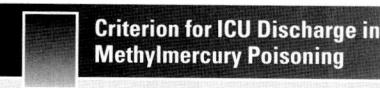

Criterion for ICU Discharge in Methylmercury Poisoning

Resolution of neurologic symptoms

Special Populations

Studies of intrauterine exposure to methylmercury have identified gross impairment of motor and mental development among infants whose mothers were exposed to high levels of methylmercury during pregnancy.[18,19] On follow-up of affected Iraqi infants over 2 years, most children showed considerable neurologic improvement; an exception was infants who were most severely affected at birth.[20]

Common Misconceptions about Methylmercury Poisoning

1. Chelation may improve clinical outcomes.
2. Toxicokinetics is similar to that with inorganic mercury.

Key Points in Methylmercury Poisoning

1. Predominant effects are neurologic (central nervous system).
2. Symptoms may develop after considerable latency.
3. No specific antidote is available.

PENTACHLOROPHENOL

Pentachlorophenol (PCP) (Fig. 89-2) and its sodium salts have been used extensively as a biocide and wood preservative in industry for many years, owing to its broad antimicrobial properties. Although its availability to the general public has been restricted in the United States, PCP continues to have wide industrial applications as a fungicide and wood preservative. There have been several historical accounts of acute poisoning caused by exposure to PCP. In 1967, a cluster of cases of critical illness in a newborn nursery occurred as a result of the misuse of sodium pentachlorophenate as an antimildew agent in the hospital laundry, resulting in nine cases and two fatalities.[21] This and other accounts of accidental occupational exposures[22,23] provide ample toxicologic evidence of the risks from acute exposure to PCP.

Biochemistry and Pharmacokinetics

Pharmacokinetics of Pentachlorophenol

Volume of distribution: >1 L/kg
Protein binding: >90%
Mechanism of clearance: renal
Active metabolites: none
Methods to enhance clearance: exchange transfusion in neonates (?)

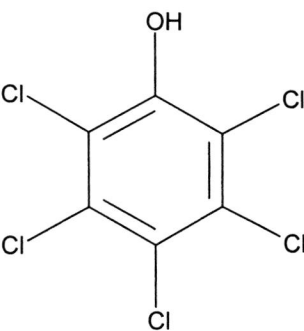

FIGURE 89-2

Chemical structure of pentachlorophenol.

PCP exists as colorless crystals that produce a sharp, phenolic odor when heated. It is insoluble in water and has considerable persistence in the environment, with a reported half-life of 5 years in soil.[22] The industrial production of PCP can yield unwanted contaminants, including dioxins. Although the detection of dioxins could be of concern for the development of chloracne, the presence of this contaminant in commercially available solutions of PCP is debatable, and suppliers in some countries, including the United States and Canada, now are required to limit the content of certain dioxins in their products.[24]

Human exposure to PCP can occur through dermal absorption, ingestion, or inhalation of vapors. Percutaneous absorption is an important route of exposure in neonates and adults. Accidental poisoning has been described in the occupational setting after dipping wood in liquid PCP formulations, immersing unprotected hands in solution, and applying PCP to wood products.[22] The epidemic of critical illness described among newborns suggests that even dermal contact with articles inappropriately treated with PCP (diapers, linens, blankets) may result in significant toxicity.

Pathophysiology

The pathophysiology observed in PCP toxicity develops as a result of the uncoupling of oxidative phosphorylation.[25] As a lipophilic weak acid, PCP can migrate across the inner mitochondrial membrane, bypassing the normal flow of protons in the electron transport chain that lead to the production of adenosine triphosphate (ATP). In this way, the normal process of capturing energy in the formation of ATP is altered, leading to the production of energy in the form of heat. This effect is most pronounced in organ systems dependent on high perfusion and oxygen delivery, including the kidneys, heart, and CNS. Vacuolization of hepatocytes, proximal tubular cells, and myocardial tissue has been shown in fatal cases involving neonates and adults, as have signs of mitochondrial injury on pathologic examination.[23,26] PCP also is an inducer of cytochrome CYP3A,[27] which could influence the metabolism of other drugs used in the critical care management of poisoned patients (e.g., diazepam, alprazolam, and midazolam).

Clinical Presentation

The uncoupling of oxidative phosphorylation best explains the clinical features that have been described as a result of PCP toxicity. Fever, tachypnea, tachycardia, and marked diaphoresis, all signs of a hypermetabolic state, are the most consistent findings.[21–23] Additional physical examination findings include hepatosplenomegaly in affected neonates.[21] Early in the clinical course, the mental status usually is normal despite the presence of moderate fever, although progression to confusion, delirium, and coma occurs at a rapid pace.[21–23] In one adult case of occupational exposure to PCP and a core temperature of 105°F, death occurred within 1 hour of presentation despite aggressive cooling measures.[23]

Diagnosis

Laboratory findings in PCP poisoning reflect the uncoupling of oxidative phosphorylation. A high anion gap metabolic acidosis commonly is observed, particularly in neonates.[21] Ketonemia and ketonuria are common findings.[26] In severe cases, rhabdomyolysis has been reported, with resultant elevation in serum creatine phosphokinase and myoglobinuria.[22] Less specific laboratory findings include elevation of the blood leukocyte count and proteinuria.[22] A consistent finding that has been described on autopsy of fatal cases is the immediate onset of extreme rigor mortis, which has been described as a hallmark of PCP poisoning.[22,23,28] PCP can be detected in serum, urine, and other body fluids by gas chromatography, although measurements obtained from cases of intentional or accidental poisoning can be comparable to levels found in unexposed controls,[23] limiting their prognostic value.

Treatment

The clinical management of PCP toxicity requires the identification of and removal from the source of exposure. The skin should be decontaminated thoroughly with soap and water if this route of exposure is suspected. Based on its physical properties, the adsorption of PCP to activated charcoal is predicted to be poor, which would limit its therapeutic benefit in single or repeated doses. Gastric lavage may be a consideration with early presentation after intentional ingestion. This therapy has not been shown to affect outcome in these patients, however, and there is a small risk of morbidity associated with the procedure (see Chapter 5). Iced gastric lavage may be of additional therapeutic benefit in the presence of hyperthermia. Successful management of PCP toxicity relies on the early recognition and aggressive management of hyperthermia and its complications. Continuous monitoring of core body temperature is necessary to monitor the response to therapy. Passive cooling techniques (administration of intravenous fluids, cooling blankets, ice bath immersion) should be instituted immediately. Given the pathophysiology of PCP toxicity, antipyretics would not be expected to be of any therapeutic benefit. Salicylates theoretically are contraindicated because they could worsen the hyperthermia by further uncoupling oxidative phosphorylation.

No effective antidote for PCP poisoning has been identified. The mainstay of therapy is aggressive supportive management in a critical care unit. Invasive hemodynamic monitoring may be used for standard indications. Exchange transfusion has been used successfully in the management of neonates with PCP toxicity.[26] In all patients treated with exchange transfusion, dramatic clinical improvement was described immediately after the procedure. One of these patients with less severe clinical signs did not undergo exchange transfusion and recovered uneventfully. In this case series, it is unclear whether the successful outcomes could be attributed to exchange transfusion or earlier

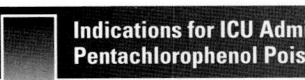

Indications for ICU Admission in Pentachlorophenol Poisoning

Fever
Tachycardia
Acidosis

Criteria for ICU Discharge in Pentachlorophenol Poisoning

Hemodynamic stability
Absence of hyperthermia

recognition of the diagnosis. Exchange transfusion should be considered a therapeutic option in infants because no other methods have been shown to have efficacy in enhancing the elimination of PCP.

Although some authors have recommended forced diuresis as a means to enhance PCP elimination,[29] the data supporting this approach are based on computer-simulated pharmacokinetic models, whereas the toxicokinetics of PCP remains poorly understood. There is no controlled evidence that forced diuresis improves clinical outcomes, and for this reason the emphasis on fluid management in PCP toxicity should focus on restoring and maintaining normal hemodynamic function.

Common Misconception about Pentachlorophenol Poisoning

Forced diuresis improves outcomes in pentachlorophenol toxicity.

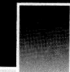

Key Points in Pentachlorophenol Poisoning

1. Hyperthermia and diaphoresis are common clinical findings.
2. Severe toxicity may develop from dermal routes of exposure.

HEXACHLOROBENZENE

Of the substituted benzene fungicides, HCB (Fig. 89-3) is the best studied. Although the acute toxicity from ingestion or inhalation exposure is low with HCB, the systemic effects from chronic exposure are well documented. Between 1955 and 1959, an epidemic of porphyria cutanea

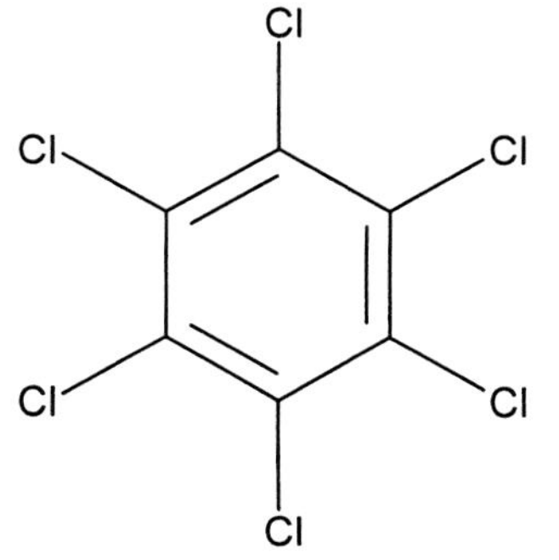

FIGURE 89-3

Chemical structure of hexachlorobenzene.

tarda (PCT) that involved 5000 cases was described in Turkey.[30] The cause was traced to the consumption of wheat that had been treated with 10% HCB as a seed protectant. HCB has been detected frequently as a contaminant in the industrial production of many chlorinated solvents, which may be important in the context of occupational and environmental exposures. Although single case reports have reported PCT in association with occupational exposure to HCB, larger-scale epidemiologic studies have not confirmed this relationship.[31] The differences in clinical manifestations between occupational exposure to HCB and the outbreak in Turkey may be related to the dose, duration, and route of exposure to the compound. Other substituted benzene formulations continue to be used as fungicides in the United States, although systemic poisonings and PCT have not been widely reported with these compounds.

Biochemistry and Pharmacokinetics

Pharmacokinetics of Hexachlorobenzene

Volume of distribution: >1 L/kg
Protein binding: 45%
Mechanism of clearance: >90% fecal
Active metabolite: pentachlorophenol (clinically insignificant)
Methods to enhance elimination: none

HCB (see Fig. 89-3) is a chlorinated aromatic hydrocarbon that is highly lipid soluble and well absorbed from the gastrointestinal tract.[32]

Pathophysiology

Animal studies have shown that when absorbed, HCB has a large volume of distribution and bioaccumulates in adipose tissue.[32] Altered heme synthesis is induced by HCB through the inhibition of uroporphyrinogen decarboxylase activity, leading to the accumulation of uroporphyrin and the induction of aminolevulinic acid synthetase. Consistent with other organochlorine compounds, HCB is capable of inducing several families of the cytochrome P-450 system. Toxicokinetic data in humans are not readily available, but an investigation of a population with a high level of HCB exposure suggested that excretion occurs predominantly through the feces.[33] A small proportion appears in the urine as chlorinated phenols, including PCP, although signs of toxicity relating to this metabolite have not been reported in individuals with high body burdens of HCB.

Clinical Presentation

The latency between exposure and the development of signs and symptoms of PCT varies depending on dose, but epidemiologic studies suggest a delay of several months after repeated ingestion.[34] In mild cases, early skin lesions consist of bullae containing clear fluid, occurring in sun-exposed areas (particularly the face and hands). The skin is unusually sensitive, and the epidermis easily rubs off from slight mechanical trauma (Nikolski's sign).[34] The bullous lesions

TABLE 89-3 Laboratory Diagnostic Patterns of Porphyria Cutanea Tarda

Urine concentration
  Porphobilinogen and aminolevulinic acid are not increased
  Uroporphyrinogen is increased greater than heptacarboxylate
Fecal porphyrins
  Isocoproporphyrinogen, heptacarboxylate present
Erythrocyte porphyrins
  Not increased

subsequently may break down and become infected, forming pigmented scars and contractures. In addition, there is marked hypertrichosis throughout the body. Weight loss and hepatomegaly frequently are present, usually without abdominal pain or neurologic symptoms.[30] These clinical findings distinguish PCT from acute intermittent porphyria, another disease associated with abnormal heme biosynthesis, in which abdominal pain and neuropsychiatric symptoms frequently are prominent.

Diagnosis

In addition to the prominent dermatologic signs of toxicity, the diagnosis of PCT can be supported on the basis of urinary findings. A dark red urine, which under Wood's light exhibits intense red fluorescence, has been described.[30] In contrast to other types of porphyria, urine concentrations of porphobilinogen and aminolevulinic acid are not increased, although elevated levels of uroporphyrinogen may be detected.[35] Table 89-3 summarizes urinary, fecal, and erythrocyte porphyrin findings suggesting PCT. Evidence of mild iron overload (elevated ferritin) frequently is present.[35] HCB may be measured in blood using gas chromatography, although a reference range is not established, and a threshold dose that corresponds with the development of PCT is not known.[31,33]

Treatment

No specific antidote for HCB-induced PCT has been identified, and no specific methods of gastric or skin decontamination have been reported. A case series has described the use of oral and intravenously administered ethylenediaminetetraacetic acid (EDTA) in the clinical management of PCT associated with HCB ingestion.[36] The administration of EDTA was reported to transiently increase the excretion of porphyrin, which was associated with improvement in skin lesions and weight gain. There have been no subsequent studies on the safety and efficacy of chelating agents for PCT since that time. Current therapeutic

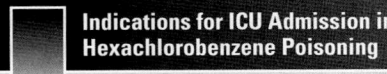
Indications for ICU Admission in Hexachlorobenzene Poisoning

Extensive skin involvement (>10% body surface area)
Superinfection of skin lesions

recommendations for PCT include avoidance of sunlight exposure and supportive management, with special attention to skin care.[35] Phlebotomy may be effective therapy in PCT to deplete excess iron stores, and the avoidance of alcohol and exogenous estrogens has been recommended.[35] Low-dose hydroxychloroquine (Plaquenil) has been investigated as a therapeutic agent for PCT in controlled studies and has been reported to be safe and effective at normalizing urinary porphyrin excretion and improving skin lesions.[37]

Criterion for ICU Discharge in Hexachlorobenzene Poisoning

Resolution of skin lesions and infection

Special Populations

In the epidemic of PCT in Turkey, a second disorder called *pembe yara,* or *pink sore,* was described in breast-fed infants of mothers who had PCT or had ingested HCB-contaminated bread.[35] Symptoms and signs included pink cutaneous lesions, fever, diarrhea, vomiting, weakness, hepatomegaly, and convulsions. The skin lesions characteristic of PCT were not observed in these infants, and the mortality rate was high (95%). No porphyrinuria was observed in these infants.

Common Misconceptions about Hexachlorobenzene Poisoning

1. Chelation is effective therapy.
2. Porphyria cutanea tarda and acute intermittent porphyria are the same disease.

Key Points in Hexachlorobenzene Poisoning

1. Skin manifestations include bullous lesions and generalized hypertrichosis.
2. Breakdown of bullous lesions can lead to scarring and contractions.
3. Urinary findings may provide important diagnostic clues.

DITHIOCARBAMATES

As a class of general- and restricted-use fungicides, the dithiocarbamates are available in a variety of formulations, including water suspensions, wettable powders, and dusts. They have many agricultural applications, including the protection of seedlings, turf, vegetables, fruits, and ornamentals from fungal growth. Compared with the known toxicity of several of the classes of fungicides that already have been described, the dithiocarbamates are of considerably lower acute toxicity owing to their rapid metabolism and lack of persistence in mammalian systems. In contrast to the *N*-methyl carbamates, dithiocarbamates have poor efficacy as insecticides because they do not have significant effects on cholinesterase activity.[38] Certain dithiocarbamates warrant further discussion, however, because of their potential for causing acute illness through several different mechanisms.

Biochemistry and Pharmacokinetics

Pharmacokinetics of Dithiocarbamate

Active metabolites: carbon disulfide (all dithiocarbamates); methyl isothiocyanate (metam-sodium)
Methods to enhance elimination: none

The chemical structure and environmental fate of the dithiocarbamates are predictive of their spectrum of toxicity (Fig. 89-4). Metam-sodium is an aqueous solution used as a soil biocide and fumigant. Although it is nonvolatile, it quickly degrades on soil or water contact to produce methyl isothiocyanate, which is responsible for its fungicidal activity. Thiram is another important dithiocarbamate because it is a known skin sensitizer and a common component of natural rubber latex. Other subclasses of the dithiocarbamate family, the metallobisdithiocarbamates and ethylene bisdithiocarbamates (EBDC compounds), are named for the metallic component in their formulation (zinc, manganese, iron). These subclasses do not interact with acetaldehyde dehydrogenase.

Pathophysiology

Metam-sodium and thiram are thiurams, in the same chemical class as disulfiram (Antabuse), and theoretically could induce a disulfiram-like reaction in a susceptible individual through inhibition of acetaldehyde dehydrogenase. Methyl isothiocyanate is a potent mucosal irritant, and effects have been observed well below the threshold for odor detection.[39] The toxicokinetics of dithiocarbamates has not been studied in humans.

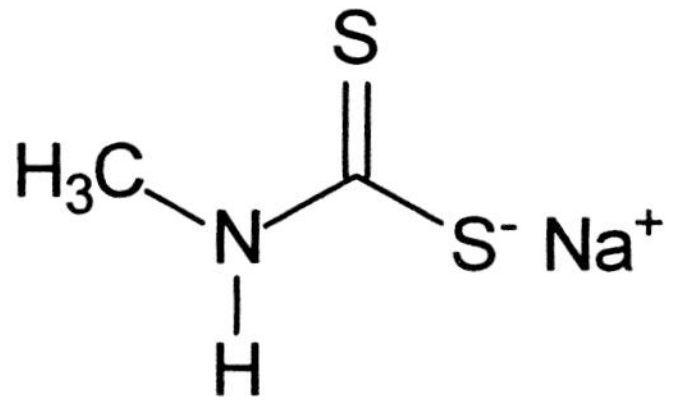

$$\underset{\text{H}_3\text{C}}{\overset{\text{S}}{\underset{|}{\underset{\text{H}}{\text{N}}}}}\text{C}-\text{S}^-\ \text{Na}^+$$

Metam-sodium (dithiocarbamate)

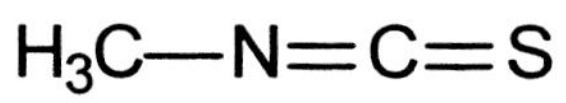

$$\text{H}_3\text{C}-\text{N}=\text{C}=\text{S}$$

Methyl isothiocyanate

FIGURE 89-4

Chemical structure of dithiocarbamate and its decomposition product, methyl isothiocyanate.

Clinical Presentation

Contact dermatitis and irritant symptoms to the upper airways are the most common clinical presentations after exposure to dithiocarbamates. Workers involved in the cleanup of an accidental metam-sodium spill into the Sacramento River developed erythema, rash, itching, and scaling of the lower extremities, areas that had come into contact with contaminated water.[40] The same chemical spill had resulted in the emergency triage of 360 individuals, most of whom had mild irritant upper airway symptoms that did not require hospitalization.[41] A follow-up study of adults living within 0.5 mile of the site of the accident identified 20 cases of persistent irritant-induced asthma and 10 cases of persistent exacerbation of asthma.[39] Although effects consistent with aldehyde dehydrogenase inhibition were not reported in this cohort, a few case reports have described signs and symptoms consistent with a disulfiram-like reaction after individuals consumed ethanol following the use of topical products containing thiram.[42]

Other systemic effects purportedly related to dithiocarbamate exposure have been described, although the results of these studies are not conclusive. A case of acute renal failure that was related temporally to the use of maneb (manganous EBDC) has been reported,[43] although the exposure history was limited, and nontoxicologic explanations for the presentation were not ruled out. A single case of Henoch-Schönlein purpura has been reported, temporally associated with thiram exposure in a tree planter.[44] The exposure history consisted of falling down a hillside while carrying a bag of seedlings treated with a solution of 42% thiram. There have been no similar cases of acute renal failure or Henoch-Schönlein purpura reported in association with dithiocarbamate exposure. Signs and symptoms consistent with manganese toxicity (muscle rigidity with cogwheeling, nervousness, memory problems) have been associated with chronic occupational exposure to maneb in a case-control study,[45] although no significant difference in blood manganese levels was noted between cases and controls.

Diagnosis

There are no validated methods for detecting dithiocarbamate fungicides in biologic fluids. The diagnosis depends on a careful exposure history and physical examination.

Treatment

When dermal exposure is suspected, decontamination with soap and water is indicated. When inhalational exposure to metam-sodium or its breakdown product, methyl isothiocyanate, is suspected, respiratory distress or signs of obstruction should be treated with supplemental oxygen, inhaled

Indications for ICU Admission in Dithiocarbamate Poisoning

Respiratory distress
Severe disulfiram (Antabuse) reaction (tachycardia, hypotension, refractory vomiting)

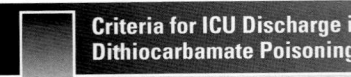

Criteria for ICU Discharge in Dithiocarbamate Poisoning

Resolution of signs of respiratory distress
Hemodynamically stable

bronchodilators, and continuous pulse oximetry monitoring in an intensive care unit. The treatment of isocyanate exposure is described further in Chapter 96. If a disulfiram-like reaction is apparent, standard supportive symptomatic management is indicated.

Common Misconception about Dithiocarbamate Poisoning

Dithiocarbamates affect cholinesterase activity.

Key Points in Dithiocarbamate Poisoning

1. Primary clinical effects are dermatologic (irritation, sensitization).
2. Decomposition product of metam-sodium is a potent mucosal irritant.
3. Disulfiram (Antabuse) reaction is possible with certain dithiocarbamates.

COPPER COMPOUNDS

Several copper compounds are available as fungicides for commercial use. Intentional and accidental ingestion of copper compounds historically has been a common cause of morbidity and mortality outside the United States, an observation that may be related to their widespread international availability and use.[46]

Biochemistry and Pharmacokinetics

Pharmacokinetics of Copper Compounds

Volume of distribution: >1 L/kg
Protein binding: >90%
Mechanism of clearance: >90% biliary
Active metabolites: none
Methods to enhance clearance: dimercaprol (?), calcium ethylenediaminetetraacetic acid (?)

The soluble copper salts (e.g., copper sulfate) are not well absorbed across the skin or gastrointestinal tract. The organic copper compounds (copper naphthenate, copper quinolinolate) have a higher bioavailability.[47]

Pathophysiology

The predominant mechanism of toxicity of copper compounds is through mucous membrane irritation and corrosive effects on the gastrointestinal tract. Corrosive injury is discussed in detail in Chapter 99.

Clinical Presentation

With massive ingestions, greenish blue emesis, hematemesis, and melena may develop.[48] Acute effects on the liver include jaundice and pathologic findings of centrilobular necrosis.[49] Intravascular hemolysis, Heinz body formation (precipitation of oxidatively denatured hemoglobin), and methemoglobinemia (see Chapter 28) also have been described.[50]

Diagnosis

Copper levels may be measured in serum, whole blood, and urine using atomic absorption spectrometry and inductively coupled plasma–atomic emission spectroscopy. There also are sensitive colorimetric assays for copper. In one case series, whole-blood concentrations greater than 2.87 mg/L (45.9 μmol/L) correlated with gastrointestinal symptoms, and levels greater than 7.98 mg/L (127.7 μmol/L) correlated with hepatorenal dysfunction or shock.[51] In this case series, whole-blood copper levels correlated better than serum copper concentrations with the severity of clinical illness. Urine levels have been investigated in the diagnosis of diseases associated with copper excess (Wilson's disease), although their diagnostic and prognostic value in copper fungicide exposures has not been evaluated.

Treatment

The role of gastrointestinal decontamination after accidental or intentional ingestion is simplified because spontaneous emesis is expected after significant ingestion of copper compounds. No data support the efficacy of activated charcoal to decrease absorption of copper compounds after accidental or intentional ingestions.

Because of the corrosive gastrointestinal injury associated with acute copper exposure, parenteral chelators, such as dimercaprol and calcium disodium edetate, theoretically would be considered the therapy of choice after acute overdose. There are few pharmacokinetic data to guide appropriate dosing of these agents,[49] and their safety and efficacy for acute copper poisonings have not been established. In one case report of intentional copper and zinc sulfate ingestion, chelation therapy with dimercaprol and penicillamine was not found to be of clinical benefit.[52] The potential therapeutic benefit of other orally available chelating agents,

Indications for ICU Admission in Copper Compound Poisoning

Hematemesis
Shock
Signs of significant hepatic injury
Renal failure

Criteria for ICU Discharge in Copper Compound Poisoning

Resolution of gastrointestinal symptoms and signs
Hemodynamic stability

such as DMSA, in acute copper toxicity has not been studied. The use of these chelators for other heavy metal poisonings is described in their respective chapters.

Common Misconception about Copper Compound Poisoning

Chelation therapy is safe and effective for copper fungicide exposures.

Key Points in Copper Compound Poisoning

1. Corrosive gastrointestinal effects develop after ingestion.
2. Hepatic injury and necrosis may develop.
3. Oxidative injury and methemoglobinemia have been described.

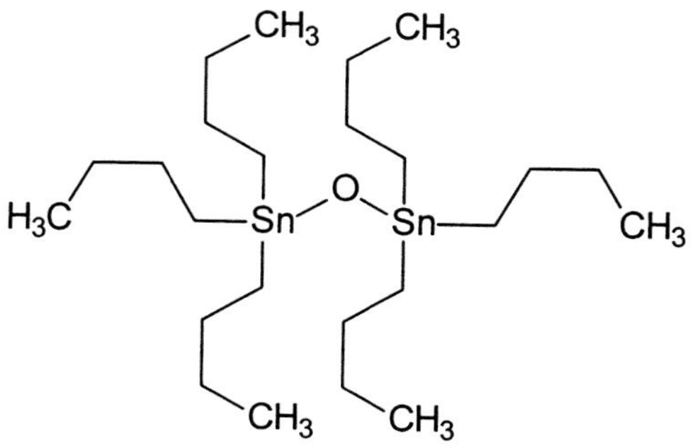

FIGURE 89-5

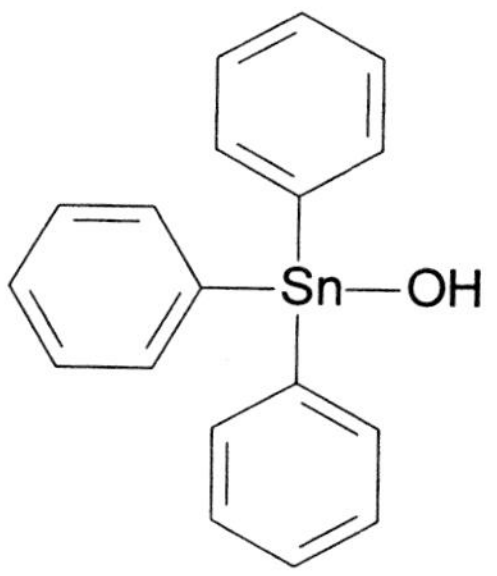

Chemical structures of organotin fungicides.

ORGANOTIN COMPOUNDS

Organotin compounds are formulated as wettable and flow-able powders and used as fungicides in a variety of agricultural and industrial settings throughout the world. Tributyltin oxide (TBTO) had been registered for use as an antimildew control agent in interior and exterior paints, but it now is severely restricted in many countries owing to its potent irritant properties. TBTO continues to be used as an antifouling agent in marine paints.

Biochemistry and Pharmacokinetics

Pharmacokinetics of Organotin

Volume of distribution: >1 L/kg
Protein binding: 80%
Mechanism of clearance: biliary, fecal
Active metabolite: trimethyltin
Methods to enhance clearance: none

In general, organotin compounds have low water solubility and are lipophilic (Fig. 89-5). Toxicokinetic data in humans are not available.[53]

Pathophysiology

TBTO is a potent skin irritant and an extreme eye irritant.[54] Triphenyltin compounds have been shown to induce irre-

versible ocular lesions in animal studies.[53] Immunotoxicity (lymphopenia, decreased spleen and thymus weights) and immunosuppressive effects (altered humoral and cellular immunity) have been described from organotin compounds in short-term and long-term animal exposure studies.[53,54] These immunotoxic effects may arise from cytoskeletal modification in addition to alterations in thymocyte calcium homeostasis.

Clinical Presentation

Symptoms from inhalational exposure to interior paints with TBTO additives include headache, nausea, mucosal irritation, watery eyes, and wheezing.[55] Dermal exposure from direct contact with TBTO compounds has resulted in severe skin irritation, contact folliculitis, and pruritic erythematous vesiculobullous rashes.[56,57]

Reports of other systemic effects from accidental or intentional ingestion of organotin compounds are rare, and limited clinical information is available. In one case of intentional ingestion of triphenyltin acetate,[58] a 19-year-old woman developed symptoms of vomiting, weakness, and nausea, followed by the development of diplopia, vertigo, bidirectional nystagmus, and disorientation. Leukopenia was noted on the sixth day postingestion. No other hematologic, renal, or hepatic abnormalities were found, and functional and radiographic studies of the CNS (including single-photon emission computed tomography and magnetic resonance imaging) were unremarkable except for nonspecific electroencephalogram changes. A full recovery was described with supportive management. A mass poisoning involving three deaths and hundreds of hospitalizations was reported in association with the misuse of industrial lard contaminated with organotin compounds as cooking oil.[59] Gas chromatography and inductively coupled plasma–mass spectrometry were used to detect and measure organotin species in blood and urine. Trimethyltin and dimethyltin were detected in urine samples at ng/mL concentrations. This report did not provide information on the clinical presentation and hospital course of the cases, which limits the utility of the biomarker findings.

Diagnosis

With inhalational and dermal routes of exposure, physical examination findings consistent with organotin exposure include skin and mucous membrane irritation. In cases of systemic intoxication, gas chromatography and inductively coupled plasma–mass spectrometry may be used to detect and quantify organotin species in blood and urine specimens, although reference ranges have not been established. A complete blood count with differential may reveal lymphopenia as an immunotoxic manifestation of systemic organotin toxicity.

Treatment

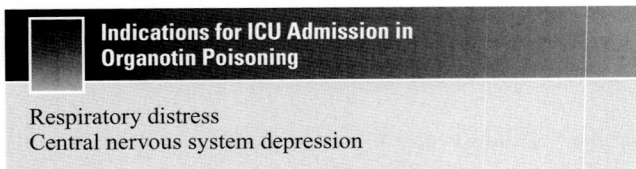

Indications for ICU Admission in Organotin Poisoning

Respiratory distress
Central nervous system depression

Identification and removal from exposure and supportive management are the mainstays of therapy after exposure to organotin compounds. No data are available on the efficacy of gastric decontamination methods after accidental or intentional human ingestions. There have been no animal studies on the efficacy of chelating agents in enhancing the elimination of organotin compounds, and there are no data supporting their efficacy in humans.

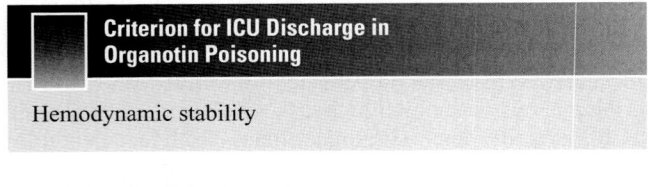

Criterion for ICU Discharge in Organotin Poisoning

Hemodynamic stability

Key Points in Organotin Poisoning

1. Organotin compounds are potent skin and mucosal irritants.
2. Immunotoxic effects have been described after acute systemic exposure.

REFERENCES

1. Litovitz TL, Klein-Schwartz W, White S, et al: 1999 Annual report of the American Association of Poison Control Centers Toxic Exposure Surveillance System. Am J Emerg Med 18:517–574, 2000.
2. Larsen AI, Larsen A, Jepsen JR, et al: Contact allergy to the fungicide benomyl? Contact Dermatol 22:278–281, 1990.
3. Spagnolo A, Bianchi F, Calabro A, et al: Anophthalmia and benomyl in Italy: A multicenter study based on 940,615 newborns. Reprod Toxicol 8:397–403, 1994.
4. Kallen B, Robert E, Harris J: The descriptive epidemiology of anophthalmia and microphthalmia. Int J Epidemiol 25:1009–1016, 1996.
5. Myers GJ, Davidson PW, Cox C, et al: Twenty-seven years studying the human neurotoxicity of methylmercury exposure. Environ Res 83:275–285, 2000.
6. Goyer RA (ed): Toxicological Effects of Methylmercury. Washington, D.C., National Academy Press, 2000.
7. Agocs MM, Etzel RA, Parrish RG, et al: Mercury exposure from interior latex paint. N Engl J Med 323:1096–1101, 1990.
8. Klaassen C: Heavy metals and heavy-metal antagonists. In Gilman AG, Rall TW, Nies AS, Taylor P (eds): Goodman and Gilman's The Pharmacological Basis of Therapeutics, 8th ed. New York, Pergamon Press, 1990, pp 1592–1614.
9. Chang LW, Verity MA: Mercury neurotoxicity: Effects and mechanisms. In Chang LW, Eyer RS (eds): Handbook of Neurotoxicology. New York, Marcel Dekker, 1995, pp 31–59.
10. Rustam H, Hamdi T: Methyl mercury poisoning in Iraq. Brain 97:499–510, 1974.
11. Bakir F, Damluji SF, Amin-Zaki L, et al: Methylmercury poisoning in Iraq: An interuniversity report. Science 181:230–240, 1973.
12. Dales LG: The neurotoxicity of alkyl mercury compounds. Am J Med 53:219–232, 1972.
13. Clarkson TW, Magos L, Cox C, et al: Tests of efficacy of antidotes for removal of methylmercury in human poisoning during the Iraq outbreak. J Pharm Exp Ther 218:74–83, 1981.
14. Environmental Health Criteria 101: Methylmercury. Geneva, International Programme on Chemical Safety, 1990.
15. Suzuki T, Hongo T, Yoshinaga J, et al: The hair-organ relationship in mercury concentration in contemporary Japanese. Arch Environ Health 48:221–229, 1993.
16. Nierenberg DW, Nordgren RE, Chang MB, et al: Brief report: Delayed cerebellar disease and death after accidental exposure to dimethylmercury. N Engl J Med 338:1672–1676, 1998.
17. Canty AJ, Kishimoto R: British anti-Lewisite and organomercury poisoning. Science 253:123–125, 1975.
18. Amin-Zaki L, Elhassani S, Majeed MA, et al: Intra-uterine methylmercury poisoning in Iraq. Pediatrics 54:587–595, 1974.
19. Kondo K: Congenital Minimata disease: Warnings from Japan's experience. J Child Neurol 15:458–464, 2000.
20. Amin-Zaki L, Majeed MA, Clarkson TW, et al: Methylmercury poisoning in Iraqi children: Clinical observations over two years. BMJ 1:613–616, 1978.
21. Smith JE, Loveless LE, Belden EA, et al: Epidemiological notes and reports: Pentachlorophenol poisoning in newborn infants—St. Louis, Missouri, April-August 1967. MMWR Morb Mortal Wkly Rep 45:545–549, 1996.
22. Jorens PG, Schepens PJ: Human pentachlorophenol poisoning. Hum Exp Toxicol 12:479–495, 1993.
23. Gray RE, Gilliand RD, Smith EE, et al: Pentachlorophenol intoxication: Report of a fatal case, with comments on the clinical course and pathologic anatomy. Arch Environ Health 40:161–164, 1985.
24. IARC Monographs on the Evaluation of Carcinogenic Risks to Humans, Vol 53: Occupational Exposures in Insecticide Application and Some Pesticides. Lyon, IARC, 1991.
25. Farquharson ME, Gage JC, Northover J: The biological action of chlorophenols. Br J Pharmacol 13:20–24, 1958.
26. Robson AM, Kissane JM, Elvick NH, et al: Pentachlorophenol poisoning in a nursery for newborn infants: I. Clinical features and treatment. J Pediatr 75:309–316, 1969.
27. Dubois M, Plaisance H, Thome JP: Hierarchical cluster analysis of environmental pollutants through P450 induction in cultured hepatic cells. Ecotoxicol Environ Saf 34:205–215, 1996.
28. Mason MF, Wallace SM, Foerster E, et al: Pentachlorophenol poisoning: Report of two cases J Forens Sci 10:136–137, 1965.
29. Young JF, Haley TJ: A pharmacokinetic study of pentachlorophenol poisoning and the effect of forced diuresis. Clin Toxicol 12:41–48, 1978.
30. Schmid R: Cutaneous porphyria in Turkey. N Engl J Med 263:397–398, 1960.
31. Currier MF, McClimans CD, Barna-Lloyd G: Hexachlorobenzene blood levels and the health status of men employed in the manufacture of chlorinated solvents. J Toxicol Environ Health 6:367–377, 1980.

32. Arnold D, Gocmen G, Jannson B, et al: International Programme on Chemical Safety Environmental Health Criteria 195: Hexachlorobenzene. Geneva, World Health Organization, 1997.
33. To-Figueras J, Barrot C, Sala M, et al: Excretion of hexachlorobenzene and metabolites in feces in a highly exposed human population. Environ Health Perspect 108:595–598, 2000.
34. Cam C, Nigogosyan G: Acquired toxic porphyria cutanea tarda due to hexachlorobenzene. JAMA 183:88–91, 1963.
35. Thadani H, Deacon A, Peters T: Diagnosis and management of porphyria. BMJ 320:1647–1651, 2000.
36. Peters HA, Johnson AM, Cam S: Hexachlorobenzene-induced porphyria: effect of chelation on the disease, porphyrin and metal metabolism. Am J Med Sci 251:314–322, 1966.
37. Wallace DJ: The use of chloroquine and hydroxychloroquine for non-infectious conditions other than rheumatoid arthritis or lupus: A critical review. Lupus 5:S59–64, 1996.
38. Machemer LH, Pickel M: Carbamate herbicides and fungicides. Toxicology 91:105–109, 1994.
39. Cone JE, Wugofski L, Balmes JR, et al: Persistent respiratory health effects after a metam sodium pesticide spill. Chest 106:500–508, 1994.
40. Centers for Disease Control: Dermatitis among workers cleaning the Sacramento River after a chemical spill—California, 1991. MMWR Morb Mortal Wkly Rep 40:825–827, 1991.
41. Koehler GA, Van Ness C: The emergency medical response to the Cantara hazardous materials incident. Prehosp Disaster Med 8:359–365, 1993.
42. Shelley WB: Golf-course dermatitis due to thiram fungicide. JAMA 188:415–417, 1964.
43. Koizumi A, Shiojima S, Omiya M, et al: Acute renal failure and maneb exposure. JAMA 242:2583–2585, 1979.
44. Duell PB, Morton WE: Henoch-Schönlein purpura following thiram exposure. Arch Intern Med 147:778–779, 1987.
45. Ferraz HB, Bertolucci PH, Pereira JS, et al: Chronic exposure to the fungicide maneb may produce symptoms and signs of CNS manganese intoxication. Neurology 38:550–553, 1988.
46. Singh D, Jit I, Tyagi S: Changing trends in acute poisoning in Chandigarh zone: A 25-year autopsy experience from a tertiary care hospital in northern India. Am J Forensic Med Pathol 20:203–210, 1999.
47. Reigart JR, Roberts JR: Recognition and Management of Pesticide Poisonings, 5th ed. Washington, DC, Environmental Protection Agency, 1999.
48. Ahasan HAMN, Chodhury MAH, Azhar MA, Rafiqueuddin AKM: Copper sulphate poisoning. Trop Doctor 24:52–53, 1994.
49. Barceleaux D: Copper. J Toxicol Clin Toxicol 37:217–230, 1999.
50. Chugh KS, Singhal PC, Sharma BK: Methemoglobinemia in acute copper sulphate poisoning. Ann Intern Med 82:226–227, 1975.
51. Chuttani HK, Gupta PS, Gulati S, Gupta DN: Acute copper sulfate poisoning. Am J Med 39:849–854, 1965.
52. Hantson P, Lievens M, Mahieu P: Accidental ingestion of a zinc and copper sulfate preparation. J Toxicol Clin Toxicol 34:725–730, 1996.
53. Sekizawa J: Concise International Chemical Assessment Document No. 13: Triphenyltin Compounds. Geneva, World Health Organization, 1999.
54. Benson R: Concise International Chemical Assessment Document No. 14: Triphenyltin Compounds, Geneva. World Health Organization, 1999.
55. Wax P, Dockstader L: Tributyltin use in interior paints: A continuing health hazard. J Toxicol Clin Toxicol 33:239–241, 1995.
56. Lyle WH: Lesions of the skin in process workers caused by contact with butyl tin compounds. Br J Ind Med 15:193–196, 1958.
57. Goh CL: Irritant dermatitis from tri-N-butyl tin oxide in paint. Contact Derm 12:161–163, 1985.
58. Lin T, Hung D, Kao C, et al: Unique cerebral dysfunction following triphenyltin acetate poisoning. Hum Exp Toxicol 17:403–405, 1998.
59. Gui-bin J, Qun-fang Z, Bin H: Tin compounds and major trace metal elements in organotin-poisoned patient's urine and blood measured by gas chromatography-flame photometric detector and inductively coupled plasma-mass spectrometry. Bull Environ Contam Toxicol 65:277–284, 2000.

CHAPTER 90

Organochlorine, Pyrethrin, and Pyrethroid Insecticides

Scott D. Phillips

The widespread use of insecticides in industry and agriculture began early in the 20th century, when naturally occurring agents were identified and structural modification and synthesis of the insecticidal components of natural pyrethrins occurred. By the 1950s, organophosphorus, methyl carbamates, and organochlorine (OC) insecticides came into widespread use, but the demand for more economical and less persistent compounds prompted the development of synthetic substances with these properties. One category of the latter used frequently is the pyrethroids.

PYRETHRIN AND PYRETHROID INSECTICIDES

Pyrethrum is the oleoresin of the dried chrysanthemum flower. The resin contains several esters with insecticidal activity, comprising approximately 50% of the ingredients. These esters are known as *pyrethrins*. Pyrethrins have been used as insecticides for centuries.[1]

In the United States, reports to poison centers regarding pyrethroid exposure have been quantitatively similar to reports regarding organophosphate insecticides, but with fewer clinically important poisonings.[2] During a more recent year of reporting, there were no deaths, and most clinical outcomes had either minor or no effects. There were 23 cases of major outcomes for pyrethrins with and without piperonyl.

Biochemistry

Pyrethrins are esters of pyrethroic and chrysanthemic acids, obtained from chrysanthemum flowers (*Chrysanthemum*). In their purified forms, each pyrethrin is a nonpolar, viscous liquid. Other esters present in the resin are cinerins and jasmolins. All of these esters are lipophilic. Pyrethrum and pyrethrins are extremely photolabile, readily decomposing in sunlight and ultraviolet light. Because of this, they typically are used indoors.

The word *pyrethrin* is a general term used for each of the six naturally occurring insecticidal compounds in pyrethrum. Pyrethrum contains a variable mixture of the six specific pyrethrins: cinerin I, cinerin II, jasmolin I, jasmolin II, pyrethrin I, and pyrethrin II (Fig. 90-1). Pyrethrins designated with *I* have a methyl group ($-CH_3$) and pyrethrins with *II* have an ester group ($-COOCH_3$) at the most significant differentiating site in these molecules. This *I* and *II* designation for pyrethrins is not related to the

type I and *type II* terminology used for the synthetic pyrethroids described in the next paragraph.

Pyrethroids, synthetic pyrethrin derivatives (see Fig. 90-1), are stable in sunlight, more potent, and of broad spectrum and hence are suitable for use in agricultural applications. The first production of pyrethroids was in the late 1940s.[3] It was not until 1973, however, that a photostable pyrethroid was developed.[4] Pyrethroids exhibit greater insecticidal activity and photostability than the natural pyrethrins. More than 1000 pyrethroids have been synthesized; each possesses different biologic activity, depending on its structure. All exhibit broad-spectrum insecticidal activity, however. The synthetic pyrethroids are divided into two types, depending on the absence (type I) or presence (type II) of a cyano (nitrile) group ($-CN$). The cyano group gives the type II pyrethroids greater insecticidal activity, greater photostability, and the potential for greater mammalian toxicity. Permethrin is an example of a type I pyrethroid that is used as a pharmaceutical scabicide in medications such as Nix and RID. Cypermethrin, deltamethrin, and fenvalerate are examples of insecticidal type II pyrethroids.

Pathophysiology

The major site of action of the pyrethrins and pyrethroids is the voltage-dependent sodium channels in excitable tissues.[5] This interaction allows a greater influx of sodium into the cell, resulting in sustained activation (depolarization) and deactivation (repolarization) in hyperexcitable tissues.[6] Some pyrethroid isomers are more potent than others. Pyrethroids have a high affinity for active sodium channels; however, they have little effect on inactive or closed channels and are known as *open channel blockers*.[7] Type I and type II pyrethroids produce sympathetic activation.

Type I (also known as *T syndrome*) pyrethroids cause brief, repetitive nerve discharges. Type II (*CS syndrome*) pyrethroids produce more sustained, repetitive nerve discharges that are due to a greater delay in sodium channel closure (Fig. 90-2). Type II pyrethroids also inhibit chloride conduction through the chloride channel in the γ-aminobutyric acid (GABA)$_A$/drug receptor–chloride channel complex, causing seizures.[8] Several other tissue targets have been described, including protein kinases, adrenergic synapses causing norepinephrine release, nicotinic receptors, mitochondrial complex I, mitochondrial adenosine triphosphatase (ATPase), and intercellular gap junctions (Table 90-1).[7]

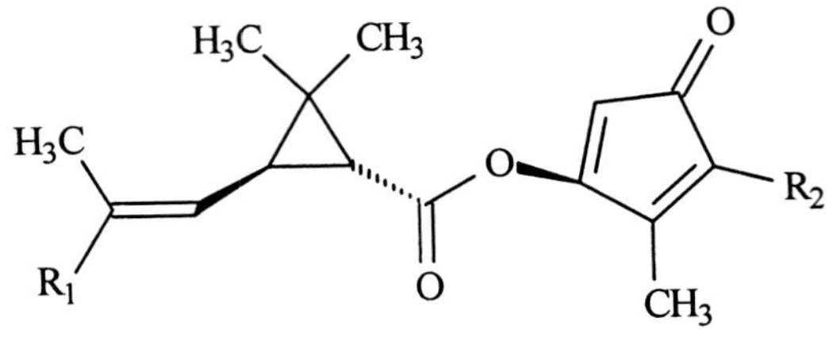

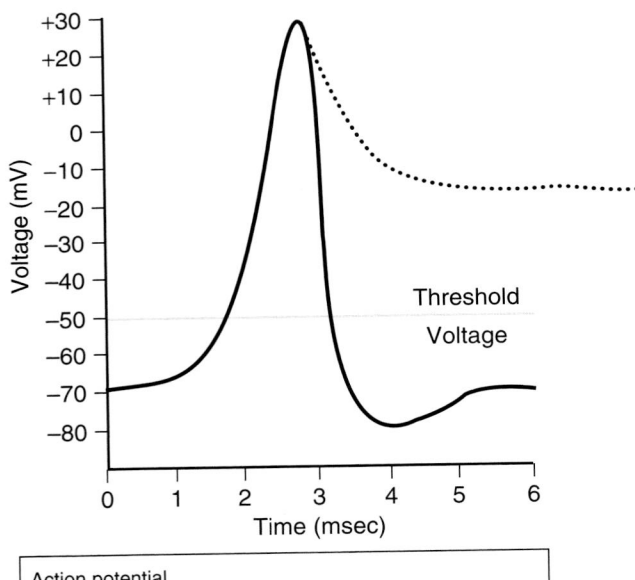

FIGURE 90-1

Chemical structures of pyrethrum isomers.

Compound Name	R_1	R_2
Pyrethrin I	$-CH_3$	$-CH_2CH=CHCH=CH_2$
Pyrethrin II	$-CO_2CH_3$	$-CH_2CH=CHCH=CH_2$
Cinerin I	$-CH_3$	$-CH_2CH=CHCH_3$
Cinerin II	$-CO_2CH_3$	$-CH_2CH=CHCH_3$
Jasmolin I	$-CH_3$	$-CH_2CH=CHCH_2CH_3$
Jasmolin II	$-CO_2CH_3$	$-CH_2CH=CHCH_2CH_3$

Toxicokinetics

Pyrethroids are lipophilic and are absorbed, to some degree, via intact skin, lungs, or intestinal tract. Depending on the specific pyrethrin or pyrethroid, this absorption may be a minor or a major route of absorption.[7,9] Skin absorption is slow.[10] Depending on the magnitude of the dose, however, the skin is the major pathway of poisoning.[11] When pyrethroids enter the vascular compartment, their half-lives range from hours to days.[12] Some metabolites have half-lives of days.[13] Pyrethroids and pyrethrins are distributed widely throughout all organ systems but with low tissue residues.[7,14]

Pyrethrins and pyrethroids are not readily metabolized by insects and other arthropods and are specifically very deadly. In mammals, rapid hydrolysis of ester bonds occurs in the digestive tract, however, before rapid liver oxidation in the microsomal monooxygenase system to primarily renally excreted inactive metabolites.[15]

Certain mixtures of pyrethroids contain modifying agents, such as piperonyl butoxide. Piperonyl butoxide acts as a

FIGURE 90-2

Effect of pyrethroids on sodium tail currents.

TABLE 90-1 Pyrethrins and Pyrethroids by Type and Prolonged Effect on Sodium Tail Currents		
COMPOUND	**SODIUM TAIL CURRENT* (msec)**	**SYNDROME**
Type I Noncyano Pyrethroids		
Allethrin	10	T
Cismethrin	21	T
Permethrin	7	T
Tetramethrin		T
Type II Cyano Pyrethroids		
Cyphenothrin (trans)	260	T
Cyphenothrin (cis)	385	CS
Cyfluthrin		CS
Fenvalerate	545	CS
Cypermethrin	1115	CS
Deltamethrin	1770	CS
Esfenvalerate		CS
Flucynthrate		CS
Fluvalinate		CS
Control Cell	1	

*Frog myelinated nerve fibers at 15°C, if determined.
CS, choreoathetosis, salivation; T, tremor.

synergist when added to pyrethroids by its inhibition of the monooxygenase enzyme system, causing the insecticidal activity to be enhanced 10-fold to 300-fold.[16,17] Oxidation and ester hydrolysis are followed by various conjugations, with low tissue residues.[14]

Clinical Presentation

The clinical presentation of pyrethrin and pyrethroid poisoning is that of hyperactivity of excitable tissues and adrenergic excess. The time to onset of clinical manifestations varies depending on the route of exposure and the dose received. The CS syndrome is seen with pyrethroids that prolong sodium currents more than 10 msec (normal is approximately 0.5 msec). The associated findings include incoordination, choreoathetosis, seizures, and salivary gland effects.[18] In poisoning with pyrethroids that cause sodium current prolongations less than 10 msec, fine tremor and hyperexcitability may be seen[19]; this is the T, or type I, syndrome. There is also an overlap syndrome, which may display tremor, choreoathetosis, and salivation. This overlap syndrome may result from pyrethroids that have intermediate sodium current prolongation approximating 10 msec and may present as type I and type II syndromes (see Table 90-1).[19]

In a series of 573 pyrethroid exposure cases, the most common findings were dizziness, nausea, vomiting, weakness, anorexia, and headache (Table 90-2).[11] Although these are relatively limited clinical findings, they may be the initial signs or symptoms of more serious conditions, such as altered consciousness, chest tightness, seizures, or pulmonary edema. The latter conditions are unexpected in the absence of intentional consumption or marked occupational exposures. One particularly interesting finding is that

of paresthesias. Paresthesias have been reported to be one of the most common findings by some authors yet were uncommon in a large case series.[11,20,21] Paresthesias from natural pyrethrins are much less intense than paresthesias from synthetic pyrethroid agents[7,22]; this is thought to be due to a direct effect of pyrethroids on the intracutaneous nerve endings. Paresthesias from synthetic pyrethroid agents occur with doses that are far lower than those required to cause systemic symptoms.[21]

Pulmonary reactions, characterized by pneumonitis, cough, dyspnea, wheezing, chest pain, and bronchospasm, may occur.[11] Rare cases of respiratory failure and cardiopulmonary arrest have been reported.[7,23] Asthma-like symptoms have been reported in susceptible individuals, especially persons with a history of asthma.[24] Wax and Hoffman[25] reported a 37-year-old woman with a history of mild asthma requiring no long-term medication who developed severe shortness of breath and died after a brief exposure to a pet shampoo containing 0.06% pyrethrin.

Case reports have suggested that asthmatic complaints may occur after inhalational exposures. These complaints may be similar to other typical asthmatic exacerbations, with cough, chest pain, dyspnea, and obstructive airflow on testing. In a single case, hypersensitivity pneumonitis was reported due to marked overuse indoors of an aerosolized pyrethrum. The patient underwent lung biopsy to confirm the diagnosis. She improved with corticosteroid therapy and was rechallenged with a pulmonary challenge 1 week after hospital discharge, with rapid recurrence of type 1 and type 3 allergic findings.[26] Patients with ragweed sensitivity are more prone to allergic reactions after pyrethrum extract administration. Fatal asthma was reported in a child, as was described previously in an adult after the use of an animal shampoo containing pyrethrin.[25,27] Another case concluded that a pyrethrin-containing pediculicide shampoo caused an anaphylactoid reaction in an adult.[28]

A potential source of an exposure that has been described more recently is from automatic insecticide disperser units. In the United States, these devices are registered by the Environmental Protection Agency for use in the restaurant industry, schools, supermarkets, hospitals, and other public buildings. Automatic insecticide disperser units usually dispense a fine mist of 50 to 100 mg of an insecticide, typically a pyrethrin with or without piperonyl butoxide, every 15 minutes, 24 hours a day. Misuse and malfunction have led to pyrethrin illness. None of the effects resulted in major medical complications.[29] For individuals who may be allergic to these substances, however, an exacerbation of asthma may occur.

Treatment

TABLE 90-2 Clinical Findings in 573 Pyrethroid Poisoning Cases	
SIGN OR SYMPTOM	PERCENT OF TOTAL
Dizziness	60.6
Nausea	59.7
Vomiting	56.8
Weakness	53.4
Anorexia	45
Headache	44.5
Fatigue	26
Leukocytosis	15
Chest tightness	13.1
Palpitations	13.1
Paresthesias	11.9
Altered consciousness	8.9
Fever	8
Blurred vision	7
Increased sweating	6.7
Seizures	5.9
Pulmonary edema	2.8
Death	1.2
Hypotension	0.8

Data from He F, Wang S, Liu L, et al: Clinical manifestations and diagnosis of acute pyrethroid poisoning. Arch Toxicol 63:54–58, 1989.

Indications for ICU Admission in Pyrethrin and Pyrethroid Insecticide Poisoning

Altered mental status
Seizures or hypotension
Respiratory failure

There are no specific treatments or antidotes. Therapy should be directed at treating objective signs and providing supportive care. During supportive therapy, careful attention must be paid to airway, breathing, and the circulatory status of the patient. If seizures occur, therapy with appropriate doses of benzodiazepines or barbiturates is indicated. Protection of the airway, control of hyperthermia from prolonged seizures, and ventilatory support are vital in cases of serious poisoning.

Special Populations

Patients with a history of seizure disorder, concomitant head injury, or coingestion of substances prone to cause seizures may increase risk of seizures after a clinically significant exposure to these insecticides.

Prevention

Keeping containers in inaccessible areas is important primary prevention. In adults, appropriate use of personal protective equipment and timely decontamination after application are important to prevent absorption.

Criteria for ICU Discharge in Pyrethrin and Pyrethroid Insecticide Poisoning

Vital sign stabilization
Minimal supplemental oxygen
Resolution of seizures

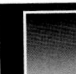

Common Errors in Pyrethrin and Pyrethroid Insecticide Poisoning

Failure to appreciate pyrethroid toxicity
Failure to control seizures and hyperthermia

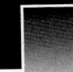

Key Points in Pyrethrin and Pyrethroid Insecticide Poisoning

1. The pyrethrin and pyrethroid agents are relatively innocuous after limited exposures. After intentional ingestions or massive accidental contact, however, central nervous system excitation, including seizures, may occur.
2. Therapy is directed at prevention of further exposure (e.g., skin decontamination), airway support, and control of seizures with benzodiazepines or barbiturates.

ORGANOCHLORINE INSECTICIDES

The OC category of substances has found use mostly as insecticides and grain protective fungicides. Three major chemical groupings are contained in this class of compounds: dichlorodiphenylethanes, cyclodienes, and cyclohexanes (Table 90-3).

Biochemistry and Pharmacology

OCs are heavily chlorinated organic (mostly aromatic) compounds with limited water solubility and low vapor pressures. Typical chemical structures for the OCs are shown in Figure 90-3.

Toxicokinetics

Dermal absorption varies widely from compound to compound. Dichlorodiphenyltrichloroethane (DDT) is poorly absorbed through the skin. Dieldrin, lindane, and chlordecone are absorbed efficiently through the skin. OCs are relatively nonvolatile.

Absorption after inhalational exposure to sprays and dusts probably occurs mainly by mucociliary trapping, followed by gastrointestinal absorption. The OC group, being fat soluble, is nearly completely absorbed. Rats convert aldrin to dieldrin in the skin after topical application, which may enhance availability for absorption.[30] Other specific examples of

TABLE 90-3 Insecticidal Classes of Organochlorines

INSECTICIDE CLASS	EXAMPLES	HALF-LIFE	WATER SOLUBILITY (g/dL)	AVERAGE DAILY INTAKE (mg/kg/day)
Dichlorodiphenylethanes	DDT	Months-years	0.000017	0.02
	Dicolfol	Months-years	<1	0.002
	Methoxychlor	Hours-days	0.00001	0.1
Cyclodienes	Aldrin	Weeks-months	0.000018	0.00001
	Dieldrin	Weeks-months	0.00002	0.00001
	Heptachlor	Weeks-months	0.000018	0.0001
	Chlordane	Hours-days	1	0.0005
	Endosulfan	Hours-days	<1	0.006
Cyclohexanes	Hexachlorobenzene	Weeks-months	0.000000062	NA
	Hexachlorocyclohexane	Weeks-months	0.0073	NA
	Lindane	Hours-days	0.00073	0.008

DDT, dichlorodiphenyltrichloroethane; NA, not available.

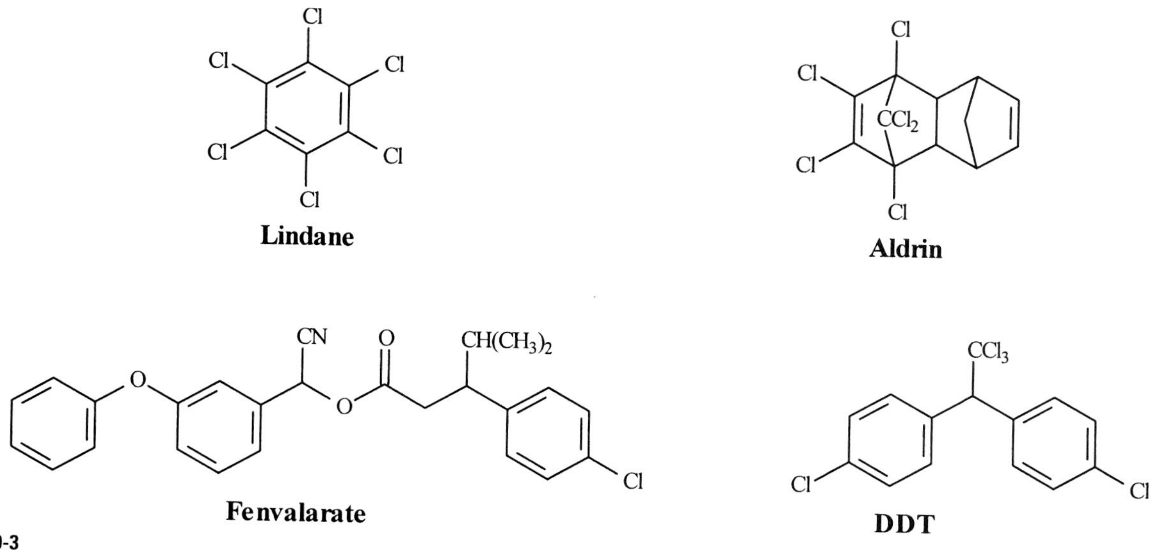

FIGURE 90-3

Chemical structures of selected organochlorines.

metabolism include heptachlor conversion to heptachlor epoxide and oxychlordane.[31]

Elimination of OC compounds does not follow classic first-order kinetics. Rather, as body stores are reduced, the half-life for the remaining fraction increases. Even with this pattern of excretion, it is useful to classify the OCs roughly in terms of the relative rates of elimination (Table 90-4).

Specific elimination kinetics data are limited. The recirculation of gut chlordecone prolongs elimination so that the half-life in blood is approximately 165 days.[32] The serum half-life of chlordane in a single case report after an acute ingestion of an unknown quantity of 45% chlordane was found to be approximately 88 days.[33]

TABLE 90-4 Elimination of Various Organochlorines

SUBSTANCE	RELATIVE RATE OF ELIMINATION
Chlordane (except the heptachlor component)	Hours-days
Chlorobenzilate	Hours-days
Endosulfan	Hours-days
Endrin	Hours-days
Kelthane	Hours-days
Methoxychlor	Hours-days
Perthane	Hours-days
Toxaphene	Hours-days
Aldrin	Weeks-months
Dieldrin	Weeks-months
Heptachlor	Weeks-months
Hexachlorobenzene	Weeks-months
Benzene hexachloride (β isomer)	Months-years
DDT	Months-years
Chlordecone	Months-years
Mirex	Months-years

DDT, dichlorodiphenyltrichloroethane.

Epidemiology

Hexachlorobenzene was responsible for an endemic poisoning event in Turkey from 1955 to 1959. During that event, an estimated 3000 to 4000 people ingested bread prepared from grain treated with hexachlorobenzene (2 kg/1000 kg wheat). Many porphyria cases arose.[34] An extremely high rate of mortality occurred in children (<1 year old) of lactating mothers known to have ingested this bread. All children born to porphyric mothers during that epidemic died, and an estimated 1000 to 2000 infants died due to a condition known as *pembe yara*, or *pink sore*, because of the associated skin lesions (blistering and epidermolysis and annular erythema).[34–37] Others have referred to the sores as "black sore." Dermal blistering, epidermolysis, pigmentation, scarring, alopecia, photosensitivity, hepatomegaly, porphyria, inflammatory arthritis, osteomyelitis, and osteoporosis characterize this toxic syndrome.[38] Although a 10% rate of mortality in exposed adults has been reported, it is not clear how that figure relates to the expected mortality rates for comparable cohorts.[34,37] An estimated dose of 0.7 to 2.9 mg/kg/day was considered to be reliable by the original investigators of the Turkey epidemic.[38] Many recovered after termination of exposure, although some remained symptomatic.[34]

Several cases of food-related poisoning with OC insecticides have been reported. Waller and colleagues[39] described five cases of multiple generalized seizures occurring within 1 hour after eating endrin-contaminated corn tortillas with meat filling. The concentration of endrin in the food was found to be approximately 100 ppm. Chugh and coworkers[40] reported 18 cases of unintentional endosulfan poisoning in northern India after crop spraying. All victims developed seizures within 24 hours after the spraying. Phenobarbital was effective seizure treatment; all patients recovered without permanent sequelae. In 1984, 21 villages in the Punjab province of Pakistan were affected by food contaminated with endrin. Eighteen of the affected villages were surveyed; 70% of the cases were in children. The mortality rate was 9.8% of all affected persons. Seizures were noted in 194, with

19 deaths.[41] The only known human effects reported after occupational exposure to chlordecone are tremulousness and a sensation of nervousness.[42]

Pathophysiology

The OC insecticides are known to prolong neuronal sodium conductance, which contributes to the clinical features observed, such as central nervous system excitation. The principal neurotoxic action of these compounds is that of "axon poison," affecting primarily central nervous system neurons. The OCs interfere with the normal flux of Na^+ and K^+ ions across the axon membrane as nerve impulses pass. This interference results in irritability, sensory aberrations, and seizures.[43] Depression of the medullary respiratory center may occur concurrently, leading to asphyxia.

Certain of these compounds are enzyme inducers of the mixed-function oxidase system. An important property of the chlorinated hydrocarbons, particularly toxaphene, chlordane, DDT, and lindane, is their capacity to induce these enzymes.[44–46] Chlordecone, no longer available in some countries, including the United States, is an inhibitor of oxidative phosphorylation and calcium-dependent ATPase. Although also an inhibitor of membrane Na^+-K^+ ATPase, mitochondrial calcium-dependent ATPase is more sensitive.[47] Chlordecone also has been reported to have a concentration-dependent effect of decreasing GABA, dopamine, and norepinephrine uptake by synaptosomes.[48] This effect may be the cause of seizures after marked exposure.

Chronic hexachlorobenzene exposure may cause porphyria cutanea tarda, which is unique among the OCs. Metabolic activation seems to be involved in porphyria, but reactive benzoquinones seem not to be involved.[49] The mechanism of endosulfan toxicity involves inhibition of the calmodulin-dependent Ca^{2+}-ATPase and inhibition *antagonism* of GABA receptors.[50–52]

Clinical Presentation

Clinical features of acute OC poisoning may include non-specific gastrointestinal symptoms, such as nausea, vomiting, and abdominal pain. The other major target organ is the nervous system. Disturbances of neurologic processes may include sensory aberrations, paresthesias of the face and tongue, tonic-clonic movements, myoclonus, seizures, and coma. Certain OCs are not as prone to cause seizures as others. Kelthane, perthane, methoxychlor, and hexachlorobenzene cause little central nervous system excitation; however, at extreme dosages, central nervous system depression may occur.

Other pertinent findings include metabolic acidosis associated with seizures. In one series, six patients who ingested endosulfan were reported with severely high anion gap acidosis, hyperglycemia, and seizures.[53] In another case report, an elderly man ingested endosulfan and was admitted with seizures and a metabolic acidosis.[54] A single case report described seizures with severe metabolic acidosis (pH 7.0, PCO_2 31 mm Hg, and HCO_3 7.8 mEq/L) after the ingestion of 6 to 8 oz of chlordane.[55] Intentional ingestion of 150 mL of methoxychlor was associated with hypoten-

sion and depressed mental status. The hypotension was responsive to intravenous fluids.[56]

After inhalational exposure, hexachlorobenzene has been noted to irritate the mucous membranes of the respiratory tract.[57] Other pulmonary changes noted include hypoventilation (aldrin, dieldrin, endrin, chlordane, toxaphene, and DDT), pulmonary infiltrates, and an increased alveolar-arterial oxygen gradient.[53]

Certain OCs, such as chlordecone, mirex, endosulfan, and chlorbenzilate, may cause tremors, ataxia, agitation, and nervousness and can cause seizures after ingestion of large quantities. These have been reported soon after ingestion. In one case, a 43-year-old man developed generalized seizures within 60 minutes of ingestion of endosulfan.[58]

Other clinical features are gastrointestinal effects, including nausea, vomiting, and diarrhea, especially when the pesticide is contained in petroleum distillates. This is a nonspecific irritant and laxative response to the ingestion. Pancreatitis, hepatitis, and acute renal failure have been reported; however, these cases had multisystem injury and significant hypotension.[53–55]

Diagnosis

Similar to the pyrethrins and pyrethroids, OC poisonings have defined toxic syndromes, as described earlier. Because these clinical findings are nonspecific, many of these features may present from drug or nondrug causes. Tremor is a nonspecific clinical sign that has many causes: rest tremor (Parkinson's disease, parkinsonism, drug induced such as lithium and stimulants), intentional tremor (multiple sclerosis, Wilson's disease), postural tremor (essential, senile, hyperthyroidism, drug or alcohol withdrawal), hysterical tremor, and mixed tremor.

The differential diagnosis of seizures is broad and includes effects from many chemical compounds. The toxins most likely to cause seizures are stimulants, antidepressants, neuroleptics, antihistamines, anticholinergics, cholinergics, antidysrhythmics, salicylates, isoniazid, and theophylline. Many pesticides may cause seizures if of sufficient dose. Most toxin-induced seizures are generalized. Chapter 20 describes the pathophysiology and treatment of toxicant-induced seizures.

Treatment

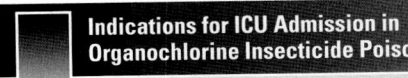

Indications for ICU Admission in Organochlorine Insecticide Poisoning

Altered mental status
Seizures or hypotension
Respiratory failure

There are no specific treatments or antidotes. Therapy should be directed at treating objective signs and providing supportive care. During supportive therapy, careful attention must be paid to airway, breathing, and the circulatory status of the patient. If seizures occur, therapy with appropriate doses of benzodiazepines or barbiturates is indicated. Protection of the airway, control of hyperthermia from prolonged seizures, and ventilatory support are vital in cases of serious poisoning.

Criteria for ICU Discharge in Organochlorine Insecticide Poisoning

Vital sign stabilization
Minimal supplemental oxygen
Resolution of seizures

Special Populations

Patients with a history of seizure disorder, concomitant head injury, or coingestion of substances prone to cause seizures may increase risk of seizures after a clinically significant exposure to these insecticides.

Prevention

Keeping containers in inaccessible areas is important primary prevention. In adults, appropriate use of personal protective equipment and timely decontamination after application are important to prevent absorption.

Common Errors in Organochlorine Insecticide Poisoning

Incorrect diagnosis of organophosphate
Failure to control seizures and hyperthermia

Key Points in Organochlorine Insecticide Poisoning

1. Organochlorines are more likely than pyrethrins to cause seizures and serious life-threatening events after intentional exposure.
2. Therapy is directed at prevention of further exposure (e.g., skin decontamination), airway support, and control of seizures with benzodiazepines or barbiturates.

REFERENCES

1. Matsui M, Yamamoto I: Pyrethroids. In Jacobson M, Crosby DG (eds): Naturally Occurring Insecticides. New York, Marcel Dekker, 1971, pp 1–70.
2. Watson WA, Litovitz TL, Rodgers GC Jr, et al: 2002 Annual Report of the American Association of Poison Control Centers Toxic Exposure Surveillance System. Am J Emerg Med 21:353–421, 2003.
3. Schecter MS, Green N, LaForge FB: Constituents of pyrethrum flowers. J Am Chem Soc 71:3165–3173, 1949.
4. Elliot M, Farnham AW, Janes NF, et al: A photostable pyrethroid. Nature 246:169–170, 1973.
5. Narahashi T: Neuronal ion channels as the target sites of insecticides. Pharmacol Toxicol 141:288–298, 1996.
6. Ginsburg KS, Narahashi T: Differential sensitivity of tetrodotoxin-sensitive and tetrodotoxin-resistant sodium channels to the insecticide

7. allethrin in rat dorsal-root ganglion neurons. Brain Res 627:239–248, 1993.
7. Ray DE, Froshaw PJ: Pyrethroid insecticides: Poisoning syndromes, synergies, and therapy. Clin Toxicol 38:95–101, 2000.
8. Bloomquist JR, Adams PM, Soderlund DM: Inhibition of gamma-aminobutyric acid-stimulated chloride flux in mouse brain vesicles by polychloroalkane and pyrethroid insecticides. Neurotoxicology 7:11–20, 1986.
9. Zhang Z, Sun J, Chen S, et al: Levels of exposure and biological monitoring of pyrethroids in spraymen. Br J Ind Med 48:82–86, 1991.
10. Zaim M, Aitio A, Nakashima N: Safety of pyrethroid-treated mosquito nets (Review). Med Vet Entomol 14:1–5, 2000.
11. He F, Wang S, Liu L, et al: Clinical manifestations and diagnosis of acute pyrethroid poisoning. Arch Toxicol 63:54–58, 1989.
12. Anadon A, Martinez-Larranaga MR, Fernandez-Cruz ML, et al: Toxicokinetics of deltamethrin and its 4′HO-metabolite in the rat. Toxicol Appl Pharmacol 141:8–16, 1996.
13. Gotoh Y, Kawakami M, Matsumoto N, et al: Permethrin emulsion ingestion: Clinical manifestations and clearance of isomers. Clin Toxicol 36:57–61, 1998.
14. Miyamoto J: Degradation, metabolism, and toxicity of synthetic pyrethroids. Environ Health Perspect 14:15–28, 1976.
15. Dorman DC, Beasley VR: Neurotoxicology of pyrethrin and pyrethroid insecticides. Vet Hum Toxicol 33:238–243, 1991.
16. Casida JE, Gammon DW, Glockman AH, Lawrence LJ: Mechanisms of selective action of pyrethroid insecticides. Ann Rev Pharmacol Toxicol 23:413–438, 1983.
17. Matsumura F: Toxicology of Insecticides. New York, Plenum Press, 1985, pp 122–128.
18. Aldridge WN: An assessment of the toxicological properties of pyrethroids and their neurotoxicity. Crit Rev Toxicol 21:89–104, 1990.
19. Wright CDP, Forshaw PJ, Ray DE: Classification of the actions of 10 pyrethroid insecticides in the rat, using the trigeminal reflex and skeletal muscle as test systems. Pestic Biochem Physiol 30:79–86, 1988.
20. Vijverberg HPM, van den Berken J: Neurotoxicological effects and the mode of action of pyrethroid insecticides. CRC Crit Rev Toxicol 1:105–126, 1990.
21. Wilks MF: Pyrethroid-induced paresthesia—a central or local toxic effect? Clin Toxicol 8:103–105, 2000.
22. Martin TY, Hester KH: Dermatitis caused by insecticidal pyrethrum flowers. Br J Dermatol Syph 53:127, 1941.
23. Fischer AB, Eikmann T: Improper use of an insecticide at a kindergarten. Toxicol Lett 88:359–364, 1996.
24. Newton JG, Breslin ABX: Asthmatic reactions to a commonly used aerosol insect killer. Med J Aust 1:378–380, 1983.
25. Wax PM, Hoffman RS: Fatality associated with inhalation of a pyrethrin shampoo. Clin Toxicol 32:457–460, 1994.
26. Carlson JE, Villaveces JW: Hypersensitivity pneumonitis due to pyrethrum: Report of a case. JAMA 237:1718–1719, 1977.
27. Wagner SL: Fatal asthma in a child after use of an animal shampoo containing pyrethrin. West J Med 173:86–87, 2000.
28. Culver CA, Malina JJ, Talbert RL: Probable anaphylactoid reaction to a pyrethrin pediculicide shampoo. Clin Pharmacokinet 7:846–849, 1988.
29. Shafey O: Illnesses associated with use of automatic insecticide disperser units—selected states and United States, 1986–1999. MMWR Morb Mortal Wkly Rep 49:492–495, 2000.
30. Graham MJ, Williams FM, Rawlins MD: Metabolism of aldrin to dieldrin by rat skin following topical application. Food Chem Toxicol 29:701–711, 1991.
31. Stehr-Green PA, Farrar JA, Burse VW, et al: A survey of measured levels and dietary sources of selected organochlorine pesticide residues and metabolites in human sera from a rural population. Am J Public Health 78:828–830, 1988.
32. Taylor JR: Neurological manifestations in humans exposed to chlordecone: Follow-up results. Neurotoxicology 6:231–236, 1985.
33. Aldrich FD, Holmes JH: Acute chlordane intoxication in a child. Arch Environ Health 19:129–132, 1969.
34. Peters HH, Gocmen A, Cripps DJ, et al: Epidemiology of hexachlorobenzene-induced porphyria in Turkey—clinical and laboratory follow-up after 25 years. Arch Neurol 39:744–749, 1982.
35. Gocmen A, Peters HA, Cripps DJ, et al: Hexachlorobenzene episode in Turkey. Biomed Environ Sci 2:36–43, 1989.

36. Cripps DJ, Peters HA, Gocmen A, Dogramici I: Porphyria turcica due to hexachlorobenzene: A 20 to 30 year follow-up study on 204 patients. Br J Dermatol 111:413–422, 1984.
37. Peters H, Cripps D, Gocmen A, et al: Turkish epidemic hexachlorobenzene porphyria: A 30-year study. Ann N Y Acad Sci 514:183–190, 1987.
38. Cam C, Nigogosyan G: Acquired toxic porphyria cutanea tarda due to hexachlorobenzene. JAMA 183:88–91, 1963.
39. Waller K, Prendergast TJ, Slagle A, et al: Seizures after eating a snack food contaminated with the pesticide endrin: The tale of toxic taquitos. West J Med 157:648–651, 1992.
40. Chugh SN, Dhawan R, Agrawal N, et al: Endosulfan poisoning in Northern India: A report of 18 cases. Int J Clin Pharmacol Ther 36:474–477, 1998.
41. Rowley DL, Rab MA, Hardjotanojo W, et al: Convulsions caused by endrin poisoning in Pakistan. Pediatrics 79:928–934, 1987.
42. Cannon SB, Veazey JM, Jackson RS, et al: Epidemic Kepone poisoning in chemical workers. Am J Epidemiol 17:529–537, 1978.
43. Morgan DP: Recognition and Management of Pesticide Poisonings, 3rd ed. Publication EPA-540/9-80-005. Washington, D.C., US Environmental Protection Agency, 1982.
44. Wells WL, Milhorn HT Jr: Suicide attempt by toxaphene ingestion: A case report. J Miss State Med Assoc 24:329–330, 1983.
45. Garrettson LK, Guzelian PS, Blanke RV: Subacute chlordane poisoning. Clin Toxicol 22:565–571, 1984–1985.
46. Klaasen CD: Nonmetallic environmental toxicants: Air pollutants, solvents and vapors, and pesticides. In Goodman A, Goodman LS, Rall TW, et al (eds): The Pharmacological Basis of Therapeutics, 7th ed. New York, MacMillan, 1985, pp 1628–1650.
47. End DW, Carchman RA, Dewey WL: Neurochemical correlates of chlordecone neurotoxicity. J Toxicol Environ Health 86:707–718, 1981.
48. Ho IK, Fujimori K, Huang TP, Chang-Tusi H: Neurochemical evaluation of chlordecone toxicity in the mouse. J Toxicol Environ Health 8:701–706, 1981.
49. denBesten C, Brouwer A, Rietjens IMCM, et al: Biotransformation and toxicity of halogenated benzenes. Hum Exp Toxicol 13:866–875, 1994.
50. Sirkanth NS, Seth PK, Desaiah D: Inhibition of calmodulin activated Ca^{2+} ATPase by endosulfan in rat brain. J Toxicol Environ Health 28:473–481, 1989.
51. Agrawal AK, Anand M, Zaidi NF, Seth PK: Involvement of serotoninergic receptors in endosulfan neurotoxicity. Biochem Pharmacol 28:3591–3593, 1983.
52. Abalis IM, Eldefrawi ME, Eldefrawi AT: Effects of insecticides on GABA-induced chloride influx into rat brain microsacs. J Toxicol Environ Health 18:13–23, 1986.
53. Blanco-Coronato JL, Repetto M, Ginestal RJ, et al: Acute intoxication by endosulfan. J Toxicol Clin Toxicol 30:575–583, 1992.
54. Lo RSK, Chan JCN, Cockram CS, et al: Acute tubular necrosis following endosulphan insecticide poisoning. Clin Toxicol 33:67–69, 1995.
55. Stipetic ME, Hobbs GD: Multi-system failure in a suicidal chlordane ingestion: A case report (Abstract). J Toxicol Clin Toxicol 36:467, 1998.
56. Thompson TS, Vorster SJ: Attempted suicide by ingestion of methoxychlor. J Anal Toxicol 24:377–380, 2000.
57. Dreisbach RH: Handbook of Poisoning. Los Altos, CA, Lange Medical Publications, 1983, pp 88–89.
58. Boereboom FTJ, van Dijk A, van Zoonen P, et al: Nonaccidental endosulfan intoxication: A case report with toxicokinetic calculations and tissue concentrations. Clin Toxicol 36:345–352, 1998.

CHAPTER 91

Organophosphorus and Carbamate Insecticides

Sally M. Bradberry ■ J. Allister Vale

ORGANOPHOSPHORUS INSECTICIDES

Organophosphorus (OP) insecticides are used widely in agriculture, horticulture, and veterinary medicine. These insecticides also are used domestically and in public hygiene to control vectors of disease. Some OP compounds (e.g., malathion) are used to treat human infestation with scabies, head lice, and crab lice. The primary action of OP insecticides on insects, and the source of their potential toxicity to humans, is a consequence of their ability to inhibit the enzyme acetylcholinesterase (AChE). The result is an acetylcholine (ACh) excess syndrome.

Epidemiology

As a result of the widespread use of pesticides, it has been estimated that the global annual incidence of acute pesticide exposures is of the order of 3 million with 220,000 associated deaths[1]; most of these exposures and fatalities occur in the developing world, and OP insecticides account for a substantial proportion. Klein-Schwartz and Smith[2] reported that in the United States over the 6-year period from 1985 through 1990, there were 338,170 exposures reported to poison control centers, 25,418 hospitalizations, and 341 fatalities from agricultural and horticultural chemicals; OP insecticides accounted for 38 deaths and 8491 hospitalizations (carbamates were included in these hospitalization data). Among nearly 2.4 million human toxic exposures recorded in 2002 by the American Association of Poison Control Centers Toxic Exposure Surveillance System (TESS), 8031 involved OP insecticides alone. Moderately severe or life-threatening clinical manifestations occurred in 466 of 8031 (5.8%) cases; four patients died.[3] Because the TESS statistics reflect only cases reported to poison centers, it is likely that they underestimate the total incidence of cases. Nearly one third of OP exposures involved children younger than 6 years old, and most of these were probably poison scares rather than true poisonings.

Biochemistry

OP insecticides are usually esters, amides, or thiol derivatives of phosphoric acid (Fig. 91-1). The R[1] and R[2] moieties are usually alkyl or aryl groups, which may be linked via oxygen (this is termed a *phosphate*) (Fig. 91-1A) or a sulfur atom to phosphorus (when bonded via sulfur the compound is called a *phosphorothiolate* or *S-substituted phosphorothioate*) (Fig. 91-1B). When the phosphorus is linked by a double bond to sulfur (P = S), this is known

as a *phosphorothioate* (Fig. 91-1C). *Phosphoramidates* (Fig. 91-1D) have a carbon atom linked to the phosphorus atom through an NH group.

X represents one of a wide range of substituted or branched aliphatic, aromatic, or heterocyclic groups linked to the phosphorus atom via an -O- or -S- to make it more labile. During the process of inhibition of the target enzyme, AChE, the phosphorus atom binds to an amino acid on the enzyme with X being eliminated; the group X often is referred to as the "leaving group." The lability of the linkage between X and the phosphorus atom is critical with regard to the reactivity of the OP with the enzyme AChE.

The P = O-containing structure sometimes is referred to as an *oxon*, and the P = S structure is referred to as a *thion*. The term *oxon* often is incorporated in the trivial name (e.g., parathion is the parent [P = S] compound of paraoxon [P = O]).

Pathophysiology of Toxic Effects

By inhibiting AChE in blood, brain, and other tissues, OP insecticides allow ACh to accumulate at autonomic and some central synapses and at the autonomic postganglionic and skeletal efferent nerve endings. The rate of spontaneous reactivation of alkyl-phosphorylated AChE depends on the chemical structure of the OP compound. Most of the commonly used OP insecticides carry either two methyl (e.g., demeton-S-methyl, dichlorvos, dimethoate, malathion) or two ethyl (e.g., chlorpyrifos, diazinon, parathion) ester groups attached to the phosphorus atom (see Fig. 91-1) so that dimethyl phosphorylated AChE or diethyl phosphorylated AChE is generated. Spontaneous reactivation of dimethyl phosphorylated AChE proceeds rapidly so that the patient's condition should improve even without oxime therapy; there is no such expectation of rapid recovery in patients intoxicated with diethyl phosphoryl insecticides (see later).

OP-induced delayed neuropathy results from phosphorylation of a nervous tissue esterase, distinct from AChE—neuropathy target esterase. The phosphorylated neuropathy target esterase becomes "aged," and axonal degeneration ensues and is followed by demyelination of nerve fibers. Only a few marketed OP insecticides (e.g., methamidophos)[4] are capable of causing this syndrome.

Toxicokinetics

Limited human toxicokinetics data are available. The aspects that are clinically important are stressed.

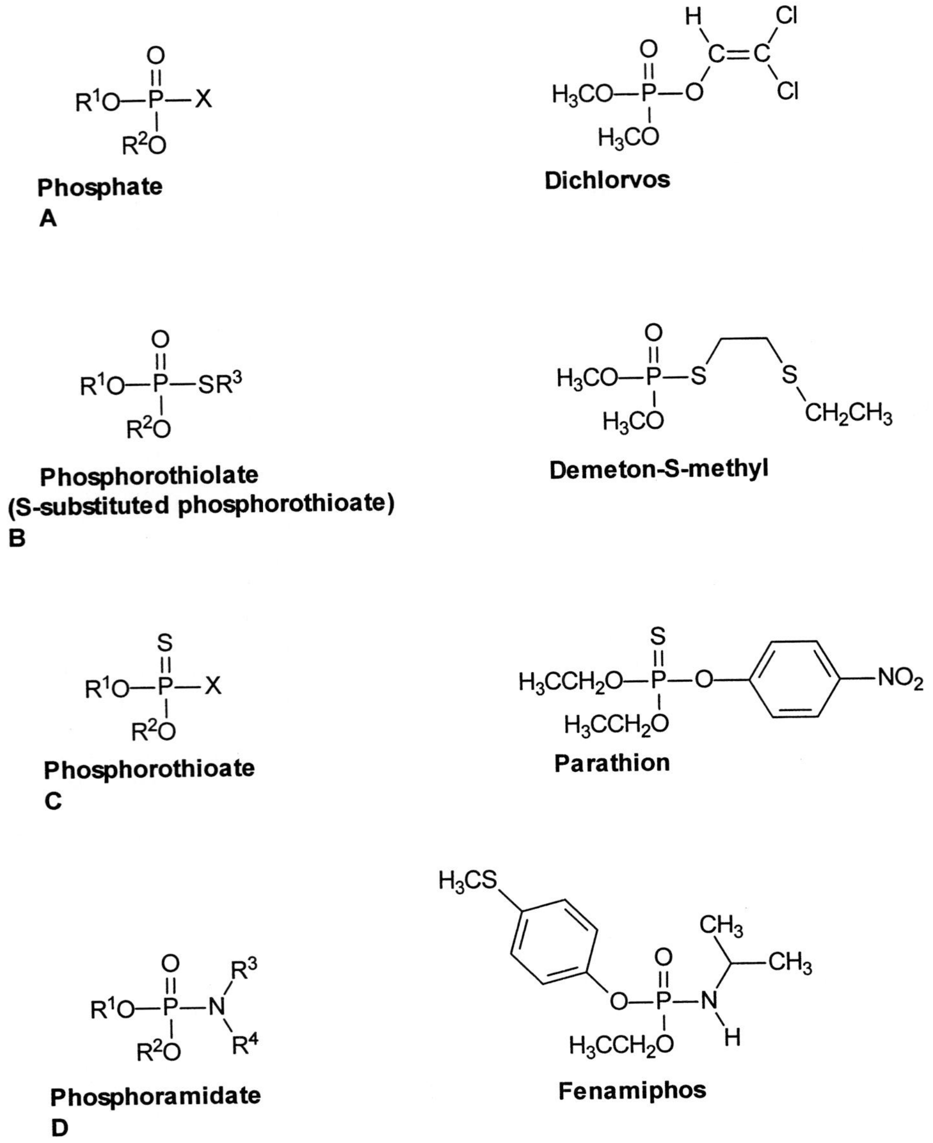

Phosphate
A

Dichlorvos

Phosphorothiolate
(S-substituted phosphorothioate)
B

Demeton-S-methyl

Phosphorothioate
C

Parathion

Phosphoramidate
D

Fenamiphos

FIGURE 91-1

A–D, Chemical structures of some organophosphorus insecticides.

ABSORPTION

As most OP insecticides are lipophilic and not ionized, they are absorbed rapidly after inhalation or ingestion. Although dermal absorption of OP compounds tends to be slow, severe poisoning still may ensue if exposure is prolonged. The degree of absorption depends on the contact time with the skin; the lipophilicity of the agent involved; and the presence of solvents (e.g., xylene) and emulsifiers in the formulation, which can facilitate absorption. For powders, the finer the powder, the more rapid and complete is skin absorption. Other important factors include the volatility of the pesticide (e.g., dichlorvos is much more volatile than malathion, although both have relatively low vapor pressures), the permeability of clothing, the extent of coverage of the body surface, and personal hygiene. The rate of absorption also varies with the skin region affected. Parathion is absorbed more readily through scrotal skin, axillae, and skin of the head and neck than it is through skin of the hands and arms. Traumatized skin or the presence of dermatitis probably allows greater absorption of OP insecticides.

DISTRIBUTION AND STORAGE

After absorption, OP compounds accumulate rapidly in fat, liver, kidneys, and salivary glands. The phosphorothioates (P = S) (e.g., diazinon, parathion, and bromophos) are more lipophilic than phosphates (P = O) (e.g., dichlorvos) and are stored extensively in fat, which may account for the prolonged intoxication and clinical relapse after apparent recovery that has been observed in poisoning from these OP insecticides. OP compounds vary in the ease with which they cross the blood-brain barrier.

BIOTRANSFORMATION

Phosphates (P = O) are biologically active, whereas phosphorothioates (P = S) need bioactivation to the corresponding metabolite (oxon) to become biologically active. As a consequence, the features of intoxication may be delayed, unless aerial oxidation of the phosphorothioate (P = S) has occurred already to generate traces of oxon. OP compounds are metabolically activated to the corresponding oxon by oxidative desulfuration mediated by cytochrome P-450 isoforms,[5] flavin-containing monooxygenase enzymes,[6] N-oxidation, and S-oxidation.[7] The oxons that inhibit AChE can be deactivated by hydrolases, such as the carboxylesterases,[8] and by A-esterases (e.g., paraoxonase). OP compounds undergo other transformations mediated by cytochrome P-450 that do not result in the production of an active metabolite, including oxidative dealkylation and dearylation.[5] OP compounds also may be transformed by enzymatic action on the side chains, including ring hydroxylation, thioether oxidation, deamination, alkyl and N-hydroxylation, N-oxide formation, and N-dealkylation.[5] The products of biotransformation may be conjugated with glucuronide, sulfate, or glycine.[9]

ELIMINATION

Elimination of metabolites occurs mostly in urine with lesser amounts in feces and expired air. Some OPs (e.g., dichlorvos, which is not stored in fat to any great extent) may be eliminated in hours, whereas the inhibitory oxon of chlorpyrifos or demeton-S-methyl may persist for days because of extensive storage in fat.

Toxicodynamics

After the formation of the Michaelis complex, the oxon phosphorylates the serine hydroxyl group located at the active site of AChE. Inhibition of AChE activity occurs in blood, brain, and other tissues in a time-dependent manner. The extent of inhibition of AChE depends on the rate constant for the reaction and the time that the enzyme is exposed to the oxon. Inhibition of AChE results in accumulation of ACh at autonomic and some central synapses and at autonomic postganglionic and skeletal afferent nerve endings. Consequently, ACh binds to and stimulates muscarinic and nicotinic receptors. Phosphorylated enzyme may become "aged" by partial dealkylation of the serine group at the active site of AChE. "Aging" of the phosphorylated enzyme leads to an inactive enzyme, after which reactivation is no longer possible. The rate of aging depends on the structure of the OP compound. The activity of any aged, inhibited enzyme returns to normal only by resynthesis of new enzyme in the liver.

The rate of spontaneous reactivation of alkylphosphorylated AChE depends on the chemical structure of the OP compound. As stated earlier, most of the commonly used OP insecticides carry either two methyl (e.g., demeton-S-methyl, dichlorvos, dimethoate, malathion) or two ethyl (e.g chlorpyrifos, diazinon, parathion) ester groups attached to the phosphorus atom so that dimethyl phosphorylated AChE or diethyl phosphorylated AChE is generated. Spontaneous reactivation of dimethyl phosphorylated AChE proceeds rapidly so that the patient's condition should improve even without oxime therapy. Unless oximes are employed, however, there is no expectation of rapid recovery for patients intoxicated with diethyl phosphoryl insecticides.

Clinical Implications of Organophosphorus Toxicokinetics and Toxicodynamics

The chemical structure of the OP insecticides and the presence of other ingredients in the formulations may have an impact on the speed of onset of features of intoxication. In addition, the fact that many OP insecticides are lipophilic means that they are distributed to and stored in body fat, and elimination takes place slowly. The severity of intoxication may increase for 12 to 36 hours after exposure, intoxication may be prolonged, or relapse may occur after apparent clinical recovery. An understanding of the toxicodynamic aspects also explains why oximes may be of particular value in intoxication due to diethyl phosphates.

Clinical Presentation

Toxicity may occur after inhalation, after ingestion, or through skin contamination. Although dermal absorption of OP compounds tends to be slow, severe poisoning still may ensue if exposure is prolonged. Skin contact and subsequent absorption is the major route of exposure occupationally. Inhalation of OP insecticides, particularly during the manufacture of formulations (e.g., because of inefficiently operating ventilation equipment) or during spraying or mixing, is a recognized occupational hazard. Ingestion is uncommon in the workplace but can occur accidentally in workers with poor personal hygiene, such as those who do not remove contaminated clothing or fail to wash their hands. This exposure is likely to lead to only mild features, whereas the deliberate ingestion of an OP insecticide is likely to result in more severe features of intoxication.

The clinical presentation and severity of OP poisoning depends not only on the pesticide and the magnitude of exposure but also on several other factors, including the route of exposure, the age of the patient, whether exposure was a suicidal attempt (when a substantial ingestion is likely), and the presence of a solvent in the formulation. Not only may skin absorption of the OP itself be enhanced by the presence of the solvent, but also ingestion of a solvent may induce vomiting with risk of aspiration; depressed consciousness may follow.

The onset and severity of toxicity depend on the speed and degree of depression of AChE activity. In addition, some OP compounds require biotransformation to become biologically active, and as a result, signs of intoxication may be delayed. Extensive occupational misuse of OP compounds may cause progressive depletion of AChE activity until toxic effects occur.

The typical features of OP poisoning are those of cholinergic excess and may be divided into muscarinic, nicotinic, and central nervous system effects (Table 91-1). Symptoms can present within 5 minutes of massive ingestion and almost always occur within 12 hours. Muscarinic symptoms rarely present more than 24 hours after ingestion, although these features can reappear if therapy with oximes and atropine is discontinued too early. Muscarinic features appear first and characterize mild-to-moderate poisoning but are not always present. In one study, no single symptom was noted in more than 60% of cases.[10] Miosis, although the most prevalent specific sign, was found in only 44% of cases.[10] In other studies, miosis was observed in 82% of 61 cases[11] and in 83% of 23 cases.[12] The first symptom of poisoning is often a feeling of exhaustion and weakness, particularly in individuals occupationally exposed. Vomiting, cramping abdominal pain, sweating, and hypersalivation may follow. Constriction of one or both pupils and a sensation of tightness in the chest during inspiration also may occur at an early stage, but these signs

TABLE 91-1 Acute Manifestations of Organophosphorus Insecticide Poisoning

EFFECT	SIGNS AND SYMPTOMS
Muscarinic	Cough, wheeze, dyspnea, bronchoconstriction, bronchorrhea, pulmonary edema, cyanosis
	Rhinitis, salivation, lacrimation, diaphoresis, sweating
	Urinary and fecal incontinence
	Nausea, vomiting, abdominal cramps, diarrhea, tenesmus
	Bradycardia, hypotension
	Blurred vision, miosis
Nicotinic	Muscle fasciculation, including diaphragm muscle weakness
	Tachycardia, pallor
	Mydriasis
	Hyperglycemia
CNS	Headaches, anxiety, dizziness, restlessness, insomnia, nightmares, drowsiness, confusion, tremor, ataxia, dysarthria, dystonic reactions
	Hypotension, respiratory depression
	Convulsions, coma

CNS, central nervous system.

TABLE 91-2 Cardiac Manifestations of Organophosphorus Insecticide Poisoning

Bradycardia, tachycardia	AV block
Ventricular arrhythmias	QT interval prolongation
Torsades de pointes	Histopathologic changes
Ventricular fibrillation	Lysis of myofibrils
Asystole	Z-band abnormalities
ECG changes	
ST-segment changes	
Peaked T waves	

AV, atrioventricular; ECG, electrocardiogram.

are not reliable indices of the severity of systemic poisoning because they may be caused by local anticholinesterase effects of spray mist on the eye or bronchi.

In cases of more severe poisoning, the nicotinic features tend to appear first. Muscle twitching affects the eyelids, tongue, face muscles, and calf muscles; respiratory muscles then become involved, and general muscle weakness ensues. Pulmonary function changes associated with OP poisoning include a decrease in dynamic lung compliance, an increase in total pulmonary resistance, and an alveolar arterial oxygen gradient. Respiratory symptoms generally are more severe in older patients with a history of respiratory disease. Convulsions also may occur.[12] Sinus tachycardia is likely to be present (although some patients may be bradycardic), and mydriasis may be observed,[13] particularly if atropine is given. Later effects may include diarrhea, tenesmus, incontinence, ataxia, and confusion. Cardiac effects (Table 91-2) include atrioventricular block, ST-segment changes, peaked T waves, and QT prolongation. Ventricular arrhythmias are a common cause of death,[14] and tachyarrhythmias of the torsades de pointes type[15,16] may progress to ventricular fibrillation or asystole or both. Bronchial hypersecretion with bronchoconstriction, cyanosis, respiratory depression, and coma supervene in severe cases, and death may follow from respiratory failure. A triad of muscarinic, nicotinic, and central nervous system symptoms is apparent in severe cases. This combination was found in 17% of patients in one series,[10] although in a further study of more severely poisoned patients requiring ventilatory support, these features occurred in 60%.[17]

Relapse after apparent resolution of cholinergic symptoms has been reported in patients who have ingested highly lipophilic OP insecticides and is termed the *intermediate syndrome*.[18] Paralysis of limb muscles, neck flexors, and cranial nerves develops approximately 24 to 96 hours after exposure and probably is best explained by combined presynaptic and postsynaptic impairment of neuromuscular transmission due to cholinergic receptor desensitization from prolonged cholinergic stimulation. Optimal use of oximes (see later) may prevent the intermediate syndrome.

Delayed mixed sensorimotor peripheral neuropathies also may result from acute exposure to some OP insecticides. Symptoms appear 1 or 2 weeks after acute exposure. Characteristically, paresthesias of the hands and feet develop, followed by sensory loss in this distribution. Bilateral and symmetric weakness follows, progressing to flaccidity of the distal skeletal muscles of the upper and lower extremities. Ataxia is often present. Gait disturbances may persist for several months and occasionally are permanent.

Diagnosis

The diagnosis of OP poisoning is based on the patient's history, clinical presentation, and laboratory tests. In a patient with a positive history, a typical odor on the breath, characteristic symptoms, and depressed erythrocyte and plasma cholinesterase activities, diagnosis is not difficult to make. The history is often unobtainable and in one study was missing in 36% of all cases.[19] The clinical features of OP poisoning may not be recognized as such if the patient presents, for example, with heart block, gastroenteritis, convulsions, or ketoacidosis. An awareness of this diversity of presentation is the first step toward accurate diagnosis. If there is a doubt regarding the diagnosis, consultation with a medical toxicologist or poison center should be considered.

Diagnosis of OP poisoning can be confirmed by showing a significantly reduced cholinesterase activity in red blood cells or plasma, preferably the former. Difficulty often arises regarding the interpretation of results of plasma cholinesterase activities because individuals can vary widely in their normal complement of plasma cholinesterase. Low plasma cholinesterase activity should be confirmed by the measurement of red blood cell cholinesterase activity. Although erythrocyte cholinesterase is invariably more specific than plasma cholinesterase activity as a marker of OP insecticide exposure, some OP insecticides (e.g., chlorpyrifos, demeton, malathion) depress plasma cholinesterase activity to a greater degree.

It is generally true that the presence of certain clinical features is more helpful in determining the severity of intoxication and prognosis than measurement of erythrocyte

TABLE 91-3 Assessment of Severity and Management of Severe Organophosphorus Insecticide Poisoning

Grade 0	Suggestive history but no features of intoxication present

Grade 1	Patient is alert and awake and has
	  Increased secretions
	  Fasciculation +

Grade 2	Patient is drowsy and has
	  Severe bronchorrhea
	  Fasciculations + + +
	  Crackles/wheezes on auscultation
	  Hypotension (systolic BP <90 mm Hg)

Grade 3	Patient is comatose and has all the features of severe intoxication Increased FiO$_2$ needed but not mechanical ventilation

Grade 4	Patient is comatose and has all the features of severe
	  intoxication
	PaO$_2$ <8 kPa (60 mm Hg) despite FiO$_2$ >40%;
	  PaCO$_2$ >6 kPa (45 mm Hg)
	Mechanical ventilation required
	Abnormal chest radiograph (circumscribed or diffuse opacities,
	  pulmonary edema)

Note. All patients ≥ grade 2 should be admitted to an intensive care unit.
BP, blood pressure; FiO$_2$, fraction of inspired oxygen.
After Johnson MK, Vale JA: Clinical management of acute organophosphate poisoning:
An overview. In Ballantyne B, Marrs TC (eds): Clinical and Experimental Toxicology of
Organophosphates and Carbamates. Oxford, Butterworth Heineman, 1992, pp 528–535.

cholinesterase activity alone soon after presentation. Patients who are moderately or severely poisoned (Table 91-3), as shown by drowsiness, hypotension, severe bronchorrhea, and marked muscle fasciculation, require treatment in a critical care unit because further deterioration may occur, and mechanical ventilation may be required.

Few laboratories can determine quantitatively the insecticide responsible for the intoxication and measurement of the parent compound or metabolite in body fluids. Such measurement has little place in the immediate diagnosis or early management of poisoning. In many cases, rapid hydrolysis prevents the detection of the parent compound, although urinary metabolites may persist for several days. The measurement of metabolites is most helpful as a measure of low-level chronic exposure.

Glycosuria and hyperglycemia[20,21] may be observed in OP insecticide poisoning. Leukocytosis and low-grade fever are noted frequently, even in the absence of infection. A low PaO$_2$ and metabolic acidosis are seen in severely poisoned patients, and creatine kinase activity may be high.

Treatment

Indications for ICU Admission in Organophosphorus Insecticide Poisoning

All cases of ingestion or substantial dermal or inhalational exposure
All patients with symptoms or signs of cholinergic excess (see Table 91-1)

All cases of OP poisoning should be dealt with as an emergency, and all patients with more than minor symptoms (grade 2 or greater; see Table 91-3) should be admitted to a critical care unit. Ventilation must be maintained. Bronchorrhea requires prompt relief with intravenous atropine (see later), and supplemental oxygen should be given to maintain PaO$_2$ greater than 10 kPa (75 mm Hg). If these measures fail, the patient should be intubated, and mechanical ventilation (with positive end-expiratory pressure) should be instituted. Careful attention must be given to fluid and electrolyte balance and adjustments to infusion fluids made as necessary. Heart rate, blood pressure, electrocardiogram, and arterial blood gases should be monitored routinely.

During and after stabilization, thorough skin decontamination should be carried out, without caregivers themselves being contaminated. All contaminated clothing should be removed, and affected skin on all exposed areas should be washed thoroughly with soap and cold water (e.g., hands, arms, face, neck, and hair).

Gastric lavage may be considered in all potentially serious cases if ingestion has occurred less than 1 hour previously, although its value is unproven. Lavage should be performed with care and with an endotracheal tube in situ if the level of consciousness is depressed because hydrocarbons are present in many OP insecticide formulations. Syrup of ipecac should be avoided because emesis is dangerous in a patient whose level of consciousness might deteriorate because of the OP or solvent in the insecticide formulation; aspiration pneumonia is a well-recognized complication in these circumstances. Aspiration also can occur in conscious patients given syrup of ipecac and is more likely to happen if hydrocarbons are present in the pesticide mixture. The capacity of activated charcoal to adsorb most OP compounds has not been shown. On theoretical grounds, a single dose of activated charcoal may be beneficial if administered less than 1 hour after OP insecticide ingestion. Caution should be exercised, however, to ensure that no cathartic is administered because this may exacerbate OP-induced gastroenteritis.

In severely poisoned patients who are hypotensive, it may be necessary not only to expand plasma volume but also to use a vasopressor (e.g., dopamine titrated to a systolic pressure >90 mm Hg) or an inotrope (e.g., dobutamine, 2.5 to 10 μg/kg/min, to maintain cardiac output). Cardiac arrhythmias should be treated conventionally, and hypoxia must be considered as a possible etiology. The management of convulsions and muscle fasciculation is discussed later.

ATROPINE

Atropine antagonizes the effects of accumulated ACh at muscarinic receptors. Atropine sulfate, 2 mg (0.02 to 0.1 mg/kg in a child) intravenously, should be given as soon as possible in moderately or severely poisoned adult patients. Repeated injections of atropine may be required over the first few hours of therapy; the dose should be titrated to control peripheral muscarinic signs, notably bronchorrhea and bronchospasm. In severe cases, particularly when oximes are not administered, 100 mg or more per day may be required to control symptoms.

RATIONALE FOR OXIMES

De Silva and colleagues[22] concluded that nothing is to be gained in cases of severe acute OP insecticide poisoning by the addition of oxime reactivators to the standard regimen of atropine plus mechanical ventilation. This conclusion, which has been challenged,[23] was based on a study in which 21 patients received atropine alone and 24 patients received atropine plus pralidoxime chloride (median doses, 4 g in the first 24 hours and 1 g daily thereafter). The mortality in both groups was 29%, which is not dissimilar to that reported from other centers managing severe cases of OP insecticide poisoning. The need for more effective treatment for OP poisoning is undeniable. The supposed failure of oxime therapy does not indicate ineffectiveness of the drug, however, and it does not necessarily indicate delay in administration; failure of treatment is usually a function of inadequate dosing.

Oximes such as pralidoxime and obidoxime are able to reverse enzyme inhibition (see Fig. 145-1) because they have a molecular structure that "fits" the surface of the inhibited AChE. The extent of reactivation by oximes depends on the chemical form of inhibited AChE, the nature and concentration of oxime present at the site, and the length of time the oxime is present and whether the inhibited AChE remains in the "unaged" form. It is commonly but erroneously believed that within 1 day of intoxication, virtually all the inhibited AChE is in the "aged" form so that oxime therapy, if employed, would be useless. There are good biochemical reasons, however, for suggesting that as soon as an effective concentration of oxime is achieved in vivo, the balance of aging and reactivation reaction rate for inhibited AChE is altered in favor of the latter.[24] Progress toward complete inhibition may be slowed markedly. It is probable that benefit would ensue even if oxime therapy were started or continued several days after intoxication occurred.[25]

Animal studies[26–33] support the value of oxime therapy, and it would be a clinical tragedy if potentially lifesaving therapy were dismissed from consideration because of the administration of inadequate doses of oxime in a clinical study[22] that did no more than confirm the known substantial morbidity and mortality in OP-poisoned patients treated supportively without the benefit of adequate oxime therapy.

Even in high dose, pralidoxime produces few side effects, whereas obidoxime may cause clinically significant hepatic damage. Pralidoxime, if available, is the oxime of choice in OP insecticide poisoning. Pralidoxime chloride or mesylate, 30 mg/kg by intravenous injection, should be administered as soon as possible in any severe or progressive case of intoxication. Repeat doses at 4- to 6-hour intervals or an intravenous infusion of 8 to 10 mg/kg/hr in an adult may be necessary. These regimens are based on reported clinical studies.[34–36] Administration of pralidoxime should continue for as long as atropine is required, that is, until clear, irreversible clinical improvement is achieved, which may take many days while residual insecticide is cleared from the body stores.

DIAZEPAM

Diazepam may be of benefit in OP-poisoned patients by

1. Reducing anxiety and restlessness
2. Reducing muscle fasciculation
3. Arresting seizures
4. Reducing morbidity and mortality when used in conjunction with pralidoxime and atropine

Diazepam, 10 mg intravenously, reduces anxiety, restlessness, and visible motor activity. Short-term, diazepam, 10 to 20 mg, is also an effective anticonvulsant, but if repeated

doses are required to suppress seizure activity, phenobarbital or phenytoin should be considered as an alternative. Potentially, respiratory depression may result from the repeated use of diazepam, although this is unlikely to be a significant clinical problem, unless OP-induced respiratory impairment also is present and the patient is breathing spontaneously. Midazolam has been employed as an alternative benzodiazepine but offers no advantages over diazepam.

Criteria for ICU Discharge in Organophosphorus Insecticide Poisoning

Absence of symptoms or signs of cholinergic excess >12 hours after ingestion or substantial dermal or inhalational exposure; normal erythrocyte or plasma cholinesterase activity after organophosphorus insecticide exposure

No recurrence of symptoms or signs of cholinergic excess 24 hours after discontinuation of oxime therapy

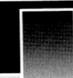

Common Misconceptions about Organophosphorus Insecticide Poisoning

1. Oximes are of no benefit in organophosphorus insecticide poisoning.
2. Oximes are of no benefit if started >24 hours after the onset of organophosphorus poisoning.

Key Points in Organophosphorus Insecticide Poisoning

1. Depending on the organophosphorus insecticide, features of cholinesterase inhibition may be delayed for 12 hours, particularly after dermal exposure.
2. The rate of spontaneous reactivation of organophosphorus-inhibited acetylcholinesterase depends on the chemical structure of the insecticide.
3. Oximes are indicated particularly in the management of poisoning due to diethyl organophosphorus insecticides.
4. Oximes must be administered in sufficient dose to reactivate inhibited acetylcholinesterase and be continued for as long as atropine is required.

CARBAMATE INSECTICIDES

Carbamate insecticides include carbaryl, aldicarb, methomyl, carbofuran, bendiocarb, benfuracarb, butoxycarboxim, carbosulfan, ethiofencarb, methiocarb, oxamyl, pirimicarb, propoxur, thiodicarb, and thiofanox. They are used extensively in agricultural, industrial, and domestic pest control, and some preparations are licensed for treatment of human parasite infestations.

Epidemiology

Carbamate insecticides are not a common cause of severe poisoning. Among nearly 2.4 million human toxic exposures recorded in 2002 by the American Association of

Poison Control Centers TESS, only 3022 were due to carbamate insecticides alone, with only 3.7% of 3022 cases recorded as developing moderately severe or life-threatening symptoms; no patients died.[3] Of these 3022 exposures, 44% involved children younger than 6 years old. Because TESS data include a substantial proportion of inquiries from members of the public, few of these cases are corroborated analytically. When severe poisoning occurs, it is usually the result of deliberate, or less commonly, accidental carbamate ingestion. Carbamate ingestion occurs predominantly in countries where agriculture is the primary industry, and pesticide ingestion is an important means of suicide. Among 228 confirmed fatal poisonings in Northern Greece between 1990 and 1995, carbamates were implicated in 24 of 85 cases of pesticide poisoning.[37] There have been occasional outbreaks of carbamate poisoning after consumption of contaminated food[38,39] or illegal use as a rodenticide[40] and as the poison in attempted murder.[41]

Biochemistry

Carbamate insecticides are derivatives of N-methyl carbamic acid and have the general formula $CH_3NHC(O)OR$, where R is an aromatic or aliphatic moiety. They are generally poorly soluble in water but highly soluble in polar organic solvents, such as methanol, ethanol, and acetone. Carbamate insecticides are susceptible to hydrolysis in alkalis, a property that is used in decontamination and clean-up after carbamate spillages.

Pathophysiology of Toxic Effects

Carbamates inhibit AChE by carbamylation of a serine hydroxyl residue at the active site of the enzyme. This process involves cleavage of the carbamate molecule, which in effect is treated by the enzyme as an alternative substrate to ACh.[42] The AChE-carbamate interaction is not truly reversible because the carbamate does not depart the encounter intact, but rather as the products of hydrolysis. AChE activity is restored when spontaneous hydrolysis of the carbamylated enzyme occurs. This spontaneous reactivation of carbamylated enzyme, expressed as half-life, varies between 2 and 240 minutes depending on the carbamate and in part explains some of the observed differences between carbamates as regards their toxicity.[43] The rate of regeneration of the carbamylated enzyme to AChE is relatively rapid compared with that of an OP phosphorylated enzyme, and aging does not occur. Many carbamates do not cross the blood-brain barrier readily, so the contributory effect on cerebral AChE is considerably less than that caused by OP insecticides. There are several mechanistic reasons why human exposure to carbamate insecticides is potentially less dangerous than exposure to an OP insecticide.

Toxicokinetics and Toxicodynamics

Carbamate insecticides are lipophilic and absorbed readily by dermal and inhalational exposure and after ingestion. Use of these agents in conditions of high temperature and humidity enhances dermal absorption because of increased exposed skin surface area and peripheral vasodilation. In addition, in high ambient temperatures, some carbamate aerosols (e.g., propoxur) are susceptible to revolatilization with increased likelihood of absorption by inhalation.

When absorbed, carbamate esters undergo rapid biotransformation via phase I and phase II detoxification reactions. Phase I detoxification involves either hydrolysis of the carbamate ester by nonspecific tissue carboxylesterases (to form a phenol or alcohol, carbon dioxide, and an amine) or oxidation by monooxygenase P-450 enzymes. Oxidative reactions predominantly involve either direct ring hydroxylation or side-chain oxidation reactions (e.g., N-dealkylation or O-dealkylation or N-methyl hydroxylation). Phase II conjugative reactions produce sulfates, glucuronides, and mercapturates of the hydrolysis products. These species are eliminated predominantly by the kidneys. Based on the limited data available, the plasma half-life of carbamate insecticides is of the order of a few hours.[43] A woman who ingested 10 g of aldicarb developed severe poisoning with a peak serum aldicarb concentration at 3 hours. The aldicarb plasma half-life in this case was 5.75 hours.[44]

Clinical Presentation

Toxicity may occur after inhalation, ingestion, or skin contamination. Inhalational and topical exposures typically are occupational. Life-threatening poisoning in these circumstances is rare, although cholinergic symptoms have occurred after equipment malfunction or inadequate protective measures.[45–47] In these cases, the rapid (often within 30 minutes) onset of mild cholinergic features, including nausea, headache, sweating, lacrimation, salivation, chest tightness, coughing, bronchorrhea, and constriction of one or both pupils causing blurred vision, serves to alert affected individuals to remove themselves from exposure.[45,46,48] Resolution of symptoms occurs typically within hours,[48] often without the need for atropinization.[46] If exposure continues, vomiting, diarrhea, abdominal pain, muscle fasciculation, and weakness develop.[46] Hypotension, sinus tachycardia or bradycardia, and dyspnea also may occur.[46] Electrocardiogram T-wave changes, including inversion, are recognized.[49] Severe sequelae after occupational carbamate exposure are rare, often involve methomyl, and include several cases involving pilots of crop-spraying aircraft exposed to carbamates in the cockpit.[50–52] One of these cases[51] proved fatal as a result of the pilot crashing the plane.

Most cases of severe carbamate poisoning occur after ingestion, which may be accidental[40,53] or deliberate.[40,54,55] These patients usually develop cholinergic symptoms within a few minutes,[55] and in most severe cases, muscle twitching, profound weakness, profuse sweating, incontinence, mental confusion, and progressive cardiac and respiratory failure ensue.[53,55] Seizures are relatively uncommon as a primary complication in severe carbamate poisoning because their penetration into the central nervous system is limited. Seizures may occur secondary to hypoxia, however. Death has occurred within a few hours in untreated cases and is usually due to respiratory failure[53,56]; pulmonary edema and evidence of cerebral hypoxia are the main findings at autopsy.[53,55] In patients who survive, coma may persist for 18 to 24 hours.[55]

In less substantial ingestions, cholinergic symptoms are evident within 2 hours in most cases and typically resolve within 24 hours.[57] There is some evidence that central nervous system depression in moderate carbamate poisoning is more common in infants than in adults, possibly as a result of a greater blood-brain barrier permeability.[57] Acute pancreatitis is reported rarely complicating acute carbamate ingestion.[58,59] Klys and associates[60] reported a case of deliberate carbofuran ingestion in a young pregnant woman, which resulted in fatal carbamate poisoning in the fetus, although the mother survived. At autopsy, the fetal liver contained 2.5 μg/g of carbofuran, which was comparable to the maternal blood carbofuran concentration of 2.6 μg/g.

Although most carbamate insecticides are less toxic than OP insecticides, they should not be considered toxicologically benign. Severe cholinergic symptoms may ensue after ingestion, and unless supportive care, often with atropinization, is instituted promptly, significant morbidity may ensue. Deaths also have been reported.

Diagnosis

Measurement of cholinesterase activity is unlikely to be helpful clinically because of the rapid course of the intoxication. Most laboratories are not acquainted with the special procedure required to assay red blood cell cholinesterase activity in the presence of carbamates. Samples must be kept on ice or frozen at −20°C during transportation to the laboratory before analysis. Spontaneous reversal of the inhibition is rapid and is accelerated by the time interval between sampling and analysis; the dilution of the sample; the addition of substrate, usually acetylcholine, at high concentration (which competes successfully for the enzymatic active site); and duration of assay time. Laboratory assay should take less than 3 minutes and employ minimal dilution and minimal amounts of substrate.[61]

Treatment

All cases of carbamate poisoning should be dealt with as an emergency, and the patient should be admitted to the hospital as quickly as possible. Gastric lavage may be considered in all potentially serious cases if ingestion has occurred less than 1 hour previously, although its value is unproven. Lavage should be performed with care and with a cuffed endotracheal tube in situ if the level of consciousness is depressed because hydrocarbon solvents are often present in the formulation. Syrup of ipecac should be avoided because emesis is dangerous in a patient whose level of consciousness might deteriorate because of the carbamate or solvent in the insecticide formulation; aspiration is a well-recognized complication in these circumstances. Aspiration pneumonia also can occur in conscious patients given syrup of ipecac and is more likely to happen if hydrocarbons are present in the pesticide mixture. The capacity of activated charcoal to adsorb most carbamate insecticides has not been shown. Theoretically a single dose of activated charcoal may be beneficial if administered less than 1 hour after carbamate insecticide ingestion. Caution should be exercised, however, to ensure that no cathartic is administered because this may exacerbate carbamate-induced gastroenteritis.

Bronchorrhea requires removal of secretions by suction and prompt relief with intravenous atropine (see next). Supplemental oxygen should be given to maintain arterial PaO$_2$ greater than 10 kPa (>75 mm Hg). If these measures fail, the patient should be intubated and mechanical ventilation instituted.

Heart rate, blood pressure, electrocardiogram, and arterial oxygen saturation or blood gas tensions should be monitored.

ATROPINE

Atropine antagonizes the effects of accumulated ACh at muscarinic receptors and is the specific antidote for carbamate poisoning. Atropine sulfate, 2 mg intravenously for an adult (0.02 mg/kg body weight for a child), should be given as soon as possible in moderately or severely poisoned patients. Repeated injections may be necessary to control features such as bronchospasm and bronchorrhea.

PRALIDOXIME

Pralidoxime has been shown in some animal studies[62–64] to increase the toxicity of the carbamate insecticide carbaryl, but there is insufficient evidence either to recommend or to prohibit its use in severe poisoning with other carbamate compounds. Pralidoxime seldom should be necessary because carbamates have a shorter duration of action than OP compounds. Pralidoxime chloride or mesylate (30 mg/kg body weight by intravenous injection over 5 to 10 minutes) should be considered in cases of serious carbamate intoxication in addition to atropine and supportive measures. Cases of mixed OP and carbamate poisoning should be treated as for OP poisoning.

Key Point in Carbamate Insecticide Poisoning

1. Severe cholinesterase inhibition after carbamate insecticide exposure usually occurs only after ingestion and typically resolves within 24 hours.

REFERENCES

1. Jeyaratnam J: Acute pesticide poisoning: A major global health problem. World Health Stat Q 43:139–144, 1990.
2. Klein-Schwartz W, Smith GS: Agricultural and horticultural chemical poisonings: Mortality and morbidity in the United States. Ann Emerg Med 29:232–238, 1997.
3. Watson WA, Litovitz TL, Rodgers GC Jr., et al: 2002 Annual report of the American Association of Poison Control Centers Toxic Exposure Surveillance System. Am J Emerg Med 21:353–421, 2003.
4. Senanayake N, Johnson MK: Acute polyneuropathy after poisoning by a new organophosphate insecticide. N Engl J Med 306:155–157, 1982.
5. Ecobichon DJ: Toxic effects of pesticides. In Klaassen CD (ed): Casarett and Doull's Toxicology: The Basic Science of Poisons, 6th ed. New York, McGraw-Hill, 2001, pp 763–810.
6. Levi PE, Hodgson E: Metabolism of organophosphorus compounds by the flavin-containing monooxygenase. In Chambers JE, Levi PE (eds): Organophosphates: Chemistry, Fate and Effects. San Diego, Academic Press, 1992, pp 141–154.
7. Mileson BE, Chambers JE, Chen WL, et al: Common mechanism of toxicity: A case study of organophosphorus pesticides. Toxicol Sci 41:8–20, 1998.
8. Maxwell DM: Detoxification of organophosphorus compounds by carboxylesterase. In Chambers JE, Levi PE (eds): Organophosphates: Chemistry, Fate and Effects. San Diego, Academic Press, 1992, pp 183–199.
9. Yang RSH: Enzymatic conjugation and insecticide metabolism. In Wilkinson CF (ed): Insecticide Biochemistry and Physiology. New York, Plenum, 1976, pp 177–225.
10. Hirschberg A, Lerman Y: Clinical problems in organophosphate insecticide poisoning: The use of a computerised information system. Fundam Appl Toxicol 4:S209–S214, 1984.

11. Bardin PG, Van Eeden SF, Joubert JR: Intensive care management of acute organophosphate poisoning: A 7-year experience in the western Cape. S Afr Med J 72:593–597, 1987.

12. Lee P, Tai DYH: Clinical features of patients with acute organophosphate poisoning requiring intensive care. Intensive Care Med 27:694–699, 2001.

13. Wyckoff DW, Davies JE, Barquet A, et al: Diagnostic and therapeutic problems of parathion poisonings. Ann Intern Med 68:875–882, 1968.

14. Saadeh AM, Farsakh NA, Al-Ali MK: Cardiac manifestations of acute carbamate and organophosphate poisoning. Heart 77:461–464, 1997.

15. Kiss Z, Fazekas T: Organophosphates and torsade de pointes ventricular tachycardia. J R Soc Med 76:984–985, 1983.

16. Ludomirsky A, Klein HO, Sarelli P, et al: Q-T prolongation and polymorphous ("torsades de pointes") ventricular arrhythmias associated with organophosphorus insecticide poisoning. Am J Cardiol 49:1654–1658, 1982.

17. Finkelstein Y, Kushnir A, Raikhlin-Eisenkraft B, Taitelman U: Antidotal therapy of severe acute organophosphate poisoning: A multihospital study. Neurotoxicol Teratol 11:593–596, 1989.

18. Senanayake N, Karalliedde L: Neurotoxic effects of organophosphorus insecticides. N Engl J Med 316:761–763, 1987.

19. Hayes MMM, van der Westhuizen NG, Gelfand M: Organophosphate poisoning in Rhodesia: A study of the clinical features and management of 105 patients. S Afr Med J 54:230–234, 1978.

20. Meller D, Fraser I, Kryger M: Hyperglycemia in anticholinesterase poisoning. Can Med Assoc J 124:745–748, 1982.

21. Namba T, Nolte CT, Jackrel J: Poisoning due to organophosphate insecticides: Acute and chronic manifestations. Am J Med 50:475–492, 1971.

22. De Silva HJ, Wijewickrema R, Senanayake N: Does pralidoxime affect outcome of management in acute organophosphorus poisoning? Lancet 339:1136–1138, 1992.

23. Johnson MK, Vale JA, Marrs TC, Meredith TJ: Pralidoxime for organophosphorus poisoning. Lancet 340:64, 1992.

24. Johnson MK, Vale JA: Clinical management of acute organophosphate poisoning: An overview. In Ballantyne B, Marrs TC (eds): Clinical and Experimental Toxicology of Organophosphates and Carbamates. Oxford, Butterworth Heineman, 1992, pp 528–535.

25. Casey PB, Blakey L, Bradberry SM, Vale JA: Late reactivation of erythrocyte cholinesterase activity by pralidoxime in a case of chlorpyrifos poisoning. Przegl Lek 52:206, 1995.

26. Bokonjic D, Jovanovic D, Jokanovic M, Maksimovic M: Protective effects of oximes HI-6 and PAM-2 applied by osmotic minipumps in quinalphos-poisoned rats. Arch Int Pharmacodyn 288:309–318, 1987.

27. Gupta RC: Acute malathion toxicosis and related enzymatic alterations in *Bubalus bubalis*: Antidotal treatment with atropine, 2-PAM, and diazepam. J Toxicol Environ Health 14:291–303, 1984.

28. Jovanovic D, Boskovic B: Current problems in the experimental treatment of dimethoate poisoning by cholinesterase reactivators. Acta Vet 33:21–28, 1983.

29. Matsubara T, Horikoshi I: Possible antidotes in severe intoxication with fenitrothion in rats. J Pharmacodynam 6:699–707, 1983.

30. O'Leary JF, Kunkel AM, Jones AH: Efficacy and limitations of oxime-atropine treatment of organophosphorus anticholinesterase poisoning. J Pharmacol Exp Ther 132:50–57, 1961.

31. Shiloff JD, Clement JG: Comparison of serum concentrations of the acetylcholinesterase oxime reactivators HI-6, obidoxime, and PAM to efficacy against sarin (isopropyl methylphosphonofluoridate) poisoning in rats. Toxicol Appl Pharmacol 89:278–280, 1987.

32. Kewitz H, Wilson IB, Nachmansohn D: A special antidote against lethal alkyl phosphate intoxication: II. Antidotal properties. Arch Biochem Biophys 64:456–466, 1956.

33. Davies DR, Willey GL: The toxicity of 2-hydroxyiminomethyl-N-methylpyridinium methanesulphonate (P2S). Br J Pharmacol 13:202–206, 1958.

34. Willems JL, Langenberg JP, Verstraet AG, et al: Plasma concentrations of pralidoxime methylsulphate in organophosphorus poisoned patients. Arch Toxicol 66:260–266, 1992.

35. Willems JL, De Bisschop HC, Verstraete AG, et al: Cholinesterase reactivation in organophosphorus poisoned patients depends on the plasma concentrations of the oxime pralidoxime methylsulphate and of the organophosphate. Arch Toxicol 67:79–84, 1993.

36. Casey PB, Gosden E, Blakey L, et al: Plasma pralidoxime concentrations following bolus injection and continuous infusion. Przegl Lek 52:203–204, 1995.

37. Tsoukali H, Tsoungas M: Fatal human poisonings in Northern Greece: 1990–1995. Vet Hum Toxicol 38:366–367, 1996.

38. Goes EA, Savage EP, Gibbons G, et al: Suspected foodborne carbamate pesticide intoxications associated with ingestion of hydroponic cucumbers. Am J Epidemiol 111:254–260, 1980.

39. Green MA, Heumann MA, Wehr HM, et al: An outbreak of watermelon-borne pesticide toxicity. Am J Public Health 77:1431–1432, 1987.

40. Lima JS, Reis CAG: Poisoning due to illegal use of carbamates as a rodenticide in Rio de Janeiro. J Toxicol Clin Toxicol 33:687–690, 1995.

41. Covaci A, Manirakiza P, Coucke V, et al: A case of aldicarb poisoning: A possible murder attempt. J Anal Toxicol 23:290–293, 1999.

42. Alvares AP: Pharmacology and toxicology of carbamates. In Ballantyne B, Marrs TC (eds): Clinical and Experimental Toxicology of Organophosphates and Carbamates. Oxford, Butterworth Heineman, 1992, pp 40–46.

43. IPCS: Environmental Health Criteria 64. Carbamate Pesticides: A General Introduction. Geneva, World Health Organization 1986.

44. Flesch F, Traqui A, Sauder P, et al: Kinetic-dynamic relationship in a case of aldicarb poisoning. EAPCCT XIX International Congress abstract. J Toxicol Clin Toxicol 37:374, 1999.

45. Simpson GR, Bermingham S: Poisoning by carbamate pesticides. Med J Aust 2:148–149, 1977.

46. Testud F, De Larquier A, Descotes J: Occupational acute poisonings with methomyl: Role of dermal exposure and need for preventive measures. J Environ Med 1:137–139, 1999.

47. McConnell R, Hruska AJ: An epidemic of pesticide poisoning in Nicaragua: Implications for prevention in developing countries. Am J Public Health 83:1559–1562, 1993.

48. Coleman AME, Smith A, Watson L: Occupational carbamate pesticide intoxication in three farm workers: Implications and significance for occupational health in Jamaica. West Ind Med J 39:109–113, 1990.

49. Saiyed HN, Sadhu HG, Bhatnagar VK, et al: Cardiac toxicity following short-term exposure to methomyl in spraymen and rabbits. Hum Exp Toxicol 11:93–97, 1992.

50. Richardson EM, Batteese RI Jr: An incident of Zectran poisoning. J Maine Med Assoc 64:158–159, 1973.

51. Driskell WJ, Groce DF, Hill RH Jr, Birky MM: Methomyl in the blood of a pilot who crashed during aerial spraying. J Anal Toxicol 15:339–340, 1991.

52. Cable GG, Doherty S: Acute carbamate and organochlorine toxicity causing convulsions in an agricultural pilot: A case report. Aviat Space Environ Med 70:68–72, 1999.

53. Liddle JA, Kimbrough RD, Needham LL, et al: A fatal episode of accidental methomyl poisoning. J Toxicol Clin Toxicol 15:159–167, 1979.

54. Ferslew KE, Hagardorn AN, McCormick WF: Poisoning from oral ingestion of carbofuran (Furadan 4F), a cholinesterase-inhibiting carbamate insecticide, and its effects on cholinesterase activity in various biological fluids. J Forensic Sci 37:337–344, 1992.

55. Miyazaki T, Yashiki M, Kojima T, et al: Fatal and non-fatal methomyl intoxication in an attempted double suicide. Forensic Sci Int 42:263–270, 1989.

56. Tsatsakis AM, Tsakalof AK, Siatitsas Y, Michalodimitrakis EN: Acute poisoning with carbamate pesticides: The Cretan experience. Sci Justice 36:35–39, 1996.

57. Lifshitz M, Shahak E, Bolotin A, Sofer S: Carbamate poisoning in early childhood and in adults. J Toxicol Clin Toxicol 35:25–27, 1997.

58. Petkovska L, Naumovski DZ, Pilovski GJ, et al: Carbamate induced pancreatitis. Arch Toxicol Kinet Xenobiot Metab 8:173–174, 2000.

59. Weizman Z, Sofer S: Acute pancreatitis in children with anticholinesterase insecticide intoxication. Pediatrics 90:204–206, 1992.

60. Klys M, Kosun J, Pach J, Kamenczak A: Carbofuran poisoning of pregnant woman and fetus per ingestion. J Forensic Sci 34:1413–1416, 1989.

61. Ecobichon DJ: Carbamate insecticides. In Krieger RI (ed): Handbook of Pesticide Toxicology Principles, 2nd ed. San Diego, Academic Press, 2001, pp 1087–1106.

62. Carpenter CP, Weil CS, Palm PE, et al: Mammalian toxicity of 1-naphthyl-N-methylcarbamate (Sevin insecticide). J Agric Food Chem 9:30–39, 1961.

63. Sterri SH, Rognerud B, Fiskum SE, Lyngaas S: Effect of toxogonin and P2S on the toxicity of carbamates and organophosphorus compounds. Acta Pharmacol Toxicol 45:9–15, 1979.

64. Harris LW, Talbot BG, Lennox WJ, Anderson DR: The relationship between oxime-induced reactivation of carbamylated acetylcholinesterase and antidotal efficacy against carbamate intoxication. Toxicol Appl Pharmacol 98:128–133, 1989.

CHAPTER 92

Paraquat and Diquat

Alan Talbot

Bipyridyl compounds are marketed as contact herbicides and desiccants.[1] Paraquat is the most widely used bipyridyl agent and is an essential component of weed control in many areas of agriculture, horticulture, and forestry.[2] Diquat is related structurally to paraquat but is much less widely used.[1]

Paraquat is toxic to green foliage when applied topically in the presence of sunlight. It exerts its herbicidal activity by interfering with the electron transfer system, inhibiting the reduction of nicotinamide adenine dinucleotide phosphate (NADP) to reduced nicotinamide adenine dinucleotide phosphate (NADPH) during photosynthesis.[3] In contrast to other herbicides, paraquat has no residual environmental activity because it is inactivated almost immediately on contact with most naturally occurring soils, forming an inert complex with clay minerals in the soil. This complex is harmless to plant and animal life.[4]

Paraquat, also known as *methyl viologen*, now is marketed in more than 130 countries.[5] It is available for home use as a 0.2% formulation or as commercial paraquat, which is sold as concentrated cation solutions (100 times more concentrated), most commonly 10% to 24% w/w liquid concentrates using the product name Gramoxone (Syngenta Crop Protection, Greensboro, NC).[4] These formulations have been reported in human poisoning in the United States,[4] Europe,[6] Australia,[7] Taiwan,[8] Korea, and Japan.[9,10] Because of its extreme toxicity and the lack of an effective treatment, the formulation in Japan was changed from 24% paraquat dichloride to 5% paraquat dichloride and 7% diquat dibromide in 1986.[11]

Diquat is used alone as a herbicide (e.g., Reglone [Syngenta Crop Protection, Greensboro, NC], an aqueous solution containing 200 g/L of diquat dibromide)[1] but occurs mainly in formulations that also contain paraquat, such as Weedol (The Scotts Company, Marysville, OH), a granular form containing approximately 2.5% of paraquat base and an equal concentration of diquat.[3] Diquat can be obtained in the United States and in several European countries.[12]

INCIDENCE OF HUMAN POISONING

Paraquat is safe when used correctly.[6] Most cases of paraquat poisoning are due to deliberate self-poisoning rather than to accidental ingestion, as may occur if the herbicide is decanted into a wine or soft drink bottle.[6] Paraquat added to food or drink has been a means of committing homicide.[13,14]

Accidental cases of poisoning occur after the concentrated formulations are decanted into poorly labeled containers and left unattended.[8]

There are wide differences from country to country in the annual numbers of deaths, ranging from 2000 in Japan and Taiwan to 0 in Sweden.[8,11,15] Exact figures are unknown because of the lack of a specific International Classification of Diseases code, the lack of standardized data collection by poison control centers, and the lack of national databases in countries where the problem is large.[16] In the United States, 4.9% of herbicide poisonings are paraquat related (an average of 264 cases/yr) with 54% mortality.[17] Most deaths in England result from ingestion of Gramoxone, with a few deaths resulting from Weedol. In France, accidental and occupational poisonings represent 74% of all cases, but suicidal poisoning is associated with the highest mortality, as are the more concentrated products. Most deaths result from ingestion.[18] In Asia, paraquat has 75% to 80% mortality.

Most cases of diquat poisoning have resulted from the intentional, usually suicidal, ingestion of concentrated solutions.[1] Accidental ingestion has occurred as a consequence of decanting diquat concentrates into soft drink bottles.[19] The mortality for cases reported in detail in the literature was 43%[1] despite a lower median lethal dose of diquat (400 mg/kg) than of paraquat (25 to 50 mg/kg). Survival has been reported after ingestion of 300 mL of 20% diquat.[20]

LEVEL OF EVIDENCE

There have been some attempts at meta-analyses for mortality against initial plasma level[21,22] and for hemoperfusion,[23,24] and there has been one randomized trial,[25,26] but otherwise most evidence comes from case reports and case series, which is level 4 for evidence-based therapy.[27] Single case reports run the risk of condemning potentially useful treatments or encouraging potentially toxic ones unnecessarily,[28] and most treatment centers see only a small number of patients, making accurate scientific study difficult. Ethical considerations limit the opportunities for cohort studies and controlled trials, but clinical trials of the sort successfully mounted in paracetamol (acetaminophen) poisoning are needed.[28] Assessment of literature reports requires information on the plasma paraquat concentration. This information often is lacking, particularly with reports before the mid-1970s.

CHEMISTRY

Paraquat

Paraquat (1,1′-dimethyl-4,4′-bipyridylium) is a bis-quaternary ammonium compound, with a molecular formula of $C_{12}H_{14}N_2$. Figure 92-1 shows the structure of paraquat and its product formulations.[14] It usually is synthesized as a dichloride salt, which is a colorless hygroscopic crystalline solid. It is a divalent cation and has a molecular weight of 186.2 (cation) and 257.2 (dichloride). Paraquat is nonvolatile, freely soluble in water, sparingly soluble in lower alcohols, and insoluble in hydrocarbons.[29] It is corrosive to metals and is stable indefinitely when stored in the original container.[30] Paraquat is strongly adsorbed to and inactivated rapidly by clay soils and anionic surfactants. It can be decomposed by ultraviolet light.[31]

In 1977, the manufacturers of paraquat (Paraquat, Syngenta Crop Protection, Greensboro, NC) added a potent emetic, the phosphodiesterase inhibitor PP796,[6] to liquid and solid formulations of paraquat to stimulate the vomiting center and reduce oral toxicity.[6] This emetic was added on the basis of studies in animals suggesting reduced mortality.[32]

Concentrations of paraquat salts should be converted to percent (w/w) of paraquat base. Otherwise, the amount of paraquat ingested in a poisoning case could be underestimated if the amount in the concentrate is based on the dichloride or dimethyl salts.[33]

Diquat

Diquat (1,1′-ethylene-2,2′-bipyridylium) is related structurally to paraquat (see Fig. 92-1). Both contain a bipyridyl ring structure and exist as divalent cations associated with anions such as bromide and chloride.[1]

PHARMACOKINETICS

Data on the pharmacokinetics of paraquat in humans are scarce because systematic studies are difficult to conduct. Paraquat is absorbed poorly from the gastrointestinal tract in humans, rats, and dogs; approximately 1% to 5% of an oral dose is absorbed systemically.[18,34,35] Most is excreted in the feces. The liquid formulations enter the small intestine rapidly, particularly if the stomach is empty. Plasma concentrations reach their peak in 0.5 to 2 hours.[18]

When absorbed, paraquat distributes to most organs in the body. The highest concentrations are found initially in the

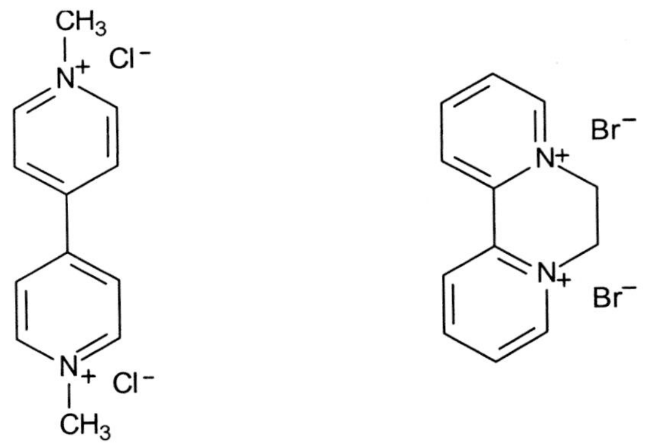

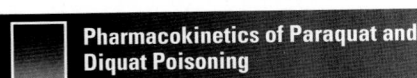

Paraquat   **Diquat**

FIGURE 92-1

Chemical structures of paraquat dichloride and diquat dibromide.

kidney, the major organ of elimination of paraquat, and the lungs.[18] Paraquat is not bound to plasma proteins. The volume of distribution has not been determined accurately in humans. In one patient to whom a tracer dose of radiolabeled paraquat was administered, the volume of distribution was estimated to be 2.74 L/kg 39.5 hours after the ingestion.[32] Several organs, including the lung and muscles, provide a reservoir for paraquat, which slowly redistributes into the bloodstream. This accounts, in part, for the continued excretion of the compound in the urine for several days to weeks after the dose.[18,34]

Most of the dose of paraquat is excreted unchanged in the urine within the first 24 hours of ingestion,[34,36] even in patients who develop renal failure. Before renal failure develops, the renal clearance of paraquat is higher than that of creatinine because of net tubular secretion.[34] As renal function deteriorates, the clearance of paraquat decreases, and the terminal plasma half-life increases from less than 12 hours to 120 hours or longer. This is the second reason why paraquat may be detected in the urine for days to weeks after ingestion.[34,36]

Paraquat is not metabolized appreciably and is excreted by glomerular filtration and renal tubular secretion.[2] Renal tubular reabsorption of paraquat is minimal. Some of the absorbed paraquat is excreted from the bile into the gastrointestinal tract. Paraquat has been detected in the urine 14 to 31 days after ingestion.[25,26] A three-compartment open model best describes the pharmacokinetics disposition of paraquat.[37] Paraquat distributes slowly; in one patient, its volume of distribution reached 2.75 L/kg.[32]

Paraquat has a relatively small diameter (0.702 nm) and does not bind to plasma proteins.[4] It is filtered freely through the glomerulus and is not metabolized by the kidney or other organs.[29] Before the onset of acute renal failure, the renal clearance exceeds that of the glomerular filtration rate, indicating that paraquat is secreted actively by an active transport system in the renal tubules.[29,38]

PATHOPHYSIOLOGY

Paraquat

Only a small amount of paraquat (5% to 10% of dose) is absorbed after oral ingestion.[33,39] Animal experiments suggest that paraquat is absorbed poorly from the stomach but

---

Pharmacokinetics of Paraquat and Diquat Poisoning

Volume of distribution: 2.75 L/kg
Protein binding: does not bind to plasma proteins
Mechanisms of clearance (hepatic, renal, both): freely filtered through the glomerulus; is not metabolized by the kidney or other organs; active secretion from renal tubules
Active metabolites: none
Methods to enhance clearance: none

that facilitated absorption takes place in the small intestine. A linear relationship was noted between the paraquat content of the small intestine and the plasma concentration of paraquat. There was no such correlation with the paraquat content of the stomach.[40,41]

Paraquat absorption from the gut may be incomplete, but it is rapid. The time at which the paraquat concentration in plasma peaks is not known in humans, but it is 60 to 75 minutes in animals.[41-43] Paraquat may be detected in the urine 1 hour after ingestion, and peak concentrations definitely are attained within 4 to 5 hours after intravenous administration and 5 to 7 hours after ingestion, provided that renal function is normal.[44] If renal failure is present, the peak pulmonary concentration is not achieved for 15 to 20 hours or even later.[45]

Administration of "tracer" doses shows exponential decrease in plasma concentrations consistent with a three-compartment model, including a central circulatory compartment, a rapid exchange zone, and a slow exchange zone.[46] Blood is assumed to be the central compartment. Concentrations in plasma and erythrocytes are approximately the same in the rat,[47] and paraquat is not bound to plasma proteins.[48] The second or superficial peripheral compartment is thought to be composed of highly vascular tissues, such as the kidneys, liver, and heart. Rapid exchanges occur between this compartment and blood. The lung is a highly vascular tissue and is exposed early to any paraquat circulating in blood. The third compartment lies within the lungs, especially the pneumocytes, whose exchanges with the central compartment are slow.[46]

The highest concentrations are found in the kidney,[49] followed by the lung and liver.[50,51] The kidney is responsible for removing almost all of the systemically absorbed paraquat,[48,52,53] possibly by an organic cation transport system. When renal damage occurs, clearance of paraquat can decrease by 10 to 20 times,[5] resulting in a dramatic slowing in the rate of decline of plasma paraquat concentrations.[46]

The lung is the primary target organ of paraquat toxicity in humans and several animal species[18,19] because of selective uptake and accumulation of paraquat by type I and type II alveolar epithelial cells. This occurs by a slow, energy-dependent active transport process, which concentrates the compound in pulmonary tissue,[54,55] reaching concentrations that may be 50 times greater than those in the plasma.

The pulmonary uptake of paraquat is virtually complete within the first 6 hours,[46,56] and there may be efflux of toxin back into the circulation as a result of parenchymal necrosis and toxin release. This efflux has been observed within 10 hours.[57]

The mechanism of paraquat uptake is also responsible for the active uptake of endogenous polyamines, such as putrescine.[36,58] The transport process seems to require the structural feature of two positively charged quaternary nitrogen ions separated by a distance of approximately 0.6 to 0.7 nm. Paraquat and the polyamines share these features.[34] The structural specification of the uptake system is shown by the observation that diquat lacks these structural features and does not accumulate in the lung or cause pulmonary injury.[20,21]

Paraquat produces degenerative lesions in the lungs[37] accompanied by biochemical and ultrastructural changes of the pulmonary capillary endothelium and damage to the alveolar epithelium.[37,59,60] Paraquat apparently stimulates the infiltration of profibroblasts, which mature into basophilic fibroblasts.[16] The coalescence of fibroblast clumps and the destruction of alveolar walls eventually obliterate the architecture of the lung parenchyma, resulting in diffuse intraalveolar fibrosis.

In the rat model, pulmonary fibrosis develops in destructive, then proliferative phases. First there is swelling and fragmentation of membranous pneumocytes (type I), followed by degenerative changes in granular pneumocytes (type II). By the third day, profibroblasts migrate into the alveolar spaces, and by day 7, the alveoli are filled with proliferating fibroblasts. Finally, the lung architecture disappears, and only the alveolar capillaries remain. Oxygen potentiates the paraquat-induced pulmonary fibrosis, but fibrotic changes still develop in rat models given room air. A reduction in antiproteases (e.g., α_1-antitrypsin) occurs as a result of superoxide generation and may promote pulmonary damage.[17]

NADPH depletion[61] and lipid peroxidation[62] have been proposed as mechanisms of paraquat toxicity.[63] Flavoenzymes, such as NADPH–cytochrome P-450 reductase,[62,64,65] xanthine oxidase,[66,67] and mitochondrial NADH–quinone oxidoreductase,[68] initiate the single electron reduction of paraquat to free paraquat radical (Fig. 92-2). This paraquat radical is extremely unstable. It transfers an electron to molecular oxygen to form a superoxide anion radical, which

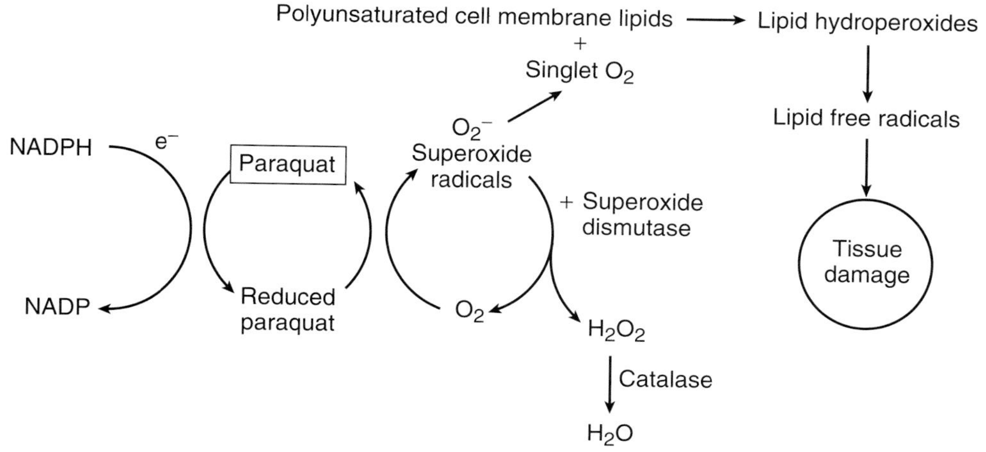

FIGURE 92-2

Proposed mechanism of paraquat toxicity. NADP, nicotinamide adenine dinucleotide phosphate; NADPH, reduced nicotinamide adenine dinucleotide phosphate. (*Adapted from Vale JA, Meredith TJ [eds]: Poisoning, Diagnosis, and Treatment. London, Update Books, 1981, p 136.*)

is thought to cause the systemic toxicity.[2,32] Paraquat continues to cycle through the process of oxidation and reduction (hence the term *redox cycling*), sustained in the lung by the plentiful supply of electrons and oxygen. The superoxide anion radicals produced react with each other, forming hydrogen peroxide and molecular oxygen, a reaction that may occur spontaneously or via the enzyme superoxide dismutase. Under normal circumstances, hydrogen peroxide is detoxified by catalase and glutathione peroxidase, but when these protective mechanisms prove inadequate, it can cause devastating effects on the cell.[1]

Experimentally, it has been shown that paraquat toxicity is enhanced by the administration of oxygen.[22] Toxicity to pulmonary artery endothelial cells is attributed at least partly to reactive oxygen species generated by xanthine oxidase because xanthine oxidase inhibitors, such as allopurinol and tungsten, reduce paraquat toxicity.[69] In the presence of iron, the superoxide anion radical reacts with hydrogen peroxide, generating the hydroxyl radical. This radical can attack the lipid chains of biologic membranes initiating lipid peroxidation, causing membrane damage and cell death. This mechanism is similar to that of oxygen toxicity.[32,33] Whether lipid peroxidation during redox cycling of paraquat is correlated to the damage in pulmonary cells is unclear, however.[37] The effect of paraquat on lipid peroxidation is independent of paraquat radical formation mediated by NADPH–cytochrome P-450 reductase.[70]

Paraquat is not metabolized and is excreted unchanged in the urine.[52] Excretion is almost exclusively renal; biliary excretion is small.[39,71,72] Paraquat renal clearance is higher than creatinine clearance and may exceed 200 mL/min when renal function is normal.[24,46,56,73–75] Large amounts (>1 g/L) are excreted within the first few hours after ingestion.[46,56,76]

Diquat

Diquat is a potent redox cycler, and its toxic effects depend on its ability to undergo a single electron addition to form a free radical; this occurs in the presence of NADPH and cytochrome P-450.[77] The oxidative stress induced by diquat is associated with the release of iron from hepatic ferritin and the depletion of reducing equivalents, including glutathione and NADPH. In experimental studies, protection against the toxic effects of diquat was provided by catalase, especially in the presence of the iron chelator deferoxamine. In contrast to paraquat, diquat is not accumulated by the lung and has a half-life in the lung five times shorter than that of paraquat.[1]

CLINICAL PRESENTATION AND LIFE-THREATENING COMPLICATIONS

Paraquat

See Table 92-1.[30]

LOCAL TOXICITY

Skin. Normally the surface epithelium of the skin is an excellent barrier to paraquat,[6] unless skin lesions are present.[78] Paraquat diluted as recommended for spraying is unlikely to irritate the skin, unless clothing soaked with spray is worn for prolonged periods,[35] the spray apparatus leaks,[35,38,79–81] or protective clothing is not worn.[78]

Aerosolized paraquat droplets have diameters exceeding 5 μm, which means that these particles do not reach the alveolar membrane to cause either direct or systemic toxicity via inhalation. The vapor pressure of paraquat is low,

TABLE 92-1 Toxicity of Dipyridylium Herbicides

	ACUTE EFFECTS	CHRONIC EFFECTS
Paraquat		
Alimentay tract	Irritation, ulceration of mucous membranes; hemorrhage	–
Respiratory tract	Irritation of upper airways, hemorrhage, lung edema, atelectasis, alveolar fibrosis	Fibrosis of the lung
Kidney	Proximal tubular degeneration	–
Liver	Focal degeneration	–
Heart	Myocarditis	–
Eye	Irritation of the conjunctiva, corneal lesions	–
Skin	Necrosis, ulcerations, erythemas, mild reactive hyperkeratosis	–
Diquat		
Alimentary tract	Ulcerations of mucosa, paralytic ileus	–
Kidney	Proximal tubular degeneration	–
Liver	Focal degeneration	–
Testis	Degeneration of seminiferous epithelium	–
Eye	–	Bilateral cataract
Morfamquat		
Kidney	Tubular, glomerular damage	–

From Manzo L, Gregotti C, DiNucci A, et al: Toxicology of paraquat and related bipyridyls: Biochemical, clinical and therapeutic aspects. Vet Hum Toxicol 21:404, 1979. Reprinted with permission.

making vapor inhalation unlikely. However, excessive inhalation of the spray may cause stomatitis, epistaxis, headache, and sore throat.[82]

Paraquat, especially in concentrated formulations, has a strong irritant action. Transverse ridging and furrowing of the fingernail progressing to gross irregular deformity of the nail plate and loss of the nail may occur. A transverse band of white discoloration affecting the nail plate may become apparent after several weeks.[83,84] Normal nail growth follows without delay when exposure has ceased.

Erythema, blistering, irritation, and ulceration of the skin occur,[2,31] and eczematous dermatitis has been reported.[84] Fatal dermal exposures have occurred.[24] A bicycle fall while the cyclist was carrying paraquat resulted in the death of the cyclist 12 days later.[85] Applied to the perineum by mistake, paraquat caused renal and respiratory failure.[86] Paraquat occasionally has been used inappropriately to treat lice and scabies.[81,87]

Eyes. Severe ocular inflammation may develop if the eyes are exposed to concentrated paraquat solution.[2] Inflammation develops gradually, reaching a maximum after 12 to 24 hours, and may progress to ulceration of the conjunctiva and cornea.[88] Although healing may be slow, recovery usually is complete.[89] Serious complications may develop if the potential seriousness of exposure is not recognized, including marked reduction in visual acuity due to either corneal edema or corneal opacity.[88] Lacrimal duct stenosis also has been described.

SYSTEMIC TOXICITY

The degree of systemic toxicity is governed by the amount of paraquat ingested.[48] Systemic toxicity has followed subcutaneous,[90] intraperitoneal, and intravenous injection[91,92] of paraquat. The oral route is the usual route for serious toxicity, however.

Gastrointestinal. Paraquat itself causes nausea, vomiting (in rare cases blood stained), and diarrhea as a result of its local irritant action on the gut. Granular preparations contain magnesium sulfate, which increases the likelihood of diarrhea. Patients who are moderately or severely poisoned develop a burning sensation, soreness, and pain in the mouth, throat, retrosternal area, and abdomen (usually epigastric and may be associated with guarding). The abdominal pain, vomiting, and diarrhea often appear soon after ingestion. Ulceration in the mouth, sloughing of the oropharyngeal mucosa, an inability to swallow saliva, dysphagia, and aphonia are common.[2,26,39] The corrosive effects become more severe as the time postingestion increases. Prominent pharyngeal membranes ("pseudodiphtheria") have been reported,[93] and perforation of the esophagus[40] may result in mediastinitis, surgical emphysema, and pneumothorax or pleural effusion in association with pleuritis.[6]

Jaundice, hepatomegaly, and central abdominal pain due to pancreatitis are frequent complications. At postmortem examination, these patients show centrilobular hepatic necrosis and cholestasis.[7,42] Serum transaminase levels also may be elevated.[26]

Renal. Oliguric or nonoliguric renal failure may supervene and usually is due to acute tubular necrosis, which becomes evident after about 24 hours. Rarely, glomerular and tubular hemorrhage may be found.[94] In other cases, proximal tubular dysfunction may develop within 2 to 6 days and may progress to anuria. Renal dysfunction commonly results in proteinuria, microscopic hematuria, glycosuria, aminoaciduria, phosphaturia, and excessive leaking of sodium and urate.[95] Histopathology may reveal proximal renal tubular and glomerular degeneration and necrosis.[2,39] Renal failure is not a common cause of death in paraquat poisoning.[32]

Pulmonary. Most patients develop a cough, which may be productive and blood stained. Dyspnea is a prominent feature and occurs early in patients who have ingested a substantial amount and, in these circumstances, is due to the development of adult respiratory distress syndrome. In less severely poisoned patients, the onset of dyspnea may be delayed and is caused by pulmonary fibrosis. Rarely, pneumothorax (in association with mediastinitis), pleural effusion, and iatrogenic pulmonary edema may precipitate dyspnea.[96]

In addition to a declining gas transfer factor and vital capacity, severely poisoned patients have a low and declining PO_2 with resultant central cyanosis. Radiologic changes do not always parallel the severity of clinical symptoms. The chest x-ray may be normal, particularly in patients dying early from multiple organ failure. More commonly, patchy infiltration occurs, which may progress to an opacification of one or both lung fields. Survivors of paraquat poisoning may be left with a restrictive type of pulmonary dysfunction.[97]

Cardiovascular. Except for sinus tachycardia, cardiovascular complications usually are not observed until the terminal phase of intoxication. Ventricular tachycardia, intraventricular conduction disturbances, and nonspecific T-wave changes on electrocardiogram occur in the terminal phase. Sinus bradycardia, hypotension, and cardiac arrest may supervene. The chest x-ray may show massive cardiomegaly, and at postmortem examination, toxic myocarditis is found histologically.[19,43]

Neurologic. Coma is a common and terminal event, although other neurologic features, such as ataxia and facial paresis,[90] occasionally are observed. Convulsions have been reported[98–100] and may be due to cerebral edema[101] precipitated by fluid overload.[102]

Endocrine. At postmortem examination, adrenal cortical necrosis often is observed,[94,103] particularly in severely poisoned patients with multiple organ failure. The clinical significance of this observation is unclear because the use of corticosteroids does not correct hypotension, which more likely is due to myocardial failure.

Hematologic. A polymorphonuclear leukocytosis is a frequent finding, but erythrocyte aplasia leading to normochromic anemia[104] and hemolytic anemia[105] has been reported. Metabolic acidosis is common. Hypocalcemia, which sometimes results in tetany, may follow forced diuresis in the presence of renal impairment[102] or charcoal hemoperfusion. Increased serum creatine kinase activity is secondary to paraquat-induced muscle damage.[6]

GENERAL TOXICITY

Three degrees of intoxication may be distinguished (Table 92-2), as follows:[6]

TABLE 92-2 Grading System for Paraquat Poisoning

Group 1	Mild poisoning (<1 g diquat ion ingested). In addition to gastrointestinal symptoms, evidence of renal impairment may develop. Recovery is invariable
Group 2	Moderate-to-severe poisoning (1–12 g diquat ion ingested). Multiple organ dysfunction is frequent, and acute renal failure in particular is common, but recovery occurs in some two thirds of cases
Group 3	Fulminant poisoning (>12 g diquat ion ingested). Multiple organ failure develops, and death eventually occurs in all cases within 24–48 hr

After Wilks MF: Diquat: Diagnosis, Treatment and Prognosis of Poisoning. Surrey, UK, Zeneca Agrochemicals, 1994.

Group 1. Mild poisoning follows the ingestion or injection of less than 20 mg of paraquat ion/kg body weight. Patients are asymptomatic or develop vomiting and diarrhea. Full recovery occurs, but there may be a transient decline in the gas transfer factor and vital capacity.

Group 2. Moderate-to-severe poisoning follows the ingestion or injection of 20 to 40 mg of paraquat ion/kg body weight (<15 mL of 20% w/v concentrate). Patients experience vomiting and diarrhea and develop generalized symptoms indicating systemic toxicity. Pulmonary fibrosis develops in all cases, but recovery may occur. In addition, renal failure due to acute tubular necrosis becomes evident after about 24 hours, and hepatic dysfunction may supervene. Death occurs in most cases but can be delayed for 2 or 3 weeks. Apart from burning and erythema, symptoms and signs of this injury may be absent if the patient is seen soon after the ingestion. The absence of symptoms and signs does not exclude the diagnosis of paraquat poisoning. A mistaken diagnosis of suppurative pharyngitis or tonsillitis has been made in some patients.

Group 3. Acute fulminant poisoning follows the ingestion of more than 40 mg of paraquat ion/kg body weight. In addition to nausea and vomiting, there is marked ulceration of the oropharynx with multiple organ failure. Damaged organs include the heart, brain (cerebral edema, convulsions), adrenals (cortical necrosis), liver, kidney (necrosis), pancreas, and lung (hemorrhagic pulmonary edema or adult respiratory distress syndrome). Mortality is 100% in this group. Death may occur within 24 hours of the overdose but is never delayed for more than 1 week. Death can occur before the results of laboratory investigations and even chest x-rays become grossly abnormal.[41]

Within 24 hours of ingestion, patients in groups 2 and 3 develop lethargy, a widespread burning sensation, generalized weakness and myalgia, giddiness, headache, anorexia, and fever. Fear and apprehension are prominent features, and restlessness sometimes is observed.

Diquat

LOCAL TOXICITY

The intact skin is an effective barrier against diquat absorption (in one human study, only 0.3% of the dose was absorbed[107]). Local toxicity has been reported after oral, dermal, inhalational, ophthalmic, and vaginal exposure to diquat-containing formulations. Corrosive damage to the oral mucosa,[19,108–110] leading to burning in the mouth and painful hemorrhagic ulceration, is a common early feature of diquat ingestion. Mucosal edema of the tongue and oropharynx[108,111] also may develop and may be severe enough to necessitate endotracheal intubation.[111]

Epistaxis and throat irritation have been reported after the inhalation of splashes or droplets caused by the careless mixing of diquat solutions.[112] Conjunctivitis and corneal scarring may occur if diquat-containing formulations are splashed directly into the eye.[113] Extensive mucosal necrosis of the vagina and vulva followed the intravaginal application of a 6% diquat solution.[114]

Nail growth disturbances followed contact of the nail base with diquat solution for a few minutes and shedding of the nail after prolonged contact with concentrated diquat.[112] Third-degree burns of the feet followed leakage from a backpack sprayer into the applicator's boots. Within 2 days, he developed partial-thickness burns, which required skin grafting.[115]

SYSTEMIC TOXICITY

Systemic toxicity usually is associated with the ingestion of diquat, although systemic toxicity followed the instillation of 20 mL of a 6% diquat solution intravaginally.[114]

Gastrointestinal. Diquat may cause severe and extensive mucosal damage not only to the mouth but also to the esophagus, stomach, and small intestine.[108,110,116,117] Consequently, generalized abdominal pain,[110,111,118,119] vomiting,[12,108,110,111,114,116,118,120] and diarrhea[12,110,111,114,118,119,121] can occur within a few minutes of ingestion.

An endoscopy performed shortly after the ingestion of a small amount of diquat showed severe panesophagitis and hemorrhagic gastritis at the fundus[110]; a second endoscopy 1 month later showed that the lesions had healed completely. First-degree and second-degree burns of the esophagus and stomach were identified after ingestion of 200 mL of diquat dibromide 1.84% (equivalent to a total of 2 g of diquat cation).[108] Hemorrhagic ulcers from the mouth to the duodenum persisted for 4 weeks in a patient who ingested 10 g.[122] Diffuse erosions and mucosal necrosis have been identified in the esophagus, stomach, and ileum at postmortem examination.[111,116]

Paralytic ileus may develop 1 to 4 days postingestion and has been reported in four cases, three of which were fatal.[12,20,123] Paralytic ileus is thought to be responsible for the accumulation or sequestration of large amounts of fluid in the gut, leading to hypovolemic shock.[12] Deranged liver function, as shown by an increase in liver transaminase activities, is reported commonly but usually is mild, is transient, and resolves spontaneously.[12,20,111,116,120,122]

Renal. Nephrotoxicity has been reported frequently and ranges from transient proteinuria[110,124] to acute renal failure.[12,19,108,111,114,116,118,119,122,125] Renal failure has developed 1 hour[116] to 5 days[126] postingestion and was invariably present in patients who died. Hypovolemia after sequestration of fluid in the gut may cause renal failure by reducing renal perfusion; however, renal failure has occurred in the absence of hypovolemia.[108,116,119] Diquat may have a direct toxic effect on the kidney, but the mechanism is not clear.

At postmortem examination, acute tubular necrosis was the typical lesion observed.[12,19,118]

Pulmonary. Bronchopneumonia has been reported at postmortem examination,[12,19,118] although it was not always diagnosed clinically.[12,19] The radiologic appearances of pulmonary infiltration and exudates observed are similar to those in adult respiratory distress syndrome. Severe pulmonary edema, without evidence of infection, also has been observed at postmortem examination.[111] Respiratory failure and the need for mechanical ventilation were reported,[19] but the pulmonary fibrosis typically seen in paraquat poisoning has not been reported.

Cardiovascular. Fatal cardiotoxic effects that lead to death within 1 to 5 days postingestion have been reported. The abnormalities were repeated attacks of ventricular fibrillation,[12] ventricular arrhythmia,[12] and no clinical features except for postmortem findings of subendocardial hemorrhages in the left ventricular wall and overlying papillary muscle.[116]

Neurologic. Coma has been reported to develop 18 hours[12] to 4 days postingestion.[123] Coma occurred in association with pontine hemorrhages in life[123] and at postmortem examination.[12,118,123] Grand mal seizures within 12 hours postingestion and sometimes progressing to status epilepticus have been reported.[111,116] The development of aggressive behavior accompanied the complication of intracerebral bleeding.[127]

Hematologic. Leukopenia,[109] pancytopenia,[122] and thrombocytopenia[20,109] have been reported, but some of these patients also received hemodialysis[128] or charcoal hemoperfusion.[20]

GENERAL TOXICITY

Of all the clinical features described, the following seem to be associated with a poor prognosis: the rapid onset of acute renal failure, intestinal ileus and subsequent fluid sequestration, ventricular arrhythmias, pulmonary complications requiring ventilation, and coma. Wilks[129] proposed that patients developing systemic features can be categorized into three groups (see Table 92-2).

DIAGNOSIS

Paraquat

The history is a good general guide. The quantity of paraquat in the specific herbicidal preparation and the volume ingested (one mouthful of a 20% solution is potentially life-threatening) is essential information and should be confirmed by examination of the container and its contents if possible.[24] The time between ingestion of paraquat and the most recent meal should be determined because of the tendency for paraquat to be absorbed and partially neutralized by food particles.[24]

A qualitative urine test should be performed with alkaline sodium dithionite.[130] Urine, 10 mL, is added to a 1% solution of 2N sodium dithionite in 1N sodium hydroxide, 1 mL. A blue color (λ maximum 603 nm)[130] indicates paraquat; a blue-green color (λ maximum 603 nm)[130] suggests diquat.[30,50,55] It is important to ensure that negative and positive controls are analyzed with each patient specimen. Failure of the test almost invariably is due to the use of sodium dithionite that has oxidized on storage.[130] This reagent may not be readily available in some laboratories. Because this method is sensitive only to concentrations of 1 mg/L or greater, a negative test does not exclude the possibility of paraquat ingestion; repeated urine tests are suggested. If this test is negative within 24 hours of the overdose, there is no need for a quantitative analysis of the blood, and the patient may be reassured accordingly.[130]

Bismuth and colleagues[24] identified several factors (Table 92-3) that indicate serious ingestions, including the ingestion of concentrated solution on an empty stomach and the presence of renal failure and esophageal and gastric mucosal lesions. Nine of 14 patients who had gastric and esophageal ulcerations observed 3 hours to 3 days after paraquat ingestion died.[23] The presence and severity of the ulceration probably reflect the extent of contact between paraquat and the mucosa and the dose ingested.

If the qualitative urine test is positive, measurement of the plasma paraquat concentration by radioimmunoassay correlates well with outcome[21,22,131] in samples taken during the first 24 hours[131] and over the ensuing 10 or 11 days.[22] The prognosis can be determined from a nomogram (Fig. 92-3),[53] which relates initial[48] and delayed[58] plasma concentrations of paraquat and the time after ingestion to the probability of survival, or by calculating an index based on serum concentrations of potassium, bicarbonate, and creatinine and the time since ingestion.[132] The Hart nomogram is valid even if hemoperfusion has been performed.[133] At present, dose

TABLE 92-3 Prognostic Factors in Paraquat Poisoning

	DEATHS/TOTAL	P*
Per os	17/24	<.05
Other routes	0/4	
Ingestion of paraquat		
Men	13/20	
Women	4/4	NS
Accidental	5/10	
Intentional	12/14	NS
1 mouthful	6/12	
>1 mouthful	11/12	.07
12% solution	1/4	
20% solution	16/20	NS
Full stomach	1/5	
Empty stomach	7/8	.06
No esophageal lesion	0/2	
Esophageal lesions	9/14	NS
No gastric lesion	0/6	
Gastric lesions	9/10	<.01
Organic renal failure	17/18	
Functional renal failure or no renal failure	0/6	<.001

*Fisher's test. NS, not significant.
Adapted from Bismuth C, Garnier R, Dally S, et al: Prognosis and treatment of paraquat poisoning: A review of 28 cases. J Toxicol Clin Toxicol 19:463, 1983. Used with permission.

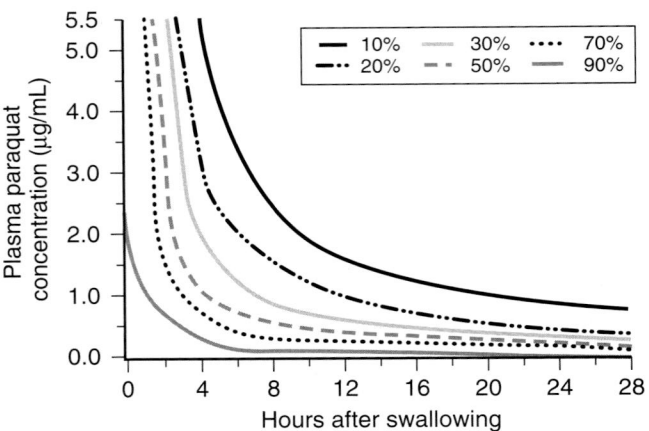

FIGURE 92-3

Contour graph shows relationships between plasma paraquat concentration (µg/mL), time after ingestion, and probability of survival (percentages). *(From Hart TB, Nevitt A, Whitehead A: A statistical approach to the prognostic significance of plasma paraquat concentrations. Lancet 2:1222, 1984.)*

rather than any subsequent treatment is the principal determinant of survival.[133]

Concentrations of paraquat in urine obtained within the first 24 hours of ingestion have also been used to determine prognosis.[58] Of 53 patients with urinary concentrations of paraquat of less than 1 mg/L within the first 24 hours, 15 survived. In patients who died within 24 hours, the urinary paraquat concentrations were 10 to 10,000 mg/L, and in patients who died later from pulmonary fibrosis, the urinary paraquat concentrations were 1 to 1000 mg/L. The development of renal impairment heralds a poor outlook. In one series, of 20 patients who developed renal failure, 19 died.[36] Toxic pulmonary concentrations possibly can be achieved only if there is concomitant renal failure.[34,36]

Additional quantitative methods of analysis in biologic fluids include spectrophotometry, ion-exchange chromatography, gas chromatography, and radioimmunoassay.[2,25,51,52] The precise toxic serum concentration has not been determined; however, values greater than 0.2 µg/mL within 24 hours of ingestion and greater than 0.1 µg/mL within 48 hours usually result in fatality.

At serum paraquat concentrations expected in overdose (i.e., <10 mg/L), little interference occurs with laboratory tests. At higher serum paraquat concentrations, false elevations of creatinine and lactate dehydrogenase occur.[54]

Diquat

Confirmation of the diagnosis can be made qualitatively and rapidly by the addition of sodium dithionite to alkalinized urine. A yellow-green color develops on reduction of diquat by sodium dithionite.[130] A disadvantage of the assay is that paraquat undergoes a similar reduction and may interfere with the analysis. The assay remains the most suitable under emergency conditions, however. Diquat also may be determined accurately in blood and urine by gas chromatography[130] and high-performance liquid chromatography.[134] At present, there are insufficient data to allow accurate determination of prognosis based on the plasma diquat concentration measured on presentation.

The International Programme on Chemical Safety[135] reviewed cases of diquat poisoning and considered the fatal dose of diquat to be 6 to 12 g for humans. Of fatal cases reported in the literature, the ingested dose ranged from 6 to 60 g.[1] One patient survived, however, without sequelae after ingestion of 60 g of diquat.[20] The time between ingestion and death ranged from 14 hours[116] to 7 days.[136] Although this did not correlate with the amount of diquat ingested, in two fatal cases in which greater than 60 g of diquat was ingested, death occurred at 14 hours and 38 hours, respectively.[116,137]

TREATMENT

Paraquat

The treatment of paraquat intoxication remains largely ineffective. Patients who ingest paraquat should be treated as medical emergencies, even if asymptomatic. In patients who claim to have had only dermal, inhalational, or ocular contact, it is imperative to ensure that ingestion has not occurred as well. The management of paraquat poisoning includes removing the chemical from the gastrointestinal tract,[138] increasing its excretion from the blood,[5] and decreasing the subsequent damage caused by tissue exposure to the poison.[5]

The severe pain of local ulceration is difficult to treat. Mouthwashes, ice-cold fluids and ice cream, local anesthetic sprays, and lozenges have been used with some success. Opiates are required eventually in most patients to relieve general and local pain and distress.

Patients are always dehydrated to some extent[139,140] because of gastrointestinal fluid losses; paraquat also may cause peripheral vasodilation.[140] This functional component of early renal failure does not indicate a poor prognosis,[24] but it should be corrected by volume expansion to maximize elimination of paraquat before the development of tubular necrosis.[48]

Forced diuresis theoretically is employed to increase the renal excretion of paraquat. Because renal tubular reabsorption is minimal, this method may act by reducing the concentration of paraquat in the renal tubular lumen.[37] Intravenous dextrose in water or normal saline solutions, along with furosemide and mannitol, may produce urine volumes of 12 to 16 L in 24 hours.[2] Some authors advise against forced diuresis because the patient may develop pulmonary edema or renal failure.[59]

Whether to refer the patient to a specialized poison treatment center depends on the nationality of the patient and the experience of the staff in the hospital of first contact. In Western countries, most physicians and nurses at local hospitals have not managed a case of paraquat poisoning.[6] A specialty center has the expertise to employ elimination techniques.[141] The time lost in transferring the patient between institutions may make the use of these techniques inappropriate, however.[6] Referral may make visiting difficult for relatives.[6]

Staff who see large numbers of paraquat poisoning cases have to cope with feelings of inadequacy leading to a tendency to minimize contact. Infrequent communication causes considerable suffering to the patient, however.[6] Cultural differences affect the decision of whether to tell the patient the prognosis, and relatives often insist that the patient not be told the truth about his or her illness.

AIRWAY AND VENTILATORY CONSIDERATIONS

Because paraquat causes hypoxemia, it seems logical that supplemental oxygen should be beneficial. Animal experiments have shown, however, that paraquat-treated rats survived longer when exposed to room air (21% oxygen) than when exposed to higher oxygen concentrations.[33,68] Formation of oxygen-free radicals, such as superoxide, may be enhanced in the presence of a high oxygen concentration.[69] Maintenance of a therapeutic hypoxemia has been suggested but has not been proved clinically. Positive end-expiratory pressure and continuous positive pressure breathing may be used to keep the inspired oxygen fraction to a minimum.[26] It is surprising how well patients tolerate hypoxemic exposure.[26] Treatment with an extracorporeal silicone membrane oxygenator was unsuccessful.[70]

DECONTAMINATION

Patients exposed to paraquat via the dermal or ophthalmic route should have any potential sites of contact extensively irrigated.

Gastrointestinal Decontamination

Gastric Lavage. Immediate induction of vomiting, gastrointestinal lavage, and administration of adsorbents and cathartics have been recommended to prevent absorption of paraquat.[39,125,142] There is little experimental[43,143] or clinical evidence, however, for the use of gastric lavage[24,144,145] or whole-gut lavage.[125,143] The role of gastric lavage in all forms of poisoning in humans has been questioned.[146] The risk of ulceration of the oropharyngeal and esophagogastric mucosal surfaces by concentrated formulations of paraquat is a theoretical contraindication.[39,40] The procedure may delay other treatment with better supporting evidence, such as the administration of oral adsorbents.

Induced Emesis. Similar to gastric lavage, there is little experimental[143] or clinical[16,32,145] evidence for induced emesis. Ingestion of the emetic formulation induces earlier vomiting, which is more likely to occur the greater the quantity of paraquat ion ingested[145]; however, no reduction in mortality has been noted.[24,143,147] There is increasing doubt about the value of induced emesis in treating any other form of intoxication.[144,148,149]

Oral Adsorbents. There is no conclusive evidence of the value of oral adsorbents. Investigation of a variety of soils showed that montmorillonite was a strong binding agent in vitro[150] and that bentonite (sodium montmorillonite) and Fuller's Earth (Oil-Dri Corp. of America, Chicago, IL) (calcium montmorillonite) were particularly effective.[43] Single[43] or repeated[40] doses reduced mortality in rats even if given after a potentially lethal dose of paraquat. This reduction in mortality was associated with a concomitant reduction in the amount of paraquat accumulated in lung tissue.[40]

In clinical practice, Fuller's Earth is preferred because it can be used as a 30% (w/v) suspension, whereas bentonite swells in water and can be used only as a 7% solution.[138] Because this treatment often induces severe diarrhea, supplemental fluids and electrolyte replacement often are required. In some cases, the clay causes hypercalcemia,

fecaliths, and fecal impaction. The use of these agents in poisoned patients[24,145,151–153] has not met with the success of the laboratory experiments.

Activated charcoal in vitro has a maximum binding capacity greater than either Fuller's Earth or bentonite,[154] and a single dose administration after paraquat ingestion was even more effective in reducing mortality in rats.[154,155] The addition of a cathartic agent (magnesium citrate) increased the survival in vivo.[155] Not all the forms of activated charcoal have the same capacity to adsorb paraquat,[138] although Ultracarbon (Norit Americas Inc., Marshall, TX) and Carbomix (DSM Copolymer Inc., Baton Rouge, LA), which are common in Asia, have maximal adsorption capacities of 8 to 10 g of paraquat/100 g.[138] Results of multiple-dose activated charcoal have not been reported for animals or humans.

Cation exchange resins, normally used for the treatment of hypercalcemia, have been suggested as an alternative means of binding paraquat in the gut. Sodium polystyrene sulfate (Kayexalate) and calcium polystyrene sulfate (Kalimate [Nikken Chemical, Tokyo, Japan]) have high maximal adsorption capacities for paraquat[138] and reduced morbidity in rats with administration 24 hours after ingestion.[156] Gastric and intestinal lavage with these materials has been used clinically,[157] but the lack of blood concentration data makes it impossible to make any judgment.[138]

Extracorporal Removal Techniques. Peritoneal dialysis is a poor means of removing paraquat.[158,159] Hemodialysis achieves good clearance when paraquat plasma concentrations are high (>10 mg/L) and can reach 150 mL/min.[160–162] Clearance decreases significantly, however, when the plasma concentration is less than 1 mg/L.

Hemoperfusion. Hemoperfusion is the most effective means of achieving extracorporeal elimination of paraquat.[44] Clearance is greater than 50 mL/min even when the plasma paraquat concentration is less than 0.2 mg/L and can be increased further by using hemodialysis and hemoperfusion in series.[162,163] Platelet counts should be measured during hemoperfusion.

 Indications and Contraindications for Hemoperfusion

Patients with paraquat plasma concentrations >3 mg/L, regardless of the time taken, died despite hemoperfusion. One should consider carefully the uniformly bad prognosis of patients within this group before subjecting them to hemoperfusion. The main considerations lie in the discomfort involved for the patient from a procedure of unproven benefit. For similar reasons, patients who clearly are going to survive should not undergo hemoperfusion.[79]

Hemoperfusion could be considered for patients whose initial plasma concentrations are <3 mg/L, patients in whom the probability of survival is 20% to 70%, and patients who present within a few hours of ingestion. Even in these groups, it is not proven that hemoperfusion, single or repeated, is useful. The likelihood of hemoperfusion being efficacious probably is greatest if it is begun within 10 to 12 hours of ingestion.[80]

When the paraquat concentrations in the venous outlet of the hemoperfusion cartridge are undetectable (indicating effective extracorporeal elimination), plasma paraquat concentrations decrease dramatically within 1 to 3 hours. The amount of herbicide removed at the end of a single session is low, even when the clearance is still good. When the procedure is stopped, a rebound in plasma concentration is observed, which is explained by the extensive tissue distribution of paraquat and its slow redistribution during the hemoperfusion process.[106,164,165] Repeat hemoperfusion was recommended[160,166] but has not proved beneficial.[24,44,133,163,167] In all large series, hemoperfusion, with or without the addition of hemodialysis, did not improve the prognosis of paraquat poisoning when plasma concentrations were above the predictive curve. There is a negative correlation between the amount of paraquat eliminated and the time of death: The larger the amount of paraquat removed from the blood, the greater the probability of early death.[44]

Other Techniques. Continuous arteriovenous hemofiltration is a new technique; sufficient data are not available to evaluate this procedure in paraquat poisoning. Plasmapheresis also has been advocated in paraquat poisoning; however, further studies are needed to determine its effectiveness.[62,63]

SPECIFIC TREATMENTS

Pharmacologic intervention in paraquat poisoning has not been successful. Many agents reduce paraquat uptake into lung in vitro[34,168,169] but fail to show significant protection in vivo.[169] Work with propranolol,[105,169,170] β-adrenoceptor antagonists,[169] and putrescine[171] has not supported any role for pump inhibitors as a mode of therapy.

Superoxide dismutase first was used on the basis that increasing the breakdown of excess superoxide would decrease paraquat toxicity. Laboratory work with animals has shown equivocal results,[172–175] and clinically, infusions of superoxide dismutase have been without apparent benefit.[28] Vitamin E is a reducing agent and could act as a free radical scavenger. The experimental evidence does not seem to support its use.[63,91,175–179] Another free radical scavenger, α-tocopherol, had no protective effect when given after paraquat.[176] Selenium is a cofactor for the enzyme glutathione peroxidase. Rats deficient in selenium are at a greater risk of paraquat damage,[180] and dietary supplementation in the chick is protective.[177] There are no clinical studies on the use of these antioxidants.

Ascorbic acid is an antioxidant, but studies have suggested that it may be protective[181,182] or may potentiate toxicity[183]; hence it does not seem to have a clinical role.[28] A combination of ascorbic acid and riboflavin in rats produced a significant improvement in paraquat mortality.[184] Niacin also decreased mortality in rats.[185] There have been no controlled human studies, although some protocols include these agents.[100]

Therapy based on manipulating the redox cycle has led to laboratory experiments with desferrioxamine,[186,187] clofibrate,[188] and N-acetylcysteine.[189,190] None of these agents have been studied in humans, however.

Immunosuppressants and antiinflammatory agents, such as azathioprine, beclomethasone dipropionate, bleomycin, cyclophosphamide, and fluorouracil, and fibrinolytics, such as potassium aminobenzoate, have been used.[7,42,43, 64,65] One reason for the lack of efficacy of many of these compounds is that they have been used after pulmonary fibrosis has developed. The ultimate value of these agents is unknown, although some degree of benefit has been observed when they were given early in the course of treatment.[66]

Pulse therapy with glucocorticoid and cyclophosphamide showed promising results in moderate-to-severe paraquat poisoning,[25,191] but the series was not analyzed on an intention-to-treat basis.[26] Further trials are required.[192,193]

Immunotherapy is a more recent approach used for reducing pulmonary accumulation of paraquat. Although prophylaxis delayed death in the rat, it did not modify overall mortality.[194] Specific antibodies reduced the accumulation of paraquat in slices of rat lung,[195] but because the efflux of paraquat was not modified, the treatment is unlikely to be effective if administered postingestion. This theory has been confirmed by in vivo experiments, which showed that immunotherapy with antiparaquat antibodies[196] on Fab$_2$ fragments[197] succeeded in sequestering paraquat in the plasma compartment but could not alter accumulation in tissues.

Hypoxic breathing mixtures do not prevent lung toxicity,[198] although oxygen has been shown to increase lung injury. In rats, total exclusion from ventilation protected lungs from the development of fibrosis after paraquat administration.[199] This kind of treatment has not been evaluated in humans.

Lung irradiation has been proposed for inhibiting fibroblastic proliferation, but the clinical role of the technique is uncertain. It would not help severely poisoned patients.[9,200–203] Other workers have suggested that nonsteroidal antiinflammatory agents, colchicines, or collagen synthesis inhibitors may prevent lung fibrosis; this has not been confirmed in humans.[179,204–206]

Transplantation is aimed at treating the fibrotic sequelae of paraquat poisoning and not the active process that leads to pulmonary fibrosis.[207] Transplantation has been employed in a few selected cases. Most patients died from fibrosis of the transplanted lung (because of too-early transplantation) or iatrogenic complication.[208–212] Lung transplantation is of theoretical interest in a few patients only.[6]

Finally, there is no effective antidote for paraquat poisoning.[28]

Diquat

The general approach to diquat intoxication is similar to that for paraquat poisoning.

GASTROINTESTINAL DECONTAMINATION

Gastric lavage and the administration of activated charcoal may be considered within 1 hour of a potentially life-threatening ingestion,[1] although no controlled studies have been performed to support the value of this approach.[138] If it is considered appropriate to undertake lavage, this must be done with extreme caution because there is a risk of perforation in the presence of corrosive mucosal damage. Vomiting, diarrhea, and massive fluid sequestration in the gut can cause clinically significant hypovolemia, so attention should be paid to fluid and electrolyte replacement. Oropharyngeal ulceration may be severe, and topical preparations, including local anesthetics, should be used to alleviate discomfort.

EXTRACORPOREAL REMOVAL TECHNIQUES

Forced Diuresis. Because renal failure is likely to develop in patients who are moderately or severely poisoned with diquat, forced diuresis is unlikely to be efficacious and may be harmful.[1] In one patient who did not develop renal damage, this technique was used for 17 days, but only 307 mg of diquat was eliminated over 13 days.[20]

Hemodialysis does not remove clinically and toxicologically relevant quantities of herbicide[125,126] at serum diquat concentrations encountered in cases of acute poisoning. Okonek and Hofmann[126] found in vitro hemodialysis clearances of 70 mL/min and 10 mL/min at serum diquat concentrations of 20 mg/L and 1 mg/L, respectively. Clearances of a maximum of 4.8 mL/min[126] and 8.5 mL/min[125] were achieved, however, with the use of hemodialysis in patients poisoned with diquat. Higher clearances (80 mL/min and 50 mL/min at serum diquat concentrations of 20 mg/L and 1 mg/L, respectively) were obtained in vitro with charcoal hemoperfusion,[125] although the amount of herbicide removed by this technique clinically appeared to be small.[119] Powell and associates[19] obtained clearances of 34 mL/min at the start of charcoal hemoperfusion and 39 mL/min 6 hours later, although the amount of diquat removed was not calculated. XAD-4 resin (Amberlite XAD-4 polymeric adsorbent, Rohm and Haas, Philadelphia, PA) did not remove diquat from serum.[19] The potential for cerebral hemorrhage dictates the cautious use of heparin during hemoperfusion.

SPECIAL POPULATIONS

Pediatric Patients

The clinical picture in children[178,214–222] follows the reported pattern of paraquat poisoning in adults. At first there is vomiting; then, after a delay of 2 to 3 days, signs of corrosive effect in the mouth and pharynx appear. Frequently the child does not give a history of ingestion or does not know what the substance ingested was. It may be concentrated solution decanted into unmarked containers and left unattended.[213,223] Often the diagnosis is delayed because of a relatively symptom-free period that occurs after the initial vomiting. This delay can be avoided if the method for rapid detection of paraquat and diquat in gastric aspirate and urine[130] is employed when the nature of the ingested fluid is not known. There are few reports of diquat poisoning in children.[19]

Pregnant Patients

Deaths from ingestion of undiluted paraquat in pregnant women have occurred, although blood levels were not available in early reports.[224,225] A patient who ingested a smaller dose of Weedol survived to complete a normal pregnancy. The authors concluded that this small dose of paraquat did not adversely affect the 20-week fetus.[226] In my series of nine patients who deliberately ingested concentrated (24% w/v) paraquat solution, all fetuses died, whether or not emergency cesarean section was performed.[227] The condition of the fetus deteriorated at delivery or in utero if the gestational age was

greater than 30 weeks. Paraquat concentrations in maternal, fetal, and cord blood in one case showed that paraquat crossed the placenta and was concentrated to levels four to six times greater than in the maternal blood. Amnioscopy in another case showed paraquat levels in amniotic fluid nearly twice that of maternal blood.[227] Breast milk contained paraquat in another case.[228] One of the two maternal survivors later had a normal pregnancy, with no evidence of teratogenicity from the earlier paraquat intoxication.[227]

Because no fetus has survived, and the placenta and fetus act as a reservoir to send paraquat back into the maternal circulation, it may be valuable to consider early removal of the fetus surgically. Although this procedure is done best as soon as possible after ingestion, it may not be possible because of the legal and ethical problems of dealing with a viable fetus. In some cases, it took 10 days for intrauterine death to occur.[227]

Elderly Patients

There is no published scientific experience specifically with paraquat poisoning in the elderly.

Key Points in Paraquat and Diquat Poisoning

1. Referral may make visiting difficult for relatives.
2. The nursing staff may be distressed by the high mortality; nursing staff may see themselves as critical care specialists and not welcome the need to practice terminal care.[48]
3. It is vital that the patient not be neglected or isolated. Frequent visits from medical and nursing staff are mandatory because infrequent communication causes considerable suffering to the patient.
4. A confident and supportive attitude reduces fear and despair.
5. Pain and distress should be reduced to a minimum, and inappropriate treatment should be avoided (e.g., cathartics, hemoperfusion).[48]

REFERENCES

1. Jones GM, Vale JA: Mechanisms of toxicity, clinical features, and management of diquat poisoning: A review. J Toxicol Clin Toxicol 38:123–128, 2000.
2. Sagar GR: Uses and usefulness of paraquat. Hum Toxicol 6:7–11, 1987.
3. Smith P, Heath D: Paraquat. CRC Crit Rev Toxicol 4:411–445, 1976.
4. Ellenhorn MJ, Barceloux DG: Medical Toxicology. New York, Elsevier, 1988.
5. Bismuth C, Garnier R, Baud FJ, et al: Paraquat poisoning: An overview of the current status. Drug Saf 5:243–251, 1990.
6. Vale JA, Meredith TJ, Buckley BM: Paraquat poisoning: Clinical features and immediate general management. Hum Toxicol 6:41–47, 1987.
7. Pond SM: Manifestations and management of paraquat poisoning. Med J Aust 152:256–259, 1990.
8. Talbot AR, Shiaw MH, Hwang JS, Randall JM: Statistics for acute poisoning seen in the emergency room. J Emerg Crit Care Med 1:55–63, 1990.
9. Talbot AR, Barnes MR: Radiotherapy for the treatment of pulmonary complications of paraquat poisoning. Hum Toxicol 7:325–332, 1988.
10. Lee SK, Ameno K, In SW, et al: Levels of paraquat in fatal intoxications. Int J Legal Med 112:198–200, 1999.
11. Yamashita M, Matsuo H, Tanaka J: Analysis of 1,000 consecutive cases of acute poisoning in the suburb of Tokyo leading to hospitalization. Vet Hum Toxicol 38:34–35, 1996.

12. Vanholder R, Colardyn F, De Reuck J, et al: Diquat intoxication: report of two cases and review of the literature. Am J Med 70:1267–1271, 1981.

13. Stephens BG, Moormeister SK: Homicidal poisoning by paraquat. Am J Forensic Med Pathol 18:33–39, 1997.

14. Teare RD: Poisoning by paraquat. Med Sci Law 16:9–12, 1976.

15. Chrome P: Paraquat poisoning. Lancet 1:333–334, 1986.

16. Onyon LJ, Volans GN: The epidemiology and prevention of paraquat poisoning. Hum Toxicol 6:19–29, 1987.

17. Klein Schwartz W, Smith GS: Agricultural and horticultural chemical poisonings: Mortality and morbidity in the United States. Ann Emerg Med 29:232–238, 1997.

18. Conso F: Paraquat poisoning: Experience of poison control centers in France. Vet Hum Toxicol 21(Suppl):112–113, 1979.

19. Powell D, Pond SM, Allen TB, Portale AA: Hemoperfusion in a child who ingested diquat and died from pontine infarction and hemorrhage. J Toxicol Clin Toxicol 20:405–420, 1983.

20. Mahieu P, Bonduelle Y, Bernard A, et al: Acute diquat intoxication: Interest of its repeated determination in urine and the evaluation of renal proximal tubule integrity. J Toxicol Clin Toxicol 22:363–369, 1984.

21. Hart TB, Nevitt A, Whitehead A: A new statistical approach to the prognostic significance of plasma paraquat concentrations. Lancet 2:1222–1223, 1984.

22. Scherrmann JM, Houze P, Bismuth C, Bourdon R: Prognostic value of plasma and urine paraquat concentration. Hum Toxicol 6:91–93, 1987.

23. Pond SM, Johnston SC, Schoof DD, et al: Repeated hemoperfusion and continuous arteriovenous hemofiltration in a paraquat poisoned patient. J Toxicol Clin Toxicol 25:305–316, 1987.

24. Bismuth C, Garnier R, Dally S, et al: Prognosis and treatment of paraquat poisoning: A review of 28 cases. J Toxicol Clin Toxicol 19:461–474, 1982.

25. Lin JL, Leu ML, Liu YC, Chen GH: A prospective clinical trial of pulse therapy with glucocorticoid and cyclophosphamide in moderate to severe paraquat-poisoned patients. Am J Respir Crit Care Med 159:357–360, 1999.

26. Buckley NA: Pulse corticosteroids and cyclophosphamide in paraquat poisoning. Am J Respir Crit Care Med 163:585, 2001.

27. Sackett DL, Straus SE, Richardson WS, et al: Evidence-Based Medicine: How to Practice and Teach EBM, 2nd ed. London, Churchill Livingstone, 2000.

28. Bateman DN: Pharmacological treatments of paraquat poisoning. Hum Toxicol 6:57–62, 1987.

29. Chan BS, Lazzaro VA, Seale JP, Duggin GG: The renal excretory mechanisms and the role of organic cations in modulating the renal handling of paraquat. Pharmacol Ther 79:193–203, 1998.

30. Haley TJ: Review of the toxicology of paraquat (1,1'-dimethyl-4,4'-bipyridinium chloride). Clin Toxicol 14:1–46, 1979.

31. Calderbank A: The bipyridilium herbicides. Adv Pest Control Res 8:127–135, 1968.

32. Denduyts-Whitehead AP, Hart TB, Volans GN: Effects of the addition of an emetic to paraquat formulations on acute poisoning in man. J Toxicol Clin Toxicol 23:422–423, 1985.

33. Dasta JF: Paraquat poisoning: A review. Am J Hosp Pharm 35:1368–1372, 1978.

34. Ross JH, Krieger RI: Structure-activity correlations of amines inhibiting active uptake of paraquat (methyl viologen) into rat lung slices. Toxicol Appl Pharmacol 59:238–249, 1981.

35. Athanaselis S, Qammaz S, Alevisopoulos G, Koutselinis A: Percutaneous paraquat intoxication. J Toxicol Cut Ocular Toxicol 2:3–5, 1983.

36. Karl PI, Friedman PA: Competition between paraquat and putrescine for accumulation by rat lung slices. Toxicology 26:317–323, 1983.

37. Bus JS, Gibson JE: Paraquat: Model for oxidant-initiated toxicity. Environ Health Perspect 55:37–46, 1984.

38. Jaros F: Acute percutaneous paraquat poisoning. Lancet 1:275, 1978.

39. Van Dijk A, Maes RAA, Drost RH, et al: Paraquat poisoning in man. Arch Toxicol 34:129–136, 1975.

40. Smith LL, Wright A, Wyatt I, Rose MS: Effective treatment for paraquat poisoning in rats and its relevance to treatment of paraquat poisoning in man. BMJ 4:569–571, 1974.

41. Bennett PN, Davies DS, Hawkesworth GM: In vivo absorption studies with paraquat and diquat in the dog (Proceedings). Br J Pharmacol 58:284P, 1976.

42. Conning DM, Fletcher K, Swan AA: Paraquat and related bipyridyls. Br Med Bull 25:245–249, 1969.

43. Clark DG: Inhibition of the absorption of paraquat from the gastrointestinal tract by adsorbents. Br J Ind Med 28:186–188, 1971.

44. Bismuth C, Scherrmann JM, Garnier R, et al: Elimination of paraquat. Hum Toxicol 6:63–67, 1987.

45. Garnier R, Efthymiou ML, Baud F: Haemoperfusion for paraquat poisoning. Lancet 2:277, 1983.

46. Hawksworth GM, Bennett PN, Davies DS: Kinetics of paraquat elimination in the dog. Toxicol Appl Pharmacol 57:139–145, 1981.

47. Sharp CW, Ottolenghi A, Posner HS: Correlation of paraquat toxicity with tissue concentrations and weight loss of the rat. Toxicol Appl Pharmacol 22:241–251, 1972.

48. Lock EA, Ishmael J: The acute toxic effects of paraquat and diquat on the rat kidney. Toxicol Appl Pharmacol 50:67–76, 1979.

49. Smith LL: Mechanism of paraquat toxicity in lung and its relevance to treatment. Hum Toxicol 6:31–36, 1987.

50. Rose MS, Lock EA, Smith LL, Wyatt I: Paraquat accumulation: Tissue and species specificity. Biochem Pharmacol 25:419–423, 1976.

51. Giri SN, Parker HR, Spangler WL, et al: Pharmacokinetics of [14C]-paraquat and associated biochemical and pathologic changes in beagle dogs following intravenous administration. Fundam Appl Toxicol 2:261–269, 1982.

52. Murray RE, Gibson JE: Paraquat disposition in rats, guinea pigs and monkeys. Toxicol Appl Pharmacol 27:283–291, 1974.

53. Chui YC, Poon G, Law F: Toxicokinetics and bioavailability of paraquat in rats following different routes of administration. Toxicol Ind Health 4:203–219, 1988.

54. Rose MS, Smith LL, Wyatt I: Evidence for energy-dependent accumulation of paraquat into rat lung. Nature 252:314–315, 1974.

55. Smith LL: Young Scientists Award Lecture 1981: The identification of an accumulation system for diamines and polyamines into the lung and its relevance to paraquat toxicity. Arch Toxicol 5(Suppl):1–14, 1982.

56. Davies DS, Hawksworth GM, Bennett PN: Paraquat poisoning. Clin Toxicol 18:21–26, 1977.

57. Baud FJ, Houze P, Bismuth C, et al: Toxicokinetics of paraquat through the heart-lung block: Six cases of acute human poisoning. J Toxicol Clin Toxicol 26:35–50, 1988.

58. Smith LL, Wyatt I, Cohen GM: The accumulation of diamines and polyamines into rat lung slices. Biochem Pharmacol 31:3029–3033, 1982.

59. Roth RA, Wallace KB, Alper RH, Bailie MD: Effect of paraquat treatment of rats on disposition of 5-hydroxytryptamine and angiotensin I by perfused lung. Biochem Pharmacol 28:2349–2355, 1979.

60. Dearden LC, Fairshter RD, Morrison JT, et al: Ultrastructural evidence of pulmonary capillary endothelial damage from paraquat. Toxicology 24:211–222, 1982.

61. Keeling PL, Smith LL: Relevance of NADPH depletion and mixed disulphide formation in rat lung to the mechanism of cell damage following paraquat administration. Biochem Pharmacol 31:3243–3249, 1982.

62. Bus JS, Aust SD, Gibson JE: Superoxide- and singlet oxygen-catalyzed lipid peroxidation as a possible mechanism for paraquat (methyl viologen) toxicity. Biochem Biophys Res Commun 58:749–755, 1974.

63. Bus JS, Cagen SZ, Olgaard M, Gibson JE: A mechanism of paraquat toxicity in mice and rats. Toxicol Appl Pharmacol 35:501–513, 1976.

64. Frank DM, Arora PK, Blumer JL, Sayre LM: Model study on the bioreduction of paraquat, MPP+, and analogs: Evidence against a "redox cycling" mechanism in MPTP neurotoxicity. Biochem Biophys Res Commun 147:1095–1104, 1987.

65. Hara S, Endo T, Kuriiwa F, Kano S: Mechanism of paraquat-stimulated lipid peroxidation in mouse brain and pulmonary microsomes. J Pharm Pharmacol 43:731–733, 1991.

66. Winterbourn CC: Production of hydroxyl radicals from paraquat radicals and H_2O_2. FEBS Lett 128:339–342, 1981.

67. Kelner MJ, Bagnell R, Hale B, Alexander NM: Methylene blue competes with paraquat for reduction by flavo-enzymes resulting in decreased superoxide production in the presence of heme proteins. Arch Biochem Biophys 262:422–426, 1988.

68. Shimada H, Hirai K, Simamura E, Pan J: Mitochondrial NADH-quinone oxidoreductase of the outer membrane is responsible for paraquat cytotoxicity in rat livers. Arch Biochem Biophys 351:75–81, 1998.

69. Sakai M, Yamagami K, Kitazawa Y, et al: Xanthine oxidase mediates paraquat-induced toxicity on cultured endothelial cell. Pharmacol Toxicol 77:36–40, 1995.

70. Hara S, Endo T, Kuriiwa F, Kano S: Different effects of paraquat on microsomal lipid peroxidation in mouse brain, lung and liver. Pharmacol Toxicol 68:260–265, 1991.

71. Daniel JW, Gage JC: Absorption and excretion of diquat and paraquat in rats. Br J Ind Med 23:133–136, 1966.

72. Hughes RD, Millburn P, Williams RT: Biliary excretion of some diquaternary ammonium cations in the rat, guinea pig and rabbit. Biochem J 136:979–984, 1973.

73. Lock EA: The effect of paraquat and diquat on renal function in the rat. Toxicol Appl Pharmacol 48:327–336, 1979.

74. Purser DA, Rose MS: The toxicity and renal handling of paraquat in cynomolgus monkeys. Toxicology 15:31–41, 1979.

75. Webb DB: Nephrotoxicity of paraquat in the sheep and the associated reduction in paraquat secretion. Toxicol Appl Pharmacol 68:282–289, 1983.

76. Scherrmann JM, Galliot M, Garnier R, Bismuth C: Acute paraquat poisoning: Prognostic significance and therapeutical interest of blood assay. Toxicol Eur Res 5:141–145, 1983.

77. Rawlings JM, Wyatt I, Heylings JR: Evidence for redox cycling of diquat in rat small intestine. Biochem Pharmacol 47:1271–1274, 1994.

78. Newhouse M, McEvoy D, Rosenthal D: Percutaneous paraquat absorption: An association with cutaneous lesions and respiratory failure. Arch Dermatol 114:1516–1519, 1978.

79. Levin PJ, Klaff LJ, Rose AG, Ferguson AD: Pulmonary effects of contact exposure to paraquat: A clinical and experimental study. Thorax 34:150–160, 1979.

80. Withers EH, Madden JJ Jr, Lynch JB: Paraquat burn of the scrotum and perineum. J Tenn Med Assoc 72:109, 1979.

81. Wohlfahrt DJ: Fatal paraquat poisonings after skin absorption. Med J Aust 1:512–513, 1982.

82. Karai I, Nakano H, Horiguchi S: [A case of lacrimal duct stenosis due to a herbicide paraquat (author's transl)]. Sangyo Igaku 23:552–553, 1981.

83. Hearn CE, Keir W: Nail damage in spray operators exposed to paraquat. Br J Ind Med 28:399–403, 1971.

84. Botella R, Sastre A, Castells A: Contact dermatitis to paraquat. Contact Dermatitis 13:123–124, 1985.

85. Okonek S, Wronkski R, Niedermayer W, et al: A near fatal percutaneous paraquat poisoning. Klin Wochenschr 61:655–659, 1983.

86. Tungsanga K, Chusilp S, Israsena S, Sitprija V: Paraquat poisoning: evidence of systemic toxicity after dermal exposure. Postgrad Med J 59:338–339, 1983.

87. Binns CW: A deadly cure for lice—a case of paraquat poisoning. P N G Med J 19:105–107, 1976.

88. Joyce M: Ocular damage caused by paraquat. Br J Ophthalmol 53:688–690, 1969.

89. Deveckova D, Mraz P, Mydlik M: [Gramoxon ocular burns]. Cesk Oftalmol 36:7–10, 1980.

90. Almog C, Tal E: Death from paraquat after subcutaneous ingestion. BMJ 16:721, 1967.

91. Harley JB, Grinspan S, Root RK: Paraquat suicide in a young woman: Results of therapy directed against the superoxide radical. Yale J Biol Med 50:481–488, 1977.

92. Hendy MS, Williams PS, Ackrill P: Recovery from severe pulmonary damage due to paraquat administered intravenously and orally. Thorax 39:874–875, 1984.

93. Stephens DS, Walker DH, Schaffner W, et al: Pseudodiphtheria: Prominent pharyngeal membrane associated with fatal paraquat ingestion. Ann Intern Med 94:202–204, 1981.

94. Kodagoda N, Jayewardene RP, Attygalle D: Poisoning with paraquat. Forensic Sci 2:107–111, 1973.

95. Vaziri ND, Ness RL, Fairshter RD, et al: Nephrotoxicity of paraquat in man. Arch Intern Med 139:172–174, 1979.

96. Chen KW, Wu MH, Huang JJ, Yu CY: Bilateral spontaneous pneumothoraces, pneumopericardium, pneumomediastinum, and subcutaneous emphysema: A rare presentation of paraquat intoxication. Ann Emerg Med 23:1132–1134, 1994.

97. Yamashita M, Ando Y: A long-term follow-up of lung function in survivors of paraquat poisoning. Hum Exp Toxicol 19:99–103, 2000.

98. Mickleson KN, Fulton DB: Paraquat poisoning treated by a replacement blood transfusion: Case report. N Z Med J 74:26–27, 1971.

99. Conradi SE, Olanoff LS, Dawson WT Jr: Fatality due to paraquat intoxication: confirmation by postmortem tissue analysis. Am J Clin Pathol 80:771–776, 1983.

100. Addo E, Ramdial S, Poon-King T: High dosage cyclophosphamide and dexamethasone treatment of paraquat poisoning with 75% survival. West Indian Med J 33:220–226, 1984.

101. Grant H, Lantos PL, Parkinson C: Cerebral damage in paraquat poisoning. Histopathology 4:185–195, 1980.

102. Fennelly JJ, Fitzgerald MX, Fitzgerald O: Recovery from severe paraquat poisoning following forced diuresis and immunosuppressive therapy. J Ir Med Assoc 64:69–71, 1971.

103. Reif RM, Lewinsohn G: Paraquat myocarditis and adrenal cortical necrosis. J Forensic Sci 28:505–509, 1983.

104. Lautenschlager J, Grabensee B, Pottgen W: [Paraquat intoxication and isolated aplastic anaemia (author's transl)]. Dtsch Med Wochenschr 99:2348–2351, 1974.

105. Fairshter RD, Rosen SM, Smith WR, et al: Paraquat poisoning: new aspects of therapy. QJM 45:551–565, 1976.

106. Siefkin AD: Combined paraquat and acetaminophen toxicity. J Toxicol Clin Toxicol 19:483–491, 1982.

107. Feldmann RJ, Maibach HI: Percutaneous penetration of some pesticides and herbicides in man. Toxicol Appl Pharmacol 28:126–132, 1974.

108. Tanen DA, Curry SC, Laney RF: Renal failure and corrosive airway and gastrointestinal injury after ingestion of diluted diquat solution. Ann Emerg Med 34(4 Pt 1):542–545, 1999.

109. Ferguson AH, Jacobsen JB, Nielsen H: [Severe diquat poisoning]. Ugeskr Laeger 144:2293, 1982.

110. Valiante F, Farinati F, Dal Santo P, et al: Upper gastrointestinal injury caused by diquat. Gastrointest Endosc 38:204, 1992.

111. Schmidt DM, Neale J, Olson KR: Clinical course of a fatal ingestion of diquat. J Toxicol Clin Toxicol 37:881–884, 1999.

112. Clark DG, Hurst EW: The toxicity of diquat. Br J Ind Med 27:51–55, 1970.

113. Cant JS, Lewis DR: Ocular damage due to paraquat and diquat. BMJ 2:224, 1968.

114. Rudez J, Sepcic K, Sepcic J: Vaginally applied diquat intoxication. J Toxicol Clin Toxicol 37:877–879, 1999.

115. Manoguerra AS: Full thickness skin burns secondary to an unusual exposure to diquat dibromide. J Toxicol Clin Toxicol 28:107–110, 1990.

116. McCarthy LG, Speth CP: Diquat intoxication. Ann Emerg Med 12:394–396, 1983.

117. Wood TE, Edgar H, Salcedo J: Recovery from inhalation of diquat aerosol. Chest 70:774–775, 1976.

118. Van den Heede M, Heyndrickx A, Timperman J: Thin layer chromatography as a routine appropriate technique for the determination of bipyridylium herbicides in post mortem human tissues. Med Sci Law 22:57–62, 1982.

119. Williams PF, Jarvie DR, Whitehead AP: Diquat intoxication: Treatment by charcoal haemoperfusion and description of a new method of diquat measurement in plasma. J Toxicol Clin Toxicol 24:11–20, 1986.

120. Buckley DA, McKiernan J: Survival after accidental ingestion of a fatal dose of diquat. Ir Med J 84:134, 1991.

121. Oreopoulos DG, McEvoy J: Diquat poisoning. Postgrad Med J 45:635–637, 1969.

122. Dodge AD, Harris N: The mode of action of paraquat and diquat. Biochem J 118:43P–44P, 1970.

123. Powell KE: A summary of pertinent medical information about paraquat in marijuana. Bull Natl Clgh Poison Control Cent Spring, 1–4, 1978.

124. Mahieu P, Hassoun A, Fautsch G, et al: Paraquat poisoning: Survival without pulmonary insufficiency after early bleomycin treatment. Acta Pharmacol Toxicol (Copenh) 41(Suppl 2):246–248, 1977.

125. Okonek S, Hofmann A, Henningsen B: Efficacy of gut lavage, hemodialysis, and hemoperfusion in the therapy of paraquat or diquat intoxication. Arch Toxicol 36:43–51, 1976.

126. Okonek S, Hofmann A: On the question of extracorporeal hemodialysis in diquat intoxication. Arch Toxicol 33:251–257, 1975.

127. Saeed SA, Wilks MF, Coupe M: Acute diquat poisoning with intracerebral bleeding. Postgrad Med J 77:329–332, 2001.

128. Ferguson DM: Renal handling of paraquat. Br J Pharmacol 42:636P, 1971.

129. Wilks MF: Diquat: Diagnosis, treatment and prognosis of poisoning. Surrey, UK, Zeneca Agrochemicals, 1994.

130. Braithwaite RA: Emergency analysis of paraquat in biological fluids. Hum Toxicol 6:83–86, 1987.

131. Proudfoot AT, Stewart MS, Levitt T, Widdop B: Paraquat poisoning: significance of plasma-paraquat concentrations. Lancet 2:330–332, 1979.

132. Yamaguchi H, Sato S, Watanabe S, Naito H: Pre-embarkment prognostication for acute paraquat poisoning. Hum Exp Toxicol 9:381–384, 1990.

133. Hart TB: When is paraquat poisoning life threatening? Lancet 1:395, 1985.

134. Fuke C, Ameno K, Ameno S, et al: Detection of two metabolites of diquat in urine and serum of poisoned patients after ingestion of a combined herbicide of paraquat and diquat. Arch Toxicol 70:504–507, 1996.

135. IPCS: Health and Safety Guide No. 52: Diquat. Geneva, World Health Organization, 1991.

136. Schonborn H, Schuster HP, Kossling FK: [Clinical and morphologic findings in an acute oral intoxication with diquat (Reglone)]. Arch Toxicol 27:204–216, 1971.

137. Narita S, Motojuku M, Sato J, Mori H: [Autopsy in acute suicidal poisoning with diquat dibromide]. Nippon Igakkai Zasshi 27:454–455, 1978.

138. Meredith TJ, Vale JA: Treatment of paraquat poisoning in man: Methods to prevent absorption. Hum Toxicol 6:49–55, 1987.

139. Webb DB, Leopold JD: Vasodilation and rehydration in paraquat poisoning. Hum Toxicol 2:531–534, 1983.

140. Williams PS, Hendy MS, Ackrill P: Early management of paraquat poisoning. Lancet 1:627, 1984.

141. Proudfoot AT, Prescott LF, Jarvie DR: Haemodialysis for paraquat poisoning. Hum Toxicol 6:69–74, 1987.

142. Vale JA, Crome P, Volans GN, et al: The treatment of paraquat poisoning using oral sorbents and charcoal haemoperfusion. Acta Pharmacol Toxicol (Copenh) 41(Suppl 2):109–117, 1977.

143. Nakamura K, Yamashita M, Naito H: Efficacy of gut lavage in the removal of paraquat in the dog. Vet Hum Toxicol 24(Suppl):157–158, 1982.

144. Kulig K, Bar-Or D, Cantrill SV, et al: Management of acutely poisoned patients without gastric emptying. Ann Emerg Med 14:562–567, 1985.

145. Vale JA, Meredith TJ, Buckley BM: Paraquat poisoning: Clinical features and immediate general management. Hum Toxicol 6:41–47, 1987.

146. Proudfoot AT: Abandon gastric lavage in the accident and emergency department? Arch Emerg Med 2:65–71, 1984.

147. Naito H, Yamashita M: Epidemiology of paraquat in Japan and a new safe formulation of paraquat. Hum Toxicol 6:87–88, 1987.

148. Neuvonen PJ, Varkainen M, Tokola D: Comparison of activated charcoal and ipecac syrup in prevention of drug absorption. Eur J Clin Pharmacol 24:557–562, 1983.

149. Curtis RA, Barone J, Giacona N: Efficacy of ipecaac and activated charcoal/cathartics: Prevention of salicylate absorption in a simulated overdose. Arch Intern Med 144:48–52, 1984.

150. Knight BAG, Tomlinson TE: The interaction of paraquat (1:1′-dimethyl 4:4′-dipyridilium dichloride) with mineral soils. J Soil Sci 18:233–243, 1967.

151. Park J, Proudfoot AT, Prescott LF: Paraquat poisoning: A clinical review of 31 cases. In Fletcher K (ed): Clinical Aspects of Paraquat Poisoning. London, ICI, 1975, pp 46–54.

152. Vale JA, Crome P, Volans GN, et al: The treatment of paraquat poisoning using oral sorbents and charcoal haemoperfusion. Acta Pharmacol Toxicol 41(Suppl 2):109–117, 1979.

153. Lee EJ, Pang M, Woo KT: Paraquat poisoning—management and prognosis. Ann Acad Med Singapore 10:233–237, 1981.

154. Okonek S, Setyadharma H, Borchert A, Krienke EG: Activated charcoal is as effective as Fuller's Earth or bentonite in paraquat poisoning. Klin Wochenschr 60:207–210, 1982.

155. Gaudreault P, Friedman PA, Lovejoy FH Jr: Efficacy of activated charcoal and magnesium citrate in the treatment of oral paraquat intoxication. Ann Emerg Med 14:123–125, 1985.

156. Nokata M, Tanaka T, Tsuchiya K, Yamashita M: Alleviation of paraquat toxicity by Kayexalate and Kalimate in rats. Acta Pharmacol Toxicol (Copenh) 55:158–160, 1984.

157. Yamashita M, Naito H, Takagi S: The effectiveness of a cation resin (Kayexalate) as an adsorbent of paraquat: experimental and clinical studies. Hum Toxicol 6:89–90, 1987.

158. Fisher HK, Humphries M, Bails R: Paraquat poisoning: Recovery from renal and pulmonary damage. Ann Intern Med 75:731–736, 1971.

159. Carson ED: Fatal paraquat poisoning in Northern Ireland. J Forensic Sci Soc 12:437–443, 1972.

160. Okonek S, Baldamus CA, Hofmann A, et al: Two survivors of severe paraquat intoxication by "continuous hemoperfusion." Klin Wochenschr 57:957–959, 1979.

161. Okonek S, Tonnis J, Baldamus CA, Hofmann A: Hemoperfusion versus hemodialysis in the management of patients severely poisoned by organophosphorus insecticides and bipyridyl herbicides. Artif Organs 3:341–345, 1979.

162. van de Vyver FL, van de Sande J, Verpooten GA, et al: Haemoperfusion ineffective for paraquat removal in life-threatening poisoning. Lancet 2:173, 1983.

163. Van de Vyver FL, Giuliano RA, Paulus GJ, et al: Hemoperfusion-hemodialysis ineffective for paraquat removal in life-threatening poisoning? J Toxicol Clin Toxicol 23:117–131, 1985.

164. De Broe ME, Bismuth C, De Groot G, et al: Haemoperfusion: A useful therapy for a severely poisoned patient? Hum Toxicol 5:11–14, 1986.

165. Mofenson HC, Greensher J, Caraccio TR, D'Agostino R: Paraquat intoxication: Report of a fatal case: Discussion of pathophysiology and rational treatment. J Toxicol Clin Toxicol 19:821–834, 1982.

166. Okonek S, Weilemann LS, Majdandzic J, et al: Successful treatment of paraquat poisoning: Activated charcoal per os and "continuous hemoperfusion." J Toxicol Clin Toxicol 19:807–819, 1982.

167. Mascie-Taylor BH, Thompson J, Davison AM: Haemoperfusion ineffective for paraquat removal in life-threatening poisoning. Lancet 1:1376–1377, 1983.

168. Lock EA, Smith LL, Rose MS. Inhibition of paraquat accumulation in rat lung slices by a component of rat plasma and a variety of drugs and endogenous amines. Biochem Pharmacol 25:1769–1772, 1976.

169. Maling HM, Saul W, Williams MA, et al: Reduced body clearance as the major mechanism of the potentiation by beta2-adrenergic agonists of paraquat lethality in rats. Toxicol Appl Pharmacol 43:57–72, 1978.

170. Patterson CE, Rhodes ML: The effect of superoxide dismutase on paraquat mortality in mice and rats. Toxicol Appl Pharmacol 62:65–72, 1982.

171. Dunbar JR, Acuff RV, Deluccia AJ: Co-administration of paraquat and putrescine to rats via miniosmotic pumps: Effects on lung glutathione antioxidant system and paraquat content. Fed Proc 44:1024, 1985.

172. Autor AP: Reduction of paraquat toxicity by superoxide dismutase. Life Sci 14:1309–1319, 1974.

173. Rhodes ML, Zavala DC, Brown D: Hypoxic protection in paraquat poisoning. Lab Invest 35:496–500, 1976.

174. Frank L: Superoxide dismutase and lung toxicity. Trends Pharmacol Sci 14:124–128, 1983.

175. Block ER: Potentiation of acute paraquat toxicity by vitamin E deficiency. Lung 156:195–203, 1979.

176. Redetzki HM, Wood CD, Grafton WD: Vitamin E and paraquat poisoning. Vet Hum Toxicol 22:395–397, 1980.

177. Combs GF Jr, Peterson FJ: Protection against acute paraquat toxicity by dietary selenium in the chick. J Nutr 113:538–545, 1983.

178. Shahar E, Barzilay Z, Aladjem M: Paraquat poisoning in a child: Vitamin E in amelioration of lung injury. Arch Dis Child 55:830–831, 1980.

179. Shahar E, Keidar I, Hertzeg E, Barzilay Z: Effectiveness of vitamin E and colchicine in amelioration of paraquat lung injuries using an experimental model. Isr J Med Sci 25:92–94, 1989.

180. Glass M, Sutherland MW, Forman HJ, Fisher AB: Selenium deficiency potentiates paraquat-induced lipid peroxidation in isolated perfused rat lung. J Appl Physiol 59:619–622, 1985.

181. Sullivan TM, Montgomery MR: The effect of ascorbic acid nutritional status on paraquat toxicity in guinea pigs. Dev Toxicol Environ Sci 11:471–474, 1983.

182. Matkovics B, Barabas K, Szabo L, Berencsi G: In vivo study of the mechanism of protective effects of ascorbic acid and reduced glutathione in paraquat poisoning. Gen Pharmacol 11:455–461, 1980.

183. Montgomery MR, Furry J, Gee SJ, Krieger RI: Ascorbic acid and paraquat: Oxygen depletion with concurrent oxygen activation. Toxicol Appl Pharmacol 63:321–329, 1982.

184. Schvartsman S, Zyngier S, Schvartsman C: Ascorbic acid and riboflavin in the treatment of acute intoxication by paraquat. Vet Hum Toxicol 26:473–475, 1984.

185. Brown OR, Heitkamp M, Song CS: Niacin reduces paraquat toxicity in rats. Science 212:1510–1512, 1981.

186. Kohen R, Chevion M: Paraquat toxicity is enhanced by iron and reduced by desferrioxamine in laboratory mice. Biochem Pharmacol 34:1841–1843, 1985.

187. Osheroff MR, Schaich KM, Drew RT, Borg DC: Failure of desferrioxamine to modify the toxicity of paraquat in rats. J Free Rad Biol Med 1:71–82, 1985.

188. Frank L, Neriishi K, Sio R, Pascual D: Protection from paraquat-induced lung damage and lethality in adult rats pretreated with clofibrate. Toxicol Appl Pharmacol 66:269–277, 1982.

189. Dawson JR, Norbeck K, Anundi I, Moldeus P: The effectiveness of N-acetylcysteine in isolated hepatocytes, against the toxicity of paracetamol, acrolein, and paraquat. Arch Toxicol 55:11–15, 1984.

190. Reference deleted.

191. Lin JL, Wei MC, Liu YC: Pulse therapy with cyclophosphamide and methylprednisolone in patients with moderate to severe paraquat poisoning: A preliminary report. Thorax 51:661–663, 1996.

192. Ayres JG, Lilford RJ: Treatment of paraquat poisoning. Thorax 52:588, 1997.

193. Newstead CG: Cyclophosphamide treatment of paraquat poisoning. Thorax 51:659–660, 1996.

194. Cadot R, Descotes J, Cuilleron CY, et al: Evaluation of active specific immunization against paraquat toxicity in rats. Vet Hum Toxicol 28:226–229, 1986.

195. Wright AF, Green TP, Robson RT, et al: Specific polyclonal and monoclonal antibody prevents paraquat accumulation into rat lung slices. Biochem Pharmacol 36:1325–1331, 1987.

196. Nagao M, Takatori T, Wu B, et al: Immunotherapy for the treatment of acute paraquat poisoning. Hum Toxicol 8:121–123, 1989.

197. Cadot R, Descotes J, Grenot C, et al: Increased plasma paraquat levels in intoxicated mice following antiparaquat F(ab′)2 treatment. J Immunopharmacol 7:467–477, 1985.

198. Chollet A, Muszynsky J, Bismuth C, et al: [Hypo-oxygenation in paraquat poisoning: Apropos of 6 cases]. Toxicol Eur Res 5:71–75, 1983.

199. Fogt F, Zilker T: Total exclusion from external respiration protects lungs from development of fibrosis after paraquat intoxication. Hum Toxicol 8:465–474, 1989.

200. Savy FP, Duval G, Her B, et al: [Failure of chemotherapy and radiotherapy in pulmonary fibrosis caused by paraquat]. Ann Fr Anesth Reanim 7:159–161, 1988.

201. Talbot AR, Barnes MR, Ting RS: Early radiotherapy in the treatment of paraquat poisoning. Br J Radiol 61:405–408, 1988.

202. Williams MV, Webb DB: Paraquat lung: Is there a role for radiotherapy? Hum Toxicol 6:75–81, 1987.

203. Franzen D, Baer F, Heitz W, et al: Failure of radiotherapy to resolve fatal lung damage due to paraquat poisoning. Chest 100:1164–1165, 1991.

204. Akahori F, Oehme FW: Inhibition of collagen synthesis as a treatment for paraquat poisoning. Vet Hum Toxicol 25:321–327, 1983.

205. Pasi A: The toxicology of paraquat, diquat and morfamquat. Bern, Hans Huber Publishers, 1978.

206. Vincken W, Huyghens L, Schandevyl W, et al: Paraquat poisoning and colchicine treatment. Ann Intern Med 95:391–392, 1981.

207. Matthew H, Logan A, Woodruff MFA, Heard B: Paraquat poisoning: Lung transplantation. BMJ 3:759–763, 1968.

208. Toronto Lung Transplant Group: Sequential bilateral lung transplantation for paraquat poisoning: A case report. J Thorac Cardiovasc Surg 89:734–742, 1985.

209. Cooke NKJ, Flenley DC, Matthew H: Paraquat poisoning: Serial studies of lung function. QJM 42:683–692, 1973.

210. Kamholz S, Veith FJ, Mollenkopf F, et al: Single lung transplantation in paraquat intoxication. N Y State J Med 84:82–84, 1984.

211. Kamholz SL: Current perspectives on clinical and experimental single lung transplantation. Chest 94:390–396, 1988.

212. Licker M, Schweizer A, Hohn L, et al: Single lung transplantation for adult respiratory distress syndrome after paraquat poisoning. Thorax 53:620–621, 1998.

213. Campbell S: Death from paraquat in a child. Lancet 1:144, 1968.

214. Gerbaka B, Hakme C, Bassil N, et al: [Paraquat poisoning in children]. J Med Liban 46:93–96, 1998.

215. Villa L, Pizzini L, Vigano G, et al: [Paraquat-induced acute dermatitis in a child after playing with a discarded container]. Med Lav 86:563–568, 1995.

216. Rivero C, Martinez E, Martinez R, et al: Paraquat poisoning in children: Survival of three cases. Vet Hum Toxicol 34:164–165, 1992.

217. Butenandt I, Mantel K, Fendel H: [Paraquat poisoning in children]. Fortschr Med 92:677–680, 1974.

218. Janssen F, Baran D, Dubois J: Paraquat poisoning in a child. Acta Paediatr Belg 29:189–192, 1976.

219. Craft AW, Sibert JR: Accidental poisoning in children. Br J Hosp Med 17(5):469–478, 1977.

220. Vlachos P, Zeis PM, Poulos L, Papadatos C: Agricultural poisons and children. Paediatrician 11:197–204, 1982.

221. Roth B, Bulla M, von Lilien T, et al: [Clinical findings and treatment of paraquat poisoning in childhood]. Monatsschr Kinderheilkd 131:458–463, 1983.

222. Mortensen ML: Management of acute childhood poisonings caused by selected insecticides and herbicides. Pediatr Clin North Am 33:421–445, 1986.

223. McDonagh BJ, Martin J: Paraquat poisoning in children. Arch Dis Child 45:425–427, 1970.

224. Fennelly JJ, Gallagher JT, Carroll RJ: Paraquat poisoning in a pregnant woman. BMJ 3:722–723, 1968.

225. Takeuchi K, Takayama K, Tomichi N, et al: [Paraquat poisoning in a pregnant woman (author's transl)]. Nihon Kyobu Shikkan Gakkai Zasshi 18:747–752, 1980.

226. Musson FA, Porter CA: Effect of ingestion of paraquat on a 20-week gestation fetus. Postgrad Med J 58:731–732, 1982.

227. Talbot AR, Fu CC, Hsieh MF: Paraquat intoxication during pregnancy: A report of 9 cases. Vet Hum Toxicol 30:12–17, 1988.

228. Goo TS, Yang SF, Talbot AR: Paraquat in breast milk (Letter). J Emerg Crit Care Med 1:67–68, 1990.

CHAPTER 93

Rodenticides

Keith K. Burkhart

Rodenticides are employed extensively worldwide. The specific type of rodenticide poisoning that a critical care physician most commonly encounters may vary from one country to another. In the United States, before 1976, anticoagulant rodenticides contained warfarin. Rodents genetically developed resistance to warfarin, however, leading to the manufacture of more potent, longer lasting products. In the United States, the most common rodenticides involved in human poisonings are the anticoagulant agents, specifically the superwarfarin products. The presence of superwarfarins is common in homes throughout the United States, and exposure to them occurs frequently in the pediatric population.[1] The amount that usually is ingested is limited, and coagulopathy from single pediatric ingestions is rare.[1,2]

The availability of various rodenticides within each country determines the types of poisoning that the critical care physician encounters. Currently, in the United States other rodenticides with high potential toxicity are available only to professional licensed exterminators. This fact has not been true historically, however. PNU (N-3-pyridymethyl-N-p-nitrophenylurea (Vacor) is an example of a highly toxic rodenticide that was available to the public. Its toxicity, although originally unknown, quickly became apparent. PNU, originally marketed by Rohm and Haas (Philadelphia; PA), lasted on the market only a few years (1975–1979) in the United States before distribution was voluntarily halted owing to the many successful suicides with this product. Patients who survived developed severe diabetes with ketoacidosis. Another highly toxic compound now used by commercial applicators in sheep collars for predator control is sodium monofluoroacetate and the metabolically related fluoroacetamide.

Aluminum phosphide was reported to be a common choice for suicide in India in the 1980s and 1990s.[3] Many reports of serious poisoning including fatalities have come from India and other countries.[4] Occupationally, phosphine (formed from phosphide) exposures and toxicity occur during grain fumigation in transport and storage areas.[5,6]

Most of the remaining rodenticides that are discussed in this chapter are primarily of historical interest, particularly in developed countries. Barium carbonate no longer is widely available as a rodenticide. It was sold as a water-soluble white powder. Many epidemics occurred when this rat poison was mistaken for flour.[7–10] ANTU (α-naphthylthiourea) remains widely available. Historically, many commercially available products contained strychnine, which at one time accounted for 30 deaths per year in the United States.[11] Only one death was reported in the 1999, 2000, and 2001 Annual Reports of the American Association of Poison Control Centers Toxic Exposure Surveillance System.[12–14] Most human exposures to strychnine resulted from its prescription as an analeptic, analgesic, aphrodisiac, appetite suppressant, cathartic, circulatory stimulant, emetic, or tonic. Other rodenticides of significance to the critical care physician are discussed in other chapters (i.e., arsenic in Chapter 76, phosphorus in Chapter 81, and thallium in Chapter 82).

BIOCHEMISTRY

Anticoagulants

A variety of anticoagulant rodenticides are available (Table 93-1).

ANTU

ANTU (molecular weight 202) is a colorless–to–white-gray powder or crystal substance (Fig. 93-1). It is odorless and bitter tasting. Bait packs contain concentrations ranging from 1% to 3%. Some trade names for ANTU are listed in Table 93-2.[11]

Barium

Barium rodenticides no longer are available for sale in many countries, including the United States, but there still may be some product stored. Barium carbonate as a powder may be inhaled and cause acute paralysis.[15]

Phosphides

Phosphides usually are found as powders or pellets and may have a rotten-fish odor. Zinc and aluminum phosphide are the most commonly available products. Calcium and magnesium phosphides also are available. In the presence of water and gastric acid, the metal is released, and phosphine gas (PH_3) is produced. This gas may have a garlic

TABLE 93-1 Available Forms of Long-Acting Anticoagulant Rodenticides

RODENTICIDE	CONCENTRATIONS (%)	FORMS	BRAND NAMES
4-Hydroxycoumarins			
Brodifacoum	0.005	Bait	D-Con Mouse Prufe II
			Talon, Talon G, Havoc
Bromadiolone	0.005	Bait	Bromone, Super-Caid
			Ratimus, Maki
Difenacoum	0.005	Bait	Ratak
Coumatetralyl			Endox, Endrocid
			Endrocide, Racumin
			Racumin 57, Rodentin
Indanediones			
Chlorphacinone	0.005	Bait	Caid, Drat, Ramucide
	0.25	Solution	Liphadione, Ratomet
	2.5	Concentrate	Microzul, Rozol
			Topitox, Raviac
Diphacinone	0.005	Cake	Diphacin
	0.05, 0.1, 0.2	Bait	Promar
	2	Concentrate	Ramik
Pindone	0.025, 0.1, 0.2, 0.5	Powder	Pival, Pivacin
	0.5, 1.5, 2	Concentrate	Pivalyn, Tri-Ban

From Burkhart KK: Anticoagulant rodenticides. In Ford MD, Delaney KA, Ling LJ, Erikson T (eds): Clinical Toxicology. Philadelphia, WB Saunders, 2001, p 849.

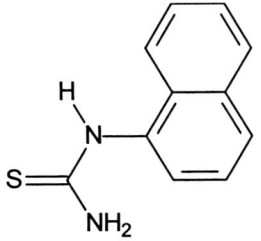

FIGURE 93-1

Chemical structure of ANTU.

odor. Examples of reactions generating phosphine from phosphides are as follows:

$$AlP + 3H_2O \rightleftharpoons PH_3 + Al(OH)_3$$

$$Ca_3P_2 + 6H_2O \rightleftharpoons 3Ca(OH)_2 + 2PH_3$$

PNU

PNU (Fig. 93-2) was sold as a yellow-green powder or cornmeal. A peanut odor may be evident. Brand names have included Vacor Rat Killer, DLP-787 2% Bait, and DLP-787 10% House Mouse Tracking Powder.

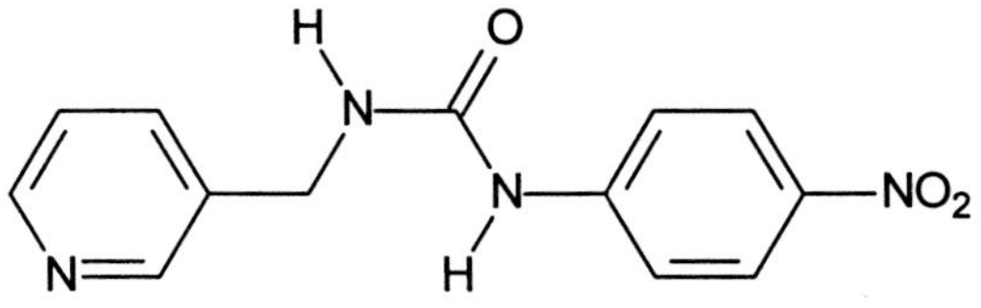

Sodium Monofluoroacetate and Fluoroacetamide

Sodium monofluoroacetate is a white, odorless and taste-less salt that is added to grain baits. It is absorbable by the gastrointestinal and pulmonary routes but not dermal routes, unless the skin is broken.[16] This product is isolated from African and Australian plants.[17,18]

TABLE 93-2 Alpha-Naphthylthiourea–Containing Products*

Bontu Prep Rat Baits
Bontu Rat Powder
Brown Rat Poison
College Brand Rodenticide
Dr. Hess Anturat
Nott's Rat Paste
Pied Piper for Rats and Mice
Ratsalt
Rat Stop
Rat Tox
Rat-X
Rateraser

*Noninclusive list.

FIGURE 93-2

Chemical structure of PNU.

Strychnine

Strychnine is an extract from the seed of Asian and Australian trees, including *Strychnos nux-vomica*. It is a bitter-tasting, odorless white powder. Table 93-3 lists strychnine-containing rodenticides.[11] Most products contain 0.5% strychnine.

TABLE 93-3 Strychnine-Containing Products

Arab Mouse Lure
Dolco Mouse Cereal
El Roy Mouse Bait
Farmite Orchard Mouse Bait
Gopher Death
Gopher Go
Hot Springs Buttons
Kilmice
Mice Doom Pellets
Mole Death
Mole-Nots
Mouse Lure
Mouse Seed
Mouse-Nots
Mouse-Rid
Mouse-Tox
Pied Piper Mouse Seed
Rat Seed
Saraseed Mouse Seed
Senco Poison Oar Kernels
Senco Special Poison Canary Seed
Sweeney's Poison Wheat

PATHOPHYSIOLOGY

Anticoagulants

Warfarin and warfarin-like anticoagulants disrupt enzymes in the liver (Fig. 93-3). These rodenticides inhibit liver vitamin K reductases, which are crucial to endogenous activation of hepatically synthesized clotting factors II, VII, IX, and X and proteins C, S, and Z. These coagulation proteins are activated by carboxylation of terminal glutamic acid groups. Vitamin K is oxidized to an epoxide during this reduction reaction. Vitamin K_1 2,3-epoxide reductase converts the epoxide to its quinone form, whereas vitamin K_1 quinone reductase changes the quinone into the active quinol form of vitamin K_1. In human overdoses, this inhibition is evident by an increased ratio of the epoxide to the quinol form.[19] Bleeding from the coagulopathy may occur when factor concentrations decline to less than 25% to 30% of baseline levels. Factor VII has the shortest half-life (approximately 5 hours). After three to four half-lives (or 15 to 24 hours), prothrombin time elevations can be seen. Bleeding complications usually manifest days after ingestion. The period of clinically significant anticoagulation for warfarin rodenticides typically lasts less than 1 week, whereas that induced by the long-acting agent brodifacoum may be months to longer than 1 year.[20–23]

ANTU

The toxicity of ANTU results from its bioactivation. Lung reduced nicotinamide adenine dinucleotide phosphate–dependent cytochrome P-450 enzymes seem to generate injurious metabolites of ANTU.[24] The thiocarbonyl group (>C=S) is most likely the site where a reactive intermediate is generated that subsequently may bind pulmonary macromolecules and produce the pulmonary injury.[24,25] Glutathione depletion seems to exacerbate the toxicity.[26] Pulmonary edema may result from the injury. Rats also may metabolize ANTU.[24] It is not known why the lung is more susceptible to this compound than the liver. Previously nonexposed or nontolerant rats are highly susceptible.

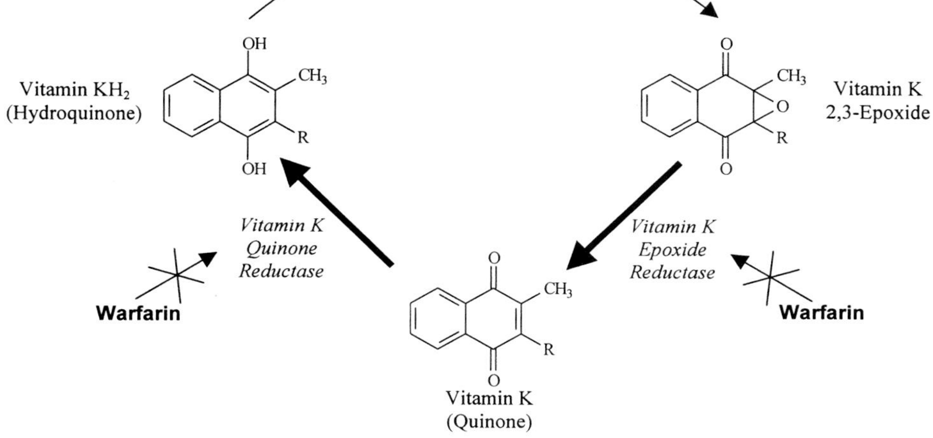

FIGURE 93-3

Graphic depiction of the actions of warfarin on the vitamin K cycle.

Barium

Barium may produce systemic illness. Life-threatening toxicity results from actions on the neuromuscular and cardiovascular systems.[27,28] Barium, after stimulating muscle, produces a depolarizing neuromuscular blockade.[27,29] Potassium is shifted intracellularly.[27,29] Profound weakness and partial paralysis result.

Phosphine

The mechanisms of phosphine toxicity are not completely understood; however, it may block cytochrome *c* and *a* oxidases.[30] Free radical generation and lipid peroxidation also seem to have a role.[31,32] Pulmonary edema is common and may develop over days.

PNU

PNU is related structurally to alloxan, streptozotocin, and 1-methyl-1-nitrosourea. These antineoplastic compounds damage pancreatic beta cells.[33–35] Because of structural similarities, these compounds may be substituted in nucleotides. A substitution for nicotinamide in the generation of nicotinamide adenine dinucleotide and possibly nicotinamide adenine dinucleotide phosphate is a proposed mechanism. Nicotinamide adenine dinucleotide depletion has been documented after streptozotocin administration.[33] Cofactors no longer can function as hydrogen carriers for enzymatic redox reactions, including oxidative phosphorylation. The pancreas is especially susceptible because beta cells are destroyed. The nervous system also may be affected, and neuropathies and encephalopathy may develop.[36–38]

Sodium Monofluoroacetate and Fluoroacetamide

Sodium monofluoroacetate blocks the tricarboxylic acid (Krebs) cycle.[17] Fluorocitrate, its metabolite, accumulates and inhibits aconitate hydratase (Fig. 93-4).[39] This inhibition disrupts cellular respiration, depleting adenosine triphosphate energy stores. The absorption, conversion, and inhibition lead to a delay of hours before effects appear.[40] This delay may be longer for fluoroacetamide because it is converted to fluoroacetate.

Strychnine

Strychnine acts on the central nervous system as a competitive antagonist at glycine receptors. Although structurally dissimilar from glycine, its charge and surface configuration seem to allow its binding at the glycine receptor site.[41] Glycine is the predominant inhibitory neurotransmitter in the brainstem and spinal cord. It acts by increased chloride conduction in postsynaptic cells, causing them to be hyperpolarized. Strychnine blocks the postsynaptic binding of glycine. Strychnine also seems to block the action of γ-aminobutyric acid (GABA) in spinal interneurons, although this inhibition is not as potent as that with glycine.[42,43] The GABAergic system provides the major neuroinhibitory pathways in the central nervous system. Benzodiazepines that are used to treat strychnine poisoning bind glycine and GABA receptor sites and increase chloride conductance.[44,45]

Barbiturates also enhance chloride conductance and have been effective in the treatment of strychnine poisoning.[46,47]

CLINICAL PRESENTATION

Anticoagulants

Critical care physicians typically assume the care of patients with superwarfarin poisoning, which results in serious bleeding complications. Most fatalities have occurred after intracranial hemorrhages. Subdural, subarachnoid, and intracerebral hemorrhages have been reported.[48–50] In addition, patients usually have bleeding from other sites or organ systems. Pulmonary hemorrhage may require ventilatory support.[22,23,51] Vaginal bleeding also has caused a fatal outcome.[52] Compartment syndromes have been reported.[22,23,51] Gastrointestinal bleeding and epistaxis should be anticipated and may be life-threatening.

ANTU

ANTU may have the potential for serious toxicity in humans. Infrequent reports of significant toxicity simply may reflect that ingestions have not been large enough to produce serious poisoning. Brewer and Haggerty[11] suggested an oral mean lethal dose of 4 g/kg in primates. Shortness of breath and rales were noted after a large ingestion of 80 g of a 30% bait pack.[53]

Barium

Facial paresthesias may be the first symptoms of barium toxicity.[7] Paresthesias may spread to the extremities.[7] Gastrointestinal symptoms usually follow and may include salivation, nausea, vomiting, abdominal pain, and diarrhea.[7,8,54] Gastrointestinal hemorrhage also has been reported.[7,8] Associated with the developing hypokalemia, profound weakness develops and may progress to paralysis. Presentations may include ptosis, monoplegia, hemiplegia, and quadriplegia.[7] Most importantly, respiratory paralysis and respiratory failure characterize severe poisoning.[28,55] The hypokalemia also is associated with cardiac conduction disturbances and dysrhythmias.[54] Electrocardiogram changes typically include QRS prolongation and flattened T waves and U waves.[8,54] Ventricular extrasystoles, hypertension, and tachycardia may follow.[28]

Ventilatory support often is needed for the respiratory paralysis.[28] Arterial blood gases may show respiratory acidosis as respiratory failure progresses. Cardiac monitoring is required to identify and treat any dysrhythmias that result from the intracellular potassium shifts and severe hypokalemia.

Phosphine

Signs and symptoms of phosphide toxicity often develop rapidly within 15 to 30 minutes, and death may occur in less than 6 hours.[56] Death seems to occur most consistently when fresh, previously unopened tablets are ingested.[57] When tablets are opened, atmospheric moisture may react with them and decrease their potency. Banjaj and Wasir[58]

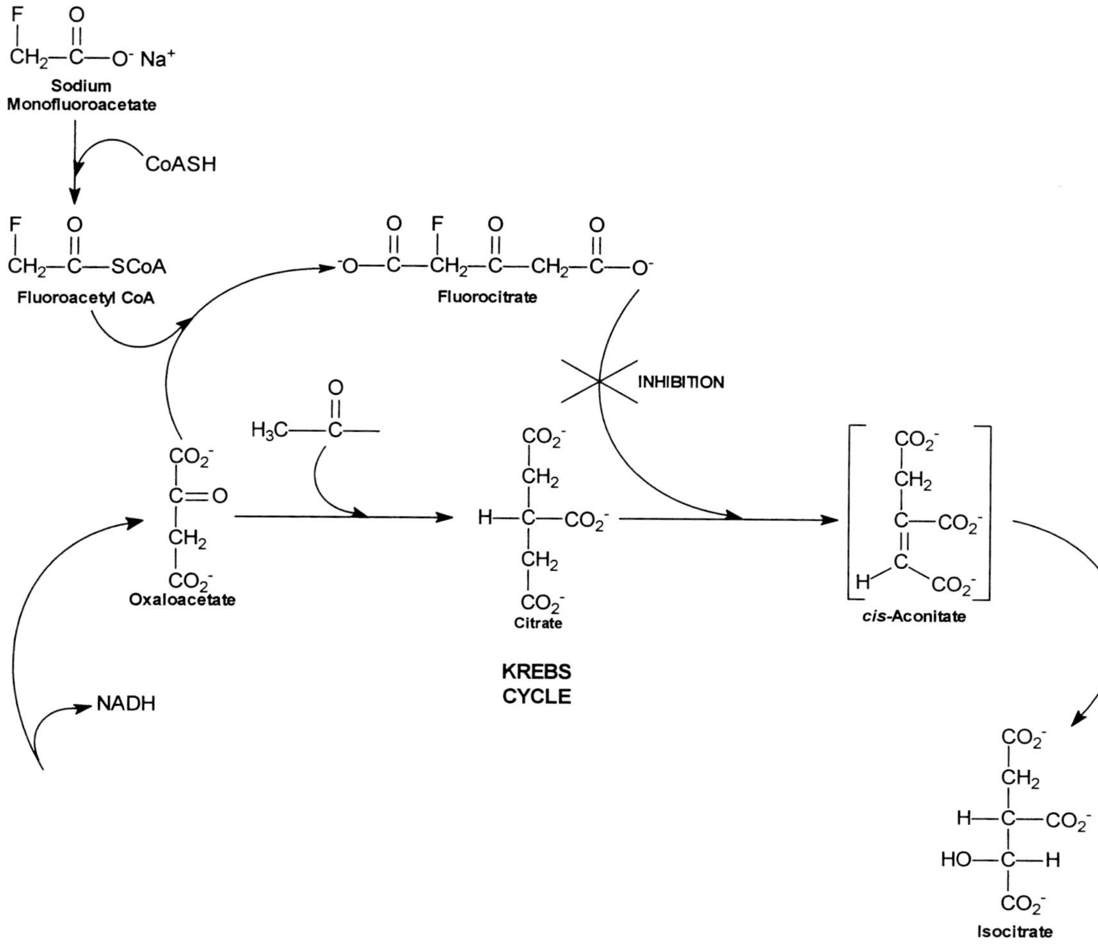

FIGURE 93-4

Interference of monofluoroacetate with the Krebs cycle.

stated that ingestions of 500 mg are usually fatal. Phosphides are potent gastric irritants; profuse vomiting and abdominal pain are often the first symptoms.[57] Tachypnea, hyperpnea, dyspnea, cough, and chest tightness usually follow. Tachycardia, hypotension, and arrhythmias may develop.[59–62] Central nervous system toxicity may include coma and delirium.[56,59]

PNU

PNU toxicity may manifest within hours or be delayed for days.[63] Anyone with a history of PNU ingestion should be observed, even if there are no manifestations of toxicity. Patients who develop signs of major toxicity should be admitted to an intensive care unit. Hyperglycemia or diabetic ketoacidosis follows the insulin deficiency from beta cell destruction, although hypoglycemia may intercede.[64] The onset of diabetes mellitus has been detected 4 hours to 7 days after exposure.[63,65] Autonomic and peripheral neuropathies causing postural hypotension, diminished gastrointestinal and bladder motility, and motor and sensory loss may develop. The onset is often acute, manifesting in the first few hours, although in some cases manifestations can be delayed for days.[65,66] These neuropathies may be reversible or irreversible.[65,66] An acute cerebral encephalopathy also may develop.[64,66] Other signs and symptoms may include delirium, confusion, lethargy, coma, memory impairment, dyskinesias, tremor, seizures, and myoclonus.[64–66] Other reported manifestations of PNU toxicity are abdominal pain, chest pain, palpitations, and hypothermia.[66] On autopsy, pancreatic beta cell destruction and neuropathic lesions of the sensory spinal roots have been documented.[66]

Sodium Monofluoroacetate and Fluoroacetamide

Neurologic and cardiovascular toxicity from sodium monofluoroacetate and fluoroacetamide has caused many fatalities, and intensive care unit admission is warranted in an exposed patient manifesting any signs of toxicity. Epigastric pain and vomiting may be the first symptom and sign to develop.[67] Mental status changes may include confusion, irritability, agitation, and coma.[16,68,69] Neuromuscular irritability may include muscle twitching, muscle spasms, and seizures.[68,69] Electrocardiogram monitoring shows nonspecific ST wave changes, prolonged QT_c intervals, ventricular ectopy and tachycardia, and rapid atrial fibrillation. Hypocalcemia and possibly hypokalemia are common manifestations that may contribute to the aforementioned life-threatening conditions.[39,68] Patients who survive beyond 24 hours usually develop renal failure.[68,69]

Gastrointestinal effects precede the life-threatening effects on the heart (ventricular dysrhythmias) and the central nervous system (coma and seizures).[16,68,69] One report suggested that subacute exposure may result in sudden death.[18] Parkin and associates[70] described a rabbiter who developed chronic toxicity with renal, hepatic, neurologic, and thyroid dysfunction.

Strychnine

Critical care admission is required to manage strychnine-poisoned patients. Stimulation of the patient should be kept to a minimum, however. Loss of motor neuron inhibition causes hyperexcitability in affected muscles. The stimulation produces muscle twitching or spasms of extensor muscle groups,[71–73] and trismus or opisthotonos has been seen.[74,75] A unique manifestation of strychnine poisoning is the appearance of seizures while the patient is awake. Such patients may manifest seizure-like activity based on spinal hyperexcitability with relative noninvolvement of the brain. Stimulation may precipitate these effects.[71] In between spasms or after recovery, patients often describe severe pain during these episodes.[72] Between seizures, the patient may be awake and relaxed. Respiratory compromise may occur secondary to spasms of the diaphragm and chest wall musculature.[71] Other complications may include rhabdomyolysis, hyperthermia, lactic acidosis, and multiorgan failure.[71,76,77] The severe spasms in addition to rhabdomyolysis may cause a compartment syndrome.[71] Because many patients are heavily sedated, frequent examinations are required to assess distal extremity temperature, capillary refill, and firmness of the compartments. If there is any question, compartment pressures should be measured. The patient must be well hydrated to avoid acute myoglobinuric renal failure. Central venous pressure monitoring should be considered if urine output decreases after appropriate volume expansion. Close monitoring of electrolytes is required. Derangements of potassium, calcium, phosphate, and magnesium may occur.[74,77,78] Hepatic and renal function should be followed in severely poisoned patients.

DIAGNOSIS

Anticoagulants

Confirming the diagnosis requires a detailed history and laboratory analyses. Most patients who present with bleeding complications do not provide the history of exposure to anticoagulant rodenticides. Many patients have presented for minor bleeding before developing a serious life-threatening bleed. A careful history first must search for liver disease or a possible cause of vitamin K deficiency in addition to bleeding disorders, such as hemophilia, von Willebrand's disease, or coagulation factor deficiencies. Hepatotoxic liver disease (e.g., from acetaminophen, hepatotoxic mushrooms, or chronic alcoholism) initially could present with a bleeding complication. The various hepatotoxins are discussed in their respective chapters in this book. A prolonged prothrombin time or international normalized ratio (INR) may be a laboratory clue to the diagnosis. Coagulation factor levels should be measured and usually confirm the clinician's suspicion. These tests should be obtained before any blood products are administered. To assess quickly for coagulation factor depletion, the patient's plasma can be mixed with known normal plasma. A 50:50 mixing of the two should correct the prothrombin time or INR if the cause of prolongation is factor deficiency.

Patients with severe hemorrhage may develop factor depletion or disseminated intravascular coagulation. D-dimer, fibrin split products, and fibrinogen levels help assess these diagnoses. Transfusions may be required. Liver function tests should be measured to rule out toxin-induced or other hepatic diseases, as mentioned earlier. Measurement of brodifacoum and other superwarfarin levels clarifies the diagnosis. Many reference laboratories now offer these assays. Often this degree of testing is required because many anticoagulant self-poisoned patients continually deny the ingestion of these products despite the above-mentioned laboratory evidence. Pediatric cases with serious bleeding complications are rare.[79] Most of these pediatric case reports are suspected to be Munchausen syndrome by proxy. In these cases, laboratory confirmation should be obtained for medicolegal reasons.

ANTU

The diagnosis of ANTU poisoning mostly relies on the history provided by the patient, family, or possibly paramedics. Care must be taken to identify the product properly when possible. This diagnosis also should be in the differential diagnosis of a patient with a history of rodenticide ingestion who presents with pulmonary edema. The laboratory is of little help in the acute management of these patients.

Barium

The diagnosis of barium intoxication is made by history, when available. The physical examination, especially paralysis coupled with hypokalemia, should confirm the diagnosis. Obtaining barium levels does not enhance patient management significantly. Although these levels have been shown to correlate with toxicity, the patients have been and can be managed appropriately without them (see treatment section).[55,80,81]

Phosphine

The clinical history coupled with the patient's clinical course make the diagnosis of phosphide poisoning. A rotten-fish odor can be an important clinical sign. One must be careful because off-gassing of the emesis theoretically can expose health care workers to phosphine fumes.[3] Laboratory tests are of limited diagnostic utility.

PNU

The diagnosis of PNU toxicity should be considered in patients with a history of rodenticide exposure and a presentation of diabetic ketoacidosis, especially with concomitant signs of neuropathy. Laboratory tests have only a confirmatory role and are not important to the acute critical care management of the patient.

Sodium Monofluoroacetate and Fluoroacetamide

The correlation of a clinical history of exposure with the onset of the clinical picture within hours of exposure is important to obtaining the diagnosis. Fluoroacetate levels can be measured, but these usually are not readily available. Laboratory consultation may provide confirmatory testing.

Strychnine

The history of exposure and rapid onset of symptoms, especially spasms or seizures, often in less than 30 minutes, is expected in strychnine poisoning. Strychnine blood levels can be obtained but are not clinically useful, only confirmatory.

TREATMENT

Anticoagulants

Gastrointestinal decontamination is of limited, if any, value in the management of the critically anticoagulant-poisoned patient. These patients present well after absorption and subsequent hepatic enzyme inhibition has developed. In the rare case of a patient presenting soon after ingestion, activated charcoal seems warranted. In one case, multiple doses of charcoal did not seem to alter the outcome, however.[82]

Critical care management decisions are based first on the bleeding complications the patient may develop and the

Indications for ICU Admission in Rodenticide Poisoning

Agent	Indication
Long-acting anticoagulants	Life-threatening hemorrhage
ANTU	Pulmonary edema
Barium	Ventilatory management, severe hypokalemia
Phosphides	Hypotension, cardiac arrhythmias, coma, status epilepticus
PNU	Autonomic neuropathy with hypotension, encephalopathy, ketoacidosis
Fluoroacetates, fluoroacetamide	Cardiac dysrhythmias, coma, status epilepticus
Strychnine	Status epilepticus or severe muscle spasms with ventilatory support, cardiac dysrhythmias, severe acidosis

severity of the coagulation defect. Control of hemorrhage should respond rapidly to the administration of whole blood, fresh frozen plasma, or factor concentrates. These blood products contain coagulation factors that stop ongoing bleeding. Whole blood additionally reverses severe anemias that may develop.

Vitamin K therapy administration allows for the conversion of the coagulation factors into their active carboxylated forms. Vitamin K_1 is the only effective form. AquaMEPHYTON is the parenteral brand available in the United States. Care must be taken with its administration because of the risk for anaphylactoid or possibly anaphylactic reactions from polyoxyethylated castor oil in its formulation.[83] To avoid these reactions, the rate of intravenous administration should not exceed 1 mg/min. The use of a dilute solution also is recommended because this step also may prevent anaphylactoid reactions. The American College of Chest Physicians published consensus guidelines for parenteral vitamin K therapy based on the INR. For patients with critical bleeding, 10 mg is recommended. If bleeding is not evident, INR results and recommended vitamin K doses are 6 to 10 (0.5 to 1.0 mg), 10 to 20 (3 to 5 mg), and greater than 20 (10 mg).[84] Some medical toxicologists believe that the subcutaneous route is safer than the intravenous route and that the efficacy may be similar. In either case, the benefits from vitamin K therapy are delayed for the approximately 6 hours it takes for the hepatic elevation of active coagulation factor levels. Oral vitamin K therapy also should be initiated as soon as possible. Although the relatively slower oral absorption delays vitamin K's effect, this route can be used to maintain elevated factor levels. Oral vitamin K doses of 100 mg to several hundred milligrams have been used.[85] Vitamin K has a half-life of less than 3 hours.[86,87] Without continued vitamin K administration, the coagulopathy may recur within 1 to 2 days. If the coagulopathy does not recur within 2 days of discontinuing therapy, vitamin K no longer should be required. When the bleeding complications are controlled, these patients can be transferred out of the intensive care unit.

ANTU

Most ANTU-exposed patients need observation rather than critical care. Gastrointestinal decontamination with activated charcoal, if done shortly after ingestion, should be sufficient. Standard management protocols for pulmonary edema should be used for patients who manifest toxicity. Experimentally, fructose-1,6-diphosphate has been shown to protect the lung from ANTU-induced injury.[88] Fructose-1,6-diphosphate is an inhibitor of oxygen free radical production by neutrophils. Additionally, the preadministration of phorone produces an elevation of glutathione levels that protects against ANTU toxicity.[26] *N*-acetylcysteine warrants testing as an antidote.

Barium

Barium carbonate is less soluble than other barium salts. Barium carbonate may have a slower onset to effect. Activated charcoal binding of barium has not been studied but is not expected to offer significant benefit.[89] Gastric lavage may be helpful if done within 1 to 2 hours postingestion; however, this has never been shown in a controlled trial. Although unproven, the administration of 30 to 60 g of magnesium sulfate or sodium sulfate has been recommended based on the theory of converting some barium into the insoluble salt barium sulfate, which would pass through the gastrointestinal tract without absorption.[90,91] If larger doses are used, frequent measurement of sodium and magnesium levels must be done, especially if renal insufficiency develops. Despite oral sulfates, there are cases in which patients' conditions continued to deteriorate.[92] Intravenous sulfates are not recommended because these may induce barium sulfate precipitates in the renal tubules and lead to renal failure.[55]

Potassium replacement is crucial. Resolution of hypokalemia reportedly has coincided with recovery from the paralysis.[80,93] Some authors believe that lowering the barium concentration is more important, however.[55,81] Intravenous routes, including central lines using rates greater than 30 mEq/hr, have been effective in elevating potassium levels in many cases.[28,55] If emesis is controlled, the intensivist also could consider nasogastric tube potassium administration.[93] Hemodialysis may be the most effective treatment, however.[55,80,81,94] Barium is removed by this procedure. The addition of a high concentration of potassium (e.g., 4 or 4.5 mEq/L) to the dialysis bath elevates the serum potassium concentration. One patient 3 hours into dialysis recovered from paralysis and was extubated successfully.[80] Hemodialysis should be considered in patients who have persistent paralysis despite adequate potassium replacement therapy, especially in patients with renal insufficiency. Hemofiltration also has been used with success.[95]

Phosphine

Gastrointestinal decontamination after exposure to phosphides has not been studied. Induced emesis is never advisable in patients who have ingested a toxin that alters the level of consciousness. Most, if not all, patients develop emesis from the irritant effects, however.[57] Health care workers should protect themselves from the emesis because it theoretically may off-gas phosphine. Jayaraman[3] reported a physician who became symptomatic when the stomach of a suicide victim was exposed. Although I recommend use of activated charcoal, it is not known how well activated charcoal binds phosphide or phosphine and prevents the development of toxicity. Historically, dilution with bicarbonate solution has been recommended, although this treatment is based on theory and unproven.[96] The bicarbonate is believed to decrease the gastric hydrochloric acid concentration, which is responsible for the conversion of phosphides to phosphine gas. Another unproven recommendation is the use of diluted potassium permanganate to remove and oxidize the phosphides.[96] Duenas and colleagues[62] described the use of trimetazidine for the treatment of cardiac toxicity. They suggested that trimetazidine may help mitigate the oxidant stress caused by phosphine.[31] Trimetazidine is not widely available, however. It is not yet available in the United States. Aggressive supportive care is the only approach that can be recommended at this time.

PNU

I recommend gastrointestinal decontamination using activated charcoal, particularly if it can be administered early. Historically, patients have not presented in a time frame for gastric lavage to be of even theoretical benefit. Management decisions depend on serum glucose determination and hemodynamic monitoring. Hypotension should be treated with volume expansion. If there is no response, a trial of fludrocortisone is warranted.[63]

Nicotinamide (vitamin B$_3$) is a specific antidote for PNU poisoning. Animal models document nicotinamide's early benefits in treating streptozotocin and N-nitromethylurea toxicity.[33,34,97] The parenteral formulation is no longer widely available, however. Historical recommendations were to give 500 mg as a loading dose followed by 100 to 200 mg every 4 hours for 2 days, not to exceed 3 g/day. Children were to receive 50% of this dose. The subsequent recommended oral dose was 100 mg three to five times per day for 2 weeks. In animal models, protection was provided only when the antidote was given before or within hours of exposure.[34] The reported experience with delayed therapy in humans is disappointing.[65] Nicotinic acid was less effective than nicotinamide in a rodent model.[98] Nicotinic acid may not be a safe alternative because its vasodilatory effects may complicate the further treatment of hypotension.[66]

Sodium Monofluoroacetate and Fluoroacetamide

Treatment of toxicity from sodium monofluoroacetate and fluoroacetamide consists of the stabilization of any cardiovascular or neurologic effect and, if it is able to be given within the first few hours postingestion, the administration of activated charcoal. Theoretical recommendations for lavage with sodium bicarbonate or magnesium sulfate are unproven and most likely would be performed too late to be of benefit. There are no proven antidotes for the management of these poisonings. Glycerol monoacetate, 0.1 to 0.5 mL/kg/hr, as a Krebs cycle substrate replacement, has prolonged survival in a primate model, but it also may aggravate toxicity and seems to be effective only early in the course.[40,99] Ethanol, metabolized to acetate, also has been studied, with inconclusive results. In a more recent mouse model, simultaneous sodium succinate and calcium gluconate, but not calcium alone, reduced mortality.[100] The mainstay of treatment remains critical care life support.

Strychnine

Signs and symptoms of strychnine poisoning can be seen within minutes depending on the route of exposure. Strychnine is absorbed rapidly through the gastrointestinal tract and mucous membranes. By the gastrointestinal route, signs and symptoms typically occur within 15 to 30 minutes. Nasal insufflation or intravenous injection can occur when strychnine is used as a substitute for drugs of abuse. In these cases effects can occur within 5 minutes.[71,75] Strychnine is cleared by hepatic elimination via cytochrome P-450 system–mediated metabolism.[78,101,102] Very little strychnine is excreted unchanged in the urine. Attempts to enhance urinary elimination are of no benefit. Half-lives of 10 to 16 hours have been reported.[78,103,104] Recovery within 12 to 24 hours is expected when patients present before complications have developed.[47,74]

Treatment interventions may precipitate seizures; if the diagnosis is known, the patient should be administered benzodiazepines immediately. Diazepam or midazolam provides a rapid onset. Propofol also may work through GABA antagonism and may be an alternative. Emesis is contraindicated because of the rapid onset of toxicity. The stimulation of gastric lavage also is contraindicated in a nonparalyzed patient. If the patient is asymptomatic, activated charcoal may be given. When a patient is intubated, activated charcoal may be given by nasogastric tube. It is doubtful that gastric lavage would provide additional benefit beyond the instillation of activated charcoal.

The patient's airway and ventilation must be monitored continually because respiratory compromise can occur at any time. Blood gases can reflect many abnormalities at different times in the poisoning.[71] Initially a patient's apprehension may produce hyperventilation and a respiratory alkalosis. When spasms compromise effective gas exchange, hypercarbia and respiratory acidosis may be seen.[71,77] Finally, the spasms can produce a severe metabolic lactic acidosis with or without a respiratory acidosis. Often the pH can become significantly less than 7.1. The acidosis precipitates multiorgan dysfunction and failure. Bradycardia and hypotension may precede cardiac arrest.[78] Lactic acidosis and hypoxia also may result in central nervous system depression. Intubation allows aggressive pharmacologic management of the neuromuscular hyperactivity. In most cases, paralysis with a nondepolarizing neuromuscular blocker, such as vecuronium or pancuronium, is recommended to facilitate intubation because the stimulation of endotracheal intubation may precipitate spasms, including trismus or convulsions.[74] In addition to tactile stimulation, auditory and visual stimuli may precipitate seizures. The resuscitation and intensive care unit atmosphere should be quiet, dark, and minimally invasive. Convulsions should be treated with benzodiazepines, phenobarbital, or possibly propofol. Continuous neuromuscular paralysis would be another option if the patient cannot tolerate high doses of the aforementioned agents.

SPECIAL POPULATIONS

Pediatric Patients

Children who present with bleeding complications indicating a significant exposure to anticoagulants warrant the consideration of Munchausen syndrome by proxy. Children rarely, if ever, of their own volition ingest enough brodifacoum to become critically ill with life-threatening hemorrhage.[1] In one report, children who had access to less than one box of the product could be managed without gastric decontamination.[1]

Common Misconceptions about Rodenticide Poisoning

1. Rodenticides other than long-acting anticoagulants are no longer a risk in the United States.
2. Gastric decontamination is useful for strychnine poisoning.
3. Potassium replacement alone reverses paralysis in barium poisoning.

Key Points in Rodenticide Poisoning

1. In most cases, avoid decontamination procedures for strychnine and late-presenting anticoagulant poisoning.
2. The rapid onset of action of most rodenticides makes decontamination procedures of little benefit.
3. Extracorporeal removal speeds recovery from barium poisoning.
4. Respiratory compromise can be multifactorial and may develop quickly or can be insidious for rodenticides.
5. Acidosis and cardiovascular instability are common after exposure to many rodenticides.
6. Many antidotes are not readily available or may be experimental; consult a medical toxicologist when available.

Criteria for ICU Discharge in Rodenticide Poisoning

Agent	Criteria
Anticoagulants	Control of hemorrhage and reduction of international normalized ratio
ANTU	Improved oxygenation, off ventilator
Barium	Resolution of paralysis, weaning parameters met
Phosphides	Hemodynamic stability, coma resolution
PNU	Hemodynamic stability, acidosis controlled
Fluoroacetates, fluoroacetamide	Cardiac rhythm stability, no respiratory compromise
Strychnine	Resolution of spasms and seizures with control of acidosis, off ventilator

REFERENCES

1. Ingels M, Lai C, Tai W, et al: A prospective study of acute, unintentional, pediatric superwarfarin ingestions managed without decontamination. Ann Emerg Med 40:73–78, 2002.
2. Smolinske SC, Scherger DL, Kearns PS, et al: Superwarfarin poisoning in children: A prospective study. Pediatrics 84:490–494, 1989.
3. Jayaraman KS: Death pills from pesticide. Nature 353:377, 1991.
4. Nocera A, Levitin HW, Hilton JMN: Dangerous bodies: A case of fatal aluminum phosphide poisoning. Med J Aust 173:133–135, 2000.
5. Garry VF, Griffith J, Danzl TJ, et al: Human genotoxicity: Pesticide applicators and phosphine. Science 246:251–255, 1989.
6. Zaebst DD, Blade LM, Burroughs GE, et al: Phosphine exposures in grain elevators during fumigation with aluminum phosphide. Appl Ind Hyg 3:146–154, 1988.
7. Lewi Z, Warsaw DM, Bar-Khayim Y: Food poisoning from barium carbonate. Lancet 2:342–343, 1964.
8. Diengott D, Rozsa O, Levy N, et al: Hypokalaemia in barium poisoning. Lancet 2:343–344, 1964.
9. Morton W: Poisoning by barium carbonate. Lancet 248:738–739, 1945.
10. Deng JF, Jan IS, Cheng H: The essential role of a poison center in handling an outbreak of barium carbonate poisoning. Vet Hum Toxicol 33:173–175, 1991.

11. Brewer E, Haggerty RJ: Toxic hazards: Rat poison: III. Thallium, strychnine, and ANTU. N Engl J Med 259:1038–1040, 1958.

12. Litovitz T, Klein-Schwartz W, White S, et al: 1999 Annual Report of the American Association of Poison Control Centers Toxic Exposure Surveillance System. Am J Emerg Med 18:517–574, 2000.

13. Litovitz T, Klein-Schwartz W, White S, et al: 2000 Annual Report of the American Association of Poison Control Centers Toxic Exposure Surveillance System. Am J Emerg Med 19:337–395, 2001.

14. Litovitz T, Klein-Schwartz W, Rodgers G, et al: 2001 Annual Report of the American Association of Poison Control Centers Toxic Exposure Surveillance System. Am J Emerg Med 20:391–452, 2002.

15. Shankle R, Keane JR: Acute paralysis from inhaled barium carbonate. Arch Neurol 45:579–580, 1988.

16. McTaggart DR: Poisoning due to sodium fluoroacetate ("1080"). Med J Aust 2:641–642, 1970.

17. Chenoweth M: Monofluoroacetic acid and related compounds. Pharmacol Rev 1:383–424, 1949.

18. Peters RA, Spencer H, Bidstrup PL: Subacute fluoroacetate poisoning. J Occup Med 23:112–113, 1981.

19. Ross GS, Zacharski LR, Robert D, et al: An acquired hemorrhagic disorder from long-acting rodenticide ingestion. Arch Intern Med 152:410–412, 1992.

20. Breckenridge AM, Cholerton S, Hart JAD, et al: A study of the relationship between the pharmacokinetics and the pharmacodynamics of the 4-hydroxycoumarin anticoagulants warfarin, difenacoum and brodifacoum in the rabbit. Br J Pharmacol 84:81–91, 1985.

21. Jones EC, Growe GH, Naiman SC: Prolonged anticoagulation in rat poisoning. JAMA 252:3005–3007, 1984.

22. Watts RG, Castleberry RP, Sadowski JA: Accidental poisoning with a superwarfarin compound (brodifacoum) in a child. Pediatrics 86:883–887, 1990.

23. Weitzel JN, Sadowski JA, Furie BC, et al: Surreptitious ingestion of a long-acting vitamin K antagonist/rodenticide, brodifacoum: Clinical and metabolic studies of three cases. Blood 76:2555–2559, 1990.

24. Lee PW, Arnau T, Neal RA: Metabolism of alpha-naphthylthiourea by rat liver and rat lung microsomes. Toxicol Appl Pharmacol 53:164–173, 1980.

25. Boyd MR, Neal RA: Studies on the mechanism of toxicity and of development of tolerance to the pulmonary toxin, alpha-naphthylthiourea (ANTU). Drug Metab Dispos 4:314–322, 1976.

26. Hardwick S, Skamarauskas J, Smith L, et al: Protection of rats against the effects of α-naphthylthiourea (ANTU) by elevation of non-protein sulphydryl levels. Biochem Pharmacol 42:1203–1208, 1991.

27. Schott GD, McArdle B: Barium-induced skeletal muscle paralysis in the rat, and its relationship to human familial periodic paralysis. J Neurol Neurosurg Psychiatry 37:32–39, 1974.

28. Johnson CH, Van Tassell VJ: Acute barium poisoning with respiratory failure and rhabdomyolysis. Ann Emerg Med 20:126–130, 1991.

29. Roza O, Berman LB: The pathophysiology of barium: Hypokalemic and cardiovascular effects. J Pharmacol Exp Ther 177:433–439, 1971.

30. Chefurka W, Kashi KP, Bond EJ: The effect of phosphine on electron transport in mitochondria. Pesticide Biochem Physiol 6:65–84, 1976.

31. Chugh SN, Arora V, Sharma A, et al: Free radical scavengers and lipid peroxidation in acute aluminum phosphide poisoning. Indian J Med Res 104:190–193, 1996.

32. Rodenberg HD, Chang CC, Watson WA: Zinc phosphide ingestion: A case report and review. Vet Hum Toxicol 31:559–562, 1989.

33. Gunnarsson R, Berne C, Hellerstrom C: Cytotoxic effects of streptozotocin and N-nitrosomethylurea on pancreatic B cells with special regard to the role of nicotinamide-adenine dinucleotide. Biochem J 140:487–494, 1974.

34. Stauffacher W, Burr I, Gutzeit A, et al: Streptozotocin diabetes: Time course of irreversible B-cell damage: Further observations on prevention by nicotinamide. PSEBM 133:194–200, 1970.

35. Kenney RM, Michaels IAL, Flomenbaum NE, et al: Poisoning with N-3-pyridylmethyl-N′-p-nitrophenylurea. Arch Pathol Lab Med 105:367–370, 1981.

36. Pont A, Rubino JM, Bishop D, et al: Diabetes mellitus and neuropathy following Vacor ingestion in man. Arch Intern Med 139:185–187, 1979.

37. Prosser PR, Karam JH: Diabetes mellitus following rodenticide ingestion in man. JAMA 239:1148–1150, 1978.

38. Watson D, Griffin J: Vacor neuropathy: Ultrastructural and axonal transport studies. J Neuropathol Exp Neurol 46:96–108, 1987.

39. Roy A, Taitelman U, Bursztein S: Evaluation of the role of ionized calcium in sodium fluoroacetate ("1080") poisoning. Toxicol Appl Pharmacol 56:216–220, 1980.

40. Chenoweth M, Kandel A, Johnson LB, et al: Factors influencing fluoroacetate poisoning—practical treatment with glyceryl monoacetate. J Pharmacol Exp Ther 102:31–49, 1951.

41. Aprison MH, Lipkowitz KB, Simon JR: Identification of a glycine-like fragment on the strychnine molecule. J Neurosci Res 17:209–213, 1987.

42. Davidoff RA, Aprison MH, Werman R: The effects of strychnine on the inhibition of interneurons by glycine and gamma-aminobutyric acid. Int J Neuropharmacol 8:191–194, 1969.

43. Curtis DR, Hosli L, Johnston GAR, et al: The hyperpolarization of spinal motoneurones by glycine and related amino acids. Exp Brain Res 5:235–258, 1968.

44. Young AB, Zukin SR, Snyder SH: Interaction of benzodiazepines with central nervous glycine receptors: Possible mechanism of action. Proc Natl Acad Sci 71:2246–2250, 1974.

45. Richter JJ: Current theories about the mechanisms of benzodiazepines and neuroleptic drugs. Anesthesiology 54:66–72, 1981.

46. Smith BA: Strychnine poisoning. J Emerg Med 8:321–325, 1990.

47. Teitelbaum DT, Ott JE: Acute strychnine poisoning. J Toxicol Clin Toxicol 3:267–273, 1970.

48. Basehore LM, Mowry JM: Death following ingestion of superwarfarin rodenticide: A case report. Vet Hum Toxicol 29:459, 1987.

49. Helmuth RA, McCloskey DW, Doedens DJ, et al: Fatal ingestion of a brodifacoum-containing rodenticide. Lab Med 20:25–27, 1989.

50. Kruse JA, Carlson RW: Fatal rodenticide poisoning with brodifacoum. Ann Emerg Med 21:331–336, 1992.

51. Swigar ME, Clemow LP, Saidi P, et al: "Superwarfarin" ingestion: A new program in covert anticoagulant overdose. Gen Hosp Psychiatry 12:309–312, 1990.

52. Routh CR, Triplett DA, Murphy MJ, et al: Superwarfarin ingestion and detection. Am J Hematol 36:50–54, 1991.

53. Cimbal G: Alpha-napthylthioharnstoff-vergiftung beim menschen. Arch Toxikol 14:2–6, 1952.

54. Schorn TF, Olbricht C, Schuler A, et al: Barium carbonate intoxication. Intensive Care Med 17:60–62, 1991.

55. Phelan DM: Is hypokalaemia the cause of paralysis in barium poisoning? BMJ 289:882, 1984.

56. Ahmad SH, Fakir S, Gupta S, et al: Celphos poisoning. Indian Pediatr 28:300–301, 1991.

57. Chopra JS, Kalra OP, Malk R, et al: Aluminum phosphide poisoning: A prospective study of 16 cases in one year. Postgrad Med J 62:1113–1115, 1986.

58. Banjaj R, Wasir HS: Epidemic aluminum phosphide poisoning in northern India. Lancet 1:820–821, 1988.

59. Misra UK, Tripathi AK, Pandey R, et al: Acute phosphine poisoning following ingestion of aluminum phosphide. Hum Toxicol 7:343–345, 1988.

60. Singh RB, Singh RG, Singh U: Hypermagnesemia following aluminum phosphide poisoning. Int J Clin Pharmacol Ther Toxicol 29:82–85, 1991.

61. Andersen TS, Holm JW, Andersen TS: Poisoning with aluminum phosphide used as a poison against moles [Danish]. Ugeskr Laeger 158:5308–5309, 1996.

62. Duenas A, Perez-Castrillon JL, Cobos MA, et al: Treatment of the cardiovascular manifestations of phosphine with trimetazidine, a new antiischemic drug [Letter]. Am J Emerg Med 17:219–220, 1999.

63. Miller LV, Stokes JD, Silpitat C: Diabetes mellitus and autonomic dysfunction after Vacor rodenticide ingestion. Diabetes Care 1:73–76, 1978.

64. Johnson D, Kubic P, Levitt C: Accidental ingestion of Vacor rodenticide. Am J Dis Child 134:161–164, 1980.

65. Gallanosa AG, Spyker DA, Curnow RT: Diabetes mellitus associated with autonomic and peripheral neuropathy after Vacor rodenticide poisoning: A review. J Toxicol Clin Toxicol 18:441–449, 1981.

66. Lewitt PA: The neurotoxicity of the rat poison Vacor. N Engl J Med 302:73–77, 1980.

67. Brockmann JL, McDowell AV, Leeds WG: Fatal poisoning with sodium fluoroacetate. JAMA 159:1529–1532, 1955.

68. Chi CH, Chen KW, Chan SH, et al: Clinical presentation and prognostic factors in sodium monofluoroacetate intoxication. Clin Toxicol 34:707–712, 1996.

69. Chung HM: Acute renal failure caused by acute monofluoroacetate poisoning. Vet Hum Toxicol 26:29–32, 1984.

70. Parkin PJ, McGiven AR, Bailey RR: Chronic sodium monofluoroacetate (Compound 1080) intoxication in a rabbiter. N Z Med J 85:93–96, 1977.

71. Boyd RE, Brennan PT, Deng JF: Strychnine poisoning: Recovery from profound lactic acidosis, hyperthermia, and rhabdomyolysis. Am J Med 74:507–512, 1983.

72. Nishiyama T, Nagase M: Strychnine poisoning: Natural course of a nonfatal case. Am J Emerg Med 13:172–173, 1995.

73. Van Heerden PV, Edibam C, Augustson B, et al: Strychnine poisoning: Alive and well in Australia. Anaesth Intensive Care 21:876–878, 1993.

74. Dickson E, Hawkins RC, Reynolds R: Strychnine poisoning: An uncommon cause of convulsions. Aust N Z J Med 22:500–501, 1992.

75. O'Callaghan WG, Joyce N, Counihan HE, et al: Unusual strychnine poisoning and its treatment: Report of eight cases. BMJ 285:478, 1982.

76. Hernandez AF, Pomares J, Schiaffino S, et al: Acute chemical pancreatitis associated with nonfatal strychnine poisoning. J Toxicol Clin Toxicol 36:67–71, 1998.

77. Gordon AM, Richards DW: Strychnine intoxication. Ann Emerg Med 8:520–522, 1979.

78. Heiser JH, Daya MR, Magnussen AR, et al: Massive strychnine intoxication: Serial blood levels in a fatal case. J Toxicol Clin Toxicol 30:269–283, 1992.

79. Katona B, Wason S: Superwarfarin poisoning. J Emerg Med 7:627–631, 1989.

80. Wells JA, Wood KE: Acute barium poisoning treated with hemodialysis. Am J Emerg Med 19:175–177, 2001.

81. Thomas M, Bowie D, Walker R: Acute barium intoxication following ingestion of ceramic glaze. Postgrad Med J 74:545–546, 1998.

82. Donovan JW, Ballard JO, Murphy MJ: Brodifacoum therapy with activated charcoal: Effect on elimination kinetics. Vet Hum Toxicol 32:350, 1990.

83. Rubia J, Grau E, Montserrat I, et al: Anaphylactic shock and vitamin K₁. Ann Intern Med 110:943, 1989.

84. Becker RC, Ansell J: Antithrombotic therapy: An abbreviated reference for clinicians. Arch Intern Med 155:149–161, 1995.

85. Bruno G, Howland MA, McMeeking A, et al: Long-acting anticoagulant overdose: Brodifacoum kinetics and optimal vitamin K dosing. Ann Emerg Med 36:262–267, 2000.

86. Choonara IA, Scott AK, Haynes BP, et al: Vitamin K₁ metabolism in relation to pharmacodynamic response in anticoagulated patients. Br J Clin Pharmacol 20:643–648, 1985.

87. Park BK, Choonora IA, Haynes BP, et al: Abnormal vitamin K metabolism in the presence of normal clotting factor activity in factory workers exposed to 4-hydroxycoumarins. Br J Clin Pharmacol 18:655–662, 1984.

88. Markov A, Causey A, Didlake R, et al: Prevention of alpha-naphthylthiourea-induced pulmonary edema with fructose-1,6 diphosphate. Exp Lung Res 28:285–299, 2002.

89. Chyka PA, Seger D: Position statement: Single-dose activated charcoal. American Academy of Clinical Toxicology; European Association of Poison Centres and Clinical Toxicologists. J Toxicol Clin Toxicol 35:721–741, 1997.

90. Mills K, Kunkel D: Prevention of severe barium carbonate toxicity with oral magnesium sulfate. Vet Hum Toxicol 35:342, 1993.

91. Jourdan S, Bertoni M, Sergio P, et al: Suicidal poisoning with barium chloride. Forensic Sci Int 119:263–265, 2001.

92. Berning J: Hypokalemia of barium poisoning. Lancet 1:110, 1975.

93. Sigue G, Gamble L, Pelitere M, et al: From profound hypokalemia to life-threatening hyperkalemia. Arch Intern Med 160:548–551, 2000.

94. Schorn T, Olbricht C, Schuler A, et al: Barium carbonate intoxication. Intensive Care Med 17:60–62, 1991.

95. Koch M, Appoloni O, Haufroid V, et al: Acute barium intoxication and hemodiafiltration. J Toxicol Clin Toxicol 41:363–367, 2003.

96. Gupta S, Ahlawat SK: Aluminum phosphide poisoning. J Toxicol Clin Toxicol 33:19–24, 1995.

97. Dulin WE, Wyse BM: Reversal of streptozocin diabetes with nicotinamide. Proc Soc Exp Biol Med 131:992–994, 1969.

98. Deckert FW, Moss JN, Sambuca AS, et al: Nutritional and drug interactions with Vacor rodenticide in rats (Abstract). Fed Proc 36:990, 1977.

99. Taitelman U, Roy A, Raikhlin-Eisenkraft B, et al: The effect of monoacetin and calcium chloride on acid-base balance and survival in experimental sodium fluoroacetate poisoning. Arch Toxicol 6(Suppl):222–227, 1983.

100. Omara F, Sisodia CS: Evaluation of potential antidotes for sodium fluoroacetate in mice. Vet Hum Toxicol 32:427–431, 1990.

101. Mishima M, Tanimoto Y, Oguri K, et al: Metabolism of strychnine in vitro. Drug Metab Dispos 13:716–721, 1985.

102. Sgaragli GP, Mannaioni PF: Pharmacokinetic observations on a case of massive strychnine poisoning. Clin Toxicol 6:533–540, 1973.

103. Edmunds M, Sheehan TMT, Hoff WV: Strychnine poisoning: Clinical and toxicological observations on a non-fatal case. J Toxicol Clin Toxicol 24:245–255, 1986.

104. Palatnick W, Meatherall R, Sitar D, et al: Toxicokinetics of acute strychnine poisoning. J Toxicol Clin Toxicol 35:617–620, 1997.

CHAPTER **94**

Carbon Monoxide

Stephen R. Thom

This chapter reviews the clinical presentation, mechanisms of toxicity, and clinical management of carbon monoxide (CO) poisoning. Emphasis is placed on the mechanisms for toxic effects of CO because this provides a demonstration of the continuum of CO-mediated effects, highlights common pitfalls in clinical management, and underscores the challenges that exist in clinical investigations.

CLINICAL IMPORTANCE

CO is one of many ubiquitous contaminants of the environment that requires prevention and control measures to ensure adequate protection of the public health. The incidence of CO-related mortality and morbidity is similar worldwide, and CO may be responsible for more than half of all fatal poisonings.[1–3] When normalized to regional population densities, fatality rates are around 0.5 to 1 per 100,000 in Belgium, Denmark, France, South Korea, Switzerland, Taiwan, United Kingdom, and the United States.[2,4–14]

CO poisoning has been estimated to cause 40,000 persons per year to seek medical attention at emergency departments in the United States.[15,16] Victims' carboxyhemoglobin (COHb) levels are sufficiently high to suspect that more than half of the 6000 deaths from fires in the United States each year may be due to CO poisoning.[18] Deaths from suicides by CO poisoning average about 2600 per year in the United States, whereas unintentional deaths seem to be decreasing.[2] Between 1979 and 1988, the rate of unintentional deaths decreased from 1513 to 878 deaths per year,[2] and in the 1990s, the rate of unintentional deaths decreased to 600 deaths annually.[15–17] The decline may be a result of increased public awareness with use of CO detectors and alarms, stronger emission controls placed on vehicles, and improvements in safety of heating and cooking appliances.

Despite efforts in prevention and in public and medical education, CO poisoning remains frequent.[19–21] Up-to-date data are difficult to obtain; this is a particular concern in developing countries.[22] Continuous surveillance is performed by monitoring all patients hospitalized in some regions,[2,23] but often individuals with CO poisoning are unaware of their exposure because symptoms are nonspecific and mimic those of viral illnesses. This situation contributes to misdiagnosis of many cases by medical professionals.[19,24–30]

BIOCHEMISTRY

The toxicity of CO is based on its propensity for forming stable complexes with transition metals. In contrast to oxygen (O_2), CO does not participate readily in reactions involving formal transfer of electrons. Its valence bond formulation is configured the same as that of nitrogen, a chemically inert gas [$:C = O:$].[31] CO exhibits a small dipole moment, which is what gives CO the tendency to form highly stable linear metal-ligand complexes.

The affinity of CO for hemoglobin is more than 200-fold greater than that of O_2, and formation of COHb is a recognized effect of CO exposure.[32] Pulmonary CO uptake and the variables that influence the body store of CO and COHb level can be estimated reliably by the Coburn-Forster-Kane equation (Fig. 94-1). The major issues of clinical relevance are that CO uptake depends on the partial pressure of CO and O_2 in the inspired gas, the ventilatory rate, and the duration of CO exposure.[33]

In the lungs, CO binds more slowly to hemoglobin than O_2 does, but this is more than offset by the extremely slow rate of dissociation of CO from hemoglobin. The CO-hemoglobin interaction exhibits cooperativity. COHb cooperativity is driven by the association of CO with hemoglobin, whereas cooperativity for oxyhemoglobin is driven by the off-reaction of O_2 from the two α and β globin chains due to the stability of the deoxy (T state) structure. CO binds to oxyhemoglobin (R state) more rapidly than to the deoxy (T state) structure; this results in two adverse effects for O_2 delivery. First, CO displaces O_2 and is bound to hemoglobin, reducing the amount of O_2 carried to the tissues. Second, the presence of CO in the heme pocket prevents modifications of hemoglobin interchain orientation and bond formation that normally occur with O_2 dissociation, the R state–to–T state conversion. The presence of CO increases the O_2 affinity of the protein, causing a left shift of the oxyhemoglobin dissociation curve. The resulting COHb dissociation curve has virtually the same shape as the O_2 dissociation curve. Because of the increased affinity of CO compared with O_2, the fraction of total hemoglobin converted to COHb increases steeply with small increases in CO partial pressure. At a CO partial pressure of only 0.16 mm Hg, 75% of the hemoglobin is combined with CO; this is why relatively small amounts (<0.1% of inspired air) of CO can inhibit the function of a large proportion of the

$$\exp(-tA/V_bB) = A[COHb]_t - BV_{CO} - PI_{CO} / A[COHb]_0 - BV_{CO} - PI_{CO}$$

$$\text{where:} \qquad A = PcO_2/M[HbO_2]$$

$$B = 1/DL_{CO} + P_L/V_A$$

FIGURE 94-1

Coburn-Forster-Kane equation. T, exposure duration; V_b, blood volume in milliliters; PcO_2, average partial pressure of oxygen in lung capillaries; M, equilibrium constant for reaction of carbon monoxide (CO) with oxyhemoglobin; $[HbO_2]$, oxyhemoglobin as milliliters of oxygen per milliliters of blood; DL_{CO}, diffusing capacity of the lungs for CO in milliliters per minute per mm Hg; P_L, barometric pressure minus vapor pressure of water at body temperature; V_A, alveolar ventilation rate per minute; $[COHb]_t$, milliliters of CO per milliliters of blood at time t after exposure; V_{CO}, rate of endogenous CO production; PI_{CO}, partial pressure of CO in inhaled air; $[COHb]_0$, carboxyhemoglobin in milliliters of CO per milliliters of blood before exposure. Units for partial pressures of gases are mm Hg.

hemoglobin in blood. When this happens, the hemoglobin concentration and O_2 partial pressure of blood may be normal, but the O_2 content of the blood is grossly reduced due to the reduced amount of oxyhemoglobin. This reduction has important clinical implications. Chromatographic measurement of oxyhemoglobin does not monitor oxygenation status adequately. Pulse oximetry commonly is used in emergency departments and intensive care units, but values do not correlate with COHb levels and overestimate arterial oxygenation.[34]

The affinity of CO varies with different heme-containing proteins because amino acid residues on the protein chains modify the binding pocket at the heme porphyrin ring. In the β chain of hemoglobin A, the E7 histidine and E11 valine residues sterically interact with the heme-bound CO and push the ligand off the heme axis. This interaction has a significant effect on the heme-CO bond and on the CO combination rate. In mutant hemoglobin A chains, or hemoglobin molecules from other animals that do not have these

types of steric hinderances, the CO combination rates are much higher.[35] Studies with synthetic iron porphyrin proteins have shown that amino acids can impede ligand binding by presenting steric hindrances to CO.[36] Other, more subtle variations in the heme binding pocket, the so-called docking site, also influence binding kinetics. The dissociation rates for CO vary markedly among different heme proteins. These rates cannot be explained based on steric hindrance, but they appear more likely to be related to alterations in the polarity within the heme pocket.[37] The amino acid residues surrounding the heme in myoglobin modulate ligand binding affinity. The binding affinity of CO compared with O_2 is reduced approximately 50-fold compared with the affinity for the free heme moiety. The difference in myoglobin is thought to be due to the characteristic geometry within the docking site, which impedes CO more so than O_2.[38]

Although clinicians may believe the details of CO chemistry have little relevance to their practice, all is not as it first would appear. Many mysteries about CO persist. These may have a substantial impact on understanding of the pathophysiology of CO poisoning. Although physiologic stresses of CO classically are related to competition between CO and O_2 for hemoproteins, more recent attention has focused on interactions between CO and another small gaseous ligand, the free radical nitric oxide ($\cdot$NO) (Fig. 94-2). Under virtually all circumstances, the affinity of $\cdot$NO for hemoproteins is vastly greater than that of either CO or O_2. Despite this fact, there are situations in which CO disturbs the association between $\cdot$NO and hemoproteins. CO increases the steady-state concentration of $\cdot$NO in and around platelets and endothelial cells.[39–41] Electron paramagnetic resonance spectroscopy has provided direct evidence that exposure to CO increases the concentration of $\cdot$NO in lung and brain.[42,43] CO does not increase activity of nitric oxide synthase (NOS) in platelets or endothelial cells, and CO does

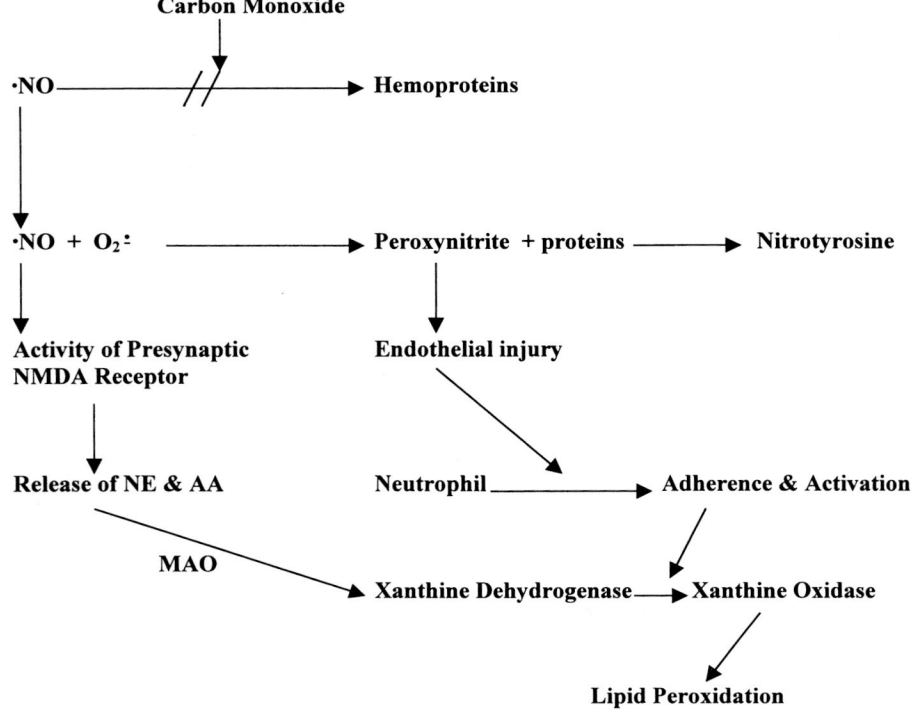

FIGURE 94-2

Interactions between carbon monoxide and the free radical nitric oxide ($\cdot$NO). AA, amino acid; MAO, monoamine oxidase; NE, norepinephrine; NMDA, *N*-methyl-D-aspartate.

not increase NOS protein concentration in tissues of CO-exposed rats at a time when they exhibit elevated ·NO levels.[39–41,43–45] CO partially inhibits NOS activity in rats exposed to 3000 ppm who have COHb levels of approximately 45%.[39] It seems that CO increases the steady-state level of unbound ·NO because it competes for intracellular sites that normally would bind ·NO. Toxic effects on cells occur because the liberated ·NO is available to undergo reactions with superoxide anion (O_2^-·), which yield the potent oxidizing and nitrating agent peroxynitrite. These events are a component to CO-mediated brain injury in some animal models,[42,46–48] and they may relate to a growing body of evidence suggesting that CO functions as a cell-signaling messenger analogous to ·NO.[49,50] Whenever CO is generated in vivo by heme oxygenase, if ·NO also is produced in the vicinity, the CO may act to increase the effective steady-state concentration of ·NO.

The mechanism behind the apparent ability of CO to increase steady-state concentration of ·NO is under investigation. The following discussion relates my current hypothesis. It is based on an assessment of potential competition between ligands using published values for the association and dissociation constants for myoglobin, which I use as a "model" intracellular hemoprotein (Table 94-1).[51]

The calculated affinity binding constant favors ·NO over CO by a factor of 10^5 when steady-state concentrations of CO and ·NO are equal (e.g., for ·NO, $1.7 \times 10^7/1.2 \times 10^{-5} = 1.4 \times 10^{12}$; for CO, $0.5 \times 10^6/1.9 \times 10^{-2} = 2.6 \times 10^7$). It is unlikely, however, for both ligands to have equal concentrations in vivo. Coburn[52] showed that a predictable relationship exists between the tissue concentration of CO and blood COHb to a level of 50%. At a COHb of 7%, the extravascular fluid CO concentration should be approximately 22×10^{-9} M.[52,53] Because CO is freely soluble, a similar concentration is expected to occur inside cells. The rate of ·NO production by endothelial cells (which I have taken as an example because these cells are physically close to delivered CO from the blood) has been estimated to be 1.1×10^{-18} M/cell/min.[54] Even in a situation in which there is a relatively low COHb, the CO concentration may be 10^9 greater than the concentration of ·NO. Competition is feasible even when considering equilibrium kinetics.

The potential for effective competition is even more favorable for CO when considering simple competition kinetics. It is more appropriate to make an assessment of competition using the association rate constants for these ligands, rather than the affinity constants. The physiologic and clinical settings where this relationship may have bearing is early during a CO exposure from exogenous sources, whenever there is a change in CO production in vivo, or when a reduction in local

·NO production occurs. Because the association constant for CO and ·NO differs by a factor of only 34, even a small increase in CO concentration relative to that of ·NO would have an impact favoring CO competition with ·NO for myoglobin. Adverse effects on endothelial cells in vitro that are mediated by ·NO-derived oxidants can be shown with exposure to a CO concentration of only 11×10^{-9} M.[45] There also may be physiologic conditions that allow favorable competition between CO and ·NO. Liver parenchyma has been estimated to generate 0.45×10^{-9} M CO/g liver/min.[55]

PATHOPHYSIOLOGY

Hypoxic effects of CO were described by Bernard[56] and Haldane.[57] An elevated COHb can precipitate tissue hypoxia, and this stress seems to be responsible for fatalities, cardiac injuries, and the acute neurologic abnormalities that develop, according to most studies, in approximately 14% of survivors of serious CO poisoning.[58–60] Clinical and animal studies have failed to establish a correlation, however, between elevated COHb levels and delayed neurologic injuries, which is the most frequent form of CO-associated morbidity.[4,61–68] Studies indicate that 23% to 47% of patients with CO poisoning develop impairments of concentration and learning, dementia, cogwheel rigidity, amnesia, or depression 6 days to 3 weeks after poisoning.[67,69–71] These events occur despite rapid and appropriate emergency care followed by careful neuropsychologic evaluations. CO poisonings that seem to be mild also may cause subtle neurologic dysfunction, which indicates that the clinical assessment of the severity of poisoning is unreliable.[67,72–74] The mechanism for delayed neurologic injuries is unknown.

Severe CO poisoning causes mitochondrial dysfunction and oxidative stress in the central nervous system. In experimental CO poisoning, mild manifestations occur when cerebral perfusion is maintained, whereas mortality and morbidity are profoundly enhanced when exposures to high CO concentrations occur in the presence of reduced cerebral perfusion.[75] The concomitant impairment of cerebral blood flow can be triggered by cardiac dysfunction due to CO or to fixed cerebrovascular lesions.[75–79]

In the presence of concomitant hypoperfusion, Coburn and associates[80] showed that 20% to 45% of CO present in circulating blood shifts into skeletal muscle and other tissues. CO impairs mitochondrial electron transport when cells sustain a reduction in O_2 delivery, as occurs when an elevated COHb level occurs concurrent with restricted perfusion.[77,78] In the setting of hypoperfusion and high CO concentrations, CO binds to cytochrome *c* oxidase, which inhibits adenosine triphosphate synthesis and causes generation of hydroxyl-like radicals.[78,81] Energy production and mitochondrial function are restored after COHb levels decrease.[78] These observations have not explained the two historical characteristics of clinical poisoning that are correlated with a high risk for delayed morbidity: (1) a prolonged exposure to CO, called a *soaking*, and (2) syncope or temporary unconsciousness.[61,82–86] It is unclear whether the transient changes observed during CO poisoning precipitate delayed neuronal dysfunction or death.[87] In some models with neuronal injuries, it has been difficult to document evidence of impaired mitochondrial function or a cellular hypoxic stress.[79]

TABLE 94-1 Rate Constants for Different Ligands with Myoglobin

GAS	ASSOCIATION RATE CONSTANT (M^{-1}/sec^{-1})	DISSOCIATION RATE CONSTANT (sec^{-1})
O_2	14×10^6	12
·NO	17×10^6	1.2×10^{-5}
CO	0.5×10^6	1.9×10^{-2}

The level of CO in tissues may have an equal or greater impact on the clinical status of patients and development of pathology than does the blood level of CO. This phenomenon is shown most clearly with regard to CO-mediated vascular injuries. When humans or experimental animals have been exposed to relatively low CO concentrations for extended periods, capillary leakage of macromolecules from the lung and systemic vasculature has been documented.[43,44,88–91] In contrast, when an hypoxic stress was established in animals by exposing them for 8 to 45 minutes to extremely high CO concentrations, sufficient to cause COHb levels of 60% to 90%, capillary leakage was not detected.[92–94] As noted in the prior section, a proposed pathologic mechanism of CO that is independent of hypoxic stress has been shown in experimental studies to be due to elevations in the steady-state concentration of the free radical ·NO (see Fig. 94-2).[43,44]

CO increases the steady-state concentration of ·NO in and around platelets and endothelial cells.[39–41] Electron paramagnetic resonance spectroscopy has provided direct evidence that exposure to CO increases the concentration of ·NO in lung and brain.[42,43] Some liberated ·NO undergoes reaction with superoxide anion ($O_2^{-·}$) to yield the potent oxidizing and nitrating agent peroxynitrite. The major product when peroxynitrite reacts with proteins is nitrotyrosine, which can be measured in tissues. Nitrotyrosine concentration is increased in aorta, lung, and brain when rats are exposed to CO for more than 40 minutes, and it is found closely associated with the vascular endothelium.[42–44] CO causes a capillary leak in skeletal muscle and in lungs that is mediated by ·NO.[43,44]

These findings have provided further insight into CO-induced neuropathology because endothelial ·NO-mediated changes are a prerequisite for neutrophil adherence to the cerebral microvasculature of CO-poisoned animals.[42,47,48] ·NO-mediated vascular stress is not sufficient by itself, however, to cause neutrophil sequestration in this model of CO-mediated brain injury. During the latter portion of the exposure, when rats breathe 3000 ppm of CO and become unconscious, they invariably sustain a period of hypotension that presumably is mediated by cardiac decompensation.[46,79,95] Cerebral blood flow, which initially is approximately 150% greater than normal due to ·NO-mediated vasodilation, decreases to about 50% below normal for 4 to 6 minutes when rats lose consciousness.[79,95] With regard to mechanisms of brain injury, in contrast to typical hypoxic-ischemic injury, there is never a time when cerebral blood flow is nil, and the interval of hypoperfusion is less than 6 minutes.[79,95] The sudden reduction in microvascular blood flow, coupled with the ·NO-mediated oxidative changes to endothelium, causes neutrophils to adhere to endothelium.

Activated neutrophils attach to the vascular wall via interactions between β_2 integrin adhesion molecules and endothelial counterreceptors.[96] β_2 integrin adhesion molecules are required for neutrophil adherence and progression of the oxidative stress cascade in CO poisoning.[42,48,97,98] This cascade occurs 45 minutes after rats are removed from CO, based on the inhibitory potential of monoclonal antibodies to β_2 integrins.[48,98] The 45-minute delay between initial adherence and β_2 integrin commitment is unusually long compared with some models of leukocyte-mediated tissue injury. The delay is due to the flux of ·NO from

platelets.[39] Nitric oxide inhibits β_2 integrin function.[99] When the animals are in fresh air and CO leaves the body, the ·NO flux decreases, and adherent leukocytes become activated. Activated leukocytes liberate proteases and reactive O_2 species that cause conversion of endothelial xanthine dehydrogenase to xanthine oxidase, and xanthine oxidase activity is required for subsequent brain lipid peroxidation.[42,46–48] These biochemical events occur within 90 minutes after CO poisoning. Metabolic defects in the basal ganglia and hippocampus appear at 5 days, and evidence of impaired learning plateaus 3 weeks after poisoning.[100] The cellular and biochemical events that occur during this 3-week period are under active investigation.[101] In other models of CO-mediated brain injury, hyperbaric oxygen (HBO_2) therapy has been shown to diminish cerebral edema, reduce mortality, and improve neurologic outcome.[102–104]

Several investigations have suggested an association between CO-induced neurotoxicity and neurotoxicity caused by excitatory amino acids.[105,106] Although this issue currently is under investigation, at least in some studies excitotoxicity is linked to elevations of intracellular calcium, ·NO, and $O_2^{-·}$.[107,108] Three types of receptors are activated by excitatory amino acids: N-methyl-D-aspartate (NMDA), D-amino-3-hydroxy-5-methyl-4-isoxazolepropionic acid, and kainic acid.[107] Agents that inhibit NMDA receptor activation attenuate CO-mediated delayed neuronal degeneration of pyramidal cells in the hippocampus and cochlear ganglion cells.[109,110]

Monoamine neurotransmitters, such as norepinephrine and dopamine, are elevated after CO exposure; enzymatic breakdown and autooxidation generate reactive O_2 species.[111,112] These agents seem to contribute to oxidative stress after CO poisoning because free radical production in the brain can be diminished by inhibiting monoamine oxidase B, an enzyme located in microglial cells.[113–115] Nitric oxide augments presynaptic release of monoamine neurotransmitters by activating NMDA receptors.[116,117] Activated microglia also can mediate neuronal injury by generating ·NO-derived oxidants.[118] Microglia can attack oligodendroglia and have been associated with demyelination processes.[119] ·NO-mediated oxidative stress may be a common biochemical link among different pathways of CO poisoning.

Neuropathology after CO poisoning may include neuronal death in the cortex, hippocampus, substantia nigra, and globus pallidus.[120] One of the most common abnormalities is demyelination of the cerebral cortex, which occurs in a perivascular distribution along with evidence of a breach in the blood-brain barrier.[120–122] Blood flow and perivascular abnormalities have been shown using several neuroimaging techniques.[123–128] Acute vascular and perivascular changes also have been found in brains of experimental animals.[42,62,66] The variability observed in lesions found in the cerebral white matter and globus pallidus of animals has been correlated with the decrease in local blood flow and metabolic acidosis.[60,129] Clinical and experimental findings suggest that the effects of CO are global, and variations in the clinical manifestations of poisoning arise because brain regions respond differently to the stresses. Acute neurologic compromise may be due to direct hypoxic stress. The syndrome of delayed neurologic sequelae seems to be a consequence of a cascade of events involving oxidative stress and inflammatory responses.

CLINICAL EFFECTS

When CO enters the body via the lungs, pulmonary cells may be injured by direct interactions, without need for delivery of CO by blood-borne hemoglobin. Elsewhere in the body, CO is delivered by hemoglobin, and concentrations found in perivascular and extravascular sites are estimated using calculations first described by Coburn (see Fig. 94-1).[52] The symptoms, signs, and prognosis of acute CO poisoning correlate poorly with the level of COHb measured at the time of arrival at the hospital.[4,63–68,107] These observations have created two concerns. The first is that investigators must be careful when attempting to study patient populations because determination of the severity of poisonings and the efficacy of treatment is difficult. The second concern is that these clinical observations raise questions regarding the mechanisms of toxicity beyond the classic perspective regarding hemoglobin binding by CO.

Neurologic symptoms of CO poisoning generally are more severe with higher COHb levels, including headache, dizziness, nausea, vomiting, weakness, confusion, disorientation, visual disturbances, and unconsciousness. Cardiac rhythm disturbances include sinus tachycardia, atrial flutter and fibrillation, premature ventricular contractions, ventricular tachycardia, and ventricular fibrillation. Myocardial infarction can occur, even among patients with normal coronary vessels.[130,131] Pulmonary edema in association with CO is relatively rare; it typically occurs as a consequence of congestive heart failure. Pulmonary edema is seen more commonly in patients with concomitant smoke inhalation, and in these patients it may be related to inhalation of the myriad toxic combustion products.[132] Skeletal muscle necrosis can occur and with it acute renal failure. Other rare complications include pancreatitis and hepatocellular injuries. Textbooks often contain tables listing symptoms associated with different COHb levels. Practicing physicians should spend little time examining these lists, however, because the relationship between clinical presentation and COHb levels is extremely poor.

Patients may sustain neurologic abnormalities that are present during the acute hospitalization and either never resolve or resolve slowly over weeks to months after poisoning. Alternatively, patients may develop a delayed neurologic syndrome in which they manifest new cognitive deficits days to weeks after apparent recovery. These manifestations include impaired judgment, poor concentration, memory loss, and a relative indifference to obvious neurologic deficits (e.g., movement disorders, incontinence, speech disturbances, parkinsonian syndrome, and, rarely, tremors).

DIAGNOSTIC TOOLS

Large clinical surveys reported a correlation between neurologic morbidity and the occurrence of an interval of unconsciousness during CO exposure.[61,84,83] This overt insult is not always necessary, however, for neurologic injuries to occur in humans.[67,72–74] Using traditional neuroimaging techniques, such as computed tomography and magnetic resonance imaging, brain lesions have been detected sporadically in severely poisoned CO patients.[133,134] The primary shortcoming with these imaging techniques is their limited sensitivity; neuroimaging has not yet provided a reliable method for assessing the severity of CO poisoning. Bianco and Floris[123] and Silverman and colleagues[128] hypothesized, however, that the initial site of injury by CO may be the vasculature, based on detection of hemosiderin deposits. These deposits are thought to result from focal hemorrhages.

More sophisticated neuroimaging techniques have been used to detect abnormalities in patients who, in some cases, exhibited only subtle neurologic impairments. Abnormalities in resting cerebral blood flow[126,127] and abnormalities in cerebral vasoactivity to CO[125] have been detected by single-photon emission computed tomography. Changes also have been detected that suggest CO causes a disturbance in coupling between neuronal O_2 demand and blood flow. DeReuck and coworkers[124] examined seven patients 5 to 7 days after CO poisoning using positron emission tomography with $^{15}O_2$. They found a global increase in cerebral O_2 extraction along with regional areas of diminished blood flow, especially in the frontal and temporal lobes. Although these observations underscore the vascular nature of CO-mediated neuropathology, they do not assist with clinical assessments of patients. To date, no objective parameters that prospectively assess the severity of poisoning have been identified. Some more recent findings with state-of-the-art neuroimaging techniques have exhibited correlations with the clinical improvement in case reports, whereas others show abnormalities when no clinical changes are noted.[135–137] In experimental studies, blood levels of glutathione, oxidized proteins, and products of lipid peroxidation offer insight into CO-mediated pathology.[138] Additional work is necessary, however, to establish if these or some other survey may be useful to stage the severity of clinical poisonings.

TREATMENT

As in any critical care setting, initial attention must be focused on restoring or maintaining vital functions. Preservation of a patent airway, ventilation, oxygenation, and adequate perfusion is the foundation for proper actions in serious CO poisoning. Emphasis is placed on O_2 treatment because the rate of COHb dissociation is proportional to the arterial O_2 partial pressure.[139]

A great deal has been written about HBO_2 therapy for CO poisoning. HBO_2 therapy is a patient treatment modality in which a person breathes 100% O_2 while exposed in a treatment chamber to increased atmospheric pressure. Treatments typically are conducted at pressures two to three times higher than normal atmospheric pressure (14.7 psi), or 2 to 3 atm absolute (ATA). The hyperbaric chamber per se is not the therapeutic agent. Oxygen is the therapeutic drug, and the chamber is used as a dosing device.

Indications for ICU Admission in Carbon Monoxide Poisoning

Persistent depressed level of consciousness
Cardiac ischemia
Intercurrent critical illness (e.g., aspiration, acidosis, cotoxicants)

Since 1960, HBO$_2$ therapy has been used with increasing frequency for severe CO poisoning because clinical recovery has seemed to be improved beyond that expected with ambient pressure O$_2$ therapy.[65,69,140] No definition has been established for staging the severity of CO poisoning, however. It is difficult to evaluate patients in a prospective manner or compare the efficacy of different treatments. For this reason, studies that have selected a discrete, presumably more homogeneous, subset of patients may provide information that is more reliable.

The initial motivation for administering HBO$_2$ therapy was to hasten removal of CO, based on the well-known relationship that COHb half-life is inversely related to the inspired partial pressure of O$_2$.[139,141] HBO$_2$ therapy also hastens dissociation of CO from cytochrome oxidase[77,78] and inhibits cerebral edema in experimental CO brain injury.[102,103] Vascular oxidative stress is prevented because HBO$_2$ therapy inhibits β$_2$ integrin–dependent leukocyte adhesion.[98,142] Neutrophils from humans exposed to HBO$_2$ exhibit the same diminished adherence as neutrophils in animal studies.[143]

Some centers have proposed using a psychometric screening test to identify patients with subtle neurologic compromise and as a method to stratify patients for treatment. When examined in a prospective study, abnormalities during the initial screening did not correlate with development of delayed sequelae, however.[67] The first prospective clinical trial involving HBO$_2$ therapy did not find it to be superior to ambient pressure treatment.[71] This study has been criticized because the authors used a low oxygen partial pressure (2 ATA versus the more usual protocols with 2.5 to 3 ATA), and because nearly half of all patients received HBO$_2$ treatments more than 6 hours after they were discovered.[144]

In 1969, a retrospective study indicated that HBO$_2$ reduced mortality and morbidity only if administered within 6 hours after CO poisoning.[145]

In a prospective trial involving patients with mild-to-moderate poisoning, 23% of patients (7 of 30) treated with ambient pressure O$_2$ developed neurologic sequelae, whereas no patients (0 of 30; $P < 0.05$) treated with HBO$_2$ (2.8 ATA) developed sequelae.[67] HBO$_2$ therapy also was found to have a significant benefit in another prospective, randomized trial.[125] Twenty-six patients were hospitalized within 2 hours of discovery and equally divided between two treatment groups: ambient pressure O$_2$ or 2.5 ATA O$_2$. Three weeks later, patients treated with HBO$_2$ had significantly fewer abnormalities on electroencephalogram, and single-photon emission computed tomography showed that cerebral vessels had nearly normal reactivity to carbon dioxide, in contrast to diminished reactivity in patients treated with ambient pressure O$_2$.

Scheinkestel and associates[146] performed a prospective trial of 191 patients and reported no benefit from relatively unorthodox administration of HBO$_2$ and ambient pressure O$_2$ therapy that extended over days. Concerns with this study include the following: There was a mean delay to treatment of 7.5 hours, symptoms of O$_2$ toxicity occurred in the experimental group, and only 46% of patients who entered the study were assessed to evaluate delayed neurologic sequelae. Acute neurologic abnormalities, which were assessed in an adequate fraction of the study population to make valid comparisons, were evaluated using an arbitrary set of psychometric tests influenced by depression. Confidence in the authors' conclusions is tempered because 67% of the study population had attempted suicide. Comatose patients accounted for 53% of the patients studied, and 44% of patients had taken additional poisons, but no specific information on these cases was provided to assess whether central nervous system insults may have been due to factors other than CO. A reevaluation of the subset of Scheinkestel's patients presumed to have mild CO poisoning presents the dilemma of patient evaluation and selection criteria. Using the "mildly" poisoned subset of patients, Kehat and Shupak[147] examined the difference in incidence of acute or persistent neurologic sequelae between the two treatment groups. Patients treated with HBO$_2$ had a significantly lower incidence of sequelae than patients treated with ambient pressure O$_2$.

Mathieu and coworkers[70] reported on a large trial of HBO$_2$ therapy for CO poisoning (n = 575 patients). Among noncomatose patients who had experienced transient unconsciousness, those treated with ambient pressure O$_2$ had a higher incidence of delayed sequelae. Most sequelae spontaneously resolved over 6 months.

Support for use of HBO$_2$ therapy comes from the aforementioned studies and from nonrandomized comparative studies.[65,69,140,145,148–151] Studies that have failed to find benefit to treatment have serious methodologic shortcomings. There is a legitimate concern over the lack of reliable methods to assess the severity of poisoning. Use of HBO$_2$ therapy in every CO-poisoned patient who has had loss of consciousness during CO exposure or who has a neurologic abnormality on clinical examination continues to be advocated. Important caveats regarding HBO$_2$ therapy include the observation that treatment efficacy may diminish if treatment is delayed for more than 6 hours after poisoning.[145] There also is discussion in the literature that patient outcome may be improved if more than a single treatment is administered.[69] The threshold for using HBO$_2$ therapy has not been established clearly. In addition to its use for patients with transient unconsciousness and neurologic signs, some centers treat patients with HBO$_2$ when they have abnormal psychometric test results and if the COHb level is greater than a certain value. Some use a COHb of 40%, whereas others use 25%, regardless of symptoms.[152,153]

HBO$_2$ therapy is reviewed in detail in Chapter 16. When arranging for treatment with HBO$_2$, probably the first consideration must be the logistical requirements of transporting a patient to a hyperbaric facility. One group examined this question in their review of 297 consecutive CO-poisoned patients and concluded that transfer need not be deferred because of a concern over cardiac or respiratory arrest, myocardial infarction, or deterioration in mental status if these events had not occurred before transfer.[154] The potential adverse effects of HBO$_2$ therapy per se are rare, and they usually are mild and self-limited. Relative risks always must be considered in any therapeutic setting, however. Preexisting conditions that require some forethought and possible management before initiating HBO$_2$ therapy include patients with claustrophobia, sinus congestion, and scarred or noncompliant structures in the middle ear (e.g., in patients with otosclerosis).[155] Middle ear barotrauma due to eustachian tube dysfunction may occur in 2% of patients and is managed easily by oral decongestants or rarely by tympanostomy tubes.[156] Transient nearsightedness, thought to be related to lenticular changes from O_2, occurs in association with treatment courses spanning weeks in approximately 33% of patients older than age 50. This risk is not a concern when treating CO poisoning because the course of therapy typically spans only one to three treatments. The visual changes resolve 3 to 6 weeks after treatments cease.[155] There are no notable pulmonary oxygen toxicity risks with therapeutic protocols[157–159] because the duration of exposure usually is kept to less than 2 hours. Patients may have central nervous system O_2 toxicity, which is manifested as a grand mal seizure. In the general population, central nervous system O_2 toxicity occurs with a frequency of approximately 1 in 10,000, but among CO poisoning victims, it may be more frequent, possibly due to the direct effects of CO or to concomitant respiratory acidosis. Regardless, if mechanical trauma can be avoided during the convulsion, there are no residual effects.[157] Vasoconstriction is a physiologic effect of hyperoxygenation; this causes negligible changes in blood pressure because of a small (about 10%) decrease in cardiac output, principally caused by vagal stimulation with a reduction in heart rate.[160] Previous exposure to the chemotherapeutic agent bleomycin is considered a relatively strong contraindication to HBO_2 therapy. Bleomycin exacerbates pulmonary oxygen toxicity.[161,162] On a case-by-case basis, careful consideration of this risk must be weighed against the potential benefits of HBO_2 therapy. The only well-recognized absolute contraindication for HBO_2 therapy is an unvented pneumothorax, based on the risk of exacerbating this condition while in the hyperbaric chamber and especially on decompression.

SPECIAL POPULATIONS

Pregnant Patients

The clinical outcomes of CO poisoning for the mother and fetus do not correlate with maternal COHb, but maternal symptoms at the time of exposure are associated with fetal morbidity and mortality.[163] Acute severe CO poisoning is associated with a maternal mortality of 19% to 24% and a fetal mortality of 36% to 67%.[164] When mother and fetus survive, many fetuses subsequently develop somatic and neurologic sequelae, including malformations of limbs, hypotonia and areflexia, persistent seizures, mental and motor disabilities, and microcephaly.[165,166]

Hypoxic stress related to impaired O_2 delivery is an obvious component to fetal distress. Normal fetal arterial PO_2 is about 20 mm Hg, versus 100 mm Hg for maternal arterial blood. The fetal O_2 exchange typically occurs near the steep portion of the oxyhemoglobin dissociation curve. A small decline in maternal PO_2 can cause a precipitous decline in fetal PO_2. This physiologic stress occurs more quickly than that associated with CO binding to fetal proteins. In studies with sheep, Longo and Hill[167] showed that fetal COHb does not reach steady state until approximately 36 to 48 hours, whereas maternal COHb reaches steady state in 7 to 8 hours. The second insult related to fetal COHb is a disturbance in the O_2-hemoglobin dissociation curve. Binding by CO causes a left shift of the curve, which increases the hypoxic stress to the fetus. Fetal COHb concentration rises

more slowly that does maternal COHb, but when steady state is reached, the fetal level is higher; this is related to the higher affinity fetal hemoglobin has for CO compared with hemoglobin A. The human fetal-maternal COHb concentration ratio is 1.1 to 1.0; that is, at steady state, the fetal COHb concentration is 10% to 15% higher than maternal COHb. Although the slow uptake kinetics may be viewed as a protective factor for the fetus, the dynamics work in reverse for CO elimination. In studies with sheep, the half-life for fetal COHb was nearly double that for maternal COHb.[167] For this reason, clinical recommendations for treating CO poisoning in pregnant women with ambient pressure O_2 suggest that pregnant women should breathe 100% O_2 five times longer than the time it takes for their own blood to register negligible residual COHb.

The current recommendations for use of HBO_2 therapy in pregnant women are essentially the same as the recommendations to treat any other patient. Some groups also treat based solely on an elevated COHb level versus only maternal symptoms (history of unconsciousness). Anecdotal clinical reports suggest that HBO_2 therapy may improve fetal outcome.[164,168–173] The only experimental study addressing the efficacy of HBO_2 for reducing fetal risk from acute CO poisoning showed a reduction in spontaneous abortion in pregnant rats.[174] There are no significant extra risks presented to the fetus or mother due to HBO_2 therapy.[175,176]

Pediatric Patients

Clinical signs and symptoms of CO poisoning in children are the same as in adults. Children may become symptomatic during CO exposures sooner than adults, however, owing to their higher metabolic rates, respiratory exchange requirements, and smaller blood volumes.[177,178] Children may present with vague symptoms of nausea, vomiting, and headache, and the condition may be misdiagnosed as gastrointestinal disease.[179] Delayed neurologic sequelae have been reported in children,[180,181] and there is a case report of hydrocephalus after CO poisoning.[182] HBO_2 therapy is recommended in pediatric CO poisoning, and intensive care support for pediatric cases is achievable.[153,183] The threshold for treating children is the same as for adults.

REFERENCES

1. National Safety Council: How people died in home accidents, 1981. In: Accident Facts, 1982 ed. Chicago, National Safety Council, 1982, pp 80–84.
2. Cobb N, Etzel RA: Unintentional carbon monoxide-related deaths in the United States, 1979 through 1988. JAMA 266:659–663, 1991.
3. Mathieu D, Mathieu-Nolf M, Wattel F: Intoxication par le monoxide de carbone: Aspects actuels [Carbon monoxide poisoning: Present aspects]. Bull Acad Natl Med (Paris) 180:965–973, 1996.
4. Meredith T, Vale A: Carbon monoxide poisoning. BMJ 296:77–79, 1988.
5. Gajdos P, Conso M, Korach JM, et al: Incidence and causes of carbon monoxide intoxication: Results of an epidemiological survey in a French department. Arch Environ Health 46:373–376, 1991.
6. Gujer H: Accidental CO poisoning caused by incomplete combustion of liquid gases. Soz Pravantivmed 27:39–42, 1982.
7. Hung D, Deng J, Yang C, et al: The climate and the occurrence of carbon monoxide poisoning in Taiwan. Hum Exp Toxicol 13:493–495, 1994.
8. Kim Y: Seasonal variation in carbon monoxide poisoning in urban Korea. J Epidemiol Community Health 39:79–81, 1985.

9. Milis L, Lagasse R: Carbon monoxide poisoning in the Brussels metropolitan area: Home survey technics and proposals for action. Arch Belg 47:24–28, 1989.

10. Saunders PJ: Surveillance of non-infectious environmental hazards in the West Midlands. Chem Incident 1:1, 1996.

11. Taudorf K, Michelsen K: The danger of CO poisoning from gas water heaters: A study of 124 systems and their uses. Ugeskr Laeger 145:3593–3598, 1983.

12. Theilade P: Carbon monoxide poisoning: Five years' experience of a defined population. Am J Forensic Med Pathol 11:219–225, 1990.

13. Thomsen JL, Kardel T: Accidents caused by gas water heaters: Fatalities and a non fatal case. Ugeskr Laeger 145:3598–3600, 1983.

14. Wilson RC, Saunders PJ, Smith G: An epidemiological study of acute carbon monoxide poisoning in the West Midlands. Occup Environ Med 55:723–728, 1998.

15. Cook M, Simon PA, Hoffman RE: Unintentional carbon monoxide poisoning in Colorado, 1986 through 1991. Am J Public Health 85:988–990, 1995.

16. Hampson NB: Emergency department visits for carbon monoxide poisoning in the Pacific Northwest. J Emerg Med 16:695–698, 1998.

17. Miller RL, Toal BF, Foscue K, et al: Unintentional carbon monoxide poisonings in residential settings—Connecticut, November 1993–March 1994. MMWR Morb Mortal Wkly Rep 44:765–767, 1995.

18. Heimbach DM, Waeckerle JF: Inhalation injuries. Ann Emerg Med 17:1316–1320, 1988.

19. Barret L, Danel V, Faure J: Carbon monoxide poisoning, a diagnosis frequently overlooked. Clin Toxicol 23:309–313, 1985.

20. Molitor L: A 45-year-old woman with flu symptoms. J Emerg Nurs 23:83–84, 1997.

21. Roy B, Crawford R: Pitfalls in diagnosis and management of carbon monoxide poisoning. J Accid Emerg Med 9:62–63, 1996.

22. Chen BH, Hong CJ, Pandey MR, et al: Indoor air pollution in developing countries. World Health Stat Q 43:127–138, 1990.

23. Litovitz TL, Holm KC, Bailey KM, et al: 1991 Annual report of the American Association of Poison Control Centers national data collection system. Am J Emerg Med 10:452–505, 1992.

24. Dolan MC, Haltom TL, Barrows GH, et al: Carboxyhemoglobin levels in patients with flu-like symptoms. Ann Emerg Med 16:782–786, 1987.

25. Fisher J, Rubin KP: Occult carbon monoxide poisoning. Arch Intern Med 142:1270–1271, 1982.

26. Grace TW, Platt FW: Subacute carbon monoxide poisoning. JAMA 246:1698–1700, 1981.

27. Heckerling PS, Leikin JB, Maturen A, et al: Predictors of occult carbon monoxide poisoning in patients with headache and dizziness. Ann Intern Med 107:174–176, 1987.

28. Heckerling PS, Leikin JB, Maturen A: Occult carbon monoxide poisoning: Validation of a prediction model. Am J Med 84:251–256, 1988.

29. Heckerling PS, Leikin JB, Terzian CG, et al: Occult carbon monoxide poisoning in patients with neurologic illness. J Toxicol Clin Toxicol 28:29–44, 1990.

30. Kirkpatrick JN: Occult carbon monoxide poisoning. West J Med 146:52–56, 1987.

31. Cotton FA, Wilkinson G: Advanced Inorganic Chemistry: A Comprehensive Text, 3rd ed. New York, Wiley, 1972, pp 684–688.

32. Douglas CG, Haldane JS, Haldane JBS: The laws of combination of haemoglobin with carbon monoxide and oxygen. J Physiol (London) 44:275–304, 1912.

33. Coburn RF, Forster RE, Kane PB: Considerations of the physiological variables that determine the blood carboxyhemoglobin concentration in man. J Clin Invest 44:1899–1910, 1965.

34. Hampson NB: Pulse oximetry in severe carbon monoxide poisoning. Chest 114:1036–1041, 1998.

35. Salhany JM, Ogawa S, Shulman RG: Correlation between quaternary structure and ligand dissociation kinetics for fully liganded hemoglobin. Biochem J 14:2180–2190, 1975.

36. Collman JP, Brauman JI, Doxsee KM: Carbon monoxide binding to iron porphyrins. Proc Natl Acad Sci U S A 76:6035–6039, 1979.

37. Sharma VS, John ME, Waterman MR: Functional studies on hemoglobin opossum. J Biol Chem 257:11887–11892, 1982.

38. Lim M, Jackson TA, Anfinrud PA: Ultrafast rotation and trapping of carbon monoxide dissociated from myoglobin. Nat Struct Biol 4:209–214, 1997.

39. Thom SR, Ohnishi ST, Ischiropoulos H, et al: Nitric oxide released by platelets inhibits neutrophil B2 integrin function following acute carbon monoxide poisoning. Toxicol Appl Pharmacol 128:105–110, 1994.

40. Thom SR, Ischiropoulos H: Mechanism of oxidative stress from low levels of carbon monoxide. Health Effect Institute Research Report 80. Cambridge, MA, 1997.

41. Thom SR, Xu YA, Ischiropoulos H: Vascular endothelial cells generate peroxynitrite in response to carbon monoxide exposure. Chem Res Toxicol 10:1023–1031, 1997.

42. Ischiropoulos H, Beers MF, Ohnishi ST, et al: Nitric oxide and perivascular tyrosine nitration following carbon monoxide poisoning in the rat. J Clin Invest 97:2260–2267, 1996.

43. Thom SR, Ohnishi ST, Fisher D, et al: Pulmonary vascular stress from carbon monoxide. Toxicol Appl Pharmacol 154:12–19,1999.

44. Thom SR, Fisher D, Xu YA, et al: Role of nitric oxide-derived oxidants in vascular injury from carbon monoxide in the rat. Am J Physiol 276(Heart Circ Physiol 45):H984–H992, 1999.

45. Thom SR, Fisher D, Xu YA, et al: Adaptive responses and apoptosis in endothelial cells exposed to carbon monoxide. Proc Natl Acad Sci U S A 97:1305–1310, 2000.

46. Thom SR: Carbon monoxide-mediated brain lipid peroxidation in the rat. J Appl Physiol 68:997–1003, 1990.

47. Thom SR: Dehydrogenase conversion to oxidase and lipid peroxidation in brain after carbon monoxide poisoning. J Appl Physiol 73:1584–1589, 1992.

48. Thom SR: Leukocytes in carbon monoxide-mediated brain oxidative injury. Toxicol Appl Pharmacol 123:234–247, 1993.

49. Verma A, Hirsch DJ, Glatt CE, et al: Carbon monoxide: A putative neural messenger. Science 259:381–384, 1993.

50. Zhuo M, Small SA, Kandel ER, et al: Nitric oxide and carbon monoxide produce activity-dependent long-term synaptic enhancement in hippocampus. Science 260:1946–1950, 1993.

51. Gibson QH, Olson JS, McKinnie RE, et al: A kinetic description of ligand binding to sperm whale myoglobin. J Biol Chem 261:10228–10239, 1986.

52. Coburn RF: The carbon monoxide body stores. Ann N Y Acad Sci 174:11–22, 1970.

53. Gothert M, Lutz F, Malorny G: Carbon monoxide partial pressure in tissue of different animals. Environ Res 3:303–309, 1970.

54. Schmidt HHHW, Nau H, Wittfoht W, et al: Arginine is a physiological precursor of endothelium-derived nitric oxide. Eur J Pharmacol 154:213–216, 1988.

55. Goda N, Suzuki K, Naito M, et al: Distribution of heme oxygenase isoforms in rat liver. J Clin Invest 101:604–612, 1998.

56. Bernard C: An Introduction to the Study of Experimental Medicine. New York, 1865, HC Greene Dover Publications. 1957 reprint.

57. Haldane J: The action of carbonic oxide on man. J Physiol 18:430–462, 1895.

58. Anderson EW, Andelman RJ, Strauch JM, et al: Effects of low-level carbon monoxide exposure on onset and duration of angina pectoris. Ann Intern Med 79:46–50, 1973.

59. Cramlet SH, Erickson HH, Gorman HA: Ventricular function following acute carbon monoxide exposure. J Appl Physiol 39:482–486, 1975.

60. Ginsberg MD: Carbon monoxide intoxication: Clinical features, neuropathology and mechanisms of injury. Clin Toxicol 23:281–288, 1985.

61. Choi S: Delayed neurologic sequelae in carbon monoxide intoxication. Arch Neurol 40:433–435, 1983.

62. Funata N, Okeda R, Takano T, et al: Electron microscopic observations of experimental carbon monoxide encephalopathy in the acute phase. Acta Pathol Jpn 32:219–229, 1982.

63. Garland H, Pearce J: Neurological complications of carbon monoxide poisoning. QJM 144:445–455, 1967.

64. Klees M, Heremans M, Doughan S: Psychological sequelae to carbon monoxide poisoning in the child. J Toxicol Clin Exp 5:301–307, 1985.

65. Myers RAM, Snyder SK, Emhoff TA: Subacute sequelae of carbon monoxide poisoning. Ann Emerg Med 14:1163–1167, 1985.

66. Okeda R, Funata N, Song SJ, et al: Comparative study pathogenesis of selective cerebral lesions in carbon monoxide poisoning and nitrogen hypoxia in cats. Acta Neuropathol 56:265–272, 1982.

67. Thom SR, Taber RL, Mendiguren II, et al: Delayed neuropsychologic sequelae after carbon monoxide poisoning: Prevention by treatment with hyperbaric oxygen. Ann Emerg Med 25:474–480, 1995.

68. Winter PM, Miller JN: Carbon monoxide poisoning. JAMA 236:1502–1504, 1976.
69. Gorman DF, Clayton D, Gilligan JE, et al: A longitudinal study of 100 consecutive admissions for carbon monoxide poisoning to the Royal Adelaide Hospital. Anaesth Intens Care 20:311–316, 1992.
70. Mathieu D, Wattel F, Mathieu-Nolf M, et al: Randomized prospective study comparing the effect of HBO versus 12 hours NBO in non-comatose CO poisoned patients. Undersea Hyperb Med 23(Suppl):7, 1996.
71. Raphael JC, Elkharrat D, Guincestre MCJ, et al: Trial of normobaric and hyperbaric oxygen for acute carbon monoxide intoxication. Lancet 2:414–419, 1989.
72. Schulte JH: Effects of mild carbon monoxide intoxication. Arch Environ Health 7:524–530, 1969.
73. Remick RA, Miles JE: Carbon monoxide poisoning: Neurologic and psychiatric sequelae. Can Med Assoc J 117:654–657, 1977.
74. Ryan CM: Memory disturbances following chronic low level carbon monoxide exposure. Arch Clin Neuropsychol 5:59–67, 1990.
75. Jiang J, Tyssebotn I: A model for acute carbon monoxide poisoning in conscious rats. Undersea Hyperb Med 23:99–106, 1996.
76. Jiang J, Tyssebotn I: Normobaric and hyperbaric oxygen treatment of acute carbon monoxide poisoning in rats. Undersea Hyperb Med 24:107–116, 1997.
77. Brown SD, Piantadosi CA: Reversal of carbon monoxide-cytochrome C oxidase binding by hyperbaric oxygen in vivo. Adv Exp Biol Med 248:747–754, 1989.
78. Brown SD, Piantadosi CA: Recovery of energy metabolism in rat brain after carbon monoxide hypoxia. J Clin Invest 89:666–672, 1991.
79. Mayevsky A, Meilin S, Rogatsky GG, et al: Multiparametric monitoring of the awake brain exposed to carbon monoxide. J Appl Physiol 78:1188–1196, 1995.
80. Coburn RF, Wallace HW, Abboud R: Redistribution of body carbon monoxide after hemorrhage. Am J Physiol 220:868–874, 1971.
81. Piantadosi CA, Zhang J, Demchenko IT: Production of hydroxyl radical in the hippocampus after CO hypoxia or hypoxic hypoxia in the rat. Free Radic Biol Med 22:725–732, 1997.
82. Bogusz M, Cholewa L, Pach J, et al: A comparison of two types of carbon monoxide poisoning. Arch Toxicol 33:141–149, 1975.
83. Min SK: A brain syndrome associated with delayed neuropsychiatric sequelae following acute carbon monoxide intoxication. Acta Psychiatr Scand 73:80–86, 1986.
84. Smith JS, Brandon S: Morbidity from acute carbon monoxide poisoning at three-year follow-up. BMJ 1:318–321, 1973.
85. Wasowski J, Myslak Z, Graczyk M, et al: An attempt at comparing the results of carboxyhemoglobin level in blood and gasometric determination in capillary blood in cases of carbon monoxide poisoning when treatment began at the place of accident. Anaesth Resusc Intens Ther 4:245–249, 1976.
86. Werner B, Back W, Akerblom H, et al: Two cases of acute carbon monoxide poisoning with delayed neurological sequelae after a "free" interval. Clin Toxicol 23:249–265, 1985.
87. Piantadosi CA, Zhang J, Levin ED, et al: Apoptosis and delayed neuronal damage after carbon monoxide poisoning in the rat. Exp Neurol 147:103–114, 1997.
88. Kjeldsen K, Astrup P, Wanstrup J: Ultrastructural intimal changes in the rabbit aorta after a moderate carbon monoxide exposure. Atherosclerosis 16:67–82, 1972.
89. Maurer FW: The effects of carbon monoxide anoxemia on the flow and composition of cervical lymph. Am J Physiol 133:170–179, 1941.
90. Parving HH, Ohlsson K, Hansen HJB, et al: Effect of carbon monoxide exposure on capillary permeability to albumin and α_2-macroglobulin. Scand J Clin Lab Invest 29:381–388, 1972.
91. Siggaard-Anderson J, Bonde-Peterson F, Hanson TI: Plasma volume and vascular permeability during hypoxia and carbon monoxide exposure. Scand J Clin Lab Invest 22:39–48, 1968.
92. Fisher AB, Hyde RW, Baue AE, et al: Effect of carbon monoxide on function and structure of the lung. J Appl Physiol 26:4–12, 1969.
93. Robinson NB, Barie PS, Halebian PH, et al: Distribution of ventilation and perfusion following acute carbon monoxide poisoning. Surg Forum 36:115–118, 1985.
94. Sugi K, Theissen JL, Traber LD, et al: Impact of carbon monoxide on cardiopulmonary dysfunction after smoke inhalation injury. Circ Res 66:69–75, 1990.
95. Meilin S, Rogatsky GG, Thom SR, et al: Effects of carbon monoxide on the brain may be mediated by nitric oxide. J Appl Physiol 81:1078–1083, 1996.
96. Von Andrian UH, Chambers JD, McEvoy LM, et al: Two-step model of leukocyte-endothelial cell interaction in inflammation: Distinct roles for LECAM-1 and the leukocyte β_2 integrins in vivo. Proc Natl Acad Sci U S A 88:7538–7542, 1991.
97. Thom SR: Antagonism of CO-mediated brain lipid peroxidation by hyperbaric oxygen. Toxicol Appl Pharmacol 105:340–344, 1990.
98. Thom SR: Functional inhibition of leukocyte β_2 integrins by hyperbaric oxygen in carbon monoxide-mediated brain injury in rats. Toxicol Appl Pharmacol 123:248–256, 1993.
99. Banick PD, Chen Q, Xu YA, et al: Nitric oxide inhibits neutrophil β_2 integrin function by inhibiting membrane-associated cyclic GMP synthesis. J Cell Physiol 172:12–24, 1997.
100. Thom SR: Learning dysfunction and metabolic defects in globus pallidus and hippocampus after CO poisoning in a rat model. Undersea Hyperb Med 23(Suppl):20, 1997.
101. Thom SR, Xu YA, Fisher DG: Autoimmune responses in carbon monoxide-mediated brain injury. Undersea Hyperb Med 2000.
102. Jiang J, Tyssebotn I: Normobaric and hyperbaric oxygen treatment of acute carbon monoxide poisoning in rats. Undersea Hyperb Med 24:107–116, 1997.
103. Jiang J, Tyssebotn I: Cerebrospinal fluid pressure changes after acute carbon monoxide poisoning and therapeutic effects of normobaric and hyperbaric oxygen in conscious rats. Undersea Hyperb Med 24:245–254, 1997.
104. Tomaszewski C, Rudy J, Wathen J, et al: Prevention of neurologic sequelae from carbon monoxide by hyperbaric oxygen in rats. Ann Emerg Med 21:1992.
105. Nabeshima T, Katoh A, Ishimaru H, et al: Carbon monoxide-induced delayed amnesia, delayed neuronal death and change in acetylcholine concentration in mice. J Pharmacol Exp Ther 256:378–384, 1991.
106. Ishimaru H, Nabeshima T, Katoh A, et al: Effects of successive carbon monoxide exposures on delayed neuronal death in mice under the maintenance of normal body temperature. Biochem Biophys Res Commun 179:836–840, 1991.
107. Choi DW: Calcium-mediated neurotoxicity: Relationship to specific channel types and role in ischemic damage. Trends Neurosci 11:465–479, 1988.
108. Mayer ML, Miller RJ: Excitatory amino acid receptors, second messengers and regulation of intracellular Ca^{2+} in mammalian neurons. Trends Neurosci 11:254–260, 1990.
109. Ishimaru H, Katoh A, Suzuki H, et al: Effects of N-methyl-D-aspartate receptor antagonists on carbon monoxide-induced brain damage in mice. J Pharmacol Exp Ther 261:349–352, 1992.
110. Liu Y, Fechter LD: MK-801 protects against carbon monoxide-induced hearing loss. Toxicol Appl Pharmacol 132:196–202, 1995.
111. Newby MB, Roberts RJ, Bhatnagar RK: Carbon monoxide and hypoxia-induced effects on catecholamines in the mature and developing rat brain. J Pharmacol Exp Ther 206:61–68, 1978.
112. Bindoli A, Rigobello MP, Deeble DJ: Biochemical and toxicological properties of the oxidation products of catecholamines. Free Rad Biol Med 13:391–405, 1992.
113. Piantadosi CA, Tatro L, Zhang J: Hydroxyl radical production in the brain after CO hypoxia in rats. Free Rad Biol Med 18:603–609, 1995.
114. Levitt P, Pintar JE, Breakfield XO: Immunocytochemical demonstration of monoamine oxidase B in brain astrocytes and serotonergic neurons. Proc Natl Acad Sci U S A 79:6385–6389, 1982.
115. Reiderer P, Konradi C, Schay V, et al: Localization of MAO-A and MAO-B in human brain: A step in understanding the therapeutic action of L-deprenyl. Adv Neurol 45:111–118, 1986.
116. Hanbauer I, Wink D, Osawa Y, et al: Role of nitric oxide in NMDA-evoked release of [³H]-dopamine from striatal slices. Neuroreport 3:409–412, 1992.
117. Montague PR, Gancayco CD, Winn MJ, et al: Role of NO production in NMDA receptor-mediated neurotrasmitter release in cerebral cortex. Science 263:973–977, 1994.
118. Chao CC, Hu S, Molitor TW, et al: Activated microglia mediate neuronal cell injury via a nitric oxide mechanism. J Immunol 149:2736–2741, 1992.
119. Merrill JE, Zimmerman RP: Natural and induced cytotoxicity of oligodendrocytes by microglia is inhibitable by TBFβ. Glia 4:327–331, 1991.

120. Lapresle J, Fardeau M: The central nervous system and carbon monoxide poisoning. In Bour H, Ledingham IM (eds): Carbon Monoxide Poisoning. Amsterdam, Elsevier, 1967, pp 31–74.

121. Courville CB: The process of demyelination in the central nervous system. J Nerv Ment Dis 125:504–546, 1957.

122. Putnam TJ, McKenna JB, Morrison LR: Studies in multiple sclerosis. JAMA 97:1591–1596, 1991.

123. Bianco F, Floris R: Transient disappearance of bilateral low-density lesions of the globi pallidi in carbon monoxide intoxication and MRI. J Neuroradiol 15:381–385, 1988.

124. DeReuck J, Deccoo D, Lemahieu I, et al: A positron emission tomography study of patients with acute carbon monoxide poisoning treated by hyperbaric oxygen. J Neurol 240:430–434, 1993.

125. Ducasse JL, Celsis P, Marc-Vergnes JP: Non-comatose patients with acute carbon monoxide poisoning: Hyperbaric or normobaric oxygenation? Undersea Hyperb Med 22:9–15, 1995.

126. Maeda Y, Kawasaki Y, Jibiki I, et al: Effect of therapy with oxygen under high pressure on regional cerebral blood flow in the interval form of carbon monoxide poisoning: Observation from subtraction of technetium-99m HMPAO SPECT brain imaging. Eur Neurol 31:380–383, 1991.

127. Shimosegawa E, Hatazawa J, Nagata K, et al: Cerebral blood flow and glucose metabolism measurements in a patient surviving one year after carbon monoxide intoxication. J Nucl Med 33:1696–1698, 1992.

128. Silverman CS, Brenner J, Murtagh FR: Hemorrhagic necrosis and vascular injury in carbon monoxide poisoning: MR demonstration. AJNR Am J Neuroradiol 14:168–170, 1993.

129. Song SY, Okeda R, Funata N, et al: An experimental study of the pathogenesis of the selective lesion of the globus pallidus in acute carbon monoxide poisoning in cats. Acta Neuropathol 61:232–238, 1983.

130. Lee D, Hsu TL, Chen CH, et al: Myocardial infarction with normal coronary artery after carbon monoxide exposure: A case report. Chin Med J 57:355–359, 1996.

131. Marius-Nunez AL: Myocardial infarction with normal coronary arteries after acute exposure to carbon monoxide. Chest 97:491–494, 1990.

132. Mathieu D, Wattel F: Oxygenotherapie hyperbare et intoxications. In Wattel F, Mathieu D (eds): Oxygenotherapie Hyperbare et Reanimation. Paris, Masson, 1990, pp 129–143.

133. Uchino A, Hasuo K, Shida K, et al: MRI of the brain in chronic carbon monoxide poisoning. Neuroradiology 36:399–401, 1994.

134. Vieregge P, Klostermann W, Blumm RG, et al: Carbon monoxide poisoning: Clinical, neurophysiological, and brain imaging observations in acute disease and follow-up. J Neurol 236:478–481, 1989.

135. Murata T, Itoh S, Koshino Y, et al: Serial cerebral MRI with FLAIR sequences in acute carbon monoxide poisoning. J Comput Assisted Tomogr 19:631–634, 1995.

136. Sakamoto K, Murata T, Omori M, et al: Clinical studies on three cases of the interval form of carbon monoxide poisoning: Serial proton magnetic resonance spectroscopy as a prognostic predictor. Psychiatr Res Neuroimaging Sect 83:179–192, 1998.

137. Yoshii F, Kozuma R, Takahashi W, et al: Magnetic resonance imaging and ¹¹C-N-methylspiperone/positron emission tomography studies in a patient with the interval form of carbon monoxide poisoning. J Neurol Sci 160:87–91, 1998.

138. Thom SR, Kang M, Fisher D, et al: Release of glutathione from erythrocytes and other markers of oxidative stress in carbon monoxide poisoning. J Appl Physiol 82:1424–1432, 1997.

139. Pace N, Strajman E, Walker EL: Acceleration of carbon monoxide elimination in man by high pressure oxygen. Science 111:652–654, 1950.

140. Mathieu D, Nolf M, Durocher A, et al: Acute carbon monoxide poisoning risk of late sequelae and treatment by hyperbaric oxygen. J Toxicol Clin Toxicol 23:315–324, 1985.

141. End E, Long CW: Oxygen under pressure in carbon monoxide poisoning. J Ind Hyg Toxicol 24:302–306, 1942.

142. Chen Q, Banick PD, Thom SR: Functional inhibition of rat polymorphonuclear leukocyte B₂ integrins by hyperbaric oxygen is associated with impaired cGMP synthesis. J Pharmacol Exp Ther 276:929–933, 1996.

143. Thom SR, Mendiguren I, Hardy KR, et al: Inhibition of human neutrophil β₂ integrin-dependent adherence by hyperbaric oxygen. Am J Physiol 272:770–771, 1997.

144. Brown SD, Piantadosi CA: Hyperbaric oxygen for carbon monoxide poisoning. Lancet 1:1032–1033, 1989.

145. Goulon M, Barois A, Rapin M, et al: Carbon monoxide poisoning and acute anoxia due to breathing coal gas and hydrocarbons. Ann Med Interne 120:335–349, 1969 [English translation in J Hyperb Med 1:23–41, 1986].

146. Scheinkestel CD, Bailey M, Myles PS, et al: Hyperbaric or normobaric oxygen for acute carbon monoxide: A randomized controlled clinical trial. Med J Aust 170:203–210, 1999.

147. Kehat I, Shupak A: Letter. Undersea Biomed Res 27, 2000.

148. Hsu LH, Wang JH: Treatment of carbon monoxide poisoning with hyperbaric oxygen. Chin Med J 58:407–413, 1996.

149. Lamy M, Hauguet M: Fifty patients with carbon monoxide intoxication treated with hyperbaric oxygen therapy. Acta Anaesthesiol Belg 1:49–53, 1969.

150. Norkool DM, Kirkpatrick JN: Treatment of acute carbon monoxide poisoning with hyperbaric oxygen: A review of 115 cases. Ann Emerg Med 14:1168–1171, 1985.

151. Roche L, Bertoye A, Vincent P, et al: Comparison de deux groupes de vingt intoxications oxycarbonees traitees par oxygenenormobare et hyperbare. Lyon Med 49:1483–1499, 1968.

152. Hampson NB, Dunford RG, Kramer CC, et al: Selection criteria utilized for hyperbaric oxygen treatment of carbon monoxide poisoning. J Emerg Med 13:227–231, 1995.

153. Waisman D, Shupak A, Weisz G, et al: Hyperbaric oxygen therapy in the pediatric patient: The experience of the Israel Naval Medical Institute. Pediatrics 102:1–9, 1998.

154. Sloan EP, Murphy DG, Hart R, et al: Complications and protocol considerations in carbon monoxide-poisoned patients who require hyperbaric oxygen therapy: Report from a ten-year experience. Ann Emerg Med 18:629–634, 1989.

155. Kindwall EP (ed): Hyperbaric Medicine Practice. Flagstaff, AZ, Best Publishing, 1994.

156. Stone JA, Loar H, Rudge FW: An eleven year review of hyperbaric oxygenation in a military clinical setting. Undersea Biomed Res 18(Suppl):80, 1991.

157. Clark JM: Oxygen toxicity. In Bennett PB, Elliott DH (eds): The Physiology and Medicine of Diving, 4th ed. Philadelphia, WB Saunders, 1993, pp 121–169.

158. Pott F, Westergaard P, Mortensen J, et al: Hyperbaric oxygen treatment and pulmonary function. Undersea Hyperb Med 26:225–228, 1999.

159. Thorsen E, Aanderud L, Aasen TB: Effects of a standard hyperbaric oxygen treatment protocol on pulmonary function. Eur Respir J 12:1442–1445, 1998.

160. Plewes JL, Farhi LE: Peripheral circulatory responses to acute hyperoxia. Undersea Biomed Res 10:123–129, 1983.

161. Comis RL: Bleomycin pulmonary toxicity: Current status and future directions. Semin Oncol 19:64–70, 1992.

162. Lazo JS, Sebati SM, Schellens JH: Bleomycin. Cancer Chemother Biol Response Modif 16:39–47, 1996.

163. Caravati EM, Adams CJ, Joyce SM, et al: Fetal toxicity associated with maternal carbon monoxide poisoning. Ann Emerg Med 17:714–717, 1988.

164. Elkharrat D, Raphael JC, Korach JM, et al: Acute carbon monoxide intoxication and hyperbaric oxygen in pregnancy. Intensive Care Med 17:289–292, 1991.

165. Ginsberg MD, Myers RE: Fetal brain injury after maternal carbon monoxide intoxication. Neurology 26:15–23, 1976.

166. Norman CA, Halton DM: Is carbon monoxide a workplace teratogen? A review and evaluation of the literature. Ann Occup Hyg 34:335–347, 1990.

167. Longo LD, Hill EP: Carbon monoxide uptake and elimination in fetal and maternal sheep. Am J Physiol 232:H324–H330, 1977.

168. Brown DB, Mueller GL, Golich FC: Hyperbaric oxygen treatment for carbon monoxide poisoning in pregnancy: A case report. Aviat Space Environ Med 63:1011–1014, 1992.

169. Gabrielli A, Layon AJ: Carbon monoxide intoxication during pregnancy: A case presentation and pathophysiologic discussion, with emphasis on molecular mechanisms. J Clin Anesth 14:876–882, 1995.

170. Hollander DI, Nagey DA, Welch R, et al: Hyperbaric oxygen therapy for the treatment of acute carbon monoxide poisoning in pregnancy: A case report. J Reprod Med 32:615–617, 1987.

171. Koren G, Sharav T, Pastusazk A, et al: A multicenter, prospective study of fetal outcome following accidental carbon monoxide poisoning in pregnancy. Reprod Toxicol 5:397–403, 1991.

172. Ledingham IM, McBride TI, Jennett WB, et al: Fatal brain damage associated with cardiomyopathy of pregnancy with notes on caesarean section in a hyperbaric chamber. BMJ 4:285–287, 1968.

173. VanHoesen KB, Camporesi EM, Moon RE, et al: Should hyperbaric oxygen be used to treat the pregnant patient for acute carbon monoxide poisoning. JAMA 261:1039–1043, 1989.
174. Cho SH, Yun DR: The experimental study on the effect of hyperbaric oxygen on the pregnancy wastage of rats with acute carbon monoxide poisoning. Seoul J Med 23:67–75, 1982.
175. Gilman SC, Greene KM, Bradley ME, et al: Fetal development: Effects of simulated diving and hyperbaric oxygen treatment. Undersea Biomed Res 9:297–304, 1982.
176. Jennings RT: Women and the hazardous environment: When the pregnant patient requires hyperbaric oxygen therapy. Aviat Space Environ Med 58:370–374, 1987.
177. Crocker PJ, Walker JS: Pediatric carbon monoxide toxicity. J Emerg Med 3:443–448, 1985.
178. Foster M, Goodwin SR, Williams C, et al: Recurrent acute life-threatening events and lactic acidosis caused by chronic carbon monoxide poisoning in an infant. Pediatrics 104:34–39, 1999.
179. Gemelli F, Cattani R: Carbon monoxide poisoning in childhood. BMJ 291:1197, 1985.
180. Binder JW, Roberts RJ: Carbon monoxide intoxication in children. Clin Toxicol 16:287–295, 1980.
181. Lacey DJ: Neurologic sequelae of acute carbon monoxide intoxication. Am J Dis Child 135:145–147, 1981.
182. So GM, Kosofsky BE, Souther JF: Acute hydrocephalus following carbon monoxide poisoning. Pediatr Neurol 17:270–273, 1997.
183. Keenan HT, Bratton SL, Norkool DM, et al: Delivery of hyperbaric oxygen therapy to critically ill, mechanically ventilated children. J Crit Care 13:7–12, 1998.

CHAPTER 95

Cyanide: Hydrogen Cyanide, Inorganic Cyanide Salts, and Nitriles

Steven C. Curry

The subject of cyanide poisoning brings consternation to most physicians because they consider it a rare disorder and are generally unfamiliar with the drugs used to treat it. Thousands of workers undergo cyanide exposure every day (Table 95-1); some victims of smoke inhalation routinely cared for by intensivists experience cyanide poisoning; and cyanide compounds are easily obtainable for use as agents of suicide, homicide, or terror.

The clinical syndrome of cyanide poisoning resembles many other illnesses, and treatment with antidotes with which most physicians are unfamiliar usually must proceed quickly without laboratory confirmation of cyanide poisoning. To provide rapid and effective therapy, the physician must become familiar with the clinical presentation of and clinical clues to the diagnosis of poisoning by cyanide.

Three main sources of cyanide exist: hydrogen cyanide (HCN); inorganic cyanide salts; and cyanogens, which are compounds that release cyanide or that undergo metabolism to cyanide after absorption. HCN and inorganic cyanide salts are discussed first and in most detail. Nitriles, the most commonly encountered cyanogens, which can produce delayed-onset and prolonged cyanide poisoning, are discussed in a separate section at the end of this chapter.

HYDROGEN CYANIDE AND INORGANIC CYANIDE SALTS

Sources and Chemistry

HYDROGEN CYANIDE

HCN (boiling point 27.7°C) exists as a gas or liquid at commonly encountered temperatures. An aqueous solution of HCN (prussic acid or hydrocyanic acid) also is available. Liquid HCN and solutions of prussic acid may release gaseous HCN into the surrounding air. Although a bitter almond odor is attributed to HCN, most persons describe the odor as pungent, musty, or metallic, and about 20% of the population does not easily detect the odor.[1] I have administered odor challenges of 30 to 50 parts per million (ppm) HCN to hundreds of firefighters; none of them thought the odor resembled almonds, and a consistent fraction of 25% were unable to detect any odor. Rapid olfactory fatigue makes it possible for large numbers of victims to be ill from HCN without any alert from a strong or bitter almond odor.

INORGANIC CYANIDE SALTS

Numerous inorganic cyanide salts are used commercially. The most common ones are sodium, potassium, and calcium cyanide. Sodium, potassium, and calcium cyanide are crystalline, white solids that are freely soluble in water.

HYDROGEN CYANIDE FORMATION FROM CYANIDE SALTS

Although cylinders or containers of HCN gas or liquid can release toxic amounts of HCN, most accidental exposures to HCN result from reactions with cyanide salts. When most inorganic cyanide salts come in contact with mineral acids, large quantities of HCN are formed and are released into the atmosphere. Using potassium cyanide (KCN) and sulfuric acid (H_2SO_4) as an example:

$$2KCN + H_2SO_4 \rightarrow 2HCN + K_2SO_4$$

Lethal amounts of HCN can result from mixing water-soluble cyanide salts with water. As an example with KCN:

$$KCN + H_2O \rightleftharpoons HCN + KOH$$

The percentage of cyanide converted to HCN (pK_a 9.3) in aqueous solutions of cyanide salts depends on the pH of the solution. The pH of a cyanide salt solution must be kept above 10.5 to 11 to prevent formation and release of significant quantities of HCN. Deaths from inhalation or dermal absorption of HCN have occurred when workers contaminated with powdered inorganic cyanide salts continued to wear wet clothing rather than completely undressing in decontamination showers.[2]

Solid cyanide salts also can react with water vapor in ambient air to form HCN. Fumigation powders containing sodium cyanide (NaCN) or calcium cyanide ($Ca(CN)_2$) are sprinkled on floors or down rodent burrows. In the presence of water or water vapor, HCN is released and reaches lethal concentrations in air. In the case of $Ca(CN)_2$:

$$Ca(CN)_2 + 2H_2O \rightarrow Ca(OH)_2 + 2HCN$$

Smoke, including that from cigarettes, commonly contains HCN.[3–5] Combustion of almost any organic compound containing carbon and nitrogen can generate HCN under the correct conditions.[6] Cyanide poisoning may be a major factor in death from smoke inhalation, especially in fires involving plastics.

TABLE 95-1 Examples of Occupations Associated with Exposure to Cyanide or Cyanogens

Jewelry making
Metal polishing
Metal plating
Metal stripping
Metal reclaiming
Metal hardening
Mining

Nylon production
Pesticide manufacturing
Pesticide applicator
Laboratory work
Products of combustion
Chemical manufacturing

PHARMACOKINETICS

Absorption. HCN is extremely well absorbed by inhalation and can produce rapid collapse and death within minutes at high concentrations.[7-9] Because HCN is nonionized and of low molecular weight, significant absorption can occur through skin if high enough concentrations are present.[10,11]

Most cyanide salts are absorbed rapidly from mucous membranes and can produce collapse within 1 minute after large ingestions. When cyanide salts are placed in capsules, peak absorption from the stomach and duodenum may be delayed for 20 to 40 minutes.

Exposures of large areas of skin to solid cyanide salts or aqueous solutions can result in absorption of lethal quantities of cyanide across skin. Dermal absorption rate of cyanide increases as the pH of a cyanide solution decreases because of increasing fractions of cyanide being found as HCN at lower pH values.[2]

Brief contact between small areas of skin and dry, powdered cyanide salts would not be expected to produce toxicity. Prolonged skin contact with smaller skin areas still can produce toxicity, however.[12] Increased absorption occurs across abraded or burned skin.[13] Onset of symptoms following large acute skin exposures has been delayed for 30 minutes if decontamination has not been effective, such as when a worker continues to wear wet, contaminated clothing.[2]

Distribution. At physiologic pH, virtually all cyanide in the body exists as HCN, and *cyanide* is used synonymously with *HCN* in this chapter when referring to cyanide in the body. Cyanide distributes widely after absorption. Measurable cyanide concentrations are found in liver, spleen, kidney, brain, heart, spinal cord, lung, and fetus after acute poisoning. Because cyanide is concentrated within erythrocytes by binding to normally low concentrations of methemoglobin (Fig. 95-1), cyanide's apparent volume of distribution varies depending on circulating methemoglobin concentrations and depending on whether such binding is saturated.[14-16]

Metabolism. Humans detoxify cyanide by transferring sulfane sulfur to cyanide to form thiocyanate (SCN^-) (see Fig. 95-1). Thiocyanate undergoes renal clearance with an elimination half-life of about 2.7 days in persons with normal renal function.[17]

The exact mechanism for cyanide's transulfuration in vivo is controversial. Two main enzymes convert cyanide to thiocyanate. Rhodanese (thiosulfate sulfurtransferase, EC 2.8.1.1) is restricted to mitochondria and found in various tissues, especially liver, kidney, and skeletal muscle.[18,19] A reaction catalyzed by rhodanese in vitro involves the transfer of a sulfur atom from thiosulfate ($S_2O_3^{2-}$) to cyanide:

$$CN^- + S_2O_3^{2-} \rightarrow SCN^- + SO_3^{2-}$$

Another enzyme, β-mercaptopyruvate–cyanide sulfurtransferase (EC 2.8.1.2), resides in liver, kidneys, and erythrocytes[19] and transfers sulfur from mercaptopyruvate to cyanide to form SCN^- by the following reaction:

$$HSCH_2COCOO^- + CN^- \rightarrow SCN^- + CH_3COCOO^-$$

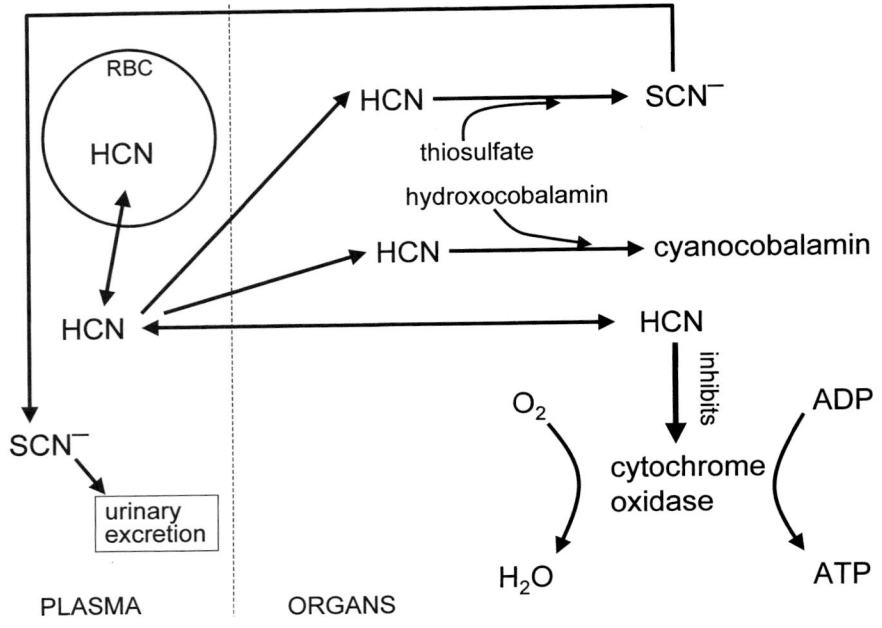

FIGURE 95-1

Schematic diagram of cyanide's distribution and elimination. At physiologic pH, virtually all cyanide is present as hydrogen cyanide (HCN). HCN that has entered plasma after absorption is concentrated within red blood cells, at least in part by binding to the normally small amount of methemoglobin, which contains ferric (Fe^{3+}) iron. HCN also easily diffuses across cell membranes into various organs, where it binds to and inhibits many enzymes, the most important being cytochrome oxidase. HCN binds to the binuclear center (copper and iron) of cytochrome oxidase to inhibit electron transport through this complex. This produces a decrease in oxygen consumption and, indirectly, a decrease in adenosine triphosphate formation. HCN is detoxified by transulfuration to thiocyanate (SCN^-), which is excreted in the urine.

The aforementioned controversy surrounding in vivo cyanide transulfuration revolves around several pieces of seemingly conflicting data. Although rhodanese was historically credited with cyanide's detoxification, thiosulfate, a substrate for rhodanese, is thought to be unable to penetrate the inner mitochondrial membrane where rhodanese is located.[20,21] Ballantyne and others[19,20,22] suggested a paradigm whereby numerous sulfur sources are acted on by various sulfurtransferases, including rhodanese and mercaptopyruvate sulfurtransferase, to form sulfane sulfur, which then complexes with albumin in blood. A nonenzymatic reaction of the sulfane-albumin complex with cyanide could account for thiocyanate formation. Other data suggest, however, that the albumin-sulfane complex seems to play a minor role in detoxification of cyanide in vivo. In rats in which blood has been replaced by a fluorocarbon emulsion, sodium thiosulfate still efficiently antagonizes cyanide.[23] In the absence of blood or circulating albumin, cyanide's detoxication can be attributed only to sulfurtransferase reactions occurring in tissue sites other than blood. Regardless of the exact mechanism explaining cyanide's transulfuration, investigators agree that sulfur sources such as thiosulfate are required for and greatly accelerate conversion of cyanide to thiocyanate.

Cyanide's affinity for the cobalt ion (Co^{2+}) causes it to combine with hydroxocobalamin to form cyanocobalamin (see Fig. 95-1), which is excreted in the urine and bile. This route of detoxification normally plays a minor role in acute cyanide poisoning. The administration of large amounts of hydroxocobalamin is used as antidotal therapy in France, however.[24] Hydroxocobalamin is not available in suitable form for this purpose in the United States.

Data on the rate at which toxic concentrations of cyanide are eliminated are limited because of inaccurate measurements of whole-blood cyanide concentrations that have been reported in poisoned patients owing to conversion of plasma thiocyanate to HCN during analysis (described later). Induction of methemoglobinemia, a treatment strategy, causes HCN to redistribute from tissues into blood (decrease in apparent volume of distribution), producing changes in blood cyanide concentrations that do not reflect absorption or elimination. Schulz[16] wrote that because of limited availability of sulfane sulfur, transulfuration of cyanide is saturable, with an average elimination rate of 1 μg HCN/kg/min in an adult. Cole and Vesey,[25] who reported decreases in elevated and accurately measured red blood cell and plasma cyanide concentrations after infusions of sodium nitroprusside were stopped, found that elimination appeared to be first order, with a half-life of about 30 minutes in the absence of sodium thiosulfate supplementation. When sodium thiosulfate was given, the elimination half-life decreased to about 10 minutes.[25] The cyanide levels were not high enough, however, to be associated with serious toxicity. The possibility of saturable elimination kinetics at higher cyanide concentrations cannot be excluded.

Pathophysiology

Cyanide inhibits more than 40 enzymes.[20,26,27] Cyanide's affinity for cytochrome oxidase in the mitochondrial inner membrane accounts for most toxicity, however. Cytochrome oxidase serves as the terminal enzyme in the electron trans-

port chain responsible for oxidative phosphorylation and transfers electrons onto oxygen to produce water. After binding to the copper-iron binuclear center of cytochrome oxidase,[28] HCN prevents electron transport, which inhibits oxidative phosphorylation and oxygen consumption.[29] Cyanide's ability to inhibit glutamate decarboxylase might produce a decrease in brain γ-aminobutyric acid concentrations and contribute to seizures.[30]

A metabolic acidosis and decrease in oxygen consumption accompany serious cyanide poisoning. The metabolic acidosis frequently is incorrectly attributed to elevated circulating lactate concentrations resulting from glycolytic conversion of glucose to lactate in the presence of impaired oxidative phosphorylation. Unquestionably the glycolytic conversion of glucose to lactate is accelerated and becomes an important source of adenosine triphosphate (ATP) during cyanide poisoning, resulting in elevated lactate concentrations. ATP production via the conversion of glucose to lactate is not significantly acidifying, however (see Chapter 57).[31-33] Although the exact amounts of ATP and lactate generated in glycolysis vary with cellular pH and concentrations of available substrates,[32] glycolytic production of lactic acid and ATP results in minimal production of protons regardless of pH.[32,34,35]

An understanding of the generation of ATP in oxidative phosphorylation and of hydrolysis of ATP in metabolic processes explains metabolic acidosis in cyanide poisoning. Cells hydrolyze ATP to adenosine diphosphate and phosphate for energy, and ATP hydrolysis results in net proton production. Conversely, in oxidative phosphorylation, there is a net consumption of protons during ATP synthesis. When homeostatic mechanisms are operating normally, a normal pH is maintained to a large extent because ATP is being hydrolyzed at the same rate that it is being synthesized via mitochondrial oxidative phosphorylation; that is, proton production from ATP hydrolysis (including from ATP produced in glycolysis) is balanced by mitochondrial proton consumption during ATP synthesis in oxidative phosphorylation.[34] Oxidative phosphorylation is an important buffer of protons for this reason. When cyanide impairs the electron transport chain, and oxidative phosphorylation slows or stops, protons created by the cellular hydrolysis of preformed ATP and of ATP produced anaerobically in glycolysis are no longer buffered by aerobic ATP synthesis.[32] Cyanide's binding to cytochrome oxidase impairs electron transport, resulting in a decrease in oxygen consumption and ATP production. Cells accelerate anaerobic glycolytic ATP production with the conversion of glucose to lactate. Although cellular and circulating lactate concentrations increase, the lactic acid is not responsible for acidosis. Rather, the acidosis occurs because cells hydrolyze ATP generated in glycolysis, producing protons, while the ability to buffer hydrogen ions via oxidative phosphorylation is impaired.

There are several reasons why cyanide poisoning is characterized mainly by dysfunction of the cardiovascular system and central nervous system. In the presence of acidosis and decreasing ATP concentrations from impaired oxidative phosphorylation, organs most sensitive to energy deprivation (brain, heart) suffer first. Cytochrome oxidase in the heart also is more sensitive to inhibition by cyanide.[36]

Finally, cyanide concentrations are higher in brain and myocardium than in other organs at the time of death.[20]

The minimal concentration of HCN in air required to produce death in humans remains ill defined because most acute fatal poisonings result from large exposures. Animal species vary in their sensitivity to cyanide, and data indicate that prolonged exposures to HCN concentrations greater than 90 ppm are incompatible with life.[37] In human cases of poisoning in which ambient HCN concentrations have been reported, headache, metallic taste, and other minor symptoms have developed after several minutes of exposure to air containing 10 to 30 ppm of HCN.[37] Death may occur within 1 hour of continuous inhalational exposure to 100 ppm of HCN[20,37] and within several minutes of breathing more than 300 ppm of HCN. Humans have survived a 90-second exposure to 453 to 557 ppm of HCN (estimated) and a 3-minute exposure to 500 ppm of HCN.[8,9] Ballantyne[20] suggested that the inhalational 5-minute median lethal concentration for HCN is 680 ppm, and the 30-minute median lethal concentration is 200 ppm.

A lethal oral dose of HCN (in solution) is estimated at 50 mg in an adult; the ingestion of 5 mL of 20% hydrocyanic acid has been fatal. The lethal oral doses of KCN or NaCN are estimated at 200 to 300 mg, but survival has followed much larger doses with intensive supportive care.[38-40]

Clinical Presentation

Onset of symptoms of cyanide poisoning may occur within seconds after the inhalation of concentrated HCN gas or mucosal contact with inorganic cyanide salts. The inhalation of moderate HCN concentrations may not produce toxicity until minutes to hours into the exposure. Persons who are asymptomatic or only moderately symptomatic after the inhalation of HCN do not worsen after exposure is terminated. Delayed onset of symptoms after the inhalation of HCN does not occur. Absorption may be delayed after ingestion of cyanide sequestered in capsules, with peak symptoms not occurring for 20 to 40 minutes or so.

The main hallmarks of acute cyanide poisoning, which are nonspecific, are central nervous system and cardiovascular dysfunction and a metabolic acidosis. Central nervous system dysfunction ranges from anxiety to confusion, delirium, lethargy, coma, convulsions, and cerebral death. Large acute exposures may result in collapse into generalized seizures. Tachypnea may occur early in cyanide poisoning from initial stimulation of carotid body receptors by relatively low concentrations of cyanide. Lethal concentrations of cyanide rapidly produce apnea.

Cardiovascular toxicity early in cyanide poisoning is characterized by tachycardia and, at times, mild transient hypertension. As the illness progresses, hypotension, tachycardia, bradycardia, heart blocks, ventricular arrhythmias, and asystole follow. Wexler and colleagues[41] described electrocardiographic changes in 16 men who received 0.2 mg cyanide/kg body weight intravenously. Sinus arrest lasting 0.88 to 4.2 seconds immediately preceded tachypnea and was thought to be vagally mediated. The periods of sinus arrest were followed by irregularities in sinus rhythms, with slowing of heart rates for periods of a few seconds to 2 minutes. There was gradual acceleration of heart rate to levels higher than control values. Wexler and colleagues[41]

also described electrocardiographic changes in four men executed by inhalation of HCN. They reported progressive shortening of the ST segment until, terminally, the T wave originated on the R wave. This "T-on-R" phenomenon has been described in other cases of cyanide poisoning.[38]

Other common signs and symptoms in patients with cyanide poisoning include diaphoresis, weakness, nausea, and vomiting.[42] In serious poisoning, additional organ systems fail, leading to rhabdomyolysis, renal failure, hepatic necrosis, and adult respiratory distress syndrome.[20,39,43]

The alkaline nature of granular cyanide salts or their aqueous solutions explains occasional corrosive injury when they come in contact with moist mucosal surfaces, including the gastrointestinal tract. Dermal injury also has followed acute skin contact with alkaline cyanide solutions.[44]

Victims of cyanide poisoning may be left with permanent neurologic sequelae, including necrosis of the basal ganglia.[45,46] Lesions in the basal ganglia are not specific for cyanide but are seen after severe hypoxemia or after poisoning by many metabolic toxins, including carbon monoxide, ethylene glycol, sodium azide, and methanol.

Diagnosis

When confronted with a case of suspected cyanide poisoning, physicians must make therapeutic decisions before results of cyanide levels are available. Certain historical points, physical findings, and general laboratory data must be used to seek evidence of cyanide poisoning.

Rapid collapse into coma or convulsions suggests the possibility of cyanide poisoning, but many patients may have gradual onset of symptoms over minutes to hours if exposures have been prolonged but not as intense, and toxicity may never become severe enough to produce coma. As noted earlier, the alleged bitter almond odor of cyanide is rarely noted, and it is possible for several persons in an exposure incident to die of cyanide poisoning without anyone's complaining of or noting an abnormal odor.

Many patients with serious cyanide poisoning are hypothermic. Depressed oxygen consumption from cyanide may produce an increased oxygen content of peripheral and mixed venous blood[47-49] if cardiac output is maintained. Bright red venous blood or retinal veins suggests the possibility of cyanide poisoning.[50] Most victims do not have unusually bright red skin or blood, however, and many victims exhibit cyanosis[46,51,52] because low cardiac output and intrapulmonary shunting in any patient with severe shock can cause arterial hypoxemia, despite low oxygen consumption. The absence of bright red skin or blood should never be used to exclude the possibility of cyanide poisoning.

An anion gap metabolic acidosis is always present in serious cyanide poisoning, unless the patient had a preexistent serious metabolic alkalosis or has received significant doses of sodium bicarbonate. Arterial lactate concentrations are elevated, but the lactate concentration does not account for the entire increase in anion gap or base deficit because lactate is not actually responsible for acidosis (discussed earlier).

Cardiovascular and metabolic parameters obtained from invasive monitoring in patients with cyanide poisoning may reveal changes compatible with many disorders, including sepsis, toxic shock syndrome, or hepatic failure. Similar to cyanide poisoning, all of these conditions can produce metabolic acidosis, hypotension, decrease in oxygen consumption, increase in mixed venous oxygen content, decrease in the arterial-venous oxygen content difference, and systemic vasodilation. Because baseline values (i.e., before cyanide poisoning) for oxygen consumption and mixed venous oxygen content are unknown for individual patients; because both parameters are influenced by cardiac output, which can vary from normal to increased early in cyanide poisoning to profound depression near death; and because both parameters depend on adequacy of oxygenation (e.g., adequate respiration, normal ventilation/perfusion), it is impossible to determine absolute cutoffs for oxygen consumption or mixed venous oxygen content that should strongly suggest cyanide toxicity. There are no studies examining the predictive values of these parameters for the diagnosis of cyanide poisoning. About the only statement that can be safely made is that a clearly normal or elevated oxygen consumption in a comatose patient does not suggest cyanide toxicity.

Claims[53,54] that cyanide combines with hemoglobin to produce cyanhemoglobin and a difference between calculated arterial hemoglobin saturation and that measured by multiwavelength cooximetry (percent saturation gap) are unfounded and have never been documented. In fact, studies have shown that erythrocytes mixed with cyanide fail to show impaired oxygen carrying capacity until after a time that death would already have occurred,[55] and cooximetry of whole blood containing lethal concentrations of cyanide does not show a percent saturation gap.[56] An unexplainable percent saturation gap is unexpected in patients with isolated and untreated (i.e., no methemoglobinemia) cyanide poisoning.

CYANIDE LEVELS

The diagnosis of cyanide poisoning can be confirmed by measurement of circulating cyanide concentrations. Plasma cyanide is in equilibrium with tissue cyanide and correlates with tissue cyanide levels.[15,57] In blood, most cyanide is concentrated within red blood cells, however, making red blood cell cyanide concentrations many times higher than concentrations in plasma. The higher levels of cyanide found in red blood cells are more easily measured, and red blood cell cyanide concentrations correlate with concentrations in plasma and tissue. Red blood cell cyanide concentrations are best used to confirm the diagnosis of cyanide poisoning.

Red blood cell cyanide concentrations of healthy adults are generally less than 29 μg/L (1 μmol/L).[16] In nonanemic patients with normal methemoglobin fractions, early metabolic disturbances from cyanide toxicity (e.g., metabolic acidosis) begin to appear at red blood cell cyanide concentrations of about 1 mg/L.[58] Obvious cyanide toxicity is apparent when red blood cell cyanide concentrations reach about 5 mg/L.

Plasma cyanide concentrations can be used to diagnose cyanide poisoning, but accurate measurement is difficult given the much lower levels and the high volatility of HCN, allowing HCN to escape into the atmosphere when the tube of blood is opened for separation of plasma and cells. Wilson and Mathews[59] reported that plasma cyanide concentrations in healthy subjects averaged 4 μg/L (0.15 μmol/L) in nonsmokers and 6 μg/L (0.22 μmol/L) in smokers. Cottrell and

colleagues[60] reported that mild metabolic acidosis developed in some patients receiving sodium nitroprusside under anesthesia when plasma cyanide concentrations reached approximately 30 to 35 μg/L (approximately 1 μmol/L). Vesey and Cole[61] estimated the minimal lethal plasma cyanide concentration to be 243 μg/L (9 μmol/L). Sheep dying from intramuscular potassium cyanide injections had plasma cyanide concentrations ranging from 900 to 2200 μg/L (33 to 81 μmol/L).[20] Because of difficulty in accurate measurement, plasma cyanide concentrations are best reserved for experimental studies in which collection, processing, and analysis are under tight quality control by personnel who regularly perform such measurements.

Measurements of *whole-blood* cyanide concentrations commonly offered by reference laboratories can fail to reflect accurate measurements of circulating cyanide. During acidification of whole blood during analysis, oxyhemoglobin released from red blood cells combines with thiocyanate in plasma to generate HCN de novo.[14] Falsely high whole-blood cyanide concentrations can result whenever plasma thiocyanate concentrations are elevated significantly above normal (but not to toxic levels), even while cyanide concentrations are quite low or within the normal range. Examples of such situations in which this occurs are in patients receiving sodium nitroprusside infusions, patients with cyanide poisoning who have been treated with sodium thiosulfate for cyanide poisoning, and patients who have been exposed to cyanide and have successfully metabolized it to thiocyanate (with or without ever having experienced cyanide poisoning). Reported whole-blood cyanide levels may be higher than actual values and may easily mislead the physician into thinking that cyanide toxicity was present when it was not. Whole-blood cyanide concentrations generally should not be ordered unless their limitations are recognized when interpreting results. The potential for falsely elevated whole-blood cyanide levels also may contribute to the relatively wide range of upper boundaries for normal concentrations reported in the literature, ranging from about 0.05 to 0.5 mg/L (1.7 to 17 μmol/L).

Finally, cyanide concentrations can change during transportation and storage of tissue.[1,7,62] Several reports describe a decrease in cyanide levels in whole blood during storage, whereas others describe increases in cyanide content. The freezing and thawing of whole-blood specimens causes whole-blood cyanide concentrations to rise compared with prefrozen values.[63] The mechanism is probably mechanical hemolysis causing HCN formation from oxyhemoglobin and plasma thiocyanate during thawing. Whole-blood specimens should not be frozen during storage and transport.

Differential Diagnosis

The toxicologic differential diagnosis of cyanide poisoning is extensive and includes asphyxiation (e.g., inert gases, methane, nitrogen, carbon dioxide); poisonings by hydrogen sulfide and sulfide salts, methanol, ethylene glycol, pentaborane, azide, arsine, stibine, phosphine, phenol, cresol, methyl halides, and carbon monoxide; and, when cyanosis is present, methemoglobinemia. Any illness characterized by sudden convulsions may be accompanied by hypotension, hypoxemia, and metabolic acidosis (e.g., poisoning by isoniazid or strychnine). Sudden unexpected collapse into unconsciousness or convulsions accompanied by metabolic acidosis and decreased oxygen consumption despite adequate oxygen delivery makes one lean toward the diagnosis of cyanide or sulfide poisoning.

Treatment

PHARMACOLOGIC BASES FOR ANTIDOTAL STRATEGIES

In the United States, the main antidotal strategy for treating cyanide poisoning comprises the combined goals of induction of methemoglobinemia with amyl nitrite or sodium nitrite and enhancement of conversion of cyanide to thiocyanate by sodium thiosulfate. Hydrogen cyanide binds to the binuclear iron-copper center of cytochrome oxidase. Cyanide expresses low affinity for ferrous iron (Fe^{2+}) in hemoglobin, however. When iron of reduced hemoglobin is oxidized to the ferric state, methemoglobin is formed, and cyanide exhibits high affinity for Fe^{3+} in methemoglobin. Induction of methemoglobinemia with nitrites serves to create a large circulating sink of ferric iron that binds cyanide, allowing cyanide to dissociate from cytochrome oxidase in tissue and redistribute into plasma and into red blood cells, where it combines with methemoglobin to form cyanmethemoglobin (Fig. 95-2).[29]

Methemoglobin cannot carry oxygen and shifts the oxygen-hemoglobin dissociation curve to the left. The body has extensive mechanisms for maintaining methemoglobin fractions within erythrocytes at less than 1% to 2% (i.e., 1% to 2% of all heme pigments are in the methemoglobin form). Methemoglobin fractions of 20% to 30% are tolerated, however, without life-threatening symptoms in otherwise healthy persons without anemia.[64]

The short-term inhalation of amyl nitrite is relatively ineffective at producing methemoglobinemia compared with intravenous sodium nitrite[65] but is meant to serve as a temporizing measure until intravenous access can be established. The historically recommended dose of sodium nitrite for nonanemic symptomatic adults with cyanide poisoning is 10 mL of a 3% solution (300 mg) intravenously over several minutes.[65] Several authors advocate methemoglobin fractions of 25% to 40% (assuming no anemia) to be most effective.[66–68] Much lower methemoglobin fractions are achieved, however, with the recommended dose of 300 mg of intravenous sodium nitrite.[65,66] Peak methemoglobin fractions of 10.1% after 400 mg of intravenous sodium nitrite and of 17.5% after 600 mg of intravenous sodium nitrite were reported by Moser.[69] Kiese and Weger[66] noted that methemoglobin fractions increased to a mean of 7% in six volunteers receiving intravenous sodium nitrite, 4 mg/kg. A single volunteer developed a methemoglobin fraction of 30% after 12 mg/kg of intravenous sodium nitrite.

Methemoglobin fractions may not peak until 30 minutes after 4 mg/kg of intravenous sodium nitrite or until 60 minutes after 12 mg/kg of intravenous sodium nitrite.[66] Despite slow onset of methemoglobinemia after 300 mg of intravenous sodium nitrite, the combination of intravenous sodium nitrite and sodium thiosulfate remains superior to more rapid methemoglobin-forming agents,[21] possibly because of a more sustained methemoglobinemia produced by sodium nitrite. The fact that dramatic improvements in symptoms have occurred well before methemoglobin levels have peaked[48,70] also suggests that mechanisms other than methemoglobin production may be important in nitrite's antidotal action.[21,71]

Indications for ICU Admission in Cyanide Poisoning

Patients symptomatic from cyanide poisoning
Patients who have been exposed to potentially toxic doses of nitriles—onset of cyanide poisoning may be delayed for longer than 12 to 15 hours

---

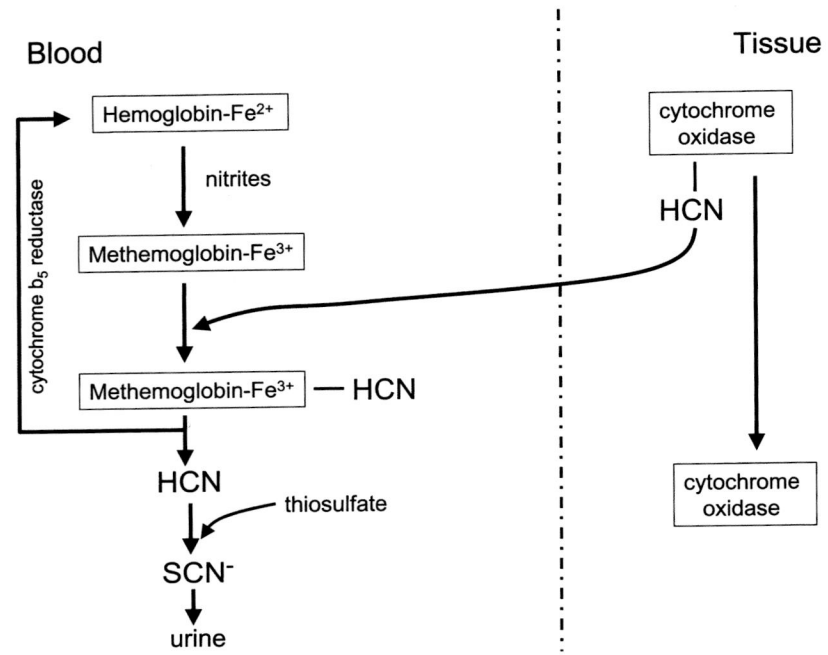

FIGURE 95-2

Antidotal strategies in the treatment of cyanide toxicity with nitrites and thiosulfate. Hydrogen cyanide (HCN) binds to tissue cytochrome oxidase to inhibit oxidative phosphorylation. Nitrite (sodium nitrite or amyl nitrite) converts some ferrous hemoglobin (Fe^{2+}) to methemoglobin (Fe^{3+}), creating a large circulating sink of ferric iron. HCN quickly dissociates from cytochrome oxidase and moves from tissue to bind to methemoglobin, forming cyanmethemoglobin and reversing inhibition of cytochrome oxidase. As cyanmethemoglobin is reduced back to Fe^{2+}, HCN is released. Sodium thiosulfate markedly enhances transulfuration of HCN to thiocyanate (SCN^-).

Sodium thiosulfate (a source of sulfane sulfur) enhances conversion of cyanide to thiocyanate. The recommended dose is 12.5 g intravenously over a few minutes. Although methemoglobinemia can rapidly reverse serious cyanide poisoning, cyanide eventually is released from cyanmethemoglobin as this pigment is reduced to hemoglobin.[72] Coadministration of sodium thiosulfate with sodium nitrite enhances transulfuration of cyanide that is unbound or that is released from cyanmethemoglobin to thiocyanate. Thiocyanate is of low-order toxicity and undergoes renal elimination with a half-life of 2.7 days in patients with normal renal function. The combination of sodium nitrite and sodium thiosulfate increases the required lethal dose for cyanide 13 times in some animal models, whereas lethal dose increases of 3 to 4 times are noted when each agent is given alone.[73]

Some animal data suggest that vasodilation from nitrites might be beneficial in treating cyanide poisoning. α-Adrenoceptor antagonist vasodilators (e.g., phenoxybenzamine, chlorpromazine) enhance antidotal effects of thiosulfate in animal models of cyanide poisoning but have little action by themselves.[74,75] Conversely, injection of erythrocytes exposed to nitrite in vitro (to produce methemoglobin) then washed free of excess nitrite provides a degree of protection equivalent to that produced by nitrite directly injected into animals poisoned with cyanide, indicating that vasodilation plays a relatively unimportant role in explaining nitrite's antidotal action compared with methemoglobin induction.[72]

Vasodilation and hypotension produced by nitrites has in part led investigators in the armed services and in other countries to use other antidotal agents in the treatment of cyanide poisoning.[67,76] No controlled trials have examined the comparative efficacy of any agents, including nitrites and thiosulfate, in humans with symptomatic cyanide poisoning. DMAP (4-dimethylaminophenol) induces methemoglobinemia more rapidly than nitrite and is routinely used in Germany.[76]

Cobalt-EDTA (ethylenediaminetetraacetic acid), used in England and Australia, chelates cyanide, which then is renally excreted.[77] It is available in 20-mL ampules, each containing 300 mg of cobalt-EDTA. The recommended dose is one ampule (300 mg) intravenously over 1 minute. Repeat doses can be given after 1 and 5 minutes if there is no response, and slower infusion rates should be allowed for non–critically ill patients. The main side effect seems to be an anaphylactoid reaction, which can be life-threatening.

Cyanide's affinity for cobalt also is exploited in France, where a concentrated aqueous solution of hydroxocobalamin is available for intravenous administration. Hydroxocobalamin combines with cyanide to form cyanocobalamin, which is excreted in the urine.[24] The recommended initial dose is 5 g intravenously, although some authorities begin with 10 g in seriously ill patients. In animal studies, hydroxocobalamin alone raises the lethal dose only three to four times (similar to nitrite alone). In some but not all animal models, the addition of intravenous sodium thiosulfate to hydroxocobalamin therapy enhances antidotal activity of hydroxocobalamin, but thiosulfate cannot be mixed with hydroxocobalamin or the cobalamin is inactivated. Intravenous sodium thiosulfate should be given as a separate infusion after dosing with hydroxocobalamin. An obvious advantage of hydroxocobalamin (and cobalt-EDTA) is the lack of methemoglobin induction, which could be advantageous in treating patients with cyanide poisoning from smoke inhalation, who also may have carbon monoxide poisoning. A disadvantage is that hydroxocobalamin dosing produces bright red discoloration of skin, urine, and plasma, and the plasma discoloration may interfere with some laboratory analyses.[78] No safe, concentrated formulation of hydroxocobalamin is commercially available in the United States.

Inhalation of 100% oxygen (along with nitrite and thiosulfate) enhances survival over breathing room air in animals, but no advantage of hyperbaric oxygen therapy over the administration of 100% oxygen at 1 atm has been shown.[79]

GENERAL MANAGEMENT

Patients who are symptomatic after the inhalation of HCN do not require decontamination. A person who has inhaled HCN without becoming seriously ill is not in danger of developing delayed onset of more serious symptoms after exposure is terminated.[7]

Patients who have undergone significant skin contamination with solid cyanide salts or solutions may serve as a threat to rescuers and treating medical personnel. *All* clothing (including shoes or boots) should be removed, and the victim should be thoroughly decontaminated with copious volumes of water before entering a hospital. Inadequate decontamination results in generation of HCN from water and remaining cyanide salts, with potential for off-gassing of HCN or delayed absorption of HCN through the skin.

Patients who have ingested cyanide salts and who have remained asymptomatic for 1 to 2 hours would not be expected to become ill. It seems unlikely that activated charcoal could be given quickly enough after oral ingestion of cyanide to change the clinical course of cyanide poisoning. Distending a patient's stomach with a solution of charcoal when the patient may become unconscious or begin convulsing at any moment may promote vomiting and pulmonary aspiration. Gastric emptying by lavage is not known to be effective and generally is not recommended.

Symptomatic patients who have ingested cyanide salts may regurgitate HCN gas. Mouth-to-mouth ventilation is not recommended in such instances. The odor (usually poorly described) of HCN can be noted sometimes around the mouth of comatose patients who have ingested cyanide compounds, but there has never been a death or severe illness from inhalation of HCN in a person who has cared for such a patient, although mild symptoms (nausea, light-headedness) have been claimed. A letter to the editor claims that mouth-to-mouth resuscitation of a cyanide-poisoned dog produced coma in the rescuer.[80] Potential for inhaling some HCN when intubating such patients should be recognized.

After addressing airway, ventilation, and circulation, efforts should be directed immediately toward antidotal therapy in symptomatic patients. A commercially available cyanide antidote kit (Taylor Pharmaceuticals/Akorn Inc., San Clemente, CA) contains breakable amyl nitrite pearls for induction of methemoglobinemia by inhalation and injectable solutions of sodium nitrite and sodium thiosulfate. Each of these agents also may be purchased individually.

Amyl nitrite inhalation is meant to be used as a temporizing measure until intravenous access is established so that sodium nitrite can be given intravenously. A crushed amyl nitrite pearl is held in front of the patient's nose and mouth or in front of an intake valve of a ventilation bag for 30 seconds of every minute. There are no controlled trials determining the best dose for the treatment of cyanide poisoning.

Antidotal Therapy for Cyanide Poisoning

1. If no intravenous line is established, break amyl nitrite pearl and hold over patient's nose/mouth or intake valve of ventilation bag for 30 seconds of every minute while intravenous line is being established.
2. As soon as intravenous line is established, give 300 mg of sodium nitrite intravenously. For critically ill patients, infuse over 2 to 3 minutes. For less severely poisoned patients, infusion can be over several minutes to limit hypotension (see separate box for pediatric doses).
3. Next infuse 12.5 g of sodium thiosulfate intravenously over 2 to 5 minutes (see separate box for pediatric doses).

As soon as intravenous access is established, 10 mL of a 3% solution of sodium nitrite (300 mg) should be given intravenously. For moribund patients, the sodium nitrite can be given over 1 to 2 minutes. For less severely ill patients, it can be given more slowly to prevent significant falls in blood pressure. The administration of an entire ampule (10 mL) of 3% sodium nitrite to a small child potentially may produce lethal methemoglobinemia.[68] The same is true for adults with severe anemia. Children without anemia can receive 0.33 mL of 3% sodium nitrite/kg body weight, up to 10 mL.

After the administration of intravenous sodium nitrite, 50 mL of 25% sodium thiosulfate should be administered intravenously to adults over several minutes. The pediatric dose is 1.65 mL of 25% sodium thiosulfate/kg body weight.[68]

Criteria for ICU Discharge in Cyanide Poisoning

Patients who were symptomatic from exposure to inorganic cyanide compounds or hydrogen cyanide:
 No antidotal therapy (nitrites or thiosulfate) given in last 12 hours
 No signs or symptoms of cyanide poisoning (e.g., no metabolic acidosis, normal vital signs)
Patients exposed to nitriles:
 If never symptomatic, at least 24 hours must have passed since exposure
 If patient developed signs and symptoms of cyanide poisoning, at least 24 hours must have passed since patient has received any cyanide antidotes, and the patient must have remained asymptomatic during this time without antidotal therapy

Doses of sodium nitrite and sodium thiosulfate can be repeated if signs of cyanide poisoning (e.g., metabolic acidosis with coma) persist for 30 minutes or recur. In my experience, methemoglobin fractions remained less than 20% in nonanemic adults who received two doses of 300 mg of sodium nitrite given within 10 minutes, and this is in keeping with data by Moser.[69] If cooximetry is available, however, total hemoglobin and methemoglobin concentrations should be measured rapidly before repeating a dose of sodium nitrite to ensure that dangerous methemoglobinemia will not occur, especially in children.

Treatment is otherwise supportive. Severe metabolic acidosis may require treatment with sodium bicarbonate. Adult respiratory distress syndrome is treated with positive-pressure ventilation and continuous positive airway pressure. Rhabdomyolysis is treated by ensuring a brisk urine output and keeping the urine pH above approximately 6.0.

Special Populations

PREGNANT PATIENTS

As a small lipophilic molecule, HCN distributes easily to most organs, including the fetus; for example, newborns of smoking mothers have higher blood cyanide concentrations than newborns of nonsmoking mothers.[81] No studies have examined the efficacy or toxicity of sodium nitrite or sodium thiosulfate in pregnant women. No guidelines exist for dosing of sodium nitrite to pregnant women with cyanide poisoning, although maternally administered sodium nitrite produces methemoglobinemia in the fetus.[82] In third-trimester gravid ewes with cyanide toxicity from sodium nitroprusside infusions, the administration of sodium thiosulfate prevented increases in circulating fetal cyanide concentrations, even though thiosulfate did not appear to cross the placenta.[83] This finding is best explained by the ability of thiosulfate to keep maternal cyanide levels low, allowing for cyanide to diffuse back out of the fetus into the maternal circulation for detoxification. Given limited available data, pregnant patients with cyanide poisoning should be treated similarly to other patients. Fetal health is best ensured by ensuring the survival of the mother.

Pediatric Doses of Cyanide Antidotes

Intravenous Sodium Nitrite

1. If child is ill and not known to be anemic, give 0.33 mL/kg 3% sodium nitrite intravenously up to initial dose of 10 mL.
2. If patient is known to be anemic, adjust for hemoglobin concentration as follows:

Hemoglobin Concentration (g/dL)	3% Sodium Nitrite Solution (mL/kg)
7	0.19
8	0.22
9	0.25
10	0.27
11	0.30
12	0.33
13	0.36
14	0.39

Intravenous Sodium Thiosulfate

1. Give 1.65 mL/kg 25% sodium thiosulfate solution.

CYANOGENS

Cyanogens are natural or synthetic compounds that, after absorption, undergo metabolism to release HCN (Table 95-2). (The term *cyanogen* also is used as a synonym for ethanedinitrile.) Nitriles (R-C-CN) and sodium nitroprusside account for most toxic exposure to synthetic cyanogens. Cyanide glycosides (e.g., amygdalin) are found naturally in many foods and plants. Because sodium nitroprusside is discussed in Chapter 37 and cyanide glycosides are discussed in Chapter 125, the toxicity of nitriles are emphasized in this section. Nitriles are used as solvents, as intermediates in chemical synthesis, in nylon production, and for other purposes. Acetonitrile was commonly used in artificial fingernail glue remover, with tragic results in children who accidentally ingested these products.

Clinical Presentation

Nitriles can be absorbed by inhalation, through dermal contact, or after ingestion. Poisonings by nitriles differ, however, from poisonings by inorganic cyanide salts and HCN in three general ways. First, there may be a delay between exposure and the onset of symptoms for many hours, because hours may be required for nitrile metabolism to release enough HCN to produce symptoms. Second, because of continued metabolism of nitriles, HCN production and symptomatic cyanide poisoning may continue for hours to days, requiring prolonged antidotal therapy. Third, nitriles themselves possess toxicologic properties beyond those of HCN production, including mucosal irritation, nephrotoxicity, and peripheral neurotoxicity. Different nitriles vary as to whether most of their toxicity is explained by HCN release or by other toxic effects. These principles are best illustrated by briefly reviewing published examples of nitrile poisoning.

Muraki and colleagues[84] described a 35-year-old man who became ill 15 hours after cleaning the inside of a reactor kiln with acetonitrile. Initial symptoms were nausea, vomiting, and weakness. More than 20 hours after exposure, he had a convulsion and depressed level of consciousness with severe metabolic acidosis (pH 6.55; PCO_2 31 mm Hg). Treatment eventually was instituted with sodium nitrite and sodium thiosulfate. The patient required mechanical ventilation and developed acute tubular necrosis from severe rhabdomyolysis (peak serum creatine kinase 325,000 IU/L) but eventually recovered completely.

Mueller and Borland[85] reported a 39-year-old woman who deliberately swallowed acetonitrile. Symptomatic cyanide poisoning developed 11 hours later and was treated successfully with repeated doses of sodium nitrite and sodium thiosulfate. The half-life of acetonitrile was 40 hours, and antidotal therapy was required for more than 24 hours, with good outcome.

Treatment

Because patients who have ingested cyanogens such as acetonitrile may experience the onset of cyanide poisoning several hours after exposure (e.g., inhalation, ingestion), they should be observed closely for 24 hours in the hospital in a monitored setting with cyanide antidotes readily available. Theoretically, activated charcoal might prevent absorption of cyanogens, and it might be reasonable to administer charcoal to such patients if they can be treated soon after ingestion. The disadvantage of distending a patient's stomach with a suspension of charcoal when the patient is at risk for rapid deterioration, convulsions, vomiting, and aspiration must be weighed against theoretical benefits that have not yet been shown in human studies.

Patients should be regularly evaluated at the bedside for evidence of cyanide poisoning. The onset of significant changes in vital signs, the onset of metabolic acidosis, or the voicing of new complaints (nausea, weakness, dyspnea) should warrant treatment of presumed cyanide poisoning with sodium nitrite and sodium thiosulfate as in acute poisoning by inorganic cyanide compounds.

No studies provide guidance as how to dose sodium nitrite or sodium thiosulfate, or both repeatedly to patients with ongoing cyanide production after nitrile exposure. After initial dosing, it seems reasonable to provide a continuous infusion of sodium thiosulfate to enhance cyanide transulfuration continually as it is being produced. At our center, we have infused 1.2 g/hr of sodium thiosulfate for 24 hours to such patients with good results and based this dose on a known safe constant infusion dose used in sodium nitroprusside therapy. More severely ill patients might require larger doses, however. If patients experience recurrence of symptoms despite sodium thiosulfate infusion, it also seems reasonable to give repeated doses of sodium nitrite so as to maintain methemoglobin fractions between 7% and 15%, but the exact dosing schedule required to achieve this has not been described.

With regard to acrylonitrile toxicity, studies suggest that an infusion of *N*-acetylcysteine, such as when used for acetaminophen toxicity, may be beneficial in promoting metabolism by a pathway that does not lead to cyanide release.[86] No controlled human studies have shown the benefit to such therapy, however.

TABLE 95-2 Examples of Cyanogens	
Acetonitrile	Lactonitrile
Acrylonitrile	Methacrylonitrile
Butyronitrile	Nitroprusside
Cyanogen	Propionitrile
Cyanogen bromide	Succinonitrile
Cyanogen chloride	

Common Errors in Cyanide Poisoning

Failure to administer antidotal therapy rapidly when cyanide poisoning seems a likely possibility

Failure to realize the potential for falsely elevated whole-blood cyanide concentrations when serum thiocyanate levels are above normal

Forgetting that patients with cyanide poisoning can be cyanotic

continued

Common Errors in Cyanide Poisoning *continued*

Failure to appreciate that cyanide poisoning can be delayed for many hours after exposure to nitriles

Believing that all victims of cyanide poisoning must have bright red skin or blood

Believing that hydrogen cyanide smells like bitter almonds to most persons

Believing that cyanide impairs oxygen transport by hemoglobin or that cyanide poisoning produces a saturation gap in arterial blood

Key Points in Cyanide Poisoning

1. In the body, virtually all cyanide exists as hydrogen cyanide (HCN).
2. HCN binds to cytochrome oxidase of the electron transport chain on the inner mitochondrial membrane to prevent oxygen consumption and electron transport, impairing adenosine triphosphate formation.
3. Rapid collapse with central nervous system dysfunction (coma, seizures, confusion), metabolic acidosis, and cardiovascular changes (hypotension, tachycardia) suggests the diagnosis of cyanide poisoning.
4. Other clues to diagnosis are hypothermia, occasionally bright red venous blood or retinal veins with cherry-red skin (but cyanosis also is common), elevated mixed venous oxygen content, and impaired oxygen consumption. Cyanide is not detected on routine urine or plasma drug screens.
5. HCN does not smell like bitter almonds to most persons, and it is possible for a group of victims to have cyanide poisoning without anyone noting a bitter almond odor.
6. In the United States, antidotal strategy is based on inducing methemoglobinemia with nitrites (to bind HCN) and enhancing cyanide's metabolism to thiocyanate with sodium thiosulfate.
7. If cyanide levels are ordered, red blood cell cyanide levels are most helpful. Plasma cyanide concentrations are difficult to measure accurately. Whole-blood cyanide concentrations, which are offered by most laboratories, can be falsely elevated in several situations. Unless specimens are handled, stored, and transported correctly and analyzed in a timely manner, reported values for cyanide may not reflect concentrations that were present when the specimen was obtained.
8. Nitriles such as acetonitrile or acrylonitrile are metabolized slowly to HCN after inhalation, ingestion, or skin contact. Cyanide poisoning may not appear for hours after exposure and may persist for 1 to 2 days.

REFERENCES

1. Ballantyne B, Marrs TC: Post-mortem features and criteria for the diagnosis of acute lethal cyanide poisoning. In Ballantyne B, Marrs TC (eds): Clinical and Experimental Toxicology of Cyanides. Bristol, England, IOP Publishing, 1987, pp 217–247.
2. Dugard PH: The absorption of cyanide through human skin in vitro from solutions of sodium cyanide and gaseous HCN. In Ballantyne B, Marrs TC (eds): Clinical and Experimental Toxicology of Cyanides. Bristol, England, IOP Publishing, 1987, pp 127–137.
3. Levine MS, Radford EP: Occupational exposures to cyanide in Baltimore fire fighters. J Occup Med 20:53–56, 1978.
4. Jones J, McMullen J, Dougherty J: Toxic smoke inhalation: Cyanide poisoning in fire victims. Am J Emerg Med 5:318–321, 1987.
5. Wetherell HR: The occurrence of cyanide in the blood of fire victims. J Forensic Sci 11:167–173, 1966.
6. Ballantyne B: Hydrogen cyanide as a product of combustion and a factor in morbidity and mortality from fires. In Ballantyne B, Marrs TC (eds): Clinical and Experimental Toxicology of Cyanides. Bristol, England, IOP Publishing, 1987, pp 248–291.
7. Peden NR, Taha A, McSorley PD, et al: Industrial exposure to hydrogen cyanide: Implications for treatment. BMJ (Clin Res) 293:538, 1986.
8. Barcroft J: The toxicity of atmospheres containing hydrocyanic acid gas. J Hyg 31:1–34, 1931.
9. Bonsall JL: Survival without sequelae following exposure to 500 mg/m³ of hydrogen cyanide. Hum Toxicol 3:57–60, 1984.
10. Drinker P: Hydrocyanic acid gas poisoning by absorption through the skin. J Ind Hyg 14:1–2, 1932.
11. Walton DC, Witherspoon MG: Skin absorption of certain gases. J Pharmacol Exp Ther 26:315–324, 1926.
12. McKelway JI: Three cases of poisoning by potassium cyanide. Am J Med Sci 129:684–688, 1905.
13. Ballantyne B: Comparative acute toxicity of hydrogen cyanide and its salts. In Lindstrom RE (ed): Proceedings of the Fourth Annual Chemical Defense Bioscience Review. Aberdeen Proving Ground, Harford County, MD, U.S. Army Medical Research Institute of Chemical Defense, 1984.
14. Vesey CJ, Wilson J: Red cell cyanide. J Pharm Pharmacol 30:20–26, 1978.
15. McMillan DE, Svoboda AC: The role of erythrocytes in cyanide detoxification. J Pharmacol Exp Ther 221:37–42, 1982.
16. Schulz V: Clinical pharmacokinetics of nitroprusside, cyanide, thiosulphate and thiocyanate. Clin Pharmacokinet 9:239–251, 1984.
17. Schulz V, Bonn R, Kindler J: Kinetics of elimination of thiocyanate in 7 healthy subjects and 8 subjects with renal failure. Klin Wochenschr 57:243–247, 1979.
18. Sorbo B: Thiosulfate sulfurtransferase and mercaptopyruvate sulfurtransferase. In Greenberg DM (ed): Metabolic Pathways: Vol VII. Metabolism of Sulfur Compounds. New York, Academic Press, 1975, pp 433–456.
19. Westley J, Adler A, Westley L, et al: The sulfur transferases. Fundam Appl Toxicol 3:377–382, 1983.
20. Ballantyne B: Toxicology of cyanides. In Ballantyne B, Marrs TC (eds): Clinical and Experimental Toxicology of Cyanides. Bristol, England, IOP Publishing, 1987, pp 41–126.
21. Way JL, Sylvester D, Morgan RL, et al: Recent perspectives on the toxicodynamic basis of cyanide antagonism. Fundam Appl Toxicol 4:S231–S239, 1984.
22. Vennesland B, Castric PA, Conn EE, et al: Cyanide metabolism. Fed Proc 41:2639–2648, 1982.
23. Piantadosi CA, Sylvia AL: Cerebral cytochrome a,a₃ inhibition by cyanide in bloodless rats. Toxicology 33:67–79, 1984.
24. Jouglard J, Nava G, Botta A, et al: A propos d'une intoxication aigue par le cyanure traitee par l'hydroxocobalamine. Marseille Med 12:617–624, 1974.
25. Cole PV, Vesey CJ: Sodium thiosulphate decreases blood cyanide concentrations after the infusion of sodium nitroprusside. Br J Anaesth 59:531–535, 1987.
26. Hartung R: Cyanides and nitriles. In Clayton GD, Clayton FE (eds): Patty's Industrial Hygiene and Toxicology, Vol II, Part D, 4th ed. New York, John Wiley & Sons, 1994, pp 3119–3172.
27. Solomonson LP: Cyanide as a metabolic inhibitor. In Vennesland B, Conn EE, Knowles CJ, et al (eds): Cyanide in Biology. London, Academic Press, 1981, pp 11–28.
28. Tsubaki M: Fourier-transform infrared study of cyanide binding to the Fea3-CuB binuclear site of bovine heart cytochrome c oxidase: Implication of the redox-linked conformational change at the binuclear site. Biochemistry 32:164–173, 1993.
29. Way JL: Cyanide intoxication and its mechanism of antagonism. Annu Rev Pharmacol 24:451–481, 1984.
30. Tursky T, Sajter V: The influence of potassium cyanide poisoning on the aminobutyric acid level in rat brain. J Neurochem 9:519–523, 1962.
31. Krebs HG, Woods HG, Alberti KGMM: Hyperlactataemia and lactic acidosis. Essays Med Biochem 1:81–103, 1975.
32. Mizock BA: Lactic acidosis. DM 35:233–300, 1989.
33. Zilva JF: The origin of acidosis in hyperlactataemia. Ann Clin Biochem 15:40–43, 1978.
34. Mizock BA: Controversies in lactic acidosis. JAMA 258:497–501, 1987.

35. Johnston DG, Alberti KGMM: Acid-base balance in metabolic acidoses. Clin Endocrinol Metab 12:267–285, 1983.

36. Ballantyne B: An experimental assessment of the diagnostic potential of histochemical and biochemical methods for cytochrome oxidase in acute cyanide poisoning. Cell Mol Biol 22:109–123, 1977.

37. National Institute for Occupational Safety and Health: Criteria for a recommended standard for occupational exposure to hydrogen cyanide and cyanide salts. NTIS PB-266-230. NIOSH, U.S. Department of Health, Education, and Welfare, Washington, DC, 1976.

38. DeBush RF, Seidl LG: Attempted suicide by cyanide. Calif Med 110:394–396, 1969.

39. Graham DL, Laman D, Theodore J, et al: Acute cyanide poisoning complicated by lactic acidosis and pulmonary edema. Arch Intern Med 137:1051–1055, 1977.

40. Miller MH, Toops TC: Acute cyanide poisoning: Recovery with sodium thiosulfate therapy. J Indiana State Med Assoc 44:1164, 1951.

41. Wexler J, Whittenberger JL, Dumke PR: The effect of cyanide on the electrocardiogram of man. Am Heart J 34:163–173, 1947.

42. Carmelo S: [New contributions to the study of subacute-chronic hydrocyanic acid intoxication in man.] Rass Med Ind 24:254–271, 1955.

43. Brivet F, Delfraissy JF, Duche M, et al: Acute cyanide poisoning: Recovery with non-specific supportive therapy. Intensive Care Med 9:33–35, 1983.

44. Tovo S: [Poisoning due to KCN absorbed through skin.] Minerva Med 75:158–161, 1955.

45. Uitti RJ, Rajput AH, Ashenhurst EM, et al: Cyanide-induced parkinsonism: A clinicopathologic report. Neurology 35:921–925, 1985.

46. Peters CG, Mundy JVB, Rayner PR: Acute cyanide poisoning. Anaesthesia 37:582–586, 1982.

47. Hall AH, Rumack B: Clinical toxicology of cyanide. Ann Emerg Med 15:1067–1074, 1986.

48. Shragg TA, Albertson TE, Fisher CJ: Cyanide poisoning after bitter almond ingestion. West J Med 136:65–69, 1982.

49. Johnson RP, Mellors JW: Arteriolarization of venous blood gases: A clue to the diagnosis of cyanide poisoning. J Emerg Med 6:401–404, 1988.

50. Buchanan IS, Dhamee MS, Griffiths FED, et al: Abnormal fundal appearances in a case of poisoning by a cyanide capsule. Med Sci Law 16:29–32, 1976.

51. Wesson DE, Foley R, Sabatini S, et al: Treatment of acute cyanide intoxication with hemodialysis. Am J Nephrol 5:121–126, 1985.

52. Lasch EE, El Shawa R: Multiple cases of cyanide poisoning by apricot kernels in children from Gaza. Pediatrics 68:5–7, 1981.

53. Hall AH, Rumack BH: Clinical toxicology of cyanide. Ann Emerg Med 15:1067–1074, 1986.

54. Hall AH, Rumack BH, Schaffer MI, et al: Clinical toxicology of cyanide: North American clinical experiences. In Ballantyne B, Marrs TC (eds): Clinical and Experimental Toxicology of Cyanides. Bristol, England, IOP Publishing, 1987, pp 312–333.

55. Vesey CJ, Krapez JR, Cole PV: The effects of sodium nitroprusside and cyanide on haemoglobin function. J Pharm Pharmacol 32:256–261, 1980.

56. Curry SC, Patrick HC: Lack of evidence of a percent saturation gap in cyanide poisoning. Ann Emerg Med 20:523–528, 1991.

57. Ballantyne B: Artifacts in the definition of toxicity by cyanides and cyanogens. Fundam Appl Toxicol 3:400–408, 1983.

58. Pasch T, Schulz V, Hoppelshauser G: Nitroprusside-induced formation of cyanide and its detoxication with thiosulfate during deliberate hypotension. J Cardiovasc Pharmacol 5:77–85, 1983.

59. Wilson J, Mathews DM: Metabolic inter-relationships between cyanide, thiocyanate and vitamin B12 in smokers and non-smokers. Clin Sci 31:1–7, 1966.

60. Cottrell JE, Casthely P, Brodie J, et al: Prevention of nitroprusside-induced cyanide toxicity with hydroxocobalamin. N Engl J Med 298:809–811, 1978.

61. Vesey CJ, Cole PV: Blood cyanide and thiocyanate concentrations produced by long-term therapy with sodium nitroprusside. Br J Anaesth 57:148–155, 1985.

62. Ballantyne B: In vitro production of cyanide in normal human blood and the influence of thiocyanate and storage temperature. Clin Toxicol 11:173–193, 1977.

63. Troup CM, Ballantyne B: Analysis of cyanide in biological fluids and tissues. In Ballantyne B, Marrs TC (eds): Clinical and Experimental Toxicology of Cyanides. Bristol, England, IOP Publishing, 1987, pp 22–37.

64. Curry SC: Methemoglobinemia. Ann Emerg Med 11:214–221, 1982.

65. Chen KK, Rose CL: Nitrite and thiosulfate therapy in cyanide poisoning. JAMA 149:113–119, 1952.

66. Kiese M, Weger N: Formation of ferrihaemoglobin with aminophenols in the human for the treatment of cyanide poisoning. Eur J Pharmacol 7:97–105, 1969.

67. Vogel SN, Sultan TR, Ten Eyck RP: Cyanide poisoning. Clin Toxicol 18:367–383, 1981.

68. Berlin CM: The treatment of cyanide poisoning in children. Pediatrics 46:793–796, 1970.

69. Moser P: Zur wirkung von nitrit auf rote blutzellen des menschen. Arch Exp Pathol Pharmakol 210:60–70, 1950.

70. Hall AH, Doutre WH, Ludden T, et al: Nitrite/thiosulfate treated acute cyanide poisoning: Estimated kinetics after antidote. J Toxicol Clin Toxicol 25:121–133, 1987.

71. Way JL, Leung P, Sylvester DM, et al: Methaemoglobin formation in the treatment of acute cyanide intoxication. In Ballantyne B, Marrs TC (eds): Clinical and Experimental Toxicology of Cyanides. Bristol, England, IOP Publishing, 1987, pp 402–412.

72. Kruszyna R, Kruszyna H, Smith RP: Comparison of hydroxylamine, 4-dimethylaminophenol and nitrite protection against cyanide poisoning in mice. Arch Toxicol 49:191–202, 1982.

73. Chen KK, Rose RL, Clowes GHA: Methylene blue (methylthionine chloride), nitrites and sodium thiosulphate against cyanide poisoning. Proc Soc Exp Biol Med 31:250–251, 1933.

74. Gurrows GE, Way JL: Antagonism of cyanide toxicity by phenoxybenzamine (Abstract). Fed Proc 36:534, 1975.

75. Way JL, Burrows GE: Cyanide intoxication: Protection with chlorpromazine. Toxicol Appl Pharmacol 36:1–5, 1976.

76. Weger NP: Treatment of cyanide poisoning with 4-dimethylaminophenol (DMAP)—experimental and clinical overview. Fundam Appl Toxicol 3:387–396, 1983.

77. Dodds C, McKnight C: Cyanide toxicity after immersion and the hazards of dicobalt edetate. BMJ (Clin Res) 291:785–786, 1985.

78. Curry SC, Connor DA, Raschke RA: Effect of the cyanide antidote hydroxocobalamin on commonly ordered serum chemistry studies. Ann Emerg Med 24:65–67, 1994.

79. Way JL, End E, Sheehy MH, et al: Effect of oxygen on cyanide intoxication: IV. Hyperbaric oxygen. Toxicol Appl Pharmacol 22:415–421, 1972.

80. Berumen U Jr: Dog poisons man. JAMA 249:353, 1983.

81. Pettigrew AR, Logan RW, Willocks J: Smoking in pregnancy—effects on birth weight and on cyanide and thiocyanate levels in mother and baby. Br J Obstet Gynaecol 84:31–34, 1977.

82. Pelclova D, Kredba V, Pokorna P, et al: Sodium nitrite intoxication in a newborn (Abstract). J Toxicol Clin Toxicol 40:352–353, 2002.

83. Graeme KA, Curry SC, Bikin DS, et al: Lack of transplacental movement of the cyanide antidote, thiosulfate, in gravid ewes. Anaesth Analg 89:1448–1452, 2000.

84. Muraki K, Inoue Y, Ohta I, et al: Massive rhabdomyolysis and acute renal failure after acetonitrile exposure. Intern Med 40:936–939, 2001.

85. Mueller M, Borland C: Delayed caynide poisoning following acetonitrile ingestion. Postgrad Med J 73:299–300, 1997.

86. Their R, Lewalter J, Bolt HM: Species differences in acrylonitrile metabolism and toxicity between experimental animals and humans based on observations in human accidental poisoning. Arch Toxicol 74:184–189, 2000.

CHAPTER 96

Isocyanates and Other Important Chemical Pulmonary Sensitizers

Ronald Balkissoon

Although there are numerous reports of severe asthma and anaphylactic episodes secondary to exposure to latex, flour, various enzymes, and diisocyanates, there have been relatively few reports in the medical literature regarding fatalities resulting from occupational asthma.[1-3] Toluene diisocyanate (TDI), the most widely studied of the diisocyanates, causes asthma in approximately 5% of exposed workers[4]; prevalence rates for other diisocyanates are presumed to be lower. Previous reports suggested that most workers affected are nonatopic and nonsmokers. The most infamous incident of accidental exposure to high levels of isocyanates occurred in 1984 in Bhopal, India, where a massive release of a methyl isocyanate was discharged from a pesticide plant.[5] The spectrum of ill health effects ranged from eye and upper respiratory tract irritation to lethal lung injury with pulmonary edema and diffuse lung inflammation.

Fabbri and colleagues[6] reported a fatality due to TDI in a 43-year-old car painter. The man had worked as a car painter for more than 26 years and was a lifelong nonsmoker. Six years before the fatal event, he was diagnosed with TDI asthma after a specific inhalational challenge with TDI. Despite recommendations to change his job or avoid the use of polyurethane paints, he continued to work in his garage as a car painter. He used regular bronchodilators, cromolyn, and steroids and reported reduced exposure to most varnishes containing TDI. Apparently he was reasonably well until the week before his death, when he used a new paint product, which led to severe and prolonged bronchospasm with significant nocturnal symptoms for the following 3 days. Seven days after his first exposure, the man used this same paint (which contained < 0.15% of TDI) without a mask. A few minutes after starting, he developed an acute fatal asthma attack. Autopsy showed mucus plugs in the airways; there were no cardiac or cerebral abnormalities. Microscopy revealed mucus plugging of small bronchi and bronchioles, sloughing and shedding of epithelium, and thickening of the basement membrane. Bronchial walls had mucosal edema with diffuse infiltration of mononuclear and polymorphonuclear leukocytes and prominent eosinophilic infiltration in the lamina propria. Bronchial smooth muscle was hypertrophic and disarrayed. These morphologic abnormalities were noted at the bronchial and alveolar levels. The concentration of isocyanate vapor at the top of the paint can that caused the fatal attack was 4 ppb.

Carino and associates[1] reported the death of a 39-year-old foundry worker secondary to exposure from mold and core processing that used resins containing diphenylmethane diisocyanate (MDI). The man was a nonsmoker and had been diagnosed with occupational asthma 5 years before his death by a specific inhalational challenge with a 0.005-ppm exposure to MDI. He had worked in this area for 6 years and had symptoms for a few years before his diagnosis. Histologic findings at time of autopsy were similar to those noted in the report by Fabbri and colleagues[6].

The only other published report of an occupational asthma fatality involved a 42-year-old bakery employee in South Africa.[2] The man had worked as an assistant baker for more than 20 years and had a 6-year history of symptoms related to work exposures. He was diagnosed with flour-related asthma after positive skin prick testing to whole-grain wheat and whole-grain maize and a positive specific inhalational challenge with flour. Despite recommendations to change his job, he continued to work at the bakery for 5 more years before his fatal asthma attack.

These cases illustrate several important features of occupational asthma. Most importantly, occupational asthma can be a severe, although rarely fatal, disease. Despite accurate diagnosis and advisement to switch jobs, many individuals with occupational asthma remain in the same employment sector and risk progression and possibly death. Ongoing exposure to the offending agent after receiving the diagnosis of occupational asthma has been shown to reduce significantly the probability that the worker will return to a nonasthmatic state after removal from exposure.

Asthma is now the most common work-related respiratory disorder in most industrialized countries, surpassing silicosis, asbestosis, and occupational lung cancer.[7-12] Estimates of the proportion of cases of adult-onset asthma due to occupational exposure range from 2% to 15%.[13-16] More than 300 agents have been identified as potential causes of occupational asthma.[17,18] The long-term sequelae from developing occupational asthma may be substantial with regard to health status and socioeconomic status. Many affected individuals require a change of job or seek workers' compensation. Individuals with severe occupational asthma often do not return to gainful employment and require long-term disability. Such outcomes emphasize the substantial socioeconomic consequences of occupational asthma.

WORK-RELATED ASTHMA

Definitions and Classifications

Work-related asthma encompasses work-aggravated asthma and occupational asthma. *Work-aggravated asthma* refers to preexisting asthma that is aggravated by irritants or physical stimuli (e.g., temperature change, dust, smoke) in the workplace. *Occupational asthma* is characterized by variable airflow limitation or airway hyperresponsiveness or both caused by exposures and conditions attributable to a particular occupational exposure.[19] Individuals with preexisting asthma may develop superimposed occupational asthma as a result of a specific workplace sensitizer. *Occupational asthma with a latency period* refers to the classic immune-mediated condition that occurs after a variable period of repeated exposure to a high-molecular-weight or low-molecular-weight antigen in the workplace. *Occupational asthma without latency* refers to irritant-induced asthma resulting from naive, unusually high concentration exposure to irritant gases, fumes, dust, or chemicals.

Reactive airways dysfunction syndrome (RADS), the prototype of irritant-induced asthma,[20] initially was defined as asthma developing after a single exposure to high levels of an irritant agent with consequent development of asthma symptoms, variable airflow limitation, and bronchial hyperresponsiveness within 24 to 72 hours of initial exposure. By definition, individuals who developed RADS did not have a history of asthma before the implicated exposure. It is now recognized that irritant-induced asthma can develop after symptomatic irritant exposures on one or several occasions[21] and may be superimposed on preexisting asthma.

There are certain forms of occupational asthma with a latency period for which the immunologic mechanism remains unknown (e.g., meat wrapper's asthma and potroom asthma). Finally, there are a group of "occupational asthma–like" disorders that show variable airflow limitation with symptoms of chest tightness associated with cross-shift changes in forced expiratory volume in 1 second (FEV_1) but without persistent bronchial hyperresponsiveness or eosinophilia.[22]

Etiologic Agents

Common low-molecular-weight agents known to cause occupational asthma include diisocyanates, acid anhydrides, amine compounds, metals such as platinum and nickel, solder flux (colophony), and wood dust extracts (e.g., plicatic acid from Western Red Cedar). Table 96-1 summarizes many of the commonly recognized agents and workplaces associated with low-molecular-weight occupational asthma. High-molecular-weight agents, such as various animal proteins and vegetable proteins from flour, natural rubber latex, and enzymes, are well-recognized causes of occupational asthma with latency. Table 96-2 lists some chemical agents that have been documented as causes of RADS. Low-molecular-weight chemical agents, pharmaceuticals, and high-molecular-weight agents reported to cause occupational asthma number greater than 300, and it

---

TABLE 96-1 Selected Examples of Low-Molecular-Weight Compounds Causing Occupational Asthma

AGENT	OCCUPATION	AGENT	OCCUPATION
Amines (Aliphatic, Aromatic, Heterocyclic)		**Metals and Metal Salts**	
Ethyleneimines	Shellac, rubber, lacquer handling industries	Aluminum pot room fumes	Pot room workers
	Photography	Chromium	Electroplating
Ethanolamines	Solderers		Printers
	Spray painters		Tanners
Paraphenylenediamine	Fur dyers	Cobalt	Hard metal workers
Piperazine hydrochloride	Chemists, chemical manufacture		Diamond polishers
Anhydrides		Nickel	Electroplating
Phthalic anhydride	Paint, plastics manufacture	Platinum	Platinum refiners
Tetrachlorophthalic anhydride	Epoxy resins, plastics manufacture	Tungsten carbide	Hard metal grinders
	Electronics workers	Zinc	Solderers
Trimellitic anhydride	Paint manufacture		Locksmiths
	Chemical workers	**Other Chemicals**	
Diisocyanates		Chloramine-T	Chemical manufacture
Toluene diisocyanate	Polyurethane manufacture	Polyvinyl chloride	Meat wrappers
	Plastics, varnish manufacture	Organophosphate insecticides	Chemical packaging plant
	Foam manufacture	Reactive dyes	Textile industry workers
Diphenylmethane diisocyanate	Foam manufacture		Reactive dye manufacture
	Foundry workers	Persulfates	Hairdressers
Hexamethylene diisocyanate	Spray painters	Hexachlorophene	Health care workers
1,5-Naphthylene diisocyanate	Rubber manufacture	Formaldehyde	Health care workers
Fluxes		Urea formaldehyde	Resin, foam manufacture
Colophony	Electronics workers	Glutaraldehyde	Hospital endoscopy technician
Zinc chloride and ammonium chloride	Metal joiners	Freon	Refrigeration workers
		Styrene	Plastics manufacture
		Acrylic	Plastics manufacture
		Latex	Glove manufacture
			Health care workers

TABLE 96-2 Chemicals Associated with Reactive Airways Dysfunction Syndrome

Acetic acid	Hydrazine
Acids (various)	Hydrochloric acid
Ammonia	Hydrogen sulfide
Bleaching agents	Isocyanates
Calcium oxide	Metal coat remover
Chlorine	Metam sodium
Cleaning agents	Paint (fumes)
Diesel exhaust	Perchlorethylene
Diethylaminoethanol	Phthalic anhydride
Epichlorohydrin	Sulfur dioxide gases (e.g., chlorine,
Ethylene oxide	phosgene, mustard)
Fire smoke (pyrolysis products)	Sulfuric acid (aromatic
Floor sealant	hydrocarbons)
Formalin	Uranium hexafluoride
Fumigating agent	Urea fumes
Glacial acetic acid	Welding fumes

is beyond the scope of this chapter to discuss all of these agents individually. For a more complete listing of presently recognized high-molecular-weight and low-molecular-weight agents, readers may consult several references.[23] As discussed earlier, there have been a few reports of fatalities, and these have involved isocyanates, flour, and more recently natural rubber latex. The specific low-molecular-weight agents that are discussed in this chapter include isocyanates and acid anhydrides because of their recognized potentially serious complications. Natural rubber latex is presented briefly as an example of a high-molecular-weight organic protein capable of causing severe asthma reactions and death.

Risk Factors for Developing Occupational Asthma

For individuals exposed to high-molecular-weight antigens, atopy is a risk factor. There is a high prevalence of skin test–proven atopy among workers with laboratory animal allergy and health care workers who develop latex asthma.[24,25] There is no increased prevalence of atopy among asthmatics who respond to the low-molecular-

weight agent plicatic acid found in Western Red Cedar[26] or isocyanate-related asthma.[4] A study of irritant-induced asthma patients showed that they were less likely to be atopic (20%) than were asthma controls (58%).[21] Tobacco smokers with atopy have an increased risk of occupational asthma. Venables and colleagues[27] showed that a greater proportion of workers with specific IgE antibody to tetrachlorophthalic anhydride were smokers compared with workers who lacked the specific antibody. Conversely, a study of sawmill workers exposed to Western Red Cedar did not indicate that smoking was associated with an increased asthma risk.[28] Tobacco smoking may contribute to the risk of irritant-induced asthma, based on the finding of higher numbers of current smokers in this group compared with other asthmatics.[21] With regard to patients who have preexisting airways hyperresponsiveness, two prospective studies of TDI manufacturing workers[4] and Western Red Cedar workers[29] showed that workers with and without prior nonspecific hyperresponsiveness were equally likely to develop occupational asthma.

CHEMISTRY

Isocyanate

Isocyanates are a group of low-molecular-weight aromatic or aliphatic organic chemical compounds formed by the reaction of amines or their hydrochlorides with phosgene that readily form esters of substituted carbamic acid or urethanes. A common structural feature of these chemicals is the presence of an —N═C═O group. The most important compounds commercially used include 2,4-TDI and 2,6-TDI, hexamethylene diisocyanate (HDI), MDI, naphthalene diisocyanate, isophorone diisocyanate, and prepolymers derived from HDI and MDI (Fig. 96-1). This chemical structure renders these compounds useful for forming plastics, adhesives, elastomers, and flexible or rigid foams. Diisocyanates are used worldwide in many important industries, including the production of foam rubber cushions, dashboards, body parts, and finish coatings in the automobile industry. Spray paints and lacquers used in a variety of applications are perhaps the most widely used source of isocyanates. It is estimated that

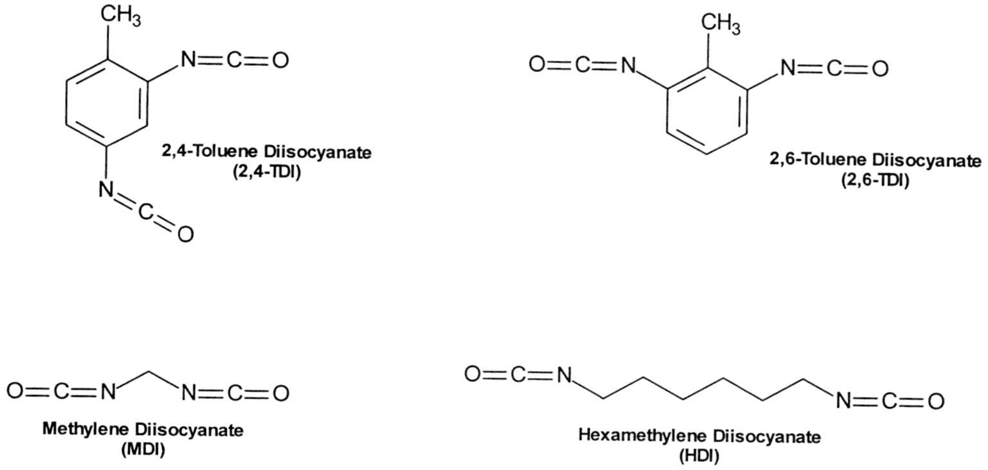

FIGURE 96-1

Chemical structures of common commercially used isocyanate compounds.

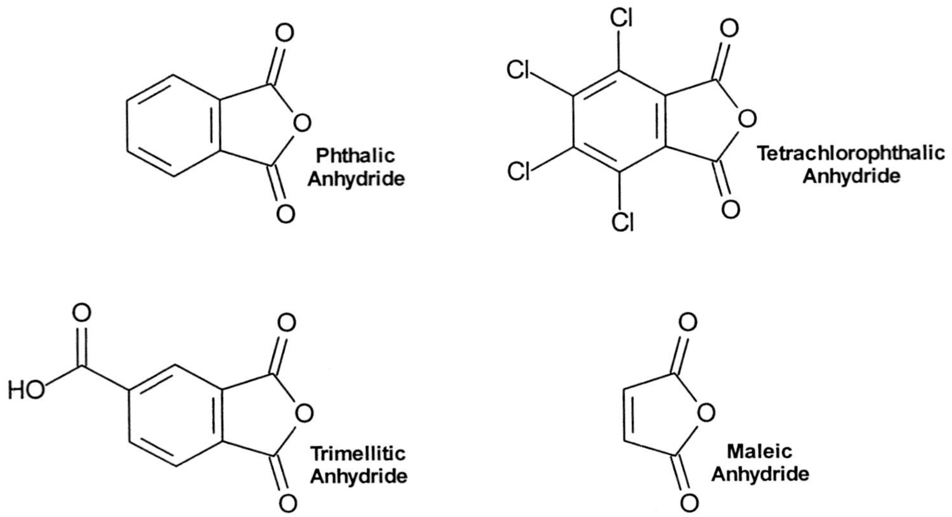

FIGURE 96-2

Chemical structures of industrially used acid anhydrides.

more than 2 million tons of isocyanates are used annually, and more than 200,000 workers are exposed in the United States. MDI is used extensively for mold and core processes in modern steel foundries. TDI and HDI are volatile at room temperature, whereas MDI needs to be heated to 60°C before becoming volatilized. Previously, monomeric isomers were considered the predominant diisocyanates to cause asthma; however, more recent studies have shown that the polyisocyanate oligomers of TDI and HDI are capable of inducing occupational asthmatic responses as proven by specific inhalational challenges.[30]

Acid Anhydrides

The chemical structure of the main acid anhydrides is shown in Figure 96-2. Acid anhydrides have many applications as intermediates in the manufacture of plastics and production of resins used in paints, varnishes, reinforced plastics, surface coatings, adhesives, encapsulation, sealants, and powder coatings. Additional applications include dyes, insecticides, pharmaceuticals, and lubricating oil additives. Attractive properties of the anhydrides, such as the trimellitates, are that they withstand high temperatures, are flexible at low temperatures, and are poorly soluble in water. The annual

world production of trimellitic anhydride (TMA) is approximately 22,500 tons produced at one site in the United States. Estimates suggest that 170,000 workers are exposed to acid anhydrides in the United States.[31] Table 96-3 lists three common commercially used acid anhydrides with their exposure limits and the health effects on which these limits have been based. Much controversy remains as to whether there is any level that truly can be protective against sensitization or exacerbation of immunologically driven responses. Table 96-4 lists health effects of acid anhydrides in general.

Natural Rubber Latex

Although the term *latex* refers to any emulsion of polymers, natural rubber latex is derived from the tree *Hevea braziliensis* and in its raw sap form is a clear odorless liquid. Natural rubber is defined as a cis-1,4-polisoprene with a molecular weight varying from 100,000 to 1 million. Typically the latex sap can be centrifuged and separated into three components: the rubber particle layer containing spherical droplets of cis-1,4-polyisoprene coated with a layer of hydrophylic colloid at the top, the "latex serum" (C-serum), and the lutoid fraction on the bottom. The lutoid fraction consists of vacuoles that have proteins that interact with the

TABLE 96-3 Major Commercial Acid Anhydrides and Recommended Exposure Limits

ACID ANHYDRIDE	TWA* (ppm or mg/m³)	STEL†/C‡ (mg/m³)	TLV§ BASIS—CRITICAL EFFECTS
Phthalic anhydride	1 ppm	—	Irritation, sensitization
Trimellitic anhydride	—	0.04	Bleeding, immunotoxicity, sensitization
Maleic anhydride	0.25 ppm	—	Irritation, sensitization

*TWA, time-weighted average airborne exposure over 8 hours.
†STEL, Short-term exposure limit/15-minute exposure limit.
‡C, ceiling—exposure level that should not be exceeded for any part of workday.
§TLV, Threshold limit value—generic term used to refer to any of the above more specific exposure limits.

TABLE 96-4 Health Effects of Acid Anhydrides

Attributed to Direct Toxicity

Skin irritation, burns, vesicles
Conjunctivitis, keratitis, corneal burns and ulcers
Rhinitis, pharyngitis
Epistaxis
Cough
Dyspnea, wheezing
Pulmonary congestion
Hemoptysis
Bronchitis, emphysema
Transient increase in airway resistance
Dyspepsia, nausea, vomiting, anorexia, weight loss
Anemia, reticulocytosis
Fever, chills, malaise, weakness, headache, dizziness

Attributed to Hypersensitivity

Asthma, rhinitis, conjunctivitis
Urticaria
Possible contact dermatitis
Hemoptysis/hemolysis
Late respiratory systemic syndrome—respiratory symptoms, fever, chills, malaise, anorexia, weight loss, myalgias

rubber particles and coagulate. Fresh natural rubber latex is 30% to 40% rubber hydrocarbon and 2% to 3% protein. Ammonia is added to freshly tapped natural rubber latex sap to prevent premature coagulation and bacterial overgrowth. Latex is processed further by adding a series of chemicals, such as antioxidants (e.g., paraphenylenediamine), accelerators (e.g., zinc oxide, thiurams, dithiocarbamates, mercaptobenzothiazole), fillers, pigments, emulsifiers, and other ingredients. Cornstarch powder has been used as a lubricant to ease donning and taking off gloves. Aside from the natural rubber latex proteins, other components of the gloves, such as the cornstarch, ethylene oxide, mercapto-

benzothiazole, and endotoxin, have been proposed to be potentially capable of causing type I hypersensitivity or "asthmatic-like" reactions. It has been shown that the powder from natural rubber latex gloves becomes aerosolized and may expose latex-sensitized individuals to significant levels of the proteins and other potentially allergenic components, leading to symptoms despite no direct personal use of the gloves.

PATHOPHYSIOLOGY

An extensive review of the pathophysiology of occupational asthma is beyond the scope of this chapter; however, a brief review of the characteristics of the inflammatory response to high-molecular-weight agents, low-molecular-weight agents, and irritants is particularly instructive. It is accepted that airway inflammation is a crucial feature in the pathogenesis of asthma. In occupational asthma, there is substantial evidence to suggest similarities and differences in the inflammatory response to high-molecular-weight agents and low-molecular-weight agents. High-molecular-weight agents have been shown to operate in part through classic IgE-mediated mechanisms that may produce immediate, delayed, or dual responses (Table 96-5).

The initiation of IgE-mediated responses is complex. Potential antigens enter the body and are processed by accessory cells or antigen presenting cells, such as macrophages, dendritic cells, epithelial cells, and B lymphocytes. The antigens are then presented into the groove of the major histocompatibility gene complex (MHC) molecule on T cells leading to a Th2 pathway cytokine response that attracts, activates, and promotes proliferation and differentiation of other white blood cells, such as neutrophils and eosinophils. CD4 helper T cells are important for stimulating B-lymphocyte IgE antibody production and subsequent hypersensitivity reactions (Fig. 96-3).

TABLE 96-5 Gell and Coombs Classification of Diseases Caused by Trimellitic Anhydride

TYPE	TERMINOLOGY	MECHANISM	IN VIVO OR IN VITRO TESTS	DISEASE
I	Anaphylactic, immediate-type IgE antibody–mediated	IgE antibody–sensitized mast cells react with TM protein and bioactive mediators are released	Immediate-type skin test: in vitro histamine release	Asthma, rhinitis, conjunctivitis
II	Cytotoxic	Antibody against hapten cell results in cell damage or destruction	Antibodies against TM-E lyse cells in the presence of complement	Anemia or pulmonary disease anemia syndrome? Other?
III	Toxic antigen-antibody complex reaction	Immune complexes fix complement, attract polymorphonuclear leukocytes, which results in tissue damage	Experimental skin reaction	Probable cause of LRSS associated with increase in total antibody and IgG and IgA antibodies against TM proteins
IV	Lymphocyte-mediated, delayed, tuberculin-type	Sensitized T lymphocytes stimulated by antigen, resulting in tissue damage	In vitro lymphocyte transformation	Uncertain: possible component of LRSS and pulmonary disease anemia syndrome

LRSS, late respiratory systemic syndrome; TM, trimellitic.
From Patterson R, Zeiss CR, Pruzansky JJ: Immunology and immunopathology of trimellitic anhydride pulmonary reactions.
J Allergy Clin Immunol 70:19–23, 1982.

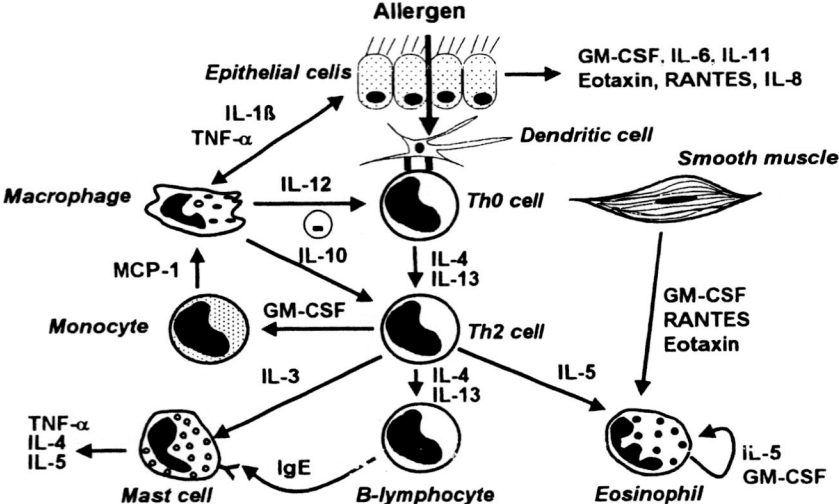

FIGURE 96-3

Pathway of allergic (Th2) immune response. GM-CSF, granulocyte-macrophage colony-stimulating factor; IL, interleukin; MCP-1, monocyte chemotactic protein-1; RANTES, regulated on activation, T-cell expressed and secreted; TNF, tumor necrosis factor.

Low-molecular-weight agents often act as haptens requiring conjugation to a host protein before initiating an immune response (Fig. 96-4). They too may lead to early (10% to 20%), late (30% to 50%), or dual (30% to 50%) responses.[32] Low-molecular-weight agents likely work through a variety of mechanisms. It has been shown that platinum salts and acid anhydrides produce substantial IgE responses and positive prick skin tests in sensitized individuals, whereas the response in diisocyanate-sensitized individuals is much less predictable.[32] Besides these classic immune-mediated pathways, there are other mechanisms that are likely operative in occupational asthma, including airway microvascular leakage, direct pharmacologic effects on smooth muscle, and neurogenic inflammation. These may be the predominant pathways in irritant-induced asthma, but this remains unknown.

The histologic features reported for occupational asthma have been shown to be similar and dissimilar to the features found in nonoccupational asthma. High-molecular-weight agents and low-molecular-weight agents can induce an inflammatory cell infiltration with eosinophil, lymphocyte, and mast cell activation.[33] Reticular basement membrane thickening also has been noted, and this has been shown to be reversible after removal from exposure to occupational sensitizers[34] or treatment with corticosteroids. The histopathologic features of irritant-induced asthma or RADS are poorly characterized. Brooks and coworkers[20] reported on two cases with RADS with bronchial epithelial cell desquamation and bronchial wall inflammation, including lymphocytes and plasma cells but not eosinophils. There was no mucous gland hyperplasia, basement membrane thickening, or smooth muscle hypertrophy. Bernstein and Zeiss[35] described more typical histopathologic features of asthma, including denuded epithelium, submucosal chronic inflammation, and collagen proliferation below the basement membrane after anhydrous ammonia exposure.

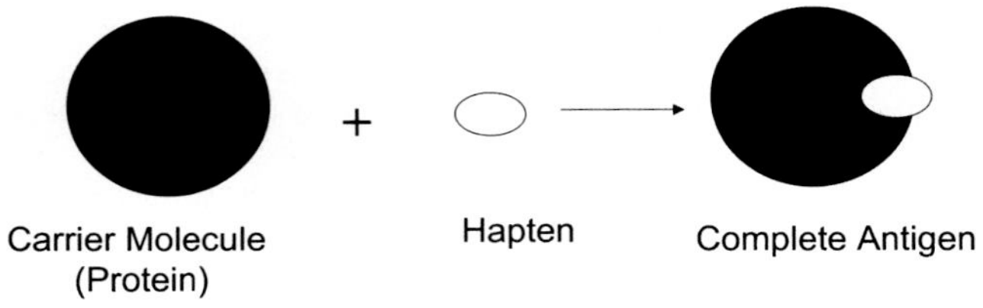

CLINICAL PRESENTATION

Clinical Features of Acute Severe Asthma
Dyspnea
Chest tightness
Anxiety
Unable to speak in complete sentences
Difficulty moving air in and out
Anxiety
Diaphoresis
Use of accessory muscles/intercostal retraction
Upright position leaning forward
Tachycardia
Pulsus paradoxus
Poor air entry/diminished breath sounds and/or wheezing

Patients with a severe asthma attack have various clinical presentations. The temporal pattern may be a gradual progression over several days or weeks that reaches a critical point or an acute onset that may be life-threatening within minutes or hours. The characteristic symptoms include shortness of breath and chest tightness, and in severe attacks, it may be as difficult to inhale as it is to exhale. The patient may or may not report audible wheezing or coughing or both. The absence of wheezing may portend a more severe asthma attack. Often patients are so short of breath that they are unable to complete full sentences before needing to take a breath. Anxiety is a common presenting symptom, and early on patients may report feeling lightheaded with numbness or tingling suggesting hyperventilation; however, as time passes and their condition worsens, patients may be more confused

Carrier Molecule (Protein)   +   Hapten   →   Complete Antigen

FIGURE 96-4

Conjugation of haptens (incomplete antigens) with carrier molecules (human proteins) to make complete antigen complexes.

or disoriented owing to hypoventilation (respiratory failure) and hypercapnia. The cardiopulmonary pathophysiologic consequences of a severe asthmatic attack are listed in Table 96-6. Severe airway inflammation and resultant bronchoconstriction lead to significant changes in intrathoracic pressures, gas exchange, and chest wall mechanics, resulting in significant cardiac and respiratory embarrassment.

Physical examination during a severe asthma attack typically reveals tachypnea, tachycardia, and hypertension. Significant pulsus paradoxus suggests fairly severe airflow obstruction and hypoxia leading to pulmonary vasoconstriction, right ventricular strain, and ballooning of the intraventricular septal wall into the left ventricle leading to left ventricular dysfunction. Patients may be slightly febrile or diaphoretic or both. Flaring of nasal alae, use of accessory muscles, and intercostal muscle retraction are signs of significant distress. Audible wheezing may be present; however, reduced or no wheezing is an ominous harbinger of pending respiratory failure. Evidence of hyperinflation, including hyperresonance on percussion and distant heart sounds, is often present with severe attacks. Confusion, altered level of consciousness, and reduced responsiveness also are signs of severe attacks.

During severe asthma attacks, it may not be possible to obtain valid spirometry or peak flow assessments. Peak flow measurements are not as reliable or instructive as FEV_1. Individuals in significant distress may have relatively well-preserved peak flows but dramatically reduced FEV_1. Individuals with severe attacks typically have spirometry values less than 25% of their normal values; however, many are so distressed that it is difficult to obtain valid spirometry. If the overall clinical scenario is consistent with a severe asthma attack, one should treat the patient accordingly regardless of the ability to obtain objective spirometric data.

Arterial blood gases generally reveal some degree of hypoxemia and initially low $PaCO_2$; however, as an attack progresses or the patient fatigues, the $PaCO_2$ increases, and hypoxemia may worsen. A low $PaCO_2$ should not engender a sense of assurance that the patient is not at risk of imminent arrest because patients have experienced respiratory arrest with relatively low or normal $PaCO_2$ levels. Low pH may reflect alveolar hypoventilation or a superimposed metabolic acidosis or both.

Isocyanates

The clinical manifestations of isocyanate exposure range from irritant effects, chronic bronchitis, and pulmonary edema to hypersensitivity reactions including mild to fatal

asthma and hypersensitivity pneumonitis. Severe RADS has been reported to occur after a single high-dose exposure due to accidental spills.[36] In addition to these effects, diisocyanates cause a dose-dependent annual decline in FEV_1.[37] A precise threshold level for sensitization has not been determined; however, it is apparent that when an individual is sensitized, levels below the threshold limit value of 20 ppb (even as low as 1 ppb) are capable of inducing reactions.[38] Reports of levels well below limits mandated by many regulatory agencies do not rule out severe work-related exacerbations of asthma in sensitized workers.

Acid Anhydrides

The anhydrides, particularly TMA, are capable of causing a variety of irritant/toxic and hypersensitivity health effects (see Tables 96-4 and 96-6). Anhydrides cause direct mucosal and skin irritation. Eye symptoms and upper respiratory tract symptoms, including epistaxis, are common. The lower respiratory tract manifestations include RADS,[39] classic IgE-mediated asthma, and allergic alveolitis.[40] The late respiratory systemic syndrome or TMA flu, similar to other inhalational fever syndromes, is characterized by cough; occasional wheezing; dyspnea; mucus production; and systemic symptoms of malaise, chills, myalgias, and arthralgias occurring 4 to 12 hours after TMA inhalational exposure but no evidence of infiltrates on chest radiograph. Immunologic studies have shown elevated levels of IgG, IgA, and IgM antibody directed against TMA human serum albumin. The pulmonary disease anemia syndrome[41] is a condition producing hemoptysis, dyspnea, pulmonary infiltrates, and restrictive lung disease. The syndrome has been described principally in TMA-exposed workers; however, cases have been attributed to pyromellitic dianhydride exposure as well.[42] Human studies have shown elevated levels of IgG, IgA, and IgM antibody to TMA protein,[43] and animal studies have shown that the response can be suppressed by cyclophosphamide.[44] Hemorrhagic rhinitis after exposure to an epoxy resin vapor containing pyromellitic dianhydride occurred in a worker who mounted an IgG response to many pyromellitic dianhydride–modified serum proteins.[42]

Natural Rubber Latex

Most cases of severe asthmatic and anaphylactic attacks associated with latex exposure have involved individuals undergoing invasive procedures in which latex-containing products, such as medical equipment including barium enema catheters or gloves, have extensive intimate contact with mucosal surfaces. More recently, there have been reports of health care workers developing severe attacks as a result of wearing latex gloves or inhaling powder containing natural rubber latex protein.

DIAGNOSIS

Isocyanates

In patients previously unrecognized to be isocyanate sensitive, measuring specific IgE antibodies to diisocyanate human serum albumin conjugate antigens may assist in linking a severe asthma exacerbation to work exposure. Few

TABLE 96-6 Pathophysiologic Consequences of Acute Severe Asthma

Respiratory	Cardiovascular
Diffuse airway inflammation	Pulmonary vasoconstriction
Inhomogeneous airway narrowing	Right ventricular strain
Air trapping and hyperinflation	Left ventricular dysfunction
Increased work of breathing	Systemic hypertension
Low ventilation/perfusion ratios— hypoxia and shunting	Pulmonary edema
	Cardiac tamponade
Increased dead space	Myocardial necrosis

TDI-sensitive workers show positive antibodies; however, 20% of MDI-sensitized and 50% of HDI-sensitized workers with occupational asthma develop positive antibody responses.[45] In vitro tests of delayed hypersensitivity, such as lymphocyte proliferation assays, remain research tools and do not have any routine clinical application to date. Confirmation of isocyanate asthma by specific inhalational challenges remains the gold standard; however, few centers are equipped to perform such testing. The metabolism and pharmocokinetics of isocyanates are poorly understood. Biologic monitoring for isocyanates is limited; however, it has been shown that diaminotoluene and 4,4-diaminodiphenylmethane can be measured in the blood and urine to detect but not quantify TDI[46] and MDI[47] exposure.

Acid Anhydrides

Zeiss and colleagues[48] followed workers who had been involved in the manufacture of TMA for more than 12 years. They noted irritant effects as most common followed by asthma/rhinitis and late respiratory systemic syndrome. The prevalence of TMA immunologic lung disease was 7% among 474 employees. Some individuals showed asthma and late respiratory systemic syndrome. There was a trend for a direct correlation between total antibody and IgE antibody titers to TMA human serum albumin and exposure levels. Zeiss and colleagues[49] reported that the latency period for development of TMA-related asthma ranged from 0.5 month to 14 years. There was a fivefold increased risk for the development of IgE antibodies to tetrachlorophthalic anhydride and a slightly increased risk if subjects were atopic. This increased risk has not been shown for other acid anhydrides. Although the absorption, distribution, metabolism, and elimination of acid anhydrides remain poorly described, it has been established that phthalic anhydride is at least partially excreted in the urine as phthalic acid with a half-life of about 14 hours.[50] Unexposed individuals may have lower but detectable levels of phthalic acid in their urine as a result of exposure to phthalate plasticizers in food, cosmetics, and plastics. Acid anhydrides avidly form conjugates with human proteins in vitro.[51]

Natural Rubber Latex

Skin prick testing and radioallergosorbent testing are the common immunologic tests used to determine natural rubber latex sensitivity.

TREATMENT

Severe Asthma Attack

Acute management of a patient with a severe asthma attack is the same regardless of whether it is caused by an occupational sensitizer, by RADS, or by nonoccupational exposures (Table 96-7). Identification of the particular inciting agent of an acute asthma attack does not affect the acute management because there are no specific measures to detoxify or reverse the effects of these agents. When the immunologic cascade has been activated, management is

TABLE 96-7 Treatment of Acute Severe Asthma

Reassurance
Oxygen
β_2-Agonist agents
    Nebulized
        Intermittent (0.5–1 mL of 0.5% solution made up in 3 mL of saline
            every 30 min)
        Continuous (10 mg over 45 min)
    Intravenous (500 μg over 1 hr, then 5–20 μg/min)
Corticosteroids
    Intravenous methylprednisolone, 40–125 mg every 6 hr
    Intravenous hydrocortisone, 100–200 mg, every 4–6 hr
Epinephrine (if suspect imminent need for intubation and ventilation)
    Subcutaneous (0.5 mg every 20 min)
    Intravenous (2–10 mL of 1:10,000 over 5 min, then intravenous infusion
        at 1–20 μg/min
    Nebulized (5 mL of 1:1000 repeated as necessary)
Other drugs
    Aminophylline
    Ipratropium bromide
    Magnesium sulfate
    Isoproterenol
Noninvasive assisted ventilation
    Continuous positive airway pressure at <10 cm H_2O, titrated to patient
        response
    Bilevel positive airway pressure
Mechanical ventilation
    Permissive hypercapnia—controlled hypoventilation
Extreme "last resort" measures
    External chest compressions
    Extracorporeal carbon dioxide removal and oxygen insufflation
    Cardiopulmonary resuscitation
    Thoracotomy

Indications for ICU Admission After a Severe Asthma Attack

Altered level of consciousness
Cyanosis or severe hypoxia (PaO_2 <60 mm Hg)
Pulsus paradoxus (≥15 mm Hg decrease in systolic blood
    pressure during inspiration)
Tachycardia (≥110 beats/min)
Bradycardia
Patient unable to complete a sentence in one breath
Silent chest on auscultation
Exhaustion
Increased respiratory rate (≥30 breaths/min)
Normal or increased $PaCO_2$
Low arterial pH

similar for all occupational sensitizers. Supplemental oxygen to provide saturations greater than 90% should be administered in all patients. Immediate administration of rapid-onset bronchodilators (via inhaler or nebulizer) and administration of intravenous corticosteroids are the cornerstones of initial therapy for a severe asthmatic attack. The addition of medications such as theophylline or magnesium sulfate has not been proved to have substantial additional benefit over β-agonists and corticosteroids alone. In certain

TABLE 96-8 Principles of Intubation and Mechanical Ventilation for Severe Asthmatics

Reassure and prepare patient
Preoxygenate
Preload with ≥300–500 mL of saline
Intubate with adequate sedation with or without muscle relaxants
Intermittent positive-pressure ventilation with following options
    Variable flow rates
    Variable inspiratory/expiratory ratios
    Pressure control or pressure limit
    Pressure support
Permissive hypercapnia ($PaCO_2$ <120 mm Hg)
Minimal peak inspiratory pressures (<50 cm H_2O)
Maintain arterial pH >7.1
Minimal low tidal volumes (5–10 mL/kg)
Start with inspiratory/expiratory ratio 1:1 and adjust to allow optimal emptying time
Sit up (angle >30 degrees)
Maximal bronchodilator and antiinflammatory treatment

patients who have not responded to initial therapy, however, one may consider adding these medications.

In patients who do not respond to initial treatment, respiratory fatigue may set in, and they may require admission to the hospital, preferably the intensive care unit. Mechanical ventilation for an acute asthmatic is a challenge (Table 96-8). As a result of the increase in airways resistance, the risk of significant barotrauma and pneumothorax is great in an acute severe asthmatic requiring mechanical ventilation. Adequate sedation is key, and temporary paralysis may reduce the chances of these complications. Permissive hypercapnia or controlled hypoventilation (using low tidal volumes, maintaining peak inspiratory pressures <50 cm H_2O and accepting $PaCO_2$ levels ≤150 mm Hg) reduces the risk of significant barotrauma in these patients. Optimizing inspiratory/expiratory ratios to allow adequate emptying time during expiration minimizes breath stacking and hyperinflation. Weaning and extubation should occur as soon as possible to avoid several of the complications known to occur in this patient population.

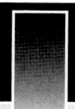

Complications of Mechanical Ventilation in Patients with Acute Severe Asthma

Pulmonary barotraumas/pneumothorax
Decreased venous return and cardiac output
Hypotension
Decreased extrathoracic organ perfusion
Mucous plugging and atelectasis
Nosocomial pneumonia
Thromboembolism
Myopathy
Electrolyte disturbances

Rarely, patients do not tolerate or improve with mechanical ventilation, at which point maneuvers such as external chest compression, extracorporeal carbon dioxide removal, and oxygen insufflation may be temporizing measures to maintain adequate gas exchange while systemic corticosteroids have time to reverse the underlying inflammation. Cardiopulmonary resuscitation and thoracotomy are reserved as absolute last-resort measures when all else has failed.

When the patient has been stabilized and is out of imminent danger, appropriate follow-up evaluation should rule out any work relationship if the patient was previously unrecognized to have occupational asthma. If the patient is known to have occupational asthma, a thorough review of work practices and conditions is essential to determine and prevent any further inadvertent reexposure. The elements of the evaluation for determining the specific occupational asthma etiologic agent are beyond the scope of this chapter; however, the key elements are obtaining a thorough occupational and environmental history; performing immunologic tests (prick skin testing, radioallergosorbent testing); and performing pulmonary physiology studies, including serial peak flows, spirometry, or methacholine testing, during times at work and away from work. In some circumstances, specific inhalational challenges are needed to establish whether there is a possible workplace etiology. Such testing is available in only a few specialized centers. Particular attention to the occupational history is warranted in examining asthmatics who are welders, electronics assemblers, laboratory technicians, health care workers, metal workers, plastics industry workers, bakers, chemical processors, and automobile and other spray painters.[8,16] There are many published occupational history questionnaire templates.[52-54] Several references provide a comprehensive review of the evaluation of occupational asthma.[55-58]

Occupational Asthma with Latency

Ultimately the goal in management of occupational asthma with latency should be avoidance of further exposure to the offending agent. Avoidance can potentially cure or significantly reverse this form of asthma, although many individuals are left with significant persistent asthma despite removal from exposure to the offending agent. Respiratory protection, using masks, is inadequate and should not be considered an option in immune-mediated occupational asthma. Low levels of ongoing exposure to sensitizers can perpetuate asthma in a sensitized individual. Pisati and colleagues[59] studied the medical outcomes of a group of 66 patients with TDI-induced asthma, some of whom remained in exposure. Despite use of respiratory protection, the 17 workers who remained assigned to jobs that had only an occasional risk of exposure to the chemical were more symptomatic, required more medication, were considered clinically unstable, and showed significant deterioration in FEV_1 and PC15 for methacholine compared with the 43 workers who no longer were exposed. No worker who had been exposed to isocyanates for more than 10 years or who continued to work for more than 3 years after onset of asthma recovered. This study emphasizes the need to recognize occupational asthma early, the inadequacy of respiratory protection, and the paramount importance of eliminating further exposure.

Nonlatent (Irritant-Induced) Asthma or RADS

In contrast, nonlatent (irritant-induced) asthma or RADS patients may be able to remain in their job, provided that there have been changes that reduce the risk of further irritant exposure or industrial accident.[60] Job process modifications include substitution of safer substances, process isolation (i.e., enclosure), improved ventilation, and the use of personal protective equipment (respirators). In certain circumstances, these individuals are unable to tolerate ongoing exposures to the offending agent even at lower levels, and attempts should be made to accommodate them in alternative locations or jobs. Respirators are the least effective option. They are uncomfortable and cumbersome to wear for a full work shift, making compliance a major problem. Some of these patients may have developed irritant-associated vocal cord dysfunction and may benefit from speech therapy instruction on throat relaxation, cough and throat clearing suppression, and breathing control techniques.[61,62]

Prognosis and Follow-up

Most patients with occupational asthma are left with some degree of permanent impairment. Several studies showed that more than 60% of subjects fail to recover completely, even after leaving exposure.[63,64] Continued exposure after the onset of symptoms often leads to more severe asthma, which persists even when exposure is eventually discontinued.[18] These studies emphasize the need for early diagnosis, removal from exposure, and appropriate treatment. To date, it is not known if there are significant differences in prognosis between latent and nonlatent occupational asthma. Brooks and associates[20] reported long-term persistent reactive airway disease in individuals who developed RADS.

To reverse the increasing prevalence of occupational asthma requires improved disease surveillance and improved physician recognition of occupational asthma. This starts with the simple but often neglected question, "What type of work do you do?" The role of the clinician is to meet the urgent care needs of the patient for his or her acute asthmatic episode and to work with industry, labor, government agencies, and specialists in occupational health to prevent disease through early identification of old and new hazards. Each time a worker is identified as having occupational asthma in a setting where no previous cases have been identified should be considered as a "sentinel health event." Such recognition should lead to consultation with individuals who can help initiate the investigative activities that will improve workplace conditions for all workers.

REFERENCES

1. Carino M, Aliani M, Licitra C, Sarns N, Ioli F: Death due to asthma at workplace in a diphenylmethane diisocyanate-sensitive subject. Respiration 64:111–113, 1997.
2. Ehrlich RI: Fatal asthma in a baker: A case report. Am J Ind Med 26:799–802, 1994.
3. Fabbri LM: Occupational factors: Asthma—what are the important experiments? Am Rev Respir Dis 138:730–744, 1988.
4. Butcher BT, et al: Longitudinal study of workers employed in the manufacture of toluene diisocyanate. Am Rev Respir Dis 116:411–421, 1977.
5. Weill H: Disaster at Bhopal: The accident, early findings and respiratory health outlook in those injured. Bull Eur Physiopathol Respir 23:587–590, 1987.
6. Fabbri LM, Danieli D, Crescioli S, et al: Fatal asthma in a subject sensitized to toluene diisocyanate. Am Rev Respir Dis 137:1494–1498, 1988.
7. Lagier F, et al: Latex as aeroallergen. Lancet 336:516–517, 1990.

8. Meredith SK, Taylor VM, McDonald JC: Occupational respiratory disease in the United Kingdom 1989: A report to the British Thoracic Society and the Society of Occupational Medicine by the SWORD project group. Br J Ind Med 48:292–298, 1991.
9. Ross DJ, Keynes HL, McDonald JC: SWORD '96: Surveillance of work-related and occupational respiratory disease in the United Kingdom. Occup Med (Oxf) 47:377–381, 1997.
10. Reilly MJ, et al: Surveillance for occupational asthma: Michigan and New Jersey, 1988–1992. MMWR Morb Mortal Wkly Rep CDC Surveill Summ 43:9–17, 1994.
11. Keskinen H, Alanko K, Saarinen L: Occupational asthma in Finland. Clin Allergy 8:569–579, 1978.
12. Contreras GR, Rousseau R, Chang-Yeung M: Occupational respiratory diseases in British Columbia, Canada in 1991. Occup Environ Med 51:710–712, 1994.
13. Brooks SM: Bronchial asthma of occupational origin: A review. Scand J Work Environ Health 3:53–72, 1977.
14. Kobayashi S: Different aspects of occupational asthma in Japan. In Frazier CA (ed): Occupational Asthma. New York, Van Nostrand-Reinhold, 1980, pp 229–244.
15. Syabbalo N: Occupational asthma in a developing country (Letter). Chest 99:528, 1991.
16. Fishwick D, et al: Occupational asthma in New Zealanders: A population-based study. Occup Environ Med 54:301–306, 1997.
17. Leonard BI, et al (eds): Asthma in the Workplace, 2nd ed. New York, Marcel Dekker, 1999.
18. Chan-Yeung M, Malo JL: Epidemiology of occupational asthma. In Busse WW, Holgate ST (eds): Asthma and Rhinitis. Boston, Blackwell Scientific Publications, 1995, pp 44–57.
19. Bernstein IL, et al: Definition and classification of asthma. In Leonard BI, et al (eds): Asthma in the Workplace. New York, Marcel Dekker, 1993, pp 1–4.
20. Brooks SM, Weiss MA, Bernstein IL: Reactive airways dysfunction syndromes (RADS): Persistent asthma syndrome after high level irritant exposures. Chest 88:376–384, 1985.
21. Tarlo SM, Broder I: Irritant-induced occupational asthma. Chest 96:297–300, 1989.
22. Merchant JA, Bernstein IL: Cotton and other textile dusts. In Leonard BI, et al (eds): Asthma in the Workplace. New York, Marcel Dekker, 1993, pp 551–576.
23. Chan Yeung M, Malo JL: Tables of major inducers of occupational asthma. In Leonard BI, et al (eds): Asthma in the Workplace. New York, Marcel Dekker, 1993.
24. Lagier F, et al: Prevalence of latex allergy in operating room nurses. J Allergy Clin Immunol 90:319–322, 1992.
25. Slovak AJM, Hill RN: Does atopy have any predictive value for laboratory animal allergy? A comparison of different concepts of atopy. Br J Ind Med 44:129–132, 1987.
26. Chan-Yeung M: Immunologic and non-immunologic mechanisms in asthma due to Western Red Cedar (Thuja plicata). Am Rev Respir Dis 70:32–37, 1982.
27. Venables KM, et al: Interaction of smoking and atopy in producing specific IgE antibody against a hapten protein conjugate. BMJ 290:201–204, 1985.
28. Chan-Yeung M, Lam S, Koener S: Clinical features and natural history of occupational asthma due to Western Red Cedar (Thuja plicata). Am J Med 72:411–415, 1982.
29. Chan-Yeung M, Desjardins A: Bronchial hyperresponsiveness and level of exposure in occupational asthma due to Western Red Cedar (Thuja plicata). Am Rev Respir Dis 146:1606–1609, 1992.
30. Séguin P, et al: Prevalence of occupational asthma in spray painters exposed to several types of isocyanates, including polymethylene polyphenylisocyanate. J Occup Med 29:340–344, 1987.
31. OSHA: Occupational Public Health Guideline for Phthalic Anhydride. Atlanta, GA US Department of Health and Human Services, Public Health Service, Centers for Disease Control and US Department of Labor, 1978.
32. Fabbri LM, et al: Pathophysiology of occupational asthma. In Leonard BI, et al (eds): Asthma in the Workplace. New York, Marcel Dekker, 1993, pp 61–92.
33. Saetta M, et al: Airway mucosal inflammation in occupational asthma induced by toluene diisocyanate. Am Rev Respir Dis 145:160–168, 1992.
34. Saetta M, et al: Effect of cessation of exposure to toluene diisocyanate (TDI) on bronchial mucosa of subjects with TDI-induced asthma. Am Rev Respir Dis 145:169–174, 1992.

35. Bernstein DI, Zeiss CR: Guidelines for preparation and characterization of chemical-protein conjugate antigens: Report of the Subcommittee on preparation and characterization of low molecular weight antigens. J Allergy Clin Immunol 84:820–822, 1989.

36. Luo JC, Nelsen KG, Fischbein A: Persistent reactive airway dysfunction syndrome after exposure to toluene diisocyanate. Br J Ind Med 47:239–241, 1990.

37. Diem JE, et al: Five-year longitudinal study of workers employed in a new toluene diisocyanate manufacturing plant. Am Rev Respir Dis 126:420–428, 1982.

38. Butcher BT, et al: Inhalation challenge and pharmacologic studies of toluene diisocyanate (TDI)-sensitive workers. J Allergy Clin Immunol 64:146–152, 1979.

39. Frans A, Pahulycz C: Transient syndrome of acute irritation of the bronchi induced by single and massive inhalation of phthalic anhydride. Rev Pneumol Clin 49:247–251, 1993.

40. Grammer LC, et al: Evaluation of a worker with possible formaldehyde-induced asthma. J Allergy Clin Immunol 92(1 Pt 1):29–33, 1993.

41. Rivera M, et al: Trimellitic anhydride toxicity: A cause of acute multisystem failure. Arch Intern Med 141:1071–1074, 1981.

42. Kaplan V, et al: Pulmonary hemorrhage due to inhalation of vapor containing pyromellitic dianhydride. Chest 104:644–645, 1993.

43. Patterson R, Zeiss CR, Pruzansky JJ: Immunology and immunopathology of trimellitic anhydride pulmonary reactions. J Allergy Clin Immunol 70:19–23, 1982.

44. Leach CL, et al: Evidence of immunologic control of lung injury induced by trimellitic anhydride. Am Rev Respir Dis 137:186–190, 1988.

45. Cartier A, et al: Specific serum antibodies against isocyanates: Association with occupational asthma. J Allergy Clin Immunol 84:507–514, 1989.

46. Persson P, et al: Biological monitoring of occupational exposure to toluene diisocyanate: Measurement of toluenediamine in hydrolysed urine and plasma by gas chromatography-mass spectrometry. Br J Ind Med 50:1111–1118, 1993.

47. Tiljander A, Skarping G, Dalene M: Chromatographic determination of amines in biological fluids with special reference to the biological monitoring of isocyanates and amines. J Chromatogr 479:145–152, 1989.

48. Zeiss CR, et al: A twelve-year clinical and immunological evaluation of workers involved in the manufacture of trimellitic anhydride (TMA). Allergy Proc 11:71–77, 1990.

49. Zeiss CR, et al: Syndromes in workers exposed to trimellitic anhydride: A longitudinal clinical and immunologic study. Ann Intern Med 98:8–12, 1983.

50. Pfaffli P: Phthalic acid excretion as an indicator of exposure to phthalic anhydride in the work atmosphere. Int Arch Occup Environ Health 58:209–216, 1986.

51. Palacian E, et al: Dicarboxylic acid anhydrides as dissociating agents of protein-containing structures. Mol Cell Biochem 97:101–111, 1990.

52. LaDou J: Approach to the diagnosis of occupational illness. In LaDou J (ed): Occupational Medicine. Los Altos, CA, Lange Medical Books, 1990, pp 5–16.

53. Rosenstock L, et al: Development and validation of a self-administered occupational health questionnaire. J Occup Med 26:50–54, 1984.

54. Schwartz DA, et al: The occupational history in the primary care setting. Am J Med 90:315–319, 1991.

55. Mapp CE: Agents, old and new, causing occupational asthma. Occup Environ Med 58:354–360, 2001.

56. Blanc PD: The association between occupation and asthma in general medical practice. Chest 115:1259–1264, 1999.

57. Quirce S, Sastre J: Occupational asthma. Allergy Eur J Allergy Clin Immunol 53:633–641, 1998.

58. Lemiere C, et al: Diagnosing occupational asthma: Use of induced sputum. Eur Respir J 13:482–488, 1999.

59. Pisati G, Baruffini A, Zedda S: Toluene diisocyanate induced asthma: Outcome according to persistence or cessation of exposure. Br J Ind Med 50:60–64, 1993.

60. Wagner GR, Wegman DH: Occupational asthma: Prevention by definition (Editorial). Am J Ind Med 33:427–429, 1998.

61. Balkissoon R, Shusterman D: Occupational upper airway disorders. Semin Respir Crit Care Med 20:569–580, 1999.

62. Perkner JJ, et al: Irritant-associated vocal cord dysfunction. J Occup Environ Med 40:136–143, 1998.

63. Chan-Yeung M: A clinician's approach to determine the diagnosis, prognosis, and therapy of occupational asthma. Med Clin North Am 74:811–822, 1990.

64. Lemiere C, et al: Closed-circuit apparatus for specific inhalation challenges with an occupational agent, formaldehyde, in vapor form. Chest 109:1631–1635, 1996.

CHAPTER 97

Irritant and Toxic Respiratory Injuries

Dorsett D. Smith

Toxic and irritating gases have been known to produce fatalities since the Athenians used a combination of pitch and sulfur to produce toxic fumes in a war against the Spartans in 428 BC. More sophisticated irritant agents were introduced during World War I, when mustard gas, chlorine, and phosgene were the primary agents of chemical warfare. These gases produced many incapacitating causalties but relatively few fatalities compared with conventional weapons. The use of mustard gas was reported in the 1988 war between Iraq and Iran, and more recently gas warfare was reported between Iraq and the Kurds.

Large amounts of irritant gases are produced; more than 0.5 million workers are exposed to anhydrous ammonia alone in the United States. In 1984, a disastrous release of large amounts of methyl isocyanate in Bhopal, India, resulted in approximately 2500 to 5000 deaths and 200,000 individuals with respiratory, eye, and other symptoms.[1] Smaller numbers are exposed to a variety of other irritant gases that are used in a multitude of industrial processes. In addition, many millions of people worldwide also are exposed to compounds related to the burning of a variety of materials that may generate toxic gases. This exposure most commonly occurs in commercial or home fires, where large amounts of hydrogen cyanide, hydrogen chloride, acrolein, sulfur dioxide, phosgene, and other irritant gases are produced (Table 97-1). Statistically the major lethal gas still is the asphyxiant gas carbon monoxide.

The magnitude of the problem is significant. In reports to poison control centers, approximately 43.6% of exposures involve an inhalational agent in the workplace, and greater than 61% of exposures are related to an environmental cause.[2] Fumes, gases, and vapors are common causes of environmental exposures and constitute the largest mortality. Hydrogen sulfide and hydrofluoric acid are the leading cause of death in the occupationally exposed group. Approximately 5% of workplace deaths are due to asphyxiation.[3]

CHEMISTRY

Exposure to toxic concentrations of inhalational agents may result in systemic injury and local injury to the respiratory system. Vapors and gases can be classified into several different types based on the physical state of the particular substance.

Dusts are a particular form of a solid organic or inorganic material that is small enough to be airborne. They usually are characterized by particles ranging from 0.1 to 25 μm in diameter.

 Characteristics of Gases and Vapors

1. A gas is a state of matter in which the molecules move freely, allowing infinite expansion.
2. A vapor is a gas below its critical temperature at which it may be liquefied by an increased pressure.
3. The density of a gas is relative to air; the more dense a gas is, the more likely it will seek low areas.
4. Cold gases are more dense and seek low areas. Nitrogen acts as an asphyxiant in low areas when cold.

Fumes are extremely fine solid particulates that usually are formed by the combustion or condensation of metals so that these metals have entered a gaseous state. These fumes usually range from 0.001 to 1.0 μm in diameter.

A *gas* is a substance that at standard conditions has a physical state in which molecules move freely, allowing infinite expansion. The vapor density of a gas by convention is expressed relative to air, which by definition has a vapor density of 1. The more dense (or the heavier) the gas, the more likely that it will seek low areas in the air column. Decreased temperature increases the density of a gas. Nitrogen may act as an asphyxiant in low areas when cold. A gas is not capable of being liquefied by pressure alone and is liquefied by lowering its temperature and increasing pressure.

A *vapor* is a gas below its critical temperature at which it may be liquefied by an increased pressure alone. It may exist as either a liquid or a solid when it is in equilibrium with its vapor. So-called industrial gases—chlorine, ammonia, propane, and butane—are actually vapors.

A *fog* is a liquid aerosol formed by a condensation from a gaseous to a liquid state.

Smoke is a mixture of airborne particles, vapors, and gases, resulting from the incomplete combustion of organic materials. These particles are usually less than 0.5 μm in diameter.

This chapter discusses primarily the health effects of gases, vapors, and fumes. A general classification of toxic inhalants is presented in Table 97-2. Table 97-3 lists the common chemical exposures and their effects and the concentrations commonly associated with a significant health hazard. Although not irritants, asphyxiants are included for completeness (Table 97-4).

Irritant gases are gases that cause respiratory tissue injury by direct contact due to their chemical reactivity. Acid and alkaline gases, such as chlorine and ammonia, may produce extreme alterations in pH, and other gases may cause chemical

TABLE 97-1 Common Pyrolysis Products of Combustion

SUBSTANCE	TOXIC PRODUCT
Acrylics	Acrolein
Batteries, paints	Metals (lead, zinc, manganese, cadmium, cobalt)
Coal, fuel, wood	Carbon monoxide
Fuels, fabrics, celluloid, nitrocellulose film	Oxides of nitrogen, cyanide, aldehydes
Fluorinated resins	Hydrogen fluoride
Melamine, silk, wool, polyurethane, nylon	Ammonia, hydrocyanic acid, hydrogen sulfide, isocyanates
Polyvinyl chloride	Chlorine, phosgene, hydrochloric acid
Rubber	Hydrogen sulfide, sulfur dioxide
Sulfur compounds	Sulfur dioxide
Wood, house fires, building fires	Acrolein, acetaldehyde, hydrocyanic acid, carbon monoxide, nitrogen dioxide, ammonia

reactions with membrane damage and release of free radicals. The site of the pulmonary injury is related largely to the water solubility of the various gases (Table 97-5). The various factors influencing the likelihood and degree of pulmonary injury are presented in Table 97-6.

PATHOPHYSIOLOGY

The early responses to the inhalation of irritant gases are primarily reduced ciliary function, increased mucus production, submucosal edema, and smooth muscle constriction. These are followed by mediator-induced airway inflammation, causing symptoms of retrosternal pain, cough, and dyspnea. Aminophylline and isoproterenol attenuate leukotriene generation by lung mast cells and prevent lysosomal degranulation of neutrophils, a key component of airway inflammation. In the lungs, swelling of type 1 pneumocytes occurs, followed later by capillary leakage due to damage of the basement membrane of epithelial cells. These changes in the cytoskeleton affect the intercellular junctions, causing them to pull apart. The role of cyclic adenosine monophosphate (cAMP) in regulating epithelial cell permeability has become an area of great interest, because it has been reported that cAMP decreases the permeability of epithelial cells by altering the structure of tight junctions.[4]

The health effects of irritant gas or vapor exposure depend on their physiochemical properties and specific host factors. The extent of adverse effects may vary among individuals when exposed to the same agent and concentration.

Oxidant-Related Injury

Oxidant-related injury causes increases in pulmonary vascular pressure and epithelial permeability. Studies with the oxidant tert-butyl hydroperoxide have shown that pulmonary phospholipid oxidation yields arachidonic acid via phospholipase A (Fig. 97-1). Arachidonic acid is a substrate of the cyclooxygenase pathway, leading to the synthesis of prostaglandin $F_{2\alpha}$ (Fig. 97-2), which is a pulmonary vasoconstrictor. Arachi-

TABLE 97-2 General Classification of Acute Inhalational Toxicants

I. Respiratory Toxicants
  A. Single agents
    1. Asphyxiants
      a. Simple
        i. Carbon dioxide
        ii. Methane
        iii. Nitrogen
      b. Chemical
        i. Agents that decrease oxygen-carrying capacity
          (a) Carbon monoxide
          (b) Hydrogen sulfide
          (c) Oxides of nitrogen
        ii. Agents that inhibit tissue oxygen utilization
          (a) Acrylonitrile
          (b) Hydrogen cyanide
          (c) Hydrogen sulfide
    2. Irritants
      a. High-solubility gases
        i. Ammonia
        ii. Methyl isocyanate
        iii. Sulfur dioxide
      b. Intermediate-solubility gases
        i. Chlorine
      c. Low-solubility gases
        i. Hydrogen sulfide
        ii. Oxides of nitrogen
        iii. Phosgene
  B. Mixtures
    1. Smoke inhalation from fires
    2. Smoke inhalation from smoke bombs
  C. Illicit drug abuse
    1. Airway burns from freebasing cocaine
    2. Asphyxia from glue sniffing and organic solvent abuse
    3. Drug-induced pulmonary edema
    4. Pulmonary hypertension, pulmonary fibrosis, bullous emphysema secondary to intravenous drug abuse
  D. War gases
    1. Lethal agents (CG, DP, CL, PS, AC)
    2. Riot control agents (CN, CS, CR, DM)

II. Systemic Toxicants
  A. Fluorinated polymers (polymer fume fever)
  B. Metal oxides (metal fume fever)
  C. Organic dusts (organic toxic dust syndrome)
  D. Poisons (arsine, stibine, carbon tetrachloride)

CG, phosgene; DP, diphosgene; CL, phosgene; PS, chloropicrin; AC, hydrogen cyanide; CN, 1-chloroacetophenone; CS, o-chlorobenzylidene malononitrile; CR, debenz (b,f):1:4-oxazepine; DM, diphenylaminearsine.
Adapted from Delclos G, Carson AI: Acute gaseous exposure. In Harber, Schenker, Balmes (eds): Occupational and Environmental Respiratory Disease. St. Louis, Mosby, 1996, p 518.

donic acid also is a substrate for the lipoxygenase pathway (Fig. 97-3), which increases vascular permeability.[5]

A variety of prooxidants produce cell injury by causing the formation of reactive oxygenate species that overwhelm the natural defense mechanisms of the cell. The reactive oxygen species include superoxides and hydrogen peroxide, which may produce highly reactive elements that damage cell membranes. Glutathione peroxidase is a key enzyme involved in the detoxification of lipid peroxides, and the maintenance of reduced glutathione is essential for glutathione peroxidase function. Several other thiol compounds have been shown to

TABLE 97-3 Commonly Used Toxic Gases and Fumes and Their Dangerous Levels of Exposure

AGENT	PRINCIPAL OCCUPATIONS EXPOSED	TIME-WEIGHTED MAIN MECHANISM OF INJURY	AVERAGE*	IDLH LEVEL†
Acetic acid	Production of cellulose, dyeing, pharmaceuticals, food processing	Severe irritation of eyes, mucous membranes, skin; RADS, bronchitis, pneumonitis	10 ppm	500 ppm
Acrolein	Plastic, rubber, textile, resin making	Direct action on mucosa of the eyes and respiratory tract, irritant effects	0.1 ppm	5 ppm
Acrylonitrile	Synthetic fiber, acrylic resin, rubber making	Asphyxiant, neurotoxicity	2 ppm	4 ppm
Ammonia	Fertilizer, refrigerator, explosive production	Direct action on mucosa of the eyes and respiratory tract; tracheitis and pulmonary edema	25 ppm	500 ppm
Antimony trichloride or pentachloride	Metallurgy	Mucous membrane irritant, eye, skin, and lung; pulmonary edema	0.5 mg/m³	—
Arsine	Smelting, refining, electronics	Systemic effects, hemolysis	0.05 ppm	6 ppm
Boron trifluoride	Fumigant, flux, catalyst	Irritant of eyes, skin, lungs; abnormal lung function	1 ppm	500 ppm
Cadmium oxide fumes	Ore smelting, alloying, welding	Tracheobronchitis, pulmonary edema, emphysema, renal effects	0.1 mg/m³ (40 μg/m³)	40 mg/m³
Carbon dioxide	Foundry work, mining	Asphyxiant	10,000 ppm	50,000 ppm
Carbon disulfide	Degreasing, electroplating, sulfur processing, insecticide	Systemic effects, cardiac disease	10 ppm (1 ppm)	500 ppm
Carbon monoxide	Foundry work, petroleum refining, mining	Asphyxiant	50 ppm	1500 ppm
Chloramine	By-product of mixture of bleach and ammonia-containing products	Common cause of pulmonary edema and pulmonary irritation in homemakers, custodians, and industrial workers	—	—
Chlorine	Bleaching, disinfectant, plastic making	Direct action on mucosa of the eyes and respiratory tract; tracheitis and pulmonary edema. Possible chronic effect and airways obstruction	0.5 ppm	100 ppm
Chloropicrin	Manufacture of pesticides	Irritation of eyes, mucous membranes, skin; pulmonary edema	0.1 ppm	100 ppm
Chromates	Electroplating	Cutaneous ulcers, dermatitis, nasal perforation, rhinitis, nose bleeds, laryngitis, tracheobronchitis, chemical pneumonitis, gingivitis, lung cancer	50 μg Cr (VI) 500 μg Cr (III)	100 mg/m³ 100 mg/m³
Chromyl chloride	Dye making, manufacturing chromium complexes	Severe irritant; second- and third-degree burns; eye, nose, throat, airway injury	0.025 ppm	1 ppm
Copper fumes	Welding	Systemic effects, "brass chills"	0.1 mg/m³	—
Dimethyl sulfate	Organic chemical manufacturing	Severe eye and skin burns, laryngeal edema, late-onset pulmonary edema	0.1 ppm	100 ppm
Dioxane	Solvent	Irritant to eyes and mucous membranes May cause pulmonary edema. Primarily systemic toxicants, hepatic necrosis, renal damage	25 ppm	1500 ppm
Ethylene oxide	Fumigant, sterilizing agent	Irritation of eyes, skin, respiratory tract; pulmonary edema, CNS depression	1 ppm	1000 ppm
Fluorine	Rocket fuel, uranium processing, manufacturing of fluorocarbons	Severe irritant of eyes, skin, mucous membranes, respiratory tract; pulmonary edema	1 ppm	25 ppm
Formaldehyde	Disinfectant, embalming fluid use, paper and photography industry	Direct action on mucosa of the eyes and respiratory tract; dermatitis, asthma (?)	1 ppm (0.8 ppm)	100 ppm
Glyphosate herbicides	Herbicide application	Acute mucosal erosions of mouth and upper respiratory tract. Damage to alveolar membrane. Gradual development of chemical pneumonitis (roundup pneumonitis)	—	—

Continued

TABLE 97-3 Commonly Used Toxic Gases and Fumes and Their Dangerous Levels of Exposure—cont'd

AGENT	PRINCIPAL OCCUPATIONS EXPOSED	TIME-WEIGHTED MAIN MECHANISM OF INJURY	AVERAGE*	IDLH LEVEL†
Halon	Fire extinguishing, refrigerant	Cardiac toxicity, asphyxiation	—	1000 ppm
Hydrogen chloride	Refining, dye making, organic chemical synthesis, pyrolysis in fires	Direct action on mucosa of the eyes and respiratory tract, tracheobronchitis	5 ppm	100 ppm
Hydrogen cyanide	Electroplating, fumigant work, steel industry	Systemic effects, asphyxiant	10 ppm	50 ppm
Hydrogen fluoride	Etching, petroleum industry, silk working, plastics, refrigerants	Direct action on mucosa of the eyes and respiratory tract, tracheitis	3 ppm	20 ppm
Hydrogen selenide	Ceramic and glass manufacturing, photocells	Irritation of eyes, nose, throat, delayed pulmonary edema	5 ppb	—
Hydrogen sulfide	Natural gas making, paper pulp, sewage treatment, tannery work, oil well prospecting	Systemic and local effects, pulmonary edema, and asphyxia	10 ppm	300 ppm
Magnesium oxide fumes	Welding, alloy, flare, filament making	Systemic effects	15 mg/m³	—
Manganese fumes	Foundry work, battery making, permanganate manufacture	Systemic effects, possible predisposition to pneumonia, neurotoxicity	5 mg/m³	—
Mercury fumes	Electrolysis	Direct action on mucosa of the eyes, gastrointestinal tract, and lung; interstitial pneumonitis, systemic effects	0.1 mg/m³ (0.05 mg/m³)	28 mg/m³
Methane	Mining	Simple asphyxiation	—	—
Methyl bromide	Fumigating, dye and refrigerant making	Direct action on mucosa of the eyes and respiratory tract	5 ppm	2000 ppm
Methyl isocyanate	Pesticide manufacturing	Direct action on mucosa of the eyes and respiratory tract; tracheitis, pulmonary edema, chronic airways obstruction	0.02 ppm	20 ppm
Methylene chloride	Solvent, paint remover, aerosol propellant	Primarily a CNS depressant, mild mucous membrane irritant, asphyxiant due to metabolism of carboxyhemoglobin	50 ppm	1000 ppm
Natural gas	Mining, petroleum refining, power	Asphyxiant	—	—
Nickel carbonyl	Metallurgy, coal gasification, petroleum refining	Pulmonary edema, delayed toxic pneumonitis	0.001 ppm	30 ppm
Nitrogen dioxide	Arc welding, dye and fertilizer making, farming, silo filling	Irritant to respiratory tract; tracheitis, pulmonary edema, bronchiolitis obliterans	5 ppm (1 ppm)	50 ppm
Osmium tetroxide fumes	Alloy making, platinum hardening	Direct irritation of respiratory tract	0.002 mg/m³	1 mg/m³
Ozone	Arc welding; air, sewage, and water	Direct irritation of respiratory tract	0.1 ppm	10 ppm
Paraquat	Herbicide	Minor irritant of mucous membranes; epistaxis, iritis, severe fatal pulmonary fibrosis. Primary absorption through skin or GI tract	0.1 µg/m³	1 mg/m³
Phosgene	Chemical industry, dye and insecticide making, refrigeration, fire fighting	Direct irritation of respiratory tract; pulmonary edema	0.1 ppm	3 ppm
Phosphine	Semiconductor manufacturing, fumigant	Severe respiratory irritant, pulmonary edema, asphyxiant. Inhibits electron transport and combination of heme to iron	0.3 ppm	100 ppm
Platinum, soluble salts (mist)	Alloy, mirror making, electroplating, catalysis, ceramic work	Asthmatic reactions	0.002 mg/m³	—
Propane	Cooking, heating	Simple asphyxiation	1000 ppm	20,000 ppm
Sulfur dioxide	Bleaching, ore smelting, paper manufacture, refrigeration industry	Direct action on the respiratory tract; bronchitis, exceptional pulmonary edema	2 ppm (0.5 ppm)	100 ppm
Sulfur pentafluoride	Production by-product of synthesis or degradation of sulfur hexafluoride	Severe pulmonary irritant, pulmonary edema	10 ppb	1 ppm
Titanium tetrachloride	Metallurgy	Highly corrosive to skin, eyes, mucous membranes—contact with water liberates hydrogen chloride and chloride. Pulmonary edema, endobronchial polyposis	—	1000 ppm

TABLE 97-3 Commonly Used Toxic Gases and Fumes and Their Dangerous Levels of Exposure—cont'd

AGENT	PRINCIPAL OCCUPATIONS EXPOSED	TIME-WEIGHTED MAIN MECHANISM OF INJURY	AVERAGE*	IDLH LEVEL†
Toluene-2,4-diisocyanate	Production of polyurethane foams, plastics, paints, wire coatings	Severe mucous membrane irritant to eyes, skin, respiratory tract; bronchitis, asthma, pulmonary edema	5 ppb	100 ppb
Trimellitic anhydride	Epoxy resins, paints, dyes, pharmaceuticals	Cough and upper airway irritation, rhinitis and asthma, flu syndrome, pulmonary disease, anemia syndrome	5 ppb	2 mg/m³
Vanadium pentoxide fumes	Glass, ceramic, alloy making, chemical industry (catalysis)	Direct action on respiratory tract; bronchitis, asthma	0.5 mg/m³ (0.05 mg/m³)	70 mg/m³
Zinc chloride fumes	Dry cell making, soldering, textile finishing, smoke grenades	Direct action on respiratory tract, irritan; pulmonary edema	1 mg/m³	2000 mg/m³
Zinc oxide fumes	Welding, cutting galvanized steel	Systemic effects, metal fume fever	5 mg/m³	—
Zirconium chloride	Metallurgy	When heated, emits chloride fumes. Can produce pulmonary edema. Damages mucous membranes	5 mg/m³	—

*Figures in parentheses are National Institute of Occupational Safety and Health (NIOSH) recommendations.
†IDLH, immediately dangerous to life or health.
CNS, central nervous system; GI, gastrointestinal; RADS, reactive airways dysfunction syndrome.
Adapted from Morgan WK, Seaton A: Occupational Lung Disease. Philadelphia, WB Saunders, 1984, pp 611–613.

TABLE 97-4 Simple Asphyxiants

HEAVIER THAN AIR	LIGHTER THAN AIR
Carbon dioxide	Methane
Ethane	Nitrogen
Natural gas	Ethylene
Butane	Neon
Propane	Acetylene
Argon	Helium
Krypton	Hydrogen
Xenon	

TABLE 97-5 Gas Solubility and Toxic Effects

1. Solubility and chemical reactivity are the major explanations for the site of action and severity of a toxic inhalation.
2. Corrosive gases, such as ammonium, sulfur hexafluoride (SF_6), mustard gas, methyl isocyanate, and silicone tetrachloride ($SiCl_4$), produce intense upper airway symptoms, such as severe coughing, conjunctivitis, burning in the nose, laryngeal edema, and facial burns.
3. Exposure to a soluble irritant gas can be estimated as significant if the conjunctivae are inflamed, the face is erythematous, and the nose and throat are red and irritated; this suggests a dose high enough to produce upper and lower airway damage.

TABLE 97-6 Determinants of Severity of Lung Injury

Duration of exposure
Minute ventilation
Proximity to source
Density of gas and height of victim
Temperature of gas
Toxicity of gas
Water solubility of gas
Particle size of mist, fog, or vapor
Breathing pattern: oronasal versus mouth breathing
Host factors such as preexisting asthma, coronary disease, or COPD
Orthopedic problems that affect the ability to evacuate quickly

COPD, chronic obstructive pulmonary disease.

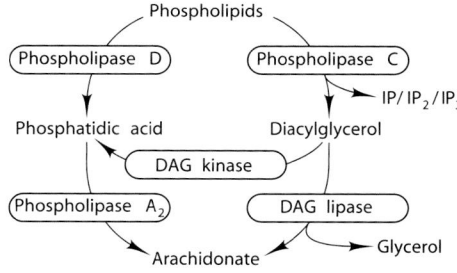

FIGURE 97-1

Pathways of release of arachidonate from phospholipids by two-step processes. DAG, diacylglycerol; IP, inositol phosphate. *(From Rang HP, Dale MM, Ritter JM, Gardner P: Local hormones, inflammation and allergy. In Pharmacology, 4th ed. New York, Churchill Livingstone, 2001, p 214.)*

be capable of protecting animals against oxygen toxicity and against lung damage from bleomycin-induced and paraquat-induced lung injury.[6-8] The discovery that glutathione constitutes the major source of a low-molecular-weight thiol in mammalian tissue for the purposes of detoxification has resulted in great interest in the substitution of other thiol compounds, such as *N*-acetylcysteine, in the treatment of phosgene and other toxic inhalations.

Studies by Miller and coworkers[9] on the inhalation of ozone in animal models suggested that the maximum dose of ozone is found in the respiratory bronchioles. Some human data from clinical studies suggest that the respiratory bronchioles

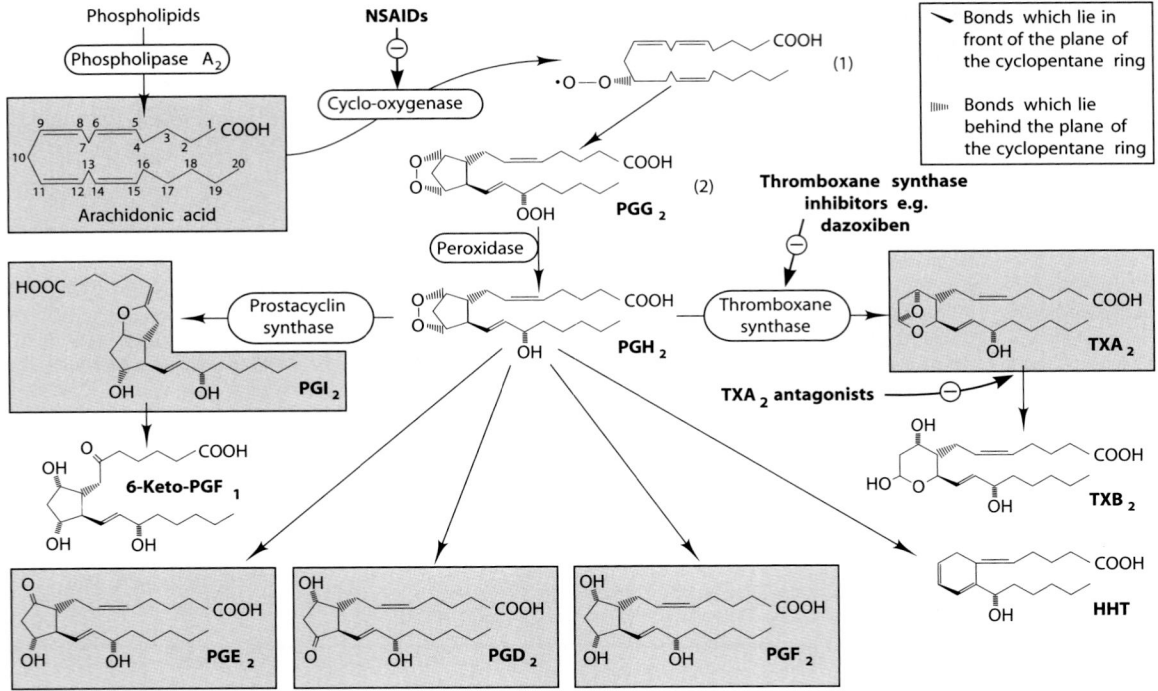

FIGURE 97-2

The biosynthesis of prostaglandins, prostacyclin, and thromboxane from arachidonate. Compounds with biologic action are shown in boxes. There are two forms of cyclooxygenase (COX): One (COX-1) is constitutive and occurs in most cell types, and the other (COX-2) is induced in inflammatory cells by inflammatory stimuli. The current nonsteroidal antiinflammatory drugs (NSAIDs) act mainly on COX-1. HHT, 17-hydroxy-heptadecatrienoic acid; IFN-γ, interferon-γ; PG, prostaglandin; TX, thromboxane. *(From Rang HP, Dale MM, Ritter JM, Gardner P: Local hormones, inflammation and allergy. In Pharmacology, 4th ed. New York, Churchill Livingstone, 2001, p 215.)*

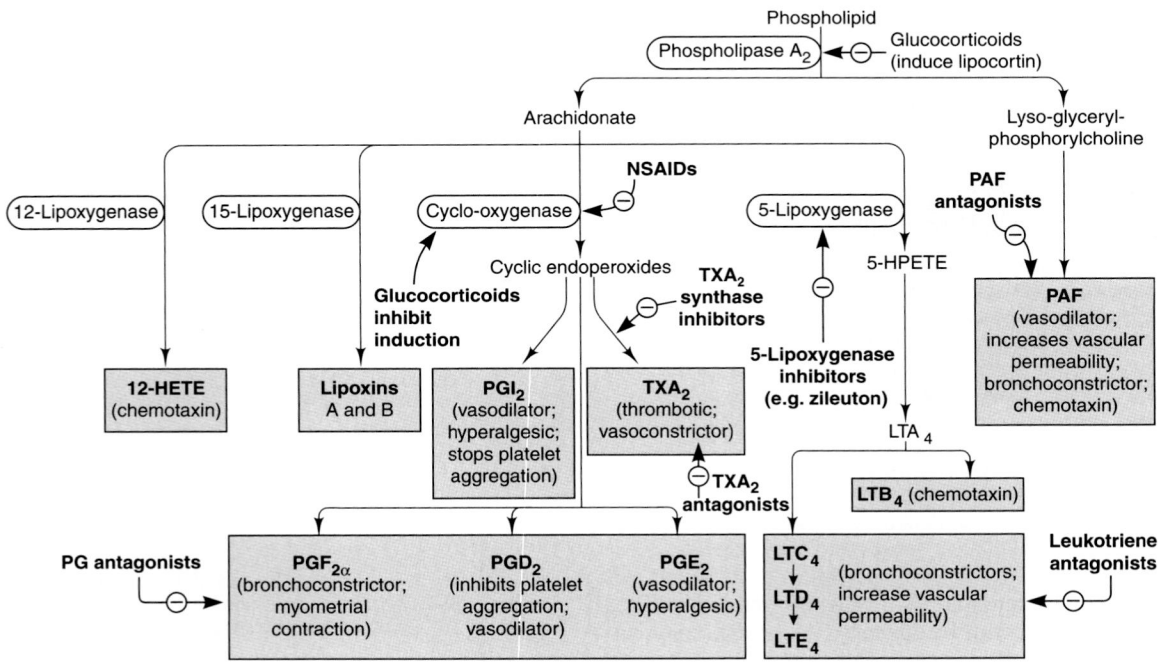

FIGURE 97-3

Summary diagram of mediators derived from phospholipids and their actions and the sites of action of antiinflammatory drugs. The arachidonate metabolites are "eicosanoids." The glucocorticoids inhibit transcription of the gene for cyclooxygenase-2, which is induced in inflammatory cells by inflammatory mediators. The effects of prostaglandin E2 (PGE2) depend on which of the three receptors for this prostanoid are activated; see text. HETE, hydroxyeicosatetraenoic acid; HPETE, hydroxyperoxyeicosotetraenoic acid; LT, leukotriene; NSAIDs, nonsteroidal antiinflammatory drugs; PAF, platelet-activating factor; PG, prostaglandin; PGI2, prostacyclin; TX, thromboxane. *(From Rang HP, Dale MM, Ritter JM, Gardner P: Local hormones, inflammation and allergy. In Pharmacology, 4th ed. New York, Churchill Livingstone, 2001, p 214.)*

are the primary target for ozone.[10] Studies suggest that there is damage to the respiratory bronchioles in many workers exposed to a variety of soluble and moderately soluble gases. Patients may be asymptomatic, but one or more years after the exposure they may have evidence of either a low residual volume or restrictive disease or reduced diffusing capacity on pulmonary function tests. Some of these patients go on to develop reactive airways dysfunction syndrome and have evidence of bronchial hyperreactivity. A list of chemical inducers and a good review of reactive airways dysfunction syndrome are provided by Alberts and do Pico.[11]

Inhalational Fevers

Metal fumes, fluorocarbon pyrolysis fumes, or organic dusts rich in endotoxins may produce a series of febrile reactions usually characterized by chills, fever, chest tightness, myalgias, joint aches, and fatigue. This group of inhalational fevers has been called a variety of names, such as *zinc welding shivers, silo unloader's disease, humidifier fever, grain fever, mill fever, polymer fume fever, metal fume fever,* and *organic dust toxic syndrome.* These conditions all are characterized by a subclinical alveolitis not apparent on chest x-ray or pulmonary function tests except in unusually severe cases. Inhalational fevers are associated with a neutrophilic predominance on bronchoalveolar lavage and a systemic leukocytosis. Their systemic effects are transient.[12] Inhalational fevers can be confused with toxic reactions to gases and vapors. Inhalational fevers are discussed in greater detail in Chapter 27.

Solubility

Water-soluble gases, such as ammonia, sulfur dioxide, formaldehyde, and methyl isocyanate, produce irritation to mucous membranes and the cornea and usually are characterized by significant ocular symptoms, such as redness of the eyes and, with heavy exposure, delayed onset of cataracts. First-degree burns of the face may be present, and there is likely to be erythema of the nose and symptoms related to the nose and posterior pharynx because most of these gases are absorbed in the mucous membranes in the upper airway. These highly water-soluble gases also are likely to cause pharyngeal injury, reflex laryngospasm, and laryngeal obstruction because of the rapid onset of laryngeal edema.[13–15]

Gases with intermediate water solubility, such as chlorine, tend to produce more upper airway irritation Because of its intermediate solubility, chlorine may produce upper and lower airway injury. Gases with low water solubility, such as phosgene or oxides of nitrogen, produce little in the way of upper airway irritation unless they are in very high concentrations, but they produce intense damage in the lower airways and pulmonary edema. Phosgene gas was used during World War I and was responsible for approximately 80% of the deaths from gassing. Its vapor density is 3.4 times that of air. Its high density made it an ideal agent in the days of trench warfare. This gas has a relatively low odor threshold and is said to smell like freshly mown hay. The low-solubility gases are more likely to produce the delayed onset of symptoms and delayed onset of pulmonary edema. Agents associated with pulmonary edema or chemical pneumonitis are listed in Table 97-7.

TABLE 97-7 Agents That Produce Pulmonary Edema/Chemical Pneumonitis	
Acetaldehyde	Nickel carbonyl
Acrolein	Nitrogen dioxide
Ammonia	Nitrogen trifluoride
Antimony trichloride or pentachloride	Nitrosyl chloride
Beryllium	Osmium tetroxide
Bismuth pentachloride	Oxygen difluoride
Boranes	Ozone
Cadmium and cadmium salts	Paraquat
Carbonyl fluoride	Perchloroethylene
Chloramine	Phosgene
Chlorine	Phosphine
Cobalt metal	Phosphorus pentafluoride
Dichlorosilane	Phosphorus trifluoride
Dimethyl sulfate	Selenium dioxide
Dioxane dimethyl sulfate	Silanes
Fire smoke	Silicone tetrachloride
Glyphosate herbicides	Silicone tetrafluoride
Hydrogen bromide	Sulfur dioxide
Hydrogen chloride	Sulfur tetrafluoride
Hydrogen fluoride	Sulfur trioxide
Hydrogen selenide	Titanium tetrachloride
Hydrogen sulfide	Toluene 2,4-diisocyanate in high concentrations
Lithium hydride	Trimellitic anhydride
Mercury vapor	Vanadium
Methyl bromide	War gases
Methyl isocyanate	Zinc oxide and chloride
Methylene chloride	Zirconium chloride

Two properties, water solubility and chemical reactivity, are the most useful in predicting the site of damage of a substance. Most water-soluble gases dissolve in the mucous lining of the upper respiratory tract; mucus contains about 95% water and acts as a sink for water-soluble gases. After dissolving in the mucus, the gas molecules can diffuse in the underlying epithelial cells of the respiratory tract, where they can cause damage. Most of the molecules that hit mucus fail to dissolve and reenter the airspace. The remaining gas molecules may be pulled farther down the airspace, where they again are exposed to more moist mucus until they get to the lower airways. There is a concentration gradient from the upper airway to the lower airway when one takes a breath of a highly soluble gas, in that it is continually being absorbed onto the mucous blanket of the respiratory tract from the upper airway through the lower airway. The concentration may be low by the time it reaches the terminal airways. This gradient is overcome, however, when the gas is inhaled in a high concentration, and this explains why lower airway damage can occur after an exposure to a highly soluble reactive gas (see Table 97-5).

The opposite is true for the fate of a gas with low water solubility because there is little uptake in the upper respiratory tract, and the most important factor is the surface area of the lower airway. The greater uptake tends to occur in regions of high surface area, such as the alveoli in terminal airways, compared with regions of lower surface area, such as the trachea and major lobar bronchi. Highly reactive low water solubility vapors are absorbed primarily in the alveolar area, and this is the site of their damage. This explains why patients with phosgene exposure may present with pulmonary edema and little in the way of upper respiratory signs or symptoms, unless the gas is present in high concentrations.

Smoke Inhalation

The pathophysiology of the acute lung injury associated with smoke inhalation suggests that the influx of neutrophils is the major source of acute lung injury via the release of a variety of cytokines resulting in increased vascular permeability. Lung injury from smoke has shown that activated neutrophils seem to play an important part in the pathogenesis of the lung injury. Depletion of neutrophils with nitrogen mustard significantly decreases smoke-induced increase in lung microvascular permeability to protein.[16] The neutrophils are recruited from the microcirculation via the up-regulation of selectin-type adherence molecules on the endothelial surface. Neutrophils adhere to the endothelium, and intercellular adhesion molecule type 1 facilitates the diapedesis of the neutrophils across the endothelium into the interstitium of the lung, where they release free oxygen radicals and proteases. Sulfo Lewis C is a compound that blocks the uptake of neutrophils out of the microcirculation.[17] These studies and other studies blocking CD-18 or CD-11b in the lung injury model of acute acid instillation in rabbits suggest that compounds that prevent neutrophil migration into the lung might be useful in certain models of inhalational injury in humans.[18] Another approach that has been evaluated is the blockage of interleukin-8, which is the major chemotactic factor for neutrophils. Pretreatment with an anti–interleukin-8 antibody reduces smoke-mediated increase in the bidirectional transport of protein across the alveolar epithelium. This suggests that interleukin-8 is important in the pathogenesis of smoke inhalational injury and probably is important in other sources of inhalational injury.

A group from Taipei showed in a wood smoke model in guinea pigs that evidence of airway injury occurs within 5 minutes after wood smoke inhalation, followed 2 hours later by parenchymal injury. The lung injury involves the release of tachykinins. Tachykinins are neuropeptides released from C-fiber nerve endings that invoke a variety of proinflammatory mediators that have the ability to increase production of oxygen radicals. The airway and late parenchymal injury is blocked by tachykinin receptor antagonists, particularly to the tachykinin NK1 receptor.[19]

TOXICOKINETICS

Inhalant gas toxicology is complex. The dose of an inhaled gas or vapor usually is expressed as the mass of the gas per unit volume, or milligrams per liter, or as the ratio of molecules of the study gas to total gas molecules; this usually is expressed as parts per million (ppm). The dose of an inhaled gas is calculated by multiplying the concentration of the gas in the breathing zone by the duration of the exposure and the minute ventilation of the individual during that exposure time:

Equation 97-1
$$\text{Dose of an inhaled gas} = C \text{ (concentration in the breathing zone)} \times \text{minute ventilation}$$

Dose-effect relationships may be expressed by Harber's rule:[20]

Equation 97-2
$$C \times T \text{ (time of exposure)} = K \text{ (biologic effect)}$$

Limitations of Harber's rule include the failure to take into account the minute ventilation, or tidal volume, which greatly affects the dose of inhalant reaching the alveoli. Harber's rule fails to recognize the exponential impact of increasing dose. With higher concentrations, the effect of concentration is far greater than the duration of exposure. In low concentration, the toxic effects are related primarily to duration of exposure, but only one or two breaths of a highly toxic concentrated irritant gas may be fatal. A more useful formula has been proposed by Baxter:[21]

Equation 97-3
$$\text{Toxic load} = \text{concentration to the exponent } n \times \text{time}$$

The exponent n is any number other than 0. This reflects an exponential increase in tissue damage with increasing dose, which varies in amount with the physical properties of that gas. In some gases, the relationship is nearly linear, whereas in other exposures, such as hydrogen sulfide, the toxic effects increase in an exponential fashion so that only a few breaths in high concentration may be fatal. The primary determinant of toxicity with hydrogen sulfide is concentration rather than duration of exposure, invalidating Harber's rule.[22]

In actuality, the estimate of exposure is much more complex than dose, duration of exposure, and chemical properties of a given gas. It is difficult to estimate the minute ventilation in an accidental exposure. The amount of gas going to the lower airways varies tremendously depending on whether the subject is breathing through the mouth or through the nose. Highly reactive gases, such as formaldehyde, would be taken up almost entirely in the nose if the patient were breathing through the nose, but some would get into the lower airways if the patient were breathing through the mouth. The distribution of the gas when it reaches the lower airways tends to be irregular if it is irritating to the bronchial mucosa. Studies in dogs by Winternitz[23] at the Department of Pathology at Yale during World War I showed severe congestion in some areas of the lungs with normal areas of the lung elsewhere, indicating irregular uptake of toxic war gases. It is believed that this irregular uptake may be related to the fact that irritant gases may induce bronchospasm, resulting in the maldistribution of toxic effects in the lung. This belief is supported clinically by the observation that patients may have patchy pulmonary infiltrates, sparing otherwise normal areas of lung, and heterogeneous abnormalities diagnosed by radionuclide imaging studies.[24] The breathing pattern affects the extent of lower airway damage. If the respiratory rate is rapid and the tidal volume is small, much of the ventilation is simply moving gas in and out of the anatomic dead space. If the patient is breathing deeply and slowly, there is a greater amount of gas taken into the lower airways; clinically, this may be seen in an industrial accident in which an individual remains calm and walks slowly out of the area versus another who panics and runs. If the gas immediately causes coughing, the patient is taking large vital capacity breaths before each cough, which causes deep inhalation of the gas into the lower airways. Similarly, another individual in the same environment who does not cough or sneeze has a lower exposure. The amount of gas inhaled into the terminal airways and alveoli can vary substantially between one individual and another. Gases that are slowly reactive or not reactive in the lung, such as carbon monoxide or arsine, simply pass through the alveolar gas exchanging surfaces into the blood. Highly reactive gases are taken up primarily by the bronchial mucosa, and there is little of the gas accessible to the circulation.

The effective dose of a gas is a function of the vapor concentration of the gas, the amount inhaled, and the amount retained in the lung. In addition, effective doses depend on the uptake of that gas in a target cell or tissue, mainly the bronchial and nasal mucosa. The effective dose is the amount of the gas that participates in a damaging reaction. This amount differs from the amount inhaled; a certain amount is going to be exhaled as dead space gas. Calculation of the effective dose of formaldehyde necessary to produce a squamous cell carcinoma of the nasal cavity in rodents is a more reliable indicator of risk than the calculation of dose simply from vapor concentration and the amount inhaled.[25]

Concentration and duration of exposure further affect the kinetics of the metabolism of a gas in various tissues. In low concentration, a gas may be taken up entirely by the mucosa in the upper airways, but at higher concentration its uptake and metabolism may be saturated, causing the effective concentration of the gas to increase with time in the lower airways. This concentration of the lower airways increases as the absorption and metabolism of the gas reaches zero order kinetics in the upper airway. The concentration also is affected by the inhalational rate; rapid, deep breaths, which occur with coughing or sneezing, overwhelm the metabolism and uptake in the upper airways.

The biologic effect of a gas depends on its water or lipid solubility. Gases that are lipid soluble, such as chloroform, ether, or other halogenated hydrocarbons, may produce central nervous system effects and little or no respiratory irritation. Methylene chloride is an exception to this rule in that it has mild irritating effects and in extremely high doses may cause pulmonary edema.[26] Water-soluble gases are taken up by the respiratory mucosa and produce their effects in the lung and upper respiratory tract and would be expected to have no systemic effects. The irritant effect of a gas is based on its reactivity or the intensity of the chemical reaction that occurs in the respiratory tissue. The reaction rate of these chemical reactions influences the site of action of the gas. A rapid reaction may occur with gases, such as formaldehyde, in which the reaction occurs so rapidly that little of the inhaled dose gets beyond the nose. Gases with moderate levels of chemical reactivity, such as chlorine, may have a greater effect on lower airways because a greater percentage of the gas bypasses the upper airway. The predominant site of action of irritant gases is influenced by the anatomy of the pulmonary airways. Miller and Kimble[25] have shown that the concentration of ozone in the airways tends to reach a maximum concentration at the 16th through 17th generation of airways. This concentration is affected predominantly by the fact that as the number of generations of airways increases, the cross-sectional diameter of the surface area of the lung increases exponentially.

There is a tremendous dilutional effect of an inhaled breath of gas by this rapid change in surface area, resulting in a maximum concentration at airway generation 16 or 17. Bates[10] suggested this idea in 1972 before the elegant studies of Miller and Kimble. Our own studies have confirmed that the smaller airways and respiratory bronchioles seem to be the major site of damage after an inhalational exposure to the reactive gas chlorine.[17]

The potential of a gas to produce a concentration high enough to be potentially injurious can be estimated by simple calculation. If one knows the vapor pressure of the gas, one can estimate the concentration at room temperature, or 25 °C, by

Equation 97-4
$$\text{ppm} = (\text{vapor pressure @ } 25° \times \text{mm Hg}/760) \times 10^6$$

A compound with a vapor pressure of less than 0.76 mm Hg at room temperature attains an air concentration of less than 1000 ppm at the saturated vapor concentration. A vapor pressure of 0.076 mm Hg would produce a concentration of 100 ppm. Using this simple formula, one can calculate the concentration of a gas in a potential exposure situation. The value of 760 mm Hg represents sea-level atmospheric pressure. At other altitudes, the relevant atmospheric pressure should be substituted.

The vapor pressure of a gas is the partial pressure exerted by that gas and is a reflection of its volatility. Factors that affect the volatility can affect the dose of an exposure greatly. Methylene disocyanate has a low vapor pressure, so it is not volatile at room temperature. When heated or mixed with an organic solvent that has a high vapor pressure, however, its vapor pressure increases, and it may be volatilized. In the case of mixture with an organic solvent, the latter serves as a carrier. Vapor pressure and density of gases are important in understanding the dynamics of a toxic exposure. Chlorine gas, which is more than 2.5 times the density of air, tends to flow into low-lying areas. This tendency explains why there can be large differences in levels of exposure in a group of exposed workers when there is only a few feet difference in elevation between one worker and another. Depending on the climatic conditions, this gas may stratify in a green cloud that flows across a floor into low areas. A worker who is in a low area may get an exposure tens of times greater than a worker who is in a location that is a few feet higher on a scaffold or walkway. This type of property of a gas explains why gas exposures tend to produce a heterogeneous degree of injury in a group of workers. I studied a group of workers involved in an accident at a paper mill where chlorine was released from a tank car. The umbilical hose that went from the tank car to the bleaching plant became detached from the bottom of the tank car. Because this occurred in the winter when the building was heated and the gas was cold, the heat of the building acted as a source of convection that drafted the dense cold chlorine to the roof, where a group of construction workers has heavily exposed. People at ground level who were working in the mill had no significant exposure despite their close proximity to the gas leak.[23] In calculating dose, temperature, humidity, wind direction, and other climatic conditions may influence the dose to a given individual. Because the upper airway acts as an absorber of water-soluble gases, any condition that causes mouth breathing, such as allergic rhinitis or an upper respiratory infection, might result in more significant lower airway injury because of the lack of absorption by the nose. The determinants of severity of lung injury are summarized in Table 97-6.

TERMINOLOGY

The following terms commonly are used to quantitate the health effects of toxic inhalants:

Dose: Dose is the quantity of the compound received by the subject.

IDLH: Immediate danger to life or health (IDLH) is commonly used as in Table 97-3 and reflects data from human experience and animal models.

LD50: The lethal dose (LD)$_{50}$ is the dose that kills 50% of the exposed population and reflects extrapolated data from animal models and therefore is only a rough estimate of human toxicity.

ID50: The incapacitating dose (ID)$_{50}$ is the dose that incapacitates 50% of the exposed population.

Ct: The concentration time (Ct) is a measure of exposure to a vapor or aerosol. The concentration in the air and the time of exposure govern the dose received, as do rate and depth of respiration. It is assumed that when the product of concentration and time is constant, so is the biologic effect over a limited range of concentration and time. This assumption may not be true except in a laboratory setting, but for purposes of making some type of estimate of exposure, a steady-state hypothetical value is used. Concentration is expressed as mg/m^3 and time as minutes so that the Ct is expressed as $mg/min/m^3$.

LCt50: The lethal concentration time (LCt)$_{50}$ is the Ct that would kill 50% of the exposed population; this reflects extrapolation from animal models.

ICt50: The incapacitating concentration time (ICt)$_{50}$ is the Ct that would incapacitate 50% of the exposed population.

RD50: The respiratory depression (RD)$_{50}$ is the concentration that would cause respiratory depression by 50% in 10 minutes of exposure.

CLINICAL PRESENTATION

Davy, a British chemist, synthesized phosgene (carbonyl chloride; CAS: 75-44-5) in 1812. Phosgene is a colorless gas. The boiling point of phosgene is 8.2 °C (47 °F); it is extremely volatile. Phosgene is hydrolyzed rapidly in the human body with the formation of hydrochloric acid and carbon dioxide ($COCl_2 \rightarrow HCl + CO_2$). Phosgene has a vapor density 3.4 times that of air, making it an ideal war gas because it accumulates in low-lying areas, such as foxholes and ditches. The first battlefield use of phosgene was at Verdun in 1917 by Germany. During and immediately after exposure, there is likely to be coughing; choking; a feeling of tightness in the chest; nausea; and occasionally vomiting, headache, and mild lacrimation. The presence or absence of these symptoms is of little value in immediate prognosis. Some patients with severe coughs fail to develop serious lung injury, whereas others with little sign of early respiratory distress develop severe delayed pulmonary edema after 2 to 24 hours. Exposure to moderate concentrations triggers lacrimation and the unique complaint that smoking tobacco produces an objectionable taste. High concentrations may trigger rapidly developing pulmonary edema with attendant severe cough, dyspnea, and frothy sputum. Onset of pulmonary edema progresses over 2 to 6 hours and is predictive of severe injury. High concentrations may produce a severe cough with laryngospasm that results in sudden death; this possibly could be due to phosgene hydrolysis, which releases free hydrochloric acid at the level of the larynx. In the first 12 hours after toxic inhalant exposure, depending on the intensity of exposure, a substernal tightness with moderate resting dyspnea and prominent exertional dyspnea becomes evident. These symptoms often are a prelude to the characteristic development of pulmonary edema. Initially small, then greater, amounts of thin airway secretions may appear. The delayed, insidious onset of severe pulmonary edema often has resulted in a patient's being medically evaluated and discharged from the medical facility, only to return some hours later with severe and occasionally lethal pulmonary edema.

Irritant gases, such as phosgene, can cause local irritation of airways, which induces bronchoconstriction, which may produce a rise in pulmonary artery pressure, increasing the pressure gradient and causing pulmonary edema.[28-31] Airway damage can affect the surfactant system, which results in destabilization of airways with atelectasis and decrease in pulmonary compliance.[32] These substances may induce transformation of the cell surface and lead to dose-related production and liberation of cytokines, which affect capillary permeability and produce pulmonary edema. Intrapulmonary shunting from ventilation/perfusion inequalities produces hypoxia, which can enhance lung injury further. The role of various mediators in the production of epithelial injury has great implications regarding treatment. Various studies have been performed on the role of arachidonate mediators in the pathogenesis of lung injury from phosgene.[5] In many other types of oxidant lung injury, there is increased synthesis of lipoxygenase products (see Fig. 97-3) after phosgene exposure, which seems to contribute to the pathogenesis of pulmonary edema.[4] Drugs that inhibit the lipoxygenase pathway possibly might reduce pulmonary edema in phosgene-exposed individuals.[33]

Nitrogen Oxides and the Risk of Bronchiolitis Obliterans

Oxides of nitrogen, such as nitrogen dioxide, characteristically produce a triphasic illness[34]; this is called *silo filler's disease* if it is related to exposure to stored silage. Initial presentation may be cough, wheeze, dyspnea, central chest pain, fever, sweating, and weakness. Physical examination at this stage may reveal wheezes and crackles, and the patient may be hypotensive and cyanotic. The patient's x-ray may be normal or may show pulmonary edema. This phase of the illness resolves, and the patient may enter the second phase of being relatively asymptomatic; 2 to 8 weeks later, the patient develops the third phase with symptoms of obliterative bronchiolitis—fevers,

TABLE 97-8 Agents That Produce Bronchiolitis Obliterans

Ammonia	Methyl isocyanate
Chlorine	Mustard gas
Cocaine freebase	Oxides of nitrogen
Fire smoke	Phosgene
Hydrogen bromide	Sulfur dioxide
Hydrogen selenide	Titanium tetrachloride
Hydrogen sulfide	

chills, wheeze, cough, dyspnea, and chest pain associated with wheezes and crackles on physical examination. The chest x-ray may be normal or may show diffuse, small nodules. The late development of bronchiolitis obliterans is a serious complication that usually responds to steroids but may progress if not treated properly and may be fatal. In cases in which there is a possibility of bronchiolitis obliterans, consideration of a course of steroids for 8 weeks seems reasonable prophylaxis for the prevention of life-threatening bronchiolitis. Table 97-8 lists toxic chemicals that are typically associated with bronchiolitis obliterans.

PATIENT EVALUATION

When evaluating a patient with an exposure to a water-soluble gas (see Table 97-2), careful examination of the upper respiratory tract may provide clues estimating whether the exposure has been sufficient enough to be associated with lower airway damage. If a patient who had been exposed to the soluble gases sulfur dioxide or ammonia presents with watery, teary eyes; red face; chronic rhinitis; red, sore nose; erythema of the posterior pharynx; hoarseness; and difficulty swallowing, one can assume that this has been a heavy exposure that may produce lower airway damage.[13–15] The corollary is that if one is exposed to highly soluble gas, such as ammonia, and there are no upper respiratory signs or symptoms, it is unlikely that the patient has inhaled a dose high enough to cause lower airway disease. This caveat applies only to individuals who are exposed to high concentrations of a highly water-soluble gas of short duration. Lower levels of exposure for longer periods may produce airway damage with minimal signs of conjunctival, cutaneous, and upper airway irritation.[35] When a patient is exposed to a low-solubility gas (see Table 97-2), such as phosgene, there would be expected to be fewer upper respiratory tract findings, and it is important to observe the patient for 6 to 24 hours because it may take several hours for pulmonary edema to develop. It is wise to observe such a patient in a closely monitored environment for at least 24 hours if there is evidence that there has been a high exposure to one of the low-solubility gases or if the patient is hypoxemic, tachypneic, or in any respiratory distress. Table 97-7 lists the common toxic gases and fumes associated with pulmonary edema and chemical pneumonitis. Referral to the list of agents that may cause pulmonary edema (see Table 97-7) should help the physician

determine if a given exposure is likely to result in acute or delayed pulmonary edema. These same principles are less reliable in evaluating fire-related inhalational injuries. Signs such as singed nasal hair, carbonaceous sputum, and soot in the posterior pharynx are not reliable predictors of lower airway damage.[36–38] Facial burns are seen frequently with and without fire-related inhalational injuries and lack specificity and sensitivity. More than 80% of patients with a fire-related inhalational injury do not have facial burns.[37,38]

Respiratory symptoms, such as severe coughing, respiratory distress, stridor, tachypnea, restlessness, wheezing, and chest tightness, suggest the possibility of significant airway injury and require prolonged observation and assessment with frequent arterial blood gases, oximetry, chest x-rays, pulmonary function tests, and possibly fiberoptic bronchoscopy or laryngoscopy.

Central nervous system symptoms, such as dizziness, headache, confusion, disorientation, hallucinations, and seizures, may reflect signs of hypoxic brain damage due to nonirritant gases, such as carbon monoxide or cyanide, or head trauma from a fall related to being overcome by toxic fumes or other problems. Drug or alcohol abuse is common in victims of industrial accidents and house fires, and a toxicologic screen may be helpful in the evaluation of the confused patient. An elevated carboxyhemoglobin level may be useful in diagnosing carbon monoxide poisoning. If a metabolic acidosis is not correctable with sodium bicarbonate, the clinician should suspect cyanide poisoning. Cardiac arrhythmias commonly accompany tissue hypoxia, and an electrocardiogram and continuous cardiac monitoring are advisable. Some patients with inhalational injuries may complain of a substernal burning chest pain that may be confused with the pain from a myocardial infarction.

Oximetry

For patients showing major signs or symptoms after gas inhalation, arterial blood gases should be obtained. Room air arterial blood gas determinations are the most useful. The PO$_2$ may be normal, however, in patients with toxic hemoglobinopathies, such as patients with high levels of methemoglobin or carboxyhemoglobin. Pulse oximetry does not detect these abnormal hemoglobins correctly and measures only normal saturated and desaturated oxyhemoglobin. An oximetry panel, which contains measurements of carboxyhemoglobin, methemoglobin, total hemoglobin, and oxyhemoglobin, is necessary to evaluate patients' levels of carboxyhemoglobin and methemoglobin and should be performed routinely in fire exposures and inhalational injuries of unknown type. Pulse oximetry may give a false sense of security in patients exposed to carbon monoxide, oxidant gases that produce methemoglobinemia, or cyanide gas from fires.

Pulmonary Function Tests

Pulmonary function tests should be obtained as a baseline as soon as the patient is stable. I obtain complete pulmonary function tests as soon as possible after the patient is admitted and again several hours later. When there is significant damage to the lower airways, spirometry may be

TABLE 97-9 Long-Term Effects of Acute Toxic Inhalation

Complete resolution of symptoms
Reactive airways dysfunction syndrome
Chronic bronchitis
Bronchiectasis (e.g., ammonia, sulfur dioxide)
Bronchiolitis obliterans (e.g., nitrogen dioxide, sulfur dioxide)
Bronchostenosis (e.g., mustard gas)
COPD or restrictive lung disease
Low residual volume

COPD, chronic obstructive pulmonary disease.

TABLE 97-10 Strategies for Managing Inhalational Injury

1. Decontaminate the victim (e.g., remove chemical-soaked clothing).
2. Obtain admission arterial blood gas and cooximetry studies.
3. Start high-flow 100% oxygen.
4. Examine the patient for eye injuries, flush eyes, and treat if inflammation is noted.
5. Record evidence of facial burns, nasal burns, and pharyngitis.
6. If the victim is hoarse and has difficulty phonating, consider immediate intubation.
7. Observe the patient for delayed pulmonary edema for 24 hr if the patient is hypoxemic or has been exposed to a low-solubility gas, such as phosgene.
8. Chest x-rays are not usually helpful unless the patient has significant hypoxemia, marked dyspnea, or basilar rales.
9. Give methylene blue, 1–2 mg/kg intravenously, or sodium nitrite, 300 mg intravenously, in patients without anemia and suspected cyanide poisoning, such as in fires. Ampules of amyl nitrate also may be inhaled, 2 ampules every 5 min, if sodium nitrite is unavailable.
10. Hydroxycobalamin (vitamin B_{12}) is used in Europe but requires high dosage, approximately 4 g of vitamin B_{12}.
11. Administer sodium bicarbonate as needed according to arterial blood gas, and avoid excessive crystalloids.
12. Hyperbaric oxygen may be helpful for carbon monoxide and cyanide toxicity.
13. Keep the patient on bed rest because low-level exercise can induce pulmonary edema in a vulnerable patient with subclinical pulmonary edema.

abnormal early in the clinical course, particularly with fire-related inhalational injury. However, normal spirometry does not exclude or predict late-onset pulmonary edema or damage to the upper airway.[39] I obtain complete pulmonary function tests again at 3, 6, 12, and 24 months after exposure in symptomatic patients. Spirometry frequently is normal in the presence of mild restrictive disease from an inhalational injury, and measurement of lung volumes is helpful when available. Airflow obstruction may be due to reactive airways dysfunction syndrome related to epithelial injury[11] or anatomic airway narrowing related to chronic scarring after airway inflammation. The most common late abnormality is an isolated reduction in residual volume.[40] After chlorine exposure, restrictive changes in lung function progress slowly and may not be detected for 2 or more years.[27] Isolated reduction in lung diffusion may occur but usually is accompanied by reduction in lung volumes. Methacholine challenge testing should be performed only in patients with signs and symptoms of bronchial hyperreactivity after the third month. Early transient bronchial hyperreactivity, which lasts only several days to weeks, is commonly seen after an irritant gas exposure. Detection of early bronchial hyperreactivity is not always predictive of long-term airway injury and irritability. Long-term consequences of irritant gas exposure are variable (Table 97-9). Most patients recover completely,[41] but others may develop long-term airway irritability, restrictive lung disease, obstructive lung disease, bronchiectasis, bronchostenosis, or bronchiolitis obliterans.

TREATMENT

The treatment of a toxic inhalation is primarily supportive, including oxygenation, bed rest, analgesia, and mechanical ventilation, if necessary. Contaminated clothing that might further increase the absorption of a substance through the skin should be removed, and the patient should be decontaminated before entering the acute care area. This care is outlined in Table 97-10. Any superficial burns should be treated conservatively. Careful attention to the eyes is important because there may be corneal burns, ulcerations, infection, anterior and posterior synechiae, corneal opacification, glaucoma, retinal atrophy, and the late development of cataracts with heavy exposures. Proper eye care, particu-

larly copious irrigation, is essential immediately after the exposure. The eye is often the forgotten organ in a patient with an acute irritant gas exposure.[42] Generally the eye needs to be irrigated for at least 20 minutes or, if this is a case of ammonia exposure, until the pH of the conjunctival sac decreases to less than 8.5. Ocular lavage needs to begin in the field at the site of injury if possible. No ointment should be applied to the eye, and contact lenses should be removed to ensure adequate irrigation. The patient should be referred to an ophthalmologist as soon as possible.[43]

The patient who presents with tachypnea and stridor, particularly with some hoarseness, is at a high risk of developing progressive laryngeal edema and complete obstruction of the airway and should be considered for emergency expectant intubation. If symptoms of upper airway damage are present, a prompt inspection of the larynx by a laryngoscope or fiberoptic bronchoscope is imperative because once sufficient edema develops, these patients are extremely difficult to intubate and may require an emergency tracheostomy.

Exercise increases cardiac output and pulmonary artery pressures. This increase may unmask latent pulmonary edema, and the patient may die quickly if medical attention is not immediately available. Sedation and bed rest are recommended for the first 24 to 48 hours.

Corticosteroids

Based on prospective trials in the management of inhalational injuries in burn patients[44] and anecdotal reports, there is probably no role for corticosteroids in the immediate emergent care of a patient with toxic inhalation.

Randomized controlled studies have been performed in other forms of adult respiratory distress syndrome (ARDS). A meta-analysis of these studies regarding prophylactic or early institution of high-dose systemic steroids suggested that steroids are not useful and may be harmful in ARDS and sepsis.[45] In patients who are likely to develop bronchiolitis obliterans or bronchiectasis at a later date, corticosteroid therapy is probably helpful. Patients with silo filler's disease or patients exposed to high doses of nitrogen dioxide particularly fall into this category. Patients with high exposure to zinc chloride may develop chronic airway disease and generally are considered candidates for systemic steroids. If the patient has been exposed to a gas in sufficient quantity and of the type commonly associated with bronchiolitis obliterans (see Table 97-8), such as nitrogen dioxide, it is recommended that the patient be kept on moderately high doses of prednisone (20 to 40 mg/day) for about 8 weeks.[46] There is suggestive evidence in an animal model of chlorine inhalation of improved lung function and reduced pathologic changes in the airways with high doses of dexamethasone given after exposure.[47] Because of the sporadic nature of acute gas inhalational injury and the heterogeneity of the human response, however, controlled studies adequate to examine the effectiveness of corticosteroids are unlikely ever to be performed in cases of acute toxic gas inhalation. The U.S. Army and Navy textbooks on acute inhalational injury recommend the early institution of systemic and aerosolized steroids in the management of acute inhalational injury.[48,49]

Pentoxifylline

The role of tumor necrosis factor (TNF)–α has been evaluated in a smoke inhalational injury model in sheep.[50] Lymph and alveolar lavage specimens failed to show elevated levels of TNF-α. These researchers were unable to establish a role for this drug in smoke-induced pulmonary injury in sheep. Pentoxifylline, a methylxanthine normally used to treat peripheral vascular disease by decreasing red blood cell rigidity, is a potent inhibitor of TNF-α.[51] It has been shown to inhibit polymorphonuclear leukocyte phagocytosis and to decrease superoxide anion production in polymorphonuclear neutrophils and monocytes. It is not found to be helpful, however, in the treatment of acute lung injury after phosgene exposure in rats.[52] Theoretically, TNF-α blockade should be useful, but the animal data have been discouraging. Human data are mixed and often confused by the fact that pentoxifylline is not used as a single agent in many clinical trials. Combination therapy with nitric oxide looks promising in the prevention of reperfusion lung injury after lung transplantation in humans.[53] The role of this type of combination therapy in smoke or irritant gas inhalation is unknown.

Aminophylline and Albuterol

Another methylxanthine, aminophylline, seems to protect against phosgene-induced acute lung injury in rabbits.[54,55] Treatment 80 to 90 minutes after exposure reduces acute lung injury. Aminophylline may protect against acute oxidant lung injury by (1) a direct antipermeability effect,

(2) inhibition of permeability-inducing sulfidopeptide leukotrienes, (3) a direct or indirect antioxidant action, (4) maintenance of cAMP concentration required to keep tight cellular junctions, and (5) possible vasodilatory mechanisms.[56] This work suggests that other drugs that increase cAMP should be explored as being useful in the treatment of irritant gas injury. The practical implication of this research is that one commonly available, reasonably safe, low-cost drug, aminophylline, may be effective in the acute management of an acute inhalational injury and should be given early in the clinical course.

N-Acetylcysteine

Glutathione is a water-soluble antioxidant that protects against free radical injury. Free radicals are thought to be the source of cytotoxic damage in many models of irritant gas injury. Chlorine gas combines with tissue water to form hypochlorous and hydrochloric acid, which diffuse into cells and react with amino groups of cytoplasm, forming N-chloral derivatives that cause nascent oxygen to be released through a series of chemical reactions. The oxidative effects are responsible for the major toxic effects and respiratory damage. Glutathione protects cells from oxidant injury via the regulation of several biologic processes. N-Acetylcysteine is a compound that maintains glutathione levels in oxidant stress and has been shown to protect against endotoxin-induced and radiation-induced damage.[57–59] It protects against bleomycin-induced damage in mice and protects alveolar type II cells from paraquat toxicity.[60,61] N-Acetylcysteine also has been shown to protect against phosgene-induced lung damage by intratracheal administration in rabbits, but it was not protective when administered by the intravascular route.[62] There is no clinical experience reported in humans other than in chronic bronchitis.[63] A dose of at least 3 mL of a 20% solution could be tried by nebulizer, but this compound can be irritating and may induce bronchospasm in humans and should be given with 2.5 mg of albuterol solution every 4 hours. There have been no clinical trials with this drug in humans for acute inhalational injury, but a short course of the drug for 24 to 48 hours in the appropriate clinical setting may be considered. A Finnish group used N-acetylcysteine in the management of a patient with zinc chloride smoke inhalation.[64]

Ibuprofen

Ibuprofen is a commonly used antipyretic and antiinflammatory compound that originally was shown to modify lung injury response to aspiration in dogs in 1982.[65] It has free radical scavenging and iron chelating mechanisms of reducing acute oxidant lung injury.[5,66,67] It has been shown to be protective against acute lung injury from paraquat in rats,[68] smoke inhalation in rabbits,[69] and burn injury in sheep.[70,71] Ibuprofen also has been shown to protect against acute lung injury from phosgene in rats and rabbits.[33] Its role in the treatment of acute inhalational injury in humans is unknown. If used in humans, a dose of 25 to 50 mg/kg of ibuprofen would be roughly compatible to the doses used in animal studies. Sciuto and coworkers[52] reported in a phosgene-exposed rat model that ibuprofen was effective alone and useful when combined with pentoxifylline. This study plus the study by Stewart and associates[69] in an animal smoke inhalational model suggest that further human trials are necessary.

Antibiotics, Chest Physical Therapy, and Bronchodilators

Prophylactic antibiotics have been suggested because the sloughing of the tracheal mucosa offers a good culture medium for bacteria; however, there is no evidence that they are beneficial.[44] Antibiotics should be withheld, unless there is clinical evidence of an infection. Chest physical therapy and high-frequency percussive ventilation may be helpful in patients with mucus plugs and thick secretions. Bronchodilators should be administered if a patient has evidence of bronchospasm.

Nitric Oxide

Nitric oxide attenuates acute lung injury in humans and animals.[72] Nitric oxide decreases release of key mediators of inflammation, down-regulates the intrapulmonary inflammatory process, decreases pulmonary artery pressure, decreases pulmonary artery remodeling, and improves oxygenation.[73–75] Nitric oxide decreases vascular permeability[76] and theoretically should be an ideal agent for the management of irritant-induced pulmonary edema. A multicenter European trial containing 268 patients from 43 university and regional hospitals showed the safety and effectiveness in reducing pulmonary artery pressure, improving oxygenation, and reducing the rate of severe respiratory failure in ARDS patients but did not produce a statistically significant improvement in survival.[77,78] Other investigators have thought that inhaled nitric oxide was useful in burn patients with respiratory failure, but this information is largely anecdotal.[79] The negative effects of nitric oxide are that in high doses (80 ppm), it paradoxically increases inflammation and activates the coagulation system in mice.[80,81]

Sodium Bicarbonate and Calcium Chloride Inhalation

The concept of neutralizing the halogen-induced acids has been suggested in animal studies, and sodium bicarbonate nebulization has been shown to improve arterial blood gases after chlorine exposure in an animal study.[82] Sodium bicarbonate also has been used successfully in humans and is recommended by some authors.[83,84] The inhalation of calcium chloride has been used to treat hydrogen fluoride inhalation.[85,86] These treatments are anecdotal, however, and there is no consensus of efficacy of this therapy.

Treatments for Smoke Inhalation

Smoke inhalational injury remains the primary determinant of burn-related mortality.[87] Smoke-related inhalational injury is complex. Exposure is to a mixture of varying concentrations of carbon particles, liquids, heat, chemicals, and toxic gases—largely carbon monoxide, hydrogen chloride,

nitrogen oxides, hydrogen cyanide, acrolein, hydrogen sulfide, hydrogen fluoride, phenol, sulfur dioxide, formaldehyde, and various other gaseous pyrolysis products. Thermal injury affects predominately the upper airway, and chemical injury from toxic gases or chemicals attached to inhaled carbon particles, such as aldehydes and organic and inorganic acids, affects the upper and lower airways. The damage to the alveolar and capillary epithelium may occur simply from the release of cytokines from peripheral tissues after a large surface area burn, without any evidence of fire-related direct effects on the airways. This cytokine release and the effects of overhydration may produce pulmonary edema not directly related to the inhalation of smoke. Smoke itself may activate a variety of hematogenous mediators that further enhance smoke-related damage. It is important to distinguish effects relating to burns and fire-related smoke inhalational injury from inhalational irritant exposures because the usual mechanisms of lower airway injury from the latter are different from the mechanisms usually occurring from the former.

Inhalational injury associated with burns from fires comprises approximately one quarter of patients admitted to a burn unit. The subglottic or supraglottic edema following this type of inhalational injury may obstruct the airway. This type of obstruction may develop slowly over the first 12 to 24 hours due to the initial hypovolemia and other factors. Chemicals in the smoke (see Table 97-1) are primarily responsible for the airway injury. Smoke particles may facilitate further airway damage via the chemicals absorbed to the surface of these particles.

Fiberoptic bronchoscopy is useful in evaluating burn patients for airway injury by showing carbonaceous material, airway edema, erythema, ulcerations, hemorrhage, blisters, or ischemia.[88] At the time of bronchoscopy, intubation, preferably over the bronchoscope, should be considered. Because the upper airway effects from smoke inhalation may progress slowly over 18 to 24 hours, consideration must be given to reevaluation by bronchoscopy or laryngoscopy at 24 to 48 hours. Tracheostomy through burn tissue generally is contraindicated because of the substantial risk of infection from the wound to the airway and the airway to the wound.[89] Xenon-133 ventilation scanning has been used in burn patients to detect airway injury missed by fiberoptic bronchoscopy.[90] It has a high sensitivity, but there are false-positive results in patients with obstructive airway disease. It has been used to assess airway injury in other types of inhalational injuries.[24]

Based on my experience, chest x-rays are valuable only in patients with heavy exposures who have respiratory symptoms, such as tachypnea, dyspnea, and hypoxemia, in acute irritant gas injuries. Chest x-rays have not been studied in a systematic fashion. It has been my observation that pulmonary infiltrates usually are not apparent without ventilation/perfusion mismatching and the consequent development of hypoxemia. The chest x-ray is unlikely to show findings that would alter management before abnormalities in gas exchange develop. It is probably not necessary in every patient, particularly after a low-level exposure and normal blood gas values. The chest x-ray is useful, however, in acute inhalational injuries related to smoke inhalation and for more severe inhalational injuries accompanied by hypoxia.[91] The chest x-ray is sensitive to changes in lung water and is useful in following severely burned patients, in whom changes in lung water are related to sepsis, hydration, pulmonary infection, and ARDS.[92]

Mortality from smoke inhalation is due mainly to the inhalation of carbon monoxide, cyanide, and other toxic gases listed in Table 97-3. Carbon monoxide is the most common cause of death from smoke inhalation.[93] Routine carboxyhemoglobin levels should be evaluated in any smoke inhalation setting. Cyanide toxicity is more difficult to diagnose but should be suspected in an obtunded victim with a blood lactate greater than 10 mmol/L. Often carbon monoxide and cyanide levels are elevated in the same victim, and dual toxicity should be considered in the obtunded smoke inhalation victim regardless of the carboxyhemoglobin level.[94]

The treatment of burn-related inhalational injury is not standardized. Early investigators tried nebulized dexamethasone and aerosolized gentamicin unsuccessfully to treat patients with inhalational burn injury.[44] Drugs that reduce free radical formation and cytokine production currently are being investigated, and inhaled nitric oxide has been tried in an effort to improve ventilation/perfusion matching and decrease pulmonary artery pressure.[95] In a sheep model of inhalational burn injury, ibuprofen reduced lung lymph flow and inhalational injury.[96] Using the same sheep model, pentoxifylline improved pulmonary function,[97] and dimethyl sulfoxide with heparin reduced lung injury.[98] These treatments are still experimental. None of these therapies can be recommended at this time for the management of non–burn-related inhalational injury or burn patients. The strategy for management of smoke inhalation is related in part to the presence or absence of direct thermal injury to the airways.

Most smoke inhalation victims do not have direct thermal injury because of the low heat transfer capacity of heated air. The trachea is an amazingly effective heat exchanger. Moritz and colleagues[99] showed in dogs that when air at 270 °C was blown into the larynx of dogs, the temperature of the inspired air declined to 50 °C in the trachea. By contrast, steam has high heat transfer capacity (approximately 4000 times that of air) and may cause intense upper and lower airway damage. The presence of large numbers of soot particles in the nose, pharynx, and sputum is another clue to possible thermal injury because carbon particles may be fairly efficient mechanisms for transfer of heat and irritating chemicals adsorbed on their surface, causing subsequent damage to the upper and lower airway.[89] The site of damage depends on particle size, with the larger (>10 μ) particles trapped in the nose and upper airway. Particles 3 to 10 μm become trapped in the tracheobronchial tree.

The site of toxic particle and gas deposition influences the type of airway injury. Airway casts and large particles may cause atelectasis. Smaller toxic particles may damage smaller airways, resulting in alveolar overdistention during mechanical ventilation and a high risk of barotraumas. The presence of irritants in the airway results in a large increase in bronchial blood flow and hyperemia of the airways. This large change in bronchial blood flow is thought to be a major factor in the development of pulmonary edema after smoke inhalation.[100,101] Currently, there is no agreed-on treatment for burn-related inhalational injury. Some centers in the United States use a combination of *N*-acetylcysteine and albuterol solution every 4 hours, then nebulized heparin, 5000 U every 4 hours, so that patients receive a

nebulized drug every 2 hours. Nebulized heparin (see later) seems to be safe and does not affect blood clotting in this dose range. Other national burn centers do not use any standard drug therapy for patients with inhalational injuries.

Nebulized Heparin Therapy in the Treatment of Respiratory Burns

Heparin is a member of a group of compounds called *glycosaminoglycans*, which are highly acidic, negatively charged polysaccharides. These are remarkable compounds with many antiinflammatory effects, including effects on toxic oxygen metabolites, cytokines, histamine, bradykinin, TNF, prostaglandins, and many other inflammatory mediators; heparin is best known as an anticoagulant.[102] Heparin influences the remodeling of collagen at the site of wound healing, which results in earlier epithelialization of burns. Pulmonary problems are less frequent in heparin-treated burn patients.[103] In 1993, Cox and associates[104] reported that heparin improves oxygenation and minimizes barotrauma after smoke inhalation in an ovine model. Nebulized heparin is being investigated in burn units in an effort to reduce bronchial cast formation.[95] A study in children with cutaneous and pulmonary burns associated with destruction of the ciliated epithelium and airway casts showed a response to nebulized heparin with a reduction in mortality compared with controls.[105] The usefulness in fire-related burns suggests that nebulized heparin might prove useful in chemical burns of the airway, particularly ammonia-related inhalational injury. My speculation is that the low pH of heparin might neutralize the alkaline pH in tissues produced by the conversion of gaseous ammonia to ammonium hydroxide in airway epithelium.

Mechanical Ventilation

Mechanical ventilation with low tidal volumes and positive end-expiratory pressure is currently the standard of care for inhalational injuries associated with severe abnormalities of gas transport.[106–108] Inhalational injuries from irritant gases or burns produce spotty areas of intense injury, leaving other areas in near-normal condition presumably protected by regional bronchospasm[109]; this originally was reported by Winternitz[23] in studies on dogs exposed to irritant gases at the end of World War I. Mechanical ventilation with high tidal volumes and positive end-expiratory pressure may improve oxygenation but at the same time may overinflate the least affected areas of lung, causing barotrauma and hyperinflation with increased pleural pressure causing reduced venous return, cardiac output, and oxygen delivery. Low tidal volume ventilation and positive end-expiratory pressure now are recommended for all types of lung injury and are associated with better survival from ARDS.[110] Low tidal volumes seem to reduce epithelial and endothelial injury.[111] Permissive hypercapnia is well tolerated as long as satisfactory oxygenation is maintained.[112] More recently, there has been interest in high-frequency percussive ventilation.[113] Some investigators believe that it helps mobilize secretions in burn patients with fibrin plugs. This treatment still is considered investigational.

REFERENCES

1. Mehta PS, Mehta AS, Mehta SJ, Makhijini AB: Bhopal tragedy's health effects. JAMA 264:2781–2787, 1990.
2. Litovitz T, Oderda G, White JD, Sheridan MJ: Occupational and enviromental exposures reported to poison centers. Am J Public Health 83:739–743, 1993.
3. Surunda A, Agnew J: Deaths from asphyxiation and poisoning at work in the United States. Br J Ind Med 46:541–546, 1989.
4. Borak J, Diller WF: Phosgene exposure: Mechanisms of injury and treatment strategies. J Occup Environ Med 43:110–119, 2000.
5. Sciuto AM, Stotts RR: Posttreatment with eicosatetraenoic acid decreases lung edema in guinea pigs exposed to phosgene: The role of leukotrienes. Exp Lung Res 24:273–292, 1998.
6. Wagner PD, Mathieu-Costello O, Bebout DE, et al: Protection against pulmonary O_2 toxicity by N-acetylcysteine. Eur Respir J 2:116–126, 1989.
7. Jamieson DD, Kerr DR, Unsworth I: Interaction of N-acetylcysteine and bleomycin on hyperbaric oxygen-induced lung damage in mice. Lung 165:239–247, 1987.
8. Hagen TM, Brown LA, Jones DP: Protection against paraquat-induced injury by exogenous GSH in pulmonary alveolar type II cells. Biochem Pharmacol 35:4537–4542, 1986.
9. Miller FJ, Menzel DB, Coffin DL: Similarity between man and laboratory animals in regional pulmonary deposition of ozone. Environ Res 17:84–101, 1978.
10. Bates DV: The respiratory bronchiole as a target organ for the effects of dusts and gases. J Occup Med 15:177–180, 1973.
11. Alberts WM, do Pico G: Reactive airways dysfunction syndrome. Chest 109:1618–1626, 1996.
12. Smith DD: Immunologic and clinical features of toxic inhalations. Immunol Allergy Clin North Am 12:267–278, 1992.
13. Caplin M: Ammonia-gas poisoning, 47 cases in a London shelter. Lancet 2:95–96, 1941.
14. Levy DM, Divertie MB, Litzow TJ, Henderson JW: Ammonia burns of the face and respiratory tract. JAMA 190:95–98, 1964.
15. Montague TJ, Macneil AR: Mass ammonia inhalation. Chest 77:496–498, 1980.
16. Traber DL, Linares HA, Herndon DN: The pathophysiology of inhalation injury—a review. Burns 14:357–364, 1988.
17. Traber DL: Effect of Sulfo Lewis C on smoke inhalation injury. Crit Care Med 26:1159, 1998.
18. Laffon M, Pittet JF, Modelska K, et al: Interleukin-8 mediates injury from smoke inhalation to both the lung endothelial and the alveolar epithelial barriers in rabbits. Am J Respir Crit Care Med 160:1443–1449, 1999.
19. Lin YS, Ho CY, Tang GJ, Kou YR: Alleviation of wood smoke–induced lung injury by tachykinin receptor antagonist and hydroxyl radical scavenger in guinea pigs. Eur J Pharmacol 425:141–148, 2001.
20. Milby TH: Hydrogen sulfide intoxication: Review of the literature and report of unusual accident resulting in two cases of nonfatal poisoning. J Occup Environ Med 4:431–437, 1962.
21. Baxter PJ: Gases. In Baxter PJ, Adams PH, Aw TC, et al (eds): Hunter's Diseases of Occupation, 9th ed. London, Arnold Press, 2000, pp 123–178.
22. Van Aalst JA, Isakov R, Polk JD, et al: Hydrogen sulfide inhalation injury. J Burn Care Rehabil 21:248–253, 2000.
23. Winternitz MC: Pathology of War Gas Poisoning. New Haven, Yale University Press, 1920.
24. Taplin GV, Chopa S, Yanda RL, Elam D: Radionuclidic lung-imaging procedures in the assessment of injury due to ammonia inhalation. Chest 69:582–586, 1976.
25. Miller FJ, Kimbell JS: Regional dosimetry of inhaled reactive gases. In McClellan RO, Henderson RF (eds): Concepts in Inhalation Toxicology, 2nd ed. Washington, D.C., Taylor & Francis, 1995, pp 257–288.
26. Buie SE, Pratt DS, May JJ: Diffuse pulmonary injury following paint remover exposure. Am J Med 81:702–704, 1986.
27. Schwartz DA, Smith DD, Lakshminarayan S: The pulmonary sequelae associated with accidental inhalation of chlorine. Chest 97:820–825, 1990.
28. Diller WF: Pathogenesis of phosgene poisoning. Toxicol Ind Health 1:7–15, 1985.
29. Diller WF: Late sequelae poisoning: A literature review. Toxicol Ind Health 1:129–136, 1985.
30. Diller WF, Zante R: A literature review: Therapy for phosgene poisoning. Toxicol Ind Health 1:117–128, 1985.
31. Mautone AJ, Katx Z, Scarpelli EM: Acute responses to phosgene inhalation and selected corrective measures (including surfactant). Toxicol Ind Health 1:37–57, 1985.
32. Regan RA: Review of clinical experience in handling phosgene exposure cases. Toxicol Ind Health 1:69–72, 1985.
33. Guo YL, Kennedy TP, Michael JR, et al: Mechanism of phosgene-induced lung toxicity: Role of arachidonate mediators. J Appl Physiol 69:1615–1622, 1990.
34. Ainsle G: Inhalational injuries produced by smoke and nitrogen dioxide. Respir Med 87:169–174, 1993.
35. Close LG, Catlin FI, Cohn AM: Acute and chronic effects of ammonia burns of the respiratory tract. Arch Otolaryngol 106:151–158, 1980.
36. Crapo RO: Smoke-inhalation injuries. JAMA 246:1694–1696, 1981.
37. Moylan JA: Inhalation injury. J Trauma 21(Suppl 8):720–721, 1981.
38. Moylan JA: Smoke inhalation and burn injury. Surg Clin North Am 60:1533–1540, 1980.
39. Cohen MA, Guzzardi LJ: Inhalation of products of combustion. Ann Emerg Med 12:628–632, 1983.
40. Charan NB, Lakshminarayan S, Meyers GC, Smith DD: Effects of accidental chlorine inhalation in pulmonary function. West J Med 143:333–336, 1985.
41. Blanc PD, Galbo M, Hiatt P, Olson KR: Morbidity following acute irritant inhalation in a population-based study. JAMA 266:664–669, 1991.
42. Levy DM, Divertie MB, Litzow TJ, Henderson JW: Ammonia burns of the face and respiratory tract. JAMA 190:873–876, 1964.
43. Jarudi NI, Golden B: Ammonia eye injuries. J Iowa Med Soc 63:260–263, 1973.
44. Levine BA, Petroff PA, Slade CL, Pruitt BA: Prospective trials of dexamethasone and aerosolized gentamicin in the treatment of inhalational injury in the burned patient. J Trauma 18:188–193, 1978.
45. Luce JM: Acute lung injury and adult respiratory distress syndrome. Crit Care Med 26:369–376, 1998.
46. Jones GR, Proudfoot AT, Hall JI: Pulmonary effects of acute exposure to nitrous fumes. Thorax 28:61–65, 1973.
47. Demnati R, Fraser R, Martin JG, et al: Effects of dexamethasone on functional and pathological changes in rat bronchi caused by high acute exposure to chlorine. Toxicol Sci 45:242–246, 1998.
48. Urbanetti JS: Toxic inhalational injury. In Zajtchuk R (ed): Textbook of Military Medicine, Medical Aspects of Chemical and Biological Warfare. Washington, D.C., Office of the Surgeon General, 1997, pp 247–270.
49. Virtual Naval Hospital: Lung-damaging agents (choking agents). In: Treatment of Chemical Agent Casualties and Conventional Military Chemical Injuries. Departments of the Army, the Navy, and the Air Force, and Commandant, Marine Corps, 1995, 2001. URL: http://www.vnh.org/.
50. Hales CA, Elsasser TH, Ocampo P, Efimova O: TNF-alpha in smoke inhalation lung injury. J Appl Physiol 82:1433–1437, 1997.
51. Ward A, Clissold SP: Drug evaluation: Pentoxifylline: A review of its pharmacodynamic and pharmocokinetic properties, and its therapeutic efficacy. Drugs 34:50–97, 1987.
52. Sciuto AM, Stotts RR, Hurt HH: Efficacy of ibuprofen and pentoxifylline in the treatment of phosgene-induced acute lung injury. J Appl Toxicol 16:381–384, 1996.
53. Thabut G, Brugiere O, Leseche G, et al: Preventive effect of inhaled nitric oxide and pentoxifylline on ischemic/reperfusion injury after lung transplantation. Transplantation 71:1295–1300, 2001.
54. Scuito AM, Strickland PT, Kennedy TP, Gurtner GH: Postexposure treatment with aminophylline protects against phosgene-induced acute lung injury. Exp Lung Res 23:317–332, 1997.
55. Post Mizus I, Summer W, Farrukh I, et al: Isoproterenol or aminophylline attenuate pulmonary edema after acid lung injury. Am Rev Respir Dis 131:256–259, 1985.
56. Kennedy TP, Michael JR, Hoidal JR, et al: Dibutyryl cAMP, aminophylline, and beta-adrenergic agonists protect against pulmonary edema caused by phosgene. J Appl Physiol 67:2542–2552, 1989.
57. Prescott LF, Illingworth RN, Critchley JAJH, et al: Intravenous N-acetylcysteine: The treatment of choice for paracetamol poisoning. BMJ 2:1097–2000, 1979.
58. Hagen TM, Brown LA, Jones DP: Protection against paraquat-induced injury by exogenous GSH in pulmonary alveolar type II cells. Biochem Pharmacol 35:4537–4542, 1986.

59. Wagner PD, Mathieu-Costello O, Bebout DE, et al: Protection against pulmonary O_2 toxicity by *N*-acetylcysteine. Eur Respir J 2:116–126, 1989.

60. Berend N: Inhibition of bleomycin lung toxicity by *N*-acetylcysteine in the rat. Pathology 17:108–110, 1985.

61. Hagiwara SI, Ischi Y, Kitamura S: Aerosolized administration of *N*-acetylcysteine attenuates lung fibrosis induced by bleomycin in mice. Am J Respir Crit Care Med 162:225–231, 2000.

62. Sciuto AM, Strickland PT, Kennedy TP, Gurtner GH: Protective effects of *N*-acetylcysteine treatment after phosgene exposure in rabbits. Am J Respir Crit Care Med 151:768–772, 1995.

63. Boman G, Backer U, Larsson S, et al: Oral acetylcysteine reduces exacerbation rate in chronic bronchitis: Report of a trial organized by the Swedish Society for Pulmonary Diseases. Eur J Respir Dis 64:405–415, 1983.

64. Peeila V, Takkunen O, Tukiainen P: Zinc chloride smoke inhalation: A rare cause of severe acute respiratory distress syndrome. Intensive Care Med 26:215–217, 2000.

65. Utsunomiya T, Krausz MM, Dunham B, et al: Modification of inflammatory response to aspiration with ibuprofen. Am J Physiol 243(Heart Circ Physiol 12):H903-H910, 1982.

66. Farrukh IS, Michael JR, Peters SP, et al: The role of cyclooxygenase and lipoxygenase mediators in oxidant-induced lung injury. Am Rev Respir Dis 137:1343–1349, 1988.

67. Kennedy TP, Rao NV, Noah W, et al: Ibuprofen prevents oxidant lung injury and in vitro lipid peroxidation by chelating iron. J Clin. Invest 86:1565–1573, 1990.

68. Lindenschmidt RC, Patterson CE, Forney RB, Rhoades RA: Selective action of prostaglandin F2 alpha during paraquat-induced pulmonary edema in the perfused lung. Toxicol Appl Pharmacol 70:105–114, 1983.

69. Stewart RJ, Yamajuchi KT, Knost PM: Effects of ibuprofen on pulmonary oedema in an animal smoke inhalation mode. Burns 16:409–413, 1990.

70. Jin LJ, LaLonde C, Demling RH: Lung dysfunction after thermal injury in relation to prostanoid and oxygen radical release. J Appl Physiol 61:103–112, 1986.

71. Kimura R, Traber L, Herndon D, et al: Ibuprofen reduces the lung lymph flow changes associated with inhalation injury. Circ Shock 24:183–191, 1988.

72. Kang J, Park W, Pack I, et al: Inhaled nitric oxide attenuates acute lung injury. J Appl Physiol 92:795–801, 2002.

73. Roberts JD, Chirche JD, Weiman J, et al: Nitric oxide inhalation decrease pulmonary artery remodeling in the injured lungs of rat pups. Circ Res 87:140–145, 2000.

74. Cuthbertson BH, Galley HF, Webster NR: Effect of inhaled nitric oxide on key mediators of inflammation. Crit Care Med 28:1736–1741, 2000.

75. Koh Y, Kang JL, Park W, et al: Inhaled nitric oxide down-regulates intrapulmonary nitric oxide production in lipopolysaccharide-induced acute lung injury. Crit Care Med 29:1169–1174, 2001.

76. Soejima K, Traber LD, Schmalstieg FC, et al: Role of nitric oxide in vascular permeability after combined burns and smoke inhalation injury. Am Rev Crit Care Med 163:745–752, 2001.

77. Lundin S, Mang H, Smithies M, et al: Inhalation of nitric oxide in acute lung injury: Results of a European multicentre study. Intensive Care Med 25:911–919, 1999.

78. Dellinger RP: Inhaled nitric oxide in acute lung injury and acute respiratory distress syndrome. Intensive Care Med 25:881–883, 1999.

79. Musgrave MA, Fingland R, Gomez M, et al: The use of inhaled nitric oxide as adjuvant therapy in patients with burn injuries and respiratory failure. J Burn Rehabil 21:551–557, 2000.

80. Nader ND, Knight PR, Bobela I, et al: High dose nitric oxide inhalation increases lung injury after gastric aspiration. Anesthesiology 91:741–749, 1999.

81. Kobayashi T, Gabazza EC, Shimizu S, et al: Long term inhalation of high dose nitric oxide increases intraalveolar activation of coagulation system in mice. Am J Crit Care Med 163:1676–1682, 2001.

82. Douidar SM: Nebulized sodium bicarbonate in acute chlorine inhalation. Pediatr Emerg Care 13:406–407, 1997.

83. Vinsel PJ: Treatment of acute chlorine gas inhalation with nebulized sodium bicarbonate. J Emerg Med 8:327–329, 1990.

84. Chisholm CD, Singeltary EM, Okerberg CV, et al: Inhaled sodium bicarbonate therapy for chlorine inhalation injuries. Ann Emerg Med 18:466, 1989.

85. Caravati EM: Acute hydrofluoric acid exposure. Am J Emerg Med 6:143–150, 1988.

86. Lee DC, Wiley JF, Snyder JW: Treatment of inhalational exposure to hydrofluoric acid with nebulized calcium gluconate. J Occup Med 35:470, 1993.

87. Taski O, Goodwin CW, Saitoh D, et al: Effects of burns on inhalation injury. J Trauma 43:603–607, 1997.

88. Masanes MJ, Legendre C, Lioret N, et al: Using bronchoscopy and biopsy to diagnose early inhalation injury. Chest 107:1365–1369, 1995.

89. Cahalane M, Demling RH: Early abnormalities from smoke inhalation. JAMA 251:771–773, 1984.

90. Agee RN, Long JM, Hunt JL, et al: Use of ^{133}xenon in early diagnosis of inhalation injury. J Trauma 16:218–224, 1976.

91. Lee MJ, O'Connell DJ: The plain chest radiograph after acute smoke inhalation. Clin Radiol 39:33–37, 1988.

92. Chrysopoulo MT, Barrow RE, Muller M, et al: Chest radiographic appearances in severely burned adults: A comparison of early radiographic and extravascular lung thermal volume changes. J Burn Care Rehabil:22:104–110, 2001.

93. Zikria BA, Weston GC, Chodoff M: Smoke and carbon monoxide-related deaths in fire victims. J Trauma 12:641–645, 1972.

94. Baud FJ, Barriot P, Toffis V, et al: Elevated blood cyanide concentration in victims of smoke inhalation. N Engl J Med 325:1761–1766, 1991.

95. Cancio LC, Mozingo DW, Pruitt BA: Strategies for diagnosing and treating asphyxiation and inhalation injuries. J Crit Illness 12:217–229, 1997.

96. Kimura R, Traber L, Niehaus G, et al: Ibuprofen reduces the lung lymph flow changes associated with inhalation injury. Circ Shock 24:183–191, 1988.

97. Ogura H, Cioffi WG, Okerberg CV, et al: The effects of pentoxifylline on pulmonary function following smoke inhalation. J Surg Res 56:242–250, 1994.

98. Brown M, Desai M, Traber LD, et al: Dimethylsulfoxide with heparin in the treatment of smoke inhalation injury. J Burn Care Rehabil 9:22–25, 1988.

99. Moritz AR, Henrigues FC, McClean R: The effects of inhaled heat on the air passages and lungs: An experimental investigation. Am J Pathol 21:311–331, 1945.

100. Saab M, Majid I: Acute pulmonary oedema following smoke inhalation. Int J Clin Pract 54:115–116, 2000.

101. Ashley KD, Sthert JCJ Jr, Traber DL, et al: Airway blood flow following light and heavy smoke inhalation. Surg Forum 41:193–195, 1990.

102. Saliba MJ: Heparin in the treatment of burns: A review. Burns 27:349–358, 2001.

103. Saliba MJ: The effects and uses of heparin in the care of burns that improves treatment and enhances the quality of life. Acta Chirurg Plast 39:13–19, 1997.

104. Cox CS, Zwischenberger JB, Traber DL, et al: Heparin improves oxygenation and minimizes barotrauma after smoke inhalation in an ovine model. Surg Gynecol Obstet 176:339–349, 1993.

105. Desi MH, Micak RRT, Richardson RCP, et al: Reduction in mortality in pediatric patients with inhalation injury with aerosolized heparin/*N*-acetylcysteine therapy. J Burn Care Rehabil 19:210–213, 1998.

106. Matthay MA, Uchida T, Fang X: Clinical acute lung injury and acute respiratory distress syndrome. Curr Treat Options Cardiovasc Med 4:139–149, 2002.

107. Meade M, Herridge M: An evidence-based approach to acute respiratory distress syndrome. Respir Care 46:1368–1391, 2001.

108. Eaton S, Martin G: Clinical developments for treating ARDS. Expert Opin Investig Drugs 11:37–48, 2002.

109. Tasaki O, Goodwin CW, Saitoh D, et al: Effects of burns on inhalation injury. J Trauma 43:603–607, 1997.

110. Brower RG, Ware LB, Rerthiaume Y, Matthay MA: Treatment of ARDS. Chest 120:1347–1367, 2001.

111. Frank J, Gutierrez J, Jones K, et al: Low tidal volume reduces epithelial and endothelial injury in rats. Am J Respir Crit Care Med 165:242–249, 2002.

112. Hickling KG: Ventilatory management of ARDS: Can it affect outcome? Intensive Care Med 16:219–226, 1990.

113. Fitzpatrick JC, Cioffi WG: Ventilatory support following burns and smoke-inhalation. Respir Care Clin N Am 3:21–49, 1997.

CHAPTER 98

Hydrogen Sulfide

Scott D. Phillips

Hydrogen sulfide (H_2S), carbon monoxide, and cyanide sometimes are referred to as *cellular asphyxiants* and are known causes of mortality and morbidity. H_2S is also known as "sewer gas," "sour gas," or "stink damp." There are many natural sources for the formation of H_2S, including bacterial decomposition of protein, putrification of organic substances (fish in holding tanks of ships), livestock, and livestock manure collection areas. Most notably, H_2S is associated with oil fields.

H_2S is liberated in other environmental situations, such as off-gassing of volcanos. A classic example occurs in the Puna District on the island of Hawaii, where an active natural volcano emits H_2S, typically in concentrations of less than 20 parts per billion (ppb).[1] Monitoring stations have been set around that geothermal area to monitor off-gassing concentrations. A similar volcanic off-gassing site exists in the City of Rotorua on the north island of New Zealand.[2]

H_2S is a common toxicant in certain settings, such as the oil and gas industry. Safety officers, industrial hygienists, and workers in those industries should be given training on the hazards of H_2S and the proper response in the event of an accident. Safe evacuation and prompt medical attention are important ingredients in the care of these patients. Real-time gas detecting devices are available, and their use should be encouraged to monitor levels of H_2S before entry into a potentially contaminated zone.

CHEMISTRY

H_2S has the odor of rotten eggs. The sense of smell for H_2S fatigues in seconds to minutes. The odor threshold is reported in the range of 1 to 130 ppb.[3] H_2S is slightly heavier than air, with a vapor density of 1.19, and is slightly less volatile than water at room temperature. It has a molecular weight of 34.08. H_2S has a solubility in water (186 mL in 100 mL of water at 40°C) between ammonia, which is highly soluble, and chlorine, which has low solubility.[4] Its metabolism is rapid; no bioaccumulation occurs.

H_2S can be anticipated to be present whenever oxygen is depleted and organic material containing sulfate is present. The major uses for H_2S include the production of elemental sulfur, inorganic sulfides, and sulfuric acid and as an additive in extremely high-pressure lubricants and cutting oils.

The principle pathway of exposure to H_2S is via inhalation. It has limited absorption through the gastrointestinal tract and intact skin.[5]

PATHOPHYSIOLOGY

H_2S causes cellular anoxia by the inhibition of mitochondrial cytochrome oxidase. This inhibition results in disruption of the electron transport chain and impaired oxidative metabolism. Tissues with high oxygen demand (e.g., brain and heart) are especially susceptible to disruption of oxidative metabolism.[6]

H_2S is metabolized by oxidation, methylation, and reactions with metalloproteins or disulfide-containing proteins.[7] The major metabolic pathway is via oxidation of sulfide to thiosulfate (Fig. 98-1), which is converted into sulfate, ultimately being excreted in the urine.[8]

H_2S toxicity seems to be related to its interaction with metalloproteins, including cytochrome oxidase. Ferritin seems to catalyze the oxidation of thiosulfate to sulfate, which may be an endogenous detoxification pathway.

Nitrites administered as an antidote create methemoglobin. The hydrosulfide anion combines with methemoglobin to form sulfmethemoglobin. Methemoglobin attracts the sulfide from cytochrome oxidase, which reactivates aerobic metabolism. This reaction also is thought to cause the binding of H_2S (in the HS^- form) with methemoglobin to form sulfmethemoglobin, a reaction exploited in the antidotal therapy of H_2S poisoning by using sodium nitrite to form methemoglobin; this is explained further in the treatment section.

H_2S also may reduce disulfide bridges in proteins, which is thought to be the mechanism of its inhibition of succinic dehydrogenase. The reduction of disulfide linkages has been tested in animal models using sodium sulfate as an antidote.[9] Mice were given either oxidized or reduced glutathione. Only the oxidized form protected from H_2S toxicity. The H_2S was thought to bind by disulfide linkage to the oxidized glutathione, which prevented toxicity.

Because of its water solubility, H_2S has irritant effects on mucous membranes but also may result in distal airway injury if exposure is of sufficient magnitude. Minimal H_2S is excreted via the lungs. Case reports have mentioned rescue personnel performing mouth-to-mouth resuscitation on H_2S victims, however, who have been victims of self-poisoning.[10]

H_2S normally is present in small amounts in the human body. In the mouth, air concentrations between 1 and 100 ppb have been reported as a component of "bad breath."[11] As a component of intestinal gas, H_2S has been found in concentrations of 1 to 4 ppb with some high levels of 18 ppm. This H_2S is detoxified or excreted. Between 40% and 90% of individuals produce H_2S, with mean values over a 4-year period of 1 to 4 ppm.[12]

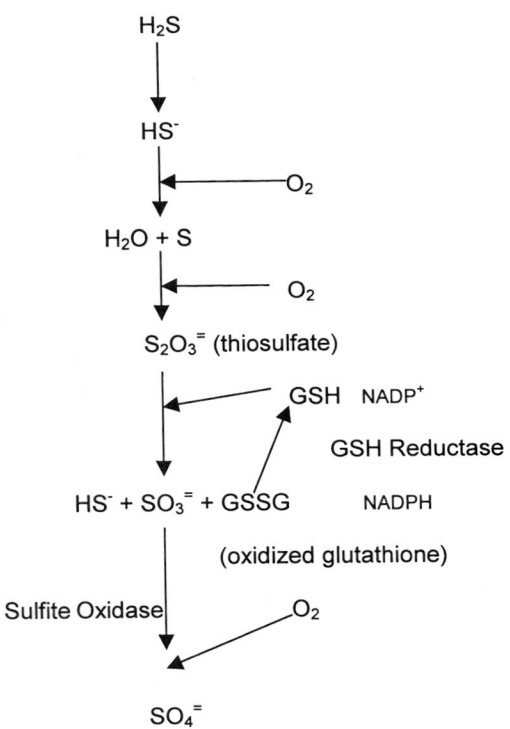

FIGURE 98-1

Oxidation of hydrogen sulfide (H_2S). *(Adapted from Beauchamp RO Jr, Bus JS, Popp JA, et al: A critical review of the literature on hydrogen sulfide toxicity. CRC Crit Rev Toxicol 13:25–97, 1984.)*

Studies in rats have found that H_2S is produced endogenously in the brain in concentrations of 1.6 ppm.[12] The brainstem was found to have the lowest endogenous concentration of H_2S but the highest uptake. This finding may explain anatomically the effect of H_2S on central respiratory drive. In rats, the lethal concentration was approximately twice that of the endogenous concentration found, showing a narrow toxicologic window.

H_2S is capable of crossing cellular membranes and ultimately may result in cellular anoxia, probably primarily through inhibition of cytochrome oxidase aa_3.[6] Electrophysiologic data obtained by Reiffenstein and colleagues[14] suggested that H_2S may cause depolarization of excitable tissue.

One of the initial physiologic effects of H_2S poisoning is the stimulation of the carotid chemoreceptors, which leads to hyperpnea and occurs after inhalation or injection of sulfides.[13] The terminal respiratory depression most likely results from H_2S's being selectively taken up by the brainstem (compared with other brain areas) with the end point similar to anoxia. The underlying mechanism is thought to be due to inhibition of monoamine oxidase.[15] H_2S also is known to inhibit cytochrome oxidase.[16] Other research has suggested that H_2S-induced reductions in sodium channel function may be responsible for respiratory failure.[17]

Concentrations of 1000 to 3000 ppm were fatal to dogs; death occurred within 15 to 20 minutes at 1000 ppm. At the higher concentration, respiration ceased after a few breaths.[18] Lund and Wieland[19] exposed Rhesus monkeys to 500 ppm of H_2S for 22 to 35 minutes. Each of three monkeys lost consciousness abruptly in approximately 15 minutes. A postmortem examination of the brain found that the motor cells of the cerebellum were the principal target organ and displayed evidence of extensive necrosis of the parietal and occipital cortex; a reduced number of Purkinje cells in the cerebellar cortex; isolated accumulation of glial cells in otherwise normal basal ganglia; and normal heart, liver, kidneys, and adrenals.[1]

CLINICAL PRESENTATION

Two well-described adverse effects may occur after H_2S poisoning: mucous membrane irritation and systemic toxicity. These occur in a classic dose-response fashion (Table 98-1). The mucous membranes are particularly susceptible to the effects of H_2S because of their moisture and anatomic proximity to the environment. The irritant effects of H_2S to the face are sensed by the trigeminal nerve distribution, and the olfactory nerve detects its odor, although there may be significant overlap between these two domains.[7] H_2S reacts with water to form irritating acid sulfides.

Membrane irritation begins to occur with H_2S exposures in the range of 4 ppm. Mild nausea, vomiting, and lacrimation tend to occur in the range of 80 to 100 ppm. Higher concentrations (500 ppm) typically are required to cause respiratory tract irritation. Obvious signs of systemic toxicity tend not to occur until H_2S concentrations of approximately 250 ppm have been attained. Findings at these concentrations may include cough, tachypnea, chest pain of cardiac and noncardiac origin, headache, dizziness, lethargy, and confusion. At still higher concentrations, anoxia-induced seizures and coma occur. The most common clinical findings after H_2S exposures are headache, nausea, vomiting, dyspnea, dysequilibrium, conjunctivitis, sore throat, and unconsciousness.[20,21]

Ocular Effects

The eyes are one of the first tissues to react because of the irritant effects of H_2S. The conjunctivae may become inflamed and swollen, resulting in chemosis. After major exposures, the cornea may develop erosions and ulcerations. Associated signs and symptoms include photophobia,

TABLE 98-1 Range of Toxicity of Hydrogen Sulfide	
CLINICAL EFFECT	**CONCENTRATION (ppm)**
Eye irritation	4–100
Respiratory irritation, possible pulmonary edema	50–500
Bronchitis, noncardiogenic pulmonary edema	250 for 24–72 hr
Symptomatic	50 for 0.5 hr
Severely toxic	200 for 1 min
Coma and death	500–1000
Fatal	800—immediate; 600—30 min
Immediate collapse	1000

lacrimation, and pain. Because both the cornea and the conjunctivae are affected, the term *keratoconjunctivitis* is used to describe the eye effects. The keratoconjunctivitis is known in industry as "gas eye," "sore eye," or "spinner's eye." Attention must be paid to the eyes of H_2S-affected patients for appropriate diagnosis and care.

Knockdown Effects

H_2S is known for its rapid "knockdown" capability.[22,23] Frequently, workers in the oil fields report this effect; after recovering, they may continue their work. This situation may result in no residual effects. Anoxic brain injury may occur, however, after significant exposure. Coma, seizures, or signs of increased intracranial pressure from edema may occur.[22,23]

Pulmonary Effects

Inhaled irritants tend to increase the respiratory rate and decrease the minute volume. Significant H_2S exposure may result in redness, inflammation, sloughing, or exfoliation of the airways. The last-mentioned may be delayed 48 hours after the poisoning in animals.[24] Exfoliation of the airways is most common in the upper portion due to its water solubility. If the patient had an overwhelming exposure or a large minute ventilation, the lower airway also may be injured. Rarely, patients may develop pulmonary edema or, more commonly, aspiration pneumonia. Hemorrhagic bronchitis has been recognized and may require ventilatory support.[25]

Cardiovascular Effects

Cardiovascular effects, believed to be related to direct cellular anoxia, are well described after H_2S exposure. Findings may include typical or atypical chest pain. Arrhythmias have been reported in the literature.[26]

Neurologic Effects

Acute high-level H_2S poisonings with resultant loss of consciousness have been associated with long-term motor dysfunction.[27] Although acute high-level exposures may result in altered neuropsychologic functioning, there is no support for chronic low-level exposures causing similar findings.[24]

Metabolic Acidosis

Metabolic acidosis, with elevated lactate concentration, may occur in individuals with serious H_2S poisoning. In exercising men, blood lactate levels were increased when inhaling H_2S for more than 16 minutes at 5 ppm, but not at 2 ppm.[28]

Death

A series of 29 deaths from 5563 exposures were evaluated over a 9-year period.[29] Most fatal cases involve exposures occurring in confined spaces, such as sewers,[30] animal-handling and processing plants,[31–33] waste dumps,[34] sludge plants,[35] tanks and cesspools,[36–40] pulp mills,[41] and other confined environments.[25,42] In case reports of deaths occurring

after acute exposure, individuals lost consciousness after only one or two breaths; this is known as the "slaughterhouse sledgehammer effect." In these fatal cases, patients seemed to succumb from respiratory failure, acute pulmonary edema, or coma. Victims exposed to only H_2S gas do not have a substantial risk of secondary contamination to personnel outside the so-called hot zone. Rescuers should be trained and attired properly with positive-pressure, self-contained breathing apparatus before entering the hot zone.

DIAGNOSIS

Important toxicologic differential diagnoses with presentation similar to H_2S poisoning include other cellular toxicants, such as carbon monoxide, cyanide, and cyanide-related substances. Carbonyl sulfide, a metabolite of disulfiram, is known to convert endogenously to H_2S. Carbonyl sulfide is metabolized to H_2S by the carbonic anhydrase. The H_2S produced may be responsible for carbonyl sulfide toxicity.[43]

Many other compounds present with a rotten egg–type odor similar to H_2S, including sulfur compounds such as mercaptans, carbon disulfide, and trimethylamine. The presence of a metabolic acidosis should be evaluated and characterized by assessment of arterial blood gases, electrolytes, lactate, salicylate, cyanide, toxic alcohols (ethylene glycol, methanol), and carboxyhemoglobin concentrations. Sulfide ion levels can be measured on whole blood; however, lack of specificity and limited availability make the test useless in initial diagnosis. Industrial hygienists, hazardous materials responders, and firefighters can measure H_2S concentrations in the ambient atmosphere around the site of an incident. In the case of an identified H_2S-related incident, H_2S concentrations need to be communicated directly with the individuals on site so that appropriate precautions can be taken and assessments made.

TREATMENT

Supportive care is the mainstay of therapy for exposures to H_2S and includes removal from exposure, supplemental oxygen, and decontamination of the eyes primarily and skin. Decontamination can be accomplished by irrigating exposed skin and eyes with normal saline. Ventilatory support, the administration of anticonvulsants if there is evidence of seizure activity, and cycloplegics and antibiotics for eye injuries also may be necessary. Later in the course, antibiotics may be indicated if there is evidence of infected aspirated pulmonary secretions.

Indications for ICU Admission in Hydrogen Sulfide Poisoning

Respiratory distress, respiratory failure, or signs of airway injury
Unconsciousness
Seizures
Electrocardiogram changes

Methemoglobin Induction

Therapy directed at the creation of methemoglobinemia has been advocated in the treatment of H_2S poisoning. Animal studies have supported the protective and antidotal effects of methemoglobinemia for sulfide and cyanide toxicity.[44]

H_2S poisoning may cause lactic acidosis by the inhibition of cytochrome c oxidase. The formation of methemoglobinemia by nitrites creates a large pool of ferric iron, which has a greater affinity for H_2S than cytochrome c oxidase. Because of this property, methemoglobin serves as a sink for the sulfide ions. This situation allows for cytochrome c to be reactivated, reestablishing aerobic metabolism.[45,46]

One method of inducing methemoglobinemia is by use of components of the cyanide antidote kit used in North America. Amyl nitrate inhalation is carried out by crushing the amyl nitrate pearls of the kit in a gauze pad, which serves as a matrix for facilitating inhalation; typically this is done for 30 seconds for each minute, for 5 minutes. The practice has limited ability to induce methemoglobinemia, however, and the use of amyl nitrite should be restricted to the time it takes to initiate intravenous sodium nitrite. The generally accepted adult dose of sodium nitrite is 10 mL of a 3% solution; the pediatric dose is 0.33 mL/kg up to 10 mL. Because sodium nitrite is a vasodilator, it should not be administered rapidly because of the possibility of hypotension. In my experience, a 10-mL dose can be administered safely over 2 to 5 minutes in a normal adult. The thiosulfate portion of the cyanide antidote kit does not form methemoglobin and is not useful in H_2S poisoning. Other methemoglobin-forming agents (see Chapter 28) also may be useful. The efficacy of methemoglobin in acute H_2S poisoning is superior to that of supplemental oxygen alone.[47] Sulfide is present in the blood only transiently, and methemoglobin therapy is not indicated in most patients. If the patient remains symptomatic, has a persistent acidosis, or is in a coma, methemoglobin formation should be considered.

Hyperbaric Oxygen

Hyperbaric oxygen is a theoretical therapy for H_2S poisoning. A few publications have reported the utility of hyperbaric oxygen for H_2S poisoning. In these cases, it was reported to be effective.[48,49] These data are uncontrolled, anecdotal, and subject to publication bias. Hyperbaric oxygen therapy, when available, should be considered for severe toxicity with persistent acidosis, altered mental status, or life-threatening dysrhythmias. Bitterman and coworkers[50] found that 3 atm was more effective in preventing death in rats than 1 atm in a pure oxygen environment. See Chapter 16 for a full discussion of hyperbaric oxygen.

Prehospital Treatment

Criteria for ICU Discharge in Hydrogen Sulfide Poisoning

Stability of clinical findings
Resolution of hypoxia and metabolic acidosis
Stable mental status

A study by Arnold and associates[20] of 250 cases of exposure to H_2S in the Alberta oil fields found that with increased awareness and improved prehospital treatment (first aid), the fatality rate was reduced by half, unconsciousness decreased from 13% to 2%, and hospitalization admission rates decreased from 51% to 22%. Prehospital treatment also resulted in an overall decrease in workers' compensation claims to 17.4%.

SPECIAL POPULATIONS

Although no definitive studies have addressed special populations, persons with cardiovascular or cerebrovascular disease may be at increased risk from cellular hypoxia related to H_2S.

Common Errors in Hydrogen Sulfide Poisoning

Failure to consider other hydrogen sulfide or cellular poisons in case of seizure, coma, or metabolic acidosis
Failure to assess trauma secondary to sudden unconsciousness
Treating based only on exposure, not on clinical presentation
Failure to decontaminate the eyes
Failure

Key Points in Hydrogen Sulfide Poisoning

1. Hydrogen sulfide causes a rapid knockdown effect.
2. Eye decontamination is essential.
3. Supportive care is the mainstay of therapy.
4. Induction of methemoglobinemia is antidotal.
5. Hyperbaric oxygen therapy may be effective.

REFERENCES

1. ATSDR: Health Consultation, Puna Geothermal Venture Pahoa (Puna District), Hawaii County, Hawaii, December 22, 1997. Available at: www.atsdr.cdc.gov\HAC\PAH\PUNA\pgv.html.
2. Bates MN, Garrett N, Graham B, et al: Cancer incidence, morbidity and geothermal air pollution in Rotorua, New Zealand. Int J Epidemiol 27:10–14, 1998.
3. American Industrial Hygiene Association: Odor Thresholds for Chemicals with Established Occupational Health Standards. Fairfax, VA, AIHA Press, 1997.
4. ATSDR: Toxicological Profile for Hydrogen Sulfide. Atlanta, GA, U.S. Department of Health and Human Services, Public Health Service, Agency for Toxic Substances and Disease Registry, 1999.
5. Laug EP, Draize JH: The percutaneous absorption of ammonium sulfide and hydrogen sulfide. J Pharmacol Exp Ther 76:179–188, 1994.
6. Ammann HM: A new look at the physiologic respiratory response to hydrogen sulfide poisoning. J Haz Mat 13:369–374, 1986.
7. Beauchamp RO Jr, Bus JS, Popp JA, et al: A critical review of the literature on hydrogen sulfide toxicity. CRC Crit Rev Toxicol 13:25–97, 1984.
8. Bartholomew TC, Powell GM, Dodgson KS, et al: Oxidation of sodium sulphide by rat liver, lungs and kidney. Biochem Pharmacol 29:1431–1437, 1980.
9. Smith RP, Abbanat RA: Protective effect of oxidized glutathione in acute sulfide poisoning. Toxicol Appl Pharmacol 9:209–217, 1966.

10. Kleinfeld, M, Giel C, Rosso A: Acute hydrogen sulfide intoxication: An unusual source of exposure. Ind Med Surg 33:656–660, 1964.
11. Rosenberg M, Septon I, Eli I, et al: Halitosis measurement by an industrial sulphide monitor. J Peridontol 62:487–489, 1991.
12. Kirk E: The quantity and composition of human colonic flatus. Gastroenterology 12:782–794, 1949.
13. Warenycia MW, Goodwin CR, Benishin CG, et al: Acute hydrogen sulfide poisoning: Demonstration of selective uptake of sulfide by the brainstem by measurement of brain sulfide levels. Biochem Pharmacol 38:973–981, 1989.
14. Reiffenstein RJ, Hulbert WC, Roth SH: Toxicology of hydrogen sulfide. Ann Rev Pharmacol Toxicol 32:109–134, 1992.
15. Warenycia MW, Smith KA, Blashko CS, et al: Monoamine oxidase inhibition as a sequel of hydrogen sulfide intoxication: increases in brain catecholamine and 5-hydroxytryptamine levels. Arch Toxicol 63:131–136, 1989.
16. Nicholls P: The effect of sulfide on cytochrome a_3, isosteric and allosteric shifts of the reduced alpha peak. Biochem Biophys Acta 396:24–35, 1975.
17. Warenycia MW, Steele JA, Karpinski E, Reiffenstein R: Hydrogen sulfide in combination with taurine or cysteic acid reversibility abolishes sodium currents in neuroblastoma cells. Neurotoxicology 10:191–199, 1989.
18. Haggard HW, Henderson Y, Charlton TJ: The influence of hydrogen sulfide upon respiration. Am J Physiol 61:289–297, 1922.
19. Lund OE, Wieland H: Pathologic: Anatomic findings in experimental hydrogen sulfide poisoning (H_2S)—a study on Rhesus monkeys. Int Arch Gewerbepathol Gewerbehyg 22:46–54, 1966.
20. Arnold IMF, Dufresne RM, Alleyne BC, et al: Health implication of occupational exposures to hydrogen sulfide. J Occup Med 27:373–376, 1985.
21. Burnett WW, King EG, Grace M, et al: Hydrogen sulfide poisoning: Review of 5 years' experience. CMAJ 117:1277–1280, 1977.
22. Ahlborg G: Hydrogen sulfide poisoning in shale oil industry. Ind Hyg Occup Med 3:247–266, 1951.
23. Hessel PA, Herbert FA, Melenka LS, et al: Lung health in relation to hydrogen sulfide exposure in oil and gas workers in Alberta, Canada. Am J Ind Med 31:554–557, 1997.
24. Lopez A, Prior M, Yong S, Lillie L: Nasal lesions in rats exposed to hydrogen sulfide for four hours. Am J Vet Res 49:1107–1111, 1988.
25. Parra O, Monso E, Gallego M, et al: Inhalation of hydrogen sulphide: A case of subacute manifestations and long term sequelae. Br J Ind Med 48:286–287, 1991.
26. Arnold IMF, Dufresne RM, Alleyne BC, et al: Health implications of occupational exposures to hydrogen sulfide. J Occup Med 27:373–376, 1985.
27. Tvedt B, Skyberg K, Aaserud O, et al: Brain damage caused by hydrogen sulfide: A follow-up study of six patients. Am J Ind Med 20:91–101, 1991.
28. Bhambhani Y, Singh M: Physiological effects of hydrogen sulfide inhalation during exercise in healthy men. J Appl Physiol 71:1872–1877, 1991.
29. Snyder JW, Safir EF, Summerville GP, et al: Occupational fatality and persistent neurological sequelae after mass exposure to hydrogen sulfide. Am J Emerg Med 13:199–203, 1995.
30. Adelson L, Sunshine I: Fatal hydrogen sulfide intoxication: Report of three cases occurring in a sewer. Arch Pathol 81:375–380, 1966.
31. Breysse PA: Hydrogen sulfide fatality in a poultry feather fertilizer plant. Am Ind Hyg Assoc J 22:220–222, 1961.
32. Audeau FM, Gnanaharan C, Davey K: Industrial medicine hydrogen sulphide poisoning: associated with pelt processing. N Z Med J 98:145–147, 1985.
33. Perry GF Jr: Occupational medicine forum. J Occup Environ Med 37:656–658, 1995.
34. Allyn LB: Notes on hydrogen sulfide poisoning. Ind Engineering Chem 23:234, 1931.
35. NIOSH: Health Hazard Evaluation Report HETA 80–13, 81–147–1644, Sclegel Tennessee, Inc, Maryville, Tennessee. Report No. HETA-85–108–1593. NITS publication No. PB86–132164. Cincinnati, OH, National Institute for Occupational Safety and Health, Hazard Evaluations and Technical Assistance Branch, 1985.
36. Campanya M, Sanz P, Reig R, et al: Fatal hydrogen sulfide poisoning. Med Lav 80:251–253, 1989.
37. Freireich AW: Hydrogen sulfide poisoning: Report of two cases, one with fatal outcome, from associated mechanical asphyxia. Am J Pathol 22:147–155, 1946.
38. Hagley SR, South DL: Fatal inhalation of liquid manure gas. Med J Aust 2:459–460, 1983.
39. Morse DL, Woodbury MA, Rentmeester K, et al: Death caused by fermenting manure. JAMA 245:63–64, 1981.
40. Osbern LN, Crapo RO: Dung lung: A report of toxic exposure to liquid manure. Ann Intern Med 95:312–314, 1981.
41. Jaakkola JJK, Vilkka V, Marttila O, et al: The South Karelia Air Pollution Study: The effects of malodorous sulfur compounds from pulp mills on respiratory and other symptoms. Am Rev Respir Dis 142:1344–1350, 1990.
42. Deng JF, Chang SC: Hydrogen sulfide poisonings in hot-spring reservoir cleaning: Two case reports. Am J Ind Med 11:447–451, 1987.
43. Chengelis CP, Neal RA: Studies of carbonyl sulfide toxicity: Metabolism by carbonic anhydrase. Toxicol Appl Pharmacol 55:198–202, 1980.
44. Smith RP, Gosselin RE: Hydrogen sulfide poisoning. J Occup Med 21:93–97, 1979.
45. Smith L, Krusyna H, Smith RP: The effect of methemoglobin on the inhibition of cytochrome c oxidase by cyanide, sulfide or azide. Biochem Pharmacol 26:2247–2250, 1977.
46. Smith RP, Gosselin RE: The influence of methemoglobinemia on the lethality of some toxic anions: II. Sulfide. Toxicol Appl Pharmacol 6:584–592, 1964.
47. Smith RP, Kruszyna R, Kruszyna H: Management of acute sulfide poisoning. Arch Environ Health 33:166–169, 1976.
48. Whitcraft DD III, Bailey TD, Hart GB: Hydrogen sulfide poisoning treated with hyperbaric oxygen. J Emerg Med 3:23–25, 1985.
49. Smilkstein MJ, Bronstein AC, Pickett HM, et al: Hyperbaric oxygen therapy for severe hydrogen sulfide poisoning. Selected Topics Toxicol 3:27–30, 1985.
50. Bitterman N, Talmi Y, Lerman A, et al: The effect of hyperbaric oxygen on acute experimental sulfide poisoning in the rat. Toxicol Appl Pharmacol 84:325–328, 1986.

CHAPTER **99**

Caustics

Joseph G. Rella ■ Robert S. Hoffman

Ingestion of caustic agents has been a difficult medical problem around the world for years. With the different types of caustic agents, varied clinical presentations, and changing recommendations for patient management, it is no wonder that many physicians consider these types of injuries complicated. Even the word *caustic* has varied interpretations and usages. *The Compact Oxford English Dictionary*[1] considers *caustic* and *corrosive* to be synonyms, both meaning something that eats away or destroys. Friedman[2] drew a distinction between caustics and corrosives, making them specifically alkalis and acids. Adding to this confusion is the fact that many people use these words to describe different agents that may be described more accurately as oxidizing agents (potassium permanganate), desiccants, vesicants (mustard gas), and protoplasmic poisons (hydrofluoric acid).[3]

DEFINITION

A caustic is any substance that can destroy tissue chemically. As already mentioned, different types of substances can cause tissue destruction by various means. Acids and alkalis are the two primary types of agents most often responsible for caustic exposures. By the classic definition, acids are proton donors, and alkalis are proton acceptors. In addition, there are caustic agents that do not fit this simple classification, such as Clinitest tablets, creosote, ingredients in electric-dishwasher detergent, phenol, zinc chloride, and surfactant.

EPIDEMIOLOGY

The number of patients exposed to caustic substances has been affected by various factors over the years. The introduction of new cleaning products to the public, notably liquid lye, which became available in 1967, increased the number of patients with caustic ingestions. At that time, the prototype of new liquid drain cleaners contained 30% sodium hydroxide. Because of the sudden increase in severe morbidity from caustic ingestions that followed the introduction of this product, however, the Poison Prevention Packing Act of 1970 and the Federal Hazardous Substance Act of 1973 were passed; these Acts mandated the use of child-resistant caps for products containing 2% or more of

an alkaline caustic and the reduction of concentration of cleaning substances. Designed to protect young children from dangerous substances found around the house, these Acts are responsible in part for a decline in the incidence of caustic ingestions in children.

The exact incidence of caustic ingestions is difficult to state due to the manner in which these data are reported. As with other poisonings, reports to poison centers involving caustic ingestions are gathered passively and likely reflect a number less than the actual number of ingestions that occur. Although treating ingestion of caustic substances is a relatively rare experience for the individual physician, caustics continue to be one of the most frequently reported substances involved in human exposures.[4] In 1998, caustic substances, which are classified under cleaning substances and chemicals in the Annual Report of the American Association of Poison Control Centers Toxic Exposure Surveillance System, accounted for more than 5000 exposures. Trowers and associates[5] estimated the number of caustic exposures in 1994 to be 26,000.

Children younger than 6 years old account for the greatest number of exposures to caustic substances, with most exposures being unintentional. Hawkins and colleagues[6] reported in 1980 that children younger than 5 years old accounted for nearly half of the caustic exposures in their series. These data closely resemble data reported from poison centers in 1998, in which 129,000 children younger than 6 years old represented nearly twice the number of all persons older than age 19 exposed to cleaning substances.[4]

Suicidal patients are the next greatest number of patients with caustic ingestions. Although the number of intentional ingestions is only 1% to 2% of the number of unintentional exposures of various caustic agents, they account for nearly 80% of all serious injury requiring a major intervention.

PATHOPHYSIOLOGY

Many factors contribute to the ability of a caustic substance to cause damage. Concentration, amount, contact time with tissue, pH, and titratable reserve all may be important in making caustics dangerous.[7–13] One ex vivo study examined damage to esophagi when exposed for 10 seconds to 4%, 10%, and 22% sodium hydroxide. Histologic damage progressed from mucosa to serosa as concentration increased.[14] People with suicidal intent more commonly ingest large amounts of caustic agents. The lesions found in these cases often are more extensive, and injury also involves stomach and duodenum.[7] Burns are more common in areas of the esophagus where passage of the caustic agent may be delayed, such as at the crossing of the aorta and the left main bronchus.[7,15] A pH of 12.5 has been cited as crucial for production of esophageal ulcerations from sodium hydroxide.[12] The contribution pH makes to the nature of a caustic substance is not straightforward, however.[16] Phenol and zinc chloride, two well-known caustic agents, have nearly neutral pHs.

Titratable reserve is defined as the volume of neutralizing substance required to bring the pH of a caustic to approximate that of a normal esophagus. In one study, titratable reserve correlated better than pH in predicting the production of esophageal injury.[17] Although titratable reserve helps explain causticity, it was not standardized for acids and bases and liquids and solids, and it does not correlate with resulting tissue strength after an exposure.[18] The best that can be said of pH and titratable reserve is that they help define the dangerous properties of a caustic agent but are only a few of the important characteristics to consider.

A caustic agent potentially can damage any tissue to which it is exposed. With the exception of hydrofluoric acid, which may have profound systemic toxicity, organs of direct contact, such as eyes, skin, lungs, gastrointestinal tract, and other intrathoracic and intraabdominal organs, all are potential sites of caustic injury. The most serious and life-threatening injuries result from ingestion of these substances because of the difficulty in establishing the diagnosis and the reduced ability to decontaminate and treat effectively compared with a topical exposure.

At one time, it was suggested that acids caused maximum damage to the stomach and minimal injury to the esophagus, whereas alkalis caused injury in the reverse pattern. Before 1965, lye was available to the public only in solid form.[19] Although there are reports of suicidal patients mixing these crystals in water before drinking, many times ingested crystals would adhere to mucosal surfaces on initial contact, injuring the pharynx and upper esophagus, whereas a less viscous acid agent would pass rapidly through the oropharynx to collect in the stomach. These types of injuries are likely at the root of this concept. In 1967, liquid lye became available to the public, and more extensive injuries were diagnosed. One study specifically addressed this question and found no difference in distribution of injury between acids and alkalis.[20] Alkalis remain available, however, as solids, as viscous liquids, and in a formula that is designed to generate a column of foam using hydrogen peroxide. Almost all acids are available exclusively as low-viscosity liquids.

Ingested liquid forms of caustics expose all mucosal surfaces to the caustic material. This tissue injury has been studied extensively over the years. Experimentally, tissue injury occurs within seconds of contact for acids and alkalis.[9,14,21] After experimental exposure to alkaline substances, esophageal mucosa grossly becomes gray and gelatinous. Fats and proteins become saponified as the tissue neutralizes the caustic in a reaction that releases heat and gas.[8,22] Microscopic evaluation of alkaline caustic injury to esophageal tissue revealed liquefactive necrosis of the mucosa with edema and inflammation.[10,21] Ulceration of

the mucosa follows, and there is widespread thrombosis of arterioles and venules.[7,9,10,21,23] Acid-induced injury is described as a coagulation necrosis with formation of a thick eschar that theoretically may limit tissue penetration and tissue damage. Despite this difference from alkaline-induced necrosis, strong acids, like strong alkalis, perforate the gastrointestinal tract and cause injury to other intraabdominal organs and death. Acid exposures to the esophagus also are characterized by edema and an acute inflammatory reaction.[5,24] At the edge of the injury, polymorphonuclear leukocytes infiltrate, and granulation tissue begins to develop.[7,10,25] Depending on the severity of the injury, inflammation may extend through the muscle layer, and perforations may occur. In these cases, periesophageal and intraabdominal tissues become affected as well.

After several days, the necrotic tissue is sloughed, edema decreases, and fibroblasts begin to proliferate. Ulcerations may persist for months, and the esophagus shortens.[10] This period also includes neovascularization and the deposition of collagen.[10] Adhesions form between pockets of granulation tissue in bands, which is where stricture formation begins.[7] With the progressive remodeling that takes place over the following weeks to months after a significant injury, the lumen of the esophagus begins to narrow. When enough scar tissue collects in a small area, it forms a stricture.[10]

The risk of stricture formation is related to depth and circumference of the injury.[26] The depth of injury can be established only by endoscopy and direct visualization of the mucosa itself. A grading system describes the various degrees of injury, which may be associated with a risk for stricture (Table 99-1).[6,19] Grade 1 injuries are characterized by superficial mucosal hyperemia and do not progress to form strictures.[19,20,27–31] Grade 2 injuries include submucosal and transmucosal ulcerations with blistering and exudate.[6,19,27,31] These injuries are divided into subtype A, which are noncircumferential and rarely develop strictures, and subtype B, which are near-circumferential or circumferential and progress to strictures in 75% of cases.[31] Grade 3 injuries are described as severe with widespread tissue destruction, deep ulcerations, and extensive necrosis.[19,27,31] These injuries progress to form strictures despite any mode of therapy provided and have a high incidence of perforation.[28,32]

TABLE 99-1 Endoscopic Grades of Esophageal Injury

GRADE	DESCRIPTION	RISK OF STRICTURE FORMATION
1	Superficial mucosal hyperemia	None
2A	Noncircumferential submucosal or transmucosal ulcerations with blistering and exudate	Rare
2B	Circumferential or near-circumferential submucosal or transmucosal ulcerations with blistering and exudate	75%
3	Severe, widespread tissue destruction with deep ulcerations and extensive necrosis	100%

Significant complications may accompany the various stages of injury and recovery. Immediately life-threatening complications include airway compromise and perforation into a great vessel.[15] Complications such as perforation may lead to periesophagitis, mediastinitis, peritonitis, infection from normal flora,[7] shock, and sepsis.[10] Other complications include esophageal dysmotility,[33] erosion into a bronchial artery, and formation of aortoesophageal and tracheoesophageal fistulae.[23,34] Survivors of lye ingestions who develop a stricture have a 1000-fold increased risk of squamous cell carcinoma of the esophagus with a latency of approximately 40 years,[35,36] although this risk assessment was not controlled for regarding alcohol abuse and smoking.[15] Additionally, acid ingestions can cause an acidemia that results from absorption of the acid itself. Ingestion of hydrochloric acid may result in a non–anion gap acidemia because hydrogen and chloride are absorbed and accounted for in measuring the anion gap, whereas ingestion of sulfuric acid might result in an anion gap acidosis because sulfate is not measured directly in the anion gap calculation. Conversely, ingestion of an alkaline substance typically does not result in alkalemia.

CLINICAL SIGNS AND SYMPTOMS

As might be expected, when a caustic agent contacts tissue, there may be severe pain. Beginning in the mouth, painful lips, tongue, and oropharynx all are well reported.[10,20,37,38] Aspiration may lead to voice change and stridor.[38] As deeper tissues become involved, dysphagia, odynophagia, chest and back pain, and vomiting may occur.[10,20,39] Abdominal pain with fever and tachycardia may suggest a potentially severe injury.[8]

Many patients who have ingested a caustic agent do not present with a classic constellation of clinical signs and symptoms, however, that allow for rapid and easy diagnosis.[40] There are many cases in which a patient is reported to appear clinically well with normal vital signs and a soft, nontender abdomen yet dies within several hours or is found to have severe injury to the gastrointestinal tract.[3,23,41,42] Many studies have found that less than half of patients with esophageal or gastric injuries diagnosed by endoscopy experience abdominal pain or have tenderness.[2,13,20,39] This finding indicates to some extent that caustic ingestions simply may not reveal the seriousness of the injury they cause by their very nature. To complicate this idea further, many other factors may modify the patient's response to an ingestion. Acids (not alkalis) are sometimes considered to be anesthetic, perhaps due to eschar formation. An ingestion of phenol, which is used commonly as a topical anesthetic agent, may not feature pain as a clinical symptom. Coingestants such as ethanol used by suicidal patients that may alter their mental status or their ability to express themselves clearly may mask any evidence of pain.

The concept that the absence of clinical signs and symptoms does not add to history has been suggested repeatedly.[11,13,20,43] When considering pediatric cases, absence of clinical findings may contribute even less.[13] It is crucial for the examining physician to be suspicious of an injury when confronted by a well-appearing patient whose history includes caustic ingestion.

PREDICTORS OF INJURY

Several studies have attempted to identify signs or symptoms that could be used to identify patients with a mucosal injury who require treatment and patients without a mucosal injury. The benefits of detecting these patients include being able to bring appropriate management to patients who require it and limiting unnecessary procedures and hospitalizations for patients who do not require them.

When the history includes a potential ingestion of a caustic substance, it is natural to examine the patient's mouth for signs of injury. The information gained by this examination has been reported to be limited.[2,7,24,44] One study found that 37% of patients who did not have burns to their cheeks, lips, or oropharynx had esophageal burns in one or more places as diagnosed by endoscopy, whereas only 50% of patients with burns to their cheeks, lips, or oropharynx were found to have visceral burns.[43] As mentioned earlier, presence or absence of abdominal pain or tenderness is also a poor predictor of gastrointestinal injury. Often less than half of patients with esophageal burns complain of abdominal pain.[27]

Several investigators have evaluated whether combinations of signs and symptoms can be used to predict injury. One study that evaluated 79 pediatric patients found that the presence of two or more of the signs vomiting, drooling, or stridor correlated to a grade 2 injury or worse by endoscopy.[45] Perhaps just as important was that no patient who had only one of these three signs had a positive finding by endoscopy. No patients in this study had only stridor as a sign. The presence of stridor should prompt emergency management of the airway. Another investigator found that all patients with an alkaline-induced injury showed some symptom of injury but that no single sign accurately predicted injury. When data from 63 patients of all ages who received esophagoscopy were examined for signs of oral burns, drooling, vomiting, abdominal pain, and dysphagia, no group of signs or symptoms could identify all patients with serious esophageal injury. The study's author found that a combination of signs had a positive predictive value of only 46%. These data may be limited in that they were gathered via poison center phone calls and because suicidal patients represented 25% of the patients who had esophagoscopy, 50% of whom had positive findings.[27] Still another author was unable to correlate injury to any signs or symptoms in a pediatric population. This study population may have been difficult to assess for dysphagia and abdominal pain or refusal to drink, however, given that 79% were 12 to 35 months old.[40]

Studying patients with caustic ingestions is difficult at best. These patients do not present frequently, requiring many years to gather substantial numbers of patients. Often children and suicidal patients compose the greater proportion of these patients and may be difficult to assess as a whole. The ideal prospective study would include communicative patients with unintentional ingestions, to reduce confounders such as coingestants and hidden agendas, and would find endoscopically a wide range of visceral injuries.

Patients with a history of caustic ingestion may present with signs of severe injury that can include severe abdominal pain or rigidity, stridor, or lactic acidosis. Patients who have obvious signs of intraabdominal injury, have an airway emergency, or have an acidosis that may indicate necrotic tissue must be presumed to have a serious injury until proved otherwise.[27,46] One study found that adults accounted for less than half of all hospital admissions for caustic ingestions but developed 81% of all esophageal injuries requiring treatment.[6] Because many of these injuries result from suicide attempts, all patients who attempted suicide must be presumed to have serious damage until this possibility is disproved by endoscopy. Conversely, asymptomatic patients with unintentional ingestions do not seem to require endoscopy.[27]

TREATMENT

As with other injuries, the initial management strategy for patients with caustic ingestions is to secure the airway, breathing, and hemodynamic stability. All patients require vital sign assessment and a rapid evaluation of the airway, including visualization of burns to the oropharynx, cheeks, and lips and so-called dribble marks. Although the absence of these signs does not exclude injuries elsewhere, their presence more strongly indicates exposure to a caustic agent.

Stridor and respiratory distress are true emergencies, given the nature of the injury. A caustic substance that contacts the respiratory mucosa causes tissue softening, edema, and, in the worst-case scenario, perforation. Direct visualization of the vocal cords may be accomplished by fiberoptic nasopharyngoscopy and can provide crucial information regarding the nature of the airway injury. As with thermal burns to the airway, edema may increase rapidly, making delayed attempts to control the airway progressively more difficult. Any signs of airway compromise or respiratory distress should prompt action to secure the airway.

For patients who require intubation, the intervening physicians should be the most skilled available for the best possible management of complications. Intubation using a fiberoptic instrument or with a laryngoscope in which the vocal cords are visualized directly may be attempted. When possible, paralytic agents should be avoided prior to intubation because edema, softened or partially dissolved tissue, and bleeding may complicate attempts to intubate and ventilate with bag-valve-mask apparatus. A surgical airway may be required depending on injury severity and the physician's ability to secure the airway by other means. A surgical airway should be considered a second choice for airway management, however, because the presence of a tracheostomy may interfere with reconstruction of the esophagus at a later stage.[46]

Along with airway management, large-bore intravenous access should be obtained. Blood analysis sufficient for the patient to go to the operating room should be sent, including hematocrit, electrolytes, coagulation studies, and a blood type and crossmatch. Hypotension should be corrected by infusion of crystalloid or blood as needed. In general, it may be useful to consider these patients similar to patients with thermal burns regarding the potential for significant shifts of fluid and changes in hemodynamic status.

Decontamination

Topical exposure to skin or eyes by a strong caustic agent has the advantage of being relatively easy to detect and treat. Lavage with copious amounts of water or saline is a safe and effective means of diluting the caustic and removing it from the exposed tissue. Specific therapies involving polyethylene glycol and a paste containing calcium salts (calcium chloride or calcium gluconate) have been recommended for exposures to phenol and hydrofluoric acid, respectively. Ocular exposures require rigorous, thorough lavage with water or saline to reduce the risk of injury.

In contrast to many other poisonings, gastrointestinal decontamination in this setting is limited. Use of an orogastric tube or nasogastric tube to remove any caustic material that has pooled in the stomach carries the risk of perforation through the softened mucosa. Activated charcoal does not adsorb caustics and obscures mucosal evaluation by endoscopy. Ipecac-induced emesis has limited use as a decontaminating agent in general. In cases of caustic ingestions, induction of emesis increases the risk of aspiration and reexposure to the caustic and increases intraabdominal pressure and the risk of perforation. At this time, the risks of conventional means of decontamination far outweigh the potential benefits, and these methods are not generally recommended.

Dilution and Neutralization

Investigations into dilution and neutralization of caustics attempted to find other means to limit the damage caused by these agents as opposed to treating the outcome. If the concentration can be decreased or the pH made more physiologic, theoretically damage is less. The potential complications of these types of therapies include the generation of heat and gas with subsequent increased intraluminal pressure. One in vitro experiment added various household items, such as lemon juice or milk, to beakers containing Clinitest tablets or crystalline sodium hydroxide and showed significantly increased temperatures.[47] Clinitest tablets previously were used to test for glycosuria and contained 37% sodium hydroxide.[48–50] Other investigations have diluted acids and alkalis with water, milk, and saline in ex vivo esophagi and shown decreased histologic damage to mucosal cells.[51–53] Yet other studies failed to show an appreciable change in pH when acid or base was diluted with water in vitro.[54] Early studies showed severe injury when ex vivo esophagi were exposed briefly to acids or alkalis, then washed copiously with either water or a dilute neutralizing agent.[9,21]

Neutralization studies have shown similar limited results. One in vitro study showed mucosal protection from acid when treated with sucralfate partly due to acid neutralization.[55] Another study found minimal temperature increases when in vivo esophagi were exposed to alkali and neutralized with orange juice.[38] Still another study showed decreased histologic damage in ex vivo esophagi when alkaline injuries were neutralized with orange juice.[56]

That this research spans 30 years indicates how difficult it is to resolve the question of how to limit damage done to patients by caustics. The existing data show that strong caustics cause tissue injury almost immediately and that dilution and neutralization might limit histologic damage when immediately applied. There are no in vivo studies, however, that show improved outcome.

All patients with caustic injuries are not the same and should not be treated as such. Pediatric patients often have limited injuries, whereas suicidal adults often have severe injuries. Administering a diluent or neutralizing agent to children at low risk may not be necessary, whereas adults at high risk may be unable to benefit. Given the risks of emesis and aspiration, which have not been well studied, and the difficulty with extrapolating the current data to ingestions in humans, more definitive studies are needed before these treatments can be recommended routinely.

Endoscopy

Endoscopy has been called the sine qua non for evaluating patients with caustic ingestions.[57] Endoscopic evaluation has many advantages.[22,31,58] Before the 1950s, the rigid esophoscope was not widely available, and the presence of severe burns could be diagnosed only after dysphagia from stricture occurred.[59] As the use of endoscopy came into the mainstream, it became widely recognized as an important tool for evaluating these patients.[3,7,8,24,30,32,58,60,61] Generally accepted guidelines for endoscopy included not passing the instrument deeper than the first serious injury. This restriction attempted to limit the number of perforations from the procedure, but it also limited the evaluation and increased the risk of underestimating the total injury. The flexible fiberoptic endoscope has a smaller outside diameter and largely has replaced the older, rigid instrument for these evaluations. Recommendations for careful, slow advancement under visual control with minimal insufflation reduce the risk of complications. The endoscope may be guided gently through areas of severe injury (Fig. 99-1), unless frank necrosis or obliteration of the lumen precludes its advancement.[31] Use of the flexible endoscope is described repeatedly as safe and necessary, and many studies report having no complications from the procedure.[31,39,62]

Controversy still exists regarding when endoscopy should proceed for a patient with a history of caustic ingestion. Although most authors are in favor of early endoscopy, the times that are recommended range from less than 6 hours to 48 hours. Older studies tend to refer to later times, which may reflect its limited availability and the relatively greater risk found with rigid esophagoscopy. Bikhazi and colleagues[32] referred to endoscopy as elective, whereas Middelkamp and associates[30,61] changed their recommendation from 24 to 48 hours in 1961 to 12 to 24 hours in 1969. Only Friedman[2] specifically recommended not performing endoscopy before 12 hours because "adequate time may not have passed for the injury to manifest, and therefore the examination may underestimate the damage." Friedman[2] recommended waiting until 24 to 48 hours pass for best results. Since the early 1980s, there has been a

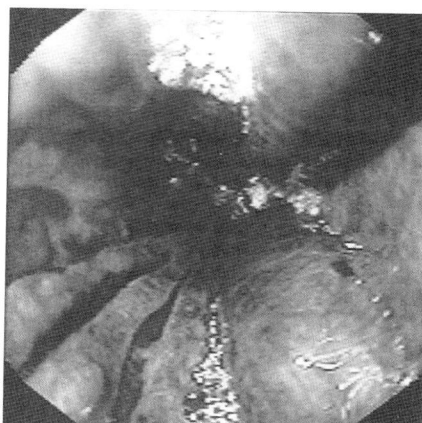

FIGURE 99-1

Endoscopy after a caustic ingestion, which shows severe necrosis in the midesophagus.

growing body of experts who recommend that endoscopy be performed as soon as the patient is stable in order for the procedure to recognize a full-thickness injury as early as possible.[3,15,34,62–65] In vitro studies showed the immediate injury these agents can cause. There is no utility in waiting to make a definitive diagnosis for these patients because to do so invites disaster in a subgroup whose injuries and outcomes are notoriously unpredictable.

Radiologic Investigations

Chest and abdominal radiographs may provide useful information rapidly in the early stages of management. The presence of a widened periesophageal stripe, pneumothorax, pneumomediastinum, pneumoperitoneum, or pleural effusion indicates a perforation in the gastrointestinal tract and may obviate the need for further studies. Although many authors advocate the use of these tests,[5,11,13,15,37,42,46] the sensitivity of radiographs seems to be low. Despite one study that showed lateral chest x-rays to be 98% sensitive compared with 80% for posteroanterior chest x-rays for finding intraperitoneal air,[66] several authors reported no visible free air despite clear perforations found at laparotomy.[42,46]

At one time, contrast swallow studies were used as a standard diagnostic tool for these patients. The generated images could find areas of esophageal dysmotility, whereas extravasation of dye could be used to indicate perforation. Swallow studies have low sensitivities as well and are accompanied by risks for aspiration and inflammation. Water-soluble solutions are even less sensitive and must be anionic to avoid the risk of pulmonary complications if such solutions are aspirated.[11,13,15] In addition, no information is gained regarding the depth of mucosal injury, limiting its utility further.

Computed tomography has never been studied as a diagnostic tool for evaluating patients with caustic injuries. Catton and associates[63] found little use for computed tomography in defining patients' injuries. Anecdotally, these authors found that computed tomography severely underestimated the injuries incurred by a patient who drank sodium hydroxide crystals mixed in water.

Advantages of Endoscopy in Caustic Ingestion

Allows for a definitive diagnosis providing a basis for treatment
Helps limit hospital stay and unnecessary treatment for patients with minimal or no injuries
Defines the degree and character of the injury and directs management
Helps to predict complications
Allows for confirmation of adequate healing

Management Plan Based on Endoscopic Findings

The character and the extent of the injury indicate the management plan and disposition of patients with caustic injuries. Because endoscopy is the best tool to establish the diagnosis, management is delineated in terms of endoscopic grade of injury. Grade 1 injuries do not develop complications of stricture or tumor. When patients tolerate oral feeding, they potentially may be discharged.[31] If endoscopy shows a grade 2A injury, patchy or linear but noncircumferential submucosal damage without stomach injury, oral feeding may be resumed cautiously as tolerated. Alternatively, a feeding tube may be passed with fiberoptic guidance to resume nutritional support. As with patients with thermal burns, patients with caustic injuries enter into a hypercatabolic state and require substantial nutritional support.[10,21] A negative nitrogen balance resulting from injury and poor nutrition inhibits healing and increases the risk of infection.[13] Patients with these injuries rarely develop stricture or other complications. Follow-up endoscopic examinations can document appropriate healing and add to disposition planning.

Patients with grade 2B or worse injuries have similar complication rates and require a longer time to heal.[31,65,66] Zargar and coworkers[31] divide grade 3 injuries into subtypes A and B. Grade 3A denotes small scattered areas of frank necrosis, and grade 3B denotes extensive necrosis.[31] For patients with grade 2B or worse injuries, oral or tube feeding may be contraindicated. Total parenteral nutrition, gastrostomy, and jejunostomy are options that may be used for these patients because nutrition continues to be a crucial factor in their healing. The risk of stricture formation for patients with grade 2B injuries is high, and the use of steroids and antibiotics may be beneficial (see the following discussion on steroids and antibiotics). In general, grade 3 injuries progress to strictures regardless of therapy, and grade 3B injuries have a high risk of infection and perforation as well. These patients require surgical consultation for early resection and should be monitored closely. Various case series in which endoscopy revealed injuries grade 2 or worse reported a mortality rate of 10% to 15%,[6,34,57] and in cases in which endoscopy discovered a grade 3B injury, a mortality rate of 66% was reported.[31]

Use of Steroids

The use of steroids in the treatment of caustic injuries has been a controversial subject since the 1950s. Steroids inhibit the inflammatory response and theoretically prevent strictures from forming. Early animal models showed a decrease in stricture formation but also showed the complications that steroid therapy could invoke. Steroids may mask infection in the patient, including a brain abscess in one report,[67] and may weaken already injured tissue, increasing the risk of perforation.

For 30 years, many authors reported using steroids as a routine part of their treatment regimen.[2,3,7,10,13,19,30,41,58,59,61,68–71] Most of these reports did not differentiate, however, between grades of injury with regard to outcome. Other case series concluded that there is no risk of stricture formation from grade 1 injuries and that grade 3 injuries progress to strictures regardless of therapy. Several reports support the use

of steroids, but only for cases with grade 2 injuries that may form a stricture but for which this outcome is not considered inevitable.[2,3,13,19,31,41,70] One well-known but often misquoted study prospectively investigated the effect of steroids on stricture formation. Sixty children were randomized over 18 years and were evaluated by rigid esophagoscopy only as far as the first serious burn. The conclusion of the study, which differs from what is stated in the abstract, is that the study lacked the statistical power to show a benefit using steroids—a type II error.[67] No other study has prospectively enrolled enough patients in a controlled investigation to answer this question adequately. One meta-analysis of 13 studies, however, found a 20% reduction in the incidence of strictures among patients with grade 2 and grade 3 injuries who received steroids and antibiotics.[28]

Since 1990, there seems to be a trend in the literature not to recommend steroid use.[11,15,65,67,72] Because many agree that the crucial factor in the development of a stricture is the degree of initial injury, a grade 2B injury is perhaps the only injury for which the use of steroids should be considered. If corticosteroids are used, the appropriate dose is 1 to 2 mg/kg/day of prednisolone, or its equivalent in children, for 2 to 3 weeks followed by a taper. Use of corticosteroids must be accompanied by the use of antibiotics because of the increased risk of infection.

Use of Antibiotics

Tissue disruption from caustic injury can increase the risk of infection from enteric organisms. This risk is increased further with corticosteroid use because corticosteroids inhibit the immune response and may mask the clinical appearance of an infected patient. Although there are no outcome studies showing a benefit for their use, antibiotics are recommended routinely with corticosteroid use to decrease the risk of infection. Prophylactic use of antibiotics generally is not recommended in favor of treating an identified source of infection in the absence of corticosteroids.

Use of Antihistamines and Proton-Pump Inhibitors

Antihistamines and proton-pump inhibitors have not been studied specifically for therapeutic use in the context of caustic injury. Gastroenterologists recommend histamine antagonists anecdotally, and occasionally use of histamine antagonists is mentioned in the literature.[73] Experimentally, serine and glycine have exhibited cytoprotective activity against chemically induced gastric lesions in rats.[74,75]

Surgical Intervention

A review of the literature presents a fascinating look at the change in the philosophy of treatment for patients with caustic injuries. In the 1960s, physicians had to wait until an injury declared itself in the form of stricture before beginning treatment. With the increased use of endoscopy, treatment with steroids and antibiotics could begin earlier, but patients with severe injuries still were treated conservatively with a watch-and-wait attitude. Various therapeutic techniques evolved only to prevent stricture formation, whereas the prevention of death was given little consideration. A certain fatalistic attitude pervades the early literature.

The conservative approach to patients with caustic injuries, including observation, hydration, nutrition, and possibly antibiotics and steroids, is appropriate for patients with minor injuries. Likewise, the decision for surgery is clear when the patient shows evidence of a perforation by endoscopy or radiography or has abdominal rigidity or hypotension.

There are many patients, however, who have serious injuries and do not present with obvious signs and symptoms that lead to an urgent operation. Several authors have reported patients who had serious injuries to the stomach, esophagus, and other intraabdominal organs and died without manifesting signs of the impending catastrophe until late in their clinical course.[41,42] These were patients whose injuries *might* have been treated surgically.

Since the late 1980s, more authors have advocated an aggressive surgical approach to patients with caustic injuries to decrease morbidity and mortality. Indications for surgery vary from group to group. One group adopted an approach that included early endoscopy, immediate laparotomy for patients with grade 2 or worse injuries, and immediate esophagogastrectomy for patients with full-thickness necrosis.[41] When using this aggressive approach, this group showed a decrease in the incidence of stricture formation in patients with grade 2 injuries and a much improved survival rate among patients with grade 3 injuries compared with their own hospital's records when a conservative approach was used. They concluded that the risk of missing a full-thickness injury was greater than that of the procedure and that the watch-and-wait attitude was too dangerous.

Other authors have advocated surgery for massive necrosis or an arterial pH less than 7.0.[34,42] Wu and Lai[46] recommended surgery for generalized abdominal pain and tenderness, continuous bleeding in the gastrointestinal tract, pleural effusion, and ascites. Although there is some debate as to whether laparoscopy provides an adequate examination of potentially injured tissues,[63] many surgeons agree that the most important factor contributing to mortality is delay to diagnosis, necessitating an aggressive surgical approach if a transmural necrosis is suspected.[15,42,64] When managing patients with extensive necrosis or patients who may have a full-thickness injury, an urgent surgical consultation should be obtained from senior surgical personnel to provide maximal possible benefit to the patient.

Lathyrogens

Lathyrogens are compounds that inhibit the activity of lysyl oxidase, the enzyme responsible for cross-linking collagen and providing tensile strength.[71] The formation of a more pliant scar can enhance dilation of the stenosis. Experimentally, many studies have attempted to attenuate stricture formation or enhance the manipulation of strictures. β-Aminopropionitrile, a potent lathyrogen, has been studied in dogs and was found to be useful in limiting stricture formation.[76,77] Similarly, penicillamine, which chelates lysine-derived aldehyde groups to prevent collagen cross-linking, was found to limit stricture formation in rats and rabbits.[78,79] Colchicine stimulates collagenase activity but was not found to alter wound fibrous response in rats and delayed healing in rabbits.[79,80] Heparin was found to decrease the incidence of stricture formation in rats, possibly through prevention of submucosal vascular thrombosis.[81] Treatment of rats with interferon gamma and epidermal growth factor also has been shown to decrease the incidence of stricture formation. N-Acetylcysteine also was shown in rats to be beneficial in restricting stricture formation.[82] All of these treatments are considered experimental, and their use currently is not supported for human exposures.

Management of Strictures

The development of a cicatricial contracture is the most important consequence for patients who survive the initial crisis of a caustic ingestion with significant injury. These debilitating complications may begin weeks to months after the initial injury and may be classified according to severity to assist in management (Table 99-2).[83] Grade 1 strictures are incomplete and noncircumferential. Grade 2 strictures are stringlike, annular, or elastic. Grade 3 strictures are dense, short strictures. Grade 4 strictures are longer than 1 cm and are divided into subtype A, which is superficial and nonprogressive, and subtype B, which is deep, tubular, and progressive.

Various procedures are used for the prevention and treatment of strictures. One group has advocated the use of intraluminal stenting for immediate and continued prophylactic bougienage of the esophagus. This group placed a stent in patients with grade 2 and some grade 3 injuries defined at celiotomy. They found that the esophageal mucosa appeared more normal when the stent was removed than other injured tissue that did not receive this treatment.[41] Most other authors recommend dilation therapy to normalize the size of the esophageal lumen. Three to 6 weeks after the initial injury, progressively larger bougies are passed over endoscopically placed guidewires for dilation. Fluoroscopy can provide an additional level of safety when strictures are tortuous. Corrosive-induced strictures are said to be more difficult to dilate than strictures resulting from other causes. The risk of dilation therapy can be high. Perforation, aspiration, and dysphagia may lead to a host of complications ranging from a general decrease in the quality of life to death.

The severity and extent of the stricture, the age of the patient, and the consideration for long-term risk of esophageal carcinoma contribute to the choice of dilation versus esophageal resection or bypass. Esophageal strictures that are resistant to dilation therapy may indicate surgery. Esophageal bypass leaves the injured esophagus in place and may reroute the gastrointestinal tract using the stomach, jejunum, or colon. Advantages to this technique include a potentially less invasive procedure and avoidance of postvagotomy sequelae. Complications, although rare, can include formation of a mucocele or esophageal abscess that may

TABLE 99-2 Stricture Description by Grade	
GRADE	**DESCRIPTION**
1	Incomplete, noncircumferential
2	Stringlike, annular, elastic
3	Dense, short
4A	>1 cm, superficial, nonprogressive
4B	>1 cm, deep, tubular, progressive

rupture into the mediastinum.[84] Resection of the esophagus has the same indications as bypass and may be accomplished by thoracotomy or by blunt dissection. Esophagoplasty is a local, in situ operation on the esophagus designed to widen the esophageal lumen. Different authors advocate these various therapies, and no comparison study has been performed to determine which procedure has a superior outcome.

Gastric stenosis may occur at any site in the stomach but is most common in the antrum. Gastrectomy and partial gastrectomies have been advocated in the past. Successful balloon dilation of gastric stenoses also is reported.[15,84]

SUMMARY

Exposure to caustic substances continues to be a leading toxicologic source of injury for adults and children. Although most childhood exposures are unintentional, often resulting in only minor injury, and adult cases are few and far between, many deaths occur each year in adults and children owing to the widespread availability of these substances and their inherent dangerous nature. Many patients die either in the acute phase from massive perforation and hemodynamic collapse or in the following few days from a wide variety of complications or multisystem organ failure. These deaths and varied forms of morbidity show the complicated nature of the injury and the comprehensive intensive care these patients require.

Today it is not sufficient to think only in terms of limiting potentially dangerous sequelae of these ingestions but to limit as far as possible the damage and complications that may result in the death of the patient, before subsequent complications arise. Despite a lack of controlled data supporting a single management plan, many authors advocate a rapid and complete evaluation of the patient with endoscopy as the most important element. Endoscopy is so useful a tool, it should be thought of in terms of which patients *should not* receive endoscopy instead of patients who should. Pediatric patients who are asymptomatic and patients who are so obviously ill that they should be in the operating room are among patients who perhaps should not undergo endoscopy. Aggressive surgical management may be considered for patients with grade 2 or worse injuries because mortality may be decreased, and endoscopic evaluation cannot evaluate the depth of mucosal injuries completely. Steroids and antibiotics may be helpful in reducing the incidence of steroids for patients with grade 2B injuries but probably are not likely to help other patients. The most skilled staff available must provide all of this treatment because infection, hemodynamic instability, organ failure, fistulae, and late perforations all contribute to patient morbidity and mortality. Caustic injuries can be deadly to patients and a formidable challenge for physicians. Only a suspicious and aggressive physician can provide the best chances for the injured patient.

REFERENCES

1. Simpson JA, Weiner ESC (eds): The Compact Oxford English Dictionary. Oxford, Clarendon Press, 1987.
2. Friedman EM: Caustic ingestions and foreign bodies in the aerodigestive tract of children. Pediatr Clin North Am 36:1403–1410, 1989.
3. Nelson R, Walson P, Kelley M: Caustic ingestion. Ann Emerg Med 12:559–562, 1983.
4. Litovitz TL, Klein-Schwartz W, Caravati EM, et al: 1998 Annual report of the American Association of Poison Control Centers toxic exposure surveillance system. Am J Emerg Med 17:435–487, 1999.
5. Trowers E, Thomas C, Silverstein FE: Chemical- and radiation-induced esophageal injury. Gastrointest Endosc Clin N Am 4:657–675, 1994.
6. Hawkins DB, Demeter MJ, Barnett TE: Caustic ingestion: Controversies in management. Laryngoscope 90:98–109, 1980.
7. Daly JF, Cardona JC: Acute corrosive esophagitis. Arch Otolaryngol 74:629–633, 1961.
8. Kirsh MM, Ritter F: Caustic ingestion and subsequent damage to the oropharyngeal and digestive passages. Ann Thorac Surg 21:74–82, 1976.
9. Leape LL, Ashcraft KW, Scarpelli DG, Holder TM: Hazard to health—liquid lye. N Engl J Med 284:578–581, 1971.
10. Postlethwait RW: Chemical burns of the esophagus. Surg Clin North Am 63:915–924, 1983.
11. Spitz L, Lakhoo K: Caustic ingestion. Arch Dis Child 68:157–158, 1993.
12. Vancura EM, Clinton JE, Ruiz E, Krenzelok EP: Toxicity of alkaline solutions. Ann Emerg Med 9:118–122, 1980.
13. Wasserman RL, Ginsburg CM: Caustic substance injuries. J Pediatr 107:169–174, 1985.
14. Krey H: On the treatment of corrosive lesions in the esophagus, an experimental study. Acta Otolaryngol 102(Suppl):1–49, 1952.
15. Hugh TB, Kelly MD: Corrosive ingestion and the surgeon. J Am Coll Surg 189:508–522, 1999.
16. Moriarty RW: Corrosive chemicals: Acids and alkalis. Drug Ther 6:143–148, 1979.
17. Hoffman RS, Howland MA, Kamerow HN, Goldfrank LR: Comparison of titratable acid/alkaline reserve and pH in potentially caustic household products. J Toxicol Clin Toxicol 27:241–261, 1989.
18. Boldt GB, Carroll RG: Titratable acid/alkaline reserve is not predictive of esophageal perforation risk after caustic exposure (Letter). Am J Emerg Med 14:106–108, 1996.
19. Friedman EM, Lovejoy FH: The emergency management of caustic ingestions. Emerg Med Clin North Am 2:77–86, 1984.
20. Zargar SA, Kochhar R, Nagi B, et al: Ingestion of corrosive acids: Spectrum of injury to upper gastrointestinal tract and natural history. Gastroenterology 97:702–707, 1989.
21. Ashcraft KW, Padula RT: The effect of dilute corrosives on the esophagus. Pediatrics 53:226–232, 1974.
22. Lowe JE, Graham DY, Boisaubin EV, Lanza FL: Corrosive injury to the stomach: The natural history and role of fiberoptic endoscopy. Am J Surg 137:803–806, 1979.
23. Ray JF, Myers WO, Lawton BR, et al: The natural history of liquid lye ingestion. Arch Surg 109:436–439, 1974.
24. Alford RR, Harris HH: Chemical burns of the mouth, pharynx and esophagus. Ann Otol Rhinol Laryngol 68:122–128, 1959.
25. Ritter FN, Newman MH, Newman DE: A clinical and experimental study of corrosive burns of the stomach. Otol Rhinol Laryngol 77:830–842, 1968.
26. Lovejoy FH: Corrosive injury of the esophagus in children: Failure of corticosteroid treatment reemphasizes prevention. N Engl J Med 323:668–669, 1990.
27. Gorman RL, Khin-Maung-Gyi MT, Klein-Schwartz W, et al: Initial symptoms as predictors of esophageal injury in alkaline corrosive ingestions. Am J Emerg Med;10:189–194, 1992.
28. Howell JM, Dalsey WC, Hartsell FW, Butzin CA: Steroids for the treatment of corrosive esophageal injury. Am J Emerg Med 10:421–425, 1992.
29. Kirsh MM, Peterson A, Brown JW, et al: Treatment of caustic injuries of the esophagus: A ten year experience. Ann Surg 188:675–678, 1978.
30. Middelkamp JN, Ferguson TB, Roper CL, Hoffman FD: The management and problems of caustic burns in children. J Thorac Cardiovasc Surg 1969;57:341–347, 1969.
31. Zargar SA, Kochhar R, Mehta S, Mehta SK: The role of fiberoptic endoscopy in the management of corrosive ingestion and modified endoscopic classification of burns. Gastrointest Endosc 37:165–169, 1991.
32. Bikhazi HB, Thompson ER, Shumrick DA: Caustic ingestion: Current status. Arch Otolaryngol 89:112–115, 1969.
33. Dantas RO, Mamede RC: Esophageal motility in patients with esophageal caustic injury. Am J Gastroenterol 91:1157–1161,1996.

34. Sarfati E, Gossot D, Assens P, Celerier M: Management of caustic ingestion in adults. Br J Surg 74:146–148, 1987.
35. Appelqvist P, Salmo M: Lye corrosion carcinoma of the esophagus. Cancer 45:2655–2658, 1980.
36. Kiviranta UK: Corrosion carcinoma of the esophagus: 381 cases of corrosion and nine cases of corrosion carcinoma. Acta Otolaryngol 42:89–95, 1952.
37. Gago O, Ritter FN, Martel W, et al: Aggressive surgical treatment for caustic injury of the esophagus and stomach. Ann Thorac Surg 13:243–250, 1972.
38. Homan CS, Singer AJ, Henry MC, Thode HC: Thermal effects of neutralization therapy and water dilution for acute alkali exposure in canines. Acad Emerg Med 4:27–32, 1997.
39. Cello JP, Fogel RP, Boland R: Liquid caustic ingestion. Arch Intern Med 140:501–504, 1980.
40. Gaudreault P, Parent M, McGuigan MA, et al: Predictability of esophageal injury from signs and symptoms: A study of caustic ingestion in 378 children. Pediatrics 71:767–770, 1983.
41. Estrera A, Taylor W, Mills LJ, Platt MR: Corrosive burns of the esophagus and stomach: A recommendation for an aggressive surgical approach. Ann Thorac Surg 41:276–283, 1986.
42. Horváth ÖP, Oláh T, Zentai G: Emergency esophagogastrectomy for treatment of hydrochloric acid injury. Ann Thorac Surg 52:98–101, 1991.
43. Previtera C, Giusti F, Guglielmi M: Predictive value of visible lesions in suspected caustic ingestion: May endoscopy reasonably be omitted in completely negative pediatric patients? Pediatr Emerg Care 6:176–178, 1990.
44. Borja AR, Ransdell HT, Thomas TV, Johnson W: Lye injuries of the esophagus. J Thorac Cardiovasc Surg 57:533–538, 1969.
45. Crain EF, Gershel JC, Mezey AP: Caustic ingestions: Symptoms as predictors of esophageal injury. Am J Dis Child 138:863–865, 1984.
46. Wu M, Lai W: Surgical management of extensive corrosive injuries of the alimentary tract. Surg Gynecol Obstet 177:12–16, 1993.
47. Rumack BH, Burrington JD: Caustic ingestions: A rational look at diluents. J Toxicol Clin Toxicol 11:27–34, 1977.
48. Burrington JD: Clinitest burns of the esophagus. Ann Thorac Surg 20:400–404, 1975.
49. Payten RJ: Clinitest tablet stricture of the esophagus. BMJ 23:728–729, 1972.
50. Warren JB, Griffin DJ, Olson RC: Urine sugar reagent tablet ingestion causing gastric and duodenal ulceration. Arch Intern Med 144:161–162, 1984.
51. Homan CS, Maitra SR, Lane BP, Geller ER: Effective treatment of acute alkali injury of the rat esophagus with early saline dilution therapy. Ann Emerg Med 22:178–182, 1993.
52. Homan CS, Maitra SR, Lane BP, et al: Histopathologic evaluation of the therapeutic efficacy of water and milk dilution for esophageal acid injury. Acad Emerg Med 2:587–591, 1995.
53. Homan CS, Maitra SR, Lane BP, et al: Therapeutic effects of water and milk for acute alkali injury of the esophagus. Ann Emerg Med 24:14–20, 1994.
54. Maull KI, Osmand AP, Maull CD: Liquid caustic ingestions: An in vitro study of the effects of buffer, neutralization, and dilution. Ann Emerg Med 14:1160–1162, 1985.
55. Orlando RC, Turjman NA, Tobey NA, et al: Mucosal protection by sucralfate and its components in acid-exposed rabbit esophagus. Gastroenterology 93:352–361, 1987.
56. Homan CS, Maitra SR, Lane BP, et al: Effective treatment for acute alkali injury to the esophagus using weak-acid neutralization therapy: An ex-vivo study. Acad Emerg Med 2:952–958, 1995.
57. Thompson JN: Corrosive esophageal injuries: I. A study of nine cases of concurrent accidental caustic ingestion. Laryngoscope 97:1060–1066, 1987.
58. Viscomi GJ, Beekhuis GJ, Whitten CF: An evaluation of early esophagoscopy and corticosteroid therapy in the management of corrosive injury of the esophagus. J Pediatr 59:356–360, 1961.
59. Aceto T, Terplan K, Fiore RR, Munschauer RW: Chemical burns of the esophagus in children and glucocorticoid therapy. J Med 1:101–109, 1970.
60. Haller JA, Andrews HG, White JJ, et al: Pathophysiology and management of acute corrosive burns of the esophagus: Results of treatment in 285 children. J Pediatr Surg 6:578–584, 1971.
61. Middelkamp JN, Cone AJ, Ogura JH, et al: Endoscopic diagnosis and steroid and antibiotic therapy of acute lye burns of the esophagus. Laryngoscope 71:1354–1362, 1961.
62. Sugawa C, Mullins RJ, Lucas CE, Leibold WC: The value of early endoscopy following caustic ingestion. Surg Gynecol Obstet 153:553–556, 1981.
63. Cattan P, Munoz-Bongrand N, Berney T, et al: Extensive abdominal surgery after caustic ingestion. Ann Surg 231:519–523, 2000.
64. Meredith JW, Kon ND, Thompson JN: Management of injuries from liquid lye ingestion. J Trauma 28:1173–1180, 1988.
65. Sugawa C, Lucas CE: Caustic injury of the upper gastrointestinal tract in adults: A clinical and endoscopic study. Surgery 106:802–807, 1989.
66. Woodring JH, Heiser MJ: Detection of pneumoperitoneum on chest radiographs: Comparison of upright lateral and posteroanterior projections. Am J Radiol 165:45–47, 1995.
67. Anderson KD, Rouse TM, Randolph JG: A controlled trial of corticosteroids in children with corrosive injury of the esophagus. N Engl J Med 323:637–640, 1990.
68. Haller JA, Bachman K: The comparative effect of current therapy on experimental caustic burns of the esophagus. Pediatrics 34:236–245, 1964.
69. Tewfik TL, Schloss MD: Ingestion of lye and other corrosive agents—a study of 86 infant and child cases. J Otolaryngol 9:72–77, 1980.
70. Webb WR, Koutras P, Ecker RR, Sugg WL: An evaluation of steroids and antibiotics in caustic burns of the esophagus. Ann Thorac Surg 9:95–101, 1970.
71. Yakshe PN, Benjamin SB: An overview of caustic ingestion. Contemp Gastroenterol 2:50–58, 1989.
72. Ulman I, Mutaf O: A critique of systemic steroids in the management of caustic esophageal burns in children. Eur J Pediatr Surg 8:71–74, 1998.
73. Rappert P, Preier L, Korab W, Neurbauer T: Diagnostic and therapeutic management of esophageal and gastric caustic burns in childhood. Eur J Pediatr Surg 3:202–205, 1993.
74. Tariq M, Al Moutaery AR: Gastric anti-ulcer and cytoprotective effect of 1-serine in rats. Res Commun Mol Pathol Pharmacol 97:171–184, 1997.
75. Tariq M, Al Moutaery AR: Studies on the antisecretory, gastric anti-ulcer and cytoprotective properties of glycine. Res Commun Mol Pathol Pharmacol 97:185–198, 1997.
76. Butler C, Madden JW, Davis WM, Peacock EE: Morphologic aspects of experimental esophageal lye strictures: II. Effect of steroid hormones, bougienage, and induced lathyrism on acute lye burns. Surgery 4:431–435, 1977.
77. Madden J, Davis WM, Butler C, Peacock EE: Experimental esophageal lye burns. Ann Surg 178:277–284, 1973.
78. Gehanno P, Guedon C: Inhibition of experimental esophageal lye strictures by penicillamine. Arch Otolaryngol 107:145–147, 1981.
79. Thompson JN: Corrosive esophageal injuries: II. An investigation of treatment methods and histochemical analysis of esophageal strictures in a new animal model. Laryngoscope 97:1191–1202, 1987.
80. Wang RY, Abrams T, Monfils P, et al: The effects of colchicine treatment on wound healing in a caustic murine injury model. J Toxicol Clin Toxicol 37:845–853, 1999.
81. Bingöl-Kologlu M, Tanyel FC, Müftüoglu S, et al: The preventative effect of heparin on stricture formation after caustic esophageal burns. J Pediatr Surg 34:291–294, 1999.
82. Liu A, Richardson M, Robertson WO: Effects of n-acetylcysteine on experimentally induced esophageal lye injury. Ann Otol Rhinol Laryngol 94:477–482, 1985.
83. Marchand P: Caustic strictures of the esophagus. Thorax 10:171–181, 1955.
84. Gossot D, Sarfati E, Celerier M: Early blunt esophagectomy in severe caustic burns of the upper digestive tract. J Thorac Cardiovasc Surg 94:188–191, 1987.

CHAPTER 100

Hydrofluoric Acid

Kennon Heard

Hydrofluoric acid (HFA) is an inorganic acid used in a wide variety of industrial and household processes. It commonly is known for its ability to etch glass and silicone. This ability has led to widespread applications in the semiconductor industry. HFA may be used as a cleaning agent in low-concentration products commonly used as household rust removers. Ammonium bifluoride has been used as a wheel-cleaning agent. It was removed from the U.S. market after several instances of life-threatening toxicity.

CHEMISTRY AND PHARMACOKINETICS

HFA is a relatively weak acid with a pK_a of 3.8. Although concentrations greater than 50% have corrosive properties, the main toxicity of HFA is related to the fluoride ion. HFA exhibits substantial dissociation at physiologic pH; the un-ionized HFA molecule can penetrate lipid tissue more easily than stronger acids.[1] Fluoride is the most electronegative of all ions and binds strongly to cations such as magnesium and calcium.

Pharmacokinetics of Hydrofluoric Acid

Volume of distribution: 0.5–0.7 L/kg
Protein binding: none
Mechanism of clearance: renal
Active metabolites: none
Methods to enhance clearance: alkalinization of urine[8] or hemodialysis[38]

Data from Baselt RC, Cravey RH: Disposition of Toxic Drugs and Chemicals in Man. Foster City, CA, Chemical Toxicology Institute, 1995, pp 327–330.

PATHOPHYSIOLOGY

Burns

Classically, HFA burns have been classified based on the concentration of the acid. Concentrations greater than 50% cause immediate pain and tissue destruction; concentrations between 20% and 50% may cause burns that are evident within several hours. Burns caused by concentrations less than 20% may not be evident for 24 hours.[2] Patients may complain of pain in the absence of visible effects. High-concentration (75%) burns start as classic corrosive injuries. Because HFA is less ionized than stronger acids,

however, it has the capacity to penetrate deeply into tissue. Damage is not limited to superficial levels by tissue coagulation, as is seen with injury from other acids. In further contrast to other acids, the damage to deep tissue is a liquefactive necrosis.[3] Affected bone may develop decalcification.[3] This injury continues as the HFA dissociates in the deep tissue.

Hypocalcemia

Severe HFA poisoning may cause profound hypocalcemia.[4] Hypocalcemia has been shown consistently in animal models of fluoride toxicity and in reports of human poisoning.[5-8] The classically accepted mechanism for HFA-induced hypocalcemia is the formation of insoluble calcium fluoride (CaF_2) salts. In vitro studies have failed to show, however, the formation of CaF_2 in solutions containing free fluoride and calcium concentrations in the range reported in fluoride poisoning deaths.[9] Other investigators have proposed that the hypocalcemia observed in overdose is from the formation of fluoroapatite, $3(Ca_3(PO_4)_2)Ca(F)_2$.[10] Fluoroapatite is formed in vitro when fluoride is added to a solution of calcium, phosphate, and hydroxyapatite. It is proposed that this is similar to what occurs in vitvo because hydroxyapatite is present in bone and certain connective tissues. In an animal model, serum calcium was shown to decrease in a 5:1 ratio with the amount of fluoride administered. This ratio is consistent with the formation of fluoroapatite rather than the 2:1 ratio that would be expected if CaF_2 is formed.[10] Regardless of the mechanism, severe hypocalcemia should be anticipated after significant HFA exposure.

Enzyme Inhibition

Fluoride is a potent inhibitor of several enzyme systems, including enzymes involved in oxidative metabolism. Adenylate cyclase is activated by fluorides.[11] Aluminum fluoride has been identified as a molecule that complexes with the enzymes responsible for deactivation of G proteins.[11] Because trace amounts of aluminum are universally present in living systems, it is likely that aluminum fluoride forms when fluoride poisoning occurs. The relative contribution of enzyme toxicity to human fluoride poisoning is unknown.

Other

Other clinical manifestations of fluoride poisoning include hyperkalemia and metabolic acidosis.[5,12]

CLINICAL PRESENTATION AND LIFE-THREATENING COMPLICATIONS

Dermal Injury

Dermal injury ranging from full-thickness burns to pain without visible injury can occur with HFA exposure.[13] Burns from high-concentration exposures (>50%) are due to the caustic effects and initially are similar to other acid burns. Because HFA tissue penetration is not limited by coagulative necrosis, there may be ongoing deeper tissue injury even after initial decontamination. Burns caused by low-concentration HFA (20% to 50%) may not have signs or symptoms for several hours but can progress to full-thickness burns. In a study of 237 patients exposed to HFA concentrations ranging from 6% to 11%, the time to onset of symptoms ranged from less than 30 minutes in 23% to more than 24 hours in 5% of patients. Slightly more than 50% of the patients had redness and swelling, 5% developed blisters, and 23% had only pain.[13]

Pulmonary Injury

Hemorrhagic pneumonitis, respiratory failure, and adult respiratory distress syndrome have been reported after inhalation of HFA. These effects are likely due to caustic pulmonary injury.[14–16] Systemic poisoning is a concern after inhalation of hydrogen fluoride. One reported death was associated with high blood fluoride levels.[17] Inhalation also was implicated after an exposure to aluminum bifluoride in a patient who developed systemic toxicity. The authors were not able to exclude ingestion of the product, however.[6]

Gastrointestinal Injury

Although HFA is a relatively weak acid, ingestion may cause caustic gastrointestinal injury. In a volunteer study of sodium fluoride ingestion, gastric mucosal erosions were noted in 70% of patients receiving therapeutic doses for 7 days.[18] Clinical reports suggest, however, that significant caustic gastrointestinal injury is not universal. Accidental ingestion of small amounts of low-concentration products caused gastrointestinal symptoms of abdominal pain, vomiting, and gagging in only 20% of patients.[19] A series of dental fluoride product ingestions also reported a benign course consisting of primarily gastrointestinal upset.[20] Life-threatening fluoride intoxication and death have been reported after HFA ingestion without significant gastrointestinal caustic injury.[4,5,21] Other investigators reported hemorrhagic gastritis but also noted no cases of perforation.[22,23] Although caustic injury can occur, it is not universal, and most importantly the absence of symptoms suggesting caustic injury cannot be used to exclude life-threatening ingestion. Severe rectal injury and perforation has been reported after rectal administration of HFA.[24,25]

Ocular Injury

Ocular HFA exposure results in a more severe burn than hydrochloric acid at a similar pH.[26] Corneal erosions, opacification, and anterior chamber reaction commonly are seen; however, most patients reported have recovered.[27–29] One case of delayed injury that developed 4 days after exposure has been reported. This patient also recovered.[30] A thorough examination of the eyes must be done in facial splash injuries.

Cardiovascular Toxicity

The most severe effects of acute fluoride toxicity are on the cardiovascular system. The major manifestations of fluoride toxicity on the cardiovascular system are QT prolongation, ventricular dysrhythmias, hypotension, and ventricular fibrillation.[12] The mechanism of this toxicity is likely multifactorial, involving hypocalcemia, hypomagnesemia, enzyme inhibition, acidosis, and hyperkalemia. Most authors consider hypocalcemia the major precipitant of cardiovascular toxicity.[5–7]

Although most authors consider hypocalcemia the underlying cause of cardiovascular toxicity after fluoride poisoning, one animal model showed that an increase in serum potassium occurs after serum calcium decreases.[31] The authors noted that cardiac arrest was related temporally to the increase in serum potassium and was not associated with the decrease in serum calcium. Fluoride is known to poison the sodium-potassium exchange pump.[32] The authors suggested that this poisoning leads to increased functioning of the sodium-calcium exchange pump and resultant intracellular hypercalcemia.[33] Ventricular irritability and dysrhythmias result. This intriguing work suggests that the exact mechanism of fluoride cardiovascular toxicity still is unknown.

DIAGNOSIS

Dermal HFA exposure should be considered in patients who present with severe pain and minimal or no dermal findings after exposure to products known to contain HFA. Patients with dermal exposures that involve more than 5% body surface area or more than 1% body surface area exposure to 50% HFA products are at risk for hypocalcemia and should be placed on cardiac monitors and have serum calcium and magnesium measurements obtained on arrival at the hospital.[34] The QT interval should be monitored. QT prolongation should be presumed to be due to hypocalcemia.

TREATMENT

Indications for ICU Admission in Hydrofluoric Acid Poisoning

Patients with dermal burns who require intraarterial infusion of calcium

Patients who develop hypocalcemia after ingestion, inhalation, or dermal exposure

Patients with symptoms of airway irritation or obstruction

Patients with a significant proportion of body surface area affected

Patients who have ingested concentrated (>50%) hydrofluoric acid

Specific Airway and Ventilatory Considerations

Patients with symptoms suggesting upper airway obstruction after inhalation or ingestion of HFA should be intubated. Patients with evidence of caustic injury to the oral pharynx or upper airway may require fiberoptic assistance or surgical airway management. Respiratory failure may occur in cases with systemic fluoride poisoning from ingestion, inhalation, and dermal exposure. Respiratory status should be monitored closely in all patients with significant exposure.

Decontamination

DERMAL

Studies of tissue cultures have shown that reduction of the fluoride concentration by dilution alone may restore tissue viability.[35] In a study of 494 cases of HFA exposures, treatment with only irrigation with cold water for 20 minutes resulted in no patients' developing deep tissue necrosis. Many of these burns were caused by HFA concentrations greater than 40%.[36] When these results are coupled with the ease and safety of irrigation, it is clear that immediate irrigation should be considered standard therapy for HFA exposures.

Hexafluorine, which has an affinity for fluoride more than 100 times greater than does calcium gluconate, has been advocated for decontamination of HFA exposures. A series of 11 patients treated with hexafluorine exposures to high-concentration HFA solutions has been published. All patients did well. Although these results are promising, the lack of adequate controls in this study prevents definitive conclusions regarding the superiority of hexafluorine over standard decontamination.[37] The clinical pharmacology of hexafluorine is discussed in Chapter 160.

ENTERAL

No prospective human trials of therapy for ingestion of fluoride poisoning have been reported. Because of the potentially caustic nature of HFA injury, gastric aspiration or lavage should be avoided. Charcoal is unlikely to be useful and is not recommended. Although experimental studies are not available, calcium or magnesium solutions (e.g., milk or antacids) administered early may convert fluoride to insoluble salts and prevent systemic absorption.[12] These solutions should be given only to patients who have no evidence of caustic injury.

INHALATION

Patients who are exposed to HFA vapors should be removed from the exposure, transported to fresh air, and administered oxygen.

OCULAR

Patients with ocular exposure to HFA should have immediate irrigation with at least 1 L of water or saline. Irrigation with other fluids is of no proven benefit, and animal studies suggest that irrigation with calcium salts may increase injury.[26]

EXTRACORPOREAL REMOVAL TECHNIQUES

Hemodialysis was used to treat one patient who developed hypocalcemia, mild hypotension, and prolongation of the QT interval. The authors reported an excellent response and fluoride clearance of 100 mL/min at a blood flow of 105 mL/min and a clearance of 188 mL/min at a blood flow of 200 mL/min. The authors used nonfluoridated water in the diasylate.[38] Although dialysis increases the clearance of fluoride, it is unlikely that severely poisoned patients would tolerate dialysis.

Antidotes

DERMAL

Classic therapies for HFA burns include magnesium oxide, ice water irrigation, and ammonium salts. Animal studies have shown, however, that calcium provides superior neutralization of fluoride ions.[39,40] Human case series also suggest that calcium provides outcomes superior to those of other therapies.[41] I recommend a stepwise approach using progressively more invasive therapies to treat dermal injuries caused by low-concentration (≤50%) HFA exposures. After irrigation, patients should be treated with topical 2.3% to 2.5% calcium gluconate gel.[13,42] The gel is formulated by the addition of 10 mL of 10% calcium gluconate solution to 30 mL of water-soluble lubricant and applied liberally to the affected areas. The gel is allowed to remain in place for 15 minutes after resolution of the pain and for a minimum of 30 minutes.[43] The gel is reapplied immediately if symptoms recur. The treatment is continued every 4 to 6 hours for the next several days.[42] Burns involving the hands may be treated by placing the gel in tight-fitting latex gloves. Successful use of this treatment has been documented in several case series.[13,44] Calcium carbonate gel also has been used successfully for treatment of low-concentration exposures.[45] Topical therapy usually is sufficient for exposure to HFA concentrations of less than 20%. The role of topical treatment for more severe exposures is not as well defined, but it was used in a patient who was completely immersed in HFA and survived.[46] Given the low toxicity of topical calcium gel, I recommend its use as an adjunct therapy to systemic calcium administration for higher concentration exposures.

Injection of HFA skin burns with calcium to bind the fluoride ion has been recommended for more than 60 years.[47] Current recommendation is injection of 0.3 to 0.5 mL/cm^2 of 10% calcium gluconate with a 27G to 30G needle.[41,43] Local calcium injection is most useful in cases in which topical therapy is not effective in providing symptomatic relief and regional perfusion therapy is not possible (i.e., head, face, trunk, perineum).[41] Because the volume that can be injected into the digits is limited to 0.3 to 0.5 mL/cm^2, this therapy is considered by many to be of limited utility if the digits are involved. If the fingers or toes are involved and do not improve with topical therapy, it is reasonable to move directly to regional perfusion techniques. Calcium chloride should not be used because it may cause local tissue necrosis.[41]

Regional intravenous perfusion using Bier's technique has been advocated as an alternative to intraarterial therapy for burns to the extremities. This treatment is well described for the upper extremity and has been used for the lower extremity.[48] The technique involves placement of an intravenous catheter (preferably a small-gauge butterfly needle) in the affected extremity. The extremity is exsanguinated using an elevation or an Esmarch bandage, and a tourniquet is inflated to 100 mm Hg above the systolic blood pressure. After inflation, calcium gluconate diluted in normal saline is infused. The dosing of calcium gluconate has ranged from 25 mL of a 2% solution to 15 mL of a 10% solution.[48,49] The largest published case series used 10 mL of a 10% solution diluted with 30 to 40 mL of normal saline.[50] No author noted symptoms suggesting hypercalcemia with any dose.[50] The tourniquet is deflated gradually over 5 minutes after 15 to 25 minutes. Relief is usually prompt, and failure to alleviate symptoms with one treatment may be an indication for intraarterial therapy,[50] although other investigators advocate repeating the Bier technique.[48] Patients often require parenteral analgesia to tolerate the tourniquet. Addition of local anesthetics to provide analgesia has been suggested[49] but is not widely accepted. Although it provides immediate relief of symptoms, the loss of pain sensation removes the best marker of tissue toxicity.

Patients with persistent pain in an extremity after regional intravenous infusion should be treated with intraarterial calcium infusion. Patients usually report prompt relief of pain, and tissue loss usually is avoided.[51] For burns involving the foot or leg, the femoral artery is cannulated with a 5F arterial catheter. The brachial artery is cannulated for hand burns involving more than the thumb and index finger, whereas burns involving only these fingers may be treated by infusion through a 20G catheter in the radial artery. To assist the infusion, the catheter is directed distally rather than proximally. Although some authors advocate an arteriogram to verify that the vessel is patent and supplies the affected area,[52] monitoring that the catheter is generating an appropriate waveform every hour seems to be sufficient. Several infusion protocols have been reported. The largest series used 10 mL of 10% calcium gluconate diluted with 40 mL of normal saline and infused over 4 hours.[51] The addition of 500 U of heparin to the infusion mixture may decrease the incidence of clotting. After the infusion, the line is flushed with an additional 10 mL of saline over 15 minutes, then flushed hourly with heparinized saline. If tenderness or pain is present after 4 hours of observation, the infusion is repeated. Using this protocol, the average number of infusions was 4.1, and no patient had significant tissue loss. Several patients required systemic magnesium replacement, and the authors recommended checking serum magnesium levels 1 hour after the completion of the infusion.[51] Other protocols have been reported.[52–54]

Adjunctive therapies for HFA burns involving the hands or feet have included fasciotomy to facilitate the injection of larger volumes of calcium gluconate into the digits and removal of the nails when there is substantial subungual involvement.[3,43] Use of the stepwise approach should allow treatment of digital injuries without resorting to either of these steps.

PULMONARY

Currently, no therapies other than standard supportive care can be recommended for pulmonary irritant exposure. Although some authors have advocated early steroid administration, this is not supported by any controlled data, and there is a theoretical potential to increase the risk of infection.[42] Thirteen patients were treated with 4 mL of nebulized 2.5% calcium gluconate.[55] No patient developed significant pulmonary toxicity or seemed to have any adverse effects. Although these results are uncontrolled and the exposure

does not appear severe, calcium gluconate may be a reasonable intervention because there seems to be minimal toxicity.

SYSTEMIC

Few experimental data are available regarding the specific treatment of systemic toxicity from HFA. Most studies instead have looked at sodium fluoride. Animal studies have resulted in variable results regarding the administration of calcium for the treatment of acute fluoride toxicity. Strubelt and colleagues[56] reported no effect of calcium administration in a rat model that used a continuous intravenous infusion of sodium fluoride. Although the results were not statistically significant, it is possible that a larger study may have achieved significance. Simultaneous administration of calcium chloride in a 1:1 molar ratio of calcium to fluoride resulted in improved survival in a mouse model of fluoride toxicity. There was no change in survival when animals were treated with magnesium sulfate.[57]

As noted earlier in the section on clinical presentation, cardiac arrest in fluoride-poisoned dogs was related temporally more closely to an increase in serum potassium than to a decrease in serum calcium. Calcium chloride, epinephrine, glucose/insulin, and lidocaine did not improve survival, whereas simultaneous administration of quinidine with calcium did. The authors hypothesized that quinidine prevents potassium efflux from fluoride-poisoned cells via calcium-mediated potassium channels and prevents fluoride toxicity. They also suggested that administration of calcium as treatment of hyperkalemia may elevate intracellular calcium levels and increase fluoride toxicity.[33] The clinical utility of quinidine in the treatment of human poisoning has not been evaluated. Because of the possibility of further prolongation of the already lengthened QT interval by quinidine, its use cannot be recommended routinely.

Infusion of isotonic sodium bicarbonate in doses to maintain arterial pH in the 7.45 to 7.50 range has been shown to improve survival in a rat model of systemic fluoride poisoning.[58] Acetazolamide administration further increased survival time and total fluoride dose. The terminal ratio of fluoride in cardiac tissue to serum was lower in treated animals. The authors hypothesized that alkalosis changes the distribution of fluoride and increases renal fluoride clearance.[58]

Human cases documenting survival of cardiac arrest after severe fluoride toxicity are rare. The administration of large doses of calcium has been associated with survival in several cases, however.[6,7] In one report, a patient presented twice after ingesting an HFA-containing rust removal agent.[59] After the initial presentation, she developed hypocalcemia and subsequently had a cardiac arrest. She was treated with a total of 111.6 mEq of calcium and 16 mEq of magnesium during her resuscitation and recovered. After discharge from a psychiatric facility, the patient presented again after ingesting what was reported to be the same amount of the same rust removal agent. This time she was treated with prophylactic calcium and magnesium (a total of 65.1 mEq calcium and 32 mEq of magnesium). She recovered uneventfully. Although only suggestive, this case suggests that early administration of calcium may prevent or attenuate the severe cardiac effects that occur after large HFA exposures.

Excision has been advocated after survival of one patient who went into cardiac arrest five times while receiving vigorous calcium replacement, then stabilized after excision of the burn site.[60] Although this case is interesting, it is not clear that the tissue excision contributed to the patient's survival. Because of the potential to cause serious injury during the excision, this treatment should be considered only for the most critically ill patients who are not responding to aggressive calcium repletion.

No treatment for systemic fluoride poisoning has been shown to improve survival in systematic human studies. In my opinion, aggressive decontamination and care of dermal exposures, supportive care with an emphasis on airway management, and early administration of large doses of intravenous calcium should be considered standard of care. McIvor and colleagues[12,33] suggested that late administration of calcium may be deleterious but still recommended early administration of calcium. Administration of an isotonic sodium bicarbonate infusion to maintain a mild systemic alkalosis (pH 7.45 to 7.50) may decrease cardiac fluoride concentrations, may increase fluoride clearance, and is of low toxicity. Moderate or severe systemic alkalosis (pH >7.50) may cause ionized calcium concentrations to fall, however, worsening systemic hypocalcemia.

SPECIAL POPULATIONS

Pediatric Patients

Pediatric patients are presumed to be at increased risk of toxicity from dermal exposure because they have high surface area–to–volume ratios such that a given percent body surface area exposure results in higher total body exposure.

Pregnant and Elderly Patients

There are no available data on the treatment of pregnant or elderly patients exposed to HFA. Standard therapy is recommended.

Common Errors in Hydrofluoric Acid Poisoning

Failure to appreciate that systemic toxicity can occur after dermal exposure

Failure to appreciate that systemic toxicity can occur after ingestion even in the absence of oral or gastrointestinal symptoms

Key Points in Hydrofluoric Acid Poisoning

1. Irrigate affected area immediately with water.
2. Dermal exposures should be treated initially with topical calcium; patients who have persistent pain should receive local injection or regional perfusion with calcium.
3. Systemic poisoning may occur after ingestion, inhalation, or dermal exposure and may result in rapid cardiovascular collapse.
4. Systemic poisoning should be treated with large doses of intravenous calcium.

REFERENCES

1. Gutnecht J, Walter A: Hydrofluoric and nitric acid transport through lipid bilayer membranes. Biochim Biophys Acta 644:153–156, 1981.
2. Division of Industrial Hygiene, NIOH: Hydrofluoric acid burns. Ind Med 12:634, 1943.
3. Dibbell DG, Iverson RE, Jones W, et al: Hydrofluoric acid burns of the hand. J Bone Joint Surg Am 52:931–936, 1970.
4. Rabinowitch IM: Acute fluoride poisoning. Can Med Assoc J 52:345–349, 1945.
5. Chan KM, Svancarek WP, Creer M: Fatality due to acute hydrofluoric acid exposure. J Toxicol Clin Toxicol 25:333–339, 1987.
6. Klasner AE, Scalzo AJ, Blume C, Johnson P: Ammonium bifluoride causes another pediatric death [Letter]. Ann Emerg Med 31:525, 1998.
7. Greco RJ, Hartford CE, Haith LR, Patton ML: Hydrofluoric acid induced hypocalcemia. J Trauma 28:1593–1596, 1988.
8. Leone NC, Geever EF, Moran NC: Acute and subacute toxicity studies of sodium fluoride in animals. Public Health Rep 71:459, 1956.
9. Mohan MS, Bates RG: Calibration of ion selective electrodes for use in biological fluids. Clin Chem 21:864–872, 1975.
10. Boink ABTJ, Werner J, Meulenbelt J, et al: The mechanism of fluoride induced hypocalcemia. Hum Exp Toxicol 13:149–155, 1994.
11. Wittinghofer A: Signaling mechanistics: Aluminum fluoride for molecule of the year. Curr Biol 7:R682–685, 1997.
12. McIvor ME: Acute fluoride toxicity: Pathophysiology and management. Drug Saf 5:79–85, 1990.
13. El Saadi MS, Hall AH, Hall PK, et al: Hydrofluoric acid dermal exposure. Vet Hum Toxicol 31:243–247, 1989.
14. Bennion JR, Franzblau A: Chemical pneumonitis following household exposure to hydrofluoric acid. Am J Ind Med 31:474–478, 1997.
15. Braun J, Stoss H, Zober A: Intoxication following inhalation of hydrogen fluoride. Arch Toxicol 56:50–54, 1984.
16. Tamura N, Shinohara N, Yamada M, et al: A case of acute respiratory failure due to nitrous fumes and hydrogen fluoride. Nihon Kyobu Shikkan Gakkai Zasshi 23:720–725, 1985.
17. Watson AA, Oliver JS, Thorpe JW: Accidental death due to inhalation of hydrofluoric acid. Med Sci Law 13:277–279, 1973.
18. Muller P, Schmid K, Warnecke G, et al: Sodium fluoride-induced gastric mucosal lesions: Comparison with sodium monofluorophosphate. Z Gastroenterol 30:252–254, 1992.
19. Kao WF, Dart RC, Kuffner E, Bogdan G: Ingestion of low-concentration hydrofluoric acid: An insidious and potentially fatal poisoning. Ann Emerg Med 34:35–41, 1999.
20. Augenstein WL, Spoerke DG, Kulig KW, et al: Fluoride ingestion in children: A review of 87 cases. Pediatr 88:907–912, 1991.
21. Bost RO, Springfield A: Fatal hydrofluoric acid ingestion: A suicide case report. J Anal Toxicol 19:535–536, 1995.
22. Manoguerra AS, Neuman TS: Fatal poisoning from acute hydrofluoric acid ingestion. Am J Emerg Med 4:362–363, 1986.
23. Menchel SM, Dunn WA: Hydrofluoric acid poisoning. Am J Forensic Med Pathol 5:245–248, 1984.
24. Cappell MS, Simon T: Fulminant acute colitis following a self-administered hydrofluoric acid enema. Am J Gastroenterol 88:122–126, 1993.
25. Foster DE, Barone JA: Rectal hydrofluoric acid exposure. Clin Pharm 8:516–518, 1989.
26. McCulley JP: Ocular hydrofluoric acid burns: Animal model, mechanism of injury and therapy. Trans Am Ophthalmol Soc 88:649–684, 1990.
27. Rubinfeld RS, Silbert DI, Arentsen JJ, Laibson PR: Ocular hydrofluoric acid burns. Am J Ophthalmol 114:420–423, 1992.
28. McCulley JP, Whiting DW, Petitt MG, Lauber SE: Hydrofluoric acid burns of the eye. J Occup Med 25:447–450, 1983.
29. Bentur Y, Tannenbaum S, Yaffe Y, Halpert M: The role of calcium gluconate in the treatment of hydrofluoric acid eye burn. Ann Emerg Med 22:1488–1490, 1993.
30. Hatai JK, Weber JN, Doizaki K: Hydrofluoric acid burns of the eye: A report of possible delayed toxicity. J Toxicol Cutan Ocular Toxicol 5:179–184, 1986.
31. Cummings CC, McIvor ME: Fluoride induced hyperkalemia: The role of Ca^{2+} dependent K^+ channels. Am J Emerg Med 6:1–3, 1988.
32. Opit J, Potter H, Charnock JS: The effect of anions on (Na^+-K^+) activated ATPase. Bichim Biophys Acta 120:159–161, 1966.
33. McIvor ME, Cummings CE, Mower MM, et al: Sudden cardiac death from acute fluoride intoxication: The role of potassium. Ann Emerg Med 16:777–781, 1987.

34. Kirkpatrick JJ, Enion DS, Burd DA: Hydrofluoric acid burns: A review. Burns 21:483–493, 1995.

35. Carney SA, Hall M, Lawrence JC, Ricketts CR: Rationale of the treatment of hydrofluoric acid burns. Br J Ind Med 31:317–321, 1974.

36. Hamilton M: OH Congress: Hydrofluoric acid burns. Occup Health (Lond) 27:468–470, 1975.

37. Mathieu L, Nehles J, Blomet J, Hall AH: Efficacy of hexafluorine for emergent decontamination of hydrofluoric acid eye and skin splashes. Vet Hum Toxicol 43:263–265, 2001.

38. Berman I, Taves D, Mitra S, Newmark K: Inorganic fluoride poisoning: Treatment by hemodialysis. N Engl J Med 289: 922, 1973.

39. Bracken WM, Cuppage F, McLaury RL, et al: Comparative effectiveness of topical treatments of hydrofluoric acid burns. J Occup Med 27:733–739, 1985.

40. Burkhart KK, Brent J, Kirk MA, et al: Comparison of topical magnesium and calcium treatment for dermal hydrofluoric acid burns. Ann Emerg Med 24:9–13, 1994.

41. Iverson RE, Laub DR, Madison MS: Hydrofluoric acid burns. Plast Reconstr Surg 48:107–112, 1971.

42. Trevino MA, Herrmann GH, Sprout WL: Treatment of severe hydrofluoric acid exposures. J Occup Med 25:861–863, 1983.

43. Anderson WJ, Anderson JR: Hydrofluoric acid burns of the hand: mechanism of injury and treatment. J Hand Surg Am 13:52–57, 1988.

44. Brown TD: The treatment of hydrofluoric acid burns. J Soc Occup Med 24:80–89, 1974.

45. Chick LR, Borah G: Calcium carbonate gel therapy for hydrofluoric acid burns of the hand. Plast Reconstr Surg 86:935–940, 1990.

46. Sadove R, Hainsworth D, Van Meter W: Total body immersion in hydrofluoric acid. South Med J 83:698–700, 1990.

47. Jones AT: The treatment of hydrofluoric acid burns. J Ind Hyg Toxicol 21:205–212, 1939.

48. Ryan JM, McCarthy GM, Plunkett PK: Regional intravenous calcium—an effective method of treating hydrofluoric acid burns to limb peripheries. J Accid Emerg Med 14:401–404, 1997.

49. Henry JA, Hla KK: Intravenous regional calcium gluconate perfusion for hydrofluoric acid burns. J Toxicol Clin Toxicol 30:203–207, 1992.

50. Graudins A, Burns MJ, Aaron CK: Regional intravenous infusion of calcium gluconate for hydrofluoric acid burns of the upper extremity. Ann Emerg Med 30:604–607, 1997.

51. Siegel DC, Heard JM: Intra-arterial calcium infusion for hydrofluoric acid burns. Aviat Space Environ Med 63:206–211, 1992.

52. Kohnlein HE, Achinger R: A new method of treatment of hydrofluoric acid burns to the extremities. Chir Plast 6:297–305, 1982.

53. Velvart J: Arterial perfusion for hydrofluoric acid burns. Hum Toxicol 2:233–238, 1983.

54. Vance MV, Curry SC, Kunkel DB, et al: Digital hydrofluoric acid burns: Treatment with intraarterial calcium infusion. Ann Emerg Med 15:890–896, 1986.

55. Lee DC, Wiley JF, Synder JW: Treatment of inhalational exposure to hydrofluoric acid with nebulized calcium gluconate. J Occup Med 35:470, 1993.

56. Strubelt O, Iven H, Younes M: The pathophysiological profile of the acute cardiovascular toxicity of sodium fluoride. Toxicol 24:313–323, 1982.

57. Heard K, Hill RE, Cairns CB, Dart RC: Calcium decreases fluoride bioavailability in a lethal model of fluoride poisoning. J Toxicol Clin Toxicol 39:349–353, 2001.

58. Reynolds KE, Whitford GM, Pashley DH: Acute fluoride toxicity: The influence of acid-base status. Toxicol Appl Pharmacol 45:415–427, 1978.

59. Stremski ES, Grande GA, Ling LJ: Survival following hydrofluoric acid ingestion. Ann Emerg Med 21:1396–1399, 1992.

60. Buckingham FM: Surgery: A radical approach to severe hydrofluoric acid burns: A case report. J Occup Med 30:873–874, 1988.

61. Baselt RC, Cravey RH: Disposition of Toxic Drugs and Chemicals in Man. Foster City, CA, Chemical Toxicology Institute, 1995, pp 327–330.

CHAPTER **101**

Overview of Snake Envenoming

Julian White

Venomous snakes are undoubtedly the most significant cause of both major morbidity and mortality among all terrestrial venomous and poisonous animals. Although poisoning by marine animals may affect large numbers of people, mortality is comparatively rare, and thus venomous snakes are the leading cause of death from venomous and poisonous animals in all environments. In some parts of the rural tropics, snakebite is in the top 10 to 15 most important health problems, but in temperate "western" countries, snakebite is often considered to be of negligible significance, a designation not necessarily in tune with reality.

TYPES OF VENOMOUS SNAKES

Even though there are approximately 3000 species of snakes globally, only about 600 species are venomous, and all of them are found in just four snake families: Colubridae, Elapidae (includes sea snakes, subfamily Hydrophiinae), Atractaspididae, and Viperidae.

Medically Important Nonvenomous Snakes

When compared with the human toll from venomous species, nonvenomous snakes cause few problems, but it should not be forgotten that a few large nonvenomous species, notably the pythons and boas (family Boidae), can cause significant bites and rarely may kill and more rarely still may eat humans.

Pythons and boas have many long, sharp, recurved teeth (Fig. 101-1) capable of penetrating deeply, even to bone in some areas such as the hand. These teeth, in addition to causing mechanical injury, may be expected to be coated with bacteria and thus may cause significant local infection. Besides the effects of the bite, large pythons and boas can potentially wrap around a human torso or neck and cause crush injuries. Such injuries may include sig-

nificant internal organ damage in addition to the lethal effects of constriction of the cardiovascular and respiratory systems.

Family Colubridae

Colubridae, the largest family of snakes, is generally considered nonvenomous and is distributed globally (Fig. 101-2). However, a few species have evolved fangs toward the back of the mouth (Fig. 101-3) that deliver venom from venom glands. Several of these species have caused human fatalities or major envenoming (Table 101-1). A further group of colubrid snakes have evolved toxic oral secretions that are inoculated during the biting process, though not with fangs. There is increasing evidence that at least some of these species can cause significant injury to humans. Some other colubrids reported to cause effects in humans are listed in Table 101-2. This list is not exhaustive, and most colubrids should be considered to have some potential of causing at least local envenoming, whether via back fangs or inoculation of toxic oral secretions.

Family Elapidae

A large and diverse family of exclusively venomous snakes covering all continents (except Antarctica) and several major oceans (Fig. 101-4), these snakes have well-developed fangs toward the front of the mouth that can deliver often highly potent venom produced in paired venom glands (Fig. 101-5). The archetypic elapid snake is the Indian cobra, but the typical cobra hood is present in only a few elapids. Some smaller species are unable or unlikely to successfully envenom humans; however, essentially all the larger species are capable of causing envenoming, and many are potentially lethal (Table 101-3). Elapids are a major cause of snakebite morbidity and mortality globally.

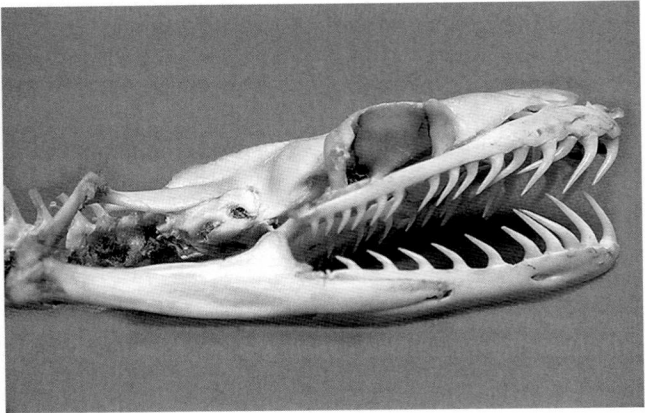

FIGURE 101-1

Boiid skull showing large array of long, sharp recurved teeth. *(Copyright © Dr. Julian White.)*

Family Atractaspididae

A small family of exclusively venomous snakes found solely in Africa and the Middle East (Fig. 101-6), atractaspids are characterized by side-striking fangs (Fig. 101-7) and unique venom components (sarafatoxins), but only a few species appear to be able to significantly envenom humans (Table 101-4).

Family Viperidae

A large and diverse family of exclusively venomous snakes covering most continents (except Australia, New Guinea, and Antarctica) (Fig. 101-8), viperids have a highly evolved fang structure. The fangs are at the front of the mouth, attached to a mobile maxilla, which enables the fangs to fold away against the roof of the mouth and thus permits longer fangs in proportion to head size (Fig. 101-9). There are two major groups of vipers; the subfamily Viperinae contains the classic vipers of the "Old World" (Fig. 101-9; Table 101-5), and the pit vipers, subfamily Crotalinae, are characterized by their anteriorly placed heat-sensitive pit organs, which can detect prey by their heat signature (Figs. 101-10 and 101-11; Table 101-6). Vipers are probably the most important cause of global snakebite morbidity and mortality.

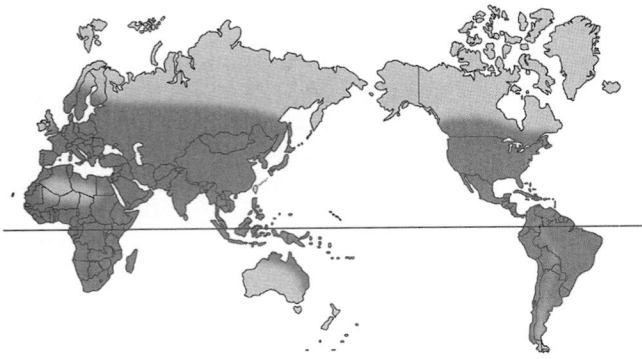

FIGURE 101-2

Approximate global distribution of colubrid snakes. *(Copyright © Dr. Julian White.)*

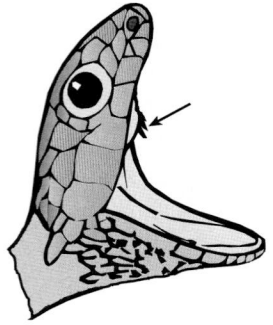

FIGURE 101-3

Diagrammatic representation of a typical colubrid snake head and fang position. *(Copyright © Dr. Julian White.)*

EPIDEMIOLOGY OF SNAKEBITE

No precise figures on the extent of global snakebite are available. The most recent estimate is 2.54 million venomous snakebites and at least 125,000 deaths per year. Certain areas are at high risk, particularly the rural tropics. Unfortunately, these areas coincide with those that have the least medical and financial resources, and thus the fatality rate is higher than would occur if modern medical care and antivenoms were universally available. Certain species groups are responsible for very high numbers of cases and deaths. Of particular note are the saw-scaled or carpet vipers of the genus *Echis* (Fig. 101-12), which are found from West Africa to the Indian subcontinent and are probably responsible for more than 100,000 bites and 10,000 deaths annually. Also important are Russell's viper *(Daboia russelii)* (Fig. 101-13), found from Sri Lanka to Southeast Asia; the puff adder *(Bitis arietans)* (Fig. 101-14); related species in many parts of Africa; and numerous cobra *(Naja)* species (Fig. 101-15) in Africa and Asia. Additional important venomous snakes are the krait species *(Bungarus)* (Fig. 101-16), found from Sri Lanka to Southeast Asia; the Malayan pit viper *(Calloselasma rhodostoma)* (Fig. 101-17) in Southeast Asia; and pit vipers of the genera *Trimeresurus* (Fig. 101-18) and *Gloydius* (Fig. 101-19) in Asia and *Bothrops* (Fig. 101-20), *Crotalus* (Fig. 101-21), and *Agkistrodon*

TABLE 101-1 Colubrid Snakes Reported to Have Caused Major or Lethal Envenoming

SCIENTIFIC NAME	COMMON NAME	EFFECT
Dispholidus typus	Boomslang	Coagulopathy and hemorrhage
Thelotornis spp.	Vine snakes	Coagulopathy and hemorrhage
Rhabdophis spp.	Yamakagashi, red-necked keelback	Coagulopathy and hemorrhage
Malpolon monspessulanus Philodryas olfersii	Montpelier snake	Mild neurotoxicity (poorly defined)
Boiga irregularis	Brown tree snake	Local swelling plus respiratory distress and possible mild paralysis in infants only

TABLE 101-2 Some Colubrid Snakes Reported Capable of Causing Mild Envenoming*

SCIENTIFIC NAME	COMMON NAME	EFFECT
Ahaetulla nasuta	Asian green whipsnake	Local swelling ± discoloration, lymphangitis
Amplorhinus multimaculatus	African many-spotted snake	Local swelling ± headache, nausea
Balanophis ceylonensis	Sri Lankan keelback	Local swelling ± discoloration, bleeding, lymphangitis
Boiga spp. (e.g., *blandingii, ceylonensis, dendrophila, forsteni*)	Tree snakes from Africa and Asia	Local swelling ± discoloration, bleeding, lymphangitis, headache, nausea
Cerberus rhynchops	Indian dog-faced water snake	Local swelling ± discoloration, lymphangitis
Coluber spp. (e.g., *ravergieri, rhodorachis*)	African racer	Local swelling ± discoloration, bleeding, lymphangitis
Crotaphopeltis hotamboeia	African herald snake	Local swelling
Enhydris enhydris	Asian rainbow water snake	Local swelling ± discoloration, lymphangitis
Madagascarophis meridionalis	Madagascan snake	Local swelling ± discoloration, bleeding, blistering, necrosis, lymphangitis, headache, nausea
Malpolon moilensis	African hooded malpolon	Local swelling ± discoloration, lymphangitis
Psammophis sibilans	African racer	Local swelling ± discoloration, bleeding, lymphangitis, headache, nausea
Psammophylax spp. (selected)	African skaapstekers	Local swelling ± discoloration, bleeding, lymphangitis, headache, nausea
Telescopus semiannulatus	African tiger snake	Local swelling ± discoloration, bleeding, lymphangitis, headache, nausea

*This list is not exhaustive.

(Fig. 101-22) in the Americas. Although Australian elapids have a fearsome reputation, they cause relatively few bites and very few deaths and are thus comparatively unimportant.

Those most at risk for snakebite are rural workers, especially while toiling in fields or rice paddies. Some areas, particularly rice-growing regions such as Southeast Asia, have a major seasonal peak of bites during harvest time. Although snakebite can occur at any time of the year in tropical regions, it tends to show a seasonal fluctuation, but in temperate climes, where venomous species may hibernate, legitimate snakebites (those not caused by deliberate handling or provocation of the snake) are a phenomenon of the summer or warmer months.

Particularly in western countries, where keeping venomous snakes attracts hobbyists, some less careful than others, illegitimate snakebites (those caused by deliberate handling or provocation of the snake or by a captive snake) are an important problem that often involves severe bites from exotic species for which no appropriate antivenom may be readily available. Such hobbyists have in the past enjoyed a reputation for recklessness and almost an encouragement of bites, the numbers of which were sometimes "worn" as a badge of honor. It is often assumed by health professionals that this attitude is as inevitable as the numerous bites. It is my experience in South Australia that such need not be the case and that with correct education and encouragement, private keepers of venomous snakes can be very careful and responsible and can work with health authorities to minimize legitimate bites and provide assistance in identifying snakes that have caused envenoming. This is therefore a plea to my medical colleagues to abandon the past, often hostile relationship between keepers and doctors and seek to establish a good, mutually respectful working relationship that reinforces an ethos among keepers that being bitten is something to be ashamed of and to be avoided at all cost.

SNAKE VENOMS

Snake venoms are generally produced in specific venom glands derived from the salivary glands, the exception being Duvernoy's glands in some colubrid species. The venom,

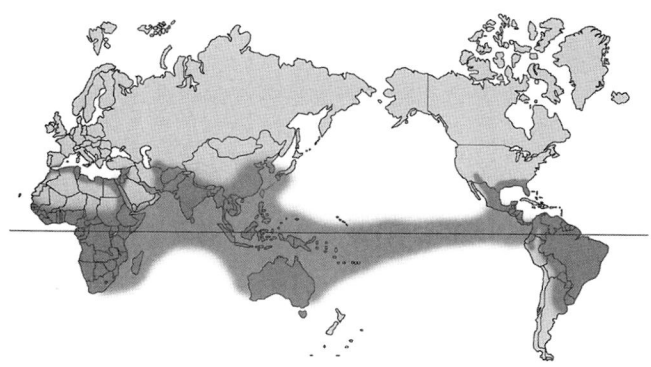

FIGURE 101-4

Approximate global distribution of elapid snakes, including sea snakes. *(Copyright © Dr. Julian White.)*

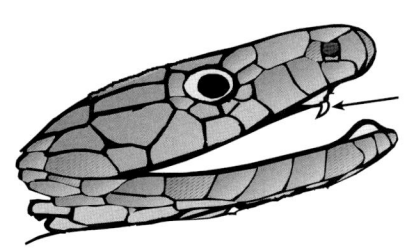

FIGURE 101-5

Diagrammatic representation of a typical elapid snake head and fang position. *(Copyright © Dr. Julian White.)*

TABLE 101-3 Major Groups of Elapid Snakes and Their Principal Clinical Effects

SCIENTIFIC NAME	COMMON NAME	EFFECT
Acanthophis spp.	Australian death adders	Neurotoxic paralysis
Austrelaps spp.	Australian copperheads	Neurotoxic paralysis
Aspidelaps spp.	African coral snakes	Neurotoxic paralysis
Bungarus spp.	Asian kraits	Neurotoxic paralysis
Boulengeria spp.	African water cobras	Neurotoxic paralysis
Calliophis spp.	Asian coral snakes	Neurotoxic paralysis
Dendroaspis spp.	African mambas	Neurotoxic paralysis and fasciculation
Elapsoidea spp.	African garter snakes	Local effects only
Hemachatus haemachatus	African rinkhals spitting cobra	Local tissue injury, paralysis
Hoplocephalus spp.	Australian broad-headed snakes	Coagulopathy and hemorrhage
Maticora spp.	Asian coral snakes	Neurotoxic paralysis
Micropechis ikaheka	New Guinea small-eyed snake	Paralysis, coagulopathy, myolysis
Micrurus spp.	American coral snakes	Depending on species, paralysis and/or myolysis
Micruroides euryxanthus	Arizona coral snake	Neurotoxic paralysis (rarely severe)
Naja spp.	African and Asian cobras	Depending on species, severe local tissue injury and/or paralysis
Notechis spp.	Australian tiger snakes	Paralysis, coagulopathy, myolysis, renal damage
Ophiophagus hannah	Asian king cobra	Paralysis, local tissue injury
Oxyuranus spp.	Australian taipans	Paralysis, coagulopathy, myolysis, renal damage
Paranaja multifasciata	African burrowing cobra	Local effects only
Pseudechis spp.	Australian mulga and black snakes	Depending on species, myolysis, coagulopathy (anticoagulant), renal damage
Pseudohaje spp.	African tree cobras	Local effects only
Pseudonaja spp.	Australian brown snakes	Coagulopathy, renal damage, rarely paralysis
Tropidechis carinatus	Australian rough-scaled snake	Paralysis, coagulopathy, myolysis, renal damage
Walterinnesia aegyptii	Middle East desert black snake	Neurotoxic paralysis
Various	Sea snakes	Paralysis and/or myolysis

once produced, is delivered by a duct to the fang base, where it is transported into the victim either by a groove in the fang or through a fang duct. Production of intraglandular pressure by contraction of muscles around the gland is the usual mode of venom transport, and this mechanism often allows the snake to "fine-tune" how much venom is expended in a given bite. This may explain, in part, why many venomous snakes exhibit the "dry bite" phenomenon whereby a bite fails to inject enough venom to cause medically significant envenoming.

Snake venoms generally consist of a complex mixture of substances, each of which may exhibit one or more distinct toxic actions. Many of the most potent snake toxins have evolved highly specific targets, such as the neuromuscular junction or components of the hemostatic system. It is

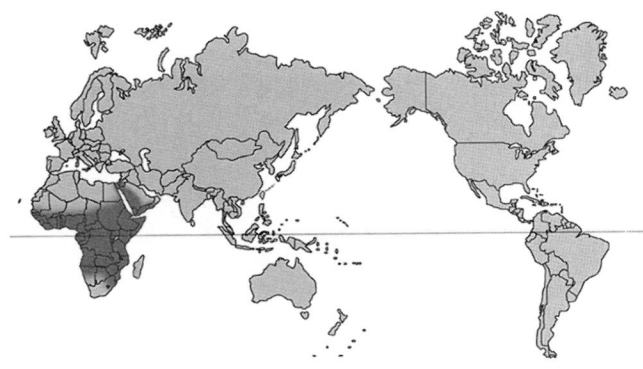

FIGURE 101-6

Approximate global distribution of atractaspid snakes. *(Copyright © Dr. Julian White.)*

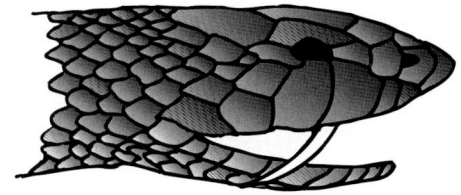

FIGURE 101-7

Diagrammatic representation of a typical atractaspid snake head and fang position. *(Copyright © Dr. Julian White.)*

TABLE 101-4 Atractaspid Snakes and Their Principal Clinical Effects

SCIENTIFIC NAME	COMMON NAME	EFFECT
Atractaspis	African mole or side-fanged vipers	Depending on species, may cause local effects, necrosis, cardiotoxicity

TABLE 101-5 Major Groups of Viperid Snakes and Their Principal Clinical Effects

SCIENTIFIC NAME	COMMON NAME	EFFECT
Atheris spp.	African bush vipers	Nothing significant
Bitis spp.	African puff adders, Gaboon vipers, etc.	Depends on species, but some cause severe local tissue injury, coagulopathy and hemorrhage, shock, cardiotoxicity
Causus spp.	African night adders	Local effects, paralysis
Cerastes spp.	African horned adders	Local effects, coagulopathy, hemorrhage, shock
Daboia russelii	Russell's viper	Local effects, coagulopathy hemorrhage, renal failure, paralysis, myolysis (Sri Lanka only)
Echis spp.	African and West Asian saw-scaled vipers	Local effects, coagulopathy, hemorrhage, shock
Macrovipera spp.	Eurasian vipers	Local effects, coagulopathy, hemorrhage, shock
Pseudocerastes spp.	Middle East horned vipers	Paralysis
Vipera	European vipers	Local effects, necrosis, shock

likely that all snake venoms fulfill multiple functions for the snake, principally

- Prey acquisition
- Prey digestion
- Defense against predators

Snake venoms may be classified in many ways, and some classifications still frequently used in medical texts are misleading or inaccurate. Foremost among these is the old aphorism that elapids are neurotoxic and viperids are hemorrhagic, a classification that is inaccurate and should be abandoned. Some of the most potent toxins active against human hemostasis are found in certain elapid venoms, whereas some other elapid species cause major local tissue injury at the bite site. Conversely, in a number of viperid species the principal clinical effect is neurotoxic paralysis, with no or minimal effect on either local tissues at the bite site or the hemostatic system. From a medical perspective, a classification based on clinical effects is generally useful (Table 101-7) and will be adopted in this chapter, but the reader should be aware that more biochemically based classifications of venoms yield a quite

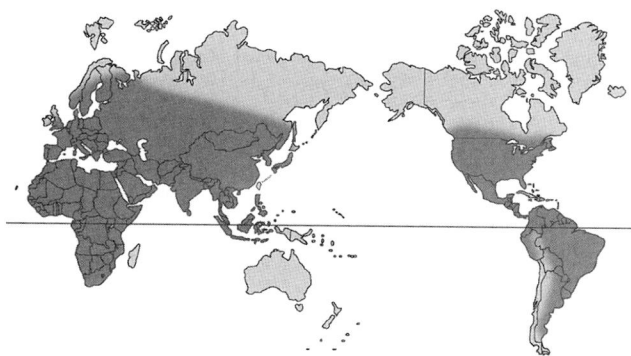

FIGURE 101-8

Approximate global distribution of viperid (including crotalid) snakes.

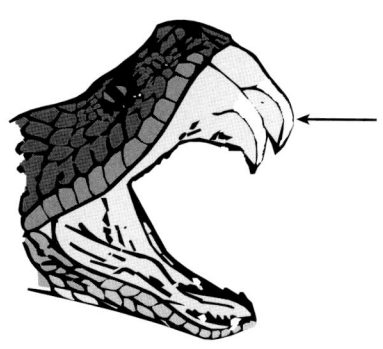

FIGURE 101-9

Diagrammatic representation of a typical viperid snake head and fang position. *(Copyright © Dr. Julian White.)*

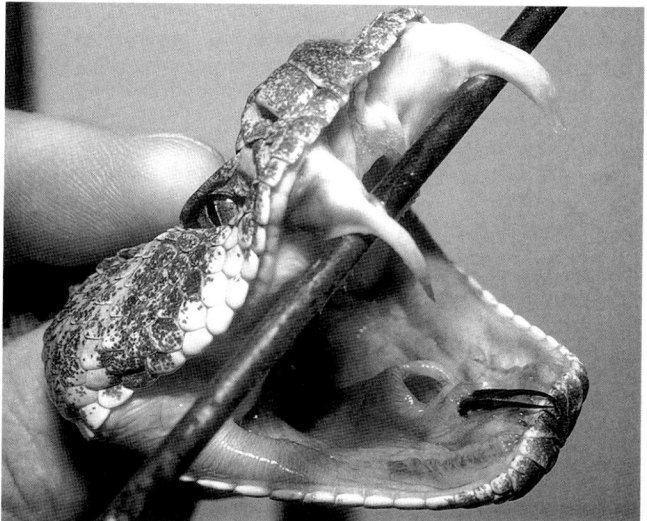

FIGURE 101-10

Crotalid snake head showing fangs in the erect position. *(Copyright © Dr. Julian White.)*

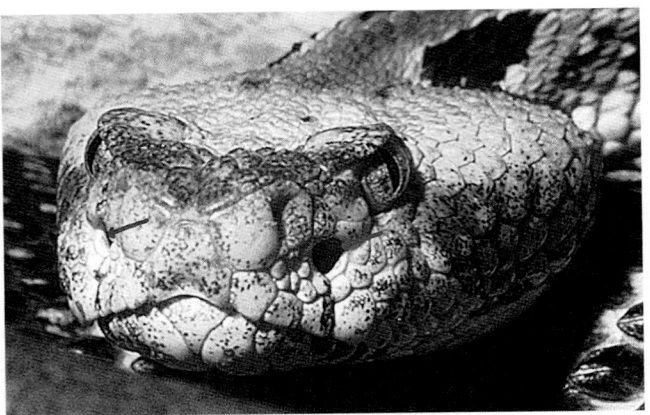

FIGURE 101-11

Typical crotalid snake head showing the position of heat-sensing pit organs. *(Copyright © Dr. Julian White.)*

different picture (Table 101-8) and that some medically important toxins from snake venoms have several physiologically distinct actions, each caused by separate regions in the toxin structure.

Neurotoxins

Snake venom neurotoxins are a diverse group of toxins that clinically cause paralytic effects mediated at the neuromuscular junction (in most cases) (Fig. 101-23). A hundred years ago, snakebite paralysis usually condemned the victim to death from respiratory failure. In the current era of intensive care unit (ICU) management, intubation, ventila-

tion, and other treatment modalities, such an outcome should be rare; however, in many regions such facilities are unavailable, and thus many snakebite victims still die annually of neurotoxic paralysis.

Presynaptic neurotoxins are generally modified phospholipase A_2 toxins that specifically target the terminal axon of the neuromuscular junction. These toxins first cause release of neurotransmitter and then extensive damage to the axonal structure culminating in complete disruption of production of transmitter synaptic vesicles and thus cessation of transmitter release. Clinically, this causes a progressive flaccid paralysis, with the onset of signs usually 1+ hours after the bite and progressive paralysis thereafter. Full respiratory paralysis, including paralysis of the diaphragm, may take 3 to 24 hours; once paralysis is complete, the recovery rate is determined by axonal repair and is not influenced by antivenom therapy. It is therefore critical in this type of envenoming to recognize the early signs of paralysis and institute effective antivenom therapy before more extensive paralysis becomes irreversibly established. Complete paralysis may take days, weeks, or rarely months to resolve. During this period the victim is dependent on external ventilatory support and is at risk for a number of potentially severe complications. Presynaptic neurotoxins are found in selected elapid and viperid venoms (Table 101-9).

Postsynaptic neurotoxins are polypeptides of varying size, usually under 12 kd, and they also target the neuromuscular junction. They act extracellularly by binding to the acetylcholine receptor on the muscle end-plate and blocking neurotransmitter binding, thus causing paralysis. The cell is not specifically damaged, and therefore this type of flaccid paralysis is often reversible with

TABLE 101-6 Major Groups of Crotalid Snakes and Their Principal Clinical Effects

SCIENTIFIC NAME	COMMON NAME	EFFECT
Agkistrodon spp.	North American copperhead, cottonmouth, cantil	Local effects, necrosis, coagulopathy, hemorrhage, shock
Atropoides spp.	Central American jumping pit vipers	Local effects, necrosis
Bothriechis spp.	Central American palm pit vipers	Local effects, necrosis, shock
Bothrops spp.	South and Central American pit vipers	Depends on species, but may include local effects, necrosis, coagulopathy, hemorrhage, renal damage, myolysis, shock
Calloselasma rhodostoma	Malayan pit viper	Local effects, necrosis, coagulopathy, hemorrhage, renal damage, shock
Cerriphidion spp.	Central American montane pit vipers	Local effects, necrosis
Crotalus spp.	Rattlesnakes	Depends on species; in North America, local effects, necrosis, coagulopathy, shock; in South America, local effects, paralysis, coagulopathy, myolysis, renal damage
Deinagkistrodon acutus	Chinese hundred pace viper	Local effects, necrosis, coagulopathy, hemorrhage, shock
Gloydius spp.	Asian terrestrial pit vipers	Local effects, necrosis, coagulopathy, hemorrhage, shock
Hypnale spp.	Sri Lankan hump-nosed vipers	Local effects
Lachesis spp.	Central and South American bushmasters	Local effects, necrosis, coagulopathy, shock
Ophryacus spp.	Central American horned pit vipers	Local effects, necrosis, shock
Ovophis spp.	Asian montane pit vipers	Local effects, coagulopathy, hemorrhage
Porthidium spp.	Central American montane pit vipers	Local effects, necrosis, shock
Sistrurus spp.	North American pygmy rattlesnakes and massasauga	Local effects, necrosis, rarely hemorrhage
Trimeresurus spp.	Asian green pit vipers	Depends on species; local effects, rarely necrosis, coagulopathy, hemorrhage
Tropidolaemus spp.	Asian tree vipers	Local effects; rarely necrosis, coagulopathy, hemorrhage

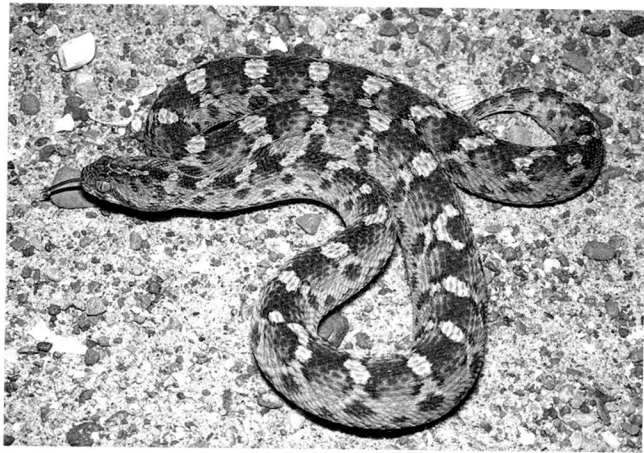

FIGURE 101-12

Saw-scaled viper (specimen from Africa). *(Copyright © Dr. Julian White.)*

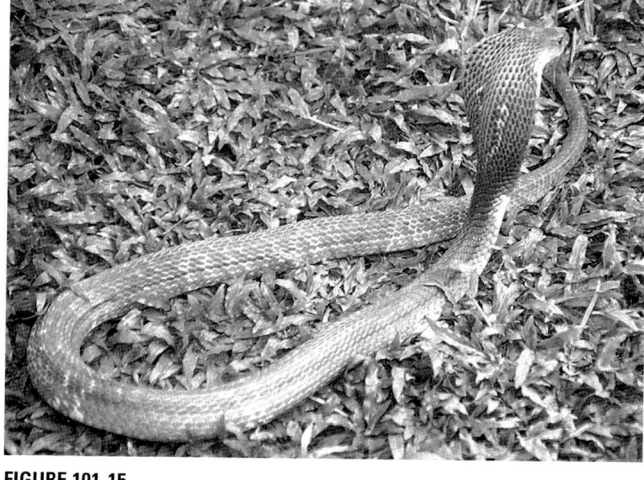

FIGURE 101-15

Typical cobra with hood displayed (specimen from Thailand). *(Copyright © Dr. Julian White.)*

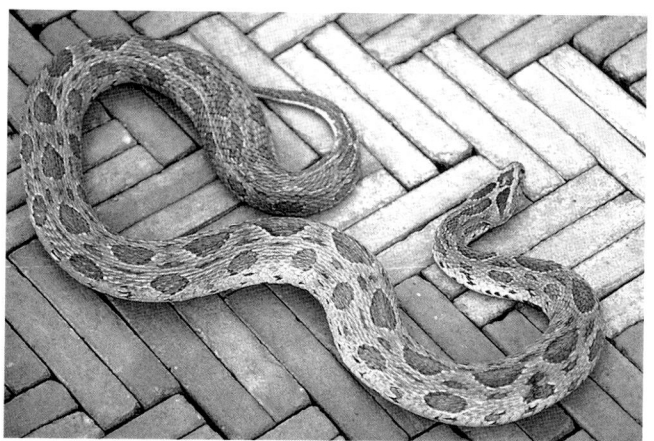

FIGURE 101-13

Russell's viper (specimen from Thailand). *(Copyright © Dr. Julian White.)*

antivenom therapy, even if very extensive. The mode of action may also allow more rapid onset and progression of paralysis, although major paralysis is uncommon earlier than 1 hour after the bite. Postsynaptic neurotoxins are present in many elapid and a few viperid venoms (Table 101-10).

Dendrotoxins and fasciculins are synergistic neurotoxins found in some African mamba venoms. Both toxins target the neuromuscular junction and cause paralysis and muscle spasms or fasciculation. Dendrotoxins target certain potassium channels in the terminal axon membrane, ultimately resulting in overrelease of neurotransmitter molecules that swamp and overstimulate the adjacent muscle end-plate receptors. Fasciculins inhibit or interfere with anticholinesterases in the junctional space, thereby significantly reducing the normal removal of synaptic acetylcholine. This decreased removal of acetylcholine enhances the effect of dendrotoxins and results in gross overstimulation

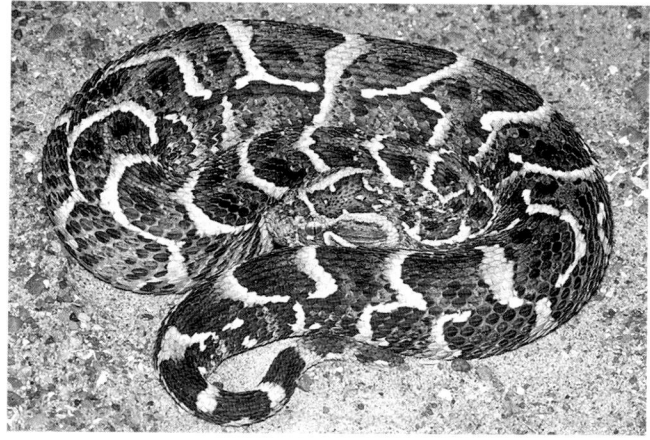

FIGURE 101-14

Puff adder (specimen from Africa). *(Copyright © Dr. Julian White.)*

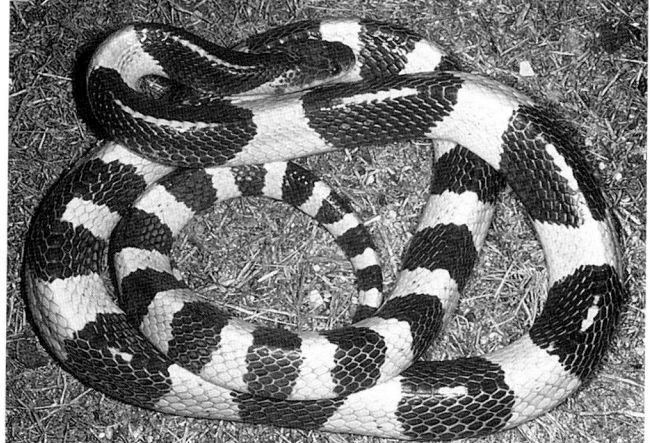

FIGURE 101-16

Asian krait (specimen from Thailand). *(Copyright © Dr. Julian White.)*

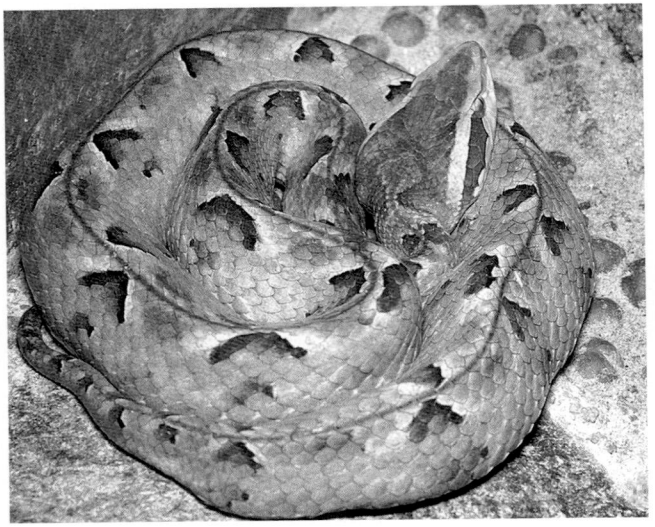

FIGURE 101-17

Malayan pit viper (specimen from Thailand). *(Copyright © Dr. Julian White.)*

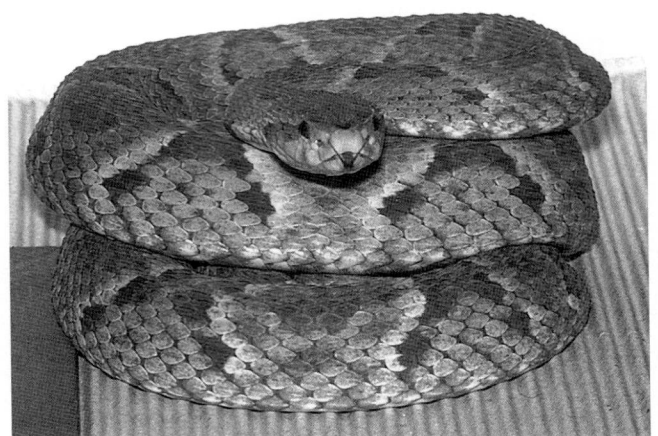

FIGURE 101-20

South American *Bothrops* pit viper (specimen from Brazil). *(Copyright © Dr. Julian White.)*

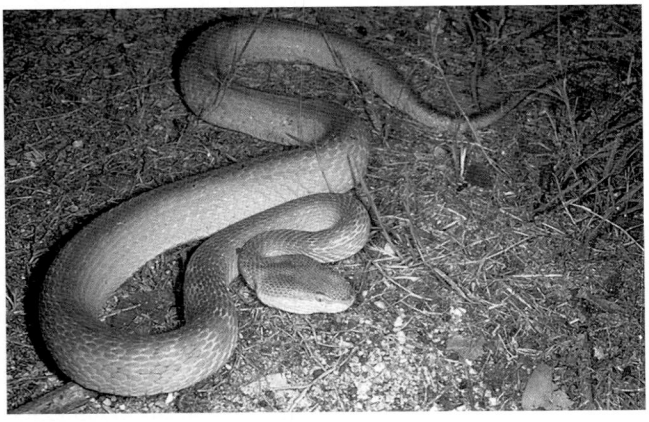

FIGURE 101-18

Green pit viper (specimen from Thailand). *(Copyright © Dr. Julian White.)*

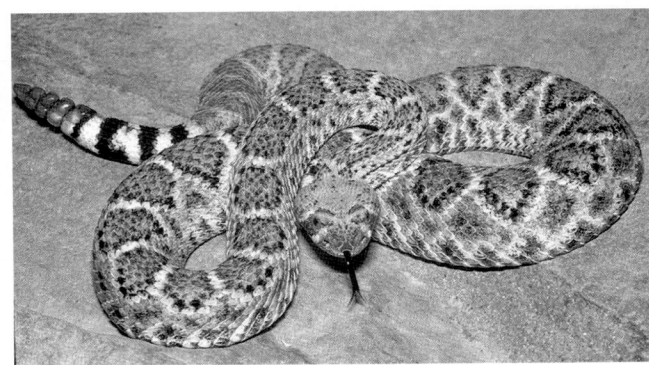

FIGURE 101-21

North American *Crotalus* pit viper (specimen from United States). *(Copyright © Dr. Julian White.)*

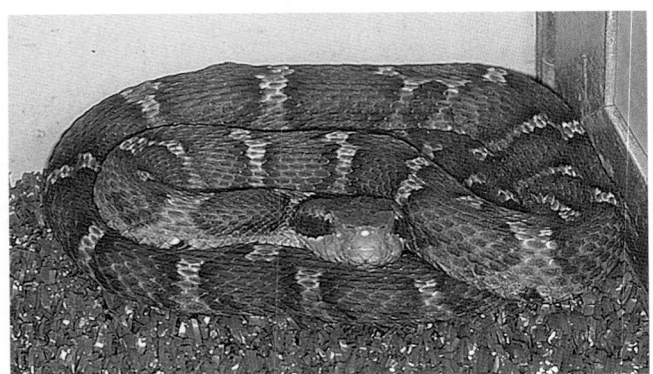

FIGURE 101-19

Asian *Gloydius* pit viper. *(Copyright © Dr. Julian White.)*

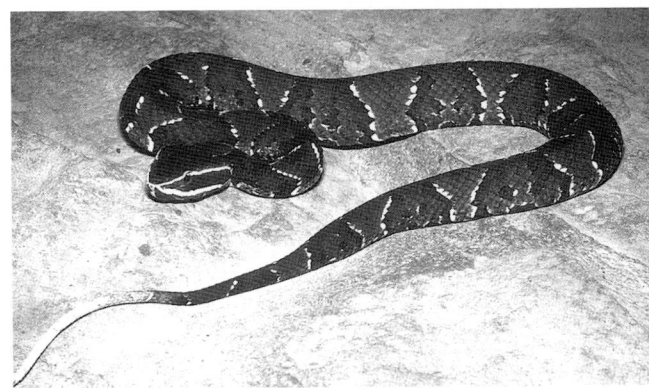

FIGURE 101-22

North American *Agkistrodon* pit viper (specimen from Mexico). *(Copyright © Dr. Julian White.)*

TABLE 101-7 Broad Medical Classification of Snake Venom Activities

TOXIN ACTIVITY TYPE	CLINICAL EFFECTS
Neurotoxin	Flaccid paralysis
Presynaptic	Resistant to late antivenom therapy
Postsynaptic	Often reversed with antivenom therapy
Anticholinesterase	Fasciculation
Myotoxin	Systemic skeletal muscle damage
Hemostatic system toxins	Interference with normal hemostasis causing either bleeding or thrombosis
Hemorrhagins	Vascular wall damage causing bleeding
Nephrotoxins	Direct renal damage
Cardiotoxins	Direct cardiotoxicity
Necrotoxins	Direct tissue injury at the bite site/bitten limb

of the muscle manifested as spasm or fasciculation, thereby effectively paralyzing the victim. Both toxins may exert their effect rapidly, and thus the clinical effects may become apparent in less than an hour after a bite.

Other types of snake neurotoxins are produced, some targeting different areas, but they either are uncommon or have limited or no significant clinical effects, particularly when compared with the foregoing toxins.

TABLE 101-8 Broad Biochemical Classification of Snake Venom Activities

TOXIN CLASS	CLINICAL EFFECTS
Polypeptide toxins	Various; autonomic, neurotoxic, cardiotoxic, myotoxic
Phospholipase toxins	Various; presynaptic neurotoxic, myolytic, procoagulant, cardiotoxic, necrotic
Enzyme toxins	Various; interfere with hemostasis, necrotic, hemolytic
Oxidoreductases	
Transferases	
Hydrolases	
Carbon-nitrogen lyases	
Metalloproteinases	
Other toxins	Various; autonomic, etc.
Lectins	
Nerve growth factors	
Phospholipase inhibitors	
Proteinase inhibitors	
Complement inhibitors	
Other components	Various or ill-defined
Amino acids	
Biogenic amines	
Carbohydrates	
Lipids	
Nucleosides and nucleotides	
Riboflavin	
Organic acids	
Anions	
Cations	

Myotoxins

Most snake venom myotoxins are based on phospholipase A_2 and cause systemic myolysis of skeletal muscle but rarely affect cardiac or smooth muscle. The damage occurs to individual muscle cells with sparing of the basement membrane; thus, regeneration of muscle usually begins about 3 days after the bite and is complete after about 28 days. Experimentally, only slow-twitch fibers regenerate, but this is still unconfirmed in human cases. In the process of muscle destruction, massive release of myoglobin, creatine kinase, and potassium occurs. The former is associated with secondary renal damage and often gross myoglobinuria. Theoretically, antivenom therapy should have no effect if muscle breakdown is already established, but experience in Australia suggests that even late antivenom treatment may reduce the severity of muscle damage. Myotoxins are found in both elapid and viperid species (Table 101-11).

Toxins Affecting Blood Coagulation

The human hemostatic system seems to be a favorite target of snake venoms. There are toxins targeting almost all parts of the system, as represented in three of the four snake families (Colubridae, Elapidae, Viperidae). Major toxin groups include procoagulants, anticoagulants, and platelet aggregation inhibitors and promoters (Table 101-12). The net effect of most of these toxins is to increase bleeding, particularly when combined with hemorrhagins, but a few venoms cause clinical thrombosis with potential for embolic problems. The mechanisms of increased bleeding vary, but most components acting as procoagulants exert their effect by consumption of fibrinogen, which results in defibrination rather than classic disseminated intravascular coagulation (DIC), and thus the thrombocytopenia associated with DIC is often absent. However, some venoms do cause thrombocytopenia via other mechanisms. Yet other venoms cause defibrination through direct action on fibrinogen by splitting fibrinopeptides inappropriately. The biochemical nature and structure of these diverse toxins vary from comparatively small molecules to large, complex multicomponent toxins that mimic normal clotting complexes such as the prothrombinase complex. The majority of viper species have toxins affecting coagulation, but only a few elapid species, notably those from Australia and New Guinea, cause similar effects (Table 101-13).

Hemorrhagins

In addition to the toxins acting on hemostasis, some venoms, notably those of certain viper species, also contain direct hemorrhagins (Table 101-14). These toxins damage the vascular endothelium, thereby promoting bleeding, and are generally zinc metalloproteinases. They are potentially lethal.

Nephrotoxins

Secondary renal damage is common in envenoming by many venomous snake species, but a few species have direct nephrotoxins (Table 101-15).

1. Signal arrives at nerve cell ending (terminal axon) from brain
2. Neurotransmitter (ACh=Acetylcholine) is released from within nerve cell ending (terminal axon)
3. ACh leaves terminal axon and crosses the gap (synapse) to the muscle cell wall
4. The ACh binds to receptors (AChR) on the muscle cell wall, causing changes in the cell, resulting in muscle contraction
5. ACh is released from the receptor and broken down by an enzyme (ChEsterase)

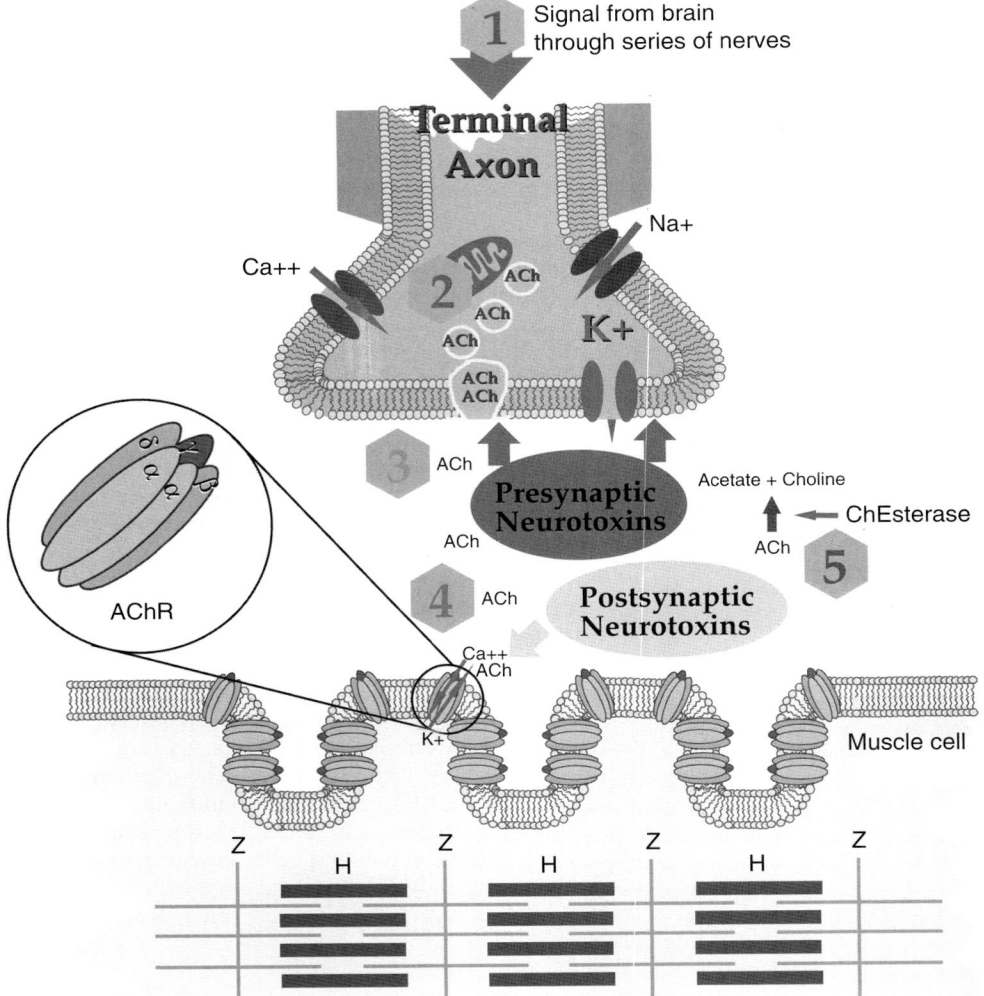

FIGURE 101-23

Diagrammatic representation of the neuromuscular junction as target site for snake neurotoxins. *(Copyright Dr. Julian White.)*

Necrotoxins

Local tissue injury around the bite site is a common feature of viperid bites, although not all vipers cause local necrosis. However, certain elapids, notably some cobra species from Africa and Southeast Asia, routinely cause local necrosis (Table 101-16). In most cases the venom components causing this damage are incompletely understood, although the ubiquitous phospholipase A_2 toxins are thought to have a major role. The misnamed "cobratoxins" also cause local tissue injury.

Other Toxins

There are, of course, many other components found in snake venoms, too numerous to list here. For many, the clinical consequences in humans are uncertain.

TABLE 101-9 Snakes Considered to Have Presynaptic Neurotoxins of Medical Significance (Postsynaptic Neurotoxins May Also Be Present in These Venoms) (Includes Mamba Dendrotoxins)

SCIENTIFIC NAME	COMMON NAME	EFFECT
Elapidae		
Bungarus spp.	Kraits	Presynaptic and postsynaptic
Dendroaspis spp.	Mambas	Dendrotoxins and fasciculins
Notechis spp.	Australian tiger snakes	Presynaptic and postsynaptic
Oxyuranus spp.	Australian taipans	Presynaptic and postsynaptic
Pseudonaja spp.	Australian brown snakes	Presynaptic and postsynaptic
Tropidechis carinatus	Rough-scaled snake	Presynaptic and postsynaptic
Viperidae		
Crotalus spp. (selected)	Selected rattlesnakes from South and Central America, plus one North American species	Presynaptic
Vipera ammodytes	European viper (Balkans)	Presynaptic

TABLE 101-10 Snakes Considered to Have Only Postsynaptic Neurotoxins of Medical Significance

SCIENTIFIC NAME	COMMON NAME	EFFECT
Elapidae		
Acanthophis spp.	Death adders	Postsynaptic only
Austrelaps spp.	Australian copperheads	Postsynaptic only
Micrurus spp.	American coral snakes	Postsynaptic only
Naja spp. (selected)	Some cobras from Africa and Asia	Postsynaptic only
Ophiophagus hannah	King cobra	Postsynaptic only
Various	Sea snakes	Postsynaptic only
Viperidae		
Daboia russelii pulchella	Sri Lankan Russell's viper	Postsynaptic only

VENOM TOXICODYNAMICS

In recent years it has been possible to measure venom or individual toxins over time in both experimental animals and human snakebite victims. Although such measurement has thus far been performed for only a very limited range of species, there is greater understanding of the toxicodynamics of envenoming (Fig. 101-24). In most cases, venom is injected fairly superficially, usually subcutaneously. Locally acting toxins causing tissue injury are placed directly at their target site and will thus begin exerting their clinical effects immediately. A significant proportion of the venom, in some species perhaps most of the venom, will not be absorbed directly into the circulation. Instead, it will be transported first via the lymphatic system and then enter the circulation through the thoracic duct. This helps explain the common

TABLE 101-11 Snakes Known to Have Systemic Myotoxins of Medical Significance

SCIENTIFIC NAME	COMMON NAME	EFFECT
Elapidae		
Micropechis ikaheka	New Guinea small-eyed snake	Moderate systemic myolysis
Micrurus spp. (selected)	Selected South American coral snakes	Moderate systemic myolysis
Notechis spp.	Australian tiger snakes	Severe systemic myolysis
Oxyuranus spp.	Australian taipans	Moderate systemic myolysis
Pseudechis spp.	Australian mulga and black snakes	Moderate-to-severe systemic myolysis
Tropidechis carinatus	Rough-scaled snake	Severe systemic myolysis
Various	Sea snakes	Moderate-to-severe systemic myolysis
Viperidae		
Bothrops spp. (selected)	Selected species of South American pit vipers	Moderate systemic myolysis
Crotalus spp. (selected)	Selected species of South American rattlesnakes	Moderate systemic myolysis
Daboia russelii pulchella	Sri Lankan Russell's viper	Moderate systemic myolysis

TABLE 101-12 Principal Types of Toxin Effects on the Hemostatic System

TOXIN TYPE	EFFECT
Procoagulants	Factor V activating
	Factor X activating
	Factor IX activating
	Prothrombin activating
	Fibrinogen clotting
Anticoagulant	Protein C activating
	Factor IX/X activating protein
	Thrombin inhibitor
	Phospholipase A$_2$
Fibrinolytic	Fibrin(ogen) degradation
	Plasminogen activation
Vessel wall interactive	Hemorrhagins
Platelet activity	Platelet aggregation inducers
	Platelet aggregation inhibitors
Plasma protein activators	Serpin inhibitors

clinical finding of enlarged or tender lymph nodes draining the bite area and also the high concentration of venom in these nodes at autopsy. Transport via the lymphatic system may be rapid or sometimes delayed, and there is a potential for sequestration of venom locally with prolonged release over a period of hours or days. Once in the circulation, those components affecting hemostasis or acting as hemorrhagins will have reached their target site and will quickly exert their effect. Similarly, nephrotoxins will quickly damage the kidneys. However, toxins that seek extravascular targets, particularly the neurotoxins and myotoxins, will need to exit the circulation in sufficient concentration to exert their effect clinically; thus, these toxins are most likely to have a delayed onset of clinically detectable action. Some venoms are quickly cleared from the circulation, but others remain detectable for days or even weeks without antivenom therapy. Knowledge of such variation is clearly relevant in determining antivenom therapy, as will be discussed later.

Venom Variability

It is often assumed by those unfamiliar with clinical toxinology that a given species of snake will have a consistent venom. Though sometimes true, probably more often there is significant intraspecies and even intraindividual venom variability. Some medically important species exhibit great variability in venom throughout their

TABLE 101-13 Snakes Considered to Cause Medically Significant Effects on the Hemostatic System

SCIENTIFIC NAME	COMMON NAME	EFFECT
Colubridae		
Dyspholidus typus	Boomslang	Coagulopathy and hemorrhage
Thelotornis spp.	Vine snakes	Coagulopathy and hemorrhage
Rhabdophis spp.	Yamakagashi, red-necked keelback	Coagulopathy and hemorrhage
Elapidae		
Hoplocephalus spp.	Australian broad-headed snakes	Coagulopathy and hemorrhage
Micropechis ikaheka	New Guinea small-eyed snake	Anticoagulant and hemorrhage
Notechis spp.	Australian tiger snakes	Coagulopathy and hemorrhage
Oxyuranus spp.	Australian taipans	Coagulopathy and hemorrhage
Pseudechis spp.	Australian mulga snakes	Anticoagulant and hemorrhage
Pseudonaja spp.	Australian brown snakes	Coagulopathy and hemorrhage
Tropidechis carinatus	Rough-scaled snake	Coagulopathy and hemorrhage
Viperidae		
Agkistrodon spp.	American copperheads	Coagulopathy and hemorrhage
Bitis spp.	African puff adders, Gaboon vipers, etc.	Coagulopathy and hemorrhage
Bothrops spp. Includes *Bothriechis, Cerriphidion, Ophryacus, Porthidium* spp.	Central and South American pit vipers	Coagulopathy and hemorrhage
Bothrops lanceolatus	Martinique viper	Coagulopathy; thrombosis with DVT and pulmonary embolism
Calloselasma rhodostoma	Malayan pit viper	Coagulopathy and hemorrhage
Cerastes spp.	North African horned vipers	Coagulopathy and hemorrhage
Crotalus spp. (selected)	North American rattlesnakes	Coagulopathy and hemorrhage
Daboia russelii	Russell's viper	Coagulopathy and hemorrhage
Echis spp.	Saw-scaled vipers	Coagulopathy and hemorrhage
Lachesis spp.	Bushmasters	Coagulopathy and hemorrhage
Trimeresurus spp.	Green pit vipers	Coagulopathy and hemorrhage
Vipera spp. (selected) Includes *Macrovipera* spp.	Selected European vipers	Coagulopathy and hemorrhage

DVT, deep venous thrombosis.

TABLE 101-14 Snakes Considered to Have Medically Significant Hemorrhagins

SCIENTIFIC NAME	COMMON NAME	EFFECT
Viperidae		
Agkistrodon spp.	American copperheads	Disintegrins and hemorrhagins
Bitis spp.	African puff adders, Gaboon vipers, etc.	Disintegrins and hemorrhagins
Bothrops spp.	Central and South American pit vipers	Disintegrins and hemorrhagins
Calloselasma rhodostoma	Malayan pit viper	Hemorrhagins
Crotalus spp. (selected)	North American rattlesnakes	Disintegrins and hemorrhagins
Daboia russelii	Russell's viper	Hemorrhagins
Echis spp.	Saw-scaled vipers	Disintegrins and hemorrhagins
Trimeresurus spp.	Green pit vipers	Disintegrins and hemorrhagins
Vipera spp. (selected)	Selected European vipers	Disintegrins and hemorrhagins

TABLE 101-15 Snakes Considered to Potentially Cause Renal Damage through Direct Nephrotoxins or Related Mechanisms (Excluding Those Causing Renal Damage through the Secondary Mechanisms of Shock, Myolysis, or Coagulopathy)

SCIENTIFIC NAME	COMMON NAME	EFFECT
Daboia russelii	Russell's viper	Direct nephrotoxin

geographic range, so significant that antivenom developed by using venom from one part of that range will be totally ineffective in treating bites by specimens from another part of the range. Classic examples are Russell's viper (*Daboia russelii*) and the South American rattlesnake (*Crotalus durrisus terrificus*). Even a single geographic location may have several distinct subpopulations of venom type. Equally, it is well established that some snake species show either or both ontogenetic and seasonal venom variability.

TABLE 101-16 Snakes Known to Potentially Cause Significant Local Tissue Injury and Necrosis at the Bite Site

SCIENTIFIC NAME	COMMON NAME	EFFECT
Elapidae		
Naja spp.	Selected cobras, especially spitting cobras	Local blistering to extensive deep necrosis
Ophiophagus hannah	King cobra	Occasional local necrosis
Atractaspididae		
Atractaspis spp.	Mole or side-fanged vipers	A few species cause only local tissue injury, occasionally necrosis
Viperidae		
Agkistrodon spp.	Cottonmouth, copperhead, cantil	Local blistering to necrosis
Atropoides spp.	Jumping pit vipers	Local blistering to necrosis
Bitis spp.	Puff adder, Gaboon viper, etc.	Local blistering to extensive deep necrosis
Bothriechis spp.	Palm pit vipers	Local blistering to extensive deep necrosis
Bothrops spp.	Lancehead vipers	Local blistering to extensive deep necrosis
Calloselasma rhodostoma	Malayan pit viper	Local blistering to extensive deep necrosis
Causus spp.	Night adders	Local blistering to necrosis
Cerastes spp.	Horned adders	Local blistering to necrosis
Cerriphidion spp.	Montane pit vipers	Local blistering to necrosis
Crotalus spp.	Rattlesnakes	North American spp.; local blistering to extensive deep necrosis
Daboia russelii	Russell's viper	Local blistering to extensive deep necrosis
Deinagkistrodon acutus	Hundred pace viper	Local blistering to extensive deep necrosis
Hypnale spp.	Hump-nosed vipers	Local blistering to necrosis
Echis spp.	Saw-scaled vipers	Local blistering to extensive deep necrosis
Lachesis spp.	Bushmasters	Local blistering to extensive deep necrosis
Ophryacus spp.	Horned pit vipers	Local blistering to necrosis
Porthidium spp.	Montane pit vipers	Local blistering to necrosis
Sistrurus spp.	Massasauga, pygmy rattlesnake	Local blistering to necrosis (uncommon)
Trimeresurus spp.	Green tree pit vipers	Local blistering to necrosis (selected species only)

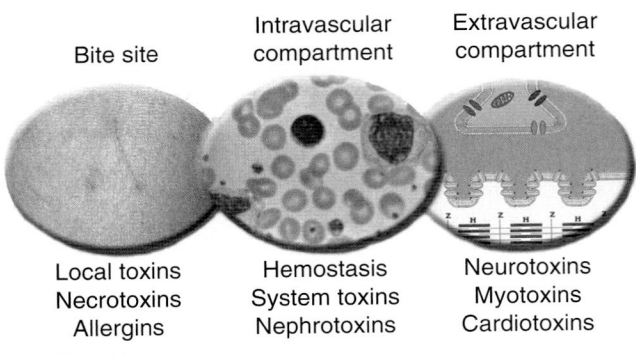

FIGURE 101-24

Diagrammatic representation of the toxicodynamics of envenoming. *(Copyright Dr. Julian White.)*

CLINICAL EFFECTS OF ENVENOMING

The clinical effects of a snakebite will vary with the species of snake; the age, size, and geographic origin of the snake; the quantity of venom injected; the route of injection; the age, size, and previous health of the victim; and past exposure to venom. Thus, although there may be typical features of envenoming for a given snake species, there will usually be significant variation between cases.

Local Effects

Snakebite may result in very obvious bite marks and a prominent local tissue response, but equally, the bite marks may be indistinct or virtually undetectable and the local response negligible. The latter is particularly true for certain elapid species, but a few viperids also cause minimal local effects and similarly exert their major clinical effects systemically.

Bite marks vary from a single fang puncture (Fig. 101-25), to classic double punctures from paired fangs (Fig. 101-26), through numerous punctures from both fangs and nonfang teeth (Fig. 101-27), to scratches where fangs have dragged through the skin (Fig. 101-28). If two or more bites have been delivered to the same region, an even more complex pattern

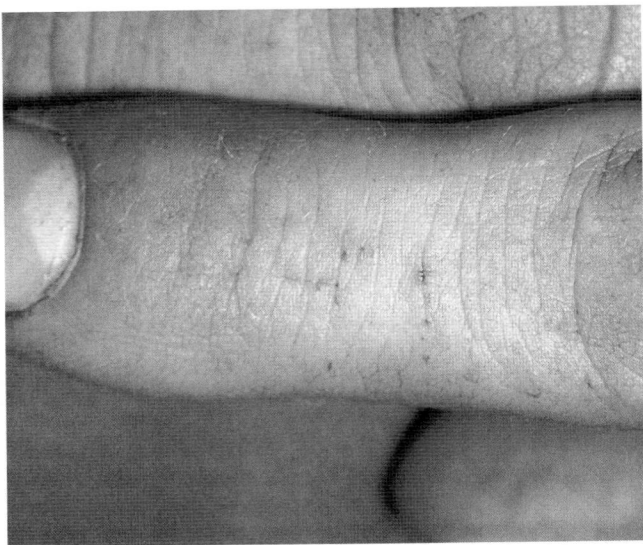

FIGURE 101-26

Classic double puncture from paired fangs. *(Copyright © Dr. Julian White.)*

may be seen (Fig. 101-29). The distance between paired fang punctures may indicate the size of the snake but depends on the species; if the snake species is unknown, interfang distance is an unreliable method of predicting snake size.

The presence of associated effects may be of value in determining the most likely culprit. Thus, there may be local swelling (Fig. 101-30), erythema, ecchymosis (Fig. 101-31), hemorrhage (Fig. 101-32), blistering (Fig. 101-33), or frank necrosis (Fig. 101-34). In general, it should never be assumed that the lack of a local response to a bite indicates a trivial bite, unless the snake species responsible is already known and is clearly associated with significant local effects in all medically noteworthy cases.

Local pain is quite variable and not always reliable as an indicator of significant envenoming.

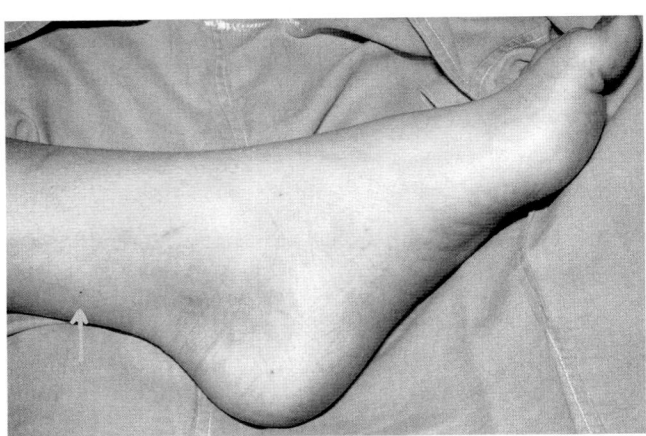

FIGURE 101-25

Single fang puncture mark. *(Copyright © Dr. Julian White.)*

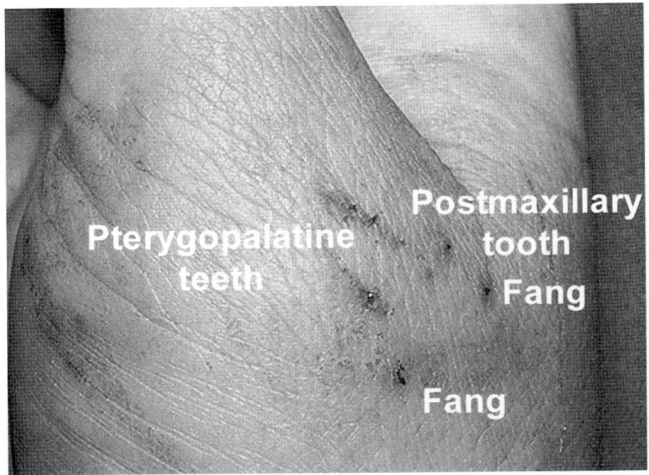

FIGURE 101-27

Multiple punctures in a single bite from both fangs and nonfang teeth. *(Copyright © Dr. Julian White.)*

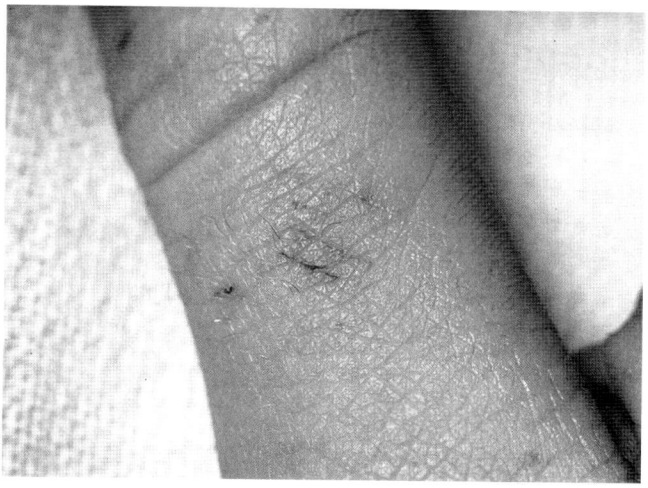

FIGURE 101-28

Scratches where fangs have dragged through skin. *(Copyright © Dr. Julian White.)*

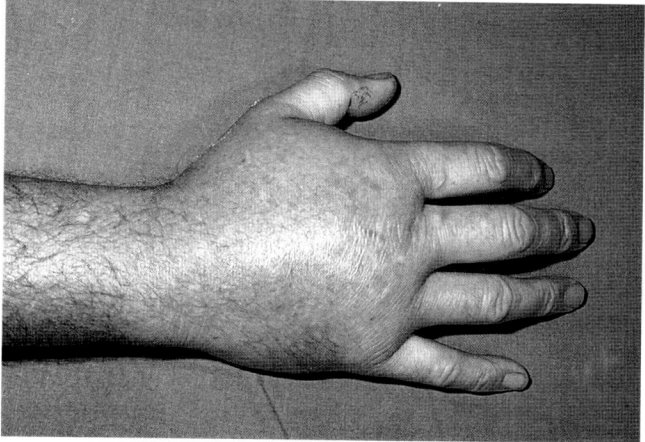

FIGURE 101-30

Local swelling in the bitten limb. *(Copyright © Dr. Julian White.)*

General Effects

General systemic symptoms vary among species and individuals but usually include some or all of the following: headache, nausea, vomiting, abdominal pain, diarrhea, dizziness, collapse, and convulsions. Particularly in children, collapse and convulsions may be the first evidence of envenoming, at least for certain species (e.g., Australian elapids). It is often assumed that hypotension will occur in response to envenoming, but hypertension is also common, and both tachycardia and bradycardia are reported.

Specific Effects

In addition to the nonspecific systemic symptoms, a variety of quite specific symptoms and signs is associated with particular venom actions. Recognition of these symptoms

and signs in the early stages is important because it allows appropriate remedial action, usually antivenom therapy, before major complications occur.

PARALYSIS

The flaccid paralysis caused by neurotoxins affects skeletal muscle and respiration, not cardiac or smooth muscle. For species with potent postsynaptic neurotoxins, paralytic symptoms can develop within 3 to 15 minutes of the bite and major paralysis within 15 to 30 minutes, but such cases are the exception. In most instances, clinically detectable paralysis will not be apparent until at least 1 hour after the bite and may be delayed up to 24 hours. The cranial nerves are usually affected first, with ptosis often being the initial sign (Fig. 101-35). Other common initial signs are dysphonia, dysphagia, drooling, and diplopia, the latter caused by partial ophthalmoplegia (Fig. 101-36). As paralysis progresses, drooling may increase and ophthalmoplegia may become total, with fixed forward gaze often associated

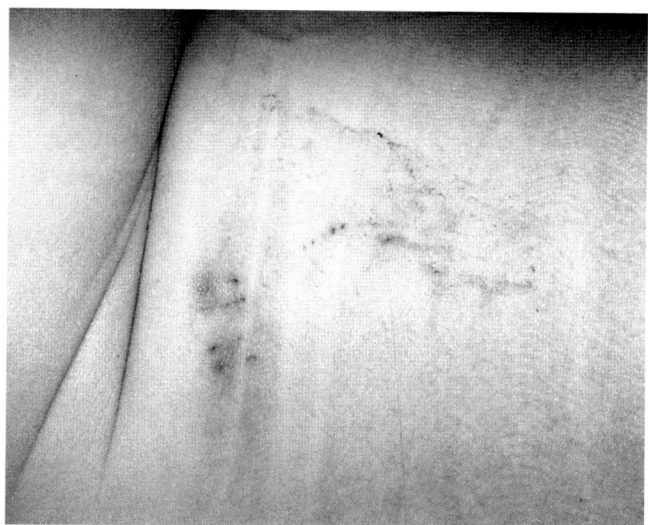

FIGURE 101-29

Complex bite marks from multiple bites. *(Copyright © Dr. Julian White.)*

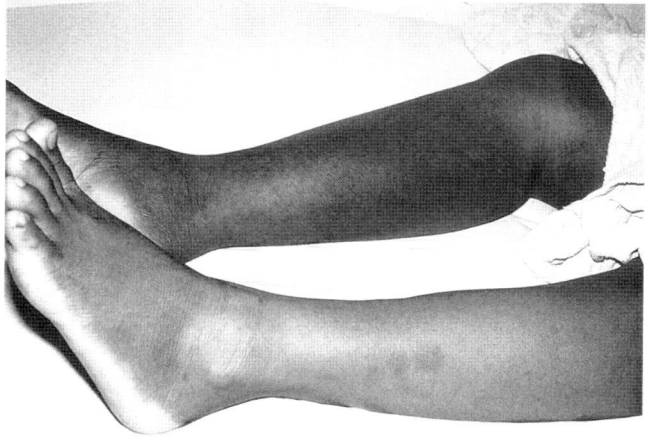

FIGURE 101-31

Erythema and ecchymosis at the bite site. *(Copyright © Dr. Julian White.)*

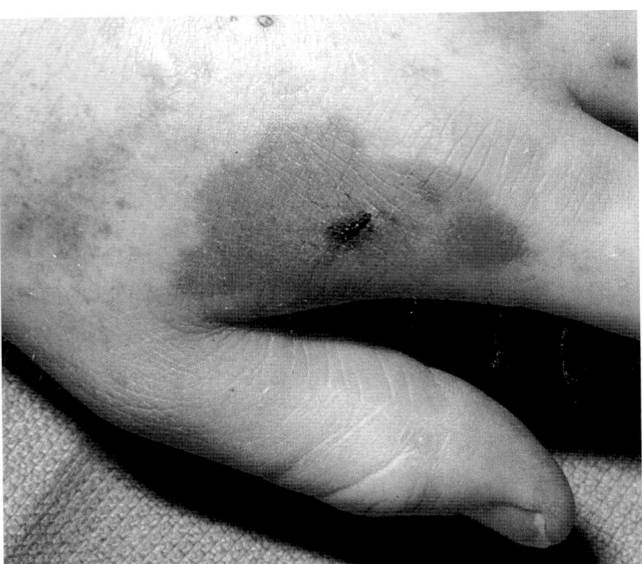

FIGURE 101-32

Local hemorrhage at the bite site. *(Copyright © Dr. Julian White.)*

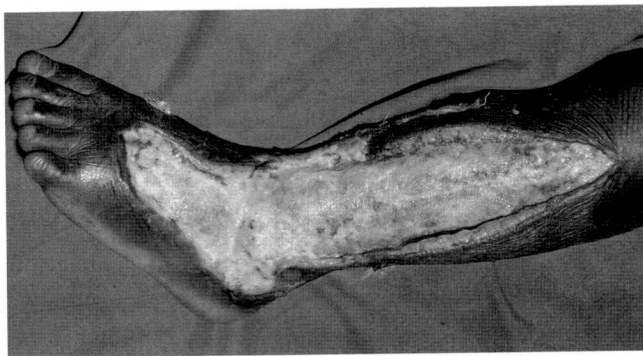

FIGURE 101-34

Necrosis of a bitten limb. *(Courtesy of David Warrell.)*

with fixed dilated pupils. Limb weakness becomes apparent, the victim usually first noticing an ataxic gait and then an inability to walk and subsequently an inability to stand or even sit up. The neck may become floppy ("broken neck" sign). Deep tendon reflexes will become reduced and then disappear. Respiratory distress develops, breathing may become shallow and rapid, and cyanosis may be apparent. Complete respiratory failure will ensue unless respiratory support is offered. The time from a bite to respiratory failure is highly variable, from as little as 30 minutes (rare) to more than 24 hours, but commonly within 6 to 12 hours. Without antivenom or anticholinesterase therapy, the period of respiratory failure may

vary from less than 24 hours to several days or even several weeks.

For species with potent presynaptic neurotoxins but low concentrations of postsynaptic neurotoxins, although the symptoms and signs are the same, the rapidity of onset is usually slower, with the first signs essentially never evident in less than 1 hour after the bite. Unless paralysis is diagnosed and halted at an early stage with antivenom therapy, this type of paralysis is not reversible, and days, weeks, or months may elapse before axonal repair is sufficient for return of neuromuscular function.

In addition to the major features just noted, several other neurotoxic effects may occur. Of particular note are transient or permanent alterations in taste or smell, sometimes leaving the victim with permanent complete anosmia.

MYOLYSIS

Muscle damage may sometimes be purely local (some rattlesnake species) but is more commonly systemic. Onset is likely to be at least 1 hour after the bite, but symptoms and signs are mostly delayed considerably longer. Symptoms include muscle pain, tenderness, and weakness, the latter possibly mimicking paralysis. The onset of symptoms is usually associated with detectable, often frank myoglobinuria,

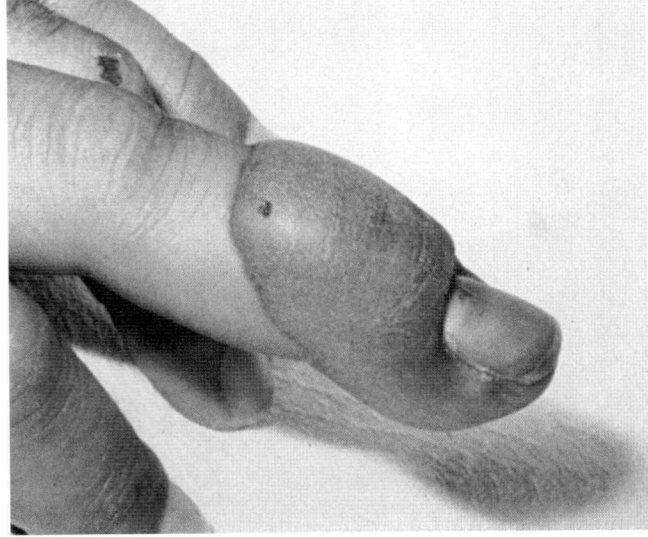

FIGURE 101-33

Blistering of a bitten limb. *(Copyright © Dr. Julian White.)*

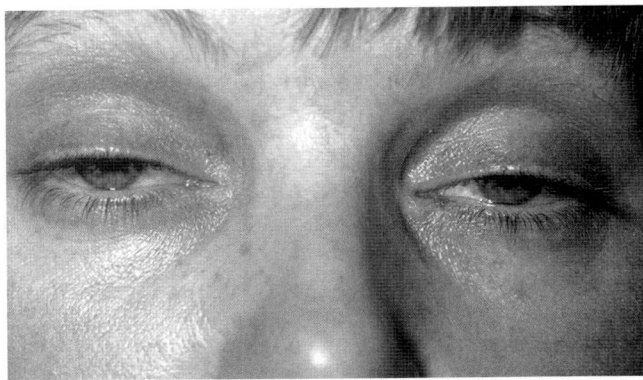

FIGURE 101-35

Bilateral ptosis, usually the earliest sign of progressive flaccid neurotoxic paralysis. *(Copyright © Dr. Julian White.)*

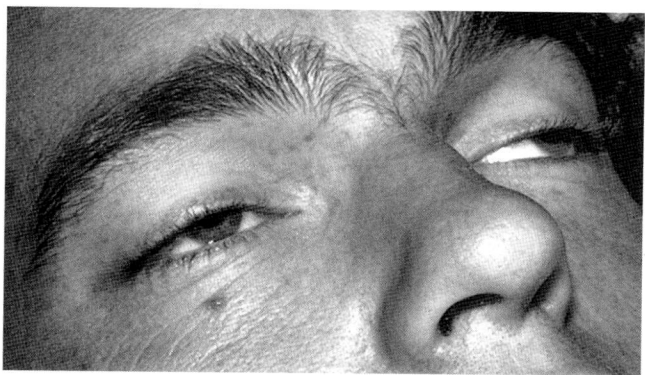

FIGURE 101-36

Partial ophthalmoplegia with divergent squinting and diplopia, as well as ptosis, indicative of progressing paralysis. *(Copyright © Dr. Julian White.)*

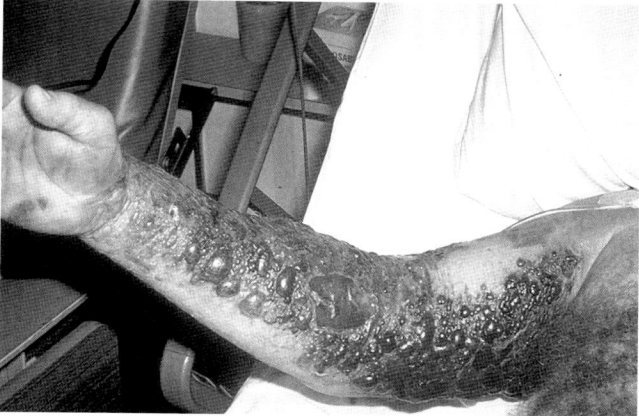

FIGURE 101-38

Marked hemorrhagic effects in a bitten limb. *(Copyright © Dr. David Hardy.)*

with the urine varying from clear red (similar to hemoglobinuria) to deep muddy brown (Fig. 101-37).

COAGULOPATHY AND HEMORRHAGIN EFFECTS

The severity and clinical manifestations of coagulopathy will be determined, in part, by the species of snake. In general, the first clinical evidence of coagulopathy is often persistent oozing of blood from the bite site, any other areas of recent trauma, venipuncture sites, and often the gums. The gums are particularly likely to bleed if hemorrhagins are present in the blood. The area around the bite site may show mild to gross and extensive ecchymosis (Fig. 101-38). Hematuria may be present; if myoglobinuria is also suspected, microscopic evidence of red cells or casts may assist in differentiation. The coagulopathy may be severe, yet the victim may be virtually symptom free and thus the severity of envenoming masked. It is particularly because of this danger that at least baseline clotting tests should be routinely performed for most types of snakebite, the exception being regions where none of the culprit species cause coagulopathy. Although full laboratory tests of coagulation might be ideal, in most parts of the world they are either unavailable or will take a long time. If detailed coagulation studies are unavailable, the whole blood clotting time (discussed later) is an invaluable bedside test in snakebite victims. In the presence of major coagulopathy, any trauma has the potential to result in major or lethal hemorrhage, particularly with head injuries.

Fibrin degradation products are cleared through the kidneys, and secondary renal failure is a potential complica-

tion of coagulopathy. A few species can cause quite specific hemorrhages; most notably, Russell's viper in Myanmar (Burma) can cause anterior pituitary hemorrhage or Sheehan's syndrome, with long-term consequences.

Although the net effect of most hemostatically active venoms is functional anticoagulation, often through consumption of fibrinogen, thrombosis is sometimes the most prominent effect. Bites by vipers in Martinique, in particular, are associated with the development of deep venous thrombosis and a significant risk for pulmonary embolism.

NEPHROTOXICITY

Renal damage is a common sequela of bites by many species of snakes and may be primary or secondary and vary from mild transient increases in creatinine and urea levels, detectable only by laboratory tests, through oliguric or anuric renal failure, to rare cases of permanent renal damage (renal cortical necrosis). Careful measurement of urine output is important to detect early evidence of functional renal problems, which are otherwise asymptomatic, at least in the critical early hours after a bite.

CARDIOTOXICITY

The cardiotoxic effects of a snakebite are primary in only a few species but may occur secondarily after bites by many species; these effects vary from mild arrhythmias to cardiac arrest. Severe myolysis, particularly when associated with secondary renal failure, may result in severe hyperkalemia, with consequent and sometimes lethal effects, as seen with other causes of hyperkalemia.

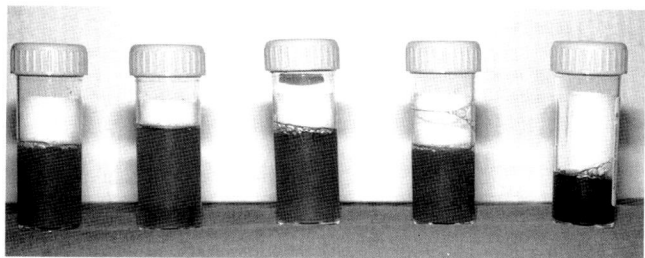

FIGURE 101-37

Myoglobinuria secondary to systemic myolysis. *(Copyright © Dr. Julian White.)*

MANAGEMENT OF SNAKEBITE

First Aid

First aid for a snakebite is controversial. Many techniques are promoted or used around the world, but most have in common a complete lack of objective evidence of efficacy and are often associated with significant adverse side effects varying from delay in obtaining appropriate care to directly related death.

The only universally approved first aid for a snakebite, applicable globally, is immobilizing the bitten area/limb and keeping the victim still. For bites by nonnecrotic species, including many elapids (but not most cobras) and a few viperids, the Australian-developed pressure immobilization method is both safe and effective. It is based on retarding venom transport in the lymphatics by applying moderate local and limb pressure sufficient to occlude the superficial lymphatics and inhibiting the muscle pump transport system by immobilizing the limb in a splint. Applied correctly, it may be safely left on for several hours and experimentally is as effective as a tourniquet in preventing venom movement, but far safer. This technique has not been subjected to clinical trials, although extensive anecdotal evidence from Australia suggests that it is safe and effective when used correctly. A modification of the technique has been tested for viper bites in Myanmar, and the initial results suggest promise, with no increase in local tissue injury. If these studies continue to be successful and are extended to other necrotic bites without evidence of increased necrosis, the pressure immobilization method may become the universally accepted first aid for all snakebites. That it is not presently accepted universally reflects concern that immobilizing necrotic venom locally may worsen the extent of necrosis and thus be counterproductive in treating the victim.

In general, the bite wound should be gently cleaned, except where bite site venom detection is available, as in Australia and New Guinea. Clear fluids may be given by mouth, but not food and certainly not alcohol.

Tourniquets are no longer recommended for snakebite because they are easily misused, are effective for too short a period, and have a high and proven potential for causing severe injury to the victim through ischemic necrosis. The resulting gangrene may prove lethal, and the personal and social cost of amputated limbs is devastating. Suction applied to the bite site is inappropriate. If mouth suction is used, active venom may be transferred to the oral cavity and bacteria instilled in the wound. Contrary to many positive claims, dedicated suction kits remove only small and often negligible quantities of venom and may disrupt local tissues and thereby promote spread and absorption of venom. Cutting the wound or, worse still, excision only adds further injury to the victim, increases the absorption of venom, and provides an avenue for major hemorrhage if a coagulopathy is present. Application of local electric shock, as used in parts of the Americas and Africa, has never been shown in either experimental studies or clinical trials to be other than a charlatan treatment. Similarly, the use of cryotherapy is without merit and associated with tissue damage. Traditional healing, such as snake stones, have no rational basis, but it is possible that certain native plant extracts may ultimately prove beneficial. However, until their safety and effectiveness have been conclusively demonstrated, they cannot be recommended.

Hospital Treatment

In regions where effective hospital care is available, it should be the cornerstone of snakebite treatment. The hospital management of specific snakebites is discussed in considerable detail in the following chapters. Unfortunately, in many snakebite-prone areas, such treatment is not reliably available.

SOME BASIC PRINCIPLES

Whenever possible, the first priority is to critically assess and stabilize the vital systems if imperiled. Thus, attention to the airway, breathing, and circulation should take priority. However, if there is a possibility of coagulopathy, attempts at cardiac compression should be circumspect and instituted only if absolutely indicated.

An intravenous (IV) line should be inserted and, in most cases, an initial IV fluid load given, especially in cases in which significant local reaction is occurring with consequent fluid shift and the potential for hypovolemic shock. The choice of IV fluids will depend on the circumstances and availability.

Particularly in victims likely to have a coagulopathy necessitating repeated assessment of coagulation, insertion of a line suitable for repeat sampling, rather than performing repeated venipunctures, should be considered. The femoral, jugular, and especially the subclavian vessels should be avoided.

DIAGNOSIS

As in other diseases, diagnosis is crucial in effective management of a snakebite. Three principal diagnostic questions should be asked: is this a snakebite or some other condition?; if it is a snakebite, is significant envenoming present and to what extent?; and finally, what type of snake was responsible?

The diagnosis of snakebite may be obvious, as in patients seen after being bitten by their pet snake, but such cases are the exception. Usually, however, it is likely that the identity of the snake is unknown. Also, there are numerous cases without a history of a bite, just a set of symptoms to be explained, where snakebite may not even be thought of initially.

History. The key features required when taking a history from a suspected snakebite victim are as follows:

- Time and geographic location where the bite did or might have occurred (time since the bite is important, and geographic location may limit the number of possible snake species)
- If a snake was seen, its description, particularly its color, pattern, and length
- If a bite was witnessed, was it a single or multiple bite? (A multiple bite is much more likely to be severe.)
- Was first aid applied, what type of first aid was it, how long after the bite was it applied, and what did the victim do between being bitten and application of first aid? (If the victim was actively chasing the snake or was escaping from the snake before application of appropriate first aid [e.g., immobilization or, for nonnecrotic species, pressure immobilization], first aid was unlikely to have been effective; thus, if the victim is not envenomed at initial hospital evaluation, it is more likely to be a dry bite. If, in contrast, the victim immediately lay still and had appropriate first aid applied, the lack of envenoming at initial hospital assessment may simply mean that the first aid was effective; in such cases, envenoming may rapidly ensue once first aid measures are removed.)
- Are there any symptoms suggestive of envenoming, such as headache, nausea, vomiting, abdominal pain, fasciculations, ptosis collapse, or convulsions?

- Are there any symptoms suggestive of ongoing major envenoming, such as blurred or double vision; difficulty speaking, swallowing, walking, or breathing; bleeding from the bite site; or muscle pain?
- Is there any relevant past history, such as past exposure to antivenoms; preexisting cardiac, respiratory, renal, or allergic disease; or recent surgery or trauma?
- Is the patient taking any medications, particularly those that might interfere with key blood tests (especially anticoagulants)?

Examination. Careful examination can often be vital in determining the extent of envenoming.

Local Signs

- Examine the bite site and look particularly for evidence of multiple bites. Fang marks may be single or double punctures or scratches when fangs have dragged through the skin, and they are sometimes very small and difficult to see, particularly with colubrids and smaller elapids. Also look for local swelling, bruising, discoloration, blistering, and developing necrosis, typical of bites by certain species. For locally active venoms, such as bites by many viperid species, the rapidity and extent of swelling may indicate the probable severity of envenoming.

General Signs

- Check the draining lymph nodes for tenderness or swelling, which may indicate absorption of venom.
- Check the pulse and blood pressure (systemic envenoming often causes hypertension).

Specific Signs

- Check for evidence of paralysis, such as ptosis, partial or complete ophthalmoplegia, fixed dilated pupils, flat facies, poor tongue protrusion, dysarthria, drooling, limb weakness, poor grip strength, reduced or absent deep tendon reflexes, paralytic-type respiratory difficulties, and cyanosis.
- Check for evidence of coagulopathy and hemorrhagin activity, such as persistent oozing of blood (not serosanguineous) from the bite site, extensive local ecchymosis, hemorrhagic blistering, and persistent bleeding from venipuncture sites, gums, recent trauma, or elsewhere. When appropriate (e.g., viper bite in Martinique), check for evidence of developing deep venous thrombosis. When appropriate (e.g., Russell's viper bite in Myanmar), check for evidence of anterior pituitary hemorrhage.
- Check for evidence of myolysis, such as muscle tenderness or weakness and red or brown urine (myoglobinuria).
- Check for evidence of renal impairment, such as oliguria or anuria.
- Check for evidence of cardiac abnormalities, particularly arrhythmias or electrocardiographic changes associated with hyperkalemia.

Laboratory Investigations. Laboratory tests are often very helpful in determining the extent of envenoming, but this does not mean that only a large hospital with a well-equipped laboratory can manage a snakebite. It is also vital to repeat tests, even if the results are initially normal. If the patient's initial examination and test results are normal and thus indicative of no current envenoming, the tests should be repeated in about 2 hours and then again 3 hours later (fifth hour after initial assessment) to ensure that the late development of envenoming, particularly coagulopathy, is not missed. In some situations, especially some viper bites causing coagulopathy (notably the Malayan pit viper bite), envenoming may persist, develop late, or recur after antivenom therapy, so retesting over a period of several days may be required. Earlier testing is indicated if symptoms or signs develop.

A Small or Rural Hospital. Many snakebite victims will initially go to a small rural hospital with no laboratories on site. However, there are some very useful tests that can easily be performed:

- Urinalysis to look for hemoglobin/myoglobin (both test positive for blood). Simple microscopy to search for red cells or casts may help differentiate between hemoglobinuria and myoglobinuria.
- Whole blood clotting time. This simple but effective test requires at least two standard *glass* test tubes or similar glass containers. A small quantity of the patient's blood is placed in one tube, a similar amount of blood from a normal control (relative or staff member) is placed in another tube, and the time taken to clot is measured. If normal, the blood should clot in 5 to 10 minutes. If just the patient's blood fails to clot or develops only a weak clot by 15 minutes, a coagulopathy is probably present. If neither the patient nor the control blood clots, there is a problem with the test system. It has been suggested that this test can be simplified by checking for clots only once, 20 minutes after taking the sample; a normal clot indicates no coagulopathy, whereas a weak or no clot indicates coagulopathy.
- Only in Australia, detection of snake venom on the bite site swab (see "Venom Detection" in Chapter 105).

A Regional or Teaching Hospital. If full laboratory facilities are available, use them! The following should be performed, labeled urgent:

- Extended coagulation studies: prothrombin time/international normalized ratio, activated partial thromboplastin time, fibrinogen level, cross-linked or D dimer degradation products of fibrin/fibrinogen
- Complete blood picture, especially platelet and absolute lymphocyte counts
- Electrolytes, urea, creatinine
- Creatinine phosphokinase
- Where appropriate, arterial blood gas determination
- Examination of a peripheral blood smear for evidence of microangiopathic hemolysis, suggestive of DIC
- Only in Australia, detection of snake venom on the bite site swab (see "Venom Detection" in the chapter on Australian snakebites)

Snake Venom Detection. Currently, the only commercial venom detection system is the Australian CSL Snake Venom Detection Kit (SVDK; CSL Ltd, Melbourne, Australia), which relies on a sensitive sandwich enzyme-linked immunosorbent assay to detect even small concentrations of snake venom. It has been in use for 20 years and can detect even nanogram concentrations of venom, but it is applicable only for snakes native to Australia and

New Guinea. The best sample is a moist swab from the bite site. If systemic envenoming has occurred, urine may be tested if a bite site is not available. Blood is the least reliable test sample and should be avoided. The kit gives only a qualitative result.

A number of experimental venom detection systems have been used in various regions of the world, and it is likely that commercial snake venom detection will become more widely available in the future. Some of these detection systems may be quantitative as well as qualitative, which will give far more scope to studying the extent of systemic envenoming and may lead to far more precise guidelines on antivenom doses.

DIFFERENTIAL DIAGNOSIS

The differential diagnosis issues surrounding snakebite are most commonly those of including snakebite in the differential diagnosis of unexplained collapse, convulsions, coagulopathy, paralysis, myolysis, or renal failure.

TREATMENT OF SNAKEBITE

Treatment of snakebite is likely to be effective only if the extent and nature of the envenoming are known, hence the importance of the diagnostic process discussed earlier.

Basic Treatment

The basics of management were listed earlier and include an IV line, initial IV fluid load, and attention to the airway, breathing, and circulation. Avoid accessing the femoral, jugular, or subclavian vessels because bleeding associated with coagulopathy may be extreme. Keep venipunctures to a minimum. Frequent blood tests are usually required, so consider insertion of a long line via the cubital fossa or even a radial arterial line, particularly if ICU facilities are available. Monitor the pulse, blood pressure, respiration, and cardiac rhythms regularly, preferably with appropriate monitors. Monitor urine output; if in any doubt, especially in adults, consider inserting a urinary catheter.

Ensure that the patient is regularly assessed for evidence of developing paralysis, coagulopathy, or myolysis, even if initially perfectly well.

Antivenom Therapy

Antivenom is the only specific therapy for envenoming. Used correctly, it is effective, comparatively safe, and cost-effective and lifesaving. Used incorrectly, it is ineffective, potentially lethal, and costly and may not save lives.

Antivenom is essentially refined antibody against venom antigens. Some newer antivenoms are Fab or F(ab′)₂ fragments of IgG molecules. Such antivenoms have a reduced rate of immediate or delayed (serum sickness) reactions when compared with whole-antibody preparations. Nevertheless, in most countries, snake antivenom is raised in horses and is thus refined horse serum. All antivenoms, particularly equine antivenoms, may cause both immediate

and delayed allergic reactions. These reactions are discussed later (see "Complications of Antivenom Therapy"). Because of these potential complications, antivenom should be used only when clearly indicated. However, the risk of antivenom reactions is usually far less than the risk of untreated envenoming; *never* withhold antivenom from a patient who needs it because of concern about reactions to antivenom!

WHEN TO USE ANTIVENOM

Antivenom should be used only if there is clear evidence of systemic envenoming, and then as soon as safely practical. Absolute indications would be

- Significant coagulopathy
- Any degree of paralysis
- Significant myolysis (generally, creatinine kinase > 5000 IU/L)
- Any degree of renal damage
- Rapidly advancing severe local effects (some vipers such as rattlesnakes)
- A patient with a known snakebite who had a period of collapse or convulsions before arrival

More difficult are the general symptoms, such as headache, nausea, vomiting, and abdominal pain, which may indicate either envenoming (though not necessarily severe) or anxiety. In general, these symptoms alone would not be an indication for antivenom.

CHOOSING THE RIGHT ANTIVENOM

A specific antivenom for the snake involved is always preferable to a polyvalent antivenom for two major reasons:

- The specific antivenom will usually be lower volume, so the risk of reactions, particularly serum sickness, is reduced and volume overload, important in small children, is less severe.
- Specific antivenoms are always cheaper than polyvalent antivenom.

However, specific antivenoms can be used only if the identity of the snake is known, which may be achieved in several ways, some more reliable than others:

- A visual description of the snake. Such identification is very unreliable in most circumstances and is generally a poor basis for choosing a specific antivenom.
- Identification of a captured or killed snake. Quite apart from the dangers posed by trying to identify a live snake or the hazards from fangs in examining a dead snake, most doctors are ill equipped to accurately or reliably identify a snake. An attempt to capture snakes is not recommended given the potential for further envenoming, even by dead snakes (whole and decapitated).
- Venom detection (only available in Australia). This method is generally preferred, where available. It is mostly reliable, but not every patient with systemic envenoming will have a positive SVDK result. Occasionally, erroneous results occur. Be sure that the clinical and laboratory pattern of envenoming fits the SVDK result. If it does not, urgently seek expert advice!

- Combination of geographic location and local and systemic effects. These criteria have been developed for some regions in recent years based on studies of the effects of envenoming by each species in the region (e.g., Australia, Southeast Asia). There will always be occasional atypical cases that will render such systems less effective, but in expert hands, this type of diagnostic algorithm is most effective.

If all the aforementioned methods fail to give a reliable result, there are two remaining choices. If the range of snake species in the area is limited, it may be possible to create a local "polyvalent" antivenom by mixing two appropriate specific antivenoms. The other alternative is to use a polyvalent antivenom. In some regions this is the only choice.

DETERMINING THE DOSE OF ANTIVENOM

The quantity of antivenom required is variable and depends on the type of snake, the size of the snake, and the number of bites. Children require the same dose as adults.

ADMINISTERING ANTIVENOM

Snake antivenoms should always be given IV. They should be diluted up to 1:10 in saline or a similar diluent and then administered over a 15- to 20-minute period. Infusions should start slowly under close medical observation and the rate gradually increased.

Before giving antivenom, have everything prepared to treat anaphylaxis should it occur, particularly epinephrine. If available, it may be advisable to have an infusion pump set up for an epinephrine infusion and ready to piggyback into an IV line if anaphylaxis develops. Premedication before administration of antivenom is no longer recommended practice. Epinephrine premedication is potentially hazardous and of uncertain value, and antihistamines and hydrocortisone are of no proven value. Pretesting for antivenom allergy, as used in North America in the past, is a useless and potentially dangerous practice because it can directly cause anaphylaxis and can fail to predict anaphylaxis, and it can sensitize the patient, causing problems on subsequent antivenom exposure; hence, pretesting for antivenom sensitivity should not be performed.

COMPLICATIONS OF ANTIVENOM THERAPY

The immediate adverse effects of antivenom therapy are threefold:

- Rash
- Biotoxin-based fever
- Anaphylaxis or anaphylactoid reaction

Rashes are the most frequent reaction, but they are still uncommon. They may herald anaphylaxis.

Febrile reactions are rare with some antivenoms, such as CSL Ltd (Australia) antivenoms, because of high manufacturing standards.

Anaphylaxis or anaphylactoid reactions, though rare (probably less than 1% of cases) with good-quality antivenoms, are potentially lethal. However, some antivenoms have high rates of adverse reaction, with rates higher than 80% noted for some products, particularly those containing unrefined IgG. Reactions to antivenom, including anaphylactic-like reactions, can occur on first exposure, and are thus clearly not mediated by IgE and are not predictable. Accord-

ingly, major life-threatening reactions to antivenom should always be anticipated and preparation for treatment made before commencing the antivenom infusion. There are three major manifestations of these major early reactions: hypotensive shock, bronchospasm, and angioneurotic edema. They should be treated the same as for any other cause of anaphylaxis, that is, with epinephrine (very cautiously IV, via an infusion pump, or subcutaneously [SC] or intramuscularly [IM]: 6 mg/100 mL at 10 mL/hr for the infusion pump or 0.5 mL SC or IM for adults, 0.01 mg/kg SC or IM for children), oxygen, IV fluids, or inhaled epinephrine for bronchospasm via a nebulizer (e.g., 2 mL of a 1:1000 solution). The antivenom infusion should be stopped while the anaphylaxis is being treated and then cautiously restarted once the reaction is controlled, with titration of epinephrine versus antivenom as required.

Delayed effects of antivenom therapy are also uncommon. The only effect of general significance is serum sickness, which may occur 4 to 14 or more days after exposure to antivenom and is characterized by rash, joint pains, fever, and malaise. It is treated with steroids. Though of unproven value, in most parts of the world it is common to prescribe a 5- to 7-day course of oral steroids to every patient who has received a significant dose of antivenom (>25 mL in total) in the hope of preventing serum sickness.

Non-antivenom Therapies

Only antivenom can neutralize venom. Few other treatments are available. For postsynaptic neurotoxins (such as bites by death adders, possibly coral snakes, Australian copperheads, selected cobras such as the Philippines cobra), temporary improvement can be achieved with an anticholinesterase (neostigmine), which is useful if paralysis is severe or antivenom is not immediately available.

Local infection after a snakebite varies with the species and region. In many areas, infection is the exception, so routine prophylactic antibiotics are inappropriate. However, some snake species, notably some of the pit vipers, seem to regularly cause local infection at the bite site. The organisms involved are variable and often atypical, and culture and sensitivity studies are advisable before commencing treatment.

As discussed later, coagulation factor replacement therapy is generally inadvisable for snakebites.

Local swelling may be absent after bites by some species, notably many elapids, but it is a common feature of envenoming by some elapids (e.g., some cobras) and most (but not all) viperids and crotalids. Although the extent of local underlying tissue injury can be severe, even for most viperids and crotalids, there is rarely any underlying compartment syndrome, and fasciotomy is hardly ever required. It should be performed only if there is absolute evidence of a compartment syndrome, such as intracompartmental pressure measurements, and any coagulopathy has been controlled.

ANTIBIOTICS

In general, antibiotics are recommended only if there is secondary infection, but every attempt should be made to target a detected organism.

OTHER

Avoid a tetanus booster IM in the presence of coagulopathy, but most patients should have their tetanus immunization status assessed.

Treating Specific Complications of Envenoming

Many potential complications are associated with envenoming, the most important being extension of major venom effects. Only the most common and important are covered here.

PARALYSIS

The paralysis associated with neurotoxins can present major management problems and secondary complications. It is therefore always best to avoid severe paralysis by detecting the early signs and giving adequate antivenom. If not possible, perhaps because the patient was initially seen late and had established major paralysis as a result of nonreversible presynaptic neurotoxins (bites by some Australian elapids, some kraits, selected other species), management must focus on maintaining adequate respiration, usually by intubation and mechanical ventilation. Intubation is preferable to tracheostomy, at least in the short term, not least because tracheostomy is a potentially lethal procedure if coagulopathy is present. Though paralyzed by the venom, the patient may be fully awake. Such patients require careful nursing and verbal reassurance during this period. It is helpful to talk to them, explain where they are and what is happening, and manually open their eyes and rotate their head so that they can see their surroundings and caregivers. Try to find some part of their body that they can move enough to indicate "yes" and "no" to establish a means of communication. Some patients will require sedation. There is a significant risk of secondary pulmonary infection. The period of complete paralysis is highly variable, from a few days to several months. Even after respiratory function has returned, there may be continued general weakness, and the cranial nerves are sometimes even slower to recover. Occasionally, permanent damage may occur and affect taste or smell, or both.

When paralysis is due to purely postsynaptic neurotoxins, antivenom may reverse this complication, but an anticholinesterase such as neostigmine may also cause a reduction in paralysis, although repeated doses will often be required.

MYOLYSIS

The major issues with myolysis often relate to secondary renal failure and hyperkalemia, which may cause lethal cardiac complications. In the early stages, before renal damage has occurred, an IV fluid load may help spare the kidneys. Alkalinization of urine has also been suggested, but it is unproven in this situation. It is uncertain whether early physical therapy speeds or hinders the muscle healing process. Experimentally, it takes about 4 weeks to recuperate from venom-induced myolysis, but it appears that only slow-twitch fibers recover, not fast-twitch fibers. This change in muscle makeup is unconfirmed in human victims of snakebite myolysis. The extent of muscle loss can be extreme and require a prolonged period of rehabilitation to rebuild normal muscle mass.

COAGULOPATHY AND HEMORRHAGE

Management of coagulopathy generally takes place in the acute stage and is achieved by neutralizing circulating procoagulant or anticoagulant with adequate antivenom, as discussed earlier. Replacement of depleted coagulation factors and fibrinogen with fresh frozen plasma or similar products while there is still active coagulopathy and circulating venom only adds fuel to the fire and increases fibrinolysis and therefore is rarely indicated. It should be performed only after it is clear that all procoagulants are neutralized, as shown by steady improvement in coagulation parameters, the exception being catastrophic bleeding. In most patients, return to safe coagulation function (not normal function) will be sufficiently rapid, within a few hours, that the need for replacement therapy is obviated. In a few cases, return to safe levels may be too slow or reach a plateau, or there may be major active bleeding. In such situations, replacement therapy is worth consideration. Some species, such as the Malayan pit viper, may cause prolonged coagulopathy, in part because of depot release of venom. Repeated doses of antivenom may be required.

Occasionally, the patient may recover from the immediate coagulopathy, only to move into a phase of thrombocytopenia with continued mild DIC. This complication is most often associated with renal failure and is not generally due to continuing envenoming, so further antivenom therapy is unlikely to be helpful.

Some species may cause thrombocytopenia in the early phases of envenoming as a direct venom effect; antivenom is generally the most effective treatment.

RENAL FAILURE

As discussed earlier, renal damage is most often secondary, although it may occasionally be primary, particularly with envenoming by snakes such as Russell's viper. Management will vary depending on the extent of damage. For a simple rise in creatinine and urea without significant oliguria or anuria, expectant treatment is often sufficient, with creatinine and urea usually showing slow improvement after 5 to 10 days. More severe renal failure, often associated with acute tubular necrosis at biopsy, may require a period of hemodialysis, but in most cases, normal renal function will eventually return. Rarely, more severe and permanent damage occurs, such as renal cortical necrosis, and requires continued renal support.

LOCAL NECROSIS

Conservative care is generally appropriate for local tissue injury to the bitten limb. It is unclear how effective antivenom will be in minimizing injury, but it should be given in most cases in the hope of at least reducing the extent of damage, if not eliminating it. Secondary infection can occur but is not routine. Antibiotics should be used only when indicated and should be preceded by culture and sensitivity studies. Fasciotomy to relieve local pressure is a much overused treatment in snakebite and frequently results in long-term functional deficits. It should be reserved only for cases in which significant compartment syndrome has occurred and been proved by intracompartmental pressure measurement (direct or Doppler). Tetanus is a risk after snakebite, but to avoid serious hematomas, an immunization booster (IM) should not be given until after reversal of any coagulopathy.

Psychological Issues

Snakebite, even without envenoming, is often a severe psychological shock for the victim, especially children and particularly if major envenoming has occurred and requires prolonged and extensive treatment. This issue should not be forgotten in the process of managing the patient's care.

Follow-up

Patients who did not sustain significant envenoming and did not require antivenom will generally not require follow-up as long as they are carefully assessed before discharge and the discharge does not occur too soon after the bite.

Patients with significant envenoming requiring antivenom therapy should not go home until it is clear that the envenoming and its complications have resolved, a follow-up plan has been determined, and the patient is made fully aware of the symptoms of serum sickness and that this complication requires immediate review. Follow-up should be arranged at approximately 1 and 2 weeks after discharge.

SPECIAL POPULATIONS

Preexisting illness may cause problems in some forms of snakebite. For instance, patients taking anticoagulants or antiplatelet drugs (even aspirin) may have a higher risk of bleeding if bitten by a snake with a venom causing coagulopathy or with a hemorrhagin-containing venom. Conversely, such medications will influence the interpretation of coagulation tests. Patients taking β-blockers, notably propranolol, may be less responsive to the epinephrine used to treat anaphylaxis. This has not been demonstrated to be a major issue in antivenom therapy, and the usual recommendation that antivenom be used only when clearly indicated applies. However, for patients receiving propranolol or similar medications, the need for antivenom therapy versus the risk of nonresponsive anaphylaxis should be carefully considered. This decision will entail a risk assessment specific for the individual patient, the type of snake, the probable degree of envenoming, and the efficacy and safety record of the chosen antivenom. Certain disease states may predispose to more severe envenoming or outcomes; renal diseases, cardiac diseases, and respiratory diseases are most prominent, but even a history of peptic ulcer may be relevant because it may increase the chance of major bleeding associated with venom-induced coagulopathy, as may liver disease associated with varices. These are but examples; for each patient, any preexisting disease or medication should be considered in relation to its interaction with the effects of the venom.

Pediatric Patients

In part because of their smaller body weight, children, especially young children, are at greater risk of severe or lethal envenoming. They may show more rapid deterioration. Conversely, despite their smaller mass, they should receive "adult" doses of antivenom, although dilution may need to be reduced to avoid fluid overload. There may also be special problems in diagnosis in that a history may often be unobtainable. Significant envenoming may result in an irritable or distraught child who may collapse or even have convulsions.

Pregnant Patients

In pregnancy, any venom-induced coagulopathy may result in bleeding affecting the fetus, and periods of hypotension may also damage the fetus. It is unclear which venom components may cross the placenta and directly affect the fetus, although most procoagulants have a large molecular weight and thus may not pass. Certainly, the health of the fetus should be closely monitored, but should major complications ensue, it may be necessary to sacrifice the fetus to save the mother. Surgical delivery should not be contemplated in the presence of coagulopathy, except when it is the only remaining course of action to save the mother. It is unclear whether paralysis affecting the mother will affect the fetus, although it may not. Similar uncertainty surrounds myolysis. Antivenom should not be withheld because of pregnancy.

Elderly Patients

The elderly and infirm are at greater potential risk from envenoming and should be managed with great caution and possibly more aggressive therapy.

SUGGESTED READINGS

Chippaux JP: Snake bites: Appraisal of the global situation. Bull World Health Organ 76:515–524, 1998.

Fan HW, Cardoso JL: Clinical toxicology of snakebite in South America. In Meier J, White J (eds): Handbook of Clinical Toxicology of Animal Venoms and Poisons. Boca Raton, FL, CRC Press, 1995, pp 667–688.

Gomez HF, Dart RC: Clinical toxicology of snakebite in North America. In Meier J, White J (eds): Handbook of Clinical Toxicology of Animal Venoms and Poisons. Boca Raton, FL, CRC Press, 1995, pp 619–644.

Gutierrez JM: Clinical toxicology of snakebite in Central America. In Meier J, White J (eds): Handbook of Clinical Toxicology of Animal Venoms and Poisons. Boca Raton, FL, CRC Press, 1995, pp 645–666.

Lundin AP, Pilkington B, Delano BG, Friedman EA: Response to inhaled beta-agonist in a patient receiving beta-adrenergic blockers. Arch Intern Med 144:1882–1883, 1984.

Meier J: Commercially available antivenoms (hyperimmune sera, antivenins, antisera) for antivenom therapy. In Meier J, White J (eds): Handbook of Clinical Toxicology of Animal Venoms and Poisons. Boca Raton, FL, CRC Press, 1995, pp 689–722.

Persson H: Clinical toxicology of snakebite in Europe. In Meier J, White J (eds): Handbook of Clinical Toxicology of Animal Venoms and Poisons. Boca Raton, FL, CRC Press, 1995, pp 413–432.

Sutherland SK, Tibballs J: Australian Animal Toxins. Melbourne, Oxford University Press, 2001.

Swaroop S, Grab B: Snakebite mortality in the world. Bull World Health Org 10:35–76, 1954.

Theakston RDG, Warrell DA: Antivenoms: A list of hyperimmune sera currently available for the treatment of envenoming by bites and stings. Toxicon 29:1419–1470, 1991.

Warrell DA: Clinical toxicology of snakebite in Africa and the Middle East. In Meier J, White J (eds): Handbook of Clinical Toxicology of Animal Venoms and Poisons. Boca Raton, FL, CRC Press, 1995, pp 433–492.

Warrell DA: Clinical toxicology of snakebite in Asia. In Meier J, White J (eds): Handbook of Clinical Toxicology of Animal Venoms and Poisons. Boca Raton, FL, CRC Press, 1995, pp 493–594.

Watson A: Don't get stung with the adrenergic blockers (beta or alpha)! Aust Fam Physician 24:1879, 1995.

White J: Elapid snakes: Aspects of envenomation. In Covacevich J, Davie P, Pearn J (eds): Toxic Plants and Animals: A Guide for Australia. Queensland Museum, Brisbane, Australia, 1987.

White J: Elapid snakes: Management of bites. In Covacevich J, Davie P, Pearn J (eds): Toxic Plants and Animals: A Guide for Australia. Queensland Museum, Brisbane, Australia, 1987.

White J: Elapid snakes: Venom production and bite mechanism. In Covacevich J, Davie P, Pearn J (eds): Toxic Plants and Animals: A Guide for Australia. Queensland Museum, Brisbane, Australia, 1987.

White J: Elapid snakes: Venom toxicity and actions. In Covacevich J, Davie P, Pearn J (eds): Toxic Plants and Animals: A Guide for Australia. Queensland Museum, Brisbane, Australia, 1987.

White J: Clinical toxinology; an Australian perspective. In Gopalakrishnakone P, Tan CK (eds): Recent Advances in Toxinology Research. Singapore, National University of Singapore, 1992, pp 722–729.

White J: Poisonous and venomous animals—the physician's view. In Meier J, White J (eds): Handbook of Clinical Toxicology of Animal Venoms and Poisons. Boca Raton, FL, CRC Press, 1995, pp 9–26.

White J: Clinical toxicology of sea snake bites. In Meier J, White J (eds): Handbook of Clinical Toxicology of Animal Venoms and Poisons. Boca Raton, FL, CRC Press, 1995, pp 159–170.

White J: Clinical toxicology of snakebite in Australia and New Guinea. In Meier J, White J (eds): Handbook of Clinical Toxicology of Animal Venoms and Poisons. Boca Raton, FL, CRC Press, 1995, pp 595–618.

White J: CSL Antivenom Handbook. Melbourne, CSL Ltd, 2001.

Williams V, White J: Snake venom and snakebite in Australia. In Thorpe RS, Wuster W, Malhotra A (eds): Ecology, Evolution and Snakebite; Venomous Snakes. London, Zoological Society of London, 1997, pp 205–217.

CHAPTER 102

Rattlesnakes and Other Crotalids

Edward W. Cetaruk

Two families of venomous snakes are native to North America: crotalids and elapids (family Elapidae). The only venomous elapid in the United States is the coral snake, which is discussed in Chapter 103. Crotalid snakes were previously categorized as members of the class Reptilia, family Crotalidae. The new classification is now class Reptilia, family Viperidae, subfamily Crotalinae.[1] Therefore, the term "crotaline" will be used here to refer to snakes in the Crotalinae subfamily. This chapter will address envenomation by snakes in the Crotalinae subfamily that are native to North America. The North American crotaline subfamily is divided into three genera: *Crotalus* (rattlesnakes), *Sistrurus* (pigmy or massasauga rattlesnakes), and *Agkistrodon* (copperheads and cottonmouths). They are found throughout the United States (except in Alaska, Hawaii, and Maine) and Canada (Table 102-1).

Crotaline snakes are also referred to as "pit vipers" because of heat-sensing organs ("pits") located anteriorly on their head between the eye and nostril (Fig. 102-1) for detection and location of their prey. They have poorly developed senses of hearing and sight. Their sense of smell, however, is highly developed. Volatile chemical compounds are sampled by olfactory sensory epithelium in their nostrils or by the flicking of their tongue, which collects and deposits these substances on Jacobsen's organ, a specialized area of olfactory sensory epithelium located on their palate. Other identifying features include a triangular head, vertical elliptical pupils, and a single row of subcaudal scales behind their anal plate. Crotaline snakes have relatively long, curved, hinged fangs that are kept folded against the roof of their mouth except when striking (Fig. 102-1). Additional pairs of replacement fangs are located in the snake's upper jaw and move forward to replace shed or broken fangs. Therefore, one may find a crotaline snake with one, two, or no fangs per side. This variable fang anatomy is important because it may result in an atypical bite wound with one to four puncture marks. Venom is delivered via these canaliculated fangs from paired venom sacs located in the snake's head. Members of the *Crotalus* and *Sistrurus* genera have the characteristic rattle appendage on their tail and are commonly referred to as "rattlesnakes." The characteristic rattle is occasionally lost during the course of a snake's life and is absent on *Agkistrodon* species. It adds another segment with each shedding (one to four times per year) of the rattlesnakes' stratum corneum.

The true number of venomous snakebites per year in the United States is difficult to determine, primarily because of underreporting. However, it is generally thought that there are several thousand bites, including 5 to 10 fatalities, per year in the United States.[2,3] A total of 1685 crotaline snake envenomations were reported to poison control centers in the United States in 1999, including 142 associated with major morbidity and 1 death.[4] Crotaline snakes typically do not strike humans unless threatened or provoked. Most often the victim is a young adult male, often intoxicated and handling a wild or pet crotaline snake. In one study, approximately 87% of snakebite victims were male, and 43% of all bites were "illegitimate" (the victim recognized an encounter with a snake and made no attempt to move away from the snake) as opposed to "legitimate" (the victim was bitten before the encounter with the snake was recognized or was bitten while attempting to move away from the snake). Ingestion of alcohol was associated with 56.5% of all illegitimate bites versus 16.7% of legitimate bites. Three fourths of all bites were to the upper extremity, 27% of which were legitimate, whereas all lower extremity bites were legitimate.[5] Envenomation has even resulted from the handling of crotaline snakes for religious practices in Christian sects found in the eastern United States that interpret the biblical verse Mark 16:17–18: *"In my name. . . they will pick up snakes with their hands. . ."* literally and routinely incorporate snake handling into their worship. The most common site of snakebite is the finger/hand, followed by the toe/foot, leg/ankle, arm/wrist, and other sites including the chest, face, tongue,[6–8] and penis.[9] Approximately 3% to 20% of crotaline snakebites are "dry bites" and do not result in envenomation.[10–12]

BIOCHEMISTRY OF CROTALINE VENOM

Crotaline snake venom is a very complex mixture of dozens of compounds, including peptides, polypeptides, enzymes, biogenic amines, and inorganic metals (Table 102-2).[13,14] The composition of venom varies greatly with the snake species, age, geographic location, and season[15–18] and includes proteins with specific activity against coagulation and fibrinolysis factors, blood vessel basement membranes, cell membranes, muscle tissue, connective tissue, platelets, inflammatory mediators, nucleic acids, and many other macromolecules. Crotaline venom is very stable and retains its toxicity after many years of storage[19] and well after the death of the snake.[20]

TABLE 102-1 Partial List of Crotaline Snakes of the United States

SCIENTIFIC NAME	COMMON NAME	GENERAL GEOGRAPHIC RANGE
Crotalus	Rattlesnakes	
C. adamanteus	Eastern diamondback rattlesnake	Southeastern U.S.
C. atrox	Western diamondback rattlesnake	Southwestern U.S., Mexico
C. cerastes spp.	Sidewinders	Southwestern U.S., Mexico
C. horridus horridus	Timber rattlesnake	Eastern U.S.
C. horridus atricaudatus	Canebrake rattlesnake	Southeastern U.S.
C. lepidus klauberi	Banded rock rattlesnake	Southwestern U.S., Mexico
C. lepidus lepidus	Mottled rock rattlesnake	Southwestern U.S., Mexico
C. mitchelli spp.	Speckled rattlesnake	Southwestern U.S., Mexico
C. molossus	Black-tailed rattlesnake	Southwestern U.S., Mexico
C. pricei	Twin-spotted rattlesnake	Southwestern U.S., Mexico
C. ruber	Red diamond rattlesnake	Southwestern U.S.
C. scutulatus	Mojave rattlesnake	Southwestern U.S.
C. tigis	Tiger rattlesnake	Southwestern U.S.
C. viridis viridis	Prairie rattlesnake	Western and southwestern U.S.
C. viridis abyssus	Grand Canyon rattlesnake	Southwestern U.S.
C. viridis cerberus	Arizona black rattlesnake	Southwestern U.S.
C. viridis decolor	Midget faded rattlesnake	Western U.S.
C. viridis helleri	Southern Pacific rattlesnake	Southern California
C. viridis lutosus	Great Basin rattlesnake	Western U.S.
C. viridis nuntius	Hopi rattlesnake	Southwestern U.S.
C. viridis oreganus	Northern Pacific rattlesnake	Northern California, northwestern U.S.
Sistrurus	Pigmy rattlesnakes and massasauga	
S. catenatus catenatus	Eastern massasauga	Great Lakes region
S. catenatus tergeminus	Western massasauga	Central, southern U.S.
S. catenatus edwardsi	Desert massasauga	Southwestern U.S.
S. milarius spp.	Pigmy rattlesnakes	Southeastern U.S.
Agkistrodon	Copperheads and cottonmouths	
A. contortix spp.	Copperheads	Southern, southeastern, eastern U.S.
A. piscivorus spp.	Cottonmouths	Southern, southeastern U.S.

From Russell FE: Snake venom poisoning. Great Neck, NY, Scholium International, 1983, pp 45–65.

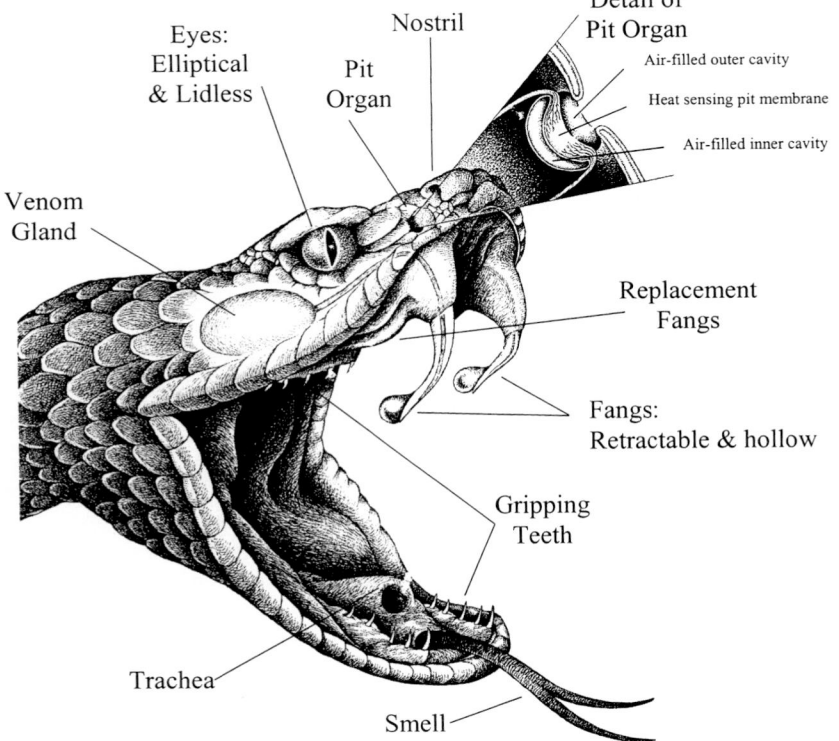

FIGURE 102-1

Anatomy of a crotaline snake head. *(Used with permission from the New York Times.)*

TABLE 102-2 Components of Crotaline Snake Venom

Acetylcholinesterase
Arginine ester hydrolase
Collagenase
DNase
Hemorrhagins
Hyaluronidase
Lactate dehydrogenase
L-Amino acid oxidase
Metalloproteinases
Myotoxins
NAD-nucleotidase
5′-Nucleotidase
Phosphodiesterase
Phosphomonoesterase
Phospholipases A_2, B, C
RNase
Thrombin-like enzymes
Inorganic metals

Data from Russell FE: Snake Venom Poisoning. Great Neck, NY, Scholium International, 1983; Russell FE, Puffer HW: Pharmacology of snake venoms. Clin Toxicol 3:433–444, 1970.

The compounds in venom can be divided into two general groups:

- Peptides and low-molecular-weight proteins that are directly toxic at specific receptors or cell types
- Enzymes that break down specific tissues, cell membranes, or other macromolecules

It is important to note that many venom components may have multiple, similar, or synergistic effects and that these effects are not necessarily mutually exclusive.

Venom metalloproteinases (VMPs) are an important class of enzymes that are responsible for much of the pathophysiology of crotaline envenomation. Their inorganic constituents include Ca, Co, Cu, Fe, K, Mg, Mn, P, and Zn. The hemorrhagic and proteolytic activity of a number of crotaline VMPs can be inhibited by ethylenediaminetetraacetate (EDTA) and restored with the addition of Mg or Zn, thus proving that the metal component is essential for metalloproteinase function.[21] They contain both catalytic and proteolytic domains; induce hemorrhage, myonecrosis, and skin necrosis; and activate the release of inflammatory mediators, including human metalloproteinases and tumor necrosis factor-α.[22–26] These enzymes are also inhibited by α-macroglobulin in vivo (Figs. 102-2 and 102-3).[27] A number of enzymes are tissue-specific digestive enzymes that are thought to initiate digestion of the prey, as well as aid in the absorption of smaller polypeptide toxins. These enzymes include

- Collagenase
- Hyaluronidase
- Proteases

PATHOPHYSIOLOGY OF CROTALINE ENVENOMATION

Individual components of crotaline snake venom target specific proteins, cellular structures, and macromolecules of the victim, some synergistically, to cause local tissue damage, myonecrosis, hemorrhage, coagulopathy, thrombocytopenia, and neurotoxicity. Some venom components may act on more than one substrate, whereas some substrates may be acted on by more than one venom component.

Hemorrhage and Coagulopathy

Local hemorrhage is a common feature of crotaline snake envenomation. Systemic or remote-site hemorrhage is relatively uncommon after a snakebite. Virtually all hemorrhagic toxins identified thus far are metalloproteinases associated with inorganic zinc in a 1:1 molar ratio. Hemorrhagic toxins are known to have both hemorrhagic and proteolytic effects, with their hemorrhagic effects dependent on their proteolytic action. Crude venom from *Crotalus atrox* (western diamondback rattlesnake) has been shown to cause hemorrhage in an experimental mouse model by breakdown of capillary endothelial cells and basement membrane proteins. Dilation of the perinuclear space and endoplasmic reticulum and cytoplasmic swelling are observable within minutes of venom injection, followed by blebbing of endothelial cell membranes into the vessel lumen, which results in loss of cytoplasm, cell thinning, and rupture. Endothelial cells separate from the basal lamina. Eventually, extravasation of erythrocytes, cellular

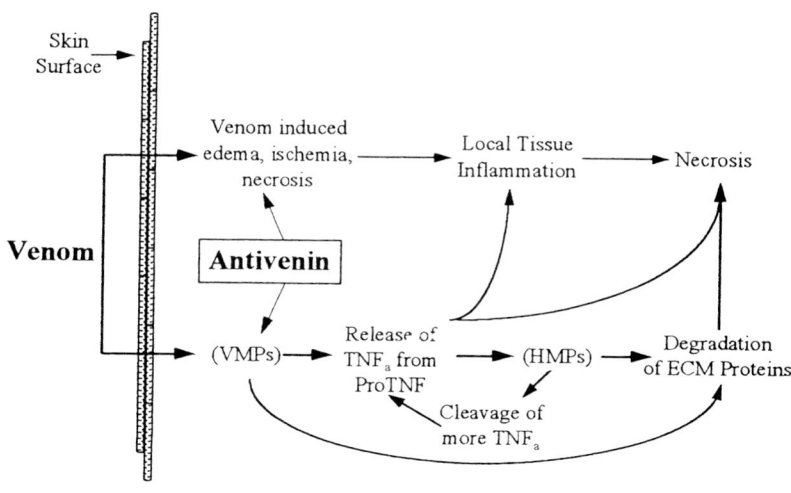

FIGURE 102-2

Venom metalloproteinases (VMPs) in venom trigger the release of tumor necrosis factor-α (TNF-α). TNF-α causes local inflammation and release of human metalloproteinases (HMPs), both of which cause muscle necrosis. Antivenom may halt this process, but only if given within minutes of the bite. (*From Holstege CP, Miller MB, Wermuth M, et al: Crotalid snake envenomation. Crit Care Clin 13:889, 1997; adapted from Moura da-Silva AM, Laing GD, Paine MJI, et al: Processing of pro-tumor necrosis factor-α by venom metalloproteinases: A hypothesis explaining local tissue damage following snake bite. Eur J Immunol 26:2000–2005, 1996.*)

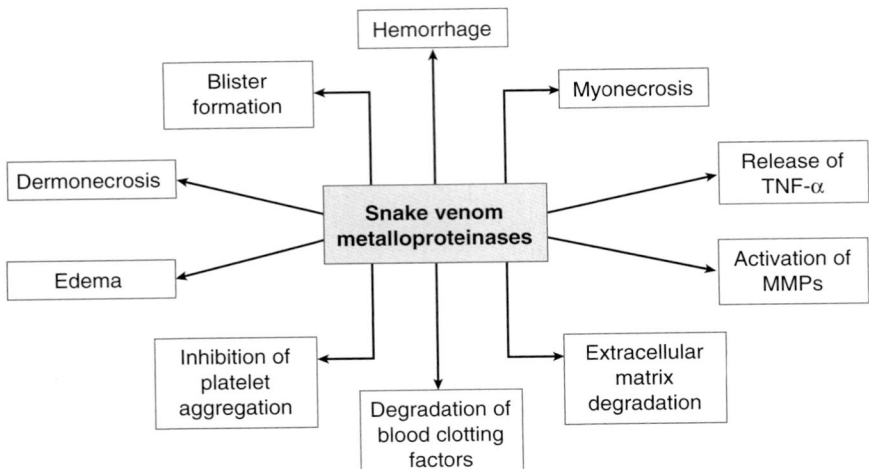

FIGURE 102-3

Summary of the roles played by snake venom metalloproteinases in the pathogenesis of local tissue damage. MMP, matrix metalloproteinases; TNF-α, tumor necrosis factor-α. *(From Gutierrez JM, Rucavado A: Snake venom metalloproteinases: Their role in the pathogenesis of local tissue damage. Biochimie 82:841–850, 2000.)*

debris, and plasma occurs through gaps in the endothelium and causes edema, ecchymosis, cyanosis, and skin blistering. Tight junctions between endothelial cells remain intact. Later, damaged capillaries are occluded by platelets.[28] Specific hemorrhagic toxins (HT) *a, b, c, d, e,* and *f* from *C. atrox* venom, also called atrolysins A, B, C, D, E, and F, respectively, have been characterized. Hemorrhagic toxins *a, b,* and *c* cause endothelial cell lysis and extravasation of capillary contents within minutes of injection. HT*b* was found to induce hemorrhage more slowly than HT*a* and HT*c* and also causes muscle necrosis.[29] All hydrolyze type IV collagen, fibronectin, nidogen, and laminin, all of which are capillary basement membrane components.[22] Hemorrhagic toxins from *C. atrox* and *Crotalus ruber ruber* have been found to be directly cytotoxic to endothelial cells, and HT-1 from *C. ruber ruber* inhibits protein synthesis in vitro.[30] The overall pathophysiologic effect of

these hemorrhagic toxins is loss of microvascular integrity and extravasation of blood cells, plasma, and cellular debris into local tissue with consequent edema, tissue ischemia, ecchymosis, and hypovolemia. Local microvascular hemorrhage at the bite site as a result of a breakdown in capillary integrity begins within minutes of envenomation. This is seen as ecchymosis locally, and it may extend to include large portions or entire limbs and trunk.

The hemorrhage seen with crotaline envenomation is usually accompanied by a coagulopathy. Crotaline snake venoms affect hemostasis at several points, including the clotting cascade and platelet function (Fig. 102-4).[31] Fibrinogen is a dimeric molecule (molecular weight [MW] 340,000) composed of two identical sets of three covalently linked polypeptide chains: Aα (MW 68,000), Bβ (MW 58,000), and γ (MW 47,000). Normally, thrombin cleaves

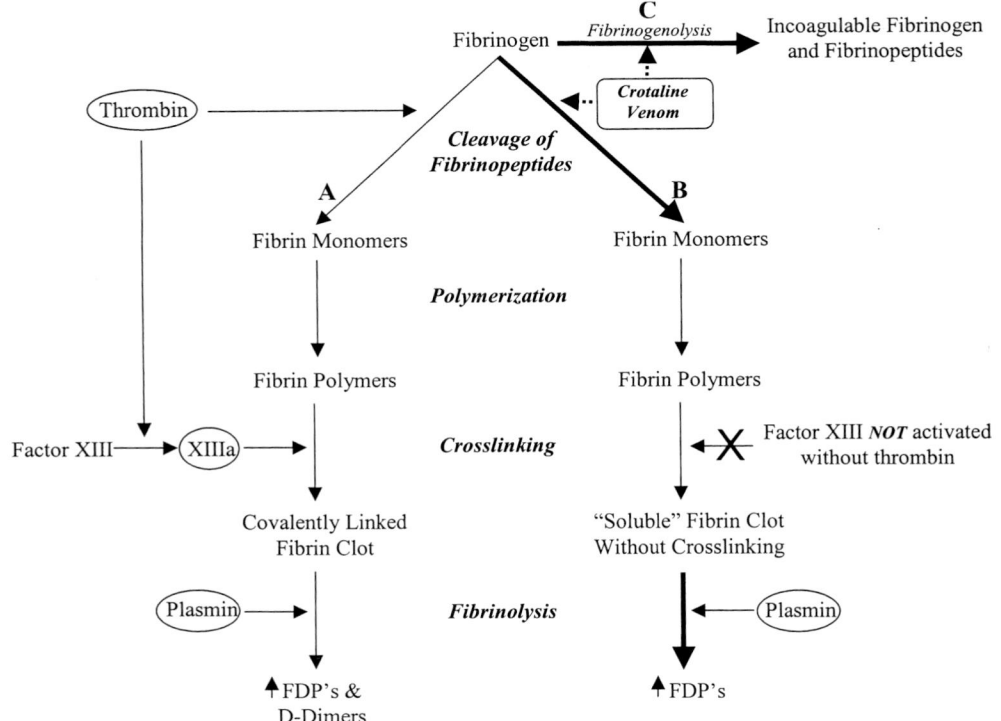

FIGURE 102-4

Comparison of a normal clotting pathway (**A**) and fibrinogenolysis and fibrinolysis by crotaline venom (**B** and **C**). The normal pathway (**A**) requires thrombin to cleave fibrinopeptides A and B to form fibrin and to activate factor XIII to form XIIIa to catalyze covalent cross-linking and thereby produce an insoluble clot. Crotaline snake venom contains enzymes that degrade fibrinogen directly to incoagulable fibrinogen and fibrinopeptides (**C**). Thrombin-like crotaline enzymes form "soluble" clots that are rapidly lysed by plasmin (**B**). Endogenous components of the coagulation system appear in *ovals*. *Boldface arrows* represent the pathway steps most affected by crotaline venom.[27,31–41] FDP's, fibrin degradation products.

fibrinopeptides A and B from *both* the α and β chains of fibrinogen, thus activating fibrinogen to fibrin, which spontaneously polymerizes to form a fibrin clot.[31] Crotaline venom contains many enzymes with fibrinogenolytic, fibrinolytic, and thrombin-like activity.[27,31–37]

Thrombin-like enzymes are a large group of metalloproteinases or serine proteases found in the venoms of North American crotaline snakes, including *Crotalus adamanteus, Crotalus horridus horridus,* and *Agkistrodon contortrix.*[27,31,32,34–38] They preferentially cleave fibrinopeptides A or B from the α and less often the β chain of fibrinogen, respectively, but have not been found to have a significant effect on the γ chain.[27,32,34,37,39] The activity of thrombin-like enzymes varies considerably within the same venom and between crotaline snake species, species of the victim, prey, or experimental model used. Venom from *C. atrox* is thought to lack a thrombin-like enzyme. However, venom collected from three captive western diamondbacks younger than 8 months clotted fibrinogen directly (i.e., a thrombin-like action) and, then, when the snake was 9 to 10 months old, could clot only plasma. From 11 months onward, the venom had no procoagulant activity at all.[15]

Multiple fibrinogenolytic and fibrinolytic enzymes are found in *C. atrox* venom. With prolonged incubation, atroxase, a metalloprotein fibrinogenase from *C. atrox,* hydrolyzes the α chain and then the β chain after the α chain is completely degraded.[27] Four unique proteases from *C. atrox* have been described, including two metalloproteinases that preferentially cleave the α chain and then the β and γ chains of purified fibrinogen and two serine proteases that cleave only the β chain, thereby rendering fibrinogen incoagulable.[35] In vitro, *C. atrox* venom has also been found to preferentially cleave the Aα chain and then the Bβ chain of purified fibrinogen, but in human plasma, the venom preferentially cleaves the Bβ chain. Both mechanisms result in the hydrolysis of fibrinogen into a variety of fibrinopeptides and no fibrin formation.[32]

The thrombin-like enzyme crotalase from *C. adamenteus* (eastern diamondback), though known to have several components, splits fibrinopeptide A from the α chain and has been shown to be a procoagulant that clots purified fibrinogen, or plasma, in vitro. However, this selective cleavage in vivo by crotalase from *C. adamenteus* and by ancrod from *Agkistrodon* species produces an improperly formed fibrin polymer.[33,36,38,40,41] Thrombin-like enzymes also fail to activate factor XIII, which would generally activate the cross-linking of normal fibrin polymers to form a clot. The result is a "soluble" fibrin clot, without cross-linking, that is readily hydrolyzed by the natural fibrinolytic system of the victim, such as plasmin, as well as degradation of fibrinogen into incoagulable fibrinogen derivatives.[37] The net effect of these enzymes is fibrinogenolysis, hypofibrinogenemia, fibrinolysis, increased fibrinopeptides, fibrin degradation products (FDPs), and anticoagulation.[36,42,43] D dimer is a specific measure of intravascular fibrin deposition and plasmin degradation. The fibrin polymers produced by venom thrombin-like enzymes are unable to correctly polymerize into stable, cross-linked fibrin clots and are degraded to FDPs. D dimer is a specific measure of cross-linked fibrin derivatives (from fibrinolysis by plasmin). Because thrombin-like enzymes from crotaline snake venom do not produce cross-linked fibrin, no elevated D

dimer is seen. However, true disseminated intravascular coagulation (DIC), which implies intravascular fibrin deposits in the microcirculation, followed by secondary fibrinolysis, red blood cell damage and hemolysis, consumption of platelets and coagulation factors, and diffuse bleeding, though rare, has been described in crotaline snake envenomation and is accompanied by elevated D dimer levels.[36,39,42,44,45] Coagulopathy can be reversed or the duration shortened with antivenom treatment.[36,39,46,47]

THROMBOCYTOPENIA

Thrombocytopenia is a common finding in crotaline envenomation. It may occur with or without accompanying coagulopathy, may occur soon after envenomation,[11,46,48,49] and may be persistent or recurrent for up to 2 weeks after envenomation.[50,51] Platelet aggregation, sequestration, and consumption, in the normal mechanisms of homeostasis, occur at the site of microvascular hemorrhage with *C. atrox* envenomation,[52] which may be in response to damaged vascular endothelium and may account for some degree of thrombocytopenia.[29] A component of *C. horridus horridus* venom, crotalocytin, has been shown to cause platelet activation and aggregation.[53,54] However, no clear mechanism for crotaline venom–induced thrombocytopenia has been described. DIC does not typically occur in crotaline snake envenomation, but it is rarely seen in severe envenomation and may also account for the thrombocytopenia in these patients.[44] Antivenom is the treatment of choice for venom-induced thrombocytopenia, although the response to antivenom may be variable.[48] Platelet aggregation inhibitors have also been described. Nucleotidases degrade adenosine diphosphate (a potent stimulator of platelet aggregation) to adenosine, thus effectively inhibiting platelet aggregation.[15,31] Phospholipase A_2 degrades negatively charged phospholipids that act as cofactors in platelet aggregation.[11,13,31] Disintegrins are low-molecular-weight polypeptides that compete with endogenous integrins and inhibit platelet aggregation.[15,31]

Myonecrosis

Myonecrosis is a major source of morbidity with crotaline snake envenomation. It begins as vacuolation of myocytes and dilation of the perinuclear space and sarcoplasmic reticulum, subsequent dissolution of the sarcomeres, and eventual complete breakdown of myofibril organization.[55] Although there are probably multiple myotoxic components in crotaline snake venom, myotoxin *a*, a specific myotoxic component of crotaline snake (*Crotalus viridis viridis*) venom, has been isolated and characterized in a mouse model. No hemorrhage, hemolysis, or damage to capillary endothelium or connective tissue was seen when using isolated myotoxin *a*, thus indicating a purely myotoxic effect.[56] Although myotoxin *a* causes skeletal muscle necrosis, additional myotoxins are also found in crude venom from *C. viridis viridis.* Animal studies have shown that polyvalent Crotalidae antivenom, unless administered immediately after envenomation, does not prevent local tissue damage well and has been found to lack specificity for myotoxin *a.* However, tissue injury decreases and survival increases as the time between experimental "envenomation" and antivenom and/or anti–myotoxin *a* serum administration decreases.[47,57,58] A 1:1 mixture of anti–myotoxin *a* serum and Wyeth antivenom was 16 times more effective than anti–myotoxin *a* serum alone and 63 times more effective than polyvalent Crotalidae antivenom alone in neutralizing the myotoxic effects of *C. viridis viridis* venom in a mouse model.[59] This finding underscores the marked complexity of the numerous components of crotaline snake venom. Disruption of intramyocellular calcium metabolism is thought to occur by several mechanisms, including inhibition of sarcoplasmic calcium-ATPase and interaction with sarcoplasmic ryanodine to allow more calcium into the cytoplasm from the sarcoplasmic reticulum. Myotoxin also opens sodium channels, which leads to the influx of extracellular calcium via the sodium-calcium exchanger. The resulting elevated intracellular calcium level is thought to cause skeletal muscle necrosis.[42,60,61]

Metalloproteinases cause hemorrhage and local tissue edema and ischemia, thereby worsening the acute injury at the time of envenomation. Hemorrhagic metalloproteinases cause significant and prolonged injury to the microvasculature that decreases capillary density and therefore the blood supply to the injured muscle. This decrease in blood supply impairs muscle cell regeneration from myogenic cells located beneath the basal lamina of the muscle fibers.[24] Although tissue and muscle necrosis is prominent local to the bite site, diffuse and severe myonecrosis with markedly elevated creatinine kinase levels have been reported after canebrake rattlesnake *(C. horridus atricaudatus)* envenomation. Histologic studies showed identical patterns and severity of myonecrosis both local and distant from the bite site.[62,63] In one experimental animal model, the intramuscular injection of southern Pacific rattlesnake *(C. viridis helleri)* venom produced marked elevations in compartment pressure. The administration of antivenom 1 hour after venom injection resulted in a dose-dependent, statistically significant, lower peak mean compartment pressure than in controls.[63]

Cardiovascular Effects

The primary effect of crotaline venom on the cardiovascular system is hypotension secondary to hypovolemia as a result of extravasation of red blood cells, blood elements, and hemorrhage.[10,11,25,42] Studies on the direct effects of venom on myocardium have described a myocardial depressant protein in *C. atrox* venom.[65] In animal studies, *C. atrox* venom had limited effect on myocardial electrophysiologic function and contractility at high doses.[66] Therefore, the hypotension seen in crotaline envenomation is probably due to a combination of hypovolemia and possibly decreased cardiac output.[25,65,66]

Neurologic Effects

Less common than the significant tissue injury and coagulopathy seen in crotaline snake envenomation are neurologic effects. Though not a pure neurotoxin, the first described neurotoxic component of rattlesnake venom was *crotoxin*, a protein component from the tropical rattlesnake *(Crotalus durissus terrificus)*.[67] In the United States, neurotoxic effects are most often attributed to the so-called Mojave toxin from the Mojave rattlesnake *(Crotalus scutulatus scutulatus)*, although this toxin has also been found in the venom of the speckled rattlesnake *(Crotalus mitchelli mitchelli)*[16] and the western diamondback *(C. atrox)*.[17] Mojave toxin has been described as a protein complex consisting of a basic phospholipase A_2 and an acidic peptide subunit with a molecular weight of 22,000.[68] Mojave toxin is a so-called β-neurotoxin that inhibits the release of acetylcholine at the neuromuscular junction, thereby causing neuromuscular paralysis. Its site of action has been localized to presynaptic neurons and specifically to noncompetitive inhibition of presynaptic calcium channels. This presynaptic calcium channel blockade inhibits the release of acetylcholine from the presynaptic membrane of the neuromuscular junction and as a result causes muscular weakness or paralysis.[69–71] The presence or concentration of Mojave toxin varies greatly with the snake species and geographic location. A distinct geographic variation in venom effects has been found among Mojave rattlesnake populations. Mojave rattlesnake venom from southern Arizona, southern Nevada, southwestern Utah, and southeastern California has a more neurotoxic venom (venom A), whereas Mojave rattlesnakes in central Arizona have more hemotoxicity and much less neurotoxicity (venom B).[72–74]

Myokymia

Myokymia, a rhythmic or semirhythmic pattern of doublet, triplet, or multiplet bursts of muscle motor unit firing producing a continuous, undulating, "wormlike" pattern of muscle contraction similar to fasciculations, has been reported after timber rattlesnake *(C. horridus horridus)*[75,76] and faded midget rattlesnake *(C. viridis decolor)* envenomation.[42] Myokymia may be localized or generalized. Low ionized calcium concentrations have been reported to cause the amplification of myokymia bursts seen in inflammatory neuropathies.[75] Myokymia associated with timber rattlesnake *(C. horridus horridus)* envenomation has resolved with intravenous calcium chloride administration, thus suggesting crotaline venom antagonism of ionized calcium at peripheral nerves as an etiology of myokymia.[76]

CLINICAL PRESENTATION

The clinical manifestations of crotaline snakebites depend on factors such as the location of the bite, the amount of venom injected, the species of the snake, and the age, weight, and underlying health of the victim. Initial findings may range from simply pain at the bite site to profound shock, altered mental status, and death.[10,11,77] Rattlesnake bites resulting in envenomation usually cause localized swelling within minutes of the bite. The incidence of signs and symptoms of crotaline envenomation are presented in Table 102-3. Approximately 3% to 20% of rattlesnake bites do not result in envenomation (defined as swelling, hematologic abnormalities, or regional lymphadenopathy) and are referred to as "dry bites." Symptoms consisting of only pain at the site, without local edema or swelling, may indicate a dry bite or an early manifestation that has yet to demonstrate local sign and symptoms of envenomation.[10–12] The severity of local signs and symptoms of envenomation may vary with the characteristics of the crotaline snake involved. Typically, envenomation by copperhead and

TABLE 102-3 Signs and Symptoms of Crotaline Snake Envenomation

SIGN OR SYMPTOM	INCIDENCE (%)
Fang marks	100
Swelling and edema	74
Weakness	70
Pain	65
Numbness or tingling of the tongue, mouth, scalp, or feet	63
Pulse rate alteration	60
Tingling or numbness of the affected part	57
Faintness or dizziness	57
Blood pressure changes	54
Ecchymosis	51
Sweating or chills	43
Nausea, vomiting, or both	42
Change in body temperature	42
Thrombocytopenia	42
Swelling of regional lymph nodes	41
Fasciculations	40
Vesiculations	40
Respiratory rate changes	40
Increased blood clotting time	37
Decreased hemoglobin	37
Thirst	34
Necrosis	27
Abnormal electrocardiogram	26
Glycosuria	20
Increased salivation	20
Sphering of red blood cells	18
Proteinuria	16
Cyanosis	16
Thrombocytosis	16
Hematemesis, hematuria, or melena	15
Unconsciousness	12
Blurring of vision	12
Swollen eyelids	7
Muscle contractions	6
Retinal hemorrhage	5
Seizures	1

Adapted with permission from FE Russell: Snake venom poisoning in the United States. Annu Rev Med 31:247–259, 1980.

cottonmouth snakes (*Agkistrodon* spp.) causes less severe tissue injury than does envenomation by rattlesnakes (*Crotalus* spp.).[13] As described earlier, the Mojave rattlesnake (*C. scutulatus scutulatus*) has been found to have two distinct venoms, depending on the geographic location.[72,73] Envenomation with venom B is likely to produce more severe local findings and coagulopathy, whereas venom A may be associated with prominent neurotoxicity and less significant local findings.

Local Effects

The appearance of the bite site itself warrants mention. The number of puncture wounds depends on the number of fangs that find their mark and the number of strikes. Because crotaline snakes shed their fangs periodically or lose them to injury and the fangs are replaced by reserve ones stored in the snake's upper jaw, a bite may have only one or multiple puncture wounds. If the strike is tangential, it may appear as a small laceration or lacerations. Thus, the absence of a classic "paired puncture wound" appearance does not rule out the possibility of a crotaline snakebite.

Typically, the initial symptom of a snakebite is pain at the bite site. If the bite has resulted in envenomation, the pain will persist and progress, whereas pain from a dry bite will gradually resolve. Local manifestations of envenomation include edema, ecchymosis, paresthesias, localized tissue necrosis, and the formation of skin bullae (bleb). Bullae are filled with serosanguineous fluid and are generally found near the bite site, although they may be seen distally as well. They develop over a number of hours to several days. Significant tissue destruction often accompanies bullae formation and may necessitate surgical débridement, prolonged wound care, and in some instances, skin grafting. Venom is usually deposited into subcutaneous tissue, outside the deep compartmental fasciae, and spreads locally with the help of enzymes such as hyaluronidase and collagenase and hemorrhagins that promote diffusion of venom away from the bite site.[13] Progression occurs regionally and proximally via lymphatic drainage. Such progression is usually appreciated clinically as an advancing front of tenderness, induration, edema, ecchymosis, and regional lymphadenopathy. Erythema may also be seen. Placing the limb in a dependent position will slow whereas elevation of the limb will promote proximal movement of the venom. Bites in central locations, such as the face, head, neck, or chest, may lead to other significant complications, including airway compromise and rapid onset of systemic toxicity.[8,62]

Overall, the severity of the local signs and symptoms of envenomation depend on a number of factors, including the snake itself (species, age, geographic location), the anatomic location of the bite,[62] and postbite interventions (position of the limb, use of tourniquets or constriction bands, time elapsed since the bite). It is important to note that progression of envenomation is a dynamic process that necessitates a sufficient period of repeated observation to adequately assess the severity of the envenomation and thus determine the need for therapy.

Penetration into muscle is uncommon but can be seen in both adults and children. However, envenomation into deep compartment muscle does increase the risk for compartment syndrome.[78] Symptoms of compartment syndrome include pain that worsens with passive movement, cyanosis, delayed capillary refill, decreased peripheral pulses, reduced sensation, and tense muscle on palpation. Clinical evidence of compartment syndrome warrants immediate evaluation of compartment pressure, either by a needle manometer technique or noninvasively.[79] Although they have no true "compartments," if significant edema and swelling develop after a bite to a finger, ischemia can develop similar to a true compartment syndrome. Therefore, careful attention should be paid to the neurovascular status of any involved digits. Management of these complications is described in the treatment section of this chapter.

Systemic Symptoms

Systemic symptoms of crotaline envenomation include nausea, vomiting, diarrhea, diaphoresis, metallic taste, and hypotension. Anaphylaxis has been reported with and without previous crotaline envenomation.[11,80–83] Systemic neurologic toxicity may include lethargy, coma, neuromuscular weakness, and rarely, seizure. The weakness may be manifested as ptosis, dysphagia, or diffuse peripheral weakness.

Rhabdomyolysis

Crotaline snake venom contains myotoxins that can cause significant rhabdomyolysis, either locally if intramuscular envenomation occurs or systemically from absorption of venom into the systemic circulation. Rhabdomyolysis may also occur secondarily as a result of compartment syndrome. Canebrake rattlesnake (*C. horridus atricaudatus*) envenomation has been reported to cause systemic rhabdomyolysis with identical degrees of myonecrosis at biopsy sites local as well as remote to the bite site.[63,84] Patients with venom-induced rhabdomyolysis may complain of muscle tenderness diffusely, as well as local to the bite site. Urinalysis may show myoglobinuria.[45,85–87]

Neurotoxicity

Though not considered a common feature of North American crotaline envenomation, neurotoxicity has occurred after bites by the Mojave rattlesnake (*C. scutulatus scutulatus*), timber rattlesnake (*C. horridus horridus*), southern Pacific rattlesnake (*C. viridis helleri*), western diamondback (*C. atrox*), and faded midget rattlesnake (*C. viridis decolor*) and can be seen as either a neuromuscular toxicity or primary neurotoxicity. Paresthesias are commonly reported.[42,75,76,85,88,89] Cranial nerve palsies manifested as dysphonia, dysphagia, blurred vision, ptosis, diplopia, and facial muscle paresis have been reported with Mojave (*C. scutulatus scutulatus*) and southern Pacific rattlesnake (*C. viridis helleri*) envenomation.[85,88] Altered mental status and generalized weakness, sometimes requiring endotracheal intubation and ventilation, have been reported.[85,88,90] Myokymia, which may be localized or diffuse, has been reported after timber rattlesnake (*C. horridus horridus*), western diamondback (*C. atrox*), and faded midget rattlesnake (*C. viridis decolor*) envenomation.[42,75,76,89] Neurotoxicity after Mojave rattlesnake (*C. scutulatus scutulatus*) envenomation has been manifested as paresthesias; generalized weakness, sometimes severe enough to cause significant difficulty with ambulation or, rarely, respiratory muscle paralysis requiring intubation; coma; and cranial nerve palsies, including dysphagia, dysphonia, ptosis, diplopia, blurred vision, and facial muscle paresis.[73,76,85,88,89] Interestingly, neurotoxicity from suspected southern Pacific rattlesnake (*C. viridis helleri*) envenomation partially improved when treated with equine-derived Crotalidae polyvalent antivenom, whereas neurotoxicity from western diamondback and Mojave rattlesnake envenomation has been reported to rapidly and completely resolve when treated with CroFab Crotalidae polyvalent immune Fab.[88,89] This could possibly be related to the fact that CroFab is produced with Mojave rattlesnake venom as one of the four venoms used to hyperimmunize sheep for its manufacture.[91] Though not native to North America, envenomation by the South American rattlesnake (*C. durissus terrificus*) has also been reported to cause ptosis, ophthalmoplegia, slurred speech, dysphagia, and generalized weakness with areflexia. This patient also presented

in coma, had a period of improvement after antivenom treatment, but then lapsed back into coma for almost 1 week.[90]

Coagulopathy

Coagulopathy is the primary hematologic toxicity of crotaline venom. Hypofibrinogenemia, either through direct fibrinogenolysis or through the action of thrombin-like enzymes, is common (see Fig. 102-4). Hypofibrinogenemia may be severe, with undetectable fibrinogen levels. Thrombocytopenia is seen in approximately 33% to 42% of envenomations.[11,12] Thrombocytosis is uncommonly seen. The result is abnormal coagulation profiles, including an elevated prothrombin time, elevated thrombin time, hypofibrinogenemia, elevated FDPs, and thrombocytopenia. Rarely, in severe envenomations with both coagulopathy and significant thrombocytopenia, spontaneous hemorrhage may occur.[77] True DIC rarely occurs but can be seen in patients with multisystem organ failure, usually related to severe or intravenous envenomation.[44] Intravascular hemolysis has rarely been reported.[92]

DIAGNOSIS

Assessment of crotaline snakebites should include a complete history and physical examination. Rarely, the patient may be too obtunded or too young to provide an adequate history, and the use of circumstantial evidence or third-party information will be necessary. A history of hearing the rattle of the snake is helpful, but its absence does not rule out a crotaline snakebite. Rattlesnakes may lose their rattle or be too young to have a rattle (juvenile or "button" rattlesnakes), or the snake may be a rattleless member of the crotaline subfamily, such as a copperhead or cottonmouth. It is *not* advisable to request that the responsible snake be brought with the patient for identification. Such practice will probably not help in the management of the patient and is more likely to result in additional envenomation. However, should the snake be provided, it should be identified by the descriptive criteria for crotaline snakes found at the beginning of this chapter and be handled with extreme care, dead or alive. Live snakes should *never* be handled, except by an experienced snake handler, and should be kept safely contained. Dead snakes should also be treated with great care because it is well documented that envenomations have resulted from dead snakes that were thought to be harmless.[20,84,93]

The major factor in the differential diagnosis of crotaline envenomation is snakebite by a noncrotaline snake. The coral snake is the only other snake in the United States with significant toxicity and should be easily distinguishable from a pit viper by its lack of local symptoms and restricted geographic distribution (see Chapter 103). Other nonvenomous snakes may cause mild local symptoms mimicking a crotaline snakebite, but local symptoms or hematologic abnormalities will not occur as one would expect with crotaline envenomation. Other causes of an "envenomation syndrome" consisting of pain, swelling, and systemic symptoms include insect stings (e.g., Hymenoptera) or bites, spider bites, and scorpion stings. Puncture wounds from thorned plants can mimic those from a crotaline snakebite. However, one should be able to differentiate all these potential clinical entities from crotaline envenomation by their failure to develop or progress through an appropriate pattern of signs and symptoms consistent with true crotaline envenomation.

The physical examination should include an overall assessment of the patient, with specific evaluation of the affected limb or bite site, and should be repeated frequently. Physical findings such as tenderness, edema, bullae, swelling, ecchymosis, tender lymphadenopathy, altered mental status, hypotension, bleeding, nausea, vomiting, and fasciculations indicate significant crotaline envenomation. Clinical assessment should be combined with laboratory evaluation for coagulopathy, thrombocytopenia, hypofibrinogenemia, and elevated FDPs. If DIC is suggested by either clinical or laboratory features, the presence of confirmatory evidence of microangiopathic hemolytic abnormalities should be assessed by examination of the peripheral blood smear.

TREATMENT

Initial Stabilization

Because crotaline envenomation can cause life-threatening complications such as hypotension, airway obstruction, and cardiorespiratory failure, initial management should always include appropriate attention to advanced life-support measures (airway, breathing, circulation) and overall resuscitation. Adequate intravenous access with normal saline or lactated Ringer's solution, cardiac monitoring, and blood pressure monitoring should be established on arrival at the hospital. Baseline laboratory parameters should be obtained, including the prothrombin time, complete blood count, platelet count, fibrinogen and FDP concentrations, electrolytes, blood urea nitrogen, and creatinine. Tourniquets, constriction bands, splints, rings, and restrictive clothing should be removed. It is recommended that if the patient has distal swelling, the tourniquet be released gradually to avoid abruptly redistributing a large dose of venom to the central vasculature compartment from the limb. It is also prudent to contact the hospital pharmacy early to determine the amount of antivenom available. It is well documented that many hospitals do not stock adequate amounts of crotaline antivenom.[82,94]

Important components of the history should include the time since the bite, previous treatment, and earlier or current symptoms, both localized and systemic. Additional history

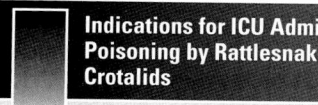

Indications for ICU Admission in Poisoning by Rattlesnakes and Other Crotalids

Any evidence of envenomation with progressing local symptoms

Significant coagulopathy, thrombocytopenia, or bleeding

Any significant systemic symptoms, such as hypotension

Any significant neurologic symptoms, such as altered mental status

Any patient receiving antivenom therapy

regarding other co-existing medical problems (especially hematologic disorders), previous envenomations and treatment with antivenom, and current medications should be obtained. A history to exclude hypersensitivity to horses, if Crotalidae equine-derived antivenom is to be used, or to papaya, papain, or sheep, if CroFab Crotalidae polyvalent immune Fab (ovine) is to be used, is essential. A history of β-blocker use or asthma should also be sought because these are at least relative contraindications to antivenom therapy.

Supportive care measures should include intravenous fluid resuscitation, analgesics, and antiemetics if needed. Fluid resuscitation should begin immediately and before antivenom therapy because envenomed patients may have significant intravascular volume depletion as a result of third spacing of fluids, vomiting, and possibly hemorrhage. Hypotensive patients should be treated with aggressive crystalloid fluid infusion and, if refractory, antivenom.

Management of the Affected Extremity

The affected limb should be elevated above the level of the heart, preferably on pillows in a fashion that does not cause localized compression of the limb. Elevation is used to encourage the absorption of venom from a distal bite site. Failure to adequately elevate a limb during the initial observation period may lead to delay in the diagnosis of significant envenomation. To determine the progression of swelling proximally, measurements of limb circumference should be taken at multiple sites distal to, near, and proximal to the bite site. Measurements should be repeated every 30 minutes at first and less frequently as changes stabilize. To maintain consistent measurements, place marks on either side of the measuring tape at each measurement site. The proximal progression of venom may also be assessed by palpating the limb in a proximal-to-distal direction and marking (with the time of measurement) the leading edge of tenderness, induration, and/or edema. Create an organized chart of the circumference measurements and other observations (e.g., distal pulses) for all sites over time (Fig. 102-5). The combination of these two methods should give the examiner an accurate estimate of the rate of progression of the local tissue effects resulting from the envenomation. Neurovascular evaluations should also be performed at regular intervals to detect signs of the development of elevated compartment pressure. (See measurement of compartment pressure later.)

Antivenom Therapy

The decision to administer antivenom treatment is based on the presence of indicators (i.e., moderate to marked local and systemic effects), balanced by contraindications (e.g., previous treatment). To determine the need for antidotal treatment with antivenom, the severity of the envenomation must be evaluated by assessing three major manifestations of crotaline envenomation: cytotoxicity, hemotoxicity, and systemic toxicity. This classification is summarized in Table 102-4. Alternatively, a quantitative snakebite severity score for the assessment of crotaline snakebite has been developed.[95] It is important to note that the effects of crotaline venom may be manifested within minutes or be delayed for hours.

TIME	Distal to Bite Site	Bite Site	Proximal to Bite Site #1	Proximal to Bite Site #2	Proximal to Bite Site #3	Distal Pulses	Capillary Refill	Neuro Check	Leading Edge (✓)

FIGURE 102-5

Sample flow sheet to document serial measurements of limb circumference and progression of local symptoms. All measurement sites should be marked with double lines between which each measurement is taken. All measurements should be taken with the same tape measure. The limb should be elevated off the bed during measurements. Document the leading edge with all measurements.

Therefore, assessment of envenomation is an ongoing process, and any patient who exhibits any signs or symptoms of envenomation should be assessed over a minimum period of 6 to 12 hours, depending on the degree of progression of local manifestations, systemic symptoms, and coagulopathy. The following are major indications for antivenom:

1. Rapid progression of local symptoms such as swelling, ecchymosis, and pain
2. Significant coagulopathy, hypofibrinogenemia, or thrombocytopenia
3. Neuromuscular toxicity
4. Shock[42]

Consulting a medical toxicologist familiar with the management of crotaline snake envenomation is encouraged if antivenom treatment is being considered. Alternatively, most poison control centers can provide timely consultations.

EQUINE-DERIVED POLYVALENT ANTIVENOM

Antivenom is the treatment of choice for crotaline snake envenomation and is indicated for moderate or severe envenomation as defined earlier. Two crotaline antivenoms are currently available in the United States: equine-derived Crotalidae polyvalent antivenom (Wyeth-Ayerst Laboratories) and CroFab, an ovine-derived Crotalidae polyvalent immune Fab. However, the former is no longer being produced and, after current stocks are depleted, will not be available. The Wyeth antivenom is a product of purified immunoglobulins from horses immunized with the venom of four crotaline snake species: *C. atrox* (western diamondback), *C. adamanteus* (eastern diamondback), *C. durissus terrificus* (tropical rattlesnake), and *Bothrops atrox* (fer-de-lance). The horse serum undergoes a crude purification process in which an antivenom is produced that contains (about 80%) components that do *not* neutralize venom.[96] It is thought to be effective in reversing coagulopathy and stopping the progression of tissue damage, ineffective in reversing local tissue damage, and inconsistent in its ability to reverse thrombocytopenia.[49] It has been shown to have little neutralizing potency for myonecrosis induced by prairie rattlesnake *(C. viridis viridis)* venom and very little activity against myotoxin A.[57,59] In addition, the neurotoxic symptoms from Mojave rattlesnake envenomation have been reported to be resistant to the Wyeth antivenom.[85] Whichever antivenom is used, reconstitution of the lyophilized product requires great care to avoid foaming. The vials should be completely filled with room-temperature sterile water or saline. Occasional gentle agitation may hasten

---

TABLE 102-4 Qualitative Grading of Crotaline Envenomation

ENVENOMATION CATEGORY	DESCRIPTION
None	Swelling, pain, and ecchymosis: pain localized only to the bite site without progression Systemic signs and symptoms: none Coagulation parameters: normal
Minimal	Swelling, pain, and ecchymosis: limited to the immediate bite site without progression Systemic signs and symptoms: none Coagulation parameters: normal with no clinical evidence of bleeding
Moderate	Swelling, pain, and ecchymosis: involving less than the full extremity or, if the bite is on the trunk, head, or neck, extending less than 50 cm Systemic signs and symptoms: present but not life-threatening, such as fasciculations, nausea, vomiting, mild hypotension and/or tachycardia, and/or tachypnea Coagulation parameters: abnormal without evidence of clinically significant bleeding
Severe	Swelling, pain, and ecchymosis: involving more than an entire extremity or threatening the airway Systemic signs and symptoms: markedly abnormal, including severe hypotension, tachycardia, tachypnea, or respiratory insufficiency Coagulation parameters: markedly abnormal with clinically significant bleeding or severe threat of bleeding

From CroFab Crotalidae Polyvalent Immune Product Information, Savage Laboratories, a division of Atlanta Inc., Melville, NY, revised December 2000.

reconstitution without denaturation of protein and loss of antivenom activity. Vigorous shaking will cause foaming and denaturation of the antivenom protein. Refrigeration or reconstitution with cold water will retard solubilization of the lyophilized material.

Though generally effective despite these limitations, the equine-derived polyvalent antivenom must be administered with great care because the risk of immunologic reaction is significant. Allergic reactions range from immediate hypersensitivity (anaphylaxis) to delayed immune complex–mediated hypersensitivity (serum sickness). However, the most common type of initial reaction is a non–IgE-mediated anaphylactoid reaction resulting from rapid administration of the antivenom. Skin testing, though routinely practiced in the United States, has been found to not be a reliable predictor of allergic reactions. Skin testing is commonly performed, however, primarily for medicolegal reasons.[97,98] Skin testing should *not* be performed on anyone with a reported allergy to Crotalidae antivenom or horses and should be performed only on patients for whom antivenom therapy is planned. The skin test is performed by injecting 0.02 to 0.03 mL of a 1:10 dilution of horse serum (provided with Crotalidae antivenom) *intradermally* on the volar aspect of the forearm. The author and others typically test with a 1:10 dilution of the antivenom itself to avoid any false-negative skin tests. Erythema or induration greater than 10 mm in diameter at the injection site, bronchospasm, or hypotension is considered a positive skin test. A negative skin test does not exclude the possibility of an acute allergic reaction to antivenom, but a positive test should preclude the use of equine-derived antivenom except in the setting of life-threatening envenomation and in locations where CroFab is not available.

Equine-derived Crotalidae antivenom should be administered only in a clinical setting capable of cardiopulmonary resuscitation. A minimum of two intravenous lines should be in place and the patient well fluid resuscitated before the administration of antivenom. Intubation equipment, epinephrine, antihistamines (e.g., hydroxyzine), and corticosteroids (e.g., Solu-Medrol) should all be at the bedside to treat any potential allergic reactions. The epinephrine should be mixed and ready to be infused via pump (1 mg in 250 mL of 5% dextrose in water). The antivenom should be started at a very low rate of infusion. The author usually begins at 10 mL/hr, with a gradual increase in increments of 10 mL/hr if no signs or symptoms of anaphylaxis are observed, eventually to deliver approximately 10 vials per hour. If allergic or anaphylactoid symptoms develop during the infusion, the infusion should be stopped and antihistamines, corticosteroids, and epinephrine administered, depending on the severity of the reaction. If epinephrine infusion is required, the solution constituted as suggested earlier (4 µg/mL) should be titrated at 30 to 60 mL/hr or 0.5 to 1.0 mL/kg/hr. The need for antivenom therapy should also be reassessed against the severity of the allergic reaction. If the decision to use equine-derived antivenom is made, a reasonable starting dose is 5 to 10 vials, with additional doses, usually in 5- to 10-vial increments, administered as needed based on the progression of signs and symptoms. Serum sickness, a type III hypersensitivity reaction, occurs in 50% to 75% of all patients treated with equine-derived antivenom. The incidence of serum sickness increases with increasing amounts

(vials) of antivenom administered. It typically occurs 1 day to 3 weeks after treatment and is seen as a diffuse maculopapular rash (Fig. 102-6), urticaria, nausea, malaise, fever, myalgias, and arthralgias. It can be treated with oral antihistamines (e.g., hydroxyzine) and oral corticosteroids such as prednisone. Glomerulonephritis and neuritis are rare complications of serum sickness.[97,99,100]

Anti-Crotalidae CroFab

CroFab (Crotalidae polyvalent immune Fab ovine) is prepared by immunizing sheep with venom from each of the following North American crotaline snakes: *C. atrox* (western diamondback rattlesnake), *C. adamanteus* (eastern diamondback rattlesnake), *C. scutulatus scutulatus* (Mojave rattlesnake), and *Agkistrodon piscivorus* (cottonmouth). Each monospecific antivenom is prepared by fractionating immunoglobulin from ovine serum, digesting it with papain, isolating the venom-specific Fab fragments by ion-exchange and affinity chromatography, and pooling them into the polyvalent final product.[91] The final CroFab product that contains all four monospecific antivenoms is a Fab fragment antivenom lacking the species-specific allergenic Fc portion of the immunoglobulin. Therefore, the risk of adverse reactions is greatly reduced, and skin testing is not generally considered necessary. As with any antivenom developed in animals, there is a remote possibility that CroFab may contain heterologous (ovine) proteins. Therefore, there still remains a theoretically finite, though probably very small risk of hypersensitivity reaction with CroFab administration. All precautions for treatment of an allergic reaction, as for the administration of equine-derived antivenom, should be taken during CroFab administration.[91]

The indications for CroFab administration are essentially the same as those for the administration of equine-derived antivenom (see earlier). The initial dose is four to six vials, followed by an observation period of 1 hour. If initial control, as defined by the complete arrest of local manifestations, reversal of coagulopathy, and resolution of systemic manifestations, is *not* achieved, additional doses of four to six vials should be repeated until the envenomation syndrome is controlled. Once initial control has been established, additional two-vial doses should be administered every 6 hours for a minimum of three doses, or more if indicated (Fig. 102-7).

Recurrent coagulopathy after antivenom treatment with both polyvalent equine-derived antivenom[50] (Crotalidae) and CroFab[51] has been reported. Patients in whom coagulopathy

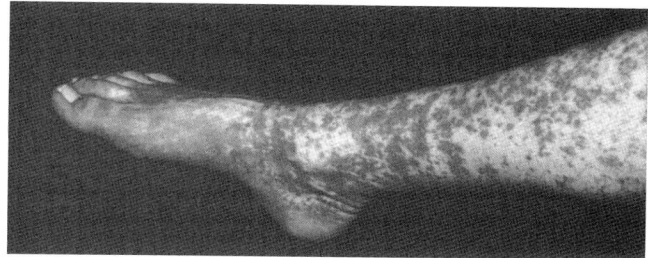

FIGURE 102-6

Serum sickness manifested as a diffuse maculopapular rash. *(Courtesy of Ken Kulig, M.D.)* See Color Fig. 102-6.

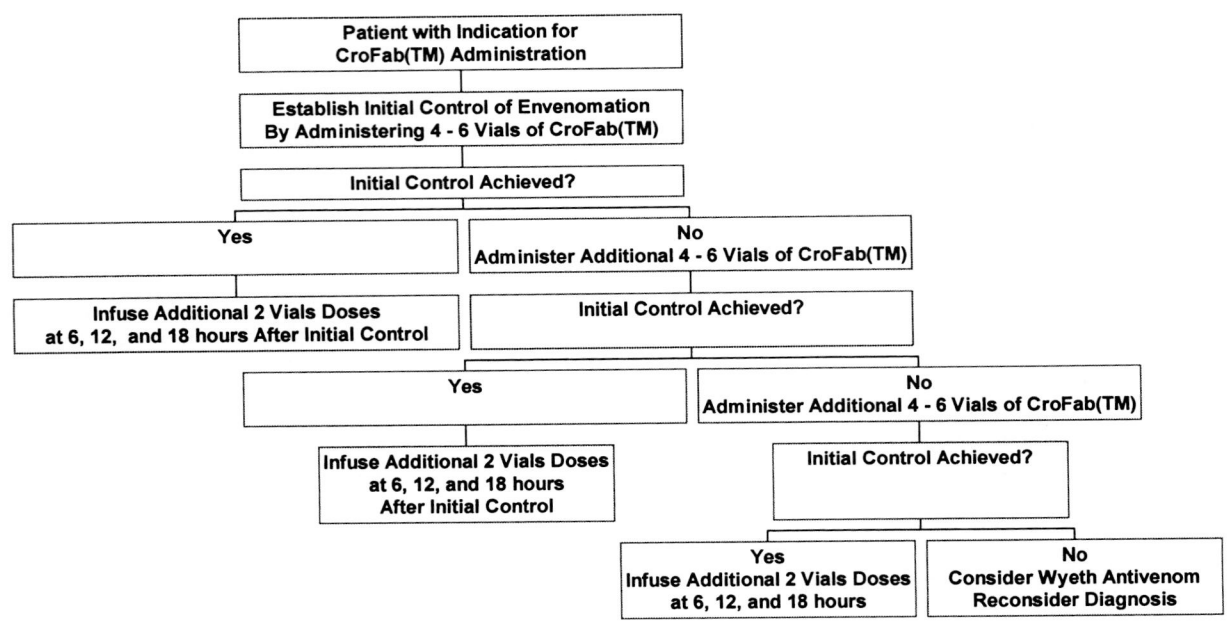

FIGURE 102-7

Dosing algorithm for CroFab. *(From Dart RC: The Clinical Use of Crotalidae Polyvalent Immune Fab (Ovine)—CroFab. Presentation, 2001. Used with permission.)*

develops within 12 hours of CroFab administration have an approximately two-thirds chance of late recurrence.[101] Because severe recurrent coagulopathy may occur after initial treatment with CroFab, close follow-up in high-risk patients (e.g., those with severe coagulopathy at initial assessment) is necessary. It has been recommended that all patients treated with CroFab be reevaluated within 5 days after treatment.[51,91,101] Patients considered to be at higher risk for recurrence (those with abnormal coagulation within the first 36 hours) should be reassessed approximately every 48 hours after the last antivenom dose until coagulation parameters are clearly stable or improving for several days.[101] If coagulation parameters become significantly abnormal or there is a definite relapsing trend, daily reassessment is recommended, and retreatment with antivenom should be considered.[101]

Compartment Syndrome

Although true compartment syndrome after a crotaline snakebite is rare, tensely swollen extremities are not. Thus, in the absence of a careful evaluation, the incorrect diagnosis of a compartment syndrome could be made. Because the envenomation is almost always limited to the subcutaneous compartment, there is little chance for a compartment syndrome, which by definition involves the deep compartments. Clinical signs and symptoms of compartment syndrome include (1) pain out of proportion to the apparent injury, (2) hypoesthesia in the distribution of nerves passing through the compartment in question, (3) pain on passive stretch of the muscles within the compartment, (4) tenseness of the compartment on palpation, and (5) weakness of muscles in the compartment.[102] Simply, if a compartment syndrome is suspected, compartment pressures *must* be measured with a needle manometer or other accurate means.

The initial treatment of crotaline snake venom–induced compartment syndrome is antivenom. It has been shown to be effective in reducing compartment pressures in animal models,[64] as well as clinical practice.[103] If compartment pressures are documented to be persistently greater than 30 to 40 mm Hg, fasciotomy is indicated.[102,104] The fingers have no true deep compartments, but elevated tissue pressure will impede distal blood flow. Because of the lack of a practical method to measure compartment pressure in the digits, a common site of envenomation, the diagnosis of elevated tissue pressure in the finger must be made on clinical grounds. The finding of a tensely swollen finger, with absent or poor capillary refill, cyanosis, or pallor, and decreased sensation is consistent with elevated "digital compartment" pressure and is an indication for surgical intervention. The recommended procedure is digital dermotomy, which consists of a longitudinal incision, through the skin only, along either the medial or lateral aspect of the affected finger, preferably performed by a physician with specialized training in surgery of the hand. Though not an emergency intervention, early rehabilitation to increase both passive and active range of motion for finger and hand bites is recommended to minimize loss of function.

Antibiotics

The use of antibiotics in the treatment of crotaline snakebite has been debated for some time. A number of organisms have been cultured from the mouth of crotaline snakes, including *Pseudomonas aeruginosa, Proteus* species, *Clostridium* species, *Bacteroides fragilis*, and *Staphylococcus* and *Streptococcus* species.[105] However, the incidence of wound infection is low. In one series of patients treated without antibiotics (n = 32), wound infection developed in 3%, whereas in patients treated with prophylactic antibiotics (n = 9), wound infection developed in 22%.[104] Therefore, it is recommended that antibiotics be used to treat infections as they occur, but not for empirical prophylaxis.[106,107] Tetanus prophylaxis is recommended.

SPECIAL POPULATIONS

Children

The treatment of children with crotaline snakebite envenomation has been studied, with varied recommendations for treatment.[108–110] Crotaline envenomation syndrome is similar in children and adults. Because it is likely that most human envenomations result from defensive bites, children and adults should receive an equivalent dose of venom. However, smaller pediatric patients may receive higher doses of venom per kilogram of body weight than adults do. Accordingly, clinical progression may be more rapid, and clinical severity (e.g., hemodynamic instability) may be more marked in young children. Infants may have difficulty providing an accurate history of the envenomation and are also unable to communicate changes in pain and sensation, systemic symptoms such as metallic taste, or paresthesias. The same indications and contraindications for antivenom treatment are applicable for pediatric envenomation patients as for adults. Therefore, the same treatment guidelines for adults may by applied to the pediatric population. The dose of antivenom, which is directed at the venom injected, should not be reduced on the basis of patient age or size.

Pregnant Patients

Crotaline envenomation in pregnant patients is a rare event. However, what little data that have been reported indicate a higher rate of fetal demise. It is thought that the overall severity of the mother's course will determine the outcome of the fetus. Therefore, treatment of a pregnant patient should be the same as for other patients.[42]

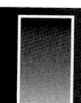

> **Common Misconceptions about Poisoning by Rattlesnakes and Other Crotalids**
>
> 1. Patients without significant symptoms on initial evaluation are not envenomated.
> 2. Surgical therapy is the treatment of choice over antivenom.
> 3. Children require "pediatric" rather than appropriate, or "adult," doses of antivenom.

> **Key Points in Poisoning by Rattlesnakes and Other Crotalids**
>
> 1. Crotaline envenomation is a dynamic, often gradually evolving process that necessitates continued reevaluation over time.
> 2. Early evaluation and intervention with antivenom can reduce morbidity and mortality.
> 3. An envenomed limb should be elevated during the initial evaluation to assess the progression of local toxicity.

continued

> **Key Points in Poisoning by Rattlesnakes and Other Crotalids** *continued*
>
> 4. Patients may need additional doses of antivenom as their symptoms progress.
> 5. Adequate preparation and close monitoring for hypersensitivity reactions are essential to the safe administration of anticrotaline antivenom.
> 6. Recurrent severe coagulopathy may occur after initial treatment with CroFab and necessitate close follow-up in high-risk patients (e.g., those with severe coagulopathy at initial evaluation).

REFERENCES

1. McDiarmid RW, Campbell JA, Toure TA: Snake Species of the World: A Taxonomic and Geographical Reference. Washington, DC, The Herpetologist's League, 1999, pp 234–351.
2. Langley RL, Morrow WE: Deaths resulting from animal attacks in the United States. Wild Environ Med 8:8–16, 1997.
3. Parrish HM: Incidence of treated snakebite in the United States. Public Health Rep 81:269–276, 1966.
4. Litovitz TL, Klein-Schwartz W, White S, et al: 1999 Annual report of the American Association of Poison Control Centers Toxic Exposure Surveillance System. Am J Emerg Med 18:517–574, 1999.
5. Curry SC, Horning D, Brady P, et al: The legitimacy of rattlesnake bites in central Arizona. Ann Emerg Med 18:658–663, 1989.
6. Seiler JG, Sagerman SD, Geller RJ, et al: Venomous snake bite: Current concepts of treatment. Orthopedics 17:707–714, 1994.
7. Wingert WA, Chan L: Rattlesnake bites in southern California and rationale for treatment. West J Med 148:37–44, 1988.
8. Gerkin R, Sergent KC, Curry SC, et al: Life-threatening airway obstruction from rattlesnake bite to the tongue. Ann Emerg Med 16:813–816, 1987.
9. Crane DB, Irwin JS: Rattlesnake bite of glans penis. Urology 26:50–52, 1985.
10. Russell FE, Carlson RW: Snake venom poisoning in the United States. Experience with 550 cases. JAMA 233:341–344, 1975.
11. Russell FE: Snake venom poisoning in the United States. Annu Rev Med 31:247–259, 1980.
12. Tanen DA, Ruha A-M, Graeme KA, et al: Epidemiology and hospital course of rattlesnake envenomations cared for at a tertiary referral center in central Arizona. Acad Emerg Med 8:177–182, 2001.
13. Russell FE: Snake Venom Poisoning. Great Neck, NY, Scholium International, 1983.
14. Russell FE, Puffer HW: Pharmacology of snake venoms. Clin Toxicol 3:433–444, 1970.
15. Reid HA, Theakston RD: Changes in coagulation effects by venoms of *Crotalus atrox* as snakes age. Am J Trop Med Hyg 27:1053–1057, 1978.
16. Glenn JL, Straight RC: Venom properties of the rattlesnakes *(Crotalus)* inhabiting the Baja region of Mexico. Toxicon 23:769–775, 1985.
17. Minton SA, Weinstein SA: Geographic and ontogenic variation in venom of the western diamondback rattlesnake *(Crotalus atrox)*. Toxicon 24:71–80, 1986.
18. Meier J: Individual and age-dependent variations in the venom of the fer-de-lance *(Bothrops atrox)*. Toxicon 24:41–46, 1986.
19. Russell FE: Snake Venom Poisoning. Great Neck, NY, Scholium International, 1983, p 156.
20. Griffen D, Donovan JW: Significant envenomation from a preserved rattlesnake head (in a patient with a history of immediate hypersensitivity to antivenin). Ann Emerg Med 15:955–958, 1986.
21. Friedrich C, Tu AT: Role of metals in snake venoms for hemorrhagic, esterase and proteolytic activities. Biochem Pharmacol 20:1549–1556, 1971.
22. Bjarnason JB, Fox JW: Hemorrhagic metalloproteinases from snake venoms. Pharmacol Ther 62:325–372, 1994.
23. Moura-da-Silva AM, Laing GD, Paine MJ, et al: Processing of pro-tumor necrosis factor-α by venom metalloproteinases: A hypothesis explaining local tissue damage following snake bite. Eur J Immunol 26:2000–2005, 1996.

24. Gutierrez JM, Rucavado A: Snake venom metalloproteinases: Their role in the pathogenesis of local tissue damage. Biochimie 82:841–850, 2000.

25. Schaeffer RC, Pattabhiraman TR, Carlson RW, et al: Cardiovascular failure produced by a peptide from the venom of the southern Pacific rattlesnake, *Crotalus viridis helleri*. Toxicon 17:447–453, 1979.

26. Rucavado A, Nunez J, Gutierrez JM: Blister formation and skin damage induced by BaP1, a haemorrhagic metalloproteinase from the venom of the snake *Bothrops asper*. Int J Exp Pathol 79:245–254, 1998.

27. Willis TW, Tu AT: Purification and biochemical characterization of Atroxase, a nonhemorrhagic fibrinolytic protease from western diamondback rattlesnake venom. Biochemistry 27:4769–4777, 1988.

28. Ownby CL, Kainer RA, Tu AT: Pathogenesis of hemorrhage induced by rattlesnake venom. Am J Pathol 76:401–414, 1974.

29. Ownby CL, Bjarnason J, Tu AT: Hemorrhagic toxins from rattlesnake *(Crotalus atrox)* venom. Am J Pathol 93:201–218, 1978.

30. Obrig TG, Louise CB, Moran TP, et al: Direct cytotoxic effects of hemorrhagic toxins from *Crotalus ruber ruber* and *Crotalus atrox* on human vascular endothelial cells, in vitro. Microvasc Res 46:412–416, 1993.

31. Braud S, Bon C, Wisner A: Snake venom proteins acting on hemostasis. Biochimie 82:851–859, 2000.

32. Pandya BV, Rubin RN, Olexa SA, et al: Unique degradation of human fibrinogen by proteases from western diamondback rattlesnake *(Crotalus atrox)* venom. Toxicon 21:515–526, 1983.

33. Bajwa SS, Markland FS, Russel FE: Fibrinolytic and fibrinogen clotting enzymes present in the venoms of western diamondback rattlesnake, *Crotalus atrox*, eastern diamondback rattlesnake, *Crotalus adamanteus*, and southern Pacific rattlesnake, *Crotalus viridis helleri*. Toxicon 19:53–59, 1981.

34. Retzios AD, Markland FS: A direct-acting fibrinolytic enzyme from the venom of *Agkistrodon contortrix contortrix*: Effects on various components of the human blood coagulation and fibrinolysis systems. Thromb Res 52:541–552, 1988.

35. Pandya BV, Budzynski AZ: Anticoagulant proteases from western diamondback rattlesnake *(Crotalus atrox)* venom. Biochemistry 23:460–470, 1984.

36. Kitchens CS, Van Mierop LH: Mechanism of defibrination in humans after envenomation by the Eastern diamondback rattlesnake. Am J Hematol 14:345–353, 1983.

37. Budzynski AZ, Pandya BV, Rubin RN, et al: Fibrinogenolytic afibrinogenemia after envenomation by western diamondback rattlesnake *(Crotalus atrox)*. Blood 63:1–14, 1984.

38. Markland FS, Damus PS: Purification and properties of a thrombin-like enzyme from the venom of *Crotalus adamanteus* (eastern diamondback rattlesnake). J Biol Chem 246:6460–6473, 1971.

39. Kitchens CS: Hemostatic aspects of envenomation by North American snakes. Hematol Oncol Clin North Am 6:1189–1195, 1992.

40. Spellman GG, Macoviak JA, Gralnick HR: Comparison of polymerization of ancrod and thrombin fibrin monomers. Blood 50:619–624, 1977.

41. Pizzo SV, Schwartz ML, Hill RL, et al: Mechanism of ancrod anticoagulation. J Clin Invest 51:2841–2850, 1972.

42. Holstege CP, Miller MB, Wermuth M, et al: Crotalid snake envenomation. Crit Care Clin 13:889–921, 1997.

43. Russell FE: Snake Venom Poisoning. Great Neck, NY, Scholium International, 1983, p 199.

44. Curry SC, Kunkel DB: Death from a rattlesnake bite. Am J Emerg Med 3:227–235, 1985.

45. Ahlstrom NG, Luginbuhl W, Tisher CC: Acute anuric renal failure after rattlesnake bite. South Med J 84:783–785, 1991.

46. Bond GR, Burkhart KK: Thrombocytopenia following timber rattlesnake envenomation. Ann Emerg Med 30:40–44, 1997.

47. Russell FE, Ruzic N, Gonzalez H: Effectiveness of antivenin (Crotalidae) polyvalent following injection of *Crotalus* venom. Toxicon 11:461–464, 1973.

48. Bush SP, Wu VH, Corbett SW: Rattlesnake venom–induced thrombocytopenia response to antivenin (Crotalidae) polyvalent: A case series. Acad Emerg Med 7:181–185, 2000.

49. Riffer E, Curry SC, Gerkin R: Successful treatment with antivenin of marked thrombocytopenia without significant coagulopathy following rattlesnake bite. Ann Emerg Med 16:1297–1299, 1987.

50. Bogdan GM, Dart RC, Falbo SC, et al: Recurrent coagulopathy after antivenom treatment of crotalid snakebite. South Med J 93:562–566, 2000.

51. Boyer LV, Seifert SA, Clark RF, et al: Recurrent and persistent coagulopathy following pit viper envenomation. Arch Intern Med 159:706–710, 1999.

52. Simon TL, Grace TG: Envenomation coagulopathy in wounds from pit vipers. N Engl J Med 305:443–447, 1981.

53. Scmaier AH, Colman RW: Crotalocytin: Characterization of the timber rattlesnake platelet activating protein. Blood 56:1020–1028, 1980.

54. Schmaier AH, Claypool W, Colman RW: Crotalocytin: Recognition and purification of a timber rattlesnake platelet aggregating protein. Blood 56:1013–1019, 1980.

55. Stringer JM, Kainer RA, Tu AT: Myonecrosis induced by rattlesnake venom. Am J Pathol 67:127–140, 1972.

56. Ownby CL, Cameron D, Tu AT: Isolation of myotoxic component from rattlesnake *(Crotalus viridis viridis)* venom. Am J Pathol 85:149–166, 1976.

57. Ownby CL, Woods WM, Odell GV: Antiserum to myotoxin from prairie rattlesnake *(Crotalus viridis viridis)* venom. Toxicon 17:373–380, 1979.

58. Ownby CL, Odell GV, Woods WM, et al: Ability of antiserum to myotoxin α from prairie rattlesnake *(Crotalus viridis viridis)* venom to neutralize local myotoxicity and lethal effects of myotoxin α and homologous crude venom. Toxicon 21:35–45, 1983.

59. Ownby CL, Colberg TR, Odell GV: Ability of a mixture of antimyotoxin α serum and polyvalent (Crotalidae) antivenin to neutralize myonecrosis, hemorrhage, and lethality induced by prairie rattlesnake *(Crotalus viridis viridis)* venom. Toxicon 23:317–324, 1985.

60. Volpe P, Damiani E, Maurer A, et al: Interaction of myotoxin α with the Ca^{2+}-ATPase of skeletal muscle sarcoplasmic reticulum. Arch Biochem Biophys 246:90–97, 1986.

61. Tu AT: Tissue damaging effects by snake venoms: Hemorrhage and myonecrosis. In Handbook of Natural Toxins, vol 5, Reptile Venoms and Toxins, New York, Marcel Dekker, 1991.

62. Moss ST, Bogdan G, Dart RC, et al: Association of rattlesnake bite location with severity of clinical manifestations. Ann Emerg Med 30:58–61, 1997.

63. Caroll RR, Hall EL, Kitchens CS: Canebrake rattlesnake envenomation. Ann Emerg Med 30:45–48, 1997.

64. Garfin SR, Castilonia RR, Mubarak SJ, et al: The effect of antivenin on intramuscular pressure elevations induced by rattlesnake venom. Toxicon 23:677–680, 1985.

65. Bonilla CA: Hypotension—a hypotensive peptide isolated from *Crotalus atrox* venom: Purification, amino acid composition and terminal amino acid residues. FEBS Lett 68:297–302, 1976.

66. Posner P, MacIntosh BR, Gerencser GA: Effects of western diamondback rattlesnake *(Crotalus atrox)* venom on heart muscle. Toxicon 19:330–333, 1981.

67. Slotta A, Fraenkel-Conrat H: Two active proteins from rattlesnake venom. Nature 142:213, 1938.

68. Cate RL, Bieber AL: Purification and characterization of Mojave *(Crotalus scutulatus scutulatus)* toxin and its subunits. Arch Biochem Biophys 189:397–408, 1978.

69. Valdes JJ, Thompson RG, Wolff VL, et al: Inhibition of calcium channel dihydropyridine receptor binding by purified Mojave toxin. Neurotoxicol Teratol 11:129–133, 1989.

70. Ho CL, Lee CY: Presynaptic actions of Mojave toxin isolated from Mojave rattlesnake *(Crotalus scutulatus)* venom. Toxicon 19:889–892, 1981.

71. Gopalakrishnakone P, Hawgood BJ, Holbrooke SE, et al: Sites of action of the Mojave toxin isolated from the venom of the Mojave rattlesnake. Br J Pharmacol 69:421–431, 1980.

72. Glenn JL, Straight R: Mojave rattlesnake *Crotalus scutulatus scutulatus* venom: Variation in toxicity with geographical origin. Toxicon 16:81–84, 1978.

73. Hardy DL: Envenomation by the Mojave rattlesnake *(Crotalus scutulatus scutulatus)* in southern Arizona, U.S.A. Toxicon 21:111–118, 1983.

74. Glenn JL, Straight RC, Wolfe MC, et al: Geographical variation in *Crotalus scutulatus scutulatus* (Mojave rattlesnake) venom properties. Toxicon 21:119–130, 1983.

75. Brick JF, Gutmann L: Rattlesnake-induced myokymia. Muscle Nerve 5:S98-S100, 1982.

76. Brick JF, Gutmann L, Brick J, et al: Timber rattlesnake venom-induced myokymia: Evidence for peripheral nerve origin. Neurology 37:1545–1546, 1987.

77. Hardy DL: Rattlesnake envenomation in Arizona: 1969–1984. Clin Toxicol 24:1–10, 1986.
78. Robert RS, Csencsitz TA, Heard CW: Upper extremity compartment syndromes following pit viper envenomation. Clin Orthop 193:184–188, 1985.
79. Curry SC, Kraner JC, Kunkel DB, et al: Noninvasive vascular studies in management of rattlesnake envenomations to extremities. Ann Emerg Med 14:1081–1084, 1985.
80. Tanen DA, Ruha A-M, Graeme KA, et al: Rattlesnake envenomations: Unusual case presentations. Arch Intern Med 161:474–479, 2001.
81. Hogan DE, Dire DJ: Anaphylactic shock secondary to rattlesnake bite. Ann Emerg Med 19:814–816, 1990.
82. Dart RC, Duncan C, McNally J: Effect of inadequate antivenin stores on the medical treatment of crotalid envenomation. Vet Hum Toxicol 33:267–269, 1991.
83. Nordt SP: Anaphylactoid reaction to rattlesnake envenomation. Vet Hum Toxicol 42:12, 2000.
84. Kitchens CS, Hunter S, Van Mierop LH: Severe myonecrosis in a fatal case of envenomation by the canebrake rattlesnake *(Crotalus horridus atricaudatus)*. Toxicon 25:455–458, 1987.
85. Jensen PW, Perkin RM, Stralen DV: Mojave rattlesnake envenomation: Prolonged neurotoxicity and rhabdomyolysis. Ann Emerg Med 21:322–325, 1992.
86. Moss ST, Bogdan G, Nordt SP, et al: An examination of serial urinalyses in patients with North American crotalid envenomation. Clin Toxicol 36:329–335, 1998.
87. Azevedo-Marques MM, Cupo P, Coimbra TM, et al: Myonecrosis, myoglobinuria and acute renal failure induced by South American rattlesnake *(Crotalus durissus terrificus)* envenomation in Brazil. Toxicon 23:631–636, 1985.
88. Bush SP, Siedenburg E: Neurotoxicity associated with suspected southern Pacific rattlesnake *(Crotalus viridis helleri)* envenomation. Wild Environ Med 10:247–249, 1999.
89. Clark RF, Williams SR, Nordt SP, et al: Successful treatment of crotalid-induced neurotoxicity with a new poly specific crotalid Fab antivenom. Ann Emerg Med 30:54–57, 1997.
90. Ekenback K, Hulting J, Persson H, et al: Unusual neurological symptoms in a case of severe crotalid envenomation. Clin Toxicol 23:357–364, 1985.
91. CroFab Crotalidae Polyvalent Immune Product Information, Savage Laboratories, a division of Atlanta Inc., Melville, NY, revised December 2000.
92. Gibly RL, Walter FG, Nowlin SW, et al: Intravascular hemolysis associated with North American crotalid envenomation. Clin Toxicol 36:337–343, 1998.
93. Suchard JR, LoVecchio F: Envenomations by rattlesnakes thought to be dead. N Engl J Med 340:1930, 1999.
94. Dart RC, Stark Y, Fulton B, et al: Insufficient stocking of poisoning antidotes in hospital pharmacies. JAMA 276:1508–1510, 1996.
95. Dart RC, Hurlbut KM, Garcia R, et al: Validation of a severity score for the assessment of crotalid snakebite. Ann Emerg Med 27:321–326, 1991.
96. Sullivan JB: Past, present, and future immunotherapy of snake venom poisoning. Ann Emerg Med 16:938–944, 1987.
97. Heard K, O'Malley GF, Dart RC: Antivenom therapy in the Americas. Drugs 58:5–15, 1999.
98. Jurkovich GJ, Luterman A, McCullar K, et al: Complications of Crotalidae antivenin therapy. J Trauma 28:1032–1037, 1988.
99. Corrigan P, Russell FE, Wainschell J: Clinical reactions to antivenin. In Rosenberg P (ed): Toxins: Animal, Plant, and Microbial. Oxford, Pergammon Press, 1978.
100. Horowitz RS, Dart RC: Antivenins and immunobiologicals: Immunotherapeutics of envenomation. In Auerbach PS (ed): Wilderness Medicine, 4th ed. St Louis, CV Mosby, 2001.
101. Boyer LV, Seifert SA, Cain JS: Recurrence phenomenon after immunoglobulin therapy for snake envenomations: Part 2. Guidelines for clinical management with crotaline Fab antivenin. Ann Emerg Med 37:196–201, 2001.
102. Hall EL: Role of surgical intervention in the management of crotaline snake envenomation. Ann Emerg Med 37:175–180.
103. Rosen PB, Leiva JI, Ross CP: Delayed antivenom treatment for a patient after envenomation by *Crotalus atrox*. Ann Emerg Med 35:86–88, 2000.
104. Downey DJ, Omer GE, Moheb MS: New Mexico rattlesnake bites: Demographic review and guidelines for treatment. J Trauma 31:1380–1386, 1991.
105. Goldstein EJ, Citron DM, Gonzalez H, et al: Bacteriology of rattlesnake venom and implications for therapy. J Infect Dis 140:818–821, 1979.
106. Clark RF, Selden BS, Furbee B: The incidence of wound infection following crotalid envenomation. J Emerg Med 11:583–586, 1993.
107. Kerrigan KR, Mertz BL, Nelson SJ, et al: Antibiotic prophylaxis for pit viper envenomation: Prospective, controlled trial. World J Surg 21:369–373, 1997.
108. Lopoo JB, Bealer JF, Mantor PC, et al: Treating the snakebitten child in North America: A study of pit viper bites. J Pediatr Surg 33:1593–1595, 1998.
109. Weber RA, White RR 4th: Crotalidae envenomation in children. Ann Plast Surg 31:141–145, 1993.
110. Wagner CW, Golladay ES: Crotalid envenomation in children: Selective conservative management. J Pediatr Surg 24:128–131, 1989.

CHAPTER 103

North American Coral Snakes and Related Elapids

Jeffrey N. Bernstein

The American Association of Poison Control Centers reported 69 coral snake bites in 2000[1]; 44 (64%) of these were reported from Florida.[2] Coral snakes belong to the family Elapidae (Fig. 103-1). Among the elapids are cobras, mambas, sea snakes, and corals. Coral snakes comprise three genera: *Leptomicrurus*, *Micrurus*, and *Micruroides*. *Micrurus* and *Micruroides* are the only endemic North American elapids.[3] *Micrurus fulvius* has five subspecies; *M. fulvius fulvius* (Eastern coral snake) and, to a lesser extent, *M. fulvius tenere* (Texas coral snake) are the most medically important. No reports exist of significant toxicity due to *Micruroides euryxanthus* (Sonoran coral snake).

The Eastern coral snake, small by comparison to the pit vipers, grows to 129.5 cm (51 inches)[4] and has a black, rounded head with a flat snout and rounded eyes. The concentric banding pattern with black, yellow, red, yellow gives rise to the mnemonic: "red on yellow, kill a fellow; red on black, venom lack." Several nonvenomous snakes in North America mimic the coral snake, most notably the king snake. Coral snakes should be distinguished easily from these, if a specimen is available for examination; however, misidentification, even by professionals at a pet store, has led to envenomation.[5]

M. fulvius is solitary except when breeding. It can be aggressive toward its own species, but it is otherwise mild mannered and does not attack humans. When disturbed, the coral snake often lays its head out of sight, rattles its flattened elevated tail, and emits a popping sound. This behavior is thought to be an evolutionary tactic, used to confuse predators. The first description of a coral snake bite by True[6] in 1883 expressed surprise that the snake did not sting with its tail. As with pit viper envenomation, most coral snake bites have been in self-defense of the animal.

VENOM BIOCHEMISTRY AND PATHOPHYSIOLOGY

The chemical components of *Micrurus* toxin still are not well understood. Dry venom itself consists of 75% protein,[7] representing a complex mixture of enzymes and nonenzymatic toxins. Phospholipase A_2, hyaluronidase, L-amino acid oxidase, phosphatases, phosphodiesterases,[8–12] adenosine triphosphatase, and deoxynucleoside phosphatase (DNPase) have been described. Other venom components include lipids, carbohydrates, riboflavin, zinc, calcium, magnesium, and potassium.

Zinc-dependent anticholinesterase may be partially responsible for effects on neuromuscular transmission.[13] A potent neurotoxin with predominantly postsynaptic curare-like effects on acetylcholine receptors at the neuromuscular junction has been described.[14] The evolutionary pressure for the neurotoxin seems to be the immobilization of prey, rather than digestion, as may be the case for the venom of crotaline species. The neurotoxin is believed to act on the presynaptic[3] and the postsynaptic receptors at the neuromuscular end plate. Cardiotoxins have been described for some of the South American elapid species.

Coral snakes have two anteriorly located fixed maxillary teeth, or fangs, attached to venom apparatus. The amount of venom injected into a victim is difficult to determine; however, this seems to be controllable by the coral snake.[15] The average amount of venom available varies from species to species and is proportionate to the size of the snake. The average yield of venom obtained from milking snakes is 12 to 20 mg for *M. fulvius* and only 6 mg from *M. euryxanthus*.[10,15,16]

The average median lethal dose for 18-g mice is reported to be 9 μg.[17] Given the average yield per snake, it is apparent that a bite from *M. fulvius* easily could be fatal to a human if the weight-adjusted median lethal dose is similar.

CLINICAL PRESENTATION

Fang marks are the most frequent initial clinical finding. Fang marks may be multiple, may appear as an abrasion, or may be absent. The finding of being able to express a small drop of blood may be present in 85% of patients[18]; however, envenomations have occurred with minimal local signs.[19] The practice of injecting lidocaine or saline into the bite site to observe expression of fluid from the fang marks has little, if any, clinical value. It has been stated that these snakes need to chew venom into the wound to inject sufficient venom. This chewing action may not be necessary for envenomation, however: Only a few patients in the Florida Poison Information Center database have given a history of the snake's "holding on."

Local swelling occurs in approximately one third of patients[18] and is typically mild compared with pit viper envenomation. The lack of local tissue injury often leads medical personnel to underestimate the severity of the injury, particularly if the patient is intoxicated. Localized pain at the bite site is common, as are paresthesias.

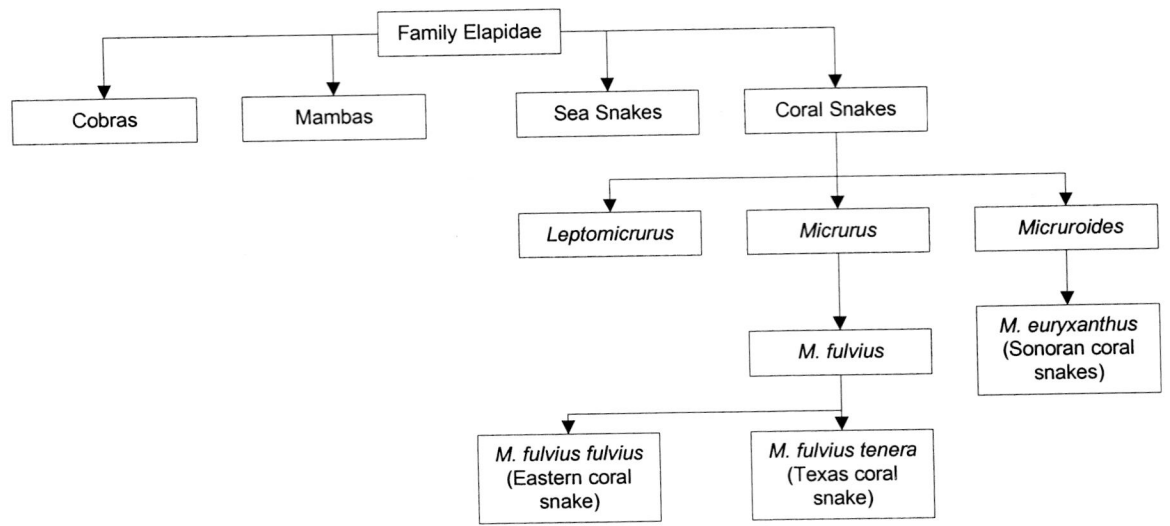

FIGURE 103-1

Family Elapidae.

The mean time to onset of symptoms is 140 minutes; however, toxicity may be delayed 13 hours.[18] Most patients who present to the hospital are asymptomatic. Asymptomatic patients, if adequately treated with antivenom before the onset of symptoms, do not go on to develop toxicity. Nausea and vomiting occur in approximately 25% of patients.[18] One patient described the following symptom to me: "It was like thousands of bees buzzing in my ears."

Cranial nerves are affected early, with the patient experiencing diplopia, ptosis, dysarthria, difficulty swallowing, and depressed gag reflex. Aspiration pneumonia is a frequent complication, particularly when early, aggressive airway protection is not maintained. Paralysis of the muscles of respiration and respiratory failure may follow, with subsequent paralysis of skeletal muscles, which is preceded by muscle fasciculations in 5% of cases.[18] Whether paralysis proceeds in ascending or descending fashion has not yet been described. Although paralysis in an untreated patient may last 2 months, long-term sequelae have not been observed. Mental status most often remains normal. Some patients with incomplete paralysis have been able to communicate through writing.

Cardiovascular toxicity has been shown in dog models with lethal doses of venom from *M. fulvius fulvius*.[20] No such toxicity has been reported in humans. Hemolytic effects on in vitro human red blood cells have been shown, but this does not seem to be clinically relevant for patients.[11]

DIAGNOSIS

The diagnosis usually is evident from the history given by the patient. In the series by Kitchens and Van Mierop,[18] nine patients who intentionally handled the snake believed they were handling a king snake. In one report of envenomation the patient was told by a local pet shop that a snake was a king snake.[5] Occasionally a patient, often intoxicated,

gives a history of having been bitten by an unknown brightly colored snake. It is often difficult to determine if a patient has been envenomed. If no snake is available for identification, the risks of antivenom administration must be weighed against the risks of untreated envenomation. Experimentally and in rare clinical circumstances, enzyme-linked immunosorbent assay has been performed on the blood of unconscious patients to diagnose coral snake envenomation. This test is not routinely commercially available, however, and can be expensive. Enzyme-linked immunosorbent assay is not indicated in cases in which the diagnosis already is known. Treatment of suspected envenomation should not be delayed for laboratory work of any kind. Routine laboratory studies may be required before intensive care unit admission per protocol and custom in many hospitals. The laboratory is not helpful, however, in making a specific diagnosis because neither coagulopathy nor rhabdomyolysis occurs in routine coral snake envenomation. A chest x-ray should be obtained, particularly if aspiration is suspected. Becauses paralysis lasts several days to months, arterial access is preferable for multiple arterial blood gas measurements.

TREATMENT

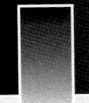
Indications for ICU Admission in Poisoning by North American Coral Snakes and Related Elapids

1. All patients with strong suspicion of coral snake bite should be treated or monitored in the intensive care unit for the first 24 hours.
2. Symptomatic patients should remain in the intensive care unit until a patent airway can be maintained by the patient.
3. Patients who have had anaphylactic symptoms from antivenom should be admitted to the intensive care unit.

Early and aggressive airway management and ventilatory support are mandatory because aspiration pneumonia is a frequent early complication. The supportive treatment of symptomatic patients mirrors the treatment of Guillain-Barré syndrome or botulism. The patient may have complete or partial paralysis of skeletal musculature but typically has normal mental status. It is important that the patient's psychological needs are met in addition to ventilatory and nutritional support.

Antivenom

The mainstay of treatment of *M. fulvius* is North American Coral Snake Antivenin (Wyeth Laboratories, Marietta, PA). This antivenom is produced by progressive immunization of horses and subsequent harvest of immune serum, presumptively rich in IgG. The immune horse serum is lyophilized for longer storage life. Because neurotoxic symptoms from *M. fulvius fulvius*, when manifest, are largely irreversible by antivenom, it is important to administer antivenom even when the diagnosis is suspected.

For asymptomatic patients with clear evidence of significant coral snake bite, a minimum of 3 to 5 vials of North American Coral Snake Antivenin generally is considered to be appropriate. The Wyeth *Micrurus* antivenom package insert recommends consideration of a repeat course of 3 to 5 vials; however, the indications for repeat treatment are left to the discretion of the practitioner. Asymptomatic patients who have received 5 vials of coral snake antivenom have not been described to display subsequent signs of envenomation, and the administration of 5 vials seems to be adequate for this population.

For patients who have developed symptoms before or during the administration of antivenom, I recommend administering 3 to 5 additional vials of antivenom. Although additional higher doses of antivenom have not been shown to reverse the effects of coral snake envenomation, the application of the higher end of the recommended therapeutic dosing range seems prudent. In my experience, a total of 18 vials may be indicated for severe cases.

The package of Wyeth *Micrurus* antivenom contains three vials: lyophilized antivenom, diluent, and diluted antivenom for skin testing. The powdered protein contained in the lyophilized antivenom vial can be reconstituted either by using the diluent that comes in the package or by filling the vials with 10 mL of 5% dextrose in water (D_5W) or normal saline from an intravenous bag. The latter process makes antivenom reconstitution and placement of the contents of the vials back into the intravenous bag easier and more efficient. The vials are warmed gradually and rolled gently (not shaken) between the hands until all powder has gone into solution. Care should be taken to ensure that all particles of the lyophilized powder are dissolved completely. This process typically takes 15 to 30 minutes.

I place 6 vials of antivenom in a weight-appropriate volume of diluent (250 to 500 mL of either D_5W or normal saline is appropriate for adults). An infusion is begun at a rate of about 3 mL/hr. The rate may be doubled every 2 minutes as tolerated. The initial goal of therapy should be the administration of 6 vials over 1 to 1.5 hours.

Pretreatment with antihistamines, steroids, or antibiotics is unnecessary for most patients. Caution should be taken with patients with a prior history of allergic reaction to horse serum. Although antivenom administration is not contraindicated in these patients, the risk-to-benefit ratio must be assessed. If therapy is deemed necessary in these patients, pretreatment with H_1 and H_2 antagonists and corticosteroids is indicated. Tetanus immunization should be updated if necessary. Because animal sera contain foreign protein, immediate hypersensitivity reactions are common. Experience with Wyeth Laboratories (Crotalidae) Antivenin Polyvalent, another equine-derived antivenom, revealed the incidence of anaphylactic, anaphylactoid, and serum sickness to be 83%.[21] Serum sickness is a delayed (days to weeks) manifestation of immune complex formation. Adverse reactions to antivenoms are described in Chapters 101 and 135.

During administration of antivenom, the patient should be observed vigilantly for type I, or immediate, hypersensitivity reactions. Hypersensitivity reactions range from a mild rash to acute bronchospasm or anaphylactic shock or both. This may be true anaphylaxis or, more commonly, a nonspecific anaphylactoid reaction (i.e., not IgE-mediated). If there is concern about the possibility of reaction, it is prudent to prepare an intravenous epinephrine infusion (1 mg in 250 mL of D_5W), which could be started immediately if necessary. The infusion rate, if needed, is typically 0.1 to 1.0 µg/kg/min for adults or 0.05 to 1.0 µg/kg/min for children. The first step in the treatment of acute allergic phenomena is to stop the antivenom infusion. Fluid administration and Trendelenburg positioning may be helpful in blood pressure support. The patient should be given weight-appropriate doses of diphenhydramine and an H_2-blocker, such as cimetidine or ranitidine. Some toxicologists prefer hydroxyzine as the H_2-blocking agent. Intravenous methylprednisolone may not be immediately helpful but may have a role if restarting the antivenom infusion is considered. β_2-Adrenergic agonists should be administered if necessary for the treatment of bronchospasm. Epinephrine should be given for hypotension or bronchospasm. Serum sickness, a type III (or immune complex) hypersensitivity reaction, occurs in many patients 3 to 21 days after antivenom administration (most commonly between days 7 and 14).[21] The risk of serum sickness is related to the number of vials of antivenom given. Serum sickness typically presents as a flulike illness, arthralgias, and rash and responds well to antihistamines and a course of prednisone. Fear of serum sickness should not be used as an argument to avoid use of antivenom.

A Costa Rican polyvalent anti–coral antivenom exists for treatment of coral snake envenomation in Central and South America. There is no literature on its effectiveness in North American coral snake bites. It was developed with venom from *Micrurus nigrocinctus*, *Micrurus carinicaudus*, and *M. fulvius*. This antivenom is not commercially available in North America; however, it occasionally may be found in local zoos and theme parks that handle poisonous animals.[22] It is prepared by immunizing sheep and digesting the IgG molecule with pepsin. The result of splitting the molecule is a 100,000 molecular weight F(ab')$_2$ and a 50,000 molecular weight Fc fraction. The Fc fragment, which is responsible for binding to and triggering degranulation of mast cells and activating the complement cascade, is removed. F(ab')$_2$ has theoretical, but untested, advantages over Fab and IgG. The product is believed to be less allergenic to humans than crude IgG preparations due to

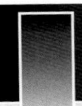

Criteria for ICU Discharge in Poisoning by North American Coral Snakes and Related Elapids

1. Asymptomatic patients may be discharged after 24 hours of observation from the time of the bite.
2. Symptomatic patients may be discharged when adequate airway and ventilation can be maintained.
3. Symptomatic patients should have absence of progression of symptoms for 24 hours before discharge.

the absence of albumin, foreign protein, and Fc fragment. The allosteric configuration of F(ab')$_2$ is closer to that of IgG and may bind to antigen more tightly than Fab. There is concern that Fab may be filtered by the glomerulus and has a short biologic half-life; this is theoretically less likely to occur with F(ab')$_2$ given the latter's greater molecular weight. An F(ab')$_2$ antivenom has been used for the treatment of coral snake bite in Mexico and Central and South America. An ovine Fab antivenom has been developed from *M. fulvius fulvius* but has not been tested in humans.[23]

It may be possible to use antivenoms from Central and South America should a shortage of North American Coral Snake Antivenom exist. Cross-neutralization of *M. fulvius fulvius* venom by anti–*Micrurus carinicauda dumerilii* serum has been shown.[24] General considerations regarding immunotherapy are discussed in detail in Chapter 135.

Neostigmine was used to improve symptoms in a single case report of a 35-year-old patient with suspected envenomation from *Micrurus*.[25] No experience with neostigmine exists for treatment of North American coral snakes, although it has been used for other elapids whose venoms exert postsynaptic neurotoxic effects on the neuromuscular junction.[26]

SPECIAL POPULATIONS

Pediatric Patients

The dosage for children should not be altered. Antivenom contains immunoglobulins, which have affinity for venom. The amount of venom to be bound by antivenom, not the weight of the patient, is the determining factor for the effective dose of antivenom.

Pregnant Patients

There is a paucity of literature on coral snake bite in pregnancy, probably because pregnant women are less likely to be exposed to the risk of envenomation. In one Brazilian study, three of eight pregnant snakebite victims developed significant obstetric complications.[27] The use of antivenom in pregnancy has been inferred from literature on other envenomations. Wyeth Laboratories *Micrurus* antivenin carries a U.S. Food and Drug Administration pregnancy C category (see Appendix A). Although no relevant human studies exist, the risk-to-benefit ratio must be weighed.[28] Because of the possible adverse fetal effects of maternal

envenomation, the indications to use antivenom in pregnant patients should be the same as for nonpregnant patients.

Patients with Late Presentation

A dilemma often exists with asymptomatic patients who have presented to the hospital many hours after a presumed coral snake bite. Although the likelihood of a significant envenomation decreases for a patient 12 hours from the time of the bite, the consequence of not treating early may be a missed opportunity to prevent a prolonged hospital course, one that often is fraught with complications. In these instances, it is usually best to err on the side of caution by giving antivenom. Expectant observation also is an acceptable option. The risks and benefits must be discussed in detail with the patient. Consultation with a clinical toxicologist is highly recommended in this situation.

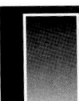

Common Errors in Treatment of Poisoning by North American Coral Snakes and Related Elapids

Delay in protecting the patient's airway
Undertreatment of pediatric patients with antivenom
Approaching the coral snake victim similar to the victim of crotaline snakebite (i.e., using symptoms or signs as an indicator for therapy)
Using Wyeth Laboratories Crotalidae antivenin for treatment of coral snake (the packages are nearly identical)

Key Points in Poisoning by North American Coral Snakes and Related Elapids

1. Victims of coral snake bite present with little, if any, local symptoms.
2. Patients with known or suspected coral snake bite should be treated before the onset of symptoms.
3. Aggressive, early airway protection in patients with evolving symptoms avoids the common complication of aspiration pneumonia.
4. There is no role for steroids (except in the treatment of reactions to antivenom).
5. There is no role for antibiotics.
6. Tetanus immunization should be updated if needed.
7. Untreated patients with full-blown toxicity have paralysis, not coma.

REFERENCES

1. Litovitz TL, Klein-Schwartz W, White S, et al: 2000 Annual Report of the American Association of Poison Control Centers Toxic Surveillance System. Am J Emerg Med 19:374, 2000.
2. Florida Statewide Annual Report, 2000. www.fpicn.org
3. Roze JA: Coral Snakes of the Americas: Biology, Identification, and Venoms. Krieger Publishing Company, Melbourne, FL, 1996, pp 131–223.
4. Parrish HM, Khan MS: Bites by coral snakes: Report of 11 representative cases. Am J Med Sci 253:561–568, 1967.
5. Pancorbo D, Leon R, et al: Eastern Coral Snake (*Micrurus fulvius fulvius*) bite of the tongue with facial swelling. J Clin Toxicol 38:465–496, 2000.

6. True FW: On the bite of the North American coral snakes (genus *Elaps*). Am Nat 17:26, 1883.

7. Stevan LJ, Seligmann EB: Agar-gel ad acrylamide-disc electrophoresis of coral snake venoms. Toxicon 8:11–14, 1970.

8. Possani LD, Alagon PL, Fletcher MJ, et al: Purification and characterization of a phospholipase A2 from the venom of the coral snake, *Micrurus fulvius microgalbineus* (Brown and Smith). Biochem J 179:603–606, 1879.

9. Rosenberg P: Pharmacology of phospholipase A2 from snake venoms. In Lee CY (ed): Snake Venoms. Handbook of Experimental Pharmacology, Vol 52. Berlin, Springer Verlag, 1979.

10. Russel FE: Snake venom poisoning. Great Neck, NY, Scholium International, 1983.

11. Jimenez-Porras JM: Pharmacology of peptides and proteins in snake venoms. Ann Rev Pharmacol 8:299–318, 1968.

12. Kocholaty WF, Boyles-Ledford E, Daly J, Bilings TA: Toxicity and some enzymatic properties and activities in the venoms of Crotalidae, Elapidae, and Viperidae. Toxicon 9:131–138, 1971.

13. Kumar V, Rejent TA, Elliott WB: Anticholinesterase activity of elapid venoms. Toxicon 11:131–138, 1973.

14. Vital Brazil O: Acao neuromuscular da peconha de Micrurus. Sao Paulo, 1963. (Tese de doutoramento—Faculdade de Medicina da Universidade de Sao Paulo), as cited in Vital Brazil O: Coral Snake Venoms: Mode of Action and Pathophysiology of Experimental Envenomation. Rev Inst Med Trop Sao Paulo 29:119–126, 1987.

15. Fix JD: Venom yield of North American Coral Snake and its clinical significance. South Med J 73:737–738, 1980.

16. Minton SA: Venom extraction and yields from the North American Coral Snake, *Micrurus fulvius*. Toxicon 14:143–145, 1976.

17. Bolanos R, Cerdas L, Abalos JW: Veneno de Micrurus (serpiente de coral) Un antiveneno multivalente de valor panamericano. Bol Ofic Sanit Panam 84:128–133, 1978.

18. Kitchens CS, Van Mierop LHS: Envenomation by the Eastern Coral Snake (*Micrurus fulvius fulvius*): A study of 39 victims. JAMA 258: 1615–1618, 1987.

19. Norris RL, Dart RC: Apparent coral snake envenomation in a patient without visible fang marks. Am J Emerg Med 7:402–405, 1989.

20. Ramsey HW, Taylor WJ, Borrichow IB, Snyder GK: Mechanism of shock produced by an elapid snake (*Micrurus fulvius fulvius*) venom in dogs. Am J Physiol 222:282–286, 1972.

21. Jurkovich GJ, Lutherman A, McCullar K, et al: Complications of crotalidae antivenin therapy. J Trauma 28:1032–1037, 1988.

22. Antivenom Index, 1994 revision. Dallas, Texas, American Zoo and Aquarium Association and American Association of Poison Control Centers, 1994.

23. Rawat S, Laing G, Smith DC, et al: A new antivenom to treat eastern coral snake (*Micrurus fulvius fulvius*) envenoming. Toxicology 32: 185–190, 1994.

24. Cohen P, Dawson JH, Seligmann EB: Cross-neutralization of *Micrurus fulvius* venom by anti-micrurus carinicauda dumerilii serum. Am J Trop Med Hyg 17:308–310, 1968.

25. Coelho LK, Silva E, Espositto C, Zanin M: Clinical features and treatment of elapidae bites: Report of three cases. Hum Exp Toxicol 11:135–137, 1992.

26. Gold BS: Neostigmine for the treatment of neurotoxicity following envenomation by the Asiatic cobra. Ann Emerg Med 28:87–89, 1996.

27. Pardal PPO, Mazzeo T, Pinheiro ACL: Snakebite in pregnancy: A preliminary study. J Venomous Animals and Toxins 3(2):280–286, 1997.

28. Fed Reg 44:37434–37467, 1980.

CHAPTER 104

European Snakes

Hans Persson ▪ Christine Karlson-Stiber

Apart from a few toxicologically less important *Colubrid* species, all naturally occurring venomous snakes in Europe are so-called vipers (family Viperidae, genus *Vipera*).

EUROPEAN VIPERS

Vipera berus, the common European adder, is considered to occupy more land area than any other venomous snake. It occurs throughout Europe except for Ireland, the southern parts of the continent, and the larger Mediterranean islands. Its range extends to the Arctic Circle and eastward to the Pacific Ocean. *Vipera aspis* is found mainly in France, Italy, southern Germany, the Pyrenees, and the Alps. The larger *Vipera ammodytes* is widespread in southeastern Europe, northern Italy, Austria, and Turkey. The smallest species, *Vipera ursinii*, has a more restricted distribution in central and eastern Europe but extends instead through Asia. *Vipera latasti* is the dominating viper on the Iberian Peninsula. *Vipera lebetina* and *Vipera xanthina* occur in Cyprus, Turkey, West Asia, and North Africa. All these snakes have subspecies in certain regions.

Incidence of Bites

The incidence of envenoming after bites by European vipers is difficult to assess. Many local and regional reports but few nationwide reports have been published. The overall picture is vague. Based on available data, estimations on the incidence have been made, more recently by Chippaux,[1] suggesting that the total number of bites in Europe amounts to around 25,000 annually (8000 of which result in envenoming) and that the number of deaths may be approximately 30, rather than 50 as indicated in the early 1990s.[2] Men are overrepresented, and in hospital records there is a relatively high incidence in children.

Circumstances

Bites generally occur outdoors when people incidentally come across the snakes in their natural habitat. Also, careless handling of snakes by private collectors may result in bite and envenoming. Bites mostly strike the extremities but also may hit the trunk, neck, and head (e.g., during swimming or when lying on the ground). *V. latasti* may stay in trees, which explains the occurrence of bites to the head and trunk in farmers harvesting fruits.

VENOM

Composition and Pathophysiology

Although the European vipers differ in appearance and size, they are related closely in terms of venom composition, and symptoms of envenoming in general are similar. The main components of the venom are proteins with enzymatic and toxic properties, such as hyaluronidase, proteolytic enzymes, peptide hydrolases, phospholipases A_2, and phosphodiesterases. Also, amino acids, polypeptides, carbohydrates, and metalloproteins occur in the venom.

The onset of venom enzyme activity is more or less immediate. Subcutaneous tissues, muscles, capillary endothelium, and basement membranes are damaged, with subsequent extravasation of plasma and erythrocytes, leading to progressive tissue swelling and discoloration of the skin. This process may not peak until 72 hours after the bite.

A wide range of systemic effects is initiated through the activity of venom enzymes. Common acute effects, such as hypotension, gastrointestinal upset, angioedema, and bronchospasm, are due to an enzyme-mediated release of potent endogenous substances, such as histamine, bradykinin, prostaglandins, and serotonin. Local and systemic hemolysis and coagulopathies can be induced by venom enzymes.

The venom likely also contains components with more specific toxic properties. This would explain the cranial and peripheral nerve disorders observed after bites by *V. ammodytes, V. aspis*, and *V. latasti*[2–4] suggesting a neurotoxic component. Similarly the early occurrence of hematuria and proteinuria in *V. berus* envenoming[5,6] indicates a specific nephrotoxicity. The presence of a cardiotoxic ingredient cannot be ruled out either, considering the many reports on electrocardiogram changes observed after bites by European vipers.[5,7–9]

Kinetics

Venom normally is injected intracutaneously or subcutaneously. Bites by the larger fanged species occasionally may result in intramuscular deposition of the venom, however, and in rare instances even in intravenous injection.[8]

Venom has been detected in blood 30 minutes after the bite and with a peak concentration at approximately 2 hours.[10] The plasma concentrations decline slowly over 1 to 2 days, but venom has been detected 1 week after the bite.[6]

The venom spreads rapidly in the local tissues, where its distribution is facilitated through the action of hyaluronidase.

The venom is transported further to the systemic circulation through the lymphatic vessels. This transport is enhanced by simultaneous muscular activity, making immobilization and rest important first-aid measures.

CLINICAL PRESENTATION

Severity

The severity of envenoming may vary. Anything from just fang marks—with no signs of envenoming—to severe systemic reactions and extensive swelling is possible. The larger species in southern and southeastern Europe often are claimed to cause more pronounced symptoms, but this is not confirmed convincingly in existing reports.

The great variation in toxic response to bites is related to several factors. The most important is the *dose injected*. Of snakebites, 30% to 50% are considered to be "dry," meaning no injection of venom; this has led to the misconception that the venom is not dangerous. The *age and weight* of the patient also is crucial, and this explains why small children are especially susceptible. Other important factors for the response are the *location of the bite* (bites on head and neck could impose a higher risk), *previous health state*, and *physical activity* after the bite. There are two reports of cardiovascular collapse following strong physical activity directly after a viper bite.[4,8]

Clinical Features

The clinical features of envenoming by European vipers have been well documented in case reports and large clinical studies.[3–8,11,12] Most bites result in only mild symptoms, but moderate or severe envenoming is reported to occur in 20% to 30% of patients treated in the hospital.[4,8,11,13]

The most common symptom is local swelling, whereas gastrointestinal disturbances and circulatory instability are the most prominent systemic effects. Many other symptoms and signs of envenoming may occur, however. It has proved logical and useful to distinguish between early symptoms and signs (within minutes or hours), late symptoms and signs (after many hours or days), and sequelae (lasting weeks, months, and years) (Table 104-1).

Psychological reactions are common after snakebites. Fright and anxiety may prevail in the early phase together with transient vegetative symptoms.

Local symptoms first include fang marks, pain, and swelling. Pain is often mild initially but may become intense, especially when the heavily swollen extremity is touched or moved. The edema may involve part of the bitten extremity (Fig. 104-1), or it may extend to involve the whole limb and significant parts of the trunk (Figs. 104-2 and 104-3). Gradually the swelling takes on a bluish, hemorrhagic discoloration, and it may not reach its maximum until after 48 to 72 hours. Lymphangitis, lymphadenitis, blisters, and ecchymoses may develop, and in children thrombophlebitis of the saphenous vein has been reported.[3]

Necrosis and gangrene with complicating infections in general are uncommon but have been reported from the more southern parts of the continent in cases of envenoming by *V. aspis, V. latasti, V. ammodytes*, and, more seldom, *V. berus*. Also a compartment syndrome may develop, but this is rare.

Early Symptoms and Signs (in the Acute Phase)
Psychological reactions
Local soft tissue injury/swelling
Gastrointestinal symptoms
Cardiovascular disturbances
Angioedema, bronchospasm, urticaria
Central and peripheral nervous system disorders
Hemoconcentration, leukocytosis, hemolysis, hematuria, proteinuria, metabolic acidosis

Late Symptoms and Signs (after Many Hours to Days)
Extensive, hemorrhagic swelling involving the whole extremity and parts of the trunk, blisters, compartment syndrome, local necrosis, infections
Pleural exudate, pulmonary edema, ascites, paralytic ileus, kidney dysfunction, bleeding
Anemia, rhabdomyolysis, coagulopathy, thrombocytopenia

Sequelae
Pain, stiffness, local circulatory disturbances, sensibility disorders, persistent or recurrent swelling of the affected limb

Bites on the face and neck are uncommon. These bites constitute a special risk, however, because they may cause considerable swelling with obstruction of the airways.

Gastrointestinal symptoms, including abdominal pain, vomiting, and diarrhea, are the most common signs of systemic envenoming. The onset is usually rapid, within minutes to a few hours, but may be delayed or recur.

Gastric perforation due to acute stress ulcer was reported in one exceptional case. Other unusual complications are hematemesis and melena, acute pancreatitis,[14] and the later development of paralytic ileus and ascites.

Cardiovascular disturbances with hypotension and circulatory shock are typical and related to hypovolemia, vasodi-

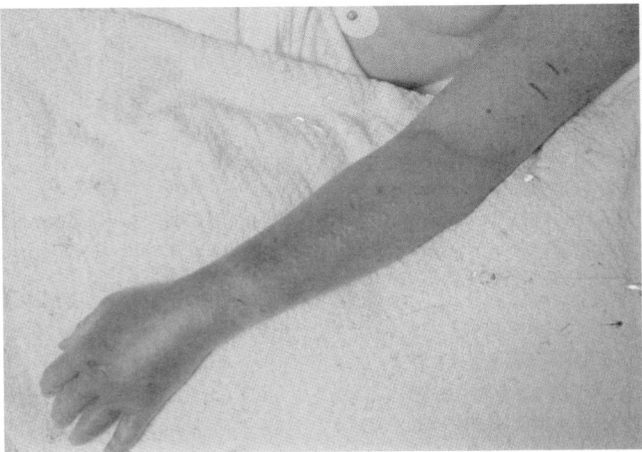

FIGURE 104-1

A 70-year-old woman who was bitten in the left hand while harvesting mushrooms. Initially, she had a severe systemic reaction with shock and impaired consciousness. She was given antivenom (ovine Fab fragments) twice with good effect. The edema never extended beyond the arm, and local bleeding was minimal.

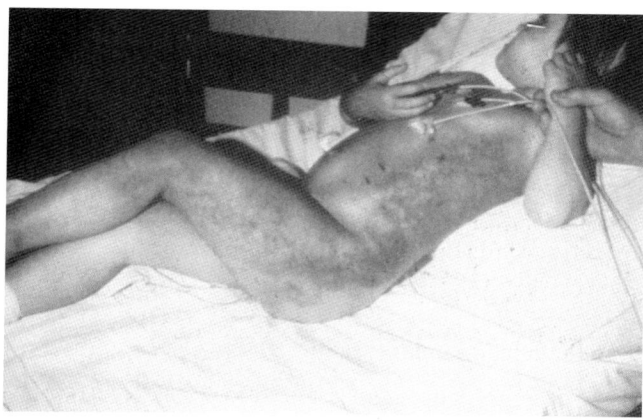

FIGURE 104-2

Envenoming after *Vipera berus* bite in a 4-year-old girl. The bite was in the left foot. No antivenom was given. On the fourth day, the edema extended over the whole extremity and the left part of the trunk up to the axillary region. There also were severe anemia, ascites, gut paralysis, pleural exudates, and eventually a complicating pulmonary edema. *(Courtesy of Karlskrona Hospital, Sweden.)*

lation, and possibly myocardial depression. An odd finding is hypertension, which is described in some *V. latasti* bites.

The most commonly reported electrocardiogram changes are T-wave flattening and inversion,[5,7,8] variably associated with severe systemic envenomation.[7] Also, transient atrial fibrillation, bradycardia, atrioventricular block II, and unspecific ST-segment elevations have been observed.[5,9] More seriously, myocardial infarction has occurred in envenomation.[16]

Neurologic symptoms occur after bites by European vipers. Central nervous system depression with dizziness, fatigue, somnolence, and coma occur in severe envenoming, particularly in children.[4,5,7,8,11] Because these symptoms usually coincide with profound hypotension, hypoxia might partly explain these symptoms. A direct neurotoxic effect cannot be ruled out, however, and in a few cases unconsciousness has persisted despite hemodynamic stabilization. Convulsions and involuntary urination and defecation also suggest some direct neurotoxic action.

A direct neurotoxic effect is obvious in patients bitten by *V. ammodytes, V. aspis*, and *V. latasti*.[2–4] These symptoms include cranial nerve engagement with ophthalmoplegia,

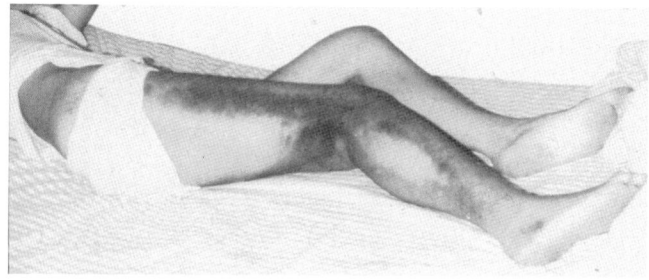

FIGURE 104-3

A 46-year-old woman bitten by *Vipera berus* at the right ankle. The local reaction was extensive; a special feature in this case was severe thrombocytopenia resulting in excessive local bleeding and dark discoloration of the leg and trunk. No antivenom was given. *(From Svensson H: Adder bite followed by pronounced thrombocytopenia, Läkartidningen 90:62–63, 1993.)*

ptosis, and speaking and swallowing difficulties and peripheral neuropathies with paralysis and paresthesia of the bitten limb.

Respiratory effects, which occur early, include mucous membrane swelling in the oropharynx and larynx and bronchospasm. These symptoms constitute an immediate threat to the airways.[5–7,11] Early respiratory distress seems more common in *V. aspis* and *V. ammodytes* envenoming than after *V. berus* bites.

A life-threatening complication seen in some cases 3 to 5 days after envenoming is the sudden onset of pulmonary edema.[12,15] This complication has occurred in small children with widespread edema (see Fig. 104-2). Reabsorption of the extravascular fluid may cause a transient but critical state of intravascular overload, which the vulnerable pulmonary capillaries cannot withstand. In cases of generalized capillary leakage, pleural effusions also may develop.

Renal dysfunction occurs but is generally mild and spontaneously resolving. Transient proteinuria and hematuria are observed commonly in significant *V. berus* envenoming.[5,6,8] Circulatory shock, rhabdomyolysis, and systemic hemolysis occasionally may cause renal tubular injury with subsequent oliguria and anuria.[3,7,8]

Hematologic disturbances are common and include early hemoconcentration and leukocytosis, which, if exceeding 15 to 20×10^9/L, indicates severe envenoming. A mild decrease in the platelet count is common,[4–6,8] and occasionally a pronounced thrombocytopenia may develop[5] and aggravate local tissue bleeding (see Fig. 104-3).

Coagulopathy, resembling consumptive coagulopathy (disseminated intravascular coagulation), is frequent but rarely of clinical significance.[5,6] Massive hematuria and pulmonary hemorrhage have been reported, however, after a *V. berus* bite,[17] and bleeding has been observed after *V. ammodytes* and *V. latasi* bites.[18,19]

Other possible effects are profuse perspiration, metabolic acidosis, and fever. Deep venous thrombosis often is suspected but in reality is rare. Damaged local tissues may become infected, resulting in impaired healing and risk of sepsis. The incidence of complicating infections seems to be higher in southern Europe than in northern Europe. Discrete elevation of liver transferases has been observed a few days after *V. berus* bites.[6]

Sequelae result mainly from extensive local tissue damage. Persistent or recurrent swelling, stiffness, lymphedema, and pain all have been present months and years after bites.[19,20] Late sensory disturbances, such as paresthesia, also have been reported (Swedish Poisons Information Centre, unpublished data).

DIAGNOSIS

Diagnosis aims at confirming the bite and assessing the severity. In most cases, the diagnosis is obvious from the actual circumstances. One to four fang punctures may be observed.

In many European regions, there is just one naturally occurring viper species around. Even if there are more than one indigenous species in a certain region, however, a precise identification is seldom necessary. The different vipers in Europe are closely enough related to respond to the same treatment—including antivenom. There seems to be an acceptable amount of cross-reactivity for most species.

Severity is assessed on the basis of careful assessment of the clinical evolution of the bite. Early signs of severe envenoming are hypotension, impaired consciousness, intense or long-lasting gastrointestinal symptoms, respiratory distress, and rapid progression of local swelling (see Table 104-1). Leukocytosis greater than 15 to 20 × 10⁹/L, pronounced hemoconcentration, metabolic acidosis, hemolysis, and coagulation disturbances similarly indicate high venom dose and a risk of further serious effects.

Based on results with enzyme-linked immunosorbent assay for detection of venom, there is evidence for a good correlation between clinical signs and the blood concentrations of venom antigen in patients bitten by *V. aspis* and *V. berus*.[10,13] This correlation has been confirmed further in a study of patients envenomed by *V. berus*. In the average clinical setting, the clinical evolution rather than venom antigen levels provides guidance to treatment, however.

TREATMENT

Initial Approach

We recommend the following initial approach:

The patient should be kept calm, at rest, and reassured.
The bitten limb is immobilized and kept in a neutral or slightly elevated position.
The site of the bite should not be manipulated (e.g., incised or suctioned) in any way.
Oral intake should be avoided initially.
Tetanus prophylaxis should be addressed.
Vital functions are supported as required.
A patient who shows no local or systemic symptoms within 6 to 8 hours after the bite is likely to remain asymptomatic (Swedish Poisons Information Centre, unpublished data). Patients with signs of envenoming, however minor, should be observed in the hospital for 24 hours.

Laboratory Studies

Some laboratory investigations are useful for initial assessment of severity and for monitoring the clinical course. The analytic data serve as an adjunct to treatment guidance.

Initially in all patients, hemoglobin concentration, hematocrit, leukocyte and platelet count, and routine urinalysis should be obtained.

Indications for ICU Admission in Envenomation by European Snakes

Symptoms of systemic envenoming (e.g., circulatory instability, gastrointestinal upset, respiratory distress, angioedema, neurologic symptoms)
Antivenom treatment
Complications (e.g., renal failure, pulmonary edema, bleeding)
Special risk groups (e.g., pregnant women, toddlers, elderly people, patients with preexisting serious illness)

Initially and repeatedly in patients with systemic symptoms or progressive edema, hemoglobin concentration, hematocrit, leukocyte and platelet count, routine urinalysis, serum electrolytes including bicarbonate (or carbon dioxide), tests for acute hemolysis (free hemoglobin), coagulation tests (e.g., prothrombin time and fibrinogen concentration), creatine kinase, and serum creatinine should be obtained.

The electrocardiogram should be monitored in systemic envenoming.

Symptomatic Treatment

Many of the treatment measures discussed subsequently can be avoided if antivenom treatment is given early.[5,6,11]

CIRCULATION

The causes of hypotension and shock are multifactorial (e.g., extravasation of plasma, vasodilation, myocardial depression). Intravenous fluids, preferably crystalloids and colloids, should be infused as indicated by the patient's clinical volume status. Vasopressors, such as dobutamine and norepinephrine, may be required, depending on the patient's hemodynamic status.

Continuous cardiac monitoring is indicated. Echocardiography, a central venous catheter, and an arterial line may prove useful when assessing and treating circulatory failure. Before invasive monitoring is instituted, however, the patient's clotting status should be assessed.

RESPIRATION

Bronchospasm and mucous membrane swelling often respond well to epinephrine. Usually a bolus dose is sufficient, and a continuous infusion is unnecessary. A dose of 0.3 to 0.5 mg in adults (children, 0.01 mg/kg) is given subcutaneously or intramuscularly and may be repeated every 10 to 15 minutes until a satisfactory clinical response is obtained. In severe cases, the epinephrine dose may be given intravenously, diluted to a concentration of 0.1 mg/mL. Corticosteroids and antihistamines may be of additional value. Pronounced swelling in the oropharyngeal and laryngeal regions occasionally may necessitate intubation or tracheotomy. Late-developing pulmonary edema, which may occur in small children with extensive swelling, may require controlled mechanical ventilation with positive end-expiratory pressure.

RENAL FUNCTION

Renal dysfunction mainly is related to hypovolemia and hypotension. Kidney function may be maintained by adequate hydration and use of diuretics as required. In cases of severe hemolysis or rhabdomyolysis, alkaline diuresis, aiming for a urine pH of 7.5, may protect kidney function.

HEMATOLOGIC DISORDERS

Anemia develops regularly in patients with extensive hemorrhagic swelling, and blood transfusions may be required. Systemic hemolysis may add to the anemia. Coagulation disorders after bites by European vipers rarely need therapeutic interventions and preferably should be treated with antivenom.

LOCAL SYMPTOMS

Immobilization and an elevated position of the bitten limb may diminish the risk of extensive swelling. The only effective treatment to prevent, or at least reduce, further progression of the edema is early administration of antivenom.[5,6] Although a rare incident, compartment syndrome may develop and require fasciotomy. This treatment should be withheld, however, unless absolutely necessary (tissue pressure >30 to 50 mm Hg). Analgesics are given liberally whenever needed, but aspirin or other antiplatelet drugs are inappropriate because of the increased risk of local bleeding.

INFECTIONS

For some southern European viper envenomations, infection often complicates bites.[2] In these cases, early antibiotic treatment is reasonable. Otherwise, antibiotics should be given only if there are signs of local or systemic infections and after appropriate cultures.

OTHER

Deep venous thrombosis is rare after viper bites. In children, thrombophlebitis of the saphenous vein has been observed,[3] but generally children are at low risk for developing deep venous thrombosis. There is no need for prophylaxis in children. Immobilized adults with a swollen limb may benefit, however, from prophylactic low-dose heparin. High doses are not indicated and may worsen bleeding in damaged tissues.

Corticosteroids do not counteract venom effects in any specific way and cannot treat severe envenoming, as was believed for many years. They might be beneficial, however, together with epinephrine, as an adjunctive agent in alleviating symptoms related to a venom-mediated histamine release.

Antivenom

Immunotherapy for European viper bites was introduced in the 1920s. The original, crude horse serum products were associated with frequent hypersensitivity reactions.[6] Antivenom treatment gradually fell into disrepute and was withheld in Europe for many years.

Over the last decades, new techniques have been developed for the production of antivenoms, resulting in products of higher quality. These new products have stimulated a reintroduction of antivenom treatment. Equine F(ab)$_2$ antivenoms have proved effective but are not without side effects.[5,11] Further progress has been achieved with the development of *V. berus*–specific ovine Fab fragments.[6,21] Their efficacy is comparable to the equine F(ab)$_2$, but the dose required is smaller, and so far no acute or delayed hypersensitivity reactions have been observed in more than 150 patients. More recently, a new equine F(ab)$_2$ product has been tested in France with promising results regarding side effects.[22]

Antivenom treatment almost invariably results in rapid dissolution of acute systemic symptoms.[5,6,11,22,23] Neutralization of venom antigen with specific antibodies, however, is the only effective way of preventing or reducing the occurrence of extensive edema and related complications (see Figs. 104-2 and 104-3).[5,6]

Indications for antivenom treatment in bites by European vipers are listed in Table 104-2. There are a few equine F(ab)$_2$ antivenoms and one ovine Fab antivenom available for treatment of envenoming by European vipers.

In severe envenoming, there are no absolute contraindications to antivenom treatment. In patients with atopic history and allergy to animals, pretreatment with antihistamines and corticosteroids may prevent or alleviate antivenom-related reactions. There are no clinical data, however, concerning pretreatment in this special population. Pretreatment usually is not necessary with Fab-based antivenoms.

DOSAGE AND ADMINISTRATION

Antivenom should be given as an intravenous infusion. Subcutaneous or intradermal test doses before administration of antivenom are not recommended. These tests are of no predictive value concerning the likelihood of a reaction due to anticomplementary activity. The currently recommended doses for some widely used antivenoms are given. Whenever antivenoms are given, there should be an immediate readiness to take care of any acute hypersensitivity reactions.

European Viper Venom Antiserum (Serum Antiviperinum). European Viper Venom Antiserum (Serum Antiviperinum) is made from purified equine F(ab')$_2$ fragments (Institute of Immunology, Zagreb, Croatia). Dose is one vial (10 mL) diluted in 200 mL of physiologic saline and given as an infusion over 60 minutes. The same dose is given to adults and children. Additional doses may be required depending on the clinical course.

Vipera Tab. Vipera Tab is made from affinity-purified ovine Fab fragments (Protherics Ltd, London, UK). Dose is 200 mg (the contents of two ampules) dissolved in 10 mL of sterile water (two ampules of 5 mL), then diluted in 100 mL of physiologic saline and given as an infusion over 30 minutes. The same dose is given to adults and children.

TABLE 104-2 Indications for Antivenom in Bites by European Vipers*

Circulatory instability that responds poorly to symptomatic treatment or recurs
Protracted or recurring gastrointestinal symptoms
Mucous membrane swelling with risk of airway obstruction
Evident progress of edema with likelihood of involving the trunk
Fluctuating level of consciousness, peripheral or cranial nerve paresis
In "borderline" cases, one or more of the following may support the indication:
    Leukocytosis >15–20 × 10^9/L
    Metabolic acidosis
    Hemolysis
    Coagulation disturbances
    ECG changes

*Small children and pregnant women are risk groups that should be given antivenom liberally.
ECG, electrocardiogram.

Criteria for ICU Discharge in Envenomation by European Snakes

Vital functions stabilized
Signs of ongoing systemic envenoming ceased
Local swelling not in progress
Further antivenom treatment not anticipated

Additional doses may be required depending on the clinical course.

Viperfav. Viperfav is made from purified equine F(ab')$_2$ fragments (Aventis Pasteur MSD, Lyon, France). For dosing, one infusion kit (2 syringes of 2 mL each = 4 mL) should be diluted in 100 mL of physiologic saline for children and in 250 mL of physiologic saline for adults. The infusion is given over 1 hour. Additional doses may be required depending on the clinical course.

SPECIAL POPULATIONS

Pediatric Patients

Small children constitute a special risk group and are over-represented in hospital populations. All children who have been bitten by a viper should be observed for at least 24 hours. Small children should be given antivenom liberally.

Pregnant Patients

Few data are available on snakebites in pregnancy, which might indicate that pregnancy is not a particular risk. Intrauterine death of the fetus, however, has occurred in late pregnancy in two women after *V. berus* bites (Swedish Poisons Information Centre, unpublished data).[8] In both cases, there was significant envenoming with systemic and local effects. It seems logical to administer antivenom early and liberally to pregnant women when signs of systemic envenoming are present.

Elderly Patients

Elderly patients may be more vulnerable, especially if they have cardiovascular disease.

Common Misconceptions about Envenomation by European Snakes

1. Viper venom is only moderately toxic because some people do not react at all.
2. Onset of severe symptoms is always early and rapid.
3. Corticosteroids have a neutralizing effect on the venom.
4. Antivenom treatment is more dangerous than the bite itself.
5. Antivenom has no effect on the local reactions.

Key Points in Envenomation by European Snakes

1. Immobilization and rest are essential.
2. Continuous observation is mandatory.
3. Life-threatening symptoms (circulatory shock, airway obstruction) may appear abruptly.
4. Onset of serious symptoms may be delayed.
5. Symptomatic and supportive care should be started immediately and given as required.
6. Indications for antivenom treatment must be considered carefully.
7. Antivenom should be given early for optimal efficacy.

REFERENCES

1. Chippaux JP: Snake bites: Appraisal of the global situation. Bull World Health Organ 78:515–524, 1998.
2. Gonzáles D: Snakebite problems in Europe. In Tu AT (ed): Reptile Venoms and Toxins, Handbook of Natural Toxins, Vol 5. New York, Marcel Dekker, 1991, pp 687–757.
3. de Haro L, Robbe-Vincent A, Saliou B, et al: Unusual neurotoxic envenomations by Vipera aspis aspis snakes in France. Hum Exp Toxicol 21:137–145, 2002.
4. Pozio E: Venomous snake bites in Italy: Epidemiological and clinical aspects. Trop Med Parasitol 39:62–66, 1988.
5. Karlson-Stiber C, Persson H: Antivenom treatment in *Vipera berus* envenoming—report of 30 cases. J Intern Med 235:57–61, 1994.
6. Karlson-Stiber C, Persson H, Heath A, et al: First clinical experiences with specific sheep Fab fragments in snake bite: Report of a multicentre study of *Vipera berus* envenoming. J Intern Med 241:53–58, 1997.
7. Reid HA: Adder bites in Britain. BMJ 2:153–156, 1976.
8. Persson H, Irestedt B: A study of 136 cases of adder bite treated in Swedish hospitals during one year. Acta Med Scand 210:433–439, 1981.
9. Moore RS: Second-degree heart block associated with envenomation by *Vipera berus*. Arch Emerg Med 5:116–118, 1988.
10. Audebert F, Sorkine M, Robbe-Vincent A, et al: Viper bites in France: Clinical and biological evaluation; kinetics of envenomations. Hum Exp Toxicol 13:683–688, 1994.
11. Stahel E, Wellauer R, Freyvogel TA: Vergiftungen durch einheimische Vipern (*Vipera berus* und *Vipera aspis*). Schweiz Med Wochenschr 115:890–896, 1985.
12. Cederholm I, Lennmarken C: *Vipera berus* bites in children—experience of early antivenom treatment. Acta Paediatr Scand 76:682–684, 1987.
13. Audebert F, Sorkine M, Bon C: Envenoming by viper bites in France: Clinical gradation and biological quantification by ELISA. Toxicon 30:599–609, 1992.
14. Kjellström BT: Acute pancreatitis after snake bite. Acta Chir Scand 155:291–292, 1989.
15. Rousselot JM, Berthier JC Roze JZ, et al: Envenomation vipérine grave. A propos de 7 opbervations pédiatriques. Arch Fr Pediatr 48:591–592, 1991.
16. Arvanis C, Ioannidis PJ, Ktena J: Acute myocardial infarction and cerebrovascular accident in a young girl after a viper bite. Br Heart J 47:500–503, 1982.
17. Gerrard M, Pugh R: An adder bite with unusual consequences. Practitioner 226:527–528, 1982.
18. Tiwari I, Johnston WJ: Blood coagulability and viper envenomation. Lancet 2:613–614, 1986.
19. Gonzáles D. Clinical aspects of bites by viper in Spain. Toxicon 20:349–353, 1982.
20. Walker CW. Notes on adder-bite (England and Wales). BMJ 2:13–14, 1945.
21. Smith DC, Krisana R, Laing G, et al: An affinity purified ovine antivenom for the treatment of *Vipera berus* envenoming. Toxicon 30:865–871, 1992.
22. de Haro L, Lang J, Bedry R, et al: Envénimations par vipères européennes: Ètude multicentrique de tolerance du Viperfav, nouvel antivenin par voie intraveneuse. Ann Fr Anesth Reanim 17:681–687, 1998.
23. Gronlund J, Vuori A, Nieminer S: Adder bites. A report of 68 cases. SJS 92:171–174, 2003.

CHAPTER 105

Australian and Pacific Snakes

Julian White

Australia and New Guinea are home to the most toxic of all the world's snakes. The snake fauna is dominated by venomous species, and most snakes that measure greater than 1 m long are potentially lethal. Snakebite is a major health issue in New Guinea, where high rates of snakebites and snakebite deaths have been reported. In Australia, with an equally deadly fauna, snakebite is uncommon, however, and fatalities are uncommon to rare. This difference reflects the urban lifestyle in Australia, the well-developed health care system, and the wide availability of intensive care units and antivenoms.

SNAKE FAUNA

In contrast to virtually all other regions, Australia, New Guinea, and the Pacific are dominated by elapid snakes, with a smattering of colubrids (none lethal) and no vipers.

Australia

Australia is home to five families of snakes (Table 105-1), of which only two contain venomous species, and only one contains species likely to cause human fatalities.

COLUBRIDS

There are only a few colubrid species in Australia, mostly confined to northern and eastern continental Australia, and only one of these is significantly venomous, the brown tree snake, *Boiga irregularis* (Fig. 105-1). Even this species does not pose a threat to human life, although infants bitten may have significant envenoming. Few bites are recorded from Australia, however.

ELAPIDS

Elapids dominate the terrestrial and aquatic Australian snake fauna. Sea snakes of numerous species abound in the waters of coastal Australia except southern waters. On land, elapids account for 81 of the 143 species of terrestrial and freshwater snakes. Although all elapids are venomous and possess fangs, only about 25 species are large enough or toxic enough to pose a significant threat to humans. This latter group is divided into five distinct groups (Table 105-2).

Brown Snakes. The brown snakes, genus *Pseudonaja*, occupy all of mainland Australia and are currently the most common cause of snakebites and fatalities. These snakes are adapting to urban habitats and are now common in

many cities. They vary widely in color and size; some exceed 2 m in length (Figs. 105-2 through 105-8).

Tiger Snake Group. The tiger snake group includes the tiger snakes, genus *Notechis* (Figs. 105-9 through 105-13); the rough-scaled snake, *Tropidechis carinatus* (Figs. 105-14 and 105-15); the copperheads, genus *Austrelaps* (Figs. 105-16 through 105-18); the broad-headed snakes, genus *Hoplocephalus* (Figs. 105-19 through 105-22); and technically, several genera of smaller elapids of little medical significance. These snakes range from northeastern mainland Australia, down the east coast, across the southern mainland, to southern islands, including Tasmania, and are the second most important cause of snakebites and fatalities.

Black Snake Group. The black snake group, genus *Pseudechis*, contains a group of larger snakes, collectively ranging across almost all of Australia and responsible for numerous snakebites but few deaths (Figs. 105-23 through 105-28). Principal species include the mulga snake and the red-bellied black snake.

Death Adders. Death adders, genus *Acanthophis*, are restricted to parts of mainland Australia; are unique in appearance, with a viper-like form (Figs. 105-29 and 105-30); but have fared poorly since European settlement and are increasingly uncommon as a cause of snakebites and fatalities.

Taipans. The two taipan species, genus *Oxyuranus*, represent the most dangerous of all snakes, combining large size (3 m), big fangs, copious amounts of toxic venom, and a rapid strike (Figs. 105-31 through 105-33). These snakes are restricted to northern and parts of eastern coastal Australia (common taipan) and sparsely populated parts of inland Australia (inland taipan) and cause relatively few snakebites and only occasional deaths. Untreated taipan bites carry a lethality rate of greater than 80%.

New Guinea

The New Guinea fauna reflects historic land bridges with Australia. Most of the venomous snake fauna is shared (see Table 105-2).

COLUBRIDS

Information about colubrids in New Guinea is essentially similar to Australia.

TABLE 105-1 Snake Families in Australia and the Pacific Islands

FAMILY	COMMON NAME	DISTRIBUTION
Typhlopidae	Blind snakes	Australia, New Guinea, some Pacific islands
Boidae	Pythons and boas	Australia, New Guinea, Samoa, Fiji, Solomon islands
Acrochordidae	File snakes	Australia, New Guinea
Colubridae	Colubrid snakes	Australia, New Guinea (including Bougainville), Solomon islands, Guam, Fiji
Elapidae (includes Hydrophiinae)	Elapid (cobra type) snakes (includes sea snakes)	Australia, New Guinea (including Bougainville), Solomon islands, Fiji. Sea snakes found throughout Pacific adjacent to islands, plus one pelagic species

ELAPIDS

Death Adders. Death adders are still common in New Guinea and are a major cause of snakebites and fatalities, particularly in highland areas.

Taipans. The New Guinea taipan is a major cause of snakebites and fatalities in the southern plains regions.

Black Snake Group. The endemic Papuan black snake and the mulga snake are found in southern plains regions but are no longer considered a common cause of bites.

Small-Eyed Snake. Unique to New Guinea and nearby islands, the small-eyed snake, *Micropechis ikaheka*, is now thought to cause significant numbers of bites and a few fatalities within its range.

Brown Snakes. A few specimens of Australian brown snakes are reported from southern New Guinea, but they are not a major cause of snakebites at present. It is unclear if they are native or if they were accidentally introduced.

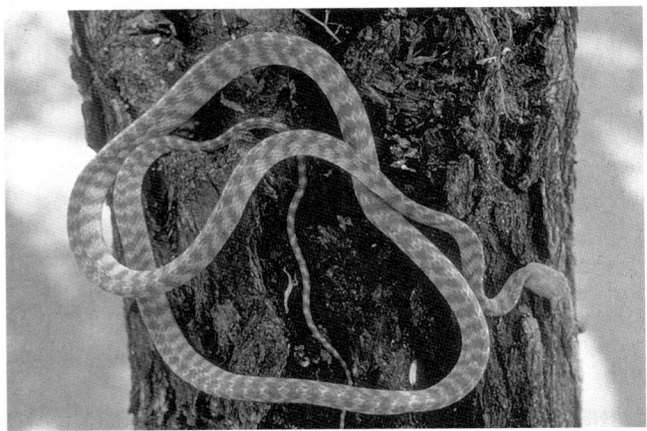

FIGURE 105-1

Brown tree snake, *Boiga irregularis. (Copyright © Dr. Julian White.)*

OTHER SPECIES

Several other species of lesser or uncertain medical significance occur in New Guinea (see Table 105-2).

Pacific

Most Pacific islands are without terrestrial snakes, or the snake fauna is limited to minor colubrid species, but sea snakes abound in most areas.

COLUBRIDS

The most important colubrid in the Pacific, the Australian brown tree snake, *Boiga irregularis*, was accidentally introduced to islands such as Guam during World War II. Although this snake is not lethal, lack of predators has resulted in a population explosion, a consequence of which is a far higher rate of bites than seen in New Guinea or Australia. Human infants, in particular, may develop significant nonlethal envenoming when bitten.

ELAPIDS

Apart from the presence of death adders and the small-eyed snake on a few islands near New Guinea and a few lesser species (see Table 105-2), medically significant elapids in the Pacific are restricted to the abundant sea snakes.

VENOMS

As with other snakes, the medically significant snakes of the Australian and Pacific region possess complex, multicomponent venoms with a variety of clinical effects. These effects are overwhelmingly systemic rather than local, however. A summary of activities for each snake is given in Table 105-3.

Neurotoxins

Neurotoxins are the classic toxins of elapid snakes, and they are well represented within the Australian and related fauna. They are all paralytic neurotoxins active at the neuromuscular junction.

PRESYNAPTIC NEUROTOXINS

Presynaptic neurotoxins are phospholipase A_2 toxins of variable size, ranging from approximately 10 to 88 kd. Some have myotoxic activity in addition to causing progressive damage to the terminal axon of the neuromuscular junction. They initially cause acetylcholine release, then destruction of synaptic vesicles and mitochondrial structures, causing irreversible cessation of signal function.

POSTSYNAPTIC NEUROTOXINS

Most venoms containing presynaptic neurotoxins also contain postsynaptic toxins, but a few snakes, notably death adders, possess only the latter. These toxins competitively bind to the acetylcholine receptor on the muscle end plate, blocking signal reception and causing paralysis, which is potentially reversible.

TABLE 105-2 Medically Important Groups of Australian and Pacific Terrestrial Venomous Snakes, Including Species of Uncertain Medical Importance

SCIENTIFIC NAME	COMMON NAME	DISTRIBUTION
Colubridae		
Boiga irregularis	Brown tree snake	Northern Australia, New Guinea, adjacent Pacific islands
Cantoria, Enhydris, Fordonia, Myron, Cerberus, Heurnia spp.	Water snakes (not sea snakes)	Northern Australia, New Guinea, adjacent Pacific islands
Elapidae		
Brown Snake Group		
Pseudonaja affinis	Dugite	Australia
Pseudonaja guttata	Spotted brown snake	Australia
Pseudonaja ingrami	Ingram's brown snake	Australia
Pseudonaja inframacula	Peninsular brown snake	Australia
Pseudonaja nuchalis	Western brown snake or gwardar	Australia
Pseudonaja textilis	Eastern brown snake	Australia, New Guinea
Tiger Snake Group		
Notechis scutatus	Common tiger snake	Australia
Notechis ater	Black tiger snake (several important subspecies)	Australia
Notechis ater occidentalis	West Australian tiger snake	Australia
Tropidechis carinatus	Rough-scaled snake	Australia
Austrelaps superbus	Lowland copperhead	Australia
Austrelaps ramsayii	Highland copperhead	Australia
Austrelaps labialis	Pygmy copperhead	Australia
Hoplocephalus bungaroides	Broad-headed snake	Australia
Hoplocephalus bitorquatus	Pale-headed snake	Australia
Hoplocephalus stephensi	Stephen's banded snake	Australia
Rhinoplocephalus nigrescens	Eastern small-eyed snake	Australia
Black Snake Group		
Pseudechis australis	Mulga snake or king brown	Australia, New Guinea
Pseudechis butleri	Butler's mulga snake	Australia
Pseudechis colletti	Collett's snake	Australia
Pseudechis guttatus	Spotted black snake	Australia
Pseudechis papuanus	New Guinea black snake	New Guinea
Pseudechis porphyriacus	Red-bellied black snake	Australia
Death Adder Group		
Acanthophis antarcticus	Common death adder	Australia, New Guinea
Acanthophis praelongus	Northern death adder	Australia
Acanthophis pyrrhus	Desert death adder	Australia
Taipan Group		
Oxyuranus scutullatus	Common taipan	Australia, New Guinea
Oxyuranus microlepidotus	Inland taipan	Australia
Miscellaneous		
Micropechis ikaheka	New Guinea small-eyed snake	New Guinea, including Bougainville
*Toxicocalamus loriae**	Loria forest snake	New Guinea
*Salomonelaps par**	Solomons coral snake	Islands North of Bougainville, Solomon islands
*Loveridgelaps elapoides**	Solomons small-eyed snake	Solomon islands
*Parapistocalamus hedigeri**	Hediger's coral snake	Bougainville Island
Aspidomorphus spp.*	New Guinea crowned snakes	New Guinea, Moluccas
Sea snakes		
	Numerous species	Throughout Indo-Pacific waters, near land or reefs; one pelagic species

*These snakes are generally small; little or nothing is known of their venom; and for most species, no bites are recorded. They are of uncertain medical importance and are not included in subsequent tables. Of the species for which bites are recorded, none were fatal, and local swelling was the most common effect. This does not exclude the possibility, however, that a large specimen might cause severe envenoming, especially in a child.

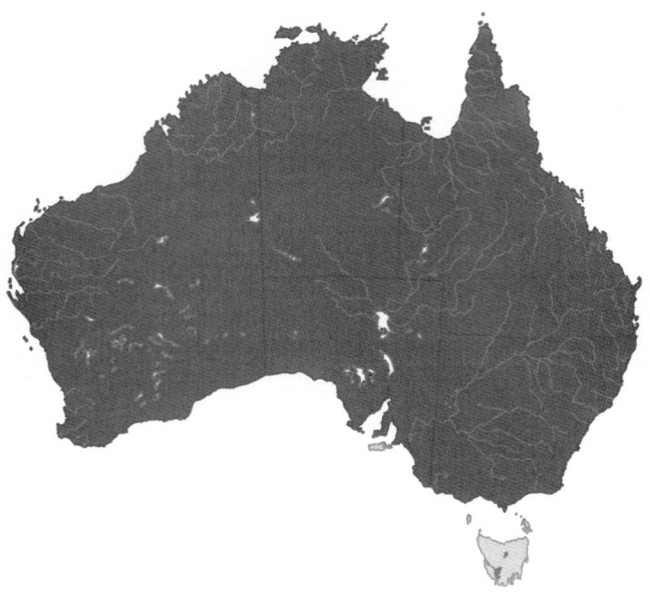

FIGURE 105-2

Distribution of Australian brown snakes, *Pseudonaja* spp. *(Copyright © Dr. Julian White.)*

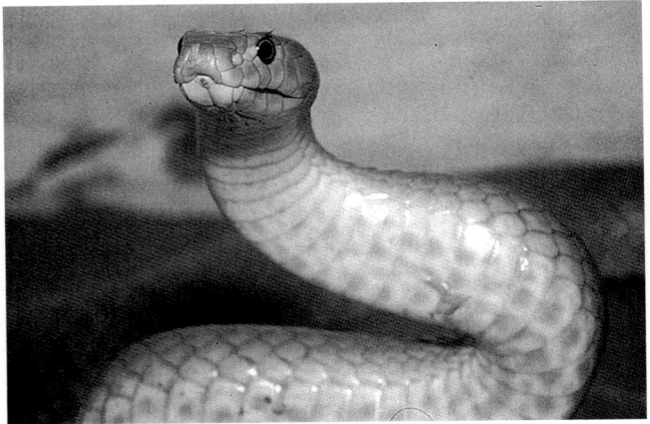

FIGURE 105-3

Eastern brown snake, *Pseudonaja textilis*. *(Copyright © Dr. Julian White.)*

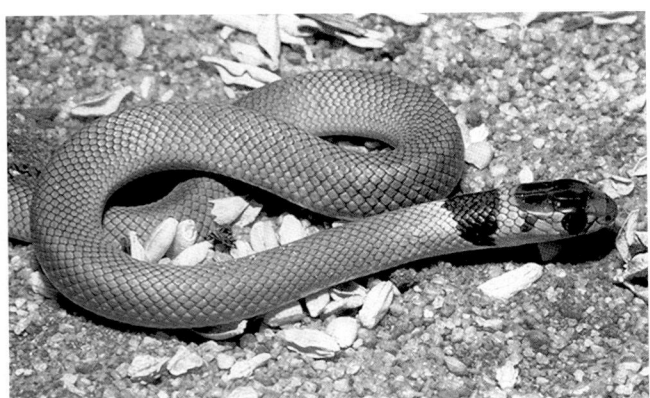

FIGURE 105-4

Juvenile eastern brown snake. Note classic black markings on the back of the head and adjacent neck. *(Copyright © Dr. Julian White.)*

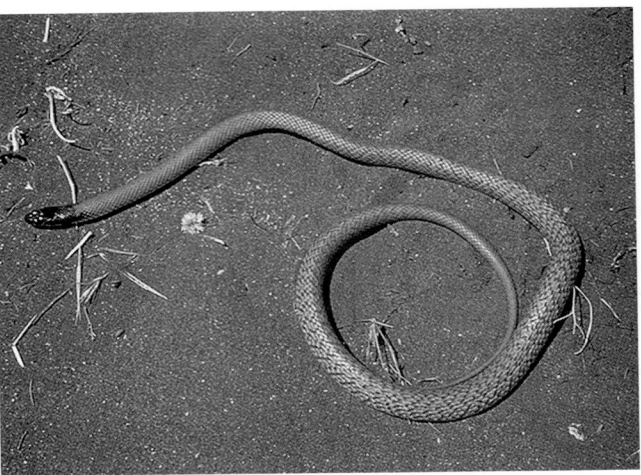

FIGURE 105-5

Western brown snake, *Pseudonaja nuchalis*. *(Copyright © Dr. Julian White.)*

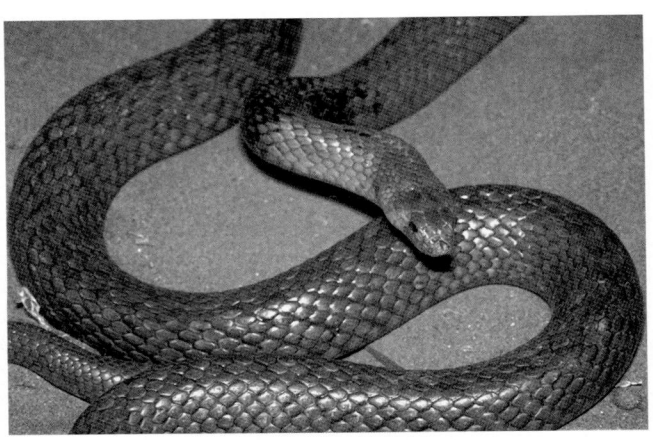

FIGURE 105-6

Western brown snake, different coloring. *(Copyright © Dr. Julian White.)*

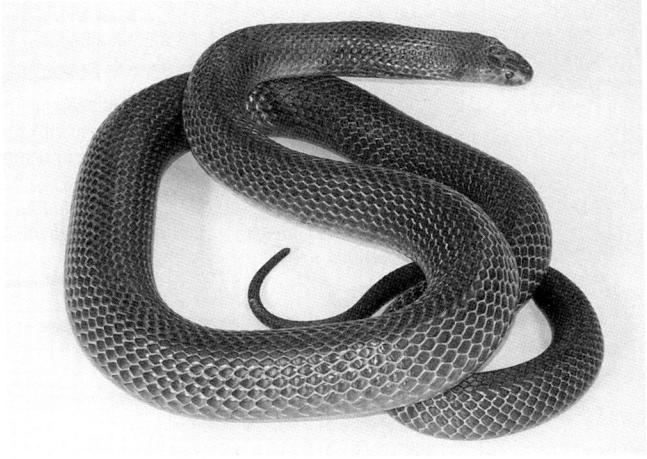

FIGURE 105-7

Dugite, *Pseudonaja affinis*. *(Copyright © Dr. Julian White.)*

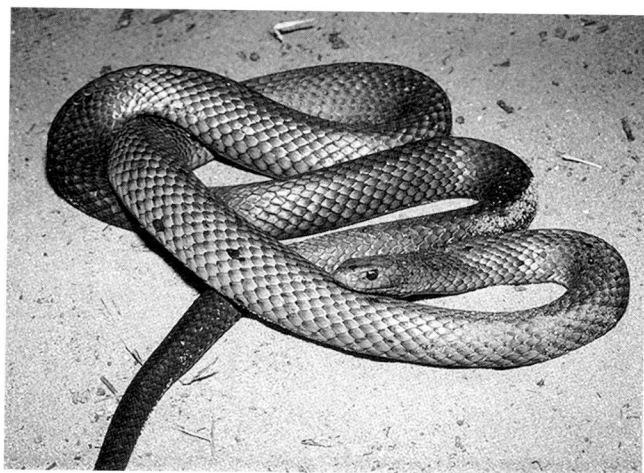

FIGURE 105-8

Peninsular brown snake, *Pseudonaja inframacula*. *(Copyright © Dr. Julian White.)*

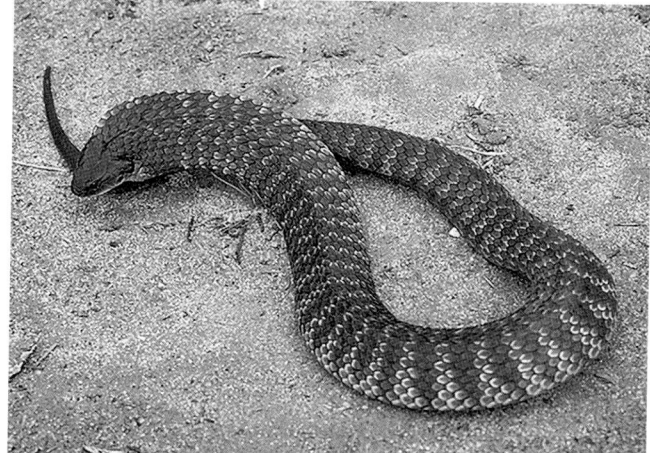

FIGURE 105-10

Common tiger snake, *Notechis scutatus*. *(Copyright © Dr. Julian White.)*

Myotoxins

The myotoxic activity in Australian snake venoms is mediated by modified phospholipase A_2 toxins, a few of which are also presynaptically active. Only skeletal muscle is affected to any significant degree, and the effect is systemic, not local in the bitten area.

Procoagulants, Anticoagulants, and Hemorrhagins

Australian snake venoms are a rich source of potent procoagulants, mostly prothrombin converters, causing a brief period of thrombosis, followed by prolonged profound defibrination. Only a few species have clinically apparent

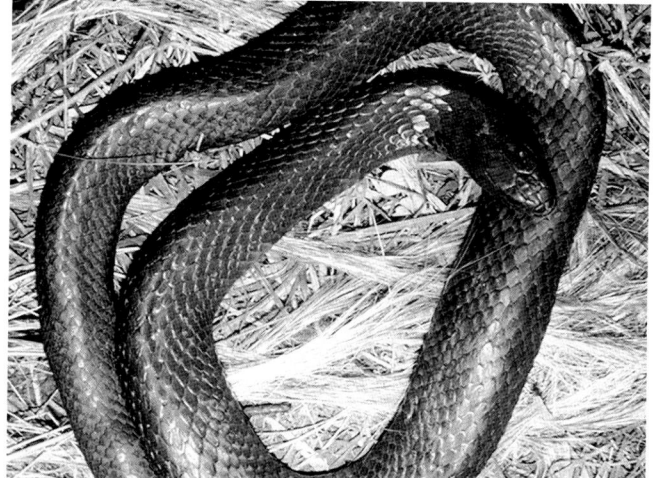

FIGURE 105-11

Common tiger snake, unbanded brown color phase. *(Copyright © Dr. Julian White.)*

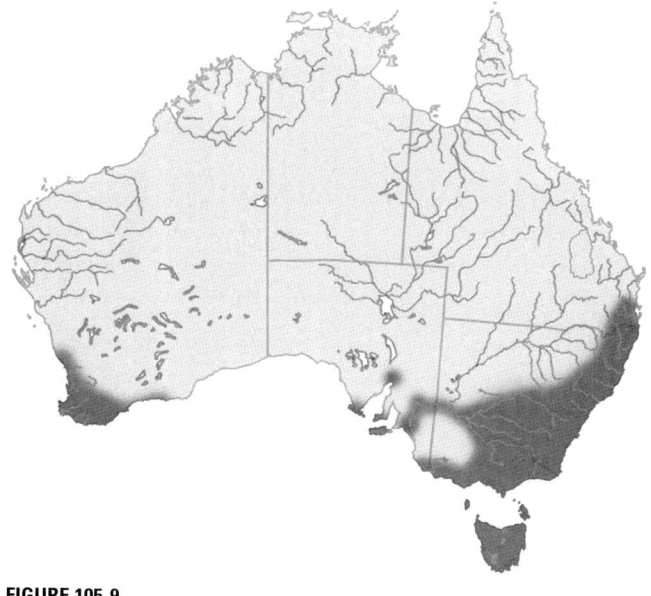

FIGURE 105-9

Distribution of tiger snakes, *Notechis* spp., in Australia. *(Copyright © Dr. Julian White.)*

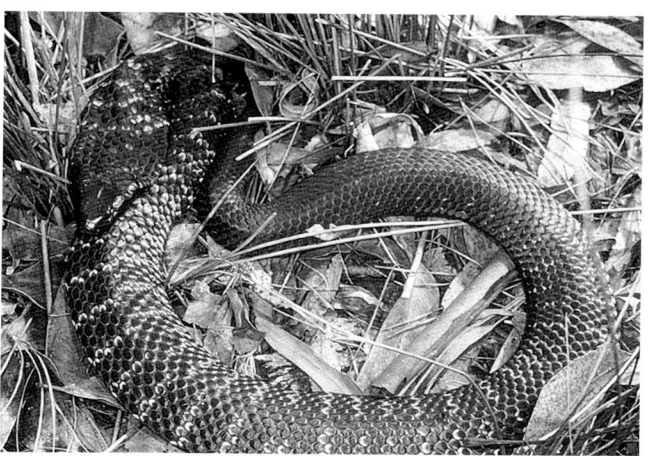

FIGURE 105-12

West Australian tiger snake, *Notechis ater occidentalis*. *(Copyright © Dr. Julian White.)*

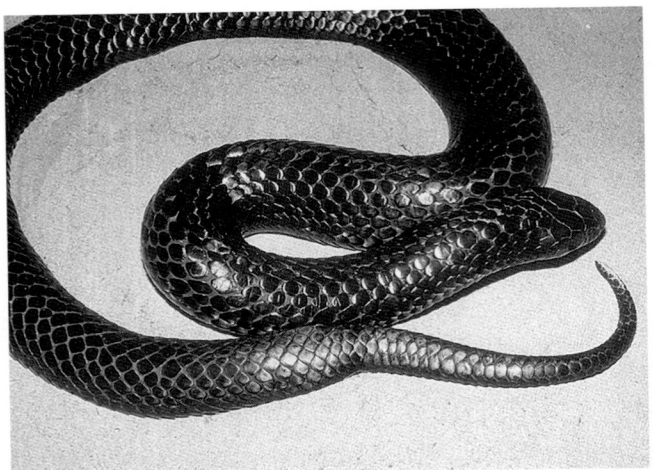

FIGURE 105-13

Black tiger snake, *Notechis ater.* (Copyright © Dr. Julian White.)

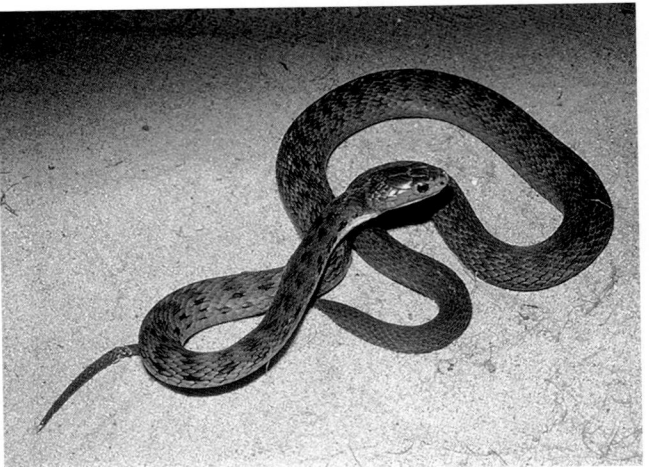

FIGURE 105-15

Rough-scaled snake, *Tropidechis carinatus.* (Copyright © Dr. Julian White.)

anticoagulants. Hemorrhagins, although suspected for some species, have not been definitively isolated so far. The massive hemorrhagic effect seen with some viper venoms is not apparent with these elapid venoms.

PROCOAGULANTS

The potent prothrombin converters in some Australian snake venoms are extraordinarily potent coagulants in vitro, but in vivo they usually are not associated with detectable thrombosis. Rather, they are associated with rapid, often complete defibrination and hyperfibrinolysis, resulting in potentially lethal bleeding from any damaged vessels. These procoagulants are of type II and III, varying in size from about 58 kd to greater than 200 kd.

ANTICOAGULANTS

Still poorly characterized, true anticoagulants of clinical significance are restricted to only some *Pseudechis* spp. and are only rarely associated with major bleeding.

HEMORRHAGINS

Hemorrhagins are unproven for any Australian venom, although they are clinically suspected for at least the New Guinea taipan venom.

Nephrotoxins

Nephrotoxins are unproven for any Australian snake venom, although they are clinically suspected for at least brown snake venom.

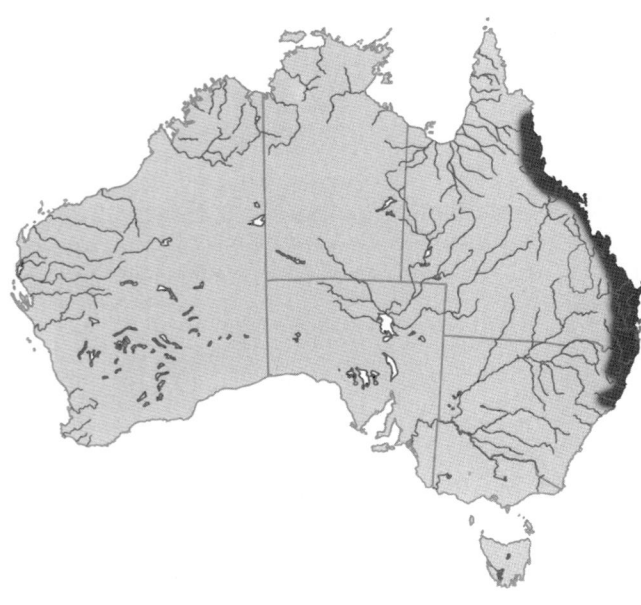

FIGURE 105-14

Distribution of rough-scaled snake, *Tropidechis carinatus.* (Copyright © Dr. Julian White.)

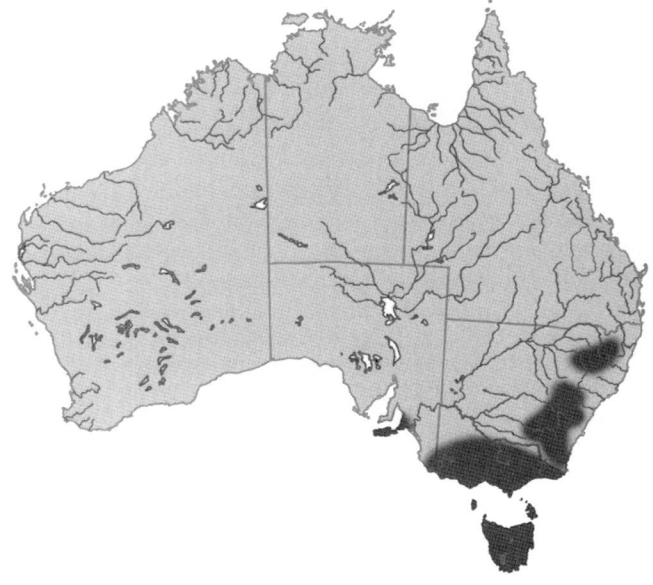

FIGURE 105-16

Distribution of Australian copperheads, *Austrelaps* spp. (Copyright © Dr. Julian White.)

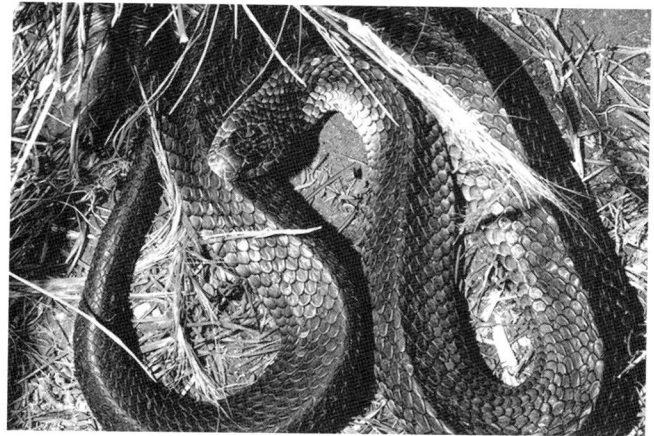

FIGURE 105-17

Common copperhead, *Austrelaps superbus.* (Copyright © Dr. Julian White.)

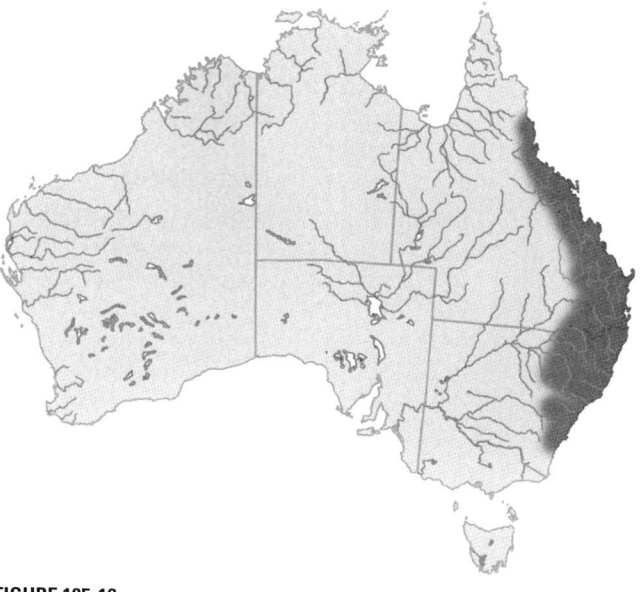

FIGURE 105-19

Distribution of broad-headed snakes in Australia, *Hoplocephalus* spp. (Copyright © Dr. Julian White.)

Necrotoxins

There is no evidence of significant necrotoxic activity in any Australian snake venom, although a few, notably *Notechis* spp., may cause minor local tissue injury in certain circumstances.

PATHOPHYSIOLOGY OF ENVENOMING

Route and Onset

Most cases of snakebite follow subcutaneous injection of venom through one or two fangs, the quantity of venom injected being highly variable within a species and between species and genera (Table 105-4). Major venom components are generally of moderate to large size, mostly greater than 10 kd, and seem to be transported principally from the bite site via lymphatics. Pressure immobilization first aid may effectively retard venom movement completely and delay onset of systemic envenoming until removed, whereupon rapid, severe systemic envenoming may ensue in less than 30 minutes. Without effective first aid, envenoming usually manifests within 30 minutes, although certain effects take longer to appear. Occasionally, envenoming may be delayed by many hours, however, even without first aid.

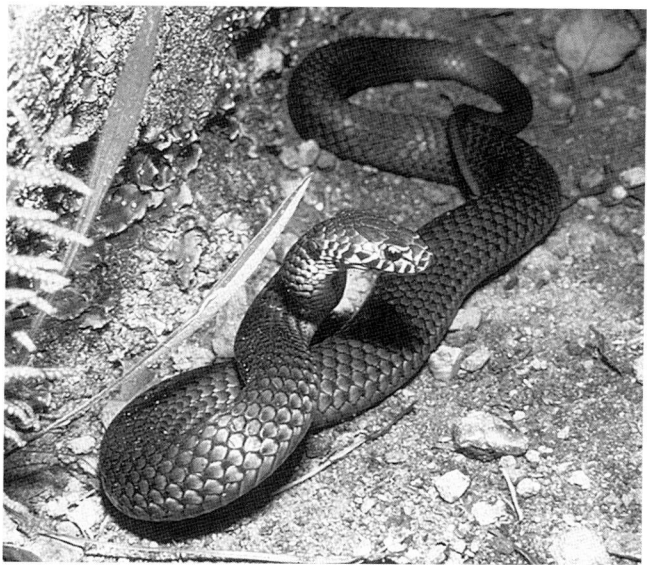

FIGURE 105-18

Pygmy copperhead, *Austrelaps labialis.* (Copyright © Dr. Julian White.)

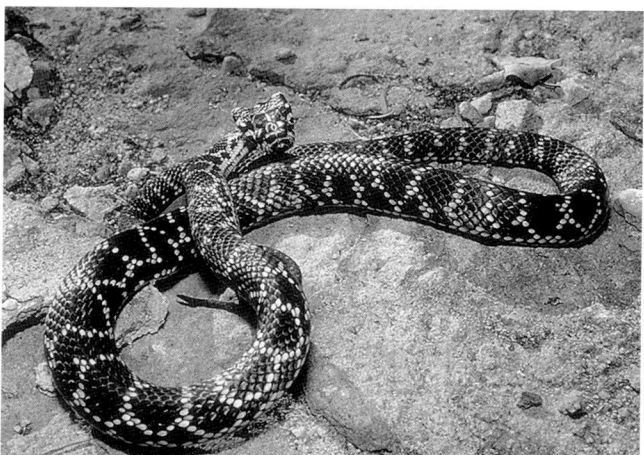

FIGURE 105-20

Broad-headed snake, *Hoplocephalus bungaroides.* (Copyright © Dr. Julian White.)

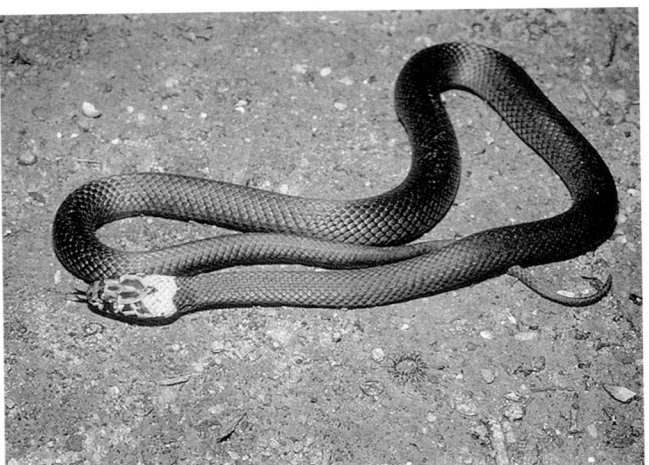

FIGURE 105-21

Pale-headed snake, *Hoplocephalus bitorquatus*. (Copyright © Dr. Julian White.)

Mechanisms

PARALYSIS

Presynaptic and postsynaptic flaccid paralysis is mediated through effects at the neuromuscular junction. The neurotoxins first must traverse from the bite site to the circulation, via the lymphatics, then exit into the extravascular space to reach their target sites, a process easily subject to delays. This may explain why paralysis is unlikely to be evident in the first 60 minutes after the bite and is often apparent only several hours later.

When paralysis has been established, the half-life of the neurotoxins, generally unknown, may have little influence anyway, particularly for presynaptic neurotoxins. When these have caused damage to the terminal axon at the neuromuscular junction, recovery depends on cell regeneration, a process that may take days, weeks, or months.

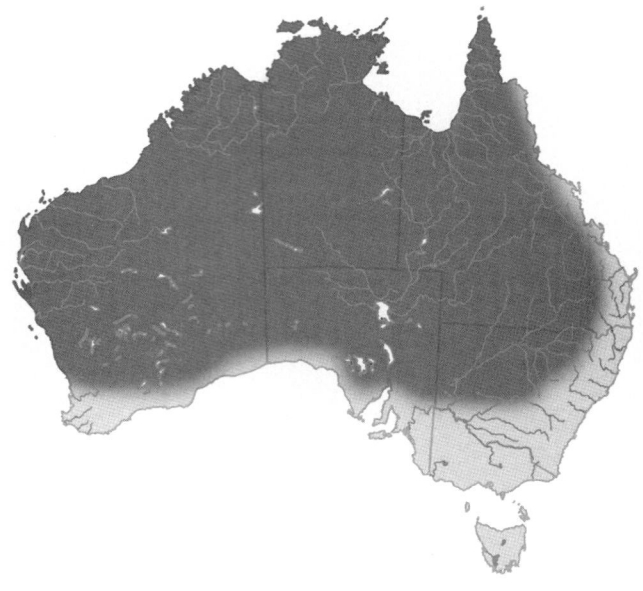

FIGURE 105-23

Distribution of mulga snakes, *Pseudechis australis* and *Pseudechis butleri*. (Copyright © Dr. Julian White.)

MYOLYSIS

The precise mechanism of myolysis induced by Australian snake venom toxins is poorly understood, but experimentally these toxins rapidly cause muscle cell damage when they have reached their target site, a process that, as with the neurotoxins, may be delayed for 1 or more hours. Complete destruction of affected muscle cells occurs within 24 to 72 hours, but the basal lamina is unaffected, and myoblasts quickly begin the rebuilding process, resulting in progressive muscle reconstitution over about 4 weeks. There is experimental evidence that only slow-twitch muscle fibers regenerate.

COAGULOPATHY

The prothrombin converters reach their target as soon as they enter the circulation, a process that may occur within

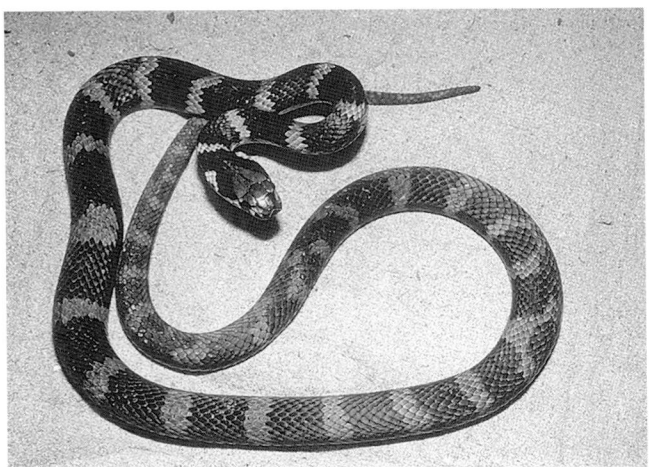

FIGURE 105-22

Stephen's banded snake, *Hoplocephalus stephensi*. (Copyright © Dr. Julian White.)

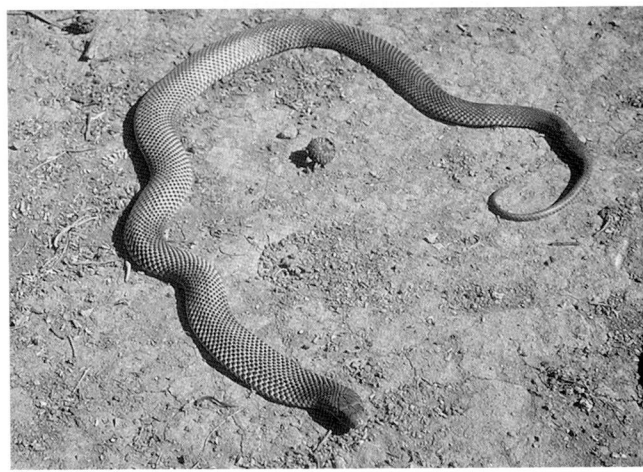

FIGURE 105-24

Mulga snake, *Pseudechis australis*. (Copyright © Dr. Julian White.)

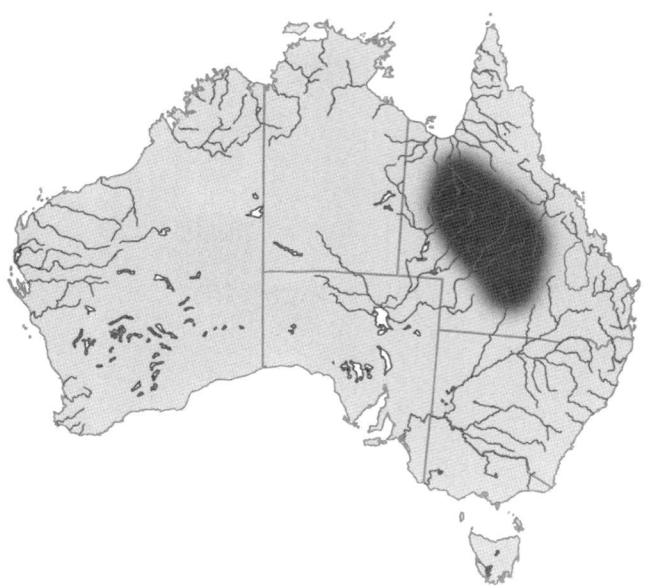

FIGURE 105-25

Distribution of Collett's snake, *Pseudechis colletti*. (Copyright © Dr. Julian White.)

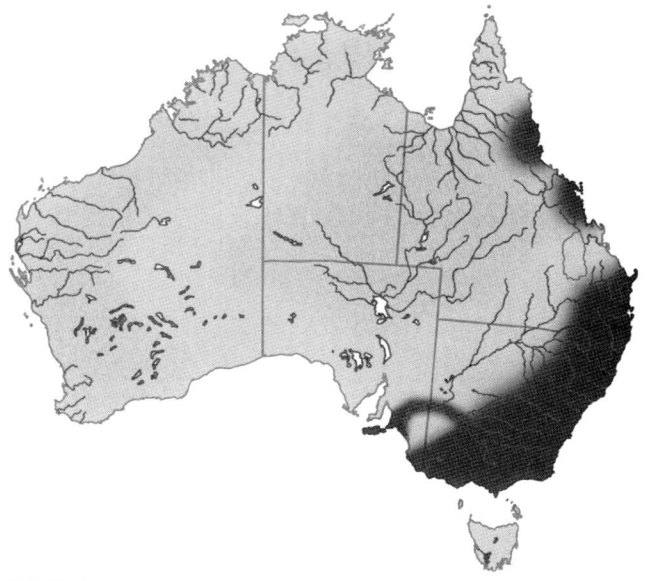

FIGURE 105-27

Distribution of Australian black snakes, *Pseudechis porphyriacus* and *Pseudechis guttatus*. (Copyright © Dr. Julian White.)

10 to 20 minutes of the bite, unless effective first aid is used. Coagulopathy, in this case defibrination, occurs in less than 30 minutes in some cases. Research in dogs suggests that with high venom loads, there may be a brief but significant period of thrombosis, before onset of prolonged and profound defibrination. Fibrinolysis takes several minutes to become established after onset of fibrin formation. During this time, significant thrombi may form, potentially occluding crucial vessels, such as coronary arteries; this may explain the apparent early, often lethal cardiac collapse associated with some severe brown snake bites. By the time an autopsy is performed, hyperfibrinolysis will have ensured removal of all thrombi.

The duration of the prolonged defibrination phase is variable. For tiger snakes, even without treatment, it may last only 15 to 18 hours, but for brown snakes and taipans, it may persist for days if not treated. Untreated coagulopathy is associated with sometimes severe, persistent bleeding from all wounds, including iatrogenic wounds, such as venipuncture sites and intravenous line insertions. Lethal intracranial haemorrhages occur, although not frequently. The addition of external coagulation factors, such as fresh frozen plasma or cryoprecipitate, as treatment can worsen the coagulopathy if active venom procoagulant is still circulating.

The true anticoagulant venoms rarely cause severe effects, although they can rapidly produce gross abnormalities in clotting tests. Because their effect is purely inhibitory, however, without destruction of clotting factors, reversal of anticoagulation is rapid after antivenom therapy. The duration of the anticoagulant effect, if left untreated, is not known, although it is unlikely to extend more than 24 to 48 hours.

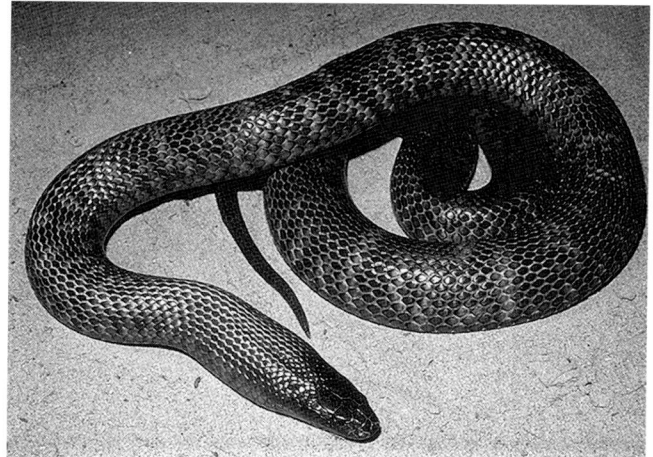

FIGURE 105-26

Collett's snake, *Pseudechis colletti*. (Copyright © Dr. Julian White.)

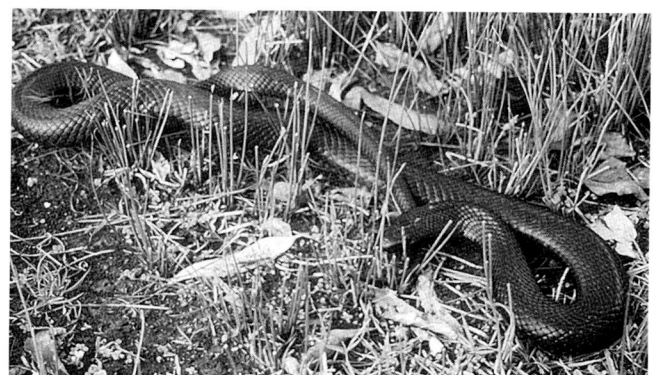

FIGURE 105-28

Red-bellied black snake, *Pseudechis porphyriacus*. (Copyright © Dr. Julian White.)

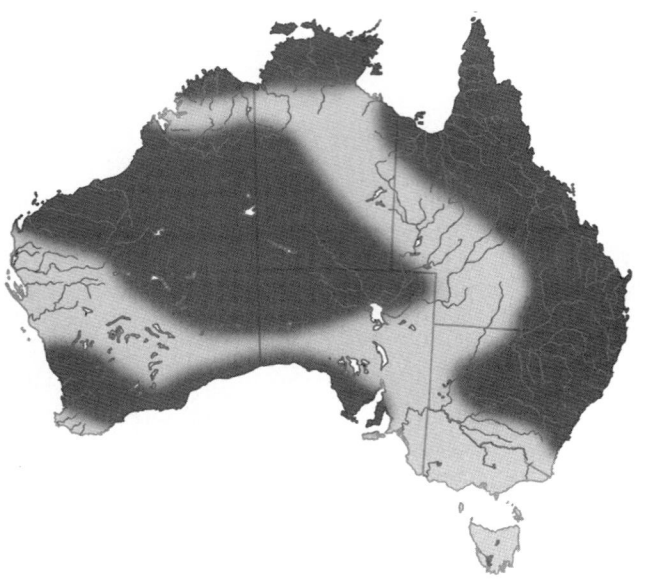

FIGURE 105-29

Distribution of Australian death adders, *Acanthophis* spp. *(Copyright © Dr. Julian White.)*

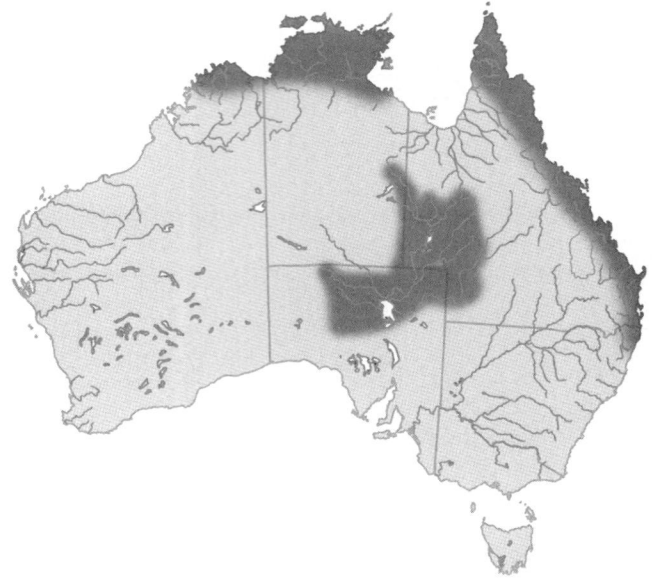

FIGURE 105-31

Distribution of Australian taipans, *Oxyuranus* spp. *(Copyright © Dr. Julian White.)*

RENAL DAMAGE

Although a primary nephrotoxic effect is suspected for brown snake venom, most cases of renal damage after Australian snakebite are probably secondary to some other process, such as myolysis with myoglobinuria, severe coagulopathy, or a hypotensive episode. The depth and duration of renal damage are highly variable, ranging from a mild-to-moderate increase in serum creatinine levels and normal urine output to oliguric or anuric renal failure, often associated with acute tubular necrosis, to rare instances of permanent renal damage, renal cortical necrosis. Only renal cortical necrosis routinely results in long-term problems.

CLINICAL PRESENTATION OF ENVENOMING

The rate of envenoming is highly variable (Table 105-5); many, if not most, Australian snakebites result in no or minimal envenoming and do not require antivenom therapy. It is difficult to determine initially, however, if the bite will be minor or major because the local effects of envenoming, in contrast to snakebite in other parts of the world, are often minor and give no indication of forthcoming systemic problems. It follows that all suspected snakebites in the Australian region should be assumed to be major until clearly shown to be otherwise.

Local Effects

Local effects vary from nil to minimal (e.g., brown snakes); to local pain, bruising, and mild edema (e.g., tiger snakes); to extensive local pain and edema (e.g., mulga and black snakes) (Table 105-6). Bite marks vary from invisible tiny punctures or scratches to obvious single or multiple fang punctures or scratches (Figs. 105-34 through 105-36).

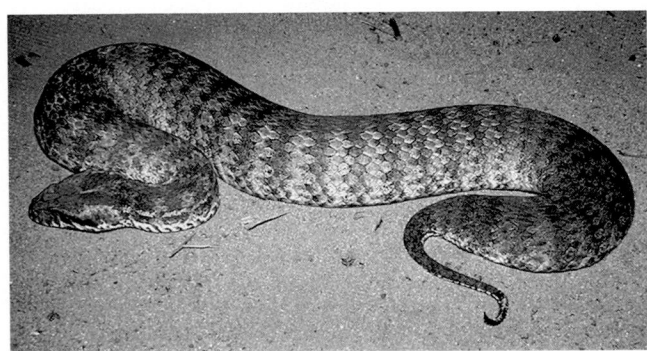

FIGURE 105-30

Common death adder, *Acanthophis antarcticus*. *(Copyright © Dr. Julian White.)*

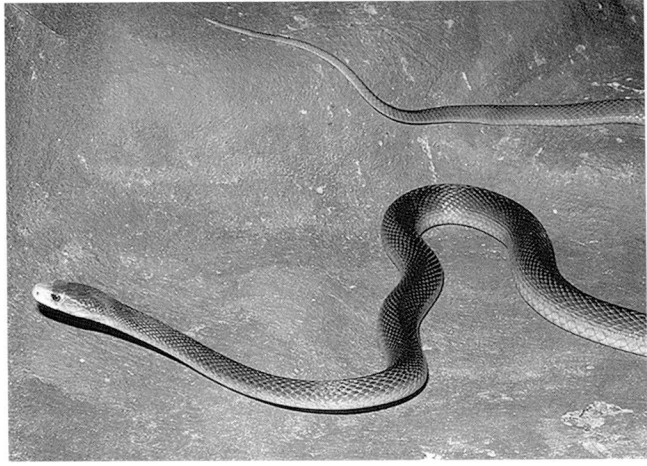

FIGURE 105-32

Common taipan, *Oxyuranus scutullatus*. *(Copyright © Dr. Julian White.)*

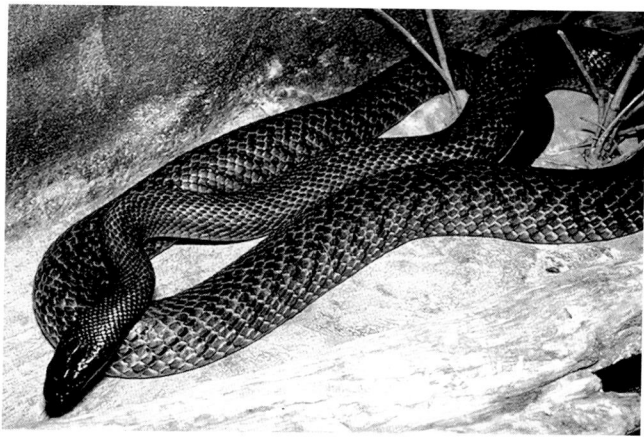

FIGURE 105-33

Inland taipan, *Oxyuranus microlepidotus. (Copyright © Dr. Julian White.)*

TABLE 105-3 Summary of Principal Venom Activities for Each Group of Snakes*

SNAKE GROUP	VENOM ACTIVITY
Colubridae	
Brown tree snake	Venom poorly characterized
Elapidae	
Brown snake group	Procoagulant, pre- and postsynaptic neurotoxin, possible nephrotoxin
Tiger snake group	Procoagulant, pre- and postsynaptic neurotoxin, myotoxin
Black snake group	Anticoagulant, myotoxin, neurotoxin (Papuan black snake)
Death adder group	Postsynaptic neurotoxin
Taipan group	Procoagulant, pre- and postsynaptic neurotoxin, myotoxin
New Guinea small-eyed snake	Anticoagulant, myotoxin, postsynaptic neurotoxin
Sea snakes	Postsynaptic neurotoxin, myotoxin

*Not all species in each group display all activities listed for that group.

TABLE 105-4 Average Venom Yields for Major Snake Groups*

SNAKE GROUP	AVERAGE VENOM YIELD (mg)
Colubridae	
Brown tree snake	1–10
Elapidae	
Brown snake group	2–>20
Tiger snake group	5–>50
Black snake group	30–>180
Death adder group	80
Taipan group	>120
New Guinea small-eyed snake	Not well characterized
Sea snakes	2–>30

*Averages vary among species within group; average milked venom in dry weight.

TABLE 105-5 Estimated Average Rate of Medically Significant Envenoming for Medically Important Snake Groups*

SNAKE GROUP	AVERAGE RATE OF ENVENOMING (%)
Colubridae	
Brown tree snake	Infants, <20; all others, <1
Elapidae	
Brown snake group	<20
Tiger snake group	>50
Black snake group	>50
Death adder group	>60
Taipan group	>80
New Guinea small-eyed snake	Not well characterized
Sea snakes	<20

*Figures are only approximate and may vary among species in group.

General Systemic Effects

The general effects of systemic envenoming are easily confused with the effects of anxiety, itself a likely response to suspected snakebite. When venom has been absorbed and traverses the lymphatics, draining lymph nodes may become enlarged or tender. The patient may develop a severe headache, nausea, persistent vomiting, abdominal pain, dizziness, blurred vision, and nonspecific (i.e., nonneurotoxic) weakness. Early collapse is common, usually associated with

TABLE 105-6 Local Effects at Bite Site for Medically Important Snake Groups

SNAKE GROUP	LOCAL EFFECT OF BITE
Colubridae	
Brown tree snake	Mild-to-moderate swelling, ± blistering, without necrosis
Elapidae	
Brown snake group	Nil or minimal local pain, swelling, or erythema. Even severe bites may be virtually invisible and the patient unaware of bite
Tiger snake group	Tiger snakes and rough-scaled snakes generally cause painful bites with local erythema, ecchymosis, and swelling. Copperhead bites are less locally severe. Broad-headed snakes usually cause few local effects
Black snake group	Locally painful, usually with moderate-to-marked local, occasionally regional swelling. Papuan black snake causes less marked local swelling
Death adder group	Locally painful, but usually little local swelling or other visible effects
Taipan group	Variable from minimal local effects to local pain, swelling, erythema, and slight ecchymosis
New Guinea small-eyed snake	Not well characterized
Sea snakes	Minimal local reaction

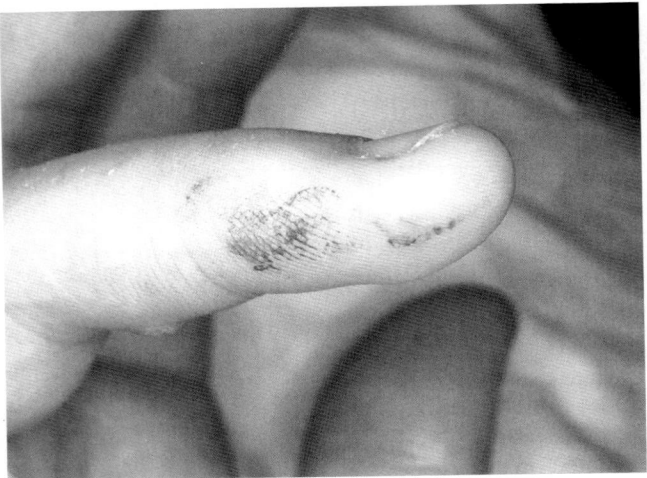

FIGURE 105-34

Minimal local reaction at the bite site, as seen with brown snake bites. Minimal local effects can be associated with life-threatening systemic envenoming. *(Copyright © Dr. Julian White.)*

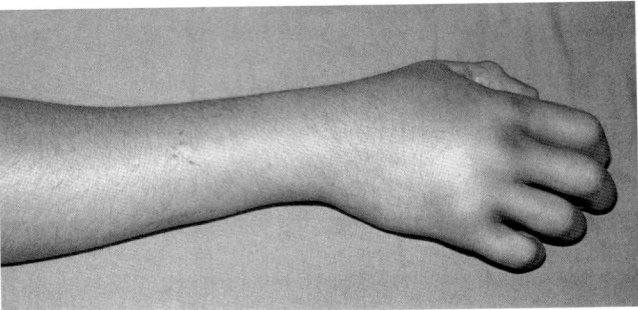

FIGURE 105-36

Extensive local swelling, typical of mulga snake bites. *(Copyright © Dr. Julian White.)*

spontaneous recovery after only a few minutes. Particularly in children, generalized convulsions may occur.

Specific Systemic Effects

Australian snakebite is strongly associated with potentially lethal specific systemic effects (Table 105-7).

NEUROTOXIC PARALYSIS

Progressive flaccid paralysis, ending after 18 to 30 hours in complete respiratory paralysis and death due to respiratory failure, previously was the classic cause of snakebite death. With modern intensive care unit facilities, such respiratory deaths should now be rare. The first signs of flaccid paralysis are seen in the cranial nerves, at least 1 hour (sometimes many hours) postbite. Ptosis usually is seen

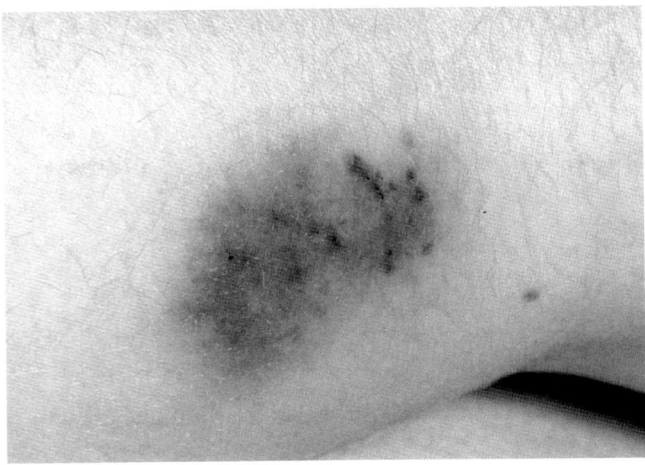

FIGURE 105-35

Local erythema and bruising at the bite site, typical of tiger snake bites. *(Copyright © Dr. Julian White.)*

first (Fig. 105-37), followed by partial ophthalmoplegia (diplopia) (Fig. 105-38), then complete ophthalmoplegia with fixed forward gaze, often with fixed dilated pupils. Ophthalmoplegia is accompanied by dysarthria, dysphagia, tongue weakness, slack facies, and drooling. Loss of airway protection at this stage may force early intubation. Untreated, the paralysis may extend to encompass limb weakness to complete paralysis, with loss of deep tendon reflexes. Paralysis of respiratory muscles, particularly the diaphragm, may take 18 to 30 hours postbite to develop (Fig. 105-39).

MYOLYSIS

Myolysis takes one or more hours postbite to become evident, as development of muscle pain, tenderness, and nonspecific weakness, usually with some degree of myoglobinuria (Fig. 105-40) and always with a major rise in plasma creatine phosphokinase (CPK). Occasionally, myolysis becomes evident only 1 to 2 days postbite. Major myolysis is associated with secondary renal failure and severe hyperkalemia, with concomitant, potentially lethal cardiac problems.

COAGULOPATHY

Coagulopathy, even complete defibrination, although usually found in association with obvious general symptoms, such as headache and vomiting, may develop silently, particularly in adults, becoming apparent only when clotting tests are performed or when major bleeding manifests unexpectedly. The classic sign of coagulopathy is a persistent oozing of blood not only from the bite site but also from venipuncture and intravenous insertion sites and from any recent wound (Fig. 105-41). Intracranial bleeds or bleeds into major organs manifest as with any other cause of such bleeding. The clinician should beware of injudicious venous or arterial line insertions if coagulopathy possibly could be present and should avoid insertion or sampling from the subclavian, femoral, or jugular vessels (Fig. 105-42). Extended coagulation tests, repeated frequently, are the most useful determinant of coagulopathy. The abnormalities detected depend not only on the severity of the envenoming but also on the type of snake and its venom constituents. Thrombocytopenia is not common and usually indicates secondary disseminated intravascular coagulation.

TABLE 105-7 Principal Systemic Effects for Medically Important Snake Groups

SNAKE GROUP	SYSTEMIC EFFECT
Colubridae	
Boiga irregularis	In infants only (Guam cases), mild flaccid paralysis (ptosis, lethargy, impaired standing/walking), rarely respiratory distress
Elapidae	
Brown Snake Group	
Pseudonaja spp.	Defibrination coagulopathy, ± renal damage, only rarely paralysis, never myolysis
Tiger Snake Group	
Notechis spp.	Defibrination coagulopathy (resolves untreated after 15–18 hr), pre- and postsynaptic flaccid paralysis (severe), severe myolysis, ± renal damage
Tropidechis carinatus	As for *Notechis* spp.
Austrelaps spp.	Poorly defined; flaccid paralysis dominant feature
Hoplocephalus spp.	Defibrination coagulopathy only
Rhinoplocephalus nigrescens	Myolysis only, ± secondary renal damage
Black Snake Group	
Pseudechis australis, Pseudechis butleri, Pseudechis colletti	Anticoagulant coagulopathy, severe myolysis, rarely mild flaccid paralysis (ptosis only)
Pseudechis papuanus	Coagulopathy, thrombocytopenia, flaccid paralysis
Pseudechis guttatus, Pseudechis porphyriacus	Occasionally mild-to-moderate myolysis
Death Adder Group	
Acanthophis spp.	Postsynaptic flaccid paralysis only
Taipan Group	
Oxyuranus spp.	Defibrination coagulopathy, hemorrhage, pre- and postsynaptic flaccid paralysis (rapid, severe), occasionally moderate myolysis, ± renal damage
Miscellaneous	
Micropechis ikaheka	Poorly defined due to paucity of reported cases, but expect coagulopathy, bleeding, flaccid paralysis, possibly myolysis, ± secondary renal damage
Sea Snakes	Varies with species, but flaccid postsynaptic paralysis and/or myolysis, ± secondary renal damage

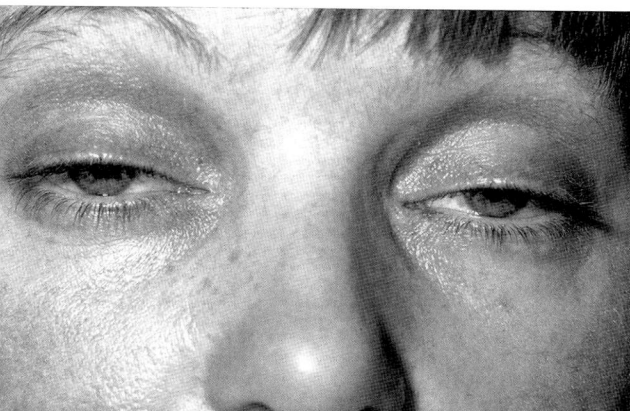

FIGURE 105-37

Early ptosis, the first sign of developing paralysis (tiger snake bite). *(Copyright © Dr. Julian White.)*

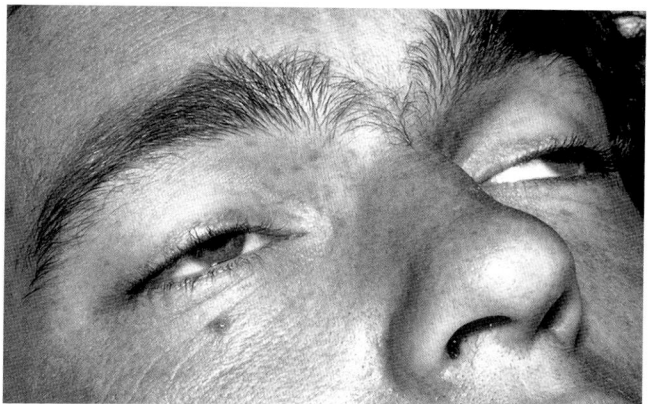

FIGURE 105-38

Partial ophthalmoplegia with divergent squint and diplopia. Ptosis is also present (death adder bite). *(Copyright © Dr. Julian White.)*

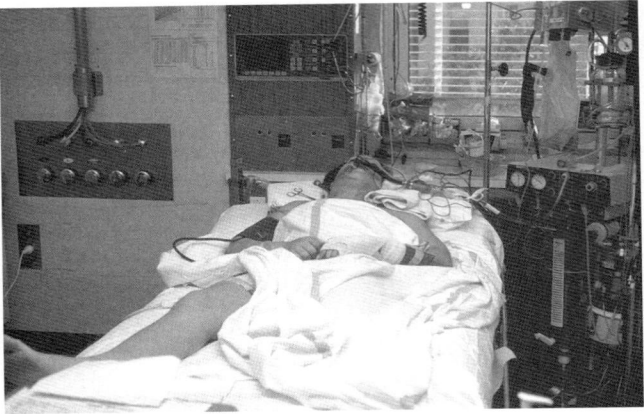

FIGURE 105-39

Complete flaccid paralysis, requiring prolonged mechanical respiratory support (on ventilator for 5 weeks; taipan bite). *(Copyright © Dr. Julian White.)*

RENAL DAMAGE

Renal damage usually is symptomatically silent. It is first announced by either a rising blood creatinine or by a falling urine output.

OTHER

Cardiac abnormalities are not common with Australian snakebite and when present are always secondary, either to coagulopathy (early temporary thrombosis) or to myolysis (hyperkalemia). Although hypotension may occur, systemic envenoming usually is associated with hypertension. An absolute lymphopenia is a common, although not universal, accompaniment of major systemic envenoming.

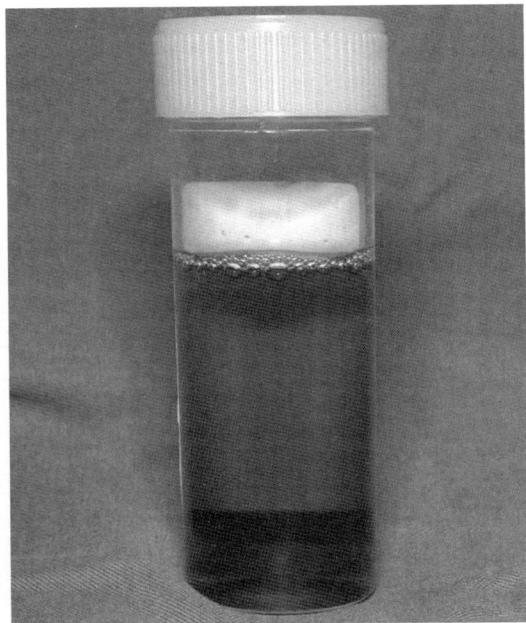

FIGURE 105-40

Red urine indicative of myoglobinuria (mulga snake bite). *(Copyright © Dr. Julian White.)*

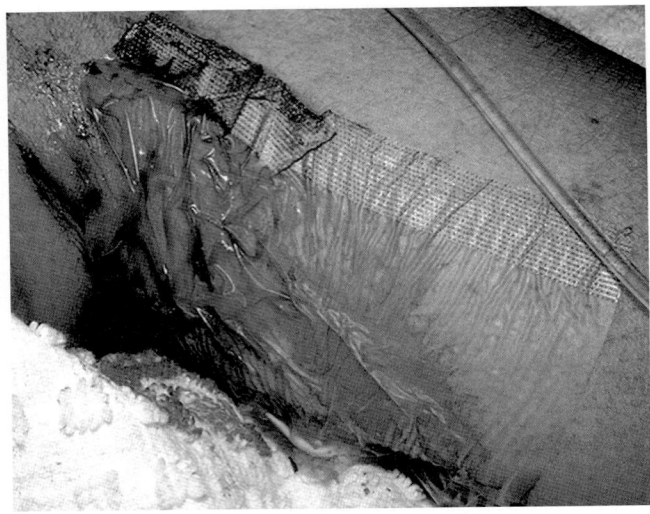

FIGURE 105-41

Persistent blood ooze from venous line site, indicating coagulopathy (inland taipan bite). *(Copyright © Dr. Julian White.)*

DIAGNOSIS OF ENVENOMING

The diagnosis of envenoming may be simple or difficult. The latter applies in children, who may not be able to give a history of a bite, and in adults, who may be bitten unawares, presenting later with general symptoms that could imply a wide array of diagnoses. The often trivial, sometimes invisible bite marks may make correct diagnosis difficult, unless a high index of suspicion is maintained for snakebite.

History

The crucial points in history are the following:

Geographic location where a bite might have occurred
Circumstances surrounding definite or suspected bite

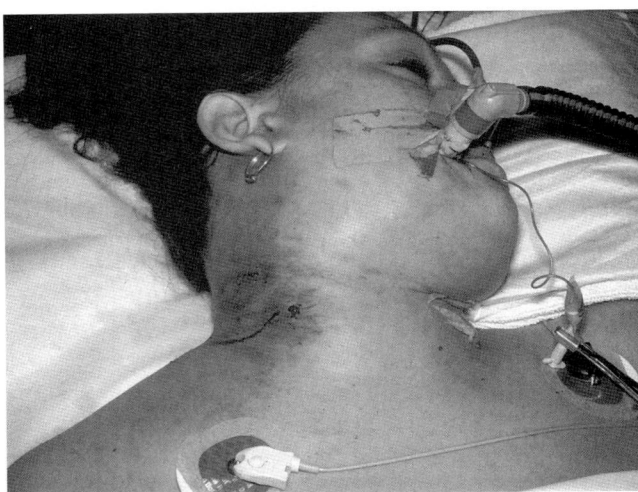

FIGURE 105-42

Extensive hematoma extending from failed jugular line insertion in the neck, in a patient with severe coagulopathy (taipan bite). *(Copyright © Dr. Julian White.)*

Number of bites

Activity before applying first aid

Type and effectiveness of first aid

Timing of onset and nature of any symptoms that might reflect envenoming

Past medical history, including any past exposure to antivenom

Medications, particularly those affecting blood clotting

Examination

The crucial points in examination are the following:

Local bite site—presence of bite marks (especially multiple bites), persistent bleeding, edema, and bruising

Tender or swollen draining lymph nodes

Presence of signs of paralysis, myolysis, or coagulopathy

Laboratory Tests

The crucial laboratory tests are the following:

Snake venom detection (Australia and New Guinea only)

Extended coagulation studies (prothrombin time or international normalized ratio [PT/INR]), activated partial thromboplastin time, fibrinogen level, and fibrin degradation products/D dimer (FDP/XDP)

Complete blood count (platelet count, absolute lymphocyte count)

Electrolytes and renal function

CPK

In a country hospital without ready access to a laboratory, a reasonable assessment can be made with the following tests:

Snake venom detection

Whole-blood clotting time

Dip-stick urine analysis

If initial tests are normal, they must be repeated to eliminate delayed envenoming. As a general rule, tests should be done on presentation, then again 2 hours and 5 hours later, and, if indicated, before discharge the following day. If tests are abnormal, a different test regimen is required (see later in treatment section).

INTERPRETING LABORATORY TESTS

Laboratory tests can be crucial in determining if systemic envenoming is present or if snakebite is likely, and it may assist in determining the type of snake.

Snake Venom Detection

Interpretation of snake venom detection tests is discussed subsequently.

Coagulation Tests

Significantly prolonged PT/INR (INR 2 to >12) and activated partial thromboplastin time plus decreased fibrinogen (often undetectable) and increased FDP/XDP (often grossly increased) usually with normal platelet count indicate defibrination coagulopathy (brown snakes, tiger snakes, rough-scaled snakes, broad-headed snakes, taipans).

Significantly prolonged PT/INR (INR 2 to >12); usually less prolonged activated partial thromboplastin time; and normal fibrinogen, FDP/XDP, and platelets indicates anticoagulant coagulopathy (mulga snake, Collett's snake, Papuan black snake).

Absolute Lymphocyte Count

Absolute lymphopenia is a feature of significant systemic envenoming by potentially all Australian dangerous snakes, but particularly tiger snakes. It is seen usually in the first 12 hours after onset of envenoming.

Electrolytes and Renal Function

Rising serum creatinine and urea indicate developing renal damage.

Hyperkalemia usually indicates severe myolysis, mostly in association with secondary renal failure.

Creatine Phosphokinase

CPK elevation may indicate myolysis; values greater than 5000 U/L almost always are due to myolysis in a snakebite patient. Values greater than 1 million U/L may occur. Peak myolysis may not be seen for 72 hours, occasionally longer.

VENOM DETECTION

The CSL Ltd. Snake Venom Detection Kit (SVDK) is an enzyme-linked immunosorbent assay–based test, unique to Australia and New Guinea, capable of detecting nanogram-quantities of major snake venoms in samples from the bite site or urine (blood is not reliable). The SVDK contains five separate wells, each one corresponding to a type of snake. The best sample is a swab from the bite site, first moistened with the SVDK fluid, but in the presence of systemic envenoming, urine also may be used. A positive result indicates that snake venom is probably present and indicates the most likely type of snake, but it is not an indication to use antivenom; it merely indicates which is the most appropriate antivenom, should this be required on clinical or laboratory grounds. A negative result indicates only the test was negative; it does not exclude snakebite. The SVDK is not readily available in New Guinea.

Diagnostic Algorithms

Diagnostic algorithms have been developed for Australia to assist in determining the most likely snake in cases with significant systemic envenoming (Figs. 105-43 and 105-44). These algorithms are useful when venom detection has failed or is not available, or when the result is suspect, they help support the SVDK result. Similar to all such diagnostic algorithms, these cannot cater to all eventualities and should be used with wisdom and caution.

Differential Diagnosis

Snakebite should be considered in the differential diagnosis of any unexplained flaccid paralysis, myolysis, coagulopathy, unexpected major hemorrhage, renal failure, cardiac collapse, general collapse, or convulsions. Snakebite is not limited to rural areas or outside buildings; dangerous snakes regularly enter gardens and homes in even the largest cities.

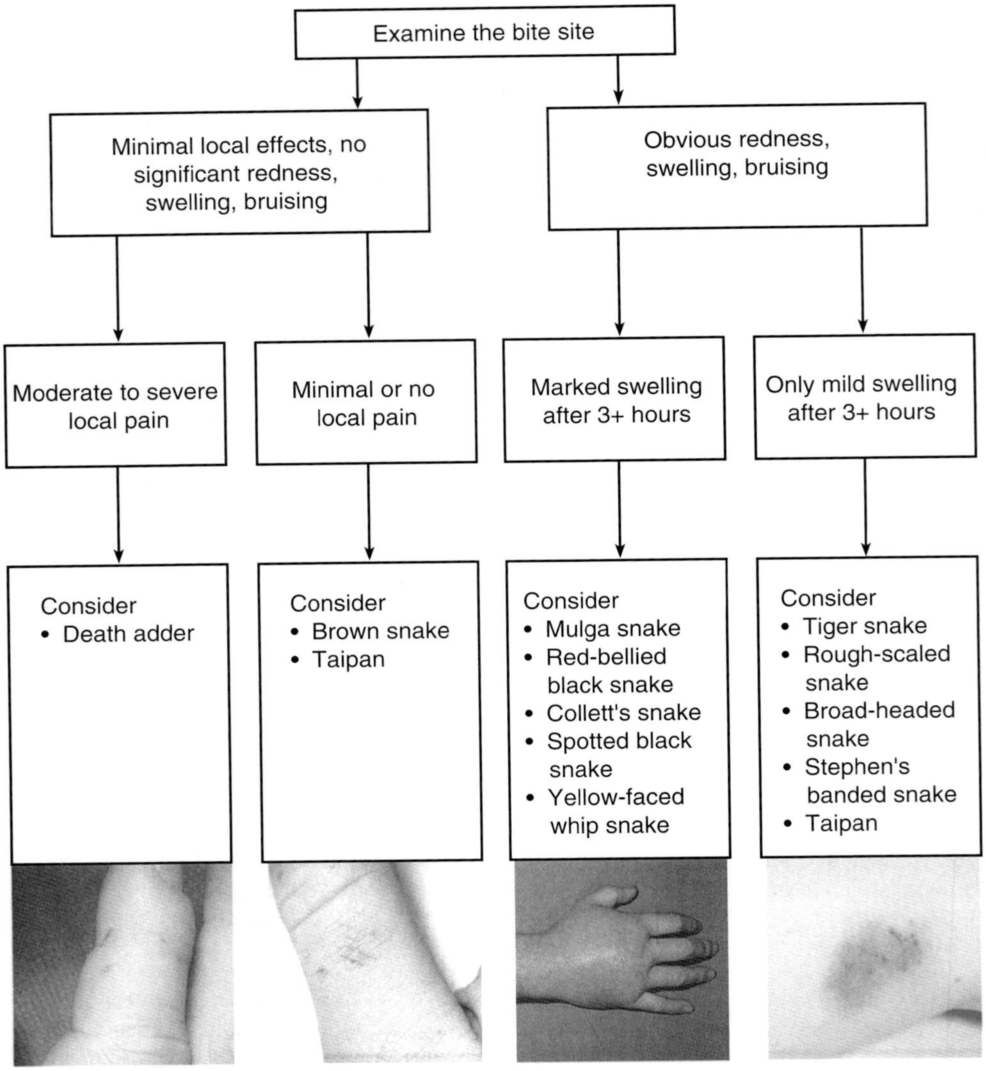

Examine the bite site

↓   ↓

Minimal local effects, no significant redness, swelling, bruising

Obvious redness, swelling, bruising

↓   ↓   ↓   ↓

Moderate to severe local pain

Minimal or no local pain

Marked swelling after 3+ hours

Only mild swelling after 3+ hours

↓   ↓   ↓   ↓

Consider
• Death adder

Consider
• Brown snake
• Taipan

Consider
• Mulga snake
• Red-bellied black snake
• Collett's snake
• Spotted black snake
• Yellow-faced whip snake

Consider
• Tiger snake
• Rough-scaled snake
• Broad-headed snake
• Stephen's banded snake
• Taipan

FIGURE 105-43

Diagnostic algorithm for Australian snakebite, based on local effects. *(Copyright © Dr. Julian White.)*

TREATMENT OF ENVENOMING

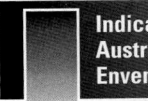

Indications for ICU Admission in Australian and Pacific Snake Envenoming

Every case of significant systemic envenoming with any of the following:
  Any degree of flaccid paralysis beyond simple ptosis
  Any established defibrination or anticoagulant coagulopathy
  Any major myolysis with creatine phosphokinase greater than 10,000 U/L
  Any major secondary problems, such as major bleeding or anuric renal failure
The following cases are best managed in a high-dependency unit setting or, if unavailable, in an intensive care unit:
  Any case of suspected snakebite, even if initially no evidence of systemic envenoming

Although most snakebites in Australia are likely to prove minor, this cannot be reliably predicted within the first few hours. All cases of definite or suspected snakebite should be considered potentially major and lethal until clearly shown to be otherwise.

First-Aid Considerations

First aid for snakebite in Australia and New Guinea is the pressure immobilization method, designed to retard venom movement via the lymphatics. It has been shown to be effective in a monkey model and anecdotally in human cases of envenoming, although the method remains unproven by clinical trial. Nevertheless, the pressure immobilization method appears comparatively safe and effective compared with the alternatives used in most other parts of the world. The technique involves the application of a broad bandage over the bitten area, at about the same pressure as used for a sprain. The bandage is extended to cover as much

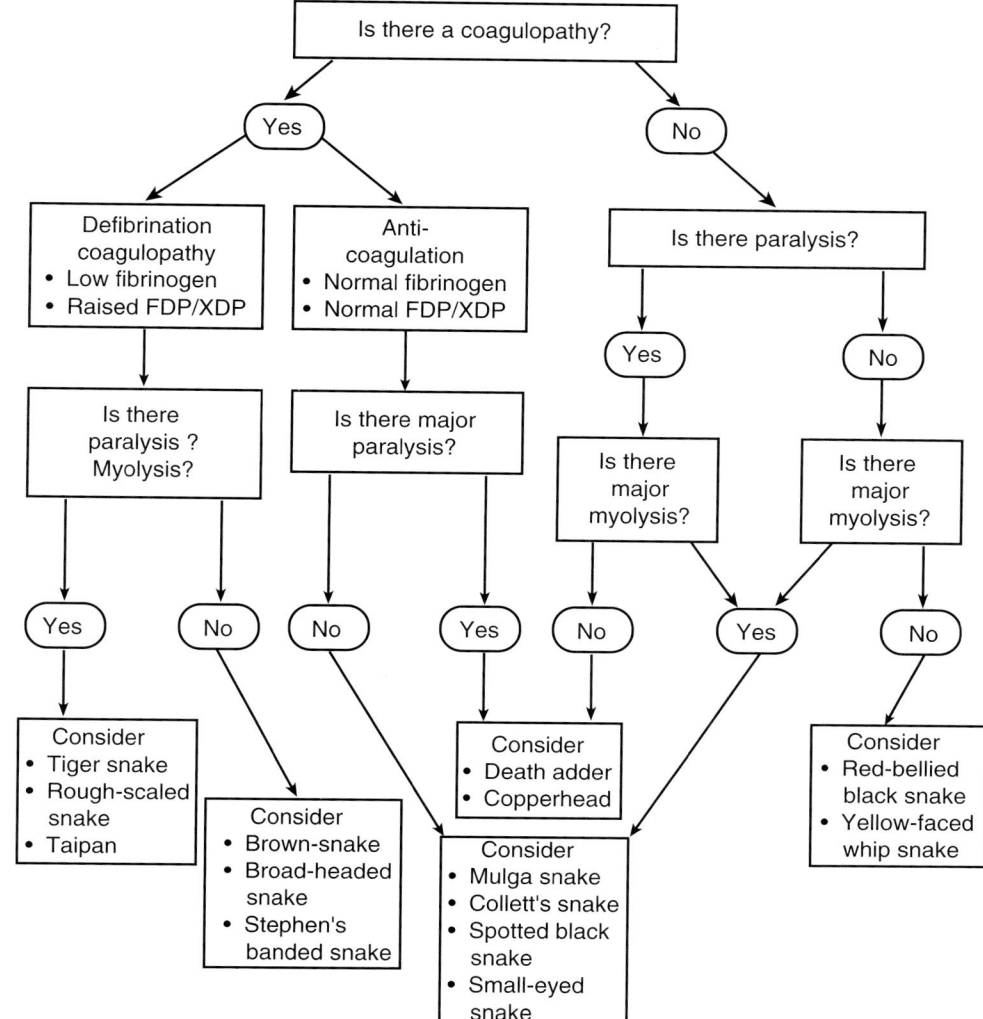

FIGURE 105-44

Diagnostic algorithm for Australian snakebite based on systemic effects. FDP/XDP, fibrin degradation product/D dimer. *(Copyright © Dr. Julian White.)*

of the limb as possible, then the limb is immobilized using a splint. Correctly applied, this first aid can be left on for several hours, until the patient is in a hospital and can be treated with appropriate antivenom, if required.

When the patient is already in the hospital, the issues with first aid are when to apply it in the hospital and, more commonly, when to remove it. First aid should be applied in a hospital only if the following apply:

1. It is less than 15 minutes postbite.
2. There are no facilities to give antivenom, and the patient will be transferred elsewhere.
3. The patient already has severe, life-threatening envenoming.

First aid should be removed in the hospital only when the following have been done:

1. An intravenous line has been inserted, with an initial intravenous fluid load.
2. The bandage over the bite site has been cut away, the wound has been inspected, and the wound has been

moist-swabbed (swab stick moistened with diluent) for venom detection.
3. Blood has been taken for relevant tests (coagulation, complete blood count, electrolytes, renal function, CPK).
4. A relevant history has been obtained.
5. The patient has been examined for signs of envenoming.
6. The results of venom detection and blood tests have been received and evaluated.
7. An expert in envenoming has been consulted (if appropriate).
8. Initial antivenom therapy has been started, if required (it is not required in most cases).

The first aid should not be left on when the above-listed requirements are fulfilled. Prolonged use of first aid may cause local skin injury (notably with tiger snake bites).

Basic Treatment

As noted earlier, after vital functions are secured (rarely an issue), initial management is based on obtaining intravenous access; ensuring adequate hydration; establishing a firm diagnosis, including assessment of the extent of any envenoming; and starting specific treatment if required. Because most cases of snakebite in Australia do not result in significant envenoming, initial tests are likely to be normal. Because delayed envenoming can occur, it is essential both that repeat tests be performed (at about 2 hours and 5 hours after the initial tests) and that vital signs be assessed frequently, including checks for early paralysis, coagulopathy, and myolysis. Renal output should be monitored; if the output is in question, the patient should be catheterized. Snakebite in New Guinea is different because a higher proportion of cases show significant envenoming, correct first aid is unlikely to have been used, laboratory testing and antivenom may be unavailable except in a few major centers, and patients frequently present many hours postbite with major problems already evident.

Antivenom

The key decision in managing snakebite is when to give antivenom, then which type and how much. All cases with significant envenoming should be considered for antivenom therapy. It is required in nearly all such cases, often proving lifesaving.

WHEN TO USE ANTIVENOM

Antivenom should be used only in the presence of significant systemic envenoming, which may be defined as the presence of one or more of the following:

Flaccid paralysis (even just ptosis, unless this is the only sign and has been present >12 hours)
Myolysis (usually a CPK >5000 U/L or a rapidly increasing CPK early after envenoming)
Coagulopathy (usually any degree of defibrination, probably an INR >2, certainly an INR >4.0, *or* any degree of true anticoagulation)
Renal damage (an elevated and rising creatinine, even if still normal urine output)
A clear history of collapse or convulsions after a witnessed snakebite by a dangerous species of snake (e.g., not a python bite).

General symptoms, such as headache, nausea, vomiting, and abdominal pain, although raising suspicions of significant envenoming, also may be due to anxiety and are not alone an indication that antivenom is required. A positive SVDK result from either the bite site or urine in isolation is not an indication that antivenom is required. Antivenom should be given as soon as safely possible when there is an indication that it is required.

CHOOSING THE RIGHT ANTIVENOM

In contrast to some other regions, the choice of snake antivenom, although limited to one producer (CSL Ltd, Melbourne), encompasses a variety of "monovalent" antivenoms, in addition to a polyvalent antivenom. The latter covers all species but is the highest volume (increased risk of adverse reactions) and the highest cost and generally is used only if the type of snake is unknown and it is not practical to cover all possible species by mixing two monovalent antivenoms. The available antivenoms and the

species they cover are listed in Table 105-8. Because envenoming by some species requires the equivalent of multiple ampules of antivenom as an initial dose, the disadvantages of routinely using polyvalent antivenom are apparent.

Identifying which type of snake is responsible for the bite is the principal function of the SVDK. This identification may be supported by the use of diagnostic algorithms, as discussed earlier. Because color is variable and an unreliable indicator of species, the patient's identification of the snake, if offered, should be used only with great caution. An exception is a herpetologist bitten by a captive snake or a wild specimen during the course of capture; however, not all herpetologists are as reliable at identifying snakes as their confidence might suggest.

In New Guinea, assuming that antivenom is even available, the range of antivenoms is often limited to Death Adder and Polyvalent. Because death adders are distinctive snakes, a patient's confident assertion that the assailant was a death adder is usually correct. In all other circumstances, polyvalent antivenom should be used. In Indonesian New Guinea (Irian Jaya) and a few islands to the east, where death adders occur, CSL antivenoms may be unavailable. Instead, local Indonesian antivenoms may be present. These are essentially useless for the snakes discussed in this chapter and should not be used, unless it is certain that the bite was from an Indonesian cobra (not likely in Irian Jaya, unless a captive specimen).

In Pacific islands with terrestrial snakes, envenoming does not warrant antivenom, or none is available (e.g., brown tree snake bite to an infant in Guam). For all areas where sea snakes are present, the optimal choice of antivenom is CSL Sea Snake. If it is unavailable, CSL Tiger Snake or Polyvalent should be tried, at a ratio of 3 ampules for each ampule of Sea Snake antivenom that would have been indicated.

CORRECT DOSE

The initial dose of antivenom depends on the type of snake and the degree of envenoming. Although there are no absolutes in determining dose, suggested guidelines are given in Table 105-8. Giving too low an initial dose is a common reason for failure of antivenom therapy. In New Guinea, where antivenom is in restricted supply, optimal doses are rarely achievable. Often only a single dose of one to two ampules is all that is possible. Children require the same dose as adults.

HOW TO GIVE ANTIVENOM

Antivenom for snakebite should always be given intravenously, preferably diluted 1:10 in saline, Hartman's, or a similar solution. The degree of dilution achievable is determined by the volume of antivenom and the size of the patient. Significant dilutions may be difficult to achieve with pediatric patients, with elderly patients with preexisting cardiac problems, or with high-volume antivenoms such as Polyvalent. The infusion should be started slowly, aiming to give the whole dose (even multiple ampules) over 15 to 20 minutes. The clinicians always should have epinephrine ready to give, should an anaphylactoid reaction occur. If available, a prepared epinephrine infusion is most suitable, with an infusion pump.

TABLE 105-8 Recommended Starting Doses of Antivenom for Patients with Significant Envenoming, Based on Type of Snake*

SNAKE	STARTING DOSE OF ANTIVENOM†
Colubridae	
Boiga irregularis	No AV available
Elapidae	
Brown Snake Group	
Pseudonaja spp.	4 vials CSL Brown Snake AV
Tiger Snake Group	
Notechis scutatus and most *Notechis ater* subspecies	3–4 vials CSL Tiger Snake AV
Notechis ater serventyi, Notechis ater humphreysi	4–6 vials CSL Tiger Snake AV
Tropidechis carinatus	4 vials CSL Tiger Snake AV
Austrelaps spp.	1–3 vials CSL Tiger Snake AV
Hoplocephalus spp.	3 vials CSL Tiger Snake AV
Rhinoplocephalus nigrescens	≥1 vials CSL Tiger Snake AV
Black Snake Group	
Pseudechis australis, Pseudechis butleri, colletti	≥1 vials CSL Black Snake AV
Pseudechis guttatus, Pseudechis porphyriacus	≥1 vials CSL Tiger Snake AV
Death Adder Group	
Acanthophis spp.	≥1 vials CSL Death Adder AV
Taipan Group	
Oxyuranus spp.	≥3 vials CSL Taipan or Polyvalent AV
Miscellaneous	
Micropechis ikaheka	1–3 vials CSL Polyvalent Snake AV
Sea Snakes	≥1 vials CSL Sea Snake AV, or if unavailable, ≥3 vials CSL Tiger Snake AV or CSL Polyvalent Snake AV

*All listed antivenoms (AV) are produced by CSL Ltd, Melbourne, Australia.
†For all snakes, if insufficient specific AV is available, consider using CSL Polyvalent Snake Antivenom at the same dose (i.e., same number of vials) as for the specific antivenom. Dose given is initial dose only. Severe cases may require higher initial doses, and many cases may require further doses after the initial dose.

WHEN TO GIVE MORE ANTIVENOM

The initial dose may not be enough, but determining when and how much more antivenom to give is not always straightforward. For defibrination coagulopathy, enough antivenom has been given when fibrinogen levels start to rise, indicated by either an increase in the absolute value or by a decrease in the PT/INR. It is not necessary to wait for return to normal values. In general, coagulation tests should be repeated at 1 hour and 3 hours after completion of the initial dose of antivenom. The first test is to indicate trends, and the second test is to decide if further antivenom is needed. If the 3-hour test shows no change from complete defibrination, further antivenom should be given in a dose similar to or slightly less than the initial dose. This cycle is repeated until resolution becomes apparent. Fresh frozen plasma or cryoprecipitate should not be given while there is active coagulopathy except if an uncontrolled and catastrophic hemorrhage is occurring.

For myolysis, laboratory tests are less helpful in guiding further therapy. If there is a persistent significant increase in CPK after initial antivenom therapy, however, giving further antivenom at a similar dose may be considered.

For postsynaptic paralysis, giving further antivenom may be considered if the initial dose fails to cause adequate reversal of signs. For presynaptic paralysis, there is little likelihood that antivenom would reverse established paralysis, so further antivenom therapy is pointless.

For renal damage, the role of antivenom is uncertain. Because most renal damage is mediated through secondary effects, further antivenom is unlikely to result in benefit.

ANTIVENOM THERAPY COMPLICATIONS

If the patient develops an early reaction of significance, such as hypotension or bronchospasm, the clinician should halt the antivenom infusion, treat the reaction, then cautiously restart the antivenom infusion, if necessary titrating the antivenom rate against the epinephrine rate, to maintain blood pressure. Usually, after a short while, the epinephrine rate can be reduced, as any reaction subsides. Antivenom therapy should not be abandoned just because the patient has an adverse reaction.

The major delayed reaction to antivenom is serum sickness. Although unproven by clinical trial, it often is recommended that patients receive a 5- to 7-day course of prophylactic oral

> **Criteria for ICU Discharge in Australian and Pacific Snake Envenoming**
>
> Evidence of resolution of significant effects of envenoming (coagulopathy, myolysis, flaccid paralysis, renal failure) to the point that major risk is no longer present
>
> In cases of suspected snakebite that develop no evidence of systemic envenoming, 18 to 24 hours postbite

steroids to reduce the incidence of serum sickness. This complication increases in rate with increased volumes of antivenom; any patient receiving greater than 25 mL of antivenom probably should be given prophylactic steroids.

Other Treatments

Tetanus rarely occurs after snakebite, but tetanus immune status should be reviewed. No injection should be given, however, until venom-induced coagulopathy is fully resolved. Routine antibiotic therapy is inappropriate because bite wound infections are uncommon. For patients with purely postsynaptic paralysis (e.g., death adder bites), neostigmine may be a useful adjunct to antivenom therapy.

SPECIAL POPULATIONS

Pediatric Patients

Young children, owing to their smaller size, are at greater risk of severe envenoming and so require even greater vigilance. Antivenom dosage is the same as for adults. Intravenous fluid therapy needs to be monitored carefully to prevent overload.

Pregnant Patients

There are few records of snakebite in pregnancy, and it is unclear which, if any, venom components might cross the placenta. Antivenom poses far less risk than envenoming in pregnancy, and there should be no reluctance to start antivenom treatment. Where practical, fetal well-being should be monitored.

Elderly Patients

The elderly are more likely to die as a result of major envenoming because they are at greater risk of secondary problems, such as renal damage and fluid overload.

Other Special Populations

The most important special population is the amateur and professional herpetologist community, whose members are at risk of repeated bites, with potential for severe allergy to antivenom and venom. Venom may cause lethal anaphylaxis within minutes of the bite, long before hospital care can be accessed. Because of the potential to develop major allergies to antivenom, its use in herpetologists should be slightly more conservative than in the general population, but even so, antivenom should never be withheld when clearly indicated.

> **Common Misconceptions about Australian and Pacific Snake Envenoming**
>
> 1. All snakebites require antivenom therapy.
> 2. A positive Snake Venom Detection Kit result indicates antivenom therapy is required.
> 3. Coagulation factor replacement is required to treat coagulopathy.
> 4. Antivenom is more dangerous than envenoming.
> 5. Intensive care unit (ICU) management of airway and respiratory function is sufficient to keep the patient alive, and antivenom is unnecessary.
> 6. ICU specialists can manage snakebite alone, as with other emergencies.

> **Key Points in Australian and Pacific Snake Envenomation**
>
> 1. Most Australian snakebites ultimately prove to be minor, or "dry" bites, not requiring antivenom therapy.
> 2. Most New Guinea snakebites are major, requiring antivenom therapy.
> 3. Diagnosis is based on venom detection or presence of specific systemic effects (as above), determined by examination and appropriate laboratory tests.
> 4. A positive Snake Venom Detection Kit on either bite site or urine indicates only that venom has been detected and the type of snake that has bitten. The requirement for antivenom is based on clinical and laboratory evidence of significant systemic envenoming.
> 5. Antivenom is the most important treatment. It should always be given intravenously, often in high doses. Always be prepared to treat an anaphylactoid adverse reaction.
> 6. If there is major presynaptic paralysis, antivenom would not help, and ICU skills are essential, but the effects of coagulopathy, myolysis, and secondary renal failure are the major causes of snakebite fatalities, and at least for the first two, antivenom is the cornerstone of treatment.
> 7. Antivenom (correct type in sufficient quantity) effectively reverses coagulopathy, abolishes general symptoms, may reduce myolysis, can reverse pure postsynaptic paralysis (e.g., death adders), but cannot reverse established presynaptic paralysis.
> 8. The type of envenoming and the most appropriate antivenom and initial dose requirements are largely determined by the type of snake; identifying the snake using venom detection or diagnostic algorithms is important.
> 9. The clinically important effects of snakebite in Australia and New Guinea are systemic, not local: flaccid paralysis, defibrination or anticoagulant coagulopathy, myolysis, and renal damage.
> 10. The extent of envenoming is not reflected in the local bite site reaction, which may be trivial despite life-threatening envenoming.
> 11. Snakebite is a potentially complicated illness that is seen infrequently in most ICUs. It is always sensible to seek outside expert assistance in managing snakebite, particularly if there is severe envenoming.

continued

Key Points in Australian and Pacific Snake Envenomation *continued*

12. Coagulopathy of the consumptive variety (defibrination) is essentially reversible only with antivenom therapy or by waiting for all venom to be cleared (the latter option prolongs the risk of lethal hemorrhage); use of coagulation factor replacement therapy (fresh frozen plasma, cryoprecipitate, whole blood) while procoagulant is still circulating merely "adds fuel to the fire," making matters worse, not better.

13. Antivenom is *not* more dangerous than envenoming. Several people die each year from snakebite envenoming, many more in New Guinea, but deaths from adverse reactions to antivenom are rare and generally occur when no provision has been made to treat anaphylactoid reactions.

SUGGESTED READINGS

Sutherland SK, Tibballs J: Australian Animal Toxins. Melbourne, Oxford University Press, 2001.

White J: Elapid snakes: Venom production and bite mechanism. In Covacevich J, Davie P, Pearn J (eds): Toxic Plants and Animals: A Guide for Australia. Brisbane, Queensland Museum, 1987, 357–367.

White J: Elapid snakes: Venom toxicity and actions. In Covacevich J, Davie P, Pearn J (eds): Toxic Plants and Animals: A Guide for Australia. Brisbane, Queensland Museum, 1987, pp 369–389.

White J: Elapid snakes: Aspects of envenomation. In Covacevich J, Davie P, Pearn J (eds): Toxic Plants and Animals: A Guide for Australia. Brisbane, Queensland Museum, 1987, pp 391–429.

White J: Elapid snakes: Management of bites. In Covacevich J, Davie P, Pearn J (eds): Toxic Plants and Animals: A Guide for Australia. Brisbane, Queensland Museum, 1987, pp 431–457.

White J: Clinical toxinology: An Australian perspective. In Gopalakrishnakone P, Tan CK (eds): Recent Advances in Toxinology Research. Singapore, National University of Singapore, 1992, pp 722–729.

White J: Poisonous and venomous animals—the physician's view. In Meier J, White J (eds): Handbook of Clinical Toxicology of Animal Venoms and Poisons. Boca Raton, FL, CRC Press, 1995, pp 9–26.

White J: Clinical toxicology of sea snake bites. In Meier J, White J (eds): Handbook of Clinical Toxicology of Animal Venoms and Poisons. Boca Raton, FL, CRC Press, 1995, pp 159–170.

White J: Clinical toxicology of snakebite in Australia and New Guinea. In Meier J, White J (eds): Handbook of Clinical Toxicology of Animal Venoms and Poisons. Boca Raton, FL, CRC Press, 1995, pp 595–618.

White J: CSL Antivenom Handbook. Melbourne, CSL Ltd, 2001.

Williams V, White J: Snake venom and snakebite in Australia. In Thorpe RS, Wuster W, Malhotra A (eds): Ecology, Evolution and Snakebite: Venomous Snakes. London, Zoological Society of London, 1997, pp 205–217.

CHAPTER 106

Asian Snakes

Michael V. Callahan

OVERVIEW

Tropical Asia is home to more than 150 venomous species, representing three snake families: the Viperidae (e.g., vipers, pit vipers, and Fea's viper), the Elapidae (e.g., kraits, cobras, king cobras, and Asian coral snakes), and the Colubridae (e.g., colubrids, including rear-fanged snakes). Kraits are discussed in detail in Chapter 107; however, important clinical aspects of krait envenoming are presented here.

Tropical Asia has the highest incidence of snakebite in the world.[1] In no other area of the world do large populations of humans live so near high concentrations of venomous snakes, and for many Asian people, snake encounters are a daily occurrence. The frequency and intensity of snake-human encounters are higher for certain occupations, such as rice farming, rubber harvesting, and forestry, and after habitat destruction and seasonal flooding, which force snakes and humans into even closer contact. In many parts of India, Sri Lanka, and Southeast Asia, snakebite has increased along with more recent agricultural development projects. The need for arable land, in particular rice fields, has destroyed habitat and displaced snakes into populated areas. In several regions, the practice of storing grain within villages has intensified snake-human encounters by attracting rodents and the snakes that prey on them. Throughout much of Asia, snake envenoming is a health problem that primarily affects the rural poor. In austere regions, inadequate and inaccessible medical care and the high cost of treatment compound the damaging effects of snakebite. When the primary wage earner of the household is disabled as a result of snakebite, the ensuing economic hardship may impoverish entire families.

The emerging economies of Asia, in particular in India, Thailand, and Vietnam, have driven improvements in medical care and in many regions have increased the number of medical intensive care units (ICUs). The availability of ICUs allows for improved care of severely envenomed patients. A correlate scenario is found in Western countries, where patients bitten by imported species benefit from ICU-level monitoring and treatment.

This chapter addresses the assessment and management of Asian snake envenoming with a focus on both treatment in resource-constrained settings typical of small hospitals in rural Asia and treatment in modern ICUs. The physician caring for patients envenomed by Asian species can benefit from an understanding of the snakes themselves. For this reason, the natural history of important Asian species and unique features of their venom are presented first. An overview of snake venoms is presented in Chapter 101.

A key principle in the effective treatment of snakebite patients requires that the therapy (e.g., antivenom) match the envenoming syndrome. Familiarity with the characteristics, range, and habits of snakes and an appreciation for the clinical effects of envenoming are beneficial in suggesting the responsible species when the snake itself is not available. Examples of this information at work include the rapid diagnosis of nonenvenoming or "dry" bites and rapid bedside determination that the bite was caused by a viper, a rear-fanged colubrid, or an elapid (e.g., coral snake, krait, or cobra). Envenoming by Asian coral snakes (*Calliophis, Maticora*) and kraits (*Bungarus*) produces minimal local reactions but results in severe systemic neurotoxicity; missing these diagnoses can have tragic consequences. In contrast, cryptic envenoming by Asian cobras is unlikely to occur because the venom of most species causes significant local reactions. In the case of Asian vipers, envenoming is *reliably confirmed* by the presence of pain, swelling, ecchymosis, or bleeding from fang marks. This finding is *not always true* for viper bites in other parts of the world. Conversely, bites by the rear-fanged yamakagashi (*Rhabdophis*) may cause minimal local symptoms but result in systemic coagulopathy. An understanding of the spectrum of these envenoming syndromes allows the physician to make decisions regarding optimal therapy for each case and to avoid mishaps in antivenom selection.

KINEMATICS OF ASIAN SNAKEBITE

Bites by venomous snakes, including the most dangerous Asian species, include cases of nonenvenoming. The observations that snakes invariably strike humans in defense and that 15% to 45% of these bites are nonenvenoming have suggested to some that the snakes regulate the amount of venom injected based on circumstance. In the field, when snakes are trod on and respond reflexively with a strike, the event seems to take the snake and the human by surprise. It is likely that the serpent's sudden and desperately delivered strike often results in incomplete fang penetration. Factors that interfere with envenoming include inefficient strike trajectories, such as when the snake delivers a backward strike to the foot that stepped on it; the large size, shape, and unfamiliarity of humans as targets; and the interference caused by clothing and footwear. The opposite scenario is also a cause for concern, such as when the patient is bitten by a captive and habituated venomous species. A high percentage of these cases occur when captive snakes smell food animals in advance and anticipate imminent feeding. Hungry, enthusiastic specimens may confuse the caretaker's hand for a food animal and respond with a venom-laden strike. Snakebites that occur during the feeding of captive specimens often produce symptoms more severe than the symptoms seen after defensive bites by wild specimens. Details surrounding snakebite involving captive specimens require close investigation because these cases may prove to be particularly severe.[2]

Representative and significant Asian terrestrial species are listed in Table 106-1. The determination of the range is derived from reports in the herpetology literature or case series of snake envenoming. The species presented are representative of the genus, are responsible for significant mortality, or possess venom with unique clinical properties.

REGIONAL DISTRIBUTION AND PATHOPHYSIOLOGY

Asia is the only region on earth where all three Viperidae subfamilies are found: the Viperinae, or Old World vipers; the more advanced Crotalidae, or pit vipers; and the Azemiopinae, containing the attractive monotypic species,

Fea's viper (*Azemiops feae*), found along the China-Laos-Vietnam border.

Physicians with experience treating snakebite in Asia generally agree that although elapids (cobras and kraits) account for the most deaths, vipers cause the most bites. The venom of Asian vipers is rich in enzymes, which induce local pain; swelling; tissue damage; coagulopathy; and, for some species, damage to the kidneys, the adrenals, or the pituitary gland. Postenvenoming sequelae after viper bites account for significant disability among certain occupational groups, such as rubber plantation workers and rice farmers.

An understanding of the habits, range, and preferred niche of certain viper species provides meaningful epidemiologic clues to the treating physician. Bite injuries to the hands of fruit and coffee plantation workers in Central Malaysia or home gardeners living in Bangkok commonly are caused by the arboreal green tree vipers (*Trimeresurus*).[3] In contrast, nocturnal bites to the feet caused by ground-dwelling vipers in Pakistan, India's arid plains, and the Shavakacheri region in Sri Lanka usually are caused by saw-scale vipers (*Echis*).

TABLE 106-1 Terrestrial Asian Venomous Snake Families and Representative Species

FAMILY	GENUS	SPECIES	COMMON NAME	RANGE
Viperidae (Viperinae)	*Azemiops*	*A. feae*	Fea's viper	Vietnam, Laos
	Cerastes	*C. gasperettii*	Horned sand viper	
	Daboia	*D. russelii* complex	Russell's viper	Asia
	Echis	*E. multisquamatus*	Tibetan saw-scaled viper	Western Asia
	Vipera	*V. xanthina*	Steppe/ottoman viper	Western Asia
Viperidae (Crotalidae)	*Agkistrodon*	*A. brevicaudus*	Chinese mamushi	Southern China
	Calloselasma	*C. rhodostoma*	Malayan pit viper	Southern Myanmar–Malaysia–Java
	Deinagkistrodon	*D. acutus*	Sharp-nosed viper	North Vietnam–central China
	Hypnale	*H. nepa*	Sri Lanka hump-nosed viper	Sri Lanka
		H. hypnale	Merrem's hump-nosed viper	Western India–Belgaum
	Ovophis	*O. convictus*	Penang pit viper	Central China
		O. monticola	Mountain pit viper	Nepal–China–Southeast Asia
	Trimeresurus	*T. stejnegeri*	Chinese bamboo pit viper	Southern China
	Tropidolaemus	*T. wagleri*	Wagler's temple viper	Indonesia
Elapidae	*Bungarus*	*B. fasciatus*	Banded krait	India-Laos
		B. caeruleus	Indian krait	Western India–Nepal–Sri Lanka
	Calliophis	*C. bibroni*	Bibron's coral snake	India-Thailand
	Maticora	*M. bivirgata*	Blue long-glanded coral snake	Malaysia-Indonesia
	Naja	*N. atra*	Taiwan-Chinese cobra	China–northern Laos, Vietnam
		N. naja	Indian cobra	Pakistan, Nepal, Sri Lanka
		N. kaouthia	Monocellate cobra	India, Thailand
		N. oxiana	Central Asian cobra	Northern India–Nepal
		N. sumatrana	Malay spitting cobra	Sumatra-Malaysia
		N. philippinensis	Philippine cobra	Philippines
	Ophiophagus	*O. hannah* (only)	King cobra	India-Philippines
	Walterinnesia	*W. aegyptia* (only)	Desert cobra	Western Asia
Colubridae	*Ahaetulla*	*A. nasuta*	Long-nosed vine snake	India, Southeast Asia
	Balanophis	*B. ceylonicus*	Sri Lankan keelback	Sri Lanka
	Boiga	*B. dendrophilia*	Mangrove snake	Thailand, Singapore-Sulawesi
		B. ceylonensis	Cat snake	Sri Lanka, southern India
	Cerebrus	*C. rhynchops*	Dog-faced watersnake	India, Southeast Asia, Philippines
	Coluber	*C. ravergieri*	Steppe racer	Northwest India, Xinjiiang province
	Enhydris	*E. enhydris*	Rainbow watersnake	Southern India–southern China
	Rhabdophis	*R. subminiatus*	Red-necked keelback	Southeast Asia–eastern China/Sulawesi
		R. tigrinus	Yamakagashi	Japan, China, Taiwan, Vietnam

NATURAL HISTORY OF IMPORTANT SPECIES AND UNIQUE FEATURES OF THEIR VENOM

Viperidae

The venoms of Asia's vipers, similar to the vipers themselves, are not without their peculiarities. The venom of most species contains a mixture of peptides with direct toxic or indirect enzymatic activity. From a clinical standpoint, the most important of the proteolytic enzymes are the phospholipases A_2 myoneurotoxins,[4] which destroy tissue and serve as presynaptic neurotoxins, and shock-inducing hemorrhagins,[5] which destroy blood vessel walls, leading to extravasation and third spacing of fluid. Additional enzymes possess procoagulant, anticoagulant, and fibrinolytic activity. More recently, unique disintegrins have been identified in the venom of several species; these disintegrins inhibit platelet aggregation by preventing von Willebrand's factor and fibrinogen from binding to platelet (glycoprotein IIb/IIIa) integrin receptors.[6]

In the first 48 hours after viper bite, death may result from the effects of defibrination-related hemorrhage, shock secondary to vascular leak, or, in several species, respiratory paralysis. Death after 72 hours is more likely to result from internal (especially intracranial) hemorrhage, renal failure, adrenal insufficiency, or secondary infection arising from necrotic tissues. Several clinical aspects of Asian viper venom require additional discussion.

LOCAL EFFECTS

Local swelling and erythema result from the combined effects of vasoactive compounds and enzymatic toxins. Tissue injury is caused by necrotoxins and phospholipase A_2 myotoxins, some of which also have neurotoxic activity, and hemorrhagins, which increase the spread of venom to extravascular targets. The presence of coagulopathy is first noted at the bite site, where incoagulable blood drains from teeth and fang marks. Local necrosis may be significant after envenoming by the Malayan pit viper (*Calloselasma*), Russell's vipers (*Daboia*), green tree vipers (*Trimeresurus*), and saw-scaled vipers (*Echis*), all of which are discussed subsequently. Minor necrosis may follow envenoming by hump-nosed vipers (*Hypnale*), hundred pace viper (*Deinagkistrodon*), habus (*Ovophis*), and Mamushis (*Agkistrodon-Gloydius*).

SYSTEMIC EFFECTS

The most common systemic symptom after envenoming by Asian *Daboia, Trimeresurus, Calloselasma,* and *Echis* spp. is coagulopathy. In the presence of hemorrhagins, local and systemic bleeding may be intense. In the hospital setting, a leading cause of death is spontaneous hemorrhage or iatrogenic hemorrhage resulting from attempts at vascular access or ill-advised attempts at fasciotomy. Bleeding into anatomic compartments, such as the muscles of the thigh and the retroperitoneum, may be missed until hypotension results.

NEUROTOXICITY

The venom of several Asian vipers—the daboia/Russell's viper group and several species of mamushis (*Agkistrodon*)—contains neurotoxins. In southern India and Sri Lanka, envenoming by local daboia subspecies (*Daboia russelii russelii*;

previously, *Daboia russelii pulchella* in Sri Lanka) can cause neurotoxic symptoms, in addition to intravascular hemolysis and myolysis seen throughout the species' range.[7] In severe cases, daboia-induced paralysis may progress to respiratory muscles.[8] The neurotoxin is a phospholipase A_2, which likely also contributes to the local tissue damage seen in daboia envenoming. In Japan, China, and South Korea, envenoming by several subspecies of mamushi (*Agkistrodon blomhoffii brevicaudus* group) also can result in neurotoxic symptoms ranging from mild ptosis to complete respiratory paralysis.[9–12] Envenoming from two other *Agkistrodon* spp., the Ussuri mamushi (*Agkistrodon ussuriensis*)[13,14] and the central Asian pit viper (*Agkistrodon intermedius*),[15] also is reported to cause neurotoxic symptoms, although these seem to be less severe.

The venom of many Asian viper species differs among regions. Asian vipers known to have geographically heterogeneous venom are *Daboia, Calloselasma, Echis* (particularly between Asia and Africa), and *Trimeresurus* spp. The variability in venom is reflected by mixed results with antivenom treatment. Economic constraints in antivenom manufacture often result in the use of venom from snakes whose collection was convenient, usually from the region where the antivenom was produced. Antivenoms are rarely prepared using pooled venom obtained from specimens from different regions. Many antivenoms may not effectively neutralize the venom of the same species from another region. The observation has implications for health centers that are purchasing antivenom from foreign manufacturers and for pharmacists who need to protect zoo and research personnel from bites by imported species.

DABOIA/RUSSELL'S VIPER (*DABOIA RUSSELII* COMPLEX)

The range of daboia vipers is discontinuous over the 10 Asian countries where it is reported (Fig. 106-1). The species is common throughout much of India, Sri Lanka, Bangladesh, Taiwan, and Myanmar. In Thailand, Cambodia, southern China, and Pakistan, hundreds of square kilometers of seemingly ideal habitat are devoid of daboia. The five subspecies of daboia were reclassified to two species: a western form, *D. russelii russelii*, found in India, Pakistan,

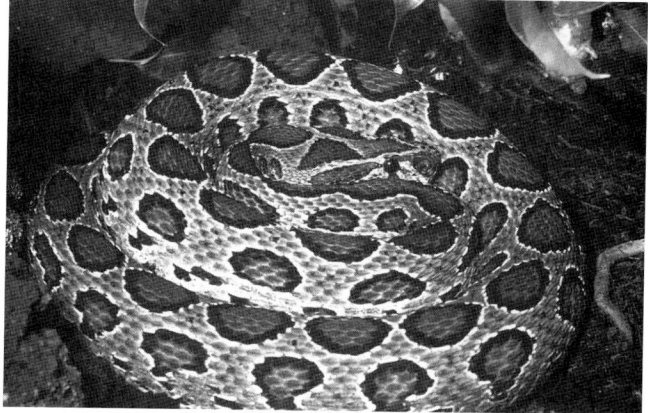

FIGURE 106-1

Daboia. This wide-ranging species possesses venom that induces largely neurotoxic symptoms, coagulopathies, and myonecrotic effects or combinations of these. *(Courtesy of Dr. Beat Akeret.)* See Color Fig. 106-1.

Sri Lanka, and Bangladesh, and an eastern form, *D. russelii siamensis*, found in Thailand, Myanmar, southern China, Taiwan, and parts of Indonesia.[16] The classification does not reflect the range of clinical effects seen in patients envenomed by species from different regions.

In addition to phospholipase A_2 myoneurotoxins, daboia venom contains hemorrhagins, platelet-aggregating factors, and venom enzymes that activate factor V, IX, and X and induce fibrinolysis.[17] In certain regions, daboia venom also possesses plasminogen and antiplasmin activity. Together, these factors induce chaotic activation of extrinsic and intrinsic coagulation pathways with simultaneous formation and destruction of blood clots. De novo thrombus formation, presenting as cortical disturbances, syncope, and sudden cardiac death, is rare but may occur soon after intravenous envenoming. The result of these clotting abnormalities is eventual defibrination with marked elevation of fibrin degradation products.[17] Intravascular hemolysis is variable after daboia envenoming.

The clinical presentation of envenomed patients may vary dramatically among regions. Throughout the range, the pro-coagulant effects of daboia venom may cause consumption of fibrinogen and incoagulable blood. In eastern Pakistan and central India, envenoming by *D. r. russelii* also causes intravascular hemolysis and excessive damage to local skeletal muscle. In Sri Lanka and southern India, however, envenoming by local *D. r. russelii* (previously *D. r. pulchella* in Sri Lanka) may result in neurotoxic symptoms that can progress to respiratory paralysis. The clinical presentation of envenoming also varies in the eastern species, *D. r. siamensis*. In Myanmar, envenoming by *D. r. siamensis* is more likely to be severe, characterized by a systemic capillary leak syndrome, conjunctival hyperemia (chemosis), pulmonary edema, and infarction of the anterior pituitary gland.[18,19] In Thailand, the most severe complications result from incoagulable blood. In Indonesia, an isolated population of *D. r. siamensis*, separated by more than 2000 km from the nearest consanguineous species, is implicated in bites with an excessively high case-fatality rate of 38.5% and a mean interval between bite and death of only 14.5 hours, far faster than that observed in other parts of the species' range.[20]

Despite the variability in presentation, all daboia venoms produce some pain and swelling within minutes of envenoming. Pain and swelling may be less significant in Madras, India, and Sri Lanka than observed elsewhere. Clinical events reflecting the activity of the venom include pain, swelling, ecchymosis, and bulla formation.[21,22] Within 1 hour of envenoming, evidence of regional coagulopathy is manifest by persistent bleeding from fang and maxillary teeth wounds. The combined loss of blood from fang marks, intravenous (IV) access sites, and the gastrointestinal and urinary tract[23] is often considerable, contributing to hypovolemia and hemorrhagic shock. Local necrosis is common in many parts of the daboia range, although it is less severe than necrosis after envenoming by *Calloselasma rhodostoma* (Malayan pit viper) and many species of cobra (*Naja naja*), which share much of the range.

In southern India, Sri Lanka, Myanmar, and Thailand, daboia envenoming is a common cause of renal failure.[23–27] In Kerala, India, daboia envenoming is the leading cause of acute renal failure in adults and children.[28] Clinical evidence that daboia venom contains a unique nephrotoxin is supported by the high incidence of renal failure in patients with negligible coagulopathy, rhabdomyolysis, or history of hypotensive episodes and with recent identification of a nephrotoxic effect.[29] Renal biopsy data indicate that nephrotoxicity is due to acute tubular necrosis. More recent investigation in India, where tissue necrosis is common after daboia bites, has characterized more fully a hemorrhagin with dermatonecrotic, fibrinolytic, and esterolytic activity.[30]

In Taiwan, bites by local *D. r. siamensis* (formerly *D. r. formosensis*) are a leading cause of acute renal failure and are implicated in neurotoxicity.[26,31] The neurotoxin of this species was found to constitute 40% of the venom and to consist of two distinct phospholipases, which combine to produce a postsynaptic neurotoxin.[32,33]

Little is known about the clinical effects of daboia envenoming in mainland China. One epidemiologic study indicated that Chinese daboia account for fewer bites than other species (e.g., *Trimeresurus*, *Agkistrodon*). Although specimens from southern China are morphologically similar to specimens in neighboring northwestern Laos, northern Thailand, and Myanmar (variant *D. r. siamensis*), few comments can be made with regard to characteristics of the venom. One case series studying bites by *Trimeresurus albolabris* mentioned a single case of envenoming by an imported Chinese daboia, resulting in defibrination, intracranial hemorrhage, acute renal failure, and death. Along the Thailand-Laos border, 18 cases of confirmed envenoming by *D. r. siamensis* treated by the author developed prolonged clotting times, hemolysis, microalbuminuria, hemoglobinuria, and hemorrhagic bulla formation. Mild necrosis was present in three bites to the hand or fingers. None of these patients developed acute renal failure. One patient developed severe pulmonary hemorrhage requiring blood transfusion, prolonged respiratory support, and antivenom therapy.

Neurotoxicity after daboia envenoming is seen most frequently in Sri Lanka, India (*D. r. russelii*), and Taiwan (*D. r. siamensis*). In one Sri Lankan series, envenoming (*D. r. pulchella*) resulted in diplopia and ptosis between 30 minutes and 7 hours after the bite.[8] Compared with envenoming by *Naja* and *Bungarus*, neurotoxicity resulting from daboia bites tends to be less severe; however, progression to respiratory paralysis is known. In western India and Bangladesh, envenoming by local daboia species induces coagulopathy, hypotension, renal failure, and anemia. In Myanmar, daboia bites may cause incoagulable blood, hemolysis, and endocrinopathies secondary to infarction of the pituitary gland[19,22,34] but no evidence of neurotoxicity. Pituitary insufficiency may manifest months after envenoming when patients return with complaints of low libido, amenorrhea, loss of pubic hair, and diabetes insipidus.[35,36] Postmortem examination of daboia victims, for which there is no shortage of opportunities, shows hyperemia and congestion of vascular beds in the anterior pituitary gland, adrenal gland, gastrointestinal tract, and alveolar beds and within the coronary vessels. The well-studied venom phospholipase A_2, VRV-PL-VIIIa, has been implicated in alveolar hemorrhage and myotoxicity, neurotoxicity, and regional edema reported previously.[37] The variability between daboia venoms from different regions has limited the usefulness of antivenoms produced in other countries.[8,38] At present, there is considerable interest in the development of polyvalent/panregional daboia antivenoms that would be effective throughout the species range.

SAW-SCALED VIPERS (*ECHIS*)

The genus *Echis* (saw-scaled viper) is widely distributed throughout northern Africa, along the southern Mediterranean coast, and eastward into southern Asia as far as Sri Lanka. Each of the 12 *Echis* spp. are characterized as small, ground-dwelling vipers with disproportionally large eyes, a blunt snout, heavily keeled scales, and a pugnacious disposition. The saw-scaled viper's name arises from the noise created when the snake becomes irritated and rubs its keeled scales together to warn other animals. In my experience, *Echis* are ill-tempered vipers, prone to striking in rapid succession and with little provocation. In captivity, *Echis* remain high-strung and prone to bite. In Asia, *Echis* bites are caused by three species: the far-ranging, prototypic *Echis carinatus*, which is found in peninsular India as far east as Maarashtra and Tamil Nadu; the largest and most dangerous species, *Echis sochureki* (Sochurek's saw-scaled viper), found in Bangladesh and northern Indian to Pakistan; and *Echis multisquamatus* (central Asian saw-scaled viper), found in eastern Pakistan and northern India. In Jammu, northern India, *E. sochureki* is the most common cause of snakebite.[39] In southern India and Sri Lanka, *Echis* (probably *E. c. sinhaleyus*) is infrequently implicated in envenoming.

The venom of *E. carinatus* activates factor X and prothrombin and inhibits thromboxane-induced platelet activation. *Echis* venom also contains hemorrhagins, which contribute to vascular leak, third spacing of fluids, hypovolemia, and shock. As with the daboia, local effects of *Echis* bites include pain, swelling, blistering, and discoloration, which often transition to ecchymosis and become necrotic. Lymphangitis and tender draining lymph nodes are common. The most important clinical feature of *Echis* envenoming is severe hemorrhage resulting from coagulopathy.

When the identity of the snake cannot be confirmed, the patient's description of the viper's unique defense behavior; time of day (night) of the bite; familiarity with the vipers' range; environmental preference; and clinical presentation of pain, blistering, and coagulopathy provide sufficient evidence to support treatment with *Echis*-specific antivenom. As with daboia, *Echis* venom is known to vary throughout the species' range. Cases of treatment failure using *Echis*-specific antivenom imported to treat bites in northern Nigeria[40] and Pakistan[41] serve as a warning for the clinician treating *Echis* bites with antivenom produced in other regions.

MALAYAN PIT VIPER (*CALLOSELASMA RHODOSTOMA*)

Adult vipers are thick-bodied, ground-dwelling, dark-colored snakes, usually covered with dark, triangular markings along the dorsum. In many countries of Southeast Asia, the Malayan pit viper *Calloselasma* is either the most common cause of snakebite[42] or the most common cause of snakebite deaths.[43] It is likely that rural environs and failure to access medical care heavily influence the number of fatalities. *C. rhodostoma* is found throughout Thailand, Kampuchea, Laos, West Malaysia, Sumatra, and Java. *Calloselasma annamensis*, a smaller species, is found in southwestern Vietnam and adjacent Kampuchea. Throughout the species range, rubber and tea plantation workers, rather than rice farmers, are most commonly bitten. This predilection reflects the species'

preference for drier, alkaline soils; partial canopy; and preference for rodents, which concentrate around farms. A crepuscular hunter, the viper is most active when workers are traveling to and from the fields. Most cases occur when the snake is stepped on and the foot and lower leg are bitten.

Calloselasma venom contains ancrod, a potent serine protease that cleaves fibrinopeptide A from fibrinogen, which is used clinically as an anticoagulant (Arvin).[44] The protease works in concert with other venom antigens to defibrinate the patient's coagulation system. The process involves thrombin formation, often with sequestration of platelets; thrombocytopenia is a common laboratory finding after bites by this species. In most cases, the thrombocytopenia, but not the coagulopathy, resolves within hours of treatment with antivenom. A second feature of *Calloselasma* venom is the presence of proteases that specifically hydrolyze vitamin K–dependent clotting factors VII, IX, and X and protein C.[45] Early after envenoming by *C. rhodostoma*, a transient increase in the prothrombin time–to–partial thromboplastin time ratio is observed. The observation is of limited utility after the first few hours because generalized activation of extrinsic and intrinsic factors results in uniform elevation of prothrombin time and partial thromboplastin time.

Patients bitten by *C. rhodostoma* may experience significant tissue destruction, which invariably extends beyond the border of bullae that form on the bitten extremity. The bullae contain bloody, rather than serous, fluid and closely resemble hemorrhagic bullae seen in New World rattlesnake (*Crotalus*) bites. The extent of blistering, bullae, and local tissue destruction is distinctive to *C. rhodostoma* envenoming, and in areas without daboia and when cobra bites are unlikely, blistering, bullae, and local tissue destruction serve as an indication for preemptive treatment with *Calloselasma*-specific antivenom. Necrosis and gangrene are a common source of secondary infection.[46] In one series, the leading cause of death after *Calloselasma* envenoming was cerebral hemorrhage followed by hemorrhagic shock.[43]

GREEN TREE VIPERS (*TRIMERESURUS* SPECIES AND *TROPIDOLAEMUS WAGLERI*)

The genus *Trimeresurus* covers an extensive range from Pakistan to Japan and south to the Philippines and the Indonesian islands. More than 36 species are recognized, including several ground-dwelling, brown-colored species (e.g., *Trimeresurus mucrosquamatus* and *Trimeresurus flavoviridis*); however, most of the species are arboreal, and most arboreal species are green (Fig. 106-2). The term *green pit viper* is used with reservation because the designation has led to confusion in herpetology and medical literature and mishaps in the preparation of antivenoms. Similarities in coloration and intergrade species have confused the taxonomy, prompting efforts to define species using molecular approaches, rather than descriptions of range, eye color, and scale counts.

In Thailand, China, Japan, and several Asian islands, green tree vipers are the leading cause of venomous snakebite.[42,47] Many *Trimeresurus* spp. are tolerant of human activity, and many bites occur in household gardens and urban parks. In parts of eastern Cambodia, the related Wagler's viper (*Tropidolaemus*) is found in Buddhist temples, where snake and monks coexist without apparent problems. Most *Trimeresurus*

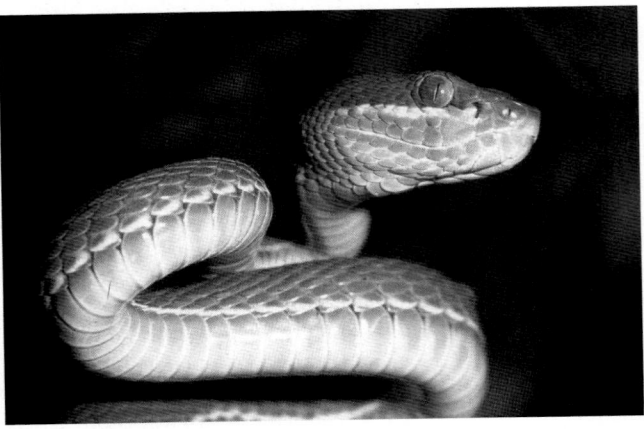

FIGURE 106-2

Trimeresurus. These Old World vipers are found throughout tropical Asia. Most species are arboreal, so bites of the hands are more common. The predominant symptoms are local tissue swelling, myonecrosis, and coagulopathy. *(Courtesy of Dr. Beat Akeret.)* See Color Fig. 106-2.

vipers are arboreal, which explains the high incidence of bites to the hands and the high occupational risk to fruit pickers, forestry workers, and gardeners. Many bites by the ground-dwelling *Trimeresurus* spp., such as the Chinese habu (*T. mucrosquamatus*)[48] and the Japanese/Okinawan habu (*T. flavoviridis*), occur in homes. In all regions, household envenoming is of great concern because it is more likely to involve children.

Similar to all vipers, the fangs of *Trimeresurus* and *Tropidolaemus* spp. are continuously replaced, although in these species, new fangs may move into position before older fangs are shed. In my experience, many *Trimeresurus* bites result in three or more fang marks at the bite site. An unpublished survey of *Trimeresurus albolabris* and *Tropidolaemus wagleri* specimens in one research colony indicated that 17 of 66 adult animals had more than two fangs present (unpublished observations).

The venom of *Trimeresurus* vipers also varies among species and within species from different regions. Several species, *T. flavoviridis*, *Trimeresurus gramineus*, and *T. mucrosquamatus*, contain high concentrations of metalloproteinases with hemorrhagin activity.[46,49–51] The physiologic activity of the hemorrhagins, notably their attack on the walls of blood vessels,[52] is shown clinically with extensive swelling and ecchymosis at the bite site. Systemic bleeding is more common in children than in adults. *T. flavoviridis* venom also contains a phospholipase A2 myotoxin,[53] which is a likely cause of myoglobinuria observed in patients envenomed by this species. Investigation has shown that the venom of the Far Eastern habu species possesses venom antigen with unusual activity. *Trimeresurus elegans* (Sakishima-habu) possesses a thrombin- like enzyme, elegaxobin, which has potent activity against mammalian systems.[54] Investigation has shown that the venom of *Trimeresurus okinavensis* (Himehabu) possesses potent hemagglutinating activity.[55] In a hospital-based series of 29 patients envenomed by *Trimeresurus* (likely *T. albolabris*) in and around Bangkok, 46% of patients developed immediate pain, swelling that involved more than half of the limb, and regional tender lymphadenopathy.[56] Although bruising was observed in 58% of

these patients, necrosis was seen in only two cases involving bites to the digits.

Elapidae

Asian elapids include the Asian cobras (*Naja*), Asian coral snakes (*Calliophis, Maticora*), king cobra (*Ophiophagus hannah*), and kraits (*Bungarus*). Sea snakes (Hydrophobidae) are specialized elapids found along Asia's tropical coasts. Kraits are discussed briefly in this chapter and in more detail in Chapter 107.

The venoms of Asian elapids are characterized by presynaptic phospholipase A2 neurotoxins, small postsynaptic peptide neurotoxins, and peptides that contribute to local tissue injury. In contrast to Australian elapids and sea snakes, the phospholipase neurotoxins found in terrestrial Asian elapid venom are not significant myotoxins; rhabdomyolysis after envenoming by these species is less common.

NEUROTOXINS

The presynaptic, or so-called β, neurotoxins found in the venoms of Asiatic kraits are class 1 phospholipase A2, remarkably homologous to mammalian pancreatic phospholipase A2. In the case of kraits, multiple isoforms of the neurotoxin may be present in the same venom; however, all activity appears to be restricted to neuromuscular junctions. Although the effect of phospholipase A2 neurotoxins is manifest at the peripheral nervous system, cases of parasympathetic inhibition and derangement have been reported. An important clinical feature of presynaptic phospholipase neurotoxins is that they *destroy* the phospholipid membranes and cholinergic synaptic vesicles at the neuromuscular junction, preventing further release of neurotransmitter.[57] When the terminal axon membrane is destroyed, antivenom and anticholinesterases are of little value (see section on treatment). Paralysis resulting from presynaptic neurotoxins may be prolonged, as recovery entails regeneration of the terminal axonal membrane. In cases of krait-induced paralysis, artificial ventilation and supportive care may be required for weeks.[58,59] The venom of several Asian cobras (*Naja kaouthia, Naja sumatrana,* and *N. naja*) also may contain phospholipases implicated in presynaptic neurotoxicity and myotoxicity.

Postsynaptic, or so-called α, neurotoxins found in Asian cobra venom (*Naja atra, N. kaouthia*), king cobra, and several kraits are nondestructive peptides less than 30 kd in size. The postsynaptic neurotoxins are small, which likely explains their fast onset of activity. Postsynaptic toxins are classified into two groups: "short" peptides (<62 amino acids) found in the cobras and "long" toxins (70 amino acids) found in the venom of king cobras and several kraits. Postsynaptic neurotoxins are the major constituents of the venom of many Asian cobras (*Naja*) and the king cobra (*Ophiophagus*).[59] The importance of this finding is that even profoundly paralyzed patients, such as patients requiring ventilator support, may recover quickly after treatment with appropriate antivenom. The clinician's familiarity with the venom of the offending snake plays a central role in differentiating paralytic cases that would respond to antivenom from cases in which antivenom stockpiles would be squandered.

LOCAL TOXINS

The venom of Asian cobras also contains destructive polypeptides implicated in tissue necrosis. With the exception of kraits and one cobra species discussed subsequently, envenoming bites from all Asian cobras (*Naja*) and the king cobra (*Ophiophagus*) are distinguished from nonenvenoming bites by the onset of local pain and minimal-to-moderate swelling. In contrast, the venom of the Philippine cobra (*Naja philippinensis*), all kraits (*Bungarus*), and Asian coral snakes (*Calliophis* and *Maticora*) produces minimal local symptoms but often causes severe neurotoxic morbidity. Bites by these species may go unnoticed or be dismissed as nonenvenoming because of the paucity of local symptoms. The point is frequently reiterated by cases involving farmers, who often sleep in the rice fields at night and occasionally roll onto questing kraits, resulting in defensive bites. The krait bite is painless and may not wake the farmer. The first evidence of envenoming may be ptosis or ophthalmoplegia when the farmer awakes the next morning. Occasionally, field biologists incorrectly identify a juvenile krait or Asian coral snake as a harmless species or dismiss any bites received as nonenvenoming, with tragic consequences.

CLINICAL PRESENTATION

Several points may be made regarding the clinical presentation of patients envenomed by Asian elapids:

1. All elapid venoms possess some degree of neurotoxin; however, envenoming by cobras often results only in local symptoms and local tissue damage.
2. Envenoming by the Philippine cobra, all kraits, and coral snakes may result in minimal local symptoms but may cause life-threatening paralysis.
3. Envenoming by most cobras (*Naja*) (except for *N. philippinensis*) and king cobras (*Ophiophagus*) results in pain, swelling, discoloration, and necrosis.
4. Neurotoxic symptoms may appear quickly or be delayed more than 18 hours.
5. Asian elapid venoms are an infrequent cause of coagulopathy.

An understanding of neurotoxic symptoms allows the physician to recognize severe cases and anticipate the need for advanced medical resources. The earliest symptoms suggesting envenoming by neurotoxic species, which may be delayed for hours, include fasciculations and tingling or aching sensation in the bitten extremity. Early systemic symptoms include drowsiness, perioral paresthesias, ophthalmoplegia (which initially may be unilateral), and ptosis. In bites by eastern Vietnamese *Bungarus multicinctus*, the earliest evidence of neurotoxicity is ptosis, usually with compensatory contraction of the frontalis muscle ("furrowed-brow" sign). These findings may be subtle, and the patient or physician may attribute them to other causes, such as alcohol or drug use. Progression of symptoms may be rapid, next affecting muscles innervated by cranial nerves IX and X, the remaining extraocular muscles, and the muscles of the upper airway. The inability to control the pharyngeal muscles may result in upper airway obstruction, which often presents before the onset of respiratory paralysis. Patients with advancing paralysis who are placed supine often have difficulties mobilizing secretions, resulting in

drooling and "gargling exhalation." Neurotoxicity also is apparent in the muscles of the neck, resulting in difficulty keeping the head upright. Progression of symptoms increases rapidly as acetylcholine neurotransmitter reserves are exhausted; the muscles of respiration may be affected with little warning. Respiratory paralysis may last hours, days, or, in the case of presynaptic neurotoxins, weeks. Patients requiring prolonged mechanical ventilation may tie up valuable ventilators, resulting in interruption of surgical and obstetric services. In austere medical settings, patients often develop iatrogenic complications as a result of a lack of skilled nursing care; clinical laboratory monitoring, in particular, blood gas analysis of ventilated patients; or adequate enteral feeding.

The effects of all elapid neurotoxins are eventually reversible. The activity of nondestructive postsynaptic neurotoxins may be quickly but temporarily reversed using anticholinesterases, which produce a transient increase in the concentration of synaptic neurotransmitter, or may be blocked using appropriate antivenom. In the case of destructive presynaptic (β) neurotoxins, reversal of symptoms is slow, occurring only after synaptic membranes and neurotransmitter receptors are regenerated. As with Asian vipers, several Asian elapids pose a significant risk and are discussed in detail subsequently.

ASIAN COBRAS (*NAJA* SPECIES)

Cobras are ubiquitous throughout tropical Asia (Fig. 106-3). The combined factors of high fecundity, toxic venom, tolerance of human activity, and close association with rice fields make cobras the leading cause of snakebite fatalities worldwide. Many cobra bites, 45% in one study,[60] are nonenvenoming. The spectrum of local and neurotoxic symptoms seen in cobra envenoming is highly variable. Cobra venom contains few enzymes, compared with the venom of vipers; however, several venoms contain cofactors that enhance migration in tissue. *N. naja* venom contains nerve growth factor, which, as implied, stimulates the growth of mammalian nerve tissue[61] but also induces degranulation of mast cells. The resulting release of histamine and proinflammatory chemokines

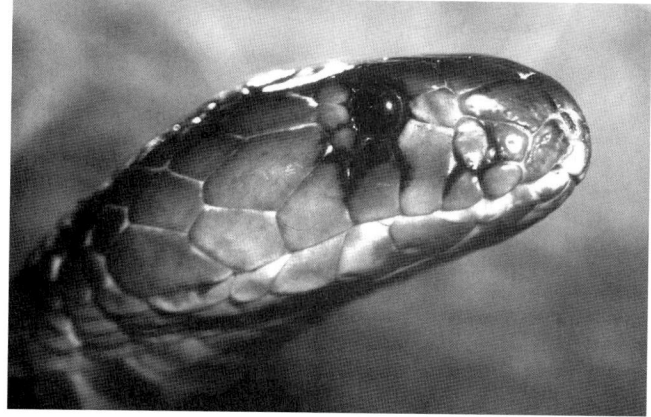

FIGURE 106-3

Naja. In contrast to many reports, members of the cobra family frequently cause significant local tissue destruction. Mixed neurotoxicity and myonecrosis is common. In contrast to kraits, few cobras possess pure neurotoxic activity. *(Courtesy of Dr. Beat Akeret.)* See Color Fig. 106-3.

induces vasodilation. *N. naja* venom also contains cobra venom factor, a glycoprotein that cleaves complement into the cytokine-inducing anaphylatoxins C3a and C5a.[62,63] The venom of several species contains varying concentrations of unique polypeptide cytotoxins, which are implicated in local tissue injury. The bites of several Asian cobras (*N. sumatrana*, *N. kaouthia*, *N. atra*) can cause significant tissue destruction, which may equal that seen after envenoming by Malayan pit vipers. In one series of 47 patients envenomed by *Naja* spp. (author note: probably *N. sumatrana* and *N. kaouthia*), 44% developed local necrosis, and 12% showed signs of neurotoxicity.[60] Laboratory studies indicate that the venom of several *N. naja* species possesses a nonenzymatic cardiotoxin that exacerbates platelet aggregation by adenosine diphosphate and thrombin activation.[64] Despite seemingly well-designed laboratory studies, procoagulant and anticoagulant activity is not observed in envenomed patients.

In India, most cobra bites are caused by *N. naja naja* (Indian spectacled cobra).[65] In Malaysia and Thailand, most cobra bites are caused by *N. kaouthia* (Monocellate cobra)[42,66] with rice farmers and aquaculturists being the most common victims.[67]

Patients envenomed by *N. kaouthia*, *N. atra*, and *N. naja* and by bites by the smaller Asian spitting cobras (see later) experience immediate pain and aching at the bite site. In the first few hours, there is soft tissue swelling and ecchymosis. Four to 60 hours after the bite, the tissue surrounding the fang marks becomes mottled and gray, and dependent migration of ecchymosis is often observed. The first systemic symptoms are drowsiness, nausea, vomiting, and ptosis. In one case, neurotoxicity developed within 30 minutes of the bite[68]; however, symptoms usually are delayed more than 3 hours and may appear 20 hours after envenoming. The delay in neurotoxicity likely reflects the time required for the neurotoxin to reach the neuromuscular junction. In children, the earliest and most common evidence of neurotoxicity after cobra bites is ptosis, drowsiness, and inability to keep the head upright.[68]

ASIAN SPITTING COBRAS

Many Asian cobras defend themselves by spitting fine droplets of venom into the eyes and mucous membranes of animals, resulting in severe contact ophthalmia. The species most frequently implicated in "spitting" venom injury are the Thai spitting cobra (*Naja siamensis*), the Javan cobra (*Naja sputatrix*), the Malay-Sumatran spitting cobra (*N. sumatrana*),[66] and the Sumar cobra (*Naja sumarensis*). During a collecting trip to obtain wild *N. siamensis*, restrained snakes would ignore the collecting bags placed directly in front of them and spit past the bag toward the researcher's face. The observation suggests that spitting cobras have the ability to target the eyes of the offending animal. Spitting cobras can spit venom 2 m; however, as the twin venom streams travel toward the target, the streams degrade into an aerosol of fine droplets. Venom that comes in contact with the eyes causes immediate pain and swelling. Within minutes, the victim experiences edema of the sclera and conjunctiva and blepharospasm. In African species, the venom of similar species may traverse the conjunctiva and enter the lymphatics, resulting in paralysis of the facial nerve.[69] Corneal erosions and secondary infection are reported after spit venom injury from several African species (ringhals). Venom sprayed onto oral and nasal mucous membranes results in tingling sensation followed by irritation, which quickly escalates in severity. The bites of Asian spitting cobras may cause local necrosis, which may be severe.

KING COBRA (*OPHIOPHAGUS HANNAH*)

The king cobra (*O. hannah*) is the world's longest venomous snake, with documented lengths greater than 5 m. The species has an extensive range, from western India to southern China, Malaysia, Indonesia, and the Philippines.[70] The species is brown-green in India, olive-green throughout most of Southeast Asia, and dull yellow on Mindoro and Negros islands. King cobras are obligate reptile predators that prey almost exclusively on other snakes, including venomous species. The species are highly evolved and are among the minority of snakes known to construct nests and to defend the eggs. This behavior may explain the reputation for aggressiveness and accounts of "unprovoked" attacks on humans. During field collection, king cobras seem more intent on escape and defend themselves only when restrained by the snake hook or when cornered. Specimens quickly acclimate to captivity, becoming tolerant of humans, and quickly learn that human activity near the cage indicates the likelihood of a meal. Many bites involving captive animals occur when snakes and snake handlers lose their fear of each other.

King cobras can deliver large amounts of venom through fixed fangs, which may exceed 9 mm in length. During venom extraction procedures, 1200 μL of venom may be obtained from a single 4-m long specimen. The venom is composed primarily of heterogeneous postsynaptic neurotoxins, and deaths usually result from respiratory paralysis. Locally active toxins include hyaluronidase; cobra-venom factor; hannahtoxin, an enzyme with hemorrhagin-like activity; and a unique protein toxin with multiple activities.[71] These factors likely explain the ecchymosis and swelling observed in the envenomed extremity. The presence of local symptoms should alert the physician to the probability of systemic envenoming. The case-fatality rate in king cobra envenoming is high. In a Myanmar series,[72] 22 of 35 (63%) bitten patients died, and in a Chinese series,[48] 7 of 13 (54%) bitten patients died. Antivenom treatment of severe bites may require many vials. Little quality research has been performed on the variability of venom from king cobras from different regions.

KRAITS (*BUNGARUS*)

Kraits (genus *Bungarus*) are a widely distributed group of snake-eating species that are found throughout the South Asian-Pacific region. These slender, fast-moving species are discussed in greater detail in Chapter 107. Many species are reportedly docile during the day but become fast moving and more prone to bite at night. In my experience, specimens collected during daylight were quick to bite, however, when lightly restrained. In many parts of India, Bangladesh, Sri Lanka, and Myanmar, humans often are bitten while sleeping in the fields or on the floors of huts. Kraits deserve special mention due to the burden that krait-bite paralysis places on ICU resources, particularly in rural hospitals. Seven of 15 krait species have been implicated in human envenoming, and each of these species possesses venom with destructive presynaptic neurotoxins. In several regions, kraits rival the cobras as the leading cause of snakebite-related fatalities.[73,74]

It is important to identify patients who are bitten by kraits because they may present before the onset of significant symptoms, when antivenom would be more effective. Early recognition of krait bites provides a crucial opportunity to make maximal use of antivenom resources and intervene in the progression of paralysis. Such efforts are advantageous for health clinics located in remote settings because they allow critical ICU resources, such as ventilators, to be conserved for other patients. Local symptoms warning of krait envenoming include numbness, paresthesias, mild discomfort, and aching of extremity muscles. Ecchymosis is uncommon and, if present, is usually confined to the immediate vicinity of the fang marks. Envenoming by several species (e.g., *Bungarus caeruleus, Bungarus candidus*) may be associated with abdominal discomfort.[75] Many patients report generalized muscle pain within hours of the bite. Laboratory evidence of envenoming is restricted to modest elevations of plasma myoglobin and marked neutrophil leukocytosis.[27,74]

Colubridae

The secretions of Duverney's gland of several colubrids is capable of producing envenoming injuries. Currently recognized physiologic effects include defibrination and disseminated intravascular coagulation–like reactions, generalized protease activity, phosphodiesterase activity, and phospholipase A_2 activity.[76] Although bites of many species produce local reactions, this discussion focuses on the two Asian colubrids implicated in severe envenoming or fatalities.

Rhabdophis tigrinus (Japanese yamakagashi) and *Rhabdophis subminiatus* (Asian keelback) are slender, fast-moving snakes that are common in many regions. Bites by *R. subminiatus* are rare throughout the species' range of Thailand, Laos, Myanmar, and Malaysia; however, imported specimens have caused fatal envenoming in several Western countries.[77–79] Lacking canaliculated fangs, the *Rhabdophis* spp. must introduce venom into puncture wounds made by a fixed pair of posterior-positioned maxillary teeth. Envenoming injuries usually involve the snake's hanging on and chewing on the patient. Local findings are distinctive for the absence of anterior fang marks. The local effects of venom may be minimal. Initial symptoms start 1 to 9 hours postbite and include nausea, vomiting, gastrointestinal discomfort, and headache. Onset of coagulopathy is indicated by return of bleeding from the teeth marks. The patient's blood may become incoagulable within hours. Laboratory studies show defibrination, with elevated degradation products, thrombocytopenia, and schistocytes appearing on peripheral blood smear, suggesting a microangiopathic hemolytic process.[80]

Envenoming by the Japanese yamakagashi, *R. tigrinus*, is more common and more severe than envenoming by *R. subminiatus*. Local reactions include swelling, which may involve the entire extremity. Coagulopathy may be severe, leading to intracranial hemorrhage.[78] In addition to severe coagulopathy, envenoming by *R. tigrinus* can cause renal failure, with postmortem studies showing acute tubular necrosis.[77] Antivenom is available for *R. tigrinus* (see Table 106-9).

TREATMENT

Prehospital Care

In many parts of rural Asia, patient transport to a medical facility often is delayed hours to days. Initial treatment by community health clinics encountered along the way may be rudimentary, may be inaccurate, or may result in injurious treatment. In recent years cellular phone networks have expanded into many of Asia's rural regions, allowing physicians to be notified of inbound emergencies. Prehospital communication also allows physicians to guide bystanders in obtaining basic vital signs, to counsel against injurious attempts at first aid, to measure for changes in swelling, and to observe for evidence of coagulopathy or neurotoxicity. By extending assessment into the prehospital period, the physician may determine the severity of symptoms and prepare in advance for the care for the patient (e.g., IV fluid, antivenom, ventilators, dialysis). In Western countries, a case of exotic snakebite invariably generates considerable interest among hospital staff—which does not translate into better medical care. In these different treatment environments, the gravity of the situation is the same: *Snake envenoming is a medical emergency until proved otherwise.* The time before the patient's arrival should be used to identify the treatment team, notify the laboratory, identify local snake experts, acquaint medical staff with management priorities and pitfalls, and transport antivenom to the treatment center.

FIRST AID

The physician should be familiar with first-aid measures for snakebite because he or she may need to make optimal use of these techniques while waiting for the arrival of antivenom or may need to address complications resulting from well-intentioned but damaging first aid. In resource-rich countries, first aid rarely is applied in the hospital setting. In Asia, rural medical clinics often can offer little to the patient except first aid. In this circumstance, simple procedures and precautions may benefit the patient by delaying the spread of venom until the patient reaches a hospital.

With the exception of lifesaving maneuvers, such as maintenance of airway, breathing, circulation, and treatment of severe hemorrhage, all first-aid measures should be considered secondary to prompt transport to medical care. *Initiation of transport* to a hospital should be considered one of the most important first-aid measures.

Results of studies evaluating the value of first-aid methods for treating snakebite are underwhelming. At best, currently recommended first-aid techniques delay the migration of venom to the systemic circulation. No first-aid measure has been shown to be therapeutic when used alone. Many previously recommended first-aid techniques are now known to be without value or dangerous to life and limb. In particular, electrical shock,[81] tourniquets,[82,83] cryotherapy, scarification, excision,[84] and prolonged suction over the fang wounds[85] have been shown to have no value or to cause additional injury. In rural Vietnam, Laos, and northeast Thailand, most patients treated in the field receive first aid that is either without value or damaging.

All victims of snakebite need reassurance. The envenomed patient is often terrorized by pain resulting from the venom or first-aid measures or by the appearance of the bitten extremity.

The experience of many traditional people is that snakebite is synonymous with death, a perception that complicates accurate history and clinical assessment. In these circumstances, the psychological stress of envenoming can be severe and is likely to compromise an accurate examination. A calm patient is more likely to provide a meaningful history and to recall events accurately. Conversely, patients bitten by kraits, coral snakes, and certain species of cobras may not realize that envenoming has occurred and may need to be encouraged to seek medical care.

The priorities of first aid are to do no harm, stabilize life-threatening conditions, delay the spread of venom, and minimize the damaging effects to the local extremity. The first-aid provider also can provide important details for the treating physician. Examples of important historical information are the local habitat, circumstances, and time of day that the bite occurred and the patient's initial symptoms. For an experienced physician, this information may help identify the snake when the animal itself was not seen. If the snake can be killed without risk or delay in patient transport, it should be attempted so that a positive identification can be made. Dead snakes should not be handled and should be transported in a rigid container to reduce the danger from reflexive postmortem bites.

Airway and Breathing. Use of an oral or nasopharyngeal airway may prevent airway obstruction in shocked or paralyzed patients. In desperate situations, when an airway cannot be improvised, the anterior third of the tongue may be pierced with a large safety pin (blanket pin), which is fastened to a cravat or sling to keep the tongue pulled forward. Patients without spontaneous respirations require continuous ventilation, which in rural settings invariably requires rescue breathing (mouth to mouth or mouth to mask). These recommendations often are made without fully appreciating the physical demands of performing rescue breathing during prolonged medical evacuation over footpaths or bumpy roads. In rural Asia, where severely envenomed patients may be carried for hours or transported in the back of bouncing utility vehicles, rescue breathing is difficult to perform and to sustain. For this reason, transport should include stops at rural medical clinics to obtain endotracheal tubes (Fig. 106-4), bag-valve-mask, and, in rare circumstances, a surgical airway (e.g., cricothyrotomy). Supplemental oxygen, if available, should be provided to any severely envenomed patient; however, the rescuer should consider how to preserve limited oxygen supplies for when they are needed most. In rural Asia, the only oxygen that is likely to be available in rural regions is from industrial sources (i.e., blue tanks), which may be contaminated with trace gases or particulate. The decision to use nonmedical oxygen should be reserved for severe cases. Smelling the vented oxygen may allow a crude assessment for contamination, and the presence of debris can be assessed by blasting the oxygen through a white cloth (e.g., a bed sheet) and examining for discoloration.

Shock. Shock is unlikely in the early minutes after envenoming except in rare cases of intravenous bites. In patients envenomed by Asian vipers, hypotension is common and may appear within 15 minutes of envenoming. Hypotensive patients should have their extremities raised and

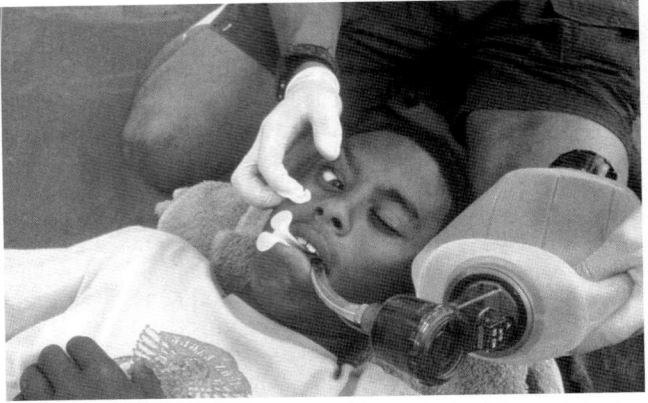

FIGURE 106-4

Severe envenoming. The patient was a 13-year-old boy with respiratory paralysis 9 hours after being bitten by an unknown krait (*Bungarus*). He received antivenom after symptoms appeared without effect, but he made a full recovery after 6 days of ventilation support. Note bulbar palsy. See Color Fig. 106-4.

antishock garments applied (if available) in an effort to increase cardiac filling and indirectly to increase cardiac afterload. Cardiac arrhythmias may occur as a result of direct cardiotoxins, hypoxia, or metabolic disturbances, such as hyperkalemia and acidosis. In a pulseless patient, cardiac compressions should be attempted; however, the prognosis of these cases, particularly when coagulopathy is present, is grim.

Local First Aid. The bite site should be inspected for retained fangs, which should be removed carefully and quickly. The skin surrounding the bite site should be forcibly irrigated with nonirritating fluid to prevent unabsorbed venom from being rubbed into fang wounds by clothing or immobilization bandages. Irrigation should be directed away from fang marks. The bite site should not be otherwise cleaned, scrubbed, massaged, or exposed to oral or mechanical suction. The extremity should be immobilized in a padded splint and placed in a dependent functional position. In the case of contact envenoming (e.g., venom ophthalmia), the eyes and mucous membranes should be irrigated immediately with available nonirritating fluid. The cornea, sclera, conjunctiva, and oral and nasal mucous membranes should be washed for a minimum of 10 minutes with fluid. Ophthalmic analgesics should not be used until symptoms of ocular-mucosal envenoming decrease. The principles of first aid for Asian snakebite are summarized in Table 106-2.

Envenoming by Asian vipers and cobras (excluding *O. hannah* and *N. philippinensis*) causes significant local injury and necrosis, and few first-aid techniques are of proven benefit. Animal studies have indicated that viper and cobra bites benefit from immobilization using a splint and sling (Fig. 106-5). Lymphatic and venous bands (e.g., low-pressure tourniquets) have been implicated in ischemia and gangrene resulting from the swelling of tissues and should not be used for envenoming by *any* Asian species (viper, elapid, or colubrid). A second problem with these bands occurs as swelling and pain increase, prompting an unsupervised patient to remove the lymphatic band.

TABLE 106-2 First Aid for Asian Snakebite

ABCs: Place patient in the lateral recumbent position. If nonbreathing, insert an oral airway or pull tongue forward. Perform rescue breathing if necessary. If hypotensive, raise extremities, or use pneumatic antishock garments

Do no harm

Transport promptly to a hospital

If patient is alert, place patient at rest and provide reassurance

Wash bite wound to remove unabsorbed venom

Immobilize the bitten extremity in a functional position at or below heart level

Remove rings, watches, and other potentially constrictive items

Delay the spread of venom

If patient is alert, without nausea, and evacuation is prolonged, provide with water

Painkillers, especially narcotic analgesia and NSAIDs, should not be used except at the recommendation of a physician familiar with snake envenoming

NSAIDs, nonsteroidal antiinflammatory drugs.

Sudden removal allows concentrated venom, lactic acid, and tissue degradation products to enter the systemic circulation quickly, with dramatic escalation of systemic symptoms.

With regard to envenoming by kraits (*Bungarus* spp.), Asian coral snakes (*Calliophis* spp., *Maticora* spp.), Philippine cobra (*N. philippinensis*), and king cobra (*O. hannah*), distinguishing between dry bites and true envenoming is initially difficult. When symptoms of neurotoxicity appear, first aid is of limited value. For this reason, all bites from these species are a medical priority, even if symptoms are not present several hours after the bite. Airway supervision is crucial to reduce the chance of aspiration or respiratory failure or both. Oral or nasopharyngeal airways should be used, if available.

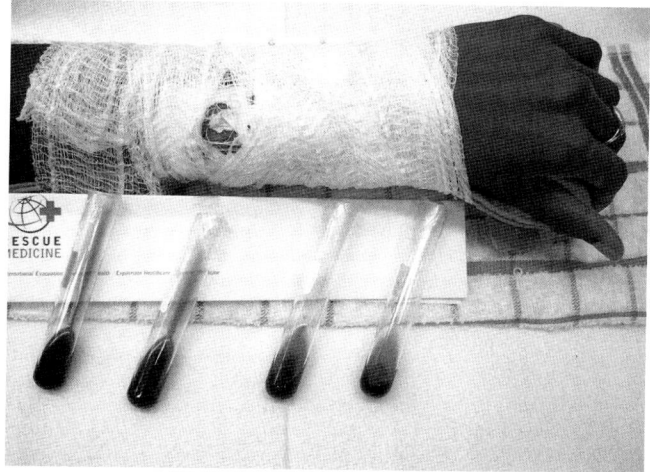

FIGURE 106-5

A 23-year-old woman with severe envenoming by *Daboia russelii*. The splint and gauze bandage help to stabilize the bitten extremity. Coagulopathy is checked using the whole-blood clotting test. The two tubes on the left, collected at 0 and 2 hours, lack clot formation. The two tubes on the right, collected at 5 and 10 hours after antivenom treatment, show return of clot formation. Note continued bleeding from the fang wounds to the forearm. See Color Fig. 106-5.

Patients bitten by kraits, coral snakes, and cobras with neurotoxic venom should be treated with pressure immobilization of the bitten extremity. The combined use of spiral pressure bandages and splint-immobilization compresses local lymphatics and microvasculature and has been shown to delay migration of venom to the central circulation. Evidence that pressure bandages are beneficial is based on experiments performed in monkeys.[86] Studies showed that pressure and immobilization decreased the movement of radiolabeled *N. naja* venom (and Australian elapid and crotalid venoms) without compromising vascular perfusion to the extremity. Evidence of efficacy in humans is limited to case reports involving Australian snakes[87] and African species, such as mambas (*Dendroaspis* spp.) and the Cape cobra (*Naja nivea*).[88] Throughout Asia, bites by most cobras and spitting cobras result in significant tissue damage and necrosis, injury potentially made worse by pressure wraps. In my experience with three patients confirmed to be envenomed by monocellate cobras (*N. kaouthia*) and treated 4 to 11 hours with pressure bandages but not immobilization, two of three hand bites developed necrosis. The area covered by the pressure wrap defined the edges of the necrotic area. This observation suggests that pressure dressings may exacerbate the necrotic effects of cobra and probably viper venom.

Another concern with treating cobra bites with pressure wrap bandages addresses the standard recommendation that when applied, the pressure dressing should be left in place until evaluation by medical personnel. Under actual conditions, most snakebites in rural regions swell well before arrival at the hospital. Swelling of tissue constrained by a tight dressing dramatically increases the pain in an already traumatized extremity. For these reasons, the universal recommendation of pressure wraps for all cobra bites is potentially harmful. In contrast, any bite by a neurotoxic species (e.g., any krait, coral snake, king cobra, or Philippine cobra) should be treated quickly with a spiral pressure bandage and immobilized. If the identity of the culprit snake cannot be established, the risks of exacerbating local damage using pressure dressing should be weighed against the benefits for a bite from a neurotoxic species. Key considerations are the probability that a neurotoxic species was responsible and the length of time required to reach medical care. Under these conditions, a smaller percentage of Asian cobra bites qualify for treatment using pressure bandages. Contraindications to pressure bandages are listed in Table 106-3. There are no

TABLE 106-3 Contraindications to Pressure Bandages

Bite by unknown species with local evidence of tissue damage
Any bite with pain, swelling, and bleeding from fang marks
Bites associated with severe coagulopathy
Bites >24 hr, without symptoms
Bites by colubrids (e.g., *Boiga, Rhabdophis*)
Bite by any Asian viper or pit viper (possible exception: *Daboia r. russelii* in southern India and Sri Lanka)
Any cobra bite with local pain, swelling, or significant discoloration

Comment: Pressure-immobilization bandages seem beneficial for envenoming by kraits, Asian coral snakes (*Calliopus, Maticora*), king cobra (*Ophiophagus hannah*), and Philippine cobra (*Naja philippinensis*) (see text).

contraindications to splint immobilization of the envenomed extremity.

Pressure bandages may be improvised from roller bandage, sports bandage, or cloth containing stretchy material such as Lycra. It is easier to start pressure compression proximally and wrap centrifugally, proceeding a short distance beyond the fang marks. If available, a sphygmomanometer inflated to a cuff pressure of 45 to 60 mm Hg also may be used. The advantage of using a blood pressure cuff is that any increase in pressure resulting from tissue swelling is easily detected, and the cuff pressure can be adjusted.

Hospital Management

HISTORY AND EXAMINATION

All patients presenting with a history of snakebite require evaluation by skilled medical personnel. The only patients not requiring admission for 24-hour observation are patients bitten by species confirmed as nonvenomous and patients bitten more than 24 hours previously *and* who have not developed symptoms. These patients still need local wound inspection and confirmation of up-to-date tetanus immunization. Because the outcome of the remaining cases is uncertain, these patients need to be observed until they remain asymptomatic for 24 hours. Physicians working in Asia need to be mindful of the costs of hospitalization, laboratory studies, and antivenom, all of which may be beyond the reach of poor families. Patients who lack resources and who present without symptoms may remain in the vicinity of the hospital until the period of observation is over. These patients require regular evaluation by either paramedical personnel or a physician, and when not being observed by medical personnel, they need to be attended by a responsible family member. Should symptoms develop, the patient needs to be admitted for treatment as described subsequently.

History. Physicians knowledgeable about local venomous snakes can obtain important information from a targeted patient history. Crucial elements of the history include age, weight, and nutritional status of the patient (particularly children); time of the snakebite; description of the snake; and presence, rate of development, and progression of any symptoms that may have developed. In many developing regions of Asia, patients often do not disclose use of traditional therapies, such as elixirs and ointments, which could complicate assessment and management.

Patients often are unable to identify the snake. If patients are alert, they should be shown full-color pictures of local species. Patients bitten by imported specimens are usually able to identify the responsible species. Many of these patients often have access to or know the location of appropriate antivenom. In the United States, many exotic snakebites involve illegally acquired animals, and the amateur reptile hobbyist may try to obtain treatment without alerting the authorities. Regardless of the treatment environment, the clinician should independently confirm the identity of the responsible species before treatment with antivenom.

In many parts of rural Asia, the snakebite victim first seeks treatment from traditional healers, which may obscure local signs of envenoming. In Laos and West Vietnam, traditional healers may administer opiate-based powders, which

can cause effects that suggest neurotoxic envenoming. Many traditional healers massage herbal compounds into the fang marks, potentially increasing the spread of venom and the risk of secondary infection. These activities also may increase the flow of bloody fluid from fang marks, suggesting coagulopathy. Table 106-4 summarizes important data to obtain from the patient history.

Local Examination. Important points of the physical examination are summarized in Table 106-5. The venoms of all Asian vipers and most cobras produce local pain, swelling, ecchymosis, and, in the case of Asian vipers, bleeding from fang marks. Local symptoms, such as pain and swelling, usually appear before the onset of systemic symptoms, such as coagulopathy and neurotoxicity.

Identification of fang marks is useful for distinguishing between the bites of vipers, elapids, and colubrids and for identifying fang and sting marks from arachnids and centipedes, which may mimic snake envenoming (see Differential Diagnosis). Locating fang marks also identifies areas for local wound care and continued observation. Fang marks from small cobras and kraits may be difficult to see and need to be located if pressure immobilization bandages are to be used. The gentle application of topical povidone-iodine to suspicious areas may help to highlight fang marks. The distance between fang marks increases with local swelling, suggesting bites by larger specimens. This differentiation is irrelevant because juvenile snakes and smaller species produce significant envenoming.

TABLE 106-4 Patient History

All Cases
Name, age, weight of victim
Size, color, shape, and distinctive feature of the snake (see Color Figs. 106-1 through 106-11)
Geographic location where bite occurred (swamp, forest, zoo)
Anatomic location of bites and number of bites received
Initial symptoms
Type of first aid or traditional therapy received
Past medical history (e.g., asthma)
Medication (prescription drugs such as β-blockers, nonprescription drugs, recreational drugs, alcohol)
Prior history of antivenom administration
Change in symptoms during transport
Presence of priority symptoms: nausea, vomiting, blurred vision, dizziness, dyspnea, syncope, weakness, chest pain, urinary retention, bleeding nares or gums, dark-colored urine, melena, hematochezia
Tetanus immunization status

For Viper and *Rhabdophis* Bites
Blood type
Recent surgery
History of cardiac disease, anemia, or hemoglobinopathy

For Cobra, Krait, and Coral Snakebites
Time of last meal
History of prior intubation
History of bronchospasm or bradyarrhythmias
Edrophonium hypersensitivity
Location of responsible family members (to assist in care of paralyzed patients)

TABLE 106-5 Physical Examination

Local Examination

Vital signs: respiratory rate, blood pressure, heart rate

Presence of fang marks, bleeding, erythema, discoloration, ecchymosis, swelling, local pain

Distal pulses (capillary refill); monitor for compartment syndrome

Lymphangitis or tender draining lymph nodes

Presence of damaging first aid methods (e.g., incisions, burns, amputations, cryotherapy, electrical burns, tourniquets)

Presence of necrosis, putrefaction, myolysis, secondary infection

Systemic Examination

Neurologic examination: Eye examination using finger count and cranial nerve examination. Assess motor strength and symmetry, and rule out respiratory abnormalities. Respiratory symptoms include dysphonia, dyspnea, use of accessory muscles of respiration, or decreasing peak expiratory flow (measured using a handheld device)

Coagulopathy: Evaluate for retinal and gingival hemorrhage; bleeding from nares or gastrointestinal tract; presence of petechiae or ecchymosis, particularly under elastic bands. Intracranial bleed should be ruled out with neurologic examination

Musculoskeletal examination: Evaluate for compartment syndrome. Palpate muscles for tenderness, which may suggest myolysis. Examine urine for color and presence of casts suggesting proximal tubular cells, hematuria, hemoglobinuria, or myoglobinuria

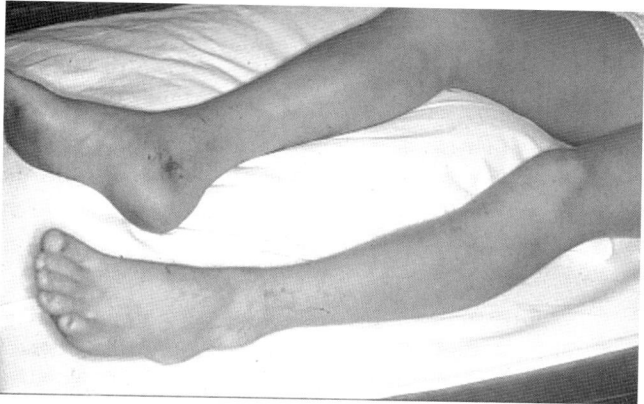

FIGURE 106-7

Moderate envenoming. The patient was a 15-year-old female tourist with bite to right ankle. Note ecchymosis and swelling involving the lower leg (species unknown). See Color Fig. 106-7.

Patients envenomed by Asian vipers experience varying degrees of pain, swelling, and ecchymosis (Figs. 106-6 and 106-7). Pain may be mild after bites by Sri Lankan daboia, but in most viper bites pain is significant. The presence of local symptoms indicates that systemic envenoming is possible, and further workup is warranted. Significant local symptoms, particularly excessive bleeding from fang marks and IV sites, marked swelling or ecchymosis, and formation of hemorrhagic bullae, are indications for close monitoring of coagulation status.

Distal pulses and capillary refill should be checked periodically to ensure adequate peripheral perfusion and to provide an early warning of compartment syndromes. Pulseless extremities should undergo intracompartment manometry using either a WIC device or a pressure transducer improvised from sterilized invasive monitoring devices. Compartment syndromes in patients with coagulopathy pose a dilemma because fasciotomy performed under these conditions may result in severe hemorrhage. The use of "prophylactic" fasciotomy is absolutely contraindicated because true compartment syndromes from snakebite are rare (Fig. 106-8). Excessive tissue swelling, particularly from viper bites, almost always is restricted to superficial muscle groups, rather than affecting muscles enclosed by deeper fascia, implicated in compartment syndrome

Systemic Examination. Envenoming by the Philippine cobra, kraits, and coral snakes, all of which may be insidious, cannot be ruled out before 24 hours of observation. This prolonged period of observation reflects experience with rare cases that present with symptoms after 21 hours of snakebite. Patients bitten by neurotoxic species need to be monitored closely for the appearance of symptoms. Initial symptoms may be nonspecific or

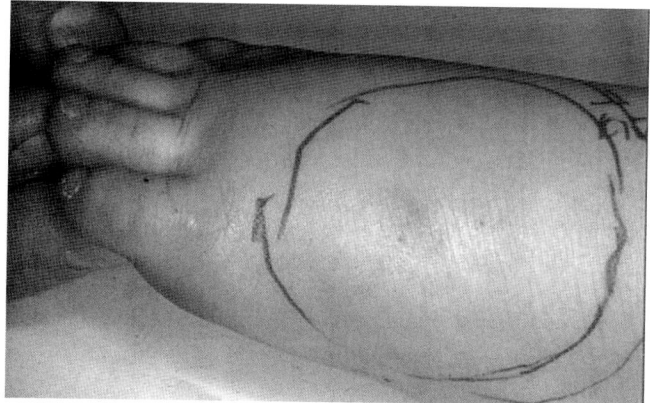

FIGURE 106-6

Minimal envenoming. The patient was a 9-year-old girl with s *Trimeresurus* bite to the foot. Note ecchymosis around fang marks and minimal swelling. The patient was observed overnight. No antivenom was given. See Color Fig. 106-6.

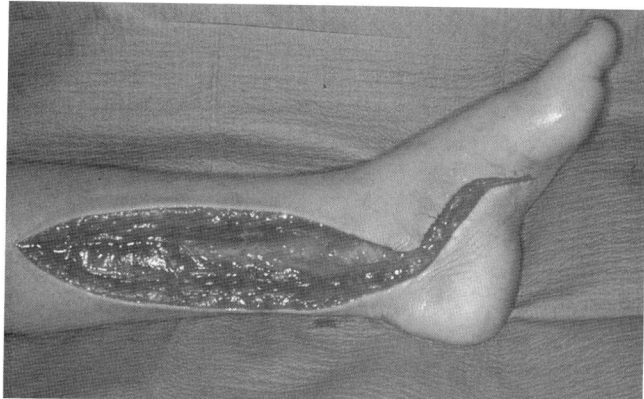

FIGURE 106-8

Fasciotomy for compartment syndrome may be suggested by excessive swelling of soft tissue; however, compartment pressures rarely are elevated significantly. Prophylactic fasciotomy is based on the belief that it protects against compartment syndrome. Such practices are unnecessary and can be catastrophic in venom-defibrinated patients. See Color Fig. 106-8.

attributed to other causes, such as traditional remedies (e.g., use of kava, opiates, or emetics) or fatigue or dehydration after prolonged transport. The earliest symptoms suggesting neurotoxicity are tingling, numbness or dull ache in the extremity, vague abdominal discomfort, restlessness, anorexia to food and fluids, drowsiness, and blurred vision (ophthalmoplegia). Ophthalmoplegia may initially be intermittent, improving when the patient continues to focus on an object. In the case of envenoming by *Bungarus* spp., patients first lose fast saccade eye movements, followed by the development of diplopia. Complete ophthalmoplegia may be delayed many hours. Other symptoms suggesting systemic neurotoxicity are perioral fasciculations or paresthesias (in a nonhyperventilating patient), metallic taste, and dizziness. In recent years, determination of neurotoxic envenoming has been facilitated by snake-venom assays, which are commercially available for diagnosing the bites of Australian elapids. In Asia, the use of molecular detection or immunoassays for diagnosing envenoming so far has been confined to research trials.[89,90]

Evidence of systemic coagulopathy may not be apparent at presentation. Early on, envenoming by Asian vipers may cause thrombotic events manifesting as transient cerebral ischemia, syncope, myocardial infarction, arrhythmias, and, rarely, pulseless extremities due to arterial thrombosis. At the time of presentation, most coagulopathies present as prolonged prothrombin time and activated partial thromboplastin time or as uncoagulable blood. Defibrination usually is first apparent at the bite site, where fang and teeth marks may continue to bleed. Spontaneous hemorrhage from the gingival sulci, retinal hemorrhage, and hematuria or hemoglobinuria suggest incoagulable blood (Fig. 106-9). The presence of incoagulable blood may be confirmed using several low-technology assays, such as the whole-blood clotting test (Fig. 106-10) with results in 20 minutes (Table 106-6).

Laboratory Studies for Asian Snake Envenoming

Bedside Studies

Whole-blood clotting test using gauze dressing, red-top glass Vacutainer, or glass slide
Urine dip-stick for proteinuria, hematuria, hemoglobinuria, and myoglobinuria (may require microscopy for confirmation)
Forced expiratory peak flow

Priority Laboratory Studies

Type and crossmatch blood for cases with severe hypotension, major ecchymosis, or swelling
Hematocrit and hemoglobin
Prothrombin time and activated partial thromboplastin time
Platelet count

Additional Studies

Complete blood count with differential
Peripheral blood smear
Fibrinogen and fibrin degradation products
Liver function test
Serum electrolytes, blood urea nitrogen, and creatinine
Urine sediment
Creatine phosphokinase
Electrocardiogram

Differential Diagnosis

Nonvenomous snakebites and bites by moderately venomous *Colubrid* spp. must be ruled out. Colubrids belonging to *Boiga* are pugnacious and capable of mild-to-moderate envenoming. Bite marks from these species have enlarged puncture wounds caused by the posterior maxillary teeth. Several arboreal green tree pythons (Pythonidae), which superficially resemble green *Trimeresurus*, possess elongated teeth suited for grasping birds; bites from these species may resemble the fang marks of vipers. Wounds from local flora, such as stinging nettle and puncture wounds from thorns, may suggest snakebite, especially when the injury occurred at night. Bites and stings from local arthropods (e.g., Hymenoptera) and

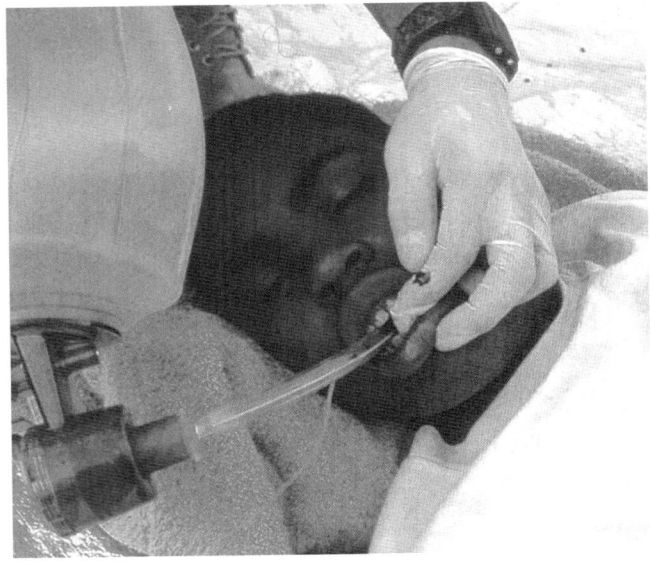

FIGURE 106-9

Caregivers should be vigilant for evidence of systemic anticoagulation, as occurred in this critically envenomed *Echis* bite. Note gingival bleeding after field intubation. See Color Fig. 106-9.

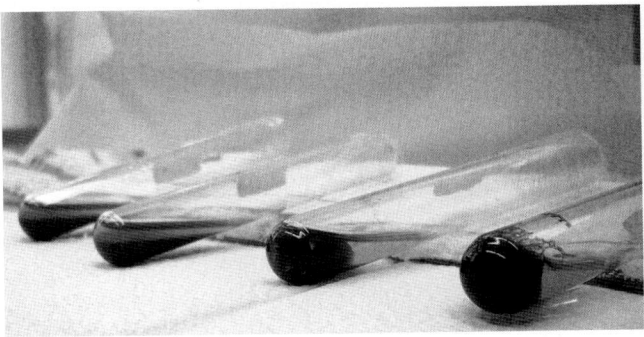

FIGURE 106-10

The whole-blood clotting test is a simple bedside test to measure anticoagulation. Clean glass tubes are filled with 5 mL of blood and left undisturbed for 20 minutes. Coagulopathy is present if blood flows down the tube (left two tubes). Antivenom usually produces a rapid but often transient return of clotting function (right two tubes). See Color Fig. 106-10.

TABLE 106-6 Bedside Tests for Coagulopathy

Whole-Blood Clotting Test

5 mL of blood is collected in a red-top Vacutainer tube or other non–silica-coated test tube and left undisturbed for 20 min at room temperature (>21°C). After 20 min, tube is tipped, allowing unclotted blood to be decanted. Unclotted blood suggests defibrination, which in Asian snakebite cases suggests envenoming by vipers or *Rhabdophis* (see Figs. 106-5 and 106-10)

Rapid Clot Test

100 μL of blood is placed carefully on an untreated microscope slide, with one edge resting on top of another slide to form a slight angle. Within 5–8 min, normal blood clots. Defibrination of blood collects at the bottom of the droplet and fails to clot or slowly rolls off the slide. After 10–12 min, slide may be tipped to evaluate further the degree of anticoagulation. The advantage of this technique is that it allows for internally controlled coagulation estimates using simple methods and inexpensive equipment (see Fig. 106-11)

arachnids may cause local pain, swelling, and inflammation that may mimic the early stages of snake envenoming. The venomous bite of Asian centipedes (*Scolopendra* spp.) may cause severe pain and local inflammation, which may mimic that seen in the early hours of viper bites. The horizontally orientated chelicerae of *Scolopendra* spp. leave a distinctive chevron-shaped puncture wound, however. Scorpion stings and bites by Asian widow spiders (*Latrodectus* spp.) may be confused with neurotoxic envenoming by elapids; however, both of these arachnids cause local pain and muscular cramping with minimal local skin changes. Envenoming by *Latrodectus* spp. also is associated with leukocytosis, moderate hypertension, and cramping of muscle groups. In central and southern India, stings by the red Indian scorpion (*Buthotus tamulus*) have been mistaken for bites by juvenile *Naja*. Important distinguishing features are that scorpion stings cause local piloerection, autonomic disturbances, and minimal local reaction. Rarely, bites by Asian running spiders (*Lycosa* spp.), sac spiders (*Chircanthium* spp.), or jumping spiders (*Phidippus* spp.) may suggest envenoming by Asian snakes. Bites from these arachnids may cause superficial necrosis, which takes several days to appear. Tick paralysis is unique in presentation, appearing as symmetric, ascending, and flaccid paralysis, and is unlikely to be confused with snake venom paralysis.

Emergency and Intensive Care

The care of a patient envenomed by an Asian elapid or viper should be viewed as a prolonged medical emergency, the intensive care management of which may last for days. A few patients are critically envenomed and present with immediate life-threatening problems. Critical envenoming may result from IV injection of venom, envenoming by highly dangerous species, or prolonged delay in reaching medical care. After initial assessment and stabilization, severely envenomed patients need to be admitted to the ICU for continued antivenom administration, close medical and laboratory monitoring, and skilled nursing care.

Before patient arrival, personnel are assigned specific roles in patient care, coordination of laboratory tests,

Indications for ICU Admission in Asian Snake Envenoming

Any patient bitten by an elapid within 24 hours who is showing symptoms

Blood loss (hemoglobin <8 mg/dL) *and* negative whole-blood clotting test or positive halo test

Heart rate >120 beats/min and diastolic blood pressure <40 mm Hg after fluid resuscitation

Swelling and intracompartment pressures >35 mm Hg

Rapidly advancing paralysis (beyond ptosis and fasciculations)

Seizure, syncope, or pulseless episode

Flaccid paralysis unresponsive to anticholinesterase treatment

Respiratory rate >24/min with use of accessory breathing muscles

Peak expiratory flow rate <80 L/min (adult)

$PaCO_2$ >45 mm Hg and pH <7.35

Creatine phosphokinase >10,000 U/L or serum potassium >6.5 mEq/L

Cortisol <15 μg/dL *and* hypotension, hyperkalemia, or abdominal pain

replenishment of IV supplies, transport and rewarming of the antivenom, and notification of the ICU. In the case of exotic bites, local antivenom repositories need to be located, institutional officers (e.g., zoo officials) contacted, and antivenom delivered to the hospital. Attempts should be

ICU Management of Asian Snake Envenoming

For All Patients

Airway and ventilation support as needed

Continuous patient monitoring (cardiac, blood pressure, oximetry)

Serial neurologic examination

Monitor urinary output; place catheter if necessary

Repeat laboratory tests within 3 hours of antivenom treatment

Repeat antivenom if coagulopathy, neurotoxicity, or local symptoms reappear

Monitor bitten extremity for thrombosis, compartment syndrome, or infection

Débridement of necrotic tissue

Early rehabilitation of damaged extremities

For Paralyzed Patients

Consider tracheostomy for krait-paralyzed cases

Atropine-neostigmine if appropriate

Sedation and analgesia

Early enteral nutrition

For Viper and Colubrid Envenoming

Avoid giving blood products if coagulopathy is ongoing; treat with antivenom instead

Monitor alveolar-arterial gradient

Avoid arterial and central line placement, unless peripheral venous access is inadequate

Nephrology consultation for acute renal failure

Monitor for endocrinopathies (adrenal or pituitary insufficiency)

made to locate an authority with experience treating envenoming by the same or a similar species. In North America and Europe, such personnel include foreign medical graduates, who often have experience treating snakebite in their home country. Familiarity with the treatment of envenoming from one species does not translate to experience treating bites from other members of the genus or family. There is variability in the clinical syndromes resulting from envenoming by different species of Asian cobras and among daboia from different regions.

On arrival, patients require primary assessment to confirm a patent airway, spontaneous respirations, and adequate oxygenation and that they are not in shock. Patients with deteriorating respiratory status should be promptly intubated with a laryngeal mask airway or endotracheal tube (see Fig. 106-4). Nasotracheal tubes should not be used for envenoming by vipers and, probably, *Rhabdophis* spp. owing to risk of bleeding and formation of compressive blood collections in the sinuses. Patients with respiratory paralysis do not require paralytics because the muscles of the upper airway are usually lax. Because patients are alert during paralysis, however, the use of benzodiazepines or other amnestic agents or haloperidol is compassionate and clinically indicated if not otherwise contraindicated by hypotension. Ketamine (1 to 2 mg/kg IV given over 2 minutes) may be used in hypotensive patients because it does not lower the blood pressure. In normotensive patients with coagulopathy, ketamine should be used with caution because it increases intracranial pressure and potentially could increase the likelihood of an intracranial bleed.

Severely envenomed patients require fluid resuscitation. The placement of IV lines also permits blood to be drawn for the bedside evaluation of coagulation and for stat blood samples to be sent to the laboratory. At least two IV lines are needed to allow the separate delivery of antivenom, ionotropes, and IV fluids. IV lines should not be placed in the envenomed extremity. Adult patients are hydrated with boluses of crystalloid as indicated by ongoing assessment of hemodynamic status. Central venous catheterization should not be attempted, unless it is found to be absolutely necessary and significant coagulopathy has been excluded. Fluid volume overload should be avoided, particularly in elderly patients and small children, because antivenom administration also requires IV fluids. In cases of envenoming with coagulopathy, saphenous vein cut-down and ligature and, in children, interosseous access are alternative hydration sites. Arterial access sites not only are unnecessary but also may prove disastrous in a patient with coagulopathy. Ionotropic agents are seldom required and should be used only when 3 to 4 L of IV hydration has failed to relieve hypotension. Volume status may be monitored by measuring urine output.

Envenoming by Asian vipers often results in shock secondary to hemorrhagin-induced extravasation of fluid. Packed red blood cells and albumin help to offset fluid extravasation by increasing oncotic pressure. In many parts of Asia, the risk of blood-borne pathogens, such as malaria, filariasis, and viral diseases, is high, however, and pathogen testing of blood supplies may be either dubious or nonexistent. Reliance on synthetic colloid replaces these risks with other concerns. The IV administration of 6% hetastarch may interfere with factor VIII activity and may increase the

---

Criteria for ICU Discharge in Asian Snake Envenoming

Reversal of coagulopathy for >12 hours
Resolution of neuromuscular symptoms for >24 hours
50% improvement in creatine phosphokinase, hyperkalemia, and fibrinogen titer
Peak expiratory flow rate >100 L/min, adequate oximetry, or arterial blood gas on room air
Stable or improving urine output

---

activated partial thromboplastin time. Dextran 40 also should be avoided because it inhibits platelet aggregation, induces fibrinolysis, and activates factor VIII.[91] In many parts of Asia, 10% pentastarch, which does not interfere with coagulation, is often available and should be considered. Many physicians favor administration of hypertonic saline; however, evidence that it is comparable to colloid fluids is lacking.[92]

Many patients are treated in the field with tourniquets, lymphatic bands, and pressure immobilization dressings. These techniques serve to compartmentalize venom and by-products of ischemia. The physician who receives patients treated with these methods (see earlier section on first aid) should remove these bands only *after* IV access is obtained, the patient is hydrated, and, ideally, antivenom therapy is started. In the cobra cases described previously, slow removal of the wrap still resulted in dramatic symptoms despite prehydration and treatment with three or more vials of appropriate antivenom (see Table 106-9). A blood pressure cuff, used to control blood return from the extremity, should be placed proximal to the tourniquet and inflated to 80 to 100 mm Hg. Significant bleeding may occur from incisions made to the fang marks, and occasionally arterial bleeding is seen. Medical care should make use of direct and indirect pressure with a sterile dressing and elevation. Wound inspection and cleaning is performed after lifesaving interventions are completed. An experienced surgeon should be consulted for convincing evidence of compartment syndrome or to identify other threats to tissue or limb. Principles of emergency care for Asian snake envenoming are summarized in Table 106-7.

IMMUNOTHERAPY

The only definitive treatment for snake envenoming is antivenom. Antivenom does more than save lives; it also conserves blood products and reduces the attendant risk of blood-borne infection; interrupts progression of paralysis, hence conserving mechanical ventilators (or personnel needed to manually ventilate patients); and shortens hospital stay. Antivenom also reduces local injury, lessening permanent disabling sequelae. It is likely that antivenom speeds convalescence, potentially allowing wage earners to return to work faster and with fewer complications (although there is no controlled trial evidence to support this). In developing regions and in resource-rich countries, antivenom treatment is cost-effective, compassionate, and usually the most important contribution made by the health care provider.

TABLE 106-7 Emergency Care of Severe Envenoming by Asian Snakes

Assign Tasks According to Medical Skill of Personnel

In the emergency department or ICU, personnel are assigned to call the laboratory; collect IV supplies; locate, transport, rewarm, and reconstitute antivenom; and identify local snakebite experts.

Airway/ventilation

Preoxygenate any patient with respiratory distress, intubate endotracheally, and provide mechanical ventilatory support. Neuromuscular blocking agents are often not necessary for venom-paralyzed patients; however, use of sedatives is appropriate, provided that caution is exercised to prevent hypotension.

Fluid Volume Resuscitation

Place 2 large-gauge IV lines in the nonenvenomed extremity, and draw blood for laboratory studies and bedside clotting tests. Hydrate adult patients with 300–500 mL fluid boluses every 5 min (children 20 mL/kg) until perfusion is restored. Use of inotropes (dopamine 10–20 μg/kg/min) should be reserved for cases that fail to respond to 3–4 L hydration (packed red blood cells or other colloid should be used in hypotensive-hypovolemic patients with severe swelling). Location of cryptic bleeding should be identified by imaging studies (e.g., CT or ultrasound).

Local Care

Fang marks should be inspected, retained fangs removed, and skin irrigated to remove unabsorbed venom. The bite site should not be otherwise manipulated. Rarely, patients present shortly after envenoming, in which case a pressure immobilization wrap may be considered (see Table 106-2). Patients with tourniquets or pressure dressings should be hydrated and pretreated with antivenom. Before removal, a blood pressure cuff must be placed proximal to the dressing and inflated to 80–100 mm Hg. The extremity should be kept immobilized in a functional position at or below heart level.

Antivenom Treatment

Prepare standby epinephrine (0.5 mL 1/10,000 in syringe taped to the IV bag, or alternatively mix 1 mg epinephrine in 250 mL D5W (4 mg/mL) and hang/place on IV pole or at bedside. Do not skin test if there is a chance antivenom will not be used. For noncritical patient, administer antivenom intravenously at a rate of 1 vial every 2–5 min. Administer monovalent antivenom in 1–2 vial aliquots and polyvalent antivenom in 3–4 vial aliquots, mixed in 250–500 mL normal saline. Start antivenom at low infusion rates, and adjust rate upward as tolerated by patient's symptoms.
Question the patient about changes in symptoms, and reassess vital signs for 5–10 min before continuing antivenom. Stop antivenom if hypersensitivity reaction (anaphylactic reaction) develops, treat with IV epinephrine, and resume antivenom at a slower rate.

Acetylcholinesterase Inhibitors

Acetylcholinesterase inhibitors should be considered in any patient with neurotoxic symptoms. Patients are first pretreated with atropine (0.6–1 mg/50 μg/kg children) and tested for edrophonium hypersensitivity (1 mg intravenously). Patients without contraindications are next treated with edrophonium, 8 mg intravenously (0.15 mg/kg in children) and evaluated for improvement. Patients showing transient improvement in symptoms (2–5 min) are treated with either edrophonium or neostigmine (0.5–1 mg intramuscularly or over 2–4 min intravenously) and atropine every 2–3 hr.

Nasogastric Tubes

Nasogastric tubes may be placed to reduce regurgitation/aspiration and in cases of extended paralysis to assist in hydration and nutrition.

CT, computed tomography; D5W, 5% dextrose in water; ICU, intensive care unit; IV, intravenous.

The first decision regarding antivenom treatment is whether the patient requires antivenom at all. Many bites are dry or result in trivial envenoming. The cases most likely to challenge the physician involve bites from kraits, coral snakes, and Philippine cobras that have not yet produced neurotoxic symptoms. Envenomings from these species are also the cases that show maximal benefit when antivenom is given early.

Antivenom should be given to any patient with symptomatic bites to the fingers or toes, severe local symptoms, rapidly progressing symptoms, or any evidence of systemic envenoming. Evidence of systemic envenoming includes prolonged prothrombin time and partial thromboplastin time; bleeding from the gums, gastrointestinal tract, or genitourinary tract; syncope; seizure; cardiac arrhythmias; perioral paresthesias; or any unusual neurologic symptom that cannot be attributed to another cause. Indications for antivenom are listed in Table 106-8.

Throughout Asia, antivenom is expensive relative to the cost of other medical services. High cost, limited shelf life, and injudicious use result in frequent shortages, particularly among the rural hospitals that treat most cases. Appropriate species-specific antivenom is often unavailable, and decisions must be made as to which alternative antivenoms may

be effective. Ideally, nonexpired, lyophilized, monospecific antivenoms provide the best results, require the lowest dosages, and have the fewest side effects. Antivenom that has exceeded the expiration date maintains neutralizing activity, even when stored at room temperature, and should

TABLE 106-8 Indications for Antivenom

Suspicion of venomous snakebite and
Progression of symptoms
Envenoming of digits
Hypotension
Moderate-to-marked swelling (e.g., involving more than half of the extremity)
Mental status changes, seizure, or syncope
Cardiac dysrhythmia
Any neurotoxic symptoms (except isolated ptosis)
Significant coagulopathy or thrombocytopenia (elevated CPK)
Rhabdomyolysis or myoglobinuria
Hematocrit <25% (with hemoglobinuria)
Potassium >6 mEq/dL or creatinine >2 mEq/dL

CPK, creatine phosphokinase.

be used if no alternative is available. In many parts of Asia, bivalent and polyvalent antivenoms are widely available. These antivenoms have neutralizing activity distributed across the different venoms used in the immunization process, and larger doses often are required compared with monovalent antivenoms. Bivalent and polyvalent antivenoms should be used when the identity of the snake is unknown or when monovalent antivenom is not available. Antivenom manufacturers may alter the method of production, including changing the venom used to immunize donor animals, and fail to update the package insert. When given a choice, the physician should select an antivenom prepared using venom from the same species and ideally from the same region. When the culprit snake is unknown, the physician should select antivenom based on the constellation of local findings, the presence of systemic symptoms, the results of clotting tests, the circumstances of the bite, and the epidemiology of bites involving local venomous species. Asian snake antivenoms available in 2003 are listed in Table 106-9.

All patients with indications for antivenom should be treated promptly. Antivenom should not be given subcutaneously or intramuscularly because absorption is erratic and delayed. Before treatment, resuscitation equipment should be placed at the bedside and epinephrine (0.5 mL 1/10,000) *predrawn* and taped to the IV bag or mixed (1 mg in 250 mL of 5% dextrose in water) and hung on an IV pump. Aliquots of 2 to 4 vials are reconstituted using sterile warm water or saline, filling each vial with as much fluid volume as it will take. Vials are gently mixed to return the antibody to its soluble phase tertiary structure. Antivenom must be completely reconstituted before administration. The ease of reconstitution varies among lyophilized preparations. Peak protein concentration, an indicator that lyophilized antibody has regained tertiary structure, is faster for F(ab)'$_2$ antivenoms (25 minutes) compared with whole immunoglobulin antivenoms (45 minutes).[93] Antivenom typically is diluted 1:5 or 1:10 in a small (250 or 500 mL) IV bag. Preferably, antivenom should be given

TABLE 106-9 Asian Snake Antivenoms

GENUS	SPECIES	SUBSPECIES	RANGE	ANTIVENOM
Agkistrodon-Gloydius (Mamushis group)		A. blomhoffi blomhoffi	Japan, eastern Japanese Island	(1) Mamushi Antivenin, The Chemo-Serotherapy. Research Institute, Kumamota, Japan, phone: ++81963441211 (2) Mamushi Antivenin, Takeda Chemical Industries Ltd., Osaka, Japan, phone: ++8162042111
		A. blomhoffi brevicaudus	Southern China to Korea	(3) Mamushi, Shanghai Institute of Biological Products, Ministry of Health, Shanghai, China, phone: ++86212513189 Alternative: (1), (2)
Deinagkistrodon	Deinagkistrodon acutus (previously A. acutus)		China, Taiwan, North Vietnam, Laos	(4) Monovalent long-nosed pit viper antiserum; Shanghai Institute of Biological Products, Shanghai, China, phone: ++86212513189 (5) Agkistrodon antivenom, National Institute of Preventative Medicine, Taipei, Taiwan, phone: ++88627857559
Hypnale	Hypnale hypnale and Hypnale nepa		Southern India, Sri Lanka	No specific antivenom; bivalent antisnake venom may be effective: Serum Institute of India Ltd., Pune-411 028 India, phone: ++91-51-240946/240973/241720
Bungarus	B. caeruleus		Eastern Pakistan, southern Nepal to Bangladesh, India, Sri Lanka	(6) Monovalent krait antiserum, Central Research Institute, Kasauli, India, phone: ++9117932060 (7) Polyvalent snake antiserum (includes D. russelii, Naja, E. carinatus), Central Research Institute, Kasauli, India, phone: ++9117932060 (8) Polyvalent antisnake venom (includes Naja, Indian Daboia, and Echis), Haffkine Biopharmaceutical Co. Ltd., Parel, Bombay, phone: ++9122-412932023/4129224
	B. multicinctus		Eastern Myanmar to Guiyang, China, northern Thailand, Laos	(9) B. multicinctus antivenom (monovalent), Shanghai Institute of Biological Products, Shanghai, China, phone: 86212513189 (10) Naja-Bungarus antivenom (N. atra), National Institute of Preventative Medicine, Taipei, Taiwan, phone: ++88627857559 Alternative: (6), (11)
	B. fasciatus		Eastern India to southern China, Southeast Asia	(11) Banded Krait Antivenin, Thai Red Cross Society, Bangkok, Thailand, phone: ++66225201614

TABLE 106-9 Asian Snake Antivenoms—cont'd

GENUS	SPECIES	SUBSPECIES	RANGE	ANTIVENOM
Calliophis and Maticora			Asia, Southeast Asia	No antivenom produced; consider antivenom for *Bungarus* (9) or a polyvalent anti-*Micrurus* (e.g., Anticoral), Instituto Clodomiro Picado, Universidad de Costa Rica, San Jose, Costa Rica, phone: ++506-290-344
Calloselasma	Calloselasma rhodostoma		Southeast Asia: from northern Thailand–Vietnam to Sumatra, Java	(12) Malayan pit viper antivenom, Thai Red Cross Society, Bangkok, Thailand, phone: ++66225201614 (13) Anti-Malayan pit viper polyvalent antivenom serum, Serum Bio Farma (Pasteur Institute), Bandung, Indonesia, phone: ++622283755
Daboia	D. russelii siamensis (China and Taiwan) (previously D. r. formosensis)		Taiwan, southern China (Kunming)	(14) Monovalent Russell viper antivenom, Central Research Institute, Kasauli, India, phone: ++9117932060 Alternative: consider (15) (monovalent) and (8) (polyvalent: includes *Naja*, Indian *Daboia*, and *Echis*)
	D. russelii siamensis (Thailand)		Thailand, Laos, Kampuchea	(15) Russell viper antivenom (Monovalent), Thai Red Cross Society, Bangkok, Thailand, phone: ++66225201614 (now using venoms isolated from throughout Southeast Asia) Alternative: (14) (monovalent); (16) (monovalent F(ab)'2), (8) (low efficacy)
	D. russelii siamensis (Indonesia) (previously D. r. limitis)		Indonesia, Komodo, Flores	(16) Russell viper antivenom (monovalent), Serum Bio Farma, Bandung Indonesia, phone: ++83755/83756 Alternative: (15), (14)
	D. russelii russelii (India)		Northern Kanpur to lowlands between the Ghats. Intergrades common	(14), (8), (16)
	D. russelii russelii (Sri Lanka) (previously D. r. pulchella)		Sri Lanka	(17) PolongaTab (anti-Daboia F(ab)'2), Protherics PLC, London, EC4V5DR, UK, phone: 44(0)2072469950 Alternative: (15) > (14) > (8)
	D. russelii russelii (Myanmar)		Myanmar, eastern Bangladesh	(18) Monovalent Russell viper antiserum, Industrie & Pharmaceutical Corporation, Rangoon, Myanmar (outdated inventory; no contact number at this time) Alternative: (15), (16), (8)
Echis	E. carinatus		Pakistan, north-western India	(19) Monovalent Echis antisnake, Central Research Institute, Kasauli, India, phone: ++9117932060 Alternative: (8) (polyvalent); (20) Monovalent Echis antivenom, Haffkine Biopharmaceutical Co. Ltd., Parel, Bombay, phone: ++9122-412932023/4129224 *Note*: In U.S. envenoming by captive Indian *Echis*, EchiTab, an anti-African *Echis* F(ab)'2 antivenom has been used with evidence of efficacy. (Protherics PLC, London, EC4V5DR, UK, phone: 44(0)2072469950)
	E. sochureki		Pakistan, northern India to southern Kashmir	As above
Naja	N. atra		China, Vietnam, northern Laos	(21) Monovalent cobra antiserum, Central Research Institute, Kasauli, India, phone: ++9117932060 (22) Cobra Antivenin, Thai Red Cross Society, Bangkok, Thailand, phone: ++66225201614 (preparation has included venom from spitting cobras)
	N. kaouthia		Eastern India–Yunnan, China, Malaysia-Vietnam	As above
	N. naja		Nepal–southeastern Pakistan to Sri Lanka	As above
	N. oxiana		Iran–southern Tajikistan, Afganistan to central Pakistan and northern India	As above

Continued

TABLE 106-9 Asian Snake Antivenoms—cont'd

GENUS	SPECIES	SUBSPECIES	RANGE	ANTIVENOM
	N. philippinensis		Manila-Mindanao	(23) "Cobra" (monovalent), Serum and Vaccine Laboratories, Rizal, Philippines
	Spitting cobras N. siamensis		Eastern Myanmar–Thailand–Cambodia–South Vietnam	(21), (22), (24), (25)
	N. sputatrix		Thailand (south of Chang Mai)–Cambodia–Laos–South Central Vietnam	(22) (see note) (24) Malayan Cobra (monovalent), Serum Bio Farma, Bandung Indonesia, phone: 83755/83756 (25) Cobra Antivenin (monovalent), Twyford Pharmaceuticals, Rhein, Germany, phone: 0621-589-2688
	N. sumatrana		Java, Flores, Bali, Malaysia to Singapore, Sumatra	(22), (24) Alternative: (21), (25)
	N. sumarensis		Philippines	No data or case studies; consider (22)
Ophiophagus	Ophiophagus hannah		India, southern Nepal, southern China, Southeast Asia–Philippines	(26) King Cobra Antivenin, Thai Red Cross Society, Bangkok, Thailand, phone: ++66225201614 Other Asian cobra antivenoms may be used as alternatives; however, efficacy seems to be much less
Rhabdophis	R. subminiatus		Western India–southern China, all of Southeast Asia	(27) Anti-Yamakagashi Antivenin, The Japan Snake Institute, Gunma Prefecture 379–23, Japan, phone: ++81277785193
	R. tigrinus		Khabarovsk (southern Russia), Japan, south-central China, Taiwan	(27)
Trimeresurus	T. albolabris		Kashmir, Bhutan–Southeast Asia	(28) Green Pit Viper Antivenin, Thai Red Cross Society, Bangkok, Thailand, phone: ++66225201614; (this antivenom will soon be prepared using an increased number of species)
	T. mucrosquamatus		Western India–southern China, Central Vietnam	(29) Habu antivenom, The Chemo-Serotherapy Research Institute, Kumamoto, Japan, phone: ++81963441211 Alternative: (28); other Trimeresurus antivenoms also have neutralizing activity

through a dedicated IV line, which allows for separate control of antivenom, other IV fluid, and medications for resuscitation. Serum antivenoms are prone to autolysis and contamination. Any vials that are cloudy, have suspended particulate matter, or have sediment are likely to contain degraded antibody or might be contaminated and should not be used.

The rate of antivenom infusion varies with the severity of the envenoming and is adjusted in response to changes in symptoms. In all but the most critical cases, antivenom should be started at a slow rate (e.g., 10 to 20 mL/hr), with gradual increase in rate of administration over the first 10 minutes. In situations in which death is not imminent, antivenom is given intravenously at a rate of 1 vial diluted 1:10, given every 5 to 10 minutes, or 2 to 4 vials in 250 to 500 mL of normal saline over 30 to 60 minutes. In most cases, antivenom treatment is completed within 1 to 2 hours. Infusion at higher rates often results in overtreatment and squanders antivenom stockpiles. Monovalent (species-specific) antivenom should be given in 1- to 2-vial aliquots, and polyvalent antivenom should be given in 3- to 4-vial aliquots. Assessment of vital signs and inquiring about symptoms should be performed before continuing

antivenom. Patients often require additional antivenom due to recrudescence of symptoms (Fig. 106-11).

The treatment of snakebite is difficult to summarize in a nomogram.[94] The enormity of variables present, including patient factors, snake factors, and differences in treatment environment, make each case unique. For this reason, reliance on treatment protocols, such as those provided in the package insert, is enthusiastically discouraged. Instead, decisions regarding the quantity of antivenom should be based on the patient's symptoms, the physician's judgment, the results of confirmatory laboratory studies, and consultation with a treatment expert, such as an experienced medical toxicologist.

Progression of symptoms and recrudescence of symptoms are the primary reasons to continue antivenom. Conditions that often respond within minutes of antivenom include syncope, hypotension, cardiac arrhythmias, fasciculations, paresthesias, and pain. Conditions that respond more slowly are blood clotting abnormalities and neurotoxic symptoms, which may take hours or days to normalize. In the case of Rhabdophis envenoming, coagulopathy may persist for weeks. Patients with respiratory paralysis should remain on the ventilator after antivenom because

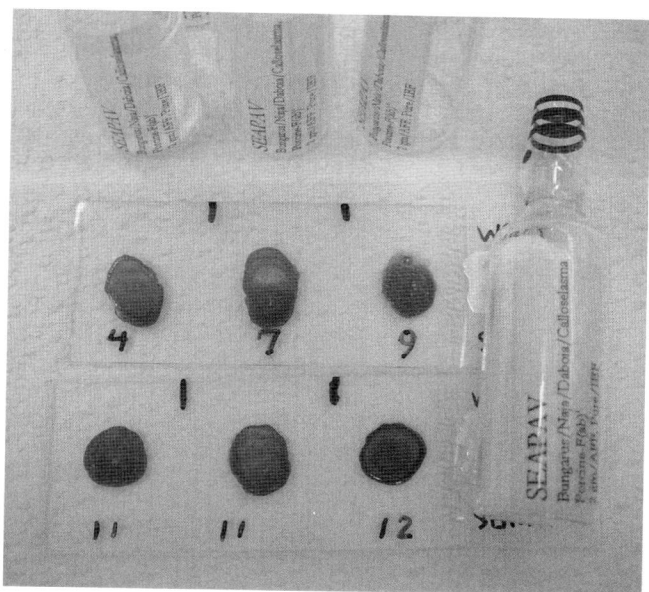

FIGURE 106-11

Rapid clot test. A simple test to guide antivenom use in austere settings. Blood (100 μL) is placed on a clean glass slide that is elevated 2 mm by resting the edge on top of another slide. Black numerals refer to the number of vials of antivenom administered. Defibrinated blood pools dependently or drips off the slide (four and seven vials). Note return of coagulopathy after 11 vials, requiring additional treatment (12 vials total). See Color Fig. 106-11.

venom continues to migrate from the bite site and may result in sudden return of neurotoxic symptoms. The practice of letting recovering patients breathe on their own through the endotracheal tube should be discouraged because the increased work of breathing combined with precarious respiratory status may lead to the sudden return of respiratory failure. Blood made coagulable by antivenom may undergo defibrination as venom continues to distribute from the bite site.

Antivenoms are prepared as either hyperimmune serum or lyophilized products, which tend to be more stable and which have a slightly reduced incidence of hypersensitivity reactions. Serum-phase antivenoms tend to have a shorter shelf life, are more prone to contamination, and have a higher concentration of coprecipitating antigens, the presence of which increases the likelihood of hypersensitivity reactions. Patients with a history of asthma, use of β-blockers, or previous antivenom administration (from the same species, e.g., horse, sheep, or pig) have a relative contraindication to antivenom therapy. Partial immunoglobulin antivenoms, composed of either F(ab) or F(ab)′₂ fragments, lack the Fc region and are less likely to activate complement or trigger mast cell degranulation. As a result, these protease-modified antivenoms tend to induce fewer hypersensitivity reactions than do whole-antibody IgG antivenoms.[38,95] A less appreciated advantage of F(ab) antivenoms is their increased volume of distribution; however, this may be offset by their shorter plasma half-life and duration of effect.

Patients presenting with rapidly deteriorating respiratory status, loss of consciousness, or shock are critically envenomed and require urgent treatment with species-specific antivenom if the snake is known or with polyvalent antivenom if the identity of the snake is unknown. For critically envenomed patients, antivenom should be given at an accelerated rate of 1 vial every 2 to 3 minutes for a total of 5 vials (in 250 to 500 mL of normal saline) followed by a 5- to 10-minute period of reassessment of respirations, blood pressure, and, in elapid bites, a repeated neurologic examination. In the case of deteriorating respiratory function resulting from *post*synaptic toxins, rapid infusion may interrupt progression of symptoms. The likelihood and severity of early hypersensitivity reactions are increased when antivenom is given at high infusion rates. When anaphylactic or anaphylactoid reactions are observed, the infusion must be stopped, the patient treated, and antivenom restarted at a slower rate.

Increasing the concentration of acetylcholine within the neuromuscular junction can alleviate the effect of venom neurotoxins on cranial and somatic motor function. Acetylcholine concentration at the neuromuscular junction can be increased either by stimulating increased release from presynaptic vesicles or by inhibiting the acetylcholinesterases. Acetylcholinesterase inhibitors (anticholinesterases) are of proven benefit in reducing the effects of postsynaptic and presynaptic neurotoxins after envenoming by several species of elapids. The goal of acetylcholinesterase inhibitor therapy is to increase the amount of neurotransmitter available for voluntary muscle activity, forestalling the onset of respiratory paralysis and buying time until antivenom can be administered.

Side effects of acetylcholinesterase inhibitor treatment include sweating, diarrhea, bronchospasm, bradyarrhythmias, and hypotension. Patients treated with an anticholinesterase first must be pretreated with atropine to prevent muscarinic excess and tested for hypersensitivity to the acetylcholinesterase inhibitor. Atropine (0.6 to 1 mg; 50 μg/kg in children) is given before a test dose of edrophonium (1 mg intravenously). Nonreacting patients are treated with edrophonium, 8 mg intravenously (0.15 mg/kg in children), and evaluated for improvement. Patients that respond will experience a transient improvement in symptoms for 2 to 5 minutes. Patients showing a positive response may be switched to a longer acting anticholinesterase, such as neostigmine (0.5 to 1 mg intramuscularly or intravenously), and atropine. Intramuscular neostigmine achieves peak activity in 30 minutes and is given every 2 to 3 hours. Atropine is given every 2 hours or when side effects of anticholinesterase treatment reappear.

Anticholinesterase therapy is more effective against postsynaptic neurotoxins typical of cobras, including the Indian cobra (*N. naja*), the Siamese/monocellate cobra (*N. kaouthia*), and the Philippine cobra (*N. philippinensis*).[96,97] In the case of krait envenoming, which involves presynaptic and postsynaptic neurotoxins, proof of efficacy is less clear. Positive results for anticholinesterases have been reported for *B. caeruleus*[98] and *B. candidus*.[99] In other regions, bites by these same species also were treated with anticholinesterase but did not show clinical improvement. There are no data reporting use of anticholinesterase in the treatment of bites by Asian coral snakes or king cobras. Testing symptomatic patients with atropine and edrophonium and then treating patients who show improvement with neostigmine makes good sense when no other therapies are available. There is no evidence that anti-cholinesterase therapy is of value in the treatment of neurotoxicity resulting from the bites of Asian vipers (*Agkistrodon* and *Daboia*).

HYPERSENSITIVITY REACTIONS

Early hypersensitivity reactions include anaphylactoid (non–IgE-mediated) reactions that are caused by antivenom complement or mast cell activation and, less commonly, anaphylactic (IgE-mediated) reactions. The symptoms of type I anaphylactic reactions appear 1 minute to 1 hour after initiation of therapy. Initial symptoms and signs include anxiety, tachycardia, pruritus of the head and neck, sensation of tightening of the throat, broncholaryngeal spasm followed by swelling of oral pharyngeal tissues, dyspnea, stridor, hypotension, and cardiac arrest. Because antivenom is administered intravenously, the onset of hypersensitivity reactions is much faster, more severe, and precipitated by lower doses than occurs when antigens are delivered by other routes. Many cases of antivenom-induced anaphylaxis require continuous infusion of IV epinephrine for correction. The physician should be particularly vigilant for hypersensitivity reactions in patients who have received antivenom in the past because anaphylactic reactions among this group are particularly severe. Skin testing before antivenom treatment is discouraged because it is of no value in predicting hypersensitivity reactions and may sensitize against future antivenom treatment.

There is debate regarding the value of antihistamines to treat antivenom-induced hypersensitivity reactions.[100] In my experience with foreign-produced, serum-phase antivenoms, diphenhydramine (50 mg intravenously) has alleviated mild hypersensitivity reactions. When given intravenously, however, diphenhydramine can cause transient hypotension. Diphenhydramine may be repeated every 4 to 6 hours.

Anaphylactoid reactions resulting from histamine release from mast cells appear 10 minutes to several hours after initiating therapy and include pruritus, angioedema, urticaria, and gastrointestinal discomfort. Late-stage type III hypersensitivity reactions, also known as immune complex–mediated or serum sickness reactions, appear days to 2 weeks after therapy. Type III reactions respond to treatment with steroids (e.g., prednisone) and antihistamines.

SPECIAL POPULATIONS

Pediatric Patients

In tropical Asia, children are likely to be envenomed by many species. Due to their smaller size, children seem to be at increased risk of intravenous envenoming. Also, children are uniquely subject to krait envenoming as a result of sleeping on the floor in rural houses. The symptoms of snakebite in children are often accelerated, more severe, and more resistant to treatment than in adults. In rural health clinics, pediatric-size oral airways and IV supplies are often unavailable. All children with indications for antivenom should receive the same treatment doses as adults, and the antivenom should be volume concentrated (e.g., 100 to 200 mL total volume) to allow for administration of the total dose. A subset of children with apparent poor prognosis after snakebite are the malnour-

ished. Many nutritionally compromised children are bitten while gathering food. In this group, close monitoring of serum electrolytes during treatment is an absolute necessity. After treatment, malnourished patients are likely to benefit from anthelmintic therapy, micronutrient repletion, and a high protein-calorie diet, all of which may support postenvenoming healing.

Pregnant Patients

Pregnant women occasionally may be envenomed and should be treated as nonpregnant patients with a few exceptions. Vaginal bleeding was an early and severe indicator of coagulopathy in one 22-week primigravida woman envenomed by a 1-m daboia. The stress of envenoming can cause premature contractions and delivery of the fetus. The distribution of venom, and likely of antivenom, in pregnant women depends on the molecular weight of venom antigen and antivenom immunoglobulin. Small proteins, including several postsynaptic neurotoxins, may be capable of traversing the placenta and entering the fetal circulation. The effects of neurotoxin on a fetus residing within a paralyzed-ventilated mother are unknown. In addition, there are no data regarding the ability of whole equine or ovine IgG immunoglobulins to traverse the human placenta in a manner akin to maternal IgG. Similarities in molecular weight and amino acid sequence suggest that this movement might be a possibility. Regardless, the pregnant patient and her fetus should be monitored closely and treated based on the mother's symptoms. Cesarean section should not be attempted unless absolutely necessary to save the mother; it should not be undertaken unless coagulopathy has not occurred or has resolved with antivenom therapy.

Elderly Patients

The elderly and patients with comorbidities also are at increased risk of severe reactions to snakebite. Bites by vipers may severely test the patient's cardiac reserve,[101] and many patients are unable to maintain adequate cardiac output during venom-induced hypovolemic episodes. All elderly patients and patients with heart disease, diabetes, and frail state require close cardiac monitoring and monitoring of serum creatine phosphokinase and creatinine.

Common Problems in Treatment of Asian Snakebite	
Problem	**Response**
Misdiagnose cobra bite as viper bite	Consider cobras in the evaluation of bites with local symptoms
Missed krait or Philippine cobra bite	These species cause minimal local symptoms and may be dismissed as dry bites. Confirm the identity of seemingly innocuous species, or admit patients with suspicious history.
Sudden respiratory failure	Reassess progression of paralysis, and intubate patient before respiratory failure is advanced

continued

Common Problems in Treatment of Asian Snakebite *continued*

Problem	Response
Missed hemolysis or hemorrhage	Extravasation leads to hemoconcentration of red blood cells, which may mask red blood cell lysis. Monitor patients with swelling, check urine output, monitor for hemoglobinuria, and obtain peripheral blood smear for evidence of hemolysis.
Delayed presentation to hospital	Monitor patients envenomed by kraits and *Naja philippinensis* and treat when first symptoms appear; locate antivenom, intravenous fluids, and emergency supplies in advance of patient arrival
Insufficient antivenom	Repeat patient and laboratory assessment to determine if more antivenom is likely to be needed. Plan in advance.
Incorrect antivenom	Match the culprit snake with the scientific name and region listed on the antivenom package insert. Attempt to locate more appropriate antivenom (zoos, poison control center, research center).
Antivenom withheld by other caregiver	Bites to the fingers and toes may result in disability; treat symptomatic bites to digits with antivenom

REFERENCES

1. Swaroop S, Grab B: Snakebite mortality in the world. Bull WHO 10:35–76, 1954.
2. Callahan MC, Pitts RM, King RE: Exotic snake envenoming in the United States. Alabama Center for Envenomation. Proceedings of the Southern Medical Society, Birmingham, Alabama, September 1986.
3. Chanhome L, Cox MJ, Wilde H, et al: Venomous snakebite in Thailand: I. Medically important snakes. Milit Med 163:310–317, 1998.
4. Kini RM, Iwanaga S: Structure-function relationships of phospholipase II: Charge density distribution and the myotoxicity of presynaptic neurotoxic phospholipases. Toxicon 24:895–905, 1986.
5. Bjarnason JB, Fox JW: Hemorrhagic metalloproteinases from snake venoms. Pharmacol Ther 62:325–372, 1994.
6. Gould RJ, Polokoff MA, Friedman PA, et al: Disintegrins—a family of integrin inhibitory proteins from viper venoms. Proc Soc Exp Biol Med 195:168–171, 1990.
7. Jayanthi GP, Gowda TV: Geographic variation in India in the composition and lethal potency of Russell's viper venom. Toxicon 26:257–264, 1988.
8. Phillips RE, Theakston RDG, Warrell DA, et al: Paralysis, rhabdomyolysis and haemolysis caused by bites of Russell's viper (*Vipera russelli pulchella*) in Sri Lanka: Failure of Indian (Haffkine) antivenom. QJM 68:691–716, 1988.
9. Moore TC: Snakebite from the Korean pit viper. Milit Med 142:546–549, 1977.
10. Sun XS: Successful treatment of 9 cases of respiratory paralysis caused by Pallas pit viper bite. Zhonghua Yi Xue Za Zhi 61:362–365, 1981.
11. Shanghai Vaccine & Serum Institute: *Agkistrodon halys* bite treated with specific antivenin: Observation of 530 cases. Chin Med J 2:59–62, 1976.
12. Tateno I, Sa Wai Y, Makino M: Current status of Mamushi snake (*Agkistrodon halys*) bite in Japan with special reference to severe and fatal cases. Jap J Exp Med 33:331–346, 1963.
13. Zhao E-M, Wu G, Yang W: Comparisons of toxicity and neutralization test among Pallas' viper and black eye-brow pit viper. Acta Herpetol Sin 1:1–6, 1979.
14. Sawai Y: Snakebites by Korean Mamushi in Japan. Snake 7:40–41, 1975.
15. Chen Y-C: Venomous snake bites and snake venom research in China. In Gopalakrishnakone P, Chou LM (eds): Snakes of Medical Importance (Asia-Pacific Region). Singapore, National University of Singapore, 1990, pp 269–279.
16. Wuster W, Otsuka S, Malhotra A, et al: Population systematics of Russell's viper: A multivariate study. Biol J Linn Soc 47:97–113, 1992.
17. Than-Than, Hutton RA, Myint-Lwin, et al: Haemostatic disturbances in patients bitten by Russell's viper (*Vipera russelli siamensis*) in Burma. Br J Haematol 69:513–520, 1988.
18. Tun-Pe, Phillips RE, Warrell DA, et al: Acute and chronic pituitary failure resembling Sheehan's syndrome following bites by Russell's viper in Burma. Lancet 2:763–767, 1987.
19. Maung-Maung-Aye: Some experience in the management of snakebite. Burma Med J 20:33–40, 1972.
20. Belt PJ, Malhotra A, Thorpe RS: Russell's viper in Indonesia: Snakebite and systematics. In Thorpe RS, Wuster W, Malhotra A (eds): Venomous Snakes: Ecology, Evolution and Snakebite. Symposia of the Zoological Society of London No. 70. Oxford, Clarendon Press, 1997, pp 219–233.
21. Wall AJ: Indian Snake Poisons, Their Nature and Effects. London, WH Allen & Co, 1883.
22. Maung-Maung-Aye: Snakes of Burma with Venomology and Envenomation. Rangoon, Arts & Science University, 1976.
23. Than-Than, Francis N, Tin-Nu-Swe, et al: Contribution of focal haemorrhage and microvascular fibrin deposition to fatal envenoming by Russell's viper (*Vipera russelli siamensis*) in Burma: Clinicopathological studies. Acta Trop Basel 46:23–28, 1989.
24. Matthai TP, Date A: Acute renal failure in children following snakebite. Ann Trop Paediatr 1:73–76, 1981.
25. Date A, Pulimood R, Jacob CK, et al: Haemolytic-uraemic syndrome complicating snake bite. Nephron 42:89–90, 1986.
26. Chen H-C, Lai Y-H, Tsai J-H: Acute renal failure following Russell's viper envenomation: A report of two cases. Kaohshiung J Med Sci 4:467–472, 1988.
27. Looareesuwan S, Vira Van C, Warrell DA: Factors contributing to fatal snake bite in the rural tropics: Analysis of 46 cases in Thailand. Trans R Soc Trop Med Hyg 82:930–934, 1988.
28. Matthai TP, Date A: Acute renal failure in children following snakebite. Ann Trop Paediatr 1:73–76, 1981.
29. Win-Aung, Khin Pa-Pa Kyaw, Baby-Hla, et al: Renal involvement in Russell's viper bite patients without disseminated intravascular coagulation. Trans R Soc Trop Hyg 92:322–324, 1998.
30. Chakrabarty D, Katta K, Gomes A: Hemorrhagic protein of Russell's viper venom with fibrinolytic and esterolytic activities. Toxicon 38:1475–1490, 2000.
31. Reference deleted.
32. Wang Y-M, Lu P-J, Ho C-L, Tsai I-H: Characterization and molecular cloning of neurotoxic phospholipases A2 from Taiwan viper (*Vipera russelli formosensis*). Eur J Biochem 209:635–641, 1991.
33. Liao WB, Lee CW, Tsai YS, et al: Influential factors affecting prognosis of snakebite patients' management: Kaohsiung Chang Gung Memorial experience. Changgeng Yi Xue Za Shi 23:577–583, 2000.
34. Kanjanajatanee J, Visutipant S: Russell's viper bite: Clinical manifestations and treatment. Thai Med Council Bull 13:25–38, 1987.
35. Eapen CK, Chandy N, Joseph JK: A study of 1000 cases of snake envenomation. Presented at XI International Congress of Tropical Medicine & Malaria, Calgary, 1984.
36. Tun-Pe, Phillips RE, Warrell DA, et al: Acute and chronic pituitary failure resembling Sheehan's syndrome following bites by Russell's viper in Burma. Lancet 2:763–767, 1989.
37. Uma B, Veerabasappa T: Molecular mechanisms of lung hemorrhage induction by VRV-PL-VIIIa from Russell's viper (*Vipera russelli*) venom. Toxicon 38:1129–1147, 2000.
38. Ariaratnam CA, Meyer WP, Perera G, et al: A new monospecific ovine Fab antivenom for treatment of envenoming by the Sri Lankan Russell's viper *Daboia russelii russelii*: A preliminary dose-finding and pharmacokinetic study. Am J Trop Med Hyg 6:259–265, 1999.
39. Bhat RN: Viperine snake bite poisoning in Jammu. J Indian Med Assoc 63:383–392, 1974.
40. Warrell DA, Arnett C: The importance of bites by the saw-scaled or carpet viper (*Echis carinatus*): Epidemiological studies in Nigeria and a review of the world literature. Acta Trop 33:307–341, 1976.

41. Weiss JR, Whatley RE, Glenn JL, et al: Prolonged hypofibrinogenemia and protein C activation after envenoming by *Echis carinatus socchureki*. Am J Trop Med Hyg 44:452–460, 1991.

42. Viravan C, Looareesuwan S, Kosakarn W, et al: A national hospital-based survey of snakes responsible for bites in Thailand. Trans R Soc Trop Med Hyg 86:100–106, 1992.

43. Warrell DA, Looareesuwan S, Theakston RDG, et al: Randomized comparative trial of three monospecific antivenoms for bites by the Malayan pit viper (*Calloselasma rhodostoma*) in southern Thailand: Clinical and laboratory correlations. Am J Trop Med Hyg 35:1235–1247, 1986.

44. Hatton MWC: Studies on the coagulant enzyme from *Agkistrodon rhodostoma* venom: Isolation and some properties of the enzyme. Biochem J 131:799, 1973.

45. Lollar P, Parker CG, Kajenski PJ, et al: Degradation of coagulation proteins by an enzyme from Malayan pit viper (*Agkistrodon rhodostoma*) venom. Biochemisty 26:7627, 1987.

46. Huang TF, Chang JH, Oyang C: Characterization of hemorrhagic principles from *Trimeresurus gramineus* venom. Toxicon 22:45–52, 1984.

47. Kawamura Y, Sawai Y, Jiang K: Comparative potency of antivenoms against Japanese and Chinese mamushi venoms. Snake 17:82–83, 1985.

48. Sawai Y, Kawamura Y, Yoriba M, et al: An epidemiologic study of snakebites in Guangxi Zhuang autonomous region, China in 1990. Snake 24:1–15, 1992.

49. Nikai T, Niikawa M, Komori Y, et al: Proof of proteolytic activity of hemorrhagic toxins, HR-2a and HR-2b, from *Trimeresurus flavoviridis* venom. Int J Biochem 19:221–226, 1979.

50. Nikai T, Mori N, Kishida M, et al: Isolation and characterization of hemorrhagic factors a and b from the venom of the Chinese habu snake (*Trimeresurus mucrosquamatus*). Biochim Biophys Acta 838:122–131, 1985.

51. Kishida, M, Nikai T, Mori N, et al: Characterization of Mucrotoxin A from the venom of *Trimeresurus mucrosquamatus* (the Chinese habu snake). Toxicon 23:637–645, 1985.

52. Tu AT: Local tissue damaging (hemorrhage and myonecrosis) toxins from rattlesnake and other pit viper venoms. J Toxicol Toxin Rev 2:205–234, 1983.

53. Mebs D, Samejima Y: Isolation and characterization of myotoxic phospholipase A2 from crotalid venoms. Toxicon 24:161–168, 1986.

54. Oyama E, Hidenobu T: Purification and characterization of thrombin-like enzyme, elegaxobin, from the venom of *Trimeresurus elegans* (Sakishima-habu). Toxicon 38:1087–1100, 2000.

55. Nikai T, Kato S, Komori H: Amino acid sequence and biological properties of the lectin from the venom of *Trimeresurus okinavensis* (Himehabu). Toxicon 38:707–711, 2000.

56. Hutton RA, Looareesuwan S, Ho M, et al: Arboreal green pit vipers (genus *Trimeresurus*) of southeast Asia: Bites by *T. albolabris* and *T. macropis* in Thailand and a review of the literature. Trans R Soc Trop Med Hyg 84:866–874, 1990.

57. Andeson DC, Paterson SM: Uncoupling of cholinergic synaptic vesicles by the presynaptic toxin β-bungarotoxin. J Neurochem 47:1305–1311, 1986.

58. Lin-Zhen-Yao, Ou-ming: The cure of a patient with respiratory paralysis for thirty days after *Bungarus multicinctus* bite. New Traditional Chin Med 4:24–28, 1976.

59. Pochanugool C, Limthongkul S, Meemano K: Clinical features of 37 non-antivenin treated neurotoxic snakebite patients. In Gopalakrishnakone P, Tan CK (eds): Progress in Venom and Toxin Research. Faulty of Medicine, National University Singapore, 1987, pp 46–57.

60. Reid HA: Cobra bites. BMJ 2:540–545, 1964.

61. Hogue-Angeletti RA, Bradshaw RA: Nerve growth factors in snake venoms. In Lee CY (ed): Snake Venoms. Berlin, Springer, 1979, pp 276–294.

62. Vogt W: Snake venom constituents affecting the complement system. In Stocker K (ed): Medical Use of Snake Venom Proteins. Boca Raton, FL, CRC Press, 1990, pp 79–96.

63. Vogel CW: Cobra venom factor: The complement-activating protein of cobra venom. In Tu AT (ed): Handbook of Natural Toxins, Vol 5. New York, Marcel Dekker, 1991, p 147.

64. Teng CM, Jy W, Ouyang G: Cardiotoxin from *Naja naja atra* venom: A potentiator of platelet aggregation. Toxicon 22:463–470, 1984.

65. Sawai Y, Honma M, Huja ML, Singh G: Snake bites in India. Indian J Med Res 42:661–686, 1954.

66. Reid HA: Cobra bites. BMJ 2:540–545, 1964.

67. Trishnananda M, Oonsombat P, Dumavibhat B, et al: Clinical manifestations of cobra bite in the Thai farmer. Am J Trop Med Hyg 28:165–166, 1979.

68. Mitrakul C, Dhamkrong AT, Futrakulp P, et al: Clinical features of neurotoxic snakebite and response to antivenom in 47 children. Am J Trop Med Hyg 33:1258–1266, 1984.

69. Warrell DA, Ormerond LD: Snake venom ophthalmia and blindness caused by the spitting cobra (*Naja nigricollis*) in Nigeria. Am J Trop Med Hyg 25:525–529, 1976.

70. Welch KRG: Snakes of the Orient: A Checklist. Malabar, FL, Robert E. Krieger Publishing Co, 1988.

71. Gomes A, Palabi D, Dasgupta SC: Occurrence of a unique protein toxin from the Indian king cobra (*Ophiophagus hannah*) venom. Toxicon 39:363–370, 2001.

72. Tin-Myint, Rai-Mra, Maung-Chit, et al: Bites by the king cobra (*Ophiophagus hannah*) in Myanmar: Successful treatment of severe neurotoxic envenoming. Q J Med 80:751–762, 1991.

73. De Silva A: Snakebites in Anuradhapura District. Snake 13:117–130, 1981.

74. Ahuja ML, Singh G: Snake bite in India. Indian J Med Res 42:661–668, 1954.

75. Theakston RDG, Phillips RE, Warrell DA, et al: Envenoming by the common krait (*Bungarus caeruleus*) and Sri Lankan cobra (*Naja naja naja*) efficacy and complications of therapy with Haffkine antivenom. Trans R Soc Trop Med Hyg 84:301–308, 1990.

76. Hill RE, Mackessy SP: Characterization of venom (Duvernoy's secretion) from twelve species of colubrid snakes and partial sequence of four venom proteins. Toxicon 38:1663–1687, 2000.

77. Mittleman MB, Goris RC: Death caused by the bite of the Japanese Colubrid snake *Rhabdophis tigrinus* (Boie) (Reptilia, Serpentes, Colubridae). J Herpetol 12:109–111, 1978.

78. Ogawa H, Sawai Y: Fatal bite of the yamakagashi (*Rhabdophis tigrinus*). Snake 18:53–54, 1986.

79. Smeets REH, Melman PG, Foffmann JJML, Mulder AW: Case report: Severe coagulopathy after a bite from a "harmless" snake (*Rhabdophis subminiatus*). J Intern Med 230:351–354, 1991.

80. De Silva A, Aloysius DJ: Moderately and mildly venomous snakes of Sri Lanka. Ceylon Med J 28:118–127, 1983.

81. Russell FE: Another warning about electrical shock for snakebite (Letter). Postgrad Med 82:32–33, 1987.

82. De Silva A, Mendis S, Warrell DA: Neurotoxic envenoming by the Sri Lankan krait (*Bungarus ceylonicus*) complicated by traditional treatment and a reaction to antivenom. Trans R Soc Trop Med Hyg 87:682–684, 1993.

83. Warrell DA: Treatment of snakebite in the Asia-Pacific region: A personal view. In Gopalakrishnakone P, Chou LM (eds): Snakes of Medical Importance (Asia-Pacific Region). Singapore, Singapore University Press, 1990, pp 641–670.

84. Callahan MV: Challenging paradigms is risky business: C.C. Snyder's A Definitive Treatment of Snakebite. Wild Environ Med 12:273–275, 2001.

85. Bush SP, Hegewald KG, Green SM, et al: Effects of a negative pressure venom extraction device (Extractor) on local tissue injury after artificial envenomation in a porcine model. Wild Environ Med 11:180–188, 2000.

86. Sutherland SK, Coulter AR, Harris RD: Rationalisation of first-aid measures for elapid snakebite. Lancet 1:183–186, 1979.

87. Currie B: Pressure-immobilization first aid for snakebite—fact and fancy. Abstracts of XIII International Congress for Tropical Medicine and Malaria, Jomtien, Pattaya, Thailand 29 Nov–4 Dec 1992. Toxicon 31:931–932, 1993.

88. Blaylock RS, Lichtman AR, Potgieter PD: Clinical manifestations of Cape cobra (*Naja nivea*) bites: Two cases. S Afr Med J 68:342–344, 1985.

89. Suntrarachun S, Pakmanee N, Tirawatnapong T, et al: Development of a polymerase chain reaction to distinguish moncellate cobra (*Naja kaouthia*) bites from other common Thai snake species using both venom extracts and bite-site swabs. Toxicon 39:1087–1090, 2001.

90. Silamut K, Ho M, Looareesuwan D, et al: Detection of venom by enzyme linked immunosorbent assay (ELISA) in patients bitten by snakes in Thailand. BMJ 294:402–404, 1987.

91. Neirmain HS, Herman ML: Toxic effects of colloids in the intensive care unit. Crit Care Clin 7:713–723, 1991.

92. Vassar MJ, Fischer RP, O'Brian PE, et al: A multi-center trial for resuscitation of injured patients with 7.5% sodium chloride. Arch Surg 128:1003–1013, 1993.

93. Hill RE, Bogdan GM, Dart RC: Time to reconstitution: Purified Fab antivenom vs. unpurified IgG antivenom. Toxicon 39:729–731, 2001.

94. Seth AK, Varma PP, Paketra R: Randomised control trial on the effective dose of anti-snake venom in cases of snake bite with systemic envenomation. J Assoc Physicians India 48:756, 2000.

95. Chen JC, Bullard MJ, Chiu TF, et al: Risk of immediate effects from F(ab)2 bivalent antivenin in Taiwan. Wilderness Environ Med 11:163–167, 2000.

96. Watt G, Theakston RDG, Hayes CG, et al: Positive response to edrophonium in patients with neurotoxic envenoming by cobra (*Naja naja philippinensis*): A placebo-controlled study. N Engl J Med 315:1444–1448, 1986.

97. Watt G, Meade BD, Theakston RDG, et al: Comparison of Tensilon and antivenom for the treatment of cobra-bite paralysis. Trans R Soc Trop Med Hyg 83:570–573, 1989.

98. Sethi PK, Rastogi JK: Neurological aspects of ophitoxemia (India krait)—a clinico-electromyographic study. Indian J Med Res 73:269–276, 1981.

99. Warrell DA, Looareesuwan S, White NJ, et al: Severe neurotoxic envenoming by the Malayan krait *Bungarus candidus* (Linnaeus): Response to antivenom and anticholinesterase. BMJ 286:678–680, 1983.

100. Seneviratne SL, Opanayaka CJ, Ratnayake NS, et al: Use of antivenin serum in snakebite: A prospective study of hospital practice in the Gampaha district. Ceylon Med J 45:65–68, 2000.

101. Upadhyaya AC, Murhty GL, Sahay RK, et al: Snakebite presenting as acute myocardial infarction, ischaemic cerebral vascular accident, acute renal failure and disseminated intravascular coagulopathy. J. Assoc Physicians India 48:1109–1110, 2000.

CHAPTER 107

Kraits

Charles Lee ■ Richard Y. Wang

Kraits are highly venomous snakes of the genus *Bungarus*. Inhabiting Southeast Asia, southern China, Indonesia, and the Indian subcontinent, they feed primarily on lizards and other snakes. Although they are not considered aggressive snakes, and the reported incidence of bites is relatively low, the 13 krait species all should be considered capable of delivering a potentially lethal envenomation. Human envenomations can involve any part of the body because kraits often enter homes and encounter sleeping humans, who inadvertently may roll onto them. In general, kraits can be found at altitudes ranging from sea level to 1600 m above, and they often inhabit lowland forest terrain.

Bungarus caeruleus, also called the *common Indian krait*, is a relatively uncommon cause of envenomation in India, Pakistan, Bangladesh, Nepal, and Sri Lanka. With mortality rates for envenoming untreated with antivenom of 77% to 100%,[1,2] *B. caeruleus* is considered one of the most dangerous snakes in the Indian subcontinent. *Bungarus multicinctus*, the *Chinese* or *many-banded krait*, is native to mainland China and Taiwan and accounts for roughly 8% of all snakebites in this region. Mortality rates were 10% and 23% in two case series.[3,4] *Bungarus candidus*, also called the *Malayan krait*, can be found throughout Southeast Asia and has been reported to be one of the most common causes of snakebite mortality in Thailand. In a case series of five patients bitten by this snake, only one patient died, and two patients never developed any signs or symptoms of envenomation.[5] *Bungarus fasciatus*, also known as the *Asian banded krait* (see Fig. 101-16), is another uncommon but significant cause of snake envenomation in China. One study reported a 7.7% mortality rate,[3] whereas another study reported two of four bitten patients dying from systemic envenomation.[6]

TAXONOMY

Kraits are snakes of the genus *Bungarus*, a subdivision of the Elapidae family that also includes cobras and coral snakes (Fig. 107-1). Thirteen species of this genus exist, although there are reported bites in humans by only seven of these, whose physical characteristics are described subsequently. In general, they tend to be slender snakes, and similar to other elapids, they have relatively short fangs mounted on the anterior maxilla.

B. caeruleus is a dark-colored snake with a white belly that grows to a maximum length of 1.5 m. The ventral portion of the snake is black, brown, or blue-black and is tra-

versed by thin, paired, white bands. *B. multicinctus* can grow to 1.84 m in length and is similar in appearance to *B. caeruleus*, with the exception of its bands, which are not paired. *B. candidus* has broad sections of black or brownish black alternating with thick bands of yellow or white. The belly also is white, and the maximum length is 1.6 m. *B. fasciatus* can exceed 2 m in length and has broad, alternating bands of black and yellow that encircle the entire circumference of the snake. *Bungarus ceylonicus*, also called the *Sri Lankan krait*, measures 1.35 m in length. It is a black snake encircled with white rings. *Bungarus flaviceps*, also called the *red-headed krait*, inhabits Southeast Asia and grows to 1.6 m. It is a dark blue-black snake that may have blue-white stripes running down the sides and is distinguished by a bright red head and tail. Finally, *Bungarus javanicus*, the *Javan krait*, is a blue-black snake with a light belly. White specks dot the vertebral scales, and the snake can grow to 860 mm. The six or so remaining krait species have not been reported to cause human envenomation, although they still should be handled with extreme caution.

BIOCHEMISTRY AND CLINICAL PHARMACOLOGY OF THE VENOMS

Krait venoms comprise a complex mixture of proteins, the most significant of which are the toxins that mediate neuromuscular junctional blockade. The most thoroughly characterized presynaptic neurotoxin is the β-bungarotoxin, isolated from *B. multicinctus*. This 21.8-kd basic protein consists of an α-chain and a β-chain linked by a disulfide bond. In in vitro studies, β-bungarotoxin has been found to effect a triphasic change in the presynaptic membrane of the neuromuscular junction. The first two phases, transient twitch inhibition followed by a prolonged facilitative phase, are mediated by the β-chain and may involve blockade of voltage-gated potassium channels.[7,8] The third phase consists of a blocking phase and is caused by α-chain–mediated phospholipase A_2 activity, which presumably destroys presynaptic phospholipid membranes.[7] The end result of β-bungarotoxin's presynaptic action is reduction in acetylcholine release into the synaptic cleft of the neuromuscular junction.

Many other toxins have been isolated from kraits, including neurotoxins with postsynaptic activity.[9,10] α-Bungarotoxin prevents acetylcholine from binding to the α-subunit of nicotinic acetylcholine receptors at the neuromuscular junction, causing a nondepolarizing neuromuscular blockade. Nicotinic receptors in the central nervous system contain

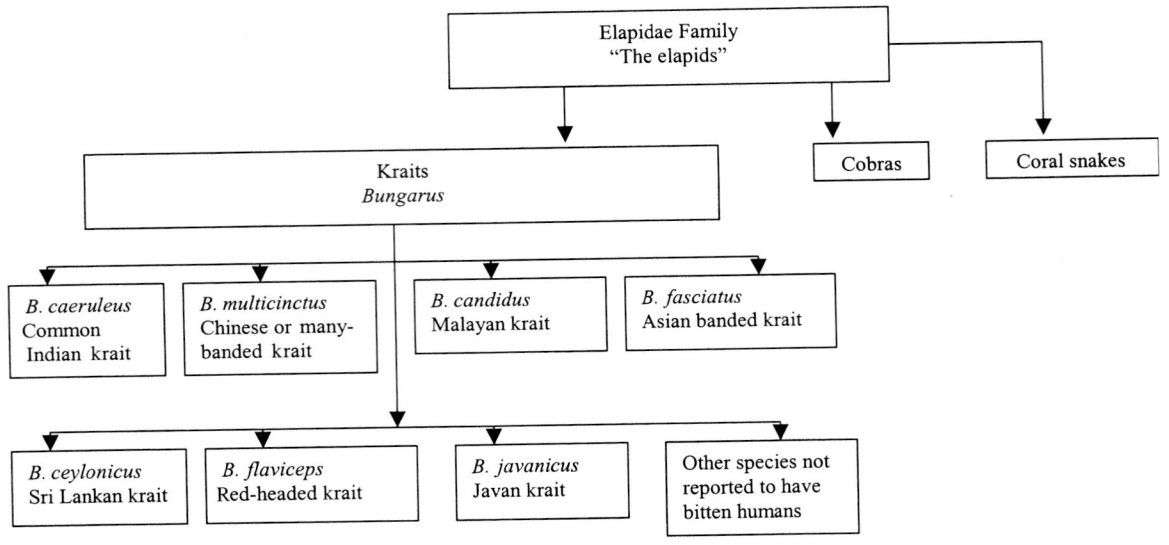

FIGURE 107-1

Simplified taxonomy of venomous snakes of the elapidae family, with emphasis on kraits reported to have envenomed humans.

different α-subunits and are not affected by α-bungarotoxin. Ceruleotoxin, which was so named because it mistakenly was thought to originate from *B. caeruleus*, affects postsynaptic neuromuscular blockade without interfering with acetylcholine binding. This dimeric protein isolated from *B. fasciatus* venom has a molecular weight of 26,000 kd and has potent phospholipase-A$_2$ activity. By hydrolyzing lipids in the postsynaptic membrane, it stabilizes the acetylcholine receptor–ionophore complex and inhibits acetylcholine release.[11] Four κ-bungarotoxins have been found; they primarily bind the subset of nicotinic acetylcholine receptors found in neuronal junctions, with markedly decreased affinity for muscular nicotinic receptors.[12] γ-Bungarotoxin, isolated from the venom of *B. multicinctus*, has been sequenced, but its pharmacology has not yet been elaborated fully.[13]

Cardiotoxins similar to those found in Asian cobra venoms also have been isolated from *B. multicinctus* and *B. fasciatus*. These toxins have been shown to cause erythrocyte hemolysis and myocardial depression in in vitro models.[14–16] The venoms of other krait species have not been as well characterized, although they have similar pathophysiologic effects and presumably contain highly homologous neurotoxins. The median lethal doses of the venoms from the various krait species are presented in Table 107-1.

PATHOPHYSIOLOGY

After snakebite, venom quickly spreads throughout the body, is carried away from the wound by the lymphatics, and then is circulated by the bloodstream.[17] As described earlier, toxin interactions with the neuromuscular junction can result in presynaptic and postsynaptic neuromuscular blockade, causing flaccid paralysis. This mechanism is consistent with neurophysiologic studies of patients envenomed by *B. caeruleus*, which have shown decreased compound muscle action potential amplitudes and decremental motor responses to repetitive nerve stimulation, with preserved distal motor latency and nerve conduction velocity. Sensation is not affected, consistent with the finding that sensory nerve action potential amplitudes and latencies remained unchanged.[18] When the venom has reached sufficient concentrations in the muscles, typically within hours of envenomation, flaccid paralysis and respiratory failure ensue. Central nervous system side effects are minimal or absent, primarily due to the fact that the major fraction of krait venom consists of toxins that exclusively bind muscular nicotinic receptors. Enzyme-linked immunosorbent assay studies in one autopsy series showed that venom concentrations in the brain tend to be about ninefold less than those

SPECIES *(BUNGARUS)*	SUBCUTANEOUS	INTRAVENOUS	INTRAPERITONEAL	VENOM YIELD
B. caeruleus	0.365	0.169	0.089	8–20 mg
B. fasciatus	3.6	1.289	1.55	20–114 mg
B. multicinctus	0.108	0.113	0.08	

TABLE 107-1 Median Lethal Doses of Various Krait Venoms in Mice (mg/kg)

Adapted from www.kingsnake.com/toxicology/LD50/LD50mrn.html, accessed Dec. 2002; and Sprawls S, Branch B: Dangerous Snakes of Africa. Sanibel, FL, R. Curtis, 1996.

present at the bite area.[19] Despite the presence of cardiotoxins in krait venoms, cardiotoxicity and hemodynamic instability typically do not occur.

CLINICAL PRESENTATION

Most cases of reported krait envenomation occur at night, while the victims are sleeping on the floor. Krait bites usually are only mildly painful and often leave little evidence of skin puncture, consisting of small, possibly multiple paired fang marks. Initially, patients usually complain of only mild local effects, which may or may not include tenderness, swelling, and erythema, although some patients develop more diffuse myalgias and abdominal pain. Numbness of the bitten extremity also has been reported. Severe localized pain and extensive tissue necrosis should prompt the clinician to consider envenomation by a different snake.[20]

The severe systemic effects of krait envenomation are mediated by the presynaptic and postsynaptic neuromuscular toxins, and generalized paresis usually starts within the first 1 to 3 hours after the bite.[20] Delays of 12 hours have been reported, however, before the onset of paralytic symptoms.[2,21,22] Conversely, direct intravenous envenomation theoretically could reduce the time to onset of action of the venom. Decreased visual acuity and oculomotor palsies are early signs of systemic toxicity and usually are followed by inability to open the jaw, masticate, or swallow. The gag reflex also may be lost. Progressive weakness of the extremities and dyspnea are hallmarks of more serious envenomation, with the most severe cases proceeding to total flaccid paralysis and respiratory failure necessitating mechanical ventilation.[20] Although transient hypotension can be seen, prolonged hemodynamic instability that does not respond to fluid resuscitation should prompt consideration of envenomation by a nonkrait snake.

Paralysis usually lasts for only a few days, although prolonged weakness may result, with one report of a patient requiring artificial ventilation for 30 days.[23] This long-term weakness probably is not due to lingering concentrations of neurotoxins. Rather, one study showed long-term depletion of presynaptic vesicles and damage to skeletal muscle motor nerve terminals and intramuscular axonal structures as a result of in vitro β-bungarotoxin administration.[24]

DIAGNOSIS

In a patient who presents with a history of snakebite, exact identification of the snake responsible usually is not possible. The victims and witnesses may not provide accurate or detailed descriptions of the snake, and attempts to kill or capture it are not recommended because a single snake can lethally envenomate several people. Because some patients who are bitten in their sleep may not even be aware of having been bitten until systemic signs and symptoms emerge, any patient who presents with signs and symptoms of neurotoxicity in areas where kraits are endemic should be suspected of having krait envenomation. If the history of snakebite has not been established firmly, the clinician also must include Guillain-Barré syndrome, botulism, and myasthenia gravis in the differential diagnosis.

In any patient bitten by a snake whose identity has not been established firmly, routine studies should include measurements of electrolytes, renal function, blood type and screen, complete blood count, coagulation parameters including fibrinogen, creatine phosphokinase, urinalysis, urine myoglobin, and 12-lead electrocardiography. In patients bitten by kraits, serum creatine phosphokinase and myoglobin levels may be mildly elevated, indicating rhabdomyolysis.[20] Leukocytosis with a neutrophilic predominance is also seen routinely.[2] Markedly abnormal indices of renal function or coagulation should prompt the suspicion of envenomation by another type of snake. Arterial blood gas measurements are essential in patients with respiratory distress to assess for hypoventilation, and any degree of hypercarbia should prompt intubation and mechanical ventilation, if available. Accurate enzyme immunoassays, although useful for diagnosis of krait bite in clinical investigations, are not commercially available in Asia.

TREATMENT

General Principles

Popular first-aid measures, such as suctioning, incision, local cryotherapy, cauterization, electric shocks, and local injection of potassium permanganate, are controversial at best and should not be administered.[25] Likewise, arterial tourniquets have not been shown to be safe and effective in humans and should not be applied. In cases in which the offending snake has not been identified, tourniquets may prove harmful. Because the venoms of many snakes where kraits are endemic have potent cytotoxic activity, application of a tourniquet may concentrate these venoms in the affected limb while limiting blood flow, increasing local tissue necrosis and the potential for limb loss.

Several effective antivenoms are available throughout the regions where kraits are endemic, and they have been shown to reverse neurotoxicity partially and to slow or stop the progression of paralysis. The clinician should not rely on antivenom, however, because its efficacy can be variable. Proper supportive therapy is crucial in patients with paralysis and respiratory compromise, with special attention being paid to airway and respiratory status.

Airway and Ventilatory Considerations

Because of the patient's risk of developing respiratory failure, the patient's airway and oxygenation must be monitored closely. The earliest manifestations of systemic neurotoxicity consist of cranial nerve palsies and subsequent dysphagia and loss of gag reflex, which also may be accompanied by

Indications for ICU Admission in Krait Envenomation

Respiratory depression or inability to protect the airway
Progressive signs of neurotoxicity or muscular weakness
Severe reaction to antivenom

difficulty in managing oral secretions.[20] Any patient who displays these signs should not receive any oral food or liquids and may require an oral airway if he or she cannot open the mouth. A patient who cannot protect the airway or who shows progressive hypoventilation should be orotracheally intubated and adequately suctioned. Although krait bites rarely cause anaphylactic reactions with airway compromise, the incidence of allergic reactions associated with antivenom administration has been reported to be 43% to 65% in various studies.[20,26] Any patient who is to receive antivenom should be viewed as a potential candidate to develop bronchospasm or laryngospasm, and this contingency should be planned for accordingly.

Patients who develop respiratory failure due to krait envenomation should be ventilated just as any other patient with neuromuscular blockade. Patients with mild respiratory compromise may be maintained adequately and comfortably on support modes of ventilation, whereas patients with complete respiratory failure may require controlled modes. Respiratory paralysis typically takes one to several days to begin to resolve.[20]

Nonantidotal Treatments

Immediately after a suspected envenomation, the patient should be brought to the nearest health care facility even if he or she is asymptomatic because toxic effects may begin one to several hours after envenomation.[5,27,28] The patient also should be instructed to remain as relaxed as possible because muscular contraction of the affected limb is likely to hasten lymphatic and venous spread of the venom. All rings, bracelets, and watches should be removed from the affected limb because these items may prove harmful if local swelling occurs. The bitten limb should be splinted and maintained below the level of the heart, and the patient should be transported immediately to a medical facility, preferably one that has critical care capabilities. As a temporizing measure, a crepe bandage may be wrapped around the entire bitten extremity, starting distal to the site of the bite. The pressure of the wrap should be approximately 55 mm Hg, or roughly the pressure achieved with a bandage applied for a ligament sprain. In animal models, this has been shown to retard venom absorption, presumably by hindering lymphatic drainage.[29] This is only a compressive wrap, not a tourniquet.

Immediately on arrival, the patient's airway and vital signs should be assessed, and reliable intravenous access should be established, preferably in a limb other than the one bitten. Removal of pressure dressings or tourniquets applied in the field may cause a surge of circulating venom and should be attempted only when the patient has been assessed neurologically and intravenous access has been obtained. Asymptomatic patients who may have been bitten by a krait must be monitored closely for signs and symptoms of systemic paresis for at least 24 hours from the time of the bite. Serial neurologic examinations should be performed throughout the hospitalization and should be done at least hourly throughout the first several hours of presentation. In patients who already have developed signs and symptoms of neurotoxicity, dressings should not be removed until the appropriate antivenom has been administered. The crepe dressing should be replaced if the patient's condition worsens during the dressing's removal. Patients who develop severe neurotoxicity and who do not already have a pressure dressing may have one placed at any time because this theoretically impedes absorption of residual venom at the injection site.

When the dressings have been removed, the bite wound can be wiped with a wet cloth to remove any venom that may be lingering on the skin, although vigorous manipulation of the wound and extremity should be avoided to minimize venom circulation. Most methods of decreasing systemic venom absorption have not proved effective, and the emphasis should be on close monitoring of the patient with prompt treatment of systemic effects. Antibiotics for prophylaxis against skin and soft tissue infection often are not needed, and we do not recommend their routine administration. As with any puncture wound, tetanus prophylaxis should be administered if indicated by the patient's immunization history.

There are reports of subjective and objective improvement of neurotoxic signs and symptoms in patients treated with anticholinesterase therapy, although with variable responses.[5,20,27,28] All patients with suspected neurotoxicity should undergo edrophonium testing, which consists of the intravenous administration of 10 mg of edrophonium for adults (0.25 mg/kg for children). A positive test consists of an immediate objective increase in muscular strength and should prompt the initiation of intravenous anticholinesterase therapy with neostigmine (0.5 mg/hr as a starting dose for adults) by continuous intravenous infusion. The muscarinic cholinergic side effects of neostigmine, such as hypersecretion and bradycardia, can be controlled with a continuous intravenous infusion of atropine (0.5 mg/hr to start and titrate to response).

Severely poisoned patients who require intubation and mechanical ventilation are at increased risk for development of gastric stress ulcer and may benefit from the administration of H_2 receptor antagonist (e.g., famotidine). Paralyzed patients also are at increased risk for deep venous thrombosis and should be treated accordingly. Sequential compression devices should not be used on the bitten limb, however, because they may aid lymphatic and venous drainage of the extremity and theoretically could mobilize the venom, resulting in increased circulating venom concentrations.

Antivenom

Aside from supportive therapy, the mainstay of treatment for a patient who develops any signs and symptoms of neurotoxicity is intravenous antivenom, which works by neutralizing circulating neurotoxins but probably has little effect on toxins that already have adhered to specific cellular binding sites, including acetylcholine receptors. Several antivenoms have been manufactured (Table 107-2), and their use is subject to differences in regional availability. Krait antivenoms are produced by isolating the hyperimmune sera from horses that have been immunized with the venom of one (monovalent antiserum) or several (polyvalent antiserum) species of snakes. When the exact identity of the offending snake is under question, polyvalent antiserum should be used. The venom-neutralizing properties of some krait antivenoms have been shown to be genus specific,[30] so that immune

TABLE 107-2 Antisera Effective Against Krait Venom

PRODUCER	VALENCY	SNAKE SPECIES
Central Research Institute, Kasauli, India	Polyvalent	*Naja naja, Bungarus caeruleus, Vipera russelli, Echis carinatus, Ophiophagus hannah, Bungarus fasciatus, Calliophis* spp., *Trimeresurus* spp., *Agkistrodon* spp.
Central Research Institute, Kasauli, India	Monovalent	*B. caeruleus, B. fasciatus, Calliophis* spp. (probably)
Haffkine Biopharmaceutical Co Ltd, Bombay, India	Polyvalent	*N. naja, B. caeruleus, V. russelli, E. carinatus, Trimeresurus* spp.
Haffkine Biopharmaceutical Co Ltd, Bombay, India	Monovalent	*B. caeruleus*
Serum Institute of India Ltd, Pune, India	Polyvalent	*N. naja, B. caeruleus, V. russelli, E. carinatus, B. fasciatus, Bungarus ceylonicus, O. hannah, Trimeresurus* spp.
National Institute of Health, Biological Production Division, Islamabad, Pakistan	Polyvalent	*N. naja* subspp., *Bungarus* spp., *V. russelli, E. carinatus, B. fasciatus, Vipera lebetina*
National Institute of Health, Biological Production Division, Islamabad, Pakistan	Monovalent	*Bungarus* spp., *B. fasciatus*
Thai Red Cross Society, Bangkok, Thailand	Monovalent	*B. fasciatus*
Pasteur Institute, Bandung, Indonesia	Monovalent	*B. fasciatus*
National Institute of Preventative Medicine, Taipei, Taiwan	Monovalent	*B. fasciatus*
Commonwealth Serum Laboratory (Tiger Snake Antivenom), Parkville, Australia	Polyvalent	*Notechis scutatus, Austrelaps superba, Austrelaps ramsayi,* genus *Pseudechis* except *P. australis* and *Hoplocephalus*

Adapted from Theakston P, Warrell DA: Antivenoms: A list of hyperimmune sera currently available for the treatment of envenomation by bites and stings. Toxicon 29:1419–1470, 1991.

serum directed against the venom of one particular krait species may be effective against the venoms of other krait species to varying degrees. The potency and purity of various antisera vary widely, and large differences can be detected among different lots of the same antivenom. Consequently, the dosages provided should be used as a guideline, with the total dose of antivenom determined by the clinical scenario.

Although it is the specific IgG fraction of hyperimmune serum that neutralizes snake toxins, current antivenoms are relatively impure and contain varying proportions of allergenic nonimmune globulin proteins.[31] Consequently, the rate of allergic reactions to antivenom is 65% and may be higher in patients with a history of atopy, previous administration of antiserum, or previous reaction to antiserum. These risk factors for allergic reaction and factors reflecting increased risk for complications, such as β-blocker use and underlying reactive airway disorder, are strong relative contraindications to antivenom treatment.

Early reactions occur within minutes of treatment and usually are caused by immune complex–mediated complement activation, although rare cases of immediate IgE-mediated (type I) hypersensitivity reactions occur. Precautionary measures including bedside preparation for hypersensitivity reactions should be taken before antivenom administration. Early reactions are characterized by pruritus, urticaria, fever, and nausea, although more than 5% of these reactions may progress to a typical anaphylactic or anaphylactoid syndrome (laryngobronchial constriction and circulatory collapse). Patients with these reactions should be treated with 0.3 mL of 0.1% epinephrine injected subcutaneously or administered as a continuous intravenous infusion at 2 to 4 μg/min (or 1 mg of epinephrine in 250 mL of 5% dextrose at 30 to 60 μL/hr) and antihistamine therapy (e.g., diphenhydramine or hydroxyzine, 50 mg intravenously, and cimetidine, 300 mg intravenously).[32] For severe reactions, copious

intravenous fluid resuscitation and further pressor therapy may be needed. Corticosteroids may be useful in controlling persistent symptoms, and methylprednisolone, 125 mg intravenously, or an equivalent can be given. We recommend that drugs used in the treatment of early reactions to antivenom be readily available at the patient's bedside.

One study showed the effectiveness of low-dose subcutaneous epinephrine in preventing early allergic reactions, with a reduction in all severities of reactions from 43% in the placebo-treated group to 11% in the group pretreated with 0.25 mg of 1:1000 epinephrine injected subcutaneously. This study excluded patients with contraindications to epinephrine and patients who had received antisera in the past or had a history of atopy.[26] Patients who do not have relative contraindications (e.g., ischemic heart disease, hypertension, or arrhythmia) may benefit from pretreatment with epinephrine; however, this is controversial. Skin sensitivity testing is neither sensitive nor specific in determining which patients will develop severe early reactions to antivenom and should not be performed.[32]

Pyrogen contamination of antivenom results in febrile reactions, which typically begin 1 to 2 hours after treatment initiation. Symptomatic relief with antipyretics is all that is needed for these reactions.[32] Serum sickness (type III hypersensitivity) reactions may occur 1 to 3 weeks after antivenom therapy and result in fever, arthralgias, vasculitis, and glomerulonephritis. These reactions typically are self-limited and can be treated with H_1 antagonists (e.g., hydroxyzine) and corticosteroids.[33]

As previously mentioned, any patient who develops signs or symptoms of systemic neurotoxicity should be treated immediately with antivenom. Although some authorities recommend concomitant injection of antivenom into the bite wound, one large retrospective study showed no benefit in this practice.[34] A typical starting dose for mild-to-moderate envenomation consists of 5 vials of polyvalent antivenom

Criteria for ICU Discharge in Krait Envenomation

Respiratory depression or inability to protect the airway resolved

Signs of neurotoxicity or muscular weakness stabilized or resolving

No requirement for vasopressor support

serum (Haffkine Laboratories, Mumbai, India) mixed in 500 mL of 0.9% normal saline solution administered over 30 to 60 minutes, beginning with a slow infusion rate (10 to 20 mL/hr) and gradually increasing over 10 to 20 minutes to a rate of 150 to 200 mL/hr. For moderate-to-severe envenomations, 10 to 20 vials of the polyvalent antivenom serum will be needed. The infusion should be paused in patients who develop early reactions to antivenom and can be restarted cautiously at a lower rate after the patient has been treated and stabilized. In any patient who develops a severe anaphylactic or anaphylactoid reaction to antivenom, the clinician must use his or her best judgment to determine whether the benefits of potential toxin reversal outweigh the risks of circulatory collapse. In facilities where modern mechanical ventilation is available, a severely envenomed patient who does not receive antivenom may be treated with supportive therapy alone.

If subjective or objective clinical improvement is not evident after a typical starting dose of antivenom, administration of additional antivenom should be considered, with some reported cases requiring several hundred milliliters of antiserum. The principle underlying this practice is the fact that antivenom does not work enzymatically, but rather inactivates circulating neurotoxins in a stoichiometric fashion. Large venom loads may require multiple administrations to neutralize the toxins, which are circulating systemically and concentrated at the bite wound.

SPECIAL POPULATIONS

Pediatric Patients

Aside from pediatric dosing of nonantidotal therapies, there are no special considerations for treating pediatric patients. The dosage and frequency of antivenom administered for neurotoxic reversal should be the same as those in adult patients. The pediatric dose of epinephrine for immediate-type hypersensitivity reactions to antivenom is 0.1 to 1.0 μg/kg/min by continuous intravenous infusion.

Pregnant Patients

There are few data regarding snakebite in pregnancy and no published data on the effects of krait envenomation in pregnancy. There have been case reports, however, of fetal hypoxia, encephalomalacia, and intrauterine demise resulting from episodes of anaphylaxis during pregnancy.[35-37] Because there is such a high incidence of anaphylactic or anaphylactoid reactions with antivenom administration, we recommend

that the use of antivenom in pregnancy probably should be reserved for cases of severe envenomation when mechanical ventilatory support is not available and the degree of maternal respiratory distress outweighs the risks of possible anaphylaxis. If anaphylaxis does occur, epinephrine remains the treatment of choice, although in prolonged hypotension, ephedrine may be preferred because its greater β-adrenergic activity theoretically leads to less uterine vasoconstriction.[38] Glucocorticoids and diphenhydramine may be administered safely, and fetal monitoring should be performed routinely.

Common Errors in Krait Envenomation

Suctioning or incising the bite wound
Applying arterial tourniquets
Relying on antivenom to reverse neurotoxicity
Thinking that skin testing can reliably determine who will develop a severe reaction to antivenom
Believing that asymptomatic patients can be discharged after a few hours of observation

Key Points in Krait Envenomation

1. Good respiratory and airway support is the mainstay of therapy.
2. All patients with signs of neurotoxicity or muscle weakness should be considered candidates for antivenom therapy.
3. If the identity of the snake is in doubt, polyvalent antivenom must be used.
4. The incidence of hypersensitivity reactions to antivenom is high; precautionary measures should be taken before antivenom treatment is initiated.
5. Relative contraindications to antivenom administration include previous antivenom treatment, history of allergy to horse serum, asthma, and recent β-adrenergic receptor antagonist treatments.

REFERENCES

1. De Silva A: Snakebites in Anuradhapura District. Snake 13:117–130, 1981.
2. Ahuja ML, Singh G: Snake bite in India. Indian J Med Res 42:661–686, 1954.
3. Sawai Y, et al: An epidemiological study on the snakebites in Guangxi Zhuang autonomous region, China, in 1990. Snake 24:1–15, 1992.
4. Kuo TP, Wu CS: Clinicopathological studies on snake bites in Taiwan. Snake 4:1–22, 1972.
5. Warrell DA, et al: Severe neurotoxic envenoming by the Malayan krait Bungarus candidus (Linnaeus): Response to antivenom and anticholinesterase. BMJ (Clin Res Ed) 286:678–680, 1983.
6. Buranasin P: Snakebites at Maharat Nakhon Ratchasima Regional Hospital. Southeast Asian J Trop Med Public Health 24:186–192, 1993.
7. Rowan EG: What does beta-bungarotoxin do at the neuromuscular junction? Toxicon 39:107–118, 2001.
8. Benishin CG: Potassium channel blockade by the B subunit of beta-bungarotoxin. Mol Pharmacol 38:164–169, 1990.
9. Kruck TP, Logan DM: Neurotoxins from Bungarus fasciatus venom: A simple fractionation and separation of alpha- and beta-type neurotoxins and their partial characterization. Biochemistry 21:5302–5309, 1982.
10. MacDermot J, Westgaard RH, Thompson EJ: Beta-Bungarotoxin: Separation of two discrete proteins with different synaptic actions. Biochem J 175:271–279, 1978.

11. Bon C, Saliou B: Ceruleotoxin: Identification in the venom of *Bungarus fasciatus*, molecular properties and importance of phospholipase A2 activity for neurotoxicity. Toxicon 21:681–698, 1983.

12. Chiappinelli VA, et al: Binding of native kappa-neurotoxins and site-directed mutants to nicotinic acetylcholine receptors. Toxicon 34:1243–1256, 1996.

13. Aird SD, et al: Primary structure of gamma-bungarotoxin, a new post-synaptic neurotoxin from venom of *Bungarus multicinctus*. Toxicon 37:609–625, 1999.

14. Chang LS, Lin J: cDNA sequence analysis of a novel cardiotoxin-like protein from Taiwan banded krait. Biochem Mol Biol Int 40:1271–1276, 1996.

15. Jiang MS, Fletcher JE, Smith LA: Factors influencing the hemolysis of human erythrocytes by cardiotoxins from *Naja naja kaouthia* and *Naja naja atra* venoms and a phospholipase A2 with cardiotoxin-like activities from *Bungarus fasciatus* venom. Toxicon 27:247–257, 1989.

16. Wu SH, Wang KT, Ho CL: Purification and pharmacological characterization of a cardiotoxin-like protein from Formosan banded krait (*Bungarus multicinctus*) venom. Toxicon 20:753–764, 1982.

17. Russell FE: Snake Venom Poisoning. New York, Schloium International, 1983, p 159.

18. Singh G, et al: Neuromuscular transmission failure due to common krait (*Bungarus caeruleus*) envenomation. Muscle Nerve 22:1637–1643, 1999.

19. Selvanayagam ZE, et al: ELISA for the detection of venoms from four medically important snakes of India. Toxicon 37:757–770, 1999.

20. Theakston RD, et al: Envenoming by the common krait (*Bungarus caeruleus*) and Sri Lankan cobra (*Naja naja naja*): Efficacy and complications of therapy with Haffkine antivenom. Trans R Soc Trop Med Hyg 84:301–308, 1990.

21. Haast WE, Winer ML: Complete and spontaneous recovery from the bite of a blue krait snake (*Bungarus cuerules*). Am J Trop Med Hyg 4:1135, 1955.

22. Sethi PK, Rastogi JK: Neurological aspects of ophitoxemia (Indian krait)—a clinico-electromyographic study. Indian J Med 73:269–276, 1981.

23. Yao LZ, Ming O: The cure of a patient with respiratory paralysis for thirty days after *Bungarus multicinctus* bite. New Traditional Chin Med 4:24–28, 1976.

24. Dixon RW, Harris JB: Nerve terminal damage by beta-bungarotoxin: its clinical significance. Am J Pathol 154:447–455, 1999.

25. Warrell DA: Treatment of snake bite in the Asia-Pacific region: A personal view. In Gopalakrishnakone P, Chou LM (eds): Snakes of Medical Importance (Asia-Pacific Region). Singapore, Singapore University Press, 1990, pp 641–670.

26. Premawardhena AP, et al: Low dose subcutaneous adrenaline to prevent acute adverse reactions to antivenom serum in people bitten by snakes: Randomised, placebo controlled trial. BMJ 318:1041–1043, 1999.

27. Pe T, et al: Envenoming by Chinese krait (*Bungarus multicinctus*) and banded krait (*B. fasciatus*) in Myanmar. Trans R Soc Trop Med Hyg 91:686–688, 1997.

28. Chan JC, et al: Envenoming by *Bungarus multicinctus* (many-banded krait) in Hong Kong. J Trop Med Hyg 98:457–460, 1995.

29. Sutherland SK, Coulter AR, Harris RD: Rationalisation of first-aid measures for elapid snakebite. Lancet 1:183–185, 1979.

30. Chanhome L, et al: Genus specific neutralization of *Bungarus* snake venoms by Thai Red Cross banded krait antivenom. J Nat Toxins 8:135–140, 1999.

31. Sullivan J Jr: Past, present, and future immunotherapy of snake venom poisoning. Ann Emerg Med 16:938–944, 1987.

32. Malasit P, et al: Prediction, prevention and mechanism of early (anaphylactic) antivenom reactions in victims of snake bites. BMJ 292:17–20, 1986.

33. Clark RF, McKinney PE, Chase PB, Walter FG: Immediate and delayed allergic reactions to Crotalidae polyvalent immune Fab (ovine) antivenom. Ann Emerg Med 39:671–676, 2002.

34. Chen JC, et al: Treatment of poisonous snakebites in northern Taiwan. J Formos Med Assoc 99:135–139, 2000.

35. Suri S, Salfield S, Baxter P: Congenital paraplegia following maternal hypotension. Dev Med Child Neurol 41:273–274, 1999.

36. Luciano R, et al: Fetal encephalopathy after maternal anaphylaxis: Case report. Biol Neonate 71:190–193, 1997.

37. Entman SS, Moise KJ: Anaphylaxis in pregnancy. South Med J 77:402, 1984.

38. Konno R, Nagase S: Anaphylactic reaction to cefazolin in pregnancy. J Obstet Gynaecol 21:577–579, 1995.

CHAPTER 108

African Snakes

Gert J. Muller

Although almost 400 snake species occur on the African continent, most are relatively harmless. Most of the venomous species of medical importance are members of the following four families:[1]

- Atractaspididae
- Colubridae
- Elapidae
- Viperidae

Although approximately 100 species are medically important, only 30 are known to have caused death.[1] Table 108-1 summarizes the specific clinical syndromes engendered by the various African snakes.[1-4] The table provides a taxonomic enumeration of significant African snakes and their geographic distribution. The geographic distribution also is shown in Color Figures 108-1 through 108-10. The composite maps have been compiled with reference to the locations published in Spawls and Branch.[1]

The highest incidence of snakebite in Africa occurs in the West African savanna region. In this region, the carpet or saw-scaled vipers (*Echis* spp.), the spitting cobras (*Naja nigricollis* and possibly *Naja katiensis*), and the puff adder (*Bitis arietans*) are commonly involved in serious envenomations.[3] The incidence of snakebite increases in parallel with agricultural activity at the start of the rainy season.[4] In East Africa, most serious bites are attributed to *B. arietans* and *N. nigricollis* and, in a few instances, to mambas.[3] Throughout eastern and southern Africa, *B. arietans* is thought to be responsible for most cases of serious envenomation, followed by the cytotoxic spitting cobras (*Naja mossambica* and *N. nigricollis*). The neurotoxic mambas and Cape cobra (southwestern regions) are responsible for relatively few bites but are associated with high fatality.[2]

Most snakebites occur during daylight hours or shortly after dusk as people walk from the fields. More than 50% of bites by the cytotoxic spitting cobras (*N. nigricollis* and *N. mossambica*) occur at night, however, while the victims are asleep in their dwellings. More than 80% of bites are inflicted on the feet and legs.[3]

CLINICAL PRESENTATION

In broad terms, the venomous snakes may be divided into neurotoxic, cytotoxic, and hemotoxic categories, although there is significant overlap of toxic effects in some snake venoms.[2] The neurotoxic snakes include the mambas and neurotoxic cobras. Some of the minor adders, such as the

berg adder, are cytotoxic and neurotoxic. The cytotoxic group is represented by the major adders (puff adder, Gaboon adder) and the minor adders or vipers, also known as the *dwarf adders* (e.g., night adder, berg adder), and the cytotoxic cobras (various spitting cobras). The hemotoxic snakes include the carpet or saw-scaled vipers, the boomslang, the vine (bird or twig) snake, and a variety of bush vipers.

TREATMENT

The priority in the management of potentially serious envenomation is to get the patient to a medical facility as soon as possible. Time must not be wasted on unnecessary treatment modalities, such as bandaging. The use of a cellular telephone or any other means of communication to alert a medical facility or physician may be lifesaving. Treatment for all snakebites should follow the general principles elaborated in Chapter 101.

There are few controlled studies on African snake envenomations. The recommendations that follow represent generally accepted practices, mostly developed through anecdotal observation. First aid should focus on the maintenance of vital functions, such as support of breathing and circulation. Unnecessary movement should be discouraged. Constricting items, such as rings or clothing distal from or proximal to the bite site, should be removed. Squeezing or incising of the wound or the use of local remedies, such as Condy's crystals and other traditional medicines, should be avoided. Electric shock treatment is of no value. Suction applied over the bite site is probably not of any therapeutic value. Application of a tourniquet may be lifesaving in cases of cobra or mamba bite, especially if the patient is far from medical help. Crepe bandaging is inappropriate in all cases of cytotoxic bites, and its efficacy in neurotoxic bites has not been firmly established.[2]

Antivenom, when indicated, should always be given intravenously (unless otherwise recommended in the antivenom package insert). The absorption of intramuscularly administered antivenom is poor. It should not be injected in or around the wound. Although uncommon, anaphylactoid reactions do occur with horse serum–derived antivenoms. The administration of antivenom in the acute phase of neurotoxic snake envenomation usually does not arrest progression of neurotoxic effects, most notably respiratory paralysis, and consequently the patient cannot survive without life support. Respiratory support is the only treatment modality that is lifesaving in this situation. Intravenous administration of an

TABLE 108-1 Venomous Snakes of Africa

FAMILY AND OTHER CLASSIFICATIONS	GENUS/SPECIES AND SUBSPECIES	COMMON NAME	DISTRIBUTION*	CLINICAL TOXICOLOGY
Atractaspididae		African burrowing snakes or asps (burrowing or mole vipers or adders, side stabbing or stiletto snakes), Natal black snake	Approximately 15 species distributed throughout sub-Saharan Africa. Limited penetration into Israel and Arabian Peninsula.	Most cause local pain, swelling, lymphadenitis only. Blistering, local necrosis described. Life-threatening and fatal cases have been recorded.
	Atractaspis aterrima (? subspecies of *Atractaspis microlepidota*)	Slender burrowing asp	Rain forest and savanna—West Africa to northwest Uganda	Local pain, swelling, lymphadenitis
	Atractaspis bibronii	Southern, Bibron's burrowing asp	Kenya, southern Africa	Local pain, swelling, lymphadenitis, necrosis
	Atractaspis corpulenta	Hallowell's burrowing, fat burrowing asp	Cameroon eastward to northern Zaire	Local pain, swelling, lymphadenitis
	Atractaspis dahomeyensis	Brown, Dahomey burrowing asp	Savanna of West Africa	Local pain, swelling, lymphadenitis
	Atractaspis engaddensis (? subspecies of *Atractaspis microlepidota*)	Ein Geddi, Israeli burrowing asp	Desert areas of Egypt	Life-threatening and fatal cases recorded. Dyspnea, respiratory failure, ECG abnormalities, collapse.
	Atractaspis irregularis	Variable, Reinhardt's burrowing asp	Forest regions of West and East Africa	Life-threatening and fatal cases recorded. See *A. engaddensis.*
	Atractaspis microlepidota	Small-scaled burrowing asp	Savanna, from Mauritania to Horn of Africa and Kenya	Local pain, swelling, necrosis. Fatalities recorded. See *A. engaddensis.*
	Macrelaps microlepidotus	Natal black snake	East coast of South Africa	Local pain, swelling. Serious cases recorded.

Atractaspididae considered potentially venomous but for which no bites have been recorded: A. battersbyi (Battersby's burrowing asp): Bolobo, Zaire River basin; A. boulengeri (Central African burrowing asp): western Zaire river basin; A. coalescens (black burrowing asp): Zaire River basin, Angola, Zambia; A. congica (Congo burrowing asp): Zaire River mouth, Angola, Zambia; A. duerdeni (Duerden's burrowing asp): northern Namibia, southeastern Botswana, northwestern South Africa; A. engdahli (Engdahl's burrowing asp): southern Somalia, northeastern Kenya; A. fallax (? subspecies of A. microlepidota): Ethiopia, Somalia, northern Kenya; A. leucomelas (Ogaden burrowing asp): eastern Ethiopia, northern Somalia, Djibouti; A. micropholis (? subspecies of A. microlepidota): West African Sahel; A. reticulata (reticulate burrowing asp): central West Africa; A. scorteccii (Somali burrowing asp): eastern Ethiopia, northern Somalia

Colubridae		Common snakes or rear-fanged snakes	Wide distribution throughout Africa	Venom of some capable of inducing fatal hemostatic defects
	Dispholidus typus	Boomslang ("tree snake")	Wide distribution throughout sub-Saharan open bushveld and savanna	Venom contains enzymes that activate prothrombin and factor X, leading to fatal bleeding if untreated
	Thelotornis capensis	Bird, twig, vine snake	Savanna and coastal bush of southern and eastern Africa	Same as for boomslang (see above)
	Thelotornis kirtlandii	Forest vine, twig snake	Rain forests of western Central Africa	Potentially dangerous (see *D. typus*). No known cases of envenomation.
	Malpolon monspessulanus	Large Montpellier snake	Semidesert, along Mediterranean coast and Atlas Mountains, North Africa	Local pain, swelling, lymphangitis. Possibly neurotoxic.

Colubridae capable of mild envenoming causing local pain, mild swelling, and lymphangitis only: Amplorhinus multimaculatus (many-spotted snake): eastern regions of southern Africa, Zimbabwe; Boiga blandingii (Blanding's tree snake): rain forests of West, East, Central Africa; Coluber rhodorhachis (Jan's desert racer): North Africa, Middle East; Crotaphopeltis hotamboeia (Herald, red-lipped or white-lipped snake): sub-Saharan Africa except rain forest and western South Africa; Malpolon moilensis (hooded malpolon): North Africa; Psammophis biseriatus (Kenyan link-marked sand snake): North and East Africa; Psammophis phillipsii (olive grass snake): sub-Saharan Africa; Psammophis sibilans: throughout Africa outside rain forests; Psammophylax rhombeatus (spotted skaapsteker): southern African grasslands; Psammophylax tri- taeniatus (striped skaapsteker): southern Africa up to southern Tanzania; Telescopus semiannulatus (tiger snake): East, Central, southern Africa

Elapidae

Neurotoxic Cobras	Cobras; rinkhals; mambas; coral, shield-nose, garter, and sea snakes	Wide distribution throughout Africa	Potently neurotoxic and cytotoxic. Common cause of fatal snakebite.
Naja haje: several subspecies:			
Naja haje haje	Egyptian cobra	Savanna, woodland (never forest): North Africa (not Morocco), West and East Africa	Potently neurotoxic, causing flaccid paralysis and respiratory depression. Fatalities due to respiratory arrest.
Naja haje legionis	Moroccan cobra	Morocco	Potently neurotoxic. See above for *Naja haje haje.*
Naja haje anchietae	Anchieta's Egyptian cobra	Namibia, Angola, northwestern Botswana, S.W. Zambia	Potently neurotoxic. See above for *Naja haje haje.*
Naja haje annulifera (? full species)	Banded cobra	Northern South Africa, eastern Botswana, Zimbabwe	Potently neurotoxic. See above for *Naja haje haje.*
Naja melanoleuca	Forest, black and white-lipped cobra	Forested areas of West and Central Africa, southern East Africa, eastern coast of South Africa	Potently neurotoxic. See above for *Naja haje haje.*
Naja nivea	Cape cobra	Western part of South Africa, southern Namibia, Botswana	Potently neurotoxic. See above for *Naja haje haje.*
Spitting Cobras (Cytotoxic)			
Naja katiensis	West African, western brown spitting cobra	Savanna of West Africa, from Senegal and southern Mauritania, eastward to Nigeria and Cameroon	Considered to be cytotoxic. No documented cases.
Naja mossambica	Mozambique spitting cobra, M'fesi	Southeast Africa, from Pemba to northern South Africa and Namibia	Potently cytotoxic. Spits and bites. Severe local pain, swelling, tissue necrosis, often extensive.
Naja pallida	Red spitting cobra	Semidesert areas of northern Kenya, Somalia, Sudan, Ethiopia, and upper Egypt	Eye envenoming. Bites not well documented
Naja nigricollis: three subspecies			
Naja n. nigricollis	Black-necked spitting cobra	Savanna, from West Africa to southern Sudan and southward, through West Africa to Angola	Potently cytotoxic. Spits and bites. As in *N. mossambica.*
Naja n. nigricincta	Barred, zebra spitting cobra	Southern coastal Angola and northern Namibia	Potently cytotoxic. Spits and bites. As in *N. mossambica.*
Naja n. woodi	Black spitting cobra	Southern Namibia, Northern Cape and down to Western Cape Province of South Africa	Potently cytotoxic. Spits and bites. As in *N. mossambica.*

Continued

TABLE 108-1 Venomous Snakes of Africa—cont'd

FAMILY AND OTHER CLASSIFICATIONS	GENUS/SPECIES AND SUBSPECIES	COMMON NAME	DISTRIBUTION*	CLINICAL TOXICOLOGY
Coral/Shield-nose Snakes				
	Aspidelaps lubricus Three coral snake subspecies recognized: *Aspidelaps lubricus lubricus* (southern race), *Aspidelaps lubricus infuscatus* (central race), and *Aspidelaps lubricus cowlesi* (northern race)		Southwestern South Africa, through Namibia to southern Angola	Local pain, swelling, lymphangitis. Mildly neurotoxic. Bites not well documented.
	Aspidelaps scutatus Three shield-nose snake subspecies (races) recognized: *Aspidelaps scutatus scutatus* (western race), *Aspidelaps scutatus fulafula* (eastern race), and *Aspidelaps scutatus intermedius* (central race)		Across northern regions of southern Africa, from Namibia across to Mozambique	Details contradictory. Local pain, swelling, and lymphangitis in some bites. Neurotoxic in others, with one fatality.
Mambas	*Dendroaspis angusticeps*	Common, eastern green, white-mouthed mamba	Forests or bush on eastern coast of Africa, from Kenya to South Africa	Local pain, swelling, lymphangitis, peripheral gangrene. Mildly neurotoxic. One fatal case.
	Dendroaspis jamesoni	Traill's, Jameson's, western green mamba	Central African forests	Local and extended swelling. Neurotoxicity prominent leading to respiratory paralysis.
	Dendroaspis polylepis	Black mamba	Savanna of eastern and southern Africa	Potently neurotoxic. Nausea, vomiting, sweating, diarrhea, involuntary muscle contractions/fasciculations. Respiratory paralysis may develop within 1 hr. High incidence of fatal cases.
	Dendroaspis viridis	Hallowell's, West African green mamba	Coastal forests of West Africa	Local swelling and neurotoxicity prominent. Same as for *D. jamesoni.*
Elapsoidea *(Garter Snakes)*	*Elapsoidea loveridgei*	East African, Loveridge's garter snake	Kenya, Ethiopia, northern Tanzania	Local pain, mild swelling, lymphangitis
	Elapsoidea semiannulata and several subspecies	Half-banded garter snake	Senegal to northern Uganda and a separate southern population from Angola to Mozambique	Local pain, swelling, lymphangitis
	Elapsoidea sundevallii	Sundevall's, southern African garter snake	Southern Africa	Local pain, swelling, lymphangitis. ? Neurotoxic.

Elapsoidea *species for which no bites have thus far been recorded: E. chelazzii* (Southern Somali garter snake): southern Somalia; *E. guentheri* (Gunther's garter snake): southern Central Africa; *E. laticincta* (Central African garter snake): Central Africa; *E. nigra,* (Usambara garter snake): northeastern Tanzania

	Species	Common name	Distribution	Clinical effects
	Hemachatus haemachatus	Rinkhals	Eastern regions of South Africa. Isolated population in southwestern Zimbabwe	Bites and spits. Local swelling and bruising. ? Mildly neurotoxic.
	Walterinnesia aegyptia	Walter Innes's, desert black snake	Northeastern Egypt	Local pain and swelling. Possibly neurotoxic.

Hydrophiidae (Sea Snakes)

	Species	Common name	Distribution	Clinical effects
	Pelamis platurus	Pelagic, yellow-bellied sea snake	East coast of Africa, from Djibouti to Cape Town	Neurotoxic. No documented cases from Africa.

Viperidae

		Adders and vipers	Approximately 45 species distributed throughout Africa	Cytotoxic, hematotoxic, and neurotoxic. Common cause of life-threatening and fatal snakebite in Africa.

Bush Vipers

	Species	Common name	Distribution	Clinical effects
	Atheris ceratophorus	Usambara bush viper	Usambara, Uzungwe, Uluguru mountains, Tanzania	Minor local pain, bruising
	Atheris chlorechis	Western bush, Schlegel's green tree viper	West African rain forests, from Guinea to Cameroon	? Hematotoxic: incoagulable blood in several cases
	Atheris desaixi	Mount Kenya bush viper	Central Kenya	Local pain, prominent swelling
	Atheris squamiger Two subspecies: *Atheris squamiger robustus* and *Atheris squamiger laeviceps*	Green tree, Hallowell's, green bush viper	West and Central Africa rain forests, from Ghana to Cameroon to Uganda, West Kenya, northern Angola	Prominent swelling, incoagulable blood, hemorrhagic shock in one fatal case
	Atheris superciliaris	Lowland, swamp, domino-bellied viper	Southwestern Tanzania, Malawi, Mozambique	Local pain, swelling, blistering

Atheris species considered venomous, but for which no bites have been recorded: *A. hindii* (Kenya montane viper): Kenya; *A. hispidus* (rough-scaled, spiny, or prickly bush viper): Zaire, Uganda, western Kenya; *A. katangensis* (Shaba bush viper): Eastern Zaire; *A. nitschei* (Great Lakes bush viper or Nitsche's bush viper): Uganda, N.W. Tanzania, Rwanda, Burundi, Zaire; *Atheris* subspecies: *A. nitschei rungweensis*: S.W. Tanzania to N.E. Zambia, northern Malawi. *Adenorhinos barbouri*, Uzungwe viper or Barber's viper, is a small adder known only from western Tanzania: no bites recorded

African Vipers (Adders)

Large Adders

	Species	Common name	Distribution	Clinical effects
	Bitis arietans	Puff adder	Widespread throughout sub-Saharan Africa, absent in African rain forests	Potently cytotoxic. Severe local pain, extensive swelling and blistering, compartmental syndrome, necrosis, hypovolemia, shock. Blood coagulation abnormalities.
	Bitis gabonica Two subspecies: *Bitis gabonica gabonica* (eastern race), *Bitis gabonica rhinoceros* (western race)	Gaboon adder or viper, forest puff adder	Tropical forests of West, Central, and East Africa; eastern parts of southern Africa	Local effects as above for *Bitis arietans*. Cardiovascular and hemostatic abnormalities may be prominent.
	Bitis nasicornis	Rhinoceros viper	Forests of West, Central, and East Africa	Not well documented. Massive local swelling, necrosis.
	Bitis parviocula	Ethiopian mountain adder	Southern Ethiopia	No documented cases, but considered highly cytotoxic

Continued

TABLE 108-1 Venomous Snakes of Africa—cont'd

FAMILY AND OTHER CLASSIFICATIONS	GENUS/SPECIES AND SUBSPECIES	COMMON NAME	DISTRIBUTION*	CLINICAL TOXICOLOGY
Small (Dwarf) Adders	*Bitis atropos*	Berg adder	Mountains of eastern Zimbabwe, Drakensberg mountains down to mountains of southwestern Cape, South Africa	Cytotoxic and neurotoxic. Local pain, swelling, lymphangitis; ophthalmoplegia; anosmia; hyponatremia; life-threatening respiratory depression in some cases.
	Bitis caudalis	Horned adder	Arid regions of South-West Africa, extending eastward through Botswana to northern South Africa and southern Zimbabwe	Local pain and swelling (may be extensive with necrosis), lymphangitis
	Bitis peringueyi	Peringuey's adder, side-winding adder	Namib desert, Namibia	Local pain, swelling, lymphangitis. Ophthalmoplegia and other minor neurotoxic effects observed.
	Bitis schneideri	Namaqua dwarf adder, Schneider's adder	Coastal regions of southern Namibia and northern Cape Province, South Africa	Local pain, swelling, lymphangitis
	Bitis worthingtoni	Kenya horned viper	Kenya	Local pain, swelling
	Bitis xeropaga	Desert mountain adder	Southern Namibia and adjacent small area across Orange River into South Africa	Local pain, swelling. Ophthalmoplegia and other minor neurotoxic effects observed.

Other small adders (vipers) considered venomous, but for which no bites have been recorded: B. cornuta (many horned adder, hornsman): coastal regions of southwestern and western South Africa to southern Namibia; B. heraldica (Angolan adder): central Angola; B. inornata (plain mountain adder): two isolated populations in Western Cape and Eastern Cape Provinces of South Africa

Carpet or Saw-Scaled Vipers	*Echis coloratus*	Burton's carpet viper, painted carpet viper	Eastern part of Egypt	Pain and severe local swelling, blistering, and necrosis, with severe hemostatic disorders leading to systemic bleeding
	Echis leucogaster	White-bellied carpet viper	West and North-West Africa	No reported cases. Presumed to cause same toxic effects as in other *Echis* spp.
	Echis ocellatus	West African, ocellated carpet viper	Savanna of West Africa, from Mauritania east to Nigeria, Chad, Cameroon	Of major medical importance in West Africa. Toxic effects as described in *E. coloratus*.
	Echis pyramidum	North-East African carpet viper, Egyptian carpet viper	North and North-East Africa	Most common cause of serious snakebite in Sudan. Toxic effects as described for *E. coloratus*.

Night Adders	*Causus defilippii*	Snouted night adder	Eastern Africa, from Kenya and Tanzania to northeastern South Africa	Local pain, swelling, lymphangitis
	Causus maculatus	West African or western rhombic night adder	Savanna and forest of West and western Central Africa	Local pain, swelling, lymphangitis
	Causus rhombeatus	Eastern rhombic night adder	From eastern Nigeria, through Central Africa, down to eastern half of South Africa	Pain, local swelling
	Causus lichtensteini	Forest or olive green night adder	Rain forests of western Central Africa	Pain, local swelling

Other night adders considered venomous, but for which no bites have been recorded: C. bilineatus (two-striped night adder): South Central Africa, from southern Zaire, West to northern Zambia, Angola; C. resimus (green night adder): scattered populations in Angola, around lake Victoria, coastal Kenya and Somalia, Sudan, eastern Cameroon–Chad border region

North African Desert Vipers			
Cerastes cerastes	Horned, Sahara horned viper	Sahara desert, from Morocco east to Egypt and Sudan	Local pain, swelling, necrosis. Some patients can develop a mild coagulopathy. Bleeding not described.
Cerastes vipera	Sahari desert, sand viper	Sahara desert from Morocco to Egypt	Local pain, swelling. See above.
Old World (or Palaearctic) Vipers			
Macrovipera mauritanica	Moorish viper	Restricted to Morocco and coastal areas of Algeria	Local swelling, bruising. Hemostatic disorders.
Macrovipera lebetina transmediterranea	Levant or blunt-nosed viper	Algeria, Tunisia	Local swelling, bruising. Hemostatic disorders mentioned.

Other old world vipers for which no bites have been recorded in Africa: Vipera latastei gaditana (Lataste's viper or Iberian viper): North African coast, from Morocco to Algeria; *V. monticola* (Atlas mountain viper): Atlas mountains of Morocco; *Macrovipera deserti* (desert adder): northern Tunisia, Libya. Water cobras: *Bonlengerina annulata* (banded water cobra): rivers and lakes of Central Africa—Cameroon, Zaire, Gabon: potentially neurotoxic, no recorded cases; *B. chrystyi* (Congo water cobra): Lower Zaire River: potentially neurotoxic, no recorded cases.

*See Color Figs. 108-1 through 108-10.
ECG, electrocardiogram.
Data from references 1–4.

adequate quantity of antivenom decreases the time course of muscle paralysis and recovery, however. Similarly, in cases of cytotoxic envenomation, administration of polyvalent antivenom does not reverse, but may well limit, tissue damage or its secondary effects (e.g., swelling, dysmobility), or both. In contrast, the hemotoxic effects of saw-scaled or carpet vipers and boomslang envenomation are reversed rapidly on administration of the specific antivenom at any time in the morbid course of events.

The following three snake antivenoms are manufactured in South Africa.*

1. *South African Institute of Medical Research (SAIMR) Polyvalent Snake Antivenom:* This is composed of pepsin-refined immunoglobulins, prepared from the serum of horses that have been hyperimmunized with snake venoms. The venoms of the following snakes are used as antigens in the preparation of the SAIMR Polyvalent Snake Antivenom: *Bitis arietans* (puff adder), *Bitis gabonica* (gaboon adder), *Hemachatus haemachatus* (rinkhals), *Dendroaspis angusticeps* (green mamba), *Dendroaspis jamesonii* (Jameson's mamba), *Dendroaspis polylepis* (black mamba), *Naja nivea* (Cape cobra), *Naja melanoleuca* (forest cobra), *Naja haje annulifera* (banded cobra), *Naja mossambica* (Mozambique spitting cobra, M'fesi). This antivenom is effective against only the venom of the snakes listed above. The Polyvalent Antivenom is supplied in 10-mL glass ampules. In neurotoxic snake bite, the average dose is 80–120 mL, and up to 200 mL in severe cases (e.g., black mamba bite). In cytotoxic snake bite, the average dose is 50–100 mL. The antivenom may be administered as a slow IV bolus over 10–15 minutes or diluted in 200-mL normal saline, or 5% dextrose in water.

2. *South African Institute of Medical Research (SAIMR) Boomslang (tree snake) Snakebite Antiserum:* This is composed of pepsin-refined immunoglobulins, prepared from the serum of horses that have been hyperimmunized with boomslang, *Dispholidus typus*, venom. This antivenom is effective against only the venom of the boomslang or tree snake. The Boomslang (tree snake) Snakebite Antiserum is supplied in 10-mL glass ampules. The average dose is 20 mL, up to 30 mL in severe cases, administered as a slow IV bolus over 5–10 minutes, or diluted in 200 mL normal saline or 5% dextrose in water.

3. *South African Institute of Medical Research (SAIMR) Echis carinatus/ocellatus Antivenom (saw-scaled viper):* This is composed of pepsin-refined immunoglobulins, prepared from the serum of horses that have been hyperimmunized with *Echis carinatus/ocellatus* snake venom. This antivenom is specifically indicated for the treatment of *E. ocellatus* bite. It also has considerable paraspecific potency against the venom of *Echis coloratus* and the two *Cerastes* species, *C. cerastes* and *C. vipera*. The antiserum is supplied in 10-mL glass ampules. The average dose is 20 mL, up to 30 mL in severe cases, administered as a slow IV bolus over 5–10 minutes, or diluted in 200 mL normal saline or 5% dextrose in water.

*South African Vaccine Producers (Pty) Ltd (a wholly owned subsidiary of the National Health Laboratory Service). 1 Modderfontein Road, Edenvale, Gauteng. P.O. Box 28999, Sandringham, 2131, South Africa. Fax +27 11 386 6016. Tel. +27 11 386 6000.

For general management and antivenom therapy, the reader is referred to chapters on general overview and dealing with general management (see Chapter 101) and on antivenoms and immunotherapy (see Chapter 135). Antivenom therapy also should be consistent with the package insert instructions applicable to each country. A bibliography of useful references concerning African snakebites is presented at the end of this chapter.

REFERENCES

1. Spawls S, Branch B: The Dangerous Snakes of Africa. London, Southern Book Publishers, 1995.
2. Schrire L, Muller GJ, Pantanowitz L: The Diagnosis and Treatment of Envenomation in South Africa. Johannesburg, South African Institute for Medical Research, 1996.
3. Warrel DA: Clinical toxicology of snakebite in Africa and the Middle East/Arabian Peninsula. In Meier J, White J (eds): Handbook of Clinical Toxicology of Animal Venoms and Poisons. New York, CRC Press, 1995, p 433.
4. Warrel DA: Snake bite in sub-Saharan Africa. Africa Health 21:5–9, 1999.

BIBLIOGRAPHY

Aitchison JM: Boomslang bite—diagnosis and management: A report of 2 cases. S Afr Med J 78:39–42, 1990.

Alkan ML, Sukenik S: Atrioventricular block in a case of snakebite inflicted by *Atractaspis engaddensis* (Letter). Trans R Trop Med Hyg 69:166, 1975.

Ariaratnam CA, Meyer WP, Perera G, et al: A new monospecific ovine Fab fragment antivenom for treatment of envenoming by the Sri Lankan Russell's viper (*Daboia russelii russelii*): A preliminary dose-finding and pharmacokinetic study. Am J Trop Med Hyg 61:259–265, 1999.

Arsura EL: Edrophonium for cobra bite. N Engl J Med 316:1608–1609, 1987.

Atkinson PM, Bradlow BA, White JAM, et al: Clinical features of twig snake (*Thelotornis capensis*) envenomation. S Afr Med J 58:1007–1011, 1980.

Barnes JM, Trueta J: Absorption of bacteria, toxins and snake venoms from the tissues: Importance of the lymphatic circulation. Ian 1:623–626, 1941.

Beiran D, Currie G: Snakebite due to *Thelotornis kirtlandii*. Cent Afr J Med 13:137–139, 1967.

Benbassat J, Shalev O: Envenomation by *Echis coloratus* (Middle-East saw-scaled viper): A review of the literature and indications for treatment. Isr J Med Sci 29:239–250, 1993.

Bey TA, Boyer LV, Walter FG, et al: Exotic snakebite: Envenomation by an African puff adder (*Bitis arietans*). J Emerg Med 15:827–831, 1997.

Blaver GT: Case history of a horned adder bite in Zimbabwe. J Herp Assoc Afr 15:23–26, 1977.

Blaylock RS: A bite from a vine snake in Bulawayo. J Herp Assoc Rhod 12:8–9, 1960.

Blaylock RS: Case history of a bite from a *Bitis arietans* in Bulawayo. J Herp Assoc Rhod 13:9, 1960.

Blaylock RSM: Snakebites at Triangle Hospital, January 1975 to June 1981. Cent Afr J Med 28:1–10, 1982.

Blaylock RSM: The treatment of snakebite in Zimbabwe. Cent Afr J Med 28:237–246, 1982.

Blaylock RS: Time of onset of clinical envenomation following snakebite. S Afr Med J 64:357–360, 1983.

Blaylock RS, Lichtman AR, Potgieter PD: Clinical manifestations of Cape cobra (*Naja nivea*) bites: A report of two cases. S Afr Med J 68:342–344, 1985.

Blaylock RS: Time of onset of clinical envenomation following snakebite in southern Africa. S Afr Med J 80:253, 1991.

Blaylock RS: Electrotherapy for snakebite. S Afr Med J 84:875, 1994.

Blaylock RSM: Pressure immobilisation for snakebite in southern Africa remains speculative. S Afr Med J 84:826–827, 1994.

Blaylock RSM: Retrospective analysis of snakebite at a rural hospital in Zululand. S Afr Med J 85:286, 1995.

Blaylock RS: Antibiotic use and infection in snakebite victims. S Afr Med J 89:874–876, 1999.

Blaylock RSM: Antibacterial properties of KwaZulu Natal snake venoms. Toxicon 38:1529–1534, 2000.

Branch WR, McCartney CJ: *Dispholidus typus*, boomslang: Envenomation. J Herp Assoc Afr 32:34–35, 1986.

Britt A, Burkhart K: Naja naja cobra bite. Am J Emerg Med 15:529–531, 1997.

Britt DP: Death following the bite of a burrowing viper. Nigerian Field 43:41–42, 1978.

Broadley DG: Fatalities from the bites of *Dispholidus* and *Thelotornis* and a personal case history. J Herp Assoc Rhod 1:5, 1957.

Broadley DG: The case history of a *Bitis atropos* bite. J Herp Assoc Rhod 2:6, 1958.

Broadley DG: Case history of a green-mamba bite in Bulawayo. J Herp Assoc Rhod 8:7, 1959.

Broadley DG: Case history of a boomslang (*Dispholidus typus*) bite. J Herp Assoc Rhod 11:7, 1960.

Brossy J: The treatment of snakebite. S Afr Med J 51:390–391, 1977.

Brossy JJ, Lewis J, Black D: Low-molecular-weight dextran and puff adder bites (Letter). S Afr Med J 62:349–350, 1982.

Campbell CH: Symptomatology, pathology and treatment of the bites of elapid snakes. In Chen-Tuan Lee (ed): Snake Venoms, Handbook of Experimental Pharmacology. New York, Springer Verlag, 1979, pp 898–921.

Chapman DS: The symptomatology, pathology and treatment of the bites of venomous snakes of central and southern Africa. In Bucherl W, Buckley E, Deaulofeau V (eds): Venomous Animals and their Venoms. New York, Academic Press, 1967, pp 463–527.

Chifundera K: Snakes of Zaire and their bites. African Study Monogr 10:137–157, 1990.

Chippaux J-P, N'Guessan G, Paris FX, et al: Spitting cobra (*Naja nigricollis*) bite (Letter). Trans R Soc Trop Med Hyg 72:106, 1978.

Chippaux J-P, Bressy C: L'endemie ophidienne des plantations de Cote-d'Ivoire. Bull Soc Pathol Exotet Fil 74:458–467, 1981.

Chippaux J-P: Snakebites epidemiology in Benin (West Africa). Toxicon 27:37, 1989.

Chippaux J-P: Antivenoms in Africa, one hundred years after Calmette. Med Afrique Noire 43:45–49, 1996.

Chippaux J-P: Snake-bites: Appraisal of the global situation. Bull WHO 76:515–524, 1998.

Chippaux J-P: The development and use of immunotherapy in Africa. Toxicon 36:1503–1506, 1998.

Chippaux J-P, Amadi-Eddine S, Fagot P: Validity of a test for diagnosis and monitoring of hemorrhagic syndrome after viper envenomation in sub-saharan Africa. Med Trop 58:369–371, 1998.

Chippaux J-P, Lang J, Amadi-Eddine SA, et al: Clinical safety of a polyvalent F(ab⁻)₂ equine antivenom in 223 African snake envenomations: A field trial in Cameroon. Trans R Soc Trop Med Hyg 92:657–662, 1998.

Chippaux J-P: Snakes of Western and Central Africa. Paris, IRD Editions, 1999.

Chippaux J-P, Lang J, Amadi-Eddine S, et al: Short report: Treatment of snake envenomations by a new polyvalent antivenom composed by highly purified F(ab⁻)₂: Results of a clinical trial in northern Cameroon. Am J Trop Med Hyg 61:1017–1018, 1999.

Christensen PA: South African Snake Venoms and Antivenoms. Johannesburg, South African Institute for Medical Research, 1955.

Christensen PA: The treatment of snakebite. S Afr Med J 43:1253–1258, 1969.

Christensen PA: Snakebite and the use of antivenom in southern Africa. S Afr Med J 59:934–938, 1981.

Cock EV: Two suspect mamba bites: Same victim, three year interval. J Herp Assoc Afr 16:2–3, 1973.

Coetzer PW, Tilbury CR: The epidemiology of snakebite in northern Natal. S Afr Med J 62:206–212, 1982.

Corkill NL, Ionides CJP, Pitman CRS: Biting and poisoning by the mole vipers of the genus *Atractaspis*. Trans R Soc Trop Med Hyg 53:95–101, 1959.

Corkill NL, Kirk R: Poisoning by the Sudan mole viper *Atractaspis microlepidota* Gunther. Trans R Soc Trop Med Hyg 48:376–384, 1954.

Cotton MF, Shahak E, Muller GJ, et al: Syndrome of inappropriate antidiuretic hormone secretion, an unusual complication of an elapid snakebite. S Afr Med J 79:735–736, 1991.

Cranko JAW: A snakebite from a burrowing adder. Cent Afr J Med 7:215, 1961.

Creighton D: Notes on a bite by the snouted night adder (*Causus defilippii*). Nyoka News 3:3–4, 1986.

Crisp HG: Black mamba envenomation (Letter). S Afr Med J 68:293–294, 1985.

Currie B: Pressure-immobilization first aid for snakebite—fact and fancy. Toxicon 31:931–932, 1993.

Daudu I, Theakston RDG: Preliminary trial of a new polyspecific antivenom in Nigeria. Ann Trop Med Parasitol 82:311–313, 1988.

Davidson RA: Case of African cobra bite. BMJ 4:660, 1970.

Delport SD, Schmid EV, Farrant PJ: Delayed neurotoxic and cytotoxic complications after snake envenomation. S Afr Med J 79:169, 1991.

Du Toit DM: Boomslang (*Dispholidus typus*) bite: A case report and a review of diagnosis and management. S Afr Med J 57:507–510, 1980.

Edington DA: Snakebite (Letter). S Afr Med J 47:364, 1973.

Edwards IR, Fleming JBM, James MFM: Management of a Gaboon viper bite: A case report. Cent Afr J Med 25:217–221, 1979.

Efrati P: Symptomatology, pathology and treatment of bites of viperid snakes. In Lee CY (ed): Snake Venoms. Berlin, Springer Verlag, 1979, pp 956–977.

Ellis CG: The berg adder: A unique snake. Practitioner 223:544–547, 1979.

Els RA: *Naja haje annulifera*, Egyption cobra: Envenomation. J Herp Assoc Afr 34:52–53, 1988.

Fainaru M, Manny N, Hershko C, Eisenberg S: Defibrination following *Echis colorata* bite in man. Isr Med J 6:720–725, 1970.

Fan HW, Marcopito LF, Cardoso JL, et al: Sequential randomised and double blind trial of promethazine prophylaxis against early anaphylactic reactions to antivenom for bothrops snake bites. BMJ 318:1451–1452, 1999.

Fitzsimons DC, Hobart MS: Another rear-fanged South African snake lethal to humans. Herpetologica 14:198–202, 1958.

Fitzsimons VFM: Snakes of Southern Africa. London, MacDonald, 1962.

Franz KH: Case of snakebite by *Atractaspis corpulenta*. Trans R Soc Trop Med Hyg 54:279–280, 1960.

French MR: Case history of a puff adder bite in Salisbury. J Herp Assoc Rhod 8:9, 1958.

Freyvogel TA: Poisonous and venomous animals in East Africa. Acta Trop 29:401–451, 1972.

Gear JHS: Non-polio causes of polio-like paralytic syndrome. Rev Infect Dis 6(Suppl 2):S379–S384, 1984.

Gerber JD, Adendorff HP: Boomslang (*Dispholidus typus*) bite: Case report. S Afr Med J 57:710–711, 1980.

Gilkes MJ: Snake venom conjunctivitis. Br J Ophthalmol 43:638–639, 1959.

Gillissen A, Theakston RDG, Barth J, et al: Neurotoxicity and haemostatic disturbances after a bite by a Tunisian saw-scaled or carpet viper (*Echis "pyramidum"* complex). Toxicon 32:937–944, 1994.

Goddard MG: Case history of a puff adder (*Bitis arietans*) bite. J Herp Assoc Rhod 17–18:15–16, 1962.

Gold BS: Neostigmine for the treatment of neurotoxicity following envenomation by the Asiatic cobra. Ann Emerg Med 29:195, 1997.

Gold BS, Pyle P: Successful treatment of neurotoxic king cobra envenomation in Myrtle Beach, South Carolina. Ann Emerg Med 32:736–738, 1998.

Gomperts ED, Demetriou D: Laboratory studies and clinical features in a case of boomslang envenomation. S Afr Med J 51:173–175, 1977.

Gray HH: Green mamba envenomation: Case report. Trans R Soc Trop Med Hyg 56:390–391, 1962.

Greenham R: Spitting cobra (*Naja mossambica pallida*) bite in a Kenyan child (Letter). Trans R Soc Trop Med Hyg 72:674–675, 1978.

Guttmann-Friedmann A: Blindness after snakebite. Br J Ophthalmol 40:57–59, 1956.

Haagner GV: *Dendroaspis angusticeps*, green mamba: Envenomation. J Herp Assoc Afr 33:32, 1986.

Haagner GV, Smit R: Case history of boomslang (*Dispholidus typus*) envenomation in the eastern Transvaal, South Africa. Br Herp Soc Bull 21:43–45, 1987.

Haagner GV, Carpenter G: Venoms and snakebite: *Aspidelaps scutatus*, shield-nosed snake. J Herp Assoc Afr 37:60, 1990.

Hadley GP, McGarr P, Mars M: The role of thromboelastography in the management of children with snake-bite in southern Africa. Trans R Soc Trop Med Hyg 93:177–179, 1999.

Hakansson T, Madsen T: On the distribution of the black mamba (*Dendroaspis polylepis*) in west Africa. J Herpetol 17:186–189, 1983.

Hall L: Investigations in a case of snake bite. E Afr Med J 39:66–68, 1962.

Hamby JA, Greybeal GE: Puff adder bite: A case presentation. Delaware Med J 55:579–581, 1983.

Harrison JR: Envenomation by a desert horned viper, *Cerastes cerastes* (Linnaeus): A case history. Contributions in Herpetology. Chicago, Greater Chicago Herpetological Society, 1992, 15–17.

Harvey AL: Twenty years of dendrotoxins. Toxicon 39:15–26, 2001.

Harvey AL, Anderson AJ, Karlsson E: Facilitation of transmitter release by neurotoxins from snake venoms. J Physiol (Paris) 79:222–227, 1984.

Harvey WR: Black mamba envenomation (Letter). S Afr Med J 67:960, 1985.

Herpetological Association of Africa: Schoolboy dies from mamba bite. Herpet Assoc Afr Newsletter 12:9, 1990.

Hilligan R: Black mamba bites: A report of 2 cases. S Afr Med J 72:220–221, 1987.

Hodgson PS, Davidson TM: Biology and treatment of the mamba snakebite. Wildern Environ Med 7:133–145, 1996.

Hoffmann LAC, De Wet Potgieter S: *Naja mossambica*. Mozambique spitting cobra or M'fezi envenomation. J Herp Assoc Afr 35:41–42, 1988.

Hurrell DP: Namaqua dwarf adder bite. S Afr Med J 59:491–492, 1981.

Hurter J: *Bitis atropos*, berg adder: Envenomation. J Herp Assoc Afr 32:33, 1986.

Hurwitz BJ, Hull PR: Berg adder bite. S Afr Med J 45:969–971, 1971.

Hutton FA, Warrell DA: Action of snake venom components on the haemostatic system. Blood Rev 7:176–189, 1993.

Hyslop S, Marsh NA: Comparison of the physiological effects in rabbits of gaboon viper (*Bitis gabonica*) venoms from different sources. Toxicon 29:1235–1250, 1991.

Ismail M, Aly MH, Abd-Elsalam MA, Morad AM: A three-compartment open pharmacokinetic model can explain variable toxicities of cobra venoms and their alpha toxins. Toxicon 34:1011–1026, 1996.

Jolkkonen M, Van Giersbergen PL, Hellman U, et al: Muscarinic toxins from the black mamba *Dendroaspis polylepis*. Eur J Biochem 234:579–585, 1995.

Kasilo OMJ, Nhachi CFB: A retrospective study of poisoning due to snake venom in Zimbabwe. Hum Exp Toxicol 12:15–18, 1993.

Krengel B, Walton J: A case of mamba bite. S Afr Med J 39:1150–1151, 1967.

Krifi MN, el Ayeb M, Ben Lasfar Z, et al: Improvement and standardization of antivenoms sera: Snake venoms preparation. Arch Inst Pasteur Tunis 70:5–12, 1993.

Laing GD, Lee L, Smith DC, et al: Experimental assessment of a new, low-cost antivenom for treatment of carpet viper (*Echis ocellatus*) envenoming. Toxicon 33:307–313, 1995.

Lake AR, Trevor-Jones TR: The venom apparatus of the boomslang or tree snake, *Dispholidus typus*. South Afr J Sci 92:167–169, 1996.

Lanoie LO, Branch WR: Venoms and snakebite: *Atheris squamiger*, green bush viper fatal envenomation. J Herp Assoc Afr 39:29, 1991.

Lath NK, Patel MM: Treatment of snake venom ophthalmia. Cent Afr J Med 30:175–176, 1984.

Laubscher HH: Snakebite: A case report. S Afr Med J 31:102–103, 1957.

Leloup P: Case history of a green mamba bite in the congo. J Herp Assoc Rhod 12:6–8, 1960.

Levine L, Wapnick S: Viperidae snakebite: Local and systemic effects. S Afr J Surg 11:19–23, 1973.

Lloyd CNV: Report on a berg adder bite. J Herp Assoc Afr 16:8–10, 1973.

Louw A: Bite by a shield-nose snake (*Aspidelaps scutatus*). Nyoka News 2:12, 1982.

Louw JX: Specific mamba antivenom—report of survival of 2 patients with black mamba bites treated with this serum. S Afr Med J 41:1175, 1967.

Mackay N, Ferguson JC, Ashe J, et al: The venom of the boomslang (*Dispholidus typus*): In vivo and in vitro studies. Thromb Diath Haemorrh 21:234–244, 1969.

Mackay N, Ferguson JC, McNicol GP: The effects of the venom of the East African green mamba (*Dendroaspis angusticeps*) on blood coagulation and platelet aggregation. East Afr Med J 43:454–463, 1966.

Macvicar N: Snake poisoning in Central Africa. J Trop Med 1–3, January, 1902.

Malasit P, Warrell DA, Chanthavanich P, et al: Prediction, prevention and mechanism of early (anaphylactic) antivenom reactions in victims of snake bites. BMJ 292:17–20, 1986.

Marais J: Case history of snouted night adder bite. J Herp Assoc Afr 26:6–7, 1980.

Mars M, Hadley GP, Aitchison JM: Direct intracompartmental pressure measurement in the management of snakebites in children. S Afr Med J 80:227–228, 1991.

Marsh NA, Whaler BC: The Gaboon viper (*Bitis gabonica*): Its biology, venom components and toxinology. Toxicon 22:669–694, 1984.

Matsen FA: Compartmental Syndromes. New York, Grune & Stratton, 1980.

Max SI, Laing JS, Potter LT: Purification and properties of M1-toxin, a specific antagonist of M1 muscarinic receptors. J Neurosci 13:4293–4300, 1993.

McNally SL, Reitz CJ: Victims of snakebite: A 5 year study at Shongwe Hospital, Kangwane, 1978–1982. S Afr Med J 72:855–860, 1987.

McNally T, Conway GS, Jackson L, et al: Accidental envenoming by a Gaboon viper (*Bitis gabonica*): The haemostatic disturbances observed and investigation of in vitro haemostatic properties of whole venom. Trans R Soc Trop Med Hyg 87:66–70, 1993.

Meyer WP, Habib AG, Onayade AA, et al: First clinical experiences with a new ovine Fab *Echis ocellatus* snake bite antivenom in Nigeria: Randomized comparative trial with Institute Pasteur Serum (Ipser) Africa antivenom. Am J Trop Med Hyg 56:291–300, 1997.

Minton SA: Venomous bites by non-venomous snakes: An annotated bibliography of colubrid envenomation. J Wildern Med 1:119–127, 1990.

Montgomery J: Two cases of ophthalmoplegia due to berg adder bite. Cent Afr J Med 5:172–177, 1959.

Moran NF, Newman WJ, Theakston RDG, et al: High incidence of early anaphylactoid reaction to SAIMR polyvalent snake antivenom. Trans R Soc Trop Med Hyg 92:69–70, 1998.

Muguti GI, Maramba A, Washaya CT: Snake bites in Zimbabwe: A clinical study with emphasis on the need for antivenom. Cent Afr J Med 40:83–88, 1994.

Murphy JB: Case history of snakebite due to the horned puff adder, *Bitis caudalis*. HISS News 1:159–160, 1973.

Naidoo DP, Lockhat HS, Naiker IP: Myocardial infarction after probable black mamba envenomation. S Afr Med J 71:388–389, 1987.

Naphade RW, Shetti RN: Use of neostigmine after snake bite. Trans R Soc Trop Med Hyg 70:78–79, 1976.

Nelson BK: Snake envenomation: Incidence, clinical presentation and management. Med Toxicol 4:17–31, 1989.

Newbery R: Bite by a Kalahari garter snake. J Herp Assoc Afr 23:10, 1980.

Newman WJ, Moran NF, Theakston RD, et al: Traditional treatments for snake bite in a rural African community. Ann Trop Med Parasitol 91:967–969, 1997.

Nhachi CF, Kasilo OM: Snake poisoning in rural Zimbabwe—a prospective study. J Appl Toxicol 14:191–193, 1994.

Oberholzer W, Oberholzer G, Dando RV, Reitz CJ: Emergency treatment of neurotoxic snakebite with a self-inflating manual bag. S Afr Med J 80:254, 1991.

Paget D, Cock EV: Case history of a berg adder bite. Cent Afr J Med 25:30–33, 1979.

Palmer NG: Bitis atropos, berg adder: Envenomation. J Herp Assoc Afr 32:31–32, 1986.

Pantanowitz L: Snakebite in children. S Afr Med J 87:77, 1997.

Payne T, Warrell DA: Effects of venom in eye from spitting cobra. Arch Ophthalmol 94:1803, 1976.

Pewtress R: The effects of a night adder (*Causus rhombeatus*) bite. Herptile 8:96–97, 1983.

Phillips LL, Weiss HJ, Christy NP: Effects of puff adder venom on the coagulation mechanism. Thromb Diath Haemorrh 30:499–508, 1973.

Pitman CRS: Bites by the saw-scaled viper (*Echis carinatus ocellatus*) in Nigeria. J Herp Assoc Afr 13:21, 1972.

Pitman CRS: The saw-scaled viper or carpet viper (*Echis carinatus*) in Africa and its bite. J Herp Assoc Afr 9:6–34, 1973.

Pugh RNH, Boudillon CCM, Theakston RDG, Reid HA: Bites by the carpet viper in the Niger valley. Lancet 2:625–627, 1979.

Pugh RNH, Theakston RDG: Incidence and mortality of snakebite in savanna Nigeria. Lancet 2:1181–1183, 1980.

Pugh NH, Theakston RDG, Reid HA, Bhar IS: Epidemiology of human encounters with the spitting cobra, *Naja nigricollis*, in the Malumfashi area of northern Nigeria. Ann Trop Med Parasitol 74:523–530, 1980.

Pugh RN, Theakston RD: A clinical study of viper bite poisoning. Ann Trop Med Parasitol 81:135–149, 1987.

Ratcliffe PJ, Pukrittayakamee S, Ledingham JG, Warrell DA: Direct nephrotoxicity of Russell's viper venom demonstrated in the isolated perfused rat kidney. Am J Trop Med Hyg 40:312–319, 1989.

Read PH, Foster DL: Case history of a brown mamba bite in Northern Rhodesia. J Herp Assoc Rhod 8:6–7, 1959.

Reid HA: Snakebite in the tropics. BMJ 3:359–362, 1968.

Reid HA: Symptomatology, pathology and treatment of the bites of sea snakes. In Chen-Tuan Lee (ed): Snake Venoms, Handbook of Experimental Pharmacology. New York, Springer Verlag, 1979, pp 922–955.

Reitz CJ, Goosen DJ, Odendaal MW, et al: Evaluation of the venom Ex apparatus in the treatment of Egyptian cobra envenomation. S Afr Med J 66:135–138, 1984.

Reitz CJ, Willemse GT, Odendaal MW, Visser JJ: Evaluation of the venom Ex apparatus in the initial treatment of puff adder envenomation. S Afr J Med 69:684–686, 1986.

Reitz CJ: Boomslang bite—time of onset of clinical envenomation (Letter). S Afr Med J 76:39–40, 1989.

Rippey JJ, Rippey E, Branch WR: A survey of snakebite in the Johannesburg area. S Afr Med J 50:1872–1976, 1876.

Russel FE, Puffer HW: African cobra bite. BMJ 2:650, 1971.

Sakier JB, Fritz VU: Consumptive coagulopathy caused by a boomslang bite. S Afr Med J 43:1052–1055, 1969.

Saunders CR: Report on a garter snake bite in Zimbabwe. J Herp Assoc Afr 11:15–16, 1972.

Saunders CR: Report on a black mamba bite of a medical colleague. Cent Afr J Med 26:121–122, 1980.

Schmid EU: Slangbyt in Suid-Africa. Geneeskunde 4:185–191, 1962.

Schulchynska-Castel H, Dvilansky A, Keynau A: *Echis colorata* bites: Clinical evaluation of 42 patients: A retrospective study. Isr J Med Sci 22:880–884, 1986.

Schwersenski J, Beatty DW: Unusual features in a case of snakebite, presumably due to a Cape cobra (*Naja nigricollis*). S Afr Med J 61:597–598, 1982.

Schweitzer G, Lewis JS: Puff adder bite—an unusual cause of bilateral carpal tunnel syndrome: A case report. S Afr Med J 60:714–715, 1981.

Servent D, Winckler-Dietrich V, Hu HY, et al: Only snake curaremimetic toxins with fifth disulphide bond have high affinity for the neuronal alpha 7 nicotinic receptor. J Biol Chem 272:24279–24286, 1997.

Servent D, Thanh HL, Antil S, et al: Functional determinants by which snake and cone snail toxins block the alpha 7 neuronal nicotinic acetylcholine receptors. J Physiol Paris 92:107–111, 1998.

Sezi CL, Alpidovsky VK, Reeve MI: Defibrination syndrome after snakebite. E Afr Med J 49:590–596, 1972.

Siemers AH: Case history of an *Atractaspis bibronii* bite. J Herp Assoc Rhod 4:5–6, 1958.

Simbotwe MP: Epidemiology and clinical study of snakebite in Kasempa district of north western Zambia. Snake 14:101–104, 1982.

Sinha AK: Cobra-venom conjunctivitis. Lancet 1:1026, 1972.

Sivilotti L: Acetylcholine receptors: Too many channels, too few functions. Science 269:1681–1682, 1995.

Smith AC: Retrospective analysis of a snakebite at a rural hospital in Zululand. S Afr Med J 85:286–287, 1995.

Smith LA, Olson MA, Lafaye PJ, Dolly JO: Cloning and expression of mamba toxins. Toxicon 33:459–474, 1995.

Snakebite in the tropics. Lancet 2:1016, 1972.

Snow RW, Bronzan R, Roques T, et al: The prevalence and morbidity of snake bite and treatment-seeking behaviour among a rural Kenyan population. Ann Trop Med Parasitol 88:665–671, 1994.

Spawls S: Notes on a bite by a West African *Atractaspis* (Colubridae: Aparallactini). J Herp Assoc Afr 28:21–22, 1980.

Spies SK, Malherbe LF, Pepler WJ: Boomslangbyt met afibrinogenemie. S Afr Med J 36:834–838, 1962.

Stahel E: Epidemiological aspects of snakebites on a Liberian rubber plantation. Acta Trop 37:367–374, 1980.

Staley FH: A case report of Gaboon viper poisoning with recovery. Bull Antivenin Inst Am 3:31–39, 1929.

Stevens-Truss R, Hinman CL: Activities of cobra venom cytotoxins toward heart and leukemic T-cells depend on localized amino acid differences. Toxicon 35:659–669, 1997.

Stewart MM: A bite by a burrowing adder (*Atractaspis bibronii*). J Herp Assoc Rhod 23–24:47–50, 1965.

Strover HM: Report on a death from black mamba bite (*Dendroaspis polylepis*). Cent Afr J Med 13:185–186, 1967.

Strover HM: Observations on two cases of snakebite by *Naja nigricollis mossambica*. Cent Afr J Med 19:12–13, 1973.

Stueven H, Aprahamian C, Thompson B, et al: Cobra envenomation: An uncommon emergency. Ann Emerg Med 12:636–638, 1983.

Sutherland SK: Pressure immobilisation for snakebite in southern Africa remains speculative. S Afr Med J 85:1039–1041, 1995.

Sutherland SK, Coulter AR, Harris RD: Rationalisation of first-aid measures for elapid snake bite. Lancet 1:183–186, 1979.

Swiecicki AW: Snakes and snakebite in the western region. Ghana J Trop Med Hyg 68:300–304, 1965.

Swinson C: Control of antivenom treatment in *Echis carinatus* (Carpet Viper) poisoning. Trans R Soc Trop Med Hyg 70:85–87, 1976.

Takahashi Y, Tu AT: Puff adder snakebite. JAMA 211:1857, 1970.

Theakston RDG, Reid HA: Epidemiology of snakebite in West Africa (Abstract). Toxicon 20:364–365, 1982.

Theakston RDG, Wyatt GB: Venom antibody levels in a patient bitten by a young puff adder (Bitis arietans) during a world record attempt. Ann Trop Med Parasitol 79:305–307, 1985.

Theakston RD, Warrell DA: Antivenoms: A list of hyperimmune sera currently available for the treatment of envenoming by bites and stings. Toxicon 29:1419–1470, 1991.

Theakston RD, Warrell DA: 1st International Congress on Envenomations and their Treatments, Institut Pasteur, Paris, 7–9 June, 1995. Biologicals 23:327–330, 1995.

Theakston RD: An objective approach to antivenom therapy and assessment of first-aid measures in snake bite. Ann Trop Med Parasitol 91:857–865, 1997.

Theakston RDG, Warrell DA: Crisis in snake antivenom supply for Africa. Lancet 356:2104, 2000.

Tilbury CR: Observations on the bite of the Mozambique spitting cobra (*Naja mossambica mossambica*). S Afr Med J 61:307–313, 1982.

Tilbury CR, Branch WR: Observations on the bite of the southern burrowing asp (*Atractaspis bibronii*) in Natal. S Afr Med J 75:327–331, 1989.

Tun-Pe, Tin-Nu-Swe, Myint-Lwin, et al: The efficacy of tourniquets as a first aid measure for Russell's viper bites in Burma. Trans R Soc Trop Med Hyg 81:403–405, 1987.

Van Egmond KC: A fatal bite by the shieldnose snake (*Aspidelaps scutatus*). S Afr Med J 66:714, 1984.

Van Wyk CW: A novel way to identify a cobra bite. S Afr Med J 87:473, 1997.

Vaughan-Scott T, Lobetti RG: Boomslang envenomation in a dog. J S Afr Vet Assoc 66:265–267, 1995.

Visser J, Carpenter G: Notes on a Gaboon adder bite. J Herp Assoc Afr 15:21–22, 1977.

Vital BO, Vieira RJ: Neostigmine in the treatment of snake accidents caused by *Micrurus frontalis*: Report of two cases (1). Rev Inst Med Trop Sao Paulo 38:61–67, 1996.

Wallach Van S: Report on bites by the west African night adder, *Causus maculatus*. J Herp Assoc Afr 22:3–8, 1979.

Wallach Van S: Report on a bite by a side-stabbing snake, *Atractaspis irregularis*, with notes on elapid bites. J Herp Assoc Afr 24:15–17, 1980.

Wapnick S, Levin L, Broadley DG: A study of snakebites admitted to a hospital in Rhodesia. Cent Afr J Med 18:137–141, 1972.

Warrell DA, Davidson N, Ormerod LD, et al: Bites by the saw-scaled or carpet viper (*Echis carinatus*): Trial of two specific antivenoms. BMJ 4:437–440, 1974.

Warrell DA, Ormerod LD, Davidson NMcD: Bites by puff adder (*Bitis arietans*) in Nigeria, and value of antivenom. BMJ 4:697–700, 1975.

Warrell DA, Arnett C: The importance of bites by the saw-scaled or carpet viper (*Echis carinatus*): Epidemiological studies in Nigeria and a review of the world literature. Acta Trop 33:307–341, 1976.

Warrell DA, Barnes HJ, Piburn MF: Neurotoxic effects of bites by the Egyptian cobra (*Naja haje*) in Nigeria. Trans R Soc Trop Med Hyg 70:78–79, 1976.

Warrell DA, Greenwood BM, Davidson NMcD, et al: Necrosis, haemorrhage and complement depletion following bites by the spitting cobra (*Naja nigricollis*). QJM 45:1–22, 1976.

Warrell DA, Ormerod LD: Snake venom ophthalmia and blindness caused by the spitting cobra (*Naja nigricollis*) in Nigeria. Am J Trop Med Hyg 25:525–529, 1976.

Warrell DA, Ormerod LD, Davidson NMcD: Bites by the night adder (*Causus maculatus*) and burrowing vipers (genus *Atractaspis*) in Nigeria. Am J Trop Med Hyg 25:517–524, 1976.

Warrell DA, Davidson NMcD, Greenwood BM, et al: Poisoning by bites of the saw-scaled or carpet viper (*Echis carinatus*) in Nigeria. QJM N S 46:33–62, 1977.

Warrell DA: Clinical snake bite problems in the Nigerian savanna region. Technische Hochschule Darmstadt Schriftenreihe Wissenschaft und Technik 14:31–60, 1979.

Warrell DA, Warrell MJ, Edgar W, et al: Comparison of Pasteur and Behringwerke antivenoms in envenoming by the carpet viper (*Echis carinatus*). BMJ 280:607–609, 1980.

Warrell DA: The global problem of snake bite: Its prevention and treatment. In Gopalakrishnakone P, Tan CK (eds): Recent Advances in Toxinology Research, Vol 1. Singapore, National University of Singapore, 1992, pp 121–153.

Warrell DA: Snake bite and snake venoms. QJM 86:351–353, 1993.

Warrell DA: Venomous bites and stings in the tropical world. Med J Aust 159:773–779, 1993.

Watt G, Theakston RD, Hayes CG, et al: Positive response to edrophonium in patients with neurotoxic envenoming by cobras (Naja naja philippinensis): A placebo-controlled study. N Engl J Med 315:1444–1448, 1986.

Watt G, Padre L, Tuazon ML, et al: Tourniquet application after cobra bite: Delay in the onset of neurotoxicity and the dangers of sudden release. Am J Trop Med Hyg 38:618–622, 1988.

Watt G, Meade BD, Theakston RD, et al: Comparison of Tensilon and antivenom for the treatment of cobra-bite paralysis. Trans R Soc Trop Med Hyg 83:570–573, 1989.

Weiser E, Wollberg Z, Kochva E, Lee SY: Cardiotoxic effects of the venom of the burrowing asp, *Atractaspis engaddensis* (Atractaspididae, Ophidia). Toxicon 22:767–774, 1984.

Wilkinson D: Retrospective analysis of snakebite at a rural hospital in Zululand. S Afr Med J 84:844–847, 1994.

Winkel KD, Hawdon GM, Levick N: Pressure immobilization for neurotoxic snake bites. Ann Emerg Med 34:294–295, 1999.

Wuster W, Golay P, Warrell DA: Synopsis of recent developments in venomous snake systematics, No. 2. Toxicon 36:299–307, 1998.

Wuster W, Golay P, Warrell DA: Synopsis of recent developments in venomous snake systematics, No. 3. Toxicon 37:1123–1129, 1999.

Yayon E, Sikular E, Keynan A: Desert black snake (*Walterinnesia aegyptia*) bites—a presentation of four cases. Harefuah 115:269–270, 1988.

Yerzingatsian KL: Snakebite—rest and elevation in the management of a selected group of patients in an urban setting. S Afr J Surg 35:188–189, 1997.

Zaltman M, Rumbak M, Rabie M, Zwi S: Neurotoxicity due to the bite of the shield-nose snake (*Aspidelaps scutatus*). S Afr Med J 66:111–112, 1984.

CHAPTER 109

South American Snakes

Anthony Wong ◼ Daisy Schwab Rodrigues ◼ João Luiz Costa Cardoso

Most snake envenomations in South America occur in Brazil because of its territorial extension, tropical climate, and natural forests. As in other regions of the world, the encroachment by humans into the natural habitats of snakes destroys their food sources and forces them from woods and forests into the fringes of civilization. Keeping dangerous species of snakes as pets has caused an increase in bites by rare species.

Snake envenomations are the major and most frequent of all accidents caused by animals and constitute an important public health problem.[1] About 23,000 snakebites are reported annually in South America. Contrary to the grossly overestimated numbers reported in the 1980s, the latest numbers reported by the Ministry of Health of Brazil indicate that annually there are only about 20,000 snakebites in Brazil (13 to 15 per 100,000 inhabitants) and a case-fatality rate of 0.43%.[2,3] More than 70% of victims are male, and snakebites occurring in the 15- to 49-year age bracket are often occupational.

Four genera are of medical importance in South America: *Bothrops*, which causes about 90% of snakebites; *Crotalus*, which causes approximately 8%; *Lachesis*, which causes 1.4%; and *Micrurus*, which causes 0.4%.[2,4–10] Certain species of the family Colubridae rarely cause bites and are generally harmless.

Identification of the poisonous snake and its genus is a crucial determinant of proper treatment of the bite. Some key differentiating features of the poisonous South American snakes are presented in Figure 109-1. In the likely circumstance that the snake is not available for identification, differential diagnosis may be obtained from certain characteristic clinical features (Fig. 109-2).[11] In addition, the patient's sera may contain antibodies to venom, which may be identified by immunoassays. These methods often may be confounding, however, or yield false-negative results.

Most of the knowledge of treating poisonous snakes in South America comes from accumulated clinical experience. Few controlled studies exist. The recommendations given in this chapter represent a consensus among regional authorities of the appropriate clinical approach.

GENERAL TREATMENT

General treatment measures include the following:[11]

1. Reassure and keep the patient as calm and comfortable as possible.
2. Ensure adequate vascular access.
3. Immobilize the affected limb, cleaning it lightly to remove the surface venom; avoid tampering with the wound or applying any form of pressure.
4. Never apply tourniquets or constricting bands because most South American snakebites are caused by members of the genus *Bothrops* (Fig. 109-3) and are associated with major limb swelling. Avoid suctioning and local incisions because most *Bothrops* wounds can cause bleeding.
5. Transport the patient as quickly as possible to a facility or hospital that stocks antivenom.
6. Monitor vital signs and extent and progression of local swelling, bleeding, and level of consciousness.
7. Provide aggressive supportive care for medical complications, including volume replacement and head-down tilt for syncope or fainting, ventilatory support for respiratory failure, and analgesics for pain (dipyrone, opioids, paracetamol; avoid salicylates).
8. Administer antivenom if available and warranted by the patient's clinical condition. Observe precautions when administering immunotherapy (antivenom) as described in Chapters 101 and 135.

Antivenoms in Latin America are generally of equine origin and composed of whole immunoglobulins. Most come lyophilized.

BOTHROPS

Snakes of the genus *Bothrops* (Fig. 109-4), which belong to the family Viperidae, are responsible for more than 80% of all snakebites in Latin America and for 90% in Brazil. Twenty species are distributed over the continent, mainly in the plateaus and lowlands, often close to water. They are popularly known as *jararaca, jararacuçu, cotiara, urutu, caiçara,* and *surucucurana.* The snake is characterized by the facial pit between the nostril and eye. The tail does not have rattles or raised scales.

Mechanism of Venom Action

The venom from *Bothrops* has the following activities:

1. *Lytic and inflammatory:* The lesions are caused by the activity of proteases, hyaluronidases, phospholipases, and proinflammatory factors. These produce swelling, hyperemia, vesicles, and tissue necrosis.

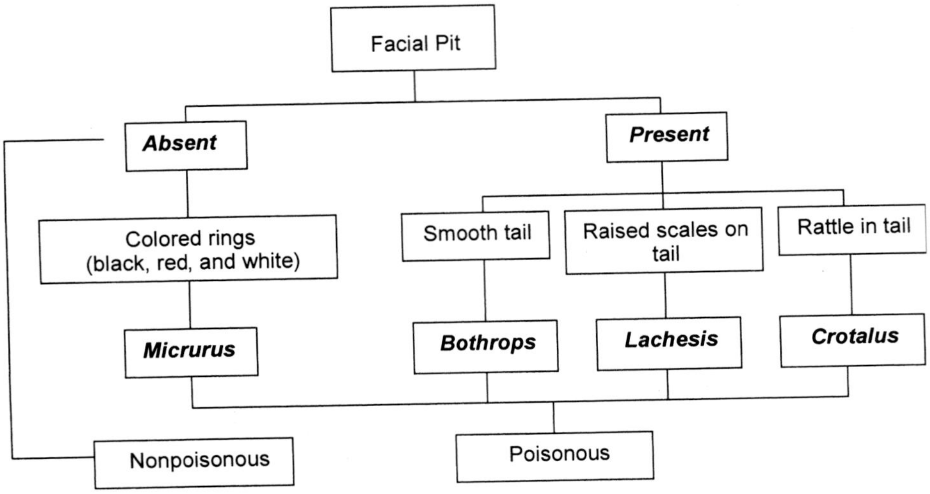

Facial Pit

Absent

Present

Colored rings
(black, red, and white)

Smooth tail

Raised scales on
tail

Rattle in tail

Micrurus

Bothrops

Lachesis

Crotalus

Nonpoisonous

Poisonous

FIGURE 109-1

Identification of poisonous snakes. False coral snakes may present the same color pattern as *Micrurus* but are toothless. Some true coral snakes do not have red rings.

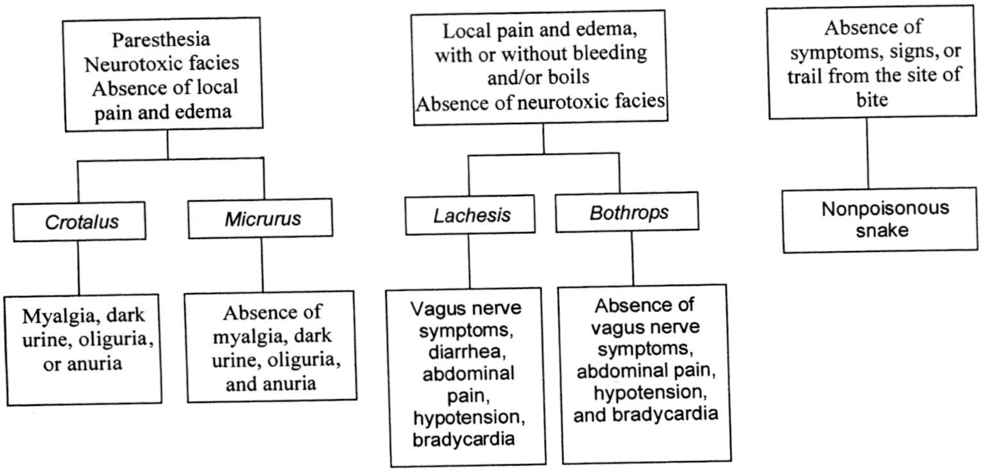

Paresthesia
Neurotoxic facies
Absence of local
pain and edema

Local pain and edema,
with or without bleeding
and/or boils
Absence of neurotoxic facies

Absence of
symptoms, signs, or
trail from the site of
bite

Crotalus

Micrurus

Lachesis

Bothrops

Nonpoisonous
snake

Myalgia, dark
urine, oliguria,
or anuria

Absence of
myalgia, dark
urine, oliguria,
and anuria

Vagus nerve
symptoms,
diarrhea,
abdominal
pain,
hypotension,
bradycardia

Absence of
vagus nerve
symptoms,
abdominal pain,
hypotension,
and bradycardia

FIGURE 109-2

Differential diagnosis of poisonous snakebites.

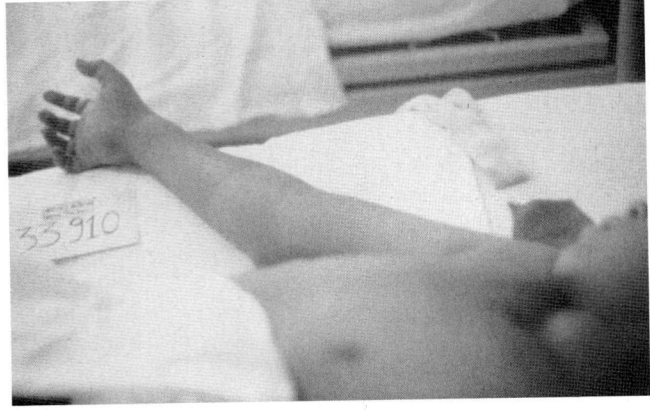

FIGURE 109-3

The right arm has a clear tourniquet mark, following a *Bothrops* bite.

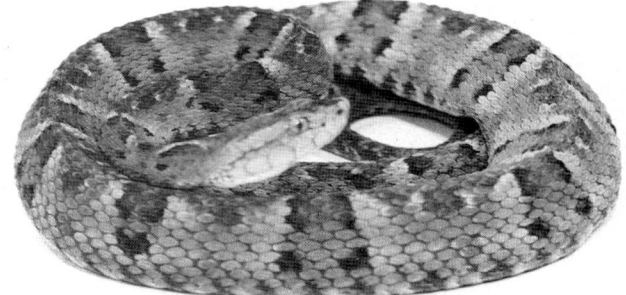

FIGURE 109-4

Bothrops jararaca. Note facial pit and smooth tail.

2. *Cardiovascular collapse:* Cardiovascular effects of the venom of *Bothrops jararaca* allowed the pioneering discovery of bradykinin by Rocha-e-Silva and colleagues[12] and of captopril by Ferreirra.[13]

3. *Coagulant: Bothrops* venom causes disseminated intravascular coagulation with activation of factor X, prothrombin, and fibrinogen and decreased concentration of factors V and VIII and platelets.[14,15]

4. *Hemorrhagic:* The action of hemorrhagins, which damage the basal membrane of the endothelium, promoting clotting and platelet consumption and tissue damage, may lead to coagulopathy.[16]

5. *Nephrotoxic:* A direct effect of the venom on the renal vascular bed, in addition to the formation of microthrombi, may cause acute renal failure and occurs in 13.8% of *Bothrops* bites. Acute tubular necrosis, renal cortical necrosis, and interstitial nephritis have been reported.[17,18]

Clinical Presentation

LOCAL

Local effects include pain of variable intensity; bleeding; and early and progressive edema affecting the whole limb, which may evolve to bullae, ecchymoses, tissue necrosis, and regional lymphadenopathy (Fig. 109-5).[19,20]

SYSTEMIC

Systemic effects include cardiovascular collapse and severe coagulopathy, with bleeding gums, epistaxis, hematuria, hematemesis, and intense bleeding from preexisting wounds. The severity of bleeding is directly related not to the hemorrhagins, but to the amount of inoculated venom and other factors, such as kinins, cytokines, and lectins. Intense bleeding is an infrequent occurrence.[21]

Treatment

General treatment of *Bothrops* envenomation includes elevation of the limb to reduce swelling, antivenom administration, local wound care, aggressive systemic fluid volume replacement, and monitoring of vital signs and urinary output. Local fasciotomy to avoid the compartment syndrome, which occurs in 1.4% of patients (Fig. 109-6); drainage or débridement of abscesses; and antitetanus vaccine should be considered. Constrictive bands and tourniquets should never be used. If they are used, extreme caution is required

for their removal to avoid sudden release of vasoactive factors and consequent shock.

It is possible that early administration of antivenom may reduce swelling and obviate the need for fasciotomy; this has not been studied, however. Our recommendations for specific treatment are based on a severity scale (Table 109-1).[11] The general management of snakebites is discusssed in Chapter 101.

GRADING

Grading of severity of snakebites is as follows:

1. *Minimal:* Mild local swelling, normal or slightly elevated clotting time (<12 minutes), and absence of systemic symptoms. Treatment is intravenous (if possible) administration of four vials of specific polyvalent anti-*Bothrops* antiserum or the combined anti-*Bothrops*/anti-*Crotalus* antiserum.
2. *Moderate:* Evident signs of progressive local swelling and possibly local hemorrhage, altered clotting time (<20 minutes), and absence of systemic symptoms. Treatment is administration of eight vials of the specific or the combined antiserum.
3. *Severe:* Intense local swelling and hemorrhage, oliguria or anuria, prolonged clotting time, or noncoagulable blood. Treatment is administration of 12 vials of the specific or the combined antiserum.

In all grades of severity, four additional vials may be given if signs of envenomation are not reversed or clotting does not return to normal.

PROGNOSIS

Death from envenomation has decreased from greater than 8% to less than 0.3% of the treated cases; better surgical

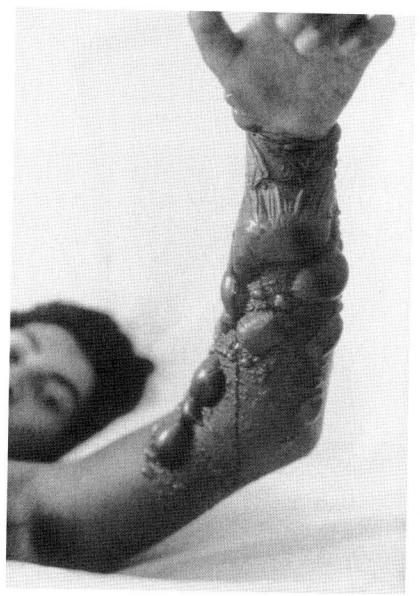 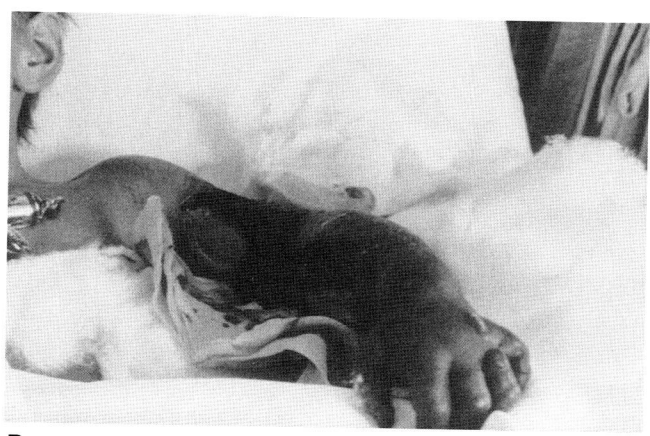

A   B

FIGURE 109-5

Severe lesions from a tourniquet, where the *Bothrops* venom has accumulated. **A,** Blood-filled boils. **B,** Intense tissue necrosis has ensued.

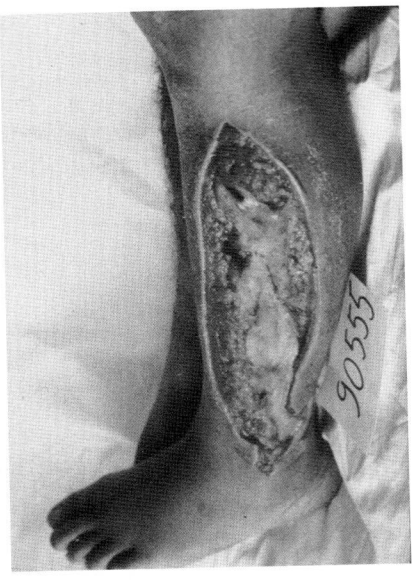 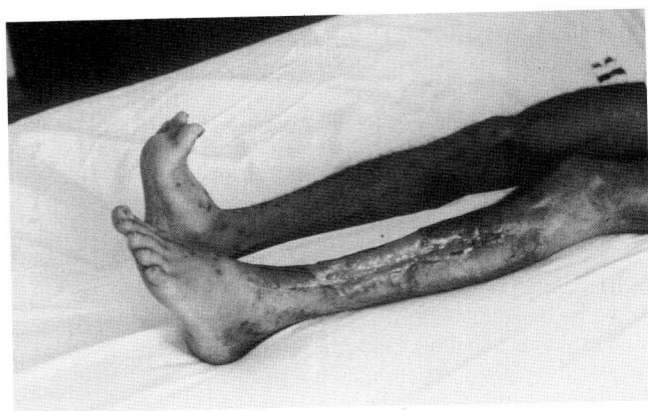

A   B

FIGURE 109-6

A, Fasciotomy of left leg to relieve pressure. **B,** The wound has closed, with satisfactory healing.

treatment and wider distribution of updated antivenom have contributed to the decreased mortality. Complications and sequelae, including affected limb dysfunction from inadequate treatment, are common. Elderly patients are especially prone to intracranial hemorrhage.[17]

LACHESIS

Snakes of the *Lachesis* genus, also called *bushmaster*, are considered to be among the largest snakes, measuring 3.7 to 4 m long. Locally, they are popularly known as *surucuçu, pico de jaca*, and *surucutinga* (Fig. 109-7). Envenomations due to *Lachesis* represent only 1.4% of the recorded snakebites in South America; there are fewer of these snakes than others, and they are less widespread geographically.[23]

Mechanism of Venom Action

The symptoms from *Lachesis* envenomations are similar to those due to *Bothrops* except that the venom seems to be more potent and is associated with additional neurotoxic

symptoms. The active components of the venom are as follows:

1. *Proteolytic:* Proteases cause cellular necrosis and vascular damage.
2. *Hemorrhagic:* The effect of hemorrhagins appears to be rapid because extensive ecchymoses, intense bleeding, and bloody vesicles are present within 5 hours.
3. *Coagulant:* The consumption of factors X, VI, and VIII and increased levels of thrombin and fibrin degradation products combined with thrombocytopenia may lead to clinically significant coagulopathy.
4. *Neurotoxic:* A specific neurotoxin has not been identified. There is parasympathetic stimulation with marked cardiovascular effects (see later).

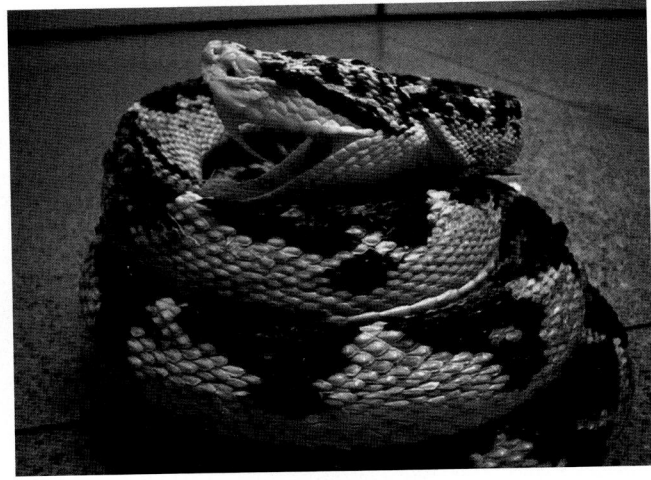

FIGURE 109-7

Lachesis spp. Note the characteristic diamond shapes and raised scales.

CLINICAL EFFECT	CLASSIFICATION		
	Mild	*Moderate*	*Severe*
Clotting time	Normal or <12 min	Normal or >12 min	>20 min
Local	Discrete	Evident	Intense
Systemic	Absent	Absent	Present

TABLE 109-1 Severity Scale of *Bothrops* Accidents

Clinical Presentation

Symptoms appear earlier and with greater intensity after *Lachesis* envenomation than with *Bothrops* and are characterized according to two grades of envenomation severity: moderate and severe (Table 109-2).

LOCAL

Intense pain and progressive edema at the envenomation site of the bite appear within 1 to 2 hours after the bite. Extensive ecchymoses, bleeding, and blebs and bullae containing serous-bloody fluid appear within 5 hours.

SYSTEMIC

The systemic signs and symptoms are similar to those of *Bothrops* envenomation but are more severe. Increased clotting time and coagulopathy develop in a shorter time frame. Tachycardia, hypotension, intense vomiting, diarrhea, colicky pain, headaches, faintness, blurred vision, anxiety, and confusion are indications of greater severity. Cardiovascular effects, including marked bradycardia, may occur within 15 minutes, as opposed to a *Bothrops* envenomation, in which cardiovascular effects appear approximately 10 hours later. Hypovolemia and hemorrhage, including gastrointestinal bleeding, may aggravate bradycardia. Increased hematocrit, creatine phosphokinase, and transaminases (alanine aminotransferase and aspartate aminotransferase) are expected.

Treatment

Envenomation by *Lachesis* is generally more serious than envenomation by *Bothrops*.[11] Snake identification is crucial, and treatment, including the administration of *Lachesis*-specific antivenom, should be aggressive and based on the severity assessment. Specific anti-*Bothrops* serum has been used for these snakes but has been shown to be generally ineffective. Besides the general treatments indicated earlier for *Bothrops* bites, additional measures include atropine sulfate for bradycardia, antispasmodics for colicky pain, and vasopressors when necessary.

MODERATE

With moderate severity of envenomation, when local symptoms are present, discrete and systemic symptoms are absent or mild, and the clotting time is elevated (<30 minutes), the generally accepted recommendation is to administer at least 10 vials of the specific anti-*Lachesis* or the combined anti-*Bothrops*/anti-*Lachesis* antivenom.

SEVERE

In severe envenomation, when local symptoms are intense, systemic symptoms are present, and the blood is nearly incoagulable, generally at least 20 vials of the specific or the combined antivenom should be administered. The precautions that apply to the administration of antivenoms to snakebite victims are discussed in Chapters 101 and 135.

CROTALUS

Bites due to the South American rattlesnake (Fig. 109-8), popularly called *cascavel*, are relatively uncommon, but mortality can be 72% in untreated cases. Treated patients have a mortality of less than 2%.[24,25] The snake measures 0.5 to 1.5 m long, with the characteristic rattle in the tail. There are 26 species of *Crotalus*, 24 of which are in Mexico; only 2 are in the rest of Latin America. In South America, *Crotalus durissus* predominates, of which there are at least five subspecies of medical importance. They are widely distributed throughout the continent (Fig. 109-9), inhabiting the higher elevations in the more arid regions, but *C. durissus* bites in rare cases may occur in the coastal areas.

Mechanism of Venom Action

Poisoning by the South American rattlesnake differs in some respects from its North and Central American cousins. Generally the effects of the venom are as follows.

NEUROTOXIC

The high lethality of Latin American *Crotalus* spp. is mainly due to crotoxin, which blocks acetylcholine release, causing neuromuscular blockade and consequent paralysis, with paresis in the distribution of cranial nerves III, IV, and VI and peripheral somatic motor nerves. Paresthesias may occur.

MYOTOXIC

Local muscular lesions may be caused by crotamine and crotoxin. The portion of the venom that causes systemic myotoxic effects has not yet been identified but is assumed to be responsible for severe effects, such as rhabdomyolysis, with elevation of serum levels of myoglobin and creatine

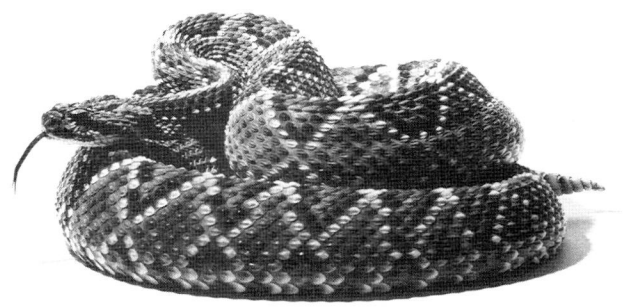

FIGURE 109-8

Crotalus durissus with the characteristic rattle.

CLINICAL EFFECT	CLASSIFICATION	
	Moderate	*Severe*
Clotting time	>12 min	>20 min
Local	Mild or evident	Intense
Systemic	Absent or present	Present

TABLE 109-2 Severity Scale of *Lachesis* Accidents

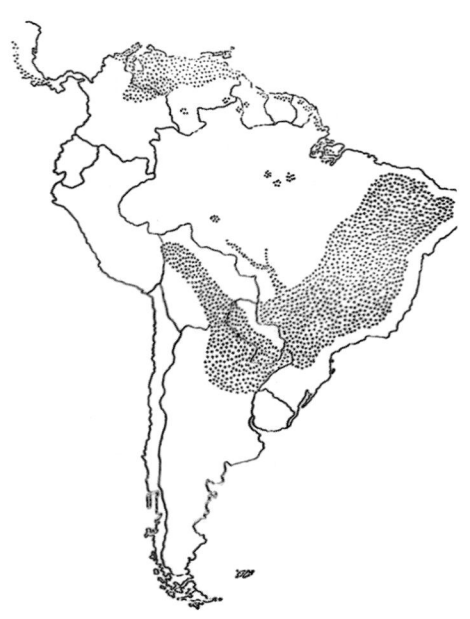

FIGURE 109-9

Geographic distribution of the South American rattlesnake (*Crotalus durissus*).

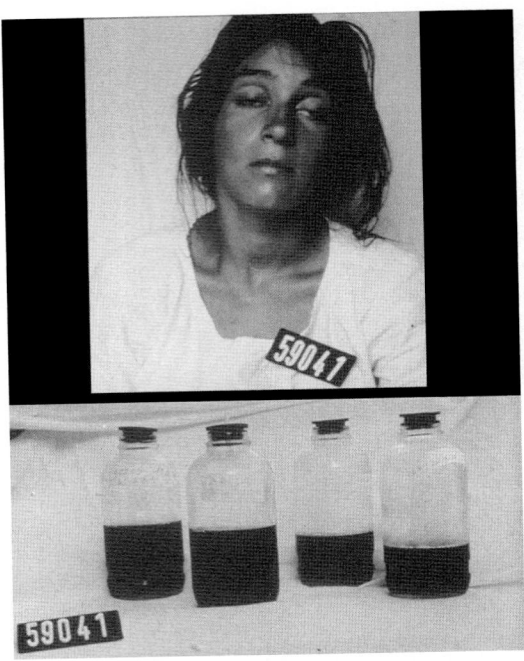

FIGURE 109-10

Woman after a bite by a South American rattlesnake (*Crotalus durissus*). Note the neurotoxic facies with ptosis and dark urine (myoglobinuria).

phosphokinase and consequent myoglobinuria and acute renal failure.[26] In contrast, envenomation by *C. durissus* from Central America has not been reported to result in acute renal failure because its venom does not cause rhabdomyolysis.[27]

COAGULANT

The activation of thrombin converts fibrinogen to fibrin but causes only moderate coagulopathy. The platelet count is typically nearly unchanged.

Clinical Presentation

LOCAL

Local effects are generally of mild intensity, with little or no pain, paresthesias, edema, and erythema.

SYSTEMIC

Systemic effects are generally the most important manifestations. Patients may have general malaise, nausea, vomiting, intense prostration, profuse sweating, restlessness, and hypotension. Neurologic manifestations, such as palpebral ptosis, myasthenic facies, ocular paralysis, mydriasis, blurred vision, and diplopia, usually appear within 6 hours. Paralysis of the velopalatine muscles, causing dysphagia, decreased gag reflex, and altered sense of smell and taste, and generalized muscle pain and acute respiratory failure also may be present.

About 40% of the patients have a coagulation disorder, which is usually mild and restricted clinically to bleeding of the gums. The most serious complication is acute renal failure from myoglobinuria and a direct nephrotoxic effect of the venom,[28] with oliguria and anuria in the first 48 hours (Fig. 109-10).

LABORATORY TESTS

Laboratory findings usually include hypocalcemia and elevation in serum creatine phosphokinase, lactic dehydrogenase, alanine aminotransferase, aspartate aminotransferase, aldolase, blood urea nitrogen, creatinine, uric acid, potassium, and phosphorus. Complete blood counts usually show leukocytosis, with neutrophilia and normal or slightly decreased platelets. Urinalysis may indicate proteinuria and myoglobinuria. Immunologic identification of the circulating venom using enzyme-linked immunosorbent assay and of a muscle biopsy specimen may be helpful, especially in distinguishing an acute myocardial infarction from a crotalic accident.

TREATMENT

General treatment includes sedation and reassurance of the patient.[11] Intravenous hydration is generally given to maintain a urinary output of at least 1 to 2 mL/kg/hr in children and 30 to 40 mL/hr in adults. Furosemide or mannitol or both may be necessary to achieve this output objective. Urinary pH should be kept alkaline (pH >7.0) because acid urine precipitates myoglobin in the tubules, increasing its nephrotoxic effect. If acute renal failure is severe, peritoneal dialysis or hemodialysis may be necessary.

Specific treatment is a key determinant of outcome and involves prompt administration of antivenom.[11] The clinical effects of South American *Crotalus* spp. may be graded as mild, moderate, or severe (Table 109-3). Specific anticrotalic antivenom should be given intravenously, but the combined anti-*Bothrops*/anti-*Crotalus* antivenom may be a suitable substitute.

TABLE 109-3 Severity Scale of *Crotalus* Accidents			
CLINICAL EFFECT	**CLASSIFICATION**		
	Mild	*Moderate*	*Severe*
Neurotoxicity	Absent or late	Discrete	Evident
Myalgia	Absent or discrete	Discrete	Intense
Dark urine	Absent	Absent or discrete	Evident
Oliguria/anuria	Absent	Absent	Absent or present
Clotting time	Normal or prolonged	Normal or prolonged	Normal or prolonged

In mild or moderate envenomations, 10 vials, which neutralize 150 mg of venom, should be administered. In severe cases, 20 vials are necessary. The antivenom serum should be diluted in 250 mL of saline or 5% dextrose and infused as rapidly as possible. In children weighing less than 10 kg, caution should be observed to avoid volume overload.

PROGNOSIS

Complications from acute renal failure and transient acute respiratory insufficiency are most likely to occur in patients treated late or inadequately. Outcome is usually favorable in patients treated within 6 hours.

MICRURUS

Elapidae are represented by the genus *Micrurus* and are popularly called *coral snakes*. Bites in humans by *Micrurus* are rare in Brazil, representing less than 1% of reported cases. They are widely distributed, from the southern United States to Argentina, but with no characteristic geographic distribution.

These snakes are usually less than 1 m long and characterized by brightly colored rings, mostly red or orange, black, and white or yellow (Fig. 109-11). In contrast to what is seen in North America (see Chapter 103), there is no clear relationship between the pattern of the ring colors and whether the snake is poisonous. The head is round, with a small mouth and no facial pit. Their habits are nocturnal. Generally, these snakes are not aggressive and attack only when threatened.

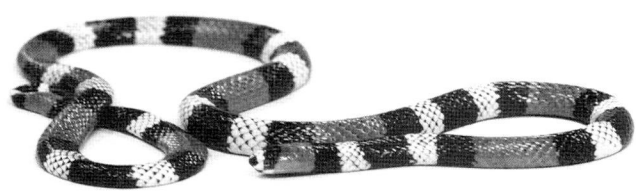

FIGURE 109-11

A true coral snake (*Micrurus*).

Mechanism of Venom Action

The toxins from Elapidae have a low molecular weight and are absorbed rapidly. Their action is generally of rapid onset and limited to neurotoxic effects. Direct proteolytic, hemorrhagic, coagulant, or nephrotoxic effects have not been identified. The neurotoxins block nicotinic transmission at the myoneural junction, by a presynaptic or postsynaptic (depending on the species) action.[29,30]

The presynaptic neurotoxins have a molecular weight of 12 to 60 kd, with phospholipase activity, and act on the presynaptic nerve terminal, preventing acetylcholine release into the neuromuscular junction. Most species of the Brazilian coral snakes have postsynaptic neurotoxins with a molecular weight of only 6 to 14 kd, without any enzymatic action. The toxins act competitively to cause nondepolarizing blockade of nicotinic cholinergic receptors of the postsynaptic membranes of the neuromuscular junction, in a manner similar to curare. Only *Micrurus corallinus* has been shown to have a presynaptic action.[29,30]

Clinical Manifestations

LOCAL

Pain, swelling, and other signs of the bite are limited or even absent.

SYSTEMIC

The characteristic signs are flaccid paralysis of the facial musculature, arms and legs, and respiratory muscles, causing blepharoptosis, ophthalmoplegia, dysphagia, drooling, pseudomyasthenia, and respiratory difficulties. Paresthesias, muscle fasciculation, somnolence, euphoria, confusion, dizziness, nausea, and vomiting are common. If the patient is untreated, death from respiratory failure usually occurs within 6 hours.

Treatment

Because of the swiftness and potency of the toxins, all cases with even minimal symptoms should be considered an extreme medical emergency. Prompt and aggressive treatment of Elapidae bites is mandatory because death may occur rapidly in untreated cases.

Pharmacologic treatment includes use of neostigmine (dose 0.05 mg/kg in children and 0.5 mg in adults), preceded by atropine sulfate (same dose), for clinical effects of postsynaptic neuromuscular block. Use of neostigmine and atropine also may prove diagnostic in distinguishing a presynaptic acting venom from a postsynaptic acting venom. The response is expected to be swift, with marked improvement within 10 minutes, and maintenance doses may be required for 24 hours. Antibiotics and tetanus prophylaxis also may be indicated.

Specific treatment is mandatory in all suspected cases of poisonous coral snake envenomations due to the severity of the outcome. Ten vials of the specific anti-Elapidae antiserum (which neutralizes 150 mg of toxin), diluted in 5% dextrose or saline, are given by intravenous infusion to adults and children alike in 20 to 60 minutes, not exceeding 8 to 12 mL/min.[31] Care to avoid fluid overload should be observed, especially in patients with cardiorespiratory signs.

PROGNOSIS

The outcome is good in adequately treated cases, and patients usually recover without sequelae. If the patient is untreated, death usually ensues.

REFERENCES

1. Fan HW, Cardoso JLC: Clinical toxicology of snakebites in South America. In Meier J, White J (eds): Handbook of Clinical Toxicology of Animal Venoms and Poisons. New York, CRC Press, 1995, pp 667–688.
2. Ministério da Saúde (Brasil), Ofidismo: Análises Epidemiológicas. Brasília-DF, Brasil, 1991.
3. Jorge MT, Ribeiro LA: Acidentes por animais peçonhentos no Brasil. Rev Assoc Med Bras 36:66–77, 1990.
4. Silva JJ: Las serpientes del genero Bothrops en la Amazonia colombiana. Acta Med Colomb 14:148–165, 1989.
5. Esteso SC: Ofidismo en la Republica Argentina. Cordoba, Argentina, Editorial Arpón, 1985.
6. Angel Mejia R: Serpientes de Colombia: Su relacion con el hombre. Medellin, Secretaria de Educacíon y Cultura de Antioquia, 1987.
7. Kerrigan KR: Venomous snakebites in Eastern Ecuador. Am J Trop Med Hyg 44:93–99, 1991.
8. Chippaux JP: Les serpents de la Guyane française. Collection Faune Tropicale XXVII, 1986.
9. Purtscher H, Burger M, Savio E, et al: Ofidismo e aracnidismo en el Uruguay. Rev Med Uruguay 7:1–37, 1983.
10. Parra MAA, La Rosa CC, Castillo FE, et al: Ofidismo en Venezuela. Valencia, Venezuela, Alpha Impressores, 1987.
11. Ministério da Saúde (Brasil): Manual de Diagnóstico e Tratamento dos Acidentes Ofídicos. Brasília-DF, Brasil, 1987.
12. Rocha-e-Silva M, Beraldo WT, Rosenfeld G: Bradykinin: A hypotensive and smooth muscle stimulating factor released from plasma globulin by snake venom and by trypsin. Am J Physiol 156:261–273, 1949.
13. Ferreirra SH: A bradykinin-potentiating factor (BPF) present in the venom of Bothrops jararaca. Br J Pharmacol Chemother 24:163–169, 1965.
14. Maruyama M, Kamiguti AS, Cardoso JLC, et al: Studies on blood coagulation and fibrinolysis in patients bitten by Bothrops jararaca. Thromb Haemost 63:449–453, 1990.
15. Sano-Martins IS, Santoro M, Castro SCB, et al: Platelet aggregation in patients bitten by the Brazilian snake Bothrops jararaca. Thromb Res 87:183–195, 1997.
16. Kamiguti AS, Rugman FP, Theakston RDG, et al: The role of venom haemorrhagin in spontaneous bleeding in Bothrops jararaca envenoming. Thromb Haemost 67:484–488, 1992.
17. Amaral CF, da Silva OA, Goody P, et al: Renal cortical necrosis following Bothrops jararaca and Bothrops jararacussu snake bite. Toxicon 23:877–885, 1985.
18. Burdmann EA, Cardoso JLC, Barcelos MAF: Insuficiência renal aguda por acidente ofídico. Rev Soc Bras Med Trop 20(Suppl):56, 1987.
19. Ribeiro LA, Jorge MT: Epidemiologia e quadro clínico dos acidentes por serpentes Bothrops jararaca adultas e filhotes. Rev Inst Med Trop São Paulo 32:436–442, 1990.
20. Nishioka SA, Silveira PVP: A clinical and epidemiological study of 292 cases of lance-headed viper bite in a Brazilian teaching hospital. Am J Trop Med Hyg 47:805–810, 1992.
21. França FOS, Málaque CMS: Acidente botrópico. In Cardoso JLC, França FOS, Fan HW, et al (eds): Animais Peçonhentos no Brasil: Biologia, Clínica e Terapêutica dos Acidentes. São Paulo, Sarvier, 2003, pp 72–86.
22. Kouyoumdjian JA, Polizelli C, Lobo SMA, et al: Fatal extradural haematoma after snakebite (Bothrops moojeni). Trans R Soc Trop Med Hyg 85:552, 1991.
23. Jorge MT, Sano-Martins IS, Ferrari RS, et al: Envenoming by Lachesis muta in Brazil. Toxicon 31:140–141, 1993.
24. A ação do Ministério da Saúde no controle dos acidentes ofídicos em âmbito nacional. Brasília, 1987 (mimeo).
25. Manual de Diagnóstico e Tratamento dos Acidentes por Animais Peçonhentos. Brasília, Ministério da Saúde, Fundação Nacional de Saúde, 1998.
26. Azevedo-Marques MM, Cupo P, Hering SE: Evidence that Crotalus durissus terrificus (South American rattlesnake) envenomation in humans causes myolysis rather than hemolysis. Toxicon 11:1163–1168, 1987.
27. Gutiérrez JM: Clinical toxicology of snakebites in Central America. In Meier J, White J (eds): Handbook of Clinical Toxicology of Animal Venoms and Poisons. New York, CRC Press, 1995, p 653.
28. Azevedo-Marques MM, Cupo P, Coimbra TM, et al: Myonecrosis, myoglobinuria and acute renal failure induced by South American rattlesnake (Crotalus durissus terrificus) envenomation in Brazil. Toxicon 23:631–636, 1985.
29. Vital Brazil O: Coral snake venoms: Mode of action and pathophysiology of experimental envenomation. Rev Inst Med Trop São Paulo 29:119–126, 1987.
30. Gutiérrez JM, Rojas G, da Silva JN Jr, et al: Experimental myonecrosis induced by the venoms of South American Micrurus (coral snakes). Toxicon 30:1299–1302, 1992.
31. Silva NJ Jr, Bucaretchi F: Mecanismo de ação do veneno elapídico e aspectos clínicos dos acidentes. In Cardoso JLC, França FOS, Fan HW, et al (eds): Animais Peçonhentos no Brasil: Biologia, Clínica e Terapêutica dos Acidentes. São Paulo, Sarvier, 2003, pp 99–107.

CHAPTER **110**

Overview of Spider Envenoming

Julian White

Spiders are ubiquitous arthropod predators, common in all habitats occupied by humans, including modern urban environments. They may achieve high population densities—greater than 1 million per hectare. Their primary interaction with humans is beneficial, as they act as biologic controls for arthropod pests, notably insects. Their medical interaction with humans is relatively minor, in comparison, but still significant because of the extent of exposure to risk.

EXTENT OF SPIDER BITE AS A MEDICAL PROBLEM

There are no accurate figures on which to gauge the global extent of spider bite. Logically, given the large numbers of spiders living in proximity to humans, bites should be common, but because most spiders are small and unlikely to inject more than miniscule quantities of venom compared with average human body mass, most bites could be expected to be trivial. Many spiders coexisting with humans are moderate to large in size, however, and at least a few of these are known to cause significant envenoming. When spider bite is considered by the human population and a venue is provided to seek advice about bites, experience in Australia suggests that bites are reported frequently. Spider bite has been the most common or second most common cause of calls to Australian poison information centers at least since 1995, usually eclipsing every pharmaceutical class, including paracetamol/acetaminophen. When consciousness of spider bite is lower or the expectation that health services can assist is not present, it can be expected that the recorded incidence of cases will be lower, underestimating the extent of spider bite incidence.

MEDICALLY IMPORTANT SPIDERS

A few spider groups or effects of spider bite stand out as clinically important (Table 110-1). Many other spiders occasionally or rarely have been reported to bite humans, although mostly with minor effects (Table 110-2). The former groups, few in number but global in extent, dominate the medical problem posed by spider bite. In Brazil,

despite a vast spider fauna, virtually all medically important spider bites are due to just three groups: banana spiders (genus *Phoneutria*—phoneutrism [Fig. 110-1]), recluse or violin spiders (genus *Loxosceles*—loxoscelism [Fig. 110-2]), and widow spiders (genus *Latrodectus*—latrodectism [Fig. 110-3]). In North America, widow spiders and recluse spiders also are responsible for most significant bites. In Europe, Africa, Asia, and Australia, widow spiders are an important source of spider bite, whereas recluse spiders also cause significant problems in parts of Africa, Europe, and possibly Australia. In Australia, widow spider envenoming occasions more use of antivenom than all other causes of envenoming combined (including snakes), a remarkable finding, given that continent's diverse, common, and highly toxic fauna. Another group of spiders also is of great relevance in Australia: the funnel-web spiders (*Atrax* and *Hadronyche* spp. [Figs. 110-4 and 110-5]), the most toxic of all the world's spiders (not to be confused with North American funnel-web spiders, which are quite different and of minor importance medically).

SPIDER TAXONOMY

Spider taxonomy is complex, and differentiating to species generally requires great expertise and the use of a microscope because it frequently involves detailed examination of male external genital organs. Most spider species are yet to receive formal scientific description and naming. Scientists undertaking this task are few in number. Although previously described common spiders were thought to belong to a single taxon, more recent research indicates that numerous species exist. This profusion of species and difficulty in assigning accurate nomenclature has ensured that the medical literature on spider bites and spider venom research is replete with inaccuracies that muddy understanding of this field.

Mygalomorphs

Order Mygalomorphae, along with the Araneomorphae (see later), currently contains most living spider species. Mygalomorphs are considered more ancient or primitive than araneomorph spiders, but neither group is recent, for spiders date back hundreds of millions of years. The basic

TABLE 110-1 Spider Groups of Major Medical Importance

SPIDER GROUP	COMMON NAME	DISTRIBUTION	CLINICAL EFFECTS
Mygalomorphae *Atrax* and *Hadronyche* spp.	Funnel-web spiders	Australia	Excitatory neurotoxic effects, catecholamine storm, potentially lethal
Araneomorphae *Latrodectus* spp.	Widow spiders	Global	Latrodectism: excitatory neurotoxic effects, pain, malaise, rarely lethal
Phoneutria spp.	Banana spiders	Brazil	Phoneutrism: excitatory neurotoxic effects, pain, malaise, rarely lethal
Loxosceles spp.	Recluse spiders	Global	Loxoscelism: local tissue necrosis, rarely major systemic effects, shock, hemolysis, DIC, occasionally fatal
Nonspecific	Various	Global	Necrotic arachnidism: spider bite resulting in local necrosis

DIC, disseminated intravascular coagulation.

TABLE 110-2 All Spiders Known to Cause Effects on Biting*

FAMILY	SCIENTIFIC NAME	COMMON NAME	DISTRIBUTION
Mygalomorphs			
Ctenizidae	*Aganippe*	Trapdoor spider	Australia
	Arabantis spp.	Trapdoor spider	Australia, East Indies
	Bothricyrtum spp.	Trapdoor spider	California
	Dyarcyops	Trapdoor spider	Australia, New Zealand
	Ummidia spp.	Trapdoor spider	North and Central America
Hexathelidae	*Atrax* spp. and *Hadronyche* spp.	Funnel-web spider	Australia
Theraphosidae	*Harpactirella*	Trapdoor spider	South Africa
	Pamphobetus spp.	Tarantula	South America
	Aphonopelma spp.	Tarantula	North America
	Dugesiella spp.	Tarantula	North America
	Selenocosmia	Tarantula	East Indies, India, Australia
Dipluridae	*Trechona* spp.	Funnel-web spider	Central and South America
Actinopodidae	*Missulena* spp.	Mouse spider	Australia
Araneomorphs			
Agelenidae	*Tegenaria agrestis*		Europe, North America
Araneidae	*Araneus* spp.	Orb weaver	Worldwide
	Argiope spp.	Orb weaver	Worldwide
	Neoscona spp.	Orb weaver	Worldwide
Clubionidae	*Chiracanthium* spp.	Sac spider	Worldwide
	Liocranoides	Running spider	Appalachia and California
	Trachelas spp.	Sac spider	North America
Ctenidae	*Cupiennius* spp.	Banana spider	Central and South America, West Indies
	Elassoctenus harpax	Hunting spider	Australia
	Phoneutria spp.	Banana spider	Central and South America
Desidae (Amaurobiidae)	*Ixeuticus (Badumna)* spp.	House spider	New Zealand, Southern California
Dysderidae	*Dysdera* spp.	Dysderid	Worldwide
Filistatidae	*Filistata* spp.	Hackled band spider	Worldwide
Gnaphosidae	*Drassodes* spp.	Running spider	Worldwide
	Lampona spp.	White-tailed spider	Australia, New Zealand
	Herpyllus spp.	Parson spider	North America

FAMILY	SCIENTIFIC NAME	COMMON NAME	DISTRIBUTION
Loxoscelidae	*Loxosceles* spp.	Recluse spiders	Worldwide
Lycosidae	*Lycosa* spp.	Wolf spiders	Worldwide
Miturgidae	*Miturga* spp.	Miturgid spiders	Australia, New Zealand
Oxyopidae	*Peucetia* spp.	Lynx spider	Worldwide
Salticidae	*Phidippus* spp.	Jumping spider	Worldwide
	Holoplatys spp.	Jumping spider	Australia
	Mopsus spp.	Jumping spider	Australia
	Thiodina spp.	Jumping spider	Americas
Siariidae	*Sicarius* spp.	Six-eyed crab spider	Africa
Sparassidae	*Heteropoda* spp.	Huntsman spiders	Worldwide
	Isopoda spp.	Huntsman spiders	Australia, New Guinea, East Indies
	Olios spp.	Huntsman spiders	Americas, Australia
Theridiidae	*Latrodectus* spp.	Widow spiders	Worldwide
	Achaeranea tepidariorum	Grey house spider	Worldwide
	Steatoda spp.	False black widow	Worldwide
Thomisidae	*Misumenoides* spp.	Crab spider	Americas
Zoridae	*Diallomus* spp.	Zorid spider	Australia

*For most (except those listed in Table 110-1), generally minor clinical effects only.

distinguishing features are shown in Figure 110-6. Mygalomorphs exist in a wide array of habitats globally, varying from small to large sized species, but in general, these are mostly large terrestrial or occasionally arboreal spiders, living most of their lives in web retreats, often a burrow in the ground, usually with traplines radiating from the retreat, such that the spider rarely ventures far from the retreat except to mate. It is generally the male that explores in search of the female, which is at least one reason bites by mygalomorphs are more likely to be caused by male spiders. In some of the most deadly species, notably the Sydney funnel-web spider, the male has venom more toxic to humans than that of the female. This phenomenon is not universal, because in some other funnel-web spiders, the female venom is as toxic as that of the male.

Araneomorphs

Araneomorph spiders, order Araneomorphae, are more diverse in numbers, range of species, size, shape, geographic distribution, and effects on humans. Their fang anatomy also is more diverse than mygalomorphs but can be distinguished from the latter moderately easily in most

cases (see Fig. 110-6). Most medically important spiders fall into just three groups of araneomorphs: widow spiders, recluse spiders, and banana spiders.

SPIDER VENOMS

As with most other venoms, spider venoms are usually complex mixtures of substances, with the most potent toxins being peptides or more complex proteins and generally falling within the class of neuroexcitatory toxins, with similarities in effect, if not structure, to the more potent scorpion toxins. There is an important significant divergence from this characterization—the necrotoxins, which are best characterized from recluse spider venoms but possibly are present much more widely than recluse spiders are.

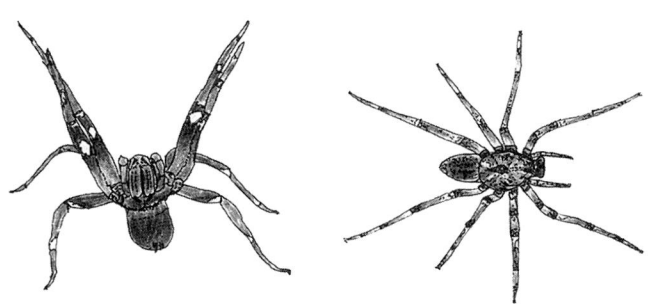

FIGURE 110-1

Banana spider, *Phoneutria nigriventer*. (Copyright © Dr. Julian White, 2001.)

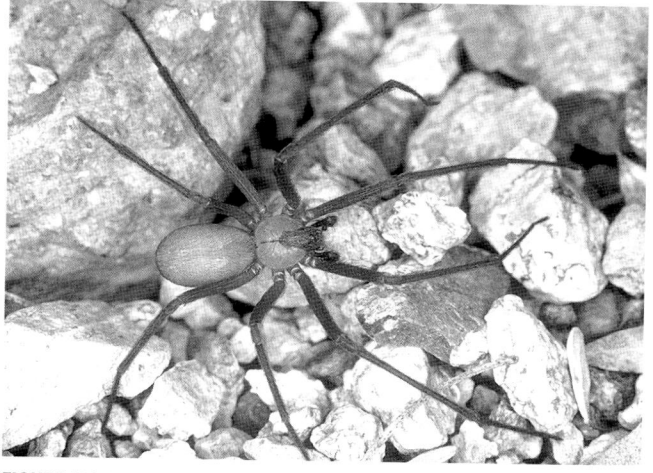

FIGURE 110-2

Recluse spider, *Loxosceles reclusa*. (Copyright © Dr. Julian White, 2001.)

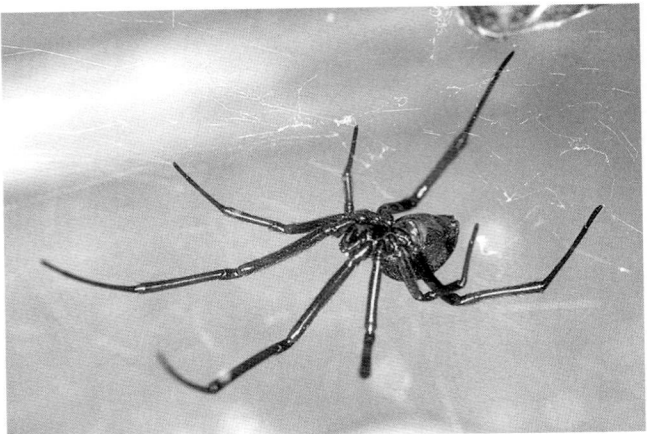

FIGURE 110-3

Female black widow spider, *Latrodectus mactans*. (Copyright © Dr. Julian White, 2001.)

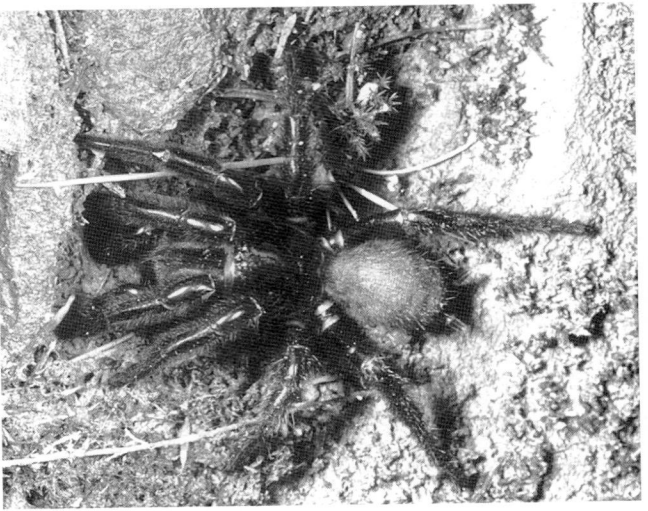

FIGURE 110-5

Female Australian tree funnel-web spider, *Hadronyche formidabilis*. (Copyright © Dr. Julian White, 2001.)

CLINICAL EFFECTS OF SPIDER BITE

The clinical effects of spider bite in humans fall into several broad categories. In most cases and for most spider species, the effects of a bite on humans are negligible. In the few cases and for the few spiders capable of inflicting injury on humans, two distinct patterns are seen: neuroexcitatory envenoming and locally necrotic envenoming. In general, these two patterns do not coexist in the same spider. Even for spiders capable of causing major envenoming in humans, the rate of dry bites is high and probably exceeds 80%. There are many factors affecting what symptoms are likely from a spider bite (Table 110-3).

Local Effects of Envenoming

For most spider species capable of causing a noticeable effect in humans, local pain, usually short-lived, sometimes accompanied by erythema or mild swelling, is the only likely effect. Fang marks may not be apparent and are most likely to be direct punctures, not the minimal lacerations seen with some snakebites (caused by fangs dragging through the skin). Double punctures are likely, mostly close together, depending on the size and type of spider.

A few species cause more notable local effects, such as formation of distinct lumps or even blistering. Fewer still occasionally cause significant local tissue injury. Foremost among the latter are the recluse spiders (see Chapter 112), whose venom contains many toxins that cause tissue necrosis, directly or indirectly. This process may begin soon after the bite but clinically is apparent only after several hours, whereas impending necrosis may take days to become discernible. There is growing, if generally inconclusive, evidence that spiders other than recluse spiders occasionally may cause tissue necrosis. This area has engendered much speculative "science," such as the speculation, raised to the level of "fact" by some, concerning tissue necrosis caused by spiders such as the wandering spider, *Tegenaria agrestis* in North America, and the white-tailed spider, *Lampona cylindrata* in Australia.

General Effects of Envenoming

Some species capable of inflicting short-term local pain or erythema also may cause general systemic symptoms, manifested as one or more of the following: headache, malaise, nausea, vomiting, abdominal pain, flulike illness, or dizziness. The toxins responsible for such symptoms are not characterized, and the effects are generally not indicative of a particular species and so have little diagnostic value. The symptoms generally resolve over a matter of a few hours, less commonly over 1 to 2 days.

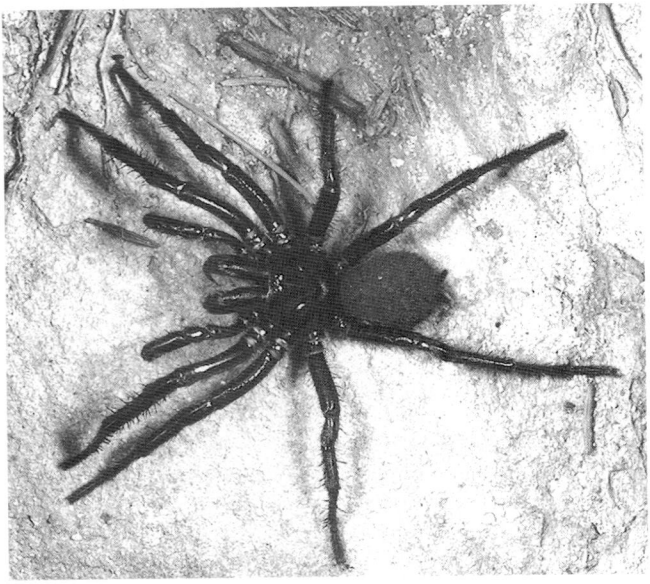

FIGURE 110-4

Male Australian Sydney funnel-web spider, *Atrax robustus*. (Copyright © Dr. Julian White, 2001.)

MYGALOMORPH
SPIDERS

ARANEOMORPH
SPIDERS

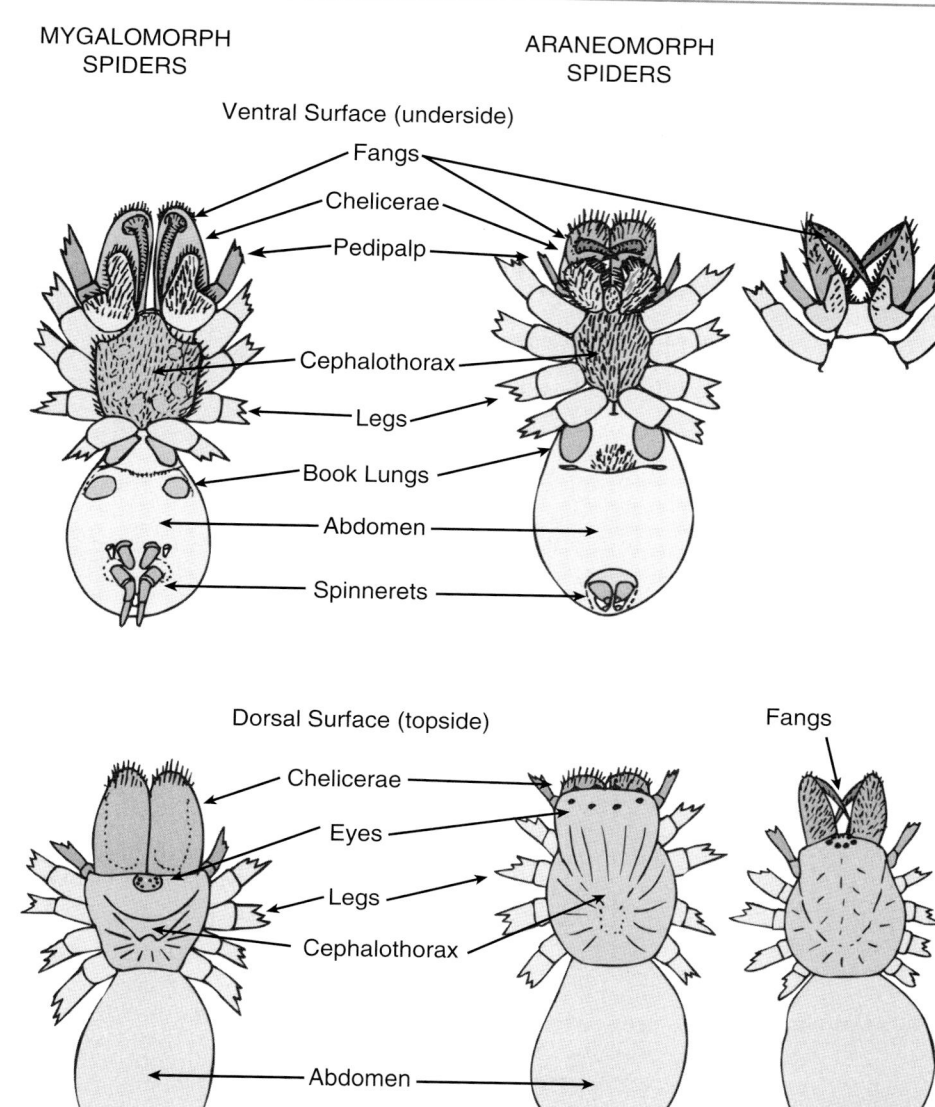

FIGURE 110-6

Diagrammatic representation of the anatomic differences between mygalomorph spiders and araneomorph spiders.

Neuroexcitatory Effects of Envenoming

Major neurologic effects generally are limited to species with potent neuroexcitatory toxins in their venom (widow spiders, banana spiders, Australian funnel-web spiders). Their presentation depends principally on the type of spider. The details of each of these groups are found in Chapters 111 and 113.

Hemolytic and Related Effects of Envenoming

A subset of patients with loxoscelism after recluse spider bite develop major, potentially life-threatening systemic envenoming, in addition to the local necrotic effects typical of these spiders. These systemic effects include hemolysis, disseminated intravascular coagulation, renal failure, shock, liver failure, multiorgan failure, and death. Death occurred in 30% of cases in the early loxoscelism literature from Chile, and fatalities still occur even in North America,

although now rarely. More detailed discussion may be found in Chapter 112.

FIRST AID FOR SPIDER BITE

Spider bite generally requires no first aid other than reassurance. For most of the remaining cases, use of local cold pack application is sufficient. Widow spiders require either no first aid or use of a cold pack. First aid is impractical for recluse spider bites because the bite is generally not apparent until many hours later. Banana spider bites may respond to cold packs.

Australian funnel-web spiders are quite different from the other spiders; funnel-web spider bite is potentially lethal, and correct first aid not only can delay envenoming but also can reduce the extent of envenoming. The reason for the latter is an observation that this venom is destroyed if restricted to the bite site for a prolonged period. The correct first aid is

TABLE 110-3 Spider and Victim Factors Affecting the Likely Symptoms of a Spider Bite

SPECIFIC FACTORS	LIKELY EFFECT OR INFLUENCE
Spider-Related Factors	
Species of spider	Most species of spider are harmless to humans
Sex of the spider	For several species known to be toxic to humans, a specific sex is more toxic (e.g., for widow spiders, only the female is clinically toxic to humans, whereas for Australian funnel-web spiders, both sexes are toxic, but only the male has caused fatalities)
Maturity of the spider	Usually only adult spiders are clinically toxic to humans
Individual spider	As with most other venomous animals, there is likely to be variation in venom components and toxicity between individuals of the same species and even for a given individual spider over time, depending on maturity, when venom was last expelled, and season
Quantity of venom injected	This varies greatly
Attack position	For any given species of spider, fang length is within a narrow range depending on the size of the spider, and angle of attack when biting a human victim determines how effectively the fangs may penetrate skin and inject venom
Gut secretions	For many species of spider, the fang tips at rest are close to the mouth parts, and it is possible that digestive secretions from the mouth may enter the wound caused by the act of biting a human with the fangs, with consequent effects being due to these digestive secretions and the venom. This may be important in causation of some clinically significant local effects of spider bite.
Bacterial flora on the fangs, mouth parts, and adjacent structures	The act of biting a human with a fang has the potential to contaminate the wound with any bacteria on adjacent areas of the spider, with the consequence that clinically significant local effects of the bite may be due at least in part to secondary infection introduced by the act of biting. The bacterial flora on relevant areas of spiders is not known.
Number of times the spider bites the human victim	Multiple bites in general are more likely to result in clinically significant effects
Length of time the spider takes to make each bite	A brief glancing strike in general is less likely to result in clinically significant effects than would occur if the spider "hangs on," taking some time to bite. This is only relative, however, because the toxicity of the spider concerned is of greater importance.
Human Victim–Related Factors	
Age of the human victim	In general, a child or an elderly adult is more likely to suffer clinically significant consequences of a spider bite than a normal healthy adult. This principle is not universal, however. In our experience in Australia with latrodectism (envenoming by widow spiders), often large, muscular men seem worst affected by the bite and require the most antivenom to reverse envenoming.
Size of the victim	In general, the larger the human, the more body mass to dilute any venom and its effects; small children are usually at greater risk (but note above caveat for latrodectism)
Position of the bite	There are some areas of the body where it would be more difficult for a spider to penetrate the skin successfully and inject venom, such as where the skin is thicker or callused. For bites causing local tissue injury, bites on peripheral or dependent areas, such as the feet and lower legs, are more likely to result in problems.
Preexisting health of the victim	Preexisting disease may make the results of any spider bite worse than might be expected in healthy people. Of concern are diseases either decreasing natural immunity to infection or reducing the capacity of local tissue at the bite site to withstand venom effects (e.g., peripheral vascular disease).
Allergic reactions	Individual inappropriate immune responses to venom may result in a far more clinically significant bite than otherwise would occur. This may be an anaphylactic-type reaction, which appears rare with spider bite, or a more localized reaction, which may result in significant and continuing tissue damage. A classic example of atypical local reaction to a bite is the development of pyoderma gangrenosum, which has been associated with loxoscelism.

After White J, Cardoso JL, Fan HW: Clinical toxicology of spider bites. In Meier J, White J (eds): Handbook of Clinical Toxicology of Animal Venoms and Poisons. Boca Raton, FL, CRC Press, 1995.

use of a pressure immobilization bandage and splint (see Chapter 105). Given that death may occur, at least in children, in 10 minutes after the bite, the importance of correct and prompt first aid is obvious.

DIAGNOSIS OF SPIDER BITE

The diagnosis of spider bite is sometimes straightforward, more commonly shrouded in some doubt, and frequently tenuous or uncertain. This situation relates to the ease with which a bite may occur without the culprit's being seen and the delayed nature of envenoming by certain species, notably species causing necrotic arachnidism, such as the recluse spiders. For certain species or groups of spiders, even in the absence of an identifiable specimen or reliable description of the culprit, a diagnosis may be made with some confidence because of the distinctive nature of presentation and symptoms and signs.

Significant envenoming by widow spiders classically is associated with a witnessed bite by a widow spider or a bite causing at least some immediate local discomfort, followed by the development of progressively more severe local pain, often with local sweating. The pain may move in focus from the bite site proximally to involve limbs or trunk, again often associated with sweating and hypertension, nausea, and malaise. The rate of progression in severity and area involved is variable, from 1 hour to more than 24 hours. Trunk pain may involve the abdomen or thorax and may mimic acute abdomen or myocardial ischemic pain. The diagnosis becomes more certain if treatment with sufficient amounts of an appropriate antivenom results in clear resolution of the symptom complex.

Significant envenoming by an Australian funnel-web spider typically is associated with immediate pain, and the spider is usually seen and sometimes may need to be pulled off the victim. Systemic symptoms ensue rapidly, first manifested in 5 to 20 minutes by tingling around the lips and twitching of the tongue, rapidly followed by signs of catecholamine storm, with piloerection, hypersalivation and hyperlacrimation, hypertension, abdominal pain, nausea, and progressive severe pulmonary edema, with secondary hypoxia and impaired conscious state. The progression from first symptoms to lethal outcome may take 20 to 30 minutes or may take 1 to 3 hours or occasionally longer. Without adequate antivenom therapy, death is likely.

Significant envenoming by a Brazilian banana spider typically is associated with a witnessed bite with marked local pain, with edema, erythema, and frequently sweating. Systemic features include tachycardia; hypertension; nausea and vomiting; increased sweating and salivation; priapism in boys; and, in severe cases, pulmonary edema, cardiac arrhythmias, and shock. A fatal outcome is rare.

Significant envenoming by recluse spiders typically presents hours or days after the presumed bite, which is usually not witnessed because the bite is painless and frequently occurs at night while the patient is asleep. A spider is rarely available for identification. Even in most published series, a spider was positively identified in less than 10% of cases. In the first 24 hours, the bite area becomes painful, erythematous, then mottled with hemorrhagic areas, often associated with systemic symptoms, such as fever, generalized erythema, and malaise. The diagnosis is usually apparent by the second day. After 4 to 7 days, an area of necrosis develops, with often severe pain. Less commonly in South American cases, rarely elsewhere, a severe systemic illness develops, with intravascular hemolysis, thrombocytopenia, disseminated intravascular coagulation, renal failure, potentially multiple organ failure, and death.

TREATMENT OF SPIDER BITE

Treatment of spider bite most often consists of reassurance and short-term follow-up to exclude development of secondary infection. For the few spiders capable of causing significant envenoming (e.g., widow spiders, Australian funnel-web spiders, Brazilian banana spiders, recluse spiders), treatment sometimes may be more significant, but even for these species, most cases ultimately prove to be minor.

Approach to Treatment

Effective treatment of spider bite relies on early diagnosis of the likely culprit—in particular, defining if it is probably one of the few spider species of medical importance. If it is likely to be a potentially dangerous species, such as an Australian funnel-web spider, assessment is urgent, and specific treatment must be instituted as soon as systemic envenoming is apparent. For most other spiders, however, even widow spiders, it is practical to observe for a period before starting definitive treatment because many cases are minor, and a delay does not endanger life in most instances.

Specific Treatment—Antivenom

When available, antivenom is the most effective treatment for systemic envenoming; this is particularly true for significant bites by Australian funnel-web spiders, where major envenoming is likely to prove lethal without antivenom. Widow spider bites rarely prove lethal but can cause prolonged and unpleasant symptoms, justifying antivenom therapy. In Australia, where widow spider bites are frequent, antivenom is used routinely and is effective and reasonably safe. The reluctance to use antivenom for widow spider bites in North America is puzzling and in my opinion ethically questionable because no other treatment is effective in severe cases. Antivenom is commonly used in moderate-to-severe cases of systemic envenoming by Brazilian banana spiders, particularly in children and the elderly. Antivenom against recluse spiders also is available in Brazil, but its effectiveness at preventing necrosis is contestable, and frequently patients present too late for antivenom to be effective. Details of specific antivenom treatments for major spider bite may be found in Chapters 111 through 113.

Other Treatments

Details of specific nonantivenom treatments for major spider bite, such as loxoscelism, may be found in Chapters 111 through 113.

Follow-up

All spider bites should be considered for follow-up, but not all require formal arrangements. For most cases, the significant and uncommon risk is secondary infection. Patients should be instructed on what symptoms and signs to look for, indicating such a complication, and to return promptly if these occur. All patients receiving antivenom should be followed, at least by phone call, to check for serum sickness.

BIBLIOGRAPHY

White J, Cardoso JL, Fan HW: Clinical toxicology of spider bites. In Meier J, White J (eds): Handbook of Clinical Toxicology of Animal Venoms and Poisons. Boca Raton, FL, CRC Press, 1995.

CHAPTER 111

Widow and Related *Latrodectus* Spiders

Frank F. S. Daly ▪ Julian White

Widow spiders (genus *Latrodectus*) are found around the world. Bites may be complicated by local pain, diaphoresis, abdominal pain, back pain, chest pain, headache, nausea, dysphoria, and mild hypertension. This clinical syndrome, called *latrodectism*, is seldom fatal but may present a diagnostic dilemma and cause significant morbidity.

It is difficult to estimate the number of patients who experience significant envenomation. In the United States, approximately 2500 cases are reported to poison centers each year.[1-3] Of these, approximately 800 require treatment in a health care facility, and 300 to 400 have pronounced or prolonged symptoms. Despite reports that mortality may reach 5%,[4-6] a death has not been reported in the United States for more than 20 years or in Australia for nearly 40 years.[7] Australia may have the highest rate of latrodectism in the world.[8] It is estimated that 5000 to 10,000 human bites occur annually, but only 20% require antivenom therapy.[9]

Latrodectism was known to Socrates and Aristotle. Italian monks wrote of the syndrome in the 9th century. Several authors described epidemics of latrodectism during military campaigns in Northern Italy in the 19th century.[10] The first detailed description of the genus *Latrodectus* was by Rossi in 1790 at the University of Pisa. Walckenaer was the first to link the genus with the clinical syndrome of latrodectism.[10]

Widow spiders occur around the world in temperate and warm climates. Clinically significant spiders include *Latrodectus mactans*, *Latrodectus hesperus*, *Latrodectus bishopi*, and *Latrodectus variolus* in North America; *Latrodectus hasseltii* (red back spider) in Australia; *Latrodectus katipo* in New Zealand; and *Latrodectus indistinctus* in South Africa. *Latrodectus geometricus* (brown widow) and *Latrodectus tredecimguttatus* are found on most continents. The taxonomy of the genus was the subject of debate throughout the 20th century. Between five species, with many allopatric (speciation that occurs when a population becomes segregated into two populations by a geographic barrier) populations being described by trinomials (e.g., *L. mactans hasseltii*), and 40 species have been described.[11]

Widow spiders are small with a protuberant abdominal section. Many species have either ventral or dorsal abdominal markings, but these are not constant. Male widow spiders are smaller than females, reach maturity earlier than females, live only 1 or 2 months, and die soon after mating. Males have a small biting apparatus and generally are considered to be unable to envenomate. We know of one unpublished case of mild envenoming after a male red-back spider bite, which did not require antivenom therapy. Female widow spiders are much larger, live several months, and are able to envenomate

humans. There is no scientific evidence to confirm the popular conception that the female spider routinely eats her mate.[10] The term *widow* probably arose from the observations that males seldom are seen in the web and that the larger females may become cannibalistic in captivity.

Widow spiders produce an irregular, untidy web to catch their prey. They are not aggressive and bite humans only when trapped against the skin. They often live in environments where they readily come into contact with humans. Human bites tend to occur in warmer months or just when the weather turns cool and the spiders migrate indoors.[7,12,13]

Hundreds of therapies have been offered for patients envenomed by widow spiders, including warm baths, alcoholic beverages, opioids, various sedative-hypnotic agents, neostigmine, physostigmine, atropine, tubocurarine, methocarbamol, dantrolene, procaine, corticosteroids, magnesium, calcium, and antivenom, to name just a few.[10] Therapies that are truly efficacious are described in the treatment section.

BIOCHEMISTRY

Latrodectus venom contains a family of high-molecular-weight proteins that lead to transmitter release from nerve endings.[14] The venoms of four black widow species (*L. mactans*, *L. variolus*, *L. bishopi*, and *L. geometricus*) were compared in a study published in 1965.[15] The electrophoretic patterns of all the venoms were similar, and one antivenom prevented the lethal effects of all venoms in a mouse model. More recently, the venom of *L. tredecimguttatus* has been studied in the most depth. The cDNAs encoding components called α-*latrotoxin*, α-*latroinsectotoxin*, and δ-*latroinsectotoxin* have been cloned and sequenced.[14] All *Latrodectus* species seem to produce α-*latrotoxin*, with a molecular weight of approximately 150,000.[14,16]

PATHOPHYSIOLOGY

It is thought that α-latrotoxin leads to the manifestations of envenomation in humans, whereas the latroinsectotoxins lead to toxicity in invertebrates.[14] In vertebrates, the existence of calcium-dependent and calcium-independent binding proteins on the presynaptic membrane has been proposed.[14] Binding of α-latrotoxin to one or more of these proteins facilitates the insertion of the α-latrotoxin tetramer into the membrane, with formation of a central transmembrane pore, leading to presynaptic transmembrane influx of calcium or other ions, which leads to vacuole release of acetylcholine. Uncontrolled release of acetylcholine in the brainstem, spinal cord, and neuromuscular junction and possibly release of catecholamines in the brain, spinal cord, or autonomic ganglia, resulting in norepinephrine discharge, lead to the clinical manifestations of envenomation. The degree to which the various neurotransmitters are released in humans is uncertain and must be inferred from in vitro studies.

CLINICAL PRESENTATION

"Robust and healthy men, torn between a feeling of approaching death and unsupportable pains, mad from horror and in a condition of psychomotor restlessness, throw themselves moaning and lamenting on the bed, roll on the floor, or perform senseless movements, seeking relief."[10] Latrodectism is similar throughout the world, but may vary slightly depending on the species involved and the amount of venom injected. *L. mactans* is notorious for causing abdominal rigidity and back pain, whereas *L. hasseltii* seems to cause more diaphoresis. *L. geometricus* tends to cause only local symptoms.[17]

The bite itself is not painful and may go unnoticed in 50% of patients.[10] Local pain becomes apparent within 10 to 60 minutes, and discomfort may spread to regional lymph nodes and beyond. A pathognomonic triad of local pain, diaphoresis, and piloerection alerts the astute clinician to the diagnosis, in addition to the presence of mild erythema around a central pale area, giving rise to the term *target lesion* (Fig. 111-1). Three quarters of patients develop only local symptoms and do not subsequently develop systemic effects.[11]

Systemic envenomation may take many hours to reach its full extent. Muscle pains occur around the bitten area and spread to become generalized. Patients may describe neck, chest, abdominal, lower back, and thigh pains. This pain often is associated with generalized diaphoresis and

dysphoria. Associated features include low-grade fever, tachycardia, hypertension, tremor, paresthesias, headache, and vomiting. A clinical grading system has been proposed,[18] based on the presence or absence of local and generalized signs and symptoms, but it has not been validated as a method to predict outcome or complications.

The term *facies latrodectismica* describes the painful grimace, general flushing, diaphoresis, trismus, and blepharoconjunctivitis[10] sometimes seen in patients with full-blown latrodectism. Altered mental status has been described, particularly in elderly patients. It is unclear whether this altered mental status is true delirium or a state of severe dysphoria. Symptoms usually peak within 12 hours of the bite and abate within 24 to 72 hours. Uncommonly, symptoms may last 1 week or more[10] if antivenom is not prescribed. Generalized muscle weakness has been described 96 hours after envenomation.[19] The older literature suggests that deaths occurred late and were secondary to respiratory failure, perhaps due to muscle weakness or pulmonary edema or both.[10] Most of these reports either lack clinical detail or lack sufficient information to determine the cause of death, however. We know of two cases with sufficient information—one associated with pulmonary edema and one with the only finding being paravertebral lymphadenopathy.[8] Chronic pain syndromes lasting weeks to months have been described.[36] In these cases, late antivenom therapy has been associated with resolution of symptoms. Rare reported complications associated with latrodectism include herpes zoster,[20] priapism,[21] and toxic epidermal necrolysis.[22] The degree to which these complications truly are related to latrodectism is unknown because these are uncontrolled observations. Older accounts from southern Europe associated latrodectism with myocardial infarction, stroke, disseminated intravascular coagulation, renal failure, and psychosis.[6,10]

DIAGNOSIS

There are no specific confirmatory laboratory tests for latrodectism, and the diagnosis is clinical. There may be a mild leukocytosis (approximately 11,000/mm³ is typical, but values of 26,000/mm³ have been described) and elevated serum glucose levels.[10] Case reports have described latrodectism being mistaken for acute abdomen with subsequent negative laparotomy, acute myocardial infarction, meningitis, psychosis, renal and biliary colic, malaria, porphyria, lead intoxication, and sickle cell crisis.[10]

TREATMENT

Since the 1980s, treatment modalities advocated for latrodectism have included opiates, benzodiazepines, muscle relaxants, calcium, and antivenom.[23] Few studies have examined the efficacy of these treatments; no studies have been published that support the routine use of calcium gluconate, methocarbamol, or dantrolene. The consensus among clinical toxicologists is that first-line treatment of patients with latrodectism in North America should be a combination of an opioid and a benzodiazepine, although this has not been

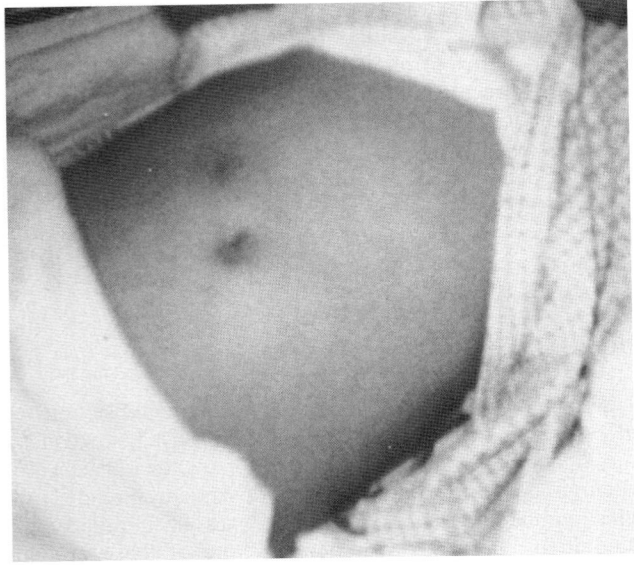

FIGURE 111-1

Target lesion after the bite of a *Latrodectus* spider. See Color Fig. 111-1.

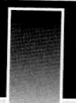

Indications for ICU Admission in Envonomation by Widow and Related *Latrodectus* **Spiders**

Requirement for continuous high-dose infusion of opioid and benzodiazepine in patients in whom antivenom is contraindicated

Rare complications, such as electrocardiogram changes, acute myocardial infarction, or pulmonary edema

Clinical monitoring during antivenom infusion (short-term admission) if safe monitoring cannot be achieved outside this setting

Anaphylactic or severe anaphylactoid reactions complicating antivenom infusion

studied prospectively. Severe systemic symptoms (e.g., muscle pain, diaphoresis, dysphoria, hypertension, prenatal labor) refractory to a combination of opioid and benzodiazepine in generous doses should prompt consideration of antivenom therapy. In Australia, where antivenom therapy is considered safe and effective, a far lower threshold for its use is accepted. It commonly is given for regional or systemic envenoming, without first using an opioid and a benzodiazepine.

Treatment of envenomation by *L. mactans* with intravenous calcium gluconate and methocarbamol was compared in a small (n = 13) prospective crossover study.[24] All four patients treated initially with methocarbamol required further treatment. Calcium gluconate also was studied in a retrospective chart review of 163 patients with latrodectism.[18] Of the 24 patients with severe envenomation who initially received calcium gluconate, 23 reported no relief of symptoms.

The use of dantrolene sodium was reported in an uncontrolled retrospective series of six patients with severe muscle pain secondary to *L. hesperus* envenomation.[25] It was reported to be effective in five of the six patients; however, the proposed prospective study has not been published.

In the series by Clark and colleagues[18] of 163 patients, 75 patients with severe envenomation received parenteral opioids. In this group, 55% of patients treated with opioids alone obtained symptomatic relief, whereas 70% of patients treated with combined opioids and benzodiazepines obtained symptomatic relief after initial treatment. It was concluded that benzodiazepines conferred an opioid-sparing effect when given with morphine. Antivenom was administered to 58 patients in Clark's series, one of whom died, apparently related to antivenom administration. This patient had a history of atopy and asthma. Antivenom led to complete resolution of symptoms within 2 hours (mean time 31 ± 26.7 minutes), and relapses did not occur, although seven patients (12%) required two doses. Patients who received antivenom had a shorter duration of symptoms (9 ± 22.7 hours compared with 22 ± 24.9 hours, $P < 0.05$) and were less likely to be admitted to the hospital (12% compared with 52%). Hypertension rarely required specific treatment, usually responding to supportive care or antivenom. Minor urticarial reactions occurred in four (7%) patients who received antivenom. Only 9 of the 58 patients treated with antivenom were followed up by telephone at a later date; however, none of these patients

reported symptoms suggesting delayed hypersensitivity reactions.

Antivenom Therapy

NORTH AMERICA

The North American black widow antivenom is an equine IgG-rich preparation. The equine serum is pooled and partially purified to produce the lyophilized antivenom. Adults and children should be treated with the contents of one vial (2.5 mL). The generally accepted indication for antivenom is severe systemic symptoms (e.g., muscle pain, diaphoresis, dysphoria, hypertension) refractory to a combination of opioids and benzodiazepines. Children, elderly patients, and pregnant patients are treated according to the same indications. Antivenom is contraindicated in patients with known hypersensitivity to equine serum. A history of asthma, a history of atopy, and the use of β-blockers are considered relative contraindications. The exact incidence of immediate hypersensitivity reactions is unknown. Delayed type III hypersensitivity (serum sickness) may occur. The exact incidence is unknown.

If antivenom is considered, the risks and benefits of this treatment should be discussed with the patient. The patient should be placed in a clinical setting where acute allergic reactions can be managed. Reliable intravenous access should be achieved, and electrocardiographic and pulse oximetry monitoring should be started. The immediate bedside availability of epinephrine and antihistamines should be ensured.

Although skin testing is commonly used, there is no good evidence that it reliably predicts reactions to antivenom. This procedure is strongly contraindicated in many other countries. Although we accept that medicolegal considerations in the United States may force its use, we do not support skin testing on medical grounds. Skin testing should never be started until after a firm decision to treat with antivenom has been made. The positive and negative predictive values of skin testing are not known but are thought to be poor. A negative skin test does not exclude the possibility of acute allergic reaction to the antivenom, which may include anaphylactic and anaphylactoid responses.[26] Skin testing typically is performed by injecting 0.01 mL of the test solution intradermally on the volar aspect of the forearm. The site should be marked and observed for 30 minutes. If the decision to use skin testing is made, we recommend that antivenom not be started until after interpretation of the skin test at 30 minutes. Erythema and induration of greater than 10 mm diameter, bronchospasm, or hypotension constitutes a positive skin test. Given the negligible mortality associated with latrodectism treated with thorough supportive care, a positive skin test should dissuade the clinician from the use of antivenom.

The product information from Merck (West Point, PA), the manufacturer of the antivenom, recommends that it be given intramuscularly, unless it is administered to a critically ill adult or a child younger than 6 years old, in which case the intravenous route is recommended. The usual practice by many specialists for many years has been to deliver the antivenom routinely to all patients by the intravenous route.[27,28] This practice may relate to the hypothesis that the intravenous route is safer because the dose may be truncated if allergic symptoms occur.[29] There is little evidence in the literature to support this hypothesis. Indirect evidence suggests that intramuscular administration of antivenom might be safer, if the route is available.[26,30,31] Premedication with subcutaneous epinephrine, antihistamines, or corticosteroids is controversial. It has not been part of routine practice for this antivenom in the United States. There is evidence that premedication with low-dose subcutaneous epinephrine reduces the incidence of acute allergic responses associated with the intravenous infusion of certain snake antivenoms with a high incidence of major adverse reactions,[32] but premedication has not been studied in latrodectus antivenom administration.

If the intravenous route is chosen, the antivenom should be diluted in 50 to 250 mL of crystalloid solution and the infusion started slowly (e.g., 10 drops per minute). Provided that no allergic symptoms occur, we recommend that the infusion rate can be doubled every few minutes so that the total volume is administered over 15 to 60 minutes. The patient should be observed closely throughout the infusion and for 30 minutes thereafter. Acute allergic reactions would not be expected to occur more than 30 minutes after cessation of the infusion, and patients may be discharged as soon as they are clinically well. Routine admission to the intensive care unit of patients with uncomplicated antivenom-treated latrodectism, even if severe, may not be required.

Patients who receive the antivenom by the intramuscular route should be observed to exclude acute allergic reactions and to ensure clinical improvement. Although not formally studied, in our experience, 2 hours of observation for allergic reaction is sufficient.

AUSTRALIA

In Australia, red-back spider (*L. hasseltii*) bite leads to signs and symptoms similar to those encountered in other parts of the world, including pronounced diaphoresis, tachycardia, hypertension, muscle cramps, tremor, vomiting, and patchy paralysis.[8,9,32] The Australian antivenom also is a purified equine-derived product.[32] More red-back antivenom is used than all the other Australian antivenoms put together.[9] No deaths due to anaphylaxis have been associated with the use of *L. hasseltii* antivenom. In a series of 2144 patients treated over 13 years, the incidence of allergic responses was 0.5%, and there were no deaths.[30] All severe acute allergic responses in this series occurred in patients who received antivenom by the intravenous route, contrary to product recommendations. Current Australian practice is to use antivenom for patients with severe local symptoms unresponsive to oral analgesics and in patients with symptoms of systemic envenomation. Benzodiazepines are used only in the rare situations when they are necessary while waiting for the antivenom to work. Most patients (66% to 97%) treated with antivenom require 1 ampule given by intramuscular injection.[12,30,33] The remaining patients require additional doses. Antivenom is uniformly effective for patients with red-back envenomation so that failure to control symptoms with antivenom brings the diagnosis into question.[34,35] Hospital admission for latrodectism is uncommon in Australia if antivenom is used; however, debilitating symptoms may continue for months if antivenom is not prescribed.[10,36]

Skin testing is not recommended in Australia,[11] and premedication is controversial.[33] Given the low risk of acute allergic reactions, it would seem reasonable to withhold premedication, unless the patient has been sensitized to horse serum or has a history of atopy. Patients should have reliable intravenous access and be placed in an environment where acute allergic reactions can be treated. If repeat doses are required, some authorities recommend the intravenous route using a technique similar to that described earlier for the North American product. We recommend that patients who receive the antivenom by the intramuscular route be observed for 2 hours to exclude acute allergic reactions and to ensure clinical improvement before discharge.

L. hasseltii antivenom has been administered by some unorthodox routes. Case reports have described local subcutaneous injection of antivenom to control severe prolonged local symptoms[37] and use of antivenom by a regional intravenous technique similar to the Bier block.[36,38] These kinds of approaches have not been validated and cannot be recommended.

The exact incidence of delayed-type hypersensitivity (serum sickness) associated with *L. hasseltii* antivenom is unknown, but it is thought to be low. Prophylactic steroid therapy is prescribed by some clinicians in an attempt to prevent serum sickness if multiple doses of antivenom are used. This practice has not been validated experimentally and is not widely adopted.

NEW ZEALAND

The New Zealand katipo spider is essentially the same as the Australian red-back spider and should be treated as such.

SOUTH AFRICA

Three members of the genus *Lacrodectus* are present in South Africa. *L. indistinctus* (black widow) and *L. geometricus* (brown widow) are thought to be chiefly responsible for human envenomation. *Latrodectus rhodesiensis* is found in Zimbabwe and the Transvaal. All of these spiders have venom that contains α-latrotoxin. The relative toxicity of *L. indistinctus* and *L. geometricus* venoms has been studied using a mouse lethality model.[39] The venom of *L. indistinctus* (black widow) seems to be three to four times more potent than that of *L. geometricus* (brown widow). In a retrospective series of 45 cases,[17] *L. indistinctus* (black widow) caused more severe envenomation with systemic signs and symptoms. The presentations of brown widow bites were mild, and local symptoms predominated.

In South Africa, antivenom is administered in severe cases to prevent a protracted course.[17] The antivenom is given as an intramuscular injection of 5 mL of equine-derived anti–spider serum globulin.

BRAZIL

Brazilian latrodectism is uncommon. Bites by *Phoneutria* are the most common spider bites. These manifest in a manner similar to that of latrodectism, but with a higher incidence of priapism. Loxoscelism occurs less frequently. Bites by the latter group of spiders are discussed in Chapter 112.

Reactions to Antivenom

As stated earlier, allergic reactions to antivenom are uncommon, especially in the Australian experience, when the antivenom is given by the intramuscular route. During intravenous infusion of antivenom, mild isolated urticaria may be treated by slowing the rate of infusion and administering an intravenous antihistamine, such as diphenhydramine. In the setting of latrodectism, airway swelling, bronchospasm, or hypotension should prompt the abandonment of antivenom therapy and aggressive therapy.

The immediate priority of management is the assessment and management of threats to the airway, breathing, and circulation. Intubation and ventilation may be required. First-line therapy consists of oxygen, epinephrine, and intravenous fluids.[40] High-flow oxygen should be given to ensure an oxygen saturation greater than 92%. Epinephrine should be administered in all cases with hypotension, airway swelling, or bronchospasm.[41] Large volumes of crystalloid or colloid may be required to maintain circulatory volume.

When the immediate threats to the airway, breathing, and circulation have been managed with airway control and first-line drugs, the use of second-line drugs, such as corticosteroids, antihistamines, H$_2$ blockers, glucagons, and aminophylline, may be considered. Antihistamines should be used in combination with H$_2$ blockers, such as cimetidine or ranitidine.[40,42] Corticosteroids are indicated to prevent prolonged symptom duration, especially bronchospasm.[43] Glucagon has been advocated for patients taking β-adrenergic blocking drugs who have an increased risk of anaphylaxis and are resistant to treatment.[40,43] Aminophylline may be appropriate for patients with bronchospasm resistant to epinephrine and steroids.[40] Tables 111-1 and 111-2 provide suggested treatment doses.

Criteria for ICU Discharge in Envenomation by Widow and Related *Latrodectus* Spiders

1. For patients who have not received antivenom, high-dose opioid and benzodiazepine infusions should be ceased. Patients who feel clinically well and have normal vital signs 4 hours after starting oral analgesia may be discharged.
2. After intravenous infusion of antivenom, patients may be discharged at the end of the infusion if there is a satisfactory clinical response (patient feels well) and there is no evidence of anaphylactic or anaphylactoid reaction.
3. After intramuscular injection of antivenom, patients may be discharged 2 hours after injection if there is a satisfactory clinical response (patient feels well) and there is no evidence of anaphylactic or anaphylactoid reaction.

Key Points in the Treatment of Envenomation by Widow and Related *Latrodectus* Spiders

1. Latrodectism is painful and associated with significant dysphoria. Initial doses of opioid and benzodiazepine should be generous and repeated as frequently as necessary. In Australia at least, antivenom may be considered as first-line treatment, rather than opioids and benzodiazepines.
2. Failure of opioids and benzodiazepines to control symptoms after 4 hours should prompt consideration of antivenom. Antivenom may be given sooner if it is clear that high doses of opioids and benzodiazepines do not afford clinical relief.

continued

Key Points in the Treatment of Envenomation by Widow and Related *Latrodectus* Spiders *continued*

3. Despite the small but finite risks associated with antivenom, prudent use in carefully selected patients is sound clinical practice.
4. Acute allergic responses occur at the time of antivenom administration. Prolonged inpatient monitoring for late reactions is not indicated.
5. Antivenom therapy is definitive; failure of antivenom to alleviate symptoms should bring the diagnosis into question.

TABLE 111-1 First-Line Therapy for Anaphylaxis

TREATMENT	DOSAGE
Oxygen	Apply high FiO$_2$ oxygen via endotracheal tube or facemask to maintain oxygen saturation >92%
Epinephrine	*Early or mild anaphylaxis*—0.3–0.5 mg (0.3–0.5 mL) 1:1000 epinephrine by intramuscular injection repeated every 5–10 min as required. *Hypotension, dyspnea, airway compromise, or patient deteriorating*—1:100,000 epinephrine 1–2 mL/min IV, repeated as necessary. 1:100,000 epinephrine may be prepared by drawing 1 mg of epinephrine (1 mL of 1:1000) in a 20-mL syringe and adding 9 mL of normal saline to make a volume of 10 mL. All but 2 mL is discarded (leaving 200 μg) before a further 18 mL of saline is added to make 20 mL (10 μg/mL)
Fluid	Give 10–20 mL/kg of crystalloid or colloid for hypotension

FiO$_2$, fraction of inspired oxygen.
Adapted from Brown AFT: Anaphylaxis. In Cameron P, Jelinek G, Kelly A-M, et al (eds): Textbook of Adult Emergency Medicine. Edinburgh, Churchill Livingstone, 2000, p 640.

TABLE 111-2 Second-Line Therapy for Anaphylaxis

TREATMENT	DOSAGE
Antihistamines	Diphenhydramine, 25–50 mg IV, or promethazine, 12.5–25 mg IV, *plus* cimetidine, 300 mg IV, or ranitidine, 50 mg IV, repeated every 6 hr as required. Oral therapy may be started when able
Corticosteroids	Hydrocortisone, 5 mg/kg (≤200 mg) IV, followed by 2.5 mg/kg IV every 6 hr, or methylprednisolone, 125 mg IV every 6 hr. Oral prednisone, 40–50 mg daily, may be started when able
Glucagon	*For patients on β-adrenergic blockers*—1 mg IV every 5 min until stable, then 5–15 μg/min as an infusion
Aminophylline	*For refractory bronchospasm*—5 mg/kg IV infused over 30 min followed by an infusion of 0.5 mg/kg/hr

Adapted from Brown AFT: Anaphylaxis. In Cameron P, Jelinek G, Kelly A-M, et al (eds): Textbook of Adult Emergency Medicine. Edinburgh, Churchill Livingstone, 2000, p 640.

SPECIAL POPULATIONS

Pediatric Patients

Infants may present with inconsolable crying, restlessness, and poor feeding. There is often an associated generalized erythematous rash. The differential diagnosis is broad. Detailed physical examination may reveal evidence of a widow bite (e.g., localized diaphoresis, target lesion) (see Fig. 111-1), or a spider may be found in bedding, in clothing, or beneath the bed. Infants and children have been said to be at increased risk of severe morbidity from latrodectism,[23] but there is little literature that specifically addresses the pediatric population. A retrospective chart review from Western Australia[44] of 156 patients presenting to a tertiary care children's hospital reported 29% showed signs of systemic envenomation, and 21% received antivenom. The authors concluded that latrodectism in children is no more severe than that found in adults and that children may be relatively resistant to venom. Experience suggests children are less likely to require multiple doses of antivenom.

Pregnant Patients

The effect of latrodectism on pregnancy is not clear. Pregnancy has been cited as an indication for antivenom therapy in case vigorous abdominal muscular contractions lead to fetal distress.[45] It is not known whether the α-latrotoxin crosses the placenta. Modern cases of latrodectism in various stages of gestation have not led to spontaneous abortion,[45,46] although there are reports of spontaneous abortion after latrodectism in 19th-century southern Russia.[45] Antivenom is not contraindicated in pregnancy.

Elderly Patients

Elderly patients have been said to be at increased risk of severe morbidity from latrodectism.[23] Patients with comorbidities, such as ischemic heart disease, might be more susceptible to the physiologic stress resulting from the high catecholamine state associated with latrodectism. Profound dysphoria may be mistaken for altered mental state. Latrodectism itself may cause chest pain, but widow bites also have been associated with acute myocardial infarction.[10] One author saw an elderly man with latrodectism who developed nonspecific ST-T wave changes in association with transient presyncope symptoms. Subsequent electrocardiograms and investigations to rule out myocardial infarction were normal. Other electrocardiogram changes associated with latrodectism include peaked P waves and prolongation of the QT interval.[10] The incidence and significance of these changes are not known.

Key Points in Envenomation by Widow and Related *Latrodectus* Spiders

1. *Latrodectism* refers to envenomation by the widow spiders (genus *Latrodectus*).
2. Latrodectism is similar throughout the world. There is structural homology of the venoms of the various *Latrodectus* species.

continued

Key Points in Envenomation by Widow and Related *Latrodectus* Spiders *continued*

3. The diagnosis is made on clinical grounds. It is based on a history of possible spider contact; local pain that migrates to other areas; autonomic changes, such as diaphoresis and hypertension; and pain or discomfort that appears disproportionate to physical signs.
4. Mortality is negligible with good supportive care.
5. Opioids and benzodiazepines improve patient comfort. There is little evidence to support the routine use of calcium gluconate or muscle relaxant agents, such as dantrolene sodium and methocarbamol.
6. Patients with symptoms refractory to a combination of opioid and benzodiazepine should be considered for antivenom therapy, especially in parts of the world where safe antivenom products are available.
7. Antivenom is the definitive therapy for latrodectism and shortens hospital stay. Most patients may be discharged from the hospital after treatment with antivenom; admission to the intensive care unit is rare, unless there are unusual complications of envenomation or treatment.
8. Antivenom raised against one *Latrodectus* species is likely to be effective treatment for envenomation by other *Latrodectus* species.
9. Contraindications to antivenom are primarily horse serum allergy, asthma, atopy, or β-blocker therapy.

REFERENCES

1. Litovitz TL, Klein-Schwartz W, Dyer KS, et al: 1997 annual report of the American Association of Poison Control Centers Toxic Exposure Surveillance System. Am J Emerg Med 16:443–497, 1998.
2. Litovitz TL, Klein-Schwartz W, Caravati EM, et al: 1998 annual report of the American Association of Poison Control Centers Toxic Exposure Surveillance System. Am J Emerg Med 17:435–487, 1999.
3. Litovitz TL, Klein-Schwartz W, White S, et al: 1999 annual report of the American Association of Poison Control Centers Toxic Exposure Surveillance System. Am J Emerg Med 18:517–574, 2000.
4. Wiener S: Red back spider antivenene. Med J Aust 2:41–44, 1961.
5. Report: Antivenin (*Latrodectus mactans*). West Point, PA, Merck Sharpe & Dohme, 1975.
6. Maretic Z, Lebez D: Araneism with special reference to Europe. Belgrade, Yugoslavia, Nolit Publishing House, 1979.
7. Weiner S: Red back spider bite in Australia: an analysis of 167 cases. Med J Aust 2:44–49, 1961.
8. White J, Cardoso JL, Hui WF: Clinical toxicology of spider bites. In Meier J, White J (eds): Handbook of Clinical Toxicology of Animal Venoms and Poisons. Boca Raton, FL, CRC Press, 1995, pp 284–302.
9. White J: Envenoming and antivenom use in Australia. Toxicon 36:1483–1492, 1998.
10. Bettini S (ed): Handbook of Experimental Pharmacology, Vol 48: Arthropod Venoms. Berlin, Springer-Verlag, 1978, pp 149–212.
11. Jelinek GA: Widow spider envenomation (latrodectism): A worldwide problem. Wilderness and Environmental Medicine 8:226–231, 1997.
12. Jelinek GA, Banham ND, Dunjey SJ: Red back spider bites at Fremantle Hospital, 1982–1987. Med J Aust 150:693–695, 1989.
13. Phillips S, personal communication, 2000.
14. Grishin EV: Black widow spider toxins: The present and the future. Toxicon 36:1693–1701, 1998.
15. McCrone JD, Netzloff ML: An immunological and electrophoretical comparison of the venoms of the North American *Latrodectus* spiders. Toxicon 3:107–110, 1965.
16. Grasso A (ed): Report and abstracts of meeting on *Latrodectus* neurotoxins from venom gland to neural receptors, Gaeta (LT), Italy. Toxicon 30:117–122, 1992.
17. Müller GJ: Black and brown widow spider bites in South Africa. S Afr Med J 83:399–405, 1993.

18. Clark RF, Wether-Kestner S, Vance MV, Gerkin R: Clinical presentation and treatment of black widow spider envenomation: A review of 163 cases. Ann Emerg Med 21:782–787, 1992.
19. O'Malley GF, Dart RC, Kuffner EF: Successful treatment of latrodectism with antivenin after 90 hours. N Engl J Med 340:657, 1999.
20. Heller AW, Kelly AP: Herpes zoster developing after a spider bite. Cutis 26:417–419, 1980.
21. Stiles AD: Priapism following a black widow spider bite. Clin Pediatr 21:174–175, 1982.
22. Welch KJ, Burke WA, Jones BE: Black widow spider poisoning as a possible cause of toxic epidermal necrolysis. Int J Dermatol 30:448–449, 1991.
23. Rees RS, Campbell DS: Spider bites. In Auerbach PS, Geehr EC (eds): Management of Wilderness and Environmental Emergencies, 2nd ed. St Louis, CV Mosby, 1989, p 549.
24. Key GF: A comparison of calcium gluconate and methocarbamol (Robaxin) in the treatment of latrodectism (black widow spider envenomation). Am J Trop Med Hyg 30:273–277, 1981.
25. Ryan PJ: Preliminary report: Experience with the use of dantrolene sodium in the treatment of bites by the black widow spider *Latrodectus hesperus*. J Toxicol Clin Toxicol 21:487–489, 1983–1984.
26. Sutherland SK: Serum reactions: An analysis of commercial antivenoms and the possible role of anticomplementary activity in de-novo reactions to antivenoms and antitoxins. Med J Aust 1:613–615, 1977.
27. Curry SC: Black widow spider envenomations. In Harwood-Nuss AL, Linden CH, Luten RC, et al (eds): The Clinical Practice of Emergency Medicine, 2nd ed. Philadelphia, Lippincott-Raven, 1996, pp 1446–1447.
28. Bernstein JN: Antidotes in depth: Antivenin (scorpion and spider). In Goldfrank LR (ed): Goldfrank's Toxicologic Emergencies, 6th ed. Stamford, CT, Appleton & Lange, 1998.
29. Otten EJ: Antivenin therapy in the emergency department. Am J Emerg Med 1:83–93, 1983.
30. Sutherland SK, Trinca JC: Survey of 2144 cases of red back spider bites: Australia and New Zealand 1963–1976. Med J Aust 2:620–623, 1978.
31. Reid H: Antivenom reactions and efficacy. Lancet 1 (8176):1024–1025, 1980.
32. Premawardhena AP, de Silva CE, Fonseka MMD, et al: Low dose subcutaneous adrenaline to prevent acute adverse reactions to antivenom serum in people bitten by snakes: randomized, placebo controlled trial. BMJ 318:1041–1043, 1999.
33. Sutherland SK: Antivenom use in Australia: Premedication, adverse reactions, and the use of venom detection kits. Med J Aust 161:701, 704–705, 1994.
34. White J: CSL Antivenom Handbook. Melbourne, CSL Ltd, 1995.
35. Winkel KD: Caution regarding Bier's block technique for redback spider bite (Letter). Med J Aust 171:220, 1999.
36. Banham NDG, Jelinek GA, Finch P: Late treatment with antivenom in prolonged red back spider envenomation. Med J Aust 161:379–381, 1994.
37. Couser GA, Wiles GJ: A red-back spider bite in a lymphoedematous arm. Med J Aust 166:587–588, 1997.
38. Fatovich DM, Dunjey SJ, Constantine CJ, Hirsch RL: Successful treatment of red-back spider bite using a Bier's block technique. Med J Aust 170:342–343, 1999.
39. Müller GJ, Koch HM, Kriegler AB, et al: The relative toxicity and polypeptide composition of the venom of two South African widow spider species: *Latrodectus indistinctus* and *Latrodectus geometricus*. S Afr J Sci 85:44–46, 1989.
40. Brown AFT: Anaphylaxis. In Cameron P, Jelinek G, Kelly A-M, et al (eds): Textbook of Adult Emergency Medicine. Philadelphia, Churchill Livingstone, 2000.
41. Fisher MM: Treating anaphylaxis with sympathomimetic drugs. BMJ 305:1107–1108, 1992.
42. Lieberman P: The use of antihistamines in the prevention and treatment of anaphylaxis and anaphylactoid reactions. J Allergy Clin Immunol 86:684–686, 1990.
43. Toogood JH: Risk of anaphylaxis in patients receiving beta blocker drugs. J Allergy Clin Immunol 1:1–5, 1988.
44. Mead HJ, Jelinek GA: Red back spider bites to Perth children 1979–1988. J Paediatr Child Health 29:305–308, 1993.
45. Russell FE, Marcus P, Streng JA: Black widow spider envenomation during pregnancy: Report of a case. Toxicon 17:188–189, 1979.
46. Handel CC, Izquierdo LA, Curet LB: Black widow spider (*Latrodectus mactans*) bite during pregnancy. West J Med 160:261–262, 1994.

CHAPTER 112

Loxosceles Spiders

Gary S. Wasserman ■ Jennifer A. Lowry

Loxoscelism, envenomation by spiders of the family Loxoscelidae, occurs in the South, Central, and North Americas; the Mediterranean area; Europe; and Africa.[1] Two clinical forms of loxoscelism are recognized: loxoscelism occurring locally involving the bite site (cutaneous or necrocutaneous form) and loxoscelism involving multiple organs (systemic or viscerocutaneous form). Local necrotic arachnidism is referred to as *gangrenous spot* or *cutaneous arachnidism* in South American countries.[2] Fatalities from *Loxosceles* envenomation, especially in children, are more common in South America than in North America, where such incidences are rare.[3–6] One article claims 54 species in the genus *Loxosceles* are found in North America.[7] The most common potent species in North America is *Loxosceles reclusa*, often called the *brown recluse, violin,* or *fiddleback* spider.

TAXONOMY OF *LOXOSCELES* SPIDERS

A taxonomy for the most common *Loxosceles* species is presented in Table 112-1.[8,9] Generally the four most notorious species are *L. reclusa, L. laeta, L. gaucho,* and *L. rufescens.* Envenomations from *L. rufipes, L. spadicea, L. deserta,* and *L. arizonica* are gaining publicity, however. *L. laeta* is presumed to be the most potent because systemic symptoms occur more frequently, and larger numbers of patients present in South America after reported *L. laeta* envenomation compared with envenomation involving the other endogenous species, *L. intermedia* and *L. gaucho.*[3]

HABITAT AND GEOGRAPHIC DISTRIBUTION

The name *reclusa* accurately describes the behavior of these spiders because they avoid areas of activity, are nocturnal, hide their webs, and are not usually seen. *Loxosceles* spiders seem to prefer warm, dry, and secluded habitats. Depending on the environmental temperature, they live outdoors or in basements, attics, and storage areas. Bites most commonly occur during the warmer seasons. Most victims are bitten while working in their yard or home, dressing, or sleeping.

Loxosceles are found throughout the world. *L. reclusa,* the brown recluse spider, has been reported in nearly half of the United States but is most prevalent in the southern Midwest. *L. deserta* and *L. arizonica* are found in the western desert regions of the United States. *L. intermedia* and

L. laeta are found in South America. *L. intermedia* and *L. laeta* mainly inhabit Peru, Bolivia, Argentina, and Uruguay but also are found in Guatemala, Honduras, and some parts of the United States and Canada. In the past, 30% of homes in Chile were infested with *L laeta*.[10] *L. rufescens* mostly resides in the Mediterranean regions of Europe and Africa but also may be found in Japan.[11–13] With modern global mobility and high-speed transportation, it is now possible for these spiders to transmigrate from continent to continent in boxes and baggage.[14]

SPIDER DESCRIPTION

Loxosceles spiders are usually a brownish to tan color, with a characteristic dark, violin-shaped marking (larger end of fiddle toward the head) on the back of its round cephalothorax (Fig. 112-1). Its abdomen is ovoid, and the eight legs are long and slender. The hairs of the body and legs are short and barely seen with the naked eye. A large spider measures 1 cm in total body length and about 0.5 cm in width, with an individual leg span of approximately 2 to 3 cm. Females are more common and slightly larger than males. A distinguishing feature is their three pairs of small eyes of equal size, differing from almost all other spiders, which normally have four eye pairs. Other hunting spiders often have one larger pair of the four sets, which is frequently located higher on the head. *Hunting spiders* refers to the few groups of spiders with fangs that are strong and long enough to puncture human skin and inject venom.

LOXOSCELES VENOM AND HISTOPATHOPHYSIOLOGIC EFFECTS

Loxosceles venom is one of the most potent natural substances known. Similar to most spiders, *Loxosceles* uses its venom to kill its insect prey. Humans are not its intended victim, and envenomation is incidental. At least 11 major components of the venom have been identified; most are enzymes with cytotoxic activity.[15,16] Important venom components include hyaluronidase (spreading factor), S-ribonucleotide phosphohydrolase, alkaline phosphatase, and sphingomyelinase D. Commercial milking of a spider by single electrical stimulation yields approximately 2 to 3 μg of venom.[17] Immunologic cross-reactivity exists among the venom components of various *Loxosceles* species, especially those of molecular weight in the range of 33 to 35 kd.[18]

TABLE 112-1 Taxonomy of *Loxosceles*	
Kingdom	Animal
Phylum	Arthropoda
Class	Arachnida
Order	Araneae
Family	Loxoscelidae
Genus	*Loxosceles*
Species	*L. adelaide*
	L. arizonica
	L. gaucho
	L. hirsuta
	L. intermedia
	L. laeta
	L. reclusa
	L. rufescens
	L. rufipes
	L. similis
	L. spinulosa
	L. unicolor
	and many other species

Major systemic manifestations of *Loxosceles* envenomation include endothelial cell damage, lysis of red blood cells, and coagulation abnormalities. These effects result from activation of calcium-dependent systems, C-reactive protein, serum amyloid P component, complement, polymorphonuclear leukocytes, antibodies, cytokines (i.e., chemokines: interleukin-8, growth-related oncogene-α, monocyte chemoattractant protein-1, granulocyte-macrophage colony-stimulating factor), and other reactants.[19–29] The major cytotoxic venom factor seems to be sphingomyelinase D (34 kd), a venom component that appears to be unique to *Loxosceles*.[20] Sphingomyelinase D reacts with cell membrane sphingomyelin, causing release of choline and *N*-acylsphingosine phosphate and, in the presence of calcium and serum amyloid protein, stimulating platelet aggregation and serotonin release.[16,20,21,25] Cutaneous

necrosis is enhanced by the resulting ischemia and marked inflammatory reaction. We have observed an irregular circular spread of venom dermal effects, with some gravitational influences noted.

Researchers in South America have shown that *Loxosceles* venom–induced erythrocyte lysis depends on activation of complement by the alternative pathway. Metalloproteinase activity induced by *Loxosceles* venom causes cleavage of glycophorins from the erythrocyte surface and facilitates complement-mediated lysis.[30] Toxins can transfer from one erythrocyte to another in vivo, allowing hemolysis-inducing activity to be transferred to a new erythrocyte population.[30] Erythrocytes become spontaneous activators of complement, causing massive hemolysis, which often leads to renal failure.

It is suggested that venom sphingomyelinase activities alter the membrane environment and fluidity, causing activation of an unknown metalloproteinase. This sequence may explain the local effects of dermonecrosis.[30] These protein toxins also may provoke a systemic cytokine response resembling that seen in endotoxic shock.[31] In rabbits, *Loxosceles*-induced dermal inflammatory markers (neutrophils and myeloperoxidase) correlate with the presence of venom.[17] Although the mechanism of *Loxosceles*-induced inflammation is indirect (via soluble mediators), the immediate tissue presence of venom is required to cause dermonecrosis.[17]

Within 3 hours of *Loxosceles* envenomation, polymorphonuclear leukocytes infiltrate the region in and around venules at the inoculation site.[32] Epidermal and dermal edema is seen within 6 hours. Histologic findings include marked infiltration of venular walls by polymorphonuclear leukocytes; vasodilation; intravascular thrombosis; and massive hemorrhage into adjoining dermis, subcutis, and occasionally underlying muscle. Also noted are fibrinoid necrosis and vacuolization of arteriolar walls with disruption of vascular integrity. Local accumulation of polymorphonuclear leukocytes continues for more than 48 hours (Fig. 112-2).[32]

A review of 23 documented *L. reclusa* bites from the surgical pathology files at a U.S. hospital noted nine histopathologic characteristics. "The lesions progressed from a polymorphonuclear perivasculitis with hemorrhage and septal edema through a phase with epidermal necrosis and ulceration with extensive eosinophils and arterial wall necrosis, and panniculitis, to persistent arterial wall necrosis with eschar-covered ulceration, extensive dermal scarring, and subcutaneous fat necrosis."[33] Finally, "gradual resolution with residual scarring of the dermis and subcutis" was reported.[33] Residual soft tissue arachnid body parts were not histologically identified.

CLINICAL PRESENTATION AND LIFE-THREATENING COMPLICATIONS

The clinical presentation of loxoscelism is summarized in Table 112-2. Patient presentation, as seen in other envenomations, depends on many variables, including the amount of venom injected; the bite site; and age, premorbid health, and immune response characteristics of the victim. Most of these cases have a relatively benign

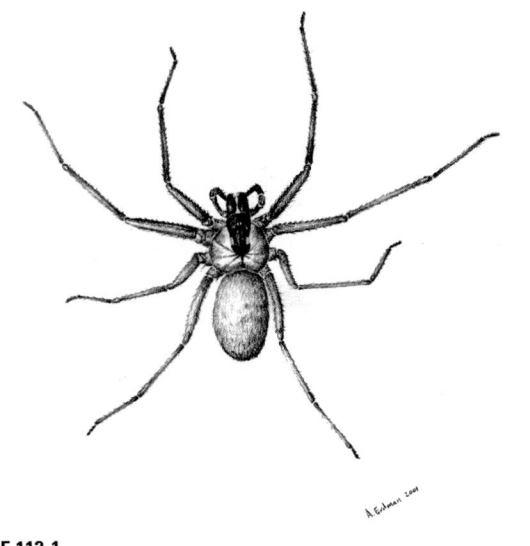

FIGURE 112-1

Loxosceles spider.

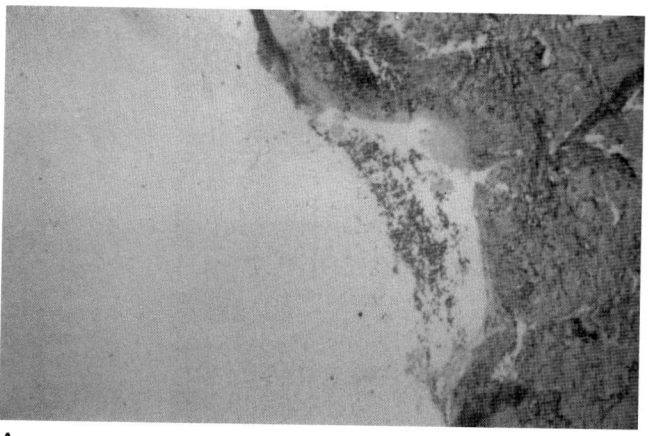

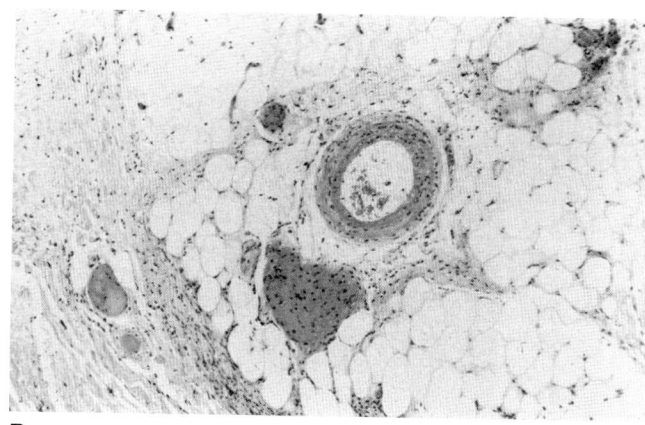

FIGURE 112-2

Dermatitis, panniculitis, and vasculitis. **A,** Skin biopsy specimen from an 18-month-old boy shows polymorphonuclear inflammatory response, 1-cm diameter necrotic crater, and probably fang mark. See Color Figure 112-2A. **B,** Skin biopsy specimen from autopsy of a 7-year-old girl who had hemolysis, disseminated intravascular coagulation, and dysrhythmias. There is superficial edema, fibrin thrombi, and moderate polymorphonuclear infiltration in the dermis, subcutaneous tissue, and large vessel wall. See Color Fig. 112-2B.

course.[34] There is usually only one bite site, although rarely two or more bites may be seen, such as when the victim swats at the spider. This is an important differential diagnostic point in contrast to many other arthropod bites or stings.

Loxoscelism may cause cutaneous or systemic manifestations or both; the systemic reactions may be more pronounced than the local lesion or vice versa. In a series of six children presenting (about third day postbite) with hemolytic anemia and a local skin lesion of erythema and induration, only one had dermonecrosis on admission.[35]

Epidemiologic studies in Chile and Brazil have shown mortality rates of 3.7% and 1.5%.[3,36]

Bite Site and Local Cutaneous Reactions

The sensation of the initial skin puncture is variable, with some victims sensing only a feeling of a mild pinprick. Many victims are bitten at night while asleep and may be unaware they have been bitten. Dermal responses vary from hours to weeks. Typically, within a few hours, the bite site progressively begins to itch and tingle and becomes indurated and

TABLE 112-2 Clinical Presentation of Loxoscelism	
Cutaneous Effects Pruritus, tingling, induration, edema, pain at site of bite Pallor/blanching or erythema Blister, bleb, purpura/ecchymosis Necrosis or eschar Ulceration, delayed wound healing Erythematous scarlatiniform eruption **Common Systemic Effects** Nausea, vomiting, abdominal distress Headache Fever Fatigue, weakness, malaise Muscle/joint pain Hepatitis, pancreatitis Other organ toxicity **Life-Threatening Systemic Effects** Hemolysis Coagulopathy Sepsis Necrotizing fasciitis Shock	**Serious Secondary Effects** Cardiac dysrhythmias Coma Congestive heart failure Pulmonary edema Renal failure Seizures **Laboratory Findings** Hemoglobinemia Hemoglobinuria, hematuria Leukocytosis, anemia, thrombocytopenia Abnormal liver and renal function tests Abnormal clotting tests (prothrombin time, partial thromboplastin time, international normalized ratio, fibrinogen, D dimer, antithrombin III) Positive antibody studies (IgG, complement, Coombs') Blood typing/matching interference Saturated haptoglobin binding capacity/decreased free haptoglobin

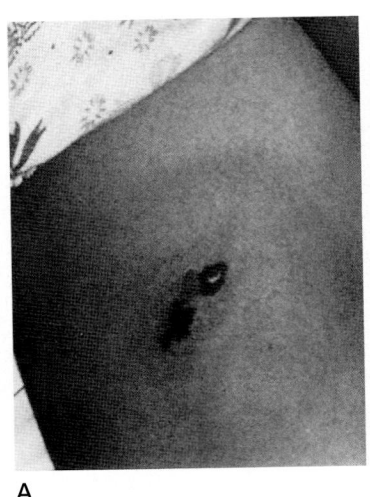
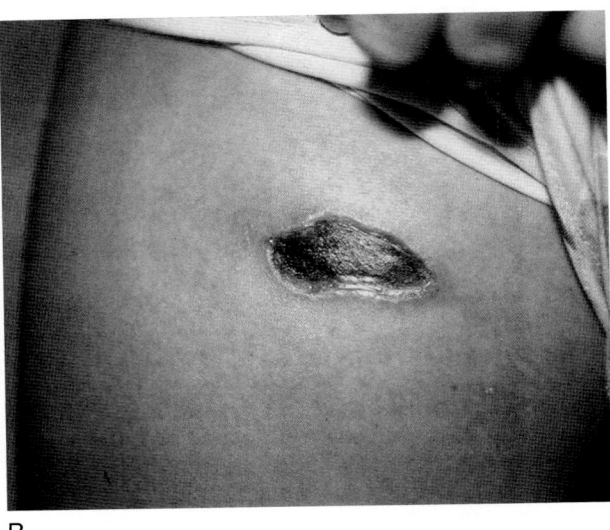

A   B

FIGURE 112-3

A, A 10-year-old girl as seen on day 2 postenvenomation. Note the blister indicating the puncture site, irregular necrosis (inferolaterally) representing venom spread by gravity, ecchymosis measuring 3.5 × 2 cm, and large area of inflammation. See Color Figure 112-3A. **B,** On day 7 postenvenomation, the entire original area of ecchymosis became necrotic and now is seen with eschar. Healing took 3 months with basic wound care. See Color Fig. 112-3B.

edematous. As ischemia and inflammation occur, the site becomes painful, becomes tender to touch, may blanch or become erythematous, and eventually becomes ecchymotic. Often within hours, many significant envenomations develop a characteristic blister or bleb, which may be normal flesh colored or purple to black (Fig. 112-3A). This lesion usually marks the exact site of venom injection. Almost always, the tissue beneath the blister or bleb becomes necrotic. The width or depth of necrosis is not predictable, however. As inflammation and ischemia/necrosis spread, pain worsens, especially during the first few days. An eschar may form within hours of the bite or be delayed for weeks (Fig. 112-3B). Eventually the eschar sloughs, revealing underlying soft tissue ulceration, which may not heal for months or, rarely, may not heal at all.

Occasionally within the first few days, a characteristic "halo," "target," or "bull's-eye" lesion develops (Fig. 112-4). The halo lesion consists of a central erythematous or violaceous area representing the initial bite site, surrounded by a ring of ischemic pallor that is further surrounded by normal or erythematous skin. Bites occurring on the neck may develop marked swelling (Fig. 112-5) and, especially in infants, can cause airway compromise with or without tracheal shifting secondary to edema of the soft tissues and aryepiglottic folds.[37] A bite to the periorbital region of an adult caused severe laryngeal edema from massive regional swelling of the neck.[38] Envenomation of the fatty areas of the body, such as abdomen, thighs, and buttocks, is associated with an especially high risk of necrosis because of relatively inadequate vascular supply.

Local wound infection almost always is a result of host streptococcal or staphylococcal flora rather than organisms transported by the spider. Rarely, sepsis, toxic shock syndrome, or necrotizing fasciitis occurs, and patients must be observed for these life-threatening complications.[39]

Systemic Manifestations

Loxoscelism involves multiple organ systems, including the skin, blood, gastrointestinal system, and musculoskeletal system. The pancreas and renal, pulmonary, and cardiovascular systems are less commonly affected. Signs and symptoms, occurring within hours to 1.5 days postenvenomation, are typically abdominal pain, nausea (and sometimes vomiting), fever often exceeding 102°F to 104°F (>39°C to 40°C), myalgias and arthralgias, headaches, and fatigue and weakness. These findings may persist for 24 to 72 hours,

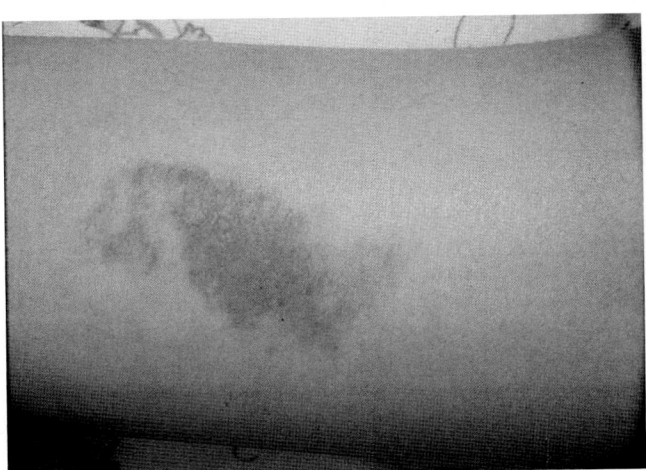

FIGURE 112-4

"Halo" skin lesion on the forearm of a 9-year-old girl, day 3 postbite. She also had fever, abdominal pain, and hemolysis. Note the small blister, surrounded by an irregular area of ecchymosis, which is outlined with pallor (ischemia), then normal skin. Only the blister site became necrotic and healed in 6 weeks. See Color Fig. 112-4.

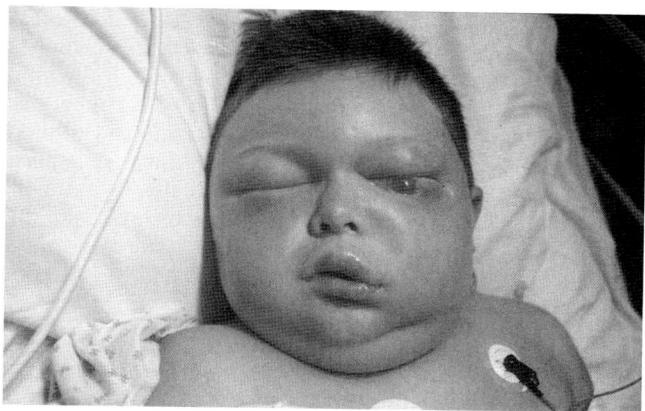

FIGURE 112-5

A 21-month-old boy bitten on the lower left eyelid. Note the extent of facial edema, which includes the neck and potentially the airway. See Color Fig. 112-5.

mimicking a viral syndrome. Worsening gastrointestinal complaints within the first few days may reflect toxic hepatitis or, rarely, pancreatitis, or both. An erythematous scarlatiniform eruption may develop. This eruption usually represents a toxic erythroderma rather than a reaction to streptococci or staphylococci. The rash may occur early and persist for many days and may be followed by epidermal sloughing. Although rarely seen, a faint lacy or speckled macular erythema of the trunk and flexor surfaces seen on days 3 to 5 often coincides with the beginning of resolution of the local ischemic lesion.[40]

Life-Threatening Complications

As loxoscelism progresses, the patient may exhibit jaundice, hemoglobinemia, hemoglobinuria, abnormal bleeding, and, rarely, pulmonary edema or effusion and congestive heart failure. The most common life-threatening reactions are hemolysis, coagulopathies (thrombocytopenia, consumptive coagulopathy, disseminated intravascular coagulation), and sepsis.[5,35,41]

Hemolysis may develop within hours or may be insidious and not appreciated until 48 to 96 hours postenvenomation. If hemolysis does not occur during the first 96 hours, it is unlikely to occur. When hemolysis does develop, it usually persists for 4 to 7 days, rarely longer. Hemolysis may be intravascular, extravascular, or both. The resulting hypoxemia contributes to lethargy, coma, shock, seizures, or possibly dysrhythmias and cardiac arrest. Hemoglobinuric renal failure or rarely death may ensue.[42] When a patient suspected of having loxoscelism is admitted to an intensive care unit, it constitutes a true medical emergency.

DIAGNOSIS

Differential Diagnosis

There are at least 14 groups of spiders capable of causing dermonecrosis (*Acanthoscurria, Argiope, Atrax, Avicularia, Chiracanthium, Loxosceles, Lycosa, Megaphobema,*

Pamphobeteus, Phidippus, Phormictopus, Tegenaria agrestis, Teraphosa, Xenesthis) (Table 112-3).[43] Only a few natural toxins cause hemolysis, however.[39] The likelihood of a patient's having moderate-to-severe consumptive coagulopathy without having some degree of hemolysis is low. The most common poisoning mimicking loxoscelism is coagulopathic (viper) snake envenomation, which should be readily distinguished by the appearance of at least one of the two fang marks, usually with some oozing of blood from the puncture site and a more rapid progression of swelling and pain.

Distinguishing a dermonecrotic lesion from a nonnecrotic skin lesion is often difficult in the early stages. The necrotic lesion typically progresses from an appearance of pallor or erythema to a violaceous macule with darkened areas. The edge of a necrotic lesion is usually uneven as the macule enlarges and the center darkens; the entire lesion tends to sink below skin level.[40,44]

Presumptive Diagnosis

Early in the course of envenomation, the presence and severity of loxoscelism are difficult to assess. Usually the diagnosis is made presumptively because the culprit spider is rarely seen, caught, and properly identified. The diagnosis is best made based on the association of characteristic local/cutaneous and systemic/visceral manifestations, a consistent skin lesion, timing of events, the known existence of *Loxosceles* spiders in the area, and the exclusion of other diagnoses. In cases without positive identification of the offending spider, the diagnosis most commonly used should be "arthropod bite or sting," "necrotizing lesion," or "presumptive *Loxosceles* envenomation."[39,44]

TABLE 112-3 Differential Diagnosis of *Loxosceles* Envenomation

Bites and stings from other arachnids, insects, and other creatures
 causing cutaneous lesions
Dermatologic conditions
Hereditary hemolytic anemias
Acquired hemolytic anemias
 Autoimmune conditions caused by medications (methyldopa, penicillin,
  quinidine), underlying diseases, idiopathic
 Nonimmune conditions caused by microangiopathic disorders,
  medications (nitrofurantoin, sulfonamides), chemicals (heavy metals),
  cardiac valve prostheses, physical agents (lightning, fresh water
  drowning)
Other natural toxins causing hemolysis
 Snakes (rattlesnakes, cobra, viper venom)
 Spiders (see text)
 Hymenoptera (e.g., bees, wasps)
 Coelenterata (Portuguese man-of-war, jellyfish)
 Infections (*Clostridium, Streptococcus* spp., *Staphylococcus* spp.)
Medical conditions causing cutaneous lesions
 Emboli
 Frostbite
 Thermal injury
 Ischemic vascular disorders
 Fat herniation/infarction
 Factitious ulcers (self-inflicted)
 Traumatic lesions

Definitive Test

There is presently no routinely available, reliable specific diagnostic test, although blood, blister fluid, and more recently tissue biopsy and hair serologic tests have been available on an investigational basis for the diagnosis of loxoscelism as late as 4 days after envenomation.[45–47]

TREATMENT

Treatment options for loxoscelism may be divided into three categories: (1) general wound care, (2) care of the ischemic necrotic lesion, and (3) treatment of systemic toxicity. The "benign neglect" approach suffices for most bites.[43] Most manifestations are determined within minutes of envenomation.

General Wound Care

Basic wound care should be provided to prevent secondary bacterial infection from the victim's endogenous staphylococci or streptococci. Prophylactic antimicrobials generally are not considered warranted, although it may be difficult to distinguish cellulitis from the common noninfected inflammatory response. In our experience, erythema appearing within the first 12 to 24 hours usually means inflammation rather than infection. Cellulitis is more apparent when lymphangitis is present or when the initial inflammatory redness has faded, then recurs with increased tenderness. There is probably no advantage to elevation or immobilization of a bitten extremity, although avoiding a dependent position is helpful; motion is self-limited by pain. Tetanus prophylaxis is indicated. Cool compresses (not ice—avoid freezing tissue) may be comforting, but heat should be avoided because it may stimulate activity of sphingomyelinase D. Analgesics and antiinflammatory drugs that affect platelet function should be avoided. Theoretically, acetaminophen should not be used if hepatotoxicity is suspected. Opioids seem to be optimal for pain control. Antipruritics or antianxiety medications may be administered as needed.

Care of the Cutaneous Lesion

Because local microvascular and tissue injury begins to occur within minutes of envenomation, medical care is directed at amelioration rather than prevention. Any further trauma to the bite site should be avoided. Palpation should be gentle and performed only as often as necessary. Restrictive bindings and needle punctures surrounding the site should be avoided except as needed for skin biopsy or leading edge aspirate for culture. No therapies (i.e., antihistamines, antimicrobials, dextran, and others) applied or injected locally or parenterally have ever been proven to reduce or prevent dermonecrosis. In animals, there were no beneficial effects of corticosteroids or the vasodilator phentolamine, even when steroids were administered before the bite or mixed in with the venom used to induce the injury.[40]

NITROGLYCERIN

A randomized, controlled therapeutic trial using 2% topical nitroglycerin ointment in rabbits experimentally envenomated with *L. reclusa* venom showed that this therapy is potentially harmful, causing increased edema, inflammation, and increased creatine phosphokinase concentrations. Skin necrosis was not significantly affected.[48]

DAPSONE

A randomized, controlled, blinded rabbit study of *Loxosceles* envenomation did not show benefit from dapsone (or either hyperbaric oxygen [HBO] or the potent antiserotonergic agent cyproheptadine).[49] Comparing dapsone with electric shock therapy and surgical excision did not show any significant beneficial effect.[46,50] Dapsone, a leukocyte inhibitor, is popular among some clinicians, although it has not been found to be effective in the treatment of loxoscelism in any human or animal controlled study. Dapsone in therapeutic and supratherapeutic doses is associated with hemolytic anemia, methemoglobinemia, or gastrointestinal distress, especially in children.[51] Even if dapsone were proven capable of lessening dermonecrosis by interrupting the leukocyte-influenced inflammatory cascade, it is doubtful that it could be administered soon enough after envenomation to be helpful. If there is any indication for dapsone for a presumed or known *Loxosceles* bite, it should be limited to use in a nonpregnant patient, bitten in a cosmetic area (i.e., face, digits), who presents with an ischemic lesion within hours of the bite. As noted earlier, however, dapsone use has never been validated. Its potential benefit is only theoretical. The adult dose is 25 to 100 mg orally, twice daily. The clinical pharmacology of dapsone is described in detail in Chapter 62. In our opinion, dapsone should never be used for children with loxoscelism.

HYPERBARIC OXYGEN

Although HBO therapy is used for a variety of tissue injuries, there is no proven benefit of HBO in loxoscelism.[49,52,53] A controlled HBO study in rabbits showed no significant effect on blood flow either at the wound center or 1 to 2 cm from the center.[54] There was a significantly decreased wound diameter noted at 10 days, however, when standard HBO was used within 48 hours of a simulated bite in contrast to normoxic pressure treatment.[54] Because HBO may promote neovascularization in necrotic tissue and reduces lipid peroxidation, it theoretically may enhance wound healing, especially in patients with vascular insufficiency (e.g., diabetes, sickle cell anemia).

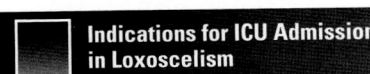

Indications for ICU Admission in Loxoscelism

Consumptive coagulopathy
Hemolysis
Dysrhythmias
Renal failure
Shock
Congestive heart failure
Pulmonary edema

SURGERY AND DÉBRIDEMENT

Early surgical intervention is not helpful because venom diffuses rapidly throughout the soft tissues surrounding a bite.[45] Some investigators have advocated wide excision of the bite site because venom can be detected in necrotic skin lesions 29 days after the bite.[55] However, excision may cause delayed wound healing, increase infection, worsen scarring, and cause disability.[44,50] Development of an abscess and suspected necrotizing fasciitis are indications for surgery. Skin grafting of a nonhealing necrotic area should be delayed for 4 to 12 weeks to allow for neovascularization at the demarcated edges.[44,45,56]

Most superficial necrotic lesions of a few centimeters in diameter or less demarcate, form an eschar, and heal completely with only basic wound care. Rarely a large necrotic area may require delayed excision with primary or secondary closure. Scar formation of smaller lesions is usually minimal, although underlying fat necrosis may produce a dimpling effect.

We have had success trimming bullae that are rapidly enlarging, stopping their progression. This layer of skin is friable and easily débrided. Usually the tissues within the borders and beneath blisters and bullae are the most necrotic. Benefit to the underlying skin from this procedure is thought to result from removal of chemotoxic substances located within the blister fluid. This fluid may be serous or hemorrhagic in appearance and on the basis of microbial culture is almost always sterile. The remaining tissue beneath the blister site may appear beefy red, friable, hemorrhagic, ischemic/necrotic, or viable. Débridement does not limit the ultimate size of necrosis.

Treatment of Systemic Toxicity

The major life-threatening effects of loxoscelism are hemolysis, disseminated intravascular coagulation, and sepsis. Systemic corticosteroid therapy seems to suppress hemolysis and usually is required for 5 to 10 days.[40,44,45] We recommend that intravenous methylprednisolone (or equivalent regimen) be administered to adults and children at a loading dose of 1 to 2 mg/kg ideal body weight and followed with 0.5 to 1 mg/kg every 6 hours. The dose may be adjusted according to patient response. Although corticosteroids may be required for 5 to 10 days, tapering usually can begin in 3 to 5 days if hemolysis/hemoglobinuria is undetectable or minimally present. Alkalization of the urine to prevent renal failure is recommended for significant hemoglobinuria. Hydration, to yield good urine output, is essential to prevent acute renal tubular necrosis from hemoglobinuria or hematuria. Extracorporeal dialysis does not remove venom but may be indicated in a supportive manner for renal failure.[44,45] If there is a potential need for blood component therapy, a blood type and screen/crossmatch should be done early in the course of events to avoid difficulties with crossmatching secondary to interfering antibodies.[57] Coombs' test and other direct antiglobulin tests may or may not be positive.[5,58,59] Severe hemolytic anemia is an indication for packed red blood cell transfusion. Transfusion of whole blood should be avoided because complement and perhaps other unknown factors in plasma

seem to react with venom and contribute to red blood cell destruction.[57]

Patients with suspected loxoscelism who are admitted to an intensive care unit should be monitored by serial evaluation of hemoglobin/hematocrit, platelet count, and urine for red blood cells or hemoglobin. Liver and renal function tests also should be followed. Pancreatic enzyme (amylase or lipase) levels should be obtained if abdominal distress is noted. A dip-stick of the urine may be negative despite significant hemolysis because the haptoglobin binding capacity must be exceeded before free hemoglobin passes into the urine. An insidious or gradual onset of hemolysis may be difficult to detect; in these instances, a serum/plasma "free" hemoglobin concentration and reticulocyte count may be helpful.

Patients presenting with significant systemic effects should be evaluated for consumptive coagulation. The coagulation workup should include the equivalent of a prothrombin and partial thromboplastin time or international normalized ratio, fibrinogen, D dimers, and platelet count. Evaluation and management of complicated disseminated intravascular coagulation may be aided by using some recently available modalities (e.g., recombinant factor VIIa [NovoSeven; Novo Nordisk Pharmaceutical Industries, Inc., Princeton, NJ]).[60] Antithrombin III is one of the most important physiologic inhibitors of coagulation and is often decreased in coagulopathies. Because antithrombin III concentrate is commercially available, an antithrombin III level is helpful when consumptive coagulopathy is documented. If the antithrombin III concentration is low, it should be replaced intravenously. Thrombocytopenia requires platelet transfusion and corticosteroids at similar doses used for hemolysis therapy.[61] Caution is needed when treating bleeding or disseminated intravascular coagulation with whole blood, fresh frozen plasma (contains all clotting factors but at relatively low concentrations), or cryoprecipitate (contains fibrin, factor VIII, factor XIII, and von Willebrand's factor) because endogenous substances in these agents may worsen hemolysis.[57] Coagulopathy is a crucial component of the pathophysiology of loxoscelism. Morbidity can occur quickly, with third-space blood loss further compromising tissue oxygen delivery caused by hemolysis.[6]

Bacteremia, septicemia, toxic shock syndrome, and necrotizing fasciitis are serious secondary bacterial infection–related complications of loxoscelism. Infections are not common, however, and usually do not occur within the first few days after the bite. Antimicrobial therapy should be selected to cover anaerobes, staphylococci, and streptococci and according to culture and sensitivity test results. Cellulitis and lymphangitis most commonly are secondary to staphylococcal or streptococcal infection.

Although *Loxosceles* antivenom is used extensively in South America, there is presently no universally available antivenom preparation. A polyvalent antiarachnidic antiserum for spider bites has been produced in Brazil by injecting horses with venom from multiple spiders. An anti-*Loxosceles* antivenom has been developed and has shown efficacy in treating *Loxosceles* envenomations.[62] Although venom from *Loxosceles* often is not detected in the serum by 12 to 24 hours after envenomation, it has been detected in necrotic skin lesions 29 days after the bite.[63] Antivenom efficacy has been noted in a few animal studies and one uncontrolled

Criterion for ICU Discharge in Loxoscelism

Resolution or stabilization of indications for intensive care unit admission (see previous box) depending on capability of other hospital resources

Key Points in Loxoscelism

1. Loxoscelism is a form of necrotic arachnidism found throughout the world.
2. Cutaneous and systemic effects can occur. Most patients do not develop significant systemic effects.
3. The severity of cutaneous effects does not indicate the severity of systemic effects and vice versa.
4. Life-threatening events (e.g., hemolysis, coagulopathy, sepsis) may occur.
5. Treatment is largely symptomatic and supportive because antivenom is not routinely available.

human study.[64–67] Anti-*Loxosceles* Fab fragments intradermally injected into rabbits showed markedly attenuated, venom-induced dermal inflammation if administered within 4 hours.[68] Infusion of a monoclonal antibody shown to neutralize interleukin-8 attenuated the development of venom-induced ulcers in rabbits injected with *Loxosceles* venom.[69] In practice, it is doubtful that antivenom could be administered soon enough after envenomation to prevent dermonecrosis because cytotoxic effects develop rapidly. It also is doubtful that antivenom could antagonize toxicity caused by cytokines, antibodies, or other mediators already elaborated. In theory, however, *Loxosceles*-specific antivenom could inactivate venom, preventing hemolysis, coagulopathy, and worsening dermonecrosis.[17,65,66]

SPECIAL POPULATIONS

Children and debilitated individuals are at a greater risk for severe systemic reactions, especially hemolysis and coagulopathy. Children seem to suffer less dermonecrosis than adults, which may be linked to the fact that they have less subcutaneous fat and better microcirculation at the bite site. Based on anecdotal reports, it has been speculated that elderly individuals who grew up in regions inhabited by *Loxosceles* spiders may be asymptomatic or experience only mild toxicity after a bite; in theory, this may be secondary to acquired immunity from prior bites in their lifetime. Women who are pregnant are not at increased risk for systemic effects and should be treated similarly to other patients; the fetus is at risk only if life-threatening maternal complications arise.[70]

A few patients with loxoscelism may develop pyoderma gangrenosum, although no common risk identifier among patients is present. Pyoderma gangrenosum is a rare disease with recurrent deep ulcerations of the skin. The etiology of the disease is unclear, but it is often associated with disorders of immune dysfunction.[71] It has been shown that impaired cell-mediated immunity with the addition of a "dermonecrotic factor" may lead to the development of the disorder.[72] As such, pyoderma gangrenosum has been seen in patients who have been diagnosed with *Loxosceles* envenomation.[73,74] This condition may occur because of the dermonecrotic effects of sphingomyelinase D. It has been seen in young and old adults after brown recluse spider bites. Treatment usually consists of long-term corticosteroid treatment because the ulcers recur when therapy is discontinued. Some authors have stated that patients who have had excision therapy for *Loxosceles* bite may be more prone to development of this rare disorder. Not all reported cases have had surgical excision, however.

REFERENCES

1. Habermehl GG: Venomous Animals and Their Toxins. Berlin, Springer-Verlag, 1981, pp 33–38.
2. Macchiavello A: La Loxosceles laeta, causa del Arachnidismo cutaneo O Mancha Gangrenosa, De Chili. Rev Chilena Hist Natl 41:11–23, 1937.
3. Sezerino UM, Zannin M, Coelho LK, et al: A clinical and epidemiological study of *Loxosceles* spider envenoming in Santa Catarina, Brazil. Trans R Soc Trop Med Hyg 92:546–548, 1998.
4. Taylor EH, Denny WF: Hemolysis, renal failure, and death presumed secondary to bite of brown recluse spider. South Med J 59:1209–1211, 1966.
5. Williams ST, Khare VK, Johnston GA, et al: Severe intravascular hemolysis associated with brown recluse spider envenomation: A report of two cases and review of the literature. Am J Clin Pathol 104:463–467, 1995.
6. Wasserman G, Garola R, Marshall J, et al: Death of a 7-year-old by presumptive Brown recluse spider bite. J Toxicol Clin Toxicol 37:614–615, 1999.
7. Gertsch WJ, Ennik F: The spider genus *Loxosceles* in North America, Central America, and West Indies (Araneae, Loxoscelidae). Bull Am Museum Natl Hist 175:265–360, 1983.
8. Lucas S: Spiders in Brazil. Toxicon 26:759–772, 1988.
9. Sams HH, Dunnick, CA, Smith ML, et al: Necrotic arachnidism. J Am Acad Dermatol 44:561–573, 2001.
10. Schenone H, Rojas A, Reyes H, et al: Prevalence of *Loxosceles laeta* in houses in central Chile. Am J Trop Med Hyg 19:564–567, 1970.
11. Costa RS, Salveraglio FJ: Nota previa sobre araneismo cutaneo en el Uruguay. Arch Urug Med 14:417, 1939.
12. Ori M: Aranea. In Sasa M, Tanaka H, Kano R, et al (eds): Animals of Medical Importance in Nansei Islands in Japan. Tokyo, Shinjuka shobo, 1977.
13. Waldron WG, Russell FE: *Loxosceles reclusa* in Southern California. Toxicon 5:57–59, 1967.
14. Hall RD, Anderson PC: Brown recluse spider bites: Can they be prevented? Mo Med 78:243–248, 1981.
15. Geren CR, Chan TK, Ward BC, et al: Composition and properties of extract of fiddleback spider venom apparatus (*L. reclusa*). Toxicon 11:471–479, 1973.
16. Rees RS, Nanney LB, Yates RA, et al: Interaction of brown recluse spider venom on cell membranes: The inciting mechanism? J Invest Derm 83:270–275, 1984.
17. Gomez HF, Greenfield DM, Miller MM, et al: Direct correlation between diffusion of *Loxosceles reclusa* venom and extent of dermal inflammation. Acad Emerg Med 8:311–314, 2001.
18. Barbaro KC, Eicksted VRD, Mota I: Antigenic cross-reactivity of venoms from medically important *Loxosceles* (Araneae) species in Brazil. Toxicon 32:113–120, 1994.
19. Babcock JL, Marmer DJ, Steele RW: Immunotoxicology of brown recluse spider (*Loxosceles reclusa*) venom. Toxicon 24:783–790, 1986.
20. Forrester LJ, Barrett JT, Campbell BJ: Red blood cell lysis induced by the venom of the brown recluse spider: The role of sphingomyelinase D. Arch Biochem Biophys 187:355–365, 1978.
21. Gates CA, Rees RS: Serum amyloid p component: Its role in platelet activation stimulated by sphingomyelinase D purified from the venom of

the brown recluse spider (*Loxosceles reclusa*). Toxicon 28:1303–1315, 1990.

22. Gertsch WJ: American Spiders, 2nd ed. New York, Van Nostrand Reinhold, 1979.

23. Huford DC, Morgan PN: C-reactive protein as a mediator in the lysis of human erythrocytes sensitized by brown recluse spider venom. Proc Soc Exp Biol Med 167:493–497, 1981.

24. Kniker WT, Morgan PN, Flanigan WJ, et al: An inhibitor of complement in the venom of the brown recluse spider, *Loxosceles reclusa*. Proc Soc Exp Biol Med 131:1432–1434, 1969.

25. Kurpiewski G, Forrester LJ, Barrett JT, et al: Platelet aggregation and sphingomyelinase D activity of a purified toxin from the venom of *Loxosceles reclusa*. Biochem Biophys Acta 678:467–476, 1981.

26. Patel KD, Modur V, Zimmerman GA, et al: The necrotic venom of the brown recluse spider induces dysregulated endothelial cell-dependent neutrophil activation. J Clin Invest 94:631–642, 1994.

27. Smith CW, Micks DW: The role of polymorphonuclear leukocytes in the lesion caused by the venom of the brown spider, *Loxosceles reclusa*. Lab Invest 22:90–93, 1970.

28. Desai A, Miller MJ, Gomez HF, et al: *Loxosceles deserta* spider venom induces NF KB-dependent chemokine production by endothelial cells. J Toxicol Clin Toxicol 37:447–456, 1999.

29. Gomez HF, Miller MJ, Desai A, et al: *Loxosceles* venom induces production of multiple chemokines by endothelial and epithelial cells. Inflammation 23:207–215, 1999.

30. Tambourgi DV, Morgan BP, de Andrade RMG, et al: *Loxosceles intermedia* spider envenomation induces activation of an endogenous metalloproteinase, resulting in cleavage of glycophorins from the erythrocyte surface and facilitating complement-mediated lysis. Blood 95:683–691, 2000.

31. Bey TA, Walters FG, Lober W, et al: *Loxosceles arizonica* bite associated with shock. Ann Emerg Med 30:701–703, 1997.

32. Futrell JM: Loxoscelism. Am J Med Sci 304:261–267, 1992.

33. Pucevich MV, Chesney TMcC: Histopathologic analysis of human bites by the brown recluse spider (Abstract). Arch Dermatol 119:851, 1983.

34. Berger SM: The unremarkable brown recluse spider bite. JAMA 225:1109–1111, 1973.

35. Wasserman GS, Mydler TT, Sharma V: Brown recluse spider envenomation as a cause of hemolysis and hemoglobinuria (Abstract). Vet Hum Toxicol 33:359, 1991.

36. Schenone H, Saaverdra T, Rojas A, et al: Loxoscelism in Chile: Epidemiologic, clinical and experimental studies. Rev Inst Med Trop Sao Paulo 31:403–415, 1989.

37. Goto CS, Abramo TJ, Ginsburg CM: Upper airway obstruction caused by brown recluse spider envenomation of the neck. Am J Emerg Med 14:660–662, 1996.

38. Edwards JJ, Anderson RL, Wood JR: Loxoscelism of the eyelid. Arch Ophthalmol 98:1997–2000, 1980.

39. Wasserman GS: Brown recluse and other necrotizing spiders. In Ford MD, Delaney KA, Ling LJ, et al (eds): Clinical Toxicology. Philadelphia, WB Saunders, 2001, pp 878–884.

40. Anderson PC: Necrotizing spider bite. Am Fam Physician 26:198–203, 1982.

41. Vorse H, Seccareccio P, Woodruff K, et al: Disseminated intravascular coagulopathy following fatal brown spider bite (necrotic arachnidism). J Pediatr 80:1035–1037, 1972.

42. Taylor EM, Denny W: Hemolysis, renal failure and death, presumed secondary to the bite of brown recluse spider. South Med J 59:1209–1211, 1966.

43. Wasserman GS: Brown recluse spider envenomations. In Harwood-Nuss A, Wolfson AB, Linden CH, et al (eds): The Clinical Practice of Emergency Medicine, 3rd ed. Philadelphia, Lippincott Williams & Wilkins, 2001, pp 1638–1640.

44. Wasserman GS, Anderson PC: Loxoscelism and necrotic arachnidism. J Toxicol Clin Toxicol 21:451–472, 1983–1984.

45. Anderson PC: What's new in loxoscelism—1978: Case report. Mo Med 74:549–552, 1977.

46. Barrett SM, Romine-Jenkins M, Blick KE: Passive hemagglutination inhibition test for diagnosis of brown recluse spider bite envenomation. Clin Chem 39:2104–2107, 1993.

47. Miller MJ, Gomez HF, Snider RJ, et al: Detection of *Loxosceles* venom in lesional hair shafts and skin application of a specific immunoassay to identify dermonecrotic arachnidism. Am J Emerg Med 18:626–628, 2000.

48. Lowry BP, Bradfield JF, Carroll RG, et al: A controlled trial of topical nitroglycerin in a New Zealand white rabbit model of brown recluse spider envenomation. Ann Emerg Med 37:161–165, 2001.

49. Philips S, Kohn M, Baker D, et al: Therapy of brown spider envenomation: A controlled trial of hyperbaric oxygen, dapsone, and cyproheptadine. Ann Emerg Med 25:363–368, 1995.

50. Rees RS, Altenbern DP, Lynch JB, et al: Brown recluse spider bites: A comparison of surgical excision versus dapsone and delayed surgical excision. Ann Surg 202:659–663, 1985.

51. Iserson KV: Methemoglobinemia from dapsone therapy for a suspected brown spider bite. J Emerg Med 3:285–288, 1985.

52. Skinner MW, Butler CS: Necrotizing arachnidism treated with hyperbaric oxygen. Med J Aust 162:372–373, 1995.

53. Hobbs GD, Anderson AR, Greene TJ, et al: Comparison of hyperbaric oxygen and dapsone therapy for *Loxosceles* envenomation. Acad Emerg Med 3:758–761, 1996.

54. Maynor ML, Moon RE, Klitzman B, et al: Brown recluse spider envenomation: A prospective trial of hyperbaric oxygen therapy. Acad Emerg Med 4:184–192, 1997.

55. Cardosa JLC, Wen FH, Franca FOS, et al: Detection by enzyme immunoassay of *Loxosceles gaucho* venom in necrotic skin lesions caused by spider bites in Brazil. Trans R Soc Trop Med Hyg 84:608–609, 1990.

56. Wasserman GS: Wound care of spider and snake envenomations. Ann Emerg Med 17:1331–1335, 1988.

57. Hardman JT, Beck ML, Hardman PK, et al: Incompatibility associated with the bite of the brown recluse spider (*Loxosceles reclusa*). Transfusion 23:233–236, 1983.

58. Eichner ER: Spider bite hemolytic anemia: Positive Coombs' test, erythrophagocytosis, and leukoerythroblastic smear. Am J Clin Pathol 81:683–687, 1984.

59. Knapp JF, Thomas KT, Mathews R, et al: Case 06–1994: A 10-year-old female with fever, jaundice and orthostatic hypotension. Pediatr Emerg Care 10:364–368, 1994.

60. Chuansumrit A, Chantarojanasiri T, Isarangkura P, et al: Recombinant activated factor VII in children with acute bleeding from liver failure and disseminated intravascular coagulation. Blood Coagul Fibrinol 11:S101–S105, 2000.

61. Levi M, de Jonge E, van der Poll T, et al: Novel approaches to the management of disseminated intravascular coagulation. Crit Care Med 28:S20–S24, 2000.

62. Braz A, Minozzo J, Abreu JC, et al: Development and evaluation of the neutralizing capacity of horse antivenom against the Brazilian spider *Loxosceles intermedia*. Toxicon 37:1323–1328, 1999.

63. Chavez-Olortegui C, Zanetti VC, Ferreira AP, et al: ELISA for the detection of venom antigens in experimental and clinical envenoming by *Loxosceles intermedia* spiders. Toxicon 36:563–569, 1998.

64. Rees R, Shack RB, Withers E, et al: Management of the brown recluse spider bite. Plast Reconstr Surg 68:768–773, 1981.

65. Bravo M, Oviedo I, Farias P, et al: Study of anti-*Loxosceles* serum action on hemolytic and ulcero-necrotic cutaneous effects of *Loxosceles laeta* venom. Rev Med Chil 122:625–629, 1994.

66. Cole HP, Wesley RE, King LE: Brown recluse envenomation of the eyelid: An animal model. Ophthalmol Plast Reconstr Surg 11:153–164, 1995.

67. Rees R, Campbell D, Rieger E, et al: The diagnosis and treatment of brown recluse spider bites. Ann Emerg Med 16:945–949, 1987.

68. Gomez HF, Miller MJ, Trachy JW, et al: Intradermal anti-*Loxosceles* Fab fragments attenuate dermonecrotic arachnidism. Acad Emerg Med 6:1195–1202, 1999.

69. Whetstone WD, Ernsting K, Warren JS, et al: Inhibition of dermonecrotic arachnidism with interleukin-8 monoclonal antibody. Acad Emerg Med 4:337, 1997.

70. Anderson PC: Loxoscelism threatening pregnancy: Five cases. Am J Obstet Gynecol 165:1454–1456, 1991.

71. Hickman JG, Lazarus GS: Pyoderma gangrenosum: A reappraisal of associated systemic diseases. Br J Dermatol 102:235–237, 1980.

72. Delescluse J, de Bast C, Achten G: Pyoderma gangrenosum with altered cellular immunity and dermonecrotic factor. Br J Dermatol 87:529–532, 1972.

73. Rees R, Fields JP, King LE: Do brown recluse spider bites induce pyoderma gangrenosum? South Med J 78:283–287, 1983.

74. Hoover EL, Williams W, Koger L: Pseudoepitheliomatous hyperplasia and pyoderma gangrenosum after a brown recluse spider bite. South Med J 83:243–246, 1990.

CHAPTER 113

Australian Funnel-Web Spiders

Julian White

Australian funnel-web spiders are arguably the world's most dangerous spiders. As with most spider bites, the bites caused by funnel-web spiders are frequently minor, but in the approximately 10% of cases in which systemic envenoming occurs, the chance of fatality is significant. Even modern interventions of intensive care medicine are insufficient to save a patient with a severe bite; only antivenom therapy is lifesaving in severe cases.[1,2]

TAXONOMY AND DISTRIBUTION

The Australian funnel-web spiders of the genera *Atrax* and *Hadronyche* are restricted to Australia, including Tasmania, as are the related mouse spiders of the genus *Missulena*.[3,4] All are mygalomorph spiders (Fig. 113-1) of the families Hexathelidae (*Atrax* and *Hadronyche*) and Actinopidae (*Missulena*). They are quite distinct from the "funnel-web spiders" of North America.

Funnel-web spiders live most of their lives in self-excavated or constructed silk-lined burrows or tubes, with traplines radiating from the entrance. The spider briefly leaves the burrow to catch prey crossing the traplines.[5] For mating to occur, however, the male must leave the burrow and roam the surrounding area in search of a female. This biologic necessity ensures that males are more likely to interact with humans than female spiders. There is significant sexual dimorphism, with females being slightly larger, more robust, with larger abdomens, and often with different coloration (particularly mouse spiders) than males.

Atrax

Currently there are three recognized species of *Atrax*, only one of which is fully described, the Sydney funnel-web spider, *Atrax robustus* (Fig. 113-2). This species has caused the most severe bites and fatalities, partly because it is distributed within a major urban conurbation (Sydney and surrounds). All three species are restricted to eastern New South Wales (Fig. 113-3).[3,4]

Hadronyche

Most of the more than 35 species of *Hadronyche* are not fully described. They are found in eastern Australia from Cape York to Tasmania (Fig. 113-3). Several *Hadronyche* spp. have

caused significant, potentially lethal bites (Table 113-1; Figs. 113-4 and 113-5).[3,4]

Missulena

The mouse spiders are of uncertain medical importance. They have a toxic venom similar to *Atrax* and *Hadronyche*, but there are virtually no cases of significant envenoming of humans, despite the Australia-wide distribution of these common spiders (Fig. 113-6).

VENOM

The venom of funnel-web spiders is a mixture of components, the most important of which is an excitatory neurotoxin, similar across species and potentially lethal for humans, but comparatively nontoxic for most other mammals.[5] This latter property has inhibited research and development of an antivenom.

Atrax

Of the three species of *Atrax*, only *A. robustus* venom has been examined in detail.[6] The venom of male spiders is approximately seven times more toxic than that of females. The principal lethal component is robustoxin,[7] a protein of molecular weight 4854 d, with 42 amino acid residues, four disulfide bridges, and subcutaneous median lethal dose of 0.16 mg/kg in newborn mice.

Hadronyche

The venom of several *Hadronyche* spp. has been examined, most notably *Hadronyche versuta*, with a principal lethal component similar to robustoxin, named *versutoxin*[8] (molecular weight 4852 d, 42 amino acid residues, four disulfide bridges, and subcutaneous median lethal dose 0.22 mg/kg in newborn mice). Venom from *H. formidabilis* and *H. infensa* appears similarly toxic, with equivalent toxicity in males and females, in contrast to *A. robustus*.

Missulena

Research has shown some *Missulena* spp. to have venom with robustoxin-like components and to be potentially lethal for humans, although no confirmed fatalities are

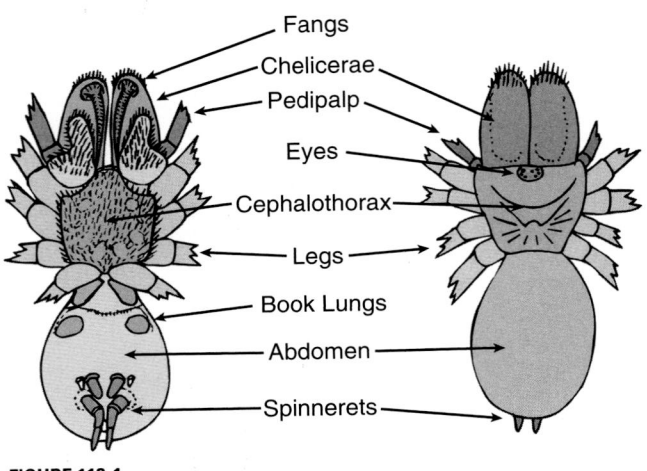

FIGURE 113-1

Diagrammatic representation of the external anatomy of mygalomorph spiders. (Copyright © Dr. Julian White, 2001.)

Labels in figure: Fangs, Chelicerae, Pedipalp, Eyes, Cephalothorax, Legs, Book Lungs, Abdomen, Spinnerets

known.[9] The similarities extend to antigenicity because antivenom against *A. robustus* appears likely to be effective against *Missulena* venom. This statement is consistent with the only reported human case of major envenoming by this genus, in which *Atrax*-specific antivenom was reported to be beneficial.[10]

CLINICAL PRESENTATION

From a clinical perspective, the effects of *Atrax* and *Hadronyche* bites on humans are essentially the same.[5] Because only one case of severe *Missulena* envenoming has been reported, the clinical features of significant envenoming from these spiders are uncertain.

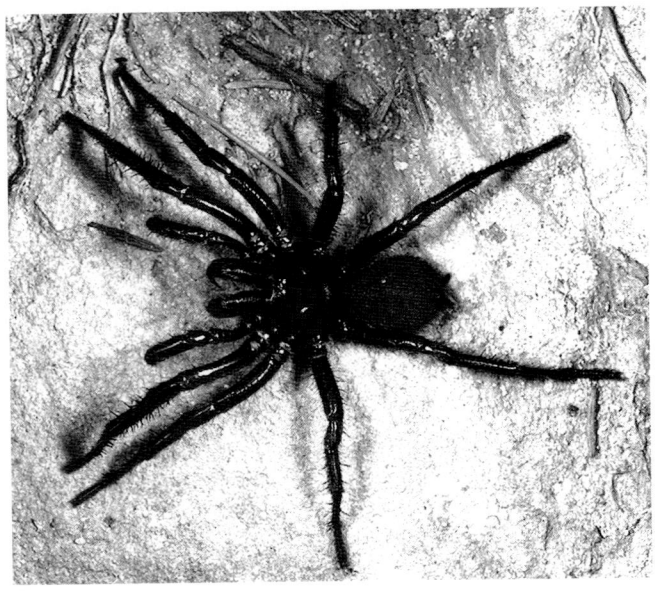

FIGURE 113-2

Male Sydney funnel-web spider, *Atrax robustus*. (Copyright © Dr. Julian White, 2001.)

Atrax

The bite is usually painful, owing to the size of the fangs (5 mm) and the acidic nature of the venom. The spider frequently hangs on. Bite marks are usually present (Fig. 113-7). In the few cases in which systemic envenoming develops, there may be rapid onset of early symptoms, such as lip paresthesias and tongue fasciculation. Time from bite to first systemic symptoms may be 10 minutes, and deaths occurring in less than 1 hour are recorded. Soon after onset of first symptoms, there is progression to more severe envenoming, which may include tachycardia, hypertension, hypersalivation and hyperlacrimation, piloerection, increased sweating, nausea, vomiting, abdominal pain, muscle fasciculation, cardiac arrhythmias, and pulmonary edema. Pulmonary edema may develop quickly, be more severe, and result in hypoxia and impaired consciousness or coma. Death in this phase is usually secondary to pulmonary edema. The pulmonary edema is considered neurogenic in origin. Should the patient survive this first phase without antivenom therapy, the untreated clinical course may progress to the second phase, in which excitatory effects subside, secretions cease, and hypertension resolves, only to evolve into a progressive and terminal hypotension, apnea, and cardiac arrest.

Hadronyche

The clinical picture for *Hadronyche* spp. is essentially the same as for *Atrax* spp. except that the former spiders are larger and it is possible, although not yet proven, that the chance of envenoming and life-threatening envenoming may be higher.[5,11–13] Virtually all well-documented deaths after funnel-web spider bite were due to *A. robustus*, however.

Missulena

The clinical picture for *Missulena* bites is uncertain. Experimentally the venom is similar to funnel-web spider venom, with similar toxicity and effects. These spiders are common, however, and many bites have occurred without deleterious effects (R. Raven: personal communication, 1994). The single case of significant envenoming, in a child, appeared similar to that of *Atrax* envenoming.[10] Nevertheless, in light of the similarity between its venom and that of *Atrax* and *Hadronyche* spp., bites by these spiders should be treated with great caution.[9]

COMPLICATIONS

The principal complications of funnel-web spider envenoming relate to the severity of direct venom effects. There may be hypoxic brain damage or other organ damage secondary to the pulmonary edema or cardiopulmonary or respiratory arrest.[1,2,5] There is a single case of prolonged status epilepticus after presumed *Hadronyche* bite, initially thought to be organophosphate poisoning (personal record; not published). In this case, there was no response to atropine, but rapid cessation of seizures occurred after administration of intravenous CSL Funnel-Web Spider Antivenom (FWSAV) (CSL Limited, Victoria, Australia). By this stage, irreversible, ultimately fatal brain damage had occurred.

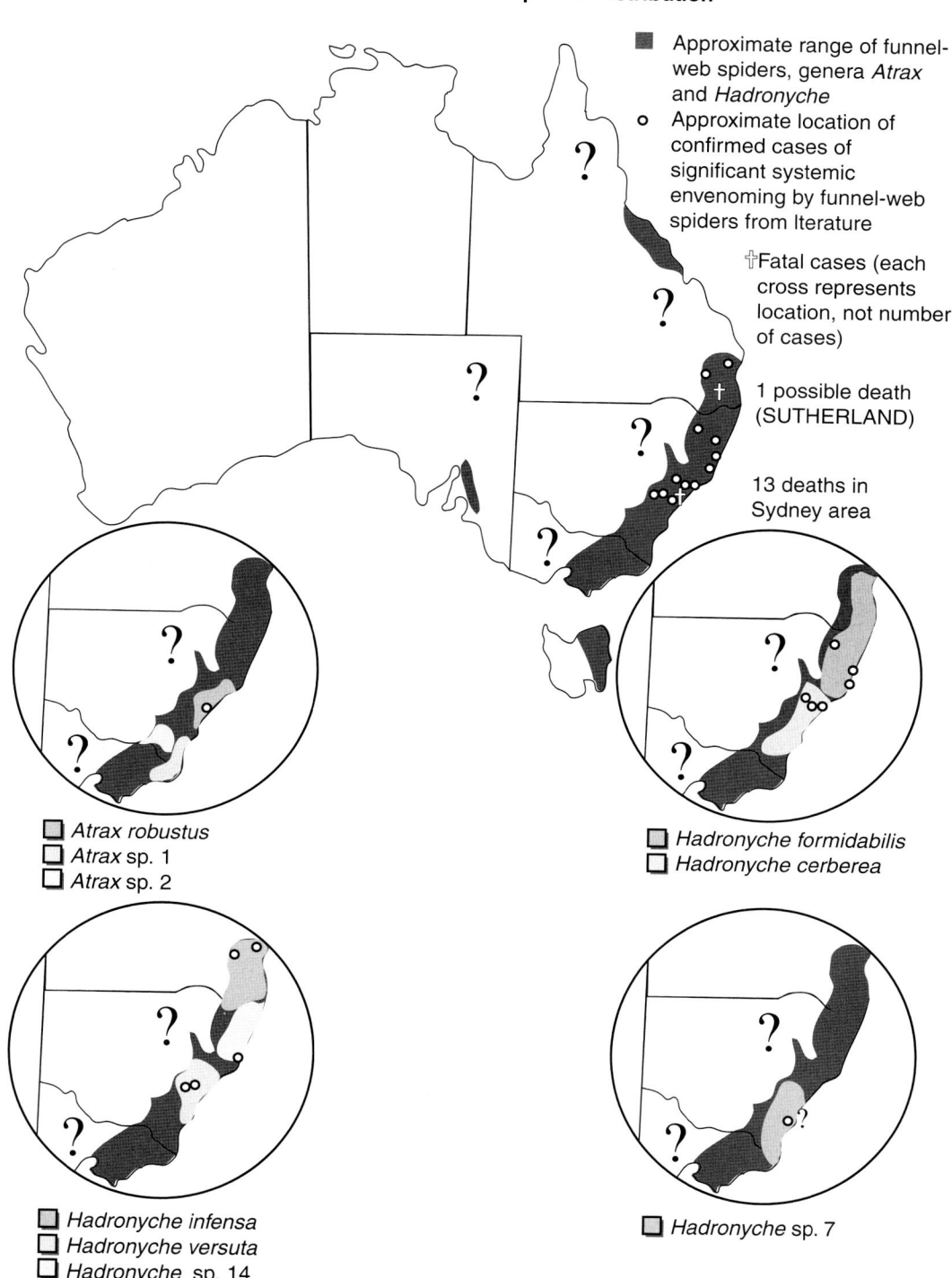

FIGURE 113-3

Distribution of Australian funnel-web spiders. *(Copyright © Dr. Julian White, 2001.)*

DIAGNOSIS

The diagnosis of funnel-web spider bite is made on clinical symptoms and signs or presentation of a funnel-web spider; currently no venom detection is available. Occasionally, patients may present in confusing circumstances, with no history of a bite and apparent exposure to a chemical (notably organophosphates), which may cause some similar clinical effects. The only known fatality due to funnel-web spider bite since introduction of antivenom occurred in such circumstances.

TABLE 113-1 Australian Funnel-Web Spiders Known to Have Caused Significant Envenoming in Humans

SPECIES	CLINICAL EFFECTS	NO. CASES WITH SIGNIFICANT EFFECTS REPORTED	NO. DEATHS REPORTED
Atrax robustus	Major systemic envenoming, known lethality	>100	13
Hadronyche cerberea	Moderate-to-severe systemic envenoming, potentially lethal	3	0
Hadronyche formidabilis	Major systemic envenoming, potentially lethal	5	0
Hadronyche infensa	Major systemic envenoming, potentially lethal	2 (4 minor cases)	? 1
Hadronyche versuta	Major systemic envenoming, potentially lethal	1	0
Hadronyche sp. 7	Moderate systemic envenoming, lethal potential uncertain	1	0
Hadronyche sp. 14	Major systemic envenoming, potentially lethal	1	0

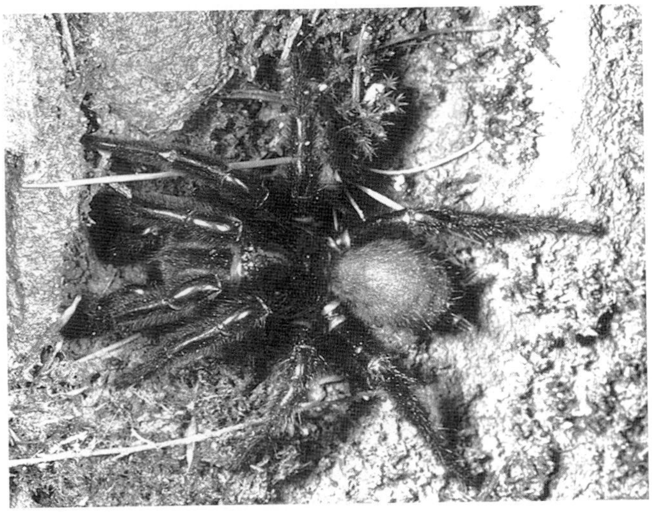

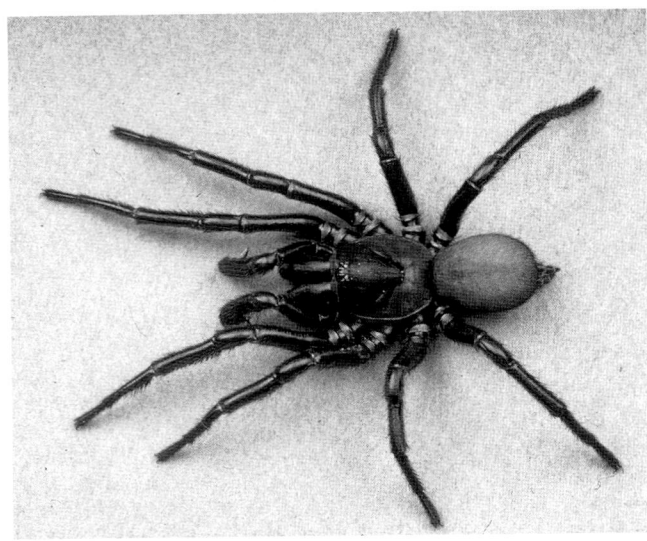

FIGURE 113-4

Female tree funnel-web spider, *Hadronyche formidabilis. (Copyright © Dr. Julian White, 2001.)*

History

In most cases, there is a history of a witnessed bite by a funnel-web spider because the spider is large and the bite generally is painful. Although patients often cannot identify a funnel-web spider confidently, these spiders are distinctive, and within their range it is appropriate that all bites by spiders of this appearance be managed initially as funnel-web bites. Conversely, outside the common range of these spiders, other mygalomorph spiders, such as trapdoor spiders (*Aganipe* spp.) and wishbone spiders (*Dekana* spp.), are frequently misidentified as funnel-web spiders. There is no evidence that these species are dangerous to humans, although also no substantial research, such as venom studies, to prove that they are harmless.

After establishing that a bite from a possible funnel-web spider has occurred, it is important to determine if systemic envenoming has developed. Major envenoming is obvious, but in initially minor cases, the clinician should determine if there has been any perioral paresthesias, tongue fasciculation, piloerection, or increased sweating or salivation. The presence of any of the aforementioned signs is strongly suspicious of development of significant systemic envenoming.

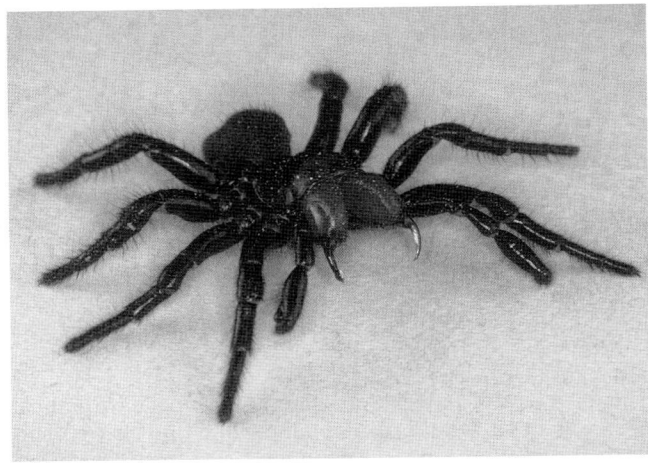

FIGURE 113-5

Male funnel-web spider, *Hadronyche cerberea. (Copyright © Dr. I. Whyte, 2000.)*

FIGURE 113-6

Male mouse spider, *Missulena insigne. (Copyright © Dr. Julian White, 2001.)*

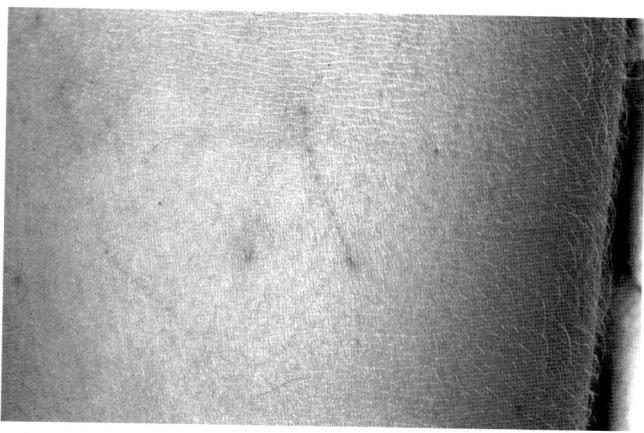

FIGURE 113-7

Local appearance of funnel-web spider bite. *(From Miller MK, Whyte IM, White J, Keir P: Clinical features and management of* Hadronyche *envenomation in man. Toxicon 38:409–427, 2000. Copyright © Dr. I. Whyte, 2000.)*

Examination

The clinician specifically should look for evidence of autonomic stimulation, such as tongue fasciculation; piloerection; increased sweating, salivation, and lacrimation; tachycardia; hypertension; and particularly pulmonary edema.

Laboratory Tests

There are no tests specific for funnel-web spider envenoming. Experimentally envenomed monkeys have developed metabolic acidosis and elevated creatine phosphokinase concentrations.

Differential Diagnosis

No other terrestrial venomous animals are likely to cause a syndrome similar to funnel-web spider envenoming. Red back spiders (widow spiders; *Latrodectus hasseltii* [latrodectism]) can cause increased sweating and occasionally piloerection and commonly cause nausea and abdominal pain and hypertension, but they virtually never cause pulmonary edema. Local, regional, or generalized pain is more prominent in most cases of latrodectism. Organophosphate poisoning may result in symptoms and signs similar to funnel-web spider envenoming—classically, tachycardia, hypertension (bradycardia and hypotension are also possible if muscarinic effects predominate), miosis, muscle fasciculation, excessive secretions, bronchospasm, vomiting, diarrhea, urinary incontinence, and occasionally pulmonary edema. The absence of bronchospasm and prominence of pulmonary edema should suggest funnel-web spider envenoming; conversely, the presence of bronchospasm and comparatively mild pulmonary edema (if present at all) should suggest organophosphate poisoning. Organophosphate poisoning is usually associated with a latent period of 1 or more hours between exposure and onset of symptoms.

TREATMENT (Fig. 113-8)

Treatment of funnel-web spider bite should focus on the needs of the few patients who develop systemic envenoming, because this is potentially lethal. All patients with definite or suspected funnel-web spider bite should be urgently hospitalized and assessed. At the first sign of systemic envenoming, antivenom therapy should be started. Most bites prove minor, however, and any patient presenting more than 6 hours postbite without symptoms or signs of systemic envenoming is unlikely to develop envenoming subsequently.

Most cases of funnel-web spider bite need no more than a period of observation because the bite is minor. Because late effects occasionally occur, observation for at least 12 hours is advisable.

First Aid

The recommended first aid for funnel-web spider bites is the pressure immobilization technique (see Chapter 105).[14,15] In contrast to snake venom, funnel-web spider venom is at least partially destroyed by prolonged immobilization at the bite site; this method not only delays envenoming but also may reduce the extent of envenoming. This technique is especially important given the rapidity of possible envenoming.

Urgent Measures

After stabilization of airway and breathing, good intravenous access is the next priority to allow rapid intravenous antivenom infusion, if indicated.

Antivenom

The only reliably lifesaving treatment in severe envenoming is intravenous antivenom therapy using specific FWSAV.[5,11,16–21] FWSAV is lyophilized rabbit IgG against male *A. robustus* venom. Since its introduction in 1980–1981, there has been only one known death after funnel-web spider bite, and in that single case, death was due to late diagnosis, not failure of antivenom. FWSAV is unlikely to cause major adverse immediate reactions, such as anaphylaxis, given the catecholamine excess that is characteristic of these envenomations, but serum sickness has occurred in at least one case (out of >50 treated cases).

WHEN TO USE ANTIVENOM

FWSAV should be used in all patients with systemic envenoming except patients who present late with no more than mild envenoming that has not progressed over several hours. At the earliest evidence of systemic envenoming, it is appropriate to consider starting antivenom therapy because progression to life-threatening envenoming may be rapid, especially in children.

DOSAGE

Initial dose depends on the degree of envenoming. For mild envenoming, the clinician should consider starting with two vials; for more severe envenoming, treatment may be started with four vials.[22] In either case, if response is incomplete, giving a further two to four vials may be considered after 15 to 30 minutes. Even severe cases usually respond to 6 to 8 vials, but occasionally more vials are required; the maximum recorded was 18 vials. There is mounting evidence that *Hadronyche* bites may require higher doses than *Atrax* bites.

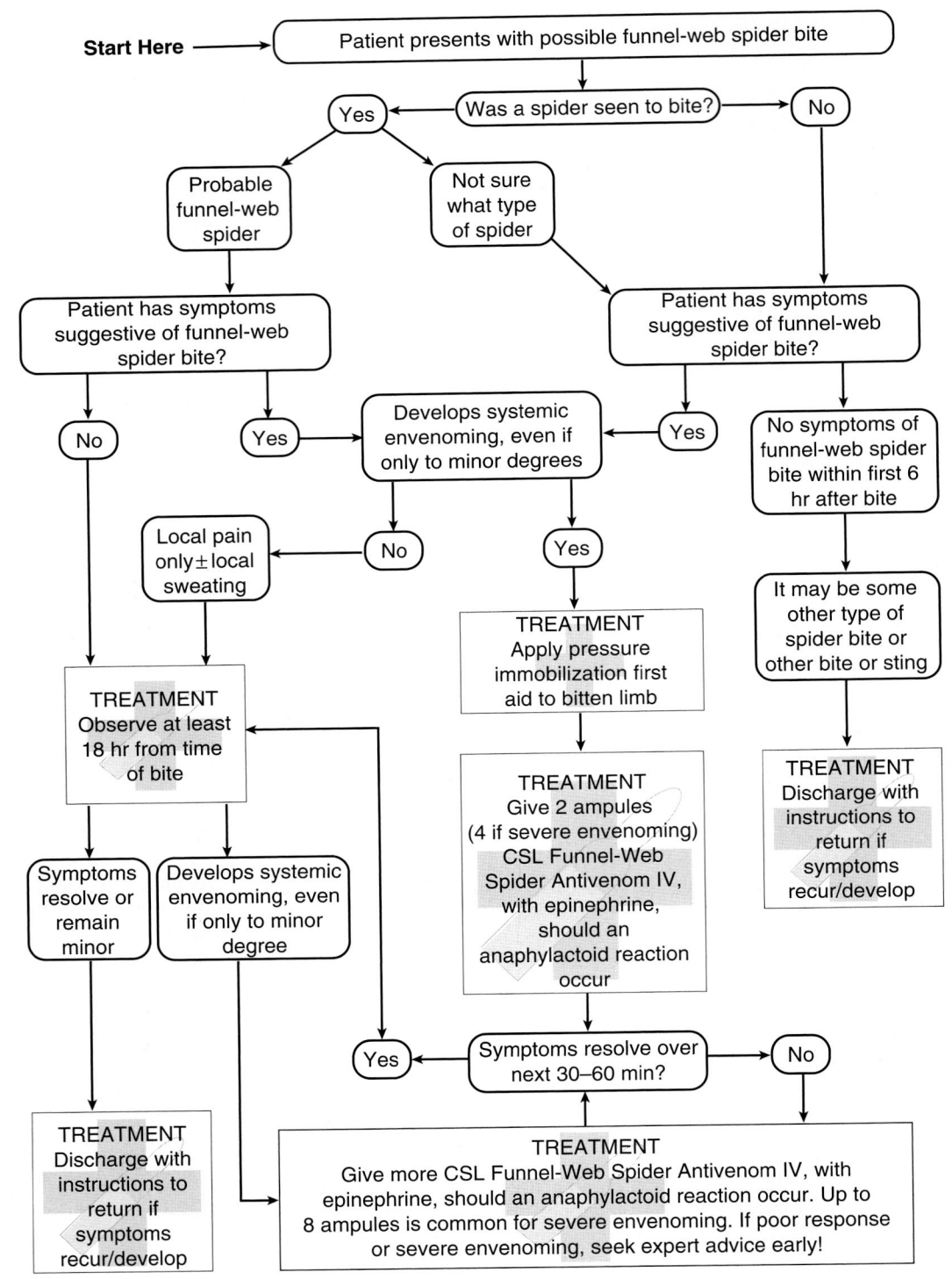

FIGURE 113-8

Outline management plan for funnel-web spider bite. *(Modified from White J: Snakebite and Spiderbite: Management Guidelines for New South Wales. Sydney: NSW Health, pp 14–15, 1998; and Miller MK, Whyte IM, White J, Keir P: Clinical features and management of* Hadronyche *envenomation in man. Toxicon 38:409–427, 2000. Copyright © Dr. Julian White, 2001.)*

There are no clinical data on requirements for *Missulena* bites. The consensus among treatment experts is to keep giving antivenom until response is complete.[22] In a few cases, there is an initial good response to FWSAV, but several hours later the patient relapses with pulmonary edema.

Although this situation occasionally may be due to intravenous fluid overload, it is more likely relapsed envenoming, and further antivenom administration is appropriate. One additional vial may be all that is required in such cases. Children require the same dose as adults.

Nonantivenom Treatment

In the absence of antivenom, the other therapeutic interventions for a patient with severe envenoming are of limited efficacy. In patients with severe pulmonary edema, intubation with intermittent positive pressure breathing and positive end-expiratory pressure has had some success.[1,2] If early hypertension and tachycardia are clinically significant, α blockade has been and may be used, but β blockade is contraindicated. Atropine has proved useful as a means of controlling secretions, as has diazepam as a sedative measure in the ventilated patient.

SPECIAL POPULATIONS

Pregnant and Breast-feeding Patients

The mother and fetus may be severely affected by funnel-web spider envenoming, requiring robust antivenom therapy. There are insufficient reported cases to determine fetal prognosis.

Pediatric Patients

Children are at higher risk of rapid, severe, even fatal envenoming, requiring a prompt therapeutic response. They require just as much antivenom as adults, but fluid overload from intravenous therapy is more likely. This situation may pose a diagnostic dilemma as to whether late-onset pulmonary edema is due to relapsing envenoming or fluid overload. Clinical circumstances may provide the answer, but if in doubt, the treating physician should consider administering more antivenom.

Elderly Patients

The elderly are at increased risk from envenoming and secondary fluid overload.

FOLLOW-UP

All patients receiving antivenom should receive follow-up, at least by telephone, to detect and monitor serum sickness. All patients with even mild systemic envenoming should be monitored closely in an intensive care setting for at least 24 hours, or at least 12 hours from complete resolution of all symptoms and signs of envenoming, whichever is longer.

REFERENCES

1. Fisher MM, Carr GA, Mcguinness R, Warden JC: *Atrax robustus* envenomation. Anaesth Intensive Care 8:410–420, 1980.
2. Torda TA, Loong E, Greaves I: Severe lung oedema and fatal consumption coagulopathy after funnel-web bite. Med J Aust 2:442–444, 1980.
3. Gray M: A guide to funnel-web spider identification. Med J Aust 22:837–839, 1984.
4. Gray M: Distribution of the funnel web spider. In Covacevich J, Davie P, Pearn J (eds): Toxic Plants and Animals: A Guide for Australia. Queensland Museum, Brisbane, 1987, pp 313–321.
5. White J, Cardoso JL, Hui WF: Clinical toxicology of spider bites. In Meier J, White J (eds): Handbook of Clinical Toxicology of Animal Venoms and Poisons. Boca Raton, FL, CRC Press, 1995, pp 259–329.
6. Duncan AW, Tibballs J, Sutherland SK: Effects of Sydney funnel-web spider envenomation in monkeys, and their clinical implications. Med J Aust 2:429–435, 1980.
7. Mylecharane EJ, Spence I, Sheumack DD, et al: Actions of robustoxin, a neurotoxic polypeptide from the venom of the male funnel-web spider (*Atrax robustus*), in anaesthetized monkeys. Toxicon 27:481–492, 1989.
8. Brown MR, Sheumack DD, Tyler MI, Howden ME: Amino acid sequence of versutoxin, a lethal neurotoxin from the venom of the funnel-web spider *Atrax versutus* [published erratum appears in Biochem J 1989 Feb 1;257(3):following 934]. Biochem J 250:401–405, 1988.
9. Rash LD, Birinyi-Strachan LC, Nicholson GM, Hodgson WC: Neurotoxic activity of venom from the Australian Eastern mouse spider (*Missulena bradleyi*) involves modulation of sodium channel gating. Br J Pharmacol 130:1817–1824, 2000.
10. Rendle Short H: Mouse spider envenomation. Proceedings of Australian and New Zealand Intensive Care Society Scientific Meeting, 1985, pp 25–25.
11. Miller MK, Whyte IM, White J, Keir P: Clinical features and management of *Hadronyche* envenomation in man. Toxicon 38:409–427, 2000.
12. Harrington AP, Raven RJ, Bowe PC, et al: Funnel-web spider (*Hadronyche infensa*) envenomations in coastal south-east Queensland. Med J Aust 171:651–653, 1999.
13. White J, Hirst D, Hender E: 36 cases of bites by spiders, including the white-tailed spider, *Lampona cylindrata*. Med J Aust 150:401–403, 1989.
14. Sutherland SK, Duncan AW: New first-aid measures for envenomation: with special reference to bites by the Sydney funnel-web spider (*Atrax robustus*). Med J Aust 1:378–379, 1980.
15. Grant SJB, Loxton EH: Effectiveness of a compression bandage and antivenene for Sydney funnel-web envenomation. Med J Aust 156:510–511, 1992.
16. Dieckmann J, Prebble J, Mcdonogh A, et al: Efficacy of funnel-web spider antivenom in human envenomation by *Hadronyche* species. Med J Aust 151:706–707, 1989.
17. Fisher MM, Bowey CJ: Urban envenomation. Med J Aust 150:695–698, 1989.
18. Fisher MM, Raftos J, Mcguinness RT, et al: Funnel-web spider (*Atrax robustus*) antivenom: 2. Early clinical experience. Med J Aust 2:525–526, 1981.
19. Hartman LJ, Sutherland SK: Funnel-web spider (*Atrax robustus*) antivenom in the treatment of human envenomation. Med J Aust 141:796–799, 1984.
20. Knight J, Sutton L: Successful treatment of *Atrax formidabilis* envenomation. Med J Aust 2:434–435, 1982.
21. Graudins AW, Wilson D, Alewood PF, et al: Cross-reactivity of Sydney funnel-web spider antivenom: Neutralization of the in vitro toxicity of other Australian funnel-web (*Atrax* and *Hadronyche*) spider venoms. Toxicon 40:259–266, 2002.
22. White J: CSL Antivenom Handbook, 2nd ed. Melbourne, CSL Ltd, 2001.

CHAPTER 114

Scorpions

Yona Amitai

Scorpions are arthropods with a hard exoskeleton, two anterior pinching claws, and a tail ending with a bulbous enlargement. The poison gland and the stinger are located at the distal part of the tail. The tail is long and able to arch over the head, allowing the stinger to hit the prey grasped between the claws (Fig. 114-1).[1] Scorpions are among the oldest creatures on earth. Their habitat is warm and arid areas, as reflected in their first mentioning in the Bible: "He led you through the vast and dreadful desert, that thirsty and waterless land, with venomous snakes and scorpions."[2] The scorpion is a nocturnal animal that hibernates in winter and is active in the warm seasons. Worldwide, there are more than 800 species of scorpions; however, only a limited number of species, belonging to six families, are toxic to humans.[3] The geographic distribution of scorpions is between latitude 45 on both sides of the equator. Infrequently, scorpion envenomation occurs in remote areas from stowaway scorpions.[4]

Scorpion species of medical importance are encountered in India,[5–10] the Middle East,[11–24] North Africa,[25–30] Brazil,[31–33] Mexico,[34–37] the southern states of the United States,[38–44] central Africa, and South Africa.[45,46] Some of the main venomous scorpions, their geographic distribution, and target organ toxicity are listed in Table 114-1.

EPIDEMIOLOGY

Scorpion sting is common and endemic in various regions. Because most envenomations occur in developing countries, where regular reporting systems often are lacking, data on scorpion stings in several countries are based on estimates. High fatality rates were reported from scorpion envenomation in India, Saudi Arabia, Israel, Tunisia, Brazil, and Mexico in the 1960s and 1970s. In recent years, there has been a marked reduction in mortality, however, owing to the improvement in supportive care and increased availability of antivenom therapy.

In a series of 119 patients reported from India in 1996, the mortality rate was 25% among patients who received supportive care only, 3.5% in patients treated with nifedipine, and 0% among those treated with prazosin.[6] In Saudi Arabia, 2240 cases of scorpion sting were recorded in the Hail region, with an incidence of 18.7 per 1000 over a 15-month period.[48] Among 7000 U.S. soldiers who served in Saudi Arabia during the Gulf War (October 1990 to January 1991), 57 cases of scorpion sting were reported.[49] These stings were sustained during the autumn and winter, whereas the peak season for scorpion stings is June through September.[48] A fatality rate of 4.8% among children was reported in one hospital in Saudi Arabia in the 1980s, before the introduction of antivenom therapy; no fatalities occurred among patients treated with antivenom.[23] In Tunisia, almost 40,000 scorpion stings in humans are recorded annually, 1000 of them with systemic manifestations requiring hospital admissions; about 100 patients die annually.[26] In Mexico, it has been estimated that 400 to 1000 people die annually as a result of 100,000 to 200,000 scorpion stings.[36] There were about 310 *documented* fatalities annually until the 1990s, when immunotherapy was introduced.[36] In Brazil, fatality rates of 1% among children and 0.28% among all subjects stung by scorpions reported in 1994.[31] There have been 15,687 exposures to scorpions reported to the American Association of Poison Control Centers Toxic Exposure Surveillance System. Of these exposures, 508 involved moderate symptoms, 28 involved major symptoms, and there were 2 fatalities, both of which occurred in todders, one of them presumably due to an adverse reaction to antivenom therapy.[44]

BIOCHEMISTRY AND PATHOPHYSIOLOGY OF SCORPION ENVENOMATION

Scorpion venom is a complex mixture of mucopolysaccharides, hyaluronidase, serotonin, histamine, protease inhibitors, histamine releasers, neurotoxins, and approximately 70 amino acids. Despite species differences, there are some similarities in venom composition; this explains some similarities among clinical manifestations in envenomation sustained from scorpion stings from different geographic locations.

Scorpion venom increases neuronal Na^+ influx by blocking inactivation of the Na^+ channel, resulting in increased duration and amplitude of the neuron action potential (Fig. 114-2). Consequently, a voltage-gated channel conductance Ca^{2+} is increased at presynaptic nerve fibers, with increased release of neurotransmitters, including acetylcholine.[50,51] The clinical effects of this enhanced neural impulse transmission include muscle fasciculations; respiratory, gastric, and pancreatic hypersecretion; and occasionally bradycardia.[18,49] Parasympathetic stimulation also may cause vascular dilation of the penile arterioles supplying the corpus cavernosus, resulting in priapism.

Scorpion venom also induces sympathetic stimulation with excessive adrenergic discharge.[19] The symptom complex of scorpion envenomation may include parasympathetic and

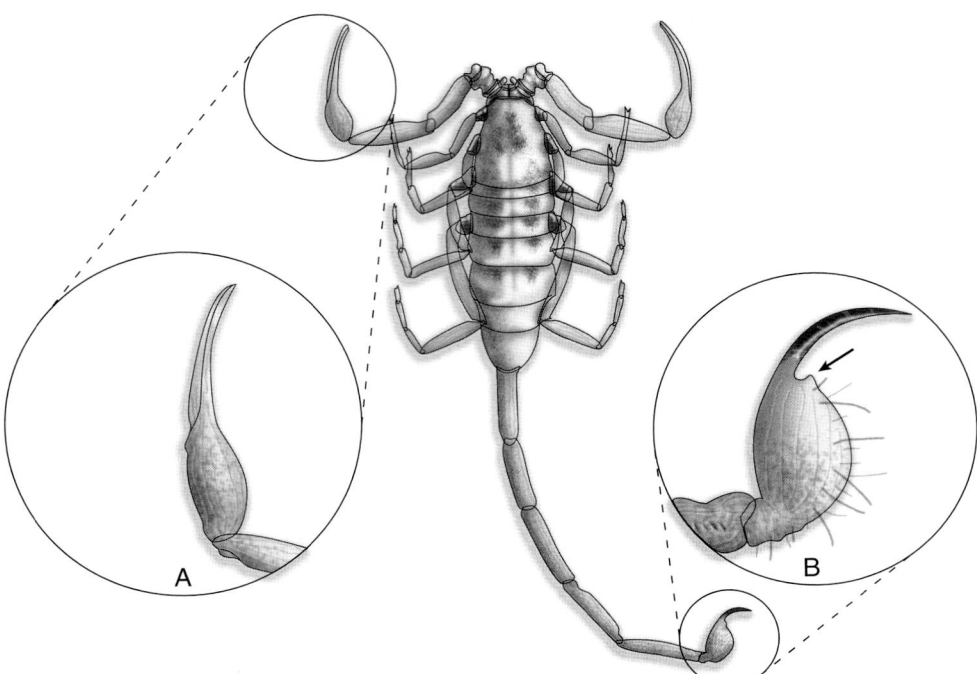

FIGURE 114-1

Bark scorpion, *Centruroides sculpturatus (exilicauda)*. **A**, Enlarged chela. **B**, Enlarged vesicle showing a tubercle below the stinger. The body length including telson is 55 mm. *(From Smith RL: Venomous Animals of Arizona. University of Arizona Cooperative Extension, Arizona Board of Regents, 1982.)*

sympathetic stimulation. The nonspecific signs of tachycardia, tachypnea, hypothermia or hyperthermia, and leukocytosis are explained by cytokine release (particularly interleukin-6[20] and interleukin-1[52]) and increased autonomic neurotransmission. In a canine model, injection of venom of the yellow scorpion *Leiurus quinquestriatus* resulted in an early stage of increased cardiac output and hypertension, followed by a second stage of reduction in cardiac output.[53] These two stages may reflect an initial catecholamine discharge and subsequently a second stage of catecholamine depletion. The mechanism of cardiotoxicity in scorpion envenomation is multifactorial: catecholamine overstimulation, causing hypertension and a transient phase of increased contractility. There is a diminished systolic performance in addition to the catecholamine effect. The combination of myocardial ischemia, excessive cate-

cholamine effect, cardiac arrhythmia, and increased oxygen demand may result in acute myocardial ischemia and infarction.[24]

Respiratory failure, caused by pulmonary edema, is a common complication of severe scorpion envenomation. It has a cardiogenic and noncardiogenic component. The latter is thought to occur as a result of increased vascular permeability induced by release of vasoactive substances.[24] Central nervous system involvement is more frequent in children with severe envenomation. In the case of *L. quinquestriatus* sting, central nervous system symptoms are explained partially on the basis of hypertension, causing hypertensive encephalopathy, and may respond to antihypertensive therapy.[54] Central nervous system manifestations, such as agitation, hyperthermia, hypertonus, seizures, and coma,[12,24,48] also occur, however, in the presence of normal blood pressure,

TABLE 114-1 Scorpion Envenomation by Species, Regions, and Characteristic Toxicity

SCORPION SPECIES	GEOGRAPHIC REGION	CARDIOTOXICITY	NEUROTOXICITY	REFERENCE
Buthus tamulus, Mesobuthus tamulus (Indian red scorpion)	India	+++	++	5–10
Leiurus quinquestriatus, Androctonus crassicauda	Middle East	+++	++	11–24, 48–50, 58, 60
A. crassicauda, Androctonus australis, Androctonus bicolor	North Africa and Middle East	+++	++	25–30, 47
Tityus serrulatus	Brazil	+++	++	31–33
Centruroides suffusus	Mexico	+	++	34–37
Centruroides sculpturatus (exilicauda)	U.S. southern states (mainly Arizona)	−	++	38–44
Parabuthus transvaalicus, Parabuthus granulatus	Central and South Africa	+	++	45, 46

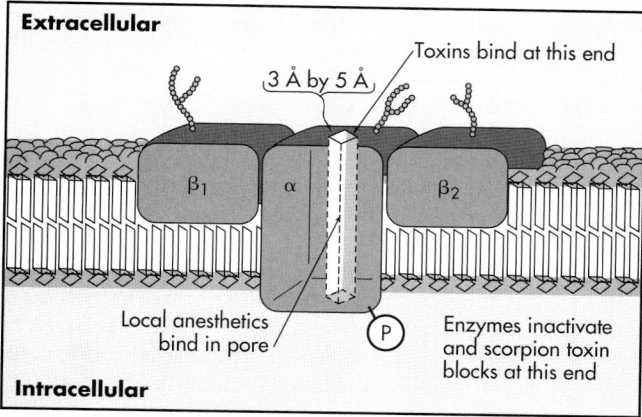

FIGURE 114-2

Schematic representation of the voltage-gated channel in a neuron showing the site of scorpion toxin binding. The channel is roughly a 0.3 mm × 0.5 nm rectangular hole formed by four of the transmembrane helices within this subunit. *(From Brody TM, Garrison JC: Sites of action: Receptors. In Brody TM, Larner J, Minneman KP (eds): Human Pharmacology: Molecular to Clinical, 3rd ed. St. Louis, Mosby, 1998, p 18.)*

suggesting a more direct central mechanism of toxicity.[24] Intraventricular injection of extremely small doses of toxic *L. quinquestriatus* venom to rabbits (1/500 to 1/100 of the intravenous lethal dose) caused complex neurotoxicity.[24] Some scorpions, such as the *Centruroides sculpturatus (exilicauda)* of the southern United States, exert neurotoxicity without cardiotoxicity.[38,39,41]

CLINICAL MANIFESTATIONS

The severity of scorpion envenomation varies with the scorpion's species, age, and size and is much greater in children. As a general rule, venomous scorpions with thin claws are more toxic than scorpions with thick claws. Clinical severity ranges from local pain to fatal cardiotoxicity and encephalopathy.

In most cases, adults stung by scorpions experience only local symptoms and signs consisting of pain, erythema, pruritus, edema, and paresthesias.[49] Paresthesias and localized percussion tenderness at the sting site are common,[14,41,46,49] occasionally involving the extremities and the perioral area.[14] Local skin necrosis of any degree is rare[55,56] and has been documented only from stings of *Hemiscorpius lepturus* in Iran.[56]

Systemic intoxication reflects stimulation or depression of the central nervous system and stimulation of the sympathetic, parasympathetic, and skeletal motor nervous systems. Skeletal motor and parasympathetic stimulation is manifested mainly as tongue and muscle fasciculation, gross skeletal motor hyperactivity (which may be involuntary), gastric and pancreatic hypersecretion, and occasionally bradycardia.[18,49] Salivation, abdominal pain, nausea, and vomiting are common and may be attributed to stimulation of salivary glands and to pancreatitis.[16] Parasympathetic stimulation also may cause priapism, even in young boys.[12,57]

In the cardiovascular system, the increased sympathetic tone prevails, as reflected by the high incidence of tachycardia and hypertension (72% and 58%) and the much lower incidence of bradycardia and hypotension (14% and 5%) in victims of scorpion envenomation.[49] In a report of 386 children with scorpion stings from Saudi Arabia, tachycardia occurred in 32% of children and bradycardia in 0.77%.[57]

Most scorpions with the potential to cause human envenomation exert cardiotoxicity and neurotoxicity (see Table 114-1). A notable exception is *C. sculpturatus (exilicauda)*, which is predominantly neurotoxic. Symptoms of envenomation in 151 patients stung by this scorpion were, in decreasing order of frequency, restlessness, nystagmus, paresthesia, hypersalivation, fasciculation, blurred vision, difficulty in swallowing, local pain, and slurred speech.[41] In the United States, a clinical gradation has been suggested for scorpion envenomation from this species. Four grades range from local pain or paresthesia or both at the site of the sting (grade 1) to involvement of cranial nerves and somatic skeletal neuromuscular dysfunction (grade 4) (Table 114-2)[39] Likewise, a grading system is used for scorpion envenomation in Tunisia. Using this grading system in one series, there were 102 patients with grade 1, consisting of local signs alone; 52 patients with grade 2, consisting of local signs and moderate general symptoms; and 26 patients with grade 3, consisting of severe symptoms.[27]

Envenomation by the main venomous scorpion species in North Africa and the Middle East (*L. quinquestriatus* and *Androctonus crassicauda*) and India (*Buthotus tamulus*) has a similar clinical course. Symptoms of mild envenomation are agitation, tachycardia, and sweating. In more severe cases, particularly in young children, additional symptoms include vomiting, abdominal pain, salivation, dehydration, priapism, extreme agitation, generalized erythema, muscle rigidity and twitching, tremor, seizures, coma, pupillary changes (miosis, mydriasis, or anisocoria), hyperthermia, tachyarrhythmia or occasionally bradyarrhythmia, hypertension (less often hypotension), cardiac and respiratory failure, and death.[12,49,57] Idiopathic dilated cardiomyopathy was found to be eight times more frequent in patients with a past history of scorpion sting in India, despite their apparently complete recovery from the acute envenomation.[10]

TABLE 114-2 Grades of Envenomation

GRADE	CLINICAL CHARACTERISTICS
1	Pain or paresthesias or both limited to sting site
2	Pain or paresthesias or both remote from sting site
3	Signs of cranial nerve or neuromuscular abnormalities*
4	Signs of cranial nerve and neuromuscular abnormalities

*Examples of neuromuscular abnormalities seen after scorpion stings are involuntary movements, motor restlessness, and severe shaking.
Adapted from Curry SC, Vance MV, Ryan PJ, et al: Envenomation by the scorpion *Centruroides sculpturatus.* J Toxicol Clin Toxicol 21:417–449, 1983–1984.

DIAGNOSIS AND LABORATORY FINDINGS

The diagnosis of scorpion envenomation is made by the characteristic clinical presentation of the patient in an area in which scorpions are endemic. Occasionally the scorpion is seen, or the bite may be witnessed.

Laboratory abnormalities have been reported mainly from scorpion stings from the Middle East, North Africa, and India. Hyperglycemia and leukocytosis are nonspecific but common.[12,20,57] Cardiac ischemia is expressed in transient elevation of cardiac enzymes[24,58] and electrocardiogram with depressed or elevated ST segment, Q waves in leads I and aVL, prolonged QT_c interval, and peaked T wave.[24] Cardiac dysfunction is evidenced by echocardiography as diminished global wall motion with decreased systolic left ventricular performance and diminished ejection fraction.[59–61] Left ventricular dysfunction also has been shown by cardiac radionuclide scan.[61] Transient elevation of pancreatic enzymes has been reported.[60]

TREATMENT

Proper general management measures are subject to controversy and not substantiated by adequate research to date. The following recommendations can be made:

1. Move the victim, particularly when the victim is an infant or small child, to a medical facility as soon as possible. If it is known or suspected that the scorpion is capable of envenoming humans, all victims of a sting should be transported to a hospital or clinic.
2. Apply a lightly constricting band just proximal to the sting site to prevent lymphatic spread of the venom. This should be removed under observation when the victim has arrived at a medical facility. Several reports emphasize the critical effect on the outcome of delay in time of arrival of the victim to medical facilities[13,24,30]; this is explained by the rapid spread of the venom.[62] Increased venom concentration at the sting site should not be a problem because local necrosis is extremely rare with scorpion stings.
3. Apply ice at the sting site, which may slow venom absorption and relieves pain.[39]

In most cases, adults stung by scorpions do not develop systemic envenomation. Close observation outside of a health care facility for 2 to 6 hours is sufficient in these cases. Analgesics may be used for pain relief, and topical application of lidocaine may be helpful. In endemic regions for cardiotoxic scorpions (see Table 114-1), an electrocardiogram should be performed.

In cases of systemic envenomation, the principles of management are observation; cardiac monitoring; supportive treatment with intravenous fluids and electrolytes, sedatives, and analgesics; and cautious use of cardiovascular agents, including vasodilators, adrenergic antagonists, or calcium channel blockers, in the hypertensive phase. Sofer and colleagues[13] advocated the use of hydralazine or nifedipine. Bawaskar and Bawaskar[5] found prazosin to be safer and more effective than nifedipine in these patients and recommended using prazosin alone in patients with hypertension and tachycardia from scorpion sting. In a controlled study, these authors reported lower complication rates (no fatalities) in patients treated with prazosin compared with patients treated with nifedipine or supportive care alone (fatality rates of 35% and 25%, respectively).[6]

Elatrous and coworkers[29] from Tunisia reported the efficacy of dobutamine infusion at 7 to 20 µg/kg/min in 19 patients with severe scorpion envenomation and acute pulmonary edema, of whom 10 also had severe hypotension. In these patients, cardiac output, blood pressure, tissue oxygenation, and clinical outcome improved significantly, but there were two fatalities.[29] Antiarrhythmics, such as lidocaine, may be required.[24] In an experimental envenomation by *L. quinquestriatus* in rabbits, lidocaine infusion significantly attenuated venom-invoked effects and reduced mortality.[63]

Use of sedatives to reduce anxiety and agitation has an important role in the treatment of symptomatic patients. Rimsza and colleagues[38] reported that phenobarbital was the most commonly used medication in a series of 24 children with scorpion envenomation in Arizona. Although there were earlier reports on adverse effects from barbiturates in some patients, they were related to the use of excessive doses.[38] Currently, sedation with benzodiazepines has replaced the use of barbiturates. At the Hadassah University Hospital, Mt. Scopus, Jerusalem, we have used diazepam or midazolam at doses titrated to control agitation and anxiety in children with scorpion envenomation, with good response.

In a retrospective study in Arizona, 104 patients, mostly children stung by *C. sculpturatus* (*exilicauda*), were treated with continuous intravenous midazolam infusion. Dosage was titrated to induce a light sleep state to control agitation and involuntary movements, with good response. This treatment seems safe and provides control of agitation as its primary benefit.[42] Steroids have no role in the treatment of scorpion envenomation.[47]

Antivenom Therapy

Specific antivenom therapy has been used for several decades. Most antivenom preparations consist of animal serum (goat, horse, and donkey). Numerous reports exist on the clinical use of specific antivenom preparations from several geographic regions.[13,22–24,26,28,30,36,37,39–41,46,57] Because of ethical considerations, most studies are retrospective, observational, or historical controls. There are only a few prospective, randomized, controlled studies.[26,28] Reports on antivenom therapy are summarized in Table 114-3. Of the 12 reports summarized there, 9 concluded that antivenom is effective,[22–24,28,30,37,39,40,46] 2 concluded that antivenom is not effective,[13,26] and 1 gave data on safety only and did not report on efficacy.[57]

Ismail[22,24] from Saudi Arabia reported robust data on 24,000 patients with scorpion envenomation treated by a national protocol. Thousands of these patients were treated with antivenom, with a reduction in the fatality rate from 4% to 6.8% to less than 0.05%.

Several reports from Mexico (not described in Table 114-3) claimed a reduction in mortality from several hundred annually to zero.[36] It was reported that not even one fatality occurred among 38,068 patients stung by scorpions, thanks to the use of antivenom.[35]

TABLE 114-3 Published Studies on Antivenom Efficacy in Scorpion Envenomation

STUDY; REGION; YEARS; SCORPION SPECIES	STUDY DESIGN; SAMPLE SIZE	ANTIVENOM TYPE; DOSE; AND ROUTE	RESULTS AND CONCLUSION	COMMENT
Sofer et al[13]; Israel; 1985–1992; *Leiurus quinquestriatus*	Retrospective, historical control; 104 children in PICU, 52 treated with AV	Specific AV, donkey's serum; 5–15 mL; IV	No effect; emphasis on supportive therapy	Treatment group in 1985–1989; controls in 1989–1992
Ismail[22,24]; Saudi Arabia; 1991–1992; *Androctonus, Leiurus quinquestriatus*	Statewide, multicenter; 24,000 patients	Specific AV; ≥5 mL; IV	Mortality reduced from 4–6.8% to <0.05%	Efficacy requires prompt IV infusion and large dose
el-Amin et al[23]; Saudi Arabia; 1988–1994; *Leiurus quinquestriatus, Androctonus*	780 hospitalized children and children treated as outpatients	Specific AV; ≥5 mL; IV	Mortality reduced from 4.8% to 0%	Very effective
Gajre and Dammas[57]; Saudi Arabia; 1991–1995; *Leiurus quinquestriatus, Androctonus*	182 children treated, 90% symptomatic	Specific AV; 5 mL (10–20 mL for severe patients); IV	Efficacy not reported; adverse reactions in 13.7%, severe in 1%	Restrict AV use to patients with systemic envenomation
Abroug et al[26]; Tunisia; 1994–1995; *Androctonus australis, Buthus occitanus*	Randomized, controlled; 825 patients >10 years old, 412 treated	Specific bivalent AV; 20 mL; IV	No effect; four (1%) developed anaphylactic reversible shock	
Krifi et al[28]; Tunisia; 1993–1997; *Androctonus australis, Buthus occitanus*	Randomized, controlled; 147 severely envenomed children, 1–2 doses IV or IM or no AV	Specific bivalent AV, Pasteur Institute, Tunisia; 5–30 mL; IV	AV given IV—effective; IM—not effective	
Ghalim et al[30]; Morocco; 1997; *Androctonus mauretanicus, Buthus occitanus*	Retrospective; 275 patients	Specific bivalent AV, Pasteur Institute, Tunisia; 2–10 mL; IV*	Effective	Prompt use and large dose important
Osnaya-Romero et al[37]; Mexico; 1997	Not controlled; 163 children		Effective	
Curry et al[39]; Arizona; 1982; *Centruroides sculpturatus (exilicauda)*	Retrospective; 670 patients, 30 treated with AV	Specific AV, goat serum; 5–10 mL; IV	Seems safe and effective	
Bond[40]; Arizona; 1987–1989; *Centruroides exilicauda (sculpturatus)*	Retrospective; 12 children treated with AV	Specific AV, goat serum; 5–10 mL; IV	Rapid response; acute reactions—0, delayed—58%	AV justified only for severely patients
Gateau et al[41]; Arizona; 1987–1989; *Centruroides exilicauda (sculpturatus)*	Retrospective; 145 patients treated with AV	Specific AV, goat serum; 5–20 mL; IV	Good response in 30 min in 71%; mild reactions in 8%	AV safe and effective
Muller[46]; South Africa; *Parabuthos transvaalicus* and *Parabuthos granulatus*	Retrospective; 42 patients			AV recommended

AV, antivenom; PICU, pediatric intensive care unit.

*Some patients received 2–5 mL of antivenom, and some received 1 mL. In those who received the higher dose, there was a higher degree of circulating venom depth.

In a study from Arizona of 116 patients, mostly children, who received *Centruroides* antivenom, only 4 developed mild, self-limited, immediate reactions, and they completed the infusion despite the reactions. In one patient, who had a history of asthma and atopy, epinephrine infusion and an inhaled β-agonist were given for transient wheezing, which resolved quickly. Of those patients who were followed, 60% developed some symptoms of serum sickness, however, which responded to oral steroids, antihistamines, or both. The mean duration of symptoms was 2.8 days. Most patients were discharged from the emergency department, and a few were admitted for 24-hour observation.[64] The high incidence of delayed hypersensitivity was in accordance with that reported by Bond[40] but was much higher than that reported by others.

Important points regarding the optimal use of antivenom can be inferred from these reports, as follows:

1. Because of regional variations in scorpion species and specific antivenom preparations, *always obtain the advice of local experts* (i.e., poison information centers, medical toxicologists, or treatment centers with expertise in the field of scorpion envenomation).
2. Reserve antivenom preparations for patients with significant systemic toxicity. A suggested guideline for treatment with antivenom is the appearance of two or more of the signs and symptoms of systemic envenomation listed in the box below or the occurrence of one of the following: arrhythmia, hypertension, hypotension, seizures, coma, and pulmonary edema.
3. When indicated, give antivenom promptly after onset of systemic signs or symptoms. In the event of a rash's appearing during antivenom administration, decrease the

Indications for ICU Admission in Scorpion Envenomation

Infants and young children (<5 years old)

Anyone with systemic manifestations consisting of two or more of the following:

Cardiovascular: tachycardia/bradycardia, hypertension/hypotension, arrhythmia

Neurologic: agitation, lethargy, coma, tremor, hypertonicity, seizures, opsoclonus, paresthesia (other than at the sting site)

Respiratory: tachypnea, respiratory distress, stridor, pulmonary edema

Dermatologic: sweating, flushed skin, dimpled goose skin

Laboratory: electrocardiogram abnormalities, elevated myocardial enzymes, echocardiogram evidence of cardiac wall dysfunction (reduced contraction)

One of the following: arrhythmia, hypertension (new), hypotension, seizures, lethargy, coma, pulmonary edema, electrocardiogram or echocardiogram abnormalities, high myocardial enzymes

infusion rate, add intravenous antihistamine, and continue the antivenom infusion, with caution and standby intravenous epinephrine.

4. Administer antivenom *intravenously only*. The intramuscular route is not effective, likely due to the slow absorption and distribution of the large antibody molecules from the intramuscular injection site.[28]

5. The volume of the dose required depends on the preparation and the initial and subsequent responses to treatment. It could vary from 4 mL to 15 to 20 mL in severe cases. Always consult with local experts about the proper preparation, dose, and precise instructions about how to administer the antivenom. At the Hadassah Hospitals in Jerusalem, we use 4 to 6 mL diluted in saline and administered intravenously over 20 to 30 minutes, starting with a slow infusion rate and increasing gradually. Skin testing generally is not performed because when antivenom is deemed necessary, there should not be a further delay in its administration. The safety of specific scorpion antivenom (i.e., low likelihood of anaphylactic or anaphylactoid reaction) given in various geographic locations is considered to be generally satisfactory.[12,24] This safety is related to the low protein content of the antivenom. Paradoxically, the theoretical likelihood of patients with severe envenomation developing an anaphylactoid reaction is lower than that of patients with mild envenomation because severe venom toxicity causes the release of massive amounts of catecholamines, inhibiting mast cell degranulation.[33]

6. The dose should not vary with the age or weight of the patient because it should be directed at neutralizing a given amount of venom introduced by the scorpion into the patient's body. At the Hadassah Hospitals, we have used antivenom therapy to treat more than 50 children with systemic scorpion envenomation. The antivenom against the yellow scorpion is prepared in donkeys as gamma globulin and specific to the venom of the yellow scorpion *L. quinquestriatus* by the Hebrew University Department of Entomology and Venomous Animals in Jerusalem: 1 mL of this antivenom neutralizes 100 median lethal doses of

the venom in 20-g mice.[62] In many instances, an impressive reversal of symptoms was observed immediately after the administration of antivenom. This specific antivenom is the only one available in Israel; however, it has been reported also to be effective in the case of envenomation by another (nonhomologous) scorpion species, *A. crassicauda*.[65] The explanation of this effect is related to the similarity in venom composition between these two scorpion species.

7. Patients who receive antivenom should be followed at home for the next few days. If serum sickness occurs, antihistamines or a short course of oral steroids should be given according to the severity of symptoms.[64]

Advances in supportive care and antivenom therapy have improved markedly the outcome of patients treated for scorpion envenomation.

Criteria for ICU Discharge in Scorpion Envenomation

Infants and young children (<5 years old) — lack of symptoms of systemic envenomation for 6 hours and normal electrocardiogram

Others—resolution of systemic manifestations of scorpion envenomation for 3 hours and no new abnormalities on electrocardiogram

SPECIAL POPULATIONS

Pregnant Patients

Data are insufficient to make conclusions about the safety of antivenom administration in pregnant women. As for poisoning by other toxins, indications for treatment should be guided by the clinical state of the pregnant woman.

Key Points in Scorpion Envenomation

1. Venomous scorpions exist in different regions, usually in warm climates, and are active in the warm season.
2. Because of marked geographic variations in scorpion species and their toxicity, the clinician *always* must consult with local experts about treatment and administration of antivenom.
3. As a rule, venomous scorpions with thin claws are more toxic than scorpions with thick claws.
4. Young children are at greater risk for severe envenomation after a sting.
5. When indicated, the dose of antivenom should be similar in children and adults.
6. After being stung, it is helpful if the patient can catch the scorpion, kill it, and bring it to the hospital for identification.
7. In contrast to bee stings, scorpions excrete only a small fraction of their venom in one sting and could cause severe toxicity immediately in repetitive stings.
8. After being stung, the patient should not run. Immobilization of the affected limb is important to slow venom distribution.
9. Incision and drainage at the site of the sting is contraindicated.

REFERENCES

1. Yarom R: Scorpion venom: A tutorial review of its effects in men and experimental animals. Clin Toxicol 3:561–569, 1970.
2. Deuteronomy 8:15.
3. Amitai Y: Clinical manifestations and management of scorpion envenomation. Public Health Rev 26:257–263, 1998.
4. Trestrail JH: Scorpion envenomation in Michigan: Three cases of toxic encounters with poisonous stow-aways. Vet Hum Toxicol 23:8–11, 1981.
5. Bawaskar HS, Bawaskar PH: Vasodilators: Scorpion envenoming and the heart (an Indian experience). Toxicon 32:1031–1040, 1994.
6. Bawaskar HS, Bawaskar PH: Severe envenoming by the Indian red scorpion *Mesobuthus tamulus*: The use of prazosin therapy. QJM 89:701–704, 1996.
7. Bawaskar HS, Bawaskar PH: Indian red scorpion envenoming. Indian J Pediatr 65:383–391, 1998.
8. Bawaskar HS, Bawaskar PH: Prazosin therapy and scorpion envenomation. J Assoc Physicians India 48:1175–1180, 2000.
9. Karnad DR: Haemodynamic patterns in patients with scorpion envenomation. Heart 79:485–489, 1998.
10. Sundararaman T, Olithselvan M, Sethuraman KR, Narayan KA: Scorpion envenomation as a risk factor for development of dilated cardiomyopathy. J Assoc Physicians India 47:1047–1050, 1999.
11. Gueron M, Yarom R: Cardiovascular manifestations of severe scorpion sting. Chest 57:156–162, 1970.
12. Amitai Y, Mines Y, Aker M, Goitein K: Scorpion sting in children. Clin Pediatr 24:136–140, 1985.
13. Sofer S, Shahak E, Gueron M: Scorpion envenomation and antivenom therapy. J Pediatr 124:973–978, 1994.
14. Bogomolski-Yahalom V, Amitai Y, Stalnikowicz R: Paresthesia in envenomation by the scorpion *Leiurus quinquestriatus*. Clin Toxicol 33:79–82, 1995.
15. Gueron M, Ilia R, Sofer S: The cardiovascular system after scorpion envenomation: A review. J Toxicol Clin Toxicol 30:245–258, 1992.
16. Sofer S, Shalev H, Weizman Z, et al: Acute pancreatitis in children following envenomation by the yellow scorpion *Leiurus quinquestriatus*. Toxicon 29:125–128, 1991.
17. Amitai Y, Katzir Z, Mann G, Amitai P: Convulsions following a black scorpion (*Buthus judaicus*) sting. Isr J Med Sci 17:1083–1084, 1981.
18. Cantor A, Wanderman KL, Ovsyshcher I, Gueron M: Parasympathetic action of scorpion venom on the cardiovascular system. Isr J Med Sci 13:908–911, 1977.
19. Gueron M, Weizmann S: Catecholamine excretion in scorpion sting. Isr J Med Sci 5:855–857, 1969.
20. Sofer S, Gueron M, White RM, et al: Interleukin-6 release following scorpion sting in children. Toxicon 34:389–392, 1996.
21. Dudin AA, Rambaud-Cousson A, Thalji A, et al: Scorpion sting in children in the Jerusalem area: A review of 54 cases. Ann Trop Paediatr 11:217–223, 1991.
22. Ismail M: The treatment of the scorpion envenoming syndrome: The Saudi experience with serotherapy. Toxicon 32:1019–1026, 1994.
23. el-Amin EO, Sultan OM, al-Magamci MS, Elidrissy A: Serotherapy in the management of scorpion sting in children in Saudi Arabia. Ann Trop Paediatr 14:21–24, 1994.
24. Ismail M: The scorpion envenoming syndrome. Toxicon 33:825–858, 1994.
25. Goyffon M, Vachon M, Broglio N: Epidemiological and clinical characteristics of the scorpion envenomation in Tunisia. Toxicon 20:337–344, 1982.
26. Abroug F, El Atrous S, Nouira S, et al: Serotherapy in scorpion envenomation: A randomized control trial. Lancet 354:906–909, 1999.
27. Krifi MN, Kharrat H, Zghal K, et al: Development of an ELISA for detection of scorpion venoms in sera of humans envenomed by *Androctonus australis Garzonii* (AAG) and *Buthus occitanus Tunetanus* (BOT): Correlation with clinical severity of envenoming in Tunisia. Toxicon 36:887–900, 1998.
28. Krifi MN, Amri F, Kharrat H, El Ayeb M: Evaluation of antivenom therapy in children severely envenomed by *Androctonus australis Garzonii* (AAG) and *Buthus occitanus Tunetanus* (BOT) scorpions. Toxicon 37:1627–1634, 1999.
29. Elatrous S, Nouira S, Besbes-Ouanes L, et al: Dobutamine in severe scorpion envenomation: Effects of standard hemodynamics, right ventricular performance and tissue oxygenation. Chest 116:748–753, 1999.
30. Ghalim N, El-Hafny B, Sebit F, et al: Scorpion envenomation and serotherapy in Morocco. Am J Trop Med Hyg 62:277–283, 2000.
31. Freire-Maia L, Campos JA, Amaral CF: Approaches to the treatment of scorpion envenomation. Toxicon 32:1009–1014, 1994.
32. Cupo P, Jurca M, Azeedo-Marques MM, et al: Severe scorpion envenomation in Brazil: Clinical, laboratory and anatomopathological aspects. Rev Inst Med Trop Sao Paulo 36:67–76, 1994.
33. Amaral CF, Dias MB, Campolina D, et al: Children with adrenergic manifestations of envenomation after *Tityus serrulatus* scorpion sting are protected from early anaphylactoid antivenom reactions. Toxicon 32:211–215, 1994.
34. Carbonaro PA, Janniger CK, Schwartz RA: Scorpion sting reactions. Cutis 57:139–141, 1996.
35. Dehesa-Davila M: Epidemiological characteristics of scorpion sting in Leon, Guanajuato, Mexico. Toxicon 27:281–286, 1989.
36. Dehesa-Davila M, Possani LD: Scorpionism and serotherapy in Mexico. Toxicon 32:1015–1018, 1994.
37. Osnaya-Romero N, de Jesus Medina-Hernandez T, Flores-Hernandez SS, Leon-Rojas G: Clinical symptoms observed in children envenomated by scorpion stings, at the children's hospital from the States of Morelos, Mexico. Toxicon 39:781–785, 2001.
38. Rimsza ME, Zimmerman DR, Bergeson PS: Scorpion envenomation. Pediatrics 66:298–302, 1980.
39. Curry SC, Vance MV, Ryan PJ, et al: Envenomation by the scorpion *Centruroides sculpturatus*. J Toxicol Clin Toxicol 21:417–449, 1983–1984.
40. Bond GR: Antivenin administration for centruroides scorpion sting: Risks and benefits. Ann Emerg Med 21:788–791, 1992.
41. Gateau T, Bloom M, Clark R: Response to specific *Centruroides sculpturatus* antivenom in 151 cases of scorpion stings. Clin Toxicol 32:165–171, 1994.
42. Gibly R, Williams M, Walter FG, et al: Continuous intravenous midazolam infusion for *Centruroides exilicauda* scorpion envenomation. Ann Emerg Med 34:620–625, 1999.
43. Ellenhorn MJ, Barceloux DG: Medical Toxicology: Diagnosis and Treatment of Human Poisoning. New York, Elsevier, 1988, pp 1152–1154.
44. Watson WH, Litovitz TL, Rodgers GC: 2002 Annual report of the American Association of Poison Control Centers Toxic Exposure Surveillance System. Am J Emerg Med 21:353–421, 2003.
45. Bergman NJ: Scorpion sting in Zimbabwe. S Afr Med J 87:163–167, 1997.
46. Muller GJ: Scorpionism in South Africa: A report of 42 serious scorpion envenomations. S Afr Med J 83:405–411, 1993.
47. Abroug F, Nouira S, Haguiga H, et al: A randomized clinical trial of high-dose hydrocortisone hemisuccinate in scorpion envenomation. Ann Emerg Med 30:245–258, 1997.
48. Mahaba HMA: Scorpion sting syndrome: Epidemiology, clinical presentation and management of 2240 cases. 3:82–89, 1997. Available at http://www.who.sci.eg/emhj/0301/10.htm
49. Groshong TD: Scorpion envenomation in Eastern Saudi Arabia. Ann Emerg Med 22:1431–1437, 1993.
50. Abdul-Ghani AS, Coutinho-Netto J, Bradford HF: In vivo release of acetylcholine evoked by brachial plexus stimulation and Tityustoxin. Biochem Pharmacol 29:2179–2182, 1980.
51. Macedo TM, Gomez MV: Effects of Tityustoxin from scorpion venom on the release and synthesis of acetylcholine in brain slices. Toxicon 20:601–606, 1982.
52. Magalhaes MM, Pereira ME, Amaral CF, et al: Serum levels of cytokines in patients envenomated by *Tityus serrulatus* scorpion sting. Toxicon 37:1155–1164, 1999.
53. Tarasuik A, Janco J, Sofer S: Effects of scorpion venom on central and peripheral circulatory response in an open-chest dog model. Acta Physiol Scand 161:141–149, 1997.
54. Sofer S, Gueron M: Vasodilators and hypertensive encephalopathy following scorpion envenomation in children. Chest 97:118–120, 1990.
55. Chanda JS, Leviav A: Hemolysis, renal failure, and local necrosis following scorpion sting. JAMA 241:1038, 1979.
56. Radmanesh M: Cutaneous manifestations of the *Hemiscorpius lepturus* sting: A clinical study. Int J Dermatol 37:500–507, 1998.
57. Gajre G, Dammas AS: Scorpion envenomation in children: Should all stings be given antivenom? Ann Saudi Med 19:444–447, 1999.
58. Sofer S, Gueron M: Respiratory failure in children following envenomation by the scorpion *Leiurus quinquestriatus*: Hemodynamic and neurological aspects. Toxicon 26:931–939, 1988.
59. Brand A, Keren A, Kerem E, et al: Myocardial damage after a scorpion sting: Long term echocardiographic follow-up. Pediatr Cardiol 9:59–61, 1988.

60. Gueron M, Margulis G, Sofer S: Echocardiographic and radionuclide angiographic observations following scorpion envenomation by *Leiurus quinquestriatus*. Toxicon 28:1005–1009, 1990.

61. Gueron M, Margulis G, Ilia R, Sofer S: The management of scorpion envenomation. Toxicon 31:1071–1076, 1993.

62. Tarasiuk A, Khvatskin S, Sofer S: Effects of antivenom serotherapy on hemodynamic pathophysiology in dogs injected with *L. quinquestriatus* scorpion venom. Toxicon 36:963–971, 1998.

63. Fatani AJ, Harvey AL, Furman BL, Rowan EG: The effects of lignocaine on actions of the venom from the yellow scorpion *Leiurus quinquestriatus* in vivo and in vitro. Toxicon 38:1787–1801, 2000.

64. LoVecchio F, Welch S, Klemens J, et al: Incidence of immediate and delayed hypersensitivity to *Centruroides* antivenom. Ann Emerg Med 34:615–619, 1999.

65. Pomeranz A, Amitai P, Braunstein I, et al: Scorpion sting: Successful treatment with nonhomologous antivenin. Isr J Med Sci 20:451–452, 1984.

CHAPTER **115**

Marine Vertebrates, Coelenterates, and Mollusks

George W. Skarbek-Borowski ■ Daniel Savitt

JELLYFISH

True jellyfish (class Scyphozoa) are members of the phylum Coelenterata, marine predators that possess venom-containing stinging chambers called *nematocysts* (Figs. 115-1 and 115-2). Hydrozoans, such as the Portuguese man-of-war, also are part of this phylum and are discussed later in the chapter. Although bites from many species of jellyfish are noxious to humans and may require medical attention, only a handful are known to cause sufficient toxicity to warrant intensive care.

The box jellyfish, *Chironex fleckeri* (named after Australian medical biologist Helen Flecker), is native to the waters off northern Queensland, Australia, although this species can be found in any Australasian waters between the Tropics of Cancer and Capricorn.[3] *Chiropsalmus*, the other cuboid jellyfish to which human fatalities have been attributed, is found in Australasian and, rarely, Caribbean (including Gulf of Mexico) waters.[2] Other highly toxic jellyfish found in these waters include *Carybdea rastoni* (jimble), *C. marsupialis* (sea wasp), and *Pelagia noctiluca*.[1]

In 1952, Flecker named a peculiar constellation of "severe systemic symptoms" (first described by Southcott) referred to as the *Irukandji syndrome*, after an aboriginal tribe local to the area of most frequent envenomation in northern Queensland. Fourteen years later, in an act reminiscent of Jennerian experimentation, Barnes captured a specimen of a yet-unnamed tiny box jellyfish. Barnes deliberately stung himself, his son, and a volunteer lifesaver, and the trio was resuscitated in a local intensive care unit for severe Irukandji syndrome; the culprit was named *Carukia barnesi*. It is found in Australian waters from Broome in the west to Rockhamptom in the east, following the northern coastline. A milder form of the syndrome has been attributed to envenomations from larger animals in more southern Australian waters.[4]

Other jellyfish are less toxic but nonetheless capable of causing concerning local and systemic reactions. *Chrysaora* and *Cynaea* spp. (sea nettles) are found in tropical and temperate waters, particularly the Chesapeake Bay on the U.S.

East Coast. *Pelagia* (purple-striped stingers) are more common off the California coast.[1]

Pharmacology

The tentacles of all coelenterates are lined with thousands of cells (cnidoblasts), each of which contains a tiny, coiled barb (nematocyst). When triggered by either physical contact or changes in the animal's chemical environment, nematocysts discharge and can penetrate human skin (even through a surgical glove) with a force of 2 to 5 psi. Venom diffuses through the epidermis and upper dermis and, particularly if dermal capillaries are inoculated directly, can enter the systemic circulation. A frightened victim often rubs or shakes the affected area while swimming or running for help, contributing inadvertently to the spread of venom locally and systemically.

A single *Chironex*, which contains one of the most potent and rapidly acting venoms known, is capable of killing three adults in less than 10 minutes. It is a completely transparent and almost invisible, cuboid-shaped animal (20 cm × 18 cm × 30 cm) with four groups of tentacles measuring as much as 100 m en masse. These animals prefer calm, shallow waters over sandy and muddy bottoms. Being photosensitive, they surface in the early mornings, late afternoons, and at night; during full sunlight, they remain well submerged. They tend to appear during summer months.[1,3] *C. fleckeri* venom contains numerous proteins with hemolytic, cardiotoxic, neurotoxic, mycotoxic, and dermonecrotic properties.[3,5–7] *Chiropsalmus quadrumanus* (box jellyfish or sea wasp) is a smaller version of *C. fleckeri*, which similarly can be rapidly fatal and is found in the Caribbean and southern U.S. waters and in Australia.

C. barnesi differs from *C. fleckeri* in that it is one tenth the size. Its cuboid body measures only 15 to 25 mm across, and its tentacles can reach lengths of 70 cm.[4,8] Standard stinger net enclosures along Australian beaches are not fine enough to prevent the entry of this animal.[9] Lulled into a false sense of security while swimming within the confines of these nets, especially given a typically mild initial stinging sensation, many bathers have inadvertently ignored

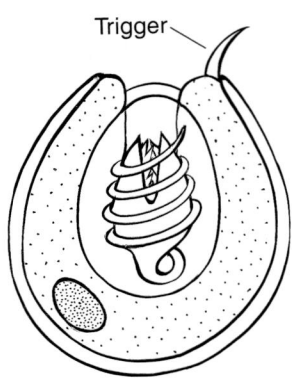

FIGURE 115-1

Nematocyst before discharge. *(From Auerbach PS: Envenomation by aquatic invertebrates. In Auerbach PS [ed]: Wilderness Medicine, 4th ed. Philadelphia, Mosby, 2001, p 1454.)*

C. barnesi envenomations until the onset of systemic symptoms. Also in contrast to *C. fleckeri*, *C. barnesi* prefer living well offshore and appear along beaches only during rough seas or due to underwater currents.[8,10] A study of 62 *C. barnesi* exposures during 1996 found, however, that 75% of stings occurred in coastal waters (63% within net enclosures), whereas only 11% occurred in people while reef diving, possibly a reflection of how many people were present in each of these areas.[9] The chemical composition of this animal's venom is still unclear.

Sea nettle venom has been shown to contain cardiotoxic, neurotoxic, and dermonecrotic proteins. Sea nettle venom also contains histamines, prostaglandins, serotonins, and kinins.[1]

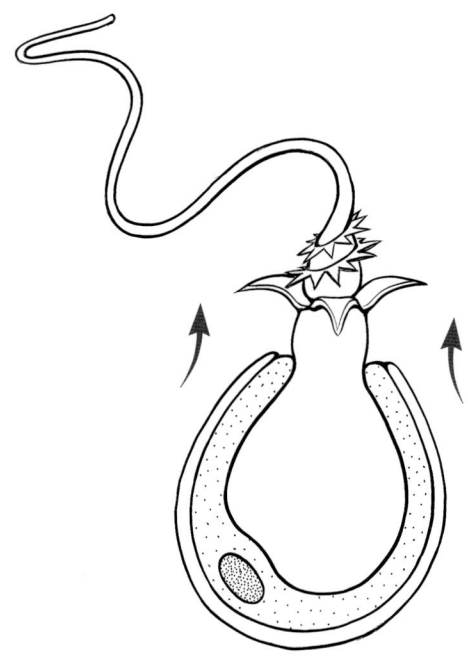

FIGURE 115-2

Nematocyst after discharge. *(From Auerbach PS: Envenomation by aquatic invertebrates. In Auerbach PS [ed]: Wilderness Medicine, 4th ed. Philadelphia, Mosby, 2001, p 1455.)*

Pathophysiology

The toxins present in *Chironex* venom may cause respiratory arrest, cardiotoxicity, and cell lysis by altering cell membrane permeability.[11] Changes in capillary wall integrity lead to edema.[7] The cardiotoxins are responsible for bradycardia, arrhythmias, decreased contractility, and a lower cardiac output. As a consequence, diminished coronary perfusion, combined with poor oxygenation because of respiratory depression and pulmonary edema, leads to cardiac ischemia. The toxins act directly to constrict coronary arteries. Lytic effects on cell membranes contribute to defects in electrical conduction and ventricular contractility, worsening myocardial hypoxia.[3,12]

Although most people who are exposed to *C. barnesi* venom and develop Irukandji syndrome can be discharged home after a brief emergency department visit, 3% to 30% develop heart failure and pulmonary edema.[4,8] The cause is still unknown, although there is support for global cardiac dilation (a direct cardiotoxic effect) and for massive α-adrenergic stimulation as instigators.[4,8,13] The former hypothesis is supported by echocardiographic evidence and the fact that some patients respond well to inotropic support. Some patients remain refractory to standard therapy, however. Advocates of the latter theory of massive α-adrenergic stimulation draw on evidence that suggests an increase in alveolocapillary membrane permeability in the setting of elevated catecholamine levels, similar to what is experienced in pheochromocytoma.[8]

Clinical Presentation and Life-Threatening Complications

Most *C. fleckeri* stings are minor, albeit always intensely painful. The toxic cutaneous reaction begins with the rapid formation of wheals and vesicles (Fig. 115-3), followed by the appearance of a dark, reddish brown or purple striped pattern, with each flare measuring 8 to 10 mm in width. More severe stings are characterized by the onset of skin blistering within 6 hours of contact and necrosis in 12 to 18 hours (Fig. 115-4). A less common but pathognomonic

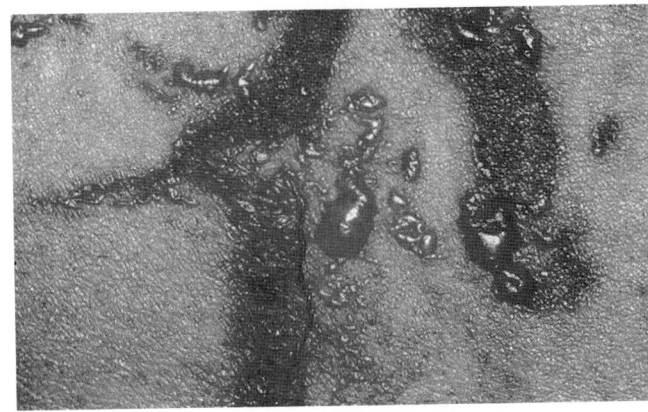

FIGURE 115-3

Incipient necrosis and blistering within 24 hours of box-jellyfish (*Chironex fleckeri*) envenomation. *(Courtesy of John Williamson, MD. From Auerbach PS: Envenomation by aquatic invertebrates. In Auerbach PS [ed]: Wilderness Medicine, 4th ed. Philadelphia, Mosby, 2001, p 1469.)* See Color Fig. 115-3.

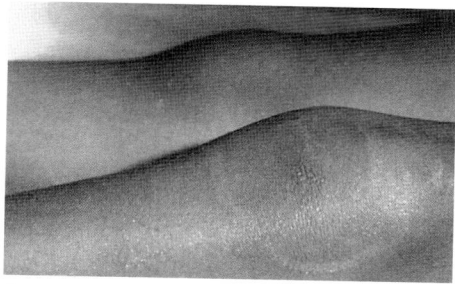

A

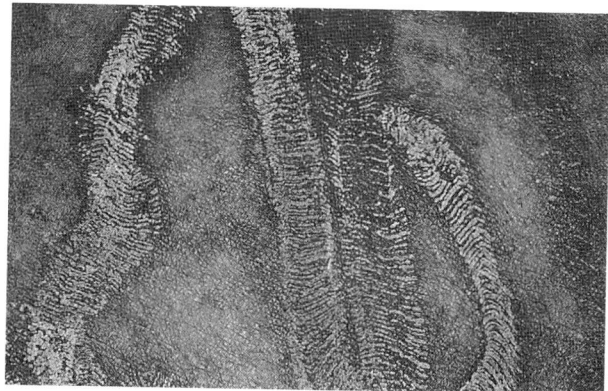

B

FIGURE 115-4

A, Frosted crosshatched pattern pathognomonic for a box-jellyfish envenomation. The victim of this sting died rapidly. See Color Fig. 115-4A. **B,** The enhanced frosted appearance is a result of application of a spray of aluminum sulfate. *(Courtesy of John Williamson, MD. From Auerbach PS: Envenomation by aquatic invertebrates. In Auerbach PS [ed]: Wilderness Medicine, 4th ed. Philadelphia, Mosby, 2001, p 1469.)* See Color Fig. 115-4B.

reaction is a "frosted" appearance with a pattern of transverse crosshatches.[1]

The reactions to major exposures can be divided by organ system. The respiratory system responds initially with tachypnea, which is followed by labored breathing and pulmonary edema, ultimately with respiratory depression and apnea. The cardiovascular system immediately shows bradycardia and decreased ventricular relaxation. After an initial increase in arterial pressure, there may be a precipitous decrease. Arrhythmias, including various conduction blocks, ventricular tachycardia, and ventricular fibrillation, are common. Effects on the central nervous system include diminished levels of consciousness and convulsive spasms. Smooth and striated muscle initially exhibit contraction but soon develop paralysis, notably affecting the diaphragm and intestinal tract.[3] Death is attributed to hypotension, muscle spasm, respiratory paralysis, acute pulmonary edema, and cardiac arrest. Overall mortality in some areas approaches 20%.[1]

Exposures to *C. fleckeri* and *C. quadrumanus* share similar local and systemic reactions.[2] The initial envenomation caused by *C. barnesi* is usually mild. Most victims, if they notice the sting at all, believe they have come into contact with an innocuous jellyfish. Although skin imprints are not always apparent, a mild blotchy redness with piloerection and local diaphoresis may be noted. Marks are more commonly left by the small bell rather than by the tentacles.

More significant local eruptions should prompt consideration of exposure to another species.[4,8]

The onset of severe systemic symptoms, characteristic of the Irukandji syndrome, usually is delayed minutes to hours (30 minutes on average). The syndrome consists of intense pain, the effects of catecholamine release, and cardiopulmonary decompensation. The first two are invariably present, and the latter occurs in 3% to 30% of patients. The pain typically consists of a severe boring sensation in the sacrum; severe muscle spasms involving the extremities, abdomen, and chest wall; and frank chest pain or tightness, sometimes accompanied by cardiac-specific enzyme elevations. The symptoms associated with catecholamine excess resemble those of pheochromocytoma and include sweating, piloerection, anxiety, restlessness, feelings of impending doom, headache, nausea, tachypnea, tremor, oliguria, tachycardia, hypertension (diastolic readings often reaching 140 mm Hg), pallor, peripheral cyanosis, and cerebral edema. Acute pulmonary edema, cardiac dilation, and reduced left ventricular function can occur 8 to 18 (average 10 to 12) hours after envenomation. We are unaware of any deaths attributed to this syndrome.[1,4,8,9]

One Australian researcher reported several cases involving the much more rapid onset of lower extremity burning and neurasthenic sensations, accompanied by priapism, periorbital edema, expiratory wheezes, and severe lethargy.[4] This previously unreported constellation of symptoms may reflect the presence of a different species of carybdeid, an area in which research is ongoing.

The clinical presentation of *Chrysaora* (sea nettle) envenomations is similar to that of *Physalia* (see later), although a greater incidence of systemic symptoms may occur. Death is exceedingly rare. *Cyanea* spp. induce local erythema, wheal formation, muscle aches, drowsiness, and nausea. *Pelagia* spp. present with a similar cutaneous reaction but can cause severe pruritus and bronchospasm.[1] One case report exists of deep venous thrombosis after envenomation in the Red Sea by an otherwise unidentified member of the Scyphozoa class.[20]

Diagnosis

As with all animal envenomations, consideration must be given to the geographic and seasonal distribution of particular species. Local maritime authorities should be questioned regarding recent sightings.

Medical personnel suspicious of possible *Chironex* or *Chiropsalmus* exposure, based on characteristic tentacle prints, the sudden onset of severe localized pain, or acute cardiopulmonary decompensation, should have a low threshold for diagnosing these envenomations. *Chironex* and *Chiropsalmus* are the only two jellyfish toxins for which an antivenom exists. Patients presenting with a history and physical examination consistent with a seemingly innocuous sting who later develop symptoms associated with the Irukandji syndrome should be suspected of having been exposed to *C. barnesi*. The differential diagnosis in these patients may include acute myocardial infarction (in a swimmer with chest pain, pulmonary edema, and elevated muscle enzyme levels) and decompression sickness (in a diver with anxiety, trouble breathing, chest pain, and backache).

Treatment

Any victim of coelenterate envenomation first must be removed from the water to protect against further envenomation and the possibility of drowning. It is important to keep the patient as still and calm as possible because movement of a stricken extremity and the catecholamine surge associated with panic can hasten systemic intoxication. Decontamination consists of nematocyst neutralization with 5% acetic acid (commercial vinegar), an important intervention that is not intended to provide analgesia and should not be interrupted if the patient complains of worsening pain. Next, all remaining tentacles are physically removed using instruments or seawater irrigation or both. Seawater irrigation may remove many of the tentacles. Health care providers must wear protective clothing until such time as the patient has been completely decontaminated; nematocyst penetration of surgical gloves has been reported. Skin irrigation with fresh water is contraindicated because this may cause massive nematocyst triggering. If acetic acid is not available, aluminum sulfate surfactant (Stingose [Pfizer, West Ryde, Australia]) may be used as a substitute, although its efficacy in specific jellyfish envenomations has not been well studied. The use of 40% to 70% isopropyl alcohol is sometimes a last resort. In vitro studies of ethanol and isopropyl alcohol have shown chemically mediated nematocyst discharge, however. Sea nettle exposures may be neutralized more effectively with the application of baking soda than with acetic acid or alcohol.[1,14,15]

Some authors recommend the use of a constricting bandage proximal to the site of *Chironex* envenomation, in an effort to limit superficial venous (never arterial) and lymphatic return. Placed immediately after exposure, the bandage should be loosened for 90 seconds every 10 minutes and completely removed after 1 hour. A technique to reduce systemic toxin absorption, supported by circumstantial evidence, involves the application of a pressure immobilization bandage over an affected extremity. Only case reports exist of the use of this technique in severe envenomations, when the theoretical benefit of arresting further toxin absorption takes precedence over the pain of this technique secondary to venom-induced local tissue damage.[15] One author recommended against its use on account of the theoretical risk of inducing a large systemic venom bolus on finally releasing the bandage.[9] Further data are needed. This technique should be applied only after neutralization, because pressure can trigger "live" nematocysts.[1,16]

Suspected or confirmed *Chironex* and *Chiropsalmus* victims should receive the Box Jellyfish Antivenom (Commonwealth Serum Laboratories, Melbourne, Australia) (Fig. 115-5) *as soon as possible.* The dose is one ampule (20,000 U) diluted 1:5 to 1:10 in isotonic crystalloid (not water) administered intravenously over 5 minutes. A less desirable alternative (too slow absorption) is three ampules intramuscularly. The antivenom can be repeated once or twice every 2 to 4 hours if the patient fails to improve in terms of cutaneous findings, pain, or systemic symptoms. The antivenom has been shown to neutralize the cardiovascular, hemolytic, and hyperkalemic effects of the venom.[17] Although it is important to be aware of the fact that this antivenom is prepared by hyperimmunizing sheep and may carry a similar risk of anaphylaxis and serum sickness as that seen with equine hyperimmune globulins, its timely

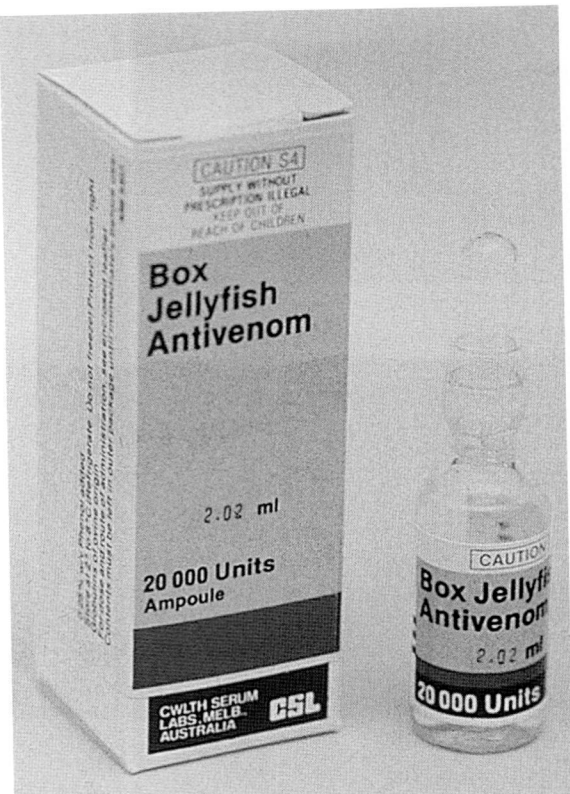

FIGURE 115-5

Box-jellyfish antivenom. *(Courtesy of John Williamson, MD. From Auerbach PS: Envenomation by aquatic invertebrates. In Auerbach PS [ed]: Wilderness Medicine, 4th ed. Philadelphia, Mosby, 2001, p 1470.)*

administration can be lifesaving. The adjuvant use of parenteral corticosteroids (e.g., hydrocortisone, 200 mg intravenously) is often recommended on theoretical grounds for their antiinflammatory properties; however, there are no data that these agents lessen the likelihood of adverse immunologic reactions. Anaphylactic or anaphylactoid reactions should be treated in the standard manner.[1]

Currently a major controversy surrounding the management of serious *Chironex* envenomations involves the use of verapamil, a calcium channel blocker and smooth muscle relaxant. Burnett and Calton[18] found that death was delayed in mice treated with verapamil before and after administration of venom obtained by tentacle milking. Burnett and colleagues[19] succeeded in reducing lethality from 21 of 21 to 16 of 22 mice treated with venom obtained from tentacle extract, by potentiating the effects of the ovine antivenom with verapamil. Tibbals and coworkers,[16] using tentacle extracts in mechanically ventilated piglets, discovered that verapamil failed to prevent any effects of the venom and worsened cardiovascular collapse and increased mortality. Bloom and associates[17] found that verapamil prolonged survival time in mice challenged with milked venom, perhaps by stabilizing the patient long enough for the antivenom to work. Different methods were used in obtaining venom in these studies. The extract method involves mechanically blending the tentacle, which may include more toxic proteins than are normally delivered during nematocyst discharge; the milking method may select certain toxic proteins that are usually present during envenomation. Given the conflicting evidence on this topic, we defer any recommendation on the use of verapamil, pending further investigation.

The Irukandji syndrome is managed in a supportive manner. The most common analgesics used are pethidine (meperidine), 0.25 to 0.5 mg/kg intravenously every 5 minutes, and morphine, 0.025 to 0.05 mg/kg intravenously every 5 minutes, or as continuous infusions. One author has raised a concern about the use of pethidine, which often is required in large quantities, because of its direct myocardial effects that in theory may worsen a patient's cardiovascular function. Pethidine has direct myocardial and respiratory depressant effects and carries the risk of seizures at high doses (often needed in these poisonings) due to the toxic metabolite norpethidine. Because the Irukandji syndrome may exhibit direct myocardial effects, too, fentanyl may be tried first (pure narcotic receptor action without myocardial effects or toxic metabolites).[9] Promethazine has been found to have analgesic and antiemetic effects in jellyfish envenomation. Phentolamine, an α-adrenergic receptor antagonist, given to adults as a 5-mg intravenous loading dose followed by 10-mg boluses as needed (or as a 5 mg/hr infusion), has been successful in blocking the effects of excess catecholamine release. Nifedipine, used to block the α-adrenergic vasoconstrictive effects seen with scorpion stings, also may be theoretically helpful. Verapamil and β-blockers may worsen heart failure or exacerbate hypotension. Patients who are asymptomatic off medications 6 hours after exposure may be discharged home with follow-up and careful discharge instructions. Patients who remain symptomatic after significant doses of parenteral analgesics should be admitted. Evaluation should include an electrocardiogram (ECG), chest radiograph, complete blood count, electrolytes, and a creatine phosphokinase level (with cardiac-specific fractionation). Patients who develop pulmonary edema should be managed in the standard fashion in a critical care setting, with central venous or pulmonary artery monitoring and inotropic support as needed.[4,8,9]

HYDROZOA

The hydrozoans comprise a range of species. The species of greatest clinical interest are the following:

- Feather hydroids (*Lytocarpus philippinus*, or "fire weed" or "fern weed")
- Hydroid corals (*Millepora*, or "fire coral")
- Floating siphonophore (*Physalia*, or Portuguese man-of-war)

Contact with *Physalia* is of most significance to intensivists,[1] although all are irritants that may necessitate medical attention.

The Physaliidae family consists of two members. *Physalia physalis* is found in the tropical and semitropical waters of the Gulf of Mexico, the Caribbean, and the entire Atlantic coast from Florida to Nova Scotia. *Physalia utriculus* is largely confined to Australia's coastal waters.[23,28] The presence of these animals depends on ocean currents; off the U.S. Atlantic coast, they first appear in October and November and return in March and April.[21] Exposures have

been reported throughout the winter and summer months, however.[9]

Physalia, rather than being a single organism, consist of four distinct entities sharing a symbiotic relationship. Two deserve mention from a toxicologic perspective. The blue or violet and iridescent float (pneumatophore), which can achieve a length of 30 cm, contains nitrogen-forming and carbon dioxide–forming glands that provide buoyancy and give this creature its distinctive ocean surface appearance. Certain species are capable of deflating their sail in rough seas and submerging to depths, where their presence might come as a surprise to divers. Dangling below the pneumatophore to lengths of up to 30 m are the nearly transparent nematocyst-bearing tentacles that capture prey and are the only part of the *Physalia* colony to harm humans. On contacting a foreign object, the stimulated nematocysts (750,000 per tentacle) not only fire but also initiate a chain reaction in which neighboring tentacles coil up, greatly increasing the potential surface area from which envenomation occurs. The nematocysts of beached *Physalia* can retain their capacity to sting for weeks if dry or even months if still moist.[1,21]

Pharmacology of *Physalia* Venom

The biologically active substances contained within each nematocyst include antigenic proteins, proteolytic enzymes, hemolytic toxins, neuromuscular toxins, kinins, histamines, and serotonins. There is anecdotal evidence, based on the months of presentation of more serious envenomations, to suggest that healthier and more venomous animals may appear early in the jellyfish season during maturation of the medusae.[22] Because the clinical effects of envenomation are dose dependent, the transfer of larger volumes of venom from bigger animals or from contact with more numerous tentacles yields greater toxicity.

Pathophysiology

As with jellyfish, fatal human envenomations can be explained by indirect inoculation into the systemic circulation via dermal capillaries at the site of nematocyst puncture. Intense localized pain is a consistent finding in jellyfish stings, and subcutaneous edema and vascular spasm without thrombosis eventually can lead to necrosis of affected digits.

Severe systemic reactions cause a sensation of chest constriction followed by vasomotor and respiratory failure, pulmonary edema, and death. Fatal stings almost always are associated with pulmonary congestion. Gross and histologic examinations have revealed visceral and cerebral congestion, pulmonary edema, minute intracranial hemorrhages, lymphoid hyperplasia, and acute toxic nephritis. Although more commonly seen with the stings of brown recluse spiders, snakes, and scorpions,[1,24,25] severe hemolysis and acute renal failure have been described after *Physalia* envenomation.[23] The case of a 4-year-old girl stung in the waters along the North Carolina coast was remarkable for hemoglobin-induced acute renal failure with oliguria that was resistant to volume expansion and diuresis, ultimately requiring five sessions of dialysis. Although the mechanism of renal vascular resistance in this otherwise healthy, well-hydrated, and nonacidotic child is unknown, it has been hypothesized that vasoactive substances in the coelenterate venom itself could produce refractory vasoconstriction.

Although life-threatening anaphylaxis has been reported,[7] it is rare compared with respiratory failure (low-dose exposure) and cardiovascular collapse (high-dose exposure).[22] Other causes of death include myocardial infarction and cerebrovascular accident, presumably consequent to pain and injury[26,27]; drowning can occur secondary to limb paralysis.[8]

Clinical Presentation and Life-Threatening Complications

Acute cutaneous reactions begin with immediate burning, stinging, or shocklike sensations, followed by the formation of painful or pruritic papules or wheals (extending proximally along an extremity to the trunk), which may progress to vesicular, hemorrhagic, necrotizing, or ulcerative lesions (Figs. 115-6 through 115-8). Chronic cutaneous reactions include erythema multiforme, erythema nodosum, granuloma annulare, and hyperpigmented or hypertrophic scars. Eczematous, urticarial, or vesicular lesions may persist or recur over weeks to months after the initial exposure.[21,28]

Acute systemic reactions to *Physalia* envenomation include nausea, vomiting, abdominal pain, headache, seizures, vertigo, ataxia, emotional lability, paresthesias, muscle cramps, arthralgias, glaucoma, hemolysis, acute renal failure, laryngospasm, dyspnea, respiratory failure, hypotension, shock, cardiac arrhythmias, cardiovascular collapse, coma, and death.[21,23,28] One case report described a 67-year-old woman with the following: normal sinus rhythm at 80 beats/min at 3 minutes postenvenomation, sinus bradycardia at 15 beats/min at 5 minutes, asystole at 26 minutes, normal sinus rhythm with evidence of ischemia on ECG and elevated creatine kinase at 60 minutes (after resuscitation).[22]

Diagnosis

When evaluating the victim of a possible coelenterate envenomation, consideration must be given to the geographic and seasonal distribution of particular species. The *Physalia*

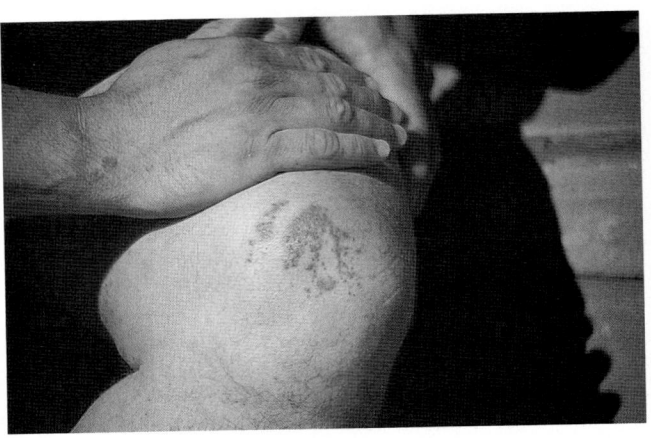

FIGURE 115-7

Fernlike hydroid print on the knee of a diver. *(Photo by Paul Auerbach, MD. From Auerbach PS: Envenomation by aquatic invertebrates. In Auerbach PS [ed]: Wilderness Medicine, 4th ed. Philadelphia, Mosby, 2001, p 1461.)* See Color Fig. 115-7.

pneumatophore is an easily identifiable marker, and local beach authorities should be questioned regarding recent sightings. Invariably, contact with this and other coelenterates produces immediate localized pain and leaves behind "tentacle prints" that consist of linear, beaded, violaceous lesions in a whiplike distribution.[27,28]

Treatment

Victims first must be removed from the water to protect against further envenomation and the possibility of drowning. It is important to keep the patient as still and calm as possible because movement of a stricken extremity and the catecholamine surge associated with panic can hasten systemic intoxication. Decontamination consists of nematocyst neutralization with 5% acetic acid (commercial vinegar) followed by physical removal of all remaining tentacles using instruments or seawater irrigation or both.[35] Health care providers should wear protective clothing until such time as the patient has been completely decontaminated.

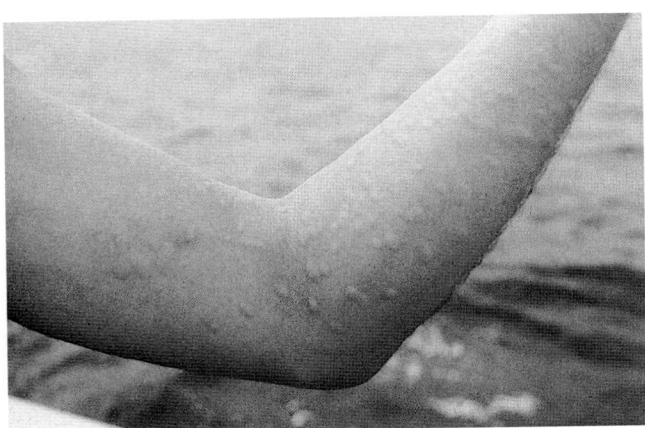

FIGURE 115-6

Hydroid sting on arm of a diver. *(Photo by Neville Coleman. From Auerbach PS: Envenomation by aquatic invertebrates. In Auerbach PS [ed]: Wilderness Medicine, 4th ed. Philadelphia, Mosby, 2001, p 1461.)* See Color Fig. 115-6.

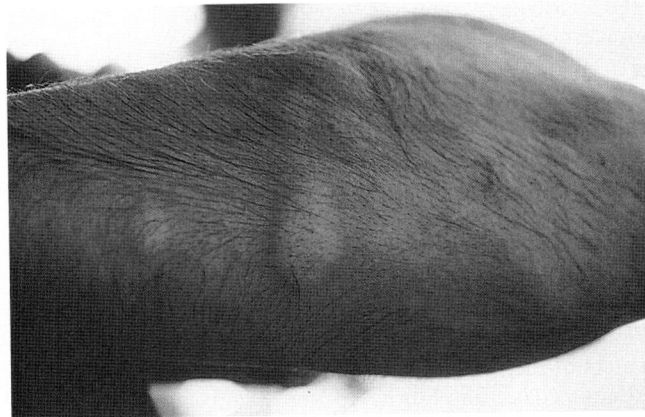

FIGURE 115-8

Fire coral sting. *(Photo by Kenneth Kizer, MD. From Auerbach PS: Envenomation by aquatic invertebrates. In Auerbach PS [ed]: Wilderness Medicine, 4th ed. Philadelphia, Mosby, 2001, p 1462.)* See Color Fig. 115-8.

The use of standard hospital gloves is not recommended because nematocysts have been shown to penetrate them. Skin irrigation with fresh water is contraindicated because this may cause massive nematocyst triggering. The use of alcohol and proteolytic meat tenderizers is controversial. In vitro studies using ethanol and isopropyl alcohol have shown chemically mediated nematocyst discharge.[29,30] One risk associated with papain use is cutaneous peeling and, conceivably, further envenomation.[31] Both of these remain popular home remedies, however.

Signs and symptoms of systemic toxicity should be managed with appropriate supportive measures. Cardiotoxicity and anaphylaxis require standard interventions, including intravenous fluid resuscitation, epinephrine, histamine receptor antagonists, and parenteral corticosteroids.[33] One author recommended that previously sensitized individuals carry an epinephrine autoinjector (EpiPen) at the beach and take antihistamines before swimming.[22] Intravenous verapamil has shown promise in mice and rats exposed to *Physalia* venom.[34] The treatment of anaphylaxis is discussed in detail in Chapter 31. Ventilatory support should be instituted according to standard indications. Of all coelenterates, only *C. fleckeri* and *C. quadrigatus* have known antivenoms, making further species identification for treatment purposes a moot point. No antivenom to hydrozoan exposures exists.

Oral or parenteral narcotic and nonsteroidal antiinflammatory medications may be given for pain relief. Severe muscle spasm may respond to 10% calcium gluconate (5 to 10 mL slow intravenous push), diazepam, or methocarbamol, although the evidence supporting their efficacy is circumstantial.[21,28] Arterial spasm has been reported to be managed successfully with intraarterial reserpine and urokinase.[32] Acute dermatosis should be treated with cold packs and, if necessary, mid-dose to high-dose topical corticosteroids. Topical anesthetics, such as benzocaine spray and lidocaine ointment, and oral antihistamines may be soothing. Although the routine use of antibiotics is not recommended, local wound care can be accomplished with daily soaks in Burow's solution.[28] Tetanus toxoid should be administered to all patients not currently immunized or in whom a history cannot be elicited.

Delayed cutaneous reactions at the site of exposure, accompanied by fever, weakness, arthralgias, and joint effusions, may recur over the course of 2 months. Each flare should be managed with a 10- to 14-day oral prednisone taper starting at 1 to 2 mg/kg/day.[1] Significant envenomations may result in permanent hyperpigmentation and keloid scarring. The former is treated with hydroquinone bleaches; the latter is treated in a standard fashion.[35]

STINGRAYS

Described by Aristotle in the 4th century BC, stingrays have come to be known as the most common fish to envenomate humans.[1,36] Stingrays are members of the class Chondrichthyes, the subclass Elasmobranchii, and the order Rajiformes. Included in this group are sharks, eagle rays, and mantas. Although the latter two species contain stinging apparatus, these are likely vestigial, and no human envenomations have been reported.[1] Stingrays

are dangerous by virtue of the trauma inflicted by their stings, the risk of infection, and the toxic effects of their venom.

Stingrays typically are found in tropical, subtropical, and temperate oceans 15 degrees of latitude north and south of the tropics. They prefer shallow waters and are a hazard in the vicinity of reefs, sheltered bays, estuaries, and lagoons. Although native to salt water oceans, they also can appear in brackish and fresh water.[1,37] Purely freshwater species exist in the rivers of the Amazon basin. Although physicians practicing along tropical and temperate coastlines handle most stingray exposures, practitioners everywhere should be aware of their toxicity because travelers and aquarium owners also are at risk.

Stingrays are nonaggressive scavengers of various sizes (from several inches to 12 feet) that respond reflexively to being disturbed as they lie camouflaged on the seabed or, less commonly, are mishandled while in an aquarium. A stingray's defensive movement consists of a whiplike upward arching of its tail on which is attached one to four serrated spines that can embed themselves into an unsuspecting victim (Figs. 115-9 and 115-10). Each spine is covered by an integumentary sheath, which, when ruptured beneath human skin (Fig. 115-11), releases venom, mucus, and pieces of sheath and spine into the wound. The spines and their neighboring retrorse (backward-facing) teeth are capable of inflicting significant soft tissue and bone injury.

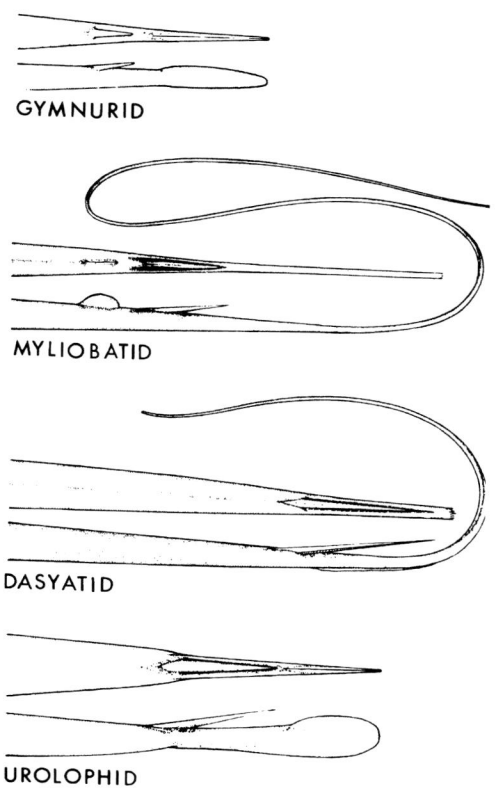

GYMNURID

MYLIOBATID

DASYATID

UROLOPHID

FIGURE 115-9

Four anatomic types of stingray venom organs. *(From Auerbach PS: Envenomation by aquatic invertebrates. In Auerbach PS [ed]: Wilderness Medicine, 4th ed. Philadelphia, Mosby, 2001, p 1489.)*

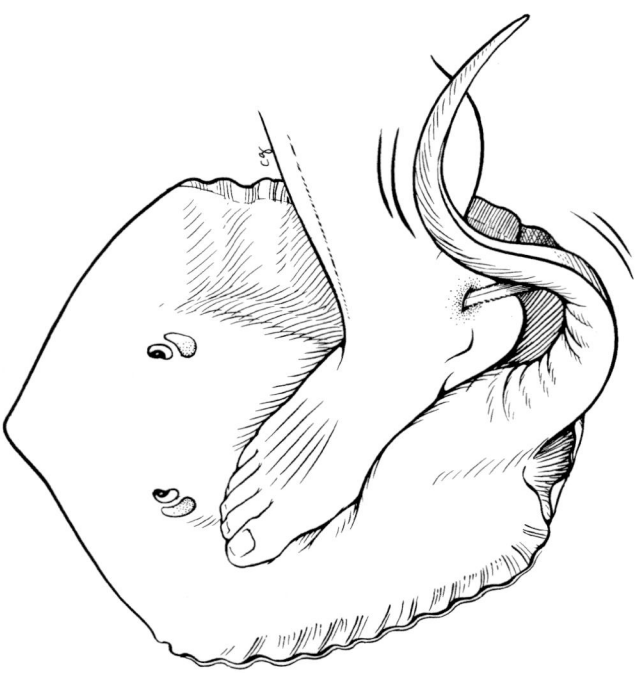

FIGURE 115-10

The stingray lashes its tail upward into the leg and generates a deep puncture wound. *(From Auerbach PS: Envenomation by aquatic invertebrates. In Auerbach PS [ed]: Wilderness Medicine, 4th ed. Philadelphia, Mosby, 2001, p 1490.)*

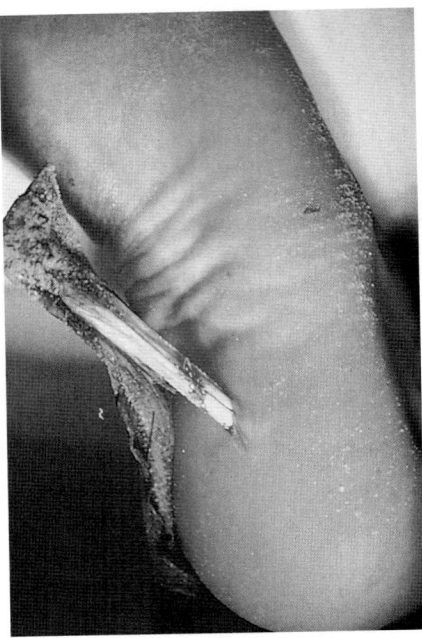

FIGURE 115-11

Stingray spine tip broken off into the heel of a victim. *(Photo by Robert D. Hayes. From Auerbach PS: Envenomation by aquatic invertebrates. In Auerbach PS [ed]: Wilderness Medicine, 4th ed. Philadelphia, Mosby, 2001, p 1490.)* **See Color Fig. 115-11.**

Pharmacology

Toxic substances contained within the venom of stingrays include phosphodiesterases, 5'-nucleotidases, and serotonin.[1,37,38]

Pathophysiology

Animal studies have shown evidence of venom-induced peripheral vasoconstriction, bradycardia, atrioventricular block, ischemic ST-T abnormalities, asystole, central respiratory depression, seizures, ataxia, coma, and death.[1,39] Monitored cats exposed to intravenous stingray (*Urolophus* spp.) venom developed bradycardia and ST-T changes consistent with ischemia. When given a lethal dose, the animals showed pupillary dilation, ataxia, salivation, incontinence, and collapse.[37,40] No evidence was found during these studies to suggest any disturbance in neuromuscular transmission.

Clinical Presentation and Life-Threatening Complications

As previously described, a stingray can cause traumatic injury, infection, and envenomation. Its powerful tail is capable of inflicting significant soft tissue lacerations and bone penetration. Bacterial infections are common, and osteomyelitis has been reported.[1,43] The lower extremities, especially the feet and ankles, are struck most frequently, followed by the upper extremities, abdomen, and thorax. Many common forms of protective clothing have failed to prevent the passage of stingray spines; this list is remark-

able for its inclusion of wetsuits and rubber and leather footwear.[1,41] Individuals who walk in shallow waters should shuffle their gait or otherwise warn nearby animals of their presence.

Envenomation typically begins with the immediate onset of excruciating pain that radiates centrally, peaks at 30 to 90 minutes, and lasts 6 to 48 hours.[1,41] Varying degrees of local edema and bleeding also may be present. The wound is initially cyanotic or dusky and rapidly progresses to erythema and petechiae, local fat and muscle necrosis, ulceration, and gangrene.[37,41] Although larger stings can cause tissue necrosis, smaller envenomations may appear simply cellulitic. The larger the spines, the more significant the trauma, and the greater the risk of deep bacterial wound infections and osteomyelitis. It is unclear whether larger animals deliver greater venom loads. The efficiency of the animal's defense mechanism is related not only to the tail length and musculature but also to the location of the spines. An animal with spines at the base of its tail is less able to inflict serious wounds, regardless of its size.[1,37] Retained integument and pieces of spine frequently have been implicated in the development of foreign-body reactions and recurrent local soft tissue and bone infections.[37,41,42]

Systemic manifestations of stingray envenomation include nausea, vomiting, diarrhea, diaphoresis, dizziness, vertigo, weakness, headache, syncope, seizures, abdominal pain, muscle cramps and fasciculations, paralysis, anaphylaxis, tachycardia, hypotension, arrhythmias, and death.[38,41] Animal studies report ischemic ST-segment changes, bradycardia, atrioventricular blocks, and asystole.[39] Reported fatalities include stab wounds to the thorax (two cases of pericardial perforation with subsequent exsanguination and one case of delayed cardiac tamponade secondary to myocardial necrosis and perforation 6 days after injury) and thigh (one case of exsanguination after traumatic rupture of a femoral artery).[37,42] Although not lethal, there have been reports of liver lacerations and bowel perforation, both necessitating surgical intervention.[37]

Diagnosis

Medical practitioners should be aware of venomous marine animals indigenous to their area. Lacerations with cyanotic borders, sustained to the lower extremities while in shallow waters, should prompt consideration of stingray envenomation.

Treatment

Therapy, the success of which depends largely on the rapidity of its delivery, is directed toward the alleviation of pain, the neutralization of toxic effects, and the prevention of infection. The wound should be irrigated immediately with copious quantities of cold water. In contrast to coelenterate attacks, stingray envenomations are not exacerbated by the application of fresh water. Any water is acceptable for decontamination as long as it is cold and capable of inducing vasoconstriction. Although controversial, suctioning the wound for 15 to 30 minutes may be beneficial in removing venom and retained stinger pieces. The use of a proximal constriction band (released for 90 seconds every 10 minutes for 30 minutes) to impede venous and lymphatic flow also is controversial.[1] Some authors attribute worsened pain and necrosis to this technique.[37,40]

Immediately after a rapid primary exploration of the wound and removal of gross contaminants (usually spine or sheath fragments), the affected area should be immersed in nonscalding hot water (45°C [113°F] or as tolerated) for 30 to 90 minutes. This immersion denatures the heat-labile components of the venom, attenuating toxicity and alleviating pain.[38,41,42] The use of ice rather than heat therapy is controversial and probably should be considered only if the latter is unavailable.[41,42] Ammonia, magnesium sulfate, potassium permanganate, and formalin should not be added to the soaking solution because these may contribute to tissue toxicity. No data exist to support to use of antihistamines or steroids.[1]

Although the removal of grossly visible foreign bodies aids in the initial therapy (retained sheath can continue to secrete venom), a thorough exploration and decontamination of the wound is crucial to successful long-term management. Chronic and recurrent wound infections are frequently attributed to retained spike fragments.[42] Analgesia should be initiated before wound exploration. Although parenteral narcotics are often needed, local infiltration or regional nerve block with 1% to 2% lidocaine is a useful adjuvant. Epinephrine should be avoided because this may worsen tissue necrosis.[42] All wounds must be evaluated radiographically for evidence of occult foreign bodies. Useful techniques include plain radiography, stereotaxic radiography, computed tomography, and ultrasound.[38,42,43] Small wounds may be conducive to débridement and cleansing in the emergency department, with careful attention to evaluating the entire puncture tract; larger wounds may require exploration in the

operating room. All wounds should be packed open for delayed primary closure, allowing for adequate drainage. If possible, suturing should be avoided.[42] Prophylactic antibiotics to cover marine microbes (trimethoprim-sulfamethoxazole is a popular choice) should be given.[37] Thorough wound débridement is important. Indolent infections should prompt the search for unusual organisms; this is recommended for all but the smallest lacerations because the incidence of secondary infection and ulceration is high.[1,42] Tetanus prophylaxis is indicated for all unimmunized victims and in victims from whom a reliable history cannot be elicited.[37,38,41,42]

Patients with penetrating thoracic injuries should be transferred to a medical center with thoracotomy capability, regardless of initial clinical presentation. Although ECG, chest radiograph, echocardiogram, and cardiac enzymes should be employed, these modalities may be insensitive to early myocardial necrosis. Technetium pyrophosphate and thallium isotope scanning have been suggested as superior techniques in detecting dying cardiac muscle early enough to permit surgical intervention before perforation.[42] Patients with punctures to the abdominal cavity should receive prophylactic antibiotics that target gram-negative and anaerobic organisms, such as cefoxitin, cefotaxime, or clindamycin-gentamicin intravenously, and appropriate radiographic and surgical evaluation to rule out intestinal perforation.[1]

SCORPAENIDAE

Members of the family Scorpaenidae, scorpaenids are considered the most dangerous of the bony fishes of the world because of the number and severity of injuries they inflict. These animals are divided into three groups according to the structure of their venom apparatus (Fig. 115-12):

1. The *Pterois* (lionfish, turkeyfish, zebrafish, butterfly cod) have long, slender spines and small venom glands.
2. The *Scorpaena* (scorpionfish, bullrout, scuplin) have long, heavy spines with medium-sized venom glands.
3. The *Synanceja* (stonefish, warty ghoul, nohu) have short and stout spines but much larger venom organs, making them the most dangerous of the scorpaenids.[44,45]

These fish are native to tropical waters but can be found, albeit less commonly, in temperate zones. Their geographic distribution is separated by genus. *Pterois* spp. are native to the Pacific, *Scorpaena* spp. can be found in the Atlantic and Pacific Oceans and the Caribbean Sea, and *Synanceja* spp. live only in Indo-Pacific waters.[44,45] In the United States, scorpaenids frequent the Florida Keys, the Gulf of Mexico, the southern California coast, and the waters around Hawaii. Despite such geographic distribution, certain scorpaenids (*Pterois* in particular) are increasingly popular as aquarium animals and constitute part of a growing import market, largely on account of their remarkable beauty.[1] Between 1979 and 1983, the San Francisco Bay Area Regional Poison Control Center in the United States reported 45 lionfish envenomations, all involving private or commercial aquariums.[44]

Synanceja are generally found in calm, shallow waters, such as tidal pools, sheltered bays, estuaries, and waters around coral reefs. They often bury themselves under rocks, in the sand or mud, or within crevices. They remain

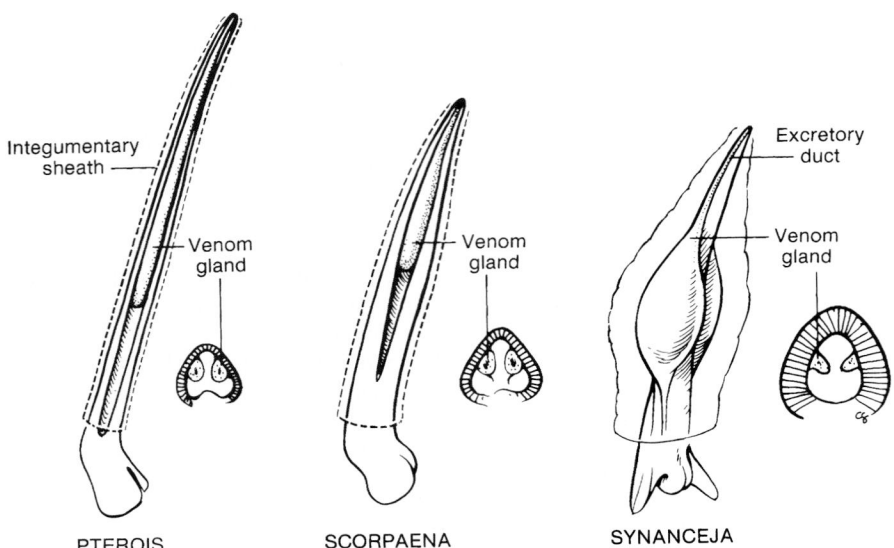

FIGURE 115-12

Lionfish, scorpionfish, and stonefish spines with associated venom glands. *(From Auerbach PS: Envenomation by aquatic invertebrates. In Auerbach PS [ed]: Wilderness Medicine, 4th ed. Philadelphia, Mosby, 2001, p 1495.)*

so motionless that algae often grow on their skin, rendering them even more camouflaged and likely to be disturbed by an unsuspecting passerby. *Scorpaena* likewise prefer shallow waters, where they blend in with the natural surroundings found on rocky bottoms and along coral reefs. *Pterois* are vividly colorful and graceful fish that, in contrast to other scorpaenids, swim freely or hover in shallow waters.[1,44,45]

The venom apparatus of the scorpaenids consists of 12 or 13 dorsal, 2 pelvic, and 3 anal spines, each of which contains venom glands and is covered with an integumentary sheath. The larger and more ornate pectoral spines are not associated with venom organs. When threatened in any way, from being handled or accidentally stepped on, these fish reflexively erect their spines. When embedded into flesh, the sheath is torn, the spine may fracture, and venom enters the wound. The venom retains its potency for 24 to 48 hours after the animal's death. Although they do not typically attack humans, stonefish have been known to do so if provoked.[44,45]

Pharmacology

Scorpaenid venom contains numerous toxic elements, the most powerful of which belongs to the stonefish. Stonustoxin is a nondialyzable, heat-labile protein of molecular weight 150,000 that is the major toxic component of stonefish venom. The potency of this venom is likened to that of the cobra.[1] When the mouse median lethal dose is extrapolated to a 60-kg adult, one finds that the lethal dose is 18 mg, or the content of six stonefish spines. In other words, a single exposure to a stonefish in which the victim steps on half the animal's spines can prove lethal.[46]

Analysis of the venom also has revealed the presence of hyaluronidase, thrombin, alkaline phosphomonoesterase, 5′-nucleotidase, acetylcholinesterase, phosphodiesterase, arginine esterase, and arginine amidase.[46] The proteases and hyaluronidase activities are probably responsible for the tissue necrosis seen in these envenomations and for the spread of venom toxicity.[45]

Pathophysiology

The principal action of *Synanceja* venom is direct muscle toxicity and subsequent paralysis of cardiac, involuntary, and skeletal muscle.[49] Animal studies have revealed massive depletion of neurotransmitters and damage to nerve and muscle fibers, which can account for the neuromuscular inhibition seen in these envenomations. The immediate response of the cardiovascular system to a lethal dose is a precipitous decline in blood pressure (with little if any reflex tachycardia) plus signs of myocardial ischemia or injury, as evidenced by T-wave flattening or inversion and ST-segment displacement. Further ECG changes include atrial and ventricular premature complexes, first-degree atrioventricular block, ventricular tachycardia, and ventricular fibrillation. The profound hypotensive action of the venom cannot be accounted for by either adrenergic or sympathetic ganglionic blockade. Direct toxicity to cardiac and involuntary muscle, coupled with peripheral vasodilation, appears to be the more likely culprit. The primary cause of death is not due to cardiac myotoxicity, however, because the heart continues to beat well beyond respiratory arrest. Rather, death seems to result from either paralysis of the diaphragm or the rapid and marked hypotension induced by the toxin.

Clinical Presentation and Life-Threatening Complications

The severity of envenomation depends on several factors, including the species of fish, the number of stings, the amount of venom released into the tissue, and the age and health of the victim. Wounds that bleed profusely tend to be associated with milder effects. Lionfish stings result in relatively mild symptoms, scorpionfish exposures may produce moderate-to-severe effects, and stonefish envenomations may be severe or life-threatening.[1,48]

Common to all scorpaenid exposures is the immediate onset of intense pain that radiates in a centripetal fashion,[1] often described as excruciating, sharp, or throbbing.[44,45]

Untreated, the intensity of the pain peaks at 60 to 90 minutes and subsides after 8 to 12 hours.[44,48] Stonefish stings can be so painful as to cause delirium and may not resolve for several days.[1] Local signs and symptoms, which may include erythema, warmth, and edema surrounding an ischemic-appearing or cyanotic-appearing puncture site, can persist for 24 hours. In the case of lionfish exposure, vesicles containing inflammatory mediators, such as prostaglandin $F_{2\alpha}$, may form around the wound (Fig. 115-13).[1] Anesthesia, hypesthesia, and paresthesias involving the affected extremity have been reported,[44,47] and tissue necrosis and sloughing at the wound site are common.[44,47]

Systemic signs and symptoms are a common feature of stonefish envenomations and are more typical of animals native to Australian rather than Asian waters.[40,45,50] Manifestations include nausea, vomiting, diarrhea, abdominal pain, anxiety, restlessness, headache, tremors, peripheral neuritis or neuropathy, lymphangitis, arthritis, fever, diaphoresis, and pallor. Severe cases can progress to bradycardia, tachycardia, atrioventricular block, ventricular fibrillation, profound hypotension, pericarditis, delirium, seizures, syncope, generalized paralysis, respiratory distress secondary to pulmonary edema and diaphragmatic paralysis, and death.[1,44,45] Death, although rare, usually occurs within the first 6 to 8 hours.[1]

Late sequelae of scorpaenid envenomations include secondary infections, deep abscesses, cutaneous granulomas, tissue defects, indolent ulcers, and peripheral neuropathies. Pain and numbness may persist for days to weeks, and wounds may take months to heal.[1,44]

Diagnosis

Clinical practitioners should be aware of the marine animals that are native to their area and should always consider the possibility of serious envenomations in patients who present after being "stung" by a "pet" fish. This consideration is of particular importance in the case of scorpaenid exposures, because a stonefish antivenom exists. Although

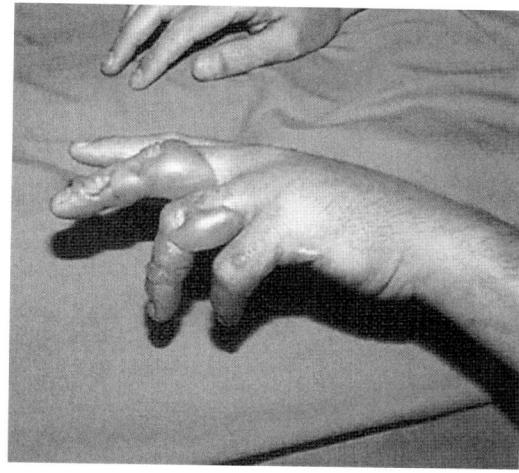

FIGURE 115-13

Vesiculation of the hand 48 hours after the sting of a lionfish. *(Photo by Howard McKinney. From Auerbach PS: Envenomation by aquatic invertebrates. In Auerbach PS [ed]: Wilderness Medicine, 4th ed. Philadelphia, Mosby, 2001, p 1495.)* See Color Fig. 115-13.

stingray and stonefish stings present in a similar fashion (typically an unsuspecting wader who complains of the acute onset of intense pain after having stepped on something), there is an important clue to distinguishing the two. Stingray wounds tend to be large and irregular. Stonefish leave relatively small punctures that initially may go unnoticed. Injecting 1% or 2% lidocaine without epinephrine near the site of pain may result in the egress of fluid and consequent discovery of a previously invisible puncture wound.

Treatment

The initial management of all scorpaenid envenomations consists of the immediate immersion of the wound in non-scalding hot water (45°C [113°F]) for 30 to 90 minutes or until analgesia is achieved.[44,45,47] This immersion inactivates the heat-labile proteins contained in the venom and may limit local sequestration by reversing vasospasm at the site of injury. Repeat immersion in hot water may be needed during the first 2 hours. If pain persists, local infiltration or regional nerve blockade with 1% or 2% lidocaine without epinephrine may be necessary.[1]

Muscle cramps can be treated with diazepam, methocarbamol, or other antispasmodics. The administration of intravenous calcium chloride and calcium gluconate has not been reported to relieve muscle spasm.[44] Infiltration with emetine, potassium permanganate, or Congo red has been largely abandoned. Although sometimes reported as effective, the success of folk remedies (e.g., meat tenderizer, mangrove sap, green papaya [papain]) and other empirical treatments (e.g., mineral spirits, organic dye, ground liver, formalin), to our knowledge, remains unproven.[1] Given the simplicity and remarkable efficacy of hot water immersion, one wonders why anyone with access to a source of heat would experiment with any other treatment. Cryotherapy is positively contraindicated,[47] as illustrated in the case of a 30-year-old woman stung on the finger by a lionfish and subsequently treated with ice water. Fibrosis and limited range of motion of the affected digit was partially treated with physical therapy, although 18 months later the patient still complained of an indurated, numb, atrophic, and stiff finger.[47]

Although the spines rarely embed in wound tissue, the puncture site must be explored carefully and all fragments of sheath removed. Punctures deep into the sole of the foot should undergo surgical exploration with magnification.[1] Vigorous irrigation with warm saline is recommended, whereas wide excision and débridement are unnecessary. Punctures should be allowed to heal by secondary intention.[44] Large wounds may require some provision for drainage. Deep wounds and wounds involving the hand or foot are at greater risk of infection and should prompt consideration of prophylactic antibiotics.[1] A tetanus booster should be administered based on the patient's current immunization status.

An antivenom to the stonefish toxin exists (Fig. 115-14). Together with standard supportive measures, such as fluid resuscitation and vasopressor therapy, antivenom is indicated in the case of severe systemic signs and symptoms that do not resolve with hot water treatment. This is rarely the case in scorpaenid envenomations other than *Synanceja* spp., (stonefish).[44,45] The initial dose depends on the number of

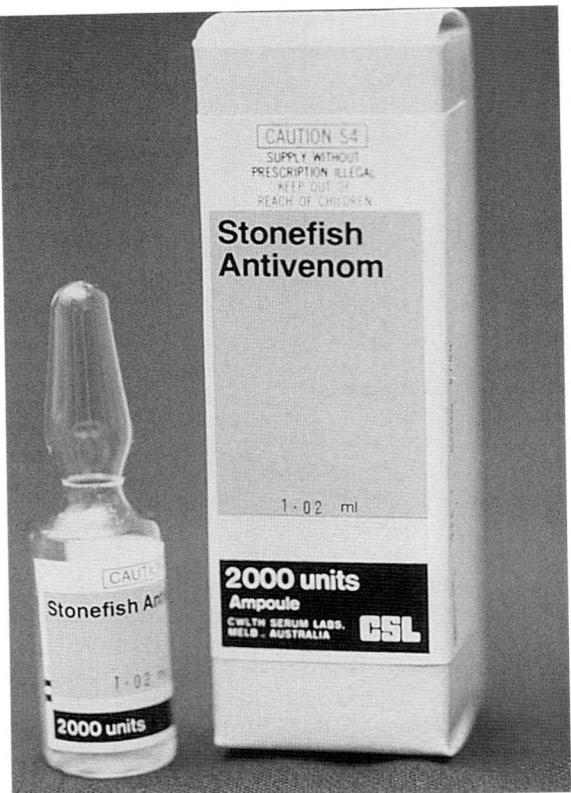

FIGURE 115-14

Stonefish antivenom. *(Courtesy of John Williamson, MD. From Auerbach PS: Envenomation by aquatic invertebrates. In Auerbach PS [ed]: Wilderness Medicine, 4th ed. Philadelphia, Mosby, 2001, p 1496.)*

puncture wounds. One or two punctures should receive 2 mL (2000 U) of antivenom; three or four punctures, 4 mL (4000 U); and so on. The initial dose can be repeated if symptoms fail to improve, although one should consider the possibility that envenomation by another animal has occurred.[45] Although some authors recommend the intramuscular route for moderately severe envenomations and the intravenous route for more severe stings,[45] others caution against intramuscular injection due to erratic absorption.[1] We direct all potential users to the manufacturer's written recommendations contained in each vial box. Because this antivenom is derived from horse serum, skin testing for possible anaphylactic reactions is recommended, although the value of this technique for the prediction of adverse effects has not been validated. The manufacturer is Commonwealth Serum Laboratories of Melbourne, Australia. In the United States, stonefish antivenom is available from Sea World in San Diego, California (619-222-6363 ext. 2201) and the Steinhart Aquarium in San Francisco, California (415-750-7145). Other locations for this antivenom can be found at www.csl.com.au.

CATFISH

Although their name often conjures up the image of slow, slimy river bottom feeders whose most threatening characteristic is their ugliness, there exist approximately 1000 species of freshwater and saltwater catfish worldwide, many of whom are capable of inflicting significant human injury. Catfish lack true scales and instead are covered by a slimy skin. Their "whiskers," to which their name is owed, are actually well-developed sensory organs. Freshwater species are typically slow-moving, nonevasive bottom dwellers. Saltwater catfish travel in large schools.

In North America, where fishing is a popular recreational sport, freshwater catfish include the brown bullhead catfish (*Noturus nebulosus*), Carolina madtom catfish (*Noturus furiosus*), channel catfish (*Noturus punctatus*), blue catfish (*Noturus furcatus*), and white catfish (*Noturus catus*). Saltwater animals include the coral catfish (*Plotatus lineatus*), common sea catfish (*Galeichthys felis*), and oriental catfish (*Plotosus lineatus*). The last species, which is often found hidden by tall seaweed, can inflict extremely painful stings.[1]

The venom apparatus of the catfish consists of three extremely sharp dorsal and pectoral fin spines and axillary venom glands. Each spine is covered by glandular tissue within an integumentary sheath, and some contain several barbed retrorse teeth.[1] Reports of envenomation after handling just the tail of certain species, including the Arabian Gulf catfish (*Arius bilineatus*) and some Mississippi River species, suggest the presence of a toxic skin substance (crinotoxin) that is secreted when the fish is excited.[55,57]

Amazonian Parasitic Catfish

The waters of the Amazon basin are home to a curious animal that has the uncanny propensity to swim up urethras of bathers (particularly when micturating), vaginas of menstruating women, ears, noses, and anuses.[60] The Amazonian parasitic catfish (genus *Vandellia*) is known locally as *candirú* in Portuguese, *canero* in Spanish, and *urethra fish* in English.[51]

Although not venomous, the Amazonian parasitic catfish can cause considerable morbidity. It is unclear why these animals enter the human urethra or other orifices, despite the common perception that they are urophilic. It does seem, however, that the act of urination is a risk factor. It has been proposed that, given their propensity to attach themselves to the gills of other swimming fish, these catfish inadvertently confuse the urinary flow of a human with the exhalant movement of water across the gills of their intended host. Regardless, these animals are exceedingly difficult to extract from the urethra when the head has entered. Their gill covers, which are adorned with sharp retrorse spines, reflexively open in an effort to breathe. Similar to tiny harpoons, these 5- to 8-cm long animals cannot be forcefully extracted from the urethra without inflicting considerable soft tissue damage.[1,51,52,53]

Pathophysiology

When the integumentary sheath of a catfish spine is broken, a heat-labile venom enters the wound and produces a localized inflammatory response.[55] Oriental catfish toxin contains various biologically active substances, including vasoconstrictive, hemolytic, dermatonecrotic, and edema-forming fractions. It manifests itself akin to a mild stingray envenomation.[1] The Arabian Gulf catfish crinotoxin causes smooth muscle contraction and stimulates the release of prostaglandins.[1]

The stings of saltwater catfish tend to be more severe and cause more local hemorrhage than the stings of freshwater animals.[1] The latter, owing to their more muddy, stagnant, and bacteria-containing environments, can produce significant soft tissue infections.[56]

Clinical Presentation and Life-Threatening Complications

Most catfish envenomations occur when the animals are handled, although waders have been known to accidentally step on the spines of fish resting on muddy river bottoms. Stings cause the immediate onset of stinging, throbbing, tingling, or scalding pain that radiates in a centripetal fashion from the site of injury. The pain often is described as being out of proportion to the mechanical injury itself. Untreated, the pain usually subsides within 30 to 60 minutes, although it may persist for 48 hours in severe envenomations, especially from saltwater species. The surrounding tissue quickly becomes ischemic; central pallor gradually becomes cyanotic before turning erythematous and edematous. Gangrene, necrosis, osteomyelitis, and secondary infection are common. Other manifestations include local muscle spasm, fasciculations, and diaphoresis. Less commonly, stings can cause peripheral neuropathy, lymphedema, adenopathy, lymphangitis, weakness, syncope, hypotension, respiratory distress, septic pulmonary emboli, and adult respiratory distress syndrome. Death has been reported, albeit rarely, after saltwater catfish envenomations.[54–56]

Secondary soft tissue and bone infections warrant special consideration because they can cause significant morbidity and mortality. Freshwater wounds are associated more often with *Aeromonas hydrophila* infections (including one death[59]), whereas their saltwater counterparts frequently grow *Vibrio* spp., especially in immunocompromised individuals.[55,56] Nine cases of *Mycobacterium marinum* have been reported in fishermen.[58] Stings inflicted in freshwater lakes and ponds also can cause *Edwardsiella tarda* infections.[55] Although catfish stings may resemble streptococcal cellulitis, the possibility of gram-negative infections always must be considered. These wounds can prove difficult to culture because of the small size of the punctures and the unique variety of marine microorganisms.[55]

Diagnosis

Practitioners should be aware of the species of marine animals that exist in their communities. Coral catfish are universally available, however, because of their popularity in the aquarium trade. Despite the fact that most catfish stings are amenable to symptomatic treatment, the risk of secondary soft tissue and bone infections and foreign-body reactions is enough to warrant the routine use of radiographs to rule out the presence of retained spines.

Treatment

There is no specific treatment for most catfish stings. Management is symptomatic, and success depends largely on the rapidity with which it is initiated. The first line of action in all catfish envenomations consists of the immediate immersion of the wound in nonscalding hot water (45°C [113°F]) for 30 to 90 minutes or until analgesia is achieved. This immersion inactivates the heat-labile proteins contained in the venom and may limit local sequestration by reversing vasospasm at the site of injury. Repeat immersion in hot water may be needed during the first 2 hours. The addition of mineral salts, solvents, antiseptics, or other chemicals to the hot water bath is of no proven efficacy. Cryotherapy is detrimental. If pain persists, local infiltration or regional nerve blockade with buffered 1% or 2% lidocaine, or a similar local anesthetic, without epinephrine may be necessary. Alkalizing the local anesthetic theoretically contributes to venom neutralization.[1] Although unstudied, a popular remedy against the sting of the Arabian Gulf catfish and various North American species involves rubbing the slimy skin of a captured specimen against the wound. Presumably the epidermal secretions of an excited animal cause local vasoconstriction and subsequent analgesia. Accelerated wound healing has similarly been reported.[1,55,61]

All wounds should be explored carefully for the presence of retained spine fragments. The routine use of radiographs is often recommended. It is generally recommended that wounds should not be sutured, but instead left to heal by secondary intention, with allowance for adequate drainage. Careful observation is necessary until healing is complete. High-risk punctures, especially punctures deep in the hand or foot, warrant prophylactic antibiotics. Many marine bacteria are penicillin resistant, and antibiotic therapy for routine soft tissue infections is often inadequate.[55] Recommended oral regimens include trimethoprim-sulfamethoxazole and tetracycline or ciprofloxacin (500 mg twice daily for 5 days). Intravenous options include ciprofloxacin, imipenem-cilastatin, ceftazidime, gentamicin, and trimethoprim-sulfamethoxazole.[54–56]

AMAZONIAN PARASITIC CATFISH

The goal in managing Amazonian parasitic catfish exposures is the careful extraction of the animal from the orifice in which it has been trapped. Forcefully pulling the fish out of the urethra is not recommended because significant soft tissue damage and hemorrhage can occur, and this approach is rarely successful. If surgical instruments are available, open urethrotomy is suggested.[53] Otherwise the common Amazonian folk remedy may be employed: the green (unripe) fruit of the jagua tree (*Genipa americana L.*), sometimes referred to as the *buitach apple*, is drunk as a hot tea. The buitach apple contains large quantities of citric acid, which theoretically dissolves the bony gills and jaw of the trapped catfish, enabling its extraction.[1,52,53] High-dose vitamin C could be a reasonable alternative for individuals without ready access to the fruit of the jagua tree. Jagua tree medicinal tea or tisane has been readily accepted by the modern local medical community as the treatment of choice for individuals who play host to the Amazonian parasitic catfish.

WEEVERFISH

The weeverfish (family Trachinidae) is considered the most venomous fish of the temperate zone.[1,62,63] The name *weever* is from the Old French (*wivre, guivre, vivre*) for "viper."

Trachinus vipera (the lesser weever) and *Trachinus draco* (the greater weever) are the better known of at least four species within this family. Common names include *adder pike, sea dragon, sea cat, black fin, scorpion fish,* and *stang* in English; *trachino vipera* in Italian; *viperqueise* in German; *petite vive* in French; and *araña del mar* or *escporpión* in Spanish.[62]

These fish are found throughout the eastern Atlantic region; Mediterranean, Baltic, North, and Black Seas; and western coastal waters of North and East Africa and are of interest primarily to the European and North African communities. The lesser weever buries itself in the sandy or muddy bottoms of shallow inshore waters, where it is a threat to waders; the greater weever is found offshore up to depths of 30 m and poses a threat to fishermen and divers.[62,63]

The weeverfish is a short, stout animal measuring roughly 10 to 50 cm in length. It typically has a yellow-gray hue with a white underbelly. Its venom apparatus consists of approximately six spines on the front dorsal fin and an additional spine on each of its gill covers. Each spine is covered by an integumentary sheath that ruptures during contact with a victim's flesh and releases its venom.[62,63] Although largely a sedentary animal, the weeverfish is capable of responding to any local disturbance by wielding its dagger-like spines with remarkable force (capable of penetrating a leather boot) and accuracy.[1] These fish can survive for hours out of water; likewise, their venom maintains its potency for hours beyond death, especially when the fish is refrigerated.[1,63]

Pharmacology

The venom secreted by the weeverfish contains several incompletely characterized, heat-labile proteins. These include 5-hydroxytryptamine (serotonin), epinephrine, norepinephrine, histamine, and a kinin-like substance. Although the lesser weeverfish venom causes no hemotoxic effects,[62] that of the greater weeverfish contains a single polypeptide, dracotoxin, of molecular weight 105,000, which has hemolytic and membrane depolarizing properties.[1,63]

Pathophysiology

The characteristic pain of a weeverfish sting is attributed to the 5-hydroxytryptamine contained in the venom. Release of histamine into the wound produces a wheal reaction with erythema.[62] Anaphylactic reactions rarely have been reported.[64]

Clinical Presentation and Life-Threatening Complications

The immediate onset of intense pain, often described as burning or crushing and out of proportion to the size of the wound, seems to be uniformly reported in weeverfish envenomations. The pain is aggravated by palpation, movement, weight bearing, and application of cold. The severity of the pain typically peaks at 30 minutes, subsides within 24 hours, but can last for days.[1,65] The folklore of Irish fishermen accurately states that the pain of weeverfish stings lasts until the tide has again reached the same height

as when the exposure occurred.[67] Pain often involves the entire limb and, over the initial 6 to 12 hours, can be accompanied by erythema, warmth, ecchymosis, edema, and numbness. Edema often lasts 10 days but has been known to persist for 1 year.[1,63] Stings, probably as a result of the pain's intensity, can acutely cause seemingly irrational behavior. Reports document delirium, psychosis, and torpidity (state of being lethargic, numbed, apathetic).[62] In 1782, a fisherman amputated his finger in an attempt at analgesia.[66]

Reported systemic manifestations of weeverfish envenomation include agitation, pallor, headaches, syncope, seizures, nausea, vomiting, diaphoresis, fever, chills, aphonia, dyspnea, cyanosis, hypotension, and cardiac arrhythmias.[62] One case report described crampy abdominal pain and vaginal bleeding in a 6-week pregnant woman who spontaneously aborted 3 weeks later.[68] Rare reports of death exist, although some authors attribute death to secondary sepsis rather than to a direct effect of the venom.[63,66]

Secondary bacterial infection occurs with varying frequency. Gangrene has been reported, and some wounds may take months to heal. Chronic musculoskeletal complaints include joint stiffness, numbness, tissue necrosis, and ankylosis.[62]

Diagnosis

As with all marine envenomations, clinical practitioners should be aware of the toxic animals that exist in their area. Weeverfish exposure must be part of the differential diagnosis of patients presenting after having been "stung" while wading or fishing in European and North African waters.

Treatment

Initial management consists of immediate immersion of the wound in nonscalding hot water (45°C [113°F]) for 30 to 90 minutes or until analgesia is achieved. This immersion inactivates the heat-labile proteins contained in the venom and may limit local sequestration by reversing vasospasm at the site of injury.[63] The application of vinegar, ammonia, urine, or mineral salts has no proven efficacy. Cooling is deleterious.[1] Parenteral narcotics are adjuvant therapy to heat, although narcotics often prove inadequate. Local or regional anesthesia with 1% or 2% lidocaine, or a similar local anesthetic, without epinephrine is frequently necessary.[63] Intravenous calcium gluconate has some reported success in cases of refractory pain.[64]

Although the spines rarely embed in wound tissue,[63] the puncture site must be explored carefully, and all fragments of sheath must be removed. Vigorous irrigation with warm saline is recommended; wide excision and débridement are unnecessary. Punctures should be allowed to heal by secondary intention. Large wounds may require some provision for drainage. Deep wounds and wounds involving the hand or foot are at greatest risk of infection and should prompt consideration of prophylactic antibiotics.[1] A tetanus booster must be administered based on the patient's current immunization status. Although no commercially available antivenom exists, the Institute of Immunology (Zagreb, Croatia) produces an effective, although experimental, *Trachinus* antivenom.[1]

STARFISH AND SEA CUCUMBERS

Although well known for their destruction of coral beds on the Great Barrier Reef, starfish also warrant mention on account of one species that is particularly venomous to humans. *Acanthaster planci*, the crown-of-thorns, is a carnivorous starfish found within the coral reefs of the Pacific and Indian Oceans, in the Red Sea, and in the Gulf of California.[69] *A. planci* are normally 25 to 35 cm in diameter but can reach sizes of 70 cm. Glandular tissue within the epidermis secretes a slimy venomous substance.[70] When the sharp, sturdy spines penetrate a victim's skin, venom is introduced into the wound. Divers should be aware that sturdy gloves may be pierced by these thorns.[1]

Sea cucumbers, also members of the phylum Echinodermata, are worm-shaped or sausage-shaped bottom scavengers that are venomous when handled or ingested. They are widely distributed in deep and shallow waters.[1] Some sea cucumbers are edible and are considered delicacies in certain countries. They are first boiled, then smoked, dried, or used to flavor soups. Common names include *trepang* and *beche-de-mer*. Sea cucumbers produce a venomous substance within their body walls. This liquid toxin is concentrated in the tentacular organs of Cuvier, which can be extended when the animal is threatened. Sea cucumbers also can secrete coelenterate venom, owing to their diet of nematocysts.[1]

Pharmacology

Analysis of *A. planci* venom has revealed the presence of potentially toxic saponins and histamine-like substances. Extracts show hemolytic, myotoxic, myonecrotic, anticoagulant, and capillary permeability–increasing properties.[1,70] A lethal factor has shown potent hepatotoxicity in experimental animals.[71] Sea cucumbers produce a cantharidin-like liquid toxin known as *holothurin*.[1]

Clinical Presentation and Life-Threatening Complications

When the starfish crown-of-thorns spine penetrates human skin, bleeding is copious, but pain and edema tend to be of only moderate severity. Untreated, pain usually resolves within 0.5 to 3 hours. The wound may become dusky or discolored. Systemic manifestations typically occur secondary to multiple punctures and are characterized by nausea, vomiting, lymphadenopathy, paresthesias, and muscle paralysis. Previously sensitized individuals may complain of edema and pruritus for weeks after the injury. Granulomatous reactions similar to reactions seen after sea urchin stings may develop in the case of retained spine fragments. Because some starfish eat poisonous shellfish, systemic toxicity should be considered in individuals who ingest starfish.[1]

Holothurin from sea cucumbers can induce toxicity through direct and indirect skin contact and from ingestion. Holothurin is a potent cardiac glycoside and may lead to severe illness or death if eaten. The toxin or even tentacle particles may diffuse through the aqueous environment surrounding the animal and cause significant damage to corneal and conjunctival surfaces. Toxicity ranges from inflammation to blindness.[72,73] Individuals who handle sea cucumbers with their bare skin may develop a papular skin irritation.[1]

Treatment

The management of crown-of-thorn stings begins with the immediate immersion of the affected body part in nonscalding hot water (113°C [45°C]) for 30 to 90 minutes or until analgesia is achieved. Rarely is the pain severe enough to warrant the use of local anesthesia, although this may be accomplished with 1% or 2% lidocaine, or similar local anesthetic, without epinephrine. The wound must be explored carefully for retained spine fragments because these may lead to the formation of granulomatous lesions, which may require excision. The use of radiographs to rule out the presence of foreign bodies is often helpful.[1]

Certain starfish, notably the sun or rose star (*Solaster papposus*), can cause indolent contact dermatitis. The dermatitis usually can be managed with topical corticosteroids or calamine lotion with 5% menthol.[1]

The contact dermatitis associated with sea cucumber exposure can be managed in a fashion similar to that described for starfish. If it is severe, systemic corticosteroids may be required. Sea cucumbers eat coelenterates, and skin irritation may respond to 5% acetic acid (commercial vinegar) irrigation. If any toxin has contacted the eyes, they should be flushed immediately with copious quantities of saline solution, preferably after local anesthesia, such as with 1 or 2 drops of 0.5% proparacaine. A fluorescein stain to look for corneal abrasions and a slit-lamp examination to rule out inflammation of the iris or anterior chamber are indicated. Inflammatory keratitis without evidence of infection can be managed with cycloplegic, mydriatic, and corticosteroid ophthalmic solutions. Any patient with ocular complaints should be referred to an ophthalmologist promptly.[1]

OCTOPUSES

Blue-ringed and blue-spotted octopuses are beautiful, nonaggressive animals that harbor one of the world's most toxic venoms, more powerful than that of the Portuguese man-of-war, the Australian box jellyfish, and any land-dwelling creature.[76] Although potentially fatal within minutes, envenomation is usually manageable with *immediate* basic life support and intensive care interventions.

Severe toxicity and fatalities have been reported with blue-ringed *Octopus (Hapalochlaena) maculosus* and blue-spotted *Octopus (Hapalochlaena) lunulata*, two species found widely throughout the Indo-Pacific (Australia, New Zealand, New Guinea, the Malay Peninsula, Japan, and Sri Lanka). The less toxic *Octopus joubini* is native to Caribbean waters. Both species are native to Indo-Pacific waters, although lunulatus may be found a little farther north. These octopuses prefer warm, shallow inshore waters with rocky bottoms. They are often found trapped in small rock pools after the tide recedes or under rocks and discarded containers. These are small animals, rarely exceeding 20 cm with tentacles extended. When at rest, the octopus' body is covered with brown–to–ochre-yellow bands over which are superimposed blue patches or rings.

When the octopus is excited, however, the entire body darkens, and the blue bands glow iridescent peacock blue.[1,74–76] Such habitats, combined with its dramatic beauty and small size, make the blue-ringed octopus an often irresistible (and occasionally fatal) attraction to children and adults alike.

The venom apparatus of the octopus consists of salivary glands and ducts, a ventral mouth at the base of the tentacles, and a powerful, parrot-like beak. It is capable of injecting venom with such force as to penetrate down to human muscle fascia.[1] It has been estimated that a single adult octopus has enough venom (25 g) to paralyze 750 kg of rabbits, which theoretically could kill 10 adult humans by causing respiratory failure.[75,76]

Pharmacology

The venom of the blue-ringed octopus, released by the salivary glands, contains the toxin "maculotoxin" (or cephalotoxin), of which one component is tetrodotoxin ($C_{11}H_{17}O_8N_3$, molecular weight 319.3), a powerful neuromuscular blocker. Tetrodotoxin is discussed in detail in Chapter 118. Although of little clinical significance, other constituents of the venom include hyaluronidase, histamine, tyramine, serotonin, and haplotoxin.[1,75]

Pathophysiology

The clinically most important toxic fraction of the salivary venom is tetrodotoxin, a paralytic agent that blocks sodium channels in excitable membranes and consequently inhibits nerve conductance (especially somatic motor nerves).[75] Depending on the dose absorbed, flaccid muscle paralysis can result, notably paralysis of the diaphragm secondary to phrenic nerve involvement. Although heat labile, this toxin remains active at 50°C, beyond the practical range for therapeutic intervention. Tetrodotoxin is also a potent depressant of vascular smooth muscle and has been shown to cause profound hypotension in experimental animals, although this effect has not been recorded in humans. No direct toxicity on the myocardium or brain has been reported.[1,75] Consciousness typically remains intact despite profound hypoxia, as evidenced by patients' recollection of remarks on the part of bystanders and caregivers.[75]

Clinical Presentation and Life-Threatening Complications

Most victims are bitten on the hand or arm while handling an octopus or allowing it to "ride" on their bodies. The most common cutaneous reaction involves the absence of symptoms, one or two tiny spots of blood, or a small blanched area.[1] Puncture wounds, which often go unnoticed, may cause a slight sting or ache. Occasionally the site may become numb or edematous 5 to 10 minutes after envenomation. Rarely, discomfort may persist for 6 hours.[75] One case of systemic allergy was reported in a woman with a history of shellfish allergy who developed a hemorrhagic vesicle at the bite site, generalized urticaria, pruritus, and joint effusions.[75] Profuse bleeding at the site is attributed to local anticoagulant effects, although may reflect other coagulation abnormalities.[1]

Serious systemic reactions follow a well-defined pattern and resolve in the reverse order of their appearance. These phenomena derive from the neurotoxicity of the venom. Within 10 to 15 minutes of envenomation, patients notice oral (classically lips and tongue) and facial numbness. This numbness may be followed rapidly by systemic progression, including diplopia, blurred vision, aphonia, dysphagia, ataxia, myoclonus, weakness, a sense of detachment, nausea, vomiting, peripheral neuropathy, flaccid muscular paralysis, respiratory failure, cardiac arrest (probably secondary to anoxia), and death.[74–76] The last muscles to become paralyzed are those of eye movements.[76] Fixed and dilated pupils in a 43-year old victim who suffered acute collapse 7 minutes after being bitten were attributed to a direct toxic effect rather than to cerebral dysfunction.[74]

Diagnosis

Practitioners not only must be aware of the geographic distribution of venomous marine animals in their area but also be cognizant of the fact that these animals exist in private and commercial aquariums. Painless or minimally symptomatic punctures rapidly followed by progressive paralysis and respiratory failure should prompt immediate consideration of blue-ringed octopus envenomation.

Treatment

Treatment is based on symptoms and is purely supportive. There is no antivenom. The key to the successful management of serious envenomations is the rapidity with which care is delivered. The onset of symptoms is swift despite their short duration (usually 4 to 10 hours). Basic life support measures (artificial ventilation and chest compressions) must be anticipated early and initiated promptly if indicated. These measures should be followed by endotracheal intubation and mechanical ventilation based on standard criteria, as soon as feasible.

Although of unproven efficacy in the management of octopus bites, an early measure to retard the spread of venom that has been suggested is the pressure immobilization technique. This technique theoretically occludes lymphatic and venous flow beneath the dressing, preventing systemic absorption of venom. A cloth of gauze pad measuring 6 to 8 cm² by 2 to 3 cm thick can be placed directly over the bite and held by a 15- to 18-cm circumferential constricting bandage, being careful not to compromise arterial circulation.[77] Removal of such a dressing should be attempted only in the acute care setting.

Care of the bite itself is controversial. Some practitioners advocate the use of a wide circular excision of the wound, down to deep fascia, with either primary closure or immediate full-thickness skin grafting. This method is intended to remove residual venom rather than manage the local soft tissue trauma, which generally tends to be minor. Others recommend a nonsurgical approach of simple observation.[1] A case of granuloma annulare of the hand 2 weeks after envenomation was treated successfully, albeit temporarily, with intralesional triamcinolone acetonide injections.[78]

CONE SNAILS

Of the roughly 300 species of these beautifully ornate mollusks, at least 18 are believed to cause human envenomation. These include *Conus aulicus* (court), *Conus gloria-maris* (glory of the sea), *Conus omaria* (marbled), *Conus striatus* (striated), *Conus textile* (textile), and *Conus tulipa* (tulip).[1] Fatalities have been reported after exposure to *Conus geographicus* and *Conus magnus*.[79] A quarter of stings of *Conus geographicus* are thought to be fatal in humans.[80] The term *mollusk* refers to members of the phylum Molluscum. These are invertebrate marine animals with unsegmented, soft bodies often covered by calcareous shells. They include squid, octopuses, scallops, snails, clams, and mussels.

Although these are tropical and subtropical animals, the most dangerous species are found in Indo-Pacific waters.[1,80] The fish-eating or mollusk-eating cones are more toxic than the cones that feed on marine worms, owing to their venom's ability to affect vertebrate neuromuscular function. Predominantly nocturnal creatures, cones tend to remain buried in sand and coral during daylight hours, making them most dangerous to divers and fossil hunters who pick up or place one in their pocket.[79,84] The remarkable beauty of their shells has contributed to a burgeoning trade in legal and smuggled specimens, transmitting this hazard to countries in which cone snails are not endemic. The venom apparatus consists of an extensible foot (proboscis), which thrusts venom-impregnated, dartlike teeth (radula) into the victim's flesh (Fig. 115-15).

Pharmacology and Pathophysiology

The venom consists of more than 100 biologically active peptides (conotoxins) that mostly target neuromuscular transmission and ion channels. The ω-conotoxins of *C. geographicus* inhibit voltage-dependent calcium uptake at the presynaptic cleft and cholinergic transmission in mammalian neuromuscular junctions. The α-conotoxins block nicotinic acetylcholine receptors. A "sleeper peptide," also of this species, causes experimental animals to enter into a deep sleeplike state. Finally, the μ-conotoxins inhibit motor end plate depolarization by modifying muscle sodium channels, similar to tetrodotoxins[1,79–83]; in other words, this is a highly redundant toxin affecting neuromuscular function.

Clinical Presentation and Life-Threatening Complications

Mild stings typically present in the form of small punctures or lacerations that resemble bee stings. These may be accompanied by local numbness, cyanosis, ischemia, nausea, blurred vision, malaise, and weakness. Signs and symptoms often resolve within a few hours.[1,80] More serious envenomations cause local paresthesias that rapidly spread periorally before generalizing. Systemic symptoms include anesthesia, numbness, stiffness, pruritus, diplopia, bilateral ptosis, dysphagia, dysarthria, aphonia, loss of the gag reflex, incoordination without cerebellar features, generalized weakness and paralysis, syncope, coma, and death. *C. geographicus* stings are often rapidly toxic and may induce cerebral edema, disseminated intravascular coagulopathy, coma, respiratory arrest, and cardiac failure. Respiratory failure is often the result of diaphragmatic paralysis, whereas death is due to cardiac failure. The first two of these clinical manifestations are a direct effect of ω-conotoxins. Complete resolution of symptoms may take 2 to 3 weeks.[1,79,80]

Treatment

There is no specific treatment for cone snail envenomations, and there is no antivenom. Management is supportive. Most authors recommend the pressure immobilization technique, although comparative studies are lacking. This technique is described above in the section on the treatment of octopus envenomations. Theoretically this technique occludes lymphatic and venous flow beneath the dressing, preventing systemic absorption of venom.[79] Removal of such a dressing should be attempted only in the acute care setting. Other approaches sometimes used include the application of a proximal lymphatic-venous occlusive dressing, incision and suction, local excision, soaking in nonscalding hot water (45°C [113°F]) until relief of pain, and local injection of

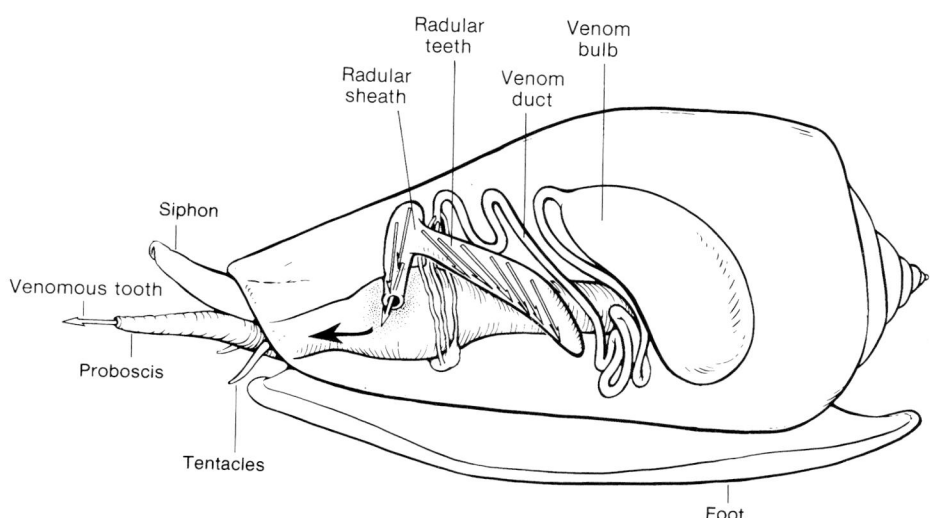

FIGURE 115-15

Venom apparatus of the cone snail. *(From Auerbach PS: Envenomation by aquatic invertebrates. In Auerbach PS [ed]: Wilderness Medicine, 4th ed. Philadelphia, Mosby, 2001, p 1481.)*

buffered 1% or 2% lidocaine or a similar local anesthetic without epinephrine.[1]

Serious envenomations may require cardiovascular and respiratory support. Generalized paralysis, necessitating a brief period of mechanical ventilation, typically reverses in 24 hours.[80] Edrophonium (10 mg intravenously in an adult) has been suggested as empirical therapy in paralysis. Naloxone (2 to 4 mg) also may be used empirically to block the β-endorphin vasodepressor response in cases of severe or persistent hypotension. The etiology of venom-induced coagulopathies, a rare complication, is not well described.[1]

SEA URCHINS

Similar to starfish and sea cucumbers, sea urchins are members of the phylum Echinodermata. They have globular or flattened bodies with hard shells and triple-jawed pedicellariae designed to capture food (Fig. 115-16). Shy and slow moving, they sit on rocks or burrow into sandy bottoms anywhere from intertidal zones to deep oceans.[1] Sea urchins are great delicacies and are not venomous when ingested. Their spines and pedicellariae are to be feared, however.

A sea urchin's venom apparatus typically consists of either venom-filled spines or a pedicellarium. Venomous spines are hollow with sharp, slender tips, whereas non-venomous spines tend to be solid with rounded ends. The former can penetrate rubber gloves and fins. When embedded in human tissue, they break off easily and are extracted only with great difficulty. Pedicellariae are small seizing organs found along the spines. Similar to a trap, they remain open at rest but quickly snap shut after making contact with a passing object, be it prey or a human finger. Pedicellariae never let go, but rather detach from the urchin's body and continue envenomating the victim for several hours.[1]

Pharmacology

Sea urchin venom contains several biologically active substances, including proteases, hemolysins, steroid glycosides, serotonin, and cholinergic fractions.

Pathophysiology

Toxopneustes pileolus causes histamine release from rat mast cells, whereas contractin A induces contraction of tracheal smooth muscle in guinea pigs.[82,85] The venom of the Pacific *Tripneustes* urchin contains a neurotoxin that targets facial and cranial nerves.[1]

Clinical Presentation and Life-Threatening Complications

After envenomation by sea urchin spines, victims complain of the abrupt onset of an intense burning sensation at the puncture site, which quickly develops into a muscle ache. Local erythema and edema also may be present (Fig. 115-17). Spines can easily be embedded beneath the skin, and spines of *Diadema setosum* and *Strongylocentrotus purpuratus* exhibit a purplish discoloration.[86] Penetration of a joint space may produce a severe arthritis, tenosynovitis, fasciitis, or bursitis.[1,88,89] Histologic specimens have revealed the presence of multinucleated giant cell granulomas surrounding optically void vacuoles.[89] Contacting a peripheral nerve may produce a neuropathy. Systemic manifestations, typically after envenomation with numerous spines, include nausea, vomiting, abdominal pain, paresthesias, numbness, muscular paralysis, syncope, delirium, hypotension, and respiratory distress.[87] Two cases involving multiple stings from a black sea urchin in Hawaii presented with bulbar polyneuritis and respiratory insufficiency 6 to 10 days after envenomation. One patient developed magnetic resonance imaging–documented meningoencephalitis, whereas the other had signs and symptoms mimicking Guillain-Barré syndrome, with hyporeflexia and

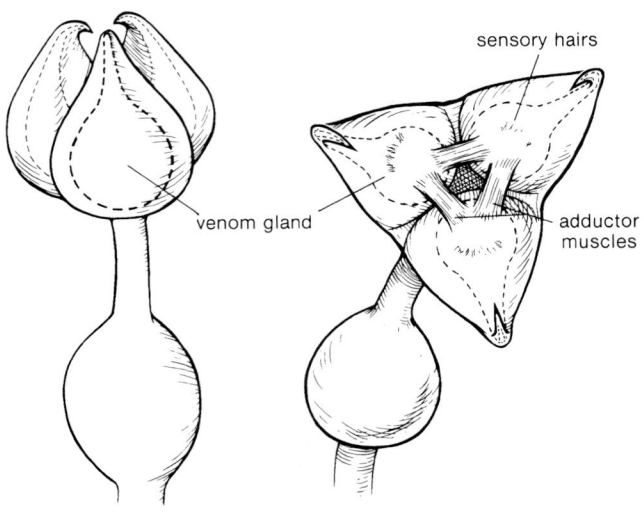

FIGURE 115-16

Globiferous pedicellaria of a sea urchin, used to hold and envenom prey. *(From Auerbach PS: Envenomation by aquatic invertebrates. In Auerbach PS [ed]: Wilderness Medicine, 4th ed. Philadelphia, Mosby, 2001, p 1476.)*

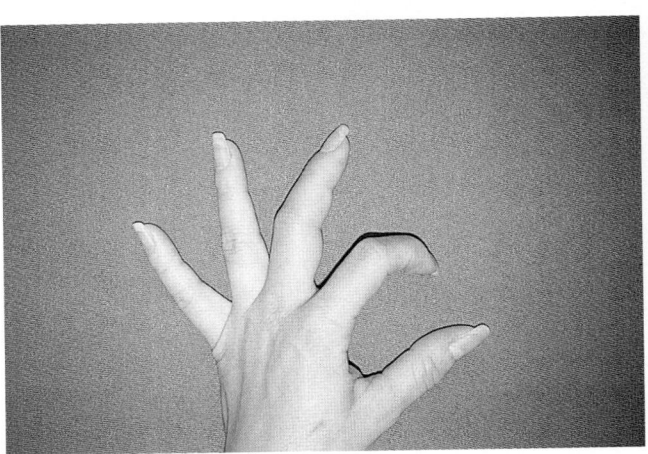

FIGURE 115-17

Finger swelling from sea urchin puncture. A single spine entered the palm over the third metacarpal bone. Swelling was severe in the second and third digits. *(Photo by Paul Auerbach, MD. Courtesy of John Williamson, MD. From Auerbach PS: Envenomation by aquatic invertebrates. In Auerbach PS [ed]: Wilderness Medicine, 4th ed. Philadelphia, Mosby, 2001, p 1478.)* See Color Fig. 115-17.

elevated cerebrospinal protein levels. Secondary infections and indolent ulcerations are common.[1] Reported infections include *Pasteurella*, atypical mycobacteria, and, most frequently, the common pyogenic organisms. Skin lesions include sarcoid-like nodules, keratomas, pseudocysts, and aseptic felon-like lesions.[89]

The stings of pedicellariae tend to cause more severe signs and symptoms. These wounds present with intense radiating pain and may bleed or become edematous. Systemic manifestations include malaise, weakness, paresthesias, hypesthesia, aphonia, arthralgias, generalized muscular paralysis, dizziness, syncope, hypotension, and, rarely, death. Although the pain sometimes resolves within 1 hour, localized muscle weakness and paralysis may persist for 6 hours.[1]

Diagnosis

Sea urchins leave relatively small punctures that initially may go unnoticed. Injecting 1% or 2% lidocaine, or a similar local anesthetic, without epinephrine near the site of pain may result in the egress of fluid and consequent discovery of a previously invisible puncture wound.[1] Because of the risk of serious complications stemming from retained spine fragments, all sea urchin wounds should be radiographed. If plain soft tissue films fail to identify a spine, one should use ultrasonography, which can identify hyperechoic foreign bodies, or computed tomography, which can show erosions. Magnetic resonance imaging is too expensive and nonspecific to warrant its use in this setting. Histology remains the gold standard in investigating chronic reactions. Specimens show either a diffuse, polymorphic inflammatory reaction or a multinucleated giant cell granuloma surrounding an optically void vacuole that may display birefringence under polarized light.[89]

Treatment

The management of sea urchin envenomations is purely symptomatic. As soon as possible, the injured area should be immersed in nonscalding hot water (45°C [113°F]) as tolerated for 30 to 90 minutes or until analgesia is achieved. Because embedded pedicellariae may continue to release venom into a wound, those at the skin surface should be removed without delay. Gentle scraping with a sharp razor, after application of shaving cream, is recommended. The spines of some sea urchin species contain a purplish dye that can be confused with retained spine fragments, but the dye should be absorbed in 24 to 36 hours.[1]

Deeply embedded spines can prove more problematic. In general, only spines that can be reached with ease should be removed because most spines readily fracture. Most of the rest should be left for dissolution, a process that typically takes 1 day to 3 weeks. Exceptions to this rule include thick calcium carbonate spines and any spine that has either entered into a joint space or lies near neurovascular structures. These should be removed promptly because of the risk of secondary infection, foreign-body encaseation, granuloma, dermoid inclusion cyst, arthritis, tenosynovitis, fasciitis, or bursitis.[1,88,89]

Casual wound exploration for spines that have not been visualized or identified radiographically should be avoided, especially if they are embedded in the hand or foot. Removal

may require the use of a surgical microscope. Any involvement of articular surfaces or neurovascular structures must be referred to the appropriate surgical specialist. Joints should be splinted in an effort to prevent further spine fragmentation, envenomation, and swelling. Scant data are available on the efficacy of local glucocorticoid injections. Although systemic antiinflammatory agents and antibiotics may help in the management of fusiform swelling of digits, focal phalangeal bone erosion, and cyanotic induration, their use is no substitute for spine removal. Secondary infections and involvement of deep structures should prompt the initiation of prophylactic antibiotics.[1] Some authors, however, have found no benefit from the use of either antibiotics or systemic antiinflammatory agents in the management of joint pathology.[89] In the case of retained spines that have prompted granulomatous reactions, the only definitive treatment is surgical excision of the spine and granuloma. When a joint is involved, partial or total synovectomy may be necessary.[1,89]

REFERENCES

1. Auerbach PS: Wilderness Medicine: Management of Wilderness and Environmental Emergencies. St. Louis, Mosby, 1995.
2. Bengston K, Nichols MM, Schnadig V, et al: Sudden death in a child following jellyfish envenomation by *Chiropsalmus quadrumanus*. JAMA 266:1404–1406, 1991.
3. Bonnet MS: The toxicology of the *Chironex fleckeri* jellyfish: The Australian sea wasp. Br Homeopath J 88:62–68, 1999.
4. Fenner P, Carney I: The Irukandji syndrome. Aust Fam Physician 28:1131–1137, 1999.
5. Endean R, Monks SA, Cameron AM: Toxins from the box-jellyfish *Chironex fleckeri*. Toxicon 31:397–410, 1993.
6. Crone HD: Further studies on the biochemistry of the toxins from the Sea Wasp *Chironex fleckeri*. Toxicon 9:145–151, 1971.
7. Freeman SE, Turner RJ: A pharmacological study of the toxin of a Cnidarian, *Chironix fleckeri*. J Pharmacol 35:510–520, 1969.
8. Martin JC, Audley I: Cardiac failure following Irukandji envenomation. Med J Aust 153:164–166, 1990.
9. Little M, Mulcahy RF: A year's experience of Irukandji envenomation in far north Queensland. Med J Aust 169:638–641, 1998.
10. Sutherland S: Australian Animal Toxins: The Creatures, Their Toxins and Care of the Poisoned Patient. Melbourne, Oxford University Press, 1983.
11. Burnett JW, Calton GJ: The chemistry and toxicology of some venomous pelagic Coelenterates. Toxicon 15:177–196, 1977.
12. Turner RJ, Freeman SE: Effect of *Chironex fleckeri* toxin on the isolated perfused guinea pig heart. Toxicon 7:277–286, 1969.
13. Fenner P, Williamson J, Burnett J, et al: The Irukandji syndrome and acute pulmonary edema. Med J Aust 149:150–156, 1988.
14. Hartwick R, Callahan V, Williamson J: Disarming the box-jellyfish. Med J Aust 1:15–20, 1980.
15. Beadnell CE, Rider TA, Williamson JA, et al: Management of a major box jellyfish (*Chironex fleckeri*) sting. Med J Aust 156:655–658, 1992.
16. Tibbals J, Williams D, Sutherland SK: The effects of antivenom and verapamil on the haemodynamic actions of *Chironex fleckeri* (box jellyfish) venom. Anaesth Intensive Care 26:40–45, 1998.
17. Bloom DA, Burnett JW, Hebel JR, et al: Effects of verapamil and CSL antivenom on *Chironex fleckeri* (box-jellyfish) induced mortality. Toxicon 37:1621–1626, 1999.
18. Burnett JW, Calton GJ: Response of the box-jellyfish (*Chironex fleckeri*) cardiotoxin to intravenous administration of verapamil. Med J Aust 2:192–194, 1983.
19. Burnett JW, Othman IB, Endean R, et al: Verapamil potentiation of *Chironex* (box-jellyfish) antivenom. Toxicon 28:242–244, 1990.
20. Al-Ebrahim K, Tahir MZ, Rustom M, et al: Jellyfish-venom-induced deep venous thrombosis. Angiology 46:449–451, 1995.
21. Schwartz S, Meinking T: Venomous marine animals of Florida: Morphology, behavior, health hazards. J Fla Med Assoc 84:433–440, 1997.
22. Stein MR, Marraccini JV, Rothschild NE, et al: Fatal Portuguese man-o'-war (*Physalia physalis*) envenomation. Ann Emerg Med 18:312–315, 1989.

23. Guess HA, Saviteer PL, Morris CR, et al: Hemolysis and acute renal failure following a Portuguese man-of-war sting. Pediatrics 70:979–981, 1982.

24. Malhotra KK, Chadha JS, Mirdehghan M, et al: Acute renal failure following scorpion sting. Am J Trop Med Hyg 27:623, 1978.

25. Reference deleted.

26. Burnett JW, Gable WD: A fatal jellyfish envenomation by a Portuguese man-o-war. Toxicon 27:823–824, 1989.

27. Ionnides G, Davis JH: Portuguese man-o-war stinging. Arch Dermatol 91:448–451, 1965.

28. Kaufman MB: Portuguese man-o-war envenomation. Pediatr Emerg Care 8:27–28, 1992.

29. Rosson C, Tolle SW: Management of marine stings and scrapes. West J Med 150:97–100, 1989.

30. Soppe GG: Marine envenomations and aquatic dermatology. Am Fam Physician 40:97–106, 1989.

31. Burnett JW, Rubinstein H, Calton GJ: First aid for jellyfish envenomation. South Med J 76:870–872, 1983.

32. Filling-Katz MR: Mononeuritis multiplex following jellyfish stings. Ann Neurol 15:213, 1984.

33. Fisher AA: Toxic versus allergic reactions to jellyfish. Cutis 34:450–454, 1984.

34. Burnett JW, Constantine JG, Calton GJ, et al: The effect of verapamil on the cardiotoxic activity of Portuguese man-o-war (*Physalia physalis*) and sea nettle venoms. Toxicon 23:681–689, 1985.

35. Turner B, Sullivan B, Pennefather J: Disarming the bluebottle: Treatment of *Physalia* envenomation, Med J Aust 2:394–395, 1980.

36. Bitseff E, Garoni W, Hardison C, et al: The management of stingray injuries of the extremities. South Med J 63:417, 1970.

37. Cooper NK: Stone fish and stingrays—some notes on the injuries that they cause to man. J R Army Med Corps 137:136–140, 1991.

38. VanOffel JF, Stevens WJ: A stingray injury in a devotee of aquarium fishes. Acta Clin Belg 55:174–175, 2000.

39. Russell FE: Comparative pharmacology of some animal toxins. Fed Proc 26:1206, 1967.

40. Sutherland SK: Australian Animal Toxins: The Creatures, Their Toxins and Care of the Poisoned Patient. Melbourne, Oxford University Press, 1983, 400–410.

41. Burk MP, Richter PA: Stingray injuries of the foot. J Am Podiatr Med Assoc 80:260–262, 1990.

42. Fenner PJ, Williamson JA, Skinner RA: Fatal and non-fatal stingray envenomation. Med J Aust 151:621–625, 1989.

43. Moyles BG, Wilson RC: Stingray spine foreign body in the foot. J Foot Surg 28:30–32, 1989.

44. Kizer KW, McKinney HE, Auerbach PS: Scorpaenidae envenomation—a five-year poison center experience. JAMA 253:807–810, 1985.

45. Gwee MC, Gopalakrishnakone P, Yuen R, et al: A review of stone fish venoms and toxins. Pharmacol Ther 64:509–528, 1994.

46. Khoo HE, Yuen R, Poh CH, et al: Biological activities of *Synanceja horrida* (stone fish) venom. Nat Toxins 1:54–60, 1992.

47. Kasdan ML, Kasdan AS, Hamilton DL: Lionfish envenomation. Plast Reconstr Surg 80:613–614, 1987.

48. Garyfallou GT, Madden JF: Lionfish envenomation. Ann Emerg Med 28:456–457, 1996.

49. Goetz CG: Pharmacology of animal neurotoxins. Clin Neuropharm 5:231, 1982.

50. Phoon WO, Alfred ER: A study of stonefish (*Synanceja*) stings in Singapore with a review of the venomous fishes of Malaysia. Sing Med J 6:158–163, 1965.

51. Breault JL: Candirú: Amazonian parasitic catfish. J Wildern Med 2:304–312, 1991.

52. Herman JR: Candirú: urinophilic catfish. Urology 1:265–267, 1973.

53. VanOphoven A, DeKernion JB: Clinical management of foreign bodies of the genitourinary tract. J Urol 164:274–287, 2000.

54. Zeman MG: Catfish stings: A report of three cases. Ann Emerg Med 18:211–213, 1989.

55. Das SK, Johnson MB, Cohly HH: Catfish stings in Mississippi. South Med J 88:809–812, 1995.

56. Baack BR, Kucan JO, Zook EG, et al: Hand infections secondary to catfish spines: Case reports and literature review. J Trauma 31:1432–1436, 1991.

57. Shiomi K, et al: Toxins in the skin secretions of the oriental catfish (*Plotosus lineatus*): Immunological properties and immunocytochemical identification of producing cells. Toxicon 26:353, 1988.

58. Chow SP, Stroebel AB, Lan JHK, et al: *Mycobacterium marinum* infection of the hand involving deep structures. J Hand Surg 8:568, 1983.

59. Hackerling PS, Stine TM, Pottage JL, et al: *Aeromonas hydrophila* myonecrosis and gas gangrene in a nonimmunocompromised host. Arch Intern Med 143:2005, 1983.

60. Gudger EW: On the alleged penetration of the human urethra by an Amazonian catfish called candiru with a review of the allied habits of other members of the family pygidiidae: Part II. Am J Surg 8:443–456, 1930.

61. Al-Hassan JM, et al: Acceleration of wound healing responses induced by preparations from the epidermal secretions of the Arabian gulf catfish (*Arius bilineatus*, Valenciennes). J Wildern Med 2:153, 1991.

62. Bonnet MS: The toxicology of *Trachinus vipera*: The lesser weeverfish. Br Homeopath J 89:84–88, 2000.

63. Davies RS, Evans RJ: Weever fish stings: A report of two cases presenting to an accident and emergency department. J Accid Emerg Med 13:139–141, 1996.

64. McGoldrick J, Marx JA: Marine envenomations: Part 1. Vertebrates, J Emerg Med 9:497–502, 1990.

65. Cain D: Weever fish sting: An unusual problem. BMJ 287:406–407, 1983.

66. Briars GL, Gordon GS: Envenomation by the lesser weever fish. Br J Gen Pract 42:213, 1992.

67. Allmann GF: On the stinging properties of the lesser weever fish: *Trachinus vipera*. Ann Mag Nat Hist 6:161–165, 1840.

68. Gonzago RA: Spontaneous abortion after a weever fish. BMJ 290:518, 1985.

69. Lucas J: The crown of thorns starfish. Oceanus 29:55, 1986.

70. Moran PJ, Williamson J: Toxic reactions to injuries caused by the spines of the crown of thorns starfish (*Acanthaster planci*). J S Pacific Underwater Med Soc 16:91, 1986.

71. Shiomi K, et al: Liver damage by the crown of thorns starfish (*Acanthaster planci*) lethal factor. Toxicon 28:469, 1990.

72. Fisher AA: Atlas of Aquatic Dermatology. New York, Grune & Stratton, 1978.

73. Freyvogel TA: Poisonous and venomous animals in East Africa. Acta Trop (Basel) 29:401, 1972.

74. Walker DG: Survival after severe envenomation by the blue-ringed octopus (*Hapalochlaena maculosa*). Med J Aust 2:663–665, 1983.

75. Williamson JA: The blue-ringed octopus bite and envenomation syndrome. Clin Dermatol 5:127–133, 1987.

76. Bonnet MS: The toxicology of *Octopus maculosa*: The blue-ringed octopus. Br Homeopath J 88:166–171, 1999.

77. Anker RL, et al: Retarding the uptake of mock venom in humans: Comparison of three first-aid treatments. Med J Aust 1:212, 1982.

78. Fulghum DD: Octopus bite resulting in granuloma annulare. South Med J 79:1434, 1986.

79. Burnett JW, Calton GJ, Morgan RJ: Cone snails. Cutis 39:107, 1987.

80. Fegan D, Andresen D: Conus geographus envenomation. Lancet 349:1672, 1997.

81. Gray WR, Olivera BM, Cruz LJ: Peptide toxins from venomous Conus snails. Annu Rev Biochem 57:665, 1988.

82. Nakagawa H, Tu AT, Kimura A: Purification and characterization of contractin A from the pedicellarial venom of sea urchin (*Toxopneustes pileolus*). Arch Biochem Biophys 284:279, 1991.

83. Olivera BM, Cruz LJ: Conotoxins, in retrospect. Toxicon 39:7–14, 2001.

84. Clark C, Olivera BM, Cruz LJ: A toxin from the venom of the marine snail *Conus geographus* which acts on the vertebral central nervous system. Toxicon 19:691–699, 1981.

85. Takei M, et al: a toxic substance from the sea urchin *Toxopneustes pileolus* induces histamine release from rat peritoneal mast cells. Agents Actions 32:224, 1991.

86. O'Neal RL, Halstead BW, Howard LD: Injury to human tissues from sea urchin spines. Calif Med 101:199–202, 1964.

87. Linaweaver PG: Toxic marine life. Milit Med 131:437, 1967.

88. Strauss MB, MacDonald RI: Hand injuries from sea urchin spines. Clin Orthop 114:216–218, 1976.

89. Guyot-Drouot M-H, Rouneau D, Rolland J-M, et al: Arthritis, tenosynovitis, fasciitis, and bursitis due to sea urchin spines: a series of 12 cases in Réunion Island. Joint Bone Spine 67:94–100, 2000.

CHAPTER 116

Ciguatera

Fergus Kerr

Ciguatera poisoning occurs after the ingestion of fish containing ciguatoxin (and other toxins) produced by marine dinoflagellates. The ingestion of substantial quantities of these toxins results in a characteristic syndrome, known since ancient times, with gastrointestinal and neurologic symptoms predominating. Captain Bligh described the symptoms of ciguatera poisoning after eating dolphin fish in 1789.[1] The mortality of ciguatera poisoning is low; however, symptoms may be persistent and incapacitating.[2] It is a common cause of food-related illness in tropical and subtropical areas. As a result of an increasingly mobile population and the rapid delivery of fish caught in endemic areas to inland and temperate regions, however, clinicians may be confronted with cases regardless of their site of practice. The incidence of ciguatera poisoning is variable depending on the location. In the United States, most cases occur in Hawaii and Florida, with reported incidence rates ranging from 8.7 to 50 per 100,000.[3,4] Globally, incidence rates vary and are not known with certainty because there is undoubtedly considerable underreporting of cases. In contrast, the South Pacific Commission reported a mean annual incidence rate of 98 per 100,000 population for the period 1979 through 1981.[5] There is increasing concern that changes in global climate and the impact of exploration and mining in tropical areas will result in the expansion of ciguatera endemic areas.[6]

Ciguatera toxins are formed by a benthic dinoflagellate, *Gambierdiscus toxicus*, which typically is found at the base of the coral reef food chain. Not all strains of *G. toxicus* are poisonous.[7] Some reports have suggested that dinoflagellates from the *Amphidinium, Coolia,* and *Ostreopsis* genera also produce these toxins and contribute to the etiology of ciguatera poisoning.[6] The dinoflagellates are ingested by small herbivorous fish, which are fed on by larger carnivorous fish. Humans may become affected by ingesting fish from any part of the food chain. More than 400 fish species have been implicated; however, the most common are snapper, barracuda, sea bass, dolphin fish, and parrotfish.[8]

CHEMISTRY AND BIOCHEMISTRY

Of the toxins involved in ciguatera poisoning, the principal and most active component is ciguatoxin. Also implicated are scaritoxin, maitotoxin, palytoxin, and okadaic acid. The ratio of these toxins in any one fish varies depending on its species and the degree of exposure to toxic dinoflagellates.[9] Ciguatoxin ($C_{60}H_{86}O_{19}$) is an odorless, tasteless, heat-stabile polyether compound.[10] Neither cooking nor freezing

destroys the toxin. It is excreted in breast milk and other body fluids.[11] Multiple subtypes of ciguatoxin with minor variations in structure have been identified. Some of these structural differences have a geographic association and have been postulated as the basis for the differences in the clinical picture of ciguatera poisoning in the Pacific compared with the Caribbean.[12,13] Maitotoxin ($C_{160}H_{225}S_2O_{74}$), scaritoxin ($C_{60}H_{24}O_{16}$), okadaic acid ($C_{44}H_{66}O_{12}$), and palytoxin ($C_{129}H_{223}N_3O_{54}$) also are polyether toxins, similar to most dinoflagellate-derived toxins.[14] The pharmacokinetics of ciguatoxin and related polyethers is largely unknown.

PATHOPHYSIOLOGY

Early studies on unpurified ciguatoxin suggested that it acted mainly as an anticholinesterase.[15] Subsequent experiments using more pure extracts failed to reproduce these findings, however.[16] In 1968, Rayner and colleagues[16,17] suggested that the toxin caused an increase in sodium permeability through its action at voltage-dependent Na^+ channels. Further study has shown that ciguatoxin binds at receptor site 5 of the Na^+ channel, resulting in prolonged firing, persistent activation,[18] and a marked and prolonged increase in axonal volume. The last-mentioned effect is reversed by mannitol.[19] Cameron and associates[20] conducted electrical studies on the sural and common peroneal nerves of 15 individuals with acute ciguatera poisoning, showing significant slowing of sensory conduction velocity and prolongation of the absolute refractory period.

Maitotoxin does not seem to have an effect at Na^+ channels. It has been shown to induce the release of norepinephrine from pheochromocytoma cells, and it results in an increase in intracellular calcium through an unknown mechanism.[6] Scaritoxin has been shown to induce the release of acetylcholine and norepinephrine and to increase the permeability of sodium channels.[21] The mechanisms by which the other toxins that have been implicated partially in ciguatera poisoning exert their effects have not been elucidated fully to date.

CLINICAL PRESENTATION
AND LIFE-THREATENING COMPLICATIONS

Symptoms generally begin within 2 to 30 hours after the ingestion of a toxic fish.[22] A plethora of symptoms and signs may result, but they can be grouped broadly into four main types—gastrointestinal, neurologic, cardiovascular, and other. Life-threatening complications are rare.

Gastrointestinal symptoms usually are first to appear, characterized by nausea, vomiting, diarrhea, and abdominal pain. These features rarely last longer than 24 hours but often necessitate fluid resuscitation.[22,23] The most noted and long lasting of all the complaints associated with ciguatera poisoning are neurologic.[2,22] Neurologic symptoms tend to appear 10 to 12 hours after ingestion and may persist for days, weeks, or months, although they usually have evolved and subsided after 2 to 5 days.[2] A typical feature is paresthesia, described as tingling or numbness in the extremities, occurring in 36% to 89% of cases with considerable geographic variability.[5,22] Myalgia, headache, ataxia, weakness, and pruritus are described commonly. Ophthalmoplegia, delirium, spasticity, and polymyositis occur less commonly.[6] Classically, ciguatera poisoning is associated with an alteration in temperature sensation, often termed *temperature reversal*, in which hot objects feel cold and vice versa.[2,3] Cameron and Capra[24] found that gross temperature perception remained intact and emphasized that the term *temperature reversal* may be misleading, suggesting instead that clinicians be more specific when describing such symptoms. Seizure and coma have been reported rarely except in life-threatening and fatal cases.[2,25]

High doses of ciguatoxin have been shown to induce atrial flutter and extrasystoles and have a negative inotropic effect on guinea pig heart muscle in vitro, an effect that was abolished by lidocaine.[26] Cardiac effects occur relatively uncommonly in clinical practice, however. Bradycardia and orthostatic hypotension were reported in only 16% of French Polynesian cases.[2,22] Electrocardiogram changes have been reported, ranging from nonspecific ST-segment changes to T-wave flattening and inversion.[26,27] Creatine phosphokinase concentrations tend to be normal.[27] In one case, a 54-year-old man developed pulmonary edema and reduced left ventricular function along with other clinical features of ciguatera poisoning, with no other causes for cardiomyopathy identified.[27]

Ciguatera poisoning may result in a mixed array of symptoms and signs. In addition to the three broad groups (gastrointestinal, neurologic, cardiovascular) described earlier, other findings associated with ciguatera poisoning include hypersalivation, photophobia, a metallic taste, and chronic fatigue.[6,28,29] In utero exposure of the fetus has variable results. A transient increase in fetal movements usually is seen.[30,31] In one case, a normal fetal outcome was reported after maternal exposure to ciguatera toxins in the second trimester.[30] Others have reported facial palsies and myotonia in newborns.[30,31] Overall, it has been shown that symptoms seem to be more common and more severe in patients who have had previous exposure.[3]

DIAGNOSIS

The diagnosis of ciguatera poisoning is a clinical one. No one feature is pathognomonic; however, the constellation of gastrointestinal and neurologic symptoms described earlier in the setting of a recent fish meal should suggest the diagnosis.

Some conditions superficially mimic ciguatera poisoning, including hallucinatory fish poisoning and scombroid fish poisoning. In the former, as the name suggests, often disturbing hallucinations are a prominent feature. In the latter, bacteria proliferate in poorly refrigerated fish, releasing histamine-like toxins. Flushing is a prominent symptom of scombroid poisoning, which is discussed in greater detail in Chapter 117. There are many folkloric tales on how to detect toxic fish, which usually involve the smearing of fish fluids or organs over one's lips and waiting for paresthesia. More scientific methods involve the feeding or injecting of fish extract into animal subjects, of which mice have become the standard, and waiting for a response, typically the percentage of subjects dead in 24 hours. Toxic samples are defined as yielding 50% to 100% mortality, whereas nontoxic samples yield less than 5% dead.[6] In recent years immunoassays have been developed with the ultimate goal being a simple robust stick test for in-the-field use.[32] Success using these tests has been variable; cross-reactivity with other toxins is a problem. There are no specific clinical laboratory profiles that aid the diagnosis.

TREATMENT

Airway and Ventilatory Considerations

There are no special airway or ventilatory considerations. Patients who present with or develop a reduced Glasgow Coma Scale score should be assessed for the need to undergo endotracheal intubation or assisted ventilation or both. Endotracheal intubation or assisted ventilation should be done for standard indications and is a rare occurrence in ciguatera poisoning.

Gastrointestinal Decontamination

Although activated charcoal has not been shown to alter the outcome in patients with ciguatera poisoning, on theoretical grounds its administration at standard doses (see Chapter 5) in patients presenting within 1 hour of ingestion is justifiable. The practicality of gastrointestinal decontamination is limited, however, because symptoms generally begin within 2 to 30 hours after the ingestion of toxic fish.

Extracorporeal Techniques

Extracorporeal techniques are not useful in ciguatera poisoning.

Indications for ICU Admission in Ciguatera Poisoning

Persisting hypotension not responsive to fluid
Persisting bradycardia not responsive to atropine
Coma not responsive to mannitol
Seizure activity not responsive to mannitol
Severe electrolyte disturbance

Specific Treatments

NONANTIDOTAL

The treatment of patients with ciguatera poisoning is mostly supportive, with initial emphasis on controlling vomiting and intravenous fluid and electrolyte replacement. Symptomatic bradycardia is usually responsive to atropine.[27,33] Patients with severe hypotension may require adjunctive inotropic support, although fluid therapy should be attempted first. Alcohol exacerbates many of the symptoms and should be avoided.[34]

ANTIDOTAL

Mannitol (in conjunction with usual supportive measures discussed earlier) has become the treatment of choice for symptomatic ciguatera poisoning. Its usefulness was discovered dramatically in 1988 when it was administered to two comatose ciguatoxic patients with suspected cerebral edema. Within minutes, both patients were awake.[35] Numerous subsequent reports have highlighted the success of mannitol treatment, not only in managing patients with coma but also in resolving relatively minor symptoms, such as paresthesia and pruritus.[36,37] Mannitol usually is given as a 20% solution (0.5 to 1 g/kg) at a rate of 500 mL/hr. It may be less effective in patients who have been symptomatic for more than 24 to 48 hours.[6,36] Caution should be used when administering mannitol to patients who are potentially hypotensive or significantly hypovolemic. Fluid balance and electrolyte status should be assessed and corrected before the initiation of mannitol therapy. Hypernatremic dehydration has been reported in a patient administered mannitol before fluid replacement.[38]

The exact mechanism by which mannitol seems to exert its beneficial effect in ciguatoxic patients is not understood fully. As noted earlier, ciguatoxin modifies the Na^+ channels, allowing for a rapid influx of Na^+ into the cell, resulting in axonal edema. Presumably, mannitol reduces this edema by its osmotic properties.[19] Lewis[39] suggested that mannitol might dissociate the ciguatoxin molecule from its binding site by its osmotic action. Purcell and associates[40] showed that nerve conduction studies were not altered in ciguatoxic rats after treatment with mannitol. This study did not assess axonal edema, however. Other authors have suggested that mannitol may act as a hydroxyl radical scavenger.[41] Although supported by anecdotal data, to my knowledge, mannitol's efficacy has not been proved by any randomized, placebo-controlled trials.

Other agents have been used in the management of ciguatoxic patients but with inconsistent results. Now outdated, cholinesterase reactivators (i.e., oximes) were used at the time it was thought that ciguatoxin possessed significant anticholinesterase activity.[15] The use of amitriptyline has resulted in partial resolution of symptoms in some cases, and this is thought possibly to be due to its blocking action at Na^+ channels.[42,43] Nifedipine may improve some of the symptoms related to maitotoxin.[43] So-called local anesthetics decrease sodium conductance in the nerve cell membrane (Fig. 116-1) and theoretically are a potential therapy for ciguatera poisoning. Lidocaine has been shown to inhibit the effects of ciguatoxin in vitro; however, there is little clinical experience in its use as an antidote in ciguatoxic patients.

Criteria for ICU Discharge in Ciguatera Poisoning

Normal vital signs
Not requiring inotropic support
Normalizing electrolytes

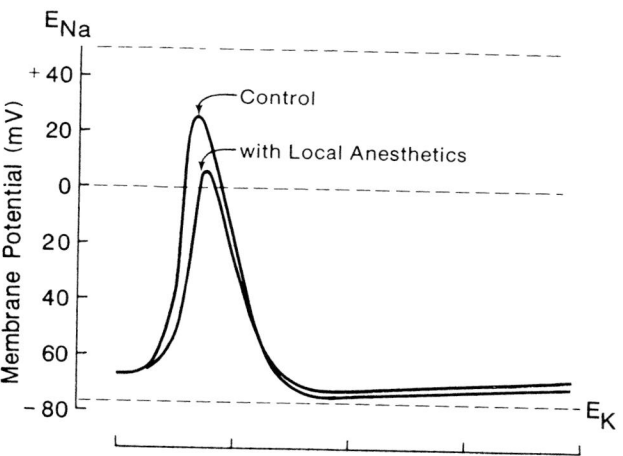

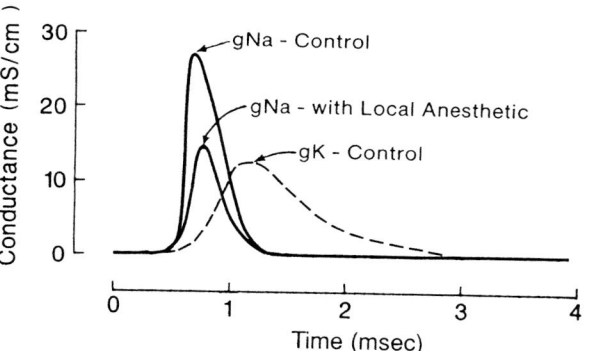

FIGURE 116-1

Action potential and associated changes in permeability of the nerve membrane to sodium and potassium ions. The ordinate of the top recording shows the nerve membrane potential recorded intracellularly, and the ordinate of the bottom recording gives the associated ion conductances. The effects of a local anesthetic show a decrease in the rate of rise and in the size of the action potential in association with a corresponding decrease in sodium permeability. (Local anesthetics have only small effects directly on potassium conductances.) This figure is a general illustration based ultimately on the pioneering work of Hodgkin and Huxley (1952) relating the membrane electrical properties and ionic permeabilities. Membrane potential is recorded as the difference in potential between the intracellular electrode and the external service expressed in millivolts (mV). E_{Na} = sodium equilibrium potential − the membrane potential at which there would be no net influx or efflux of sodium ions; E_K = potassium equilibrium potential. Conductance is expressed as gNa = sodium conductance; gK = potassium conductance. *(From Smith CM, Reynaud AM: Textbook of Pharmacology. Philadelphia, WB Saunders, 1992, p 214.)*

SPECIAL POPULATIONS

Infants and Elderly Patients

Because of the possibility of dehydration, care should be taken to ensure adequate fluid balance and electrolyte correction in infants and elderly patients before treatment with mannitol.

Pregnant Patients

Pregnant patients should be warned that there are some reports of transient neurologic abnormalities in infants born to mothers who have had ciguatera fish poisoning.[31] There are other reports of spontaneous abortion and premature labor.[22] Nursing mothers with ciguatera poisoning should be advised against breast-feeding because there are some reports of diarrheal illness in infants breast-fed by ciguatoxic mothers.[22]

Other Patients

Patients who have been affected previously by ciguatera fish poisoning may have more severe symptoms on reexposure.[3]

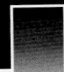

Common Errors in Ciguatera Poisoning

Forgetting to inform the other dinner guests about the poisoning incident
Inadequate volume replacement before giving mannitol
Assuming that mannitol cures everyone
Not realizing that symptoms cannot be prolonged
Believing that alcohol causes clinical improvement

Common Misconceptions about Ciguatera Poisoning

1. Ciguatera occurs only in the tropics.
2. Only carnivorous fish cause ciguatera fish poisoning.
3. Cooking or freezing the fish renders it safe.

Key Points in Ciguatera Poisoning

1. Ciguatera fish poisoning is a worldwide phenomenon.
2. Poisoning occurs after the ingestion of fish containing ciguatoxin, which is derived from dinoflagellates.
3. Initial symptoms are gastrointestinal, with neurologic symptoms following.
4. Neurologic symptoms may be delayed in onset and prolonged.
5. Life-threatening features are rare, but may include coma, seizure, bradycardia, and hypotension.
6. Management is essentially supportive, although mannitol anecdotally seems beneficial in some patients.

REFERENCES

1. Steinfeld AD, Steinfeld HJ: Ciguatera and the voyage of Captain Bligh. JAMA 228:1270–1271, 1974.
2. Bagins R, Kuberski T, Laugier S: Clinical observations on 3009 cases of ciguatera (fish poisoning) in the South Pacific. Am J Trop Med Hyg 28:1067–1073, 1979.
3. Lawrence DN, Enriquez MB, Lumish RM: Ciguatera fish poisoning in Miami. JAMA 244:254–258, 1980.
4. Gollop JH, Pon EW: Ciguatera: A review. Hawaii Med J 51:91–99, 1992.
5. Glaziou P, Legrand A: The epidemiology of ciguatera fish poisoning. Toxicon 32:863–873, 1994.
6. Swift AEB, Swift TR: Ciguatera. Clin Toxicol 31:1–29, 1993.
7. Holmes MJ, Lewis RJ, Poli MA, et al: Strain dependent production of ciguatoxin precursors (Gambier toxins) by G. toxicus (Dinophyceae) in culture. Toxicon 29:761–775, 1991.
8. Halstead BW: Poisonous and Venomous Marine Animals of the World, Vertebrates. Washington, D.C., U.S. Government Printing Office, 1967.
9. Lewis RJ, Sellin M: Short communications: Multiple ciguatoxins in the flesh of fish. Toxicon 30:915–919, 1992.
10. Murata M, Legrand AM, Ishibashi Y, et al: Structure of ciguatoxin and its congener. J Am Chem Soc 111:8929–8931, 1989.
11. Blythe DG, de Sylva DP: Mother's milk turns toxic following fish feast. JAMA 264:2074, 1990.
12. Lewis RJ, Sellin M, Poli MA, et al: Purification and characterisation of ciguatoxins from moray eel (Lycodontis javaincus, Muraenidae). Toxicon 29:1115–1127, 1991.
13. Vernoux J, Lewis RJ: Isolation and characterisation of Caribbean ciguatoxins from Horse-eye Jack (Caranx latus). Toxicon 35:889–900, 1997.
14. Hokama Y, Miyahara JT: Ciguatera poisoning: Clinical and immunological aspects. J Toxicol Toxin Rev 5:25–53, 1986.
15. Li KM: Fish poisoning: A potent cholinesterase inhibitor. Science 147:1580–1581, 1965.
16. Rayner MD, Kosaki TI, Fellmeth EL: Ciguatoxin: More than an acetylcholinesterase. Science 160:70–71, 1968.
17. Rayner MD: Mode of action of ciguatoxin. Fed Proc 31:1139–1145, 1972.
18. Lombet A, Bidard JN, Lazdunski M: Ciguatoxin and brevetoxins share a common receptor site on the neuronal voltage-dependent Na+ channel. FEBS Letts 219:355–359, 1987.
19. Mattei C, Dechraoui M-Y, Molgo J, et al: Neurotoxins targeting receptor site 5 of voltage-dependent sodium channels increase the nodal volume of myelinated axons. J Neurosci Res 55:666–673, 1999.
20. Cameron J, Flowers AE, Capra MF: Electrophysiological studies on ciguatera poisoning in man (Part II). J Neurol Sci 101:93–97, 1991.
21. Tatsumi M, Kajiwara A, Yasumto T, et al: Potent excitatory effect of Scaritoxin on the guinea-pig vas deferens, taenia caeci and ileum. J Pharmacol Exp Ther 235:783–787, 1985.
22. Bagnis R, Legrand AM: Clinical features on 12890 cases of ciguatera (fish poisoning) in French Polynesia. In Gopalakrishnakone P, Tan CK (eds): Progress in Venom and Toxin Research. Singapore, National University of Singapore and International Society of Toxicology, Asia-Pacific Section, 1987, pp 372–377.
23. Engleberg NC, Morris JG, Lewis J, et al: Ciguatera fish poisoning: A major common source outbreak in the US Virgin Islands. Ann Intern Med 98:336–337, 1983.
24. Cameron J, Capra MF: The basis of the paradoxical disturbance of temperature perception in ciguatera poisoning. Clin Toxicol 31:571–579, 1993.
25. Ho AMH, Fraser IM, Todd ECD: Ciguatera poisoning: A report of three cases. Ann Emerg Med 15:1225–1228, 1986.
26. Lewis RJ: Negative inotropic and arrhythmic effects of high doses of ciguatoxin on guinea-pig atria and papillary muscles. Toxicon 26:639–649, 1988.
27. Miller RM, Pavia S, Keary P: Cardiac toxicity associated with ciguatera poisoning. Aust N Z J Med 29:373–374, 1999.
28. Stommel EW, Parsonnet J, Jenkyn LR: Polymyositis after ciguatera toxin exposure. Arch Neurol 48:874–877, 1991.
29. Pearn JH: Chronic fatigue syndrome: Chronic ciguatera poisoning as a differential diagnosis. Med J Aust 166:309–310, 1997.
30. Senecal PE, Osterloh JD: Normal fetal outcome after maternal ciguateric toxin exposure in the second trimester. Clin Toxicol 29:473–478, 1991.
31. Pearn J, Harvey P, De Ambrosis W, et al: Ciguatera and pregnancy. Med J Aust 1:57–58, 1982.
32. Hokama Y: Simplified solid-phase immunobead assay for detection of ciguatoxin and related polyethers. J Clin Lab Anal 4:213–217, 1990.
33. Geller RJ, Benowitz NL: Orthostatic hypotension in ciguatera fish poisoning. Arch Intern Med 152:2131–2133, 1992.
34. Sims JK: Theoretical discourse on the pharmacology of toxic marine ingestions. Ann Emerg Med 16:1006–1015, 1987.
35. Palafox NA, Jam LG, Pinano AZ, et al: Successful treatment of ciguatera fish poisoning with intravenous mannitol. JAMA 259:2740–2742, 1988.
36. Pearn JH, Lewis RJ, Ruff T, et al: Ciguatera and mannitol: Experience with a new treatment regimen. Med J Aust 151:77–80, 1989.

37. Stewart MPM: Ciguatera fish poisoning: Treatment with intravenous mannitol. Trop Doct 21:54–55, 1991.
38. Williams RK, Palafox NA: Treatment of pediatric fish poisoning. Am J Dis Child 144:747–748, 1990.
39. Lewis RJ: Mannitol reverses the action of ciguatoxin in vitro. Proc Austr Physiol Pharmacol Soc 19:237, 1988.
40. Purcell CE, Capra MF, Cameron J: Action of mannitol in ciguatoxin-intoxicated rats. Toxicon 37:67–76, 1999.
41. Magovern GJ, Bolling SF, Casale AS, et al: The mechanism of mannitol in reducing ischemic injury: hyperosmolarity or hydroxyl scavenger? Circulation 70(Suppl 1):1–91, 1984.
42. Dais RT, Villar LA: Symptomatic improvement with amitriptyline in ciguatera fish poisoning. N Engl J Med 315:65, 1986.
43. Calvert GM, Hryhorczuk DO, Leikin JB: Treatment of ciguatera fish poisoning with amitriptyline and nifedipine. Clin Toxicol 25:423–428, 1987.

CHAPTER 117

Scombroid

Henrietta Harrison ▪ Nicola Bates

Scombroid fish poisoning is a food-borne chemical intoxication caused by eating spoiled or bacterially contaminated fish containing high concentrations of histamine.[1] Fish with a relatively high concentration of red meat, which turns brown when cooked, contain high concentrations of free histidine in their muscle tissue. When these fish are refrigerated improperly or refrigeration is delayed, bacteria containing histidine decarboxylase convert histidine to histamine.[2]

Scombroid fish poisoning has been recognized since 1799, although the first reference to a scombrotoxin outbreak appeared in the literature in 1830. Five crew members on board the *Triton of Leith* had violent headaches, swollen and flushed faces, and shivering after eating bonito.[3]

Histamine is tasteless, odorless, and heat stabile; cooking, drying, canning, smoking, freezing, salting, or marinating does not alter fish that already are contaminated. Effective prevention of scombroid poisoning requires proper handling and storage of fish (rapid refrigeration). Histamine formation is usually negligible in fish stored at 0°C.[4,5] Implicated fish may have a normal taste or may be described as tasting sharp or peppery.

The term *scombroid poisoning* originates from the fact that spoiled fish from the families Scombridae and Scomberesocidae (e.g., tuna, mackerel, and bonito) originally were implicated in incidents of this type of poisoning. Nonscombroid fish (e.g., pilchards, herring, sardines) also have been implicated, however. Table 117-1 summarizes sources of scombroid fish poisoning.

Scombroid poisoning is a common form of fish poisoning that appears throughout the world; cases have been reported in Africa, Asia, Australia, New Zealand, Canada, Europe, and the United States. Many incidents or cases go unreported because of the mildness of the disease or misdiagnosis. Scombroid poisoning is a significant global public health and safety concern due to the large network for harvesting, processing, and distributing fish. Because scombroid poisoning is a consequence of improper handling or storage of fish, however, and there are effective methods of identifying toxic fish, control and prevention are possible.[1]

Scombroid fish are distributed widely throughout all temperate and tropical seas, and some are found occasionally in Arctic and Antarctic waters. They are largely oceanic fish, migrating long distances through the open seas.[6] Fig. 117-1 shows the bluefin tuna and its fishing grounds.

Generally, scombrotoxic fish poisoning is not serious but may be alarming and unpleasant. Most cases are mild and self-limiting and require no treatment. Serious complications are rare, and no deaths have been reported in recent years.[2] It is not an allergic reaction, and it does not result from ingestion of fresh, unspoiled fish.

Occasionally, cheese, particularly Swiss cheese, has been implicated in outbreaks of scombroid poisoning. Cheddar cheese and Gouda cheese also have been implicated in single incidents of scombroid poisoning.[7,8]

BIOCHEMICAL BASIS OF SCOMBROID POISONING

As mentioned earlier, fish with a relatively high concentration of red flesh, which turns brown when cooked, contain high concentrations of free histidine in their muscle tissue. When these fish are refrigerated improperly or refrigeration is delayed, bacteria containing histidine decarboxylase convert histidine to histamine.[2] Fig. 117-2 shows the pathways of biosynthesis and metabolism of histamine after conversion from histidine.[9]

PATHOPHYSIOLOGY

Histamine is produced in the fish by the action of bacterial decarboxylase enzymes (histidine decarboxylase) on the amino acid histidine. The latter is available in the free state in scombroid fish, but not in most other varieties. Many bacterial species possess these enzymes, but the most active and common are *Klebsiella pneumoniae*, *Klebsiella oxytoca*, *Proteus (Morganella) morganii*, *Serratia marcescens*, *Enterobacter intermedium*, and *Plesiomonas shigelloides*.[10] These bacteria form part of the normal microflora of fish skin, gut, and gills or may be present secondary to contamination from handlers.[5] The conversion of histidine to histamine can occur at varying temperatures, depending on the bacteria involved, but generally does not occur with storage at less than 0°C.[4,5]

Histamine is a naturally occurring substance in mammalian physiology. It is contained in mast cells and basophils, and its biologic effects are usually seen only when it is released in large amounts in the course of allergic and other reactions. Histamine exerts its effects by binding to receptors on cellular membranes in the respiratory, cardiovascular, gastrointestinal, and hematologic/immunologic systems and the skin.[1]

Scombrotoxic poisoning results from eating fish containing high concentrations of histamine. Levels of 5 mg/100 g are considered normal in fish flesh. Concentrations of 20 mg/100 g

TABLE 117-1 Fish Implicated in Scombroid Fish Poisoning

FAMILY	COMMON NAME	GENUS AND SPECIES
Arripidae	Australian salmon	*Arripis trutta*
Clupeidae	Pilchard	*Sardinops sagax*
Clupeidae	Spotted sardines	*Amblygaster sirm*
Coryphaenidae	Dolphin fish (mahi-mahi)	*Coryphaena hippurus*
Scomberesocidae	Saury	*Cololabis saira*
Scombroidae	Frigate mackerel	*Auxis thazard*
	Little tuna	*Euthynnus affinis*
	Little tunny	*Euthynnus alletteratus*
	Skipjack tuna	*Euthynnus pelamis* or *Katsuwonas pelamis*
	Striped bonito	*Sarda orientalis*
	Bonito	*Sarda sarda*
	Pacific mackerel	*Scomber japonicus*
	Atlantic mackerel	*Scomber scombrus*
	King mackerel	*Scomberomorus cavalla*
	Spanish mackerel	*Scomberomorus maculatus*
	Cero	*Scomberomorus regalis*
	Albacore	*Thunnus alalunga*
	Yellowfin tuna	*Thunnus albacares*
	Bigeye tuna	*Thunnus obesus*
	Bluefin tuna	*Thunnus thynnus*
Xiphiidae	Swordfish	*Xiphias gladius*

Data from references 2, 8, and 18.

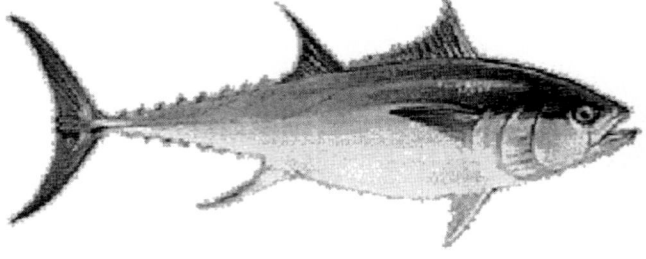

A

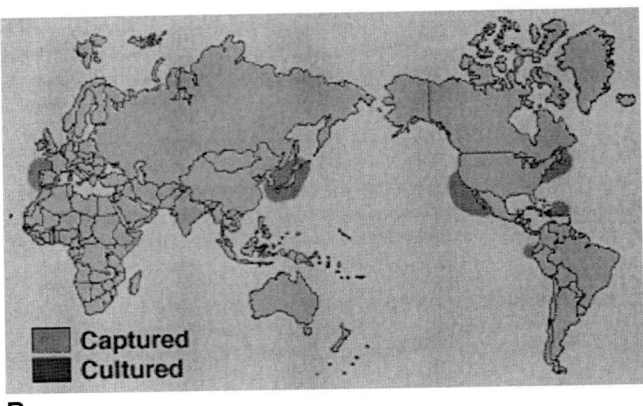

Captured
Cultured

B

FIGURE 117-1

A and **B**, Bluefin tuna (*Thunnus thynnus*) and its fishing grounds. All tuna belong to the Scombroidea family of mackerels, with the bluefin tuna being one of five varieties of tuna that has been harvested for centuries. Bluefins are the largest of the commercially important tuna species and are marketed at sizes around 68 kg (150 lb), although they can grow to greater than 675 kg (>1500 lb).

have been associated with mild symptoms of the disease and suggest slight mishandling of the fish, whereas severe cases have resulted from the consumption of fish containing more than 100 mg/100 g.[4] The tissue histamine concentration is a good indicator of fish spoilage and is a key to the diagnosis of scombrotoxin. Most histamine is produced in the flesh around the intestines, then diffuses into the tissues so that distant tissue can have misleadingly low concentrations.[11]

There is some controversy as to whether histamine itself is responsible for the symptoms and the mechanism of the histamine-like reaction. Histamine is not always found in the fish involved, and some fish contain high concentrations of histamine but do not cause this type of poisoning. Also, pure histamine given orally is metabolized rapidly by gut enzymes and generally causes mild poisoning, but it has not been possible to reproduce the clinical picture of scombrotoxicity.[12] This may be because histamine is poorly absorbed and because the liver and intestinal mucosa inactivate histamine. It has been suggested that there are substances, perhaps other amines, in the fish that enhance the pharmacologic activity of histamine, facilitate its absorption, or interfere with its metabolism. Another suggested mechanism is that some other toxin in the fish is absorbed from the gastrointestinal tract and causes endogenous histamine release, perhaps from basophils.[1]

Morrow and colleagues[12] found that urinary concentrations of histamine and its metabolite, *N*-methylhistamine, were respectively 9 to 20 times and 15 to 20 times the normal limit in three patients who developed symptoms of scombrotoxicity. These increased concentrations occurred without a change in the concentration of PGD-M (a metabolite of prostaglandin D_2, a mast cell secretory product). This mast cell had not been activated to release histamine, so the fish must have been the source. It was concluded that histamine was the causative agent.[12] However, Clifford and associates[13] found that ingestion of fresh and spoiled mackerel with added histamine did not induce scombrotoxicity. Only fish previously associated with illness produced the clinical features of toxicity. They suggested that the unidentified scombrotoxin is a substance that causes basophil degranulation, mast cell degranulation without the release of prostaglandins, or both.

CLINICAL PRESENTATION

Symptoms of scombroid poisoning develop typically within 10 minutes to 3 hours after ingestion and are consistent with a mildly to moderately severe histamine-mediated reaction. The initial symptoms and signs suggest an allergic response with flushing (particularly of the

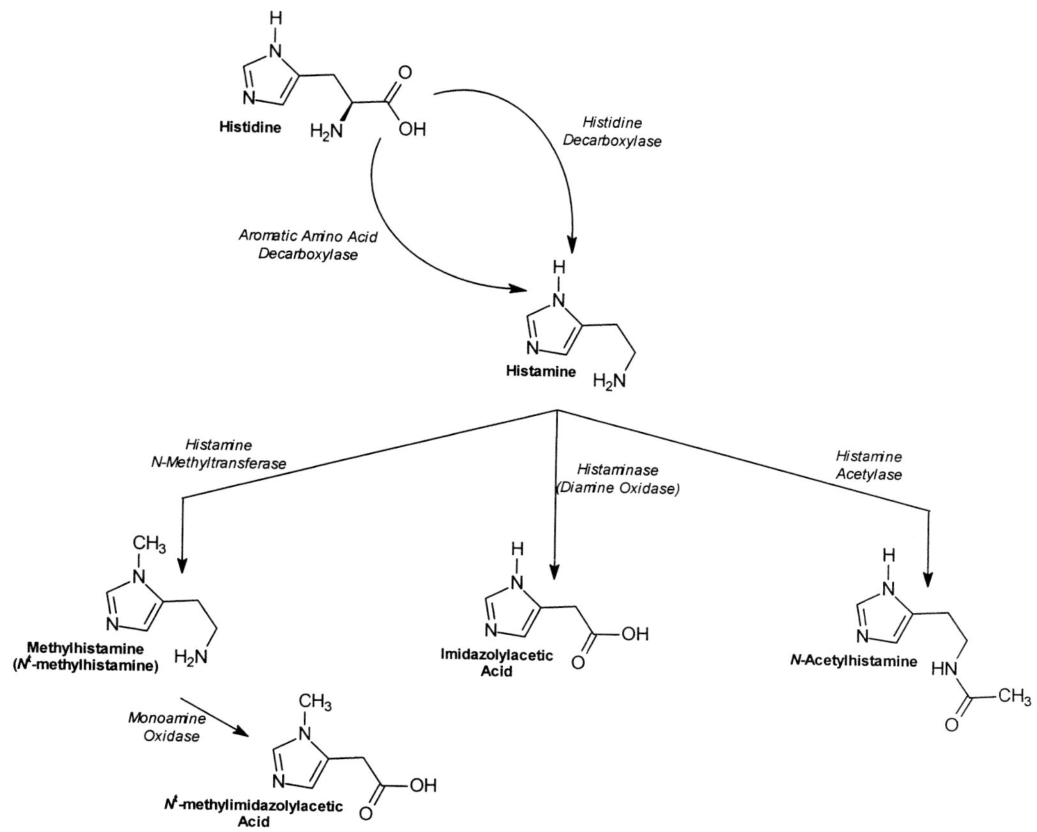

FIGURE 117-2

Pathways in the biosynthesis and metabolism of histamine.

face, neck, and upper trunk), burning of the mouth or a peppery taste, and sweating. These symptoms may be accompanied by a throbbing headache, palpitations, nausea, vomiting, abdominal cramps, and diarrhea. The initial reaction may progress to diffuse erythema with itching or a hot burning sensation; pruritus and urticaria, with mouth blistering, also may occur. Localized swelling, particularly around the mouth and the tongue, may occur secondary to angioedema. Hypotension, dizziness, and dysphagia have been reported.[14]

In severe cases, bronchospasm, respiratory distress, vasodilatory shock, and atrial flutter may occur. These conditions are seen more often in patients with preexisting cardiac or pulmonary disease.[12] Transient vision loss, atrial tachycardia, and atrioventricular block were reported in an adult with a history of diabetes and hypertension after scombroid poisoning from tuna. Symptoms resolved within 1 hour of diphenhydramine administration. It was suggested that vision loss was secondary to cerebral blindness caused by either vasospasm or an exacerbation of hypertension due to the effects of histamine.[15] Histamine is metabolized by amine oxidases (Fig. 117-2). Patients taking drugs that inhibit these enzymes (e.g., isoniazid or nonselective monoamine oxidase inhibitors) may be at risk of more severe effects.

The clinical presentation of scombroid poisoning may be classified as mild, moderate, or severe according to Smart (Table 117-2).[16]

DIAGNOSIS

The symptoms of scombrotoxicity generally are self-limiting and usually subside in 3 to 12 hours. Recovery usually occurs within 8 to 12 hours if untreated and 2 to 3 hours if antihistamines are given. Occasionally, effects can persist for 24 to 48 hours.

The diagnosis of scombroid poisoning is based on the clinical presentation, the rapid onset of illness, and ingestion of incriminating food shortly before the onset of illness. Symptoms of scombroid poisoning can be confused with allergic reactions or other forms of food poisoning. Scombroid poisoning can be distinguished from an allergic reaction by inquiring into any history of previous reactions when eating the implicated food. The diagnosis is supported further if other individuals ate the same food and developed a similar reaction.

The diagnosis of scombroid poisoning can be confirmed by analysis of the suspect food and detection of high concentrations of histamine. When cases of scombroid poisoning are suspected, samples of the incriminated food should be sought immediately. Local health departments can be helpful in obtaining the appropriate sample. Food samples should be stored frozen if prompt analysis cannot be done.[8]

Concentrations of 20 mg of histamine/100 g of flesh or more may be associated with toxicity[17]; however, toxicity has occurred with lower concentrations. Bacterial counts

TABLE 117-2 Recommended Classification and Treatment of Scombroid Poisoning

SEVERITY	CLINICAL FEATURES	TREATMENT
Mild poisoning	Rash only or brief flushing; tachycardia	Observe for 2 hours
		Consider parenteral antihistamines if condition fails to improve or worsens
Moderate poisoning	Rash and persistent flushing; tachycardia; headache and/or gastrointestinal symptoms	Overnight admission if symptoms slow to resolve
		Basic life support (ABCs, oxygen)
		IV access
		Parenteral antihistamines (H$_1$ and H$_2$ antagonists); repeat if necessary
Severe poisoning	Any of the above And/or bronchospasm	Hospital admission
		Basic life support (ABCs, oxygen) and/or advanced life support
	And/or hypotension And/or airway compromise And/or angioedema	IV fluids
		Epinephrine
		Parenteral antihistamine (H$_1$ and H$_2$ antagonists); repeat as necessary
		Nebulized bronchodilators

ABCs, airway, breathing, and circulation; IV, intravenous.
Adapted from Smart DR: Scombroid poisoning: A report of seven cases involving the Western Australian salmon, *Arripis truttaceus*. Med J Aust 157:748–751, 1992.

are not useful because processing the flesh subsequent to spoilage may destroy the responsible organisms. When food samples are not available, vomitus and stomach contents can be analyzed, but baseline control data on histamine concentrations in these body fluids are not readily available.

TREATMENT

Because vomiting frequently occurs in scombroid poisoning and symptoms generally are mild and of rapid onset, gastric lavage and the use of activated charcoal are not indicated. Treatment generally is symptomatic and supportive. Patients may require rehydration and antiemetics. Although symptoms are short lived, administration of H$_1$ antagonists

(e.g., promethazine, chlorpheniramine, or diphenhydramine) or H$_2$ antagonists (e.g., cimetidine) lessens discomfort and reduces the duration of effects.[8,10]

H$_1$ receptor antagonists are used widely in the management of scombroid fish poisoning. H$_2$ receptor antagonists also have been shown to be useful. The efficacy of cimetidine has been found to be equivalent to or to exceed that achieved with H$_1$ antagonists alone. H$_2$ antagonists are easy to administer and lack the sedating side effects of H$_1$ antagonists, reducing delay in hospital discharge.[8,10]

In severely poisoned patients, bronchodilators may be necessary in the presence of bronchospasm, and intravenous fluids may be required. Patients with preexisting cardiac disorders should have cardiac monitoring until their symptoms resolve. In atopic patients, in whom bronchospasm or other severe histamine reactions may occur, the use of β-adrenergic agonists and even corticosteroids should be considered.[2] Table 117-2 outlines the recommended treatment and admission criteria for scombroid poisoning.

Indications for ICU Admission in Scombroid Poisoning

Admission may be considered for any patient with underlying cardiac or respiratory disease because of the risk of severe effects such as bronchospasm, respiratory distress, vasodilatory shock, and atrial flutter.

Criteria for ICU Discharge in Scombroid Poisoning

Discharge may be considered when the severe effects have resolved or have been treated successfully.

SPECIAL POPULATIONS

Scombroid fish poisoning is mild and self-limited in most cases. Individuals with a history of allergic diseases, concurrent use of certain drugs (e.g., isoniazid, nonselective monoamine oxidase inhibitors), or preexisting cardiac or respiratory conditions may have more severe effects, however. Bronchospasm, respiratory distress, vasodilatory shock, and atrial flutter are seen more often in patients with preexisting cardiac or pulmonary disease.[12] Russell and Maretic[18] described the case of a young child with a history of asthma who developed respiratory collapse after scombroid poisoning.

Scombroid poisoning in pregnancy is unlikely to affect the growth or development of the fetus. Symptoms should be treated symptomatically and supportively, ensuring adequate hydration.

Children do not seem to be more susceptible to scombroid poisoning. They should be treated symptomatically and supportively, checking for preexisting cardiac and respiratory conditions.

Common Misconceptions about Scombroid Poisoning

1. Scombroid poisoning is an allergic reaction.
2. Scombroid poisoning is due to ingestion of a toxin.
3. Scombroid poisoning occurs only from scombroid fish.

Key Points in Scombroid Poisoning

1. Scombrotoxin poisoning is not an allergic reaction.
2. Scombroid poisoning is caused by ingestion of food, usually fish, containing high concentrations of histamine following bacterial conversion to histamine of histidine present in tissue.
3. Scombroid poisoning may occur with nonscombroid fish and, more rarely, with cheese or beer.
4. Often, multiple patients have ingested the same meal.
5. Onset usually is 30 to 60 minutes after ingestion but can be delayed for 2 hours.
6. Most cases are mild and self-limiting, resolving within 2 to 3 hours if antihistamines are given or 8 to 12 hours if untreated.

continued

Key Points in Scombroid Poisoning *continued*

7. Occasionally, effects can persist for 24 to 48 hours.
8. Common symptoms include dermal flushing, throbbing headache, nausea, dizziness, diarrhea, and vomiting.
9. Respiratory distress or cardiac problems may occur, usually in patients with preexisting pulmonary or cardiac disease.
10. Shock and death have been reported in the past but not in recent years.

REFERENCES

1. Lehane L, Oliey J: Histamine poisoning revisited. Int J Food Microbiol 58:1–37, 2000.
2. Muller GJ, Lamprecht JH, Barnes JM, et al: Scombroid poisoning. South Afr Med J 81:427–430, 1992.
3. Henderson PB: Case of poisoning from the bonito (*Scomber pelamis*). Edinb Med J 34:317–318, 1830.
4. Scoging AC: Illness associated with seafood. Communicable Dis Rep 1:R117-122, 1991.
5. Stell IM: Trouble with tuna: Two cases of scombrotoxin poisoning. J Accid Emerg Med 14:110–117, 1997.
6. Wu M-L, Yang C-C, Yang G-Y, et al: Scombroid fish poisoning: An overlooked marine food poisoning. Vet Hum Toxicol 39:236–241, 1997.
7. Doeglas HMG, Huisman J, Nater JP: Histamine intoxication after cheese. Lancet 2:1361–1362, 1967.
8. Taylor SL, Stratton JE, Nordlee JA: Histamine poisoning (scombroid fish poisoning): An allergy-like intoxication. Clin Toxicol 27:225–240, 1989.
9. Bowman WC, Rand MJ: Textbook of Pharmacology, 2nd ed. Oxford, Blackwell Scientific, 1968.
10. Guss DA: Scombroid fish poisoning: Successful treatment with cimetidine. Undersea Hyperb Med 25:123–125, 1998.
11. Bedry R, Gabinski C, Paty M-C: Diagnosis of scombroid poisoning by measurement of plasma histamine. N Engl J Med 342:520–521, 2000.
12. Morrow JD, Margolies GR, Rowland J, Roberts LJ II: Evidence that histamine is the causative toxin of scombroid-fish poisoning. N Engl J Med 324:716–720, 1991.
13. Clifford MN, Walker R, Ijomah P, et al: Is there a role for amines other than histamines in the aetiology of scombrotoxicosis? Food Addit Contam 8:641–651, 1991.
14. Etkind P, Wilson ME, Gallagher K, Cournoyer J: Bluefish associated scombroid poisoning: An example of the expanding spectrum of food poisoning from seafood. JAMA 258:3409–3410, 1987.
15. McInerney J, Sahgal P, Vogal M, et al: Scombroid poisoning. Ann Emerg Med 28:235–238, 1996.
16. Smart DR: Scombroid poisoning: A report of seven cases involving the Western Australian salmon, *Arripis truttaceus*. Med J Aust 157:748–751, 1992.
17. Gilbert RJ, Hobbs G, Murray CK, et al: Scombrotoxic fish poisoning: Features of the first 50 incidents to be reported in Britain (1976–1979). BMJ 2:71–72, 1980.
18. Russell FE, Maretic Z: Scombroid poisoning: Mini-review with case histories. Toxicon 24:967–973, 1986.

CHAPTER **118**

Tetrodotoxin

Chen-Chang Yang ■ Jou-Fang Deng

Tetrodotoxin (TTX), with a toxicity more than 1000 times deadlier than sodium cyanide (median lethan dose approximately 10 μg/kg, versus 10 mg/kg for sodium cyanide), is one of the most potent marine poisons known to toxicologists.[1–3] It also may be the best known marine toxin because it is responsible for puffer fish poisoning (fugu or *Tetraodon* poisoning), which has caused many fatalities, particularly in Japan. Although puffer fish poisoning has been associated with a high fatality rate in Japan for centuries, the danger of puffer fish consumption also has long been recognized in other countries, including China and Egypt.[3,4] The first Chinese pharmacopoeia, the *Book of Herbs* (*Pen-T'so Chin*), usually attributed to the legendary Emperor Shun Nung (2838–2698 BC), listed puffer eggs as one of the 120 medium drugs that were believed to have tonic effects but could be toxic depending on the dose.[3] A detailed description of the appearance and general toxic properties of a puffer fish (known as "piglet of the river" in Chinese, likely representing *Tetraodon oscellatus*) was given in the most authoritative pharmacopoeia of traditional Chinese medicine, *The Great Herbal* (*Pen-T'so Kang Mu*), by Li Shih-Chen in 1596 AD.[3] A puffer fish identified as *Tetraodon lineatus* is shown on an Egyptian tomb from 2500 BC, and there is evidence that the Egyptians knew the poisonous nature of this fish.[4]

Despite biblical admonitions prohibiting the consumption of scaleless fishes,[5,6] Europeans probably were unaware of puffer fish poisoning until they began to visit the Orient in the 17th century. In his classic work *History of Japan*, published in 1727, Engelbert Kaempfer, a physician to the Dutch embassy in Japan, described the lethality of puffer fish and its use in suicide attempts.[3] Direct and well-documented European experiences of puffer fish poisoning first occurred during the second voyage of Pacific explorer Captain James Cook.[1,3] In 1774, he and two naturalists, J.R. and G. Forster, on the *Resolution*, experienced various neurologic manifestations after eating a fish traded with a native in New Caledonia. According to his journal record and the Forsters' description of the fish, it is believed that they had been served puffer fish.

Puffer fish also are known as *blowfish, swellfish, globefish, porcupine fish, balloonfish*, and *toadfish* because they can take large quantities of water into the stomach when they are frightened or injured and assume an enlarged, globular shape. The skin of puffer fish is distinct because it is smooth or prickly and is covered partially by bristly or hairlike spines. Most puffer fish live in shallow warm waters. Puffer fish belong to the order *Tetraodontiformes*,

which includes the families Tetraodontidae, the puffer fish; Diodontidae, the porcupine fish; Canthigasteridae, the sharp-nosed puffer fish; Molidae, the mola or ocean sunfish; Triodontidae, the three-toothed puffer fish; and others. Currently, there are at least 40 species of puffer fish that have been shown to be poisonous, most belonging to the family Tetraodontidae.[1,5] The term *puffer fish poisoning* has been reserved largely for intoxications caused by ingestions of members of the family Tetraodontidae or, on some occasions, of other aforementioned families. In puffer fish, TTX is found mainly in the liver, ovaries, intestines, and skin.[4,5] The musculature usually is safer to eat than other parts of the fish (especially when it is prepared by a licensed chef), but for some species (e.g., *Lagocephalus lunaris*), it can be toxic as well.[7] The testes almost always are safe to eat, although they can be weakly toxic in certain puffer fish (e.g., *Spheroides niphobles*).[3] Female puffer fish generally are more toxic than males, and the level of toxicity seems to be related to the reproductive cycle, with the toxicity increasing from the beginning of the puffer fish season (usually October through March) and reaching its peak during the spawning season (May and June for most puffer fish).[3,5]

In Japan, puffer fish have long been considered an epicurean delight, and it is believed that eating *sashimi*, thin slices of raw puffer fish meat, can give a peculiar tingling oral sensation, sensation of warmth, and euphoria induced by minute amounts of TTX contained in the flesh.[5,6] For this reason, many Japanese regard eating fugu as a "must-have" experience despite the potentially severe toxicity of the fish. Some Japanese also believe that drinking a mixture of hot sake and fugu testes can contribute to virility and that adding a small amount of puffer fish liver can impart a particularly piquant flavor to certain dishes.[1] All of these eating behaviors may incur various risks of TTX poisoning.

Compared with the frequency of other food poisonings or the amount of fish consumed annually in Japan, the incidence of puffer fish poisoning is small; it is not considered a major public health hazard.[3,8] Puffer fish poisoning is remarkable, however, for its dramatically severe course and for the multiple deaths that may occur in the same household.[3] Data obtained from the Ministry of Health and Welfare of Japan indicate that the overall case-fatality rate of puffer fish poisoning, excluding the 6-year period of 1943–1948, was 59.4% in the period 1886–1963[5] and was 36.7% in the period 1967–1976.[8] Puffer fish poisoning accounted for more deaths than all other types of food poisoning combined in Japan.[8] Because of the popularity of eating fugu and the high case-fatality rate, legislative controls, such as licensing of chefs in special restaurants requiring them to be knowledgeable regarding the species and seasonal variations in toxicity and education of the public, have been implemented in Japan to prevent puffer fish poisoning. As a result of these efforts and better therapeutic measures, the number of deaths caused by puffer fish poisoning per year declined from more than 100 persons in the late 19th and early 20th centuries to approximately 20 during the period 1974–1979.[3,4] Nevertheless, because the cost of the fugu delicacy is usually high in Japan, people of low socioeconomic status continue to eat puffer fish that is prepared or sold privately by unlicensed peddlers, a behavior that increases the likelihood of poisoning.[3,5] The statistics in 1957 showed that there were 119 incidents of puffer fish poisoning involving 176 persons.[3] Of these, only two incidents occurred after the eating of fugu in a licensed restaurant, neither of which had a fatal outcome. Of the remaining 176 persons, 90 died. Similar statistics also have been noted in other countries. In an analysis of Taiwan Poison Control Center data over the period 1988–1995, Yang and colleagues[9] found that among 18 incidents of puffer fish poisoning that involved 36 persons, only 1 victim purchased the fish from a restaurant, whereas the others collected the fish directly from the offshore waters by themselves or purchased them from fishmongers.

Puffer fish have a worldwide distribution and may extend from latitudes 63°N to 47°S. Although many cases have been reported from Japan, poisonings may be encountered wherever these fish occur.[5] Poisonings have been reported in many countries other than Japan, including the United States,[10–12] Mexico,[13] Australia,[14,15] Papua New Guinea,[16] China,[5,17] Taiwan,[9,18] and several Southeast Asian countries.[5,19–24] Accidental poisoning due to consumption of mislabeled or improperly processed puffer fish also has occurred in Italy[6] and the United States.[11] Outside of Japan, accurate statistics of puffer fish poisonings generally are not available because reporting this poisoning is not required.[5] Currently available, albeit incomplete, statistics from Taiwan revealed a case-fatality rate of 16.7% for puffer fish poisoning in that country during the period 1988–1995,[8] at an average of 1 to 2 deaths yearly.[9,18]

Although TTX poisoning previously was thought to occur almost exclusively from puffer fish poisoning, more recent evidence has shown that the toxin also can be found in a wide variety of seemingly unrelated aquatic organisms and amphibians, including the Australian blue-ringed octopus (*Hapalochlaena maculosa*),[25] other gastropod mollusks (Japanese ivory shell [*Babylonia japonica*], trumpet shell *Charonia sauliae*], and several species of *Nassariidae*),[5,26,27] Indo-Pacific goby (*Gobius criniger*),[28] starfish (*Astropecten latespinosus* and *Astropecten scoparius*),[5,29] crabs (xanthid crabs [*Atergatis floridus*], *Zozymus aeneus*, and horseshoe crab [*Carcinoscorpius rotundicauda*]),[5,30–33] ribbon worms (*Lineus fuscoviridis* and *Tubulanus punctatus*),[34] frogs (*Atelopus chiriquiensis* and *Atelopus varius*),[35] and salamanders and newts (Salamandridae family [true newts], e.g., true salamander [*Cynops ensicauda*], Oregon newt [*Taricha granulosa*], and California newt [*Taricha torosa*]).[5,36–38] Human cases of TTX poisoning also have been reported after the ingestion of goby fish,[5,9,39,40] gastropod mollusks,[27] and salamanders[41,42] and after being bitten by a blue-ringed octopus.[43–45] Among these species, the finding of TTX in salamanders and a blue-ringed octopus merits further discussion.

In 1932, Twitty serendipitously found that the larvae of striped salamanders (*Ambystoma tigrinum*) became paralyzed after receiving grafted eye and limb buds from embryos of the California newt (*T. torosa*).[1] No further extensive studies of the compound were carried out until the 1960s. In 1962, a potent nonprotein toxin, of which 1 mg was capable of killing 7000 mice, was crystallized and was named *tarichatoxin*. To the investigators' astonishment, it was found later that tarichatoxin and TTX were identical in their infrared and nuclear magnetic resonance spectra and in their characteristics in various chromatographic systems. Newts did not become intoxicated after exposure to TTX. It is apparent that the two biologically different species—puffer fish and newts—contain the same toxin.

The isolation of TTX from the posterior salivary gland of the blue-ringed octopus was the first instance that TTX was found in extracts of the venom glands, in contrast to the identification of toxin in the skin, muscle, liver, ovaries, or eggs in other species.[25] The chemistry and pharmacology of extracts of the blue-ringed octopus were investigated after the occurrence of many human fatalities in Australia.[42,43] The principal toxin present in the venom glands was found to be a neurotoxin, which initially was named *maculotoxin*. Although it now is believed that toxic components other than maculotoxin also are present in octopus venom (e.g., haplotoxin, histamine),[5,45] there is little doubt that maculotoxin is TTX.[25,45]

The origin of TTX remains a mystery. The erratic distribution of TTX in widely different species suggests that the toxin is acquired through the food chain as a consequence of consuming toxic marine algae. Evidence supporting this hypothesis has come from the discovery of a TTX-producing *Pseudomonas* species isolated from a red alga *Jania*[5,46] and the skin of puffer fish,[47] the observed difference in toxicity between cultured and wide puffer fish,[8,48] the documented transmission of TTX from one fish to the next in a feeding experiment,[5] and the regional variation in toxicity of puffer fish.[5] Some investigators proposed, however, that the ability to synthesize TTX in various marine organisms and amphibians may be simply a coincidental genetic development because of its survival value.[35] The finding of unique exocrine glands for the secretion of TTX in puffer fish supports the possibility that puffer fish and other species actively produce the toxin.[49]

BIOCHEMISTRY AND PHARMACOLOGY

In the 1950s, Yokoo and Tsuda independently crystallized TTX in a relatively pure form.[1,5] TTX is an amino perhydroquinazoline compound with a molecular formula of $C_{11}H_{17}N_3O_8$ (Fig. 118-1) and a molecular weight of 319.[1,3,5] It forms a colorless crystal and is a monoacidic base with a pK_a of 8.5 in aqueous solution.[3] It is soluble in water if a trace of acid is added but readily decomposes in strongly acidic or alkaline conditions.[1,3,5,50,51] The toxicity of TTX reportedly has been destroyed by the action of 2%

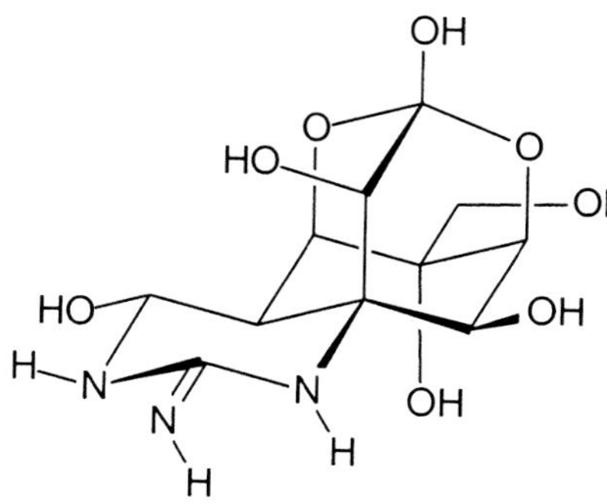

FIGURE 118-1

Chemical structure of tetrodotoxin.

sodium hydroxide treatment for 90 minutes.[5] Because TTX is a nonprotein toxin, it is relatively heat stable; frying, stewing, baking, or boiling for hours does not destroy the toxin.[5] Storage at $-15°C$ for 12 hours or exposure to sunlight for 20 days also does not change its activity.[5] Commercial canning processes do not significantly reduce the lethality of the toxin. In contrast to its heat stability, TTX is found to lose its activity markedly even after minor alterations of its chemical structure.[2]

Although TTX is one of the most potent marine toxins, little is known about its mode of action. Current evidence indicates that TTX abolishes propagated action potentials through its selective blockade of voltage-gated neuronal sodium channels.[1–3,5] In some animal experiments, TTX also has been shown to reduce the production of acetylcholine[52,53] and to depress cytochrome oxidase and acetylcholinesterase at high concentrations.[5] There is no universal agreement, however, on whether the toxin acts on cytochrome oxidase[3]; in most experiments, the toxin does not inhibit, or only slightly affects, acetylcholinesterase, even in high concentrations.[53–56]

Pharmacokinetics of Tetrodotoxin Poisoning

Volume of distribution: widely distributed; more specific data not available

Protein binding: low; specific data not available

Mechanism of clearance: renal

Active metabolites: none

Methods to enhance clearance: none

PATHOPHYSIOLOGY

The main pharmacologic effect of TTX is to block the propagation of nerve and muscle action potentials by a nondepolarizing blockade of sodium channels.[2,3,5,51] As a consequence, the neuromuscular effects are prominent, and rapidly progressive skeletal muscle paralysis, including muscles associated with respiratory function, is characteristic of TTX poisoning. Although TTX primarily inhibits the transmission of nerve impulses, it also has a direct action on skeletal muscle. This blockade of neuromuscular transmission generally is believed to occur on motor nerve axons and on muscle fiber membranes, rather than at the motor end plates.[3,54,57] After administration, the time required to inhibit muscle fiber function is usually longer, however, than that for nerve block, except in the case of diaphragmatic muscle.[3,57] Slow muscle fibers are more susceptible to TTX than are fast fibers. Because TTX generally does not act on the motor end plate, the administration of anticholinesterase drugs, such as neostigmine or edrophonium, is not likely to antagonize TTX-induced neuromuscular blockade effectively.[3] The axonal blockade caused by TTX is not limited to somatic motor nerves because disturbance of sensory nerve function is seen frequently in the early phase of poisoning.[3,5] TTX is approximately 160,000 times more potent than cocaine in blocking axonal conduction in sensory neurons.[5]

Respiratory depression is the most prominent and serious toxic effect of TTX intoxication and is usually the cause of death among poisoned patients.[3,5,57,58] Despite considerable controversy over how TTX produces respiratory paralysis and the belief of some investigators that depression of the medullary respiratory center is responsible for respiratory arrest,[5,58,59] more recent work has shown conclusively that TTX causes respiratory depression predominantly through direct paralysis of the diaphragmatic muscles.[3,51,57] The respiratory musculature is extraordinarily sensitive to TTX, and low doses of TTX (4% of the lethal dose) can depress respiration markedly in experimental animals.[3] Respiratory muscles may be more vulnerable to TTX than are other skeletal muscles or the phrenic nerve because of their greater blood supply, resulting in a more rapid and proportionately greater distribution of toxin to the diaphragm.[57] Although central depressant effects are unlikely to be important in most instances of TTX poisoning, their role in the terminal stage of severe TTX poisoning or after rapid intravenous absorption of the toxin cannot be dismissed.[3,51,57] Besides the inhibition of the respiratory musculature, TTX also causes depression of the cough reflex and relaxes bronchial smooth muscles.[3]

Profound hypotension is a characteristic manifestation of TTX poisoning, which may or may not be associated with bradycardia.[3,56] Hypotension has been noted further to be the cause of death in certain animal TTX poisonings.[45] Although a central vasomotor depressant effect previously was thought by many Japanese investigators to be the mechanism of TTX-induced hypotension,[3,5] the experimental evidence supporting this view was weak and unconvincing.[3,51] Kao,[2,3] in a series of head-body cross-perfusion experiments, showed that hypotension did not develop in the recipient's body when TTX, in a dose large enough to cause hypotension in the donor, was administered to the recipient's head via the donor's circulation. In other studies, the decrease in blood pressure was not accompanied by slowed heart rate or decreased cardiac output, which suggests that hypotension is attributable to direct peripheral vasodilation by TTX rather than to cardiac depression.[54,58] Large doses of TTX cause prolonged cardiac depression[2,3,56,60] or conduction disturbances (e.g., bradycardia)[54,60]; however, hypotension occurs before the cardiac depression at such doses.[51,60]

Most investigators now agree that TTX-induced hypotension is caused primarily by decreased peripheral vascular resistance rather than affecting the heart or the vasomotor center,[2,3,51,60] but the exact mechanism for this vasodilation is unclear. Some investigators believe that TTX causes hypotension by blocking sympathetic vasomotor nerves, causing relaxation of vascular smooth muscles[3,51,60]; others propose that TTX also has a direct effect on arterial smooth muscles.[2,61] Kao[2] showed that the systemic hypotension seems to be due to a combination of a direct relaxant effect of TTX on vascular smooth muscle at low doses and blockade of vasomotor nerve conduction at high doses. Li[58] found that the TTX-related vasodilatory action had a histamine-like component because pretreatment with an antihistamine prevented the decrease in blood pressure caused by a sublethal dose of the toxin.

The effect of TTX on blood pressure seems to be dose dependent. In dogs, Nomiyama[5] found that small doses of puffer fish toxin produced an initial increase in blood pressure and heart rate followed by a decrease in blood pressure, whereas large doses produced immediate hypotension followed by a gradual increase in heart rate. Duce and colleagues[62] noted that nonlethal doses of TTX (0.6 to 2.4 μg/kg) resulted in an increase in heart rate and mean arterial blood pressure in unanesthetized dogs; higher concentrations of TTX caused moderate hypotension, apnea, and death. These investigators also reported that TTX produced persistent hypotension and bradycardia in all anesthetized dogs and suggested that the difference between unanesthetized and anesthetized animals may be attributable to an indirect effect of TTX on the activation of the sympathetic nervous system or on a reduction in vagal tone. Hypertension has been noted in some human cases of TTX poisoning; almost all of them were of mild severity.[9,11,18,27] It seems likely that in nonlethal TTX poisoning, hypertension can be caused by an exaggerated reaction to sympathetic stimuli.

The primary systemic action of TTX is to block the nerve conduction. Although TTX acts primarily on peripheral nerves, it also can cause central nervous system effects in sufficient doses. As previously mentioned, TTX may exert effects on medullary respiratory and vasomotor centers. TTX also is known to induce vomiting, a frequent manifestation of TTX poisoning.[3,5] Because surgical ablation of the medullary chemotrigger receptor zone in dogs and cats abolishes this emetic action, vomiting seems to represent a central action of TTX.[3,63] Nicotinic antagonism by TTX also has been suggested to be responsible for vomiting because tetraethylammonium (a nicotinic agonist), but not chlorpromazine or hexamethonium (a nicotinic antagonist), prevented the emetic action.[5,63]

In experimental animals, TTX causes a sustained decrease in rectal temperature,[3,59,62] but little is known about the mechanism of this action. Anecdotal reports also suggested that TTX may have a central narcotic or sedative effect; TTX has been used as a sedative in the treatment of opioid addiction.[5] Nevertheless, currently available data about the efficacy of TTX in the treatment of this addiction are inconclusive. Paralysis of the motor and sensory components of the spinal cord and indirect central actions of TTX, such as hypoxia-related convulsions, are among the other central nervous system manifestations that have been reported in TTX poisonings.[5]

TTX blocks the neurally elicited responses of the autonomic nervous system[3,5,54] and may cause a decrease in gastric secretory volume, mydriasis, salivation, and hyperglycemia.[5] It has been suggested that TTX may cause a pathologic state that is similar to the pathologic states of organophosphate or carbamate insecticide poisonings.[64] These toxic effects are not consistently observed, however, in animal or human TTX poisonings; the autonomic nerves seem to be more resistant to the effects of the toxin than are the somatic nerves.[5] It also has been suggested that parasympathetic nerves are blocked by TTX before the sympathetic nerves[5] and that the postganglionic nerves are affected less severely than are the preganglionic cholinergic nerves.[54] Although TTX does affect autonomic nerves and probably vascular smooth muscle as well, it is unclear whether it also has direct effects on other smooth muscle or autonomic effector cells.

Few data regarding the pathology of human TTX poisoning are available. In reported cases,[5,8,12,18,41] fatalities caused by TTX poisoning have been characterized by pulmonary edema and generalized congestion of the viscera. Localized changes in the gastric mucosa also have been noted occasionally. There are no reported human neuropathologic alterations based on autopsy findings, although significant changes have been observed in experimental animals.[5] Fig. 118-2 summarizes the pathophysiology of TTX poisoning.

Impure TTX was used widely as an analgesic in Japan in the early 20th century.[1] There currently is no clinical utility for TTX, however, in any practice because its anesthetic properties generally are attained only with near-lethal doses.[5]

CLINICAL PRESENTATION

There have been numerous reports of human TTX poisoning,[5,8–12,14–24,27,32,39–44,65,66] and most humans were intoxicated by ingesting puffer fish. Typically, symptoms begin within 10 to 45 minutes of ingestion because TTX is absorbed rapidly from the gastrointestinal tract[3]; however, this may be delayed for 3 or more hours.[5,10,14] TTX poisoning usually manifests first with a tingling sensation involving the tongue and inner surface of the mouth and throat.[5,7,9,11,12] General malaise, pallor, dizziness, headache, ataxia, constricted pupils, nausea, vomiting, and sweating also are likely to be present early.[5,9,11,14] Paresthesias subsequently may involve the fingers and toes and spread to other parts of the limbs.[5] In more severe poisonings, severe limb numbness, hypotension, cardiac arrhythmia, dyspnea, and generalized weakness may develop, followed by respiratory paralysis, fixed and dilated pupils, and convulsions over the ensuing 4 to 24 hours.[5,7,9,11] Patients with severe TTX poisoning may become or look comatose, yet in most instances their sensorium is intact.[5,14,16] Death in TTX poisoning generally occurs within the first 6 to 24 hours[5,7,11,14] and usually is the result of progressive respiratory paralysis.[1,5,7,9,12] Less frequently, death may result from profound hypotension[1,5] or other complications, such as hypertensive congestive heart failure among hypertensive patients[18] or aspiration pneumonia.[27] Death occurring 17 minutes after TTX poisoning has been reported.[3]

The onset and types of signs and symptoms of TTX poisoning can be diverse because they depend on the individual and the amount of toxin consumed.[5,7,9] Toxic features that have been reported are as follows:

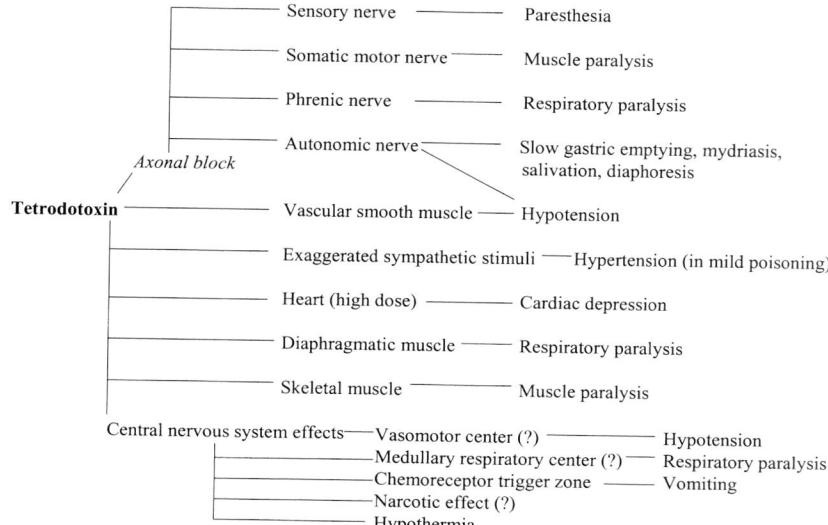

FIGURE 118-2

Pathophysiology of tetrodotoxin poisoning.

1. *Neuromuscular*:[5,9–12,14–18,20,22,27,32,39–41,43,65–67] circumoral numbness, paresthesia of phalanges and extremities, constrictive sensation of throat, dry mouth, floating sensation, generalized paresthesia, extreme weakness with walking difficulty, muscle twitching, tremor, incoordination, extensive limb paralysis, aphonia, dysarthria, dysphagia, backache

2. *Cardiovascular/pulmonary*:[5,9–12,14–20,22,27,32,39,43,65–67] hypotension, rapid and weak pulse, hypertension, cardiac arrhythmias (sinus bradycardia, tachycardia, conduction block, asystole), chest tightness/pain, cyanosis, pallor, chilliness, facial flush, dyspnea, tachypnea, shallow respiration, aspiration pneumonia, acute pulmonary edema, acute respiratory failure, sudden death

3. *Central nervous system (direct or indirect effects)*:[5,8–11,14–20,22,27,32,39–41,65–68] dizziness, vertigo, headache, drowsiness, lethargy, anxiety, transient/prolonged ataxia, blurred vision, hyporeflexia/areflexia, muscle fasciculation, convulsion, peculiar taste sensation, cranial nerve palsy, hypothermia, diabetes insipidus, reversible locked-in syndrome, coma

4. *Autonomic*:[5,9,10,12,14–17,27,32,39,65–67] diaphoresis, initial miosis followed by mydriasis (or, rarely, prolonged constricted pupils), irregular pupils, reflex change of pupils, hypersalivation, urinary incontinence, bronchorrhea

5. *Peripheral sensorimotor nerve functions*:[5,9,15,16,65] diffuse reduction of conduction velocities and amplitudes of sensory and motor nerve action potentials in nerve conduction studies

6. *Gastrointestinal*:[5,8–12,14,17,19,20,27,32,39,41,43,65–67] nausea, vomiting, retching, hyperemesis, hematemesis, increased/decreased gastrointestinal motility, diarrhea, epigastric/abdominal pain

7. *Dermatologic (rare)*:[5,67] exfoliative dermatitis, petechiae, blister, itching

8. *Miscellaneous*:[5,9,10,14,15,17,22,39,67] delayed coagulation of blood, hypokalemia, hypocalcemia, elevated hepatic transaminase levels, hyperglycemia, leukocytosis

Anecdotal reports also suggest that TTX might cause a "living dead" phenomenon; two patients recovered hours or days after they were pronounced dead in the late 19th century.[5] It is unclear, however, how the "death" diagnoses in these two patients were made and whether they were confirmed by any objective tests. TTX has been found in some voodoo potions used to transform a person into a creature of living death (zombi) of Haitian folklore[69,70]; however, its role in zombification is questionable.[71]

In 1941, Fukuda and Tani proposed a severity measure of TTX poisoning (Table 118-1).[5] This scoring system still is used today.

DIAGNOSIS

The diagnosis of TTX poisoning is based largely on clinical manifestations (i.e., the presence of typical neurologic manifestations, such as paresthesia and motor paralysis) and a history of exposure to puffer fish or other TTX-containing organisms. An accurate exposure history may not be available, however, and the clinical presentations of TTX poisoning may be atypical. Some TTX-containing organisms also possess toxins other than TTX (e.g., saxitoxin).[5,26,31,33,44,67,72–74] It is important to formulate a careful differential diagnosis that includes other neurotoxic

TABLE 118-1 Severity Classification of Tetrodotoxin Poisoning	
DEGREE OF POISONING	**CLINICAL MANIFESTATIONS**
First degree	Oral paresthesia with or without gastrointestinal symptoms (e.g., vomiting)
Second degree	Advanced paresthesia and limb paralysis with intact reflexes
Third degree	Presence of gross muscular incoordination, dysphonia, dysphagia, respiratory depression, chest pain, cyanosis, and hypotension, with clear consciousness
Fourth degree	Coma, respiratory paralysis, and severe hypotension, followed by cardiac arrest in the absence of prompt treatment

Data from Fukuda and Tani (1941).[5]

exposures and nontoxic acute paralytic disorders. Among various marine poisonings, paralytic shellfish poisoning (saxitoxin) and ciguatera poisoning (ciguatoxin) are least likely to be distinguished easily clinically from TTX intoxication.[6] An accurate and detailed history is crucial because the species harboring these other neurotoxins usually are different from TTX-containing organisms.[67] A complete physical examination, including a thorough neurologic examination, and electrophysiologic studies are helpful in making the final diagnosis of TTX poisoning; routine laboratory tests are not useful. TTX poisoning should be differentiated from anticholinesterase poisonings, such as those caused by organophosphate or carbamate pesticides or nerve agents. The differential diagnosis is unlikely to be difficult because TTX does not affect cholinesterases significantly,[53–56] and cholinergic features usually are minor and transient in TTX poisoning.

The definitive diagnosis of TTX poisoning relies on the detection of TTX in poisoned patients or in the incriminating poisoning source. Specific methods for detecting TTX (e.g., gas chromatography–mass spectrometry) have been developed.[8,65,72] The procedures are complicated, however, and the assay is rarely available. The clinical utility of these assays is extremely limited. More commonly, bioassay methods can be used to determine the toxicity of a suspected TTX source. These methods are reasonably specific when properly performed.[3] A commonly employed method involves the injection of dilute crude toxin intraperitoneally into mice; the toxicity is expressed semiquantitatively in mouse units (mu) per gram of specimen[3,8,9]; 1 mu is defined as the amount of toxin that kills a 20-g mouse in a standard period of time. It has been said that 200,000 mu of toxicity is the minimal lethal dose for humans,[8,18,27] yet deaths after ingestion of lower doses of TTX have been reported.[18,27] Although these bioassay methods can be performed easily, they are unlikely to be helpful in the early management of TTX-poisoned patients because they are generally unavailable in acute care settings. Nevertheless, these methods can serve as a useful tool in confirming the diagnosis, especially when the exposure history is unclear or there is uncertainty about the incriminating source (e.g., in cases of mixed ingestion of various seafoods). Repeated exposure to TTX does not produce immunity.

TREATMENT

Indications for ICU Admission in Tetrodotoxin Poisoning

Respiratory paralysis or marked respiratory depression (i.e., difficulty in dealing with saliva or bronchial secretions, increasing dyspnea, rising respiratory rate, or worsening arterial blood gases)

Hypotension with impaired perfusion (e.g., oliguria, abnormal renal function, shock)

Symptomatic or significant cardiac dysrhythmia or conductive disturbance

Extensive neurologic dysfunction (e.g., coma, areflexia, fixed and dilated pupils)

Seizures

Other life-threatening complications (e.g., congestive heart failure, severe aspiration pneumonia)

There is no specific antidote for TTX poisoning.[5,51] Treatment is mainly symptomatic and supportive. After exposure to TTX, rapid removal of unabsorbed toxin is theoretically important. If spontaneous vomiting does not occur, an emetic (often apomorphine)[5,10] frequently is given, provided that there is no risk of aspiration.[5,6,14] This practice has not been shown to improve outcome, however, or alter the clinical course. Induction of emesis may be contraindicated because of an increased risk of aspiration. Gastric lavage may be used shortly after TTX poisoning (1 to 3 hours)[5,10,14,15] in an attempt to remove toxin still in the stomach. This technique also has not been shown to improve outcome or affect the patient's clinical course. Although it is uncertain whether gastric lavage would be effective, theoretically it may remove some toxin even more than 3 hours after ingestion because TTX can slow gastric emptying.[5] Because TTX is less stable in an alkaline environment, Sims and Ostman[10] suggested the use of 2% sodium bicarbonate solution in gastric lavage. The efficacy of this intervention is unproven, however. Activated charcoal is reportedly effective in early TTX poisoning.[9,10] Some investigators even recommend endoscopy as a measure to remove the ingested toxin.[39,75]

After the occurrence of systemic manifestations, treatment should be aimed at the maintenance of adequate ventilation and circulation because respiratory arrest and profound hypotension are the two major causes of death.[5,14] Supplemental oxygen is indicated in patients with hypoxia, hypoventilation, or respiratory distress. Early endotracheal intubation and mechanical ventilation, which are potentially lifesaving interventions,[9,23] are indicated in patients with difficulty handling saliva or respiratory secretions, increasing dyspnea, hypoventilation or hyperventilation, or worsening arterial blood gases.[5,14] Because patients usually are conscious, a full explanation of all procedures and sedation should be provided if they need intubation.[14] Tracheostomy is not necessary because recovery from TTX poisoning usually is rapid and complete within 24 hours.[5] Antibiotics may be required in patients whose clinical courses are complicated by aspiration pneumonia.[9,20]

In patients with hypotension, fluid resuscitation should be given as indicated based on arterial blood pressure, urinary output, cardiac output, systemic vascular resistance, or central venous pressure.[5,14] Vasopressor agents, inotropic agents, or both also may be required to alleviate hypotension if cardiac output, systemic vascular resistance, or both decrease or if central venous pressure increases without restoration of urine output. A target urine output of equal to or greater than 40 mL/hr has been suggested.[5] Maintenance of a brisk production of urine is theoretically important in speeding recovery because TTX is eliminated mainly unchanged by the kidney within a few hours of ingestion.[3,51]

Among various inotropic agents, it has been shown in experimental animals that amphetamine, phenylephrine, and norepinephrine are the most effective in treating hypotensive effects of TTX, possibly due to their ability to stimulate directly or indirectly postsynaptic α-adrenergic receptors.[45] Epinephrine, probably because of its predominantly β-adrenergic effects, is less effective or in some instances detrimental.[5,45] It is unclear whether these observations can be applied to human TTX poisonings. Some investigators have suggested the use of dopamine as the first-line inotropic agent.[10] Atropine can be given to patients with bradycardia, but its efficacy is controversial.[10,14,15,56] Because bradycardia is rarely a serious problem in TTX poisoning, atropine is not routinely necessary. The electrocardiogram should be monitored continuously for cardiac dysrhythmias, however, and a temporary pacemaker may have to be inserted in cases of severe conduction disturbance.[5,14] Hypertension in TTX poisoning is usually mild and transient[9] but may require treatment with antihypertensive medications in severe cases or in patients with preexisting hypertension.[18] Because of the possibility of the patient's progressing from hypertension to hypotension, only short-acting antihypertensive agents, such as sodium nitroprusside, should be used.

Several experimental therapeutic modalities have been suggested in the management of human TTX poisoning but their roles are controversial, and none have been scrutinized by large-scale prospective clinical studies.[10,17] Anticholinesterase drugs (e.g., edrophonium), which can increase the concentration of acetylcholine at the neuromuscular junction, have been shown to be promising in some reports[14,22] but not in others.[3,5,9,15] Because TTX probably does not act on the motor end plate until its concentration reaches a high level,[76] anticholinesterase drugs are not likely to be useful treatments.[3] Cysteine also has been claimed to be potentially effective in the management of TTX poisoning,[5,10] and several possible mechanisms have been proposed.[17] Nevertheless, its benefit in human poisonings has not been documented. Other possible, yet unproven, therapeutic strategies for TTX poisoning are antihistamines, steroids, naloxone, veratrine-like agents, calcium, and hyperbaric oxygenation.[5,6,17,23,67] Antiserum and monoclonal antibodies against TTX have been developed and tested successfully in experimental animals,[77–79] but their role in human TTX poisoning needs further research.

Hemodialysis instituted 21 hours after TTX poisoning was reported to be effective in a uremic patient who manifested profound neurologic dysfunction.[40] It is not clear, however, whether the relationship of this intervention to clinical outcome was more than a coincidence. TTX is only slightly water soluble under normal circumstances,[3,5,51] and hemodialysis may not be an effective treatment. TTX has a low molecular weight and is minimally bound, however, which are properties often found in toxins amenable to hemodialysis. Despite these considerations, the short course of TTX poisoning and the effectiveness of mechanical ventilation and supportive measures undermine the potential benefits of hemodialysis.

The prognosis of TTX poisoning usually is favorable if adequate supportive measures can be instituted before cardiopulmonary arrest occurs. Because TTX can cause coma, areflexia, dilated pupils, or other signs of extensive brain damage early in the course of poisoning, resuscitation should not be abandoned prematurely even in the presence of the above-noted signs.[15,19] If a patient survives beyond 24 hours, the recovery is likely to be complete unless complicated by other life-threatening conditions.[5,6,9,14,17]

Common Misconceptions about Tetrodotoxin Poisoning

1. Tetrodotoxin is found only in puffer fish.
2. The musculature of puffer fish always is safe to eat.
3. It is not difficult to differentiate between poisonous and edible puffer fish.
4. A puffer fish that previously was safe to eat always is non-toxic.
5. Puffer fish or other tetrodotoxin-containing organisms contain only tetrodotoxin.
6. Tetrodotoxin has a major effect on the acetylcholine-cholinesterase system.
7. Tetrodotoxin causes respiratory depression and hypotension mainly through its central depressant effects.
8. Tetrodotoxin poisoning always manifests hypotension.
9. The presence of extensive neurologic dysfunction in a patient with tetrodotoxin poisoning often indicates severe hypoxic brain damage, and aggressive resuscitation is unnecessary.

Key Points in Tetrodotoxin Poisoning

1. Tetrodotoxin is a heat-stable nonprotein toxin.
2. Tetrodotoxin can be found in a wide variety of totally unrelated aquatic organisms and amphibians.
3. Tetrodotoxin poisoning most commonly is caused by consumption of puffer fish, which has a worldwide distribution.
4. Puffer fish poisoning usually is the result of improper handling of the fish (e.g., private sale and preparation by fishmongers or vagabonds).
5. In puffer fish, tetrodotoxin is found mainly in the liver, ovaries, intestines, and skin.
6. The toxicity of puffer fish varies according to sex, species, season of the year, geographic locality, and organ of the animals.
7. The main pharmacologic mechanism of tetrodotoxin is to block the propagation of nerve action potentials by non-depolarizing blockade through its selective inhibition on the sodium channel.
8. Tetrodotoxin mainly affects the neuromuscular system, especially respiratory muscles.
9. Respiratory depression and hypotension are the two characteristic manifestations and the leading causes of death from tetrodotoxin poisoning.
10. Tetrodotoxin poisoning is not common; however, it has high mortality if proper treatment is not instituted promptly.
11. The treatment of tetrodotoxin poisoning is largely symptomatic and supportive. Treatment should be aimed primarily at the maintenance of adequate ventilation and circulation.
12. If a patient survives the first 24 hours, a complete recovery should be anticipated unless complicated by other life-threatening conditions.

Criteria for ICU Discharge in Tetrodotoxin Poisoning

Successful weaning from ventilatory support
Normal blood pressure in the absence of inotropic agents
Adequate control of life-threatening complications

REFERENCES

1. Fuhrman FA: Tetrodotoxin. Sci Am 217:61–71, 1967.
2. Kao CY: Pharmacology of tetrodotoxin and saxitoxin. Fed Proc 31:1117–1123, 1972.
3. Kao CY: Tetrodotoxin, saxitoxin and their significance in the study of excitation phenomena. Pharmacol Rev 18:997–1049, 1966.
4. Mills AR, Passmore R: Pelagic paralysis. Lancet 1:161–164, 1988.

5. Halstead BW: Poisonous and Venomous Marine Animals of the World, 2nd ed. Princeton, NJ, Darwin Press, 1988.

6. Lange WR: Puffer fish poisoning. Am Fam Physician 42:1029–1033, 1990.

7. Yang CC, Deng JF: Overview of marine toxins: I. Tetrodotoxin. Clin Med 38:125–135, 1996.

8. Tsunenari S, Uchimura Y, Kanda M: Puffer poisoning in Japan—a case report. J Forensic Sci 25:240–245, 1980.

9. Yang CC, Liao SC, Deng JF: Tetrodotoxin poisoning in Taiwan. Vet Hum Toxicol 38:282–286, 1996.

10. Sims JK, Ostman DC: Pufferfish poisoning: Emergency diagnosis and management of mild human tetrodotoxication. Ann Emerg Med 15:1094–1098, 1986.

11. Anonymous: Tetrodotoxin poisoning associated with eating puffer fish transported from Japan—California, 1996. JAMA 275:1631–1632, 1996.

12. Benson J: Tetraodon (blowfish) poisoning: A report of two fatalities. J Forensic Sci 1:119–125, 1956.

13. Sierra-Beltran AP, Cruz A, Nunez E, et al: An overview of the marine food poisoning in Mexico. Toxicon 36:1493–1502, 1998.

14. Torda TA, Sinclair E, Ulyatt DB: Puffer fish (tetrodotoxin) poisoning: Clinical record and suggested management. Med J Aust 1:599–602, 1973.

15. Tibballs J: Severe tetrodotoxic fish poisoning. Anaesth Intens Care 16:215–217, 1988.

16. Trevett AJ, Mavo B, Warrell DA: Tetrodotoxic poisoning from ingestion of a porcupine fish (Diodon Hystrix) in Papua New Guinea: Nerve conduction studies. Am J Trop Med Hyg 56:30–32, 1997.

17. Sun K, Wat J, So P: Puffer fish poisoning. Anaesth Intensive Care 22:307–308, 1994.

18. Deng JF, Tominack RL, Chung HM, et al: Hypertension as an unusual feature in an outbreak of tetrodotoxin poisoning. Clin Toxicol 29:71–79, 1991.

19. Tambyah PA, Hui KP, Gopalakrishnakone P, et al: Central-nervous-system effects of tetrodotoxin poisoning. Lancet 343:538–539, 1994.

20. Laobhripatr S, Limpakarnjanarat K, Sangwonloy O, et al: Food poisoning due to consumption of the freshwater puffer Tetraodon fangi in Thailand. Toxicon 28:1372–1375, 1990.

21. Kanchanapongkul J: Puffer fish poisoning: Clinical features and management experience in 25 cases. J Med Assoc Thai 84:385–389, 2001.

22. Chew SK, Chew LS, Wang KW, et al: Anticholinesterase drugs in the treatment of tetrodotoxin poisoning. Lancet 2:108, 1984.

23. Lyn PC: Puffer fish poisoning: Four case reports. Med J Malaysia 40:31–34, 1985.

24. Kan SK, Chan MK, David P: Nine fatal cases of puffer fish poisoning in Sabah, Malaysia. Med J Malaysia 42:199–200, 1987.

25. Sheumack DD, Howden MEH, Spence I, et al: Maculotoxin: A neurotoxin from the venom glands of the octopus Hapalochlaena maculosa identified as tetrodotoxin. Science 199:188–189, 1978.

26. Hwang DF, Lin LC, Jeng SS: Occurrence of a new toxin and tetrodotoxin in two species of the gastropod mollusk Nassariidae. Toxicon 30:41–46, 1992.

27. Yang CC, Han KC, Lin TJ, et al: An outbreak of tetrodotoxin poisoning following gastropod mollusc consumption. Hum Exp Toxicol 14:446–450, 1995.

28. Hashimoto Y, Noguchi T: Occurrence of a tetrodotoxin-like substance in a goby Gobius criniger. Toxicon 9:79–84, 1971.

29. Maruyama J, Noguchi T, Jeon JK, et al: Occurrence of tetrodotoxin in the starfish Astropecten latespinosus. Experientia 40:1395–1396, 1984.

30. Inoue A, Noguchi T, Konosu S, et al: A new toxic crab, Atergatis floridus. Toxicon 6:119–123, 1968.

31. Noguchi T, Uzu A, Daigo K, et al: A tetrodotoxin-like substance as a minor toxin in the xanthid crab Atergatis floridus. Toxicon 22:425–432, 1984.

32. Kanchanapongkul J, Krittayapoositpot P: An epidemic of tetrodotoxin poisoning following ingestion of the horseshoe crab Carcinoscorpius rotundicauda. Southeast Asian J Trop Med Public Health 26:364–367, 1995.

33. Tsai YH, Hwang DF, Chai TJ, et al: Occurrence of tetrodotoxin and paralytic shellfish poison in the Taiwanese crab Lophozozymus pictor. Toxicon 33:1669–1673, 1995.

34. Miyazawa K, Higashiyama M, Ito K, et al: Tetrodotoxin in two species of ribbon worm (nemertini), Lineus fuscoviridis and Tubulanus punctatus. Toxicon 26:867–874, 1988.

35. Kim YH, Brown GB, Mosher HS, et al: Tetrodotoxin: Occurrence in atelopid frogs of Costa Rica. Science 189:151–152, 1975.

36. Wakely JF, Fuhrman GJ, Fuhrman FA, et al: The occurrence of tetrodotoxin (tarichatoxin) in amphibian and the distribution of the toxin in the organs of newts (Tacha). Toxicon 3:195–203, 1966.

37. Levenson CH, Woodhull AM: The occurrence of a tetrodotoxin-like substance in the red-spotted newts, Notophthalmus viridescens. Toxicon 17:184–187, 1979.

38. Brown MS, Mosher HS: Tarichatoxin: Isolation and purification. Science 140:295–296, 1963.

39. Fong VH, Chow SY: Electrophysiological studies on acute tetrodotoxin poisoning: A case report. Chin Med J (Taipei) 58:299–302, 1996.

40. Lan MY, Lai SL, Chen SS, et al: Tetrodotoxin intoxication in a uraemic patient. J Neurol Neurosurg Psychiatry 67:127–128, 1999.

41. Bradley SG, Klika LJ: Fatal poisoning from the Oregon rough-skinned newt (Taricha granulosa). JAMA 246:247, 1981.

42. King BR, Hamilton RJ, Kassutto Z: "Tail of newt": An unusual ingestion. Pediatr Emerg Care 16:268–269, 2000.

43. Flecker H, Cotton BC: Fatal bite from octopus. Med J Aust 26:329–331, 1955.

44. Sutherland SK, Lane WR: Toxins and mode of envenomation of the common ringed or blue-banded octopus. Med J Aust 1:893–898, 1969.

45. Flachsenberger WA: Respiratory failure and lethal hypotension due to blue-ringed octopus and tetrodotoxin envenomation observed and countered in animal models. Clin Toxicol 24:485–502, 1986–1987.

46. Yasumoto T, Yasumura D, Yotsu M, et al: Bacterial production of tetrodotoxin and anhydrotetrodotoxin. Agric Biol Chem 50:793–795, 1986.

47. Yotsu M, Yamazaki T, Meguro Y, et al: Production of tetrodotoxin and its derivatives by Pseudomonas sp. isolated from the skin of a pufferfish. Toxicon 25:225–228, 1987.

48. Matsui T, Sato H, Hamada S, et al: Comparison of toxicity of the cultured and wide puffer fish Fugu-niphobles. Bull Jpn Soc Sci Fish 48:253–254, 1982.

49. Kodama M, Sato S, Ogata T, et al: Tetrodotoxin secreting glands in the skin of puffer fishes. Toxicon 24:819–829, 1986.

50. Nagai J, Ito T: On the chemical study of fugu (spheroides) poison. J Biochem (Tokyo) 30:235–238, 1939.

51. Evans MH: Mechanism of saxitoxin and tetrodotoxin poisoning. Br Med Bull 25:263–267, 1969.

52. Fleisher JH, Killos PJ, Harrison CS: Effects of puffer poison on neuromuscular transmission (Abstract). Fed Proc 19:264, 1960.

53. Fleisher JH, Killos PJ, Harrison CS: Effects of puffer poison on neuromuscular transmission. J Pharmacol Exp Ther 133:98–105, 1961.

54. Kao CY, Fuhrman FA: Pharmacological studies on tarichatoxin, a potent neurotoxin. J Pharmacol Exp Ther 140:31–40, 1963.

55. Dettbarn WD, Higman HB, Rosenberg P, et al: Rapid and reversible block of electrical activity by powerful marine biotoxins. Science 132:300–301, 1960.

56. Yudkin WH: The occurrence of a cardio-inhibitor in the ovaries of the puffer, Spheroides maculates. J Cell Comp Physiol 25:85–95, 1945.

57. Cheng KK, Ling YL, Wang JCC: The failure of respiration in death by tetrodotoxin poisoning. Q J Exp Physiol 53:119–128, 1968.

58. Li KM: Action of puffer fish poison. Nature 200:791, 1963.

59. Borison HL, McCarthy LE, Clark WG, et al: Vomiting, hypothermia, and respiratory paralysis due to tetrodotoxin (puffer poison) in the cat. Appl Pharmacol 5:350–357, 1963.

60. Bernstein ME: Pharmacologic effects of tetrodotoxin: Cardiovascular and antiarrhythmic activities. Toxicon 7:287–302, 1969.

61. Lipsius MR, Siegman MJ, Kao CY: Direct relaxant actions of procaine and tetrodotoxin on vascular smooth muscles. J Pharmacol Exp Ther 164:60–74, 1968.

62. Duce BR, Feldman HS, Smith ER: Acute cardiovascular, antiarrhythmic and toxic effects of tetrodotoxin (TTX) in unanesthetized dogs. Toxicol Appl Pharmacol 23:701–712, 1972.

63. Hayama T, Ogura Y: Site of emetic action of tetrodotoxin in dog, I. Pharmacol Exp Ther 139:94–96, 1963.

64. Mackenzie CF, Smalley AJ, Barnas GM, et al: Tetrodotoxin infusion: nonventilatory effects and role in toxicity models. Acad Emerg Med 3:1106–1112, 1996.

65. Oda K, Araki K, Totoki T, et al: Nerve conduction study of human tetrodotoxication. Neurology 39:743–745, 1989.

66. Wilson SF, Collins N: Ataxia and toadfish poisoning. Aust N Z J Med 30:637, 2000.

67. Sims JK: A theoretical discourse on the pharmacology of toxic marine ingestions. Ann Emerg Med 16:1006–1015, 1987.
68. Udaka F, Kameyama M: A case of reversible "locked-in syndrome" like state due to pufferfish poisoning. Clin Neurol (Tokyo) 21:762–766, 1981.
69. Davis W: Tetrodotoxin and the zombi phenomenon. J Ethnopharmacol 25:119–122, 1989.
70. Benedek C, Rivier L: Evidence for the presence of tetrodotoxin in a powder used in Haiti for zombification. Toxicon 27:473–480, 1989.
71. Booth W: Voodooscience. Science 240:274–277, 1988.
72. Suenaga K: Verification of tetrodotoxin by instrumental analysis. Japan J Legal Med 32:97–111, 1978.
73. Sato S, Ogata T, Borja V, et al: Frequent occurrence of paralytic shellfish poisoning toxins as dominant toxins in marine puffer from tropical water. Toxicon 38:1101–1109, 2000.
74. Mahmud Y, Arakawa O, Noguchi T: An epidemic survey on freshwater puffer poisoning in Bangladesh. J Natural Toxins 9:319–326, 2000.
75. Goldfrank L, Lewin N, Weisman R: The red snapper. Hosp Physician 5:36–51, 1981.
76. Matsumura M, Yamamoto S: The effect of tetrodotoxin on the neuromuscular junction and peripheral nerve of the toad. Jpn J Pharmacol 4:62–68, 1954.
77. Fukiya S, Matsumura K: Active and passive immunization for tetrodotoxin in mice. Toxicon 30:1631–1634, 1992.
78. Matsumura K: A monoclonal antibody against tetrodotoxin that reacts to the active group for the toxicity. Eur J Pharmacol 293:41–45, 1995.
79. Rivera VR, Poli MA, Bignami GS: Prophylaxis and treatment with a monoclonal antibody of tetrodotoxin poisoning in mice. Toxicon 33:1231–1237, 1995.

CHAPTER **119**

Overview of Mushroom Poisoning

Michael Beuhler ■ Kimberlie A. Graeme

Mushroom ingestions often evoke fear in clinicians because of the lethality of certain species and the difficulty differentiating between types of mushrooms. Modern methods of intensive care medicine have reduced mushroom mortality and morbidity substantially. Nearly all mushroom fatalities are due to amatoxin, but there are some notable exceptions.[1] It is often difficult to determine the exact species ingested. Understanding of the anatomy of a mushroom is important for this determination (Fig. 119-1).[2]

Even if the allegedly culpable mushroom is brought to the emergency department along with the patient, often it was not the actual mushroom that was consumed. Multiple species often grow together. Some mushrooms contain multiple pharmacologically active compounds. Laboratory tests to identify toxins may not be available for days to weeks or may be completely unavailable.

It is important to focus initially on the patient's examination, clinical presentation in relation to the time of consumption, and emergent supportive treatment, rather than on mushroom identification. As a general guideline, mushroom ingestions may be separated into two groups: mushrooms that produce symptoms within 4 hours and mushrooms that produce symptoms after 6 hours (Table 119-1). These times are far from being absolutely reliable, however, because there is significant individual variability. This chapter and Chapters 120 and 121 delineate symptom onset and treatment for each of these groups of mushrooms. There are many variations on the "classic" presentations, however.

Universal treatment recommendations for mushroom ingestions do not exist. Administration of ipecac is no longer recommended because it may mask the presence of gastroin-

testinal irritation (a possible clue to the identity of the mushroom ingested) and has never been shown to alter outcome. Gastric lavage is not risk free and has not been shown to alter outcome. Lavage tubes often have become blocked by mushroom fragments.[3] Activated charcoal may be used for gastrointestinal decontamination if there is a concern for amatoxins, but caution should be used because of the risk of aspiration, especially in the presence of altered mental status. Treatment of any mushroom ingestion with atropine is no longer recommended because toxicity from some types of mushroom ingestions may worsen with atropine. Because of the overall paucity of information on mushroom toxicity, it is particularly difficult to give specific recommendations for treatment of pregnant women and pediatric patients.

Criteria for ICU Discharge in Mushroom Poisoning

Patient's signs and symptoms have resolved
Patient has stabilized for non–intensive care unit treatment

Common Misconceptions about Mushroom Poisoning

1. Gastric lavage is risk free.
2. Gastric lavage has been shown to alter outcome after mushroom ingestion.
3. If a patient is ill early (<4 hours) after mushroom ingestion, the patient will not become critically ill later.

Indications for ICU Admission in Mushroom Poisoning

Patient has evidence of end-organ damage (e.g., renal insufficiency or failure, elevated liver transaminases, rhabdomyolysis)
Patient has persistent altered mental status or status epilepticus
Patient has unstable or significantly abnormal vital signs

Key Points in Mushroom Poisoning

1. Identification of mushrooms and their toxins is generally not readily available.
2. The focus should be on the clinical course and supportive care of patients.

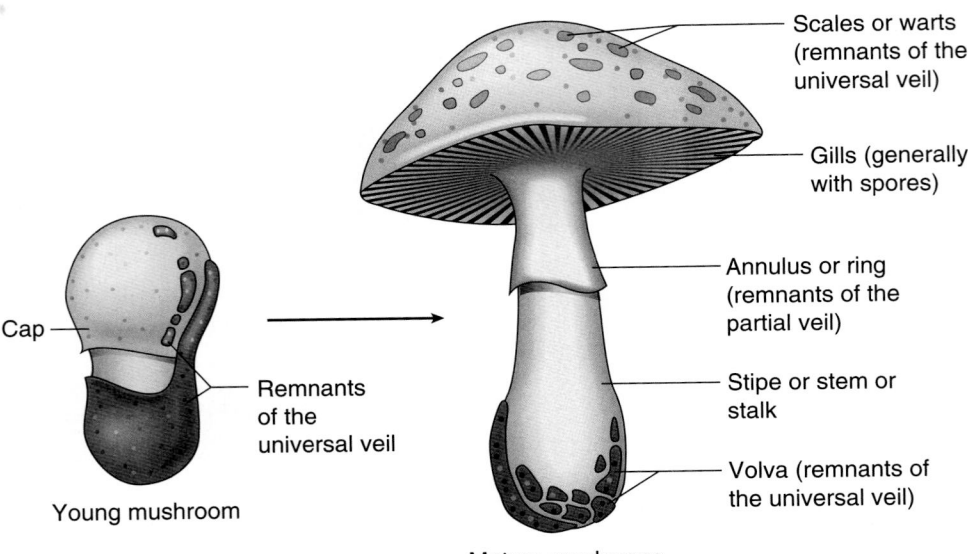

Scales or warts
(remnants of the
universal veil)

Gills (generally
with spores)

Annulus or ring
(remnants of the
partial veil)

Stipe or stem or
stalk

Volva (remnants of
the universal veil)

Cap

Remnants
of the
universal veil

Young mushroom

Mature mushroom

FIGURE 119-1

Anatomy of a mushroom.

NEPHROTOXIC MUSHROOMS

 Nephrotoxic Mushrooms

Include *Cortinarius* spp. and *Amanita smithiana*
Cortinarius spp. ingestion associated with delay of days
  before symptom onset
May need hemodialysis for renal failure

The genus *Cortinarius* grows in semimountainous forests and is usually found from the end of summer through early autumn.[4] The *Cortinarius* genus is common in Europe. Nephrotoxic species include *Cortinarius orellanus, Cortinarius gentilis, Cortinarius speciosissimus*, and *Cortinarius splendens*.[5,6] They are found occasionally in Australia and less commonly in North America.[7] *C. orellanus* is difficult to identify because of a lack of distinctive mor-phologic characteristics. The caps are medium sized (2 to 5 cm) with orange or orange-brown to dark gray-yellow coloration with fine scales. The gills are rusty orange to dark orange-yellow, the stalk is thick with a yellow-to-orange color, and the spores are rust brown.[2,4]

The nephrotoxicity of *C. orellanus* was first described in Poland in 1956. The toxicity was not recognized initially because of the long delay between ingestion and the development of renal failure.[8]

The nephrotoxicity of *Amanita smithiana* has been recognized more recently. *A. smithiana* was implicated in a series of patients with renal failure who presented with clinical effects similar, but not identical, to those arising from ingestion of *Cortinarius* mushrooms.[9,10] *A. smithiana* is found in the Pacific Northwest of the United States and is commonly mistaken for the pine mushroom *Tricholoma magnivelare*.[9,11] *A. smithiana* usually is found growing under conifers and is a light-colored mushroom that changes from a light brown to yellow-brown with age and handling. It has a large (5 to 12 cm) cap with white gills and spores and a long white, rough, bulbous (10 to 20 cm) stem with a ring.[9,11] Part of the stem, which may be helpful in later identification, occasionally remains behind when picked.[10] Older specimens of *A. smithiana* may have a strong unpleasant odor.[10]

Biochemistry

The toxic compound in *Cortinarius* mushrooms is orellanine, a cationic bipyridine similar to paraquat, present in amounts up to 1.4% by weight (Fig. 119-2).[12,13] It is a resilient toxin, resistant to heat, freezing, and drying.[12,14] Orellanine is concentrated in renal tissue, possibly due to active cellular uptake. The exact mechanism of toxicity of orellanine is unknown, but available evidence indicates that it causes a disruption of cytoskeleton actin filaments and inhibits protein synthesis in cell culture after 24 hours.[14–16] Orellanine requires activation by mitochondria (or possibly light) before cytotoxicity.[5,16] *Cortinarius* spp. also contain cortinarin A and B, cyclopeptides that may contribute to nephrotoxicity.[5,6,13]

TABLE 119-1 Onset of Symptoms of Various Mushroom Ingestions

GENERALLY PRODUCE SYMPTOMS WITHIN 4 HOURS	GENERALLY PRODUCE SYMPTOMS AFTER 6 HOURS
Gastrointestinal irritant mushroom species (e.g., *Chlorophyllum molybdites*)	Monomethylhydrazine-containing mushrooms (e.g., *Gyromitra* spp.)
Amanita smithiana (nephrotoxic)	Mushrooms that contain amatoxin (some *Amanita* spp.)
Mushrooms containing coprine (ethanol reaction)	*Cortinarius* (nephrotoxic)
Mushrooms containing muscarine	
Mushrooms containing psilocybin	
Mushrooms containing ibotenic acid and muscimol	

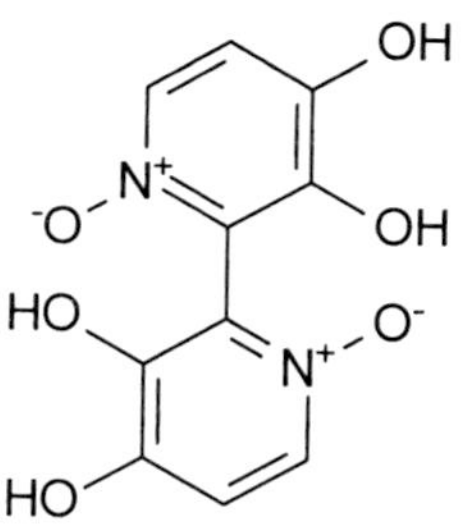

FIGURE 119-2

Chemical structure of orellanine.

A. smithiana contains aminohexadienoic acid, which is believed to be responsible for its toxicity.[9,17,18] The injury from aminohexadienoic acid observed in cell culture and animal models is similar to that seen after ingestion of *A. smithiana* and occurs after a latency period of 12 hours.[10,18,19]

Clinical Presentation

Ingestion of one fruiting body of *C. orellanus* or *A. smithiana* has been reported to cause renal injury in otherwise healthy individuals; however, a dose of 100 g usually is required.[8,10,20] Acute renal failure develops in about 30% to 45% of orellanine-poisoned patients, but this percentage has been found to depend on the amount eaten, the age of the mushrooms, and the environmental conditions.[21] Neither *C. orellanus* nor *A. smithiana* causes clinically significant hepatic injury.

The onset of *C. orellanus* toxicity is delayed, with no early symptoms. Patients who ingest *C. orellanus* typically are asymptomatic for 2 to 14 days (average 6 days and maximum 17 days) before symptoms develop.[7,10,21] Symptoms consist of nausea, vomiting, abdominal pain, chills, malaise, dizziness, paresthesias, myalgias, headache, polydipsia, and polyuria followed by oliguria or anuria.[8,21] Renal failure occurs in approximately one third of all ingestions and is usually the reason for presentation. Severely poisoned patients tend to present earlier. The onset of symptoms coincides with the clinical manifestations of renal failure, rather than occurring as a separate prodrome of symptoms as with *A. smithiana*.[22,23] Recovery of renal function after poisoning may occur over several weeks. Patients occasionally are left with residual hypertension.[7] Of patients poisoned with *C. orellanus*, 30% to 66% do not have complete recovery of renal function and have chronic renal insufficiency or failure.[4,5,15,21] Transplantation has been successful in some patients.[22,23]

Patients ingesting *A. smithiana* mushrooms have a short, but variable, asymptomatic delay, ranging from 30 minutes to 12 hours (average 6 hours). The onset of symptoms occurs more rapidly than with orellanine-containing mushrooms. This rapidity of effect also is observed in cell culture.[10,18] Symptoms of nausea, vomiting, diarrhea, abdominal cramps, rash, myalgias, fatigue, headache, and weakness are characteristic and can last for days. These symptoms occasionally may improve before the onset of renal failure. Patients intoxicated with *A. smithiana* tend to develop renal failure 2 to 5 days after ingestion.

Occasionally, clinically insignificant hepatic transaminase elevations ensue.[9,10] A greater percentage of patients poisoned by *A. smithiana* recover renal function than do patients poisoned by *C. orellanus*. It is believed that patients with preexisting renal insufficiency are at greater risk for developing renal failure from *A. smithiana*.

Diagnosis

Overall the diagnosis of mushroom-induced nephrotoxicity usually is made retrospectively based on descriptions of the ingested mushrooms and the clinical presentation. After ingestion of *C. orellanus*, leukocyturia, proteinuria, and hematuria are typically observed early in the clinical course.[5,24] If an appropriate sample is available, microscopic identification of the spores of *Cortinarius* or *A. smithiana* possibly can be made by an experienced mycologist. A poison control center or botanical garden may be of assistance in identifying a local mycologist. Orellanine may be found in urine for 24 hours after ingestion but cannot be found in urine, plasma, or dialysis fluid after onset of symptoms.[20,25,26] Orellanine may be assayed by high-performance liquid chromatography or thin-layer chromatography.[26,27]

A qualitative test for orellanine in a mushroom sample using ferric chloride is accomplished by crushing fresh or dried mushrooms in 5 volumes of water and filtering after standing for 10 minutes at room temperature. The filtrate is mixed with an equal amount of 3% ferric chloride hexahydrate dissolved in 0.5 normal hydrochloric acid. The presence of orellanine is suspected if a dark gray-blue color appears.[28]

Renal biopsy findings of patients with *C. orellanus* poisoning have shown acute tubular necrosis with interstitial fibrosis, mitochondrial injury, and inflammatory edema; tubulointerstitial nephritis is the most common biopsy finding, developing within 4 days of ingestion.[7,15,16,24,25,29] Rat studies show interstitial and tubular epithelial pathology beginning within 12 hours of poisoning; however, rats exhibit great interanimal variability in sensitivity to orellanine-induced renal injury.[20] Orellanine has been detected in small quantities in some renal tissue samples weeks after ingestion.[26]

Treatment

ORELLANINE-CONTAINING MUSHROOMS

Treatment options for orellanine are limited because the patient is unlikely to present early after the ingestion, during the asymptomatic period. Gastrointestinal decontamination with activated charcoal may be beneficial in early presenting patients but has not been studied. Patients in renal failure should be admitted for monitoring and possibly hemodialysis. Although some advocate early, aggressive dialysis, the benefit of this intervention is questionable because the toxin seems to be dialyzable only for 24 hours, the injury occurs subclinically as early as 12 hours, and clinical presentation is typically delayed.[20,23,25] Orellanine crosses the dialysis membrane and has been shown to adsorb onto hemoperfusion resin.[23,25] Some clinicians have tried hemoperfusion and plasmapheresis to eliminate serum protein-bound toxins. There is extremely limited clinical experience using hemoperfusion, but some anecdotal data suggest improved outcome.[25,30] Other treatments have been tried on an individual basis, including corticosteroids, acetylsalicylic acid, diltiazem, and dopamine, but none have any demonstrated effect on clinical outcome.[25] Furosemide has worsened outcome in animals.[31] Some patients have received renal transplantation.[15,20]

AMANITA SMITHIANA

No specific treatment for *A. smithiana* has been proposed. Most patients (80%) recover renal function after 4 weeks but may need dialysis in the interim. The more rapid onset of injury with aminohexadienoic acid, compared with orellanine, suggests that early dialysis is unlikely to be beneficial.

Special Populations

Elderly and diabetic patients intoxicated with *A. smithiana* or *C. orellanus* tend to develop renal failure more rapidly than other patients.[10] In addition, elderly patients tend to have less renal improvement after poisoning by *C. orellanus* and require dialysis longer than younger patients.[7] With *A. smithiana*, the elderly may develop renal failure sooner and require dialysis longer.[10] There are no published data regarding toxicity of either mushroom in pregnancy.

MUSCARINE-CONTAINING MUSHROOMS

Muscarine-Containing Mushrooms
Include *Clitocybe* spp. and *Inocybe* spp.
Agonists at acetylcholine muscarinic receptors
Cholinergic syndrome seen
Antidote is atropine or possibly glycopyrrolate

Muscarine is found in a broad range of mushroom species, but the two genera of greatest importance are *Clitocybe* and *Inocybe*. In addition, the mushroom *Rhodophyllus rhodopolius*, found in Japan, has been shown to contain muscarine in quantities sufficient to produce human illness.[32] Multiple other species, including *Amanita muscaria*, contain small amounts of muscarine but not enough to produce muscarine poisoning.[33]

The genus *Clitocybe* includes edible species and multiple inedible muscarine-containing species, including *Clitocybe dealbata*, *Clitocybe cerrusata*, *Clitocybe rivulosa*, and *Clitocybe candicans*.[2,34,35] These mushrooms are found worldwide, usually growing in forests or grasslands, and may be found in fairy ring formations. The mushrooms often have white-to-brown, small, funnel-shaped caps with light gray, white, or cream-colored gills. The spores are white to grayish yellow, pink, or violet. The flesh may have a pleasant smell. No veil or ring is present. There are substantial differences in morphology among species.[2]

The genus *Inocybe* includes many different species, and most contain muscarine.[35–37] These mushrooms are found worldwide and usually grow in soil under trees. The conical caps have a surface pattern similar to a bicycle wheel with streaks radiating from the center. Gills are light when young and become brown at maturity. The spores are brown to yellowish brown. The flesh has an earthy to unpleasant smell. The veil is fragile. There are minor differences in morphology among species.[2]

Biochemistry and Pathophysiology

Muscarine is a quaternary ammonium compound (Fig. 119-3). Four stereoisomers are found in nature, but only L-(+)-muscarine has significant physiologic activity.[33,34] Muscarine is not degraded by either boiling or peptic digestion.[38] It is usually found in concentrations of 0.1% to 0.3% dry weight in *Inocybe* and *Clitocybe* spp., but the amount may vary by three orders of magnitude among species.[34,36,37] Its gastrointestinal absorption appears to be limited and erratic. The median lethal dose in humans is unknown but has been suggested to be around 200 mg.[38,39]

Muscarine is a small, charged molecule that has specific agonist activity at acetylcholine muscarinic receptors (see Chapter 23), a property used experimentally to define these receptors. This agonism produces a cholinergic muscarinic syndrome. As a result of its positive charge, muscarine has limited ability to cross the blood-brain barrier, and its toxicity is limited to peripheral effects.[33] Muscarine has no affinity for and is not metabolized by acetylcholinesterase.[33] Some muscarine is renally excreted and may be detectable in urine.[40]

Clinical Presentation

Symptoms from ingestion of muscarine-containing mushrooms are primarily cholinergic and typically begin 0.5 to 2.5 hours after ingestion. Among the various mushroom poisonings, the constellation of signs that are characteristic of muscarine intoxication are lacrimation, perspiration, and salivation. Other commonly reported clinical manifestations are nausea and vomiting (seen in nearly all patients), abdominal pain, anxiety, wheezing, headache, fatigue, chills, perioral paresthesias, diplopia, urinary urgency, and diarrhea.[41] Muscarine-intoxicated patients occasionally are bradycardic and hypotensive and have miotic pupils. Their symptoms usually last approximately 2 hours, although symptoms may persist for 24 hours if untreated.[35,42]

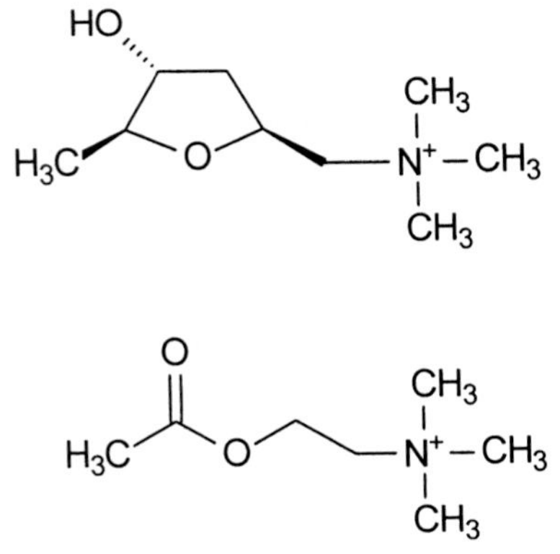

FIGURE 119-3

Chemical structures showing homology between muscarine (*top*) and acetylcholine (*bottom*).

The clinical presentation of muscarine poisoning is similar to that of some other mushroom ingestions, such as the gastrointestinal irritants; however, the triad of perspiration, salivation, and lacrimation also is seen. Central nervous system effects, such as confusion, vertigo, and hallucinations, are not expected because muscarine does not cross the blood-brain barrier. If patients are confused, they may have ingested a mushroom with centrally active compounds, such as ibotenic acid, or alternatively are dehydrated from vomiting and diarrhea. It is unproven, but suspected, that there are mushrooms containing muscarine and ibotenic acid that produce a mixed clinical picture.[41]

Diagnosis

The diagnosis of muscarine mushroom ingestion is clinical, based on the time course of the signs and symptoms and the description or identification of the ingested mushrooms. With an actual mushroom sample, testing for muscarine can be performed if the laboratory is equipped with liquid chromatography.[37] Gas chromatographic methods are technically difficult and are not commonly performed.[43]

Treatment

Muscarine is one of the few toxins that has an almost perfect antidote. Atropine was recommended in the past to reverse muscarinic cholinergic symptoms. The generally recommended treatment consists of sequential intravenous doses of 0.1 mg in adults and 0.02 mg/kg in children (minimum 0.1 mg per dose). The goal of treatment is the resolution of symptoms; however, atropine is not an ideal antidote because it crosses the blood-brain barrier and may cause central anticholinergic symptoms.

Although not studied, glycopyrrolate is a more selective antidote and may have an advantage over atropine. It antagonizes peripheral acetylcholine muscarinic receptors, but being a quaternary amine it does not penetrate the blood-brain barrier the way atropine does. Sequential intravenous doses of 0.1 mg in adults and 0.005 mg/kg in children seem to be safe.[44] When patients present with significant bronchospasm, inhaled ipratropium, an anticholinergic quaternary amine that has limited systemic absorption, can be considered.

Intravenous volume replacement may be required if patients are significantly dehydrated from vomiting and diarrhea. Fluids also may help correct hypotension. Patients with an unclear diagnosis or significant clinical manifestations should be admitted. Mildly symptomatic or asymptomatic patients may be discharged from the emergency department after a period of observation and clinical recovery, provided that there is assurance that the patient has not ingested a more toxic mushroom. The possibility of a mixed mushroom ingestion always should be considered, and close follow-up should be ensured.

Special Populations

Children and elderly individuals are at increased risk of dehydration from the cholinergic effects of muscarine. In addition, the dose of atropine or glycopyrrolate must be titrated carefully to effect. A more prolonged period of observation is warranted for these populations to ensure that there is no recurrence. It is unknown whether muscarine crosses the placenta. Data are limited regarding the safety of glycopyrrolate in pregnancy, but it has significantly less placental transfer than atropine and does not alter fetal hemodynamics.[39]

COPRINUS MUSHROOMS

Coprinus Mushrooms

Contain a protoxin
Produce a disulfiram-like reaction with concurrent or delayed ethanol consumption
Alcohol dehydrogenase inhibitors (e.g., fomepizole) may be beneficial

Toxicity from *Coprinus* mushrooms occurs only with temporally proximate coingestion of ethanol, producing a disulfiram-like interaction.[45-47] *Coprinus atramentarius* is known as the "inky cap" because at maturity the cap and gills autodigest, or deliquesce, into a black, inklike liquid. The mature mushroom has a gray-to-brown, bell-shaped cap 4 to 6 cm across, with small brown scales or fibrils located primarily in the center of the cap. The stalk is slender with a hollow center and false ring. The stalk is white above the ring and gray below. The gills are crowded, and the spores are black to brown-black. The mushrooms are widely distributed in the fall and spring, usually growing in clumps at the base of trees or over buried wood.[2]

Biochemistry and Pathophysiology

C. atramentarius contains the nonessential amino acid coprine (N[5]-[1-hydroxycyclopropyl]-L-glutamine) (Fig. 119-4).[48,49] Coprine has been found in several other *Coprinus* spp. that are too tiny to be eaten in clinically significant amounts.[50] Other mushroom genera have been reported to produce similar symptoms when combined with ethanol, but none have been found to contain coprine. The symptoms of gastrointestinal upset, possibly arising from a concomitantly ingested gastrointestinal irritant mushroom or other systemic illness, with ethanol ingestion may mimic a disulfiram-like reaction.[50] Cooking does not generally change the concentration of coprine significantly.[48,50] There are reports that cooking may increase toxicity.[51]

Coprine is a protoxin that is metabolized to the active toxin, 1-aminocyclopropanol (ACP), after ingestion. ACP inhibits the activity of aldehyde dehydrogenase, an enzyme required for the metabolism of the ethanol metabolite acetaldehyde.[46,52,53] ACP irreversibly inactivates aldehyde dehydrogenase by forming a covalent bond with the active site, resulting in an accumulation of acetaldehyde, which is thought to contribute to the disulfiram-like syndrome.[50,52,54,55]

Although clinically similar to disulfiram, coprine does have some important differences. It is an alkylating agent and has been shown to be mutagenic and to be able to cause

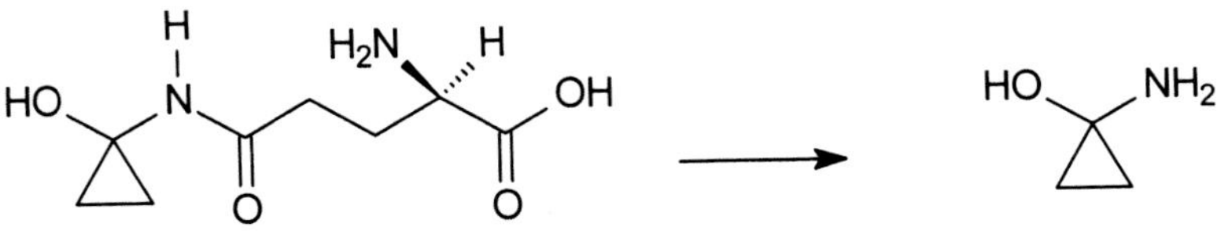

FIGURE 119-4

Chemical structure of coprine (*left*) and conversion to the metabolite, 1-aminocyclopropanol.

bone marrow depression in dogs.[56] Coprine ingestion seems to result in inhibition of aldehyde dehydrogenase to a greater degree than disulfiram. Coprine does not inhibit dopamine β-hydroxylase, the enzyme responsible for norepinephrine synthesis, in contrast to disulfiram.[55,57]

Clinical Presentation

The disulfiram-like reaction that occurs after coprine mushroom ingestion promptly occurs when ethanol is consumed within 24 to 48 hours of eating the mushroom meal.[50,51,58] Symptoms can recur if alcohol is consumed again within 72 hours after mushroom ingestion.[50] The intensity of the reaction is related to the timing and quantity of the mushrooms and the ethanol ingested. The reaction is more pronounced if ethanol is consumed several hours after the mushrooms are consumed, rather than at the same time.[59] Ingestion of ethanol before the mushrooms does not produce a reaction if sufficient time passes for the ethanol to be metabolized completely before the coprine is metabolized to ACP. Typical symptoms occur within a few minutes of the ethanol ingestion. Facial flushing, a blotchy, erythematous rash extending over the arms and chest, dyspnea, headache, metallic taste, diaphoresis, nausea and vomiting, tachycardia, premature ventricular contractions, atrial fibrillation, hypotension, hypothermia, vertigo, confusion, and coma may occur.[60–62] Esophageal rupture is a reported complication of the forceful emesis that can occur.[61] Coprine/ethanol reactions typically cause more tachycardia than disulfiram/ethanol interactions.[57] Symptoms usually last 30 minutes to a few hours. Recovery usually occurs within 24 hours, even when reactions are severe.[47,50,60]

Diagnosis

A history of mushroom and ethanol ingestion followed by a rapid onset of a disulfiram-like reaction is diagnostic. A careful history eliciting any other exposures capable of producing a disulfiram-like reaction should be obtained (e.g., metronidazole, trichloroethylene, disulfiram). A serum ethanol assay may be obtained if confirmation of alcohol ingestion is warranted.

Treatment

Treatment is primarily symptomatic and supportive. There is no role for gastrointestinal decontamination with lavage, ipecac, or charcoal. In addition, there is no evidence that antihistamines reduce the flushing associated with this poisoning. Propranolol has been proposed to treat the hyperadrenergic-like state; however, this has not been well studied and may be risky in patients who are seriously ill.[63] Because the symptoms are caused by acetaldehyde accumulation, an alcohol dehydrogenase inhibitor, such as

fomepizole, administered while blood ethanol concentrations are elevated may reduce the severity of the symptoms by limiting acetaldehyde production.

Hypotension occasionally develops and usually responds to fluids but may require intravenous pressor agents. In contrast to disulfiram, there is no inhibition of dopamine β-hydroxylase by coprine or its metabolites, and dopamine may be effective.[57]

If the patient is critically ill, hemodialysis could be used to remove ethanol and acetaldehyde; this treatment would not be expected to limit the effects of coprine or ACP because at the time of dialysis the patient already would have undergone significant irreversible inhibition of aldehyde dehydrogenase. The administration of any ethanol-containing preparation or product should be avoided for at least 72 hours after ingestion of coprine-containing mushrooms.

Special Populations

The scenario of coingestion of mushrooms and ethanol is unlikely in children. Fomepizole has not been evaluated in pregnancy.[64] The elderly are more likely to have greater morbidity from a reaction, especially elderly individuals with cardiovascular disease. Treatment for these groups is as outlined earlier.

IBOTENIC ACID– AND MUSCIMOL–CONTAINING MUSHROOMS

Ibotenic Acid/Muscimol–Containing Mushrooms
Include *Amanita muscaria* and *Amanita pantherina*   Inebriating mushrooms   Toxins have similar structures to glutamate and γ-aminobutyric acid   Rare seizures may be treated with benzodiazepines

Ibotenic acid and muscimol are structurally related isoxazole compounds present in certain *Amanita* spp. These substances are known for their sensorium-altering effects. Hundreds of years ago, Siberian and Eskimo tribes ingested these mushrooms for their intoxicating properties; the urine from intoxicated individuals was consumed as well, causing inebriation.[65] The most important mushrooms containing ibotenic acid and muscimol are *A. muscaria* and *A. pantherina*.[66–68]

A. muscaria ("fly agaric") is found worldwide except for the tropics, often growing under trees such as pine, beech, and aspen. It is the classic mushroom from fairy tales, with a distinctive cap having a color ranging from red to orange,

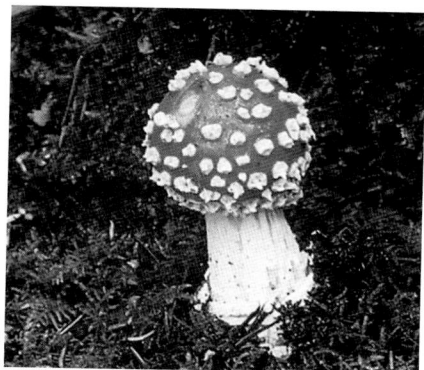

FIGURE 119-5

Amanita muscaria. (From Schneider S, Donnelly M: Mushroom toxicity. In Auerbach PS [ed]: Wilderness Medicine, 4th ed. Philadelphia, Mosby, 2001, p 1148.) See Color Fig. 119-5.

yellow, or white, as the color may fade with age (Fig. 119-5). The cap, about 7 to 15 cm in diameter, is covered with pale yellow–to–white spots or warts. The stalk is white with a persistent membranous ring; the gills and spores are also white. The volva tissue is intergrown with the bulb, and there are characteristic rings along the volva from the universal veil.[2]

A. pantherina ("panther mushroom") has a brown–to–dull yellow cap about 5 to 12 cm in diameter with white or yellow warts. It grows alone or in small groups and commonly is found under conifers. It has a white stalk with a white membranous ring, pale gills, and white spores.[2] Generally, *A. pantherina* has greater concentrations of toxins than *A. muscaria*.[66]

Biochemistry and Pathophysiology

Ibotenic acid and muscimol are false neurotransmitters; their structures are similar to the excitatory neurotransmitter glutamate and the inhibitory neurotransmitter γ-aminobutyric acid (GABA) (Fig. 119-6), respectively. The major structural difference between the mushroom toxins and the true neurotransmitters is the presence of an isoxazole ring involving the

terminal carboxylic acid residue on the former. In contrast to their true neurotransmitter counterparts, ibotenic acid and muscimol readily cross the blood-brain barrier, producing inebriation. The amino acids stizolobic and stizolobinic acid also are found in relatively large amounts in *A. smithiana* and *A. pantherina*; their physiologic effects, if any, are unknown.[69]

Muscimol is an agonist at GABA-A receptors.[70] This GABAergic activity is likely responsible for the somnolence and inebriation seen in poisoning by mushrooms in this group. Ibotenic acid is an agonist at N-methyl-D-aspartate–glutamate receptors, causing neuronal excitation. Ibotenic acid is decarboxylated to muscimol in a manner analogous to the enzymatic conversion of glutamate to GABA. The decarboxylation of ibotenic acid is spontaneous, whereas the conversion of glutamate to GABA requires glutamate decarboxylase (see Fig. 119-6).

Ibotenic acid and muscimol are not effectively removed from the neuronal synapse by the uptake systems that remove glutamate and GABA. About one third of the muscimol and almost all of the ibotenic acid absorbed after mushroom ingestion are excreted in the urine unchanged, with peak excretion of ibotenic acid occurring within 60 minutes. The remainder of muscimol is excreted as oxidative and conjugated metabolites.[71]

Ibotenic acid and muscimol are present at a concentration between 0.03% and 0.5% in some *Amanita* spp., in roughly equal quantities.[66,71] The total toxin content varies greatly, even among mushrooms of the same species, collected at the same time from the same area.[72] Their toxicity also depends on growth substrates, methods of preparation, and length of storage before use. Ibotenic acid spontaneously converts to muscimol. Ibotenic acid is much less potent than muscimol. Drying the mushroom increases the muscimol content and the potency. The yellow pigments of *A. muscaria* have been shown to possess a significantly larger amount of ibotenic acid than the rest of the mushroom. Although it is not recommended, people do eat *A. muscaria* after peeling off the skin and parboiling the mushroom.

The median lethal dose of muscimol varies greatly in rats but is approximately 25 mg/kg. It is unusual for

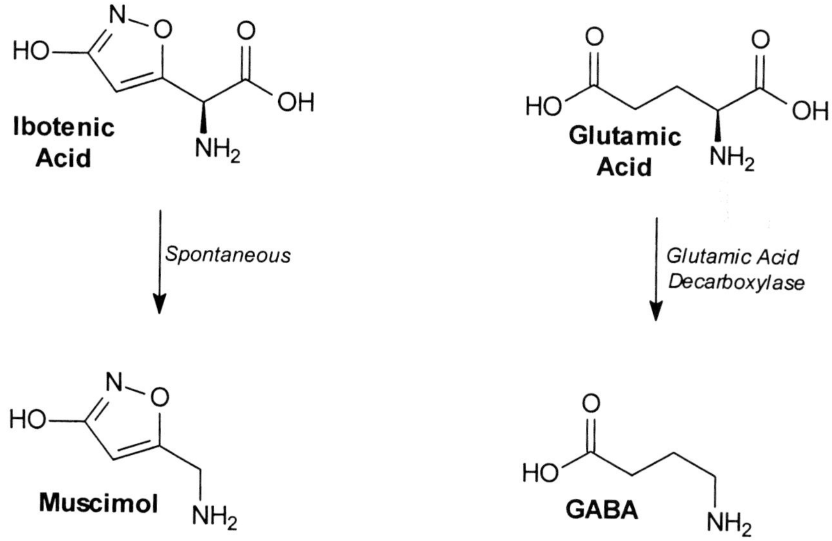

FIGURE 119-6

Comparison of isoxazole toxins with endogenous neurotransmitter structures and metabolic pathways.

Ibotenic Acid

Spontaneous

Muscimol

Glutamic Acid

Glutamic Acid Decarboxylase

GABA

humans to ingest enough *A. muscaria* to cause death. Human toxicity usually occurs with ingestion of 6 mg of muscimol, or two to four mushrooms, but a single mushroom has produced toxicity.[72]

Clinical Presentation

Signs and symptoms begin 0.5 to 2 hours after ingestion.[72] Experimentally, clinical manifestations begin within 1 hour of ingestion of 10 mg of muscimol or 75 mg of ibotenic acid. Symptoms consist of nausea and vomiting (in about half of patients), diarrhea, cramps, increased reflexes, tremor, myoclonic jerking, fasciculations, ataxia, extremity paresthesias, incoordination, visual changes, and altered mental status.[68,72] The pupillary response is variable. The skin has been described as flushed and diaphoretic. Respiratory depression, bradycardia, and hypotension are rarely reported. Seizures rarely occur but may be more common in children.[72] Deaths have been reported after large ingestions (>10 mushrooms) or in association with comorbidities.[73]

The usual clinical presentation of toxicity by these mushrooms is an altered mental status or inebriation, without airway compromise. The clinical course is characterized by a waxing and waning sensorium, alternating between agitation and obtundation. This effect is especially pronounced in children. Patients often exhibit bizarre behavior—elation with disorientation, depersonalization, and increased motor activity.[72] Perceptual illusions are common.[74] As the effects resolve, lethargy usually develops followed by deep protracted sleep. Patients often are amnestic to events occurring during intoxication.

Occasionally, patients exhibit muscarinic-like symptoms, including salivation, bradycardia, perspiration, vomiting, and diarrhea.[72] It is not known whether these symptoms are due to the isoxazoles, to the presence of abnormally large amounts of muscarine,[65] or to an unidentified compound.[68] Most patients have improvement of symptoms within 8 hours, with major toxic effects lasting 12 hours.[72] Residual symptoms of headache, paresthesias, and fatigue occasionally are reported 48 hours afterward.[74–76]

Diagnosis

No specific laboratory tests are required. Identification of the offending mushroom and its associated toxic syndrome usually is based on the description of the mushroom and the patient's clinical presentation.

Treatment

Treatment is primarily supportive, with symptomatic patients requiring observation in a quiet environment. Most toxicologists recommend that the patient be observed until the clinical manifestations resolve. Severely intoxicated patients may require admission to the intensive care unit (see the earlier box on "Indications for ICU Admission in Mushroom Poisoning").

Patients poisoned with these mushrooms should be monitored for seizures, central nervous system depression, and aspiration. Activated charcoal may be considered, but the risk of aspiration may outweigh its theoretical benefits, especially if significant time has passed after ingestion.

Carefully titrated benzodiazepines may be considered to control agitation and seizures. The respiratory depressant effect of benzodiazepines is potentially increased with muscimol intoxication; small doses should be used to prevent apnea.[74] Volume replacement should be initiated for patients with significant gastrointestinal losses or hypotension, with vasoactive agents reserved for hypotension refractory to fluid resuscitation.

Although these patients may manifest features similar to cholinergic or anticholinergic toxidromes, there is no role for either atropine or physostigmine. Muscimol and ibotenic acid do not have significant activity at the muscarinic receptors, and there is no role for atropine. Because these patients do not have a true anticholinergic syndrome, physostigmine should not be used. For a mixed ingestion, including a cholinergic mushroom, glycopyrrolate may be considered instead of atropine because the former does not alter mental status.

Special Populations

Seizures are much more likely to occur in children.[72] Mortality increases with age and the presence of significant comorbidities, including coronary artery disease and chronic obstructive pulmonary disease. There should be a reduced threshold for admission to the intensive care unit for these patients. There are no data relating to isoxazole-containing mushroom toxicity in pregnancy.

PSILOCYBIN-CONTAINING MUSHROOMS

> **Psilocybin-Containing Mushrooms**
>
> Include *Psilocybe* spp. and *Panaeolus* spp.
> Hallucinogenic mushrooms
> Toxins have similar structure to serotonin
> Meixner's test (nonspecific)
> Rare seizures may be treated with benzodiazepines

Psilocybin and psilocin are present in many different genera and species of mushroom, with the genus *Psilocybe* being the most frequently encountered. *Psilocybe semilanceata* ("liberty cap"), *Psilocybe stuntzii, Psilocybe cubensis, Psilocybe cyanescens,* and *Psilocybe baeocystis* are some of the more commonly encountered species.[77] Other genera containing psilocybin include *Panaeolus, Stropharia, Conocybe, Gymnopilus, Inocybe,* and *Pluteus.*[77,78] These mushrooms are sometimes referred to as "magic mushrooms."

The morphology of psilocybin-containing mushrooms is varied; generally, they have smooth, light-colored caps, elongated stalks, dark gills, and dark spores. A characteristic of psilocybin-containing mushrooms is that the flesh stains a bluish green color when bruised.[2] This color change is found consistently only in some of the *Psilocybe* and *Panaeolus* spp.; it is absent in others. The reaction is thought to be due to the conversion of psilocin to a bluish pigment.[79,80]

The major danger inherent in consumption of these mushrooms is misidentification and consumption of other toxic species. This danger is especially worrisome in areas where the prevalent hallucinogenic mushroom has a relatively low concentration of psilocybin, prompting consumption of many mushrooms. Examples of mushrooms similar in appearance to some *Psilocybe* spp. that have been inadvertently ingested include *Galerina autumnalis* (contains amatoxin),[77] *Inocybe geophylla* (contains muscarine),[81] *Cortinarius* spp. (contain orellanine),[82] and *Chlorophyllum molybdites* (produces gastroenteritis).[83]

Biochemistry and Pathophysiology

The pharmacologically active compounds present in these mushrooms are psilocybin (Fig. 119-7), a serotonin-like indole compound with similarities to LSD (lysergic acid diethylamide), and its dephosphorylated metabolite psilocin. Both are 4-substituted tryptamine compounds, which are present in variable amounts. Psilocin is never found without psilocybin. Other biologic amines are present, including baeocystin and norbaeocystin, but their exact physiologic effects are unknown.[84,85] Phenylethylamine, found in *P. semilanceata*, has been suggested as a cause of tachycardia and flushing; others suggest that phenylethylamine is essentially inactive in humans.[86,87]

There is great variability in the interspecies concentration of psilocybin, with an average of approximately 2 mg/g of dry flesh. *P. semilanceata* often contain large amounts of psilocybin, usually greater than 10 mg/g of dried tissue,[77] whereas other species may have only 0.1 mg/g. There is even a substantial difference in the content between subsequent growths of the same species on the same culture media.[88] Because of the great variation in psilocybin concentrations, ingestion of collected wild mushrooms may result in overdose, as usually 20 to 100 mushrooms are eaten at one time, any one of which may have an unexpectedly large amount of psilocybin.[89–91] Occasionally users make a tea from multiple mushrooms.

Psilocybin is approximately 50% absorbed orally and is rapidly dephosphorylated to psilocin.[92] Psilocin is responsible for the central nervous system effects because it is more lipid soluble and crosses the blood-brain barrier. Approximately 65% of a psilocybin dose is excreted in the urine, 25% is excreted as psilocin, and the rest is excreted as 4-hydroxyindolacetic acid and conjugated derivatives.[93] Tolerance to the hallucinogenic effects of psilocybin develops rapidly and is hypothesized to occur even during its continued absorption.[90]

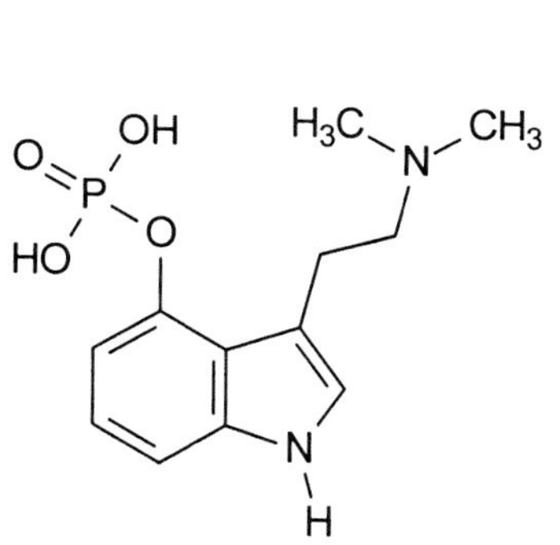

FIGURE 119-7

Chemical structure of psilocybin.

Psilocin is believed to stimulate serotonin receptors in the raphe nuclei of the reticular formation, among other areas. This stimulation is thought to decrease negative feedback on sensory input (i.e., disinhibit), causing increased stimulation of cognitive, emotional, and visual areas.[84] This reduction in negative feedback also may contribute to seizures and hyperthermia in children. A dose of 6 to 12 mg of psilocybin causes symptoms in most individuals.[93]

Clinical Presentation

Euphoria is common, and "bad trips" are the exception after the ingestion of these mushrooms. Most people ingesting psilocybin-containing mushrooms never seek medical attention. The onset of effects generally occurs approximately 15 minutes after ingestion, depending on the preparation. A full stomach may delay onset. The peak hallucinogenic activity lasts 1 hour, and the effects generally resolve after 12 hours.[93–95] Symptoms persisting greater than 12 hours are atypical and should prompt a search for alternative explanations, although clinical manifestations may persist beyond this time frame.[90,96]

Central nervous system effects of these mushrooms include optical, auditory, and tactile illusions, with true hallucinations occurring much less commonly.[90] Most patients remain aware that they are having altered perceptions or are hallucinating and remain able to engage in limited conversation.[89] The degree of perceptual alteration seems to be dose related. Depersonalization or body image distortion occurs infrequently. Racing thoughts, difficulty concentrating, and the experience of time distortions have been reported.[93] Other effects include delayed mydriasis that lasts much longer than the acute CNS effects, nausea, abdominal pain, yawning, anxiety, upper trunk flushing, tachycardia, hypertension, hyperreflexia, and paresthesias, which are usually unilateral and transient, involving the face and occasionally the extremities.[84,90,91,93,95,96] Tachycardia and hypertension are likely due to agitation rather than a direct physiologic effect of psilocybin or psilocin.[90,93]

As the symptoms resolve, exhaustion and depression may ensue. Mild cognitive alteration may persist for days. Although persistent psychotic symptoms have been reported with repeated large ingestions, flashbacks are not a well-documented real phenomenon.[96,97] Rare reported effects have included cerebral demyelination resulting in focal weakness, visual changes, and deafness 2 weeks after ingestion of *Psilocybe* mushrooms. Rechallenge in this case caused recurrence of symptoms and clinical findings.[98]

The hyperadrenergic agitated state induced by psilocybin has caused paroxysmal supraventricular tachycardia and cardiac arrest in a patient with Wolff-Parkinson-White syndrome.[99] Patients with preexisting heart disease may be more likely to have ischemic injury or arrhythmias as a consequence of ingestion of these mushrooms.

Intravenous injection of mushroom material was not reported to cause hallucinations but instead to produce hyperpyrexia, rigors, hypoxemia, facial paresthesias, headache, vomiting, and myalgias. The cause of these effects is likely secondary to contaminants because injection of pure psilocybin does not produce these effects.[93,100,101]

Psilocybin-containing mushrooms are not hepatotoxic; however, two cases of transient elevation of aspartate transaminase, lactate dehydrogenase, and alkaline phosphatase after ingestion of *Psilocybe* and *Conocybe* mushrooms have been described. In the same report, seizures were described.[102] Another case series detailed seizures in several children, with a 6-year-old developing status epilepticus and hyperthermia resulting in death.[103]

Diagnosis

Urine assay for psilocin is not routinely available. Psilocin may be detected in urine and blood after derivatization using gas chromatography–mass spectrometry or may be detected in the mushroom itself.[104,105] Small amounts of psilocin are excreted in the urine days after ingestion.[92] The presence of phenylethylamine has caused positive amphetamine screens using polyclonal antibodies.[86]

The Meixner test is performed by squashing mushroom tissue against a piece of newsprint, allowing it to dry, and adding one or two drops of concentrated hydrochloric acid to the residue. A bluish color change is a positive result for mushrooms in this class. This is a nonspecific test, producing positive results for amatoxin-containing mushrooms as well.[106] Identification of the mushroom through morphologic and microscopic characteristics is possible.[81] Identification of the toxins or mushroom is rarely available or of clinical utility.

Treatment

Agitated patients should be observed in a quiet, safe environment; if agitation persists, benzodiazepines are often the only further intervention required. Neuroleptic agents should be avoided on theoretical grounds because their side effects may confuse the clinical picture, worsen hyperthermia, or increase the risk of seizures. Seizures induced by psilocybin should respond to high doses of benzodiazepines or barbiturates. Gastric emptying and administration of activated charcoal have not been shown to alter outcome and are not recommended. Additionally, most patients will have vomited before presentation.[94,107] It is important to evaluate patients for injuries that may have been sustained as a result of their altered perceptual state and to monitor for evidence of rhabdomyolysis.

Because of the short duration of effect, admission to the hospital usually is not required. Most patients are improving by the time they reach medical attention, and a short observation period in the emergency department is usually sufficient. Admission to the intensive care unit is recommended for patients who present with rhabdomyolysis, prolonged agitation, hyperthermia, status epilepticus, or traumatic injuries. Recovery generally occurs within 12 hours of presentation if psilocybin was the sole ingested toxicant.

Special Populations

Younger children rarely may develop seizures after psilocybin ingestion.[103] Seizures are extremely rare in adults.

GASTROINTESTINAL IRRITANT MUSHROOMS

Gastrointestinal Irritant Mushrooms
Include *Omphalotus olearius* and *Chlorophyllum molybdites* and many others Intravenous hydration may be necessary

Gastrointestinal irritant mushrooms are the largest and least well-defined group of mushrooms; there are hundreds of species that produce gastrointestinal irritation primarily, including *Omphalotus olearius* and *C. molybdites*. The toxins responsible for gastrointestinal irritation are varied and in many cases have not been identified. There is great individual variability in response to these toxins. Some people become very ill after ingestion; others do not become ill at all.[108] Clinical onset of nausea, vomiting, or diarrhea occurs within several hours after ingestion, an important distinguishing feature that commonly allows differentiation from cyclopeptide-containing mushroom poisoning, unless a coingestion of multiple mushroom types has occurred (see Chapter 120).

The symptoms of poisoning by this class of mushrooms are abdominal pain, nausea, vomiting, and diarrhea. Generally, only supportive care is required. Significant electrolyte disturbances and volume depletion with hypotension may occur. Children and the elderly are more likely to require medical treatment and admission to the hospital. Treatment consists of intravenous hydration, electrolyte supplementation, and antiemetics. An antiemetic 5-hydroxytryptamine serotonin agonist, such as ondansetron, is theoretically preferred to a phenothiazine, which may produce symptoms mistaken for a component of mushroom toxicity. The possibility of a hepatotoxic or nephrotoxic mushroom coingestion always should be considered, and close follow-up is essential.

Omphalotus olearius

The mushroom *O. olearius* (*Clitocybe olearia* or jack-o-lantern mushroom) has sometimes been classified with muscarine-containing mushrooms, but it does not contain muscarine.[109] The symptoms of abdominal pain, diarrhea, vomiting, rare sweating, weakness, and visual changes may be similar, but patients do not consistently report salivation and lacrimation.[110–112] It is more useful clinically to classify *O. olearius* as a gastrointestinal irritant mushroom. European reports of toxicity describe a more severe syndrome than that seen in North America. European reports of toxicity include elevated hepatic transaminases and prolonged duration of illness.[113]

Chlorophyllum molybdites

C. molybdites has worldwide distribution and is commonly found on lawns, occasionally growing in fairy rings. The mature mushroom has a large white cap 7 to 30 cm in diameter that is covered with scales, frequently with a hint of pink-to-brown color at the center of the cap and scale tips. The stalk is smooth, tall (10 to 15 cm), and slender (2 to 2.5 cm at apex, 4 to 6 cm at base) with a thick ring. The flesh has a pleasant taste. The gills are pale yellow when young, turning green with age. The spore print is a distinctive green color (Fig. 119-8).[2]

The toxins have not been isolated. Cooking may reduce the potency of the toxins. A few people remain asymptomatic after ingesting *Chlorophyllum* mushrooms, an observation that is consistent with interindividual variation in response to the toxin.

C. molybdites is a gastrointestinal irritant mushroom that is renowned for its rapid onset. Ingestion of a portion of a single mushroom generally produces nausea and vomiting within 1 to 2 hours of ingestion and rarely beyond that time limit. Vomiting is copious. Diarrhea also is common, it is often explosive, and it can be heme positive. Other symptoms commonly reported are diaphoresis, chills, dizziness, and abdominal pain.[114–116] Hypovolemia and electrolyte disturbances from the gastrointestinal losses may be severe and accompanied by other complications (e.g., seizures) if not treated. Gastrointestinal bleeding associated with disseminated intravascular coagulation has been reported rarely.[117] *C. molybdites* ingestion has not been reported to cause hepatic or renal injury.

Most patients improve within 4 to 6 hours, but severely poisoned patients may not improve for 2 to 3 days. Patients with diarrhea and vomiting should be observed until symptoms subside. Patients should be monitored closely for laboratory evidence of fluid or electrolyte depletion. Typing and screening for blood is recommended for patients with evidence of significant bleeding. Patients with refractory vomiting or bloody diarrhea should be admitted to the hospital. Intensive care unit admission is warranted for children, elderly individuals, patients with significant fluid losses, and patients with significant comorbidities.[116]

Analysis of the vomitus or stool may be done to determine the presence of *Chlorophyllum* spores.[118] The green spore print is pathognomonic and if possible should be obtained. A spore print is made by placing the mushroom cap spore-bearing surface (gill-side) down on a piece of paper and covering the cap with a cup. The spore print generally takes at least 4 hours to process. *C. molybdites* caps leave a residue of green spores on the paper in the shape of the mushroom cap and underlying gills.

Treatment

Treatment primarily consists of aggressive intravascular volume replacement with careful monitoring and replacement of electrolytes. Antiemetics may be indicated. Fluid losses can be severe, necessitating several liters of intravenous fluid replacement in adults; pressors may be used if the patient continues to be hypotensive after adequate resuscitation. Invasive monitoring may be employed to guide treatment, if needed.[116] Deaths have occurred in pediatric patients, and intubation has been required.[116] There is no role for gastrointestinal decontamination; activated charcoal is unlikely to be of clinical benefit.

RHABDOMYOLYSIS-PRODUCING MUSHROOMS

Rhabdomyolysis induced by mushroom ingestion has recently been been reported. The mushroom *Russula subnigricans* caused nausea, vomiting, and diarrhea within 2 hours of a single ingestion in nine patients. In most of these patients, symptoms were self-limited and resolved within 1 day, but two patients became progressively ill. They developed muscle pain, weakness, dark urine, and rhabdomyolysis. One required dialysis; both survived.[119]

In another case series, the mushroom *Tricholoma equestre* (or yellow-knight fungus) was ingested for at least three consecutive meals in 12 patients. They did not experience gastrointestinal symptoms but developed fatigue, myalgias, nausea, and dark urine associated with rhabdomyolysis 1 to 3 days after their last meal. Three of these patients developed myocarditis, acidosis, and renal failure and died despite aggressive intensive care unit support.[120]

For both mushrooms, the toxins responsible have not been well characterized, although compounds called *russuphelins* may be responsible for the toxicity of *R. subnigricans*.[121,122] Treatment of both toxins centers on recognition and early aggressive care.

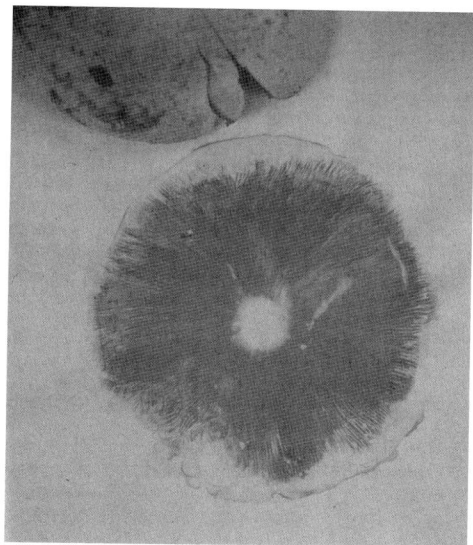

FIGURE 119-8

Chlorophyllum molybdites spore print. See Color Fig. 119-8.

REFERENCES

1. Giusti GV, Carnevale A: A case of fatal poisoning by *Gyromitra esculenta*. Arch Toxicol 33:49–54, 1974.
2. McKnight KH, McKnight VB: A Field Guide to Mushrooms, North America. Boston, Houghton Mifflin, 1987.
3. Peden N, Pringle S: Hallucinogenic fungi. Lancet 1:396–397, 1982.
4. Calvino J, Romero R, Pintos E, et al: Voluntary ingestion of *Cortinarius* mushrooms leading to chronic interstitial nephritis. Am J Nephrol 18:565–569, 1998.
5. Michelot D, Tebbett I: Poisoning by members of the genus *Cortinarius*—review. Mycol Res 94:289–298, 1990.
6. Tebbett IR, Caddy B: Mushroom toxins of the genus *Cortinarius*. Experientia 40:441–446, 1984.
7. Horn S, Horina JH, Krejs GJ, et al: End-stage renal failure from mushroom poisoning with *Cortinarius orellanus*: Report of four cases and review of the literature. Am J Kidney Dis 30:282–286, 1997.

8. Grzymala S: Massenvergiftung durch den Orangefuchsigen Hautkopf. Z Pilzkd 23:139–142, 1957.
9. Warden CR, Benjamin DR: Acute renal failure associated with suspected *Amanita smithiana* mushroom ingestions: A case series. Acad Emerg Med 5:808–812, 1998.
10. Leathem AM, Purssell RA, Chan VR, et al: Renal failure caused by mushroom poisoning. Clin Toxicol 35:67–75, 1997.
11. Tulloss RE, Lindgren JE: *Amanita smithiana*—taxonomy, distribution and poisonings. Mycotaxon 45:373–387, 1992.
12. Prast H, Werner ER, Pfaller W, et al: Toxic properties of the mushroom *Cortinarius orellanus*: I. Chemical characterization of the main toxin of *Cortinarius orellanus* (Fries) and *Cortinarius speciosissimus* (Kuhn and Romagn) and acute toxicity in mice. Arch Toxicol 62:81–88, 1988.
13. Holmdahl J, Ahlmen J, Bergek S, et al: Isolation and nephrotoxic studies of orellanine from the mushroom *Cortinarius speciosissimus*. Toxicon 25:195–199, 1987.
14. Richard JM, Louis J, Cantin D, et al: Nephrotoxicity of orellanine, a toxin from the mushroom *Cortinarius orellanus*. Arch Toxicol 62:242–245, 1988.
15. O'Donnell M, Fleming S: The renal pathology of mushroom poisoning. Histopathology 30:280–282, 1997.
16. Richard JM, Creppy EE, Benoit-Guyod JL, et al: Orellanine inhibits protein synthesis in Madrin-Darby canine kidney cells, in rat liver mitochondria, and in vitro: Indication for its activation prior to in vitro inhibition. Toxicology 67:53–62, 1991.
17. Chilton WS, Ott J: Toxic metabolites of *Amanita pantherina, A. cothurnata, A. muscaria* and other *Amanita* species. Lloydia 39:150–157, 1976.
18. Pelizarri V, Feifal E, Rohrmoser MM, et al: Partial purification and characterization of a toxic component of *Amanita smithiana*. Mycologia 86:555–560, 1994.
19. Chilton WS, Tsou L, Decato L Jr, et al: The unsaturated norleucines of *Amanita solitaria*: Chemical and pharmacological studies. Lloydia 36:169–173, 1973.
20. Prast H, Pfaller W: Toxic properties of the mushroom *Cortinarius orellanus*: II. Impairment of renal function in rats. Arch Toxicol 62:81–88, 1988.
21. Bouget J, Bousser J, Pats B, et al: Acute renal failure following collective intoxication by *Cortinarius orellanus*. Intensive Care Med 16:506–510, 1990.
22. Schumacher T, Hoiland K: Mushroom poisoning caused by species of the genus *Cortinarius fries*. Arch Toxicol 53:87–106, 1983.
23. Holmdahl J, Mulec H, Ahlmen J: Acute renal failure after intoxication with *Cortinarius* mushrooms. Hum Toxicol 3:309–313, 1984.
24. Eigler A, Neman I, Schiffl H: Orellanus syndrome: A rare cause of uremia. Nephron 76:485–486, 1997.
25. Andary C, Raptor S, Delpech N, et al: Laboratory confirmation of *Cortinarius* poisoning. Lancet 1:213, 1989.
26. Rohrmoser M, Kirchmair M, Feifel E, et al: Orellanine poisoning: Rapid detection of fungal toxin in renal biopsy material. Clin Toxicol 35:63–66, 1997.
27. Tebbett IR, Caddy B: Analysis of *Cortinarius* toxins by reversed-phase high pressure liquid chromatography. J Chromatogr 283:417–420, 1984.
28. Spoerke DG, Rumack BH (eds): Handbook of Mushroom Poisoning: Diagnosis and Treatment. Boca Raton, FL, CRC Press, 1994.
29. Holzl B, Regele H, Kirchmair M, et al: Acute renal failure after ingestion of *Cortinarius speciosissimus*. Clin Nephrol 48:260–262, 1997.
30. Holmdahl J, Blohme I: Renal transplantation after *Cortinarius speciosissimus* poisoning. Nephrol Dial Transplant 10:1920–1922, 1995.
31. Nieminen L, Pyy K, Hirsimaki Y: The effect of furosemide on the renal damage induced by the toxic mushroom *Cortinarius speciosissimus* in the rat. Br J Exp Pathol 57:400–405, 1976.
32. Maki T, Takahashi K, Shibata S: Isolation of vomiting principles from the mushroom *Rhodophyllus rhodopolius*. J Agric Food Chem 33:1204–1205, 1985.
33. Waser PG: Chemistry and pharmacology of muscarine, muscarone and some related compounds. Pharm Rev 13:465–515, 1961.
34. Genest K, Hughes DW, Rice WB: Muscarine in *Clitocybe* species. J Pharm Sci 57:331–333, 1968.
35. Köppel C: Clinical symptomatology and management of mushroom poisoning. Toxicon 31:1513–1540, 1993.
36. Malone MH, Robichaud RC: Relative muscarinic potency of thirty *Inocybe* species. Lloydia 25:231–237, 1962.
37. Stijve T: High perfomance thin-layer chromatographic determination of the toxic principles of some poisonous mushrooms. Mitt Gebiete Lebensm Hyg 72:44–54, 1981.
38. Fraser PJ: Pharmacological actions of pure muscarine chloride. Br J Pharmacol 12:47–52, 1957.
39. Briggs GG, Freeman RK, Yaffe SJ: A Reference Guide to Fetal and Neonatal Risk Drugs in Pregnancy and Lactation, 4th ed. Baltimore, Williams & Wilkins, 1994.
40. Eisen TD: Mushrooms: Part II. J Toxicol Clin Toxicol 10:1–2, 1988.
41. Stallard D, Edes TE: Muscarinic poisoning from medications and mushrooms, a puzzling system complex. Postgrad Med 85:341–345, 1989.
42. McCormick DJ, Avel AJ, Gibbons RB: Nonlethal mushroom poisoning. Ann Intern Med 90:332–335, 1979.
43. Cunningham LV: Microanalytical determination of muscarine in *Amanita muscaria* (L. Ex Fr.) Hooker by gas chromatography. PhD Thesis, University of Connecticut, 1974.
44. Glycopyrrolate package insert. Robins Company, Richmond, VA.
45. Chifflot MJ: Sur un cas de rubefaction de la face, tendant a se generaliser a la suite de l'ingestion de Corprinus atramentaricus. Fr Bull Soc Mycol Fr 32:63, 1916.
46. Coldwell BB, Genest K, Hughes DW: Effect on *Coprinus atramentarius* on the metabolism of ethanol in mice. J Pharm Pharmacol 21:176–179, 1969.
47. Barkman R, Perman ES: Supersensitivity to ethanol in rabbits treated with *Coprinus atramentarius*. Acta Pharm Toxicol 20:43–46, 1963.
48. Lindenberg P, Bergman R, Wickberg B: Isolation and structure of coprine, the in vivo aldehyde desthydrogenase inhibitor in *Coprinus atramentarius*: Syntheses of coprine and related cyclopropa4one derivatives. J Chem Soc [Perkin I] 6:684–691, 1977.
49. Hatfield GM, Schaumberg JP: Isolation and structural studies of coprine, the disulfiram-like constituent of *Coprinus atramentarius*. Lloydia 38:489–496, 1975.
50. Michelot D: Poisoning by *Coprinus atramentarius*. Nat Toxins 1:73–80, 1992.
51. List PH, Reith H: Der Faltentintling, *Coprinus atramentarius* Bull. und seine dem tetraethylthiuramdisulf ahnliche wirkung. Arzneimittel Forschung 10:34–40, 1960.
52. Tottmar O, Lindberg P: Effects on rat liver acetaldehyde dehydrogenases in vitro and in vivo by coprine, the disulfiram-like constituent of *Coprinus atramentarius*. Acta Pharmacol Toxicol 40:476–481, 1977.
53. Hellstrom E, Tottmar O: Effects of aldehyde dehydrogenase inhibitors on enzymes involved in the metabolism of biogenic aldehydes in rat liver and brain. Biochem Pharm 31:3899–3905, 1982.
54. Marchner H, Tottmar O: Studies in vitro on the inactivation of mitochondrial rat liver aldehyde dehydrogenase by the alcohol sensitizing compounds cyanamide, 1-aminocyclopropanol and disulfiram. Biochem Pharmacol 32:2181–2188, 1983.
55. Tottmar O, Hellstrom E: Blood pressure response to ethanol in relation to acetaldehyde levels and dopamine-beta-hydroxylase activity in rats pretreated with disulfiram, cyanamide and coprine. Acta Pharmacol Toxicol 45:272–281, 1979.
56. Jonsson M, Lindquist NG, Ploen L, et al: Testicular lesions of coprine and bezcoprine. Toxicology 12:89–100, 1979.
57. Carlson A, Henning M, Lindberg P, et al: On the disulfiram-like effect of coprine, the pharmacologically active principle of *Coprinus atramentrius*. Acta Pharmacol Toxicol 42:292–297, 1978.
58. Lampe KF: Toxic fungi. Ann Rev Pharmacol Toxicol 18:85–104, 1979.
59. Genest K, Coldwell BB, Hughes DW: Potentiation of ethanol by *Coprius atramentarius* in mice. J Pharm Pharmacol 20:102–106, 1968.
60. Reynolds WA, Lowe FH: Mushrooms and a toxic reaction to alcohol: Report of four cases. N Engl J Med 272:630–631, 1965.
61. Mayer JH, Herlocher JE, Parisian J: Esophageal rupture after mushroom alcohol ingestion. N Engl J Med 285:1323, 1971.
62. Caley MJ, Clark RA: Cardiac arrhythmia after mushroom ingestion. BMJ 2:1633, 1977.
63. Rappolt RT, Rappolt N, Ratlift B: *Coprinus atramentarius* (cooked inky top mushroom) and ethanol; acetaldehyde storm controlled by propanolol (Inderal). Presented at National Drug Abuse Conference, San Francisco, 1977.
64. Fomepizol package insert. Orphan Medical Inc, Minnetonka, MN.
65. von Strahlenburg FJ: An Historic-Geographic Description of the North and Eastern Parts of Europe and Asia. Stockholm, 1730.

66. Benedict RG, Tyler VE, Brady LR: Chemotaxonomic significance of isoxazole derivative in *Amanita* species. Lloydia 29:333–342, 1966.

67. Chilton WS, Ott J: Toxic metabolites of *Amanita pantherina, A. cothumata, A. muscaria,* and other *Amanita* species. Lloydia 31:150–157, 1976.

68. Elonen E, Tarssanen L, Harkonen M: Poisoning with brown fly agaric, *Amanita regalis*. Acta Med Scand 205:121–123, 1979.

69. Chilton WS, Hsu CP, Zdybak WT: Stizolobic and stizolobinic acids in *Amanita pantherina*. Phytochemistry 13:1170–1181, 1974.

70. DeFeudis FV: Binding studies with muscimol: relation to synaptic gamma-aminobutyrate receptors. Neurosci 5:675–688, 1980.

71. Ott J, Wheaton PS, Chilton WS: Fate of muscimol in the mouse. Physiol Chem Physics 7:381–384, 1975.

72. Benjamin DR: Mushroom poisoning in infants and children: The *Amanita pantherina/muscaria* group. J Toxicol Clin Toxicol 30:13–22, 1992.

73. Hotson JW: Mushroom poisoning at Seattle. Mycologia 26:194–195, 1934.

74. Theobald W, Buch O, Kunz H, et al: Pharmakologische und experimental-psychologishe untersuchungen mit 2 inhaltsstoffen des fliegenpilzes (*Amanita muscaria*). Arzneim Forsch 18:311–315, 1968.

75. Chilton WS: The course of an intentional poisoning. McIlvaninea 2:17–18, 1975.

76. Hanrahan JP, Gordon MA: Mushroom poisoning case reports and a review of therapy. JAMA 251:1057–1061, 1984.

77. Beug MW, Bigwood J: Psilocybin and psilocin levels in twenty species from seven genera of wild mushrooms in the Pacific Northwest, U.S.A. J Ethnopharm 5:271–285, 1982.

78. Antkowiak R, Antkowiak WZ: Alkaloids from mushrooms, ill indole alkaloids. In Brossi A (ed): The Alkaloids: Chemistry and Pharmacology, Vol 40. San Diego, Academic Press, 1991.

79. Weber LF, Horita A: Oxidation of 4 and 5-hydroxyindole derivatives by mammalian cytochrome oxidase. Life Sci 1:44–49, 1963.

80. Blocks SM: Fungal metabolism: IV. The oxidation of psilocin by p-diphenol oxidase (laccase). Phytochemistry 6:1629–1631, 1967.

81. Watling R: Hallucinogenic mushrooms. J Forensic Sci Soc 23:53–66, 1983.

82. Calvino J, Romero R, Pintos E, et al: Voluntary ingestion of *Cortinarius* mushrooms leading to chronic interstitial nephritis. Am J Nephrol 18:565–569, 1998.

83. Blayney D, Rosenkranz E, Zettner A: Mushroom poisoning from *Chlorophyllum molybdites*. West J Med 132:74–77, 1980.

84. Beck JE, Gordon DV: Psilocybin mushrooms. Pharm Chem News 11:1–5, 1982.

85. Leung AY, Paul AG: Baeocystin and norbaeocystin: New analogs of psilocybin from *Psilocybe baeocystis*. J Pharm Sci 57:1667–1671, 1968.

86. Beck O, Helander A, Karlson-Stiber, et al: Presence of phenylethylamine in hallucinogenic *Psilocybe* mushroom: Possible role in adverse reactions. J Anal Toxicol 22:45–49, 1998.

87. Shulgin A, Shulgin A: PHILKKAL: A Chemical Love Story. Berkeley, Transform Press, 1991.

88. Bigwood J, Beug M: Variation of psilocybin and psilocin levels with repeated flushes (harvest) of mature sporocarps of *Psilocybe cubensis* (earle) Singer. J Ethnopharm 5:287–291, 1982.

89. Mills PR, Lesinskas D, Watkinson G: The danger of hallucinogenic mushrooms. Scot Med J 24:316–317, 1979.

90. Peden NR, Pringle SD, Crooks J: The problem of psilocybin mushroom abuse. Hum Toxicol 1:417–424, 1982.

91. Penden NR, Bissett AF, Macaulay KEC, et al: Clinical toxicology of 'magic mushroom' ingestion. Postgrad Med J 57:543–545, 1981.

92. Kalberer F, Kreis W, Rutschmann J: The fate of psilocin in the rat. Biochem Pharmacol 11:261–269, 1962.

93. Maltiz S, Esecover H, Wilkens B, et al: Some observations on psilocybin, a new hallucinogen in volunteer subjects. Compr Psychiatry 1:8–17, 1960.

94. Penden NR, Pringle SD: Hallucinogenic fungi. Lancet 1:396–397, 1982.

95. Harries AD, Evans V: Sequelae of a 'magic mushroom banquet.' Postgrad Med J 57:571–572, 1981.

96. Hyde C, Glancy G, Omerod P, et al: Abuse of indigenous psilocybin mushrooms: A new fashion and some psychiatric complications. Br J Psychiatry 132:602–604, 1978.

97. Benjamin C: Persistent psychiatric symptoms after eating psilocybin mushrooms. BMJ 1:1319–1320, 1979.

98. Spengos K, Schwartz A, Hennerici M: Multifocal cerebral demyelination after magic mushroom abuse. J Neurol 247:224–225, 2000.

99. Borowiak KS, Ciechanowski K, Waloszczyk P: Psilocybin mushroom (*Psilocybe semilanceata*) intoxication with myocardial infarction. J Toxicol Clin Toxicol 36:47–49, 1988.

100. Sivyer G, Dorrigion L: Intravenous injection of mushroom. Med J Aust 140:182, 1984.

101. Curry S, Rose M: Intravenous mushroom poisoning. Ann Emerg Med 14:900–902, 1985.

102. McCormick D, Avbel AJ, Gibbons RB: Nonlethal mushroom poisoning. Ann Intern Med 90:332–335, 1979.

103. McCawley EL, Brummett RE, Dana GW: Convulsions from *Psilocybe* mushroom poisoning. Proc West Pharmacol Soc 5:27–33, 1962.

104. Sticht G, Kaferstein H: Detection of psilocin in body fluids. Forensic Sci Int 113:403–407, 2000.

105. Repke DB, Leslie DT, Mandell DM, et al: GLC-mass spectral analysis of psilocin and psilocybin. J Forensic Sci 66:743–744, 1977.

106. Beuhler M, Lee DC Gerkin R: The Meixner test in the detection of alpha-amanitin and false-positive reactions caused by psilocin and 5-substituted tryptamines. Ann Emerg Med 44:114–120, 2004.

107. Francis J, Murray VS: Review of enquiries made to the NPIS concerning *Psilocybe* mushroom ingestion. Hum Toxicol 2:349–352, 1983.

108. Spoerke DG, Rumack BH: Handbook of Mushroom Poisoning: Diagnosis and Treatment. Ann Arbor, CRC Press, 1994.

109. Bresinsky A, Besl H: A Color Atlas of Poison Fungi. London, Wolfe Publishing, 1990.

110. Vanden Hoek TL, Erickson T, Hryhorczuk D: Jack o'lantern mushroom poisoning. Ann Emerg Med 20:559–561, 1991.

111. French AL, Garrettson LK: Poisoning with the North American Jack O'Lantern mushroom, *Omphalotus illudens*. J Toxicol Clin Toxicol 26:81–88, 1988.

112. Maretic Z, Russell FE, Golobic V: Twenty-five cases of poisoning by the mushroom *Pleurotus olearius*. Toxicon 13:379–381, 1975.

113. Maretic Z: Poisoning by the mushroom *Clitocybe olearia marie*. Toxicon 4:263–267, 1967.

114. Blayney D, Rosenkranz E, Zettner A: Mushroom poisoning from *Chlorophyllum molybdites*. West J Med 132:74–77, 1980.

115. Lehmann PF, Khazan U: Mushroom poisoning by *Chlorophyllum molybdites* in the Midwest United States, case and a review of the syndrome. Mycopathologia 118:3–13, 1992.

116. Stenklyft PH, Augenstein WL: Chlorophyllum molybdites—severe mushroom poisoning in a child. Clin Toxicol 28:159–168, 1990.

117. Levitan D, Macy JI, Weissman J: Mechanism of gastrointestinal hemorrhage in a case of mushroom poisoning by *Chlorophyllum molybdites*. Toxicon 19:179–180, 1981.

118. Eilers FI, Barnard BL: A rapid method for the diagnosis of poisoning caused by the mushroom *Lepiota morgani*. Am J Clin Pathol 60:823–825, 1973.

119. Lee PT, Wu ML, Tsai WJ, et al: Rhabdomyolysis: An unusual feature with mushroom poisoning. Am J Kidney Disease 38:1–5, 2001.

120. Bedry R, Baudrimont I, Deffieux G, et al: Wild-mushroom intoxication as a cause of rhabdomyolysis. N Engl J Med 345:798–802, 2001.

121. Takahashi A, Agatsuma T, Matsuda M, et al: Russuphelin A, a new cytotoxc substance from the mushrroom *Russula subnigricans* Hongo. Chem Pharm Bull 40:3185–3188, 1992.

122. Takahashi A, Agatsuma T, Ohta T, et al: Russuphelins B, C, D, E and F, new cytotoxic substances from the mushroom *Russula subnigricans* Hongo. Chem Pharm Bull 41:1726–1729, 1993.

CHAPTER 120

Cyclopeptide-Containing Mushrooms: The Deadly *Amanita* Mushrooms

Mark Donnelly ■ Paul Wax

In contrast to many of the man-made toxins found in the world today, the toxins present in amanitine-containing mushrooms probably have been afflicting humans for as long as they have been picking mushrooms from their varied habitats and consuming them as a readily available and tasty food source. Treatments have been tried and accepted over time based on anecdotal evidence. Often the offending source mushroom is not well identified. Despite its notoriety for lethality, survival from "deadly" mushroom poisoning without specific therapy has been reported to be 40%.[1] One of the treatments for amatoxin poisoning that evolved in the 1800s and lasted until the 1930s was based on the observation that rabbits consumed these mushrooms with impunity. This led to the development of an antidote consisting of the stomachs of three rabbits and the brains of seven rabbits, with addition of sweeteners for palatability. The ingredients were finely chopped to mask their origins. Because many individuals who received this regimen survived, the use of this remedy persisted for many years.[1]

Mushrooms that contain amatoxin are largely from the following three genera:

- *Amanita*
- *Galerina*
- *Lepiota*

Amatoxin-containing mushrooms can be found on all continents with temperate climates. The genus *Amanita* contains the best-known poisonous mushroom species, including *Amanita phalloides*, which is probably responsible for 90% to 95% of the cyclopeptide fatalities worldwide.[2] Other *Amanita* spp. that contain these toxins include *Amanita virosa, Amanita ocreata, Amanita verna*, and *Amanita bisporigera*.[3] *Amanita* mushrooms are usually large in size and often fruit in sufficient numbers to invite picking. *A. phalloides* bears enough resemblance to a widely cultivated mushroom of southern Asia, *Vovariella volvacea* (paddy straw mushroom), that groups of immigrants in California, Oregon, and New York have mistakenly harvested and been poisoned by them. Nontoxic *Amanita* spp., including *Amanita caesarea, Amanita calyptrata*, and *Amanita velosa*, are sought by knowledgeable collectors for their fine taste.[3] Two other *Amanita* spp., *Amanita pantherina* and *Amanita muscaria*, do not contain cyclopeptides but are toxic owing to the presence of ibotenic acid, which when eaten is decarboxylated to muscimol. *Amanita pantherina* and *Amanita muscaria* cause a transient and nonlethal syndrome primarily involving the central nervous system (see Chapter 119).

Galerina spp., the other amatoxin-containing genus, are small brown mushrooms growing most frequently on decaying wood and are unlikely to be picked by the food gatherer. Because *Galerina* mushrooms may be mistaken for the hallucinogenic *Psilocybe* mushrooms, misidentification between these genera by the hallucinogenic mushroom hunter potentially may lead to amatoxin poisoning. Amatoxin-containing *Galerina* spp. include *Galerina autumnalis, Galerina marginata*, and *Galerina venenata*.[3] Some samples of *Conocybe filaris* also have been shown to contain the toxin.[1]

Certain *Lepiota* spp. also contain amatoxins. The poisonous *Lepiota* mushrooms tend to be small and may be confused by the indiscriminate picker with larger edible *Lepiota* spp. *Lepiota helveola, Lepiota josserandii, Lepiota brunneolilacea*, and *Lepiota castanea* have been implicated in fatalities, primarily in Europe and North America. Among amatoxin-containing mushrooms, *Lepiota* spp. tend to be more potent than *Amanita* spp. *Lepiota* spp. may contain 3.5 mg of amanitine per gram of dry mushroom compared with 1.75 mg/g to 2.5 mg/g in *A. phalloides*.[3]

CHEMISTRY OF ACTIVE TOXINS

Amanitine was first isolated in 1940 by Hallermayer from the mushroom *A. phalloides* after 10 years of work at the Ludwig-Maximilian University in Munich.[4] Continued elucidation of the relevant chemical structures has resulted in the identification of at least three subtypes of amanitine: α, β, and γ amanitine. These thermostable cyclic octapeptides are collectively known as *amatoxins*. Other cyclopeptides found in these mushrooms include heptapeptides referred to as *phallotoxins* and *virotoxins*. Phalloidin, one of the phallotoxins, previously was thought to be responsible for the gastroenteritis that develops after cyclopeptide mushroom ingestion.[5] The rapid activity of phalloidin on susceptible cells and the delayed onset in gastrointestinal symptoms suggest, however, that phalloidin most likely does not play a crucial role.[1] It is unknown if virotoxins play a role in human toxicity. Phallolysins are another group of compounds found in amatoxin-containing mushrooms. These chemicals have hemolytic properties but are heat labile, break down in the presence of the low gastric pH, and are not believed to contribute to toxicity.[1] A lethal dose of amatoxins may be 0.1 mg/kg body weight and may be contained in a single mushroom.[6]

> **Pharmacokinetics of Cyclopeptides**
>
> *Volume of distribution:* 0.2 L/kg
> *Protein binding:* none
> *Mechanism of clearance:* renal clearance 83% to 89%
> *Active metabolites:* none
> *Methods to enhance clearance:* charcoal hemoperfusion

PATHOPHYSIOLOGY

Amatoxin-containing mushrooms are most often consumed cooked, but given the heat stability of the cyclopeptides, cooking has no effect on their toxicity.[4] The subtype α amanitine is absorbed through the intestinal epithelium with little or no serum protein binding. Transport into the hepatocytes is by the same mechanism used by bile salts. Toxicity and cell death occur when amanitine binds to a subunit of RNA polymerase II, interfering with messenger RNA synthesis and ultimately halting protein production. Hepatic cell necrosis follows this inhibition of protein synthesis.[5] Injury to gastrointestinal mucosa, kidney, pancreas, and testes also may occur.[7] The slow depletion of a reservoir of already formed messenger RNA accounts for the 24- to 48-hour delay in symptoms attributed to hepatic necrosis.[4] Gastrointestinal symptoms, such as vomiting and diarrhea, occur earlier and result from the effects of amanitines on rapidly dividing cells, such as gastrointestinal epithelial cells.[1,2]

Amatoxins undergo enterohepatic recirculation, which effectively prolongs the hepatic insult.[4] Most amatoxins are cleared by the kidneys during the first several hours after ingestion.[8] The gastrointestinal symptoms that occur 6 to 24 hours after ingestion are most likely related to direct effects of amatoxins on mucosal cells. Amatoxin-containing *Lepiota* mushrooms lack the phallotoxins yet produce the same type of gastrointestinal symptoms as the *Amanita* mushrooms. Significant fluid depletion and electrolyte abnormalities may result from vomiting and diarrhea.

Clinical evidence of hepatic injury usually begins approximately 48 hours after ingestion, but in some cases may be delayed for 96 hours or occasionally longer. In some cases, the gastrointestinal symptoms resolve before the onset of symptoms directly attributable to hepatic damage. Liver injury causes a variety of life-threatening systemic problems. Coagulopathy is caused by the decreased synthesis of clotting factors. Hypoglycemia occurs as a result of impaired gluconeogenesis and glycogenolysis. Mental status changes usually represent the onset and progression of hepatic encephalopathy.

Varying degrees of renal failure often occur late in the course of amatoxin poisoning. It is not clear if renal failure is due to a direct effect of amatoxin on renal tubular cells, a secondary effect from hepatorenal syndrome, or acute tubular necrosis from dehydration and shock from the gastroenteritis. Pancreatitis develops in 50% of serious poisonings.[5]

Postmortem or explant studies of damaged liver from amatoxin poisoning may show reduced mass (median 825 g in one case series,[7] normal liver weight being 1400 to 1600 g), a nutmeg pattern with focal lesions on gross inspection, and massive necrosis with centrilobular hemorrhage histologically.[5] The lobular architecture is often intact, and in some cases regenerative changes are found.

CLINICAL PRESENTATION AND LIFE-THREATENING COMPLICATIONS

The clinical presentation of amatoxin poisoning follows one of a few typical scenarios. Most commonly, patients present after the onset of symptoms, usually at least 6 to 24 hours after ingestion. Only rarely do patients present less than 6 hours after ingestion. Such an early presentation before the onset of symptoms would suggest that the patient knew that the mushrooms were poisonous. In one documented suicide attempt, a 15-year-old boy ate a variety of mushrooms from a wooded area and reported his actions within 30 minutes. He was admitted to an intensive care unit (ICU) immediately before the onset of symptoms. Within 2 hours of ingestion, he had measurable amatoxin (by radioimmunoassay) in his stomach contents and his urine. The boy was treated aggressively (see section on treatment) and never developed the typical symptoms associated with amatoxin poisoning.[9]

The more usual presentation is for a patient to present within 6 to 24 hours of ingestion complaining of crampy abdominal pain, vomiting, and profuse watery diarrhea.[1,5] The patient sometimes fails to make an association between a previous meal and the current symptoms; this may delay the diagnosis further, and in some cases the patient may be discharged home with a presumed diagnosis of viral gastroenteritis. There may be evidence of dehydration and electrolyte abnormality associated with these fluid losses. In severe cases, hypotension, tachycardia, hypoglycemia, and acid-base disturbances may be present.[1,7]

During the next 24 to 48 hours the gastroenteritis symptoms may resolve, and some patients may feel well enough to resume normal activity for a brief period if not hospitalized. An elevation in hepatic transaminases may first become apparent during this quiescent period. Subsequently an increase in prothrombin time may be noted.[5]

By 48 to 96 hours after ingestion, the patient may develop signs and symptoms of fulminant hepatic failure (FHF). Coagulopathy and renal insufficiency may appear during this final stage. Lethargy, obtundation, and seizures may develop. Hepatic encephalopathy may progress rapidly to coma.[5] Death after ingesting cyclopeptide-containing mushrooms typically occurs between days 6 and 16.[8]

Not all of the clinical features are present in every poisoning. In milder cases, the patient may show signs of recovery after gastrointestinal symptoms resolve and does not develop clinical evidence of hepatic injury, although in some cases a mild increase in hepatic transaminases still may occur.[1] In severe poisonings, the patient may progress through these stages more rapidly regardless of treatment.[5] Life-threatening complications are the same as those with any patient experiencing FHF and include increased intracranial pressure, intracranial hemorrhage from coagulopathy, sepsis, pancreatitis, renal failure, aspiration, and cardiorespiratory arrest.[2,5,7]

DIAGNOSIS OF CYCLOPEPTIDE MUSHROOM POISONING

The diagnosis of cyclopeptide mushroom poisoning is made largely based on history, clinical presentation, and knowledge of local endogenous mushroom species. In some cases, the ingestion of amatoxin-containing mushrooms may be confirmed by identifying the type of mushrooms used in the mushroom meal; this can be accomplished by sending someone who is skilled in mushroom identification to visit the site where the mushrooms were harvested or to examine additional mushrooms that were picked and not consumed. Spore analysis of mushroom fragments from the stomach also may be useful in facilitating positive identification of amatoxin-containing species. Although identification of the ingested mushroom species may confirm the diagnosis, waiting for such proof should never delay treatment.

It is important for the clinician to maintain a suspicion of mushroom poisoning when a patient presents with severe gastroenteritis, particularly where the season and locale are favorable for the growth of mushrooms. Although symptoms of cyclopeptide poisoning usually begin more than 6 hours after ingestion, one cannot rule out toxicity from these mushrooms if the symptoms occur earlier because the patient may have ingested other types of mushrooms along with amatoxin-containing species. Many types of mushrooms can cause gastrointestinal symptoms within 2 to 3 hours of consumption, well before the symptoms of amatoxin poisoning occur. The *Agaricus* spp. with a phenol odor and *Chlorophyllum molybdites* are often the culprits because of their ubiquity and their similarity in appearance to edible species.[3]

Serum levels of amatoxins have been detected 30 hours after ingestion but may no longer be present by 48 hours after ingestion. The presence of detectable serum concentrations at any level has been associated with more severe poisoning.[8] Becauses many patients do not present until at least 2 days after the ingestion, testing for amatoxin in the blood is usually not helpful. The absence of amatoxin from the blood does not rule out cyclopeptide poisoning. In addition, amatoxin assays generally are not readily available.

If one suspects amatoxin poisoning by the clinical presentation alone and there is no supporting history or physical evidence, it is important to consider other hepatotoxins and nontoxic causes, such as infectious hepatitis. Acetaminophen toxicity shares many of the same clinical and laboratory findings seen with amatoxin poisoning and must be considered by performing a careful history and checking a serum acetaminophen concentration. Similar to cyclopeptides, however, acetaminophen may not be detectable in the blood when hepatotoxicity is evident. Because acetaminophen poisoning is much more common than cyclopeptide mushroom poisoning, owing to acute intentional overdoses and chronic ingestions, and is the most common cause of acute liver injury, one should always consider acetaminophen toxicity as a potential cause. Other potentially toxic agents that may cause similar clinical and pathologic findings include carbon tetrachloride, chloroform, isoniazid, halothane, and yellow phosphorus.

TREATMENT

Patients with cyclopeptide mushroom poisoning should be admitted to an ICU for close monitoring and observation. Given the propensity toward rapid deterioration in patients with worsening liver failure, ICU admission is crucial until the patient is truly stabilized. Supportive treatment for progressive encephalopathy (grade III or IV [Table 120-1]),

Indications for ICU Admission in Cyclopeptide Mushroom Poisoning

Suspected cyclopeptide mushroom ingestion in pediatric, pregnant, elderly, or chronically ill patient
Known cyclopeptide mushroom ingestion in all patient populations until stable resolution of symptoms
Suspected cyclopeptide mushroom ingestion with elevated hepatic transaminases (>1000 IU/L), coagulopathy, metabolic acidosis, mental status changes, hypoglycemia, elevated bilirubin, vomiting, or diarrhea

Treatment of Cyclopeptide Mushroom Ingestion

Aggressive supportive care and close monitoring
Multiple doses of activated charcoal (orally or through gastric tube) to adsorb toxin and reduce enterohepatic recirculation for 24 to 48 hours after suspected ingestion
Fluids and bicarbonate to treat acidosis, if needed
Vitamin K, fresh frozen plasma, or other needed blood replacement products to treat coagulopathy
Glucose solutions to treat hypoglycemia
Forced diuresis to eliminate toxin early in course
Antibiotic and antifungal prophylaxis
Charcoal hemoperfusion to adsorb toxin
Duodenal drainage to reduce enterohepatic recirculation
Intubation for airway protection or for hyperventilation
Intracerebral pressure monitoring for encephalopathic patient
Osmotic diuretic for increased intracerebral pressure
Hemodialysis/hemoperfusion for renal failure
Antidotal treatments, including high-dose penicillin, silibinin/silymarin, and *N*-acetylcysteine
Liver transplant or liver-sustaining therapies

Diagnosis of Cyclopeptide Mushroom Poisoning*

History of ingestion of mushrooms known to contain cyclopeptides (*Amanita, Lepiota, Galerina*)
History of ingestion of unknown mushrooms and symptoms consistent with cyclopeptide mushroom ingestion
Initial onset of vomiting and diarrhea 6 to 24 hours after mushroom ingestion
Signs and symptoms of acute hepatic injury 1 to 3 days after mushroom ingestion

*Identification of mushrooms is best made by mycologists.

TABLE 120-1 Grades of Hepatic Encephalopathy

GRADE	
0	Normal level of consciousness but abnormal liver function; no asterixis
I	Drowsy, but easily arousable, oriented; asterixis present
II	Sleeping continuously, difficult to rouse, slurred speech, disoriented
III	Confused, agitated, often aggressive, incomprehensible speech
IV	Coma, does not open eyes, no speech, ± response to pain

cardiovascular instability, fluid and electrolyte management, or coagulopathy may be needed.

Although many treatment regimens are used worldwide, there are no controlled trials to establish efficacy of any of the therapies often employed to treat cyclopeptide poisoning. Reasons for the lack of controlled studies are the following: (1) Cases of amatoxin poisoning are relatively infrequent and isolated—it is difficult to treat a large group of people under similar conditions. (2) Individual mushrooms can vary in the amount of toxin they contain, and people seldom know precisely how much they have eaten; establishing the dose consumed is impossible. (3) Different people seem to metabolize the toxins in different ways; it is not clear why one person in a group can consume larger quantities than others in the group yet suffer fewer ill effects. (4) Patient presentation is variable. (5) Seldom is a single treatment employed—it is difficult to discern the benefit of a single agent when most patients are treated with multiple therapies. Despite these limitations, gains have been made in survival that are probably attributable to aggressive intensive care and to a few specific therapies that are discussed subsequently.

In the treatment of amatoxin poisoning, the therapeutic goals can be summarized as follows:

1. Evacuation of mushroom from the gastrointestinal tract before toxins are absorbed
2. Fluid and electrolyte resuscitation
3. Elimination of amatoxins from blood and tissues
4. Prevention of enterohepatic recirculation
5. Protection of liver and other organs from the toxic effects of amanitine
6. Prevention and treatment of sepsis, coagulopathy, encephalopathy, and renal failure[5]

There are no controlled, randomized, double-blinded clinical trials to support any single treatment option. Instead, clinicians have had to rely on suggestions garnered from case reports and limited case series regarding treatment efficacy. Ideally the treatment should have minimal adverse effects. Many older treatment recommendations have fallen out of favor. Most of these have been based on anecdotal evidence or animal models that are poorly representative of human physiologic responses.

Nonantidotal Treatments

Self-protection of the airway is usually adequate early in the course of amatoxin poisoning. During the phase with predominantly gastrointestinal symptoms, there is an increased chance of aspiration, but intubation generally is not considered to be indicated unless there are accompanying mental status changes. Tachypnea may develop as a compensatory response to metabolic acidosis. Later in the course, when hepatic encephalopathy develops, it is advisable to intubate the patient and assist ventilations because self-protective mechanisms may be lost, and hyperventilation may be beneficial in the management of cerebral edema. Severe aspiration, leading to adult respiratory distress syndrome, may render an otherwise appropriate candidate too unstable for transplantation.

GASTROINTESTINAL DECONTAMINATION

The theoretical efficacy of gastrointestinal decontamination is greatest immediately after cyclopeptide mushroom ingestion, when undigested mushroom matter still may be amenable to removal. No studies have compared gastric lavage or activated charcoal or both with no decontamination for decreasing mushroom absorption. By the time the patient develops gastrointestinal symptoms, it may be too late to gain much benefit from decontamination.

Despite the presence of gastrointestinal symptoms, activated charcoal administration is generally recommended in late presentations because it may enhance amatoxin elimination by interrupting its enterohepatic recirculation. A dosing regimen of 0.5 g/kg of activated charcoal given each hour has been suggested to enhance elimination.[8] It is not clear how long after ingestion that enterohepatic recirculation continues to deliver toxin to the liver. Multiple-dose activated charcoal frequently is administered in an attempt to interrupt this enterohepatic recirculation of amatoxins. This therapy has not been shown to enhance amatoxin elimination, however. Based on theoretical considerations, it would be predicted that multiple-dose charcoal therapy would be beneficial, and we recommend its use for at least up to 24 hours postingestion. Beyond this time frame, the theoretical likelihood of benefit decreases.[8,9] When using multiple-dose activated charcoal, it is important to ensure that the charcoal is an aqueous suspension and that multiple-dose cathartics, such as sorbitol or magnesium salts, are not given. The administration of multiple-dose cathartics can cause serious volume depletion and electrolyte abnormalities. Nasoduodenal suction also has been recommended as a means to reduce enterohepatic recirculation.[10] In one case of suspected amatoxin poisoning, a nasobiliary diversion drain was placed endoscopically approximately 24 hours after ingestion. Using high intermittent suction for 48 hours, 290 mL of dark green viscous bile was collected. The only other treatments were intravenous fluids and intramuscular vitamin K. The patient remained asymptomatic throughout his hospital stay.[10] As with many logical but isolated, infrequently applied therapies, there is no way of discerning whether this treatment truly made a difference in the patient's outcome.

EXTRACORPOREAL AMATOXIN REMOVAL

Extracorporeal removal techniques using charcoal hemoperfusion to reduce amatoxin load potentially may provide some benefit when the patient presents to the hospital soon after ingestion. The intent of such a therapy is to reduce the serum load of amatoxin before distribution to peripheral tissues. Most patients do not present during the time period immediately after mushroom ingestion, when extracorporeal removal would provide maximal benefit. In one case series, charcoal hemoperfusion used within 24 hours of ingestion (along with penicillin and vitamin C therapy) was associated with a benign course in four patients who may have ingested lethal amounts of amatoxin.[11] It is difficult to draw conclusions about the benefits of such an intervention given the lack of controlled outcome and analytical data. Hemodialysis, plasmapheresis, peritoneal dialysis, and hemofiltration have not been shown to be helpful in removing amatoxin from the serum or tissues.

FORCED DIURESIS

Forced diuresis to enhance amatoxin elimination also has been suggested by some authors, although efficacy data for this modality by itself are lacking. Urine concentrations of amanitine have been shown to be high within the first few hours after ingestion. In a 4-year experience with 39 patients, forced diuresis (along with at least four other interventions) resulted in complete recovery of all patients.[12] Forced diuresis typically is accomplished by administering normal saline or Ringer's lactate and a loop diuretic, such as furosemide, in an attempt to maintain a urine output of at least 150 to 200 mL/hr. With the use of forced diuresis, amanitine has been recovered 3 days after cyclopeptide mushroom ingestion. There are no controlled data, however, validating the efficacy of forced diuresis in amatoxin poisoning. Patients with persistent vomiting and diarrhea should receive additional fluid resuscitation as needed.

GLUCOSE AND ELECTROLYTES

Hypoglycemia may present early with amatoxin-induced hepatic injury and may worsen significantly with FHF. Serum glucose monitoring should be performed frequently. Glucose replacement using 5% to 20% solutions is indicated to maintain euglycemia.

Electrolyte abnormalities may result from vomiting and diarrhea and should be corrected. Aggressive fluid resuscitation to replace fluid losses may be required. Correction of refractory metabolic acidosis, if severe, with sodium bicarbonate may be warranted.

COAGULOPATHY

Because significant hepatic injury often is associated with reduction in clotting factor synthesis, treatment of coagulopathy may become important. When the amount of liver injury reaches a critical threshold, the failure to synthesize additional clotting factors leads to the development of coagulopathy and the possibility of frank hemorrhage. Factor VII has the shortest half-life of the vitamin K–dependent clotting factors at 6 hours. Coagulopathy first may be observed 24 hours (four half-lives) after clotting factor synthesis failure. Vitamin K and fresh frozen plasma have been given to help avoid bleeding complications that may develop. Although clotting factor replacement (e.g., fresh frozen plasma) may provide benefit, the short duration of action precludes long-term benefit. We recommend that factor replacement be used only in patients with frank hemorrhage or in patients needing an invasive procedure, such as arterial or central venous line placement. Although vitamin K is given frequently, its administration to patients with FHF is probably of marginal benefit. However, because the degree

of coagulopathy may serve as a marker of liver failure progression, the administration of either fresh frozen plasma or vitamin K may limit the usefulness of prothrombin time or international normalized ratio as a prognostic marker. Such therapies should be used sparingly.

HEPATIC TRANSPLANTATION

The therapy that has probably saved more lives than any other since the 1980s is orthotopic liver transplantation (OLT). First performed in 1983[5] for a case of amatoxin-caused FHF, OLT has become the standard salvage procedure at transplant centers. As with any other organ transplant, its utility depends on an adequate supply of donor organs.

It is important early in the evaluation of suspected cyclopeptide mushroom poisoning to recognize that what appears to be a case of viral gastroenteritis may soon require ICU admission and transport to a facility that performs liver transplants. Earlier recognition of the progressive signs and symptoms of amatoxin poisoning allows a slightly longer time frame in which to procure an organ. In contrast to chronic hepatic failure, when transplant decisions may be made over weeks to months, the decision to undertake OLT after cyclopeptide mushroom ingestion may need to be made within hours to just a few days from the time of presentation.

At present, there are no universal indications for referral to liver transplant centers after cyclopeptide mushroom ingestion. Given the potential for rapid deterioration, patients identified at risk for FHF should be transferred to a liver transplant center. Patients with significant transaminase elevation (aspartate aminotransferase >1000 IU/L) and, particularly, evidence of coagulopathy may benefit from transfer to a liver transplant center. The transfer of a patient to a liver transplant center should not be interpreted to mean that the patient definitely needs a liver transplant. Given the regenerating capabilities of the liver, recovery still may occur despite markedly elevated transaminases and other evidence of liver injury. More stringent criteria (see later) should be used to assess need for actual transplantation.

INFECTION

Infection is a major concern in a patient with acute liver failure. Increased risk for infectious complications is associated with impaired phagocytic function, reduced complement levels, and invasive procedures. Bacterial infections have been found in 80% of acute liver failure patients (not specifically caused by cyclopeptide mushrooms), and fungal infections have been found in 32%.[13] Pneumonia may be found in 50% of these infections.[13] Early treatment with parenteral antibiotics (including antifungals) has been shown to increase survival, reduce progression to encephalopathy, and increase opportunity for transplantation.[13] Enteral decontamination has not been shown to be beneficial.[14] Candidiasis is the most common fungal infection.[13] Bacterial sources are highly variable and warrant broad-spectrum prophylaxis.

In patients who undergo transplantation, postoperative infection is a significant cause of mortality. Candidiasis is the most common fungal infection, whereas aspergillosis is difficult to treat effectively and has a high mortality rate.[15] Gram-positive cocci, including *Staphylococcus aureus* and *Enterococcus faecium*, are common bacterial pathogens that may cause bacteremia or wound infection. Bacterial infection is more likely with patients experiencing acute rejection and in patients with prolonged hospitalization. Risk factors for postoperative fungal infection include low pretransplantation hemoglobin, high pretransplantation bilirubin, return to surgery, and prolonged ciprofloxacin therapy.[16]

CEREBRAL EDEMA

Acute hepatic failure often causes mental status changes as a result of increasing intracranial pressure secondary to cerebral edema. The resulting ischemia and herniation may account for 50% of deaths in patients with acute liver failure[17] and may preclude a patient's consideration for transplantation. Intracranial pressure monitoring is warranted when the patient shows progression of encephalopathy. Hyperventilation, diuretics, barbiturates, or a combination of these interventions may be used with a goal of maintaining a cerebral perfusion pressure greater than 50 mm Hg (cerebral perfusion pressure = mean arterial pressure − intracranial pressure). Failure to maintain the cerebral perfusion pressure may lead to irreversible neurologic damage.[18] Mannitol frequently is used as an osmotic diuretic in this situation. Barbiturates are thought to lower intracranial pressure by cerebral vasoconstriction and decreasing neuronal metabolic activity, reducing cerebral oxygen demand.[18]

RENAL FAILURE

Renal failure develops in 55% of patients with acute hepatic failure.[19] This renal failure may represent direct renal injury caused by amatoxin or may be a component of a hepatorenal syndrome secondary to the hepatic failure. Renal failure as evidenced by increasing serum creatinine or decreasing urine output or both may require hemodialysis as a supportive measure. The hepatorenal syndrome usually resolves if hepatic function improves.

INDICATIONS FOR TRANSPLANTATION

The decision to pursue transplantation is not to be made lightly. There are surgical risks common to all liver transplantations. With a lifetime of immunosuppression to follow a successful transplant, one must be relatively confident that the patient would not survive without the surgery. Different criteria have been used to help make this decision. Serum transaminase elevations that are rapid and severe suggest worsening hepatic failure, but there is no definite correlation between the amount of elevation and the severity of injury. Serum transaminase concentrations may decline after near-complete destruction of the liver. Factor V levels decreasing to less than 10% to 20% of control have been used as an indication to pursue transplantation. Floersheim and associates[20] reported an 84% fatality rate in *A. phalloides*–poisoned patients with factor V values less than 10%.

Although the King's College criteria for OLT are commonly used in the much more common acetaminophen-induced FHF, criteria have not been developed for FHF resulting from cyclopeptide mushroom ingestion. The King's College criteria for acetaminophen suggest that the most predictive marker for lethality—and OLT consideration—is a serum pH less than 7.30[21] despite fluid resuscitation and bicarbonate replacement. In cases without acidosis, the next best predictor is the combination of grade III or IV hepatic encephalopathy (see Table 120-1) and coagulopathy

(prothrombin time >100 seconds) and renal failure (serum creatinine >300 μmol/L [>3.39 mg/dL]).[22,23] In addition, the transplant, if it is to be performed, should be done before the onset of conditions that contraindicate transplantation, such as sepsis and increased intracranial pressure. Although it may make intuitive sense to use the acetaminophen criteria for cyclopeptide cases, such an approach has not been validated, given the paucity of cyclopeptide cases. What makes the transplantation decision even more difficult are the cases in which patients have met commonly accepted indications for OLT but were not transplanted and survived without sequelae anyway.[24]

Other indications for transplantation have included hypofibrinogenemia, gastrointestinal hemorrhage, and evidence of bone marrow toxicity.[7] Worsening hepatic encephalopathy is a grave sign and may be a valid indication for transplantation. Patients with grade III or IV encephalopathy have had complete neurologic recovery soon after receiving a transplant.[5] It is important to monitor intracranial pressure preoperatively, intraoperatively, and postoperatively in patients with signs of cerebral edema or grade III or IV encephalopathy. Persistent neurologic damage is common in patients with increased ICP.[7,18]

Even when there are strong indications that a liver transplant may be lifesaving, it is not always possible to obtain a suitable liver on short notice. In Japan, where OLT from brain-dead donors is rarely performed, living donor partial liver transplantation has been tried in emergent cases of FHF.[25] Although postsurgical mortality is high, this method provides for a greater number of potential transplants. There is a theoretical advantage of partial liver transplantation, from either a live or a dead donor. Because patients with amatoxin-induced hepatic failure have an acute toxic insult to the liver, it is possible that their liver would regenerate if given significant time. Partial liver transplantation allows for a portion of the patient's liver to stay in place while a lobe of a donor liver supports hepatic function. If the patient's liver regenerates to the point of being able to support hepatic function, the donor lobe can be removed, eliminating the need for lifelong immunosuppression. The feasibility of this approach has not been prospectively assessed in amatoxin-poisoned patients.

ARTIFICIAL DETOXIFICATION SYSTEMS AND THE BIOARTIFICIAL LIVER

Other methods of extending life while awaiting liver transplantation or while allowing native liver to regenerate are being used now or are being developed. These include bioartificial livers, which typically are based on porcine hepatocytes and a charcoal column. Six-hour treatments with these devices have allowed patients with acute hepatic failure to recover with their native livers or to survive until an orthotopic transplant was available.[26] Extracorporeal liver-assist devices, extracorporeal whole-organ perfusion (human and transgenic pig), and hepatocyte transplantation have been tried, but further clinical trials are needed to prove their effectiveness.[27]

Antidotal Treatments

The idea of simply treating a poisonous mushroom ingestion with a single antidote is appealing and has led to experimental treatments with several substances. As with other interventions, it has been difficult to measure the success of any single treatment because the treatments are seldom used alone and because of the other limitations on human experimentation. Mouse and dog models to study this problem have been used extensively; however, such data cannot always be generalized to humans. None of the antidotes used in the treatment of human cyclopeptide mushroom poisoning have undergone randomized, prospective clinical trials. Two agents that have been well tested in dogs and have been associated with improved outcomes in humans are silymarin and penicillin.[28]

SILYMARIN

Silymarin is isolated from the milk thistle plant *Silybum marianum*. It is available for use in Europe in oral (silymarin) and parenteral (silibinin) forms and has been used extensively, although most commonly in combination therapy. Oral dosing is 140 mg two to three times a day; intravenous dosing is 20 to 80 mg/kg/day in four divided doses given as an infusion over 2 hours.[29] The mechanism of action is uncertain, but it has been hypothesized to prevent amatoxin penetration into hepatocytes. Such an effect suggests that silymarin's greatest benefit would be found when administered as soon as possible after cyclopeptide mushroom ingestion. Silymarin has not been approved by the Food and Drug Administration for use in the United States but has been marketed as a food supplement and may be available through health food stores. (There are no randomized, controlled, clinical trials showing the efficacy of silymarin as a single agent in the treatment of amatoxin ingestion. In Europe, it has been used extensively, often in combination with penicillin, with anecdotal reports of improved survival.[1]

PENICILLIN

Penicillin G also has been shown in experiments with dogs given sublethal doses of amatoxin to prevent the increase of liver enzymes and may show an hepatoprotective effect.[28] In human case studies, it has been shown to be associated with increased survival, but most of the experiences with penicillin in the treatment of cyclopeptide mushroom poisoning have been as part of combination therapies. Recommended dosing is 300,000 to 1 million U/kg/day as an intravenous infusion.[30] At such high doses, penicillin may precipitate seizures, necessitating careful monitoring. As with silymarin, penicillin should be given as soon after ingestion as possible.

N-ACETYLCYSTEINE

N-Acetylcysteine, routinely used in the treatment of acetaminophen overdose, has shown promise in combination with other therapies in treating victims of *A. phalloides* poisoning.[31] *N*-Acetylcysteine and prostacyclin, a vasodilator, are hypothesized to work by increasing oxygen usage in the microcirculation.[32] *N*-Acetylcysteine seems to have antioxidant properties and may help slow the progression of hepatic encephalopathy, nephropathy, and coagulopathy.[33] It has been used without adverse effects and warrants further study to clarify its role in the treatment of cyclopeptide-induced liver failure. The clinical pharmacology of *N*-acetylcysteine is discussed in Chapter 136.

THIOCTIC ACID

Thioctic (α-lipoic) acid, first used in humans in the treatment of heavy metal–induced hepatic injury, also has been used in the treatment of cyclopeptide mushroom ingestion. Given intravenously as a continuous infusion, it was reported to reduce mortality in 40 cases of *A. phalloides* poisoning in Czechoslovakia in 1968.[34] There have been other reports showing higher mortality with its use.[35] Its mechanism is unknown, and although it has minimal inherent toxicity and is still used sporadically, it cannot be recommended at this time.

PICRORRHIZA

Picrorrhiza kurro'a is a plant that traditionally has been used in Asian Indian folk medicine for treating liver disorders. Experiments with the alcoholic extract of the root and rhizome have shown a strong protective effect and a weak curative effect in the mouse model after intraperitoneal injection of lyophilized *A. phalloides*.[36] This mixture of iridoid glycosides (called *kutkin*) has not been tested in dog models or humans and has the same limitations as other antidotes that need to be given before an ingestion of hepatotoxin to provide maximal benefit.

HYPERBARIC OXYGEN THERAPY

Hyperbaric oxygen therapy has been suggested in cyclopeptide mushroom poisoning because it has been used in treating poisoning caused by hepatotoxins that undergo biotransformation, such as carbon tetrachloride. A mouse model with high-dose amanitine and low-dose amanitine and hyperbaric (2.5 atm) versus normobaric conditions showed no benefit to hyperbaric treatment and the expected increase in liver damage with higher doses of amanitine under both pressures.[37] Empirical treatment of experimental human poisoning victims is limited and has been employed along with other interventions, making it difficult to prove any benefit.

CIMETIDINE

Cimetidine, a potent inhibitor of the P-450 cytochrome system,[38] has been shown to be hepatoprotective when the liver was exposed to acetaminophen,[39] carbon tetrachloride,[40] and halothane.[41] Mouse models were used to see if this cimetidine-induced hepatoprotection also would prevent the hepatotoxic effects of amatoxins. In these studies, cimetidine was administered 1 hour before or 4 hours after amatoxin exposure. In both cases, the treatment with cimetidine resulted in a decrease in microscopic liver injury compared with controls.[42] Because amanitine metabolites have never been identified, the proposed mechanism that cimetidine prevents the conversion of α-amanitine to a toxic metabolite is suspect. Another speculative mechanism of cimetidine's action is that it may facilitate a reduction in amanitine hepatic circulation. This mechanism also remains to be proven. Cimetidine is used occasionally as part of multitherapy, but we do not recommend its use.

MISCELLANEOUS THERAPIES

Cytochrome *c*,[43] steroids,[44] vitamin C,[45] and ethanol[46] have been tried in combination with other therapies but have not shown any significant improvements that would recommend their further use.

Criteria for ICU Discharge in Cyclopeptide Mushroom Poisoning*

Self-protection of airway
Resolution of coagulopathy and metabolic acidosis
Euglycemia
Ability to tolerate oral feedings
Resolution of altered mental status
Resolving bilirubin and hepatic transaminases
Resolving renal function abnormalities (or ability to provide dialysis in non–intensive care setting)

*All should be present.

Common Errors in Cyclopeptide Mushroom Poisoning

Missing the initial diagnosis owing to insufficient history or inadequate suspicion
Discounting the possibility of amatoxin poisoning because *Amanita* mushrooms were not consumed (other mushrooms contain these toxins)
Discounting the possibility of amatoxin poisoning because the symptoms appeared "too soon" (other mushrooms, such as those with predominantly gastrointestinal irritant properties, may have been consumed also, causing earlier onset of symptoms)
Discharging the patient after initial resolution of gastrointestinal symptoms
Waiting too long to transfer the patient to a liver transplant center

SPECIAL POPULATIONS

Pediatric Patients

Cyclopeptide mushroom ingestion in children is less common than in adults. Nonetheless, children are at greater risk of experiencing lethal hepatic injury after a cyclopeptide mushroom meal because, given the apparent 0.1 mg/kg lethal dose, a child would need to consume far less than an adult. A case in which, unknown to the parent or guardian, a young child ingests a cyclopeptide mushroom from the backyard or neighborhood park would be particularly challenging to diagnose, and such diagnostic confusion may delay further the onset of appropriate therapy. Adolescent ingestions have been reported after misidentification of hallucinogenic mushrooms or as suicide attempts.

Pregnant Patients

There have been a few case reports of amatoxin-containing mushroom consumption during pregnancy. In one case, a 25-year-old woman was at 9 weeks' gestation when she developed mushroom poisoning after ingesting *A. phalloides*. She survived the ingestion and had a therapeutic abortion at 12 weeks' gestation. The fetus showed hepatocellular damage, which suggested that amatoxin can cross the placenta.[47] There have been other case reports, however, showing no damage to the infant, questioning whether amatoxin does actually cross the placenta.[48] In a retrospective review of 22 cases (from 1960 to 1993) of pregnant women in Hungary with mild to moderate mushroom poisoning thought to be caused by *A. phalloides* or related species (including 5 during the first trimester), the mean birth weight was lower than in controls, but there was no difference in major and minor anomalies compared with controls.[49] No recommendations have been made for special protection of the fetus other than optimizing care of the mother. There is currently not enough evidence to recommend therapeutic abortion because of cyclopeptide mushroom poisoning in the mother.

Other Special Populations

The elderly and patients with serious comorbidities are theoretically at increased risk primarily because of the lack of reserve to survive the many systemic insults of cyclopeptide mushroom poisoning.

Key Points in Cyclopeptide Mushroom Poisoning

1. Keep cyclopeptide mushroom poisoning in the differential diagnosis for a patient with gastrointestinal complaints, and consider the possibility of an ingestion when obtaining the history.
2. Contact regional poison control center for help in diagnosing and treating suspected cyclopeptide mushroom ingestions.
3. Provide initial and continuing aggressive treatment of fluid and electrolyte abnormalities, acid-base disturbances, coagulopathies, and encephalopathy.
4. Make early contact with regional liver transplant center, and consider early transfer to a transplant center.
5. Report cyclopeptide mushroom ingestion cases to local and regional surveillance centers.

REFERENCES

1. Benjamin DR: Mushrooms: Poisons and Panaceas: A Handbook for Naturalists, Mycologists, and Physicians. New York, WH Freeman & Company, 1995.
2. Hanrahan JP, Gordon MA: Mushroom poisoning: Case reports and a review of therapy. JAMA 251:1057–1061, 1984.
3. Arora D: Mushrooms Demystified, 2nd ed. Berkeley, CA, Ten Speed Press, 1986.
4. Wieland T, Faulstich H: Fifty years of amanitin. Experientia 47:1186–1193, 1991.
5. Klein AS, Hart J, Brems J, et al: *Amanita* poisoning: Treatment and the role of liver transplantation. Am J Med 86:187–193, 1989.
6. Faulstich H: New aspects of Amanita poisoning. Klin Wochenschr 57:1143–1152, 1979.
7. Pinson CW, Daya MR, Benner KG, et al: Liver transplantation for severe *Amanita phalloides* mushroom poisoning. Am J Surg 159:493–499, 1990.
8. Vesconi S, Langer M, Iapichino G, et al: Therapy of cytotoxic mushroom intoxication. Crit Care Med 13:402–406, 1985.
9. Homann J, Rawer P, Bley H, et al: Early detection of amatoxins in human mushroom poisoning. Arch Toxicol 59:190–191, 1986.
10. Frank IC, Cummins L: Case review: *Amanita* poisoning treated with endoscopic biliary diversion. J Emerg Nurs 13:132–134, 1987.
11. Wauters JP, Rossel C, Farquet JJ: *Amanita phalloides* poisoning treated by early charcoal haemoperfusion. BMJ 2:1465, 1978.
12. Piqueras J, Duran-Suarez JR, Massuet L, et al: Mushroom poisoning: Therapeutic apheresis or forced diuresis. Transfusion 27:116–117, 1987.
13. Rolando N, Philpott-Howard J, Williams R: Bacterial and fungal infection in acute liver failure. Semin Liver Dis 16:389–402, 1996.

14. Rolando N, Wade JJ, Stangou A, et al: Prospective study comparing the efficacy of parenteral antimicrobials, with or without enteral decontamination, in patients with acute liver failure. Liver Transplant Surg 2:8–13, 1996.
15. Daas M, Plevak DJ, Wijdicks EF, et al: Acute liver failure: Results of a 5-year clinical protocol. Liver Transplant Surg 1:210–219, 1995.
16. Wade JJ, Rolando N, Hayllar K, et al: Bacterial and fungal infections after liver transplantation: an analysis of 284 patients. Hepatology 21:1328–1336, 1995.
17. Lee WM: Acute liver failure. Am J Med 96(1A):3S-9S, 1994.
18. Donovan JP, Shaw BW Jr, Langnas AN, et al: Brain water and acute liver failure: The emerging role of intracranial pressure monitoring. Hepatology 16:267–268, 1992.
19. Moore K: Renal failure in acute liver failure. Eur J Gastroenterol Hepatol 11:967–975, 1999.
20. Floersheim GL, Weber O, Tschumi P, et al: Clinical death cap (*Amanita phalloides*) poisoning: Prognostic factors and therapeutic measures: Analysis of 205 cases. Schweiz Med Wochenschr 112:1164–1177, 1982.
21. Mitchell I, Bihari D, Chang R, et al: Earlier identification of patients at risk from acetaminophen-induced acute liver failure. Crit Care Med 26:279–284, 1998.
22. O'Grady JG, Alexander GJ, Hayllar KM, Williams R: Early indicators of prognosis in fulminant hepatic failure. Gastroenterology 97:439–445, 1989.
23. Anand AC, Nightingale P, Neuberger JM: Early indicators of prognosis in fulminant hepatic failure: An assessment of the King's criteria. J Hepatol 26:62–68, 1997.
24. Lopez A, Jerez V, Rebollo J, et al: Fulminant hepatitis and liver transplantation. Ann Int Med 108:769, 1988.
25. Uemoto S, Inomata Y, Sakurai T, et al: Living donor liver transplantation for fulminant hepatic failure. Transplantation 70:152–157, 2000.
26. Chen SC, Mullon C, Kahaku E, et al: Treatment of severe liver failure with a bioartificial liver. Ann N Y Acad Sci 831:350–360, 1997.
27. Ostapowicz G, Lee WM: Acute hepatic failure: A Western perspective. J Gastroenterol Hepatol 15:480–488, 2000.
28. Floersheim GL, Eberhard M, Tschurni P, et al: Effects of penicillin and silymarin on liver enzymes and blood clotting factors in dogs given a boiled preparation of *Amanita phalloides*. Toxicol Appl Pharmacol 46:455–462, 1978.
29. Parish RC, Doering PL: Treatment of *Amanita* mushroom poisoning: A review. Vet Hum Toxicol 28:318–322, 1986.
30. Floersheim GL: Treatment of human amatoxin mushroom poisoning: Myths and advances in therapy. Med Toxicol 2:1–9, 1987.
31. Montanini S, Sinardi D, Pratico C, et al: Use of acetylcysteine as the life-saving antidote in *Amanita phalloides* (death cap) poisoning: Case report on 11 patients. Arzneimittel-Forschung 49:1044–1047, 1999.
32. Ellis A, Wendon J: Circulatory, respiratory, cerebral, and renal derangements in acute liver failure: Pathophysiology and management. Semin Liver Dis 16:379–388, 1996.
33. Ben-Ari Z, Vaknin H, Tur-Kaspa R: N-acetylcysteine in acute hepatic failure (non-paracetamol-induced). Hepatogastroenterology 47:786–789, 2000.
34. Plotzker R, Jensen DM, Payne JA: Case report: *Amanita virosa* acute hepatic necrosis: Treatment with thioctic acid. Am J Med Sci 283:79–82, 1982.
35. Floersheim GL, Weber O, Tschumi P, et al: Die Klinsche Knollenblatterpilzverg: Ftung: prognistische faktoren und therapeutische massnahmen. Schweiz Med Wochenschr 112:1164–1177, 1982.
36. Floersheim GL, Bieri A, Koenig R, et al: Protection against *Amanita phalloides* by the iridoid glycoside mixture of Picrorhiza kurroa (kutkin). Agents Actions 29:386–387, 1990.
37. Thomas J, Tomaszewski C, Gordon B, et al: Effect of hyperbaric oxygen on alpha amanitin hepatotoxicity in mice (Abstract). J Toxicol Clin Toxicol 35:557, 1997.
38. Speeg KV, Patwardhan RV, Arvant GR, et al: Inhibition of microsomal drug metabolism in histamine H2-receptor antagonists studied in vivo and in vitro in rodents. Gastroenterology 82:89–96, 1975.
39. Mitchell MG, Schenker S, Arvant GR, et al: Cimetidine protects against acetaminophen toxicity in rats. Gastroenterology 81:1052–1060, 1981.
40. Homann J, Rotter, Schneider S, et al: Influence of cimetidine on CC14-induced liver injury and survival in rats. Biochem Pharm 34:415–416, 1985.
41. Plummer JL, Wanwimolruk S, Jenner MA, et al: Effects of cimetidine and ranitidine on halothane metabolism and hepatotoxicity in an animal model. Drug Metab Dispos 12:106–110, 1984.
42. Schneider SM, Borochovitz D, Krenzelok EP: Cimetidine protection against alpha-amanitin hepatotoxicity in mice: A potential model for the treatment of *Amanita phalloides* poisoning. Ann Emerg Med 16:1136–1140, 1987.
43. Floersheim GL: Curative potencies against alpha-amanitin poisoning by cytochrome C. Science 177:808–809, 1972.
44. Floersheim GL: Antagonistic effects against single lethal doses of *Amanita phalloides*. Naunyn Schmiedeberg Arch Pharmacol 293:171–174, 1976.
45. Schneider SM, Vanscoy GJ, Michelson EA: Combination therapy with cimetidine, penicillin, and ascorbic acid for alpha amanitin toxicity in mice. Ann Emerg Med 18:482, 1989.
46. Floersheim GL: Ethanol and tolerated doses of *Amanita phalloides* protect against lethal doses of the mushroom. Agents Actions 7:171–173, 1977.
47. Kaufmann M, Muller A, Paweletz N, et al: Fetal damage due to mushroom poisoning with *Amanita phalloides* during the first trimester of pregnancy. Geburtshilfe und Frauenheilkunde 38:122–124, 1978.
48. Belliardo F, Massano G, Accomo S: Amatoxins do not cross the placental barrier (Letter). Lancet 1:1381, 1983.
49. Timar L, Czeizel AE: Birth weight and congenital anomalies following poisonous mushroom intoxication during pregnancy. Reprod Toxicol 11:861–866, 1997.

CHAPTER 121

Gyromitra Mushrooms

Daniel E. Brooks ■ Kimberlie A. Graeme

The mushroom species *Gyromitra* (formerly *Helvella*) *esculenta* grows throughout the northern hemisphere and is found in North America, Europe, and Asia. It is common in coniferous and hardwood forests, growing solitary or in groups. The species fruits only in early spring (later at higher elevations), often at edges of receding snow banks or where snow has recently melted. These mushrooms are moderately sized, brown to reddish brown, with wrinkled or folded caps 3 to 10 cm across, and have a brainlike or saddle shape (Fig. 121-1). *G. esculenta* is a member of the fungus class Ascomycetes, meaning that it has no gills, tubes, or spines but develops its spores in saclike structures called *asci*. The stalk is white to brown in color, thick, and hollow, usually with a single chamber.

G. esculenta often is misidentified as Morchellaceae due to similar appearance. Morchellaceae (genera *Disciotis*, *Morchella*, and *Verpa*) or "true morels," are highly sought for consumption. True morels may cause significant gastrointestinal (GI) distress if consumed raw.[1] *G. esculenta*, or "false morel," contains the toxin gyromitrin, which is metabolized to the toxin monomethylhydrazine (MMH) (Fig. 121-2). Other mushrooms that contain gyromitrin are listed in Tables 121-1 and 121-2.[1–6]

Almost 9000 mushroom exposures were reported to the American Association of Poison Centers in 1999; 36 of these involved gyromitrin-containing species.[7] *G. esculenta* was second only to *Amanita* spp. for mushroom-induced deaths during the first 72 years of the 20th century.[8] A European review of 513 cases of gyromitrin toxicity reported a 14% mortality rate.[9] In northern Europe, false morels may be identified correctly but incorrectly regarded as nontoxic and ingested. *G. esculenta* is canned and sold in Europe and can be purchased raw for consumption in some European markets.

Poisoning occurs after the ingestion of either raw or cooked mushrooms. These mushroom toxins are volatile; the boiling point of gyromitrin is 64°C (147.2°F) and of MMH is 87°C (188.6°F). Cooking decreases the toxin content. Parboiling is a technique used to prepare *G. esculenta* and decrease its toxicity. It involves repeated boiling of the mushroom with water changes. This process is not proven to remove all toxin completely, however, and gyromitrin can be detected in dried, boiled, and lyophilized specimens.[10,11] Several specific gyromitrin homologues have been identified in the steam during boiling. Toxicity from inhaling the steam or drinking the cooking water has been reported.[10] Drying the mushrooms in outdoor air at 20°C (68°F) removed 98.9% of an intermediate metabolite, *N*-methyl-*N*-formylhydrazine (MFH) (see Fig. 121-2), in 14 days, and boiling 100 g of *G. esculenta* in 300 mL of water, pH of 7.8, for 10 minutes removed 81.3% of the toxin. Parboiling and decreasing the water's pH further aid in the removal of toxin.[10]

BIOCHEMISTRY OF *GYROMITRA* TOXINS: METABOLISM OF GYROMITRIN

In the 19th century, Bohm and Kulz[12] falsely identified helvellic acid as the compound responsible for the toxicity of *G. esculenta*. List and Luft[13] were the first to identify gyromitrin correctly (acetaldehyde MFH) in 1967 with subsequent structural confirmation via direct synthesis.

Under physiologic conditions, gyromitrin is metabolized rapidly to acetaldehyde and MFH (see Fig. 121-2). This reaction has been reproduced experimentally under conditions mimicking the gastric environment.[14] Subsequently, and more slowly, MFH is hydrolyzed to MMH and formic acid. Alternative metabolism of MFH by the hepatic mixed-function oxidase system has been studied and might explain gyromitrin's hepatotoxic effects.[15] At this time, at least 11 structurally similar hydrazones (hydrazine homologues) have been identified in *G. esculenta*.[10,16]

PATHOPHYSIOLOGY

Effect on Pyridoxine Metabolism

γ-Aminobutyric acid (GABA), the major inhibitory neurotransmitter in the central nervous system (CNS), is synthesized from the excitatory neurotransmitter glutamate by glutamic acid decarboxylase. This reaction requires pyridoxal phosphate, the activated form of pyridoxine (vitamin B$_6$), as a cofactor (Fig. 121-3). MMH inhibits glutamic acid decarboxylase, causing increased concentrations of glutamate and decreased concentrations of GABA. MMH blocks the phosphorylation of pyridoxine by inhibiting pyridoxine phosphokinase. MMH also binds phosphorylated pyridoxine, inhibiting its role in various reactions.[17] These effects on GABA synthesis account for the CNS excitation (e.g., seizures) seen with poisoning by gyromitrin-containing mushrooms.

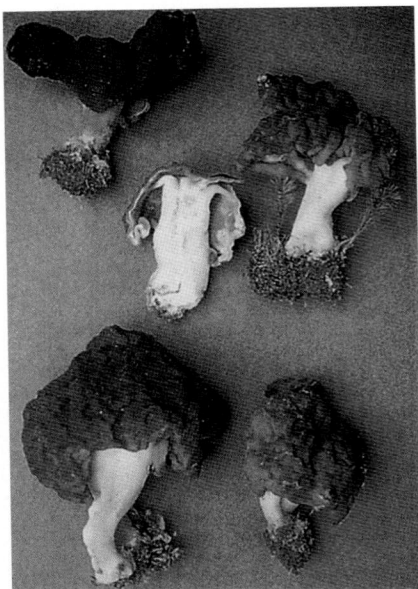

FIGURE 121-1

Gyromitra esculenta, which contains the hepatoxin gyromitrin. *(From Phillips R: Mushrooms of North America. Boston, Little Brown, 1991.)* **See Color Fig. 121-1.**

Fast versus Slow Acetylators and Difference in Toxicity

The ability to acetylate xenobiotics via hepatic metabolism varies within the human population and is genetically determined.[18,19] There is a dichotomous distribution of acetylator phenotypes in humans, referred to as *slow* and *rapid* acetylators. After ingestion of *G. esculenta,* hydrazine compounds may be acetylated, which seems to protect against neurologic effects but enhances hepatotoxicity. Formation of acetylhydrazine is the first step in the biotransformation of the hydrazines, ultimately resulting in formation of hepatotoxic alkylating radicals.[19-23]

Oxidative Stress

Gyromitrin toxicity can cause an oxidative stress that overwhelms the endogenous antioxidant systems normally used to maintain methemoglobin (MetHb) concentrations at less than 3%. MetHb is formed by oxidation of hemoglobin's iron from the ferrous (Fe^{2+}) to ferric (Fe^{3+}) state. MetHb is incapable of carrying oxygen and shifts the oxygen dissociation curve to the left, hindering oxygen delivery and producing cyanosis and tissue hypoxia. Methemoglobinemia is discussed in detail in Chapter 28.

Inhibition of Diamine Oxidase

Diamine oxidase (histaminase) is a regulatory enzyme responsible for the metabolism of histamine. It is found in rapidly proliferating tissue, such as intestinal mucosa and bone marrow. MFH noncompetitively inhibits diamine oxidase in human and animal tissues in vitro.[24] This inhibition may lead to elevated histamine concentrations, which produce cramping abdominal pain, nausea, vomiting, diarrhea, headache, and flushing; this explains the similarity between the gyromitrin and scombroid syndromes.

Mixed-Function Oxidase Inhibition

During the oxidation of gyromitrin and MFH, highly reactive nitrosamide intermediates that decrease hepatic cytochrome P-450 concentrations in rat microsomes are formed.[25] These nitrosamide metabolites may account for some of the hepatotoxicity and destruction of the mixed-function oxidase system.

Inhibition of Folate Conversion to Folinic Acid

Folate is the inactive form of a B-complex vitamin essential for protein synthesis and erythropoiesis. Dihydrofolate reductase (Fig. 121-4), the enzyme that converts folate to folinic acid (the active form), is inhibited by the hydrazones in *G. esculenta.* Folinic acid (leucovorin) administration may maintain normal cellular catabolism.

Carcinogenicity and Embryotoxicity

There have been significant increases in neoplasm development reported in animals fed fresh *G. esculenta* or its

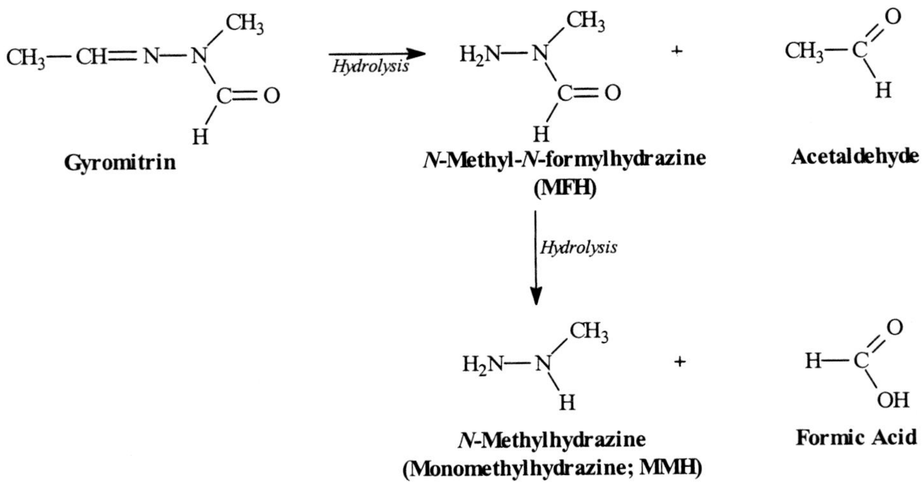

Gyromitrin   →(*Hydrolysis*)   **N-Methyl-N-formylhydrazine (MFH)**   +   **Acetaldehyde**

↓ *Hydrolysis*

N-Methylhydrazine (Monomethylhydrazine; MMH)   +   **Formic Acid**

FIGURE 121-2

Metabolism of gyromitrin.

TABLE 121-1 Mushrooms Known to Contain Gyromitrin*

SCIENTIFIC NAMES	COMMON NAMES
Gyromitra ambigua and *Gyromitra infula*	Hooded false morel
Gyromitra esculenta	False morel, beefsteak (brain) mushroom, elephant ears, turban fungus, lorchel

*This list is composed cognizant of the low consensus among authors with respect to nomenclature and classification of these mushrooms.[1–6]

TABLE 121-2 Mushrooms Thought to Contain Gyromitrin*

SCIENTIFIC NAMES	COMMON NAMES
Cudonia circinans	
Cyathipodia macropus	
Gyromitra brunnea or *Gyromitra fastigiata*	Brown false morel
Gyromitra californica	California false morel, umbrella false morel
Gyromitra caroliniana	Carolina false morel, big red mushroom
Gyromitra gigas (including *Gyromitra montana*)	Giant false morel, snow (snowbank) false morel
Gyromitra korfii	Bullnose
Gyromitra sphaerospora	Round-spored gyromitra
Helvella crispa	Common white helvella
Helvella lacunosa	Black helvella
Leoptopodia elastica	
Leotia lubrica	Slippery cap
Neobulgaria pura	Beech jelly-drop cup
Otidea onotica	Lemon-peel cup
Sarcophaere crassa	Violet star cup
Spathularia flavida	

*This list is composed cognizant of the low consensus among authors with respect to nomenclature and classification of these mushrooms.[1–6]

prepared hydrazones.[26–40] MMH causes teratogenic effects in toad embryos[41] and has shown a dose-dependent decrease in pregnancy rates of exposed rats.[42] More research is required to better understand the possible carcinogenic and mutagenic potential of these compounds after human mushroom ingestion.

CLINICAL PRESENTATION AND LIFE-THREATENING COMPLICATIONS

Interpersonal Differences in Dose Response— the Individual Threshold Dose

Individual responses to *G. esculenta* are varied and range from no toxicity to severe poisoning resulting in rapid death. Dose-dependent and interpersonal differences in response determine the minimal amount of ingested mushroom necessary to cause toxicity in any given patient. This phenomenon is known as the *individual threshold dose*.[1,43,44] Patient factors, such as age, size, health, and metabolic capability (i.e., slow versus fast acetylators); amount ingested; preparation technique; and amount of coingested food may affect a person's clinical course. Toxicity also has been reported to occur only after repeated exposure, suggesting a kindling or sensitizing mechanism. Others have suggested that bioaccumulation of gyromitrin may lead to poisoning.[20] It has been

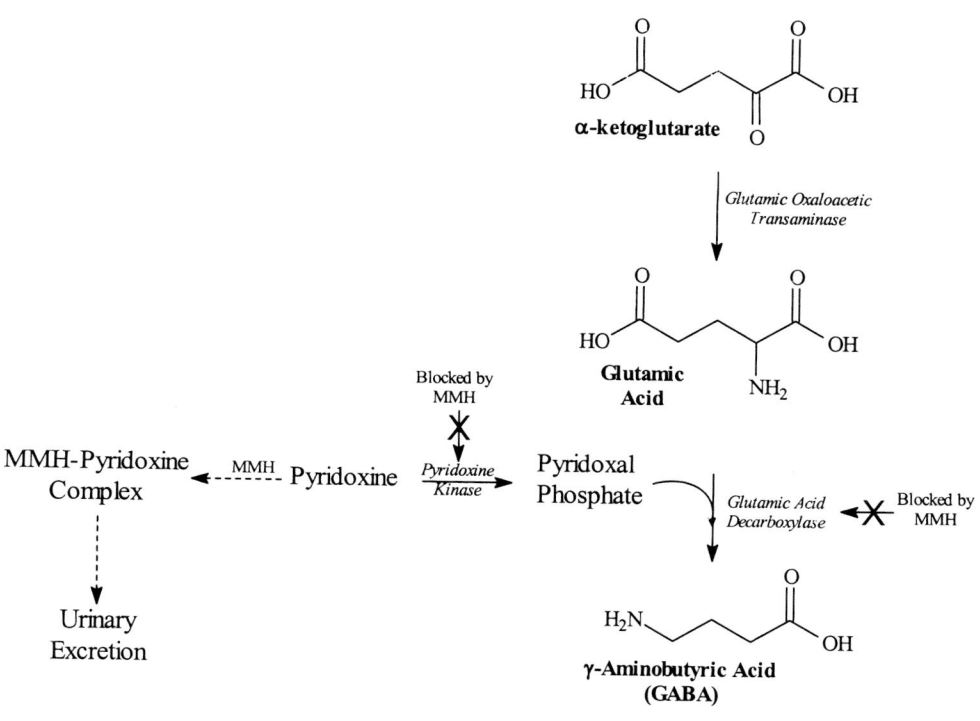

FIGURE 121-3

Inhibition of γ-aminobutyric acid synthesis by monomethylhydrazine.

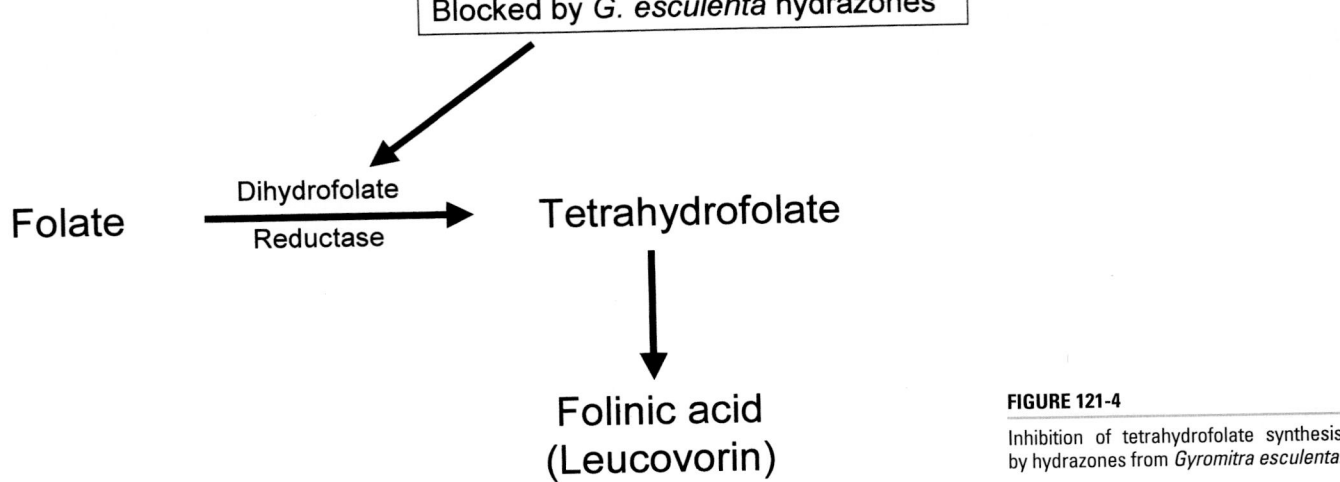

FIGURE 121-4

Inhibition of tetrahydrofolate synthesis by hydrazones from *Gyromitra esculenta*.

observed that a person may eat *G. esculenta* for years but develop poisoning only after consuming a large, threshold amount.

There also is considerable variation in the potential of any gyromitrin-containing mushroom to cause toxicity. The toxicity of an individual mushroom is determined by several factors, including genetic strain, hybridization, environment (soil, temperature, light), age, and internal distribution of toxin. The altitude at which the mushrooms grow has been identified as a potent determinant of toxin content. Mushrooms sampled from "middle" altitudes often contain more than five times the amount of MMH as samples from higher elevations.[45] It has been reported, but not confirmed, that within the United States *G. esculenta* is toxic east of the Rocky Mountains only, being safe to consume on the western side.[1]

Systems Approach to Signs and Symptoms and Complications

Clinical findings of *G. esculenta* toxicity are varied. Symptoms typically are delayed for 6 to 12 hours, with reported onset ranging from 2 to 48 hours. Time until onset of symptoms may be explained in part by variations in the concentrations of the various mushroom toxins.[46] The gyromitrin syndrome normally starts with GI symptoms, including abdominal pain and bloating, nausea, vomiting, and occasionally watery or bloody diarrhea. Most patients manifest GI symptoms only and make a complete recovery within several days. Severe toxicity may develop, however, progressing from GI distress to neurologic, hepatic, and renal dysfunction. An asymptomatic interval between resolution of GI symptoms and the onset of neurologic or hepatorenal toxicity may occur. It is imperative to maintain a high index of suspicion for severe, protracted illness when caring for a gyromitrin-poisoned patient. The gyromitrin syndrome typically involves the onset of gastroenteritis within 12 hours of mushroom ingestion, accompanied by headache, myalgias, and fever. Hemolysis, neurologic complications, and hepatorenal failure may follow.

Systemic Effects of Gyromitrin

The GI symptoms of gyromytrin poisoning can last for several days, with excessive fluid losses causing hypovolemia, hypotension, shock, and acidosis. Patients may develop tachycardia and hypotension secondary to hypovolemia from GI losses. Cardiovascular instability may indicate significant multiorgan dysfunction or shock. Neurologic symptoms appear later, often after resolution of gastric complaints, with or without an asymptomatic period. Patients may exhibit labile emotions or report headache, dizziness, vertigo, delirium, seizures, or coma.

Hepatic failure usually develops within 48 hours of ingestion, if at all, and is manifested by elevated transaminases, coagulopathy, and jaundice. Abdominal examination may reveal right upper quadrant tenderness. Biopsy samples of rat liver and kidney tissue after death from gyromitrin poisoning reveal discoloration of tissue, inflammatory changes, and focal necrosis.[46]

Infrequently, renal failure develops as a result of hemolysis, rhabdomyolysis, or prolonged hypotension.[47] Renal failure also may occur as a result of a gyromitrin-induced hepatorenal syndrome. Patients may also report diffuse myalgias secondary to rhabdomyolysis.

Hypoglycemia and electrolyte abnormalities may develop from significant gastrointestinal losses and lack of intake before seeking medical treatment. Fever may develop as a manifestation of a systemic inflammatory response or as a consequence of hepatic injury.

Gyromitrin-induced oxidative stress may precipitate intravascular hemolysis and methemoglobinemia. Hemolysis can be assessed by measuring plasma free hemoglobin, haptoglobin, and hemoglobinuria. Significant hemolysis may cause splenomegaly. The skin may appear jaundiced (from hepatotoxic effects), pale (from dehydration, hypovolemia, or hemolysis), or cyanotic (from methemoglobinemia). Methemoglobinemia should be suspected in any patient who develops cyanosis unresponsive to supplemental oxygen. Although symptoms and clinical findings do not correlate well with cooximetry-derived MetHb concentrations, most patients develop significant symptoms at MetHb levels 30%

or greater. Methemoglobinemia is discussed in detail in Chapter 28.

DIAGNOSIS

A history of *G. esculenta* consumption greatly assists the diagnosis and management of gyromitrin poisoning. When this history is not available, other disease processes should be considered.

Differential Diagnosis of Gyromitrin Poisoning

Hydrazine (monomethylhydrazine) poisoning from nonmushroom source (rocket fuel)
Poisoning from other mushroom toxins (amatoxin, coprine, ibotenic/muscimol)
Bacterial food poisoning
Other toxic ingestions (acetaminophen, salicylate, iron, isoniazid, organophosphates)
Methemoglobinemia from nonmushroom source (benzocaine)
Gastritis/gastroenteritis
Biliary disease/cholelithiasis
Hepatitis
Sepsis
Encephalopathy or seizure disorder

Laboratory testing should include evaluating liver and renal function, electrolytes, blood glucose, complete blood count, creatine kinase (or myoglobin), coagulation profiles, methemoglobin, serum haptoglobin, and plasma free hemoglobin. Gyromitrin concentrations can be quantitated by gas chromatography–mass spectrometry but have not been shown to correlate with clinical status and are not available in a timely fashion.[48]

Patients should be placed on a cardiac monitor and have vital signs and oxygen saturation assessed frequently. Pulse oximetry uses sensors with only two wavelengths and does not reliably differentiate between different hemoglobin species. Pulse oximetry also is unreliable after the use of methylene blue, when falsely decreased saturations occur.

TREATMENT

Treatment is mainly supportive, with emphasis on controlling gastroenteritis and replacing fluid and electrolyte losses. Patients typically present at least 4 hours after ingestion, which limits the utility of GI decontamination. If patients present within 1 hour of ingestion, however, activated charcoal theoretically may be beneficial and should be given without cathartic because these patients already are prone to developing diarrhea. No study has assessed the effect of activated charcoal administration on the outcome of gyromitrin-poisoned patients. All symptomatic patients should be admitted for supportive care, observation, and treatment for progression of symptoms.

Indications for ICU Admission in Gyromitrin Poisoning

Severe gastrointestinal symptoms with significant fluid imbalance
Neurologic instability (coma or seizure)
Hemodynamic compromise
Hemolysis (especially in patients with glucose-6-phosphate dehydrogenase deficiency)
Significant or symptomatic methemoglobinemia (dyspnea, tachypnea, dysrhythmias, mental status changes, seizures, or cyanosis)
Signs of toxicity in patients with significant comorbidity (ischemic heart disease or renal failure)

Antidotes

METHYLENE BLUE

All patients with signs or symptomatic of methemoglobinemia (or MetHb levels >30%) should be treated with supplemental oxygen and methylene blue, unless contraindicated. The dose of methylene blue is 1 to 2 mg/kg by intravenous push. Reversal of symptoms is expected to occur within 15 minutes. If necessary, a second dose can be administered, with a maximal total dose of 7 mg/kg. At higher doses, methylene blue can induce oxidative stress and worsen methemoglobinemia. Methylene blue is contraindicated in patients with known glucose-6-phosphate dehydrogenase deficiency because of increased risk of methylene blue–induced hemolysis.[49] If clinically indicated, these patients should undergo exchange transfusion to correct methemoglobinemia. The treatment of methemoglobinemia and the clinical pharmacology of methylene blue are discussed in Chapters 28 and 155.

FOLINIC ACID (LEUCOVORIN)

Hydrazines inhibit the conversion of folate to its active form, and patients should receive the active formulation, folinic acid or leucovorin. The usual dose is 5 to 15 mg/day intravenously, intramuscularly, or orally for 5 to 7 days. Higher doses (≤1 mg/kg intravenously every 4 hours) can be given for severely poisoned patients. Because the inhibition of dihydrofolate reductase is transient, it is generally thought that after 24 hours folate can be used instead of folinic acid.

THIOCTIC ACID AND *N*-ACETYLCYSTEINE

A case series from 1968 mentions the use of thioctic acid (α-lipoic acid) in the successful treatment of *G. esculenta*–poisoned patients.[50] This compound, similar to *N*-acetylcysteine, is reported to have antioxidant effects. Although there is a theoretical advantage to using these compounds, to date there are no studies showing improved clinical outcome. *N*-acetylcysteine was shown to be ineffective at reversing methemoglobinemia produced by other oxidants in human volunteers.[50] Neither thioctic acid nor *N*-acetylcysteine is routinely recommended.

PYRIDOXINE

The use of pyridoxine (vitamin B_6) has been shown to limit the severity of hydrazine-induced neurologic dysfunction from isoniazid and gyromitrin.[19,51–55] The optimal dose for gyromitrin-induced neurotoxicity is unknown; recommendations range from 1 to 70 mg/kg.[52] The empirical intravenous administration of 5 g of pyridoxine to patients who convulse after ingesting an unknown quantity of the hydrazine compound isoniazid or who fail to respond to conventional anticonvulsant therapy is well established.[55]

It seems reasonable to administer 25 mg/kg intravenously once to all patients with known or suspected acute gyromitrin toxicity and to repeat doses if seizures occur or continue. Administration of pyridoxine at doses greater than 500 mg/day for extended periods (≥6 months) is associated with the development of sensory neuropathy and other adverse effects.[54,56,57] This should not become an issue in the treatment of acute gyromitrin poisoning. The clinical pharmacology of pyridoxine is discussed in Chapter 147.

Other Treatments

HEMODIALYSIS

Gyromitrin-induced renal failure should be managed in a standard fashion, including the use of hemodialysis. Usual guidelines for initiating hemodialysis in acute-onset renal failure should be followed.

INTRAVENOUS FLUIDS AND SERUM ALKALINIZATION

Patients may develop significant dehydration secondary to GI losses and decreased fluid intake. Barring contraindications, aggressive fluid resuscitation should be provided to replace fluid deficits, compensate for ongoing losses, and ensure adequate urine output (>0.5 mL/kg/hr). A Foley catheter should be placed to assess urine output accurately. Hypovolemia should be managed with normal saline or lactated Ringer's solutions, with close monitoring of electrolytes and renal function. Rhabdomyolysis should be treated with urinary alkalinization to a urine pH greater than 6.5 to prevent the renal tubular deposition of myoglobin–Tamm-Horsfall protein complexes and acute renal failure.[58] Urinary alkalinization usually can be accomplished by placing 2 or 3 ampules of sodium bicarbonate in 1 L of 5% dextrose in water, infusing this at approximately 200 mL/hr in adults. Adding this amount of sodium bicarbonate to saline-containing fluids would create a hypertonic solution, leading to hypernatremia.

TREATMENT OF SEIZURES

Treatment of gyromitrin-induced seizures includes the administration of pyridoxine, benzodiazepines, or barbiturates (with the possible exception of phenobarbital). All three agents are GABA-agonists that increase CNS concentrations of GABA, decreasing neuronal excitation. Pyridoxine overcomes the gyromitrin-induced inhibition of GABA synthesis (see Fig. 121-3). Benzodiazepines bind to the GABA_A chloride channel and increase GABA binding to its receptor and increase the rate of channel opening. Barbiturates enhance GABA's actions at these chloride channels by prolonging the duration of opening. At high concentrations, some barbiturates can directly open these chloride channels. Phenobarbital induces hepatic P-450 enzymes and increases the microsomal metabolism of gyromitrin, theoretically causing more hepatotoxicity.[25] The use of phenobarbital in the treatment of a gyromitrin-poisoned patient should be avoided.

Criteria for ICU Discharge in Gyromitrin Poisoning

Clinical improvement with no evidence of end-organ disease
Withdrawal of care

Phenytoin blocks voltage-gated sodium channels and inhibits the spread or propagation of seizure activity but does not increase GABA concentrations within the CNS.[59] This mechanism is effective at preventing the spread of abnormal focal CNS electrical activity but is not expected to abort the diffuse neuronal involvement in gyromitrin-induced seizures. The use of phenytoin is not recommended in the treatment of these patients.

VITAMIN K

Gyromitrin-induced hepatotoxicity can decrease vitamin K–dependent coagulation factors (factors II, VII, IX, and X and proteins C and S). Pharmacologic correction for this effect can be administered in the form of vitamin K, at doses of 0.5 to 10 mg intravenously, intramuscularly, or orally, depending on the severity of the hepatotoxicity. A dose of only 0.5 mg intravenously should be used for patients requiring medical anticoagulation because reversal of vitamin K effects, which are long lasting, can be difficult.[60] The prophylactic use of vitamin K in patients with hepatotoxicity but no coagulopathy is controversial.

Observation Time

Patients presenting after known or suspected *G. esculenta* ingestion should be observed clinically for the onset of gastroenteritis for at least 12 hours after ingestion. Asymptomatic or minimally symptomatic patients can be discharged home if they have appropriate social support, outpatient follow-up, and strict instructions to return if symptoms progress. However, all patients with signs and symptoms of toxicity (gastroenteritis, liver or renal dysfunction, seizures), patients with comorbidities (cardiac disease or renal failure), and the very young or very old should be admitted to the hospital for observation and supportive care. Severely ill patients need intensive monitoring and care.

SPECIAL POPULATIONS

Theoretically, patients at increased risk are patients with smaller body surface areas (i.e., children and small adults) and patients with significant comorbidities (i.e., hepatitis, anemia, cardiac disease, dehydration). A pregnant patient who ingests *G. esculenta* places the fetus at risk because of maternal stress caused by dehydration, shock, hepatotoxicity, methemoglobinemia, and other sequelae of the gyromitrin syndrome. The treatment of pregnant patients should focus on the mother, given the potential benefits to fetal and maternal outcome. The teratogenic and embryotoxic risks of *G. esculenta* are unknown.

Patients with glucose-6-phosphate dehydrogenase deficiency are at increased risk for hemolysis. They may develop significant hemolysis, anemia, methemoglobinemia, and hypovolemic shock from either gyromitra poisoning or the use of methylene blue. As previously reviewed, symptomatic methemoglobinemia in known glucose-6-phosphate dehydrogenase–deficient patients should not be treated with methylene blue and may require exchange transfusion.

Common Errors in Gyromitrin Poisoning

Failure to consider the diagnosis
Failure to recognize potential severity of poisoning
Failure to recognize methemoglobinemia
Interpreting asymptomatic interval as resolution of poisoning
Failure to identify patients with G6PD deficiency
Treating G6PD-deficient patients with methylene blue
Giving excessive or prolonged pyridoxine

G6PD, glucose-6-phosphate dehydrogenase.

Key Points in Gyromitrin Poisoning

1. Gyromitrin can lead to significant morbidity and death.
2. Clinical onset generally in 6 to 12 hours.
3. Gastrointestinal symptoms predominate early.
4. Most patients develop gastrointestinal complaints only and recover within several days.
5. A transient asymptomatic period may occur.
6. Occasional progression to hepatorenal or neurologic disease (or both) within 48 hours may occur.
7. Hemolysis, methemoglobinemia, hepatorenal failure, jaundice, seizures, and coma can occur.

REFERENCES

1. Benjamin DR: Mushrooms, Poisons and Panaceas. New York, WH Freeman & Company, 1995.
2. Koppel C: Clinical symptomatology and management of mushroom poisoning. Toxicon 31:1513–1540, 1993.
3. Spoerke DG, Rumack BH (eds): Handbook of Mushroom Poisoning, Diagnosis and Treatment. Ann Arbor, CRC Press, 1994.
4. McKnight KH, McKnight VB: Peterson Field Guide: Mushrooms. Boston, Houghton Mifflin, 1987.
5. Toth B: Carcinogenic fungal hydrazines. In Vivo 5:95–100, 1991.
6. Læssøe T, Lincoff G: Mushrooms. New York, DK Publishing, 1998.
7. Litovitz TL, Klein-Schwartz W, White S, et al: 1999 Annual report of the American Association of Poison Control Centers Toxic Exposure Surveillance System. Am J Emerg Med 18:517–574, 2000.
8. Buck RW: Acute encephalopathy in children after eating wild mushrooms. In Rumack B, Salzman E (eds): Mushrooms Poisoning: Diagnosis and Treatment. West Palm Beach, FL, CRC Press, 1978, pp 191–197.
9. Franke S, Freimuth U, List PH: Uber die giftigkeit der fruhjahrslorchel, *Gyromitra (Helvella) esculenta*. Arch Toxikol 22:293–332, 1967.
10. Pyaysalo H, Niskanen A: On the occurrence of N-methyl-N-formylhydrazones in fresh and processed false morel, *Gyromitra esculenta*. J Agric Food Chem 25:644–647, 1977.
11. Schmidon-Meszaros J: Gyromitrin in trockenloercheln (*Gyromitra esculenta sicc.*). Mitt Gebiete Lebensm Hyg 65:453–465, 1974.
12. Bohm RV, Kulz E: Uber den giftigen bestandtheil der essbaren morchel (*Helvella esculenta*), naunyn-schmeidebergs. Arch Exp Pathol Pharmak 19:403–414, 1885.
13. List PH, Luft P: Gyromitrin, das gift des fruhjashrslorchel. Arch Pharm 301:294–305, 1968.
14. Nagel D, Wallcave L, Toth B, Kupper R: Formation of methylhydrazine from acetaldehyde N-methyl-N-formylhydrazone, a component of *Gyromitra esculenta*. Cancer Res 37(9):3459–3460, 1997.
15. Braun R, Greeff U, Netter KJ: Indications for nitrosamide formation from the mushroom poison gyromitrin by rat liver microsomes. Xenobiotica 10:557–564, 1980.
16. Toth B, Gannett P: *Gyromitra esculenta* mushroom: A comparative assessment of its carcinogenic potency. In Vivo 8:999–1002, 1992.
17. Biehl JP, Vilter RW: Effects of isoniazid on pyridoxine metabolism. JAMA 165:1549–1552, 1954.
18. Evans DAP, Manley KA, McKusick VA: Genetic control of isoniazid metabolism in man. Br Med J 2:485–491, 1960.
19. Hein DW, Weber WW: Relationship between N-acetylator phenotype and susceptibility towards hydrazine-induced lethal central nervous system toxicity in the rabbit. J Pharmacol Exp Ther 228:588–592, 1984.
20. Coulet M, Guillot J: Poisoning by *Gyromitra*: A possible mechanism. Med Hypothesis 8:325–334, 1982.
21. Mitchell JR, Thorgeirsson UP, Black M, et al: Increased incidence of isoniazid hepatitis in rapid acetylators: Possible relation to hydrazine metabolites. Clin Pharmacol Ther 18:70–79, 1975.
22. Mitchell JR, Jollow DJ: Biochemical basis for drug-induced hepatotoxicity. Isr J Med Sci 10:312–318, 1974.
23. Peters JH, Miller KS, Brown P: Studies on the metabolic basis for the genetically determined capacities for isoniazid inactivation in man. J Pharmacol Exp Ther 150:298–304, 1965.
24. Bieganski T, Braun R, Kuschel J: N-methyl-N-formylhydrazine: A toxic and mutagenic inhibitor of the intestinal diamine oxidase. Agents Actions 14:351–355, 1984.
25. Braun R, Greef U, Netter KJ: Indications for nitrosamide formation from the mushroom poison gyromitrin by rat liver microsomes. Xenobiotica 10:557–564, 1980.
26. Toth B: Hydrazine, methylhydrazine and methylhydrazine sulfate carcinogenesis in Swiss mice: Failure of ammonium hydroxide to interfere in the development of tumors. Int J Cancer 9:109–118, 1972.
27. Toth B, Nagel D: Tumors induced in mice by N-methyl-N-formylhydrazine of the false morel *Gyromitra esculenta*. J Natl Cancer Inst 60:201–204, 1978.
28. Toth B, Patil K, Erickson J, Kupper R: False morel mushroom *Gyromitra esculenta* toxin: N-methyl-N-formylhydrazine carcinogenesis in mice. Mycopathologia 68:121–128, 1979.
29. Toth B, Patil K: The tumorigenic effect of low dose levels of N-methyl-N-formylhydrazine in mice. Neoplasma 27:25–31, 1980.
30. Toth B, Smith J, Patil K: Cancer induction in mice with acetaldehyde methylformylhydrazone of the false morel mushroom. J Natl Cancer Inst 67:881–887, 1981.
31. Toth B, Patil K: Tumorigenicity of minute dose levels of N-methyl-N-formylhydrazine of *Gyromitra esculenta*. Mycopathologia 78:11–16, 1982.
32. Toth B, Raha CR: Carcinogenesis by pentanal methylformylhydrazone of *Gyromitra esculenta*. Mycopathologia 98:83–89, 1987.
33. Toth B, Gannett P: Carcinogenesis study in mice by 3-methylbutanal methylformylhydrazone of *Gyromitra esculenta*. In Vivo 4:283–288, 1990.
34. Toth B, Taylor J, Gannett P: Tumor induction with hexanal methylformylhydrazone of *Gyromitra esculenta*. Mycopathologia 115:65–71, 1991.
35. Toth B, Patil K, Pyysalo H, et al: Cancer induction in mice by feeding the raw false morel mushroom *Gyromitra esculenta*. Cancer Res 52:2279–2284, 1992.
36. Hawks A, Magee PN: The alcylation of nucleic acids of rats and mouse in vivo by the carcinogen 1,2-dimethylhydrazine. Br J Cancer 30:440–447, 1974.
37. Wright VA, Niskanen A, Pyysalo H: The toxicities and mutagenic properties of ethylidene gyromitrin and N-methylhydrazine using *Escherichia coli* as a test organism. Mutat Res 56:105–110, 1977.
38. Toth B, Shimizu H: Methylhydrazine tumorigenesis in Syrian golden hamsters and the morphology of malignant histiocytomas. Cancer Res 33:2744–2753, 1973.
39. Toth B, Patil K: Carcinogenic effects in the Syrian golden hamster of N-methyl-N-formylhydrazine of the false morel mushroom *Gyromitra esculenta*. J Cancer Res Clin Oncol 93:109–121, 1979.
40. Toth B: Hepatocarcinogenesis by hydrazine mycotoxins of edible mushrooms. J Toxicol Environ Health 5:193–202, 1979.

41. Greenhouse G: Evaluation of the teratogenic effects of hydrazine, methylhydrazine, and dimethylhydrazine on embryos of *Xenopus laevis*, the South American clawed toad. Teratology 13:167–178, 1976.

42. Slanina P, Cekan E, Halen B, et al: Toxicological studies of the false morel (*Gyromitra esculenta*): Embryotoxicity of monomethylhydrazine in the rat. Food Addit Contam 10:391–398, 1993.

43. Giusti GV, Carnevale A: A case of fatal poisoning by *Gyromitra esculenta*. Arch Toxicol 33:49–54, 1974.

44. Hendericks HC: Poisoning by false morels (*Gyromitra esculenta*). JAMA 114:1625, 1940.

45. Andary C, Privat G, Bourrier M-J: Variations of monomethylhydrazine content in *Gyromitra esculenta*. Mycologia 77:259–264, 1985.

46. von Wright AV, Niskanen A, Pyysalo H, Korpela H: The toxicity of some N-methyl-N-formylhydrazones from *Gyromitra esculenta* and related compounds in mouse and microbial tests. Toxicol Appl Pharmacol 45:428–434, 1978.

47. Braun R, Kremer J, Rau H: Renal functional response to the mushroom poison gyromitrin. Toxicology 13:187–196, 1979.

48. Michelot D, Toth B: Poisoning by *Gyromitra esculenta*—a review. J Appl Toxicol 11:235–243, 1991.

49. Kirsh IR, Cohen HJ: Heinz body hemolytic anemia from the use of methylene blue in neonates. J Pediatr 96:276–278, 1980.

50. Mittman W: Zur klinik und therapie der lorchelvergiftungen (*Gyromitra esculenta*). Z Aerztl Forbild 67:710–711, 1968.

51. Tanen DA, LoVecchio F, Curry SC: Failure of intravenous N-acetylcysteine to reduce methemoglobin produced by sodium nitrite in human volunteers: A randomized controlled trial. Ann Emerg Med 35:369–373, 2000.

52. von Wright A, Niskanen A, Pyysalo H: Amelioration of toxic effects of ethylidene gyromitrin (false morel poison) with pyridoxine chloride. J Food Saf 3:199–203, 1981.

53. Toth B, Erickson J: Reversal of the toxicity of hydrazine analogues by pyridoxine hydrochloride. Toxicology 7:31–36, 1977.

54. Biehl JP, Vilter RW: Effects of isoniazid on pyridoxine metabolism. JAMA 156:1549–1552, 1954.

55. Wason S, Lacouture PG, Lovejoy FH Jr: Single high-dose pyridoxine treatment for isoniazid overdose. JAMA 246:1102–1104, 1981.

56. Cohen M, Bendich A: Safety of pyridoxine-a review of human and animal studies. Toxicol Lett 34:129–139, 1986.

57. Schaumburg H, Kaplan J, Windebank A, et al: Sensory neuropathy from pyridoxine abuse. N Engl J Med 309:445–448, 1983.

58. Visweswaran P, Guntupalli J: Rhabdomyolysis. Crit Care Clin 15:415–428, 1999.

59. Saad SF, el Masry AM, Scott PM: Influence of certain anticonvulsants on the concentration of GABA in the cerebral hemispheres of mice. Eur J Pharmacol 76:386–392, 1972.

60. Hung A, Singh S, Tait RC: A prospective randomized study to determine the optimal dose of intravenous vitamin K in reversal of over-warfarinization. Br J Haematol 109:537–539, 2000.

CHAPTER **122**

Overview of Plant and Herbal Toxicity

Anthony J. Scalzo

Critical care physicians are often experienced in the management of overdoses of common pharmaceuticals, such as tricyclic antidepressants. Toxins of plant origin, including herbal products, may present challenging and often unfamiliar territory, however. Medical toxicologists and poison centers are consulted frequently for common household plant ingestions by children, but only a few of such ingestions result in serious toxicity.[1] Nevertheless, plant poisonings have been associated with admission to intensive care units (ICUs) around the world.

In one retrospective study of plant poisonings, 56 medical records, from 29 adults and 27 children, treated at a Tunisian toxicologic ICU were evaluated. Eleven species of plants were identified, and the toxic alkaloids were analyzed by thin-layer and gas chromatography.[2] The following plants, which are discussed in this and other chapters, were among the plant species reported: *Datura stramonium* (Jimson weed), *Ricinus communis* (castor bean), *Nerium oleander* (oleander), *Urginea maritima* (red squill), and *Solanum nigrum* (black nightshade). These poisonings involved the neurologic (91%), gastrointestinal (GI) (73%), and cardiovascular (18%) systems. Sixteen were fatalities from liver failure secondary to *Atractylis gummifera* (white cameleon). The rhizomes of *A. gummifera* plants are poisonous and contain the toxic glycosides atractyloside and carboxyatractyloside. These toxic components induce hepatic necrosis by blocking conversion of adenosine diphosphate (ADP) to adenosine triphosphate (ATP) and inhibition of cytochromes, specifically cytochrome b_5. Atractyloside and carboxyatractyloside are potent inhibitors of oxidative phosphorylation in rat liver mitochondria.[3] They inhibit ADP transport into mitochondria by binding to the ADP carrier protein in the inner mitochondrial membrane.[4] These toxins create a negative cellular energy balance with resultant cellular necrosis. The concept that there are toxic principles, such as alkaloids or glycosides, in plants that may interfere with normal cellular processes, such as energy production, is central to the understanding of plant toxicology. Poisonings resulting from the major plant syndromes are discussed in subsequent chapters. This chapter provides an introductory overview of plant-induced toxic syndromes and highlights major issues regarding herbal toxic agents.

The American Association of Poison Control Centers reported a total of 71,009 plant ingestions in 1999.[5] Plants were the fourth most common ingestant in children younger than 6 years old. Only nine deaths were reported.

It has been recognized that herbal products and their interaction with conventional medications (e.g., St. John's wort and retroviral agents) may pose a more prevalent problem than classic plant poisonings, such as castor bean, oleander, aconitine, and the hemlocks. Herbal products are obtained easily without prescription at health food stores, pharmacies, general department stores, neighborhood groceries, and the Internet. The World Health Organization estimated that 4 billion people (80% of the world's population) use herbal preparations.[6]

CLASSIFICATION OF PLANT SYNDROMES BY TOXIC PRINCIPLES

Although there are a myriad of different species of plants, only a few have the potential to result in serious toxicity. This chapter presents an introduction to plant species containing the following:

- Toxalbumins
- Anticholinergic alkaloids
- Cardiac glycosides
- Amygdalin and cyanogenic glycosides
- Solanine
- Oxalates, soluble and insoluble

Table 122-1 provides a detailed summary of plant toxins. Additionally, selected herbal products with potential for serious drug interactions in ICUs are considered in this chapter.

Toxalbumins

Toxalbumins are derived primarily from the castor bean plant (*Ricinus* spp.), which is native to tropical Africa. This plant has been cultivated for the production of castor oil. Despite poor GI absorption, oral exposures to toxalbumins are characterized by acute gastroenteritis. Dehydration can occur as a result of fluid loss. Acute renal failure, hepatocellular necrosis, rhabdomyolysis, and multiorgan failure may be late complications. Toxalbumins are also allergens and may precipitate symptoms such as dermatitis, rhinitis, and asthma or rarely anaphylactic shock. Because toxalbumins

TABLE 122-1

SCIENTIFIC NAMES	COMMON NAMES (REPRESENTATIVE PLANTS FROM TOXIC GROUPS)	TOXIC PRINCIPLES	PREDOMINANT SIGNS OR SYMPTOMS OF TOXICITY AND TARGET ORGANS
Abrus precatorius	Jequirty (rosary) pea	Toxalbumins (lectins): abrin and ricin	Delayed gastroenteritis, hepatic failure, cytotoxicity
Ricinus communis	Castor bean		
Jatropha curcas	Physic nuts		
Philodendron spp.	Philodendron	Insoluble oxalates (oxalic acid)	Local (mouth and throat edema, bullae, salivation, dysphagia) and GI irritation
Dieffenbachia spp.	Dumbcane		
Rheum rhaponticum	Rhubarb	Soluble oxalates; anthraquinones (glycosides) also have been implicated	Oxalic acid poisoning with acidosis and cytotoxicity: nephropathy, hepatotoxicity, CNS injury
Parthenocissus tricuspidata	Boston ivy		
Rumex crispus	Garden sorrel		
Taxus cuspidata and other spp.	Yew (Japanese)	Taxine (cardiac glycosides)	Cardiac rhythm disturbances; GI irritation
Phytolacca americana	Pokeweed	Phytolaccine (saponin glycosides) and pokeweed mitogen	Severe GI irritation; mitosis of lymphoid cells
Atropa belladonna	Belladonna, deadly nightshade	Hyoscyamine (atropine) and scopolamine	Anticholinergic symptoms (peripheral and central)
Datura stramonium	Jimson weed		
Hyocyamus niger	Henbane		
Solanum nigrum	Black nightshade	Glycoalkaloids solanine, solasodine, chaconine	Nausea, vomiting, diarrhea, muscular weakness
Solanum pseudocapsicum	Jerusalem cherry	Solanine, solanocapsine	
Nerium oleander	Oleander	Oleandrin	Cardiac rhythm disturbances, degrees of AV block, hyperkalemia
Thevetia peruviana	Yellow oleander	Thevetin	
Digitalis purpurea	Foxglove	Digitoxin	
Urginea maritima	Red squill	Scillaren-A/B, scillaridin	
Aconitum napellus	Monkshood (aconite, wolfsbane)	Aconitine and other (C19) norditerpinoids	Nausea, vomiting, bradycardia, hypotension, polymorphous ventricular arrhythmias, respiratory failure
Rhododendron spp.	Rhododendron	Andromedotoxins (grayanotoxins)	Respiratory depression, bradycardia, hypotension, generalized weakness
Rhododendron spp.	Azalea		
Kalmia spp.	Mountain laurel		
Hydrangea macrophylla	Hydrangea	Cyanogenic glycosides (amygdalin)	Dyspnea, dizziness, cyanosis, hypotension, shock. Signs of cyanide poisoning
Prunus spp.	Almond, apricot		
Manihot esculenta	Tapioca plant		
Cicuta maculata	Water hemlock	Cicutoxin	GI symptoms (nausea, vomiting, abdominal pain), intractable seizures
Conium maculatum	Poison hemlock	Conine	Tachycardia, GI symptoms, ascending paralysis, coma
Symphytum officinale	Comfrey (knitbone)	Pyrrolizidine alkaloids	Anorexia, vomiting, abdominal pain, venoocclusive hepatic disease, hepatomegaly
Laurea tridentata	Chaparral (creosote bush)		

AV, atrioventricular; CNS, central nervous system; GI, gastrointestinal.

are highly toxic, one immediately should focus on rapid initial assessment and decontamination.

INITIAL ASSESSMENT AND MANAGEMENT

Initial assessment and management of toxalbumin ingestion should focus on the following:

1. Cardiopulmonary stability is established by administering life support as needed.

2. Prevention of absorption may be beneficial. If seeds are swallowed whole and intact, toxicity is unlikely due to the durable seed husk, which contains the toxic principle. The severity of toxalbumin intoxication is generally proportional to the degree of mastication (i.e., whether the beans were chewed or were not chewed)[7,8] and the amount of seed material (i.e., number of beans) ingested.[9] There are differences in the quantity of the toxic component in each plant as determined by seasonal

changes and species variation.[10] GI decontamination procedures should be guided by the American Academy of Clinical Toxicologists and European Association of Poison Centres and Clinical Toxicologists position statements,[11] which are reviewed in detail in Chapter 5. Methods to be considered include gastric lavage and activated charcoal. It is advisable to avoid cathartics with charcoal because toxalbumins may cause diarrhea. There have been no randomized trials showing a beneficial effect of GI decontamination after toxalbumin ingestion.

3. Fluids, electrolytes, and glucose should be replaced.
4. If the diagnosis is uncertain, emesis and stool should be examined for the presence of seeds and seed fragments.
5. Blood glucose should be monitored because of the possibility of hypoglycemia.
6. Administration of oral antacids or other GI protective agents may have theoretical benefit, although rigorous evidence-based studies supporting their use are lacking.
7. Alkalinization of the urine may be useful to prevent deposition of crystals from hemoglobinuria in cases of hemolysis.
8. Toxalbumins are not eliminated through extracorporeal techniques, such as hemodialysis or alkaline diuresis.

TOXICOLOGY OF TOXALBUMINS

Toxalbumins are large glycoproteins that interfere with protein synthesis, ultimately resulting in cell death. Ricin and abrin, the two main toxalbumins, each consist of an A and a B subunit bound by a disulfide linkage (Fig. 122-1). The molecular weights of ricin and abrin (A and B chains together) are approximately 66,000 and 65,000, respectively.[12] When the disulfide link is eliminated, the toxicity to intact cells is virtually eliminated. The B part of the toxin binds to galactose-containing receptors in the cell wall, and the intact (A and B) toxin is actively transported into the cell. Toxalbumins disrupt DNA synthesis and protein synthesis at the 60S ribosomal subunit. Toxalbumin-containing plants of the greatest toxicologic significance are the following:

- Castor bean plant (*R. communis*)
- Jequirty bean plant (*Abrus precatorius*)
- Black locust tree (*Robinia pseudoacacia*)
- European mistletoe (*Viscum album*)

These plants contain the glycoproteins ricin, abrin, robin, and viscumin. Castor oil, prepared by cold pressing castor seeds, does not contain ricin and does not impart toxicity other than a laxative effect.[13]

Ingestion of seeds or other plant material, such as the leaves, may induce toxicity. When toxalbumin-containing seeds are ingested, resulting symptoms rarely have included oropharyngeal or esophageal burns. Acute gastroenteritis is the hallmark presentation of toxalbumin exposure.[8] Patients initially may have severe symptoms but often recover, highlighting the extreme toxicity of pure ricin and the lower mortality for castor seed ingestions.[14] Hepatorenal dysfunction and death may be due to persistent hypovolemia.

One case series and subject review discussed reports of 424 cases of castor bean intoxication in the literature. Delayed toxicity was not reported. Of the 424 patients, 14 died (mortality 8.1% of untreated and 0.4% of treated). Because this was a review of existing reports, some of which dated back to 1900, it is unclear what therapies the patients received. Where it was able to be determined, the patients received intravenous (IV) fluids as supportive therapy. Deaths were attributed to hypovolemic shock.[7]

Toxalbumins also can cause erythrocyte agglutination, which may result in hemolysis. Although the mechanism of hemolysis is unclear, it seems that ricin induces a glomerular thrombotic microangiopathy in rats with resultant hemolysis

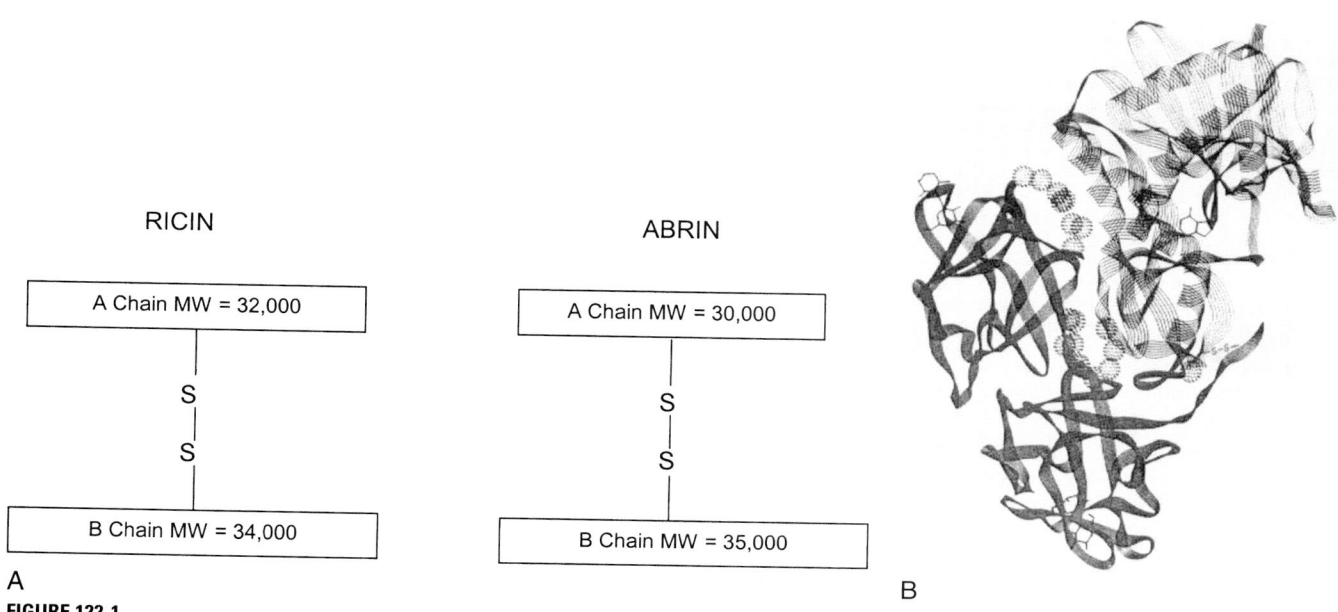

A, Schematic structure of A and B chains of ricin and abrin showing disulfide bonds between chains. **B,** Ribbon structure of ricin showing A and B chains. MW, molecular weight. *(**B** from http://www.ansci.cornell.edu/ plants/toxicagents/ricin/ricin.html#ricstruc.)*

FIGURE 122-1

closely resembling *Escherichia coli*–induced hemolytic ure-mic syndrome.[15]

Hepatic effects have been reported secondary to toxalbu-mins. Deterioration in liver function may be a late compli-cation. Disturbances in carbohydrate metabolism may precipitate hypoglycemia, and hepatic glycogen stores may become depleted. Hepatocellular damage may be a late complication. A 20-month-old infant ingested an unknown amount of castor bean seeds; vomited four times, producing two partially chewed seeds; and developed reversible hepa-totoxicity at 48 to 72 hours postingestion.[16] Delayed hyper-sensitivity and immediate anaphylactic reactions have been reported after exposure to castor beans and their dust.[17] Toxalbumins may precipitate allergic symptoms, such as dermatitis, rhinitis, and asthma.[18] It seems that castor oil may cause hypersensitivity reactions, and the allergen in castor oil has been found to be ricinoleic acid.[19] Despite the above-described effects, castor bean ingestions are associ-ated with severe toxicity only infrequently.[9]

RANGE OF TOXICITY

Death has followed the ingestion of a single jequirity bean that has been chewed. Toxicity with other members of this group may occur after ingestion of just a few seeds. If the seed is swallowed with the seed coat intact, there is a mini-mal risk of toxicity. Seeds from these plants are used in jew-elry making because of their colorful and shiny appearance and similarity to beads.[20] Drilling into the seed coat to pass a thread or wire to create necklaces and bracelets renders the toxin available for GI absorption if the seed is ingested. The natural curiosity of children makes them particularly vulner-able to ingesting these appealing-looking seeds. Many cases of abrus or ricinus exposure result in few or no clinical effects.[9,20] This lack of clinical manifestations may be due to variations in toxicity or poor GI absorption or both.

The ricin content of castor beans varies from plant to plant but averages approximately 3%. Ingestion is hundreds of times less toxic than parenteral exposure to ricin. The estimated lethal dose by the latter route is less than 3 mg/kg. The mortality rate for ricin ingestions has been reported at 6%, or slightly higher for symptomatic cases devoid of sig-nificant medical intervention. After medical support, the mortality rate for symptomatic patients has been reported at 0.4%.[7] The potential toxic effects of ricin may have implica-tions for law enforcement personnel, who may encounter such exposure in clandestine methamphetamine laboratories because drug traffickers have been known to coat their equipment with highly toxic ricin powder in an attempt to thwart attempts at raiding their supplies.

Although no formal guidelines have been studied, it is recommended that asymptomatic patients who have chewed one or more raw beans should have emergency department evaluation, administration of activated charcoal, observa-tion until 4 to 6 hours postingestion, and discharge instruc-tions to return if symptoms develop.[7] If there are signs of toxicity, such as gastroenteritis with vomiting and diarrhea, abdominal pain, GI bleeding, hematuria, dehydration, or shock, the patient should be observed and treated in a mon-itored unit or critical care unit. There is no known antidote for toxalbumins. Toxalbumin poisoning is discussed in detail in Chapter 127.

Anticholinergic Plant Poisoning

Numerous plants contain toxic principles that result in anti-cholinergic effects (see Table 122-1). The signs and symp-toms of anticholinergic poisoning can be divided into central and peripheral effects. Central anticholinergic effects are anxiety, agitation, delirium, myoclonus, seizures, and hallucinations, which may progress to lethargy, somno-lence, coma, respiratory failure, and circulatory collapse. Peripheral effects are mydriasis, hyperthermia, vasodilation, decreased salivation, urinary retention, tachycardia, hyper-tension, and arrhythmias. The pathophysiology of anti-cholinergic syndrome is discussed in detail in Chapter 22. Common plants that contain anticholinergic alkaloids are Jimson weed (*D. stromonium*), deadly nightshade (*Atropa belladonna*), matrimony vine (*Lycium barbarum*), and night blooming jessamine (*Cestrum nocturnum*).

Plants with anticholinergic properties generally contain belladonna alkaloids, primarily atropine, hyoscyamine, or scopolamine. Signs and symptoms of toxicity from anti-cholinergic plants are the result of antagonism of the actions of acetylcholine at muscarinic receptors. These alkaloids have no effect on the nicotinic anticholinergic receptors, which occur at neuromuscular junctions and in the central nervous system. The most commonly affected organs are heart, brain, exocrine glands, and smooth mus-cle, particularly in the bladder, iris, and bowel. Predominant anticholinergic principles and the plant species associated with them are summarized in Table 122-2.

An example of anticholinergic alkaloid poisoning is a report of five adolescents who presented to an emergency department manifesting hallucinations, tachycardia, and dilated pupils after ingesting an angel trumpet lily mixed with a cola soft drink concoction.[21] Other mass ingestions of anticholinergic plants, such as Jimson weed, have been reported.[22] Ingestion and smoking of Jimson weed have resulted in atropine intoxication.[23] The critical care physi-cian caring for such patients should consider this possibility when taking a history. Anticholinergic poisoning also may arise from unsuspected sources, such as certain bee and wasp honeys, and should be included in the differential diagnosis of delirium and hallucinations. Honey-induced poisoning from grayanotoxin (a sodium channel toxin) may occur when bees obtain the toxin inadvertently from the nectar of some species of rhododendron, a plant known to cause grayanotoxin intoxication. In one report, 15 cases of atropine poisoning were associated with ingestion of wasp honey in a rural area in Venezuela.[24] *Datura* spp. plants were found in the area, and their nectar likely served as sources of atropine and scopolamine.

The anticholinergic syndrome produced by plant alka-loids may be rapid in onset and continue for 24 to 48 hours, possibly owing to delayed gastric motility induced by the alkaloids. As described earlier, central anticholinergic effects include anxiety, agitation, delirium, hyperactivity, myoclonus, seizures, aphasia, dysarthria, amnesia, disorien-tation, confusion, hallucinations (particularly lilliputian), choreoathetoid movements, lethargy, somnolence, coma, respiratory failure, circulatory collapse, and death. Periph-eral effects due to muscarinic blockade are mydriasis, hyperpyrexia, vasodilation, dysphagia, decreased salivation causing intense drying of the mouth and intense thirst

TABLE 122-2 Predominant Anticholinergic Toxic Principle by Plant Species

SCIENTIFIC NAME	COMMON NAME	TOXIC PART	PREDOMINANT TOXIC PRINCIPLE*
Datura stramonium	Jimson weed, loco weed	Seeds (highest concentration of toxin found in seeds)	Hyoscyamine
Brugmansia suaveolens	Angel's trumpet	Roots	Hyoscyamine, hyoscine
		Leaves	Hyoscyamine
Hyoscyamus niger	Henbane, black henbane	All plant parts	Hyoscyamine, hyoscine
Atropa belladonna	Deadly nightshade, belladonna	All plant parts	Hyoscyamine, hyoscine, atropine
Lycium halimfolium	Matrimony vine	All plant parts	Hyoscyamine
Cestrum nocturnum	Night blooming jessamine	All plant parts	Atropine, gastroenterotoxin, also has solanine properties

*Atropine is an isomer of hyoscyamine. Scopolamine is the l-isomer of hyoscine and is much more physiologically active than the d-isomer.

(drying of secretions may not be apparent in a severely agitated patient), dry skin (may be absent in an agitated patient), decreased bronchial and nasal secretions, decreased GI motility (Jimson weed seeds have been recovered from the stomach 16 to 36 hours postingestion), urinary retention, hypertension, and arrhythmias. Cardiac effects may consist of abnormal conduction, such as bundle-branch block and atrioventricular dissociation. Unless hemodynamic instability results, sinus tachyarrhythmias do not pose a severe hazard. The electrocardiogram (ECG) may display an increased QT interval, decreased ST segments, and increased QRS intervals. Rarely, anticholinergic plant poisoning may result in lethal arrhythmias, such as ventricular fibrillation.[25]

The range of anticholinergic toxicity depends on the alkaloid content of plants and varies secondary to factors that affect plant growth from year to year, making it difficult to anticipate the severity of symptoms based on the amount of plant material ingested. All parts of the *Datura* spp. are poisonous. Young *Datura* plants contain mainly scopolamine, whereas mature plants contain mainly hyoscyamine. Toxic effects have been seen after ingestion of leaves or flowers, ingestion of tea brewed from various plant parts, and smoking of stramonium cigarettes.[23] The most common exposure is from ingestion of the seeds or teas for mind-altering effects. Each Jimson weed seed contains the approximate equivalent of 0.1 mg of atropine. The estimated adult lethal doses of atropine and scopolamine are approximately 10 mg and greater than 2 to 4 mg, respectively. Analysis of the alkaloid content of a wine made from *Datura suaveolens* (angel's trumpet, also known as *Brugmansia suaveolens*) found that it contained 29 mg of scopolamine/mL. Ingestion of 15 to 20 mL of this wine in a man caused respiratory distress, partial body paralysis, and muscular weakness within 90 minutes of exposure.[26] Although this case report is not a classic case of anticholinergic syndrome, the ganglionic blocking effects of scopolamine and its derivatives may have accounted for the presentation in this patient. The seeds and unripe fruit of *A. belladonna* contain primarily l-hyoscyamine. The ripe fruit contains almost entirely racemic atropine (98% of the alkaloids in the plant).[27] Atropine intoxication from the ingestion and the smoking of Jimson weed also has been reported.

Other reported sources of anticholinergic alkaloids have included herbal remedies, such as lupine seeds. There are about 100 different species of lupine plant in the United States alone, but not all are toxic. Lupine beans are used commonly in Southern Europe and the Middle East, but occurrences of toxicity have been reported mainly in the United States.[28] Although not all species are toxic, all parts of the plants are toxic in the poisonous varieties. Generally, dried lupine beans are soaked in water overnight, then boiled to leach out their bitterness. They are soaked further in water and after several days they are ready for consumption. In one case report, a 72-year-old woman drank a glassful of the bitter water in which the beans had been soaked under the assumption that it would lower her blood sugar. She presented with dilated and minimally reactive pupils (7 mm) and sinus tachycardia but normal temperature. The compounds oxo-sparteine and sparteine (an alkaloid found in lupine plants) were found in the extract by gas chromatography–mass spectrophotometry.[28]

Management of patients intoxicated with anticholinergic alkaloids involves hemodynamic stabilization, control of seizures, and most commonly control of agitation, which may be severe. Benzodiazepines (e.g., diazepam or midazolam) have been used for treatment of agitation. Physostigmine may be used for extreme agitation (see later). When one is confronted with an anticholinergic crisis from plants or other sources, butyrophenones and phenothiazines are not recommended because of their additive anticholinergic properties.

Patients with severe manifestations of anticholinergic poisoning, such as agitation unresponsive to benzodiazepine or hemodynamically significant tachyarrhythmias, may require specific management with physostigmine, which is an effective antidote for significant anticholinergic poisonings. The clinical pharmacology of physostigmine is discussed in Chapter 153. Its use in the treatment of anticholinergic plant syndromes is discussed in Chapters 22 and 126.

Anticholinergic alkaloid–induced cardiac arrhythmias should be treated with standard advanced life support measures. Sinus tachycardia generally does not require treatment. Severe tachyarrhythmias due to anticholinergic overdose may respond only to physostigmine. A short-acting β-receptor antagonist, such as esmolol, may be considered to treat tachycardia, but true anticholinergic poisoning probably responds best to physostigmine.

After GI decontamination, length of observation or need for admission is based on the severity of symptoms. Although not systematically studied, based on the existing literature, I recommend that patients exhibiting significant tachyarrhythmias or central nervous system manifestations, such as disorientation, hallucinations, or delusions, should be observed until symptoms resolve. Patients who require physostigmine should be considered for admission for several hours of observation. With anticholinergic ingestion, it is theoretically possible that delayed absorption of undigested plant product might occur with further symptoms. Many patients have resolution of their symptoms after treatment with physostigmine.

Supportive care in an ICU is effective in most cases for other manifestations of anticholinergic poisoning. Hyperthermia should be treated by standard techniques, including placing the patient in a cool room, decreasing muscular activity, sponging the patient with tepid to cool water, or possibly applying ice or use of a hypothermia blanket device. It is unknown whether standard antipyretics, such as acetaminophen (paracetamol), would be effective. A presumed anticholinergic syndrome unresponsive to physostigmine should prompt a reconsideration of the diagnosis.

The efficacy and safety of physostigmine have been studied by Burns and associates[29] in 52 patients with anticholinergic agitation and delirium. Physostigmine controlled agitation and reversed delirium in 96% and 87% of patients compared with benzodiazepines, in which case agitation was controlled in only 24% of patients. Benzodiazepines did not control delirium. Physostigmine has a tainted reputation due mostly to adverse events reported with its use in combination with tricyclic antidepressant overdose. Outside of these infrequent negative reports, physostigmine remains an excellent antidote for the treatment of severe anticholinergic syndrome. Peritoneal dialysis and hemodialysis are not effective in treating patients with plant-induced anticholinergic syndrome.[30]

Laboratory abnormalities that have been noted in patients with anticholinergic poisoning include elevations in liver enzymes, particularly aspartate aminotransferase and lactate dehydrogenase. Prolongation of prothrombin time also has been reported. Elevation of the white blood cell count has been noted in some cases. Some anticholinergic agents can be detected in the urine (e.g., atropine, hyoscyamine) but usually cannot be quantified. Such urinary assays are of minimal use in guiding clinical management. Scopolamine may be detected with high-performance liquid chromatography. Anticholinergic plant poisoning is discussed in greater detail in Chapter 126.

Cardiac Glycosides

Critical care physicians typically are familiar with the use of cardiac glycosides for the management of cardiac failure and tachyarrhythmias. They may encounter toxicity from digitalis glycosides frequently due to dosage errors, electrolyte disturbances, or frank overdose. Most cardiac glycosides that are used in practice today were initially derived from plants belonging to the genus *Digitalis* (i.e., *Digitalis purpurea*, or foxglove). Common plants that contain cardiac glycosides are oleander (*N. oleander*), yellow oleander (*Thevetia peruviana*), lily of the valley (*Convallaria majalis*), red squill (*Urginea maritima*), and foxglove. Toxicity may result from routes of exposure other than ingestion. Even inhalation of smoke from burning plants has caused toxicity.[31] A case of ingestion of two bulbs of *U. maritima* (squill) was reported in a 55-year-old woman who presented with nausea and vomiting followed by seizures, hyperkalemia, atrioventricular block (9 hours postingestion), and ventricular tachycardia (24 hours after admission).[32]

Herbal products may contain cardiac glycosides. A prominent example is a traditional Chinese patent medicine, Chan Su. Chan Su contains bufotenin, a cardiac glycoside. In one reported exposure, analyses of the Chinese medication Chan Su, a product derived from toads, showed that it contained the same bufadienolides as a West Indian aphrodiasiac known as "Love Stone."[33]

An aphrodisiac called Love Stone that is similar to Chan Su resulted in severe toxicity and deaths in a case series from New York City, in which secretions from a Colorado River toad, *Bufo alvarius*, and the cane toad, *Bufo marinus*, intended to be used as a topical preparation, were ingested.[34] These products contained the toxin bufadenisolide.

N. oleander is probably one of the most common causes of toxic exposures in this category. The oleandrin derived from common oleander and thevetin from yellow oleander are toxic glycosides that are structurally similar to digitoxin (Fig. 122-2).

These toxins act like digitoxin or digoxin, attaching to the α subunit of the Na^+, K^+-ATPase pump and inhibiting the latter's action. In toxic amounts, the resulting intracellular increases in sodium and calcium depolarize cardiac cells and cause late afterdepolarizations and increased automaticity, typical of cardiac glycoside poisoning.[35] Hyperkalemia may accompany and exacerbate these effects, similar to severe digoxin poisoning.

Patients presenting with ingestion of these plant glycosides may display GI irritation, with vomiting being the most common presenting complaint.[35] They also may have diarrhea; abdominal pain; dizziness; and numbness of the tongue, throat, and lips. Physical examination may reveal bradycardia and hypotension. ECG changes are myriad and are similar to changes encountered with digoxin toxicity, including PR prolongation, atrioventricular block of varying degrees including complete heart block, QT shortening, P- and T-wave flattening, premature ventricular contractions, and tachyarrhythmias including ventricular tachycardia and fibrillation. Cardiac glycoside poisoning is discussed in detail in Chapter 33. Cardiotoxic plants are discussed further in Chapter 125.

Amygdalin and Cyanogenic Glycosides

Cyanogenic glycosides are found in the trees of the *Prunus* spp., which contain the toxin amygdalin. Amygdalin itself is not harmful until it is metabolized by emulsin, an

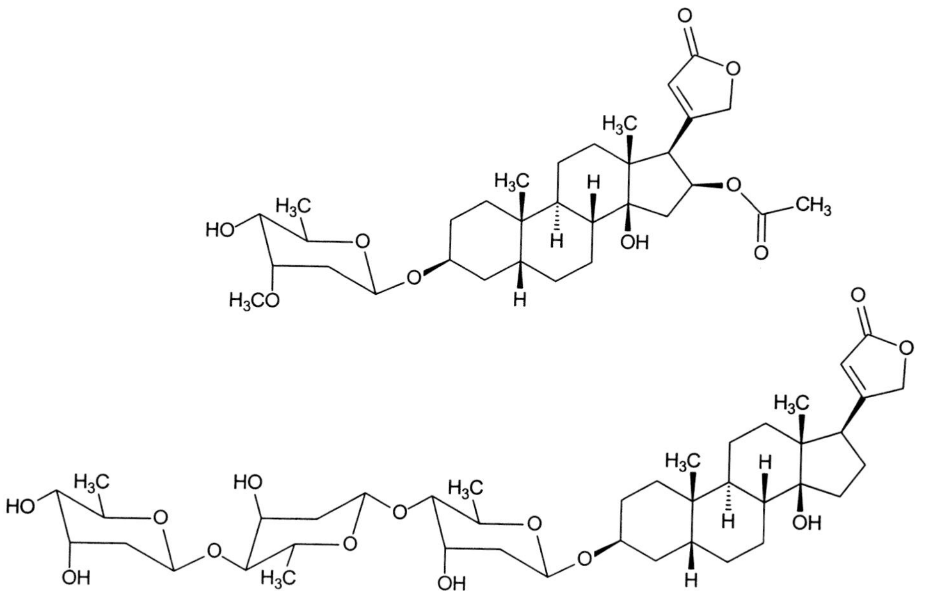

FIGURE 122-2

Chemical structures of oleandrin (*top*) and digitoxin (*bottom*).

enzyme in the plant seeds, or by certain bacteria in intestinal flora, liberating cyanide.[36]

The cyanogenic glycosides, composed of an α-hydroxynitrile type of aglycon and a sugar moiety (mainly D-glucose), are widely distributed in the plant kingdom, with at least 2500 taxa.[37] Common plants (mainly *Prunus* spp.) that contain cyanogenic glycosides are listed in Table 122-3.

The widespread use of amygdalin-containing seeds (primarily almond and apricot) has gained popularity with some patients seeking alternative cures for cancer (i.e., Laetrile). Although trials in cancer patients in the early 1980s and further studies in the 1990s for the most part debunked the efficacy of Laetrile, some patients continue to seek this "therapy." A study in mice showed the lack of antitumor activity against lymphocytic leukemia and mast cell leukemia despite doses of amygdalin (Laetrile) varying from 200 mg/kg to 2000 mg/kg.[38]

Several reports document cases in which Laetrile has caused life-threatening toxicity when taken in large doses. In one report by Kalyanaraman and colleagues,[39] a 67-year-old woman with lymphoma presented with a neuromyopathy after treatment with Laetrile. The authors found significant elevation of blood and urinary thiocyanate and cyanide levels. Sural nerve biopsy revealed a mixed pattern of demyelination and axonal degeneration. Other causes were excluded.

TABLE 122-3 Common Cyanogenic Glycoside Plants

Apple (seeds)	Elderberry
Apricot (pit)	Hydrangea (leaves)
Bitter almond	Lima beans
Cassava (beans and rhizomes)	Peach (pit)
	Pear (seeds)
Cherry laurel	Plum
Chokecherry	Wild black cherry
Crab apple (seeds)	Western chokecherry

Despite this controversy, some research on this topic has been conducted in the last few years. A group in London has used a novel technique to harness the potential cytotoxicity of amygdalin-generated cyanide using antibody-directed enzyme prodrug therapy (ADEPT), combining it with the use of amygdalin as prodrug.[40] Their hypothesis was that if amygdalin could be activated specifically at the tumor site by the enzyme β-glucosidase, malignant cells would be killed without the systemic toxicity usually associated with chemotherapy. They conjugated β-glucosidase to a tumor-associated monoclonal antibody (HMFG1). Amygdalin was cytotoxic to HT1376 bladder cancer cells only at high concentrations, whereas the combination of amygdalin with HMFG1-β-glucosidase enhanced the cytotoxic effect of amygdalin by 36-fold. The investigators concluded that ADEPT was more effective than nondirected enzyme activation of the prodrug and possibly could result in a nontoxic cancer therapy. Their approach has not been widely tested, however.

Prunus spp. seeds, such as peach pits, when crushed or warmed, liberate a bitter almond odor, often attributed to cyanide poisoning. Hydrocyanic acid, the likely toxic product that is released, accounts for the toxicity of amygdalin. The degree of toxicity is directly related to the amount of plant or seed ingestion. Significant ingestion may lead to the classic signs and symptoms of cyanide poisoning, such as dizziness, agitation, confusion, headache, lethargy, coma, seizures, bradycardia with initial hypertension, and terminal hypotension. The pathophysiology of cyanide poisoning is described in detail in Chapter 95.

The amount of hydrocyanic acid production depends on the biosynthesis of cyanogenic glycosides and the presence or absence of degrading enzymes, such as β-glucosidase and α-hydroxynitrilase.[37] The production of these cyanogenic glycosides is thought to play a role in plant defense mechanisms, and conversely their production is affected by ecologic factors. Human poisoning with cyanogenic glycoside–containing plants has been clustered in areas of the world where certain plants serve as major food sources.

Konzo, a disorder involving acute symmetric spastic paraparesis in association with the ingestion of cassava, is caused by insufficient processing of bitter cassava and low intake of essential amino acids.[41] This disorder is not a trivial concern because cassava (*Manihot esculenta*) is an important tropical root crop providing food for approximately a half a billion people in the world. One report documented three patients who were admitted after consuming a cassava-based meal and died shortly after admission.[42] The patients had complained of abdominal pain and had emesis immediately after ingestion of the meal and were unconscious on presentation. They developed renal failure and died of cardiopulmonary arrest. Blood cyanide levels averaged 1.12 mg/L (43 μmol/L).

Other investigators question the fate of dietary cyanogenic glycosides in humans. A group in Cuba studied the consumption of boiled fresh roots from sweet cassava varieties grown locally.[43] Nonsmoking adults consumed 1 to 4 kg of cassava over 2 days, and their urine was analyzed for thiocyanate and linamarin, the main cyanogenic glucoside in cassava. The mean thiocyanate levels increased from 12 ± 2 μmol/L to 22 ± 2 μmol/L (0.07 to 0.13 mg/dL), which the authors reported as negligible. Their mean urinary linamarin levels increased, however, from 2 ± 1 μmol/L to 68 ± 16 μmol/L. In a second experiment, five of the subjects consumed one meal of 0.5 kg of boiled cassava that contained 105 μmol of linamarin and 8 μmol of hydrocyanic acid. Quantitative urine collections before and after consumption showed that 28% of the linamarin was excreted within 24 hours, and there was only a modest increase in urinary thiocyanate. Although these results are reassuring that ingestion of cassava may not cause cyanide poisoning, the amount of cyanogen production of a given plant or species depends on local environmental and plant biologic factors. This situation may account for the descrepancy between data derived from Cuban-grown cassava versus other areas of the world.

Detoxification of cassava around the world centers on processing techniques that include drying by oven and by sun exposure. Sun exposure eliminates more cyanide because of prolonged time of the enzyme linamarase and the cyanogenic glucosides. Soaking followed by boiling is superior to soaking or boiling alone.[44] Traditional African food products, such as *gari* and *fufu*, are made by a series of processing steps, such as grating, dewatering, fermenting, and roasting, which remove about 80% to 95% of the cyanide. The best processing method for the use of cassava leaves as human food seems to be drying the leaves in the sun, pounding the leaves, and cooking the mash in water.

Treatment of cyanide poisoning from cyanogenic plants or amygdalin is similar to the treatment of this poisoning from any source and is discussed in detail in Chapter 95.

Solanine

The genus of plants known as *Solanum* includes 1700 species that can induce toxicity when ingested in sufficient quantities. Most notably, this includes the potato (*Solanum tuberosum*), which can cause significant symptoms after the consumption of tubers that have been damaged or stored under improper conditions. Other common plants that can contain significant amounts of solanine alkaloids include Jerusalem cherry (*Solanum pseudocapsicum*), bittersweet (*Solanum dulcamara*), black nightshade (*S. nigrum*), ground cherry (*Physalis peruviana*), tomato plant (*Lycopersicon lycopersicum*), and eggplant (*Solanum melongena*).

All parts of the potato can contain two major glycoalkaloids, α-solanine and α-chaconine, which may be synthesized by the potato as protection from viral or bacterial infection when stored under adverse conditions. Normal potatoes contain a small amount of the alkaloids in the peel but none in the flesh. Excess formation of alkaloids is favored when potatoes are damaged or are improperly stored with exposure to light (ultraviolet radiation) or when they are sun-greened or allowed to sprout. There can be a 10-fold increase in the amount of solanine present in the tuber and the flesh of the potato when any of these conditions exist. Although the stems and foliage of the tomato plant are toxic, the ripe fruit of the tomato is edible.

A characteristic bitter taste may accompany solanine ingestion. Symptoms of solanine toxicity are initially characterized by hyperthermia and a cluster of symptoms that mimic acute gastroenteritis, including nausea, vomiting, diarrhea, and abdominal cramps, which may progress to hemorrhagic injury of the GI tract. Other signs and symptoms from severe solanine poisoning are neurologic effects, such as headache, dizziness, drowsiness, mental confusion, hallucination, and seizures. Mild bradycardia or hypotension may result from the weak cardiac activity of solanine. Additionally, some of the plants in this group may have anticholinergic activity, which initially may dominate the clinical picture.

Nightshade plant ingestion is a common cause of solanine poisoning. Severe nightshade toxicity may manifest with tachycardia or bradycardia, weakness, headache, fever, diaphoresis, central nervous system depression, and respiratory depression. Some cases manifest classic anticholinergic toxicity. In one case report, a 4-year-old girl ingested multiple orange and red berries from a climbing vine in her backyard. She presented with tachycardia (190 beats/min), temperature of 39.5°C (103.7°F), rigidity, tremor, and mydriatic pupils (7 to 8 mm). She was administered 0.2 mg of physostigmine (0.02 mg/kg) intravenously, which was repeated twice over 50 minutes. She was admitted to the ICU and was monitored for 36 hours.[45] Results of gas chromatography–mass spectrophotometry in this patient revealed peaks of solasodine and diosgenin, alkaloids that are characteristically found in *Solanum dulcamara* (woody nightshade or bittersweet), but no atropine or hyoscyamine, as found in *A. belladonna* (deadly nightshade). The authors concluded that in their cases the responsible anticholinergic principles were likely not detected by their analysis.[45]

The onset of symptoms after ingestion of plants containing solanine may take 4 to 24 hours. Hyperthermia may be an early sign of solanine toxicity.[46] Neurologic effects often predominate in the initial clinical presentation and may include headache, apathy, dizziness, drowsiness that may progress to mental confusion, hallucinations, and seizures in severe exposures. Excitement, delirium, and hallucinations are particularly likely in young children. Solanaceous plants often contain anticholinergic alkaloids also, which may lead to a confusing clinical picture. Some patients exhibit prominent anticholinergic symptoms, such as hallucinations and delirium.

Solanine has weak cardiac effects because of its structural similarity to cardiac glycosides, causing mild bradycardia and mild hypotension. There are no reports, however, of successful use of digoxin-specific antibodies in this setting. Supportive care and fluid resuscitation usually suffice. Rarely the use of chronotropic or inotropic agents may be required. Some of the plant material in this group may contain an atropine component, which can mask initial solanine-induced bradycardia, confusing the clinical picture. The atropine component typically causes toxic effects before the solanine component. Onset of illness after ingestion of plants containing predominantly atropine is usually within a few hours of ingestion and is initially dominated by anticholinergic effects. One plant that contains both alkaloids is the trumpet flower (*Solandra longiflora*).

Solanine toxicity is extremely variable and depends on the individual plant species and the amount of plant material ingested. Other variables that can affect toxicity include the plant part ingested and the developmental growth stage of the plant. The toxic dose of solanine in humans is unknown but has been reported to be in the range of 20 to 25 mg (3 mg/kg).[47,48] For purposes of comparison, the normal solanine content of properly stored potatoes is 7 mg/100 g of potato. In most of the members of this group, a small amount of plant material is generally all that is required to induce toxicity.

Solanine-induced hyperthermia may occur similar to anticholinergic plant ingestion. Conservative treatment is effective in most cases, including the use of a hypothermia blanket or application of cold compresses or ice. Dantrolene may be theoretically beneficial, especially if the patient required general anesthesia to control seizures. For clinicians unfamiliar in the use of dantrolene, consultation with an anesthesiologist, medical toxicologist, or poison center may be advisable. Anesthesiologists are experienced in the use of this agent in the management of malignant hyperthermia. The clinical pharmacology of dantrolene is described in detail in Chapter 156. Dantrolene typically is administered at a dose of 1 to 1.5 mg/kg by a rapid IV infusion push. Doses may be repeated until symptoms subside or a maximal cumulative dose of 10 mg/kg has been administered.

Few laboratories are capable of identifying solanine in body fluids or plant material. A history of ingestion of a solanine-containing plant and clinical presentation are important clues to diagnosis. Atropine alkaloids usually can be identified in the urine in toxicologic laboratories.

Oxalic Acid–Containing Plants

Oxalic acid ($C_2H_2O_4$) in plants is present in two forms: insoluble and soluble. Plants containing insoluble oxalate crystals may cause pain or irritation in the mouth and throat. Edema of the mouth, tongue, and throat with increased salivation and blistering may occur. In contrast, plants containing soluble oxalates do not produce oral discomfort when ingested and are more likely to be ingested in amounts that may result in systemic toxicity. Hypocalcemia with resultant tetany, seizures, and ventricular arrhythmias has been reported. Renal injury with a delayed onset of 24 to 48 hours may occur.[49]

Insoluble salts include calcium and magnesium oxalates, which occur as needle-like structures (raphides) located in ampule-shaped raphide ejector cells in the plant (Fig. 122-3). Irritation or slight pressure on the cap causes swelling of the ejector cell contents, resulting in a simultaneous, sudden expulsion of the raphides and free oxalic acid. The sharp ends of the raphides are the immediate cause of tissue injury, followed by further damage from proteolytic enzymes that coat the raphide. The proteolytic enzymes may stimulate bradykinin and histamine release with resultant local swelling and pain. Because of the immediate oral symptoms they provoke, the insoluble oxalates usually are not ingested in sufficient quantities to produce systemic toxicity. Although these ingestions occur commonly, they are rarely fatal. Mrvos and colleagues[50] retrospectively studied philodendron or dieffenbachia cases (insoluble oxalate–containing plants) reported to a regional poison center, identifying 188 cases. The integrity of the leaf had been broken in all cases. Philodendrons accounted for 67.5% and dieffenbachias for 32.5% of the cases. Children age 4 to 12 months were involved in 72.8% of the cases. Only 2.1% (four) of the patients were symptomatic (three dieffenbachia, one philodendron). All symptoms occurred within 5 minutes of the exposure and were of short duration, and the outcome was classified as minor. No severe oral complications or delayed development of symptoms was observed. Although other literature has ascribed significant morbidity to dieffenbachia exposures, the American Association of Poison Control Centers reports from poison centers would suggest less serious symptoms.[51]

Nevertheless, isolated case reports of serious exposures to oxalates such as in philodendron have been reported. McIntire and coworkers[52] reported an 11-month-old infant who chewed the leaves of a philodendron plant (*Araceae*) and developed oropharyngeal erosions and dysphagia. Esophageal erosions of the middle third of the esophagus and an esophageal stricture at the cricoid level were diagnosed 16 days after ingestion. Unexpected sudden death

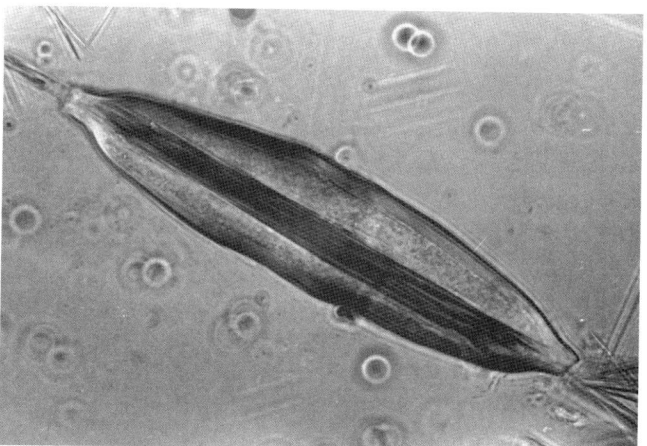

FIGURE 122-3

Insoluble salts include calcium and magnesium oxalates, which occur as needle-like structures (raphides) located in ampule-shaped raphide ejector cells in the plant. *(From Gardner DG: Injury to oral mucous membranes caused by the common houseplant, dieffenbachia. Oral Surg Oral Med Oral Pathol 78:632, 1994.)*

occurred on day 17 and was attributed to vagotonia secondary to the esophageal lesions.

Soluble compounds, including sodium, potassium, and ammonium oxalate, do not cause local pain or irritation but may result in systemic effects. Because of the lack of immediate discomfort, there is a greater likelihood that these plants may be ingested in sufficient quantity to cause systemic toxicity. When absorption of significant quantities of oxalic acid occurs, evidence of systemic intoxication usually develops in 2 to 12 hours. Gastroenteritis may occur. Oxalate reacts with calcium in plasma to form insoluble calcium oxalate, which may precipitate in organs such as the kidney, brain, blood vessels, heart, lungs, and liver and cause hypocalcemia. Hypocalcemic tetany and seizures may result.[53] Common plants containing insoluble or soluble oxalates are listed in Table 122-4.

INSOLUBLE OXALATES

Ingestion of plant material containing insoluble oxalate salts may result in symptoms of oral irritation. In significant exposures, edema of the mouth, tongue, and throat with increased salivation and blistering may occur.[52,54] Partial airway obstruction or difficulty breathing secondary to edema of the tongue, oropharynx, and larynx may occur.[52] Ocular exposure may cause immediate pain, lacrimation, photophobia, corneal abrasion, and deposition of calcium oxalate crystals on the corneal epithelium. Local necrosis of the cornea and keratitis have been reported with ocular exposure to the white, milky sap of dieffenbachia.[55,56] One infant death has been reported after ingestion of philodendron leaves. Death was attributed to cardiorespiratory arrest secondary to vagotonia due to esophageal erosions.[52]

SOLUBLE OXALATES

Respiratory depression was reported in a comatose patient who ingested soup prepared with *Rumex crispus*. Pulmonary edema was noted in a fatality due to the ingestion of *R. crispus*. Ventricular arrhythmias and fibrillation presumably secondary to hypocalcemia were seen.[57] Hypocalcemia and tetany may develop after ingestion of large quantities of plants containing sodium or potassium oxalates. Cerebral edema and coma also may occur. Metabolic acidosis was seen after

ingestion of 500 g of sorrel.[53] Renal damage may occur after ingestion of plants that contain soluble oxalates.[49]

Systemic poisoning from rhubarb leaves and sorrel has been reported when these were used as a food source, especially in soups.[53] In one case report, a 53-year-old man died after ingestion of soup containing 500 g of sorrel (*R. crispus*). Autopsy revealed extensive liver cell necrosis. It was estimated that he ingested 6 to 8 g of oxalic acid.[57] Insoluble and soluble oxalates may cause gastroenteritis with hematemesis and bloody stools.

Treatment is largely supportive, but systemic effects from soluble oxalates may require cardiac monitoring and serial laboratory studies, such as serum calcium, creatinine, electrolytes, and routine urinalysis to detect hypocalcemia and systemic organ damage requiring specific management. The initial approach to ingestion of oxalate-containing plants includes dilution and decontamination. Immediate dilution with milk or water is recommended by Poisindex for ingestion of plant material containing insoluble oxalate crystals. Emesis for ingestion of plants containing insoluble salts is never recommended because of the lack of systemic toxicity and the potential for edema of the airway. Decisions regarding GI decontamination should follow American Academy of Clinical Toxicologists and European Association of Poison Centres and Clinical Toxicologists guidelines (see Chapter 5) but should also take into account the presence or absence of insoluble oxalate crystal/raphide damage to the upper airway. When dealing with soluble oxalate plant ingestion, GI decontamination with activated charcoal may be advisable for ingestions of a significant or unknown quantity of plant material containing soluble oxalate salts. The use of cathartics routinely in overdose cases has been questioned (see Chapter 5). Most poison centers and toxicologists do not recommend the routine use of cathartics in this type of overdose.

Cold water, Popsicles, or ice pack applications may ease local oral pain. Analgesics may be required if the pain is intense. The exposed skin should be irrigated twice with soap and water. A close examination of the skin may be required if pain or irritation exists after decontamination. Close examination of the eyes may be needed if pain or irritation exists after initial irrigation with water or saline. This may require fluorescein staining to uncover corneal abrasions. Maintenance of adequate hydration with IV fluids may be necessary if oral fluids cannot be tolerated or if GI symptoms are severe.

If plant material containing soluble oxalate crystals has been ingested, one should monitor blood urea nitrogen, serum creatinine, and urine for calcium oxalate crystals. If renal function remains normal, adequate urine flow should be established to prevent deposition of calcium oxalate crystals in the renal tubules.

Hypocalcemia and tetany should be treated with IV calcium gluconate or diluted calcium chloride, unless administered through a central line. Continuous ECG monitoring is recommended during bolus calcium infusions. Adults may receive 0.5 to 2 g (5 to 20 mL of 10% calcium gluconate) by slow IV infusion. Children may be administered 100 to 200 mg/kg of 10% calcium gluconate by slow IV infusion.

Significant metabolic acidosis also may occur secondary to oxalic acid formation. Correction of acidosis should be guided by blood gases, electrolytes, and clinical judgment.

TABLE 122-4 Insoluble and Soluble Oxalates

INSOLUBLE OXALATES	SOLUBLE OXALATES
Philodendron (*Philodendron* spp.)	Rhubarb leaves (*Rheum rhaponticum*)
Caladium (*Caladium hortulanum*)	Boston ivy (*Parthenocissus tricuspidata*)
Dieffenbachia (*Dieffenbachia* spp.)	Virginia creeper (*Parthenocissus quinquefolia*)
Calla lily (*Zantedeschia aethiopica*)	Garden sorrel (*Rumex crispus*)
Elephant ear (*Colocasia*)	Shamrock (*Oxalis* spp.)
Jack-in-the-pulpit (*Arisaema triphyllum*)	

Note: A regional poison center may be instrumental in identifying plants that may contain soluble versus insoluble oxalates.

Attention should be directed to volume status and correction of poor perfusion in mild cases. Sodium bicarbonate may be used to correct the acidosis in severe cases with an initial infusion of 1 to 2 mEq/kg intravenously (not to exceed adult doses if administered to children). Infusion of bicarbonate in an appropriate fluid for the patient's size and age may be guided by the base deficit on blood gases. Usually this requires 1 to 2 ampules of sodium bicarbonate per liter of IV fluids administered at a rate appropriate for the patient's weight. Additional bicarbonate or slow boluses may be required. A hypertonic solution with respect to sodium content should not be made. Sodium content generally should not exceed that of normal saline. There are no data supporting a beneficial effect of correcting the metabolic acidosis in cases of oxalate poisoning.

HERBAL TOXICITY

Herbal preparations and "medicines" have become one of the fastest growing markets for alternative health products. Herbal and alternative medicines are now used worldwide. All practitioners, including critical care physicians, should have a working knowledge of these products because significant herb-drug interactions are possible.[58] Patients who seek conventional health care also frequently use herbal remedies. In 1997, 60 million Americans used herbs for medicinal purposes and spent $3.24 billion in doing so.[59] Other authors estimate the out-of-pocket expenditure to be much higher. Total 1997 U.S. out-of-pocket expenditures relating to alternative therapies were conservatively estimated at $27 billion.[60] There are an estimated 20,000 or more herbal products on the market. In 1997, sales increased by 59% and are growing at a rate of 15% per year. The most common herbs sold in the United States are listed in Table 122-5.

Seventy percent of patients do not reveal their use of herbal preparations to their allopathic physicians.[61] Consequently, there is a great potential for misuse of these

TABLE 122-5 Thirteen Best-Selling Herbs*

Ginkgo (*Ginkgo biloba*)
Ginseng (*Panax quinquefolium* and *Panax ginseng*)
Echinacea (*Echinacea purpurea* and other species)/goldenseal (*Hydrastis canadensis*)
Kava (*Piper methysticum*)
Cranberry (*Vaccinium macrocarpon*)
Evening primrose (*Oenothera caespitosa*)
Milk thistle (*Silybum marianum*)
St. John's wort (*Hypericum perforatum*)
Garlic (*Allium sativum*)
Saw palmetto (*Serenoa* spp.)
Pycnogenol (*Pinus* spp.)/grape seed (*Vitus* spp.)
Valerian root (*Valeriana officinalis*)
Bilberry (*Vaccinium myrtillus*)

*1998 ranking in mainstream market sales.
Data from Blumenthal M: Herb market levels after five years of boom: 1999 sales in mainstream market up only 11% in first half of 1999 after 55% increase in 1998. Herbalgram 47:64–65, 1999.

products and herb-drug interactions. There is no standardization of active constituents. In 1994, the U.S. Congress passed the Dietary Supplement and Health Education Act (DSHEA) that reduced the U.S. Food and Drug Administration (FDA) oversight of products classified as dietary supplements. An example of how DSHEA affected U.S. society has been the proliferation of products containing sympathomimetic alkaloids and caffeine and the attendant possibility of misuse of these products if they are not taken as labeled. Because the FDA is hampered by DSHEA, it is imperative that physicians, including intensivists, take an active role in reporting herbal agent toxicity. In the United States, all adverse events associated with herbal preparations should be reported to the U.S. FDA Medwatch at 1–800-FDA-1088.

Herbs are sold as teas, foods, or food supplements but are packaged similar to drugs and vitamins. Because they are not categorized as "drugs," no proof of efficacy or warnings about side effects and interactions are required in the United States. Patients can access some correct, but also erroneous, information from numerous Websites on the Internet. Although there are many reputable companies selling legitimate herbal preparations, many products are fraught with misidentification, adulteration, contamination, and lack of standardization.

Herbal toxicity can be viewed in terms of inherent toxicity versus chemical interactions with drugs. Examples of inherent toxicity include the following:

1. *Chaparral*—used as an antioxidant but linked with acute hepatitis, subacute hepatocellular necrosis, cholestatic hepatitis, and hepatic failure.[62–64]
2. *Pennyroyal oil*—used as an abortifacient but linked with hepatic necrosis similar to acetaminophen in toxic amounts.[65]
3. *Pyrrolizidine alkaloids* (comfrey tea, ragwort, coltsfoot)—used as poultices for joint pain but linked with hepatic veno-occlusive disease.[66]

Sources of toxicity in herbal preparations include incorrect dosing guidelines; acute overdose of toxic constituents of agents, such as the above-listed herbs; chronic accumulation of toxins; use in children, in whom dosing is excessive or there is no experience; and use in pregnancy. It is widely accepted by clinical toxicologists that some herbal preparations often vary in potency. Correct preparation is necessary to decrease intrinsic toxicity. The combination of herbs in so-called herbal cocktails may enhance toxicity further if used incorrectly. Examples of combination products are "herbal Fen-Phen," which is ephedra and St. John's wort, and ma huang, which contains ephedra (approximately 20 mg) and guarana extract (caffeine approximately 200 mg).

No formal regulation or organized tracking of herb-related adverse effects occurs in any society worldwide. Some herbal preparations, including patented Chinese herbal medications, may contain other pharmaceuticals as adulterants. Nelson and colleagues[67] reported a case of aplastic anemia induced by an herbal medication adulterated with phenylbutazone. The product label did not list phenylbutazone as an ingredient. The authors performed extensive laboratory evaluation of the patient and found no other plausible cause. Phenylbutazone is known to be associated with such hematologic abnormalities. Toxins including arsenic, lead, and mercury may arise from manufacturing processes. Patients in the ICU with symptoms consistent with heavy metal poisoning should have appropriate testing performed. Not only chemical but also microbial contamination may occur from bacteria and fungi. This contamination may occur during preparation or from improper storage.

Toxicity from herbal products may be due in part to lack of safety information. The knowledge base for possible toxic effects is limited. There are approximately 7000 species of plants used in China for herbal preparations, but only 230 have been studied in depth. Clinical trials with many of these agents in humans either are nonexistent or involve small numbers of volunteers and lack statistical power with regard to toxicity and therapeutic efficacy. There is no effective tracking system to detect isolated reports (e.g., autoimmune hepatitis triggered by herbal medicines such as Dai-Saiko-to[68]). Some adverse effects have long latency (i.e., carcinogenicity), further compounding the difficulty of tracking adverse effects.

There is a paucity of stringent quality assurance for herbal remedies. This paucity has been partially remedied by the production of herbal preparations by well-known reputable drug and vitamin companies. Nevertheless, the lack of warnings on these products, as typically would be mandated for drugs, contributes to possible adverse effects and herb-drug interactions. There are also instances of erroneous substitutions of active constituents. Active pharmaceuticals in some Chinese herbal medicines have included dexamethasone, diazepam, diclofenac, indomethacin, mefenamic acid, and hydrochlorothiazide. Proprietary (patent) herbal "medicines" in tablet, capsule, powder, or liquid form pose other problems (undeclared conventional drugs).

Clinical Toxicology of Herbal Preparations

CLASSES OF HERBAL PREPARATIONS

Herbal preparations can be categorized into five classes: (1) volatile (essential) oils, (2) resins, (3) alkaloids, (4) glycosides, and (5) fixed oils.[69] With the possible exception of fixed oils (e.g., olive oil), these classes of agents may be responsible for significant adverse effects at the right dose. For essential oils, it is apparent that even these so-called natural products have inherent toxicity. Essential oils are any of a class of volatile oils composed of a mixture of complex hydrocarbons (usually terpenes) and other chemicals extracted from a plant that give the plant its characteristic aroma. Examples of essential oils are the following:

1. Nutmeg (*Myristica fragrans*) is used for toothache, GI upset, and halitosis. The toxic principles are myristicin, a hallucinogen, and eugenol, which is used by some dentists as a topical anesthetic for the gums.
2. Garlic (*Allium sativum*) is used for lipid-lowering, antithrombotic, antihypertensive, and anticancer effects. The FDA considers garlic safe. It is possible, however, to encounter enhanced bleeding tendency in patients using large quantities of garlic who also are on antithrombotic therapy. This is likely due to the inhibition of platelet aggregation by garlic.
3. Pennyroyal (*Hedeoma pulegeoides*) is used as an abortifacient, emmenagogue, and carminative and is found in some animal insect repellants, such as aloe herbal horse spray and spray-on dog shampoo.

A popular method of pennyroyal ingestion is to make a tea by steeping about 1 to 2 teaspoonfuls of the dried herb or leaves with 1 cup of warm water. This tea should not be used more than twice a day. About 50 to 100 g of leaves yields about 1 mL of oil. The main toxic constituents of pennyroyal are terpenes (pulegone, isopulegone, menthol, isomenthone, limonene, piperitone, neomenthol, tannins, 3-methylcyclohexanone). The toxic principle pulegone undergoes bioactivation to menthofuran, which is hepatotoxic. The α-isopropylidene ketone unit is required for hepatic damage. The 5-methyl ketone group also contributes to toxicity. Cytochrome P-450 oxidizes pulegone and can be affected by inducers or inhibitors contributing to the likelihood of toxicity in a rat model. Dose-related toxicity occurs, with 10 mL causing GI distress; 30 mL has caused centrilobular hepatic necrosis. Symptoms and signs of pennyroyal toxicity include nausea, vomiting, dizziness, abdominal pain, throat burning, coagulopathy, liver dysfunction, renal failure, and seizures.

Treatment involves decontamination and supportive care. Observation for at least 24 hours is recommended to detect any hepatic effects. There are a few case reports of use of *N*-acetylcysteine therapy to prevent hepatotoxicity from pennyroyal ingestion.[70] Although no randomized controlled trials have been performed to assess the efficacy of *N*-acetylcysteine in this setting, one may consider its use in a significant ingestion of pennyroyal. Dosing similar to that in acetaminophen poisoning seems reasonable, but the duration of treatment is unclear at this time.

Other significantly toxic herbs are derived from plants and used as teas, including comfrey, chaparral, germander, *Gordolobo yerba*, and *Senecio*, which contain toxic pyrrolizidine alkaloids. These alkaloids generally are found in foliage of 6000 species (3% of flowering plants). Pyrrolizidine alkaloids are found primarily in three major plant families: (1) borage family (e.g., *Symphytum* spp., such as comfrey and *Heliotropium*), (2) aster family (e.g., *Senecio* spp. responsible for loss of livestock), and (3) bean or legume family (e.g., *Crotalaria* spp. or "rattlebox" [toxic alkaloid is found in seeds]).

Comfrey is the most common source of pyrrolizidine alkaloids. It is used as a tea (made from roots) with the leaves prepared for salads or dried and powderized into tablets. Traditionally, comfrey has been used to heal broken bones. There are several historical accounts of toxic exposures involving individual or mass poisonings due to pyrrolizidine alkaloids. In 1954, hepatic venoocclusive disease ("Bush tea disease") was reported in Jamaican children from *Senecio* spp. and others. In 1974, there was a massive human outbreak of poisoning in Afghanistan (7000 poisonings and many deaths from liver failure) from contaminated wheat (found to have *Heliotropium* seeds, which contained the pyrrolizidine alkaloid heliotrine).[71] Poisoning from contaminated wheat also occurred in 1976 in India. In 1984, comfrey was made a restricted drug in Australia, requiring a license to prescribe. The toxicologic mechanism for pyrrolizidine alkaloids involves the conversion to toxic active principles, which likely occurs in vivo by hepatic metabolism to pyrroles (biologic alkylating agents). Monocrotaline and other cyclic diesters are the most toxic, and their toxic principle depends on a 1,2-double bond plus an esterified branched chain (Fig. 122-4). The

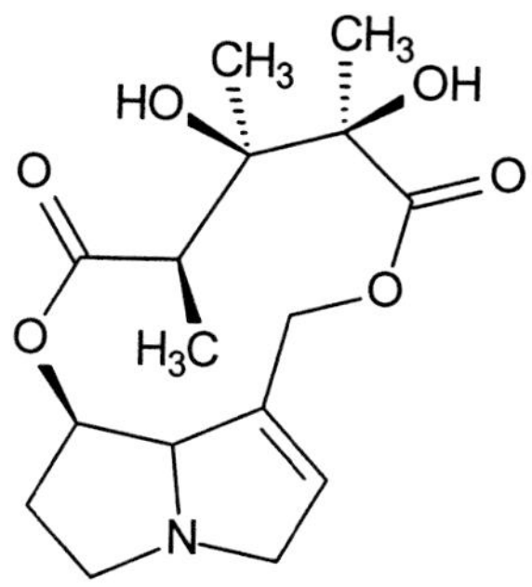

FIGURE 122-4

Chemical structure of monocrotaline.

toxic effect on hepatocytes and sinusoidal cells is a result of collapse of the reticulin network surrounding the central vein and associated hemorrhage. This effect leads to occlusion of the small branches of the hepatic vein, resulting in a Budd-Chiari–like syndrome. Fibrosis develops with a pattern of centrilobular necrosis. Clinically, patients may present with nausea and vomiting, hepatomegaly, portal hypertension, ascites, jaundice (rare), and only modestly elevated hepatic transaminases.[72] Hepatotoxicity may progress to cirrhosis, unless the course is fatal. Care is largely supportive.[73]

TYPES OF REACTIONS

In addition to the categories of toxins discussed earlier, reactions to herbal preparations can be classified based on effect. The types of reactions are as follows:[74]

- *Type A*—pharmacologically predictable, generally dose dependent (e.g., yohimbine with resultant hypertension)
- *Type B*—idiosyncratic reactions occur in a small percentage of patients and can be serious or life-threatening
- *Type C*—reactions develop during long-term use (e.g., hypokalemia and muscle weakness from herbal laxatives or misuse of ipecac syrup)
- *Type D*—delayed effects of herb use, such as carcinogenicity or teratogenicity (e.g., safrole from *Sassafras albidum* is hepatocarcinogenic in mice)

INTERACTIONS WITH PRESCRIBED MEDICATIONS

Numerous herbal products have serious potential for interaction with medications used by allopathic physicians. Concurrent use of herbs may lead to pharmacologic interactions with each other (i.e., combined effect on platelets increasing bleeding, such as garlic with other herbs) or with prescribed drugs. Examples of herb-drug interactions include the following:

1. Increased bleeding when warfarin is combined with ginkgo (*Ginkgo biloba*), garlic (*Allium sativum*), dong quai (*Angelica sinensis*), or danshen (*Salvia miltiorrhiza*)
2. Mild serotonin syndrome in patients who mix St. John's wort (*Hypericum perforatum*) with serotonin reuptake inhibitors, such as paroxetine, or other serotonergic agents (serotonin syndrome is discussed in Chapter 24)
3. Decreased bioavailability of digoxin, theophylline, and cyclosporine when these drugs are combined with St. John's wort

4. Development of mania in depressed patients who mix antidepressants and *Panax ginseng*
5. Exacerbation of extrapyramidal effects with neuroleptic drugs and betel nut (*Areca catechu*)
6. Increased risk of hypertension when tricyclic antidepressants are combined with yohimbine (*Pausinystalia yohimbe*) and hypertension with excessive doses of yohimbine by itself
7. Potentiation of mineralocorticoid effects of oral and topical corticosteroids by licorice (*Glycyrrhiza glabra*)

Some herbal products contain alkaloids, which may decrease the absorption of drugs. Examples are the anthranoid-containing plants including senna (*Cassia senna*) and cascara (*Rhamnus purshiana*) or soluble fibers (including guar gum and psyllium).[58] Other herbal products that may have practice implications for the intensivist include milk thistle (*Silybum marianum*), aconitum, and goldenseal (*Hydrastis canadensis*).

Effects of Frequently Used Herbal Preparations

GOLDENSEAL

Goldenseal (*H. canadensis*) is used by herbalists as an antidiarrheal, antiseptic, and unproven cold remedy. It is erroneously thought to mask illicit drugs, and drug abusers still may ingest it in an attempt to mask detection. Investigationally, goldenseal is used as an antineoplastic and anti–human immunodeficiency virus (HIV) (berberine) agent. Side effects include GI tract disturbances, neonatal jaundice, and central nervous system stimulation.

MILK THISTLE

Milk thistle (*S. marianum*) is used as antioxidant and hepatoprotectant. The active principle is silymarin. For more than 2000 years, the seeds have been used to treat liver disorders. A randomized, double-blind, placebo-controlled trial in patients with cirrhosis revealed that 4-year mortality decreased by 30% in patients treated for 2 years with 140 mg three times a day.[75] In another trial in 200 patients with alcoholic cirrhosis, the authors found no difference after 2 years of treatment with 150 mg of silymarin three times a day.[76]

ST. JOHN'S WORT

St. John's wort (*H. perforatum*) is one of the top-selling herbal products (see Table 122-5). It is used most often to treat depression (referred to as "herbal Prozac"). It is a potent inducer of cytochrome P-450 3A4 (CYP3A4),[77] which accounts for 60% to 70% of the cytochrome activity in the liver.

CYP3A4 is the P-450 enzyme implicated in most clinically significant drug-drug interactions. Roby and associates[77] determined the in vivo effect of reagent-grade St. John's wort extract on CYP3A4 activity through evaluation of ratios of urinary 6-β-hydroxy cortisol to cortisol. The investigators studied 13 subjects (age range 18 to 25 years) in an unblinded, multiple-dose, single-treatment, before-and-after trial conducted in a university-based pharmacokinetics and biopharmaceutics laboratory. Each subject ingested a 300-mg tablet of reagent-grade St. John's wort extract standardized to 0.3% hypericin three times a day for

14 days. Baseline and posttreatment CYP3A4 activity was assessed with the urinary 6-β-hydroxy cortisol-to-cortisol ratio after a 24-hour urine collection. The mean ± standard deviation urinary 6-β-hydroxy cortisol-to-cortisol ratio increased significantly ($P = .003$) from a baseline value of 7.1 ± 4.5 to 13 ± 4.9 in all but one subject. Treatment with St. John's wort for 14 days resulted in significant increases in the urinary 6-β-hydroxy cortisol-to-cortisol ratio suggesting that St. John's wort is a CYP3A4 inducer.

In another study, St. John's wort reduced the area under the curve of the HIV-1 protease inhibitor indinavir by a mean of 57% with a standard deviation of 19 and decreased the extrapolated 8-hour indinavir trough level by 81% (standard deviation 16) in healthy volunteers. The authors concluded that a reduction in indinavir exposure of this magnitude could lead to the development of drug resistance and treatment failure.[78]

Use of St. John's wort also has implications for the intensivist caring for transplant patients. Many immunosuppressive agents, including lidocaine, tacrolimus, and cyclosporine, are metabolized via CYP3A4. Reduction in cyclosporine levels and actual heart transplant rejection have been reported.[79,80]

YOHIMBE

Cardiovascular and neurologic complications of herbal product and alternative medicine use can be dramatic. Herbal products such as yohimbe can exert potent α-adrenergic agonism.[81] Yohimbe contains the principle yohimbine, a central α_2-adrenergic antagonist. Yohimbine is an indolealkylamine alkaloid derived from the West African yohimbe tree (*Coryanthe yohimbe*).[58,82-84] It is structurally similar to reserpine. Yohimbine is used extensively either by prescription or in extracts of "health food" products marketed as virulizing agents for men. The literature is replete with references reporting the beneficial effects of yohimbine in erectile dysfunction. Adverse effects of yohimbine are tachycardia, hypertension, nausea, vomiting, diaphoresis, mydriasis, and lacrimation.[85]

ACONITINE

Aconitine is another potent alkaloid. Herbal drugs such as chuanwu made from the dried roots of *Aconitum* plants are used widely in several populations worldwide, most notably the Chinese. In April 2001, a U.S. FDA warning was released regarding autumn monkshood (*Aconitum carmichaelii*). A Canadian nursery located in British Columbia is known to have distributed the plants with the incorrect labels to other nurseries in British Columbia, Washington State, and Idaho, but full distribution was not known. The packages were mistakenly labeled with the statement, "All parts of this plant are tasty in soup," instead of indicating that the plant is poisonous. Distribution started on March 4, 2001, and the first plants had been received by accounts in mid-April. Approximately 1500 plants were believed to have been sold.[86]

The dried rhizomes of *Aconitum* spp. contain varying amounts of aconitine and other aconite alkaloids, such as mesaconitine and hypaconitine.[87] Ingestion of aconitine-containing plants (*Aconitum* spp.) may result in profound cardiovascular symptoms. These effects are not dissimilar to another family of alkaloid toxins called *grayanotoxins*. The grayanotoxins veratrine and andromedotoxin derive from the rhododendron species, azalea, and mountain laurel. These toxins share with aconitine clinical effects including vomiting, weakness, bradycardia (presumably via muscarinic M_2-receptor stimulation), and hypotension.[88,89]

The aconitum alkaloids are C19 diterpenoids. Their toxicity includes cardiovascular features, notably hypotension and ventricular arrhythmias; neurologic effects, including numbness, muscle weakness, and paresthesias; and GI disturbances, such as nausea, vomiting, abdominal pain, and diarrhea. Other signs include hyperventilation, sweating, and confusion. Aconitine is neurotoxic and cardiotoxic, acting on voltage-sensitive sodium channels, resulting in persistent activation and prolonged depolarization; this prevents repolarization of excitable membranes. Aconitine alkaloids result in an increase in intracellular calcium concentration via sodium/calcium exchange, which enhances automaticity. They also result in vagally mediated cardiodepressant effects. Enhanced automaticity coupled with increased vagal activity and slowed atrioventricular conduction most likely leads to observed arrhythmias. The lethal dose of pure aconitine is estimated to be about 3 to 6 g. In 18 patients reported in one series, the latent period between ingestion and occurrence of symptoms ranged from 0.3 to 1.5 hours (mean 0.9 hours). All except 5 of 18 patients developed symptoms and signs of toxicity after taking the first dose of the aconitine-containing Chinese herb products chuanwu and caowu.[87]

In another case report, a 61-year-old, previously healthy man was admitted for precipitous onset of severe palpitations, chest pain, and perioral paresthesia.[90] He had taken some Chinese herbal medicine purported to alleviate back pain and arthralgias, which he prepared by boiling a combination of herbs, including rootstocks of *Aconitum*. His presenting ECG revealed polymorphic ventricular tachycardia with occasional bidirectional configurations. IV lidocaine was unsuccessful, and 150 mg of amiodarone was administered over 15 minutes. The arrhythmias resolved 1 hour after initiation of the amiodarone bolus while on a continuous infusion. Before discharge, the patient had a normal ECG, echocardiogram, and coronary angiogram. Cardiotoxic plants are discussed in detail in Chapter 125.

ARISTOLOCHIC ACID

In April 2001, the FDA received reports of two patients in the United States who developed serious kidney disease associated with the use of botanical products that were shown by laboratory analysis to contain aristolochic acid. In addition, the agency analyzed a sample of 38 botanical products available in the United States that were labeled as containing aristolochia or other herbs that might contain aristolochic acid and found that 18 of these products contained aristolochic acid. Based on these analytic results, the FDA requested that the involved U.S. manufacturers or distributors initiate recalls of these products. Because of the potential serious public health risk, the FDA now is advising consumers to stop using any products that may contain aristolochic acid; this includes products with *aristolochia, bragantia,* or *asarum* listed as ingredients on the label and any of the products the FDA has found to contain aristolochic acid.

Aristolachia fangchi (fang-ji) contains the toxic alkaloid aristocholine, which also may cause tachycardia, weak pulses, constipation, polyuria, and an acute inflammation of the urogenital tract. One case of reversible hepatitis has been reported. Schmeiser and colleagues[91] reported on possible DNA mutation responsible for kidney-destructive fibrotic processes in patients with aristolochia nephropathy. Persistence of specific DNA adducts months after discontinuation of aristolochia herbs suggests nonreparable lesions in many tissues exposed to carcinogens. These authors further suggested the possibility that aristolochic acid DNA adducts also initiated a renal fibrotic process. The fibrotic process extended from the kidney to the pelvis and ureter in one patient.

REFERENCES

1. Ogzewalla CD, Bonfiglio JF, Sigell LT: Common plants and their toxicity. Pediatr Clin North Am 34:1557–1598, 1987.
2. Hamouda C, Arnamou M, Thabet H, et al: Plant poisonings from herbal medication admitted to a Tunisian toxicologic intensive care unit, 1983–1998. Vet Hum Toxicol 42:137–141, 2000.
3. Hedili A, Warnet JM, Thevenin M, et al: Biochemical investigation of *Atractylis gummerifera L.* hepatotoxicity in the rat. Arch Toxicol 13(Suppl):312–315, 1989.
4. Brandolin G, Meyer C, Defaye G, et al: Partial purification of an atractyloside-binding protein from mitochondria. FEBS Lett 46:149–153, 1974.
5. Watson WA, Litovitz, TL, Rogers GC, et al: 2002 Annual Report of the American Association of Poison Control Centers Toxic Exposure Surveillance System. Am J Emerg Med 21:353–421, 2003.
6. Akerele O: Summary of WHO Guidelines for the Assessment of Herbal Medicines. Herbalgram 28:13–16, 1993.
7. Challoner KR, McCarron MM: Castor bean intoxication. Ann Emerg Med 19:1177–1183, 1990.
8. Wedin GP, Neal JS, Everson GW, Krenzelok EP: Castor bean poisoning. Am J Emerg Med 4:259–261, 1986.
9. Rauber A, Heard J: Castor bean toxicity re-examined: A new perspective. Vet Hum Toxicol 27:498–502, 1985.
10. Scarpa A, Guerci A: Various uses of the castor oil plant (*Ricinus communis* L.): A review. J Ethnopharmacol 5:117–137, 1982.
11. American Academy of Clinical Toxicology and European Association of Clinical Toxicologists and Poison Control Centres: Position Statement on Gastrointestinal Decontamination. J Toxicol Clin Toxicol 35:695–762, 1997.
12. Olsnes S, Refsnes K, Pihl A: Mechanism of action of the toxic lectins abrin and ricin. Nature 249:627–631, 1974.
13. Hebel SK (ed): Castor. In: The Lawrence Review of Natural Products—Monograph System. St. Louis, Facts & Comparisons, 1992.
14. Aplin PJ, Eliseo T: Ingestion of castor oil plant seeds. Med J Aust 167:260–261, 1997.
15. Taylor CM, Williams JM, Lote CJ, et al: A laboratory model of toxin-induced hemolytic uremic syndrome. Kidney Int 55:1367–1374, 1999.
16. Palatnick W, Tenenbein M: Hepatotoxicity from castor bean ingestion in a child. J Toxicol Clin Toxicol 38:67–69, 2000.
17. Kanerva L, Estlander T, Jolanki R: Long-lasting contact urticaria from castor bean. J Am Acad Dermatol 23:353–355, 1990.
18. Heger MR, Wahl R, Cromwell O, et al: Seasonal occupational asthma in an agricultural products merchant—a case report. Allergy 49:897–901, 1994.
19. Andersen KE, Nielsen R: Lipstick dermatitis related to castor oil. Contact Derm 11:253–254, 1984.
20. Kinamore PA, Jaeger RW, deCastro FJ, et al: *Abrus* and *Ricinus* ingestion: Management of three cases. J Toxicol Clin Toxicol 17:401–405, 1980.
21. Francis PD, Clarke CF: Angel Trumpet lily poisoning in five adolescents: Clinical findings and management. J Paediatr Child Health 35:93–95, 1999.
22. Tiongson J, Salen P: Mass ingestion of Jimson Weed by eleven teenagers. Del Med J 70:471–476, 1998.
23. Guharoy SR, Barajas M: Atropine intoxication from the ingestion and smoking of Jimson Weed (*Datura stramonium*). Vet Hum Toxicol 33:588–589, 1991.
24. Ramirez M, Rivera E, Ereu C: Fifteen cases of atropine poisoning after honey ingestion. Vet Hum Toxicol 41:19–20, 1999.
25. Rauber-Luthy C, Guirguis M, Meier-Abt AS, et al: Lethal poisoning after ingestion of a tea prepared from the angel's trumpet (*Datura suaveolens*) (Abstract). J Toxicol Clin Toxicol 37:414, 1999.
26. Smith EA, Meloan CE, Pickell JA, Oehme FW: Scopolamine poisoning from homemade "Moon Flower" wine. J Anal Toxicol 15:216–219, 1991.
27. Schneider F, Lutun P, Kintz P, et al: Plasma and urine concentrations of atropine after the ingestion of cooked deadly nightshade berries. J Toxicol Clin Toxicol 34:113–117, 1996.
28. Tsiodras S, Shin RK, Christian M, et al: Anticholinergic toxicity associated with lupine seeds as home remedy for diabetes mellitus. Ann Emerg Med 33:715–717, 1999.
29. Burns MJ, Linden CH, Graudins A, et al: A comparison of physostigmine and benzodiazepines for the treatment of anticholinergic poisoning. Ann Emerg Med 35:373–381, 2000.
30. Worth DP, Davison AM, Roberts TG, et al: Ineffectiveness of haemodialysis in atropine poisoning. BMJ 206:2023–2024, 1983.
31. Khasigian P, Everson G, Bellinghausen R, et al: Poisoning following oleander smoke inhalation. J Toxicol Clin Toxicol 36:456, 1998.
32. Tuncok Y, Kozan O, Cavdar C, et al: *Urginea maritima* (Squill) toxicity. J Toxicol Clin Toxicol 33:83–86, 1995.
33. Barry TL, Petzinger G, Zito SW: GC/MS comparison of the West Indian aphrodisiac "Love Stone" to the Chinese medication "chan su": Bufotenine and related bufadienolides. J Forensic Sci 41:1068–1073, 1996.
34. Brubacher JR: Deaths associated with a purported aphrodisiac—New York City, February 1993-May 1995. MMWR Morb Mortal Wkly Rep 44:853–855, 1995.
35. Furbee B, Wermuth M: Life-threatening plant poisoning. Crit Care Clin North Am 13:849–888, 1997.
36. Strugala GJ, Rauws AG, Elbers R: Intestinal first pass metabolism of amygdalin in the rat in vitro. Biochem Pharmacol 35:2123–2128, 1986.
37. Vetter J: Plant cyanogenic glycosides. Toxicon 38:11–36, 2000.
38. Chitnis MP, Adwankar MK, Amonkar AJ: Studies on high-dose chemotherapy of amygdalin in murine P388 lymphocytic leukaemia and P815 mast cell leukaemia. J Cancer Res Clin Oncol 109:208–209, 1985.
39. Kalyanaraman UP, Kalyanaraman K, Cullinan SA, et al: Neuromyopathy of cyanide intoxication due to "laetrile" (amygdalin): A clinico-pathologic study. Cancer 51:2126–2133, 1983.
40. Syrigos KN, Rowlinson-Busza G, et al: In vitro cytotoxicity following specific activation of amygdalin by beta-glucosidase conjugated to a bladder cancer-associated monoclonal antibody. Int J Cancer 78:712–719, 1998.
41. Cliff J, Nicala D: Long-term follow-up of konzo patients. Trans R Soc Trop Med Hyg 91:447–449, 1997.
42. Akintonwa A, Tunwashe OL: Fatal cyanide poisoning from cassava-based meal. Hum Exp Toxicol 11:47–49, 1992.
43. Hernandez T, Lundquist P, Oliviera L, et al: Fate in humans of dietary intake of cyanogenic glycosides from roots of sweet cassava consumed in Cuba. Nat Toxins 3:114–117, 1995.
44. Padmaja G: Cyanide detoxification in cassava for food and feed uses. Crit Rev Food Sci Nutr 35:299–339, 1995.
45. Ceha LJ, Presperin C, Young E, et al: Anticholinergic toxicity from nightshade berry poisoning responsive to physostigmine. J Emerg Med 15:65–69, 1997.
46. Hopkins J: The glycoalkaloids: Naturally of interest (but a hot potato?) Food Chem Toxicol 33:323–339, 1995.
47. McMillan M, Thompson JC: An outbreak of suspected solanine poisoning in schoolboys. QJM 190:227–243, 1979.
48. Dalvi RR, Bowie WC: Toxicology of solanine: A review. Vet Hum Toxicol 25:13–15, 1983.
49. Sanz P, Reig R: Clinical and pathological findings in plant oxalosis: A review. Am J Forensic Med Pathol 13:342–345, 1992.
50. Mrvos R, Dean BS, Krenzelok EP: Philodendron/dieffenbachia ingestions: Are they a problem? J Toxicol Clin Toxicol 29:485–491, 1991.
51. Pedaci L, Krenzelok EP, Jacobsen TD, Aronis J: *Dieffenbachia* species exposures: An evidence-based assessment of symptom presentation. Vet Hum Toxicol 41:335–338, 1999.
52. McIntire MS, Guest JR, Porterfield JF: Philodendron—an infant death. J Toxicol Clin Toxicol 28:177–183, 1990.
53. Farre M, Xirgu J, Salgado A, et al: Fatal oxalic acid poisoning from sorrel soup. Lancet 2:1524, 1989.
54. Gardner DG: Injury to oral mucous membranes caused by the common houseplant, dieffenbachia. Oral Surg Oral Med Oral Pathol 78:631–633, 1994.

55. Lim KH: External eye allergy from sap of *Dieffenbachia picta*. Singapore Med J 18:176–177, 1977.

56. Seet B, Chan WK, Ang CL: Crystalline keratopathy from Dieffenbachia plant sap. Br J Ophthalmol 79:98–99, 1995.

57. Reig R, Sanz P, Blanche C, et al: Fatal poisoning by *Rumex crispus* (Curled Dock): Pathological findings and application of scanning electron microscopy. Vet Hum Toxicol 32:468–470, 1990.

58. Fugh-Berman A: Herb-drug interactions. Lancet 355:134–138, 2000.

59. Johnston BA: One third of nation's adults use herbal remedies: Market estimated at 3.2 billion. Herbalgram 40:52, 1997.

60. Eisenberg DM, Davis RB, Ettner SL, et al: Trends in alternative medicine use in the United States, 1990–1997: results of a follow-up national survey. JAMA 280:1569–1575, 1998.

61. Eisenberg DM, Kessleer RC, Foster C, et al: Unconventional medicine in the United States. Prevalence, costs, and patterns of use. N Engl J Med 328:246–252, 1993.

62. Shad JA, Chinn CG, Brann OS: Acute hepatitis after ingestion of herbs. South Med J 92:1095–1097, 1999.

63. Alderman S, Kailas S, Goldfarb S, et al: Cholestatic hepatitis after ingestion of chapparal leaf: Confirmation by endoscopic retrograde cholangiopancreatography and liver biopsy. J Clin Gastroenterol 19:242–247, 1994.

64. Brent J: Three new herbal hepatotoxic syndromes. J Toxicol Clin Toxicol 17:715–719, 1999.

65. Bakerink JA, Gospe SM Jr, Dimand RJ, Eldridge MW: Multiple organ failure after ingestion of pennyroyal oil from herbal tea in two infants. Pediatrics 98:944–947, 1996.

66. Stickel F, Seitz HK: The efficacy and safety of comfrey. Public Health Nutr 3:501–508, 2000.

67. Nelson L, Shih R, Hoffman R: Aplastic anemia induced by an adulterated herbal medication. J Toxicol Clin Toxicol 33:467–470, 1995.

68. Kamiyama T, Nouchi T, Kojima S, et al: Autoimmune hepatitis triggered by administration of an herbal medicine. Am J Gastroenterol 92:703–704, 1997.

69. Kunkel DB, Spoerke DG: Evaluating exposures to plants. Emerg Med Clin North Am 2:133–144, 1984.

70. Anderson IB, Mullen WH, Meeker JE, et al: Pennyroyal toxicity: Measurement of toxic metabolite levels in two cases and review of the literature. Ann Intern Med 124:726–734, 1996.

71. Tandon HD, Tandon BN, Mattocks AR: An epidemic of veno-occlusive disease of the liver in Afghanistan: Pathologic features. Am J Gastroenterol 70:607–613, 1978.

72. Ridker PM, Okhuma S, McDermott WW: Hepatic venoocclusive disease associated with the consumption of pyrrolizidine containing dietary supplements. Gastroenterology 88:1050–1054, 1985.

73. Pillans PI: Toxicity of herbal products. N Z Med J 108:469–471, 1995.

74. De Smet PA: Health risks of herbal remedies. Drug Saf 13:81–93, 1995.

75. Ferenci P, Dragorics B, Dettrich H, et al: Randomized controlled trial of silymarin treatment in patients with cirrhosis of the liver. J Hepatol 9:105–113, 1989.

76. Pares A, Planas R, Torres M, et al: Effects of silymarin in alcoholic patients with cirrhosis of the liver: Results of a controlled, double-blind, randomized and multicenter trial. J Hepatol 28:615–621, 1998.

77. Roby CA, Anderson GD, Kantor E, et al: St John's wort: Effect on CYP3A4 activity. Clin Pharmacol Ther 57:451–457, 2000.

78. Piscitelli SC, Burstein AH, Chaitt D, et al: Indinavir concentrations and St John's wort. Lancet 355:547–548, 2000.

79. Breidenbach T, Kliem V, Burg M, et al: Profound drop of cyclosporin A whole blood trough levels caused by St. John's wort. Transplantation 69:2229–2230, 2000.

80. Ruschitzka F, Meier PJ, Turina M, et al: Acute heart transplant rejection due to Saint John's wort. Lancet 355:548–549, 2000.

81. Ruck B, Shih RD, Marcus SM: Hypertensive crisis from herbal treatment of impotence. Am J Emerg Med 17:317–318, 1999.

82. Riley AJ: Yohimbe in the treatment of erectile disorder. Br J Clin Pract 48:133–136, 1994.

83. Lin SC, Hsu T, Fredrickson PA, Richelson E: Yohimbine and tranylcypromine-induced postural hypotension. Am J Psychiatry 144:119, 1987.

84. Linden CH, Vellman WP, Rumack B: Yohimbine: A new street drug. Ann Emerg Med 14:1002–1004, 1985.

85. Holmberg G, Gershon S: Autonomic and psychic effects of yohimbe hydrochloride. Psychopharmacologia 2:93–106, 1961.

86. FDA Talk Paper, April 26, 2001. www.fda.gov/bbs/topics/ANSWERS/2001/ANS01080.html

87. Chan TYK, Tomlinson B, Tse LKK, et al: Aconitine poisoning due to Chinese herbal medicines: A review. Vet Hum Toxicol 36:452–455, 1994.

88. Onat FY, Yegen BC, Lawrence R, et al: Mad honey poisoning in man and rat. Rev Environ Health 9:3–9, 1991.

89. Shih RD, Goldfrank LR: Plants. In: Goldfrank's Toxicologic Emergencies, 6th ed. Stamford, CT, Appleton & Lange, 1998

90. Yeih D-F, Chiang F-T, Huang SKS: Successful treatment of aconitine induced life threatening ventricular tachyarrhythmia with amiodarone. Heart 84:E8, 2000.

91. Schmeiser HH, Bieler CA, Wiessler M, et al: Detection of DNA adducts formed by aristolochic acid in renal tissue from patients with Chinese herbs nephropathy. Cancer Res 56:2025–2028, 1996.

CHAPTER 123

Water Hemlock

Edward W. Cetaruk

Water hemlock belongs to the family Apiaceae (Umbelliferae). The genus *Cicuta* includes the species spotted water hemlock (*C. maculata* L); western water hemlock (*C. douglasii*); northern water hemlock, also known as European water hemlock (*C. virosa*); *C. bolanderi* Wats; *C. bulbifera* L; *C. californica* Gray; *C. curtissii* Coult. and Rose; *C. mackenziana* Raup.; *C. occidentalis* Greene; and *C. vagans* Greene. The hemlock water dropwort (*Oenanthe crocata*) belongs to the family Umbelliferae, genus *Oenanthe*. It is native to Europe but has been introduced to some parts of the United States. *O. crocata* lacks the chambered root of the *Cicuta* spp. and produces oenanthotoxin, an isomer of cicutoxin, the active substance in water hemlock.

The various species of *Cicuta* and *Oenanthe* have approximately equivalent toxicity at similar stages of plant growth and produce virtually identical clinical manifestations in poisoning and are discussed as a single group. Common names of these plants include *cowbane, children's bane, poison parsnip, five-fingered root, dead men's fingers, death-of-man, wild parsnip, snakeroot, snakeweed, beaver poison, muskrat weed, spotted hemlock, spotted cowbane, musquash root, false parsley, poison hemlock, wild carrot, fever root, mock-eel root, spotted parsley, cigue vireuse,* and *carotte à moreau.*

Water hemlock species are biennial or perennial plants that grow to a height of 6 to 8 feet with narrow, compound leaves that have serrated edges (Fig. 123-1). Purple spots ("macules") may be visible on the stalk, which is hollow and chambered. Small fragrant white flowers develop as compound umbrella-like formations (umbels) that typically blossom in June or July. *Cicuta* spp. and *Oenanthe* spp. grow only in habitats with continuous water such as swamps, lakesides, stream banks, drainage ditches, and marshes. *Cicuta* spp. have thick, tuberous roots, which are often bundled with five or six roots. When cut, the roots yield an oily yellow sap that has an odor of parsnips and rapidly turns brown on contact with air. When the thickened underground portions of the stem and roots are sectioned sagittally, characteristic multilayered air chambers separated by pith diaphragms are seen (Fig. 123-2).[1] These chambers are not as distinct in the spring as they are later in the season.[2] All parts of the plant are considered poisonous. The tuberous roots are the most toxic part, especially in the spring before flowering, when they are typically the most developed. *O. crocata* roots are usually more bulbous than the roots of the *Cicuta* spp. and are solid rather than chambered. They also produce a sticky, oily yellow sap when cut.[3,4]

It is important not to confuse water hemlock with the closely related poison hemlock (*Conium maculatum*), which has a similar appearance (see Fig. 124-1). Poison hemlock also belongs to the family Umbelliferae and has small white flowers in umbellate clusters similar to the flowers of water hemlock. Poison hemlock has wider leaves that have three to five divisions and a single tap root that is nonchambered. The root of poison hemlock also yields an oily yellow sap when cut. *C. maculatum* was imported to North America from Europe and is now found in the same geographic range as water hemlock, throughout the United States and southern Canada. Its habitat differs from water hemlock in that it is typically drier (e.g., roadsides, fields, and ditches). The active toxic principles in poison hemlock, including coniine, *N*-methyl coniine, conhydrine, λ-coniceine, and pseudoconhydrine, produce a different spectrum of clinical effects than the toxins found in water hemlock. Poisoning from water hemlock manifests primarily as vomiting and seizures that occur within 1 hour of ingestion, whereas poisoning from poison hemlock presents with initial gastrointestinal upset, then autonomic and somatic stimulatory features that are followed by central nervous system (CNS) depression, ascending paralysis, and bradycardia (see Chapter 124).

Water hemlock has been mistaken for other members of the Umbelliferae family that are edible, such as *Daucus carota* (carrots); *Pastinaca sativa* (parsnip); "wild parsnips"; and many other wild tuberous plants that are objects of human foraging, including artichokes, celery, sweet potatoes, and sweet anise.[2-16] Fatal poisonings have resulted from the ingestion of *C. maculata* that was mistakenly identified as American ginseng.[17,18] Livestock poisoning also occurs, frequently in the spring, because water hemlock is usually located near water sources where animals graze and emerges early in the season before other forage becomes available.

BIOCHEMISTRY

The compounds responsible for water hemlock's toxicity vary depending on the species, but all belong to a class of conjugated C_{17}-polyacetylenes. These are highly unsaturated, polyacetylenic alcohols that are isomers or analogues of a 17-carbon skeleton that includes a conjugated polyacetylene system, a terminal hydroxyl group at C_1, and an allylic hydroxyl group at C_{14}.[19] Cicutoxin, isocicutoxin, cicutol, oenanthotoxin, oenanthetol, oenanththetone, and virols A, B, and C have been isolated from *Cicuta* spp. and *Oenanthe* spp. Cicutoxin was first described by Boehm in 1876[20] and has been extensively characterized since in multiple subsequent works. The principle toxic members of this

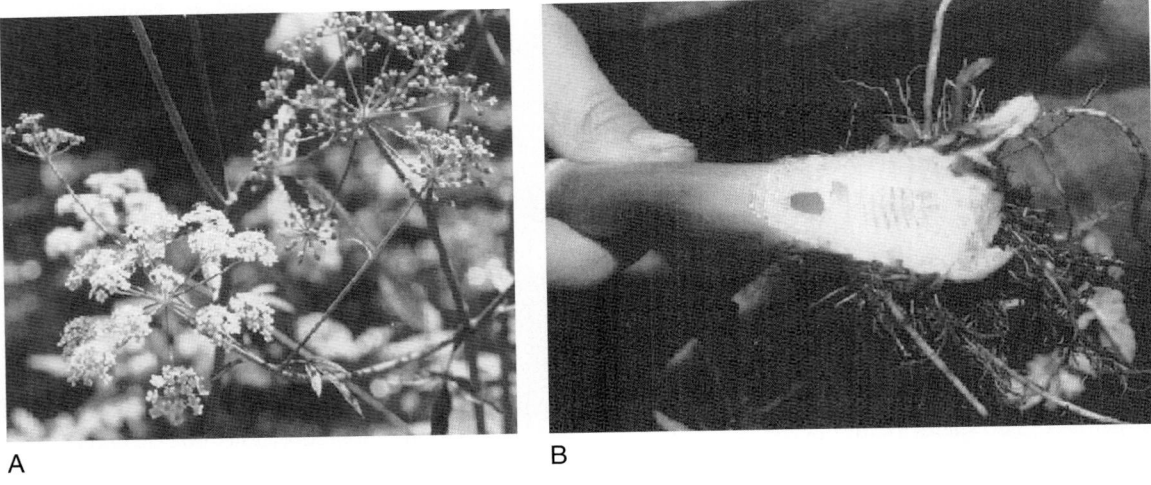

A

B

FIGURE 123-1

A, *Cicuta* spp. umbels typical of the Umbelliferea family. See Color Fig. 123-1A. **B,** Chambered root characteristic of *Cicuta* spp. See Color Fig. 123-1B. *(Photos courtesy of Steven Curry, MD. From Graeme KA, Braitberg G, Kunkel DB, Adler M: Toxic plant ingestions. In Auerbach PS [ed]: Wilderness Medicine. St. Louis, Mosby, 2001.)*

group are *oenanthotoxin* (*trans*-heptadeca-2:8:10-triene-4:6-diyne-1:14-diol), *cicutoxin* (*trans*-heptadeca-8:10:12-triene-4:6-diyne-1:14-diol), and *virol A* (*trans*-heptadeca-8:10-diene-4:6-diyne-1:11-diol) (Fig. 123-3).[19,21–23]

These C_{17}-polyacetylenes are found in all parts of the plants. The tuberous roots contain the highest concentra-

tion of toxins and are the portion of the plant most commonly ingested. As is typical with naturally occurring toxins, the concentration and variety of active compounds in a given plant vary with season, environmental conditions such as water supply, and which plant species or plant part is being considered. Although cicutoxin and oenanthotoxin

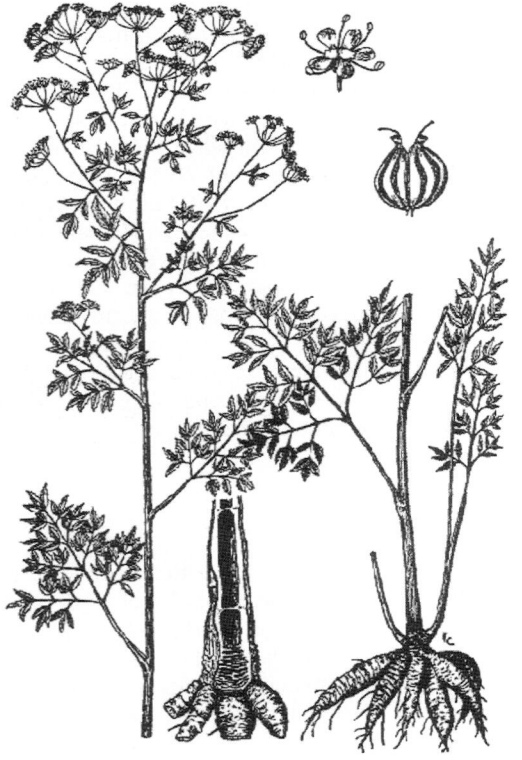

FIGURE 123-2

Cicuta maculata. Lower and upper portions of flowering stem, with details of chambered stalk and root, flowers in umbel formations, and fruit. *(From Kingsbury JM: Poisonous Plants of the United States. Englewood Cliffs, NJ, Prentice-Hall, 1964, p 375.)*

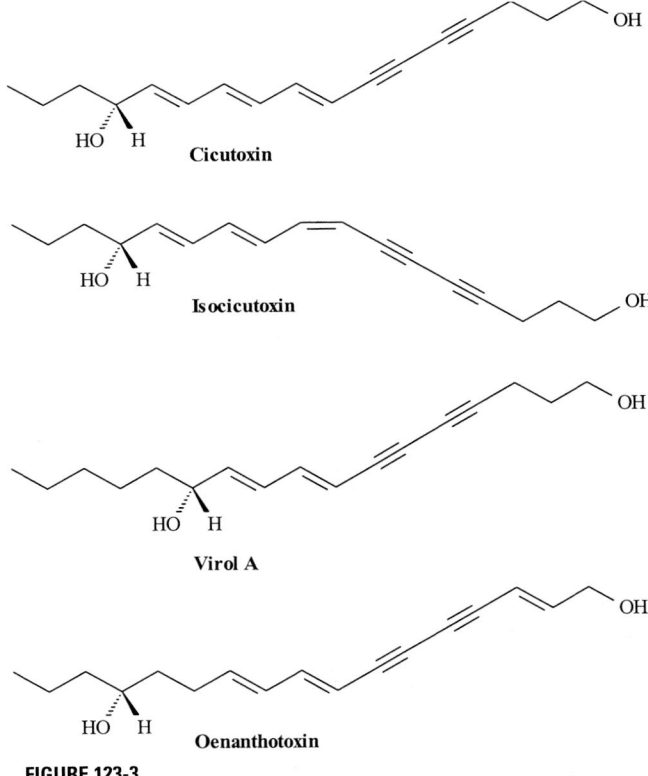

Cicutoxin

Isocicutoxin

Virol A

Oenanthotoxin

FIGURE 123-3

Chemical structures of C_{17}-polyacetylenes from water hemlock.

are relatively unstable compounds on exposure to air, light, and heat, poisonings after ingestion of dried or cooked roots of *O. crocata* and *C. maculata* have been reported.[3,4,24,25] Pharmacologic studies by Grundy and Howarth[26] showed marked toxicity with dried and powdered tubers of *O. crocata.*

The C_{17}-polyacetylenes are water soluble but can be readily extracted with organic polar solvents, such as methanol, ethanol, and ethers. They can be studied in biologic and environmental samples using high-performance liquid chromatography, thin-layer chromatography, and mass spectrometry.[19,21,25,26]

The structure-activity relationship between C_{17}-polyacetylenes found in *C. virosa* and γ-aminobutyric acid A (GABA$_A$) receptors in rat brain cortex has been studied. Eleven C_{17}-polyacetylenes have been isolated from water hemlock root, including cicutoxin, isocicutoxin, and virol A, B, and C.[19,22,23] By synthesizing more chemically stable structural analogues, the structural requirements for toxicity have been determined. The length of the π-bond conjugation system and the geometry of the double bonds are critical for toxicity; this is exemplified by comparing the median lethal dose (LD$_{50}$) of cicutoxin, with all *trans* double bonds, and that of isocicutoxin, which has a *cis* configuration at its C_8-C_9 double bond (Fig. 123-4). The LD$_{50}$ values of cicutoxin, isocicutoxin, virol A, and picrotoxin in a mouse model (intraperitoneal) are 2.8 mg/kg, 38.5 mg/kg, 9.5 mg/kg, and 9.8 mg/kg, respectively.[19,22,23] Other C_{17}-polyacetylene analogue studies showed that the terminal *O*-functional group and the allylic alcohol also were essential for toxicity.[19]

PATHOPHYSIOLOGY

The primary toxic effects of water hemlock—severe and recurrent seizures—result from its GABA antagonist action in the CNS. Normally, agonism of GABA$_A$ receptor–linked ion channels results in the influx of chloride into the neuron. This influx hyperpolarizes the neuron, inhibiting depolarization. Cicutoxin and the other toxic C_{17}-polyacetylenes are believed to inhibit this hyperpolarization, allowing depolarization of neurons to go unchecked, leading to seizures. This effect is dose dependent, as the severity of poisoning has been found to be directly related to the amount of the plant (usually the root) ingested.

Grundy and Howarth[26] noted that seizures produced by oenanthotoxin were indistinguishable from seizures produced by picrotoxin. Picrotoxin is a noncompetitive indirect GABA antagonist and binds to a specific site, distinct from the GABA itself, on the GABA$_A$ chloride channel.[27] Pretreatment with one tenth the convulsive dose of an extract of *C. douglasii* decreased the convulsive dose of picrotoxin in a dose-dependent manner but did not significantly decrease the convulsive dose of pentylenetetrazol, supporting a picrotoxin-like mechanism for cicutoxin's proconvulsant activity.[28]

The potency of each C_{17}-polyacetylene compound as a GABA$_A$ antagonist was determined by comparing the compound's ability to inhibit the specific binding of [^{3}H]EBOB (ethynylbicycloorthobenzoate), a specific noncompetitive inhibitor of GABA-gated chloride channels) to the GABA$_A$ receptor complex in rat brain cortex.[19] Binding studies showed that virol A reversibly reduced GABA-induced chloride current in a noncompetitive, concentration-dependent manner. The [^{3}H]EBOB 50% inhibitory concentrations values (μM) for cicutoxin, virol A, and picrotoxin were 0.54, 1.15, and 1.81, respectively. In addition, there was a correlation between the potency of the compounds in inhibiting the specific binding of [^{3}H]EBOB to GABA-gated chloride channels of GABA$_A$ receptors in rat brain cortex and their LD$_{50}$ values.[19]

Binding studies have been performed to measure virol A's effect on the GABA-induced inhibitory chloride current (I_{GABA}). Virol A reversibly reduced I_{GABA} and muscimol-induced chloride current (I_{MUS}) (muscimol is a GABA$_A$ receptor agonist) in rat brain hippocampal CA1 neurons in a concentration-dependent manner. It inhibited I_{GABA} in a competitive manner at lower concentrations, however, and in a noncompetitive manner at high concentrations.[29] Other studies showed that virol A further reduced the I_{GABA} already reduced by lower doses of picrotoxin, but not at high doses of picrotoxin, indicating that picrotoxin and virol A may recognize a common binding site.[29] Virol A did not decrease the glycine-induced (glycine is an inhibitory neurotransmitter) current, indicating that it selectively inhibits the GABA response.[29] Virol A was not displaced by [^{3}H]muscimol or by [^{3}H]flunitrazepam in rat brain membrane preparations. Virol A apparently binds to a site that is distinct from GABA agonist and benzodiazepine binding sites.[29] Mice pretreated with subconvulsive doses of cicutoxin had a lower convulsive threshold to picrotoxin, further suggesting a common, possibly synergistic, mode of action.[28] Neuroanatomic studies in animals in which the CNS was either destroyed or severed at different levels suggest a GABA antagonism–induced seizure origin in the brainstem.[26]

Cardiovascular effects, including hypotension, hypertension, bradycardia, tachycardia, ventricular fibrillation, and cardiac arrest, have been reported in water hemlock

FIGURE 123-4

General structure activity relationship of C_{17}-polyacetylenes from hemlock. Cicutoxin is the *trans*-isomer, and isocicutoxin is the *cis*-isomer. (Modified from Uwai K, Ohashi K, Takaya Y, et al: Exploring the structural basis of neurotoxicity in C_{17}-polyacetylenes isolated from water hemlock. J Med Chem 43:4508–4515, 2000.)

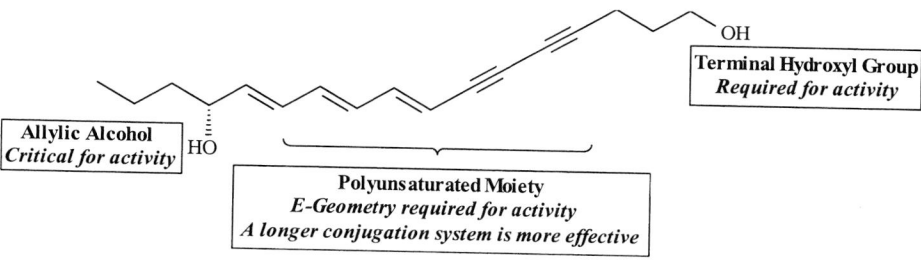

poisoning.[6,7,11,12,18,30] It is unclear from these case reports, however, whether these cardiovascular effects are secondary to severe seizures or are due to a primary cardiotoxic effect of cicutoxin or related toxins found in water hemlock. Studies in anesthetized, nonseizing animals showed that these toxins can cause marked hypotension, usually followed by a hypertensive phase.[26,31] Bilateral vagotomy or destruction of the CNS prevented the bradycardia seen in one of these experiments but did not affect blood pressure, suggesting a centrally mediated mechanism for bradycardia.[31] In human case reports and animal experiments, these cardiovascular effects have been variable, and a mechanism of action has yet to be elucidated.

Parts of C. maculata have been used as herbal remedies for scirrhous mammary cancer and scirrhous tumors.[32] Cicutoxin itself has been studied as a potential chemotherapeutic agent. An extract of C. maculata was found to have significant in vitro cytotoxic effects against a human nasopharyngeal cancer cell culture line. Structure-activity relationship studies showed that the same structural moieties responsible for cicutoxin's toxicity (the conjugated double and triple bonds and the two hydroxyl groups) also are responsible for its cytotoxic antileukemic activity.[32]

Cicutoxin also has been shown to have activity at voltage-gated potassium channels in stimulated T lymphocytes. Cicutoxin reversibly, and in a potent manner, blocked n-type potassium current in a dose-dependent fashion, inhibiting potassium current–dependent T-cell proliferation.[33]

The toxic C_{17}-polyacetylenes responsible for water hemlock's neurologic toxicity inhibit the GABAergic inhibitory chloride current, resulting in decreased inhibitory tone and leading to seizures. They apparently do not have effects at the benzodiazepine and glycine receptors, may share a common binding site with picrotoxin, and may act primarily in the brainstem to cause seizures. They have variable effects on the cardiovascular system. They block voltage-gated potassium channels, are cytotoxic in vitro, and inhibit T-cell proliferation. It is unclear, however, how each of these effects may contribute to their clinical toxicity.

CLINICAL PRESENTATION

Water hemlock poisoning typically occurs in persons, often in groups, foraging for edible wild plants. The clinical presentation of water hemlock poisoning was first reported by Wepfer in 1679, when he described five children who were poisoned after they ingested the plant.[34] The first report of poisoning in North America is attributed to Stockbridge, who published a case of fatal water hemlock poisoning in 1814.[35] Poisoning has since been reported in adults and children and often occurs in the spring when the plants have not yet developed to their full size and are more likely to resemble other edible wild plants, such as ginseng or wild parsnips, carrots, and turnips. Fatal poisoning in a young woman who ingested hemlock water dropwort roots in the hope that they would be hallucinogenic also has been reported.[25] Egdahl[7] reported a case of water hemlock poisoning as the means of a murder attempt. Egdahl[7] also cited Chevallier in reporting five cases, including two fatalities, of dermal water hemlock poisoning when a family rubbed their skin with the roots of Cicuta aquatica in an effort to

treat pruritus. It has even been reported that placing slices of C. virosa root on the backs of frogs can induce seizures.[7]

The clinical presentations of water hemlock poisoning for Cicuta spp. and Oenanthe spp. are essentially identical. Initial symptoms are generally gastrointestinal complaints, including nausea, vomiting, and abdominal cramping. Symptoms often begin within a few minutes and nearly always within 30 to 45 minutes of ingesting the root, but onset may be delayed several hours.[11–13,15,16,18,30] Typically, as the amount of the root ingested increases, the time to onset of symptoms decreases, and the severity increases. Vomiting may be significant and repetitive. Other early signs and symptoms include diaphoresis, mydriasis, increased salivation, confusion, dizziness, diarrhea, weakness, ataxia, and hypotension.[11–13,15,16,18,24,30] Although mydriasis is typical, miosis also has been reported.[30] Respiratory distress is common, and rales and wheezing have been reported.[6,7] The initial symptoms of nausea, vomiting, diarrhea, abdominal cramping, diaphoresis, altered mental status, increased salivation, and weakness suggest a cholinergic toxidrome. Conversely, mydriasis and seizures are consistent with an anticholinergic toxidrome. There are many poisonous plants that produce cholinergic or anticholinergic toxidromes. A careful and complete physical examination is important to avoid mistaking water hemlock poisoning for either cholinergic or anticholinergic poisoning from another cause. The typical presentation is abrupt onset of seizures accompanied by cholinergic-like signs with the notable exception of mydriasis.

The hallmark of water hemlock poisoning is severe, recurrent, and often refractory generalized seizures. Seizures may occur before or after vomiting and may be the initial sign of poisoning. They are most often described as grand mal, tonic, tonic-clonic, or status epilepticus. Opisthotonos and hemiballismus also have been reported.[6,12,36] Coma, hypotonia, and decreased deep tendon reflexes usually follow seizures.[3,4,15] If seizures persist, cyanosis and acidosis develop, and cardiac or respiratory arrest (or both) may follow. Other reported neurologic symptoms include amnesia,[2,12,30] paresthesias,[24] neuropsychologic abnormalities,[6] and hallucinations.[12] Electroencephalograms show diffuse abnormalities that may be persistent.[6,12,13,24,30] Coagulopathy has been reported on multiple occasions.[9,30]

I consulted on a group of five boys who ingested varying amounts of the root from a water hemlock plant. They were removing winter overgrowth from a drainage ditch in the springtime. All five developed gastrointestinal symptoms, and two had seizures. One patient reported visual hallucinations and an "out-of-body" experience en route to the hospital. All patients survived, including the most severely poisoned patient, who had multiple seizures over approximately 45 minutes before arrival at the hospital. He was treated with benzodiazepines, phenobarbital, intubation, and mechanical ventilation and eventually recovered.

Rhabdomyolysis is common in water hemlock poisoning.[5,6,24] Patients may complain of muscle pain and tenderness, and creatine phosphokinase values are elevated; this has been noted many times in patients with recurrent seizures and has been seen in patients in the absence of seizures, although to a much lesser degree. The etiology of rhabdomyolysis has not yet been determined. It is likely multifactorial, resulting from seizure-induced muscle activity and breakdown and possibly direct myotoxicity. Creatine phosphokinase and renal function monitoring is recommended in all patients with water hemlock poisoning. Acute renal failure has been reported after water hemlock poisoning.[5]

Case-fatality rates have been reported to range from 30% to 70%. Cardiopulmonary arrest during status epilepticus is the primary cause of death. This wide mortality range likely reflects in part publication bias and the fact that many cases reported in the literature occurred before the development of effective anticonvulsant therapy and before the use of modern critical care techniques and advanced life-support protocols.[7,9,10,21] Despite such advances in treatment, however, water hemlock is still considered the most toxic plant in North America and can be rapidly fatal if not diagnosed early and treated agressively.[11,13,25]

DIAGNOSIS

The diagnosis of water hemlock poisoning must be made on the basis of history and clinical presentation. There are no readily available diagnostic tests. Table 123-1 lists critical features that should be elucidated in the history of possible water hemlock ingestion.

The cholinergic-like manifestations, such as emesis, abdominal cramping, excessive salivation and lacrimation, diaphoresis, and seizures, may lead some clinicians to suspect poisoning by grayanotoxin-containing plants, such as death camas (*Zigadenus* spp.), mountain laurel (*Kalmia latifolia*), azalea, or rhododendron (*Rhododendron* spp.). Death camas has been mistaken for wild onion by people foraging for edible wild plants. Identification of the ingested plant should help differentiate water hemlock from these species. Other poisonous plants found in the United States that cause seizures include black cherry (*Prunus serotina*), Jimson weed (*Datura stramonium*), black nightshade (*solanum nigrum*), and sneezeweed (*Helenium autumnale*).[7] Jimson weed and nightshade present with an anticholinergic syndrome, including marked mydriasis, but should not have the cholinergic symptoms reported with water hemlock poisoning. Black cherry is a cyanogenic plant and produces significantly delayed symptoms, including vomiting, abdominal pain, coma, and seizures, whereas water hemlock poisoning typically develops soon after ingestion of the plant.

Water hemlock often grows in drainage ditches, which may contain irrigation runoff contaminated with organophosphate pesticides. Organophosphate (or similarly carbamate) pesticide poisoning produces a cholinergic toxidrome similar to the symptoms seen in water hemlock poisoning. Organophosphate poisoning should be considered in the differential diagnosis of a poisoned patient with cholinergic symptoms in an agricultural setting. The marked mydriasis seen in water hemlock poisoning is inconsistent with a cholinergic agent, however. Also, these pesticides produce profuse *atropine-responsive* bronchorrhea, a feature that is not seen in water hemlock poisoning.

As discussed earlier, it is important not to confuse the water hemlock plant with the closely related poison hemlock (*Conium maculatum*), which has a similar appearance. The active toxins in poison hemlock, coniine, *N*-methyl coniine, conhydrine, λ-coniceine, and pseudoconhydrine, are structurally similar to nicotine and bind to nicotinic receptors. Toxicity from water hemlock manifests primarily as vomiting and seizures within 1 hour of ingestion. Although poison hemlock poisoning may present initially with nausea, vomiting, and abdominal cramping, similar to water hemlock, this initial stimulatory phase is followed by an ascending paralysis, CNS depression, bradycardia, and death from respiratory paralysis. Poison hemlock poisoning is discussed in detail in Chapter 124.

The diagnosis of water hemlock poisoning is based on the identification of the plant ingested and a clinical presentation that includes signs and symptoms suggesting cholinergic poisoning, mydriasis, and abrupt onset of severe seizures. The differential toxicologic diagnosis should include other toxic plants that produce similar manifestations, organophosphate/carbamate pesticide poisoning if the ingestion occurs in an agricultural setting, and other conditions that suggest such a pesticide exposure.

TREATMENT

There is no specific antidote for water hemlock poisoning. Management should focus on cardiopulmonary stabilization, control of seizures, and gastrointestinal decontamination. Aggressive airway management should be the initial treatment priority because these seizing patients are at high risk for aspiration, hypoxia, and anoxia. Stability and security of the airway should be ensured to minimize the risk of aspiration before the oral administration of activated charcoal or performance of gastric lavage.

Patients often partially self-decontaminate with repeated bouts of vomiting that may occur after water hemlock ingestions. Given the extremely high toxicity of even a

TABLE 123-1 Historical Features Important in the Diagnosis of Water Hemlock Poisoning

Detailed description of ingested plant, including the locale in which it was found (if possible, the plant itself should be obtained for identification)
Part and amount of the plant ingested
Time of ingestion
History of any coingestants
History of all signs and symptoms since ingestion (patient may present obtunded and unable to provide history)
Other possible victims

Indications for ICU Admission in Water Hemlock Poisoning

Any symptomatic patient with a history of water hemlock ingestion
Any patient requiring anticonvulsant treatment after water hemlock ingestion

small amount of ingested plant material, if the patient presents for treatment early, decontamination including gastric lavage or the administration of activated charcoal should be performed without delay. However, these measures have not been shown to alter the outcome or clinical course of water hemlock–poisoned patients or even poisoned patients in general. Theoretically, gastric lavage becomes less effective as the time since ingestion increases and should be considered only in a patient presenting early after poisoning. If lavage were to provide any benefit, it almost certainly would require that it be completed within the first hour postingestion. The usual dose of activated charcoal is 50 g orally in adults and 1 g/kg in children. Because these patients are prone to develop diarrhea, cathartics should not be administered with the activated charcoal. The airway must be protected before either method of gastric decontamination.

Although not studied in clinical trials, benzodiazepines or barbiturates or both generally are recommended for the treatment of water hemlock–induced seizures. This recommendation is based on cicutoxin's stimulatory effect on $GABA_A$ receptors. The seizures seen in water hemlock poisoning are often refractory to treatment. Anticonvulsants should be administered aggressively and as promptly as possible after onset of seizures or possibly even as a prophylactic measure if other clinical manifestations of poison hemlock toxicity are already apparent. Anticonvulsant dose should be titrated to effect with the end point of seizure control. Intubation also should be considered early with the use of high-dose or repeated dosing of benzodiazepines or barbiturates or both. Phenytoin has been shown to be less effective than phenobarbital in controlling cicutoxin-induced seizures in an animal model and is not recommended.[28] Although water hemlock poisoning has many features of a cholinergic toxidrome, an animal study found that water hemlock–induced seizures were not suppressed by pretreatment with the anticholinergic agents benztropine or biperiden, nor were they worsened by the cholinergic agonist physostigmine, but they were well controlled with diazepam.[37,38]

Rhabdomyolysis may be severe and may be treated with intravenous fluids or urine alkalinization or both to maintain good urine output and to minimize the risk of myoglobin-induced renal failure. Urine alkalization (to pH >6.5) can be achieved by adding 50 to 100 mEq of sodium bicarbonate to 1 L of dextrose in water, or half-normal saline, and administering this intravenously at approximately 1.5 to 2 times the maintenance rate. Acute oliguric renal failure due to water hemlock poisoning with rhabdomyolysis has been treated with short-term hemodialysis.[5]

The use of hemodialysis and hemoperfusion as treatment for water hemlock poisoning was reported in a 30-year-old man who also was treated with gastric lavage, oral activated charcoal, urine alkalization, forced diuresis, paralysis, mechanical ventilation, and physostigmine.[12] The patient recovered, although it is unclear what impact, if any, the use of extracorporeal elimination techniques had on his outcome. Except for the supportive treatment of acute renal failure, there are insufficient data to recommend hemodialysis or hemoperfusion in the treatment of water hemlock poisoning.

Criteria for ICU Discharge in Water Hemlock Poisoning

Resolution of seizure activity without ongoing anticonvulsant administration
Resolution of acidosis (if previously present)
Normal mental status

SPECIAL POPULATIONS

Water hemlock poisoning should be suspected in patients with vomiting and recurrent seizures with a history of wild plant ingestion, camping, or foraging. No populations have been reported as either more or less susceptible to water hemlock poisoning.

Common Errors in Water Hemlock Poisoning

Misdiagnosis as either anticholinergic poisoning (due to mydriasis) or cholinergic poisoning (due to increased secretions, nausea, vomiting, diarrhea, abdominal cramping, and seizures)
Failure to manage the patient's airway and cardiorespiratory status aggressively
Failure to use benzodiazepine and barbiturate anticonvulsant medications (e.g., lorazepam, phenobarbital) aggressively

Key Points in Water Hemlock Poisoning

1. Ingested plants should be identified rapidly, if possible.
2. Early and aggressive management of airway and cardiopulmonary status is important.
3. Early and aggressive management of seizures is important.
4. The patient should be monitored for rhabdomyolysis.

REFERENCES

1. Kingsbury JM: Poisonous Plants of the United States. Englewood Cliffs, NJ, Prentice-Hall, 1964.
2. Stratton MR: Water hemlock poisoning. Colorado Med 16:104–111, 1919.
3. Mitchell MI, Routledge PA: Poisoning by hemlock water dropwort. Lancet 1:423–424, 1977.
4. Mitchell MI, Routledge PA: Hemlock water dropwort poisoning—a review. Clin Toxicol 12:417–426, 1978.
5. Carlton BE, Tufts E, Girard DE: Water hemlock poisoning complicated by rhabdomyolysis and renal failure. Clin Toxicol 14:87–92, 1979.
6. Costanza DJ, Hoversten VW: Accidental ingestion of water hemlock. Calif Med 119:78–82, 1973.
7. Egdahl A: A case of poisoning due to eating poison-hemlock (*Cicuta maculata*). Arch Intern Med 7:348–356, 1911.
8. Furbee B, Wermuth M: Life-threatening plant poisoning. Crit Care Clin North Am 13:849–888, 1997.
9. Gompertz LM: Poisoning with water hemlock (*Cicuta maculata*). JAMA 87:1277–1278, 1911.
10. Haggarty DR, Conway JA: Report of poisoning by *Cicuta maculata*. N Y State J Med 36:1511–1514, 1936.

11. Heath KB: A fatal case of water hemlock poisoning. Vet Hum Toxicol 43:35–36, 2001.

12. Knutsen OH, Paszkowski P: New aspects in the treatment of water hemlock poisoning. Clin Toxicol 22:157–166, 1984.

13. Landers D, Seppi K, Blauer W: Seizures and death on a white river float trip. West J Med 142:637–640, 1985.

14. Mulligan GB, Munro DB: The biology of Canadian weeds: 48. *Cicuta maculata L., C. douglasii* (D.C.) Coult. and Rose and *C. virosa L.* Can J Plant Sci 61:93–105, 1981.

15. Robson P: Water hemlock poisoning. Lancet 2:1274–1275, 1965.

16. Rork LE: Plant poisoning in a child. Rocky Mtn Med J 66:47–49, 1969.

17. Campell EW: Plant poisoning umbelliferae (parsley family). J Maine Med Assoc 20:40–41, 1966.

18. Sweeney K, Gensheimer KF, Knowlton-Field J, et al: Water hemlock poisoning—Maine, 1992. MMWR Morb Mortal Wkly Rep 43:229–231, 1994.

19. Uwai K, Ohashi K, Takaya Y, et al: Exploring the structural basis of neurotoxicity in C_{17}-polyacetylenes isolated from water hemlock. J Med Chem 43:4508–4515, 2000.

20. Boehm R: Archiv fur Experimentelle Pathologie und Phamakologie. Bd. 5, Heft 4–5:279–310, 1876.

21. Anet EFLJ, Lythgoe B, Silk MH, et al: Oenanthotoxin and cicutoxin: Isolation and structure. J Chem Soc 62:355–364, 1953.

22. Ohta T, Uwai K, Nozoe S, et al: Absolute stereochemistry of cicutoxin and related toxic polyacetylenic alcohols from *Cicuta virosa*. Tetrahedron 55:12087–12098, 1999.

23. Uwai K, Oshima Y: Syntheses and stereochemical assignment of toxic C_{17}-polyacetylenic alcohols virols A, B, and C, isolated from water hemlock (*Cicuta virosa*). Tetrahedron 55:9469–9480, 1999.

24. Ball MJ, Flather ML, Forfar JC: Hemlock water dropwort poisoning. Postgrad Med J 63:363–365, 1987.

25. King LA, Lewis MJ, Parry D, et al: Identification of oenanthotoxin and related compounds in hemlock water dropwort poisoning. Hum Toxicol 4:355–364, 1985.

26. Grundy HF, Howarth F: Pharmacological studies on hemlock water dropwort. Br J Pharmacol 11:225–230, 1956.

27. Akaike N, Hattori K, Oomura Y, et al: Bicuilline and picrotoxin block γ-aminobutyric acid-gated Cl⁻ conductance by different mechanisms. Experimentia 41:70–71, 1985.

28. Nelson RB, Cole FR: The convulsive profile of *Cicuta douglasii* (water hemlock). Proc West Pharmacol Soc 19:193–197, 1976.

29. Uwai K, Ohashi K, Takaya Y, et al: Virol A, a trans-polyacetylenic alcohol of *Cicuta virosa*, selectively inhibits the GABA-induced Cl⁻ current in acutely dissociated rat hippocampal CA1 neurons. Brain Res 889:174–180, 2001.

30. Starrveld E, Hope CE: Cicutoxin poisoning (water hemlock). Neurology 25:730–734, 1975.

31. Withers LM, Cole FR, Nelson RB: Water hemlock poisoning. N Engl J Med 281:566–567, 1969.

32. Konoshima T, Lee KH: Antitumor agents, 85. Cicutoxin, an antileukemic principle from *Cicuta maculata,* and the cytotoxicity of the related derivatives. J Nat Prod 49:1117–1121, 1986.

33. Strauss U, Wittstock U, Schubert R, et al: Cicutoxin from *Cicuta virosa:* A new and potent potassium channel blocker in T lymphocytes. Biochem Biophys Res Commun 219:332–336, 1996.

34. Wepfer JJ: Cicutae Aquatica historia et noxae. SM 4° Basiloe, JR Konig, 1679.

35. Stockbridge J: Account of the effects of a poisonous plant called *Cicuta maculata*. Boston Med Surg J 3:334–337, 1814.

36. Miller MM: Water hemlock poisoning. JAMA 101:852–853, 1933.

37. Nelson RB, North DS, Kaneriya M, et al: The influence of biperiden, benztropine, physostigmine and diazepam on the convulsive effects of *Cicuta douglasii*. Proc West Pharmacol Soc 21:137–139, 1978.

38. North DS, Nelson RB: Anticholinergic agents in cicutoxin poisoning. West J Med 143:250, 1985.

39. Rizzi D, Basile C, Di Maggio A, et al: Clinical spectrum of accidental hemlock poisoning: Neurotoxic manifestations, rhabdomyolysis and acute renal failure. Nephrol Dial Transplant 6:939–943, 1991.

40. Smith RA, Lewis D: *Cicuta toxicosis* in cattle: Case history and simplified analytical method. Vet Hum Toxicol 29:240–241, 1987.

41. Undine CA: Poisoning with *Cicuta maculata* or water hemlock. Minn Med 21:262–263, 1938.

CHAPTER 124

Poison Hemlock

Frederick W. Fiesseler ■ Richard D. Shih

Poison hemlock (*Conium maculatum*) is regarded as one of the most poisonous plants worldwide. This plant is a member of the family of Umbelliferae. The term *Umbelliferae* originates from *umbellula*, which means "little shade," referring to the parasol-shaped clusters of flowers. Other members of this family include celery (*Apium graveolens*), lovage (*Levisticum officianale*), angelica (*Angelicu archagelice*), carrots (*Daucus carota*), and parsnip (*Pastinaca sativa*). Poison hemlock has been misidentified as one of the aforementioned edible species and consumed, leading to toxic exposure. However, this misidentification occurs infrequently because of the plant's "mousy" odor, bitter taste, and burning in the mouth after ingestion.

Poison hemlock was the official poison of ancient Greece and was used by executioners during this period.[1] It typically was mixed into a concoction containing conium juice, opium, and other alkaloids. This type of extract is believed to have been administered to Socrates in 399 BC, when he was sentenced to death for presumed political reasons. The ability of the hemlock to induce a motor paralysis was elegantly documented by Socrates' student Plato, who was at his bedside during his death: "The man who administered the poison kept his hand upon Socrates, and after a little while examined his feet and legs; then pinched his foot hard and asked if he felt it. Socrates said no. Then he did the same to his legs; and moving gradually upwards in this way let us see that he was getting cold and numb."[2]

Poison hemlock typically grows to a height of about 2 m. The stem is large and hollow and contains purple spots that are considered an identifying characteristic—hence one of its common names, *spotted hemlock*.[3] Its foliage and leaves are three times divided (tripinnate), similar to a fern (Fig. 124-1). Poison hemlock develops white flowers that are organized into a flowering head in which the pedicle, individual flower stems, all spring from one point; this is called an *umbel*. Its long, solid white taproot also is characteristic of this species. Poison hemlock can grow anywhere adequate moisture is supplied; it is often found in pastures and meadows and alongside streets and streams. Hemlock can be found throughout the world, although most ingestions occur in North and South America, Europe, western Asia, and Australia. *C. maculatum* is native to Europe and Asia and was introduced to America as an ornamental plant.[4] Poison hemlock growing in the southern climates is thought to be more poisonous than that in temperate regions. Ancient Greeks considered the poison hemlock growing in Macedonia to be the most toxic substance.[5]

Toxicity can follow ingestion of any anatomic part of the plant, including leaves, stem, root, flowers, or seeds. Severe toxicity has occurred in children, when the stems were used as whistles.[6] Toxicity has occurred after the consumption of small birds (skylarks, chaffinches, robins) that recently ingested hemlock buds.[7] Overall, most exposures are unintentional and dose related, and exposures are more frequent in children.

The active alkaloids in poison hemlock are physiologically and structurally related to nicotine. The syndrome they cause is the result of direct effects on nicotinic receptors. Other plants, such as those of the genus *Nicotiana*, which includes tobacco plants, act in a similar fashion.

Poison hemlock has many common names throughout the world, such as *cicuta* (Argentina, Colombia, Chile), *hemlock* (England), *grande cique* (France), *giftjeks* (Norway), *odort* (Sweden), *wild carrot* (Australia), *cigue maculee* (Canada), and *doku-ninjin* (Japan).[8] Poison hemlock should be distinguished from water hemlock (*Cicuta maculate*).

BIOCHEMISTRY

The biologic activity originates from the simple alkaloids found within poison hemlock. Alkaloids are nitrogenous compounds, physiologically active, and usually insoluble in water. Hemlock, similar to other alkaloids, is bitter tasting. Eight piperidinic alkaloids have been identified from *C. maculatum*: λ-coniceine, coniine, *N*-methyl coniine, conhydrine, pseudoconhydrine, conhydrinone, *N*-methyl pseudoconhydrine, and 2-methylpiperidine.[4]

The two principal toxins, λ-coniceine and coniine, are thought to be responsible for the acute and chronic clinical manifestations of poison hemlock intoxication. These alkaloids are found in greatest concentrations within the plant and are the focus of this discussion (Fig. 124-2).[4] They are synthesized from an eight-acetate unit. Reduced nicotinamide-adenine dinucleotide phosphate–dependent λ-coniceine reductase catalyzes the synthesis of coniine.[9] This is a reversible reaction, allowing for the interconversion between the two alkaloids.[10] These substances are structurally similar to nicotine (see Fig. 124-2), a pyrrolidine alkaloid, and stereospecifically bind to cholinergic ligand-gated sodium channels at so-named nicotinic sites. Although pyrrolidine alkaloids contain a five-member *N*-containing ring, the piperidine alkaloids differ in that they incorporate a heterocyclic six-member *N*-containing

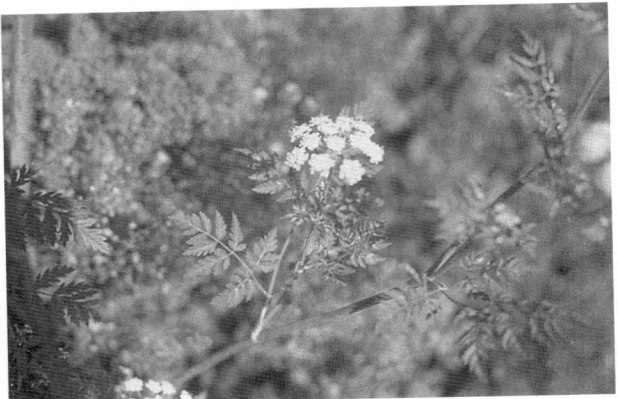

FIGURE 124-1

Poison hemlock (*Conium maculatum*). *(From Graeme KA, Braitberg G, Kunkel DB, et al: Toxic plant ingestions. In Auerbach PS [ed]: Wilderness Medicine, 4th ed. Philadelphia, Mosby, 2001, p 1114.)* See Color Fig. 124-1.

ring. Similar to nicotine, coniine and related alkaloids have an initially excitatory effect followed by a depressant effect on the central nervous system.

Coniine and λ-coniceine can be found in varying concentrations and proportions depending on the season, nutrients available, and amount of rainfall. During dry, sunny seasons, the average fruit size and amount of toxins increase. During rainy seasons, the λ-coniceine alkaloid predominates.[11] The relative concentrations of these two alkaloids also change as the plant matures.[10] λ-Coniceine is the predominant alkaloid in the leafy parts of poison hemlock and in the early stages of development from flower to fruit.[10] The overall change in λ-coniceine to coniine is associated with rapid growth of the fruit. The peak in λ-coniceine concentration precedes the peak of coniine concentration. As the fruit approaches the final stage of maturation, the coniine content declines, and there is another slight increase in the λ-coniceine concentration.[10] The percentage of total alkaloid weight compared with plant weight varies from 0.009 in dry stems to 0.750 in dry seeds harvested in the midwinter. Fresh secondary

growth material is midway between, at 0.075%.[12] This makes the determination of the median lethal dose based on weight variable depending on the season, part of plant, and degree of maturation.

Conhydrine, similar to λ-coniceine, is an oxidation product of coniine.[11] Conhydrine concentrations peak at approximately the same time as λ-coniceine, which is during the rainy season. N-methyl coniine, another minor alkaloid, is found to increase in concentration when coniine is at its peak. It is not clear how coniine is converted to N-methyl coniine. Coniine and N-methyl coniine predominate in mature seeds, however.[10]

PATHOPHYSIOLOGY

Pharmacokinetics of Poison Hemlock
Volume of distribution: 1 L/kg
Protein binding: <5%
Mechanism of clearance: excretion in the kidneys and lungs; metabolized in the liver
Active metabolites: none known
Methods of enhanced clearance: gastric lavage, activated charcoal

The physiologic effects of coniine are complex and dose dependent. Most toxicity occurs when coniine and related alkaloids enhance the nicotinic actions of acetylcholine with depolarization of voltage-gated nicotinic acetylcholine receptors. Muscarinic effects of acetylcholine are generally unaffected. Nicotinic receptors are in the central nervous system, at neuromuscular junctions, postganglionic autonomic nerves, and the adrenal medulla. There are two major categories of nicotinic receptors: The N_M type is found at the skeletal neuromuscular junction, and the N_N variety is found at nerve terminals (Fig. 124-3). The alkaloids' agonist properties on nicotinic receptors are the predominant mechanism responsible for the clinical effects. Receptor stimulation results in sodium channel influx, leading to membrane depolarization and action potential propagation. Although the effect on the nicotinic receptor–controlled structures is initially stimulatory, it is followed shortly thereafter by depressant, curare-like, antagonistic effects, similar to the clinical effects of nicotine.[1] The resulting effects have been referred to as the *nicotinic syndrome* (Table 124-1).

The striking effect of these alkaloids can be seen in terms of the action on spinal reflexes. Convulsive activity, induced by local application of coniine to the spinal cords of frogs, was thought to be the result of direct agonist action on the motor neurons within the cord.[13] Based on these kinds of initial experiments, it was previously believed that the main action of coniine was strychniniform, causing convulsive activity of spinal origin.[1] Experiments with intact animals have shown, however, that hemlock alkaloids and strychnine have predominantly antagonistic properties.[13] The paralyzing effect of hemlock

γ-Coniceine

Coniine

Nicotine

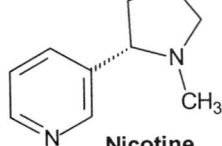

FIGURE 124-2

Chemical structures of major alkaloids in poison hemlock. The chemical structure of nicotine is shown for comparison.

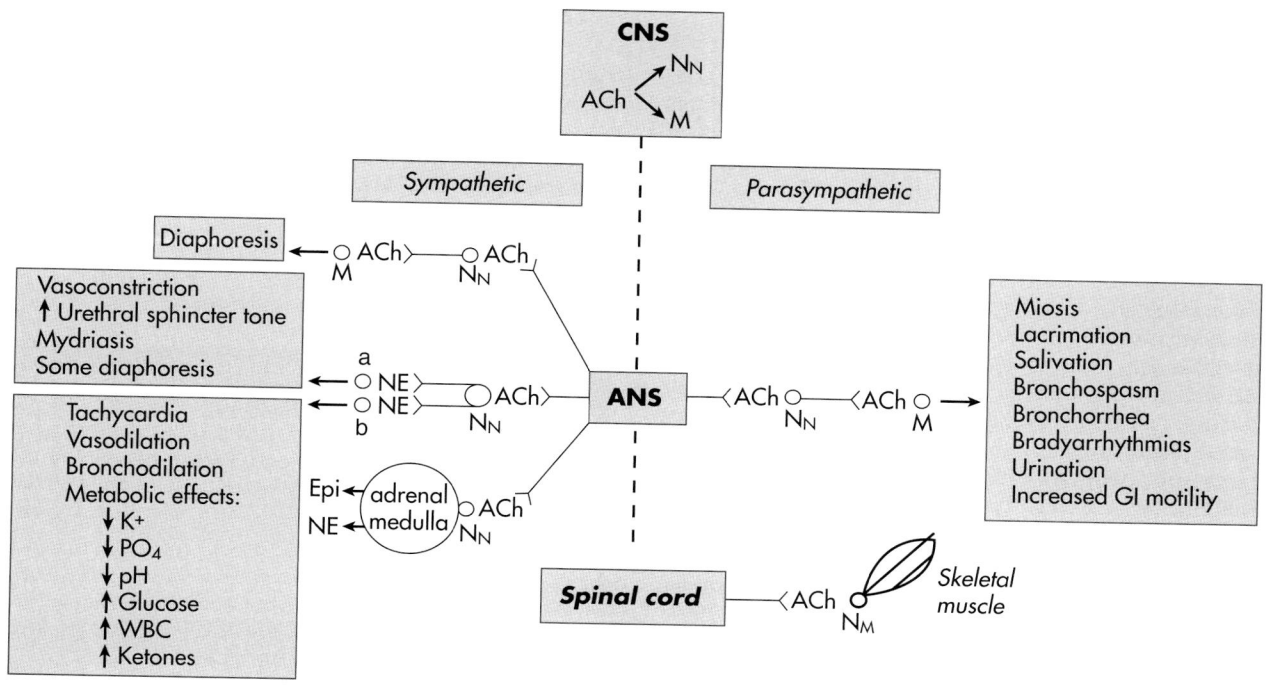

FIGURE 124-3

Nicotinic and muscarinic receptors of the central nervous system (CNS), autonomic nervous system (ANS), and peripheral skeletal muscles. Direct nicotinic agonists (e.g., arecoline, coniine, cytisine, lobeline, nicotine) stimulate nicotinic receptors; however, prolonged depolarization at the receptor causes eventual blockade of nicotinic receptors. ACh, acetylcholine; Epi, epinephrine; GI, gastrointestinal; M, muscarinic receptor; N_M, nicotinic receptor at skeletal muscle; N_N, nicotinic receptor in nervous system; NE, norepinephrine; WBC, white blood cell count. *(From Graeme KA, Braitberg G, Kunkel DB, et al: Toxic plant ingestions. In Auerbach PS [ed]: Wilderness Medicine, 4th ed. Philadelphia, Mosby, 2001, p 1111.)*

alkaloids is the result of the ascending neuromuscular blockade, similar to that of curare.[1]

Reportedly the toxic dose in humans is approximately 60 mg of coniine, and the fatal dose is approximately 150 to 300 mg.[14] Ingestion of a piece of hemlock 1 inch square has been reported to be lethal in a child.[2]

CLINICAL PRESENTATION AND LIFE-THREATENING COMPLICATIONS

The symptoms after poison hemlock ingestion are biphasic. There is an initial stimulatory phase, followed by a more pronounced state of skeletal motor depression, associated

TABLE 124-1 Nicotinic Syndrome	
EARLY STAGE	**LATE STAGE**
Hypertension	Hypotension
Tachycardia	Bradyarrhythmias
Vomiting	Paralysis
Diarrhea	Coma
Muscle fasciculations	
Convulsions	

From Graene KA, Braitberg G, Kunkel DB, et al: Toxic plant ingestions.
In Auerbach PS (ed): Wilderness Medicine, 4th ed. Philadelphia, Mosby, 2001, p 1114.

with muscle weakness, paralysis, and respiratory arrest (see Table 124-1).

Immediately after ingestion, there is usually a short latent period before the onset of clinical manifestations. The first symptoms to occur are typically direct gastrointestinal irritation of the mucosa of the oropharynx, esophagus, and stomach. Gastrointestinal irritation is followed in approximately 30 minutes by profuse salivation, nausea, and vomiting,[15] manifestations of initial cholinergic nicotinic stimulation. These episodes of emesis theoretically help to limit further exposure and toxicity.

Cardiovascular effects from these toxins are generally minor. Large doses of coniine, λ-coniceine, and *N*-methyl coniine in isolated animal heart preparations cause decreased inotropy.[13] However, these effects are not seen in intact animals. In the late stages of significant poison hemlock ingestion, bradycardia, hypotension, and shock may occur.

Fasciculations of skeletal muscle and tonic-clonic contractions of separate limbs are characteristic during the initial excitatory phase. These skeletal motor effects are mediated by spinal cord and neuromuscular junction stimulation and may lead to rhabdomyolysis.[1,7]

The excitatory phase is followed by ascending muscular weakness and paralysis. The skeletal muscles are typically painful and hypotonic.[7] Affected individuals are often lethargic, and their muscle weakness may lead to respiratory arrest, requiring mechanical ventilation. Death is usually from progressive paralysis and respiratory arrest. Severe toxicity treated with ventilatory support and supportive care has led to recovery without sequelae.[2]

DIAGNOSIS

Poisoning by poison hemlock should be a diagnostic consideration in any patient with nicotinic signs and symptoms (see prior section) or ascending paralysis after ingestion of "plant material." No specific diagnostic tests are routinely available.

Signs of rhabdomyolysis (myoglobinuria and serum creatine phosphokinase elevations) are often present.[16] Transient elevations in liver enzymes often occur but typically resolve as the patient recovers.[16]

Alkaloids from poison hemlock are excreted by the lungs and kidneys, giving the breath and urine of poisoned animals a "mousy" odor characteristic of the plant. Analysis for coniine can be performed on urine or serum samples. The most commonly useful method for diagnostic confirmation is obtaining a portion of the plant that has been ingested. Analysis of the plant specimen by gas chromatography– mass spectrometry for the presence of the piperidine alkaloids confirms the diagnosis. In cases in which poisoning has occurred after ingestion of toxic bird flesh, coniine has been isolated from the animal specimens.[7]

TREATMENT

There is no specific antidote for poison hemlock. Supportive care is the mainstay of treatment. If the patient presents early after ingestion, gastrointestinal decontamination with orogastric lavage may be considered because of the potency of these toxins. Orogastric lavage reasonably may be contemplated if the patient presents within 1 hour of the poisoning; however, the efficacy of this intervention is questionable (see Chapter 5). Most clinical toxicologists generally recommend a dose of activated charcoal (see Chapter 5), although there are no data showing that this alters the clinical course or outcome. Mechanical ventilation may be required for patients who are severely poisoned. In one case series of 11 poison hemlock–poisoned patients, 3 patients required ventilatory support, and all 3 subsequently died.[7] The use of forced diuresis, hemoperfusion, and hemodialysis has been reported, but no clinical or experimental support is available for these techniques.[7] Aggressive volume replacement with maintenance of brisk urine output is indicated in patients at risk for rhabdomyolysis. Vasopressor agents are required when there has been an inadequate response to volume resuscitation. Bradycardia should be treated per standard protocols. Patients not exhibiting systemic toxicity after 6 hours of observation may be discharged home safely.

Indications for ICU Admission in Poison Hemlock Toxicity

Respiratory depression
Seizure-like activity
Change in mental status
Large ingestion
Pediatric patients with signs of ingestion

SPECIAL POPULATIONS

Animal studies suggest potential teratogenic effects associated with chronic exposure to poison hemlock. Observations in different animal species have found malformations predominantly of the limbs, including limb rotation; permanent flexure of the carpal or elbow joints, with or without scoliosis; and sometimes cleft palate and lip.[12] No human data are available regarding teratogenicity.

Common Misconceptions about Poison Hemlock

1. Poison hemlock is nontoxic.
2. Poison hemlock is the same as water hemlock (see Chapter 123).

Key Points in Poison Hemlock Toxicity

1. Ingestion of any part of the plant can lead to severe toxicity.
2. The main alkaloids are coniine and λ-coniceine.
3. Patients with overdoses present with nicotinic and curare-like symptoms.
4. No specific antidote is available.
5. Treatment is supportive without specific antidotes.
6. If the patient survives, usually there are no long-term sequelae.
7. There are possible teratogenic effects.

REFERENCES

1. De Boer J: The death of Socrates: A historical and experimental study of the action of coniine and conium maculatum. Arch Int Pharmacodyn 83:473–490, 1950.
2. Davies ML, Davies TA: Hemlock: Murder before the lord. Med Sci Law 34:331–333, 1994.
3. Frank BS, Michelson WB, Panter KE, et al: Ingestion of poison hemlock (*Conium maculatum*). West J Med 163:573–574, 1995.
4. Lopez TA, Cid MS, Bianchini ML: Biochemistry of hemlock (*Conium maculatum*) alkaloids and their acute and chronic toxicity in livestock. Toxicon 37:843–865, 1999.
5. Redwood TD: Gray's Supplement to the Pharmacopeia. London, Longmans, 1848.
6. Everist S (ed): Umbelliferae. In Poisonous Plants of Australia, 2nd ed. Sydney, Angus & Robertson Publishers, 1981, pp 717–729.
7. Rizzi D, Basile L, Dimaggio A, et al: Rhabdomyolysis and acute tubular necrosis in coniine (hemlock) poisoning. Lancet 2:1461–1462, 1989.
8. Holm L, Doll E, Pancho J, Herberger L (eds): *Conium maculatum*. In World Weeds: Natural History and Distribution. New York, J. Wiley & Sons, 1997, pp 221–225.
9. Roberts MF: λ-coniceine reductase in *Conium maculatum*. Phytochemistry 14:2393–2397, 1975.
10. Fairbairn JW, Suwal PN: The alkaloids of hemlock (*Conium maculatum L*): II. Evidence for the rapid turnover of the major alkaloids. Phytochemistry 1:38–46, 1961.
11. Fairbairin JW, Challin SB: The alkaloids of hemlock (*Conium maculatum L*). Biochem J 72:556–561, 1958.

12. Keeler RF: Coniine, a teratogenic principle from *Conium maculatum* producing congenital malformations in calves. Clin Toxicol 7:195–206, 1974.

13. Bowman W, Sanghi I: Pharmacological action of hemlock (*Conium maculatum*) alkaloids. J Pharm Pharmacol 15:1–25, 1963.

14. Thienes CH, Haley TJ: Clinical Toxicology, 2nd ed. Philadelphia, Lea & Febiger, 1948.

15. Ober WB: Did Socrates die of hemlock poisoning? N Y State J Med 77:254–258, 1977.

16. Scatizzi A, Maggio A, Rizzi D, et al: Acute renal failure due to tubular necrosis caused by wildfowl-mediated hemlock poisoning. Ren Fail 15:93–96, 1993.

CHAPTER **125**

Cardiotoxic Plants

Barbarajean Magnani ■ Alan D. Woolf

When Withering wrote his classic *An Account of the Foxglove and Some of Its Medicinal Uses* in 1785,[1] he recognized the beneficial uses of foxglove (*Digitalis purpurea*); but in the section "Effects, Rules and Cautions," he described what is now the well-known toxicity of digitalis: "occasions sickness, vomiting, purging, giddiness, confused vision, objects appearing green or yellow; increased secretion of urine, with frequent motions to part with it, and sometimes inability to retain it; slow pulse, even as slow as 35 in a minute, cold sweats, convulsions, syncope, death."

Intoxication from cardiotoxic plants may result from direct ingestion of plant parts, such as leaves, flowers, nectars, seeds, or roots, or may result from teas (decoctions and infusions) brewed from the plant. In some cases, toxicity has occurred from drinking water from a vase that contained the cut flowers of foxglove or lily of the valley or, according to common folklore, from roasting hot dogs on a branch from oleander.[2] Herbal products, especially those contained in traditional medicines, may contain cardiac glycosides[3–5] or alkaloids from *Aconitum* spp.[6,7] Cardiotoxic alkaloid–containing toxic honey was implicated in poisonings in 400 BC. Xenophon reported the poisoning of Greek soldiers by honey made by bees from the nectar of wild rhododendron.[8]

TYPE AND ACTIVITY OF PLANT TOXIN

Plants producing cardiac toxins may be separated into characteristic groups based on the type and the activity of the plant toxin. These groups include (1) digitalis and digitalis-related compounds, (2) aconitine and related alkaloids, (3) grayanotoxins, and (4) *Veratrum* alkaloids. Table 125-1 lists common plants and the nature of their cardiotoxic components.[2,9–14]

Digitalis and Digitalis-like Glycosides

Digitalis, digoxin, and related cardiac glycosides are found naturally in several plant species around the world (see Table 125-1).[15] Medicinally important glycosides are obtained from the foxglove plant. Other plants, such as oleander, lily of the valley, Christmas rose, and sea onion, also contain potentially toxic cardiac glycosides.

Foxglove (*Digitalis* spp.) is a biennial plant commonly grown in North American gardens, but it originates from southern Europe and Central Asia. During the first year of growth, the plant produces a basal rosette of large oval leaves. In the second year, flowers are borne on a large stalk that matures from the bottom to the top. Each flower is cup-shaped with darker spots on the lower inside of the tubular-shaped flower. Blooms vary in color from dark pink or purple (*Digitalis purpurea*) to yellowish or whitish (*Digitalis lanata*). The entire plant is toxic, and poisoning has resulted from consumption of teas brewed from foxglove leaves.[16,17] In some cases, the leaves during the first-year growth were mistaken for comfrey (*Symphytum officinale*).[2]

Oleander is native to tropical and subtropical climates and comprises two related plants, *Nerium oleander* and *Thevetia peruviana*. *N. oleander* is a tall evergreen shrub frequently grown indoors as an ornamental plant in temperate North America, but it also can be grown outdoors, where it may reach heights of 25 feet. The dark, leathery leaves are arranged in whorls of three, and the flowers, borne in clusters with five petals each, are usually pink, peach, red, or white. Yellow oleander (*T. peruviana*) is similar in shape, with yellow or orange flowers, and produces black fruits with a central stone (seeds). Oleander is particularly enticing to small children because of its lovely flowers and seed pods that are easily accessible.[18] All parts of the plant are toxic; reported cases of toxicity include consumption of oleander tea derived from the leaves[19] and the ingestion of seeds. In some countries (e.g., Sri Lanka), the ingestion of the seeds ("lichy nuts") of yellow oleander is a common means of suicide.[20]

Lily of the valley (*Convallaria majalis*) is a small perennial plant with two elliptical, pointed leaves and flowers borne on a single, small stalk. Blooms are small, cup-shaped, white, and fragrant and are located along only one side of the flower stem. Bright red berries form later in the season along the flower stalks. Lily of the valley is reported by the Poison Information Center as a common plant exposure for children in Helsinki,[21] and accidental ingestion has resulted in intoxication.[22]

Hellebore, or Christmas rose (*Helleborus niger*), is an herbaceous perennial from the buttercup family, with compound leaves and white or sometimes purplish flowers that bloom in the spring or winter. Although the plant contains cardiac glycosides, reported poisonings are rare.[2] This plant should not be confused with the *Veratrum* spp., which sometimes are called *false hellebore* (see later).

Squill (*Urginea maritima*) or sea onion is a perennial plant with lily-like leaves and small white flowers borne off terminal clusters. Ingestion of the bulbs has produced effects consistent with cardiac glycoside toxicity.[23]

TABLE 125-1 Cardiotoxic Plants

CLASS	COMMON NAME	SCIENTIFIC NAME	TOXIN
Cardiac glycosides	Purple foxglove	*Digitalis purpurea*	Digitoxin
	Grecian foxglove; wooly foxglove	*Digitalis lanata*	Digitoxin, digoxin
	Oleander	*Nerium oleander*	Oleandrin
	Yellow oleander; be still tree	*Thevetia peruviana (T. neriifolia)*	Thevetin A and B
	Christmas rose	*Helleborus niger*	Helleborin, helleborein
	Lily of the valley	*Convallaria majalis*	Convallotoxin, convallarin, convallamarin
	Squill or sea onion	*Urginea maritima*	Scillaren, scillarenin
Aconitum alkaloids	Monkshood; wolfsbane	*Aconitum* spp. *(A. napellus)*	Aconitine alkaloids
	Larkspur	*Delphinium* spp.	Delphinine
Grayanotoxins	Rhododendron, azalea	*Rhododendron* spp.	Grayanotoxin 1 or andromedotoxin
	Japanese pieris; lily of the valley bush	*Pieris japonica*	Grayanotoxin 1 or andromedotoxin
	Mountain laurel	*Kalmia latifolia*; other *Kalmia* spp.	Andromedotoxin
Veratrum alkaloids	Indian hellebore; American white hellebore; false hellebore; green hellebore	*Veratrum viride*	Germidine, germitrine, veratridine, veratrosine, veratramine
	Corn lily	*Veratrum californicum*	
	Death camass; black snakeroot	*Zygandenus venenosus*	Zygacine, zygadenine, protoveratrine

Aconitum and Related Alkaloids

Monkshood, aconite, or wolfsbane (*Aconitum* spp., e.g., *Aconitum napellus*) is a perennial plant found within North America, originally native to Europe, with deeply divided palmate leaves. The plant grows 3 to 4 feet tall from a tuberous root. The flowers are borne off a long spike, each flower containing five petaloid septals, with one shaped in the form of a monk's hood. Blooms vary in color, including purple, blue, and combination of purple and white. Related species are grown in China and Japan. *Aconitum carmichaelii* and *Aconitum kusnezoffii* are the main source of medicinal aconite drugs, *ts'ao wu (wu t'ou)* and *fu tzu (ch'uan wu)*.[10]

Delphinium and larkspur (*Delphinium* spp.) are perennial, biennial, or annual plants similar in appearance to monkshood with deeply divided leaves; various species grow from 6 inches to 6 feet tall. The flowers are usually borne off multiple racemes or flower clusters, each flower, commonly blue, containing a long "spur" off the back, hence the name *larkspur*.

Aconitine and delphinium alkaloids are under investigation as potential analgesic and antiinflammatory drugs,[24,25] and *Aconitum* roots currently are used in preparations of Chinese and Japanese medicines for the treatment of rheumatic and neurologic diseases.[26,27] This usage frequently results in unintentional, potentially fatal, toxicity.[6,7,26–30]

Grayanotoxins

Rhododendrons (*Rhododendron* spp.) are large evergreen shrubs with leathery leaves and large, showy flower clusters, each flower containing protruding stamens. Bloom colors are highly variable, depending on the hybrid, but can be pink, purple, maroon, or red. The related azaleas are either evergreen or deciduous small shrubs, with additional flower colors of white, orange, salmon, or crimson. Japanese pieris (*Pieris japonica*), also known as the *lily of the valley bush*, is an evergreen with dark, leathery leaves, bearing chains of white, urn-shaped flowers in the spring. Although native to Japan, this small shrub is found frequently in gardens of North America. Mountain laurel, *Kalmia latifolia* and other *Kalmia* spp., are small, evergreen shrubs that produce clusters of white to pinkish, bell-shaped flowers.

Toxic diterpenoids (grayanotoxins), mainly grayanotoxin I or andromedotoxin, are responsible for poisonings attributed to toxic honey, which is produced by bees collecting pollen from *Rhododendron* spp.[31,32] Toxic honey, known in Turkey as *deli bal* or *tutan bal*, is ingested as a treatment for gastritis and peptic ulcers.[8] Sucking azalea nectar from the flower may pose less of a hazard.[33]

Veratrum Alkaloids

Indian hellebore, also called *American white hellebore, false hellebore,* or *green hellebore (Veratrum viride)*, is an herbaceous perennial with oval, alternately arranged leaves. Each leaf has prominent parallel veins, and the flowers, borne in terminal clusters, are greenish white. Related species, such as *Veratrum californicum* (or corn lily), have white flowers.[2] Confusion of *Veratrum* spp. with other plants, particularly gentian, has led to ingestion of the plant or of wine made from *Veratrum album*.[34–37] Death camass (black snakeroot, *Zygandenus venenosus*, and other species) is a perennial plant in the lily family with grasslike leaves grown from a bulb. Creamy white flowers are clustered together and borne off a single central stalk. Toxicity arises from ingestion of the bulbs,[38] frequently mistaken for wild onion.[39]

BIOCHEMISTRY OF CARDIOTOXIC SUBSTANCES IN PLANTS

Plant Cardiac Glycosides

The plant cardiac glycosides, known as *cardenolides*, have a characteristic chemical structure consisting of an aglycone or genin (i.e., a steroid nucleus joined to a lactone ring) attached to one to four sugar moieties (Fig. 125-1). The aglycone is essential for the pharmacologic activity

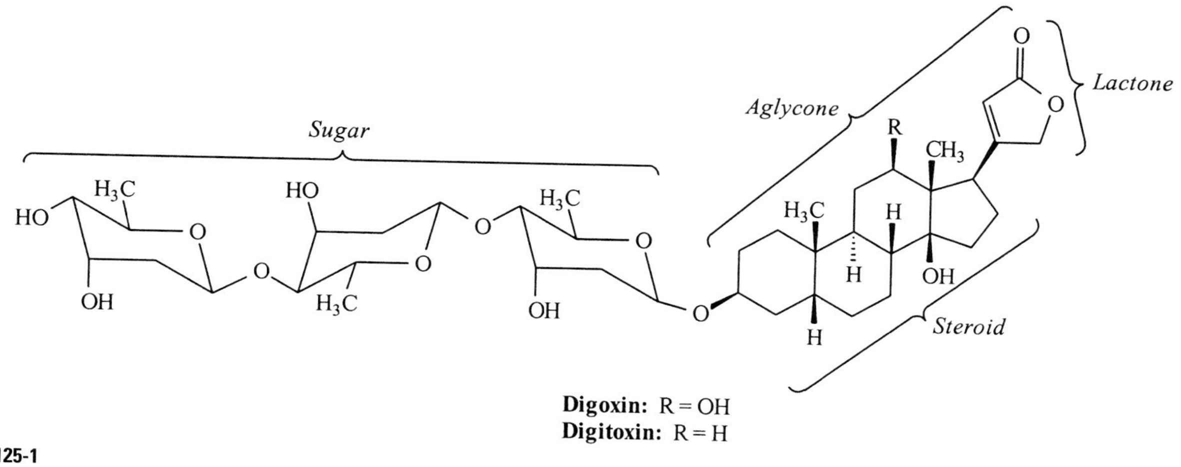

FIGURE 125-1

Chemical structures of plant glycosides, including major component divisions.

of the glycoside, whereas the sugar moieties, specific for each cardenolide, affect the water and lipid solubility and the potency.[18,40]

The foxglove plant produces several cardiac glycosides, most notably digoxin from the Grecian foxglove (*D. lanata*) and digitoxin from the purple foxglove (*D. purpurea*) and from *D. lanata*.[12]

D. lanata contains the precursor glycosides, lanatoside A, B, and C. After mild alkaline hydrolysis to remove an acetyl group and enzymatic hydrolysis to remove glucose, digitoxin and digoxin are produced from lanatoside A and C. *D. purpurea* contains the precursor purpurea-glycoside A, which contains no acetyl groups, and enzymatic hydrolysis is sufficient to produce digitoxin.[12] Because digitoxin is less polar than digoxin, it avidly binds to serum albumin, which results in a longer distribution phase than digoxin.[12]

Oleandrin and thevetin A have a structure similar to digitoxin but with varying sugar residues attached at the number three carbon of the "A" ring on the steroid nucleus.[18] The genins for thevetin B and digitoxin are identical, with the only difference being that in thevetin B a thevetose and gentiobiose are conjugated to oxygen at the number three carbon.[14] Oleandrin and, to a lesser extent, oleandrigenin bind to albumin.[41]

Aconitine and Related Cardiotoxic Alkaloids

Compounds derived from *Aconitum* spp. (principally the tubers or root stock) are diterpenoid alkaloids (i.e., a nitrogenous base formed from some C20-terpenoid precursors) (Fig. 125-2).[26] The most toxic alkaloids are aconitine, mesaconitine, and 3-acetylaconitine. The presence of a benzoylester side chain at carbon 14 produces the arrhythmic effects attributed to these three alkaloids.[26] The alkaloids contained within the plant vary depending on the species and the geographic location, with some species being more toxic than others.[42] Raw tubers are "processed" by boiling or steaming *bushi* under high pressure in Japan and China to produce *Kako-bushi*. This process reduces the toxicity of the parent alkaloids by producing less toxic pyro-type aconitine alkaloids.[43]

Grayanotoxins

Grayanotoxins are diterpenoids with a perhydroazulene skeleton[44] found primarily in the leaves of shrubs in the heather family (e.g., rhododendrons, azaleas, and mountain laurel). Grayanotoxins I, II, and III differ by virtue of (1) an OH group off carbon 10 in grayanotoxins I and III, which is a carbonyl in grayanotoxin II, and (2) an OH moiety at carbon 14 in grayanotoxins II and III, which is esterified to an acetyl in grayanotoxin I (Fig. 125-3). The content of grayanotoxin I in a fresh leaf from *Rhododendron ponticum* was estimated at 0.024%.[45]

Veratrum Alkaloids

Veratrum alkaloids are steroid-like, polycyclic, nitrogen-containing structures.[11] Veratrine is a mixture of alkaloids, with veratridine being one of the major components. All *Veratrum* alkaloids are based on a steroid nucleus, with a fused two-ring, *N*-containing heterocycle added across the 13–17 bond (Fig. 125-4). Protonation of this nitrogen makes these drugs primarily cationic at physiologic pH. The steroid 3-position oxygen exists as an OH, in weakly active cevine, esterified to veratric acid in moderately potent veratridine and to methyl-butenoic acid in the highly

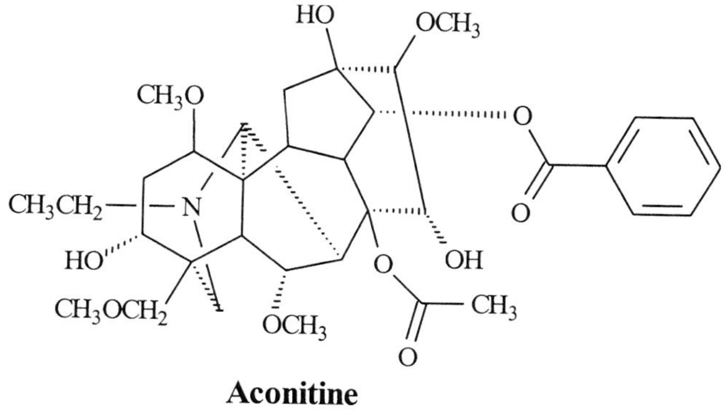

Aconitine

FIGURE 125-2

Chemical structure of aconitine.

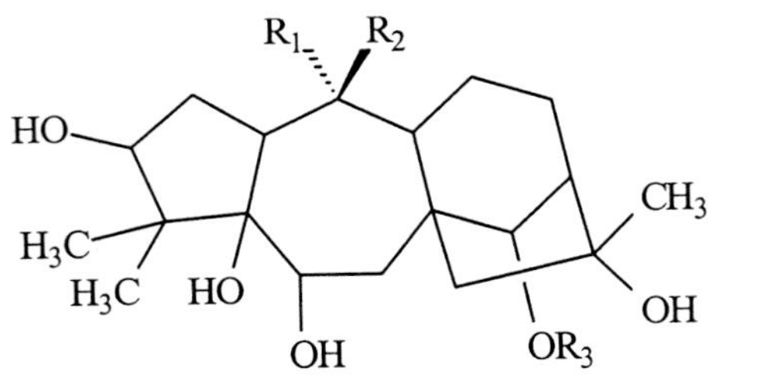

Grayanotoxin I: $R_1 = OH$; $R_2 = CH_3$; $R_3 = COCH_3$
Grayanotoxin II: $R_1R_2 = H_2C$⚌; $R_3 = H$
Grayanotoxin III: $R_1 = OH$; $R_2 = CH_3$; $R_3 = H$

FIGURE 125-3

Chemical structures of grayanotoxins.

potent cevadine. The 6–7 OH groups on these molecules account for their (limited) aqueous solubility, whereas differences in potency result primarily from varied substituents at the 3-OH position.

PATHOPHYSIOLOGY

Plant Digitalis Glycosides

Digitalis compounds exert a positive inotropic effect on the heart and have arrhythmogenic activity. Cardioactive steroids are specific inhibitors of the membrane protein sodium pump (Na^+,K^+-ATPase).[46] Na^+,K^+-ATPase effectively moves ions across membranes and maintains transmembrane Na^+ and K^+ gradients with energy generated from the hydrolysis of adenosine triphosphate (ATP). The enzyme is composed of three subunits (α, β, and γ), with the α subunit containing the Na^+,K^+, and ATP binding sites and the binding site for cardiac glycosides.[46] Inhibition of the pump by cardiac glycosides reduces active Na^+ efflux, resulting in increased intracellular $[Na^+]$ and effectively lowering the Na^+ gradient–dependent driving force that powers plasmalemmal sodium-calcium exchange. The net effect is an increased intracellular calcium concentration,

leading to an elevated amount of calcium released during cardiac systole and increased force development, the positive inotropic effect (Fig. 125-5). By a totally different mechanism, these cardiotoxic steroids are thought to modify the ion selectivity of the voltage-gated Na^+ channel to a state of "promiscuous permeability" or "slip-mode conductance" (meaning calcium follows sodium), allowing the usually impermeant Ca^{2+} to enter cells through Na^+ channels. This Ca^{2+} influx promotes Ca^{2+} release from the sarcoplasmic reticulum.[47] The steroidal alkaloid veratridine also increases the calcium conductance of voltage-gated Na^+ channels, suggesting the possibility of a generalized action of steroid-containing drugs on this ion channel. The positive inotropic effect of cardiac glycosides results from the increases in intracellular calcium effected by both of these mechanisms because more calcium is now available for the myocardial contractile elements.

With toxicity, cardiac glycosides can cause many possible arrhythmias (see Chapter 33). Junctional pacemakers can discharge at an increased rate, leading to nonparoxysmal atrioventricular junctional tachycardia.[46] Enhanced automaticity and impaired conduction, such as an atrioventricular block with an accelerated junctional pacemaker, is consistent with digitalis toxicity. Sinus bradycardia, sinoatrial arrest, and heart block (second-degree or third-degree atrioventricular block) also are associated with toxicity. Oleandrin, the major cardiac glycoside found in oleander, also functions as a Na^+,K^+-ATPase pump inhibitor (see Fig. 125-4) and produces pathophysiologic changes similar to those of digoxin overdose (see Chapter 33). As with digitalis, severe poisoning produces conduction defects in the sinus node (sinus bradycardia, sinus arrest, or exit block), atrioventricular node (second-degree or third-degree heart block), or both. Higher serum cardiac glycoside levels correlate with involvement of both nodes.[48] There may be decreased atrioventricular conduction and bradycardia secondary to increased vagal tone resulting from increased carotid sinus baroreceptor firing in response to sodium/calcium influx and increased vagal outflow. Acute cardiac glycoside toxicity produces systemic hyperkalemia secondary to Na^+,K^+-ATPase pump inhibition because there is a shift of potassium extracellularly from all tissues in the body (e.g., release from skeletal muscle).

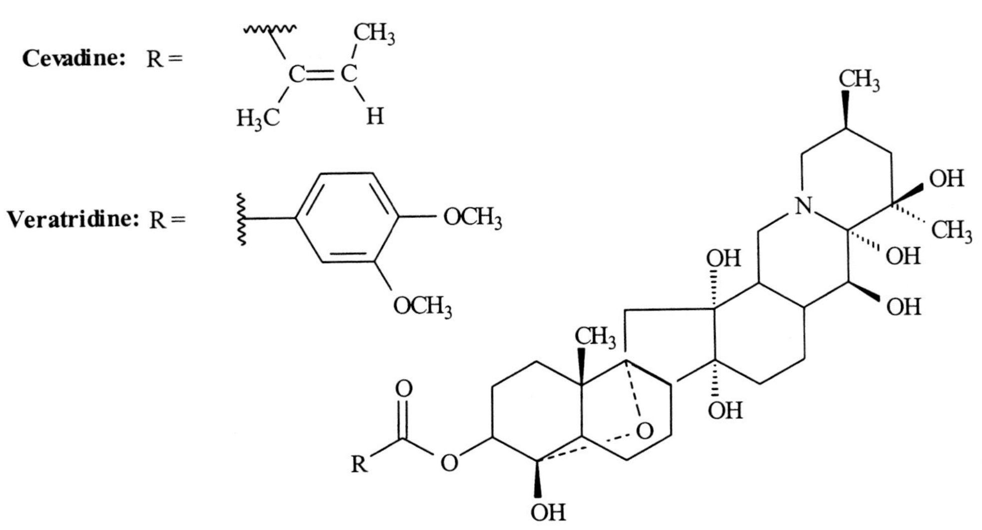

FIGURE 125-4

Chemical structures of veratrum alkaloids.

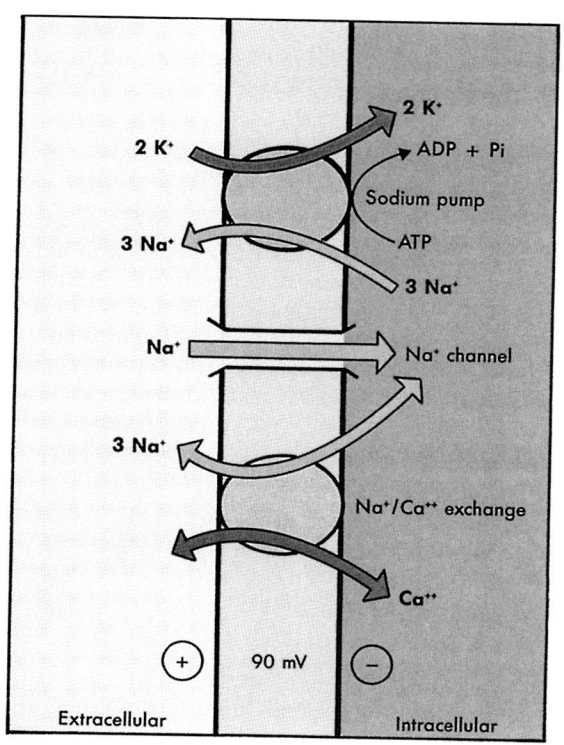

FIGURE 125-5

Membrane ion flux of Na+ and Ca2+ in heart. Glycoside-induced inhibition of Na+,K+-ATPase secondarily inhibits the Na+ influx–Ca2+ efflux exchange reaction. *(From Brody TM, Larner J, Minneman KP [eds]: Human Pharmacology: Molecular to Clinical, 3rd ed. St Louis, Mosby, 1998, p 217.)*

Aconitine, Grayanotoxins, and Veratridine

Although digitalis and digitalis-like compounds primarily inhibit the Na+,K+-ATPase pump, aconitine, grayanotoxins, and veratridine are "activator" agents that open

sodium channels.[49] The cardiac conduction tissues and the autonomic nerves innervating the heart are affected by these activators, and both of these actions contribute to the clinical presentation. Aconitine and veratridine bind within the transmembrane region, known as *neurotoxin receptor site 2*.[50] This binding produces persistent activation of the voltage-gated Na+ channel (Fig. 125-6) at the resting membrane potential and concomitant inhibition of channel inactivation. A persistent Na+ permeability, a relatively constant inward current, and depolarization of the excitable cardiac membrane result. Persistent channel opening also produces prolonged phase 3 depolarization in cardiac myocytes, inducing afterpotentials with generated automaticity.

Similarly, grayanotoxin I and α-dihydrograyanotoxin and *Veratrum* alkaloids in general increase the resting sodium permeability by holding transmembrane sodium channels open at rest.[44] As a result of this permeability increase, the resting membrane depolarizes, resulting in spontaneous action potentials that produce neurotransmitter release and cardiac dysrhythmias. This persistent, toxin-modified sodium permeability, if present in cardiac membranes, results in prolonged atrial and ventricular action potentials, often followed by oscillatory afterpotentials.[51] If enough of the sodium channels are bound by toxin, the resulting depolarization is so large that the remaining toxin-free channels become inactivated, and the membrane becomes refractory, preventing further conduction.

Specific diterpenoid alkaloids from *Aconitum* and *Delphinium* spp. most likely cause hypotension and bradycardia through activation of autonomic reflexes.[52] This activation produces an end result at the level of the carotid sinus similar to that of digoxin: reflex stimulation of vagal tone manifested chiefly as decreased heart rate and atrioventricular block. *Veratrum* intoxication also produces vagal reflex hypotension and bradycardia through a similar mechanism, most likely secondary to withdrawal of peripheral α-adrenergic tone.[53]

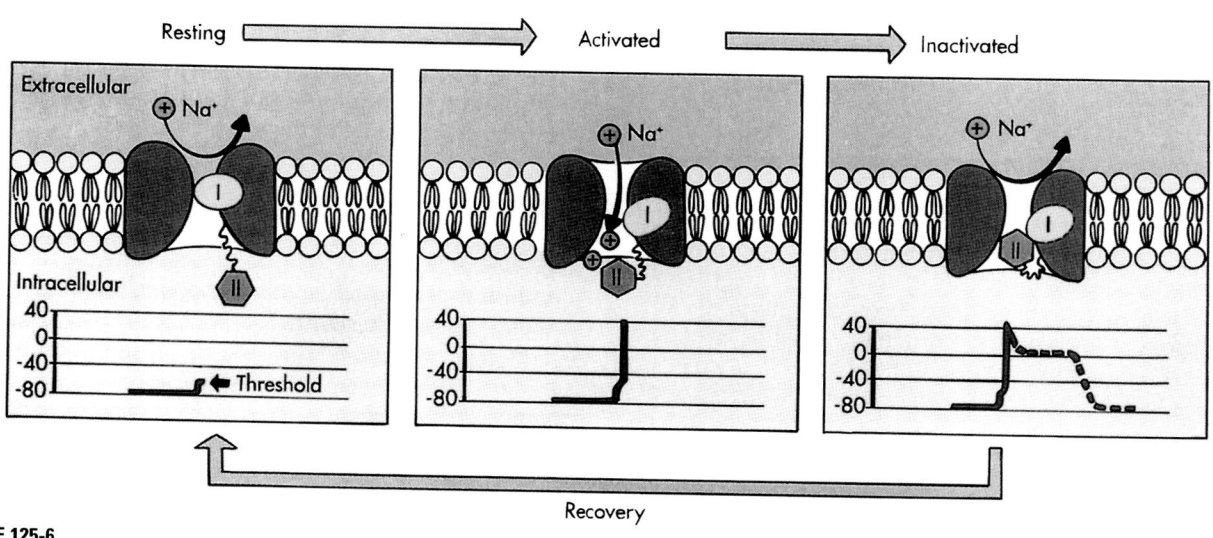

FIGURE 125-6

Postulated conformational arrangements of cardiac Na+ channels compatible with the concept of resting, activated, and inactivated states. Transitions between resting, activated, and inactivated states depend on membrane potential and time. Aconitine, veratridine, and related toxins maintain the channel in the activated state. Potentials for each state are shown under each channel schema as a function of time. *(From Brody TM, Larner J, Minneman KP [eds]: Human Pharmacology: Molecular to Clinical, 3rd ed. St Louis, Mosby, 1998, p 198.)*

Neuronal responses to systemic activator alkaloids include a range of positive and negative symptoms as nerves that are "weakly affected" show spontaneous repetitive firing and exaggerated transmitter release, whereas "strongly affected" nerves show depolarizing block. Perioral innervation manifests both effects, with paresthesia (positive) and numbness (negative) occurring simultaneously in the lips and tongue. Aconitine also is thought to have other ion (e.g., K^+) channel effects that produce a prolonged QT interval and possibly torsades de pointes.

CLINICAL PRESENTATION AND LIFE-THREATENING COMPLICATIONS

Plant Cardiac Glycosides

Manifestations of oleander poisoning are the same as manifestations of digitalis glycosides poisoning (see Chapter 33), although differences in bioavailability of the plant-derived glycosides make the clinical course less predictable. Early after an overdose, oleander poisoning causes nausea, vomiting, decreased appetite, and diarrhea. Patients often present with weakness and evidence of dehydration. Patients may have changes in consciousness, with lethargy progressing to confusion and coma. Seizures also have been described after oleander ingestion.[54] Visual disturbances and yellow-green vision may occur.[55,56]

Cardiac dysrhythmias and conduction disturbances may supervene at any time; bradydysrhythmias and tachydysrhythmias may be seen.[5,54,57] Bradycardia may be more common; in one review of 170 cases of yellow oleander poisoning, atrioventricular block was seen in 52.4% of patients, and bradycardia was seen in 49.5%.[58] Atrioventricular block or complete dissociation may produce complex junctional or reentrant dysrhythmias,[55,57,59] which may degenerate into life-threatening ventricular tachycardia or fibrillation or sudden cardiac arrest.[56] Electrolyte disturbances, related to paralysis of the cellular Na^+,K^+-ATPase pump, are manifest as hyperkalemia with peaked T waves on electrocardiogram.

Aconitine and Related Cardioactive Plant Alkaloids

Aconite is one of the most potent plant-derived toxins known, with severe poisoning caused by 5 mL of the tincture, 0.2 mg of aconitine, or 1 g of the cured plant.[28] Aconitine has systemic toxicity, with gastrointestinal disturbances present within hours after poisoning, including the early onset of nausea, hypersalivation, and vomiting. Neurotoxicity may include numbness, ataxia, dysarthria, perioral paresthesias, weakness of the extremities, and deteriorating consciousness leading to seizures and coma.[60]

Characteristic bradydysrhythmias and hypotension support the diagnosis. Ventricular ectopy can be life-threatening, with ventricular tachycardia or fibrillation or both preceding asystole. Cardiac conduction disturbances include QRS widening, a prolonged QT interval, and bundle-branch block. Toxicity progresses rapidly, with life-threatening cardiotoxicity evident often within 2 hours of the ingestion. Death results from direct myocardial depression and cardiovascular collapse or from a malignant dysrhythmia.[30,60]

Metabolic disturbances, such as metabolic acidosis, hypokalemia, and hyperglycemia, are sometimes seen.[30] Blood creatine phosphokinase (cardiac isoenzymes) may be elevated.[30]

Grayanotoxins

Grayanotoxins cause dose-dependent manifestations that are similar to the manifestations associated with poisoning by *Veratrum* alkaloids. In one report of 23 victims of grayanotoxin-contaminated honey in Turkey, the most common symptoms included hypotension, bradycardia, nausea, and vomiting. Sweating, faintness, weakness, dizziness, chills, exhaustion, impaired consciousness, and blurred vision also were common.[61] Victims of massive overdoses may develop seizures, severe cardiac conduction delays, and life-threatening ventricular ectopy.[62]

Grayanotoxins are rapidly metabolized and excreted.[63] Patients who are supported through the severe gastrointestinal and cardiovascular toxicity usually survive and become symptom-free 1 to 5 days later.[8]

Veratrum Alkaloids

Poisoning by the glycoalkaloids from ingestion of hellebore causes symptoms within 30 to 60 minutes of the exposure. Nausea and repeated vomiting with intense abdominal pain and sometimes diarrhea herald the onset of toxicity. Paresthesias, salivation, sweating, dilated pupils, blurred vision, respiratory depression, lightheadedness, headache, and syncope are reported commonly by victims.[64] Myalgias, weakness, muscle spasms, paresthesias, and myoclonus have been reported.[65] Cardiovascular effects include hypertension or hypotension, bradycardia, and sinoatrial or atrioventricular blocks. Ventricular arrhythmias may occur with massive overdoses.[64,65]

DIAGNOSIS

Laboratory Detection of Plant Toxins

Detection of cardiac glycosides from plants is possible with existing instrumentation.[66] Routine clinical laboratories capable of performing immunoassay procedures can detect digitalis compounds because they cross-react with assays currently on hand for therapeutic drug monitoring. Other cardiac glycosides, such as oleandrin, cross-react with a fluorescent polarization immunoassay for digitoxin and show a linear correlation with concentration.[67] Newer assays using monoclonal chemiluminescent methods, however, show that oleandrin has little cross-reactivity with existing digitoxin and digoxin assays.[68] Detection of oleandrin and oleandrigenin (the aglycone metabolite) varies among different immunoassay procedures, and each assay method used should assess cross-reactivity independently.[41] Squill ingestion has produced serum "digoxin" levels of 1.59 ng/mL by enzyme immunoassay.[23]

Specific identification of cardiac glycosides, such as digoxin, digitoxin, deslanoside, digoxigenin, and digitoxigenin, may require sophisticated applications, such as high-performance liquid chromatography tandem mass spectrometry (HPLC-MS)[69] or HPLC-ionspray–mass spectrometry.[70] Similarly, oleandrin has been assayed in cases of oleander poisoning using HPLC[71] or HPLC-MS with serum concentrations of 1.1 ng/mL.[72] Because many clinical laboratories do not have sophisticated chromatography mass spectrophotometry equipment available, however, they may rely on the more readily available immunoassay procedures. Chromatography methods have been used to detect grayanotoxins (andromedotoxins) in material obtained from the rumen contents of poisoned sheep and goats[73] and in honey responsible for poisoning humans.[8] Similarly, thin-layer chromatography and ionization spectrometry have been used to detect *Veratrum* alkaloids in wine produced from *V. album*.[37] Although these methods may confirm the presence of one of these toxins, they are unavailable in most clinical laboratories.

TREATMENT

Resuscitation and Supportive Care

Patients with life-threatening poisoning from plant cardiotoxins may require advanced cardiac life support. The initial approach should be carried out according to current algorithms established by the American Heart Association in collaboration with the International Liaison Committee on Resuscitation.[74] Certain specific interventions that should be undertaken in addition to the standard American Heart Association guidelines are described here.

Decontamination

If the patient presents to medical care in a timely fashion, he or she should have gastrointestinal decontamination in an attempt to reduce absorption of cardiotoxins. Activated charcoal is the preferred agent because it should effectively adsorb cardiac glycosides, aconitine, veratrine, and other active toxicants while they are still in the stomach. See Chapter 5 for details on the administration of activated charcoal. There has been no role or benefit to outcome defined for repetitive doses of charcoal in the context of plant poisoning.

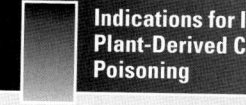

Indications for ICU Admission in Plant-Derived Cardiac Glycoside Poisoning

History of massive overdose and early onset of symptoms
History of overdose and unusually susceptible patient (e.g., extremes of age, underlying congenital or acquired cardiac disease)
Life-threatening cardiac rhythm disturbances (or potentially life-threatening with evidence of progression)
Life-threatening cardiac conduction disturbances or asystole
Life-threatening hemodynamic instability
Severe metabolic disturbances (e.g., hyperkalemia)
Progressive deterioration in level of consciousness
Seizures or coma

Ipecac-induced vomiting, with its potential for exacerbating the toxic effects through exaggerated vagal tone and negative chronotropy, is not recommended. Orogastric lavage should be approached cautiously for the same reason.

Extracorporeal Removal Techniques

Patients are unlikely to derive any benefit from hemodialysis in cardiotoxic plant poisoning, given the large molecular size of these alkaloids and other natural compounds. The value of hemoperfusion has not been established.

Specific Treatments

Cardioversion or transcutaneous cardiac pacing may be lifesaving for patients with cardiac toxicity from plants. In the series by Eddleston and associates of 66 patients with yellow oleander poisoning, 6 patients had a temporary pacemaker inserted as part of their management.[59]

Antiarrhythmic agents, such as amiodarone, have been suggested for malignant arrhythmias associated with aconite poisoning.[30] Atropine may be effective in the treatment of bradyarrhythmias associated with aconite and *Veratrum* toxicity. Successful management of hyperkalemia also may resolve cardiac conduction disturbances.

Vasopressors, such as dopamine, may be needed in addition to intravenous fluids to treat refractory hypotension. Standard anticonvulsants, such as benzodiazepines, are a rational choice of treatment for aconite-associated seizures.

Antidotes

Digoxin Fab-specific antibodies have been used successfully to treat patients with significant poisoning by oleander or other cardiac glycoside–containing plants.[75,76] In a randomized controlled trial, Eddleston and associates[59] showed that Fab fragments resolved arrhythmias and bradycardia after yellow oleander poisoning rapidly, often within 2 hours of administration. These authors pointed out that the relatively short half-life of Fab fragments (16 hours) and continued absorption of cardiac glycosides from ingested oleander seeds may account for recrudescent symptoms. Lower affinity of the Fab fragments for oleandrin and other natural toxicants than for digoxin may account for recurrent dysrhythmias seen in some patients. In Eddleston's series, recrudescence of oleander-related bradycardia was noted in three patients 48 hours after the initial administration of Fab antibodies.[59] In the context of oleander poisoning, an empirical dose of 800 mg of Fab fragments may be given as a starting dose. This is a larger dose than is typically used in the initial treatment of pharmaceutical digoxin poisoning and is recommended because of the lower binding affinity of the antibody to the natural cardiac glycosides. Suggested indications for the administration of digoxin immune Fab are listed in Table 125-2. Although this has not been formally studied, it is suggested that the pediatric dose should be similar to that for adults.

TABLE 125-2 Indications for Digoxin Immune FAB in Plant-Derived Cardiac Glycoside Poisoning

For the treatment of life-threatening complications of history-confirmed oleander, foxglove, or other plant-derived cardiac glycoside poisoning:
Severe ventricular arrhythmias (e.g., ventricular tachycardia or fibrillation)
Progressive bradyarrhythmias (e.g., severe sinus bradycardia or second-degree or third-degree heart block not responsive to atropine)
Potassium concentrations >5 mEq/L in the context of severe poisoning

Note: Each vial of Digibind contains 38 mg of digoxin-specific Fab fragments, which bind approximately 0.5 mg of digoxin or digitoxin. Plant-derived cardiac glycosides have lower binding affinities for the Fab, however. Patients poisoned by plant-derived cardiac glycosides may require a substantially increased dose of the antidote over that conventionally used in the treatment of digitalis poisoning.

Criteria for ICU Discharge in Plant-Derived Cardiac Glycoside Poisoning

With coma, seizures, or gastrointestinal upset: normalization of consciousness, resolution of gastrointestinal symptoms, and no evidence of progressive cardiac disturbances after at least 24 hours of monitoring
After administration of the antidote: stable heart rate and rhythm for at least an additional 48 hours of continuous cardiac monitoring with no evidence of recrudescent cardiac toxicity
After administration of the antidote: resolution of hyperkalemia and associated electrocardiogram findings and, on monitoring for at least an additional 48 hours, no evidence of rebound hypokalemia or recrudescent hyperkalemia

SPECIAL POPULATIONS

Pediatric Patients

Because of their smaller size and lower weight, children receive larger doses of the toxins when they ingest poisonous plants. Because most of the life-threatening symptoms associated with aconite, *Veratrum* alkaloids, grayanotoxins, and cardiac glycosides are dose dependent, children are theoretically a more vulnerable group. In addition to their smaller size, the oral behaviors and developmental immaturity of toddlers place them at a higher risk for inadvertent poisoning by plants. Oral exploration of plant parts is likely to produce inadvertent poisoning in young children.

Elderly Patients

The relative instability of the cardiovascular system of the elderly and their diminished capacity to detoxify and eliminate toxins place them at high risk for toxic effects from plants. The elderly already may be on cardiac medications and have underlying cardiac disease, which may compound the adverse effects of poisoning from plant cardiotoxins.

Other Special Populations

Immigrant populations and others who practice herbal medicine constitute a group at higher risk for inadvertent poisoning by cardiotoxic plants.

Key Points in Plant-Derived Cardiac Glycoside Poisoning

1. Cardiotoxic plant poisoning can occur in suicidal individuals, individuals experimenting with herbal tea or alternative therapies, or in children.
2. Plant-derived alkaloid toxins may or may not be detected by conventional laboratory assays. Management of symptomatic patients with a history of poisoning should not be delayed.
3. Digoxin Fab antibody administration may be helpful in the management of patients with significant oleander or foxglove poisoning.
4. Multiple and varying cardiac rhythms, with conduction disturbances, ventricular excitability, and ST-segment depression, and poor response to atropine and other initial management measures are poor prognostic signs.

REFERENCES

1. Withering W: An Account of Foxglove and Some of Its Medicinal Uses. Birmingham, G.G.J. and J. Robinson, Pasternoster-Row, 1785.
2. Turner NJ, Szczawinski AF: Common Poisonous Plants and Mushrooms of North America. Portland, Oregon, Timber Press, 1991.
3. Pantanowitz L, Naude TW, Leisewitz A: Noxious toads and frogs of South Africa. South Afr Med J 88:1408–1414, 1998.
4. McVann A, Havlik I, Joubert PH, et al: Cardiac glycoside poisoning involved in deaths from traditional medicines. South Afr Med J 81:139–141, 1992.
5. Brewster D: Herbal poisoning: A case report of a fatal yellow oleander poisoning from the Solomon Islands. Ann Trop Paediatr 6:289–291, 1986.
6. Kolev ST, Leman P, Kite GC, et al: Toxicity following accidental ingestion of *Aconitum* containing Chinese remedy. Hum Exp Toxicol 15:839–842, 1996.
7. Dickens P, Tai YT, But PP, et al: Fatal accidental aconitine poisoning following ingestion of Chinese herbal medicine: A report of two cases. Forensic Sci Int 67:55–58, 1994.
8. Sutlupinar N, Mat A, Satganoglu Y: Poisoning by toxic honey in Turkey (Letter). Arch Toxicol 67:148–150, 1993.
9. Karawya MS, Balbaa SI, Khayyal SE: Estimation of cardenolides in *Nerium oleander*. Planta Med 23:70–73, 1973.
10. Bisset NG: Arrow poisons in China: Part II. *Aconitum*—botany, chemistry, and pharmacology. J Ethnopharmacol 4:247–336, 1981.
11. Reed JK, Gerrie J, Reed KL: Purification of veratridine from veratrine using high-performance liquid chromatography. J Chromatogr 356:450–454, 1986.
12. Smith TW, Antman EM, Friedman PL, et al: Digitalis glycosides: Mechanisms and manifestations of toxicity. Prog Cardiovasc Dis 26:413–458, 1984.
13. Tallent WH, Riethof ML, Horning EC: Studies on the occurrence and structure of acetylandromedol (andromedotoxin). J Am Chem 79:4548–4554, 1957.
14. Uber-Bucek E, Hamon M, Pham Huy C, et al: Determination of thevetin B in serum by fluorescence polarization immunoassay. J Pharmaceut Biomed Anal 10:413–419, 1992.
15. Radford DJ, Gillies AD, Hinds JA, et al: Naturally occurring cardiac glycosides. Med J Aust 144:540–544, 1986.
16. Dickstein ES, Kunkel FW: Foxglove tea poisoning. Am J Med 69:167–169, 1980.
17. Simpkiss M, Holt D: Digitalis poisoning due to the accidental ingestion of foxglove leaves. Ther Drug Monit 5:217, 1983.
18. Langford SD, Boor PJ: Oleander toxicity: An examination of human and animal toxic exposures. Toxicology 109:1–13, 1996.
19. Haynes BE, Bessen HA, Wightman WD: Oleander tea: Herbal draught of death. Ann Emerg Med 14:350–353, 1985.
20. Eddleston M, Anaratnam CA, Meyer WP, et al: Epidemic of self-poisoning with seeds of the yellow oleander tree (*Thevetia peruviana*) in northern Sri Lanka. Trop Med Int Health 4:266–273, 1999.
21. Lamminpaa A, Kinos M: Plant poisonings in children. Hum Exp Toxicol 15:245–249, 1996.

22. Edgerton PH: Symptoms of digitalis-like toxicity in a family after accidental ingestion of lily of the valley plant. J Emerg Nurs 15:220–223, 1989.
23. Tuncok Y, Kozan O, Cavdar C, et al: *Urginea maritima* (squill) toxicity. J Toxicol Clin Toxicol 33:83–86, 1995.
24. Heubach JF, Schule A: Cardiac effects of lappaconitine and N-deacetyllappaconitine, two diterpenoid alkaloids from plants of the *Aconitum* and *Delphinium* species. Planta Med 64:22–26, 1998.
25. Friese J, Gleitz J, Gutser UT, et al: *Aconitum* sp. alkaloids: The modulation of voltage-dependent Na+ channels, toxicity and antinociceptive properties. Eur J Pharmacol 337:165–174, 1997.
26. Ameri A: The effects of *Aconitum* alkaloids on the central nervous system. Prog Neurobiol 56:211–235, 1998.
27. Zhu YP, Woerdenbag HJ: Traditional Chinese herbal medicine. Pharm World Sci 17:103–112, 1995.
28. But PP, Tai YT, Young K: Three fatal cases of herbal aconite poisoning. Vet Hum Toxicol 36:212–215, 1994.
29. Fatovich DM: Aconite: A lethal Chinese herb. Ann Emerg Med 21:309–311, 1992.
30. Tai YT, But PP, Young K, et al: Cardiotoxicity after accidental herb-induced aconite poisoning. Lancet 340:1254–1256, 1992.
31. Gossinger H, Hruby K, Pohl H, et al: [Poisoning with andromedotoxin-containing honey]. Deutsche Med Wochenschr 108:1555–1558, 1983.
32. Gossinger H, Hruby K, Haubenstock A, et al: Cardiac arrhythmias in a patient with grayanotoxin-honey poisoning. Vet Hum Toxicol 25:328–329, 1983.
33. Klein-Schwartz W, Litovitz T: Azalea toxicity: An overrated problem? J Toxicol Clin Toxicol 23:91–101, 1985.
34. Festa M, Andreetto B, Ballaris M, et al: [A case of Veratrum poisoning]. Min Anestesiol 62:195–196, 1996.
35. Quatrehomme G, Bertrand F, Chauvet C, et al: Intoxication from *Veratrum album*. Hum Exp Toxicol 12:111–115, 1993.
36. Jaffe AM, Gephardt D, Courtemanche L: Poisoning due to ingestion of *Veratrum viride* (false hellebore). J Emerg Med 8:161–167, 1990.
37. Garnier R, Carlier P, Hoffelt J, et al: [Acute dietary poisoning by white hellebore (*Veratrum album* L.): Clinical and analytical data: A propos of 5 cases]. Ann Med Int 136:125–128, 1985.
38. Spoerke DG, Spoerke SE: Three cases of *Zigadenus* (death camus) poisoning. Vet Hum Toxicol 21:346–347, 1979.
39. Heilpern KL: *Zigadenus* poisoning. Ann Emerg Med 25:259–262, 1995.
40. Shah AN, Shaw LA, Shah S: Digoxin and other cardiac glycosides. In Shaw LM (ed): Contemporary Practice in Clinical Toxicology. St. Paul, MN, AACC Press, 2000.
41. Jortani SA, Helm RA, Valdes R Jr: Inhibition of Na,K-ATPase by oleandrin and oleandrigenin, and their detection by digoxin immunoassays. Clin Chem 42:1654–1658, 1996.
42. Mizugaki M, Ito K, Ohyama Y, et al: Quantitative analysis of *Aconitum* alkaloids in the urine and serum of a male attempting suicide by oral intake of aconite extract. J Analyt Toxicol 22:336–340, 1998.
43. Murayama M, Mori T, Bando H, et al: Studies on the constituents of *Aconitum* species: IX. The pharmacological properties of pyro-type aconitine alkaloids, components of processed aconite powder "kako-bushi-matsu": Analgesic, antiinflammatory and acute toxic activities. J Ethnopharmacol 35:159–164, 1991.
44. Narahashi T: Modulation of nerve membrane sodium channels by chemicals. J Physiol 77:1093–1101, 1981.
45. Humphreys DJ, Stodulski JBJ: Detection of andromedotoxins for the diagnosis of *Rhododendron* poisoning in animals. J Appl Toxicol 6:121–122, 1986.
46. Hauptman PJ, Kelly RA: Digitalis. Circulation 99:1265–1270, 1999.
47. Santana LF, Gomez AM, Lederer WJ: Ca2+ flux through promiscuous cardiac Na+ channels: Slip-mode conductance. Science 279:1027–1033, 1998.
48. Eddleston M, Ariaratnam CA, Sjostrom L, et al: Acute yellow oleander (*Thevetia peruviana*) poisoning: Cardiac arrhythmias, electrolyte disturbances, and serum cardiac glycoside concentrations on presentation to hospital. Heart 83:301–306, 2000.
49. Kosower EM: A hypothesis for the mechanism of sodium channel opening by batrachotoxin and related toxins. FEBS Lett 163:161–164, 1983.
50. Catterall WA: Structure and function of voltage-sensitive ion channels. Science 242:50–61, 1988.
51. Brown BS, Akera T, Brody TM: Mechanism of grayanotoxin III-induced afterpotentials in feline cardiac Purkinje fibers. Eur J Pharmacol 75:271–281, 1981.
52. Ameri A: Structure-dependent differences in the effects of the *Aconitum* alkaloids lappaconitine, N-desacetyllappaconitine and lappaconidine in rat hippocampal slices. Brain Res 769:36–43, 1997.
53. Hintze TH: Reflex regulation of the circulation after stimulation of cardiac receptors by prostaglandins. Fed Proc 46:73–80, 1987.
54. Osterloh J, Herold S, Pond S: Oleander interference in the digoxin radioimmunoassay in a fatal ingestion. JAMA 247:1596–1597, 1982.
55. Kaojarern S, Sukhupunyarak S, Mokkhavesa C: Oleander yee tho poisoning. J Med Assoc Thai 69:108–111, 1986.
56. Haynes BE, Bessen HA, Wightman WD: Oleander tea: Herbal draught of death. Ann Emerg Med 14:350–353, 1985.
57. Shumaik GM, Wu AW, Ping AC: Oleander poisoning: Treatment with digoxn-specific Fab antibody fragments. Ann Emerg Med 17:732–735, 1988.
58. Saravanapavananthan N, Ganeshammoorthy J: Yellow oleander poisoning—a study of 170 cases. Forens Sci Int 36:247–250, 1988.
59. Eddleston M, Rajapakse S, Rajakanthan S, et al: Anti-digoxin Fab fragments in cardiotoxicity induced by ingestion of yellow oleander: A randomised controlled trial. Lancet 355:967–972, 2000.
60. Fatovich DM: Aconite: A lethal Chinese herb. Ann Emerg Med 21:309–311, 1992.
61. Yavuz H, Ozel A, Akkus I, Erkul I: Honey poisoning in Turkey. Lancet 337:789–890, 1991.
62. Gossinger H, Hruby K, Haubenstock A: Cardiac arrhythmias in a patient with grayanotoxin-honey poisoning. Vet Hum Toxicol 25:328–329, 1983.
63. Moran NC, Dresel PE, Perkins ME, Richardson AP: The pharmacological actions of andromedotoxin, an active principle from *Rhododendron maximon*. J Pharmacol Exp Ther 110:415–432, 1954.
64. Quatrehomme G, Bertrand F, Chauvet C, Ollier A: Intoxication from *Veratrum album*. Hum Exp Toxicol 12:111–115, 1993.
65. Jaffe AM, Gephardt D, Courtemanche L: Poisoning due to ingestion of *Veratrum viride* (false hellebore). J Emerg Med 8:161–167, 1990.
66. Cheung K, Hinds JA, Duffy P: Detection of poisoning by plant-origin cardiac glycoside with the Abbott TDx analyzer. Clin Chem 35:295–297, 1989.
67. Dasgupta A, Hart AP: Rapid detection of oleander poisoning using fluorescence polarization immunoassay for digitoxin: Effect of treatment with digoxin-specific Fab antibody fragment (ovine). Am J Clin Pathol 108:411–416, 1997.
68. Datta P, Dasgupta A: Interference of oleandrin and oleandrigenin in digitoxin immunoassays: Minimal cross reactivity with a new monoclonal chemiluminescent assay and high cross reactivity with the fluorescence polarization assay. Therap Drug Monit 19:465–469, 1997.
69. Guan F, Ishi A, Seno H, et al: Identification and quantification of cardiac glycosides in blood and urine samples by HPLC/MS/MS. Analyt Chem 71:4034–4043, 1999.
70. Tracqui A, Kintz P, Ludes B, et al: High-performance liquid chromatography-ionspray mass spectrometry for the specific determination of digoxin and some related cardiac glycosides in human plasma. J Chromatog B Biomed Sci Appl 692:101–109, 1997.
71. Namera A, Yashiki M, Okada K, et al: Rapid quantitative analysis of oleandrin in human blood by high-performance liquid chromatography. Nippon Hoigaku Zasshi Jpn J Legal Med 51:315–318, 1997.
72. Tracqui A, Kintz P, Branche F, et al: Confirmation of oleander poisoning by HPLC/MS. Int J Legal Med 111:32–34, 1998.
73. Humphreys DJ, Stodulski JB: Detection of andromedotoxins for the diagnosis of *Rhododendron* poisoning in animals. J Appl Toxicol 6:121–122, 1986.
74. Proceedings of the International Guidelines 2000 Conference for Cardiopulmonary Resuscitation and Emergency Cardiovascular Care. Ann Emerg Med 37(Suppl):s1–s200, 2001.
75. Rich SA, Libera JM, Locke RJ: Treatment of foxglove extract poisoning with digoxin-specific Fab fragments. Ann Emerg Med 22:1904–1907, 1993.
76. Safadi R, Levy I, Amitai Y, Caraco Y: Beneficial effect of digoxin-specific Fab antibody fragments in oleander intoxication. Arch Intern Med 155:2121–2125, 1995.

CHAPTER 126

Anticholinergic Plants

J. Ward Donovan

Exposure to plants with anticholinergic properties can result in emergency department and intensive care unit (ICU) admissions due to delirium, hallucinations, hyperpyrexia, and other associated adverse effects (e.g., rhabdomyolysis). Alkaloid-containing plants of the Solanaceae (nightshade) family, especially *Datura* spp., have been used since antiquity for their analgesic, hypnotic, aphrodisiac, hallucinogenic, and herbal properties. Homer referred to *Datura* as a poison in the *Odyssey*. Dioscorides in *De Materia Medica* described dose-dependent *Datura* toxicity; Cleopatra lured Caesar with this plant, and Marc Antony's troops suffered confusion and fatalities after eating the plant when retreating from Parthia in 38 AD.[1,2] Medieval European witches were said to apply *Datura* extract ointments from the handle of a broom to their genitals for hallucinogenic effect.[3] This application would result in imaginary flights and visions of festive banquets and objects flying in the air, providing the modern symbol of Halloween witches riding a broom.[2,3] Yaqui Indians in Mexico applied crushed *Datura* leaves to their genitals and legs for hallucinogenic effects, and American Algonquin Indians used it in the initiation of boys into manhood.[4] Sometimes these plants were used for their sedating effects, such as the Colombian Chiba Indians' use to drug widows and slaves before burying them alive with their dead warrior masters.[1] Thornapple (*Datura stramonium*) in Russia and China, the mandrake plant in Egypt, and henbane in Middle Europe were added to beer to increase its potency.[2]

The first documented poisoning episode from *Datura* in the United States occurred in Jamestown, Virginia, in 1676, among British troops.[1,2,4] The soldiers inadvertently prepared a salad of *D. stramonium*, and many experienced acute poisoning. The original description of the result is an accurate depiction of some of the clinical effects: "...they turned natural fools upon it for several days; one would blow up a feather in the air; another would dart straws at it with much fury; and another, stark naked, was sitting in a corner like a monkey grinning and making mows at them ... after eleven days returned to themselves again, not remembering anything that had passed."[4] This episode spawned the common name *Jamestown weed*, eventually being corrupted to *Jimson weed*.

In addition to their use in religious rituals, accidental ingestions, and hallucinogen-inducing practices, Solanacea alkaloids have been used for criminal purposes. Numerous deaths in the upper echelons of French society were ascribed to intentional poisoning by nightshade alkaloids in the 1600s; Catherine Voison was known then as the "palace deliverer" of the anticholinergic plants henbane and thornapple in poison

drinks.[2] Two physicians were convicted in the late 19th and early 20th centuries of using hyoscine extracted from plants to poison their wives.[2] *Datura* seeds and powder sometimes are used to facilitate robbery.[4] In 1991, a gardener rendered a female acquaintance and two others helpless with thornapple seeds and sexually abused them.[2]

Herbal medicines also have been prepared for centuries from the Solanaceae plants. Aboriginal tribes use an anticholinergic plant called *pituri* for its narcotic-like properties, and Chinese herbal medicines are often made from the anticholinergic plant *Datura metel* L (yangjinhua) for treatment of asthma and chronic bronchitis.[5,6] Herbal cigarettes containing the dried leaves of *D. stramonium* have been used as traditional asthma remedies, especially in Britain and India.[7] The Pueblo Indians of Mexico used Nacazcul seeds, a South American variant of *D. stramonium*, as an analgesic for orthopedic procedures.[4] Other herbal preparations sometimes are contaminated with belladonna alkaloids, resulting in mini-epidemics of poisoning.[8] Foods also may be mistakenly prepared with anticholinergic berries or leaves or be ingested as food contaminants.[3,9-13] Cooking does not destroy the toxic alkaloids.[13]

Modern exposure to anticholinergic plants usually results from accidental ingestion by children and more commonly from their recreational use as hallucinogens.[14-17] The American Association of Poison Control Centers reported 1144 anticholinergic plant exposures in 2001, 623 (54%) accidental and 489 (43%) intentional.[18] Children younger than age 6 accounted for 380 (33%) of the exposures, and adolescents accounted for 496 (43%). This reporting system likely overrepresents accidental childhood exposures and underreports intentional recreational uses and resulting hospitalizations. Although *Datura* plants are not among the top 20 most frequent plant exposures in the United States, they are the most likely to require medical care.[16,17,19]

Intentional use for recreation first began to occur in the 1960s, especially among adolescents and young adults seeking an inexpensive and natural hallucinogen.[19] Since then, there have been many episodic reports of group recreational experiences with anticholinergic plants.[1,7,9,10,16,17,19-30] These experiences tend to occur in clusters due to seasonal episodes of discovery of these agents, spread by word of mouth in a school or neighborhood. In Florida in 1994, abuse of *Datura sauveolens* (angel's trumpet) increased 10-fold as a result of enhanced awareness of its effects publicized by the media and public health officials.[1] Most recreational exposures occur in the summer and fall, when the plants mature.[19,31] In one series of 73 Jimson weed exposures, 95%

1335

were recreational abuse, and the mean age was 17.3 years (range 11 to 28 years), with a male-to-female ratio of 5.4:1.[19]

TAXONOMY

Anticholinergic plants are members of the Solanaceae family. This family includes a wide variety of other plants, such as foods (tomatoes, potatoes, paprika, eggplants, red pepper), tobacco, and ornamentals (petunias).[2] These plants grow in temperate and tropical climates and include the genera *Datura, Hyoscyamus, Atropa, Mandragora,* and *Duboisia*.[5] The genus names *Datura* and *Brugmansia* are used interchangeably, especially when referring to *D. sauveoloens* (angel's trumpet).[1] The pharmacologically active components are the tropane (also called *belladonna*) alkaloids, atropine, hyoscyamine, and scopolamine. Table 126-1 lists the anticholinergic plants of the Solanaceae family, including their locale, their common names, and some of their uses.

D. stramonium is the most widespread of the potentially toxic Solanaceae, especially in the United States. This woody, large annual shrub is found throughout the United States growing in cultivated soybean fields and cornfields and in weedy roadsides, particularly in the eastern and midwestern states from Florida north into Canada.[26] The plant grows to 5 feet and is malodorous, especially at night, with large, dark green, ovate-oblong leaves.[30] A white, tubular flower blooms from July to September, followed by the growth of a fruit consisting of a four-lobed spinous capsule. Each of these golf ball–size pods contains 50 to 100 kidney-shaped, 2- to 3-mm seeds, which change from yellow to tan to black as they mature in the fall. All parts of the plant are toxic, but the seeds have a concentration of 0.4% alkaloids compared with 0.25% in the leaves and flowers.[11,12] Each seed contains about 0.05 to 0.1 mg of atropine (*D/L*-hyoscyamine), or about 6 mg per pod.[11,12,19] Immature plants contain mostly scopolamine, and mature plants contain mostly hyoscyamine.[32]

D. stramonium is known as *Jimson weed, locoweed, thornapple, mad apple,* and other names reflecting its effects (see Table 126-1). It is used most often as a hallucinogen by ingesting the seeds or sometimes by smoking the leaves or brewing the plant into a tea.[19,20] It also has been mixed with

TABLE 126-1 Anticholinergic Plants: Family Solanaceae (Nightshade)

SCIENTIFIC NAME	COMMON NAME	GEOGRAPHIC DISTRIBUTION/USE
Datura		
D. stramonium	Jamestown weed	Throughout United States
	Jimson weed	Disturbed ground
	Locoweed	Soybean fields
	Devil's weed	Cultivated fields
	Stinkweed	Barnyards
	Apple of Peru	Roadsides
	Devil's apple	Canada
	Thornapple	South America
	Locoseed	Asia
	Green dragon	Africa
	Mad apple	
	Moon weed	
	Tolguacha	
	Samura	Asthma cigarettes
D. sauveolens	Angel's trumpet	Southeast United States
(D. candida)	Sacred datura	South America
(D. meteloides)	Trompetero	Caribbean
(Brugmansia candida)	Borrachero	Common garden shrub
	Magic drink	Hallucinogenic tea
D. arborea	Trumpet lilly	
D. metel L	Datura folium	Asia
	Hindu datura	China
	Unmatel	
	Flos daturae	
	Yangjinhua	Chinese herbal medicine
D. innoxia Mill		Chinese herbal medicine
D. fastuosa		Chinese herbal medicine
D. tabula		Chinese herbal medicine
Hyoscyamus		Northern Rocky Mountains
H. niger	Henbane	
	Old World nightshade	
	Black henbane	
	Fetid nightshade	
	Insane root	
	Poison tobacco	

TABLE 126-1 Anticholinergic Plants: Family Solanaceae (Nightshade)—cont'd

SCIENTIFIC NAME	COMMON NAME	GEOGRAPHIC DISTRIBUTION/USE
Cestrum		
C. nocturnum	Willow-leaved jasmine	Coastal Plains in South/Southwest United States
C. diurnum	Night-blooming jasmine Day-blooming jasmine	
Atropa		
A. belladonna	Deadly nightshade Sorcerer's herb	Europe Cultivated in eastern United States
Duboisia		
D. hopwoodii	Pituri	Australia
Mandragora		
M. officinarum	Mandrake Mandragos Satan's apple	Mediterranean Basin
Lycium		
L. halimifolium	Matrimony vine	Eastern/northern United States

marijuana in cigarettes, known as "green dragons," to enhance the hallucinogenic effect.[30] Accidental poisoning sometimes still occurs in modern times from use as an herbal tea, when mistaken as an edible food, and when asthma cigarettes are misused.[7,20,33,34]

Angel's trumpet, or sacred *Datura*, is another abused anticholinergic plant. It grows wild throughout the southeastern United States, the Caribbean, and South America and is a common garden ornamental plant.[21] It is referred to variously as *D. sauveolens, D. candida, D. innoxia, D. meteloides, B. candida*, and *B. sauveolens*.[1] It is an evergreen bush 2 to 8 m high, with trumpet-shaped, purplish-to-white flowers measuring 20 to 50 cm that hang straight down.[1,35,36] Alkaloid content is 0.25% to 0.7%, or 0.2 mg of atropine and 0.65 mg of scopolamine per blossom.[1] Exposure is typically from abuse as a hallucinogen by brewing or ingesting the leaves and flowers or steeping the leaves and blossoms in water and alcohol to yield a "magic drink." It also may be mistaken for a vegetable root or herbal tea.[1,3,21,24,28,35–37]

Atropa belladonna (deadly nightshade) contains 98% atropine and only small amounts of hyoscyamine and scopolamine. It is native to continental Europe and Great Britain and is cultivated in the United States as an ornamental plant.[15] It grows as a bush with purple-black berries and got its name during the Italian Renaissance when it was used to dilate pupils for cosmetic purposes. There is 2 mg of atropine per berry, and these may be mistaken for edible berries, such as bilberries, also known as whortleberries or hurtleberries (*Vaccinum myrtillus*) in Great Britain and Europe.[9,10,13] Anticholinergic alkaloid-containing plants also include *H. niger* (henbane, fetid nightshade), which is used rarely as a hallucinogen by eating its dirty-yellow flowers or seed-filled pods.[11,12] The *Cestrum* genus includes jasmine (or jessamine) plants of the southern United States, which have trumpet-shaped fragrant flowers and berries. They are rare causes of poisoning. *Mandragora officinarum* (mandrake, Satan's apple) grows in the Mediterranean Basin and contains hyoscyamine, scopolamine, and mandragorine. It

should not be confused with the American mandrake, which is also known as mayapple and contains podophyllum.

Some Chinese herbal medications are from *Datura* spp. that are native to South Asia and China,[6] including *D. metel, D. innoxia, D. tabula*, and *D. fastuosa*. They are used in the treatment of asthma, chronic bronchitis, seizures, and psychosis and as analgesics; their toxic effects account for 0.2% of all acute medical admissions in Hong Kong.[35] Yangjinhua is the most common herb, made from the dried flowers of *D. metel*, containing 85% scopolamine and 15% hyoscyamine.[6] They may be smoked or given orally or intravenously. The recommended oral dose of Yangjinhua is 0.3 to 0.6 g, with 0.3% to 0.43% alkaloid.[6]

PHARMACOLOGIC PROPERTIES

The anticholinergic plants contain the so-called tropane alkaloids atropine, scopolamine, and hyoscyamine, with scopolamine (*l*-hyoscine) being present in higher concentrations than hyoscyamine in most *Datura* spp. (Fig. 126-1). Atropine is a racemic mixture of the *d*- and *l*-forms of hyoscyamine, with the *l*-isomer possessing greater pharmacologic (antimuscarinic) potency.[22] These alkaloids, often also referred to as *belladonna alkaloids*, competitively block the binding of acetylcholine to cholinergic muscarinic receptors on postganglionic parasympathetic neurons, on sympathetic postganglionic sweat gland receptors, and in the cortex and subcortical regions of the brain.[3] The postganglionic sites are found in autonomic receptor cells in smooth muscle, cardiac muscle, exocrine glands, and sinoatrial and atrioventricular nodes. Antimuscarinic agents have little effect on the actions of acetylcholine at nicotinic receptor sites of autonomic ganglia or skeletal muscle junctions. High doses may cause competitive blockade of these receptors, however, and this curare-like action of high concentrations of scopolamine in particular may account for reports of muscle weakness and flaccidity.[3,21]

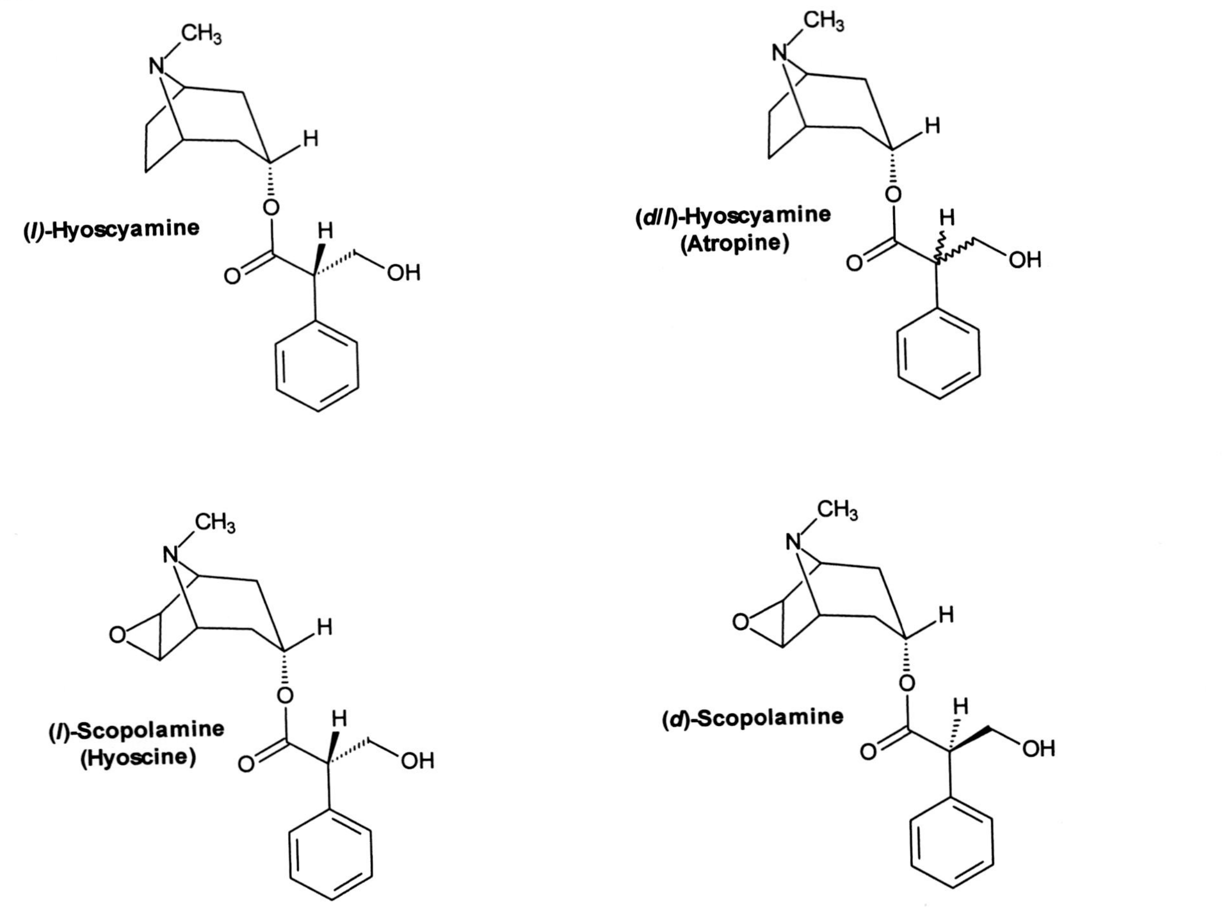

FIGURE 126-1

Chemical structures of the belladonna alkaloids. The importance of chirality is shown by the fact that the *l*-enantiomer of hyoscyamine possesses most antimuscarinic activity. Atropine is composed of equal amounts of *d*- and *l*-hyoscyamine (i.e., atropine is a racemate). Scopolamine also is chiral, and the *l*-enantiomer is commonly known as *hyoscine*. The enantiomeric designations deserve mention. The uppercase *D*- and *L*-, and similarly, *R*- and *S*-, refer to absolute configuration, which is assigned by examining the three-dimensional representation of a given stereocenter. The lowercase letters, *d*- and *l*-, which in this setting are equivalent in meaning to the arithmetic symbols, + and −, refer to the optical rotation of a solution of the pure enantiomer. Optical rotation is the direction in which a solution of the pure enantiomer rotates plane polarized light. An enantiomerically pure solution with an optical rotation that is to the right of center (clockwise) is designated as positive (+) or *dextrorotatory* (*d*-), whereas an enantiomerically pure solution with a leftward (anticlockwise) optical rotation is designated as negative (−) or *levorotatory* (*l*-). When the two enantiomerically pure solutions are compared, their optical rotations are equal in magnitude but opposite in direction. In the case of a racemate, the clockwise rotation imparted by the *d*-enantiomer is exactly balanced by an equal but opposite contribution imparted by the *l*-enantiomer resulting in a net optical rotation of zero. In short, D/L and R/S can be assigned empirically to a specific stereocenter based on a three-dimensional drawing of that stereocenter. Conversely, *d/l* (or, +/−) refers to the optical rotation properties of the molecule as a whole, which may contain multiple stereocenters and must be determined experimentally. There is no consistent relationship between *D/L* (*R/S*) and *d/l* (+/−). It is common for an enantiomer of a given compound to have a *D*- absolute configuration at a stereocenter but simultaneously have a negative, or *l*-, optical rotation. Such is the case for the pharmacologically more active *d*-isomer of methamphetamine, which actually has an *S*- absolute configuration at its single stereocenter. By convention, pharmacologists typically refer to isomeric compounds in terms of optical rotation (*d/l* or +/−) rather than absolute configuration (*D/L* or *R/S*), whereas organic chemists frequently describe the absolute configuration of each specific stereocenter in a compound.

The various tropane alkaloids have prominent effects on the central nervous system (CNS), with quantitative differences between them. Scopolamine exhibits greater brain penetration than atropine and is a depressant even in therapeutic doses. It also has amnestic properties, favoring its earlier use as a preanesthetic. High doses of these alkaloids, especially scopolamine, antagonize central muscarinic neurotransmission, resulting in depression of the inhibitory portion of the reticular activating system.[21] The CNS effects may be exacerbated by inhibition of the central response to histamine, 5-hydroxytryptamine (serotonin), and norepinephrine, by acting as receptor antagonists for these neurotransmitters.[21]

The muscarinic receptor antagonists block the cholinergic actions on the sphincter muscle of the iris and the cil-

iary muscle of the lens, resulting in mydriasis and loss of accommodation. In contrast to atropine, even usual therapeutic doses of scopolamine exert this effect. Cardiovascular effects at low doses of anticholinergic alkaloids are initial blockade of inhibitory postganglionic parasympathetic receptors, resulting in slowed heart rate.[21] At higher doses, postsynaptic vagal effects on the sinoatrial nodal pacemaker are blocked, resulting in sinus tachycardia. High doses of these alkaloids dilate cutaneous blood vessels but have little or no effect on blood pressure. Blockade of postganglionic cholinergic receptors in the gastrointestinal tract results in reduced motility and secretions. Anticholinergic agents decrease the tone and contractile force of the ureter, bladder, and gallbladder but have little effect on the uterus. Blockade of sympathetic cholinergic neurons of sweat glands, combined with a central hyperthermic response and increased basal metabolic rate, can elevate body temperature.

PHARMACOKINETICS

The belladonna alkaloids are rapidly absorbed, with onset of symptoms typically within 5 to 10 minutes after the ingestion of teas and 1 to 3 hours after ingestion of leaves or seeds.[1,30,32] Slow dissolution of the plant parts, coupled with

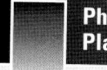

Pharmacokinetics of Anticholinergic Plants

Atropine
Volume of distribution: 2.3 to 3.6 L/kg
Half-life: 2.5 to 4 hours
Elimination: 20% to 50% renal

Scopolamine
Volume of distribution: 1.4 to 2 L/kg
Half-life: 1 to 3 hours
Elimination: 95% hepatic

the anticholinergic slowing of the gastrointestinal tract, prolongs their absorption, however.[25,38] Unabsorbed alkaloids have been found in the stomach 24 hours after ingestion, and effects last much longer than expected from known absorption and elimination rates of the extracted forms of these agents.[19,23,25] Their distribution is widespread throughout the body, but scopolamine penetrates the CNS more readily than the others. Elimination of belladonna alkaloids is by hepatic metabolism and renal excretion. Twenty percent to 50% of atropine is excreted unchanged in the urine, in contrast to only about 1% to 5% of scopolamine.[9,10,23,30,39] Half-lives of the various alkaloids range from 2.5 to 8 hours.[9,10]

CLINICAL PRESENTATION

The Solanaceae family of plants causes central and peripheral manifestations of the anticholinergic syndrome (see Chapter 22). Common peripheral effects include mydriasis, skin flushing, tachycardia, dry skin and mouth, and hyperpyrexia, and central effects are usually delirium and hallucinations. Victims may truly be "hot as a hare, red as a beet, dry as a bone, blind as a bat, and mad as a hatter."[19]

The severity and duration of clinical effects depend on the route, form (e.g., tea ingestion, flower/leaf smoking), and dose, with some variation in content among the different plants within this class. The progression of symptoms can be related to the equivalent dose of atropine, with 0.5 mg causing dry mouth, thirst, and slight cardiac slowing. Mydriasis and increasing heart rate, skin flushing, and CNS excitation occur after ingestion of 1 to 2 mg of atropine, or about 20 to 40 Jimson weed seeds. Fever, hallucinations, extreme agitation, and possibly seizures and coma typically occur with

TABLE 126-2 Effects of Atropine in Relation to Dose

DOSE (mg)	EFFECTS
0.5	Slight cardiac slowing; some dryness of mouth; inhibition of sweating
1	Definite dryness of mouth; thirst; acceleration of heart, sometimes preceded by slowing; mild dilation of pupil
2	Rapid heart rate; palpitation; marked dryness of mouth; dilated pupils; some blurring of near vision
5	All the above symptoms marked; difficulty in speaking and swallowing; restlessness and fatigue; headache; dry, hot skin; difficulty in micturition; reduced intestinal peristalsis
≥10	Above symptoms more marked; pulse rapid and weak; iris practically obliterated; vision blurred; skin flushed, hot, dry, and scarlet; ataxia, restlessness, and excitement; hallucinations and delirium; coma

From Brown JH, Taylor P: Muscarinic receptor agonists and antagonists. In Hardman JG, Limbird LE (eds): Goodman and Gilman's The Pharmacologic Basis of Therapeutics, 9th ed. New York, McGraw-Hill, 1996, p 148.

exposure to 5 to 10 mg of atropine, equivalent to the contents of one pod of *D. stramonium* (Jimson weed) or 5 to 10 *D. sauveolens* (angel trumpet) blossoms.[11,12,30] Table 126-2 lists the clinical effects in relation to dose of atropine, but CNS effects occur even at lower doses than listed because of the presence of scopolamine, especially in *Datura* spp., which more readily penetrates the CNS than atropine and exaggerates the CNS effects. Time of onset of clinical effect varies with the route and with the plant involved, beginning within 5 to 10 minutes if a tea or broth is ingested or delayed for 1 to 3 hours if seeds or leaves are used.[1,21] Signs and symptoms may last 1 to 6 days (average 2 days), and mydriasis is frequently the last to resolve.[19] Table 126-3 lists a compilation of symptoms and signs present in 134 cases from eight case series.[16,17,21–27] Not all findings were noted in each series, so the numbers in the table reflect totals reported.

TABLE 126-3 Clinical Effects in 134 Cases

SYMPTOM/SIGN	NUMBER	FREQUENCY (%)
Mydriasis	80/89	90
Hyperreflexia	14/16	88
Skin flush	39/45	87
Delirium	96/116	83
Hallucinations	72/89	81
Tachycardia	78/118	66
Dry skin/membranes	40/63	63
Weakness	5/10	50
Hypertension	48/104	46
Ataxia	4/10	40
Amnesia	4/10	40
Fever	16/67	24
Clonus	6/43	14
Urinary retention	2/32	6
Seizures	3/94	3
Coma	2/103	2

Altered mental status is ordinarily the most prominent and frequent manifestation, being present in all 27 patients in one report.[25] Specific CNS effects are restlessness, bizarre behavior, delirium, disorientation, and combative behavior, but seizures and coma are unusual. Patients characteristically pick at imaginary objects in the air, clothing, and bed sheets and have fragmented, mumbling, rapid, and incomprehensible speech.[19,30] They may be able to answer questions appropriately with one to two words, but their disorientation and confusion are revealed when responding in sentences. Severely affected patients may be mute.[32] Hallucinations occur in about 50% of patients and commonly feature the appearance of family or friends, natural colors, simple objects, visual misperceptions, and the sensation of flying.[30] The hallucinations are sometimes described as *Lilliputian*.[11,12] The colors are not as brilliant as with hallucinogens such as the indole alkaloids (e.g., lysergic acid diethylamide [LSD], psilocybin), and patients often are amnestic for the events on recovery.[3,26,30] Auditory hallucinations are less common. Particularly characteristic of belladonna alkaloid intoxication is undressing behavior, presumably due to the subjective symptoms associated with flushing and hyperpyrexia combined with loss of inhibitions.[21,26,29,32] Neurologic examination may reveal hyperreflexia, clonus, myoclonus, and sometimes dorsiflexor Babinski responses and decerebrate posturing.[26] Convulsions and flaccid paralysis might occur in severe cases, especially with *D. sauveolens* owing to its high scopolamine content.[21]

Cardiovascular abnormalities ordinarily are limited to sinus tachycardia. This may not occur in elderly patients, patients taking β-receptor antagonists, or patients presenting late.[19,21,23] Ventricular arrhythmias and cardiovascular collapse rarely may occur as a consequence of seizures and hyperpyrexia.[1,28] Mild hypertension and widened pulse pressure are seen in some cases.[21,22,37]

Other noteworthy peripheral effects are hyperpyrexia, which is rarely life-threatening, and mydriasis, which is early in onset and long-lasting. Blurred vision and dilated pupils may present as the only manifestations of a minor exposure or as anisocoria from monocular contact with plant parts (Gardener's mydriasis).[24,40] Urinary retention and gut hypomotility may present as early or late complications, and ileus may result in seeds' being retrieved from the stomach 16 to 36 hours after ingestion.[22,25] Vomiting may be present early, particularly with accidental ingestion of large amounts, such as in foods and teas.[8,13] Dysphagia and dysarthria result from severe mouth and throat dryness. Renal failure may occur as a consequence of the combination of rhabdomyolysis and dehydration.

Complications of severe anticholinergic plant poisoning include aspiration pneumonitis due to loss of airway protection, particularly in patients with seizures, and respiratory failure.[9,10,36] Severe agitation, myoclonus, and seizures, coupled with fever and dehydration, create a risk of rhabdomyolysis and resultant renal failure.[13,41]

Death is rare, but it may occur as a result of dangerous behavior or impaired judgment.[30] There are a few isolated reports of death due to hyperpyrexia to 43°C, with prolonged seizures, ventricular arrhythmias, and cardiovascular collapse.[28,33,42] Autopsy findings have included multiple epicardial and endocardial petechiae, hyperemia, and pulmonary and cerebral edema.[33,42]

DIAGNOSIS

Diagnostic Tests

The diagnosis of anticholinergic plant poisoning is made by careful history and physical examination, with no routinely available test to confirm the diagnosis. Clusters of cases, simultaneous onset in family or friends, and especially onset of the anticholinergic syndrome in a group of adolescents or young adults suggest the diagnosis.[13] Routine immunoassays for drugs of abuse and even comprehensive drug screens do not detect the belladonna alkaloids. Qualitative and quantitative assays of blood, urine, gastric contents, and plants for atropine, scopolamine, and hyoscyamine by gas chromatography–mass spectrometry or thin-layer chromatography may be reliably applied but are time-consuming and not routinely available.[3,8–10,21,25,32,33,43] Detectable alkaloid may remain in the urine for 3 days after exposure, but only for 1 day in plasma.[9,10]

Nonspecific laboratory abnormalities in anticholinergic plant toxicity have included transient elevations of lactate dehydrogenase, hepatic transaminases, calcium, phosphorus, and prothrombin time and leukocytosis[1,25,26]; these may occur as a result of fever and agitation.[26] Serum creatine kinase levels, renal function tests, and urinalysis may reveal rhabdomyolysis, myoglobinuria, and renal failure.[13] Electrocardiograms typically show sinus tachycardia and rarely ventricular arrhythmias.[8,11,12]

Electroencephalograms have shown increased high amplitude, slow-wave activity, prominent lambda activity, and epileptiform high-voltage sharp and spike waves.[26] The changes may be due to fever or to the antagonistic actions of toxic alkaloids on cholinergic pathways in the reticular activating system.[26]

Differential Diagnosis

The differential diagnosis of the agitated, delirious, sometimes febrile, and tachycardic patient includes a multitude of toxic, metabolic, infectious, and psychiatric causes (see Chapter 22). These especially include anticholinergic plant, mushroom, and drug exposure; amphetamine, alcohol, and cocaine abuse; withdrawal from alcohol and sedatives; functional psychoses; and CNS infections. The presence of peripheral and central manifestations should aid in the diagnosis (Table 126-4).[9,11,12,24]

Ataxia, aggression, and slurred speech may be confused with alcohol intoxication, and hyperthermia and agitation might mimic cocaine, amphetamine, sympathomimetic, or salicylate drug intoxication and tobacco or nicotinic plant exposure. These conditions typically cause diaphoresis, however, which is distinctly unusual for anticholinergics. Toxicity from hallucinogens (e.g., indole alkaloid) may cause different types of hallucinations than with anticholinergics, with more brilliant colors and less aggressiveness than in the anticholinergic state, and the hallucinogens cause less disorientation but more memory loss.[11,12] The mumbling, rapid, incomprehensible speech

TABLE 126-4 Differential Diagnosis of Anticholinergic Plant Poisoning

DRUG RELATED	PLANTS/MUSHROOMS	METABOLIC/OTHER
Amphetamines	Hallucinogens	Encephalitis
Alcohol withdrawal	Marijuana	Hypoglycemia
Anticholinergic drugs	Nutmeg	Hepatic encephalopathy
Antihistamines	Morning glory seeds	Meningitis
Carbamazepine	Khat	Intracranial bleed
Antidepressants	Peyote	Psychosis
Muscle relaxants	Argyreia nervosa	Schizophrenia
Neuroleptics	Ololiuqui	Uremia
Phenothiazines	Piptadenia	
Cocaine	Plants causing seizures	
Hallucinogens	Golden chain	
LSD	Tobacco	
Mescaline	Mescal beans	
Phencyclidine	Glory lilly	
Lithium	Water hemlock	
Neuroleptic malignant	Mushrooms	
syndrome	*Amanita muscaria*	
Salicylates	*Amanita pantherina*	
Sedative withdrawal	*Panaeolus campanulatus*	
Serotonin syndrome	*Paneolus foenisecii*	
Sympathomimetics	*Psilocybe*	
Theophylline	*Gymnopilus*	
Caffeine	*Conocybes*	
	Cortinarius	

pattern is particularly characteristic of the anticholinergic syndrome, as is the undressing behavior. Patients with serotonin syndrome (see Chapter 24) and neuroleptic malignant syndrome (see Chapter 26) typically have more adrenergic manifestations (e.g., diaphoresis, hypertension) and greater extremity rigidity than in the anticholinergic syndrome, but the history of medication use is essential in the diagnosis.

Mushrooms also are used for hallucinogenic purposes and may be difficult to differentiate from abuse of anticholinergic plants (see Chapter 126). Such mushrooms include *Amanita muscaria* and *Amanita pantherina*, which contain botenic acid, muscimol, muscazone, and stizolobic acid, the last-mentioned having anticholinergic properties.[11,12] *Psilocybe* (or "magic mushrooms"), *Paneolus*, and *Gymnopilus* mushrooms also cause hallucinations and alterations in perception.[11,12] Generally, hallucinogenic mushrooms do not cause the intense delirium and agitation, severe thirst, and dry throat, which are characteristic of anticholinergic plant poisoning.

Diagnostic studies may be helpful in the differential, and these should include a urine drugs-of-abuse screen, complete blood cell count, blood glucose, and electrocardiogram. Suspicion for CNS infection may require a lumbar puncture when the diagnosis of a poisoning is not established. As discussed in the treatment section, a diagnostic trial of physostigmine may be the most reliable tool in the differential diagnosis. Failure of physostigmine to improve delirium dramatically should prompt reconsideration of the diagnosis.

TREATMENT

Treatment in most cases must focus initially on management of the delirium and agitated behavior of these patients. Consideration also must be given to gastric decontamination, airway protection in patients with coma or seizures, rehydration, and protection from complications such as myoglobinuric renal tubular injury.

A common presenting scenario is a patient being restrained by several emergency or security personnel and confused enough that there is concern for the patient's safety. Soft physical restraints may be needed temporarily but should be avoided for prolonged periods because of the risk of rhabdomyolysis. Immediate administration of a rapid-acting benzodiazepine, such as diazepam or midazolam, is warranted to calm the patient and prevent seizures in

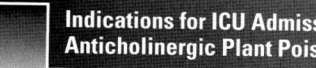

Indications for ICU Admission in Anticholinergic Plant Poisoning

Delirium unresponsive to mild sedatives
Hallucinations
Physostigmine administration required
Associated respiratory failure
Associated renal failure
Airway compromise
Seizures or symptomatic dysrhythmias (both rare)

these cases. In my experience, dosages need to be higher than usually prescribed for sedation, such as 5 to 10 mg of diazepam (0.1 to 0.2 mg/kg) or 2 to 5 mg of midazolam (0.5 to 1 mg/kg) intravenously, repeated approximately every 10 minutes as needed. Lorazepam may be used alternatively, but it has a slightly slower onset of action. Benzodiazepines have the advantage of being a nonspecific means of controlling agitation when the diagnosis is unclear. In cases of severe anticholinergic plant poisoning, even large doses of benzodiazepines may not control the patient.[41] Neuroleptics are used sometimes, but they do not prevent seizures, and some (e.g., chlorpromazine) have the theoretical potential of exacerbating anticholinergic effects and causing hypotension owing to their α-blocking properties.[21]

Gastric decontamination is theoretically useful for prolonged periods after ingestion because of slow absorption of seeds and anticholinergic reduction in gastric motility. Intact Jimson weed seeds have been found in gastric lavage fluid 12 to 23 hours after ingestion.[25,44] Activated charcoal effectively binds anticholinergic agents and is considered the decontamination therapy of choice.[11,12,27,32] Its use was shown in one case series to reduce inpatient length of stay compared with patients not receiving charcoal.[38] Introduction of oral lavage tubes into these patients is difficult and potentially dangerous and can increase agitation. In addition, lavage and induced emesis with ipecac syrup risk aspiration in patients with altered mental status.[11,12]

Dehydration and hypotension can develop secondary to agitation, vomiting, hyperthermia, and decreased intake and should be treated aggressively with intravenous fluids. Rhabdomyolysis also requires vigorous rehydration and urinary alkalization if myoglobinuria is present. Hyperthermia is managed best with external cooling with fans, cool mist, or cooling blankets.[19,27] Seizures, although unusual in isolated anticholinergic toxicity, should be treated aggressively with benzodiazepines. Phenytoin is not likely to be useful and is not indicated (see Chapter 20).

Physostigmine is indicated and rational for diagnostic and therapeutic purposes, as initial therapy or after sedation, and is used to reverse agitated delirium and stupor.[3,25,30,32] Physostigmine is a methyl carbamate compound that is obtained from dried ripe seeds of *Physostigma venenosum* (Calabar bean).[15] It is an acetylcholinesterase inhibitor, increasing the concentration of acetylcholine at the muscarinic receptors (see Chapter 153).[1,3] In contrast to other cholinesterase inhibitors, it is a tertiary amine and crosses the blood-brain barrier, reversing the peripheral and the central effects of the anticholinergic plants. Many authors caution against its use or advise that it be used only for the most severe cases of uncontrollable hallucinations, hyperthermia, hemodynamic instability, seizures, or extreme delirium.[9,10,12,13,20,21] These concerns are based on isolated case reports of bradycardia, asystole, seizures, cholinergic crisis, and hypotension, temporally associated with physostigmine administration. These fears seem unfounded, however, based on its reported consistent effectiveness without untoward consequences. In 16 published case reports and case series totaling use in 90 patients with anticholinergic plant poisoning, 85 (94%) had successful reversal of delirium or otherwise uncontrollable agitation, without any reports of adverse effects.[8,10,13,19,21–23,26,28,29,36,45–48] Of the five patients who did not respond to physostigmine, three were adults given a

subtherapeutic dose, and another already had progressed to multisystem failure.[10,28] The remaining case involved an extraordinarily large ingestion of a deadly nightshade berry pie, so the dose still may have been relatively subtherapeutic.[13] Physostigmine not only controls agitation but also reverses delirium, potentially prevents seizures, and rarely causes adverse effects. In a retrospective comparison of therapy with physostigmine versus benzodiazepines in anticholinergic toxicity, physostigmine controlled agitation in 96% of cases (versus only 24% with benzodiazepines) and reversed delirium in 86% of patients (versus no reversal with benzodiazepines).[41] Side effects were limited to diaphoresis, vomiting, diarrhea, and asymptomatic sinus bradycardia. In another retrospective review of 225 patients treated with physostigmine, none with anticholinergic toxicity alone had adverse effects.[48]

The dose of physostigmine is 0.5 to 1 mg intravenously in small children and 2 mg in adolescents and adults. Standard recommendations are that physostigmine be diluted in saline or dextrose and given slowly over 4 minutes or at a rate no greater than 0.5 mg/min. I have routinely administered it undiluted over 2 minutes, however, without any adverse effects. Full onset of action requires 10 to 15 minutes due to slow distribution into the brain.[41,46] Because physostigmine's half-life is only 16 minutes and its clinical effect may last only 30 to 60 minutes, repeat doses may be necessary and have been used without untoward effects.[3,15,19,25,26,41] Tacrine hydrochloride, a cholinesterase inhibitor available in parenteral form in Europe, was used to reverse *Datura* toxicity in one report.[24] It has the advantage of a longer half-life than physostigmine (2 to 4 hours versus 16 minutes), but experience in therapy of anticholinergic poisoning is limited.

Patients with delirium, seizures, hallucinations, or hyperpyrexia and patients who receive physostigmine require either ICU care or a prolonged stay in the emergency department. Of 86 patients poisoned by anticholinergic plants, 57 were admitted to an ICU, and the remaining 29 were held in the emergency department for an average length of stay of 14 hours.[19,25] ICU stays averaged 2 days (range of 1 to 6 days).

Criteria for ICU Discharge in Anticholinergic Plant Poisoning

Resolution of delirium and hallucinations
No physostigmine or sedatives required for at least 4 hours
Resolution of associated respiratory or renal failure

Common Errors in Anticholinergic Plant Poisoning

Misdiagnosis as psychosis or anxiety
Use of physical restraints rather than sedatives
Failure to use adequate sedative doses
Failure to recognize and treat hyperthermia
Failure to rehydrate adequately
Failure to use physostigmine when indicated despite its relative safety and efficacy
Failure to monitor patient closely for repeat doses of physostigmine

Key Points in Anticholinergic Plant Poisoning

1. Anticholinergic plants are used by adolescents and young adults as hallucinogens.
2. Anticholinergic plants may be mistaken for edible berries or foods.
3. Delirium, hallucinations, tachycardia, dry mouth, and mydriasis are the most common clinical effects.
4. Seizures, rhabdomyolysis, respiratory failure, and renal failure are potential serious complications.
5. There is no routinely available diagnostic test to confirm the diagnosis.
6. Physostigmine may be safe and effective therapy.

REFERENCES

1. Greene GS, Patterson SG, Warner E: Ingestion of angel's trumpet: An increasingly common source of toxicity. South Med J 89:365–369, 1996.
2. Müller JL: Love potions and the ointment of witches: Historical aspects of the nightshade alkaloids. J Toxicol Clin Toxicol 36:617–627, 1998.
3. Hanna JP, Schmidley JW, Braselton WE: Datura delirium. Clin Neuropharmacol 15:109–113, 1992.
4. Jennings RE: *Stramonium* poisoning: Review of the literature and report of two cases. J Pediatr 6:657–664, 1935.
5. Aronson SM: The deadly nightshades. Conn Med 59:35–37, 1995.
6. Chan TYK: Anticholinergic poisoning due to Chinese herbal medicines. Vet Hum Toxicol 37:156–157, 1995.
7. Ballantyne A, Lippiett P, Park J: Herbal cigarettes for kicks. BMJ 2:1539–1540, 1976.
8. Hsu CK, Leo P, Shastry D, et al: Anticholinergic poisoning associated with herbal tea. Arch Intern Med 155:2245–2248, 1995.
9. Schneider SM, Krenzelok E: Toxic plant ingestions: Optimizing the course of treatment. Emerg Med Rep 13:141–148, 1992.
10. Schneider F, Lutun P, Kintz P, et al: Plasma and urine concentrations of atropine after the ingestion of cooked deadly nightshade berries. Clin Toxicol 34:113–117, 1996.
11. Spoerke DG, Hall AH, Dodson CD, et al: Mystery root ingestion. J Emerg Med 5:385–388, 1987.
12. Spoerke DG, Hall AH: Plants and mushrooms of abuse. Emerg Med Clin North Am 4:579–593, 1990.
13. Southgate HJ, Egerton M, Dauncey EA: Lessons to be learned: A case study approach. J R Soc Promotion Health 120:127–130, 2000.
14. Rosen CS, Lechner M: Jimson-weed intoxication. N Eng J Med 267:448–450, 1962.
15. Ceha LJ, Presperin C, Young E, et al: Anticholinergic toxicity from nightshade berry poisoning responsive to physostigmine. J Emerg Med 15:65–69, 1997.
16. CDC: Anticholinergic poisoning associated with an herbal tea—New York City, 1994. MMWR Morb Mortal Wkly Rep 44:193–195, 1995.
17. CDC: Jimson weed poisoning—Texas, New York, and California, 1994. MMWR Morb Mortal Wkly Rep 44:41–44, 1995.
18. Litovitz TL, Klein-Schwartz W, Rodgers GC, et al: 2001 Annual report of the American Association of Poison Control Centers Toxic Exposure Surveillance System. Am J Emerg 20:391–452, 2002.
19. Klein-Schwartz W, Oderda GM: Jimsonweed intoxications in adolescents and young adults. Am J Dis Child 138:737–739, 1984.
20. Coremans P, Lambrecht G, Schepens P, et al: Anticholinergic intoxication with commercially available thorn apple tea. Clin Toxicol 32:589–592, 1994.
21. Hall RCW, Popkin MK, McHenry LE: Angel trumpet psychosis: A central nervous system anticholinergic syndrome. Am J Psychiatry 134:312–314, 1977.
22. O'Grady TC, Brown J, Jacamo J: Outbreak of jimson weed abuse among Marine Corps personnel at Camp Pendleton. Milit Med 148:732–734, 1983.
23. Shervette RE, Schydlower M, Lampe RM, et al: Jimson "Loco" weed abuse in adolescents. Pediatrics 63:520–523, 1979.
24. Francis PD, Clarke CF: Angel trumpet lily poisoning in five adolescents: Clinical findings and management. J Paediatr Child Health 35:93–95, 1999.
25. Levy R: Jimson seed poisoning—a new hallucinogen on the horizon. J Am Coll Emerg Physicians 6:58–61, 1977.
26. Mikolich JR, Paulson GW, Cross CJ: Acute anticholinergic syndrome due to jimson seed ingestion: Clinical and laboratory observation in six cases. Ann Intern Med 83:321–325, 1975.
27. Tiongson J, Salen P: Mass ingestion of jimson weed by eleven teenagers. Del Med J 70:471–476, 1998.
28. Rauber-Luthy C, Guirguis M, Meier-Abt AS, et al: Lethal poisoning after ingestion of a tea prepared from the angel's trumpet (*Datura suaveolens*). J Toxicol Clin Toxicol 37:414, 1999.
29. Shenoy RS: Pitfalls in the treatment of jimsonweed intoxication. Am J Psychiatry 151:1396–1397, 1994.
30. Schreiber W: Jimson seed intoxication: recognition and therapy. Milit Med 144:329–336, 1979.
31. Krenzelok EP, Jacobsen TD, Aronis JM: Jimsonweed (*Datura stramonium*) poisoning and abuse: An analysis of 1,458 cases (Abstract). J Toxicol Clin Toxicol 33:500, 1995.
32. Furbee B, Wermuth M: Life-threatening plant poisoning. Med Toxicol 13:849–887, 1997.
33. Urich RW, Bowerman DL, Levisky JA, et al: *Datura stramonium*: A fatal poisoning. J Forensic Sci 27:948–954, 1982.
34. Smidt N, Bieder L, Thomas RG: Datura intoxication. N Z Med J 87:61–62, 1978.
35. Chang TYK, Chan JCN, Tomlinson B, et al: Chinese herbal medicines revisited: A Hong Kong perspective. Lancet 342:1532–1534, 1993.
36. Chang SS, Wu ML, Deng JF, et al: Poisoning by datura leaves used as edible wild vegetables. Vet Hum Toxicol 41:242–245, 1999.
37. Finlay P: Anticholinergic poisoning due to *Datura candida* (Letter). Trop Doctor 28:183–184, 1998.
38. Burkhart KK, Magalski AE, Donovan JW: A retrospective review of the use of activated charcoal and physostigmine in the treatment of jimson weed poisoning. Am J Emerg Med 16:443–447, 1998.
39. Baselt RC, Cravey RH (eds): Disposition of Toxic Drugs and Chemicals in Man, 4th ed. Foster City, CA, Chemical Toxicology Institute, 1995.
40. Voltz R, Hohfeld R, Liebler M, et al: Gardener's mydriasis (Letter). Lancet 339:752, 1992.
41. Burns MJ, Linden CH, Graudins A, et al: A comparison of physostigmine and benzodiazepines for the treatment of anticholinergic poisoning. Ann Emerg Med 35:374–381, 2000.
42. Michalodimitrakis M, Koutselinis A: Discussion of *Datura stramonium*: A fatal poisoning. J Forensic Sci 29:961–962, 1984.
43. Nogue S, Pujol L, Sanz P, et al: *Datura stramonium* poisoning: Identification of tropane alkaloids in urine by gas chromatography–mass spectrometry. J Int Med Res 23:132–137, 1995.
44. Salen P, Shih R, Sierzenski P, Reed J: Effect of physostigmine and gastric lavage in a *Datura stramonium*–induced anticholinergic poisoning epidemic. Am J Emerg Med 21:316–317, 2003.
45. Walker WE, Levy RC, Hanenson IB: Physostigmine—its use and abuse. J Am Coll Emerg Physicians 5:436–439, 1976.
46. Beaver KM, Gavin TJ: Treatment of acute anticholinergic poisoning with physostigmine. Am J Emerg Med 16:505–507, 1998.
47. Cheng SW, Hu WH, Hung DZ, et al: Anticholinergic poisoning from a large dose of scopolia extract. Vet Hum Toxicol 44:222–223, 2002.
48. O'Donnell SJ, Burkhart KK, Donovan JW, Holland MJ: Safety of physostigmine use for anticholinergic toxicity. J Toxicol Clin Toxicol 40:684, 2002.

CHAPTER 127

Toxalbumins

Melissa DiIanni Lee ■ Richard Y. Wang

Toxalbumins are complex proteins found in certain plant species that are toxic when ingested or administered parenterally. The most common plants containing toxalbumins are *Ricinus communis, Abrus precatorius*, and *Robinia pseudoacacia*. Although *R. communis* and *A. precatorius* concentrate the toxin within their seeds, the toxic lectins of *R. pseudoacacia* are found in the bark, seeds, leaves, and roots of the plant. The toxalbumins are summarized in Table 127-1.

RICINUS COMMUNIS (CASTOR BEAN)

R. communis is native to Mexico and Africa and is cultivated in the southern temperate regions of the United States for castor oil. These large, leafy plants can grow 10 to 12 feet and produce brown capsules, each containing three hard, shiny, almond-colored seeds (Fig. 127-1). The seed is composed of three components: oil, which contains ricinoleic acid; pulp, which is rich in glycoproteins; and fibrous portion, which contains the toxalbumin ricin.

Stillmark, who found that the seed extract caused red blood cell agglutination, originally identified ricin in 1888. Ricin toxin gained notoriety in 1978, when a Bulgarian writer for the British Broadcasting Company, Georgi Markov, was fatally stabbed in the thigh with the point of an umbrella at a bus stop near Waterloo Bridge. On autopsy, in Markov's leg, a small, perforated, metallic pellet was found that presumably contained ricin toxin.[1] Also that year, a second Bulgarian émigré is said to have experienced a similar attack, with a ricin pellet removed from his skin.[2]

R. communis is grown in ornamental gardens and as a houseplant but is cultivated primarily for the production of castor oil, with more than 1 million tons of seeds harvested each year.[3,4] The seeds also are incorporated into necklaces, rosaries, and other decorative items imported from South America and Africa.[5,6] Most cases of ricin poisoning result from children accidentally ingesting these colorful beans.[1]

Castor seeds have been used for centuries in the treatment of various medical conditions. Some cultures have used this seed to treat leprosy, to treat syphilis, or as a cathartic. Modern medicine has experimented with ricin in pain control and in the prevention of graft-versus-host disease.[7]

Because ricin is one of the most potent poisons in the plant kingdom, it has been produced by governments for use in biologic weapons.[2,8,9] In 1989, 10 L of concentrated ricin was made in Iraq for payload in artillery shells.[9] Owing to this threat, the United States Army Medical Research Institute of Infectious Disease, congressional hearings, and government warnings have implicated ricin as a potential biologic warfare agent.

ABRUS PRECATORIUS

A. precatorius is a green vine native to India, South America, Florida, and the Caribbean. This vine produces light purple or white flowers and 3-cm-long pods each containing three to five oval, hard, glossy seeds approximately 5 mm in diameter. The seeds may be red with a black center, black with a white center, or white with a black center (Fig. 127-2). *Abrus* seeds, also called *jequirity pea, Indian bean, crab's eye, rosary pea, and Buddhist's rosary*, are used primarily in ornaments, jewelry, and other decor. The bean contains *N*-methyltryptophan, abric acid, and the toxin abrin.[5,1]

ROBINIA PSEUDOACACIA (BLACK LOCUST TREE)

R. pseudoacacia, commonly known as the *black locust tree*, grows to 30 m tall and 3 m in diameter and has deeply furrowed bark that is gray on the outside and creamy yellow on the inside. This tree is native to the U.S. Appalachian and Ozark Mountains, Canada, and Mexico. The genus *Robinia* originally was named after Jean Robin, the herbalist to the kings of France during the 16th century who introduced this hardwood to Europe. Because of the strong bark, these trees are used primarily for furniture, mine timbers, boat ribs, fencing, and strip mine reclamation. The Cherokee Indians used this plant as a purgative, as a laxative, and for toothaches. The bark and roots contain five major flavonoids, including the toxalbumin robin.[10]

BIOCHEMISTRY AND PHARMACOLOGY

The toxalbumins ricin, abrin, and robin destroy cells by inactivating eukaryotic ribosomes. Their structure, similar to those of botulinum, tetanus, diphtheria, and cholera toxins, consists of two subunits that, in the case of ricin and abrin, are joined by a disulfide bond. Ricin has a total weight of 66 kd divided into a 34-kd B subunit and a 32-kd A subunit. The B subunit binds to glycoproteins on the surface of the cell, enabling the toxin to enter, then the A subunit depurinates

TABLE 127-1 Toxalbumins

SCIENTIFIC NAME	COMMON NAME	TOXIN	LOCATION OF TOXIN	GEOGRAPHY	SYMPTOMS
Abrus precatorius	Crab's eye, jequirity bean, rosary pea	Abrin	Seeds	India, South America, Florida, Caribbean	GI, pulmonary, shock
Ricinus communis	Castor bean plant, mole bean	Ricin	Seeds	Mexico, Africa, southern United States	GI, pulmonary, shock
Robinia pseudoacacia	Black locust	Robin, phasin	Bark, leaves, buds	United States, Canada, Mexico	GI, CNS
Jatropha multifida	Coral plant, physic nut	Ricin	Seeds, fruit	Mexico, Brazil, Central America, Florida	GI
Jatropha curcas	Barbados nut, curcas bean	Curcin	Seeds, fruit	India, Central America, South America	GI
Hura crepitans	Sandbox tree, monkey's dinner bell	Hurin	Bark juice, seeds	South America, Central America	GI, blindness

CNS, central nervous system; GI, gastrointestinal.
Adapted from references 30–35.

residues on the robosomal RNA, ultimately inhibiting protein synthesis, adenosine triphosphate depletion, and finally cell death.[1,5,11–14] A total of 108 ricin molecules can bind per cell, but less than 10 molecules are needed to induce cell death.[13]

R. communis has two toxins in the fibrous portion of its seed: *R. communis* agglutinin and ricin, each with 66-kd domains.[4] In contrast to ricin, *R. communis* agglutinin is a weak cytotoxin but a powerful hemagglutinin that is not absorbed enterally, but intravenous administration can result in red blood cell agglutination hemolysis.[13]

Abrin is a water-soluble mixture of five complex toxic proteins labeled α-1, α-2, α-3, β-1, and β-2. The α-3 fraction, composed primarily of cystine, methionine, and tyrosine amino acids, is the most toxic, producing 100% mortality at a dose comparable to the median lethal dose (LD_{50}) of unfractionated abrin aqueous extract.[15] Table 127-2 lists the LD_{50} of the toxalbumins.

tional or injection exposures are possible, particularly in the setting of biologic warfare or homicide. Hypersensitivity reactions can occur by either inhaled or dermal exposure to the seed's pulp.

Oral ingestion of abrin and ricin can produce biphasic toxicity. The first, or local, phase starts with corrosive burns in the oropharyngeal mucosa, producing lesions resembling alkali burns within hours of ingestion.[8,16] After 2 to 24 hours, many patients develop nausea, vomiting, diarrhea with or without hematochezia, and colicky abdominal pain. Challoner and McCarron,[17] in a review of documented ricin ingestions, found that most patients experienced primarily gastrointestinal complaints (Table 127-3). The second phase of toxicity, the systemic phase, is characterized by hypovolemic shock and multiorgan involvement. In a study of 424 cases of castor bean ingestion, 14 developed fatal hypovolemic shock from intestinal fluid losses.[5] Liver failure can result from direct hepatotoxicity and shock liver.[1,13,18,19] Hemolysis, kidney failure,

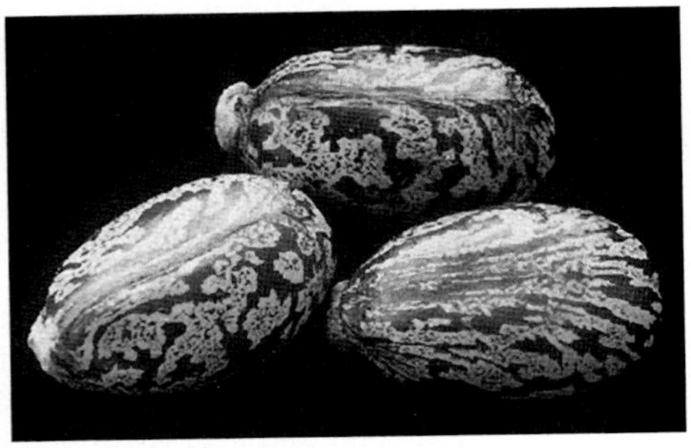

CLINICAL PRESENTATION

The clinical presentation of abrin and ricin toxicity depends on the route and magnitude of exposure. The most common route is oral, by accidental ingestion of ornamental or jewelry beans or eating seeds found along the beach. Inhala-

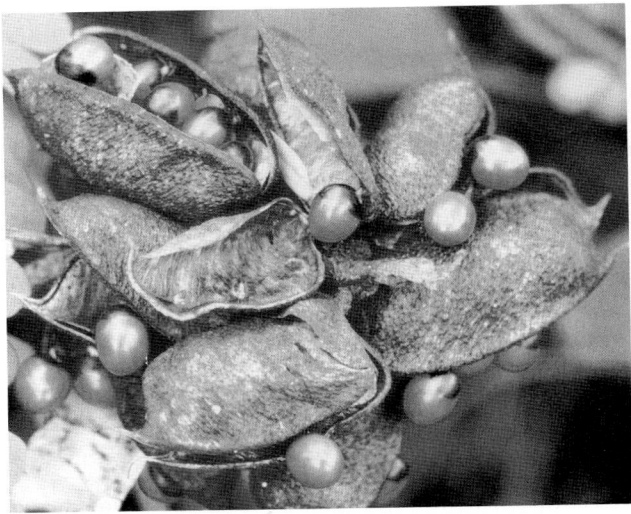

FIGURE 127-1

Ricinus communis seeds. *(From New Leaf Graphics, Port St. Lucie, FL.)*

FIGURE 127-2

Abrus precatorius seeds. *(From New Leaf Graphics, Port St. Lucie, FL.)* See Color Fig. 127-2.

TABLE 127-2 Comparative Median Lethal Dose of Toxins in Laboratory Mice

TOXIN	MEDIAN LETHAL DOSE (μg/kg, IV)
Botulinum	0.001
Tetanus	0.002
Abrin	0.04
Ricin	3
Ricin (inhaled)	3–5
Sarin	100

IV, intravenous.

Adapted from Eitzen E (ed): Medical Management of Biological Casualties Handbook, 3rd ed. Fort Detrick Frederick, MD, United States Army Medical Research Institute of Infectious Disease, 1998.

splenic necrosis, seizures, and cardiac arrhythmias have been described.[1,4,16,19,20]

Variations of this biphasic presentation have occurred, with case reports of only mild gastroenteritis and one case of an infant developing fulminant liver failure without previous gastrointestinal manifestations.[18,19] Which patients progress to the second phase of toxicity is difficult to predict on the basis of the number of seeds ingested; however, patients who have 3 to 4 days of progressive diarrhea and large fluid losses are more likely to develop shock.[1,5,17]

Inhalational exposures, primarily in settings of biologic warfare, produce a different presentation. Based on data collected during a sublethal accidental aerosol exposure in the 1940s, fever, cough, dyspnea, chest tightness, and arthralgias develop after 4 to 8 hours. Development of profuse sweating is usually the hallmark of resolution.[4] In animals exposed to large doses, noncardiogenic pulmonary edema develops, with death occurring due to hypoxia in 36 to 72 hours.[8]

Injection of crystalline or liquid abrin and ricin can produce local pain, mild dyspnea, and cough or wheeze. Progression to multiorgan failure and death can occur.[4,13]

Ingestion of *R. pseudoacacia* bark results primarily in gastroenteritis, similar to that described for ricin and abrin.

TABLE 127-3 Frequency of Symptoms after Ricin Ingestion, 1900–1985

SYMPTOM	CASES (%)
Vomiting	84
Diarrhea	83
Dehydration	35
Shock	27
Abdominal pain	13
Diarrhea with bleeding	3
Abnormal kidney function	9
Abnormal liver function tests	5
Hemolysis	3

Adapted from Challoner KR, McCannon MM: Castor bean intoxication. Ann Emerg Med 19:1177–1183, 1990.

Some reports of central nervous system involvement have been described. In accidental ingestion by two horses, one showed alternating phases of somnolence and excitation, mydriasis, and decreased sensation to the head.[21] Vertigo, muscle twitches, cardiac arrhythmia, and weakness also have been described.[10,22]

Hypersensitivity reactions to *R. communis* seeds have been well described in response to contact and inhalational exposures. Garcia-Gonzalez and colleagues[23] showed the role of *R. communis* as a pneumoallergen, causing primarily respiratory and nasal symptoms. In sensitized industrial castor bean workers, allergic dermatitis, rhinitis, asthma, and anaphylaxis have been recognized.[5] One representative case report described facial itching and periorbital edema with complete eyelid closure and urticarial wheals after touching the powder in a broken ricin bean from a necklace.[24] Diagnosis depends primarily on history of exposure and is important for the avoidance of subsequent, more severe anaphylactic reactions.

PATHOPHYSIOLOGY

The effects of ricin and abrin exposure can range from mild gastroenteritis to multiorgan failure and death. The type and severity of a patient's response depend on the method of exposure—ingestion, inhalation, or injection. Each can evoke specific early symptoms, but all can result in multisystem failure.

When ricin is injected intramuscularly, local necrosis of the soft tissue or regional lymph nodes can occur. If the toxin is absorbed systemically or injected intravenously, however, multiorgan failure can ensue. *R. communis* agglutinin causes hemagglutination and intravascular hemolysis by binding to glycoproteins on red blood cells.[6] The by-products of hemolysis can crystallize in the kidney's tubules, resulting in acute renal failure. Ricin can bind and damage the lung's vascular endothelium, resulting in noncardiogenic pulmonary edema and hypoxia. Fulminant liver failure may result from direct hepatotoxicity or indirectly from hypovolemic shock.[18,19] In vitro experiments with mice have shown that peritoneal injection of ricin at low doses results in multifocal necrosis in parenchymal organs, and larger doses produce hemorrhage in visceral and serous cavities with subsequent death from organ failure and shock.[13]

Ingestion of ricin, abrin, or robin can result in a syndrome similar to that of *Shigella sonnei* and *Escherichia coli* 0157:H7. Direct toxin contact with the gastrointestinal mucosa causes corrosive burns and gut endothelial damage, resulting in ulceration and seepage of fluid, blood, and cells.[1,11,17] The ensuing bowel wall edema and decreased intestinal absorption can lead to diarrhea, dehydration, and hypovolemic shock. When systemic, these toxins can cause direct cytotoxicity to any organ—damage to the pancreas, spleen, liver, heart, and kidney.[1,4–6,11]

Inhalation of ricin is another method of exposure that is potentially dangerous. The airways may develop necrotizing lesions resulting in tracheitis, bronchitis, bronchiolitis, or interstitial pneumonia. These conditions can progress to perivascular and alveolar edema and subsequent hypoxia requiring mechanical ventilation.[4,19]

LETHALITY

Compared with other well-known poisons, ricin and abrin are highly lethal, with a mortality rate of 8.1% in untreated symptomatic patients.[17] Specifically, ricin is 6000 times more poisonous than cyanide and 12,000 times more poisonous than rattlesnake venom.[6] Intravenous administration can produce death more quickly and at lower doses than can ingestion or inhalation.

For oral administration, data have been variable on the number of seeds required for serious sequelae. Eight to 20 ricin seeds in adults and 3 seeds in children have been reported to produce death.[5,6,19] In one case report, a patient swallowed more than 30 ricin seeds and survived, whereas other authors have reported ingestions of 3 berries that resulted only in a mild gastroenteritis.[17,19] This variability in toxicity may depend on how well masticated the bean is, whether the patient has developed immunity, or possible variation in bean toxin concentration in different climates. Animal models have provided quantitative data for ricin toxicity. In cattle, 0.2% of body weight in seeds can prove lethal; 0.01% can be lethal in horses.[20] *Abrus* seeds have been reported to be more potent, with only one seed required for a lethal dose, corresponding to 0.00015% of body weight.[25] For ricin and abrin, only one seed is necessary to produce severe anaphylaxis in sensitized individuals.[12]

When lyphophilized into a powder, ricin toxin can be inhaled. The aerosolized dose that was fatal in 50% of exposed mice (LD_{50}) is 3 to 5 μg/kg. Based on this, 8 tons of toxin would have to be produced and deployed to affect significantly a human population living in an area of 100 km².

Injectable forms of ricin and abrin are available when prepared in a liquid or crystallized form. In vitro experiments with mice show that the LD_{50} for intraperitoneal administration of ricin and abrin are 100 ng and 40 ng, producing death within days. Subcutaneous administration of 0.13 to 0.2 mg of abrin into mice resulted in death within 24 to 48 hours, and 0.2 mL can induce red blood cell agglutination.[15] Because a lethal dose of these toxins can be delivered in a small concentration, there is concern for their homicidal potential.

DIAGNOSIS

Diagnosis of toxalbumin intoxication depends primarily on the history of illness. If the patient presents with the beans for identification, protective gloves should be used when handling these seeds to avoid possible contact dermatitis. There are many causes of bloody and nonbloody diarrhea, so exposure to these seeds is important to document. Because of this difficulty, the diagnosis often is delayed or not made correctly at all.[5,8] Serum and tissue polymerase chain reaction tests are marketed, although not widely available, for patients suspected of having been exposed to ricin toxin. Within 18 to 24 hours of ingestion, the toxin assay can be applied to nasal swab; serum; or spleen, lung, and kidney tissue. After 36 hours, acute and convalescent serum antibodies can be measured.[4,6]

TREATMENT

If only one or two castor beans have been ingested, we believe that discharge is reasonable if the patient is asymptomatic after a 4- to 6-hour observation period. If more than two seeds were eaten or if symptoms have developed, the patient should be admitted. Because of abrin's higher potency, any amount of oral exposure to this seed is potentially lethal, and patients should be admitted.

If a patient presents within 2 hours of oral ingestion, gastric decontamination with activated charcoal may be helpful and should be administered. If diarrhea already has started, cathartics should be withheld.[5,6] It is unknown whether activated charcoal administration affects outcome or alters the clinical course. Whole-bowel irrigation after *Abrus* ingestion has not been shown to be helpful, although this has not been studied extensively.[6] Abrin-induced caustic buccal lesions can be treated symptomatically with topical anesthetics.[16]

Supportive measures are the mainstay of treatment of abrin, robin, or ricin toxicity. Aggressive fluid resuscitation should be started as early as possible for treatment of dehydration and prevention of hypovolemic shock and pigment-mediated acute tubular necrosis. Admitted patients should be observed for 24 to 48 hours for evidence of hypovolemia, hepatotoxicity, renal failure, and hemolysis with daily or twice-daily laboratory evaluation. For inhalational exposure, the patient's respiratory status and pulse oximetry should be monitored. Patients with diarrhea persisting for more than 3 to 4 days, hepatotoxicity, or respiratory compromise should be monitored in an intensive care unit. Patients who have been injected with ricin or abrin have a higher risk for systemic toxicity and should be monitored in an intensive care unit. Hypovolemic shock should be treated with intravenous colloid or crystalloid resuscitation and vasopressor support if necessary. Pulmonary edema may require intubation and mechanical ventilation. Owing to toxin-induced arrhythmias, continuous cardiac monitoring should be employed. Brisk urine output should be maintained to prevent acute tubular necrosis. In the setting of massive intravascular hemolysis, urinary alkalinization, with a goal urinary pH of 6 of 7, and aggressive fluid management should be started to avoid hemoglobin precipitation and schistocyte-mediated renal tubular damage.[26,27] There are no data to support the use of loop diuretics, atrial natriuretic peptide, or mannitol in the treatment of heme compound–induced acute tubular necrosis. Low-dose dopamine (3 to 5 μg/kg/min) can improve renal blood flow and glomerular filtration rate, but prospective controlled

Indications for ICU Admission in Toxalbumin Poisoning

Significant hepatotoxicity
Diarrhea for >3 to 4 days with dehydration
Respiratory distress, failure, or significant hypoxia
Exposure by injection
Shock
Massive hemolysis

trials have not shown this to alter the course of or prevent ischemic or nephrotoxic acute tubular necrosis.[27,28] Dialysis may be required if uremia or refractory acidosis ensues.

Ricin and abrin are water soluble and excreted by the liver; consequently, hemodialysis or forced diuresis does not promote elimination. An antidote in the form of a monoclonal antibody to the ricin A chain has been manufactured but is not available. Other therapies have been studied on mice, including dexamethasone and the antioxidant vitamin E. Although neither agent prevented death, both extended survival time and may be considered in the management of ricin toxicity. Nucleoside analogues, including acyclovir, potentiate the toxicity of ricin in mice.[29]

SPECIAL POPULATIONS

Pediatric Patients

- Incidence of toxalbumin exposure is higher among children, given their attraction to the decorative, colorful beans.
- Caustic alkaline oral mucosa burns seen with ricin exposure resemble viral exanthems and may be misdiagnosed easily.
- As a result of the higher respiratory rate seen in children, an aerosolized ricin exposure may deliver a higher toxin dosage and increase the risk of pulmonary manifestations.
- Children may progress to hypovolemic shock more readily than adults after gastrointestinal fluid losses.

Key Points in Toxalbumin Poisoning

1. The most common route of toxicity is accidental ingestion; intravenous delivery can produce death more quickly and at lower doses.
2. Diagnosis of toxalbumin toxicity is primarily by history.
3. Hypersensitivity reactions have been described for dermal and inhalational exposures.
4. Gastroenteritis, after seed ingestion, is the most common and usually the first symptom; multiorgan failure can ensue.
5. Supportive measures are the mainstay of treatment.

REFERENCES

1. Goldfrank LR (ed): Goldfrank's Toxicologic Emergencies, 6th ed. Stamford, CT, Appelton & Lange, 1998, pp 1254–1259.
2. Simon J: Biological terrorism: Preparing to meet the threat. JAMA 278:428–430, 1997.
3. Brown D: *Ricinus communis* (castor bean). Available at: http://www.ansci.cornell.edu/plants/castorbean/html. Accessed November 11, 2000.
4. Eitzen E (ed): Medical Management of Biological Casualties Handbook, 3rd ed. Fort Detrick Frederick, MD, United States Army Medical Research Institute of Infectious Disease, 1998.
5. Ellenhorn MJ (ed): Ellenhorn's Medical Toxicology, 2nd ed. Baltimore, Williams & Wilkins, 1997, pp 1847–1859.
6. NPS Herbs: Castor bean. Available at: http://www.ny2aap.org/npsherbs.html. Accessed November 20, 2000.
7. Friedrich MJ: Loss of nerve: A molecular approach to better treatment of chronic pain. JAMA 283:187–188, 2000.
8. Committee on Environmental Health and Committee on Infectious Disease: Chemical biological terrorism and its impact on children: A subject review. Pediatrics 105:662–670, 2000.
9. Zilinskas RA: Iraq's biological weapons: The past or future. JAMA 278:418–424, 1997.
10. Duke JA: *Robinia pseudoacacia L.* 1983. Available at: http://www.hort.purdue.edu/newcrop/duke_energy/Robinia_pseudoacacia.html. Accessed March 27, 2000.
11. Heyworth MF: Pathogenesis of bacterial colitis (Letter). Gut 36:154–155, 1995.
12. Nobukazu K, Masami N, Tatsuya O, et al: Depletion of intracellular NAD$^+$ and ATP levels during ricin-induced apoptosis through the specific ribosomal inactivation results in the cytolysis of U937 cells. J Biochem 128:463–470, 2000.
13. Olsnes S, Refsnes K, Pihl A: Mechanism of action of the toxic lectins abrin and ricin. Nature 249:627–631, 1974.
14. Endo Y, Mitsui K, Motizuki M, et al: The mechanism of action of ricin and related toxic lectins on eukaryotic ribosomes: The site and the characteristics of the modification in 28 S ribosomal RNA caused by the toxins. J Biol Chem 262:5908–5912, 1987.
15. Niyogi SK: The toxicology of *Abrus precatorius linnaeus*. J Forensic Sci 15:529–536, 1970.
16. Haddad L: Clinical Management of Poisoning and Drug Overdose, 3rd ed. Philadelphia, Saunders, 1998, 376–387.
17. Challoner KR, McCarron MM: Castor bean intoxication. Ann Emerg Med 19:1177–1183, 1990.
18. Palatnick W, Tenenbein M: Hepatotoxicity from castor bean ingestion in a child. J Toxicol 38:67–69, 2000.
19. Mera V: Traveller's diarrhoea (Letter). Lancet 356:1446, 2000.
20. Williams M: Castor bean (*Ricinus communis*). 1996. Available at: http://www.library.uiuc.edu/vex/toxic/castor/castor5.htm. Accessed November 20, 2000.
21. Landolt G, Feige K, Schoeberl M: Poisoning due to the bark of *Robinia pseudoacacia* in two horses. Schweiz Arch Tierheilkd 139:363–366, 1997.
22. Black locust (*Robinia pseudoacacia*). Available at: http://www.ansci.cornell.edu/courses/as625/1997term/Kevin/black11.htm. Accessed March 27, 2001.
23. Garcia-Gonzalez JJ, Bartolome-Zavala B, DelMar Trigo-Perez M, et al: Pollinosis to *Ricinus communis*: An aerobiological, clinical and immunochemical study. Clin Exp Allergy 29:1265–1275, 1999.
24. Lockey SD: Anaphylaxis from an Indian necklace (Letter). JAMA 206:2900, 1968.
25. Munro D: *Abrus precatorius* poisoning. 1996. Available at: http://res.agr.ca/cgi-bin/brd/poisonpl/ddplant5?plant=abrus+precatorius&info=all&name=sci. Accessed November 20, 2000.
26. Vanholder R, Sukuru Sever Y, Ekrem E, et al: Rhabdomyolysis. J Am Soc Nephrol 11:1553–1561, 2000.
27. Bone RC (ed): Bone's Pulmonary and Critical Care Medicine. St Louis, Mosby, 1998.
28. Brenner B (ed): Brenner and Rector's the Kidney, 6th ed. Philadelphia, WB Saunders, 2000.
29. Muldoon DF, Stohs SJ: Modulation of ricin toxicity in mice by biologically active substances. J Appl Toxicol 14:81–86, 1994.
30. Ahmed OM, Adam SE: Toxicity of *Jatropha curcas* in sheep and goats. Res Vet Sci 27:89–96, 1979.
31. Floridata: *Jatropha multifida*. 2000. Available at: http://www.florida.com/ref/j/jatr_mul.cfm. Accessed March 27, 2001.
32. Duke JA (1983) Jatropha curcas L. http://www.hort.purdue.edu/newcrop/duke_energy/Jatropha_curcas.html (27 March 2001)
33. Clarke JH (2000) Hura crepitans. http://www.homeoint.org/clarke/h/hura_cre.htm (29 March 2001)
34. Levin Y, Sherer Y, Bibi H, et al.: Rare Jatropha multifida intoxication in two children, J. Emer Med 19(2):173–5, 2000.
35. Abdu-Aguye I, Sannusi A, Alafiya-Tayo RA, et al: Acute toxicity studies with *Jatropha curcas L.* Hum Toxicol 5:269–274, 1986.

CHAPTER **128**

Botulism

Hernan F. Gomez

The toxin produced by the spore-forming bacterial organism *Clostridium botulinum* is one of the deadliest poisons known to humans.[1,2] Ingestion of minute amounts of botulinum toxin may result in respiratory failure and death by muscular paralysis. It has been encountered commonly as a cause of food poisoning (other forms of botulism are outlined subsequently).[3] The potential use of botulinum toxin as a biologic weapon has been highlighted as a major public health concern[4,5]; this is due in part to the remarkable resilience and potency of this toxin. It is estimated that 1 g of evenly dispersed and inhaled crystalline botulinum toxin in a major urban center could kill more than 1 million people.[5,6] Botulism is characterized by four distinct presentations: (1) foodborne (classic), (2) wound, (3) infant, and (4) undetermined[1,7] All forms of botulism are characterized by toxin-induced neuromuscular paralysis, potentially resulting in death.[1,7]

Botulism received its name from the Latin term *botulus*, which means "sausage," because many early cases of this disease occurred from the consumption of contaminated blood sausages.[1,8] The elucidation of the etiology and scientific basis of botulism began in the 19th century when Van Ermengem isolated the clostridial organism responsible for botulism.[1,8] His investigative efforts were conducted as a response to an epidemic of botulism in a group of musicians at a funeral in 1896 in Belgium.[3,8] As a result of his investigations, the organism, the toxin, and the observation that the illness is toxin mediated were established.[3,8]

Most preserved foods have been implicated in foodborne botulism, but the usual offenders are foods with a low acid content (pH ≥ 6.0), such as home-canned vegetables.[9] Home-canned fruits containing citric acid provide a less conducive environment for spore and toxin production. The spores of *C. botulinum* are heat resistant and can withstand 100°C for hours,[1] although 30 minutes of moist heat at 120°C heat usually destroys them.[10] The toxins are heat labile and can be destroyed by boiling for 10 minutes or heating at 80°C for 30 minutes.[1,10] Changes in the epidemiology of botulism have emerged in the past few decades.[7] More recently identified vehicles for foodborne botulism include baked potatoes sealed in aluminum foil,[11] homemade salsa,[12] cheese sauce,[13] and sautéed onions held under a layer of butter.[14] From 1976 through 1984, restaurant-associated outbreaks accounted for a large proportion of botulism cases.[7,15] Food sources for some of the largest restaurant-related outbreaks include jalapeno peppers in Michigan in 1977[16] and potato salad in New Mexico in 1978.[16]

In 1950, the U.S. Centers for Disease Control and Prevention (CDC) began surveillance of this disease. Infant botulism originally was described in 1976 and is currently the most common form of this illness.[17] From 1973 through 1996, more than 2310 cases of botulism were reported to the CDC in the United States.[7] These include 724 cases of foodborne botulism (median 24 cases annually), 103 cases of wound botulism (median 3 cases annually), 1444 cases of infant botulism (median 71 cases annually), and 39 cases of botulism of undetermined etiology (Fig. 128-1).[7]

CHEMISTRY AND BIOCHEMISTRY

At least seven serologically distinct but structurally similar types of botulinum toxin have been described: A, B, C, D, E, F, and G. The nucleotide sequences for all seven toxin types have been sequenced.[7,18–26] These types are defined by the International Standards for botulinum antitoxin.[27] Serotypes A, B, E, and F affect humans, whereas types C and D cause illness in other animals.[1,2] Type G has not been established as a cause of either human or animal disease.[9] Most botulism cases in the continental United States have resulted from either serotype A or serotype B strains. In the United States, type A botulinum toxin is found predominantly west of the Mississippi River,[14] whereas type B is more common in the eastern states.[28] Alaskan foodborne outbreaks have resulted from type E stains in Native American foods (e.g., "fermented whale blubber").[29] Type E is found in association with seafood products and is implicated more frequently in areas with higher rates of fish and marine mammal consumption.[30] Botulism outbreaks can occur anywhere around the world and have been reported in a variety of countries, such as Iran, the former Soviet Union, Japan, France, Belgium, and Portugal.[10,31] Type B is found most commonly in all European countries except the Baltic states, where type E is the most common form.[10,31,32] Overall the botulinum serotype distribution implicated in disease outbreaks is similar to the endogenous spore types.[33]

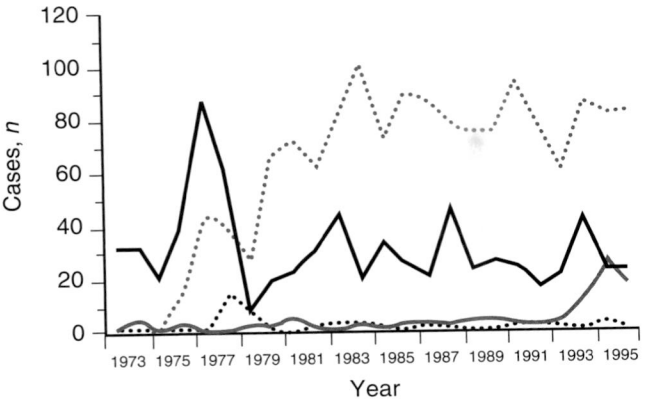

FIGURE 128-1

Annual incidence of botulism in the United States, 1973 to 1996. The line interspersed with dots indicates botulism in infants, the solid line indicates foodborne botulism, the short-dashed line indicates wound botulism, and the long-dashed line indicates botulism from an undetermined source. *(From Shapiro RL, Hatheway C, Swerdlow DL: Botulism in the United States: A clinical and epidemiologic review. Ann Intern Med 129:211–225, 1998.)*

Botulinum toxin is a protein consisting of a single polypeptide chain, with a molecular weight of 900 kd, including the nontoxic protein hemagglutinin and the active neurotoxic 150-kd component.[34] The toxin binds rapidly and irreversibly to a specific cell membrane receptor on the nerve terminal at the neuromuscular junction and at peripheral ganglia.[34] To become fully active, the single-chain molecule must be cleaved to generate a 100-kd heavy chain joined to a 50-kd light chain by a disulfide bond (Fig. 128-2).[35] The dichain form of the molecule is responsible for its toxicity and for the therapeutic benefits of selective administration by local injection.[36]

Pharmacokinetics of *Clostridium Botulinum* Toxins

Volume of distribution: unknown
Protein binding: irreversible binding to presynaptic nerve terminals
Incubation period: generally 12–36 hours (initial symptoms reported up to 96 hours)
Half-life: unknown—reportedly detectable in circulation for weeks
Mechanism of clearance: unknown
Active metabolites: none
Methods to enhance clearance: adsorbed to activated charcoal

PATHOPHYSIOLOGY OF THERAPEUTIC AND TOXIC EFFECTS

The main site of action of botulism toxin is the neuromuscular junction, where it binds and inhibits the release of acetylcholine.[34,37] The pathogenesis of clinical botulism begins when the dichain form of the protein enters the junctional nerve terminal by endocytosis (see Fig. 128-2).[34,37]

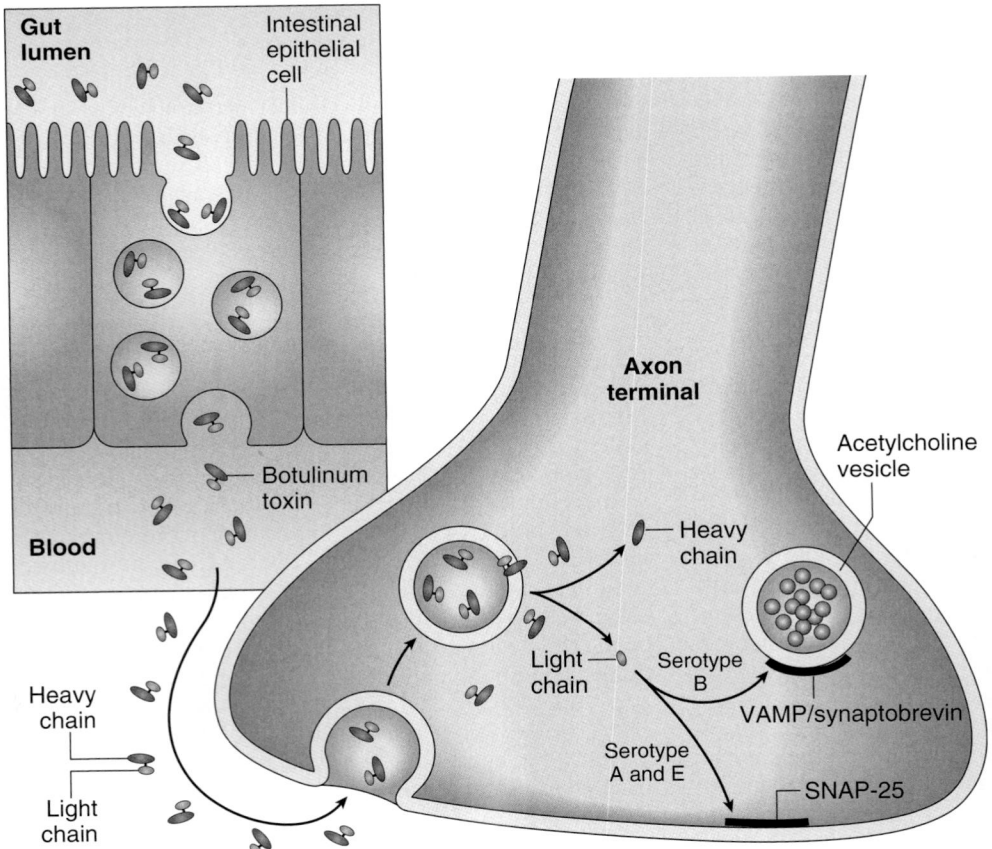

FIGURE 128-2

The potency of botulinum toxin is linked to the ease with which it passes from the gut into the circulation. Receptor-mediated membrane transport depends on the toxin's heavy chain. The enzymatically active part of the molecule is the light chain. The various serotypes have different substrates. Type B cleaves VAMP/synaptobrevin, a polypeptide associated with acetylcholine storage vesicles. Type A and type E cleave SNAP-25, a component of the neuronal membrane. Both polypeptides are essential for exocytosis of acetylcholine. *(From Simpson LL: Botulinum toxin: Potent poison, potent medicine. Hosp Pract (Off Ed) 34:87–91, 1999.)*

Receptor-mediated membrane transport depends on the toxin's heavy chain.[34,37] Internalization of the catalytic portion of the toxin molecule (residing in the light chain) occurs with subsequent cleavage of protein components of the calcium-dependent acetylcholine neuroexocytosis apparatus.[34,37] The various serotypes act on different substrates. Serotype B cleaves VAMP/synaptobrevin, a polypeptide associated with acetylcholine storage vesicles, and serotypes A and E cleave SNAP-25, a component of the neuronal membrane (see Fig. 128-2).[38,39] Ultimately the presynaptic release of acetylcholine is inhibited at all acetylcholine-dependent synapses in the peripheral nervous system.[34] There is no effect on the central nervous system or on axonal conducton.[34,40] Mental status is unaffected.

The recovery period is variable and is directly related to the extent of the neuromuscular blockade and nerve ending and presynaptic membrane regeneration rates.[40]

CLINICAL PRESENTATION AND LIFE-THREATENING COMPLICATIONS

Botulism is characterized by an acute, afebrile, symmetric, descending flaccid paralysis that always begins in bulbar musculature.[41,42] It should be suspected in a patient who presents with acute onset of gastrointestinal, autonomic, and cranial nerve dysfunction (Table 128-1 and Fig. 128-3).[1,17,35,43] The

TABLE 128-1 Symptoms and Physical Findings of Botulism

FOODBORNE	TYPE A*	TYPE B*	P VALUE†	Type A or B‡ (%)
Symptoms				
Neurologic				
Dysphagia	24/25	28/29	NS	96
Dry mouth	15/18	25/25	NS	93
Diplopis	18/20	24/26	NS	91
Dysarthria	26/26	20/29	0.002	84
Upper extremity weakness	18/21	18/28	NS	73
Lower extremity weakness	16/21	18/28	NS	69
Blurred vision	16/16	10/24	<0.001	65
Dyspnea	21/23	10/29	<0.001	60
Paresthesia	2/10	3/25	NS	14
Gastrointestinal				
Constipation	8/11	19/26	NS	73
Nausea	16/22	16/28	NS	64
Vomiting	16/23	14/28	NS	59
Abdominal cramps	4/12	11/24	NS	42
Diarrhea	6/17	2/26	0.04	19
Miscellaneous				
Fatigue	12/13	18/26	NS	77
Sore throat	12/16	9/23	0.05	54
Dizziness	12/14	7/23	0.002	51
Physical Findings				
Upper extremity weakness	21/23	18/29	0.02	75
Ptosis	22/23	16/29	0.001	73
Lower extremity weakness	18/22	17/29	NS	69
Hypoactive gag reflex	17/21	15/28	NS	65
Extraocular muscle weakness	20/23	13/28	0.003	65
Facial nerve dysfunction	16/19	13/27	0.02	63
Tongue weakness	20/22	8/26	<0.001	58
Pupils fixed or dilated	6/18	10/18	NS	44
Nystagmus	8/18	1/23	0.005	22
Ataxia	4/17	3/24	NS	17
Initial mental status				
Alert	22/25	25/27	NS	90
Lethargic	1/25	1/27	NS	4
Obtunded	2/25	1/27	NS	6
Deep tendon reflexes				
Normal	8/24	20/28	0.01	54
Hypoactive or absent	13/24	8/28	NS	40
Hyperactive	3/24	0/28	NS	6

*Number of patients with symptoms or findings per number in whom data were available.
†NS, not significant.
‡Percent of patients with symptoms or findings.
Data from botulism reported in the United States in 1973–1974. Adapted from Hughes JM, Blumenthal JR, Merson MH, et al: Clinical features of types A and B food-borne botulism. Ann Intern Med 95:442–445, 1981.

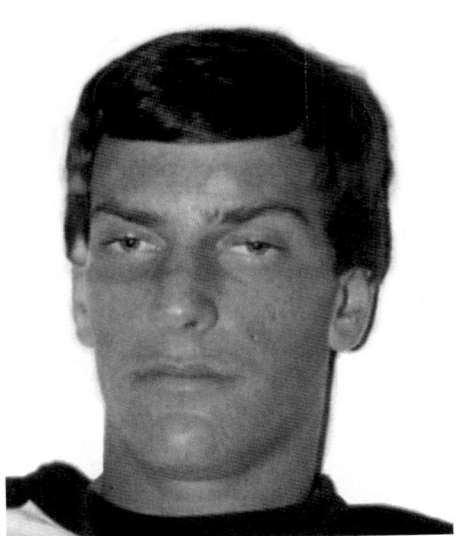

FIGURE 128-3

Patient at rest. Note bilateral mild ptosis, dilated pupils, disconjugate gaze, and symmetric facial muscles. *(From Arnon SS, Schechter R, Inglesby TV, et al: Botulinum toxin as a biological weapon: Medical and public health management. JAMA 285:1062, 2001.)*

patient frequently presents with visual complaints and difficulty speaking or swallowing (see Table 128-1).[1,40,43] Additional common complaints in the initial presentation of foodborne botulism include constipation, dry or sore mouth and throat, difficulty with visual accommodation, dysphonia, and diplopia.[1,10,43] The diagnosis is even more likely if the patient has recently eaten home-canned foods and if family members or companions have shared meals and are similarly ill. There may or may not be a time lag (12 hours to several days) before the signs and symptoms appear.[1,12,40] Characteristic findings on physical examination include descending, bilaterally symmetric motor paralysis beginning with abducens (cranial nerve VI) or oculomotor (cranial nerve III) nerve palsy; dysphagia (at times predominant and severe); mydriasis (often fixed) (see Fig. 128-3); respiratory insufficiency; and urinary retention.[1,40] When medial rectus palsy, ptosis, and sluggish pupillary reactivity occur, there is a high correlation with subsequent respiratory insufficiency and failure.[1,40]

Many of the initial signs and symptoms are anticholinergic, whereas mental status, sensory examination, and reflexes all usually remain normal.[1,3,40] The normal mental status, absence of fever, and presence of ophthalmoplegia seen with botulism, but not anticholinergic poisoning, should allow the clinician to move rapidly toward appropriate management.[44] Other typical nonanticholinergic findings are a frequently normal or slow pulse and normal temperature.[1,2]

In severe cases, life-threatening complications of botulism ultimately occur from extensive paralysis of respiratory muscles.[45] This paralysis may result in death from respiratory failure unless close monitoring and appropriate ventilatory support are instituted.[1,43] Patients most commonly require mechanical ventilatory support for 2 to 8 weeks. In severe cases, patients have remained venti-

lator dependent for 7 months, which may lead to secondary medical complications from prolonged ventilator use, such as nosocomial infection.[1,43] Death now occurs in 5% to 10% of cases of foodborne botulism.[7] Early deaths result from a failure to recognize the severity of the disease, whereas deaths after 2 weeks usually result from complications of long-term mechanical ventilatory management.[7,45,46]

DIAGNOSIS

The diagnosis of botulism is primarily a clinical one; key medical decisions in terms of respiratory support and administration of antitoxin are optimally made before the results of serum and stool assays are known.[1] The clinician's index of suspicion for this diagnosis should be raised in the setting of temporal and physical clustering of related clinical presentations. Botulism is generally underdiagnosed because most clinicians lack familiarity with the disease and because symptoms can be mistaken for more common clinical entities, such as stroke or Guillain-Barré syndrome.[7,47,48] In addition, because the initial presentation of botulism is often subtle, serious delays may occur in the diagnosis and initiation of botulism-specific management. The diagnosis of botulism is not difficult in most cases, however, once it has been considered.[7]

The role of the laboratory is limited to confirmation of a clinically based diagnosis. Botulinum toxin may be detected in serum or gastric contents in an affected patient.[1,27] If the food source has been identified, the mouse bioassay (neutralization test) is considered the optimal (most sensitive) assay in detecting botulinum toxin. In the United States, food source cultures, toxin detection assays, and mouse bioassays of suspect foods generally are performed by local Food and Drug Administration laboratories or by the CDC in Atlanta, Georgia. Other diagnostic studies include neuromuscular testing using electromyography.[45,49] The characteristic electromyography findings of botulism are normal nerve conduction velocity; normal sensory nerve function; a pattern of brief, small-amplitude motor potentials; and, most distinctively, an incremental response (facilitation) to repetitive stimulation often seen only at 50 Hz (Fig. 128-4).[49]

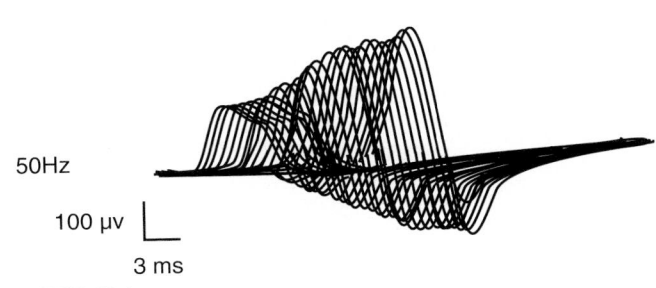

50Hz

100 µv

3 ms

FIGURE 128-4

Repetitive stimulation of the left median innervated abductor pollicis brevis in infantile botulism. Note the characteristic incremental response to repetitive stimulation noted at 50 Hz. *(From Cornblath DR, Sladky JT, Sumner AJ: Clinical electrophysiology of infantile botulism. Muscle Nerve 6:448–452, 1983.)*

Botulism **1355**

TREATMENT

The major emphasis in the initial care of botulism is serial neurologic and respiratory evaluations of suspected cases. Clinicians should observe patients carefully for progression

Indications for ICU Admission in Botulism Poisoning

Deteriorating respiratory parameters
Progressive cranial nerve dysfunction
Known exposure to contaminated food
Compromised gag reflex
Diminished cough reflex
Significant comorbidities

of limb and respiratory muscle weakness. Respiratory failure is the usual cause of death from botulism; serial assessments using objective parameters, such as vital capacity, peak expiratory flow rate, negative inspiratory force, and gag reflex, are required to determine progression of the disease and assess the potential need for endotracheal intubation.[1,3,34,40] Activated charcoal has been shown to bind botulinum toxin and may be administered in suspected cases of foodborne botulism to bind any remaining toxin in the gastrointestinal tract.[50] Tracheostomy generally is required for long-term management of these patients because the illness in severe cases may last weeks or months.[42]

In the United States, a trivalent equine-derived antitoxin is available through the CDC (weekdays 404-639-3356 or 404-639-3670 after hours). International botulinum antitoxin manufacturers are listed in Table 128-2. The antitoxin generally is used for cases of foodborne botulism, although in theory it would be an effective antidote in the event of an aerosolized release of botulinum toxin. Animal experiments have shown that the antitoxin may be effective if administered early after an aerosolized release of lethal concentrations of botulinum toxin.[51] The antitoxin limits progression of the disease via prevention of further binding of botulinum toxin to the neuromuscular junction. Recovery results from new motor axon

TABLE 128-2 International Manufacturers of *Clostridium Botulinum* Antitoxin

MANUFACTURER	CONTACT INFORMATION
Biomed (CIECH)	ul. Chelmska 30/34, 00-725 Warsaw, Poland; telephone: 22-41-06-06
Behringwerka AG	P.O. 1140, D3500 Hamburg, Germany; fax: 49-6421-394723
Chiba Serum Institute	2-6-1 Konodai, Ichikawa, Chiba 272, Japan; telephone: 81-473-72-3571
Aventis Pharmaceuticals Inc.	Route 611, P.O. Box 187, Bridgewater, NJ, 08807; USA; 1-800-981-2491
Instituto Butantan	Av. Vital Brazil 1500, Caixa Postal 65, Sao Paulo, Brazil; telephone: 55-11-8137222

Source: Centers for Disease Control and Prevention, Atlanta, GA.

twigs that sprout and reinnervate paralyzed muscle tissue in a process that may take months to complete.[41,52]

No controlled studies have been done in humans to evaluate the usefulness of antitoxin therapy. Tacket and coworkers[53] retrospectively reviewed 132 cases of type A botulism reported to the CDC between 1963 and 1980. After controlling for age and incubation period, Tacket and coworkers[53] showed that administration of antitoxin within 24 hours after onset of symptoms was associated with a lower mortality rate and shorter course of illness. Although the antitoxin is most effective when administered early, more delayed use (>24 hours after clinical onset) still may be beneficial. The toxin has been found in the blood of some patients 30 days after botulinum ingestion.[53]

Botulinum antitoxin is manufactured and stored in a limited number of facilities in the United States (Anchorage, Atlanta, Chicago, Honolulu, Los Angeles, New York, Miami, San Francisco, and Seattle) and around the world (see Table 128-2). Most commercially available botulinum antitoxins are equine derived, and clinicians should prepare for possible adverse immunologic reactions. Allergic responses are attributable to foreign proteins contained in antibody products of nonhuman origin. It has been reported that 20% of patients have untoward reactions from the antitoxin preparations.[54-56] Black and Gunn[54] reported a 9% rate of either acute or delayed hypersensitivity reactions collected over 10 years in 268 patients. Serum sickness was significantly more frequent in patients treated with more than 40 mL of antitoxin, suggesting a dose-response relationship phenomenon.[54]

The antitoxin used in North America is trivalent ABE and is produced by Aventis Pharmaceuticals (Bridgewater, NJ) (formerly Connaught Medical Research Laboratories); each vial contains at least 7500 IU of type A, 5500 IU of type B, and 8500 of type E specific antigen. Previous recommendations for treatment were two vials to be given initially, followed by two additional vials in 4 hours if the patient's condition continued to deteriorate. The CDC currently releases one vial of trivalent ABE for the treatment of patients with suspected botulism. This change is based on published and unpublished clinical data showing that the administration of one vial of antitoxin results in circulating antitoxin levels 100-fold greater than that needed to neutralize the largest amount of circulating toxin ever measured at the CDC.[57]

Other therapeutic modalities are considered to be experimental. Guanidine has been used in the past to enhance acetylcholine release.[58,59] However, placebo-controlled studies failed to show an acceleration in the rate of improvement when patients received guanidine, and a regression in the disease progress has not been shown when the drug was stopped.[58,59] Other therapies, including steroids,[60] 4-aminopyridine,[61] and plasmapheresis,[62] have been tried, with no proven benefit.

Criteria for ICU Discharge in Botulism Poisoning

Stabilized respiratory status
Stabilized neurologic status
Improvement in respiratory parameters
Extubation or presence of ventilator floor
Controlled comorbidities

SPECIAL TYPES OF BOTULISM

Infant Botulism

In 1976, it was first reported that infection with *C. botulinum* could produce the syndrome of the hypotonic ("floppy") infant.[45] Infant botulism now is recognized as a distinct clinical entity in which *C. botulinum* spores enter and colonize the gastrointestinal tract and produce toxin, which is absorbed systemically.[45] The disease most commonly occurs during the first 3 months of life, with an average pediatric intensive care unit stay lasting 29 days.[63] Constipation is usually the earliest clinical sign, but this usually is not serious enough to be brought to medical attention. The spectrum of disease is wide, ranging from mild constipation to sudden death.

Several days after onset of infant botulism, the infant's suck becomes weak, the cry becomes feeble and altered in tone, and oral secretions and food may pool in the pharynx. This is followed by poor feeding, lethargy, a weak cry, decreased sucking, and generalized lack of muscle tone, notably characterized by a floppy head.[63,64] The source of ingestion is unknown in approximately 85% of cases; in 15% of cases, honey contaminated with *C. botulinum* spores is the implicated source of colonizing botulinum spores.[65] An important message of prevention to mothers is to avoid feeding honey to infants.

The mainstay of therapy for infant botulism is meticulous supportive care, including respiratory support and nutritional support through enteral feeding. Recovery is a gradual process that (similar to other forms of botulism) generally occurs over weeks to months.[63,65] A 5-year, randomized, double-blind, placebo-controlled treatment trial of human-derived botulinum antitoxin (formally known as *botulinum immune globulin*) in infant botulism showed a significant reduction in length of hospital stay, requirements for mechanical ventilation and tube feedings in botulinum immune globulin recipients, and a $70,000 reduction in hospital cost per case.[66] The California Department of Health Services (24-hour telephone number, 510-540-2646) may be contacted about the procurement of botulinum immune globulin even for cases outside of that state.[66]

Wound Botulism

Wound botulism is defined as botulism occurring in any person with an antecedent wound and no history suggesting foodborne botulism.[67] Typically, on a worldwide basis, these patients are young men with open extremity injuries sustained outside the home during work or play.[68] In this form of botulism, spores of *C. botulinum* are embedded in an open wound after a traumatic injury. This local anaerobic tissue environment allows for spore germination, bacterial replication, and subsequent release of botulinum toxin.[68] The incubation period between the time of injury and the onset of symptoms is 4 to 14 days.[68] In addition to traumatic wounds, botulism has been identified as an unusual complication of wounds caused by intravenous or nasal drug abuse.[69] Since 1982, when the first drug abuse–related case was reported, the number of cases associated with drug use has grown to surpass the cases of wound botulism related to trauma.[70,71] The number of

reported cases of wound botulism has increased dramatically, from 1 case in 1990 to 25 in 1995, with 23 occurring in California alone. In California, greater than 97% of the cases of wound botulism reported since 1990 have involved infected drug users.[72] Most of these cases of wound botulism have been associated with the subcutaneous injection of black tar heroin, a dark, gummy crudely processed (and less expensive) form of heroin produced in Mexico.[70,72]

The treatment of patients with wound botulism involves aggressive respiratory support (as with foodborne botulism) in addition to extensive wound irrigation, débridement, and prompt administration of botulinum antitoxin.[72–74] Aggressive surgical wound débridement is needed to remove the source of toxin production. Débridement and irrigation ideally should occur after the administration of botulinum antitoxin.[70] The use of antibiotics in the treatment of wound botulism is controversial. Penicillin G is considered the antibiotic of choice, but its efficacy has not been firmly established.[72] No formal CDC recommendations exist regarding the use of antibiotics in treating wound botulism at this time.[72]

Classification Undetermined Etiology (Adult Infectious Botulism)

Botulism in adults also can occur (albeit rarely) as a result of intestinal colonization with *C. botulinum* and in vivo toxin production in a manner similar to that of infant botulism.[7,75] This class of botulism as defined by the CDC includes any patient older than 1 year of age for whom it has been impossible to implicate a particular food source. The general risk factors that favor organism persistence and *C. botulinum* colonization include a history of abdominal surgery, achlorhydria, inflammatory bowel disease, or recent antibiotic therapy that may have altered the gastrointestinal flora.[1,76] The finding of *C. botulinum* in feces of adult patients almost always is associated with clinical botulism.[77]

Terrorism

Botulinum toxin poses a major biologic weapon threat because of its extreme potency, ease of production and transport, and need for prolonged intensive care among affected persons.[5] The potential for botulinum toxin as a weaponized agent is related in part to this toxin's being considered the most potent lethal substance known. It is estimated to be 15,000 to 100,000 times more toxic than sarin, the potent organophosphate nerve agent used in a terrorist attack perpetrated by the Aum Shinrikyo cult in the Tokyo subway system.[7,51,78] Terrorists from this Japanese cult already have attempted to use botulinum toxin as a biologic weapon. Botulinum toxin was aerosolized and dispersed in several sites in downtown Tokyo, Japan, and at U.S. military installations on three occasions between 1990 and 1995 by the Aum Shinrikyo cult. The *C. botulinum* was obtained from soil collected from northern Japan.[78,79] In addition, four countries listed by the U.S. government as "state sponsors of terrorism" (Iran, Iraq, North Korea, and Syria)[80] have developed or are believed to be developing botulinum toxin as a weapon.[5,81,82]

The aim in minimizing the potentially devastating outcome of botulinum toxin dispersal is to achieve early detection of foodborne or aerosolized forms of the toxin with the goal of early notification and treatment. Early detection would allow the prevention of further exposure and alert public health departments to ship botulinum antitoxin where needed. A biologic terrorist attack should be suspected if multiple casualties simultaneously present with progressive descending bulbar, muscular, and respiratory weakness.[51] Timely recognition of a botulism outbreak begins with an astute clinician who quickly notifies public health officials.[5]

Common Misconceptions about Botulism

1. Antitoxin reverses paralysis.
2. Antitoxin is locally available.
3. Multiple vials of antitoxin are required.
4. Foodborne botulism requires antibiotics.
5. Botulism affects mental status.
6. Contaminated foods smell rancid.

Key Points in the Diagnosis and Management of Botulism

1. Botulism presents with bulbar palsies and descending motor paralysis.
2. Serial pulmonary function testing is indicated for all suspected cases.
3. Aggressive respiratory support is the mainstay of treatment.
4. Diagnostic tests include electromyography and serum, stool, and food assays.
5. Botulinum antitoxin is most effective when administered early.
6. Botulinum toxin is a potential biologic weapon of terror.
7. Antitoxin halts progression of the disease.
8. Antitoxin stocks are limited and stored in designated areas.
9. One vial (manufacturer Aventis, available from Centers for Disease Control and Prevention) neutralizes circulating toxin.
10. Antibiotics are not effective because the toxin is preformed.
11. Botulism patients are fully alert and oriented.
12. Appearance and odor of contaminated food may be entirely normal.

REFERENCES

1. Schaffner W: *Clostridium botulinum* (botulism). In Mandell GL, Douglas RG, Bennett JE (eds): Principles and Practice of Infectious Diseases, 5th ed. New York, John Wiley & Sons, 2002, pp 2543–2547.
2. Gill MD: Bacterial toxins: A table of lethal amounts. Microbiol Rev 46:86–94, 1982.
3. Botulism: The Organism, Its Toxins, the Disease. Springfield, IL, Charles C Thomas, 1977.
4. Hallet M: One man's poison—clinical applications of botulinum toxin. N Engl J Med 341:118–120, 1999.
5. Arnon SS, Schechter R, Inglesby TV, et al: Botulinum toxin as a biological weapon: medical and public health management. JAMA 285:1059–1070, 2001.
6. Patrick, Spertzel, 1992: Based on Cader KL, BWL Tech Study #3, Mathematical models for dosage and casualty resulting from single point and line source release of aerosol near ground level, DTIC#AD3 10–361, Dec 1957.
7. Shapiro RL, Hatheway C, Swerdow DL: Botulism in the United States: A clinical and epidemiologic review. Ann Intern Med 129:221–228, 1998.
8. Van Ermengem E: Classics in infectious disease: A new anaerobic bacillus and its relation to botulism. Originally published as "Über einen neuen anaeroben Bacillus und seine Beziehungen zum Botulismus," in Zeitschrift für Hygiene und Infektionskrankheiten 26:1–56, 1897. Rev Infect Dis 1:701–719, 1979.
9. Schechter R, Arnon S: Botulism. In Behrman RE, Kliegman RM, Jenson HB (eds): Nelson Textbook of Pediatrics, 16th ed. Philadelphia, WB Saunders, 2000, pp 875–878.
10. Goldfrank LR, Flomenbaum NE: Botulism. In Goldfrank LR, Flomenbaum NE, Lewin NA, et al (eds): Goldfrank's Toxicologic Emergencies, 7th ed. Stamford, CT, Appleton & Lange, 2002, pp 1100–1113.
11. Seals JE, Snyder JB, Edell TA, et al: Restaurant-associated type A botulism: Transmission by potato salad. Am J Epidemiol 113:436–444, 1981.
12. Hughes JM, Hatheway CL, Ostroff SM: Botulism. In Scheld WM, Whitley RJ, Durack DT (eds): Infections of the Central Nervous System, 2nd ed. Philadelphia, Lippincott-Raven, 1997, pp 615–617.
13. Townes JM, Cieslak PR, Hatheway CL, et al: An outbreak of type A botulism associated with a commercial cheese sauce. Ann Intern Med 125:558–563, 1996.
14. MacDonald KL, Spengler RF, Hatheway CL, et al: Type A botulism from sautéed onions: Clinical and epidemiologic observations. JAMA 253:1275–1278, 1985.
15. MacDonald KL, Cohen ML, Blake PA: The changing epidemiology of adult botulism in the United States. Am J Epidemiol 124:794–799, 1986.
16. Botulism (foodborne)—by year, United States, 1975–1994. MMWR Morb Mortal Wkly Rep 43:22–23, 1995.
17. Pickett J, Berg B, Chaplin E, et al: Syndrome of botulism in infancy: Clinical and electrophysiologic study. N Engl J Med 295:770–772, 1976.
18. Thompson DE, Brehm JK, Oultram JD, et al: The complete amino acid sequence of the *Clostridium botulinum* type A neurotoxin, deduced by nucleotide sequence analysis of the encoding gene. Eur J Biochem 189:73–81, 1990.
19. Binz T, Kurazono H, Willie M, et al: The complete sequence of botulism neurotoxin type A and comparison with other clostridial neurotoxins. J Biol Chem 265:9153–9158, 1990.
20. Whelan SM, Elmore MJ, Bodsworth NJ, et al: Molecular cloning of the *Clostridium botulinum* structural gene encoding the type B neurotoxin and determination of its entire nucleotide sequence. Appl Environ Microbiol 58:2345–2354, 1992.
21. Hauser D, Eklund MW, Kurazono H, et al: Nucleotide sequence of *Clostridium botulinum* C1 neurotoxin. Nucleic Acids Res 18:4924, 1990.
22. Binz T, Kurazono H, Popoff MR, et al: Nucleotide sequence of the genes encoding *Clostridium botulinum* neurotoxin type D. Nucleic Acids Res 18:5556, 1990.
23. Whelan SM, Elmore MJ, Bodsworth NJ, et al: The complete amino acid sequence of *Clostridium botulinum* type-E neurotoxin derived by nucleotide-sequence analysis of the encoding gene. Eur J Biochem 204:657–667, 1992.
24. Elmore MJ, Hutson RA, Collins MD, et al: Nucleotide sequence of the gene encoding for proteolytic (group 1) *Clostridium botulinum* type F neurotoxin genealogical comparison with other clostridial neurotoxins. System Appl Microbiol 18:23–31, 1995.
25. East AK, Richardson PT, Allaway D, et al: Sequence of the gene encoding type F neurotoxin of *Clostridium botulinum*. FEMS Microbiol Lett 75:225–230, 1992.
26. Campbell K, Collins MD, East AK: Nucleotide sequence of the gene coding for *Clostridium botulinum (Clostridium argentinense)* type G neurotoxin: Genealogical comparison with other clostridial neurotoxins. Biochem Biophys Acta 1216:487–491, 1993.
27. Bowmer EJ: Preparation and assay of the international standards for *Clostridium botulinum* types A, B, C, D, and E antitoxins. Bull World Hearth Organ 29:701–709, 1963.
28. Barker WH, Weissman MD, Dowell VR, et al: Type B botulism outbreak caused by a commercial food product. JAMA 237:456–459, 1977.
29. Wainwright RB, Heyward WL, Middaugh JP, et al: Food-born botulism in Alaska, 1947–1985: Epidemiology and clinical findings. J Infect Dis 157:1158–1162, 1988.
30. Weber JT, Hibbs RG, Darwish A, et al: A massive outbreak of type E botulism associated with traditional salted fish in Cairo. J Infect Dis 167:451–454, 1993.

31. LeCour H, Ramos H, Almeida B, Barbosa R: Food borne botulism: A review of 13 outbreaks. Arch Intern Med 148:578–580, 1988.
32. Koenig M, Spickard A, Cardella M, et al: Clinical and laboratory observations on type E botulism in man. Medicine 43:517–545, 1964.
33. Smith LDS: The occurrence of *Clostridium botulinum* and *Clostridium tetani* in the soil of the United States. Health Lab Sci 15:74–80, 1978.
34. Kao I, Drachman DB, Price DL: Botulinum toxin: Mechanism of presynaptic blockade. Science 193:1256–1258, 1976.
35. Hatheway CL: Toxigenic clostridia. Clin Microbiol Rev 3:66–98, 1990.
36. Simpson LL: Botulinum toxin: A deadly poison sheds its negative image. Ann Intern Med 125:616–617, 1996.
37. Halpern JL, Neale EA: Neurospecific binding, internalization, and retrograde axonal transport. In Monecucco C (ed): Clostridial Neurotoxins. Current Topics in Microbiology and Immunology, Vol 195. New York, Springer, 1995, pp 221–241.
38. Schiavo G, Santucci A, Dasgupta BR, et al: Protein botulinum neurotoxins serotypes A and E cleave SNAP-25 at distinct COOH-terminal peptide bonds. FEBS Lett 335:99–103, 1993.
39. Lalli G, Herreros J, Osborne SL, et al: Functional characterization of tetanus and botulinum neurotoxins binding domains. J Cell Sci 112:2715–2724, 1999.
40. Gutmann L, Pratt L: Pathophysiologic aspects of human botulism. Arch Neurol 33:175–179, 1976.
41. Arnon SS, Schechter R, Inglesby TV, et al: Botulinum toxin as a biological weapon: Medical and public health management. JAMA 285:1059–1069, 2001.
42. Duchen LW, Strich SJ: The effects of botulism toxin on the pattern of innervation of skeletal muscle in the mouse. Q J Exp Physiol 53:84–89, 1968.
43. Hughes JM, Blumenthal JR, Merson MH, et al: Clinical features of types A and B food-borne botulism. Ann Intern Med 95:442–445, 1981.
44. Terranova W, Palumbo JN, Breman JG: Ocular findings in botulism type B. JAMA 241:475–477, 1979.
45. Pickett J, Berg B, Chaplin E, et al: Syndrome of botulism in infancy: Clinical and electrophysiologic study. N Engl J Med 295:770–772, 1976.
46. Schmidt-Nowara WW, Samet JM, Rasario PA: Early and late pulmonary complications of botulism. Arch Intern Med 143:451–456, 1983.
47. Griffin PM, Hatheway CL, Rosenbaum RB, Sokolow R: Endogenous antibody production to botulism toxin in an adult with intestinal colonization of botulism and underlying Crohn's disease. J Infect Dis 175:633–637, 1997.
48. St Louis ME: Botulism. In Evans AS, Brachman PS (eds): Bacterial Infections of Humans: Epidemiology and Control, 2nd ed. New York, Plenum Medical, 1991, pp 115–117.
49. Cornblath DR, Sladky JT, Sumner AF: Clinical electrophysiology of infantile botulism. Muscle Nerve 6:448, 1983.
50. Gomez HF, Johnson R, Guven H, et al: Adsorption of botulinum toxin to activated charcoal with a mouse bioassay. Ann Emerg Med 25:818–822, 1995.
51. Botulinum toxins. In Eitzen E, Pavlin J, Cieslak T, et al (eds): Medical Management of Biological Casualties Handbook, 3rd ed. Fort Detrick, MD, U.S. Army Medical Research Institute of Infectious Diseases, 1998.
52. Duchen LW: Motor nerve growth induced by botulinum toxin as a regenerative phenomenon. Proc R Soc Med 65:196–197, 1972.
53. Tacket CO, Shandera WX, Mann JM, et al: Equine antitoxin use and other factors that predict outcome in type A foodborne botulism. Am J Med 76:794–798, 1984.
54. Black RE, Gunn RA: Hypersensitivity reactions associated with botulinal antitoxin. Am J Med 69:567–570, 1980.
55. Hibbs RG, Weber JT, Corwin A, et al: Experience with the use of an investigational F(ab′)2 heptavalent botulism immune globulin of equine origin during an outbreak of type E botulism in Egypt. Clin Infect Dis 23:337–340, 1996.
56. Hughes JM: Botulism. In Scheid WM, Whitley RJ, Durack DT (eds): Infections of the Central Nervous System. New York, Raven Press, 1991, pp 150–153.
57. Hatheway CH, Snyder JD, Seals JE, et al. Antitoxin levels in botulism patients treated with trivalent equine botulism antitoxin to toxin types A, B, E. J Infect Dis 150:407–412, 1984.
58. Faich GA, Greegher RW, Sato S: Failure of guanidine therapy in botulism A. N Engl J Med 285:773–776, 1971.
59. Kaplan JE, Davis LE, Narayan V, et al: Botulism, type A, and treatment with guanidine. Ann Neurol 6:69–71, 1979.
60. Cherington M, Schultz D: Effect of guanidine, germine, and steroids in a case of botulism. J Toxicol Clin Toxicol 11:19–25, 1977.
61. Davis LE, Johnson JK, Bicknell JM, et al: Human type A botulism and treatment with 3,4 diaminopyridine. Electromyogr Clin Neurophysiol 32:379–383, 1992.
62. Rapoport S, Watkins PB: Descending paralysis resulting from occult wound botulism. Ann Neurol 16:359–361, 1984.
63. Schreiner MS, Field E, Ruddy R: Infant botulism: A review of 12 years' experience at the Children's Hospital of Philadelphia. Pediatrics 87:159–165, 1991.
64. Wilson R, Morris JG Jr, Snyder JD, Feldman RA: Clinical characteristics of infant botulism in the United States: A study of the non-California cases. Pediatr Infect Dis 1:148–150, 1982.
65. Arnon SS: Infant botulism. In Feigin RD, Cherry JD (eds): Textbook of Pediatric Infectious Diseases, 4th ed. Philadelphia, WB Saunders, 1998, pp 1570–1577.
66. Schecter R, Arnon SS: Botulism. In Behrman RE, Kliegman RM, Jenson HB (eds): Nelson Textbook of Pediatrics, 17th ed. Philadelphia, WB Saunders, 2004, pp 947–950.
67. MacDonald KL, Cohen ML, Blake PA: The changing epidemiology of adult botulism in the United States. Am J Epidemiol 124:794–799, 1986.
68. Merson MH, Dowell VR: Epidemiologic, clinical and laboratory aspects of wound botulism. N Engl J Med 289:1005–1010, 1973.
69. MacDonald KL, Rutherford GW, Friedman SM, et al: Botulism and botulism-like illness in chronic drug abusers. Ann Intern Med 102:616–618, 1985.
70. Anderson MW, Sharma K, Feeney CM: Wound botulism associated with black tar heroin. Acad Emerg Med 4:805–809, 1997.
71. CDC: Wound botulism associated with parenteral cocaine abuse, New York City. MMWR Morb Mortal Wkly Rep 31:87–88, 1982.
72. Werner SB: Wound botulism—California, 1995. JAMA 275:95–96, 1996.
73. Mechem CC, Walter FG: Wound botulism. Vet Hum Toxicol 36:233–237, 1994.
74. Burningham MD, Walter FG, Mechem C, et al: Wound botulism. Ann Emerg Med 24:1184–1187, 1994.
75. Griffin PM, Hatheway CL, Rosenbaum RB, Sokolow R: Endogenous antibody production to botulism toxin in an adult with intestinal colonization botulism and underlying Crohn's disease. J Infect Dis 175:633–637, 1997.
76. McCroskey LM, Hatheway CL: Laboratory findings in four cases of adult botulism suggest colonization of the intestinal tract. J Clin Microbiol 26:1052–1054, 1988.
77. Dowell VR, McCroskey LM, Hatheway CL, et al: Coproexamination for botulinal toxin and *Clostridium botulinum*. JAMA 238:1829–1832, 1977.
78. Tucker JB (ed): Toxic Terror: Assessing the Terrorist Use of Chemical and Biological Weapons. Cambridge, MA, MIT Press, 2000.
79. WuDunn S, Miller J, Broad WJ: How Japan germ terror alerted world. New York Times, May 26, 1998, pp A1, A10.
80. United States Department of State: Patterns of Global Terrorism 1999. Department of State publication no. 10687. Washington, DC, US Department of State, 2000. Available at: http://www.state.gov/global/terrorism/annual_reports.html.
81. Cordesman AH: Weapons of Mass Destruction in the Gulf and Greater Middle East: Force Trends, Strategy, Tactics and Damage Effects. Washington, DC, Center for Strategic and International Studies, November 9, 1998.
82. Bermudez JS: The Armed Forces of North Korea. London, 1B Tauris, 2001.

CHAPTER 129

Massive Hymenopteran Envenomation

Hugo Kupferschmidt

The order Hymenoptera includes many important groups of stinging insects—bees, vespids, and ants. Medically the most important of the Hymenoptera are honeybees; vespids, including wasps, hornets, yellow jackets, and paper wasps; and ants, particularly fire ants. The main components of hymenopteran venoms are melittin, phospholipases, hyaluronidase, acid phosphatases, mast cell degranulation factors (mastoparans, MCD-peptide), kinins, biogenic amines (histamine, serotonin, dopamine), and a variety of low-molecular-weight substances. Their effects in massive human envenomation include cytolysis (hemolysis, rhabdomyolysis, renal and hepatocellular injury), cardiovascular toxicity, neurologic toxicity, respiratory failure, and metabolic sequelae. Multiorgan failure may result. The treatment of massive hymenopteran envenomation is entirely supportive. In contrast to the nonimmunologic toxic effects of massive envenomation, most hymenopteran sting–related deaths are due to allergic reactions (anaphylaxis).

Many species of the insect order Hymenoptera have stingers. These organs originally have served as ovipositors and still are used for this purpose by many species. In other species, the stingers have transformed into venom delivery apparatus designed to paralyze or kill the prey or, in the case of the social Hymenoptera (honeybees, social wasps, ants), to defend their colonies against intruders and predators. Hymenoptera of medical importance are the bees (family Apidae), wasps (Vespidae), and ants (Formicidae). The most important species include the honeybees (*Apis*), hornets (*Vespa* and *Dolichovespula*), yellow jackets (*Vespula*), paper wasps (*Polistes*), and fire ants (*Solenopsis*). A common trait of all these species is a high degree of socialization associated with strong defensive behavior, which is important to protect the colonies and hives. The venoms of these insects may cause considerable morbidity and mortality,[1–7] which derive from (1) local reactions (toxic and allergic), (2) systemic immunologic reactions, and (3) systemic toxicosis (envenomation).

Local reactions after single stings include pain, swelling, and pruritus, which are more annoying than dangerous, unless they compromise vital functions, such as by airway obstruction if the victim is stung in the oral cavity, throat, or trachea. The most dangerous immunologic systemic reaction is anaphylaxis, the most common cause of fatal outcome after single hymenopteran stings. Systemic toxicosis results only from multiple stings with massive envenomation. A fatal outcome from massive envenomation is rare (less than a few percent), however, compared with allergic reactions after single stings.[5,7,8] An exception may be geographic regions where Africanized honeybees (*Apis mellifera scutellata*) have been introduced,[9] leading to a higher incidence of multiple stings with increased morbidity and mortality.

Allergic reactions including anaphylaxis are discussed in depth in Chapter 31. Nevertheless, patients with massive hymenopteran envenomation may have allergic reactions and systemic toxicosis. Similarities between some of the features of anaphylaxis and systemic toxic effects, such as skin flushing or hypotension, can make differentiation difficult. Signs such as urticaria and bronchospasm after only a few stings indicate an allergic reaction, whereas hemolysis, rhabdomyolysis, and renal and hepatic damage indicate toxic effects rather than anaphylaxis (Table 129-1).

BEE STINGS

Most cases of massive hymenopteran envenomation occur from honeybee stings rather than stings from vespids or ants. Analysis of hymenopteran sting–associated mortality shows differences, however, in the proportion of wasp and bee stings in different countries.[5,7] A particular problem has emerged since the importation of African bees into the Americas. Queens of the African honeybee (*A. mellifera scutellata*) were introduced to Brazil in 1957, where they escaped and hybridized with the indigenous European honeybee (*Apis mellifera mellifera*). The Africanized honeybee has spread gradually from Brazil to the North, at a rate of some 300 miles per year, and invaded the southern United States in 1992. In Latin America and the southern United States, where these Africanized "killer" bees have spread, the chances of mass envenomation and the incidence of fatal cases have increased 5 to 10 times or more.[9] There were more than 190 deaths from Africanized bee attacks in Mexico between 1988 and 1993.[10] The mortality rate from massive attacks by bees in Mexico has been estimated to be more than 15%. The Africanized bees are particularly aggressive, attack their victims more quickly and in greater numbers than European honeybees when disturbed, and continually sting and pursue a victim over distances of up to 0.6 mile.[11] Victims typically are stung by hundreds to thousands of bees. The European honeybee and its Africanized counterpart cannot be distinguished by sight. Individual species can be differentiated only by morphometry or DNA analysis, particularly of mitochondrial DNA.[12–16] The individual sting of both types of bees is nearly identical, and there is no significant difference in their venoms.[17,18]

TABLE 129-1 Clinical Features of Systemic Envenomation and Systemic Allergic Reaction

SYSTEMIC TOXICITY	ALLERGIC REACTIONS
Early or delayed onset	Early onset
Diffuse and widespread edema	Large local reaction with an appearance of diffuse and extensive cellulitis
Burning sensation in the skin	
Headache, fever, weakness, dizziness, fatigue	Generalized urticaria
Vomiting, diarrhea	Symptoms of anaphylaxis with stridor, wheezing, sweating, shock, abdominal pain, loss of consciousness
Shock	
CNS depression	
Thrombocytopenia	
Hemolysis, hemoglobinuria	
Rhabdomyolysis	
Renal failure	

CNS, central nervous system.
Data from Schumacher MJ, Egen NB: Significance of Africanized bees for public health: A review. Arch Intern Med 155: 2038–2043, 1995.

It is the multiple stinging, and not increased venom potency or delivery, that poses the principal risk to victims of Africanized bees.[11,19]

After a bee has buried its stinger into the skin and pulled away, the stinging apparatus becomes extruded from the insect's abdomen, a process known as *autotomization (autotomy)*, which leads to the death of the bee. After denervation by autotomization, the barbed stylets of the stinger perform reciprocal axial movements effected by rhythmic action of the motor apparatus at the base of the stinger. The autotomized stinger embeds itself progressively deeper over approximately 30 seconds; at the end, at least two thirds of the length of the stinger are embedded. By this mechanism, venom delivery is rapid and complete in less than 30 seconds. Substantial amounts of venom are delivered in the first 5 to 10 seconds. To try to prevent anaphylaxis, it is theoretically necessary to remove the stinger within a few seconds of implantation.

VESPID STINGS

The family Vespidae includes three main types of venomous wasps—hornets, paper wasps, and yellow jackets. The genus *Vespa* and *Dolichovespula* comprise the large wasps, which are referred to as *hornets* or *vespid wasps*. Although most species of wasps are solitary and pose no hazard to humans, attacks by colonies of social wasps can result in envenomation with life-threatening toxicity. Social wasps form large colonies with nests that contain several thousand individuals. The proximity of a human to a colony may provoke a severe attack in defense of the nest. The size of the colony, among other factors, determines the average number of stings in hymenopteran mass attacks. Because of the different sizes of their colonies, mass stinging events with social wasps include tens to hundreds of individual insects, whereas swarms of honeybees consist of hundreds to thousands of individual bees.

ANT STINGS

Ants have a greater diversity in venom composition between different species than vespids and bees. In addition, there are differences in their modes of venom administration. Although most of the subfamilies of ants are capable of stinging, species in the subfamily Formicinae, which possess an atrophied stinger, spray their poisonous gland products into the wounds made by the abrasive action of their mandibles.[20]

Medically important ant species are the fire ants (*Solenopsis*) (Fig. 129-1) and harvester ants (*Pogonomyrmex*) in the Americas and jumper ants (*Myrmecia pilosula*) in Australia. In the United States, there are imported and native fire ant species. The native species include *Solenopsis xyloni* and *Solenopsis geminata*, whereas the imported species include *Solenopsis richteri* and *Solenopsis invicta*. The latter species were imported from South America[21] and exhibit a more aggressive behavior than the native ones. The imported fire ant possesses a unique method of stinging. It first secures itself with its mandibles, causing pain, then, using its head as a pivot, swings its abdomen in an arc, repeatedly stinging with its abdominal stinger. This characteristic clustering of stings is useful in identifying a lesion as a fire ant sting.[21–23]

BIOCHEMISTRY OF HYMENOPTERAN VENOMS

Bee and vespid venoms have little in common regarding their biochemistry.[24] Ant venoms exhibit an important diversity in composition among the different species. There are even larger differences between ant venoms and bee/vespid venoms in that the latter are protein rich due to their content of enzymes and peptides, whereas some of the ant venoms contain only traces of proteins (0.01%) dissolved in the aqueous phase of the venom (<5% of the volume), with alkaloids being the important constituents instead.

Bee Venom

The composition of bee venom from different strains, and even individual bees, can vary considerably.[17,19] The average venom protein content was reported to be 57 ± 7 μg in honeybees and 10 to 31 μg in bumblebees and carpenter bees.[25] The average venom sac content in a bee has been found to be 146.6 μg for European bees and 93.5 μg for Africanized

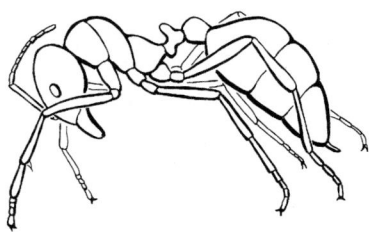

FIGURE 129-1

One species of the imported fire ant (*Solenopsis saevissima*). The ant can bite and sting simultaneously. *(From Carlson RW: Injuries by venomous and poisonous animals. In Carlson RW, Geheb MA [eds]: Principles and Practice of Medical Intensive Care. Philadelphia, WB Saunders, 1993, p 1681.)*

bees.[19] Because the venom sac usually is emptied completely with a sting, the amount of venom delivered by one sting corresponds to the contents of the venom sac.

Bee venom comprises at least 40 components, including enzymes, peptides, and low-molecular-weight components (Table 129-2).[26] The major components are melittin (50% of dry weight), a peptide of 26 amino acids and a molecular weight of 2840 d, and phospholipase A_2, an enzyme with 128 amino acids and a molecular weight of 15,800 d.[27] Their main effect is cytolytic. Other important toxic constituents of bee venom are hyaluronidase, MCD-peptide, and active amines (see Table 129-2).

Vespid Venoms

Vespid venoms contain biologically active amines, peptides, and proteins, including enzymes and neurotoxins. The main biogenic amines are histamine, serotonin, tyramine, and dopamine; minor components are adrenaline, noradrenaline, and polyamines. Hornet venom contains high concentrations of acetylcholine. Active peptides in wasp venom include kinins, mastoparans, and a chemotactic peptide. The venom of *Vespa mandarina* contains a proteinaceous component called *mandaratoxin*, a potent neurotoxin. Vespid venoms contain various enzymes, including phospholipases, hyaluronidases, and cholinesterase, and show proteolytic activity (Table 129-3). Hornet (*Vespa orientalis*) venom exerts anticholinesterase-like activity.[28]

When venom was collected from *V. mandarina*, the average yield per worker hornet was 3.5 to 4.7 μL, with a maximum of 7 to 12.5 μL and a dry weight of 6.69 mg from 25 μL of fresh venom.[29] The protein content of a single sting (0.5 to 2 μL) was determined to be 1.7 to 3.1 μg in yellow jackets, 2.4 to 5 μg in hornets, and 4.2 to 17 μg in paper wasps.[25]

With respect to the biochemical characteristics of peptides and proteins, social vespid venom differs greatly from bee venom. Vespid venom, in contrast to bee venom, contains wasp kinin.[24] Mastoparans, the peptides that degranulate

TABLE 129-2 Bee Venom, Its Composition, and Its Effects

COMPONENTS	PERCENT IN DRY VENOM	PHARMACOLOGIC EFFECTS IN HUMANS
Enzymes (15–17%)		
α-Glucosidase (invertase), MW 170 kd	0.6%	Antigenicity
Acid phosphomonoesterase, MW 55 kd	1%	Antigenicity
Hyaluronidase, MW 40 kd	1.5–2%	"Spreading factor," anaphylaxia
Lysophospholipase, MW 22 kd	1%	
Phospholipase A_2, MW 15.8 kd	10–12%	Cytolysis (enhanced by melittin), antigenicity
Other proteins and peptides (48–58%)		
Adolapin, MW 11.1 kd	1%	Inhibition of prostaglandin biosynthesis, antiinflammatory activity, analgesia
Protease inhibitor, MW 9 Kd	0.8%	Unknown
Melittin, MW 2.84 kd	50%	Cytolysis (i.e., hemolysis, rhabdomyolysis, renal and hepatocellular injury), in combination with phospholipase A_2 leading to inflammatory reactions, increased capillary permeability, smooth muscle contraction. Inhibition of CNS acetylcholinesterase and Na^+K^+-ATPase
Secapin	0.5%	Nontoxic
MCD (mast cell degranulating, syn. 401 peptide), MW 5–6 kd	2%	Mast cell degranulation, binding to basophil granulocytes; systemically antiinflammatory, local inflammatory action
Tertiapin	0.1%	Mast cell degranulation
"Melittin F"	0.01%	Melittin fragment without cytolytic properties
Apamin, MW 2 kd	3%	Neurotoxicity, binding to K^+ channels
Procamine A, B	1.4%	
Active amines (3%)		
Histamine	0.6–1.6%	
Dopamine	0.13–1%	
Norepinephrine	0.1–0.7%	
Amino acids (0.8–1%)		
γ-Aminobutyric acid	0.4%	
β-Aminoisobutyric acid	0.02%	
Other		
Carbohydrates (glucose, fructose)		
Lipids		

CNS, central nervous system; MW, molecular weight.
Data from references 27, 30, and 32.

TABLE 129-3 Vespid Venom, Its Composition, and Its Effects

COMPONENTS	PHARMACOLOGIC EFFECTS IN HUMANS
Enzymes	
Phospholipase activity	
Hyaluronidase activity	"Spreading factor"
Cholinesterase activity	
Antigen 5 (in *Dolichovespula* and *Vespula* spp.), MW 25 kd	Antigenicity
Mandaratoxin (*in V. mandarina*), MW 19–21 kd	Neurotoxicity
Anticholinesterase activity (in *V. orientalis*)	
Peptides	
Wasp kinins, hornet kinin, MW 1.2 kd (1%)*	Bradykinin-like activity
Mastoparans	Mast cell degranulation, catecholamine release, increase in ion permeability, reduction of membrane conductance
Chemotactic peptide	Macrophage chemotaxis
Active amines	
Histamine	Neurotoxicity
Serotonin	Neurotoxicity
Acetylcholine (only in hornet, not in wasp and yellow jacket venoms)	Neurotoxicity
Tyramine	
Dopamine	
Epinephrine	
Norepinephrine	
Polyamines (including putrescine, spermidine, spermine)	

*Percent in dry venom.
MW, molecular weight.
Data from references 24, 30, and 32.

mast cells and release histamine, although similar in action to MCD-peptide in bee venom, have different structures.[24,27,30] Vespid venoms do not contain melittin or apamin as does bee venom.[24,27]

Ant Venoms

The composition of the venoms of the different ant families and species exhibit broad variability. Ant venoms of the *Monomorium* and *Solenopsis* spp. are almost devoid of proteins and consist mainly of alkaloids. Fire ant venom consists of an alkaloid fraction that is more than 95% of the volume and an aqueous fraction that accounts for approximately 5% of the venom and contains dissolved proteins that are responsible for the allergic reactions (Table 129-4).[22] Venoms of other species contain enzymes, proteins, and peptides, including hyaluronidase, phospholipase, phosphatase, esterases, lipase, and smaller molecules such as histamine and amino acids. The venom of some *Formicinae* spp. contains formic acid. The *Myrmicaria* spp. venom is different from the venoms of all other ant species in that it contains limonene and many other monoterpene hydrocarbons. The volume of venom delivered by one fire ant sting ranges from 0.04 to 0.11 μL.[21,31]

PATHOPHYSIOLOGY

The clinically important toxic effects of Hymenoptera venoms are cytolytic, antiinflammatory, myotoxic, and neurotoxic. Their clinical effects in humans can be classi-

fied as cytolytic, neurologic, cardiovascular, or metabolic toxicity.

Cytolysis caused by various venoms occurs as a result of actions of direct and indirect cytolytic factors.[30] The direct cytolytic activities in honeybee and social wasp venoms are associated with basic polypeptides and are heat stabile, whereas the indirect cytolytic activities are associated with enzymes and are heat labile. The best-known direct-acting cytolytic compound in hymenopteran venom is honeybee melittin. Cytolytic effects are coagulation disturbances, hemolysis, lysis of mast cells, and mast cell degranulation.[30] Hyaluronidase (also known as "spreading factor") cleaves the intercellular matrix at the sting site, and phospholipase and protease release by local mast cells causes a breakdown of cellular and extracellular components in the skin. Both principles facilitate the propagation of the venom within the tissue.

There is a cooperative effect of melittin and phospholipase A_2 with regard to cytolysis, which is considered the main toxic action of bee venom. Melittin has an affinity for the phospholipid bilayer of the cell membranes and, together with phospholipase A_2, causes membrane disruption (see Table 129-2). The consequences are lysis of red blood cells, leukocytes, and platelets and damage to vascular endothelium. This cytolytic action also accounts for rhabdomyolysis (skeletal and myocardial), myotoxicity, and hepatocellular damage seen in severe envenomation and may contribute to acute tubular necrosis.[6]

A third mast cell degranulating principle is the MCD-peptide (peptide 401) in bee venom. This is a strongly basic polypeptide composed of 22 amino acids. Its counterparts in wasp venom are the mastoparans and bradykinin-like

TABLE 129-4 Ant Venom, Its Composition, and Its Effects	
COMPONENTS	**PHARMACOLOGIC EFFECTS IN HUMANS**
Proteins	
Hyaluronidase activity (in Myrmeciinae,* *Myrmica* spp., *Solenopsis*, and *Pogonomyrmex*)	
Phospholipase A activity (in Myrmeciinae, *Solenopsis*)	
Phospholipase A and B (the venom of the genus *Pogonomyrmex* contains high activities)	Cytolysis (i.e., hemolysis)
Melittin-like substance (in Myrmeciinae)	
Convulsive component (in Myrmeciinae), MW 15 kd	Smooth muscle stimulation
Esterases (in *Pogonomyrmex* spp.)	
Lipase (in *Pogonomyrmex* spp.)	
Peptides	
Small peptides (in *Formicinae* spp.)	
Active amines	
Histamine (in Myrmeciinae, *Myrmica* spp., *Pogonomyrmex* spp.)	
Alkaloids	
Pyrrolidines and pyrroline alkaloids (in *Monomorium* spp., *Solenopsis* spp.)	Formation of pruritic pustules and epidermal necrosis
Piperidine alkaloids (in *Solenopsis* spp.), mainly 2-alkyl-6-methylpiperidines (syn. solenopsin)	Cytolysis, histamine release, inhibition of N^+, K^+-ATPase, reduction of mitochondrial respiration, uncoupling of oxidative phosphorylation, postsynaptic block of neuromuscular transmission
Indolizidine alkaloids (in *Monomorium* spp.)	
Low-molecular-weight substances	
Formic acid (in some *Formicinae* spp.)	
Monoterpene hydrocarbons (in *Myrmicaria natalensis*)	
Amino acids	

*Myrmeciinae = family containing Australian bulldog ants.
Data from references 20 and 30.

substances. These substances cause vascular dilation (erythema) and increased capillary permeability leading to edema. In contrast to its properties as an inducer of mast-cell degranulation, MCD-peptide has shown antiinflammatory activity in rats.[30] A second peptide with antiinflammatory activity is adolapin.[30]

Neurotoxic actions include afferent somatosensory effects (e.g., pain) or efferent effects with actions at the sites of synaptic or neuromuscular transmission. Pain is evoked by substances including histamine, serotonin, acetylcholine, bradykinin, wasp kinins, and a variety of mediators released during cytolysis. Apamin, a bee venom component, causes excitation in the mammalian central nervous system. In vertebrates, it blocks most hyperpolarizing-inhibitory effects, including α-adrenergic, cholinergic, purinergic, and neurotensin-induced relaxation, but not β-adrenergic relaxation. It blocks the Ca^{2+}-dependent K^+ channels in neurons, myocytes, and hepatocytes.[30] The small molecules melittin, apamin, and MCD-peptide may pass the blood-brain barrier and cause central nervous system depression or seizures. The inhibitory actions of melittin on acetylcholinesterase and Na^+, K^+-ATPase may induce cholinergic effects, including diarrhea, bradycardia, hypotension, miosis, bronchoconstriction, and depolarizing blockade of nicotinic neurotransmission.[32]

Kinins are peptides with effects on muscle fibers causing contraction or relaxation.[30] Wasp venom contains bradykinin-like substances, called *wasp kinins*. They have potent pain-inducing activity, and their hemodynamic effects are believed to play a significant role in anaphylactic (IgE-mediated) reactions.[24,30] Important antigenic determinants of allergic reactions to hymenopteran stings include

enzymes, such as α-glucosidase (invertase), acid phosphatase, hyaluronidase, phospholipase, and antigen 5, whereas the smaller peptide components of hymenopteran venom have only minor immunogenicity.[24,30,32]

Fire Ants

Local reactions associated with fire ant envenomation are most often due to the direct toxic effect of dialkylpiperidine alkaloids on mast cell membranes, leading to mast cell lysis.[23] The in vitro biologic activities of piperidine include hemolytic, insecticidal, and cytotoxic properties, which can activate the alternative complement pathway.[33] The proteinaceous substances in fire ant venom are responsible for allergic reactions despite their small amount (0.1% of total venom).

CLINICAL PRESENTATION AND LIFE-THREATENING COMPLICATIONS

Although the components of the bee and vespid venoms differ chemically, their clinical effects are similar and are discussed together. The clinical presentation of envenomation by ant stings is different and is described separately.

Bee and Vespid Stings

LOCAL EFFECTS

Single stings from honeybees or vespids commonly produce only a local nonallergic reaction with pain, irritation, itching, and erythema at the site of the sting without systemic reaction. Stings in the mouth and throat may cause soft tissue edema severe enough to result in airway obstruction.

SYSTEMIC EFFECTS

The risk of systemic reactions to a massive envenomation is increased after more than approximately 50 stings. Massive envenomation with more than 500 stings is potentially fatal, although victims surviving 1000 stings have been reported.[34,35] The median lethal dose for honeybee venom is estimated to be about 19 stings per kg of body weight,[11] corresponding to approximately 1.3 mg/kg body weight.[6] Assuming a median lethal dose of 3.5 mg/kg and an average venom delivery of 140 µg per sting, one could speculate that a 70-kg human would have a 50% risk of death from 1750 stings.[36]

Reactions to massive bee envenomation can be immediate or delayed for several days. They can develop so rapidly that it may be difficult to differentiate them from an anaphylactic reaction.[37] Immediate signs and symptoms can be mild or totally absent[38] and nevertheless may be followed by delayed toxicity. Early symptoms typically include diffuse and widespread edema, a burning sensation of the skin, diaphoresis, conjunctivitis, headache, nausea, abdominal pain, weakness, dizziness, and fatigue. Allergic reactions including anaphylaxis may occur together with or precede systemic toxic reactions. Victims of more numerous stings experience vomiting, diarrhea, shock, coma, hemolysis with hemoglobinuria, thrombocytopenia, rhabdomyolysis with elevated serum levels of creatine kinase, and acute renal failure. Renal failure has been explained by the direct toxic effect of the circulating venom (histologically as nephritis) or by pigment nephropathy (histologically as acute tubular necrosis) secondary to hemolysis and rhabdomyolysis.[7,8,19,34,35,39–77] In a report from Brazil,[53] adult respiratory distress syndrome, hepatic dysfunction, myocardial infarction, serum sickness, and disseminated intravascular coagulation also were observed. Hemorrhagic pancreatitis, cerebral infarction, and a myasthenia gravis–like syndrome have been reported.[40,61,62] Other systemic complications in hymenopteran envenomation include superinfection of the sting site with *Staphylococcus aureus* potentially leading to toxic shock syndrome.[49,50] Laboratory abnormalities include neutrophilic leukocytosis; elevated serum creatinine levels; and elevated serum enzyme concentrations, including aspartate aminotransferase, alanine aminotransferase, lactate dehydrogenase, creatine kinase.[6,63]

Ant Stings

LOCAL EFFECTS

Most ant stings result in self-limited, painful, pruritic, wheal-and-flare reactions, but fatal anaphylaxis may occur.[78,79] Most (96%) patients develop characteristic lesions at sting sites with minor superficial skin necrosis. A vesicle containing clear fluid forms at the sting site in about 4 hours. Subsequently the fluid becomes cloudy, and after 24 hours a white pustule, which is characteristic of fire ant sting, forms. The pustule is invariably sterile and remains for 3 to 10 days before rupturing, after which a small scar may be noticeable at the site of the sting; secondary infections may develop.[80]

Harvester ants (*Pogonomyrmex* spp.) generally are regarded as producing the most painful stings of all North American species. In addition to the potent allergenicity of their venoms, characteristic reactions of humans stung by these ants include extensive sweating and prolonged pain and tenderness at the most proximate lymph nodes.[20]

SYSTEMIC EFFECTS

Systemic reactions after fire ant stings may include drowsiness and central nervous system involvement with confusion, coma, seizures, blurred vision, and peripheral neuropathy. Nephrotic syndrome has been reported.[81] Severe systemic reactions are estimated to occur in 0.6% to 2% of cases.[21] Massive fire ant envenomation may be fatal, particularly in the elderly, small children, and neonates. These patients are at increased risk for multiple stings due to their limited ability to escape attack.[21,33,78,79,81]

EVALUATION

Evaluation of a stung patient should assess the number of stings and the victim's venom-allergy status, body size, and general health. Important historical information includes any previous episode consistent with insect sting allergy; other complicating medical conditions (e.g., cardiovascular disease, pulmonary disease including asthma, immunosuppression, systemic mastocytosis); and use of medications, particularly β-blockers. The anatomic location of stings may increase the risk. Multiple stings involving the mouth, throat, or tongue may cause upper airway obstruction,[11] and stings involving the eyes can lead to retinal damage and optic neuropathy.[56,77] In single stings manifesting local reaction only, no further diagnostic evaluation is needed. Laboratory tests suggested for evaluation of multiple sting incidents are enumerated in Table 129-5.

TABLE 129-5 Laboratory Tests Useful in Multiple Sting Incidents

Total blood count
Platelets
Hemoglobin
Prothrombin time
Creatinine
Urea/BUN
Glucose
Electrolytes
Enzymes (AST, ALT, CK, LDH)
C-reactive protein
Troponin
Albumin
Bilirubin
Blood gas analysis
Ammonia
Urinalysis for protein, blood, hemoglobin, myoglobin, casts

ALT, alanine aminotransferase; AST, aspartate aminotransferase; BUN, blood urea nitrogen; CK, creatine kinase; LDH, lactate dehydrogenase.

TREATMENT

Airway and Ventilatory Considerations

Airway compromise may occur after stings to the head and neck or in the oral cavity, throat, esophagus, or trachea with consequent edema of soft tissue and mucous membranes; tracheal intubation may be difficult for this reason. Mechanical ventilatory support should be provided according to the clinical situation and the oxygenation and ventilatory needs of the patient. There are no envenomation-related particulars in ventilator settings.

Bee and Vespid Stings

Children with greater than 10 honeybee stings and adults with greater than 100 stings should seek immediate emergency medical attention even in the absence of allergy.[11] In single stings with only local reaction, appropriate treatment is limited to use of analgesics and cold compresses. In massive envenomations, clinical care is guided by signs and symptoms, which reflect the degree of systemic toxicity.[82] Involvement of several organ systems in massive honeybee or wasp envenomation poses a significant risk for multiorgan failure,[83] which makes aggressive supportive treatment paramount. Treatment of severe toxic reactions to multiple stings usually includes management of shock, hypoxia, and other effects of organ damage.

Many authors recommend that bee stingers should be scraped from the patient's skin without pinching or pulling of stingers because the remaining venom in the sac could be squeezed into the patient.[11] More recent studies have shown that removal of a bee stinger that has been embedded for more than 1 minute has little or no effect in reducing envenomation because most of the venom empties from detached honeybee stings within 10 to 20 seconds.[36]

In massive envenomation, it has been recommended that epinephrine (0.3 to 0.5 mL of 1:1000 dilution intramuscu-

larly or subcutaneously) and an antihistamine (e.g., 50 mg of diphenhydramine parenterally) should be given immediately because it may be difficult to distinguish systemic toxic effects from anaphylaxis when relatively small numbers of stings are sustained. Also, anaphylaxis and toxic effects could occur simultaneously in a venom-allergic patient (Table 129-6).[6]

When large numbers of stings are sustained, transportation to an emergency department and treatment for the toxic effects of venom must be started immediately, even if the initial presentation suggests an allergic reaction. Airway management and ensurance of adequate ventilation are the first priorities. Aggressive initial fluid volume resuscitation with continual attention to ongoing increased fluid requirements may be necessary, given the potential for gastrointestinal and distributive intravascular volume decline. H_1 and H_2 antagonists should be given intravenously to treat the vascular effects of histamine in bee venom because the combination of the two types of antihistamine is more effective than either alone.[6] Intravenous vasopressor administration and mechanical ventilation may be indicated in severe cases, whereas corticosteroids should be considered for adjunctive control of the inflammatory response. Intravenous glucagon should be considered a potentially efficacious alternative or adjunct to epinephrine in a patient who has been treated with a β-blocker. The need for tetanus vaccination is controversial, but vaccination may be considered.[11] Newer approaches to reduce the blood concentration of venom components, including hemodialysis and plasmapheresis[51] or production of a bee antivenom,[84] require further study.[6]

Within 2 to 3 days of massive hymenopteran envenomation, acute renal failure may occur due to myoglobinuria (rhabdomyolysis), hemoglobinuria, renal ischemia, or immune mechanisms. Close monitoring of urine output and serum electrolytes, creatinine, and urea nitrogen concentrations is indicated, as is repeated urinalysis assaying for the presence of hemoglobin and myoglobin.[6]

A patient with massive envenomation also should be assessed for evidence of intravascular hemolysis, rhabdomyolysis, and disseminated intravascular coagulation. Maintenance

---

Indications for ICU Admission in Massive Hymenopteran Envenomation

Anaphylaxis
Impaired vital signs
Impaired mental status
Signs of renal, pulmonary, hepatic, neurologic, or hematologic toxicity
>500 stings in adults; >7 stings per kilogram body weight in children
Adults with >50 stings (children with >10) should be monitored (blood pressure, heart rate, respiration, urinary output, mental status) in an emergency department for at least 6 hours, including laboratory workup (complete blood count, serum creatine kinase, serum creatinine, serum urea, serum potassium, liver enzymes, coagulation parameters, urinary hemoglobin and protein).
Patients with medical conditions (cardiovascular or renal history, allergies, pulmonary affections, mastocytosis), elderly patients, and pediatric patients should be monitored for an extended period (>24 hours).

TABLE 129-6 Administration Guidelines for Epinephrine

Mild reactions
  0.3–0.5 mL 1:1000 (0.3–0.5 mg) SC
  May repeat every 5–10 min
  Consider 0.1–0.2 mL (0.1–0.2 mg) at site of sting or entry
Moderate-to-severe reactions
  Slow IV infusion of 0.1–0.2 mL 1:1000 in 10 mL NS or 1–2 mL of 1:10,000 in 10 mL NS (1:100,000)
For persistent hypotension consider
  Continuous infusion of 1–2 mg in 250 mL D_5W or NS (4–8 μg/mL) at 2+ μg/min

D_5W, 5% dextrose in water; IV, intravenously; NS, normal saline; SC, subcutaneously. From Haupt MT, Fujii TK, Carlson RW, et al: Anaphylactic reactions. In Grenuik A, Ayres SM, Holbrook PR, et al (eds): Textbook of critical care, 4th ed. Philadelphia, WB Saunders, 2000.

of blood pressure, renal perfusion, urine output, and urinary alkalinization may minimize pigment nephropathy. In severe cases, hemodialysis should be considered, not only for the treatment of renal failure but also for removal of circulating low-molecular-weight venom components, such as melittin.[51,53]

Continuous electrocardiogram monitoring should be done routinely because of the possibility of myocardial damage, arrhythmia, and hyperkalemia. Individuals who develop systemic anaphylactic reactions to envenomation have a 35% to 60% risk of recurrent anaphylaxis and should be considered for desensitization treatment (venom immunotherapy).[11]

Fire Ant Stings

Anaphylaxis should be treated in a standard fashion, including parenteral epinephrine, histamine antagonists, corticosteroids, and possibly glucagon (in the setting of β-blocker use). In patients without anaphylaxis, a conservative approach consisting of observation and symptomatic (e.g., analgesic and antipruritic) treatment is recommended. Based on a report of two cases, care probably should be taken not to rupture the sterile pustules because of a risk of superinfection.[81]

Decontamination

As discussed earlier, there is no practical benefit to stinger removal.[6,36]

Extracorporeal Techniques

Peritoneal dialysis, hemodialysis, or plasmapheresis[35,51] may assist correction of volume, electrolyte, and acid-base abnormalities and enhance the clearance of circulating venom components.[35,51]

Immunotherapy

Ovine antibody Fab fragment–based antivenom has shown neutralizing effects in vitro and protection against the effects of bee venom in mice.[84] Antibodies from beekeepers and immunized rabbits have been incubated with bee venom, and effects on survival from envenoming were studied in intravenously injected mice.[85] Beekeeper serum antibodies were found to be protective in mice challenged with whole bee venom, and serum from rabbits hyperimmunized with bee venom phospholipase A_2 was protective against the lethal effects of phospholipase A_2. Serum antibodies from rabbits immunized with whole bee venom or melittin were found ineffective in neutralizing whole venom in vivo and were observed to be present in low titers in immune serum by enzyme-linked immunosorbent assay.[85] Persistence of circulating venom in fatal or near-fatal victims of multiple stings for many hours or days suggests that delay in antivenom administration would not contraindicate its potential use. The Fab or (Fab′) digestion fragments of antivenom antibodies may be more effective than whole immunoglobulin because of the enhanced tissue distribution of the smaller molecules.[6]

Criteria for ICU Discharge in Massive Hymenopteran Envenomation

Acute systemic toxicity (hemolysis, rhabdomyolysis, renal or hepatic failure) resolved
Normal hemodynamic parameter with no vasopressors (catecholamines) required
Normal or near-normal pulmonary function (patient extubated and not requiring large oxygen supplements)
Hemodialysis discontinued
Normal mental status

SPECIAL POPULATIONS

Pediatric Patients

Children are potentially at increased risk for the toxic effects of massive attacks by Africanized honeybees due to their limited ability to recognize and take appropriate evasive actions in potential stinging situations and the size-based increased dose of venom. Children with 10 to 20 honeybee stings should undergo emergency medical evaluation even in the absence of a history of hymenopteran allergy. Bee envenomation resulted in mild systemic illness in a series of children receiving 1 to 4.5 stings/kg body weight. Nausea, vomiting, and diarrhea, particularly in this age group, do not always portend a poor prognosis or involvement of other organ systems.[8,11,39,47,48,53,58–60,71,75,76]

Elderly Patients

Elderly individuals and individuals with severe underlying diseases are at increased risk because of their relative intolerance to large toxic exposures. Another common risk factor of the elderly is their relative inability to escape a dangerous situation quickly.[11] The prevalence of comorbid conditions is increased in the elderly, a fact that increases their risk for severe effects. Individuals of any age with significant cardiovascular and pulmonary disease are at an increased risk.[11] In Mexico, 71% of the reported deaths occurred in people older than 50 years, but it is not known whether the mortality rate from massive envenomation is higher in this age group or whether older people are less able to escape from a massive attack.[6,86]

Other Special Populations

Workers who clear vegetation or cut tall weeds and grass are at increased risk of an encounter with Hymenoptera nests.[6] As described earlier, individuals unable to withdraw from fire ant attacks, including neonates or poorly mobile nursing home residents, eventually may experience multiple stings indoors.[31,81,87] Individuals with mastocytosis have an increased risk for allergic reactions, including anaphylaxis.[88,89]

Common Misconceptions about Massive Hymenopteran Envenomation

1. Systemic toxicosis from multiple Hymenoptera stings develops immediately.
2. Most fatalities from Hymenoptera stings occur after multiple stings.
3. Removal of bee stingers in the emergency department is important in the prevention of systemic toxicosis because the attached venom sac delivers venom into the victim for an extended period.
4. The venom of the Africanized bee is more toxic than the venom of the common honey bee.

Key Points in Massive Hymenopteran Envenomation

1. The most important Hymenoptera species that cause massive envenomations include honeybees, wasps, yellow jackets, hornets, paper wasps, and fire ants.
2. Systemic toxicosis may result after >50 stings from honeybees or wasps. Fatalities may occur after >500 stings.
3. Symptoms of systemic toxicosis from bee or wasp stings include hemolysis, thrombocytopenia, rhabdomyolysis, renal and hepatic failure, cardiovascular and neurologic toxicity (shock, myocardial infarction, coma), and respiratory failure. General symptoms are headache, nausea, vomiting, diarrhea, and abdominal pain.
4. Symptoms of systemic toxicosis from fire ant stings are mainly neurologic, including drowsiness, confusion, coma, seizures, blurred vision, and peripheral neuropathy.
5. Anaphylaxis can occur in addition to systemic toxicosis.
6. Treatment is entirely supportive.

REFERENCES

1. Barnard J: Studies of 400 Hymenoptera sting deaths in the United States. J Allergy Clin Immunol 52:259–264, 1973.
2. Rubenstein HS: Bee-sting diseases: Who is at risk? What is the treatment? Lancet 1:496–499, 1982.
3. Lockey RF, Turkeltaub PC, Baird-Warren IA, et al: The Hymenoptera venom study: I. 1979–1982: Demographics and history-sting data. J Allergy Clin Immunol 82:370–381, 1988.
4. Reisman RE: Insect stings. N Engl J Med 331:523–527, 1994.
5. Sasvary T, Müller U: Todesfälle an Insektenstichen in der Schweiz 1978 bis 1987. Schweiz Med Wochenschr 124:1887–1894, 1994.
6. Schumacher MJ, Egen NB: Significance of Africanized bees for public health: A review. Arch Intern Med 155:2038–2043, 1995.
7. McGain F, Harrison J, Winkel KD: Wasp sting mortality in Australia. Med J Aust 173:198–200, 2000.
8. Gädeke R, Helwig H, Otto M, et al: Tödliche Vergiftungskrankheit eines Kindes nach massenhaften Wespenstichen. Med Klin 72:1487–1492, 1977.
9. Winston ML: The Africanized 'killer' bee: Biology and public health. QJM 87:263–267, 1994.
10. Guzman-Novoa E, Page RE: The impact of Africanized bees on Mexican beekeeping. Am Bee J 134(Suppl 2):101–106, 1994.
11. Kim KT, Oguro J: Update on the status of Africanized honey bees in the Western states. West J Med 170:220–222, 1999.
12. Smith DR, Brown WM: Polymorphisms in mitochondrial DNA of European and Africanized honeybees. Experientia 44:257–260, 1988.
13. Smith DR, Taylor OR, Brown WM: Neotropical Africanized honey bees have African mitochondrial DNA. Nature 339:213–215, 1989.
14. Crozier YC, Koulianos S, Crozier RH: An improved test for Africanized honeybee mitochondrial DNA. Experientia 47:968–969, 1991.
15. Arias MC, Sheppard WS: Molecular phylogenetics of honey bee subspecies (Apis mellifera L.) inferred from mitochondrial DNA sequence. Mol Phylogenet Evol 5:557–566, 1996.
16. Clarke KE, Oldroyd BP, Javier J, et al: Origin of honeybees (Apis mellifera L.) from the Yucatan peninsula inferred from mitochondrial DNA analysis. Mol Ecol 10:1347–1355, 2001.
17. Schumacher MJ, Schmidt JO, Egen NB, et al: Biochemical variability of venoms from individual European and Africanized honeybees (Apis mellifera). J Allergy Clin Immunol 90:59–65, 1992.
18. Nelson DR, Collins AM, Hellmich RL, et al: Biochemical and immunochemical comparison of Africanized and European honeybee venoms. J Allergy Clin Immunol 85:80–85, 1990.
19. Schumacher MJ, Schmidt JO, Egen NB, et al: Quantity, analysis, and lethality of European and Africanized honey bee venoms. Am J Trop Med Hyg 43:79–86, 1990.
20. Blum MS: Poisonous ants and their venoms. In Tu AT (ed): Handbook of Natural Toxins, Vol 2, Insect Poisons, Allergens, and Other Invertebrate Venoms. New York, Marcel Dekker, 1984, pp 225–242.
21. Freeman TM: Imported fire ants: The ants from hell! Allergy Proc 15:11–15, 1994.
22. Diaz JD, Lockey RF, Stablein JJ, et al: Multiple stings by imported fire ants (Solenopsis invicta), without systemic effects. South Med J 82:775–777, 1989.
23. Ginsburg CM: Fire ant envenomation in children. Pediatrics 73:689–692, 1984.
24. Nakajima T: Biochemistry of vespid venom. In Tu AT (ed): Handbook of Natural Toxins, Vol 2, Insect Poisons, Allergens, and Other Invertebrate Venoms. New York, Marcel Dekker, 1984, pp 109–133.
25. Hoffman DR, Jacobson RS: Allergens in Hymenoptera venom XII: How much protein is in a sting? Ann Allergy 52:276–278, 1984.
26. Tu AT (ed): Handbook of Natural Toxins, Vol 2, Insect Poisons, Allergens, and Other Invertebrate Venoms. New York, Marcel Dekker, 1984.
27. Shipolini RA: Biochemistry of bee venom. In Tu AT (ed): Handbook of Natural Toxins, Vol 2, Insect Poisons, Allergens, and Other Invertebrate Venoms. New York, Marcel Dekker, 1984, pp 49–85.
28. Ishay JS: Anticholinesterase-like activity by oriental hornet (Vespa orientalis) venom and venom sac extract. Experientia 35:636–639, 1979.
29. Schmidt JO, Yamane S, Matsuura M, et al: Hornet venoms: Lethalities and lethal capacities. Toxicon 24:950–954, 1986.
30. Piek T: Pharmacology of Hymenoptera venoms. In Tu AT (ed): Handbook of Natural Toxins, Vol 2, Insect Poisons, Allergens, and Other Invertebrate Venoms. New York, Marcel Dekker, 1984, pp 135–185.
31. Hardwick WE, Royall JA, Petitt BA, et al: Near fatal fire ant envenomation of a newborn. Pediatrics 90:622–624, 1992.
32. Kroegel C: Insektenstiche. Deutsch Med Wochenschr 111:1157–1164, 1986.
33. Fox RW, Lockey RF, Bukantz SC: Neurologic sequelae following the imported fire ant sting. J Allergy Clin Immunol 70:120–124, 1982.
34. Beccari M, Castiglione A, Cavaliere G, et al: Unusual case of anuria due to African bee stings. Int J Artif Organs 15:281–283, 1992.
35. Diaz-Sanchez CL, Lifshitz-Guinzberg A, Ignacio-Ibarra G, et al: Survival after massive (>2000) Africanized honeybee stings. Arch Intern Med 158:925–927, 1998.
36. Schumacher MJ, Tveten MS, Egen NB: Rate and quantity of delivery of venom from honeybee stings. J Allergy Clin Immunol 93:831–835, 1994.
37. Rodriguez-Lainz A, Fritz CL, McKenna WR: Animal and human health risks associated with Africanized honeybees. J Am Vet Med Assoc 215:1799–1804, 1999.
38. Kolecki P: Delayed toxic reaction following massive bee envenomation. Ann Emerg Med 33:114–116, 1999.
39. Munoz-Arizpe R, Valencia-Espinoza L, Velasquez-Jones L, et al: Africanized bee stings and pathogenesis of acute renal failure. Nephron 61:478, 1992.
40. Daisley H: Acute haemorrhagic pancreatitis following multiple stings by Africanized bees in Trinidad. Trans R Soc Trop Med Hyg 92:71–72, 1998.
41. Hommel D, Bollandard F, Hulin A: Multiple African honeybee stings and acute renal failure. Nephron 78:235–236, 1998.
42. Bourgain C, Pauti MD, Fillastre JP, et al: Envenimation massive après piqûres d'abeilles Africaines. Presse Med 27:1099–1101, 1998.
43. Mejia G, Arbelaez M, Henao JE, et al: Acute renal failure due to multiple stings by Africanized bees. Ann Intern Med 104:210–211, 1986.

44. dos Reis MA, Costa RS, Coimbra TM, et al: Acute renal failure in experimental envenomation with Africanized bee venom. Ren Fail 20:39–51, 1998.

45. Beccari M, Castiglione A, Cavaliere G, et al: Direct tubular toxicity of Hymenoptera venom (Letter). Nephron 65:159, 1993.

46. Sert M, Tetiker T, Paydas S: Rhabdomyolysis and acute renal failure due to honeybee stings as an uncommon case (Letter). Nephron 65:647, 1993.

47. Desmukh LS, Borse BT: Acute renal failure following multiple stings by honeybees. Indian Pediatr 33:781–783, 1996.

48. Tumwine JK, Nkrumah FK: Acute renal failure and dermal necrosis due to bee stings: Report of a case in a child. Cent Afr J Med 36:202–204, 1990.

49. Klug R, Immerman R, Giron JA: Bee bite and the toxic shock syndrome (Letter). Ann Intern Med 96:382, 1982.

50. Truskinovsky AM, Dick JD, Hutchins GM: Fatal infection after a bee sting. Clin Infect Dis 32:E36–38, 2001.

51. Beccari M: Dialysis or plasmapheresis for acute renal failure due to Africanized honeybee stings (Letter). Arch Intern Med 159:1255–1256, 1999.

52. Ceyhan C, Ercan E, Tekten T, et al: Myocardial infarction following a bee sting (Letter). Int J Cardiol 80:251–253, 2001.

53. Franca FOS, Benvenuti LA, Fan HW, et al: Severe and fatal mass attacks by "killer" bees (Africanized honey bees—*Apis mellifera scutellata*) in Brazil: Clinicopathological studies with measurements of serum venom concentrations. QJM 87:269–282, 1994.

54. Hiran S, Pande TK, Pani S, et al: Rhabdomyolysis due to multiple honey bee stings (Letter). Postgrad Med J 70:937, 1994.

55. Law DA, Beto RJ, Dulaney J, et al: Atrial flutter and fibrillation following bee stings. Am J Cardiol 80:1255, 1997.

56. Maltzman JS, Lee AG, Miller NR: Optic neuropathy occurring after bee and wasp sting. Ophthalmology 107:193–195, 2000.

57. Moret C, Enzel C, Leclercq M, et al: Un cas d'envenimation mortelle par piqûres multiples d'abeilles (*Apis mellifera L.*). Rev Med Liege 38:815–822, 1983.

58. Ariue BK: Multiple Africanized bee stings in a child. Pediatrics 94:115–117, 1994.

59. LoVecchio F, Graeme KA, Gerkin R, et al: Bee swarmings in children (Abstract). J Toxicol Clin Toxicol 36:460, 1998.

60. Tasic V: Nephrotic syndrome in a child after a bee sting. Pediatr Nephrol 15:245–247, 2000.

61. Brumlik J: Myasthenia gravis associated with wasp sting. JAMA 235:2120–2121, 1976.

62. Crawley F, Schon F, Brown MM: Cerebral infarction: A rare complication of wasp sting. J Neurol Neurosurg Psychiatry 66:550–551, 1999.

63. Lim P, Tan IK, Feng PH: Elevated serum enzymes in patients with wasp/bee sting and their clinical significance. Clin Chim Acta 66:405–409, 1976.

64. Bousquet J, Huchard G, Michel FB: Toxic reactions induced by Hymenoptera venom. Ann Allergy 52:371–374, 1984.

65. Chao SC, Lee YY: Acute rhabdomyolysis and intravascular hemolysis following extensive wasp stings. Int J Dermatol 38:131–141, 1999.

66. Gale AN: Insect-sting encephalopathy. BMJ 284:20–21, 1982.

67. Levine HD: Acute myocardial infarction following wasp sting: Report of two cases and critical survey of the literature. Am Heart J 91:365–374, 1976.

68. Schulte KL, Kochen MM: Haemolytic anaemia in an adult after a wasp sting (Letter). Lancet 2:478, 1981.

69. Thiruventhiram T, Goh BK, Leong CL, et al: Acute renal failure following multiple wasp stings. Nephrol Dial Transpl 14:214–217, 1999.

70. Zhang R, Meleg-Smith S, Batuman V: Acute tubulointerstitial nephritis after wasp stings. Am J Kidney Dis 38:E33, 2001.

71. Vachvanichsanong P, Dissaneewate P, Mitarnun W: Non-fatal acute renal failure due to wasp stings in children. Pediatr Nephrol 11:734–736, 1997.

72. Barss P: Renal failure and death after multiple stings in Papua New Guinea: Ecology, prevention and management of attacks by vespid wasps. Med J Aust 151:659–663, 1989.

73. Chugh KS, Sharma BK, Singhal PC: Acute renal failure following hornet stings. J Trop Med Hyg 79:42–44, 1976.

74. Shilkin KB, Chen BTM, Khoo OT: Rhabdomyolysis caused by hornet venom. BMJ 1:156–157, 1972.

75. Watemberg N, Weizman Z, Shahak E, et al: Fatal multiple organ failure following massive hornet stings. J Toxicol Clin Toxicol 33:471–474, 1995.

76. Weizman Z, Mussafi H, Ishay JS, et al: Multiple hornet stings with features of Reye's syndrome. Gastroenterology 89:1407–1410, 1985.

77. Kitagawa K, Hayasaka S, Setogawa T: Wasp sting-induced retinal damage. Ann Ophthalmol 25:157–158, 1993.

78. Bloom FL: Imported fire ants and death: A documented case report. J Fla Med Assoc 71:87–89, 1984.

79. Prahlow JA, Barnard JJ: Fatal anaphylaxis due to fire ant stings. Am J Forensic Med Pathol 19:137–142, 1998.

80. Adams CT, Lofgren CS: Red imported fire ants (Hymenoptera: formicidae): Frequency of sting attacks on residents of Sumter County, Georgia. J Med Entomol 18:378–382, 1981.

81. deShazo RD, Williams DF, Moak ES: Fire ant attacks on residents in health care facilities: A report of two cases. Ann Intern Med 131:424–429, 1999.

82. Vetter RS, Visscher PK, Camazine S: Mass envenomations by honey bees and wasps. West J Med 170:223–227, 1999.

83. Tsain BJ, Leung J, Chen JB, et al: Mortality in wasp stings: A report of three cases (Abstract). Seventeenth International Congress of the EAPCCT, Marseille, June 4–7, 1996.

84. Jones RGA, Corteling RL, To HP, et al: A novel Fab-based antivenom for the treatment of mass bee attacks. Am J Trop Med Hyg 61:361–366, 1999.

85. Schumacher MJ, Egen NB, Tanner D: Neutralization of bee venom lethality by immune serum antibodies. Am J Trop Med Hyg 55:197–201, 1996.

86. Camazine S, Morse RA: The Africanized honeybee. Am Sci 76:465–471, 1988.

87. deShazo RD, Williams DF: Multiple fire ant stings indoors. South Med J 88:712–715, 1995.

88. Marshall H: What makes a bee sting deadly? Trends Immunol 22:183, 2001.

89. Geerlings SE, Canninga-van Dijk MR: A patient resuscitated after an insect sting. Neth J Med 58:45–51, 2001.

PART 7

Agents of Chemical and Biologic Terrorism

CHAPTER 130

Chemical and Biologic Terrorism Incidents and Intensive Care

R. Steven Tharratt ▪ Timothy E. Albertson

The events of 2001, including the terrorist bombing of the World Trade Centers and the deliberate introduction of anthrax spores into the U.S. postal system, mark a watershed in the medical planning for and response to an attack using a chemical or biologic weapon. Although much planning has focused on the prehospital and emergency department phases of these disasters, toxicology and intensive care are among the key resources in the management of the actual uses of these weapons.

Despite the popular notion of the inevitability of the threat posed by the terrorist use of chemical and biologic agents, few systematic scientific studies of mitigation efforts appropriate for civilian use have been published in the open literature. An Institute of Medicine study outlined priorities for research to improve the civilian medical response to terrorist incidents.[1] Successful management of an incident involving these weapons requires the coordinated efforts and response of a multidisciplinary team of fire, law enforcement, and medical and public health professionals and an emergency response at the federal, state, regional, and local levels. In the medical community, expertise in toxicology, emergency medicine, critical care, infectious diseases, and public health is required to successfully manage the medical response to these incidents. This chapter focuses on the planning for and the medical management of the severely intoxicated victims of a chemical or biologic (or both) incident.

FRAMING THE PROBLEM

Terrorism has many different definitions and can manifest in many different forms and venues. A simple definition of *terrorism* for our purposes is "violence, or the threat of violence, calculated to create an atmosphere of fear and alarm, through acts designed to coerce others into actions they otherwise would not undertake or into refraining from

actions that they desired to take."[2] The use of a chemical, biologic, radiologic, or nuclear (CBRN) weapon as a component of a terrorist act is an extremely rare event in the United States. Most terrorist incidents in the United States have involved conventional explosives. Because most non–scientifically trained people do not understand chemical and biologic agents, they appeal to the public's psychological fear of destruction by a powerful, imperceptible force. This fundamental fear of destruction, coupled by the intense media attention surrounding a CBRN event, fulfills the need for attention to the cause espoused by the terrorist.

Misconceptions about Chemical, Biologic, Radiologic, or Nuclear Planning

1. Medical management of a terrorist use of a CBRN weapon is the same as medical management of a military use of a CBRN weapon.
2. Chemical terrorism incidents are the same as biologic terrorism incidents.
3. It is impossible to plan for events of this type.
4. Intensive care unit planning is the same as emergency planning in other areas of the hospital.

CBRN, chemical, biologic, radiologic, or nuclear.

To plan appropriately for terrorist incidents, a local risk assessment must be made. Incidents involving CBRN weapons may be classified appropriately as a "low-frequency/high-consequence event." Planning for a low-frequency/high-consequence event is more successful when these contingencies are built into the framework of existing emergency plans for more common events. CBRN medical planning focuses on the similarities of patient management to the typical management of patients in intensive care units

(ICUs). Several fallacies pervade planning for CBRN events. These fallacies significantly impede appropriate ICU planning. Appropriate medical planning requires an understanding of the challenges posed by the following principles.

1. Civilian medical response is not the same as military medical response.

In 1975, the United States ratified the Biological Warfare Convention, which bans the development, production, stockpiling, acquisition, and retention of biologic agents and toxins. However, during the mid-20th century, the United States pursued a defensive and an offensive military chemical and biologic weapons program. During this time, potentially effective medical response measures to chemical and biologic agents were developed. Although most of the experience and scientific data concerning medical management of CBRN incidents have been conducted by or under the sponsorship of the U.S. military, the goals and use of a CBRN weapon by a terrorist are fundamentally different from the military use of these weapons. The civilian population is a more heterogeneous population, chronologically and medically, than a military force. Additional planning needs are introduced by the unknown time and location of a terrorist use of a CBRN weapon coupled with the lack of psychological preparation of the civilian population. A large amount of military medical response is predicated on minimally affecting the readiness of the military force and rapidly returning to battle as many exposed soldiers as medically possible. These concerns generally are not appropriate in the civilian population. Military doctrine refers to the concept of *acceptable losses*; terrorist use of a CBRN weapon produces *unavoidable losses* in the civilian population. From these differences, it can be seen that, despite basing medical care on the data developed by the military, medical care of civilian victims of a terrorist use of a CBRN weapon requires unique planning efforts and perhaps different treatment regimens.

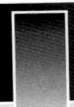

Differences Between Military Use and Civilian Use of Chemical, Biologic, Radiologic, or Nuclear Weapons

Goals

Military use—efficiency degradation of opponent, denial of tactical or strategic objectives, demoralization of enemy
Terrorist use—infliction of terror or death or both, media attention to cause

Other Differences

Age and medical heterogeneity of a civilian population
Physical and psychological preparation of potential victim
Known location and time (war zone) versus use at safe locations
Acceptable versus unavoidable losses

2. Chemical incidents are not the same as biologic incidents.

A common pitfall equates the planning needs and management principles for these two classes of agents. Several fundamental differences exist between chemical and biologic agents (Table 130-1). These differences alter the latency period and the presenting signs and symptoms of victims in events involving these agents.

TABLE 130-1 Differences Between Biologic and Chemical Agents

BIOLOGIC AGENTS	CHEMICAL AGENTS
Naturally exist	Man-made
Production difficult (scientific)	Production difficult (industrial)
None volatile	Many volatile
Among most toxic agents known	Less toxic than many biologics
Infectious agents reproduce	Do not reproduce
Cannot penetrate intact skin (most)	Can penetrate intact skin
Odorless and tasteless	Odor or taste or both when exposed (most)
Effects require incubation (days)	Effects immediate
Aerosol delivery (HEPA filters protect)	Aerosol/mist/droplet delivery (self-contained breathing apparatus and vapor-tight ensembles protect)

HEPA, high-efficiency particulate air.

Chemical agents refer to man-made chemicals designed to kill or incapacitate. Several classes of common industrial chemicals produce intoxications similar to the chemical threat agents, and patient management is similar to the management of victims exposed to these industrial chemicals. Emergency medical response and hazardous material response teams are important to the management of a chemical incident.

Biologic agents refer to living organisms or their biologic products that are intended to kill or incapacitate. A successful covert use of a weapon of this type is likely to occur as an "unusual outbreak of an unusual disease." This outbreak is likely to be recognized initially by an astute clinician or inferred via the public health and poison control reporting infrastructures. Use of biologic weapons heavily involves public health resources and not directly emergency response/hazardous materials teams. Although the differentiation between a natural and man-made outbreak of disease may be difficult in the early stages of the incident, the ICU management of the patients is similar.

3. It is not impossible to plan for a terrorist use of a CBRN weapon.

It seems daunting to plan for a terrorist attack that leaves hundreds to thousands of victims requiring intensive care. It is possible to construct extreme scenarios that can overwhelm any response plan. However, a response plan that builds on existing daily capacity, emergency plans, and procedures to respond effectively to an incident can be developed. As a general rule, it is not a prudent use of medical resources to provide for a standby capability to manage a major CBRN incident in most locations in the United States. It is the unusual hospital system in today's medical environment that can manage even a minor CBRN incident without relying on a regional or statewide "mutual aid" and patient disbursement capability. Certain high-risk potential targets, identified through a locally based risk assessment, may require a more extensive commitment of personnel and resources. The capabilities to provide intensive care, although scalable to a certain degree, are fixed by equipment and personnel availability. When these capabilities are exceeded by the magnitude of an incident, some combination of triage and regional/national patient transfer assistance is required. It still is possible to provide for the basic management principles as outlined subsequently as part of an intensive care plan for the medical management of victims of a terrorist use of a CBRN weapon.

4. ICU planning is not the same as emergency planning in other areas of the hospital.

The needs and planning requirements of the ICU are different from those of other areas of the hospital. Intensive care is concerned with the *successful* use of a CBRN device. These events are significantly less frequent than the *threat* or false claim of use. In 1998–1999, more than 100 hoaxes claiming the release of anthrax occurred in cities throughout the United States. These incidents triggered a significant emergency response and resulted in a major improvement in various emergency response plans.[3] None of these hoaxes proved to involve a pathologic strain of *Bacillus anthracis*, and no victims required intensive care services. Emergency departments have to plan for decontamination of victims and triage of the nonexposed "worried well" from the truly exposed. Although these plans do affect intensive care planning, these concerns are less prominent in the ICU. ICUs are more concerned with the procurement of pharmaceuticals, life-support equipment such as ventilators, and staffing for a prolonged high-acuity patient population. Issues such as triage of scarce resources, provision of intensive care in nontraditional areas of the hospital, and forgoing or terminating futile therapy all assume significant planning needs for ICUs. There are key planning considerations in the development of a critical care response plan.

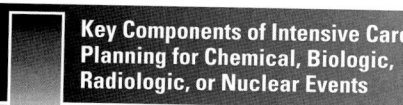

Key Components of Intensive Care Planning for Chemical, Biologic, Radiologic, or Nuclear Events

Provision of high acuity–level staffing for prolonged periods
Procurement of pharmaceuticals and equipment (e.g., ventilators)
Provision of appropriate personnel protective equipment
Indications for cohort nursing
Interface with hospital epidemiology and community public health
Provision of critical care in nontraditional areas of the hospital
Austere critical care
Triage within the intensive care unit
Termination of futile therapy
Psychological support for caregivers

CHEMICAL AGENTS

The chemical threat agents of interest to ICUs include the organophosphate nerve agents, the cyanides, the vesicants, and industrial chemicals with predominantly respiratory effects, including phosgene and chlorine. Each of these chemical threat agents is clinically similar to more commonly encoun-

tered industrial chemical analogues and has similar management strategies (Table 130-2). The medical management of exposures to these more common chemical agents is discussed in depth elsewhere in this book. This chapter focuses on the clinically significant differences in the medical management of these chemical threat agents versus their more commonly encountered industrial analogues.

Nerve Agents

Nerve agents are among the most toxic of the chemical threat agents. Although they are referred to in the popular literature as *nerve gases*, all are liquid at room temperature. Although these agents were originally synthesized by the Germans during World War II in search of alternatives to the embargoed insecticide nicotine, their toxicity for mammalian nervous systems soon was appreciated. All of these agents (sometimes referred to as *G agents*) are organophosphate compounds. They differ from the more commonly encountered organophosphate pesticides in that the organic side chains are relatively short (ethyl and methyl moieties), and they differ in the electronegativity of the leaving group (usually containing fluorine or a cyano group). The volatility of these agents is slightly less than that of water. Volatility determines in part the onset of symptoms and the persistence of these agents in the environment. Another nerve agent, O-ethyl S-diisopropylaminomethyl methylphosphonothiolate, usually referred to as *VX*, has a significantly lower volatility and vapor pressure, resulting in more persistence in the environment and on clothing. The nerve agents all are potent irreversible inhibitors of acetylcholinesterase and butyrocholinesterase in humans.

Although it is claimed that several "recipes" for the synthesis of nerve agents circulate on the Internet, a review of these pages showed little more than reaction equations. The chemistry involved in the actual synthesis of these agents, together with knowledge of the appropriate reaction conditions, requires a significant background in synthetic chemistry. This background, the tight controls placed on the likely precursor materials, the reactivity of several of the intermediate products, the requirement for specialized reaction containers, and the need for containment of the resulting agent make the actual successful synthesis of nerve agents beyond all but the most sophisticated, well-funded terrorist groups. The production of sarin by the Aum Shinrikyo cult was estimated to cost $30 million, involved 80 persons led by a Ph.D.-level scientist, and took at least 1 year to synthesize.[2]

TABLE 130-2 Typical Chemical Threat Agents		
THREAT AGENTS	**MILITARY IDENTIFICATION**	**INDUSTRIAL CHEMICAL WITH SIMILAR NATURE**
Nerve agents	Nerve agents	Organophosphate pesticides
Cyanide	Blood agents	Cyanides
Phosgene	Pulmonary (choking) agents	Chlorine
Vesicants	Blister agents	Acids

CLINICAL EFFECTS

Exposure to nerve agents occurs usually via respiratory exposure to vapor, although skin exposure to a liquid agent may occur. The few case reports of industrial exposure to sarin vapor described significant miosis, rhinorrhea, mild respiratory distress, and wheezing in the victims.[4] These symptoms also were observed in the victims of the Japan sarin incident. Victims who have continued exposure to the agent rapidly progress to unconsciousness, fine motor fasciculations, respiratory failure, and cardiovascular collapse. The timing and progression of symptoms depend on the dose delivered and the exposure circumstances. Symptoms develop almost immediately after vapor exposure; they can be delayed several minutes if cutaneous exposure to a liquid agent occurs. Cutaneous exposure also may produce local sweating and muscle fasciculations at the site of contamination followed by nausea and vomiting.

DECONTAMINATION

Rapid scene decontamination of victims is required for any contact with a liquid nerve agent. Because of the toxicity of these agents and the time required for patients to arrive to the ICU, it is unlikely that any nerve agent remains on the skin when victims are admitted to the ICU. It is possible that an agent could be present in the hair, nail beds, and other areas where it has not been adsorbed. It is vital to confirm that adequate decontamination has occurred on arrival of the victim in the ICU. If any doubt about the adequacy of decontamination exists, careful skin cleansing with soap and water by ICU personnel clothed in personal protective equipment equivalent to universal (barrier/splash) precautions is required. Particular attention should be directed to the poorly adsorbed areas of the scalp and nail beds and other areas commonly missed in rapid scene or emergency department decontamination, including armpits, perineum, interdigital areas, and feet. Although nerve agents hydrolyze more rapidly in the presence of sodium hypochlorite, the potential toxicity of this agent on ocular tissue and mucous membranes makes the use of specialized decontamination solutions unnecessary in the ICU.

Stabilization

Stabilization of a patient exposed to a nerve agent is identical to the management of an organophosphate-exposed patient. Rapid decontamination, aggressive airway control, and respiratory support with assisted ventilation usually are accomplished in the prehospital area and emergency department. A significant difference between nerve agent and other organophosphate intoxications is the amount of atropine required to modulate the muscarinic symptoms. Atropine doses of 2 to 20 mg usually stabilize a victim exposed to a nerve agent.[4] This dose is significantly less than the hundreds of milligrams of atropine often required in some cases of pesticide intoxication.[5] The relative smallness of the doses of atropine required to reverse the muscarinic effects of nerve agents is not understood completely; it may be due in part to the potency of the agents compared with industrial organophosphate agents.

OXIME THERAPY

After decontamination, stabilization of the patient, and reversal of muscarinic symptoms with atropine, regeneration of the organophosphate-inhibited cholinesterase by oxime therapy is required. When acetylcholinesterase is inactivated by a nerve agent, the enzyme can be reactivated either by spontaneous hydrolytic cleavage (a minor pathway with nerve agents) or by use of a nucleophilic oxime antidote. If neither occurs, the nerve agent–acetylcholinesterase complex undergoes dealkylation—a process referred to as *aging*—rendering the enzyme irreversibly inactivated. The speed of the aging process depends on the specific nerve agent. The aging half-lives range from a few minutes with soman (GD)[4] to 48 hours with VX.[6] Sarin and tabun are intermediate, with aging half-lives of 3 hours and 14 hours, respectively.[3] Oxime therapy is most effective when administered within these half-lives. The implication is that successful oxime therapy likely requires prehospital or emergency department use of oximes to be most effective in cases of soman and sarin exposures. Some prehospital providers have access to Military Mark I kits, which contain 2 mg of atropine and 600 mg of pralidoxime chloride in autoinjectors for intramuscular injection. These providers are trained to administer the contents of three Military Mark I kits to victims exhibiting severe nerve agent poisoning.

Pralidoxime chloride (Protopam Chloride) is the only oxime available for use in the United States. Ideally, it is infused intravenously at a dose of 15 to 25 mg/kg. Hypertensive effects of this drug are minimized by slow (over 30 minutes) infusion. Pralidoxime chloride is formulated in 600-mg autoinjectors for intramuscular use in the field (Military Mark I kit). These devices may be the only source of pralidoxime chloride available in the early hours after a significant incident because few hospitals that do not see organophosphate-intoxicated patients on a regular basis stock sufficient supplies of pralidoxime chloride to treat more than one or two patients.

CARE IN THE ICU

Patients who survive to be admitted to the ICU are at risk of developing seizures. Control of seizure activity induced by nerve agents is identical to control of other chemically induced seizures and may include benzodiazepines, barbiturates, and propofol. Diazepam is used widely by the military for seizure control; it is packaged in 10-mg autoinjectors for field intramuscular injection. There are no data to suggest, however, that diazepam is any more effective than the newer benzodiazepines. The recommendation for diazepam use probably reflected its sole availability when drug therapy for nerve agent exposure was developed by the military.

Considerable anxiety and uncertainty may surround the need for isolation of critically ill victims and respiratory protection of the health care team. This anxiety is extrapolated in part from the uncertainty of the appropriate levels of protective equipment required for field health care workers and emergency department personnel. Assuming that emergency field decontamination with complete clothing removal, followed by additional skin decontamination in the emergency department, has occurred, the risk of significant contamination of the ICU is small. These agents do not off-gas from victims, so the standard barrier protective equipment available to the ICU should suffice to protect the health care team. The development of miosis or rhinorrhea in any members of the ICU team should trigger a reassessment of the adequacy of patient decontamination.

Cyanide

The physiochemical properties of cyanide make successful mass casualty use of this chemical weapon by a terrorist difficult. Cyanides are not an effective weapon in outdoor use and are more likely to be encountered as an agent of product tampering, homicide, suicide, or assassination. Law enforcement personnel are familiar with the use of cyanide salts in booby trap–type devices. Cyanide vapors are highly toxic in closed space encounters, prolonged vapor exposures, and ingestions. If vapor exposure is terminated rapidly, recovery can be rapid, even without antidote use. The management of victims exposed to cyanide fumes is identical to the management of victims exposed industrially to cyanide and is covered in Chapter 95.

Vesicants

Vesicants have the capability to produce severe cutaneous, ocular, and respiratory damage. Formation of large blisters after vesicant exposure is classic. During World War I, the vesicants resulted in the largest numbers of chemical casualties. Although considered a major chemical threat agent by the military, there has been little use of vesicants by classic terrorist groups. The principal agents in this class include mustard and lewisite.

MUSTARD

Chemistry and Pathophysiology. Mustard, bis-(2-chloroethyl) sulfide, distantly related to the alkylating chemotherapeutic agents, is a highly reactive electrophilic molecule that alkylates cellular DNA immediately on contact. Mechanisms involving cellular depletion of glutathionine and free radical–induced cellular damage also have been proposed to explain the toxicity of mustard. Mustard exists as an oily liquid with a high vapor density and relatively low volatility. Exposure to mustard is likely through direct contact with the liquid agent or inhalation of vapor. The target organs of mustard exposure include the skin, eyes, and respiratory tract. Mustard does not produce immediate pain or symptoms, even though the cellular damage occurs within minutes after exposure. It is unique among the chemical agents in its lack of immediate symptoms of exposure. Cutaneous exposure to mustard produces erythema approximately 4 to 8 hours after exposure. The development of fluid-filled blisters occurs 2 to 18 hours later. Ocular exposure initially produces a conjunctivitis that progresses in approximately 12 hours to blepharospasm, corneal ulcerations, and occasionally panophthalmitis. Mustard produces dose-dependant inflammation and necrosis of the upper and lower respiratory tracts. This necrosis can result in pseudomembrane formation and obstruction of the tracheobronchial tree and secondary bacterial infection. Cough, hoarseness, and sinus tenderness may be present.

Decontamination and Treatment. Because of the speed by which mustard produces cellular damage, decontamination must occur within 1 to 2 minutes after contact to be effective. Thorough decontamination of the victim is required to protect the health care team from secondary contamination resulting from residual mustard liquid on skin or clothing. Treatment of mustard exposure is supportive and is similar to the management of other chemically induced burns. Respiratory support and bronchoscopy may be required for significant respiratory system involvement. Because of the alkylating effects of these agents, severe exposures may result in bone marrow suppression and require blood product or factor support.

LEWISITE

Lewisite, chlorovinyldichloroarsine, an arsinical vesicant, differs from mustard in its ability to produce immediate pain and stinging on contact. Lewisite produces clinical effects similar to those of mustard, although the onset of symptoms is much faster than with mustard. The development of immediate pain and irritation after contact with lewisite reduces the duration of ocular and respiratory exposures. Large exposures to lewisite may produce an increased capillary permeability syndrome with resultant shock. A specific antidote, British antilewisite, reduces the severity of injury when applied topically and ocularly. Preparations of British antilewisite for ocular and cutaneous use no longer are manufactured. Intramuscular British antilewisite may reduce systemic effects for lewisite exposure, although clinical studies are lacking.

Chemicals with Predominantly Respiratory Effects

A wide variety of chemicals potentially available for terrorist use produce toxic vapors or gases. These include the traditional chemical threat agents phosgene and chlorine, the non-traditional toxic by-products of conventional explosives, and the pyrolysis products of Teflon (perfluoroisobutylene). These chemical agents may produce toxicity via asphyxiation, direct corrosive effects on the respiratory system, or systemic toxicity. A key physiochemical property determining the location and extent of injury is the water solubility of the compound. Because the respiratory system is lined with a water-rich mucosa, chemicals with low water solubility are able to penetrate farther into the lower respiratory system. These compounds also have poor warning properties because eye, nose, and upper airway irritation may be minimal or absent. Management of exposures to these chemicals follows standard medical approaches to industrial chemical exposures. Termination of exposure, scene decontamination, aggressive management of the airway, and respiratory support should be accomplished in the prehospital or emergency department setting. Noncardiogenic pulmonary edema or adult respiratory distress syndrome or both may supervene within 24 hours. Management is identical to management of adult respiratory distress syndrome induced by other etiologies. There are no data to support the prophylactic use of corticosteroids or inhaled sodium bicarbonate.

High-temperature pyrolysis of Teflon-containing substances produces perfluoroisobutylenes. Inhalation of this chemical produces a syndrome of fever and rapid development of pulmonary edema within 1 to 4 hours (polymer fume fever). This edema may be worsened by significant exertion in the immediate postexposure period. Treatment is supportive.

BIOLOGIC AGENTS

Recognition

Biologic agents present more of a planning challenge to intensive care because the toxicity of these agents results in victims who require prolonged critical care services and because of the geographic dispersion of victims that occurs during the incubation period. The delay from agent exposure to disease manifestation (due to the incubation period of most biologics) in the setting of worldwide rapid transportation systems makes it possible for a victim to be exposed to a biologic agent on one continent and manifest disease on another. The lack of immediate symptoms after exposure is a significant difference between chemical and biologic agents. This distinction is crucial because a successful covert use of a biologic agent is likely to manifest as an unusual outbreak of an unusual disease. The initial recognition of a terrorist event is likely to be made by an astute clinician recognizing an unusual outbreak of disease. The investigation of an outbreak of this type follows basic epidemiologic investigative principles, although there is tremendous pressure to accelerate the process. Most of the biologic threat agents exist naturally in the environment as zoonoses (e.g., anthrax and plague), represent rare intoxications (e.g., botulism), or typically present in geographically defined epizootic outbreaks (e.g., hemorrhagic fever viruses). Table 130-3 lists the biologic agents believed to present the highest threat for terrorist use.

The requirements for successful use of a biologic agent arguably have been oversimplified in the popular press. Although much is written about the "ease" with which pathologic bacteria or viruses may be obtained or isolated, the difficulty of producing large volumes of infective material and converting this material into a form and size suitable for delivery to victims is underestimated. The Aum Shinrikyo cult apparently tried unsuccessfully to deliver biologic agents on multiple occasions without any evidence of successful infection.[7] In 1346 in the siege of Caffa, the corpses of plague victims were hurled into the city via catapult. This story illustrates the importance of the delivery system in the successful use of a biologic weapon!

Because many of the threat biologic infections present with similar nonspecific early symptoms and rapidly progress to a clinical picture indistinguishable from septic shock, it is likely that the initial victims would reach the ICU without a specific diagnosis being established. Because most of these threat infections are rare and because most physicians have never seen a case of plague, inhalational anthrax, or tularemia, they often are not included in the differential diagnosis of septic shock. Multiple cases of unexplained sepsis occurring in previously healthy young individuals should trigger the suspicion of a possible biologic attack. Further complicating the ability to reach a specific diagnosis rapidly is that many of the threat agents are not cultured in the microbiology laboratory because they resemble contaminants that routinely are discarded or not worked up further (*Bacillus*) or because the appropriate medium is not plated routinely (tularemia and some *Salmonella* species). Because few case series of antimicrobial therapy of these uncommon diseases have been reported, and randomized trials of treatment regimens are nonexistent, antibiotic recommendations are largely anecdotal, derived from in vitro sensitivities of antimicrobials to the organism or extrapolated from animal models of disease.

Level of Isolation

Among the earliest decisions to be made in the ICU is the appropriate level of isolation of victims. This level is determined largely by the identification of the infecting organism. Early uncertainty as to the etiologic organism or fear and emotional reaction to the terrorist event often lead to maximal isolation—"just in case." This irrational isolation may have adverse effects on personnel and resources. Most biologic threat agents either have no person-to-person transmission potential (anthrax) or have minimal and limited transmission potential (plague and hemorrhagic viruses). The major exception to this is smallpox, which has significant secondary transmission potential. Cohort care and quarantine procedures may be appropriate if an outbreak of smallpox is suspected. Because skin adsorption of these organisms does not occur, barrier isolation (universal precautions) with high-efficiency particulate air (HEPA) level air filtration, respirators, and masks is sufficient to care for most patients in the emergency situation of an ICU with multiple victims. Additional patient decontamination beyond the emergency field decontamination is of a lower priority with biologic agent exposure compared with chemical agents. Because of static electrical charge, most crude biologic weapons likely constructed by a terrorist group do not resuspend back into the air or produce secondary contamination of the health care team. A thorough shower or bed bath with antiseptic soap should suffice to decontaminate ICU patients adequately and should reassure the health care team.

Chemoprophylaxis and Vaccination of the Health Care Team

The need for prophylactic antibiotic and vaccine administration for members of the health care team must be considered carefully. This need must be based on the transmission

---

> **TABLE 130-3 Critical Biologic Agents**

Bacterial Agents
Bacillus anthracis (anthrax)
Yersinia pestis (plague)
Francisella tularensis (tularemia)

Bacterial Toxins
Clostridium botulinum toxin (botulism)

Viral Agents
Variola (smallpox)
Filoviruses
    Ebola hemorrhagic fever
    Marburg hemorrhagic fever
Arenaviruses
    Lassa fever
    Argentine hemorrhagic fever

Adapted from Biological and Chemical Terrorism: Strategic Plan for Preparedness and Response: Recommendation of the CDC Strategic Planning Workgroup. MMWR Morbid Mortal Wkly Rep 49(RR-4), 2000.

potential of the agent together with the ability of prophylactic antimicrobial therapy to prevent or attenuate disease. It is not reasonable to ask health care providers to care for patients at personal risk if an appropriate prophylactic regimen is available but not used. Fear and uncertainty regarding appropriate chemoprophylaxis can lead to inappropriate self-medication. The directors of one hospital in California, when informed of the imminent arrival of victims from a purported anthrax exposure, immediately ordered dosing of the entire emergency department staff with ciprofloxacin, a totally unnecessary measure (JA Alsop, personal communication, 2000). Firm recommendations for prophylactic treatment of health care team members who have *not* been exposed in the terrorist incident have not been reported. Smallpox requires vaccination of treating personnel as soon as possible with vaccinia vaccine. If possible until arrival of the vaccine, victims should be cared for by previously vaccinated caregivers, who may be afforded at least partial immunity. Anthrax, because of lack of person-to-person transmission, probably requires no prophylaxis for caregivers. Cases of plague, particularly the pneumonic form, may be appropriate for health care team prophylaxis with a fluoroquinolone or doxycycline. Effective prophylactic antivirals currently do not exist for the viral hemorrhagic fevers.

Specific Agents

ANTHRAX

Anthrax (*B. anthracis*) is a gram-positive, nonmotile, spore-forming bacillus that has a worldwide distribution. Because of its ability to form long-lived, environmentally resistant spores, anthrax has significant potential as a biologic threat agent. Anthrax naturally exists primarily as a zoonotic disease of cattle that become infected by ingestion of spores. Humans become infected by contact with infected animals or their contaminated products, such as wool, meat, or hides. Virulence factors in *B. anthracis* include an antiphagocytic capsule and two exotoxins, lethal and edema. Clinical disease in humans usually manifests as cutaneous anthrax, gastrointestinal anthrax, or inhalational anthrax. Inhalation of anthrax spores produces a hemorrhagic mediastinitis after an incubation period of 1 to 6 days. Although this incubation period is cited widely, an epidemiologic investigation of an anthrax outbreak in Swerdlovsk, Russia, in 1979, ascribed to an airborne release of weaponized anthrax, suggested that the incubation period may be as long as 45 days.[8] The mediastinitis rapidly progresses to septic shock. Meningitis may occur and manifest as seizures. When symptoms develop, even with aggressive supportive care, mortality of inhalational anthrax is estimated at 85%. The mortality of the inhalational anthrax series in the eastern United States in 2001–2002 was 36%.

Consensus recommendations for the medical management of a terrorist use of anthrax exist.[9] Anthrax infection is treated with high-dose penicillin. Tetracycline, chloramphenicol, and erythromycin also can be used. In vitro activity has been shown against anthrax by the fluoroquinolones, gentamicin, first-generation cephalosporins, vancomycin, and clindamycin—although there is not as much clinical experience with these drugs. In the early stages of an

anthrax outbreak, the scarcity of antibiotics may require use of a variety of treatment regimens until the arrival of one of the predeployed national pharmaceutical caches. These caches, controlled by the U.S. Public Health Service, are intended to supply a medical community rapidly with sufficient pharmaceuticals to treat the victims of a chemical or biologic incident.

Prophylactic antimicrobial treatment beginning within 24 hours after exposure to anthrax aerosol confers protection against the development of disease in a primate model.[10] Ciprofloxacin, doxycycline, and penicillin were the antibiotics used in conjunction with active immunization with the human anthrax vaccine. This vaccine is produced from filtrates of an attenuated *B. anthracis* and contains predominantly protective antigen. Exposed victims not manifesting signs of illness need to receive prophylaxis with antibiotics as soon as possible after exposure and continue on oral antibiotics until vaccination with anthrax vaccine can be accomplished.

PLAGUE

The causative agent of plague, *Yersinia pestis*, a gram-negative, nonsporulating, non–lactose-fermenting bacillus, exists worldwide. Transmitted by fleas to rodents, *Y. pestis* normally produces enzootic infection in rodents. Intermittent epizootic outbreaks in rodents, particularly in rural areas, allow for human infection, usually from bites by infected fleas. Several virulence factors of *Y. pestis* have been identified and are coded for chromosomally and on three plasmids. Because natural outbreaks of human disease sporadically occur, distinguishing a natural epizootic infection from a deliberate act may be difficult in the early stages of the outbreak.

Plague manifests in humans in the bubonic form, a suppurative lymphadenitis in the regional nodes draining the fleabite site; a primary septicemic form, similar in clinical presentation to other gram-negative septic states; and a primary pneumonic form, contracted from inhalation of an infectious *Y. pestis* aerosol. Septicemic plague also can develop into secondary pneumonic plague by involving the respiratory system. Plague often is suspected when a patient presents with the bubonic form, but less so when patients present with primary plague septicemia. A review of naturally occurring epizootic plague cases in New Mexico revealed that the correct diagnosis was suspected in 69% of bubonic patients but only 17% of the primary septicemic patients. Diagnosis of these septicemic patients took 1 day longer (5 days), and the overall mortality was 33%.[11] Diagnosis of plague is made by Gram stain or direct fluorescent antibody stains of aspirates from the buboes and is confirmed by culture.

Because of the potential for person-to-person transmission of plague, plague patients with pneumonia and suspected primary pneumonic plague patients need strict isolation for the first 4 days of antibiotic therapy. Antibiotics of choice for plague include streptomycin and chloramphenicol. It is unlikely that large amounts of these antibiotics would be available for treatment of multiple patients early in an outbreak. Gentamicin also has been used clinically. In vitro activity against *Y. pestis* has been shown by cefotaxime and levofloxacin.[12] A murine model of pneumonic plague showed the efficacy of ciprofloxacin and high-dose (20 mg/kg) gentamicin.[13]

TULAREMIA

Tularemia, a zoonotic disease with worldwide distribution, is produced by *Francisella tularensis*, a gram-negative aerobic bacterium. Its principal animal reservoir is in several species of tick. Rabbits and other small mammals maintain the infection in nature. Humans become infected either via inhalation of an infectious aerosol or via breaks in the skin. Extremely low numbers of bacteria, on the order of 10 to 50 organisms, are sufficient to produce disease.[14] Most patients who cutaneously contract tularemia present with ulcers on the skin or mucus membranes, together with lymphadenopathy. Inhalational infection results in a nonspecific syndrome of fever, chills, headache, and myalgias. Pulse-temperature disassociation may be present, having being described as typhoidal tularemia. Diagnosis of tularemia is made by serologic evidence of infection or culture of the organism from fluids. Streptomycin is the current antibiotic of choice for treatment; however, it is unlikely that a hospital would have sufficient stores of this antibiotic to treat multiple patients. Clinical experience supports the use of gentamicin. Ciprofloxacin and doxycycline have afforded protection in animal challenge studies.[15]

BOTULISM

The neurotoxins produced by clostridial organisms rank among the most potent toxins known. *Clostridium botulinum*, an anaerobic, spore-forming bacterium, elaborates seven neurotoxins that are capable of producing a flaccid descending paralysis with prominent bulbar symptoms. The bacterium has a worldwide distribution and usually produces intoxication via ingestion of contaminated food products. Direct multiplication of the agent in infants results in infant botulism.[16] Intravenous drug abusers can contract botulism via injection of contaminated illicit drugs[17]; in rare cases, direct contamination of open wounds produces wound botulism. These routes of exposure constitute the "typical" cases of botulism. In addition to these routes, direct inhalation of the purified toxin is a potential terrorist route of exposure.

Bulbar symptoms, including diplopia, ptosis, dysphagia, and dysarthria, are among the earliest manifestations of botulism. Muscle weakness progresses in a descending fashion until respiratory failure supervenes. The absence of convulsions can differentiate botulism from nerve agent exposure. Botulism differs from the other biologic agents discussed in the absence of fever and a nonspecific viral-like syndrome. Because of the small amount of botulinum toxin needed to produce disease from inhalation, it is unlikely that serologic examination of blood would yield the diagnosis. Enzyme-linked immunosorbent assay identification of the toxin from samples obtained from nasal mucosa identifies inhalational botulism in primate models.

Early administration of botulinum immune globulin can attenuate symptoms; however, it is less effective after the disease manifests. With the exception of Alaska and California, which control their own supplies of immune globulin, botulinum immune globulin is controlled by the Centers for Disease Control and Prevention (CDC). A toxoid exists for preexposure prophylactic use and is available under an Investigational New Drug (IND) protocol held by the CDC.

SMALLPOX

Variola virus, the causative agent of smallpox, is a member of the Poxviridae family of double-stranded DNA viruses. Because of the absence of an animal reservoir, natural smallpox was eradicated worldwide in 1977. Currently, smallpox virus exists officially in only two locations—the CDC in the United States and laboratories in Russia. Several illicit, clandestine stockpiles of variola virus are thought to exist in several other countries, however. The high contagion rate of smallpox together with the virtual absence of immunity to the natural disease makes smallpox the most dangerous of the biologic threat agents.

Smallpox is infectious by aerosol and through contact with infectious lesions. Mortality in unvaccinated victims is approximately 30%. Immunity conferred by vaccinia vaccination wanes after approximately 10 years. Persons previously vaccinated would be expected to have an attenuated form of variola with an estimated mortality of 3%.

The lesions of variola resemble other vesicular exanthems, especially varicella (chickenpox). Because most clinicians practicing today have never seen a case of variola, the possibility exists of delay in recognizing the disease. Table 130-4 highlights some key differences distinguishing varicella and variola lesions. Consensus recommendations for management of terrorist use of smallpox have been published.[18]

Even a small suspicion of smallpox infection requires immediate strict isolation. The suspected diagnosis must be reported immediately by telephone to public health personnel because this disease has international quarantine requirements. Even one case of smallpox would strongly suggest that a bioterrorism event has occurred. Treatment of smallpox is supportive; no effective antiviral therapy currently exists.

VIRAL HEMORRHAGIC FEVERS

Several RNA viruses from diverse families share the ability to induce an acute febrile illness in humans with profound increased vascular permeability and shock. These syndromes all have high morbidity and mortality. Most of these viruses have an animal host, although some (e.g., Ebola) have not had the animal reservoir identified. Table 130-5 lists the hemorrhagic viral agents considered to be threats.

TABLE 130-4 Key Features for Distinguishing Between Variola and Varicella

FEATURE	VARIOLA (SMALLPOX)	VARICELLA (CHICKEN POX)
Incubation	7–17 days	14–21 days
Prodrome	Fever 2–4 days before rash	None
Pock aging	Synchronous	Asynchronous
Pock spread	Centrifugal	Centripetal
Pock location	Involves palms and soles	Seldom involves palms and soles
Infectivity	From exanthem until vesicles scab	1 day before exanthem until vesicles scab

TABLE 130-5 Threat of Viral Hemorrhagic Viruses

DISEASE	VIRUS (FAMILY)	NATURAL DISTRIBUTION
Ebola hemorrhagic fever	*Filovirus*	Africa
Marburg hemorrhagic fever	*Filovirus*	Africa
Lassa fever	*Arenavirus*	Africa
Argentine hemorrhagic fever	*Arenavirus*	South America

The development of clinical illness varies with each agent and depends on the route of exposure, viral virulence factors, and host responses to infection. The onset of a viral prodrome, with fever, malaise, conjunctival injection, and myalgias, rapidly develops into shock with generalized bleeding from the mucous membranes. The degree of hemorrhagic manifestations is variable, being less in Lassa fever and more prominent in Ebola hemorrhagic fever. Diagnosis of a hemorrhagic fever is made initially on a clinical basis with confirmation by immunologic identification of antibodies to the virus. The patient's travel history usually is a key part of the history to suggest the particular etiologic virus. This history is not present with a terrorist use of one of these agents. Although the virus usually can be isolated from the patient, the virulence of these agents requires special containment procedures, and viral culture attempts are carried out only in highly specialized and secured laboratories.

Treatment of hemorrhagic fevers is supportive; volume replacement, correction of reversible coagulation abnormalities, and blood product support are crucial. Ribavirin has been shown to have activity against Lassa fever[19] and hemorrhagic fever with renal syndromes produced by viruses in the Hantavirus genus.[20] A loading dose of 33 mg/kg, 16 mg/kg every 6 hours for 4 days, and 8 mg/kg every 8 hours for 3 additional days seems effective. Person-to-person transmission of these viruses has been reported, but human-to-human propagation of the virus does not seem to be sustained. Barrier precautions seem to be sufficient for naturally occurring outbreaks of these diseases. No vaccine exists for these viruses except for yellow fever vaccine.

REFERENCES

1. Committee on R&D Needs for Improving Civilian Medical Response to Chemical and Biological Terrorism Incidents: Chemical and Biological Terrorism—Research and Development to Improve Civilian Medical Response. Washington, D.C., National Academy Press, 1999.
2. Advisory Panel to Assess Domestic Response Capabilities for Terrorism Involving Weapons of Mass Destruction: First Annual Report to the President and the Congress: I. Assessing the Threat. 1999. Available at: http://www.rand.org/organization/nsrd/terrpanel/terror.pdf 1–123. Accessed April 27, 2000.
3. Centers for Disease Control: Bioterrorism alleging use of anthrax and interim guidelines for management—United States 1998. MMWR Morbid Mortal Wkly Rep 48:69–74, 1999.
4. Sidell F: Soman and sarin: Clinical manifestations and treatment of accidental poisoning by organophosphates. Clin Toxicol 7:2–6, 1974.
5. Singh S, Batra YK, Singh SM, et al: Is atropine alone sufficient in acute severe organophosphorus poisoning? Experience of a North West Indian Hospital. Int J Clin Pharmacol Ther 33:628–630, 1995.
6. Dunn MA, Sidell FR: Progress in medical defense against nerve agents. JAMA 262:649–652, 1989.
7. Kaplan DE, Marshall A: The Cult at the End of the World: The Incredible Story of Aum., London, Hutchinson, 1996.
8. Meselson M, Guillemin J, Hugh-Jones M, et al: The Sverdlovsk anthrax outbreak of 1979. Science 266:1202–1208, 1994.
9. Inglesby TV, Henderson DA, Bartlett JG, et al: Anthrax as a biological weapon: Medical and public health management. Working Group on Civilian Biodefense. JAMA 281:1735–1745, 1999.
10. Friedlander AM, Welkos SL, Pitt MLM, et al: Postexposure prophylaxis against experimental inhalation anthrax. J Infect Dis 167:1239–1243, 1993.
11. Hull HF, Montes JM, Mann JM: Septicemic plague in New Mexico. J Infect Dis 155:113–118, 1987.
12. Frean JA, Arntzen L, Capper T, et al: In vitro activities of 14 antibiotics against 100 human isolates of *Yersinia pestis* from a Southern African plague focus. Antimicrob Agents Chemother 40:2646–2647, 1996.
13. Byrne WR, Welkos SL, Pitt ML, et al: Antibiotic treatment of experimental pneumonic plague in mice. Antimicrob Agents Chemother 42:675–681, 1998.
14. Saslaw S, Eigelsbach HT, Wilson HE, et al: Tularemia vaccine study I and II. Arch Intern Med 107:121–146, 1961.
15. Russell P, Eley SM, Fulop MJ, et al: The efficacy of ciprofloxacin and doxycycline against experimental tularaemia. J Antimicrob Chemother 41:461–465, 1998.
16. Glatman-Freedman A: Infant botulism. Pediatr Rev 17:185–186, 1996.
17. Passaro DJ, Werner SB, McGee J, et al: Wound botulism associated with black tar heroin among injecting drug users. JAMA 279:859–863, 1998.
18. Henderson DA, Inglesby TV, Bartlett JG, et al: Smallpox as a biological weapon: Medical and public health management. Working Group on Civilian Biodefense. JAMA 281:2127–2137, 1999.
19. McCormick JB, King IJ, Webb PA, et al: Lassa fever: Effective therapy with ribavirin. N Engl J Med 314:20–26, 1986.
20. Huggins JW, Hsiang CM, Cosgriff TM, et al: Prospective, double-blind, concurrent, placebo-controlled clinical trial of intravenous ribavirin therapy of hemorrhagic fever with renal syndrome. J Infect Dis 164:1119–1127, 1991.

CHAPTER 131

Nerve Agents

Mahdi Balali-Mood ■ Kia Balali-Mood

HISTORY OF THE USE OF NERVE AGENTS

Nerve agents are organophosphate (OP) compounds, similar to OP pesticides, and are a group of potentially lethal chemical warfare agents. They are extremely potent inhibitors of the enzyme acetylcholinesterase (AChE), a key regulator of cholinergic neurotransmission. Early attempts in the synthesis of OP were made by Von Hofman, who developed methylphosphor chloride in 1873. Michaelis in 1903 introduced a compound with P—CN bond, which led to the synthesis of many insecticides, including the nerve agent tabun. Lang and Von Kreuger synthesized compounds with P—F linkage in 1932. Schrader developed sarin and tabun in 1937; in 1944, Germans developed soman. British scientists developed VX in 1952.[1]

Exposure of nerve agents to humans was restricted to one prospective study with VX and sarin and to case reports of treatment of accidental exposure to sarin and soman.[2] The first reported use of nerve agents in a war occurred in February 1984 in Majnoon Island, by the Iraqi army against Iranian troops. The nerve agent tabun was found in the environmental samples and in the postmortem examination of the patients who died soon after exposure. More than 300 patients died within 30 minutes of exposure in the field, and several thousands were poisoned by tabun.[3] Toxicologic analyses of the blood, urine, skin, and gastric juice of the chemical war gas victims revealed tabun and sulfur mustard.[4] Later in 1987 and 1988, particularly during the Halabjah massacre, another nerve agent (sarin) also was identified.[5]

A presumed terrorist attack with sarin occurred in a residential area of the city of Matsumoto, Japan, on June 27, 1994. About 600 residents and rescue staff were poisoned; 58 were admitted to hospitals, and 7 died.[6] On March 20, 1995, terrorists released sarin at several points in the Tokyo subway, killing 11 and poisoning more than 5500 people.[7]

RELEVANT CHEMISTRY

Nerve agents are divided into two groups of G and V agents. The G agents (except for tabun, which is a cyanide derivative) are fluorinated OP compounds. The V agents are sulfur-containing OP compounds. The principal G agents, GA, GB, and GD, have the common names of tabun, sarin, and soman, respectively. The other G agents and V agents do not have common names. The oldest and most common V agent is called VX. The names and chemical structures of all nerve agents are summarized in Table 131-1.

Although G agents and V agents commonly are called nerve gases, they exist under temperate conditions as clear, colorless, viscous liquids with high boiling points. They become aerosolized when dispersed by spraying or by an explosive blast from a shell or bomb. The G agents are only moderately volatile (vapor pressure of <2 mm Hg at 20°C), but owing to their great toxicity, the vapors pose a significant inhalational hazard. Vapor pressure of the G agents is sufficiently high for the vapor to be disseminated rapidly. GB is mainly a vapor hazard. VX is less volatile and is normally a liquid contact hazard. Delivery systems of nerve agents include bombs, missiles, cluster spray, and spray tanks. G agents spread rapidly on surfaces such as skin and in the lungs. They are dispersed within hours and are described as *nonpersistent agents*, whereas VX spreads slowly and remains in the place for weeks or longer after exposure and is called a *persistent nerve agent*. Clothing releases G agents for about 30 minutes after contact with vapor.[8] If G agents are released into the air, they are degraded rapidly by reaction with photochemically produced hydroxyl radicals and have an estimated half-life of 10 hours.

Nerve agents are four to six times denser than air. As a result, they tend to remain close to the ground and pose a risk particularly to people in low areas and below-ground shelters. They are soluble in water, organic solvents, and fat. After contact with water, they are hydrolyzed to products that are less toxic than the parent compounds.[9]

PATHOPHYSIOLOGY

Mechanism of Action

The well-known mechanism of action of OP compounds is the inhibition of cholinesterases. Two types of cholinesterase are involved:

1. AChE is a specific enzyme useful for the diagnosis of OP poisoning; it also is called *true cholinesterase*. It usually is estimated in red blood cells and called *RBC AChE* or *erythrocyte AChE*.
2. Butyrylcholinesterase (BChE) is less specific but more sensitive than AChE for the diagnosis of OP poisoning. It also is called *pseudocholinesterase*. BChE is usually estimated in plasma and is called *plasma cholinesterase*.

The reaction between OP compounds and AChE occurs in three steps, as shown in Figure 131-1.[9] The toxic manifestations and lethality after nerve agent exposure seem to follow the irreversible phosphorylation of the serine-containing

TABLE 131-1 Names and Chemical Structures of Nerve Agents

SHORT NAME	COMMON NAME	SYNONYM	PROPER NAME AND CHEMICAL STRUCTURE
GA	Tabun	mLe-100	Ethyl dimethylphosphoramidocyanidate
GB	Sarin	Zarin	Isopropyl Methylphosphonofluoridate
GD	Soman	Zoman	Pinacolyl methylfluorophosphonate
GE	—	—	Isopropyl Ethylphosphonofluoridate
GF	—	—	Cyclohexyl Methylphosphonofluoridate
VX	—	—	O-Ethyl-S-(2-diisopropylaminoethyl)methylphosphonothioate
VE	—	—	O-Ethyl-S-(2-diethylaminoethyl)ethylphosphonothioate

TABLE 131-1 Names and Chemical Structures of Nerve Agents—cont'd

SHORT NAME	COMMON NAME	SYNONYM	PROPER NAME AND CHEMICAL STRUCTURE
VG	—	—	O,O-Diethyl-S-(2-diethylaminoethyl)phosphonothioate 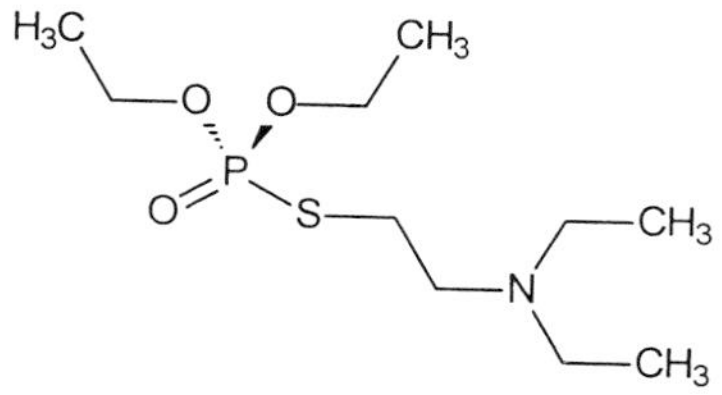
VM	—	—	O-Ethyl-S-(2-diethylaminoethyl)methylphosphonothioate 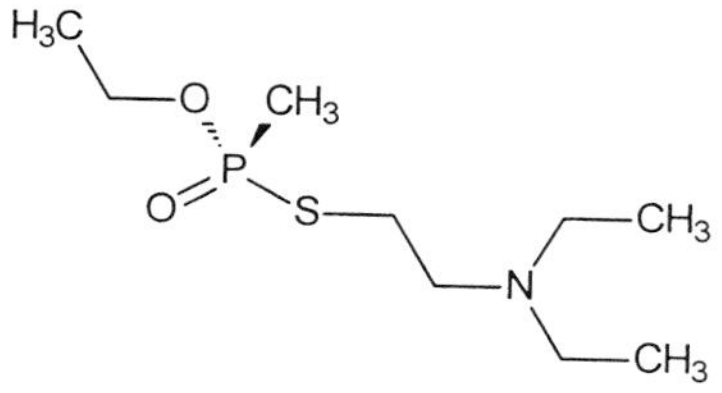

active site of AChE. BChE also is inhibited. People with BChE genetic variation deficiencies may be at risk. The clinically most important variant is atypical (D70G) BChE because people with this variation have 2 hours of apnea after receiving a dose of succinylcholine that is intended to paralyze muscle for 3 to 5 minutes.[10]

Different aging mechanisms are involved. Tabun and butyl-tabun seem to be accommodated similarly in the active center, as suggested by molecular modeling via kinetic studies of phosphorylation and aging with a series of HuAChE mutants (E202Q, F338A, F295A, F297A, and F295L/F297V).[11] A variety of proteolytic enzymes (e.g., chymotrypsin, trypsin) also may be inhibited by OP. Soman and sarin are detoxified in part via a two-step pathway involving bioactivation of the parent compound by the cytochrome P-450 system, then hydrolysis of the resulting oxygenating metabolite (oxon) by serum and liver paraoxygenase (PON1). Serum PON1 has been shown to be polymorphic in humans.[12]

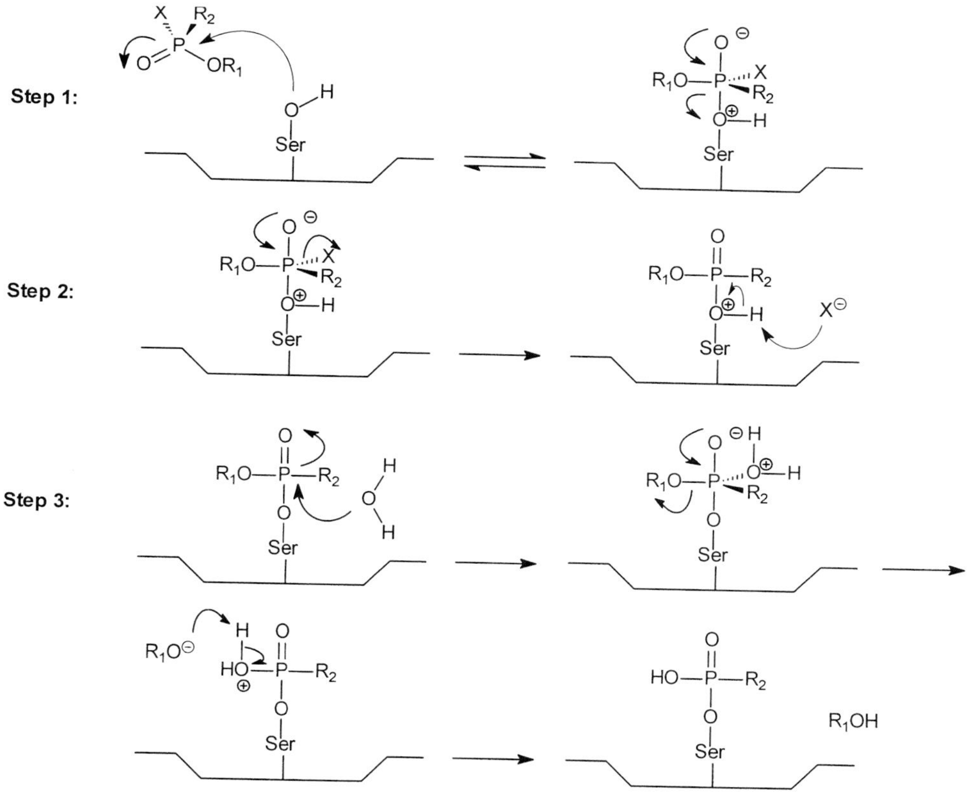

FIGURE 131-1

Three-step reaction mechanism for the inactivation of acetylcholinesterase (AChE) by an organophosphate compound. Step 1 depicts the formation of a reversible complex between a serine residue in the AChE active site and the organophosphate. Step 2 shows the elimination of the organophosphate leaving group (X⁻). In step 3, the aging of the AChE is completed, forming a phosphorylated AChE.

Biochemical Changes

Acetylcholine accumulation is involved in the calcium flux into skeletal muscle fibers during OP poisoning.[13] Bright and coworkers[14] reported a histochemical demonstration of sarin-induced calcium influx in mouse diaphragm, which may be linked with OP-induced myopathy. Sarin may induce myonecrosis. Significant increase in alkaline phosphatase and creatine phosphokinase activity and minor changes in coagulation parameters (prothrombin time, activated partial thromboplastin time, fibrinogen) were observed after soman poisoning in rabbits.[15] Significant increases in creatine phosphokinase, lactate dehydrogenase, alanine aminotransferase, aspartate aminotransferase, and serum potassium, associated with damage to striated muscle and metabolic acidosis, occurred 2 days after GF poisoning in 20 male rhesus monkeys.[16]

Toxicity

The vapor pressure of the three G agents (GA, GB, and GD) makes them significant inhalational hazards, especially at warmer temperatures or when droplets are created by explosion or spray. Based on information from animal studies, the lethal inhaled dose of G agents in humans may be about 1 mg. The G agents also represent a skin contact hazard, particularly when evaporation is minimized and contact is prolonged by contamination of clothing. The percutaneous absorption of G agents is much less rapid and complete, however, than the inhalational form.[8]

VX does not pose a major inhalational hazard under usual circumstances, but it is well absorbed through the skin.[8] The relative lethality as determined in animal studies is VX > soman > sarin > tabun.[17] Acute toxic values of nerve agents in humans are summarized in Table 131-2.

The acute toxicity of nerve agents is due primarily to irreversible inactivation of AChE leading to an accumulation of toxic levels of acetylcholine. Similar to other OP compounds, these agents act by binding to a serine residue at the active site of a cholinesterase molecule, forming a phosphorylating protein that is inactive and incapable of breaking down acetylcholine. The resulting accumulation of toxic levels of acetylcholine at the synapse initially stimulates, then paralyzes cholinergic synaptic transmission. Cholinergic synapses are found in the central nervous system, at the termination of somatic nerves, in the ganglionic synapses of autonomic nerves, and at the parasynaptic nerve endings, such as those in the sweat glands.[9]

The rate of aging varies greatly among the nerve agents. The half-time of aging is within minutes after soman exposure, about 5 hours after sarin exposure, and more than 40 hours after exposure to tabun and VX.[17]

OP compounds also bind to other esterases and cholinergic receptors. Inactivation of neurotoxic esterase by some OP pesticides can lead to delayed peripheral neuropathic effects (OPIND). At many times the median lethal dose (LD_{50}), the nerve agents inhibit neurotoxic esterase to some extent, although the activity of VX is much less than that of G agents.[18] Possible involvement of neurotrophic factor (growth-related enzyme ornithine decarboxylase) during early stages of OPIND, particularly after diisopropylfluorophosphate, has been reported.[19] Nerve agents also bind quickly to cardiac muscarinic (M_2) receptors at higher than physiologic concentrations, but whether this contributes to cardiac toxicity is unknown.[20] They also interact with the nicotinic acetylcholine receptor–ion channel complexes, but only at tissue concentrations of 10 to 100 times greater than the concentrations fully inhibiting AChE. Sarin, soman, and tabun are partial agonists of these channel complexes, whereas VX acts as an antagonist.[21] There also is evidence that nerve agents affect noncholinergic mechanisms in the central nervous system at a dose approaching LD_{50}.[22] Antagonistic effects of γ-aminobutyric acid (GABA)–ergic systems may explain convulsive activity after OP poisoning. Effects of soman and tabun on the uptake and release of GABA and glutamate in the synaptosomes of guinea pig cerebral cortex did not support the previous belief that nerve agents cause convulsions by affecting the uptake or release of GABA or glutamine. Indirect evidence that soman and tabun inhibit catabolism of GABA and glutamine was obtained, however.[23]

Acute exposure to tabun, sarin, or soman alters brain levels of cyclic adenosine monophosphate and cyclic guanosine monophosphate as a result of effects of adenylyl

---

TABLE 131-2 Summary of Available Acute Toxic Values of Nerve Agents in Humans

TERM	UNIT	ROUTE	TABUN	SARIN	SOMAN	VX
LD_{50}	mg/kg	PC		28		
LD_{50}	mg/m³	Inhale		70		
LCLo	μg/kg	PC				86
LDLo	mg/kg	PC	23		18	
LDLo	mg/m³	Inhale	150			70
TDLo	μg/kg	IV	14	2		1.5
TDLo	μg/kg	Oral				30
TDLo	μg/kg	SC				3.2

IV, intravenous; LCLo, lethal concentration at the lowest dose; LD_{50}, median lethal dose; LDLo, lethal dose at the lowest concentration; PC, percutaneous; SC, subcutaneous; TDLo, toxic dose at the lowest concentration.
Based on Grob[27] and Sidell.[28]

cyclase and phosphodiesterase systems.[6,24] VX at 10 μM produced a significant reduction in cell metabolism within 2 minutes as measured by changes in the acidification rate of medium after 4 hours of exposure. Two alkali degradation products of VX produced no cytotoxicity.[25]

Toxicokinetics

Few data are available on the toxicokinetics of nerve agents. A two-compartment model, with a biologic half-life of 1 to 1.5 minutes, described toxicokinetics of the four stereoisomers of soman in atropinized rats. The extremely toxic C(±) P(−) isomers could be followed in rat blood samples for more than 4 and 2 hours at doses of 6 and 3 LD$_{50}$ (82 μg/kg). The toxicokinetics of P(−) isomers was described with a three-compartment model, with terminal half-lives of 40 to 64 minutes and 16 to 22 minutes at doses of 6 and 3 LD$_{50}$, respectively.[26]

CLINICAL PRESENTATION AND COMPLICATIONS

The nerve agents cause pathologic effects mainly by interfering with cholinergic synaptic function. This effect occurs at cholinergic neuroeffector functions (muscarinic effects), at the skeletal myoneural junctions and autonomic ganglia (nicotinic effects), and in the central nervous system. The signs and symptoms of nerve agent poisoning are classified according to whether they are due to overstimulation of muscarinic, nicotinic, or central nervous system receptors.

Muscarinic effects of acetylcholine stimulation include miosis; blurred vision; eye pain; hypersecretion by salivary, sweat, lachrymal, and bronchial glands; bronchoconstriction; cough; cyanosis; pulmonary edema; nausea; vomiting; diarrhea; crampy abdominal pains; tenesmus; urinary and fecal incontinence; hypotension; and bradycardia (see Chapter 23). Nicotinic effects include easy fatigue, weakness, muscle cramping, fasciculations, skeletal muscle twitching, convulsions, and flaccid paralysis. Nicotinic stimulation also can obscure muscarinic parasympathetic effects and produce mydriasis, tachycardia, and hypertension by stimulation of the adrenal medulla. Central nervous system effects include irritability; nervousness; giddiness; ataxia; fatigue; generalized weakness; depression of respiratory and circulatory centers with dyspnea, cyanosis, hypoventilation, and hypotension; lethargy; impairment of memory; confusion; convulsions; coma; and respiratory depression.[6,7,9,27,28] The main toxic effects of nerve agents at various sites in the body are summarized in Table 131-3.

Clinical Manifestations by Routes of Exposure

The effects of nerve agent exposure occur via inhalation, contact with skin and eye, and, rarely, ingestion. Most often, exposure is to vapor (inhalation) or liquid (percutaneous). After small-to-moderate doses, initial effects and their time of onset are determined by the route of exposure. In contrast, large doses cause similar effects by all exposure routes, although the time of onset varies.[9] Gastrointestinal absorption rarely may occur through ingestion of contaminated food.

INHALATION

Exposure to low vapor concentrations may affect only the eyes, nose, and airways. Miosis, visual disturbances,

TABLE 131-3 Main Toxic Effects and Clinical Manifestations of Nerve Agent Poisoning

RECEPTOR	TARGET ORGAN	SYMPTOMS AND SIGNS
Muscarinic	Glands	
	Nasal mucosa	Rhinorrhea, nasal hyperemia
	Bronchial mucosa	Bronchorrhea
	Sweat	Sweating
	Lacrimal	Lacrimation
	Salivary	Salivation
	Smooth muscle	
	Iris	Miosis, blurred vision, decreased eye field
	Ciliary muscle	Failure of accommodation, eye pain
	Bronchial tree	Breathing difficulties, tightness of breath, bronchospasm (wheezing)
	Stomach	Nausea and vomiting
	Gut	Abdominal cramp, diarrhea
	Bladder	Frequency, involuntary micturition
	Heart	Bradycardia, hypotension
Nicotinic	Autonomic ganglia	Sympathetic effects, pallor, tachycardia, hypertension, mydriasis
	Skeletal muscle	Weakness, fasciculation, muscle twitching, convulsions, muscle paralysis, flaccid paralysis
Central	Central nervous system	Giddiness, anxiety, restlessness, headache, tremor, confusion, failure to concentrate, convulsions, respiratory depression, cyanosis, coma, apnea, death

rhinorrhea, and some degree of dyspnea develop within seconds to several minutes. The severity of dyspnea is dose dependent. Usually, these effects do not progress significantly when the patient is removed from contamination. After inhalation of high vapor concentrations, victims lose consciousness within 1 or 2 minutes, then have seizures, flaccid paralysis, and apnea. Other early effects of high vapor concentrations include miosis and copious secretions. Involuntary micturition and defecation also may occur. Unless medical assistance is immediate, victims die within 30 minutes.[6,7,9,27,28]

SKIN ABSORPTION

Percutaneous absorption of nerve agents varies according to the body site exposed and the ambient temperature. VX was absorbed nearly eight times more rapidly from facial skin than it was from the volar forearm, and absorption increased markedly as surrounding temperature increased from 18°C to 46°C.[24] Initial local effects of liquid, which seldom are noticed, include muscular fasciculations and sweating at the contamination site. A large droplet also may cause gastrointestinal effects and complaints of malaise and weakness. Droplets containing near-lethal or lethal doses cause loss of consciousness, seizures, flaccid paralysis, and apnea. The onset of these effects is sudden, usually after a symptomatic interval of 10 to 30 minutes.[9,27,28]

EYES

Miosis rapidly occurs after splash exposure or eye contact with vapor and later, if at all, after systemic poisoning. Unilateral miosis can occur if only one eye has been exposed. Miosis may be accompanied by deep, aching eye pain; conjunctival irritation; and visual disturbances. Dim vision may be due to constricted pupils or inhalation of cholinergic fibers of the retina or central nervous system. The miotic pupil may improve vision (the pinhole effect), although complaints of blurred vision are common.[29] Direct installation of diluted nerve agent into the eye does not produce tissue damage.[9]

Life-Threatening Complications

The most life-threatening complication is respiratory failure, which is due mainly to the effect of the nerve agents on the central nervous system,[30,31] although in one animal experiment with sarin, respiratory paralysis could be purely central, peripheral, or both, depending on the doses of sarin and atropine antidote employed.[32] Hypoxia also is a major problem in the nerve agent poisoning, as it may cause cerebral edema and convulsions and may induce histopathologic brain damage.

Cardiovascular complications sometimes are severe and life-threatening.[33,34] The nerve agents tabun, sarin, soman, or VX at 5 to 10 times the LD_{50} administered to guinea pigs induced circulatory arrest a few minutes after apnea in nontreated animals. Antidote treatment by atropine (10 mg/kg) and HI-6 or HLo-7 (30 mg/kg) 2 minutes later rapidly restored heart rate and arterial pressure and respiratory function to various extents. The nerve agent injection caused marked sinus bradycardia and a subsequent complete atrioventricular block within 1 to 2 minutes. In guinea pigs with depressed respiratory function (<50%), intermittent ST-T wave alterations and second-degree atrioventricular heart

block were observed.[33] Other reported electrocardiogram abnormalities in animal experiments and in humans exposed to nerve agents include torsades de pointes, atria fibrillation, idioventricular dysrhythmias, complete heart block, and ventricular fibrillation.[6,9,33,34] Histopathologic changes compatible with toxic myocarditis were observed after sarin and soman in animal experiments,[33] but myocarditis has not been reported in humans.

Intermediate Syndrome

The intermediate syndrome consists of marked weakness of the proximal skeletal musculature (including the muscles of respiration) and cranial nerve palsies and occurs 1 to 4 days after acute poisoning. This syndrome, which was observed after certain OP poisoning,[35] has not been reported yet after nerve agent poisoning. Intermediate syndrome may be a consequence of cholinergic overactivity at the neuromuscular junction, and a connection has been made between the intermediate syndrome and OP-induced myopathy or undertreatment. Myopathy has been observed histologically in experimental animals with the nerve agents tabun, soman, and sarin.[13,14] It can be anticipated that the intermediate syndrome occurs in some cases of nerve agent poisoning.

Delayed Neuropathy

OPIND is a symmetric sensorimotor axonopathy, tending to be most severe in long axons and occurring 7 to 14 days after exposure. In severe cases, it is an extremely disabling condition.[36] Inhibition of neuropathy target esterase seems to be necessary for OPIND to develop. Other mechanisms may be involved, however. The trophic factor ornithine decarboxylase, a growth-related enzyme, was decreased in the spinal cord after the neuropathic agent diisopropylfluorophosphate.[19] Although OPIND was not observed after nerve agent poisoning in experimental studies[37,38] and in accidental nerve agent poisoning, a case of sensory polyneuropathy 7 months after sarin poisoning has been reported.[39]

Temporary psychological effects, such as depression, fatigue, insomnia, irritability, nervousness, and impairment of memory, have been described after nerve agent exposure.[28] Electroencephalography in a person who was severely intoxicated with sarin showed marked slowing with bursts of high-voltage waves at a rate of five per second.[27] Epileptic-type changes of electroencephalography were observed after sarin poisoning 11 months after exposure.[6]

Course and Prognosis

Victims with heavy exposure to nerve agents may die within a few minutes in the field. Persons with physical and chemical protection (pyridostigmine) who remain in a heavily contaminated area may become intoxicated after 30 minutes. A patient with moderate-to-severe intoxication who receives first aid and emergency medical treatment may survive a few days to a few weeks, according to the severity of intoxication and type of treatment.

Hypoxia, coma, convulsions, and respiratory failure are signs of a poor prognosis. Patients who remain severely hypoxic and cyanotic may develop cardiac arrhythmias and die quickly. Patients who develop apnea and do not receive assisted ventilation immediately may incur brain damage and either die or become vegetative. It is unlikely that nerve agents possess the potential to give rise to OPIND.

Soldiers who are caught unaware and who are exposed to large amounts of nerve agent before donning respirators and other protective clothing and who rapidly develop severe symptoms and signs are unlikely to survive. Soldiers who rapidly develop respiratory failure and who become incapable of self-administrating their own autoinjector systems/devices also have a poor prognosis, unless emergency medical treatment is provided rapidly.

DIAGNOSTIC CONSIDERATIONS

Initial diagnosis of nerve agent poisoning can be made based on the exposure history (accidental, terrorism, chemical warfare attack) and clinical manifestations. In low-level exposure, the route of absorption may affect the clinical features, but in high-level exposure, severe intoxication occurs. Absorption is faster through inhalation than through skin contact. Estimation of AChE in erythrocytes is required to confirm the anticholinesterase diagnosis and to estimate the severity of intoxication. BChE estimation also may help, although it is not specific and may be low due to genetic variations.[10]

Certain diagnosis of nerve agent exposure requires toxicologic analyses of the environment, blood sampling, or both. A biosensor, which is a potentiometer enzyme electrode for direct determination of OP nerve agent, has been developed.[40]

A fiberoptic enzyme biosensor for the direct measurement of OP nerve agents also has been developed. Concentrations of 2 μM can be measured in less than 2 minutes using the kinetic response. When stored in buffer at 4°C, the biosensor shows long-term stability.[41] A new method for retrospective detection of exposure to OP nerve agents was applied to estimate serum sarin concentrations of the Matsumoto incident. The concentrations ranged from 0.2 to 4.1 ng/mL serum.[42] Definitive evidence for the acute sarin poisoning of the Tokyo subway was obtained by detecting sarin-hydrolyzed products from erythrocytes of four victims in postmortem examinations.[43]

Intravenous administration of atropine can be used as a diagnostic test for anticholinesterase poisoning, whereas oximes are used only for treatment.[44] Cholinesterase activity in postmortem blood as a screening test for OP nerve agent exposure was performed in 53 nonpreserved postmortem whole-blood specimens. There was a negligible loss of cholinesterase activity by the 7th day of the study. Cholinesterase activity could be applied as the screening test for anticholinesterase nerve agents.[45]

Diagnosis of the delayed neurotoxic effects can be made by estimation of neuropathy target esterase, although it is unlikely to occur after nerve agent poisoning. Marked reduction of neurotrophic factor (ornithine decarboxylase) during the early stages of neurotoxicity also may be helpful when it is possible to perform it.[19] Measurement of nerve conduction velocity and electromyography may be useful for the diagnosis of the delayed neuropathy of OPs (Balali-Mood M, unpublished data).

Toxicologic Analyses

CHOLINESTERASES AND NEUROPATHY TARGET ESTERASE DETERMINATION

Estimation of BChE in plasma is widely available and should be performed as soon as possible. Erythrocyte AChE is more specific, however, and has more quantitative value than BChE, although both enzymes usually are measured spectrophotometrically. Inhibition of greater than 50% activity of either enzyme confirms the diagnosis of an anticholinesterase poisoning. Reactivation of BChE is relatively more rapid, depending on the agent, severity of intoxication, and use of oximes, taking 1 to 4 weeks. In contrast, reactivation of AChE may take 3 months.[6] Neuropathy target esterase also may be assayed, particularly when there would be clinical features of delayed neuropathy.

NERVE AGENT DETECTION

Detection and estimation of nerve agents are easier in environmental samples than in blood and urine samples from patients. By using new technology, such as biosensors and fiberoptic bioenzyme, and new methods for detection and determination of nerve agents (e.g., sarin) in the serum and erythrocytes, identification and estimation of common nerve agents are possible.[40–44]

OXIME ESTIMATION

Estimation of pralidoxime concentration in blood may be required, although it is not necessary for the routine management of the patient. To achieve a maximal therapeutic effect, however, a blood pralidoxime concentration of 4 mg/L should be reached. Estimation of other oximes is not recommended for patient management.

Biochemical and Hematologic Analyses

Acid-base and electrolyte disturbances are common during severe nerve agent poisoning. Arterial blood gas analysis, estimation of serum electrolytes, liver and kidney function tests, amylase, creatine phosphokinase, and lactate dehydrogenase may be required for patient management. Hypokalemia and hyperglycemia are common and should be considered and corrected. Elevation of serum amylase may reveal acute pancreatitis. Transient elevation of liver enzymes, hematuria, leukocyturia, and proteinuria may be observed during nerve agent poisoning. Blood cell count and other hematologic tests may be performed as clinically indicated. Transient leukocytosis, particularly in polymorphonuclear neutrophils, may be observed during severe nerve agent poisoning.

Other Investigations

Chest x-ray, electrocardiogram, electroencephalogram, electromyogram, nerve conduction velocity, spirometry, computed tomography, magnetic resonance imaging, and other investigations may be performed in nerve agent poisoning as clinically indicated.

Severity Grading of Intoxication

Severity grading of nerve agent poisoning can be done based on clinical manifestations, cholinesterase activity, and initial atropine dose required for atropinization.

CLINICAL SYMPTOMS AND SIGNS

Patients with OP nerve agent poisoning can be divided into four groups—mild, moderate, severe, and fatal—according to symptoms and signs of poisoning (Table 131-4).

INHIBITION OF CHOLINESTERASES

Patients with nerve agent poisoning may be divided into three groups according to cholinesterase activities (Table 131-5).

ATROPINE DOSE

Patients with OP nerve agent poisoning can be divided into three groups according to the initial atropine dose required for atropinization:

1. Mild: less than 2 mg
2. Moderate: 2 to 10 mg
3. Severe: greater than 10 mg

Causes of Death

Death after nerve agent exposure is mainly due to respiratory failure resulting from depression of the respiratory center, paralysis of respiratory muscles, and obstruction caused by bronchospasm and bronchial secretions. Some animal studies suggest that lack of central drive is the major factor.[30,31] Cardiomyopathy in soman-intoxicated and sarin-intoxicated rats has been reported[33] and may be a contributory cause of death.

Status seizures occurred in animals after high doses of sarin, soman, or VX despite early treatment with atropine and pralidoxime. Prolonged seizures may cause anoxia and morphologic brain damage, which induces more morbidity and mortality.[37,38]

TREATMENT

Priorities

The first rule for managing chemical casualties is that the emergency responders must protect themselves from contamination resulting from contact with casualties and the environment (Fig. 131-2). This can be done by wearing personal protective equipment or by thoroughly decontaminating the patient. At minimum, rescuers should wear a protective mask (or mask containing a charcoal filter for a self-contained breathing apparatus device, not a surgical or similar mask) and heavy rubber gloves (surgical gloves offer negligible protection) and avoid skin contact with victims until decontamination has been carried out.[9,46]

As soon as possible, victims should be removed from the contaminated place and decontamination must be initiated. Antidotes should be given at the onset of effects as appropriate (e.g., autoinjector containing atropine, obidoxime, and diazepam). For unconscious or severely intoxicated patients, priorities must follow the ABCs (airway, breathing, and circulation) of resuscitation. Oxygen administration and assisted ventilation should be undertaken as soon as possible in patients with respiratory distress. Because atropine reverses bronchoconstriction within minutes, one could hesitate to intubate a dyspneic, conscious patient who is likely to improve

---

TABLE 131-4 Symptoms and Signs of Organophosphate Nerve Agent Poisoning

GRADE	SYMPTOMS	SIGNS
1—mild	Dizziness, anxiety, headache, nausea, weakness, tightness of breath	Failure of accommodation, rhinorrhea, sweating, salivation, coughing, lacrimation
2—moderate (worsening of the above features plus the following)	Restlessness, confusion, dyspnea, disorientation, abdominal pain, diarrhea	Pallor, miosis, failure of concentration, tachycardia, hypertension, muscle twitching, fasciculation, respiratory depression, bronchorrhea, loss of consciousness, bronchospasm
3—severe (worsening of the above features plus the following)	—	Convulsions, respiratory failure, pulmonary edema, flaccid paralysis, involuntary micturition/defecation, cyanosis, deep coma
4—fatal	—	Coma, convulsions, miosis, hypersecretions, apnea within a few minutes after exposure

---

TABLE 131-5 Cholinesterase Activities*

GRADE	BUTYRYLCHOLINESTERASE ACTIVITY (%)	ACETYLCHOLINESTERASE ACTIVITY (%)
1—mild	40–50	50–90
2—moderate	10–40	10–50
3—severe	<10	<10

*Butyrylcholinesterase activity has less quantitative value than acetylcholinesterase activity.

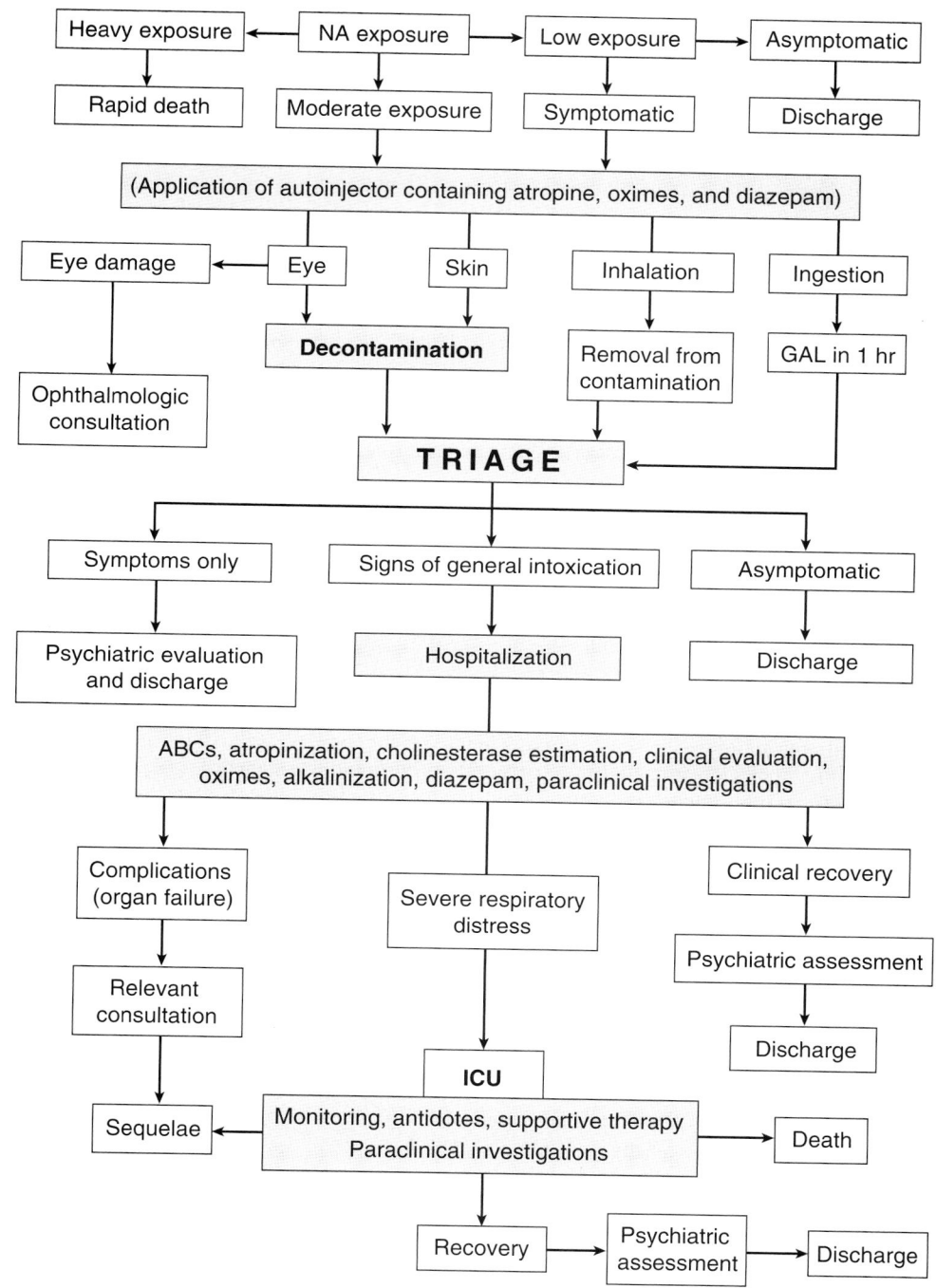

FIGURE 131-2

Management of nerve agent (NA) poisoning. ABCs, airway, breathing, circulation; GAL, gastric aspiration and lavage; ICU, intensive care unit.

quickly. In a severely poisoned, unconscious, apneic patient, however, endotracheal intubation with assisted ventilation should be undertaken as quickly as possible.

Airway resistance may be high initially, causing some mechanical ventilators to malfunction, but this should return to normal after atropine administration. Frequent airway suctioning may be required for copious bronchial secretions. Supplemental oxygen through an endotracheal tube with positive end-expiratory pressure is indicated for severely hypoxic patients. It is important to improve tissue oxygenation before atropine administration to minimize the risk of

ventricular fibrillation. Advanced life support, including intravenous line placement, should be provided to all victims with evidence of respiratory compromise or other signs of severe exposure.[9]

Decontamination

Decontamination must be carried out at the earliest opportunity to limit skin absorption of the agent and prevent contamination of the rescuers. Thorough decontamination is essential before casualties enter an emergency department

Indications for ICU Admission in Nerve Agent Poisoning

1. Patients with severe nerve agent intoxication (see section on Severity Grading of Intoxication), particularly patients with respiratory failure who need mechanical ventilation, should be admitted to the intensive care unit.
2. Although intermediate syndrome has not been reported in nerve agent poisoning, it may occur in some cases. Patients with moderate-to-severe intoxication even without assisted ventilation should be monitored, preferably in the intensive care unit, for possible sudden respiratory arrest due to muscle paralysis.

or other site of medical care to avoid contamination of staff and other patients.

If the eyes have been exposed, they should be irrigated as soon as possible with running water or saline. Skin should be decontaminated by pouring on large amounts of a chlorine-liberated solution, such as 5% hypochlorite solution (household bleach), followed by copious water rinsing. If bleach is not available, the skin should be blotted gently (without rubbing) with generous amounts of alkaline soap and water followed by a water rinse. Generous amounts of water alone can be used if nothing else is available. Water dilutes and physically washes away nerve agents, but it does not hydrolyze them. Contaminated clothing and jewelry should be removed, and the underlying skin should be decontaminated thoroughly. Care should be taken to clear under the nails, the intertriginous areas, the axillae, the groin, and the hair.[9]

Experimental Antidotes

Fetal bovine serum AChE protected mice from multiple LD_{50} doses of OP nerve agents.[47] BChE purified from human plasma also was effective in vitro and in vivo in mice and rats as a single prophylactic antidote against the lethal effects of nerve agents.[48] Addition of the oxime HI-6 to fetal bovine serum AChE as a pretreatment drug amplified the efficacy of enzyme as a scavenger of nerve agents.[49]

Recombinant DNA–derived AChEs showed a great improvement over wild-type AChEs as bioscavengers; they can be used to develop effective methods for the safe disposal and storage of OP nerve agents and are potential candidates for preexposure or postexposure treatment for OP toxicity.[50] By the use of cell immobilization technology, immobilized *Escherichia coli* with surface-expressed organophosphorus hydrolase was made to detoxify nerve agents.[51] By protein engineering techniques, one BChE mutant, G117H, was made to hydrolyze V and G agents, but it reacted much too slowly.[52]

OP acid hydrolyses from two species of *Alteromonas* were cloned and sequenced to detoxify G agents, which was effective.[53] Cholinesterases that are covalently linked to a polyurethane matrix can be used effectively to remove nerve agents from and decontaminate surface biologic areas (skin or wounds) or other areas (clothing or medical equipments) or the environment. These cholinesterases could protect medical personnel from secondary contamination while attending chemical casualties and civilians exposed to highly toxic nerve agents.[54]

A reactive skin decontamination lotion active against classic nerve agents and mustard was developed. The inactivation process was time and agent dependent and related to the ratio of OP to reactive skin decontamination lotion.[55]

Pretreatment

In animal studies, pretreatment with reversible carbamate AChE inhibitors, such as pyridostigmine and physostigmine, enhances the efficacy of postexposure treatment of soman exposure or soman poisoning with atropine and pralidoxime chloride and permits survival at higher agent challenges. This protection apparently is due to the fact that the more lethal nerve agents cannot attack AChE molecules bound by carbamates. Carbamoylation of 20% to 40% of the erythrocyte AChE is associated with antidotal enhancement. Carbamate pretreatment does not reduce the effects of the agents, and by themselves carbamates provide no benefit. Pretreatment is not effective against sarin and VX challenge and should not be considered a panacea for all nerve agents. It is of value for soman intoxication when agent challenge is followed by atropine and an oxime. Pretreatment is ineffective unless standard therapy is administered after the exposure.

Because physostigmine is toxic at the amounts required, pyridostigmine is the drug of choice for pretreatment. The standard dosage is 30 mg orally every 8 hours for impending nerve agent attack. Because pyridostigmine does not cross the blood-brain barrier, it causes no central nervous system toxicity of nerve agents. Carbamates must never be used after nerve agent exposure; in that setting, carbamate administration worsens, rather than protects from, toxicity. Excessive doses cause many of the same toxic effects as do the nerve agents, and the recommended amounts caused annoying side effects in more than half of the population in a war zone. Eptastigmine treatment given intravenously protected mice better than physostigmine against soman exposure[56]; eptastigmine is not available in the United States.

Pretreatment with a drug mixture (pyridostigmine, benactyzine, and trihexyphenidyl) and antidotal treatment (HI-6 and benactyzine) were investigated in rats. This cholinergic-anticholinergic pretreatment in restoring respiratory and circulatory changes induced by soman is important.[57]

Antidotes

Available antidotes (atropine, oximes) do not prevent respiratory failure or incapacitation.[58] Early aggressive medical therapy with antidotes and intensive care management are the keys, however, to prevention of morbidity and mortality associated with nerve agent poisoning.

ATROPINE

Atropine should be titrated with the goal of drying secretions and resolving bronchoconstriction and bradycardia.[59] There is no actual dose for atropine. The dose (2 mg) of atropine available in an autoinjector is not adequate for moderate-to-severe exposure to nerve agents. Atropine should be given intravenously in doses to produce mild-to-moderate atropinization (dryness of tongue, oropharyngeal and bronchial tree, tachycardia, mydriasis, and flushing) as soon as possible. At least the same amount as the initial atropinization dose should be infused in 500 mL of dextrose 5% constantly to sustain the atropinization and should be repeated as needed until the patient becomes asymptomatic. Continuous infusion of atropine effectively antagonizes the muscarinic effects and some of the central nervous system effects of nerve agent poisoning, but it has no effect on skeletal muscle weakness, seizures, unconsciousness, or respiratory failure.[9] Large doses of atropine require higher concentrations of atropine preparation (e.g., 100 mg/10 mL made in Germany) or at least a vast amount of atropine (10 to 100 mg) in dextrose 5% solution, readymade for intravenous infusion in severely nerve agent–intoxicated patients. Based on clinical experience of the first author (M.B.-M.), much lower atropine doses are required for nerve agents than for the severe OP pesticides poisoning.

Atropine should not be given intravenously to a hypoxic patient. If the patient is hypotensive, atropine can be given through an endotracheal tube or intratracheally for more rapid absorption through the peribronchial vessels.[9] Aerosolized atropine has also been used and can be administered quickly by inhalation. Studies suggest that in addition to the local effects in the lungs, it is absorbed systemically.[60]

OXIMES

Oximes are mainly pyridinium compounds, which are divided into mono-Pyridium and bis Pyridium oximes. Names and suppliers of the common oximes are presented in Table 131-6. Although oximes have been designed to reactivate the inhibited AChE, clinical experience has indicated that they are not always effective as reactivators, and at this time, none of them can be regarded as a broad-spectrum antidote.[61] The choice of oximes based on the data presently available also may depend on factors other than protection against lethality, such as cost and availability of the oxime and its side effects. Obidoxime (Toxogonin, Merck, Germany) is likely to cause more toxic effects (particularly with high doses) than pralidoxime and HI-6.[62] HI-6 is the least toxic, but it is less stable in solution and is not commercially available in many parts of the world.

Pralidoxime, HI-6, and HGG-12 were used in dogs with soman and tabun poisoning. Pralidoxime (in conjunction with atropine and diazepam) showed the best protective effects in soman-poisoned dogs: The protective indices were 9 for pralidoxime, 6.3 for HI-6, and 3.5 for HGG-12.

None of these agents was effective against tabun poisoning.[63] Efficacy of two other oximes, HLo-7 and pyrimidoxime (an analogue of trimedoxime), in three times the LD_{50} of sarin, soman, and GF and two times the LD_{50} of tabun, was tested in mice. HLo-7 produced significant ($P < .05$) reactivation of phosphorylated AChE, resulting in 47%, 38%, 27%, and 10% reactivation of sarin-inhibited, GF-inhibited, soman-inhibited, and tabun-inhibited mouse diaphragm AChE, respectively.[64] In a comprehensive study, the order of effectiveness against soman was HI-6, HLo-7, and pyrimidoxime. HLo-7 was extremely effective against tabun poisoning, whereas HI-6 and pyrimidoxime were of moderate value. Against GF, HI-6 and HLo-7 were extremely effective, obidoxime was moderately effective, and pralidoxime and pyrimidoxime were least effective.[65] In soman-intoxicated guinea pigs, HI-6 was therapeutically slightly more effective than HLo-7; HLo-7 was more effective than HI-6 against tabun intoxication.[66]

Pharmacokinetics and effects of HI-6 in blood and brain of soman-intoxicated rats were studied. High doses of HI-6 can reach the brain in sufficient amounts to reactivate inhibited brain AChE. Signs of soman poisoning correlated positively to AChE inhibition and negatively to the concentration of inbound HI-6 in the brain, and soman intoxication significantly decreased uptake of HI-6 into the brain.[67] Reactivating potency of obidoxime, pralidoxime, HI-6, and HLo-7 in human erythrocyte AChE inhibited by soman, sarin, cyclosarin, and VX was studied in vitro. After soman, sarin, cyclosarin, and VX inhibition, the reactivating potency decreased in the following order: HLo-7 > HI-6 > obidoxime > pralidoxime.[68] Dose-response effects of atropine and HI-6 treatment in soman and tabun poisonings were studied in guinea pigs. Atropine had a large effect on the efficacy of HI-6 against both the nerve agents. They also were more effective against soman than against tabun. Adjunctive treatment with diazepam enhanced the efficacy of HI-6 and atropine against soman.[69] The effects of common oximes in different nerve agent poisonings are summarized in Table 131-7.

Despite many oximes tested in animal experiments, the human experience in war or terrorism is limited to pralidoxime and obidoxime. Pralidoxime should be administered intravenously at a dose of 30 mg/kg initially over 30 minutes followed by constant infusion of 8 mg/kg/hr in dextrose 5%. Pralidoxime can be continued until full recovery or until atropine is required. Obidoxime was hepatotoxic at high recommended doses of 8 mg/kg initially and

TABLE 131-6 Common Oximes Used in the Treatment of Organophosphate Nerve Agent Poisoning

TYPE OF OXIME	GENERIC NAME	TRADE NAME	SUPPLIER/COUNTRY
Monopyridinium	Pralidoxime chloride (2-PAM)	Protopam	Ayerst/U.S./Canada
	Pralidoxime methylsulfate	Contrathion	SERB/France
	Pralidoxime methanesulfonate	P2S	U.K. government
Bispyridinium	Trimedoxime	TMB-4	
	Obidoxime	Toxogonin	Merck/Germany
	HI-6		
	HLo-7		
	HGG-12		

TABLE 131-7 Relative Effects of Oximes in Organophosphate Nerve Agent Poisoning

OXIMES	GA (SARIN)	GB (SOMAN)	GD (TABUN)	GF	VX
Pralidoxime*	+++[†]	++	+	+	+++
Pyrimidoxime	++	++	++	+	++
Obidoxime	++	+++	++	++	+++
HI-6	+++	++++	++	++++	+++
HLo-7	++++	+++	++++	++++	++
HGG-12	NA	+++	+	NA	NA

*proPAM, the tertiary amine analogue of pralidoxime, penetrates the central nervous system more readily than pralidoxime. Consequently, proPAM would be expected to have greater beneficial effect in nerve agent poisoning than pralidoxime. This expectation has not in general been realized in experimental studies.
[†]Key: + = least effective; ++ = partially effective; +++ = moderately effective; ++++ = most effective.
NA, no data available.

3 mg/kg/hr.[5] It may be given at a dose of not more than 500 mg initially and about 750 to 1000 mg/day. Liver function tests should be checked regularly during obidoxime therapy.

Diazepam

Behavioral efficacy of diazepam against nerve agents in rhesus monkeys was studied. The results showed that diazepam would be an excellent adjunct to traditional nerve agent therapy to facilitate behavioral recovery from nerve agent intoxication that might be encountered by medical military personnel on the battlefield.[70] Despite the introduction of diazepam as a symptomatic anticonvulsant, many studies indicate that the effects of diazepam may be more specific. These studies mainly have investigated the effects on cholinergic and GABAergic systems.

Gacyclidine

Gacyclidine is an antiglutaminergic compound that was studied as a complement to the available emergency therapy in OP poisoning. It was used in conjunction with atropine, pralidoxime, and diazepam in nerve agent poisoning in primates.

Gacyclidine prevents the mortality observed after early administration of the aforementioned classic emergency medications. Electroencephalogram recordings and clinical observations revealed that gacyclidine prevented soman-induced seizures and motor convulsions. It also markedly accelerated clinical recovery of soman-challenged primates. Gacyclidine prevented the neuropathology observed 3 weeks after soman exposure in animals.[72] In a case of severe nerve agent poisoning, gacyclidine represented a promising adjuvant therapy to the currently available polymedication to ensure optimal management of OP nerve agent poisoning in humans. This drug currently is being evaluated in human clinical trials for different neuroprotective indications.[73]

Serum Alkalization

Effects of sodium bicarbonate in OP pesticide poisoning were investigated in patients with moderate-to-severe intoxication. The goal of the investigation was to make an alkalization to reach and sustain the arterial blood pH between 7.45 and 7.55. Sodium bicarbonate was administered intravenously first to correct the metabolic acidosis, then as a constant infusion of 3 to 5 mg/kg/24 hr until recovery or until atropine was required. Arterial blood gas analysis was performed at certain intervals to adjust the dosing. The preliminary results were promising.[74] Because alkalization products of nerve agents, particularly soman, are less toxic, it seems that administration of intravenous infusion of sodium bicarbonate to produce moderate alkalization may be effective in nerve agent poisoning.

Drug Interactions

Drugs reported as contraindicated in severe OP nerve agent poisoning are morphine and its derivatives, aminophylline, theophylline, and chlorpromazine. Drugs known to be hydrolyzed by the enzyme cholinesterase, such as suxamethonium (succinylcholine) and procaine, may have sustained effects.

Hemoperfusion

Effects of hemoperfusion through coated resin adsorbent synachrome E-5 were studied in five anesthetized dogs after intoxication by two to six times the LD_{50} of VX and another four dogs after intoxication by two to three times the LD_{50} of sarin. Hemoperfusion therapy prevented the development of serious signs of intoxication, provided that the dose of both nerve agents was only two times the LD_{50}. It was concluded that hemoperfusion therapy in poisoning by the nerve agents sarin and VX is only partially successful.[75] Clinical experience of the first author with the management of OP nerve agents and pesticides in humans revealed that hemoperfusion may be effective in patients with severe OP intoxication.

SPECIAL POPULATIONS

Pediatric Patients

Children are more susceptible to OP nerve agents, as was seen during the Halabjah massacre. Mortality was higher in children than in adults. Children also are more sensitive to atropine and oximes. Atropine should be administered with care, by monitoring vital signs, particularly pulse rate. If the pulse rate exceeds more than 160 beats/min, atropine infusion should be stopped and restarted when the pulse rate decreases to less than 140 beats/min. Based on clinical experience with children poisoned by OP pesticides, pralidoxime should be administered at 25 mg/kg as an initial loading dose and be infused over 15 to 30 minutes followed by 10 to 20 mg/kg/hr to provide a plasma concentration of greater than 4 mg/L.

Pregnant Patients

OP nerve agents may cross the placenta and induce fetal intoxication. The fetus is more sensitive to OP nerve agents than the mother and more sensitive to atropine than the mother. Based on clinical experience with pregnant women exposed to sarin during the Iran-Iraq war in Sardasht and Halabjah, mortality also was higher in the fetus than the mother. Some pregnant women survived after sarin poisoning, but the fetus died within a few hours to a few days. Atropine and oximes should be administered with caution and at lower doses to pregnant women. Obstetric consultation may be required.

OP nerve agents may be excreted in the mother's milk. It would be advisable to stop breast-feeding at least for a few days after exposure.

Elderly Patients

Elderly people also are more susceptible to OP nerve agents. Experience with sarin poisoning during the Iran-Iraq War in Sardasht and Halabjah revealed that morbidity and mortality were higher among elderly people. Multiple organ failure and complications were more common among the elderly than other adult age groups. Atropine, oxime, diazepam, and any other medication should be administered with caution. Depending on the age and clinical condition of the patient, critical care therapy should be initiated more rapidly. Elderly patients with OP nerve agent poisoning should be treated as the same priority group as children.

Rescue Staff and Hospital Personnel

Rescue staff and hospital personnel who are in contact with victims of OP nerve agent poisoning may become intoxicated due to secondary exposure. Among 59 rescuers and duty physicians, 8 had mild symptoms of sarin poisoning during the Matsumoto incident. All the rescue activities had taken place without gas masks or decontamination procedures.[76]

Secondary contamination of house staff that treated victims occurred during the sarin Tokyo subway incident. More than 20% of the house staff had symptoms, including ocular pain, headache, sore throat, dyspnea, nausea, dizziness, and nasal pain, but none were seriously affected.[7] Rescue staff and medical personnel in the field, during transportation, and in the hospital should be protected by proper gas masks, clothing, and thick gloves (not surgical gloves).

EXPERIENCE IN WAR AND TERRORISM

Observations during the nerve gas attack of the Iraqi army against the Iranian troops in Majnoon Island revealed that the heavily exposed people died within 30 minutes after onset of coma, convulsions, hypersecretion, respiratory failure, and apnea. Although the medical facilities were not adequate in Majnoon Island, first-aid treatment and decontamination were performed. The victims with moderate-to-severe intoxication were transferred from the field hospital to medical centers in big cities for further management.

Recorded clinical manifestations include miosis, hypersecretions, hypotension, nausea, vomiting, abdominal cramps, diarrhea, loss of consciousness, respiratory depression, cyanosis, pulmonary edema, muscle twitching, and convulsions. Bradycardia and hypotension were observed more before treatment with atropine, whereas tachycardia, normal hypertension, mydriasis, and dryness of the tongue were recorded more after atropinization. Morbidity and mortality were higher in patients with severe respiratory distress and cyanosis who received large doses of atropine. It is vital to correct the severe hypoxemia and cyanosis before atropinization (see section on Treatment). Suctioning of nasooropharyngeal and bronchial secretions (clear airway) and establishing adequate ventilation are the first priority. Intermediate syndrome, which was described after OP pesticide poisoning,[35] has not been observed with nerve agent poisoning.

Sulfur mustard was the most common chemical warfare agent that was used by the Iraqi army. Mixed poisoning by tabun and sulfur mustard also was common. No exact quantitative records of the nerve agent exposure are available. It has been estimated that greater than 2000 patients with nerve agent (later on diagnosed as tabun) poisoning were treated in March 1984. Another massive nerve agent poisoning occurred during the Halabjah massacre. It also was diagnosed as sarin and mixed with sulfur mustard.[40,41]

Two main terrorist attacks with sarin occurred in Japan. The first one occurred on June 27, 1994, in Matsumoto with about 600 casualties and 7 deaths.[6] The second attack occurred on March 20, 1995, in the Tokyo subway system, killing 11 and injuring more than 5500 people.[7] Diagnosis of sarin on both occasions was made based on the chemical analysis of environmental samples similar to the diagnosis of tabun in Majnoon Island and sarin in Halabjah.[4] Confirmative tests of serum sarin concentrations of the Halabjah massacre, Matsumoto incident, and Tokyo subway incident[42] and detection of sarin hydrolysis products from erythrocytes of four victims of the Tokyo subway incident[43] were performed after the incidents.

Preparation for a chemical incident resulting from an accident, war, or terrorism is important in every community. Because the rescue staff and medical personnel usually are from different departments, coordination between them is required. Guidelines and protocols should be available to all personnel. Teaching the staff and performing a simulation exercise at certain intervals is also necessary. Public awareness through the mass media and even written instructions to the public are valuable and may prevent chaos during the incident.

Key Points in the Diagnosis and Management of Nerve Agents

1. Although plasma cholinesterase activity is given as percentages or U/mL, it should be valued qualitatively rather than quantitatively. Because of genetic variation in plasma cholinesterase, lower activity may be observed in 5% to 20% of normal individuals.

2. Hypokalemia and metabolic acidosis, which occur during organophosphate nerve agent poisoning, should be corrected near to the upper limit of normal range.

3. Administration of atropine in single repeated doses is mentioned in other textbooks. Mild-to-moderate atropinization must be produced and sustained until the patient's recovery.

4. Mydriatic eye drops are not needed; mydriasis should be induced by intravenous atropine.

5. Aminophylline and theophylline should not be administered for bronchospasm during organophosphate nerve agent poisoning. Anticholinergic bronchodilators and β_2-agonists (salbutamol, terbutaline) should be administered.

6. Although pulmonary edema is less common in organophosphate nerve agent poisoning than in pesticide organophosphate poisoning, it should be treated only by atropine and not by morphine, aminophylline, furosemide, or digoxin. Morphine and aminophylline are contraindicated in organophosphate poisoning; furosemide might induce dehydration and electrolyte imbalance.

REFERENCES

1. Holmsted B: The third symposium on prophylaxis and treatment of chemical poisons, April 22–24, 1985, Stockholm, Sweden. Fundam Appl Toxicol 5:S1-S9, 1985.

2. Sidell FR, Groff WA: The reactivability of cholinesterase inhibited by VX and sarin in man. Toxicol Appl Pharmacol 27:241–252, 1974.

3. Foroutan A: Report of the specialist appointed by the Secretary-General of the United Nations to investigate allegation by the Islamic Republic of Iran concerning the use of chemical weapons. Proceedings of the First World Congress on Biological and Chemical Warfares, Ghent, May 21–23, 1984, pp 302–310.

4. Hendrickx B: Report and conclusion of the biological samples of men, intoxicated by war gases, sent to the Department of Toxicology of the State University of Ghent, for toxicological investigation. Proceedings of the Second World Congress on Biological and Chemical Warfares, Ghent, August 24–27, 1986, pp 553–582.

5. Balali-Mood M, Shariat M: Treatment of organophosphate poisoning: Experience of nerve agents and acute pesticide poisoning on the effects of oximes. J Physiol (Paris) 92:375–378, 1998.

6. Morita H, Yanagisawa N, Nakajima T, et al: Sarin poisoning in Matsumoto, Japan. Lancet 346:290–293, 1995.

7. Ohbu S, Yamashina A, Takasu N, et al: Sarin poisoning on Tokyo subway. South Med J 90:587–593, 1997.

8. Dunn MA, Sidell FR: Progress in medical defense against nerve agents. JAMA 262:649–652, 1998.

9. Sidell FR, Borak J: Nerve agents. Ann Emerg Med 21:865–871, 1992.

10. Lockridge O, Masson P: Pesticides and susceptible populations: People with butyrylcholinesterase genetic variants may be at risk. Neurotoxicology 21:113–126, 2000.

11. Barak D, Ordentlich A, Kaplan D, et al: Evidence for P-N bond scission in phosphoramidate nerve agent adducts of human acetylcholinesterase. Biochemistry 39:1156–1161, 2000.

12. Furlong CE, Li WF, Richter RJ, et al: Genetic and temporal determinants of pesticide sensitivity: Role of paraoxonase (PON1). Neurotoxicology 21:91–100, 2000.

13. Inns RH, Tuckwell NJ, Bright JE, Marrs TC: Histochemical demonstration of calcium accumulation in muscle fibres after experimental organophosphate poisoning. Hum Exp Toxicol 9:245–250, 1990.

14. Bright JE, Inns RH, Marrs TC, Tuckwell NJ: Histochemical demonstration of sarin-induced calcium influx in mouse diaphragm. Hum Exp Toxicol 9:245–250, 1990.

15. Lee MJ, Clement JG: Effect of soman poisoning in haematology and coagulation parameters and serum biochemistry in rabbits. Milit Med 155:244–249, 1990.

16. Young GD, Koplovitz I: Acute toxicity of cyclohexylmethylphosphonofluoridate (CMPF) in rhesus monkeys: Serum biochemical and hematologic changes. Arch Toxicol 69:379–383, 1995.

17. Rickell DJ, Glenn JF, Houston WE: Medical defense against nerve agents: New direction. Milit Med 152:35–41, 1987.

18. Gordon JJ, Inns RH, Johnson MK, et al: The delayed neuropathic effects of nerve agents and other organophosphate compounds. Arch Toxicol 52:82–86, 1983.

19. Pope C, Dilorenzo K, Ehrich M: Possible involvement of a neurotrophic factor during the early stages of organophosphate-induced delayed neurotoxicity. Toxicol Lett 75:111–117, 1995.

20. Silveria CL, Eldefrawi AT, Eldefrawi ME: Putative M2 muscarinic receptors of rat heart have high affinity for organophosphorous anticholinesterases. Toxicol Appl Pharmacol 103:474–481, 1990.

21. Albuquerque EX, Deshpande SS, Kawabuchi M, et al: Multiple actions of anticholinesterase agents on chemoreceptive synapses: Molecular basis for prophylaxis and treatment of organophosphate poisoning. Fundam Appl Toxicol 5:S182–S203, 1985.

22. Sivam SP, Hoskins B, Ho IK. An assessment of comparative acute toxicity of diisopropyl-fluorophosphate, Tabun, Sarin and soman in relation to cholinergic and GABAergic enzyme activities in rats. Fundam Appl Toxicol 19:23–32, 1984.

23. Szilagyi M, Gray PJ, Dawson RM: Effects of the nerve agents soman and tabun on the uptake and release of GABA and glutamate in synaptosomes of guinea pig cerebral cortex. Gen Pharmacol 24:663–668, 1993.

24. Liu DD, Watanabe HK, Ho IK, et al: Acute effects of soman, sarin and tabun on cyclic nucleotide metabolism in rat striatum. J Toxicol Environ Health 19:23–32, 1986.

25. Cao CJ, Mioduszewski RJ, Menking DE, et al: Cytotoxicity of organophosphate anticholinesterases. In Vitro Cell Dev Biol Anim 35:493–500, 1999.

26. Benschop HP, Bijleved EC, deJong LPA, et al: Toxicokinetics of the four stereoisomers of the nerve agent soman in atropinized rats, influence of soman simulator. Toxicol Appl Pharmacol 90:490–500, 1987.

27. Grob D: The manifestations and treatment of poisoning due to nerve gas and other organic phosphate anticholinesterase compounds. Arch Intern Med 98:221–239, 1956.

28. Siddell FR: Soman and sarin: Clinical manifestations and treatment of accidental poisoning by organophosphates. Clin Toxicol 7:1–17, 1974.

29. Rengstoff RH: Accidental exposure to sarin: Vision effects. Arch Toxicol 56:201–203, 1985.

30. Rickett DL, Glenn JF, Beers ET: Central respiratory effects versus neuromuscular actions of nerve agents. Neurotoxicology 8:466–475, 1953.

31. Decandole CA, Duglas WW, Evans CL, et al: The failure of respiration in death by anticholinesterase poisoning. Br J Pharmacol 8:466–475, 1953.

32. Stewart WC: The effects of sarin and atropine on the respiratory center and neuromuscular junctions of the rat. Can J Biochem Physiol 37:651–660, 1959.

33. Singer AW, Jaax NK, Graham JS, et al: Cardiomyopathy in soman and sarin intoxicated rat. Toxicol Lett 36:243–249, 1987.

34. Worek F, Kleine A, Falke K: Arrhythmias in organophosphate poisoning: Effect of atropine and bispyridinium oximes. Arch Int Pharmacodyn Ther 3:418–435, 1995.

35. Senanayake N, Karalliede L: Neurotoxic effects of organophosphorous insecticides: An intermediate syndrome. N Engl J Med 316:761–763, 1987.

36. DeBleecker J, Van Den Neucker K, Willems J: The intermediate syndrome in organophosphate poisoning: Presentation of a case and review of the literature. J Toxicol Clin Toxicol 30:321–329, 1992.

37. McLeod CG, Singer AW, Harrington DG: Acute neuropathology in soman poisoned rats. Neurotoxicology 5:53–58, 1984.

38. Anzueo A, Berdine GG, Moore GT, et al: Pathophysiology of soman intoxication in primates. Toxicol Appl Pharmacol 86:56–68, 1986.

39. Sekijima Y, Morita H, Yanagisawa N: Follow-up of sarin poisoning in Matsumoto. Ann Intern Med 127:1042–1046, 1997.

40. Mulchandani P, Mulchandani A, Kaneva I, et al: Biosensor for direct determination of organophosphate nerve agents: 1. Potentiometric enzyme electrode. Biosens Bioelectron 14:77–85, 1999.

41. Mulchandani A, Pan S, Chen W: Fiber-optic enzyme biosensor for direct determination of organophosphate nerve agents. Biotechnol Prog 15:130–134, 1999.

42. Polhuijs M, Langenberg JP, Benschop HP: New method for retrospective detection of exposure to organophosphorous anticholinesterases: Application to alleged sarin victims of Japanese terrorists. Toxicol Appl Pharmacol 146:156–161, 1997.

43. Nagao M, Takatori T, Matsuda Y, et al: Definitive evidence for the acute sarin poisoning diagnosis in the Tokyo subway. Toxicol Appl Pharmacol 144:198–203, 1997.

44. Nozaki H, Aikawa N, Fujishima S, et al: A case of VX poisoning and the difference from sarin. Lancet 346:698–699, 1995.

45. Klette KL, Levine B, Dreka C, et al: Cholinesterase activity in post-mortem blood as a screening test for organophosphate/chemical weapon exposure. J Forensic Sci 38:950–955, 1993.

46. Munro N: Toxicity of the organophosphate chemical warfare agents GA, GB, and VX: Implications for public protection. Environ Health Perspect 102:18–37, 1994.

47. Wolfe AD, Rush RS, Doctor BP, et al: Acetylcholinesterase prophylaxis against organophosphate toxicity. Fundam Appl Toxicol 9:266–270, 1987.

48. Ravesh L, Grunwald J, Marcus D, et al: Human butyrylcholinesterase as a general prophylactic antidote for nerve agent toxicity: In vitro and in vivo quantitive characterization. Biochem Pharmacol 45:2465–2474, 1993.

49. Caranto GR, Waibel KH, Asher JM, et al: Amplification of the effectiveness of acetylcholinesterase for detoxification of organophosphorous compounds by bis-quatenary oximes. Biochem Pharmacol 47:347–357, 1994.

50. Saxena A, Maxwell DM, Quinn DM, et al: Mutant acetylcholinesterase as potential detoxification agents for organophosphate poisoning. Biochem Pharmacol 54:269–274, 1997.

51. Mulchandani A, Kaneva I, Chen V: Detoxification of organophosphate nerve agents by immobilized Escherichia coli with surface expressed organophosphate hydrolase. Biotechnol Bioeng 63:216–223, 1999.

52. Broomfield CA, Lockridge O, Millard CB: Protein engineering of a human enzyme that hydolyzes V and G nerve agents: design, construction and characterization. Chem Biol Interact 119–120:413–418, 1999.

53. Cheng TC, DeFrank JJ, Rastogi VK: Alteromonas prolidase for organophosphorous G-agent decontamination. Chem Biol Interact 119–120:455–462, 1999.

54. Gordon RK, Feaster SR, Russell AJ, et al: Organophosphate skin decontamination using immobilized enzymes. Chem Biol Interact 119–120:463–470, 1999.

55. Sawyer TW, Parker D, Thomas N, et al: Efficacy of an oximate-based skin decontaminant against organophosphate nerve agents determined in vivo and in vitro. Toxicology 67:267–277, 1991.

56. Tuovinen K, Hannien O: Protection of mice against soman by pretreatment with eptastigmine and physostigmine. Toxicology 139:233–241, 1999.

57. Kassa J, Fusek J: The positive influence of a cholinergic-anticholinergic pretreatment and antidotal treatment on rats poisoned with supralethal doses of soman. Toxicology 128:1–7, 1998.

58. Munro NB, Watson AP, Ambrose KR, et al: Treating exposure to chemical warfare agents: Implications for health care providers and community emergency planning. Environ Health Perspect 89:205–215, 1990.

59. Holstege CP, Kirk M, Sidell FR: Chemical warfare: Nerve agent poisoning. Crit Care Clin 13:923–942, 1997.

60. Orma PS, Middleton RK: Aerosolized atropine as an antidote to nerve gas. Ann Pharmacother 26:937–938, 1992.

61. van Helden HPM, Busker RW, Melchers BPC, et al: Pharmacological effects of oximes: How relevant are they? Arch Toxicol 70:779–786, 1996.

62. Dawson RM: Review of oximes available for treatment of nerve agent poisoning. J Appl Toxicol 14:317–331, 1994.

63. Boskovic B, Kovacevic V, Jovanovic D: PAM-2, HI-6 and HGG-12 in soman and tabun poisoning. Fundam Appl Toxicol 4:S106–115, 1984.

64. Clement JG, Hansen AS, Boulet CA: Efficacy of HLo-7 and pyrimidoxime as antidotes of nerve agent poisoning in mice. Toxicology 66:216–219, 1992.

65. Lundy PM, Hansen AS, Hand BT, et al: Comparison of several oximes against poisoning by soman, tabun and GF. Toxicology 72:99–105, 1992.

66. Melchers BP, Philippens IH, Wolthuis OL: Efficacy of HI-6 and HLo-7 in preventing incapacitation following nerve agent poisoning. Pharmacol Biochem Behav 49:781–788, 1994.

67. Cassel G, Karlsson L, Waara L, et al: Pharmacokinetics and effects of HI-6 in blood and brain of soman-intoxicated rats: A microdialysis study. Eur J Pharmacol 332:43–52, 1997.

68. Worek F, Widmann R, Knopff O, et al: Reactivating potency of obidoxime, pralidoxime, HI 6 and Hlo7 in human erythrocyte acetylcholinesterase inhibited by highly toxic organophosphorous compounds. Arch Toxicol 72:237–243, 1998.

69. Kopolovitz I, Menton R, Matthews C: Dose-response effects of atropine and HI-6 treatment of organophosphorous poisoning in guinea pigs. Drug Chem Toxicol 18:119–136, 1995.

70. Castro CA, Larsen T, Finger AV, et al: Behavioral efficacy of diazepam against nerve agent exposure in rhesus monkeys. Pharmacol Biochem Behav 41:159–164, 1992.

71. Volans AP: Sarin: Guidelines on the management of victims of a nerve gas attack. J Accid Emerg Med 13:202–206, 1996.

72. Lallement G, Clarencon D, Masqueliez C, et al: Nerve agent poisoning in primates: Antilethal, anti-epileptic and neuroprotective effects of GK-11. Arch Toxicol 72:84–92, 1998.

73. Lallement G, Clarencon D, Galonnier M, et al: Acute soman poisoning in primates neither pretreated nor receiving immediate therapy: Value of gacyclidine (GK-11) in delayed medical support. Arch Toxicol 73:115–122, 1999.

74. Balali-Mood M, Salimifar H, Shariate M: Effects of sodium bicarbonate in human organophosphate poisoning. Proceedings of the Third International Chemical and Biological Medical Treatment Symposium, Spiez, Switzerland, May 7–12, 2000.

75. Monhart V, Fusek J, Brndiar M, et al: Use of hemoperfusion in experimental intoxication with nerve agents. Artif Organs 18:770–772, 1994.

76. Okudera H, Morita H, Iwashita T, et al: Unexpected nerve gas exposure in the city of Matsumoto: Report of rescue activity in the first sarin gas terrorism. Am J Emerg Med 15:526–530, 1997.

CHAPTER **132**

Anthrax

Edward W. Cetaruk

A brief discussion of biologic agents as weapons of mass destruction is essential to the understanding, recognition, and treatment of victims of such attacks. Although this chapter addresses anthrax only, these concepts are applicable to all biologic warfare agents, including plague, smallpox, the viral encephalitides, and the viral hemorrhagic fevers, which are discussed in other chapters. Biologic weapons may be lethal, with high case-fatality rates (e.g., plague, smallpox, anthrax) or incapacitating (e.g., Venezuelan equine encephalitis, Q fever), with relatively low case-fatality rates. All potential biologic warfare agents must have several common characteristics, however, to be effective biologic weapons: (1) The organism chosen for weaponization must be highly virulent, with a high attack rate; (2) the organism must be stable in a weaponized form (preferably a dry powder); (3) the organism must be able to withstand environmental stressors, such as desiccation, ultraviolet light, disinfectants, and extremes of temperature; (4) the organism possibly may possess antibiotic resistance; and (5) the organism must have a susceptible population. This last concept led the U.S. armed forces to institute an anthrax vaccination program and has rekindled interest in large-scale smallpox immunization.

Biologic weapons are best disseminated by aerosolization because it is the most efficient technique to deliver enough agent to affect a large area or population. Ideally a biologic agent is weaponized as dry particles, 1 to 5 μ in diameter, that have been engineered to overcome electrostatic forces (that cause clumping) and are resistant to environmental stressors. When properly prepared and disseminated, aerosolized particles of this size remain suspended in air for prolonged periods. Particles smaller than 1 μ are likely to be exhaled after being inhaled, and particles larger than 5 μ are likely to affect the upper airways and nasopharynx, greatly reducing the likelihood of establishing an infection. Particles in the 1- to 5-μ range, when inhaled, are carried to the distal airways, where they can best establish an infection, become absorbed parenterally, or initiate toxic actions. Particle size is the most important determinant of an aerosolized biologic warfare agent's effectiveness (William C. Patrick, III, personal communication). The successful use of the mail as a means to deliver *Bacillus anthracis* as a biologic weapon in the United States in 2001 illustrates, however, that biologic weapon attacks may take place on any scale, via unlikely routes, and against unsuspected targets.

Natural anthrax is endemic to many areas of the world, with episodic outbreaks occasionally involving humans (epizootics).[1] In 1876, Koch proved his postulates by showing that *B. anthracis* was the microbiologic etiology of the clinical disease anthrax. Bell[2] showed that aerosolized anthrax was the cause of woolsorters' disease. In 1881, Pasteur developed a capsule-null anthrax strain by growing *B. anthracis* cultures at 42°C, producing the first effective live, attenuated bacterial vaccine and concurrently showing the importance of the capsule as a virulence factor.

Japan's infamous biologic weapons program during the 1930s and 1940s, known as Unit 731, directed by General Shiro Ishii, conducted experiments on thousands of human victims during their occupation of mainland China.[3] Biologic agents used included *B. anthracis, Neisseria meningitides, Vibrio cholerae, Shigella* spp., *Salmonella* spp., *Yersinia pestis*, smallpox, and others.

Although it was never deployed, anthrax was developed as a potential defense against an Axis invasion of Britain during World War II.[3–5] Between 1942 and 1943, anthrax bomblets were tested in open-air releases on Gruinard Island, off the northwest coast of Scotland. Although the entire island was burned bare after the war, viable anthrax spores were still abundant more than 40 years later.[4] The island was finally decontaminated successfully in 1986 using several hundred tons of a 5% formaldehyde and seawater solution.[4–6] Anthrax has been a first-line agent in the biologic weapon arsenals of the United States, the former Soviet Union, the United Kingdom, and Iraq, among others.

The United States abandoned its offensive biologic weapons program in 1969. The Biological Weapons Convention was established in 1972, prohibiting the development and stockpiling of offensive biologic weapons. Although a signatory to the Biological Weapons Convention, the former Soviet Union continued its offensive biologic warfare program, *Biopreparat*, well into the 1990s. The latter grew to the point of employing tens of thousands of scientists at dozens of biologic weapon facilities, developing technologies and processes to produce massive quantities of highly virulent biologic agents, including anthrax (estimated annual production capacity = 4500 metric tons), smallpox (estimated annual production capacity = 200 tons), plague, tularemia, and Marburg virus. The dissolution of the Soviet Union and *Biopreparat* has made a great deal of expertise, technology, and possibly microbiologic cultures of biologic warfare agents potentially available to terrorist and state-sponsored biologic weapon programs.

The Aum Shinrikyo cult of Japan released aerosolized anthrax spores and botulinum toxin in Japan on multiple occasions. In June 1993, they weaponized and disseminated a nonvirulent strain of *B. anthracis* from a rooftop in Kameido, Japan.[7,8] Although no one was made ill, the attack was not recognized until well after the fact. An investigation of the Aum cult led to a retrospective microbiologic analysis of the material released from the rooftop of their headquarters, which yielded the Sterne strain of anthrax. This is a nonvirulent, nonencapsulating *B. anthracis* strain used for animal immunizations.[8] The cult successfully executed many nerve agent attacks between 1990 and 1995, however, culminating with a sarin nerve agent attack in the Tokyo subway that sent thousands to local hospitals, caused hundreds of casualties, and resulted in 12 deaths.[7] The successful use of anthrax sent through the mail as a bioterrorist weapon in the United States in 2001 has underscored the need to be able to recognize and treat victims of a biologic weapon attack.

The spore form of *B. anthracis* is used for weaponization because it is extremely resistant to environmental stressors. Viable anthrax spores have been recovered at sites, such as tanneries and slaughterhouses, many decades after their introduction into the soil. Historically, humans become infected by contact with infected animals or contaminated animal products, such as wool, hides, and bones. Typically, there are a few zoonotic outbreaks of animal anthrax per year in the United States.[7] The anthrax spore is highly infectious, amenable to weaponization, and stable for long-term storage and deployment in munitions. Other biologic weapons, such as plague and smallpox, lack the anthrax spore's innate stability in the environment and require more extensive weaponization to withstand environmental stressors.

MICROBIOLOGY

B. anthracis is a toxigenic, spore-forming, nonmotile, aerobic, encapsulating, gram-positive bacillus that causes the disease anthrax. It usually is found as the spore form in the environment and as the vegetative bacillus form when causing infection in an animal host.

The anthrax spore begins as an endospore within the vegetative bacillus and is usually visible in either a central or a paracentral location. It is essentially a dormant form of *B. anthracis*, which must germinate into the vegetative bacillus to complete its reproductive life cycle and to cause infection (Fig. 132-1). The anthrax spore comprises a central protoplast, which contains the essential constituents of a future vegetative cell, encased by several peptidoglycan and phospholipid layers that protect it from environmental stressors.[9,10] As mentioned earlier, the soil is the natural reservoir of *B. anthracis* spores, resulting in areas of endemic anthrax. The spores are extremely stable in the environment, remaining viable for decades when protected from ultraviolet light.[4] Anthrax most often exists as a zoonotic infection of herbivores, such as sheep, cattle, other domesticated livestock, and wild grazing animals. Animals may either ingest or inhale spores while grazing, especially when vegetation is sparse, forcing them to forage closer to

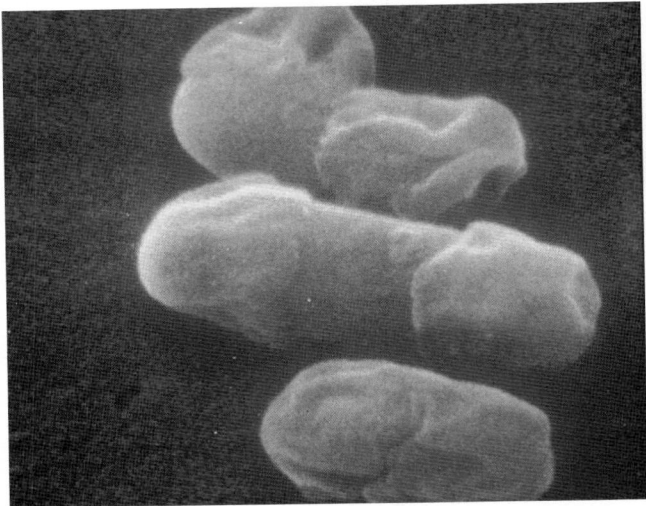

FIGURE 132-1

Electron micrograph of *Bacillus anthracis* spores in multiple stages of germination. *(Courtesy of U.S. Army Medical Research Institute of Infectious Diseases, Fort Detrick, Frederick, MD.)*

or in contact with the soil. When introduced into the body of a susceptible host, the spore germinates into a vegetative bacillus and causes disease. All mammals are susceptible, although some have significant resistance.[11]

Sporulation, the release of a spore on the death and lysis of the vegetative bacillus, typically occurs under nutrient-limiting conditions, such as when an infected animal dies. As the animal's carcass dries, vegetative anthrax bacilli rapidly sporulate on exposure to oxygen and contaminate the surrounding area, effectively returning *B. anthracis* spores back into the soil reservoir. Each vegetative bacillus produces one spore. The soil acts as a reservoir for the organism. Although rare in North America (owing to human and livestock vaccination programs), anthrax still is endemic to areas of South America, Africa, Asia, and the Mediterranean region.

When conditions are favorable for germination from the spore into the bacillus, the spore coat layers alter their structural morphology, allowing the protoplast to develop into a *B. anthracis* bacillus (see Fig. 132-1).[9,10,12] In vitro studies have shown that *B. anthracis* spores germinate optimally at 22°C (71.6°F). This low temperature may be important for the establishment of cutaneous anthrax infection where the body temperature is lower.[10] Other promoters of germination include L-alanine, tyrosine, adenosine, and low pH.[9,10] The vegetative form is a nonmotile, rod-shaped, gram-positive, aerobic or facultative anaerobic bacillus measuring 1 to 1.2 μm × 3 to 5 μm. The bacillus multiplies readily in infected animals and in laboratory media and causes the clinical disease anthrax (Fig. 132-2).

Vegetative anthrax bacilli produce several virulence factors, including an antiphagocytic capsule and three exotoxins: protective antigen (PA), lethal factor (LF), and edema factor (EF). Although susceptibility may vary, the capsule is essential for virulence. Pasteur's nonencapsulated *B. anthracis* variant, produced by incubating wild-type *B. anthracis* at 42°C (107.6°F), was nonvirulent and used as an effective vaccine. The Aum Shinrikyo's 1993 anthrax attack in Kameido, Japan,

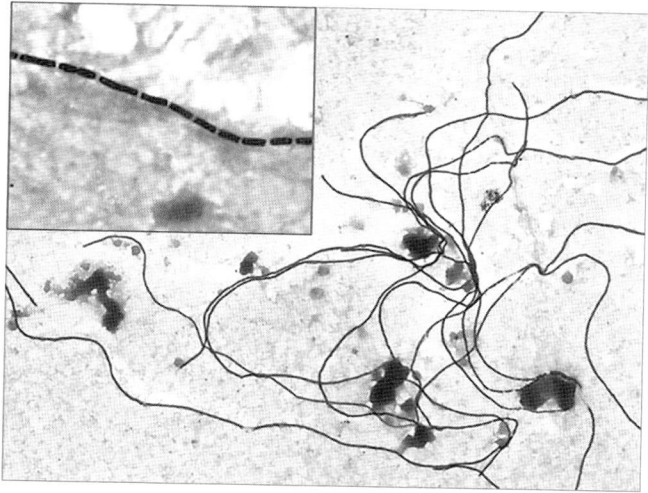

FIGURE 132-2

Gram-positive vegetative *Bacillus anthracis* growing in characteristic long chains in culture (original magnification 20%). *Inset,* Enlargement shows "jointed bamboo rod" of *B. anthracis* in culture (original magnification 100%). *(From Borio L, Frank D, Mani V, et al: Death due to bioterrorism-related inhalational anthrax: Report of 2 patients. JAMA 286:2554–2559, 2001.)* See Color Fig. 132-2.

failed because they weaponized the nonvirulent, nonencapsulated Sterne 34F2 strain used for vaccinations.[8] Capsule formation by *B. anthracis* produces characteristic mucoid-appearing colonies when grown on bicarbonate-containing media. It also is antigenic, which is the basis for direct fluorescence antibody capsule staining to identify *B. anthracis.*

PATHOPHYSIOLOGY

Weaponized anthrax spores are disseminated most effectively by an aerosolization, which may take place as a large-scale, open-air attack or as a more limited attack, such as introducing anthrax spores into the ventilation system of a building. As was shown in the bioterrorist anthrax attacks in the United States in 2001, however, a less likely, or less "efficient," means of dissemination (the postal system) still may cause casualties.[13–20] Depending on the munitions efficiency of the weaponization process used (e.g., particle size, virulence, agent viability), a percentage of inhaled spores reaches the bronchioles, alveolar ducts, and alveoli.

Animal studies have shown that when anthrax spores reach the alveoli, they are phagocytosed and transported to the mediastinal lymph nodes via the pulmonary lymphatics.[21,22] In a guinea pig study, most anthrax spores were phagocytosed in the alveoli within 35 minutes when introduced into the respiratory system by transtracheal injection of a liquid spore suspension, and within 3 hours after an aerosol inhalational exposure.[22] All spores reaching the alveoli and alveolar ducts were taken up by the septal cells lining the alveoli or by free alveolar macrophages derived from these cells. These spore-containing macrophages then migrated to the mediastinal and peribronchial lymph nodes via peribronchial, perivascular, and subpleural lymphatic channels. Spores were found in the tracheobronchial lymph nodes at 4 hours postimplantation. No free spores or anthrax bacilli were seen in transit. Most spores are phagocytosed

and transported to the regional lymph nodes, although vegetative bacilli were found in alveoli damaged by the experimental methods, creating small foci of bronchopneumonia. Anthrax spores also underwent phagocytosis by polymorphonuclear leukocytes, although to a much lesser degree than macrophages, and none were found in lymph nodes on biopsy.[21–23]

Germination of the spore is the essential first step for the growth of the organism into the vegetative bacillus form, establishing an infection and the production of anthrax exotoxins. Germinating spores and vegetative bacilli were seen within macrophages in lymph nodes within 17 hours of inhalational exposure.[22] Inhaled anthrax spores are phagocytosed in the alveoli and undergo germination within alveolar macrophages[9] en route to the mediastinal lymph nodes via lymphangioles. They multiply rapidly in the lymph nodes as vegetative bacilli, then spread hematogenously to the local tissues (mediastinum, lungs), causing vasculitis, edema, pneumonia, necrosis, and toxemia.

Pathologic findings similar to the above-described experimental findings have been seen in cases of human anthrax. A detailed study[24] of 41 postmortem tissue samples from the 1979 Soviet Sverdlovsk anthrax epidemic[25] found vegetative *B. anthracis* in nearly all tissue specimens, with the heaviest burden being found in the pulmonary microvasculature, mediastinal lymph nodes, and alveoli. There appeared to be a gradient in the tissue burden of vegetative bacilli: More than 50% were found in alveolar septal capillaries and venules, less than 20% were in the extravascular interstitium of the alveolar septa, and approximately 18% were in the alveolar airspaces.[24]

Anthrax's two virulence factors, its antiphagocytic capsule and exotoxins, are encoded on plasmids pOX1 and pOX2. Full virulence requires the presence of both plasmids and of their respective gene products. Anthrax toxin is a three-part protein exotoxin consisting of PA, LF, and EF, which are individually nontoxic.[26] Strains lacking plasmid pOX1 do not produce exotoxin and are essentially avirulent, whereas strains lacking the pOX2 plasmid are 10,000 times less virulent than wild-type *B. anthracis* that has both plasmids.[8] *B. anthracis* virulence in mice was reduced more than 1000-fold in mutants lacking either LF or PA and about 10-fold in mutants lacking EF.[27] A spontaneous nonvirulent, nonencapsulated variant that lacked the pXO2 plasmid (pOX1+, pOX2−) was the basis for the live Sterne anthrax vaccine.[28]

Carbon dioxide is thought to be a positive molecular environmental signal that increases expression of genes coding for PA and the antiphagocytic capsule. The synthesis of anthrax toxin proteins and capsule is induced and enhanced in the presence of bicarbonate and serum, under conditions with elevated (>5%) levels of carbon dioxide, and at physiologic temperatures (37°C [98.6°F]).[29,30] In the presence of serum and elevated carbon dioxide, germinating spores release a poly-γ-D-glutamic acid polymer antiphagocytic capsule through openings in the spore surface. The capsule appears exterior to the S layer of the vegetative cell, confers resistance to phagocytosis by macrophages, and allows anthrax bacilli to multiply virtually unchecked by the host's immune system. The capsule is synthesized by three membrane-associated polymerases of 44 kd, 16 kd, and 46 kd, encoded on three genes, arranged in the order *capB, capC*, and *capA*, on the 95.3 kbp plasmid, pXO2. A fourth gene, *dep*, located downstream and adjacent to the *cap* region on pXO2, encodes a capsular depolymerase.[31,32] This enzyme catalyses the hydrolysis of poly-γ-D-glutamic acid polymers into lower-molecular-weight polyglutamates and seems to be essential for replication in vivo.[33] Two regulator proteins, encoded by *acpA* on pXO2 and *atxA* on pXO1, also enhance transcription of capsule genes.[31,34–36]

Anthrax toxin was first demonstrated when sterile plasma from guinea pigs dying of anthrax was injected into healthy guinea pigs and caused a clinical condition identical to the toxemia of an anthrax infection.[37] Three structural genes, *pag, lef*, and *cya*, located on plasmid pXO1, encode anthrax's three exotoxin proteins, PA, LF, and EF. *atxA*, a fourth gene also located on pXO1, codes for a 56-kd positive gene regulator protein that increases the transcription of all three toxin genes and many other genes on pXO1 and is essential for virulence.[34,36] Transcription of *pag, lef*, and *cya* is enhanced during growth in 5% or greater atmospheric carbon dioxide. This carbon dioxide–induced gene transcription is dependent on *atxA*, which increases transcription 10-fold from an otherwise silent start site associated with the anthrax toxin structural genes.[29,38] These three protein gene products combine after secretion to form two binary or AB toxins.[39] *Binary toxins* are secreted as individual monomeric protein moieties that later assemble into toxin complexes. *AB toxins* have two distinct functional components: the enzymatic A moiety, which exerts its effects in the cytosol, and the receptor-binding B moiety, which binds to a cell surface receptor and translocates the active A moiety through the cell membrane into the cytosol. Anthrax toxin is a unique binary AB toxin in that it has two alternate A moieties—LF and EF—and a single B moiety—PA. Lethal factor and EF competitively bind to the same site on PA. The final toxins, edema toxin (ET) and lethal toxin (LT), are heterooligomers of PA bound to either EF or LF (Fig. 132-3).[27,39]

Protective antigen (735 amino acids, 82.7 kd) is the central, receptor-binding component that mediates the internalization of LF and EF into the cytosol of macrophages and has four functional domains.[40] The amino-terminus *domain 1* (amino acids 1 to 249) includes a large, flexible polypeptide loop with the protease recognition sequence $_{164}$Arg-XX-Arg$_{167}$[41]; *domain 2* forms the membrane insertion channel and is involved in oligomerization; *domain 3* has no known function; and *domain 4* is loosely associated with the other three domains and is involved in receptor binding.[40]

In vivo binding studies have shown that PA binds to a specific eukaryotic cell membrane anthrax toxin receptor (ATR) in a specific, concentration-dependent, saturable, and reversible manner.[42] This receptor has not been completely described, but enzymatic and chemical cross-linking studies strongly suggest that a cell surface protein of 85 to 90 kd is, or constitutes a portion of, ATR.[42] Cloning studies of the human ATR have produced a 368-amino acid type I membrane protein with an extracellular von Willebrand factor A (VWA) domain between amino acid residues 44 and 216.[43] VWA domains are type I domains, which are common in the extracellular regions of cell surface proteins and are important for protein-protein interactions, such as ligand-receptor binding. The ATR also includes a *MIDAS* (metal ion-dependent adhesion site) motif, which is required for

domain I ligand binding.[43] A soluble version of the ATR's binding domain was created by synthesizing a polypeptide of amino acid residues 41 to 227 of the anthrax receptor (ATR$_{41–227}$) with a hexahistidine tag (T7).[43] This fusion protein (T7-ATR$_{41–227}$) was used to study the direct binding between PA and the ATR. Maximal binding required the presence of calcium,[44] and ethylenediaminetetraacetic acid impaired the in vivo interaction of PA and ATR, showing that PA-ATR binding requires divalent cations and the MIDAS site.[43] A mutant form of PA, with an amino acid substitution in the ATR-binding region, was unable to bind to the "soluble ATR" fusion protein, T7-ATR$_{41–227}$, in vitro and was impaired in its ability to intoxicate cells in vivo. Finally, soluble T7-ATR$_{41–227}$ also was shown to be an effective inhibitor of PA-ATR binding, protecting CHO-K1 cells from lysis by a PA+LF$_N$-DTA (lethal factor-diphtheria toxin A chain) fusion protein.[44] These studies show that there is a specific ligand-receptor interaction between the VWA domain of ATR and domain 4 of PA and that this interaction is important for the anthrax toxin pathogenicity.[45] Inhibitors of PA binding to the macrophage ATR may represent future treatment modalities.[46,47]

After binding to the ATR on the macrophage cellular membrane,[42,43] PA is cleaved at the amino acid sequence $_{164}$Arg-XX-Arg$_{167}$ by cell-surface furin, or a furin-like protease, yielding a 63-kd carboxy-terminal fragment (PA63) and a 20-kd amino-terminal fragment (PA20) that dissociate into the medium.[38,41,48] Receptor-bound PA63 undergoes oligomerization to yield ring-shaped PA63 heptamers.[49,50] The proteolytic activation of PA reveals a binding site in domain 1 with high affinity for EF or LF.[27,48,50,51] Binding studies have shown that the PA63 heptamer competitively binds three to seven A toxin moieties (EF or LF).[38,40,50,52,53] The resulting heterooligomeric complex (PA$_7$·EF$_n$ or PA$_7$·LF$_n$) is internalized by the macrophage via receptor-mediated endocytosis.[50,54] The PA63 heptamer is capable of forming channels through planar phospholipid bilayers in vitro.[55] After endocytosis, acidification of the endolysosome by membrane-associated proton pumps induces a conformational change in PA63, allowing the PA heptamer to form a pore with a negatively charged lumen and a hydrophobic exterior surface that inserts into the endolysosomal membrane, forming a channel for the translocation of LF or EF into the cytosol.[27,53,56–58]

Bacterial proliferation leads to increased production of protective antigen and lethal and edema toxins. The combination of PA+LF and LT kills cells by the intracellular delivery and action of LF. LF is the major virulence factor produced by *B. anthracis*.[26] It is a 90-kd, highly specific, zinc-dependent metalloprotease[59–61] that triggers a series of events in sensitive macrophages that causes cell death within 2 hours.[27,62] Early events include increased cell membrane permeability to sodium and rubidium and adenosine triphosphate (ATP) depletion. Cell membrane permeability for other ions and molecules increases, followed by inhibition of macromolecule synthesis and finally cell lysis.[35,62] LF was found to have a proteolytic activity profile similar to that of PD09859, a selective inhibitor of the mitogen-activated protein kinase (MAPK) signal transduction pathway.[63,64] In response to specific extracellular signals, mitogen-activated protein kinase kinase 1 and 2 (MAPKK1 and MAPKK2) phosphorylate

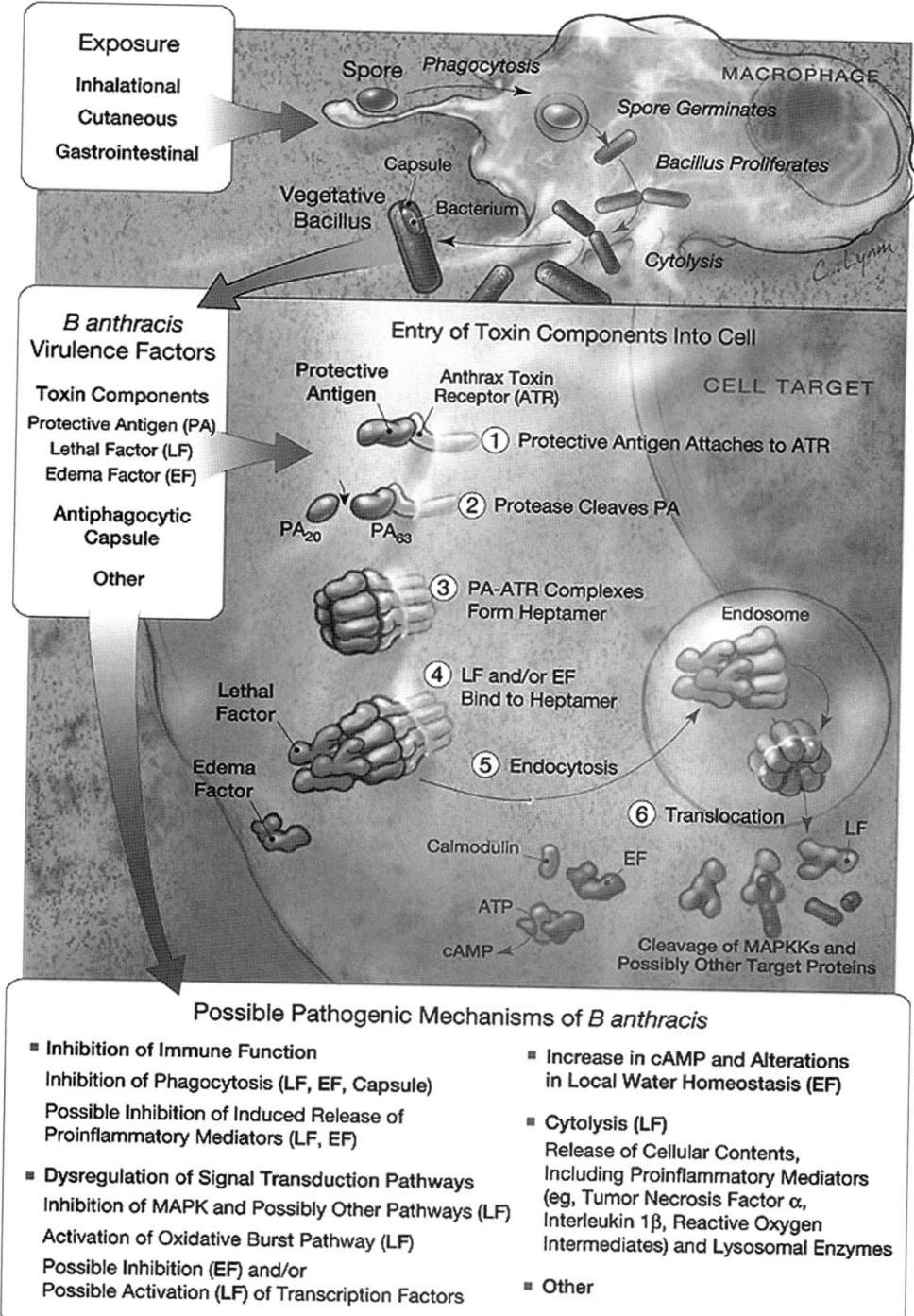

FIGURE 132-3

Pathogenesis of Bacillus anthracis. *(From Inglesby TV, O'Toole T, Henderson DA, et al: Anthrax as a biological weapon, 2002: Updated recommendations for management. JAMA 287:2236–2252, 2002.)*

and activate MAPKs.[17,32,65–67] These pathways control cell proliferation and differentiation.[68]

Deletion mutant studies and amino acid sequence analysis have shown that LF proteolytically cleaves the NH$_2$-terminal seven and the NH$_2$-terminal nine, amino acids of MAPKK1 and MAPKK2.[64,69,70] The NH$_2$-terminal 32 amino acids of MAPKK1 contain a MAPK binding site, suggesting that LF's proteolytic activity blocks MAPKK's ability to phosphorylate its substrate, MAPK.[69] Although the exact role that inhibition of the MAPK pathways plays in LF's cytotoxicity

is unknown, it has been shown to induce apoptosis in human melanoma cells[71] and lymphocytes[24] and to inhibit cell growth and differentiation.[68]

Edema factor is a potent calmodulin-dependent adenylate cyclase similar to that of *Bordetella pertussis*.[72,73] EF and LF share significant sequence homology at their amino-terminus regions (amino acid residues 1 to 250), and both bind by this region to the same site on PA63.[40,51,56] This supports the binary AB toxin motif, with PA being the membrane-translocating B moiety and EF and LF as alternate enzymatically active

A moieties. Inhibitors of receptor-mediated endocytosis or endosome acidification protect cells from EF.[54] After endocytosis and translocation out of the endolysosome, EF remains membrane bound with a cytosolic half-life of about 2 hours in Chinese hamster ovary (CHO) cells.[73,74] After a lag period of 10 minutes, EF causes markedly increased intracellular cyclic adenosine monophosphate (camp) levels in CHO cells.[73] It reversibly increases intracellular cAMP levels 1000-fold, leading to ATP depletion and activation of cAMP-dependent protein kinase. EF also blocks priming of polymorphonuclear leukocytes by lipopolysaccharide and by muramyl dipeptide, resulting in decreased release of superoxide anion on later stimulation.[75] Although not as toxic as LF, EF seems to disrupt multiple cellular pathways, leading to inhibition of macrophage phagocytosis, impairment of neutrophil function (including the inhibition of opsonized vegetative *B. anthracis*), and impaired water homeostasis.[27,38,54,56,72]

The macrophage inflammatory response plays a central role in the pathogenesis of anthrax.[23,35,62,76] MAPKKs are involved with the production of inflammatory cytokines, including tumor necrosis factor (TNF)-α, interleukin (IL)-1, and IL-6. LT induces the overproduction of proinflammatory cytokines, including IL-1b and TNF-α, by macrophages[23,35,53] that stimulate the production of reactive oxygen intermediates, leading to lysis of the macrophage.[76] Treatment with antisera to IL-1 and TNF-α protected anthrax toxin–treated animals, showing that the excessive production and release of these cytokines from macrophages causes death.[23,27] Proinflammatory cytokines, reactive oxygen intermediates, and bacteremia all induce sepsis, leading to septic shock and death. Gene mutation studies producing *B. anthracis* strains that consisted of every combination of the three toxin components have been done. Only the mutant strain that produced PA and LF retained any significant virulence. These studies show that reactive oxygen intermediates mediate LT's cytolytic activity and are involved in the overall pathophysiology of anthrax and that LT is the more important virulence factor, with EF making a lesser contribution.[23,26,31,35,76]

CLINICAL PRESENTATION

Clinical human anthrax occurs in three forms, classified by the organism's portal of entry into the host: cutaneous, gastrointestinal (including oropharyngeal), and inhalational. Cutaneous anthrax is the most common naturally occurring form of the disease. Its course may be less acute and is typically less severe than the often-fulminant presentation seen with the inhalational and gastrointestinal forms. Cutaneous anthrax is acquired by direct contact with anthrax spores, infected animals, or animal products through an abrasion or open wound in the skin.[17,77–81] The cutaneous anthrax cases resulting from the 2001 bioterrorist attacks in the United States had a mean incubation period of 5 days (range 1 to 10 days), based on estimated dates of exposure to anthrax-contaminated letters.[17] Lesions occurred on the forehead, chest, face, forearm, and fingers.[17,79–81] In the anthrax outbreak in Sverdlovsk, cutaneous anthrax lesions presented 12 days after the suspected time of the aerosol release.[25]

After the incubation period, a small papule appears at the site of inoculation. These lesions are typically not painful but may be pruritic and evolve into fluid-filled vesicles within 1 or 2 days. Gram stain of the vesicular fluid may show many *B. anthracis* organisms. These vesicles rupture and ulcerate, leaving the characteristic black eschar of cutaneous anthrax that gives *B. anthracis* its name (*anthrakos* is a Greek term meaning "coal, black"). Histologic studies of the lesions show skin necrosis, *B. anthracis* bacilli, and lymphocytic infiltration without suppuration or abscess formation. The surrounding tissue becomes markedly edematous, sometimes involving the entire limb. Lymphangitis with tender, local lymphadenopathy also may be seen.[17,77–79] Patients with cutaneous anthrax may develop systemic disease, including fever, lymphadenopathy, septic shock, and death.[78,79]

The pulmonary form of anthrax results from inhalation of aerosolized anthrax spores and is the most fulminant clinical form of the disease. The median incubation period in the 2001 bioterrorism-related cases in the United States from known time of exposure in six cases was 4 days (range 4 to 6 days).[18] This range is similar to that seen in the 1979 Sverdlovsk anthrax outbreak. At Sverdlovsk, many patients presented 43 days after the date of the release, however.[25,83] Initially, patients are likely to have relatively nonspecific symptoms, including fever, fatigue, nausea, vomiting, myalgias, abdominal pain, sore throat, shock, and coma.[14,18,25,84,85] Respiratory complaints, including nonproductive cough, shortness of breath, chest pain, and dyspnea, soon develop (Table 132-1).[13,14,19,25,62,85] This initial presentation is distressingly nonspecific given the grave nature of the disease. As vegetative bacilli multiply, producing marked mediastinal lymphadenopathy, anthrax toxins cause severe tissue hemorrhage, necrosis, and edema, often causing stridor. Edema of the chest wall also may be seen with advanced cases of mediastinal anthrax. Approximately half of patients with inhalational anthrax also develop hem-

TABLE 132-1 Symptoms for 10 Patients with Bioterrorism-Related Inhalational Anthrax, October–November 2001

SYMPTOMS	n = 10
Fever, chills	10
Fatigue, malaise, lethargy	10
Cough (minimally or nonproductive)	9
Nausea or vomiting	9
Dyspnea	8
Sweats, often drenching	7
Chest discomfort or pleuritic pain	7
Myalgias	6
Headache	5
Confusion	4
Abdominal pain	3
Sore throat	2
Rhinorrhea	1

From Jernigan JA, Stephens DS, Ashford DA, et al: Bioterrorism-related inhalational anthrax: The first 10 cases reported in the United States. Emerg Infect Dis 7:933–944, 2001.

orrhagic meningitis. These patients may present with fever, headaches, confusion, and mental status changes.[14,18,80,83,85] The index case of inhalational anthrax from the 2001 bioterrorist attacks initially presented with fever, confusion, vomiting, myalgias, and malaise and *without* any respiratory complaints.[14] The diagnosis was made by isolating *B. anthracis* from cerebrospinal fluid obtained to rule out meningitis (Table 132-2).[14,18]

Gastrointestinal anthrax is caused by the ingestion of insufficiently cooked contaminated meat. It is thought to occur from the ingestion of vegetative bacilli rather than anthrax spores. It is a relatively rare form of human anthrax, but carries a high case-fatality rate (>90%) and may be seen after the use of an anthrax biologic weapon. It is found in two forms: oropharyngeal and abdominal. Oropharyngeal anthrax may produce significant edema of the soft tissues of the mouth, oropharynx, head, and neck. Gastrointestinal anthrax involving the intestines presents with abdominal pain, nausea, vomiting, gastrointestinal hemorrhage, and ascites.[77] Similar to inhalational anthrax, gastrointestinal anthrax may present as generalized sepsis and may mimic other abdominal catastrophes, such as peritonitis, perforated viscus, diverticulitis, and invasive infectious gastroenteritis. As with the other clinical forms of anthrax, gastrointestinal

TABLE 132-2 Initial Clinical Findings in 10 Patients with Bioterrorism-Related Inhalational Anthrax, October–November 2001

Physical findings	
Fever (>37.8°C)	7/10
Tachycardia (heart rate >100 beats/min)	8/10
Hypotension (systolic blood pressure <110 mm Hg)	1/10
Laboratory results	
White blood cell count (median, range)	$9.8 \times 10^3/mm^3$
Differential—neutrophilia (>70%)	7/10
Neutrophil band forms (>5%)	4/5
Elevated transaminases (SGOT or SGPT >40)	9/10
Hypoxemia (alveolar-arterial oxygen gradient >30 mm Hg on room air oxygen saturation <94%)	6/10
Metabolic acidosis	2/10
Elevated creatinine (>1.5 mg/dL)	1/10
Chest x-ray findings	
Any abnormality	10/10
Mediastinal widening	7/10
Infiltrates/consolidation	7/10
Pleural effusion	8/10
Chest computed tomography findings	
Any abnormality	8/8
Mediastinal lymphadenopathy, widening	7/8
Pleural effusion	8/8
Infiltrates, consolidation	6/8

SGOT, serum glutamic oxalacetic transaminase; SGPT, serum glutamic pyruvic transaminase.
From Jernigan JA, Stephens DS, Ashford DA, et al: Bioterrorism-related inhalational anthrax: The first 10 cases reported in the United States. Emerg Infect Dis 7:933–944, 2001.

anthrax progresses to fatal sepsis and toxemia if not treated early and aggressively.[64]

DIAGNOSIS

As long as there is a credible risk of a bioterrorism, it is crucial to consider the possibility of a bioterrorism-related infectious disease in the differential diagnosis of a patient with a syndrome comprising the features of anthrax. As mentioned earlier, the clinical presentation of bioterrorism-related anthrax may be nonspecific. It is important to be alert to local epidemiologic trends and patterns of febrile illness. The diagnosis of a bioterrorism-related illness is likely to be made by considering the specific presentation (e.g., fever, dyspnea, confusion) and the situational presentation (e.g., multiple patients presenting to area hospitals with similar severe illnesses and a common history of attending a parade the preceding weekend).

The highly distinctive appearances of cutaneous anthrax lesions simplify their diagnosis. Characteristically, they are painless lesions that eventually ulcerate into a black eschar with associated tissue edema (Fig. 132-4). Because they can be recognized early, these more visible cutaneous cases may lead to early detection of an anthrax bioterrorist attack. These patients typically should not require intensive care unit admission unless they have progressed to the septicemic or toxemic form of the infection. It is likely, however, that an aerosolized anthrax release would produce multiple forms of the illness.[17,66,79,80,83]

History regarding the patient's place and type of employment, recent local and distant travel, and all other information should be obtained to reconstruct the patient's activities and whereabouts for at least the previous 2 weeks. History of employment in an occupation that may have increased risk from a bioterrorist attack (e.g., mail handler, government official) also should prompt the clinician to include a bioterrorism event in the differential diagnosis.[13,15,16] As multiple patients present with an undiagnosed febrile illness within a hospital, a hospital system, or a community, a careful review of their recent activities may reveal a pattern of common events (e.g., recent sporting event, concert) or locations linking patients to the site where a biologic weapon release took place days earlier (i.e., the incubation period of the agent).[25]

As discussed earlier, the clinical presentation of inhalational anthrax may be varied, but respiratory symptoms are likely to be common. Pulmonary findings include chest wall edema, rhonchi, wheezing, pleural effusions, stridor, and hypoxemia. Other systemic symptoms include confusion, fever, headache, vomiting, diarrhea, abdominal pain, and fatigue.[13,14,18,82]

Radiologic studies can help confirm the diagnosis of inhalational anthrax. In a case series (n = 42), perihilar interstitial pneumonia was present in all cases, and nearly half (n = 17) had acute bronchopneumonia. Of these, 3 cases had panlobar bronchopneumonia, 3 had two lobes involved, and the remaining 11 cases had single-lobe involvement.[83] Pulmonary infiltrates (multilobar in three of four) were present in 40% of the initial 10 cases of inhalational anthrax in the 2001 anthrax attacks in the United States.[18] All computed tomography scans of the chest (n = 8) showed some

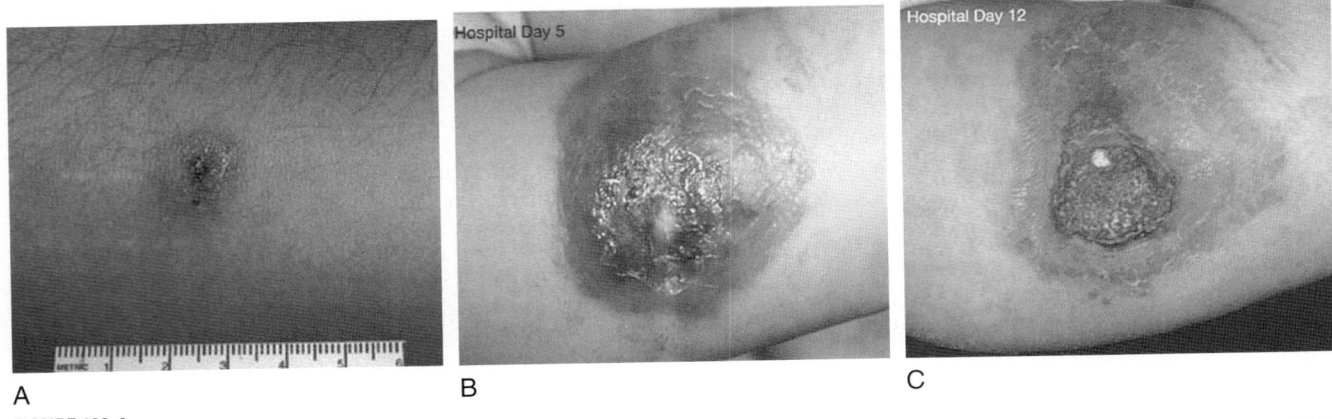

FIGURE 132-4

A, Cutaneous anthrax on forearm of a 34-year-old mail handler. **B,** Cutaneous anthrax on upper arm of a 7-month-old infant. **C,** Same patient as in **B** after antibiotic therapy. *(**A** from Gallagher TC, Strober BE: Cutaneous Bacillus anthracis infection. N Engl J Med 345:1646, 2001. **B** and **C** from Freedman A, Afonja O, Chang MW, et al: Cutaneous anthrax associated with microangiopathic hemolytic anemia and coagulopathy in a 7-month-old infant. JAMA 287:869–874, 2002.)* See Color Fig. 132-4A through C.

abnormality (mediastinal lymphadenopathy, pleural effusion, or infiltrates) (Figs. 132-5 and 132-6).[18]

Initial laboratory testing of suspected cases of anthrax should include sputum, blood, and body fluid cultures (e.g., cerebrospinal fluid, pleural effusion fluid). *B. anthracis* was isolated from the cerebrospinal fluid of the index case of the 2001 bioterrorism-related anthrax attacks within 7 hours and presumptively confirmed within 18 hours.[14,18] Admission blood cultures from inhalational anthrax patients (obtained

before the initiation of antibiotics) (n = 7) grew *B. anthracis* at a median of 18 hours (range 12 to 24 hours).[18] Blood cultures rapidly become sterile, however, after antibiotic administration (n = 4).[18,86] Cutaneous lesions can be biopsied for polymerase chain reaction analysis and immunohistologic studies.[26,29] White blood cell counts at presentation ranged from 7500 to 13,300 white blood cells/mm^3,[7] and hepatic aminotransferase levels were elevated and hypoxemia was present in 91% and 64% of bioterrorism-related cases of inhalational anthrax.[18,87]

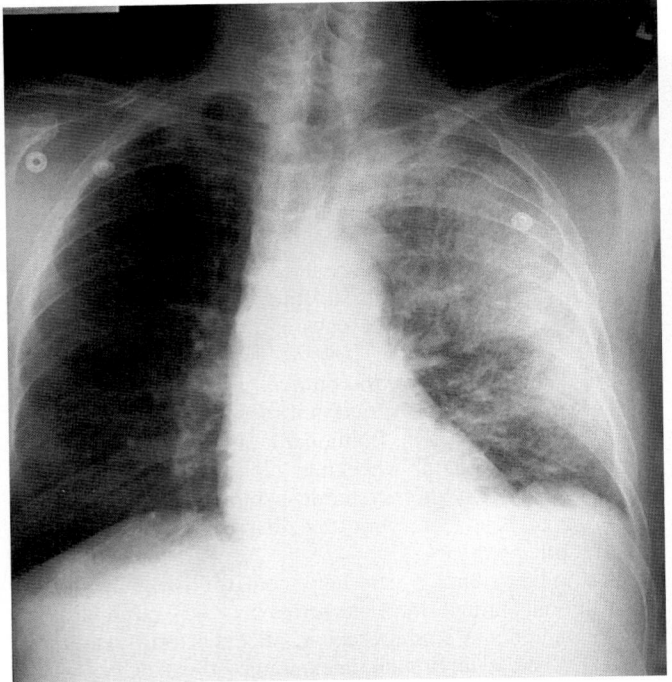
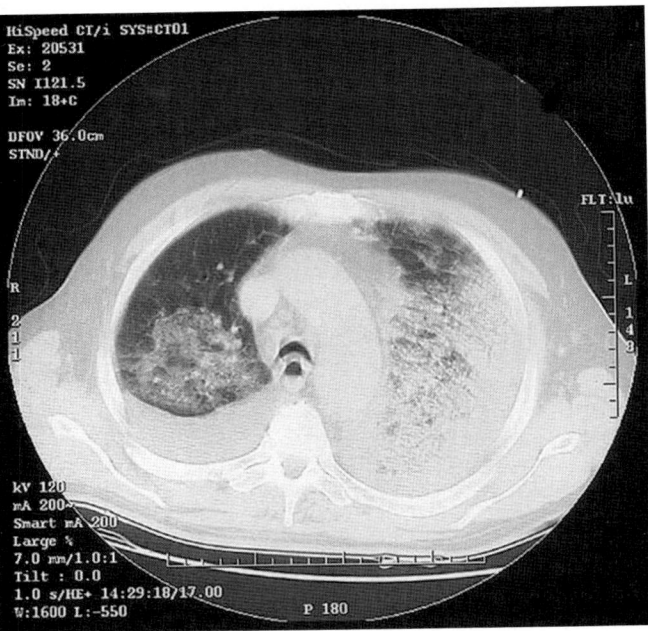

FIGURE 132-5

A, Chest x-ray of a 73-year-old man who was the second case of bioterrorist-related inhalational anthrax reported in the United States in 2001. Note diffuse consolidation with pneumonia throughout the left lung and no mediastinal widening. **B,** Computed tomography scan of the same patient shows bilateral pulmonary consolidation and pleural effusions. *(From Jernigan JA, Stephens DS, Ashford DA, et al: Bioterrorism-related inhalational anthrax: The first 10 cases reported in the United States. Emerg Infect Dis 7:933–944, 2001.)*

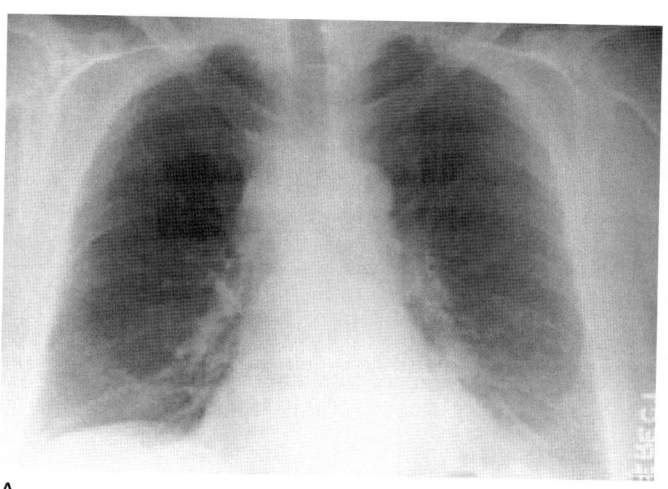
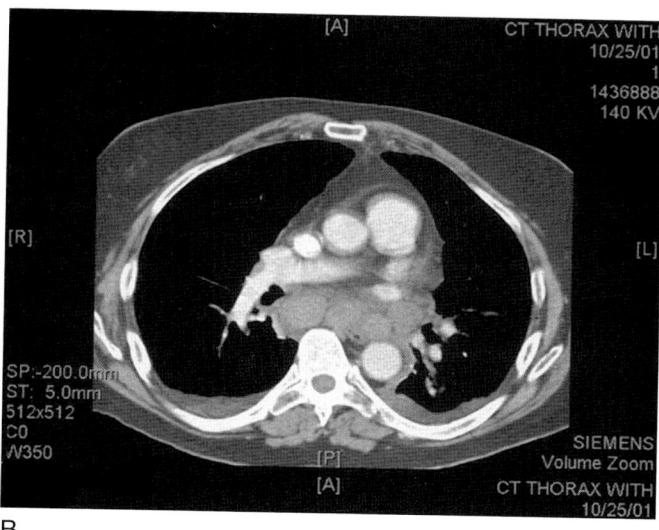

FIGURE 132-6

A, Chest x-ray of a 59-year-old mail handler with bioterrorist-related inhalational anthrax from the United States 2001 anthrax attacks. Note mediastinal widening and small left pleural effusion. **B,** Computed tomography scan of the same patient shows mediastinal adenopathy and small bilateral pleural effusions. *(From Jernigan JA, Stephens DS, Ashford DA, et al: Bioterrorism-related inhalational anthrax: The first 10 cases reported in the United States. Emerg Infect Dis 7:933–944, 2001.)*

Confirmatory identification of *B. anthracis* is done by a combination of laboratory tests including gamma-phage lysis, growth on blood and bicarbonate agar, capsule and cell wall antigen detection by direct fluorescence antibody, and *B. anthracis* polymerase chain reaction. Hospital microbiology laboratories should be capable of doing primary culturing of clinical specimens. Additional testing is available from laboratories in the United States by the National Bioterrorism Laboratory Response Network, including immunohistochemical testing of clinical specimens using *B. anthracis* capsule and cell-wall antibodies, *B. anthracis*–specific polymerase chain reaction, and serologic detection of immunoglobulin IgG to *B. anthracis* PA.[17,18]

TREATMENT

A high index of suspicion and rapid administration of antibiotic therapy are crucial for the timely and effective treatment of anthrax.[17,54,84] The pathogenesis of anthrax affords several potential targets for antimicrobial therapy. Being gram positive, *B anthracis* has potential sensitivity to

Indications for ICU Admission in Anthrax Poisoning

Any patient with a febrile illness, pulmonary complaints (e.g., dyspnea or chest pain), mental status changes or meningeal signs, or significant gastrointestinal complaints (e.g., abdominal pain and vomiting), with a history of exposure to *Bacillus anthracis*

Any patient with cutaneous anthrax who develops systemic signs and symptoms of sepsis and toxemia (e.g., fever, mental status changes, hypotension)

many antibiotic classes, including penicillins, cephalosporins, quinolones, macrolides, and inhibitors of DNA synthesis.[88] Cell wall synthesis is inhibited by β-lactams, which inhibit peptidoglycan polymerization, and by vancomycin, which forms a complex with the carboxy-terminal D-alanine residues of peptidoglycan precursors. These two antibiotic classes act synergistically. DNA gyrase relieves the torsional strain during replication of circular bacterial chromosomes. Quinolones, such as ciprofloxacin, norfloxacin, and ofloxacin, bind to the bacterial DNA-DNA gyrase complex, blocking DNA replication. Several antibiotic classes inhibit bacterial protein synthesis. Rifampin blocks RNA synthesis by binding to DNA-directed RNA polymerase. Aminoglycosides and tetracycline interfere with the 30S ribosome subunit, whereas chloramphenicol, erythromycin, and clindamycin all interfere with 50S ribosome function. Penicillin, fluoroquinolones, tetracyclines, chloramphenicol, clindamycin, imipenem, clarithromycin, aminoglycosides, rifampin, vancomycin, and cefazolin all have shown in vitro activity against *B. anthracis*.[17]

Historically, penicillin has been the drug of choice for naturally occurring anthrax and is the only antimicrobial agent that has been studied for the treatment of human anthrax infection. There are no controlled studies of the treatment of inhalational anthrax in humans, however. The Ames strain of *B. anthracis* used in the 2001 anthrax bioterrorist attacks was found to have an inducible β-lactamase and a constitutive cephalosporinase.[13,17,84] Monotherapy with a penicillin, or a penicillin derivative, is not recommended.[17,84] Naturally occurring strains of *B. anthracis* have been found to have resistance to sulfamethoxazole, trimethoprim, aztreonam, and several cephalosporins, including cefuroxime, ceftazidime, and cefotaxime.[88] These antibiotics are *not* recommended.[17,84]

Current treatment recommendations are based on animal studies and limited clinical human experience.[17,65,84] Penicillin, doxycycline, and ciprofloxacin are the only antibiotics currently approved by the U.S. Food and Drug Administration for the treatment of inhalational anthrax.[17] The U.S. Centers for Disease Control and Prevention recommendations include using either ciprofloxacin or doxycycline as first-line drugs in a multidrug regimen until antimicrobial sensitivities are known (Table 132-3).[17,18,84] When antimicrobial sensitivities are determined, antibiotic regimens can be adjusted appropriately.[17,77,84] Although based on a small series (n = 11), the survival rate for the United States 2001 bioterrorist-related inhalational anthrax cases treated with multidrug regimens (55%)[17,18] is significantly higher than previously reported survival rates.[77,84,85,89] Antibiotics that inhibit protein synthesis, such as clindamycin, can inhibit the release of exotoxins, such as *Streptococcus pyogenes* exotoxin,[90] and are recommended as part of the multidrug regimen for the treatment of inhalational anthrax.[17]

Antibiotic resistance is a significant concern in the management of naturally occurring pathogens and biologic warfare agents. Although it is the consequence of adaptive genetic evolution in a naturally occurring pathogen, it may likely be the result of genetic engineering by a terrorist biologic weaponeer to produce a more virulent biologic weapon in a biologic warfare agent.[91] The possibility of a terrorist's using multiple strains of a biologic agent simultaneously or a multidrug-resistant strain of *B. anthracis*[56] as a biologic weapon also supports the use of a multidrug antimicrobial regimen for treatment.

Immunotherapy has been used for treatment of anthrax.[46,47,86,92–94] *B. anthracis* antisera have been derived from horses, cattle, sheep, donkeys, and mules (e.g., Sclavo's serum). Although fraught with limitations, including anaphylaxis and serum sickness, such passive immunization was an

---

TABLE 132-3 Recommended Therapy for Inhalational Anthrax in the Contained Casualty Setting

CATEGORY	INITIAL THERAPY (INTRAVENOUS)[§,¶]	DURATION
Adults	Ciprofloxacin 400 mg every 12 hr* **or** Doxycycline 100 mg every 12 hr[††] **and** One or two additional antimicrobials[¶]	IV treatment initially.** Switch to oral antimicrobial therapy when clinically appropriate: Ciprofloxacin 500 mg PO BID **or** Doxycycline 100 mg PO BID Continue for 60 days (IV and PO combined)[§§]
Children	Ciprofloxacin 10–15 mg/kg every 12 hr[¶¶,***] **or** Doxycycline:[†††,§§] >8 yr and >45 kg: 100 mg every 12 hr >8 yr and ≤45 kg: 2.2 mg/kg every 12 hr ≤8 yr: 2.2 mg/kg every 12 hr **and** One or two additional antimicrobials[¶]	IV treatment initially.** Switch to oral antimicrobial therapy when clinically appropriate: Ciprofloxacin 10–15 mg/kg PO every 12 hr*** **or** Doxycycline:[†††] >8 yr and >45 kg: 100 mg PO BID >8 yr and ≤45 kg: 2.2 mg/kg PO BID ≤8 yr: 2.2 mg/kg PO BID Continue for 60 days (IV and PO combined)[§§]
Pregnant women[§§§]	Same for nonpregnant adults (the high death rate from the infection outweighs the risk posed by the antimicrobial agent)	IV treatment initially. Switch to oral antimicrobial therapy when clinically appropriate.[†] Oral therapy regimens same for nonpregnant adults
Immunocompromised persons	Same for nonimmunocompromised persons and children	Same for nonimmunocompromised persons and children

*For gastrointestinal and oropharyngeal anthrax, use regimens recommended for inhalational anthrax.

[†]Ciprofloxacin or doxycycline should be considered an essential part of first-line therapy for inhalational anthrax.

[§]Steroids may be considered as an adjunct therapy for patients with severe edema and for meningitis based on experience with bacterial meningitis of other etiologies.

[¶]Other agents with in vitro activity include rifampin, vancomycin, penicillin, ampicillin, chloramphenicol, imipenem, clindamycin, and clarithromycin. Because of concerns of constitutive and inducible β-lactamases in *Bacillus anthracis*, penicillin and ampicillin should not be used alone. Consultation with an infectious disease specialist is advised.

**Initial therapy may be altered based on clinical course of the patient; one or two antimicrobial agents (e.g., ciprofloxacin or doxycycline) may be adequate as the patient improves.

[††]If meningitis is suspected, doxycycline may be less optimal because of poor central nervous system penetration.

[§§]Because of the potential persistence of spores after an aerosol exposure, antimicrobial therapy should be continued for 60 days.

[¶¶]If intravenous ciprofloxacin is not available, oral ciprofloxacin may be acceptable because it is rapidly and well absorbed from the gastrointestinal tract with no substantial loss by first-pass metabolism. Maximum serum concentrations are attained 1 to 2 hours after oral dosing but may not be achieved if vomiting or ileus is present.

***In children, ciprofloxacin dosage should not exceed 1 g/day.

[†††]The American Academy of Pediatrics recommends treatment of young children with tetracyclines for serious infections (e.g., Rocky Mountain spotted fever).

[§§§]Although tetracyclines are not recommended during pregnancy, their use may be indicated for life-threatening illness. Adverse effects on developing teeth and bones are dose related; doxycycline might be used for a short time (7–14 days) before 6 months of gestation.

Malecki J, Wiersma S, Cahill K, et al: Update: Investigation of bioterrorism-related anthrax and interim guidelines for exposure management and antimicrobial therapy, October 2001. MMWR Morb Mortal Wkly Rep 50:909–919, 2001.

effective treatment for anthrax before the antibiotic era,[92,94] and an antianthrax globulin was used to treat victims of the 1979 Sverdlovsk anthrax outbreak.[17] New forms of immunotherapy have focused on the development of monoclonal and polyclonal antibodies to anthrax toxin components.[47,93,97] As mentioned earlier, the binding of either LF or EF to $[(PA63)_7]$ produces the final dimeric toxins, LT and ET,[95] which cause massive tissue necrosis, edema, and death. Toxin-specific inhibitors and antibodies have been developed to block the binding of LT and ET to PA63. Polyclonal antibodies raised against recombinant PA are protective in a guinea pig model.[93,96] Multiple copies of a synthetic polypeptide, with weak affinity to the heptameric cell-binding subunit of anthrax toxin $[(PA63)_7]$, were covalently linked to a flexible backbone, producing a synthetic polyvalent inhibitor of anthrax toxin that binds to heptameric PA63 $[(PA63)_7]$. This polyvalent inhibitor prevented assembly of the toxin complex in vitro by blocking PA63's interaction with EF and LF and blocked toxin action in a rat model.[97] Human antibody fragments have been developed that block binding of PA83 (PA before being cleaved to PA63 by cell surface proteases) to its cell surface receptor. PA32, a recombinant 32-kd carboxy-terminal PA fragment, was an effective and competitive inhibitor of PA binding to its cell surface receptor.[46]

Corticosteroid therapy has been used and is recommended for the treatment of extensive edema, meningitis, or swelling of the head and neck region.[17,77] Finally, aggressive general medical care, such as the drainage of pleural or pericardial effusions, is crucial.[17] The United States anthrax vaccine (Bioport Corporation, Lansing, MI) is a cell-free filtrate, including PA as the primary immunogenic antigen. It is administered as a six-dose series over 18 months. Although not effective as monotherapy in the postexposure treatment of inhalational anthrax, the anthrax vaccine adsorbed prevented latent cases of anthrax after cessation of antibiotic treatment and protected against an anthrax rechallenge in an animal model.[65]

New research has focused on developing a new class of antibacterial agents that employ bacteriophage-derived lysins.[98,99] A bacteriophage is an obligate intracellular virus pathogen that requires the nucleic acid and protein synthesizing machinery of a host bacterium to complete its life cycle. Lysins are lytic enzymes with high affinities for specific cell wall carbohydrate structures, encoded on the bacteriophage genome. They hydrolyze covalent bonds essential for peptidoglycan integrity, causing bacterial cell wall lysis. In their natural role in the bacteriophage's life cycle, lysins cause rupture of the host bacterium's cell membrane to release bacteriophage progeny. The *B. anthracis* γ phage produces phage lysin γ (PlyG) that has been shown to kill *B. anthracis* bacilli in vitro and in vivo.[99] PlyG also was shown to be specific and sensitive enough to be used as a method for detection of *B. anthracis* in the environment.[99] Although they would have to be administered before fatal blood/circulating levels of anthrax toxin developed, *B. anthracis* lysins soon may find a role in the treatment of anthrax.

SPECIAL POPULATIONS

Fluoroquinolones are not approved for use in young children. Doxycycline is recommended.

Common Misconceptions about Anthrax Poisoning

1. Cutaneous anthrax cannot cause life-threatening illness.
2. Treatment of inhalational anthrax is futile.
3. Anthrax is contagious.
4. Antimicrobial therapy can be delayed until cultures are positive.

Key Points in Anthrax Poisoning

1. The diagnosis of anthrax and the prompt initiation of antimicrobial therapy should be based on clinical presentation and before definitive laboratory testing.
2. Antimicrobial therapy must be initiated as soon as anthrax is suspected.
3. Pulmonary and pericardial effusions should be managed aggressively.
4. Bioterrorist agents may have antibiotic resistance; a multidrug antimicrobial regimen, including either ciprofloxacin or doxycycline, with one or two additional antibiotics, is the first-line choice of therapy.

International Classification of Disease (ICD) Codes for Anthrax

ICD Codes	ICD-9-CM	ICD-10
Anthrax	022	A22
Cutaneous anthrax	022.0	A22.0
Pulmonary anthrax	022.1	A22.1
Gastrointestinal anthrax	022.2	A22.2
Anthrax septicemia	022.3	A22.7
Other specified manifestations of anthrax	022.8	A22.8
Anthrax, unspecified	022.9	A22.9

REFERENCES

1. Shireley L, Dwelle T, Streitz D, et al: Human anthrax associated with an epizootic among livestock—North Dakota, 2000. Morb Mortal Wkly Rep 50:677–680, 2001.
2. Bell JH: On woolsorter's disease. Lancet 1:871, 1880.
3. Christopher GW, Cieslak TJ, Pavlin JA, et al: Biological warfare: A historical perspective. JAMA 278:412–417, 1997.
4. Manchee RJ, Broster MG, Melling J, et al: *Bacillus anthracis* on Gruinard Island. Nature 294:254–255, 1981.
5. Manchee RJ, Broster MG, Stagg AJ, et al: Formaldehyde solution effectively inactivates spores of *Bacillus anthracis* on the Scottish Island of Gruinard. Appl Environ Microbiol 60:4167–4171, 1994.
6. Manchee RJ, Stewert R: The decontamination of Guinard Island. Chem Br 24:690–691, 1988.
7. Anonymous: A chronology of Aum Shinrikyo CBW activities. Monterey WMD terrorism database, Monterey Institute of International Studies, Monterey, CA, 2001.
8. Keim P, Smith KL, Keys C, et al: Molecular investigation of the Aum Shinrikyo anthrax release in Kameido, Japan. J Clin Microbiol 39:4566–4567, 2001.

9. Guidi-Rontani C, Weber-Levy M, Labruyère E, et al: Germination of *Bacillus anthracis* spores within alveolar macrophages. Mol Microbiol 31:9–17, 1999.

10. Titball RW, Manchee RJ: Factors affecting the germination of spores of *Bacillus anthracis*. J Appl Bacteriol 62:269–273, 1987.

11. Watters JW, Dewar K, Lehoczky J, et al: Kif1C, a kinesin-like motor protein, mediates mouse macrophage resistance to anthrax lethal factor. Curr Biol 11:1503–1511, 2001.

12. Aronson AI, Fitz-James P: Structure and morphogenesis of the bacterial spore coat. Bacteriol Rev 40:360–402, 1976.

13. Borio L, Frank D, Mani V, et al: Death due to bioterrorism-related inhalational anthrax: Report of 2 patients. JAMA 286:2554–2559, 2001.

14. Bush LM, Abrams BH, Beall A, et al: Index case of fatal inhalational anthrax due to bioterrorism in the United States. N Engl J Med 345:1607–1610, 2001.

15. Dewan PK, Fry AM, Larerson K, et al: Inhalational anthrax outbreak among postal workers, Washington, DC, 2001. Emerg Infect Dis 8:1066–1072, 2002.

16. Greene CM, Reefhuis J, Tan C, et al: Epidemiologic investigations of bioterrorism-related anthrax, New Jersey, 2001. Emerg Infect Dis 8:1048–1055, 2002.

17. Inglesby TV, O'Toole T, Henderson DA, et al: Anthrax as a biological weapon, 2002: Updated recommendations for management. JAMA 287:2236–2252, 2002.

18. Jernigan JA, Stephens DS, Ashford DA, et al: Bioterrorism-related inhalational anthrax: The first 10 cases reported in the United States. Emerg Infect Dis 7:933–944, 2001.

19. Mayer TA, Bersoff-Matcha S, Murphy C, et al: Clinical presentation of inhalational anthrax following bioterrorism exposure: Report of 2 surviving patients. JAMA 286:2549–2553, 2001.

20. Nelson LS, Hanner R, Hoffmas RS: Cutaneous anthrax infection. N Engl J Med 346:945–946, 2002.

21. Lincoln RE, Hodges DR, Klein F, et al: Role of the lymphatics in the pathogenesis of anthrax. J Infect Dis 115:481–494, 1965.

22. Ross JM: The pathogenesis of anthrax following the administration of spores by the respiratory route. J Pathol Bacteriol 73:485–494, 1957.

23. Hanna PC, Acosta D, Collier RJ: On the role of macrophages in anthrax. Proc Natl Acad Sci U S A 90:10198–10201, 1993.

24. Grinberg LM, Abramova FA, Yampolskaya OV, et al: Quantitative pathology of inhalational anthrax: I. Quantitative microscopic findings. Mod Pathol 14:482–495, 2001.

25. Meselson M, Guillemin J, Hugh-Jones M, et al: The Sverdlovsk anthrax outbreak of 1979. Science 266:1202–1208, 1994.

26. Pezard C, Berche P, Mock M: Contribution of individual toxin components to virulence of *Bacillus anthracis*. Infect Immun 59:3472–3477, 1991.

27. Leppla SH: The bifactorial *Bacillus anthracis* lethal and oedema toxins. In: Moss J, Iglewski B, Vaughan M, Tu A (eds): Bacterial Toxins and Virulence Factors in Disease. Handbook of Natural Toxins, vol 8. New York, Marcel Dekker, 1995.

28. Sterne M: Variation in *Bacillus anthracis*. Onderstepoort J Vet Sci Anim Ind 8:271–349, 1937.

29. Hoffmaster AR, Koehler TM: The anthrax toxin activator gene atxA is associated with CO_2-enhanced non-toxin gene expression. Infect Immun 65:3091–3099, 1997.

30. Sirard J-C, Mock M, Fouet A: The three *Bacillus anthracis* genes are coordinately regulated by bicarbonate and temperature. J Bacteriol 176:5188–5192, 1994.

31. Little SF, Ivins BE: Molecular pathogenesis of *Bacillus anthrax* infection. Microbes Infect 2:131–139, 1999.

32. Uchida I, Makino S, Sasakawa C, et al: Identification of a novel gene, dep, associated with depolymerization of the capsular polymer in *Bacillus anthracis*. Mol Microbiol 9:487–496, 1993.

33. Makino S, Watarai M, Cheun HI, et al: Effect of lower molecular weight capsule released from the cell surface of *Bacillus anthracis* on the pathogenesis of anthrax. J Infect Dis 186:227–233, 2002.

34. Ezzell JW, Welkos SL: The capsule of *B. anthracis*, a review. J Appl Microbiol 87:250–268, 1999.

35. Hanna PC: Anthrax pathogenesis and host response. Curr Topics Microbiol Immunol 225:13–35, 1998.

36. Uchida I, Makino S, Sekizaki T, et al: Cross-talk to the genes for *Bacillus anthracis* capsule synthesis by atxA, the gene encoding the trans-activator of anthrax toxin. Mol Microbiol 23:1229–1240, 1997.

37. Smith H, Keppie J, Stanley JL: The chemical basis of the virulence of *Bacillus anthracis*: V. The specific toxin produced by *B. anthracis* in vivo. Br J Exp Pathol 36:460–472, 1955.

38. Leppla SH: Anthrax toxins. In Alouf JE, Freer JH (eds): The Comprehensive Sourcebook of Bacterial Protein Toxins, 2nd ed. New York, Academic Press, 1999.

39. Gill DM: Seven toxin peptides that cross cell membranes. In Jeljaszewicz J, Wadstrom T (eds): Bacterial Toxins and Cell Membranes. New York, Academic Press, 1978, pp 291–332.

40. Brossier F, Weber-Levy M, Mock M, et al: Role of functional domains in anthrax pathogenesis. Infect Immun 68:1781–1786, 2000.

41. Molloy SS, Bresnahan PA, Leppla SH, et al: Human furin is a calcium-dependent serine endoprotease that recognizes the sequence Arg-X-X-Arg and efficiently cleaves anthrax protective antigen. J Biol Chem 267:16396–16402, 1992.

42. Escuyer V, Collier RJ: Anthrax protective antigen interacts with a specific receptor on the surface of CHO-K1 cells. Infect Immun 59:3381–3386, 1991.

43. Bradley KA, Modridge J, Mourez M, et al: Identification of the cellular receptor for anthrax toxin. Nature 414:225–229, 2001.

44. Bhatnagar LJ, Singh Y, Leppla SH, et al: Calcium is required for the expression of anthrax lethal factor activity in the macrophage-like cell line J774A.1. Infect Immun 57:2107–2114, 1989.

45. Milne JC, Blanke SR, Hanna PC, et al: Protective antigen-binding domain of anthrax lethal factor mediates translocation of a heterologous protein fused to its amino- or carboxy-terminus. Mol Microbiol 15:661–666, 1995.

46. Cirino NM, Sblattero D, Allen D, et al: Disruption of anthrax toxin binding with the use of human antibodies and competitive inhibitors. Infect Immun 67:2957–2963, 1999.

47. Casadevall A: Passive antibody administration (immediate immunity) as a specific defense against biological weapons. Emerg Infect Dis 8, 2002.

48. Klimpel KR, Molloy SS, Thomas G, et al: Anthrax toxin protective antigen is activated by a cell surface protease with the sequence specificity and catalytic properties of furin. Proc Natl Acad Sci U S A 89:10277–10281, 1992.

49. Milne JC, Furlong D, Hanna PC, et al: Anthrax protective antigen forms oligomers during intoxication of mammalian cells. J Biol Chem 269:20607–20612, 1994.

50. Singh Y, Klimpel KR, Goel S, et al: Oligomerization of anthrax toxin protective antigen and binding of lethal factor during endocytic uptake into mammalian cells. Infect Immun 67:1853–1859, 1999.

51. Arora N, Leppla SH: Residues 1-254 of anthrax toxin lethal factor are sufficient to cause cellular uptake of fused polypeptides. J Biol Chem 268:3334–3341, 1993.

52. Modridge J, Cunningham K, Collier RJ: Stoichiometry of anthrax complexes. Biochemistry 41:1079–1082, 2002.

53. Rossetto O, Montecucco C: Bacterial toxins with metalloprotease activity. In Ménez A (ed): Perspectives in Molecular Toxinology. West Sussex, John Wiley & Sons, 2002.

54. Gordon VM, Leppla SH, Hewlett EL: Inhibitors of receptor-mediated endocytosis block the entry of *Bacillus anthracis* cyclase toxin but not that of *Bordetella pertussis* adenylate cyclase toxin. Infect Immun 56:1066–1069, 1988.

55. Blaustein RO, Koehler TM, Collier RJ, et al: Anthrax toxin: Channel-forming activity of protective antigen in planar phospholipid bilayers. Proc Natl Acad Sci U S A 86:2209–2213, 1989.

56. Bhatnagar R, Batra S: Anthrax toxin. Crit Rev Microbiol 27:167–200, 2001.

57. Menard A, Altendorf K, Breves D, et al: The vacuolar ATPase proton pump is required for the cytotoxicity of *Bacillus anthracis* lethal toxin. FEBS Lett 386:161–164, 1996.

58. Petosa C, Collier RJ, Klimpel KR, et al: Crystal structure of the anthrax toxin protective antigen. Nature 385:833–838, 1997.

59. Hammond SE, Hanna PC: Lethal factor active-site mutations affect catalytic activity in vitro. Infect Immun 66:2374–2378, 1998.

60. Klimpel KR, Arora N, Leppla SH: Anthrax toxin lethal factor contains a zinc metalloprotease consensus which is required for lethal toxin activity. Mol Microbiol 13:1093–1100, 1994.

61. Pannifer AD, Wong TY, Schwarzenbacher R, et al: Crystal structure of the anthrax lethal factor. Nature 414:229–233, 2001.

62. Hanna PC, Kochi S, Collier RJ: Biochemical and physiological changes induced by anthrax toxin in J774 macrophage-like cells. Mol Biol Cell 3:1269–1277, 1992.

63. Alessi DR, Cuenda A, Cohen P, et al: PD 098059 is a specific inhibitor of the activation of mitogen-activated protein kinase kinase in vitro and in vivo. J Biol Chem 270:27489–27494, 1995.

64. Duesbery NS, Webb CP, Leppla SH, et al: Proteolytic inactivation of MAP-kinase-kinase by anthrax lethal factor. Science 280:734–737, 1998.

65. Friedlander AM, Welkos SL, Pitt MLM, et al: Postexposure prophylaxis against experimental inhalational anthrax. J Infect Dis 167:1239–1242, 1993.

66. Gallagher TC, Strober BE: Cutaneous *Bacillus anthracis* infection. N Engl J Med 345:1646, 2001.

67. Singh Y, Leppla SH, Bhatnagar R, Friedlander AM: Internalization and processing of *Bacillus anthracis* lethal toxin by toxin-sensitive and -resistant cells. J Biol Chem 264:11099–11102, 1989.

68. Duesbery NS, Reseau J, Webb CP, et al: Suppression of ras-mediated transformation and inhibition of tumor growth and angiogenesis by anthrax lethal factor, a proteolytic inhibitor of multiple MEK pathways. Proc Natl Acad Sci U S A 98:4089–4094, 2001.

69. Duesbery NS, Vande Woude GF: Anthrax lethal factor causes proteolytic inactivation of mitogen-activated protein kinase kinase. J Appl Microbiol 87:289–293, 1999.

70. Vitale G, Pellizzari, Recchi C, et al: Anthrax lethal factor cleaves the N-terminus of MAPKKs and induces tyrosine/threonine phosphorylation of MAPKs in cultured macrophages. Biochem Biophys Res Commun 248:706–711, 1998.

71. Han-Mo K, VanBrocklin M, McWilliams MJ, et al: Apoptosis and melanogenesis in human melanoma cells induced by anthrax lethal factor inactivation of mitogen-activated protein kinase kinase. Proc Natl Acad Sci U S A 99:3052–3057, 2002.

72. Gordon VM, Young WW, Lechler SM, et al: Adenylate cyclase toxins from *Bacillus anthracis* and *Bordetella pertussis*: Different processes for interaction with and entry into target cells. J Biol Chem 264:14792–14796, 1989.

73. Leppla SH: Anthrax toxin edema factor: A bacterial adenylate cyclase that increases cyclic AMP concentrations in eukaryotic cells. Proc Natl Acad Sci U S A 79:3162–3166, 1982.

74. Guidi-Rontani C, Weber-Levy M, Mock M, et al: Translocation of *Bacillus anthracis* lethal and oedema factors across endosome membranes. Cell Microbiol 2:259–264, 2000.

75. Wright GG, Mandell GL: Anthrax toxin blocks priming of neutrophils by lipopolysaccharide and by muramyl dipeptide. J Exp Med 164:1700–1709, 1986.

76. Hanna PC, Kruskal BA, Ezekowitz RAB, et al: Role of macrophage oxidative burst in the action of anthrax toxin. Mol Med 1:7–18, 1994.

77. Dixon TC, Meselson M, Guillemin J, et al: Anthrax. N Engl J Med 341:815–826, 1999.

78. Freedman A, Afonja O, Chang MW, et al: Cutaneous anthrax associated with microangiopathic hemolytic anemia and coagulopathy in a 7-month-old infant. JAMA 287:869–874, 2002.

79. Gallagher TC, Strober BE: Cutaneous *Bacillus anthracis* infection. N Engl J Med 345:1646, 2001.

80. Macher A: An industry-related outbreak of human anthrax: Massachusetts, 1868. Emerg Infect Dis 8, 2002.

81. Roche KJ, Chang MW, Lazarus H: Cutaneous anthrax infection. N Engl J Med 345:1611, 2001.

82. Mackey TA, Page EH, Martinez KF, et al: Suspected cutaneous anthrax in a laboratory worker—Texas, 2002. MMWR Morb Mortal Wkly Rep 51:279–281, 2002.

83. Abramova FA, Grinberg LM, Yampolskaya OV, et al: Pathology of inhalational anthrax in 42 cases from the Sverdlovsk outbreak of 1979. Proc Natl Acad Sci U S A 90:2291–2294, 1993.

84. Malecki J, Wiersma S, Cahill K, et al: Update: Investigation of bioterrorism-related anthrax and interim guidelines for exposure management and antimicrobial therapy, October 2001. MMWR Morb Mortal Wkly Rep 50:909–919, 2001.

85. Plotkin SA, Brachman PS, Utell M, et al: An epidemic of inhalation anthrax, the first in the twentieth century: I. Clinical features. Am J Med 29:992–1001, 1960.

86. Gold H: Treatment of anthrax. Fed Proc 26:1563–1568, 1967.

87. Barakat LA, Quentzel HL, Jernigan JA, et al: Fatal inhalational anthrax in a 94-year-old woman. JAMA 287:863–868, 2002.

88. Doganay M, Aydin N: Antimicrobial susceptibility of *Bacillus anthracis*. Scand J Infect Dis 23:333–335, 1991.

89. Jackson PJ, Hugh-Jones ME, Adair DM, et al: PCR analysis of tissue samples from the 1979 Sverdlovsk anthrax victims: The presence of multiple strains in different victims. Proc Natl Acad Sci U S A 95:1224–1229, 1998.

90. Sriskandan S, McKee A, Hall L, et al: Comparative effects of clindamycin and ampicillin on superantigenic activity of *Streptococcus pyogenes*. J Antimicrob Chemother 40:275–277, 1997.

91. Stepanov AV, Marinin LI, Pomerantsev AP, et al: Development of novel vaccines against anthrax in man. J Biotechnol 44:155–160, 1996.

92. Knudson GB: Treatment of anthrax in man: History and current concepts. Milit Med 151:71–77, 1986.

93. Little SF, Ivins BE, Fellows PF, et al: Passive protection by polyclonal antibodies against *Bacillus anthracis* infection in guinea pigs. Infect Immun 65:5171–5175, 1997.

94. Mitchell W: Anthrax and fatalism. BMJ 1:751–752, 1911.

95. Brossier F, Mock M: Toxins of *Bacillus anthracis*. Toxicon 39:1747–1755, 2001.

96. Kobiler D, Gozes Y, Rosenberg H, et al: Efficiency of protection of guinea pigs against infection with *Bacillus anthracis* spores by passive immunization. Infect Immun 70:544–560, 2002.

97. Mourez M, Kane RS, Mogridge J, et al: Designing a polyvalent inhibitor of anthrax toxin. Nat Biotech 19:958–961, 2001.

98. Rosovitz MJ, Leppla SH: Virus deals anthrax a killer blow. Nature 418:825–826, 2002.

99. Schuch R, Nelson D, Fischetti VA: A bacteriolytic agent that detects and kills *Bacillus anthracis*. Nature 418:884–889, 2002.

CHAPTER 133

Plague

Edward W. Cetaruk ■ Jeffrey Brent

Among the many biologic agents that have been developed as weapons, *Yersinia pestis*, the causative agent of plague, is unique. The disease plague has been known for 2 or 3 millennia. It is mentioned in ancient Hindu writings and the Bible. The word *plague* originates from the Latin word, *plaga*, which means "to blow." Ancient Romans believed plague epidemics were the result of an angry blast of the wrath of the Gods. Their fear was with good reason because the first great pandemic, the Justinian pandemic, which occurred between 542 AD and 546 AD, caused epidemics in Asia, Africa, and Europe, killing an estimated 40 to 100 million people.[1]

Plague is arguably the first biologic agent used as a weapon of war. Although the origin of plague is uncertain, it was first reported in the modern era in Central Asia between 1339 and 1340 and is thought to have been brought west along trade routes and with traveling Tartar armies. Caffa, now Feodosia, Ukraine, was established in 1266 as a port city for trading between European merchants and the Asian Mongols. A series of wars in the early 14th century between the Tartars and the Genoese followed, with the city being periodically destroyed and rebuilt. The Tartars laid siege to the city again in 1345 but were forced to abandon their attack in late 1346 due to devastation of their troops by an epidemic of plague.[2,3] As their losses due to plague mounted, the Tartar forces hurled the diseased cadavers of their dead comrades over the defensive walls of Caffa and into the city. Although there was no understanding of microbiology or the contagious nature of an infectious disease such as plague at this point in history, it was a common belief that the stench of corpses (which was likely overwhelming given that thousands were dying daily) could transmit the plague to the inhabitants of Caffa. The unpleasant but essential task of removing the accumulating corpses from the city was likely a sufficient means to spread *Y. pestis* among the city's inhabitants, and Caffa became overwhelmed by plague.

Ultimately the Tartar army was forced to withdraw as the plague rendered it an ineffective fighting force, and Caffa remained under Genoese control. As occurs with many epidemics, however, many of Caffa's inhabitants fled the city. Because of Caffa's location on the Crimean peninsula, with access to the Black and Mediterranean Seas, many who fled, including people infected with plague, did so by ship. Epidemics reached Europe when Genoese vessels docked in Messina, Genoa, and Marseilles. It is also thought that this exodus was instrumental in the spread of plague to the Middle East and Northern Africa.[3] These events led to the second plague pandemic, also known as the *Black Death*, which killed an estimated 17 to 28 million Europeans (30% to 40% of the total population) between the years 1347 and 1351. Smaller plague epidemics continued to occur periodically in Europe over the next few centuries. It is unclear how great a role the use of plague as a biologic weapon played during the 1346 siege of Caffa or in creating the second plague pandemic. These events are illustrative, however, of the far-reaching and devastating potential a plague biologic weapon might have.

The third, or modern, pandemic began in the Canton region of China and Hong Kong in 1894. It was spread rapidly throughout the world, carried by plague-infected rats aboard swifter steamships that had replaced slow-moving sailing vessels. Within 10 years (1894 to 1903), plague entered 77 ports on five continents and became widespread in many countries. In India, there were more than 6 million deaths between 1898 and 1908.

In the modern era, many countries, including the United States, the former Soviet Union, and Japan, have studied the use of plague as a biologic weapon.[2] Japan is the only country, however, known to have used plague as a biologic weapon. During World War II, Japan established Unit 731 under the command of General Shiro Ishii. Officially designated as a water purification unit, Unit 731 established the Ping Fan prison on the outskirts of Harbin, in Manchuria, China.[4] Here some of the most gruesome atrocities of World War II took place, including the experimental infection of thousands of Chinese, Russian, and American prisoners of war and thousands of Chinese men, women, and children. These victims experienced horrible deaths, including vivisection, as part of Japan's effort to develop biologic weapons. Among the many pathogens investigated, a great deal of time was devoted to the development of plague as a weapon. At the height of the program, Unit 731 was able to produce 660 pounds of *Y. pestis* per month. It was cultivated in prisoners, who were bled to death to yield plague-infected blood, which was used to cultivate hundreds of pounds of infected fleas in "plague nurseries." Although unable to weaponize isolated *Y. pestis* successfully, Unit 731 did develop a plague-infected flea weapon that was released in airborne attacks over Manchuria at least five times between 1940 and 1941, successfully causing localized plague outbreaks.[2] Japanese army "doctors" would visit these areas under the guise of providing medical care to victims. In actuality, many of their "patients" unknowingly became research subjects in Unit 731's biologic weapons program. Reportedly, Japan also developed plans to attack the American mainland by submarine-launched aircraft and balloons armed with plague-infected fleas; other biologic agents, including anthrax; and livestock and agricultural pathogens. At the end of the war, the occupying American forces exempted General Ishii from prosecution as a war criminal in exchange for his biologic weapons research data because of fear that it would fall into the hands of the Soviet Union.[4] Ironically, although it carefully chronicled Unit 731's horrific practice of human experimentation, the data were crude and not of any significant scientific value to the American biologic weapons program (William C. Patrick, III, personal communication). Ultimately the Soviets did acquire blueprints of Unit 731's facilities, which they used to build their own biologic weapon factories.

Decades later, the Soviet biologic weapons program, *Biopreparat*, grew to the point of employing tens of thousands of scientists and technicians at scores of secret biologic weapon facilities throughout the former Soviet Union.[5] They successfully developed highly virulent viral and bacterial biologic weapons, including smallpox, Marburg virus, tularemia, anthrax, and plague. They also perfected the technology to produce many tons of these pathogens per year and to deliver them by intercontinental ballistic missile. More concerning, however, is that the dissolution of the Soviet Union, and *Bio-*

preparat with it, has made biologic weapon development and weaponization expertise, and possibly even biologic weapon–grade *Y. pestis*, potentially available to terrorist entities around the world.[5]

EPIDEMIOLOGY

Naturally occurring plague is a zoonotic disease that is maintained within a mammalian reservoir (Fig. 133-1), particularly in wild rodents, in endemic foci worldwide with the exception of Australia.[6] During the 1990s, there were human plague outbreaks in Africa, Asia, South America, and India and sporadic cases in many countries, including the United States.[7,8] Typically the number of human cases in a geographic area correlates with the number of animal cases.[9] Outbreaks of human plague often follow plague epizootics, sometimes called *rat falls* or *die-offs*, in the mammalian animal reservoirs.[8,10–12]

Plague is transmitted between rodents and to humans primarily by fleabite. Animals also may become infected by grazing in areas contaminated by plague-infected rodent feces or by preying on plague-infected animals. The most common form of the disease in humans is bubonic plague.[8]

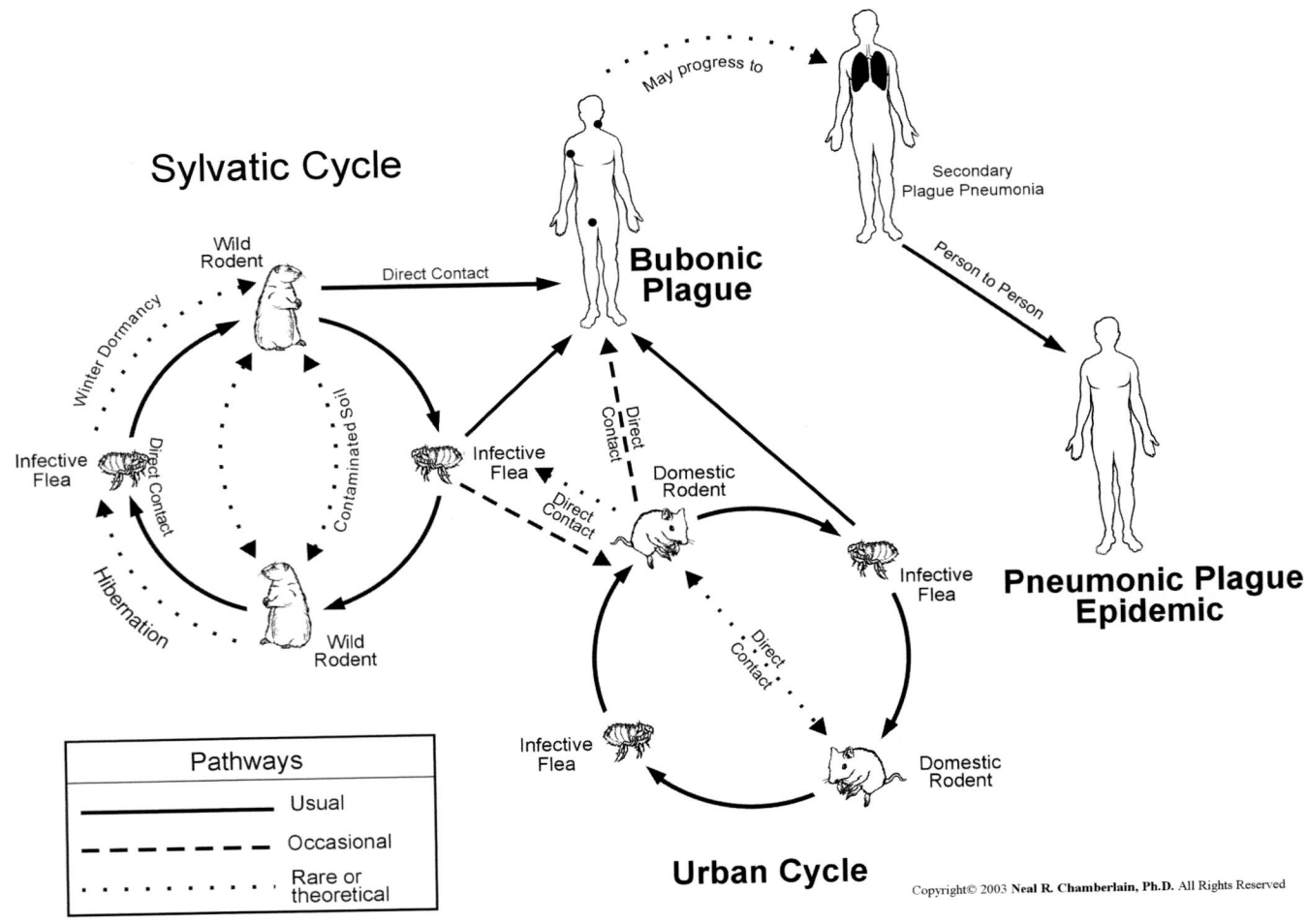

FIGURE 133-1

Epidemiologic patterns of naturally occurring plague. *(Copyright 2002, Neal R. Chamberlain, PhD.)*

It usually is spread by biting fleas that regurgitate blood from previously-fed-on infected rodents into the bite wound; this introduces thousands of *Y. pestis* organisms into the bite wound, effectively inoculating the new mammalian host with plague. The pathogen also may cause a cutaneous infection, leading to bubonic plague, if plague-infected feces contaminate an open skin lesion.[1,6]

A second important mode of plague transmission is the aerosol route. Aerosolization of infectious *Y. pestis* may occur in two ways. In a natural outbreak, bubonic or septicemic cases usually occur first. Some of these patients develop pneumonic plague via hematogenous spread of the infection to the lungs. These patients can transmit plague directly from person to person by droplet infection due to coughing, causing additional cases of pneumonic plague.[13] Any case of plague, regardless of the clinical form, should be considered a public health emergency.[14,15] Appropriate measures to treat and isolate the patient should be taken immediately, and public health authorities should be notified as soon as possible.

Alternatively, the intentional aerosolization of weaponized *Y. pestis* by a bioterrorist produces the pneumonic form without any preceding cases of bubonic plague. This epidemiologic pattern is a crucial clue to the early recognition of an intentional plague outbreak.[14,16] A bioterrorist attempts to maximize the size of the outbreak and the speed at which it spreads. Early recognition and response to a bioterrorist-related plague outbreak may have enormous impact on the course of the outbreak, potentially preventing thousands of cases or deaths.[3,14,17]

More than 200 species of rodents, including the common brown rat, *Rattus rattus*, and the Norwegian rat, *Rattus norvegicus*, are reservoirs for *Y. pestis*.[6,8] Outbreaks affecting large numbers of people can occur in cities when plague infects urban rodent populations, particularly of the genus *Rattus*.[1] In the United States, ground squirrels, rock squirrels, prairie dogs, chipmunks, bats, rabbits, and domestic animals may become infected.[10,18] Animals have differing susceptibility to developing the disease, however. Many carnivores, such as domestic dogs, bears, coyotes, and raccoons, appear to be resistant to plague.[6] Domestic cats are extremely susceptible,[18] have a high mortality rate, and can effectively transmit bubonic[19] and pneumonic plague to humans.[11,20] Arthropod vectors include 85 species of fleas and the tick, *Hyalomma detritium*. The vector efficiency (ability to transmit plague) of a flea is determined by three factors: (1) infection potential, the percentage of fleas taking a blood meal from an infected mammalian host that becomes infected; (2) vector infective potential, the percentage of infected fleas that become capable of transmitting infection; and (3) transmission potential, the observed ability of each flea to transmit plague before its death. These factors are determined by the size and shape of the proventriculus (a sphincter-type organ between the flea's esophagus and stomach), feeding frequency, and survival time after infection. The most important flea vectors are *Xenopsylla cheopis* (Oriental rat flea) (Fig. 133-2), *Ceratophyllus fasciatus* (rat flea in temperate climates), and *Ctenocephalus canis. Ctenocephalus felis* (which bites dogs, cats, and humans) and the human flea, *Pulex irritans*, are relatively poor vectors.[6,8,21]

Flea behavior has a significant impact on its role as a plague vector. Although fleas can survive months between feeding, fleas require mammalian hosts for a regular source of blood meals. An Oriental rat flea (*X. cheopis*) typically ingests 0.03 to 0.5 µL of blood per feeding. Although no quantitative studies have been done, the level of bacteremia in the infected host correlates with the percentage of fleas that become infected. Because fleas leave a dead rat as its body cools and quickly seek out the nearest warm mammal to feed on, the infection is transmitted continually within a mammalian reservoir. Humans living near rodents are at high risk to become infected. When *Y. pestis* multiplies at room temperature, it produces a coagulase that clots blood. Given that the body temperature of a flea approximates room temperature, when a flea feeds on a plague-infected mammal, the ingested blood clots in the flea's proventriculus. Within several days of feeding, a solid fibrous mass of multiplying *Y. pestis* bacilli and coagulated blood obstructs the proventriculus, preventing the flea from digesting its blood meal (see Fig. 133-2). The fed but unsatiated flea continues to feed, only to regurgitate repeatedly the infectious contents of its proventriculus into the bite wound of its next host. By this pattern of feeding, the plague-infected flea efficiently transfers *Y. pestis* among multiple mammalian hosts (called the *sylvatic cycle*). Although this mammalian reservoir does not play a central role in the use of plague as a biologic weapon, the deliberate release of *Y. pestis* may introduce the organism into a potential animal reservoir, as a "collateral infection," in addition to the intended human target population.

Japan's Unit 731 used infected fleas as part of the delivery system for a plague biologic weapon used against targets in mainland China during World War II.[4] Although this method is not as "efficient" as delivering a highly weaponized and aerosolized plague biologic weapon, it is still a potential mode of delivery and should be considered part of a biologic terrorist's armamentarium. Also, by using a natural plague vector, the initial cases are predominantly of the bubonic form, resembling a natural epizoonotic outbreak. This natural vector may serve to delay recognition of the outbreak as a biologic attack.

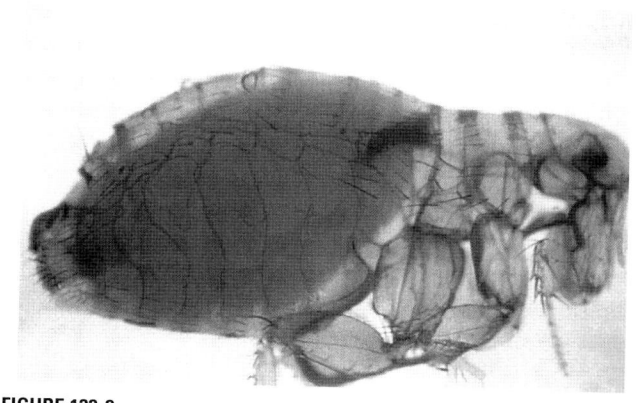

FIGURE 133-2

Xenopsylla cheopis, Oriental rat flea, with a proventricular plague mass. During feeding, the flea draws viable *Yersinia pestis* organisms into its esophagus, which multiply and block the proventriculus just in front of the stomach, later forcing the flea to regurgitate infected blood onto the host when it tries to swallow. *(From U.S. Centers for Disease Control, Public Health Image Library ID 2025.)* See Color Fig. 133-2.

Should *Y. pestis* be released as a biologic weapon, the resultant disease outbreak and the clinical presentation of the victims might or might not resemble patterns of naturally occurring plague.[14] If an outbreak consisting of primarily bubonic plague occurs after a die-off of local rodents, a natural outbreak is more likely. Conversely, if a plague outbreak includes a predominance of early pneumonic cases, a large aerosol release of *Y. pestis* should be suspected.

In May 2000, the U.S. Department of Justice, in cooperation with numerous other agencies, conducted a large-scale drill to test the preparedness of the United States to respond to terrorist attacks. The exercise, called *TOPOFF*, included a chemical weapons event in Portsmouth, New Hampshire; a radiologic event in Washington, D.C.; and a biologic event in Denver, Colorado.[22] The biologic scenario included the covert release of aerosolized *Y. pestis* at a local performing arts center during a show. In the scenario, large numbers of victims began seeking medical attention within 3 days of the "attack." As the exercise progressed over 4 days, there were 3000 to 4000 cases of pneumonic plague, with 1000 to 2000 deaths. Cases eventually were found in 11 other states and in distant cities such as Tokyo and London. During this time, the local medical resources (including hospital beds, antibiotics, ventilators, and staff) were overwhelmed. Many outside assets, including the U.S. Centers for Disease Control and Prevention (CDC), many emergency response agencies, and the Strategic National Stockpile (formerly the National Pharmaceutical Stockpile), were brought in to help manage the explosive outbreak. Although this exercise included many artificial aspects, it effectively showed how a biologic attack with *Y. pestis* could produce a massive outbreak of plague rapidly overwhelming most medical systems.

The epidemiologic patterns of naturally occurring plague are well known (see Fig. 133-1). It is important to be familiar with these normal patterns to be able to detect patterns that may suggest an intentional plague biologic weapon release. If an aerosolized plague weapon is used, the pneumonic, contagious form of plague is likely to predominate.

MICROBIOLOGY

Y. pestis is a small, gram-negative, nonmotile, non–spore-forming, invasive, pathogenic coccobacillus of the family Enterobacteriaceae.[6] It was first isolated as the causative agent of plague by Yersin, who had been sent to Hong Kong by Louis Pasteur from the Institut Pasteur to study plague during the epidemic in 1894. Yersin's description of the bacillus fits the now-known characteristics of *Y. pestis*, and he identified the link between rats and plague.[23] The organism originally was named *Bacterium pestis* by Yersin in 1900; the name was changed to *Bacillus pestis* in 1903, to *Pasteurella pestis* in 1923 (after Pasteur, Yersin's mentor), and finally to *Yersinia pestis* in 1970.[6,24] Other human pathogens in the *Yersinia* genus include *Yersinia enterocolitica* and *Yersinia pseudotuberculosis*. *Y. pestis* measures 0.5 to 0.8 μm wide by 1 to 3 μm long, is capable of aerobic and anaerobic growth, and is a facultative intracellular organism. It typically shows strong bipolar staining ("closed safety pin") with Giemsa, Wright, or Wayson staining. Pleomorphic and club-shaped

forms are not unusual, however. *Y. pestis* may remain viable for days in water or moist soil, can resist drying if protected by mucus or similar compounds, but is quickly killed by exposure to direct sunlight. *Y. pestis* can maintain viability on environmental surfaces for 5 days under controlled conditions.[25] Depending on the sophistication of the dissemination methods used by a bioterrorist, a plague biologic weapon may be relatively persistent. Overall, the geographic range and persistence of a plague biologic weapon, often referred to as its "footprint," is determined by the environmental stability of the *Y. pestis* strain used, the weaponization measures employed, and the meteorologic conditions at the time of its release (William C. Patrick, III, personal communication). Weaponization techniques are discussed in more detail in the introductory portion of Chapter 132.

Although primarily of historical importance, three classic *biovars* of *Y. pestis* have been described based on their ability to convert nitrate to nitrite and to ferment glycerol: *Biovar antiqua* is positive for both characteristics and is thought to have originated in Africa, southwestern Russia, and central Asia and to have caused the first (Justinian) pandemic; *biovar medievalis* can convert nitrate to nitrite, does not ferment glycerol, and is thought to have originated in the Caspian sea region and been the cause of the second (Black Death) pandemic; *biovar orientalis* does not convert nitrate to nitrite but can ferment glycerol, is found in Asia and the Western hemisphere, and is the cause of the third (Modern) pandemic.[6] Many strains of *Y. pestis* have been described by molecular biology, including many variants of these classic *biovars*.

Y. pestis grows best at 28°C. It has greater nutritional requirements when grown at 37°C, but at that temperature *Y. pestis* also produces specific virulence factors that allow it to evade the immune system of its mammalian host.[26,27] *Y. pestis* has adapted to two distinct host environments—its arthropod vector at room temperature and its mammalian host at approximately 37°C. Freshly isolated cultures often exhibit substantial slime production, owing to a so-called capsular or envelope antigen, which is heat labile and is readily lost when the organism is growing in vitro or in the insect vector. Individual colonies are described as having a "fried egg" or "beaten copper" appearance.

PATHOGENESIS

Y. pestis has features of a typical enteric bacterium, including a cell wall, an enterobacterial antigen, and lipopolysaccharide side chains. It also encodes many additional virulence factors, on chromosomal DNA and on the three plasmids,[28] which allow it to combat the immune system of its mammalian host and to propagate its infection. These include a capsular antigen (F1), plasminogen activator, pH 6 antigen, V antigen, and a large and complex system of *Yersinia* outer proteins (Yops), their secretion apparatus (Ysc), and intracellular chaperones (Syc).[26,29–31]

The *Y. pestis* genome consists of a single circular 4.65-Mb chromosome and three plasmids: pPCP1 (*pesticin, coagulase, plasminogen*, 9.6 kb), pCD1 (*calcium dependence*, 70.5 kb), and pMT1 (*murine toxin*, 100.9 kb).[32,33] There is a great deal of DNA sequence homology among *Y. pestis*, *Y. enterocolitica*, and *Y. pseudotuberculosis*.[34] Plasmid CD1 is designated pYV227 and pIB1 in *Y. enterocolitica* and *Y. pseudotuberculosis* and is required for virulence of all three *Yersinia* spp. pathogenic to humans.[6] Only *Y. pestis* has all three of these plasmids, however.[28,32,33]

Plasmid CD1 encodes certain regulatory functions that mediate growth and virulence factor synthesis. At 37°C, in vitro vegetative growth of *Y. pestis* depends on the addition of calcium to the culture medium at a concentration that approximates mammalian vascular fluid (2.5 mM). Conversely, cultivation at 37°C in calcium-deficient medium is characterized by decreased adenylate energy charge, reduced stable RNA synthesis, and inhibition of cell division.[35] This condition (termed *growth restriction*) is referred to as the *low calcium response* (LCR) and is thought to approximate in vivo conditions when *Yersinia* is in contact with eukaryotic cells of a mammalian host. This restricted cellular metabolism is accompanied, however, by the selective synthesis of the virulence factors LcrV (also called the *V antigen*) and Yops encoded on the Yop virulon of pCD1.[6,30,36] The Yop system is a complex group of proteins that are potent mediators of *Y. pestis* virulence.[37] It includes *effector* proteins that are translocated from the plague bacillus into the cytosol of target eukaryotic cells, *chaperone* proteins that bind effector Yops in the bacterial cytosol until they are secreted, *secretory* and *translocator* proteins that facilitate the delivery of the effector proteins into the cytosol of target host cells, and *regulatory* proteins to control the entire process.[38,39]

The delivery of the effector Yops depends on a type III secretion apparatus (also called the *Ysc* [*Yop secretion complex*] injectisome) (Fig. 133-3).[36,38–40] At the temperature of its mammalian host (37°C), *Y. pestis* begins synthesis of the secretory portion of the Ysc and a cytosolic pool of Yops.[34,41] This structure comprises many membrane-based hydrophobic structural proteins that span the bacterial peptidoglycan layer and inner and outer membranes.[41] A final hollow needle-like portion at the tip *translocates* the effec- tor Yops across the membrane of the target eukaryotic cell into its cytosol.[36,38–40,42] This process requires *Y. pestis* to be in contact with the target cell and binding of specific cell surface membrane receptors on the target cell.[38] By this mechanism, the plague bacillus can "inject" cytotoxic effector Yops into the macrophage of the mammalian host immune system to inhibit phagocytosis and kill the macrophage. YscN is a 47.8-kd protein similar to the catalytic subunits of F_0F_1 adenosine triphosphatase and contains two consensus nucleotide-binding motifs (Walker boxes A and B). It localizes to the bacterial cytosolic side of the secretion apparatus and hydrolyzes adenosine triphosphate to energize the secretion process (see Fig. 133-3).[43]

Translocator proteins, YopB, YopD, and LcrV, form a hydrophobic transmembrane pore through the bacterial outer membrane and into the eukaryotic cell membrane.[30,36] YopB and YopD act as protein translocases and have hydrophobic domains within their amino acid structure, consistent with their putative transmembrane role.[38] They are not translocated into the target cell, but they are required for the formation and stability of the translocation pore. The type III secretion mechanism transports them to the bacterial cell surface, where they remain during the translocation process. YopB induces 1.2- to 3.5-nm-diameter pores in red blood cell membranes and disrupted purified lipid membranes in vitro, supporting its role as a transmembrane pore for the translocation of effector Yops.[41,44] *Yersinia yopBD⁻* mutants, which do not synthesize Yops B and D, are avirulent. They are able to transport Yops to the bacterial surface but are not able to translocate them into the target cell. As a result, effector Yops (e.g., YopE, YopH) accumulate at the zone of contact between the *Yersinia* bacterium and the target eukaryotic cell. When the plague bacillus contacts the host cell, it also triggers the polymerization of YscF, a 6-kd protein, forming a hollow "needle" with an internal diameter of approximately 2 nm. This supplies the necessary force to perforate the cell membrane and provide the final conduit that the Yops use to enter the host cell cytosol.[42]

FIGURE 133-3

When yersinia are placed at 37°C in a rich environment, the Ysc secretion apparatus is installed, and a stock of Yop proteins is synthesized. As long as there is no contact with a eukaryotic cell, a stop-valve, possibly made of YopN, TyeA, and LcrG, blocks the Ysc secretion channel. On contact with the eukaryotic target cell, a sensor interacts with a receptor on the cell surface, which results in the opening of the secretion channel at the zone of contact. The Yops are transported through the secretion channels, and the Yop effectors are translocated across the plasma membrane guided by YopB and YopD. During their intrabacterial stage, Yops are capped with their specific Syc chaperone, presumably to prevent premature associations. *(From Cornelis GR: Yersinia type III secretions: Send in the effectors. J Cell Biol 158:401–408, 2002.)*

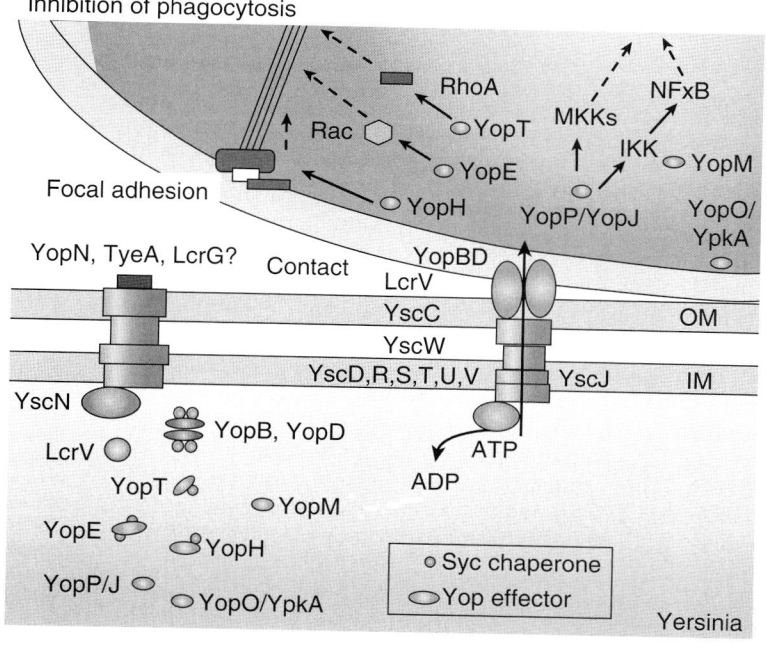

Yops and LcrV expression is regulated by the temperature-sensitive transcriptional activator LcrF (which also is encoded in the Yop virulon on pCD1) that controls transcription of most of the genes involved in Yop synthesis and secretion.[6,30,36] Before contact with a host eukaryotic cell, the type III secretion channel is blocked by regulatory proteins YopN, LcrG, and TyeA.[36,38,39] Also, cytosolic accumulation of the negative regulary factor, LcrQ, causes repression of *yop* gene transcription.[39] TyeA (*t*ranslocator of *Y*ops into *e*ukaryotic cells *A*) has been found to interact with YopN and with YopD. It also has been shown to be required for the translocation of YopE and YopH but not for the remaining effector Yops.[45] On interaction of *Y. pestis* outer membrane adhesins and eukaryotic cell integrins, YopN is released, the Ysc apparatus opens, and Yop secretion takes place.[39] The secretion of LcrQ and the dissociation of YopN from the Ysc apparatus allow Yop synthesis and secretion to proceed (see Fig. 133-3).[38,46]

Several Yops require specific Yop chaperone proteins (e.g., SycE) to complex with specific Yops (e.g., YopE) in the bacterial cytosol before their secretion via the Yop secretion apparatus.[47] These are small (13.6- to 19-kd) acidic proteins that are encoded on pCD1 adjacent to their respective Yop and are required for Yop secretion but not synthesis.[36] Specific chaperones have been found for YopB, YopD, YopE, YopH, YopN, and YopT.[30,36,38,39,47] It is thought that these chaperones prevent premature interactions between different secreted proteins with each other and parts of the secretion and translocation machinery. They also may prevent Yop degradation in the bacterial cytosol[3] and protect the plague bacillus from the cytotoxic effects of Yops.[48] They also maintain a specific Yop conformational structure to facilitate its delivery to and secretion by the Ysc apparatus.[36]

Yops secretion occurs when *Y. pestis* contacts a eukaryotic cell or when calcium is removed from its growth medium in vitro.[36,49] The in vitro condition of low calcium has given rise to the LCR designation for these Yops-associated genes.[50] Secretion of the effector Yops proteins is negatively and positively regulated by the pCD1 gene products, LcrG and LcrV, also called the V antigen.[50,51] LcrG has been shown to block the assembly of Ysc. Conversely, LcrV is thought to induce Yops secretion positively by inactivating the inner membrane LcrG-mediated Ysc block.[52] On contact with a eukaryotic cell, LcrG and LcrV interact in the bacterial cytoplasm, which removes LcrG from its secretion-blocking role, allowing full induction of the LCR.[44,50]

Resistance to phagocytosis is one of the primary defenses used by *Y. pestis* to overcome the host immune response. Dedicated phagocytic cells, such as macrophages and neutrophils, phagocytose pathogens by a complex interaction of membrane receptors, intracellular signaling pathways, and cytoskeletal rearrangement.[53] When a macrophage contacts a plague bacillus, several phagocytic pathways intended to engulf and kill it are triggered.[54] When contact between the two cells is made, however, *Y. pestis* also rapidly establishes its type III secretion apparatus and translocates at least six known Yop effector proteins (YopE, YopH, YopM, YpkA/YopO, YopJ, and YopT).[46,55] These proteins specifically target host cell intracellular macromolecules to disrupt intracellular cell signaling pathways,[56] block phagocytosis,[55,57] inhibit the immune response by suppressing secretion of interferon-γ and tumor necrosis factor-α,[58,59] and

induce apoptosis.[60] This form of close-quarter cellular combat allows *Y. pestis* to disable the mammalian host immune system one cell at a time.[38,46] Individual Yop virulence components are discussed subsequently.

YopJ is a 32.5-kd, 288-amino acid residue effector protein that is translocated into eukaryotic cells by the Ysc. It inhibits the activation of the NF-κB and MAPK kinases, disrupting multiple intracellular signaling pathways (Fig. 133-4).[61] This inhibition prevents synthesis of cytokines (interleukin-8, tumor necrosis factor-α) and anti-apoptotic factors, resulting in a significantly impaired inflammatory response and cell death (see Fig. 133-4).[30,36,38,59–63] These combined effects allow *Y. pestis* to eliminate its primary immune system adversary and inhibit an inflammatory response.[64]

Four Yop effectors (YpoH, YopE, YopT, YpkA/YopO) inhibit phagocytosis.[34,36,57] *YopH* is a potent phosphotyrosine phosphatase injected into the cytosol of the macrophage via the Ysc.[39] Within the target cell, it rapidly catalyzes the specific tyrosine dephosphorylation of several proteins whose tyrosine phosphorylation appears to be an early intracellular signal that occurs during phagocytosis.[65] These proteins include the χ subunit of the Fcχ receptor (which is required for Fc-mediated phagocytosis), paxillin (a 68-kd, cytoskeleton-associated tyrosine phosphoprotein that associates with F-actin in the cytoplasm immediately beneath nascent

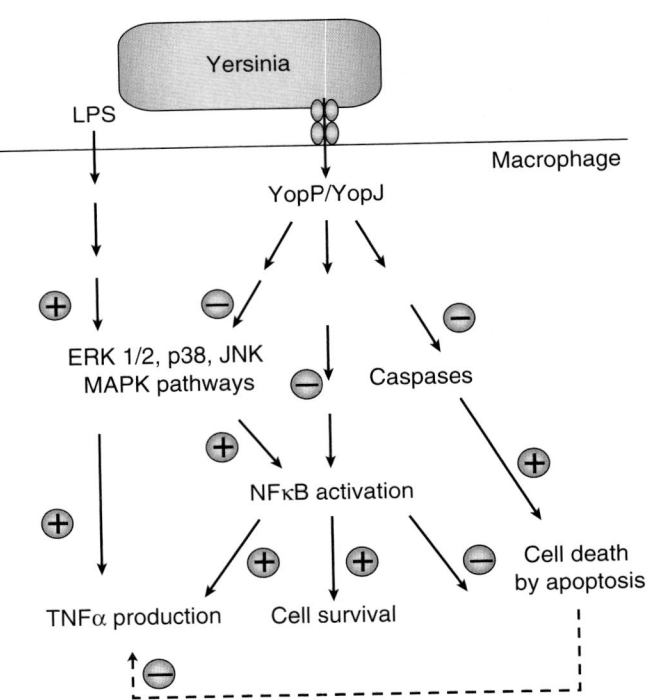

FIGURE 133-4

Model showing the effects of YopP/YopJ on the macrophage intracellular cascades. Lipopolysaccharide (LPS) activates the ERK1/2, JNK, and p38 MAPK pathways, which leads to increased tumor necrosis factor (TNF)-α production. Activated MAPKs can lead to NFκB activation; activated NFκB can enhance TNF-α transcription. Translocated YopP/YopJ induces macrophage apoptosis by a mechanism involving caspase activation. It also down-regulates MAPKs and impairs NFκB activation, two effects that could explain the YopP/YopJ-induced reduction of TNF-α production. *(From Cornelis GR: Minireview: The Yersinia deadly kiss. J Bacteriol 180:5495–5504, 1998.)*

phagosomes), p130^cas, and the tyrosine kinase syk.[39,65] The coordinated tyrosine phosphorylation of these proteins appears to be an important step in integrating signals between Fc receptors and the underlying cytoskeleton.[65] Dephosphorylation of these same proteins by YopH may interrupt Fc receptor signaling and the formation or maintenance of F-actin–rich pseudopods, which impairs phagocytosis and inhibits the oxidative burst.[36,38,66] YopH inhibits phagocytosis mediated by complement and Fc receptors in polymorphonuclear leukocytes and macrophages.[30,38] YopH also participates in the down-regulation of the immune response by inhibiting the production of the monocyte chemoattractant protein, MCP-1, by dephosphorylating key enzymes in its synthetic pathway.[36]

YopE also is injected into the eukaryotic cell cytosol via Ysc when *Yersinia* species is in contact with the target cell membrane. It acts on monomeric guanosine triphosphatases (GTPases) of the Rho family, which are known to control cytoskeleton dynamics.[67] More specifically, it acts as a GTPase-activating protein, accelerating GTP hydrolysis.[36] This activity inhibits phagocytosis by causing collapse of the cytoskeleton via indirect disruption of actin microfilaments.[68] *YopT* is a 35.5-kd cysteine protease that cleaves Rho family GTPases and causes cell death by disrupting the actin filament structure and cell cytoskeleton.[30,55] *YpkA/YopO* is a serine-threonine protein kinase that binds actin and RhoA and Rac1 GTPases. Although these binding activities likely inhibit phagocytosis, no specific target protein or mode of action for YpkA/YopO has been shown yet.[36]

YopM has α-thrombin binding activity that may provide a local antiinflammatory effect. It localizes to the macrophage nucleus after translocation and influences gene expression. Very little is known, however, about its intended role.[69,70]

In contrast to *Bacillus anthracis, Y. pestis* does not have a true capsule. However, when grown at temperatures greater than 33°C, it does produce a gellike antiphagocytic glycoprotein envelope, called the *capsular antigen*, or fraction 1 (F1).[6,71] F1 is encoded by the *caf1* gene on the pMT1 plasmid.[30,32] It is a protein linked to a polysaccharide (fraction 1A) and a free protein (fraction 1B) complexed into the glycoprotein subunit, Caf1, with a molecular weight of 15.5 kd.[27,72] These 15.5-kd monomers form seven-membered chains in open-ring structures with a molecular weight of 114 kd. Mass spectroscopy studies have shown that these open-ring heptamers join end-to-end to form high-molecular-weight helical, heptamer oligomers, similar to the structures of adhesive pili on other bacteria.[73] These long coiled structures remain attached to the outer membrane of the plague bacillus and constitute the gel matrix of *Y. pestis'* antiphagocytic envelope. Maximal synthesis of F1 occurs at 37°C, the typical body temperature of a mammalian host. Fraction F1 is not synthesized at temperatures less than 33°C and is not expressed by *Y. pestis* found in fleas or other arthropod vectors.[74] This envelope has been shown to be important in the ability of *Y. pestis* to resist phagocytosis by neutrophils and monocytes during the initial phase of infection.[75] Although not present at the time of inoculation (e.g., fleabite), capsular antigen is produced by plague bacilli replicating in macrophages and in regional lymph nodes. The importance of the antiphagocytic envelope in the pathogenesis of plague infection varies significantly among species.[6]

The pH 6 antigen is encoded on chromosomal DNA. As its name suggests, it is a pH-dependent virulence factor that is synthesized at temperatures greater than 35 °C between pH 5 and 6.7. Sites where pH 6 is expressed include the acidic phagolysosomes of macrophages or the acidic environments of abscesses, such as in buboes or necrotic lesions in the liver and spleen. The pH 6 antigen has been shown to be a 15-kd structural protein that forms a fibrillar structure on the bacterial surface, which has been shown to promote adherence to eukaryotic cells and may participate in the delivery of Yops into phagocytic target cells.[6,33,76,77] Although its complete role in *Y. pestis* virulence is unknown, mutants lacking the pH 6 gene have been shown to be 100-fold less virulent.

Y. pestis encodes a 34.6-kd outer membrane–bound serine protease called *plasminogen activator* (Pla) on pPCP1 with coagulase and fibrinolytic activity. This fibrinolytic action is temperature dependent, being more active at 37°C than 28°C.[78] It also has specific binding affinity for type IV collagen.[79] Pla inhibits the local immune response by cleaving and inactivating complement component C3, reducing chemoattractants at the site of infection.[80,81] This virulence factor's primary pathogenic function is thought to be the proteolytic activation of a host serine protease, plasminogen, into plasmin.[6,80,82] Plasmin is a broad-spectrum serine protease that degrades fibrin and noncollagenous proteins of extracellular matrices and activates latent procollagenases. The Pla surface protease of *Y. pestis* resembles mammalian activators in function and converts plasminogen to plasmin by limited proteolysis. It activates plasminogen by cleaving the same Arg_{560}-Val_{561} bond, as does mammalian tissue plasminogen activator.[82] Through this capacity to generate plasmin, *Y. pestis* indirectly degrades fibrin and extracellular matrix proteins such as laminin and fibronectin and activates procollagenases to active collagen-degrading enzymes.[82] Pla also proteolytically inactivates $α_2$-antiplasmin, the main endogenous inhibitor of plasmin, potentiating the invasive process.[82,83] Plasminogen activation has been shown to enhance bacterial metastasis in vitro through reconstituted basement membrane or epithelial cell monolayers. Animal studies have shown that Pla is essential for *Y. pestis* acquired by the cutaneous route to cause disseminated infection, and the inactivation of the *pla* gene on pPCP increased the median lethal dose of bacteria 1 million–fold.[81] This aggressive proteolytic attack by *Y. pestis* degrades the usual tissue barriers (e.g., basement membranes) that bacteria must penetrate to reach the lymphatic or circulatory systems, resulting in an extremely invasive infection, with rapid dissemination throughout the body.

Pla also promotes *Y. pestis* adherence to components of basement membranes.[79] Some Pla⁻ *Y. pestis* strains have reduced virulence significantly via peripheral routes of infection (e.g., fleabite).[80] In vitro studies also have shown that Pla increases *Y. pestis* adherence to and degradation of extracellular matrices, including matrices found in human lung. In animal studies, plasmin has been found to increase the release of interleukin-1 from endotoxin-stimulated monocytes.[84] Interleukin-1 is a proinflammatory mediator that increases the permeability of cell layers to allow migration of inflammatory cells to the site of infection. This increased tissue permeability may increase the migration of *Y. pestis* away from the site of infection.[84] It is likely that Pla activity increases the invasiveness of plague infection by the peripheral and possibly the pulmonary routes of infection.[80] Plague Pla also causes formation of intravascular thrombi, causing areas of tissue necrosis due to arteriole and capillary occlusion.

Similar to infection with *B. anthracis*, the clinical pathogenesis of *Y. pestis* infection varies with the route of infection.[37] The plague bacillus gains entry by inoculation of the skin, either by fleabite or by the introduction of *Y. pestis*–infected material, such as flea feces, into an open wound. The organism also may be inhaled secondary to exposure to a person with pneumonic plague and a productive cough or secondary to the release of an aerosolized plague biologic weapon. Although not a common route of human infection, predacious mammalians may become infected by feeding on plague-infected mammals (e.g., cats feeding on plague-infected rock squirrels). This is an important route of secondary infection, however, because humans may become infected on exposure to these animals (e.g., human plague due to exposure to plague-infected cat).[11,12,18,19,85]

Pneumonic Plague

Pneumonic plague occurs in *primary* and *secondary* clinical forms. The route of infection determines which pathologic form develops. Primary pneumonic plague results from the inhalation of plague bacilli. Inhalation may occur after the intentional release of weaponized plague bacilli or the aerosolization of plague-infected sputum by a person or animal[12,18,20,21,85] with plague pneumonia.[6,7,21,86] An important pathologic characteristic of primary pneumonic plague is that the pneumonia is a bronchoalveolar pneumonia, with bacilli localized to the airspaces of the lung. The same virulence mechanisms that allow plague bacilli to evade the immune system and invade local tissue at the site of infection in bubonic plague enable the organism to establish and propagate infection in the lung rapidly. The pathologic result is a rapidly progressive necrotizing pneumonia.[12,21,85]

Experimental inhalational exposure of nonhuman primates to aerosolized *Y. pestis* (mean dose 3×10^4 bacilli) generally produced a focus of lobular consolidation in the peripheral portion of one lobe, most often a lower lobe. Rarely, a second focus of consolidation was found in the same or another lobe.[87] On section, these areas of lung consolidation showed hepatization and occasionally liquefaction necrosis and hemorrhage. Microscopically, hemorrhages were common, with vascular inflammation and alveolar polymorphonuclear leukocyte infiltration. Alveoli were filled with edema fluid and large numbers of *Y. pestis* bacilli. Lymphatics in edematous areas of lung were dilated and heavily colonized with plague bacilli. Splenic findings included hemorrhages with foci of necrosis and abundant plague bacilli. Fibrin thrombi were seen in glomerular capillaries, lungs, adrenal glands, sinusoids of the spleen, and occasionally sinusoids of the liver.[87] Postmortem studies of fatal human cases of primary plague pneumonia showed areas of consolidation ranging from patchy foci to involving the entire lung, severe bronchopneumonia, purulent exudates on the pleural surfaces, and pleural effusions.[12,20]

Secondary pneumonic plague develops due to hematogenous seeding of the lungs with plague bacilli from either primary septicemic plague or secondary septicemia due to bubonic plague.[6,9,21,85,86] Initially the organism localizes to

the lung interstitium, where it multiplies, causing microabscesses. These may enlarge to cause areas of necrosis and cavitation.[88] The same tissue-destroying and immune system–inhibiting mechanisms described for bubonic plague are active in pneumonic plague, allowing the infection to progress. Compared with primary plague pneumonia, secondary pneumonic plague is a more diffuse, often bilateral process due to the initial widespread interstitial distribution of the organism in the lung.[86]

Bubonic Plague

In bubonic plague, when a plague-infected flea or other arthropod vector bites a human, it disgorges an estimated tens of thousands of organisms into the bite wound, initiating a local infection. Because these bacilli had been living and multiplying in the flea vector at approximately room temperature, they do not have the antiphagocytic glycoprotein envelope at the time of inoculation into the skin and are susceptible to phagocytosis.[6,27] For *Y. pestis* to establish an infection after inoculation, it must evade the host immune mechanisms, including phagocytosis by polymorphonuclear leukocytes and macrophages. As the organism grows and multiplies at body temperature, the antiphagocytic envelope is expressed.[30,37] Soon after a localized infection is established at the site of inoculation, plague bacilli migrate via cutaneous lymphatics to the regional lymph nodes, where they may be phagocytosed but not killed.[89,90] Early in the course of the infection, lymph nodes develop congestion and edema without necrosis. As the disease progresses, growing numbers of bacilli cause necrosuppurative inflammation and destruction of the nodal architecture with localized tissue necrosis and hemorrhage, producing the characteristic buboes of bubonic plague.[88,91] As this process continues, it causes suppuration of the bubo and breakdown of the local anatomic structures that otherwise would contain the infection within the abscess. *Y. pestis* bacteremia (secondary septicemic plague) ensues and seeds organs such as the liver, spleen, and lungs. The first detectable pathologic manifestation in these organs is the development of areas of focal necrosis. Plague bacilli undergo linear growth up to 1 million organisms per gram of tissue. Abscesses may coalesce, causing organ necrosis.[27] Histopathologic studies of *Y. pseudotuberculosis* (which employs many of the same virulence mechanisms as *Y. pestis*) show that multiplying organisms localize to extracellular sites (e.g., liver sinusoids), but despite rapid growth and tissue necrosis, no significant inflammatory response was seen, and there was little or no interaction with professional phagocytes.[92]

Septicemic Plague

Septicemic plague occurs in two forms: *primary*, which occurs due to direct introduction of *Y. pestis*, usually by fleabite, into the blood, and *secondary*, in which *Y. pestis* is introduced into the blood by hematogenous extension from either bubonic or pneumonic plague. Primary septicemic plague occurs without palpable lymphadenopathy or focal pneumonia. Because the organism bypasses the lymphatic system, no characteristic buboes are seen, and the patient develops septicemia more rapidly than the secondary septicemia due to bubonic plague. After the development of generalized septicemia, the course of primary septicemic plague is pathophysiologically the same as that for secondary plague septicemia due to bubonic plague. There is diffuse seeding of organs with plague bacilli, which continue to multiply rapidly, causing high levels of bacteremia in the tissues and blood. These high levels of bacteremia, whether in primary or secondary septicemic plague, produce an overall clinicopathologic picture of gram-negative sepsis.[1,14,88,93]

Although seen most often in septicemic plague, disorders of coagulation can be found in all major clinical forms of plague. The pathophysiologic mechanism likely involves YopM, a 41.5-kd virulence protein of *Y. pestis* believed to have an antiinflammatory role in bubonic plague and Pla. It has been shown that YopM binds human α-thrombin (but not prothrombin) and inhibits ristocetin-induced and thrombin-induced platelet activation in vitro. YopM also shares significant sequence homology with the von Willebrand factor–binding and thrombin-binding domains of the α chain of human platelet membrane glycoprotein Ib.[69,70,94–96] Although the contribution of Pla to plague-associated coagulopathy has not been described clearly, it is likely that endotoxin-mediated disseminated intravascular coagulation,[97] in combination with effects of Pla, contributes to the coagulopathy seen in plague.[98,99] Plague interferes with the coagulation system at multiple sites, including the inflammatory cascade, platelet function, and clotting cascade.

CLINICAL PRESENTATION

Similar to anthrax, plague may present in several clinical forms, including pneumonic plague, bubonic plague, septicemic plague, pharyngeal plague, and plague meningitis. Also similar to anthrax, several clinical types of plague may result from a single biologic weapon attack with *Y. pestis*. Most information regarding clinical plague is the result of studying the naturally occurring form of the disease. Incubation periods, clinical presentation, and response to treatment are affected, however, by innate and bioengineered characteristics of the *Y. pestis* used in an attack. If the strain of *Y. pestis* used has been manipulated to be especially virulent or resistant to antibiotics,[100] one would expect a relatively short incubation period and a high mortality rate. Patients may present with nonspecific findings, such as fever, cough, dyspnea, gastrointestinal symptoms such as abdominal pain and nausea and vomiting, and headache. Some patients may present with characteristic clinical signs, such as buboes or acral gangrene. It is important for the critical care clinician to consider plague and other potential biologic weapons when unusual patterns of illness are noticed or an intentionally caused outbreak is suspected.[14]

Bubonic Plague

The incubation period for bubonic plague lasts 1 to 8 days in a patient after being bitten by an infected flea.[6,14,27] Incubation periods may vary with size of inoculum, virulence of the organism, and underlying health of the patient. Ulcerating lesions at the site of the inoculation (fleabite) may develop but are not common. Initial systemic symp-

toms are nonspecific, with sudden onset of fever, chills, generalized weakness and malaise, chest pain, cough, skin rash, nausea, vomiting, diarrhea, abdominal pain, myalgias, arthralgias, sore throat, and headache.[1,14,88,93,101,102] Fever develops quickly, is present in virtually all cases,[8,93,98,99] and ranged from 100°F to 105.8°F (37.8° to 41°C) in one case series.[99] Patients are often tachycardic and hypotensive and may be tachypneic if there is pulmonary involvement. Conjunctivitis also has been seen in bubonic plague. Within a day and often within hours of the fleabite, the infection spreads from the inoculation site via the lymphatics to regional lymph nodes, which become swollen and painful (buboes).[8,98] Buboes develop most commonly in the groin (Fig. 133-5) (*bubo* is derived from the Greek word *boubon*, for "groin") because fleas often bite the legs. Because buboes develop in the regional lymph nodes that provide lymphatic drainage to the anatomic site of *Y. pestis* inoculation, however, they can be seen in femoral or inguinal nodes in the groin and axillary nodes (Fig. 133-6).[19,98] One occasionally may see cervical or submandibular buboes with plague pneumonia or plague pharyngitis.[88] These buboes may appear as single, smooth ovoid masses or as an irregular cluster of multiple infected nodes and range in size from 1 to 15 cm in diameter. They are nonfluctuant, painful, warm, and extremely tender on palpation. Patients usually position the affected limb so as to relieve pressure on the buboes and often resist examination of the buboes because of severe tenderness on palpation. Buboes rarely develop at lymph nodes distant from the inoculation site. They often are associated with a significant amount of surrounding edema and erythema, but rarely lymphangitis. They also may point and drain spontaneously.[10,88,93,98,99]

If treated early and appropriately, the course of bubonic plague usually includes rapid defervescence and overall

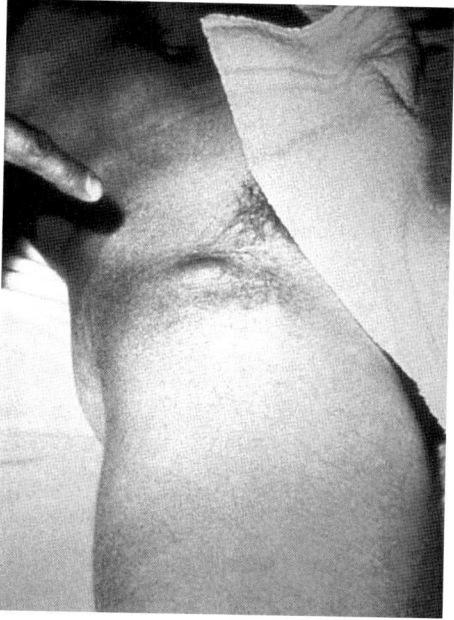

FIGURE 133-5

This plague patient shows symptoms that include a swollen inguinal lymph node, or bubo. *(From U.S. Centers for Disease Control, Public Health Image Library ID 2044.)* See Color Fig. 133-5.

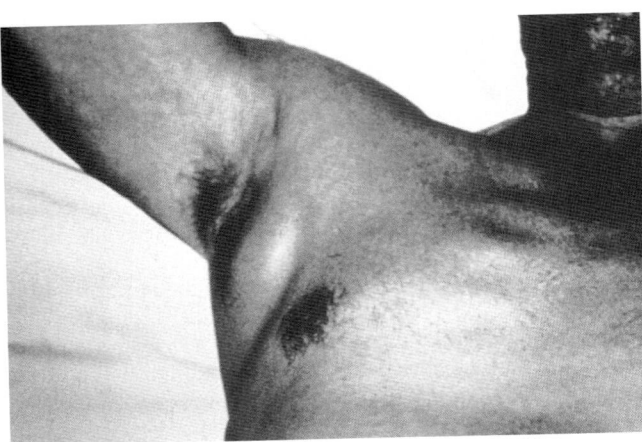

FIGURE 133-6

Plague patient displaying a swollen axillary lymph node. *(From U.S. Centers for Disease Control, Public Health Image Library ID 2045.)* See Color Fig. 133-6.

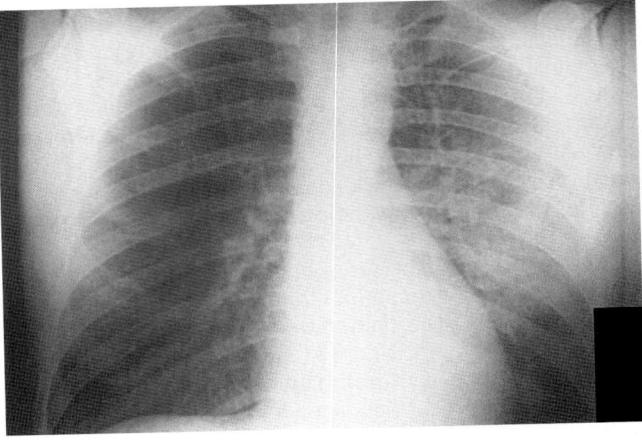

FIGURE 133-7

Anteroposterior chest x-ray of a plague patient. *(From U.S. Centers for Disease Control, Public Health Image Library ID 1955.)*

clinical improvement over 3 to 5 days. Buboes typically remain tender for about 1 week, becoming fluctuant as they resolve. If untreated, bubonic plague can progress rapidly, however, to *septicemic plague*, causing fulminant gram-negative sepsis and death within 2 to 4 days.[88,93,98,99]

Gastrointestinal symptoms may be prominent in all forms of plague and include nausea, vomiting, diarrhea, anorexia, and abdominal pain.[10,12,19,20,95,102] A review of 71 cases of human plague showed that gastrointestinal symptoms occurred in 57% of cases, with vomiting being the most common (39%) symptom, followed by nausea (43%), diarrhea (28%), and abdominal pain (17%).[102] The liver and spleen may become palpable or tender or both, and liver function test results may be elevated.[102] Intraabdominal buboes also may develop, with severe abdominal pain mimicking an acute abdomen. Upper and lower gastrointestinal hemorrhages also have been reported.

Pneumonic Plague

Pneumonic plague, also called *plague pneumonia*, can occur as either a *primary* or *secondary* process. Primary pneumonic plague results from inhalation of aerosolized plague bacilli, which may result from an intentional bioterrorist release or from the productive cough of a person with plague pneumonia.[86] As mentioned earlier, inhaled aerosolized plague bacilli localize to the alveolar space after inhalation.[87] Cough is productive of copious purulent sputum that is frothy, watery, and often blood-tinged.[21,86] The incubation period for pneumonic plague is generally much shorter (1 to 4 days) than either the bubonic or the septicemic forms of the disease.[14] Onset of illness is sudden with fever and chills. The primary manifestations of pneumonic plague include fever, chest pain, and productive cough of purulent sputum, often with hemoptysis, dyspnea, and shortness of breath.[21,86] Sputum with primary pneumonic plague is typically watery or mucoid, frothy, and blood tinged, although it may become frankly bloody.[86] It is a bronchopneumonia, usually starting in a single lobe, with rapid spreading to other lobes (Fig. 133-7). As areas of consolidation develop, they may develop liquefaction necrosis

and cavitation. Primary pneumonic plague begins as a lobular pneumonia, rapidly extending to lobar, multilobar, and often bilateral pneumonia. Chest radiographs typically show patchy bronchopneumonia, cavities, or consolidation.[12,21] This pattern is in contrast to secondary plague pneumonia, which begins as a diffuse process with an interstitial appearance on chest radiographs. Patients also are likely to have additional symptoms, including nausea, vomiting, abdominal pain, and weakness.[8,14,21]

Under *natural* conditions, exposure to aerosolized *Y. pestis* bacilli is most likely to occur from exposure to victims with plague pneumonia who cough and aerosolize the *Y. pestis*. Although rare compared with the bubonic form, naturally occurring pneumonic plague is considered highly contagious and responsible for the person-to-person transmission of plague that caused the great plague pandemics of history.[2] In the setting of a bioterrorist attack, *Y. pestis* may be disseminated as an aerosol, in which case there may be many cases of pneumonic plague. Given the technologic challenges of weaponizing *Y. pestis* into an effective 1- to 5-μm-particle-size aerosol, however, a bioterrorist could use a less efficient aerosol. Although the challenge of maintaining organism viability remains, and the aerosol would have a short range, plague is spread effectively and naturally by droplets of greater size. Using plague-infected fleas as a "low-tech" delivery system was employed successfully by Japan's Unit 731 to cause several epidemics in China during World War II.[2,4]

Secondary plague pneumonia occurs as a result of hematogenous seeding of the lungs with *Y. pestis* from either bubonic or septicemic plague. The bacilli are diffusely distributed in the lungs localizing to the interstitium, producing the clinical presentation of an interstitial pneumonia with scant sputum production. Also the sputum seen in secondary pneumonic plague is thicker and inspissated than that seen in primary pneumonic plague.

Septicemic Plague

Differentiation of patients with septicemic plague from patients with other types of gram-negative sepsis is often difficult because of the similarity of signs and symptoms. Septicemic plague patients may present with fever, tachycardia, tachypnea, and hypotension. Systolic blood pressures are usually less than 100 mm Hg. The constitutional symptoms are similar to bubonic plague, but gastrointestinal symptoms are more common in septicemic plague (72%) than in bubonic plague (51%).[14,102] The absence of palpable buboes differentiates the two forms, and meningitis is more common in septicemic plague than in bubonic plague. Additionally, secondary plague pneumonia occurs twice as often in septicemic plague than in the bubonic form. Septicemic patients are often older than 60 years, are usually less febrile, and have a higher mortality.[8,14] Bacteremia may be so great that organisms can be seen on peripheral blood smears.[103]

Overall, septicemic plague patients appear extremely ill and toxic. As the disease progresses, patients develop shock, delirium, coma, and rapid clinical deterioration similar to the course seen with other causes of overwhelming gram-negative sepsis. Although not absolutely specific for plague, cutaneous manifestations, including petechiae, ecchymoses, spontaneous hemorrhage, acral gangrene (Fig. 133-8), and increased bleeding due to trauma such as venipuncture, are the hallmarks of overwhelming *Y. pestis* sepsis.[13,14,98] Confluent ecchymoses, sometimes covering large areas of body surface area, gave plague its famous moniker, the *Black Death*.

Pestis Minor

A milder form of bubonic plague, *pestis minor* (also called *abortive bubonic plague*), may occur in patients with some degree of *Y. pestis* immunity. They present with buboes but without signs of systemic illness except fever. Lymphadenopathy resolves, and patients recover without treatment. In extremely mild cases, the only clinical finding may be vesiculation at the site of inoculation (e.g., fleabite).[8,14]

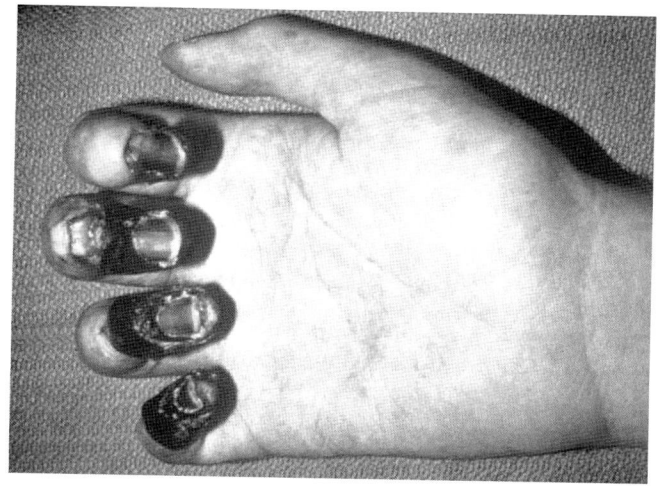

FIGURE 133-8

Right hand of a plague patient displaying acral gangrene. *(From U.S. Centers for Disease Control, Public Health Image Library ID 1957.)* See Color Fig. 133-8.

Plague Meningitis

Plague meningitis occurs as a result of hematogenous seeding of the meninges. Patients present with typical signs and symptoms of meningitis, including fever, headache, meningismus, seizures, and mental status changes.[10,93] Additional symptoms include the nonspecific symptoms described earlier for all forms of plague. Specific symptoms, such as buboes, depend on the primary clinical form of plague that caused the meningitis. It often occurs approximately 1 week after inadequately treated bubonic plague but may occur in any of the clinical forms and is more common after septicemic plague. Cerebrospinal fluid may show an elevated white blood cell count with a pleocytosis of primarily polymorphonuclear leukocytes and gram-negative bacilli.[8,10,14,93]

Plague Pharyngitis

Plague pharyngitis resembles acute bacterial tonsillitis or pharyngitis. It occurs after inhalation or ingestion of the organism. Cervical lymphadenopathy is common and may progress to forming characteristic buboes. Although it is generally considered a minor clinical form of plague, patients still may develop secondary septicemic plague with all of its clinical features, complications, and prognosis as mentioned earlier. Cervical lymphadenopathy also is seen occasionally with pneumonic plague.[8]

DIAGNOSIS

Because it is an unusual disease, plague easily may be inadvertently omitted from the consideration of the differential diagnosis of a patient presenting with pneumonia, sepsis, or suppurative lymphadenitis. The various forms of plague have distinctly different clinical manifestations, although because there can be an evolution of one form into another, there may be considerable overlap between stages. It is paramount to determine the primary form in a patient with plague. This assessment may have profound ramifications in terms of how the patient acquired the disease. A patient presenting with the primary bubonic form in a plague endemic area where multiple rodents such as prairie dogs have been dying likely has naturally occurring disease. In contrast, otherwise healthy young individuals in a non–plague-infected area presenting with primary plague pneumonia would be so unusual as to prompt immediate consideration of a biologic weapon–induced disease. This consideration would be virtually proven by more than one such individual case. It is only with early recognition of an intentionally induced outbreak that effective measures can be instituted, attenuating the impact of the disease.

The diagnosis of plague requires the recognition of the clinical syndrome by an astute clinician. The most effective response to a bioterrorist attack includes rapid recognition of the event and identification of the agent, treatment of the victims, and containment of the outbreak. Many epidemiologic surveillance systems have been established to assist in the rapid recognition of a bioterrorist attack. More importantly, the individual clinician must be vigilant for unusual epidemiologic patterns of illness in the community. When a suspicious illness has been identified, clinical samples must be sent to the nearest clinical laboratory as soon as possible to begin confirmatory testing. Empirical antibiotic treatment should not be delayed, however, while awaiting laboratory results.

Because microbiology laboratory personnel are at risk for occupationally acquired *Y. pestis*,[104] it has been recommended that routine culturing and manipulation of potential colonies should be done with biosafety level (BSL)–2 precautions as a minimum.[105,106] It has been recommended further that procedures that may lead to high droplets or aerosolization of this organism should be done under BSL-3 precautions.[106] Such activities include agitation of cultures, centrifugation, or working with animals that can generate droplets.

Theoretically, any biologic sample may be assayed for *Y. pestis*. The most common sources are blood, bubo aspirate, cerebrospinal fluid, and sputum.[99] Histochemical and serologic tests can be useful adjuncts to the establishment of the definitive diagnosis.

Histologic Appearance

Y. pestis should be suspected if gram-negative coccobacilli are detected by standard staining techniques. This suspicion should be heightened if the so-called safety pin bipolar staining pattern is seen. If there is a clinical suspicion of plague, the identification of organisms with these characteristics should markedly heighten the concern for this diagnosis. There are no data, however, available on the sensitivity, specificity, or predictive values of these morphologic characteristics in the diagnosis of plague. Other organisms that may show this safety pin pattern are *Pasteurella*, *Klebsiella*, *Streptococcus* spp., and *Escherichia coli*. *Y. pestis* may not always have this morphologic appearance, however. Despite these uncertainties, the detection of gram-negative coccobacilli should raise the suspicion for *Y. pestis*. Gram, Wright-Giemsa, and Wayson staining are useful for detecting *Y. pestis*.[103]

Immunochemical Staining

Although not published in an original research paper, a direct fluorescent antibody technique, which stains *Y. pestis* capsular antigen, F1, has been described.[107] Sensitivity and predictive values of this technique have not been established. It is anticipated, however, that this test has more specificity for detecting the plague bacillus than the traditional histochemical staining approach described previously.

Serologic Assays

Serologic assays are useful retrospectively for confirming the diagnosis of plague. These assays are not generally commercially available, and they are not done at standard microbiology laboratories. In the case of a suspected case or outbreak of *Y. pestis* infection, local public health authorities should be consulted. This practice not only makes the appropriate authorities aware of the possible existence of such a case but also expedites and facilitates the obtaining of appropriate serologic assays. In the United States, such assays are available from the CDC and

from the U.S. Military Medical Research Institute of Infectious Diseases (USAMRIID). A fourfold increase in serum antibody to *Y. pestis* is considered to be diagnostic.[107] In addition to the assays described subsequently, research programs are ongoing at several laboratories worldwide aimed at the development of rapid diagnostic assays.

Fraction One Antigen Assay

There are two assays based on antibodies to F1 of *Y. pestis*. An older passive hemagglutination assay measured circulating antibodies to F1 antigen. This test has largely been replaced, however, because of its relative insensitivity. A more sensitive immunologic assay to F1 antigen[108] was field tested in a plague outbreak in Namibia, after which 16% of the cases were confirmed by F1 antigenemia.[109] A rapid diagnostic test, using a monoclonal antibody enzyme-linked immunosorbent assay for the F1 antigen of *Y. pestis*, has been assessed against a range of bacterial cultures and clinical samples from plague outbreaks in Madagascar.[110,111] One assay yielded positive and negative predictive values of 90.6% and 86.7%.[110]

Polymerase Chain Reaction Assay

A polymerase chain reaction test for the detection of *Y. pestis* in fleas has been described.[112] This test is potentially useful for field surveillance of rodents for *Y. pestis* and theoretically could have utility in the diagnosis of plague in humans. There is no published experience with the use of this assay for the diagnosis of human *Y. pestis* infection, however.

Culture

Y. pestis can be cultured in standard media, although its growth is slow. It has been cultured most commonly from blood, sputum, and bubo aspirates. A portion of the culture should be used to detect F1 antigen. One authoritative source[107] states that automated culture methods may misidentify *Y. pestis*. No primary reference was provided for this observation, however. There is ongoing research on culture techniques for *Y. pestis*, and in some countries laboratory personnel are being trained specifically in the microbiologic assay of this organism. In one case series, blood cultures were positive in 24 of 25 cases (96%), and bubo aspirates were positive in 10 of 13 cases (77%).[93]

Public health authorities may be helpful in directing samples to the appropriate laboratories for *Y. pestis* culture. The U.S. Laboratory Response Network (LRN) has been established to create an organized laboratory system for bioterrorism-related specimen testing and referral. The LRN is a system of public and private laboratories, linked with local, state, and federal agencies, which test suspected bioterrorism-related clinical samples by established consensus protocols to provide timely and accurate testing and reporting. It is composed of four levels of laboratories: A, B, C, and D, which perform testing and refer samples to the next higher level laboratory. The largest, and lowest, tier of the LRN, level A, comprises BSL-2 designated clinical laboratories. Their role is to *rule in and refer* presumptive early cases of bioterrorism-related illness. The critical care clinician should become familiar with the readiness and capabilities of his or her local laboratory *before* an actual event takes place. Level B comprises public health laboratories, which usually operate at BSL-3 conditions and perform isolation, identification, and susceptibility testing of samples and *rule in and refer*. Level C also comprises public health laboratories but with more advanced typing and identification capabilities. They also *rule in and refer* to the final level, level D, where additional high-level characterization studies can be performed under BSL-4 conditions. Presently, there are two level D laboratories in the United States: the CDC and the USAMRIID. A complete discussion of the LRN is beyond the scope of this chapter. The reader is urged to consult the CDC, U.S. public health service, and local laboratories for additional information on using this system. Detailed guides and instructions for the selection, collection, storage, and shipping of specimens for analysis and additional information regarding bioterrorism preparedness are available from the CDC website bioterrorism page (www.bt.cdc.gov). There are presently no generally accepted and validated antibiotic susceptibility protocols for this organism, and it is unknown whether standard assays are reliable.

Bubonic Plague

The diagnosis of bubonic plague is primarily based on clinical suspicion with laboratory confirmation. Although patients initially may present with rapid onset of severe fever, chills, malaise, and headache, followed by gastroenteritis, it is not until buboes becomes apparent that the diagnosis may become apparent. In a few cases, a small ulcer or pustule may be identified at the site of inoculation.[93,113] The differential diagnosis of plague buboes encompasses several common conditions (Table 133-1).

The patient with a bubo may have it aspirated as a source of potential organism for stain and culture.[93] The described technique for bubo aspiration is to use a 20G needle on a 10-mL syringe containing 1 mL of sterile saline. The needle is inserted into the bubo, saline is

injected, and the plunger is used to withdraw and reinject the saline several times. This process should be continued until the saline is tinged with blood. The irrigation of a surgically opened bubo (abscess) has the potential to aerosolize plague bacilli, creating a significant respiratory hazard. Buboes should not be incised and drained unless clinically indicated and then only under conditions to minimize environmental release of the plague bacilli (e.g., negative pressure, BSL-3 conditions).

Pneumonic Plague

Patients with plague pneumonia tend to present with the clinical picture of a fulminant pneumonia with systemic symptoms followed by cough and blood-tinged sputum approximately 24 hours later. Although pneumonia can occur primarily or secondary to hematogenous dissemination from other forms of plague, as noted earlier, cases of primary plague pneumonia always should raise concern for a biologic weapon–induced disease.

The chest x-ray in plague pneumonia most commonly shows bilateral alveolar infiltrates, but many other patterns are possible as well.[93,114] An extremely suggestive finding is a predominance of gram-negative rods in the sputum, particularly in individuals who are not at posterior risk for the development of gram-negative pneumonia.

Septicemic Plague

Patients with septicemic plague present with the typical picture of gram-negative sepsis, although meningococcemia and rickettsiae should be included in the differential diagnosis.[13] This form of plague can be primary, or it may represent hematogenous spread of bubonic plague. In the latter case, a bubo should be easily identifiable, expediting the diagnosis. In the latter stages, patients with septicemic plague develop peripheral cyanosis and necrosis, causing the tips of end organs such as fingers, toes, penis, ear lobes, or nose to become necrotic—hence the term *Black Death*. Laboratory confirmation of septicemic plague is by the above-described staining, serologic, and culture methods.

Plague Meningitis

Patients with plague meningitis typically present with a typical picture of bacterial meningitis. Plague meningitis occurs almost exclusively in children.[115] It is unlikely to be a presenting form of plague for biologic weapon–induced disease, but it may be seen among cases of primary septicemic or pneumonic plague.

Pharyngeal Plague

Patients with pharyngeal plague can present as asymptomatic carriers of plague in the pharynx[15,24] or with symptoms of plague pharyngitis. These patients can present with cervical buboes, peritonsillar abscesses, or what appears to be uncomplicated bacterial tonsillitis. Similar to plague meningitis, this too would be an unlikely presentation for biologic weapon–induced disease, but it may be seen among cases of primary septicemic or pneumonic plague.

TABLE 133-1 Differential Diagnosis of Buboes

Cat-scratch disease	Much fewer systemic symptoms and possibility of detectable scratch distal to the bubo
Chancroid	Fewer systemic symptoms, little local pain, history of genital lesions and sexual contact
Tuberculous cervical lymphadenitis	Few systemic symptoms and little local pain
Streptococcal lymphadenitis	Significant systemic symptoms but not as severe as with plague, and the involved lymphadenopathy is not as tender
Tularemia	Much fewer systemic symptoms, and frequently a distal inoculation site can be identified
Lymphogranuloma venereum	Presence of genital lesions and history of sexual contact
Scrub typhus	Some degree of generalized lymphadenopathy, identifiable inoculation site, diffuse rash, limited geographic distribution

TREATMENT

Public health officials should be notified immediately of any suspected plague patient. If a bioterrorist event occurs, the agent may not be initially known or correctly identified, or multiple agents may be employed. Initial management of any suspected bioterrorism victim should include immediate isolation of the patient in a negative-pressure room (minimum six air exchanges per hour), strict universal precautions (gloves, gowns, N95 or N100 masks), and respiratory isolation. In pneumonic plague, bacilli are transmitted by large particle droplets (generally >5 μm) that can be generated by the infected patient during coughing, sneezing, or talking or during respiratory care procedures. When pneumonic plague is confirmed and other pathogens are ruled out, respiratory droplet precautions, patient isolation, and standard universal precautions should be maintained until the patient has completed 48 hours of appropriate antimicrobial therapy. Droplet precautions include a surgical-type mask, although some authors have raised concern that a higher level of respiratory protection is warranted.[116] Plague-infected patients should be placed in private rooms when possible. Patients with the same presumptive diagnosis (i.e., pneumonic plague) may be cohorted, however, when private rooms are not available. Movement and transport of patients on droplet precautions should be limited to that for essential medical purposes only. To minimize dispersal of droplets, a surgical-type mask should be placed on the patient when transport is necessary. All infectious waste and contaminated protective clothing should be disposed of properly in biohazard containers or sterilized in an appropriate manner.[8,14,116,117]

Treatment for the various forms of plague involves supportive cardiopulmonary management and the administration of antibiotics. Almost all of the research and published experience regarding the treatment of plague involves antibiotic administration. Despite optimal supportive care, the expected mortality for untreated pneumonic, septicemic, and meningitic plague is 100%. The expected survival rate for untreated bubonic plague is approximately 60%.[118]

High-efficiency particulate air filters are recommended for all exhaust vents and air recirculation systems servicing treatment areas for pneumonic plague cases. If the patient requires mechanical or bag-valve ventilation, all tube connections and fittings should be taped to avoid aerosolization of plague bacilli from a leaking or accidentally disconnected ventilation system. High-efficiency particulate air filters should be fitted to all ventilator and bag-valve exhaust ports.

There are no prospective clinical trials on antibiotic treatment of plague, and animal data are limited.[119–121] The recommendations that have been promulgated for the treatment of plague derive from consensus based on anecdotal, in vitro, and animal data. The recommendations described herein come from two major sources: The USAMRIID and the U.S. Working Group on Civilian Bio Defense (WGCB). The former is one of the major research laboratories in the world dealing with biologic weapon exposures and a LRN level D laboratory. The WGCB represents a group from major academic medical centers, government, the military, public health, research institutes, and emergency management institutions. WGCB recommendations are based on a comprehensive review of the medical literature and have been published in a major peer-reviewed journal.[19]

As with any biologic weapon, there is a military advantage to developing multiple drug–resistant strains. No such strains of *Y. pestis* are known to have been developed, although there have been reports that such organisms were developed in the *Biopreparat* biologic weapons laboratories of the former Soviet Union.[122] This chapter considers the spectrum of antimicrobial agents available for the treatment of plague syndromes and assesses their utility in various scenarios. Recommendations of USAMRIID and the WGCB are provided.

Aminoglycosides

STREPTOMYCIN

Used since 1948 in the treatment of plague, streptomycin traditionally has been considered to be the treatment of choice for most *Y. pestis* syndromes. Although never prospectively studied, observations by the CDC[123] and other authorities[36,61] are that streptomycin seems to dramatically reduce the mortality of plague syndromes when started in a timely fashion. The usually recommended dose is 30 mg/kg intramuscularly in two divided doses for a typical duration of 10 days.[14,107]

GENTAMICIN

Several publications have reported the successful use of gentamicin in the treatment of various forms of plague.[14,93,124,125] Gentamicin has the advantage of being widely available and can be administered once a day, which would simplify the management of cases in a mass-casualty situation. The WGCB views streptomycin and gentamicin as appropriate first-line agents, and the committee on infections of the American Academy of Pediatrics recommends similarly that gentamicin is a suitable alternative to streptomycin. In vitro antimicrobial susceptibility studies indicate that, at least in the laboratory, *Y. pestis* is sensitive to gentamicin. It also has been shown to be effective in an experimental study of *Y. pestis* infection in mice.[119] The typical 30-mg/kg parenteral dose of gentamicin is the same as that for streptomycin, although, as noted, it can be dosed on a once-a-day basis.

Tetracyclines

Y. pestis seems to be sensitive to the tetracyclines.[14] They have been used in plague treatment and prophylaxis, although they are generally considered to be primarily prophylactic agents. Numerous publications have supported the role of the tetracyclines as second-line agents for the treatment of plague syndromes.[14] The WGCB recommends that the tetracyclines be considered second-line agents for the treatment of pneumonic plague and be administered when gentamicin and streptomycin are not available or are contraindicated.[14] Publications from the USAMRIID indicate that in mild cases of bubonic plague, primary therapy with tetracyclines (2 g/day of tetracycline) is acceptable.[126] For sicker patients who have been treated with parenteral antibiotics, publications from the USAMRIID indicate that if the patient is stable after 5 days, he or she can be changed to an oral tetracycline for an additional 5 days.[126]

TETRACYCLINE

Although tetracycline's primary plague-related indication is for prophylaxis, it has been used successfully for treatment. Antibiotic susceptibility testing done during the 1991 plague outbreak in Tanzania found that the sensitivity of *Y. pestis* to tetracycline was similar to that of aminoglycosides. The recommended dose for prophylaxis is 500 mg orally four times a day for 7 days.[107]

DOXYCYCLINE

There are no published data on the efficacy of doxycycline for the treatment of plague in humans. Two studies have documented an in vitro susceptibility of *Y. pestis* similar to that of aminoglycosides.[127,128] In Madagascar, 13% of *Y. pestis* cases show, however, at least some degree of resistance to tetracycline.[129] The WGCD considers doxycycline preferable to tetracycline because of its superior absorption characteristics after oral administration, good tissue penetration, and relatively long half-life.[14] Three studies in mice showed the efficacy of doxycycline for the treatment and prophylaxis of plague.[128,130,131] Two additional studies, from one laboratory, failed to verify doxycycline's efficacy in the mouse model.[121,132] As Inglesby and colleagues[14] pointed out, however, the dose used in one of these studies was inadequate to expect efficacy. In the second study,[132] the mice were infected with 290,000 times the median lethal dose of *Y. pestis*, and any potential efficacy of doxycycline may have been masked.

Publications from USAMRIID recommend that the therapeutic dose of doxycycline for the treatment of plague should be 200 mg intravenously followed by 100 mg every 12 hours for 10 to 14 days. Their dosing recommendation for prophylaxis is 100 mg orally every 12 hours for 7 days.[107]

Fluoroquinolones

Fluoroquinolones have broad bactericidal activity against gram-positive and gram-negative aerobes. They have little activity against anaerobes. Most are absorbed well when taken orally, and they have a side-effect profile that renders them well tolerated. There are few data on fluoroquinolone use in the treatment of human plague. Fluoroquinolones are efficacious in animals, however.[68,121,122,132–135]

CIPROFLOXACIN

Two separate laboratories have reported the efficacy of ciprofloxacin in mouse models of pneumonic plague.[121,128,132] In these studies, ciprofloxacin seemed to have similar efficacy to that of aminoglycosides. Similar results have been reported for in vitro susceptibility tests.[14]

OFLOXACIN

Ofloxacin has been shown to be efficacious in the treatment of a mouse model of *Y. pestis* septicemia.[122] There are no data on its efficacy in humans.

LEVOFLOXACIN

The WGCD has pointed out that there are in vitro studies showing *Y. pestis* has a susceptibility to this agent similar to that of aminoglycosides or tetracyclines.[14]

Chloramphenicol

Chloramphenicol seems to be active against *Y. pestis*, and because of its ability to cross the blood-brain barrier, it is generally thought of as an agent of significant potential utility in the treatment of plague and meningitis. Recommendations from USAMRIID are to add chloramphenicol to the treatment regimens of patients who are hemodynamically unstable with plague infection.[107,126] There are no published studies formally supporting this recommendation, however. The recommended dose of chloramphenicol by USAMRIID is 1 g intravenously every 6 hours for 10 to 14 days.[107,126]

Sulfonamides

Representing the oldest class of systemically administered antibiotics, sulfonamides are active by virtue of their structural similarity to paraaminobenzoic acid. The latter is a precursor for the synthesis of folic acid, and organisms that are dependent on their own endogenous folate synthesis are sensitive to sulfonamides.

SULFATHIAZOLE

Sulfathiazole was used, with apparent success, in the treatment of pneumonic plague during the outbreak in Madagascar.[136]

SULFADIAZINE

Sulfadiazine is a biphenyl sulfa derivative that was reported to be successful in the treatment of plague in Vietnam. A report from the World Health Organization expert committee on plague concluded that sulfadiazine is efficacious in the treatment of bubonic plague but not of pneumonic plague.[137] In general, it was considered to be less effective than tetracycline.

SULFAMERAZINE

Sulfamerazine also has been reported to be effective for the treatment of bubonic plague in Vietnam.[138]

TRIMETHOPRIM-SULFAMETHOXAZOLE

Trimethoprim and sulfamethoxazole act synergistically in their effects on folate synthesis in sensitive bacteria. Worldwide, this drug combination is known as *co-trimoxazole*. The trimethoprim component of co-trimoxazole inhibits the reduction of dihydrofolate to tetrahydrofolate, the active form of folic acid (see Fig. 157-2). This combination has been used with apparent success in the treatment of bubonic and septicemic plague.[139] Based on the experience in Vietnam, however, it has seemed less efficacious than streptomycin.[138] The WGCD points out that co-trimoxazole is generally recommended to be only a second-line agent.

Cephalosporins

Ceftazidime, cefotetan, and cefazolin have relatively poor activity against *Y. pestis* infection in animals.[119] Ceftriaxone does seem to have efficacy, however, in the treatment of murine experimentally induced septicemic plague.[122]

Rifampin

Studies on murine experimental pneumonic plague have failed to show significant activity of rifampin.

Aztreonam

Based on studies of experimentally induced murine pneumonic plague, aztreonam does not seem to be highly active.

Contained-Casualty Situation

The recommended treatment of cases in a contained-casualty situation is with parenteral streptomycin or gentamicin. As noted earlier, USAMRIID recommends the addition of chloramphenicol to hemodynamically unstable patients. It is further recommended by USAMRIID that treatment be carried out for a minimum of 10 days or 3 to 4 days after the resolution of clinical signs, whichever is longest.[126]

Mass-Casualty Situation

Given the practicalities of treating mass casualties, the WGCD recommends that primarily oral treatment should be given. Recommended agents are doxycycline, tetracycline, and ciprofloxacin.

Bubonic Plague

USAMRIID recommendations call for the use of streptomycin, tetracycline, chloramphenicol, or gentamicin for the treatment of bubonic plague.[126] Based on experience in Vietnam, untreated bubonic plague is expected to have a 60% mortality.[119]

Pneumonic Plague

The experience in Vietnam has shown that untreated pneumonic plague has 100% mortality. This mortality could be reduced by antibiotic therapy, but only if treatment is started within 18 hours of the onset of symptoms.[119]

WGCD recommends that parenteral aminoglycosides be first-line treatment against pneumonic plague, with tetracycline or doxycycline being used as a second-line agent. Co-trimoxazole is not generally recommended for this form of the disease.

Consensus guidelines recommend that disposable surgical masks should be used to prevent droplet spread of plague.[140,141] The WGCD recommends that this practice be continued until at least 48 hours of antibiotic therapy and clinical improvement is obvious.

Y. pestis is not a spore-forming organism and does not persist for long periods in the environment. The World Health Organization, cognizant that plague could be spread as an aerosol of droplets, estimated that these could remain infectious for 1 hour as an aerosol.[142]

Septicemic Plague

Based on the experience of Vietnam, septicemic plague is uniformly fatal if untreated.[119] Although there are no formal recommendations for specific antibiotic therapy of septicemic

plague, USAMRIID publications indicate that streptomycin should be the first-line agent, with gentamicin being an acceptable alternative. Patients who are hemodynamically unstable also should receive intravenous chloramphenicol (50 to 75 mg/kg/day in four to five doses).[126] A critically ill patient with septicemic plague and peripheral gangrene was treated successfully with ciprofloxacin. Peripheral gangrene of this patient's feet was managed with the use of sympathetic blockade; the patient's toes seem to have been saved by this approach.[143]

Postexposure Prophylaxis

The WGCD guidelines call for parenteral antibiotic therapy for anyone developing a new cough or fever greater than 38.5°C in the setting of a pneumonic plague outbreak.[14] In a mass-casualty scenario, oral antibiotic therapy could be substituted.[14]

The WGCD recommends that asymptomatic persons who have been within 2 m of a patient with pneumonic plague should receive postexposure prophylaxis with doxycycline for 7 days. Other potential agents that can be used include tetracycline, a sulfonamide, a chloramphenicol, and a fluoroquinolone. If there is belief that there has been exposure through the dissemination of an aerosol as in a biologic weapon attack, potentially exposed individuals also should be treated.

The recommended dose of doxycycline is 100 mg twice a day. The recommended prophylactic dose of tetracycline is 15 to 30 mg/kg/day in four divided doses, also for 7 days. This works out to be 1 to 2 g/day for an adult. Patients given prophylaxis with a sulfonamide should receive co-trimoxazole in a dose of 40 mg sulfa/kg/day taken orally in two divided doses, also for 7 days.

SPECIAL POPULATIONS

Pediatric Patients

The WGCD recommends that the first-line agents for treatment of plague be streptomycin or gentamicin.[14] In a mass-casualty setting, doxycycline could be used as an alternative. There is concern about using tetracycline in children younger than 8 years old because of potential discoloration of teeth and an adverse effect on skeletal development. The American Academy of Pediatrics Committee on Infectious Diseases reported, however, that in their opinion tetracycline is safe to use in children older than age 8.

The AAP Committee on Infectious Diseases also recommends the use of chloramphenicol in children who are older than 2 years of age. Younger children may be at risk for the gray syndrome, which is a potentially fatal reaction after exposure to high doses of this agent. The gray syndrome has been reported primarily in premature infants and neonates. This syndrome is a multisystem disease causing the development of an ashen or gray hue to the skin.

The USAMRIID recommendations for pediatric patients younger than age 8 who have been exposed to pneumonic plague or plague aerosols are for co-trimoxazole at a dose of 20 mg sulfa/kg/day, given twice a day for 7 days. The WGCD endorses the American Public Health Association recommendation that infants with tachypnea who live in a community in which there is a pneumonic plague epidemic also are candidates for treatment.

Pregnant and Breast-feeding Patients

The WGCD recommends that gentamicin be the drug of choice for pregnant women with pneumonic plague. It is further recommended that streptomycin not be given in pregnancy because of the possibility of congenital deafness. The WGCD recommends that tetracycline be avoided in pregnancy because of adverse skeletal effects. Citing a large epidemiologic study indicating that there was no demonstrable fetal risk associated with taking doxycycline in pregnancy, the WGCD recommends this agent as a second-line agent. The WGCD also recommends doxycycline for postexposure prophylaxis, although USAMRIID recommends that pregnant women receive co-trimoxazole at the same dose as recommended for children (see earlier). Because of concern for the lack of efficacy of co-trimoxazole in pneumonic plague, the WGCD recommends postexposure prophylaxis of pregnant women with a fluoroquinolone,[14] citing the consensus report of the International Society of Chemotherapy Commission on the use of fluoroquinolones in children[144] that these agents have been used to treat infections in pediatric patients. Intravenous tetracycline should not be used in pregnant women because of the possibility of hepatotoxicity.

The WGCD recommends that the best treatment for breast-feeding women is to treat the mother and infant with the most appropriate antibiotic for the infant. This typically would be gentamicin, but doxycycline would be used if there was a mass-casualty scenario. WGCD recommends that fluoroquinolones could be used as second-line agents.

Hospital Personnel

Although person-to-person spread of pneumonic plague via droplet aerosols is theoretically possible, it is rare.[14,116] The Hospital Advisory Committee for Infectious Control recommends that the patient and staff should wear surgical masks, and these precautions should be continued until there are clear-cut signs of objective clinical improvement, and the patient has been on antibiotics for at least 48 hours.[105,137,140,141] The USAMRIID isolation recommendations are more stringent, recommending that patients with all forms of plague should be isolated for 48 hours and that for patients with pneumonic plague this must be continued until at least 4 days of antibiotic therapy.[126]

REFERENCES

1. Ranga S, Gulati I, Pandey J, et al: Plague—a review. Indian J Pathol Microbiol 38:213–222, 1995.
2. Roffey R, Tegnell A, Elgh F: Biological warfare in a historical perspective. Clin Microbiol Infect 8:450–454, 2002.
3. Wheelis M: Biological warfare at the 1346 siege of Caffa. Emerg Infect Dis 8:971–979, 2002.
4. Harris SH: Factories of Death: Japanese Biological Warfare, 1932–45, and the American Cover-up. London, Routledge, 1994.
5. Alibek K: Biohazard. New York, Random House, 1998.
6. Perry RD, Fetherston JD: *Yersinia pestis*: Etiologic agent of plague. Clin Microbiol Rev 10:35–66, 1997.
7. Campbell GL: Plague in India: A new warning from an old nemesis. Ann Intern Med 122:151–153, 1995.
8. Dennis DT, Gage KL, Gratz N, et al: World Health Organization Plague Manual: Epidemiology, Distribution, Surveillance, and Control. WHO/CDS/CSR/EDC/99.2. Geneva, World Health Organization, 1999.
9. Centers for Disease Control: Human plague—United States, 1983. MMWR Morb Mortal Wkly Rep 32:329–330, 1983.
10. Tenborg M, Davis B, Smith D, et al: Fatal human plague—Arizona and Colorado, 1996. MMWR Morb Mortal Wkly Rep 46:617–620, 1997.
11. Werner SB, Murray R, Reilly K, et al: Human plague—United States, 1993–1994. MMWR Morb Mortal Wkly Rep 43:242–246, 1994.
12. Opulski A, MacNeill E, Rosales C, et al: Plague pneumonia—Arizona, 1992. MMWR Morb Mortal Wkly Rep 41:737–739, 1992.
13. McGovern TW, Christopher GW, Eitzen E: Cutaneous manifestations of biological warfare and related threat agents. Arch Dermatol 135:311–322, 1999.
14. Inglesby TV, Dennis DT, Henderson DA, et al: Plague as a biological weapon. JAMA 283:2281–2290, 2000.
15. Chang M-H, Glynn MK, Groceclose SL: Endemic, notifiable bioterrorism-related diseases, United States, 1992–1999. Emerg Infect Dis 9:556–564, 2003.
16. Cunha BA: Anthrax, tularemia, plague, ebola, or smallpox as agents of bioterrorism: Recognition in the emergency department. Clin Microbiol Infect 8:489–503, 2002.
17. Barbera J, Macintyre A, Gostin L, et al: Large-scale quarantine following biological terrorism in the United States: Scientific examination, logistic and legal limits, and possible consequences. JAMA 286:2711–2717, 2001.
18. Gage KL, Dennis DT, Orloski KA, et al: Cases of cat-associated plague in the western United States, 1977–1998. Clin Infect Dis 30:893–900, 2000.
19. Weniger BG, Warren AJ, Forseth V, et al: Human bubonic plague transmitted by a domestic cat scratch. JAMA 251:927–928, 1984.
20. Werner SB, Weidmer CE, Nelson BC, et al: Primary plague pneumonia contracted from a domestic cat at South Lake Tahoe, Calif. JAMA 251:929–931, 1984.
21. Cleri DJ, Vernaleo JR, Lombardi LJ, et al: Plague pneumonia disease caused by *Yersinia pestis*. Semin Respir Infect 12:12–23, 1997.
22. Inglesby T, Grossman R, O'Toole T: A plague on your city: Observations from TOPOFF. Biodefense Q 2, 2000.
23. Gross L: How the plague bacillus and its transmission through fleas were discovered: Reminiscences of my years at the Pasteur Institute in Paris. Proc Natl Acad Sci U S A 92:7609–7611, 1995.
24. Butler T: *Yersinia* infections: Centennial of the discovery of the plague bacillus. Clin Infect Dis 19:655–663, 1994.
25. Rose LJ, Donlan R, Banerjee SN, et al: Survival of *Yersinia pestis* on environmental surfaces. Appl Environ Microbiol 69:2166–2171, 2003.
26. Cornelis GR: Molecular and cell biology aspects of plague. Proc Natl Acad Sci U S A 97:8778–8783, 2000.
27. Brubaker RR: Factors promoting acute and chronic diseases caused by Yersiniae. Clin Microbiol Rev 4:309–324, 1991.
28. Ferber DM, Brubaker RR: Plasmids in *Yersinia pestis*. Infect Immun 31:839–841, 1981.
29. Brubaker RR: The genus *Yersinia*: Biochemistry and genetics of virulence. Curr Top Microbiol Immunol 57:111–158, 1972.
30. Cornelis GR, Boland A, Boyd AP, et al: The virulence plasmid of *Yersinia*, an antihost genome. Microbiol Mol Biol Rev 62:1315–1352, 1998.
31. Burrows TW, Bacon GA: The basis of virulence in *Pasteurella pestis*: An antigen determining virulence. Br J Exp Pathol 37:481–493, 1956.
32. Hu P, Elliott J, McCready P, et al: Structural organization of virulence-associated plasmids of *Yersinia pestis*. J Bacteriol 180:5192–5202, 1998.
33. Parkhill J, Wren BW, Thomson NR, et al: Genome sequence of *Yersinia pestis*, the causative agent of plague. Nature 413:523–527, 2001.
34. Straley SC, Skrzypek E, Plano GV, et al: Yops of *Yersinia* spp: Pathogenesis for humans. Infect Immun 61:3105–3110, 1993.
35. Zahorchak RJ, Charnetzky WT, Little RV, et al: Consequences of Ca^{2+} deficiency on macromolecular synthesis and adenylate energy charge in *Yersinia pestis*. J Bacteriol 139:792–799, 1979.
36. Cornelis GR: Yesinia type III secretion: Send in the effectors. J Cell Biol 158:401–408, 2002.
37. Koornhof HJ, Smego RA, Nicol M: Yersiniosis: II. The pathogenesis of *Yersinia* infections. Eur J Clin Microbiol Infect Dis 18:87–112, 1999.

38. Cornelis GR: Minireview: The *Yersinia* deadly kiss. J Bacteriol 180:5495–5504, 1998.
39. Hueck CJ: Type III protein secretion systems in bacterial pathogens of animals and plants. Microbiol Mol Biol Rev 62:379–433, 1998.
40. Galán JE, Collmer A: Type III secretion machines: Bacterial devices for protein delivery into host cells. Science 284:1322–1328, 1999.
41. Tardy F, Homblé F, Neyt C, et al: Yersinia enterocolitica type III secretion-translocation system: Channel formation by secreted Yops. EMBO J 18:6793–6799, 1999.
42. Hoiczyk E, Blobel G: Polymerization of a single protein of the pathogen *Yersinia enterocolitica* into needles punctures eukaryotic cells. Proc Natl Acad Sci U S A 98:4669–4674, 2001.
43. Woestyn S, Allaoui A, Wattiau P, et al: YscN, the putative energizer of the *Yersinia* Yop secretion machinery. J Bacteriol 176:1561–1569, 1994.
44. Neyt C, Cornelis GR: Insertion of a Yop translocation pore into the macrophage plasma membrane by *Yersinia enterocolitica*: Requirement for translocators YopB and YopD, but not LcrG. Mol Microbiol 22:971–981, 1999.
45. Iriarte M, Sory M-P, Boland A, et al: TyeA, a protein involved in control of Yop release and in translocation of *Yersinia* Yop effectors. EMBO J 17:1907–1918, 1998.
46. Silhavy TJ: Death by lethal injection. Science 278:1085–1086, 1997.
47. Wattiau P, Bernier B, Deslée P, et al: Individual chaperones required for Yop secretion Yersinia. Proc Natl Acad Sci U S A 91:10493–10497, 1994.
48. Neyt C, Cornelis G: Role of SycD, the chaperone of the *Yersinia* Yop translocators YopB and YopD. Mol Microbiol 31:143–156, 1999.
49. Fowler JM, Brubaker RR: Physiologic basis of the low calcium response in *Yersinia pestis*. Infect Immun 62:5234–5241, 1994.
50. Matson JS, Nilles ML: Interaction of the *Yersinia pestis* type III regulatory proteins LcrG and LcrV occurs at the hydrophobic interface. BMC Microbiol 2:16–28, 2002.
51. Sarker MR, Sory M-P, Boyd AP, et al: LcrG is required for efficient translocation of *Yersinia* Yop effector proteins into eukaryotic cells. Infect Immun 66:2976–2979, 1998.
52. Nilles ML, Fields KA, Straley SC: The V antigen of *Yersinia pestis* regulates Yop vectorial targeting as well as Yop secretion through effects on YopB and LcrG. J Bacteriol 179:1307–1316, 1998.
53. May RC, Machesky LM: Phagocytosis and the actin skeleton. J Cell Sci 114:1061–1077, 2001.
54. Gruenheid S, Finlay BB: Microbial pathogenesis and cytoskeletal function. Nature 422:775–781, 2003.
55. Iriarte M, Cornelis GR: YopT, a new *Yersinia* Yop effector protein, affects the cytoskeleton of host cells. Mol Microbiol 29:915–929, 1998.
56. Fällman M, Persson C, Wolf-Watz H: Yersinia proteins that target host cell signaling pathways. J Clin Invest 99:1153–1157, 1997.
57. Grosdent N, Maridonneau-Parini I, Sory M-P, et al: Role of Yops and adhesions in resistance of *Yersinia enterocolitica* to phagocytosis. Infect Immun 70:4165–4176, 2002.
58. Boland A, Cornelis GR: Role of YopP in suppression of tumor necrosis factor alpha release by macrophages during *Yersinia* infection. Infect Immun 66:1878–1884, 1998.
59. Nakajima R, Brubaker RR: Association between virulence of *Yersinia pestis* and suppression of gamma interferon and tumor necrosis factor alpha. Infect Immun 61:23–31, 1993.
60. Monack DM, Mecsas J, Ghori N, et al: *Yersinia* signals macrophages to undergo apoptosis and YopJ is necessary for this cell death. Proc Natl Acad Sci U S A 94:10385–10390, 1997.
61. Orth K, Palmer LE, Bao ZQ, et al: Inhibition of the mitogen-activated protein kinase superfamily by a *Yersinia* effector. Science 285:1920–1923, 1999.
62. Donnenberg MS: Pathogenic strategies of enteric bacteria. Nature 406:768–774, 2000.
63. Ruckdeschel K, Harb A, Roggenkamp A, et al: Yersinia enterocolitica impairs activation of transcription factor NF-κB: involvement in the induction of programmed cell death and in the suppression of the macrophage TNF-α production. J Exp Med 187:1069–1079, 1998.
64. Mills SD, Boland A, Sory M-P, et al: *Yersinia enterocolitica* induces apoptosis in macrophages by a process requiring functional type III secretion and translocation mechanisms and involving YopP, presumably acting as an effector protein. Proc Natl Acad Sci U S A 94:12638–12643, 1997.
65. Greenberg S, Chang P, Silverstein SC: Tyrosine phosphorylation of the χ subunit of Fcχ receptors, p72^{syk}, and paxillin during Fc receptor-mediated phagocytosis in macrophages. J Biol Chem 269:3879–3902, 1994.

66. Bliska JB, Black DS: Inhibition of the Fc-mediated oxidative burst in macrophages by the *Yersinia enterocolitica* tyrosine phosphatase. Infect Immun 63:681–685, 1995.
67. Von Pawel-Rammingen U, Telepnev MV, Schmidt G, et al: GAP activity of the *Yersinia* YopE cytotoxin specifically targets the Rho pathway: a mechanism for the disruption of actin microfilament structure. Mol Microbiol 36:737–748, 2000.
68. Rosqvist R, Forsberg A, Wolf-Watz H: Intracellular targeting of the *Yersinia* YopE cytotoxin in mammalian cells induces actin microfilament disruption. Infect Immun 59:4562–4569, 1991.
69. Skrzypek E, Cowan C, Straley SC: Targeting of the *Yersinia pestis* YopM protein into HeLa cells and intracellular trafficking to the nucleus. Mol Microbiol 30:1051–1065, 1998.
70. Nemeth J, Straley SC: Effect of *Yersinia pestis* YopM on experimental plague. Infect Immun 65:924–930, 1997.
71. Andrews GP, Heath DG, Anderson GW, et al: Fraction 1 capsular antigen (F1) purification from *Yersinia pestis* CO92 and from an *Escherichia coli* recombinant strain and efficacy against lethal plague challenge. Infect Immun 64:2180–2187, 1996.
72. Du Y, Rosqvist R, Forsberg Å: Role of Fraction 1 of *Yersinia pestis* in inhibition of phagocytosis. Infect Immun 70:1453–1460, 2002.
73. Tito MA, Miller J, Griffin KF, et al: Macromolecular organization of the *Yersinia pestis* capsular F1 antigen: Insights from time-of-flight spectroscopy. Protein Sci 10:2408–2413, 2001.
74. Cavanaugh D: Specific effect of temperature upon transmission of the plague bacillus by the oriental rat flea, *Xenopsylla cheopis*. Am J Trop Med Hyg 20:264–272, 1971.
75. Abramov VM, Vasiliev AM, Khlebnikov VS, et al: Structural and functional properties of *Yersinia pestis* Caf1 capsular antigen and their possible role in fulminant development of primary pneumonic plague. J Proteome Res 1:307–315, 2002.
76. Cowan C, Jones HA, Kaya YH, et al: Invasion of epithelial cells by *Yersinia pestis*: Evidence for a *Y. pestis*-specific invasion. Infect Immun 68:4523–4530, 2000.
77. Straley SC: Adhesins in *Yersinia pestis*. Trends Microbiol 1:285–286, 1993.
78. Mcdonough KA, Falkow S: A *Yersinia-pestis*-specific DNA fragment encodes temperature-dependent coagulase and fibrinolysin-associated phenotypes. Mol Microbiol 3:767–775, 1989.
79. Kienle Z, Emody L, Svanborg C, et al: Adhesive properties conferred by the plasminogen activator of *Yersinia pestis*. J Gen Microbiol 138:1679–1687, 1992.
80. Lähteenmäki K, Virkola R, Sarén A, et al: Expression of plasminogen activator Pla of *Yersinia pestis* enhances bacterial attachment to the mammalian extracellular matrix. Infect Immun 66:5755–5762, 1998.
81. Sodeinde OA, Subrahmanyam YV, Stark K, et al: A surface protease and the invasive character of plague. Science 258:1004–1007, 1992.
82. Lähteenmäki K, Kuusela P, Korhonem TK: Bacterial plasminogen activators and receptors. FEMS Microbiol Rev 25:531–552, 2001.
83. Kukkonen M, Lähteenmäki K, Suomalainen M, et al: Protein regions important for plasminogen activation and inactivation of α$_2$-antiplasmin in the surface protease Pla of *Yersinia pestis*. Mol Microbiol 40:1097–1111, 2001.
84. Matsushima K, Taguchi M, Kovacs EJ, et al: Intracellular localization of human monocyte associated interleukin 1 (IL 1) activity and release of biologically active IL 1 from monocytes by trypsin and plasmin. J Immunol 136:2883–2891, 1986.
85. Johnson B, Almas J, Salkin M, et al: Plague pneumonia—California. MMWR Morb Mortal Wkly Rep 3:481–483, 1984.
86. Heddurshetti R, Pumpradit W, Lutwick LI: Pulmonary manifestations of bioterrorism. Curr Infect Dis Rep 3:249–257, 2001.
87. Finegold MJ, Petery JJ, Berendt RF: Studies on the pathogenesis of plague: Blood coagulation and tissue responses of Macca mulatto following exposure to aerosols of *Pasteurella pestis*. Am J Pathol 53:99–114, 1968.
88. Finegold MJ: Pathogenesis of plague: A review of plague deaths in the United States during the last decade. Am J Med 45:549–554, 1968.
89. Straley SC, Harmon PA: *Yersinia pestis* grows within phagolysosomes in mouse peritoneal macrophages. Infect Immun 45:655–659, 1984.
90. Cavanaugh DC, Randall R: The role of multiplication of *Pasteurella pestis* in mononuclear phagocytes in the pathogenesis of flea-borne plague. J Immunol 84:348–363, 1959.
91. Watson RP, Blanchard TW, Mense MG, et al: Histopathology of experimental plague in cats. Vet Pathol 38:165–172, 2001.

92. Simonet M, Richard S, Berche P: Electron microscope evidence for in vivo extracellular localization of *Yersinia pseudotuberculosis* harboring the pYV plasmid. Infect Immun 58:841–845, 1990.

93. Crook LD, Tempest B: Plague: A clinical review of 27 cases. Arch Intern Med 152:1253–1256, 1992.

94. Reisner BS, Straley SC: *Yersinia pestis* YopM: Thrombin binding and overexpression. Infect Immun 60:5242–5252, 1992.

95. Leung KY, Reisner BS, Straley SC: YopM inhibits platelet aggregation and is necessary for virulence of *Yersinia pestis* in mice. Infect Immun 58:3262–3271, 1990.

96. Leung KY, Straley SC: The yopM gene of *Yersinia pestis* encodes a released protein having homology with the human platelet surface protein GPUba. J Bacteriol 171:4623–1632, 1989.

97. Ten Cate H: Pathophysiology if disseminated intravascular coagulation in sepsis. Crit Care Med 28(Suppl):S9–S11, 2000.

98. Butler T: A clinical study of bubonic plague: Observations of the 1970 Vietnam epidemic with emphasis on coagulation studies, skin histology and electrocardiograms. Am J Med 53:268–276, 1972.

99. Butler T, Bell WR, Linh NN, et al: *Yersinia pestis* infection in Vietnam: I. Clinical and hematologic aspects. J Infect Dis 129(Suppl):S78–S84, 1974.

100. Galimand M, Guiyoule A, Gerbaud G, et al: Multidrug resistance in *Yersinia pestis* mediated by a transferable plasmid. N Engl J Med 337:677–680, 1997.

101. Gage KL, Dennis DT, Tsai TF: Prevention of plague: Recommendations of the Advisory Committee on Immunization Practices (ACIP). MMWR Morb Mortal Wkly Rep 45(RR-14):1–15, 1997.

102. Hull HF, Montes JM, Mann JM: Plague masquerading as gastrointestinal illness. West J Med 145:485–487, 1986.

103. Mann JF, Hull HF, Schmid GP, et al: Plague and the peripheral smear. JAMA 251:953, 1984.

104. Burmeister RW, Tigertt WD, Overhold EL: Laboratory-acquired pneumonic plague. Ann Intern Med 56:1–26, 1962.

105. Centers for Disease Control and Prevention: Prevention of plague: Recommendations of the Advisory Committee on Immunizations Practice (ACIP). MMWR Morb Mortal Wkly Rep 45:1–15, 1996.

106. Morse S, McDade J: Recommendations for working with pathogenic bacteria. Methods Enzymol 235:1–26, 1994.

107. Franz DR, Jahrling PG, Friedlander AM, et al: Clinical recognition and management of patients exposed to biological warfare agents. JAMA 278:399–411, 1997.

108. Williams JE, Gentry MK, Braden CA, et al: Use of an enzyme-linked immunosorbent assay to measure antigenaemia during acute plague. Bull WHO 62:463–466, 1984.

109. Williams JE, Arntzen L, Tyndal GL, et al. Application of enzyme immunoassays for the confirmation of clinically suspect plague in Namibia. Bull WHO 64:745–752, 1986.

110. Chanteau S, Rahalison L, Ralafiarisoa L, et al: Development and testing of a rapid diagnostic test for bubonic and pneumonic plague. Lancet 361:211–216, 2003.

111. Ratsitorahine M, Chanteau S, Rahalison L: Epidemiological diagnostic aspects of the outbreak of pneumonic plague in Madagascar. Lancet 355:111–113, 2000.

112. Hinnebusch J, Schwan TG: New method for plague surveillance using polymerase chain reaction to detect *Yersinia pestis* in fleas. J Clin Microbiol 31:1511–1514, 1993.

113. Welty TK: Plague. Am Fam Physician 33:159–164, 1986.

114. Alsofrom DJ, Mettler FA Jr, Mann JM: Radiographic manifestations of plague in New Mexico, 1975–1980: Review of 42 proved cases. Radiology 139:561–565, 1981.

115. Becker TM, Poland JD, Quan TJ, et al: Plague meningitis: A retrospective analysis of cases reported in the United States 1970–1979. West J Med 147:554–557, 1987.

116. Nolte KB, Levison ME, Inglesby TV, et al: Safety precautions to limit exposure from plague-infected patients (Letters). JAMA 284:1648–1649, 2000.

117. Garner JS: Hospital infection control practices advisory committee guideline for isolation precautions in hospitals. Infect Control Hosp Epidemiol 17:53–80, 1996.

118. Legters LJ, Cottingham AJ Jr, Hunter DH: Clinical and epidemiologic notes on a defined outbreak of plague in Vietnam. Am J Trop Med Hyg 19:639–652, 1970.

119. Byrne WR, Welkos SL, Pitt ML, et al: Antibiotic treatment of experimental pneumonic plague in mice. Antimicrob Agents Chemother 42:675–681, 1998.

120. Wong JD, Barash JR, Sandfort RF, et al: Susceptibilities of *Yersinia pestis* strains to 12 antimicrobial agents. Antimicrob Agents Chemother 44:1995–1996, 2000.

121. Russell P, Eley SM, Green M, et al: Efficacy of doxycycline and ciprofloxacin against experimental *Yersinia pestis* infection. J Antimicrob Chemother 41:301–305, 1998.

122. Hughes J: Nation's Public Health Infrastructure Regarding Epidemics and Bioterrorism (Congressional Testimony). Washington, DC, Appropriations Committee, US Senate, June 2, 1998.

123. Centers for Disease Control and Prevention. Fatal human plague. MMWR Morb Mortal Wkly Rep 278:380–382, 1997.

124. Wong TW: Plague in a pregnant patient. Trop Doct 16:187–188, 1986.

125. Welty TK, Grabman J, Kompare E, et al: Nineteen cases of plague in Arizona. West J Med 142:641–646, 1985.

126. McGovern TW, Friedlander AM: Plague. In Sidell FR, Takafuji ET, Franz DR (eds): Medical Aspects of Chemical and Biological Warfare. Falls Church, VA, Office of the Surgeon General, US Army, 1997, pp 479–502.

127. Smith MD, Vinh SX, Hoa NT, et al: In vitro antimicrobial susceptibilities of strains of *Yersinia pestis*. Antimicrob Agents Chemother 39:2153–2154, 1995.

128. Bonacorsi SP, Scavizzi MR, Guiyoule A, et al: Assessment of a fluoroquinolone, three B-lactams, two aminoglycosides, and a cycline in the treatment of murine *Yersinia pestis* infection. Antimicrob Agents Chemother 38:481–486, 1994.

129. Rasoamanana B, Coulanges P, Michel P, et al: Sensitivity of *Yersinia pestis* to antibiotics: 277 strains isolated in Madagascar between 1926 and 1989. Arch Inst Pasteur Madagascar 56:37–53, 1989.

130. Makarovskaia LN, Shcherbaniuk AL, Ryzhkova VV, et al: Effectiveness of doxycycline in experimental plague. Antibiot Khimioter 38:48–50, 1993.

131. Samokhodkina ED, Ryzhko IVM, Shcherbaniuk AI, et al: Doxycycline in the prevention of experimental plague induced by plague microbe variants. Antibiot Khimioter 37:26–28, 1992.

132. Russell P, Eley SM, Bell DL, et al: Doxycycline or ciprofloxacin prophylaxis and therapy against experimental *Y. pestis* infection in mice. J Antimicrob Chemother 37:769–774, 1996.

133. Ehrenkranz NF, Meyer KF: Studies on immunization against plague: VIII. Study of three immunizing preparations in protection primates against pneumonic plague. J Infect Dis 96:138–144, 1955.

134. Speck RS, Wolochow H: Studies on the experimental epidemiology of respiratory infections: VIII. Experimental pneumonic plague in *Macacus rhesus*. J Infect Dis 100:58–68, 1957.

135. Conrad FG, LeCocq FR, Krain R: A recent epidemic of plague in Vietnam. Arch Intern Med 3:193–198, 1968.

136. Brygoo ER, Gonon M: Une epidemie de peste pulmonaire dans le Nor-Est de Madagascar. Bull Soc Pathol Exot 51:47–66, 1958.

137. WHO Expert Committee on Plague: Third Report. Technical Report Series 447. Geneva, World Health Organization, 1970.

138. Butler TJ, Levin J, Linh NN, et al: *Yersinia pestis* infection in Vietnam. J Infect Dis 133:493–499, 1976.

139. Nguyen VI, Nguyen DDH, Pham VD, et al: Peste bubonique et septicemique traitee avec success par du trimethoprime-suylfamethoxazole. Bull Soc Pathol Exot 769–779, 1972.

140. American Public Health Association: Plague In Benenson AS (ed): Control of Communicable Diseases Manual. Washington, DC, American Public Health Association, 1995, pp 353–358.

141. Garner JS: Guidelines for isolation precautions in hospitals: Hospital infection Control Practices Advisory Committee. Infect Control Hosp Epidemiol 17:53–80, 1996.

142. World Health Organization: Health Aspects of Chemical and Biological Weapons. Geneva, World Health Organization, 1970, pp 98–109.

143. Kuberski T, Robinson L, Schurgin A: A case of plague successfully treated with ciprofloxacin and sympathetic blockade for treatment of gangrene. Clin Infect Dis 36:521–523, 2003.

144. Consensus Report of the International Society of Chemotherapy Commission: Use of fluoroquinolones in pediatrics. Pediatr Infect Dis J 14:1–9, 1995.

CHAPTER 134A

Smallpox

Edward W. Cetaruk

Historically, smallpox has been responsible for more human deaths that any other single pathogen. It has affected nearly every culture, in all geographic regions of the world, over many centuries. Among the many potential biologic agents that have been weaponized or are amenable to weaponization, it ranks as one of the most worrisome. The biologic agent characteristics, weaponization process, and environmental conditions necessary to carry out an effective biologic weapon attack are discussed in detail in the introductory section of Chapter 132. Briefly stated, the causative agent of smallpox, variola virus, makes an effective biologic weapon for the following reasons: (1) Variola virus is infectious via aerosol exposure; (2) smallpox vaccination has been discontinued, leaving the general population susceptible to infection; (3) clinical inexperience of health care providers, limited availability of vaccine, and lack of effective antiviral medications limit therapeutic options; (4) infection causes severe morbidity and mortality; (5) smallpox is extremely communicable; and (6) its reputation as one of the most feared diseases of humankind makes it an effective terrorist agent. Efforts such as renewed production of vaccine and health care education are under way to mitigate some of these factors.

As with many of the viral biologic warfare agents, smallpox is difficult to weaponize in large quantities. The former Soviet Union's biologic weapons program, *Biopreparat*, succeeded in this endeavor, however, developing the capacity to produce 200 metric tons of smallpox per year.[1] This program is thought to be responsible for a smallpox outbreak in Aralsk, Kazakhstan, a small city that was downwind from Vozrozhdeniye Island in the Aral Sea, where *Biopreparat* conducted open-air tests of its biologic weapons.[2] More concerning, however, is that the demise of the Soviet Union and *Biopreparat* with it has made their weaponization expertise and possibly even variola virus potentially available to terrorist entities around the world. For these reasons, critical care clinicians must be able to recognize that a bioterrorist attack has taken place, what agents have been employed, and how to respond. Still more crucial, clinicians must recognize cases involving highly contagious agents, such as plague (*Yersinia pestis*) (see Chapter 133) and smallpox (variola virus).

MICROBIOLOGY

Variola virus is a member of the family Poxiviridae, subfamily Chordopoxvirinae, genus *Orthopoxvirus*. *Orthopoxvirus* also includes vaccinia virus, monkeypox, cowpox, ectromelia, rabbitpox, raccoonpox, camelpox, buffalopox, taterapox, and

Uasin Gishu disease.[3] Among this group, variola, vaccinia, cowpox, and monkeypox viruses can infect humans. Although variola has a restricted host range under experimental laboratory conditions, including monkeys, its only natural host is humans, and it has no animal reservoir. This fact made the worldwide eradication of smallpox by the containment and vaccination program of the World Health Organization successful.[3] Although its common name, *chickenpox*, suggests that varicella virus belongs in the poxvirus family, it is a herpesvirus.

Variola virus strains traditionally have been classified as variola major and variola minor on the basis of clinicoepidemiologic criteria, such as the severity of the outbreak, but strains also can be differentiated by laboratory methods.[4] Major and minor strains typically produce case-fatality rates of 30% to 40% and less than 1%, respectively.[5] Recognized variola minor strains include the alastrim, amass, and kaffir strains. A DNA sequencing study compared the genome of an alastrim strain of variola isolated from skin lesions on a patient in Sao Paulo during a mild smallpox outbreak in 1966 with two strains from variola major outbreaks in India in 1967 and Bangladesh in 1975 and a vaccinia virus strain from Copenhagen.[6] The alastrim (variola minor) strain genome sequence was 98.24% and 98.02%, identical to the variola major strains from India (IND) and Bangladesh (BSH). This study shows that a small yet crucial amount of genomic genotype may determine phenotype; in the case of smallpox, this is seen in the severity of the clinical illness. It is unlikely, however, that a single change in a single gene corresponds to the milder course of variola minor smallpox, but rather that a variety of DNA mutations or substitutions that produce modified gene protein products affect the ultimate virulence of the strain.

A comparison of open reading frames showed that the alastrim strain contained many truncated interrupted variants of longer ones found in variola major and that these open reading frames were truncated variants of open reading frames found in vaccinia and cowpox viruses. This finding suggests that the variola minor strain likely derived from variola major, and variola major likely derived from a "precursor" virus, such as cowpox.[7] These relationships underscore the close genetic overlap found within the orthopox genus.

Variola virus has one of the largest viral genomes known. It has a linear, double-stranded DNA genome 186 kb in length with its ends closed by terminal hairpin loops.[7] The genome is associated with at least four proteins, forming DNA-protein globular structures within the virus core, and is organized into a nucleosome. The genomes of vaccinia (Copenhagen strain,

191,636 bp) and several strains of smallpox (IND-1967, 185,578 bp, and BSH-1975, 186,102 bp) have been completely sequenced and coded for 187 proteins.[3] Of these proteins, 150 are shared by variola and vaccinia virus. The remaining 37 are variola-specific proteins. The variola virus genome has a large conserved central DNA region, predominantly containing genes for virus structure and replication, including viral DNA–dependent RNA polymerase subunits; DNA polymerase, helicase, ligase, and topoisomerase; DNA transcription factors; and DNA core proteins, ankyrin, envelope, and surface membrane proteins. These enzymes enable poxviruses to replicate in the cytoplasm of infected cells rather than their nucleus, making them unique from other DNA viruses. Hypervariable terminal regions that contain arrays of near-terminal repeats, genes that contribute to phenotypic variation, and covalently closed hairpin ends flank this central region.[8–11]

Much of the morphology, molecular genetics, life cycle, and pathogenesis of variola are common to other members of the poxvirus genus.[7] Given its high pathogenicity and strong human tropism and its potential for weaponization, however, variola virus is not available for open research. Although current molecular biology techniques have advanced to the point of being able to synthesize a viable infectious virus[12] or complex viral proteins[13] de novo, most of what is known about variola virus has been the result of research on other members of the poxvirus genus, primarily vaccinia virus. Variola's genome shares a great deal of homology with many of the other poxviruses.[3,7] There is extensive immunologic cross-neutralization between orthopoxviruses, which accounts for the protection against smallpox infection afforded by vaccination with cowpox and vaccinia viruses.

The variola virus is the largest of the animal viruses, measuring approximately 260 × 150 nm, and is usually described as "brick-shaped." It is often called a *complex virus* because it is neither icosahedral nor helical in shape. Poxviruses are extremely complex and typically contain more than 100 proteins. Their basic anatomy, including variola virus, comprises a nucleosome, containing the viral DNA genome encased within a core membrane. This core is compressed into a biconcave shape by two lateral bodies of unknown function. The virion core and the lateral bodies are enclosed within a lipoprotein bilayer outer membrane. The outer membrane exterior is covered with surface tubules composed of polymers of a 58,000-kd protein, which appear to be embedded in the virion outer membrane, giving the nonenveloped, or "naked," virion a textured surface.[3,14,15]

The vaccinia virus can be found as two distinct types of infectious particles: an extracellular enveloped virion (EEV), and the naked nonenveloped intracellular mature virion (IMV). The EEV is formed from the IMV in a process involving the Golgi apparatus of the host cell.[16–18] Although most extracellular virions are found as EEVs, extracellular IMVs also may be found. IMVs represent most infectious progeny and usually remain in the cytoplasm of the host cell until released by cell lysis, but occasionally they may be released individually from the cell surface.[15]

Poxviruses have not been shown to have a major binding site for receptor-mediated binding to cells. The EEV and the *extracellular* nonenveloped virions (eIMV) gain entry into host cells via a pH-independent fusion with the cell plasma membrane. In an in vitro study using vaccinia virus,

EEV fused more efficiently and approximately 50% faster than eIMV. Fusion of eIMV and EEV was strongly temperature dependent; fusion was decreased by 50% at 34°C and by 90% at 28°C.[19] Several virion membrane and envelope proteins play a crucial role in this process, and entry may be blocked by monoclonal antibodies to these proteins.[20] After fusion, the virion core penetrates the cell membrane by pinocytosis, and host cell enzymes release the viral core into the cytoplasm.

On entry into the host cell cytoplasm, the virion particle undergoes a two-stage disassembly process. The first step involves the loss of virion proteins and membranes, exposing the viral core. Viral transcriptase immediately begins transcription of viral DNA to produce "early enzymes" and "early viral proteins." Viral mRNA can be found in the cytoplasm within a few minutes of infection. Some early viral enzymes complete the second stage of virion disassembly by releasing the entire viral genome from the virion core, making it available for replication. Viral DNA polymerase, thymidine, thymidylate kinases, and ribonucleotide reductase are required for viral DNA replication. Other early events include modification of the host cell's cytoplasmic cytoskeleton, with the development of a microtubule network to facilitate the assembly of the IMVs, and inhibition of host cell macromolecule synthesis.[21] Vaccinia virus also has been shown to synthesize and secrete many early proteins that interfere with the host immune response by blocking the action of interferon, complement, and other chemokines.[5,22–27] Early gene products are crucial for the successful initiation and completion of the intracellular life cycle of the virus and the pathogenesis of the viral infection within the host animal.

Poxviruses rapidly inhibit host cell metabolism soon after infection.[25] Host nuclear DNA synthesis is progressively inhibited, possibly by a viral endonuclease, within hours of infection. Similarly, host RNA synthesis and processing also is inhibited, leading to the cessation of protein synthesis as well.[20]

Late transcription of newly synthesized viral DNA produces "late proteins" that include most of the structural components of the progeny virions. These proteins undergo posttranslational modifications, such as glycosylation, acylation, phosphorylation, and proteolytic cleavage by "late enzymes." The assembly of newly synthesized DNA and many structural components into progeny vaccinia virions is a complex process that occurs in juxtanuclear cytoplasmic "virus factories." These areas exclude host cell organelles and appear as B-type inclusion bodies on microscopy within 2.5 hours postinfection.[3] At these sites, lipoprotein bilayer "cupules," which appear as crescents studded with spicules on two-dimensional microscopy, assemble into spherical membrane structures and acquire nucleocapsids to become immature virions (IVs) within 6 to 8 hours postinfection. These IVs subsequently go through a series of biochemical and morphologic changes to yield single-membrane, IMVs.[3,20,28] After their formation, IMV particles may become wrapped by a double layer of membrane to form an intracellular enveloped virus (IEV), or they may remain in the cell until cell lysis or, with some orthopoxviruses, become sequestered in A-type inclusion bodies.[29] Late in infection, some IMVs bud through the plasma membrane.[15]

IMVs consist of a nucleocapsid enclosed within a single-lipid bilayer outer membrane and are functional and infectious.[28] As mentioned earlier, most IMVs remain in the cytoplasm until released by cell lysis, or they may be released by direct plasma membrane "budding."[15] Some IMVs are transported via microtubules,[21,30] however, to the *trans*-Golgi network[16,18] or tubular endosomes,[31] where they are enwrapped in a double-lipid bilayer membrane to form a *three-membrane* IEV. The assembly of the enveloped virion is a critical point where host-encoded and virus-encoded proteins are incorporated into the virion envelope.[16–18,29,31–33] These proteins are important for the final localization and movement of the IEV within the cell, its interaction with and translocation through the cell's plasma membrane,[32,34,35] and its interaction with the host's immune system when it leaves the cell.[32,33,36] The IEV is wrapped in three-lipid bilayers (outer membrane, inner envelope membrane, and outer envelope membranes) because specific membrane proteins are incorporated into each membrane layer and may be localized on the luminal side (facing the interior of the IEV) of the envelope membrane or on the exterior surface, exposed to the cytosol.[18] Transport proteins encoded by genes *A27L* and *F12L* are found on the outer membrane and envelope membrane and facilitate intracellular microtubule–associated movement of vaccinia IMVs and IEVs. Early during infection, most IMV particles are wrapped to form IEV, whereas later during infection, IMVs predominate possibly due to depletion of wrapping membranes.[29]

Proteins A33R, A34R, and A36R are membrane-associated viral proteins found on the cytosolic face of the IEV outer envelope membrane. On reaching the plasma membrane, the outer envelope of the IEV membrane, with these three membrane proteins, fuses with and is incorporated into the host cell's plasma membrane (Fig. 134A-1).[20] This action yields a cell surface–associated enveloped virion

(CEV), with these membrane-associated proteins remaining localized beneath it on the cytoplasmic surface of the cell membrane. The vaccinia A36R protein is a type Ib integral membrane protein with a cytoplasmic domain of about 200 amino acid residues that plays an essential, but undefined role in the actin-based motility of vaccinia. It is phosphorylated at tyrosine residue 112 (tyr_{112}) by plasma membrane tyrosine kinase. This phosphorylation results in an interaction between the CEV and the cellular adapter protein Nck and the recruitment of N-WASP (an actin-depolymerizing protein) to a site on the cytoplasmic surface of the cell membrane immediately below the CEV.[37] This sequence of events is similar to those in normal cell signal-transduction pathways that control actin polymerization. In this setting, polymerization of "actin tails" produces microvilli, however, which extend from the cell surface and project, or push, the CEV toward neighboring cells. This CEV projection greatly increases local cell-to-cell spreading of vaccinia virus, which is shown by increased plaque size in cultured cells.[38] If enveloped virions were released from the cell surface immediately, to become free EEVs, the actin-driven microvilli may not form, limiting the infection of neighboring cells. Vaccinia virus protein A36R shared significant homology with the variola virus protein A39R, indicating that variola virus also uses actin-based motility to spread infection among cells.[39,40] Rapid cell-to-cell spreading of infection in the epidermis and vascular endothelium is an important poxvirus characteristic and produces the characteristic poxvirus skin eruption.

As much as CEVs are crucial for localized vaccinia virus spread, EEVs are important for long-range virus spread. When released from the host cell, EEVs can travel great distances from the infected primary host cell to infect distant cells in culture. Payne[41] found that high in vitro EEV-yielding vaccinia strains were able to cause long-range spread of infection, bypassing the CEV-mediated, cell-to-cell mechanism

FIGURE 134A-1

Poxvirus nucleocapsids are formed and acquire envelopes in virus factories, producing intracellular mature virus (IMV), which subsequently acquire two additional membranes by budding into the *trans*-Golgi network (TGN), forming intracellular enveloped virus (IEV). Microtubules are involved in the transport of IMV and IEV to the plasma (cellular) membrane (PM). There is fusion of the outer envelope with PM, and cell-associated enveloped virus (CEV) (bound to the cell surface) rest on platforms, composed in part of A33R, A34R, and A36R (viral proteins), that sit at one pole of the virus particle. A36R promotes the nucleation of actin filaments through interactions with Nck and recruitment of WIP, N-WASP, and Arp2/3 (*inset*), leading to actin polymerization. Actin tails produce microvilli that project CEV toward adjacent cells, promoting virus entry. CEV also may be released to form EEV. IV, immature virus. *(From Smith VP, Alcami A: Inhibition of interferons by ectromelia viruses. J Virol 76:1124–1134, 2002.)*

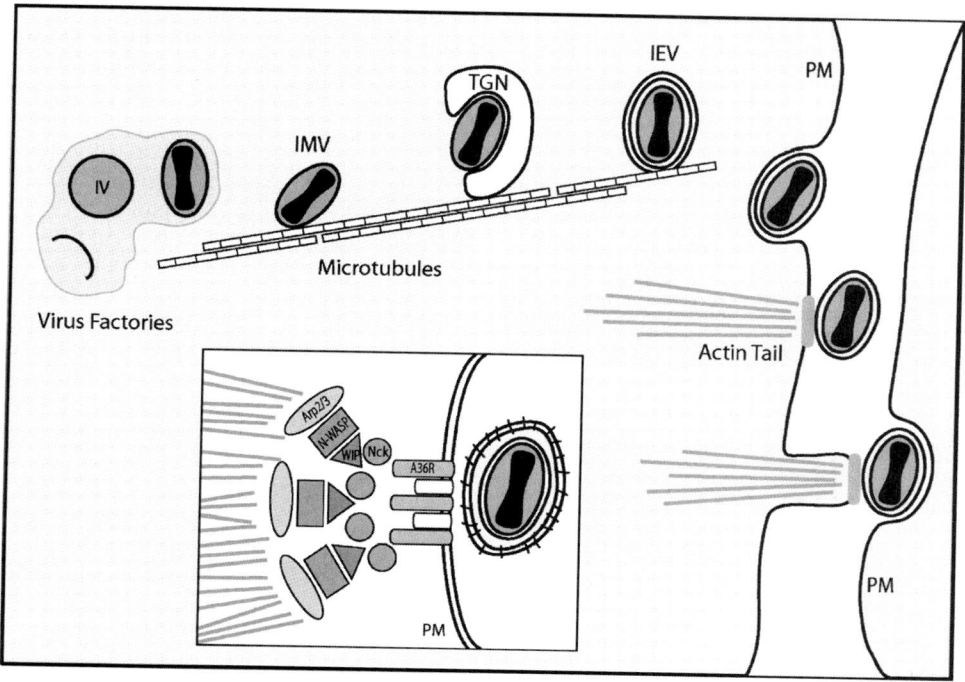

of spreading. In cell culture, this spread of infection is shown by formation of "comets" (polar projections of infected cells from the plaque) extending from infected plaques.[3] These in vitro high EEV–yielding vaccinia strains also were found to spread vaccinia virus infection effectively from the respiratory tract to the brains of mice, causing death.[42] In vitro low EEV–yielding vaccinia strains generally were not able to disseminate in vivo or cause mouse death, with the notable exception of the western reserve vaccinia strain, which released only small amounts of EEV in vitro, but nevertheless could spread in vivo effectively, causing a high rate of mouse mortality. These results indicate that the in vitro dissemination of vaccinia infection is mediated by EEV and has a role in in vivo dissemination.[41]

There are four forms of vaccinia poxvirus and presumably variola. The IMV form is the most abundant form and is environmentally stable, making it well suited for transmission of virus between hosts (i.e., aerosol). IEV is an intermediate form between IMV and CEV/EEV required for the incorporation of viral and host encoded membrane proteins into the viral envelope and for transporting the virions to the cell surface. CEVs facilitate the efficient cell-to-cell spread of virus. Finally, EEVs are released from the infected host cell to mediate the distant spread of infection within a host.

Virion envelope–associated proteins include hemagglutinin, proteins that enhance virus growth in human cells, thymidine kinase, and poxvirus antigens that are thought to be important in eliciting an immune response that can protect against a poxvirus challenge and mediate immune system evasion by the poxvirus.[20,43,44] Host interactive proteins include epidermal growth factor, probably for increasing cell numbers around the site of infection; zinc RING finger protein[45] and protein kinases, which may influence viral and host cell metabolism; and cellular ankyrin-related proteins, which may specify tissue tropism. Variola also synthesizes many proteins that could alter host defenses, such as superoxide dismutase homologue and binding proteins for interferon (IFN)-α, IFN-β,[5] IFN-γ,[22] interleukin (IL)-1β, tumor necrosis factor,[26] chemokines,[23] and complement.[13,20,27,44,46]

EPIDEMIOLOGY

The epidemiology of smallpox is concerned with the movement of variola virus particles between humans (i.e., the spread of infection in populations). Potential routes of infection include the upper respiratory tract, conjunctiva, and skin. Infection via the skin is relatively uncommon and historically has been either by accidental inoculation with variola virus in certain occupations, such as health care providers or morticians, or by variolation. The practice of variolation involved *intentional* dermal inoculation with a small amount of smallpox scab material that contained viable variola virus. Although the recipient of variolation ran the risk of developing a fatal case of smallpox, the practice conferred lifelong immunity. Variolation is discussed in more detail in the treatment section later. The predominant route of transmission is by aerosol.

After an asymptomatic incubation period (7 to 17 days), clinical smallpox presents with an initial fever spike,

followed by an enanthem consisting of ulcerative lesions in the oropharynx. These lesions release large amounts of virus into oropharyngeal secretions, and spreading of variola virus occurs primarily by the aerosolization of these virus-laden secretions by coughing, sneezing, or simply talking.[47] Human-to-human transmission usually occurs by inhalation of droplet nuclei of these secretions from an infected person.[3,48,49] The principal route of entry is via the oropharynx, the nasopharynx, occasionally the lower respiratory tract, and rarely the conjunctiva. Variola virus in these airborne droplets infects the epithelial cells of the mucous membranes of a susceptible individual, who becomes infected and repeats the cycle of virus aerosolization, which propagates spread of the virus among the population.[48,49]

There are three possible mechanisms of transmission: direct personal contact with an infected person, contact with contaminated fomites (e.g., patient bed linens), and airborne spread.[3,50] Transmission of smallpox most often occurs as the result of direct face-to-face contact with an infected person, usually among household members[49] or hospital workers.[51,52] There have been smallpox outbreaks, however, resulting from the dissemination of variola virus over considerable distance. Two hospital outbreaks, Monschau in 1961[3] and Meschede in 1969,[38,53] were the result of airborne transmission of virus particles. The outbreak at Meschede began when a 20-year-old man returned from Pakistan and developed a febrile illness 10 days later. He initially was diagnosed with typhoid fever and was restricted to his room. It quickly became apparent, however, that he had smallpox when he developed a rash 3 days after admission. This case resulted in 17 secondary cases and 2 tertiary cases of smallpox. One case occurred in a hospital visitor who spent 15 minutes in the hospital lobby, well away from the index patient's room or any of the identified contacts. Several factors were identified that may have favored the airborne transmission of virus: The index patient had a densely confluent rash and severe cough, there was low humidity in the hospital (outbreak occurred in January),[54] and smoke diffusion studies identified air current patterns within the hospital that correlated with the location of the additional cases.[53] Although most cases of smallpox transmission occur as a result of face-to-face contact, it is possible to have transmission over much longer distances. This possibility underscores the need for careful evaluation of isolation practices and facilities to limit the possible dissemination of virus.[51] There is no evidence that ingestion of smallpox-contaminated food causes smallpox or that arthropods are involved in the transmission of smallpox.

The last case of variola major was on Bhola Island, Bangladesh, in 1975. The last case of variola minor was in Somalia in 1977. Although never as common as in Asia and Africa, variola major was endemic in the United States[55] until 1926; variola minor persisted until the late 1940s.[56] The last U.S. epidemic occurred in the lower Rio Grande valley of Texas in 1949.[57] On August 24, 1978, the world's last case of smallpox was diagnosed in a medical photographer who worked in the anatomy department of Birmingham University Medical School in England.[58] Although smallpox had not yet been declared eradicated by the World Health Organization, the medical photographer had not traveled abroad during the previous year and had no known contact with any smallpox patients. This final case, which was fatal and also caused a secondary case, was the result of variola virus escaping from a laboratory within the building where she worked.[59] She had never entered the laboratory in question, meaning the virus had traveled a significant distance, likely through the building's ventilation system, similar to the outbreak that occurred in Meschede, West Germany, in 1969.[38,53] It also has been shown that health care facilities, such as this one in Birmingham, and health care workers are often major amplifiers of smallpox outbreaks via nosocomial transmission of virus and disseminating virus out of the facility into the community.[51] Successful infection containment and control are crucial epidemiologic measures essential to combating a smallpox outbreak.

Studies by Sarkar and colleagues[48] and Downie and associates[60] quantified the amount of virus from oropharyngeal secretions, conjunctiva, and urine of patients. These investigators reported that viral titers in oropharyngeal secretions were highest 3 to 4 days after the onset of fever and were highest and persisted the longest in the most clinically severe cases. Virus was usually still present in throat swabs of fatal cases at the time of death, 14 days in confluent ordinary-type smallpox, and 7 to 9 days in discrete ordinary-type smallpox. Sarkar and colleagues[49] also collected throat swabs on 328 household contacts of 52 smallpox patients. They found that 10.4% (n = 34) were positive for variola virus when collected 4 to 8 days after onset of illness in the family member. A higher percentage of unvaccinated contacts (27.1%) were positive for the virus than were vaccinated contacts (6.7%). Four of the positive contacts (11.8%) went on to develop clinical smallpox. Although secretion of virus titers were much lower in the contacts than in the index patients with clinical smallpox, virus still was detected in the throats of these four secondary patients 5 to 6 days *before* they developed clinical smallpox (i.e., during the incubation period). This finding raises the question: Do infected individuals spread smallpox while it is still in the incubation period? This finding is contradicted by other published studies, leaving the question unresolved.

Viruses shed by aerosolization of oropharyngeal secretions may infect persons nearby (e.g., family members, caregivers) while still airborne or by direct contact with infected secretions. These secretions also may settle on bed linens, where they may readily be reaerosolized and inhaled.[47,52,60] The viability of vaccinia and variola is longest at low temperatures and low humidities.[47,54] In naturally occurring smallpox, this fact produced seasonal fluctuations in incidence, with most cases and outbreaks occurring during the spring and summer.[3]

Another potential route of virus dissemination is shedding of virus from skin lesions or from the separated scabs of rash lesions.[61] Although separated scabs often contaminate the patient's bed linens and the floors, these virions typically remained encased within a fibrous matrix, decreasing the likelihood of these viruses' being transmitted effectively by an aerosol route.[52] It is well known, however, that Lord Jeffrey Amherst distributed blankets and handkerchiefs collected from smallpox infirmaries to North American Indians during the French and Indian War of the 1760s. This use of smallpox as a biologic weapon by the English literally wiped out entire tribes, showing that smallpox scab debris in blankets can effectively disseminate variola virus. A study of smallpox rash crusts showed that virus viability was highly affected by temperature and relative humidity. Virus viability was 3 weeks at 35°C (95°F), 8 weeks at room temperature, and 11 weeks at room temperature with relative humidity less than 10%. Virus viability extended beyond 16 weeks at 4°C and −20°C.[54] Mitra and coworkers[61] showed that the virus content of smallpox scabs was not affected by vaccination status, length of clinical illness, or severity of clinical illness. A case of smallpox in the former Soviet Union in 1959 was attributed to an imported variola virus–contaminated carpet.[3] Although aerosolization of secretions is a more effective means of transmission, it is reasonable to conclude that smallpox scab or crust debris, either airborne or on fomites, may be sources of infectious variola virus, and infection control precautions should include measures to limit such exposures.

Naturally occurring smallpox outbreaks often occur in communities as the result of a single infected person's (index case) returning from an area where smallpox was endemic and subsequently infecting multiple persons. In the case of a bioterrorist attack using smallpox, however, one may not see this "natural" epidemiologic pattern of transmission. In June 2001, the federal government, in cooperation with many academic and defense organizations, held a table-top exercise entitled "Dark Winter" that simulated a covert smallpox attack on the United States.[62] The scenario was based on an attack that simultaneously disseminated approximately 30 g of weaponized smallpox in three separate shopping malls in Atlanta, Oklahoma City, and Philadelphia, causing 3000 primary infections. The model used known epidemiologic data, such as transmission rates from naturally occurring smallpox outbreaks of the pre–eradication era, and allowed for the increased mobility of today's population. The exercise progressed through four generations of virus transmission. In the absence of adequate outbreak containment measures and with limited vaccine supply, the worst-case scenario projected 3 million cases with 1 million deaths over a simulated 8 weeks.[63] The lessons of this exercise and the impact of the anthrax bioterrorist attacks of 2001 have resulted in the development of a national bioterrorism response plan that encompasses prevention, detection, response, and recovery capabilities.[64]

Case-fatality rates for smallpox vary depending on several factors, including strain of variola, patient age, previous vaccination history, time since vaccination, and nutritional status and underlying health of the patient. Pregnant women were especially susceptible, having higher case-fatality rates for variola major and minor compared with men and nonpregnant women of comparable age.[50] Pregnant women also had a higher incidence of developing hemorrhagic-type smallpox (HTS). In persons with a history of only a primary vaccination, susceptibility increased with the interval since vaccination. Age was an important determinant of case-fatality rates. Case-fatality rates were highest in the very young (<1 year old) at 43.5%, versus 24.5% in ages 1 to 4, 11.4% in ages 5 to 14, 9% in ages 15 to 39, 20.1% in ages 40 to 49, and 37.4% in ages 50 and older.[3,50]

PATHOGENESIS

Variola virus infection begins with implantation of the virus on the oropharyngeal or respiratory mucosa. Other portals of virus entry include skin, as in variolation by scarification; mucous membranes, such as the conjunctiva; and the placenta, in cases of congenital variola infection. The actual infectious dose is unknown but may be only a few virions. The virus gains entry into these cells and enters its replication phase.

During the incubation period, the virus establishes an infection in epithelial cells of the nasopharyngeal, oropharyngeal, and respiratory tract mucosa.[39,48,65,66] Virions are released from epithelial cells as enveloped virions, or as undeveloped virions in the case of epithelial cell death and lysis. They are quickly phagocytosed by macrophages and transported to the regional lymph nodes, where intense viral replication begins. After replication in the regional lymphoid tissues (approximately 3 to 4 days), enveloped and unenveloped progeny virions are released, causing an asymptomatic viremia. Virions also spread via a cell-associated viremia, in which they are hematogenously disseminated within infected leukocytes.[59] Virions infect endothelial cells throughout the body, seeding major organs, such as the spleen, liver, bone marrow, and reticuloendothelial system.[3,67,68]

A secondary, major viremia occurs about 12 days (range 4 to 17 days) after infection, followed by the initial enanthem (mucosal lesions) and the onset of fever. In ordinary-type smallpox (OTS), viremia is thought to be primarily cell associated because virus was only rarely recovered from blood or serum.[3] HTS, especially early HTS, typically produces marked viremia, with virus being recovered from blood or serum in high titers at all stages of the illness.[68,69]

Autopsy studies have shown diffuse organ system involvement.[2,68] Large quantities of virus can be isolated from all organs, including the spleen, lymph nodes, kidney, bone marrow, and liver. Kidney histologic studies have shown endothelial cell degeneration, interstitial edema, and lymphocytic infiltration consistent with acute tubulointerstitial nephritis. Renal pelvis hemorrhages can be seen in cases of early HTS.[3,65,68] Encephalitis was an occasional complication of smallpox, but studies of the pathologic features of central nervous system infection by variola are varied and limited. Perivascular infiltration, demyelination, and cerebral edema have been reported, however. Liver involvement typically included parenchymal cell swelling, degeneration, and lysis; vascular congestion; and infiltration by lymphocytes and macrophages.[68]

The skin lesions of smallpox have been extensively studied. As a result of the secondary viremia, virus localizes in the capillaries of the dermis and oropharyngeal mucosa. This is followed by capillary dilation, infection of local endothelial and dermal papillary layer cells, and lymphocytic and histiocytic infiltration.[68] The infection extends to the adjacent stratum germinativum of the overlying epidermis. These cells become swollen and vacuolated, develop characteristic B-type cytoplasmic inclusions, and undergo "ballooning" degeneration. They then undergo "reticular degeneration" with the coalescence of vacuoles forming papules, followed by vesiculation.[3] Pustulation occurs with the migration of polymorphonuclear leukocytes into the vesicle. Sebaceous glands are the only dermal appendage destroyed by variola. Because sebaceous glands tend to be found at greater density in the skin of the face, scarring left by healed smallpox lesions is typically worst on the face.

Lungs of smallpox patients show signs of viral interstitial pneumonitis, including hyperemia and degeneration of alveolar lining cells and congestion of alveoli with sloughed epithelial cells of the upper respiratory tract.[2,68] Although the viral pneumonia caused by smallpox contributes to the cause of death, it also may be complicated by secondary bacterial bronchopneumonia. A postmortem study of post–antibiotic era smallpox cases showed less than 15% had bronchopneumonia as a contributing cause of death.[68]

Although the precise cause of death in smallpox is the topic of debate, current data suggest that it is likely multifactorial. The cumulative effect of the destruction of respiratory, capillary, and renal tubular epithelium leads to multisystem organ failure. Respiratory failure as a result of viral or bacterial pneumonia, complicated by systemic hypotension, dehydration, malnutrition, and generalized toxemia, is usually the final fatal pathway. Circulating immune complexes are thought to contribute to overwhelming toxemia.[3,39,68,70]

The presentation of virus to lymphocytes in the lymph nodes after the initial infection elicits an immune response, including cellular and humoral mechanisms. Vaccinia virus and other poxviruses express a wide variety of proteins that help the virus evade the host immune response to infection.[44] Poxviruses evade many of the host immune system's defenses by blocking the antiviral effects of IFN, downregulating cytotoxic cellular immunity and the expression of ILs, and affecting the differentiation of T lymphocytes. Examples include soluble receptors for tumor necrosis factor,[26] IL-1β, IFN-γ,[22,27,43] IFN-α/β,[5,44] chemokines,[23,44,46] and complement.[13]

HOST RESPONSE

The host immune response to viral infections includes the production of ILs and IFNs and the differentiation and activation of T lymphocytes and natural killer (NK) cells.[24] NK cells are considered "natural killers" because they have cytoplasmic granules containing perforins and granzymes that are cytolytic when released. They comprise approximately 5% to 10% of the circulating lymphocyte population and produce many immunomodulators, such as IFN-γ, and are involved in the early response to viral infection.[71]

IFNs are a large group of cytokines that inhibit virus replication and spread by inducing a host antiviral response.[72] IFNs are the first defense against virus infections. Early in the course of a viral infection, type I or viral IFNs, including IFN-α (leukocyte), IFN-β (fibroblast), and IFN-γ, are synthesized and secreted by virus-infected cells.[71] They bind to a single IFN-α/β cellular receptor to stimulate the production of an "antiviral state" in virus-infected cells, which limits viral replication and signals the adaptive arm of the immune response to the presence of the virus.[43]

IFN-γ is secreted only by NK cells, CD4 Th1 cells, and CD8 cytotoxic suppressor cells on antigenic recognition of a virus-infected cell.[71,73] IFN-γ binds to a specific IFN-γ receptor and acts by several mechanisms, including the activation of an endoribonuclease that degrades viral RNA, to induce antiviral activity in infected cell. Its antiviral activity also may be mediated by inducing cellular production of nitric oxide by nitric oxide synthase.[72] Many poxviruses produce soluble IFN receptors.[5,20,22,43,44,73] Vaccinia virus also has been found to encode a protein inhibitor of the IFN-induced, double-stranded, RNA-dependent protein kinase, which further inhibits the antiviral action of IFN by blocking its intracellular effects.[74]

Chemokines are chemoattractant cytokines that regulate leukocyte migration and activity in the immune response to an infection. Poxviruses produce soluble chemokine binding proteins that have significant protein sequence homology with the extracellular domains of host cellular cytokine receptors.[23,44]

IL-18 is produced by activated macrophages and induces IFN-γ production in antigen-stimulated T-cell lines and NK cells and stimulates NK cell cytotoxicity. The ectromelia (mousepox) poxvirus encodes a soluble IL-18 receptor (p13 protein) that binds and inactivates IL-18, resulting in impaired NK cell cytotoxicity, and is one mechanism by which poxviruses evade the host immune system.[24]

NK cell activity is regulated by a combination of soluble cytokines, including IFN-α, IFN-β, tumor necrosis factor-α, IL-2, IL-12, IL-15, and IL-18, which stimulate NK cell activity and the "opposing signal" model of stimulatory and inhibitory receptor binding. NK cells have an activation receptor that interacts with a membrane ligand on potential target cells and stimulates the NK cell to kill the target cell. This cell can be a normal or altered self (e.g., virus-infected cell or tumor cell). Normal cells express class I major histocompatibility complex (MHC) molecules, identifying them as normal host cells, which also bind to a receptor on the NK cell, inhibiting its cytolytic action. The balance of these two binding interactions regulates NK cell activity. Virus-infected host cells have decreased expression of cell surface membrane class I MHC, allowing the activation receptor interaction to stimulate the NK cell to kill the virus-infected cell. In this way, NK cells help contain the viral infection, while the cytotoxic T-lymphocyte population is stimulated.[44]

Most poxviruses encode a growth factor homologue with significant amino acid sequence homology with epidermal growth factor. Vaccinia virus growth factor competes with epidermal growth factor for binding to epidermal growth factor membrane receptors.[44] These growth factors are not essential for virus replication and induce proliferation of infected and noninfected cells, although their exact role in poxvirus pathogenesis is not clear.[20,44]

The complement system is a complex system of enzymes important for the innate and the adaptive response to viral infection. Although three different pathways can initiate complement activation in part, they all lead to the activation of the terminal pathway and the formation of membrane attack complexes. Membrane attack complexes cause membrane disruption and death of virus-infected cells and enveloped virions. Other components of complement mediate the inflammatory response, such as mast cell degranulation, chemotaxis of leukocytes, platelet aggregation, and opsonization of antigens, to increase their phagocytosis. Complement activation is closely regulated by host inhibitory proteins, such as factors I, H, and S, which interfere with the classic, alternative, and terminal complement pathways. Poxviruses evade these complement defenses by incorporating the host complement regulatory proteins into virion

envelopes or up-regulating the expression of these proteins on infected cell membranes or both.[33,44] These proteins down-regulate the host complement activity by inhibiting the formation of and accelerating the decay of complement at several steps in the activation pathway.[33,46] Vaccinia virus secretes a complement-control protein similar to the naturally occurring complement inhibitor C4b binding protein.[75] Variola virus secretes a complement-control protein called smallpox inhibitor of complement enzymes (SPICE).[13,46] Both of these viral proteins promote the activity of physiologic complement regulator factor I and inactivate human C3b and C4b. Perhaps reflecting its increased virulence in humans, SPICE is nearly 100-fold and 6-fold more potent at inactivating human C3b and C4b.[13]

These mechanisms of immune system evasion used by poxviruses have evolved via natural selection over millennia. Understanding the immune response to viral infection and the development of advanced recombinant molecular biology techniques have led, however, to the development of viruses that can overwhelm the immune system, even after vaccination.[76,77] Using only recombinant DNA techniques and published genomic sequences, infectious poliovirus has been synthesized entirely de novo.[12] These developments and the former Soviet Union's efforts to develop a smallpox biologic weapon[1,2] are worrisome reminders that biologic agents used as biologic weapons today may be much more virulent than the naturally occurring organisms of the past.

CLINICAL PRESENTATION

The clinical presentation of smallpox varies by clinical type and at which point in the illness the patient presents. The incubation period is the time between implantation of infectious virus on the respiratory mucosa and the onset of fever. All patients experience an asymptomatic incubation period lasting 7 to 17 days (mean 10 to 12 days). The length of the incubation period can be affected by virulence of the variola virus strain, number of infectious particles received, and underlying health of the patient. The incubation period for OTS is usually around 12 days (range 7 to 19 days).[3,50] After multiplying in the regional lymph nodes for 3 to 4 days, a brief asymptomatic viremia occurs, seeding the reticuloendothelial system (including liver, spleen, bone marrow, and lymphoid organs), followed by an asymptomatic latent period during which viral replication continues.

The abrupt onset of a febrile prodrome marks the beginning of the second viremia and the end of the incubation period. The fever is often as high as 105°F, although the height of fever does not correlate well with the severity of the illness that follows. The fever typically decreases 4 or 5 days after the eruption of the rash, but rises again by 7 or 8 days and may remain high throughout the vesicular and pustular stages, until scabs form.[67,68] Other symptoms include severe malaise, chills, headache, backache, vomiting, pharyngitis, abdominal pain that is sometimes severe, and diarrhea.[3,39,50,67,79] This prodrome typically lasts several days and is followed quickly by the development of an enanthem (ulcerative lesions on mucous membranes) and the characteristic smallpox rash. Studies have shown that there is a significant amount of virus released into the oropharyngeal secretions from the enanthem lesions between the time of the prodrome and appearance of the rash, making the patient highly infectious during this period.[47–49]

Smallpox is divided into two major types: variola major and variola minor. Variola minor has relatively low mortality and is discussed separately from the forms of variola major.

Variola Major

Rao[50] established five major clinical forms of variola major, based primarily on rash characteristics: OTS; flat-type smallpox (FTS), also called malignant type; HTS, which is subdivided into early and late forms; modified-type smallpox (MTS); and variola sine eruptione. The rashes of OTS, MTS, and FTS are subdivided further into confluent, semiconfluent, and discrete forms. In the discrete subtype, lesions are distinct with normal skin between all lesions, and lesions are typically fewer in number than the other two subtypes. As the name suggests, in the confluent subtype, skin lesions are confluent on the face and extremities, whereas in the semiconfluent subtype, they are confluent on the face but not the extremities. These clinical distinctions have prognostic value for variola major.[50,79]

The rash that follows the prodrome erupts in a characteristic pattern, although there is patient-to-patient variation, and a history without a classic rash evolution is common.[3,50,67] Patients typically remain febrile throughout the development of the rash. The rash usually begins as macules on the face, often around the mouth and nares, although the appearance of "herald spots" or "herald lesions," especially

on the forehead, have been reported.[3] The rash spreads to the trunk and proximal, then distal, extremities in a centrifugal pattern (Fig. 134A-2A).[50] The pustular lesions of the rash are typically painful as they grow and expand.[67,70] These lesions are more deeply embedded in the skin, compared with the more superficial lesions of varicella (chickenpox).[67] Vesicles are multilocular with fibrinous threads dividing the interior of the lesions into compartments. Loss of vesicular fluid and retraction of the fibrinous threads causes a dimpling at the apex of the lesion, referred as *umbilication* (Fig. 134A-2B).[50,67] In OTS, the characteristic evolution of the rash is seen as a progression through an order of appearance of focal lesions: macules → papules → vesicles → pustules → umbilication → scabbing → scab separation and scarring. The complete course of evolution of the rash in OTS usually takes 3 to 4 weeks, and patients remain infectious until all scabs separate.[50,79]

The rash erupts in a synchronous pattern, with all lesions appearing within 24 hours. This is an important distinction from the rash associated with varicella, which typically develops in an asynchronous pattern, or in "crops," with lesions of varying ages present at a given point in time on a given anatomic area.[79] The distribution of the classic smallpox rash is well described by Rao[50]: "It would almost seem that the patient, during the stage of viremia, had been fixed on a centrifuge with outstretched limbs and spun." The rash is denser on the extremities than on the trunk. On the extremities, it is more dense distally than proximally and denser on the flexor surfaces compared with the extensor surfaces. On the trunk, it is denser on the back

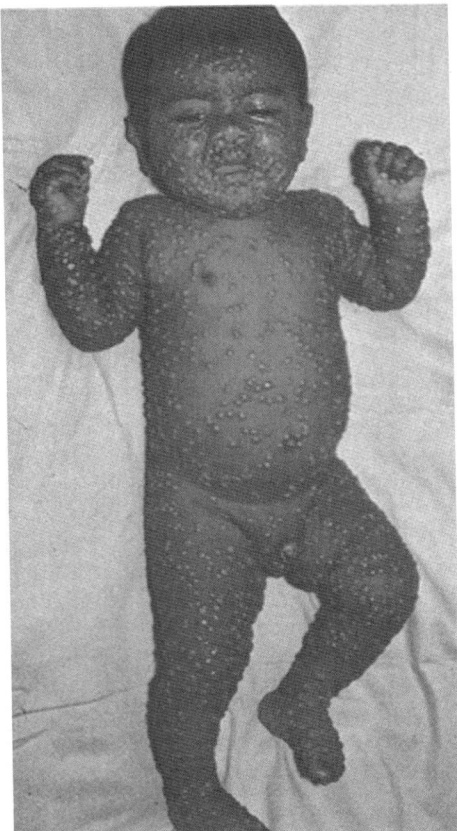

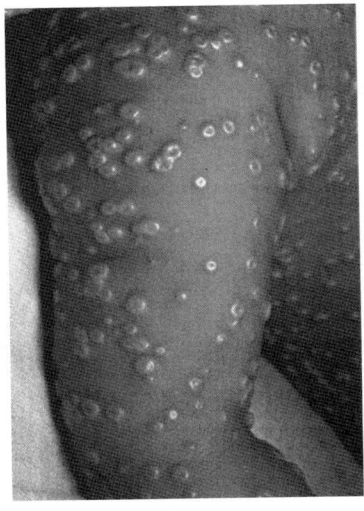

A

B

FIGURE 134A-2

A, A 9-month-old infant with discrete ordinary-type smallpox, day 9 of rash. **B,** Umbilicated lesions from the same patient, day 8 of rash. *(Fom Senkevich T, Wolffe EJ, Buller ML: Ectromelia virus RING finger protein is localized in virus factories and is required for virus replication in macrophages. J Virol 69:4103–4111, 1995.)* See Color Figs. 134A-2A and 134A-2B.

compared with the front and denser on the lower half of the abdomen compared with the upper half (Gaspirini's sign). The apex of axilla is free of lesions compared with the folds (Rickett's sign). On the face, the rash is denser on the upper half than on the lower half. Rao[50] also noted that approximately 10% of patients do not follow this classic pattern of lesion distribution.

ORDINARY-TYPE SMALLPOX

OTS was the most common form of variola major infection, accounting for more than 90% of cases during the global smallpox eradication program.[3,50] After the prodrome described previously, an enanthem appears 1 day before or concomitantly with the skin rash (exanthem). It has been reported that fair-skinned patients may have a brief erythematous rash that precedes the development of discrete lesions. Lesions cover the trunk but are more densely distributed on the extremities, including the palms and soles (Fig. 134A-3A). The rash of OTS can be classified further as confluent (Fig. 134A-3B), semiconfluent, or discrete (see Fig. 134A-2).[3,50]

The overall clinical picture of a patient with OTS is one of sepsis or toxemia or both. Patients may develop significant dehydration, with or without hypotension, and electrolyte abnormalities due to decreased oral fluid intake and vomiting and increased insensible losses due to fever, sepsis, and third spacing of fluid into the skin during the vesicular and pustular stages of the rash.[3,50] Significant skin desquamation may occur in patients with confluent disease, causing clinical and metabolic complications similar to those seen in burn victims. Patients may present in considerable respiratory distress secondary to viral pneumonia or secondary bacterial pneumonia or both. The overall case-fatality rate for OTS was 15% to 45%, with an average of approximately 30% in unvaccinated patients and 3% in vaccinated patients. There is a continuum of severity of illness, however, between confluent and discrete subtypes. The case-fatality rates for the confluent, semiconfluent, and discrete subtypes of OTS in unvaccinated individuals were 62%, 37%, and 9%, respectively.[50]

FLAT-TYPE SMALLPOX

FTS, also called *malignant smallpox*, is relatively uncommon, constituting only 6.7% of all unvaccinated cases in Rao's series,[50] although 72% of cases occurred in children. FTS acquires its name from the fact that its characteristic lesions remain relatively flush with the skin at a time when vesicles normally form in OTS (Fig. 134A-4A). Its prodrome precedes the exanthem; is usually prolonged to 3 to 4 days; includes severe constitutional symptoms; includes fever as high as 105°F; and continues after the rash develops, usually until the patient dies.[50,67]

The rash of FTS may not develop in the classic centrifugal pattern of smallpox and lacks the characteristic pustules seen in OTS. If the patient survives the initial stage of the exanthem, the rash develops slowly, reaching the papulovesicular

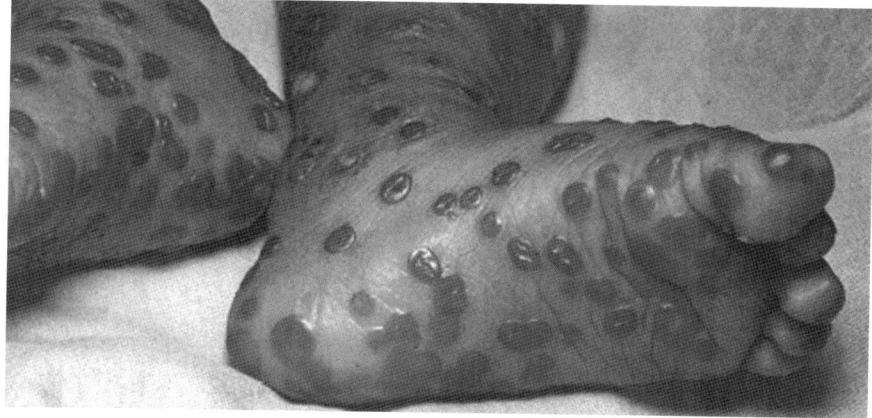

A

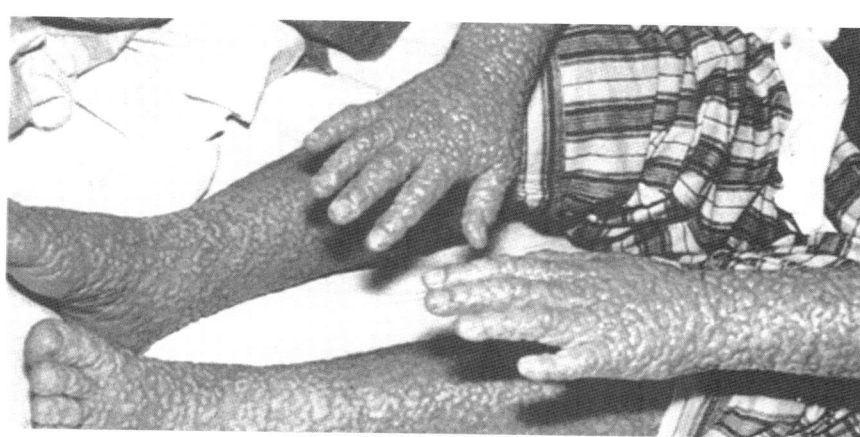

B

FIGURE 134A-3

A, Smallpox lesions on soles of feet. **B,** Confluent ordinary-type smallpox. *(Fom Senkevich T, Wolffe EJ, Buller ML: Ectromelia virus RING finger protein is localized in virus factories and is required for virus replication in macrophages. J Virol 69:4103–4111, 1995.)* See Color Figs. 134A-3A and 134A-3B.

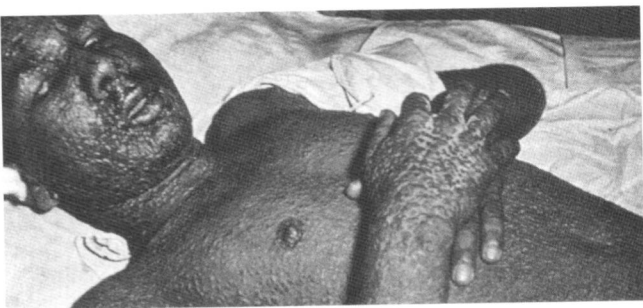

A

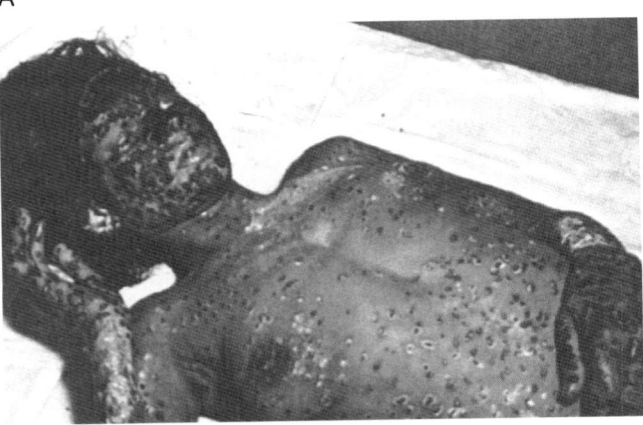

B

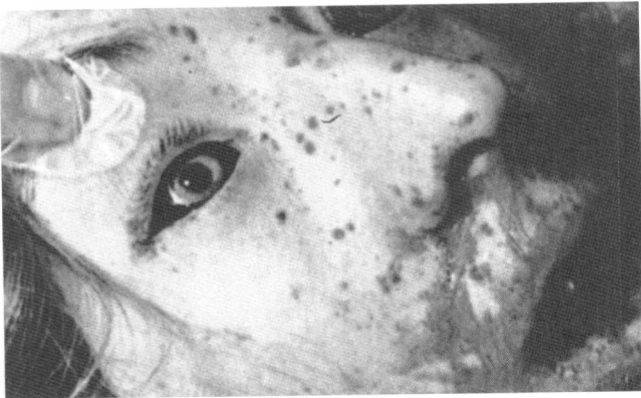

C

FIGURE 134A-4

A, Confluent flat-type smallpox; note lack of papular or vesicular lesions and severely toxic appearance. **B,** Late hemorrhagic-type smallpox; note well-evolved lesion with hemorrhages into lesions and severely toxic appearance. **C,** Early hemorrhagic-type smallpox; note conjunctival hemorrhages, poorly evolved lesions, and severely toxic appearance. *(From Senkevich T, Wolffe EJ, Buller ML: Ectromelia virus RING finger protein is localized in virus factories and is required for virus replication in macrophages. J Virol 69:4103–4111, 1995.)* See Color Figs. 134A-4A, 134A-4B, and 134A-4C.

stage approximately 1 week after the onset of fever. It does not progress through the normal evolution of lesions seen in OTS, however, and frank pustules are rarely seen.[50] The initial papulovesicular lesions level out by 7 or 8 days, producing the characteristic flat lesions of FTS. Skin texture often is described as "velvety" or "crepe rubber" and is fragile, peeling and leaving raw areas of desquamation after only minor trauma.[3] Not to be confused with HTS, the lesions of FTS

often have hemorrhages into their base, but FTS lacks the other systemic hemorrhages usually seen in HTS. The flattened lesions of FTS can develop in discrete, semiconfluent, or confluent distributions. As with OTS, prognosis worsens with the more confluent form. In Rao's series,[50] which included 281 cases of FTS, overall mortality was 66.7% and 96.5% in vaccinated and unvaccinated patients, respectively. The case-fatality rates for discrete, semiconfluent, and confluent forms in unvaccinated patients were 95.6%, 95.3%, and 100%, respectively. Vaccination offered some protection, with case-fatality rates for these same forms of 42.1%, 60%, and 85.7%, respectively.

The enanthem of FTS is also quite severe. It is often confluent, with mucous membrane sloughing that leaves extensive raw areas in the oropharynx and upper airway. The enanthem also can involve the rectal mucous membranes, causing passage of blood and mucus during the course of the illness. Rao[50] also reported sloughing of significant sections of rectal mucosa as a tubular cast immediately before death.

Overall the clinical course for FTS can be described as a severely toxic febrile syndrome, with an atypical flattened smallpox exanthem and a severe enanthem. Respiratory complications, which may include viral pneumonitis or frank pneumonia or both, set in by 7 or 8 days and are often considered a major contributor to the cause of death. Death usually occurs between 8 and 12 days. Rao[50] also reported that unvaccinated patients, mostly children, develop acute gastric dilation 1 to 2 days before death.

HEMORRHAGIC-TYPE SMALLPOX

HTS is relatively rare, occurring primarily in adults and in less than 3% of all patients in Rao's series of smallpox patients.[50] HTS is subdivided into early and late forms, also classified as hemorrhagic type I and II (Fig. 134A-4B and C).[3,50] Compared with OTS, in which case-fatality rates for vaccinated and unvaccinated patients are approximately 3% and 30%, respectively, vaccination does not seem to be as protective against HTS. Several case series report that 26% to 50% of HTS patients had a history of previous immunization. Case-fatality rates for all patients invariably exceeded 90%, however.[3,50,67,69] Early and late forms of HTS in unvaccinated patients carry mortality rates of 100% and 96.8%, respectively.[50] In all case series of early HTS, the case-fatality rate was 100%.[3,50,69]

In a study of 77 patients with HTS, Downie and associates[69] found that 57 had been previously vaccinated, 38 were male, and 39 were female. In Rao's series, HTS was more common in adults, and two thirds of all cases were in women.[50] Pregnancy seemed to be a risk factor for HTS. One third (n = 13) of the women were pregnant, 10 of whom developed early HTS and 3 late HTS.[50]

The prodrome for both forms of HTS is usually prolonged to 3 to 6 days. Toxic symptoms, including fever, prostration, headache, and backache, are usually more severe than the prodrome seen with OTS and may continue after the appearance of the rash.[3,50] Patients may develop generalized erythema, petechiae, hemorrhages, and ecchymoses; patients often did not survive long enough to develop a rash (Table 134A-1). Because of its atypical appearance, the rash of HTS may be difficult to diagnose. This is exemplified by an outbreak of smallpox

NATURE OF HEMORRHAGES	EARLY HEMORRHAGIC-TYPE SMALLPOX (%)	LATE HEMORRHAGIC-TYPE SMALLPOX (%)
Skin	85	16
Conjunctiva	65	52
Hematuria	25	29
Gingiva	20	29
Hemoptysis	12	30
Melena	10	8
Epistaxis	2	3
Hematemesis	1	4
Vagina (women only)	80	58

TABLE 134A-1 Hemorrhagic-Type Smallpox

Adapted from Feery BJ: Adverse reactions after smallpox vaccination. Med J Aust 2:180–183, 1977.

in Yugoslavia in 1972, which began when an infected 38-year-old Muslim priest returned from a pilgrimage to Iraq, where smallpox was endemic at the time. Although the local outbreak was recognized relatively early, a second-generation case was misdiagnosed when he presented to a local medical center with a fever. He was treated with penicillin, and when he developed a rash soon thereafter again was misdiagnosed as having an unusual drug reaction to penicillin. Subsequently, he was transferred between four medical treatment facilities and was used as a case presentation to the medical staff before he died 7 days after developing fever. Only after this patient's death and 38 people, including 8 who subsequently died, developed smallpox from contact with the patient was it retrospectively realized that he had early HTS.[3] Hematologic studies in many HTS case series of early and late forms have shown increased lymphocyte counts, granulocytopenia, thrombocytopenia, hypofibrinogenemia, prolonged prothrombin time, and clotting factor deficiency.[50,59,80–83]

Early Hemorrhagic-Type Smallpox. In Rao's case series,[50] 88% of early HTS cases were in patients older than 14 years, two thirds were women, and pregnant women were most susceptible. Previous vaccination did not offer significant protection against infection with HTS or death. The onset of the prodrome of early HTS is sudden and accompanied by high fever (105°F to 106°F), chills, severe headache, and backache and is prolonged 4 to 6 days.[50] Early HTS is characterized by hemorrhages into the skin or mucous membranes early in the course of the illness, before the development of a skin rash (see Fig. 134A-4C). By the second day of fever, patients have whole-body flushing and erythema, petechiae, and ecchymoses. Subconjunctival hemorrhages are most common, but no intracranial hemorrhages have been reported.[50] Other sites of bleeding and their frequency are listed in Table 134A-1. Areas of subcutaneous hemorrhage may become confluent, leading to extremely friable skin, large serosanguineous bullae formation, and desquamation.[50,69,82]

In a case series (n = 24) of early HTS by Downie and associates,[69] death occurred an average of 5 to 6 days (range

3 to 11 days) after the onset of fever. Rao[50] reported that death occurs suddenly about day 6 of fever. Patients may complain of dyspnea, chest pain, and severe anxiety but remain conscious until death. The cause of death is unknown but is thought to be due to toxemia or viremia or both.[50,69,79]

Late Hemorrhagic-Type Smallpox. Late HTS has a severe, prolonged febrile prodrome similar to that of early HTS. Approximately 80% of cases occur in patients older than 14 years of age; there is equal occurrence between males and females. Among pregnant women with smallpox, 6% develop late HTS compared with 2% of nonpregnant women and 2.1% of men. Fevers usually reach 104°F to 105°F. The late form differs from the early form, however, in that hemorrhages typically develop after the eruption of the rash. The rash begins as macules, progresses to papules, but matures slowly thereafter. Skin lesions have bleeding into their bases, giving them a flattened appearance (see Fig. 134A-4B). These flattened lesions usually do not progress beyond the vesicular stage, but remain flattened and turn black, giving this form the name *black pox*. Patients with flat lesions experience a higher fatality than patients with ordinary lesions.[50,69]

Patients with late HTS also have abnormal bleeding elsewhere, although typically not as severe as seen in early HTS, and bleeding may occur at any stage of the disease. In a case series of late HTS by Downie and associates,[69] death occurred an average of 10 to 11 days (range 7 to 19 days) after the onset of fever. This same series (n = 2) also included three survivors.

MODIFIED-TYPE SMALLPOX

All cases of smallpox in which scabs are formed on all lesions by day 10 of the illness are empirically classified as *modified*. In Rao's series,[50] MTS accounted for 2.1% of cases in unvaccinated persons and for 25.3% in previously vaccinated persons. Patients may develop MTS after exposure to one of the more severe forms of smallpox and vice versa. The prodrome of MTS includes moderate-to-high fever, headache, backache, body aches, and vomiting and usually lasts 2 to 3 days. Enanthem is uncommon in MTS. In its mildest form, MTS may run its course with only the constitutional symptoms without any rash following.[3,50]

Lesions are fewer (sometimes only one or two lesions), smaller, and more superficial than the lesions in patients with OTS, may be pleomorphic, do not umbilicate, and evolve more rapidly than the lesions seen in the other clinical forms of smallpox. The discrete form of MTS was most common in Rao's series[50]—24.3% and 2% of vaccinated and unvaccinated cases, respectively. The semiconfluent form constituted 0.5% of unvaccinated cases of MTS in Rao's series. Rarely, cases of confluent MTS can be seen (0.1% of unvaccinated cases in Rao's series were this type). Although the rash is densely distributed, the patient is not toxic, and all lesions form scabs by day 10 of illness. The modified cases were rarely fatal; no deaths were reported in Rao's series,[50] which included 937 cases of MTS.

VARIOLA SINE ERUPTIONE

As the name suggests, the *variola sine eruptione* form of smallpox does not develop a rash. It usually occurs in well-vaccinated persons but can occur in unvaccinated persons and in infants with maternal antibodies.[79] The transmission of smallpox has not been documented in variola sine eruptione.[79] Diagnosis is possible only by laboratory tests. Patients typically have a febrile prodrome similar to the other clinical forms, but their fever resolves within a few days, does not recur, and is not followed by a rash.

Variola Minor

Variola minor is a much milder form of smallpox, also called *alastrim* or *kaffir* smallpox, that was found primarily in the Americas, Africa, and Europe. The constitutional symptoms are mild. The rash of variola minor is less dense than the OTS rash, lesions are usually discrete, and it resolves over 1 to 2 weeks (Fig. 134A-5). The hemorrhagic form of variola minor is rare, occurring in less than 0.5% of cases. The case-fatality rate for variola minor is less than 1%.[3,50]

DIAGNOSIS

Differential Diagnosis

The differential diagnosis of smallpox varies with the type of smallpox that a patient has and the stage at which the patient presents. Typical illnesses in the differential diagnosis include other rash-associated diseases. Varicella virus infection either as a primary infection (chickenpox) or as disseminated herpes zoster (shingles) is probably the most commonly encountered infection in the differential diagnosis of smallpox (Table 134A-2). Varicella variants may be hemorrhagic, appearing similar to the lesions of HTS.[79,84] The lesions of disseminated varicella zoster also may have a hemorrhagic appearance and are typically painful (similar to the lesions of smallpox). Additional clinical features, such as the distribution and morphology of the lesions and characteristics of the prodrome, if present, are helpful in discriminating between these illnesses. The most important distinctions between the rash of smallpox and that of chickenpox are that the rash of smallpox erupts synchronously, in contrast to the asynchronous eruption (cropping) characteristic of chickenpox, and the lesions of smallpox are more densely distributed to the extremities (centrifugal pattern), whereas chickenpox lesions are more densely distributed to the trunk (centripetal pattern).[67] Also, the characteristic umbilication seen on smallpox vesicles is uncommon in chickenpox lesions. Crusting of chickenpox lesions begins within 24 hours of the initial eruption and is complete within 4 to 6 days. Although the classic rashes of these two infections are readily distinguished, smallpox and chickenpox have variants that are more challenging to differentiate.

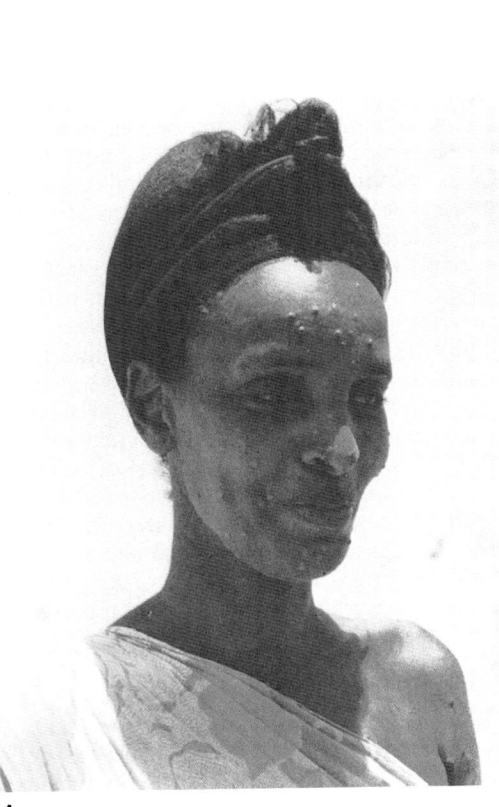

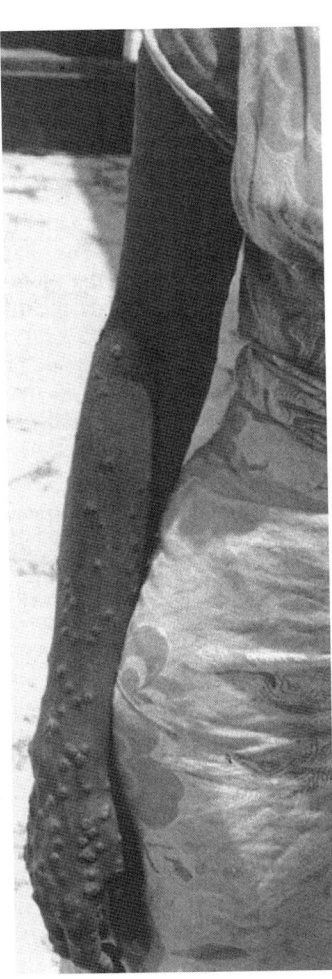

FIGURE 134A-5

Variola minor in an unvaccinated 30-year-old woman (12 days after rash eruption). The patient was not toxic throughout course of illness. Lesions are sparse on the face **(A)** and evolved more rapidly than lesions on the extremities **(B)**. *(Fom Senkevich T, Wolffe EJ, Buller ML: Ectromelia virus RING finger protein is localized in virus factories and is required for virus replication in macrophages. J Virol 69:4103–4111, 1995.)* See Color Figs. 134A-5A and 134A-5B.

A   B

TABLE 134A-2 Differential Diagnosis of Smallpox and Chickenpox

	VARIOLA MAJOR (OTS)	VARICELLA (CHICKENPOX)
Incubation period*	7–19 days (mean 12 days)	14–21 days
Pock characteristics	Enanthem present Synchronous eruption "Shotty" Deep dermally based Painful	Enanthem absent Asynchronous (cropping) Pleomorphic Superficial Pruritic

Lesion evolution	Macules → papules → vesicles →
	  pustules → umbilication → scabbing
	  → scab separation → scarring
		Macules → papules → vesicles →
		  pustules → scabbing → scab
		  separation

Scab formation	10–14 days after rash onset	1–7 days after rash onset
Scab separation	14–28 days after rash onset	Within 14 days of rash onset

Infectivity	From onset of enanthem to
	  scab separation
		From 1 day *before* rash eruption until
		  scab formation

*May vary with form of smallpox.
OTS, ordinary-type smallpox.

The critical care clinician must maintain a high degree of clinical suspicion and consider the other clinical features of the illness and epidemiologic data to make the correct diagnosis as expeditiously as possible to limit additional cases. The electronic transmission of digital photographs of suspect rashes to appropriate consultants and public health agencies, such as the U.S. Centers for Disease Control and Prevention (CDC), to assist in diagnosis has been used.[84] The CDC has established criteria for determining the risk that a febrile illness associated with a rash is smallpox (Table 134A-3).

Monkeypox is an orthopoxvirus closely related to variola and causes human illness that probably most resembles smallpox.[85–87] It is an enzootic disease of mammals, including squirrels and primates, in the rainforests of central and western Africa. Humans usually become infected through contact with infected animals,[87] although studies have shown that monkeypox is infectious via the aerosol route.[88,89] Immunization with vaccinia virus is approximately 85% protective.[86] Because routine smallpox immunization has not been practiced for many years, however, the population at large is susceptible. Monkeypox is considered a potential biologic weapon as a surrogate for variola virus.[90] Outbreaks of human monkeypox[86,91,92] continue to occur in Africa, providing a potential source of the infectious agent for weaponization by bioterrorists. Although not as infectious as smallpox, monkeypox can be transmitted between humans, and multiple generation transmission has been reported.[88] The clinical presentation includes a vesiculopustular exanthem that erupts in a centrifugal, synchronous pattern, including the palms and soles, and an ulcerating enanthem. The rash lesions are usually discrete or semiconfluent, although typically not as densely distributed as smallpox, and last 2 to 4 weeks. Of cases, 98% reported fever; 11%, diarrhea; 41%, cough; 69%, cervical lymphadenopathy (inguinal lymphadenopathy also has been reported)[90]; 63%, sore throat; and 50%, mouth ulcers.[91] Monkeypox's prominent lymphadenopathy is not typical of smallpox and produces a much less severe illness. Case-fatality rates reported in several case series ranged from

1.5% to 11%.[86,87,91,92] Overall, naturally occurring human monkeypox is not likely to be found outside of Africa except from research laboratories. Given its similarity to smallpox, however, and the theoretical potential that it

TABLE 134A-3 Centers for Disease Control and Prevention Vesicular or Pustular Rash Protocol

High Risk for Smallpox (all 3 of the following *major criteria* are present)

Febrile prodrome occurring 1–4 days before rash onset with fever >102°F *and* at least one of the following:
  Prostration
  Headache
  Backache
  Chills
  Vomiting
  Severe abdominal pain
Classic smallpox lesions
  Deeply embedded in the dermis
  Firm/hard
  Well circumscribed
  Round
  May be umbilicated
  May be discrete, semiconfluent, confluent
Synchronous eruption; all lesions in the same stage of development

Moderate Risk for Smallpox

Febrile prodrome *and* one of the "High Risk for Smallpox" criteria, *or*
Febrile prodrome and at least 4 of the 5 following *minor criteria*:
  Centrifugal distribution
  First lesions appear on the oral mucosa/palate, face, or forearms
  Patient appears toxic or moribund
  Slow evolution of lesions from macules to papules to pustules over several days
  Lesions on the palms and soles

Low Risk for Smallpox

No viral prodrome, *or*
Febrile prodrome with fewer than 4 of the 5 minor criteria for "Moderate Risk for Smallpox"

could be used as a biologic weapon, monkeypox should be included in the differential diagnosis of smallpox.

Other rash-causing illnesses included in the differential diagnosis of smallpox include cocksackievirus infection (hand-foot-and-mouth disease), disseminated herpes simplex, disseminated herpes zoster, secondary syphilis, impetigo, acne, measles, rickettsialpox (*Rickettsia akari*), and rubella. Meningococcemia, severe acute leukemia, gram-negative sepsis, or other conditions that cause a petechial rash may resemble the poorly differentiated rash of HTS. Immunosuppressed patients may develop severe disseminated molluscum contagiosum (another orthopoxvirus), which may resemble smallpox.

Vaccinia virus is the live viral agent in the "smallpox vaccine" that confers immunity to infection by variola virus. If the threat of a bioterrorist attack increases or a smallpox attack occurs, there likely would be widespread smallpox immunization. Conversely, because vaccinia virus is much more readily available to a would-be bioterrorist and can be genetically engineered to produce a virulent biologic agent,[76,77] it may be employed as a biologic weapon. It is likely that generalized vaccinia, eczema vaccinatum, may be seen in both of these settings and needs to be included in the differential diagnosis.[3,39,70,79] Noninfectious conditions that may appear similar to smallpox include drug eruptions, erythema multiforme, Stevens-Johnson syndrome, insect bites, and pemphigus.[79]

The differential diagnosis of smallpox includes infection with other viruses, bacterial infections, and noninfectious clinical conditions. Careful attention to the distribution and lesions of the rash and other clinical manifestations, such as hemorrhages and prodrome, is the mainstay of the diagnosis. Laboratory testing is an essential adjunct for the confirmation of smallpox. Many techniques can be employed, and collaboration with the LRN provides expanded access to specialized methods and hasten arrival at the correct diagnosis.

Response to Bioterrorist Attack

The most potent defense against a bioterrorist attack is the rapid identification of the event and agent, treatment of the victims, and containment of the infection. Many epidemiologic surveillance systems have been established to assist in the rapid identification of a bioterrorist attack. The clinician still must be vigilant, however, for unusual patterns of illness in the community. When a suspicious illness has been identified, clinical samples must be sent to the nearest clinical laboratory as soon as possible to begin confirmatory testing. Empirical treatment should not be delayed while awaiting laboratory results.

The Laboratory Response Network (LRN) has been established to create an organized system of bioterrorism-related specimen testing and referral. The LRN is a system of public and private laboratories, linked with local, state, and federal agencies, that test suspected bioterrorism-related clinical samples by established consensus protocols to provide timely and accurate testing and reporting. It comprises four levels of laboratories—A, B, C, and D—which perform testing and refer samples to the next higher level laboratory. The largest and lowest tier of the LRN comprises biosafety level (BSL)–2 clinical laboratories des-

ignated *level A*. Their role is to *rule in and refer* presumptive early cases of bioterrorism-related illness. The critical care clinician should become familiar with the readiness and capabilities of his or her local laboratory *before* an actual event takes place. Level B comprises public health laboratories that usually operate at BSL-3 conditions and perform isolation, identification, and susceptibility testing of samples and *rule in and refer*. Level C also is made up of BSL-3 public health laboratories, but with more advanced typing and identification capabilities. They also *rule in and refer* to the final level, level D, where additional high-level characterization studies can be performed under BSL-4 conditions. Presently, there are two level D laboratories in the United States: the CDC and the United States Army Institute of Infectious Diseases. A complete discussion of the LRN is not within the scope of this chapter. The reader is urged to consult the CDC, public health service, and local laboratories for additional information on using this system. Detailed guides and instructions for the selection, collection, storage, and shipping of specimens for analysis and additional information regarding bioterrorism preparedness are available from the CDC Website bioterrorism page (www.bt.cdc.gov).

Laboratory Testing

The clinical laboratory is an important asset to establish or rule out the diagnosis of smallpox. Many techniques have been developed to confirm the presence of variola virus in biologic samples, such as material from skin lesions, including culture on chick embryo chorioallantoic membrane culture, agar gel precipitation, tissue culture, immunofluorescence, and electron microscopy.[14,93,94] Variola virus can be isolated from blood during the preeruptive viremia; from saliva, blood, and skin lesions during the maculopapular stage of the rash; and from the blood and skin lesions until the crusting stage of the rash. A presumptive diagnosis of smallpox can be made with Giemsa-stained clinical specimens in which Guanieri inclusion bodies can be seen.[95] Electron microscopy is a powerful method that allows rapid morphologic identification and differential diagnosis of different agents contained in a specimen.[95] It can identify intracellular and extracellular viral particles with characteristic orthopoxvirus morphology and can be performed in parallel with other methods, such as cell culture, to hasten and confirm results. Electron microscopy requires specialized technicians, however, to prepare and examine specimens.[14] Plans and protocols should be established before an event to incorporate electron microscopy efficiently into the laboratory diagnostic armamentarium. Polymerase chain reaction gene amplification for nucleic acid detection and identification is a sensitive method for detecting the DNA of specific biologic agents in specimens.[40,96] It is usually available at level B and higher LRN laboratories and is useful for differentiating smallpox from other orthopoxviruses and for assaying limited quantities of specimen. Additional indirect serologic testing, such as complement fixation, hemagglutination inhibition, and neutralizing antibody testing, also are helpful clinical tests that can be performed with lower risk than culturing or handling potentially infectious variola virus–containing samples.

TREATMENT

Isolation

Public health officials should be notified immediately of any suspected smallpox patient. Unless the diagnosis of smallpox is confirmed, all patients who will be isolated with other suspected or confirmed cases of smallpox should be vaccinated. Vaccination is done to prevent accidental transmission of smallpox virus to any *suspected* smallpox patients who have been misdiagnosed and placed in quarantine with "true" smallpox patients. Initial management of any suspected smallpox patient should include immediate isolation of the patient in a negative-pressure room (minimum six air exchanges per hour), strict contact and respiratory isolation (gloves, gowns, N95 or N100 masks, protective eyewear, shoe covers), and immediate quarantine of all contacts. Health care workers should remove and dispose of all protective clothing in biohazard waste containers before leaving the isolation area and reentering other areas of the hospital. All infectious waste and contaminated protective clothing should be disposed of properly in biohazard containers or sterilized in an appropriate manner. All personnel entering the isolation area and handling infectious waste or clinical specimens from the patients should be vaccinated or have documentation of successful vaccination within the previous 3 years.

High-efficiency particulate air (HEPA) filters are recommended for all exhaust vents and air recirculation systems. If the patient must be transported between isolation settings, all lesions should be covered and a mask should be placed on the patient. If possible, patients should be encapsulated in a portable isolation chamber for transport. If the patient requires mechanical or bag-valve ventilation, all tube connections and fittings should be taped to avoid aerosolization of virus from a leaking, or accidentally disconnected, ventilation system. HEPA filters should be fitted to all ventilator and bag-valve exhaust ports. Simple measures, such as limited personnel in contact with the patient and keeping doors and windows closed, should not be overlooked. All linen and medical waste must be placed in biohazard bags and autoclaved before being laundered or incinerated. Outbreaks have occurred when laundry workers handled improperly-disposed-of linens and blankets from smallpox patients.[67] When possible, patients who die of smallpox should be cremated. All hospital personnel, medical staff, and mortuary workers should be vaccinated as soon as smallpox has been diagnosed.

Supportive Care

Treatment for smallpox is largely supportive because no effective antiviral therapies have yet been adequately tested as safe and effective. Ensuring adequate fluid and nutrition intake is important because the enanthem typically makes it impossible for severely ill patients to take sufficient amounts of liquids and food. Patients during the vesicular and pustular stages of smallpox are at high risk for hypovolemic shock because of fluid losses from fever, vomiting, decreased oral fluid intake due to painful enanthem, fluid shifts into the skin, and skin desquamation in patients with confluent lesions. Patients with HTS are at risk for additional blood loss due to hemorrhage. Control of pain and fever with appropriate analgesics and antipyretics is indicated.

Keeping lesions clean and dressed and taking care to avoid rupturing vesicles and pustules can reduce risk of secondary infection of the rash lesions. Salves and ointments are not recommended. The desquamation sometimes seen with the most severe forms of smallpox, such as HTS, may necessitate dressing changes and treatment comparable to that employed in the management of major burns. Secondary bacterial skin infections should be treated with appropriate antibiotics and guided by culture and sensitivity testing.

Viral bronchitis and pneumonitis are common complications in severe cases of smallpox. Treatment is supportive with supplemental oxygen, intubation, and mechanical ventilation as indicated. Secondary bacterial pneumonia can occur and should be treated with appropriate antibiotics and guided by culture and sensitivity testing. Pulmonary edema also is common in severe cases of smallpox and should be treated with careful fluid management, ventilation, and pressor support.

Other, less common complications include acute arthritis (1.7% in Rao's series) and orchitis (0.1% in Rao's series).[50] These conditions usually resolved spontaneously without treatment. Corneal ulcers and variola keratitis also were reported in Rao's series, usually in HTS, but occasionally in OTS.[50] There are no studies to support the use of topical ophthalmic antiviral agents. Recommended management for ocular complications may be helpful (see Table 134A-4). Encephalitis was reported to occur in 1 of every 500 cases of smallpox and occasionally was fatal. No treatment is available.

Variolation

Variolation, a cutaneous infection by variola virus caused by scarification and the first use of inoculation as a preventive treatment for smallpox, was introduced in Egypt in the 13th century.[3] The modern technique of vaccination was developed in 1796 by Jenner, who recognized that prior infection with cowpox virus was protective against smallpox.[97] More than 300 years later, his concept of inoculation by scarification with vaccinia virus is still the primary defense used against smallpox. Vaccination exploits the cross-immunizing characteristics of poxviruses. When introduced into the dermal layer by a multiple puncture technique, vaccinia virus multiplies in the basilar epithelium, causing a local cellular immune

---

Indications for ICU Admission for Smallpox

1. Any patient with a suspected case of smallpox should be admitted to an isolation room until the diagnosis can be ruled out or the patient's rash resolves.
2. *All* smallpox patients require isolation; *however*, if the number of patients exceeds intensive care unit (ICU) capacity, alternative isolation facilities should be used and ICU facilities reserved for critically ill smallpox patients.
3. Any smallpox patient with respiratory distress or hypotension should be admitted.
4. Any patient with postvaccination progressive vaccinia, eczema vaccinatum, or postvaccinial encephalitis should be admitted.

reaction. A lesion develops at the site and evolves through the same progression seen with smallpox lesions. The result is a Jennerian pustule (Fig. 134A-6) that is referred to as a *take*, indicating that an adequate immune response has occurred. Typically the vaccination lesion should progress through all stages within 3 weeks, leaving a dark crust, or scab, that separates, leaving a scar. This scar is considered evidence that a person has been previously, successfully immunized against smallpox.[3]

Vaccination

Worldwide, different vaccinia strains have been used for production of smallpox vaccine, but all current U.S. vaccine formulations contain the New York City Board of Health vaccinia strain. Dryvax (Wyeth Laboratories Inc, Marietta, PA) is the vaccine being administered in the current U.S. smallpox vaccination effort. Dryvax contains polymyxin B, streptomycin, chlortetracycline, and neomycin. It is contraindicated for vaccination in persons with known allergies to these medications. Development of new smallpox vaccines is ongoing.[64,98] Two newly developed vaccines from Acambis/Baxter Pharmaceuticals (Cambridge, MA), ACAM1000, which is grown in human embryonic lung cell culture (MRC-5), and ACAM2000, which is grown in African green monkey cells (VERO cells), are being stockpiled in the United States.[99]

During the period January 24, 2003, to March 21, 2003, 25,645 civilian health care workers received the smallpox vaccination in the United States. Six cases of vaccinia transmission from military personnel to civilian contacts have been reported, including two cases of ocular vaccinia.[100] Ophthalmologic examination on one of these patients revealed severe right scleral injection and chemosis, a small pustule at the right palpebral lower lid margin, and tender right preauricular and submandibular lymphadenopathy. No evidence of keratitis, iritis, or periocular lesions was found. The patient improved within 24 hours after treatment with trifluridine eyedrops and a single dose of intravenous vaccinia immune globulin (VIG).[100] No cases of transmission from civilian vaccinees to close contacts have been reported. There have been 15 moderate-to-severe events reported and 16 severe events reported, including 3 myocardial infarctions, 2 cases of angina, and 2 cases of myopericarditis. All three patients with myocardial infarction had two or more cardiac risk factors, and two of the patients died.[101] Ten cases of myocarditis or myopericarditis or both, 29 case of autoinoculation, and 25 cases of generalized vaccinia have been reported among approximately 350,000 primary vaccinees in the military smallpox program.[101] No cases were reported in personnel who previously had been vaccinated. None of these cases were clinically severe, and all personnel recovered fully and returned to duty; two were treated with VIG. A 55-year-old male National Guard soldier with a history of cardiac risk factors, who was called to active duty, had a myocardial infarction on March 25, 2003, 5 days after smallpox vaccination. He died late on March 26, 2003. Autopsy showed that coronary artery disease existed before vaccination and showed evidence of prior heart disease. Cardiac complications after smallpox vaccination have been previously reported.[102–104] These reports suggest that smallpox vaccination may cause myocarditis, pericarditis, and myopericarditis. A causal relationship between smallpox vaccination and ischemic cardiac complications has yet to be shown, however. At the time of this writing, the CDC recommends that persons with a history of heart disease, with or without symptoms, including previous myocardial infarction, angina, congestive heart failure, and cardiomyopathy, should not receive smallpox vaccine. All vaccinees should be instructed to seek medical attention if they develop chest pain, shortness of breath, or other symptoms of cardiac disease after smallpox vaccination.[101,105]

Should smallpox immunization become necessary, the critical care clinician may be faced with caring for major complications of vaccination (Table 134A-4). Minor

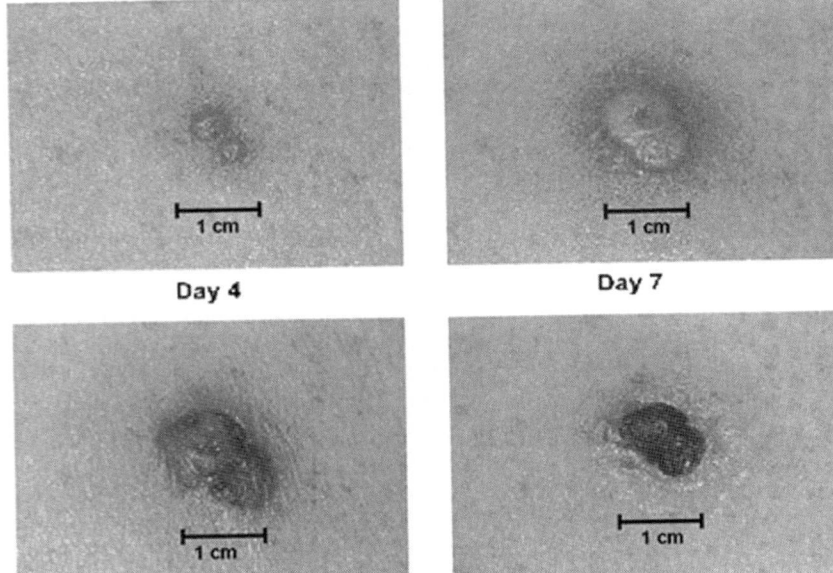

Day 4

Day 7

Day 14

Day 21

FIGURE 134A-6

Major (primary) reaction. Expected vaccine site reaction and progression after primary smallpox vaccination or revaccination after a prolonged period between vaccinations. Multiple pressure vaccination technique was used. *(From U.S. Centers for Disease Control and Prevention. Available at: http://www.bt.cdc.gov/agent/smallpox/vaccineimages.asp.)* See Color Fig. 134A-6.

TABLE 134A-4 Complications of Vaccination

ADVERSE EVENT	DESCRIPTION	RISK FACTOR OR PREDISPOSITION	TREATMENT
Eczema vaccinatum	High fever Generalized lymphadenopathy with extensive vesicular and pustular eruption Onset: concurrently or shortly after local vaccinial lesion in vaccinee, or in contacts, 5–19 days after suspected exposure Risk for secondary bacterial or fungal infections Virus recovered from lesions High mortality rate with poor prognosis	History of eczema or atopic dermatitis regardless of disease activity or severity Less frequently, persons without a history of dermatologic conditions	Prompt evaluation and diagnosis Infection-control precautions Might require multiple doses of VIG (cidofovir, second-line therapy) Hemodynamic support Volume and electrolyte repletion Observe for secondary skin infections
Progressive vaccinia	Nonhealing vaccination site Painless progressive (central) necrosis at the vaccination site Occasional metastatic lesions in skin, bones, and viscera No inflammation initially Absence of inflammatory cells on histopathologic examination Inflammation weeks later Bacterial infection might develop Differential diagnosis: severe bacterial infection, severe chickenpox, disseminated herpes simplex, and other necrotic conditions Prognosis: poor, despite therapy	Humoral and cellular immunocompromise (e.g., malignancy, human immunodeficiency virus–acquired immunodeficiency syndrome, severe combined immunodeficiency syndrome, or hypogammaglobulinemia) Protective level of T-cell count or humoral immunity unknown	Prompt evaluation and diagnosis Infection-control precautions Might require multiple doses of VIG (cidofovir second-line therapy) Surgical débridement of progressive necrotic lesions not proven useful
Postvaccinial encephalitis or encephalomyelitis	Diagnosis of exclusion Appears similar to postinfectious encephalomyelitis or toxic encephalopathy caused by other agents Abrupt onset of symptoms: fever, headache, malaise, lethargy, vomiting, meningeal signs, seizures, paralysis, drowsiness, altered mental status, or coma Age <2 yr (encephalopathy): cerebrovascular changes occuring 6–10 days postvaccination Age ≥2 yr (encephalomyelitis): demyelinating changes occurring 11–15 days postvaccination Cerebrospinal fluid: normal or nonspecific; monocytosis, lymphocytosis, or elevated protein Prognosis: mortality, 25%; neurologic sequelae, 25%; complete recovery, 50%	Age <1 yr	Intensive supportive care Anticonvulsants as needed VIG not recommended Antiviral role unclear Use of modern imaging studies has not been evaluated
Fetal vaccinia	Incidence: rare (<50 reported cases) Route of transmission: unknown Outcomes: premature birth, fetal loss, high mortality Not associated with congenital anomalies	Cases in all trimesters of pregnancy Greatest risk, third trimester	Efficacy of VIG unknown Antivirals not recommended
Generalized vaccinia	Maculopapular or vesicular rash Onset: 6–9 days postvaccination Nontoxic, with or without fever	Hematogenous spread Lesions contain vaccinia More serious among immunocompromised persons	Usually self-limited in immunocompetent person Infection-control precautions VIG usually not indicated

Continued

TABLE 134A-4 Complications of Vaccination—cont'd

ADVERSE EVENT	DESCRIPTION	RISK FACTOR OR PREDISPOSITION	TREATMENT
Inadvertent inoculation	Differential diagnosis: erythema multiforme, varicella, inadvertent inoculation, progressive vaccinia, and smallpox Most common complication Physical transfer of vaccinia virus from a vaccination site to second site on the vaccinee or to a close contact of vaccinee	Manipulation of vaccination site Children aged <4 yr Conditions that disrupt the epidermis (e.g., burns, severe acne, or psoriasis)	Antiinflammatory medications Antipruritic medications Antivirals usually not indicated Usually self-limited Resolution in 3 wk Infection-control precautions VIG if extensive body surface involved or severe ocular disease (cidofovir, second-line therapy)
Ocular vaccinia Inadvertent periocular or ocular implantation with vaccinia virus; can range from mild to severe	Keratitis Marginal infiltration or ulceration with or without stromal haze/infiltration Conjunctivitis Hyperemia, edema, membranes, focal lesions, fever, lymphadenopathy Blepharitis Lid pustules on or near the lid margin, edema, hyperemia, lymphadenopathy, cellulitis, fever	Manipulation of vaccination site, followed by eye rubbing More likely with conditions that cause eye itching and scratching (conjunctivitis, corneal abrasion/ulceration)	Ophthalmologic consultation Certain ophthalmologists consider off-label topical antiviral medications Topical prophylactic antibacterial medications for keratitis VIG for severe blepharitis and blepharo-conjunctivitis (without keratitis) VIG not indicated for isolated keratitis VIG considered for keratitis with vision-threatening conditions VIG indicated for keratitis with life-threatening conditions that require VIG
Erythema multiforme and SJS	Typical bull's eye (target) lesions Hypersensitivity reaction Pruritus Onset: 10 days postvaccination Can progress to SJS	No known risk factors	Antipruritic medications VIG not indicated Hospitalization and supportive care for SJS Steroid use for SJS is controversial
Pyogenic infections of vaccination site	Uncommon Onset: 5 days postvaccination Fever not specific for bacterial infection Fluctuance at vaccination site	More frequent in children (touching vaccination site)	Gram stain Bacterial culture Antibacterial medications, if clinically indicated No topical medications
Robust take	>7.5 cm with swelling, warmth, and pain at vaccination site Fluctuant lymph nodes not expected Peak symptoms: 8–10 days postvaccination Nonprogressive Improvement in 24–72 hr	Might be more likely among first-time vaccinees	Observation most important Antibacterial medications not indicated Rest affected limb Antipruritic medications Antiinflammatory medications No salves or ointments
Tape adhesive reactions	Sharply demarcated raised lines of erythema that correspond to adhesive placement Local pruritus No systemic illness	Sensitivity to adhesives	No salves, ointments, or topical/oral steroids Frequent bandage changes Periodic bandage removal

SJS, Stevens-Johnson syndrome; VIG, vaccinia immune globulin.
From Saraiva M, Alcami A: CrmE, a novel soluble tumor necrosis factor receptor encoded by poxviruses. J Virol 75:226–233, 2001.

complications are more common but usually do not require treatment and are limited to local findings or mild systemic illness (Fig. 134A-7). Studies of vaccination adverse effects during smallpox eradication in the United States found that there were 1254 complications and approximately 1 death per 1 million primary vaccinations.[78,106] A review of 68 vaccinia-related deaths during a 9-year period revealed that deaths occurred among first-time vaccinees as a result of postvaccinial encephalitis (36 cases) and progressive vaccinia (vaccinia necrosum) (19 cases), eczema vaccinatum (12 cases), and Stevens-Johnson syndrome (1 case). Of the deaths, 24 (35%) were in infants, although they constituted only 12% of all primary vaccinees. All deaths from eczema vaccinatum were in secondary contacts, and all deaths due to vaccinia necrosum were in vaccinees with underlying immunodeficiencies.[107] Secondary bacterial infections at the vaccination site are relatively uncommon if the site is kept clean and dressed (Fig. 134A-8A). The most common organisms are *Staphylococcus* spp. and *Streptococcus* spp. Treatment is with appropriate antibiotics as guided by culture and sensitivities. Erythema multiforme also occurs, although it generally does not require treatment beyond antihistamines (Fig. 134A-8B).

Progressive vaccinia, also called *vaccinia gangrenosum* or *vaccinia necrosum*, can occur in persons with deficiencies in cellular immunity. Although rare, occurring in approximately 1 person per 1 million vaccinees, it is the most serious complication of vaccination and is often fatal. It is characterized by continual enlargement of the primary vaccination site, progressive necrosis at the site, and minimal inflammation with little or no axillary lymphadenopathy.[108] Patients may have secondary lesions at other body sites with the same characteristics (see Fig. 134A-8D). VIG is indicated for the treatment of progressive vaccinia. Codofovir also is indicated

for the treatment of this complication under the conditions of the investigational drug protocol established by the CDC.

Postvaccination encephalitis is an unpredictable complication that occurs only in primary vaccinees. Its incidence seemed to be related to the strain of vaccinia virus, although most cases occurred in primary vaccinees younger than 1 year of age. In the national survey, there were 12 cases with 1 death among 13 million vaccinees.[106] Patients develop high fever, seizures, vomiting, drowsiness, occasional spastic paralysis, meningeal signs, and coma. It typically occurs 8 to 15 days postvaccination at a rate of 1 case per 300,000 vaccinations. Approximately 15% to 25% of cases were fatal, and another 25% of patients had permanent neurologic sequelae. VIG is not effective in treating this complication and is not recommended.[99]

Inadvertent inoculation occurs when the live vaccinia virus is transferred from the primary site of inoculation to either a second site on the vaccinee (autoinoculation) or a close contact.[109,110] The most common sites involved are the face, eyelid, nose, mouth, lips, genitalia, and anus (see Fig. 134A-8C).[99]

Ocular vaccinial infections account for most inadvertent inoculations and can occur in different forms, including blepharitis (see Fig. 134A-8C), conjunctivitis, keratitis, and iritis.[111] Treatment of vaccinia keratitis with VIG has been associated with increased corneal scarring, however, and is *contraindicated* for the treatment of isolated vaccinial keratitis.[99] Because of the potential for severe morbidity due to vaccinia ocular complications, specific CDC recommendations for its management are included here, as follows:

1. VIG should be considered for use in severe ocular disease when keratitis is not present.
2. VIG should not be withheld if a severe comorbid condition exists that requires administration of VIG

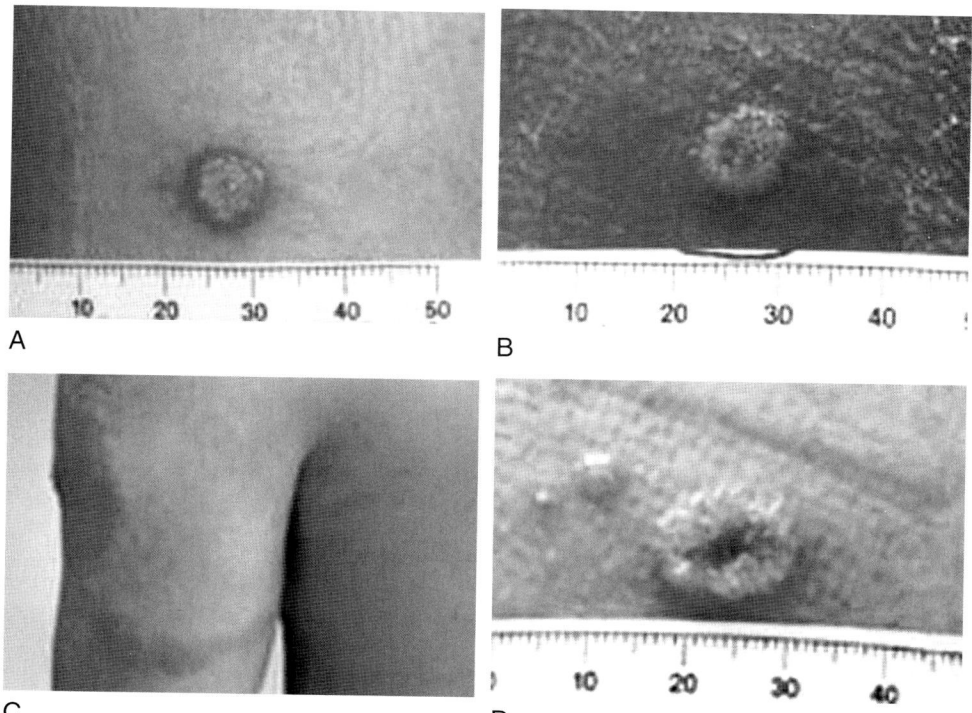

FIGURE 134A-7

A and **B,** Normal vaccination reactions. **C,** Normal reaction with lymphangitis. **D,** Normal reaction with satellite lesions. *(From U.S. Centers for Disease Control and Prevention. Available at: http://www.bt.cdc.gov/training/smallpoxvaccine/reactions/default.htm.)* See Color Figs. 134A-7A through 134A-7D.

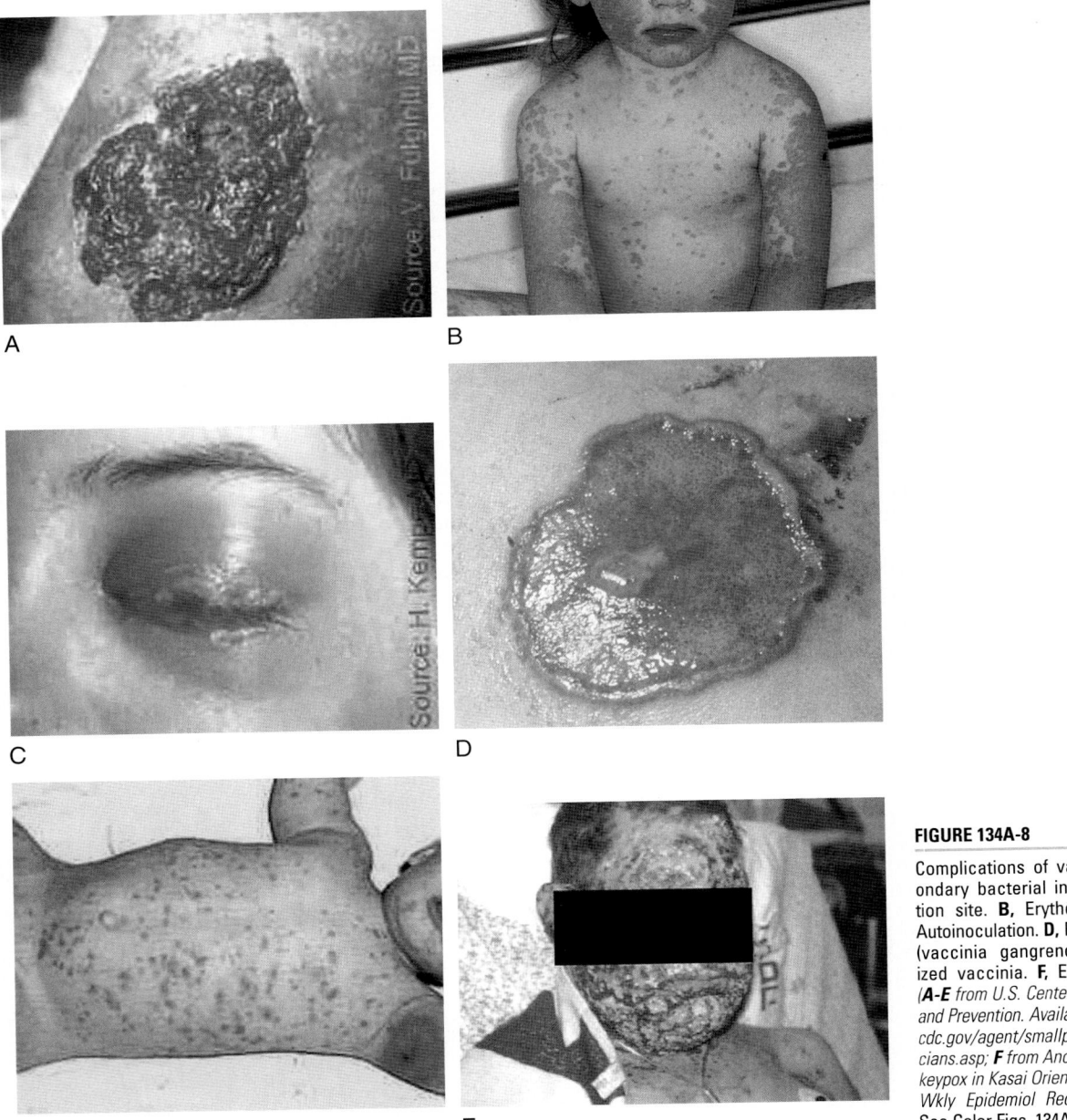

FIGURE 134A-8

Complications of vaccination. **A,** Secondary bacterial infection at vaccination site. **B,** Erythema multiforme. **C,** Autoinoculation. **D,** Progressive vaccinia (vaccinia gangrenosum). **E,** Generalized vaccinia. **F,** Eczema vaccinatum. (*A-E* from U.S. Centers for Disease Control and Prevention. Available at: http://www.bt.cdc.gov/agent/smallpox/vaccination/clinicians.asp; *F* from Anonymous: Human monkeypox in Kasai Oriental, Zaire [1996–1997]. Wkly Epidemiol Rec 72:101–104, 1997.) See Color Figs. 134A-8A through 134A-8F.

(e.g., vaccinia necrosum) and should be considered for severe ocular disease *except isolated keratitis*.

3. Complications of vaccination should be comanaged with an ophthalmologist.
4. Off-label use of topical ophthalmic trifluridine or vidarabine can be considered for treatment of vaccinia infection of the conjunctiva or cornea.
5. Prophylactic therapy with these drugs also might be considered to prevent spread to the conjunctiva and cornea if vaccinia lesions are present on the eyelid, including near the lid margin or adjacent to the eye.
6. Topical antivirals should be continued until all periocular or lid lesions have healed and the scabs have fallen off; however, topical trifluridine usually is not used for

more than 14 days to avoid possible toxicity (when used for >14 days, trifluridine can lead to superficial punctate keratopathy).
7. VIG can be considered if the ocular disease is severe enough to pose a substantial risk of impaired vision as a long-term outcome.
8. If VIG is administered specifically to treat ocular disease in the presence of keratitis, treatment usually should be limited to one dose, and the patient or guardian should be informed of the possible risks and benefits before its use.
9. Topical ophthalmic antibiotics should be considered for prophylaxis of bacterial infection in the presence of keratitis, including if a corneal ulcer is present or steroids are used.

10. In severe cases of keratitis (e.g., with an ulcer and stromal haze or infiltrate) and in iritis, topical steroids should be considered after the corneal epithelium is healed to decrease immune reaction.
11. Mydriatics also are indicated.
12. Topical steroids should not be used without ophthalmologic consultation and should not be used acutely without topical antiviral therapy.
13. All patients with ocular vaccinia infection should receive careful follow-up evaluation by an ophthalmologist.[99]

Generalized vaccinia is a diffuse maculopapular or vesicular rash, usually occurring 6 to 9 days after vaccination (see Fig. 134A-8E). The individual lesions resemble the lesion at the vaccination site. As mentioned earlier, generalized vaccinia is in the differential diagnosis of smallpox because its lesions may resemble the lesions of smallpox. The rash of generalized vaccinia is not distributed in the centrifugal pattern characteristic for smallpox, however, and patients are not typically toxic. This postvaccination complication is not typically associated with immunodeficiency, although it has been reported[112] and has a good prognosis. During smallpox immunization in the United States in the 1960s, there were 9.7 cases per 1 million vaccinees, 2 cases among several million of their contacts, and no deaths. In general, VIG treatment is not required except in patients who appear toxic or have serious underlying conditions.[78,106]

Eczema vaccinatum can occur in vaccinees or contacts of vaccines who have active or healed eczema or other chronic skin conditions, such as atopic dermatitis, severe acne, chickenpox, burns, varicella zoster (shingles), herpes, or psoriasis. The skin of atopic dermatitis patients is known to produce higher levels of IL-4 and lower levels of IFN-γ than the skin of normal individuals. It also is known that IL-4 effectively diminishes the cellular immune response to viral infection[76] and that IFN-γ has antiviral activity.[71,73] It is thought that this dermal immunologic environment may promote the overgrowth of vaccinia virus in the skin of these patients.[113] This complication is usually self-limiting but occasionally can be fatal. It can be treated effectively with VIG (see Fig. 134A-8F).[99,114]

The recommended agents for treatment of certain vaccine-associated severe adverse reactions are VIG as the first-line therapy and cidofovir as the second-line therapy. These agents are available under investigational new drug protocols from the CDC and the U.S. Department of Defense.[99]

VIG has been shown to be an effective prophylactic agent against smallpox in exposed patients.[115] Because of its limited availability, it has never widely been used in this fashion. VIG has been used successfully, however, for the treatment of complications of vaccination and for smallpox prophylaxis in individual patients in whom vaccination is contraindicated (Table 134A-5). VIG (Baxter) is available from the CDC for treatment of complications of vaccination as an investigational drug, because its efficacy has not yet been shown in controlled clinical trials. VIG is administered intramuscularly, in the buttocks or anterolateral thigh, in doses of 0.6 mL/kg, usually over 24 hours, and can be repeated every 2 to 3 days for severe, prolonged complications.[116] Efforts are under way to produce new lots of VIG

TABLE 134A-5 Vaccinia Immune Globulin

ADVERSE REACTIONS	VIG TREATMENT
Mild to moderate	
Inadvertent inoculation	Usually not required; might be indicated for ocular implantation*
Erythematous or urticarial rashes	Not indicated†
Bullous erythema multiforme (Stevens-Johnson syndrome)	Not indicated†
Moderate to severe	
Eczema vaccinatum	Indicated in severe cases
Generalized vaccinia	Usually not required but might be indicated if patient is severely ill or has serious underlying illness
Progressive vaccinia (vaccinia necrosum)	Might be effective, depending on immune defect
Postvaccinial encephalitits	Not indicated†
Vaccinial keratitis	Contraindicated*

*VIG contraindicated if vaccinial keratitis present because increased scarring can occur.
†VIG is not effective in treatment of these adverse reactions.
VIG, vaccinia immune globulin.

that meet standards for intravenous administration.[99] VIG is indicated for the treatment of eczema vaccinatum, progressive vaccinia, severe generalized vaccinia if the patient is toxic or has a serious underlying illness, and inadvertent inoculation of the eye *without vaccinial keratitis*.[75] VIG is *not* indicated for the treatment of postvaccination encephalitis and is *contraindicated* for vaccinial keratitis because it may increase corneal scarring.[99]

An initial evaluation of approximately 274 compounds identified 27 agents with significant anti–variola virus activity. The most promising antiviral medication under investigation to date is cidofovir (Vistide), a nucleotide analogue. It is currently approved for treatment of acquired immunodeficiency syndrome–associated cytomegalovirus infection. Cidofovir inhibits a wide variety of DNA viruses, including orthopoxviruses.[117] The mechanism of action of this drug is through selective inhibition of viral DNA polymerase. It is renally cleared, and renal tubular secretion contributes to its elimination. It must be administered with probenecid to maintain clinically effective serum levels. Cidofovir has significant renal toxicity, however, and is contraindicated in patients with serum creatinine greater than 1.5 mg/dL, a calculated creatinine clearance less than 55 mL/min, or a urine protein greater than 100 mg/dL. Patients must be prehydrated before its administration, all other nephrotoxic agents must be discontinued before its administration, and renal function must be monitored before and after its administration. It is classified as category C for use in pregnancy.

Cidofovir inhibits vaccinia virus and 35 different isolates of variola virus in vitro, and it has demonstrable activity against cowpox in mice and against monkeypox in monkeys.[118–121] Work is in progress to improve the formulation of cidofovir so that it can be delivered orally in a prodrug form.[117,122] It has been shown that coadministration of cidofovir with vaccinia vaccine did not affect the efficacy of the vaccine preparation. The United States currently allows cidofovir to be used as an investigational new drug in emergencies to treat adverse effects after immunization with the current smallpox vaccine and in the event of smallpox reemerging.[120,121]

Ribavirin (Virazole, Rebetol, Copegus) has been shown to have activity against variola virus and vaccinia virus in vitro.[6] In one case report, ribavirin and VIG were used to treat progressive vaccinia. To date, no clinical trials have been performed to recommend ribavirin for the treatment of either smallpox or complications of smallpox vaccination.

The CDC provide cidofovir for civilian use or for military use if a patient fails to respond to VIG treatment, a patient is near death, or all inventories of VIG have been exhausted. The benefit of cidofovir therapy for vaccinia-related complications is uncertain, and insufficient information exists to determine the appropriate dosing and accompanying hydration and probenecid dosing, if it is needed to treat smallpox vaccine–related adverse events among children. Dosages for these patients should be determined in consultation with specialists at the CDC.[99]

Physicians at civilian medical facilities may request consultation regarding adverse reactions to smallpox vaccinations, VIG, or cidofovir by calling the CDC's Smallpox Vaccinee Adverse Events Clinician Information Line at 877-554-4625. Military physicians at military medical facilities may request consultation regarding adverse reactions to smallpox vaccinations, VIG, or cidofovir by calling the U.S. Army Medical Research Institute of Infectious Diseases at 301-619-2257 or 888-USA-RIID. Additional information regarding dosing and administration of cidofovir is included in the *Investigator's Brochure* that accompanies the release of this product to the clinician when cidofovir is used under the investigational new drug protocol (Table 134A-6).

SPECIAL POPULATIONS

Approximately 7% of children younger than age 5 years develop febrile seizures.[78] Children younger than age 1 year had higher case-fatality rates than older children and adults.

Pregnant women develop HTS more frequently than other populations: 16% compared with 0.9% in nonpregnant women and 0.8% in men.[5] Vaccination is contraindicated in pregnancy, however, owing to the possibility of fetal vaccinia (disseminated and usually fatal vaccinia infection acquired in utero when the mother is vaccinated during pregnancy). Vaccination of pregnant women is indicated only when the woman has been exposed to a confirmed case of smallpox because the risk of fetal vaccinia is outweighed by the risk of developing smallpox.

Immunocompromised patients are at high risk for progressive vaccinia and should be vaccinated only when they have been exposed to a confirmed case of smallpox. Also, all potential vaccinees should be asked if they would be exposed to an immunocompromised person during the course of their vaccination, either at work if they are involved in health care or at home. Such exposure would be a relative contraindication to vaccination, necessitating strict procedures to keep the vaccination site covered at all times. Potential vaccinees with a history of heart disease, with or without symptoms, including previous myocardial infarction, angina, congestive heart failure, and cardiomyopathy, should not receive smallpox vaccine.

Common Misconceptions about Smallpox

1. Smallpox is not a communicable disease.
2. Smallpox is uniformly fatal.
3. The smallpox vaccination contains variola virus.
4. Smallpox vaccination provides 100% immunity against smallpox.
5. Smallpox vaccination provides lifelong immunity.

Key Points in Smallpox

1. Smallpox is a public health emergency—all cases of suspected smallpox must be reported immediately to public health officials.
2. All smallpox patients must be isolated immediately.
3. All smallpox patients and their contacts must be vaccinated immediately.
4. Hospitalized smallpox patients must be isolated from the rest of the hospital.
5. Preparation and planning for the effective management of a smallpox emergency must occur *before* an actual bioterrorist attack occurs.
6. Management of a smallpox emergency should focus on rapid identification, isolation, and immunization of suspected smallpox patients and their contacts.

TABLE 134A-6 International Classification of Disease (ICD) Codes*	
DISEASE	**ICD-9-CM**
Smallpox	050
Variola major	050.1
Alastrim	050.2
Smallpox, unspecified	050.9

*There is no ICD-10 classification for smallpox.

REFERENCES

1. Alibek K: Biohazard. New York, Random House, 1998.
2. Tucker JB, Zilinskas RA (eds): The 1971 Smallpox Epidemic in Aralsk, Kazakhstan, and the Soviet Biological Warfare Program. Occasional Paper No. 9. Monterey, CA, Monterey Institute of International Studies, 2002.
3. Fenner F, Henderson DA, Arita I, et al: Smallpox and Its Eradication. Geneva, World Health Organization, 1988.
4. Wollfe EJ, Weisberg AS, Moss B: Role for the vaccinia virus A36R outer envelope protein in the formation of virus-tipped actin- containing microvilli and cell-to-cell virus spread. Virology 244:20–26, 1998.

5. Alcami A, Symons JA, Smith GL: The vaccinia virus soluble alpha/beta interferon (IFN) receptor binds to cell surface and protects cells from the antiviral effects of IFN. J Virol 74:11230–11239, 2000.

6. Baker RO, Bray M, Huggins JW: Potential antiviral therapeutics for smallpox, monkeypox and other orthopoxvirus infections. Antiviral Res 57:13–23, 2003.

7. Cowley R, Greenway PJ: Nucleotide sequence comparison of homologous genomic regions from variola, monkeypox, and vaccinia viruses. J Med Virol 31:267–271, 1990.

8. Dumbell KR, Harper L, Buchan A, et al: A variant of variola virus, characterized by changes in polypeptide and endonuclease profiles. Epidemiol Infect 122:287–290, 1999.

9. Massung RF, Esposito JJ, Liu L, et al: Potential virulence determinants in terminal regions of variola smallpox virus genome. Nature 366:748–751, 1993.

10. Massung RF, Loparev VN, Knight JC, et al: Terminal region sequence variations in variola virus DNA. Virology 221:291–300, 1996.

11. Shchelkunov SN: Functional organization of variola major and vaccinia virus genomes. Virus Genes 10:53–71, 1995.

12. Cello J, Aniko P, Wimmer E: Chemical synthesis of poliovirus cDNA: Generation of infectious virus in the absence of natural template. Science 297:1016–1018, 2002 (published online July 11, 2002; 10.1126/science.1072266).

13. Rosengard AM, Liu Y, Nie Z, et al: Variola virus immune evasion design: Expression of a highly efficient inhibitor of human complement. Proc Natl Acad Sci U S A 99:8808–8813, 2002.

14. Hazelton PR, Gelderblom HR: Electron microscopy for rapid diagnosis of infectious agents in emergent situations. Emerg Infect Dis 9:294–303, 2003.

15. Tsutsui K, Uno F, Akatsuka K, et al: Electron microscopic study of vaccinia virus release. Arch Virol 75:213–218, 1983.

16. Hiller G, Weber K: Golgi-derived membranes that contain an acylated viral polypeptide are used for vaccinia virus envelopment. J Virol 55:651–659, 1985.

17. Risco C, Rodriguez JR, Lopez-Iglesias C, et al: Endoplasmic reticulum-Golgi intermediate compartment membranes and vimentin filaments participate in vaccinia virus assembly. J Virol 76:1839–1855, 2002.

18. Schmelz M, Sodeik B, Ericsson M, et al: Assembly of vaccinia virus: The second wrapping cisterna is derived from the trans Golgi network. Virology 68:130–147, 1994.

19. Doms RW, Blumenthal R, Moss B: Fusion of intra- and extracellular forms of vaccinia virus with the cell membrane. J Virol 64:4884–4892, 1990.

20. Buller RM, Palumbo GJ: Poxvirus pathogenesis. Microbiol Rev 55:80–122, 1991.

21. Ward BM, Moss B: Vaccinia virus intracellular movement is associated with microtubules and independent of actin tails. J Virol 75:11651–11663, 2001.

22. Alcami A, Smith GL: Vaccinia, cowpox, and camelpox viruses encode soluble gamma interferon receptors with novel broad species specificity. J Virol 69:4633–4639, 1995.

23. Alcami A, Symons JA, Collins PD, et al: Blockade of chemokine activity by a soluble chemokine binding protein from vaccinia virus. J Immunol 160:624–633, 1998.

24. Born TL, Morrison LA, Esteban DJ, et al: A poxvirus protein that binds to and inactivates IL-18, and inhibits NK cell response. J Immunol 164:3246–3254, 2000.

25. Moss B: Inhibition of HeLa cell protein synthesis by the vaccinia virion. Virol 2:1028–1037, 1968.

26. Saraiva M, Alcami A: CrmE, a novel soluble tumor necrosis factor receptor encoded by poxviruses. J Virol 75:226–233, 2001.

27. Seregin SV, Babkina IN, Nesterov AE, et al: Comparative studies of gamma-interferon receptor-like proteins of variola major and variola minor viruses. FEBS Lett 382:79–83, 1996.

28. Hollinshead M, Vanderplasschen A, Smith GL, et al: Vaccinia virus intracellular mature virions contain only one lipid membrane. J Virol 73:1503–1517, 1999.

29. Smith GL, Vanderplasschen A, Law M: The formation and function of extracellular enveloped vaccinia virus J Gen Virol 83:2915–2931, 2002.

30. Ward BM, Moss B: Visualization of intracellular movement of vaccinia virus virions containing a green fluorescent protein-B5R membrane protein chimera. J Virol 75:4802–4813, 2001.

31. Tooze J, Hollinshead M, Reis B, et al: Progeny vaccinia and human cytomegalovirus particles utilize early endosomal cisternae for their envelopes. Eur J Cell Biol 60:163–178, 1993.

32. Engelstad M, Smith GL: The vaccinia virus 42-kDa envelope protein is required for the envelopment and egress of extracellular virus and for virus virulence. Virology 194:627–637, 1993.

33. Vanderplasschen A, Mathew E, Hollinshead M, et al: Extracellular enveloped vaccinia virus is resistant to complement because of incorporation of host complement control proteins into its envelope. Proc Natl Acad Sci U S A 95:7544–7549, 1998.

34. Sanderson M, Frischknecht F, Way M, et al: Roles of vaccinia virus EEV-specific proteins in intracellular actin tail formation and low pH-induced cell-cell fusion. J Gen Virol 79:1415–1425, 1998.

35. van Eiji H, Hollinshead M, Rodger G, et al: The vaccinia virus F12L protein is associated with intracellular enveloped virus particles and is required for the egress to the cell surface. J Gen Virol 83:195–207, 2002.

36. Vanderplasschen A, Hollinshead M, Smith GL: Antibodies against vaccinia virus do not neutralize extracellular enveloped virus but prevent virus release from infected cells and comet formation. J Gen Virol 78(Pt 8):2041–2048, 1997.

37. Frischknecht F, Moreau V, Röttger S, et al: Actin-based motility of vaccinia virus mimics receptor tyrosine kinase signaling. Nature 401:926–929, 1999.

38. Gelfand HM, Posch J: The recent outbreak of smallpox in Meschede, West Germany. Am J Epidemiol 93:234–237, 1971.

39. Henderson DA, Inglesby TV, Bartlett JG, et al: Smallpox as a biological weapon: Medical and public health management. JAMA 281:2127–2137, 1999.

40. Higgins JA, Ibrahaim MS, Knauert FK, et al: Sensitive and rapid identification of biological threat agents. Ann N Y Acad Sci 894:130–148, 1999.

41. Payne LG: Significance of extracellular enveloped virus in the in vitro and in vivo dissemination of vaccinia. J Gen Virol 50:89–100, 1980.

42. Payne LG, Kristensson K: Extracellular release of enveloped vaccinia virus from mouse nasal epithelial cells in vivo. J Gen Virol 66(Pt 3):643–646, 1985.

43. Grandvaux N, tenOever BR, Servant MJ, et al: The interferon antiviral response: From viral invasion to evasion. Curr Opin Infect Dis 15:259–267, 2002.

44. Seet BT, Johnston JB, Brunetti CR: Poxviruses and immune evasion. Annu Rev Immunol 21:377–423, 2003.

45. Senkevich T, Wolffe EJ, Buller ML: Ectromelia virus RING finger protein is localized in virus factories and is required for virus replication in macrophages. J Virol 69:4103–4111, 1995.

46. Favoreel HW, Van de Walle GR, Nauwynck HJ, et al: Virus complement evasion strategies. Gen Virol 84:1–15, 2003 (published ahead of print on October 22, 2002 as DOI 10.1099/vir.0.18709-0).

47. Downie AW, Saint Vincent L, Meiklejohn G, et al: Studies on the virus content of mouth washings in the acute phase of smallpox. Bull World Health Organ 25:49–53, 1961.

48. Sarkar JK, Mitra AC, Mukherkee MK, et al: Virus excretion in smallpox: 1. Excretion in the throat, urine, and conjunctiva of patients. Bull World Health Organ 48:517–522, 1973.

49. Sarkar JK, Mitra AC, Mukherkee MK, et al: Virus excretion in smallpox: 2. Excretion in the throats of household contacts. Bull World Health Organ 48:523–527, 1973.

50. Rao AR: Smallpox. Bombay, India, The Kothari Book Depot, 1972.

51. Arita I, Shafa E, Kader MA: Role of hospital in smallpox outbreak in Kuwait. Am J Public Health 60:1960–1966, 1970.

52. Meiklejohn G, Kempe CH, Downie AW, et al: Air sampling to recover variola virus in the environment of a smallpox hospital. Bull World Health Organ 25:63–67, 1961.

53. Wehrle PF, Posch J, Richter KH, et al: An airborne outbreak of smallpox in a German hospital and its significance with respect to other recent outbreaks in Europe. Bull World Health Organ 43:669–679, 1970.

54. Huq F: Effect of temperature and relative humidity on variola virus in crusts. Bull World Health Organ 54:710–712, 1976.

55. Albert MR, Ostheimer KG, Bremen JG: The last smallpox epidemic in Boston and the vaccination controversy, 1901–1903. N Engl J Med 344:375–379, 2001.

56. Weinstein I: An outbreak of smallpox in New York City. Am J Public Health 37:1376–1384, 1947.

57. Irons JV, Sullivan TD, Cook EBM, et al: Outbreak of smallpox in the lower Rio Grande valley of Texas in 1949. Am J Public Health 43:24–29, 1953.

58. Shooter RA: Report of the Investigation into the Cause of the 1978 Birmingham Smallpox Occurrence. London, Her Majesty's Stationery Office, 1980.

59. Robert JF, Coffee G, Creel SM, et al: Haemorrhagic smallpox: 1. Preliminary haematological studies. Bull World Health Organ 33:607–613, 1965.

60. Downie AW, Meiklejohn M, Saint Vincent L, et al: The recovery of smallpox virus from patients and their environments in a smallpox hospital. Bull World Health Organ 33:615–622, 1965.

61. Mitra AC, Sarkar JK, Mukherkee MK: Virus content of smallpox scabs. Bull World Health Organ 51:106–107, 1974.

62. O'Toole T, Inglesby T, Larsen R, DeMier M: Dark Winter: A Bioterrorism Exercise. Baltimore, Johns Hopkins Center for Civilian Biodefense, Center for Strategic and International Studies, Analytic Services, Inc., and Memorial Institute for the prevention of Terrorism, 2001. Available at: http://www.hopkins-biodefense.org/index.html.

63. O'Toole T, Mair M, Inglesby TV: Shining light on "Dark Winter." Clin Infect Dis 34:972–983, 2002.

64. Leduc JW, Jahrling PB: Strengthening national preparedness for smallpox: An update. Emerg Infect Dis 7:155–157, 2001.

65. Hahon N, Wilson BJ: Pathogenesis of variola in *Macaca irus* monkeys. Am J Hyg 71:69–80, 1969.

66. Noble J, Rich JA: Transmission of smallpox by contact and aerosol routes in *Macaca irus*. Bull World Health Organ 40:279–286, 1969.

67. Dixon CW: Smallpox. London, Churchill, 1962.

68. Martin DB: The cause of death in smallpox: An examination of the pathology record. Milit Med 167:546–551, 2002.

69. Downie AW, Fedson DS, St Vincent L, et al: Haemorrhagic smallpox. J Hyg 67:619–629, 1969.

70. Henderson DA: Smallpox: Clinical features and epidemiological features. Emerg Infect Dis 5:537–539, 1999.

71. Samuel CE: Antiviral actions of interferons. Clin Microbiol Rev 14:778–809, 2001.

72. Karupiah G, Xie Q, Buller ML, et al: Inhibition of viral replication by interferon-gamma-induced nitric oxide synthase. Science 261:1445–1448, 1993.

73. Smith VP, Alcami A: Inhibition of interferons by ectromelia viruses. J Virol 76:1124–1134, 2002.

74. Chang H-W, Watson JC, Jacobs BL: The E3L gene of vaccinia virus encodes an inhibitor of the interferon-induced, double-stranded RNA-dependent protein kinase. Proc Natl Acad Sci U S A 89:4825–4829, 1992.

75. Isaacs SN, Kotwal GJ, Moss B: Vaccinia virus complement-control protein prevents antibody-dependent complement-enhanced neutralization of infectivity and contributes to virulence. Proc Natl Acad Sci U S A 89:628–632, 1992.

76. Jackson RJ, Ramsay AJ, Christensen CD, et al: Expression of mouse interleukin-4 by a recombinant ectromelia virus suppresses cytolytic lymphocyte responses and overcomes genetic resistance to mousepox. J Virol 75:1205–1210, 2001.

77. Sharma DP, Ramsay AJ, Maguire DJ, et al: Interleukin-4 mediates down regulation of antiviral cytokine expression and cytolytic T-lymphocyte responses and exacerbates vaccinia virus infection in vivo. J Virol 70:7103–7107, 1996.

78. Lane JM, Ruben FL, Neff JM: Complications of smallpox vaccination, 1968: Results of ten statewide surveys. J Infect Dis 122:303–309, 1970.

79. Breman JG, Henderson DA: Diagnosis and management of smallpox. N Engl J Med 346:1300–1308, 2002.

80. McKenzie PJ, Githens JH, Harwood ME, et al: Haemorrhagic smallpox: 2. Specific bleeding and coagulation studies. Bull World Health Organ 33:773–782, 1965.

81. Mehta BC, Doctor RG, Purandare NM, et al: Hemorrhagic smallpox: A study of 22 cases to determine cause of bleeding. Indian J Med Sci 21:518–523, 1967.

82. Mitra M, Bhattacharya DK: Some observations on hemorrhagic smallpox (type I). J Indian Med Assoc 67:237–240, 1976.

83. Sarkar JK, Chatteriee SN, Mitra AC, et al: Antibody response in hemorrhagic smallpox. Indian J Med Res 55:1143–1149, 1967.

84. Hanrahan JA, Jakubowycz M, Davis BR: A smallpox false alarm. N Engl J Med 348:467–468, 2003.

85. Crandell RA, Casey HW, Brumlow WB: Studies of a newly recognized poxvirus of monkeys. J Infect Dis 119:80–88, 1969.

86. Hutin YJF, Williams RJ, Malfait P, et al: Outbreak of human monkeypox, Democratic republic of Congo, 1996–1997. Emerg Infect Dis 7:434–438, 2001.

87. Jezek Z, Szczeniowski M, Paluku KM, et al: Human monkeypox: Clinical features of 282 patients. J Infect Dis 156:293–298, 1987.

88. Jaezek Z, Mutombo M, Dunn C, et al: Four generations of probable person-to-person transmission of human mokeypox. Am J Epidemiol 123:1004–1012, 1986.

89. Zaucha GM, Jahrling PB, Geisbert GW, et al: The pathology of experimental aerosolized monkeypox virus infection cynomolgus monkeys (*Macaca fascicularis*). Lab Invest 81:1581–1600, 2001.

90. Breman JG, Henderson DA: Poxvirus dilemmas—monkeypox, smallpox, and biologic terrorism. N Engl J Med 339:556, 1998.

91. Anonymous: Human monkeypox in Kasai Oriental, Democratic Republic of Congo (former Zaire). Wkly Epidemiol Rec 72:369–372, 1997.

92. Anonymous: Human monkeypox in Kasai Oriental, Zaire (1996–1997). Wkly Epidemiol Rec 72:101–104, 1997.

93. Nakano JH: Evaluation of virological laboratory methods for smallpox diagnosis. Bull World Health Organ 48:529–534, 1973.

94. Tarantola DJM, Huq F, Nakano JH, et al: Immunofluorescence staining for detection of variola virus. J Clin Microbiol 13:723–725, 1981.

95. Klietmann WF, Ruoff KL: Bioterrorism: Implications for the clinical microbiologist. Clin Microbiol Rev 14:364–381, 2001.

96. Ropp SL, Jin Q, Knight JC, et al: PCR strategy for identification and differentiation of smallpox and other orthopoxviruses. J Clin Microbiol 33:2069–2076, 1995.

97. Jenner E: An Inquiry into the Causes and Effects of the Variolae Vaccinae, or Cow-Pox. Berkeley, Gloucestershire, England, 1798.

98. Rosenthal SR, Merchlinsky M, Kleppinger C, et al: Developing new smallpox vaccines. Emerg Infect Dis 7:920–926, 2001.

99. Cono J, Casey CG, Bell DM: Smallpox vaccination and adverse reactions: Guidance for clinicians. MMWR Morb Mortal Wkly Rep 52(RR04):1–28, 2003.

100. CDC: Smallpox vaccine adverse events among civilians—United States, February 25-March 3, 2003. MMWR Morb Mortal Wkly Rep 52:181–182, 191, 2003.

101. CDC: Cardiac events following smallpox vaccination—United States, 2003. MMWR Morb Mortal Wkly Rep 52:248–250, 2003.

102. Feery BJ: Adverse reactions after smallpox vaccination. Med J Aust 2:180–183, 1977.

103. Finlay-Jones LR: Fatal myocarditis after vaccination against smallpox: Report of a case. N Engl J Med 270:41–42, 1964.

104. Helle EP, Koskenvuo K, Keikkila J, et al: Myocardial complications of immunisations. Ann Clin Res 10:280–287, 1978.

105. CDC: Smallpox vaccine information statement (VIS): Smallpox vaccine and heart problems. March 27, 2003. Available at: http://www.bt.cdc.gov/agent/smallpox/vaccination/heartproblems-vis.asp.

106. Lane JM, Ruben FL, Neff JM, Millar JD: Complications of smallpox vaccination: National surveillance in the United States, 1968. N Engl J Med 281:1201–1208, 1969.

107. Lane JM, Ruben FL, Abrutyn El, et al: Deaths attributable to smallpox vaccination, 1959 to 1966, and 1968. JAMA 212:441–444, 1970.

108. Bray M, Wright ME: Progressive vaccinia. Clin Infect Dis 36:766–774, 2003.

109. Chaudhuri AKR, Cassie R, Douglas WS: Contact vaccinia from recently vaccinated British soldiers. BMJ 282:1797, 1981.

110. Williams WL, Cook HT, Slidell CT: Contact spread of vaccinia from a recently vaccinated marine—Louisiana. MMWR Morb Mortal Wkly Rep 33:37–38, 1984.

111. Fulginiti VA, Winograd LA, Jackson M, et al: Therapy of experimental vaccinal keratitis: Effect of idoxuridine and VIG. Arch Ophthalmol 74:539–544, 1965.

112. Redfield RR, Wright DC, James WD, et al: Disseminated vaccinia in a military recruit with human immunodeficiency virus (HIV) disease. N Engl J Med 316:673–676, 1987.

113. Engler RJM, Kenner J, Leung DYM: Smallpox vaccination: Risk considerations for patients with atopic dermatitis. J Allergy Clin Immunol 110:357–365, 2002.

114. Moses AE, Cohen-Poradosu R: Eczema vaccinatum—a timely reminder. N Engl J Med 346:1287, 2002.

115. Kempe CH, Bowles C, Meiklejohn G, et al: The use of hyperimmune gamma-globulin in the prophylaxis of smallpox. Bull World Health Organ 25:41–48, 1961.

116. Abramowicz M (ed): Smallpox vaccine. Med Lett 45:1–3, 2003.

117. Kern ER, Hartline C, Harden E, et al: Enhanced inhibition of orthopoxvirus replication in vitro by alkoxyalkyl esters of cidofovir and cyclic cidofovir. Antimicrob Agents Chemother 46:991–995, 2002.

118. Bray M, Martinez M, Smee DF, et al: Cidofovir protects mice against lethal aerosol or intranasal cowpox virus challenge. J Infect Dis 181:10–19, 2000.

119. De Clerq E: Vaccinia virus as a paradigm for the chemotherapy of poxvirus infections. Clin Microbiol Rev 14:382–397, 2001.

120. Huggins J: Review of antiviral candidate drugs "Interim report on joint DHHS-DoD research project: Antiviral therapy of smallpox and other orthopoxvirus infections from terrorist or biological warfare release." Presented at the WHO Advisory Committee on Variola Virus Research: Report of WHO Second Meeting, Geneva, February 15–16, 2001. Available at: http://www.who.int/csr/resources/publications/viral/whocdscsredc200017.pdf.

121. Huggins JW, Bray M, Smee DF, et al: Potential antiviral therapeutics for smallpox, monkeypox, and other orthopoxvirus infections. Presented at the WHO Advisory Committee on Variola Virus Research: Report of WHO Third Meeting, Geneva, December 3–4, 2001. Available at: http://www.who.int/csr/resources/publications/viral/whocdsc-srgar20023.pdf.

122. Clarke T: Smallpox pill promising. Nature Science Update, March 20, 2002. Available at: http://www.nature.com/nsu/020318/020318-3.html.

Encephalitis and Hemorrhagic Fever Viruses

Andrew Erdman ■ Edward W. Cetaruk

This chapter addresses certain viral agents that may be used as weapons of biologic terrorism or warfare. These agents are discussed in a medical toxicology text because toxicologists may become involved in such events for a variety of reasons: (1) The development of early, nonspecific symptoms in multiple patients may mimic an environmental or occupational chemical exposure; (2) toxicologists frequently are involved in mass casualty incidents or disaster plans for the community, which can be adapted to a bioterrorist event; (3) toxicologists are often familiar with clinical problem solving and disease management on a community level; (4) toxicologists are typically versed in risk communication to the general public; (5) toxicologists generally work closely with poison centers, which are ideally suited for recognition of a bioterrorist event and assistance in its subsequent management; and (6) toxicologists frequently work closely with various laboratory, public health, and law enforcement personnel. Consequently, many medical toxicologists have begun to play an integral and proactive role in biologic and chemical terrorism.

To date, there have been no documented attacks with any of the agents discussed in this chapter. Most of the information regarding transmission, clinical effects, and treatment comes from studying the natural disease form. It is possible that these features would differ in the setting of an attack with a biologic weapon.[1] For example, the virus may be genetically altered, increasing its virulence or resistance to treatment, and the mode of infection is likely to be different (e.g., aerosolized versus vector transmitted). The resulting disease and its epidemiology differ from outbreaks in the wild.

This chapter discusses what is known about natural encephalitis and hemorrhagic fever (HF) viruses and their respective diseases. The potential differences between the natural and biologic weapon strains are emphasized, and any existing data are extrapolated as well as possible. Terrorist events have heightened collective awareness of biologic terrorism and undoubtedly will lead to new research and scientific developments in the near future. As a result, recommendations may evolve as knowledge and experience are accumulated rapidly.

ENCEPHALITIS VIRUSES

Viruses causing human encephalitis are often grouped together and termed *encephalitis viruses*. However, the individual viruses composing this group are taxonomically different. Included are the equine encephalitis viruses (eastern equine encephalitis [EEE], western equine encephalitis [WEE], and Venezuelan equine encephalitis [VEE]), Japanese encephalitis virus, the tick-borne encephalitis viruses, St. Louis encephalitis virus, and others. The viruses most commonly considered agents of concern for use as biologic weapons are the equine encephalitis viruses, particularly VEE.[1–4] Lists of concerning agents have been compiled by the World Health Organization (WHO), U.S. Army Medical Research Institute of Infectious Diseases, North Atlantic Treaty Organization (NATO), and the Biological Weapons Convention Protocol. Inclusion is based on individual pathogen characteristics, evidence of previous use or development as a weapon, and intelligence suggesting that the agent currently may be under development or stockpiled.[2,5]

The equine encephalitis viruses have been weaponized successfully, or they were candidates for weaponization, by several nations, and they were part of the U.S. biologic warfare program until its dismantling in 1969.[1,4,6] The equine encephalitis viruses are divided into three categories: WEE, EEE, and VEE. Over the last century, all three viruses have been responsible for periodic outbreaks of encephalitis in humans and livestock throughout the Americas. Several features make these viruses good candidates for biologic warfare: (1) They are highly infectious; (2) they are active and environmentally stable in aerosol form; (3) they have been studied extensively, and technical information and biologic expertise may be available to bioterrorists; (4) natural outbreaks with a variety of different strains are relatively frequent, providing a regular source of starting material; (5) they are inexpensive to produce in large quantities; and (6) they are amenable to genetic alteration, creating the potential for development of a more virulent or resistant strain.[1,7–15]

Microbiology and Epidemiology

WEE, EEE, and VEE are members of the *Alphavirus* genus, in the Togaviridae family. Rather than individual viruses, WEE, EEE, and VEE actually represent three separate groups of viruses, also known as *complexes*. Each complex comprises several antigenically related viral subtypes (Table 134B-1). Alphaviruses contain a single-stranded RNA genome complexed with several core proteins, forming a nucleocapsid. The nucleocapsid is enveloped in a spherical lipid bilayer, approximately 60 nm in diameter, which is derived from the host cell membrane. In this envelope are embedded several virally encoded glycoproteins,

TABLE 134B-1 Constituents of the Western Equine Encephalitis, Eastern Equine Encephalitis, and Venezuelan Equine Encephalitis Virus Complexes	
Western Equine Encephalitis Virus Complex	**Venezuelan Equine Encephalitis Virus Complex**
Aura virus	AG80-663 virus
Fort Morgan virus	Bijou Bridge virus
Buggy Creek virus	Cabassou virus
Highlands J virus	Mucambo virus
Sindbis virus	Tonate virus
Babanki virus	Pixuna virus
Kyzylagach virus	Venezuelan equine encephalitis virus
Ockelbo virus	Venezuelan equine encephalitis virus (3880 strain)
Sindbis virus (HRSP strain)	Venezuelan equine encephalitis virus (Everglades
Sindbis virus (wild-type strain derived from AR339)	FE3-7C strain)
Sindbis-like virus	Venezuelan equine encephalitis virus (Mena II
Sindbis-like virus YN87448	strain)
Western equine encephalomyelitis virus	Venezuelan equine encephalitis virus (P676 strain)
Whataroa virus	Venezuelan equine encephalitis virus (TC-83 strain)
	Venezuelan equine encephalitis virus
Eastern Equine Encephalitis Virus Complex	(Trinidad/Donkey strain)
Eastern equine encephalitis virus	71D1252
Eastern equine encephalitis virus (VA33 strain)	78V3531

which mediate viral adhesion to host target cells and subsequent uptake.[13,14,16,17] These glycoproteins may also mediate virulence and serve as target sites for neutralizing antibodies.[12,17–19]

All of the equine encephalitis viruses are *arboviruses,* meaning that under natural circumstances they are transmitted through arthropod vectors, primarily mosquitoes. Each viral strain seems to "prefer" a particular animal species as host reservoir—most prefer birds or rodents, but some, such as certain strains of VEE, prefer horses. Natural virus strains can be *enzootic* or *epizootic.* The enzootic strains reside chronically in the "reservoir" of a certain animal population over time, cycling between mosquito and animal. These strains are generally less virulent, and humans and equines are infected only incidentally in sporadic, relatively small outbreaks. Epizootic strains probably arise from enzootic viruses that have mutated or otherwise evolved. They are much more virulent, causing widespread outbreaks among horses and humans.

Outbreaks of viral equine encephalitis in horses have been documented for nearly 200 years. The first confirmed human cases were not noted until 1938, however, with the isolation of EEE and WEE in patients with encephalitis.[20] VEE first was described in Venezuelan livestock around 1939, and it soon became clear that humans also were being infected.[21–24] Today, outbreaks of WEE, EEE, and VEE continue to occur every few years in livestock and humans throughout the Americas.[25,26] Invariably, natural human epidemics are preceded by an outbreak of disease in local equines or other livestock.[4,25,29] The equine encephalitides occur most commonly in the summer and in rural areas (closely paralleling mosquito proliferation).

Although natural transmission to humans occurs via mosquito bite, the encephalitis viruses can be extremely infective as an aerosol, either by inhalation or by mucous membrane contact.[7,10,28] Aerosol dispersion, as either a wet

or a lyophilized, dry particulate, is considered the most likely route of transmission during a biologic attack. The infectious aerosol dose in humans is not known, but all the equine encephalitis viruses are considered to be highly infectious.[1] The median lethal dose (LD$_{50}$), by aerosol, for VEE in mice was 8 to 11 plaque-forming units in one study.[29] Infection rates after exposure vary, and many who are exposed do not go on to develop clinically detectable infection. During natural outbreaks of WEE, attack rates generally are low (0.001% to 1.7%), but many more patients may seroconvert without developing clinical disease.[25,30,31] It has been estimated that only about 1 person out of every 1000 who seroconvert develops clinically detectable disease. Infants seem particularly susceptible to developing clinically significant infections after exposure. In contrast, EEE seroconversion rates generally are low during natural outbreaks. The likelihood of an infected person's developing clinical disease is much higher, however, suggesting that EEE may be more virulent in general than WEE. Attack rates during natural EEE outbreaks are about 3%.[32] For VEE, seroconversion rates during natural epidemics are fairly high (approximately 20%).[33] The incidence of clinical illness is also impressive (approximately 10% to 18% among the general exposed population).[23,34] The Trinidad Donkey and P-676 strains of VEE are considered particularly virulent, often resulting in explosive outbreaks among humans and animals. In contrast to patients with the other equine encephalitides, patients with VEE are almost always symptomatic to some degree; however, severe disease and encephalitis are rare.[35–37]

These figures represent natural outbreaks with wild viral strains. It is not known if similar seroconversion and clinical disease rates would be seen after a terrorist attack given a different, possibly more effective route of infection and the potential for more virulent strains. There have been no documented cases of direct transmission from human to human or from equine to human with any of the natural viral strains, meaning that secondary transmission is improbable.

Pathophysiology

The precise host target cells for the equine encephalitis viruses in humans have not been established, but based on animal data, a wide variety of tissues seem to be involved, including cells of the immune system and central nervous system (CNS).[38–40] Glycoproteins (particularly the E2 glycoprotein) embedded in the viral envelope probably mediate the virus' tissue tropism and help it to bind to host cell surface receptors.[16,17,33,41,42] The identity of the specific host cell receptors is unclear, but it may be a type of laminin-binding protein.[43] After binding, the virus is engulfed by the cell via endocytosis. Once inside the endocytic vesicle, the viral envelope fuses with the vesicle membrane, releasing its nucleocapsid into the host cell's cytoplasm.[16,44,45] The nucleocapsid is disassembled, and the free viral RNA is released. The viral genome is essentially a functional mRNA, and as such it is translated by the host cell's ribosomal apparatus. Initial translation generates copies of viral RNA polymerase. This RNA polymerase, using the free viral genome as its template, generates a negative sense strand of RNA. This negative strand becomes a template for making multiple copies of the viral genome via the action of RNA polymerase. It also serves as a template for generating smaller, subgenomic, positive RNA sections that are transcribed and translated to yield a single precursor polypeptide that is cleaved proteolytically by virally encoded or host peptidases, to generate all the precursor components for the necessary viral structural proteins (C, E3, E2, 6K, and E1).[46–49] Many of these precursor proteins undergo posttranslational modification and glycosylation before assembly, however, a complex process involving the host's endoplasmic reticulum, Golgi apparatus, and cytosol.[46,48,49] Assembly of the final multimeric glycoproteins seems to occur simply by physical interaction of the various components.[49]

The final glycoproteins are inserted into the host plasma membrane, where they assume their final orientation on the exterior surface. The progeny nucleocapsids, consisting of genomic RNA and structural proteins, are assembled, then they make their way through the cytosol to the host plasma membrane, where they bind to the previously embedded E2 glycoproteins. The viral envelope subsequently is acquired by budding: The host cell's lipid membrane wraps around the nucleocapsid, with the interaction of E2 glycoprotein and nucleocapsid C protein, completing the formation of a mature viral particle.[50–54] Completed progeny virions are released systemically, where they can infect other cells.[40,55–57] Meanwhile, the original host cell typically perishes, probably as a result of apoptosis.[58,59]

The course of infection seems to be bimodal. First, the virus replicates and proliferates in cells of the lymphoid tissues and then is released, causing viremia and distribution of the virus to the CNS and various other nonneural organs. The process begins, under natural circumstances, with the bite of an infected mosquito, which introduces the virus into the human skin.[60] In the skin, it invades the dendritic Langerhans' cells of the epidermis, which, when activated by viral invasion, migrate via the lymphatic system to local draining nodes, where the virus can spread to other cells of the immune system.[55,57,61] This initial sequence of events applies only to natural viral transmission.

The pathogenesis after inhalational exposures is less clear. Studies in laboratory workers suggest that the clinical disease caused by inhalation is similar to the natural vector-acquired disease, and the general pathophysiology is likely to be similar.[7,28] Few data are available. Infection after aerosol exposure probably begins with viral invasion of the respiratory epithelial or mucous membrane cells, then is followed by migration into draining lymphatic nodes or direct invasion of the neuroepithelial cells of the olfactory nerve, giving it access to the CNS.[62,63] The host's mucosal immunity seems to play a significant role in defense against aerosol exposures.[63] With viral replication in the cells of the lymph nodes and their subsequent release, viremia ensues, and the pathogen is distributed hematogenously to various cells of the peripheral nervous system (especially the olfactory and trigeminal nerves), which it invades. The virus can spread directly to the CNS, via retrograde axonal transport, resulting in meningoencephalitis and gliosis.[39,64] Alternatively, it may gain access to the CNS through fenestrated capillaries of the nasal mucosa or damaged vasculature.[64–67]

Nonneural tissues also may become infected with hematogenous spread, including the lymphoid, bone marrow, and reticuloendothelial systems and various glandular structures.[57,68–71] Viral replication in these neural and nonneural cells leads to direct cellular necrosis, inflammation, edema, vascular congestion, and organ dysfunction. The exact mechanisms of cellular and organ dysfunction may include the disruption of cellular homeostasis or normal function by replicating virion particles, the induction of cell death by apoptosis, the induction of inflammation and the local and systemic effects of various inflammatory mediators triggered by cellular invasion (e.g., nitric oxide synthetase and tumor necrosis factor-α), and localized edema as a result of inflammation and vascular compromise.[69,72,73] Inadequate host interferon-α and interferon-β production or sensitivity also may enhance viral pathogenicity and disease severity.[74,75] The host's immunocompetency, particularly the activation of various cells such as macrophages, also may determine pathogenicity to some extent.[40] Viral invasion of lymphoid tissues, in and of itself, causes an impairment in host immunity, which may enhance the disease severity.[71,76]

Histopathologic changes of viral CNS infection, based primarily on animal data, include vascular inflammation with perivascular cuffing; gliosis; neuronal demyelination, necrosis, edema, and hemorrhage; and meningeal inflammation.[69,71,77] Viral antigens have been identified in the dendrites and perikaryon of CNS neurons. Anatomically, lesions may involve the spinal cord, brain, or both. The basal ganglia and thalami seem to be particularly susceptible.[71,78]

Clinical Presentation

Human infection with the encephalitis viruses can result in an asymptomatic carrier state, an acute subclinical infection, or a febrile syndrome of varying severity that can progress to frank encephalitis. A variety of host and viral factors determines the clinical presentation and its severity. The victim's age, underlying immune status (particularly mucosal immunity), previous vaccinations, and concurrent medical problems may affect disease severity and mortality.[23] Some viral strains are more neurotropic and hence more likely to lead to encephalitis; other viral strains may be more virulent overall, causing severe or rapidly progressive systemic effects.[63,67,79] Patients with WEE infections are less likely to develop severe encephalitis compared with patients infected by the other equine encephalitis viruses. Rates of progression to encephalitis after WEE infection are low for adults (about 0.1%) but much higher for infants and children (approaching 100%).[1] On the other hand, case-fatality rates for WEE are around 3% to 8% for adults but lower in children.[17,25] For VEE, rates of neurologic progression are variable (0.5% to 6% in adults and 3% to 4% in children).[23,34] Case-fatality rates range from 0.05% to 1.5% but are 20% in patients who develop encephalitis.[25,34] Children are more likely to develop severe disease during VEE outbreaks. EEE has a higher likelihood of progressing to severe encephalitis and death. Approximately 5% of patients with clinical EEE infections go on to develop encephalitis, and case-fatality rates in patients who develop encephalitis have ranged from 36% in adults to 55% in the elderly and 100% in infants.[27,32,78] These figures are based on natural disease outbreaks with wild viral strains. Little is known about the neurotropism and virulence of weapon-grade pathogens and what the infection, encephalitis, and mortality rates would be.

The prodromal phase of clinical illness typically begins after an incubation period of several days to 2 weeks. The incubation period may be shorter (i.e., 1 to 5 days), with aerosol-acquired infections.[10] Initial symptoms include fever, chills, headache, malaise, nausea, vomiting, abdominal pain, myalgias, and sore throat (Table 134B-2).[24,78,80–85] Occasionally, photophobia or respiratory symptoms may be present. Based on the limited data currently available (e.g., case reports of lab workers who acquired the disease occupationally), the clinical syndrome after an aerosol exposure seems

to be similar to the naturally acquired disease, suggesting that such a clinical picture would be seen in victims of a biologic attack.[7,28] It is not known whether such victims are more likely to develop respiratory symptoms.

Physical examination during the prodromal phase usually reveals little more than pharyngeal erythema, conjunctival injection, or muscle tenderness.[24,35–37,86] Laboratory findings are typically nonspecific and include leukopenia or leukocytosis and elevated serum transaminases.[24,78] Viremia is greatest during this phase of the disease, and it generally follows the fever curve.[87,88]

In most patients, the viremia and symptoms begin to fade after several days, and the illness resolves without further sequelae. In patients who do not go on to develop encephalitis, improvement seems to correlate with a rise in antibody titers against the offending virus.[24,68,89] In patients who do go on to develop neurologic sequelae, antibody titers often rise to similar levels. However, some authors have noted a lack of serum or spinal fluid IgM antibodies in fatal cases of encephalitis.[90] The significance of this finding is uncertain.

Progression to encephalomyelitis is variable and depends on the patient and viral strain. Patients with VEE rarely develop encephalitis (<0.5% to 4%).[23,25] EEE viral infections also are unlikely to progress to encephalitis (<5%), but when they do, the resulting CNS involvement tends to be severe, with high rates of mortality (50% to 70%) and long-term neurologic sequelae.[25,78] The WEE virus tends to be much less virulent, and most patients remain asymptomatic or develop only mild symptoms. Encephalitis with WEE virus infections is also rare (<0.1% in adults).[1] With all of the equine encephalitis viruses, CNS involvement is more likely and tends to be more severe in patients at the extremes of age, particularly children.[23,25,27,91,92]

CNS involvement, if it occurs, typically manifests within a few days of illness onset and is usually heralded by clinical deterioration and the development of confusion, delirium, drowsiness, coma, seizures, ataxia, or focal neurologic deficits.[24,27,28,78,85,93] On physical examination at this stage, patients may appear ill, with fever, tachycardia, altered consciousness, nuchal rigidity, hyporeflexia or hyperreflexia, tremors, muscle twitching, or neurologic deficits. Viremia has typically subsided, but antibody titers are likely to be detectable. Lumbar puncture in patients with CNS invasion often reveals elevated cerebrospinal fluid pressure, cerebrospinal fluid lymphocytic pleocytosis (hundreds to thousands of WBCs/μL), and elevated cerebrospinal fluid protein levels. Radiographic manifestations of encephalitis are common on computed tomography or magnetic resonance imaging of the brain and include focal lesions in the basal ganglia, thalami, or brainstem; cortical lesions; meningeal enhancement; and periventricular white matter changes.[78] Data on electroencephalograms in equine encephalitis are limited to a few scattered reports. If an electroencephalogram is performed, it should reveal generalized slowing; a disorganized background with or without epileptiform discharges[78]; or focal abnormalities.[85]

Overall mortality is low for equine encephalitis virus infections. Mortality increases significantly with CNS involvement. For example, in VEE virus infections, case-fatality rates average about 0.6% overall, but they increase to 10% to 35% if encephalitis develops.[25] Death usually

TABLE 134B-2 Common Signs and Symptoms of Western Equine Encephalitis, Eastern Equine Encephalitis, and Venezuelan Equine Encephalitis and Their Approximate Reported Incidence in Hospitalized Patients

SIGN/SYMPTOM	INCIDENCE (%)
Fever	98–100
Seizures	74–98
Drowsiness/stupor/coma	67–92
Headache	30–95
Neck stiffness	54–62
Nausea/vomiting	48–52
Myalgias	37–56
Photophobia	19–56
Diarrhea	48
Sore throat	31
Irritability	20
Conjunctivitis	9
Rash	5

Data from references 17, 27, and 34.

occurs in the first or second week of illness. Long-term or permanent consequences are rare except in patients who develop encephalitis. Such patients may be left with cognitive deficits, behavioral changes, emotional lability, memory problems, weakness or paralysis, recurrent seizures, parkinsonism, chronic fatigue, headaches, or impaired concentration.[23,27,28,93] Sequelae are more common in children and after severe cases of encephalitis, as with EEE.[78,91]

Diagnosis

There are two relevant diagnostic goals: making the diagnosis of an equine encephalitis virus infection in individual patients presenting for treatment and, perhaps more importantly, identifying a biologic attack. Recognizing an infection with any of the equine encephalitis viruses can be problematic. These diseases are uncommon, and the early symptoms are both nonspecific and protean. As a result, they may be confused with a wide variety of more common infectious and noninfectious diseases. Furthermore, infections from a biologic attack may lack the usual epidemiologic, environmental, or geographic clues that otherwise help in making the diagnosis of naturally acquired disease. With the onset of CNS symptoms, however, the differential diagnosis narrows considerably (Table 134B-3). The diagnosis is typically made using a combination of clinical features, radiographic findings, and the results of lumbar puncture. The most important initial task in patients suspected of having encephalitis is ruling out treatable causes (e.g., bacterial meningoencephalitis, herpes simplex virus infection). Efforts can then focus on determining the specific etiology. Every effort should be made to determine the causative pathogen, particularly if there are multiple cases within a geographic area. This may help identify a natural outbreak or biologic attack, for which measures can be taken to reduce exposure and to identify and treat cases. There are no routine historical, clinical, or laboratory findings to distinguish the equine encephalitides from other causes of encephalitis. Specialized diagnostic tests need to be performed.

The gold standard for confirming an infection with one of the equine encephalitis viruses is isolation of the offending virus from symptomatic patients. During the initial febrile phase of illness, the virus may be cultured from blood, cerebrospinal fluid, or other body fluids using specialized techniques (usually by plating onto Vero cells).[94] The pathogen can be identified by electron microscopy or immunohistochemical assay. Tissue specimens can also be examined for virion particles using similar methods.[95] Direct isolation tends to be difficult and time-consuming. It also may yield negative results, despite an active infection, because the virus is present only for a limited time in certain tissues.[28] As a result, most clinical infections are diagnosed using serologic assays.

Serologic tests for viral antigens or antiviral antibodies can be performed on almost any body fluid, but blood and cerebrospinal fluid are the tissues of choice. Measurements of IgM or IgG antiviral antibodies are the most commonly used serologic tests. Serum titers of IgM antiviral antibodies usually rise within a few days of illness onset and can be measured by a variety of methods, including enzyme-linked immunosorbent assay (ELISA), immunofluorescence, hemagglutinin inhibition, and plaque reduction neutralization.[68,89,90,96,97] ELISA is the current standard. Generally, a strong clinical suspicion combined with a positive IgM titer should be adequate for a presumptive diagnosis. IgG titers usually begin to rise several days after IgM.[68,89] Serologic confirmation using IgG is typically based on a fourfold increase in titers between paired sera (about 2 weeks apart). Serial samples over time, samples from different body fluids, and the use of multiple assays may help to confirm the diagnosis. Most state public health departments can perform or arrange for the necessary tests, and they should be contacted immediately if equine encephalitis is suspected. Communication with laboratory personnel, public health officials, and infectious disease specialists is important so that the appropriate studies are performed.

Determining that a biologic attack has occurred is a more difficult task. This determination should be left to law enforcement and public health officials, who have the capacity to investigate all of the epidemiologic, forensic, and intelligence evidence. The role of the physician should be relegated to recognizing a possible attack and contacting the appropriate authorities.

Treatment

There are no specific treatments for the equine encephalitides or other alphavirus infections, and no antimicrobial agents have yet been shown to alter the clinical course. Management rests on aggressive supportive care and the recognition and treatment of complications. Airway management is important, especially if patients have significant alterations in mental state, and it should take precedence over all other measures. Seizures should be treated with benzodiazepines or phenobarbital in the usual doses. However, anticonvulsants should not be given prophylactically, because this may worsen clinical outcome.[78] Corticosteroids do not seem to be helpful and may lead to complications.[78] Fluid and electrolytes should be monitored closely and corrected if necessary.

TABLE 134B-3 Differential Diagnosis for Viral Equine Encephalitides

Other viral causes of meningoencephalitis
Enteroviral
Herpes simplex virus
West Nile
St. Louis
La Crosse
Japanese
Dengue fever
Paramyxovirus
Lymphocytic choriomeningitis virus
Machupo
Junin
Colorado tick fever
Rabies
Cytomegalovirus
Epstein-Barr virus
Human immunodeficiency virus
Infectious, nonviral causes of meningoencephalitis (e.g., bacterial, fungal, parasitic, mycobacterial, rickettsial)
Brain abscess
Postinfectious encephalomyelitis
Autoimmune disease (e.g., lupus cerebritis, arteritis, Behçet's syndrome, sarcoidosis)
Neoplasia
Acute multiple sclerosis
Intracerebral hemorrhage
Reye's syndrome
Cerebrovascular disease
Toxic encephalopathy

Decontamination measures are unlikely to be helpful or necessary for victims of a biologic attack, particularly if symptoms have already developed. The exposure will have occurred days to weeks before the development of symptoms. If the physician is aware of a very recent biologic attack, basic decontamination measures may be attempted, but their efficacy is unproven. Basic decontamination measures include the removal of a patient's clothing and personal belongings (with appropriate bagging and disposal as hazardous waste) and a thorough irrigation of all potentially exposed areas with soap and water or dilute bleach.

Basic universal precautions should be followed by all health care workers caring for these patients. There is no evidence of person-to-person transmission with naturally acquired equine encephalitis infections, so isolation of symptomatic patients suspected of having equine encephalitis is not necessary. Data on the epidemiology and secondary transmission of viruses engineered for biologic weapons are virtually nonexistent, and there is a possibility that virulence and mode of transmission may differ. Protective equipment and isolation procedures may need to be intensified in such an instance, after discussion with local, state, or federal epidemiologists or public health personnel.

There are inactivated vaccines for WEE, EEE, and VEE viruses (the inactivated VEE vaccine is sometimes called C-84), and there is a live attenuated vaccine for VEE (called TC-83).[1,98–101] These vaccines are currently considered investigational, and their use is limited to humans at a high baseline risk for infection (i.e., laboratory workers).[1]

Traditionally the VEE vaccines were considered to be poorly immunogenic in humans.[99,102] More recent studies in human volunteers suggest otherwise, however.[68,99,103] A single dose (0.5 mL subcutaneously) of TC-83 resulted in an 82% successful response rate, as measured by achievement of antibody titers equal to or greater than 1:20 on 80% reduction plaque neutralization assay.[99] Of the subjects vaccinated, 60% maintained this level of immunity for about 5 years. A booster injection using the C-84 vaccine (0.5 mL subcutaneously) was effective in inducing immunity among initial nonresponders to TC-83 and in restimulating immunity in infected responders with waning antibody titers. The vaccines were found to be relatively safe, but minor reactions occurred in about 6% of C-84 vaccinations and 23% of TC-83 vaccinations (e.g., fever, chills, malaise, symptoms of upper respiratory infection).[99] One case of hydrops fetalis has been associated with maternal inoculation using the live-attenuated vaccine.[104] The question remains as to whether these vaccines could prevent disease transmission from a genetically manipulated viral strain or whether they would be effective against an aerosol exposure. There are little data to assess the former question, although in animal studies of the vaccines, some cross-protection to a variety of viral strains was noted.[105,106] With regard to the latter issue, studies in animals have shown that TC-83 vaccines may confer some immunity (as measured by viral challenge tests and mucosal antiviral IgA levels) against aerosol exposures of the VEE virus.[105,106] C-84 does not seem to confer the same protection against airborne exposure, however, unless it is given in three successive doses (at days 0, 7, and 28).[107,108] Mucosal IgA antibody seems to be an important factor for protection against aerosol attacks.[106,109] Although adequate immunity can be induced by subcutaneous vaccination,

aerosolization and inhalational delivery of the vaccine may be more effective.[106,109–111] This route needs further evaluation and testing before it can be recommended widely. TC-83 and C-84 vaccines are currently limited to use in laboratory personnel working with VEE. There is no evidence that postexposure vaccination with either vaccine prevents or ameliorates the subsequent clinical illness.[4]

There are no known plans to initiate widespread public vaccination as a prophylactic measure against an attack. The decision to initiate such campaigns would remain a public health decision, in which the likelihood of a release and its effect are weighed against the risks and costs of widespread immunization. Because VEE does not seem to be transmitted from person to person, there is no indication for vaccinating secondary contacts. These vaccines can be obtained through the Department of Defense's Joint Program Office for Bio-Defense, but their availability for civilian use is not clear. Many genetically engineered VEE vaccines are currently under development and testing.[109]

The existing inactive EEE and WEE vaccines may be able to protect patients from infection by aerosol exposure, but limited response rates, immunologic interference, strain specificity, and rapidly waning immunity limit their effectiveness for widespread vaccination campaigns in the general public.[102,103] As with the VEE vaccines, there is no evidence that postexposure prophylaxis or treatment is of any value. There is similarly no reason to inoculate contacts of infected patients given the lack of person-to-person transmission for these viruses.

The use of passive immunization to treat victims of an equine encephalitis viral infection is controversial. A few animal studies have demonstrated efficacy with neutralizing antisera.[20,112] However, other studies have suggested that the administration of immune serum may actually lead to a more severe infection or, at best, delay the onset of symptoms.[63,113] The use of serotherapy in humans has been reported in only two cases. One of these victims survived, but it is not clear from the report whether passive immunization truly affected the outcome.[7,28] Based on the current evidence, passive immunization could be considered in individual patients early in the course of illness, but its efficacy in humans is clinically unproven, and its lack of availability would likely limit its use. Studies on a novel recombinant antibody suggest there may be a more readily available and effective immunotherapy on the horizon.[47] Passive delivery of antiviral antibodies to the respiratory or nasal mucosa, by direct application (e.g., via nasal spray), may enhance mucosal immunity and protect against an aerosol attack.[63]

When a biologic attack is suspected by a clinician, he or she should contact local or state public health, infectious disease, and law enforcement personnel immediately. Their early involvement can help make the diagnosis of a biologic attack, assist with management of individual patients, help design strategies to reduce the number of infected victims, and mobilize the necessary resources.

HEMORRHAGIC FEVER VIRUSES

Viral HF is defined as an acute, virally mediated febrile illness accompanied by signs of vascular involvement. The clinical course of viral HF can be severe, depending on the

TABLE 134B-4 Viral Families and Specific Agents Capable of Causing Hemorrhagic Fever

Arenaviridae	**Filoviridae**
Lassa	Marburg
Argentine hemorrhagic	Ebola
fever (Junin)	
Bolivian hemorrhagic fever (Machupo)	**Flaviviridae**
Venezuelan hemorrhagic fever (Guanarito)	Dengue hemorrhagic
Brazilian hemorrhagic fever (Sabia)	fever
	Yellow fever
Bunyaviridae	Omsk hemorrhagic fever
Rift Valley fever	Kyasanur Forest disease
Crimean-Congo hemorrhagic fever	
Hantavirus	

etiology, and may result in high mortality rates. A wide variety of viral agents from four different taxonomic families can cause HF: Arenaviridae, Bunyaviridae, Filoviridae, and Flaviviridae (Table 134B-4). Several of these agents are considered significant biologic threats by the U.S. Army, the WHO, and the U.S. Centers for Disease Control and Prevention, particularly the filoviruses Ebola and Marburg and the arenaviruses Lassa, Machupo, and Junin.[2-4,114] Dengue is not transmitted by aerosol and does not make for an effective biologic weapon. Crimean-Congo HF (CCHF) and the agents that cause HF with renal syndrome (HFRS) are considered poor candidates for weaponization.[115,116] Scientists in the Soviet Union are reported to have weaponized or experimented with the weaponization of Ebola, Marburg, Junin, Machupo, and Lassa viruses.[115,117,118] The United States is reported to have weaponized yellow fever and Rift Valley fever before the dismantling of its offensive biologic weapons program in 1969.[115] Yellow fever may have been weaponized by North Korea.[115] The Aum Shinrikyo cult in Japan is reported to have tried, unsuccessfully, to obtain Ebola.[115] It is not known to what extent these and other HF agents have been pursued or developed by other countries or terrorist groups.

CCHF was one of the first HFs ever described. Although the agent would not be identified for centuries to come, the clinical syndrome was well documented in Russia during the 12th century.[119] Yellow fever was described in the 17th century, and the underlying virus was isolated in 1927.[120] The rarest, and perhaps most notorious, of the HF viruses, the Filoviridae, were not described in humans until the latter half of the 20th century. In 1967, Marburg virus was isolated from biomedical researchers in Germany who developed a severe form of viral HF after working with infected African monkeys.[121-123] Secondary cases also occurred in some of the initial patients' contacts. Smaller outbreaks of Marburg have been reported in Kenya and South Africa since then.[124,125] Ebola first was discovered in 1976, during two separate major epidemics of viral HF in Zaire and Sudan.[126,127] Outbreaks of Ebola have occurred sporadically since then, in animals and humans in various African countries such as Gabon, Uganda, Côte d'Ivorie, and the Democratic Republic of Congo.[128-133] There was another recent human epidemic of Ebola in the Democratic Republic of Congo.[134] Various strains of *Hantavirus* have been known to cause epidemics of HFRS throughout Asia, Europe, and

Russia for more than a century. Another *Hantavirus* strain (called *Sin Nombre virus*) was identified and described in the mid-1990s in the United States; it causes a unique and more severe form of *Hantavirus* disease called *Hantavirus pulmonary syndrome* (HPS).[135] Small HPS outbreaks have occurred in the Four Corners region of the United States, but also in South America and Canada.[136-139]

Because of their high lethality, HF viruses have the capacity for significant clinical and psychological impact on a population. Several additional features make these agents particularly attractive to terrorists: their high infectivity by aerosol; the severity of their resulting illnesses, which can overwhelm existing resources; the potential for secondary human-to-human transmission (at least by several of the agents, such as Marburg, Ebola, and Lassa), which could amplify the number of victims and necessitate strict isolation precautions; and the lack of effective treat-, ments or vaccines.[126,140-147]

As with most biologic weapons, the viral HF agents would likely be disseminated as aerosols. The possibility of human-to-human transmission means that terrorists theoretically could infect themselves, then proceed to expose others. Information on the HF viruses comes primarily from reports of naturally occurring disease outbreaks and laboratory investigations in animals. Transmission, infectivity, and clinical features of the disease may differ in a biologic attack owing to differences in the route of exposure, dose, or manipulations of the pathogen.

Despite varying etiologies, clinical features of the various types of viral HF are similar. After a brief incubation period, patients generally develop nonspecific, influenza-like symptoms followed later by vascular manifestations. The illness may progress to shock, multiorgan failure, and death. The diagnosis can be confirmed by serology or viral isolation. There also are two variant syndromes to consider: HPS and HFRS.

The treatment for all forms of viral HF is primarily supportive, but some viral strains may respond to ribavirin. Vaccines are available for a couple of the viral HF agents, but their clinical use is limited, and their role in the management of a biologic attack is not yet defined.

Epidemiology and Microbiology

The filoviruses, Marburg and Ebola, are diseases native to rural sub-Saharan Africa, and epidemics in humans are relatively rare. The Arenaviridae cause human illnesses primarily limited to Africa (e.g., Lassa fever) and South America (Junin and Machupo). HFRS or variants thereof are common to Europe, Asia, and Russia but essentially may occur worldwide. Outbreaks of HPS so far have been limited to the United States, Canada, and South America. Outbreaks of human disease by mosquito-borne Flaviviridae (e.g., Dengue HF and yellow fever) occur in the tropical regions of Africa, Asia, and South America, whereas tick-borne Flaviviridae cause epidemics primarily in India and Russia. There may be several strains or subtypes for any given agent (e.g., Zaire, Sudan, Reston, and Côte d'Ivoire subtypes of Ebola).

All of the HF viruses exist primarily in *zoonotic* life cycles. Humans are generally infected only incidentally. Animal reservoirs for the different viruses vary, but each virus tends to "prefer" a specific host species. The Arenaviridae primarily inhabit various rodents.[148] The Bunyaviridae reside in ungulates, rabbits, hedgehogs, birds, domestic animals, or rodents.[31] The Flaviviridae favor primate hosts, including humans.[149] The reservoir for Filoviridae (Marburg and Ebola) has not been determined yet, but bats are believed to be the most likely candidates.[150]

All of the HF viruses contain a single-stranded RNA genome surrounded by a host cell–derived lipid envelope. Many also express virally encoded proteins embedded in this outer membrane. The Flaviviridae are the smallest pathogens with spherical particles that measure approximately 30 to 50 nm in diameter. Bunyaviridae and Arenaviridae are also spherical but tend to be slightly larger, with diameters ranging from 90 to 130 nm. The Filoviridae are elongated, filamentous structures about 1000 nm in length.

Pathophysiology

Natural disease transmission to humans depends on the specific agent. Some of the HF viruses (e.g., most Bunyaviridae and several of the Flaviviridae) are *arboviruses*, carried by ticks or mosquito vectors.[31,149,151,152] Others (e.g., Arenaviridae, some Flaviviridae, and the *Hantaviruses* in the Bunyaviridae family) are transmitted to humans primarily by aerosolization and subsequent inhalation or mucosal contact (e.g., oral, nasal, conjunctival) of virion particles from the urine, feces, or other material of infected animals or their carcasses. They may also be acquired by ingestion or dermal/mucosal contact with infected material.[153–159] Little is known about the transmission of Ebola or Marburg, but inhalation or mucosal exposure during close contact with infected subjects (animals or humans) is believed to be the most likely method.[124,126,127] Most of these viruses can be spread parenterally, either from the bite of an infected animal or from contaminated needles or sharp instruments, but this is not the primary route of natural transmission.

Transmission during a biologic weapons attack is likely to occur via inhalation of or mucosal contact with disseminated wet or dry aerosol particles. Although most viruses do not seem to survive long (e.g., more than several minutes to an hour) in aerosol form, this time period varies greatly depending on environmental conditions and on the vehicle and mechanism of viral particulate suspension.[144,160] Experiments in animals have demonstrated the efficacy of aerosol delivery for Ebola, Marburg, Lassa, and Junin viruses.[143,144,161–164] Even viruses that are normally transmitted only through arthropod vectors can be successfully deployed as an aerosol.[141,165] It is not clear whether cutaneous exposures with infected materials can lead to infection through open wounds or breaks in the skin.[166] Secondary transmission from human to human may occur with some of the viral HF agents. It has been well documented for Ebola and Marburg and occurs with Lassa fever and possibly certain *Hantaviruses*.[124–127,156,157,167–171] Secondary transmission typically occurs only among close physical contacts of acutely ill individuals or after direct contact with infected body fluids, such as blood, urine, excreta, or semen. It is unclear whether secondary transmission via the airborne route is possible for any of the viruses (e.g., via oral, conjunctival, or respiratory mucosal contact with infective airborne droplets). Epidemiologic data and

some experiments with Ebola in primates are suggestive.[142,171–173] Epidemiologic data in Lassa fever patients also are suggestive.[168] If it occurs, however, it is rare.

Secondary transmission appears to occur only from patients with active symptoms.[170,174,175] There is little evidence to suggest that any of the major HF viruses (Ebola, Marburg, Lassa, Junin, or Machupo) may be transmitted during the incubation period. Persistence of the virus in the body fluids of recovering victims suggests the possibility, at least theoretical, of transmission during the convalescent phase, however, and a few sporadic cases in humans are suggestive.[174,176,177] Secondary transmission after a biologic attack theoretically could occur via arthropod vectors, under the right conditions.[115] If the appropriate animal and arthropod populations were present in the location of a biologic attack, the aerosolized virus could infect livestock, establishing a reservoir of viremic hosts for vectors to feed on and subsequently infect humans. Vertical transmission to the fetus of an infected mother has been described for a few of the viruses, such as Ebola and some Bunyaviridae.[127,178]

Little is known about the infectious dose and pathophysiology after inhalation exposures for most of the important HF viral agents. The limited data suggest that the clinical features of inhalational infection are similar, if not identical, to naturally acquired disease.[118,141,143,144,163,165] For the filoviruses, Ebola and Marburg, the specific mechanisms underlying cellular uptake or invasion have yet to be elucidated fully, but the vascular endothelial cells of the lungs may serve as the initial site of invasion.[164] In these cases, the virus has easy access to the systemic circulation. With regard to the other HF viruses, little is known regarding their invasion and distribution in the victim, after inhalational exposures.

Once inside the host, the pathophysiology of HF varies significantly depending on the specific etiologic agent. A complete and detailed discussion of the pathophysiologic mechanisms underlying each specific agent is beyond the scope of this chapter, but a few general mechanisms are discussed. With Ebola and probably Marburg, glycoproteins on the viral cell surface probably mediate tissue tropism.[179] Most of the initial viral replication takes place in the mononuclear phagocytic cell system (e.g., monocytes and macrophages).[179,180] The same process appears to occur with some of the Arenaviridae.[181,182] As the infected cells rupture, viremia ensues, and the virus is disseminated to a variety of secondary organs, where further cellular invasion by the virus leads to cellular necrosis and to organ injury or dysfunction.[124–127,180,183] Histologically, areas of necrosis have been observed in organs such as the spleen, kidney, and liver.[124–127,184,185] The mechanism of necrosis may be apoptosis, cellular rupture with virion release, or the secondary effects of inflammation.[126,180] Hemorrhages, edema, vascular congestion, and inflammation also have been observed in the kidneys, heart, muscle, adrenal glands, and other tissues.

Vascular involvement is a primary feature of viral HF infections. Direct viral invasion of vascular fibroblasts and endothelial cells, and the effects of inflammatory mediators, immune complexes, and the complement system, all contribute to vascular injury.[135,179,186–197] This injury results in increased vascular permeability with fluid extravasation. The weakened vessels are also more susceptible to breakage, leading to hemorrhages, petechiae, and ecchymoses. Thrombocytopenia and dysfunctional platelets have been associated with almost all of the viral HFs, and platelet abnormalities may play a role in the bleeding manifestations common to these illnesses.[188,193,194,196] Some viruses may cause the elaboration of a factor that inhibits platelet or clotting function, as in Junin infections.[198,199] A decrease in activity or concentration of the various clotting factors, owing to hepatic injury or frank disseminated intravascular coagulation, may contribute to any bleeding diathesis, as is common with Rift Valley fever and yellow fever.[124,187,188,196] A combination of vascular injury, fluid loss, and cellular mediators accounts for the hypotension seen in many patients.

In some syndromes, particularly HPS, Dengue HF, and HFRS, immune mechanisms may play a prominent pathophysiologic role.[200–203] In HFRS, a tubulointerstitial nephritis caused by viral invasion of renal cells and subsequent inflammation or complement deposition seems to be the primary cause of renal injury.[201]

Depending on the virus, host recovery may depend primarily on humoral immunity, cellular immunity, or both.[183,204,205] The cause of death in most patients with viral HF is uncontrolled bleeding or shock, producing multiple organ failure.[124–127,157,169,170,174,206–213]

Clinical Presentation

The clinical presentation of patients with viral HF varies based on viral etiology, route of exposure, dose, and host factors such as susceptibility and comorbid illnesses. Not every patient follows the classic disease pattern, develops all the clinical manifestations listed here, or develops full-blown HF.[115] Information on the clinical aspects of various viral HFs is based primarily on studies of natural outbreaks. It is difficult to predict what the clinical picture would be after a biologic weapons attack, in which the exposure route and viral characteristics may be different. Nonetheless, the limited existing data suggest that the clinical picture after aerosol exposure would be similar.[118,141,143,144,163,165]

It is difficult to distinguish the exact viral etiology based on clinical manifestations alone, but certain features are more suggestive of a particular agent (Table 134B-5). After a

TABLE 134B-5 Differential Diagnosis for Patients with Viral Hemorrhagic Fever

Other Infectious Diseases
Bacterial (e.g., typhoid fever, meningococcemia, salmonellosis, shigellosis, toxic shock syndrome, sepsis)
Viral (e.g., influenza, viral hepatitis)
Parasitic (e.g., malaria, trypanosomiasis)
Rickettsial (e.g., Rocky Mountain spotted fever)
Leptospiral

Noninfectious Diseases
Thrombotic thrombocytopenic purpura
Idiopathic thrombocytopenic purpura
Hemolytic uremic syndrome
Disseminated intravascular coagulation
Vasculitis/collagen vascular diseases (e.g., lupus)
Acute leukemia

variable incubation period averaging a few days (range 48 hours to 3 weeks), the syndrome of viral HF generally begins with nonspecific influenza-like symptoms, such as high fever, myalgias, arthralgias, malaise, and headache.[124–127,157,169,170,174,206–214] The onset of symptoms is typically abrupt for the filoviruses and most other HF viruses but is often more insidious with Lassa fever, Junin, and Machupo. Other symptoms and signs may include nausea, vomiting, diarrhea, abdominal or back pain, pharyngitis, cough, chest discomfort, a diffuse maculopapular rash (e.g., particularly with Marburg and Ebola) or erythematous flushing (e.g., particularly with some Arenaviridae), and conjunctival injection.[124,125] Physical examination generally reveals fever; tachycardia or relative bradycardia; diaphoresis; muscle tenderness; conjunctivitis; pharyngitis; lymphadenopathy; rash; and occasionally meningismus, rales, and evidence of dehydration. At this point in the illness, laboratory studies show little more than leukopenia or leukocytosis. This prodromal phase typically lasts less than a week before signs of vascular involvement and clinical deterioration develop.

Evidence of vascular involvement heralds the onset of full-blown viral HF, but the extent of involvement may vary.[124–127,157,169,170,174,206–214] Vascular manifestations almost always include some degree of bleeding (gastrointestinal, pulmonary, mucosal, genitourinary, or at venipuncture sites) and often include petechiae, ecchymoses, edema, and hypotension or shock. In patients with Lassa fever, bleeding complications are less common, though they may be progressive and severe. In some patients, organ dysfunction also becomes evident at this point. Which organs are involved and to what extent varies. Neurologic manifestations, including mood changes, somnolence, delirium, or coma, are more common with infection by certain Arenaviridae, such as Junin or Machupo. Hepatic involvement, including jaundice or elevated serum transaminases, is more common with infections by Marburg or Ebola and with yellow fever, Rift Valley fever, and CCHF. Renal injury is common in severely affected individuals. It is usually the result of hypovolemia (except in HFRS, when immune mechanisms play a role) and typically presents with oliguria, elevated serum creatinine, and abnormal serum electrolytes. Pulmonary involvement is typified by an adult respiratory distress syndrome (ARDS)–type clinical picture with dyspnea, rales, hemoptysis, or chest radiographic findings. It is common in early HPS, but it often occurs late in the course of many other viral HFs. Varying degrees of hematologic involvement, including thrombocytopenia, elevated prothrombin or partial thromboplastin times, increased bleeding time, and frank disseminated intravascular coagulation, are common with all of the viral HFs. Other tissues, such as the retina, pancreas, testes, and uvea, may rarely be involved.

After about 1 to 2 weeks of clinical illness, patients who ultimately will survive generally begin to show signs of improvement. Others continue to progress to intractable shock, overwhelming multiple organ failure, and death. In some cases, recovery is prolonged, with symptoms such as fatigue, arthralgias, and anorexia persisting for several weeks to months.[209] Specific long-term sequelae are rare after recovery from most of the viral HFs but may include orchitis, transverse myelitis, recurrent hepatitis, pericarditis, uveitis, and, with Lassa fever, permanent deafness.[169,170,173,174,215] Recovery may confer immunity with some viruses.

Overall, the severity of illness varies greatly among individual patients.[124–127,157,196,214] Some develop only mild or even asymptomatic infections, whereas others exhibit a rapidly progressive and overwhelming course. Mortality rates for hospitalized patients with viral HF are generally about 5% to 20%, but they may be much lower or higher with certain viruses. For example, case-fatality rates in Ebola outbreaks can reach 50% to 90%, whereas they rarely exceed 1% for Omsk HF.[115,127,216] Death usually occurs 1 to 2 weeks into the clinical illness and is generally the result of excessive bleeding, shock, or multiple organ failure.

HPS, a unique type of HF caused by a *Hantavirus* strain found in the United States, begins after an incubation period of 1 to 6 weeks, with fever, malaise, headache, myalgias, and, occasionally, gastrointestinal symptoms.[135,217,218] After several days, pulmonary signs and symptoms rapidly emerge, with cough, dyspnea, tachypnea, and rales representing the development of diffuse noncardiogenic pulmonary edema. Many patients require supplemental oxygen or mechanical ventilation. Hypotension and shock are common during this period, and cardiopulmonary arrest can occur. Hemorrhage and other vascular manifestations are rare, but laboratory evidence of coagulopathy is common. Mortality can be high in HPS. If patients survive the pulmonary and cardiovascular manifestations, recovery generally begins a few days later.

HFRS is another, generally milder, variant of HF caused by four different strains of *Hantavirus*.[178,219,220] HFRS is often described as occurring in five phases: febrile, hypotensive, oliguric, diuretic, and convalescent.[220] After a 1- to 5-week incubation period (average 2 weeks), clinical disease begins with the development of fever, chills, headache, malaise, and myalgias.[220–222] Gastrointestinal or upper respiratory symptoms and back pain may also occur, and an erythematous, blanching rash is common over the torso and face. Physical examination generally reveals little more than a fever, rash, injected mucous membranes, and back or abdominal tenderness. Leukocytosis is the only common laboratory finding at this point. After a few days to a week, patients develop the same vascular manifestations seen with other HFs, particularly hypotension. Other organ systems may become involved (CNS, pulmonary, hepatic). Clinical shock generally resolves in a couple of days, at which time varying degrees of oliguric renal failure become a prominent feature. The renal failure sometimes necessitates hemodialysis, but it is usually reversible. After about 1 week, the oliguric phase gives way to a diuretic phase, with impressive urinary fluid losses and electrolyte abnormalities but an overall general systemic improvement.[223] The diuretic phase can last a few days to several weeks. Mortality in HFRS ranges from 5% to 15%. A milder form of the disease common to Scandinavia is sometimes referred to as *nephropathia epidemica*.[201]

Diagnosis

The diagnosis of viral HF is difficult to make during the prodromal phase given the nonspecific and protean nature of symptoms. With the development of vascular manifestations, the differential diagnosis narrows considerably but still includes a variety of more common illnesses.

Viral HF should be considered in any patient with a severe febrile illness accompanied by evidence of vascular involvement. The WHO uses the following surveillance standards for early clinical identification of a viral HF: patients with a fever of less than 3 weeks' duration, who are severely ill, and have at least two of the following bleeding manifestations: hemorrhagic or purpuric rash, epistaxis, hematemesis, melena, hematochezia, hemoptysis, or other hemorrhagic symptoms, in the absence of any preexisting hemorrhagic predisposition (e.g., coagulopathy, anticoagulant medications, vasculitis). Rapid development of pulmonary edema or adult respiratory distress syndrome in patients with an influenza-like syndrome who are otherwise healthy should prompt a search for *Hantavirus* and HPS. The characteristic five-phase progression of HFRS may make the diagnosis more apparent. Prominent renal failure, especially in the absence of significant or prolonged hypotension or if followed by a significant diuretic phase, should suggest the possibility.

There are no specific routine laboratory abnormalities to help make the diagnosis of viral HF. Thrombocytopenia and leukocytosis or leukopenia are common but vary in severity and are nonspecific.[124,125,135,196,209] Hemoconcentration and acidosis, typically the result of fluid losses, can occur. Proteinuria and an elevated serum creatinine are common during the later stages of HFRS but also can be seen in many of the other viral HFs, especially among severely ill patients.[220–222] Serum transaminase elevation is common with all of the HF viruses, but hepatic involvement is both more common and more severe with certain viral HFs (e.g., Ebola, Marburg, yellow fever, Lassa fever, Rift Valley fever, CCHF).[124,125,209,214] Radiographic studies are rarely helpful except in diagnosing pulmonary edema, typical with HPS, or complications of severe illness, such as adult respiratory distress syndrome and pneumonia.[135]

Confirmation of a suspected case of viral HF can be made by viral isolation or serologic studies.[114,115] Viral isolation during the acute illness is often considered the gold standard for confirmation, but it requires biosafety level 4 (BSL-4) precautions, seriously limiting its value and feasibility, and several days are usually required for results.[224] Isolation involves culturing the virus from various tissues or blood using special plates (e.g., Vero cells), then identifying it using electron microscopy or immunofluorescence.[124–127,183] The viremia associated with many HFs allows for isolation and culture of the pathologic agent from serum or plasma. Most patients, with the exception of patients with *Hantavirus* infections, have viremia at the time of presentation, and it typically lasts days to weeks.[124–127,183] Attempts at viral isolation from the blood may be unsuccessful later in the course of an illness as the viremia fades. The pathogen can also be identified in various histopathologic specimens by microscopy or immunofluorescence, but the same safety considerations apply.

Serologic tests, involving the assay of specific viral antigens or antiviral antibodies, can be performed on inactivated blood samples and usually have a quicker turnaround time. Thus, serologic tests are more useful for making an initial diagnosis in most cases.[115,224] Viral antigens can be detected in sera or tissues by reverse-transcriptase polymerase chain reaction techniques, immunohistochemistry, or ELISA, during the acute illness.[135,225–227] Later, antibodies can be detected in patients' blood using a variety of techniques, such as ELISA, complement fixation, or immunofluorescence.[124,125,127,178,183,194,228,229] IgM antibodies are typically detectable within several days of the onset of clinical illness, whereas IgG titers may take days or weeks to rise. Antibody detection is the most common and rapid method for diagnosing viral HF agents. The presence of antiviral IgM during the acute illness or a fourfold rise in antiviral IgG titers between acute and convalescent sera by any method is sufficient for diagnosis.[115] Currently, local hospital and even Public Health Department laboratories are not equipped to test for most of the viral HF agents (except perhaps for agents that normally occur in the United States, such as some hantaviruses). The Centers for Disease Control, U.S. Army Medical Research Institute of Infectious Diseases, or WHO should be contacted for assistance in ordering and handling of the appropriate tests.[115] All suspected cases should be reported immediately to the local or state health departments.

Determination of a biologic attack is based on the factors listed in the previous section and must be made in coordination with the appropriate public health and law enforcement personnel. Natural cases of the disease can often be distinguished from biologic terror cases by a history of travel to epidemic/endemic areas (e.g., Africa, Asia, South America), of working with infected animals or humans, or an arthropod bite within the previous several weeks.[115] Because most of the HF viruses are not endemic to the United States (with the exception of certain *Hantaviruses*, Dengue HF, and yellow fever virus strains), any patient confirmed to have one of the viral HFs should essentially be considered a victim of a biologic attack, unless recent travel to an endemic area or contact with an infected case has occurred.

Treatment

There is no specific treatment for most of the viral HFs, although the antiviral drug ribavirin seems to exhibit limited in vitro and in vivo activity against some Arenaviridae and Bunyaviridae. The management of viral HF depends primarily on good supportive and symptomatic care. Treatment for victims of a viral HF biologic attack is similar to the treatment of patients who have acquired the disease naturally. Because of the possibility of human-to-human transmission for some viruses (e.g., Marburg, Ebola, Arenaviridae), strict protective precautions are needed in all suspected viral HF cases until confirmation of the specific agent has been obtained (Table 134B-6).

SUPPORTIVE CARE

Most patients suspected of having viral HF should receive close monitoring, preferably in an intensive care unit, if resources permit. General supportive care is similar to that for other patients in the intensive care unit with multiple organ failure. Patients with pulmonary edema or hypoxia may need supplemental oxygen or intubation and mechanical ventilation. Hypotension should be treated aggressively with fluids and pressors, with care being taken to avoid fluid overload, especially in patients with HPS, evidence of pulmonary edema, or renal failure (e.g., HFRS).[135,193,230] Pulmonary arterial catheters or other invasive monitors of fluid status may help manage these patients. Many patients do not respond to fluids alone, and pressors should be added early in the course in these cases. There is no evidence that colloidal solutions are more beneficial than crystalloids.

Intravenous lines and procedures should be minimized, if possible, to avoid sites for potential bleeding. Electrolytes should be monitored regularly and corrected if necessary. Patients in the diuretic phase of HFRS are especially susceptible to life-threatening fluid and electrolyte abnormalities. Monitoring for bleeding is extremely important and can be accomplished by using serial measures of hematocrit and regularly inspecting for blood in the stool, emesis, urine, mucosal surfaces, and sputum. If evidence of significant hemorrhage (e.g., gastrointestinal bleeding or intracerebral hemorrhage) occurs, the appropriate blood, factor,

TABLE 134B-6 Clinical Characteristics and Treatment of Some Viral Hemorrhagic Fevers

AGENT	NATURAL DISTRIBUTION	UNIQUE CLINICAL CHARACTERISTICS	PERSON-TO-PERSON TRANSMISSION POSSIBLE?	TREATMENT
Filoviridae (Ebola, Marburg)	Africa	High mortality (70–90%)	Yes	Supportive care
Arenaviridae (Lassa, Junin, Machupo)	Africa (Lassa); Americas (Junin, Machupo)	More gradual onset of prodromal symptoms; hemorrhagic complications less common (Lassa); CNS dysfunction may occur (Junin, Machupo)	Yes	Ribavirin, supportive care
Rift Valley fever	Africa	Eye symptoms common; hepatitis, encephalitis, and retinitis infrequent complications	No	Ribavirin, supportive care
Yellow fever	Africa, South America	Prodromal symptoms may be followed by remission before hemorrhagic fever develops; hepatitis and jaundice common	No	Supportive care
Dengue hemorrhagic fever	Asia, Americas, Africa	Hemorrhagic complications rare	No	Supportive care

or platelet transfusions should be administered—similar to other patients with coagulopathy and bleeding. Mild bleeding rarely requires replacement therapy and generally responds to direct pressure and conservative measures alone. Bed rest is important to minimize the risk of trauma and subsequent bleeding. Coagulation parameters, platelet counts, and bleeding times should be monitored regularly, along with serial complete blood counts. Heparin for disseminated intravascular coagulation is controversial but may be considered.[124,231,232] Evidence of secondary infection should be sought and the infection treated with appropriate antimicrobials. Hemodialysis is sometimes necessary in patients with HFRS or other viral HFs.[193,219] The usual indications for dialysis apply, except that some authors have advocated earlier dialysis in the hope of preventing uremia-induced platelet dysfunction from contributing to hemorrhagic complications.[193]

INFECTION PRECAUTIONS

Nosocomial viral transmission and secondary infection of close contacts have been well documented with the filoviruses and certain arenaviruses, primarily after direct dermal or mucosal contact with blood or bodily fluids from infected patients.[124–127,233,234] Such transmission may also occur with certain strains of *Hantavirus* causing HPS.[167] It is not yet clear that airborne person-to-person transmission can be excluded for some agents. Consequently, all hospital staff should observe strict barrier and airborne precautions, including double gloving, masks (e.g., N-95 masks or powered air-purifying respirators), face and eye protection, impermeable gowns, and leg/shoe covers. All hospital staff should wash hands regularly.[115,235] If resources permit, patients suspected of having viral HF should be kept in a room with a negative airflow system and dedicated medical equipment. Patient contact and unnecessary laboratory tests and procedures should be minimized as much as possible to prevent further spread or potential exposures.

Although, in general, lipid-enveloped viruses are not environmentally stable, certain agents (e.g., Marburg) have been shown to survive on surfaces for several days, making fomite transmission theoretically possible and highlighting the need for surface decontamination.[116,160] Regular decontamination of all environmental surfaces with a hospital disinfectant or dilute bleach solution should be performed. In addition, the hospital's epidemiologist and local/state public health agencies should be notified immediately when a patient is suspected to have viral HF. All biologic specimens from infected patients should be labeled as hazardous, and personnel should be notified about the necessary handling precautions (e.g., barrier and airborne precautions) because these viruses can be transmitted by direct contact with the infected material or via small-particle aerosols that can be generated during certain procedures (e.g., centrifugation, pipetting, or spills). Specimens should be treated using at least BSL-3 safety precautions. The same precautions should be observed among pathology, autopsy, and burial personnel, given that postmortem transmission has been documented with certain viruses.[171,173] Prompt management of deceased patients should be done by burial or cremation and with a minimum of postmortem procedures. All other contaminated materials should be autoclaved or sterilized with disinfectant or dilute bleach solutions, or discarded by incineration; linens should

be washed with bleach and hot water.[236] The addition of bleach or disinfectant to patient excreta or fluids before disposal is currently not recommended by most experts.[115] Although only a few of the natural HF viruses are known to exhibit person-to-person transmission, when viral HF is suspected in a patient, these precautions should be maintained until the exact viral etiology is known and confirmed not to be acquired through close contact. In the event of a biologic attack, the risk for altered or manipulated pathogen characteristics warrants extra caution, at least until more information regarding the epidemiology and transmission is known. This imperative must be balanced with the availability of resources.

The duration of the contagious period is not clear for most of the viral agents. People with close contact of infected patients within 3 weeks of the illness onset (and in the absence of appropriate infection control measures) should be observed closely for development of the disease.[115] Patients should be instructed to avoid direct bodily fluid contact with others for at least 3 months after recovering from the illness, given the persistence of active virus in certain specimens and the theoretical risk of subsequent transmission.[174,176,177]

ANTIVIRAL AGENTS

The only specific drug shown to have any benefit in the course of certain viral HFs (HFs associated with Arenaviridae and some Bunyaviridae infections) is ribavirin. This nucleoside analogue has proved to be efficacious in improving mortality in patients with Lassa fever and to a lesser extent in patients with Junin or Machupo viral infections or HFRS.[237–245] Although ribavirin has not been well studied in HPS, it is used commonly, and anecdotal reports seem promising.[219,246,247] Although less convincing, animal data and some human data indicate a potential benefit for patients with CCHF and Rift Valley fever.[234,240,242,248] Ribavirin is of no benefit for patients with *Filovirus* and *Flavivirus* infections. Because the exact etiologic agent may not be known at the time of presentation, all patients with suspected viral HF should be treated with ribavirin until HF is ruled out or the underlying pathogen has been identified as one that generally does not respond to the drug.[236] The recommended regimen is a loading dose of 30 mg/kg intravenously, followed by 15 mg/kg intravenously every 6 hours for 4 days, followed by 7.5 mg/kg every 8 hours for 6 days.[115] Ribavirin should be administered as soon as possible, because it seems to be more effective if given earlier in the disease course (within 1 week). Its main side effects include anemia and hemolysis, which are generally mild and reversible. It is classified as pregnancy category X (see Appendix A).[249] However, use of ribavirin may still be appropriate in certain pregnant patients with viral HF, if the benefits outweigh its risk to the developing fetus.[115] In a mass casualty situation, intravenous ribavirin may not be feasible. In this case, oral ribavirin should be given, although efficacy by this route is unproven.[115] The following oral regimen is recommended for adults: 2 g orally as a loading dose, followed by 600 mg orally twice daily for 10 days in patients weighing more than 75 kg (or 400 mg orally every morning and 600 mg orally every evening for 10 days in patients weighing <75 kg). The recommended regimen for children is 30 mg/kg orally as a loading dose, followed by 7.5 mg/kg orally twice daily for 10 days.[115]

Prophylactic use of oral ribavirin could be considered for high-risk contacts of patients with certain viral HFs, particularly Lassa fever and perhaps other Arenaviridae, based largely on limited animal data.[239,250] The efficacy of ribavirin for this indication has not been established in humans, however, and other authors have advised against postexposure prophylaxis with ribavirin in asymptomatic patients.[115]

OTHER DRUGS

Interferon alfa has been tried for some of the viral HFs, and a few case reports suggest it might be helpful as an adjunctive measure in filoviral infections or Rift Valley fever.[251-253] Given the lack of adequate data, use of interferon alfa should still be considered experimental. There is no evidence that corticosteroids have any value for the management of patients with viral HF.[114]

PASSIVE IMMUNOTHERAPY

The use of convalescent serum from survivors as a method of conferring passive immunity to acutely affected individuals has been attempted with several viral HFs. Although case reports and animal data are encouraging, at least for patients with *Filovirus*, Machupo, Junin, Rift Valley fever, and CCHF infections, good clinical data are lacking.[204,252,254-257] The data are conflicting for patients with Lassa fever.[169,238,245,258,259] Immune serum is rarely available in sufficient quantities (especially in the United States or other nonendemic areas), and it carries certain inherent risks, such as the transmission of other infections. Passive immunization may increase viral replication in some cases. Finally, it requires that the specific causative pathogen has been identified. As a result, the widespread use of convalescent serum after a biologic attack in most cases would not be feasible or recommended.[115] It may be considered, however, on a limited and individualized basis for victims with the aforementioned viral HFs. Two or more units of convalescent plasma or its equivalent in immunoglobulin should be given early in the disease course (within 1 week) if it is to be used. Recombinant human antibodies may prove useful as a treatment in the future.[260]

VACCINES

Vaccines are available clinically or experimentally for a few of the viruses, including yellow fever, Machupo, Junin, dengue HF, and Rift Valley fever. The yellow fever vaccine, a live-attenuated product, is the only vaccine commercially available and widely used.[206] World stocks are insufficient for a widespread vaccination program.[115] The U.S. Army is currently experimenting with Marburg, Ebola, and Lassa vaccines.[261,262] To date, there is no evidence that the vaccines would be useful in a postexposure situation either preventively or therapeutically.

REFERENCES

1. Smith J, Davis K, Hart M, et al: Viral encephalitides. In Zajtchuk R (ed): Textbook of Military Medicine, Part I: Medical Aspects of Chemical and Biological Warfare. Washington, D.C., Office of the Surgeon General, U.S. Army, 1997, pp 561–589.
2. Biological and chemical terrorism: Strategic plan for preparedness and response. Recommendations of the CDC Strategic Planning Workgroup. MMWR Morb Mortal Wkly Rep Recomm Rep 49(RR-4):1–14, 2000.
3. U.S. Army Medical Research Institute of Infectious Diseases: Medical Management of Biological Casualties: Handbook. Frederick, MD, Fort Detrick, 1996.
4. World Health Organization: Public Response to Biological and Chemical Weapons, 2nd ed. Annex 1 (Prepublication Issue). Geneva, WHO, 2001.
5. Khan AS, Morse S, Lillibridge S: Public-health preparedness for biological terrorism in the USA. Lancet 356:1179–1182, 2000.
6. Huxsoll DL, Patrick WC 3rd, Parrott CD: Veterinary services in biological disasters. J Am Vet Med Assoc 190:714–722, 1987.
7. Helwig F: Western equine encephalitis following accidental innoculation with chick embryo virus. JAMA 115:291–292, 1940.
8. Ryzhikov AB, Ryabchikova EI, Sergeev AN, Tkacheva NV: Spread of Venezuelan equine encephalitis virus in mice olfactory tract. Arch Virol 140:2243–2254, 1995.
9. Ryzhikov AB, Tkacheva NV, Sergeev AN, Ryabchikova EI: Venezuelan equine encephalitis virus propagation in the olfactory tract of normal and immunized mice. Biomed Sci 2:607–614, 1991.
10. Slepushkin AN: An epidemiological study of laboratory infections with Venezuelan equine encephalomyelitis. Vopr Virusol 3:311–314, 1959.
11. Strauss JH, Strauss EG: The alphaviruses: gene expression, replication, and evolution. Microbiol Rev 58:491–562, 1994.
12. Brault AC, Powers AM, Holmes EC, et al: Positively charged amino acid substitutions in the e2 envelope glycoprotein are associated with the emergence of Venezuelan equine encephalitis virus. J Virol 76:1718–1730, 2002.
13. Davis NL, Powell N, Greenwald GF, et al: Attenuating mutations in the E2 glycoprotein gene of Venezuelan equine encephalitis virus: Construction of single and multiple mutants in a full-length cDNA clone. Virology 183:20–31, 1991.
14. Davis NL, Willis LV, Smith JF, Johnston RE: In vitro synthesis of infectious Venezuelan equine encephalitis virus RNA from a cDNA clone: Analysis of a viable deletion mutant. Virology 171:189–204, 1989.
15. Spotts DR, Reich RM, Kalkhan MA, et al: Resistance to alpha/beta interferons correlates with the epizootic and virulence potential of Venezuelan equine encephalitis viruses and is determined by the 5′ noncoding region and glycoproteins. J Virol 72:10286–10291, 1998.
16. Anthony RP, Brown DT: Protein-protein interactions in an alphavirus membrane. J Virol 65:1187–1194, 1991.
17. Davis NL, Fuller FJ, Dougherty WG, et al: A single nucleotide change in the E2 glycoprotein gene of Sindbis virus affects penetration rate in cell culture and virulence in neonatal mice. Proc Natl Acad Sci U S A 83:6771–6775, 1986.
18. Dalrymple JM, Schlesinger S, Russell PK: Antigenic characterization of two sindbis envelope glycoproteins separated by isoelectric focusing. Virology 69:93–103, 1976.
19. Pereboev AV, Razumov IA, Svyatchenko VA, Loktev VB: Glycoproteins E2 of the Venezuelan and eastern equine encephalomyelitis viruses contain multiple cross-reactive epitopes. Arch Virol 141:2191–2205, 1996.
20. Howitt B: Equine encephalomyelitis. J Infect Dis 51:493–510, 1932.
21. Beck C, Wyckoff RWG: Venezuelan equine encephalomyelitis. Science 88:530, 1938.
22. Kubes V, Rios F: The causative agent of infectious equine encephalomyelitis in Venezuela. Science 90:20–21, 1939.
23. Leon CA: Sequelae of Venezuelan equine encephalitis in humans: A four year follow-up. Int J Epidemiol 4:131–140, 1975.
24. Sanmartin-Barberi C, Groot H, Osorno-Mesa E: Human epidemic in Columbia caused by the Venezuelan equine encephalomyelitis virus. Am J Trop Med Hyg 3:283–293, 1954.
25. Monath TP: Arthropod-borne encephalitides in the Americas. Bull World Health Organ 57:513–533, 1979.
26. Vaupel M, Dietz H, Linder D, Thauer RK: Primary structure of cyclohydrolase (Mch) from *Methanobacterium thermoautotrophicum* (strain Marburg) and functional expression of the *mch* gene in *Escherichia coli*. Eur J Biochem 236:294–300, 1996.
27. Feemster R: Equine encephalitis in Massachusetts. N Engl J Med 257:701–705, 1957.
28. Gold H, Hampil B: Equine encephalomyelitis in a laboratory technician with recovery. Ann Intern Med 16:556–569, 1942.

29. Stephenson EH, Moeller RB, York CG, Young HW: Nose-only versus whole-body aerosol exposure for induction of upper respiratory infections of laboratory mice. Am Ind Hyg Assoc J 49:128–135, 1988.

30. Western equine encephalitis—United States and Canada, 1987. MMWR Morb Mortal Wkly Rep 36:655–659, 1987.

31. Peters CJ, Johnson KM: California encephalitis viruses, hantaviruses, and other Bunyaviridae. In Mandell G, Bennet J, Dolin R (eds): Principles and Practice of Infectious Diseases, 4th ed. New York, Churchill Livingstone, 1995, pp 1567–1572.

32. Goldfield M, Welsh JN, Taylor BF: The 1959 outbreak of Eastern encephalitis in New Jersey: 5. The inapparent infection:disease ratio. Am J Epidemiol 87:32–33, 1968.

33. Hinman AR, McGowan JE Jr, Henderson BE: Venezuelan equine encephalomyelitis: Surveys of human illness during an epizootic in Guatemala and El Salvador. Am J Epidemiol 93:130–136, 1971.

34. Update: Venezuelan equine encephalitis—Colombia, 1995. MMWR Morb Mortal Wkly Rep 44:775–777, 1995.

35. Franck PT, Johnson KM: An outbreak of Venezuelan encephalitis in man in the Panama Canal Zone. Am J Trop Med Hyg 19:860–865, 1970.

36. Sanchez JL, Takafuji ET, Lednar WM, et al: Venezuelan equine encephalomyelitis: Report of an outbreak associated with jungle exposure. Milit Med 149:618–621, 1984.

37. Martin DH, Eddy GA, Sudia WD, et al: An epidemiologic study of Venezuelan equine encephalomyelitis in Costa Rica, 1970. Am J Epidemiol 95:565–578, 1972.

38. Charles PC, Trgovich J, Davis NL, Johnston RE: Immunopathogenesis and immune modulation of Venezuelan equine encephalitis virus-induced disease in the mouse. Virology 284:190–202, 2001.

39. Schoneboom BA, Fultz MJ, Miller TH, et al: Astrocytes as targets for Venezuelan equine encephalitis virus infection. J Neurovirol 5:342–354, 1999.

40. Grieder FB, Nguyen HT: Virulent and attenuated mutant Venezuelan equine encephalitis virus show marked differences in replication in infection in murine macrophages. Microb Pathog 21:85–95, 1996.

41. Wahlberg JM, Bron R, Wilschut J, Garoff H: Membrane fusion of Semliki Forest virus involves homotrimers of the fusion protein. J Virol 66:7309–7318, 1992.

42. Woodward TM, Miller BR, Beaty BJ, et al: A single amino acid change in the E2 glycoprotein of Venezuelan equine encephalitis virus affects replication and dissemination in Aedes aegypti mosquitoes. J Gen Virol 72(Part 10):2431–2435, 1991.

43. Ludwig GV, Kondig JP, Smith JF: A putative receptor for Venezuelan equine encephalitis virus from mosquito cells. J Virol 70:5592–5599, 1996.

44. Bron R, Wahlberg JM, Garoff H, Wilschut J: Membrane fusion of Semliki Forest virus in a model system: Correlation between fusion kinetics and structural changes in the envelope glycoprotein. EMBO J 12:693–701, 1993.

45. Corver J, Bron R, Snippe H, et al: Membrane fusion activity of Semliki Forest virus in a liposomal model system: Specific inhibition by Zn2+ ions. Virology 238:14–21, 1997.

46. Liljestrom P, Garoff H: Internally located cleavable signal sequences direct the formation of Semliki Forest virus membrane proteins from a polyprotein precursor. J Virol 65:147–154, 1991.

47. Lubiniecki AS: Replication of eastern equine encephalitis viruses (New Jersey and Louisiana strains and the Ets-4 mutant) in rabbit kidney cells. Arch Virol 47:21–29, 1975.

48. Sefton BM: Immediate glycosylation of Sindbis virus membrane proteins. Cell 10:659–668, 1977.

49. Ziemiecki A, Garoff H, Simons K: Formation of the Semliki Forest virus membrane glycoprotein complexes in the infected cell. J Gen Virol 50:111–123, 1980.

50. de Curtis I, Simons K: Dissection of Semliki Forest virus glycoprotein delivery from the trans-Golgi network to the cell surface in permeabilized BHK cells. Proc Natl Acad Sci U S A 85:8052–8056, 1988.

51. Gliedman JB, Smith JF, Brown DT: Morphogenesis of Sindbis virus in cultured Aedes albopictus cells. J Virol 16:913–926, 1975.

52. Lopez S, Yao JS, Kuhn RJ, et al: Nucleocapsid-glycoprotein interactions required for assembly of alphaviruses. J Virol 68:1316–1323, 1994.

53. Metsikko K, Garoff H: Oligomers of the cytoplasmic domain of the p62/E2 membrane protein of Semliki Forest virus bind to the nucleocapsid in vitro. J Virol 64:4678–4683, 1990.

54. Paredes AM, Brown DT, Rothnagel R, et al: Three-dimensional structure of a membrane-containing virus. Proc Natl Acad Sci U S A 90:9095–9099, 1993.

55. Aronson JF, Grieder FB, Davis NL, et al: A single-site mutant and revertants arising in vivo define early steps in the pathogenesis of Venezuelan equine encephalitis virus. Virology 270:111–123, 2000.

56. Simons K, Garoff H: The budding mechanisms of enveloped animal viruses. J Gen Virol 50:1–21, 1980.

57. Grieder FB, Davis NL, Aronson JF, et al: Specific restrictions in the progression of Venezuelan equine encephalitis virus-induced disease resulting from single amino acid changes in the glycoproteins. Virology 206:994–1006, 1995.

58. Jackson AC, Rossiter JP: Apoptotic cell death is an important cause of neuronal injury in experimental Venezuelan equine encephalitis virus infection of mice. Acta Neuropathol (Berl) 93:349–353, 1997.

59. Levine B, Huang Q, Isaacs JT, et al: Conversion of lytic to persistent alphavirus infection by the bcl-2 cellular oncogene. Nature 361:739–742, 1993.

60. Turell MJ, Tammariello RF, Spielman A: Nonvascular delivery of St. Louis encephalitis and Venezuelan equine encephalitis viruses by infected mosquitoes (Diptera: Culicidae) feeding on a vertebrate host. J Med Entomol 32:563–568, 1995.

61. MacDonald GH, Johnston RE: Role of dendritic cell targeting in Venezuelan equine encephalitis virus pathogenesis. J Virol 74:914–922, 2000.

62. Bulychev LE, Sergeev AN, Ryzhikov AB, et al: [Course of infection in white rats, infected with Venezuelan equine encephalomyelitis virus by a respiratory route]. Vopr Virusol 40:79–82, 1995.

63. Elvin SJ, Bennett AM, Phillpotts RJ: Role for mucosal immune responses and cell-mediated immune functions in protection from airborne challenge with Venezuelan equine encephalitis virus. J Med Virol 67:384–393, 2002.

64. Charles PC, Walters E, Margolis F, Johnston RE: Mechanism of neuroinvasion of Venezuelan equine encephalitis virus in the mouse. Virology 208:662–671, 1995.

65. Danes L, Kufner J, Hruskova J, Rychterova V: The role of the olfactory route on infection of the respiratory tract with Venezuelan equine encephalomyelitis virus in normal and operated Macaca rhesus monkeys: I. Results of virological examination. Acta Virol 17:50–56, 1973.

66. Danes L, Rychterova V, Kliment V, Hruskova J: Penetration of Venezuelan equine encephalomyelitis virus into the brain of guinea pigs and rabbits after intranasal infection. Acta Virol 17:138–146, 1973.

67. Dropulic B, Masters CL: Entry of neurotropic arboviruses into the central nervous system: An in vitro study using mouse brain endothelium. J Infect Dis 161:685–691, 1990.

68. Coates DM, Makh SR, Jones N, Lloyd G: Assessment of assays for the serodiagnosis of Venezuelan equine encephalitis. J Infect 25:279–289, 1992.

69. de la Monte S, Castro F, Bonilla NJ, et al: The systemic pathology of Venezuelan equine encephalitis virus infection in humans. Am J Trop Med Hyg 34:194–202, 1985.

70. Jackson AC, SenGupta SK, Smith JF: Pathogenesis of Venezuelan equine encephalitis virus infection in mice and hamsters. Vet Pathol 28:410–418, 1991.

71. Gleiser C, Gochenour W, Berge T, Tigert W: The comparative pathology of experimental Venezuelan equine encephalomyelitis infection in different animal hosts. J Infect Dis 110:80–97, 1962.

72. Schoneboom BA, Catlin KM, Marty AM, et al: Inflammation is a component of neurodegeneration in response to Venezuelan equine encephalitis virus infection in mice. J Neuroimmunol 109:132–146, 2000.

73. Goldfield M, Taylor BF, Welsh JN: The 1959 outbreak of Eastern encephalitis in New Jersey: 6. The frequency of prior infection. Am J Epidemiol 87:39–49, 1968.

74. Grieder FB, Vogel SN: Role of interferon and interferon regulatory factors in early protection against Venezuelan equine encephalitis virus infection. Virology 257:106–118, 1999.

75. Grieder FB, Davis BK, Zhou XD, et al: Kinetics of cytokine expression and regulation of host protection following infection with molecularly cloned Venezuelan equine encephalitis virus. Virology 233:302–312, 1997.

76. Levitt NH, Miller HV, Edelman R: Interaction of alphaviruses with human peripheral leukocytes: In vitro replication of Venezuelan equine encephalomyelitis virus in monocyte cultures. Infect Immun 24:642–646, 1979.

77. Schoneboom BA, Fultz MJ, Miller TH, et al: Astrocytes as targets for Venezuelan equine encephalitis virus infection. J Neurovirol 5:342–354, 1999.

78. Deresiewicz RL, Thaler SJ, Hsu L, Zamani AA: Clinical and neuro-radiographic manifestations of eastern equine encephalitis. N Engl J Med 336:1867–1874, 1997.

79. Ludwig GV, Turell MJ, Vogel P, et al: Comparative neurovirulence of attenuated and non-attenuated strains of Venezuelan equine encephalitis virus in mice. Am J Trop Med Hyg 64:49–55, 2001.

80. Hart KL, Keen D, Belle EA: An outbreak of eastern equine encephalomyelitis in Jamaica, West Indes, Nov-Dec 1962: I. Description of human cases. Am J Trop Med Hyg 13:331–334, 1964.

81. Sciple GW, Ray CG, Holden P, et al: Encephalitis in the high plains of Texas. Am J Epidemiol 87:87–98, 1968.

82. Farber S, Hill A, Connerly DJH: Encephalitis in infants and children caused by the virus of the eastern variety of equine encephalitis. JAMA 114:1725–1731, 1940.

83. Leech RW, Harris JC, Johnson RM: 1975 encephalitis epidemic in North Dakota and western Minnesota: An epidemiologic, clinical, and neuropathologic study. Minn Med 64:545–548, 1981.

84. Franck PT, Johnson KM: An outbreak of Venezuelan encephalitis in man in the Panama Canal Zone. Am J Trop Med Hyg 19:860–865, 1970.

85. Bia FJ, Thornton GF, Main AJ, et al: Western equine encephalitis mimicking herpes simplex encephalitis. JAMA 244:367–369, 1980.

86. Bowen GS, Fashinell TR, Dean PB, Gregg MB: Clinical aspects of human Venezuelan equine encephalitis in Texas. Bull Pan Am Health Organ 10:46–57, 1976.

87. Goldfield M, Taylor BF, Welsh JN: The 1959 outbreak of Eastern encephalitis in New Jersey: 3. Serologic studies of clinical cases. Am J Epidemiol 87:18–22, 1968.

88. Clarke DH: Two non-fatal human infections with the virus of eastern encephalitis. Am J Trop Med Hyg 10:67–70, 1961.

89. Calisher CH, Emerson JK, Muth DJ, et al: Serodiagnosis of western equine encephalitis virus infections: Relationships of antibody titer and test to observed onset of clinical illness. J Am Vet Med Assoc 183:438–440, 1983.

90. Calisher CH, Berardi VP, Muth DJ, Buff EE: Specificity of immunoglobulin M and G antibody responses in humans infected with eastern and western equine encephalitis viruses: Application to rapid serodiagnosis. J Clin Microbiol 23:369–372, 1986.

91. McGowan JE Jr, Bryan JA, Gregg MB: Surveillance of arboviral encephalitis in the United States, 1955–1971. Am J Epidemiol 97:199–207, 1973.

92. Monath TP: Arthropod-borne encephalitides in the Americas. Bull World Health Organ 57:513–533, 1979.

93. Gold H, Hampil B: Equine encephalomyelitis in a laboratory technician with recovery. Ann Intern Med 16:556–569, 1942.

94. Bowen GS, Calisher CH: Virological and serological studies of Venezuelan equine encephalomyelitis in humans. J Clin Microbiol 4:22–27, 1976.

95. Bastian FO, Wende RD, Singer DB, Zeller RS: Eastern equine encephalomyelitis: Histopathologic and ultrastructural changes with isolation of the virus in a human case. Am J Clin Pathol 64:10–13, 1975.

96. Frazier CL, Shope RE: Detection of antibodies to alphaviruses by enzyme-linked immunosorbent assay. J Clin Microbiol 10:583–585, 1979.

97. Rosato RR, Macasaet FF, Jahrling PB: Enzyme-linked immunosorbent assay detection of immunoglobulins G and M to Venezuelan equine encephalomyelitis virus in vaccinated and naturally infected humans. J Clin Microbiol 26:421–425, 1988.

98. Engler RJ, Mangiafico JA, Jahrling P, et al: Venezuelan equine encephalitis-specific immunoglobulin responses: Live attenuated TC-83 versus inactivated C-84 vaccine. J Med Virol 38:305–310, 1992.

99. Pittman PR, Makuch RS, Mangiafico JA, et al: Long-term duration of detectable neutralizing antibodies after administration of live-attenuated VEE vaccine and following booster vaccination with inactivated VEE vaccine. Vaccine 14:337–343, 1996.

100. Strizki JM, Repik PM: Differential reactivity of immune sera from human vaccinees with field strains of eastern equine encephalitis virus. Am J Trop Med Hyg 53:564–570, 1995.

101. Edelman R, Ascher MS, Oster CN, et al: Evaluation in humans of a new, inactivated vaccine for Venezuelan equine encephalitis virus (C-84). J Infect Dis 140:708–715, 1979.

102. Cieslak TJ, Christopher GW, Kortepeter MG, et al: Immunization against potential biological warfare agents. Clin Infect Dis 30:843–850, 2000.

103. Burke DS, Ramsburg HH, Edelman R: Persistence in humans of antibody to subtypes of Venezuelan equine encephalomyelitis (VEE) virus after immunization with attenuated (TC-83) VEE virus vaccine. J Infect Dis 136:354–359, 1977.

104. Casamassima AC, Hess LW, Marty A: TC-83 Venezuelan equine encephalitis vaccine exposure during pregnancy. Teratology 36:287–289, 1987.

105. Phillpotts RJ, Wright AJ: TC-83 vaccine protects against airborne or subcutaneous challenge with heterologous mouse-virulent strains of Venezuelan equine encephalitis virus. Vaccine 17:982–988, 1999.

106. Phillpotts RJ: Immunity to airborne challenge with Venezuelan equine encephalitis virus develops rapidly after immunization with the attenuated vaccine strain TC-83. Vaccine 17:2429–2435, 1999.

107. Pratt WD, Gibbs P, Pitt ML, Schmaljohn AL: Use of telemetry to assess vaccine-induced protection against parenteral and aerosol infections of Venezuelan equine encephalitis virus in non-human primates. Vaccine 16:1056–1064, 1998.

108. Jahrling PB, Stephenson EH: Protective efficacies of live attenuated and formaldehyde-inactivated Venezuelan equine encephalitis virus vaccines against aerosol challenge in hamsters. J Clin Microbiol 19:429–431, 1984.

109. Hart MK, Caswell-Stephan K, Bakken R, et al: Improved mucosal protection against Venezuelan equine encephalitis virus is induced by the molecularly defined, live-attenuated V3526 vaccine candidate. Vaccine 18:3067–3075, 2000.

110. Greenway TE, Eldridge JH, Ludwig G, et al: Induction of protective immune responses against Venezuelan equine encephalitis (VEE) virus aerosol challenge with microencapsulated VEE virus vaccine. Vaccine 16:1314–1323, 1998.

111. Charles PC, Brown KW, Davis NL, et al:. Mucosal immunity induced by parenteral immunization with a live attenuated Venezuelan equine encephalitis virus vaccine candidate. Virology 228:153–160, 1997.

112. Griffin DE, Johnson RT: Role of the immune response in recovery from Sindbis virus encephalitis in mice. J Immunol 118:1070–1075, 1977.

113. Seamer JH, Boulter EA, Zlotnik I: Delayed onset of encephalitis in mice passively immunised against Semliki Forest virus. Br J Exp Pathol 52:408–414, 1971.

114. Jahrling PB: Viral hemorrhagic fevers. In Zajtchuk R (ed): Textbook of Military Medicine: Part I. Medical Aspects of Chemical and Biological Warfare. Washington, D.C., Office of the Surgeon General, United States Army, 1997, pp 591–602.

115. Borio L, Inglesby T, Peters CJ, et al: Hemorrhagic fever viruses as biological weapons: Medical and public health management. JAMA 287:2391–2405, 2002.

116. Peters CJ, Jahrling PB, Khan AS: Patients infected with high-hazard viruses: Scientific basis for infection control. Arch Virol Suppl 11(Suppl):141–168, 1996.

117. Klietmann WF, Ruoff KL: Bioterrorism: Implications for the clinical microbiologist. Clin Microbiol Rev 14:364–381, 2001.

118. Alibek K: Biohazard: The Chilling True Story of the Largest Covert Biological Weapons Program in the World—Told from the Inside by the Man Who Ran It. New York, Random House, 1998.

119. Chumakov MP, Smirnova SE, Tkachenko EA: Relationship between strains of Crimean haemorrhagic fever and Congo viruses. Acta Virol 14:82–85, 1970.

120. Markoff L: Alphaviruses. In Mandell G, Bennet J, Dolin R (eds): Principles and Practice of Infectious Diseases, 4th ed. New York, Churchill Livingstone, 1995, pp 1455–1459.

121. Luby JP, Sanders CV: Green monkey disease ("Marburg virus" disease): A new zoonosis. Ann Intern Med 71:657–660, 1969.

122. Martini GA, Knauff HG, Schmidt HA, et al: A hitherto unknown infectious disease contracted from monkeys: "Marburg-virus" disease. Geriatr Med Mon 13:457–470, 1968.

123. Malherbe H, Strickland-Cholmley M: Human disease from monkeys (Marburg virus). Lancet 1:1434, 1968.

124. Gear JS, Cassel GA, Gear AJ, et al: Outbreak of Marburg virus disease in Johannesburg. BMJ 4:489–493, 1975.

125. Smith DH, Johnson BK, Isaacson M, et al: Marburg-virus disease in Kenya. Lancet 1:816–820, 1982.

126. Ebola haemorrhagic fever in Sudan, 1976. Report of a WHO/International Study Team. Bull World Health Organ 56:247–270, 1978.

127. Ebola haemorrhagic fever in Zaire, 1976. Bull World Health Organ 56:271–293, 1978.

128. Okware SI, Omaswa FG, Zaramba S, et al: An outbreak of Ebola in Uganda. Trop Med Int Health 7:1068–1075, 2002.

129. Le Guenno B, Formenty P, Boesch C: Ebola virus outbreaks in the Ivory Coast and Liberia, 1994–1995. Curr Top Microbiol Immunol 235:77–84, 1999.

130. Georges AJ, Leroy EM, Renaut AA, et al: Ebola hemorrhagic fever outbreaks in Gabon, 1994–1997: Epidemiologic and health control issues. J Infect Dis 179(Suppl 1):S65–75, 1999.

131. Khan AS, Tshioko FK, Heymann DL, et al: The reemergence of Ebola hemorrhagic fever, Democratic Republic of the Congo, 1995. Commission de Lutte contre les Epidemies a Kikwit. J Infect Dis 179(Suppl 1):S76–86, 1999.

132. Jahrling PB, Geisbert TW, Dalgard DW, et al: Preliminary report: Isolation of Ebola virus from monkeys imported to USA. Lancet 335:502–505, 1990.

133. Rollin PE, Williams RJ, Bressler DS, et al: Ebola (subtype Reston) virus among quarantined nonhuman primates recently imported from the Philippines to the United States. J Infect Dis 179(Suppl 1):S108–114, 1999.

134. World Health Organization (WHO): Ebola hemorrhagic fever in the Republic of Congo—Update 6. WHO Website: Communicable Disease Surveillance and Response, 2003. www.who.int/csr/en/

135. Duchin JS, Koster FT, Peters CJ, et al: Hantavirus pulmonary syndrome: A clinical description of 17 patients with a newly recognized disease. The Hantavirus Study Group. N Engl J Med 330:949–955, 1994.

136. Rhodes LV 3rd, Huang C, Sanchez AJ, et al: Hantavirus pulmonary syndrome associated with Monongahela virus, Pennsylvania. Emerg Infect Dis 6:616–621, 2000.

137. Verity R, Prasad E, Grimsrud K, et al: Hantavirus pulmonary syndrome in northern Alberta, Canada: Clinical and laboratory findings for 19 cases. Clin Infect Dis 31:942–946, 2000.

138. Gonzalez Della Valle M, Edelstein A, Miguel S, et al: Andes virus associated with hantavirus pulmonary syndrome in northern Argentina and determination of the precise site of infection. Am J Trop Med Hyg 66:713–720, 2002.

139. Castillo C, Naranjo J, Sepulveda A, et al: Hantavirus pulmonary syndrome due to Andes virus in Temuco, Chile: Clinical experience with 16 adults. Chest 120:548–554, 2001.

140. Fisher-Hoch SP, Tomori O, Nasidi A, et al: Review of cases of nosocomial Lassa fever in Nigeria: The high price of poor medical practice. BMJ 311:857–859, 1995.

141. Smithburn KC, Mahaffy AF, Haddow AJ, et al: Rift Valley fever: Accidental infections among laboratory workers. J Immunol 62:213–227, 1949.

142. Jaax N, Jahrling P, Geisbert T, et al: Transmission of Ebola virus (Zaire strain) to uninfected control monkeys in a biocontainment laboratory. Lancet 346:1669–1671, 1995.

143. Johnson E, Jaax N, White J, Jahrling P: Lethal experimental infections of rhesus monkeys by aerosolized Ebola virus. Int J Exp Pathol 76:227–236, 1995.

144. Stephenson EH, Larson EW, Dominik JW: Effect of environmental factors on aerosol-induced Lassa virus infection. J Med Virol 14:295–303, 1984.

145. Ryabchikova E, Strelets L, Kolesnikova L, et al: Respiratory Marburg virus infection in guinea pigs. Arch Virol 141:2177–2190, 1996.

146. Monath TP, Mertens PE, Patton R, et al: A hospital epidemic of Lassa fever in Zorzor, Liberia, March-April 1972. Am J Trop Med Hyg 22:773–779, 1973.

147. Gear JS, Cassel GA, Gear AJ, et al: Outbreak of Marburg virus disease in Johannesburg. BMJ 4:489–493, 1975.

148. Peters CJ, Johnson KM: Lymphocytic choriomeningitis virus, Lassa virus, and other Arenaviruses. In Mandell G, Bennet J, Dolin R (eds): Principles and Practice of Infectious Diseases, 4th ed. New York, Churchill Livingstone, 1995, pp 1572–1579..

149. Monath TP: Flaviviruses (yellow fever, dengue, dengue hemorrhagic fever, Japanese encephalitis, St. Louis encephalitis, tick-borne encephalitis). In Mandell G, Bennet J, Dolin R (eds): Principles and Practice of Infectious Diseases, 4th ed. New York, Churchill Livingstone, 1995, pp 1465–1474.

150. Monath TP: Ecology of Marburg and Ebola viruses: Speculations and directions for future research. J Infect Dis 179(Suppl 1):S127–138, 1999.

151. Meegan JM: The Rift Valley fever epizootic in Egypt 1977–78: 1. Description of the epizootic and virological studies. Trans R Soc Trop Med Hyg 73:618–623, 1979.

152. Hoogstraal H: The epidemiology of tick-borne Crimean-Congo hemorrhagic fever in Asia, Europe, and Africa. J Med Entomol 15:307–417, 1979.

153. Johnson KM, Mackenzie RB, Webb PA, Kuns ML: Chronic infection of rodents by Machupo virus. Science 150:1618–1619, 1965.

154. Johnson KM, Kuns ML, Mackenzie RB, et al: Isolation of Machupo virus from wild rodent Calomys callosus. Am J Trop Med Hyg 15:103–106, 1966.

155. Calisher CH, Sweeney W, Mills JN, Beaty BJ: Natural history of Sin Nombre virus in western Colorado. Emerg Infect Dis 5:126–134, 1999.

156. Wells RM, Young J, Williams RJ, et al: Hantavirus transmission in the United States. Emerg Infect Dis 3:361–365, 1997.

157. McCormick JB, Webb PA, Krebs JW, et al: A prospective study of the epidemiology and ecology of Lassa fever. J Infect Dis 155:437–444, 1987.

158. Hjelle B, Torrez-Martinez N, Koster FT, et al: Epidemiologic linkage of rodent and human hantavirus genomic sequences in case investigations of hantavirus pulmonary syndrome. J Infect Dis 173:781–786, 1996.

159. Childs JE, Kaufmann AF, Peters CJ, Ehrenberg RL: Hantavirus infection—southwestern United States: Interim recommendations for risk reduction. Centers for Disease Control and Prevention. MMWR Morb Mortal Wkly Rep Recomm Rep 42(RR-11):1–13, 1993.

160. Belanov EF, Muntianov VP, Kriuk VD, et al: [Survival of Marburg virus infectivity on contaminated surfaces and in aerosols]. Vopr Virusol 41:32–34, 1996.

161. Simpson DI: Marburg agent disease: in monkeys. Trans R Soc Trop Med Hyg 63:303–309, 1969.

162. Lub MIu, Sergeev AN, P'iankov OV, et al: [Certain pathogenetic characteristics of a disease in monkeys in infected with the Marburg virus by an airborne route]. Vopr Virusol 40:158–161, 1995.

163. Kenyon RH, McKee KT Jr, Zack PM, et al: Aerosol infection of rhesus macaques with Junin virus. Intervirology 33:23–31, 1992.

164. Jaax NK, Davis KJ, Geisbert TJ, et al: Lethal experimental infection of rhesus monkeys with Ebola-Zaire (Mayinga) virus by the oral and conjunctival route of exposure. Arch Pathol Lab Med 120:140–155, 1996.

165. Banerjee K, Gupta NP, Goverdhan MK: Viral infections in laboratory personnel. Ind J Med Res 69:363–373, 1979.

166. Shu HL, Siegert R, Slenczka W: The pathogenesis and epidemiology of the "Marburg-virus" infection. Geriatr Med Mon 14:7–10, 1969.

167. Wells RM, Sosa Estani S, Yadon ZE, et al: An unusual hantavirus outbreak in southern Argentina: Person-to-person transmission? Hantavirus Pulmonary Syndrome Study Group for Patagonia. Emerg Infect Dis 3:171–174, 1997.

168. Carey DE, Kemp GE, White HA, et al: Lassa fever: Epidemiological aspects of the 1970 epidemic, Jos, Nigeria. Trans R Soc Trop Med Hyg 66:402–408, 1972.

169. White HA: Lassa fever: A study of 23 hospital cases. Trans R Soc Trop Med Hyg 66:390–401, 1972.

170. Peters CJ, Kuehne RW, Mercado RR, et al: Hemorrhagic fever in Cochabamba, Bolivia, 1971. Am J Epidemiol 99:425–433, 1974.

171. Outbreak of Ebola hemorrhagic fever Uganda, August 2000-January 2001. MMWR Morb Mortal Wkly Rep 50:73–77, 2001.

172. Dalgard DW, Hardy RJ, Pearson SL, et al: Combined simian hemorrhagic fever and Ebola virus infection in cynomolgus monkeys. Lab Anim Sci 42:152–157, 1992.

173. Roels TH, Bloom AS, Buffington J, et al: Ebola hemorrhagic fever, Kikwit, Democratic Republic of the Congo, 1995: Risk factors for patients without a reported exposure. J Infect Dis 179(Suppl 1):S92–97, 1999.

174. Slenczka WG: The Marburg virus outbreak of 1967 and subsequent episodes. Curr Top Microbiol Immunol 235:49–75, 1999.

175. Dowell SF, Mukunu R, Ksiazek TG, et al: Transmission of Ebola hemorrhagic fever: A study of risk factors in family members, Kikwit, Democratic Republic of the Congo, 1995. Commission de Lutte contre les Epidemies a Kikwit. J Infect Dis 179(Suppl 1):S87–91, 1999.

176. Buckley SM, Casals J, Downs WG: Isolation and antigenic characterization of Lassa virus. Nature 227:174, 1970.

177. Rodriguez LL, De Roo A, Guimard Y, et al: Persistence and genetic stability of Ebola virus during the outbreak in Kikwit, Democratic Republic of the Congo, 1995. J Infect Dis 179(Suppl 1):S170–176, 1999.

178. Lee HW: Hemorrhagic fever with renal syndrome in Korea. Rev Infect Dis 11(Suppl 4):S864–876, 1989.
179. Feldmann H, Volchkov VE, Volchkova VA, Klenk HD: The glycoproteins of Marburg and Ebola virus and their potential roles in pathogenesis. Arch Virol Suppl 15(Suppl):159–169, 1999.
180. Ryabchikova EI, Kolesnikova LV, Luchko SV: An analysis of features of pathogenesis in two animal models of Ebola virus infection. J Infect Dis 179(Suppl 1):S199–202, 1999.
181. Ambrosio AM, Enria DA, Maiztegui JI: Junin virus isolation from lympho-mononuclear cells of patients with Argentine hemorrhagic fever. Intervirology 25:97–102, 1986.
182. Gonzalez PH, Cossio PM, Arana R, et al: Lymphatic tissue in Argentine hemorrhagic fever: Pathologic features. Arch Pathol Lab Med 104:250–254, 1980.
183. Johnson KM, McCormick JB, Webb PA, et al: Clinical virology of Lassa fever in hospitalized patients. J Infect Dis 155:456–464, 1987.
184. McCormick JB, Walker DH, King IJ, et al: Lassa virus hepatitis: A study of fatal Lassa fever in humans. Am J Trop Med Hyg 35:401–407, 1986.
185. Kissling RE, Murphy FA, Henderson BE: Marburg virus. Ann N Y Acad Sci 174:932–945, 1970.
186. Peters CJ, Jahrling PB, Liu CT, et al: Experimental studies of arenaviral hemorrhagic fevers. Curr Top Microbiol Immunol 134:5–68, 1987.
187. McKay DG, Margaretten W: Disseminated intravascular coagulation in virus diseases. Arch Intern Med 120:129–152, 1967.
188. Chen JP, Cosgriff TM: Hemorrhagic fever virus-induced changes in hemostasis and vascular biology. Blood Coagul Fibrinolysis 11:461–483, 2000.
189. Cosgriff TM, Lewis RM: Mechanisms of disease in hemorrhagic fever with renal syndrome. Kidney Int 35(Suppl):S72–79, 1991.
190. Cosgriff TM: Mechanisms of disease in Hantavirus infection: Pathophysiology of hemorrhagic fever with renal syndrome. Rev Infect Dis 13:97–107, 1991.
191. Murphy FA, Simpson DI, Whitfield SG, et al: Marburg virus infection in monkeys: Ultrastructural studies. Lab Invest 24:279–291, 1971.
192. Baskerville A, Fisher-Hoch SP, Neild GH, Dowsett AB: Ultrastructural pathology of experimental Ebola haemorrhagic fever virus infection. J Pathol 147:199–209, 1985.
193. Guang MY, Liu GZ, Cosgriff TM: Hemorrhage in hemorrhagic fever with renal syndrome in China. Rev Infect Dis 11(Suppl 4):S884–890, 1989.
194. Fisher-Hoch SP, Mitchell SW, Sasso DR, et al: Physiological and immunologic disturbances associated with shock in a primate model of Lassa fever. J Infect Dis 155:465–474, 1987.
195. Ignatyev G, Steinkasserer A, Streltsova M, et al: Experimental study on the possibility of treatment of some hemorrhagic fevers. J Biotechnol 83:67–76, 2000.
196. Lee M, Kim BK, Kim S, et al: Coagulopathy in hemorrhagic fever with renal syndrome (Korean hemorrhagic fever). Rev Infect Dis 11(Suppl 4):S877–883, 1989.
197. Schnittler HJ, Mahner F, Drenckhahn D, et al: Replication of Marburg virus in human endothelial cells: A possible mechanism for the development of viral hemorrhagic disease. J Clin Invest 91:1301–1309, 1993.
198. Heller MV, Marta RF, Sturk A, et al: Early markers of blood coagulation and fibrinolysis activation in Argentine hemorrhagic fever. Thromb Haemost 73:368–373, 1995.
199. Cummins D, Molinas FC, Lerer G, et al: A plasma inhibitor of platelet aggregation in patients with Argentine hemorrhagic fever. Am J Trop Med Hyg 42:470–475, 1990.
200. Settergren B, Ahlm C, Alexeyev O, et al: Pathogenetic and clinical aspects of the renal involvement in hemorrhagic fever with renal syndrome. Ren Fail 19:1–14, 1997.
201. Collan Y, Mihatsch MJ, Lahdevirta J, et al: Nephropathia epidemica: Mild variant of hemorrhagic fever with renal syndrome. Kidney Int Suppl 35(Suppl):S62–71, 1991.
202. Penttinen K, Lahdevirta J, Kekomaki R, et al: Circulating immune complexes, immunoconglutinins, and rheumatoid factors in nephropathia epidemica. J Infect Dis 143:15–21, 1981.
203. Halstead SB: Antibody, macrophages, dengue virus infection, shock, and hemorrhage: A pathogenetic cascade. Rev Infect Dis 11(Suppl 4):S830–839, 1989.
204. Enria DA, Briggiler AM, Fernandez NJ, et al: Importance of dose of neutralising antibodies in treatment of Argentine haemorrhagic fever with immune plasma. Lancet 2:255–256, 1984.
205. Peters CJ, Liu CT, Anderson GW Jr, et al: Pathogenesis of viral hemorrhagic fevers: Rift Valley fever and Lassa fever contrasted. Rev Infect Dis 11(Suppl 4):S743–749, 1989.
206. Monath TP: Yellow fever: An update. Lancet Infect Dis 1:11–20, 2001.
207. Bwaka MA, Bonnet MJ, Calain P, et al: Ebola hemorrhagic fever in Kikwit, Democratic Republic of the Congo: clinical observations in 103 patients. J Infect Dis 179(Suppl 1):S1–7, 1999.
208. Frame JD, Baldwin JM Jr, Gocke DJ, Troup JM: Lassa fever, a new virus disease of man from West Africa: I. Clinical description and pathological findings. Am J Trop Med Hyg 19:670–676, 1970.
209. Formenty P, Hatz C, Le Guenno B, et al: Human infection due to Ebola virus, subtype Cote d'Ivoire: Clinical and biologic presentation. J Infect Dis 179(Suppl 1):S48–53, 1999.
210. Keane E, Gilles HM: Lassa fever in Panguma Hospital, Sierra Leone, 1973–6. BMJ 1:1399–1402, 1977.
211. Re-emergence of Bolivian hemorrhagic fever. Epidemiol Bull 15:4–5, 1994.
212. Harrison LH, Halsey NA, McKee KT Jr, et al: Clinical case definitions for Argentine hemorrhagic fever. Clin Infect Dis 28:1091–1094, 1999.
213. Laughlin LW, Meegan JM, Strausbaugh LJ, et al: Epidemic Rift Valley fever in Egypt: Observations of the spectrum of human illness. Trans R Soc Trop Med Hyg 73:630–633, 1979.
214. McCormick JB, King IJ, Webb PA, et al: A case-control study of the clinical diagnosis and course of Lassa fever. J Infect Dis 155:445–455, 1987.
215. Kuming BS, Kokoris N: Uveal involvement in Marburg virus disease. Br J Ophthalmol 61:265–266, 1977.
216. Muyembe-Tamfum JJ, Kipasa M, Kiyungu C, Colebunders R: Ebola outbreak in Kikwit, Democratic Republic of the Congo: Discovery and control measures. J Infect Dis 179(Suppl 1):S259–262, 1999.
217. Outbreak of acute illness—southwestern United States, 1993. MMWR Morb Mortal Wkly Rep 42:421–424, 1993.
218. Moolenaar RL, Breiman RF, Peters CJ: Hantavirus pulmonary syndrome. Semin Respir Infect 12:31–39, 1997.
219. McCaughey C, Hart CA: Hantaviruses. J Med Microbiol 49:587–599, 2000.
220. Sheedy JA, Froeb HF, Batson HA, et al: The clinical course of epidemic hemorrhagic fever. Am J Med 16:619–628, 1954.
221. Bruno P, Hassell LH, Brown J, et al: The protean manifestations of hemorrhagic fever with renal syndrome: A retrospective review of 26 cases from Korea. Ann Intern Med 113:385–391, 1990.
222. Giles RB, Sheedy JA, Ekman CN, et al: The sequelae of epidemic hemorrhagic fever: With a note on causes of death. Am J Med 16:629–638, 1954.
223. Antoniadis A, LeDuc JW, Acritidis N, et al: Hemorrhagic fever with renal syndrome in Greece: Clinical and laboratory characteristics. Rev Infect Dis 11(Suppl 4):S891–896, 1989.
224. Centers for Disease Control (CDC): Management of patients with suspected viral hemorrhagic fever. MMWR Morb Mortal Wkly Rep 37(S-3):1–16, 1988.
225. Ksiazek TG, Rollin PE, Jahrling PB, et al: Enzyme immunosorbent assay for Ebola virus antigens in tissues of infected primates. J Clin Microbiol 30:947–950, 1992.
226. Trappier SG, Conaty AL, Farrar BB, et al: Evaluation of the polymerase chain reaction for diagnosis of Lassa virus infection. Am J Trop Med Hyg 49:214–221, 1993.
227. Yao ZO, Yang WS, Zhang WB, Bai XF: The distribution and duration of hantaan virus in the body fluids of patients with hemorrhagic fever with renal syndrome. J Infect Dis 160:218–224, 1989.
228. Jenison S, Yamada T, Morris C, et al: Characterization of human antibody responses to four corners hantavirus infections among patients with hantavirus pulmonary syndrome. J Virol 68:3000–3006, 1994.
229. Saijo M, Niikura M, Morikawa S, et al: Enzyme-linked immunosorbent assays for detection of antibodies to Ebola and Marburg viruses using recombinant nucleoproteins. J Clin Microbiol 39:1–7, 2001.
230. Franz DR, Jahrling PB, Friedlander AM, et al: Clinical recognition and management of patients exposed to biological warfare agents. JAMA 278:399–411, 1997.
231. Corrigan JJ Jr, Jordan CM: Heparin therapy in septicemia with disseminated intravascular coagulation. N Engl J Med 283:778–782, 1970.
232. Katz J, Lurie A, Kaplan B: Haemolytic-uraemic syndrome and heparin therapy. Lancet 2:700, 1969.

233. Monath TP, Mertens PE, Patton R, et al: A hospital epidemic of Lassa fever in Zorzor, Liberia, March-April 1972. Am J Trop Med Hyg 22:773–779, 1973.

234. van de Wal BW, Joubert JR, van Eeden PJ, King JB: A nosocomial outbreak of Crimean-Congo haemorrhagic fever at Tygerberg Hospital: Part IV. Preventive and prophylactic measures. S Afr Med J 68:729–732, 1985.

235. Kerstiens B, Matthys F: Interventions to control virus transmission during an outbreak of Ebola hemorrhagic fever: Experience from Kikwit, Democratic Republic of the Congo, 1995. J Infect Dis 179(Suppl 1):S263–267, 1999.

236. Update: Management of patients with suspected viral hemorrhagic fever—United States. MMWR Morb Mortal Wkly Rep 44:475–479, 1995.

237. McKee KT Jr, Huggins JW, Trahan CJ, Mahlandt BG: Ribavirin prophylaxis and therapy for experimental argentine hemorrhagic fever. Antimicrob Agents Chemother 32:1304–1309, 1988.

238. Jahrling PB, Peters CJ: Passive antibody therapy of Lassa fever in cynomolgus monkeys: Importance of neutralizing antibody and Lassa virus strain. Infect Immun 44:528–533, 1984.

239. Jahrling PB, Hesse RA, Eddy GA, et al: Lassa virus infection of rhesus monkeys: Pathogenesis and treatment with ribavirin. J Infect Dis 141:580–589, 1980.

240. Canonico PG, Kende M, Luscri BJ, Huggins JW: In-vivo activity of antivirals against exotic RNA viral infections. J Antimicrob Chemother 14(Suppl A):27–41, 1984.

241. Huggins JW, Hsiang CM, Cosgriff TM, et al: Prospective, double-blind, concurrent, placebo-controlled clinical trial of intravenous ribavirin therapy of hemorrhagic fever with renal syndrome. J Infect Dis 164:1119–1127, 1991.

242. Huggins JW: Prospects for treatment of viral hemorrhagic fevers with ribavirin, a broad-spectrum antiviral drug. Rev Infect Dis 11(Suppl 4):S750–761, 1989.

243. Kilgore PE, Ksiazek TG, Rollin PE, et al: Treatment of Bolivian hemorrhagic fever with intravenous ribavirin. Clin Infect Dis 24:718–722, 1997.

244. Enria DA, Maiztegui JI: Antiviral treatment of Argentine hemorrhagic fever. Antiviral Res 23:23–31, 1994.

245. McCormick JB, King IJ, Webb PA, et al: Lassa fever: Effective therapy with ribavirin. N Engl J Med 314:20–26, 1986.

246. Hallin GW, Simpson SQ, Crowell RE, et al: Cardiopulmonary manifestations of hantavirus pulmonary syndrome. Crit Care Med 24:252–258, 1996.

247. Murphy ME, Kariwa H, Mizutani T, et al: Characterization of in vitro and in vivo antiviral activity of lactoferrin and ribavirin upon hantavirus. J Vet Med Sci 63:637–645, 2001.

248. Fisher-Hoch SP, Khan JA, Rehman S, et al: Crimean Congo-haemorrhagic fever treated with oral ribavirin. Lancet 346:472–475, 1995.

249. Chapman LE, Mertz GJ, Peters CJ, et al: Intravenous ribavirin for hantavirus pulmonary syndrome: Safety and tolerance during 1 year of open-label experience. Ribavirin Study Group. Antivir Ther 4:211–219, 1999.

250. Kenyon RH, Canonico PG, Green DE, Peters CJ: Effect of ribavirin and tributylribavirin on argentine hemorrhagic fever (Junin virus) in guinea pigs. Antimicrob Agents Chemother 29:521–523, 1986.

251. Jahrling PB, Geisbert TW, Geisbert JB, et al: Evaluation of immune globulin and recombinant interferon-alpha2b for treatment of experimental Ebola virus infections. J Infect Dis 179(Suppl 1):S224–234, 1999.

252. Emond RT, Evans B, Bowen ET, Lloyd G: A case of Ebola virus infection. BMJ 2:541–544, 1977.

253. Morrill JC, Jennings GB, Cosgriff TM, et al: Prevention of Rift Valley fever in rhesus monkeys with interferon-alpha. Rev Infect Dis 11(Suppl 4):S815–825, 1989.

254. Peters CJ, Jones D, Trotter R, et al: Experimental Rift Valley fever in rhesus macaques. Arch Virol 99:31–44, 1988.

255. Mupapa K, Massamba M, Kibadi K, et al: Treatment of Ebola hemorrhagic fever with blood transfusions from convalescent patients. International Scientific and Technical Committee. J Infect Dis 179(Suppl 1):S18–23, 1999.

256. Sadek RF, Khan AS, Stevens G, et al: Ebola hemorrhagic fever, Democratic Republic of the Congo, 1995: Determinants of survival. J Infect Dis 179(Suppl 1):S24–27, 1999.

257. Maiztegui JI, Fernandez NJ, de Damilano AJ: Efficacy of immune plasma in treatment of Argentine haemorrhagic fever and association between treatment and a late neurological syndrome. Lancet 2:1216–1217, 1979.

258. Monath TP, Maher M, Casals J, et al: Lassa fever in the Eastern Province of Sierra Leone, 1970–1972: II. Clinical observations and virological studies on selected hospital cases. Am J Trop Med Hyg 23:1140–1149, 1974.

259. Leifer E, Gocke DJ, Bourne H: Lassa fever, a new virus disease of man from West Africa: II. Report of a laboratory-acquired infection treated with plasma from a person recently recovered from the disease. Am J Trop Med Hyg 19:677–679, 1970.

260. Maruyama T, Parren PW, Sanchez A, et al: Recombinant human monoclonal antibodies to Ebola virus. J Infect Dis 179(Suppl 1):S235–239, 1999.

261. Pushko P, Geisbert J, Parker M, et al: Individual and bivalent vaccines based on alphavirus replicons protect guinea pigs against infection with Lassa and Ebola viruses. J Virol 75:11677–11685, 2001.

262. Hevey M, Negley D, VanderZanden L, et al: Marburg virus vaccines: Comparing classical and new approaches. Vaccine 20:586–593, 2001.

CHAPTER **135**

Immunotherapy

Steven A. Seifert

Immunotherapy of drug and chemical toxicity and toxin envenomations involves the administration of specific immunoglobulin antibodies or antibody fragments (IgG, Fab, F(ab′)$_2$, or sFv). Binding of the antibody to the target molecules (antigens of toxicant, toxin, or extracellular or intracellular mediators of injury)[1] is intended to result in partial or complete neutralization of the toxic effect of the target, a concentration gradient of free target molecules encouraging efflux into the vascular compartment, and ultimate elimination of the antibody/target complex by renal or reticuloendothelial system routes.[2–4]

Specific therapeutic antibodies have been developed for cardiac glycosides,[5–9] colchicine,[10,11] and phencyclidine[12–14]; paraquat[15–17]; tricyclic antidepressants[18–22]; amantadine[23,24]; botulinum toxin[25–27]; verapamil[28]; and snake,[29–34] scorpion,[35–39] spider,[40–42] and bee venoms.[43,44] In the United States, currently approved therapeutic immunoglobulins are available for Crotalinae snake envenomations (antivenin [Crotalidae] polyvalent, an equine IgG, and Crotalidae polyvalent immune Fab, an ovine Fab), coral snake envenomations (*Micrurus fulvius* antivenom, an equine IgG), cardiac glycosides (Digibind, an ovine Fab), scorpion envenomations (*Centruroides sculpturatus* antivenom, a caprine IgG available in Arizona only), and black widow spider envenomations (*Latrodectus mactans* antivenom, an equine IgG). In addition, an experimental ovine Fab to tricyclic antidepressants has reached human clinical trials.[22] Antivenoms to nonnative venomous animals often are kept at zoos under U.S. Food and Drug Administration (FDA) Investigational New Drug license.[45]

This approach offers the promise of a family of therapeutic immunoglobulins with the ability to bind, neutralize, and eliminate molecules that produce toxic effects without having to devise specific, metabolically based antidotal therapies. The use of heterologous and homologous proteins carries certain risks, however, and the pharmacokinetics and pharmacodynamics of these agents pose significant challenges in the development and clinical application of these antidotal agents.

HISTORY

One of the first immunoglobulin antivenoms in clinical practice was anti-Crotalidae polyvalent (ACP), an equine IgG, in widespread use since 1954. Based on decades of compelling case experience and experimental data, ACP is effective at stopping the progression of local effects and reversing the systemic effects of Crotalinae envenomations. The occurrences of sometimes severe immediate and delayed hypersensitivity reactions to heterologous whole IgG[37,46,47] have led to a search for safer alternatives, however. In the 1970s and 1980s, it was shown that F(ab′)$_2$ and Fab fragments (Fig. 135-1) could be produced by enzymatic treatment of IgG, resulting in immunoglobulin fragments that retained binding specificity.[48–50] Because of the removal of the Fc chain and immunoglobulin and other non–target-specific proteins by affinity purification and other techniques,[51] F(ab′)$_2$ and Fab fragments were shown generally to have fewer immediate and delayed hypersensitivity reactions than whole IgG,[32,52–55] and it was shown that ovine-derived sera were less likely to result in immediate hypersensitivity reactions than equine-derived sera.[32,33,54,56,57] F(ab′)$_2$ and Fab antivenoms from a variety of source animals have been developed to venoms from snakes, scorpions, and spiders in many countries. Target-specific, single-chain Fv fragments (sFv) (see Fig. 135-1) have been developed to a variety of agents and have been produced in a variety of host cell lines.[6,16,58–60]

PROPERTIES

Chemical

IgG is one of a family of structurally related antibodies. In response to an immunologically recognizable antigen, ultimately an antigen-specific IgG is produced. IgG has a molecular weight of approximately 150,000 d and comprises an Fc chain of amino acids of about 50,000 d. The Fc chain

1473

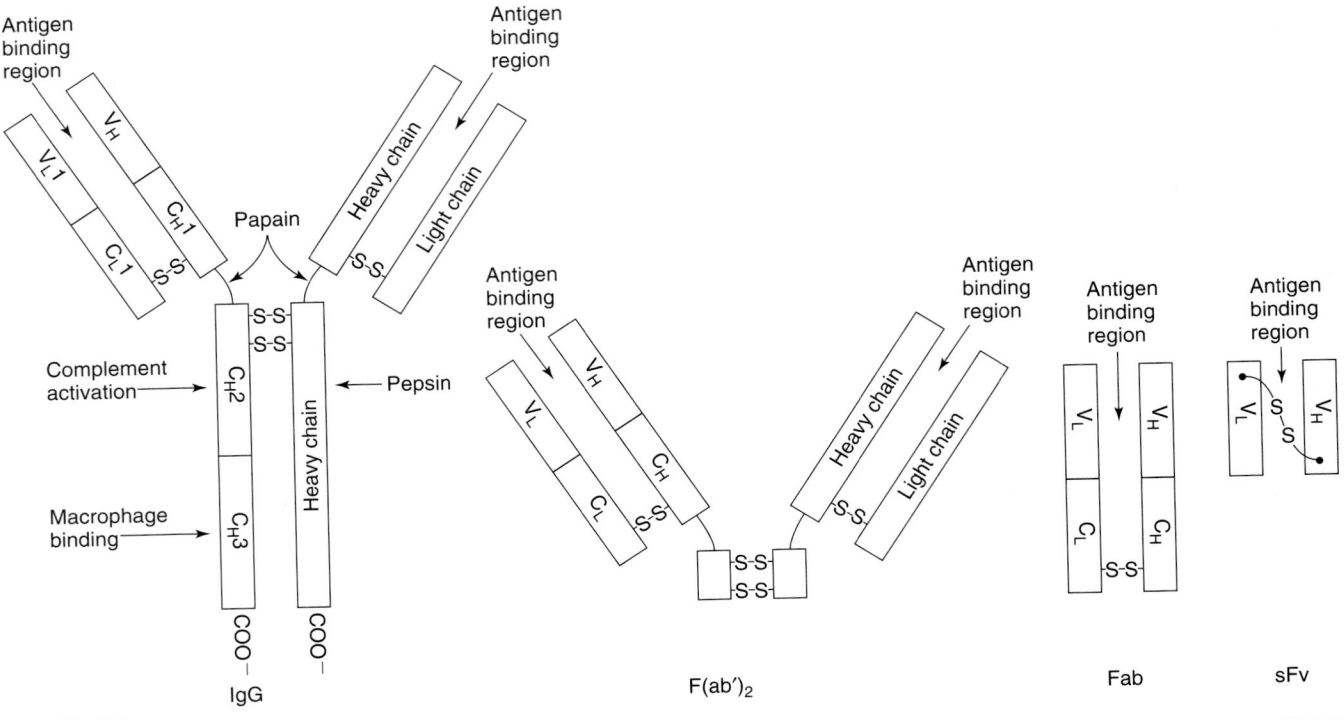

FIGURE 135-1

Chemical structure of immunoglobulin.

produces many effector functions, which may be activated by conformational changes induced by immunoglobulin/antigen binding.[61,62] Two antigen-binding chains attach to the Fc chain at a hinge region (see Fig. 135-1).[47,50] The amino acid sequences in the Fc chain are species specific, and as such, whole IgG is relatively immunogenic. Depending on the source animal and other factors, it may be complement fixing in humans.[61,63,64]

IgG may be cleaved between the Fc chain and the hinge region, and the Fc component may be eliminated, resulting in a fragment containing both antigen-binding arms, $F(ab')_2$. This fragment is about 100,000 d and retains excellent antigen-binding specificity. The $F(ab')_2$ fragment may be cleaved further at the hinge, resulting in two Fab fragments of about 50,000 d each, also retaining antigen-binding specificity.[31,50] Fab itself comprises three portions, a constant proximal portion and two variable distal chains covalently linked; the conformational relationships of the portions are responsible for the binding specificity. Elimination of the proximal portion of the Fab results in a single variable-chain Fv fragment of about 25,000 d, which contains the target-specific binding region. Currently, this is the smallest immunoglobulin fragment that retains sufficient antigen-binding specificity for clinical purposes.[6,65] In addition, there are associated oligosaccharide moieties that contribute to the conformational structure and binding of immunoglobulins and may vary based on the cell type in which the immunoglobulin is produced, on the culture methods, and on nutrient depletion states; these moieties may be responsible for variability not predicted from studies of protein or DNA sequences alone.[62]

Physical

In general, immunoglobulins are concentrated or otherwise purified from the source animal's serum or from a cell line culture. Antivenin polyvalent Crotalidae, *Micrurus* antivenin, CroFab, Digibind, and others are lyophilized, resulting in an off-white pellet that retains binding specificity for years. Heat may result in denaturation, as do shear forces and polymerization from shaking, foaming, and bubbling that may occur in the process of reconstitution.[66,67]

PHARMACOKINETICS

Immunoglobulin kinetics is source, recipient, and target dependent, making extrapolation from animal studies difficult and giving each therapeutic immunoglobulin a relatively unique kinetic and dynamic profile. Kinetics is stable over a wide dose range but may be affected by factors such as source animal, valence (monovalent, mixed monovalent, polyvalent), route of administration, ionic charge, nonspecific binding, analytic methods, and study design. Individuals display varying kinetics based on renal function and other physiologic parameters. Interaction with the target molecule also can alter the kinetics of the immunoglobulin.

Immunoglobulin kinetics generally fits a two-compartment model with a biexponential curve on a log-linear plot.[68] Generally, the larger the immunoglobulin molecule, the smaller the volume of distribution and the longer the half-life. IgG is distributed to a volume roughly equivalent to the vascular space (approximately 90 mL/kg) and is eliminated predominantly by the reticuloendothelial system, with a relatively long

Ig Type	Valence	Target	Source	Recipient	Wt (kg)	Route	Dose	Vdss (Vdβ)	$T_{1/2\alpha}$ (h)	$T_{1/2\beta}$ (h)	Clearance (mL/min)	Special Notes
IgG₁	Monovalent	Cytomegalovirus	Human	Human		IV	5/10/20/40/80 mg	79.7 mL/kg	31	581	0.0017	16 patients. No antiidiotypic antibody for up to 57 days[68]
IgG	Polyvalent	Sepsis	Human	Human	2.8	IV	250/500/1000 mg/kg	42.1 mL/kg		581	0.0059	15 neonates with sepsis[73]
IgG	Polyvalent	None	Human	Human		IV	400 mg/kg			619.2		8 patients with primary immunodeficiency[74]
IgG	Monovalent	rh-D	Human	Human		IV				507.2		3 patients[75]
IgG	Monovalent	anti-Rh	Human	Human		IM/SC	18 mg			528		20 patients. Absorption rate (%/day) = 0.22 (SC); 0.43 (IM)[76]
IgG	Polyvalent	Crotalus, Agkistrodon	Horse	Human		IV	100 mL			158.4		Single patient with Crotalus atrox envenomation[77]
IgG	Monovalent	C. rhodostoma	Horse	Human	50	IV	1081 μL/kg	90 mL/kg	0.46	82	0.525	7 patients; unpurified horse serum[69]
IgG	Monovalent	C. rhodostoma	Goat	Human	51.5	IV	216 μL/kg	92.5 mL/kg	1.96	45.5	1.118	6 patients. Processing to minimize aggregate formation[69]
IgG	Monovalent	rCD4	Hamster	Human	70	IV	1-300 μg/kg	70 mL/kg			57	26 patients[78]
IgG	Monovalent	CD4	Hamster	Human	82	IV	1000 μg/kg	76.5 mL/kg			2.62	2 patients[78]
IgG	Monovalent	rhGH	Hamster	Human	73.7	IV	20 μg/kg	56.3 mL/kg			152.4	18 patients[78]
IgG	Monovalent	rt-PA	Hamster	Human	76	IV	250–500 μg/mL	105.9 mL/kg			620	12 patients[78]
IgG	Monovalent	Synthetic Relaxan	Hamster	Human	62.4	IV	10 μg/kg	278 mL/kg			175	25 patients[78]
F(ab')₂	Monovalent	C. rhodostoma	Horse	Human	46	IV	1087 μL/kg	233 mL/kg	0.3	96	1.279	5 patients; pepsin-digested serum[69]
F(ab')₂	Polyvalent	Echis	Horse	Human		IV				18		17 patients with Echis ocellatus envenomation[54]
F(ab')₂	Polyvalent	MOv18/CD3	Mouse	Human		IV			1	18.1		5 patients with ovarian cancer; HAMA seen as early as 1 wk[79]

continued

Human Pharmacokinetic Parameters of Specific IgG, F(ab')₂, and Fab Antibodies* *continued*

Ig Type	Valence	Target	Source	Recipient	Wt (kg)	Route	Dose	Vdss (Vdβ)	$T_{1/2\alpha}$ (h)	$T_{1/2\beta}$ (h)	Clearance (mL/min)	Special Notes
Fab	Polyvalent	*Crotalus, Agkistrodon*	Sheep	Human	70	IV	3000–6000 mg	110 mL/kg	2.7	18	5.7	4 patients with *Crotalus* snakebite[80]
Fab	Monovalent	Digoxin	Sheep	Human		IV	800 mg	10.8 L		12.1	23.4	1 patient with digoxin toxicity[81]
Fab	Monovalent	*Echis ocellatus*	Sheep	Human		IV					4.3	22 patients with *Echis ocellatus* envenomation[54]
Fab	Monovalent	Digoxin	Sheep	Human		IV		430 mL/kg (Vdβ)	14	0.324 mL/kg/min		7 patients with toxicity and normal renal function—CrCl = 103 mL/min[72]
Fab	Monovalent	Digoxin	Sheep	Human		IV		369 mL/kg (Vdβ)	9.3	0.389 mL/kg/min		4 patients with digoxin toxicity and impaired renal function—CrCl = 38 mL/min[72]
Fab	Monovalent	Digoxin	Sheep	Human	44	IV	121 mg	669 mL/kg (Vdβ)		23.9	7.1	Treatment of digoxin toxicity in patient with serum creatinine = 1.4 mg/dL[82]
Fab	Monovalent	Digoxin	Sheep	Human	70	IV	80 mg	2751 mL/kg (Vdβ)		56.3	6.3	Treatment of digoxin toxicity in patient with serum creatinine = 1.8 mg/dL[82]
Fab	Monovalent	Digoxin	Sheep	Human	61	IV	160 mg	95 mL/kg (Vdβ)		71.8	2.6	Treatment of digoxin toxicity in patient with serum creatinine = 4 mg/dL[82]
Fab	Monovalent	Digoxin	Sheep	Human	47	IV	120 mg	163 mL/kg (Vdβ)		45.6	2.3	Treatment of digoxin toxicity in patient on hemodialysis[82]
Fab	Monovalent	Digoxin	Sheep	Human		IV			290 mL/kg	82	0.049	4 patients with digoxin toxicity, ESRD, and hemodialysis[5]
Fab	Monovalent	Digoxin	Sheep	Human		IV	80 mg	36.2 L	49.9	138.6	3.02	1 patient with digoxin toxicity, ESRD (CrCl = 8 mL/min), and peritoneal dialysis[83]

*Significant variability in kinetic parameters can be seen within and between classes depending on source animal, target antigen, renal function, immunoglobulin structure, route, and other factors.

CrCl, creatinine clearance; ESRD, end-stage renal disease; HAMA, human antimurine antibody; IM, intramuscular; IV, intravenous; SC, subcutaneous.

half-life (approximately 60 to 194 hours).[69,70] F(ab')$_2$, Fab, and sFv are distributed to volumes closer to the extracellular volume and are eliminated more rapidly: F(ab')$_2$, 18 to 96 hours; Fab, 15 to 25 hours; sFv, 1.5 hours. As their size decreases, proportionate renal elimination increases.[69–71] Elimination ultimately depends on the size and charge of the unbound immunoglobulin and immunoglobulin/target molecule complex, affecting renal or reticuloendothelial system clearance or both.[5,71,72] Interaction between the target molecule and immunoglobulin may affect the target molecule's kinetics, resulting in altered tissue and vascular compartment concentrations.[12,15,23]

PHARMACODYNAMICS

Clinical efficacy depends on many factors. In general, the immunoglobulin locates and binds to its target and neutralizes its physiologic interaction. Target specificity and binding affinities of immunoglobulins are high (10^8 to 10^{10} M^{-1})[84,85] and usually greater than tissue affinities for most drugs. Specific IgG, F(ab')$_2$, Fab, and sFv with similar target specificity and affinity or given in equivalent neutralizing doses should display similar acute neutralization of a target molecule that is localized in the central circulation or must pass through the central circulation to exert its toxicity,[86,87] excluding half-life differences. Theoretically, compared with IgG, the progressively smaller sizes and larger volumes of distribution of F(ab')$_2$, Fab, and sFv should allow progressively increasing tissue penetration and target binding and neutralization there. Mean tissue residence time still may be greater, however, for IgG than for smaller immunoglobulin fragments, because its long half-life[71] and destructive tissue effects, as in the case of snake envenomation, may limit immunoglobulin access to the site, allowing venom there to remain unneutralized,[80,88,89] or may result in equal tissue accumulation of immunoglobulins regardless of size and similar neutralization profiles.[64,90,91] Because small-molecular-weight toxins and toxicants may assume the kinetic profiles of their specific antibodies and are redistributed to the vascular compartment or other tissues, if there is only partial neutralization of the target molecules or if immunoglobulin/target dissociation occurs, it may result in increased tissue toxin/toxicant concentrations, variable efficacy, and potentially increased toxicity.[12,15,17,23,24]

Disparity may exist between the half-life of the target and the target-specific immunoglobulin, resulting in clearance of unbound immunoglobulin while there still is a body depot of unneutralized target.[80,88,89] This situation may result in recurrence of toxicities after most of the unbound immunoglobulin has been eliminated.[57,92] Degradation of the immunoglobulin may occur, with some F(ab')$_2$ having instability at the hinge region. Conversion of a F(ab')$_2$ to a Fab alters distribution and elimination kinetics, although immunoglobulins seem to retain the ability to bind their targets as long as they are in circulation.[5] Manipulation of cross-linking of sulfhydryl bonds between cysteine residues can increase resistance to degradation of F(ab')$_2$.[93] Theoretically, the target/immunoglobulin complex may dissociate if it remains in circulation for prolonged periods, although there has been no evidence of this in ovine Fab–treated digoxin toxicity in patients with renal failure.[5] Antiidiotypic antibodies (antibodies the patient makes to the target-specific immunoglobulin), which develop one to several weeks after exposure, may decrease therapeutic immunoglobulin efficacy in subsequent treatments.[52,94] Because IgG and F(ab')$_2$ antibodies bind to their targets in a 1:2 molar ratio and Fab and sFv bind in a 1:1 ratio, the quantity of target molecules in certain overdoses (e.g., tricyclic antidepressants) may exceed the amount of immunoglobulin that can be given safely or practicably. Clinical efficacy in these circumstances still may be shown if the life-threatening toxicities are abated by partial neutralization of toxin body burdens.[22,34]

In the United States, decades of experience have shown clinical efficacy for immunoglobulin treatment of snake (*Crotalus* and *Micrurus*), scorpion (*Centruroides*), and spider (*Latrodectus*) envenomations and cardiac glycosides. Because of similarities of venom components across genera and species, specific antibodies raised to one venomous species often show clinical efficacy against others.[40,47,95] Similarly, antidigoxin antibodies show efficacy against other plant and animal cardiac glycosides.[7–9] Clinical efficacy of this immunotherapy in humans has yet to be shown convincingly for bee envenomation, colchicine, tricyclic antidepressants, phencyclidine, paraquat, and diquat. Future developments include possibly complexing immunoglobulin fragments with molecules that alter their kinetics and dynamics[96,97] and ultimately the production of "humanized" immunoglobulins by recombinant DNA technology, allowing the creation and selection of the appropriate immunoglobulin for a given toxicologic setting.[61,62,98]

SPECIAL POPULATIONS

Neonatal and Pediatric Patients

Generally the dose of immunoglobulin is related to the quantity of target molecules to be neutralized. Children usually receive more immunoglobulin per body weight than adults, especially for antivenoms.[99] The dose adjustment for body size generally made for pharmaceuticals is not appropriate for immunotherapeutic agents. Attention also should be paid to fluid volumes. Snake antivenom should be reconstituted in a fluid volume of 20 mL/kg total to be infused ($\leq$250 mL).[45]

Elderly Patients

Unbound sFv and Fab, some F(ab')$_2$, and immunoglobulin/target complexes of less than 70,000 d are eliminated in part by renal excretion.[2,71,100] Impaired renal function results in prolonged half-lives of unbound immunoglobulin and immunoglobulin/target complexes.[5,82,83] This situation may prevent or delay recurrence of toxicity by delaying the elimination of unbound immunoglobulin when there is a large disparity between its half-life and that of the target.

Pregnant Patients

Immunoglobulins generally have not been tested in pregnant patients. F(ab')$_2$ and smaller fragments may cross the placental barrier. The effects of the immunoglobulin and immunoglobulin/target complex on the developing fetus are unknown.

All of the FDA-approved immunoglobulin antibodies are FDA pregnancy category C, which is defined as follows: "Studies have shown that the drug exerts animal teratogenic or embryocidal effects, but there are no controlled studies in women, or no studies are available in either animals or women."[101] These immunoglobulin antibodies include antivenin (Crotalidae) polyvalent (equine; Wyeth-Ayerst, Philadelphia, PA), antivenin *Latrodectus mactans* (equine; Merck & Co, West Point, PA), CroFab (ovine; Protherics, London, UK), and *M. fulvius* antivenin (equine; Wyeth-Ayerst).

CONTRAINDICATIONS

Contraindications to the use of therapeutic immunoglobulins include a perceived risk-to-benefit ratio that does not favor treatment. This determination must be made on a case-by-case basis. Because type I (anaphylactic) reactions are common, particularly with whole immunoglobulin preparations, and may be fatal,[47,102–104] indications and contraindications for use have varied.[33] A *Crotalinae* envenomation of moderate or greater severity generally has been accepted as an indication for antivenom,[105] but because of the rapidity of onset of respiratory paralysis with Eastern coral snake envenomations, it has been recommended that antivenom be given before signs and symptoms appear.[47,106] Special caution should be used when administering immunoglobulin treatment to patients with a history of prior immediate hypersensitivity reactions to that antivenom or to the serum of the source animal, although such patients have been treated successfully with antivenom.[107–109]

PRECAUTIONS

Type I hypersensitivity reactions are immediately occurring reactions to an antigenic stimulus, usually because specific immunoglobulins to that antigen were produced during a previous exposure. Anaphylactic reactions occur when the antigen (in this case, heterologous immunoglobulin) binds to tissue-bonded, basophil-bonded, or mast cell–bonded, specific IgE. An explosive degranulation of mast cells occurs with release of histamine and other vasoactive amines and other factors producing symptoms, such as bronchiolar smooth muscle contraction and bronchospasm, increased capillary permeability, angioedema including laryngeal edema, urticaria, hypotension, and cardiovascular collapse; this degranulation may be fatal.[102,104] Anaphylactoid reactions are type I hypersensitivity reactions that are not IgE mediated and may occur on first exposure to an antigen. They are thought to result from activation of complement and direct histamine and other vasoactive amine release. The clinical picture is similar to that of IgE-mediated reactions but does not usually result in the explosive degranulation of mast cells and less commonly produces severe bronchospasm, angioedema, or hypotension. Often these anaphylactoid reactions are related to the rate of administration of the antivenom.

Skin tests are recommended by the manufacturers of ACP, *Micrurus*, and *Latrodectus* antivenoms as a way to test for the patient's risk of developing a type I hypersensitivity

reaction. The sensitivity and specificity of skin tests to predict subsequent hypersensitivity reactions are poor,[33,47] however, and the main advantage to skin testing seems to be the medicolegal position of having followed the manufacturer's recommendations. Skin testing should be performed only when the decision has been made to use an antivenom, to avoid potentially needlessly sensitizing someone to the source animal's serum, and should not delay administration of antivenom in life-threatening situations.[47] It has been recommended that a positive result be used as an indication for pretreatment with H₁- and H₂-receptor blockers.[47] In general, smaller immunoglobulin fragments have fewer and milder reports of type I reactions. Reports of the incidence of type I reactions to various IgGs have ranged from 8% to 87% and to various Fab and F(ab')₂ immunoglobulins from 6.3% to 20%.[47,110] In one large study, type I reactions to ACP in Crotalinae envenomations were reported in 23% of cases, with half of them severe reactions.[102] In contrast, type I reactions to CroFab, a Crotalinae ovine Fab, were reported in 19% of cases, with two thirds of them mild, one third moderate, and none severe.[57] Because venom and other toxins and toxicants are themselves antigens, patients may have a type I hypersensitivity reaction to the offending agents that, depending on the timing of administration, may be confused with a reaction to a therapeutic immunoglobulin.[111]

Type III (delayed) hypersensitivity reactions (serum sickness) typically may occur 1 day to 3 weeks after treatment with an immunoglobulin. Type III reactions result from the formation of circulating immunoglobulin/target complexes, usually in the context of antigen excess and associated with complement activation.[112] These complexes are deposited in endothelial vessels, where they produce widespread vascular injury and complement activation. Clinical symptoms are persistent urticaria, arthralgias, myalgias, angioedema, swollen lymph nodes, vomiting, and fever.[47,102] Type III reactions typically are seen much more frequently and are more severe with IgG snake antivenoms than with other antivenoms[47]; this is thought to reflect the higher doses associated with treatment of snakebites and the relatively greater immunogenic reactivity of whole IgG preparations, which may predispose to vascular injury. The incidence of type III reactions after equine IgG has been reported to be 15% to 86% with ACP[33,47] and 61% with *Centruroides* antivenom.[37] CroFab had an incidence of type III reactions of 6% after patients exposed to a batch contaminated with high levels of Fc were excluded.[57]

RECURRENCE PHENOMENA

A phenomenon of recurrent toxicity (recurrence of toxicity after initial reversal or stabilization) has been reported in patients treated with therapeutic immunoglobulins and is believed to be the result of disparities in the pharmacokinetics and pharmacodynamics between the target and its specific immunoglobulin.[89] In the treatment of Crotalinae envenomations with a Fab antivenom, local symptoms may recur in 50% of patients, and coagulopathy (abnormal platelet counts, fibrinogen, prothrombin time, and activated thromboplastin time) may recur in 69% of patients after initial control with the antivenom.[57,113] The mechanisms of recurrence are believed to be a kinetic disparity between the half-life of venom components and unbound immunoglobulin and a dynamic disparity in which not all venom is neutralized initially. This situation allows local injury to recur when protective serum levels are lost at the interface between normal tissue and the local venom depot and likewise allows coagulopathy to recur when unneutralized venom from a depot reenters the vascular compartment after protective Fab concentrations have been lost.[57] Coagulopathy recurrence with IgG antivenom, usually mild and subclinical but occasionally severe, also has been reported and is likely due to the same mechanism.[92,113,114] Local recurrence with Fab antivenom, consistent with the time course of local injury,[115] typically occurs within the first 24 hours.[57,115] Because coagulopathy recurrence likely results from recurrence of venom antigenemia from a depot of unneutralized venom, it is similar in kind and degree to the presenting coagulopathy, is typically seen 2 to 4 days after treatment, and may persist for more than 2 weeks.[57,88,114]

A similar recurrence phenomenon has been reported with digoxin toxicity treated with an ovine Fab. Recurrence of free digoxin concentrations usually occurs 12 to 24 hours after initial treatment. In patients with renal failure, this recurrence may be delayed 12 to 130 hours.[5] Other kinetic and dynamic mismatches between targets and target-specific immunoglobulins may result in decreased therapeutic benefit or other adverse effects.

TREATMENT OF ADVERSE EFFECTS

Anaphylactic and anaphylactoid reactions should be treated in the standard manner. If an immunoglobulin is being given intravenously and is suspected of being the cause of the reaction, the infusion should be stopped. Epinephrine, H_1- and H_2-blockers, and corticosteroids should be given as indicated. The treatment of anaphylaxis is discussed in detail in Chapter 31. The decision to restart the infusion in severe reactions should be made on the basis of the risk-to-benefit ratio to the patient. If the infusion is restarted, consideration should be given to diluting the infusion further and restarting it slowly. It is uncertain, however, whether the incidence of severe type I reactions can be reduced by slower infusion.[45,116] Simultaneous infusion of antivenom along with intravenous epinephrine may be instituted and maintained cautiously if the patient is showing signs of an anaphylactic reaction, but it still is deemed clinically essential that the patient receive the antivenom.[107,108,111,117]

Late hypersensitivity reactions (serum sickness) usually produce pruritic and sometimes painful urticaria or purpuric skin rashes. These reactions may be treated with H_1- and H_2-blockers, nonsteroidal antiinflammatory agents, or corticosteroids, which have been recommended for moderate-to-severe symptoms.[118] Although patients have been reported to improve after these medications,[102,118] no controlled studies have established their utility firmly. Some patients may require readmission for symptomatic care.[102] Corticosteroids are recommended for patients with severe symptoms or evidence of nephritis or other significant vasculitides.

Prevention of recurrence of local effects in ovine Fab–treated Crotalinae envenomation can be accomplished by following the initial control of local symptoms with additional scheduled doses of antivenom (two vials of

antivenom every 6 hours for three additional doses).[57] Although it is theoretically possible to prevent coagulopathy recurrences by maintaining a constant protective level of antivenom,[80] no such studies have been performed. The need for and efficacy of late use of antivenom in these cases are uncertain.[113] Although the risk of spontaneous bleeding from recurrent coagulopathy is considered small, there almost certainly is an increased risk with surgery or trauma in patients with low platelet counts or fibrinogen.[113] Recommendations for posttreatment monitoring of Fab-treated patients and for consideration of retreatment with antivenom are presented in Figure 135-2 and Table 135-1.[113] Similarly, significant recurrence of toxic effects from digoxin toxicity after treatment with ovine Fab may be retreated with additional digoxin-specific Fab.[5]

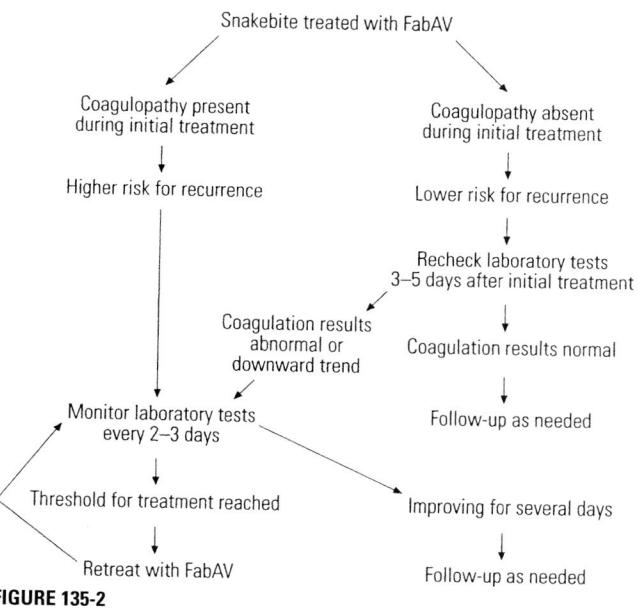

FIGURE 135-2

Monitoring for coagulopathy in patients treated with Crotalidae polyvalent immune Fab (ovine). *(From Boyer LV, Seifert SA, Cain JS: Recurrence phenomena after immunoglobulin therapy for snake envenomations: Part 2. Guidelines for clinical management with Crotaline Fab Antivenom. Ann Emerg Med 37:199, 2001.)*

TABLE 135-1 Recommendations for Indications for Retreatment of Recurrent Coagulopathy with FabAV

Fibrinogen <50 μg/mL
Platelet count <25,000/mm^3
INR >3.0
aPTT >50 sec
Multicomponent coagulopathy
Worsening trend in patient with prior severe coagulopathy
High-risk behavior for trauma
Comorbid conditions that increase hemorrhagic risk

From Boyer LV, Seifert SA, Cain JS: Recurrence phenomena after immunoglobulin therapy for snake envenomations: Part 2. Guidelines for clinical management with crotaline Fab antivenom. Ann Emerg Med 37:199, 2001.

REFERENCES

1. Kelly KJ, Meehan SM, Colvin RB, et al: Protection from toxicant-mediated renal injury in the rat with anti-CD54 antibody. Kidney Int 56:922–931, 1999.
2. Arend WP, Silverblatt FJ: Serum disappearance and catabolism of homologous immunoglobulin fragments in rats. Clin Exp Immunol 22:502–513, 1975.
3. Sabouraud A, Scherrmann JM: Immunotherapy of drug poisoning. Therapie 49:41–48, 1994.
4. Riviere G, Choumet V, Saliou B, et al: Absorption and elimination of viper venom after antivenom administration. J Pharmacol Exp Ther 285:490–495, 1998.
5. Ujhelyi MR, Robert S: Pharmacokinetic aspects of digoxin-specific Fab therapy in the management of digitalis toxicity. Clin Pharmacokinet 28:483–493, 1995.
6. Lemeulle C, Chardes T, Montavon C, et al: Anti-digoxin scFv fragments expressed in bacteria and in insect cells have different antigen binding properties. FEBS Lett 423:159–166, 1998.
7. Clark RF, Selden BS, Curry SC: Digoxin-specific Fab fragments in the treatment of oleander toxicity in a canine model. Ann Emerg Med 20:1073–1077, 1991.
8. Cummins RO, Haulman J, Quan L, et al: Near-fatal Yew Berry intoxication treated with external cardiac pacing and digoxin-specific Fab antibody fragments. Ann Emerg Med 19:38–43, 1990.
9. Brubacher JR, Ravikumar PR, Bania T, et al: Treatment of toad venom poisoning with digoxin-specific Fab fragments. Chest 110:1282–1288, 1996.
10. Sabouraud A, Urtizberea M, Cano NJ, et al: Colchicine-specific Fab fragments alter colchicine disposition in rabbits. J Pharmacol 260:1214–1219, 1992.
11. Baud FJ, Sabouraud A, Vicaut E, et al: Brief report: Treatment of severe colchicine overdose with colchicine-specific Fab fragments. N Engl J Med 3:642–645, 1995.
12. Owens SM, Mayersohn M: Phencyclidine-specific Fab fragments alter phencyclidine disposition in dogs. Drug Metab Disp 14:52–58, 1986.
13. McClurkan MB, Valentine JL, Arnold L, Owens SM: Disposition of a monoclonal anti-phencyclidine Fab fragment of immunoglobulin G in rats. J Pharmacol Exp Ther 266:1439–1445, 1993.
14. Valentine JL, Arnold LW, Owens SM: Anti-phencyclidine monoclonal Fab fragments markedly alter phencyclidine pharmacokinetics in rats. J Pharmacol Exp Ther 269:1079–1085, 1994.
15. Chen N, Bowles MR, Pond SM: Prevention of paraquat toxicity in suspensions of alveolar type II cells by paraquat-specific antibodies. Hum Exp Toxicol 13:551–557, 1994.
16. Devlin CM, Bowles MR, Gordon RB, Pond SM: Production of a paraquat-specific murine single chain Fv fragment. J Biochem 118:480–487, 1995.
17. Nagao M: Production and toxicological application of anti-paraquat antibodies. Nippon Hoigaku Zasshi 43:134–147, 1989.
18. Pentel PR, Ross CA, Sidki A, et al: Reversal of desipramine toxicity in rats with polyclonal drug-specific antibody Fab fragments. J Lab Clin Med 123:387–393, 1994.
19. Pentel PR, Scarlett W, Ross CA, et al: Reduction of desipramine cardiotoxicity and prolongation of survival in rats with the use of polyclonal drug-specific antibody Fab fragments. Ann Emerg Med 26:334–340, 1995.
20. Keyler DE, Le Couteur DG, Pond SM, et al: Effects of specific antibody Fab fragments on desipramine pharmacokinetics in the rat and in the isolated perfused liver. J Pharmacol Exp Ther 272:1117–1123, 1995.
21. Lin G, Pentel PR, Shelver W, et al: Bacterial expression and characterization of an anti-desipramine single-chain antibody fragment. Int J Immunopharmacol 18:729–738, 1996.
22. Heard K, O'Malley GF, Dart RC: Treatment of amitriptyline poisoning with ovine antibody to tricyclic antidepressants. Lancet 354:1614–1615, 1999.
23. Chen N, Bowles MR, Pond SM: Polyclonal amanitin-specific antibodies: Production and cytoprotective properties in vitro. Biochem Pharmacol 46:327–329, 1993.
24. Faulstich H, Kirchner K, Derenzini M: Strongly enhanced toxicity of the mushroom toxin α-amanitin by an amatoxin-specific Fab or monoclonal antibody. Toxicon 26:491–499, 1988.
25. Metzger JF, Lewis GE Jr: Human-derived immune globulins for the treatment of botulism. Rev Infect Dis 1:689–692, 1979.
26. Hatheway CH, Snyder JD, Seals JE, et al: Antitoxin levels in botulism patients treated with trivalent equine botulism antitoxin to toxin types A, B and E. J Infect Dis 150:407–412, 1984.
27. Pless DD, Torres ER, Reinke EK, Bavari S: High-affinity protective antibodies to the binding domain of boulinum nuerotoxin Type A. Infect Immun 69:570–574, 2001.
28. Hill RE, Heard K, Bogdan GM, et al: Attenuation of verapamil-induced myocardial toxicity in an ex-vivo rat model using a verapamil-specific ovine immunoglobin. Acad Emerg Med 8:950–955, 2001.
29. Russell RE, Ruzic N, Gonzales H: Effectiveness of antivenin (Crotalidae polyvalent) following injection of Crotalus venom. Toxicon 11:461–464, 1973.
30. Bolanos R, Cerdas L, Taylor R: The production and characteristics of a coral snake (Micrurus mipartitus hertwigi) antivenin. Toxicon 12:139–142, 1975.
31. Sullivan JB Jr, Russell FE: Isolation and purification of antibodies to rattlesnake venom by affinity chromatography. Proc West Pharmacol Soc 25:185–192, 1982.
32. Karlson-Stiber C, Persson H, Heath A, et al: First clinical experiences with specific sheep Fab fragments in snake bite: Report of a multicentre study of Vipera berus envenoming. J Intern Med 241:53–58, 1997.
33. Dart RC, McNally J: Efficacy, safety, and use of snake antivenoms in the United States. Ann Emerg Med 37:181–188, 2001.
34. Dart RC, Sidki A, Sullivan JB Jr, et al: Ovine desipramine antibody fragments reverse desipramine cardiovascular toxicity in the rat. Ann Emerg Med 27:309–315, 1996.
35. Borges A, Tsushima RG, Backx PH: Antibodies against Tityus discrepans venom do not abolish the effect of Tityus serrulatus venom on the rat sodium and potassium channels. Toxicon 37:867–881, 1999.
36. Calderon-Aranda ES, Riviere G, Choumet V, et al: Pharmacokinetics of the toxic fraction of Centruroides limpidus limpidus venom in experimentally envenomed rabbits and effects of immunotherapy with specific F(ab')2. Toxicon 37:771–782, 1999.
37. LoVecchio F, Welch S, Klemens J, et al: Incidence of immediate and delayed hypersensitivity to Centruroides antivenom. Ann Emerg Med 34:669–670, 1999.
38. Devaux C, Moreau E, Goyffon R, et al: Construction and functional evaluation of a single-chain antibody fragment that neutralizes toxin AahI from the venom of the scorpion Androctonus australis hector. Eur J Biochem 268:694–702, 2000.
39. Ghalim N, El-Hafny B, Sebti F, et al: Scorpion envenomation and serotherapy in Morocco. Am J Trop Med Hyg 62:277–283, 2000.
40. Graudins A, Padula M, Broady K, Nicholson GM: Red-black spider (Latrodectus hasselti) antivenom prevents the toxicity of widow spider venoms. Ann Emerg Med 37:154–160, 2001.
41. Clark RF: The safety and efficacy of antivenin Latrodectus mactans. J Toxicol Clin Toxicol 39:125–127, 2001.
42. Daly FF, Hill RE, Bodgan GM, Dart RC: Neutralization of Latrodectus mactans and L. hesperus venom by redback spider (L. hasseltii) antivenom. J Toxicol Clin Toxicol 39:119–123, 2001.
43. Schumacher MJ, Egen NB, Tanner D: Neutralization of bee venom lethality by immune serum antibodies. Am J Trop Med Hyg 55:197–201, 1996.
44. Jones RG, Coreling RL, Bhogal G, Landon J: A novel Fab-based antivenom for the treatment of mass bee attacks. Am J Trop Med Hyg 61:361–366, 1999.
45. Rumack BH, Rider PK, Gelman CR (eds): Snakes: Crotalinae (management/treatment protocol): In POISINDEX System. Englewood, CO, MICROMEDEX, 2002.
46. LoVecchio F, DeBus DM: Snakebite envenomation in children: A 10-year retrospective review. Wildern Environ Med 12:184–189, 2001.
47. Heard K, O'Malley GF, Dart RC: Antivenom therapy in the Americas. Drugs 58:5–15, 1999.
48. Fey H: A simple procedure for the production of Fab from bovine IgG as an absorbent in the preparation of class-specific anti-immunoglobulin. Immunochemistry 12:235–239, 1975.
49. Prince HE, Folds JD, Spitznagel JK: In vitro production of a biologically active Fab₂-like fragment by digestion of human IgG rheumatoid factor with human polymorphonuclear leukocyte elastase. Mol Immunol 16:975–978, 1979.
50. Dos Santos MC, D'Imperio MR, Furtado GC, et al: Purification of F(ab')2 anti-snake venom by caprylic acid: A fast method for obtaining IgG fragments with high neutralization activity, purity and yield. Toxicon 27:297–303, 1989.

51. Russell FE, Sullivan JB, Egen NB, et al: Preparation of a new antivenin by affinity chromatography. Am J Trop Med Hyg 34:141–150, 1985.

52. Smith TW, Lloyd BL, Spicer N, Haber E: Immunogenicity and kinetics of distribution and elimination of sheep digoxin-specific IgG and Fab fragments in the rabbit and baboon. Clin Exp Immunol 36:384–396, 1979.

53. Otero-Patino R, Cardose JLC, Higashi HG, et al: A randomized, blinded, comparative trial of one pepsin-digested and two whole IgG antivenoms for *Bothrops* snake bites in Uraba, Colombia. Am J Trop Med Hyg 58:183–189, 1998.

54. Meyer WP, Habib AG, Onayade AA, et al: First clinical experiences with a new ovine Fab *Echis ocellatus* snake bite antivenom in Nigeria: Randomized comparative trial with Institute Pasteur serum (Ipser) Africa antivenom. Am J Trop Med Hyg 56:291–300, 1997.

55. Karlson, EW, Sudarsky L, Ruderman E, et al: Treatment of stiff-man syndrome with intravenous immune globulin. Arthritis Rheum 37: 915–918, 1994.

56. Ariaratnam CA, Sjostrom L, Raziek Z, et al: An open, randomized comparative trial of two antivenoms for the treatment of envenoming by Sri Lankan Russell's viper (*Diaboia russelii russelii*). Trans R Soc Trop Med Hyg 95:74–80, 2001.

57. Dart RC, Seifert SA, Boyer LV, et al: A randomized multicenter trial of Crotalinae polyvalent immune Fab (ovine) antivenom for the treatment for crotaline snakebite in the United States. Arch Intern Med 161:2030–2036, 2001.

58. Milenic DE, Yokota T, Filpula DR, et al: Construction, binding properties, metabolism and tumor targeting of a single-chain Fv derived from the pancarcinoma monoclonal antibody CC49. Can Res 51:6363–6371, 1991.

59. Brinkmann U, Reiter Y, Jung S-H, et al: A recombinant immunotoxin containing a disulfide-stabilized Fv fragment. Proc Natl Acad Sci U S A 90:7538–7542, 1993.

60. Shelver WL, Keyler DE, Lin G, et al: Effects of recombinant drug-specific single chain antibody Fv fragment on [3H]-desipramine distribution in rats. Biochem Pharmacol 51:531–537, 1996.

61. Nydegger UE, Mohacsi PJ, Escher R, Morell A: Clinical use of intravenous immunoglobulins. Vox Sang 78(Suppl 2):191–195, 2000.

62. Jefferis R, Lund J, Pound JD: IgG-Fc-mediated effector functions: Molecular definition of interaction sites for effector ligands and the role of glycosylation. Immunol Rev 163:59–76, 1998.

63. Nydegger UE, Sturzenegger M: Adverse effects of intravenous immunoglobulin therapy. Drug Saf 21:171–185, 1999.

64. Leon G, Monge M, Rojas E, et al: Comparison between IgG and F(ab′)(2) polyvalent antivenoms: Neutralization of systemic effects induced by *Bothrops asper* venom in mice, extravasation to muscle tissue, and potential for induction of adverse reactions. Toxicon 39:793–801, 2001.

65. Colcher D, Pavlinkova G, Beresford G, et al: Pharmacokinetics and biodistribution of genetically-engineered antibodies. Q J Nucl Med 42:225–241, 1998.

66. Grainger RJ, Ko S, Koslov E, et al: Effect of shear on human insulin in zinc suspension. Appl Biochem Biotechnol 84–86:761–768, 2000.

67. Inazu K, Shima K: Freeze-drying and quality evaluation of protein drugs. Dev Biol Stand 74:307–322, 1992.

68. Azuma J, Kurimoto T, Tsuji S, et al: Phase I study on human monoclonal antibody against cytomegalovirus: Pharmacokinetics and immunogenicity. J Immunother 10:278–285, 1991.

69. Ho M, Silamut K, White NJ, et al: Pharmacokinetics of three commercial antivenoms in patients envenomed by the Malayan pit viper, *Calloselasma rhodostoma*, in Thailand. Am J Trop Med Hyg 42:260–266, 1990.

70. Bazin-Redureau MI, Renard CB, Scherrmann J-MG: Pharmacokinetics of heterologous and homologous immunoglobulin G, F(ab′)2 and Fab after intravenous administration in the rat. J Pharm Pharmacol 49:277–281, 1997.

71. Covell DG, Barbet J, Holton OD, et al: Pharmacokinetics of monoclonal immunoglobulin G1, F(ab′)2, and Fab′ in mice. Cancer Res 46:3969–3978, 1986.

72. Schaumann W, Kaufmann B, Neubert P, Smolarz A: Kinetics of the Fab fragments of digoxin antibodies and of bound digoxin in patients with severe digoxin intoxication. Eur J Clin Pharmacol 30:527–533, 1986.

73. Weisman LE, Fischer GW, Marinelli P, et al: Pharmacokinetics of intravenous immunoglobulin in neonates. Vox Sang 57:243–248, 1989.

74. Mankarious S, Lee M, Fischer S, et al: The half-lives of IgG subclasses and specific antibodies in patients with primary immunodeficiency who are receiving intravenously administered immunoglobulin. J Lab Clin Med 112:634–640, 1988.

75. Callaghan TA, Fleetwood P, Contreras M, Mollison PL: Human monoclonal anti-D with a normal half-life. Transfusion 33:784–785, 1993.

76. Smith GN, Mollison D, Griffiths B, Mollison PL: Uptake of IgG after intramuscular and subcutaneous injection. Lancet 1:1208–1212, 1972.

77. Sorensen HNH, Faber V, Svehag S-E: Circulating immune complexes, complement activation kinetics and serum sickness following treatment with heterologous anti-snake venom globulin. Scand J Immunol 7:25–33, 1978.

78. Mordenti J, Chen SA, Moore JA, et al: Interspecies scaling of clearance and volume of distribution data for five therapeutic proteins. Pharmaceut Res 8:1351–1359, 1991.

79. Tibben JG, Boerman OC, Massuger LFAG, et al: Pharmacokinetics, biodistribution and biological effects of intravenously administered bispecific monoclonal antibody OC/TR F(ab)2 in ovarian carcinoma patients. Int J Cancer 66:477–483, 1996.

80. Seifert SA: Pharmacokinetic analysis of a crotalid Fab antivenom and theoretical considerations for the prevention of coagulopathic recurrence. J Toxicol Clin Toxicol 36:526–527, 1998.

81. Thanh-Barthet CV, Urtizberea M, Sabouraud AE, et al: Development of a sensitive radioimmunoassay for Fab fragments: Application to Fab pharmacokinetics in humans. Pharmaceut Res 10:692–695, 1993.

82. Allen NM, Dunham GD, Sailstad JM, Findlay JWA: Clinical and pharmacokinetic profiles of digoxin immune Fab in four patients with renal impairment. DICP 25:1315–1320, 1991.

83. Caspi O, Zylber-Katz E, Gotsman O, et al: Digoxin intoxication in a patient with end-stage renal disease: Efficiency of digoxin-specific Fab antibody fragments and peritoneal dialysis. Therap Drug Monit 19:510–515, 1997.

84. Polymenis M, Stollar BD: Domain interactions and antigen binding of recombinant anti-Z-DNA antibody variable domains: The role of heavy and light chains measured by surface plasmon resonance. J Immunol 154:2198–2208, 1995.

85. Cohen P, Laune D, Teulon I, et al: Interaction of the octapeptide angiotensin II with a high-affinity single-chain Fv and with peptides derived from the antibody paratope. J Immunol Methods 254:147–160, 2001.

86. Lomonte B, Leon G, Hanson LA: Similar effectiveness of Fab and F(ab′)2 antivenoms in the neutralization of hemorrhagic activity of *Vipera berus* snake venom in mice. Toxicon 34:1197–1202, 1996.

87. Consroe P, Egen NB, Russell FE, et al: Comparison of a new ovine antigen binding fragment (Fab) antivenin for United States *Crotalidae* with the commercial antivenin for protection against venom-induced lethality in mice. Am J Trop Med Hyg 53:507–510, 1995.

88. Seifert SA, Boyer LV, Dart RC, et al: Relationship of venom effects to venom antigen and antivenom serum concentrations in a patient with *Crotalus atrox* envenomation treated with a Fab antivenom. Ann Emerg Med 30:49–53, 1997.

89. Seifert SA, Boyer LV: Recurrence phenomena after immunoglobulin therapy for snake envenomations: Part 1. Pharmacokinetics and pharmacodynamics of immunoglobulin antivenoms and related antibodies. Ann Emerg Med 37:189–195, 2001.

90. Leon G, Rojas G, Lomonte B, Gutierrez JM: Immunoglobulin G and F(ab′)2 polyvalent antivenoms do not differ in their ability to neutralize hemorrhage, edema and myonecrosis induced by *Bothrops asper* (Terciopelo) snake venom. Toxicon 35:1627–1637, 1997.

91. Gutierrez JM, Leon G, Bojas G, et al: Neutralization of local tissue damage induced by *Bothrops asper* (Terciopelo) snake venom. Toxicon 36:1529–1537, 1998.

92. Bogdan GM, Dart RC, Falbo SC, et al: Recurrent coagulopathy after antivenom treatment of crotalid snakebite. South Med J 93:562–566, 2000.

93. Humphreys DP, Vetterlien OM, Chapman AP, et al: F(ab′)2 molecules made from *Escherichia coli* produced Fab′ with hinge sequences conferring increased serum survival in an animal model. J Immunol Methods 217:1–10, 1998.

94. Chatenoud L: Humoral immune response against OKT3. Transplant Proc 25:68–73, 1993.

95. Bolanos R, Cerdas L, Abalos JW: Venoms of coral snakes (*Micrurus spp.*): Report on a multivalent antivenin for the Americas. Bull Pan Am Health Organ 12:23–27, 1978.

96. Fagnani R, Halpern S, Hagan M: Altered pharmacokinetic and tumour localization properties of Fab' fragments of a murine monoclonal anti-CEA antibody by covalent modification with low molecular weight dextran. Nucl Med Commun 16:362–369, 1995.

97. Kobayashi H, Kim I-S, Drumm D, et al: Favorable effects of glycolate conjugation on the biodistribution of humanized antiTac Fab fragment. J Nucl Med 40:837–845, 1999.

98. Renner C, Hartmann F, Pfreundschuh M: The future of monoclonal antibody engineering. Ann Hematol 80(Suppl 3):B127-B129, 2001.

99. Buntain WL: Successful venomous snakebite neutralization with massive antivenin infusion in a child. J Trauma 23:1012–1014, 1983.

100. Jacobson HR, Striker GE, Klahr S (eds): The Principles and Practice of Nephrology. Philadelphia, BC Decker, 1991, pp 249–251.

101. Rumack BH, Rider PK, Gelman CR (eds): Alternative health consults: Pregnancy categories. In MICROMEDEX Healthcare Series Integrated Index. Englewood, CO, MICROMEDEX, 2002.

102. Jurkovich GJ, Luterman A, McCullar K, et al: Complications of *Crotalidae* antivenin therapy. J Trauma 28:1032–1037, 1988.

103. Sutherland SK, Lovering KE: Antivenoms: Use and adverse reactions over a 12-month period in Australia and Papua New Guinea. Med J Aust 2:671–674, 1979.

104. Clark RF, Wethern-Kestner S, Vance MV, et al: Clinical presentation and treatment of black widow spider envenomation: A review of 163 cases. Ann Emerg Med 21:782–787, 1992.

105. Ellenhorn MJ (ed): Envenomations—bites and stings. In Ellenhorn's Medical Toxicology, 2nd ed. Baltimore, Williams & Wilkins, 1997, p 1762.

106. Kitchens CS, Mierop LHS: Envenomation by the eastern coral snake (*Micrurus fulvius fulvius*). JAMA 258:1615–1618, 1987.

107. Loprinzi CL, Hennessee J, Leonard T, et al: Snake antivenin administration in a patient allergic to horse serum. South Med J 76:501–503, 1983.

108. Russell FE: Snake Venom Poisoning. Great Neck, NY, Scholium, 1980.

109. Griffen D, Donovan JW: Significant envenomation from a preserved rattlesnake head (in a patient with a history of immediate hypersensitivity to antivenin). Ann Emerg Med 15:955–958, 1986.

110. Chippaux JP, Lang J, Edine SA, et al: Clinical safety of a polyvalent F(ab')2 equine antivenom in 233 African snake envenomations: A field trial in Cameroon. Trans R Soc Trop Med Hyg 92:657–662, 1998.

111. Davidson TE: Intravenous rattlesnake envenomation. West J Med 148:45–57, 1988.

112. Nielsen H, Sorensen H, Faber V, Svehag S-E: Circulating immune complexes, complement activation kinetics and serum sickness following treatment with heterologous anti-snake venom globulin. Scand J Immunol 7:25–33, 1978.

113. Boyer LV, Seifert SA, Cain JS: Recurrence phenomena after immunoglobulin therapy for snake envenomations: Part 1. Pharmacokinetics and pharmacodynamics of immunoglobulin antivenoms and related antibodies. Ann Emerg Med 37:196–201, 2001.

114. Boyer LV, Seifert SA, Clark RF, et al: Recurrent and persistent coagulopathy following pit viper envenomation. Arch Intern Med 159:706–710, 1999.

115. Burch JM, Agarwal R, Mattox KL, et al: The treatment of crotalid envenomation without antivenin. J Trauma 28:35–43, 1988.

116. Malasit P, Warrell DA, Chanthavanich P, et al: Prediction, prevention and mechanism of early (anaphylactic) antivenom reactions in victims of snakebites. BMJ 292:17–20, 1986.

117. Hasiba U, Rosenbach LM, Rockwell D, Lewis J: DIC-like syndrome after envenomation by the snake *Crotalus horridus horridus*. N Engl J Med 292:505–507, 1975.

118. Otten EJ, McKimm D: Venomous snakebite in a patient allergic to horse serum. Ann Emerg Med 12:624–627, 1983.

CHAPTER 136

N-Acetylcysteine

Anthony S. Manoguerra

N-Acetylcysteine (NAC) was first marketed for use by inhalation as a mucolytic agent for the management of abnormal, viscid, or inspissated mucus secretions in chronic bronchopulmonary disease. It subsequently was discovered to be an antidote for acetaminophen (paracetamol) poisoning, for which it has become the standard of care. In addition, NAC has potential usefulness as an antidote for a range of other toxins.

HISTORY OF USE

In 1973, Mitchell and coworkers[1] reported on the metabolism of acetaminophen (see Fig. 55-1) and postulated that the acute toxicity of this drug was related to the bioactivation of acetaminophen to a chemically reactive arylating agent. This highly reactive intermediate is conjugated by glutathione, which prevents tissue damage. When glutathione is depleted, the reactive intermediate binds to hepatocytes, leading to hepatocellular necrosis.[2] This discovery led to a search for agents that could modify the metabolism of acetaminophen or interrupt the binding of the toxic metabolite to liver cells. Agents such as cysteamine and methionine had been tried with varying degrees of success.[3,4] While screening potential antidotes, Piperno and Berssenbruegge[5] showed in experimental animals that NAC provided protection against a fatal dose of acetaminophen. Before this time, NAC, sold in the United States and elsewhere under the brand name of Mucomyst, had been used by inhalation as an adjunct in the removal of abnormally thick, excessive mucus secretions from the lungs. Rumack and Peterson[6] obtained a New Drug Application from the U.S. Food and Drug Administration (FDA) in 1976 to study the effectiveness of the oral administration of NAC in the management of acetaminophen poisoning and reported in 1978 the results of the treatment of the first 416 patients. At the same time, the efficacy of intravenous NAC was under investigation in the United Kingdom, with the results reported in 1977.[7] In 1985, NAC received FDA approval for the treatment of acetaminophen poisoning. Extensive use of NAC in the treatment of acetaminophen poisoning since that time has resulted in this antidote's becoming the standard of care worldwide. In the United States, oral administration is the only approved route, whereas the intravenous route is prevalent in most other countries.

Although not as well studied as in the treatment of acetaminophen poisoning, NAC also has been advocated in the treatment of mercury toxicity,[8,9] carbon tetrachloride hepatotoxicity,[10,11] gold toxicity,[12] arsenic toxicity,[13] zinc chloride smoke inhalation,[14] and *Amanita phalloides* mushroom poisoning[15] and to reduce the adverse effects of many cancer chemotherapy drugs.[16,17] The enthusiasm for the free radical scavenging properties of NAC has extended into the treatment of non–toxicology-related illnesses, such as septic shock,[18] coronary artery disease,[19] hepatic failure,[20] and respiratory distress syndrome.[21] In addition, more recently NAC has been promoted as a dietary supplement; it is marketed as a free radical scavenger capable of enhancing immune function, specifically for prevention of colds and influenza and as an adjunct to mainstream therapy for patients with human immunodeficiency virus infection and chronic lung disease.[22]

PROPERTIES

Chemical

The chemical structure of NAC is shown in Figure 136-1. Other chemical names synonymous with NAC are *N*-acetyl-L-cysteine, L-α-acetamido-β-mercaptoproprionic acid, and *N*-acetyl-3-mercaptoalanine.

Physical

The molecular weight of NAC is 163.2. It is a crystalline solid at room temperature with a melting point of 110°F (43°C). It has a strong, disagreeable, "rotten egg" odor.

PHARMACODYNAMICS

The exact mechanism by which NAC protects from acute acetaminophen toxicity is not known. Several possible mechanisms have been proposed, however. NAC is deacetylated to cysteine, which can be incorporated into the synthesis of glutathione, raising the intracellular concentration of glutathione and providing protection.[23] The availability of cysteine seems to be the rate-limiting step in the synthesis of glutathione, and NAC administration replenishes depleted supplies. Alternatively, NAC may act as a glutathione substitute and provide thiol groups to bind to the acetaminophen reactive metabolite, *N*-acetyl-p-benzoquinone imine, or encourage the reduction of this metabolite to acetaminophen, sparing hepatocytes from injury.[24] Animal experiments failed to show, however, that NAC formed significant amounts of conjugate with the

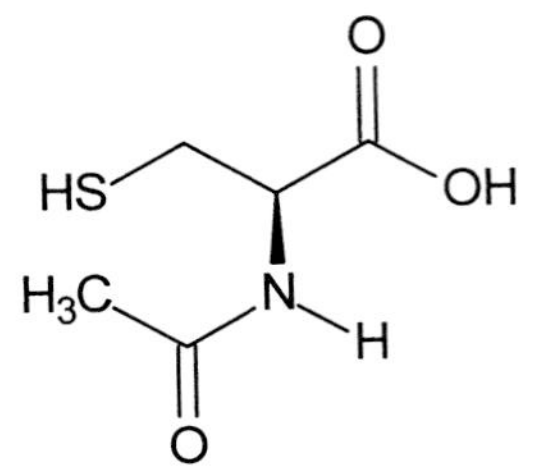

FIGURE 136-1

Chemical structure of *N*-acetylcysteine.

reactive metabolite of acetaminophen. In this model, NAC provided a source of sulfate, reduced *N*-acetyl-p-benzoquinone imine back to acetaminophen, and increased the synthesis of glutathione.[25]

In acute acetaminophen poisoning, NAC, if given within 8 hours of ingestion, is highly effective.[26,27] Between 8 and 15 hours, NAC may be less effective but still provides some protection. Considerable controversy exists as to the effectiveness of administration of NAC more than 15 hours after ingestion or in the event of chronic poisoning.[28] NAC may be effective at modulating the cascade of inflammation that occurs in hepatic necrosis, limiting further injury to unaffected liver cells. It also has been postulated that NAC increases hepatic and cerebral microvascular blood flow in patients with liver failure.[19] The clinical significance of these findings is not clear. There is no conclusive evidence that the use of NAC is effective in altering the outcome in these situations. Clinicians may argue, however, that the use of NAC carries such a low risk of adverse consequences that use of the drug, even without good evidence of efficacy, may be justified. The efficacy of NAC in acetaminophen poisoning is discussed more fully in Chapter 55.

PHARMACOKINETICS

The pharmacokinetics of NAC is difficult to study because the drug exists in the plasma in a multitude of forms—oxidized, reduced, and protein bound. Analytic techniques may detect some but not all of the forms, making comparisons between studies impossible.[29]

Oral absorption of NAC seems to be rapid, with peak blood concentrations occurring at 30 to 90 minutes after ingestion.[30–32] The bioavailability of oral NAC may be 10% because of significant first-pass extraction or metabolism by the liver.[33] With such a large first-pass effect and the fact that the target organ for protection is the liver, the clinical relevance of this low bioavailability is unclear. The volume of distribution of unchanged NAC has been estimated to be 0.3 to 0.5 L/kg.[31,32] Metabolism of NAC is extensive, with the following oxidized metabolic products found in the plasma: N,N'-diacetylcystine, *N*-acetylcysteine cysteine, *N*-acetylcysteine protein, and *N*-acetylcysteine glutathione. The major metabolic products after complete metabolism are cysteine, cystine, inorganic sulfate, and glutathione.[34]

After an intravenous loading dose of 150 mg/kg administered over 15 minutes, peak plasma NAC concentrations averaged 554 mg/L. Using Prescott and colleagues'[35] 20-hour

intravenous protocol (150 mg/kg loading dose, followed by 50 mg/kg for 4 hours, followed by 100 mg/kg for 16 hours), a mean steady-state concentration of 35 mg/L (range 10 to 90 mg/L) was achieved at 12 hours. North and associates[31] reported peak NAC plasma levels of 9.3 to 16.2 µg/mL after the oral administration of 140 mg/kg of NAC.

Controversy exists over the effect of concurrently administered oral activated charcoal on the bioavailability of oral NAC. Ekins and coworkers,[36] using 19 healthy volunteers, reported a 39% reduction in the oral absorption of NAC when immediately followed by a 100-g dose of activated charcoal. North and associates[31] reported no decrease in peak plasma NAC concentrations or area under the curve and a slight delay in time to peak when 50 g of oral activated charcoal was given 15 minutes before a 140-mg/kg oral dose of NAC in three healthy volunteers. Renzi and colleagues[37] found similar results in six volunteers given activated charcoal and NAC in the same fashion as in the North study. None of these studies considered the total amount of NAC that must be supplied to prevent acetaminophen-induced cell injury effectively. Because the oral dose of NAC used (140 mg/kg loading dose followed by 17 doses of 70 mg/kg every 4 hours) seems to be effective for even large acetaminophen overdoses, there is an apparent "margin of safety" built into the dose.

SPECIAL POPULATIONS

There is preliminary evidence that the pharmacokinetics of NAC may be altered in patients with severe hepatic failure. Jones and coworkers[38] compared the pharmacokinetics of NAC in nine biopsy-proven cirrhotic patients with six controls. In the patients with cirrhosis, the area under the serum concentration versus time curve was increased substantially when they were given 600 mg intravenously compared with controls given the same dose. In addition, clearance of NAC was reduced significantly. The authors warned that the increased levels seen in these patients may increase the likelihood of anaphylactoid reactions.

NAC has not been studied for potential teratogenic effects in humans. It does seem, however, that there is a greater risk from delays in treatment with NAC in pregnant women with acute acetaminophen poisoning. Although few cases have been reported, deaths of the mother and fetus have occurred when NAC treatment either has not been given or has been delayed.[39,40] Horowitz and colleagues[41] showed that NAC concentrations equal to concentrations seen in adults being treated with NAC are found in the cord blood of infants whose mothers are being treated with NAC.

CONTRAINDICATIONS

The only absolute contraindication to the use of NAC is a well-documented history of a prior severe allergic reaction. In these cases, the benefits of treatment must be weighed against the potential severity of an allergic reaction. True allergic reactions to NAC are rare because most individuals do not have prior exposure and are not sensitized. With the use of NAC as a dietary supplement, the number of people with prior exposure and the possibility of sensitization may increase.

ADVERSE EFFECTS

Oral NAC is generally well tolerated and considered an extremely safe treatment. As a result of the strong rotten egg odor and the gastrointestinal upset commonly seen after acetaminophen overdose, vomiting is the most common side effect observed. In one study, 51% of 515 acetaminophen overdose patients experienced vomiting while receiving oral NAC.[42] Administration of NAC through an enteral tube minimizes the nausea caused by the unpleasant odor. If vomiting remains a problem, antiemetics may be helpful. Scharman[43] reported in a retrospective review of 78 patients with acute acetaminophen poisoning and vomiting that the vomiting could not be controlled with antiemetic agents in only 3 patients. Allergic skin reactions were reported in 13 of 515 acetaminophen overdose patients while receiving NAC.[42] Anaphylactoid reactions to oral administration of NAC have not been reported except for a case of angioedema.[44] A serum sickness–like disorder with fever, arthritis, adenopathy, rash, and thrombocytopenia occurred in a young man 3 days after starting oral NAC treatment.[45]

Intravenous NAC is associated with more concerning adverse events. Anaphylactoid reactions characterized by sudden onset of respiratory distress with dizziness, rash, nausea, bronchospasm, angioedema, and apnea have been reported with intravenous infusion and are thought to be due to high plasma concentrations of NAC resulting from overdose or rapid infusion.[35,46–48] In two instances, these reactions were associated with hypotension and death.[49,50] The mechanism of this anaphylactoid reaction is believed to be NAC-induced histamine release. Anaphylactoid reactions to NAC can be managed by discontinuing the infusion. Some clinicians have advocated the administration of H_1-receptor blocking agents, but the role of histamine in these reactions is unclear. In many patients, if it is determined that intravenous therapy is required to prevent acetaminophen-induced hepatic injury, the infusion may be restarted at a slower rate,[51] or oral therapy may be substituted. Some authorities recommend routinely administering the initial infusion over 1 hour rather than over 15 minutes as a strategy to decrease the risk for an anaphylactoid reaction.

DOSAGE AND ADMINISTRATION

According to Rumack (personal communication, September 11, 2001), the traditional U.S. dosing protocol (see below) for oral NAC was based on the amount needed to protect experimental animals from acetaminophen toxicity extrapolated to humans with an added safety factor. At the time NAC use first was being studied, it was thought that the drug acted primarily as a glutathione surrogate. From the early animal work, it was known that liver injury occurred after the depletion of hepatic glutathione by 70%. Extrapolating from animals, it was estimated that the typical 70-kg human had approximately 6 mmol of glutathione in the liver. The dose of NAC necessary to compensate for a 70% level

of depletion was calculated and multiplied by a threefold safety factor to produce the dose that currently is in use. The duration of treatment was determined by taking a 4-hour elimination half-life for acetaminophen, multiplying it by 5 to account for total disappearance, then multiplying by a threefold safety factor. Because of the concern that some patients, particularly patients with severe hepatic injury, could have half-lives longer than 4 hours, an additional safety factor of 12 hours was added, resulting in the 72-hour treatment protocol. This was the best information available at the time that could be used to develop an acceptable protocol for the FDA. With time and experience, the dose and duration have proved effective. The lowest effective dose of NAC for most acetaminophen overdose situations and the optimal duration of treatment are not known, however. It is likely in most cases that far more NAC is being given for a longer time than is needed.

In the United States, the traditional dosing schedule for NAC is an oral loading dose of 140 mg/kg followed by 17 70-mg/kg doses given every 4 hours. The solution of NAC should be diluted to a 5% concentration with juice or a soft drink to attempt to enhance palatability. It is either ingested orally or placed in the stomach through an enteral tube. If vomiting occurs within 1 hour of administration, the dose should be repeated. As stated previously, the duration of treatment probably is longer than necessary in most cases, and alternative protocols have been advocated. Woo and colleagues[52] reported that in patients who do not show evidence of hepatotoxicity within 36 hours of an acetaminophen overdose, treatment with NAC may be stopped when the acetaminophen serum concentration no longer is detectable.

Prescott and colleagues' intravenous protocol[53] is preferred in most countries other than the United States. Use of the intravenous route and this protocol is becoming more popular in the United States, however. Another intravenous protocol has been studied in the United States,[54] but it does not have regulatory approval. Prescott's protocol is 150 mg/kg given intravenously over 15 minutes followed by 50 mg/kg over 4 hours, then 100 mg/kg over 16 hours. This regimen has been shown to be effective if started within 10 hours of ingestion.[53] The other intravenous protocol uses a 140-mg/kg loading dose followed by 70 mg/kg every 4 hours for 48 hours.[54] It is the most commonly used intravenous protocol in the United States, although the data of Woo and colleagues[52] support a shorter course. Typically the 20% NAC solution is diluted to a 3% solution in 5% dextrose in water and infused over 1 hour. The Prescott protocol was recently approved in the United States, and it may supplant the every-4-hour dosing regimen that is currently used in this country.

The question of which route is more effective is unresolved. There likely is no clinically important difference. Clinicians who routinely use the intravenous route point out that it results in shorter hospital stays, provides better patient and physician convenience, and allays any concerns over decreased effectiveness or concurrent activated charcoal administration.[55] The advantage of the intravenous route is for patients who are intolerant of the oral route.[56] Perry and Shannon[57] reported a study of acute acetaminophen poisoning in adolescents comparing the usual 72-hour oral versus a 52-hour intravenous NAC protocol. They showed equal efficacy. Although a definitive answer cannot be found in the current literature, it seems that the oral and the intravenous routes of administration are equally effective at reducing acetaminophen-induced liver injury.

REFERENCES

1. Mitchell JR, Jollow DJ, Potter WZ, et al: Acetaminophen induced hepatic necrosis: I. Role of drug metabolism. J Pharmacol Exp Ther 187:185–194, 1973.
2. Potter WZ, Davis DG, Mitchell JR, et al: Acetaminophen induced hepatic necrosis: IV. Protective role of glutathione. J Pharmacol Exp Ther 187:203–210, 1073.
3. Prescott LF, Newton RW, Swainson CP, et al: Successful treatment of severe paracetamol overdosage with cysteamine. Lancet 1:588–592, 1974.
4. Crome P, Vale JA, Volans GN, et al: Oral methionine in the treatment of severe paracetamol (acetaminophen) poisoning. Lancet 1:111–115, 1976.
5. Piperno E, Berssenbruegge DA: Reversal of experimental paracetamol toxicosis with N-acetylcysteine. Lancet 2:738–739, 1976.
6. Rumack BH, Peterson RG: Acetaminophen overdose: Incidence, diagnosis and management in 416 patients. Pediatrics 62:898–903, 1978.
7. Prescott LF, Park J, Ballantyne A, et al: Treatment of paracetamol (acetaminophen) poisoning with n-acetylcysteine. Lancet 2:432–434, 1977.
8. Lund ME, Clarkson TW, Banner W: Treatment of acute methylmercury poisoning. Vet Hum Toxicol 25:280, 1983.
9. Livardjani F, Ledig M, Kopp P, et al: Lung and blood superoxide dismutase activity in mercury vapor exposed rats: Effect of N-acetylcysteine treatment. Toxicology 66:289–295, 1991.
10. Ruprah M, Mant TG, Flanagan RJ: Acute carbon tetrachloride poisoning in 19 patients: Implications for diagnosis and treatment. Lancet 1:1027–1029, 1985.
11. Valles EG, deCastro CR, Castro JA: N-Acetylcysteine is an early but also a late preventive agent against carbon tetrachloride-induced liver necrosis. Toxicol Lett 71:87–95, 1994.
12. Godfrey NF, Peter A, Simon TM, Lorber A: IV. N-Acetylcysteine treatment of hematologic reactions to chrysotherapy. J Rheumatol 9:519–526, 1982.
13. Flora SJS: Arsenic-induced oxidative stress and its reversibility following combined administration of N-acetylcysteine and meso-2,3-dimercaptosuccinic acid in rats. Clin Exp Pharmacol Physiol 26:865–869, 1999.
14. Pettila V, Takkunen O, Tukiainen P: Zinc chloride smoke inhalation: A rare cause of severe acute respiratory distress syndrome. Intensive Care Med 26:215–217, 2000.
15. Montanini S, Sinardi D, Pratico C, et al: Use of acetylcysteine as the life-saving antidote in amanita phalloides (death cap) poisoning: Case report of 11 patients. Arzneimittel-Forshung 49:1044–1047, 1999.
16. Jiminez JJ, Huang HS, Yunis AA: Treatment with ImuVert/N-acetylcysteine protects rats from cyclophosphamide/cytarabine induced alopecia. Cancer Invest 10:271–276, 1992.
17. Schwartsmann G, Sander EB, Vinholes J, et al: N-acetylcysteine protects skin lesion induced by local extravasation of doxorubicin in a rat model. Am J Pediatr Hematol Oncol 14:280–281, 1992.
18. Bakker J, Ahang H, Depierreux M, et al: Effects of N-acetylcysteine in endotoxic shock. J Crit Care 9:236–243, 1994.
19. Sochman J, Peregrin JH: Total recovery of left ventricular function after acute myocardial infarction: Comprehensive therapy with streptokinase, N-acetylcysteine and percutaneous transluminal coronary angioplasty. Int J Cardiol 35:116–118, 1992.
20. Harrison PM, Wendon JA, Gimson AE, et al: Improvement by N-acetylcysteine of hemodynamics and oxygen transport in fulminant hepatic failure. N Engl J Med 324:1852–1857, 1991.
21. Suter PM, Domenighetti G, Schaller MD, et al: N-acetylcysteine enhances recovery from acute lung injury in man: A randomized, double-blind, placebo-controlled clinical study. Chest 105:190–194, 1994.
22. Project Inform Hotline Handout on N-acetylcysteine. December 1998. Available at: http://www.thebody.com/pinf/nac.html.
23. Ruffman R, Wendel A: GSH rescue by N-acetylcysteine. Klin Wochenschr 69:857–862, 1991.
24. Buckpitt AR, Rollins DE, Mitchell JR: Varying effects of sulfhydryl nucelophiles on acetaminophen oxidation and sulfhydryl adduct formation. Biochem Pharmacol 28:2841–2946, 1979.
25. Lauterberg BH, Corcoran GB, Mitchell JR: Mechanism of action of N-acetylcysteine in the protection against the hepatotoxicity of acetaminophen in rats in vivo. J Clin Invest 71:980–991, 1983.
26. Smilkstein MJ, Bronstein AC, Linden CH, et al: Acetaminophen overdose: A 48 hour intravenous N-acetylcysteine protocol. Ann Emerg Med 20:1058–1063, 1991.
27. Smilkstein MJ, Knapp GI, Kulig KW, et al: Efficacy of oral N-acetylcysteine in the treatment of acetaminophen overdose: Analysis of the national multicenter study (1976–1985). N Engl J Med 319:1557–1562, 1988.
28. Harrison PM, Keays R, Bray GP, et al: Improved outcome of paracetamol-induced fulminant hepatic failure by late administration of acetylcysteine. Lancet 3:1572–1573, 1990.
29. Jones AL: Mechanism of action and value of N-acetylcysteine in the treatment of early and late acetaminophen poisoning: A critical review. Clin Toxicol 36:277–285, 1998.
30. De Caro L, Ghizzi A, Costa R, et al: Pharmacokinetics and bioavailability of oral acetylcysteine in healthy volunteers. Arzneim-Forsch/Drug Res 39:382–386, 1989.
31. North DS, Peterson RG, Krenzelok EP: Effect of activated charcoal administration on acetylcysteine serum levels in humans. Am J Hosp Pharm 38:1022–1024, 1981.
32. Borgstrom L, Kagedal B, Paulsen O: Pharmacokinetics of N-acetylcysteine in man. Eur J Clin Pharmacol 31:217–222, 1986.
33. Olsson B, Johanson M, Gabrielsson J, et al: Pharmacokinetics and bioavailability of reduced and oxidized N-acetylcysteine. Eur J Clin Pharmacol 34:77–82, 1988.
34. Toll LL, Hurlbut KM (eds): N-acetylcysteine Management, POISINDEX System, Volume 110. Greenwood Village, CO, MICROMEDEX, Inc, 2001.
35. Prescott LF, Donovan JW, Jarvie DR, et al: The disposition and kinetics of intravenous N-acetylcysteine in patients with paracetamol overdosage. Eur J Clin Pharmacol 37:501–506, 1989.
36. Ekins B, Ford D, Thompson M, et al: The effect of activated charcoal on N-acetylcysteine absorption in normal subjects. Am J Emerg Med 5:483–487, 1987.
37. Renzi F, Donovan J, Morgan L, et al: Concomitant use of activated charcoal and N-acetylcysteine. Ann Emerg Med 14:568–572, 1985.
38. Jones AL, Jarvie DR, Simpson D, et al: Pharmacokinetics of N-acetylcysteine are altered in patients with chronic liver disease. Aliment Pharmacol Ther 11:787–791, 1997.
39. Riggs BS, Bronstein AC, Kulig KW, et al: Acute acetaminophen overdose during pregnancy. Obstet Gynecol 74:247–253, 1989.
40. Wang PH, Yang MJ, Lee WL, et al: Acetaminophen poisoning in late pregnancy: A case report. J Reprod Med 42:367–371, 1997.
41. Horowitz RS, Dart RC, Jarvie DR, et al: Placental transfer of N-acetylcysteine following human maternal acetaminophen toxicity. J Toxicol Clin Toxicol 35:447–451, 1997.
42. Miller LF, Rumack BH: Clinical safety of high oral doses of acetylcysteine. Semin Oncol 10(Suppl 1):76–85, 1983.
43. Scharman EJ: Use of ondansetron and other antiemetics in the management of toxic acetaminophen ingestions. J Toxicol Clin Toxicol 36:19–25, 1998.
44. Mrvos R, Benitez JG, Krenzelok EP: Angioedema with oral N-acetylcysteine (Letter). Ann Emerg Med 30:240–241, 1997.
45. Mohammed S: Serum sickness-like illness associated with N-acetylcysteine therapy (Letter). Ann Pharmacother 28:285, 1994.
46. Bonfiglio M, Traeger S, Hulisz D, et al: Anaphylactoid reaction to IV acetylcysteine associated with electrocardiographic abnormalities. Pharmacotherapy 26:22–25, 1992.
47. Bateman DN, Woodhouse KW, Rawlins MD: Adverse reactions to N-acetylcysteine. Hum Toxicol 3:393–398, 1984.
48. Dawson A, Henry D, McEwen J: Adverse reactions to N-acetylcysteine during treatment for paracetamol poisoning. Med J Aust 150:329–331, 1989.
49. Mant TG, Tempowski JH, Volans GN, et al: Adverse reactions to acetylcysteine and effects of overdose. BMJ 289:217–219, 1984.
50. Death after N-acetylcysteine (Notes and News). Lancet 1:142, 1984.
51. Bailey B, McGuigan MA: Management of anaphylactoid reactions to intravenous N-acetylcysteine. Ann Emerg Med 31:710–715, 1998.

52. Woo OF, Mueller PD, Olson KR, et al: Shorter duration of oral N-acetylcysteine therapy for acute acetaminophen overdose. Ann Emerg Med 35:363–368, 2000.

53. Prescott LF, Illingworth RN, Critchley JA, et al: Intravenous N-acetylcysteine: The treatment of choice for paracetamol poisoning. BMJ 2:1097–1100, 1979.

54. Smilkstein MJ, Bronstein AC, Linden CH, et al: Acetaminophen overdose: A 48 hour intravenous N-acetylcysteine protocol. Ann Emerg Med 20:1058–1063, 1991.

55. Buckley NA, Whyte IM, O'Connell DL, et al: Oral or intravenous N-acetylcysteine: Which is the treatment of choice for acetaminophen (paracetamol) poisoning. J Toxicol Clin Toxicol 37:759–767, 1999.

56. Yip L, Dart RC, Hurlbut KM: Intravenous administration of oral N-acetylcysteine. Crit Care Med 26:40–43, 1998.

57. Perry HE, Shannon MW: Efficacy of oral versus intravenous N-acetylcysteine in acetaminophen overdose: Results of an open-label, clinical trial. J Pediatr 132:149–152, 1998.

CHAPTER **137**

Opioid Antagonists

In-Hei Hahn ■ Lewis S. Nelson

Despite the long history of opioid use, opioid antagonists were not developed until the 20th century. The impetus for their development was, at least in part, the increasing incidence of abuse and overdose, coinciding with the understanding that minor structural alterations to certain opioid agonists impart antagonist activity. In the 1940s, *N*-allylnormorphine (nalorphine) became widely used to reverse the adverse effects of opioid agonists, but its agonist-antagonist nature was not defined until 1954.[1] Further refinements led to the subsequent development of naloxone, naltrexone, and nalmefene (Fig. 137-1), the opioid antagonists currently in routine clinical use.

PHARMACODYNAMICS

Opioid antagonists are structural analogues of opioid agonists and are effective at the μ, κ, and δ receptors. These agents antagonize most competitively at the μ receptor; higher doses are required to affect the κ and δ receptors. As competitive antagonists, they have no significant effect in the absence of opioid agonists.

Opioid antagonists reverse all the effects of endogenous and exogenous opioid agonists at the μ, κ, and δ receptors if an adequate dose has been administered. Reversal of opioid agonism corrects most signs of opioid poisoning, including respiratory and CNS depression, analgesia, miosis, inhibition of baroreceptors, muscular rigidity, vasodilation, and gastrointestinal immobility. Opioid antagonists do not reverse opioid-associated histamine release (morphine, meperidine, and codeine)[2,3] and the sodium channel antagonist effects of propoxyphene.

Opioid antagonists can also prevent opioid agonism if given as pretreatment. Their most consequential effects are at the μ receptor subtype, where they may precipitate opioid withdrawal symptoms (yawning, rhinorrhea, lacrimation, nausea, vomiting, diaphoresis, piloerection, mydriasis, abdominal cramping, diarrhea, and insomnia) in opioid-tolerant patients. Opioid withdrawal is not in itself life-threatening, although morbidity and mortality occur. Most concerning is precipitating withdrawal-associated emesis in a patient whose mental status is altered concomitantly by another substance (e.g., ethanol) or another condition (e.g., head injury), leading to catastrophic effects. Specifically, pulmonary aspiration and its sequelae may occur owing to the inability to clear or protect the airway. To that end, the lowest dose necessary to reverse the patient's respiratory depression should be administered initially (e.g., 0.05 mg of naloxone) and titrated upward to clinical effect. The goal of administration is alleviation of respiratory depression and avoidance of precipitation of withdrawal. It rarely is necessary to administer higher doses (≥0.2 mg) of naloxone initially because the primary desired effect of naloxone, the reversal of respiratory depression, may be provided by exogenous ventilation with a bag-valve-mask apparatus. Dosing in this manner may prevent the effect of precipitation of opioid withdrawal yet allow the larger dose ultimately to be administered in the rare instances in which it is required.

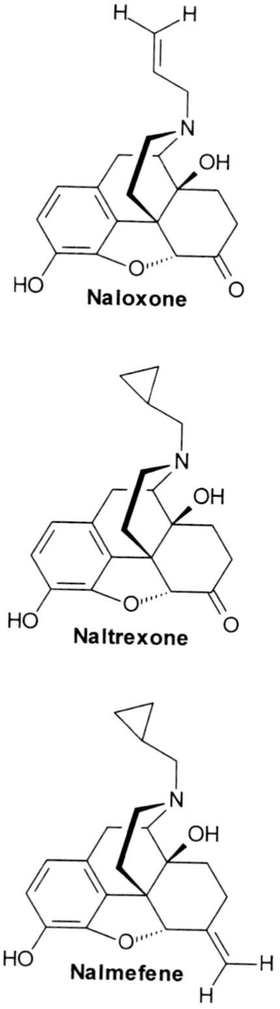

FIGURE 137-1

Chemical structures of naloxone, naltrexone, and nalmefene.

PHARMACOKINETICS

Although opioid antagonists are remarkably similar in clinical effects, they differ markedly in their pharmacokinetic profile. The durations of action of nalmefene (4 to 6 hours) and naltrexone (approximately 24 hours) are substantially longer than that of naloxone (20 to 30 minutes). The practical implication of their pharmacokinetic differences is that the opioid poisoning may recur, particularly if a short-acting opioid antagonist (e.g., naloxone) is administered to a patient exposed to a long-acting agonist (e.g., methadone). Although an agent with a longer duration of action is preferable to promote abstinence and prevent resedation, a short-acting agent is preferred initially to allow resolution of inadvertently precipitated withdrawal.

CONTRAINDICATIONS

Opioid antagonists should not be used in certain populations, specifically opioid-dependent neonates and patients using cocaine in combination with opioids, colloquially known as a speedball. Reversal of a heroin-cocaine overdose with naloxone may result in the unopposed effects of cocaine and lead to a cardiac dysrhythmia.[4] Opioid-dependent neonates who develop withdrawal may have life-threatening seizures (see Chapter 56).

TREATMENT

In the event that naloxone is administered in excess to a patient presenting with an opioid overdose (which is seen frequently when naloxone is administered in the field by paramedics or iatrogenically in the hospital), the treatment recommended during the period of withdrawal is first an explanation, which should include the reassurance that the symptoms of withdrawal are not life-threatening and will wane rapidly and that symptomatic care, such as antiemetic therapy for severe nausea and vomiting, will be provided. We do not recommend treating iatrogenically induced withdrawal symptoms with an opioid agonist because it is difficult to titrate an individual's opioid needs, and naloxone's short effects wane rapidly (duration of action is 30 minutes) without any intervention.

ADMINISTRATION

Naloxone and nalmefene must be given by a parenteral route owing to their extensive first-pass hepatic elimination. Naltrexone may be administered orally and typically is used for detoxification and maintenance of opioid abstinence secondary to its long duration of action.

Pharmacokinetics of Opioid Antagonists

Drug	Route	Dose	Elimination Half-life	Duration of Effect
Naloxone*	IM, IV, ET, SC	Neonate, 0.01 mg/kg	60–90 min	20–90 min
		Adult with opioid dependence, start 0.05 mg and titrate as necessary to avoid withdrawal symptoms and to preserve ventilation	—	—
		Adult without opioid dependence, start at 0.4 mg	—	—
Nalmefene†	IV, IM, SC	0.1 mg IV/IM for opioid-dependent subjects	11 hr	4–6 hr
		0.5 mg if no signs of withdrawal, followed by 1 mg q 2–5 min if necessary	—	—
		Postoperative opioid depression, start at 0.25 µg/kg and redose at 0.25 µg/kg q 2–5 min to desired effect up to 1 µg/kg	—	—
Naltrexone†	PO	50 mg PO daily	10 hr	24 hr

ET, endotracheal; IM, intramuscular; IV, intravenous; PO, oral; SC, subcutaneous.

*From Reisine T, Pasternak G: Opiod analgesics and antagonists. In Hardman JG, Limbird LE, Molinoff PB, et al (eds): Goodman and Gilman's The Pharmacological Basis of Therapeutics, 9th ed. New York, McGraw-Hill, 1996, pp 521–555.

†From Howland MA: Opioid antagonists. In Goldfrank LR, Flomenbaum NE, Lewin BA, et al (eds): Goldfrank's Toxicological Emergencies, 6th ed. Stamford, CT, Appleton & Lange, 1998, pp 996–1000.

REFERENCES

1. Hart ER, McCauley EL: The pharmacology of n-allylnormorphine as compared with morphine. J Pharmacol Exp Ther 82:339–348, 1944.
2. Levy JH, Brister NW, Shearin WA, et al: Wheal and flare responses to opioids in humans. 70:756–760, 1989.
3. Ballantyne JC, Loach AB, Carr DB: Itching after epidural and spinal opiates. Pain 33:149–160, 1988.
4. Merigian KS: Cocaine-induced ventricular arrhythmias and rapid atrial fibrillation temporally related to nalozone administration. Am J Emerg Med 1:96–97, 1993.
5. Howland MA: Opioid antagonists. In Goldfrank LR, Flomenbaum NE, Lewin NA, et al (eds): Goldfrank's Toxicological Emergencies, 6th ed. Stamford, CT, Appleton & Lange, 1998, pp 996–1000.

CHAPTER **138**

Flumazenil

Stephen Munday ▪ Kevin L. Wallace

Flumazenil (Romazicon) is a specific benzodiazepine receptor antagonist that has generated debate regarding its clinical indications since its initial release in the United States in 1991. A major argument against the use of flumazenil in the management of benzodiazepine intoxication is the relatively high safety index (i.e., toxic-to-therapeutic dose ratio) of benzodiazepines. In addition, the anticonvulsant effects of benzodiazepines may be advantageous in individuals simultaneously poisoned by other substances with proconvulsant actions, such as tricyclic antidepressants. Another significant concern regarding the clinical use of flumazenil in the emergent management of poisoning is the possibility of precipitating acute withdrawal in individuals who have developed pharmacodynamic tolerance to benzodiazepine receptor agonist drugs. In contrast to naloxone-induced opioid withdrawal, which causes symptomatic distress but is not life-threatening, sedative-hypnotic withdrawal from benzodiazepines is associated with significant morbidity and mortality. These safety concerns have prevented flumazenil from gaining widespread clinical acceptance as a component of the initial pharmacologic management of coma (see Chapters 3 and 19).

CHEMICAL PROPERTIES

Flumazenil is an imidazobenzodiazepine similar in structure to midazolam (Fig. 138-1). It is formulated for intravenous administration primarily because it undergoes extensive first-pass metabolism after oral administration.[1]

PHARMACODYNAMICS

Pharmacokinetics of Flumazenil

Volume of distribution: approximately 1 L/kg
Protein binding: approximately 50%
Oral bioavailability: 16%
Onset of effects: 1–2 min
Peak effects: approximately 5 min
Mechanism of clearance: hepatic metabolism to inactive metabolites
Elimination half-life: 0.8 hr

Flumazenil was discovered during the screening of compounds for effects at the central nervous system benzodiazepine site on the γ-aminobutyric acid (GABA) receptor complexes of the $GABA_A$ subtype. The latter functions as ligand-gated chloride (Cl^-) channels (see Chapter 47 for a detailed discussion of $GABA_A$ receptor physiology).[2] Ligand interactions at the benzodiazepine receptor are of three types. Agonists, such as benzodiazepines, bind to the receptor and, as described, enhance the $GABA_A$-mediated Cl^- influx. Inverse agonists, such as certain β-carboline derivatives (Fig. 138-2), on binding decrease $GABA_A$-mediated Cl^- cell entry.[3] Competitive antagonists, such as flumazenil, prevent the binding of agonists and inverse agonists in a dose-dependent manner, suppressing both agonist and inverse agonist effects on the $GABA_A$ receptor (Fig. 138-3).[4]

Flumazenil has been shown to bind the benzodiazepine receptor based on displacement of radiolabeled diazepam and other benzodiazepines in vitro.[5] Subsequent in vivo animal and human studies with flumazenil have failed to reveal most of the expected benzodiazepine $GABA_A$ neuroinhibitory effects.[5–7] Although it initially was postulated that flumazenil might not penetrate the central nervous system, this subsequently was disproved, and flumazenil's antagonist properties were confirmed when it prevented or reversed the effects of concurrently administered benzodiazepines.[5] Flumazenil does not reverse the $GABA_A$ agonist–related sedative effects of meprobamate or phenobarbital or the inverse agonist–induced proconvulsant effects of picrotoxin because none of these agents exert their effects by binding to benzodiazepine receptors.[8]

Although initial studies suggested that flumazenil antagonizes the benzodiazepine receptor, some discrepancies have been noted.[7] Most compelling are animal and human data that hint at possible benzodiazepine agonist effects.[9] Studies of flumazenil in several animal models have shown anticonvulsant activity in the absence of exposure to benzodiazepines, despite the finding that in benzodiazepine-dependent animals flumazenil can precipitate convulsions.[10–13] Also, limited human studies of flumazenil have shown anticonvulsant activity.[14] Flumazenil-induced inverse agonism also may occur because some rodent studies have revealed evidence of increased anxiogenic effect under certain circumstances of flumazenil exposure.[15,16] Despite these findings, few data suggest that any weak inverse agonist activity is relevant at clinically appropriate doses.

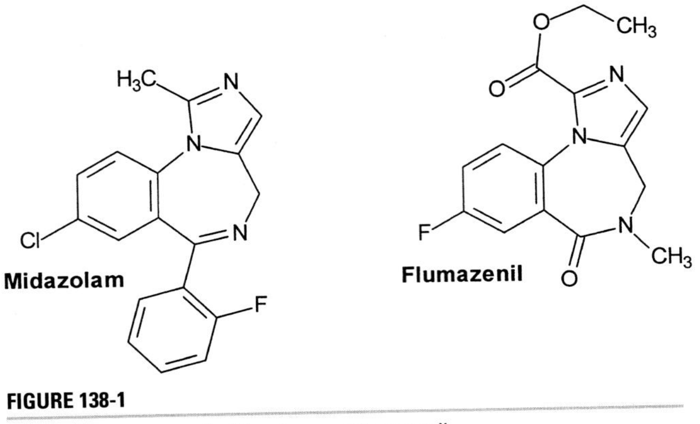

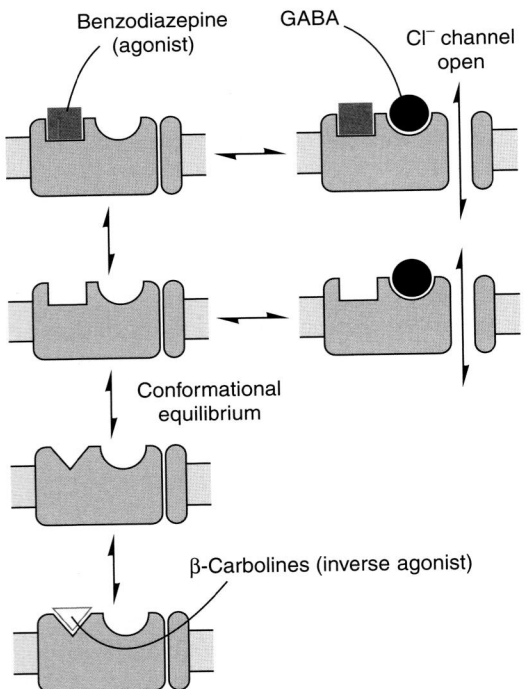

FIGURE 138-1

Chemical structures of midazolam and flumazenil.

Acute toxicity studies in rodents revealed oral median lethal dose values of 4300 to 6000 mg/kg.[6] Evaluation in human volunteers showed no serious toxicity in doses of 600 mg orally[17] and 100 mg intravenously.[18–20] Positron emission tomography has shown essentially complete benzodiazepine receptor occupancy in human adults after an intravenous flumazenil dose of 1.5 mg.[21]

FIGURE 138-2

Model of benzodiazepine/γ-aminobutyric acid (GABA) receptor interaction. Benzodiazepine agonists (e.g., diazepam) and antagonists (e.g., flumazenil) are believed to bind to a site on the GABA receptor distinct from the GABA-binding site. A conformational equilibrium exists between states in which the benzodiazepine receptor exists in its agonist-binding conformation *(above)* and in its antagonist binding conformation *(below)*. In the latter state, the GABA receptor has a greatly reduced affinity for GABA, and as a result the chloride (Cl−) channel remains closed. *(From Rang HP, Dale MM, Ritter JM, Gardner P: Other transmitters and modulators. In: Pharmacology, 4th ed. Philadelphia, Churchill Livingstone, 2001.)*

CLINICAL USE

Initial use of flumazenil was limited to reversal of benzodiazepine effects after conscious sedation and regional or general anesthesia.[22–34] One early randomized, double-blind study administered flumazenil, 0.1 mg/kg, or placebo to anesthetized patients. There was a significant improvement in level of consciousness in the flumazenil-treated patients compared with placebo-treated patients, and no serious side effects were reported. Many of the patients who received the flumazenil developed anxiety severe enough to require diazepam for sedation.[28] Subsequent studies have used lower doses—typically 1 mg or less.[26,27,32,33] In studies that limited flumazenil dose to 0.5 mg or less, no anxiety was noted.[23,24,34] Numerous evaluations in patients undergoing endoscopy, bronchoscopy, and cardiac catheterization have shown effective reversal of sedation. It also has been effective after orthopedic, urologic, and other surgical procedures, including studies that enrolled elderly and other high-risk patients.[35]

Although flumazenil has been effective at reversal of benzodiazepine-induced sedation, there is some evidence that other effects were not reversed fully. One study revealed minor residual memory deficit after flumazenil was administered to antagonize diazepam-induced sedation.[27] Controversy regarding flumazenil reversal of benzodiazepine-induced respiratory depression has been generated by the diversity of findings in the few studies that have been performed.[36] Much of the lack of scientific consensus in this regard seems to relate to the fact that a variety of respiratory parameters have been used as outcome measures, making direct comparisons among studies extremely difficult. In general, studies of effort-dependent respiratory function,[37–39] such as vital capacity, have been supportive of flumazenil-induced improvement. It is unclear, however, whether this improvement is due merely to improved conscious control of breathing, because studies of effort-independent respiratory parameters, such as the carbon dioxide respiratory response curve, have not shown consistent improvement in benzodiazepine-induced respiratory depression after administration of flumazenil.[4,30,40]

After studies showed flumazenil's efficacy in reversing benzodiazepine-induced sedation, reports began to emerge describing its use to reverse the effects of benzodiazepine overdose. The first report included nine patients in coma from excessive doses of benzodiazepines. The group was diverse and included four patients who were iatrogenically oversedated, four patients who were treated for status epilepticus, and one patient who had attempted suicide. All patients had improvement in mental status and improvement in electroencephalogram patterns after being treated with 10 mg of flumazenil intravenously. Several patients became resedated after 3 to 5 hours. One patient who had been treated for status epilepticus developed focal seizures, but no other significant side effects were reported.[41]

Subsequent published reports have shown efficacy in poisoning involving diazepam, oxazepam, midazolam, flunitrazepam, flurazepam, nitrazepam, and triazolam.[4,19,42–44] Although, as previously mentioned, large flumazenil doses were used in early studies (in some instances, >0.1 mg/kg), further evaluation has shown that doses of 0.1 mg may be effective in reversing benzodiazepine-induced sedation. In

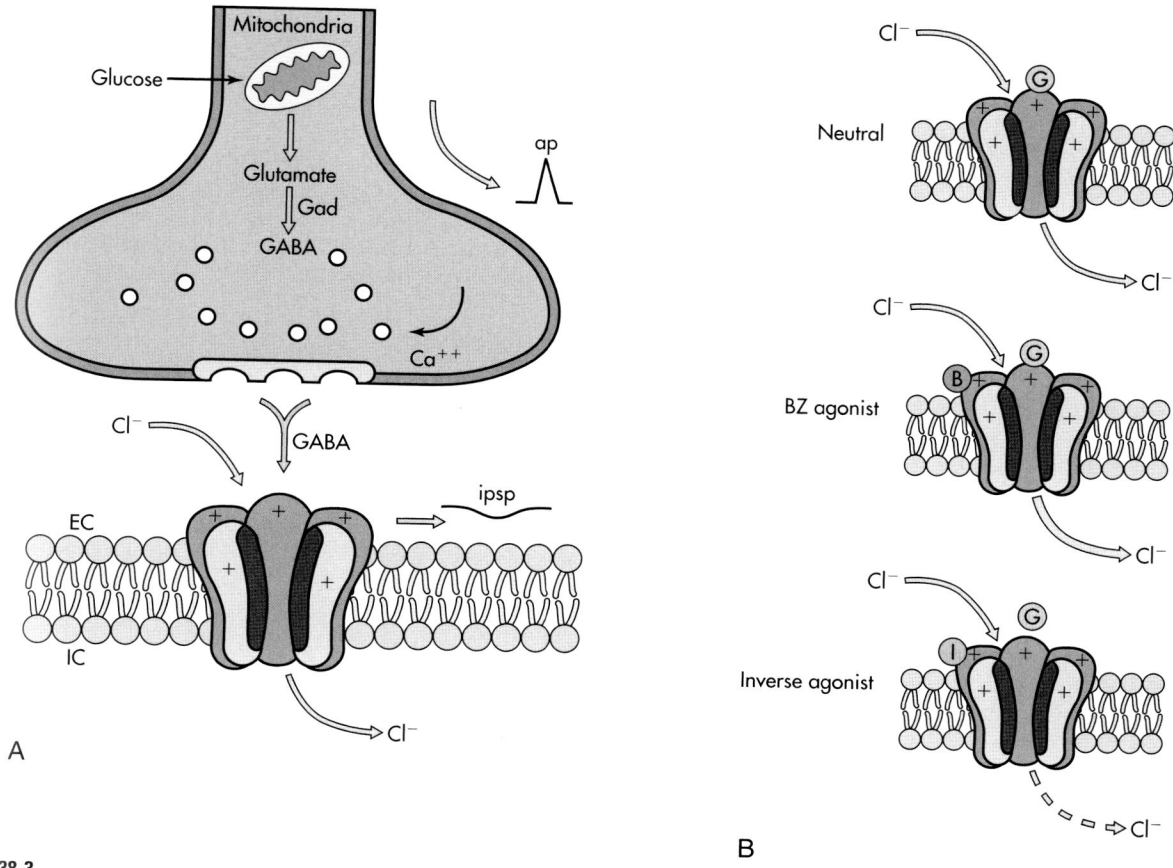

FIGURE 138-3

Idealized model of γ-aminobutyric acid (GABA)-benzodiazepine (BZ)-chloride (Cl⁻) channel at axosomatic (postsynaptic) inhibitory synapses. **A**, Presynaptic and postsynaptic elements. ap, Action potential; EC, extracellular; Gad, glutamic acid decarboxylase; IC, intracellular; ipsp, inhibitory postsynaptic potential. **B**, GABA-BZ receptor interactions influencing permeability of Cl⁻ channels. *Neutral:* GABA receptor binds GABA (G) with moderate affinity in the absence of BZ ligand. *BZ agonist:* Direct BZ agonist (B) enhances GABA affinity for its receptor, resulting in maximal Cl⁻ permeability. *Inverse agonist:* Inverse agonists bound to BZ receptor result in poor GABA affinity and markedly reduced Cl⁻ permeability. *(From Rech RH: Drugs to treat anxieties and related disorders. In Brody TM, Larner J, Minneman KP [eds]: Human Pharmacology: Molecular to Clinical, 3rd ed. St. Louis, Mosby, 1998, p 367.)*

one large study, more than half of benzodiazepine-poisoned patients responded to 3 mg, and nearly three quarters responded to 5 mg; a single patient required 8 mg for a measurable response.[45] Because the interaction between benzodiazepines and flumazenil is competitive, however, the larger the benzodiazepine dose, the higher the dose of flumazenil that would be required to reverse the former's central nervous system depressant effects.[46,47]

Patients at risk for adverse effects of flumazenil administration include patients who are benzodiazepine dependent. Acute benzodiazepine withdrawal, manifested by agitation, peripheral hyperadrenergic signs (e.g., tachycardia, hypertension, diaphoresis), or convulsions, may occur after flumazenil administration.[48–51]

Another population of concern comprises patients who present after concomitant overdose of benzodiazepines and proconvulsant drugs, such as tricyclic antidepressants. Reports of seizure occurrence in temporal association with the empirical use of flumazenil in the management of suspected benzodiazepine overdose rapidly emerged during the early postmarketing surveillance period.[25,45,52–58] One clearly plausible explanation for this phenomenon is flumazenil-induced removal of benzodiazepine-mediated anticonvulsant protection against the proconvulsant effects

of other drugs, such as tricyclic antidepressants.[59] Animal data that support this supposition have been reported.[54]

Iatrogenic convulsions as a complication of the intended antidotal use of flumazenil also have been reported in a case of combined diazepam and baclofen poisoning[60] and in combined propoxyphene and benzodiazepine overdose.[45] Reported cardiac complications of flumazenil administration have included cardiac arrest in a patient who was 5 days status post anterior myocardial infarction and had been excessively sedated with diazepam[61] and complete heart block in a 79-year-old woman who was self-poisoned by acetaminophen and temazepam.[9] Although there is a temporal association between these reported complications and the use of flumazenil, other operational criteria used to assess the likelihood of a cause-and-effect relationship, such as response to drug rechallenge, are not fulfilled in these cases.

Flumazenil has been shown to reverse the sedative-hypnotic effects of zolpidem, another benzodiazepine receptor agonist.[62] It also has been studied for its ability to reverse ethanol intoxication, with uncontrolled human studies suggesting possible efficacy in this setting.[59,63] Carefully performed controlled studies in ethanol-toxic animals and humans have not shown significant benefit, however.[50,54,64,65] Evidence to suggest a role for flumazenil in the management of carbamazepine poisoning is limited to a single case report.[66]

The clinical application of flumazenil in fulminant hepatic failure also has been studied. The lethargy and sedation in patients with hepatic encephalopathy seems to be related, to some extent, to increased levels of endogenous, centrally active benzodiazepine receptor ligands.[67] Initial animal data and subsequent human case reports of improvement in hepatic encephalopathy with the use of flumazenil have been confirmed by a double-blind, placebo-controlled trial.[68] In none of the enrolled subjects in this and other studies did mental status return to normal, however, and in subjects who responded, the improvement was temporary.[69–71]

ADMINISTRATION

Flumazenil generally is available only as an intravenous preparation. In the United States, it is formulated as a 10-mL vial containing 0.1 mg of flumazenil per mL of normal saline and small amounts of methylparaben, propylparaben, edetate sodium, and acetic acid. Sodium hydroxide or hydrochloric acid or both are used to adjust the pH of the solution to 7.4.

The product insert recommends that the smallest effective dose of the drug be given and that for reversal of conscious sedation it should be administered at an intravenous rate of 0.2 mg/min to an initial dose of 1 mg or less. In patients treated for benzodiazepine poisoning, the recommendation is 0.5 mg/min to a total of 5 mg. Flumazenil doses of 10 mg have been well tolerated, however, in acutely benzodiazepine-poisoned patients with no contraindications,[45,72] and much larger doses have been used in volunteers without significant sequelae.[17–19,73] In children 1 year old or older, the recommended intravenous flumazenil dose for reversal of conscious sedation with benzodiazepines is 0.01 mg/kg (maximum 0.2 mg) over 15 seconds, with repeat administration of bolus doses of 0.01 mg/kg (maximum 0.2 mg) at 1-minute intervals, as needed for adequate clinical reversal, up to four times or a maximal total dose of 0.05 mg/kg or 1 mg, whichever is lower.

Absolute contraindications to flumazenil administration include allergies to flumazenil or any components of its formulation. Relative contraindications include (1) use in patients poisoned by proconvulsant agents (e.g., tricyclic antidepressants, propoxyphene) because this may remove the desirable anticonvulsant effects of coingested benzodiazepines and (2) use in patients at risk of benzodiazepine or other sedative-hypnotic withdrawal.[45]

REFERENCES

1. Whitwan G, Amrein R: Pharmacology of flumazenil. Acta Anaesthesiol Scand 39(Suppl 108):3–14, 1995.
2. Haefely W, Hunkelr W: The story of flumazenil. Eur J Anaesthesiol 2(Suppl):3–13, 1988.
3. Mehta AK, Ticku MK: Benzodiazepine and beta-carboline interactions with GABA$_A$ receptor-gated chloride channels in mammalian cultured spinal cord neurons. J Pharmacol Exp Ther 249:418–423, 1989.
4. Brogden RN, Goa KL: Flumazenil: A reappraisal of its pharmacological properties and therapeutic efficacy as a benzodiazepine antagonist. Drugs 42:1061–1089, 1991.
5. Hunkeler W, Mohler H, Pieri L, et al: Selective antagonists of benzodiazepines. Nature 290:514–516, 1981.
6. Dunton AW, Schwam E, Pitman V, et al: Flumazenil: US clinical pharmacology studies. Eur J Anaesth 2:81–95, 1988.
7. File SE, Pellow S: Intrinsic actions of the benzodiazepine receptor antagonist Ro 15-1788. Psychopharmacology 88:1–11, 1986.
8. Bonetti EP, Pieri L, Cumin R, et al: Benzodiazepine antagonist Ro 15-1788L neurological and behavioral effects. Psychopharmacology 78:8–18, 1982.
9. Herd B, Clarke F: Complete heart block after flumazenil. Hum Exp Toxicol 10:289, 1991.
10. Cole SO: Dose-dependent reversal of chlordiazepoxide-induced discrimination impairment by Ro-15-1788. Psychopharmacology 96:458–461, 1988.
11. Grockseh G, Prado De Carvalbo L, Venault P, et al: Convulsions induced by submaximal dose of pentylenetetrazol in mice are antagonized by the benzodiazepine antagonist Ro 15-1788. Life Sci 32:2579–2584, 1983.
12. Loscher W, Honack D, Fassbender CP: Physical dependence on diazepam in the dog: Precipitation of different abstinence syndromes by the benzodiazepine receptor antagonists Ro 15-1788 and ZK 93426. Br J Pharmacol 97:843–852, 1989.
13. Nutt DI, Cowen PI: Unusual interactions of benzodiazepine receptor antagonists. Nature 295:436–438, 1982.
14. Scollo-Lavizzari G: The clinical anti-convulsant effects of flumazenil, a benzodiazepine antagonist. Eur J Anaesth 2(Suppl):129–138, 1988.
15. File SE, Pellow S: The anxiogenic action of Ro 15-1788 is reversed by chronic, but not by acute treatment with chlordiazepoxide. Brain Res 310:154–156, 1984.
16. Wagner IA, Katz RI: Anxiogenic action of benzodiazepine antagonists Ro 15-1788 and CGS 8216 in the rat. Neurosci Lett 48:317–320, 1984.
17. Darragh A, Lambe R, Brick I, et al: Antagonism of the central effects of 3-methylclonazepam. Br J Clin Pharmacol 14:871–872, 1982.
18. Bosman DK, Van Den Buijs CACG, De Haan JC, et al: The effects of benzodiazepine-receptor antagonists and partial inverse agonists on acute hepatic encephalopathy in the rat. Gastroenterology 101:772–781, 1991.
19. Breheny FX: Reversal of midazolam sedation with flumazenil. Crit Care Med 20:736–739, 1991.
20. Darragh A, Lambe R, Kenny M, et al: Tolerance of healthy volunteers to intravenous administration of the benzodiazepine antagonist Ro-15-1788. Eur J Clin Pharmacol 24:569–570, 1983.
21. Persson A, Pauli S, Halldin C, et al: Saturation analysis of specific ^{11}C Ro 15-1788 binding to the human neocortex using positron emission tomography. Hum Psychopharmacol 4:21–31, 1989.
22. Alon E, Baitella L, Hossli G: Double-blind study of the reversal of midazolam supplemented general anesthesia with Ro 15-1788. Br J Anaesth 59:455–458, 1987.
23. Dimitriou B, Kottis G, Bathrelou S, et al: Flumazenil in reversal of central effects of midazolam used as induction agent in general anesthesia. Drug Res 39:399–400, 1989.

Indications and Contraindications for Flumazenil Administration

Indications

Reversal of benzodiazepine-induced conscious sedation or general anesthesia

Isolated severe benzodiazepine poisoning (e.g., with respiratory failure)

Contraindications

ABSOLUTE

Allergy to flumazenil or any coformulant

RELATIVE

Benzodiazepine receptor agonist (e.g., ethanol, benzodiazepine drug, zolpidem) dependence

Concomitant proconvulsant (e.g., tricyclic antidepressant, propoxyphene, bupropion) overdose or toxicity

Underlying life-threatening disorder (e.g., status epilepticus) for which benzodiazepines have been administered

24. Fisher GC, Hutton P: Cardiovascular responses to flumazenil-induced arousal after arterial surgery. Anesthesiology 44:104–106, 1989.

25. Geller E, Niv D, Matzkin C, et al: The antagonism of midazolam sedation by Ro 15-1788 in 50 postoperative patients. Anesthesiology 63:A369, 1985.

26. Geller E, Niv D, Nevo Y, et al: Early clinical experience in reversing benzodiazepine sedation with flumazenil after short procedures. Resuscitation 16(Suppl):549–556, 1988.

27. Ghoneim MM, Dembo JB, Block RI: Time course of antagonism of sedative and amnesic effects of diazepam by flumazenil. Anesthesiology 70:899–904, 1989.

28. Louis M, Forster A, Suter PM, et al: Clinical and hemodynamic effects of a specific benzodiazepine antagonist (Ro-15-1788) after open heart surgery. Anesthesiology 61:A61, 1984.

29. Marty J, Nitenberg A, Phillip I, et al: Coronary hemodynamic responses following reversal of benzodiazepine-induced sedation with flumazenil in patient with coronary artery disease. Anesthesiology 69:A110, 1988.

30. Mora CT, Torjman M, White PF: Effects of diazepam and flumazenil on sedation and hypoxic ventilatory response. Anesth Analg 68:473–478, 1989.

31. Ricou B, Forster A, Brückner A, et al: Clinical evaluation of a specific benzodiazepine antagonist (Ro-15-1788). Br J Anaesth 58:1005–1011, 1986.

32. Rosenbaum NL, Hooper PA: The effects of flumazenil, a new benzodiazepine antagonist, on the reversal of midazolam sedation and amnesia in dental patients. Br Dent J 65:400–402, 1985.

33. White PF, Shafer A, Boyle WA, et al: Benzodiazepine antagonism does not provoke a stress response. Anesthesiology 70:636–639, 1989.

34. Wolff J, Carl P, Clausen TG, et al: Ro 15-1788 for postoperative recovery. Anesthesiology 41:1001–1006, 1986.

35. Katz JA, Fragen RJ, Dunn KL: Flumazenil reversal of midazolam sedation of the elderly. Reg Anesth 16:247–252, 1991.

36. Shalansky SJ, Naumann TL, Englander FA: Therapy update: Effect of flumazenil on benzodiazepine-induced respiratory depression. Clin Pharm 12:483–487, 1993.

37. Jensen S, Kirkegaard L, Anderson BN: Randomized clinical investigation of Ro-15-1788, a benzodiazepine antagonist, in reversing the central effects of flunitrazepam. Eur J Anaesth 4:113–118, 1987.

38. Jensen S, Kirkegaard L, Anderson BN: Randomized clinical investigation of Ro-15-1788, a benzodiazepine antagonist, in reversing the central effects of flunitrazepam. Acta Anaesth Scand 88(suppl):89–90, 1985.

39. Radakovic D, Toia D, Bentzinger C: Double-blind, placebo-controlled study of the effects of Ro 15-1788 (flumazenil, Anexate) on recovery of ventilatory function after total intravenous anaesthesia with midazolam-alfentanyl. Eur J Anaesth 2(Suppl):279–282, 1988.

40. Hunkeler W: Preclinical research findings with flumazenil (Ro 15-1788, Anexate): Chemistry. Eur J Anaesth 2(Suppl):37–62, 1988.

41. Scollo-Lavizzari G: First clinical investigation of the benzodiazepine antagonist (Ro-15-1788) in comatose patients. Eur Neurol 22:7–11, 1983.

42. Carter AS, Bell GD, Coady T, et al: Speed of reversal of midazolam-induced respiratory depression by flumazenil: A study in patients undergoing upper GI endoscopy. Acta Anaesth Scand 34:59–64, 1990.

43. Gross JB, Weller RS, Conard P: Flumazenil antagonism of midazolam-induced ventilatory depression. Anesthesiology 75:179–185, 1991.

44. Klotz U, Kant J: Pharmacokinetics and clinical use of flumazenil. Clin Pharmacokinet 14:1–12, 1988.

45. Spivey WH: Flumazenil and seizures: Analysis of 43 cases. Clin Ther 14:292–305, 1992.

46. Paul S, Marangos PJ, Skolnick P: The benzodiazepine GABA-chloride ionophore receptor complex. Biol Psychiatry 16:213–229, 1981.

47. Twyman RE, Rogers CJ, MacDonald RL: Differential regulation of GABA receptor channels by diazepam and phenobarbital. Ann Neurol 25:213–220, 1989.

48. Amrein R, Hetzel W, Hartmann D, Lorscheid T: Clinical pharmacology of flumazenil. Eur J Anaesth 2:65–80, 1988.

49. Amrein R, Leishman B, Bentzinger C, Roncari G: Flumazenil in benzodiazepine antagonism: Actions and clinical use in intoxications and anaesthesiology. Med Toxicol 2:411–429, 1987.

50. Flückiger A, Hartmann D, Leishmann B, et al: Lack of effect of the benzodiazepine antagonist flumazenil (Ro 15-1788) on the performance of healthy subjects during experimentally induced ethanol intoxication. Eur J Clin Pharmacol 34:273–276, 1988.

51. Lukes SE, Griffiths RR: Precipitated withdrawal by a benzodiazepine receptor antagonist (Ro-15-1788) after 7 days of diazepam. Science 217:1161–1163, 1982.

52. Gueye PN, Hoffman JR, Taboulet P, et al: Empiric use of flumazenil in comatose patients: Limited applicability of criteria to define low risk. Ann Emerg Med 27:730–735, 1996.

53. Haverkos GP, DiSalvo RP, Imhoff TE: Fatal seizures after flumazenil administration in a patient with mixed overdose. Ann Pharmacother 28:1347–1349, 1994.

54. Lheureux P, Vranckx M, Leduc D, Askenasi R: Flumazenil in mixed benzodiazepine/tricyclic antidepressant overdose: A placebo controlled study in the dog. Am J Emerg Med 10:184–188, 1992.

55. Lim AG: Death after flumazenil. BMJ 299:858–859, 1989.

56. Mordel A, Winkler E, Almog S, et al: Seizures after flumazenil administration in a case of combined benzodiazepine and tricyclic antidepressant overdose. Crit Care Med 20:1733–1734, 1992.

57. Weinbroum A, Halpern P, Geller E: The use of flumazenil in the management of acute drug poisoning: A review. Intensive Care Med 17:S32–S38, 1991.

58. Winkler E, Shlomo A, Kriger D, et al: Use of flumazenil in the diagnosis and treatment of patients with a coma of unknown etiology. Crit Care Med 21:538–542, 1993.

59. Martens F, Köppel C, Ibe K, et al: Clinical experience with the benzodiazepine antagonist flumazenil in suspected benzodiazepine or ethanol poisoning. J Toxicol Clin Toxicol 28:341–356, 1990.

60. Chern TY, Kwan A: Flumazenil-induced seizure accompanying benzodiazepine and baclofen intoxication. Am J Emerg Med 14:231–232, 1996.

61. Katz Y, Boulos, M, Singer P, et al: Cardiac arrest associated with flumazenil. BMJ 304:1415, 1992.

62. Naef MM, Forster A, Nahory A, et al: Flumazenil antagonizes the sedative action of zolpidem, a new imidazopyridine hypnotic. Anesthesiology 71:A297, 1989.

63. Scollo-Lavizzari G, Matthis H: Antagonist (Ro 15-1788) in ethanol intoxication pilot study. Eur Neurol 24:352–354, 1985.

64. Clausen TG, Wolff J, Carl P, Theilgaard A: The effect of the benzodiazepine antagonist, flumazenil, on psychometric performance in acute ethanol intoxication in man. Eur J Clin Pharmacol 38:233–236, 1990.

65. Linowiecki K, Paloucek F, Donnelly A, Leikin JB: Reversal of ethanol-induced respiratory depression by flumazenil. Vet Hum Toxicol 34:417–419, 1992.

66. Zuber M, Elsasser R, Ritz R, et al: Flumazenil (Anexate) in severe intoxication with carbamazepine (Tegretol). Eur Neurol 28:161–163, 1988.

67. Basile AS, Hughes RD, Harrison PM, et al: Elevated brain concentrations of 1,4-benzodiazepines in fulminant hepatic failure. N Engl J Med 325:473–478, 1991.

68. Pomier-Layrargues G, Giguére JF, Lavoie J, et al: Flumazenil in cirrhotic patients in hepatic coma: A randomized double-blind placebo-controlled crossover trial. Hepatology 19:32–37, 1994.

69. Ferenci P, Grimm G, Meryn S, Gangl A: Successful long-term treatment of portal-systemic encephalopathy by the benzodiazepine antagonist flumazenil. Gastroenterology 96:240–243, 1989.

70. Howard CD, Seifert CF: Flumazenil in the treatment of the hepatic encephalopathy. Ann Pharmacother 27:46–47, 1993.

71. Van der Rijt CC, de Knegt RJ, Schalm SW, et al: Flumazenil does not improve hepatic encephalopathy associated with acute ischemic liver failure in the rabbit. Metab Brain Dis 3:131–141, 1990.

72. Skolnick P: The γ-aminobutyric acid A (GABA$_A$) receptor complex. In: Jones EA (moderator): The γ-aminobutyric acid A (GABA$_A$) receptor complex and hepatic encephalopathy: Some recent advances. Ann Intern Med 100:532–546, 1989.

73. Darragh A, Lambe R, Kenny M, et al: Tolerance of healthy volunteers to intravenous administration of the benzodiazepine antagonist Ro-15-1788. Eur J Clin Pharmacol 24:569–570, 1983.

CHAPTER 139

Dimercaprol (BAL)

Michael J. Kosnett

Dimercaprol is the generic term for 2,3-dimercaptopropranol. Because British investigators developed dimercaprol during World War II as an antidote to the war gas lewisite, it also came to be known as *British antilewisite* or *BAL*.

HISTORY

The development of dimercaprol as an antidote to the organoarsenical agent lewisite (dichloro [2-chlorovinyl] arsine) extended earlier observations that the action of arsenoxide drugs involved biochemical interaction with the thiol groups of enzymes and that this process could be mitigated by a large excess of sulfhydryl reagents. After screening many monothiol and dithiol chemicals, Peters and coworkers[1] found that the dithiol compound 2,3-dimercaptopropranol was most effective at preventing lewisite-induced inhibition of pyruvate oxidase and protecting experimental animals from lewisite's vesicant and lethal effects. A penetrating oily liquid, dimercaprol initially was conceived of as a topical treatment for lewisite burns to the eyes and skin. Subsequent studies found that topical and intramuscular injections of dimercaprol alleviated severe dermatologic and systemic complications associated with organoarsenical antibiotics used in the treatment of syphilis.[2] Within 3 years, the use of dimercaprol extended to treatment of poisoning by inorganic heavy metals, particularly inorganic arsenic and mercuric salts.[3] It still is used for this purpose today.

CHEMICAL AND PHYSICAL PROPERTIES

Dimercaprol (Fig. 139-1) ($C_3H_8OS_2$; molecular weight 124.2) is an oily, colorless liquid with a skunk-like mercaptan odor. Although soluble in water to 6% (weight/volume), the vicinal thiol groups are readily oxidized in aqueous solutions. To achieve greater stability, the pharmaceutical product is prepared as a 10% solution (100 mg/mL) in peanut oil that also contains 20% (200 mg/mL) benzyl benzoate. Dimercaprol forms 1:1 or 2:1 complexes with several metals in vitro; however, the nature of metal complexes formed by dimercaprol or its metabolites in vivo has not been determined.

PHARMACODYNAMICS

Dimercaprol increases the urinary excretion of certain toxic metals (particularly arsenic, lead, and mercury). In animal studies, it has been shown to redistribute mercury and arsenic to the brain, however.[4,5] Dimercaprol increases elimination of copper, an essential trace mineral. In human studies, dimercaprol injection results in a transient increase in blood pressure and heart rate, but it otherwise has no clinically significant pharmacodynamic impact on cardiovascular, hepatic, or renal function.

PHARMACOKINETICS

In humans exposed to arsenicals, intramuscular dimercaprol is associated with an increase in urinary arsenic excretion that peaks in 2 to 4 hours,[6] then quickly declines. Pharmacodynamic effects, such as increased blood pressure and pulse, peak at approximately 30 minutes and resolve within 2 hours.[7] Limited observations such as these imply that dimercaprol is absorbed, distributed, and excreted rapidly. After intramuscular injection of radiolabeled dimercaprol to rats, 80% of the radioactivity entered the bloodstream within 1 hour.[8] The radiolabel was distributed rapidly and widely to most soft tissues, with the highest levels measured in the kidneys and the liver. Some intracellular distribution has been inferred from the ability of dimercaprol to traverse cell membranes in vitro,[9] but the drug's volume of distribution has not been determined. After injection in animals, an altered form of dimercaprol is excreted in the urine, with minor amounts in the bile or feces, within 6 to 12 hours.[8,10] It was observed consistently in rats and rabbits that unchanged dimercaprol was not excreted in the urine. In rabbits, dimercaprol seemed to be metabolized partly to an unspecified thiol compound[11]; in rats, no free thiols were excreted.[12]

CONTRAINDICATIONS AND PRECAUTIONS

Because it is dissolved in peanut oil, dimercaprol should not be administered to patients who are allergic to peanuts. Dimercaprol has been associated with hemolysis in two patients with glucose-6-phosphate dehydrogenase

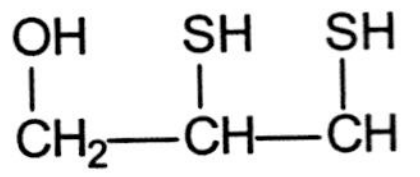

$$\begin{array}{ccc} OH & SH & SH \\ | & | & | \\ CH_2 & -CH & -CH \end{array}$$

FIGURE 139-1

Chemical structure of dimercaprol (2,3-dimercaptopropanol).

deficiency[13]; susceptible patients should be monitored for hemolysis during treatment.

Because the metabolites of dimercaprol and the metals it mobilizes are excreted predominantly in the urine, caution should be exercised in administering dimercaprol to patients with severe renal insufficiency. A few reports suggest that dimercaprol or its metabolites may be dialyzable and that dimercaprol may increase the dialysis clearance of mercury in patients with renal failure.[14–16] Although increased mortality was found when massive doses of dimercaprol were given to animals with acute hepatic damage from carbon tetrachloride,[17] no relevant clinical experience implicates hepatic insufficiency as a contraindication.

Dimercaprol (0.3 mg/kg) did not redistribute radiolabeled mercury to the fetus when administered to pregnant mice concurrently exposed to mercuric chloride.[18] Dimercaprol was teratogenic and embryotoxic, however, at a dose of 125 mg/kg/day in a mouse model, and it seems less effective than succimer or unithiol in averting the adverse reproductive effects of arsenic or mercury.[19,20] Dimercaprol is rated pregnancy category C by the U.S. Food and Drug Administration (see Appendix A).

ADVERSE EFFECTS

The adverse effects of dimercaprol are dose dependent. Reactions are relatively mild and infrequent at doses of 3 mg/kg intramuscularly or less but occur in two thirds of patients receiving 5 mg/kg intramuscularly. Transient elevation in blood pressure, with an increase in diastolic pressure of 10 to 40 mm Hg, is common at doses of 4 or 5 mg/kg intramuscularly. The blood pressure usually normalizes within 2 hours.[7] Compared to adults, children are prone to tachycardia rather than blood pressure elevation after dimercaprol injections.[21] In 60 healthy adults and 61 adults with complications of organoarsenical antisyphilitic therapy, dimercaprol doses of 4 to 5 mg intramuscularly were associated with the following adverse effects, in decreasing order of frequency: nausea, vomiting, and headache; a burning sensation of the lips, mouth, throat, and eyes, sometimes with accompanying lacrimation, rhinorrhea, or salivation; generalized muscular aches; burning and tingling of the extremities, with sweating of the forehead and hands; pain in the teeth; and a sense of constriction in the chest, with a feeling of anxiety and general agitation. These symptoms appeared within 10 to 30 minutes of the injection and subsided within 30 to 50 minutes. Fever was observed after the second or third dimercaprol injection in two thirds of children receiving doses greater than 3 mg/kg,[21] but this seems to be uncommon in adults. Convulsions and transient coma occurred in 3 children who accidentally received dimercaprol injections of 25 mg/kg.[21]

One anecdotal report suggested that 25 mg of ephedrine administered (to an adult) 0.5 hour before dimercaprol injection may diminish the severity of subsequent adverse effects.[22] This has not been a consistent observation, however, and ephedrine conceivably might aggravate the pressor response of dimercaprol. Intramuscular injections of dimercaprol frequently are perceived as painful and may be complicated by sterile or pyogenic abscesses. Prior local injection of procaine has been suggested as a means to diminish the pain associated with intramuscular dimercaprol injection.[23]

ADMINISTRATION

Dimercaprol (BAL in Oil) is supplied as 3-mL ampules containing dimercaprol (100 mg/mL) and benzyl benzoate (200 mg/mL) in peanut oil. For the treatment of systemic poisoning by relevant heavy metals, it can be administered only as a deep intramuscular injection. The initial dose ranges from 2.5 to 4 mg/kg intramuscularly every 4 to 6 hours depending on the nature and severity of the poisoning being treated. It is common to progressively taper the amount and frequency of dimercaprol administered during the initial days of therapy. Dimercaprol inunctions have been used as an experimental topical treatment for vesicant burns to the skin and eye induced by lewisite.

REFERENCES

1. Peters RA, Stocken LA, Thompson RHS: British Anti-Lewisite (BAL). Nature 156:616–619, 1945.
2. Eagle H, Magnuson HJ: The systemic treatment of 227 cases of arsenic poisoning (encephalitis, dermatitis, blood dyscrasia, jaundice, fever) with 2,3-dimercaptopropanol (BAL). Am J Syph Gon Ven Dis 30:420–441, 1946.
3. Longcope WT, Luetscher JA: The use of BAL (British Anti-Lewisite) in the treatment of the injurious effects of arsenic, mercury and other metallic poisonings. Ann Intern Med 31:545–553, 1949.
4. Berlin M, Lewander T: Increased brain uptake of mercury caused by 2,3-dimercaptopropanol (BAL) in mice given mercuric chloride. Acta Pharmacol Toxicol 22:1–7, 1965.
5. Hoover TD, Aposhian HV: BAL increases the arsenic-74 content of rabbit brain. Toxicol Appl Pharmacol 70:160–162, 1983.
6. Wexler J, Eagle H, Tatum HJ, et al: Clinical uses of 2,3-dimercaptopropanol (BAL): II. The effect of BAL on the excretion of arsenic in normal subjects and after minimal exposure to arsenical smoke. J Clin Invest 25:467–473, 1946.
7. Modell W, Gold H, Cattell M: Clinical uses of 2,3-dimercaptopropanol (BAL): IV. Pharmacologic observations on BAL by intramuscular injection in man. J Clin Invest 25:480–487, 1946.
8. Peters RA, Spray GH, Stocken LA, et al: The use of British Anti-Lewisite containing radioactive sulfur for metabolism investigations. Biochem J 41:370–373, 1947.
9. Muckter H, Liebl B, Reichl FX, et al. Are we ready to replace dimercaprol (BAL) as an arsenic antidote? Hum Exp Toxicol 16:460–465, 1997.
10. Simpson SD, Young L: Biochemical studies of toxic agents: I. Experiments with radioactive 2:3-dimercaptopropanol (British Anti-Lewisite). Biochem J 46:634–640, 1950.
11. Spray GH, Stocken LA, Thompson RHS: Further investigations on the metabolism of 2:3-dimercaptopropanol. Biochem J 41:362–366, 1947.
12. Tamboline B, Matheson AT, Zbarsky SH: Radioactive compounds excreted by rats treated with 35S-labelled British Anti-Lewisite: Preliminary studies. Biochem J 61:651–657, 1956.
13. Janakiraman N, Seeler RA, Royal JE, et al. Hemolysis during BAL chelation therapy for high blood lead levels in two G6PD deficient children. Clin Pediatr 17:485–487, 1978.
14. Doolan PD, Hess WC, Kyle LH: Acute renal insufficiency due to bichloride of mercury: Observations on gastrointestinal hemorrhage and BAL therapy. N Engl J Med 249:273–276, 1953.

15. Maher J, Schreiner GE: The dialysis of mercury and mercury-BAL complex. Clin Res 7:298–299, 1959.
16. Khan A, Denis R, Blum D: Accidental ingestion of mercuric sulphate in a 4-year-old child: Management with BAL and peritoneal dialysis. Clin Pediatr 16:956–958, 1977.
17. Cameron GR, Burgess F, Trenwith VS: The possibility of toxic effects from 2,3-dimercaptopropanol in conditions of impaired renal or hepatic function. Br J Pharmacol 2:59–64, 1947.
18. Berlin M, Lewander T: Increased brain uptake of mercury caused by 2,3-dimercaptopropanol (BAL) in mice given mercuric chloride. Acta Pharmacol Toxicol 22:1–7, 1965.
19. Domingo JL: Prevention by chelating agents of metal-induced developmental toxicity. Reprod Toxicol 9:105–113, 1995.
20. Domingo JL: Developmental toxicity of metal chelating agents. Reprod Toxicol 12:499–510, 1998.
21. Woody JT, Kometani JT: BAL in the treatment of arsenic ingestion of children. Pediatrics 1:372–378, 1948.
22. Tye M, Siegel JM: Prevention of reaction to BAL. JAMA 134:1477, 1947.
23. Stafford BT, Crosby WH: Late onset of gold-induced thrombocytopenia: With a practical note on the injections of dimercaprol. JAMA 239:50–51, 1978.

CHAPTER 140

Calcium Edetate (Calcium Disodium EDTA)

Michael J. Kosnett

Calcium edetate (calcium disodium ethylenediaminetetraacetic acid [ETDA]) is the generic name for the chelating agent calcium disodium ethylenediaminetetraacetate. The drug also has been called *calcium disodium edathamil* and *edetate calcium disodium*. It is marketed in the United States under the brand name Calcium Disodium Versenate. (*Note*: Calcium edetate should not be confused with the disodium, trisodium, or tetrasodium salts of EDTA, which do not contain calcium and which can cause dangerous hypocalcemia).

HISTORY

In 1950, EDTA (edetic acid), an industrial chemical widely employed to control cations in solution, was used clinically in the treatment of hypercalcemia. In 1952, investigators reported the first use of the calcium disodium salt of ethylenediaminetetraacetate (calcium edetate) in the treatment of lead intoxication in children[1] and in adults.[2] Use of calcium edetate was associated with large increases in the urinary excretion of lead without the risk of hypocalcemia that had been encountered with the use of edetic acid. Within a few years, numerous accounts of the clinical utility of calcium edetate in the treatment of lead poisoning appeared in the medical literature. Its clinical use for this purpose has continued to the present.

CHEMICAL PROPERTIES

Calcium edetate ($C_{10}H_{10}CaNa_2O_8 \bullet \chi \ H_2O$; molecular weight 374.27 [anhydrous]) (Fig. 140-1) is a white, crystalline powder that is freely soluble in water. The compound forms stable, water-soluble complexes, or chelates, with numerous cations. Because the stability constant of the lead EDTA chelate ($K_{K2} = 18.2$) greatly exceeds that of the calcium EDTA chelate ($K_{K2} = 10.59$), lead ions react with calcium edetate in vivo to form a lead chelate that is excreted in the urine.

PHARMACODYNAMICS

On absorption, calcium edetate forms complexes not only with lead but also with zinc, an essential trace metal. During the course of calcium edetate treatment, serum zinc levels may decline to approximately 60% to 70% of pretreatment values, and urinary zinc excretion may increase approximately 5-fold to 20-fold.[3–5] This increase may be associated with partial inhibition of zinc metalloenzymes (e.g., alkaline phosphatase). These indices of zinc status return to normal within a few days of cessation of calcium edetate treatment; their clinical significance is uncertain. Calcium edetate exerts no significant pharmacodynamic effects on cardiovascular, hepatic, or renal function.

PHARMACOKINETICS

Calcium edetate may be administered by either intramuscular injection or intravenous infusion. Oral absorption is poor, and oral administration is not recommended because it may increase absorption of lead that may be present in the intestinal tract. The volume of distribution is 0.19 L/kg, consistent with distribution in extracellular water.[6] The serum half-life is approximately 2 hours in subjects with normal renal function. Calcium edetate is excreted unchanged in the urine, predominantly as a result of glomerular filtration. Some data indicate that relatively greater metal excretion is achieved when the total daily dose is administered by continuous infusion over all or most of the day, as opposed to short-term infusion over 1 hour.[7] Renal clearance of calcium edetate and the mobilization of lead into the urine occur more slowly in patients with renal insufficiency.[6,8]

CONTRAINDICATIONS AND PRECAUTIONS

Because calcium edetate and the metals it mobilizes are excreted in the urine, caution should be exercised in administering the drug to patients with renal insufficiency. In patients with moderate renal insufficiency, a reduction in dose proportionate to the deficit in creatinine clearance should be considered. Some case reports suggest that calcium edetate can be used in conjunction with peritoneal dialysis, hemodialysis, or hemofiltration to enhance lead decorporation in lead-poisoned patients with renal failure.[9–11]

Calcium edetate was teratogenic when administered to pregnant rats at a dose of 4 mmol/m²/day (comparable to a therapeutic adult human dose of approximately 40 mg/kg/day).[12] This teratogenicity may have been a consequence of zinc depletion, because the administration of a

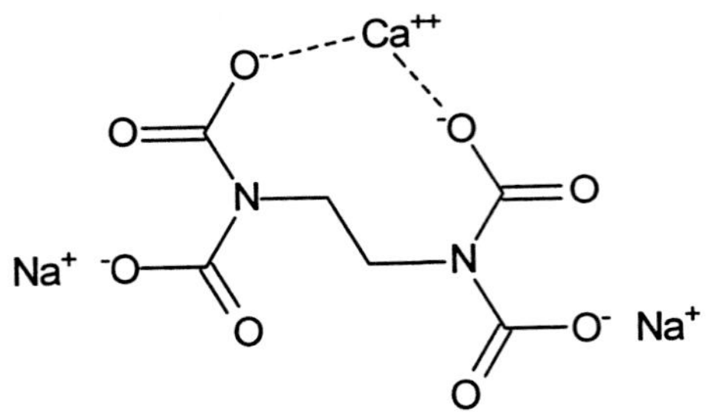

FIGURE 140-1

Chemical structure of calcium disodium edetate.

zinc chelate of EDTA was not teratogenic. Calcium edetate has diminished the adverse reproductive effect of lead in pregnant experimental animals[13] and in two isolated reports has been used to treat lead poisoning in the late stages of human gestation without apparent adverse effect.[14,15] Calcium edetate is rated pregnancy category B by the U.S. Food and Drug Administration (see Appendix A). If its use in pregnancy is necessary, maternal supplementation with zinc should be considered.

ADVERSE EFFECTS

Calcium edetate generally is well tolerated, and adverse effects are rare. The drug has been associated with nephrotoxic damage to the proximal tubule in humans and animals, usually after administration of high or protracted doses.[16,17] Moel and Kumar[18] reported four pediatric cases of oliguric acute renal failure among 207 courses of lead chelation that consisted of 5 days of combined treatment with calcium edetate, 50 mg/kg/day, *and* dimercaprol, 18 mg/kg/day. The oliguria developed 1 to 2 days after chelation was discontinued and lasted 2 to 4 days. Moderate elevations in serum creatinine (3.9 to 8.4 mg/dL) normalized after 11 to 22 days. Although such nephrotoxicity from calcium edetate is uncommon, it is reasonable to monitor renal function (urinalysis, blood urea nitrogen, serum creatinine) at the onset of treatment and every 24 to 48 hours during therapy. A course of calcium edetate treatment should not exceed 5 consecutive days, and repeat courses should be separated by at least a 2-day interval. Maintaining urine output of approximately 1 to 2 mL/kg may optimize lead elimination and diminish the risk of nephrotoxicity, but care must be taken to avoid fluid overload in patients with lead encephalopathy and cerebral edema. Calcium edetate has been associated with mild reversible increases in hepatic transaminases, which are of minimal or no clinical significance.[5]

ADMINISTRATION

Continuous intravenous infusion is the preferred route of calcium edetate administration. The drug should be diluted to a concentration of 2 to 4 mg/mL in normal saline or 5% dextrose. In adults with severe lead poisoning, the recom-

mended dose is 2 to 4 g (30 to 50 mg/kg) intravenously per 24 hours, as a continuous infusion. The pediatric dose is 1000 to 1500 mg/m2/24 hours as a continuous intravenous infusion. To diminish the risk of nephrotoxicity, a course of treatment should not exceed 5 consecutive days.

Although intravenous administration is preferable, the daily dose of calcium edetate also can be administered by deep intramuscular injection in divided doses spaced 8 to 12 hours apart. To minimize pain at the injection site, lidocaine can be added to the calcium edetate injection solution to achieve a final lidocaine concentration in the injectate of 5 mg/mL (0.5%). Calcium Disodium Versenate (edetate calcium disodium injection, USP) is supplied as 5-mL ampules containing 200 mg/mL of calcium edetate (1 g per ampule).

REFERENCES

1. Bessman SP, Ried H, Rubin M: Treatment of lead encephalopathy with calcium disodium versenate. Med Ann Dist Columbia 21:312–315, 1952.
2. Belknap EL: EDTA in the treatment of lead poisoning. Ind Med Surg 21:305–306, 1952.
3. Graziano JH, Siris ES, LoIacono N, et al: 2,3-Dimercaptosuccinic acid as an antidote for lead intoxication. Clin Pharmacol Ther 37:431–438, 1985.
4. Thomas DJ, Chisolm JJ: Lead, zinc, copper decorporation during calcium disodium ethylenediamine tetraacetate treatment of lead-poisoned children. J Pharm Exp Ther 239:829–835, 1986.
5. Chisolm JJ: Evaluation of the potential role of chelation therapy in treatment of low to moderate lead exposures. Environ Health Perspect 89:67–74, 1990.
6. Osterloh J, Becker CE: Pharmacokinetics of CaNa2EDTA and chelation of lead in renal failure. Clin Pharmacol Ther 40:686–693, 1986.
7. Leckie WJ, Tompsett SL: The diagnostic and therapeutic use of edathamil calcium disodium (EDTA, Versene) in excessive inorganic lead absorption. QJM 27:65–82, 1958.
8. Emmerson BT: Chronic lead nephropathy: The diagnostic use of calcium EDTA and the association with gout. Aust Ann Med 12:310–324, 1963.
9. Mehbod H: Treatment of lead intoxication: Combined use of peritoneal dialysis and edetate calcium disodium. JAMA 201:152–154, 1967.
10. Roger SD, Yiannikas C, Crimmins D, et al: Lead intoxication in an anuric patient: Management by intraperitoneal EDTA. Aust N Z J Med 20:814–817, 1990.
11. Kessler M, Durand PY, Huu TC, et al: Mobilization of lead from bone in end-stage renal failure patients with secondary hyperparathyroidism. Nephrol Dial Transplant 14:2731–2733, 1999.
12. Brownie CF, Brownie C, Noden D, et al: Teratogenic effect of calcium edetate (CaEDTA) in rats and the protective effect of zinc. Toxicol Appl Pharmacol 82:426–443, 1986.
13. McClain RM, Siekierka JJ: The effects of various chelating agents on the teratogenicity of lead nitrate rats. Appl Pharmacol 31:434–442, 1975.
14. Angle CR, McIntire MS: Lead poisoning during pregnancy: Fetal tolerance of calcium disodium edetate. Am J Dis Child 108:436–439, 1964.
15. Timpo AE, Amin JS, Casalino MB, et al: Congenital lead intoxication. J Pediatr 94:765–767, 1979.
16. Foreman H, Finnegan C, Lushbaugh CC: Nephrotoxic hazard from uncontrolled edathamil calcium-disodium therapy. JAMA 160:1042–1046, 1956.
17. Rueber MD, Bradley JE: Acute versenate nephrosis occurring as the result of treatment for lead intoxication. JAMA 174:263–269, 1960.
18. Moel DI, Kumar K: Reversible nephrotoxic reactions to a combined 2,3-dimercapto-1-propanol and calcium disodium ethylenediamine-tetraacetic acid regimen in asymptomatic children with elevated blood lead levels. Pediatrics 70:259–262, 1982.

CHAPTER 141

Succimer (DMSA)

Michael J. Kosnett

Succimer is the generic name for meso-2,3-dimercaptosuccinic acid (DMSA).

HISTORY

In 1954, Froitzheim and Olligs[1] described the utility of the dimercaprol analogue DMSA in the chelation treatment of experimental mercuric chloride poisoning in mice. In 1957, Liang and associates[2] reported experimental evidence of the antidotal effects of the sodium salt of DMSA (sodium dimercaptosuccinate) against the toxicity of antimony-containing parasitic drugs, and in 1958, these Chinese investigators began the first clinical trials in humans.[3] Additional investigations showed the value of sodium dimercaptosuccinate in the treatment of other metal poisonings. In 1965, Wang and colleagues[4] reported its clinical use as an intravenous therapy for occupational lead and mercury intoxication. Okonishnikova[5] reported the utility of DMSA in experimental arsenic poisoning in the Soviet literature. A stable formulation of DMSA for the oral chelation of heavy metal poisoning was introduced in China in 1977.[6] The clinical use of oral DMSA for lead poisoning was the subject of a report in the Western literature in 1978.[7] Phase I clinical trials of DMSA were begun in the United States in 1980, and Graziano and coworkers[8] reported a dose-ranging study of DMSA in occupational plumbism in 1985. Phase II trials were conducted in lead-poisoned children.[9]

The generic name of DMSA is *succimer*. It has been approved for use in many countries. Under the trade name Chemet, oral DMSA was approved by the U.S. Food and Drug Administration in 1991 as an orphan drug for the treatment of childhood lead poisoning.

CHEMICAL PROPERTIES

Succimer ($C_4H_6O_4S_2$; molecular weight 182.2) (Fig. 141-1) is a white crystalline powder that is soluble in aqueous alkaline solutions, such as 5% sodium bicarbonate. The vicinal thiol groups of the crystalline solid are relatively stable at room temperature. The drug has a mercaptan-like odor. Although succimer forms stable complexes with several metals in vitro, it may be several disulfide biotransformation products that are responsible for metal complexing action in vivo. A preformed complex of 1.2 mg of succimer and ^{99m}Tc

has been licensed in the United States as a diagnostic agent for scintigraphic imaging of the renal parenchyma. The form of succimer marketed as a chelating agent (Chemet) is supplied as capsules containing 100 mg of succimer absorbed onto inactive beads.

PHARMACODYNAMICS

In addition to increasing excretion of toxic metals, such as lead, mercury, and arsenic, in human and animal studies, succimer has been associated with small increases (approximately twofold) in the urinary excretion of zinc in human trials. Pharmacodynamic effects on cardiovascular, hepatic, or renal function have not been noted after oral administration.

PHARMACOKINETICS

Approximately 20% of orally administered succimer is recovered in the urine as the parent compound or metabolites in human studies.[10,11] Although not definitive, the data on urine and fecal recovery are consistent with an oral bioavailability of approximately 20%. After absorption, greater than 90% of succimer in the blood is found in the plasma fraction, where it is highly bound (92% to 95%) to plasma proteins (mainly albumin) by disulfide linkages.[12] Peak blood concentrations are reached in approximately 3 hours. Most succimer seems to be distributed extracellularly. Minor amounts may penetrate erythrocytes,[13] and some succimer transformation products are excreted in the bile and undergo enterohepatic circulation.[11] Succimer is excreted predominantly in the urine, where 80% to 90% appears as mixed disulfides.[10,14] Approximately 70% of the mixed disulfide occurs as a 2:1 cysteine-DMSA adduct, 20% occurs as a 1:1 cysteine-DMSA adduct, and 10% occurs as cyclic disulfides of DMSA.[14] The increased urinary excretion of metals such as lead that follows administration of succimer parallels the urinary excretion of the mixed disulfides.[10,11] The collective data suggest that it is a biotransformation product (or products) of succimer, and not the unaltered parent drug, that is responsible for its metal mobilizing activity. The elimination half-life of transformed succimer is approximately 2 to 4 hours. Some evidence suggests that renal clearance of the drug and its metabolites may be diminished in lead intoxication.[13]

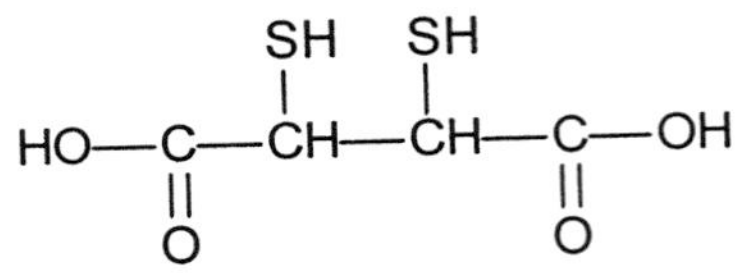

FIGURE 141-1

Chemical structure of succimer (*meso*-2,3-dimercaptosuccinic acid).

CONTRAINDICATIONS AND PRECAUTIONS

Because succimer and its metabolites are excreted predominantly in the urine, the safety and utility of the drug in patients with severe renal insufficiency are uncertain. Limited experience yields no evidence that succimer can increase the hemodialysis clearance of toxic metals in anuric patients.

Succimer should not be administered to patients with a history of allergy to the drug. One case report[15] linked succimer with hemolysis in an adult with glucose-6-phosphate dehydrogenase deficiency. In an open-label clinical trial,[16] five children with glucose-6-phosphate dehydrogenase deficiency tolerated succimer without incident.

Succimer has exerted fetotoxic effects when administered to pregnant rats at oral doses of 100 mg/kg/day[17] and teratogenic effects in pregnant mice at oral doses of 400 mg/kg/day.[18] Chelation with succimer also has mitigated the adverse reproductive effects of several heavy metals in animal models, however.[19,20] A report[21] described succimer chelation in a pregnant woman with a blood lead concentration of 44 μg/dL (2.1 μmol/L) at 29 weeks' gestation and subsequent succimer chelation of the neonate. The child exhibited no evidence of teratogenicity or overt drug toxicity. Oral chelation with succimer was used successfully to lower blood lead concentration in an asymptomatic 6-month-old infant with a blood lead concentration of 84 μg/dL (4.1 μmol/L).[22]

ADVERSE EFFECTS

Succimer chelation generally is well tolerated. Patients should be advised that the drug may impart a mercaptan-like odor to the urine. During clinical trials, gastrointestinal symptoms (e.g., nausea, vomiting, or diarrhea) or mild, reversible serum transaminase elevation was observed in approximately 10% of patients. There were isolated reports of mild-to-moderate neutropenia. These adverse effects were not associated with succimer, however, in an open-label trial of 59 children[16] or a randomized, placebo-controlled, double-blind clinical trial of 780 children.[23] Rashes, some necessitating discontinuation of therapy, have been observed in approximately 4% of patients. One documented case of a drug-related mucocutaneous vesicular rash has been encountered.[24] A 3-year-old child tolerated a succimer overdose of 185 mg/kg without adverse effects.[25] During clinical testing in adults, succimer doses of 80 mg/kg were associated with an occasional report of mild-to-moderate drowsiness and mild abdominal disturbance.[26] An adult experienced no significant adverse effects after an intentional succimer overdose of 43 to 87 mg/kg.[27]

ADMINISTRATION

In accordance with the Food and Drug Administration–approved regimen for lead poisoning, succimer has most often been administered at an oral dose of 10 mg/kg (pediatric dose, 350 mg/m^3) every 8 hours for 5 days, decreasing to 10 mg/kg (pediatric dose, 350 mg/m^3) every 12 hours for another 14 days. Repeat courses and extended dosing have been performed in some cases, depending on the patient's clinical status. Although sodium dimercaptosuccinate is not available in parenteral form elsewhere, in China it has been administered intravenously (10% solution in normal saline) at daily adult doses of 1 to 2 g.[4]

REFERENCES

1. Froitzheim G, Olligs H: Tierexperimentelle Untersuchungen zur Behandlung der Quecksilbervergiftung mit α,α1-Dimercaptobernsteinsaure. Dermat Wschr 129:497–500, 1954.
2. Liang YI, Chu CC, Tsen YL, et al: Studies on the antibilharzial drugs: VI. The antidotal effects of sodium dimercaptosuccinate and BAL-glucoside against tartar emetic. Acta Physiol Sin 21:24–32, 1957.
3. Ding GS, Liang YY: Antidotal effects of dimercaptosuccinic acid. J Appl Toxicol 11:7–14, 1991.
4. Wang SC, Ting KS, Wu CC: Chelating therapy with Na-DMS in occupational lead and mercury intoxications. Chin Med J 84:437–439, 1965.
5. Okonishnikova IE: Experimental therapy and prophylaxis of acute poisonings with arsenic compounds [in Russian]. Gig Truda Prof Zabolev 9:38–43, 1965.
6. Wang S, Liu J, Shi Z: Chelating therapy in occupational metal intoxications in China. Plzen lek Sborn 56(Suppl):111–113, 1988.
7. Friedheim E, Graziano JH, Popovac D, et al: Treatment of lead poisoning by 2,3-dimercaptosuccinic acid. Lancet 2:1234–1236, 1978.
8. Graziano JH, Siris ES, LoIacono N, et al: 2,3-Dimercaptosuccinic acid as an antidote for lead intoxication. Clin Pharm Ther 37:432–438, 1985.
9. Graziano JH, LoIacono NJ, Meyer P: Dose-response study of oral 2,3-dimercaptosuccinic acid in children with elevated blood lead concentrations. J Pediatr 113:751–757, 1988.
10. Aposhian HV, Maiorino RM, Dart RC, et al: Urinary excretion of meso-2,3-dimercaptosuccinic acid in human subjects. Clin Pharmacol Ther 45:520–526, 1989.
11. Asiedu P, Moulton T, Blum CB, et al: Metabolism of meso-2,3-dimercaptosuccinic acid in lead-poisoned children and normal adults. Environ Health Perspect 103:734–739, 1995.
12. Maiorino RM, Akins JM, Blaha K, et al: Determination and metabolism of dithiol chelating agents: X. In humans, meso-2,3-dimercaptosuccinic acid is bound to plasma proteins via mixed disulfide formation. J Pharm Exp Ther 254:570–577, 1990.
13. Dart RC, Hurlbut KM, Maiorino RM, et al: Pharmacokinetics of meso-2,3-dimercaptosuccinic acid in patients with lead poisoning and in healthy adults. J Pediatr 125:309–316, 1994.
14. Maiorino RM, Bruce DC, Aposhian HV: Determination and metabolism of dithiol chelating agents: VI. Isolation and identification of the mixed disulfides of meso-2,3-dimercaptosuccinic acid with L-cysteine in human urine. Toxicol Appl Pharmacol 97:338–349, 1989.
15. Gerr F, Frumkin H, Hodgins P: Hemolytic anemia following succimer administration in a glucose-6-phosphate dehydrogenase deficient patient. Clin Toxicol 32:569–575, 1994.
16. Chisolm JJ: Safety and efficacy of meso-2,3-dimercaptosuccinic acid (DMSA) in children with elevated blood lead concentrations. Clin Toxicol 38:365–375, 2000.
17. Domingo JL, Ortega A, Paternain JL, et al: Oral meso-2,3-dimercaptosuccinic acid in pregnant Sprague-Dawley rats: Teratogenicity and alterations in mineral metabolism: I. Teratological evaluation. J Toxicol Environ Health 30:181–190, 1990.
18. Taubeneck MW, Domingo JL, Llobet JM, et al: Meso-2,3-dimercaptosuccinic acid (DMSA) affects maternal and fetal copper metabolism in Swiss mice. Toxicology 72:27–40, 1992.

19. Domingo JL: Prevention by chelating agents of metal-induced developmental toxicity. Reprod Toxicol 9:105–113, 1995.
20. Chen S, Golemboski KA, Sanders FS, et al: Persistent effect of in utero meso-2,3-dimercaptosuccinic acid (DMSA) on immune function and lead-induced immunotoxicity. Toxicology 132:67–79, 1999.
21. Horowitz BZ, Mirkin DB: Lead poisoning and chelation in a mother-neonatal pair. Clin Toxicol 39:727–731, 2001.
22. Speranza V, Gaar G, Chambers-Emerson J, et al: The successful management of serious lead intoxication in a six-month old child with oral chelation (Abstract). Clin Toxicol 38:549, 2000.
23. Treatment of Lead Poisoned Children (TLC) Trial Group: Safety and efficacy of succimer in toddlers with blood lead levels of 20–44 µg/dL. Pediatr Res 48:593–599, 2000.
24. Chemet product Information. New York, Sanofi Pharmaceuticals, 1999.
25. Sigg T, Leiken JB, Grossman W, et al: A report of pediatric succimer overdose. Vet Hum Toxicol 40:90–91, 1998.
26. U.S. Food and Drug Administration: Chemet: Summary Basis for Approval. Rockville, MD, U.S. FDA, 1991.
27. Buchwald AL: Intentional overdose of dimercaptosuccinic acid in the course of treatment for arsenic poisoning. Clin Toxicol 39:113–114, 2001.

CHAPTER 142

Unithiol (DMPS)

Michael J. Kosnett

Unithiol and *DMPS* are the commonly used generic terms for the compound 2,3-dimercaptopropane-1-sulfonic acid, sodium salt monohydrate.

HISTORY

The synthesis and metal binding properties of 2,3-dimercaptopropane-1-sulfonic acid were reported by Petrunkin[1] in Kiev in 1956. By 1958, the agent had become available in the former Soviet Union as a pharmaceutical known as *unithiol* for the treatment of poisoning by certain heavy metals, particularly arsenic and mercury, and for other medical applications. In 1976, Heyl (Berlin, Germany) began marketing oral capsules of unithiol under the trade name Dimaval. Heyl has produced DMPS as a solution for injection (DMPS-Heyl) since 1991. Although it has not been approved as a pharmaceutical by the U.S. Food and Drug Administration, DMPS has been included on the Food and Drug Administration's "list of bulk drug substances that may be used in pharmacy compounding."[2] It is legally available for medicinal purposes in the United States.

CHEMICAL PROPERTIES

Unithiol ($C_3H_7NaO_3S_3$; molecular weight 210.27) (Fig. 142-1) is a crystalline solid that is freely soluble in water. It normally crystallizes as a monohydrate. The thiol groups are relatively stable but become increasingly subject to oxidation under alkaline conditions (pH >7). In addition to their role in the formation of complexes with numerous metals, the vicinal thiol groups contribute antioxidant activity under certain conditions. The polar sulfonate group is responsible for the agent's water solubility, in contrast to the low water solubility of 2,3-dimercaptopropanol (dimercaprol), which has a terminal hydroxyl group. Although unithiol forms stable binary complexes with many heavy metals in vitro, the precise structure of its complexes with metals in vivo is uncertain.

PHARMACODYNAMICS

Rapid intravenous injection may have a vasodilatory effect that results in transient hypotension; for this reason, intravenous injections should be administered slowly over 15 to 20 minutes. A moderate diuretic effect has been observed in animal studies. Unithiol has not been shown otherwise to interact with renal or with hepatic function at therapeutic doses. Unithiol has increased the urinary excretion of copper and zinc in several animal and human studies. Prolonged high-dose administration to dogs (150 mg/kg/day for 6 months) decreased the copper content of many visceral organs and was associated with anemia.[3]

PHARMACOKINETICS

The oral bioavailability of DMPS is approximately 50%.[4] Peak blood concentrations occur at approximately 3.7 hours.[5] Almost all of absorbed unithiol undergoes transformation in the plasma, mostly to DMPS-albumin complexes and to a lesser extent nonprotein-associated DMPS disulfides.[6] A small amount of DMPS may enter erythrocytes. Greater than 80% of an intravenous dose is excreted in the urine, with an elimination half-life of 20 hours. The form recovered in the urine exists as 10% unaltered DMPS and 90% transformed products, the latter consisting mostly (97%) of cyclic polymeric DMPS sulfides, with minor amounts (2.5%) as a DMPS-cysteine (1:2) mixed disulfide and acyclic DMPS disulfides (0.5%).[6] Experimental animal studies suggest that renal elimination of DMPS may occur via tubular secretion and that metals such as mercury are extracted from the renal tubular epithelium during this process.[7] In normal human volunteers treated with DMPS, urinary mercury excretion correlated well with urinary excretion of DMPS and its disulfide metabolites.[4]

CONTRAINDICATIONS AND PRECAUTIONS

Because DMPS and its metal complexes seem to be excreted predominantly via the kidney, caution should be exercised when administering unithiol to patients with severe renal insufficiency. Unithiol has been used as an adjunct to hemodialysis in patients with anuric renal failure from mercury salts.[8,9]

Unithiol has not been associated with teratogenicity. In a murine model, doses of 300 mg/kg/day during gestational days 6 to 15 showed no evidence of developmental toxicity. Unithiol has averted or diminished adverse reproductive effects of certain toxic metals in experimental studies.[10]

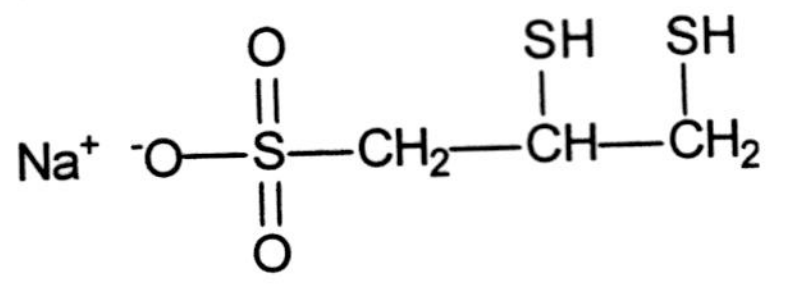

FIGURE 142-1

Chemical structure of unithiol (DMPS; 2,3-dimercaptopropane-1-sulfonic acid, sodium salt).

Clinical experience in the use of unithiol during human pregnancy is unavailable.

ADVERSE EFFECTS

Unithiol is generally well tolerated, with a low incidence (<4%) of adverse side effects.[11] The most common adverse effects are allergic cutaneous reactions, such as exanthems or urticaria, which have resolved on discontinuation of the drug or lowering of the dose. Isolated cases of major allergic reactions, including Stevens-Johnson syndrome and erythema multiforme, have been reported.

ADMINISTRATION

Unithiol can be administered by oral, intramuscular, or intravenous routes. In general, the intravenous route should be reserved for treatment of severe acute intoxications by heavy metals (e.g., arsenic, mercury, or lead) in which compromised cardiovascular or gastrointestinal status may interfere with rapid or efficient absorption by the oral route. The daily intravenous dose for acute heavy metal poisoning is 20 to 30 mg/kg/day. One sixth of the daily dose should be administered every 4 hours by slow intravenous infusion over 20 minutes. For oral chelation, a daily dose of 20 to 30 mg/kg/day can be administered in four divided doses

(i.e., every 6 hours). In some cases, protracted long-term treatment has been administered at a dose of 100 mg orally three times daily in adults or 50 mg orally three times daily in small children.[11] The pharmacokinetic and clinical database that forms the basis for various dosing regimens is limited.

REFERENCES

1. Petrunkin VE: Synthesis and properties of dimercapto derivatives of alkylsulfonic acids: I. Synthesis of sodium 2,3-dimercaptopropylsulfonate (Unithiol) and sodium 2-mercaptoethyl-sulfonate. Ukrainskii Khimicheskii Zhurnal 22:603–607, 1956.
2. Food and Drug Administration: List of drug substances that may be used in pharmacy compounding. Fed Reg 64:996–1003, 1999.
3. Szinicz L, Wiedemann P, Haring H, et al: Effects of repeated treatment with sodium 2,3-dimercaptopropane-1-sulfonate in beagle dogs. Arzneim-Forsch/Drug Res 33:818–821, 1983.
4. Hurlbut KM, Maiorino RM, Mayersohn M, et al: Determination and metabolism of dithiol chelating agents: XVI. Pharmacokinetics of 2,3-dimercapto-1-propanesulfonate after intravenous administration to human volunteers. J Pharmacol Exp Ther 268:662–668, 1994.
5. Maiorino RM, Dart RC, Carter DE, et al: Determination and metabolism of dithiol chelating agents: XII. Metabolism and pharmacokinetics of sodium 2,3-dimercaptopropane-1-sulfonate in humans. J Pharmacol Exp Ther 259:808–814, 1991.
6. Maiorino RM, Xu ZF, Aposhian HV: Determination and metabolism of dithiol chelating agents: XVII. In humans, sodium 2,3-dimercapto-1-propanesulfonate is bound to plasma albumin via mixed disulfide formation and is found in the urine as cyclic polymeric disulfides. J Pharmacol Exp Ther 277:375–384, 1996.
7. Zalups RK, Parks LD, Cannon VT, et al: Mechanisms of action of 2,3-dimercaptopropane-1-sulfonate and the transport, disposition, and toxicity of inorganic mercury in isolated perfused segments of rabbit proximal tubules. Mol Pharmacol 54:353–363, 1998.
8. Nadig J, Knutti R, Hany A: DMSP-Behandlung bei einer akuten Sublimat-(Quecksilberchlorid-) Vergiftung. Schweiz Med Wochenschr 115:507–511, 1985.
9. Toet AE, van Dijk A, Savelkoul TJ, et al: Mercury kinetics in a case of severe mercuric chloride poisoning treated with dimercapto-1-propane sulfonate (DMPS). Hum Exp Toxicol 13:11–16, 1994.
10. Domingo JL: Prevention by chelating agents of metal-induced developmental toxicity. Reprod Toxicol 9:105–113, 1995.
11. Ruprecht J: Dimaval (DMPS). DMPS-Heyl scientific monograph. Berlin, Heyl, 1997.

CHAPTER 143

Deferoxamine

Jeffrey Brent

Deferoxamine is a chelator that is used for acutely ill iron-poisoned patients. It also can be used as an aluminum chelator and for the treatment of transfusional iron overload states. Its use in critically ill patients almost always is confined to patients who have had an acute iron overdose, however. The treatment of acute iron toxicity is discussed in detail in Chapter 65. This chapter focuses on the clinical pharmacology of deferoxamine for the treatment of acute iron poisoning.

HISTORY

In 1964, ferrioxamine D, which is an iron chelate of deferoxamine, was isolated from *Streptomyces pilosus*.[1] Several animal studies verified deferoxamine's efficacy in iron poisoning.[2] In 1966, a clinical series of 172 children treated with deferoxamine was published.[3] Five years later, the same author published a series of 472 patients, providing the largest clinical series available on the treatment of iron poisoning with this agent.[4]

PROPERTIES

Chemical

Deferoxamine (Fig. 143-1) has a molecular weight of 561 d. It typically is supplied as desferoxamine mesylate (*N*-[5-[3-[(5-aminopentyl) hydroxycarbamoyl] propionamido] pentyl]-3-[(5-(*N*-hydroxyacetamido) pentyl] carbamoyl] propionhydroxamic monomethane sulfonate (salt). Its molecular formula is $C_{25}H_{48}N_6O_8$.

Physical

Deferoxamine usually is supplied as a lyophilized powder with a white to off-white color. It is highly water soluble. It has no odor, or its odor is subtle. The melting point of deferoxamine is 148°C to 149°C (280°F to 300°F).

PHARMACODYNAMICS

Deferoxamine binds ferric iron in a 1:1 molar ratio with an affinity constant approximating 10^{31}.[1,4] Deferoxamine has low affinity for other common ions (with the exception of aluminum), including ferrous iron.[1] The structure of the deferoxamine-iron chelate is shown in Figure 143-1.

There is some uncertainty regarding the compartment from which deferoxamine removes iron. Given its hydrophilic nature and molecular weight of 561, its cellular permeability is limited.[1,5–7] In addition to the various molecules for which it has a physiologic function, such as hemoglobin, myoglobin, and cytochrome oxidase, iron is stored in the form of ferritin and transported in the blood primarily bound to transferrin. After absorption from the gastrointestinal tract as ferrous iron, it is oxidized to the ferric form and bound to transferrin. Under normal conditions, almost all circulating iron is bound to transferrin. Routine serum iron determinations generally reflect this bound iron. Transferrin has a molecular weight of approximately 90,000, and each molecule can bind two ferric ions. Typically, only approximately one third of transferrin's iron-binding sites are occupied, and it serves as a natural chelator when free serum iron is present. Normally, there is some iron release, particularly from the reticuloendothelial system, where hemoglobin and red blood cells are broken down. In this situation, the iron is released in the form of ferritin in small amounts.

In cases of iron toxicity, the ability of transferrin to bind iron is exceeded. Deferoxamine does not remove significant amounts of transferrin-bound iron.[8] Non–transferrin-bound iron usually has a serum half-life of 60 to 120 minutes. It is assumed that deferoxamine's major mode of action is in its ability to chelate non–transferrin-bound serum iron.[9] It is intuitively apparent that deferoxamine has the capacity to chelate the fraction of serum iron that may be most likely to be responsible for intercellular transport and toxicity. A dose of 100 mg of deferoxamine has the capacity to bind 8.5 mg of iron. That fraction of deferoxamine that enters cells may chelate nonbound or weakly bound intracellular iron.

There are no prospective controlled studies verifying deferoxamine's efficacy in the treatment of iron poisoning. Considerable data exist, however, in patients treated for iron overload states, indicating that iron reduces serum ferritin and, when given on a long-term basis, reduces intracellular iron deposition.[10]

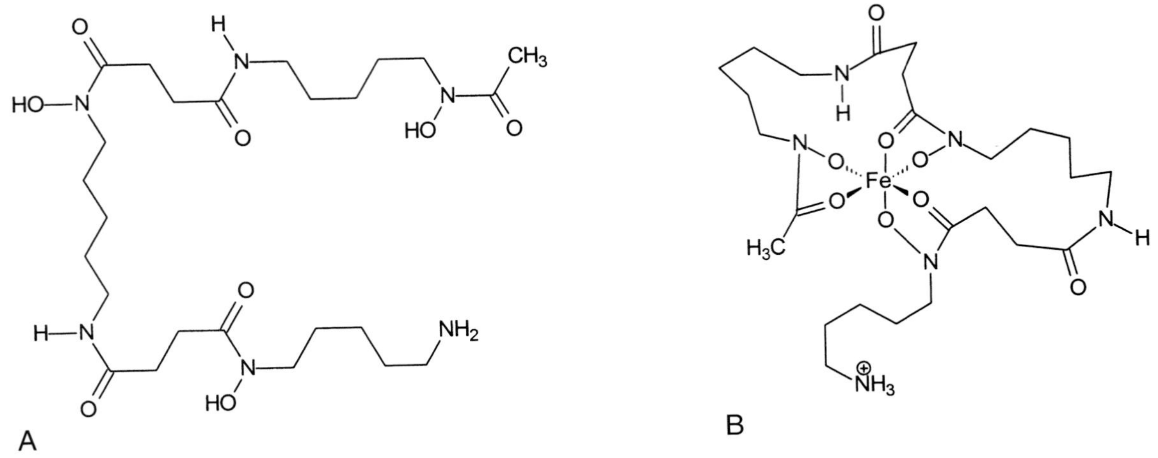

FIGURE 143-1

Chemical structures of deferoxamine (**A**) and the ferrioxamine B chelate (**B**).

PHARMACOKINETICS

> **Pharmacokinetics of Deferoxamine**
>
> *Oral absorption:* poor
> *Volume of distribution:* 0.6–1.33 L/kg
> *Excretion in breast milk:* unknown
> *Mode of clearance:* metabolism followed by renal metabolite
>   elimination
> *Elimination half-life:* 3–6 hr
> *Cleared by extracorporeal techniques:* yes

The pharmacokinetics of deferoxamine in acute iron poisoning has been poorly characterized. There is a small body of data from patients with transfusional iron overload states and from studies with volunteers, however, which allows for some conclusions concerning the relevant pharmacokinetics. Deferoxamine is poorly absorbed orally and should not be given by that route. In the case of an acute iron ingestion, it is possible for ferrioxamine, the deferoxamine–iron chelate, to form in the gastrointestinal tract after absorption of deferoxamine. This situation may enhance iron toxicity because of the greater absorption of iron and the intrinsic toxicity of ferrioxamine.

Although clinically significant deferoxamine concentrations are achievable by all parenteral routes, only the intravenous route generally is used in the case of acute iron poisoning. The pharmacokinetics of deferoxamine in relation to the hemodynamic perturbations associated with acute iron poisoning has not been characterized for the intramuscular and subcutaneous routes. These routes should be avoided if possible. After intravenous administration, deferoxamine follows a two-component elimination profile consisting of a fast initial distribution half-life of 5 to 10 minutes followed by an elimination half-life of approximately 3 hours.[11] A steady-state concentration was achieved in 6 to 12 hours in volunteers receiving an intravenous deferoxamine infusion.[11] In a canine infusion model, a steady-state serum concentration of 10.7 μg/mL was achieved with a dose of 10 mg/kg/hr.[12]

Deferoxamine that is not renally cleared has two potential fates when absorbed. One is to complex with iron to form ferrioxamine; the other is to be metabolized hepatically.[11,13–15] The degree of metabolism depends on the chelatable iron status of the patient. The primary metabolite of deferoxamine is called *metabolite B*. When formed, deferoxamine metabolites are excreted renally. In healthy volunteers, renal clearance accounts for 30% of total deferoxamine clearance.[16]

Deferoxamine has been reported to have a volume of distribution of 0.6 to 1.33 L/kg.[1,13,17] It distributes into the intracellular compartment and can chelate intracellular iron.[1,5–8] Deferoxamine is removable by hemodialysis and other extracorporeal drug removal techniques.[18,19]

Ferrioxamine has a volume of distribution of only 0.2 L/kg and has an initial half-life of 2.3 hours, followed by a terminal half-time of 5.8 hours in volunteers.[16] Similar to deferoxamine, ferrioxamine can be removed by extracorporeal techniques.[20–22]

SPECIAL POPULATIONS

Pregnant and Breast-feeding Patients

There have been several cases of treatment of iron-poisoned pregnant women with deferoxamine without an evident harmful effect to the fetus.[23–25] As in women with thalassemia being treated with deferoxamine, there seemed to be no adverse effects on the fetus.[25,26] Deferoxamine is a highly charged molecule and is unlikely to cross the placenta, a prediction verified in an ovine model.[28] Iron poisoning in pregnancy should be treated in a fashion similar to that in nonpregnant patients. It is unknown whether deferoxamine is excreted in breast milk; it is prudent to suspend breast-feeding during administration of this agent.

CONTRAINDICATIONS

As with all agents, a known allergic reaction to deferoxamine should be considered to be a contraindication. Because deferoxamine and ferrioxamine are excreted renally, patients with renal failure should receive this agent only in association with hemodialysis. If the renal failure is prerenal, aggressive fluid resuscitation can be followed by standard deferoxamine therapy.

PRECAUTIONS

The precautions associated with deferoxamine therapy for acute iron poisoning relate to the potential adverse effects described in detail next.

ADVERSE EFFECTS

The major adverse effects associated with the use of deferoxamine in the treatment of iron poisoning are hypotension, acute renal failure, a pulmonary syndrome, *Yersinia* sepsis, and allergy. Many additional effects have been reported with long-term use of deferoxamine as an iron chelator for the treatment of iron overload states, such as thalassemia major, hemosiderosis, or hemochromatosis. These effects have little relevance to the use of deferoxamine in the treatment of acute iron intoxication and are not discussed further in this chapter. For additional information regarding these toxicities, the reader is referred to an excellent review on this topic by Bentur and colleagues.[29]

Hypotension and Shock

There have been several reports of hypotension and shock associated with intravenous deferoxamine therapy.[4,30,31] Most sources recommend that hypotension can be avoided if doses of deferoxamine do not exceed 15 mg/kg/hr. It is likely, however, that the intravascular volume depletion associated with iron poisoning may contribute to the hypotension, and substantially higher doses may be tolerated. The dose rate is best determined based on the clinical response in an appropriately volume-resuscitated patient. It also is possible that histamine release may contribute to the hypotension.[31,32] One article reported, however, that the use of H_2 antagonists did not prevent deferoxamine-induced hypotension.[31]

Acute Renal Failure

Acute renal failure has been reported after deferoxamine administration.[33–35] It seems that this renal injury is related to decreased renal perfusion associated with intravascular volume depletion as seen in acute iron poisonings. A study of intravenous deferoxamine administration to dogs showed that it causes decreased renal perfusion independent of changes in systemic blood pressure, an effect preventable in this model by intravascular volume expansion.[33] Intravascular volume resuscitation should be started before deferoxamine administration; this should be accomplished by a bolus rather than delaying therapy by a slow infusion.

Adult Respiratory Distress Syndrome

Beginning around 1990, several reports[36–38] described a pulmonary syndrome in patients who received high doses of deferoxamine for prolonged periods for the treatment of iron overload states[36,37] or iron poisoning.[38] This syndrome occurred within 32 hours to 9 days of continuous high-dose deferoxamine therapy and was associated with noncardiogenic pulmonary edema, tachypnea, hypoxia, fever, eosinophilia, cough, and diffuse pulmonary infiltrates. Some of the patients had urticaria before the development of the syndrome. Pulmonary function tests in one of the patients being treated for thalassemia major showed a restrictive pattern; however, the interpretation is confused by the high incidence of pulmonary abnormalities in patients with thalassemia.[37] In the early 1990s, several reports appeared of fatalities in patients with acute respiratory distress syndrome after deferoxamine treatment for iron poisoning.[38] Subsequently, several other reports also described acute respiratory distress syndrome in patients who had received prolonged or high-dose deferoxamine therapy.[34,39,40] Because these patients generally were treated for prolonged periods, it is unlikely that 24 hours of deferoxamine therapy, even at high doses, is a risk for the development of acute respiratory distress syndrome. If treatment is continued for more than 48 hours, patients should be monitored carefully for the development of this syndrome.

Yersinia Sepsis

There have been several reports[41,43] of patients being treated with deferoxamine for acute iron poisoning or iron overload secondary to thalassemia major who developed infections due to *Yersinia enterocolitica*. Although patients with thalassemia have increased susceptibility to *Y. enterocolitica*, it is likely that the deferoxamine enhances the possibility of sepsis by this organism.[42,44–46] Normally, *Yersinia* proliferation is limited by its iron dependency. Ferrioxamine can substitute for iron, however.[42] It also is possible that the excess iron from an iron overdose may stimulate *Yersinia* virulence even in the absence of deferoxamine therapy.

Allergy

Several reports of apparent allergic and anaphylactoid reactions to deferoxamine therapy have been published. The early studies by Whitten and associates[31] reported that deferoxamine induces release of histamine, which may play a role in these reactions. A patient with an apparent anaphylactic reaction, including laryngospasm,[48] subsequently was desensitized and was able to continue receiving deferoxamine therapy for thalassemia.

Interference with Iron Assays

Deferoxamine interferes with iron determinations by several routine assays[49,50]; this occurs not because of deferoxamine-related interfering color but because its chelating qualities interfere with the iron-binding reagents used in the assays. Atomic absorption and plasma emission spectrophotometric assays are unaffected by the presence of deferoxamine and should be used during deferoxamine therapy. A deferoxamine-insensitive modification of the routine aca method of iron determination has been published.[51]

ADMINISTRATION

As reviewed previously and in Chapter 65, deferoxamine should be administered by the intravenous route in all patients with acute systemic iron poisoning. Because of the concern for hypotension in these often volume-depleted patients, it is important to administer fluid resuscitation aggressively to these patients as soon as possible. It is not necessary to complete fluid resuscitation before starting deferoxamine therapy; both can be accomplished simultaneously.

The rate of deferoxamine infusion, as described earlier, is best individualized on the basis of patient tolerability. Although a maximal rate of intravenous infusion of 15 mg/kg/hr is often cited, there is little empirical justification for this recommendation. In a severely iron-poisoned patient who is able to tolerate higher doses, there is no reason to restrict the rate of infusion to this parameter. Most acutely iron-poisoned patients require less than 48 hours of deferoxamine treatment.[52] Because of concerns for deferoxamine-induced acute respiratory distress syndrome, as described earlier, treatment with this agent should be restricted to less than 48 hours if possible.

REFERENCES

1. Keberle H: The biochemistry of desferrioxamine and its relation to iron metabolism. Ann N Y Acad Sci 119:758–768, 1964.
2. Moeschlin S, Schnider U: Treatment of primary and secondary hemochromatosis and acute iron poisoning with a new potent iron eliminating agent (desferrioxamine-B). N Engl J Med 269:57–66, 1963.
3. Westlin W: Deferoxamine in the treatment of acute iron poisoning: Clinical experiences with 172 children. Clin Pediatr 5:531–535, 1966.
4. Westlin W: Deferoxamine as a chelating agent. Clin Toxicol 4:597–602, 1971.
5. Hershko C, Konijn AM, Ling G: Iron chelators for thalassemia. Br J Haematol 101:399–406, 1998.
6. Cabantchik ZL, Milgram P, Glickstein H, et al: A method for assessing iron chelation in membrane model systems and in living mammalian cells. Anal Biochem 233:221–227, 1995.
7. Zannineli G, Glickstein H, Breuer W, et al: Chelation and mobilization of cellular iron by different classes of chelators. Mol Pharmacol 51:842–852, 1997.
8. Pollack S, Vanderhoff G, Lasky F: Iron removal from transferrin—an experimental study. Biochim Biophys Acta 497:481–487, 1977.
9. Breuer W, Marieke J, Ermers J, et al: Desferrioxamine-chelatable iron, a component of serum non-transferrin-bound iron, used for assessing chelation therapy. Blood 97:792–798, 2001.
10. Barry M, Flynn DM, Letsky EA, et al: Long-term chelation therapy in thalassemia major: Effect on liver iron concentration, liver histology, and clinical prograss. BMJ Clin Res 2:16–20, 1974.
11. Porter JB: Deferoxamine pharmacokinetics. Semin Hematol 38:63–68, 2001.
12. Bentur Y, Koren G, Klein J, et al: Pharmacokinetics of deferoxamine with and without iron load. Vet Hum Toxicol 31:156–157, 1989.
13. Lee P, Mohammed N, Abeysinghe RD, et al: Intravenous infusion pharmacokinetics of desferrioxamine in thalassaemia patients. Drugs Metab Disp 21:640–644, 1993.
14. Singh S, Hider RC, Porter JB: Separation and identification of desferrioxamine and its iron chelating metabolites by high-performance liquid chromatography and fast atom bombardment mass spectrometry. Anal Biochem 187:1–8, 1990.
15. Singh S, Mohammed N, Ackerman R, et al: Quantification of desferrioxamine and its iron chelating metabolites by high-performance liquid chromatography and simultaneous ultraviolet-visible/radioactive detection. Anal Biochem 203:116–120, 1992.
16. Allain P, Mauras Y, Chaleil D, et al: Pharmacokinetics and renal elimination of desferrioxamine and ferrioxamine in healthy subjects and patients with haemochromatosis. Br J Clin Pharmacol 24:207–212, 1987.
17. Peter G, Keberle M, Schmid K: Distribution and renal excretion of desferrioxamine and ferrioxamine in the dog and in the rat. Biochem Pharmacol 15:93–109, 1966.
18. Richardson JR, Sugerman DL, Hulet WH: Extraction of iron by chelation with desferrioxamine and hemodialysis. Clin Res 15:368, 1967.
19. Banner W Jr, Vernon DD, Ward RM, et al: Continuous arteriovenous hemofiltration in experimental iron intoxication. Crit Care Med 17:1187–1190, 1989.
20. Ceriati F, Pomponi M, Cavicchioni C, et al: Continuous intra-venous (CIV) infusion of deferoxamine (DF) in a hemodialysed patient with transfusion or siderosis (Letter). Int J Artif Organ 4:409, 1981.
21. McGonigle RJS, Keogh AM, Weston MJ, et al: Iron status in chronic hemodialysis patients: Treatment of transfusional iron overload with desferrioxamine. Dial Transplant 13:214, 1984.
22. Hilfenhaus M, Koch KM, Bechstein PB, et al: Therapy and monitoring of hypersiderosis in chronic renal insufficiency. Contrib Nephrol 38:167–174, 1984.
23. Rayburn WF, Donna SM, Wulf ME: Iron overdose during pregnancy: Successful therapy with deferoxamine. Am J Obstet Gynecol 147:717–718, 1983.
24. Blanc P, Hryhorczuk D, Danel I: Deferoxamine treatment of acute iron intoxication in pregnancy. Obstet Gynecol 64:125–145, 1984.
25. Thomas RM, Skalicka AE: Successful pregnancy in transfusion-dependent thalassaemia. Arch Dis Child 55:572–574, 1980.
26. Singer ST, Vichinsky EP: Deferoxamine treatment during pregnancy: Is it harmful? Am J Hematol 60:24–26, 1999.
27. Martin K: Successful pregnancy in β-thalassaemia major. Aust Pediatr J 19:182–183, 1983.
28. Curry SC, Bond GR, Raschke R, et al: An ovine model of maternal iron poisoning in pregnancy. Ann Emerg Med 19:632–638, 1990.
29. Bentur Y, McGuigan M, Koren G: Deferoxamine (desferrioxamine) new toxicities for an old drug. Drug Saf 6:37–46, 1991.
30. Howland MA: Risks of parenteral deferoxamine. J Toxicol Clin Toxicol 34:491–497, 1996.
31. Whitten CF, Gibson GW, Good MH, et al: Studies in acute iron poisoning: I. Desferrioxamine in the treatment of acute iron poisoning. Pediatrics 36:322–335, 1965.
32. Brunner H, Peters G, Jaques R: Wirkungen ven desferrioxamine-methansulfonat auf kreislauf und nierenfunktion. Helv Physiol Pharmacol Acta 21:C3–6, 1963.
33. Koren G, Bentur Y, Strong D, et al: Acute changes in renal function associated with deferoxamine therapy. Am J Dis Child 143:1077–1080, 1989.
34. Tenenbein M: Benefits of parenteral deferoxamine for acute iron poisoning. J Toxicol Clin Toxicol 34:485–489, 1996.
35. Bentur Y, Koren G, Klein J, et al: Pharmacokinetics and nephrotoxicity of deferoxamine. Vet Hum Toxicol 30:371, 1988.
36. Scanderbeg AC, Izzi GC, Butturini A, et al: Pulmonary syndrome and intravenous high-dose desferrioxamine. Lancet 336:1511, 1990.
37. Freedman MH, Grisaru D, Olivieri N, et al: Pulmonary syndrome in patients with thalassemia major receiving intravenous deferoxamine infusions. Am J Dis Child 144:565–569, 1990.
38. Tenenbein M, Kowalski S, Sienko A, et al: Pulmonary toxic effects of continuous desferrioxamine administration in acute iron poisoning. Lancet 379:699–701, 1992.
39. Douglas D, Smilkstein M: Deferoxamine-iron induced pulmonary injury and N-acetylcysteine. J Toxicol Clin Toxicol 33:495, 1995.
40. Rego EM, Neto EB, Simoes BP, Zago MA: Dose-dependent pulmonary syndrome in patients with thalassemia major receiving intravenous deferoxamine (Letter). Am J Hematol 58:340–341, 1998.
41. Melby K, Slordahl S, Gutteberg TJ, et al: Septicemia due to Yersinia enterocolitica after oral doses of iron. BMJ 285:487–488, 1982.
42. Gallant T, Freedman MH, Velland H, et al: Yersinia sepsis in patients with iron overload treated with deferoxamine. N Engl J Med 314:1643, 1986.
43. Mofenson HC, Caraccio TR, Sharieff N: Iron sepsis: Yersinia enterocolitica septicemia possibly caused by an overdose of iron. N Engl J Med 316:1092–1093, 1987.
44. Bouza A, Dominguez A, Meseguer M, et al: Yersinia enterocolitica septicemia. Am J Clin Pathol 74:404–409, 1980.
45. Rabson AR, Halett AF, Koornhof HJ: Generalised Yersinia enterocolitica infection. J Infect Dis 131:447–451, 1975.
46. Robins-Browne RM, Rabson AR, Koornhof HJ: Generalized infection with Yersinia enterocolitica and the role of iron. Contrib Microbiol Immunol 5:277–282, 1979.
47. Brock JH, Ng J: The effect of desferrioxamine on the growth of Staphylococcus aureus, Yersinia enterocolitica and Streptococcus

faecalis in human serum: Uptake of desferrioxamine-bound iron. Fed Eur Microbiol Soc Microbiol Lett 2:439–442, 1983.

48. Authanosiou A, Shepp MA, Nechles H: Anaphylactic reaction to deferoxamine. Lancet 2:616, 1977.

49. Gevirtz NR, Wasserman LR: The measurement of iron and iron-binding capacity in plasma containing deferoxamine. J Pediatr 68:802–804, 1966.

50. Helfer RE, Rogerson DO: The effect of deferoxamine on the determination of serum iron and iron-binding capacity. J Pediatr 68:804–806, 1966.

51. Steinmetz WL, Glick MR, Oei TO: Modified aca method for determination of iron chelated by deferoxamine and other chelators. Clin Chem 26:1593–1597, 1980.

52. Fine JS: Iron poisoning. Curr Probl Pediatr 30:71–90, 2000.

CHAPTER 144

Atropine

Kia Balali-Mood ■ Mahdi Balali-Mood

GENERIC NAME

The most common name for atropine is *dl*-hyoscyamine. Other names are tropic acid with tropine and tropine tropate. The chemical names of atropine are endo-($\pm$)-α-(hydroxymethyl)benzene-acetic acid 8-methyl-8-azobicyclo[3.2.1]oct-3-yl ester and 1αH,5αH-tropan-3α-ol ($\pm$)-tropate.[1]

HISTORY

Atropine is an alkaloid, which may be obtained from *Atropa belladonna, Datura stramonium*, and other solanaceous plants.[2] The ancient Hindus were aware of preparations of belladonna, and Hindus have used these preparations for centuries. The deadly nightshade plant was used frequently in the Middle Ages to poison individuals. Linne named the shrub *Atropa belladonna*, after the mythical figure Atropos, who cut the thread of life. The origin of the term *belladonna* is linked to the use of this agent by Italian women to dilate their pupils. Inhaled smoke derived from burning Jimson weed was used to treat asthma in India. British colonists introduced this treatment into Western medicine in the early 19th century. Mein isolated pure atropine in 1831, and the study of its actions ensued. Soon thereafter, atropine's blocking of the cardiac effects of vagal stimulation and its prevention of salivary secretion were shown.

Atropine has been used in a variety of disorders, including bradydysrhythmias of multiple etiologies. It has been used to treat bradycardia of acute myocardial infarction. It has been given before the induction of general anesthesia to diminish the risk of vagal inhibition of the heart and to reduce salivary and bronchial secretions. It has been administered by inhalation via a nebulizer for the treatment or prevention of bronchospasm. Other muscarinic agents, such as ipratropium bromide, are preferred now, however. Atropine also was used to treat vertigo, but other agents now supersede it. Although atropine sulfate was used as a mydriatic and cycloplegic, because of its long mydriatic action (7 to 12 days), shorter acting agents are preferred.[2]

PHYSICAL AND CHEMICAL PROPERTIES

Atropine is a naturally occurring antimuscarinic tertiary amine, which also is prepared synthetically. The chemical structure of atropine is shown in Figure 144-1.

Atropine is an organic ester that is formed by combining tropic acid, an aromatic acid, with tropine, an organic base. The antimuscarinic action of atropine requires this intact ester because neither tropic acid nor tropine has significant antimuscarinic activity. The presence of the free hydroxyl group in the acid moiety of the ester also is important for activity. The antimuscarinic activity is not lost with the substitution of other aromatic acids for tropic acid, but it may be modified. After parenteral administration, the muscarinic receptor and the ganglionic blocking activities of the quaternary ammonium derivative of atropine are more intense than those of its parent compound. It lacks central nervous system activity, however, because of poor brain penetration. Similar to other quaternary ammonium compounds, atropine is poorly absorbed after oral administration.[3] The extraction of atropine results in a mixture of its *d*- and *l*- isomers. The antimuscarinic activity resides in its naturally occurring *l*- form, however.[4]

Different salts of atropine, such as sulfate, methobromide, and methonitrate, have been synthesized, but atropine sulfate has been used most commonly, particularly as an antidote for organophosphate poisoning. The chemical abstract number of atropine is 51-55-8 and of atropine sulfate is 55-48-1. The chemical formula of atropine sulfate is $(C_{17}H_{35}NO_3)_2$, H_2SO_4, H_2O. Its molecular weight is 694.8.

Atropine sulfate is a bitter, colorless, odorless crystal or white crystalline powder. It effloresces in dry air. It is soluble in water and freely soluble in alcohol and glycerol but particularly insoluble in chloroform and ether. Its USP solubilities are 1:0.5 in water, 1:2.5 in boiling water, 1:5 in alcohol, and 1:2.5 in glycerol. The British Pharmacopoeia states that 2% solution in water has a pH of 4.5 to 6.2. The British Pharmacopoeia injectable form has a pH of 2.8 to 4.5. The USP injectable form and the ophthalmic solution have a pH of 3.0 to 6.5 and 3.5 to 6.0. Atropine sulfate should be stored in single-dose or multiple-dose containers between 15°C and 30°C (59°F and 85°F) and protected from light. Freezing should be avoided. The shelf life is 24 months from the date of manufacture if it is kept under the above-mentioned conditions.[5]

When atropine is heated to decomposition, toxic fumes of nitrogen oxides and sulfur oxides are emitted. Atropine sublimes under high vacuum at 93°C to 110°C (199.4°F to 230°F) and has a melting point of 114°C to 116°C (237.2°F to 240.8°F). Hydrated atropine sulfate has a melting point of 190°C to 196°C (374°F to 384.4°F). Incompatibility between atropine sulfate and hydroxybenzoate preservatives has resulted in a total loss of atropine activity in 2 to 3 weeks.[6]

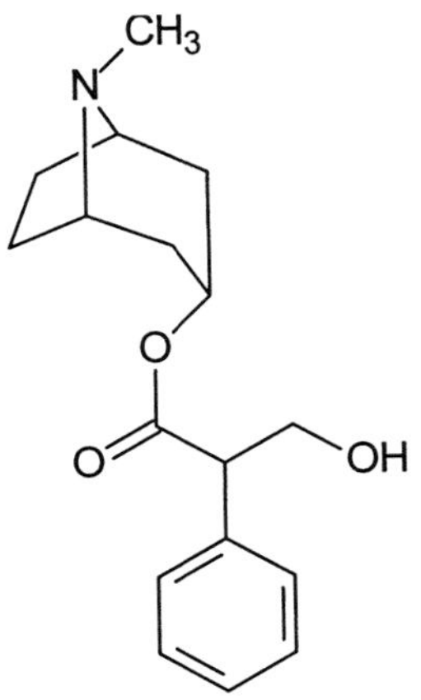

FIGURE 144-1

Chemical structure of atropine.

PHARMACODYNAMICS

Atropine is a competitive muscarinic receptor antagonist. It competes with acetylcholine and other muscarinic agonists for a common binding site on the muscarinic receptor.[7] The binding site on the muscarinic receptor consists of a cleft formed by a series of transmembrane helices. The aspartic acid moiety present within the third transmembrane helix of the receptor is believed to be the binding site for either receptor activation by an endogenous agonist, such as acetylcholine, or blockade by a competitive antagonist, such as atropine.[8] All five muscarinic receptor subtypes are believed to have a similar binding site. The aspartic acid moiety bonds with the quaternary nitrogen in acetylcholine, which is the first step toward the pharmacologic response produced by the endogenous agonist. This ability to induce a change in the resting physiology of a living organism is referred to as *efficacy*. Atropine and other antagonists have no efficacy. With atropine, the receptor antagonism can be overcome by a larger concentration of acetylcholine. All muscarinic receptors are blocked by atropine. Muscarinic receptors are located throughout the body. All known muscarinic receptors are prototypical members of the superfamily of G protein–coupled receptors. The odd-numbered receptor subtypes M_1, M_3, and M_5 are coupled preferentially to G proteins of the Gq/G11 family, resulting in the hydrolysis of phosphoinositide lipids mediated by activation of different phospholipase isoforms.[9] The even-numbered receptor subtypes (M_2 and M_4) are linked primarily to G proteins of the Gi/Go class, which at a biochemical level mediate the inhibition of adenylate cyclase.

In vitro receptor studies have shown that muscarinic acetylcholine receptors activate many downstream signaling pathways, some of which can lead to mitogen-activated protein kinase phosphorylation and activation, in particular in quiescent PC12 cells. Further analysis by Western blotting revealed that the M_4 receptor was responsible for 95% of activity; the remaining 5% were M_1 and M_5 receptor subtypes. These findings are yet to be confirmed in vivo.[10] Much work has been done to understand the structure and functions of the muscarinic cholinoceptor and its subtypes. More recent discoveries include a radioligand binding assay in human peripheral blood lymphocytes, in which it was found that M_3 and M_5 receptors were more abundant than any other receptor subtype.[11] After the M_4 receptor was up-regulated, it was identified as a potential target for new memory-enhancing drugs to be developed for the treatment of Alzheimer's disease.[12] Further work was performed to identify the specific locations of the receptor subtypes M_1 through M_4 in the brain and in particular the hippocampus.[13] Other studies identified muscarinic receptors in epidermal keratinocytes mainly of the M_4 and M_5 varieties. More work needs to be done to detect whether these muscarinic receptors play a specific role in keratinocyte regulation.[14] Another study performed comparative pharmacology of recombinant M_3 and M_5 muscarinic receptors that were expressed in Chinese hamster ovary cells. The investigators concluded that the M_3 and M_5 muscarinic receptors have similar pharmacologic profiles. They showed that in the absence of a high-affinity M_5 selective antagonist, affinity data for a large range of antagonists are crucial to define operationally the M_5 receptor subtype.[15] Table 144-1 summarizes the distribution and actions of muscarinic receptors in the human body.

PHARMACOKINETICS

Pharmacokinetics of Atropine
Volume of distribution: 1–1.7 L/kg
Peak plasma concentration: 30 min after intramuscular administration; 60 min after oral administration
Renal plasma flow: 712 ± 38 mL/min
Distribution half-life: 1 min
Hepatic plasma clearance: 519 ± 147 mL/min
Renal plasma clearance: 656 ± 118 mL/min
Elimination half-life: 2.6–4.3 hr

Atropine is absorbed rapidly from the gastrointestinal tract and across mucous membranes. It also is absorbed after ophthalmologic administration and to a lesser extent through intact skin. Systemic absorption of inhaled aerosolized atropine is minimal. In adults, atropine is absorbed mainly in the duodenum and the jejunum, as opposed to the stomach. After the ingestion of radiolabeled ^3H atropine, maximal radioactivity occurred at 1 hour.[16] Atropine also is absorbed after rectal administration. In children, the ratio between intramuscular and rectal peak plasma concentrations is 3.2:1.[17] Atropine can be absorbed via the lacrimal ducts.[18] Peak plasma concentrations are reached after 30 minutes when atropine is administered intramuscularly. The plasma concentration 1 hour after intramuscular administration is virtually equal to the plasma concentration seen with the intravenous route. Animal studies performed in anesthetized monkeys show that mean plasma concentrations after intraosseous administration correspond to concentrations seen at 2 minutes after intravenous administration. Endotracheal and intraosseous routes are feasible means of administration if intravenous access is delayed.[19] The endotracheal route could prove to be valuable in a military setting (e.g., soon after a nerve gas attack); the intraosseous route can be

TABLE 144-1 Distribution and Actions of Muscarinic Receptor Subtypes

RECEPTOR SUBTYPE	LOCATION	TRANSDUCTION SYSTEM	MAIN FUNCTIONS	RECEPTOR ANTAGONISTS
M_1	Neural: cerebral cortex, hippocampus, ganglia (enteric and autonomic); gastric: parietal cells	IP_3; DAG; depolarization excitation (slow EPSP)	CNS excitation; gastric acid secretion and gastrointestinal motility	Atropine, pirenzepine, dicyclomine
M_2	Cardiac: atria, conducting tissue; neural: presynaptic terminals	Inhibition of cAMP; slow IPSP; lowered intracellular Ca^{2+}	Cardiac, neural, and presynaptic inhibition	Atropine, gallamine, AF-DX 116*
M_3	Glandular: exocrine glands (lacrimal and sweat glands); vascular: smooth muscle and vascular endothelium; immune system: blood lymphocytes	IP_3; increased intracellular Ca^{2+}; stimulation via DAG	Secretion; smooth muscle contraction; vasodilation via nitric oxide; regulation of blood lymphocytes (?)	Atropine, HHSD
M_4	Neural: cerebral cortex, amygdala, hippocampus; skin: keratinocytes	Inhibition of cAMP; slow IPSP followed by decrease in intracellular Ca^{2+}	Cell-to-cell communication in keratinocytes; involved in memory/thought processes	Atropine, piperinidyl, tryptamine
M_5	Skin: keratinocytes; immune system: peripheral blood lymphocytes	Increase in IP_3 followed by increase in intracellular Ca^{2+}	Cell-to-cell communication in keratinocytes; possible role in lymphocyte function (?)	Atropine, tolterodine, oxybutynin, pirenzepine

*A test compound of selective M_2-receptor antagonist.

cAMP, cyclic adenosine monophosphate; DAG, diacylglycerol; EPSP/IPSP, excitatory/inhibitory postsynaptic potential; HHSD, hexahydrosiladifendiol; IP_3, inositol triphosphate.

recommended as a last-resort emergency route of administration in children.[5]

Only 5% of intravenously administered atropine remains within the circulatory system after 5 minutes.[20] Atropine has an initial distribution half-life of approximately 1 minute.[21] Elimination kinetics of atropine could be fitted to a two-compartment model after therapeutic doses. The apparent volume of distribution is 1 to 1.7 L/kg, with a clearance of 5.9 to 6.8 mL/kg/min.[22] Atropine crosses the placenta rapidly. Concentrations in the umbilical vein were 93% of the maternal level 5 minutes after intravenous administration.[23] Penetration into the lumbar cerebrospinal fluid is less complete, particularly after a single intravenous injection.[24] It has been suggested that the cerebrospinal fluid behaves as a deep compartment with a slow rate of drug penetration.[21] Penetration of atropine into the central nervous system is significantly greater than into lumbar cerebrospinal fluid, however, accounting for its known central anticholinergic effects.

Atropine is metabolized predominantly in the liver by microsomal monooxygenases. High-performance liquid chromatography separation of urine has identified five compounds: atropine, noratropine, tropine, equatorial N-oxide, and tropic acid. Atropine is metabolized partially in the urine, which is its main route of excretion.[25] Its excretion half-life is 2.6 to 4.3 hours, and its hepatic plasma clearance is 519 ± 147 mL/min with an extraction ratio of 0.32. The elimination of atropine is blood flow dependent.[26]

After intravenous administration, 57% of the dose is found in the urine as unchanged atropine and 29% as tropine. The renal plasma clearance, 656 ± 118 mL/min, is similar to renal plasma flow, 712 ± 38 mL/min. Because the liver and the kidneys are crucial in the metabolism and excretion of atropine, any diseases affecting these organs influence the kinetics of atropine.[26]

SPECIAL POPULATIONS

Neonatal Patients

Atropine crosses the placenta and reaches the fetal circulation.[23] Neonates may show a mild bradycardia after premedication of mothers with atropine, but it seems to be of little clinical significance.[23] Atropine administration in lactating mothers may impair milk production, although the evidence for this is inconclusive. Small quantities of atropine appear in breast milk when the drug is given to lactating mothers. No adverse effects have been reported, however, in nursing infants whose mothers were taking atropine.[27]

Pediatric Patients

Children absorb atropine percutaneously and per rectum more efficiently than adults. In children, plasma atropine concentration after intramuscular administration is 3.2 times greater than after rectal administration. Plasma elimination half-life in children is longer than in adults.[21] In emergency situations, the intraosseous route can be used in young children when the intravenous route is unavailable.[28]

Infants and children are particularly susceptible to the central nervous system toxic effects of atropine. They are better able to tolerate the cardiac effects, however.[29] In 1990, 268 Israeli children were given atropine accidentally or inappropriately from autoinjectors issued to the population for use in the event of a chemical nerve gas attack. Doses 17 times the standard dose for age were used, and plasma levels of 61 ng/mL were measured. Only 48% of the children showed systemic signs of atropinization, and 8% had severe toxicity. There were no fatalities.[30] Children with Down syndrome or convulsive disorders seem to be especially sensitive to atropine.[31]

Elderly Patients

The plasma elimination half-life is longer in elderly patients.[21] They are particularly at risk for adverse effects on the central nervous system. Urinary retention, constipation, and paralytic ileus are other potential adverse effects. The prevalence of acute glaucoma increases with age, and atropine may precipitate it.[31] Although the cardiac response to atropine is often less in the elderly, central nervous system effects are a particular problem. In addition, urinary retention and constipation are the side effects of atropine that are more troublesome in the elderly.

Pregnant Patients

Atropine rapidly crosses the placenta. In one study, concentrations in the umbilical vein were 93% of maternal values 5 minutes after intravenous injection.[23] Atropine has a negligible effect on the human uterus. There is no evidence that it is teratogenic. With organophosphate poisoning one always should use the dose required by the mother. Not using the appropriate dose increases the risk to the mother and the fetus.

Patients with Concurrent Disease

Many conditions, such as glaucoma, pyloric stenosis, and prostatic hypertrophy, can be exacerbated by atropine. The amount of atropine given as a single dose needs to be reduced in patients with renal and hepatic impairment. If further doses are required for conditions such as bradycardia and organophosphate poisoning, renal or hepatic dysfunction is not a contraindication, and the dose given should be titrated against clinical therapeutic end points.[31]

CONTRAINDICATIONS

Atropine is contraindicated in patients with glaucoma, chronic lung disease, unstable cardiac rhythm, prostatic hypertrophy, reflux esophagitis, and pyloric stenosis. Local and systemic use of atropine can precipitate acute glaucoma, particularly in patients predisposed to narrow-angle glaucoma. Prolonged mydriasis occurred after administration of Lamaline (atropine derivative containing belladonna, acetaminophen, opium, and caffeine) suppositories in one patient.[32] If mydriasis is prolonged, blindness may ensue. The risk is greatest with high-dose or parenteral use.[2,31] Because of the reduction of bronchial secretions, there may be a marked increase in viscosity resulting in inspissation of residual secretions.[31]

If the cardiac rhythm is unstable or if there already is tachycardia, atropine should not be administered. Sick sinus syndrome, thyrotoxicosis, and cardiac failure with tachycardia are specific contraindications for atropine.[2,31] Atropine antagonizes parasympathetic action on the bladder, reducing bladder contractions. In patients with prostatic hypertrophy, atropine may produce acute urinary retention.[31] Atropine lowers esophageal sphincter tone and reduces gastric emptying. Esophageal reflux is a relative contraindication to atropine.[31] Atropine may convert partial organic pyloric stenosis into complete obstruction.

ADVERSE EFFECTS

Atropine, similar to other muscarinic receptor antagonists, produces many adverse effects. Dryness of the mouth results in thirst, difficulty with swallowing, and difficulty with speech. Ophthalmologic effects include cycloplegia resulting in photophobia and blurred vision. Dermatologic adverse effects include flushing and dryness of the skin. Cardiac effects include initial transient bradycardia followed by tachycardia, palpitations, and dysrhythmias. Because of decreased smooth muscle tone, difficulty in micturition and constipation may result. Vomiting also may occur. Hypersensitivity reactions may occur as well. Anaphylactic shock developed in a 38-year-old woman after an intravenous injection of atropine.[33]

At higher doses, atropine may cause the following symptoms: tachycardia, tachypnea, hyperpyrexia, and central nervous system stimulation (marked by restlessness, confusion, excitement, ataxia, incoordination, paranoia, psychotic reactions, hallucinations, and delirium). Seizures also rarely can occur. Flushing may appear on the face or upper trunk. If the patient is severely intoxicated, the initial stimulation of the central nervous system may revert to a depressive effect, followed by coma, circulatory and respiratory failure, and eventual death.

As a result of the variation of the numbers and nature of receptors, considerable variation exists in susceptibility to atropine. Recovery has occurred even after 1 g, whereas deaths have been reported from doses of 100 mg or less in adults and 10 mg in children. Quaternary ammonium antimuscarinic compounds, such as atropine methobromide, have some ganglion-blocking action, and in larger doses postural hypotension may occur. Impotence also may occur. In toxic doses, nondepolarizing neuromuscular block may develop.

Systemic toxicity may be produced by instillation of antimuscarinic eye drops, particularly in children. Atropine poisoning occurred in a patient who had been given 10 atropine sulfate aerosol treatments in the preceding 24 hours and in children who had taken overdoses of a preparation containing diphenoxylate and atropine.[34] Atropine can cause hyperpyrexia as a result of inhibition of sweating; there was a report of hypothermia in a 14-year-old feverish patient after administration of atropine.[35]

In overdoses of atropine that have been taken by mouth, activated charcoal should be administered if less than one hour has elapsed. Supportive therapy should be given as required. Physostigmine has been tried for atropine poisoning, but its value is limited, and it generally is not recommended. Physostigmine may cause cardiac arrhythmias and higher morbidity and mortality. Diazepam may be given to control marked excitement and convulsions. Phenothiazines should not be administered because they may exacerbate the antimuscarinic effects.[2]

Although atropine intoxication causes severe morbidity and potentially life-threatening effects, particularly on the heart, mortality is rare after treatment of atropine poisoning.[2] Inducing mild-to-moderate atropine poisoning (atropinization) is required in the treatment of organophosphate poisoning.

ADMINISTRATION

Dosage Forms

Atropine sulfate is available from several manufacturers as oral, parenteral, nebulizing, and ophthalmic preparations. In the United States, tablets containing 400 mg and soluble tablets containing 400 μg or 600 μg of atropine sulfate are available. In the United Kingdom, tablets containing 600 μg of atropine sulfate may be available. Different preparations for injections ranging from 0.5 to 10 mg/mL are available in many countries.

Indications

Atropine sulfate has been used for the treatment of brady-arrhythmias, mushroom poisoning, and organophosphate poisoning. It also has been used as anesthetic premedication and ophthalmic eye drops for various ophthalmologic conditions and after cataract surgery. Atropine has been used as an adjunct in the treatment of diarrhea, irritable colon syndrome, myasthenia gravis, vestibular disorders, asthma, and tetanus. Other anticholinergic agents, such as ipratropium bromide, are used now rather than atropine for asthma.

Doses

Apart from organophosphate and carbamate poisonings, atropine normally is used in low doses, not exceeding 1.2 mg as a single parenteral dose. In the case of bradyasystolic cardiac arrest in adults, atropine is recommended in a single intravenous dose of 3 mg if there is no response to epinephrine.[36,37] Atropine may be given via an endotracheal tube in a dose that is two to three times the intravenous dose in 10 mL of isotonic saline.[38] Doses of atropine greater than 100 mg may be needed to treat severe organophosphate poisoning as an initial dose to induce atropinization. Doses greater than 1000 mg over the first 24 hours may be required.

REFERENCES

1. Budavari S: Atropine. In The Merck Index, 11th ed. Rahway, NJ, Merck & Co, 1989, p 138.
2. Reynolds JFF: Martindale—the Extra Pharmacopoeia, 31st ed. London, Royal Pharmaceutical Society, 1996, pp 490–493.
3. Ali-Melkkila A, Kanto J, Iisalo E: Pharmacokinetics and related pharmacodynamics of anticholinergic drugs. Acta Anesthesiol Scand 37:633–642, 1993.
4. Brown JH, Taylor P: Muscarinic receptor antagonists. In Goodman and Gilman's the Pharmacological Basis of Therapeutics, 9th ed. New York, McGraw-Hill, 1996, pp 148–154.
5. Heath AJW, Meredith T: Atropine in the management of anti-cholinesterase poisoning. In Ballantyne B, Marrs T (eds): Clinical and Experimental Toxicology of Organophosphate Poisoning. New York, Macmillan, 1993, pp 543–554.
6. Deeks T: Oral atropine sulphate mixtures. Pharm J 230:481, 1983.
7. Yamamura HI, Snyder SH: Muscarinic cholinergic receptor binding in the longitudinal muscle of the guinea pig ileum with [3H]quinuclidinyl benzilate. Mol Pharmacol 10:861–867, 1974.
8. Caulfield MP: Muscarinic receptors—characterization, coupling and function. Pharmacol Ther 58:319–372, 1993.
9. Kostensis E, Zeng FY, Wess J: Structure-function analysis of muscarinic acetylcholine receptors. J Physiol (Paris) 92:265–268, 1998.
10. Berkeley JL, Levey AI: Muscarinic activation of mitogen-activated protein kinase in PC12 cells. J Neurochem 75:487–493, 2000.
11. Tayebati SK, Codini M, Gallai V, et al: Radioligand binding assay of M1-M5 muscarinic cholinergic receptor subtypes in human peripheral blood lymphocytes. J Neuroimmunol 29:224–229, 1999.
12. Flynn DD, Ferrari-DiLeo G, Mash DC, et al: Differential regulation of molecular subtypes of muscarinic receptors in Alzheimer's disease. J Neurochem 64:1888–1891, 1995.
13. Rouse ST, Marino MJ, Potter LT, et al: Muscarinic receptor subtypes involved in hippocampal circuits. Life Sci 64:501–509, 1999.
14. Ndoye A, Buchli R, Greenberg B, et al: Identification and mapping of keratinocyte muscarinic acetylcholine receptor subtypes in human epidermis. J Invest Dermatol 111:410–416, 1998.
15. Watson N, Daniels DV, Ford AP, et al: Comparative pharmacology of recombinant human M3 and M5 muscarinic receptors expressed in CHO-K1 cells. Br J Pharmacol 127:590–596, 1999.
16. Beerman B, Hellstrom K, Rosen A: The gastrointestinal absorption of atropine in man. Clin Sci 40:95–106, 1971.
17. Olsson GL, Bejersten A, Feytching H, et al: Plasma concentration of atropine after rectal administration. Acta Anaesthesiol Scand 29:782–784, 1985.
18. Reynolds JFF: Martindale—the Extra Pharmacopoeia, 29th ed. London, Royal Pharmaceutical Society, 1989.
19. Prete MR, Hannan CJ, Bunce FM: Plasma atropine concentrations via intravenous, endotracheal and intraosseous administration. Am J Emerg Med 5:101–104, 1987.
20. Berghem L, Bergman U, Schildt B, et al: Plasma atropine concentrations determined by radioimmunoassay after single dose iv and im administration. Br J Anaesth 52:597–601, 1980.
21. Kanto J, Klotz U: Pharmacokinetic implications for the clinical use of atropine, scopolamine and glycopyrrolate. Acta Anaesthesiol Scand 32:69–78, 1988.
22. Aaltonen L, Kanto J, Iisalo E, et al: Comparison of radioreceptor assay and radioimmunoassay for atropine pharmacokinetic application. Eur J Clin Pharmacol 26:613–617, 1984.
23. Kivalo I, Saarikoski S: Placental transmission of atropine at full term pregnancy. Br J Anaesth 49:1017–1021, 1977.
24. Virtanen R, Kanto J, Iisalo E, et al: Pharmacokinetic studies on atropine with special reference to age. Acta Anaesthesiol Scand 26:297–300, 1982.
25. Van der Meer MJ, Hundt HKL, Muller FO: Inhibition of atropine metabolism by organophosphate pesticides. Hum Toxicol 2:637–640, 1983.
26. Hinderling PH, Gundert-Remy U, Schmidlin O: Integrated pharmacokinetics and pharmacodynamics of atropine in healthy humans. J Pharm Sci 74:703–710, 1985.
27. Committee on Drugs, American Academy of Pediatrics: The transfer of drugs and other chemicals into human milk. Paediatrics 93:137–150, 1994.
28. Prete MR, Hannan CJ, Burkle FM: Plasma atropine concentrations via intravenous, endotracheal, and intraosseous administration. Am J Emerg Med 5:101–104, 1987.
29. Rumack BH: Anticholinergic poisoning: Treatment with physostigmine. Pediatrics 52:449–451, 1973.
30. Amitai Y, Almog S, Singer R, et al: Atropine poisoning in children during the Persian Gulf crisis: A national survey in Israel. JAMA 268:630–632, 1992.
31. Dollery C: Therapeutic Drugs, 2nd ed. Edinburgh, Churchill Livingstone, 1999, pp A240–A244.
32. Maizoub S, Autret E, Furet Y, et al: Prolonged mydriasis caused by Lamaline. Bull Soc Ophtalmol Fr 89:421–422, 1989.
33. Aguilera L: Anaphylactic reaction after atropine. Anaesthesia 43:955–957, 1988.
34. McCarron MM: Diphenoxylate-atropine (Lomotil) overdose in children: An update (report of eight cases and review of the literature). Pediatrics 87:694–700, 1991.
35. Lacouture PG: Acute hypothermia associated with atropine. Am J Dis Child 137:291–292, 1983.
36. McAuliffe G, Bissonnette B, Boutin C: Should the routine use of atropine before succinylcholine in children be reconsidered? Can J Anaesth 42:724–729, 1995.
37. Shorten GD, Bissonette B, Hartley E, et al: It is not necessary to administer more than 10 g·kg⁻¹ of atropine to older children before succinyl choline. Can J Anaesth 48:8–11, 1995.
38. Hapnes S, Robertson C: CPR-drug delivery routes and systems. Resuscitation 24:137–142, 1992.

CHAPTER 145

Oximes

J. Allister Vale

Studies performed in North America[1-7] and in Great Britain[8-19] in the 1950s led to the introduction and assessment of several pralidoxime salts for military purposes (nerve agent exposure). Pralidoxime was used first in humans to treat organophosphorus insecticide poisoning in 1956.[20]

HISTORY

Pralidoxime was synthesized originally as the iodide salt, but this preparation was poorly soluble in water and produced iodism.[21] Alternatives were sought, although pralidoxime iodide remains in some pharmacopoeias and was used in Japan to treat some victims of the sarin releases.[22,23] Pralidoxime chloride and pralidoxime mesylate (P2S) have largely superseded the iodide salt because they are soluble in water and produce fewer undesirable side effects. P2S was introduced for clinical use in the United Kingdom in 1961, and pralidoxime chloride first was licensed for use in the United States in 1964.[24] Pralidoxime methylsulfate (Contrathion) is licensed in France and Italy. Subsequently, obidoxime was developed in an attempt to provide more effective treatment than pralidoxime for some types of nerve agent poisoning, such as tabun and soman poisoning. Obidoxime also has been employed in the treatment of organophosphorus insecticide poisoning in some countries (e.g., Germany).[25] In addition to pralidoxime salts and obidoxime, the Hagedorn (H) oximes, particularly HI-6 and HLö-7, have been studied mostly in a military context.[26,27]

In clinical practice, oximes usually are administered intravenously because this is the most rapid way of achieving and maintaining satisfactory plasma concentrations. Oximes also may be given intramuscularly, which is the route employed for self-administration (using an autoinjector) when it is not possible to give intravenous injections either because of lack of medical expertise or because of special circumstances such as arise in war. This chapter focuses on pralidoxime because this is the most widely available oxime.

SHELF-LIFE OF PREPARATIONS

The rate and degree of degradation of pralidoxime solutions depend on several factors, including the initial and final pH of the solution and the type of container in which the solution is stored. Calculated shelf-lives allowing for 10% degradation of 50% (w/v) pralidoxime chloride solution are 37 years, 7 years, and 1.6 years at 10°C (50°F), 20°C (68°F), and 30°C

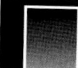

Commercially Available Preparations of Oximes

Pralidoxime Chloride

Synonyms: 2-PAM, 2-PAM chloride, 2-pyridine aldoxime methylchloride
Formula: $C_7H_9ClN_2O$
Molecular weight: 172.6
Trade names: Protopam Chloride (Ayerst, United States; Wyeth-Ayerst, Canada)
Pharmaceutical preparation: Pralidoxime chloride, 1 g, suitable for parenteral use

Pralidoxime Mesylate

Synonyms: P2S, pralidoxime methanesulphonate, 2PAMM
Formula: $C_8H_{12}N_2O_4S$
Molecular weight: 232.3
Pharmaceutical preparation: Pralidoxime mesylate, 1 g, suitable for parenteral use (license holder: United Kingdom Departments of Health)

Pralidoxime Methylsulfate

Synonym: 2-Pyridine aldoxime methylsulfate
Formula: $C_8H_{12}N_2O_5S$
Molecular weight: 248.3
Trade name: Contrathion (SERB, France; Rhone-Poulenc Rorer, Italy)
Pharmaceutical preparation: Pralidoxime methylsulfate, 200 mg, suitable for parenteral use

Pralidoxime Iodide

Synonyms: 2-PAM iodide, protopam iodide, 2-pyridine aldoxime methiodide
Formula: $C_7H_9IN_2O$
Molecular weight: 264.1

Obidoxime Chloride

Synonym: Obidoxime dichloride
Formula: $C_{14}H_{16}Cl_2N_4O_3$
Molecular weight: 359.2
Trade names: Toxigonin (Australia, Germany, Netherlands, South Africa, Sweden); Toxigonine (Switzerland)
Pharmaceutical preparation: Obidoxime chloride, 250 mg, suitable for parenteral use

(86°F), respectively.[28] P2S can be stored for at least 5 years at 5°C (41°F) with less than 7% decomposition.[29] Schroeder and colleagues[30] showed that an autoinjector solution (pralidoxime chloride, 300 mg/mL) stored at 5°C for more than 10 years contained more than 90% pralidoxime chloride.

GENERAL PROPERTIES

Oximes act primarily as acetylcholinesterase reactivators, although newer oximes, such as HI-6 (which is not yet commercially available), may exert pharmacologic effects unrelated to reactivation of inhibited acetylcholinesterase that could lead to survival of the poisoned patient, even when the enzyme is "aged."[31] After exposure either to an organophosphorus insecticide or to a nerve agent, acetylcholinesterase is inactivated by a process of alkylphosphorylation (Fig. 145-1); this leads to the accumulation of acetylcholine and the development of the characteristic signs of poisoning (see Chapter 91). Oximes bind to the phosphate to form an oxime-phosphate complex, which splits off, leaving the enzyme regenerated. The speed of the reactivation varies, depending on the nature of the organophosphorus compound and whether the phosphorylated enzyme is "aged." (For a fuller discussion, see Chapter 91.)

Clinically the main benefit of oximes is to reverse cholinergic effects at peripheral nicotinic sites so that muscle strength may improve within 10 to 30 minutes of oxime administration. Oximes are much less effective than atropine at peripheral muscarinic sites, and their effects on central nervous system–mediated symptoms and signs may not be clinically significant.[32] The therapeutic combination of oxime and atropine is well established in the treatment of organophosphorus insecticide and nerve agent poisoning.

PHARMACODYNAMICS

The dose of oxime to produce the appropriate area-under-the-curve (AUC) of (concentration) × (time) required to achieve the desired reactivation of phosphorylated enzyme is not known with certainty. The AUC to reactivate a certain

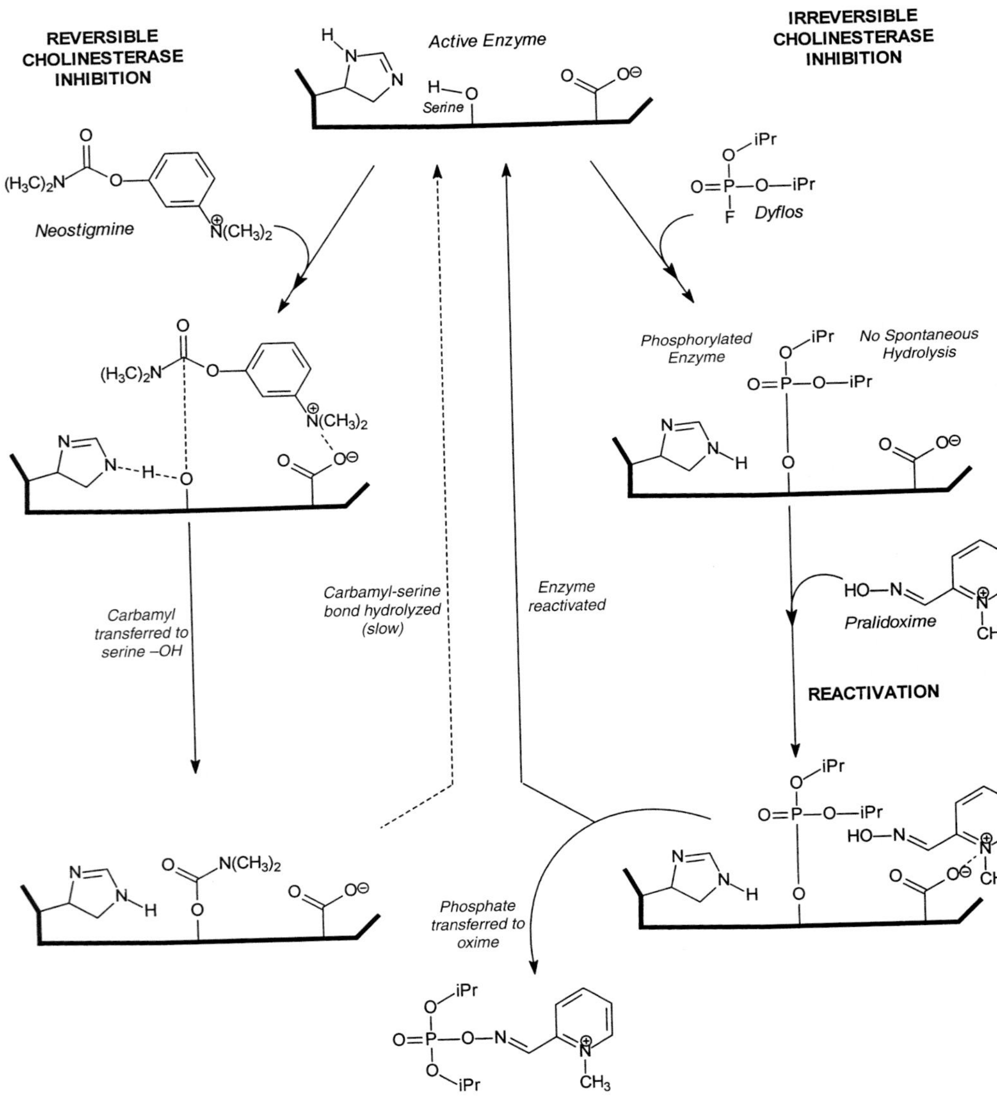

FIGURE 145-1

The action of anticholinesterase agents and reactivation by the oxime pralidoxime. For comparison, the actions of a reversible (neostigmine) agent and an irreversible (dyflos) acetylcholinesterase inhibitor are shown. In the case of dyflos, the reactivation of the enzyme by pralidoxime is illustrated. iPr, isopropyl.

percentage of human acetylcholinesterase may be different for human dimethyl and diethyl phosphorylated enzyme. Estimates of appropriate AUCs often are derived from animal or in vitro studies with nerve agents, which are chemically distinct from organophosphorus insecticides.

Oximes are cleared rapidly from the body, and although some reactivation may be achieved, another cycle of inhibition (and possibly of aging of inhibited acetylcholinesterase) may follow. This is particularly so in the case of massive overdose, in which residual insecticide may persist in the body for many days, causing a continuous release of inhibitory oxon (active metabolite) in the circulation.[33] The initial benefit of an effective dose of oxime may be overcome by such a process, and only persistent treatment can be expected to bring about a lasting clinical improvement.

It is commonly, but erroneously, believed that 1 day after intoxication with an organophosphorus insecticide virtually all the phosphorylated enzyme is in the aged inhibited form so that oxime therapy would be ineffective after this time. This interpretation derives from in vitro studies, however, in which acetylcholinesterase is inhibited rapidly and is maintained fully inhibited thereafter by the presence of an excess of inhibitor and in the absence of oxime throughout the experiment. These experiments do not represent the case in vivo, however, and should not be used as a reason to abandon the use of oxime therapy after 24 hours.

The beneficial effect of continuous oxime therapy has been shown experimentally. Oxime was delivered by continuous infusion from implanted minipumps to rats intoxicated orally with quinalphos, a diethyl phosphorothioate with prolonged action. Treated rats received only one small dose of atropine and diazepam plus continuous oxime for 2 to 4 days and were able to survive more than 30 times the usual median lethal dose.[34] The value of prolonged oxime therapy has also been shown in human poisoning.[25,35-38]

Animal Studies

Pralidoxime alone can reduce mortality in organophosphorus intoxication,[4,39-41] although in combination with atropine the protection is far greater.[4,11,34,41-44] The addition of diazepam to pralidoxime and atropine may add further benefit.[34]

Early experiments in anesthetized cats (possibly only seven animals) given lethal doses of intravenous sarin and P2S, 10 mg/kg intramuscularly, but not atropine, established that plasma pralidoxime concentrations of greater than 4 mg/L were required to counteract neuromuscular block in vitro and bradycardia, hypotension, and respiratory failure in vivo.[45] Crook and associates[46] gave dogs oral pralidoxime (P2S and lactate), 30 to 115 mg/kg body weight, 1 to 5 hours before exposure to sarin vapor. Atropine, 5 mg/kg body weight, was administered 1 minute after the dogs were exposed to sarin. The authors extrapolated from this study in dogs to humans and concluded that a plasma pralidoxime concentration of at least 3 mg/L would be required "for reasonably protective attenuation of the toxic effects of organophosphorus anticholinesterases."

The relationship between plasma oxime concentrations after dosing with pralidoxime and obidoxime and protection against sarin poisoning has been investigated by Shiloff and Clement[47] in rats (Table 145-1) and by Bokonjic and colleagues[34] in quinalphos-poisoned rats given pralidoxime (Table 145-2). Taken together, these studies support the recommendation that plasma oxime concentrations of more than 4 mg/L are required to produce a significant reduction in mortality in experimental organophosphorus poisoning.

Human Studies

Grob and Johns[48] conducted a series of experiments in volunteers in whom neuromuscular block was produced by the intraarterial administration of many anticholinesterase compounds, including sarin. Pralidoxime was administered either intraarterially or intravenously. The neuromuscular block induced by sarin was "promptly and strikingly reversed in the injected extremity immediately after the intraarterial injection" of pralidoxime iodide. The prophylactic intraarterial administration of the oxime protected against the action of sarin on neuromuscular transmission. Intravenous therapy was less effective than intraarterial therapy, although generalized weakness was "ameliorated" to a moderate degree after the injection of pralidoxime iodide, 500 to 2000 mg. Muscular fasciculations also were reduced to a lesser degree than after intraarterial injection. Approximately 20 minutes after pralidoxime administration, there

TABLE 145-1 Relationship Between Plasma Oxime Concentrations and Mortality in Sarin-Poisoned Rats also Given Atropine*

OXIME	n	MEAN (± SD) OXIME CONCENTRATION (mg/L)	% MORTALITY
Pralidoxime	5	0.7 ± 0.1	100
Pralidoxime	4	2.0 ± 0.4	80
Pralidoxime	5	3.3 ± 2.3	20
Obidoxime	10	3.6 ± 0.2	90
Obidoxime	8	9.2 ± 0.6	62.5
Obidoxime	5	19.7 ± 3.7	0

*Atropine dose, 17.4 mg/kg.

After Shiloff JD, Clement JG: Comparison of serum concentrations of the acetylcholinesterase oxime reactivators HI-6, obidoxime, and PAM to efficacy against sarin (isopropyl methylphosphonofluoridate) poisoning in rats. Toxicol Appl Pharmacol 89:278–280, 1987.

TABLE 145-2 Relationship Between Plasma Pralidoxime Concentrations and LD$_{50}$ in Quinalphos-Poisoned Rats also Given Atropine and Diazepam*

MEAN (± SEM) PLASMA PRALIDOXIME CONCENTRATION (mg/L)	MEAN (± SEM) LD$_{50}$ (mg/kg)	PROTECTIVE INDEX
0	10.5 ± 3.8	—
0.8	353.6 ± 33.6	33.7
1.5 ± 0.6	457.9 ± 121.6	43.6
2.9 ± 0.7	498.7 ± 137.9	47.5

*Atropine dose, 10 mg/kg; diazepam, 2.5 mg/kg.
LD$_{50}$, median lethal dose.
Modified from Bokonjic D, Jovanovic D, Jokanovic M, Maksimovic M: Protective effects of oximes HI-6 and PAM-2 applied by osmotic minipumps in quinalphos-poisoned rats. Arch Int Pharmacodyn 288:309–318, 1987.

was usually some return of weakness and fasciculation, but not to the original level.

Studies in poisoned patients have shown that reactivation of dimethoate-inhibited enzyme was not achieved with a plasma pralidoxime concentration of 6.37 mg/L.[49] In the same study, it was shown that reactivation of inhibited enzyme did not occur even in the presence of a plasma pralidoxime concentration of 14.6 mg/L when plasma ethyl and methyl parathion concentrations were greater than 30 μg/L.[49] Data from case reports suggest that pralidoxime concentrations of greater than 40 mg/L may be required in severe cases of organophosphorus insecticide poisoning to produce reactivation of inhibited acetylcholinesterase.[37,38] The modest doses of pralidoxime that often have been recommended in the past (to achieve plasma oxime concentrations of approximately 4 mg/L) would be insufficient to produce reactivation of phosphorylated enzyme and a lasting clinical improvement, unless the patient is only mildly poisoned. Clinically effective pralidoxime concentrations need to be maintained as long as inhibitory oxons (active organophosphorus metabolites) are circulating.

PHARMACOKINETICS

Pralidoxime

Most kinetic studies on pralidoxime have been performed in healthy, nonpoisoned subjects. There is evidence from animal[50,51] and human[52] studies that organophosphorus compounds can alter pralidoxime kinetics in a complex manner; this may be due to the cardiovascular changes and reduced blood flow seen in organophosphorus insecticide poisoning. It may be inappropriate to extrapolate the results of volunteer studies to severely intoxicated individuals.

Being quaternary amines, pralidoxime salts and obidoxime are not well absorbed after oral administration, although pralidoxime chloride tablets remain commercially available. Ethanol does not seem to interfere with the absorption of pralidoxime.[53]

The distribution of pralidoxime is determined largely by its small molecular size and quaternary amine structure. It is distributed widely in most body fluids and is not significantly bound to plasma proteins.[54] Pralidoxime penetrates the erythrocyte membrane by simple diffusion and does not bind either to red blood cell stroma or to hemoglobin.[55] Pralidoxime does not pass readily into the central nervous system.[56] The values for the apparent volume of distribution in the central compartment, in the peripheral compartment, and at steady state in volunteers are given in Table 145-3; the values at steady state were 0.6 to 0.8 L/kg. In poisoned patients treated with the methylsufate and the chloride salts, the mean (± SD) volumes of distribution were 2.77 ± 1.45 L/kg[57] and 2.8 ± 2.2 L/kg.[52]

Pralidoxime is metabolized only to a minor extent in humans.[58] It is excreted rapidly in urine,[53,54,59–65] and there is no evidence of dose-dependent kinetics. Because urinary clearance of pralidoxime exceeds simultaneously measured creatinine clearance, pralidoxime is probably secreted by the renal tubules at least in part by mechanisms shared by several other strong bases.[64] Josselson and Sidell[66] investigated the effect of intravenous thiamine hydrochloride on the elimination of pralidoxime chloride, 5 mg/kg body weight administered intravenously. The addition of thiamine lengthened the elimination half-life, and the oxime concentration increased, whereas the intercompartment clearances and rate constant for elimination of oxime decreased. The authors suggested that either thiamine and pralidoxime compete for a common secretory mechanism or thiamine alters the membrane transport of pralidoxime. Pralidoxime is excreted preferentially in an acid urine,[67] and intravenous sodium bicarbonate markedly reduces pralidoxime excretion.

Most studies, whether performed in humans or animals, have seemed to show first-order disappearance of pralidoxime from the plasma,[54,59,68] but more complex models have been proposed.[62] In several volunteer studies, the pralidoxime half-life varied from 67 to 84 minutes (see Table 145-3) after intravenous dosing of pralidoxime, 5 to 10 mg/kg body weight. In poisoned patients treated with the methylsulfate and chloride salts, the mean (± SD) elimination half-lives were found to be 3.44 ± 0.9 hours[57] and 2.9 ± 1.18 hours, respectively.[52]

Swartz and Sidell[64] observed that in six volunteers given pralidoxime chloride, 5 mg/kg body weight (but not atropine), exercise alone and exercise plus heat stress significantly (P < .05) increased the pralidoxime elimination half-life and increased the volumes of distribution

TABLE 145-3 Pralidoxime Kinetics After Intravenous Dosing in Volunteers

DOSE (mg/kg) (SALT)	HALF-LIFE β (min)	VOLUME OF DISTRIBUTION (L/kg)			STUDY
		V_1	V_2	$(Vd)_{ss}$	
5 (chloride)	78	0.27	0.54	0.82	Sidell et al[54]
5 (chloride)	71	0.37	0.39	0.76	Swartz and Sidell[76]
5 (chloride)	67	0.18	0.42	0.60	Josselson and Sidell[66]
5 (P2S)	84	0.20	0.58	0.78	Sidell et al[62]
10 (chloride)	79	0.30	0.46	0.76	Sidell and Groff[61]

V_1, central compartment; V_2, peripheral compartment; Vd_{ss}, volume of distribution at steady state.

for central and peripheral compartments. This finding suggests that exercise and heat not only reduced the renal elimination of pralidoxime but also changed oxime distribution.

Obidoxime Chloride

Obidoxime chloride is absorbed poorly after oral administration and is given parenterally. Sidell and Groff[69] reported in volunteers that the mean plasma half-life was 1.38 hours after obidoxime, 2.5 to 10 mg/kg intramuscularly. Within 24 hours, 84% of the total administered dose was excreted via the urine.[69] In another study in volunteers, a mean (± SD) of 68 (± 8)% of the administered dose (0.5 to 1 mg/kg intravenously) was recovered in the urine in 24 hours.[54] The mean (± SD) elimination half-life was 1.2 ± 0.16 hours, the mean (± SD) volume of distribution at steady state was 0.173 (± 0.022) L/kg, and the mean (± SD) plasma clearance was 133 (± 12) mL/min.[54]

In keeping with the difference in molecular weight between obidoxime and pralidoxime, the plasma concentrations versus time curves were almost identical after intravenous administration of obidoxime, 1 mg/kg, and pralidoxime chloride, 5 mg/kg.[54]

SPECIAL POPULATIONS

Pharmacokinetic data have not been collected in neonates, children, pregnant women, or elderly patients. Experimental studies are insufficient with respect to the effects of pralidoxime in pregnancy and on fetal development. The risk to mother and fetus is likely to be considerable, however, if adequate treatment for organophosphorus insecticide poisoning with oxime is not instituted promptly, and this consideration should override the minor possibility that fetal damage may ensue.

CONTRAINDICATIONS

There are no absolute contraindications to the use of oximes, although it is possible that in patients with renal impairment, dosage adjustment of pralidoxime and obidoxime may need to be considered if the glomerular filtration rate is less than

30 mL/min; further data are required to support this recommendation. Caution also is required when pralidoxime is administered to patients with myasthenia gravis because it may precipitate a myasthenic crisis.

ADVERSE EFFECTS

Pralidoxime

Sidell and coworkers[70] gave military personnel pralidoxime chloride, 3 to 9 g orally; only individuals receiving 8 to 9 g experienced diarrhea. Volunteers were administered pralidoxime chloride, pralidoxime iodide, and P2S, 1.5 to 10 g orally.[68] The subjects receiving the iodide salt experienced the signs and symptoms of iodism, including coryza, pharyngeal burning, and painful parotid glands; consequently the iodide salt now is used only rarely. No subjective complaints were made by the volunteers who ingested pralidoxime chloride and P2S in this study.

Jager and associates[71] found that medical students given a single dose of pralidoxime iodide, 15 to 20 mg/kg body weight intravenously, experienced dizziness, blurred vision, diplopia, impaired accommodation, headache, and nausea. Single oral doses of pralidoxime chloride, 1, 2, or 4 g, did not lead to changes in blood pressure or pulse, whereas the intramuscular administration of pralidoxime chloride, 30 mg/kg, produced a pressor response and T-wave elevation on the electrocardiogram.[53] Clinically significant electrocardiogram changes due to pralidoxime have not been observed in clinical practice. The same dose of pralidoxime chloride given intravenously had similar effects, but pralidoxime chloride, 45 mg/kg body weight, also produced prolongation of the PR interval. Headache, disturbance of accommodation, and epigastric discomfort also were noted.

Volunteers who received pralidoxime chloride daily for 6 months tolerated the oxime well, although elevation of transaminase (aminotransferase) activity, transient lymphocytosis, and clinically insignificant electrocardiogram changes were noted in some subjects.[53] The same workers found that oral P2S was less well tolerated than pralidoxime chloride because it produced more gastrointestinal disturbance. Soldiers given repeated *oral* doses of pralidoxime for 48 hours experienced diarrhea (often recurrent), anorexia, and malaise.[70]

Obidoxime

It has been recognized since the introduction of obidoxime that treatment for several days, particularly in high dosage, may result in liver damage, which is usually transient. Finkelstein and coworkers[72] showed an association between liver dysfunction and the cumulative dose of obidoxime. The liver damage usually manifests as an increase in hepatic enzyme activities and hyperbilirubinemia.[25]

ADMINISTRATION

Clinical Use: Choosing Which Oxime to Use

Choosing which oxime to use is largely an academic discussion because a choice usually is not available to critical care physicians. Various experimental studies in animals have claimed the superiority of one or another oxime in the treatment of poisoning by a particular organophosphorus compound (usually a short-lived nerve agent), but comparative studies in humans have not been reported. Between-study comparisons should recognize that plasma concentrations measured by weight for unit volume need to be converted to molar units because the molecular weights of the available oxime salts are markedly different. The molecular weights of pralidoxime chloride, P2S, and obidoxime chloride are 172, 232, and 359 d, respectively. The potency of a particular oxime depends in part on the "goodness-of-fit" of its molecule to the region of the active site of the inhibited acetylcholinesterase molecule. This "fit" is influenced by the chemistry of the particular inhibitor and varies among compounds. Conclusions drawn from studies with one organophosphorus insecticide cannot be applied automatically to all others (or to nerve agent poisoning), although class comparisons (i.e., for diethyl phosphates) may be valid.

Organophosphorus Insecticide Poisoning: Dose and Route

The wide availability of pralidoxime chloride, P2S, and obidoxime chloride, together with experimental evidence showing efficacy particularly when these oximes are used in conjunction with atropine, makes these oximes the appropriate choice for immediate treatment of organophosphorus insecticide poisoning. Prolonged, high-dose treatment with pralidoxime iodide and with obidoxime chloride should be avoided, if possible, because of potential adverse effects.

Pralidoxime chloride or P2S should be administered as soon after exposure as possible in a dose of 30 mg/kg body weight (2 g in an adult) every 4 to 6 hours preferably by intravenous injection, although intramuscular dosing is possible. Alternatively, pralidoxime chloride or P2S can be given as an intravenous infusion at a rate of 8 to 10 mg/kg/hr, after pralidoxime has been administered in a loading dose of 30 mg/kg body weight parenterally. This dosing regimen should ensure continued reactivation of inhibited enzyme, regardless of the organophosphorus insecticide involved, until recovery has occurred (see Chapter 91).

The dose of obidoxime often employed is 4 mg/kg intravenously followed by a continuous infusion of 0.5 mg/kg/hr until clinical recovery is observed. Alternatively, continued administration of obidoxime may be by intermittent intravenous doses of 2 mg/kg every 4 hours. In severely poisoned patients, doses greater than the aforementioned doses may be necessary to achieve enzyme reactivation.[73]

Nerve Agent Poisoning: Dose and Route

It is unlikely that it will be known with certainty in a clinically relevant period which nerve agent has been released. The oxime most readily available should be administered in the appropriate therapeutic dose. Experimental studies in guinea pigs and monkeys have shown that pralidoxime plus atropine and obidoxime plus atropine were less effective in soman poisoning than HI-6 plus atropine, although pralidoxime plus atropine was more effective than obidoxime plus atropine.[74] Studies have shown invariably that higher oxime doses, together with atropine, have increased survival further, regardless of the nerve agent.[74] HI-6 also was more effective in GF nerve agent poisoning than obidoxime plus atropine.[75] Overall, however, pralidoxime is the first-choice oxime for civilian use in many countries because it is the most widely available, it is cheaper to synthesize than HI-6, and it produces fewer adverse effects than obidoxime in equimolar concentrations.

If pralidoxime is available (either as the chloride or mesylate salts), it should be administered as soon after exposure as possible to moderately or severely poisoned patients in a dose of 30 mg/kg body weight (2 g in an adult) intravenously over 4 minutes to reactivate phosphorylated enzyme. Early administration is a priority to ensure that enzyme reactivation occurs before substantial "aging" ensues. In severe cases, pralidoxime chloride or P2S, 30 mg/kg body weight intravenously, is required every 4 to 6 hours, depending on the clinical features and erythrocyte cholinesterase activity. Alternatively an infusion of P2S or pralidoxime chloride, 8 to 10 mg/kg/hr, may be administered. Obidoxime chloride, 4 mg/kg intravenously, should be administered as soon as possible after exposure, and further doses of obidoxime, 2 to 4 mg/kg, should be given as required to maintain clinical improvement.

REFERENCES

1. Wilson IB, Meislich EK: Reactivation of acteylcholinesterase inhibited by alkylphosphates. J Am Chem Soc 75:4628–4629, 1953.
2. Wilson IB, Ginsburg S: A powerful reactivator of alkylphosphate-inhibited acetylcholinesterase. Biochim Biophys Acta 18:168–170, 1955.
3. Kewitz H, Wilson IB: A specific antidote against lethal alkylphosphate intoxication. Arch Biochem 60:261–263, 1956.
4. Kewitz H, Wilson IB, Nachmansohn D: A special antidote against lethal alkyl phosphate intoxication: II. Antidotal properties. Arch Biochem Biophys 64:456–466, 1956.
5. Wills JH, Kunkel AM, Brown RV, Groblewski GE: Pyridine-2-aldoxime methiodide and poisoning by anticholinesterases. Science 125:743–744, 1957.
6. Wilson IB, Sondheimer F: A specific antidote against lethal alkyl phosphate intoxication: V. Antidotal properties. Arch Biochem Biophys 69:468–474, 1957.
7. Poziomek EJ, Hackley BE, Steinberg GM: Pyridinium aldoximes. J Org Chem 23:714–717, 1958.
8. Childs AF, Davies DR, Green AL, Rutland JP: The reactivation by oximes and hydroxamic acids of cholinesterase inhibited by organophosphorus compounds. Br J Pharmacol 10:462–465, 1955.

9. Askew BM, Davies DR, Green AL, Holmes R: The nature of the toxicity of 2-oxo-oximes. Br J Pharmacol 11:424–427, 1956.
10. Askew BM: Oximes and hydroxamic acids as antidotes in anticholinesterase poisoning. Br J Pharmacol 11:417–423, 1956.
11. Askew BM: Oximes and atropine in sarin poisoning. Br J Pharmacol 12:340–343, 1957.
12. Hobbiger F: Protection against the lethal effects of organophosphates by pyridine-2-aldoxime methiodide. Br J Pharmacol 12:438–446, 1957.
13. Davies DR, Willey GL: The toxicity of 2-hydroxyiminomethyl-N-methylpyridinium methanesulphonate (P2S). Br J Pharmacol 13:202–206, 1958.
14. Hobbiger F, O'Sullivan DG, Sadler PW: New potent reactivators of acetocholinesterase inhibited by tetraethyl pyrophosphate. Nature 182:1498–1499, 1958.
15. Ladell WSS: Treatment of anticholinesterase poisoning. BMJ 2:141–142, 1958.
16. Berry WK, Davies DR, Green AL: Oximes of diquaternary alkane salts as antidotes to organophosphate anticholinesterases. Br J Pharmacol 14:186–191, 1959.
17. Creasey NH, Green AL: 2-Hydroxyiminomethyl-n-methylpyridinium methanesulphonate (P2S), an antidote to organophosphorus poisoning: Its preparation, estimation and stability. J Pharm Pharmacol 11:485–490, 1959.
18. Davies DR, Green AL: The chemotherapy of poisoning by organophosphate anticholinesterases. Br J Ind Med 16:128–134, 1959.
19. Hobbiger F, Sadler PW: Protection against lethal organophosphate poisoning by quaternary pyridine aldoximes. Br J Pharmacol 14:192–201, 1959.
20. Hiraki K, Namba Y, Taniguchi Y, et al: Effect of 2-pyridine aldoxime methiodide (PAM) against parathion (Folidol) poisoning: Analysis of 39 cases. Naika Ryoiki 6:84, 1958.
21. Kondritzer AA, Ellin RI, Edberg LJ: Investigation of methyl pyridinium-2-aldoxime salts. J Pharm Sci 50:109–112, 1961.
22. Nozaki H, Aikawa N: Sarin poisoning in Tokyo subway. Lancet 345:1446–1447, 1995.
23. Suzuki T, Morita H, Ono K, et al: Sarin poisoning in Tokyo subway. Lancet 345:980, 1995.
24. Hayes WJ: Parathion poisoning and its treatment. JAMA 192:135–136, 1965.
25. Thiermann H, Mast U, Klimmek R, et al: Cholinesterase status, pharmacokinetics and laboratory findings during obidoxime therapy in organophosphate poisoned patients. Hum Exp Toxicol 16:473–480, 1997.
26. Van Helden HPM, Van der Wiel HJ, Zijlstra JJ, et al: Comparison of the therapeutic effects and pharmacokinetics of HI-6, HLoe-7, HGG-12, HGG-42 and obidoxime following non-reactivatable acetylcholinesterase inhibition in rats. Arch Toxicol 68:224–230, 1994.
27. Worek F, Kirchner T, Szinicz L: Treatment of tabun poisoned guinea-pigs with atropine, HLö-7 or HI 6: effect on respiratory and circulatory function. Arch Toxicol 68:231–239, 1994.
28. Ellin RI: Stability of concentrated aqueous solutions of pralidoxime chloride. J Pharm Sci 71:1057–1059, 1982.
29. Barkman R, Edgren B, Sundwall A: Self-administration of pralidoxime in nerve gas poisoning with a note on the stability of the drug. J Pharm Pharmacol 15:671–677, 1963.
30. Schroeder AC, DiGiovanni JH, von Bredow J, Heiffer MH: Pralidoxime chloride stability-indicating assay and analysis of solution samples stored at room temperature for ten years. J Pharm Sci 78:132–136, 1989.
31. Van Helden HPM, Busker RW, Melchers BPC, Bruijnzeel PLB: Pharmacological effects of oximes: How relevant are they? Arch Toxicol 70:779–786, 1996.
32. Taylor P: Anticholinesterase agents. In Hardman JG, Limbird LE, Molinoff PB, et al (eds): Goodman and Gilman's the Pharmacological Basis of Therapeutics, 9th ed. New York, McGraw-Hill, 1996, pp 161–176.
33. Worek F, Bäcker M, Thiermann H, et al: Reappraisal of indications and limitations of oxime therapy in organophosphate poisoning. Hum Exp Toxicol 16:466–472, 1997.
34. Bokonjic D, Jovanovic D, Jokanovic M, Maksimovic M: Protective effects of oximes HI-6 and PAM-2 applied by osmotic minipumps in quinalphos-poisoned rats. Arch Int Pharmacodyn 288:309–318, 1987.
35. de Kort WLAM, Kiestra SH, Sangster B: The use of atropine and oximes in organophosphate intoxications: A modified approach. J Toxicol Clin Toxicol 26:199–208, 1988.
36. Tush GM, Anstead MI: Pralidoxime continuous infusion in the treatment of organophosphate poisoning. Ann Pharmacother 31:441–444, 1997.
37. Casey PB, Gosden E, Blakey L, et al: Plasma pralidoxime concentrations following bolus injection and continuous infusion. Przegl Lek 52:203–204, 1995.
38. Casey PB, Blakey L, Bradberry SM, Vale JA: Late reactivation of erythrocyte cholinesterase activity by pralidoxime in a case of chlorpyrifos poisoning. Przegl Lek 52:206, 1995.
39. Kopecky J, Gut I, Nerudová J, et al: Acrylonitrile metabolism in the rat. Arch Toxicol 4(Suppl):322–324, 1980.
40. Davies DR, Green AL, Willey GL: 2-Hydroxyiminomethyl-N-methylpyridinium methanesulphate and atropine in the treatment of severe organophosphate poisoning. Br J Pharmacol 14:5–8, 1959.
41. Clement JG: Efficacy of pro-PAM (N-methyl-1,6-dihydropyridine-2-carbaldoxime hydrochloride) as a prophylaxis against organophosphate poisoning. Toxicol Appl Pharmacol 47:305–311, 1979.
42. O'Leary JF, Kunkel AM, Jones AH: Efficacy and limitations of oxime-atropine treatment of organophosphorus anticholinesterase poisoning. J Pharmacol Exp Ther 132:50–57, 1961.
43. Das Gupta S, Ghosh AK, Moorthy MV, et al: Comparative studies of pralidoxime, trimedoxime, obidoxime and diethyxime in acute fluostigmine poisoning in rats. Pharmazie 37:605, 1982.
44. Jovanovic D, Boskovic B: Current problems in the experimental treatment of dimethoate poisoning by cholinesterase reactivators. Acta Vet 33:21–28, 1983.
45. Sundwall A: Minimum concentrations of N-methylpyridinium-2-aldoxime methanesulphonate (P2S) which reverse neuromuscular block. Biochem Pharmacol 8:413–417, 1961.
46. Crook JW, Goodman AI, Colbourn JL, et al: Adjunctive value of oral prophylaxis with the oximes 2-PAM lactate and 2-PAM methane-sulfonate to therapeutic administration of atropine in dogs poisoned by inhaled sarin vapor. J Pharmacol Exp Ther 136:397–399, 1962.
47. Shiloff JD, Clement JG: Comparison of serum concentrations of the acetylcholinesterase oxime reactivators HI-6, obidoxime, and PAM to efficacy against sarin (isopropyl methylphosphonofluoridate) poisoning in rats. Toxicol Appl Pharmacol 89:278–280, 1987.
48. Grob D, Johns RJ: Use of oximes in the treatment of intoxication by anticholinesterase compounds in normal subjects. Am J Med 24:497–511, 1958.
49. Willems JL, De Bisschop HC, Verstraete AG, et al: Cholinesterase reactivation in organophosphorus poisoned patients depends on the plasma concentrations of the oxime pralidoxime methylsulphate and of the organophosphate. Arch Toxicol 67:79–84, 1993.
50. Green MD, Talbot BG, Clark CR: Pharmacokinetics of pralidoxime chloride in the rat. Life Sci 39:2263–2269, 1986.
51. Green MD, Jones DE, Hilmas DE: Sarin intoxication elevates plasma pralidoxime. Toxicol Lett 28:17–21, 1985.
52. Jovanovic D: Pharmacokinetics of pralidoxime chloride: A comparative study in healthy volunteers and in organophosphorus poisoning. Arch Toxicol 63:416–418, 1989.
53. Calesnick B, Christensen JA, Richter M: Human toxicity of various oximes: 2-Pyridine aldoxime methyl chloride, its methane sulfonate salt, and 1,1′-trimethylenebis-(4-formylpyridinium chloride). Arch Environ Health 14:599–608, 1967.
54. Sidell FR, Groff WA, Kaminskis A: Toxogonin and pralidoxime: Kinetic comparison after intravenous administration to man. J Pharm Sci 61:1765–1769, 1972.
55. Ellin RI, Groff WA, Sidell FR: Passage of pyridinium oximes into human red cells. Biochem Pharmacol 23:2663–2670, 1974.
56. Uehara S, Hiromori T, Isobe N, et al: Studies on the therapeutic effect of 2-pyridine aldoxime methiodide (2-PAM) in mammals following organophosphorus compound-poisoning (report III): Distribution and antidotal effect of 2-PAM in rats. J Toxicol Sci 18:265–275, 1993.
57. Willems JL, Langenberg JP, Verstraet AG, et al: Plasma concentrations of pralidoxime methylsulphate in organophosphorus poisoned patients. Arch Toxicol 66:260–266, 1992.
58. Gibbon SL, Tong H, de Miranda PMS, Way JL: Metabolism of pralidoxime (2-PAM) in man. J Anal Toxicol 3:14–17, 1979.
59. Jager BV, Stagg GN: Toxicity of diacetyl monoxime and of pyridine-2-aldoxime methiodide in man. Bull Johns Hopkins Hosp 102:203–211, 1958.
60. Loomis TA: Distribution and excretion of pyridine-2-aldoxime methiodide (PAM): Atropine and PAM in sarin poisoning. Toxicol Appl Pharmacol 5:489–499, 1963.

61. Sidell FR, Groff WA: Intramuscular and intravenous administration of small doses of 2-pyridinium aldoxime methochloride to man. J Pharm Sci 60:1224–1228, 1971.

62. Sidell FR, Groff WA, Kaminskis A: Pralidoxime methanesulfonate: plasma levels and pharmacokinetics after oral administration to man. J Pharm Sci 61:1136–1141, 1972.

63. Rivero González A, Navarro González JF, Macía Heras ML, et al: Intoxicación por paraquat: presentación de dos casos y revisión de la literatura. Ann Med Int 18:208–210, 2001.

64. Swartz RD, Sidell FR: Effects of heat and exercise on the elimination of pralidoxime in man. Clin Pharmacol Ther 14:83–89, 1973.

65. Vojvodic VB, Maksimovic M: Absorption and excretion of pralidoxime in man after intramuscular injection of PAM-2Cl and various cholinolytics. Eur J Clin Pharmacol 5:58–61, 1972.

66. Josselson J, Sidell FR: Effect of intravenous thiamine on pralidoxime kinetics. Clin Pharmacol Ther 24:95–100, 1978.

67. Berglund F, Elwin C-E, Sundwall A: Studies on the renal elimination of N-methylpyridinium-2-aldoxime. Biochem Pharmacol 11:383–388, 1962.

68. Kondritzer AA, Zvirblis P, Goodman A, Paplanus SH: Blood plasma levels and elimination of salts of 2-PAM in man after oral adminstration. J Pharm Sci 57:1142–1146, 1968.

69. Sidell FR, Groff WA: Toxogonin: Blood levels and side effects after intramuscular administration in man. J Pharm Sci 59:793–797, 1970.

70. Sidell FR, Groff WA, Ellin RI: Blood levels of oxime and symptoms in humans after single and multiple oral doses of 2-pyridine aldoxime methochloride. J Pharm Sci 58:1093–1098, 1969.

71. Jager BV, Stagg GN, Green N, Jager L: Studies on distribution and disappearance of pyridine-2-aldoxime methiodide (PAM) and of diacetyl monoxime (DAM) in man and in experimental animals. Bull Johns Hopkins Hosp 102:225–234, 1958.

72. Finkelstein Y, Kushnir A, Raikhlin-Eisenkraft B, Taitelman U: Antidotal therapy of severe acute organophosphate poisoning: a multihospital study. Neurotoxicol Teratol 11:593–596, 1989.

73. Johnson MK, Jacobsen D, Meredith TJ, et al: Evaluation of antidotes for poisoning by organophosphorus pesticides. Emerg Med 12:22–37, 2000.

74. Dawson RM: Review of oximes available for treatment of nerve agent poisoning. J Appl Toxicol 14:317–331, 1994.

75. Clement JG: Efficacy of various oximes against GF (cyclohexyl methylphosphonofluoridate) poisoning in mice. Arch Toxicol 66:143–144, 1992.

CHAPTER 146

Bromocriptine

Michael J. Burns

Bromocriptine, a semisynthetic ergot alkaloid structurally similar to dopamine, is a dopamine receptor agonist that results in the inhibition of prolactin secretion.[1,2] Compared with other ergot derivatives, bromocriptine has significantly less cardiovascular, oxytocic, adrenergic, and serotonergic effects.[2,3] Although the drug is marketed primarily for the treatment of hyperprolactinemia and Parkinson's disease, medical toxicologists currently use it as an adjunct medication to treat neuroleptic malignant syndrome (NMS). It also is used occasionally to treat cocaine craving and withdrawal dysphoria.[4,5]

HISTORY

During the ergotism epidemics of the Middle Ages, it was observed that women failed to lactate when they ate ergot-contaminated grain. It was not until 1968, however, that this ergot characteristic was used therapeutically when the semisynthetic ergoline bromocriptine was developed as an inhibitor of prolactin secretion.[6] In 1973, bromocriptine was approved in the United States to treat amenorrhea, galactorrhea, and infertility associated with hyperprolactinemia.[7] In 1978, bromocriptine (Parlodel) was approved in the United States for the treatment of Parkinson's disease and to inhibit puerperal lactation.[7,8] Bromocriptine first was used for NMS in 1983.[9] Since that time, its use has been reported in more than 100 cases of NMS.[10–12] In 1995, the U.S. Food and Drug Administration (FDA) withdrew approval of bromocriptine for physiologic lactation prevention due to reports of serious adverse effects (e.g., hypertension, seizures, myocardial infarction, and cerebrovascular accident) associated with its use.[1,13] At the same time, the U.S. manufacturer (Sandoz, Princeton, NJ) of bromocriptine agreed voluntarily to withdraw this indication from its package labeling.[1]

Currently, bromocriptine is indicated primarily for the treatment of Parkinson's disease and conditions associated with hyperprolactinemia (e.g., amenorrhea, galactorrhea, and infertility).[1,14,15] Hyperprolactinemia may be physiologic, drug induced (e.g., associated with a neuroleptic), or pathologic (e.g., due to a pituitary adenoma). Bromocriptine also is effective in the treatment of acromegaly and NMS (see Chapter 26).[1,4,16] Although data to date are insufficient to make recommendations, bromocriptine additionally may play a role in the selective treatment of cocaine withdrawal, premenstrual symptoms, Cushing's disease, chronic hepatic encephalopathy, tardive dyskinesia, depression, mania, and schizophrenia.[1,4,5]

PROPERTIES

Bromocriptine (2-bromo-α-ergocryptine) is an amino acid, alkaloid derivative of lysergic acid.[2,3,15] It consists of a heterocyclic nucleus to which a single bromine and peptide side chain is attached (Fig. 146-1).[3] The structure of dopamine is embedded within its heterocyclic nucleus. This structural characteristic probably imparts dopamine receptor agonism to the compound.[3,17] The common pharmaceutical preparation is bromocriptine mesylate, which exists as a yellowish white crystalline powder that is slightly soluble in water and sparingly soluble in alcohol.[1] Bromocriptine mesylate is available as tablets and capsules, containing 2.5 mg (tablets) and 5 mg (capsules) of bromocriptine.[1]

PHARMACODYNAMICS

The therapeutic and certain adverse effects of bromocriptine are mediated by central and peripheral dopamine receptor binding.[4,18–20] Bromocriptine is a potent agonist of D_2-dopamine receptors and a partial antagonist of D_1-dopamine receptors.[1–4,17–20] In vitro, bromocriptine has approximately 30 times greater affinity at D_2- compared with D_1-receptors.[17–20] Dopamine receptors are found in a variety of central and peripheral locations (Table 146-1). Centrally, nigrostriatal and mesolimbic regions have presynaptic D_2-autoreceptors, which diminish the release of dopamine when stimulated.[4,17,18] Peripherally, sympathetic ganglia and postganglionic sympathetic nerve terminals have presynaptic D_2-autoreceptors, which diminish the release of norepinephrine when stimulated.[22] These autoreceptors are more sensitive to dopamine than are postsynaptic receptors (D_1 and D_2 subtypes) and are stimulated preferentially at low doses of agonist.[4] At low doses, bromocriptine acts predominantly at the autoreceptor, whereas at higher doses, it acts predominantly at the postsynaptic receptor (similar to dopamine).

Bromocriptine binds to postsynaptic D_2-dopamine receptors on anterior pituitary cells to inhibit their release of prolactin.[1,2] For patients with hyperprolactinemia, bromocriptine reduces prolactin to low levels and restores gonadal function and fertility. For patients with pituitary adenomas, bromocriptine restores endocrinologic function and may cause tumor regression and reverse visual field deficits.[23] For patients with acromegaly, bromocriptine binds to postsynaptic D_2-dopamine receptors on anterior pituitary cells to inhibit their release of growth hormone.[1,2]

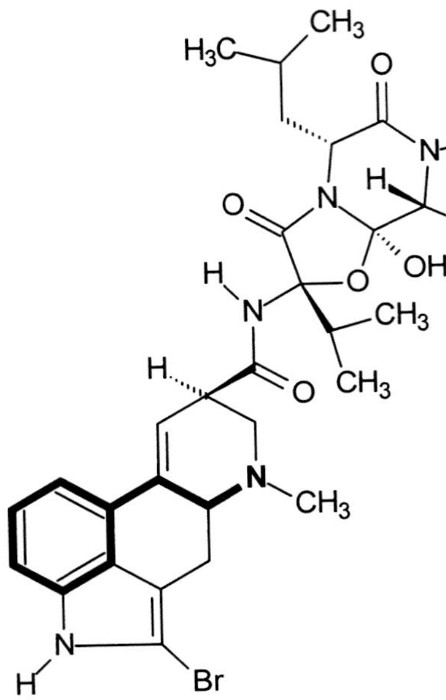

FIGURE 146-1

Chemical structure of bromocriptine. A significant portion of the structure of dopamine (highlighted) is embedded in the heterocyclic ring system of bromocriptine.

Core temperature regulation is mediated partly by D_2-receptors in the anterior hypothalamus.[4,24] D_2-receptor antagonists, such as neuroleptics, may disrupt thermoregulation to produce hyperthermia, whereas D_2-agonists, such as bromocriptine, may result in hypothermia.[24] Neuroleptic blockade of D_2-receptors in the striatum often produces muscle rigidity and parkinsonism, whereas receptor stimulation by bromocriptine may produce choreic and dystonic movements.[25] NMS is an uncommon, life-threatening condition that results from neuroleptic blockade of D_2-receptors in the hypothalamic, striatal, mesocortical, mesolimbic, and

TABLE 146-1 Predominant Sites of Dopamine Receptors

CENTRAL NERVOUS SYSTEM*	PERIPHERAL NERVOUS SYSTEM†
Area postrema of medulla oblongata (chemoreceptor trigger zone)	Sympathetic nerve terminals
Tuberoinfundibular pathway (connects hypothalamus to pituitary)	Vascular smooth muscle (predominantly renal, mesenteric, coronary, and cerebral vascular beds)
In certain hypothalamic neurons (link various hypothalamic nuclei)	
Thermoregulatory center of hypothalamus	
Medullary periventricular neurons	
Nigrostriatal pathway	
Mesocortical pathways	
Mesolimbic pathways	
Retina and olfactory tubercle	

*Data from references 4 and 18 through 20.
†Data from reference 21.

sympathetic nerve terminals (see Chapter 26).[24] Bromocriptine is thought to counteract such D_2-receptor antagonism and hasten recovery from NMS.[26]

Bromocriptine activates postsynaptic D_2-receptors in the striatum and offsets decreased dopamine release that occurs from degenerating nigrostriatal neurons in patients with Parkinson's disease.[15,18–20] Bromocriptine also seems to serve a neuroprotective function by activating D_2-autoreceptors of nigrostriatal neurons, which results in a reduction of presynaptic dopamine synthesis and turnover. As a consequence, there is a reduction in the oxidative breakdown of striatal dopamine and formation of neurotoxic free radicals.[15,18] Early treatment with bromocriptine for patients with Parkinson's disease also allows a cumulative reduction in levodopa doses and reduces the long-term motor complications (e.g., dyskinesias and motor response fluctuations) associated with levodopa therapy.[15,18–20]

Bromocriptine has been used to treat cocaine craving and withdrawal dysphoria. It also may have a role in maintaining abstinence from cocaine.[1,4,5,27] Short-term cocaine use blocks dopamine reuptake and provides increased stimulation of the pleasure or reward centers of the brain through mesocortical and mesolimbic dopamine pathways. Long-term cocaine use results in decreased presynaptic dopamine production and release coupled with postsynaptic dopamine receptor up-regulation. In the absence of cocaine, dopaminergic neurotransmission in mesocortical and mesolimbic pathways is decreased, and craving and abstinence symptoms result.[5,27] By stimulating postsynaptic central nervous system dopamine receptors directly, bromocriptine may simulate cocaine effects centrally and reduce craving and withdrawal dysphoria.[5,27] Bromocriptine also may block the euphoric effects of cocaine by occupying postsynaptic dopamine receptors during cocaine use. Bromocriptine could be used to maintain abstinence in an active cocaine user.

The most frequent adverse effects from bromocriptine therapy result from central and peripheral dopamine receptor stimulation; effects are dose, duration, and age dependent.[1,18–20,28] Low-dose, early adverse effects include nausea, vomiting, dizziness, and orthostasis.[1,2,28] Bromocriptine directly stimulates D_2-dopamine receptors in the area postrema of the medulla oblongata to produce nausea and vomiting.[20] Stimulation of postsynaptic D_2-receptors of vasculature (renal, mesenteric, coronary, and cerebral blood vessels) and presynaptic D_2-autoreceptors of sympathetic nerve terminals (diminished release of norepinephrine) result in vasodilation, orthostatic hypotension, dizziness, and headache[21,22,29]; these latter effects are experienced most commonly after bromocriptine initiation. Adverse effects that result from large doses and long-term treatment with bromocriptine include agitation, confusion, psychosis (e.g., delusions and hallucinations), and involuntary movements (e.g., chorea and dyskinesia).[1,2,20,28,30,31] Bromocriptine-associated psychosis likely is mediated by stimulation of mesocortical and mesolimbic dopamine pathways; discontinuing bromocriptine or initiating dopamine-receptor antagonists (e.g., clozapine) may reverse symptoms.[1,4,28,30,31] Dyskinesias reflect bromocriptine stimulation of supersensitive postsynaptic D_2-receptors.

Although bromocriptine shows selective binding for dopamine receptors, this selectivity may be lost at higher drug doses. Bromocriptine has low affinity for α-adrenergic (α_1 and α_2) and serotonergic (5-HT_1 and 5-HT_2) receptors.[3,15,17,18] In vitro, bromocriptine is a weak antagonist at these receptors. In vivo, the effects may be stimulatory, however, because receptor effects depend on dose, target organ, individual host factors, and physiologic conditions.[3] Although small doses of bromocriptine are expected to result in vasodilation from dopamine agonism, large doses of bromocriptine may produce peripheral vasoconstriction from α-adrenergic and serotonergic receptor stimulation.[3] This vasoconstriction may result in hypertension, cerebrovascular accidents, and myocardial infarction, particularly for patients with predisposing factors (e.g., patients with a history of pregnancy-induced hypertension, migraine headaches, or Raynaud's phenomenon).[1,13,28,32–37]

Long-term bromocriptine therapy, similar to other ergot alkaloids, uncommonly may result in Raynaud's phenomenon, erythromelalgia (erythema and edema of lower extremities), and pleuropulmonary fibrosis.[1,30,38–40] Vasoconstriction of microvasculature and perivascular inflammatory changes and fibrosis occur in the latter two conditions.[38,39] The mechanisms mediating these effects are not well understood; α-adrenergic and serotonergic receptor–mediated effects or a drug hypersensitivity reaction is plausible.

EFFICACY

Medical toxicologists use bromocriptine to treat NMS (see Chapter 26). Evidence to support the efficacy of bromocriptine comes from more than 100 case reports in the literature and a few uncontrolled retrospective studies.[10–12,26] In one retrospective study, the use of bromocriptine significantly reduced the time to clinical improvement and resolution from NMS to a mean of 1 and 9.9 days, respectively, compared with 6.8 and 15.8 days for supportive care alone.[26] In another retrospective study, bromocriptine significantly reduced mortality associated with NMS from 21% to 7.8% compared with supportive care alone.[11] Because it has not been evaluated prospectively in a controlled fashion, further studies are necessary to determine definitively the efficacy of bromocriptine for the treatment of NMS. One prospective uncontrolled study found that bromocriptine in combination with dantrolene resulted in a more prolonged illness and greater complication rates than with supportive care alone.[41] The efficacy data concerning the use of bromocriptine in NMS are discussed in further detail in Chapter 26.

PHARMACOKINETICS

Pharmacokinetics of Bromocriptine

Volume of distribution: 1–4 L/kg
Bioavailability: 6%
Maximum threshold: 1.7 hr
Protein binding: 90–96%
Elimination half-life (α phase): 3–6 hr
Elimination half-life (β phase): 44–50 hr
Metabolism: hepatic
Active metabolites: none
Peak plasma concentration range: 1.3–24.6 ng/mL (1–8.4 mmol/L)
Recommended daily dose range: 2.5–40 mg

Bromocriptine is absorbed poorly from the gastrointestinal tract (28%) and has significant first-pass hepatic metabolism (93%).[1,2,18,19,42,43] After oral administration, systemic bioavailability is 6%. After oral administration of doses of 2.5 to 100 mg, plasma concentrations peak at 0.5 to 3.5 hours (mean 1.7 hours) and range from 1.3 to 24.6 ng/mL (1 to 18.4 mmol/L).[42] Peak plasma concentrations correlate poorly with the dose given; substantial interindividual variability exists.[1,42,43] Clinical effects are observed within a couple of hours of oral administration.[1] Peak clinical response does not correlate with peak plasma concentrations.[1] Plasma concentrations typically are measured by radioimmunoassay.[42,43] Bromocriptine is highly protein bound (90% to 96%) to serum albumin. Its volume of distribution is 1 to 4 L/kg. During long-term administration, bromocriptine accumulates in the plasma.[42] Bromocriptine is metabolized extensively in the liver to numerous inactive metabolites. Bromocriptine and its metabolites are excreted principally into bile and feces. Only a small amount of parent drug (≤5%) is excreted unchanged in the urine.[1,42,43] The terminal elimination half-life of bromocriptine is 44 to 50 hours.[42]

SPECIAL POPULATIONS

Neonatal and Pediatric Patients

The safety and efficacy of bromocriptine have not been established in neonates and children younger than 15 years old.[1] Although bromocriptine has been administered without adverse effects to children with NMS, macroadenomas, and acromegaly, most of these children were adolescents.[12,44–46] Young children may be more sensitive to the adverse effects of this drug. Accidental ingestion of 7.5 mg of bromocriptine in two young children resulted in lethargy.[47]

Elderly Patients and Patients with Hepatic and Renal Disease

Bromocriptine has been used safely and effectively in many elderly patients with Parkinson's disease. The elderly seem more likely, however, to develop nausea, vomiting, dizziness, orthostasis, and neuropsychiatric adverse effects from bromocriptine therapy.[1,2,28] Although data are lacking, patients with hepatic disease are likely to have an impaired total body clearance of bromocriptine. The initial bromocriptine dose should be small, and dose escalation should proceed slowly in these patients. Patients with renal disease should not have impaired total body clearance of bromocriptine. Dose adjustment in this group of patients is not likely to be necessary.

Pregnant and Breast-feeding Patients

The use of bromocriptine during pregnancy was not associated with an increased risk of spontaneous abortion or congenital malformations in one study of 2587 pregnancies.[30,48] In addition, postnatal development has been normal in children exposed in utero to bromocriptine.[49] Despite its apparent safety, bromocriptine should be discontinued in women who discover that they are pregnant while taking the drug, unless the benefits of continued treatment outweigh theoretical risks.[1,49] One animal study showed an increased risk of fetal abnormalities when pregnant rabbits were exposed to 30 mg/kg or more of bromocriptine a day.[30] Because bromocriptine suppresses lactation, women who wish to breast-feed should discontinue the drug. No adverse effects have been reported from bromocriptine secreted in breast milk.[1]

CONTRAINDICATIONS AND PRECAUTIONS

According to the manufacturer (Novartis, East Hanover, NJ), bromocriptine is contraindicated for patients with uncontrolled hypertension, toxemia of pregnancy, and sensitivity to ergot alkaloids.[1] These contraindications are based largely on a theoretical increased risk of serious adverse effects (e.g., cerebrovascular accident, seizure, myocardial infarction) occurring in these patients. Supporting evidence is limited to a few case reports.[32–37] Use of bromocriptine for the prevention of postpartum lactation is no longer recommended by the FDA or the drug manufacturer.[1,13] To date, 63 cases of seizures, 31 cases of stroke, and 4 cases of acute myocardial infarction have been reported in women taking bromocriptine for postpartum lactation suppression.[1,13,32–37] Although the absolute incidence and relative risk of these adverse effects are unknown, accumulated evidence from case reports suggests that the possibility of adverse effects outweighs the limited benefits of such therapy. Many patients who experienced seizures and stroke from bromocriptine developed severe headache, visual disturbances, hypertension, or a combination of these symptoms before these adverse effects.[13,32–37] Bromocriptine therapy should be discontinued immediately when these signs or symptoms occur.[1]

Bromocriptine also is not recommended for women with a history of pregnancy-induced hypertension, patients with severe ischemic heart disease or peripheral vascular disease, and patients taking other ergot alkaloids concomitantly.[1] These recommendations are based on a few case reports that associate bromocriptine use with serious adverse effects in these patients.[2,13,32–37] Certain preparations of bromocriptine contain sodium bisulfite (e.g., Parlodel, 5-mg capsules). These preparations are not recommended for use in patients with known sulfite sensitivity due to the risk of severe allergic reactions.[1] Large doses of bromocriptine may produce confusion and psychosis. This drug should be used with caution in elderly patients and patients with baseline dementia or psychotic illness.[30,31]

Drug Interactions

Bromocriptine should be used with caution in patients who take antihypertensive agents because additive hypotensive effects may occur. Bromocriptine may reduce tolerance to ethanol and may reduce the effectiveness of certain antiemetics and antipsychotics.[1] Conversely, antiemetics and antipsychotics may reduce the efficacy of bromocriptine.

Adverse Effects

Adverse effects are often dose related and occur in 60% of patients treated with bromocriptine.[20,28] The incidence of adverse effects is greatest when treatment is initiated

and when doses exceed 20 mg daily.[20,28] Starting with small doses and increasing doses gradually can minimize early adverse effects. The most commonly reported adverse effects from bromocriptine include nausea and vomiting (60% of patients), dizziness, and postural hypotension (25%).[28] Tolerance to these effects usually occurs after a few days of therapy. Symptomatic orthostasis is minimized by administering bromocriptine at night or when the patient is recumbent.[20,28] Other early adverse effects include dry mouth, dyspepsia, abdominal pain, constipation, headache, lethargy, leg cramps, flushing, and nasal congestion.[20,28]

Neuropsychiatric, pleuropulmonary, and vascular adverse effects are associated with high-dose and long-term bromocriptine therapy.[28,30,31] Neuropsychiatric effects include agitation, confusion, delusions, hallucinations, chorea, dyskinesias, and myoclonus. These effects occur in 1% to 2% of patients receiving lower doses, but the incidence is higher in elderly patients and patients with advanced Parkinson's disease.[1,2] These side effects resolve within 2 to 3 weeks when bromocriptine therapy is discontinued.[20,28,30] Pleuropulmonary and retroperitoneal fibrosis, pleural effusion, pleuritic chest pain, and pulmonary infiltrates have been reported in 2% to 6% of patients who take 20 to 100 mg of bromocriptine over an extended period.[28,30,39] Use of bromocriptine has been associated with Raynaud's phenomenon, erythromelalgia, and livedo reticularis.[38–40] Bromocriptine therapy also has been associated with transient asymptomatic increases in serum transaminases, alkaline phosphatase, creatine kinase, and blood urea nitrogen.[30]

Overdose

There are few reported cases of bromocriptine overdose. Signs and symptoms reflect dopamine receptor overstimulation and include nausea, vomiting, dizziness, lethargy, sweating, hypotension, agitation, hallucinations, and dyskinesias.[47,50] Seizures have occurred in animal toxicity studies.[51]

DOSAGE AND ADMINISTRATION

Bromocriptine is available for oral administration only. For most indications, the usual initial adult dosage is 1.25 to 2.5 mg twice daily.[2,4,28] The dose is increased by 2.5 mg daily every 3 to 7 days until the desired therapeutic effect is achieved.[2,19,20,28] Dosages up to 100 mg/day are administered to patients with acromegaly and Parkinson's disease.[2] For the treatment of NMS, bromocriptine initially is administered in dosages of 2.5 to 10 mg three to four times daily.[9–12,16,45,46] Dosages of 20 mg four times daily have been used.[9–12] Bromocriptine is administered until signs and symptoms of NMS resolve. The appropriate dose in children is not well established. Toxic effects with therapeutic doses are most likely to occur when treatment is initiated; significant effects are more likely to occur when doses exceed 40 mg. Adults have taken therapeutic doses of 300 mg without adverse effects.[51] No fatal dose has been determined.[51]

REFERENCES

1. McEvoy GK, Litvak K, Welsh OH, et al (eds): Bromocriptine mesylate. In American Hospital Formulary Service Drug Information. Bethesda, MD, American Society of Health-System Pharmacists, 1998, pp 3045–3049.
2. Parkes D: Bromocriptine. N Engl J Med 301:873–878, 1979.
3. Peroutka SJ: Drugs effective in the therapy of migraine. In Hardman JG, Limbird LE, Molinoff PB, et al (eds): Goodman and Gilman's the Pharmacological Basis of Therapeutics, 9th ed. New York, McGraw-Hill, 1996, pp 491–496.
4. Sitland-Marken PA, Wells BG, Froemming JH, et al: Psychiatric applications of bromocriptine therapy. J Clin Psychiatry 51:68–82, 1990.
5. Dackis CA, Gold MS, Davies RK, Sweeney DR: Bromocriptine treatment for cocaine abuse: The dopamine depletion hypothesis. Int J Psychiatry Med 15:125–135, 1985–6.
6. Flückiger ER: Effects of bromocriptine on the hypothalamic-pituitary axis. Acta Endocrinol (Copenh) 216(Suppl):111–117, 1978.
7. McGregor A: Bromocriptine. Practitioner 225:1471–1475, 1981.
8. Factor SA: Dopamine agonists. Med Clin North Am 83:415–443, 1999.
9. Mueller PS, Vester JW, Fermaglich J: Neuroleptic malignant syndrome: Successful treatment with bromocriptine. JAMA 249:386–388, 1983.
10. Addonizio G, Susman VL, Roth SD: Neuroleptic malignant syndrome: Review and analysis of 115 cases. Biol Psychiatry 22:1004–1020, 1987.
11. Sakkas P, Davis JM, Janicak PG, Wang Z: Drug treatment of the neuroleptic malignant syndrome. Psychopharmacol Bull 27:381–384, 1991.
12. Silva RR, Munoz DM, Alpert M, et al: Neuroleptic malignant syndrome in children and adolescents. J Am Acad Child Adolesc Psychiatry 38:187–194, 1999.
13. Postpartum hypertension, seizures, strokes reported with bromocriptine. FDA Drug Bull 14:3–4, 1984.
14. Jenner P: The rationale for the use of dopamine agonists in Parkinson's disease. Neurology 45(Suppl 3):S6–S12, 1995.
15. Blanchet PJ: Rationale for use of dopamine agonists in Parkinson's disease: Review of ergot derivatives. Can J Neurol Sci 26(Suppl 2): S21–S26, 1999.
16. Dhib-Jalbut S, Hesselbrock R, Mouradian MM, Means ED: Bromocriptine treatment of neuroleptic malignant syndrome. J Clin Psychiatry 48:69–73, 1987.
17. Tulloch IF: Pharmacologic profile of ropinirole: A nonergoline dopamine agonist. Neurology 49(Suppl 1):S58–S62, 1997.
18. Watts RL: The role of dopamine agonists in early Parkinson's disease. Neurology 49(Suppl 1):S34–S48, 1997.
19. Montastruc JL, Tascol O, Senard JM: Current status of dopamine agonists in Parkinson's disease management. Drugs 46:384–393, 1993.
20. Goetz CG, Diederich NJ: Dopaminergic agonists in the treatment of Parkinson's disease. Neurol Clin 10:527–538, 1992.
21. Goldberg LI, Rajkes SI: Dopamine receptors: Applications in clinical cardiology. Circulation 72:245–248, 1985.
22. Stoof JC, Kebabian JW: Two dopamine receptors: Biochemistry, physiology and pharmacology. Life Sci 34:2281–2286, 1984.
23. Colao A, Annunziato L, Lombardi G: Treatment of prolactinomas. Ann Med 30:452–459, 1998.
24. Ebadi M, Pfeiffer RF, Murrin LC: Pathogenesis and treatment of neuroleptic malignant syndrome. Gen Pharmacol 21:367–386, 1990.
25. Jackson DM, Jenkins OF, Ross SB: The motor effects of bromocriptine—a review. Psychopharmacology 95:433–446, 1988.
26. Rosenberg MR, Green M: Neuroleptic malignant syndrome: Review of response to therapy. Arch Intern Med 149:1927–1931, 1989.
27. Hall WC, Talbert RL, Ereshefsky L: Cocaine abuse and its treatment. Pharmacotherapy 10:47–65, 1990.
28. Webster J: A comparative review of the tolerability profiles of dopamine agonists in the treatment of hyperprolactinaemia and inhibition of lactation. Drug Saf 14:228–238, 1996.
29. Lindvall O, Bjorklung A, Skagerberg G: Dopamine-containing neurons in the spinal cord: Anatomy and some functional aspects. Ann Neurol 14:255–260, 1983.
30. Weil C: The safety of bromocriptine in long-term use: A review of the literature. Curr Med Res Opin 10:25–51, 1986.
31. Boyd A: Bromocriptine and psychosis: A literature review. Psychiatr Q 66:87–95, 1995.
32. Loewe C, Dragovic LJ: Acute coronary artery thrombosis in a postpartum woman receiving bromocriptine. Am J Forensic Med Pathol 19:258–260, 1998.
33. Iffy L, TenHove W, Frisoli G: Acute myocardial infarction in the puerperium in patients receiving bromocriptine. Am J Obstet Gynecol 155:371–372, 1986.
34. Katz M, Kroll D, Pak I, et al: Puerperal hypertension, stroke, and seizures after suppression of lactation with bromocriptine. Obstet Gynecol 66:822–824, 1985.
35. Ruch A, Duhring JL: Postpartum myocardial infarction in a patient receiving bromocriptine. Obstet Gynecol 74:448–451, 1989.
36. Watson DL, Bhatia RK, Normal GS, et al: Bromocriptine mesylate for lactation suppression: A risk for postpartum hypertension? Obstet Gynecol 74:573–576, 1989.
37. Gittelman DK: Bromocriptine associated with postpartum hypertension, seizures, and pituitary hemorrhage. Gen Hosp Psychiatry 13:278–280, 1991.
38. Eisler T, Hall RP, Kalavar KAR, Calne DB: Erythromelalgia-like eruption in parkinsonian patients treated with bromocriptine. Neurology 31:1368–1370, 1981.
39. McElvaney NG, Wilcox PG, Churg A, Fleetham JA: Pleuropulmonary disease during bromocriptine treatment of Parkinson's disease. Arch Intern Med 148:2231–2236, 1988.
40. Quagliarello J, Barakat R: Raynaud's phenomenon in infertile women treated with bromocriptine. Fertil Steril 48:877–878, 1987.
41. Rosebush PI, Stewart T, Mazurek MF: The treatment of neuroleptic malignant syndrome: Are dantrolene and bromocriptine useful adjuncts to supportive care? Br J Psychiatry 159:709–712, 1991.
42. Kanto J: Clinical pharmacokinetics of ergotamine, dihydroergotamine, ergotoxine, bromocriptine, methysergide, and lergotrile. Int J Clin Pharmacol Ther Toxicol 21:135–142, 1983.
43. Aellig WH, Nuesch E: Comparative pharmacokinetic investigations with tritium-labeled ergot alkaloids after oral and intravenous administration in man. Int J Clin Pharmacol Biopharm 15:106–112, 1977.
44. Tyson D, Reggiardo D, Sklar C, David T: Prolactin-secreting macroadenomas in adolescents: Response to bromocriptine therapy. Am J Dis Child 147:1057–1061, 1993.
45. Tenenbein M: The neuroleptic malignant syndrome: Occurrence in a 15-year-old boy and recovery with bromocriptine therapy. Pediatr Neurosci 12:161–164, 1985–6.
46. Trasmonte J, Dayner J, Barron TF: Neuroleptic malignant syndrome in an adolescent head trauma patient. Clin Pediatr 38:611–613, 1999.
47. Vermund SH, Goldstein RG, Romano AA, et al: Accidental bromocriptine ingestion in childhood. J Pediatr 105:838–840, 1984.
48. Krupp P, Monka C: Bromocriptine in pregnancy: Safety aspects. Klin Wochenschr 65:823–827, 1987.
49. Raymond JP, Goldstein E, Konopka P, et al: Follow-up of children born of bromocriptine-treated mothers. Horm Res 22:239–246, 1985.
50. Tunca Z, Alkiin T, Guven H: A case of bromocriptine poisoning that resembles Pickwick syndrome. Pharmacol Toxicol 73(Suppl):78, 1993.
51. Hurlbut KM, Rumack BH: Bromocriptine mesylate and related drugs. In Poisondex. Englewood, CO, Micromedex, 1998.

CHAPTER 147

Pyridoxine

K. Sophia Dyer ▪ Michael Shannon

Because they have similar biologic properties, the related compounds pyridoxine, pyridoxal, and pyridoxamine fall under the common name of *vitamin B₆*.[1] Pyridoxine is found in several dietary sources, including eggs, meat, liver, legumes, vegetables, and grain cereals. It is used as an antidote for poisoning by isoniazid, monomethylhydrazine, and other hydrazines for seizure control and possibly to reverse the depressed mental status induced by these compounds. It also is possibly efficacious as an adjunct therapy for ethylene glycol poisoning. Pyridoxine has been used in the treatment of insomnia, premenstrual syndrome, nausea of pregnancy, and diabetic neuropathy, all with varying degrees of efficacy.

PROPERTIES

The most common pyridoxine product available, pyridoxine hydrochloride, is available in either tablet or parenteral formulations. This white crystalline powder is slightly bitter. The parenteral formulation has a pH of 2.0 to 3.8.[2] It can degrade when exposed to light.

PHARMACODYNAMICS

Pyridoxine is essential for the production of γ-aminobutyric acid (see Fig. 61-3). In vivo, the active molecule is pyridoxal-5′-phosphate for this and many other biologic reactions. Pyridoxal-5′-phosphate is the sole known active form of the vitamin.

PHARMACOKINETICS

Pyridoxine has good oral bioavailability and is absorbed in the jejunum. Time to peak concentration after oral administration is 1.25 hours.[3] Circulating pyridoxal phosphate is bound to serum albumin, and small amounts can be stored in liver and muscle tissue. The conversion of pyridoxine to pyridoxal-5′-phosphate occurs in the liver, with release of active vitamin in the circulating blood volume. Of circulating vitamin B₆, 60% is pyridoxal-5′-phosphate.[1] The half-life of pyridoxine is up to 20 days. A major inactive metabolite is 4-pyridoxal acid, which is excreted in the urine.[4] Biliary excretion accounts for only 2% of drug elimination.

CONTRAINDICATIONS

Known allergy to pyridoxine or components of the preparation is a contraindication to its use.

ADVERSE EFFECTS

Prolonged use of excessive doses of pyridoxine, administered orally or intravenously, is not without risk. Most of the adverse effects seem to be on the central and peripheral nervous systems. Sedation, hypotonia, dyspnea, and apnea all have been reported in oral and parenteral administration. Of great concern is pyridoxine-induced peripheral sensory neuropathy. In a report of two patients treated with 2 g/kg over 3 days, this effect seemed to be permanent. Other effects observed in these patients were transient autonomic dysfunction, nystagmus, lethargy, and respiratory depression.[5] In a group of women with chronic excessive pyridoxine intake, symptoms included paresthesias, hyperesthesia, muscle weakness, numbness, and fasciculation. The average dose was 117 ± 92 mg in the affected group of 103 women with a duration of treatment of 2.9 ± 1.9 years longer than in the unaffected women. Complete recovery occurred in 6 months for these women.[6] Finally, pyridoxine can affect levodopa therapy by increasing the peripheral decarboxylation of levodopa, reducing its effectiveness in the treatment of Parkinson's disease.

ADMINISTRATION

Pyridoxine therapy of poisoning by isoniazid or other hydrazines is recommended for the treatment of seizures and may be efficacious for the reversal of coma (see Chapter 61) In adults, the standard accepted dosing recommendation for isoniazid poisoning is gram-for-gram administration of pyridoxine. If the amount of isoniazid is unknown, the generally accepted dose is 5 g (maximum initial dose of 70 mg/kg), given intravenously at a rate of 0.5 g/min in adults.[7] Pyridoxine dosing may be repeated later in the patient's hospital course if coma persists. In a report of three cases, pyridoxine was used for the latter indication in doses of 3 to 5 g given up to 42 hours after isoniazid ingestion with apparent awakening.[8] For seizures unresponsive to initial pyridoxine administration, repeat dosing at 20-minute intervals until seizure activity stops has been recommended.[9] If repeat dosing is indicated for either reversal of coma or persistent seizure activity, it is crucial to be cognizant of the total dose administered to the patient. In two cases of pyridoxine use for *Gyromitra* mushroom poisoning, adult patients were given 132 and 183 g of pyridoxine (>2 g/kg) over 2 days. Both patients experienced irreversible sensory and peripheral neuropathy.[5] Animal data suggest a synergistic effect between diazepam and pyridoxine.[10] Addition of a benzodiazepine may be helpful in such a situation. Other authors have suggested that if intravenous pyridoxine is unavailable, the oral formulation of the drug can be crushed and administered via a nasogastric tube as a slurry in the similar gram-for-gram dosing (for isoniazid poisoning) that is recommended for intravenous dosing.[11]

REFERENCES

1. Marcus R, Coulston AM: Water-Soluble vitamins. In Hardman JG, Linbird LE, Molinoff PB, Ruddon RW (eds): Goodman and Gilman's the Pharmacologic Basis of Therapeutics, 9th ed. New York, McGraw-Hill, 1996, pp 1561–1563.
2. McEvoy GK, Litvak K, Welsh OH, et al: Pyridoxine. In: American Hospital Formulary Service. Bethesda, MD, American Society of Health Care Pharmacist, 1999, pp 3186–3189.
3. Thakker KM, Sitren HS, Gregory JF, et al: Dosage form and formulation effects on the bioavailability of vitamin E, riboflavin and vitamin B_6 from multiple preparations. Am J Clin Nutr 45:1472–1479, 1987.
4. Ink SL, Henderson LM: Vitamin B_6 metabolism. Ann Nutr 4:455–470, 1984.
5. Albin RL, Alber JW, Greenberg HS, et al: Acute sensory neuropathy-neuronopathy from pyridoxine overdose. Neurology 37:1729–1732, 1987.
6. Dalton K, Dalton MJ: Characteristics of pyridoxine overdose neuropathy syndrome. Acta Neurol Scand 76:8–11, 1987.
7. Wason S, Lacouture PG, Lovejoy FH: Single high-dose pyridoxine treatment for isoniazid overdose. JAMA 246:1102–1104, 1981.
8. Brent J, Vo N, Kulig K, Rumack BH: Reversal of prolonged isoniazid-induced coma by pyridoxine. Arch Intern Med 150:1751–1753, 1990.
9. Siever ML, Herrier RN: Treatment of acute isoniazid toxicity. Am J Hosp Pharm 32:202–206, 1975.
10. Chin L, Sievers ML, Laird HE, et al: Evaluation of diazepam and pyridoxine as antidotes to isoniazid intoxication in rats and dogs. Toxicol Appl Pharmacol 45:713–727, 1978.
11. Romero JA, Kuczler FJ: Isoniazid overdosage: Recognition and management. Am Fam Physician 57:749–752, 1988.

CHAPTER 148

Nitrites

Bruce D. Anderson

Nitrites have been used in a variety of food packaging, manufacturing, and medical settings for more than 150 years. The therapeutic benefit of nitrites has been investigated since the mid-1800s, when nitroglycerin was first used as a treatment for angina.[1] Antidotal use of nitrite currently is reserved for cyanide poisoning. Two nitrite agents are packaged together in the Taylor Cyanide Antidote Kit (Buffalo Grove, IL), amyl and sodium nitrite. These agents have been used for the treatment of cyanide overdose since the 1930s. Despite the long history of nitrite use for management of cyanide exposures, efforts to find newer and better cyanide antidotes continue.

HISTORY

Nitroglycerin first was synthesized in 1847 by Sombrero. Subsequent studies of amyl nitrite by Guthrie in 1859 were undertaken for the treatment of angina.[2] Initial descriptions of the actions of amyl nitrite inhalation included profound vasodilatory effects: "When inhaled in doses of from 5 to 10 drops, nitrite of amyl produces in man violent flushing of the face, associated with a feeling as though the head would burst, and a very excessive action on the heart."[2] At the time, inhaled amyl nitrite was recommended for a variety of conditions, including angina, asthma, tetanus, seizures, strychnine poisoning, and hysterical convulsions. The earliest described use of amyl nitrite as a potential cyanide antagonist was in 1888 by Pedigo.[3]

These findings were followed by Mladoveanu and Gheorhiu[4] in 1929 with sodium nitrite being used to block lethal doses of cyanide in dogs. In 1932, Geiger[5] used methylene blue as a methemoglobin former in experimental cyanide poisoning. In 1933, Mota[6] published the first human case of cyanide poisoning successfully managed with sodium nitrite alone. That same year, Chen and colleagues[7,8] showed dramatic improvements in survival when nitrites were paired with sodium thiosulfate in a canine model of cyanide poisoning. These studies led to the development of the original Lilly Cyanide Antidote kit (now manufactured by Taylor), which contains sodium thiosulfate and amyl and sodium nitrites. In many parts of the world, this kit is the only available specific treatment for cyanide poisoning. It still is the only cyanide antidote approved by the U.S. Food and Drug Administration.

PROPERTIES

Amyl Nitrite

Amyl nitrite's (Fig. 148-1) molecular weight is 110.14. It is a clear, yellow, volatile, flammable liquid with an unpleasant, fruity odor that is nearly insoluble in water but is miscible with alcohol and ether.[9]

Sodium Nitrite

Sodium nitrite ($NaNO_2$) has a molecular weight of 69. It exists as white or slightly yellow, hygroscopic granules, rods, or powder with a mild saline taste and has a pH of 9 in aqueous solution.[10]

PHARMACOKINETICS

Absorption

Amyl nitrite is absorbed rapidly via inhalation. Its clinical effects may be seen within seconds and continue for 5 to 10 minutes.

Sodium nitrite is absorbed rapidly when administered intravenously. Vasodilation may occur rapidly after administration.

Metabolism

Nitrite is converted almost completely to nitrate within 1 hour and is largely excreted in urine; 33% of the dose is excreted as unchanged nitrate. Urinary nitrite and nitrate concentrations in normal healthy volunteers average 0.2 mg/L and 61 mg/L.[11,12]

In unexposed persons, plasma nitrite and nitrate concentrations average 0.19 mg/L and 1.22 mg/L, respectively.[12] Serum nitrite concentrations have not been assessed during treatment for cyanide poisoning. Because nitrites induce methemoglobinemia, indirect monitoring generally takes place by measuring the hemoglobin fraction present as methemoglobin.

PHARMACODYNAMICS

The cyanide antidote kit and the mechanism of action of nitrites in cyanide poisoning were described in the classic publication of Chen and colleagues in 1933.[8] Cyanide

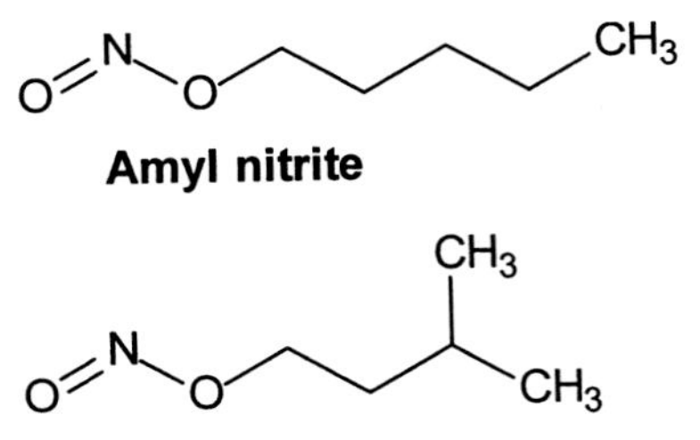

Amyl nitrite

Isoamyl nitrite

FIGURE 148-1

Chemical structures of the two primary constituents of amyl nitrite.

blocks the activity of cytochrome oxidase, preventing use of oxygen for cellular respiration (see Fig. 95-1). Nitrites oxidize hemoglobin to form methemoglobin. Because of its high affinity for methemoglobin, cyanide preferentially binds to it, forming cyanmethemoglobin (see Fig. 95-2). Further elimination of cyanide occurs by conversion of cyanide to thiocyanate via rhodanase. Sodium thiosulfate (the third therapeutic component in the Taylor Cyanide Antidote Kit) serves as a substrate for rhodanase and enhances cyanide clearance.

Despite these findings and demonstrated clinical benefit from nitrite administration, other pathways for cyanide detoxification likely are present.[13,14] In clinical settings, methemoglobin formation lags behind the clinical response to nitrite treatment.[14–16] In experimental studies, animals exposed to cyanide and treated with nitrite have had methemoglobin formation blocked by administration of methylene blue, yet still retained an antidotal response.[17] Questions remain regarding the exact mechanism of action of nitrites in cyanide overdose.

Similar to many poisonings, patients with cyanide exposures have effects that range along a continuum. Wurzburg[18] described a series of patients acutely exposed to cyanide in an occupational setting who were managed successfully with amyl nitrite and supplemental oxygen alone. In this setting, some workers underwent treatment and were able to return to work to complete their shifts. There also are cases of patients surviving cyanide poisoning with aggressive supportive therapy alone.[19,20] Patients have survived higher whole-blood cyanide concentrations with supportive therapy plus antidotal therapy.[14,15,21]

Although some references have recommended administration of adequate amounts of nitrite to produce "therapeutic" methemoglobin levels of 20% to 25%, an absolute level of methemoglobinemia has not been determined in humans. The often-quoted figure of 20% to 25% generally is considered to be higher than what is truly desirable, however, because methemoglobin is not oxygen carrying. Most patients treated with standard doses of sodium nitrite achieve methemoglobin fractions of 10% to 15%,[26] although exceptions are common. The literature reports that patients have had dramatic clinical responses to nitrite administration despite methemoglobin levels of less than or equal to 10%.[14–16] Overaggressive nitrite use is associated with hypotension, tachycardia, syncope, and cyanosis. One death has been reported secondary to excessive nitrite use.[22] Nitrites should not be given indiscriminately.

SPECIAL POPULATIONS

Amyl nitrite and sodium nitrite are listed as Food and Drug Administration Pregnancy Risk Category C (see Appendix A).[23] Patients who are anemic should have the nitrite dose adjusted based on blood hemoglobin concentration (Table 148-1).[22] The formation of any amount of methemoglobin in these patients causes a proportionally higher percentage of methemoglobin. Concerns have been raised regarding the administration of nitrites to victims of smoke inhalation. Nitrite-induced methemoglobin formation may further limit the oxygen-carrying capacity of blood when carbon monoxide is present.[24] This limitation is unlikely to be of clinical significance, however.[26]

CONTRAINDICATIONS

Cyanide poisoning is potentially life-threatening. Although there are populations of patients, such as patients with anemia, who have an added risk for developing toxic effects from nitrite administration, there are few absolute contraindications to nitrite therapy for cyanide poisoning.

PRECAUTIONS

Patients with Profound Hypotension

Nitrite therapy may produce vasodilation and hypotension. Hypotension is not a contraindication for nitrite therapy, however, because cyanide poisoning is life-threatening, and its treatment is expected to improve the patient's hemodynamic parameters.

Patients Taking Sildenafil

Although there is no clinical experience with patients who have taken sildenafil and who have been given amyl nitrite or sodium nitrite for cyanide overdose, a pronounced hypotensive effect would be expected based on reactions of sildenafil and other nitrites.[10]

TABLE 148-1   Adjustment of Sodium Nitrite Dose with Hemoglobin Concentration

HEMOGLOBIN (g/dL)	INITIAL DOSE OF SODIUM NITRITE (mg/kg)
7	5.8
8	6.6
9	7.5
10	8.3
11	9.1
12	10.0
13	10.8
14	11.6

Adapted from Berlin CM: Treatment of cyanide poisoning in children. Pediatrics 46:793–796, 1970.

Other Patients

Patients who co-ingest alcohol may have an additional hypotensive response from nitrite exposure. Amyl nitrite is extremely flammable. It should be kept away from any source of an open flame or spark.

ADVERSE EFFECTS

Signs and symptoms of hypotension (dizziness, fainting, mental status changes) are common with cyanide exposures and with nitrite administration. Headache is a commonly encountered side effect, especially with exposure to amyl nitrite. This effect generally is short lived.

ADMINISTRATION

Amyl Nitrite

Pearls may be broken in gauze, cloth, or a sponge and held close to the nose and mouth of the spontaneously breathing patient. In patients requiring assisted ventilation, the pearl may be placed into the lip of the facemask, inside the resuscitation bag, or in port access to the endotracheal tube. Amyl nitrite should be inhaled for 30 seconds out of each minute. The pearls should be replaced with a fresh one every 2 to 4 minutes, and their use should be considered at best a temporary measure until sodium nitrite is administered.[25]

Sodium Nitrite

A determination of the need for additional nitrite therapy should be made when intravenous access has been established. The sodium nitrite should be considered to be the primary possible lifesaving antidote, however, when the nitrite/thiosulfate combination approach is used. It is possible that patients who have responded positively to amyl nitrite and supportive care and are doing well clinically may not need sodium nitrite. For patients with serious cyanide poisoning, sodium nitrite and thiosulfate should be administered as soon as possible.

The usual adult dose of sodium nitrite is 300 mg (one 10-mL vial of a 3% solution). The pediatric dose is 0.12 to 0.33 mL/kg to a maximum of 300 mg (10 mL).[22] The dose should be given intravenously over at least 5 minutes or diluted in 50 to 100 mL of intravenous fluid and infused slowly. Blood pressure monitoring is essential during nitrite administration.[25]

Early animal studies showed the superiority of the combination of nitrite and thiosulfate over either agent alone.[7,8] Use of sodium nitrite plus sodium thiosulfate provided pro-

tection 18 times the median lethal dose of cyanide in dogs. If sodium nitrite is given, it should be followed by a dose of sodium thiosulfate.

REFERENCES

1. Murell W: Lancet 1:80–81, 113–115, 151–152, 225–227, 1879.
2. Wood GB, Bache F: Nitrite of amyl. In United States Dispensatory, Vol 15. Philadelphia, JB Lippincott, 1883, pp 185–186.
3. Pedigo LG: Antagonism between amyl nitrite and prussic acid. Tr Med Soc Virginia 19:124–131, 1888.
4. Mladoveanu C, Gheorhiu P: Le nitre de sou de comme antidote de l'empoisonnement experimental pa le cyanure de potassium. Compt Rend Soc Biol 102:164–166, 1929.
5. Geiger JC: Cyanide poisoning in San Francisco. JAMA 99:1944–1945, 1932.
6. Mota MM: Sobre un caso de intoxicacion por cianuro de potasio tratado con exito por el nitrito de sodio. Rev Med Rossario 23:670–674, 1933.
7. Chen KK, Rose CL, Clowes GH: Methylene blue, nitrites, and sodium thiosulfate against cyanide poisoning. Proc Soc Exp Biol Med 31:250–252, 1933.
8. Chen KK, Rose CL, Clowes GH: Amyl nitrite and cyanide poisoning. JAMA 100:1920–1922, 1933.
9. Baselt RC: Disposition of Toxic Drugs and Chemicals in Man, 5th ed. Foster City, CA, Chemical Toxicology Institute, 2000.
10. Toll LL, Hurlbut KM (eds): Nitrites. In Klasco RK (ed): POISINDEX System. Thompson MICROMEDEX, Greenwood Village, CO. Edition expires 6/2004.
11. Moshage H, Kok B, Huizenga JR, Jansen PLM: Nitrite and nitrate determinations in plasma. Clin Chem 41:892–896, 1995.
12. Rath MM, Kratz JC: Nitrites: IX. A further study of the mechanism of the action of organic nitrates. J Pharm Exp Ther 76:33–38, 1942.
13. Way JL: Cyanide intoxication and its mechanism of antagonism. Ann Rev Pharmacol Toxicol 24:451–458, 1984.
14. Hall AH, Rumack BH, Shaffer MO, et al: Clinical toxicology of cyanide: North American clinical experiences. In Ballantyne B, Marrs TC (eds): Clinical and Experimental Toxicology of Cyanides. Bristol, UK, John Wright and Sons, 1987, p 312.
15. Hall AH, Doutre WH, Ludden T, et al: Nitrite/thiosulfate treated acute cyanide poisoning: Estimated kinetics after antidote. Clin Toxicol 25:121–133, 1987.
16. Johnson WS, Hall AH, Rumack BH: Cyanide poisoning successfully treated without "therapeutic methemoglobin levels." Ann Emerg Med 7:437–440, 1989.
17. Way JL, Sylvester D, Morgan RL, et al: Recent perspectives on the toxicodynamic basis of cyanide antagonism. Fundam Appl Toxicol 4:S231–S239, 1984.
18. Wurzburg H: Treatment of cyanide poisoning in an industrialized setting. Vet Hum Toxicol 38:44–47, 1996.
19. Graham DL, Laman D, Theodore J, et al: Acute cyanide poisoning complicated by lactic acidosis and pulmonary edema. Arch Intern Med 137:1051–1055, 1977.
20. Yen D, Tsai J, Wang LM, et al: The clinical experience of acute cyanide poisoning. Am J Emerg Med 13:524–528, 1995.
21. Hall AH, Rumack BH: Clinical toxicology of cyanide. Ann Emerg Med 15:1067–1074, 1986.
22. Berlin CM: Treatment of cyanide poisoning in children. Pediatrics 46:793–796, 1970.
23. Briggs GG, Freeman RK, Yaffe SJ: Drugs in Pregnancy and Lactation, 4th ed. Baltimore, Williams & Wilkins, 1994.
24. Kulig K: Cyanide antidotes and fire toxicology. N Engl J Med 325:1801–1802, 1991.
25. Holland MA, Kozloski LM: Clinical features and management of cyanide poisoning. Clin Pharm 5:737–741, 1986.

CHAPTER 149

Thiosulfate

Christine M. Stork

Thiosulfate is a unique inorganic compound that is used in a variety of medical and nonmedical settings. The antidotal use of thiosulfate stems largely from its powerful reducing capabilities along with its ability to enhance endogenous enzymatic activity. Thiosulfate also exists naturally in humans but at much lower concentrations than those found when used therapeutically. When used medicinally, it is virtually always in the form of sodium thiosulfate.

HISTORY

Thiosulfate has a long history of use in industrial and medical settings. In industry, thiosulfate is used as an inorganic reducing agent for the production of finished materials.[1] Medical treatments using thiosulfate are quite diverse. Best known for the enhancement of rhodanase enzymatic activity in the mitigation of cyanide toxicity, thiosulfate is also studied and used in the treatment of toxic effects stemming from a variety of chemicals, including acrylonitrile, bromate, cisplatin, hypochlorous acid, paraquat, and platinum.[2–9] It is used topically in the treatment of selenium dioxide burns and is used as a treatment for cytotoxic drug extravasation.[10] A small amount of animal evidence supports the use of thiosulfate in hydrogen sulfide toxicity, although the mechanism is not clarified.[11] Finally, thiosulfate has been studied and used in the treatment of several medical disorders, including tumor calcifications, thromboangiitis, calcium nephrolithiasis, and tinea versicolor.[11–14]

PROPERTIES

Thiosulfate is a white, transparent crystal or powder.[15–17] In nature it occurs in the anhydrous form, but it is found most often in the pentahydrate form and is unstable as a powder unless maintained under dry conditions.[1] When solubilized as a 1.5% or 9.76% solution, thiosulfate is stable in normal saline, dextrose 5% water, and dextrose 5%/0.45% sodium chloride for at least 24 hours.

Biochemically, this naturally occurring sulfur compound has strong nucleophilicity and appreciable redox activity. In humans, it is produced as a systemic metabolic intermediate derived from the amino acid cysteine, where it serves to protect against the depletion of reduced glutathione.[18–20]

PHARMACODYNAMICS

Exogenous administration of thiosulfate results in a rapid elevation in serum concentrations. The pharmacologic activity of sodium thiosulfate is hypothesized to develop more slowly, however, and to last far longer than the biologic half-life. The increased duration of effect currently is shown in a swine model in which pretreatment resulted in 4 hours of protection from hydrogen cyanide after a single dose.[21] The delay in pharmacologic effect is hypothesized to be due to the occurrence of thiosulfate activity in the mitochondria and the slow intramitochondrial diffusion of $S_2O_3^{2-}$ ions. The mitochondria are the location of enzymatic rhodanase activity.[22] Thiosulfate, when in the mitochondria, donates a sulfane sulfur group (a divalent form of sulfur that is joined to one or more sulfur atoms to enhance the activity of rhodanase) (Fig. 149-1).[23]

PHARMACOKINETICS

Thiosulfate exists naturally in healthy humans at a plasma concentration of 1.1 ± 0.1 mg/dL. After exogenous intravenous administration in healthy humans, its calculated volume of distribution is 151 mL/kg into extracellular fluid space, with a distribution half-life of 23 minutes.[17,24]

Sodium thiosulfate is metabolized partially in the liver to sulfate and is excreted partially unchanged by the kidneys.[25] The renal excretion data are contradictory. Some authors report that it is filtered solely through the glomerulus.[26,27] Others report additional tubular secretion and reabsorption.[28,29]

Thiosulfate is reported to be eliminated using a one-compartment and a two-compartment model.[29,30] Its reported elimination half-life ranges from 16 to 182 minutes.[29,31,32] Using a one-compartment model, $28.5\% \pm 9.4\%$ of the drug was recovered in the urine, with 95% recoverable in the urine within 4 hours. The mean total body clearance was 190 ± 76 mL/min/m^2, and renal clearance was 50.4 ± 11 mL/min/m^2.[30] Using a two-compartment model, clearance was 1.39 mL/min, with urinary excretion of $42.6\% \pm 3.5\%$ of the dose at 180 minutes postdose and $47.4\% \pm 2.4\%$ at 18 hours postdose.[29] The renal clearance of thiosulfate sometimes is used as a marker for inulin or glomerular filtration rate.

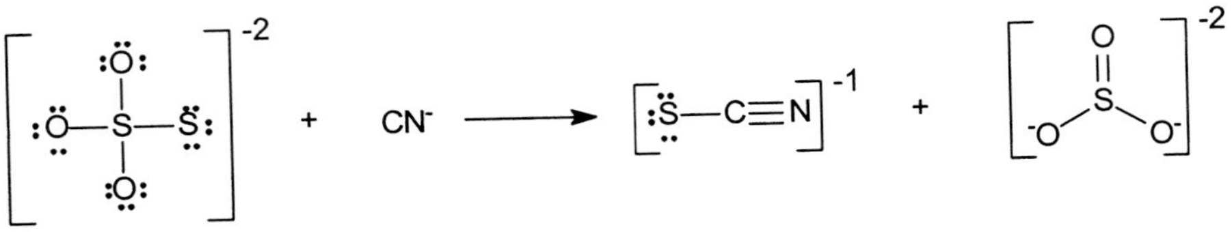

FIGURE 149-1

Reaction of thiosulfate in the detoxification of cyanide.

SPECIAL POPULATIONS

Pediatric Patients

Thiosulfate is used successfully to treat cyanide toxicity in newborns and children with sodium nitroprusside–associated cyanide toxicity.[33] There is no reason that this population would respond differently than adults after administration of thiosulfate.

Pregnant Patients

The use of thiosulfate was studied in animal models in terms of thiosulfate's ability to cross the placenta and its ability to improve outcome clinically after poisoning. Although sodium thiosulfate did decrease toxicity from cyanide in the mother and fetus of gravid ewes, thiosulfate did not cross the placenta in the same animal model.[34,35] The implications of this finding are not clear but may include the contribution of improvement of maternal outcome to the well-being of the fetus. Based on these data, thiosulfate should not be withheld.

ADVERSE EFFECTS

Thiosulfate is generally well tolerated, even when administered to healthy patients in large doses. In dogs, hypotension is seen after overdoses of 500 mg/kg, but this has never been reported in humans.[36] Intravenous infusion of sodium thiosulfate can cause nausea, vomiting, localized burning, muscle cramping, and twitching at the injection site.[37] A single case of allergic contact dermatitis has been reported.[38] Large oral doses are reported to result in a cathartic effect due to osmotic gradient changes.[39]

ADMINISTRATION

There are no unusual contraindications or precautions when administering sodium thiosulfate. Thiosulfate must be administered intravenously because absorption from the gastrointestinal tract is poor.[17] For cyanide toxicity in adults, the usual dose is 12.5 g administered intravenously over 10 minutes, repeated at half of the initial dose if required.[40] In France, a combination hydroxycobalamin/sodium thiosulfate kit is available for cyanide toxicity in which 8 g of thiosulfate is administered (see Fig. 150-2).[41] Practically, caution is required when administering the combination of hydroxycobalamin and thiosulfate because if given concurrently, they combine to form an inactive complex.[42] In addition, although all current dosing information relies on bolus dosing, animal data suggest that an infusion may be more effective.[43] For protection of cisplatin nephrotoxicity, 12 g of thiosulfate is administered intravenously over 6 hours, or 9 g/m^2 is administered as an intravenous bolus, followed by 1.2 g/m^2/hr intravenously for 6 hours.[44]

In children, the dose of thiosulfate depends on the hemoglobin concentration and is variable. For a 25% thiosulfate solution, the usual recommended dose is 1.10 mL/kg if the hemoglobin concentration is 8 g, 1.35 mL/kg if the hemoglobin concentration is 10 g, 1.65 mL/kg if the hemoglobin concentration is 12 g, and 1.95 mL/kg if the hemoglobin concentration is 14 g.[45]

REFERENCES

1. Budavari S (ed): The Merck Index, 12th ed. Whitehouse Station, NJ, Merck & Co, 1996.
2. Hall AH, Rumack BH: Hydrocobalamin/sodium thiosulfate as a cyanide antidote. J Emerg Med 5:115–121, 1987.
3. Muldoon LL, Pagel MA, Kroll RA, et al: Delayed administration of sodium thiosulfate in animal models reduces platinum ototoxicity without reduction of antitumor activity. Clin Cancer Res 6:309–315, 2000.
4. Warshaw BL: Treatment of bromate poisoning (Letter). J Pediatr 115:660–661, 1989.
5. Goel R, Cleary SM, Horton C, et al: Effect of sodium thiosulfate on the pharmacokinetics and toxicity of cisplatin. J Natl Cancer Inst 81:1552–1560, 1989.
6. Robbins KT, Storniolo AM, Kerber C, et al: Phase 1 study of highly selective supradose cisplatin infusions for advanced head and neck cancer. J Clin Oncol 12:2113–2120, 1994.
7. Yamamoto H: Protection against paraquat-induced toxicity with sulfite or thiosulfate in mice. Toxicology 79:37–43, 1993.
8. Kozumbo WJ, Agarwal S, Koren HS: Breakage and binding of DNA by reaction products of hypochlorous acid with aniline, 1-naphthylamine, or 1-naphthol. Toxicol Appl Pharmacol 115:107–115, 1992.
9. Mehta C: Antidotal effect of sodium thiosulfate in mice exposed to acrylonitrile. Res Commun Mol Path Pharmacol 87:155–165, 1995.
10. Finkel AJ (ed): Hamilton and Hardy's Industrial Toxicology, 4th ed. Boston, John Wright, PSG, 1983, p 125.
11. Scheler W, Kabisch R: Uber die antagonistische beeinflussung der akuten H2S-Vergiftung bei der maus durch methamoglobinbildner. Acta Biol Med Ger 11:194–199, 1963.
12. Papadakis JT, Patrikarea A, Digenis GE, et al: Sodium thiosulfate in the treatment of tumoral calcification in a hemodialysis patient without hyperparathyroidism. Nephron 72:308–312, 1996.
13. Theis FV, Freeland MR: Thromboangiitis obliterans. Surgery 11:101, 1942.
14. Yatzidis H: Successful sodium thiosulfate treatment for recurrent calcium urolithiasis. Clin Nephrol 23:63–67, 1985.
15. HSDB: Hazardous Substances Data Bank. Bethesda, MD, National Library of Medicine (Internet Version); Englewood, CO, Micromedex, 2000.
16. Persson H, Walter J: Sodium Thiosulfate Monograph (Preliminary Version). Geneva, International Programme on Chemical Safety, 1987.
17. ITI: Toxic and Hazardous Industrial Chemicals Safety Manual. Tokyo, International Technical Information Institute, 1985, pp 490–491.
18. Yamamoto H: Protection against paraquat-induced reactive metabolites. Toxicology 79:37–43, 1993.
19. Kedderis GL, Sumner SC, Held SD, et al: Dose dependent urinary excretion of acrylonitrile metabolites by rats and mice. Toxicol Appl Pharmacol 12:288–297, 1993.
20. Vesey CJ, Krapez JR, Varley JG, et al: The antidotal action of thiosulfate following acute nitroprusside infusion in dogs. Anaesthesiology 62:415–421, 1985.

21. Mengel K, Kramer W, Isert B, et al: Thiosulfate and hydroxycobalamin prophylaxis in progressive cyanide poisoning in guinea-pigs. Toxicology 54:335–342, 1989.
22. Harth O, Wasserhaushalt, Stoff, et al: In Schmidt RF, Thews G (eds): Physiologie des Menschen, 21 Auflage. Berlin Heidelberg-NY, Springer-Verlag, 1983, p 707.
23. Way JL, Sylvester D, Morgan RL, et al: Recent perspectives on the toxicodynamic basis of cyanide antagonism. Fundam Appl Toxicol 4:S231–239, 1984.
24. Dennis DL, Fletcher WS: Toxicity of sodium thiosulfate (NSC-45624), a nitrogen mustard antagonist, in the dog. Cancer Chemother Rep 50:255–257, 1966.
25. Schulz V: Clinical pharmacokinetics of nitroprusside, cyanide, thiosulfate and thiocyanate. Clin Pharmacokinet 9:239–251, 1984.
26. Newman EV, Gilman A, Philips FS: The renal clearance of thiosulfate in man. Bull Johns Hopkins Hosp 79:229, 1946.
27. Gilman A, Philips FS, Koelle ES: The renal clearance of thiosulfate with observations on its volume distribution. Am J Physiol 146:48, 1946.
28. Bucht H: On the tubular excretion of thiosulfate and creatinine under the influence of caronamide. Scand J Clin Lab Invest 1:270, 1949.
29. Ivankovich AD, Braverman B, Stephens TS, et al: Sodium thiosulfate disposition in humans: Relation to sodium nitroprusside toxicity. Anesthesiology 58:11–17, 1983.
30. Shea M, Koziol JA, Howell SB: Kinetics of sodium thiosulfate, a cisplatin neutralizer. Clin Pharmacol Ther 35:419–425, 1984.
31. Schulz V, Gross R, Pasch T, et al: Cyanide toxicity of sodium nitroprusside in therapeutic use with and without sodium thiosulfate. Klin Wochenschr 60:1393–1400, 1982.
32. Ritschel WA: Biologic half-lives of drugs. Drug Intell Clin Pharm 4:332–347, 1970.
33. Schulz V, Roth B: Detoxification of cyanide in a new-born child. Klin Wochenschr 60:527–528, 1982.
34. Curry SC, Carlton MW, Raschke RA: Prevention of fetal and maternal cyanide toxicity from nitroprusside with coinfusion of sodium thiosulfate in gravid ewes. Anesth Analg 84:1121–1126, 1997.
35. Graeme KA, Curry SC, Bikin DS, et al: The lack of transplacental movement of the cyanide antidote thiosulfate in gravid ewes. Anesth Analg 89:1448–1452, 1999.
36. Mizoule J: Etude de l'action de l'hydroxocobalamine a l'egard de l'intoxication cyanhydrique. Thesis. Paris, Faculte de Pharmacie de l'Universite de Paris, 1966.
37. Forsyth JC, Mueller PD, Becker CE, et al: Hydroxycobalamin as a cyanide antidote: Safety, efficacy and pharmacokinetics in heavily smoking normal volunteers. J Toxicol Clin Toxicol 31:277–294, 1993.
38. Rudzki E: Dermatitis from sodium hyposulfite. Contact Dermatitis 6:148, 1980.
39. Reynolds JEF (ed): Martindale: The Extra Pharmacopoeia (electronic version). Denver, CO, Micromedex, 1990.
40. Olin BR (ed): Facts and Comparisons. St Louis, Facts and Comparisons, 2000.
41. Hall AH, Rumack BH: Hydroxycobalamin/sodium thiosulfate as a cyanide antidote. J Emerg Med 5:115–121, 1987.
42. Friedberg KD, Shukla UR: The efficiency of aquacobalamine as an antidote in cyanide poisoning when given alone or combined with sodium thiosulfate. Arch Toxicol 33:103–113, 1975.
43. Gonzales J, Sabatini S: Cyanide poisoning: Pathophysiology and current approaches to therapy. Int J Artif Organs 12:347–355, 1989.
44. Abe R, Akiyoshi T, Koba F, et al: "Two-route chemotherapy" using intra-arterial cisplatin and intravenous sodium thiosulfate, its neutralizing agent, for hepatic malignancies. Eur J Cancer Oncol 24:1671–1674, 1988.
45. Henretig FM, Shannon M: Toxicologic emergencies. In Fleisher GR, Ludwig S (eds): Textbook of Pediatric Emergency Medicine, 3rd ed. Baltimore, Williams & Wilkins, 1993.

CHAPTER 150

Cyanide Binding Antidotes: Dicobalt Edetate and Hydroxocobalamin

George Braitberg

Death from cyanide is one of the most rapid and dramatic seen in medicine.[1] Serious acute cyanide poisoning is rare. More recent events have highlighted the need for preparedness against possible chemical terrorist attacks. There is currently no single treatment that is used for the management of cyanide poisoning worldwide. The lack of evidence-based treatment regimens is one major barrier to the lack of universal acceptance of a single antidote. The availability of antidotal therapy also is subject to a combination of market and regulatory forces.[2]

In Australia, the National Occupational Health and Safety Commission (NOHSC) Guide on Cyanide Poisoning (1993) recommends dicobalt edetate (Kelocyanor) as the cyanide poisoning antidote. Dicobalt edetate also is used in the United Kingdom. In the United States, the cyanide antidote kit (CAK), also called the Lilly Cyanide Kit, is the only available treatment (Eli Lilly, Inc., Indianapolis, IN). In Europe, hydroxocobalamin and 4-dimethylaminophenol (4-DMAP) are used. The treatment of cyanide poisoning is discussed in detail in Chapter 95.

Cyanide is used in a variety of commercial processes. Exposure can be in the form of hydrogen cyanide gas, produced when inorganic cyanide comes in contact with mineral acids as in electroplating or accidentally when cyanide solutions are poured into acid waste containers. Cyanide is used in metal extraction and recovery, in metal hardening, and in the production of agricultural and horticultural pest control compounds.[3] Cyanide off-gassing in house fires is well documented, and in one study significant blood concentrations occurred in 59% of smoke inhalation patients.[4]

PHARMACODYNAMICS

Cyanide inhibits aerobic metabolism. The uptake of cyanide into cells is rapid and follows first-order kinetics. Cyanide, or its ion, CN^-, may enter the body through inhalation, ingestion, or skin and mucous membrane absorption. After it is absorbed, it is rapidly distributed. Most cyanide (60%) is protein bound.[5] Its half-life is 2 to 3 hours. Although the precise in vivo action of cyanide is yet to be determined, it is thought that its major effect is due to binding with the ferric ion (Fe^{3+}) of cytochrome oxidase, the last cytochrome in the respiratory chain. This binding results in inhibition of oxidative phosphorylation, leading to a net accumulation of hydrogen ions and a change in the nicotinamide adenine

dinucleotide:reduced nicotinamide adenine dinucleotide ratio, with greatly increased lactic acid production. Other processes involving catalase, superoxide dismutase, and glutathione may contribute to toxicity.[6] Cyanide also is a potent stimulator of neurotransmitter release in the central and peripheral nervous systems.[7] The pathophysiology of cyanide poisoning is discussed in detail in Chapter 95.

Humans detoxify cyanide by transferring sulfane sulfur (R-Sx-SH) to cyanide to form thiocyanate. The availability of R-Sx-SH is the rate-limiting step. This reaction is thought to be catalyzed by the liver enzyme rhodanese. Other enzymes, such as β-mercaptopyruvate sulfur transferase, may be important, however. Other routes of biotransformation include oxidative detoxification.[6] The mode of action of the CN^- binding antidotes is given in Table 150-1 (Figs. 150-1 and 150-2).

Cyanide antidotes bind CN^-, form methemoglobin (which then binds CN^-), or, in the case of thiosulfate, provide a substrate for enzymatic detoxification. Although this chapter focuses on cyanide binding antidotes, a comparison is made with other antidotes. The various antidotes are summarized in Tables 150-1 through 150-3.

ADVERSE EFFECTS

In life-threatening situations in which cyanide toxicity is suspected, the antidote must be given before any confirmatory tests can be performed. In this situation, the potential for antidote-induced morbidity and mortality is particularly significant because some patients receive the antidote unnecessarily. In smoke inhalation victims with suspected combined carbon monoxide and cyanide poisoning, the availability of an antidote that does not exacerbate any oxygen carriage or delivery problem (as with the methemoglobin-forming agents) or cause toxicity by its own action is theoretically desirable.[16,17]

Dicobalt Edetate

The current recommended antidote for clinically severe cyanide toxicity in Australia and the United Kingdom is dicobalt edetate.[18] Significant adverse effects are associated with the use of this drug (see Table 150-1), many of which are life-threatening. These effects are exacerbated in individuals treated for suspected cyanide poisoning who are not cyanide poisoned. Administration of glucose may mitigate some of these adverse effects.

TABLE 150-1 Cyanide Ion Binding Antidotes

ANTIDOTE*	TYPICAL DOSE	MECHANISM OF ACTION	ADVERSE EFFECTS
Dicobalt edetate (Kelocyanor)	300 mg IV	Chelation of cyanide. Dicobalt edetate complexes with cyanide forming cobalt cyanide, removing cyanide from the circulation and reducing toxicity. Unless cyanide is forced into the extra-cellular fluid, however, tissue concentrations are minimally affected.	Severe hypotension, cardiac arrhythmias, convulsions.[8,9] Gross edema after treatment with dicobalt edetate also has been reported.[10] These effects are most noted when given in the absence of cyanide.[9] Intravenous glucose may mitigate some of these reactions.[18]
Hydroxocobalamin†	5–15 g IV	Chelation of cyanide. Cobalt complexes with cyanide to form cyanocobalamin (vitamin B_{12}). Antidotal doses of hydroxocobalamin (vitamin B_{12a}) are approximately 5000 times the physiologic dose.[25]	Minimal, transient reddish discoloration of the skin, mucous membranes, and urine, producing a mean elevation in systolic blood pressure of 13.6% with a concomitant decrease in heart rate.[11] Allergic reactions have been noted.[23]

*See Figure 150-1.
†See Figure 150-2.
IV, intravenously.

4-Dimethylaminophenol

In Germany, 4-dimethylaminophenol (4-DMAP) is used as the methemoglobin generator because of its rapid onset of action.[19] The problems associated with methemoglobin formation, as described earlier for nitrites, apply to 4-DMAP to an even greater extent. It has poor dose-response curve reproducibility.[20] Hemolysis as a result of 4-DMAP therapy has been observed in overdose and after a correct therapeutic dose.[8] The dose is typically 5 mL of 5% 4-DMAP solution (250 mg [or 3 to 4 mg/kg]) intravenously for 1 minute.[21] 4-DMAP is discussed in detail in Chapter 160.

Cyanide Antidote Kit (Sodium Thiosulfate)

The clinical effects of sodium nitrite are observed before significant levels of methemoglobinemia are detected,

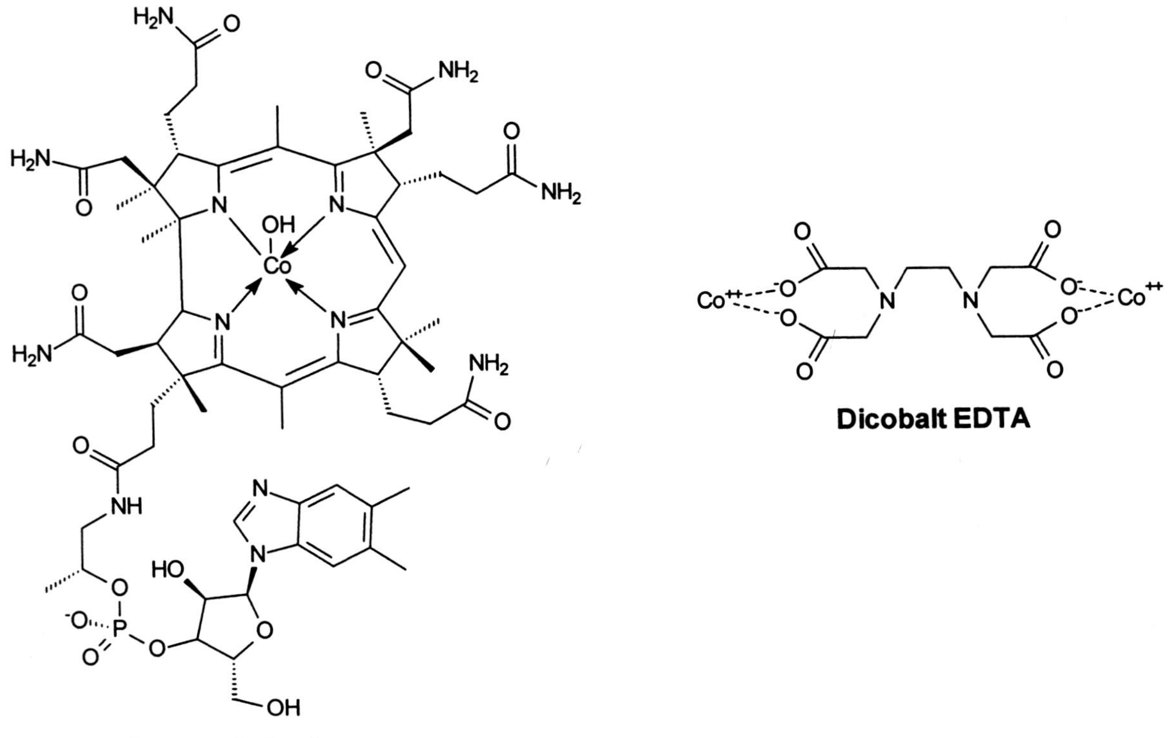

Hydroxocobalamin

Dicobalt EDTA

FIGURE 150-1

Chemical structures of hydroxocobalamin and dicobalt edetate (EDTA).

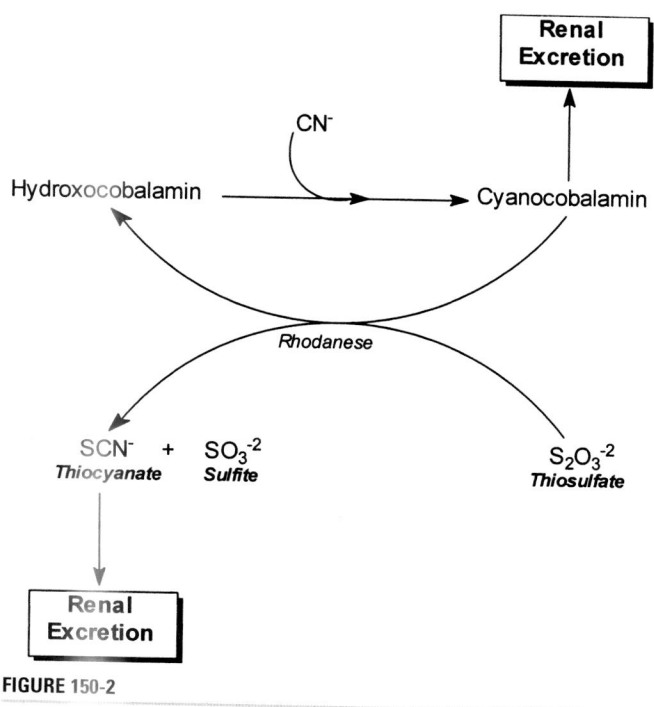

FIGURE 150-2

Interconversion of hydroxocobalamin and cyanocobalamin.

suggesting an alternative mode of action.[8,14] After administration of 300 mg of sodium nitrite, the mean of the peak methemoglobin levels was 10.5%.[22,23] Although this amount is less than the once thought "ceiling therapeutic" methemoglobin level of 30%, it seems that the latter degree of methemoglobinemia is not required. Such high methemoglobin concentrations may seriously impair oxygen carrying in patients with anemia. Although there is a theoretical concern about additive effects on oxygen carrying capacity in smoke inhalation patients who also may be poisoned with carbon monoxide,[24,25] this does not seem to be a problem in actual clinical practice if patients are treated with supplemental oxygen.[15]

Elevated methemoglobin concentrations rarely have been reported in fire victims,[24] adding a further note of caution. On a practical note, Marrs[8] pointed out that the trivalent iron of methemoglobin cannot reversibly bind oxygen, and common methods for measuring the amount of methemoglobin after nitrite administration are unable to measure the amount of cyanmethemoglobin produced.

Hydroxocobalamin

In Europe, hydroxocobalamin is used. Extensive research has shown the safety of this drug in experimental and clinical practice (Baud FJ: unpublished data).[23,25–30] There is substantial evidence of the efficacy of hydroxocobalamin in

TABLE 150-2 Methemoglobin-Inducing Agents			
ANTIDOTE	**TYPICAL DOSE**	**MECHANISM OF ACTION**	**ADVERSE EFFECTS**
4-Dimethylaminophenol (4-DMAP)	5 mL of 5% 4-DMAP solution (250 mg or 3–4 mg/kg) IV for 1 min	Generates a methemoglobin concentration of 30–50% within a few minutes at these doses	Poor dose-response curve reproducibility. Hemolysis has been shown at therapeutic doses.[21]
Amyl nitrite pearls		Methemoglobin formation, which promotes a concentration-dependent movement of cyanide out of mitochondria	Decreases oxygen carrying capacity. This may be important if there is coexistent carbon monoxide poisoning.[12,13]
Sodium nitrite	10 mL (30 mg/mL) IV	Methemoglobin formation, which promotes movement of cyanide out of mitochondria. Clinical effects are observed before significant levels of methemaglobinemia, however, suggesting an alternate mode of action.[14]	The mean of the peak amount of methemoglobin concentrations is 10.5% after administration of 300 mg of sodium nitrite.[15] This may be significant in conditions of oxygen deficit, severe anemia, or preexisting cardiorespiratory morbidity.[4] Hypotension may occur.[2]

IV, intravenously.

TABLE 150-3 Sodium Thiosulfate			
	TYPICAL DOSE	**MECHANISM OF ACTION**	**ADVERSE EFFECTS**
CAK (sodium thiosulfate)	50 mL (250 mg/mL) IV or 12.5 g/50 mL	Thiosulfate is intravenously injected. It has a higher affinity for cyanide than methemoglobin. Thiosulfate reacts with cyanide ion to form thiocyanate. Thiocyanate is nearly nontoxic and rapidly secreted by the kidneys.	High thiocyanate concentrations (>10 mg/dL) have been associated with vomiting, psychosis, arthralgias, and myalgia. Anaphylaxis is a rare event.[5]

CAK, cyanide antidote kit; IV, intravenously.

cyanide poisoning (Baud FJ: unpublished data).[25,31] Hydroxo-cobalamin, when given to humans receiving sodium nitroprusside infusions, has been shown significantly to prevent cyanide accumulation.[32] Other studies have shown the safety and efficacy of hydoxocobalamin in sodium nitroprusside–induced cyanide toxicity.[33]

In clinical practice, hydroxocobalamin has been given successfully to patients with much higher concentrations of cyanide than the concentrations achieved by a sodium nitroprusside infusion.[23,27,34] Proponents of hydroxocobalamin therapy caution that in cases of ingestion of cyanide with suicidal intent (in which blood cyanide concentrations may be >150 μmol/L [0.4 mg/dL], or plasma lactate concentrations may be >20 mmol/L), the usual 5- to 10-g dose of hydroxocobalamin may be insufficient, and an additional antidote or higher concentrations of hydroxocobalamin may be useful in such cases.[8,27]

The required dose of hydroxocobalamin theoretically may be reduced by the concomitant administration of sodium thiosulfate. There are no controlled clinical trials with the adjutant use of sodium thiosulfate; however, there is in vitro and anecdotal evidence supporting its use. Sodium thiosulfate, 2 mmol/kg given intravenously after potassium cyanide, doubled the median lethal dose in rabbits. Case reports, such as that reported by Tassan and colleagues,[34] document successful outcomes in patients with extremely high concentrations of cyanide (494 μmol/L [1.3 mg/dL]) with combination therapy. In 1987, Hall and Rumack[35] reviewed several case reports detailing the French experience from 1970 to 1984. They reported cases in which hydroxocobalamin/sodium thiosulfate combination therapy was used in patients who recovered from severe, life-threatening poisoning with cyanide.

Baud, in an open trial conducted in 69 patients to assess the efficacy and safety of hydroxocobalamin in smoke inhalation victims (unpublished data), documented 42 patients with cyanide levels of greater than 39 μmol/L (>0.1 mg/dL). The median concentration of cyanide was 96.1 μmol/L (0.2 mg/dL) (six patients had levels >200 μmol/L [0.5 mg/dL]). These poisoned patients had a median concentration of carbon monoxide of 2.86 μmol/L. Many of these patients were symptomatic; 28 of 42 patients survived, including 11 of 19 patients with blood cyanide levels greater than 100 μmol/L (>0.3 mg/dL). A mean dose of 8 g of hydroxocobalamin was given. In patients who had cyanide levels less than 39 μmol/L (<0.1 mg/dL), the administration of hydroxocobalamin led to no adverse effects. Fourteen patients presented with initial cardiorespiratory arrest, and although the administration of a mean dose of 8 g of hydroxocobalamin was associated with restoration of pulse and blood pressure, 13 died as a result of decerebration. The mean cyanide value in these patients was 121.5 μmol/L (0.32 mg/dL) with a mean carbon monoxide level of 2.63 μmol/L. Hydroxocobalamin in all groups was given as an infusion over 20 to 30 minutes.

Baud[27] reported a case series of nine patients treated with hydroxocobalamin. Using a dose range of 5 to 15 g of hydroxocobalamin (average 8.1 g) to treat patients with an average cyanide concentration of 171 μmol/L (0.4 mg/dL) from intentional and accidental exposure, the investigators showed marked improvement in blood pressure for all patients presenting with shock or hypotension and in two of five com-

atose patients showed complete normalization of consciousness. Overall, the administration of hydroxocobalamin enabled six of nine patients to recover. Recovery occurred in one patient with a level of 217 μmol/L (0.6 mg/dL).

Hyperbaric Oxygen

The role of hyperbaric medicine in the management of cyanide toxicity is controversial, with conflicting animal data. In most published human reports, hyperbaric oxygen is offered after a combination of modalities, and it is not possible to discern the effect of one treatment over another.[36–40]

ADMINISTRATION

In cyanide poisoning from smoke inhalation or self-poisoning in patients with clinical signs and associated lactic acidosis (or in whom semiquantitative bedside testing for cyanide in blood is available and the result suggestive of cyanide poisoning)[41] and in patients in whom one is suspicious that cyanide poisoning is the cause of unknown coma or cardiovascular instability, the following regimen is recommended.[42] The treatment of cyanide poisoning is discussed more thoroughly in Chapter 95.

Hydroxocobalamin

A dose of 5 to 15 g of hydroxocobalamin, repeated if necessary, is typically given over 30 minutes (70 mg/kg in a child), but it may be given as an intravenous push as needed. Hydroxocobalamin is contraindicated in patients allergic to vitamin B_{12}. In addition, sodium thiosulfate, 12.5 g, 50 mL of a 25% solution at 2.5 to 5 mL/min (i.e., over 10 to 20 minutes), is given.

Dicobalt Edetate

Typical dosing of dicobalt edetate is 300 mg by intravenous injection over 1 to 5 minutes. This dose can be repeated if necessary; however, it is best to wait approximately 5 minutes to assess the degree of clinical improvement and to reduce the likelihood of adverse effects. As described earlier, the coadministration of glucose (50 mL of 50% solution for adults) may reduce some of the adverse effects associated with this agent.

CONCLUSION

There is a paucity of scientific data comparing the efficacy of hydroxocobalamin and dicobalt edetate, precluding any definitive conclusion about which antidote is better. More is known, however, about the fate of hydroxocobalamin in humans and its safety. In the emergency situation, hydroxocobalamin seems to offer a greater margin of safety. Hydroxocobalamin is well recognized as a safe, easily administered cyanide antidote. Because of its extremely low adverse effect profile, it is ideal for out-of-hospital use in suspected cyanide intoxication. To prepare effectively for a cyanide disaster, we must investigate, adopt, manufacture, and stockpile hydroxocobalamin to prevent needless morbidity and mortality.[2]

REFERENCES

1. Gonzales J, Sabatini S: Cyanide poisoning: Pathophysiology and current approaches to therapy. Int J Artif Org 12:347–355, 1989.
2. Sauer SW, Keim ME: Hydroxocobalamin: Improved public health readiness for cyanide disasters. Ann Emerg Med 37:635–641, 2001.
3. Hall AH, Rumack BH: Cyanide and related compounds. In Haddad LM, Shannon MW, Winchester JF (eds): Clinical Management of Poisoning and Drug Overdose, 3rd ed. Philadelphia, WB Saunders, 1998, pp 899–905.
4. Baud FJ, Barriot P, Toffis V, et al: Elevated blood cyanide levels in victims of smoke inhalation. N Engl J Med 325:1761–1766, 1991.
5. Ellenhorn MJ, Barceloux DG (eds): Ellenhorn's Medical Toxicology, 2nd ed. Baltimore, Williams & Wilkins, 1997.
6. Curry SC: Hydrogen cyanide and inorganic salts. In Sullivan JB, Krieger GR (eds): Hazardous Materials Toxicology: Clinical Principles of Environmental Health. Baltimore, Williams & Wilkins, 1992, pp 698–709.
7. Isom GE, Borowitz JL: Modification of cyanide toxicodynamics mechanistic based antidote development. Toxicol Lett 82/83:795–799, 1995.
8. Marrs TC: Anidotal treatment of acute cyanide poisoning. Adv Drug React Acute Poisoning Rev 4:179–206, 1988.
9. Vogel SN, Sultan RT, Teneyck RP: Cyanide poisoning. Clin Toxicol 18:367–383, 1981.
10. Dodds C, McKnight C: Cyanide toxicity after immersion and the hazards of dicobalt edetate. BMJ 291:785–786, 1985.
11. Forsyth JC, Mueller PD, Becker CE, et al: Hydroxocobalamin as a cyanide antidote: Safety, efficacy and pharmacokinetics in heavily smoking normal volunteers. J Toxicol Clin Toxicol 31:277–294, 1993.
12. Moore SJ, Norris JC, et al: Antidotal use of methemoglobin-forming cyanide antagonists in concurrent carbon monoxide/cyanide intoxication. J Pharm Exp Ther 242:70–73, 1987.
13. Hall AH, Kulig KW, Rumack BH: Suspected cyanide poisoning in smoke inhalation: Complications of sodium nitrite therapy. J Toxicol Clin Exp 9:3–9, 1989.
14. Shragg TA, Albertson TE, et al: Cyanide poisoning after bitter almond ingestion. West J Med 6:401–404, 1982.
15. Kirk MA, Gerace R, Kulig KW: Cyanide and methaemaglobin kinetics in smoke inhalation victims treated with the cyanide antidote kit. Ann Emerg Med 22:1413–1418, 1993.
16. Baud J, Richter F, et al: Pre hospital strategy for therapeutic intervention of fire victims. Toxicol Lett 64/65:273–281, 1992.
17. Hall AH, Kulig KW, Rumack BH: Suspected cyanide poisoning in smoke inhalation: Complications of sodium nitrite therapy. J Toxicol Clin Exp 9:3–9, 1989.
18. Hillman B, Bardan KD, Bain JTB: The use of dicobalt edetate (Kelocyanor) in cyanide poisoning. Postgrad Med J 50:171–174, 1974.
19. Kiese M, Weger N: Formation of ferrihaemaglobin with aminophenols in the human for the treatment of cyanide poisoning. Eur J Pharmacol 7:97–105, 1969.
20. Van Dijk A, Glerum JH, Van Heijst ANP, Douze JMC: Clinical evaluation of the cyanide antagonist 4-DMAP in a lethal cyanide poisoning case. Vet Hum Toxicol 29(Suppl 2):38–39, 1987.
21. Weger N: Aminophenols as antidotes to prussic acid [in German]. Arch Toxikol 24:49–50, 1968.
22. Kirk MA, Gerace R, Kulig KW: Cyanide and methaemaglobin kinetics in smoke inhalation victims treated with the cyanide antidote kit. Ann Emerg Med 22:1413–1418, 1993.
23. Borron SW, Baud FJ: Acute cyanide poisoning: Clinical spectrum, diagnosis and treatment. Arh Hig Rada Toksikol 47:307–322, 1996.
24. Lui D, Olsen KR: Smoke inhalation. In Hoffman RS, Goldfinger CR (eds): Critical Care Toxicology. London, Churchill Livingstone, 1991, pp 203–224.
25. Houeto P, Borron SW, et al: Pharmacokinetics of hydroxocobalamin in smoke inhalation victims. J Toxicol Clin Toxicol 34:397–404, 1996.
26. Riou B, Berdeaux A, et al: Comparison of the hemodynamic effects of hydroxocobalamin and dicobalt edetate at euipotent cyanide doses in conscious dogs. Intensive Care Med 19:26–32, 1993.
27. Baud FJ: Intoxication aigue par les cyanures (ingestion, inhalation): Traitement par l'hydroxocobalamin. Presented at the Congres de la Societe de Toxicologie Clinique, Grenoble, October 12–13, 1995.
28. Riou B, Baud FJ, et al: In vitro demonstration of the antidotal efficacy of hydroxocobalamin in cyanide poisoning. J Neurosurg Anaesth 2:296–304, 1990.
29. Posner MA, Tobey RE, McElroy H: Hydroxocobalmin therapy of cyanide intoxication in guinea pigs. Anesthesiology 44:157–160, 1976.
30. Ivankovich AD, Braverman B, et al: Cyanide antidotes and methods of their administration in dogs: A comparative study. Anaesthesiology 52:210–216, 1980.
31. Mushett CW, Kelley KL, et al: Antidotal efficacy of vitamin B12a (hydroxo-cobalamin) in experimental cyanide poisoning. Proc Soc Exp Biol 18:234–237, 1952.
32. Cottrell JE, Casthely P, et al: Prevention of nitroprusside-induced cyanide toxicity with hydroxocobalamin. N Engl J Med 298:809–811, 1978.
33. Zerbe NF, Wagner BKJ: Use of vitamin B12 in the treatment and prevention of nitroprusside induced cyanide toxicity. Crit Care Med 21:465–467, 1993.
34. Tassan H, Joyon D, et al: Potassium cyanide poisoning treated with hydroxocobalamin. Ann Fr Anesth Reanim 4:383–385, 1990.
35. Hall AH, Rumack BH: Hydroxocobalamin/sodium thiosulfate as a cyanide antidote. J Emerg Med 5:115–121, 1987.
36. Sheehy M, Way JL: Effect on oxygen on cyanide intoxication: III. Mithridate. J Pharmacol Exp Ther 161:163–168, 1968.
37. Skee WG, Norman JN, et al: Effect of hyperbaric oxygen in cyanide poisoning. National Academy of Sciences—National Research Council Publication 1404:705–710, 1966.
38. Takano T, Miyazaki Y, et al: Effect of hyperbaric oxygen on cyanide intoxication: In situ changes in intracellular oxidation reduction. Undersea Biomed Res 7:191–197, 1990.
39. Hart GB, Strauss MB, et al: Treatment of smoke inhalation by hyperbaric oxygen. J Emerg Med 3:211–215, 1985.
40. Litovitz TL, Larkin RF, et al: Cyanide poisoning treated with hyperbaric oxygen. Am J Emerg Med 3:211–215, 1983.
41. Fligner CL, Luthi R, et al: Paper strip screening method for detection of cyanide in blood using the CYANOTESTMO test paper. Am J Forensic Med Pathol 13:81–84, 1992.
42. Braitberg G, Vanderpyl MMJ: Treatment of cyanide poisoning in Australasia. Emerg Med 12:232–240, 2000.

CHAPTER 151

Ethanol

Daniel J. Cobaugh

Significant toxicity can occur after exposure to methanol and ethylene glycol.[1,2] Along with gastrointestinal decontamination, hemodialysis, and intensive supportive care, ethanol has a long history of use in the treatment of ethylene glycol and methanol poisoning.[3–6] Despite this extensive use, the U.S. Food and Drug Administration has never approved ethanol for this indication. Although fomepizole has been used as an antidote in some other countries for many years, and the Food and Drug Administration more recently approved its use as an antidote for ethylene glycol and methanol poisoning, ethanol still plays a significant role in the therapeutic approach to toxicity from these substances. Although fomepizole has been shown to be efficacious and safe,[7] in some situations ethanol may be more readily available than fomepizole. Given the need to inhibit rapidly the formation of the toxic metabolites of ethylene glycol and methanol, initial use of ethanol may be necessary until fomepizole is available.

Initiation of ethanol therapy often occurs in the emergency department or before transfer of the patient from another facility. Ethanol therapy generally mandates an intensive care unit admission regardless of the patient's clinical status. The critical care medicine physician should be familiar with many issues related to the efficacious and safe use of ethanol in this clinical situation. Ethylene glycol and methanol poisoning are discussed extensively in Chapters 83 and 86. The clinical pharmacology of fomepizole is addressed in Chapter 152.

HISTORY

In 1946, Roe[8] described anecdotal experiences with the use of ethanol to treat methanol poisoning. Animal studies regarding use of ethanol in the treatment of methanol and ethylene glycol poisoning date back to the early 1950s. In 1950, Bartlett[4] described the use of ethanol to inhibit the oxidation of methanol in a rat model. Peterson[9] and vonWartberg and colleagues[10] reported use of ethanol to inhibit metabolism of ethylene glycol by hepatic alcohol dehydrogenase. In 1965, Wacker and colleagues[6] published case reports in which ethanol was used to treat two ethylene glycol–poisoned men. Along with extensive supportive care, including serum alkalinization and peritoneal dialysis, these patients received intravenous ethanol to treat ethylene glycol toxicity successfully. The literature contains numerous other reports of the use of ethanol to treat ethylene glycol and methanol toxicity.[3,5] Between 1983 and 2000, the American Association of Poison Control Centers reported the use of ethanol in 8821 patients.[11] The World Health Organization's International Programme on Chemical Safety and the American Academy of Clinical Toxicology have discussed the role of ethanol in the treatment of ethylene glycol and methanol poisoning.[12,13]

PROPERTIES

Ethanol (C_2H_5OH) is a colorless, hygroscopic, volatile two-carbon alcohol (Fig. 151-1) with a molecular weight of 46.07. Ethanol is synthesized from carbohydrates by the enzyme zymase, found in yeast cells. Ethanol also can be formed through the hydration of ethylene or through the hydration of acetylene to form acetaldehyde, which is hydrogenated further to form ethanol.[14]

PHARMACODYNAMICS

Figure 151-1 provides the metabolic pathways for ethanol, ethylene glycol, and methanol. The figure shows that alcohol dehydrogenase is the principal enzyme that catalyzes the initial step of metabolism for each of these substances. The toxicities of ethylene glycol and methanol are due primarily to the toxic metabolites that are formed. In the presence of sufficient concentrations of ethanol, the metabolism of ethylene glycol and methanol to these toxic metabolites is inhibited because of competitive inhibition of alcohol dehydrogenase. When compared with methanol, ethanol has approximately 20 times the affinity for alcohol dehydrogenase. Ethylene glycol has an even weaker affinity for alcohol dehydrogenase than methanol, and its metabolism can be blocked through administration of ethanol. In clinical practice, ethanol concentrations of 100 to 150 mg/dL (21.7 to 32.5 mmol/L) have been targeted for therapeutic effect. This ethanol concentration range did not result from dose-response studies. It is an empirical range that dates back to early investigations of ethanol as an antidote.[15]

The most prominent clinical effect of ethanol is central nervous system excitation and inebriation, followed by depression. The mechanism of ethanol's effect on the central nervous system is a matter of some debate. Being a lipophilic solvent, ethanol increases the fluidity of cellular membranes. It is not known, however, if this alteration in membrane fluidity is related to the observed effects at clinically relevant concentrations. Ethanol also modulates the activities of multiple ion channels in the central nervous system. The specific channels affected and the ethanol concentrations necessary to do so are provided in Table 151-1.

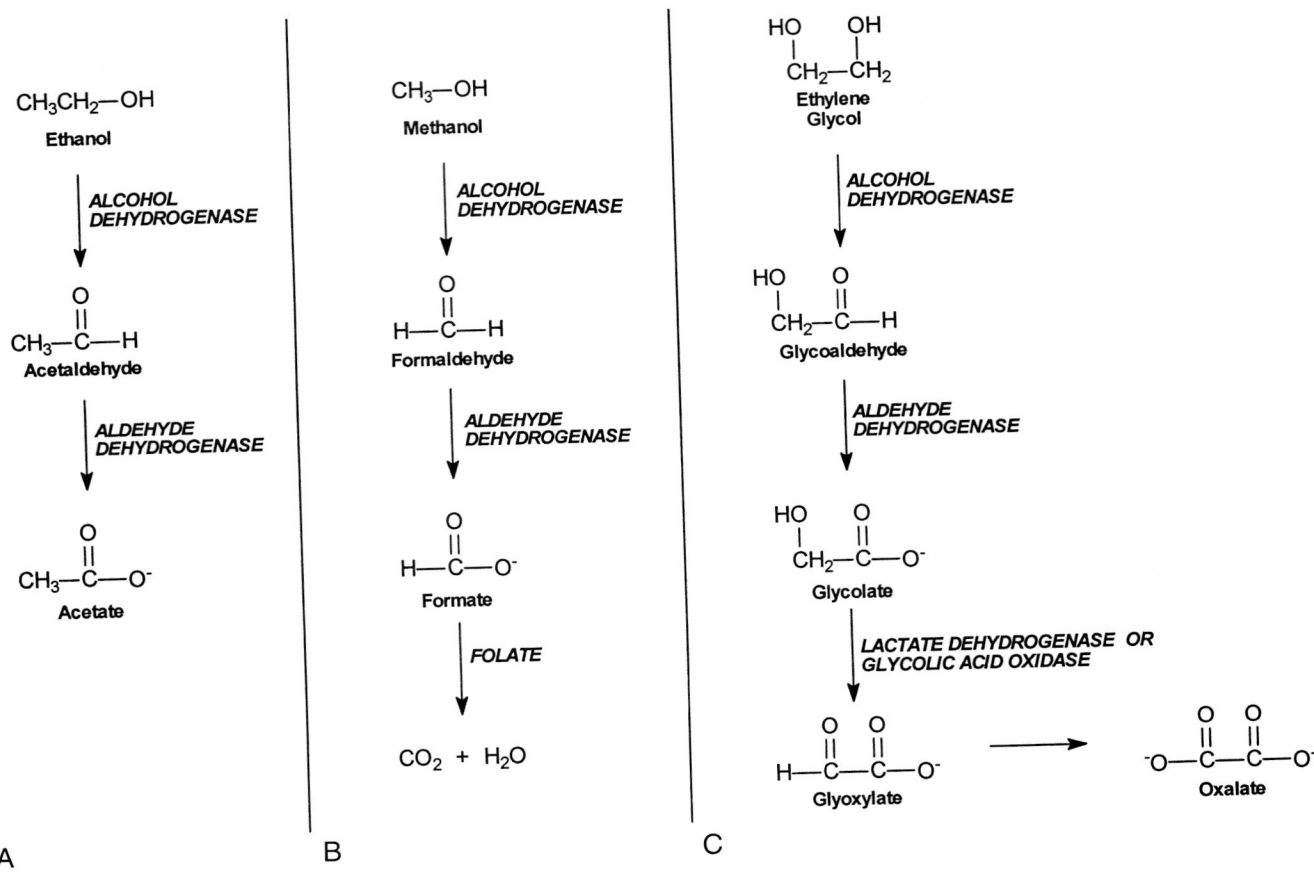

FIGURE 151-1

Metabolic pathways for ethanol (**A**), methanol (**B**) and ethylene glycol (**C**).

TABLE 151-1 Ion Channels Functionally Altered by Ethanol

CHANNEL	EFFECT	ETHANOL CONCENTRATION (mM)*
Sodium (voltage-gated)	Inhibited	$\geqslant 100$
Potassium (voltage-gated)	Facilitated	50–100
Calcium (voltage-gated)	Inhibited	$\geqslant 50$
Calcium (glutamate-activated)	Inhibited	20–50
Chloride (GABA-gated)	Facilitated	10–60
Chloride (glycine-gated)	Facilitated	10–50
Sodium-potassium (5-HT₃-gated)	Facilitated	10–50

*100 mM ethanol is 460 mg/dL.
GABA, γ-aminobutyric acid; 5-HT₃, 5-hydroxytryptamine.
From Deitrich RA, Palmer JD: Alcohol. In Brody TM, Lerner J, Minneman KP (eds): Human Pharmacology: Molecular to Clinical, 3rd ed. St. Louis, Mosby, 1998.

PHARMACOKINETICS

Absorption

Ethanol is absorbed from the stomach and the small intestine.[15] In two studies in healthy volunteers, peak absorption of ethanol was shown to occur at 104 minutes after a 700-mg/kg ethanol dose in men and 84 minutes after administration of the same dose in women.[16,17] Large amounts of ethanol are absorbed directly from the stomach after an oral dose.[16] Many factors, including gender, presence of food, gastritis, presence of other medications, and ethanol concentration, may alter the absorption kinetics of ethanol. Cobaugh and colleagues[18] showed that women achieve higher serum concentrations of ethanol than men after oral administration of equivalent doses. These authors attributed this difference to increased levels of gastric alcohol dehydrogenase in men.[18] A study comparing breath alcohol concentrations after administration of 690 mg/kg of ethanol after either a large meal or a 6-hour fast showed that ethanol absorption was delayed by the presence of food in the stomach.[19] Roine and coworkers[20] studied the effect of ethanol concentration on absorption and determined that higher concentration ethanol products were absorbed more slowly. In two different phases, 300 mg/kg of ethanol was administered as either a 4% solution or a 40% solution after a meal. Higher peak ethanol concentrations were observed after administration of the 4% solution. This phenomenon was not observed when different concentrations of ethanol were administered in a fasting state.[20]

Distribution

Ethanol is well distributed to tissue sites; its volume of distribution is approximately 0.6 L/kg. Differences in volume of distribution may exist between men and women. Using a linear regression model, Cowan and associates[21] calculated a mean volume of distribution of 0.64 L/kg in women and 0.72 L/kg in men.[21]

Metabolism

The primary route of ethanol metabolism is via hepatic alcohol dehydrogenase (see Fig. 151-1). Debate continues about the extent of gastric first-pass metabolism of ethanol in humans. Caballeria and associates[22] compared areas under the curve after intravenous, oral, and duodenal administration of ethanol, reporting that after oral administration, the area under the curve was 17% of that observed after intravenous and duodenal administration. The authors attributed this difference to gastric alcohol dehydrogenase activity. Cobaugh and colleagues[18] reported similar findings in a comparison of men and women. Ammon and colleagues[23] did not observe significant first-pass metabolism of ethanol in men or women, however, when intravenous and oral ethanol administration were compared with intravenous and duodenal administration. It is thought that in chronic alcoholics a small amount of ethanol also is metabolized via a microsomal ethanol oxidizing system.

Elimination

In nonalcoholics presenting to the emergency department, ethanol has been shown to be eliminated at a *mean* rate of approximately 20 mg/dL/hr, although there is considerable interindividual variation.[24,25] In alcoholics, ethanol often is metabolized more rapidly. Winek and Murphy[26] reported that in nondrinkers the elimination rate was 12 ± 4 mg/dL/hr (2.6 ± 0.9 mmol/L/hr); in social drinkers, it was 15 ± 4 mg/dL/hr (3.3 ± 0.9 mmol/L/hr); and in alcoholics, it was 30 ± 9 mg/dL/hr (6.4 ± 2 mmol/L/hr). Similarly, ethanol elimination rates may be decreased in ethanol-naive patients. Women tend to eliminate ethanol more rapidly than men.[23,27] Although ethanol elimination frequently is described as a zero-order process, some authors have concluded that it undergoes Michaelis-Menton kinetics with dose-dependent elimination occurring at higher ethanol concentrations.[28]

LABORATORY STUDIES

Ethanol can be measured quantitatively by several methods, typically from blood, breath, saliva, and urine. The most frequently used methods involve blood and breath. During therapeutic use of ethanol for ethylene glycol and methanol poisoning, frequent monitoring (every 1 to 2 hours) of blood ethanol concentrations is mandatory to ensure that concentrations are maintained at greater than 100 mg/dL (>21.7 mmol/L) and to avoid development of toxicity. There have been reports in the literature regarding use of saliva to measure ethanol.[29] Determination of ethanol in urine specimens usually is qualitative rather than quantitative.

PRECAUTIONS

During intravenous administration of ethanol, efforts should be made to avoid local vein irritation, phlebitis, and extravasation. Maximal concentrations of ethanol of 10% generally are recommended. The loading dose of ethanol should be administered over 30 to 60 minutes. Although less concentrated solutions, such as 5%, may be helpful in decreasing the risk of vein irritation, fluid overload can occur, given the large volume required. When oral ethanol is used, it generally is recommended that solutions should be diluted to 20% and administered over 30 minutes to decrease the risk of gastritis and vomiting. This is particularly important in children and other ethanol-naive patients.

ADVERSE EFFECTS

This discussion focuses on the adverse effects associated with acute exposure to ethanol rather than on the numerous adverse effects reported with chronic abuse of ethanol and alcoholism (the latter is discussed in Chapter 14). Blood ethanol concentrations of 100 mg/dL (21.7 mmol/L) result in inebriation in many patients. The most concerning sequelae of inebriation are decreased level of consciousness, loss of airway control, and respiratory compromise. These patients may require intubation, airway management, and assisted respiration. Hypoglycemia also is a life-threatening effect of ethanol, with young children being at greatest risk. Although there are many anecdotal case reports describing hypoglycemia after exposure to ethanol,[30–32] retrospective medical record reviews and case series have questioned its incidence.[33–35] Sporer and associates[33] measured blood glucose in 378 nondiabetic patients with a blood ethanol greater than 100 mg/dL (>21.7 mmol/L) and reported that 1% of patients had a blood glucose concentration less than 50 mg/dL (<2.7 mmol/L), and 4% had a blood glucose less than 67 mg/dL (<3.7 mmol/L). Frequent monitoring of blood glucose measurements is beneficial in preventing and recognizing hypoglycemia. For profound hypoglycemia, 50% dextrose should be administered. Supplemental infusions of 5% dextrose may be helpful in decreasing the risk of hypoglycemia.

Gastritis, nausea, and vomiting after exposure to ethanol have been well described. There is an increased risk for vomiting after oral administration of therapeutic amounts of ethanol in children and other ethanol-naive patients, given the high concentrations and frequent doses administered. This risk can be complicated further by concurrent decreases in level of consciousness and the potential for development of aspiration pneumonitis. If vomiting occurs after oral ethanol doses, the treatment should be converted to intravenous ethanol or, preferably, fomepizole. If intravenous ethanol and fomepizole are not available, nonsedating antiemetics, such as ondansetron, should be administered, and a nasogastric tube should be inserted for ethanol administration. Lactic acidosis has been reported after exposure to ethanol.[36] It is frequently difficult to attribute the lactic acidosis to ethanol alone, however, given other potential causes in these patients. In the setting of ethylene glycol and methanol poisoning, it is practically impossible to differentiate ethanol-induced lactic acidosis from the lactic acidosis known to occur with these poisons. Allergic reactions, described as anaphylactoid, have been described after ethanol administration.[37]

ADMINISTRATION

To reach a serum concentration of 100 mg/dL (21.7 mmol/L), loading doses of 600 mg/kg (13 mmol/kg or 6 mL/kg of ethyl alcohol [EtOH] 10%) have been recommended by McCoy and Peterson and others based on pharmacokinetic calculations.[38–40] These authors also recommended maintenance doses of 109 mg/kg/hr (2.4 mmol/kg/hr or 1.1 mL/kg/hr of EtOH 10%) and doses during hemodialysis of 237 mg/kg/hr (5.1 mmol/kg/hr or 2.4 mL/kg/hr of EtOH 10%). Many clinicians use doses greater than 600 mg/kg (>13 mmol/kg or >6 mL/kg of EtOH 10%) to reach blood ethanol concentrations of 100 mg/dL (21.7 mmol/L).[38] A popular but non–evidence-based approach is to administer an ethanol loading dose of 700 mg/kg (15.2 mmol/kg or 7 mL/kg of EtOH 10%) followed by a maintenance dose of 125 to 150 mg/kg/hr (2.7 to 3.3 mmol/kg/hr or 1.25 to 1.5 mL/kg/hr of EtOH 10%) with the hope of achieving ethanol serum concentrations of 100 mg/dL (21.7 mmol/L).[41] If the patient also is being hemodialyzed, the maintenance dose generally is increased to 250 to 275 mg/kg/hr (5.4 to 6 mmol/kg/hr or 2.5 to 2.75 mL/kg/hr of EtOH 10%).

In the original work by Peterson and McCoy and others,[38–40] the authors suggested that equivalent doses of oral and intravenous ethanol could be administered. In two human volunteer studies of the bioavailability of ethanol after oral and intravenous administration in men and women, differences in peak ethanol serum concentrations and time to peak were observed when the routes were compared. In the study in men, intravenous and oral ethanol doses, 700 mg/kg (15.2 mmol/kg or 7 mL/kg of EtOH 10%), were administered in two different phases. A similar method was used in the study in women.[16,17] In men, the peak blood ethanol concentration was 71.3 mg/dL (15.5 mmol/L) after oral administration and 103.6 mg/dL (22.5 mmol/L) after intravenous administration. In women, the peak blood concentration was 98.1 mg/dL (21.3 mmol/L) after oral administration and 146.9 mg/dL (31.9 mmol/L) after intravenous administration. Although blood ethanol concentrations of less than 100 mg/dL (<21.7 mmol/L) may inhibit alcohol dehydrogenase effectively, these differences need to be considered especially in men patients. In these studies, peak blood ethanol concentrations were achieved immediately after intravenous administration and delayed well beyond 60 minutes after oral administration. When ethanol is used, intravenous ethanol is preferred over oral ethanol. In the absence of fomepizole or intravenous ethanol, oral ethanol therapy should be initiated promptly. In the absence of pharmaceutical-grade ethanol, other alcohol sources, such as vodka, can be used to prepare an oral ethanol solution; 80 proof alcohol provides a 40% ethanol solution. An example of calculations used to determine a loading dose of ethanol is presented in the accompanying box.

 Calculation of Ethanol Loading Dose and 10% Solution Preparation

Commercially available 10% ethanol solutions provide 100 mg/mL of ethanol. If a commercially available solution is not available, the following formula can be used to prepare a 10% ethanol solution using 100% ethanol.

Loading Dose

Patient weight = 70 kg
EtOH dose = 0.7 g/kg
Total dose = 70 kg × 0.7 g/kg = 49 g

10% Solution Preparation Using 100% EtOH

EtOH specific gravity = 0.8 g/mL
1 g EtOH = 1.25 mL
49 g × 1.25 mL/g = 61.3 mL

For an EtOH 10% solution, dilute 61.3 mL of EtOH 100% to 613 mL with 5% dextrose. This provides 61.3 mL/613 mL (10% V/V).

EtOH, ethyl alcohol.

REFERENCES

1. Burkhart KK, Kulig KW: The other alcohols: Methanol, ethylene glycol and isopropanol. Emerg Med Clin North Am 8:913–928, 1990.
2. Litovitz T: The alcohols: Ethanol, methanol, isopropanol, ethylene glycol. Pediatr Clin North Am 33:311–323, 1986.
3. Agner K, Hook O, vonPorat B: The treatment of methanol poisoning with ethanol. Q J Stud Alcohol 9:512–522, 1949.
4. Bartlett GR: Inhibition of methanol oxidation by ethanol in the rat. Am J Physiol 163:619–621, 1950.
5. Kowalczyk M, Halvorsen S, Ovrebo S, et al: Ethanol treatment in ethylene glycol poisoned patients. Vet Hum Toxicol 40:225–228, 1998.
6. Wacker WE, Haynes H, Druyan R, et al: Treatment of ethylene glycol poisoning with ethyl alcohol. JAMA 194:173–175, 1965.
7. Brent J, McMartin K, Phillips S, et al: Fomepizole for the treatment of methanol poisoning. N Engl J Med 344:424–429, 2000.
8. Roe O: Methanol poisoning: Its clinical course, pathogenesis and treatment. Acta Med Scand 126:1–253, 1946.
9. Peterson DI: Experimental treatment of ethylene glycol poisoning. JAMA 186:955–957, 1963.
10. vonWartberg JP, Bethune JL, Vallee BL: Human liver alcohol dehydrogenase: Kinetic and physiochemical. Biochemistry 3:1775–1782, 1964.
11. Litovitz TL, Klein-Schwartz W, White S, et al: 2000 annual report of the American Association of Poison Control Centers Toxic Exposure Surveillance System. Am J Emerg Med 19:337–394, 2001.
12. Jacobsen D, McMartin KE: Antidotes for methanol and ethylene glycol poisoning. J Toxicol Clin Toxicol 35:127–143, 1997.
13. Barceloux DG, Krenzelok EP, Olson K, et al: American Academy of Clinical Toxicology Practice guidelines on the treatment of ethylene glycol poisoning. J Toxicol Clin Toxicol 37:537–560, 1999.
14. Swinyard EA, Lowenthal W: Pharmaceutical necessities. In Osol A, Chase GD, Gennaro AR, et al (eds): Remington's Pharmaceutical Sciences. Easton, PA, Mack, 1980, pp 1225–1267.
15. Palatnick W, Redman LW, Sitar DS, et al: Methanol half-life during ethanol administration: Implications for management of methanol poisoning. Ann Emerg Med 26:202–207, 1995.
16. Watkins RL, Adler EV: The effect of food on alcohol absorption and elimination patterns. J Forensic Sci 38:285–291, 1993.
17. Cobaugh DJ, Gibbs M, Shapiro D, et al: A comparison of the bioavailabilities of oral and intravenous ethanol in healthy male volunteers. Acad Emerg Med 6:984–988, 1999.
18. Cobaugh DJ, Goldberg JW, Wax PM, et al: A comparison of the bioavailabilities of oral and intravenous ethanol in healthy female volunteers (Abstract). J Toxicol Clin Toxicol 36:452, 1998.

19. Frezza M, DiPadova C, Pozzato G, et al: High blood alcohol levels in women: The role of decreased gastric alcohol dehydrogenase activity and first-pass metabolism. N Engl J Med 322:95–99, 1990.
20. Roine RP, Gentry RT, Lim RT, et al: Effect of concentration of ingested ethanol on blood alcohol levels. Alcohol Clin Exp Res 15:734–738, 1991.
21. Cowan JM, Weathermon A, McCutcheon JR, et al: Determination of volume of distribution for ethanol in male and female subjects. J Anal Toxicol 20:287–290, 1996.
22. Caballeria J, Frezza M, Hernandez-Munoz R, et al: Gastric origin of the first-pass metabolism of ethanol in humans: Effect of gastrectomy. Gastroenterology 97:1205–1209, 1989.
23. Ammon E, Schafer C, Hofmann U, et al: Disposition and first-pass metabolism of ethanol in humans: Is it gastric or hepatic and does it depend on gender? Clin Pharmacol Ther 59:503–513, 1996.
24. Brennan DF, Betzelos S, Reed R, et al: Ethanol elimination rates in an ED population. Am J Emerg Med 13:276–280, 1995.
25. Gershman H, Steeper J: Rate of clearance of ethanol from the blood of intoxicated patients in the emergency department. J Emerg Med 9:307–311, 1991.
26. Winek CL, Murphy KL: The rate and kinetic order of ethanol elimination. Forensic Sci Int 25:159–166, 1984.
27. Mishra L, Savitri S, Potter JJ, et al: More rapid elimination of alcohol in women as compared to their male siblings. Alcohol Clin Exp Res 13:752–754, 1989.
28. Rango RE, Kreeft JH, Sitar DS: Ethanol dose-dependent elimination: Michaelis-Menten v classical kinetic analysis. Br J Clin Pharmacol 12:667–673, 1981.
29. Christopher TA, Zeccardi JA: Evaluation of the QED saliva alcohol test: A new, rapid, accurate device for measuring ethanol in saliva. Ann Emerg Med 21:1135–1137, 1992.
30. Gillam DM, Harper JR: Hypoglycaemia after alcohol ingestion. Lancet 14:829–830, 1973.
31. Moss MH: Alcohol-induced hypoglycemia and coma caused by alcohol sponging. Pediatrics 46:445–446, 1970.
32. Salaspuro MP, Pikkarainen P, Lindros K: Ethanol-induced hypoglycemia in man: Its suppression by the alcohol dehydrogenase inhibitor 4-methylpyrazole. Eur J Clin Invest 7:487–490, 1977.
33. Sporer KA, Ernst AA, Conte R, et al: The incidence of ethanol-induced hypoglycemia. Am J Emerg Med 10:403–405, 1992.
34. Sucov A, Woolard RH: Ethanol-associated hypoglycemia is uncommon. Acad Emerg Med 2:185–189, 1995.
35. Ernst AA, Jones K, Nick TG, et al: Ethanol ingestion and related hypoglycemia in a pediatric and adolescent emergency department population. Acad Emerg Med 3:46–49, 1996.
36. MacDonald L, Kruse J, Levy DB: Lactic acidosis and acute ethanol intoxication. Am J Emerg Med 12:32–35, 1994.
37. Kelso JM, Keating MU, Squillace DL, et al: Anaphylactoid reaction to ethanol. Ann Allergy 64:452–454, 1990.
38. McCoy HG, Cipolle RJ, Ehlers SM, et al: Severe methanol poisoning: Application of a pharmacokinetic model for ethanol therapy and hemodialysis. Am J Med 67:804–807, 1979.
39. Peterson CD: Oral ethanol doses in patients with methanol poisoning. Am J Hosp Pharm 38:1024–1027, 1981.
40. Peterson CD, Collins AJ, Himes JM, et al: Ethylene glycol poisoning: Pharmacokinetics during therapy with ethanol and hemodialysis. N Engl J Med 304:21–23, 1981.
41. Gurell M, Cobaugh D: Utilization guidelines for ethanol as an antidote: A survey of toxicologists (Abstract). J Toxicol Clin Toxicol 34:634, 1996.

CHAPTER 152

Fomepizole

Kenneth McMartin

Fomepizole is the generic drug name for the chemical 4-methyl-1H-pyrazole (4-MP). It is a potent inhibitor of alcohol dehydrogenase (ADH) activity with demonstrated efficacy in vivo against the conversion of methanol and ethylene glycol to their toxic metabolites. Because of its high safety profile and ease of use, fomepizole is rapidly replacing ethanol as the standard of care for the inhibitory therapy of methanol and ethylene glycol poisoning.[1] Fomepizole currently is marketed for these indications in the United States as a parenteral solution under the trade name Antizol (Orphan Medical, Inc, Minnetonka, MN). Fomepizole also may be useful in the therapy of other similar intoxications, such as glycol ethers, diethylene glycol, and propylene glycol.[2–4]

HISTORY

Fomepizole was developed in Sweden in the late 1960s as one of a series of ADH inhibitors, with the potential goal of treating alcohol-related pathologies. Blomstrand and Theorell[5] first used fomepizole to inhibit ethanol metabolism in humans in vivo and to reduce the ethanol-induced increase in the lactate-to-pyruvate ratio. These changes reversed various metabolic effects of ethanol, such as hypoglycemia and inhibition of fatty acid oxidation.[6,7] Fomepizole also was shown in humans to block the accumulation of acetaldehyde from ethanol ingestion after the use of aldehyde dehydrogenase inhibitors or from genetic polymorphism (reduced aldehyde dehydrogenase activity).[8,9]

In a landmark 1969 paper by Li and the Nobelist Theorell,[10] fomepizole was shown to be a powerful competitive inhibitor of human liver ADH in vitro. These authors made the insightful suggestion that "whether or not the pyrazole derivatives can serve as clinically useful agents (for poisoning by methanol and ethylene glycol) remains to be examined experimentally." Fomepizole first was shown experimentally in 1975 to be useful in the treatment of lethal doses of methanol in monkeys by McMartin and coworkers.[11] Fomepizole at 50 mg/kg rapidly reversed the formate accumulation and the severe metabolic acidosis, without any dialysis.[12] Subsequent studies showed that lower doses of fomepizole were effective in returning formate levels to background within several hours.[13] The minimal plasma concentration of fomepizole to prevent any accumulation of formate was determined to be 10 μM. An initial dose of 15 mg/kg, followed by supplemental doses of 5 to 10 mg/kg every 12 hours, seemed to be sufficient to reverse and prevent methanol toxicity. Fomepizole was also shown to reverse ocular signs associated

with methanol toxicity in monkeys, such as the decreased b wave of the electroretinogram.[14]

Fomepizole was first shown to be effective at reversing the toxicity of lethal doses of ethylene glycol in monkeys in 1977.[15] Fomepizole at 50 mg/kg reversed the acidosis and the accumulation of glycolate. Similar results were obtained in rats and dogs.[16,17] In the dog study, fomepizole was compared with ethanol. Although both inhibitors displayed similar efficacy against the metabolism of ethylene glycol, fomepizole was shown to be superior in clinical usefulness because of its lesser degree of central nervous system depression and because ethanol-treated animals needed intravenous fluid therapy to maintain hydration. Fomepizole subsequently has been confirmed to be therapeutically effective as a veterinary antidote.[18]

Fomepizole officially was designated as an orphan drug in the United States in 1988 and has been an excellent example for that developmental strategy. Phase I clinical studies of the safety and metabolism of fomepizole in human volunteers were conducted from 1986 through 1988, and the results have been published.[19–22] Concurrently, fomepizole was being used in France in the treatment of ethylene glycol poisoning, with the first case reports appearing in 1987 and 1988.[23,24] The first case report of the use of fomepizole in methanol poisoning appeared in 1997.[25] Subsequent to these initial studies, a multicenter prospective clinical trial (phases II/III) was conducted in the United States. The results of the ethylene glycol arm of the META (Methylpyrazole for Toxic Alcohols) trial were published in 1999,[26] and the results for the methanol arm appeared in 2001.[27] Based on these trials, fomepizole was approved initially by the U.S. Food and Drug Administration for marketing in the United States for the treatment of ethylene glycol toxicity in late 1997; the added indication for methanol was approved in 2000. In other countries, fomepizole is available under certain conditions or has received marketing approval for methanol or ethylene glycol poisoning or both.

PROPERTIES

Chemical

Fomepizole is the parenteral preparation of the freebase 4-MP, with the formula $C_4H_6N_2$ (Fig. 152-1) and a molecular weight of 82.1. 4-MP also is available chemically as the hydrochloride, with a molecular weight of 118.6. The base form is soluble in water and ethanol.

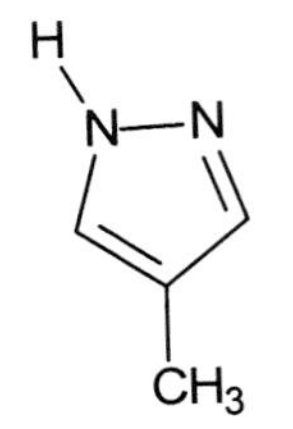

FIGURE 152-1

Chemical structure of fomepizole.

Physical

4-MP base is stable in light and at 4°C. Its melting point is 16°C, and its boiling point is 99°C. Its density is 0.993 g/mL. Light wavelength (λ_{max}) is 219 nm. The parenteral preparation (Antizol) contains 1.5 g per vial and is a slightly yellow liquid that may solidify at room temperature.

PHARMACODYNAMICS

Mechanism of Action

Fomepizole is an inhibitor of ADH that forms a ternary complex with that enzyme and its coenzyme nicotinamide-adenine dinucleotide (oxidized form), competitively inhibiting the enzyme complex formation with alcohols. Among the pyrazole derivatives, fomepizole is one of the most potent, with an inhibitory constant (K_I) versus horse liver ADH less than 0.1 μM.[28] The K_I for fomepizole in vitro with liver ADH from the rat, monkey, and human was reported as 1 μM, 7.5 μM, and 0.2 μM, respectively.[10,29,30] Fomepizole also inhibits the metabolism of methanol by human ADH in vitro.[31] Its initial metabolite, 4-hydroxymethylpyrazole (4-OHMP), is also an inhibitor but is 66-fold less potent, whereas its secondary metabolite, 4-carboxypyrazole (4-CP), has no inhibitory activity. The affinity of fomepizole for ADH is about 500 to 1000 times that of ethanol[10,29]—about 5000 to 10,000 times that of methanol or ethylene glycol.[31] Fomepizole should compete substantially with either methanol or ethylene glycol, reducing their metabolism by ADH.

Because the major route of elimination of most alcohols is by ADH, inhibition of this enzyme in vivo is characterized best by a decreased alcohol elimination rate. In rats, fomepizole doses of less than 40 mg/kg decrease the rate of ethanol elimination by greater than 25%.[32] In monkeys, fomepizole 50 mg/kg inhibits the metabolism of methanol to carbon dioxide by 75%,[11] whereas 20 mg/kg lowers the elimination rate of methanol by 50%,[13] eliminating any formate accumulation. Studies with smaller doses (5 to 15 mg/kg) have shown that the minimal plasma fomepizole concentration necessary to prevent formate accumulation is 10 μM.[13] In dogs, a loading dose of fomepizole of 20 mg/kg at 3 hours, followed at 24 hours by 15 mg/kg and at 36 hours by 5 mg/kg, increases the area under the concentration curve of the ethylene glycol elimination curve, indicating an inhibition of ethylene glycol metabolism in vivo.[17] Analysis of data from the META trial confirmed that fomepizole inhibits ethylene glycol elimination in humans in vivo.[33]

Other Effects

Acute administration of fomepizole inhibits rat liver cytochrome P-450 activity, especially the isozyme CYP2E1 (which metabolizes ethanol, acetaminophen, and nitrosamines), but at much higher doses (100 mg/kg) than necessary to inhibit ADH.[34,35] The K_I for this inhibition is about 0.5 to 1 mM, or about 1000 times higher than that for liver ADH. In vivo, fomepizole inhibits the clearance of cytochrome P-450–related substrates, such as antipyrine.[36] The ability to inhibit certain cytochrome P-450 isozymes may have therapeutic usefulness, including action as an adjunct therapy in the treatment of acetaminophen overdose.[37,38] Repeated administration of fomepizole over several days also is known to induce hepatic cytochrome P-450 activity, including total levels and activity of specific isozymes.[39] As such, fomepizole can increase the oxidation of several different classes of drugs and maybe its own metabolism.[21,40] The initial conversion to 4-OHMP may be catalyzed by cytochrome P-450 because it is known that fomepizole binds to cytochrome P-450 to produce a type II substrate binding spectrum.[41] Other actions of fomepizole that may be important include its abilities to scavenge hydroxyl free radicals,[42] to block the disulfiram-ethanol reaction,[8] and to protect against the gastric lesions induced by high concentrations of ethanol, probably due to an ability of fomepizole to decrease lipid peroxidation.[43]

PHARMACOKINETICS

Absorption, Distribution, Metabolism, and Elimination

Given orally, fomepizole is absorbed rapidly, producing peak plasma levels at 2 hours in rats given doses of 5 to 20 mg/kg.[44] Similarly, in humans ingesting doses of 10 to 100 mg/kg, the peak plasma levels of fomepizole are reached within 2 hours.[20] In humans given equivalent doses of fomepizole intravenously or orally, the bioavailability of fomepizole is essentially 1, indicating complete absorption. These results suggest that although fomepizole is marketed as an intravenous preparation, it would be equally effective if given orally.

Fomepizole is distributed rapidly to total body water; the volume of distribution in human volunteers given fomepizole intravenously was 0.74 L/kg at 5 mg/kg body weight and 0.59 L/kg at 7 mg/kg.[22] When identical intravenous and oral doses are administered to human volunteers, the plasma fomepizole elimination curves are identical after 30 minutes, indicating its rapid absorption and distribution. In dogs, the plasma protein binding of fomepizole is reported as low.[45]

The renal clearance of unchanged fomepizole is low, about 1 mL/min in human volunteers.[20] Total urinary excretion of fomepizole is only about 3% of the dose in humans and only 1% at similar doses in rats.[20,44] Fomepizole is eliminated primarily by metabolism.

Fomepizole is metabolized primarily by oxidation, presumably by cytochrome P-450, as noted earlier, to 4-OHMP and 4-CP. These metabolites represent greater than 70% of the dose that is excreted in the urine of mice and rats within 24 hours.[46,47] A minor metabolic pathway seems to be formation of an N-glucuronide conjugate of fomepizole itself.[46] In monkeys, levels of 4-OHMP in the plasma represent about 10% of the 4-MP levels; however, no indication of the total mass of 4-OHMP excretion was reported.[13] In humans, 4-CP is the major urinary metabolite, representing more than 50% of the total dose in volunteer studies.[22]

Elimination Kinetics

At doses in the therapeutic range, fomepizole is eliminated by saturation kinetics. Mayersohn and colleagues[45] showed that intravenous doses of 1 and 10 mg/kg in dogs produce a downward curve of the log-linear plot and an area under the concentration curve ratio significantly greater than the dose ratio, two indications of saturation kinetics. The apparent zero-order elimination rate at 10 mg/kg is 5 μmol/L/hr, and an estimate of the Michaelis constant (K_m) is 6 μM. In rats, oral doses of 10 to 20 mg/kg produce similar elimination kinetics, with a zero-order rate of about 10 μmol/L/hr.[44] In human volunteers, oral doses of 10 to 20 mg/kg show definite saturation kinetics, with an elimination rate of about 4 to 5 μmol/L/hr.[20] At higher doses of 50 mg/kg and 100 mg/kg, the elimination kinetics also seems to be nonlinear, although the plasma levels were not followed long enough to confirm this. The elimination rates are increased to 15 μmol/L/hr at the highest dose, possibly because a secondary elimination pathway becomes important. Elimination of fomepizole after intravenous dosing in humans also is saturable, with a zero-order rate of 4.2 μmol/L/hr at 5 mg/kg.[22] The apparent K_m for fomepizole elimination is 2.4 to 2.5 μM with a maximal velocity of 4.2 to 6.5 μmol/kg/hr, showing that elimination of therapeutic doses (producing blood fomepizole levels >10 μM) always should follow saturation or nonlinear kinetics. The kinetics in treated patients seems to be similar to that in human volunteers. Vu and associates[48] reported nonlinear elimination kinetics after intravenous doses of 16 mg/kg and 8 mg/kg in one case, with a zero-order elimination rate of 7 μmol/kg/hr.

The alcohols seem to decrease the elimination of fomepizole, suggesting a mutual inhibition of metabolism. In rats, blood ethanol levels in the range of 350 mg/dL (76 mmol/L) decreased the rate of elimination of fomepizole by 50%.[44] In human volunteers, blood ethanol levels of 50 to 150 mg/dL (11 to 33 mmol/L) also decreased the elimination by about 50%.[22] Ethanol does not alter the volume of distribution of fomepizole or the urinary excretion of unchanged fomepizole; rather, it decreases the urinary excretion of 4-CP.[22] These data indicate that ethanol inhibits some step in the conversion of fomepizole to 4-CP. In monkeys, high doses of methanol (2 to 3 g/kg) decrease the rate of fomepizole elimination by 25%.[13] In patients exposed to ethanol and methanol (possibly ethylene glycol, but not studied), one could expect the rate of fomepizole elimination to be slower than that reported in human volunteers because of this interaction.

Dialysis Kinetics

Studies in pigs showed that fomepizole is removed by hemodialysis, with a dialysance of 56 mL/min, similar to that of urea (51 mL/min) in the same study.[49] About 20% of the dose is removed during a 4-hour dialysis. Similar dialysis clearance rates have been reported in two ethylene glycol–poisoned patients (52 mL/min and 80 mL/min), with higher rates in two other patients (117 mL/min and 127 mL/min).[50,51] These studies show the need to replace the fomepizole that is lost when hemodialysis is carried out in fomepizole-treated patients (see subsequent dosing guidelines).

SPECIAL POPULATIONS

Pediatric Patients

In the United States, fomepizole has not been approved officially for use in children, and no controlled studies have been conducted. No matter what the age of the patient, however, the use of fomepizole obviates the need for intravenous ethanol therapy with its various problems. In addition to the problems of ethanol in poisoned adults (discussed elsewhere), the adverse effects of ethanol in children make it dangerous and difficult to use (added central nervous system depression, hypothermia, hypoglycemia). Fomepizole has been used in several cases of pediatric poisoning, with apparently excellent results. In two cases of ethylene glycol ingestion and one of methanol ingestion (in an 8-month-old infant), fomepizole was well tolerated and useful therapeutically.[52–54]

Pregnant Patients

Fomepizole is considered a U.S. Food and Drug Administration class C drug, meaning that its effects on reproduction and development have not been determined adequately in animal studies. Fomepizole should be used with care in pregnant or breast-feeding women, considering the risks and benefits of use and nonuse. Also, one must consider that the alternative, ethanol, is a known teratogen. Although fetal alcohol syndrome generally is associated with long-term ethanol use (not likely in methanol or ethylene glycol therapy), short-term use of ethanol at a crucial period of organogenesis in gestation is controversial.

CONTRAINDICATIONS

Fomepizole should not be administered to patients with known hypersensitivity reactions to pyrazole compounds.

PRECAUTIONS

Fomepizole must be administered intravenously as a properly diluted formulation (see later) to avoid producing venous irritation. It should be administered as an intravenous infusion over 30 minutes to be able to monitor for anaphylactic reactions. Animal studies indicate that acute fomepizole inhibits and repeated fomepizole (similar to the recommended treatment protocol) induces cytochrome P-450, including specific isozymes.[34,35,39,40] Because fomepizole seems to be metabolized by cytochrome P-450,[41] other inhibitors of this enzyme may interact with fomepizole metabolism. Physicians need to be aware of possible drug interactions due to fomepizole.

ADVERSE EFFECTS

The acute median lethal dose for fomepizole in rodents is 310 mg/kg (intravenous) and 500 to 650 mg/kg (oral).[55] The subacute oral toxicity of fomepizole has been studied in rats (100 mg/kg for 3 weeks, then 200 mg/kg for the fourth week) and monkeys (100 mg/kg for 5 weeks, then 200 mg/kg for the sixth week).[55,56] There is no indication of toxicity in rats or monkeys in terms of clinical signs, clinical chemical measures, or pathology. The plasma fomepizole concentrations in the latter study reached 2000 μM in week 6. No visual effects are noted in monkeys treated with fomepizole at 100 mg/kg for 9 days.[56] After a 12-week drinking water exposure in rats, no abnormal liver histology was noted, with plasma fomepizole levels at 85 μM (in the therapeutic range).[57] At high doses of 400 mg/kg in mice, central nervous system depression is observed.[58]

In the human studies done in the 1970s and 1980s, 10 subjects were given oral doses of fomepizole equal to or less than 10 mg/kg,[5,7] and 54 subjects were given intravenous doses of fomepizole of 7 mg/kg.[6,8,9,59,60] Other than irritation of the peripheral vein in the intravenous studies, no adverse effects were reported.

In randomized, blinded, placebo-controlled human volunteer studies, 31 subjects received single oral or intravenous doses in the therapeutic range, with no significant adverse effects reported.[19,21,22] During the intravenous administration, about half of the subjects reported an abnormal smell or taste sensation (fomepizole per se emits an odor). In 2 of 6 initial intravenous subjects, when the preparation was not diluted suitably and was given as a bolus over 5 minutes, venous irritation and transient phlebosclerosis were noted near the site of injection. Four of 6 subjects also reported a transient lightheadedness, probably due to high plasma fomepizole concentrations during the brief distribution phase after the bolus injection. At high single oral doses (50 mg/kg and 100 mg/kg), 6 of 7 subjects experienced dizziness and nausea, with objective signs of central nervous system depression at 100 mg/kg.[19] Despite these effects, vital signs were not affected, and clinical chemical and hematologic parameters remained within normal limits in all subjects. In repeated-dose studies, 15 subjects were treated with oral fomepizole (loading doses of 10 to 15 mg/kg, maintenance doses of 3 to 10 mg/kg every 12 hours for 5 days).[21] Mildly intense subjective side effects such as nausea, headache, and dizziness were reported, but with a similar frequency in treated subjects as in placebos. No changes in vital signs were noted in any subject or in most laboratory parameters. In 40% of the subjects in the two lower dose groups, there was a slight transient increase in either serum ALT or AST activity. This mild increase in transaminases resolved by the end of the study and was not dose related because no subject in the high-dose group was affected.

In the META trial, adverse effects of fomepizole have been infrequent and minor.[26,27] Four of 19 patients in the ethylene glycol arm reported effects possibly related to fomepizole, including bradycardia, headache (in two patients) and a seizure after one dose (but not after subsequent dosing). Six of 11 patients in the methanol arm of the trial reported effects possibly related to fomepizole, including phlebitis, dyspepsia, anxiety, agitation (in two patients), transient tachycardia, and a transient rash (only after initial doses).

Two case summaries have been published from the experience with fomepizole use in the treatment of ethylene glycol and methanol poisoning in France.[61,62] Adverse effects in 11 ethylene glycol patients included pain or inflammation at the site of injection (in 2 patients); transient eosinophilia and cutaneous eruption; and, in 14 methanol patients, fever, nausea, headache, and a burning-skin sensation. During the clinical studies, various clinical laboratory parameters remained stable, suggesting that fomepizole is well tolerated in these cases.

ADMINISTRATION

The dosing schedule for fomepizole is designed to maintain therapeutic plasma levels during the necessary treatment course. In contrast to ethanol, no monitoring of plasma fomepizole concentrations is needed to ensure efficacy. Fomepizole is available as a parenteral solution that may solidify on storage.[63] It should be warmed slightly to liquefy and then diluted in at least 100 mL of sterile 0.9% sodium chloride or 5% dextrose solution. Dilution is important to minimize venous irritation during infusion. Diluted solutions remain stable for 24 hours when stored refrigerated or at room temperature.

Dose

The loading dose of fomepizole is 15 mg/kg, followed by 10 mg/kg every 12 hours for four doses and then 15 mg/kg every 12 hours until methanol or ethylene glycol levels have been reduced to less than 20 mg/dL (6.2 mmol/L or 3.2 mmol/L, respectively).[63] All doses should be administered as intravenous infusions over 30 minutes.

Dosing During Hemodialysis

Fomepizole is dialyzed, and its frequency of dosing should be increased during hemodialysis. The current recommendations for the administration of additional doses related to dialysis times are as follows: If dialysis begins more than 6 hours after the last dose of fomepizole, the next scheduled dose should be administered before dialysis.[1] During dialysis, the scheduled dose of fomepizole is administered at 4-hour intervals. At the end of the dialysis period, if 1 to 3 hours have elapsed since the last dose and the end of dialysis, half of the next scheduled dose is administered, and if more than 3 hours have elapsed, the next scheduled dose is administered. After dialysis, the next scheduled dose is administered 12 hours after the last dose (including any during dialysis). This protocol has been validated in the META study.[26,27] Alternatively, it has been recommended to infuse fomepizole at 1.5 mg/kg/hr during dialysis to maintain therapeutic plasma levels of fomepizole.[50]

Route

An oral preparation of fomepizole is not available in the United States but is available in some other countries. As described earlier, phase I studies indicate that oral and intravenous routes of administration have nearly identical elimination kinetics.

REFERENCES

1. Barceloux DG, Krenzelok EP, Olson K, Watson W: American Academy of Clinical Toxicology practice guidelines on the treatment of ethylene glycol poisoning. J Toxicol Clin Toxicol 37:537–560, 1999.
2. Ghanayem BI, Burka LT, Matthews HB: Metabolic basis of ethylene glycol monobutyl ether (2-butoxyethanol) toxicity: Role of alcohol and aldehyde dehydrogenases. J Pharmacol Exp Ther 242:222–231, 1987.
3. Herold DA, Keil K, Bruns DE: Oxidation of polyethylene glycols by alcohol dehydrogenase. Biochem Pharmacol 38:73–76, 1989.
4. Van de Weile B, Rubinstein E, Peacock W, Martin N: Propylene glycol toxicity caused by prolonged infusion of etomidate. J Neurosurg Anesthesiol 7:259–262, 1995.
5. Blomstrand R, Theorell H: Inhibitory effects on ethanol oxidation in man after administration of 4-methylpyrazole. Life Sci 9:631–640, 1970.
6. Salaspuro MP, Pikkarainen P, Lindros K: Ethanol-induced hypoglycemia in man: Its suppression by the alcohol dehydrogenase inhibitor 4-methylpyrazole. Eur J Clin Invest 7:487–490, 1977.
7. Blomstrand R, Kager L: The combustion of triolein-1-14C and its inhibition by alcohol in man. Life Sci 13:113–123, 1973.
8. Lindros KO, Stowell A, Pikkarainen P, Salaspuro M: The disulfiram (Antabuse)-alcohol reaction in male alcoholics: Its efficient management by 4-methylpyrazole. Alcohol Clin Exp Res 5:528–530, 1981.
9. Inoue K, Fukunaga M, Kiriyama T, Komura S: Accumulation of acetaldehyde in alcohol-sensitive Japanese: Relation to ethanol and acetaldehyde oxidizing capacity. Alcohol Clin Exp Res 8:319–322, 1984.
10. Li TK, Theorell H: Human liver alcohol dehydrogenase: Inhibition by pyrazole and pyrazole analogs. Acta Chem Scand 23:892–902, 1969.
11. McMartin KE, Makar AB, Amat GM, et al: Methanol poisoning: 1. The role of formic acid in the development of metabolic acidosis in the monkey and the reversal by 4-methylpyrazole. Biochem Med 13:319–333, 1975.
12. McMartin KE, Martin-Amat G, Makar AB, Tephly TR: Methanol poisoning: Role of formate metabolism in the monkey. In Thurman RG, Williamson JR, Drott H, Chance B (eds): Alcohol and Aldehyde Metabolizing Systems, Vol 2. New York, Academic Press, 1977, pp 429–440.
13. McMartin KE, Hedstrom KG, Tolf BR, et al: Studies on the metabolic interactions between 4-methylpyrazole and methanol using the monkey as an animal model. Arch Biochem Biophys 199:606–614, 1980.
14. Ingemansson SO: Studies on the effect of 4-methylpyrazole on retinal activity in the methanol poisoned monkey by recording the electroretinogram. Acta Ophthalmol Suppl 158:5–24, 1983.
15. Clay KL, Murphy RC: On the metabolic acidosis of ethylene glycol intoxication. Toxicol Appl Pharmacol 39:39–49, 1977.
16. Chou JY, Richardson KE: The effect of pyrazole on ethylene glycol toxicity and metabolism in the rat. Toxicol Appl Pharmacol 43:33–44, 1978.
17. Grauer GF, Thrall MA, Henre BA, Hjelle JJ: Comparison of the effects of ethanol and 4-methylpyrazole on the pharmacokinetics and toxicity of ethylene glycol in the dog. Toxicol Lett 35:307–314, 1987.
18. Dial SM, Thrall MA, Hamar DW: 4-Methylpyrazole as treatment for naturally acquired ethylene glycol intoxication in dogs. J Am Vet Med Assoc 195:73–76, 1989.
19. Jacobsen D, Sebastian S, Blomstrand R, McMartin KE: 4-Methylpyrazole: A controlled study of safety in healthy human subjects after single, ascending doses. Alcohol Clin Exp Res 12:516–522, 1988.
20. Jacobsen D, Barron SK, Sebastian CS, et al: Non-linear kinetics of 4-methylpyrazole in healthy human subjects. Eur J Clin Pharmacol 37:599–604, 1989.
21. Jacobsen D, Sebastian CS, Barron SK, et al: Effects of 4-methylpyrazole, methanol/ethylene glycol antidote, in healthy humans. J Emerg Med 8:455–461, 1990.
22. Jacobsen D, Sebastian CS, Dies DF, et al: Kinetic interactions between 4-methylpyrazole and ethanol in healthy humans. Alcohol Clin Exp Res 20:804–809, 1996.
23. Baud FJ, Bismuth C, Garnier R, et al: 4-Methylpyrazole may be an alternative to ethanol therapy for ethylene glycol intoxication in man. J Toxicol Clin Toxicol 24:463–483, 1987.
24. Baud FJ, Galliot M, Astier A, et al: Treatment of ethylene glycol poisoning with intravenous 4-methylpyrazole. N Engl J Med 319:97–100, 1988.
25. Burns MJ, Graudins A, Aaron CK, et al: Treatment of methanol poisoning with intravenous 4-methylpyrazole. Ann Emerg Med 30:829–832, 1997.
26. Brent J, McMartin K, Phillips S, et al: Fomepizole for the treatment of ethylene glycol poisoning. N Engl J Med 340:832–838, 1999.
27. Brent J, McMartin KE, Phillips S, et al: Fomepizole for the treatment of methanol poisoning. N Engl J Med 444:424–429, 2001.
28. Theorell H, Yonetani T, Sjoberg B: On the effects of some heterocyclic compounds on the enzymatic activity of liver alcohol dehydrogenase. Acta Chem Scand 23:255–260, 1969.
29. Reynier M: Pyrazole inhibition and kinetic studies of ethanol and retinol oxidation catalyzed by rat liver alcohol dehydrogenase. Acta Chem Scand 23:1119–1129, 1969.
30. Makar AB, Tephly TR: Inhibition of monkey liver alcohol dehydrogenase by 4-methylpyrazole. Biochem Med 13:334–342, 1975.
31. Pietruszko R: Human liver alcohol dehydrogenase—inhibition of methanol activity by pyrazole, 4-methylpyrazole, 4-hydroxymethylpyrazole and 4-carboxypyrazole. Biochem Pharmacol 24:1603–1607, 1975.
32. Lester D, Keokosky WZ, Felzenberg F: Effect of pyrazole and other compounds on alcohol metabolism. Q J Stud Alcohol 29:449–454, 1968.
33. Sivilotti MLA, Burns MJ, McMartin KE, Brent J: Toxicokinetics of ethylene glycol during fomepizole therapy: Implications for management. Ann Emerg Med 36:114–125, 2000.
34. Feiermann DE, Cederbaum AI: Inhibition of microsomal oxidation of ethanol by pyrazole and 4-methylpyrazole in vitro. Biochem J 239:671–677, 1986.
35. Feiermann DE, Cederbaum AI: Increased sensitivity of the microsomal oxidation of ethanol to inhibition by pyrazole and 4-methylpyrazole after chronic ethanol treatment. Biochem Pharmacol 36:3277–3283, 1987.
36. Chow HH, Hutchaleelaha A, Mayersohn M: Inhibitory effect of 4-methylpyrazole on antipyrine clearance in rats. Life Sci 50:661–666, 1992.
37. Brennan RJ, Mankes RF, Lefevre R, et al: 4-Methylpyrazole blocks acetaminophen hepatotoxicity in the rat. Ann Emerg Med 23:487–493, 1994.
38. Burk RF, Hill KE, Hunt RW Jr, Martin AE: Isoniazid potentiation of acetaminophen hepatotoxicity in the rat and 4-methylpyrazole inhibition of it. Res Commun Chem Pathol Pharmacol 69:115–118, 1990.
39. Feiermann DE, Cederbaum AI: Interaction of pyrazole and 4-methylpyrazole with hepatic microsomes: Effect on cytochrome P-450 content, microsomal oxidation of alcohols and binding spectra. Alcohol Clin Exp Res 9:421–428, 1985.
40. Krikun G, Feierman DE, Cederbaum AI: Rat liver microsomal induction of the oxidation of drugs and alcohols, and sodium dodecyl sulfate-gel profiles after in vivo treatment with pyrazole or 4-methylpyrazole. J Pharmacol Exp Ther 237:1012–1019, 1986.
41. Feiermann DE, Cederbaum AI: Increased content of cytochrome P-450 and 4-methylpyrazole binding spectra after 4-methylpyrazole treatment. Biochem Biophys Res Commun 126:1076–1081, 1985.
42. Cederbaum AI, Berl L: Pyrazole and 4-methylpyrazole inhibit oxidation of ethanol and dimethylsulfoxide by hydroxyl radicals generated from ascorbate, xanthine oxidase and rat liver microsome. Arch Biochem Biophys 216:530–543, 1982.
43. Iaquinto G, Del Tacca M, Cuccurullo L, et al: Gastroprotection by 4-methylpyrazole against ethanol in humans. Dig Dis Sci 43:816–825, 1998.
44. McMartin KE, Collins TD: Distribution of oral 4-methylpyrazole in the rat: Inhibition of elimination by ethanol. J Toxicol Clin Toxicol 26:451–466, 1988.
45. Mayersohn MI, Owens SM, Anaya AL, et al: 4-Methylpyrazole disposition in the dog: Evidence for saturable elimination. J Pharmacol Sci 74:895–896, 1985.
46. Murphy RC, Watkins WD: Pharmacology of pyrazoles: I. Structure elucidation of metabolites of 4-methylpyrazole. Biochem Biophys Res Commun 49:283–291, 1972.
47. Blomstrand R, Ohman G: Studies on the metabolites of the ADH inhibitor 4-methylpyrazole in the rat. Life Sci 13:107–112, 1973.
48. Vu BD, Crouzier C, Hubert I, et al: Etude analytique et pharmacocinetique du 4-methylpyrazole, nouvel antidote pour le traitement de l'intoxication a l'ethylene glycol. Ann Fals Exp Chim 85:99–110, 1992.
49. Jacobsen D, Østensen J, Bredesen L, et al: 4-Methylpyrazole (4-MP) is effectively removed by hemodialysis in the pig model. Hum Exp Toxicol 15:494–496, 1996.

50. Jobard E, Harry P, Turcant A, et al: 4-Methylpyrazole and hemodialysis in ethylene glycol poisoning. J Toxicol Clin Toxicol 34:373–377, 1996.

51. Faessel H, Houze P, Baud FJ, Scherrmann JM: 4-Methylpyrazole monitoring during hemodialysis of ethylene glycol intoxicated patients. Eur J Clin Pharmacol 49:211–213, 1995.

52. Harry P, Jobard E, Briand M, et al: Ethylene glycol poisoning in a child treated with 4-methylpyrazole. Pediatrics 102:31–33, 1998.

53. Baum CR, Langman CB, Oker EE, et al: Fomepizole treatment of ethylene glycol poisoning in an infant. Pediatrics 106:1489–1491, 2000.

54. Brown MJ, Shannon MW, Woolf A, Boyer EW: Childhood methanol ingestion treated with fomepizole and hemodialysis. Pediatrics 108:77–79, 2001.

55. Magnusson G, Nyberg J-A, Bodin N-O, Hansson E: Toxicity of pyrazole and 4-methylpyrazole in mice and rats. Experientia 28:1198–1200, 1972.

56. Blomstrand R, Ingemansson S-O, Jensen M, Hedstrom C-G: Normal electroretinogram and no toxicity signs after chronic and acute administration of the alcohol dehydrogenase inhibitor 4-methylpyrazole to the cynomolgus monkey. Drug Alcohol Depend 13:9–20, 1984.

57. Lindros KO, Stowell L, Vaananen H, et al: Uninterrupted prolonged ethanol oxidation as a main pathogenetic factor of alcoholic liver damage: Evidence from a new liquid diet animal model. Liver 3:79–91, 1983.

58. MacDonald E: Effect of pyrazole, 4-methylpyrazole, 4-bromopyrazole and 4-iodopyrazole on brain noradrenaline levels of mice and rats. Acta Pharmacol Toxicol 39:513–524, 1976.

59. Salaspuro MP, Lindros KO, Pikkarainen PH: Effect of 4-methylpyrazole on ethanol elimination rate and hepatic redox changes in alcoholics with adequate or inadequate nutrition and in nonalcoholic controls. Metab Clin Exp 27:631–639, 1978.

60. Kupari M, Lindros K, Hillbom M, et al: Cardiovascular effects of acetaldehyde accumulation after ethanol ingestion: Their modification by β-adrenergic blockade and alcohol dehydrogenase inhibition. Alcohol Clin Exp Res 7:283–288, 1983.

61. Borron SW, Megarbane B, Baud FJ: Fomepizole in treatment of uncomplicated ethylene glycol poisoning. Lancet 354:831, 1999.

62. Megarbane B, Borron SW, Trout H, et al: Treatment of acute methanol poisoning with fomepizole. Intensive Care Med 27:1370–1378, 2001.

63. Antizol (fomepizole) Product Monograph. Minnetonka, MN, Orphan Medical, 2001.

CHAPTER 153

Physostigmine

Thomas G. Martin ■ William D. Morris

Physostigmine (eserine) salicylate (Antilirium) is a short-acting, lipid-soluble, nonselective, carbamate cholinesterase (ChE) inhibitor used to increase acetylcholine (Ach) concentrations at cholinergic receptors. In the 1970s, physostigmine was used commonly to reverse central anticholinergic toxicity of many drugs and natural substances and less often to reverse nonanticholinergic sedation.[1] Following reports in the 1980s of serious adverse effects after physostigmine's use in tricyclic antidepressant (TCA) overdoses, its use has diminished (Table 153-1). In 2004, except in certain well-defined circumstances, it is used cautiously by medical toxicology, critical care, and emergency medicine specialists.[2]

HISTORY

Physostigmine was the first known anticholinesterase used by humans. Natives of tropical West Africa used dried, ripened Calabar beans (*Physostigma venenosum*) containing the alkaloid physostigmine in their "trial by ordeal."[3,4] In a "trial by ordeal," a person accused of a crime was forced to drink a potion made from the Calabar bean. If the accused were innocent, he or she purportedly would swallow the potion, develop acute toxicity resulting in vomiting, regurgitate unabsorbed physostigmine, and survive. If the accused were guilty, he or she would be reluctant to swallow the potion. Instead, the person would hold it in the mouth, allowing a lethal amount of physostigmine to be absorbed through the oral mucosa.

In 1863, the ophthalmologist Robertson described the first clinical use of Calabar bean extract to reverse the mydriatic effects of atropine. In 1864, the first clinical use of physostigmine as a systemic antidote was described in four prisoners who were cleaning the rooms of a local hospital.[3] They broke into a locked box containing three bottles of atropine in a solution, which they believed to be alcohol, so they drank them. Two of the prisoners developed severe anticholinergic toxicity. Knowing its ability to reverse the ophthalmic effects of atropine, Kleinwachter gave the most severely poisoned patient Calabar bean extract orally as an experiment. Although the physostigmine extract made him vomit promptly, it also decreased his elevated temperature and increased his pulse rate (from 60 beats/min) and strength, alertness, and ability to answer questions appropriately. The less severely poisoned of the two took longer to recover and experienced greater signs of anticholinergic toxicity than his Calabar-treated partner.

The clinical use of physostigmine as an antidote did not become popular until nearly a century later. In 1958, 4 mg of physostigmine by injection was reported to be "entirely effective" in reversing iatrogenic coma induced by 32 to 212 mg of atropine intramuscularly, where "by 20 minutes there was complete restoration of the patient's pretreatment psychophysiological status."[5] This recovery lasted 30 to 45 minutes, when manifestations of atropine toxicity returned. To prevent relapse of atropine toxicity in this group, 2 mg of physostigmine orally was given hourly for 4 hours. In 1967, physostigmine (0.05 mg/kg intramuscularly) given for iatrogenic scopolamine toxicity reportedly resulted in "dramatic, rapid improvement, which was noticeable at 10 minutes and maximal at 30 minutes, at which time they were alert, coherent and well oriented."[6] Also in 1967, 1 to 2 mg of physostigmine parenterally was reported to reverse central anticholinergic effects of antiparkinsonian drugs promptly in 26 consecutive patients.[7,8] In 1970, successful use of physostigmine for a TCA overdose first was reported,[9] but the safety and necessity of this TCA overdose treatment still is debated.

PROPERTIES

Chemical

Physostigmine (Fig. 153-1) is a carbamate anticholinesterase with a tertiary amine structure, which enables it to cross the blood-brain barrier.[4,9] In contrast, neostigmine methylsulfate and pyridostigmine bromide, the other injectable anticholinesterases, have a charged quaternary amine structure, which inhibits their penetration across the blood-brain barrier.

Physical

Physostigmine has a pK_a of 7.9.[10] A 0.5% aqueous solution has a pH of 5.8.[11] At physiologic pH, it exists primarily as a cation. Physostigmine is unstable at room temperature and should be stored in light-resistant packages at temperatures between 15°C and 30°C.[9] Physostigmine solution develops a red tint when exposed to metals or with prolonged exposure to heat, light, or air.[10] It should not be injected if it is more than slightly colored.

TABLE 153-1 Anticholinergic Toxicity–Related Hospitalizations and Physostigmine Use in the United States

YEAR	ANTICHOLINERGIC PLANTS	ANTICHOLINERGIC DRUGS	ANTIHISTAMINE DRUGS	TOTAL*	PHYSOSTIGMINE USE (%)†
1983	55	679	726	1460	6.6
1984	134	1855	2852	4841	7.6
1985	114	2356	4127	6597	3.7
1986	192	2226	5412	7830	4.8
1987	143	2137	6476	8756	3.5
1988	237	1836	9924	11,997	2.2
1989	259	2169	11,254	13,682	1.8
1990	329	2233	12,922	15,484	1.6
1991	422	2424	15,088	17,934	1.3
1992	516	2543	16,445	19,504	1.3
1993	498	2417	15,702	18,617	1
1994	715	2535	17,394	20,644	0.9
1995	586	2729	18,581	21,896	1
1996	585	2778	18,804	22,167	1.2
1997	555	2789	19,166	22,510	0.8
1998	607	2575	18,326	21,508	0.8
1999	537	2384	17,781	20,702	0.9
2000	511	2809	21,895	25,215	0.8

*Total = Anticholinergic drugs and plants and antihistamine drug exposures per year.
†Use = (Number of cases in which physostigmine used/total) × 100%.
From Litovitz TL, Klein-Schwartz W, White S, et al: 2000 Annual reports of the American Association of Poison Control Centers Toxic Exposure Surveillance System. Am J Emerg Med 19: 337–395, 2001.

PHARMACOLOGY

ACh is the neurotransmitter for all preganglionic autonomic neurons and postganglionic parasympathetic neurons and some postganglionic sympathetic neurons. During basal states, there is a low level of ACh release from these neurons. After release, ACh is catabolized by synaptic ChE. There are two types of ChE: (1) tissue or acetyl (AChE) and (2) plasma, pseudo, or butyryl (BuChE). Circulating ACh from ingested foods and various medications, such as various choline esters, succinylcholine, and cocaine, are BuChE substrates. Synaptic ACh is the primary substrate for AChE and is deacetylated rapidly by it.[12] ACh and physostigmine bind to the same site on ChE. ACh acetylates ChE and physostigmine carbamoylates ChE. After hydrolysis (deacetylation or decarbomoylation) of the enzyme, the ChE is regenerated. Because hydrolysis occurs rapidly (150 μsec) for acetylated ChE, the effect of ACh is dissipated before the end of the refractory period of the postsynaptic potential.

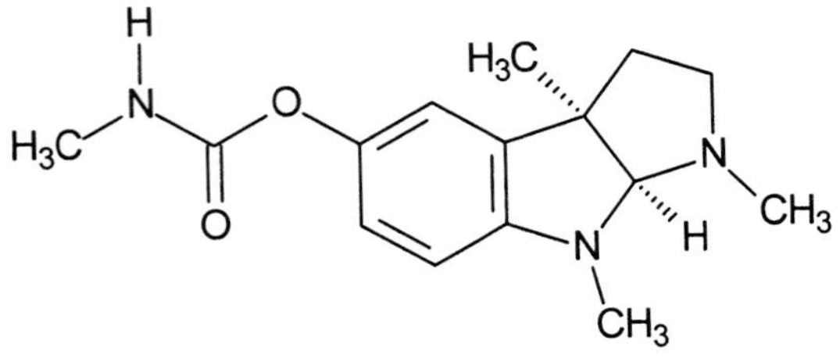

Decarbamoylation takes 15 to 30 minutes.[4] Physostigmine reversibly inhibits the degradation of ACh, resulting in synaptic accumulation and repetitive, asynchronous stimulation of neighboring cholinergic receptors. Excess postsynaptic cholinergic receptor stimulation may result in sustained depolarization and subsequent blockade, leading to weakness or paralysis. Excess presynaptic cholinergic receptor stimulation may induce antidromic firing of the motor neuron, leading to fasciculations.[4] Clinically, reversible inhibition of ACh metabolism by carbamoylation lasts 3 to 4 hours.[4] In the setting of anticholinergic toxicity, the intended function of physostigmine is to reverse cholinergic receptor antagonism and normalize cholinergic stimulation.

The primary pharmacologic, toxicologic, and antidotal effects of physostigmine result from increased ACh stimulation of muscarinic, nicotinic, and central nervous system (CNS) cholinergic receptors. Physostigmine is a nonselective ChE inhibitor, effective on ChE throughout the body. The physiologic effects of physostigmine, which are the result of decreased ACh breakdown, are listed in Table 153-2. Physostigmine's cardiac properties are complex, owing to mixed effects from muscarinic and nicotinic stimulation.[9] Muscarinic stimulation leads to increased conduction time at the sinoatrial and atrioventricular nodes, bradycardia, and diminished cardiac output, whereas nicotinic stimulation has the opposite effects. In one study of "anticholinergic" overdoses, physostigmine led to significantly increased mean arterial pressure and cardiac output.[13] In a dog model of amitriptyline poisoning treated with physostigmine, cardiac output was increased, but systolic blood pressure and heart rate largely remained unchanged.[14]

FIGURE 153-1

Chemical structure of physostigmine.

TABLE 153-2 Physiologic Effects of Physostigmine

RECEPTORS	ORGAN SYSTEM	CLINICAL EFFECTS
Muscarinic	Exocrine	Salivation, lacrimation, perspiration, bronchorrhea
	Gastrointestinal	Nausea, vomiting, abdominal cramps, diarrhea, fecal incontinence
	Ocular	Miosis, ptosis, blurred vision, eye ache
	Respiratory	Dyspnea, pulmonary edema, bronchospasm
	Cardiovascular	Bradycardia, hypotension
	Urinary	Micturition, urinary incontinence
Nicotinic	Cardiovascular	Tachycardia, hypertension
	Ocular	Mydriasis
	Skeletal	Muscle cramps, weakness, fasciculations, tremor, flaccid or rigid paralysis
Brain	Central nervous system	Restlessness, emotional lability, ataxia, lethargy, confusion, amnesia, headache, hallucinations, convulsions, respiratory depression, seizures, coma

Physostigmine's vasodilatory effects are mediated by ACh-stimulated presynaptic inhibitory receptors on vascular sympathetic fibers and inhibitory vascular cholinergic receptors. Stimulation of the inhibitory vascular cholinergic receptors leads to release of endothelium-derived relaxing factor, leading to smooth muscle relaxation and vasodilation.[12] In patients treated with methscopolamine, then given 0.022 mg/kg (≤2 mg) of physostigmine intravenously over 10 minutes, significant increases in blood pressure, heart rate, and serum epinephrine levels were observed.[12,15] Physostigmine's catecholamine-releasing effects seem to be centrally mediated.[15] Neostigmine is an anticholinesterase that does not cross the blood-brain barrier and does not increase serum epinephrine levels. Scopolamine, a centrally acting anticholinergic, blocks physostigmine's ability to increase serum epinephrine levels.

Physostigmine has nonspecific CNS arousal properties, possibly due to ACh-induced stimulation of the reticular activating system or inhibition of neural phosphodiesterase, leading to increased CNS levels of cyclic adenosine monophosphate or both.[16] Muscarinic stimulation of the midbrain increases alertness, making the individual more responsive to internal and external stimuli.[17] Many volatile anesthetics antagonize muscarinic systems through interference with either ACh receptor binding or G-protein functioning.[17] Physostigmine has been reported in animal studies, case reports, and case series to reverse sedation from hepatic encephalopathy and many nonanticholinergic drugs, including barbiturates, benzodiazepines, ethanol, droperidol, volatile anesthetics, ketamine, opiates, and propofol. Results from randomized clinical trials have been conflicting, with some supporting[18–25] and others refuting[26–29] physostigmine's nonspecific arousal properties.

PHARMACOKINETICS

Hydrolytic cleavage by ChEs destroys physostigmine and is the major form of physostigmine metabolism.[30] Renal excretion is only a minor factor in physostigmine clearance. The pharmacokinetics of 1.5 mg of physostigmine given intravenously over 1 hour to subjects with Alzheimer's disease and 1 mg of physostigmine given postoperatively is listed in the accompanying box.[31,32]

Pharmacokinetics of Intravenous Physostigmine*

	Asthana[31] (SEM)	Hartvig[32] (SD)
Volume of distribution:	186.1 L (53.7)	46.5 L (19.2)
Plasma half-life:	16.4 min (3.2)	21.7 min (8.3)
Clearance:	7.7 L/min (0.9)	1.54 L/min (0.63)

*1.5 mg of physostigmine given intravenously over 1 hour to subjects with Alzheimer's disease and 1 mg of physostigmine given postoperatively.

SD, standard deviation; SEM, standard error of the mean.

Physostigmine easily penetrates the blood-brain barrier; it has an onset of action of 2 minutes after intravenous use and time to peak effect averaging 20 to 30 minutes after intramuscular and 5 minutes after intravenous use.[34] Because of its short blood elimination half-life (15 to 20 minutes), one might expect physostigmine's duration of action to be no more than 30 to 60 minutes. The ChE inhibition half-life (84 minutes) is much longer than the blood elimination half-life, however.[31,33] Clinical reports suggest a duration of action of 30 minutes to several hours.[6,7,34,35]

SPECIAL POPULATIONS

Pediatric Patients

Physostigmine has been used successfully in a variety of pediatric anticholinergic ingestions.[36,37] Physostigmine has been given to a 30-day-old infant with atropine toxicity without apparent adverse effects.[38]

Elderly Patients

The safety and efficacy of physostigmine use in elderly patients has not been studied specifically. All patients, but especially the elderly, should be screened for premorbid conditions, including cardiovascular and pulmonary disease; long-term medications; and contraindications before physostigmine administration.

Pregnant Patients

The safety and efficacy of physostigmine use in pregnancy has not been studied specifically. In 15 pregnant patients given physostigmine to reverse the effects of scopolamine at the time of delivery, it was well tolerated.[39] Physostigmine is classified in pregnancy category C by the U.S. Food and Drug Administration (see Appendix A). In one chick embryo model, physostigmine led to embryo paralysis and skeletal anomalies.[40]

INDICATIONS

The Food and Drug Administration labeled indication is reversal of central anticholinergic toxicity.[11] The American Psychiatric Association's "Practice Guidelines for Treatment of Patients with Delirium" recommend the use of physostigmine in severe cases of anticholinergic delirium.[40a] Successful use of physostigmine to reverse central anticholinergic toxicity in more than 600 and 700 different anticholinergic drugs and plants has been reported anecdotally.[1,41] In a retrospective comparative review of 52 anticholinergic poisonings, physostigmine was reported to be more effective than benzodiazepines for control of agitation and reversal of delirium and had a lower incidence of aspiration, lower rate of endotracheal intubation, and shorter mean time to recovery.[42] The usual cited indications for the use of physostigmine are anticholinergic toxicity with hyperthermia, hemodynamically significant sinus tachycardia, and marked delirium or coma. The goals of physostigmine therapy in these cases are to treat hyperthermia and to avoid emergent intubation (needed to protect the airway), artificial ventilation (in order to treat excess respiratory depression from sedatives), and rhabdomyolysis (caused by restraints). The uses of physostigmine as a general analeptic, as a treatment of overdose patients at high risk of cardiovascular toxicity or seizures, or as a treatment of patients with anticholinergic-induced cardiovascular toxicity or seizures are addressed subsequently.

Central anticholinergic toxicity usually, but not always, is accompanied by signs of peripheral anticholinergic toxicity and may be difficult to diagnose clinically (see Chapter 22). In cases of suspected anticholinergic toxicity, a diagnostic test with carefully titrated physostigmine doses may be attempted if contraindications are not present.[43] In these cases, physostigmine would be given until at least a mild degree of excess cholinergic stimulation was observed before one concluded that anticholinergic toxicity was not present.

Tricyclic Antidepressant Overdose

In the early 1970s, physostigmine was considered by many to be the drug of choice for TCA poisoning.[44,45] Although there have been many successful uses of physostigmine to reverse the CNS toxicity from TCA overdose, the safety and necessity of this use have been questioned.[46,47] When seizures or cardiovascular deterioration are observed after physostigmine use in TCA overdose, it is difficult to know whether they were due to the TCA overdose or to the physostigmine. Also, in TCA overdose, the prevalence of seizures varies from 3% to 30%.[48–50] In TCA overdose, seizures occur infrequently after physostigmine.[46,51,52] The peak effects of physostigmine are usually seen within 5 to 10 minutes.[46] Seizures or cardiovascular deterioration may be considered to be more likely due to physostigmine when they occur within 10 minutes of administration. Seizures often lead to significant cardiovascular deterioration in TCA overdose.[53–55] A collective review of 16 case series revealed that clinical deterioration often occurred rapidly, yet death in hospitalized TCA overdose patients was uncommon (2.6% mortality rate).[56] In 81 TCA overdose patients admitted from the "casualty" ward but who later died in the hospital (most within 20 hours), 16 had a sudden cardiac arrest, 9 developed a tachydysrhythmia, and 8 developed bradycardia.[57] These authors concluded, "the incidence of tachydysrhythmias has been overrated." Of the 11 of 81 who seized, 6 had a cardiac arrest shortly thereafter.[57] In four published TCA overdoses in which asystole occurred within minutes of physostigmine administration, significant QRS prolongation was seen in three cases, and seizures were seen in all four cases before physostigmine; administration was reported as slow in three and was not reported in one; and successful resuscitation with complete recovery was reported in three, but death occurred in one of these cases.[58–60] Significant cardiovascular toxicity or seizures generally are considered to be a contraindication to physostigmine in TCA overdose.

Methodologic differences confound the interpretation of animal studies of physostigmine use in TCA poisoning. These differences include use of different animal types; amounts, rates, and modes of TCA administration; physostigmine doses; and study end points. One possible reason for the conflicting results in animal studies is the use of excessive amounts of physostigmine. The lethal dose in all exposed subjects for physostigmine in a rat model is 0.75 mg/kg.[61] In a rat model of poisoning from several different TCA agents, physostigmine reduced lethality, with the most effective doses of physostigmine found to be 0.02 to 0.1 mg/kg intraperitoneally.[62] In a dog model of amitriptyline poisoning, physostigmine doses of 0.06 to 0.25 mg/kg intramuscularly had favorable effects on heart rate and neurologic toxicity.[63] In a dog model of amitriptyline poisoning, physostigmine (0.33 mg/kg intravenously) improved cardiac output, systolic blood pressure, intraventricular conduction, and maximal rate of increase of arterial blood pressure.[14] In a mouse model of amitriptyline and imipramine poisoning, physostigmine (0.3 mg/kg intraperitoneally) significantly increased the incidence of seizures and death.[64] In a rat model of imipramine poisoning, physostigmine (0.5 mg/kg intravenously) had no effect on cardiac toxicity.[61] In a rabbit model of amitriptyline poisoning, a large dose of physostigmine (0.66 to 0.8 mg/kg intravenously) had no effect on QRS prolongation within the first 5 minutes.[65]

Based on the infrequent yet potentially serious adverse effects (seizure and brady-asystolic arrest) and rare fatal outcomes associated with the use of physostigmine, most medical toxicologists believe that physostigmine is contraindicated in TCA overdose. Although its use in TCA overdose cases without signs of serious toxicity and no sooner than 12 hours postingestion is probably safe, the benefit at that point is less likely.[66]

Seizure-Inducing Antidepressant Overdose

Maprotiline is a tetracyclic antidepressant with less peripheral anticholinergic toxicity and a greater propensity for causing seizures (which may occur without concomitant cardiovascular toxicity) than with TCAs.[67] In one series, 15 of 41 patients with maprotiline overdose experienced a seizure, 6 shortly after physostigmine was administered.[68] In an animal study, maprotiline failed to counteract the lethal effect of physostigmine, suggesting that maprotiline has little to no central anticholinergic effect.[69] Physostigmine should not be used to treat overdoses of seizure-prone antidepressants, such as maprotiline, dothiepin,[70] loxapine[71] and amoxapine.[72]

Gamma Hydroxybutyrate Overdose

Because gamma hydroxybutyrate (GHB) abuse currently is widespread throughout the United States, the reports of rapid reversal by physostigmine of GHB-induced sedation in five emergency department cases are of great interest.[73,74] In the 1970s, two poorly designed studies reported that physostigmine could be used safely and effectively to reverse GHB that was used as an anesthetic agent.[75,76] To facilitate emergence from GHB, 2-mg increments of intravenous physostigmine up to 6 mg were used.[75] Although most patients awoke rapidly, 4 of 42 experienced prolonged sedation despite physostigmine. Of particular concern is the potential for physostigmine to increase the risk of two well-known adverse effects of GHB overdose—seizures and hemodynamically significant bradycardia. One author anecdotally reported, however, the safe and effective use of physostigmine in reversing 50 cases of GHB overdose.[77] More peer-reviewed data verifying the safety and efficacy of physostigmine treatment of GHB overdose is required before it can be recommended.

CONTRAINDICATIONS

Although some authors recommend physostigmine only for anticholinergic toxicity without serious cardiovascular toxicity,[42] others recommend it only for cases of anticholinergic toxicity with serious cardiovascular toxicity.[78,79] Although the cautious approach is to consider seizures, hypotension, intraventricular or atrioventricular heart block, bradycardia, and ventricular dysrhythmias to be contraindications to physostigmine use, the following cases argue against this position. In three "anticholinergic" overdoses with QRS and QT$_c$ interval prolongation, no dysrhythmias were observed during aggressive physostigmine therapy.[13] A wide-complex rhythm at a rate of 110 beats/min developed 4 hours after an imipramine and trifluoperazine overdose and responded within 90 seconds of 0.5 mg of physostigmine administered intravenously with dramatic narrowing of the QRS complex.[80] Within 20 minutes, the QRS gradually widened again but responded with narrowing with each subsequent repeat physostigmine dose. After an acute, large total ingestion (9850 mg) of several types of TCAs, recurrent wide-complex tachycardia was treated effectively over a 4-hour period by multiple doses of physostigmine, 5 to 10 mg slow intravenous administration.[81] Wide-complex tachycardia

from a dibenzazepine-type TCA overdose responded to physostigmine therapy.[50] At 2 hours after orphenadrine overdose, a 3-year-old child developed wide-complex tachycardia resistant to a precordial thump, two synchronized cardioversions (30 j), and three boluses of lidocaine (1 mg/kg) but responded to physostigmine (0.02 mg/kg).[82] A 68-year-old man who ingested 1600 mg of sustained-release thioridazine and developed torsades de pointes and monomorphic wide-complex tachycardia 17 hours later was treated with physostigmine, 3 mg, with termination of the ventricular rhythm but development of complete sinus node arrest requiring temporary pacing.[83] Because supraventricular rhythms with aberrant conduction can be confused with ventricular tachycardia, one must interpret these reports with caution.

Asthma

Asthma long has been considered a relative contraindication to physostigmine. Bronchial hyperreactivity has occurred when physostigmine was given via nebulization to asthmatic subjects.[84] In a series of 45 patients with anticholinergic poisonings given physostigmine, however, none of the 8 patients with a history of asthma developed bronchospasm.[42] One possible explanation is that reversal of anticholinergic toxicity by physostigmine in these cases was incomplete and not associated with bronchospasm in these asthmatic patients. It generally is accepted that physostigmine should not be given to anyone who is actively wheezing and should be used with caution in asthmatic patients who are not actively wheezing.

Sodium Bisulfite Sensitivity

Because the vehicle for parenteral physostigmine salicylate contains sodium bisulfite, allergic-like reactions, including anaphylactic symptoms and severe asthma exacerbations, may occur.[11] Physostigmine should not be used in patients with known sensitivity to sulfur or sulfites.

Other Contraindications

Other traditional contraindications to cholinergic agents include coronary artery disease, gangrene, gastrointestinal or urogenital obstruction, diabetes, and use of other cholinergic medications.[11] Recent seizures observed in association with other signs of serious anticholinergic toxicity are not a contraindication to physostigmine use.[85] In these situations, one must weigh the risk versus the benefit of physostigmine therapy.

PRECAUTIONS

Physostigmine should be given only in a controlled setting, with intravenous access and continuous cardiac and frequent blood pressure monitoring. Anticholinergic agents, such as atropine, should be available to reverse excess muscarinic effects of physostigmine when indicated. Slow administration of physostigmine is important to minimize the risk of arrhythmia or seizures.[86] The manufacturer recommends an intravenous or intramuscular dose of 0.5 to 1 mg, with an intravenous rate of no more than 1 mg/min.[11] Some authors recommend a more cautious approach and give no more than 2 mg every 5 minutes. Physostigmine infusions have been reported by some[13,50,51,114] but not recommended by others.[41] Theoretically, infusions may minimize the recurrence of central anticholinergic toxicity and avoid repeat bolus injections, but insufficient data are available to judge the safety of this approach.

ADVERSE EFFECTS

Except in large doses, physostigmine's main adverse effects result from excess muscarinic, nicotinic, or CNS stimulation. Excess muscarinic stimulation may result in excess secretions (diaphoresis, drooling, bronchorrhea), smooth muscle contraction (diarrhea, urinary incontinence, bronchospasm), vasodilation (hypotension), and decreased myocardial conduction (heart block and bradycardia). Excess nicotinic stimulation at first may lead to fasciculations and tremor, which may be followed by weakness and paralysis. CNS toxicity from physostigmine includes nausea, headache, ataxia, and seizures. Serious adverse effects usually are a result of physostigmine given improperly (in excess amount, at an excessive rate, or in the absence of anticholinergic toxicity) or despite contraindications. When used appropriately, physostigmine has a relatively low incidence of side effects, most of which are not serious or life-threatening. In two large reports of physostigmine use, there were no adverse effects in one group of 707 patients and one seizure in the other group of 255 patients.[1,87] This patient also had ingested sertraline and valproic acid, drugs that may cause seizures. In another 45 cases of anticholinergic poisoning treated with physostigmine, adverse effects were recorded in 5 (11%) and consisted of one case each of diaphoresis, emesis, diarrhea, bradycardia (hemodynamically nonsignificant), and bronchorrhea.[42] In 21 TCA-poisoned patients treated with physostigmine, one patient seized, and two others developed cholinergic excess requiring therapy.[46] When used aggressively in 83 overdoses of various types, physostigmine was associated with two major adverse outcomes, frequent monofocal premature ventricular contractions in one patient and a grand mal seizure in another.[88] When physostigmine was used inappropriately or in conditions now recognized as contraindications, hemodynamically significant bradycardia or heart block, asystole, and seizures have been reported, as discussed subsequently.

In high doses, physostigmine may block autonomic ganglia directly, causing muscle fasciculation and paralysis. Tremor, ataxia, and hallucinations have been reported. Extremely high doses may produce profound CNS depression and fatal respiratory depression. After an intentional ingestion of 1 g of physostigmine, diaphoresis, vomiting, and severe abdominal cramps occurred within minutes followed by muscle twitching, weakness, seizures, visual hallucinations, copious bronchorrhea, and coma.[89]

Seizures

Seizures and seizure-like abnormal motor activity occur commonly with anticholinergic toxicity.[90–96] Seizures also may occur from an excessive dose or rate of physostigmine administration. Seizures may be more likely to occur when physostigmine is used to treat overdoses of seizure-prone drugs. Although individual case reports imply otherwise, animal studies question the efficacy of physostigmine to treat seizures secondary to antihistamine or antimuscarinic toxicity.[97–99]

Cardiovascular

Cardiovascular abnormalities temporally related to physostigmine administration have been reported. It is sometimes difficult to distinguish between the effects due to the underlying drug toxicity or cardiovascular disease and the effects due to physostigmine. Ventricular fibrillation occurred in a 62-year-old man soon after 2 mg of physostigmine was given intravenously over 5 minutes for excess postoperative sedation despite a heart rate of 60 beats/min and known cardiovascular disease.[100] In a study of reversal of diazepam sedation, one subject developed vomiting and bradycardia after intravenous physostigmine, 1.5 mg.[18] After atropine was given to reverse the bradycardia, atrial flutter occurred in this patient, then resolved spontaneously within 4 hours. Severe hypertension (240/140 mm Hg) occurred after 2 mg of physostigmine was given intravenously for a mixed diazepam and methyprylon (sedative-hypnotic) ingestion.[18]

Drug Interactions

Several cases of prolonged neuromuscular blockade have been reported when succinylcholine was given after physostigmine administration.[101] Physostigmine slows the metabolism of succinylcholine by BuChE, prolonging its effect, although other mechanisms also may be involved.[102]

Treatment of Adverse Effects

Anticholinergic agents may be used to treat excessive muscarinic stimulation due to physostigmine. Atropine and scopolamine cross the blood-brain barrier, however, and may induce or worsen central anticholinergic toxicity. Glycopyrrolate and propantheline do not cross the blood-brain barrier and would not worsen the central anticholinergic syndrome, but also would not reverse CNS cholinergic adverse effects. Propantheline is available in the United States only in an oral formulation. Glycopyrrolate is the preferred anticholinergic agent for peripheral muscarinic manifestations of physostigmine toxicity (i.e., bradycardia, wheezing, bronchorrhea).[41,51,103] Glycopyrrolate is administered in titrated doses beginning with 0.1 mg intravenously and repeated every 2 to 3 minutes as needed. When seizures (possible CNS cholinergic effects) occur after use of physostigmine, benzodiazepines have been recommended as first-line therapy.[104] For benzodiazepine-refractory seizures, animal studies suggest that scopolamine may be more effective than atropine because of its greater CNS penetration.[105,106] In a controlled study of induced central anticholinergic syndrome, scopolamine had a "central potency" eight to nine times greater, slightly less peripheral effects, and more rapid onset than atropine.[107] Atropine may be used for physostigmine toxicity when more selective agents (i.e., glycopyrrolate for peripheral effects or scopolamine for central effects) are not readily available.[108] In a case of intentional massive physostigmine overdose, tachycardia and multiple ventricular ectopic beats were seen after low-dose atropine administration.[89] In a mouse model of physostigmine toxicity, a single dose of atropine plus escalating doses of diazepam was safer and more effective than a single dose of atropine alone.[109] Some authors have described concomitantly administering glycopyrrolate,[110] propantheline,[51] or methylscopolamine[111] along with physostigmine rather than waiting for excessive peripheral cholinergic toxicity to occur, but this is not recommended without further data.

Most authors do not recommend pralidoxime in the treatment of physostigmine toxicity. In a murine model, atropine plus pralidoxime had no added protective effect from high doses of physostigmine over atropine alone.[109] In a study of bovine erythrocyte (AChEs), Dawson[112] reported that pralidoxime lowered the rate constant (slowed) of carbamoylation by physostigmine and increased its median lethal dose. There are no human studies of pralidoxime use in physostigmine toxicity.

ADMINISTRATION

Adult

Physostigmine salicylate is available in 2-mL ampules in a concentration of 1 mg/mL. The solution contains sodium bisulfite 0.1% and benzyl alcohol 2%.[11] In adults, the usual recommended dose is 1 to 2 mg intravenously or intramuscularly. When given intravenously, it should be given at a rate of 1 mg/min. The dose may be repeated in 5 to 10 minutes until the desired clinical response is achieved or adverse effects are seen.

Pediatric

In children, the recommended dose is 0.02 mg/kg intravenously or intramuscularly. When given intravenously, it should be given at a rate of 0.5 mg/min. The dose may be repeated in 5 to 10 minutes until the desired clinical response is achieved or adverse effects are seen.

Dosing Regimens

Because physostigmine is relatively short acting, repeat dosing in 30 to 120 minutes may be required. When the desired clinical response has been achieved, it can be maintained with intermittent doses. In 45 cases of anticholinergic poisonings treated with physostigmine, central anticholinergic symptoms recurred in 32 (78%) cases, and 26 cases required multiple doses.[42] Oral, subcutaneous, transdermal, nebulized, and continuous intravenous forms of administration of physostigmine have been reported but are not recommended in acute overdose management.

A wide variation in the total doses of physostigmine required to maintain arousal and coherence has been reported. In 45 cases of anticholinergic poisonings treated with physostigmine, the mean initial dose (given in first 30 minutes), was 2.2 mg and mean total dose was 3.9 mg.[42] By comparison, in the 26 patients treated with benzodiazepines in this report, the mean total doses were diazepam, 53.1 mg; lorazepam, 35.5 mg; and midazolam, 31.7 mg. In a series of 8 patients with "anticholinergic" overdose in which 4 mg of physostigmine was given every 15 minutes until either marked arousal or adverse effects were noted, the average total physostigmine dose was 5 mg (range 6.5 to 14.5 mg).[13] In a series of 35 "anticholinergic" overdoses (74% TCA overdoses) in which 2 mg of physostigmine was given every 5 to 10 minutes until either marked arousal or adverse effects were noted, the average total physostigmine dose was 5.5 mg (range 2 to 24 mg).[88] Because the average arousal physostigmine dose in the two previously cited studies was 5 to 5.5 mg, failure to respond to total doses below this range may be secondary to underdosing.

Several cases have been reported in which large doses of physostigmine were administered. A 7-year-old girl who had ingested imipramine received 260 mg of physostigmine over 30 hours (reported via personal communication to reference author).[113] A 55-year-old woman who had ingested a large amount of amitriptyline received 196 mg of physostigmine over 36 hours.[111] Because this patient did not receive her first dose of physostigmine until 64 hours postingestion, it is questionable whether central anticholinergic toxicity was causing her sedation at that point. A 27-year-old woman who had ingested 9850 mg of a TCA received 74 mg of physostigmine (in 5- to 10-mg doses) over 6 hours for recurrent ventricular tachycardia.[81] A 20-year-old woman who had ingested 70 mg of benztropine and an unknown amount of amitriptyline received 77 mg of physostigmine over 52 hours through a combination of intravenous bolus and infusion (1 to 3 mg/hr) and intramuscular routes.[114] In 15 TCA overdoses, an initial bolus of 2 to 6 mg of physostigmine was followed by an infusion of 2 mg/hr for 30 ± 6 hours.[50]

Management of patients with increasing delirium and sedation presenting within the first 2 hours after an anticholinergic overdose is controversial. Some authors have suggested using physostigmine to arouse the patient and avoid the need for prophylactic endotracheal intubation if gastric lavage is contemplated.[115] In a patient with a substantial amount of anticholinergic drugs in the stomach, however, physostigmine theoretically could increase the rate of gastric emptying and enhance drug absorption and toxicity. In the initial hours after an anticholinergic ingestion, it is theoretically more prudent to use routine gastrointestinal decontamination procedures (gastric lavage or activated charcoal or both) and airway protection before physostigmine.

FUTURE THERAPIES

Longer acting and more selective ChE inhibitors may be preferred for treating the central anticholinergic syndrome. Alzheimer's disease is an important health problem in many parts of the world, and research on effective therapies is widely supported. ChE inhibitors have been found to be useful in symptomatic treatment of this disease.[116] The more CNS-selective inhibitors (greater effect on AChE than BuChE) are less likely to produce adverse effects for these ChE inhibitors in this use. Some of the ChE inhibitors studied and used in Alzheimer's disease may be useful in treating the central anticholinergic syndrome. Galantamine (Reminyl) is a tertiary amine–type ChE inhibitor shown to be more

CNS selective and with an elimination half-life of approximately 5 hours.[117] Galantamine has been used successfully in two cases of central anticholinergic syndrome due to poisoning and in one volunteer study of 10 patients given scopolamine.[118–120] Rivastigmine tartrate (Exelon) is also a tertiary amine shown to be more CNS selective and with an elimination half-life of 10 hours.[121] These ChE inhibitors are available only in oral formulations in the United States, but they are examples of possible future therapies. They cannot be recommended for general use until further studies have been completed.

SUMMARY

When used appropriately, physostigmine can effectively reverse confusion, agitation, delirium, coma, hemodynamically significant sinus tachycardia, and hyperthermia secondary to the central anticholinergic syndrome, while avoiding the risks associated with excess sedation, physical restraints, and "crash" intubations. Physostigmine is contraindicated in patients with active wheezing, hypotension, heart block, or bradycardia. Use of physostigmine is not recommended in overdoses at increased risk of cardiovascular or CNS toxicity (i.e., TCA or seizure-inducing drug overdoses). One must avoid giving physostigmine too quickly and be prepared to treat signs of excess central or peripheral cholinergic toxicity or both.

REFERENCES

1. Rumack BH: 707 cases of anticholinergic poisoning treated with physostigmine (Abstract). Presented at the Annual Meeting of the American Academy of Clinical Toxicology, Montreal, Quebec, 1975.
2. Sivilotti MLA, Burns MJ, Linden CH: The attitudes of US regional poison centers toward physostigmine for anticholinergic delirium (Abstract). J Toxicol Clin Toxicol 35:653, 1999.
3. Nickalls RW, Nickalls EA: The first use of physostigmine in the treatment of atropine poinsoning. Anaesthesia 43:776–779, 1988.
4. Taylor P: Anticholinesterase agents. In Hardman JG, Limberd LE, Molinoff PB, et al (eds): Goodman and Gilman's the Pharmacological Basis of Therapeutics, 9th ed. New York, McGraw-Hill, 1996.
5. Forrer GR, Miller JJ: Atropine coma: A somatic therapy in psychiatry. Am J Psychiatry 115:455–456, 1958.
6. Crowell EB, Ketchum JS: The treatment of scopolamine-induced delirium. Clin Pharmacol Ther 8:409–414, 1967.
7. Duvoisin RC: Cholinergic-anticholinergic antagonism in Parkinsonism. Arch Neurol 17:124–136, 1967.
8. Duvoisin RC, Katz R: Reversal of central anticholinergic syndrome in man by physostigmine. JAMA 206:1963–1965, 1968.
9. Ecobichon DJ: Toxic effects of pesticides. In Klassen CD (ed): Casarett and Doull's Toxicology: The Basic Science of Poisons, 5th ed. New York, McGraw-Hill, 1996.
10. Somani SM, Dube SN: Physostigmine—an overview as pretreatment drug for organophosphate intoxication. Int J Clin Pharm Ther Toxicol 27:367–387, 1989.
11. Physostigmine salicylate injection (Product insert). Decatur, IL, Taylor Pharmaceuticals, 1998.
12. Lefkowitz RJ, Hoffman BB, Taylor P: The autonomic and somatic motor nervous systems. In Hardman JG, Limberd LE, Molinoff PB, et al (eds): Goodman and Gilman's the Pharmacological Basis of Therapeutics, 9th ed. New York, McGraw-Hill, 1996.
13. Nilsson E, Meretoja OA, Neuvonen P: Hemodynamic responses to physostigmine in patients with a drug overdose. Anesth Analg 62:885–888, 1983.
14. O'Keefe DB, Crome P, Medd RK: The effects physostigmine on amitriptyline induced cardiotoxicity in dogs. Vet Hum Toxicol 21(Suppl):58–60, 1979.
15. Janowsky DS, Risch SC, Ziegler MG, et al: Physostigmine-induced epinephrine release in patients with affective disorder. Am J Psychiatry 143:919–921, 1986.
16. Anderson JA: Reversal agents in sedation and anesthesia: A review. Anesth Prog 35:43–47, 1988.
17. Durieux ME: Muscarinic signaling in the central nervous system. Anesthesiology 84:173–198, 1996.
18. Avant GR, Speeg KV, Freemon FR, et al: Physostigmine reversal of diazepam-induced hypnosis. Ann Intern Med 92:53–55, 1979.
19. Toro-Matos A, Rendon-Platas AM, Avila-Valdez E, et al: Physostigmine antagonizes ketamine. Anesth Analg 59:764–767, 1980.
20. Snir-Mor I, Weinstock M, Davidson JT, et al: Physostigmine antagonizes morphine-induced respiratory depression in human subjects. Anesthesiology 59:6–9, 1983.
21. Rupreht J, Dworacek B: Physostigmine versus naloxone in heroin overdose. Clin Toxicol 21:387–397, 1983–1984.
22. Spaulding BC, Choi SD, Gross JB, et al: The effect of physostigmine on diazepam-induced ventilatory depression: A double-blind study. Anesthesiology 61:551–554, 1984.
23. Kesecioglu J, Rupreht J, Telci L, et al: Effect of aminophylline or physostigmine on recovery from nitrous oxide-enflurane anaesthesia. Acta Anaesthesiol Scand 35:616–620, 1991.
24. Fassoulaki A, Sarantopoulos C, Derveniotis C: Physostigmine increases the dose of propofol required to induce anaesthesia. Can J Anaesth 44:1148–1151, 1997.
25. Meuret P, Backman SB, Bonhomme V, et al: Physostigmine reverses propofol-induced unconsciousness and attenuation of the auditory steady state response and bispectral index in human volunteers. Anesthesiology 93:708–717, 2000.
26. Drummond JC, Brebner J, Galloon S, et al: A randomized evaluation of the reversal of ketamine by physostigmine. Can Anaesth Soc J 26:288–295, 1979.
27. Bourke DL: Physostigmine: effectiveness as an antagonist of respiratory depression and psychomotor effects cause by morphine or diazepam. Anesthesiology 61:523–528, 1984.
28. Garber JG: Physostigmine-atropine solution fails to reverse diazepam sedation. Anesth Analg 59:58–60, 1980.
29. Pandit UA, Kothary SP, Samra S, et al: Physostigmine fails to reverse clinical, psychomotor, or EEG effects of lorazepam. Anesth Analg 62:679–685, 1983.
30. Aquilonius SM, Hartvig P: Clinical pharmacokinetics of cholinesterase inhibitors. Clin Pharmacokinet 11:236–249, 1986.
31. Asthana S, Greig NH, Hegedus L, et al: Clinical pharmacokinetics of physostigmine in patients with Alzheimer's disease. Clin Pharmacol Ther 58:299–309, 1995.
32. Hartvig P, Wiklund L, Lindstrom B: Pharmacokinetics of physostigmine after IV, IM and subcutaneous administration in surgical patients. Acta Anaesthesiol Scand 30:177–182, 1986.
33. Knapp S, Wardlow ML, Albert K, et al: Correlation between plasma physostigmine concentrations and percentage of acetylcholinesterase inhibition over time after controlled release of physostigmine in volunteer subjects. Drug Metab Dispos 19:400–404, 1991.
34. Natel S, Bayne L, Ruedy J: Physostigmine in coma due to drug overdose. Clin Pharmacol Ther 25:96–102, 1979.
35. Snyder BD: Reversal of amitriptyline intoxication by physostigmine. JAMA 230:1433–1434, 1974.
36. Rumack BH: Anticholinergic poisoning: Treatment with physostigmine. Pediatrics 52:449–451, 1973.
37. Magera BE, Betlach CJ, Sweatt AP, et al: Hydroxyzine intoxication in a 13-month-old child. Pediatrics 67:280–283, 1981.
38. Gillick JS: Atropine toxicity in a neonate. Br J Anaesth 46:793–794, 1974.
39. Smiler BG, Bartholomew EG, Sivak BJ, et al: Physostigmine reversal of scopolamine delirium in obstetric patients. Am J Obstet Gynecol 116:326–329, 1972.
40. Sullivan GE: Proceedings: Paralysis and skeletal anomalies in chick embryos treated with physostigmine. J Anat 116:463–464, 1973.
40a. American Psychiatric Association. Practice Guidelines for Treatment of Patients with Delirium. Am J Psychiatry 156(5 Suppl):1–20, 1999.
41. Daunderer M: Physostigmine salicylate as an antidote. Int J Clin Pharmacol Ther Toxicol 18:523–535, 1980.
42. Burns MJ, Linden CH, Graudins A, et al: A comparison of physostigmine and benzodiazepines for the treatment of anticholinergic poisoning. Ann Emerg Med 35:374–381, 2000.

43. Heindl S, Binder C, Desel H, et al: Etiology of initially unexplained confusion of excitability in deadly nightshade poisoning with suicidal intent: Symptoms, differential diagnosis, toxicology and physostigmine therapy of anticholinergic syndrome. Dtsch Med Wochenschr 125:1361–1365, 2000.

44. Heiser JF: Reversal of delirium induced by tricyclic antidepressant drugs with physostigmine. Am J Psychiatry 127:1050–1054, 1971.

45. Munoz RA: Treatment of tricyclic intoxication. Am J Psychiatry 133:1085–1087, 1976.

46. Newton RW: Physostigmine salicylate in the treatment of tricyclic antidepressant overdosage. JAMA 231:941–943, 1975.

47. Walker WE, Levy RC, Hanenson IB: Physostigmine—its use and abuse. J Am Coll Emerg Physicians 5:436–439, 1976.

48. Lavoie FW, Gansert GG, Weiss RE: Value of initial ECG findings and plasma drug levels in cyclic antidepressant overdose. Ann Emerg Med 19:696–700, 1990.

49. Boehnert MT, Lovejoy FH: Value of the QRS duration versus the serum drug level in predicting seizures and ventricular arrhythmias after an acute overdose of tricyclic antidepressants. N Engl J Med 313:474–497, 1985.

50. Pall H, Czech K, Kotzaurek R, et al: Experiences with physostigmine salicylate in tricyclic antidepressant poisoning. Acta Pharmacol Toxicol 14(Suppl 2):171–178, 1977.

51. Aquilonius SM, Hedstrand U: The use of physostigmine as an antidote in tricyclic anti-depressant intoxication. Acta Anaesth Scand 22:40–45, 1978.

52. Ordiway MV: Treating tricyclic overdose with physostigmine. Am J Psychiatry 135:1114, 1978.

53. Ellison DW, Pentel PR: Clinical features and consequences of seizures due to cyclic antidepressant overdose. Am J Emerg Med 7:5–10, 1989.

54. Lipper B, Bell A, Gaynor B: Recurrent hypotension immediately after seizures in nortriptyline overdose. Am J Emerg Med 12:452–453, 1994.

55. Taboulet P, Michard F, Muszynski J, et al: Cardiovascular repercussions of seizures during cyclic antidepressant poisoning. J Toxicol Clin Toxicol 33:205–211, 1995.

56. Callaham M, Kassel D: Epidemiology of fatal tricyclic antidepressant ingestion: Implications for management. Ann Emerg Med 14:1–9, 1985.

57. Crome P, Newman B: Fatal tricyclic antidepressant poisoning. J R Soc Med 72:649–653, 1979.

58. Tong TG, Benowitz NL, Becker CE: Tricyclic antidepressant overdose. Drug Int Clin Pharm 10:711–713, 1976.

59. Pentel P, Peterson CK: Asystole complicating physostigmine treatment of tricyclic antidepressant overdose. Ann Emerg Med 9:588–590, 1980.

60. Shannon M: Toxicology reviews: Physostigmine. Pediatr Emerg Care 14:224–226, 1998.

61. Zandberg P, Sangster B: The influence of physostigmine on respiratory and circulatory changes caused by overdoses of orphenadrine or imipramine in the rat. Acta Pharmacol Toxicol 50:185–195, 1982.

62. Fleck CH, Braunlich H: Failure of physostigmine in intoxications with tricyclic antidepressants in rats. Toxicology 24:335–344, 1982.

63. Torchiana ML, Wenger HC, Lagerquist B, et al: Pharmacological antagonism of the toxic manifestations of amitriptyline and protriptyline in dogs. Toxicol Appl Pharmacol 21:383–389, 1972.

64. Vance MA, Ross SM, Millington WR, Blumberg JB: Potentiation of tricyclic antidepressant toxicity by physostigmine in mice. J Toxicol Clin Toxicol 11:413–421, 1977.

65. Goldberger AL, Curtis GP: Immediate effects of physostigmine on amitriptyline-induced QRS prolongation. J Toxicol Clin Toxicol 19:445–454, 1982.

66. Burns MJ, Linden CH, Graudins A: Physostigmine versus diazepines for anticholinergic poisoning (In reply). Ann Emerg Med 37:239–241, 2001.

67. Northup L, Reed G, McAnalley B, et al: Seizures due to maprotiline overdose. Ann Emerg Med 13:468–470, 1984.

68. Knudsen K, Heath A: Effects of self poisoning with maprotiline. BMJ 288:601–603, 1984.

69. Ueki S, Fujiwara M, Inoue K, et al: Behavior pharmacology of maprotiline, a new antidepressant. Nippon Yakurigaku Zasshi 71:789–815, 1975.

70. Buckley NA, Dawson AH, Whyte IM, et al: Greater toxicity in overdose of dothiepin than of other tricyclic antidepressants. Lancet 343:159–162, 1994.

71. Peterson CD: Seizures induced by acute loxapine overdose. Am J Psychiatry 138:1089–1091, 1981.

72. Litovitz TL, Troutman WG: Amoxapine overdose: Seizures and fatalities. JAMA 250:1069–1071, 1983.

73. Yates SW, Viera AJ: Physostigmine in the treatment of γ-hydroxybutyric acid overdose. Mayo Clin Proc 75:401–402, 2000.

74. Caldicott DG, Kuhn M: Gamma-hydroxybutyrate overdose and physostigmine: Teaching new tricks to an old drug. Ann Emerg Med 37:99–102, 2001.

75. Henderson RS, Holmes CM: Reversal of the anaesthetic action of sodium gamma-hydroxybutyrate. Anaesth Intensive Care 4:351–354, 1976.

76. Holmes CM, Henderson RS: The elimination of pollution by a non inhalational technique. Anaesth Intensive Care 6:120–124, 1978.

77. Kuhn M, Caldicott D: Use of physostigmine in the management of gamma-hydroxybutyrate overdose (In reply). Ann Emerg Med 38:347–348, 2001.

78. Rumack BH: Physostigmine: Rationale use (Editorial). J Am Coll Emerg Physicians 5:541–542, 1976.

79. Slang RD: Ponder physostigmine use (Editorial). J Emerg Med 3:485–486, 1985.

80. Weisdorf D, Kramer J, Goldbarg A, et al: Physostigmine for cardiac and neurologic manifestations of phenothiazine poisoning. Clin Pharmacol Ther 24:663–667, 1978.

81. Munoz RA, Kuplic JB: Large overdose of tricyclic antidepressants treated with physostigmine salicylate. Psychosomatics 16:77–78, 1975.

82. Danze LK, Langdorf, MI: Reversal of orphenadrine-induced ventricular tachycardia with physostigmine. J Emerg Med 9:453–457, 1991.

83. Schmidt W, Lang K: Life-threatening dysrhythmias in severe thioridazine poisoning treated with physostigmine and transient atrial pacing. Crit Care Med 25:1925–1930, 1997.

84. Miller MM, Fish JE, Patterson R: Methacholine and physostigmine airway reactivity in asthmatic and nonasthmatic subjects. J Allergy Clin Immunol 60:116–120, 1977.

85. Brunner GA, Fleck S, Pieber TR, et al: Near fatal anticholinergic intoxication after routine fundoscopy. Intensive Care Med 24:730–731, 1998.

86. Levy R: Arrhythmia following physostigmine administration in jimson weed poisoning. J Am Coll Emerg Physicians 6:107–108, 1977.

87. O'Donnell SJ, Burkhart KK, Donovan JW, et al: Safety of physostigmine use for anticholinergic toxicity. J Toxicol Clin Toxicol 40:634, 2002.

88. Nilsson E: Physostigmine treatment in various drug-induced intoxications. Ann Clin Res 14:165–172, 1982.

89. Cummings G, Harding LK, Prowse K: Treatment and recovery after massive overdose of physostigmine. Lancet 20:147–149, 1968.

90. Koppel C, Ibe K, Tenczer J: Clinical symptomatology of diphenhydramine overdose: An evaluation of 136 cases in 1982 to 1985. J Toxicol Clin Toxicol 25:53–70, 1987.

91. Schneck HJ, Rupreht J: Central anticholinergic syndrome (CAS) in anesthesia and intensive care. Acta Anaesthesiol Belg 40:219–228, 1989.

92. Dziukas LJ, Vohra J: Tricyclic antidepressant poisoning. Med J Aust 154:344–350, 1991.

93. Benjamin DR: Mushroom poisoning in infants and children: The *Amanita pantherina/muscaria* group. J Toxicol Clin Toxicol 30:13–22, 1992.

94. Dailey JW, Naritoku DK: Antidepressants and seizures: Clinical anecdotes overshadow neuroscience. Biochem Pharmacol 52:1323–1329, 1996.

95. Lader M: Some adverse effects of antipsychotics: prevention and treatment. J Clin Psychiatry 60(Suppl 12):18–21, 1999.

96. Radovanovic D, Meier PJ, Guirguis M, et al: Dose-dependent toxicity of diphenhydramine overdose. Hum Exp Toxicol 19:489–495, 2000.

97. Enginar N, Nurten A, Yamanturk P, et al: Scopolamine-induced convulsions in food given fasted mice: Effects of physostigmine and MK-801. Epilepsy Res 28:137–142, 1997.

98. Kamei C, Ohuchi M, Sugimoto Y, et al: Mechanism responsible for epileptogenic activity by first-generation H1-antagonists in rats. Brain Res 887:183–186, 2000.

99. Holger JS, Harris CR, Engebretsen KM: Physostigmine, sodium bicarbonate, or hypertonic saline to treat diphenhydramine toxicity. Vet Hum Toxicol 44:1–4, 2002.

100. Boon J, Prideaux PR: Cardiac arrest following physostigmine. Anaesth Intensive Care 8:92–93, 1980.
101. Kopman AF, Strachovsky G, Lichtenstein L: Prolonged response to succinylcholine following physostigmine. Anesthesiology 49:142–143, 1978.
102. Sunew KY, Hicks RG: Effects of neostigmine and pyridostigmine on duration of succinylcholine action and pseudocholinestrase activity. Anesthesiology 49:188–191, 1978.
103. Granacher RP, Baldessarini RJ: Physostigmine: Its use in acute anticholinergic syndrome with antidepressant and antiparkinson drugs. Arch Gen Psychiatry 32:375–379, 1975.
104. Domino EF: Comparative seizure inducing properties of various cholinesterase inhibitors: Antagonism by diazepam and midazolam. Neurotoxicology 8:113–122, 1987.
105. Janowsky DS, Drennan M, Berkowitz A, et al: Comparative effects of scopolamine and atropine in preventing cholinesterase inhibitor induced lethality. Milit Med 150:693–695, 1985.
106. Janowsky DS, Berkowitz A, Turken A, et al: Antagonism of physostigmine induced lethality by a combination of scopolamine and methscopolamine. Acta Pharmacol Toxicol 56:154–157, 1985.
107. Ketchum JS, Sidell FR, Crowell EB Jr, et al: Atropine, scopolamine, and ditran: Comparative pharmacology and antagonists in man. Psychopharmacologia 28:121–145, 1973.
108. Weiss S: Persistence of action of physostigmine and the atropine-physostigmine antagonism in animals and man. J Pharmacol Exp Ther 27:181–188, 1925.
109. Klemm WR: Efficacy and toxicity of drug combinations in treatment of physostigmine toxicosis. Toxicology 27:41–53, 1983.
110. Snyder BD: Reversal of amitriptyline intoxication by physostigmine. JAMA 230:1433–1434, 1974.
111. Holinger PC, Klawans HL: Reversal of tricyclic-overdose-induced central anticholinergic syndrome by physostigmine. Am J Psychiatry 133:1018–1023, 1976.
112. Dawson RM: Oxime effects on the rate constants of carbamylation and decarbamylation of acetylcholinesterase for pyridostigmine, physostigmine and insecticidal carbamates. Neurochem Int 26:643–654, 1995.
113. Brier RH: Physostigmine dose for tricyclic antidepressant overdose. Ann Intern Med 89:579, 1978.
114. Stern TA: Continuous infusion of physostigmine in anticholinergic delirium: Case report. J Clin Psychiatry 44:463–464, 1983.
115. Brashares ZA, Conley WR: Physostigmine in drug overdose. J Am Coll Emerg Physicians 5:46–48, 1975.
116. Grutzendler J, Morris JC: Cholinesterase inhibitors for Alzheimer's disease. Drugs 61:41–52, 2001.
117. Harvey AL: The pharmacology of galanthamine and its analogues. Pharmacol Ther 68:113–128, 1995.
118. Cozanitis DA, Toivakka E: Treatment of respiratory depression with the anticholinesterase drug galanthamine hydrobromide. Anaesthesia 29:581–584, 1974.
119. Cozanitis DA: Galanthamine hydrobromide, a longer acting anticholinesterase drug, in the treatment of the central effects of scopolamine (Hyoscine). Anaesthetist 26:649–650, 1977.
120. Baraka A, Harik S: Reversal of central anticholinergic syndrome by galanthamine. JAMA 238:2293–2294, 1977.
121. Polinsky RJ: Clinical pharmacology of rivastigmine: A new-generation acetylcholinesterase inhibitor for the treatment of Alzheimer's disease. Clin Ther 20:634–647, 1998.
122. Litovitz TL, Klein-Schwartz W, White S, et al: 2000 Annual Reports of the American Association of Poison Control Centers Toxic Exposure Surveillance System. Am J Emerg Med 19:337–395, 2001.

CHAPTER 154

Anti-Digitalis Fab Fragments

Bruno Mégarbane ▪ Stephen W. Borron ▪ Frédéric J. Baud

Digitalis poisoning is rare but may be responsible for life-threatening complications.[1,2] Intoxication may result from suicidal or unintentional ingestion of a single large dose or from accumulation during long-term dosing. Immunotoxicotherapy with anti-digitalis Fab fragments now is the first-line treatment in cases of severe digitalis poisoning. Several concerns remain, however, including indications, minimal efficient dose, and the optimal mode of administration. Despite being an expensive therapy, anti-digoxin Fab was considered beneficial in a cost-effectiveness analysis for the treatment of digoxin toxicity.[3] It also seemed useful in poisonings with digitoxin and plants containing cardiac glycosides, such as oleander, foxglove, and lily of the valley.[4–6] The commercial products, Digidote (80 mg) and Digibind (40 mg) are safe and effective digitalis antitoxins.

HISTORY

Assessment of anti-digoxin Fab fragments for the treatment of cardiac glycoside toxicity began with the development of specific antibodies for immunoassay. Subsequent experimental and clinical studies on anti-digoxin Fab allowed determination of the fundamental mechanisms of modern immunotoxicotherapy. Butler and Chen[7] first suggested that purified anti-digoxin antibodies with high affinity and specificity should be developed to treat human digoxin poisonings. Digoxin, with a molecular weight of 781 d, was too small to be immunogenic, however, so it was necessary to link it to serum bovine albumin to generate antibodies in immunized sheep. Highly purified antibodies were obtained by separation techniques, and in vitro and animal studies were employed to assess their ability to bind cardiac glycosides avidly.[7–12] Intact IgG anti-digoxin antibodies reversed digoxin toxicity in dogs, but excretion of the digoxin/IgG complexes was delayed, and risks of hypersensitivity reactions or secondary digoxin release were postulated. Fab fragments of 50 kd were obtained by treating these IgG anti-digoxin antibodies with papain, yielding a safer and more effective therapy.[9]

In 1976, Smith and colleagues[13] described the first clinical use of digoxin-specific antibody fragments in a human. Thereafter, clinical studies dealing with large numbers of poisoned patients allowed the assessment of the safety of Fab fragments. Since 1976, large series of cardiac glycoside poisonings treated with anti-digoxin Fab fragments have been published, including 717 cases by Hickey and colleagues,[14] 150 cases by Antman and associates,[15] 34 cases by Smolarz

and coworkers,[16] and 28 cases by Taboulet and coworkers.[17,18] In the observational surveillance study of 717 cases, 50% of the poisoned patients exhibited full resolution of all symptoms of digitalis toxicity, 24% exhibited a partial response, and 12% exhibited no response.[14] Lack of response was explained by an insufficient dose of Fab fragments, the presence of a moribund state, or a diagnosis other than digitalis poisoning. None of the patients without heart disease who ingested a single overdose was a nonresponder. In this study, 54% of the 56 patients who had had a cardiac arrest survived, compared with 100% mortality before the advent of Fab.[15,19] No clear relationship was established, however, between the initial dose and the response to treatment, rendering it difficult to establish an effective dose. After this report, recrudescent toxicity (atrioventricular block, ventricular arrhythmias, or asystole) was reported, with rates varying from 2.8% in the series of 717 cases[14] to 11% in the series of 28 cases (which included many digitoxin poisonings).[17,18] More recently, earlier use of Fab therapy, before cardiac pacing or treatment with antiarrhythmic agents, has been advocated.[18]

PROPERTIES

Anti-digoxin Fab fragments are derived by papain cleavage (Fig. 135-1) of all the heterologous IgG sheep-derived digoxin-specific antibodies, leading to the removal of the F_c fragment and a substantial reduction in the molecular weight (50 kd) and the risk of hypersensitivity. As shown by radioimmunoassay of digoxin levels, anti-digoxin Fab showed high affinity for digoxin and sufficient cross-reactivity with digitoxin to be clinically useful.[5] Because of structural similarities among all cardiac glycosides, anti-digoxin Fab can neutralize lanatoside C, proscillaridin, and scilliroside toxins and other glycosides found in *Nerium oleander* and toad venom.[4,6] Higher doses may be needed in these other glycoside poisonings, however, because of the lower affinity binding of Fab to these toxins.

PHARMACODYNAMICS

Immunotoxicotherapy is a toxicokinetic treatment inducing redistribution of the cardiac glycoside to the extracellular compartment.[20] Affinity of digoxin for Fab (10^9 to 10^{11} M^{-1}) is greater than its affinity for the membrane-bound Na^+,K^+-ATPase receptors. The redistribution is so rapid and complete that symptoms usually resolve within a few minutes.

So-called cardiac glycosides inhibit Na$^+$,K$^+$-ATPases located on the external membrane of myocardial cells. In patients with chronic exposures, compared with patients with acute overdoses, less digoxin is necessary for the development of symptoms.[21] Reversibility of the binding of these glycosides to this molecular target has been shown with Fab fragments. Clinical studies have shown that the onset of Fab action is rapid when the Fab fragments are infused over 20 to 30 minutes. Reversal of the toxic clinical effects of digitalis occurred within 1 hour after administration. Most patients who responded had clinically evident improvement by 1 hour after termination of infusion and had a complete response, including the resolution of hyperkalemia, by 4 hours.[15] Anti-digoxin Fab also quickly improved digitalis intoxication–related gastrointestinal disturbances, including ischemic colitis.[22]

PHARMACOKINETICS

Pharmacokinetics of Digoxin-Specific Fab Fragments

Apparent volume of distribution: 25–54 L
Distribution: biphasic or triphasic
Elimination half-life: 10–20 hr in patients with normal renal function, 10-fold in patients with renal failure
Total body clearance: 24.5 mL/min
Renal clearance: 13.6 mL/min

Anti-digoxin Fab fragments are effective in digitalis poisoning by causing (1) induction of an extracellular redistribution of the toxin, (2) its sequestration in extracellular spaces, and (3) the renal elimination of the antibody/toxin complex.[13,20,23] Administered intravenously, these fragments bind immediately to circulating free digitalis molecules, forming complexes unable to bind to tissue digitalis receptors. After infusion of a dose containing equimolar binding sites, total serum digoxin concentration increases 5 to 20 times, whereas unbound serum digitalis decreases to 0 within minutes. By mass action resulting from the concentration gradient from their target tissue to the interstitial and intravascular spaces, free intracellular digitalis and receptor-bound digitalis are displaced, and reactivation of membrane ATPases ensues. Ultimately, bound toxin/Fab elimination depends on renal function.[24]

Serum Fab concentrations exhibit a biphasic or triphasic decline, reflecting their distribution into different compartments and their excretion and nonrenal elimination. The elimination half-life of Fab/digoxin complexes is about 10 to 20 hours in patients with normal renal function, compared with spontaneous half-lives of 39 hours for digoxin and 160 hours for digitoxin. The elimination half-life of Fab/digoxin complexes is prolonged 10-fold in the case of renal failure, with no changes in the volume of distribution.[24] Schaumann and associates[25] calculated a volume of distribution ranging from 25.4 to 54 L for anti-digoxin Fab. The total body clearance of Fab was estimated at 24.5 mL/min, of which 13.6 mL/min was renal clearance.

The advantages of anti-digoxin Fab compared with the whole IgG antibody are a threefold increase in volume of distribution, more rapid onset of action, smaller risk of adverse immunologic effects, and more rapid elimination.[26] More recent data, based on comparisons of the volume of distribution of immunoglobulins and Fab fragments, suggested that Fab fragments might enter cells despite their molecular weight. The apparent volume of distribution of Fab fragments is greater than the volume of extracellular water.[25]

After acute massive ingestion, serum digoxin concentration does not correlate with myocardial concentrations, and tissue distribution occurs with a delay of about 4 to 6 hours. After anti-digoxin administration, standard serum digoxin concentration determinations measure unbound and bound digoxin. Methods using ultrafiltration make free digoxin measurements possible. After infusion of sufficient doses of Fab, the unbound digoxin concentration decreases to an undetectable level, with a reappearance 5 to 24 hours later, depending on the dose, the infusion technique, and the patient's renal function. There is no evidence of dissociation of the Fab/digoxin complex over time. The rebound in free digoxin concentrations is secondary to Fab's leaving the vascular space, digoxin's effluxing from the tissues, and possibly continued gastrointestinal absorption.

The institution of a maintenance infusion after the loading dose reduces the early reappearance of free digoxin. The loading dose immediately binds digoxin present in the vascular space and the digoxin that is redistributed rapidly to the vascular space. The maintenance dose provides enough Fab to capture digoxin redistributed from the tissues into the serum. The risk of too rapid an infusion is that elimination of Fab occurs before redistribution of digoxin from its binding sites. In this case, the total amount of Fab effectively bound to digoxin is less than that predicted.[25]

SPECIAL POPULATIONS

Neonatal and Pediatric Patients

Pediatric patients with no underlying heart disease generally tolerate higher doses of digoxin than do adults. The administration of Fab is indicated in infants and young children with ingested digoxin doses of greater than or equal to 0.3 mg/kg, underlying heart disease, serum digoxin concentration greater than or equal to 6.4 nmol/L ($\geq$5 ng/mL), life-threatening arrhythmia, hemodynamic instability, hyperkalemia ($\geq$6 mmol/L), or rapidly progressive toxicity.[27–31] Pediatric patients with chronic exposure may be treated successfully with small doses of Fab because of their small body burden of digoxin, whereas acute overdose requires quantities similar to those in adults.

Elderly Patients

The elderly are at relatively greater risk for severe digitalis intoxication.[32] Age 55 years and older has been shown to be associated with an increase in mortality rate.[21] Fab fragments are also useful for digoxin-induced acute psychosis (digitalis delirium), characterized by severe agitation, delusional thinking, and assaultive behavior.

Pregnant and Breast-feeding Patients

Although digitalis passes through the placenta, few data are available on embryonic or fetal toxicity. Fab transplacental passage is poorly understood. Pregnant patients with acute digitalis overdose should be treated similarly to nonpregnant patients. In case of in utero exposure, the efficacy and safety of anti-digoxin Fab for the fetus are not documented. Fetal cardiac rhythm should be monitored, and, if necessary, the fetus can be delivered and Fab administered to the neonate, as indicated by clinical signs and blood levels. Digitalis compounds are excreted in breast milk.

Renal Insufficiency Patients

Patients with renal failure on dialysis respond to Fab treatment in a manner similar to that in patients with normal renal function.[15] A theoretical possibility exists, however, that digoxin could be released with recurrence of toxicity because of decreased clearance of digoxin Fab. In the case of anephric patients, Fab fragments are effective, although symptoms may recur 7 to 14 days later, indicating the need for an additional dose. Among 18 patients with a pretreatment serum creatinine of greater than or equal to 4 mg/dL, including 5 patients on dialysis, recurrence of toxicity was observed only in 1 dialyzed patient. A multivariate analysis performed on the series of 717 cases did not show an increased risk of recrudescent toxicity in patients with renal failure.[14] The rebound in digoxin concentration is delayed in patients with renal dysfunction, presumably secondary to a prolonged distribution phase, and serum Fab concentrations remain detectable for 2 to 3 weeks, with a parallel decline in total digoxin serum concentration.[24]

CONTRAINDICATIONS

There are no known contraindications, apart from allergy to sheep immunoglobulin. No interactions with other medications have been reported.

PRECAUTIONS

Considering the risk of allergy, particularly in cases of repeated administration, manufacturers recommend intracutaneous or conjunctival allergy tests before Fab administration. Most toxicologists believe that the risk of sensitization to sheep Fab fragments is low, however, and that such testing is unnecessary. After infusion, patients require close monitoring because a second dose may be necessary if toxicity recurs or fails to resolve. In nondigoxin digitalis poisoning, required doses of Fab may be higher, as reported in the case of a child poisoned after ingesting yew berries, which contain taxine, a cardiac glycoside.[10] Recurrence of toxicity is infrequent, and its exact mechanism still is not understood fully. There is no evidence to support a dissociation of the Fab/digoxin complexes over extended periods.[33,34] Recrudescent toxicity seems to be related to redistribution of free digoxin into the serum. Compatible clinical signs are not always accompanied by an increase in unbound digoxin concentrations, however.

ADVERSE EFFECTS

Safety of a single low dose of Fab fragments was assessed in multiple case series involving approximately 900 patients, with rare adverse effects.[14–16,18] Mild hypersensitivity reactions, including pruritic rash, facial swelling and flushing, urticaria, thrombocytopenia, shaking, and chills, occurred in only 0.8% of the treated patients. Because anti-digoxin Fab fragments are obtained from ovine serum, there is a theoretical possibility of sensitization.[35] The likelihood of allergic reaction was greater in patients with allergy or asthma history.[14] Results of skin testing before Fab treatment were reported in 94 patients and were uniformly negative except for one patient who developed erythema without wheal or induration.[15] One patient received Fab three separate times over the course of 1 year as treatment for attempted suicide by digitalis ingestion, with no evidence of adverse effects.[36] No cross-reactivity was noted with endogenous steroids that have structural similarities to digoxin.

Adverse reactions caused by rapid reversal of the effects of digitalis, such as accelerated ventricular rate in atrial fibrillation, worsened left ventricular function, or hypokalemia, were noted in 7% of 717 treated patients.[14] In a several-hour-old neonate, hypokalemia, worsening of congestive heart failure, and transient apnea were reported.[15]

ADMINISTRATION

The efficacy of anti-digitalis Fab fragments in decreasing the mortality rate of digitalis intoxication has not been proved by prospective controlled clinical trials. The mortality rate ranged from 4.6% to 41% before availability of Fab fragments[2] and 6% to 29% after their availability.[15,16] These results raise questions regarding the accuracy of diagnosis, the selection of patients to receive Fab, and the amount and dosage regimen of Fab administration.

Fab administration initially was restricted to patients exhibiting actual or potentially life-threatening cardiac rhythm disturbances or hyperkalemia caused by digitalis intoxication when these conditions were refractory to treatment with conventional therapeutic modalities. The notion of administering conventional therapy, which results in delays in Fab administration, has been called into question, however.[17,18] Delaying the administration of Fab fragments by waiting for the appearance of life-threatening symptoms may preclude their benefit. The decision to administer digoxin Fab fragments should take into account their known safety and the persistently high mortality of digitalis poisoning. Because many adult overdoses are polypharmaceutical, it is important to consider other toxicants in patients not responding to this antidote.

Dose

The dose of Fab fragments is calculated on a molar basis to be equal to the amount of digoxin or digitoxin in the body.[15] The body burden of cardiac glycoside may be calculated using either the supposed ingested dose or the serum digitalis concentration. Experimental data show the efficiency of Fab doses in full stoichiometric equivalence. The

Calculation of Dosage of Fab Fragments from Body Load of Glycoside

From the ingested amount, if the amount and type of digitalis are known:

$$Q = IA \cdot A$$

Q = Body load of glycoside (mg)
IA = Ingested amount of glycoside (mg)
A = Digoxin bioavailability (0.6) or digitoxin bioavailability (1)

From the serum glycoside concentration, if the steady-state serum concentration is known:

$$Q = SGC \cdot Vd \cdot Wt \, 10^{-3}$$

Q = Body load of glycoside (mg)
SGC = Serum glycoside concentration (ng/mL)
Vd = Distribution volume: 5.61 L/kg (digoxin) or 0.56 L/kg (digitoxin)
Wt = Patient weight (kg)

Conversion factors:
SGC (nmol/L) × 0.781 = SGC (ng/mL) for digoxin
SGC (nmol/L) × 0.765 = SGC (ng/mL) for digitoxin

Determination of the number of 40-mg vials needed*:

$$Q/0.6$$

Empirical dosing recommendations with 40-mg vials:
Acute ingestion: adult—10 to 20 vials
Chronic toxicity: adult—3 to 6 vials

*Fab fragment dose (mg) = [molecular weight Fab (50 kd)/molecular weight digoxin (781 d)] × body load (mg). Using this calculation, 0.6 mg of digoxin is neutralized by each 40-mg vial of Fab fragments.

accuracy of these calculations is questionable, however, for many reasons. The ingested dose frequently is not known with accuracy. Calculation of the number of vials from the ingested amount also may overestimate the dose of needed Fab because loss of digitalis may result from vomiting, gastric lavage, or activated charcoal administration. The measured plasma concentration of digoxin accurately reflects the body load, but only after equilibration, which requires at least 6 hours after the last dose. The volume of distribution of digoxin also may be smaller in certain disease states (e.g., renal disease, hypothyroidism). It is unclear whether the theoretical equimolar dose is attained or exceeded. The necessity of administering an equimolar dose of Fab to obtain an initial beneficial response is not supported by the literature.[14] Initial response to therapy generally is favorable, with doses below the equimolar ratio, whereas the risk of recrudescent toxicity is more frequent if less than 50% of the estimated full neutralizing dose was administered. If initial administration of Fab fails to reduce digitalis-induced arrhythmias, another dose should be administered.

Route of Administration

Anti-digitalis Fab fragments should be diluted in sterile isotonic saline solution and administered intravenously in a monitored setting. When reconstituted, the preparation should be used immediately or, if refrigerated, within 4 hours. The dosage regimen initially proposed included the administration of the dose of Fab fragments over 15 to 30 minutes. More recent data suggested that the duration of Fab infusion should be increased to optimize the binding of digoxin to Fab fragments.[25,37] Schaumann and colleagues[25] recommended a loading dose of four to six vials, followed by 0.5 mg/min for 8 hours. The optimal dosage regimen using the minimal effective dose remains to be determined.

REFERENCES

1. Bayer MJ: Recognition and management of digitalis intoxication: Implications for emergency medicine. Am J Emerg Med 9(2 Suppl 1):29–32, 1991.
2. Kelly RA, Smith TW: Recognition and management of digitalis toxicity. Am J Cardiol 69:108G-118G, 1992.
3. Mauskopf JA, Wenger TL: Cost-effectiveness analysis of the use of digoxin immune Fab (ovine) for treatment of digoxin toxicity. Am J Cardiol 68:1709–1714, 1991.
4. Hess T, Stucki P, Barandun S, et al: Treatment of a case of lanatoside C intoxication with digoxin-specific F(ab')2 antibody fragments. Am Heart J 98:767–771, 1979.
5. Kurowski V, Iven H, Djonlagic H: Treatment of a patient with severe digitoxin intoxication by Fab fragments of anti-digitalis antibodies. Intensive Care Med 18:439–442, 1992.
6. Shumaik GM, Wu AW, Ping AC: Oleander poisoning: Treatment with digoxin-specific Fab antibody fragments. Ann Emerg Med 17:732–735, 1988.
7. Butler VP Jr, Chen JP: Digoxin-specific antibodies. Proc Natl Acad Sci U S A 57:71–78, 1967.
8. Butler VP Jr, Schmidt DH, Smith TW, et al: Effects of sheep digoxin-specific antibodies and their Fab fragments on digoxin pharmacokinetics in dogs. J Clin Invest 59:345–359, 1977.
9. Butler VP Jr, Smith TW, Schmidt DH, Haber E: Immunological reversal of the effects of digoxin. Fed Proc 36:2235–2241, 1977.
10. Curd J, Smith TW, Jaton JC, Haber E: The isolation of digoxin-specific antibody and its use in reversing the effects of digoxin. Proc Natl Acad Sci U S A 68:2401–2406, 1971.
11. Schmidt DH, Butler VP Jr: Immunological protection against digoxin toxicity. J Clin Invest 50:866–871, 1971.
12. Schmidt DH, Butler VP Jr: Reversal of digoxin toxicity with specific antibodies. J Clin Invest 50:1738–1744, 1971.
13. Smith TW, Haber E, Yeatman L, Butler VP Jr: Reversal of advanced digoxin intoxication with Fab fragments of digoxin-specific antibodies. N Engl J Med 294:797–800, 1976.
14. Hickey AR, Wenger TL, Carpenter VP, et al: Digoxin immune Fab therapy in the management of digitalis intoxication: Safety and efficacy results of an observational surveillance study. J Am Coll Cardiol 17:590–598, 1991.
15. Antman EM, Wenger TL, Butler VP Jr, et al: Treatment of 150 cases of life-threatening digitalis intoxication with digoxin-specific Fab antibody fragments: Final report of a multicenter study. Circulation 81:1744–1752, 1990.
16. Smolarz A, Roesch E, Lenz E, et al: Digoxin specific antibody (Fab) fragments in 34 cases of severe digitalis intoxication. J Toxicol Clin Toxicol 23:327–340, 1985.
17. Taboulet P, Baud FJ, Bismuth C, Vicaut E: Acute digitalis intoxication—is pacing still appropriate? J Toxicol Clin Toxicol 31:261–273, 1993.
18. Taboulet P, Baud FJ, Bismuth C: Clinical features and management of digitalis poisoning—rationale for immunotherapy. J Toxicol Clin Toxicol 31:247–260, 1993.
19. Bismuth C, Motte G, Conso F, et al: Acute digitoxin intoxication treated by intracardiac pacemaker: Experience in sixty-eight patients. Clin Toxicol 10:443–456, 1977.
20. Baud FJ, Borron SW, Bismuth C: Modifying toxicokinetics with antidotes. Toxicol Lett 82–83:785–793, 1995.
21. Borron SW, Bismuth C, Muszynski J: Advances in the management of digoxin toxicity in the older patient. Drugs Aging 10:18–33, 1997.
22. Bourhis F, Riard P, Danel V, et al: [Digitalis poisoning with severe ischemic colitis: A favorable course after treatment with specific antibodies]. Gastroenterol Clin Biol 14:95, 1990.
23. Urtizberea M, Sabouraud A, Baud F, et al: Concepts for toxicokinetic-toxicodynamic modelling in clinical toxicology: Application to acute

cardiac glycoside intoxications. Arch Toxicol 15(Suppl):253–256, 1992.

24. Renard C, Grene-Lerouge N, Beau N, et al: Pharmacokinetics of digoxin-specific Fab: Effects of decreased renal function and age. Br J Clin Pharmacol 44:135–138, 1997.
25. Schaumann W, Kaufmann B, Neubert P, Smolarz A: Kinetics of the Fab fragments of digoxin antibodies and of bound digoxin in patients with severe digoxin intoxication. Eur J Clin Pharmacol 30:527–533, 1986.
26. Lloyd BL, Smith TW: Contrasting rates of reversal of digoxin toxicity by digoxin-specific IgG and Fab fragments. Circulation 58:280–283, 1978.
27. Berkovitch M, Akilesh MR, Gerace R, et al: Acute digoxin overdose in a newborn with renal failure: Use of digoxin immune Fab and peritoneal dialysis. Ther Drug Monit 16:531–533, 1994.
28. Gittelman MA, Stephan M, Perry H: Acute pediatric digoxin ingestion. Pediatr Emerg Care 15:359–362, 1999.
29. Kaufman J, Leikin J, Kendzierski D, Polin K: Use of digoxin Fab immune fragments in a seven-day-old infant. Pediatr Emerg Care 6:118–121, 1990.
30. Schmitt K, Tulzer G, Hackel F, et al: Massive digitoxin intoxication treated with digoxin-specific antibodies in a child. Pediatr Cardiol 15:48–49, 1994.
31. Woolf AD, Wenger T, Smith TW, Lovejoy FH Jr: The use of digoxin-specific Fab fragments for severe digitalis intoxication in children. N Engl J Med 326:1739–1744, 1992.
32. Wofford JL, Ettinger WH: Risk factors and manifestations of digoxin toxicity in the elderly. Am J Emerg Med 9(2 Suppl 1):11–15, 1991.
33. Ujhelyi MR, Robert S, Cummings DM, et al: Influence of digoxin immune Fab therapy and renal dysfunction on the disposition of total and free digoxin. Ann Intern Med 119:273–277, 1993.
34. Ujhelyi MR, Robert S: Pharmacokinetic aspects of digoxin-specific Fab therapy in the management of digitalis toxicity. Clin Pharmacokinet 28:483–493, 1995.
35. Kirkpatrick CH: Allergic histories and reactions of patients treated with digoxin immune Fab (ovine) antibody. The Digibind Study Advisory Panel. Am J Emerg Med 9(2 Suppl 1):7–10, 1991.
36. Bosse GM, Pope TM: Recurrent digoxin overdose and treatment with digoxin-specific Fab antibody fragments. J Emerg Med 12:179–185, 1994.
37. Keyler DE, Salerno DM, Murakami MM, et al: Rapid administration of high-dose human antibody Fab fragments to dogs: Pharmacokinetics and toxicity. Fundam Appl Toxicol 17:83–91, 1991.

CHAPTER **155**

Methylene Blue

Jack Clifton II ▪ Jerrold B. Leikin

Methylene blue was one of the first antimalarial agents to be used clinically. It was also used as an intestinal and urinary antiseptic since the 19th century.[1] Since that time, methylene blue has mostly been abandoned for these clinical indications owing to the discovery of much more effective agents. Today, however, methylene blue continues to be a component of certain medications, used to treat urinary tract infections, including Atrosept, Dolsed, UAA, Uridon Modified, Urised, Uritin, and Prosed/DS. Methylene blue also has many nontoxicologic medical uses. A major use of methylene blue by clinical toxicologists is in the treatment of methemoglobinemia, a condition discussed in detail in Chapter 28. Methylene blue was reported to have been administered as an antidote in the United States 85 times last year by poison centers.[2] It is likely that this report represented a fraction of its total antidotal use.

Nontoxicologic Medical Uses for Methylene Blue

Urinary tract infections, antiseptic,[1] antimalarial agent[1]
Nasolacrimal dust patency[73]
Topical ophthalmic medication[74]
Detection of cerebrospinal fluid leaks after intrathecal administration[75]
Detection of enteroperitoneal fistulas[76]
Evaluation of fallopian tube patency after cervical administration[64,77]
Component of cancer chemotherapeutic regimens[78–84]
Histochemical staining reagent[85]
Priapism treatment[86]
Viral inactivation[87–94]
Treatment for septic shock[95]
Management of condylomata acuminata[96]
Reduction of intraperitoneal surgical adhesions[97]
Treatment of hepatopulmonary syndrome[98]
Inhibition of postintervention restenosis of vessels[99]
Use in multiple indicator dilution studies of in situ pulmonary endothelium[100]
Multidrug-resistant reverser in cells[101]
Component of protein solder for vascular anastomoses[102]
Intraoperative parathyroid gland identification[103]
Targeting of melanomas[104]
Supravital stain[105]
Detection of prepartum leakage in the presence of twins after intraamniotic infusion (rarely used)[27,28,46–57]

HISTORY

Before its use in the treatment of methemoglobinemia, methylene blue was used as an antidote for cyanide and carbon monoxide poisoning. After the studies of Sahlin in 1926 and Eddy in the early 1930s as reported by Hanzlik,[3] Geiger[4] was the first to use methylene blue clinically as an antidote for cyanide poisoning. Geiger, the director of public health in San Francisco at that time, reported the demise of three patients from cyanide poisoning treated with supportive care only. A fourth patient, following an attempted suicide by potassium cyanide ingestion, was resuscitated successfully, however, using 50 mL of 1% methylene blue solution. At the same time, numerous cases of the successful treatment of patients with carbon monoxide poisoning with methylene blue were reported.[5–7] Today, more effective and appropriate therapies are available for carbon monoxide and cyanide poisoning.

The first reported case showing the use of methylene blue to treat methemoglobinemia was by Williams and Challis,[8] who described their treatment of a male university student exposed to parabromaniline and who presented with a skin color of "mauve lavender." Spectrophotometric evaluation confirmed the disappearance of methemoglobin from the blood after treatment with methylene blue. Animal experimentation with two rabbits by these authors, published in conjunction with this case report, showed that 5 to 6 mg/kg of a 1% methylene blue solution was effective in treating methemoglobinemia. The reported patient was treated with 1000 mg of methylene blue as an intravenous 1% solution. Williams and Challis[8] chose to use methylene blue in their reported case and animal studies because of the previous literature suggesting the utility of this dye in cyanide and carbon monoxide poisoning. Steele and Spink[9] reported a similar reversal of methemoglobinemia in two cases, one aniline induced and the other caused by acetanilid intoxication, after the administration of methylene blue at a dose of approximately 4 mg/kg. The reversal of methemoglobinemia by methylene blue reported by these authors did not elicit enthusiasm at the time because it was thought of as the antidote for cyanide toxicity. In addition, there were reports that warned of the potential problem of methylene blue paradoxically inducing methemoglobinemia.[10–12]

Nadler and colleagues[13] examined the possible induction of methemoglobinemia by intravenous methylene blue (50 mL of 1% solution) administered to 18 healthy adult volunteers. This was the same dose reported by Geiger to be effective in the treatment of his cyanide-poisoned patient. Assuming that the volunteers weighed 50 to 70 kg, this would constitute a 5- to 7-mg/kg dose of methylene blue. Neither Geiger nor Nadler provided the actual weights of the patient or volunteers treated; however, a letter to the editor of the *Journal of the American Medical Association* by Bodansky[14] in 1950 stated that the dose was approximately 7 mg/kg. Nadler and colleagues[13] showed that in their volunteers methemoglobin concentrations never exceeded 1.3 g/dL and that the side effects, including electrocardiogram changes, "a sense of oppression in the chest," dysuria, nausea, and blue discoloration of the skin and mucous membranes, were due not to the presence of methemoglobin, but rather to the direct effects of the dye itself.

Wendel,[15] who had shown that methylene blue's mode of action in cyanide toxicity derived from its ability to form methemoglobin, initially expressed disbelief in the ability of methylene blue to reduce the concentrations of methemoglobin in the blood. His own later studies in dogs with sulfanilamide-induced methemoglobinemia showed, however, that intravenous administration of methylene blue at 5 mg/kg would increase the normal conversion rate of methemoglobin to hemoglobin by 8-fold to 10-fold, and a dose of only 1 mg/kg intravenously would increase this rate 3-fold to 4-fold.[16] Gutmann and coworkers[17] later elucidated the mechanism by which methylene blue reduces methemoglobin levels.

Further refinement of the dosage of methylene blue required for the treatment of methemoglobinemia arose from the work of Hartmann and colleagues.[18] This was a case series of six patients, ranging from 3.5 to 11 years of age, admitted to the hospital with an infection and treated with sulfanilamide. Four patients developed methemoglobinemia, which was treated successfully with methylene blue at doses of 1 to 2 mg/kg intravenously or 65 to 130 mg/day orally (3.8 to 4.7 mg/kg/dose; 18.9 to 23.9 mg/kg/day). Two of the six children were given methylene blue orally concomitant with the sulfanilamide administration and had no methemoglobinemia. This series suggested that elevated methemoglobin concentrations could be treated successfully with a methylene blue dose of 1 to 2 mg/kg and that the higher doses administered in earlier studies were unnecessary. Additional reported cases of methemoglobinemia confirmed the safety and efficacy of intravenous methylene blue administered at 1 to 2 mg/kg.[19–21]

Etteldorf[22] reported eight premature infants, ages 6 to 26 days, all of whom developed methemoglobinemia after being placed in new cloth diapers with the name of the hospital recently stamped on them with an aniline-containing ink. Seven of the eight infants were discovered to be neurologically depressed, with cyanosis of the nail beds and mucous membranes, and with methemoglobin concentrations ranging from 10% to 60%. These infants received methylene blue intravenously at a dose of 1.5 mg/kg (0.1% via a scalp vein). All had clinical responses within 15 to 30 minutes, simultaneous with the resolution of the methemoglobinemia. Strauch and colleagues[23] published a report of the development of methemoglobinemia in a 2-year-old girl with burns over 50% of her body after treatment with topical 0.5% silver nitrate. Her methemoglobin concentration of 59% and clinical findings resolved 15 to 30 minutes after the initiation of intravenous methylene blue at a dose of 2 mg/kg. Wendel[15] reported that dogs with sodium nitrite–induced methemoglobinemia responded rapidly to the intravenous

administration of 2 mg/kg of methylene blue, which also reportedly increased the rate of conversion of methemoglobin to hemoglobin by fourfold to fivefold. This report also described 100 cyanotic patients receiving sulfanilamide; 90 of these had methemoglobin concentrations of greater than 3%, and 35 had methemoglobin levels of 15% to 40%. The administration of 1 to 2 mg/kg of intravenous methylene blue to these patients was associated with rapid clinical improvement and resolution of methemoglobinemia.[24]

The generally recommended dose of methylene blue for the treatment of methemoglobinemia is 1 to 2 mg/kg intravenously. Continuous intravenous administration of methylene blue, in doses ranging from 0.1 mg/kg/hr for 96 hours to 3 to 7 mg/kg/hr for 7 days, has been reported in the treatment of dapsone intoxication. Acute Heinz body hemolytic anemia, as a result of either the dapsone or the methylene blue treatment, was reported in both patients. Until further evidence of its safety and efficacy can be attained, methylene blue therapy via continuous intravenous administration is not recommended.[25,26]

PROPERTIES

Chemical

Methylene blue (Fig. 155-1), with its polycyclic, planar ring structure, is a chromophore possessing the ability to absorb photons (λ_{max} 665 nm) with consequent transformation to a short-lived excited state. The chromophore character of methylene blue is essential for the important role this cationic dye assumes in the treatment of methemoglobinemia because it allows the molecule to accept electrons from the nicotinamide-adenine dinucleotide phosphate (reduced form) (NADPH)–dependent methemoglobin reductase and subsequently donate them to methemoglobin with the resultant reduction back to hemoglobin. This same characteristic is also the basis of the methylene blue–associated phototoxicity reactions that have been noted in neonates having been exposed to it intraamniotically and who then were placed under phototherapy lights for hyperbilirubinemia.[27,28]

Physical

Methylene blue, tetramethyl thionine chloride (anhydrous form, CAS* no. 61-73-4; trihydrate form, CAS no. 7220-79-3), is a water-soluble and alcohol-soluble compound with a

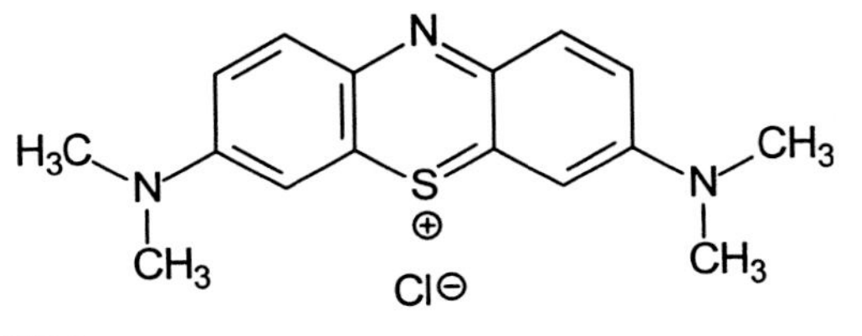

FIGURE 155-1

Chemical structure of methylene blue (tetramethylthionine chloride).

---

*Chemical Abstracts Service number.

molecular weight of 373.90 and a maximum absorption at wavelength of 665 nm. First prepared by Caro in 1876, this compound now is usually prepared from dimethylaniline and thiosulfuric acid. The trihydrate form usually is found as dark green crystals with a bronzelike luster and a slight odor or as a crystalline powder.

PHARMACODYNAMICS

Methylene blue's role in the treatment of methemoglobinemia arises from its ability to interact with methemoglobin and specific enzyme systems within the erythrocyte. Even in the absence of any additional chemically induced oxidative stress, the hemoglobin within the red blood cells (RBCs) slowly tends to oxidize in the presence of normal concentrations of oxygen. The enzyme system responsible for the endogenous reduction of methemoglobin to hemoglobin is NADH-dependent cytochrome-b_5 reductase, which actually consists of the cytochrome b_5 and the flavin-containing cytochrome-b_5 reductase (Fig. 155-2).[29,30] This is a first-order process that occurs at a rate of approximately 15% of total methemoglobin per hour. Under normal circumstances, this enzyme system is capable of maintaining the methemoglobin concentration at less than 1% of the total hemoglobin.[31] The reducing agent NADH is a normal product of glycolysis (see Fig. 155-2) and acts as an electron source to reduce cytochrome-b_5 reductase. This reduced enzyme acts as an electron donor for oxidized cytochrome b_5. The now reduced cytochrome b_5 reduces the ferric (Fe^{3+}) iron of methemoglo-

bin to the ferrous (Fe^{2+}) form, generating hemoglobin. In the presence of a sufficient exogenous oxidative stress, the amount of methemoglobin formed may exceed the reducing capacity of this cytochrome-b_5 reductase system, resulting in methemoglobinemia.

A second enzyme system within the RBC, the NADPH-dependent methemoglobin reductase, normally has a minimal role in the reduction of methemoglobin (Fig. 155-3). Under usual conditions, the absence of this system or its activity does not result in clinical methemoglobinemia.[30,32] This enzyme system, which apparently usually functions to reduce exogenous substances other than methemoglobin, in the presence of methylene blue can enhance the reduction of methemoglobin to hemoglobin.[17,33,34] NADPH, produced by the hexose monophosphate shunt, reduces NADPH-dependent methemoglobin reductase, an enzyme that has an affinity for methylene blue, among other dyes, and reduces methylene blue to the form leukomethylene blue, which has a high affinity for methemoglobin (see Fig. 155-3). The leukomethylene blue reduces the ferric (Fe^{3+}) iron of methemoglobin, forming hemoglobin. The NADPH-dependent methemoglobin reductase, which under usual conditions is responsible for less than 5% of the reduction of methemoglobin to hemoglobin, assumes a major role in the pharmacotherapy of methemoglobinemia. Oxidation of hemoglobin to methemoglobin can occur at high doses of methylene blue due to a reversal of the NADPH-dependent methemoglobin reductase pathway.

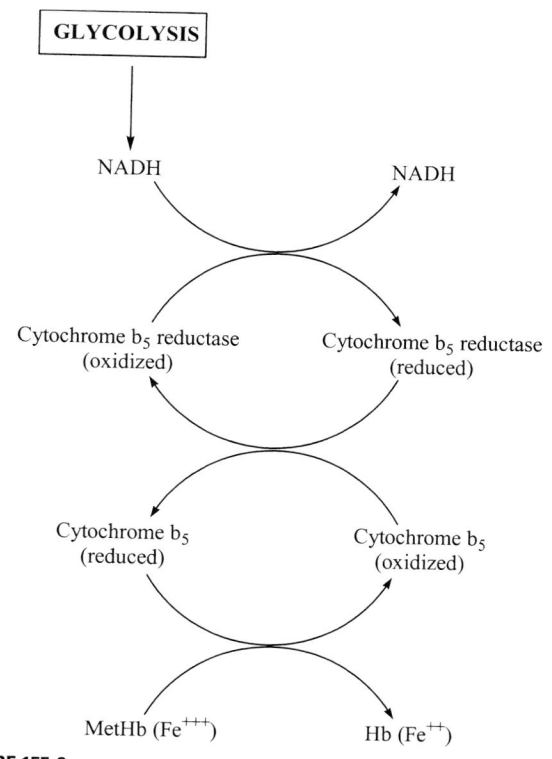

FIGURE 155-2

Predominant pathway for endogenous methemoglobin (MetHb) reduction. NADH, nicotinamide-adenine dinucleotide (reduced form).

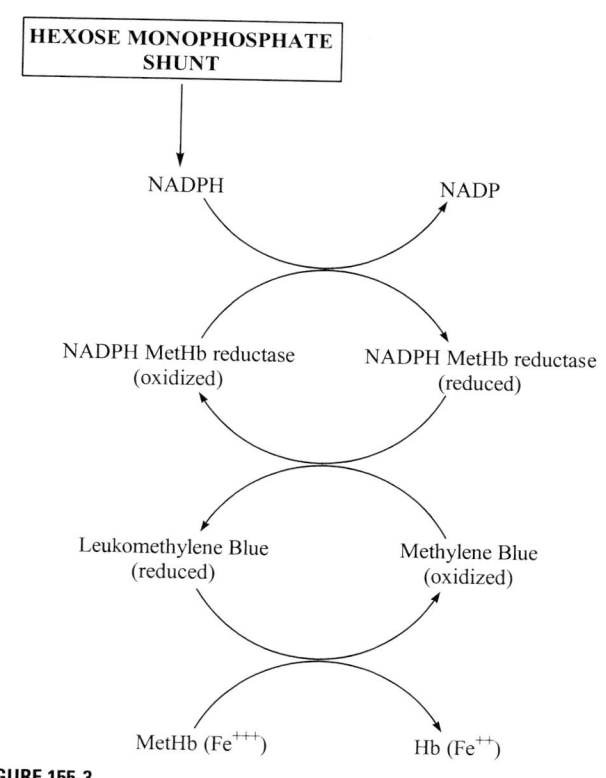

FIGURE 155-3

Minor pathway for methemoglobin (MetHb) reduction, which is increased in the presence of methylene blue. NADP, nicotinamide-adenine dinucleotide phosphate; NADPH, nicotinamide-adenine dinucleotide phosphate (reduced form).

PHARMACOKINETICS

Pharmacokinetics of Methylene Blue

Volume of distribution: 0.222–0.876 L/kg
pK_a: 0 to −1
Clearance: 1.98–2.65 L/kg/hr
Half-life: 5–6.5 hr
Time of maximal concentration: 1–2 hr

After developing a spectrophotometric assay to measure methylene blue and leukomethylene blue in blood, urine, and tissues, DiSanto and Wagner[35–37] examined the pharmacokinetics of methylene blue in humans, dogs, and rats. In a study of seven adult male volunteers who received 10 mg of methylene blue orally, with subsequent urinary methylene blue determinations for 120 hours, 74% (range 53% to 97%) of the administered material was recovered; 78% (range 65% to 85%) in the leukomethylene blue form was recovered, showing that methylene blue is well absorbed orally in humans. In the same study, two dogs (one female and one male) received methylene blue orally, with blood concentrations assayed in both animals and urine concentrations assayed in one animal. After receiving 15 mg/kg of methylene blue orally, the male dog had undetectable blood methylene blue 6.9 hours after administration. No urine was sampled from this animal. The female dog received 15 mg/kg of methylene blue orally, with urine sampled every hour for 10 hours. Only 2.4% of the methylene blue was excreted in the urine over 10 hours. This same female dog also received a total of 10 mg of methylene blue orally followed by methylene blue measurements in the blood at 2.5 and 3.5 hours and in the urine every hour for 14 hours after the administration. Only 3.8% of the methylene blue was recovered in the urine, and essentially undetectable levels of methylene blue were reported in the blood. The authors concluded that in contrast to humans, dogs have poor gastrointestinal absorption of methylene blue.

In a second study by the same authors, one dog was administered each of five doses of methylene blue (2 to 15 mg/kg) at least 2 to 3 weeks apart followed by measurement of the compound in the blood. A semilog plot revealed a biexponential relationship between blood concentration of methylene blue and time after administration, which was consistent with a linear two-compartment open model. The data also were well fitted to the nonlinear single-compartment model, however, with even less variability noted in the volumes of distribution, elimination rate constants, and clearance rates. Using the linear two-compartment model, the average volume of distribution was found to be 0.876 L/kg, with a plasma clearance rate of 2.65 L/kg/hr. The nonlinear one-compartment model yielded an average volume of distribution of 0.222 L/kg, with a plasma clearance rate of 1.98 L/kg/hr.

In rat studies of intravenous administration of methylene blue, six doses ranging from 2 to 25 mg/kg were given, and methylene blue was measured spectrophotometrically in the blood, lungs, liver, kidney, and heart after the rats were killed 3 minutes after the injection. An average of 29.8% (range 25.3% to 35.8%) of the administered dose of methylene blue

was present in the four tissues 3 minutes after intravenous administration. This finding provided support to the nonlinear one-compartment model. The pharmacokinetics of methylene blue after oral and intravenous administration also has been studied in humans.[38] After the administration of 100 mg of methylene blue via either the oral or the parenteral route in seven human volunteers, the time course of methylene blue in the blood was measured by high-pressure liquid chromatography, and the urinary excretion was determined spectrophotometrically. After oral administration, the maximal methylene blue blood concentration was reached at 1 to 2 hours, with the levels being an order of magnitude lower than that attained after intravenous administration of the same dose. The time course displayed by methylene blue blood concentrations after intravenous administration was multiphasic, requiring an equation containing three exponential terms to fit the data. The urinary excretion of methylene blue at 24 hours was approximately 28% and 18% after intravenous and oral administration, respectively, with one third excreted as leukomethylene blue. The half-life of methylene blue was calculated to be 5 to 6.5 hours.

These same authors studied the organ distribution of methylene blue after oral and intravenous administration in eight rats. One hour after the administration of 10 mg/kg of methylene blue intravenously or intraduodenally, the animals were killed, and the distribution of methylene blue into the blood, brain, intestinal wall, liver, and bile was measured by high-pressure liquid chromatography. These studies revealed that greater than 97% of the dose administered intraduodenally was absorbed in this period. Little methylene blue could be detected in the blood 1 hour after intraduodenal administration compared with the significantly higher level after intravenous administration; however, there was a 50-fold greater concentration of methylene blue in the intestinal wall after intraduodenal administration than that measured after intravenous administration. The authors offer this "first pass distribution" as the explanation for the order-of-magnitude difference in the methylene blue blood concentrations and area under the concentration curve found after intravenous and intraduodenal administration. As a result of the experimental differences noted between species and within the same species, as attested to by previous studies in humans, dogs, and rats, the pharmacokinetics of methylene blue requires further elucidation.

SPECIAL POPULATIONS

Neonatal Patients

Neonates, especially premature ones, are expected to be more vulnerable to the formation of methemoglobinemia and to the development of side effects from methylene blue therapy if appropriate doses are not used. Neonates may be more vulnerable to the oxidant stresses of the environment for the following reasons: (1) NADH-dependent methemoglobin reductase activity or levels or both are not fully acquired until age 3 to 6 months (perhaps longer in premature infants)[39–42]; (2) although this idea is controversial, the fetal hemoglobin may be oxidized more readily into methemoglobin than the adult type[43,44]; and (3) the skin of infants (especially premature infants) is much more permeable to some external toxicants than the skin of children or adults. Heinz body hemolytic anemia has been noted in premature infants in whom methylene blue was instilled to ensure proper placement of a nasojejunal tube.[45]

Exposure of an infant during intraamniotic infusion of methylene blue to determine prepartum leakage or the presence of twins may result in methemoglobinemia, acute hemolytic anemia with Heinz body formation, hyperbilirubinemia, photosensitization of the skin with subsequent desquamation in the newborn, and possibly intestinal obstruction.[27,28,46–57] Methylene blue used in the treatment of methemoglobinemia in an infant first was reported to cause hemolytic anemias by Goluboff and Wheaton.[58] The doses used were excessive, however: a total of greater than 26 mg/kg in one infant and greater than 35 mg/kg in the second infant. Many reports showed that newborn infants, including premature ones, with methemoglobinemia from an intoxicant may be treated safely with intravenous methylene blue at a dose of 1 to 2 mg/kg without adverse effects.[19–22] The 1- to 2-mg/kg dose may not be required, however. Hjelt and colleagues[59] treated 13 infants with a mean gestational age of 28 weeks and birth weight average of 895 g with methylene blue for methemoglobinemia. In these neonates, intoxicated via the skin and respiratory tract by parachloraniline produced by the heating of chlorhexidine, the mean methemoglobin concentration was 19% (range 6.5% to 45.5%). Intravenous methylene blue administered at a dose of 0.3 to 0.9 mg/kg was found to be as effective as the 1 to 1.6 mg/kg initially used in this group. In the treatment of neonates with methemoglobinemia, a lower dose of intravenous methylene blue may be effective. A problem commonly encountered in small infants is intravenous access. Methylene blue at a dose of 1 mg/kg administered by the intraosseous route over 3 to 5 minutes has been shown to be effective in the treatment of methemoglobinemia in a 6-week-old infant without adverse effects.[60]

Glucose-6-Phosphate Dehydrogenase Deficiency Patients

Glucose-6-phosphate dehydrogenase (G6PD) deficiency is an X-linked disorder that results in an altered primary structure of G6PD with a subsequent reduction in the enzyme's functional activity.[32,61] A male with the disorder or a female homozygous for the mutant gene would be expected to express the defect fully. Numerous variants of this enzyme deficiency exist. The African type, the G6PD A variant, is estimated to be present in approximately 11% of African Americans. The G6PD activity level within the erythrocyte of unaffected individuals normally decreases as the RBCs age. An accelerated rate of activity loss is seen in the African type of G6PD, with only 10% residual activity present mostly in the younger RBCs; an even greater rate of loss is found in the Mediterranean type of the deficiency, which may be present in 2.5% to 25% of that population.[62,63] Heinz body hemolytic anemias and methemoglobinemias may be produced by the administration of methylene blue to patients with G6PD deficiency.[64–66] An absence of G6PD, the first enzyme in the hexose monophosphate shunt pathway, results in the absence of

NADPH production within the RBCs. Without NADPH, the RBC is unable to reduce methylene blue to leukomethylene blue. The resultant proportionately higher levels of the electron acceptor (oxidizing agent) methylene blue may produce hemolysis and, paradoxically, methemoglobinemia in the G6PD-deficient patient.

Methylene blue administered to a G6PD-deficient patient with methemoglobinemia would not be expected to be effective because of the absence of sufficient NADPH. A G6PD-deficient patient may possess only a partial deficiency of the enzyme, however; this is true especially in a heterozygous female, who may possess nearly normal activity levels and display some lowering of methemoglobin levels after methylene blue therapy.[67,68] Methylene blue administration remains the first-line therapy for methemoglobinemia, even in G6PD-deficient individuals; however, if the recommended dose of 1 to 2 mg/kg of intravenous methylene blue does not produce a response in these individuals, additional doses of methylene blue are not recommended owing to the possibility of escalating further the already elevated levels of methemoglobin and inducing a hemolytic anemia.

Other Patients

Patients not expected to respond to methylene blue include those with sulfhemoglobinemia, fully expressed G6PD deficiency (X-linked), NADPH-dependent methemoglobin reductase deficiency,[69] NADH-dependent cytochrome-b_5 reductase deficiency,[70] cytochrome b_5 deficiency (autosomal recessive),[71] and hemoglobin M (autosomal dominant).[72] Patients already treated with extreme doses of methylene blue who have developed methemoglobinemia may experience an escalation of methemoglobin concentration with further methylene blue administration. Lastly, patients poisoned with an overwhelming amount of intoxicants or poisons characterized by continual gastrointestinal absorption or metabolite formation may seem not to respond to methylene blue.

REFERENCES

1. Goodman LS, Gilman A: The Pharmacological Basis of Therapeutics, 4th ed. New York, Macmillan, 1970.
2. Litovitz TL, Klein-Schwartz WF, White S: 2000 Annual Report of the American Association of Poison Control Centers Toxic Exposure Surveillance System. Am J Emerg Med 19:337–395, 2001.
3. Hanzlik PJ: Methylene blue as an antidote for cyanide poisoning. JAMA 100:357, 1933.
4. Geiger JC: Cyanide poisoning in San Francisco. JAMA 99:1944–1945, 1932.
5. Geiger JC: Methylene blue solution in the treatment of carbon monoxide poisoning. JAMA 100:1103, 1933.
6. Nass J: Treatment of a case of illuminating gas poisoning with methylene blue solution. JAMA 100:1862, 1933.
7. Christopherson AW: Report of cases of carbon monoxide poisoning treated by methylene blue injection. JAMA 100:2008, 1933.
8. Williams JR, Challis FE: Methylene blue as an antidote for poisoning. J Lab Clin Med 19:166–171, 1933.
9. Steele CW, Spink WW: Methylene blue in the treatment of poisonings associated with methemoglobinemia. N Engl J Med 208:1152, 1933.
10. Wendel WB: Role of methemoglobin in methylene blue catalysis of lactic acid oxidation. J Biol Chem 97:ixxv–bcxvi, 1932.
11. Haggard HW, Greenberg LA: Methylene blue: a synergist, not an antidote for carbon-monoxide. JAMA 100:2001, 1933.
12. Mangelsdorff AF: Treatment of methemoglobinemia. Arch Ind Health 14:148, 1956.

13. Nadler JE, Green H, Rosenbaum A: Intravenous injection of methylene blue in man with reference to its toxic symptoms and effect on the electrocardiogram. Am J Med Sci 188:15–21, 1934.
14. Bodansky O: Mechanism of action of methylene blue in treatment of methemoglobinemia (Letter). JAMA 142:923, 1950.
15. Wendel WB: Methylene blue, methemoglobin, and cyanide poisoning. J Pharmacol Exp Ther 54:283, 1935.
16. Wendel WB: Use of methylene blue in methemoglobinemia from sulfanilamide poisoning. JAMA 109:1216, 1937.
17. Gutmann HR, Jandorf BJ, Bodansky O: Role of pyridine nucleotides in reduction of methemoglobin. J Biol Chem 169:145–152, 1947.
18. Hartmann AF, Perley AM, Barnett HL: A study of some of the physiological effects of sulfanilamide: II. Methemoglobin formation and its control. J Clin Invest 17:699–710, 1938.
19. Comly HH: Cyanosis in infants caused by nitrates in well water. JAMA 129:112–116, 1945.
20. Faucett RL, Miller HC: Methemoglobinemia occurring in infants fed milk diluted with well water of high nitrate content. J Pediatr 29:583–596, 1946.
21. Ferrant M: Methemoglobinemia: Two cases in newborn infants caused by nitrates in well water. J Pediatr 29:585–592, 1946.
22. Etteldorf JN: Methylene blue in the treatment of methemoglobinemia in premature infants caused by marking ink. J Pediatr 38:24–27, 1951.
23. Strauch B, Buch W, Grey W, et al: Successful treatment of methemoglobinemia secondary to silver nitrate therapy. N Engl J Med 281:257–258, 1969.
24. Wendel WB: The control of methemoglobinemia with methylene blue. J Clin Invest 18:179–185, 1939.
25. Southgate HJ, Masterson R: Lessons to be learned: A case study approach: Prolonged methemoglobinemia due to inadvertent dapsone poisoning; treatment with methylene blue and exchange transfusion. J R Soc Health 119:52–55, 1999.
26. Berlin G, Brodin B, Hilden J-O, et al: Acute dapsone intoxication: A case treated with continuous infusion of methylene blue, forced diuresis and plasma exchange. Clin Toxicol 22:537–548, 1984–85.
27. Porat R, Gilbert S, Magilner D: Methylene blue-induced phototoxicity: An unrecognized complication. Pediatrics 97:717–721, 1996.
28. Sills MR, Zinkham WH: Methylene blue-induced Heinz body hemolytic anemia. Arch Pediatr Adolesc Med 148:306–310, 1994.
29. Finch CA: Treatment of intracellular methemoglobinemia. Bull N Engl J Med Ctr 6:241–245, 1947.
30. Jaffe ER, Hultquist DE: Cytochrome b5 reductase deficiency and enzymopenic hereditary methemoglobinemia. In Scriver CR, Beaudet AL, Sly WS, et al (eds): The Metabolic and Molecular Basis of Inherited Disease, 7th ed. New York, McGraw-Hill, 1995, pp 2267–2280.
31. Coleman MD, Coleman NA: Drug-induced methaemoglobinaemia: Treatment issues. Drug Saf 14:394–405, 1996.
32. Beutler E: G6PD: Population genetics and clinical manifestations. Blood Rev 10:45–52, 1996.
33. Metz EN, Balcerzak SP, Sagon LR: Mechanism of methylene blue stimulation of the hexose monophosphate shunt in the erythrocyte. J Clin Invest 58:797–802, 1976.
34. Curry S: Methemoglobinemia. Ann Emerg Med 2:214–221, 1982.
35. DiSanto AR, Wagner JG: Pharmacokinetics of highly ionized drugs: I. Methylene blue—whole blood, urine, and tissue assays. J Pharm Sci 61:598–602, 1972.
36. DiSanto AR, Wagner JG: Pharmacokinetics of highly ionized drugs: II. Methylene blue—absorption, metabolism, and excretion in man and dog after oral administration. J Pharm Sci 61:1086–1090, 1972.
37. DiSanto AR, Wagner JG: Pharmacokinetics of highly ionized drugs: III. Methylene blue—blood levels in the dog and tissue levels in the rat following intravenous administration. J Pharm Sci 61:1090–1094, 1972.
38. Peter C, Hongwan D, Kupfer A, et al: Pharmacokinetics and organ distribution of intravenous and oral methylene blue. Eur J Clin Pharmacol 56:247–250, 2000.
39. Bartos HR, Desforges JF: Erythrocyte DPNH-dependent diaphorase levels in infants. Pediatrics 37:991–993, 1966.
40. Nilsson A, Engberg G, Henneberg S, et al: Inverse relationship between age-dependent erythrocyte activity of methaemoglobin reductase and prilocaine-induced methaemoglobinaemia during infancy. Br J Anaesth 64:72–76, 1990.
41. Choury D, Reghis A, Pichard AL, et al: Endogenous proteolysis of membrane-bound red cell cytochrome b5 reductase in adults and newborns: Its possible relevance to the generation of soluble "methemoglobin reductase." Blood 61:894–898, 1983.
42. Lukens JN: The legacy of well-water methemoglobinemia. JAMA 257:2793–2795, 1987.
43. Feig SA: Methemoglobinemia. In Nathan DG, Oski FA (eds): Hematology of Infancy and Childhood. Philadelphia, WB Saunders, 1981, pp 654–686.
44. Martin T, Huisman THJ: Formation of ferrihaemoglobin of isolated human hemoglobin types by sodium nitrite. Nature 200:898–899, 1963.
45. Kirsch I, Cohen M: Heinz body hemolytic anemia from the use of methylene blue in neonates. J Pediatr 96:276–278, 1980.
46. McEnerney JK, McEnerney LN: Unfavorable neonatal outcome after intra-amniotic injection of methylene blue. Obstet Gynecol 61:35S–37S, 1983.
47. Cowett RM, Hakanson DO, Kocon RW, et al: Untoward neonatal effect of intra-amniotic administration of methylene blue. Obstet Gynecol 48(Suppl):74S, 1976.
48. Plunkett GD: Neonatal complications (Letter). Obstet Gynecol 14:476, 1973.
49. Crooks J: Haemolytic jaundice in a neonate after intra-amniotic injection of methylene blue. Arch Dis Child 57:872–886, 1982.
50. Spahr RC, Salsburey DJ, Krissberg A, et al: Intra-amniotic injection of methylene blue leading to methemoglobinemia in one of twins. Int J Gynaecol Obstet 17:477–478, 1980.
51. Nicolini U, Monni G: Intestinal obstruction in babies exposed in utero to methylene blue. Lancet 336:1258–1259, 1990.
52. Dolk H: Methylene blue and atresia or stenosis of the ileum and jejunum. Lancet 338:1021–1022, 1991.
53. Van Der Pol JG, Wolf H, Kees B, et al: Fetal and neonatal medicine: Jejunal atresia related to the use of methylene blue in genetic amniocentesis in twins. Br J Obstet Gynaecol 99:141–143, 1992.
54. Serota FT, Bernbaum JC, Schwartz E: The methylene-blue baby. Lancet 2:1142–1143, 1979.
55. Troche BI: The methylene-blue baby. N Engl J Med 320:1756–1757, 1989.
56. Fish WH, Chazen EM: Toxic effects of methylene blue on the fetus. Am J Dis Child 146:1412–1413, 1992.
57. Vincer MJ, Allen AC, Evans JR, et al: Methylene blue induced hemolytic anemia in a neonate. Can Med Assoc J 136:503–504, 1987.
58. Goluboff N, Wheaton R: Methylene blue induced cyanosis and acute hemolytic anemia complicating the treatment of methemoglobinemia. J Pediatr 58:86–89, 1961.
59. Hjelt K, Lund JT, Scherling B, et al: Methaemoglobinaemia among neonates in a neonatal intensive care unit. Acta Paediatr 84:365–370, 1995.
60. Herman MI: Methylene blue by intraosseous infusion for methemoglobinemia. Ann Emerg Med 33:11–13, 1999.
61. Weatherall DJ: The thalassaemias. BMJ 314:1675–1678, 1997.
62. Meloni T, Forteleoni G, Dore A, et al: Favism and hemolytic anemia in glucose-6-phosphate dehydrogenase deficient subjects in North Sardinia. Acta Haematol 70:83–90, 1983.
63. Cin S, Akar N, Arcasoy A, et al: Prevalence of thalassemia and G-6-PD deficiency in North Cyprus. Acta Hematol 71:69–70, 1984.
64. Bilgin H, Ozcan B, Bilgin T: Methemoglobinemia induced by methylene blue perturbation during laparoscopy. Acta Anaesthesiol Scand 42:594–595, 1998.
65. Harvey JW, Keitt AS: Studies of the efficacy and potential hazards of methylene blue therapy in aniline-induced methaemoglobinaemia. Br J Haematol 54:29–41, 1983.
66. Rosen PJ, Johnson C, McGehee WG, et al: Failure of methylene blue treatment in toxic methemoglobinemia: Association with glucose-6-phosphate deficiency. Ann Intern Med 75:83–86, 1971.
67. Smith CL, Snowdon SL: Anesthesia and glucose-6-phosphate dehydrogenase deficiency: A case report and review of the literature. Anaesthesia 42:281–288, 1987.
68. Ashmun RA, Hultquist DE, Schultz JS: Kinetic analysis in single, intact cells by microspectrophotometry: Evidence for two populations of erythrocytes in an individual heterozygous for glucose-6-phosphate dehydrogenase deficiency. Am J Hematol 23:311–316, 1986.
69. Sass MD, Caruso CJ, Farhangi M: TPNH-methemoglobin reductase deficiency: A new red cell enzyme defect. J Lab Clin Med 70:760–767, 1967.
70. Kobayashi Y, Fukumaki Y, Yubisui T, et al: Serine-proline replacement at residue 127 of NADH-cytochrome b5 reductase causes hereditary methemoglobinemia, generalized type. Blood 75:1408–1413, 1990.

71. Hegesh E, Hegesh J, Kraftory A: Congenital methemoglobinemia with a deficiency of cytochrome b₅. N Engl J Med 314:757–761, 1986.
72. Bunn HF: Human hemoglobins: Normal and abnormal. In Nathan DG, Orkin SH (eds): Hematology of Infancy and Childhood, 5th ed. Philadelphia, WB Saunders, 1998, pp 749–761.
73. Kushner BJ: Solutions can be hazardous for lacrimal system irrigation. Arch Ophthalmol 111:904–905, 1993.
74. Brownstein S, Liszauer AD, Jackson WB: Ocular complications of a topical methylene blue-vasoconstrictor-anesthetic preparation. Can J Ophthalmol 24:317–324, 1989.
75. Schultz P, Schwarz GA: Radiculomyelopathy following intrathecal instillation of methylene blue. Arch Neurol 22:240–244, 1970.
76. Macia M, Gallego E, Garcia-Cobaleda I, et al: Methylene blue as a cause of chemical peritonitis in a patient on peritoneal dialysis. Clin Nephrol 43:136–137, 1995.
77. Koh CH: Laparoscopic microsurgical tubal anastomosis. Obstet Gynecol Clin North Am 26:189–200, 1999.
78. Kupfer A, Aeschlimann C, Wermuth B, Cerny T: Prophylaxis and reversal of ifosfamide encephalopathy with methylene-blue. Lancet 343:763–764, 1994.
79. Pelgrims J, DeVos F, Vanden BJ, et al: Methylene blue in the treatment and prevention of ifosfamide-induced encephalopathy: Report of 12 cases and a review of the literature. Br J Cancer 82:291–294, 2000.
80. Kupfer A, Aeschlimann C, Cerny T: Methylene blue and the neurotoxic mechanisms of ifosfamide encephalopathy. Eur J Clin Pharmacol 4:249–252, 1996.
81. Zulian GB, Tidlen E, Maton B: Methylene blue for ifosfamide-associated encephalopathy. N Engl J Med 332:1239–1240, 1995.
82. Alonso JL, Nieto Y, Lopez JA, et al: Ifosfamide encephalopathy and methylene-blue: A case report. Ann Oncol 7:643–644, 1996.
83. Dourthe LM, Coutant G, Desrame J, et al: Ifosfamide-related encephalopathy: Report of two cases. Rev Med Intern 20:264–266, 1999.
84. Link EM, Costa DC, Dominic L, et al: Targeting disseminated melanoma with radiolabelled methylene blue: Comparative biodistribution studies in man and animals. Acta Oncol 35:331–341, 1996.
85. Gangarosa LM: Methylene blue staining and endoscopic ultrasound evaluation of Barrett's esophagus with low-grade dysplasia. Dig Dis Sci 45:225–229, 2000.
86. Martinez PF, Hoang-Boehm J, Weiss J, et al: Methylene blue as a successful treatment alternative for pharmacologically induced priapism. Eur Urol 39:20–23, 2001.
87. Schneider JE Jr, Tabatabaie T, Maidt L, et al: Potential mechanisms of photodynamic inactivation of virus by methylene blue: I. RNA-protein crosslinks and other oxidative lesions in Q beta bacteriophage. Photochem Photobiol 67:350–357, 1998.
88. Schneider JE Jr, Phillips JR, Pye Q, et al: Methylene blue and rose bengal photoinactivation of RNA bacteriophages: Comparative studies of 8-oxoguanine formation in isolated RNA. Arch Biochem Biophys 301:91–97, 1993.
89. Schneider JE Jr, Pye Q, Floyd RA: Q beta bacteriophage photoinactivated by methylene blue plus light involves inactivation of its genomic RNA. Photochem Photobiol 70:902–909, 1999.
90. Aznar JA, Bonanad S, Montoro JM, et al: Influence of methylene blue photoinactivation treatment on coagulation factors from fresh frozen plasma, cryoprecipitates and cryosupernatants. Vox Sang 79:156–160, 2000.
91. Wainwright M: Methylene blue derivatives—suitable photoantimicrobials for blood product disinfection? Int J Antimicrob Agents 16:381–394, 2000.
92. Yamada-Ohnishi Y, Owada T, Abe H, et al: Cell-associated virus infectivity of primary HIV-1 isolate can be eliminated by a filtration/methylene blue photoinactivation system. Transfusion 40:1542–1543, 2000.
93. Owada T, Yamada Y, Abe H, et al: Elucidation of the HIV-1 virucidal mechanism of methylene blue photosensitization and the effect on primary isolates. J Med Virol 62:421–425, 2000.
94. Skripchenko AA, Wagner SJ: Inactivation of WBCs in RBC suspensions by photoactive phenothiazine dyes: Comparison of dimethylmethylene blue and MB. Transfusion 40:968–975, 2000.
95. Keaney JF Jr, Puyana JC, Francis S, et al: Methylene blue reverses endotoxin-induced hypotension. Circ Res 74:1121–1125, 1994.
96. Holcombe RG Jr: Methylene blue dye in the management of condylomata acuminata. J La State Med Soc 133:68–69, 1981.
97. Kluger Y, Weinbroum A, Ben-Avraham R, et al: Reduction in formation of peritoneal adhesions by methylene blue in rats: A dose response study. Eur J Surg 166:568–571, 2000.
98. Schenk P, Madl C, Rezaie-Majd S, et al: Methylene blue improves the hepatopulmonary syndrome. Ann Intern Med 133:701–706, 2000.
99. Heckenkamp J, Adili F, Kishimoto J, et al: Local photodynamic action of methylene blue favorably modulates the postinterventional vascular wound healing response. J Vasc Surg 31:1168–1177, 2000.
100. Audi SH, Olson LE, Bongard RD, et al: Toluidine blue O and methylene blue as endothelial redox probes in the intact lung. Am J Physiol 278:H137–150, 2000.
101. Trindade GS, Farias SL, Rumjanek VM, et al: Methylene blue reverts multidrug resistance: Sensitivity of multidrug resistant cells to this dye and its photodynamic action. Cancer Lett 151:161–167, 2000.
102. Birch JF, Mandley DJ, Williams SL, et al: Methylene blue based protein solder for vascular anastomoses: An in vitro burst pressure study. Laser Surg Med 26:323–329, 2000.
103. Traynor S, Adams JR, Andersen P, et al: Appropriate timing and velocity of infusion for the selective staining of parathyroid glands by intravenous methylene blue. Am J Surg 176:15–17, 1998.
104. Blower PJ, Clark K, Link EM: Radioiodinated methylene blue for melanoma targeting: Chemical characterisation and tumour selectivity of labelled components. Nucl Med Biol 24:305–310, 1997.
105. Muller T: Supravital uptake of methylene blue by dendritic cells within stratified squamous epithelia: A light and electron microscope study. Biotech Histochem 71:96–101, 1996.

CHAPTER 156

Dantrolene

Blaine E. Benson

Dantrolene is a unique, non–centrally acting, nondepolarizing muscle relaxant used primarily to treat malignant hyperthermia and chronic muscle spasticity caused by upper neuron disorders, such as stroke, spinal cord injury, cerebral palsy, and multiple sclerosis.

HISTORY

Snyder and colleagues[1] first described the possible muscle-relaxing properties of dantrolene in 1967, while studying the ability of substituted furans to inhibit hind-limb flexor reflexes in cats. Shortly thereafter, dantrolene was shown to alleviate muscle spasticity effectively in animals[2] and humans.[3] In 1972, Ellis and colleagues[4,5] showed that dantrolene uncoupled the excitation-contraction process during skeletal muscle stimulation. Because malignant hyperthermia was thought to result from continuous muscle contraction, perhaps through an abnormality in the excitation-contraction coupling mechanism, the compound was tested as treatment for this condition. In 1982, the first human data showing that dantrolene could reduce the mortality of malignant hyperthermia from 50% to 0% were published.[6] Since then, dantrolene has been tried in the treatment of other medical conditions associated with muscle spasm, such as tetanus,[7] neuroleptic malignant syndrome,[8] lethal catatonia,[9] amphotericin-induced rigors,[10] black widow spider envenomation,[11] 3,4-methylenedioxymethamphetamine (Ecstasy) overdose,[12,13] phenelzine poisoning,[14] theophylline poisoning,[15] muscle rigidity associated with carbon monoxide poisoning,[16] and organophosphate poisoning.[17] Dantrolene protected mice envenomated with *Androctonus australis hector* scorpion venom.[18] It also has been used as a treatment for neurogenic bladder obstruction associated with external urethral sphincter spasm.[19]

PROPERTIES

Dantrolene (1-[[[5-(4 nitrophenyl)-2-furanyl] methylene] amino]-2,4-imidazolidinedione) is a hydantoin derivative with structural similarities to phenytoin and nitrofurantoin (Fig. 156-1). Anhydrous dantrolene sodium has a molecular weight of 336. Medicinal dantrolene is an orange hemiheptahydrate sodium salt with a molecular weight of 399. It is a weak acid (pK_a 7.5) that is only slightly soluble in water. Sodium hydroxide and mannitol (3 g/20 mg vial) are added to the intravenous product to enhance solubility.[20]

PHARMACODYNAMICS

Dantrolene relaxes skeletal muscle by decreasing release of calcium from the sarcoplasmic reticulum. Normally, nerve impulses reach the neuromuscular junction and are carried across the surface membrane of the myofiber to transverse tubules (T tubules) (Fig. 156-2). T tubule activation releases calcium from the sarcoplasmic reticulum into the surrounding myofibrils. Calcium binds to troponin C, which allows actin and myosin to interact to cause muscle contraction. Dantrolene interferes with the triggering of calcium release through T tubules and the actual release of calcium from the sarcoplasmic reticulum. Dantrolene does not affect reuptake of sarcoplasmic calcium, and it does not affect pretubular steps of skeletal muscle excitation-contraction. It has weak muscle relaxant effects on smooth muscle and depresses cardiac contractility when used in higher than therapeutic doses.[21-23]

PHARMACOKINETICS

Approximately 70% of an oral dose of dantrolene is absorbed in humans. In animals, dantrolene is absorbed primarily in the small intestine.[24] Peak blood concentrations occur 4 to 8 hours after ingestion in healthy human volunteers.[25] Therapeutic blood concentrations are 0.3 to 0.6 µg/mL (1 to 1.9 µmol/L) for treatment of spasticity[25-27] and 2 to 3 µg/mL (6.4 to 9.5 µmol/L) for treatment of malignant hyperthermia.[28,29] The volume of distribution and protein binding for dantrolene have not been determined in humans. In animal models, dantrolene is widely distributed.[21] It crosses the placenta in humans with a fetal-to-maternal serum concentration ratio of 0.4 to 0.7.[30,31]

When distributed, dantrolene is metabolized in the liver by 5-hydroxylation of the hydantoin ring, resulting in 5-hydroxydantrolene (Fig. 156-3), which is about half as potent in inhibiting twitch contractions as the parent compound. In children, steady-state concentrations of 5-hydroxydantrolene are 30% to 50% those of dantrolene.[33] Dantrolene also may undergo reduction of the nitro moiety on the benzene ring to form aminodantrolene. Aminodantrolene is acetylated further to an inactive metabolite, called *reduced aminodantrolene* (see Fig. 156-3).[32]

Approximately two thirds of the absorbed dose of dantrolene appears in bile. The remaining one third appears in the urine, with 79% as the 5-hydroxydantrolene metabolite, 17% as the reduced acetylated metabolite, and 4% unchanged.[21,24,33] The renal clearance of dantrolene in

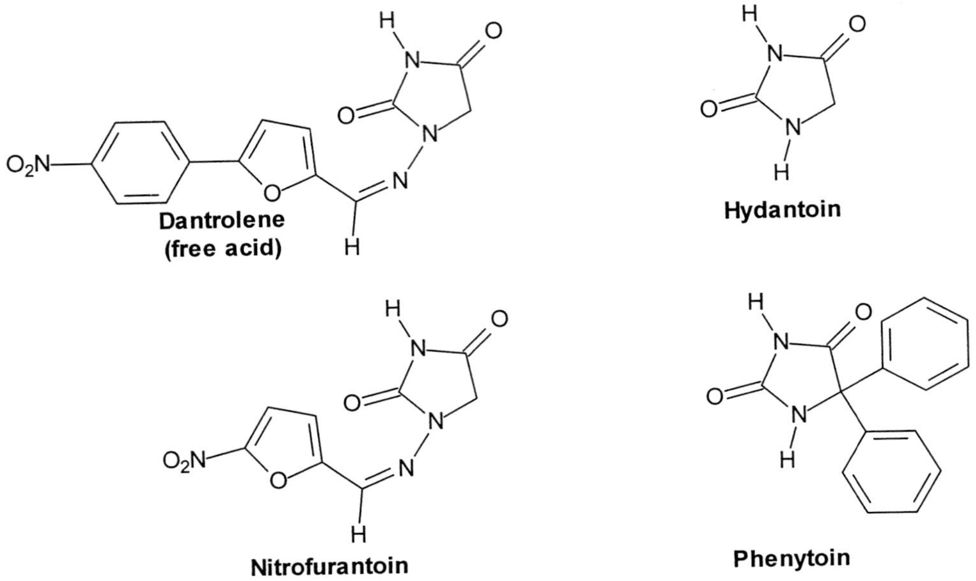

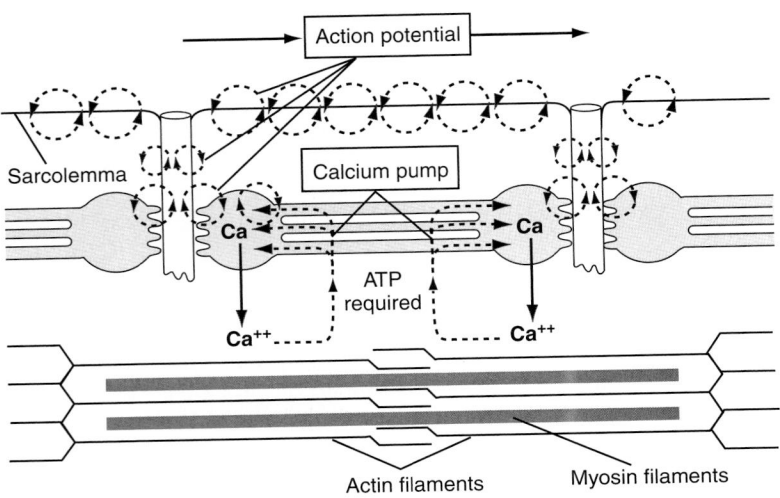

Dantrolene (free acid)

Hydantoin

Nitrofurantoin

Phenytoin

FIGURE 156-1

Chemical structures of dantrolene, and, for comparison, hydantoin, nitrofurantoin, and phenytoin.

Action potential

Sarcolemma

Calcium pump

Ca

Ca

ATP required

Ca^{++}

Ca^{++}

Actin filaments

Myosin filaments

FIGURE 156-2

Excitation-contraction coupling in muscle, showing an action potential that causes release of calcium ions from the sarcoplasmic reticulum, then reuptake of calcium ions by a calcium pump. The perpendicular cylindrical objects next to the sarcolemmas are T tubules. ATP, adenosine triphosphate. *(From Guyton AC, Hall JE: Textbook of Medical Physiology, 10th ed. Philadelphia, WB Saunders, 2000, p 85.)*

healthy volunteers is 1.8 to 7.8 L/hr. Dantrolene's serum half-life is 6 to 9 hours in adults with spasticity.[21,27] The mean half-life of dantrolene in patients with malignant hyperthermia is 12 hours.[34] In children, the half-life is 7 to 10 hours.[33,35] In neonates, the half-life is 20 hours.[33]

Pharmacokinetics of Dantrolene

Volume of distribution: unknown
Oral bioavailability: 70%
Time to peak blood levels: 4–8 hr
Therapeutic range: 0.1–0.6 μg/mL (spasticity); 2–3 μg/mL (malignant hyperthermia)
Metabolism: extensively metabolized in liver by hydroxylation or acetylation
Route of clearance: 70% biliary, 30% renal
Clearance: 1.8–7.8 L/hr
Half-life: Healthy adults, 6–9 hr; adults with malignant hyperthermia, 12 hr; children, 7–10 hr; neonates, 20 hr

---

SPECIAL POPULATIONS

Pediatric and Geriatric Patients

There is little published dosing experience with dantrolene in neonatal or geriatric populations. Current dosing guidelines apply to children 5 years old and older. It is likely that dantrolene accumulates in patients with renal, hepatic, or biliary impairment. Dosage reductions should be considered in these patients, especially if the drug must be continued for more than 2 or 3 days. Signs of dantrolene poisoning include muscle weakness, lethargy, vomiting, diarrhea, and crystalluria.

Pregnant and Breast-feeding Patients

The safety of dantrolene use during pregnancy has not been established. Minor skeletal abnormalities not attributable to teratogenicity were observed in offspring of rats and mice given 60 mg/kg of dantrolene by mouth.[36,37] No adverse effects were observed in sheep given therapeutic doses or in

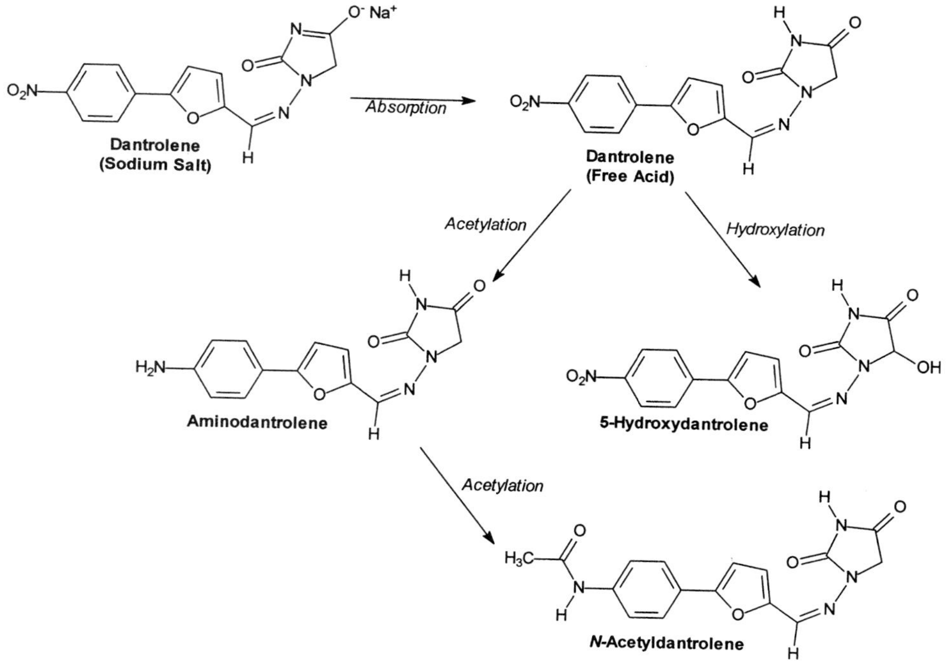

FIGURE 156-3

Metabolic pathway for dantrolene sodium.

their offspring.[38] In two small case series involving pregnant women, dantrolene crossed the placenta but caused no apparent harm to the mothers or the neonates. Neonatal dantrolene serum concentrations were 40% to 70% those of the mothers.[30,31] Dantrolene also has been detected in breast milk of a mother who was being treated for malignant hyperthermia after an emergency cesarean section. Her peak breast milk concentration was 1.2 μg/mL (3.8 μmol/L) 36 hours after birth. The half-life of dantrolene passing through breast milk was 9 hours.[39]

CONTRAINDICATIONS

Other than prior allergic reactions, there are no contraindications for short-term intravenous use of dantrolene. Long-term oral therapy (>45 days) is contraindicated in patients with active hepatic disease because of the possibility of exacerbating liver damage. Dantrolene also is contraindicated in patients who depend on spasticity to maintain posture or locomotion.

PRECAUTIONS

Intravenous dantrolene has a pH of 9.5. It can cause significant tissue loss if extravasation occurs. During the infusion, care must be taken to ensure that the catheter tip is placed within a nonmovable vein and that the solution is infused slowly enough to prevent backflow into surrounding tissue.

Each 20-mg vial of dantrolene contains 3 g of mannitol. This source of mannitol should be considered when a patient receives additional mannitol to preserve renal function. Patients should be monitored carefully for evidence of dehydration and pulmonary edema while receiving dantrolene. Patients with impaired cardiac or pulmonary function may be particularly susceptible to developing pulmonary edema during intravenous therapy.

On the day of intravenous administration, patients may experience difficulty swallowing, so they must be monitored carefully during meals for choking. Because dantrolene's muscle relaxant effects may last 48 hours after intravenous administration, patients who recover quickly should be told to avoid ethanol and sedative drugs and should be cautioned not to drive or operate heavy machinery.

Dantrolene should be avoided in patients taking verapamil. Anesthetized swine given therapeutic intravenous doses of verapamil and dantrolene developed rapid-onset atrioventricular block, hyperkalemia, and cardiovascular collapse.[40] Similar results were seen in dogs.[41] There is a single human case report of hyperkalemia and myocardial depression after concomitant administration of dantrolene and verapamil. A 60-year-old man treated with verapamil for coronary artery disease was given dantrolene 30 minutes before surgery. At 2.5 hours after the infusion finished (45 minutes after surgery was completed), his cardiac index decreased from 2.1 to 1.9 L/min/m^2 and his serum potassium increased to 7.1 mmol/L, despite an otherwise uneventful hemicolectomy. He was treated with insulin, and his condition improved over 4 hours. Six months later, the same patient received dantrolene before another surgical procedure. He had been switched to nifedipine 2 weeks before surgery and this time did not develop hyperkalemia or myocardial depression.[42] The exact mechanism responsible for this adverse effect is unknown. It is possible that myocardial depression results from a combination of slow calcium channel blockade and suppressed calcium release within the myocardium. Hyperkalemia may result from an enhanced release of potassium from muscle secondary to a direct effect of dantrolene on muscle or from decreased potassium uptake by the liver, skeletal muscle, and kidneys secondary to decreased cardiac output. It is unknown whether this interaction would occur with all calcium channel blockers.

Dantrolene also may potentiate vecuronium-induced muscle block. A 60-year-old woman given dantrolene and vecuronium before a breast biopsy had a longer recovery period, based on 75% recovery of evoked twitch tension, compared with eight control subjects.[43] Dantrolene may prevent presynaptic neurotransmitter release at the neuromuscular junction through a calcium-mediated process.

ADVERSE EFFECTS

The adverse effects of dantrolene depend on the dose, route, and duration of therapy. For short-course (3 to 5 days) intravenous or oral therapy, typical during treatment or prophylaxis of malignant hyperthermia, patients often develop transient muscle weakness, drowsiness, dizziness, lightheadedness, diarrhea, nausea, malaise, and fatigue (30% incidence of combined findings).[24] These side effects subside within 2 to 4 days of continued therapy and are alleviated by reducing the daily dose.[45,46] Patients receiving intravenous dantrolene also may experience phlebitis near the infusion site. The most serious side effects associated with short-course intravenous therapy are anaphylaxis and pulmonary edema. There has been one case of anaphylaxis and "rare reports" of dantrolene-associated pulmonary edema, according to the manufacturer. Large diluent and mannitol doses may have contributed to the development of pulmonary edema. The true incidence of anaphylaxis and pulmonary edema is unknown.

Long-term oral therapy has been associated with drowsiness (30%), dizziness (14%), nausea (9%), vomiting (9%), fatigue, and malaise.[24] In addition, patients may experience either constipation (4%) or persistent diarrhea (2.5%). Other, less frequent side effects include skin rash, acne-like dermatosis, headache, light-headedness, insomnia, feeling of inebriation, nervousness, dysarthria, anorexia, dysphagia, sialorrhea, gastric irritation, enuresis, visual disturbances, and blood dyscrasias.[44] The two most serious side effects associated with chronic dantrolene therapy are hepatotoxicity and pulmonary effusion; neither side effect occurs with short-course therapy.

Dantrolene-associated hepatotoxicity tends to occur after 1 to 6 weeks of long-term therapy, usually in patients taking more than 200 to 300 mg/day. Fatalities have clustered in patients older than 35 years of age, women, and patients taking dantrolene longer than 6 to 10 months.[47,48] These observations are based on two overlapping case series composed almost entirely of voluntary reports to the U.S. Food and Drug Administration. It is impossible to characterize true risk of dantrolene-associated hepatotoxicity without knowing the size and characteristics of the chronic dantrolene user population and without comparing the dantrolene population with a similarly matched control population.

The best estimate of the incidence of dantrolene-associated hepatotoxicity is derived from a review of safety data from premarketing clinical trials involving 1044 patients taking dantrolene for at least 60 days. In this group, 1.8% of patients taking dantrolene on a long-term basis developed hepatotoxicity, 0.6% showed clinical manifestations of hepatotoxicity, and 0.3% died as a direct result of hepatotoxicity.[47] Large doses were used regularly in these trials, so it is possible that the true incidence of hepatotoxicity is lower with current dosing.

Clinical manifestations are not sensitive indicators of hepatotoxicity during long-term dantrolene therapy. In four patients undergoing liver biopsy after suspected dantrolene-induced hepatotoxicity, two patients had no clinical symptoms but had marked hepatic necrosis on biopsy specimen.[49] Liver biopsy specimens usually show changes consistent with chronic active hepatitis, submassive necrosis, massive necrosis, or bridging necrosis.[47–50] The underlying mechanism for dantrolene-associated hepatotoxicity is poorly understood. Studies in rats have shown that dantrolene or one of its metabolites inactivates mixed-function oxidase and binds strongly to hepatic proteins. This activity is enhanced when glutathione is depleted.[51,52]

The treatment for dantrolene-induced hepatotoxicity is discontinuation of the drug. In most instances, serum transaminases and bilirubin return to normal within 1 to 12 months.[47]

Another rare, but serious, side effect of long-term dantrolene therapy is pleural effusion. Six cases have been published to date.[53–55] In two instances, the patients also had drug-induced pericarditis. Patients ranged in age from 20 to 53 years. All took oral dantrolene for longer than 60 days and presented with symptoms or shortness of breath. In all instances, the patient recovered after discontinuation of the drug. None of the patients were rechallenged. There is no discernible pattern in dose, gender, or age. Although the patients may have had pleural and peripheral eosinophilia, serum IgE concentrations were normal in all patients in whom IgE titers were checked, making it unlikely that pleural effusion was immunologically mediated.

ADMINISTRATION

The dosage of dantrolene for treating suspected malignant hyperthermia is 1 mg/kg/min intravenously until temperature, muscle stiffness, and heart rate decline. No more than 10 mg/kg should be used over a 15-minute period using this regimen. The loading dose may be repeated every 15 minutes if hyperthermia recurs. When an appropriate loading dose has been infused, the patient should be started on a maintenance infusion of 1 to 2 mg/kg over 3 to 4 hours, then switched to oral maintenance therapy (4 to 8 mg/kg/day) as soon as possible. This regimen works best if started within 6 hours of detection of malignant hyperthermia.[22]

The prophylactic oral preoperative dosage for children and adults known to be susceptible to malignant hyperthermia is 4 to 8 mg/kg/day divided into three or four doses given 1 to 2 days before surgery. The last dose should be given 3 to 4 hours before surgery begins. Alternatively a single intravenous dose of 2.5 mg/kg administered over 1 hour can be given 1.25 hours before surgery.[20] Malignant hyperthermia is discussed in detail in Chapter 25.

Intravenous dantrolene is prepared by adding 60 mL of sterile water for injection to each 20-mg vial of lyophilized product. It should not be reconstituted or administered with any other solution. The final reconstituted product should be transferred to a plastic administration bag (not glass) and shielded from light. Intravenous dantrolene must be used within 6 hours of reconstitution.

A dantrolene oral suspension can be prepared by mixing the contents of an appropriate number of dantrolene capsules into a simple syrup containing citric acid (150 mg/100 mL final product) with or without preservative (0.15% methyl hydroxybenzoate). This suspension is stable at 5°C, 25°C, and 40°C (104°F, 41°F, and 77°F) for 150 days. It should be dispensed in high-density polyethylene bottles and should be shaken before use. Fawcett and associates[56] recommended assuming a shelf-life of 30 days for the suspension.

The oral dosage used for treating spasticity in adults is 25 mg/day initially. The dose should be increased in 7-day increments until limb functionality is improved. Dosage should not exceed 400 mg/day. Typically the progression is as follows:

25 mg once daily for 7 days
25 mg three times daily for 7 days
50 mg three times daily for 7 days
100 mg three times daily for 7 days

In pediatric patients, the dosage progression is as follows:

Starting dose, 0.5 mg/kg/dose once daily for 7 days
0.5 mg/kg three times daily for 7 days
1 mg/kg three times daily for 7 days
2 mg/kg three times daily, if needed

The lowest effective dose always should be used.[44]

Dosages used to treat neuroleptic malignant syndrome are 3 to 10 mg/kg intravenously followed by repeat oral doses of 25 to 600 mg/day depending on response. Most patients respond within 12 hours.[21] Neuroleptic malignant syndrome is discussed in detail in Chapter 26.

REFERENCES

1. Synder HR, Davis CS, Bickerton RK, et al: 1-[(5-Arylfurfurylidene) amino] hydantoins: A new class of muscle relaxants. J Med Chem 10:807–810, 1967.
2. Honkomp LJ, Halliday RP, Wessels FL: Dantrolene, 1-[5-(p-nitrophenyl) furfurylidene] amino hydantoin: A unique skeletal muscle relaxant. Pharmacologist 12:301, 1970.
3. Chyatte SB, Birdsong JH, Bergman BA: The effect of dantrolene sodium in spasticity and motor performance in hemiplegia. South Med J 64:180–185, 1971.
4. Ellis KO, Bryant SH: Excitation-contraction uncoupling in skeletal muscle by dantrolene sodium. Naunyn Schmiedebergs Arch Pharmacol 274:107–109, 1972.
5. Ellis KO, Carpenter JF: Studies on the mechanism of action of dantrolene sodium: A skeletal muscle relaxant. Naunyn Schmiedebergs Arch Pharmacol 275:83–94, 1972.
6. Kolb ME, Horne ML, Martz R: Dantrolene in human malignant hyperthermia. Anesthesiology 56:254–262, 1982.
7. Bernal ORA, Bender MA, Lacey ME: Effficacy of dantrolene sodium in management of tetanus in children. J R Soc Med 79:277–281, 1986.
8. Tsutsumi Y, Yamamoto K, Matsuura S, et al: The treatment of neuroleptic malignant syndrome using dantrolene sodium. Psychiatr Clin Neurosci 52:433–438, 1998.
9. Pennati A, Sacchetti E, Calzeroni A: Dantrolene in lethal catatonia (Letter). Am J Psychiatry 148:268, 1991.
10. Gross MH, Fulkerson WJ, Moore JO: Prevention of amphotericin B-induced rigors by dantrolene. Arch Intern Med 146:1587–1588, 1986.
11. Ryan PJ: Preliminary report: Experience with the use of dantrolene sodium in the treatment of bites by the black widow spider Latrodectus hesperus (Abstract). J Toxicol Clin Toxicol 21:487–489, 1984.
12. Singarajah C, Lavies NG: An overdose of ecstasy: A role for dantrolene. Anaesthesia 47:686–687, 1992.
13. Hall AP, Lyburn ID, Spears FD, et al: An unusual case of Ecstasy poisoning. Intensive Care Med 22:670–671, 1996.
14. Kaplan RF, Feinglass NG, Webster W, et al: Phenelzine overdose treated with dantrolene sodium. JAMA 255:642–644, 1986.
15. Parr MJA, Willatts SM: Fatal theophylline poisoning with rhabdomyolysis: A potential role for dantrolene treatment. Anaesthesia 46:557–559, 1991.
16. Ten Holter JBM, Schellens RLLAM: Dantrolene sodium for treatment of carbon monoxide poisoning. BMJ 296:1772–1773, 1988.
17. Ochi G, Watanabe K, Tokuoka H, et al: Neuroleptic malignant-like syndrome: A complication of acute organophosphate poisoning. Can J Anaesth 42:1027–1030, 1995.
18. Guieu R, Kopeyan C, Sampieri F, et al: Use of dantrolene in experimental scorpion envenomation by Androctonus australis hector. Arch Toxicol 69:575–577, 1995.
19. Hackler RH, Broecker BH, Klein FA, et al: A clinical experience with dantrolene sodium for external urinary sphincter hypertonicity in spinal cord injured patients. J Urol 124:78–81, 1980.
20. Dantrium Intravenous (dantrolene sodium). Product Information. Mason, OH, Proctor & Gamble Pharmaceuticals, 2001.
21. Ward A, Chaffman MO, Sorkin EM: Dantrolene—a review of its pharmacodynamic and pharmacokinetic properties and therapeutic use in malignant hyperthermia, the neuroleptic malignant syndrome, and an update of its use in muscle spasticity. Drugs 32:130–168, 1986.
22. Britt BA: Dantrolene. Can Anaesth Soc J 31:61–75, 1984.
23. Harrison GG: Dantrolene—dynamics and kinetics. Br J Anaesth 60:279–286, 1988.
24. Dykes MHM: Evaluation of a muscle relaxant: Dantrolene sodium (Dantrium). JAMA 231:862–864, 1975.
25. Herman R, Mayer N, Mecomber SA: Clinical pharmaco-physiology of dantrolene sodium. Am J Phys Med 51:296–311, 1972.
26. Monster AW, Herman R, Meeks S, et al: Cooperative study for assessing the effects of a pharmacological agent on spasticity. Am J Phys Med 52:163–188, 1973.
27. Meyler WJ, Mols-Thürkow HW, Wesseling H: Relationship between plasma concentration and effect of dantrolene sodium in man. Eur J Clin Pharmacol 16:203–209, 1979.
28. Flewellen EH, Nelson TE, Jones WP, et al: Dantrolene dose response in awake man: Implications for management of malignant hyperthermia. Anesthesiology 59:275–280, 1983.
29. Allen GC, Cattran CB, Peterson RG, et al: Plasma levels of dantrolene following oral administration in malignant hyperthermia-susceptible patients. Anesthesiology 69:900–904, 1988.
30. Morison DH: Placental transfer of dantrolene (Letter). Anesthesiology 59:265, 1983.
31. Shime J, Gare D, Andrews J, et al: Dantrolene in pregnancy: Lack of adverse effects on the fetus and newborn infant. Am J Obstet Gynecol 159:831–834, 1988.
32. Ellis KO, Wessels FL: Muscle relaxant properties of the identified metabolites of dantrolene. Naunyn Schmiedebergs Arch Pharmacol 301:237–240, 1978.
33. Leitman PS, Haslam RHA, Walcher JR: Pharmacology of dantrolene sodium in children. Arch Phys Med Rehabil 55:388–392, 1974.
34. Flewellen EH, Nelson TE: Intravenous dantrolene pharmacokinetics in malignant hyperthermia suspect patients. Anesthesiology 63(Suppl 3A):300, 1985.
35. Lerman J, McLeod ME, Strong HA: Pharmacokinetics of intravenous dantrolene in children. Anesthesiology 70:625–629, 1989.
36. Nagaoka T: Reproductive test of dantrolene: Teratogenicity test on rats. Clin Rep 11:2218–2230, 1977.
37. Nagaoka T: Reproductive studies of dantrolene: Teratogenicity study in rabbits. Clin Rep 11:2212–2217, 1977.
38. Craft JB, Goldberg NH, Lim M, et al: Cardiovascular effects and placental passage of dantrolene in the maternal-fetal sheep model. Anesthesiology 68:68–72, 1988.
39. Fricker RM, Hoerauf KH, Drewe J, et al: Secretion of dantrolene into breast milk after acute therapy of a suspected malignant hyperthermia crisis during Cesarean section. Anesthesiology 89:1023–1025, 1998.
40. Saltzman LS, Kates RA, Corke BC, et al: Hyperkalemia and cardiovascular collapse after verapamil and dantrolene administration in swine. Anesth Analg 63:473–478, 1984.
41. Lynch C, Durbin CG, Fisher NA, et al: Effects of dantrolene and verapamil on atrioventricular conduction and cardiovascular performance in dogs. Anesth Analg 65:252–258, 1986.
42. Rubin AS, Zablocki AD: Hyperkalemia, verapamil, and dantrolene. Anesthesiology 66:246–249, 1987.
43. Driessen JJ, Wuis EW, Gielen MJM: Prolonged vecuronium neuromuscular blockade in a patient receiving orally administered dantrolene. Anesthesiology 62:523–524, 1985.

44. Dantrium Capsules (dantrolene sodium). Product information. Mason, OH, Proctor & Gamble Pharmaceuticals, 2001.

45. McEvoy G, Litvak K, Welsh OH, et al (eds): Dantrolene. In: AHFS Drug Information. Bethesda, MD, American Society of Health-System Pharmacists, 2001.

46. Pinder RM, Brogden RN, Speight TM, et al: Dantrolene sodium: A review of its pharmacological properties and therapeutic efficacy in spasticity. Drugs 13:3–23, 1977.

47. Utili R, Boitnott JK, Zimmerman HJ: Dantrolene-associated hepatic injury. Gastroenterology 72:610–616, 1977.

48. Chan CH: Dantrolene sodium and hepatic injury. Neurology 40:1427–1432, 1990.

49. Wilkinson SP, Portmann B, Williams R: Hepatitis from dantrolene sodium. Gut 20:33–36, 1979.

50. Schneider R, Mitchell D: Dantrolene hepatitis. JAMA 235:1590–1591, 1976.

51. Roy S, Francis KT, Born CK, et al: Interaction of dantrolene with the hepatic mixed function oxidase system. Res Commun Chem Pathol Pharmacol 27:507–520, 1980.

52. Arnold TH, Epps JM, Cook HR, et al: Dantolene sodium: Urinary metabolites and hepatoxicity. Res Commun Chem Pathol Pharmacol 39:381–398, 1983.

53. Petusevsky M, Faling LJ, Rocklin RE, et al: Pleuropericardial reaction to treatment with dantrolene. JAMA 242:2772–2774, 1979.

54. Miller DH, Haas LF: Pneumonitis, pleural effusion, and pericarditis following treatment with dantrolene. J Neurol Neurosurg Psychiatry 47:553–554, 1984.

55. Mahoney JM, Bachtel MD: Pleural effusion associated with chronic dantrolene administration. Ann Pharmacother 28:587–589, 1994.

56. Fawcett JP, Stark G, Tucker IG, et al: Stability of dantrolene oral suspension prepared from capsules. J Clin Pharm Ther 19:349–353, 1994.

CHAPTER 157

Folic and Folinic Acid

S. Rutherfoord Rose ■ Christopher P. Holstege

Folic acid is a water-soluble, B-complex vitamin that is essential for nucleoprotein synthesis. It traditionally is administered for the treatment of megaloblastic anemias, and more recent data have confirmed its ability to reduce fetal neural tube defects when administered as a vitamin supplement or through food fortification. Subsequently, folic acid supplementation has been associated with decreases in blood homocysteine concentrations and decreased risk of cardiovascular disease. Folic or folinic acid is used in the treatment of drug-induced toxicity due to folic acid antagonists and methanol. This chapter focuses on the use of folate as an antidote.

HISTORY

Research in anemias in the early to mid 20th century showed that extracts of crude liver had hematopoietic properties and could be used to treat macrocytic anemia. These observations led to the discovery of cyanocobalamin (vitamin B_{12}) and folic acid (formerly known as vitamins Bc, B_9, B_{10}, B_{11}, or M), water-soluble vitamins necessary for the maturation of erythrocytes. Folic acid first was isolated from spinach in the early 1940s and received its name from the word *foliage* (dark green leaf). Other common dietary sources include green leafy vegetables, liver, beans, peas, asparagus, beets, broccoli, and citrus fruits. Subsequent work showed that dietary folate (pteroylpolyglutamate) is not metabolically active but must be converted in vivo to the active 5-formyl tetrahydrofolate (folinic acid or leucovorin).

Folic acid is now recognized as a necessary cofactor not only for hematopoiesis but also for normal growth and development. Periconceptional treatment with multivitamins containing folic acid has reduced the incidence around the world of infants born with neural tube defects, such as spina bifida, encephalocele, and anencephaly.[1,2] The U.S. Food and Drug Administration mandated the fortification of enriched grain products with folic acid by 1998, and more recent data suggest that birth prevalence of neural tube defects is reduced with food fortification of 140 μg of folic acid per 100 g of grain (approximately 100 μg in an average daily diet).[3]

Folate and other B vitamins also are cofactors in the metabolism of homocysteine, an amino acid formed during the metabolism of methionine, an essential dietary amino acid. The relationship between hyperhomocysteinemia and vascular disease was identified in the late 1960s, and more recent data suggest that elevated plasma homocysteine levels are associated with increased mortality in patients with coronary artery disease.[4,5] Folic acid fortification resulting in increased plasma folate concentrations has been shown to reduce total blood homocysteine concentrations and to reduce the rate of restenosis after coronary angioplasty.[6,7]

The ability of leucovorin (the active form of folic acid) to attenuate the toxicity of high-dose methotrexate therapy first was shown in mice in the 1960s.[8] The concept of "leucovorin rescue" is to take advantage of the cytotoxicity of high-dose methotrexate against malignant cells and spare the toxic effects from normal cells.[8,9] The use of leucovorin also is approved for the treatment of toxicity from other folate antagonists (trimethoprim, pyrimethamine), but two more recent trials found no benefit and possibly worse outcomes in patients with human immunodeficiency virus–associated infections.[10,11]

Today, commercially available folic acid (pteroylmonoglutamic acid) is prepared synthetically and is used in vitamin supplements (alone or in multivitamin preparations) and in food fortification. Commercial products that contain more than 0.4 mg (or 0.8 mg for prenatal use) of folic acid require a prescription in the United States, as does the parenteral formulation. Folic acid is used in the treatment of megaloblastic and macrocytic anemias that result from folate deficiency.

Folinic acid is the active, reduced form of folic acid. It is commercially available as the calcium salt leucovorin. It is marketed primarily as an antidote for the hematologic toxicity of folic acid antagonists, such as methotrexate, trimethoprim, and pyrimethamine.

PROPERTIES

The term *folic acid* refers to dihydrofolic acid, a B-complex vitamin that in pure form appears as a yellow-orange crystalline powder. It is slightly soluble in water, soluble in dilute alkaline solutions, and insoluble in alcohol. The pharmaceutical folic acid products are prepared synthetically and consist of a central *p*-aminobenzoic acid molecule that is linked to a pteridine ring on one end and a glutamate molecule on the other end (Fig. 157-1). Folic acid's chemical formula is $C_{18}H_{19}N_7O_6$; its molecular weight is 441.40. It is heat sensitive and decomposes rapidly in light. Dietary folates occur naturally as polyglutamates and must be hydrolyzed (reduced) before absorption.

Folinic acid is the highly water-soluble product of the reduction of folic acid by dihydrofolic acid reductase (DHFR) (Fig. 157-2). Its chemical formula is $C_{19}H_{22}N_7O_7$, and its

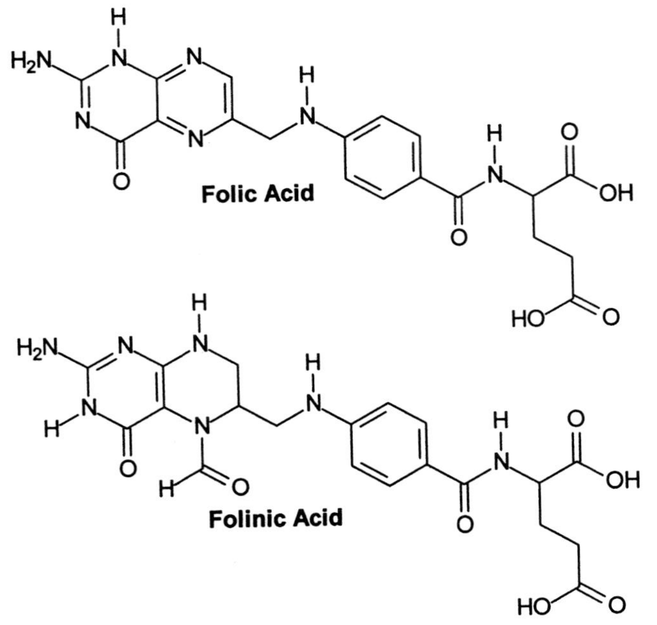

Folic Acid

Folinic Acid

FIGURE 157-1

Chemical structures of folic and folinic acids.

structure is shown in Figure 157-1. It is commercially available as the calcium salt (leucovorin), a 50% racemic mixture of the *d* and *l* isomers; only the *l*-isomer (*l*-folinic acid or citrovorum factor) is metabolically active.

PHARMACODYNAMICS

Folic acid is an essential vitamin necessary for nucleoprotein synthesis and the maintenance of normal erythropoiesis (see Fig. 157-2). Folic acid itself is not metabolically active but rather is activated by reduction and catalyzed by DHFR to 5-methyltetrahydrofolic acid and other tetrahydrofolate

derivatives. Each of the reduced folate congeners can acquire 1-carbon moieties that can be donated in the biosynthesis of nucleic acids, amino acids, proteins, or lipids.[9] Specific reactions (and the specific congener) in amino acid metabolism that require reduced folic acid coenzymes include the metabolism of homocysteine to methionine (5-methyltetrahydrofolate), the formation of glutamic acid from histidine (tetrahydrofolic acid), and the interconversion of glycine and serine (tetrahydrofolic acid). The methylation of deoxyuridylate to thymidylate, a crucial step in the synthesis of DNA, uses 5,10-methylenetetrahydrofolic acid. In folic acid–deficient patients or patients with inhibited DHFR, a futile cycle of faulty DNA replication occurs and subsequently leads to clinical effects such as megaloblastic anemias.

Folic acid (as tetrahydrofolate and 10-formyltetrahydrofolate) is also a cofactor that is necessary for the metabolism of formic acid. Methanol poisoning results in the accumulation of formic acid in humans. Plasma formic acid concentrations have been shown in animal models and in human case series to correspond closely to the development of the metabolic acidosis seen after methanol poisoning.[12–16] The development of metabolic acidosis and depletion of serum bicarbonate that coincide with the accumulation of formic acid after methanol poisoning are unique to primates. Other species, such as rats, do not accumulate formic acid and subsequently do not develop metabolic acidosis because of their differences in the rate of formic acid oxidation to carbon dioxide, which is folate dependent.[17] The rate of formic acid metabolism and subsequent resolution of metabolic acidosis are decreased during states of folic acid deficiency and increased with folic or folinic acid therapy in primates.[18] Folic or folinic acid therapy is an integral component in the treatment of methanol toxicity. The treatment of methanol poisoning is discussed in detail in Chapter 86.

Folinic acid also is used in the treatment of methotrexate toxicity.[19,20] Methotrexate competitively inhibits the enzyme DHFR (Fig. 157-3). Subsequently, no reduced folate is formed, and the biosynthesis of nucleic acids,

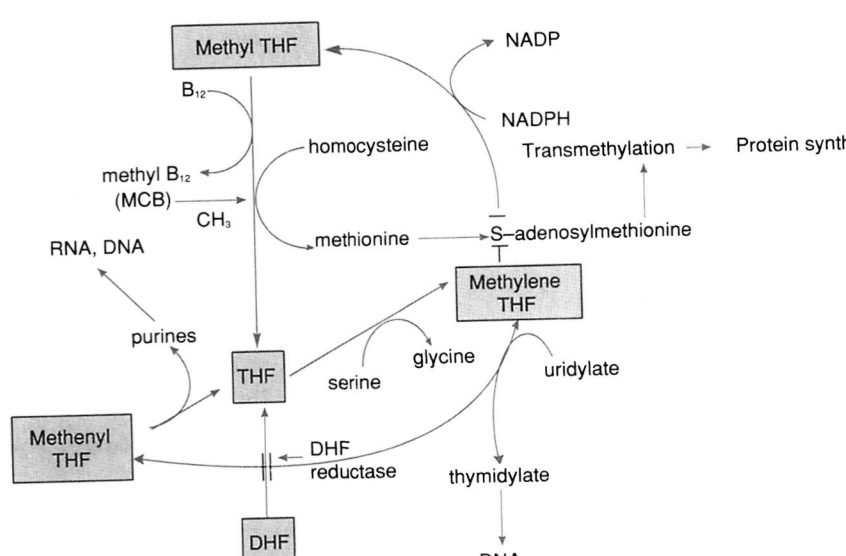

FIGURE 157-2

Folate metabolism. DHF, folic acid; NADP, nicotinamide-adenine dinucleotide phosphate; NADPH, nicotinamide-adenine dinucleotide phosphate, reduced form; THF, folinic acid. *(From Ballen KK: Drugs to treat anemia. In Brody TM, Larner J, Minneman KP [eds]: Human Pharmacology: Molecular to Clinical, 3rd ed. St. Louis, Mosby, 1998, p 892.)*

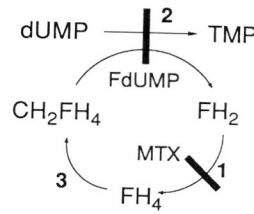

FIGURE 157-3

Sites of action of methotrexate (MTX) and the fluoropyrimidine antimetabolite fluorodeoxyuridylate (FdUMP): (1) DHFR, dihydrofolate reductase; (2) TS, thymidylate synthase; (3) SHM, serine hydroxymethylate; FH_2, dihydrofolate; FH_4, tetrahydrofolate; CH_2FH_4, N^5,N^{10}-methylenetetrahydrofolate. *(From Bertino JR: Antineoplastic drugs. In Smith CM, Reynard CM [eds]: Textbook of Pharmacology. Philadelphia, WB Saunders, 1992, p 944.)*

amino acids, proteins, and lipids is inhibited (see Fig. 157-2). Clinically, methotrexate toxicity results in a triad of mucositis, renal failure, and myelosuppression. Gastrointestinal symptoms may be pronounced and consist of stomatitis, pharyngitis, anorexia, nausea, emesis, diarrhea, gastrointestinal hemorrhage, and hepatotoxicity. Pancytopenia can develop and may lead to life-threatening bleeding disorders, anemia, and sepsis. Nephrotoxicity can result in oliguria, azotemia, and acute renal failure. This nephrotoxicity may exacerbate systemic toxicity because the kidneys primarily eliminate methotrexate. The management of methotrexate toxicity, which is discussed in detail in Chapter 60, focuses on administration of folinic acid. Folinic acid administration allows purine and subsequent DNA synthesis to resume. Folic acid administration is not effective because of the methotrexate-induced inhibition of DHFR. Even if methotrexate concentrations are not detectable, intracellular inhibition of DHFR still may be occurring in methotrexate toxicity. Folinic acid should be administered until signs of systemic toxicity resolve. Theoretically, folinic acid rescue also can be employed when toxicity occurs from other weaker DHFR inhibitors, such as trimethoprim, trimetrexate, pentamidine, and pyrimethamine.

PHARMACOKINETICS

Reduced dietary folate and pharmaceutical folic acid are absorbed rapidly from the proximal small intestine, regardless of the presence of malabsorption syndromes. Absorbed folic acid is methylated rapidly by dihydrofolate reductase to active tetrahydrofolate metabolites, including 5-methyltetrahydrofolate, the primary transport and storage form of folate. The active tetrahydrofolates are distributed widely throughout the body, with the highest concentrations found in the liver (approximately 50% of body stores) and in cerebrospinal fluid. Urinary recovery of folate is dose dependent, with only trace amounts of folate found in urine after low doses (<1 mg) and 90% of folate found in urine after a dose of 15 mg. Excretion generally is complete within 24 hours.

In contrast to folic acid, leucovorin does not require reduction (activation) and is converted easily to other

Pharmacokinetics of Folic Acid and Folinic Acid

Folic Acid

Absorption: 90–100% (synthetic)
Time to peak serum concentration: 30–60 min
Normal serum concentration (total folate): 5–15 ng/mL
Normal red blood cell concentration (total folate): 175–316 ng/mL
Metabolites: 5-methyltetrahydrofolate (active)
Excretion (total folate): via urine as metabolites; generally complete by 24 hr

Folinic Acid

Absorption: 97% of 25 mg; 37% of 100 mg
Time to peak serum concentration: 1–2 hr
Normal serum concentration (total folate): 5–15 ng/mL
Normal red blood cell concentration (total folate): 175–316 ng/mL
Metabolites: 5-methyltetrahydrofolate (active); L-formyltetrahydrofolate (active); D-formyltetrahydrofolate (inactive)
Excretion (total folate): via urine as metabolites; generally complete by 24 hr

tetrahydrofolate derivatives. The absorption of leucovorin administered orally becomes saturated with doses greater than 25 mg, making bioavailability dose limited. The *l*-isomer of leucovorin is converted more rapidly to 5-methyltetrahydrofolate when administered orally than when injected (see Fig. 157-2). In addition, oral and parenteral doses of leucovorin result in different kinetic profiles for the various metabolites, but these differences are not known to affect efficacy.[21] The inactive *d*-isomer is excreted renally as unchanged drug. The various reduced serum folate metabolites are removed by hemodialysis.

SPECIAL POPULATIONS

Neonatal Patients

Recommended dietary allowances of folate are 25 μg/day and 35 μg/day for infants 0 to 6 months and 6 to 12 months of age, respectively. Folate is distributed to breast milk, and infant requirements should be met if the mother is healthy. There is no published experience with the use of folate as an antidote in neonates, but there should be no reason not to administer folate if necessary in this population.

Pediatric Patients

Recommended dietary allowances of folate are 50 to 100 μg/day for children age 1 to 10 years. There are no special dosing precautions in children who require emergent leucovorin therapy.

Pregnant Patients

Dietary requirements of folate are highest in pregnant women, particularly women with a history of previous pregnancies complicated by infants with neural tube defects. Theoretically, treatment with folate as an antidote for drug toxicity should be particularly aggressive in these patients.

Alcoholic Patients

Alcoholics who are malnourished may have relative deficiencies of all B vitamins, including folic acid.

CONTRAINDICATIONS

Folic or folinic acid preparations should not be administered to patients with previous hypersensitivity reactions. Folic acid and leucovorin should be administered with extreme caution to patients with undifferentiated anemia because folate alleviates hematologic but not neurologic complications associated with pernicious anemia secondary to vitamin B_{12} deficiency.

PRECAUTIONS

Rare cases of allergic reactions to oral and parenteral folic acid have been reported. Symptoms have included erythema, pruritus, rash, and bronchospasm.

Intravenous leucovorin infusions should not exceed 160 mg/min of leucovorin because of the calcium concentration of the solution. Folic acid for injection contains benzyl alcohol as a preservative and should be administered with caution to (premature) infants because a potentially fatal "gasping syndrome" has been associated with benzyl alcohol administration in this age group.

Treatment using high-dose methotrexate with leucovorin rescue therapy should be administered only by physicians who are experienced in cancer chemotherapy. Leucovorin may enhance the toxicity of 5-fluorouracil by causing increased inhibition of thymidylate synthetase (see Fig. 157-3). In addition, in patients diagnosed with a high-grade malignancy, such as a blast crisis from acute leukemia, the disease process may be accelerated if folic or folinic acid alone is administered without antineoplastic therapy.[9]

DRUG INTERACTIONS

Several antiepileptic drugs, specifically phenytoin, phenobarbital, primidone, and carbamazepine, may result in a lowering of erythrocyte folic acid concentrations. Phenytoin has been the most extensively studied antiepileptic drug showing this interaction, with reports of abnormally low erythrocyte folic acid concentrations in 25% of patients receiving phenytoin therapy.[22,23] Conversely, reports of oral folic acid therapy causing a decrease in serum phenytoin concentrations with subsequent breakthrough seizures have been published.[23,24] Clinicians should consider monitoring antiepileptic drug serum concentrations in patients taking antiepileptic drugs who subsequently receive folic or folinic acid supplementation.

ADVERSE EFFECTS

Folic acid administered orally or parenterally is generally well tolerated. Repeated high oral doses (>10 mg/day) may cause nausea, abdominal pain, anorexia, or flatulence. Central nervous system effects associated with high oral doses include irritability, depression, impaired judgment, difficulty in concentration, and altered sleep. Adverse consequences related to folate therapy have not been reported in patients treated for acute methanol poisoning. Patients should be monitored for allergic reactions, with supportive care provided as needed.

ADMINISTRATION

There are no controlled data evaluating the dose and administration of folate for acute poisoning; however, in these patients, it generally is accepted that doses of leucovorin calcium and folic acid should be administered intravenously. Folic acid for injection (5 mg/1 mL) should be diluted with 49 mL of sterile water for injection to a final concentration of 0.1 mg/mL of folic acid and administered by injection. Leucovorin calcium powder, after reconstitution with sterile water for injection, should be infused at a rate not exceeding 160 mg/min owing to the calcium content of the leucovorin solution.

REFERENCES

1. Smithells RW, Sheppard S, Schorah CJ, et al: Possible prevention of neural-tube deficits by periconceptional vitamin supplementation. Lancet 1:339–340, 1980.
2. Berry RJ, Li Z, Erickson JD, et al: Prevention of neural-tube defects with folic acid in China. N Engl J Med 341:1485–1490, 1999.
3. Honein MA, Paulozzi LJ, Mathews TJ, et al: Impact of folic acid fortification of the US food supply on the occurrence of neural tube defects. JAMA 285:2981–2986, 2001.
4. Welch GN, Loscalzo J: Homocysteine and atherothrombosis. N Engl J Med 338:1042–1050, 1998.
5. Nygard O, Nordrehaug JE, Refsum H, et al: Plasma homocysteine levels and mortality in patients with coronary artery disease. N Engl J Med 337:230–236, 1997.
6. Jacques PF, Selhub J, Bostom AG, et al: The effect of folic acid fortification on plasma folate and total homocysteine concentrations. N Engl J Med 340:1449–1454, 1999.
7. Schnyder G, Roffi M, Pin R, et al: Decreased rate of coronary restenosis after lowering of plasma homocysteine levels. N Engl J Med 345:1593–1600, 2001.
8. Treon SP, Chabner BA: Concepts in use of high-dose methotrexate therapy. Clin Chem 42:1322–1329, 1996.
9. Bleyer WA: New vistas for leucovorin in cancer chemotherapy. Cancer 63:995–1007, 1989.
10. Bozzette SA, Forthal D, Sattler FR, et al: The tolerance for zidovudine plus thrice weekly in daily trimethoprim-sulfamethoxazole with and without leucovorin for primary prophylaxis in advanced HIV disease. Am J Med 98:177–182, 1995.
11. Safrin S, Lee BL, Sande MA: Adjunctive folinic acid with trimethoprim-sulfamethoxazole for *Pneumocystis carinii* pneumonia in AIDS patients is associated with an increased risk of therapeutic failure and death. J Infect Dis 170:912–917, 1994.

12. McMartin KE, Makar AB, Martin-Amat G, et al: Methanol poisoning: I. The role of formic acid in the development of metabolic acidosis in the monkey and the reversal by 4-methylpyrazole. Biochem Med 13:319–333, 1975.

13. Clay KL, Murphy RC, Watkins WD: Experimental methanol toxicity in the primate: Analysis of metabolic acidosis. Toxicol Appl Pharmacol 34:49–61, 1975.

14. McMartin KE, Martin-Amat G, Makar AB, et al: Methanol poisoning: V. Role of formate metabolism in the monkey. J Pharmacol Exp Ther 201:564–572, 1977.

15. McMartin KE, Ambre JJ, Tephly TR: Methanol poisoning in human subjects—role for formic acid accumulation in the metabolic acidosis. Am J Med 68:414–418, 1980.

16. Sejersted OM, Jacobsen D, Øvrebø S, et al: Formate concentrations in plasma from patients poisoned with methanol. Acta Med Scand 213:105–110, 1983.

17. Palese M, Tephly TR: Metabolism of formate in the rat. J Toxicol Environ Health 1:13–24, 1975.

18. Noker PE, Eells JT, Tephly TR: Methanol toxicity: Treatment with folic acid and 5-formyl tetrahydrofolic acid. Alcohol Clin Exp Res 4:378–383, 1980.

19. Grimes DJ, Bowles MR, Buttsworth JA, et al: Survival after unexpected high serum methotrexate concentrations in a patient with osteogenic sarcoma. Drug Saf 5:447–454, 1990.

20. Flombaum CD, Meyers PA: High-dose leucovorin as sole therapy for methotrexate toxicity. J Clin Oncol 17:1589–1594, 1999.

21. McGuire BW, Sia LL, Leese PT, et al: Pharmacokinetics of leucovorin calcium after intravenous, intramuscular, and oral administration. Clin Pharm 7:52–58, 1988.

22. Tamura T, Aiso K, Johnston KE, et al: Homocysteine, folate, vitamin B-12, and vitamin B-6 in patients receiving antiepileptic drug monotherapy. Epilepsy Res 40:7–15, 2000.

23. Lewis DP, Van Dyke DC, Willhite LA, et al: Phenytoin-folic acid interaction. Ann Pharmacother 29:1303–1304, 1995.

24. Seligmann H, Potasman I, Weller B, et al: Phenytoin-folic acid interaction: A lesson to be learned. Clin Neuropharmacol 22:268–272, 1999.

CHAPTER **158**

Thiamine

William A. Watson

Thiamine (vitamin B$_1$, thiamin) is a water-soluble vitamin used primarily to treat patients either with thiamine deficiency or at risk for thiamine deficiency. Plants synthesize thiamine; grains, vegetables, and, to a lesser extent, meats are the primary dietary sources for humans. Adults require a daily dietary intake of at least 1 mg. Although bacteria synthesize thiamine, this pathway does not play a significant role in providing thiamine because it occurs in the large bowel, where there is minimal absorption. Inadequate dietary intake is the most common cause of thiamine deficiency worldwide. The addition of thiamine to food (e.g., baking flour) minimizes the prevalence of thiamine deficiency, unless other risk factors are present. Cooking results in the degradation of varying amounts of thiamine content.[1]

The most common toxicologic reason for thiamine deficiency is decreased dietary thiamine and impaired absorption of oral thiamine resulting from ethanol abuse; this is particularly likely in individuals consuming greater than 30% of their total calories in the form of ethanol.[2] Decreased thiamine absorption also is seen with malabsorption syndromes, hepatic disease, folate deficiency, renal dialysis, eating disorders, cancer, and severe infection and during parenteral alimentation.[3,4] Less commonly, thiamine deficiency is secondary to increased clearance associated with diuretic administration.[5] In addition to thiamine deficiency, Wernicke's disease in some patients is associated with a hereditary decrease in the affinity of transketolase for thiamine pyrophosphate.[6] The clinical presentation of thiamine deficiency is beriberi, which can include polyneuritis, high-output cardiac failure, and, in severe cases, the syndrome of Wernicke's disease and Korsakoff's psychosis (Wernicke-Korsakoff syndrome). Thiamine deficiency often is not diagnosed clinically and most commonly is identified at autopsy.[7] The clinical syndromes of thiamine deficiency occur because of thiamine's role as a cofactor in various metabolic reactions (see Pharmacodynamics).[1,8]

In ethylene glycol toxicity, thiamine is a potential antidote; it is a coenzyme in the conversion of glyoxylic acid (an ethylene glycol metabolite) by α-ketoglutarate:glyoxylate carboligase to α-hydroxy-β-ketoadipate (see Fig. 83-1).[9] This is a minor pathway of glyoxylic acid metabolism, and there is no direct evidence that thiamine administration enhances glyoxylic acid metabolism or decreases ethylene glycol toxicity.

HISTORY

In 1885, the role of dietary supplementation in the prevention of beriberi was described, and thiamine was isolated in 1926. Synthesis of thiamine was described in 1936, and adverse effects associated with parenteral thiamine administration were described soon after.[1,10] The routine administration of parenteral thiamine in patients with risk factors for thiamine deficiency is associated with the recommendation in the mid-1970s to administer glucose to patients with depressed mental status of unknown cause. The administration of hypertonic glucose without prior thiamine administration was believed to precipitate Wernicke's disease, although this was based on incomplete background information. The clinical evidence supports the worsening of Wernicke's disease after the administration of glucose, as opposed to the precipitation of disease. The worsening of Wernicke's encephalopathy by glucose administration has been reported in only a few cases in which large amounts of glucose were administered over a prolonged period in the absence of concomitant thiamine supplementation.[8,11,12]

PROPERTIES

Thiamine is 3-[(4-amino-2-methyl-5-pyrimidinylchloride)-methyl]-5-(2-hydroxyethyl)-4-methylthiazolium (Fig. 158-1). It is most commonly available as the hydrochloride salt C$_{12}$H$_{18}$CL$_2$N$_4$OS, with a molecular weight of 337.28. It is water soluble, with 1 g of thiamine hydrochloride dissolving in 1 mL of water.

PHARMACODYNAMICS

Thiamine is a coenzyme in numerous metabolic pathways that generate and use cellular energy. In humans, thiamine is phosphorylated and is found as monophosphate, diphosphate, and triphosphate. The diphosphate (pyrophosphate) is the active coenzyme. The presence of thiamine pyrophosphate is required for the conversion of pyruvate to acetyl coenzyme A, which is the gateway to the Krebs cycle, allowing aerobic adenosine triphosphate production. Decreased enzyme activity causes increased pyruvate conversion to lactate, resulting in lactic acidosis.

Thiamine also is a coenzyme for α-ketoglutarate dehydrogenase in the Krebs cycle. In the pentose phosphate

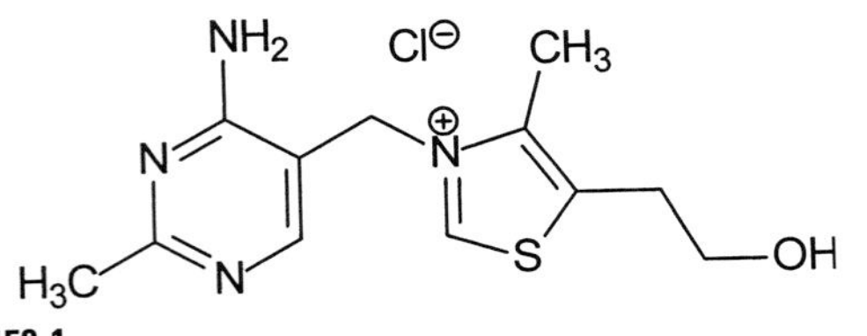

FIGURE 158-1

Chemical structure of thiamine chloride.

cycle, thiamine is a coenzyme for transketolase in the synthesis of nucleotides and reduced nicotinamide-adenine dinucleotide phosphate.[1,3]

In the central nervous system, thiamine is present as the diphosphate and triphosphate forms. Although the mechanisms are not understood, thiamine is necessary for normal brain metabolism, blood-brain barrier integrity, and neuronal conduction. Thiamine content is maintained relatively constant in the brain.[13] It also is believed to have a role in lipid elaboration and membrane transport. As noted earlier, in ethylene glycol toxicity, thiamine may play a role in the conversion of glyoxylic acid by α-ketoglutarate:glyoxylate carboligase to α-hydroxy-β-ketoadipate (see Fig. 83-1). This pathway seems to be of little significance, however.

Thiamine use is relatively rapid compared with body stores. With no thiamine source, clinical findings of thiamine deficiency start to develop within 2 to 3 weeks. The minimal daily thiamine requirement is 0.5 mg per 4200 J of energy (0.5 mg/1000 kcal).[1,3]

Wernicke-Korsakoff Syndrome

Evaluation of patients with acute Wernicke's disease shows small petechial hemorrhages in the medial portions of the thalamus and hypothalamus, brainstem, and periventricular structures. Chronic Wernicke's disease additionally has atrophy of mammillary bodies and degeneration of the cerebellar cortex.[7,14] Microscopic changes and atrophy in mammillary bodies are the most common findings at necropsy. Patients with Korsakoff's psychosis have been shown to have wider third ventricles and more dilated lateral ventricles. The clinical findings seem to be secondary to the combination of damage to the blood-brain barrier, decreased central nervous system glucose use, and localized cerebral hypoperfusion. Glutamate concentrations have been shown to increase significantly in thiamine-deficient rats and may be the cause of neuronal damage.[14] Glutamate is a major excitatory neurotransmitter in the central nervous system.

The classic clinical triad of Wernicke's disease is ophthalmoplegia, ataxia, and global confusion. This triad is rarely present.[6] The triad is found infrequently in patients who later have an autopsy diagnosis of Wernicke's disease, which may explain why the diagnosis is difficult.[3,7] Clinical diagnosis is important because the mortality rate is 10% to 20%.[6]

A range of clinical abnormalities is described in Wernicke's disease. Ocular signs are considered the hallmark findings.[5] The ophthalmoplegia includes nystagmus, paralysis of lateral conjugate gaze, diplopia, and internal strabismus.[3,15] Ataxia of stance and gait can be seen in acute Wernicke's disease secondary to vestibular paresis.[6] Loss of equilibrium may prevent the patient from being able to stand or walk without support.

Incoordination of movement is infrequent. Global confusion is common, with apathy, inattentiveness, and infrequent spontaneous speech.[7,14] Temperature regulation is disrupted, and patients can be hypothermic.[6]

Korsakoff's psychosis is a group of findings including antegrade and retrograde amnesia, confabulation, hypofrontality, peripheral neuropathy, and impaired distinction of odors. Confabulation and confusion are the hallmark of acute Korsakoff's psychosis.[7] Korsakoff's psychosis has a relatively poor prognosis, with approximately 20% recovery.[6]

Cardiovascular Effects

The cardiovascular effects of thiamine deficiency are peripheral edema, vasodilation, and congestive heart disease.

PHARMACOKINETICS

Thiamine is absorbed from the duodenum, jejunum, and ileum. Absorption from the gastrointestinal tract seems to be an energy-dependent, rate-limited process, with maximal absorption of 5 to 8 mg of a single dose. With large doses, there is passive uptake. Ethanol inhibits the rate-limited absorption but not the passive absorption of thiamine.[16] Peak serum concentrations are observed at approximately 2 hours after a 10-mg oral dose. Thiamine absorption is decreased in the presence of ethanol, chronic alcohol abuse, cirrhosis, hypoadrenalism, and malabsorption syndromes.[1]

Thiamine is highly bound to serum albumin, and free thiamine is excreted in urine. Total urinary clearance is dose dependent and correlates with creatinine clearance.[17] Transport of thiamine across cell membranes seems to require specific phosphatases. It is widely distributed into body tissue. Its volume of distribution is not described. Body stores in adults are approximately 30 mg. Thiamine is metabolized hepatically, and many different metabolites are excreted in the urine. The half-life is reported to be approximately 1.8 days in healthy, non–thiamine-deficient individuals and is described by a three-compartment model.[17] The daily body turnover is approximately 1 mg.

SPECIAL POPULATIONS

Neonatal Patients

From birth to 3 years of age, the recommended daily thiamine intake is 0.3 to 0.7 mg. Thiamine deficiency most likely is caused by inadequate dietary thiamine or malabsorption. Decreased thiamine intake secondary to gastrointestinal disease and severe food and milk allergy has been described in neonates and infants.[4]

Pediatric Patients

From 4 years to adulthood, the generally recommended daily thiamine intake ranges from 0.9 to 1.5 mg. In this group, thiamine deficiency most likely is secondary to inadequate dietary thiamine or malabsorption. Decreased thiamine intake secondary to malignancy, gastrointestinal disease, and various eating disorders has been described in children.[4]

Elderly Patients

Elderly populations may be at increased risk for thiamine deficiency. The most likely causes in this age group are alcohol abuse, hepatic insufficiency, and chronic diminished intake and absorption. The generally recommended daily thiamine intake is higher in elderly men (1.2 to 1.5 mg) than in women (1 to 1.1 mg).

Pregnant and Breast-feeding Patients

Pregnancy is associated with increased thiamine requirements. The generally recommended daily thiamine intake in pregnant patients is 1.5 mg. Thiamine requirements are increased during breast-feeding.

CONTRAINDICATIONS

The only contraindication to the administration of parenteral thiamine is sensitivity to thiamine or any of the components of the parenteral product. This history is often difficult to obtain because of the patient's altered mental status. Anaphylaxis has been described with intravenous, intramuscular, and subcutaneous administration.[18] In the case of a history of sensitivity to parenteral thiamine, oral administration is an alternative, although oral administration has been reported as associated with anaphylaxis.[18,19]

PRECAUTIONS

The precautions for the administration of parenteral thiamine include headache, weakness, tremors, and central nervous system stimulation. These findings generally are associated with excessive rather than therapeutic doses of thiamine.[20,21] Patients should be observed for signs and symptoms of anaphylaxis after parenteral thiamine administration, especially if they have a past history of thiamine administration. The early literature suggests that patients who received multiple doses of thiamine might have an increased risk of anaphylaxis.[22]

ADVERSE EFFECTS

The adverse effects associated with parenteral thiamine administration are infrequent. They include irritability, tremors, palpitations, and anorexia. These adverse effects seem to be dose related, and it has been stated that they resolve after cessation of thiamine administration.[20,21] The frequency of these adverse effects is not documented. Extremely high-dose thiamine produces central nervous system depression and peripheral neuromuscular blockade (for which reason it was previously evaluated as an anesthetic agent).[13,23] A case of cardiovascular collapse and ventricular fibrillation immediately after the intravenous dose of a vitamin preparation containing thiamine, vitamin B_2, vitamin B_6, vitamin C, and nicotinamide was attributed to thiamine. Although other signs of anaphylaxis were not seen, it is possible that this was an anaphylactic or anaphylactoid reaction rather than a direct effect of the preparation on myocardial conduction.[24]

Anaphylaxis, though infrequent, has been described with all parenteral routes of administration and ranges in severity from mild to fatal. The common symptoms of anaphylaxis include coughing, difficulty swallowing, hives, pruritus, swelling of the face and lips, wheezing and respiratory embarrassment, hypotension, and cardiovascular collapse. Evidence suggests that thiamine may act as a hapten, and IgG and IgE antibodies are induced.[19,21,25] The English Committee on Safety of Medicines received 90 reports of adverse reactions probably associated with parenteral thiamine when a combination of B vitamins and vitamin C was evaluated. There were 41 cases classified as anaphylaxis, 13 cases of dyspnea or bronchospasm, and 22 cases of rash or flushing. Approximately 85% of the cases were associated with intravenous administration, with the remainder occurring after intramuscular dosing. This was a rate of approximately four reports after intravenous administration for every 1 million ampules sold.[26] In a series of 989 patients who received 1070 doses of 100 to 1000 mg thiamine intravenously, the prevalence of general pruritus was 0.09%, and transient burning on injection was reported in 1.1%.[27] In one case of intravenous thiamine administration associated with immediate cardiovascular collapse, subsequently administered oral thiamine was well tolerated.[19] At least one author stated, however, that anaphylaxis has been described previously with oral thiamine.[18] The treatment of anaphylaxis (reviewed in detail in Chapter 31) secondary to thiamine administration is the same as that for anaphylaxis from other causes: administration of epinephrine, intravenous fluids, parenteral antihistamines, and corticosteroids.

ADMINISTRATION

Dose

The most effective adult dose of parenteral thiamine is not well defined. In critically ill patients, a dose range of 5 to 100 mg three times daily is common. In patients with Wernicke's disease, 100 mg daily is commonly recommended, although this dose is empirical and likely more than necessary.[3,6-8] Dosing should continue until the patient tolerates a balanced oral diet. It is unlikely, however, based on total body stores, that amounts greater than approximately 30 mg would be used. In children, the recommended total daily thiamine dose is unresolved, with recommendations ranging from 1.8 mg/1000 kcal daily to 0.35 to 0.5 mg/kg daily.[4]

Route

In critically ill patients, the intravenous route of administration generally is considered to be appropriate. Intramuscular and oral therapies are unlikely to be effective.

REFERENCES

1. Davis RE, Icke GC: Clinical chemistry of thiamin. Adv Clin Chem 23:93–140, 1983.
2. Lieber CS: Hepatic, metabolic, and nutritional disorders of alcoholism: From pathogenesis to therapy. Crit Rev Clin Lab Sci 37:551–584, 2000.
3. Heye N, Terstegge K, Sirtle C, et al: Wernicke's encephalopathy—causes to consider. Intensive Care Med 20:282–286, 1994.

4. Vasconcelos MM, Silva KP, Vidal G, et al: Early diagnosis of pediatric Wernicke's encephalopathy. Pediatr Neurol 20:289–294, 1999.

5. Suter PM, Vetter W: Diuretics and vitamin B_1: Are diuretics a risk factor for thiamin malnutrition? Nutr Rev 58:319–323, 2000.

6. Reuler JB, Girard DE, Cooney TG: Wernicke's encephalopathy. N Engl J Med 312:1035–1039, 1985.

7. Zubaran C, Fernandes JG, Rodnight R: Wernicke-Korsakoff syndrome. Postgrad Med J 73:27–31, 1997.

8. Hoffman RS, Goldfrank LR: The poisoned patient with altered consciousness—controversies in the use of a "coma cocktail." JAMA 274:562–569, 1995.

9. Barceloux DG, Krenzelok EP, Olson K, Watson WA: American Academy of Clinical Toxicology Practice guidelines on the treatment of ethylene glycol poisoning. Clin Toxicol 37:537–560, 1999.

10. Schiff L: Collapse following parenteral administration of solution of thiamine hydrochloride. JAMA 117:609, 1941.

11. Doyon S, Roberts JR: Reappraisal of the "coma cocktail": Dextrose, flumazenil, naloxone, and thiamine. Emerg Med Clin N Am 12:301–315, 1994.

12. Watson AJS, Walker JF, Tomkin GH, et al: Acute Wernicke's encephalopathy precipitated by glucose loading. Irish J Med Sci 50:301–303, 1981.

13. Spector R: Thiamin homeostasis in the central nervous system. Ann N Y Acad Sci 378:344–354, 1982.

14. Butterworth RF: Pathophysiology of cerebellar dysfunction in the Wernicke-Korsakoff syndrome. Can J Neurol Sci 20(Suppl 3): S123–S126, 1993.

15. Kumar PD, Nartsupha C, West BC: Unilateral internuclear ophthalmoplegia and recovery with thiamine in Wernicke syndrome. Am J Med Sci 320:278–280, 2000.

16. Royer-Morrot MJ, Zhire A, Paille F, et al: Plasma thiamine concentrations after intramuscular and oral multiple dosage regimens in healthy men. Eur J Clin Pharmacol 42:219–222, 1992.

17. Weber W, Nitz M, Looby M: Nonlinear kinetics of the thiamine cation in humans: Saturation of nonrenal clearance and tubular reabsorption. J Pharmacokinet Biopharm 18:501–523, 1990.

18. Stephen JM, Grant R, Yeh CS: Anaphylaxis from administration of intravenous thiamine. Am J Emerg Med 10:61–63, 1992.

19. Proebstle TM, Gall H, Jugert FK, et al: Specific IgE and IgG serum antibodies to thiamine associated with anaphylactic reaction. J Allergy Clin Immunol 95(5 Part 1):1059–1060, 1995.

20. DiPalma JR, Ritchie DM: Vitamin toxicity. Ann Rev Pharmacol Toxicol 17:133–148, 1977.

21. Van Haecke P, Ramaekers D, Vanderwegen L, et al: Thiamine-induced anaphylactic shock. Am J Emerg Med 13:371–372, 1995.

22. Weigand CG: Reactions attributed to administration of thiamin chloride. Geriatrics 5:274–279, 1950.

23. Valenti F, Sauli M, D'Alessandro R: High doses of thiamine in clinical anesthesia. Acta Anaesthesiol 19(Suppl 1):55–66, 1968.

24. Falk RH, Protheroe DE: Ventricular fibrillation following high potency intravenous vitamin injection. Postgrad Med J 55:201–202, 1979.

25. Fernandez M, Barcelo M, Munoz C, et al: Anaphylaxis to thiamine (vitamin B_1). Allergy 52:958–960, 1997.

26. Thomson AD, Cook CCH: Parenteral thiamine and Wernicke's encephalopathy: The balance of risks and perception of concern. Alcohol Alcoholism 32:207–209, 1997.

27. Wrenn KD, Murphy F, Slovis CM: A toxicity study of parenteral thiamine hydrochloride. Ann Emerg Med 18:867–870, 1989.

CHAPTER 159

Octreotide

Christopher H. Linden

Octreotide (Sandostatin) is a synthetic analogue of somato-statin that has similar, if not identical, pharmacologic activity to this endogenous hormone but is longer acting and more potent.[1–11] Somatostatin was first isolated from the hypothalamus and characterized as an inhibitor of pituitary growth hormone secretion in 1973.[12] It is now known that it is synthesized and widely distributed throughout the body (particularly in neurons, pancreas, and gastrointestinal tract, but also in immune and inflammatory cells); that it modulates neurotransmission (primarily in the central nervous system); and that it has more generalized inhibitory effects on paracrine function. With respect to the last-mentioned, somatostatin inhibits the release of the following:

Thyrotropin
Prolactin
Gastrin
Motilin
Vasoactive intestinal peptide
Pancreatic polypeptide
Glicentin
Glucagon
Insulin
Insulin-like growth factors (somatomedins)
Parathyroid hormone
Luteinizing hormone
Calcitonin
Renin
Adrenocorticotropic hormone
Growth hormone

Somatostatin also inhibits exocrine secretions from the pancreas, gut, gallbladder, and salivary glands. Current research in this area is intense, with results suggesting that somatostatin is involved in the regulation of most, if not all, physiologic processes.

It also is known that "somatostatin" is not one entity, but a group or family of related cyclic polypeptides with internal disulfide bonds accounting for their cyclic structures. Hypothalamic somatostatin (S-14) consists of 14 amino acids. A larger, more potent 28–amino acid analogue (S-28) is found in gut tissue and may be the physiologically active parent compound of S-14. As the name suggests, octreotide is a cyclic octapeptide. Many other somatostatin analogues (e.g., lanreotide, vapreotide, and many yet to be named) have been synthesized, but octreotide is the only one currently in widespread clinical use. Octreotide is the only somatostatin analogue approved for use in the United States.

Indications for the use of octreotide currently sanctioned by the U.S. Food and Drug Administration are limited to the treatment of acromegaly, carcinoid tumors, and vasoactive intestinal peptide tumors.[11] Clinical experience also supports its use in the treatment of nonsecretory, corticotropin-secreting, and thyrotropin-secreting pituitary adenomas; pancreatic islet cell tumors; congenital and acquired hyper-insulinism; nesidioblastosis; acute pancreatitis; pancreatic fistulas and pseudocysts; bleeding from esophageal varices and peptic ulcers; and diarrhea associated with ileostomies, short bowel syndrome, intestinal graft-versus-host disease, radiation colitis, intestinal fistulas, and acquired immuno-deficiency syndrome (AIDS).[6–10,13,14] Its effects on other endocrine disorders, nonendocrine tumors, hematologic function, immunologic function, neurologic function, vascular disease, and a host of other processes, including aging, are under investigation.

The ability of octreotide to inhibit the secretion of insulin, glucagon, and other insulin counterregulatory hormones makes it a rational choice for the treatment of poisoning due to sulfonylureas and other drugs that cause hyperinsulinemia (see Chapter 70). With proven efficacy, low cost, ease of administration, and a highly favorable safety profile, it has virtually all the properties that characterize an ideal antidote. Although much more is known about the pharmacology of octreotide (and somatostatin), the remainder of this chapter focuses only on the actions relevant to the understanding and treatment of drug-induced hyperinsulinemic hypoglycemia.

PHARMACODYNAMICS

Physiologically, somatostatin acts as a gastrointestinal and pancreatic counterregulatory hormone.[1,3,15] It is secreted from pancreatic islets of Langerhans delta cells in response to increases in blood glucose, amino acids, fatty acids, and gastrointestinal hormones that occur after the ingestion of food. Systemic effects include decreased gastrointestinal and gallbladder motility and secretory activity with consequent slowing of the digestion and absorption of food. Locally, somatostatin inhibits the pancreatic secretion of insulin from islet beta cells and of glucagon from islet alpha and intestinal alpha-like or L cells, decreasing the uptake and use of absorbed nutrients. Although pancreatic alpha cells are about 50 times more sensitive to somatostatin than beta cells, their effect on insulin secretion is more prolonged than that on glucagon secretion. Teleologically, by preventing the rapid assimilation and consequent exhaustion of ingested food, somatostatin lessens inequalities between the intermittent supply and continuous demand for nutrients and increases the overall efficiency of food processing.

Sulfonylurea drugs counteract hyperglycemia by enhancing the release of insulin from pancreatic islet beta cells in response to glucose, the principal stimulus and an essential permissive factor for insulin secretion.[3,16,17] Their mechanism of action is similar to that of high plasma glucose concentrations: inhibition of the pancreatic islet beta cell membrane adenosine triphosphate (ATP)–sensitive potassium (K^+) channels leading to membrane depolarization with consequent calcium (Ca^{2+}) influx through voltage-sensitive Ca^{2+} channels, mobilization of Ca^{2+} from the endoplasmic reticulum, increased intracellular Ca^{2+}, and insulin secretion. Sulfonylureas bind to specific receptors associated with K^+ channels on the beta cell membrane, whereas glucose generates ATP through its oxidative metabolism by glucokinase within beta cells. Intracellular Ca^{2+} is the ultimate insulin secretagogue, with increases in intracellular calcium promoting the synthesis and release of insulin (Fig. 159-1) (see Chapter 70).

The action of octreotide (and of somatostatin and other analogues) on beta cell Ca^{2+} disposition is diametrically opposite to that the sulfonylureas, and the mechanism is slightly different.[3,18,19] Octreotide binds to specific somatostatin membrane receptors (SST receptors or SSTRs) associated with Ca^{2+} channels, resulting in decreased calcium conductance, decreased intracellular Ca^{2+}, and inhibition of insulin secretion. Opening of potassium channels with subsequent membrane hyperpolarization also may be involved. Somatostatin receptors are coupled to G proteins. To date,

five SSTR subtypes have been identified. Receptor affinity and selectivity differ from one somatostatin analogue to another. Subtypes 2 and 5 mediate insulin secretion. Suppression of insulin secretion by octreotide has been documented in experimental[20] and spontaneously occurring[21,22] human sulfonylurea poisoning (see Fig. 159-1).

Congenital hyperinsulinism secondary to inherited defects in genes regulating the expression of sulfonylurea receptors and ATP-sensitive K^+ channels, both mapped to the short arm of chromosome 11, have been described.[23,24] This condition suggests that an as yet unidentified endogenous sulfonylurea-like substance exists. Treatment of these conditions with diazoxide, which inhibits insulin secretion through interactions with sulfonylurea receptors or K^+ channels (see Fig. 159-1 and Chapter 70), has been ineffective. The fact that octreotide has been only partly successful supports the notion that effects on potassium channels also are involved in its mode of action.

The antidotal effects of octreotide in sulfonylurea poisoning also may be due to its antagonism of glucagon and possibly other counterregulatory hormones. Octreotide not only inhibits the secretion of glucagon in response to hypoglycemia but also inhibits the actions of glucagon.[1,3] Glucagon activates adenylyl cyclase, which catalyzes the synthesis of cyclic adenosine monophosphate (AMP), whereas octreotide inhibits this enzyme. In the absence of octreotide, this action of glucagon increases cyclic AMP levels, and this stimulates phosphorylase (the rate-limiting enzyme in glycogenolysis), inhibits glycogen synthase, and increases intracellular Ca^{2+}, effects that may lead to hyperglycemia,

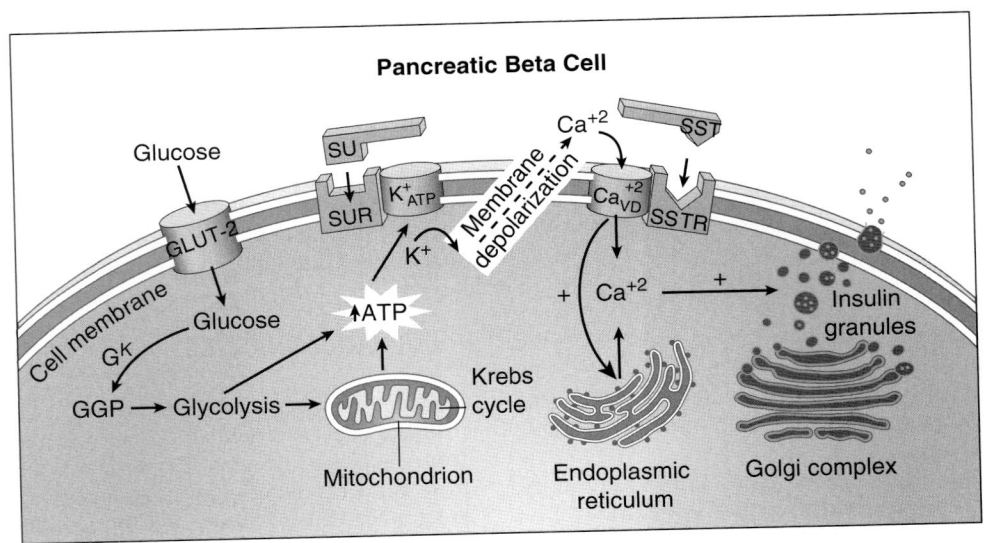

Pancreatic Beta Cell

FIGURE 159-1

Schematic diagram of a pancreatic beta cell showing the regulation of insulin secretion. Glucose is transported into the beta cell by a glucose-transporter protein (GLUT-2). The enzyme glucokinase (GK) initiates glycolysis by catalyzing the transfer of phosphate from adenosine triphosphate (ATP) to glucose, resulting in the formation of glucose-6-phosphate (G-6-P). ATP generated by subsequent steps in the glycolytic pathway and by the Krebs (citric or tricarboxylic acid) cycle leads to closure of ATP-sensitive potassium channels (K^+_{ATP}) and membrane depolarization. Membrane depolarization results in opening of voltage-dependent calcium channels (Ca^+_{VD}), influx of extracellular calcium, and subsequent release of calcium from intracellular (endoplasmic reticulum) stores. Increased intracellular calcium promotes the exocytosis of insulin granules (Golgi vesicles) with release of insulin into extracellular fluid and the systemic circulation. Although the phosphorylation of glucose is a rate-limiting step, beta cell GK has a high Michaelis constant (K_M, the substrate concentration at which the reaction rate is half of the maximal value) for glucose. Glucose metabolism and ATP production, potassium and calcium channel activity, intracellular calcium concentration, and insulin release are controlled primarily by the intracellular glucose concentration. Sulfonylureas (SU) inhibit potassium efflux by binding to specific receptors (SUR) associated with K^+_{ATP} channels and enhance the release of insulin. Somatostatin (SST) and its analogues, such as octreotide, inhibit calcium influx by binding to receptors (SSTR) associated with Ca^+_{VD} channels, inhibiting the release of insulin.

rebound hyperinsulinemia, and recurrent hypoglycemia after glucose administration (see Fig. 159-1 and Chapter 70). As with insulin, SSTR subtypes 2 and 5 mediate glucagon secretion.[18,19] Octreotide has been shown to decrease epinephrine and norepinephrine and glucagon levels in experimental glipizide overdose.[20]

Octreotide also is likely to be effective in treating hyperinsulinemic hypoglycemia due to other drugs, including insulin itself (see Chapter 70). To date, its use has been reported in only one such case, which involved quinine.[25] The drug also is remarkably inexpensive, costing only about $11 for a 100-μg dose.

PHARMACOKINETICS

Octreotide is well absorbed after subcutaneous administration, with peak plasma concentrations averaging 5.2 ng/mL 0.4 hour after a 100-μg dose in healthy volunteers.[11] It is about 65% bound to plasma lipoproteins, has a small volume of distribution (approximately 0.2 L/kg), and a half-life of about 1.7 hours, which is much longer than that of somatostatin (1 to 3 minutes). About one third of the dose is excreted unchanged in the urine, and the half-life is doubled in renal dialysis patients and the elderly. The metabolic fate of the remaining fraction has not been determined.

Octreotide is also absorbed after oral administration. Its bioavailability by this route is low; a 2-mg oral dose results in peak plasma drug levels similar to a 50-μg subcutaneous dose, with the time to peak level delayed about 1.5 hours.

CONTRAINDICATIONS AND ADVERSE EFFECTS

Except for hypersensitivity, there are no contraindications to octreotide.[1,3,5–11] No adverse effects have been reported during its use in the treatment of sulfonylurea poisoning. Common adverse effects after its short-term use in acromegaly include nausea, abdominal cramps, diarrhea, and flatulence. A high incidence of bradycardia (19% to 25%), cardiac conduction abnormalities (10%), and arrhythmias (3% to 9%) has been reported during long-term therapy in patients with carcinoid syndrome and acromegaly, but not in other conditions. None of these abnormalities has had a significant hemodynamic effect. Other adverse effects, primarily constitutional, occur in less than 2% of patients treated.

Octreotide has been used in all age groups, including neonates and pregnant women. Although no adverse effects on fertility or fetal development have been noted in experimental animals, because octreotide has not been studied extensively in pregnant women, it has a Food and Drug Administration category B use-in-pregnancy rating (no evidence of risk in humans; the chance of fetal harm is remote but remains a possibility).

ADVERSE EFFECTS

Adverse effects usually are transient and require no treatment except for monitoring, dosage adjustment or discontinuation of therapy, and supportive care.

ADMINISTRATION

Dose

Based on clinical experience and data from volunteer studies and the manufacturer (see later), a subcutaneous dose of 1 to 2 μg/kg every 8 hours can be expected to be effective for the treatment of sulfonylurea-induced hypoglycemia. A continuous intravenous infusion of the same dose on an hourly basis also is likely to be effective. Intravenous administration is more expensive and more difficult to prepare and administer (and more susceptible to dosing errors). Because there is no evidence that this route and method of dosing are superior or necessary, intermittent subcutaneous dosing is recommended as the preferred treatment regimen.

Therapeutic doses of octreotide vary widely and depend on the condition being treated.[1,5–11,13,14] Doses used in children generally range from 1 to 40 μg/kg/day, and doses in adults range from 50 to 3000 μg/day, although doses of 120,000 μg over 8 hours have been used to treat secretory diarrhea associated with AIDS. Dose-response relationships with respect to the treatment of sulfonylurea poisoning have not been studied formally, but the fact that low-end doses have been consistently effective indicates that octreotide is extremely potent in this regard. The manufacturer reports a variable duration of action—averaging about 12 hours after subcutaneous administration.

A continuous octreotide infusion (30 ng/kg/min or 126 μg/hr for a 70-kg person) was effective in lessening the severity of hypoglycemia in nondiabetic human volunteers (n = 8) who ingested an overdose of glipizide (1.45 mg/kg).[20] This therapy reduced the need for exogenous glucose in all subjects and entirely eliminated it in half of them. It also was more effective than diazoxide (300 mg intravenously every 4 hours), which was no more effective than treatment with dextrose alone. Infusions of 50 to 125 μg/hr have been used to treat adults with nonexperimental, nonaccidental sulfonylurea overdose.[26,27]

Lower doses seem to be effective when octreotide is administered subcutaneously. A single 25-μg dose was successful in a 5-year-old child with an accidental exposure to a therapeutic dose of glipizide,[22] and doses of 50 to 100 μg once to every 6 to 12 hours have been used successfully in adults with accidental and nonaccidental poisoning by chlorpropamide, glyburide, and glipizide.[21,26,28] A depot effect resulting in prolonged absorption and action after subcutaneous administration and similar to that which occurs with insulin (see Chapter 70) is the likely explanation for the apparently greater efficacy of octreotide when given by this route. It would be a mistake to assume that the same doses given intravenously would be therapeutically equivalent.

Route of Administration

Octreotide is administered parenterally for the treatment of hyperinsulinemic hypoglycemia due to drug overdose. Solutions containing 50 μg/mL, 100 μg/mL, 200 μg/mL, 500 μg/mL, or 1000 μg/mL are available for subcutaneous injection or intravenous infusion. Long-acting, sustained-release preparations containing 10 mg/2 mL, 20 mg/2 mL, or 30 mg/2 mL for intramuscular (intragluteal) injection at monthly intervals (e.g., Sandostatin LAR Depot) are used for the treatment of chronic conditions. No oral formulations are commercially available.

UNANSWERED QUESTIONS

The optimal dose and frequency of administration of octreotide for the treatment of sulfonylurea poisoning are unknown. Lower doses and less frequent dosing intervals than those cited earlier may be effective. Similar doses probably would be effective for the treatment of other drug-induced states of hyperinsulinism (see Chapter 70), but there is little experience with its use in this setting. It is also possible that a single intramuscular injection (e.g., 90 mg) of the depot formulation of octreotide would be effective in the treatment of drug-induced hypoglycemia. If this is true, such therapy could obviate the need for hospitalization, particularly in those with unintentional poisoning.

Indications for octreotide treatment are not well defined. Although it is generally agreed that octreotide is indicated for recurrent hypoglycemia due to sulfonylurea poisoning, whether it should be given after the first episode of hypoglycemia is controversial. Doing so is reasonable in patients who are likely to develop further episodes (e.g., patients with large or intentional overdoses), but it may prolong unnecessarily the period of observation for patients who are not (e.g., patients with therapeutic misadventures). As always, the reliability of the history must be assessed when making such decisions. Given that the overdose history is often inaccurate, incomplete, or unobtainable, I prefer to reserve treatment for patients with a documented second episode of hypoglycemia. Treatment recommendations for these patients are discussed in detail in Chapter 70.

REFERENCES

1. Reichlin S: Somatostatin. N Engl J Med 309:1495–1501, 1556–1563, 1983.
2. Ascoli M, Segaloff DL: Adenohypophyseal hormones and their hypothalamic releasing factors. In Hardman JG, Limbird LE, Molinoff PB, et al (eds): Goodman and Gilman's The Pharmocological Basis of Therapeutics, 9th ed. New York, McGraw-Hill, 1996, pp 1369–1370.
3. Davis SN, Granner DK: Insulin, oral hypoglycemic agents, and the pharmacology of the endocrine pancreas. In Hardman JG, Limbird LE, Molinoff PB, et al (eds): Goodman and Gilman's The Pharmocological Basis of Therapeutics, 9th ed. New York, McGraw-Hill, 1996, pp 1512–1513.
4. Underwood LE: Growth hormone and insulin-like growth factors. In Munson PL, Mueller RA, Breese GR (eds): Principles of Pharmacology: Basic Concepts and Clinical Applications. New York, Chapman & Hall, 1996, p 904.
5. McEvoy GK, Litvak K, Welsh OH, et al (eds): American Hospital Formulary Service Drug Information. Bethesda, MD, American Society of Health-System Pharmacists, 2000, pp 3431–3435.
6. Rosenberg JM: Octreotide: A synthetic analog of somatostatin. Drug Intell Clin Pharm 22:748–754, 1988.
7. Battershill PE, Clissold SP: Octreotide: A review of its pharmacodynamic and pharmacokinetic properties, and therapeutic potential in conditions associated with excessive peptide secretion. Drugs 38:658–702, 1989.
8. Chanson P, Timsit J, Harris AG: Clinical pharmacokinetics of octreotide: Therapeutic applications in patients with pituitary tumours. Clin Pharmacokinet 25:375–391, 1993.
9. Proceedings: Sandostatin, "State of the Art." Metabolism 41(Suppl 2): 1–122, 1992.
10. Lamberts SWJ, van der Lely AJ, de Herder WW, et al: Octreotide. N Engl J Med 334:246–253, 1996.
11. Sandostatin Prescribing Information (package insert). East Hanover, NJ, Sandoz Pharmaceuticals Corporation/Summit, NJ, Novartis Concomer Health, 1999.
12. Brazeau P, Vale WW, Burgess R, et al: Hypothalamic polypeptide that inhibits the secretion of immunoreactive ptiuitary growth hormone. Science 179:77–79, 1973.
13. Barrons RW: Octreotide in hyperinsulinism. Ann Pharmacother 31: 239–241, 1997.
14. Stanley CA: Hyperinsulinism in infants and children. Pediatr Clin North Am 44:363–374, 1997.
15. Guyton AC, Hall JE: Textbook of Medical Physiology, 10th ed. Philadelphia, WB Saunders, 2000, p 893.
16. Gerich JE: Oral hypoglycemic agents. N Engl J Med 321:1231–1245, 1989.
17. Panten U, Schwantecher M, Schwantecher C: Pancreatic and extrapancreatic sulfonylurea receptors. Horm Metab Res 24:549–554, 1992.
18. Patel YC, Srikant CB: Subtype selectivity of peptide analogs for all five cloned human somatostatin receptors (hsstr 1–5). Endocrinology 135:2814–2817, 1994.
19. Benali N, Ferjoux G, Puente E, et al: Somatostatin receptors. Digestion 62(Suppl 1):27–32, 2000.
20. Boyle PJ, Justice K, Krentz AJ, et al: Octreotide reverses hyperinsulinemia and prevents hypoglycemia induced by sulfonylurea overdoses. J Clin Endocrinol Metab 76:752–756, 1993.
21. Graudins A, Linden CH, Ferm RP: Diagnosis and treatment of sulfonylurea-induced hyperinsulinemic hypoglycemia. Am J Emerg Med 15:95–96, 1997.
22. Mordel A, Sivilotti MLA, Old AC, Ferm RP: Octreotide for pediatric sulfonylurea poisoning. Clin Toxicol 36:437, 1998.
23. Aquilar-Bryan L, Nichols CG, Wechsler SW, et al: Cloning of the β cell high-affinity sulfonylurea receptor: A regulator of insulin secretion. Science 268:423–426, 1995.
24. Thornton PM, Alter CA, Levitt-Katz LE, et al: Short and long term use of octreotide in the treatment of congenital hyperinsulism. J Pediatr 123:637–643, 1993.
25. Phillips RE, Looaresuwan S, Bloom SR, et al: Effectiveness of SMS 201-995, a synthetic, long-acting somatostatin analogue, in treatment of quinine-induced hyperinsulinemia. Lancet 1:713–716, 1986.
26. McLaughlin SA, Crandall CS, McKinney PE: Octreotide: An antidote for sulfonylurea-induced hypoglycemia. Ann Emerg Med 36:133–138, 2000.
27. Bui L, Adler D, Keller KH: Prolonged octreotide infusion to treat glyburide-induced hypoglycemia (Abstract). Clin Toxicol 38:576, 2000.
28. Hung O, Eng J, Ho J, et al: Octreotide as an antidote for refractory sulfonylurea hypoglycemia (Abstract). Clin Toxicol 35:540, 1997.

CHAPTER 160

4-Dimethylaminophenol (4-DMAP) as an Antidote for Poisoning by Cyanide

Thomas Zilker ■ Peter Eyer

In normal intermediary metabolism, six adenosine triphosphates (ATPs) are created by passing two pairs of electrons down the respiratory chain from two reduced nicotinamide-adenine dinucleotides to molecular oxygen. In the course of this mitochondrial ATP synthesis, the iron in cytochrome aa_3, the terminal oxidative respiratory enzyme, is oxidized from the ferrous (Fe^{2+}) to the ferric (Fe^{3+}) form. Cyanide has a special affinity for the ferric heme, blocking oxygen consumption and oxidative phosphorylation. Blood contains a great quantity of ferrous heme within hemoglobin that can be converted to the ferric form (methemoglobin) by the use of methemoglobin-generating agents. If methemoglobin is formed in excess of total body cytochrome aa_3, the cyanide ion binds to methemoglobin, restoring normal cellular respiration (Fig. 160-1).

The use of nitrite for this purpose was suggested by Chen and colleagues[1] in 1933, and nitrite is still used to treat cyanide poisoning in the United States. A theoretical disadvantage of nitrite therapy, however, is that methemoglobinemia is induced slowly. The originally suggested dose of 4 mg/kg intravenously results in 6% of methemoglobin after only 40 minutes.[2] A high dose of nitrite, if given too quickly, may lead to vasomotor relaxation and hypotension.[3] Amyl nitrite, which is administered by inhalation, creates little methemoglobin,[4] but similar to nitrite it has a vasodilating effect. Another cyanide antidote, dicobalt ethylenediamine tetraacetic acid (cobalt EDTA) can cause severe reactions, such as urticaria, hypotension, convulsions, and laryngeal edema.[5,6]

The antidote with the least side effects is hydroxocobalamin, which is discussed in Chapter 150.[7] It is expensive, however, and has practical disadvantages. It can be given only in a large volume (500 mL), and the lyophilized powder must be reconstituted first. This process may be too time-consuming in a critically poisoned patient. A compound that quickly creates sufficient methemoglobin with few adverse effects would be preferable. 4-Dimethylaminophenol (4-DMAP) may have advantages regarding these criteria. For severe cases of cyanide poisoning, 4-DMAP is the antidote of choice in Germany, and most ambulances in that country are equipped with it.

HISTORY

4-DMAP was developed and studied in the laboratories of the Walther Straub Institute of the Ludwig Maximilia University in Munich, Germany. The German army supported its development because it was thought that hydrogen cyanide might be used as a chemical warfare agent.

In 1969, Kiese and Weger[8] reported that 4-DMAP was the most potent methemoglobin-forming agent among a series of aminophenols tested in humans for the treatment of cyanide poisoning. 4-DMAP was used in human cyanide poisoning successfully by Daunderer et al in 1972.[9] Because severe cyanide poisoning has become a rare incident, only single case reports have been published since. A series of 13 cases in which 4-DMAP was given to humans between 1973 and 1979 has been described in a thesis from our department; however, these cases have not been published elsewhere.[10] A further series of nine cases from our department, from 1981 to 1991, was published as an abstract.[11] We are aware of use of 4-DMAP in Austria and the Netherlands.[12] 4-DMAP is registered as a pharmaceutical by the German authorities (BfArM). Permission for its use was extended in 1991. The producer of this drug is the company Dr. Franz Koehler Chemie, Alsbach-Hähnlein, Germany.

PROPERTIES

The properties of 4-DMAP are summarized as follows:

Chemical name: Dimethyl (para) aminophenol hydrochloride (Fig. 160-2)
Chemical formula: $C_8H_{11}ON$ HCl
Relative molecular mass: 173.5
Appearance: White crystals
CAS* number: 619-60-3
Raw material: White colorless crystals
Melting point: 145°C ± 1°C
Solubility: Soluble in water. The solution is oxidized by contact with air and changes from colorless to black-brown.

PHARMACODYNAMICS

4-DMAP produces methemoglobin by catalytic transfer of electrons from ferrohemoglobin to oxygen. This process is terminated by binding of oxidized 4-DMAP to compounds that possess free SH-groups (see Fig. 160-1).

---

*Chemical Abstracts Service.

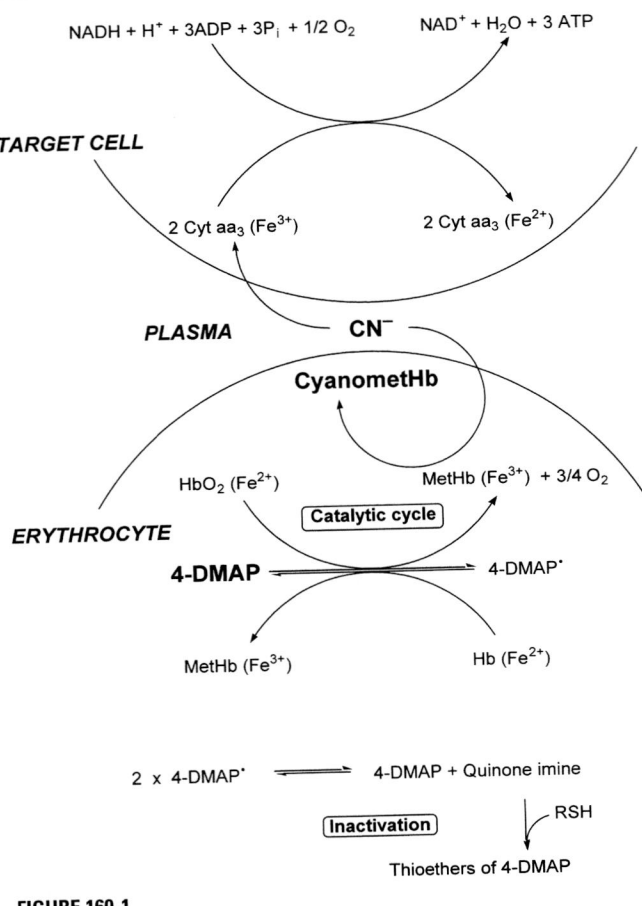

FIGURE 160-1

Mechanism of action of cyanide, 4-DMAP, and methemoglobin. Cyta₃, cytochrome aa_3.

In human volunteers, 3.25 mg/kg of 4-DMAP given intravenously oxidized about 30% of the total hemoglobin to methemoglobin (Fig. 160-3).[13] The spontaneous reduction of methemoglobin back to ferrohemoglobin was 8% per hour at 30% to 20% of methemoglobin levels.[14] In vivo, 1 molecule of 4-DMAP is capable of converting 15 molecules of hemoglobin to methemoglobin.[13] Methemoglobin formation by 4-DMAP occurs rapidly. In experiments on seven volunteers,[2] an intravenous bolus of 3.25 mg/kg of 4-DMAP resulted in 15% methemoglobin after 1 minute and 28.5% after 10 minutes. The peak of 30% was attained after 20 minutes. 4-DMAP can be administered intramuscularly or orally. The intramuscular injection of 3.5 mg/kg of 4-DMAP in human volunteers (n = 6) resulted in a maximal measured methemoglobin concentration of 30% after 45 minutes. The administration of 12 mg/kg of 4-DMAP orally (n = 5) created 27% methemoglobin within 30 minutes, but the actual oral bioavailability is uncertain.[13]

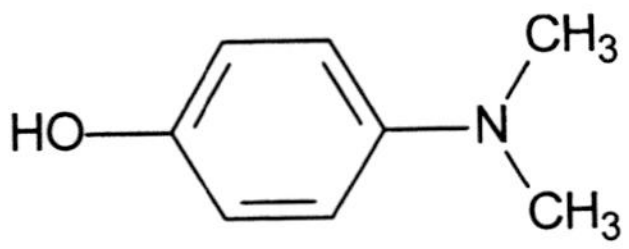

FIGURE 160-2

Chemical structure of 4-dimethylaminophenol.

4-DMAP (3.25 mg/kg) given intravenously to dogs 1 minute after poisoning with potassium cyanide (4 mg/kg) that is twice the lethal dose in dogs[15] resulted in the survival of all dogs.[16] The peak concentration of methemoglobin was 32% ± 1.9%.[16]

4-DMAP has other effects on physiologic functions. Although the venous lactate concentration did not change, the pyruvate concentration increased by 30% after 4-DMAP administration. This effect also was found in canine blood in vitro, most probably caused by the lactate-induced methemoglobin reduction.[14,17]

In dogs,[17] the mean arterial pressure after 4-DMAP (3.25 mg/kg intravenously) increased by 15% within 5 minutes, and the effect was maintained for 1 hour. The respiratory minute volume increased by 30%. Both effects may be advantageous in cyanide poisoning. The arterial PO_2 increased within 1 minute from 95 to 190 mm Hg, after which it normalized by 10 minutes. This increase has been attributed to the release of oxygen from oxyhemoglobin during the formation of methemoglobin. It is possible that in a critically ill, cyanide-poisoned patient, this may improve tissue oxygenation.[17] When cerebral blood flow was measured in canine brain,[18] 4-DMAP evoked a dose-dependent increase in cerebral blood flow. The positive cerebral blood flow response did not occur until at least 10% methemoglobin was formed. As long as the methemoglobin concentration was less than 40%, the canine brain could compensate for the diminished oxygen transport capacity by elevating oxygen use as indicated by a decrease of PO_2 in the sinus sagittalis. At higher methemoglobin concentrations, oxygen use no longer could be improved.[18] A 4-DMAP dose producing more than 40% methemoglobin is not advisable. As long as methemoglobin is less than 40%, most physiologic reactions to 4-DMAP seem to be favorable for treating cyanide poisoning.

PHARMACOKINETICS

In humans and dogs, 4-DMAP (3.25 mg/kg intravenously) is cleared rapidly from the blood with a half-life of less than 1 minute.[19] This rapid clearance is due to various first-pass effects.[13] Using ^{14}C-labeled 4-DMAP in canine experiments, approximately one third of 4-DMAP equivalents were found in red blood cells, and two thirds were found in plasma and the extracellular space (apparent volume of distribution 0.17 L/kg).[20] To understand the particular pharmacokinetics of 4-DMAP, one must differentiate between the metabolism in erythrocytes and elsewhere, mainly in the liver.

Metabolism of 4-DMAP in Erythrocytes

The distribution of 4-DMAP between plasma and erythrocytes is not known because of the ultrashort lifetime of 4-DMAP within red blood cells. 4-DMAP is cooxidized quickly with oxyhemoglobin to form methemoglobin and a phenoxyl radical. The phenoxyl radical oxidizes deoxyhemoglobin, sustaining the catalytic cycle of methemoglobin formation.[21] Alternatively, the phenoxyl radical disproportionates to form 4-DMAP and a quinone imine that is bound covalently to hemoglobin SH groups.[22] In the presence of high glutathione concentrations, such as occurs in erythrocytes, the quinone imine undergoes sequential addition/oxidation

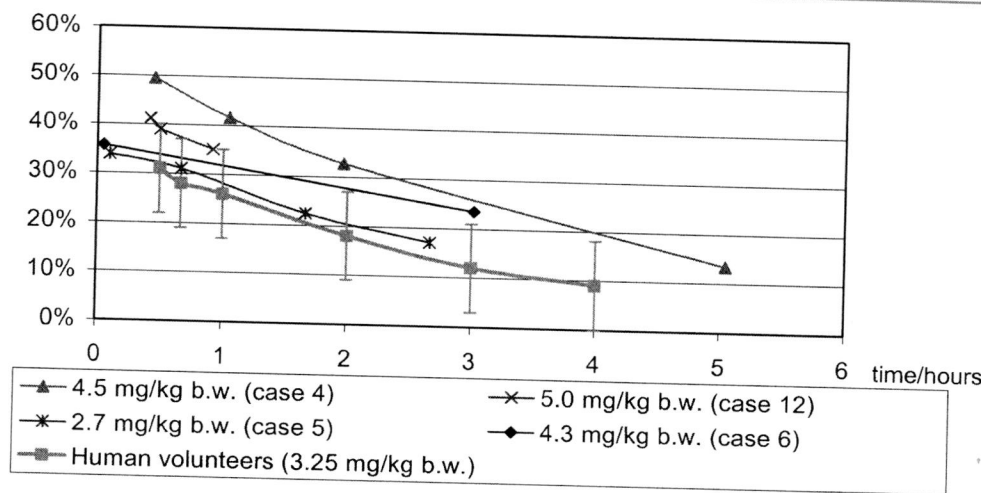

FIGURE 160-3

Course of methemoglobin concentrations in cyanide-poisoned patients and human volunteers after intravenous administration of 4-DMAP.[10] b.w., body weight.

reactions with formation of mono-glutathione, bis-glutathione, and tris-glutathione adducts of 4-DMAP.[23] The trisubstituted conjugate is not oxidized further but is actively excreted from the erythrocyte into plasma.[24] This conjugate has a half-life of about 1 hour in plasma and is processed further by the kidneys and excreted mainly as a tris-cysteinyl derivative of DMAP[25], as has also been observed in dogs.[20] It has been calculated that probably all 4-DMAP thioethers excreted (15% of the dose) originate from the metabolism of 4-DMAP within the red blood cells. About the same amount of 4-DMAP is bound covalently to the hemoglobin SH groups.

Metabolism of 4-DMAP in Liver

About 50% of the 4-DMAP administered intravenously to humans is transformed in the liver to the glucuronide and sulfate conjugate. In urine, 41% 4-DMAP glucuronide and 12% 4-DMAP sulfate were detected.[13,25] This conjugation seems to occur rapidly, as shown in the isolated, hemoglobin-free perfused rat liver, in which covalent binding to liver proteins or formation of glutathione conjugates were of no importance.[26] The first-pass effect in the liver may be the reason for the much higher oral dose compared with the parenteral dose of 4-DMAP required to obtain an equivalent degree of methemoglobin.[13]

TOXICITY

The toxicity of 4-DMAP has been studied in the mouse, rat, and dog. The median lethal doses are listed in Table 160-1.

TABLE 160-1 Median Lethal Doses in Mice, Rats, and Dogs	
ROUTE/SPECIES	**MEDIAN LETHAL DOSE (mg/kg)**
Intravenous/mouse	50–70[27,28]
Oral/mouse	946[28]
Intravenous/rat	57[29]
Oral/rat	689–780[28]
Intravenous/dog	26[30]

In all studies, the cause of death was severe methemoglobinemia. Single intravenous injection of 4-DMAP (100 mg/kg) to rats was followed by a large amount of necrosis and inflammation of the convoluted tubules without affecting the glomeruli and papillae. No changes were found in liver, heart, and spleen.[27] In isolated, hemoglobin-free perfused rat kidneys, 4-DMAP underwent a sharp increase of covalent binding to kidney proteins at concentrations greater than 15 μM. Microautoradiograms (^{14}C) showed that the high binding was particularly prominent in the proximal convoluted tubules.[31]

SPECIAL POPULATIONS

No data for neonates or children are available. In our series of 23 patients in whom 4-DMAP was used, the eldest person was 66 years old (case 13) (Tables 160-2 and 160-3). This patient received 9.3 mg/kg of 4-DMAP. He developed mild hemolysis, with an increase in lactate dehydrogenase to 378 U/L, a decrease in hemoglobin from 13.8 to 10 g/dL within 5 days, and an increase in bilirubin to 3 mg/dL. Because this was nearly three times the recommended dose and hemolysis occurs in younger patients at similar doses, we could not detect a difference between elderly and younger people in reacting to this dose.

CONTRAINDICATIONS

Patients with glucose-6-phosphate dehydrogenase deficiency who are unable to reduce methemoglobin by the pentose phosphate shunt are at risk of developing long-lasting methemoglobinemia after 4-DMAP and may have severe hemolysis. To our knowledge, the drug was never used in such a case. On theoretical grounds, glucose-6-phosphate dehydrogenase deficiency is a contraindication for the use of 4-DMAP. Given the desperate situation of a potentially fatally poisoned patient, we recommend that this be considered only a relative contraindication in cyanide poisoning. If a glucose-6-phosphate dehydrogenase–deficient patient were treated with 4-DMAP, because the

TABLE 160-2 Data in 23 Patients in Whom 4-DMAP Was Administered*

CASE NO./YEAR	CAUSE/ROUTE OF POISONING	4-DMAP DOSE/INTERVAL BEFORE ADMINISTRATION	INDICATION	ADVERSE EFFECTS	OUTCOME
1/1975	Accident/transdermal	250 mg/12 min	None; not in coma	None	Recovery
2/1976	Accident/inhalation	250 mg/55 min	None; not in coma	None	Recovery
3/1976	Accident/transdermal	125 mg/2.5 hr	None; not in coma	None	Recovery
4/1976	Accident/oral	250 mg/1.5 hr	None; not in coma	None	Recovery
5/1977	Accident/inhalation	250 mg/5.5 hr	None; not in coma	None	Recovery
6/1978	Accident/almond type with high amygdaline content (cyanogenic glycoside)	250 mg/9.5 hr	None; not in coma	None	Recovery
7/1979	Accident/bitter almond	500 mg/2 hr	None; not in coma	Severe hemolysis, Hb from 13 to 5.9 within 3 days	Recovery
8/1973	Suicidal/oral	250 mg/15 min	Questionable somnolence	None	Recovery
9/1978	Suicidal/oral	250 mg/15 min	Questionable blood level 3 mg/L	None	Recovery
10/1972 (published 1974)	Accident	250 mg/45 min	Yes; deep coma	Circulatory suppression due to additional cobalt EDTA	Recovery
11/1973	Suicidal/oral	250 mg/5 hr	Yes; deep coma	None	Recovery
12/1977	Accident/transdermal	250 mg/2 hr	Coma	None	Recovery
13/1979	Suicidal/oral	500 mg/?	Yes; coma	Mild hemolysis, Hb from 13.8 to 10 bilirubin (maximum): 3	Recovery
14/1985	Suicidal, oral	250 mg/10 min; 250 mg/3 hr	Yes; deep coma	Mild hemolysis. Hb from 13.3 to10.3 bilirubin (maximum): 4.7	Recovery
15/1987	Suicidal, oral	500 mg/1.5 hr	Yes; coma	Mild hemolysis, Hb from 15 to 13.4 bilirubin (maximum): 4.4	Recovery
16/1989	Suicidal, oral	500 mg/20 min	Yes; deep coma	Hemolysis, Hb from 13.6 to 9 bilirubin (maximum): 9.3	Recovery
17/1991	Suicidal, oral	250 mg/15 min	Yes; deep coma	None	Recovery
18/1986	Accident, inhalation	1000 mg/15 min; 73% MetHb	Yes; deep coma	Severe hemolysis, Hb from 13.9 to 7.3 bilirubin (maximum): 8.9	Recovery
19/1977	Suicidal, oral	250 mg/1.5 hours; 125 mg/5 hr	Yes; deep coma	Severe hemolysis, Hb from 16.4 to 10.9 bilirubin (maximum): 18.4	Death after 4 days
20/1986	Suicidal, oral	125 mg (only)/1.5 hr	Yes; resuscitation after 4-DMAP successful	None	Death after 4 days
21/1987	Suicidal, oral	250 mg/2 hr	Yes; resuscitation after 4-DMAP successful	Mild hemolysis, Hb from 15.7 to 13.7 bilirubin (maximum): 4.4	Death after 5 days
22/1989	Suicidal, oral	250 mg/1 hr	Yes; resuscitation after 4-DMAP successful	Too short to judge	Death after 3 hr
23/1981	Suicidal, inhalation	500 mg/?	Dead for unknown time	Not possible to judge	Found dead

*Sodium thiosulfate was administered after 4-DMAP in all patients.
Hb, hemoglobin; MetHb, methemoglobin.

enzyme deficiency was unrecognized or it was thought that the treatment was mandated because of life-threatening cyanide poisoning, the induced hemolysis could be treated by transfusion or blood exchange. In whites in Europe, glucose-6-phosphate dehydrogenase deficiency is a rare disease.

CLINICAL EXPERIENCES WITH USE OF 4-DMAP IN CYANIDE POISONING

Limited data are available for the use of 4-DMAP in cyanide poisoning because of the rarity of such poisonings and because few such poisoned persons are found alive. Some

TABLE 160-3 Whole-Blood Cyanide and Methemoglobin Levels in 23 Patients in Whom 4-DMAP Was Administered

PATIENT	CYANIDE LEVEL/TIME AFTER INTOXICATION	DOSE 4-DMAP	METHEMOGLOBIN/TIME AFTER 4-DMAP
1	Negative/1 hr	250 mg	23%/13 min
2	Not measured	250 mg; 4.38 mg/kg	Not measured
3	Negative/150 min	125 mg; 2.7 mg/kg	Not measured
4	Positive in breath/90 min	250 mg; 4.5 mg/kg	49.5%/27 min
5	Positive in breath/5.25 hr	250 mg; 2.7 mg/kg	33%/9 min
6	0.18 mg/L/9 hr	250 mg; 4.3 mg/kg	35.6%/3 min
7	Not measured	500 mg; 8.3 mg/kg	35%/72 hr
8	1.5 mg/L/15 min	250 mg	Not measured
9	3 mg/L/15 min	250 mg; 4 mg/kg	14.7%/1 hr
10	Not measured	250 mg	Not measured
11	Not measured	250 mg; 3.57 mg/kg	22%/13 min
12	2 ppm in breath/2 hr	250 mg; 5 mg/kg	41.2%/25 min
13	Not measured	500 mg; 9.3 mg/kg	Not measured
14	2.4 mg/L/2 hr	250 mg/10 min; 250 mg/3 hr	15.8%/1 hr; 37.7%/155 min after second administration
15	6.0 mg/L/2.25 hr	500 mg	Not measured
16	25 mg/L/1 hr	500 mg	33.4%/130 min
17	1.46 mg/L/130 min	250 mg	Not measured
18	Positive in breath	1000 mg	73%/1 hr; 46%/3.5 hr
19	2.65 mg/L	250 mg; 125 mg	Not measured
20	34 mg/L/1.5 hr	125 mg	Not measured
21	10.9 mg/L/2 hr	250 mg	19%/15 min
22	14 mg/L	250 mg	14.8%/45 min
23	Not measured	500 mg	Not measured

single case reports are published.[9,12,32–34] All but one of these case reports describe patients who survived, probably reflecting a publication bias.

Since 1972, our department has accumulated 23 cases of cyanide poisoning treatment by 4-DMAP either before or at the time of admission and one case in which 4-DMAP was used by mistake (see Tables 160-2 and 160-3): 13 cases were published in a thesis by Werner in 1979,[10] 1 case (number 10) was published by Daunderer and coworkers,[9] and 9 additional cases were published in an abstract.[11]

In the original Werner series, the indications for administering 4-DMAP were less strict than they are today. Of the 13 patients, only 4 (see Table 160-2), found in coma, seemed to meet the absolute indications we use today. Three of these four patients survived. In two further cases (cases 8 and 9 in Table 160-2), the indications for 4-DMAP were questionable. One patient was somnolent and still arousable. The other patient was in a coma, but 5 hours had elapsed since the poisoning. In 1981 (when the first author joined the department), the indications for 4-DMAP administration were clarified. Cases of mild cyanide poisoning were treated with sodium thiosulfate. Since 1981, nine patients received 4-DMAP: five survived, three died, and one was dead for an unknown period before he was found. From the eight remaining cases, three had to be resuscitated at the scene. In all three cases, it was possible to restore circulation after the administration of 4-DMAP. Two of the patients died of irreversible brain damage or edema after brain death had ensued, and one fatally rearrested after 3 hours. All patients who were found

in deep coma without cardiac arrest or without severe circulatory failure survived. Of the group of 12 patients (excluding the one who was found dead, the one who got the antidote after 5 hours, and all the cases in which the indication was doubtful), 8 survived and 4 died. 4-DMAP has not been studied in a controlled trial comparing its efficacy with other cyanide antidotes.

DOSE

Considering the optimal 4-DMAP dose for a severely poisoned patient, the clinician has to keep in mind that exact dosing is difficult for a physician who finds the patient in extremis; the exact weight or height of the patient is unknown, and calculations under stress are difficult. We recommend that a standard dose, based on animal studies and clinical experience, be 1 ampule (equivalent to 3.25 mg/kg of 4-DMAP in a 76-kg person). As can be seen from Table 160-2, 125 mg was administered in 2 cases (cases 3 and 20), and 250 mg was administered in 13 cases. One patient (case 21) who could not be saved had mild hemolysis. One patient received 375 mg of 4-DMAP (case 19) in two divided doses and died on day 5 with severe hemolysis. All five patients (cases 7, 13, 14, 15, and 16) who were given 500 mg showed mild-to-severe hemolysis. One patient (case 18) received 1000 mg and developed severe hemolysis with a peak methemoglobin content of 73%; the patient survived. Another patient treated with 1000 mg of 4-DMAP was poisoned with parathion. This patient also survived with severe hemolysis and renal failure (not shown in Table 160-2 or 160-3).

Methemoglobin Formation

A dose of 250 mg of 4-DMAP (see Table 160-3, cases 4, 5, 6, and 12) seems to create methemoglobin concentrations between 33% and 49.5%, which disappeared with a half-life of around 140 minutes (see Fig. 160-3). The half-life is not influenced by the dose. In our patients, it was a little bit longer than in normal controls (117 minutes). As seen in case 7, 500 mg of 4-DMAP can lead to long-lasting methemoglobin formation. It is likely that most of the methemoglobin found in this case after 72 hours stemmed from extracellular methemoglobin due to hemolysis.

From this limited experience, we conclude that in a healthy adult, 250 mg is theoretically sufficient, yet safe. Repeated 4-DMAP administrations do not seem to be necessary if sodium thiosulfate administration is administered subsequently.

PRECAUTIONS

Before 4-DMAP is used in a patient, it should be certain to the degree practically possible that the patient is poisoned by cyanide. We recommend that 4-DMAP should be used only if the patient is in a coma. It should not be used in smoke inhalation because carboxyhemoglobin and methemoglobin jointly may impair oxygen transport and delivery.

ADVERSE EFFECTS

Two major adverse effects are related to the desired action of 4-DMAP: excessive methemoglobinemia and hemolysis. Our cases suggest that significant hemolysis does not occur at doses of 5 mg/kg body weight. The suggested dose of 3.25 mg/kg did not produce excessive methemoglobinemia. Only in one fatal case of cyanide poisoning was excessive methemoglobinemia observed using the recommended dose of 4-DMAP.[12] In vitro, the methemoglobin production rate at atmospheric oxygen pressure was only 60% of that at 40 mm Hg, similar to that in venous blood[35]; this may be important in hypoxic patients when cardiopulmonary insufficiency is present. In our opinion, this fact should not lead to reducing the dose in such circumstances as long as the patient is ventilated with a fraction of inspired oxygen of 1.

Some minor adverse effects are of little relevance in severely poisoned patients. Phlebitis was observed 6 to 7 days after 4-DMAP was infused in the antecubital vein. After an intramuscular injection of 4-DMAP, slight pressure was felt after 5 to 10 minutes at the site of injection, slowly growing in intensity and finally resulting in severe pain in one patient. In another patient, shivering, sweating, and fever occurred approximately 10 hours after the injection. In volunteers, after the intravenous injection of 4-DMAP (3.25 mg/kg), the total bilirubin concentration increased by 140%, conjugated bilirubin increased by 180%, and iron increased by 200%. Within 24 hours of an intramuscular injection of this dose, the total bilirubin increased by 270%, then declined rapidly, whereas the conjugated bilirubin concentration increased by 120% and iron increased by 50%.[13]

TREATMENT OF ADVERSE EFFECTS

Excess methemoglobinemia may be corrected by 2 mg/kg of toluidine blue or by 1 mg/kg of methylene blue intravenously.[36] We suggest that this should be done only if within 1 hour after the administration of 4-DMAP the methemoglobin level exceeds 50%. Otherwise, cyanide is released again, and thiosulfate infusion is mandatory. Exchange tranfusion is needed if the methemoglobin level remains high. Because this methemoglobin comes from hemolysis, it cannot be reduced.

ADMINISTRATION

4-DMAP should be administered in a dose of 3.25 mg/kg intravenously in a comatose, cyanide-poisoned person. In adults, it seems reasonable to administer one ampule of 4-DMAP, which contains 250 mg, if the exact weight is not known. It is possible to administer 4-DMAP in the same dose intramuscularly in mass poisoning.

REFERENCES

1. Chen KK, Rose CL, Clowes GHA: Amyl nitrite and cyanide poisoning. JAMA 100:1920–1922, 1933.
2. Weger N: Aminophenols as antidotes to prussic acid. Arch Toxicol 24:49–50, 1969.
3. Hall AH, Rumack BH: Clinical toxicology of cyanide. Ann Emerg Med 15:1067–1074, 1986.
4. Bastian G, Mercker H: The efficacy of amyl nitrite inhalation in the treatment of cyanide poisoning. Naunyn-Schmiedeberg Arch Exp Pathol 237:285–295, 1959.
5. McKiernan MJC: Emergency treatment of cyanide poisoning. Lancet 2:86, 1980.
6. Tyrer FH: Treatment of cyanide poisoning. J Soc Occup Med 31:65–66, 1981.
7. Mushett CW, Kelly KL, Boxer EG, Rickards JC: Antidotal efficacy of vitamin B₁₂a (hydroxocobalamin) in experimental cyanide poisoning. Proc Soc Exp Biol Med 81:234–237, 1952.
8. Kiese M, Weger N: Formation of ferrihemoglobin with aminophenols in the human for the treatment of cyanide poisoning. Eur J Pharmacol 7:97–105, 1969.
9. Daunderer H, Theml H, Weger N: Treatment of prussic acid poisoning with 4-dimethylaminophenol (4-DMAP). Med Klin 69:1626–1631, 1974.
10. Werner H: Die Behandlung von Vergiftungen mit Blausäure, ihrer Salze und Derivate mit 4-Dimethylaminophenol. Thesis München, 1979.
11. Zilker T, Felgenhauer N: 4-DMAP as cyanide antidote: Its efficacy and side effects in human poisoning. Clin Toxicol 38:217, 2000.
12. Van Dijk A, Glerum JH, Van Heijst CNP, et al: Clinical evaluation of the cyanide antagonist 4-DMAP in a lethal cyanide poisoning case. Vet Hum Toxicol 29(Suppl 2):38–39, 1987.
13. Klimmek R, Krettek C, Szinicz L, et al: Effects and biotransformation of 4-dimethylaminophenol in man and dog. Arch Toxicol 53:275–288, 1983.
14. Kiese M, Methemoglobinemia: A Comprehensive Treatise. Cleveland, CRC Press, 1974.
15. Paulet G: Valeur des sels organiques de cobalt dans le traitement de l'intoxication cyanhydrique. C R Soc Biol 151:1932–1935, 1957.
16. Klimmek R, Fladerer H, Weger M: Circulation, respiration, and blood homeostasis in cyanide-poisoned dogs after treatment with 4-dimethylaminophenol or cobalt compounds. Arch Toxicol 43:121–133, 1979.

17. Klimmek R, Fladerer H, Szinicz L, et al: Effects of 4-dimethyl-aminophenol and Co2 EDTA on circulation, respiration, and blood homeostasis in dogs. Arch Toxicol 42:75–84, 1979.
18. Klimmek R, Roddewig C, Weger N: Effects of 4-dimethylaminophenol on blood flow and blood gases in the brain. Res Exp Med 179:141–151, 1981.
19. Eyer P, Kiese M, Lipowsky G, Weger N: Metabolism of 4-dimethyl-aminophenol. Arch Pharmacol 270(Suppl R):29, 1971.
20. Eyer P, Gaber H: Biotransformation of 4-dimethylaminophenol in the dog. Biochem Pharmacol 27:2215–2221, 1978.
21. Eyer P, Lengfelder E: Radical formation during autoxidation of 4-dimethylaminophenol and some properties of the reaction products. Biochem Pharmacol 33:1005–1013, 1984.
22. Eyer P, Lierheimer E, Strosar M: Site and mechanism of covalent binding of 4-dimethylaminophenol to human hemoglobin, and its implications to the functional properties. Mol Pharmacol 24:282–290, 1983.
23. Ludwig E, Eyer P: Oxidation versus addition reactions of glutathione during the interactions with quinoid thioethers of 4-(dimethylamino)phe-nol. Chem Res Toxicol 8:302–309, 1995.
24. Eckert KG, Eyer P: Formation and transport of xenobiotic glutathione-S-conjugates in red cells. Biochem Pharmacol 35:325–329, 1986.
25. Jancso P, Szinicz L, Eyer P: Biotransformation of 4-dimethylamino-phenol in man. Arch Toxicol 47:39–45, 1981.
26. Eyer P, Kampffmeyer H: Biotransformation of 4-dimethylaminophenol in the isolated perfused rat liver. Biochem Pharmacol 27:2223–2228, 1978.
27. Kiese M, Weger N: The treatment of experimental cyanide poisoning by ferrihemoglobin formation. Arch Toxicol 21:89–100, 1965.
28. Marrs TC, Scawin J, Swanson DW: The acute intravenous and oral tox-icity in mice, rats and guinea pigs of 4-dimethylaminophenol (DMAP) and its effects on hematological variables. Toxicology 31:165–173, 1984.
29. Kiese M, Szinicz L, Thiel N, et al: Ferrihemoglobin and kidney lesions in rats produced by 4-aminophenol or 4-dimethylaminophenol. Arch Toxicol 34:337–340, 1975.
30. Weger N: Cyanide poisoning and therapy. Wehrmed Monatschr 191:6–11, 1975.
31. Elbers FR, Kampffmeyer HG, Rabes H: Effects and metabolic path-way of 4-dimethylaminophenol during kidney perfusion. Xenobiotica 10:621–632, 1980.
32. Jakobs K: Report on experience with the administration of 4-DMAP in severe prussic acid poisoning: Consequences for medical practice. Zentralbl Arbeitsmed 34:274–277, 1984.
33. Van Heijst ANP, Douze JMC, Van Kesteren RG, et al: Therapeutic problems in cyanide poisoning. Clin Toxicol 25:383–398, 1987.
34. Zilker Th, Schweizer W: Zyankali-Intoxikation. Der Notarzt 3:59–60, 1987.
35. Eyer P, Hertle H, Kiese M, Klein G: Kinetics of ferrihemoglobin for-mation by some reducing agents, and the role of hydrogen peroxide. Mol Pharmacol 11:326–334, 1975.
36. Kiese M, Lörcher W, Weger N, Zierer A: Comparative studies on the effects of toluidine blue and methylene blue on the reduction of ferri-hemoglobin in man and dog. Eur J Clin Pharmacol 4:115–118, 1972.

U.S. Food and Drug Administration Pregnancy Risk Categories

Jeffrey Brent

Currently the U.S. Food and Drug Administration (FDA) rates the risk of taking pharmaceuticals during pregnancy on a five-category scale,* as follows:

A. Controlled studies in pregnant women fail to show a risk to the fetus in the first trimester with no evidence of risk in later trimesters. The possibility of fetal harm seems remote.

B. Either animal reproduction studies have not shown a fetal risk, but there are no controlled studies in pregnant women, or animal reproduction studies have shown an adverse effect (other than a decrease in fertility) that was not confirmed in controlled studies in women in the first trimester, and there is no evidence of a risk in later trimesters.

C. Studies in animals have revealed adverse effects on the fetus (teratogenic or embryocidal effects or other), and the drug should be used only if the potential benefits justify the potential risk to the fetus.

D. There is positive evidence of human fetal risk, but the benefits from use in pregnant women may be acceptable despite the potential risk to the patient.

X. Studies in animals or humans have shown fetal abnormalities, or there is evidence of fetal risk.

It is important to be aware of the limitations in this grading system. The FDA determines a drug's rating at the time that it is approved. If adverse information becomes available after drug approval, the rating may change. If favorable information or experience is available after drug approval, however, there is no automatic mechanism for changing the rating, and many of the pregnancy ratings do not reflect such new information. Assessments of pregnancy effects of pharmaceuticals should not be made based on FDA ratings alone, but rather should derive also from an examination of the recent published scientific literature.

*Adapted from Leikin JB, Paloucek FP (eds): Leikin and Paloucek's Poisoning and Toxicology Handbook, 3rd ed. Hudson, OH, Lexi-comp, 2002.

Sympathomimetic Pressors

Jeffrey Brent

DOPAMINE

Action and Structure

Dopamine (Fig. B-1) exerts its action predominantly through the following three mechanisms:

1. *Dopamine receptor agonism*: Dopamine is an agonist for the dopamine receptor. Dopamine administration causes dopamine$_1$ (D$_1$) receptor–mediated vasodilation.
2. *β$_1$-receptor agonism*: At doses higher than those required for D$_1$ receptor agonism (see subsequently), dopamine may cause stimulation of β$_1$-receptors.
3. *Generation of norepinephrine*: As shown in Figure B-2, dopamine is a precursor in the biosynthetic pathway of epinephrine and norepinephrine. Approximately 75% of an administered dose of dopamine is inactivated by either monoamine oxidase (MAO) or catechol O-methyl transferase (COMT), and only about 25% is stoichiometrically converted to norepinephrine. Because of this, norepinephrine-mediated α-receptor agonism is seen only when high doses (see subsequently) of dopamine are administered.

Based on animal data, it seems that dopamine does not cross the placenta, and it does not cross the blood-brain barrier except in preterm infants. Its volume of distribution has been reported to range from 1.81 to 2.45 L/kg, and dopamine's primary metabolite by MAO and COMT is homovanillic acid. Its half-life is approximately 2 minutes in adults, although it can be significantly longer in small children. Plasma dopamine concentrations are normally less than 100 pg/mL.

Dosage and Administration

Dopamine should be administered intravenously. Solutions may be prepared by mixing 200 to 800 mg of dopamine in 250 to 1000 mL of any standard intravenous solution.

Because of the various mechanisms by which dopamine acts, its effects depend on the dose administered. There are several possible ranges of doses, as follows:

1. *Low dose*: Doses ranging from 1 to 3 μg/kg/min act primarily to dilate renal, intracerebral, mesenteric, and coronary vascular beds through activation of the D$_1$ receptor. At these doses, there tends to be little observed effect on most monitored hemodynamic parameters, although in some cases the vasodilation of these beds may cause a decrease in mean and diastolic blood pressure.
2. *Intermediate dose*: At doses ranging from 3 to 10 μg/kg/min, predominantly β$_1$-receptor effects are seen. There is still an increase in D$_1$-mediated blood flow in the above-described vascular territories and in the β$_1$-receptor effects on the heart, resulting in an increase in heart rate, cardiac contractility, cardiac index, and conduction. At these doses, there may be modest increases in blood pressure but generally few effects on systemic vascular resistance (SVR), although small decreases in SVR may be seen.
3. *High dose*: At doses greater than 10 μg/kg/min, the α-adrenergic effects from norepinephrine synthesis tend to predominate and may overwhelm the D$_1$ receptor–mediated vasodilation of the above-described vascular beds. Doses greater than 50 μg/kg/min predictably cause severe vasoconstriction and generally should not be used.

Precautions and Contraindications

Because MAO is a major enzyme in the catabolism of dopamine, patients taking an inhibitor of this enzyme (see Chapter 43) are expected to have a substantially exaggerated effect. It is

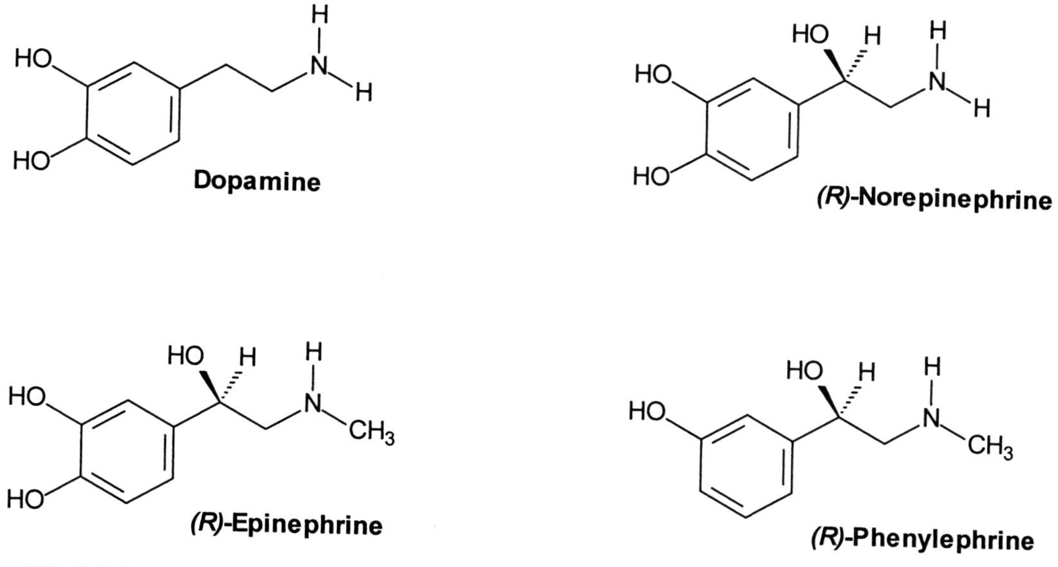

FIGURE B-1

Chemical structures of dopamine, norepinephrine, epinephrine, and phenylephrine. Where indicated, the (*R*)-isomer, which possesses the most adrenergic activity, is shown.

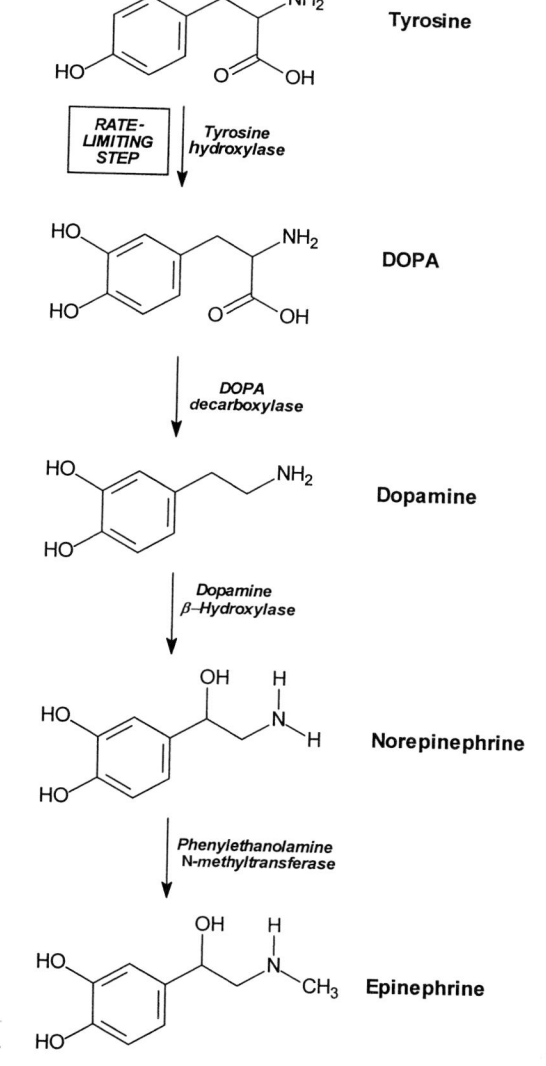

FIGURE B-2

Biosynthesis of catecholamines.

generally recommended that doses of dopamine approximating one tenth of standard doses be administered in patients taking these agents. If these doses are ineffective, the dose can be titrated to the desired clinical effect. Because many dopamine preparations contain sodium metabisulfite, patients with sulfite allergies may develop allergic reactions to dopamine administration.

EPINEPHRINE

Action and Structure

Epinephrine (see Fig. B-1), a term applicable only to the L-isomer of 1-(3,4-dihydroxy phenyl)-2-methylamino ethanol, exerts its action predominantly through the following two mechanisms:

1. *β-Receptor agonism*: Epinephrine is an agonist at β-receptors causing an increase in cardiac index, contractility, conduction, and heart rate. At low doses (see subsequently), the vasodilating effects of β-receptor agonism predominate, resulting in a decrease in SVR and widening of the pulse pressure. Epinephrine is not an ideal first-line vasopressor except in cases of anaphylactic shock.
2. *α-Receptor agonism*: At higher doses (see subsequently), epinephrine has significant α-receptor agonism resulting in an increase in SVR and mean arterial blood pressure. These effects may result in a reflex decrease in heart rate.

Plasma epinephrine concentrations normally are 15 to 55 pg/mL. It is metabolized by MAO and COMT (Fig. B-3). Its half-life is 2 to 3 minutes.

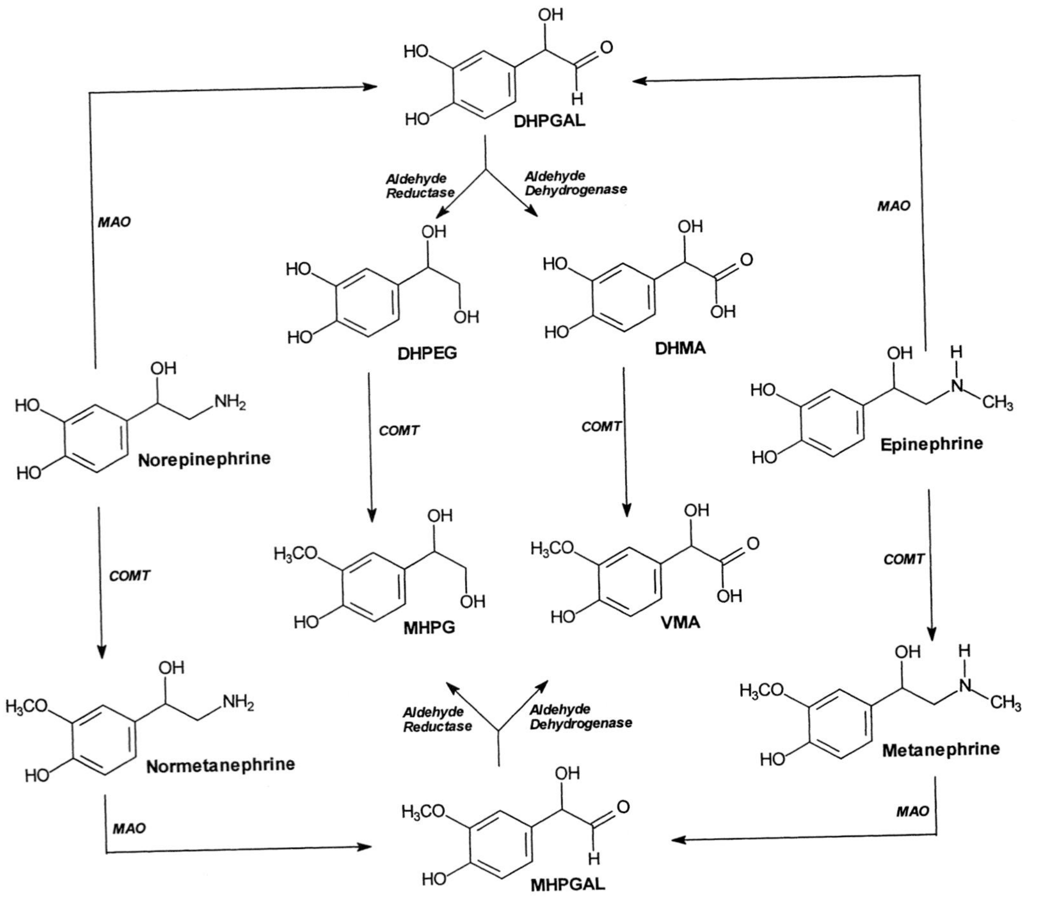

FIGURE B-3

Metabolism of norepinephrine and epinephrine by monoamine oxidase (MAO) and catechol *O*-methyltransferase (COMT). DHPGAL, 3,4-dihydroxyphenylglycolaldehyde; DHPEG, 3,4-dihydroxyphenylethylene glycol; DHMA, 3,4-dihydroxymandelic acid; MHPG, 3-methoxy-4-hydroxyphenylethylene glycol; VMA, 3-methoxy-4-hydroxymandelic acid; MHPGAL, 3-methoxy-4-hydroxyphenylglycol aldehyde.

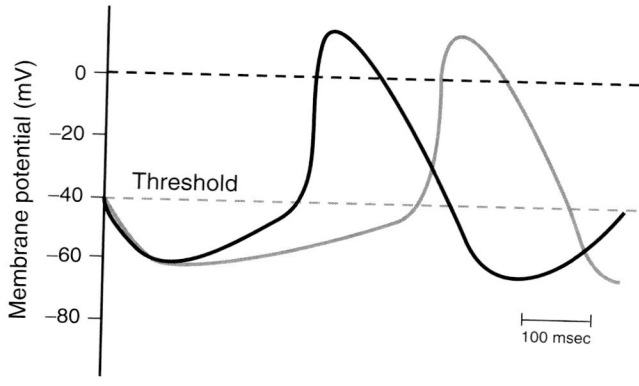

FIGURE B-4

Transmembrane potentials of pacemaker cells of mammalian heart illustrating slowing the rate of diastolic depolarization produced by vagus nerve stimulation (darker curve). Threshold is the potential for generation of an action potential. *(From Smith CM, Reynard AM [eds]: Textbook of Pharmacology. Philadelphia, WB Saunders, 1995.)*

Dosage and Administration

Epinephrine is compatible with most standard intravenous fluid solutions. Autooxidation may occur in bicarbonate-containing solutions, however. It is generally constituted as a 1:1000 (1 mg/mL) or 1:10,000 (100 μg/mL) solution; 10 mL of 1:10,0000 is equivalent to 1 mg. When given as a constant infusion, typically 1 to 2 mg is diluted into 250 mL (i.e., 4 to 8 μg/mL) of 5% dextrose in water or normal saline.

Epinephrine is best administered intravenously. If access is not immediately available, other routes are possible. It can be given subcutaneously, typically as a 1:1000 solution, but the effects are delayed and variable, particularly because of the local vasoconstriction it causes. Epinephrine also can be administered via an endotracheal tube in an emergent situation, whereby its pharmacologic effect is approximately half of that which would be achieved by intravenous administration.

In almost all circumstances in a critically ill patient, epinephrine should be infused intravenously, typically at doses ranging from 1 to 10 μg/min (0.02 to 0.2 μg/kg/min) and subsequently titrated to the desired effect. At the lower end of this dose spectrum, β-adrenergic effects predominate. As the dose is increased, α-adrenergic effects become evident and eventually predominate (Fig. B-4). The exact doses at which these effects occur in the individual patient are variable and should be determined based on the assessment of the clinical response.

Precautions and Contraindications

Patients on β-receptor antagonist therapy may have an exaggerated hypertensive effect after the administration of epinephrine due to unopposed α-receptor agonism. In patients taking these agents, epinephrine should be used at the lowest possible doses, which can be titrated as necessary. This effect potentially is seen even with patients using β-receptor antagonist eye drops. Because patients taking tricyclic antidepressants or venlafaxine have reduced reuptake of sympathomimetic amines, their response to epinephrine may be exaggerated. Here too doses should start low and be titrated gradually to the desired clinical effect.

Because of a possible "catecholamine-sensitizing" effect of halogenated hydrocarbons on the heart, epinephrine and other β-receptor agonists should be used cautiously in patients poisoned by these agents. If it is necessary to use sympathomimetics such as epinephrine in these patients, therapy should be initiated at the lowest possible dose and titrated as necessary.

For patients with circulatory shock, the β2-adrenergically mediated decrease in SVR of epinephrine may be detrimental. Agents with predominantly α-adrenergic activity and few β2-adrenergic effects, such as norepinephrine or phenylephrine, are preferable.

NOREPINEPHRINE

Action and Structure

Norepinephrine (levarterenol) (see Fig. B-1), a term applicable only to the L-isomer of 1-(3,4 dihydroxy phenyl)-2-amino ethanol, exerts its action predominantly through the following two mechanisms:

1. *α-Receptor agonism*: Norepinephrine is a direct-acting agonist at α-receptors and is predominantly used for this effect. Although it is a less potent α-receptor agonist than epinephrine, the lack of β_2-agonism makes norepinephrine a preferable α-adrenergic vasoconstrictor (see later).
2. *β_1-Receptor agonism*: Norepinephrine is a direct-acting agonist at the β_1-receptor. Its agonistic properties at this receptor are roughly equal in potency to that of epinephrine.

Norepinephrine generally is used primarily for its α-receptor–mediated vasoconstrictive properties. As described earlier, it is preferable to epinephrine in this regard despite norepinephrine's lower potency at the α-receptor because of epinephrine's vasodilating effect secondary to its agonist properties at the β_2-receptor. The net result of the administration of norepinephrine is an increase in SVR and mean arterial blood pressure.

Norepinephrine is metabolized by COMT and MAO. The product of COMT metabolism is normetanephrine, which is inactive. MAO action forms norepinephrine aldehyde, which is subsequently methylated by COMT to the inactive vanillylmandelic acid.

Norepinephrine generally is supplied as the bitartrate (Levophed); 2 mg of the bitartrate is equivalent to 1 mg of norepinephrine base. When specifying doses, it is important to be unambiguous about the bitartrate versus the base. It is preferable to express dosage in terms of norepinephrine base, and that convention is followed here.

Dosage and Administration

It is best to dilute norepinephrine bitartrate in dextrose-containing solutions because the latter inhibits its oxidation. It is generally prepared by adding 1 ampule (4 mg of norepinephrine base) to 250 to 1000 mL. Infusions should start at 0.5 to 1 μg/min and should be titrated to the desired clinical effect. Pediatric infusion should begin at 0.05 to 0.1 μg/kg/mL (or approximately 2 μg/m^2). Because of the powerful vasoconstricting effect of norepinephrine, it should not be given subcutaneously or intramuscularly, and precautions should be taken to prevent extravasation by its administration into large peripheral or central veins.

Precautions and Contraindications

As described earlier, it is important to avoid extravasation of norepinephrine. In the event of an extravasation, the local vasoconstriction should be treated by α-receptor blockade, which can be accomplished by the administration of phentolamine. A typical dose is 5 to 10 mg of phentolamine diluted in 10 to 15 mL of normal saline administered through a fine needle; this should be infiltrated diffusely in the area of extravasation.

Patients taking guanethidine may have an exaggerated hypertensive effect from norepinephrine or other direct-acting α-adrenergic agonists because guanethidine decreases the uptake of these agents and may induce receptor supersensitivity. Patients taking amine uptake–inhibiting antidepressants, such as tricyclic antidepressants, also can be expected to have an exaggerated effect of direct-acting sympathomimetic amines such as norepinephrine secondary to decreased uptake. Patients taking any of the aforementioned agents should be treated with minimal doses of norepinephrine initially, which can be titrated to the desired clinical effect.

PHENYLEPHRINE

Action

Phenylephrine (Neo-Synephrine) (see Fig. B-1) is primarily a direct-acting α_1-adrenergic agonist and is devoid of activity at β-adrenergic receptors. It also seems to have a component of indirect action causing the release of dopamine and norepinephrine. The latter activity is probably not responsible for its pressor effects, although it can have some significance for potential drug interactions, which are explained subsequently.

When administered as a vasopressor, phenylephrine can be given intravenously, subcutaneously, or intramuscularly. The intravenous route is always preferred and except in extraordinary circumstances should be used exclusively when seeking a vasopressor effect. Phenylephrine's duration of action after intravenous use is approximately 15 minutes, in contrast to hours after subcutaneous or intramuscular injection. The long duration of action for these routes is probably the result of the delayed release from these sites because of phenylephrine's α-adrenergic vasoconstricting properties.

Approximately 16% of an intravenous dose is excreted unchanged. It is not appreciably protein bound. Its volume of distribution is reported to be 4.9 L/kg. Peak serum concentrations are generally in the vicinity of 200 ng/mL.

Dosage and Administration

Phenylephrine infusions generally are administered at a rate of 40 to 360 μg/min, although it is unusual to require dose rates greater than 180 μg/min. The usual pediatric dose is 0.1 to 0.5 μg/kg/min. If needed, an initial bolus of 200 to 500 μg (5 to 20 μg/kg) can be given before the infusion.

If it is necessary to use the subcutaneous or intramuscular route, the usual adult dose is 2 to 10 mg repeated every 10 to 15 minutes. The pediatric dose is typically 0.05 to 1 mg/10 kg or 0.1 mg/kg (3 mg/m²) as a single dose. Because of the long duration of action of phenylephrine given by these routes, it should be administered only every 1 to 2 hours.

Phenylephrine solutions for infusion generally are prepared by mixing 10 mg with 500 mL of any standard intravenous solution. For a more concentrated solution, 20 mg/500 mL may be used. When mixed with phenytoin, the solution may form precipitates.

Precautions and Contraindications

An enhanced pressor effect may be expected in patients taking guanethidine because of guanethidine's inhibition of phenylephrine uptake from the neuromuscular junction or possibly by adrenergic receptor hypersensitivity. Patients taking MAO inhibitors may be anticipated to have an exaggerated response to phenylephrine secondary to its indirect effects. In patients taking these agents, it is best to start with the lowest possible dose and titrate the dose as clinically indicated. Patients taking tricyclic antidepressants also may have an exaggerated response to phenylephrine, and they too should be treated with the lowest possible doses followed by a titration to clinical effect.

Pharmacokinetic Data and Guidelines for Adjusting Drug Dosage in Adults with Renal Failure

MAINTENANCE DOSE ADJUSTMENTS FOR KIDNEY FAILURE*

DRUG	MW	PROTEIN BINDING (%)	V_d (L/kg)	$t_{1/2}$ (hr) NORMAL/ESRD	RENAL EXCRETION (%) (INTACT DRUG AND ACTIVE METABOLITE)	USUAL DOSE IN NORMAL RENAL FUNCTION	METHOD	Estimated Creatinine Clearance (mL/min)			HD	CAPD/CCPD	CRRT	COMMENTS
								>50	>10 < 50	<10				
Antibacterial Antibiotics														
Aminoglycosides														
Amikacin	585.6	<5	0.25	2–3/80	95	15 mg/kg q24h	D and I	7.5–12 mg/kg q24h	1.5–6 mg/kg q24h	1.5–3 mg/kg q48h	5–7 mg/kg AD	150–200 mg IV/IP qd	Dose for Cl_{CR} = UFR + 0.5 Q_D†	Nephro/ototoxic; monitor levels
Gentamicin	496.6	<5	0.25	2–3/60	95	4.5 mg/kg q24h	D and I	2.4–3.6 mg/kg q24h	0.5–2.3 mg/kg q24h	0.5–1 mg/kg q48h	1–1.5 mg/kg AD	30–40 mg IV/IP qd	Dose for Cl_{CR} = UFR + 0.5 Q_D	Nephro/ototoxic; monitor levels
Netilmicin	475.6	<5	0.22	2–3/72	95	6 mg/kg q24h	D and I	3.1–4.8 mg/kg q24h	0.6–3.0 mg/kg q24h	0.6–1.2 mg/kg q48h	1.2–1.8 mg/kg AD	30–40 mg IV/IP qd	Dose for Cl_{CR} = UFR + 0.5 Q_D	Nephro/ototoxic; monitor levels
Streptomycin	581.6	30	0.26	2–3/110	70	15 mg/kg q24h + AD	D and I	7.5 mg/kg q24h	7.5 mg/kg q24–72h	7.5 mg/kg q72–96h	5–7 mg/kg AD	150–200 mg IV/IP qd	Dose for Cl_{CR} = UFR + 0.5 Q_D	Ototoxic
Tobramycin	467.5	<5	0.25	2–3/60	95	4.5 mg/kg q24h	D and I	2.4–3.6 mg/kg q24h	0.5–2.3 mg/kg q24h	0.5–1 mg/kg q48h	1–1.5 mg/kg AD	30–40 mg IV/IP qd	Dose for Cl_{CR} = UFR + 0.5 Q_D	Nephro/ototoxic; monitor levels
Carbapenem														
Imipenem/ cilastatin	317.4	20	0.38	1/4	70	0.5 g q6h	D and I	250–500 mg q6–8h	250–500 mg q8–12h	125–250 mg q12h	125–250 mg q12h + AD	125–250 mg q12h	Dose for Cl_{CR} = UFR + 0.5 Q_D	↑Risk of seizures in ESRD
Cephalosporins														
Cefazolin	454.5	80	0.20	1.9/70	80	1–2 g q8h	D and I	1–2 g q8 h	1–2 g q12–24h	0.5–1 g q24h	0.5–1 g q24h + AD	0.5 g q12h	Dose for Cl_{CR} = UFR + 0.5 Q_D	

Continued

MAINTENANCE DOSE ADJUSTMENTS FOR KIDNEY FAILURE*

DRUG	MW	PROTEIN BINDING (%)	V_d (L/kg)	$t_{1/2}$ (hr) NORMAL/ESRD	RENAL EXCRETION (%) (INTACT DRUG AND ACTIVE METABOLITE)	USUAL DOSE IN NORMAL RENAL FUNCTION	METHOD	Estimated Creatinine Clearance (mL/min) >50	>10 < 50	<10	HD	CAPD/CCPD	CRRT	COMMENTS
Cefepime	534.5	16	0.30	2.2/14	85	1–2 g q12h	D and I	1–2 g q12h	1–2 g q24h	0.5–1 g q24h	0.5–1 g q24h + AD	0.5–1 g q24h	Dose for Cl_{CR} = UFR + 0.5 Q_D	
Cefotaxime	455.5	37	0.25	1.7/11	60	1–2 g q8h	D and I	1–2 g q8-12h	1–2 g q12-24h	1 g q24h	1 g q24h + AD	1 g q24h	Dose for Cl_{CR} = UFR + 0.5 Q_D	
Cefoxitin	427.5	70	0.20	1/23	85	1–2 g q8h	D and I	1–2 g q8-12h	1–2 g q12-24h	1–2 g q24-48h	0.5–1 g q24h + AD	1 g q24h	Dose for Cl_{CR} = UFR + 0.5 Q_D	
Ceftazidime	546.6	15	0.25	1.7/25	85	1–2 g q8h	D and I	1–2 g q8-12h	1–2 g q12-24h	1–2 g q24-48h	0.5–1 g q24h + AD	0.5–1 g q24h	Dose for Cl_{CR} = UFR + 0.5 Q_D	
Cefuroxime	242	33	0.30	1.3/22	95	0.75–1.5 g q8h	I	0.75–1.5 g q8h	0.75–1.5 g q8-12h	0.75–1.5 g q24h	0.75–1.5 g q24h + AD	0.75–1.5 g q24h	Dose for Cl_{CR} = UFR + 0.5 Q_D	
Penicillins Ampicillin	349.4	15–25	0.30	1.3/20	70	0.5–2 g q6h	I	0.5–2 g q6-8h	0.5–2 g q8-12h	0.5–2 g q12-24h	0.5–1 g q24h + AD	0.5–1 g q24h	Dose for Cl_{CR} = UFR + 0.5 Q_D	
Methicillin	380.4	30–50	0.30	0.5-1/4-6	80	1–2 g q4h	I	1–2 g q4-6h	1–2 g q6-8h	1–2 g q8-12h	1–2 g q12h	1–2 g q12h	Dose for Cl_{CR} = UFR + 0.5 Q_D	
Mezlocillin	539.6	16–42	0.20	1.2/6	60–70	1.5–4 g q4-6h	I	1.5–4 g q4-6h	1.5–4 g q6-8h	1.5–4 g q8-12h	1.5–4 g q12h	1.5–4 g q12h	Dose for Cl_{CR} = UFR + 0.5 Q_D	
Penicillin G	334.4	45–68	0.35	0.6/6-12	85	$0.5–4 \times 10^6$ U q4h	I	$0.5–4 \times 10^6$ U q4-6h	$0.5–4 \times 10^6$ U q6-12h	$0.5–4 \times 10^6$ U q12-24h	$0.5–4 \times 10^6$ U q12-24h + AD	Dose for Cl_{CR} <10	Decrease dose for liver disease	
Piperacillin	517.6	16–22	0.25	0.6-1.3/5	80–90	3–4 g q4-6h	I	3–4 g q4-6h	3–4 g q6-8h	3–4 g q8-12h	3–4 g q12h + AD	3–4 g q12h	Dose for Cl_{CR} = UFR + 0.5 Q_D	

Continued

Ticarcillin-clavulanate	384.4	45–65	0.21	0.9–1.3/16	80–90	3.1 g q4h	D and I	3.1 g q4-6h	2 g q6-8h	2 g q12h	2 g q12h + 3.1 g AD	2 g q12h	Dose for Cl_{CR} = UFR + 0.5 Q_D
Quinolones													
Ciprofloxacin	331.4	20–40	2.5	3–5/6–12	50–70	400 mg IV q12h	D and I	400 mg IV q12h	200–300 mg IV q12h	200 mg IV q12h	400 mg IV q24h	200 mg IV q12h	Dose for Cl_{CR} = UFR + 0.5 Q_D
Ofloxacin	361.4	25	2.5	4–8/25–48	>90	200–400 mg IV q12h	D and I	200–400 mg IV q12h	100–200 mg IV q12h	100 mg IV q12h	200 mg IV q24h	100 mg IV q12h	Dose for Cl_{CR} = UFR + 0.5 Q_D
Miscellaneous													
Aztreonam	435.4	56	0.15	1.3–2.2/8	58–74	1–2 g q8h	D and I	1–2 g q8h	1–1.5 g q8-12h	0.5–1 g q12h	0.5–1 g q12h + AD	0.5–1 g q12h	Dose for Cl_{CR} = UFR + 0.5 Q_D
Clarithromycin	748	70	3.0	6/22	15	0.5–1 g q12h	D	0.5–1.0 g q12h	0.25–0.75 g q12h	0.25–0.5 g q12h	0.25–0.5 g q12h	0.25–0.5 g q12h	Dose for Cl_{CR} = UFR + 0.5 Q_D
Erythromycin	733.9	70–85	0.8	2/5	15	250–500 mg q6-12h	D	250–500 mg q6-12h	250–500 mg q6-12h	125–250 mg q6-12h	125–250 mg q6-12h	125–250 mg q6-12h	Dose for Cl_{CR} = UFR + 0.5 Q_D; Ototoxic with high dose in ESRD
Metronidazole	171.2	<20	0.75	6–8/12–20	<20	7.5 mg/kg q6h	I	7.5 mg/kg q6h	7.5 mg/kg q6-8h	7.5 mg/kg q12h	7.5 mg/kg q12h + AD	7.5 mg/kg q12h	Dose for Cl_{CR} = UFR + 0.5 Q_D; Metabolites ↑ in ESRD
Teicoplanin	934	90	0.76	20–70/240–380	>50	6 mg/kg q24h	I	6 mg/kg q24h	6 mg/kg q48h	6 mg/kg q72h	6 mg/kg q72h	6 mg/kg q72h	Dose for Cl_{CR} = UFR + 0.5 Q_D; Ototoxic
Tetracycline	444.4	25–65	1.5	6–12/57–120	48–60	250–500 mg q6h	I	250–500 mg q8-12h	250–500 mg q12-24h	Avoid	Avoid	Avoid	Avoid

MAINTENANCE DOSE ADJUSTMENTS FOR KIDNEY FAILURE*

DRUG	MW	PROTEIN BINDING (%)	V_d (L/kg)	$t_{1/2}$ (hr) NORMAL/ESRD	RENAL EXCRETION (%) (INTACT DRUG AND ACTIVE METABOLITE)	USUAL DOSE IN NORMAL RENAL FUNCTION	METHOD	Estimated Creatinine Clearance (mL/min)			HD	CAPD/ CCPD	CRRT	COMMENTS
								>50	>10 < 50	<10				
Trimethoprim/ Sulfamethoxazole	290.3/ 253.3	40–70/ 65	1.6/0.25	8–11/ >26/ 10–13/ >50	50–60/ 10–25	2.5–5 mg/kg/ 12.5–25 mg/kg IV q6-12h	I	2.5–5 mg/kg/ 12.5–25 mg/kg IV q6-12h	2.5–5 mg/kg/ 12.5–25 mg/kg IV q12-24h	2.5–5 mg/kg/ 12.5–25 mg/kg IV q24h	2.5–5 mg/kg/ 12.5–25 mg/kg IV q24h	2.5–5 mg/kg/ 12.5–25 mg/kg IV q24h	Dose for Cl_{CR} = UFR + 0.5 Q_D/ Dose for Cl_{CR} = UFR + 0.5 Q_D	Nephrotoxic; monitor levels
Vancomycin	1449.2	30	0.65	4–8/>150	>95	1 g q12h	I	1 g q12-24h	1 g q24-96h	1 g q4-7d	1 g q4-7d	1 g q4-7d	Dose for Cl_{CR} = UFR + 0.5 Q_D	Nephrotoxic; monitor levels
Antifungal Antibiotics														
Amphotericin	924.1	95	4	24/24	<10	0.3–0.8 mg/kg q24h	I	0.3–0.8 mg/kg q24h	0.3–0.8 mg/kg q24-36h	0.3–0.8 mg/kg q48h	Dose for Cl_{CR} <10	Dose for Cl_{CR} <10	Dose for Cl_{CR} <10	Nephrotoxic
Fluconazole	303.6	12	0.85	22–30/ 100	80	200–400 mg q24h	D	200–400 mg q24h	100–200 mg q24h	100 mg q24h	200 mg AD	100 mg q24h	Dose for Cl_{CR} = UFR + 0.5 Q_D	
Flucytosine	129.1	<10	0.6	3–6/ 75–250	80–90	37.5 mg/kg q6h	D and I	37.5 mg/kg q8-12h	37.5 mg/kg q12-24h	20 mg/kg q24h	20 mg/kg q24h	20 mg/kg q24h	Dose for Cl_{CR} = UFR + 0.5 Q_D	Monitor levels
Antiparasitic Antibiotics														
Pentamidine	340.4	69	3	29/118	<5	4 mg/kg q24h	I	4 mg/kg q24h	4 mg/kg q36-48h	4 mg/kg q48h	4 mg/kg q48h	4 mg/kg q48h	4 mg/kg q48 h	Nephrotoxic
Sulfadiazine	250.3	20–55	0.3	5–7/32	40–60	0.5–2 g q6h	I	0.5–2 g q6h	Avoid	Avoid	Avoid	Avoid	Avoid	ARF from crystal deposition
Antituberculous Antibiotics														
Cycloserine	102.1	<5	0.19	10/>25	60–70	250 mg q12 h	I	250 mg q12h	250 mg q18-24h	250 mg q24-36h	ND	ND	ND	CNS toxicity; monitor levels
Ethambutol	204.3	8–22	2.3	3.3/7–15	80	15 mg/kg q24 h	I	15 mg/kg q24h	15 mg/kg q24-36h	15 mg/kg q48h	15 mg/kg AD	15 mg/kg q48h	Dose for Cl_{CR} = UFR + 0.5 Q_D	Optic neuritis

Antiviral Agents

Drug	MW	% Protein binding	V_d	$t_{1/2}$ (normal/ESRD)	% Excreted	Dose	Method	GFR >50	GFR 10–50	GFR <10	Hemodialysis	CAPD	CRRT	Comments
Acyclovir	225.2	9–33	0.8	2–3/20	75–85	5–10 mg/kg IV q8h	D and I	5–10 mg/kg q8–12h	5–10 mg/kg q12–24h	2.5–5 mg/kg q24h	2.5–5 mg/kg q24h	2.5–5 mg/kg q24h	Dose for Cl_{CR} = UFR + 0.5 Q_D	ARF from crystal deposition
Amantadine	151.3	67	5–7	12–24/200	>90	200 mg q24h	D and I	100–200 mg q24–36h	100 mg q36–72h	100 mg q7d	100 mg q7d	100 mg q7d	100 mg q7d	
Didanosine	236	<5	54	1.5/4.5	20–55	200 mg q12h	D and I	200 mg q12h	200 mg q24h	100 mg q24h	100 mg q24h + AD	100 mg q24h	Dose for Cl_{CR} = UFR + 0.5 Q_D	
Ganciclovir	204.2	<5	0.55	3.1/30	>90	5 mg/kg q12h	D and I	2.5–5 mg/kg q12h	1.25–2.5 mg/kg q24h	1.25 mg/kg q48–72h	1.25 mg/kg AD	1.25 mg/kg q48–72h	Dose for Cl_{CR} = UFR + 0.5 Q_D	Monitor levels
Lamivudine	229.3	36	1.3	6/15–35	70	150 mg q12h	D and I	150 mg q24h	100–150 mg q24h	25–50 mg q24h	ND	ND	ND	
Zalcitabine	211.2	<4	0.55	1.6/>8	60–80	0.75 mg q8h	I	0.75 mg q8h	0.75 mg q24h	0.75 mg q24h	ND	ND	ND	
Zidovudine	267.3	36	1.5	1.1/1.4–3	15–25	200 mg q8h	I	200 mg q8h	200 mg q8h	100 mg q8h	100 mg q8h + AD	100 mg q8h	Dose for Cl_{CR} = UFR + 0.5 Q_D	

Cardiovascular Agents

ACE Inhibitors

Drug	MW	% Protein binding	V_d	$t_{1/2}$ (normal/ESRD)	% Excreted	Dose	Method	GFR >50	GFR 10–50	GFR <10	Hemodialysis	CAPD	CRRT	Comments
Benazepril	424	95	1.5	20/30	85	10–40 mg q24h	D	10–40 mg q24h	10–30 mg q24h	5–20 mg q24h	5–20 mg q24h	5–20 mg q24h	Dose for Cl_{CR} = UFR + 0.5 Q_D	
Captopril	217.3	30	0.7	1–3/40	80	12.5–25 mg q8h	D and I	12.5–25 mg q8–12h	12.5–25 mg q12–24h	12.5–25 mg q24h	12.5–25 mg q24h	12.5–25 mg q24h	Dose for Cl_{CR} = UFR + 0.5 Q_D	
Enalapril	368.4	55	—	11–24/34–60	80	10–40 mg q24h	D	10–40 mg q24h	5–20 mg q24h	2.5–10 mg q24h	2.5–10 mg q24h	2.5–10 mg q24h	Dose for Cl_{CR} = UFR + 0.5 Q_D	
Lisinopril	405.5	<5	1.4	12.6/40–50	90	10–40 mg q24h	D	10–40 mg q24h	5–20 mg q24h	2.5–10 mg q24h	2.5–10 mg q24h	2.5–10 mg q24h	Dose for Cl_{CR} = UFR + 0.5 Q_D	
Quinapril	475	97	—	1–2/6–15	60	10–40 mg q24h	D	10–40 mg q24h	10–30 mg q24h	5–20 mg q24h	2.5–10 mg q24h	2.5–10 mg q24h	Dose for Cl_{CR} = UFR + 0.5 Q_D	

Continued

MAINTENANCE DOSE ADJUSTMENTS FOR KIDNEY FAILURE*

DRUG	MW	PROTEIN BINDING (%)	V_d (L/kg)	$t_{1/2}$ (hr) NORMAL/ESRD	RENAL EXCRETION (%) (INTACT DRUG AND ACTIVE METABOLITE)	USUAL DOSE IN NORMAL RENAL FUNCTION	METHOD	>50	>10 < 50	<10	HD	CAPD/CCPD	CRRT	COMMENTS
								Estimated Creatinine Clearance (mL/min)						
Ramipril	416.5	55–70	—	6–10/ 15–30	35	2.5–20 mg q24h	D	2.5–20 mg q24h	2.5–10 mg q24h	2.5–5 mg q24h	2.5–5 mg q24h	2.5–5 mg q24h	Dose for Cl_{CR} = UFR + 0.5 Q_D	LD unchanged; adjust MD
Antiarrhythmia Agents														
Bretylium	414.4	<10	1.3	5–10/>30	>90	LD: 5–30 mg/kg MD: 5–10 mg/kg q6h	D	MD: 5–10 mg/kg q6h	2.5–5 mg/kg q6h	1.25–2.5 mg/kg q6h	1.25–2.5 mg/kg q6h	1.25–2.5 mg/kg q6h	Dose for Cl_{CR} = UFR + 0.5 Q_D	
Disopyramide	339.5	50–65	0.9	4–9/17–43	42–62	150 mg q6h	D and I	100 mg q6h	100 mg q8–12h	100 mg q24h	100 mg q24h	100 mg q24h	Dose for Cl_{CR} = UFR + 0.5 Q_D	Active metabolite ↑ in ESRD
Procainamide (NAPA)	235.3	15 (10)	2.2 (1.6)	3–5/6–10 (6–8/>40)	50–60 (15–35)	12.5 mg/kg q6h	D and I	12.5 mg/kg q6–8h	6–9 mg/kg q8–12h	3–6 mg/kg q12–24h	3–6 mg/kg q12–24h + AD	3–6 mg/kg q12–24h	Dose for Cl_{CR} = UFR + 0.5 Q_D	Monitor NAPA and procainamide levels
Tocainide	192.3	10–20	2.2	13/>20	30–50	400–600 mg q8h	D and I	400–600 mg q8–12h	400–600 mg q12–24h	200–300 mg q24h	200–300 mg q24h	200–300 mg q24h	Dose for Cl_{CR} = UFR + 0.5 Q_D	
β-Blocking Agents														
Acebutolol (active metabolite: diacetolol)	236.4	11–25	1.2	3–4/6–12 (7–11/ 17–54)	10–17 (65)	200–400 mg q12–24h	D and I	200–400 mg q12–24h	100–200 mg q12–24h	100–200 mg q24–48h	100–200 mg q24–48h	100–200 mg q24–48h	Dose for Cl_{CR} = UFR + 0.5 Q_D	Active metabolite ↑ in ESRD
Atenolol	266.3	<5	0.7	6/>27	>90	50–100 mg q12–24h	D and I	50–100 mg q12–24h	25–50 mg q12–24h	25–50 mg q24–48h	25–50 mg q24–48h	25–50 mg q24–48h	Dose for Cl_{CR} = UFR + 0.5 Q_D	
Nadolol	309.4	20–30	1.9	14–24/45	70	80–160 mg q24h	D	80–160 mg q24h	40–80 mg q24h	20–40 mg q24h	20–40 mg q24h	20–40 mg q24h	Dose for Cl_{CR} = UFR + 0.5 Q_D	
Sotalol	272.4	0	2.0	7.5–15/ >30	>90	80–160 mg q12h	D and I	80–160 mg q12h	40–80 mg q12–24h	20–40 mg q24–48h	20–40 mg q24–48h	20–40 mg q24–48h	Dose for Cl_{CR} = UFR + 0.5 Q_D	

Cardiac Glycosides / *H₂-Blocking Agents* / *Miscellaneous Drugs*

Drug	MW	Protein binding (%)	V_d (L/kg)	$t_{1/2}$ normal/ESRD (hr)	Excreted unchanged (%)	Dose for normal renal function	Method	Dose for ClCR >50	Dose for ClCR 10–50	Dose for ClCR <10	Dose for ClCR <10	Dose for ClCR <10	Dose for ClCR = UFR + 0.5 QD	Comments
Cardiac Glycosides														
Digoxin	780.9	20–30	5–8	34–44/>100	70	LD: 10–15 µg/kg; MD: 2.5–5.25 µg/kg/day	D and I	MD: 2–4 µg/kg q24h	0.6–2.6 µg/kg q24-48h	0.6–1.3 µg/kg q48-72h			Dose for ClCR = UFR + 0.5 QD	↓ LD in RF; monitor levels
H₂-Blocking Agents														
Cimetidine	252.3	15–20	1.0	1.5-2/5	50–75	300 mg IV q6-8h	D	300 mg IV q6-8h	300 mg IV q8-12h	300 mg IV q12h	300 mg IV q12h	300 mg IV q12h	Dose for ClCR = UFR + 0.5 QD	Inhibits liver microsomal enzymes
Famotidine	337.4	15–20	1.3	2.5-4/12-24	65–80	20 mg IV q12h	D and I	20 mg IV q12h	20 mg IV q24h	10 mg IV q24h	10 mg IV q24h	10 mg IV q24h	Dose for ClCR = UFR + 0.5 QD	
Ranitidine	314.4	10–20	1.6	2-3/7-14	40–70	50 mg IV q6-8h	I	50 mg IV q6-8h	50 mg IV q12-16h	50 mg IV q24h	50 mg IV q24h	50 mg IV q24h	Dose for ClCR = UFR + 0.5 QD	
Miscellaneous Drugs														
Allopurinol (active metabolite: oxypurinol)	136.1	<5	0.5	1-3/1-3 (18-30/125)	10 (50-60)	300 mg q24h	D	200–300 mg q24h	100–200 mg q24h	100 mg q48h	100 mg AD	100 mg q48h	Dose for ClCR = UFR + 0.5 QD	
Phenobarbital	232.2	20–45	0.85	48-144/160	20–25	100–300 mg q24h	D	100–300 mg q24h	75–200 mg q24h	50–150 mg q24h	50–150 mg q24h + AD	50–150 mg q24h	Dose for ClCR = UFR + 0.5 QD	Monitor levels

*The recommended maintenance dose adjustments assume that the patient receives a standard loading dose.

†This formula is valid only for dialysate flow rates of 3 L/hr or less.

MW, molecular weight; V_d, volume of distribution; t_{1/2}, half-life of drug in plasma; ESRD, end-stage renal disease; D, dose reduction method; I, interval prolongation method; HD, conventional hemodialysis; CAPD, continuous ambulatory peritoneal dialysis; CCPD, continuous cycling peritoneal dialysis; CRRT, continuous renal replacement therapies (see text); ClCR, creatinine clearance; UFR, ultrafiltration rate; QD, dialysate flow rate; LD, loading dose; MD, maintenance dose; ACE, angiotensin-converting enzyme; ARF, acute renal failure; CNS, central nervous system; RF, renal failure; AD, after hemodialysis; ND, no data; IP, intraperitoneal.

Adapted from Kaloyanides GJ: Drug-kidney interactions. In Shoemaker WC, Ayres SM, Grenvik A, Holbrook PR (eds): Textbook of Critical Care, 4th ed. Philadelphia, WB Saunders, 2000.

Drugs Useful in Poisoned Patients

DRUG	PEDIATRIC DOSE	ROUTE
Anticonvulsants		
Diazepam	0.1–0.5 mg/kg/dose; may repeat every 10–15 min	IV/IO
	0.5–0.7 mg/kg/dose	Oral
Lorazepam	0.05–0.15 mg/kg/dose; may repeat every 10–15 min	IV/IO
Paraldehyde	0.3 mL/kg every 2–4 hr in equal amounts of oil	PR
Phenobarbital	Loading dose: 20 mg/kg; maintenance 4–8 mg/kg/day	IV/IO
Phenytoin	Loading dose: 20 mg/kg; maintenance 5–10 mg/kg/day	IV/IO
Antidotes		
N-Acetylcysteine	Loading dose: 140 mg/kg, followed by 70 mg/kg every 4 hr for 17 doses	Oral
Activated charcoal	1 g/kg	Oral
Antivenin, Crotalidae polyvalent immune fab	Initially 4–6 vials, followed by 2 vials every 6 hr for 3 doses	IV
Antivenin, *Latrodectus mactans*	Generally 1 vial	IV
Antivenin, *Micrurus fulvius*	Generally 4–10 vials, depending on severity	IV
BAL in oil (dimercaprol)	3–5 mg/kg every 4 hr, usually for 5–10 days	Deep IM
Benztropine	0.02 mg/kg (1 mg maximum)	IV/oral
Botulinum antitoxin	1–2 vials every 4 hr for 4–5 doses	IV
Cyanide antidote kit	Amyl nitrite: 1 crushable ampule	Inhalation
	Sodium nitrite: 0.33 mL/kg of 3% solution if hemoglobin level not known, otherwise based on tables with product	IV
	Sodium thiosulfate: 1.6 mL (400 mg)/kg of 25% solution, may be repeated every 30–60 min to a maximum of 50 mL	IV
Dantrolene (Dantrium)	1 mg/kg every 10 min to maximum 10 mg/kg, then switch to oral administration	IV
Deferoxamine	15 mg/kg/hr CI (maximum 6 g/day)	IV (preferred)
	Loading dose: 1 g, then 0.5 g every 4 hr	IM
Digoxin-specific Fab antibodies (Digibind)	1 vial binds 0.6 mg of digitalis glycoside; ingested dose may be estimated from serum level (see table with product)	IV
Diphenhydramine	0.5–1 mg/kg every 4–8 hr; 300 mg/24 hr maximum	IV/oral
Dimercaptosuccinic acid (succimer, DMSA, Chemet)	10 mg/kg every 8 hr for 5 days, then 10 mg/kg every 12 hr for 14 days	Oral
EDTA, calcium	1–1.5 g/m^2/day in divided doses every 4–12 hr for 5 days	IM
Ethanol	Loading dose: 750 mg/kg; followed by 100–150 mg/kg/hr infusion of 5% or 10% ethanol	IV/oral
Flumazenil	0.3 mg every 1 min to a maximum of 3 mg	IV
Folic acid	1 mg/kg every 4 hr	IV
Glucagon	Loading dose: 0.15 mg/kg bolus followed by infusion of 0.05–0.1 mg/kg/hr	IV
Hydroxocobalamin (vitamin B$_{12a}$)	50 times the amount of cyanide	IV
Ipecac syrup	Age 6 mo-1 yr: 10 mL	Oral
	Age 1–12 yr: 15 mL	
	Age >12 yr: 30 mL	
	May repeat dose once if no emesis in 30 min	
Methylene blue	0.1–0.2 mL/kg of 1% solution, slow infusion, may be repeated every 30–60 min	IV
Naloxone	0.01 mg/kg; if no effect, give 0.1 mg/kg; may be repeated as needed; may give continuous infusion	IV
Penicillamine	25–100 mg/kg/day divided 4 times a day (maximum 1 g)	Oral
Physostigmine	0.02 mg/kg, slow IV push	IV

DRUG	PEDIATRIC DOSE	ROUTE
Pralidoxime	25–50 mg/kg over 5–10 min (maximum 200 mg/min); can be repeated every 1 hr as needed	IV
Pyridoxine	Isoniazid: dose = dose of isoniazid; gyromitrin-containing mushrooms, 25 mg/kg; ethylene glycol, 50 mg/kg	IV
Sodium polystyrene sulfonate (Kayexalate)	1 g/kg as a suspension	Oral/PR
Vitamin K	1–5 mg repeated every 6–8 hr as needed	SC or IM
Cardiac Drugs		
Adenosine	50–100 μg/kg/dose rapid push (maximum dose 12 mg) or 5–20 μg/kg/min CI	IV/IO
Amiodarone	5 mg/kg over 20–60 minutes (may repeat if needed), then 5–10 mg/kg/day CI	IV
Amrinone	Loading dose: 2–4 mg/kg over 20–60 min, then 5–20 μg/kg/min CI	IV
Atropine	0.02 mg/kg/dose (minimum 0.1 mg; maximum 2 mg)	IV/IO
	0.04 mg/kg	ETT
Calcium chloride	20–25 mg/kg/dose over 20–30 min via central venous catheter (maximum 1 g)	IV/IO
Calcium gluconate	100 mg/kg/dose (maximum 3 g)	IV/IO
Diazoxide	1–6 mg/kg (maximum 150 mg); repeat every 5–15 min × 3 as needed	IV
Dobutamine	5–20 μg/kg/min CI	IV
Dopamine	3–20 μg/kg/min CI	IV
Epinephrine (1:10,000)	0.01–0.1 mg/kg/dose	IV/IO
Epinephrine (1:1000)	0.1–6.0 μg/kg/min CI	IV/IO
	0.1 mg/kg/dose	ETT
Esmolol	Loading dose: 100–500 μg/kg over 1 min, then 100–300 μg/kg/min CI	IV
Hydralazine	0.1–0.3 mg/kg (maximum 20 mg); repeat every 0.5–4 hr (maximum 3.5 mg/kg/day)	IV
Isoproterenol	0.1–2 μg/kg/min CI	IV
Labetalol	0.1–0.5 mg/kg over 2 min; repeat every 10 min or 1–3 mg/kg/hr CI	IV
Lidocaine	1 mg/kg/dose or 10–50 μg/kg/min CI	IV/IO/ETT
Nitroglycerin	0.2–3 μg/kg/min CI	IV
Nitroprusside	0.5–10 μg/kg/min CI	IV
Norepinephrine	0.1–2 μg/kg/min CI	IV
Procainamide	Loading dose: 15 mg/kg (maximum 300 mg) over 1 hr, then 1–4 mg/kg/hr CI (maximum daily dose 2 g)	IV
Diuretics		
Bumetanide	0.035–0.05 mg/kg/dose (maximum 2 mg) or 8–10 μg/kg/hr CI	IV
Ethacrynic acid	1 mg/kg/dose	IV
Furosemide	0.5–2 mg/kg/dose (maximum 20 mg) or 0.05–0.1 mg/kg/hr	IV
Mannitol	0.25–1 g/kg/dose	IV
Metolazone	0.2–0.4 mg/kg every 12–24 hr	Oral
Respiratory Drugs		
Albuterol (nebulization)	0.1–0.15 mg/kg/dose (maximum 10 mg) or 0.2–0.5 mg/kg/hr continuous nebulization	Inhalation
Aminophylline	Loading dose: 6 mg/kg over 20 mins, then 0.7 mg/kg/hr (6 mo-1 yr), 1–1.2 mg/kg/hr (1–9 yr), or 0.8 mg/kg/hr (>9 yr)	IV
Atracurium	0.5–1 mg/kg/dose, then 1 mg/kg/hr CI	IV
Doxacurium	0.05–0.1 mg/kg/dose, then 0.1 mg/kg/hr CI	IV
Ipratropium	250 μg/dose every 1–6 hr	Inhalation
Succinylcholine	1–2 mg/kg/dose with pretreatment with atropine	IV/IO
Terbutaline	Loading dose: 10 μg/kg over 3–10 min, then 0.5–10 μg/kg/min CI	IV
Vecuronium	0.1 mg/kg/dose, then 0.1 mg/kg/hr CI	IV
Sedatives/Analgesics		
Chloral hydrate	25–100 mg/kg/dose	PR/oral
Fentanyl	1–5 μg/kg/dose, then 1–10 μg/kg/hr CI	IV
Midazolam	0.05–0.2 mg/kg/dose, then 0.05–0.2 mg/kg/hr CI	
Morphine	0.05–0.15 mg/kg/dose, then 0.1–0.15 mg/kg/hr CI	IV
Propofol	1–3 mg/kg/dose, repeat as needed, or 7–10 mg/kg/hr CI	IV

CI, continuous infusion; ETT, endotracheal tube; IM, intramuscular; IO, intraosseous; IV, intravenous; PR, per rectum; SC, subcutaneous.

Index

Hydrogen chloride, fumes of, dangerous exposure levels of, 1014t
Hydrogen cyanide
  chemistry of, 987
  formation of from inorganic cyanide salts, 987
  fumes of, dangerous exposure levels of, 1014t
  metabolism of, 988f, 988–989
  pharmacokinetics of, 988f, 988–989
  poisoning with
    antidotes for, 994b
    clinical presentation of, 990
    common errors in, 995b, 996b
    diagnosis of, 990–991
    differential diagnosis of, 991–992
    in pregnant patients, 994
    key points in, 996b
    lethal dose of, 990
    pathophysiology of, 989–990
    treatment of, 992–994
  sources of, 987
Hydrogen fluoride, fumes of, dangerous exposure levels of, 1014t
Hydrogen peroxide
  in irritant gas injury, 1012
  in paraquat toxicity, 950
Hydrogen selenide, fumes of, dangerous exposure levels of, 1014t
Hydrogen sulfide, 1029–1032
  chemistry of, 1029
  fumes of, dangerous exposure levels of, 1014t
  poisoning with
    clinical presentation of, 1030t, 1030–1031
    common errors in, 1032b
    diagnosis of, 1031
    first aid for, 1032
    key points in, 1032b
    pathophysiology of, 1029–1030, 1030f
    treatment of, 1031–1032
Hydroid coral, 1225, 1226f
Hydromorphone
  chemical structure of, 612f
  vs. other opioid analgesics, 615t
Hydrophiidae snakes, African, distribution and clinical toxicology of, 1163t
Hydroxocobalamin
  chemical structure of, 1548f
  for cyanide poisoning, 993, 1549–1550, 1609
    dose and administration of, 1550, 1632t
    mechanism of action and adverse effects of, 1548t
  in metabolism of cyanide, 989
γ-Hydroxybutyrate. *See* Gamma-hydroxybutyrate.
Hydroxychloroquine, for porphyria cutanea tarda, 922
5-Hydroxydimethyltryptamine, 755, 757
l-Hydroxyhexamide, chemical structure of, 731f
5-Hydroxyindoleacetic acid
  in serotonin synthesis and metabolism, 282, 284f
  MDMA effects on, 767
Hydroxyl radicals
  free, in iron poisoning, 688
  in paraquat toxicity, 950
7-Hydroxymethotrexate, chemical structure of, 650f
5-Hydroxytryptamine, 755, 756f. *See also* Serotonin.
  chemical structure of, 756f
  receptors for
    hallucinogen cross-tolerance and, 757, 758–759
    indolealkylamine affinity for, 757
    neuroleptic antagonism to, 509–510, 511
  synthesis and metabolism of, 281, 283f, 284f
5-Hydroxytryptophan, in serotonin synthesis and metabolism, 281, 283f, 284f
Hydroxyzine
  for anaphylaxis, 380
  structure of, 450f
Hydrozoa, poisoning with, 1225–1227
Hymenoptera
  envenomation by, 1359–1367
    clinical presentation of, 1363–1364
    common misperceptions about, 1367b
    evaluation of patient with, 1364, 1364t
    in special populations, 1366
    key points in, 1367b
    pathophysiology of, 1362, 1363
    treatment of, 1365t, 1365–1366
  species of, 1359

Hyoscyamine
  chemical structure of, 1338f
  pharmacologic properties of, 1337–1339, 1338f
  plant origin of, 1337
    toxicity of, 1298–1300, 1299t
Hyoscyamus species, 1336, 1336t
dl-Hyoscyamine, 1517. *See also* Atropine.
Hyperadrenergic crisis
  in amphetamine toxicity, 767
  MAO inhibitor overdose and, 490t
Hyperaldosteronism, in cirrhosis, 166
Hyperattentiveness, sympathomimetic agents and, 386, 387
Hyperbaric oxygen therapy
  defibrillation ability and, 183
  definition of, 181
  equipment for, 183
  for carbon monoxide poisoning, 979–981
  for critically ill patients, 181–186
  for cyanide poisoning, 1550
  for cyclopeptide-containing mushroom poisoning, 1283
  for hydrogen sulfide toxicity, 1032
  for *Loxosceles* spider bite, 1200
  for maternal carbon monoxide poisoning, 133
  for methemoglobinemia, 341
  history of, 181
  in pregnant women, 981
  indications for, 182, 182t
  monitoring of, 183, 184
  patient management during, 185–186
  patient preparation for, 184
  PEEP use and, 183–184
  physiologic effects of, 181–182, 183f
  relative risks with, 182–183, 980–981
  staff members providing, 183
  types of chambers used for, 181, 182f, 183f
Hyperbilirubinemia, in acetaminophen toxicity, 602
Hypercalcemia
  in rhabdomyolysis, 81
  in salicylate intoxication, 623
  malignant hyperthermia and, 296
Hypercapnia, permissive
  for adult respiratory distress syndrome, 76
  in mechanical ventilation, 114–115
Hyperchloremia, drugs and toxins inducing, 22
Hyperglycemia
  calcium channel antagonist effects and, 416
  in chronic alcoholism, postprandial, 167
  in isopropyl alcohol ingestion, 890
  in organophosphorus insecticide toxicity, 941
  in PNU toxicity, 967
  in theophylline toxicity, 459
Hyperinsulinemia
  quinine-induced, 677, 679
  rebound, 738
Hyperkalemia
  drugs and toxins inducing, 22
  in acute renal failure, 78–79, 211
  in digitalis toxicity, 257, 398
  in rhabdomyolysis, 81
  in theophylline poisoning, 460
  malignant hyperthermia and, 296, 297
Hyperlactatemia
  clinical features of, 683–684
  definition of, 683
Hypermagnesemia, in treatment for digitalis toxicity, 398
Hypermetabolism, malignant hyperthermia and, 296, 297
Hypernatremia, drugs and toxins inducing, 22
Hyperphosphatemia
  anion gap interpretation and, 349
  in rhabdomyolysis, 81
Hyperprolactinemia, bromocriptine for, 1531
Hyperreactivity, bronchial, in irritant gas inhalation, 1022
Hyperreflexia
  in serotonin syndrome, 285, 286t
  lithium toxicity and, 525
Hypersensitivity pneumonitis
  agents associated with, 322t
  diagnosis of, 322t, 325
  differential diagnosis of, 323
  drug-related, pulmonary syndromes with, 322, 322f, 322t
  immune-mediated, 375
  in pyrethroid toxicity, 931
  methotrexate overdose and, 652

occupational causes of, 154
pathophysiology of, 154
toxic agents and occupational exposures associated with, 156t–157t
treatment of, 154, 326
vs. inhalational fever, lung injury with, 153
Hypersensitivity reactions, 371
  delayed, 374
    to antivenom, 1478, 1479
    to antivenom for *Latrodectus* spiders, 1189, 1190
    to antivenom for widow spiders, 1189
  drug-related, pulmonary syndromes with, 321–322
  fulminant hepatic failure and, 192
  to antivenom, 1146
    coral snake, 1093
    IgE-mediated, 1155
    IgG-mediated, 1473
    skin tests for, 1478
  to phenytoin, 556
  to *Ricinus communis* seeds, 1347
  type IV, inorganic mercury exposure and, 839
Hypersensitivity syndrome
  antiepileptic drug, 376
  phenytoin, idiosyncratic, 556
Hypertension
  amphetamine-induced, 768
  approach to, 32, 33t
  causes of, 32
  cocaine-induced, 788, 789, 791, 792, 793
  common toxins causing, 33t
  imidazoline for, 441–446. *See also* Imidazoline.
    intoxication with, 443, 444
  in α-adrenergic agonist poisoning, 472
  in anticholinergic syndrome, 264
  in baclofen overdose, 573, 574
  in cyanide toxicity from sodium nitroprusside, 436
  in ergot alkaloid poisoning, 726
  in levodopa toxicity, 587
  in MAO inhibitor overdose, 488, 491
  in phencyclidine toxicity, 778, 782, 782t
  in poisoned children, 108–110
    drugs producing, 109t
  in poisoned patients, 17, 17t, 18
  in tetrodotoxin poisoning, 1256, 1257, 1259
  intracranial, brain death and, 174
  MDMA-induced, 769
  portal, in chronic alcoholism, 164–165
  pulmonary, with appetite-suppressant agents, 324
  rebound, clonidine cessation and, 443
  sympathomimetic-induced, 32
  treatment of, 32
Hypertensive crisis, spontaneous, MAO inhibitor overdose and, 488
Hyperthermia
  fulminant hepatic failure and, 194
  GABA receptors and, 571
  in amphetamine toxicity, 768, 772
  in anticholinergic syndrome, 264, 267
    from plant alkaloids, 1300
  in baclofen overdose, 571
  in cocaine toxicity, 787, 792
  in elderly, adverse drug effects and, 145
  in gamma-hydroxybutyrate toxicity, 747
  in imidazoline intoxication, 444
  in indolealkylamine poisoning, 758
  in MAO inhibitor overdose, 490t, 492
  in neuroleptic malignant syndrome, 308
  in NSAID overdose, 636
  in pentachlorophenol toxicity, 920
  in salicylate intoxication, 623
  in serotonin syndrome, 288
  in solanine poisoning, 1302, 1303
  indolealkylamine hallucinogen activity and, 757, 759
  malignant, 291–303
    anesthetic drugs safe and unsafe for, 296t
    clinical presentation of, 296–297, 297t
    conditions related to, 297–299
    dantrolene for. *See* Dantrolene.
    diagnosis of, 300
      hotline for, 300
      tests for, 294f, 294–296, 295f, 295t, 298, 299, 300
    differential diagnosis of, 299t, 299–300
    history of, 291, 292t
    in awake patients, 297, 298
    incidence of, 291–292